American Medical Association

Physicians dedicated to the health of America

Also Available on CD-ROM!

Graduate Medical Education Directory

1999 2000

Including programs accredited by the Accreditation Council for Graduate Medical Education

ACGME

Comments or Inquiries

Fred Donini-Lenhoff
Medical Education Products
American Medical Association
515 N State St
Chicago, IL 60610
312 464-4635
312 464-5830 Fax
E-mail: fred_lenhoff@ama-assn.org
Internet: http://www.ama-assn.org

Order Information

The Graduate Medical Education Directory is available for $64.95 ($48.95 AMA members) from
American Medical Association
Order Department OP416799
PO Box 7046
Dover, DE 19903-7046
800 621-8335
312 464-5600 Fax

ISBN 0-89970-984-2

Table of Contents

11 **Section I—Graduate Medical Education Information**

11 Review and Accreditation of Graduate Medical Education Programs
11 Introduction
12 Application and Site Visit
12 Review and Accreditation
14 Notification of Accreditation Status
15 Procedures for Proposed Adverse Actions and Procedures for Appeal of Adverse Actions
16 Program Organization
16 Institutional Review
16 Fees for Evaluation and Accreditation
17 Information and Inquiries
18 Entry of Foreign-born Medical Graduates to the United States
22 Fifth Pathway Program
22 Appointment to US Armed Services Graduate Medical Education Programs
22 Electronic Residency Application Service (ERAS)
22 National Resident Matching Program (NRMP)
24 Information on Unfilled Positions
24 Information on Canadian Residency Programs

25 **Section II—Essentials of Accredited Residencies in Graduate Medical Education: Institutional and Program Requirements**

25 **Preface**
25 I. The Education of Physicians
26 II. Accreditation of GME Programs
27 III. A Glossary of Selected Terms Used in GME Accreditation
28 **Institutional Requirements**
28 I. Institutional Organization and Commitment
30 II. Residents
32 **Program Requirements for Residency Education**
32 Allergy and Immunology
35 Clinical and Laboratory Immunology
38 Anesthesiology
42 Policies and Procedures for Subspecialties of Anesthesiology
42 Subspecialties of Anesthesiology
44 Anesthesiology Critical Care Medicine
46 Pain Management
48 Pediatric Anesthesiology
51 Colon and Rectal Surgery
53 Dermatology
56 Dermatopathology
59 Emergency Medicine
65 Subspecialties of Emergency Medicine
66 Pediatric Emergency Medicine
68 Medical Toxicology
70 Sports Medicine
72 Family Practice
80 Family Practice Geriatric Medicine and Family Practice Sports Medicine
82 Family Practice Geriatric Medicine
85 Family Practice Sports Medicine
86 Internal Medicine

95 Policies and Procedures for Subspecialties of Internal Medicine
95 Subspecialties of Internal Medicine
100 Cardiovascular Disease
101 Clinical Cardiac Electrophysiology
103 Critical Care Medicine
105 Endocrinology, Diabetes, and Metabolism
106 Gastroenterology
108 Geriatric Medicine
110 Hematology
111 Hematology and Oncology
112 Infectious Disease
113 Interventional Cardiology
115 Nephrology
116 Oncology
117 Pulmonary Disease
119 Pulmonary Disease and Critical Care Medicine
121 Rheumatology
122 Sports Medicine
124 Medical Genetics
128 Neurological Surgery
134 Neurology
137 Policies and Procedures for Subspecialties of Neurology
138 Child Neurology
142 Clinical Neurophysiology
145 Nuclear Medicine
150 Obstetrics and Gynecology
157 Ophthalmology
161 Orthopaedic Surgery
164 Adult Reconstructive Orthopaedics
167 Foot and Ankle Orthopaedics
170 Hand Surgery
173 Musculoskeletal Oncology
176 Orthopaedic Sports Medicine
178 Orthopaedic Surgery of the Spine
181 Orthopaedic Trauma
184 Pediatric Orthopaedics
186 Otolaryngology
191 Otology-Neurotology
194 Pediatric Otolaryngology
198 Pathology—Anatomic and Clinical
202 Blood Banking/Transfusion Medicine
204 Chemical Pathology
206 Cytopathology
208 Dermatopathology
210 Forensic Pathology
212 Hematology
214 Immunopathology
216 Medical Microbiology
218 Neuropathology
220 Pediatric Pathology
223 Pediatrics
232 Subspecialties of Pediatrics
234 Adolescent Medicine
235 Neonatal-Perinatal Medicine

236 Pediatric Cardiology
238 Pediatric Critical Care Medicine
240 Pediatric Emergency Medicine
241 Pediatric Endocrinology
242 Pediatric Gastroenterology
243 Pediatric Hematology/Oncology
245 Pediatric Infectious Diseases
246 Pediatric Nephrology
247 Pediatric Pulmonology
248 Pediatric Rheumatology
250 Pediatric Sports Medicine
251 Physical Medicine and Rehabilitation
256 Policies and Procedures for Subspecialties of Physical Medicine and Rehabilitation
256 Spinal Cord Injury Medicine
262 Plastic Surgery
267 Subspecialties of Plastic Surgery
268 Craniofacial Surgery
271 Hand Surgery
275 Preventive Medicine
282 Medical Toxicology
284 Psychiatry
291 Addiction Psychiatry
296 Child and Adolescent Psychiatry
300 Forensic Psychiatry
305 Geriatric Psychiatry
310 Radiology—Diagnostic
314 Policies and Procedures for Subspecialties of Diagnostic Radiology
314 Subspecialties of Diagnostic Radiology
316 Abdominal Radiology
318 Musculoskeletal Radiology
319 Neuroradiology
321 Nuclear Radiology
321 Pediatric Radiology
324 Vascular and Interventional Radiology
326 Radiation Oncology
330 Surgery—General
334 Subspecialties of General Surgery
337 Surgical Critical Care
339 Hand Surgery
342 Pediatric Surgery
344 Vascular Surgery
346 Thoracic Surgery
350 Urology
354 Pediatric Urology
357 Transitional Year

361 Section III—Accredited Graduate Medical Education Programs

363 Specialties/Subspecialties with ACGME Program Requirements
364 Addiction Psychiatry (Psychiatry)
367 Adolescent Medicine (Pediatrics)
368 Adult Reconstructive Orthopaedics (Orthopaedic Surgery)
369 Allergy and Immunology
375 Anesthesiology

386 Blood Banking/Transfusion Medicine (Pathology—Anatomic and Clinical)
390 Cardiovascular Disease (Internal Medicine)
404 Chemical Pathology (Pathology—Anatomic and Clinical)
405 Child and Adolescent Psychiatry (Psychiatry)
414 Child Neurology (Neurology)
420 Clinical and Laboratory Immunology (Allergy and Immunology)
422 Clinical Cardiac Electrophysiology (Internal Medicine)
427 Clinical Neurophysiology (Neurology)
433 Colon and Rectal Surgery
436 Critical Care Medicine (Anesthesiology)
440 Critical Care Medicine (Internal Medicine)
444 Cytopathology (Pathology—Anatomic and Clinical)
450 Dermatology
459 Dermatopathology (Dermatology and Pathology)
462 Emergency Medicine
473 Endocrinology, Diabetes, and Metabolism (Internal Medicine)
483 Family Practice
521 Foot and Ankle Orthopaedics (Orthopaedic Surgery)
522 Forensic Pathology (Pathology—Anatomic and Clinical)
525 Forensic Psychiatry (Psychiatry)
527 Gastroenterology (Internal Medicine)
540 Geriatric Medicine (Family Practice)
542 Geriatric Medicine (Internal Medicine)
550 Geriatric Psychiatry (Psychiatry)
555 Hand Surgery (Surgery—General)
555 Hand Surgery (Orthopaedic Surgery)
560 Hand Surgery (Plastic Surgery)
561 Hematology (Internal Medicine)
564 Hematology (Pathology—Anatomic and Clinical)
569 Hematology and Oncology (Internal Medicine)
578 Immunopathology (Pathology—Anatomic and Clinical)
578 Infectious Disease (Internal Medicine)
590 Internal Medicine
622 Medical Genetics
626 Medical Microbiology (Pathology—Anatomic and Clinical)
627 Musculoskeletal Oncology (Orthopaedic Surgery)
628 Musculoskeletal Radiology (Radiology—Diagnostic)
628 Neonatal-Perinatal Medicine (Pediatrics)
637 Nephrology (Internal Medicine)
647 Neurological Surgery
656 Neurology
667 Neuropathology (Pathology—Anatomic and Clinical)
670 Neuroradiology (Radiology—Diagnostic)
677 Nuclear Medicine
683 Nuclear Radiology (Radiology—Diagnostic)
686 Obstetrics and Gynecology
706 Oncology (Internal Medicine)
709 Ophthalmology
720 Orthopaedic Sports Medicine (Orthopaedic Surgery)
724 Orthopaedic Surgery
739 Orthopaedic Surgery of the Spine (Orthopaedic Surgery)
740 Orthopaedic Trauma (Orthopaedic Surgery)
741 Otolaryngology
751 Otology-Neurotology (Otolaryngology)

752 Pain Management (Anesthesiology)
760 Pathology—Anatomic and Clinical
774 Pediatric Anesthesiology (Anesthesiology)
775 Pediatric Cardiology (Pediatrics)
779 Pediatric Critical Care Medicine (Pediatrics)
784 Pediatric Endocrinology (Pediatrics)
789 Pediatric Gastroenterology (Pediatrics)
793 Pediatric Hematology/Oncology (Pediatrics)
799 Pediatric Infectious Diseases (Pediatrics)
803 Pediatric Nephrology (Pediatrics)
807 Pediatric Orthopaedics (Orthopaedic Surgery)
810 Pediatric Otolaryngology (Otolaryngology)
810 Pediatric Pathology (Pathology—Anatomic and Clinical)
812 Pediatric Pulmonology (Pediatrics)
816 Pediatric Radiology (Radiology—Diagnostic)
820 Pediatric Rheumatology (Pediatrics)
822 Pediatric Surgery (Surgery—General)
825 Pediatric Urology (Urology)
826 Pediatrics
843 Physical Medicine and Rehabilitation
851 Plastic Surgery
860 Preventive Medicine
868 Psychiatry
884 Pulmonary Disease (Internal Medicine)
887 Pulmonary Disease and Critical Care Medicine (Internal Medicine)
896 Radiation Oncology
903 Radiology—Diagnostic
919 Rheumatology (Internal Medicine)
928 Selective Pathology (Pathology—Anatomic and Clinical)
929 Spinal Cord Injury Medicine (Physical Medicine and Rehabilitation)
930 Sports Medicine (Emergency Medicine)
930 Sports Medicine (Family Practice)
934 Sports Medicine (Internal Medicine)
934 Surgery—General
956 Surgical Critical Care (Surgery—General)
961 Thoracic Surgery
969 Transitional Year
981 Urology
992 Vascular and Interventional Radiology (Radiology—Diagnostic)
999 Vascular Surgery (Surgery—General)

1007 Section IV—New and Withdrawn Programs

1007 New Programs
1013 Withdrawn Programs

1019 Section V—Graduate Medical Education Teaching Institutions

1091 Appendix A—Combined Specialty Programs

1094 Internal Medicine/Emergency Medicine
1095 Internal Medicine/Family Practice
1095 Internal Medicine/Neurology
1097 Internal Medicine/Pediatrics

1106 Internal Medicine/Physical Medicine and Rehabilitation
1107 Internal Medicine/Preventive Medicine
1108 Internal Medicine/Psychiatry
1111 Neurology/Diagnostic Radiology/Neuroradiology
1111 Neurology/Physical Medicine and Rehabilitation
1112 Pediatrics/Emergency Medicine
1112 Pediatrics/Medical Genetics
1113 Pediatrics/Physical Medicine and Rehabilitation
1113 Pediatrics/Psychiatry/Child and Adolescent Psychiatry
1114 Psychiatry/Family Practice
1116 Psychiatry/Neurology

1117 Appendix B—Medical Specialty Board Certification Requirements

1118 Member Boards of the American Board of Medical Specialties
American Board of:
1119 Allergy and Immunology
1123 Anesthesiology
1133 Colon and Rectal Surgery
1135 Dermatology
1139 Emergency Medicine
1141 Family Practice
1145 Internal Medicine
1152 Medical Genetics
1156 Neurological Surgery
1159 Nuclear Medicine
1161 Obstetrics and Gynecology
1169 Ophthalmology
1177 Orthopaedic Surgery
1185 Otolaryngology
1188 Pathology
1196 Pediatrics
1213 Physical Medicine and Rehabilitation
1221 Plastic Surgery
1235 Preventive Medicine
1238 Psychiatry and Neurology
1250 Radiology
1254 Surgery
1260 Thoracic Surgery
1263 Urology

1269 Appendix C—Medical Licensure Information

1269 Obtaining a Medical License: The Basics
1270 Examinations Used for Entry to Residency Education and the Practice of Medicine
1273 Licensure Policies and Regulations of State Medical Boards
1275 Contact Information for State Medical Boards

1279 Appendix D—Medical Schools in the United States

1283 Appendix E—Graduate Medical Education Glossary

Preface

The *1999-2000 Graduate Medical Education Directory* (84th edition), published by the American Medical Association (AMA), lists programs accredited by the Accreditation Council for Graduate Medical Education (ACGME).

The *Directory* provides medical students with a list of accredited graduate medical education (GME) programs in the United States, which aids them in making important professional decisions. State licensing boards, specialty societies, and hospitals refer to the *Directory* to verify the authenticity of programs presented by physicians who wish to qualify for licensure, certification, or hospital privileges. The *Directory* provides a unique historical record of accredited GME programs and background information about the ACGME accreditation process.

Section I—Graduate Medical Education Information—summarizes the accreditation policies and procedures followed by the ACGME. Also included is information on regulations for entry of international medical graduates to the United States and admission to US residency programs, appointment to US armed services GME programs, the Educational Commission for Foreign Medical Graduates, and the National Resident Matching Program.

Section II—Essentials of Accredited Residencies in Graduate Medical Education: Institutional and Program Requirements—provides information on the ACGME accreditation process, requirements for institutions sponsoring GME programs, and Program Requirements for each of the medical specialties and subspecialties. The Program Requirements describe curricular content for GME programs and may also address program resources and personnel, program length, and other specifications.

Section III—Accredited Graduate Medical Education Programs—lists GME programs accredited by the ACGME. Section III provides program name, sponsoring institution, major participating institution(s), program director name, address, and phone/fax numbers, e-mail address, program web address, accredited program length, program size, and program identification number. Specialties and subspecialties are listed in alphabetical order. Programs within each specialty or subspecialty are listed in alphabetical order by state and city. A list of accredited transitional year programs offered by hospitals or groups of hospitals is also included. (*Note:* The *Directory* may include programs that are on probation. For information on a program's current accreditation status, contact the ACGME, 515 N State St/Ste 2000, Chicago, IL 60610; 312 464-4920; http://www.acgme.org.)

Section IV—New and Withdrawn Programs—lists GME programs newly accredited since the publication of the 1998-1999 edition of the *Directory* and programs that are no longer accredited to offer GME training as of June 30, 1999, or earlier.

Section V—Graduate Medical Education Teaching Institutions—lists institutions and organizations that sponsor or participate in GME programs. Teaching institution listings include type of affiliation (sponsor and/or participant) and are listed alphabetically by state and city. Institution listings include the name and address of the institution, medical school affiliations (as verified biennially by the deans of accredited US medical schools), a list of the specialties and subspecialties in which the institution provides training, and the institution identification number.

Appendix A—Combined Specialty Programs—provides information on programs that offer combined specialty training. These combined programs are approved by each respective medical specialty board, and physicians completing combined training programs are eligible for board certification. Although the ACGME has accredited each program separately, neither the ACGME nor the Residency Review Committees have reviewed these combined programs.

Appendix B—Medical Specialty Board Certification Requirements—contains information about the American Board of Medical Specialties (ABMS) and the certification requirements for each of the 24 member boards of the ABMS. Certification is the process by which a medical specialty board grants recognition to a physician who has met certain predetermined qualifications, as specified by the board. Certification requirements are also published by and available from each medical specialty board. Questions concerning certification requirements should be directed to the particular specialty board office listed in Appendix B.

Appendix C—Medical Licensure Information—contains information on the licensure requirements of state medical boards, as published in the AMA's *Licensing and Credentialing: What Physicians Need to Know* and *US Medical Licensure Statistics and Requirements by State*. Licensure is the process by which a state government agency grants permission to a physician to practice medicine within that state's jurisdiction. Inquiries concerning licensure should be directed to the individual state licensure offices listed in Appendix C.

Appendix D—Medical Schools in the United States—contains a list of US medical schools accredited by the Liaison Committee on Medical Education (LCME). Appendix D provides the identification number, name, and location of each LCME-accredited medical school.

Appendix E—Graduate Medical Education Glossary—defines various terms commonly used in GME.

AMA Annual Survey of Graduate Medical Education Programs

Each summer, the AMA distributes the Annual Survey of GME Programs to almost 7,600 programs accredited by the ACGME and more than 200 programs in combined specialties. This electronic survey (on computer disk) collects data on program characteristics, such as clinical and research facilities and the curriculum and workload residents can expect. GME program directors also provide detailed information about individual residents, which are stored in the AMA Enterprise Information Base (see below).

Role of the Accreditation Council for Graduate Medical Education (ACGME)

The work of the ACGME's Residency Review Committees (RRCs), which review and evaluate programs, provides a basis for program and institution information included in the *Directory*. Through regular electronic data transfers, the ACGME shares with the AMA information about accreditation actions and other changes. The *Directory* contains a list of ACGME-accredited programs, generally reflecting accreditation actions completed by December of the previous year.

The ACGME also provides the Institutional Requirements and Program Requirements listed in Section II of this Directory ("Essentials of Accredited Residencies in Graduate Medical Education"). Accreditation of a residency program indicates that the program and its sponsoring and affiliated institutions are judged to be in substantial compliance with the Essentials.

Back issues of the *Directory*

Copies of the last 10 editions of the *Directory* are available for purchase at $25 per copy. For more information or to order, please call 312 464-5333.

FREIDA Online (Fellowship and Residency Electronic Interactive Database Access)

FREIDA Online provides Internet access to extensive information on ACGME-accredited residency programs and combined specialty programs. FREIDA Online allows users to search all ACGME-accredited programs by program identifier, specialty/subspecialty, state/region, program size, and educational requirements, among other variables. All program listings include program director name, address, and phone number, as well as program length and number of positions offered. In addition, the majority of programs listed include expanded variables, such as program benefits (including compensation), resident-to-faculty ratio, work schedule, policies, and educational environment.

FREIDA Online is available through the AMA home page at http://www.ama-assn.org/freida.

AMA Enterprise Information Base (EIB)

The AMA Enterprise Information Base (EIB), a comprehensive and authoritative database on resident and licensed physicians, is used to produce portions of the *Directory* as well as of FREIDA Online and AMA Physician Select. The EIB data track physicians' entire educational and professional careers, from medical school and graduate medical education to practice.

Medical Education Data Service

The AMA Medical Education Data Service provides published information, existing tables, custom tables, electronic data, and mailing labels to educational institutions, professional associations, government agencies, foundations, and others interested in collecting, analyzing, and disseminating medical education data. Written requests for data must state the purpose of the project, describe the specific data service requested, include expected due date for data, and provide the name, address, phone, and fax number of the project contact. When requests require staff contribution or organizational overhead, a fee is assessed. Some data requests (custom tables) require a letter of agreement; others (electronic data) require a licensure agreement.

Individuals interested in obtaining medical education data should contact Rebecca Miller, AMA, 515 N State St, Chicago, IL 60610; 312 464-4680.

Special Acknowledgment to the ACGME

The AMA gratefully acknowledges the cooperation of the Accreditation Council for Graduate Medical Education (ACGME) in supplying the ACGME accreditation standards, the list of programs accredited by the ACGME, and relevant information about the ACGME accreditation process. Particularly helpful have been the contributions of the RRC Executive Secretaries and Accreditation Administrators, who provided corrected copy of Program Requirements for residency education and notification of the most recent actions of the RRCs and ACGME.

Finally, the AMA thanks ACGME staff personnel Ingrid Philibert, PhD, Marvin Dunn, MD, Philip Kenny, PhD, and John Nylen, MBA, for their many ongoing contributions to the *Directory*.

Acknowledgments

Many people contributed to the publication of the 1999-2000 *Graduate Medical Education Directory*. In addition to collaborative efforts with the ACGME (see "Special Acknowledgment"), program directors and medical education and housestaff affairs staff provided updated information on the programs they administer through the AMA Annual Survey of GME Programs. The ABMS and the individuals who staff the member boards of the ABMS provided requirements for certification in each of the medical specialties and subspecialties. Staff from the National Resident Matching Program and the Educational Commission for Foreign Medical Graduates also provided updated information. Information on licensure was provided by state medical boards and Arthur Osteen, PhD, of the AMA Office of Physician Credentials and Qualifications. Updated information for entry of foreign-born medical graduates to the United States was provided by Cathryn Cotten of the Duke University Medical Center International Office.

Special acknowledgment is given to Pam Rosinski, P J Shoulders, Andrea Creswell, Todd Feinstein, and Chris Matthews for data collection and information resources management; to Florence Steels, Selby Toporek, Ronnie Summers, Denise Bryson, and Boon Ai Tan of the AMA and Rod Hill of North Coast Associates for production support; to Tim Ryan and Suzanne Fraker for assistance in disseminating this product; and to survey, database, and publication staff, including Sylvia Etzel, Rebecca Miller, Tom Richter, Dorothy Grant, and Enza Messineo.

Communications concerning this *Directory* should be addressed to

Editor, Medical Education Products
American Medical Association
515 N State St
Chicago, IL 60610
312 464-4635
312 464-5830 Fax
E-mail: fred_lenhoff@ama-assn.org

Fred Donini-Lenhoff, Editor
Hannah Hedrick, PhD, Director, Medical Education Products

Section I

Graduate Medical Education Information

Review and Accreditation of Graduate Medical Education Programs

Note: This summary of the process of review and accreditation of graduate medical education programs was adapted from official policies of the Accreditation Council for Graduate Medical Education (ACGME); for the official *Manual of Policies and Procedures for Graduate Medical Education Review Committees,* contact the ACGME office of the Executive Director.

Introduction

The Accreditation Council for Graduate Medical Education (ACGME) is jointly sponsored by the American Board of Medical Specialties, the American Hospital Association, the American Medical Association, the Association of American Medical Colleges, and the Council of Medical Specialty Societies. Each sponsoring organization appoints four representatives. The federal government names a representative to serve in a nonvoting capacity, and the ACGME chooses two public representatives. There is also a resident representative, and the chair of the Residency Review Committee Council sits as a nonvoting representative.

The mission of the ACGME is to improve the quality of health in the United States by ensuring and improving the quality of graduate medical education experience for physicians in training. The ACGME establishes national standards for graduate medical education by which it approves and continually assesses educational programs under its aegis. It uses the most effective methods available to evaluate the quality of graduate medical education programs. It strives to develop evaluation methods and processes that are valid, fair, open, and ethical.

In carrying out these activities the ACGME is responsive to change and innovation in education and current practice, promotes the use of effective measurement tools to assess resident physician competency, and encourages educational improvement. As part of this response, the ACGME recently established the Institutional Review Committee (IRC) which is composed of ten members who are appointed by the Chair of the ACGME in conjunction with the Executive Committee. This committee reviews institutions sponsoring training programs in graduate medical education for compliance with the Institutional Requirements.

Under the aegis of the ACGME, the accreditation of graduate medical education programs is carried out by review committees with delegated accreditation authority. A Residency Review Committee (RRC) consists of representatives appointed by the American Medical Association, the appropriate specialty board, and, in some cases, a national specialty organization. The Transitional Year Review Committee is composed of nine members who are appointed by the chair of the ACGME in conjunction with the Executive Committee. The term "review committee" is used to denote a Residency Review Committee and the Transitional Year Review Committee.

Graduate medical education programs are accredited when they are judged to be in substantial compliance with the *Essentials of Accredited Residencies in Graduate Medical Education*. The *Essentials* consist of (a) the Institutional Requirements, which are prepared by the ACGME, approved by its sponsoring organizations, and apply to all programs, and (b) the Program Requirements, which are prepared by a review committee for its area(s) of competence and approved by the ACGME. The activities of the ACGME extend only to those institutions within the jurisdiction of the United States of America.

A list of programs accredited by the ACGME, including detailed information about each program, is published by the American Medical Association annually in the *Graduate Medical Education Directory*. With the exception of that information, the contents of program files are confidential, as are all other documents regarding a program used by a review committee.

Application and Site Visit

The accreditation review process is set in motion in one of two ways, depending upon whether the program under consideration is seeking initial accreditation, reaccreditation, or continued accreditation.

Application

In the case of a program seeking initial accreditation or reaccreditation, the process begins when the program director sends an application to the executive director of the review committee. Review and evaluation of an application involves several steps and usually requires 8 to 12 months from the time the application is received by the review committee executive director until an accreditation action is taken.

The review committee executive director checks the application for completeness and forwards the document to the director of field staff, who schedules a site visit of the program. The scheduling and completion of the site visit take approximately 6 months. In some specialties, a member of the review committee or a specialist will review the application to identify areas requiring clarification by the site visitor.

Reaccreditation following loss of accreditation involves the same process described above. A program cannot apply for reaccreditation while engaged in the appeals process described in this document.

Review of Accredited Programs

Accredited programs undergo site visits and reviews on cycles determined by the review committee, as described below in the sections on actions regarding accreditation of general specialty and subspecialty programs. Program directors are notified well in advance of the site visit, at which time they receive the appropriate forms for completion. Program directors may request forms earlier.

A review committee may elect to review a program outside the usual cycle. A program director also may request an early review. However, a program will not be reviewed while it is in the appeals process.

Function of Site Visitor

There are two types of site visits: those conducted by ACGME field staff and those conducted by specialists. In either case, the site visitor does not participate in the final accreditation decision or recommendation of the review committee beyond providing a written report. It is the site visitor's primary responsibility to verify the information that has been provided by the program director. The site visitor also conducts interviews with administrators, faculty, and residents in order to report accurately on the various aspects of the educational program. The site visitor, whether field staff or specialist, should not be viewed as a consultant to the program and should not be expected to provide feedback to the program or to conduct a formal exit interview.

After the site visit has been completed, the site visitor's report is submitted to the review committee executive director, who prepares the program file for evaluation by the review committee. The site visitor is not present when the review committee evaluates the program.

Review and Accreditation

The review committee reviews the program information in detail, evaluates the program, and determines the degree to which it meets the published educational standards (*Essentials*). The review committee decides upon an accreditation status for the program and identifies areas of noncompliance with the *Essentials*.

Actions Regarding Accreditation of General Specialty Programs

The following actions may be taken by a review committee regarding the accreditation status of general specialty programs and by the Transitional Year Review Committee regarding the status of transitional year programs.

Withhold Accreditation

A review committee may withhold accreditation when it determines that the proposal for a new program does not substantially comply with the *Essentials*. The review committee will cite those areas in which the proposed program does not comply with the *Essentials*.

Provisional Accreditation

Provisional accreditation is granted for initial accreditation of a program or for a previously accredited program that had its accreditation withdrawn and has subsequently applied for reaccreditation. Provisional accreditation may also be used in the unusual circumstance in which separately accredited programs merge into one or an accredited program has been so altered that in the judgment of the review committee it is the equivalent of a new program.

When a program is accredited on a provisional basis, the effective date of accreditation will be stipulated. Under special circumstances, the effective date may be made retroactive; however, unless specifically justified, it should not precede the beginning of the academic year during which the program is accredited.

Provisional accreditation implies that a program is in a developmental stage. It remains to be demonstrated that the proposal for which accreditation was granted will be implemented as planned. A review committee will monitor the developmental progress of a program accredited on a provisional basis. Following accreditation, programs should undergo a site visit in approximately 2 years in preparation for review by the respective committee. The interval between accreditation and the next review of the program should not exceed 3 years. In the course of monitoring a program's development, a review committee may continue provisional accreditation; however, the total period of provisional accreditation should not exceed 5 years for programs of 4 years' duration or less, or the length of the program plus 1 year for programs of 5 years' duration or longer. With the exception of special cases as determined by a review committee, if full accreditation is not granted within either of these time frames, accreditation of the program should be withdrawn.

Full Accreditation

A review committee may grant full accreditation in three circumstances:

A. When programs holding provisional accreditation have demonstrated, in accordance with ACGME procedures, that they are functioning on a stable basis in substantial compliance with the *Essentials*;

B. When programs holding full accreditation have demonstrated, upon review, that they continue to be in substantial compliance with the *Essentials*; and

C. When programs holding probationary accreditation have demonstrated, upon review, that they are in substantial compliance with the *Essentials*.

The maximum interval between reviews of a program holding full accreditation is 5 years; however, a review committee may specify a shorter cycle.

Probationary Accreditation

This category is used for programs holding full accreditation that are no longer considered to be in substantial compliance with the *Essentials*. The normal interval for review of programs holding probationary accreditation is 2 years; however, a review committee may specify a shorter cycle. In reviewing a program holding probationary accreditation, a committee may exercise the following options: grant full accreditation; withdraw accreditation; or, in special circumstances, continue probationary accreditation. A program should not hold probationary accreditation for more than 4 consecutive years until it is returned to full accreditation or the review committee acts to withdraw accreditation. This period may be extended for procedural reasons, as when a program exercises the right to appeal procedures or the review schedule exceeds 4 years. The probationary period is calculated from the date of the initial decision for probation. The *Procedures for Proposed Adverse Actions* and *Procedures for Appeal of Adverse Actions*, in subsequent text, provide further details on adverse actions.

Withdrawal of Accreditation

Accreditation of a program may be withdrawn under the following conditions:

A. Noncompliance with *Essentials*. Accreditation of programs holding either provisional accreditation or probationary accreditation may be withdrawn as follows:
   1. For programs holding provisional accreditation, once a review committee has notified a program director that the program has not developed as proposed to establish and maintain substantial compliance with the *Essentials*, the program will be subject to withdrawal of accreditation for failure to be in substantial compliance with the *Essentials*.
   2. For programs holding probationary accreditation, once a review committee has notified a program director that the program is accredited on a probationary basis, the program will be subject to withdrawal of accreditation for continued failure to be in substantial compliance with the *Essentials*.
   3. In giving notification, as indicated in 1 and 2 above, a review committee must indicate the areas in which the program is judged not to be in substantial compliance with the *Essentials*. It is understood that these areas may change in the course of multiple reviews conducted from the time a program is first given notice that it is not in compliance until withdrawal of accreditation may occur.

B. Request of Program. Voluntary withdrawal of accreditation may occur at the request of the program director in the following ways:
   1. A program director may request voluntary withdrawal of accreditation of a program, without prejudice. It is expected that if a program is deficient for one or more of the reasons set forth in E below, the director will seek voluntary withdrawal of accreditation. Normally such requests would come from the program director, with a letter of confirmation from the sponsoring institution's chief executive officer.
   2. Two or more programs may be merged into a single new program. If the review committee accredits the new program, it will take concurrent action for withdrawal of accreditation, without prejudice, of the previously separate programs. The review committee will consider the expressed preference of the program director in establishing the effective date for withdrawal of accreditation of the program(s).

C. Delinquency of Payment. Programs that are judged to be delinquent in payment of fees are not eligible for review and shall be notified by certified mail, return receipt requested, of the effective date of withdrawal of accreditation. On that date, the program will be removed from the list of ACGME-accredited programs.

D. Noncompliance with Accreditation Actions and Procedures. A program director may be deemed to have withdrawn from the voluntary process of accreditation and a review committee may take appropriate action to withdraw accreditation if that director refuses to comply with the following actions and procedures:
   1. To undergo a site visit and program review;
   2. To follow directives associated with an accreditation action; and
   3. To supply a review committee with requested information.

E. Program Inactivity or Deficiency. A review committee may withdraw accreditation from a program, regardless of its current accreditation status, under the following circumstances:
   1. The program has been inactive for 2 or more years.
   2. The program has incurred a catastrophic loss or complete change of resources, eg, faculty, facilities, or funding, such that the program is judged not accreditable.

F. Withdrawal of accreditation for reasons noted in the above paragraphs (Delinquency of Payment, Noncompliance with Accreditation Actions and Procedures, and Program Inactivity or Deficiency) is an administrative action and is not subject to the appeals process.

G. The following policies apply when action is taken to withdraw accreditation (except for establishment of an effective date in the case of voluntary withdrawal of accreditation or withdrawal of accreditation because of inactivity or deficiency):
   1. The effective date of withdrawal of accreditation shall not be less than 1 year from the date of the final action taken in the procedures to withdraw accreditation.
   2. The effective date of withdrawal of accreditation shall permit the completion of the training year in which the action becomes effective.
   3. Once notification has been made of the effective date of withdrawal of accreditation, no residents may be appointed to the program.
   4. When action has been taken by a review committee to withdraw accreditation of a residency program and the program has entered into appeal procedures, an application for reaccreditation of the program will not be considered until the appeal action is concluded.

The *Procedures for Proposed Adverse Actions* and *Procedures for Appeal of Adverse Actions,* provided in this document, contain further details.

Actions Regarding Accreditation of Subspecialty Programs

There are two procedural models for the accreditation of subspecialty programs:

A. When the accreditation status of a subspecialty program is not directly related to, or dependent upon, the status of a general specialty/parent program, the subspecialty programs are accredited in accordance with the same procedures used for general specialty programs as heretofore described.

B. When the accreditation status of a subspecialty program is directly related to, or dependent upon, the status of a general specialty/parent program, the following accreditation actions are used:

1. Withhold Accreditation. A review committee may withhold accreditation when it determines that the proposal for a new subspecialty program does not substantially comply with the *Essentials*. The review committee will cite those areas in which the proposed program does not comply with the *Essentials*.
2. Accreditation. The subspecialty program has demonstrated substantial compliance with the *Essentials* and is attached to a general specialty program that holds full accreditation or is otherwise deemed satisfactory by the review committee.
3. Accreditation With Warning. The accredited subspecialty program has been found to have one or more areas of noncompliance with the *Essentials* that are of sufficient substance to require correction.
4. Accreditation With Warning, Administrative. The general specialty program to which the subspecialty program is attached has been granted accreditation on a probationary basis. This action simultaneously constitutes an administrative warning of potential loss of accreditation to any subspecialty program that is attached to the general specialty program.
5. Withdraw Accreditation. An accredited subspecialty program is considered not to be in substantial compliance with the *Essentials* and has received a warning about areas of noncompliance.
6. Withdraw Accreditation, Administrative. If a general specialty program has its accreditation withdrawn, simultaneously the accreditation of any subspecialty program that is attached to the general specialty program is administratively withdrawn.
7. Other Actions by a Review Committee. The policies and procedures on withdrawal of accreditation of general specialty programs, as well as those on deferral of action, resident complement, participating institutions, and progress reports governing general specialty programs, also apply to the actions concerning subspecialty programs.

Warning Notices

A review committee may use a special procedure to advise a program director that it has serious concerns about the quality of the program and that the program's future accreditation status may be in jeopardy. In keeping with the flexibility inherent in the accreditation process, each review committee may use this procedure in accordance with its own interpretation of program quality and the use of the different accreditation categories. This procedure is not considered an adverse action and therefore is not subject to the appeal procedures.

The warning procedure may be used as follows:

A. For a program with provisional accreditation. A review committee may elect to continue provisional accreditation, but include in the letter of notification a statement that the program will be reviewed in approximately 1 year, following a site visit, at which time withdrawal of accreditation will be considered if the program has not achieved satisfactory development in establishing substantial compliance with the *Essentials*.

B. For a program with full accreditation. A review committee may elect to continue full accreditation, but include in the letter of notification a statement that the program will be reviewed in approximately 1 year, following a site visit, at which time probationary accreditation will be considered if the program is not in substantial compliance with the *Essentials*.

C. Review committees may extend the interval before the next review to 2 years, as in cases where program improvements may be addressed more appropriately within 2 years rather than 1 year.

Deferral of Accreditation Action

A review committee may defer a decision on the accreditation status of a residency program. The primary reason for deferral of accreditation action is lack of sufficient information about specific issues, which precludes an informed and reasonable decision. When a committee defers accreditation action, the residency program retains its current accreditation status until a final decision is made.

Size of Resident Complement

The complement of residents in a program must be commensurate with the total capacity of the program to offer each resident an educational experience consistent with accreditation standards; thus, a review committee may indicate that a residency program is accredited to train a specific number of residents as a maximum at any one time. In addition, a committee may indicate the number of residents to be trained in each year of the program. A review committee may also indicate that a minimum number of residents is considered necessary in each program to provide an effective learning environment.

Participating Institutions

The sponsoring institution of a residency program may utilize one or more additional institutions to provide necessary educational resources. In such cases, a review committee may evaluate whether each participating institution contributes meaningfully to the educational program.

Progress Reports

A review committee may request a progress report from a program director. The committee should specify the exact information to be provided and a specific due date for the report.

Notification of Accreditation Status

Letters of Notification

Accreditation actions taken by a review committee are reported to program directors by formal letters of notification. The accreditation status of any program will change only by subsequent action of the review committee. The notification letters usually contain reference to the approximate time of the next site visit and review of the program.

Notifying Residents and Applicants

All residents in a program, as well as applicants (that is, all candidates invited to come for an interview), should be aware of the accreditation status of the program and must be notified of any change in the accreditation status. When an adverse action is taken, program directors must notify all current residents as well as applicants to the program in writing. For applicants, the information on accreditation status must be provided in writing prior to having candidates come to the program for an interview. Copies of the letters to residents and applicants must be kept on file by the program director and a copy must be sent to the executive director of the review committee within 50 days of receipt of the notification of the adverse action. Additional information regarding notification letters is contained in the *Procedures for Proposed Adverse Actions* and *Procedures for Appeal of Adverse Actions*.

Duration of Accreditation

When a residency program is initially accredited, accreditation commences with the date specified in the letter of notification. A program remains accredited until formal action is taken by a review committee to withdraw accreditation. The action to withdraw accreditation will specify the date on which accreditation ends. ACGME accreditation does not lapse merely because of the passage of time. The time interval specified in the letter of notification is the time of the next site visit and review; it does not imply that accreditation will end when the time of next review occurs.

Identification of Programs in ACGME Records

Because numerous users consult and reference ACGME records, the ACGME retains the right to identify programs in a way that is consistent and will not give unfair advantage to any program.

The following standards are followed:

a. The program title clearly identifies the sponsoring institution.
b. Only one sponsoring institution is identified.
c. Participating institutions are identified in the program listing only if they provide major teaching sites for resident education. This means that, in a 1-year program, residents must spend at least 2 months in a required rotation at the site for it to be listed; in a 2-year program, the rotation must be 4 months, and in a program of 3 years or longer, the rotation must be at least 6 months. Review committees retain the right to grant exceptions to this formula.
d. Outpatient facilities and ambulatory clinics are not listed.
e. Units that do not operate under a separate license are not listed as discrete training sites.

Procedures for Proposed Adverse Actions and Procedures for Appeal of Adverse Actions

Procedures for Proposed Adverse Actions (Effective January 1, 1993, Editorial Revision: June 1995)

The following procedures will be implemented when a Residency Review Committee (RRC) determines that a program is not in substantial compliance with the *Essentials of Accredited Residencies in Graduate Medical Education (Essentials).* [*Note*: Here and elsewhere in these *Procedures for Proposed Adverse Actions*, reference to "Residency Review Committee" also includes the ACGME's Transitional Year Review Committee.]

A. When an RRC determines that an adverse action is warranted, the RRC will first give notice of its proposed adverse action to the program director, the chief administrative officer, and the educational coordinator, if one is identified, of the sponsoring institution. This notice of proposed adverse action will include the citations that form the basis for the proposed adverse action, a copy of the site visitor's report, and the date by which the program may submit, in writing, its response to each of the citations and to the proposed adverse action. [*Note*: Here and elsewhere in these *Procedures for Proposed Adverse Actions*, the word "action" reflects delegation of accreditation authority to the RRC. In the event of a decision by an RRC not holding delegated authority, read "recommendation of an RRC and action by the ACGME" throughout the procedures.]

B. The program may provide to the RRC written information revising or expanding factual information previously submitted; challenging the findings of the site visitor; rebutting the interpretation and conclusions of the RRC; demonstrating that cited areas of noncompliance with the published standards did not exist at the time when the RRC reviewed the program and proposed an adverse decision; and contending that the program is in compliance with the standards. The RRC will determine whether the information may be considered without verification by a site visitor.

C. The RRC will complete its evaluation of the program at a regularly scheduled meeting, as indicated to the program director in the notice of proposed adverse action. The RRC may confirm the adverse action or modify its position and take a nonadverse action.

D. If an RRC confirms the adverse action, it will communicate to the program director the confirmed adverse action and the citations, as described above, including comments on the program director's response to these citations.

E. The letter of notification, which will include information on the right of the program to appeal the RRC's decision to the ACGME, will be sent to the program director, as well as to the persons or agencies entitled to receive copies. The program director may appeal the decision; otherwise, it is final. If the decision is accepted as final, the program director may subsequently request a new review in order to demonstrate that the program is in compliance with the standards.

F. Upon receipt of notification of a confirmed adverse accreditation action, the program director must inform, in writing, the residents and any applicants who have been invited to interview with the program that the adverse action has been confirmed, whether or not the action will be appealed. A copy of the written notice must be sent to the executive director of the RRC within 50 days of receipt of the RRC's letter of notification.

ACGME Procedures for Appeal of Adverse Actions (Effective Date: June 10, 1997)

A. If a Residency Review Committee (RRC) takes an adverse action, the program may request a hearing before an appeals panel. [*Note:* Here and elsewhere in these *Procedures for Appeal of Adverse Actions*, reference to "Residency Review Committee" also includes the ACGME's Transitional Year Review Committee.] [*Note:* Here and elsewhere in these *Procedures for Appeal of Adverse Actions*, the word "action" reflects delegation of accreditation authority to an RRC. In the event of a decision by an RRC not holding delegated authority, read "recommendation of an RRC and action by the ACGME" throughout the procedures.] If a written request for such a hearing is not received by the executive director of the ACGME within 30 days following receipt of the letter of notification, the action of an RRC will be deemed final and not subject to further appeal.

Requests for a hearing must be sent express mail to: Executive Director, Accreditation Council for Graduate Medical Education, 515 North State Street, Suite 2000, Chicago, Illinois 60610.

If a hearing is requested, the appeals panel will be appointed according to the following procedures:

1. The ACGME shall maintain a list of qualified persons in each specialty as potential appeals panel members.
2. For a given hearing, the program shall receive a copy of the list of potential appeals panel members and shall have an opportunity to delete a maximum of one-third of the names from the list of potential appeals panel members. Within 15 days of receipt of the list, the program shall submit its revised list to the executive director of the ACGME.
3. A three-member appeals panel will be constituted by the ACGME from among the remaining names on the list.

B. When a program requests a hearing before an appeals panel, the program reverts to its status prior to the appealed adverse action until the ACGME makes a final determination on the status of the program. Nonetheless, at this time residents and any applicants who have been invited to interview with the program must be informed in writing as to the confirmed adverse action by an

RRC on the accreditation status. A copy of the written notice must be sent to the executive director of the RRC within 50 days of receipt of the RRC's letter of notification.

C. Hearings conducted in conformity with these procedures will be held at a time and place to be determined by the ACGME. At least 25 days prior to the hearing, the program shall be notified of the time and place of the hearing.

D. The program will be given the documentation of the RRC action in confirming its adverse action.

E. The documents comprising the program file, the record of the RRC's action, together with oral and written presentations to the appeals panel, shall be the basis for the recommendations of the appeals panel.

F. The appeals panel shall meet and review the written record and receive the presentations. The appropriate RRC shall be notified of the hearing and a representative of the RRC may attend the hearing to be available to the appeals panel to provide clarification of the record.

Proceedings before an appeals panel are not of an adversary nature as typical in a court of law, but rather, provide an administrative mechanism for peer review of an accreditation decision about an educational program. The appeals panel shall not be bound by technical rules of evidence usually employed in legal proceedings.

The program may not amend the statistical or narrative descriptions on which the decision of the RRC was based. The appeals procedures limit the appeals panel's jurisdiction to clarification of information as of the time when the adverse action was proposed by the RRC. Information about the program subsequent to that time cannot be considered in the appeal. Furthermore, the appeals panel shall not consider any changes in the program or descriptions of the program that were not in the record at the time when the RRC reviewed the program and confirmed the adverse decision. [*Note:* Option: When there have been substantial changes in a program and/or correction of citations after the date of the proposed action by the RRC, a program may forego an appeal and request a new evaluation and accreditation decision. Such an evaluation will be done in accordance with the ACGME procedures, including an on-site survey of the program. The adverse status will remain in effect until a reevaluation and an accreditation decision have been made by the RRC.] Presentations shall be limited to clarifications of the record, arguments to address compliance by the program with the published standards for accreditation, and the review of the program in the context of the administrative procedures governing accreditation of programs. Presentations may include written and oral elements. The appellant may make oral arguments to the appeals panel, but the oral argument will be limited to 2 hours in duration.

The appellant shall communicate with the appeals panel only at the hearing or in writing through the executive director of the ACGME.

The appeals panel shall make recommendations to the ACGME whether there is substantial, credible, and relevant evidence to support the action taken by the RRC in the matter that is being appealed. The appeals panel, in addition, will make recommendations as to whether there has been substantial compliance with the administrative procedures governing the process of accreditation of graduate medical education programs.

G. The program may submit additional written material within 15 days after the hearing. The intention to submit such material must be made known to the appeals panel at the hearing.

H. The appeals panel shall submit its recommendations to the ACGME within 20 days after receipt of additional written material. The ACGME shall act on the appeal at its next regularly scheduled meeting.

I. The decision of the ACGME in this matter shall be final. There is no provision for further appeal.

J. The executive director of the ACGME shall, within 15 days following the final ACGME decision, notify the program under appeal of the decision of the ACGME.

K. Expenses of the appeals panel members and the associated administrative costs shall be shared equally by the appellant and the ACGME.

Program Organization

The organization of a program may involve any of several administrative forms. For example, a program may be conducted within a single institution, that is, the assignment of residents is limited to that institution; or a program may involve more than one institution, that is, the resident assignments are not limited to the sponsoring institution.

Some RRCs have specific requirements relating to program organization. These may be found in the appropriate *Program Requirements* (see Section II). In all cases, however, a single, clearly identified sponsoring organization must exercise oversight over the educational program.

Institutional Review

Procedures for review of sponsoring institutions for compliance with the *Institutional Requirements* of the *Essentials* have been established, in addition to the process of review and accreditation of programs in graduate medical education.

The purpose of the review is to determine whether the sponsoring institution has established, documented, and implemented institutional policies as required by the *Institutional Requirements* of the *Essentials* for the governance of all residency programs under its sponsorship.

Institutions that sponsor two or more programs will undergo an institutional site visit and will have formal review by the Institutional Review Committee of the ACGME. Institutions that sponsor only one residency program will undergo an institutional review as part of their program site visit and will be reviewed by the appropriate RRC.

Results of institutional review evaluation for institutions with two or more programs are reported as either favorable or unfavorable in a formal letter of report. The date of the next institutional review will be identified in this letter. Results of institutional review for institutions with a single residency are incorporated into the letter of notification concerning program accreditation.

An institution that has received an unfavorable evaluation can request another institutional review earlier than the specified review cycle. Two successive unfavorable reviews of an institution will lead to a warning and a third successive unfavorable review to the withdrawal of accreditation of all the residency programs sponsored by the institution. An appeals mechanism has been established for the latter contingency.

Fees for Evaluation and Accreditation

Fees charged for the accreditation of programs are determined annually by the ACGME. As of January 1, 1999, the following fee schedule is in effect.

Application Fee

A fee is charged for processing applications for programs seeking initial accreditation or reaccreditation, including subspecialty programs. The charge for applications is $3,000. It is normally billed at the time the application is received.

Program Site Visit and Review

A fee is charged for the site visit and review of programs.

The charge for a site visit and review by an ACGME field representative is $3,100, and by a specialist in the appropriate discipline, $3,250. This fee applies to all accredited programs, including subspecialty programs. This fee applies also to site visits for institutional review.

Annual per Resident Fee

An annual fee is charged for each position filled in an accredited residency training program. The fee is calculated on the number of residents/fellows/trainees in each program as of September 1 of the given academic year. Programs are billed around January 1 of each academic year. The fee charged in 1998-1999 was $50 per resident.

Information and Inquiries

Inquiries regarding the accreditation of residency programs should be directed to ACGME staff members listed below. The educational standards (Essentials of Accredited Residencies in Graduate Medical Education: Institutional and Program Requirements) published in this edition of the *Graduate Medical Education Directory* have an effective date as indicated for each document. Please consult with the ACGME for changes in those standards that occur throughout the year. Copies of the Institutional Requirements and of the Program Requirements for each specialty/subspecialty may be obtained through the Internet at http://www.acgme.org or through the ACGME FAXBACK system at (312) 245-9174. Other documents pertaining to the accreditation process are also available through either of these sources.

The address for the ACGME is as follows:

ACGME
515 N State St/Ste 2000
Chicago, IL 60610

Inquiries regarding fees should be directed to:

Barbara J Warren
ACGME Credit Manager (invoices, vouchers)
515 N State St/Ste 2000
Chicago, IL 60610
312 464-4939

ACGME staff members may be contacted for information as follows:

David C Leach, MD
Executive Director, ACGME
312 464-4920
E-mail: dcl@acgme.org

Judith S Armbruster, PhD
Executive Director, RRCs for
Anesthesiology
Nuclear Medicine
Radiation Oncology
Radiology-Diagnostic
312 464-4642
E-mail: jsa@acgme.org

John T Boberg, PhD
Executive Director, RRCs for
Ophthalmology
Surgery
Thoracic Surgery
312 464-4687
E-mail: jtb@acgme.org

Larry D Sulton, PhD
Executive Director, RRCs for
Emergency Medicine
Neurological Surgery
Preventive Medicine
Psychiatry
312 464-5404
E-mail: lds@acgme.org

Steven P Nestler, PhD
Executive Director, RRCs for
Dermatology
Medical Genetics
Orthopaedic Surgery
Pathology
312 464-4692
E-mail: spn@acgme.org

Paul O'Connor, PhD
Executive Director, RRCs for
Colon and Rectal Surgery
Neurology
Obstetrics and Gynecology
Physical Medicine and Rehabilitation
312 464-4683
E-mail: poc@acgme.org

Mary Alice Parsons
Executive Director, RRCs for
Family Practice
Pediatrics
312 464-4947
E-mail: map@acgme.org

William E Rodak, PhD
Executive Director, RRC for
Internal Medicine
312 464-4953
E-mail: wer@acgme.org

Karen L Lambert
Associate Executive Director, RRC for
Internal Medicine
312-464-5472
E-mail: kll@acgme.org

Doris A Stoll, PhD
Executive Director, RRCs for
Allergy and Immunology
Otolaryngology
Plastic Surgery
Urology
312 464-5505
E-mail: das@acgme.org

Linda Thorsen
Executive Director for
Transitional Year Review Committee
RRC for Psychiatry - Child and Adolescent Psychiatry Subcommittee
312 464-5366
E-mail: lmt@acgme.org

Marsha A Stojek
Associate Executive Director, RRCs for
Anesthesiology
Diagnostic Radiology
Pediatrics
312 464-4940
E-mail: mas@acgme.org

Cynthia Taradejna
Executive Director for
Institutional Review Committee
312 464-4685
E-mail: cat@acgme.org

Ingrid Philibert
Director of Field Staff (site visits)
312 464-4948
E-mail: iphilibert@acgme.org

Barbara J Warren
Office Manager
312 464-4939
E-mail: bjw@acgme.org

Tami S Walters
ACGME Accreditation Appeals Administrator
312 464-5584
E-mail: tsw@acgme.org

John H Nylen, MBA
Director of Information Services
312 464-4962
E-mail: jhn@acgme.org

Sheri A Bellar
Help Desk Specialist
Department of Information Services
312 464-5393
E-mail: sab@acgme.org

Susan R Swing, PhD
Director of Research
312 464-5402
E-mail: srs@acgme.org

Marvin R Dunn, MD
Director of Residency Review Committee Activities
312 464-5405
E-mail: mrd@acgme.org

Entry of Foreign-born Medical Graduates to the United States

The entry of foreign-born graduates of non-US medical schools to the United States is governed by the US Immigration and Nationality Act (INA), as amended, which is administered by the US Immigration and Naturalization Service (INS) of the Department of Justice, by the Department of State, and by other departments and agencies specified in the Act. It is a violation of federal law to provide employment to a non-US citizen who does not hold a visa permitting employment or other appropriate work authorization documents from the INS. Thus, residency program directors considering foreign-born international medical graduates (IMGs) should appoint only those whose visa classification or status in the US permits employment and participation in a training program. The most common of these are exchange visitor (J-1), temporary worker (H-1B), immigrant visa or "green card," or an INS-issued or -approved work permit. These foreign-born IMGs must also hold the Standard Certificate of the Educational Commission for Foreign Medical Graduates.

The Educational Commission for Foreign Medical Graduates (ECFMG), through its program of certification, assesses the readiness of IMGs to enter US residency or fellowship programs that are accredited by the Accreditation Council for Graduate Medical Education (ACGME). The ECFMG and its sponsoring organizations define an IMG as a physician whose basic medical degree or qualification was conferred by a medical school located outside the United States, Canada, and Puerto Rico. The medical school must be listed at the time of graduation in the *World Directory of Medical Schools* published by the World Health Organization. US citizens who have completed their medical education in schools outside the United States, Canada, and Puerto Rico are considered IMGs, while foreign nationals who have graduated from medical schools in the United States, Canada, and Puerto Rico are not.

ECFMG certification provides assurance to ACGME-accredited residency and fellowship program directors and to the people of the United States that IMGs have met minimum standards of eligibility required to enter such programs. ECFMG certification is also a prerequisite required by most states for licensure to practice medicine in the United States and is one of the eligibility requirements to take Step 3 of the United States Medical Licensing Examination (USMLE).

To meet the *medical education credential requirements* for ECFMG certification, applicants must document the completion of all requirements for, and receipt of, the final medical diploma. All documents provided to ECFMG are sent by ECFMG to the foreign medical schools for verification by the appropriate officials. ECFMG medical education credential requirements are not fulfilled until such verifications are received directly from the medical school and accepted by the ECFMG.

To meet the *examination requirements* for ECFMG certification, an applicant must:

1. Pass the basic medical and clinical science components of the medical science examination within a 7-year period. Step 1 and Step 2 of the USMLE are currently administered for this purpose. The ECFMG also accepts a passing performance on the following former medical science examinations for the purpose of ECFMG certification: ECFMG Examination, Visa Qualifying Examination (VQE), Foreign Medical Graduate Examination in the Medical Sciences (FMGEMS), and Part I and Part II Examinations of the National Board of Medical Examiners (NBME). Additionally, ECFMG accepts, for the purpose of its certification, a score of 75 or higher on each of the 3 days of a single administration of the

former Federation Licensing Examination (FLEX), if taken prior to June 1985.

Certain combinations of examinations are also acceptable. Applicants who have passed only part of the former VQE, FMGEMS, or the NBME Part I or Part II may combine a passing performance on the basic medical science component of one of these examinations or USMLE Step 1 with a passing performance on the clinical science component of one of the other examinations or USMLE Step 2, provided that the components are passed within the period specified for the examination program. While these examination combinations are accepted by the ECFMG for its certification, applicants should be aware that after December 31, 1999, use of portions of FLEX or portions of the Part examination sequence of the NBME to fulfill the eligibility requirements for USMLE Step 3 will no longer be accepted. Additionally, although the ECFMG Examination and FLEX, if taken prior to June 1985, satisfy the medical science examination requirement for ECFMG certification, they have not been recognized by the US Secretary of Health and Human Services as meeting the medical science examination requirement to obtain a visa to enter the United States (see below).

2. Pass the English Language Proficiency Test.

Through March 3, 1999
A passing performance on the ECFMG English Test is accepted by ECFMG to meet this requirement. The only alternative English test that the ECFMG will accept is a paper-based Friday or Saturday (formerly special or international) administration or a computer-based administration of the Test of English as a Foreign Language (TOEFL), provided that applicants have previously taken an ECFMG English Test.

After March 3, 1999
The last administration of the ECFMG English Test is scheduled for March 3, 1999. After this date, applicants will be required to demonstrate a performance acceptable to the ECFMG on one of the TOEFL administrations described above. (Applicants who have not fulfilled the English language proficiency requirement by March 3, 1999, will no longer be required to have taken the ECFMG English Test prior to taking TOEFL.) For applicants who have not taken a prior ECFMG English Test, the administration date of the TOEFL submitted in fulfillment of this requirement must be after March 3, 1999. A passing performance on the ECFMG English Test will continue to be accepted by ECFMG to fulfill the English language proficiency requirement after March 3, 1999.

Passing performance on the English language proficiency test is valid for 2 years from the date passed for the purpose of entry into graduate medical education.

3. Pass the ECFMG Clinical Skills Assessment (CSA). Passing performance is valid for 3 years from the date passed for the purpose of entry into graduate medical education.

The Standard ECFMG Certificate is issued to applicants who meet the examination requirements (medical science examination, English language proficiency test, and Clinical Skills Assessment), fulfill the medical education credential requirements, and clear their financial accounts with ECFMG. The Standard ECFMG Certificate may be used for entry into accredited graduate medical education programs so long as the program start date is not later than either of the "valid through" dates (English test and Clinical Skills Assessment) indicated on the Standard ECFMG Certificate. If the holder of the certificate has entered such a program in the United States before the expiration of the "valid-through" dates, the dates are no longer subject to expiration. In order for an applicant to obtain permanent validation for the certificate, the ECFMG must receive a *Request for Permanent Validation of Standard ECFMG Certificate* (Form 246). On receipt of such official documentation, the ECFMG will provide "valid indefinitely" sticker(s) to the holder of the certificate. The English test "valid-through" date may also be revalidated for a period of 2 years by passing a subsequent TOEFL; the CSA "valid-through" date may be revalidated for a period of 3 years by passing a subsequent CSA.

For further information on ECFMG examinations and certification, contact:

ECFMG
3624 Market St
Philadelphia, PA 19104-2685
215 386-5900
215 386-9196 Fax
Internet: http://www.ecfmg.org

Visas That Permit Graduate Medical Education or Training

Exchange Visitor J-1

Foreign national physicians use the exchange visitor J-1 nonimmigrant visa class most often for graduate medical education and training. The Exchange Visitor Program is regulated by the United States Information Agency (USIA), which designates various organizations and educational institutions as Exchange Visitor Program sponsors. Each designation is designed for a specific purpose appropriate to that sponsor. The USIA has designated the ECFMG as the only organization authorized to sponsor foreign national physicians to engage in graduate medical education or training. Such education or training is defined in the US Code of Federal Regulations as participation in a program in which the foreign national physician will receive graduate medical education or training, which generally consists of a residency or fellowship program involving the provision of health care services to patients. This program may consist of a medical specialty, a directly related medical subspecialty, or both.

To be eligible for ECFMG exchange visitor sponsorship for graduate medical education, the foreign national physician must pass specific examinations and meet certain other requirements. ECFMG's application and instructions for J-1 visa sponsorship are available via the Internet at http://www.ecfmg.org.

Examinations. The INA requires that the physician pass either the National Board of Medical Examiners (NBME) Part I and Part II examinations, or an examination determined to be equivalent to the NBME examinations by the Secretary of the US Department of Health and Human Services. The following examinations have been determined to be equivalent to the NBME Part 1 and Part 2 examinations for this purpose:

Day 1 and Day 2 of the former Visa Qualifying Examination;

Day 1 and Day 2 of the former Foreign Medical Graduate Examination in the Medical Sciences; and

Step 1 and Step 2 of the United States Medical Licensing Examination.

(*Note:* The former 1-day ECFMG examination does *not* meet the requirements for J-1 visa sponsorship.)

Other Requirements. The foreign national physician must hold a valid Standard ECFMG Certificate or be eligible for the certificate and awaiting its issue (see "Certification by the ECFMG").

The physician must have a contract to train in an accredited graduate medical education program that is affiliated with a Liaison Committee on Medical Education (LCME)-accredited medical school or affiliated hospital.

The physician must provide a written statement from the Ministry of Health in the country of most recent legal permanent residence that attests to the need for physicians trained in the exchange visitor's specialty and that verifies that the exchange visitor has filed written assurance that he/she will return to the country upon completion of training.

Upon establishing an applicant's eligibility, the ECFMG issues Form IAP-66, Certificate of Eligibility for Exchange Visitor (J-1) status. Associated training/employment authorization is specific to approved sponsorship stated on Form IAP-66. A Form IAP-66 obtained for a particular program may be used only for that program and is not transferrable to another institution or program. Unauthorized employment outside the approved training program is a violation of J-1 status.

The duration of participation for exchange visitors in graduate medical education is the time typically required to complete the program. The director of the USIA establishes the limit, which is usually the time required to meet the educational requirements for certification by an American specialty board that has been recognized by the American Board of Medical Specialties. The maximum duration of participation is further limited to 7 years and is available for those exchange visitor physicians who progress in programs of graduate medical education. Extensions beyond 7 years may be granted by the director of the USIA when exceptional need in the home country is demonstrated.

Exchange visitor physicians who enter the United States for the purpose of graduate medical education are automatically subject to the 2-year home country physical presence requirement of the Immigration and Nationality Act as amended. This means that prior to obtaining H (temporary worker), L (intracompany transferee), permanent resident, or immigrant status, the exchange visitor must reside and be physically present in the country of most recent legal permanent residence for an aggregate of at least 2 years.

Foreign nationals who are graduates of LCME-accredited US and Canadian medical schools and who wish to enter the United States for the purpose of graduate medical education are also eligible for ECFMG sponsorship. They are *not required* to hold a Standard ECFMG Certificate or pass the examinations required under PL94-484 to obtain an Exchange Visitor visa. However, they must meet the other requirements for Exchange Visitor sponsorship and are held to the 2-year home country physical presence requirement.

An uncommon, but possible, case occurs when an exchange visitor is a medical student in J-1 student status at a US college or university. Such students who graduate from US LCME-accredited medical schools are eligible for up to 36 months of postdoctoral academic training in the field of study. Graduates of US medical schools may, therefore, use academic training authorization to undertake a residency. This work must be authorized by the school from which the student graduated. (The USIA has indicated that it is reviewing internally whether this kind of academic training is appropriate, but the Agency has not, so far, moved to change its regulations in this regard.) The J-1 "responsible officer" at the US medical school can usually provide information necessary to make employment eligibility determinations for these graduates. If the training will take longer than 3 years, some other visa class must be sought for the additional years. The 2-year home country physical presence requirement does not automatically apply to these individuals because they are not under ECFMG sponsorship for clinical training. However, the requirement may apply on one of the other grounds such as US or foreign government funding or a home country "skills list."

Foreign national physicians who wish to enter the United States for advanced training may do so in programs involving observation, consultation, teaching, or research with or without patient contact incidental to one or more of these activities. The ECFMG is authorized to sponsor foreign national physicians for this purpose. The USIA may also authorize universities and other health science institutions to sponsor foreign national physicians for this purpose.

It is important to note that J-1 (exchange visitor) status physicians who enter the United States in a J-1 visa category other than the trainee category of "alien physician" under ECFMG sponsorship may not, as a matter of course, change their J-1 visa category to alien physician to allow them to engage in graduate medical education or training sponsored by the ECFMG. The ECFMG, as the proposed new sponsor, must present a request for visa category change to the USIA for review and decision. The request must demonstrate unusual and extenuating circumstances. Similarly, an attempt to exit in a nonclinical J-1 category and return under ECFMG sponsorship for clinical training is likely to be unsuccessful. Although the USIA has not published a change in its regulations, it appears that it has instructed the ECFMG to withhold Form IAP-66 from physicians who have held J-1 status during the year immediately preceding the beginning of the intended training program. This is, in fact, an extra-regulatory imposition of a 1-year bar to the J-1 for training purposes. Exchange visitors in programs involving observation, consultation, teaching, or research may remain in the United States for a maximum of 3 years with a possible 6-month extension under specific circumstances. Although it has the authority to do so, the USIA rarely grants extensions beyond 3.5 years.

Temporary Worker H-1B

The H-1B visa is for temporary workers in specialty occupations who hold professional level (bachelor's degree minimum) appropriate to the employment in which they will be engaged. Between 1976 and 1991, graduates of foreign medical schools were not permitted to use the H-1B for residencies, except in cases where individuals were of national or international renown. The Immigration Act of 1990, and subsequent technical amendments, made the H-1B available to graduates of foreign medical schools who have passed FLEX or the equivalent, have passed an English language exam, and hold a license appropriate to the activity. The Secretary of the Department of Health and Human Services has determined that the USMLE Steps 1, 2, and 3 or the former NBME Parts I, II, and III are equivalent to FLEX for this purpose. Combinations of the USMLE and NBME are not acceptable for this purpose; only the full series of one or the other meets the H-1B requirement. The level of licensure required is determined by the state and by the activity. For example, in many states a limited or training license is sufficient for a residency and would be acceptable for the H-1B.

Because of the FLEX or equivalent examination requirement and the requirement in most states that physicians complete a certain amount of US training prior to admission to the third or final portion of the licensure exam, it is likely that only a small number of physicians will qualify for and use the H-1B visa for residencies. Because the purpose of the J-1 (exchange visitor) visa is to provide foreign nationals with opportunities to participate in educational and cultural programs in the United States, many individuals and organizations believe that the J-1 visa is the appropriate visa for the purpose of graduate medical education. This is a matter of philosophy, not law. Any training program may, for its own reasons, elect to file or refrain from filing H-1B petitions for trainees. At the request of the trainee, some training programs will sponsor H-1B status, and others will not. Training programs are subject neither to prohibition nor obligation in this regard.

H-1B employment authorization is employer-specific, so that the training program must file an H-1B petition on behalf of the international medical graduate. An H-1B visa obtained for a particular program may be used only for that program and is not transferrable to another institution or program. Each new institution/employer must file a new petition. The total amount of continuous time permitted in H-1B classification is 6 years; no extensions are permitted. An absence from the United States of 1 year or more restarts the 6-year period.

There are some exceptions and special circumstances. Graduates of LCME-accredited US medical schools are exempt from the FLEX and English language examination requirements. Graduates of LCME-accredited Canadian medical schools are exempt from the English language exam, but not the FLEX exam. Interestingly, full licensure in Canada based on Canadian examinations, which may be reciprocal for full licensure in a US state, is not equivalent to FLEX for H-1B purposes. The FLEX, or its equivalent, is still required even if these physicians hold full licensure in the state in which training will occur. Physicians of national or international renown are exempt from the special examination requirements for the H-1B, but must meet the usual examination and certification requirements described in the *Essentials of Accredited Residencies in Graduate Medical Education* (see Section II) for admission to a GME program and must meet licensure requirements for the intended training. Certain physicians admitted to subspecialty or upper-level GME programs may have an established reputation at the specialty level and may qualify for this exemption.

F-1 Student Optional Practical Training

Students in F-1 status may be authorized for up to 12 months of practical training after completion of studies for an appointment that can be completed in 12 months. This is appropriate for the first or matched year, which is a 1-year contract. IMGs who receive US medical degrees while in F-1 status may apply to the INS for practical training work authorization. If employment authorization is granted, the individual may use that authorization for residency education for a period of 12 months. The F-1 "designated school official" at the US medical school can usually provide information necessary to make employment eligibility determinations for these graduates. Note that graduation from a US PhD program does not permit practical training in graduate medical education, since the PhD prepares one for research, but not for clinical practice.

Persons of Extraordinary Ability O-1

The O-1 is for persons of extraordinary ability demonstrated by sustained national or international acclaim. Although rare at the GME level, it is possible and not unknown. In medicine, most often this is someone who, as the definition indicates, has an established and exceptional reputation in a particular field based on original research or on development of specialized techniques for patient care. These people come into or remain in GME programs to apply their research clinically or to enhance or improve their techniques by acquiring related skills. For J-1 physicians at or near the end of the J-1 time limits, it provides an avenue for continuing training beyond those limits. Another important characteristic is that the J-1 2-year home country physical presence requirement does not prevent one from obtaining O-1 status. That requirement's restrictions apply only to obtaining H, L, and immigrant visas. For example, one can depart from the United States as a J-1 and return almost immediately as an O-1 provided an appropriate O-1 petition has been approved and an O-1 visa obtained at a post abroad. (See "Exchange Visitor J-1" for information on time limits and the home residence requirement.) Similar to the H-1B, the O-1 petition must be filed with the INS for a particular GME program at a particular location, and employment is limited to work for the employer who filed the petition in the capacity described in the petition. Unlike the H-1B, no special examination requirements apply. The physician must meet the usual examination and certification requirements described in the *Essentials of Accredited Residencies in Graduate Medical Education* (see Section II) for admission to a GME program and must meet licensure requirements for the intended training. Obtaining the O-1 does not waive the 2-year home country physical presence requirement of the J-1 Exchange Visitor status. Regardless of how long one remains in the United States in O-1 status, the requirement continues to attach to the physician's immigration status until it has been met or waived. Nothing in the O-1 status ameliorates the prohibition against H, L, or permanent resident status.

Employment Authorization From the US Immigration and Naturalization Service

The INS is empowered to grant employment authorization to certain nonimmigrants or intending immigrants. Such authorization is usually temporary and may have conditions.

A common employment authorization in academic institutions is that given to the J-2 spouse or child of a J-1 exchange visitor. J-2 dependents may apply to the INS for work authorization provided it is not to support the principal J-1. When granted, it permits any employment for which the individual is qualified, including residency training. Residency program directors are cautioned that this employment authorization is absolutely dependent upon the J-1 exchange visitor maintaining status. If the J-1 leaves the United States, or fails to maintain status, the J-2 work authorization ends, even though he/she may hold a J-2 employment authorization document that appears to be valid.

Other classifications or circumstances under which the INS may grant work authorization include, but are not limited to, G-4 dependent of a foreign government employee in the United States, temporary protected status, voluntary departure, refugee, asylee, or certain lawful permanent resident applicants. These must be evaluated case by case.

Lawful Permanent Resident (Immigrant) Status

Persons who hold lawful permanent resident or "green card" status are permitted to remain in the United States permanently and to accept any employment for which they qualify. All physicians, regardless of visa status, must meet the usual examination and certification requirements described in the *Essentials of Accredited Residencies in Graduate Medical Education* (see Section II) for admission to a GME program and must meet licensure requirements of the intended training.

Foreign-born international medical graduates may immigrate to the United States based on relationship to a US citizen, lawful permanent resident, or employment and skills. In general, the rules for immigration are the same for international medical graduates as for any other immigrant, but special rules apply to physicians who immigrate based on their intention and ability to practice the profession of medicine, including practice at the residency level. Employment-based immigration based on a job offer for the practice of medicine requires that the physician pass the NBME Parts I and II examinations, or the equivalent as determined by the Secretary of the US Department of Health and Human Services. These are the same examinations needed for ECFMG sponsorship for clinical training and for ECFMG certification described earlier. Certain exceptions apply to physicians who are of national or international renown.

Information and Inquiries

ECFMG Certification and J-1 Visa Sponsorship

Educational Commission for Foreign Medical Graduates
3624 Market St
Philadelphia, PA 19104-2685
Internet: http://www.ecfmg.org

Certification
215 386-5900
215 386-9196 Fax
Exchange Visitor Sponsorship Program (J-1 Visa)
215 823-2121
215 386-9766 Fax

F-1 Student Practical Training and J-1 Student Academic Training

NAFSA: Association of International Educators
1307 New York Ave NW
Washington, DC 20005-4701
202 462-4811
Internet: http://www.nafsa.org

H-1B, O-1, Lawful Permanent Resident Status, and Other Temporary Work Authorization

American Immigration Lawyers Association
1400 Eye St NW/Ste 1200
Washington, DC 20005
202 371-9377
http://aila.org

Catheryn Cotten, Director
Duke University International Office
Box 3882 DUMC
Durham, NC 27710
919 681-8472
919 681-8492 Fax
E-mail: cotte002@mc.duke.edu

Fifth Pathway Program

The Fifth Pathway Program, an academic year of supervised clinical education provided by a Liaison Committee on Medical Education (LCME)-accredited medical school, is available to persons who meet all of the following conditions:

A. Have completed, in an accredited US college or university, undergraduate premedical work of the quality acceptable for matriculation in an accredited US medical school;
B. Have studied medicine in a medical school located outside the United States, Puerto Rico, and Canada that is listed in the *World Directory of Medical Schools,* published by the World Health Organization;
C. Have completed all of the formal requirements of the non-US medical school except internship and/or social service. (Those who have completed all of these requirements, including internship and/or social service, are not eligible for the Fifth Pathway program.)

Students who have completed the academic curriculum in residence at a non-US medical school and who meet the above conditions may be offered the opportunity to substitute, for an internship and/or social service required by a non-US medical school, an academic year of supervised clinical training provided in a medical school accredited by the LCME.

Before beginning the supervised clinical training, students must pass an examination acceptable to the sponsoring medical school.

Physicians who have a Fifth Pathway Certificate and have passed Steps I and II of the United States Medical Licensing Examination (USMLE), the Foreign Medical Graduate Examination in the Medical Sciences (FMGEMS), or the Visa Qualifying Examination (VQE) are eligible for appointment to a residency program. They must also meet requirements established by the state medical board in the state where the residency program is located and must be accepted for appointment by the director of the residency program. Any medical school accredited by the LCME can provide Fifth Pathway education. As of the printing of this *Directory*, the only medical school known to provide such education is New York Medical College in Valhalla, New York. For more information, contact Dolores Ercole at 914 993-4000.

Appointment to US Uniformed Services Graduate Medical Education Programs

US Uniformed Services (Army, Navy, Air Force, Public Health Service) first-year GME positions are filled by graduates of accredited schools of medicine and osteopathic medicine. Only those individuals who have graduated from accredited US medical schools are eligible to apply for these first-year GME positions. The majority of the Uniformed Services' first-year GME positions are filled by individuals with an existing active duty service obligation. In most cases, only those individuals already serving in the Uniformed Services are eligible for appointment to military postgraduate year 2 and beyond residency positions. Graduates of non-US or non-Canadian medical schools are eligible to apply for postgraduate year 2 positions if they possess the standard ECFMG Certificate and have completed 1 year of GME training at an ACGME-accredited program.

It is important to note that an individual seeking to be trained in a Uniformed Services medical treatment facility **must** be qualified for appointment as a commissioned officer in the Uniformed Services. **An active duty service obligation is required for participation in Uniformed Services GME training.** Acceptance of GME applications from civilian applicants may vary among the four services. Selection priorities for Uniformed Services positions for year 2 and beyond are given to officers on active duty. For more information, interested individuals should contact their local Uniformed Services recruiting office.

Electronic Residency Application Service (ERAS)

ERAS is the Electronic Residency Application Service from the Association of American Medical Colleges (AAMC). It is being used for 1999-2000 applications by most residency programs in emergency medicine, family practice, internal medicine, obstetrics and gynecology, orthopaedic surgery, pediatrics, physical medicine and rehabilitation, general surgery, and radiology, as well as transitional year, combined internal medicine/pediatrics, and US Army programs. For more information about ERAS, students and graduates of US medical schools should contact the student affairs office at their medical schools of graduation. Students and graduates of foreign medical schools should contact the Educational Commission for Foreign Medical Graduates (ECFMG). General information about ERAS is available through the Internet at *http://www.aamc.org/eras*.

National Resident Matching Program

The National Resident Matching Program (NRMP) has been matching the preferences of applicants and programs for residency positions since 1952. The program was created to provide both applicants and residency program directors a fair opportunity to consider their options for appointment, to make reasoned decisions, and to have their decisions announced at a specified time. Participants in the NRMP agreed to honor the commitment to offer or to accept an appointment if a match resulted.

In 1998, in addition to 15,914 US medical students, another 19,909 "independent" applicants competed for 20,299 first graduate year positions and 2,152 second graduate year positions offered in the NRMP. Independent applicants include US physicians and eligible students/graduates of osteopathic, Canadian, and foreign medical schools, and Fifth Pathway programs. The numbers of applicants and programs participating in the 1998 match was virtually unchanged from the previous year.

The NRMP is not a centralized application service. Applicants apply directly to residency programs and the programs administer their own selection process, including requests for interviews. Programs that participate in the NRMP require applicants to register with the NRMP. In February, after interviewing has been completed, applicants and programs submit to the NRMP Rank Order Lists indicating their choices in order of preference.

Beginning with the 1999 Match, all participants will submit their Rank Order Lists to the NRMP via the Web. The disk-based Rank Order List Input and Confirmation (ROLIC) system will be replaced by a Web-based ROLIC system. The new WebROLIC system will be updated daily with current information on applicants and programs participating in the match.

Both applicants and programs must agree that neither will ask the other to make a commitment before the Match Day, although a high level of interest may be expressed. Verbal or written contracts prior to Match Day should not be expected or made. The final preferences of program directors and applicants as reflected on the submitted Rank Order Lists will determine the offering of positions and the placement of applicants.

Through the NRMP process, each applicant and program submits a list of their preferences in rank order. Through the matching process, an applicant is matched into a program he or she prefers that has ranked the applicant and has not been matched with an applicant ranked higher on the program's list. Traditionally, match results are announced in mid-March. Applicants who fail to obtain a position and programs that do not fill all their offered positions are informed 2 days before the general announcement so that they may contact one another to secure appointments. The majority of appointments to residency programs begin on or about July 1.

Positions Offered Through the NRMP

The positions offered by programs participating in the NRMP are typically those sought by US seniors; that is, positions that provide the first year of graduate training. In addition, specialties that start their training at the second graduate year offer positions in the NRMP, so that applicants may link their first and second years of training.

Categorical (C) positions are offered by programs that expect applicants who enter in their first graduate year to continue until completion of training required for specialty certification, provided their performance is satisfactory (normally 3 to 4 years).

Preliminary (P) positions provide 1 or 2 years of prerequisite training for entry into advanced programs that require 1 or more years of clinical training. Internal medicine, surgery, and transitional year programs commonly offer preliminary positions.

Advanced (S) positions at the second graduate year, which do not commence until a year after the match, are in specialty programs that require completion of 1 or more years of preliminary training. Applicants without prior graduate medical training may apply for these positions while also applying for preliminary positions that are compatible with their plans.

Resident (R) positions at the second graduate year, which begin in July of the NRMP year, are reserved for physicians who have had prior graduate medical education. These positions are not available to senior US medical students.

Couples and Shared Residency Positions

Applicants who are members of a couple may link their program choices together. In creating pairs of program choices, couples can mix specialties, program types, and geographic locations.

Some programs offer shared residency positions. In a shared residency, two residents share one position, usually alternating months on clinical rotations, with time off to devote to family, research, or other interests. Obtaining a shared residency position through the NRMP requires that two applicants who have enrolled separately in the NRMP become partners to be matched together in a single position.

Specialties Matching Services

In addition to the conduct of the match for first and second graduate year residency positions, the NRMP conducts matches for advanced residency or fellowship positions through the Specialties Matching Services. These specialty matches occur throughout the year, and each requires its own registration with the NRMP.

Specialty matches currently include the following:

- Combined Musculoskeletal Matching Program (participating subspecialties of orthopaedic surgery)
- Child and adolescent psychiatry
- Colon and rectal surgery
- General vascular surgery
- Medical Specialties Matching Program (participating subspecialties of internal medicine)
- Obstetrics-Gynecologic Fellowship Match (including gynecologic oncology, maternal-fetal medicine, and reproductive endocrinology)
- Ophthalmic plastic and reconstructive surgery
- Pediatric cardiology
- Pediatric emergency medicine
- Pediatric pathology
- Pediatric surgery
- Primary care sports medicine
- Thoracic surgery

Important Dates

May	The NRMP disseminates information and materials for the following spring's match to the Liaison Committee for Medical Education (LCME) medical schools and teaching hospitals.
June	NRMP agreement materials are made available to independent applicants. Independent applicants are defined as students from and/or graduates of non-LCME schools (osteopathic physicians, international medical graduates) and/or LCME graduates from earlier years.
July	Students and institutions return their agreements to the NRMP. Concurrently, students request applications and program information from teaching institutions.
October	The NRMP provides to participants information on all institutions, programs, and positions registered for the following year's Match.
January	WebROLIC is opened on the Web at aamc.org/nrmp in mid-January and the submission of Rank Order Lists begins.
February	The ranking process culminates with the closing of WebROLIC in the third week of February.

March Applicants and institutions receive the match results the third week of March. Unmatched applicants and unfilled specialty positions are released that Tuesday at noon Eastern Standard Time.

July 1 Most appointments to residency programs begin.

Information and Inquiries

The National Resident Matching Program is sponsored by the Council of Medical Specialty Societies, American Board of Medical Specialties, American Hospital Association, American Medical Association, and Association of American Medical Colleges. The NRMP is managed and operated by the Association of American Medical Colleges.

Inquiries regarding the NRMP should be directed to:

National Resident Matching Program
2501 M St NW/Ste 1
Washington, DC 20037-1307
202 828-0566
Internet: http://www.aamc.org/nrmp

Information on Unfilled Positions

Applicants to residency positions who did not match to a program through the NRMP should contact individual programs to ascertain the availability of unfilled positions. **The AMA does not have a list of unfilled post-Match positions.**

Applicants for positions in a given specialty should also contact the appropriate specialty society. Applicants for positions in obstetrics and gynecology can call the following number for regularly updated information on GY1 through GY4 positions:

American College of Obstetricians and Gynecologists
202 863-2559 or 800 673-8444 ext 2559

Information on Canadian Residency Programs

Residency programs in Canada are not accredited by the ACGME but by the Royal College of Physicians and Surgeons of Canada. For more information, contact

Royal College of Physicians and Surgeons of Canada
774 promenade Echo Dr
Ottawa, ON K1S 5N8
Canada
613 730-8177 or 800 668-3740
613 730-8830 Fax
http://medical.org/rcpsc.html

Section II

Essentials of Accredited Residencies in Graduate Medical Education: Institutional and Program Requirements

Section II—Essentials of Accredited Residencies in Graduate Medical Education: Institutional and Program Requirements—begins with a preface containing general information about the three major phases of the education of physicians, the accreditation of graduate medical education programs, and a glossary of selected terms, followed by a copy of the Institutional Requirements effective July 1997. The bulk of Section II consists of Program Requirements organized by specialty/related subspecialty.

Preface

I. The Education of Physicians

Medical education in the United States occurs in three major phases.

A. Undergraduate Medical Education

Undergraduate medical education is the first or "medical school" phase. The medical school curriculum provides instruction in the sciences that underlie medical practice and in the application of those sciences to health care. Students learn basic information-gathering, decision-making, and patient-management skills in rotations through the various clinical services. Students are granted the MD or DO degree on the successful completion of the medical school curriculum and are eligible to undertake the next phase of medical education.

Accreditation of educational programs leading to the MD degree is the responsibility of the Liaison Committee on Medical Education (LCME). Accreditation of educational programs leading to the DO degree is the responsibility of the American Osteopathic Association.

B. Graduate Medical Education

Graduate medical education (GME), the second phase, prepares physicians for practice in a medical specialty. GME focuses on the development of clinical skills and professional competencies and on the acquisition of detailed factual knowledge in a medical specialty. This learning process prepares the physician for the independent practice of medicine in that specialty. The programs are based in hospitals or other health care institutions and, in most specialties, utilize both inpatient and ambulatory settings, reflecting the importance of care for adequate numbers of patients in the GME experience. GME programs, including Transitional Year programs, are usually called residency programs, and the physicians being educated in them, residents.

The single most important responsibility of any program of GME is to provide an organized educational program with guidance and supervision of the resident, facilitating the resident's professional and personal development while ensuring safe and appropriate care for patients. A resident takes on progressively greater responsibility throughout the course of a residency, consistent with individual growth in clinical experience, knowledge, and skill.

The education of resident physicians relies on an integration of didactic activity in a structured curriculum with diagnosis and management of patients under appropriate levels of supervision and scholarly activity aimed at developing and maintaining life-long learning skills. The quality of this experience is directly related to the quality of patient care, which is always the highest priority. Educational quality and patient care quality are interdependent and must be pursued in such a manner that they enhance one another. A proper balance must be maintained so that a program of GME does not rely on residents to meet service needs at the expense of educational objectives.

A resident is prepared to undertake independent medical practice within a chosen specialty on the satisfactory completion of a residency. Residents in a program accredited by the Accreditation Council for Graduate Medical Education (ACGME) typically complete educational requirements for certification by a specialty board recognized by the American Board of Medical Specialties (ABMS).

The accreditation of GME programs is the responsibility of the ACGME, its associated Residency Review Committees (RRCs) for the various specialties, and the Transitional Year Review Committee (TYRC)(hereafter referred to as "review committees"). Further information on the ACGME and the review committees is provided below.

C. Continuing Medical Education

Continuing medical education (CME) is the third phase of medical education. This phase continues the specialty education begun in graduate training; it reflects the commitment to life-long learning inherent in the medical profession.

The Accreditation Council for Continuing Medical Education (ACCME) is responsible for accrediting the providers of CME.

II. Accreditation of GME Programs

A. Accreditation, Certification, Licensure

In the context of GME, accreditation is the process for determining whether an educational program is in substantial compliance with established educational standards as promulgated in the institutional and program requirements. Accreditation represents a professional judgment about the quality of an educational program. Decisions about accreditation are made by the review committees under the authority of the ACGME.

Certification is the process for determining whether an individual physician has met established requirements within a particular specialty. The standards for certification are determined by the appropriate member specialty board recognized by the ABMS.

Licensure is distinct from both accreditation and certification. Licensure is a process of government through which an individual physician is given permission to practice medicine within a particular licensing jurisdiction. Medical licenses are granted by the Board of Medical Examiners (or the equivalent) in each licensing jurisdiction (the 50 states, the District of Columbia, Guam, Puerto Rico, and the Virgin Islands).

B. Accreditation of Residency Programs

Accreditation of residency programs is a voluntary process. By participating in the process, residency programs undergo regular review. The review helps programs in their goals of attaining and maintaining educational excellence. The review also serves to inform the public, specialty boards, residents, and medical students whether specific residency programs are in substantial compliance with the standards that have been established for GME.

For a program to become accredited, the sponsoring institution must demonstrate a commitment to GME. The sponsoring institution must be in substantial compliance with the Institutional Requirements and must assume responsibility for the educational quality of its sponsored program(s). (Further information concerning a "sponsoring institution" is provided below.)

The Institutional Requirements, which have been established by the ACGME, apply to all institutions that seek to sponsor programs in GME. An assessment of whether institutions fulfill these requirements is made by the ACGME through its institutional review process and by the review committees through their program review process.

The program must demonstrate to its RRC that it is in substantial compliance with the Program Requirements for its particular discipline and that it is sponsored by an institution in substantial compliance with the Institutional Requirements. Materials used by the review committees in making this determination include the results of the most recent institutional review conducted by the ACGME.

The Program Requirements are developed by each review committee for programs in its specialty. The Program Requirements specify essential educational content, instructional activities, responsibilities for patient care and supervision, and the necessary facilities of accredited programs in a particular specialty. In developing and updating Program Requirements, a review committee obtains comments on the proposed documents from interested parties and agencies. The review committee then decides on the final proposal to be submitted to the ACGME. The ACGME has final authority for approving all Program Requirements.

Accreditation actions taken by the review committees are based on information submitted by program directors and on the reports of site visitors. Actions of the committees, under the authority of the ACGME, determine the accreditation status of residency programs.

The ACGME is responsible for adjudication of appeals of adverse decisions and has established policies and procedures for such appeals.

Current operating policies and procedures for review, accreditation, and appeal are contained in the ACGME *Manual of Policies and Procedures for Graduate Medical Education Review Committees*. The *Manual* is reviewed annually and is revised as appropriate. (A copy of the *Manual*, as well as copies of the Institutional Requirements and of the Program Requirements, may be obtained from the Office of the Executive Director, ACGME, 515 N State St/Ste 2000, Chicago, IL, 60610.)

Information about the accreditation status of a residency program may be obtained by contacting the executive director of the ACGME.

C. Structure of the ACGME and of the RRCs

1. The ACGME is a voluntary association formed by five member organizations. Its member organizations are national professional bodies, each of which has major interests in and involvement with residency education.

   The five member organizations of the ACGME are as follows:

   American Board of Medical Specialties (ABMS)
   American Hospital Association (AHA)
   American Medical Association (AMA)
   Association of American Medical Colleges (AAMC)
   Council of Medical Specialty Societies (CMSS)

   Each member organization selects four representatives to the ACGME. The ACGME appoints two public members.

   The Resident Physician Section of the AMA, with the advice of other national organizations that represent residents, selects a resident representative to the ACGME.

   The Chair of the RRC Council, an advisory body of the ACGME, represents that group on the ACGME.

   The Secretary of the US Department of Health and Human Services designates a nonvoting representative of the federal government to the ACGME.
2. There is an RRC for each of the specialties in which certification is offered by a specialty board that is a member of the ABMS. Each RRC is sponsored by the AMA's Council on Medical Education, by the board that certifies physicians within that specialty, and in most cases, by the professional college or other professional association within the specialty.

Residency Review Committee Sponsoring Organizations

Residency Review Committee	Sponsoring Organizations
Allergy and Immunology	American Board of Allergy and Immunology (A Conjoint Board of the American Board of Internal Medicine and the American Board of Pediatrics) AMA Council on Medical Education
Anesthesiology	American Board of Anesthesiology American Society of Anesthesiologists AMA Council on Medical Education
Colon and Rectal Surgery	American Board of Colon and Rectal Surgery American College of Surgeons AMA Council on Medical Education
Dermatology	American Board of Dermatology AMA Council on Medical Education
Diagnostic Radiology	American Board of Radiology American College of Radiology AMA Council on Medical Education
Emergency Medicine	American Board of Emergency Medicine American College of Emergency Physicians AMA Council on Medical Education
Family Practice	American Academy of Family Physicians American Board of Family Practice AMA Council on Medical Education
Internal Medicine	American Board of Internal Medicine American College of Physicians AMA Council on Medical Education
Medical Genetics	American Board of Medical Genetics American College of Medical Genetics AMA Council on Medical Education
Neurological Surgery	American Board of Neurological Surgery American College of Surgeons AMA Council on Medical Education
Neurology	American Academy of Neurology American Board of Psychiatry and Neurology AMA Council on Medical Education
Nuclear Medicine	American Board of Nuclear Medicine AMA Council on Medical Education Society of Nuclear Medicine
Obstetrics-Gynecology	American Board of Obstetrics and Gynecology American College of Obstetricians and Gynecologists AMA Council on Medical Education
Ophthalmology	American Academy of Ophthalmology American Board of Ophthalmology AMA Council on Medical Education
Orthopaedic Surgery	American Academy of Orthopaedic Surgeons American Board of Orthopaedic Surgery AMA Council on Medical Education
Otolaryngology	American Board of Otolaryngology American College of Surgeons AMA Council on Medical Education
Pathology	American Board of Pathology AMA Council on Medical Education
Pediatrics	American Academy of Pediatrics American Board of Pediatrics AMA Council on Medical Education
Physical Medicine and Rehabilitation	American Academy of Physical Medicine and Rehabilitation American Board of Physical Medicine and Rehabilitation AMA Council on Medical Education
Plastic Surgery	American Board of Plastic Surgery American College of Surgeons AMA Council on Medical Education
Preventive Medicine	American Board of Preventive Medicine AMA Council on Medical Education
Psychiatry	American Board of Psychiatry and Neurology American Psychiatric Association AMA Council on Medical Education
Radiation Oncology	American Board of Radiology American College of Radiology AMA Council on Medical Education
Surgery	American Board of Surgery American College of Surgeons AMA Council on Medical Education
Thoracic Surgery	American Board of Thoracic Surgery American College of Surgeons AMA Council on Medical Education
Urology	American Board of Urology American College of Surgeons AMA Council on Medical Education

The Transitional Year Review Committee, which accredits 1 year of GME consisting of rotations in multiple clinical disciplines, is appointed directly by the ACGME.

The established RRCs and their respective sponsors are listed in the chart above.

III. A Glossary of Selected Terms Used in GME Accreditation

Applicants: Persons invited to come for an interview for a GME program.

Consortium: Two or more organizations or institutions that have come together to pursue common objectives (eg, GME). A consortium may serve as a "sponsoring institution" for GME programs if it is formally established as an ongoing institutional entity with a documented commitment to GME.

Desirable: A term, along with its companion "highly desirable," used to designate aspects of an educational program that are not mandatory but are considered to be very important. A program may be cited for failing to do something that is desirable or highly desirable.

Essential: (See "Must.")

Fellow: A term used by some sponsoring institutions and in some specialties to designate participants in subspecialty GME programs. The *Graduate Medical Education Directory* and the ACGME use "resident" to designate all GME participants in ACGME-accredited programs.

Institution: An organization having the primary purpose of providing educational and/or health care services (eg, a university, a medical school, a hospital, a school of public health, a health department, a public health agency, an organized health care delivery system, a medical examiner's office, a consortium, an educational foundation).

A. Major Participating Institution: An institution to which residents rotate for a required experience and/or those that require explicit approval by the appropriate RRC prior to utilization. Major participating institutions are listed as part of an accredited program in the *Graduate Medical Education Directory*.

B. Participating Institution: An institution that provides specific learning experiences within a multi-institutional program of

GME. Subsections of institutions, such as a department, clinic, or unit of a hospital, do not qualify as participating institutions.

C. Sponsoring Institution: The institution that assumes the ultimate responsibility for a program of GME.

Institutional Review: The process undertaken by the ACGME to judge whether a sponsoring institution offering GME programs is in substantial compliance with the Institutional Requirements.

Intern: Historically, "intern" was used to designate individuals in the first year of GME; less commonly it designated individuals in the first year of any residency program. Since 1975 the *Graduate Medical Education Directory* and the ACGME have not used the term, instead referring to individuals in their first year of GME as residents.

Internal Review: The formal process conducted by a sponsoring institution to assess the educational effectiveness of its sponsored residency programs.

Must (Shall, Essential): Terms used to indicate that something is required, mandatory, or done without fail. These terms indicate absolute requirements.

Program: The unit of specialty education, comprising a series of graduated learning experiences in GME, designed to conform to the program requirements of a particular specialty.

Resident: A physician at any level of GME in a program accredited by the ACGME. Participants in accredited subspecialty programs are specifically included.

Scholarly Activity: Educational experiences that include active participation of the teaching staff in clinical discussions, rounds, and conferences in a manner that promotes a spirit of inquiry and scholarship; active participation in journal clubs, research conferences, regional or national professional and scientific societies, particularly through presentations at the organizations' meetings and publications in their journals; participation in research, particularly in projects that are funded following peer review and/or result in publications or presentations at regional and national scientific meetings; offering of guidance and technical support, eg, research design, statistical analysis, for residents involved in research; and provision of support for resident participation as appropriate in scholarly activities. May be defined in more detail in specific Program Requirements.

Shall: (See "Must.")

Should: A term used to designate requirements that are so important that their absence must be justified. The accreditation status of a program or institution is at risk if it is not in compliance with a "should."

Substantial Compliance: The judgment made by experts, based on all available information, that a sponsoring institution or residency program meets accreditation standards.

Suggested: A term, along with its companion "strongly suggested," used to indicate that something is distinctly urged rather than required. An institution or a program will not be cited for failing to do something that is suggested or strongly suggested.

Institutional Requirements

I. Institutional Organization and Commitment

The purpose of GME is to provide an organized educational program with guidance and supervision of the resident, facilitating the resident's professional and personal development while ensuring safe and appropriate care for patients. Sponsoring institutions, therefore, must be appropriately organized for the conduct of GME in a scholarly environment and be committed to excellence in both education and medical care. This commitment is exhibited by the provision of leadership and resources to enable the institution to achieve substantial compliance with the Institutional Requirements and to enable the educational programs to achieve substantial compliance with Program Requirements. This includes providing an ethical and professional environment in which the educational curricular requirements, as well as the applicable requirements for scholarly activity, can be met. The regular assessment of the quality of the educational programs is an essential component of this commitment.

A. Sponsoring Institution

1. A residency program must operate under the authority and control of a sponsoring institution (see definition for sponsoring institution in the Glossary under "Institution").
2. There must be a written statement of institutional commitment to GME that is supported by the governing authority, the administration, and the teaching staff.
3. Sponsoring institutions must be in substantial compliance with the Institutional Requirements and must ensure that their ACGME-accredited programs are in substantial compliance with the Program Requirements.
4. An institution's failure to comply substantially with the Institutional Requirements may jeopardize the accreditation of all of its sponsored residency programs.

B. Educational Administration

There must be an organized administrative system to oversee all residency programs sponsored by an institution. In addition, there must be a designated institutional official who has the authority and the responsibility for the oversight and administration of the GME programs.

1. Institutions must have a GME Committee (GMEC) that has the responsibility for monitoring and advising on all aspects of residency education. Voting membership on the committee must include residents nominated by their peers, appropriate program directors, other members of the faculty, and the accountable institutional official or his or her designee.
2. The committee must meet at least quarterly; minutes must be kept and be available for inspection by accreditation personnel.
3. The responsibilities of the committee must include
   a. establishment and implementation of policies that affect all residency programs regarding the quality of education and the work environment for the residents in each program.
   b. establishment and maintenance of appropriate oversight of and liaison with program directors and assurance that program directors establish and maintain proper oversight of and liaison with appropriate personnel of other institutions participating in programs sponsored by the institutions.
   c. regular review of all residency programs to assess their compliance with both the Institutional Requirements and Program Requirements of the relevant ACGME RRCs.
      1. The review must be conducted by the GMEC or a body designated by the GMEC, which should include faculty, residents, and administrators, both within and outside the depart-

ment in which the residency exists. The review must follow a written protocol approved by the GMEC. External reviewers may also be utilized as determined by the GMEC.

2. Reviews must be conducted between the ACGME program surveys.
3. While assessing the residency program's compliance with each of the program standards, the review should also appraise the following:
   a. The educational objectives of each program;
   b. The adequacy of available educational and financial resources to meet these objectives;
   c. The effectiveness of each program in meeting its objectives; and
   d. The effectiveness in addressing citations from previous ACGME letters of accreditation and previous internal reviews.
4. Examples of materials and data to be used in the review process should include the following:
   a. Institutional and Program Requirements from the Essentials of Accredited Residency Programs;
   b. Letters of accreditation from previous ACGME reviews;
   c. Reports from previous internal reviews of the program; and
   d. Interviews with the program director, faculty, and residents in the program and individuals outside the program deemed appropriate by the committee.
5. There must be documentation of the review, including recorded mechanisms to correct identified deficiencies. In addition, succinct summaries of each review are required as part of the ACGME institutional review document.
6. Although departmental annual reports are often important sources of information about a residency program, they do not in themselves necessarily meet the requirement for a periodic review.

d. Assurance that each residency program establishes and implements formal written criteria and processes for the selection, evaluation, promotion, and dismissal of residents in compliance with both the Institutional and relevant Program Requirements.

e. Assurance of an educational environment in which residents may raise and resolve issues without fear of intimidation or retaliation. This includes:

1. Provision of an organizational system for residents to communicate and exchange information on their working environment and their educational programs. This may be accomplished through a resident organization or other forums in which to address resident issues.
2. A process by which individual residents can address concerns in a confidential and protected manner.
3. Establishment and implementation of fair institutional policies and procedures for academic or other disciplinary actions taken against residents.
4. Establishment and implementation of fair institutional policies and procedures for adjudication of resident complaints and grievances related to actions which could result in dismissal or could significantly threaten a resident's intended career development.

f. Collecting of intra-institutional information and making recommendations on the appropriate funding for resident positions, including benefits and support services.

g. Monitoring of the programs in establishing an appropriate work environment and the duty hours of residents.

h. Assurance that the residents' curriculum provides a regular review of ethical, socioeconomic, medical/legal, and cost-containment issues that affect GME and medical practice. The curriculum must also provide an appropriate introduction to communication skills and to research design, statistics, and critical review of the literature necessary for acquiring skills for lifelong learning. There must be appropriate resident participation in departmental scholarly activity, as set forth in the applicable Program Requirements.

C. Institutional Agreements

When resident education occurs in a participating institution, the sponsoring institution continues to have responsibility for the quality of that educational experience and must retain authority over the residents' activities.

Therefore, current interinstitutional agreements must exist with all of its major participating institutions.

The sponsoring institution must ensure that for each accredited program appropriate letters of agreement exist between the sponsoring institution and the participating institution. These agreements should

1. identify the officials at the participating institution or facility who will assume administrative, educational, and supervisory responsibility for the resident(s);
2. outline the educational goals and objectives to be attained within the participating institutions;
3. specify the period of assignment of the residents to the participating institution, the financial arrangements, and the details for insurance and benefits;
4. determine the participating institution's responsibilities for teaching, supervision, and formal evaluation of the residents' performances; and
5. establish with the participating institution the policies and procedures that govern the residents' education while rotating to the participating institution.

D. Accreditation for Patient Care

Institutions sponsoring or participating in GME programs should be accredited by the Joint Commission on the Accreditation of Healthcare Organizations (JCAHO), if such institutions are eligible. If an institution is eligible for JCAHO accreditation and chooses not to undergo such accreditation, then the institution should be reviewed by and meet the standards of another recognized body with reasonably equivalent standards. If the institution is not accredited, it must provide a satisfactory explanation of why accreditation has not been either granted or sought.

E. Quality Assurance

Institutions participating in GME must conduct formal quality-assurance programs and review complications and deaths.

1. All residents should receive instruction in quality-assurance/performance improvement. To the degree possible and in conformance with state law, residents should participate in appropriate components of the institution's performance improvement program.
2. As part of the educational program, it is important that autopsies be performed whenever possible and appropriate. A sufficient number of autopsies representing an adequately diverse spectrum of diseases should be performed to provide an adequate educational experience and to enhance the quality of patient care.
3. Institutions participating in GME must have a medical records system that is available at all times and documents the course of each patient's illness, and care. The medical records system must be adequate to support the education of residents and quality-assurance activities and provide a resource for scholarly activity.

F. Compliance with ACGME Policies and Procedures

Sponsoring institutions must ensure that their ACGME-accredited programs are in substantial compliance with ACGME policies and procedures as defined in the ACGME *Manual of Policies and Procedures for Graduate Medical Education Review Committees*. Of particular note are those policies and procedures that govern "Administrative Withdrawal of Accreditation," an action that is not subject to the appeals process:

1. A program may be deemed to have voluntarily withdrawn from the ACGME accreditation process, and an RRC may withdraw accreditation, if the program is not in substantial compliance with:
   a. site visit and program review policies and procedures;
   b. directives associated with an accreditation action; or
   c. requests by the RRC for information.
2. A program that is judged to be delinquent in payment of fees is not eligible for review and will be notified by certified mail, return receipt requested, of the effective date of the withdrawal of accreditation. On that date, the program will be removed from the list of ACGME-accredited programs.

II. Residents

A. Resident Eligibility and Selection

The sponsoring institution must have written policies and procedures for the recruitment and appointment of residents that comply with the requirements listed below, and it must monitor the compliance of each program with these procedures.

1. Resident Eligibility
   Applicants with one of the following qualifications are eligible for appointment to accredited residency programs:
   a. Graduates of medical schools in the United States and Canada accredited by the Liaison Committee on Medical Education (LCME.)
   b. Graduates of colleges of osteopathic medicine in the United States accredited by the American Osteopathic Association (AOA).
   c. Graduates of medical schools outside the United States and Canada who meet one of the following qualifications:
      1. Have received a currently valid certificate from the Educational Commission for Foreign Medical Graduates or
      2. Have a full and unrestricted license to practice medicine in a US licensing jurisdiction.
   d. Graduates of medical schools outside the United States who have completed a Fifth Pathway program provided by an LCME-accredited medical school. [*Note:* A Fifth Pathway program is an academic year of supervised clinical education provided by an LCME-accredited medical school to students who meet the following conditions: (1) have completed, in an accredited college or university in the United States, undergraduate premedical education of the quality acceptable for matriculation in an accredited United States Medical school; (2) have studied at a medical school outside the United States and Canada but listed in the *World Health Organization Directory of Medical Schools*; (3) have completed all of the formal requirements of the foreign medical school except internship and/or social service; (4) have attained a score satisfactory to the sponsoring medical school on a screening examination; and (5) have passed either the foreign Medical Graduate Examination in the Medical Sciences, Parts I and II of the examination of the National Board of Medical Examiners, or Steps 1 and 2 of the United States Medical Licensing Examination (USMLE).]
2. Resident Selection
   a. The sponsoring institution must ensure that programs select from among eligible applicants on the basis of their preparedness, ability, aptitude, academic credentials, communication skills, and personal qualities such as motivation and integrity. Programs must not discriminate with regard to sex, race, age, religion, color, national origin, disability, or veteran status.
   b. In selecting from among qualified applicants, it is strongly suggested that institutions and all of their sponsored programs participate in an organized matching program, where available, such as the National Resident Matching Program (NRMP).
3. Enrollment of Noneligibles
   The enrollment of noneligible residents may be a cause for withdrawal of accreditation of the involved program.

B. Resident Participation in Educational Activities

Institutions must ensure that residents have the opportunity to

1. develop a personal program of learning to foster continued professional growth with guidance from the teaching staff.
2. participate in safe, effective, and compassionate patient care, under supervision, commensurate with their level of advancement and responsibility.
3. participate fully in the educational and scholarly activities of their program and, as required, assume responsibility for teaching and supervising other residents and students.
4. participate as appropriate in institutional programs and medical staff activities and adhere to established practices, procedures, and policies of the institution.
5. participate on appropriate institutional committees and councils whose actions affect their education and /or patient care.
6. submit to the program director or to a designated institutional official at least annually confidential written evaluations of the faculty and of the educational experiences.

C. Resident Support, Benefits, and Conditions of Employment

Sponsoring and participating institutions should provide all residents with appropriate financial support and benefits. Compensation of residents and distribution of resources for the support of education should be carried out with the advice of the GMEC.

1. Financial Support: Adequate financial support of residents is necessary to ensure that residents are able to fulfill the responsibilities of their educational programs.
2. Applicants: Applicants for GME programs must be informed in writing of the terms and conditions of employment and benefits including financial support, vacations, professional leave, parental leave, sick leave, professional liability insurance, hospital and health insurance, disability insurance, and other insurance benefits for the residents and their family, and the conditions under which living quarters, meals and laundry or their equivalents are to be provided.
3. Contracts: Sponsoring institutions must provide residents with a written agreement or contract outlining the terms and conditions of their appointment to an educational program, and the institutions must monitor the implementation of these terms and conditions by the program directors.
   The agreement must contain or reference at least the following:
   a. Financial support
   b. Vacation policies
   c. Professional liability insurance in conformity with II.C.5, below
   d. Disability insurance and other hospital and health insurance benefits for the residents and their family in conformity with II.C.6, below
   e. Professional, parental, and sick-leave benefits in conformity with II.C.7, below

f. Conditions under which living quarters, meals, and laundry or their equivalents are to be provided
g. Counseling, medical, psychological, and other support services in conformity with II.C.8 and 9, below
h. Institutional policies covering sexual and other forms of harassment.

4. The agreement must also delineate or reference specific policies regarding
   a. resident's responsibilities
   b. duration of appointment and conditions for reappointment
   c. professional activities outside the educational program
   d. grievance procedures in conformity with I.B.e.4.
5. Liability Insurance: Residents in GME must be provided with professional liability coverage for the duration of training. Such coverage must provide legal defense and protection against awards from claims reported or filed after the completion of GME if the alleged acts or omissions of the residents are within the scope of the education program. The coverage to be provided should be consistent with the institution's coverage for other medical/professional practitioners. Each institution must provide current residents and applicants for residency with the details of the institution's professional liability coverage for residents.
6. Disability Insurance: Institutions sponsoring GME must provide access to insurance, where available, to all residents for disabilities resulting from activities that are part of the educational program.
7. Leave of Absence: There must be a written institutional policy on leave (with or without pay) for residents that complies with applicable laws. The institution must provide residents with a written policy concerning the effect of leaves of absence, for any reason, on satisfying the criteria for completion of a residency program.
8. Counseling Services: GME places increasing responsibilities on residents and requires sustained intellectual and physical effort. Therefore, institutions should facilitate resident access to appropriate and confidential counseling, medical and psychological support services.
9. Physician Impairment: Institutions must have written policies that describe how physician impairment, including that due to substance abuse, will be handled. In addition, institutions should provide an educational program for residents regarding physician impairment, including substance abuse.
10. Residency Closure/Reduction: If an institution intends to reduce the size of a residency program or to close a residency program, the institution must inform the residents as soon as possible. In the event of such a reduction or closure, institutions must allow residents already in the program to complete their education or assist the residents in enrolling in an ACGME-accredited program in which they can continue their education.
11. Restrictive Covenants: ACGME-accredited residencies must not require residents to sign a non-competition guarantee.

D. Resident Supervision, Duty Hours, and Work Environment

Institutions must ensure that their GME programs provide appropriate supervision for all residents, as well as a duty hour schedule and a work environment, that is consistent with proper patient care, the educational needs of residents, and the applicable Program Requirements.

1. Supervision: There must be sufficient institutional oversight to assure that residents are appropriately supervised. Residents must be supervised by teaching staff in such a way that the residents assume progressively increasing responsibility according to their level of education, ability, and experience. On-call schedules for teaching staff must be structured to ensure that supervision is readily available to residents on duty. The level of responsibility accorded to each resident must be determined by the teaching staff.
2. Duty Hours: The sponsoring institution must ensure that each residency program establishes formal policies governing resident duty hours that foster resident education and facilitate the care of patients.
   a. The educational goals of the program and learning objectives of residents must not be compromised by excessive reliance on residents to fulfill institutional service obligations. Duty hours, however, must reflect the fact that responsibilities for continuing patient care are not automatically discharged at specific times. Programs must ensure that residents are provided appropriate backup support when patient care responsibilities are especially difficult or prolonged.
   b. Resident duty hours and on-call time periods must not be excessive. The structuring of duty hours and on-call schedules must focus on the needs of the patient, continuity of care, and the educational needs of the resident. Duty hours must be consistent with the Institutional and Program Requirements that apply to each program.
3. Work Environment: Sponsoring institutions must provide services and develop systems to minimize the work of residents that is extraneous to their educational programs, ensuring that the following conditions are met:
   a. Residents on duty in the hospital must be provided adequate and appropriate food services and sleeping quarters.
   b. Patient support services, such as intravenous services, phlebotomy services, and laboratory services, as well as messenger and transporter services, must be provided in a manner appropriate to and consistent with educational objectives and patient care.
   c. An effective laboratory, medical records, and radiologic information retrieval system must be in place to provide for appropriate conduct of the educational programs and quality and timely patient care.
   d. Appropriate security and personal safety measures must be provided to residents in all locations including but not limited to parking facilities, on-call quarters, hospital and institutional grounds, and related clinical facilities (eg, medical office building).

ACGME: September 1998 Effective: September 1998

Program Requirements

Program Requirements for Residency Education in Allergy and Immunology

I. Introduction

A. Definition and Scope of the Specialty

Graduate medical education programs in allergy and immunology should be designed to prepare specialists in the delivery of skilled medical or consultative care to patients with allergic and immunologic disorders, including asthma and other related disorders.

B. Duration and Scope of Education

1. Residents admitted to allergy and immunology programs should have successfully completed a program in Internal Medicine or Pediatrics accredited by the Accreditation Council for Graduate Medical Education (ACGME).
2. The length of the educational program is 24 months of full-time education. Before entry into the program, each resident must be notified in writing of the required length of the allergy and immunology educational program. The required educational program may be spread over a longer time if the program documents the required 24 months of education consistent with the goals, objectives, educational content, and policies as referenced in these Program Requirements, Section IV.
3. Residents must receive education in both pediatric and adult allergic and immunologic disorders, including asthma and other related disorders, and cross-training and experience with both inpatients and outpatients.
4. The program must provide documentation that each resident receives the following components in the 24-month course of study:
   a. Twenty-five percent of the program, or 6 months, must be devoted to research and scholarly activities as referenced in the Program Requirements, Section IV. D;
   b. Fifty percent of the program must be devoted to direct patient care activities. Direct patient care is defined as both inpatient and outpatient care, clinical care conferences, and record reviews;
   c. Twenty-five percent of the program, or 6 months, must be devoted to other educational activities as referenced in these Program Requirements, Section IV.

II. Institutional Organization

A. Sponsoring Institution

1. Allergy and immunology programs should be conducted principally in institutions with accredited graduate medical education programs in pediatrics and internal medicine.
2. The sponsoring institution must provide sufficient faculty, financial resources, clinical resources, research opportunities, and library facilities to meet the educational needs of the residents and to enable the program to comply with the requirements for accreditation.

B. Participating Institutions

1. Affiliations with other institutions may be necessary to ensure graduate education in the broad fields of both pediatric and adult allergy and immunology. Participation by any institution providing more than 4 months of resident education must be approved by the Residency Review Committee (RRC).
2. There must be an appropriately executed interinstitutional agreement that conforms to the ACGME Institutional Requirements between the sponsoring institution and each participating institution.

C. Appointment of Residents

1. The program director must comply with the requirements for resident eligibility as listed in the ACGME Institutional Requirements.
2. The number of residents appointed must be consistent with the adequacy of program resources for resident education.

III. Faculty Qualifications and Responsibilities

The program director and faculty are responsible for the general administration of the program, including those activities related to the recruitment, selection, instruction, supervision, counseling, evaluation, and advancement of residents, and the maintenance of records related to program accreditation.

A. Program Director

1. Qualifications
   a. A single program director with the requisite and documented clinical, educational, and administrative experience must be responsible for the program. In a conjoint program, one codirector must be designated as the single responsible administrator. The program director must be experienced as a clinician, teacher, and administrator in the specialty. The program director must possess leadership qualities and must devote sufficient time and effort to the program to provide day-to-day continuity of leadership and to fulfill all of the responsibilities of meeting the educational goals of the program.
   b. The program director must develop a sound organizational framework and an effective faculty as essential elements of the educational program. Continuity of leadership is important to the stability of the program. Frequent changes of leadership or long periods of temporary leadership may adversely affect an educational program and will be cause for concern.
   c. The program director must be licensed to practice medicine in the state where the institution that sponsors the program is located. (Certain federal programs are exempted.)
   d. The program director must be certified by the American Board of Allergy and Immunology or possess suitable equivalent qualifications, as determined by the RRC. Recertification in allergy and immunology at appropriate intervals is encouraged.
   e. The program director must be appointed in good standing to the medical staff of an institution participating in the program.
2. Responsibilities
   a. Preparation of a written statement outlining the educational goals of the program with respect to the knowledge, skills, and other attributes of residents at each level of education for each major rotation or other program assignment. This statement must be distributed to residents and faculty. It should be readily available for review.
   b. Selection of residents for appointment to the program in accordance with institutional and departmental policies and procedures.
   c. Selection and supervision of the faculty and other program personnel at each institution participating in the program.
   d. Supervision of residents through explicit written descriptions of supervisory lines of responsibility for the care of patients. Such guidelines must be communicated to all members of the faculty. Residents must be provided with prompt, reliable systems for communication and interaction with supervisory physicians.

e. Regular evaluation of resident knowledge, skills, and overall performance, including the development of professional attitudes consistent with being a physician.
f. Implementation of fair procedures, as established by the sponsoring institution, regarding academic discipline and resident complaints or grievances.
g. Monitoring of resident stress, including mental or emotional conditions inhibiting performance or learning, and drug- or alcohol-related dysfunction. Program directors and faculty should be sensitive to the need for timely provision of confidential counseling and psychological support services to residents. Educational situations that consistently produce undesirable stress on residents must be evaluated and modified.
h. Preparation of an accurate statistical and narrative description of the program as requested by the RRC.
i. Notification of the executive director of the RRC of changes in the program, ie, changes in the program director, faculty appointments, participating institutions, or facilities.

B. Faculty

1. There must be sufficient faculty with suitable academic and practice qualifications to ensure proper teaching and supervision in the disciplines of the field. The faculty must include qualified allergists and immunologists with a background in internal medicine, qualified allergists and immunologists with a background in pediatrics, and faculty with a background in the basic and clinical science aspects of allergy and immunology. One mechanism to satisfy the requirements would be to incorporate from both basic and clinical science departments a number of faculty who can provide expert education in each discipline. All faculty must demonstrate a commitment to the educational program and possess those special competencies in teaching and research needed to provide a broad educational experience.
2. All members of the faculty should be willing to give the necessary time and effort to the program, demonstrate a strong interest in the education of residents, evidence sound clinical and teaching abilities, support the goals and objectives for the program, and be committed to their own continuing education.
3. A faculty member at each participating institution, appointed by and responsible to the program director, must be designated to assume responsibility for the day-to-day activities of the program at that institution, with overall coordination by the program director.
4. The faculty must be organized and have regular documented meetings to review program goals and objectives and program effectiveness in achieving them.
5. The faculty should at least annually evaluate the utilization of resources available to the program, the contribution of each institution participating in the program, the financial and administrative support for the program, the volume and variety of patients available to the program for educational purposes, the performance of members of the faculty, and the quality of resident supervision.
6. Allergy and immunology faculty are encouraged to seek recertification in allergy and immunology at appropriate intervals.

C. Scholarly Activities

Graduate medical education must take place in an environment of inquiry and scholarship in which residents participate in the development of new knowledge, learn to evaluate research findings, and develop habits of inquiry as a continuing professional responsibility. The responsibility for establishing and maintaining an environment of inquiry and scholarship rests with the program director and faculty. While not all faculty can be investigators, the faculty as a whole must demonstrate broad involvement in scholarly activity, including

1. participation in clinical discussions, rounds, and conferences in a manner that promotes a spirit of inquiry and scholarship;
2. participation in journal clubs and research conferences;
3. participation in regional or national professional and scientific societies;
4. participation in research, particularly in projects funded following peer review that result in presentations at regional and national scientific meetings and/or publication in journals;
5. offering of guidance and technical support, eg, research design and statistical analysis for residents involved in research or other scholarly activities; and
6. provision of support for resident participation in scholarly activities.

A faculty that does not exhibit such characteristics will be cause for concern as to its adequacy and suitability for conducting a program of graduate education in allergy and clinical immunology.

D. Other Program Personnel

Programs must be provided with the additional professional, technical, and clerical personnel needed to support the administration and educational conduct of the program.

IV. The Educational Program

The course of study must include allergic and immunologic disorders, including asthma and other related disorders. All residents must be provided with opportunities to apply immunologic theories, principles, and techniques to the investigation, diagnosis, and treatment of a broad spectrum of allergic and immunologic diseases. The required education in the various aspects of the clinical program may involve supervised patient care; rotations through cooperating services; attendance at conferences, lectures, journal clubs, demonstrations, or seminars; reading; and preparation and conduct of teaching assignments.

A. Program Goals and Objectives

1. The program director and faculty must prepare and comply with written educational goals for the program. All educational components of the program should be related to program goals.
2. The program design and/or structure must be approved by the appropriate review committee as a part of the regular review process.

B. Clinical Program

Clinical education is defined as direct patient contact in both the outpatient and inpatient settings, clinical care conferences, and record reviews. To ensure a sufficient experience for each resident, the program must provide a sufficient number of patients in the pediatric and adult age groups to provide education in the varying manifestations of allergic and immunologic disorders, including asthma and other related disorders. It is particularly important that residents be provided with continuing responsibility for the care of patients with chronic allergic and immunologic disorders, including asthma and other related disorders.

1. Fifty percent of the resident's time must be devoted to direct patient care activities.
2. Ambulatory experience: The ambulatory experience must include a sufficient number of adult and pediatric patients for each resident during the 24-month program. A patient listing containing a unique patient identifier, age, and diagnosis must be available for verification by the site visitor. There must be sufficient diversity of patient ages and diagnoses to reflect the breadth of the specialty.
3. Inpatient experience: The inpatient experience must include a sufficient number of adult and pediatric patients for each resi-

dent during the 24-month program. These inpatient experiences should include direct patient care such as primary patient care, consultation, or teaching rounds. These activities may be accomplished through educational liaisons with other specialties or services. There must be sufficient diversity of patient ages and diagnoses to reflect the breadth of the specialty. A patient listing consisting of a unique patient identifier, age, and diagnosis for each patient seen by each resident must be available for verification by the site visitor.

4. Cross-training in internal medicine and pediatrics:
   a. Residents must receive cross-training in both pediatric and adult allergy and immunology because specialists in allergy and immunology, whatever their primary specialties, are called on to diagnose and treat individuals of all ages. The equivalent of 40 full days of cross-training experience with a combination of adequate ambulatory and inpatient experience must be documented for each resident caring for patients in the crossover specialty.
   b. Residents should be provided with inpatient experiences both initially and through follow-up as an educational experience in the crossover specialty.

C. Academic Content for the Course of Study

1. Patient base
   a. Residents must be exposed to patients with rhinitis, sinusitis, nasal polyposis, asthma, urticaria, angioedema, anaphylactic and anaphylactoid reactions, atopic dermatitis, contact dermatitis, insect sensitivity, drug reactions, adverse reactions to foods and food additives, and primary and secondary immunodeficiency diseases, as well as to patients receiving immunomodulatory therapy.
   b. Resident experience is highly desirable for patients with hypersensitivity diseases of the lung, eg, hypersensitivity pneumonitis, allergic bronchopulmonary aspergillosis, disorders of occupational exposure, autoimmune disorders, ocular allergic diseases, mastocytosis, and eosinophilic disorders.
2. Residents must be provided with the following:
   a. Opportunity to develop skills in history and physical examination; skin testing, both immediate and delayed; interpretation of pulmonary function tests; oral and bronchial challenges; desensitization to pharmacological agents; interpretation of in vitro methods to measure total and specific IgE antibodies; and the safe practice of immunotherapy.
   b. Knowledge of the etiology, immunopathogenesis, differential diagnosis, therapy, and complications of those diseases referenced in these Program Requirements, Section IV.C.1. The following areas should be emphasized: aerobiology; cellular and molecular immunobiology; humoral and cellular immunology; pulmonary physiology; mechanisms of inflammation; pharmacology and pharmacokinetics, drug metabolism, drug side effects, and drug interactions, the scientific basis of the methodology, indications, and interpretation of laboratory tests and imaging procedures used in the diagnosis and follow-up of patients with asthmatic, allergic, immunologic, and other diseases; preparation and standardization of allergen extracts; means to measure indoor allergens and the institution of environmental control measures in the home and other sites; transplantation medicine and tumor immunology; reproductive immunology; the costs of therapy and diagnostic testing; and the psychological effects of chronic illness.
   c. Knowledge of applied immunology, to include the principles and techniques of clinical immunology laboratory procedures such as tests for humoral immunity, cellular immunity, neutrophil function, cytokines, immune complexes, cryoprecipitable proteins, total serum complement activity and individual complement components, and histocompatibility, and procedures for the preparation and use of monoclonal antibodies.
3. Resident experience with rhinoscopy, nasal challenges, and patch testing is highly desirable.

D. Resident Research and Scholarly Activity

1. Twenty-five percent of the educational program, or 6 months, must be devoted to research and scholarly activities.
2. Residents must be provided with a structured research experience sufficient to result in an understanding of the basic principles of study design, performance, analysis, and reporting.
3. Resident scholarly activities must include participation in clinical discussions, rounds and conferences, journal clubs or research conferences; participation and/or presentations at regional or national professional societies; or participation in either clinical or basic research.
4. Residents must be provided with the opportunity to communicate their knowledge to others, both orally and in written form; to conduct lectures, seminars, and clinical conferences; and to prepare written reports of their research activities either for faculty review or for publication.

E. Resident Policies

1. Supervision: Appropriately qualified faculty must supervise all patient care services. The program director must ensure, direct, and document the proper supervision of residents at all times. Residents must be provided with rapid, reliable systems for communicating with faculty. Appropriate supervision must be available at all times on site. This is particularly necessary for patients with severe and/or complex disease.
2. Duty hours and conditions of work: It is the responsibility of the program director to ensure enforcement of reasonable policies with respect to work hours. Those services requiring in-hospital on-call periods should require no more than 80 hours of hospital duties per week when averaged over 4 weeks. Residents should have, on the average, the opportunity to spend at least 1 full day out of 7 free of hospital duties, and should be on-call in the hospital no more often than every third night. Physicians must have personal responsibility for continuing patient care and must recognize that their obligation to patients is not automatically discharged at any given hour of the day or on any particular day of the week. In no case should residents go off duty until the proper care and welfare of the patients have been ensured. There should be adequate backup if sudden and unexpected needs create resident fatigue sufficient to jeopardize patient care during or following on-call periods. Schedules must be structured to ensure that consultation is readily available to residents. An on-call room to provide rest and privacy must be available for each resident assigned night duty in the hospital.
3. Graded responsibility: The program must provide residents with direct experience and progressive responsibility for patient management as they advance through the educational program. The program must ensure that the graduating resident has achieved the ability to formulate and carry out appropriate management plans.

V. Evaluation

A. Resident Evaluation

The program director and faculty must

1. at least semiannually evaluate the knowledge, skills, and professional growth of the residents, using appropriate criteria and procedures;
2. communicate each evaluation to the resident in a timely manner;

3. advance residents to positions of higher responsibility only on the basis of evidence of their satisfactory progressive scholarship and professional growth;
4. maintain a permanent record of evaluation for each resident and have it accessible to the resident and other authorized personnel;
5. provide a final written evaluation for each resident who completes the program that includes a review of the resident's performance during the final period of education and verifies that the resident has demonstrated sufficient professional ability to practice competently and independently. This final evaluation should be a part of the resident's permanent record maintained by the institution.

B. Program Evaluation

1. The educational effectiveness of the program must be evaluated at least annually in a systematic manner. In particular, the quality of the curriculum and the extent to which educational goals have been met by the residents must be assessed. Written and confidential evaluations by residents should be utilized in this process.
2. A review of the performance of program graduates on the written examination of the American Board of Allergy and Immunology will be employed by the RRC as one measure of the quality of an educational program.

VI. Certification

Residents who plan to seek certification by the American Board of Allergy and Immunology should communicate with the executive secretary of the board, as listed in the *Graduate Medical Education Directory,* to ascertain the requirements for certification.

ACGME: September 1996 Effective: July 1997

Program Requirements for Residency Education in Clinical and Laboratory Immunology (Allergy and Immunology)

I. Introduction

A. Scope and Duration of Education

A graduate medical education program in clinical and laboratory immunology (CLI) must be designed to train individuals to become fully versed in all aspects of the direction of a clinical immunology laboratory. These programs must be 1 year in duration.

B. Sponsoring and Participating Institutions

The CLI program must be conducted in institutions with accredited graduate medical education programs in allergy and immunology or in the various relevant subspecialties of internal medicine and pediatrics.

Affiliations with other institutions and existing laboratories may be necessary to ensure a full educational experience in CLI. When the resources of two or more institutions are utilized, letters of agreement must be approved by the institutional governing boards. Affiliations should be avoided with institutions that are at such a distance from the parent institution as to make attendance at rounds and conferences difficult and/or that do not add to the educational value of the program.

C. Trainees

Candidates for these programs should have successfully completed an accredited residency program in internal medicine or pediatrics and should have additional training in an immunologically related subspecialty.

The number of residents should not exceed the educational resources available in the program. It is desirable that each program have at least one resident at all times to keep the educational process current.

Residents must have a keen sense of personal responsibility for continuing patient care and must recognize that their obligation to patients is not automatically discharged at any given hour of the day or any particular day of the week. In no case should residents go off duty until the proper care and welfare of the patients have been ensured. When averaged over 4 weeks, residents should spend no more than 80 hours per week in hospital duties; should have, on the average, the opportunity to spend at least 1 full day out of 7 free of hospital duties; and should be on call no more often than every third night. It is the responsibility of the program director to ensure enforcement of reasonable policies with respect to work hours.

D. Objectives

A CLI training program must provide a structured educational experience that allows the resident to become proficient in the basic science, laboratory procedures, and technical management underlying the operation of the clinical immunology laboratory. In addition, the program must provide an appropriate clinical background that will prepare the resident to act as a consultant in the application and interpretation of diagnostic immunology tests. The program director and faculty must prepare and comply with written educational goals for the program.

1. Program Design

All educational components of the program should be related to program goals.

a. The program design and/or structure must be approved by the Residency Review Committee (RRC) as part of the regular review process.

b. Participation by any institution providing more than 2 months of education must be approved by the RRC.

2. Program Evaluation

The educational effectiveness of a program and faculty must be evaluated in a systematic manner. In particular, the quality of the curriculum and the extent to which the educational goals have been met by residents must be assessed. Written evaluations by residents should be utilized in this process.

II. Personnel

A. Program Director

The program director and faculty are responsible for the general administration of a program, including those activities related to the recruitment, selection, instruction, supervision, counseling, evaluation, and advancement of residents and the maintenance of records related to program accreditation.

There must be a single program director responsible for the program.

1. Qualifications of the program director include:

a. Competence as a scientist, clinician, and teacher in the field of CLI. The director must possess leadership qualities and have the authority to organize the program. This individual must maintain close contact with the program participant(s), contributing sufficient time to ensure adequate teaching and guidance. The director, or a qualified designee, must be available to provide advice and instruction to the resident(s) on a day-to-day basis.

b. Certification by the American Board of Allergy and Immunology or by a board in an immunologically related subspecialty of internal medicine or pediatrics or possession of suitable equivalent qualifications. In addition, the director should have a certificate in CLI or must demonstrate suitable equivalent qualifications.
c. Licensure to practice medicine in the state where the institution that sponsors the program is located. (Certain federal programs are exempted.)
d. Appointment in good standing to the medical staff of an institution participating in the program.
2. Responsibilities of the program director include:
a. Preparation of a written statement outlining the educational goals of the program with respect to knowledge, skills, and other attributes of residents at each level of training and for each major rotation or other program assignment. This statement must be distributed to residents and members of the teaching staff. It should be readily available for review.
b. Selection of residents for appointment to the program in accordance with institutional and departmental policies and procedures.
c. Selection and supervision of the faculty and other program personnel at each institution participating in the program.
d. Supervision of residents through explicit written descriptions of supervisory lines of responsibility for the care of patients. Such guidelines must be communicated to all members of the program staff. Residents must be provided with prompt, reliable systems for communication and interaction with supervisory physicians.
e. Evaluation of residents' knowledge, skills, and overall performance, including the development of professional attitudes consistent with being a physician.
f. Implementation of fair procedures, as established by the sponsoring institution, regarding academic discipline and resident complaints or grievances.
g. Monitoring residents' stress, including mental or emotional conditions inhibiting performance or learning and drug- or alcohol-related dysfunction. Program directors and teaching staff should be sensitive to the need for timely provision of confidential counseling and psychological support services to residents. Training situations that consistently produce undesirable stress on residents must be evaluated and modified.
h. Preparation of an accurate statistical and narrative description of the program as requested by the RRC.

B. Faculty

1. There must be a sufficient number of faculty with documented qualifications to instruct and supervise adequately all the residents in the program. The faculty must possess special competencies in the laboratory procedures currently used in clinical immunology and be able to provide the broad educational experience necessary for the interpretation of laboratory results. Members of the faculty must be able to devote sufficient time to meet their supervisory and teaching responsibilities.
2. All members of the faculty must demonstrate a strong interest in the education of residents, sound clinical and teaching abilities, support of the goals and objectives of the program, a commitment to their own continuing medical education, and participation in scholarly activities.
3. A member of the faculty of each participating institution must be designated to assume responsibility for the day-to-day activities of the program at that institution, with overall coordination by the program director.
4. The faculty must be organized and have regular documented meetings to review program goals and objectives as well as program effectiveness in achieving them. At least one resident representative should participate in these reviews.
5. The faculty should periodically evaluate the utilization of the resources available to the program, the contribution of each institution participating in the program, the financial and administrative support of the program, the volume and variety of patients available to the program for educational purposes, the performance of members of the faculty, and the quality of supervision of residents.

C. Other Program Personnel

Programs must be provided with the additional professional, technical, and clerical personnel needed to support the administration and educational conduct of the program.

III. Institutional Resources

A. Facilities

The CLI program must be supported by an adequate administrative and technical staff and have appropriate laboratory space available. In most instances this means the presence of an ongoing and operational diagnostic immunology laboratory in which a wide variety of immunologic tests are being performed on a routine basis employing state-of-the-art equipment. The laboratory should employ modern record-keeping procedures to ensure timely return of laboratory results and adequate storage of data.

B. Clinical Resources

The program should be in a setting in which there are sufficient clinical resources to ensure a large enough pool of patients to contain the full spectrum of immunologic disorders, and these patients should be available to the trainees for teaching purposes.

C. Library

1. Residents must have ready access to a major medical library, either at the institution where the residents are located or through arrangement with convenient nearby institutions.
2. Library services should include the electronic retrieval of information from medical databases.
3. There must be access to an on-site library or to a collection of appropriate texts and journals in each institution participating in a residency program. On-site libraries and/or collections of texts and journals must be readily available during nights and weekends.

IV. Educational Program

A. Curriculum

1. The educational goals must be defined in appropriate documents and must be available to prospective and current residents as well as to all faculty members involved in the program. Such goals must be defined not only for broad objectives but also for individual rotations, both inside and outside the main teaching laboratory. These goals must address the question of graded responsibility within the program, methods of resident evaluation, and means of involving trainees in diagnostic immunology consultation.
2. The curriculum should include a combination of practical and didactic training that addresses a number of different areas of CLI. The core areas forming a central part of every CLI program must involve training in the theoretical and practical aspects of quantifying immunoglobulins, immunoserologic testing, detection of autoantibodies, immunofluorescent and immunoperoxidase techniques, the study of lymphocyte phenotypes and functions, the use of monoclonal antibodies, ELISA (enzyme-linked immunosorbent assay) and radioimmunoassay techniques, and the use of

serologic methods for the detection of HIV (human immunodeficiency virus) infections.

3. In addition, there must be training in assays of immune complexes and the procedures for the measurement of complement components. These core areas should be supplemented by several additional important areas, which may be covered by organized conferences. These include training in methods of in vitro allergy testing, molecular genetic techniques as applied to immunologic diagnosis, immunohematology, procedures for the rapid diagnosis of infectious diseases, evaluation of phagocyte functions, histocompatibility testing, and the detection and quantification of tumor antigens. The resident must gain experience in the proper selection of laboratory procedures for the most efficient evaluation of immunologic disease.
4. Such education should include discussion of controversial immunodiagnostic techniques so that the resident will be able to make a rational determination regarding the scientific merit of such tests. In addition, the program must include education in the principles of quality control, laboratory management, and interaction with regulatory agencies.

B. Seminars and Conferences

Residents must attend seminars and conferences that are conducted on a regular basis and that must be of adequate quantity and quality to ensure an interchange of teaching within the various disciplines of clinical immunology. These conferences must include discussions of basic immunology; allergy; immunodeficiency disorders; and the immunologic aspects of rheumatology, pulmonology, gastroenterology, nephrology, hematology-oncology, endocrinology, cardiology, neurology, and infectious diseases.

C. Teaching Rounds/Clinical and Basic Science/ Didactic Teaching

Residents in CLI should attend appropriate clinical rounds and other didactic teaching sessions outside the CLI program itself. In addition, they should have access to prepared teaching materials on clinical and basic immunology.

D. Program Research and Scholarly Activity

Graduate medical education must take place in an environment of inquiry and scholarship in which residents participate in the development of new knowledge, learn to evaluate research findings, and develop habits of inquiry as a continuing professional responsibility. The responsibility for establishing and maintaining an environment of inquiry and scholarship rests with the faculty. While not all members of a faculty must be investigators, the faculty as a whole must demonstrate broad involvement in scholarly activity. This activity should include:

1. Active participation of the faculty in clinical discussions, rounds, and conferences in a manner that promotes a spirit of inquiry and scholarship. Scholarship implies an in-depth understanding of basic mechanisms of normal and abnormal states and the application of current knowledge to practice.
2. Participation in journal clubs and research conferences.
3. Active participation in regional or national professional and scientific societies, particularly through presentations at the organizations' meetings and publication in their journals.
4. Participation in research, particularly in projects that are funded following peer review and/or result in publications or presentations at regional and national scientific meetings.
5. Offering of guidance and technical support (eg, research design, statistical analysis) for residents involved in research.
6. Provision of support for resident participation in scholarly activities.

V. Evaluation

A. Resident Evaluation

The program director, with participation of members of the faculty, shall:

1. Semiannually evaluate the knowledge, skills, and professional growth of the resident, using appropriate criteria and procedures.
2. Communicate each evaluation to the resident in a timely manner.
3. Advance resident to positions of higher responsibility only on the basis of evidence of his/her satisfactory progressive scholarship and professional growth.
4. Maintain a permanent record of evaluation for each resident and have it accessible to the resident and other authorized personnel.
5. Provide a written final evaluation for each resident who completes the program. The evaluation must include a review of the resident's performance during the final period of training and should verify that the resident has demonstrated sufficient professional ability to practice competently and independently. This final evaluation should be part of the resident's permanent record maintained by the institution.

B. Program Evaluation

1. There should be formal provision for evaluation of the educational program by the faculty and residents.
2. Review of performances of past residents on the written examination of CLI will be employed by the RRC as one measure of the quality of the program.

C. Miscellaneous

Programs are required to notify the committee of major programmatic change, ie, change in program director, addition or deletion of participating institutions, and changes in numbers of trainees. The committee retains the prerogative to assess the impact of such change(s) upon the quality of the education offered to the trainees.

VI. Certification

Residents who plan to seek certification by the American Board of Allergy and Immunology in Clinical Laboratory Immunology should communicate with the executive secretary of the board to ascertain the full requirements.

ACGME: February 1990 Effective: July 1995

Program Requirements for Residency Education in Anesthesiology

I. Introduction

A. Definition and Scope of the Specialty

Anesthesiology, a discipline within the practice of medicine, specializes in the management of patients rendered unconscious or insensible to pain and stress during surgical, obstetric, and certain other medical procedures. This involves the perioperative evaluation and treatment of these patients and specialized care in (a) pain management, (b) cardiopulmonary resuscitation, (c) respiratory care problems, and (d) the management of critically ill and/or injured patients in special care units. Subspecialty training within the discipline plus investigative efforts are vital to the progress of the specialty.

B. Duration and Scope of Education

The Residency Review Committee (RRC) for Anesthesiology and the Accreditation Council for Graduate Medical Education (ACGME) accredit programs only in those institutions that possess the educational resources to provide 3 years of training in clinical anesthesia. The capability to provide the Clinical Base Year within the same institution is desirable but not required for accreditation.

C. Goals and Objectives

An accredited program in anesthesiology must provide education, training, and experience in an atmosphere of mutual respect between instructor and resident so that residents will be stimulated and prepared to apply acquired knowledge and talents independently.

The program must provide an intellectual environment for the acquisition of the knowledge, skills, clinical judgment, and attitudes essential to the practice of anesthesiology. This objective can be achieved only when the program leadership, faculty, supporting staff, and administration demonstrate a commitment to the educational program and provide appropriate resources and facilities. Service commitments must not compromise the achievement of educational goals and objectives.

The director and teaching staff of a program must prepare and comply with written educational goals for a program. All educational components of a residency program should be related to the program goals. The program design must be approved by the RRC as part of the regular review process. A written statement of the educational objectives must be given to each resident.

The institution sponsoring an accredited program in anesthesiology must also sponsor or be affiliated with ACGME-approved residencies in at least the specialties of general surgery and internal medicine.

II. Institutional Organization

Participating Institutions

No more than 6 months during the first 2 clinical anesthesia years and a maximum of 12 months during the 3 years of clinical anesthesia may be spent outside the parent institution in affiliated institutions.

Affiliation means that a formal written agreement exists between an accredited program and another institution to make facilities, clinical experience, supervision, and teaching sessions available to residents of the program who will rotate through the affiliated institution. Rotations to affiliates are limited, as noted above.

An integrated relationship exists when the program director (a) appoints the members of the teaching staff and makes recommendations for the appointment of the chief of service at the integrated institution, (b) determines all resident rotations and assignments at the integrated institution, and (c) has responsibility for the overall conduct of the educational program in the integrated institution. The amount of time residents may spend in integrated institutions is not limited.

The program director must seek prior approval from the RRC for the participation by any institution that provides more than 6 months of training. Prior approval also must be obtained for participation of an institution on an integrated basis, regardless of the duration of the rotation(s).

III. Faculty Qualifications and Responsibilities

A. Program Director

There must be a single program director responsible for the program. The department chair must be the program director.

1. Qualifications of the Program Director:
   The program director shall be certified by the American Board of Anesthesiology or have equivalent qualifications in anesthesiology. The program director also must be licensed to practice medicine in the state where the institution that sponsors the program is located (certain federal programs are exempted) and have an appointment in good standing to the medical staff of an institution participating in the program.
   The program director must possess faculty experience, leadership, organizational and administrative qualifications, and the ability to function effectively within an institutional governance. The program director must have significant academic achievements in anesthesiology, such as publications, the development of educational programs, or the conduct of research. Frequent changes in leadership or long periods of temporary leadership may adversely affect an educational program and may present serious cause for concern. When a new director, either permanent or acting, has been appointed, the RRC must be notified immediately. The RRC may initiate an inspection of the program in conjunction with this change when it deems it necessary to ensure continuing quality.
2. Responsibilities of the Program Director:
   a. Preparation, periodic review, and, if necessary, revision of a written outline of the educational goals of the program with respect to knowledge, skills, and other attributes of residents at each level of training and for each major rotation or other program assignment. This statement must be distributed to residents and members of the teaching staff. It should be readily available for review.
   b. Selection of residents for appointment to the program in accordance with institutional and departmental policies and procedures.
   c. Selection and supervision of the teaching staff and other program personnel at each institution participating in the program.
   d. Supervision of residents through explicit written descriptions of supervisory lines of responsibility for the care of patients. Such guidelines must be communicated to all members of the program staff. Residents must be provided with prompt, reliable systems for communication and interaction with supervisory physicians.
   e. Implementation of fair procedures, as established by the sponsoring institution, regarding academic discipline and resident complaints or grievances.
   f. Preparation of an accurate statistical and narrative description of the program as requested by the RRC.

B. Faculty

The faculty should have varying interests, capabilities, and backgrounds, and must include individuals who have specialized expertise in a significant majority of the recognized subspecialties. Didactic and clinical teaching must be provided by faculty with documented interests and expertise in the subspecialty involved. Fellowship training; several years of practice, primarily within a subspecialty; and membership and active participation in national organizations related to the subspecialty may signify expertise.

There must be a sufficient number of teaching staff with documented qualifications to instruct and supervise adequately all the residents in the program. The number of faculty must be sufficient to provide each resident with adequate supervision, which shall not vary substantially with the time of day or day of the week. In the clinical setting, faculty members should not direct anesthesia for more than two locations anesthetizing simultaneously.

All members of the teaching staff must demonstrate a strong interest in the education of residents, sound clinical and teaching abilities, support of the goals and objectives of the program, a commitment to their own continuing medical education, and participation in scholarly activities.

A member of the teaching staff of each participating institution must be designated to assume responsibility for the day-to-day activities of the program at that institution, with overall coordination of the program.

Teaching by residents of medical students and junior residents represents a valid learning experience. However, the use of a resident as an instructor of junior residents must not substitute for experienced faculty.

C. Other Program Personnel

Programs must be provided with the additional professional, technical, and clerical personnel needed to support the administration and educational conduct of the program.

The integration of nonphysician personnel into a department with an accredited program in anesthesiology will not influence the accreditation of such a program unless it becomes evident that such personnel interfere with the training of resident physicians. Interference may result from dilution of faculty effort, dilution of the available teaching experience, or downgrading of didactic material. Clinical instruction of residents by nonphysician personnel is inappropriate, as is excessive supervision of such personnel by resident staff.

IV. Facilities and Resources

There must be adequate space and equipment for the educational program, including meeting rooms, classrooms with visual and other educational aids, study areas for residents, office space for teaching staff, diagnostic and therapeutic facilities, laboratory facilities, and computer support. The institution should provide appropriate on-call facilities for male and female residents and faculty.

There must be a department library. This may be complemented, but not replaced, by private faculty book collections and hospital and/or institutional libraries. Journals, reference books, and other texts must be readily available to residents and faculty during nights and weekends. Residents must also have ready access to a major medical library, either at the institution where the residents are located or through arrangements with convenient nearby institutions. Library services should include electronic retrieval of information from medical databases. There must be access to an on-site library or to a collection of appropriate texts and journals in each institution participating in a residency program. On-site libraries and/or collections of texts and journals must be readily available during nights and weekends.

V. The Educational Program

Graduate medical education must take place in an environment of inquiry and scholarship in which residents participate in the development of new knowledge, learn to evaluate research findings, and develop habits of inquiry as a continuing professional responsibility. The responsibility for establishing and maintaining an environment of inquiry and scholarship rests with the teaching staff.

A. Program Design

The program must demonstrate a judicious balance between didactic presentations and clinical care obligations. Clinical responsibilities must not prevent the resident from participating in the requisite didactic activities and formal instruction. The ultimate goal is to produce a consultant anesthesiologist who relates confidently and appropriately to other specialists in addition to being a competent clinical anesthesiologist.

1. Clinical Base Year. A minimum of 4 years of graduate medical education is necessary to train a physician in the field of anesthesiology. Three years of the training must be in clinical anesthesia. One year of the total training must be the Clinical Base Year, which should provide the resident with 12 months of broad clinical education in medical disciplines, of which a maximum of only 1 month may involve the administration of anesthesia. The Clinical Base Year is usually the first year of graduate medical education. If an accredited anesthesiology program offers this year of training, the RRC will verify that the content is acceptable, ie, training in internal medicine, pediatrics, surgery or a surgical specialty, obstetrics and gynecology, neurology, family practice, or any combination of these. When the parent institution provides the Clinical Base Year, the anesthesiology program director should approve the rotations for individual residents and should have general oversight for rotations on the services that are used for the Clinical Base Year.
2. CA-1 to CA-3 Years. These 3 years, usually the second through the fourth years of graduate medical education, consist of training in basic and advanced anesthesia. They must include preoperative evaluation and management, intraoperative care and postoperative evaluation, and all aspects of perioperative care. The clinical training must progressively challenge the resident's intellect and technical skills and must provide experience in direct and progressively responsible patient management. As the resident advances through training, she or he should have the opportunity to learn to plan and to administer anesthesia care for patients with more severe and complicated diseases as well as patients who undergo more complex surgical procedures. The training must culminate in sufficiently independent responsibility for clinical decision making and patient care so that the program is assured that the graduating resident has achieved the ability to execute sound clinical judgment and function as a consultant in anesthesiology.

   Experience in basic anesthesia training must emphasize the fundamental aspects of anesthesia. At least 12 months of the CA-1 and CA-2 years should be spent in basic anesthesia training, with the majority of this time occurring during the CA-1 year. Residents should receive training in the complex technology and equipment associated with the practice of anesthesiology. There must be documented evidence of direct faculty involvement with tutorials, lectures, and clinical supervision of beginning residents.

   Anesthesiology encompasses the theoretical background and clinical practice of a variety of subspecialty disciplines. Exposure to these should occupy a minimum of 7 months in the CA-1 and CA-2 years. There must be identifiable 1-month rotations in obstetric anesthesia, pediatric anesthesia, neuroanesthesia, cardiothoracic anesthesia, and pain management, and a 2-month rotation in critical care. In addition, a delineated experience is required for anesthesia for ambulatory surgical patients and for the postanesthesia care unit, not necessarily in a continuum but equivalent to 1 month for each. The program director may determine the sequencing of these rotations. The resident should be evaluated following each rotation, and the written evaluations should be maintained in each resident's file. There must be a written description of each rotation in the CA-1 and CA-2 years. The goals and objectives for the CA-1 and CA-2 experience must be separate and distinct from those designed for the CA-3 year training.

The CA-3 year consists of experience in advanced anesthesia training. The program must have the resources and an organized plan to provide the Advanced Clinical Track, the Subspecialty Clinical Track, and the Clinical Scientist Track. The program director, in collaboration with the resident, will select one of the three tracks. Regardless of the track selected, resident assignments in the CA-3 year must include difficult or complex anesthesia procedures and the care of seriously ill patients. These tracks must not compromise the learning opportunities for the CA-1 and CA-2 residents.

a. Description of the Three Tracks:
   1. The Advanced Clinical Track. The track must provide a minimum of 6 months' experience in advanced and complex anesthesia assignments. The remaining 6 months may be in one to three selected subspecialty rotations; alternatively, additional complex clinical anesthesia assignments may be offered. A curriculum describing the goals and objectives of this track must be on file in the department.
   2. The Subspecialty Clinical Track. Nine to 12 months' experience in one subspecialty rotation along with up to 3 months of advanced experience may be offered. Alternatively, 6 months' experience in each of two subspecialty rotations may be offered. Such rotations may include some time assigned to medical or surgical activities directly related to the anesthesia subspecialty. The curriculum must be distinct from the CA-1 and CA-2 years' subspecialty curricula and reflect increased responsibility and opportunity. A curriculum specific to each of the subspecialty programs offered must be on file in the department.
   3. The Clinical Scientist Track consists of a combination of advanced clinical assignments and investigative work. It must offer 6 months' experience in advanced and complex clinical anesthesia assignments or, alternatively, in one selected anesthesia subspecialty rotation. The curriculum for the 6 months of clinical experience must comply and be consistent with the Advanced or Subspecialty Clinical Track rotations. The remaining 6 months will be devoted to laboratory or clinical investigation. A curriculum describing the goals and objectives of this track must be on file in the department.

B. Clinical Components

A wide spectrum of disease processes and surgical procedures must be available within the program to provide each resident with a broad exposure to different types of anesthetic management. The following list represents the minimum clinical experience that should be obtained by each resident in the program. Although the minimum requirements are for the CA-1 through CA-3 years, the majority of these should be accomplished in the CA-1 and CA-2 years.

1. Forty anesthetics for vaginal delivery personally performed by residents; evidence of direct involvement in cases involving high-risk obstetrics, as well as a minimum of 20 cesarean sections, including some administered under general anesthesia
2. Anesthesia for 100 children under the age of 12, including anesthesia for 15 infants less than 1 year of age, including infants less than 45 weeks postconceptual age
3. Anesthesia for 20 patients undergoing surgical procedures involving cardiopulmonary bypass
4. Twenty other major vascular cases
5. Twenty intrathoracic (thoracotomy, thoracoscopy) noncardiac cases
6. Twenty procedures involving an open cranium, some of which must include intracerebral vascular procedures
7. Management of a minimum of 100 patients undergoing ambulatory surgery
8. Fifty epidural anesthetics for patients undergoing surgical procedures, including cesarean sections
9. Fifty subarachnoid blocks performed for patients undergoing surgical procedures
10. Forty peripheral nerve blocks for patients undergoing surgical procedures other than those described above
11. Twenty-five nerve blocks for management of patients with acute, chronic, and cancer pain disorders
12. Documented involvement of anesthesia residents in the management of acute postoperative pain, including familiarity with patient-controlled intravenous techniques, neuraxial blockade, and other pain-control modalities
13. Significant experience with certain specialized techniques for airway management (such as fiberoptic intubation, double lumen endotracheal tube placement, and laryngeal mask airway management), central vein catheter placement, pulmonary artery catheter placement, peripheral artery cannulation, evoked potentials, and electroencephalography
14. Structured postanesthesia care experience of at least 1 month's duration; must involve direct care of patients in the postanesthesia-care unit and responsibilities for management of pain, hemodynamic changes, and emergencies related to the postanesthesia-care unit; designated faculty must be readily and consistently available for consultation and teaching
15. Critical care rotation, to include active participation in patient care by anesthesia residents in an educational environment in which participation and care extend beyond ventilatory management; active involvement by anesthesiology faculty experienced in the practice and teaching of critical care (This training must take place in units in which the majority of patients have multisystem disease. The postanesthesia-care unit experience does not satisfy this requirement.)
16. Appropriate didactic instruction and sufficient clinical experience in managing problems of the geriatric population

C. Didactic Components

Didactic instruction should encompass clinical anesthesiology and related areas of basic science, as well as pertinent topics from other medical and surgical disciplines. Practice management should be included in the curriculum and should address issues such as operating room management, types of practice, job acquisition, financial planning, contract negotiations, billing arrangements, and issues of professional liability. The material covered in the didactic program should demonstrate appropriate continuity and sequencing to ensure that residents are ultimately exposed to all subjects at regularly held teaching conferences. The number and types of such conferences may vary among programs, but a conspicuous sense of faculty participation must characterize them. The program director should also seek to enrich the program by providing lectures and contact with faculty from other disciplines and other institutions.

D. Resident Policies

1. Programs will be reviewed for assurance that they provide an appropriate balance between the number of residents in training and the educational resources available to them. Appointment of a minimum of nine residents with, on average, three appointed each year is required. Any proposed increase in the number of residents must receive prior approval by the RRC. Such approval will require documentation that the available clinical resources and faculty remain in compliance with the requirements.
2. Duty Hours and Conditions of Work
While the actual number of hours worked by residents may vary, residents should have sufficient off-duty time to avoid undue fatigue and stress. The program director must monitor on-duty schedules for residents to ensure that these assignments do not interfere with education, performance, or clinical care and judgment. The monitoring should ensure
   a. 1 full day out of 7 free of program duties;
   b. on average, on call no more than every third night;
   c. adequate backup if patient care needs create resident fatigue sufficient to jeopardize patient care or resident welfare during or following on-call periods;
   d. that residents do not administer anesthesia on the day after in-house overnight call;
   e. that during on-call hours, residents are provided with adequate sleeping, lounge, and food facilities;
   f. that support services are such that residents do not spend an inordinate amount of time in noneducational activities that can be properly discharged by other personnel.

   Formal written policies on these matters should be established. Formal educational activity shall have high priority in the allotment of the resident's time and energies.
3. Substance Abuse
The residency program must have a written policy specifically addressing the needs of anesthesiology and an educational program regarding substance abuse.

   The program director should monitor resident stress, including mental or emotional conditions inhibiting performance or learning, and drug- or alcohol-related dysfunction. Program directors and teaching staff should be sensitive to the need for timely provision of confidential counseling and psychological support services to residents. Training situations that consistently produce undesirable stress on residents must be evaluated and modified.

E. Scholarly Activity

While not all members of a teaching staff must be investigators, the staff as a whole must demonstrate broad involvement in scholarly activity. This activity should include

1. active participation of the teaching staff in clinical discussions, rounds, and conferences in a manner that promotes a spirit of inquiry and scholarship. Scholarship implies an in-depth understanding of basic mechanisms of normal and abnormal states and the application of current knowledge to practice;
2. participation in journal clubs and research conferences;
3. participation in research, particularly in projects funded following peer review and/or that result in publications or presentations at regional and national scientific meetings;
4. active participation in regional or national professional and scientific societies, particularly through presentations at the organizations' meetings and publication in their journals;
5. offering of guidance and technical support (eg, research design, statistical analysis) for residents involved in scholarly activities.

VI. Internal Evaluation

A. Resident Evaluation

The program director is responsible for regular evaluation of residents' knowledge, clinical competence, skills specific to anesthesiology management, and overall performance, including the development of professional attitudes consistent with being a physician. Evaluations of each resident's progress and competence must be conducted at the end of each 6-month period of training. The subspecialty evaluations as described above are in addition to this minimum requirement. There must be provision for appropriate and timely feedback of the content of the evaluations to the trainee. The program must maintain a permanent record of the evaluation and counseling process for each resident. Such records must be accessible to only the resident and other authorized personnel. Residents should be advanced to positions of higher responsibility only on the basis of their satisfactory progressive scholarship and professional growth. When a resident fails to progress satisfactorily, a written plan identifying the problems and addressing how they can be corrected must be placed in his or her individual file. The plan should be communicated in writing and in a timely manner to the resident and should be signed by the resident.

A written final evaluation for each resident who completes the program must be provided. The evaluation must include a review of the resident's performance during the final period of training and should verify that the resident has demonstrated sufficient professional ability to practice competently and independently. This final evaluation should be part of the resident's permanent record maintained by the institution.

B. Program Evaluation

The educational effectiveness of the program must be evaluated in a systematic manner. In particular, the quality of the curriculum and the extent to which the educational goals have been met must be assessed. There must be opportunity for trainees to evaluate confidentially faculty performance and the educational program. Written evaluations by residents should be utilized in this process at least annually. The teaching staff must be organized and have regular documented meetings to review program goals and objectives as well as program effectiveness in achieving them. At least one resident representative must participate in these reviews.

The teaching staff should evaluate periodically the utilization of the resources available to the program, the contribution of each institution participating in the program, the financial and administrative support of the program, the volume and variety of patients available to the program for educational purposes, the performance of members of the teaching staff, and the quality of supervision of the residents.

Resident participation in the periodic evaluation of patient care (continuous quality improvement) is mandatory.

The record of its graduates in obtaining certification by the American Board of Anesthesiology represents one measure of the quality of a program. The RRC will consider this information as part of the overall evaluation of the program.

C. Records

A comprehensive anesthesia record must be maintained for each patient as an ongoing reflection of the drugs administered, the monitoring employed, the techniques used, the physiologic variations observed, the therapy provided as required, and the fluids administered. The patient's medical record should contain evidence of preoperative and postoperative anesthesia assessment. When residents participate in patient care outside the operating room, they should receive instruction in proper recordkeeping for the activity involved and the faculty should review their records.

VII. Additional Information

A. Accreditation may be withdrawn from a program that has been without a resident for 2 years. Reactivation of a program following withdrawal of accreditation will require a new application.
B. Questions relating to educational programs and communication for the ACGME should be directed to the Executive Secretary, Residency Review Committee for Anesthesiology, 515 N State St, Chicago, IL 60610. Inquiries relating to the credentials of individual applicants for certification should be directed to the secretary of the American Board of Anesthesiology.

ACGME: June 1995 Effective: July 1996

Policies and Procedures for Subspecialties of Anesthesiology

Anesthesiology subspecialty programs will be surveyed and reviewed in conjunction with the survey and review of the core anesthesiology programs to which they are attached. In the case of a new application or in special cases determined by the Residency Review Committee (RRC), a subspecialty program may be reviewed separately. For an initial application, a survey will not be required when the application is reviewed without the core program.

Applications for accreditation of new subspecialty programs will not be considered if the core residency program in anesthesiology is accredited on a provisional or probationary basis, or if it has been accredited with a warning that adverse action will be taken if it is not in substantial compliance with the Essentials of Accredited Residencies at the time of the next review.

The RRC will designate the subspecialty programs as being accredited or not accredited. No further delineation of accreditation categories will be utilized. The accreditation of a subspecialty program will be directly tied to that of the core. If the core program is subsequently accredited on a probationary basis, this is simultaneously a warning to the related subspecialty program that accreditation is in jeopardy. Withdrawal of accreditation of the core program will result in the simultaneous loss of accreditation of the subspecialty program that functions in conjunction with it.

If the core program remains in good standing but the RRC judges a subspecialty program to be in noncompliance with the Program Requirements, a warning will be issued. If suitable improvement is not demonstrated in the time specified by the RRC, accreditation may be withdrawn from the subspecialty program. The *Procedures for Proposed Adverse Actions* and the *Procedures for Appeal of Adverse Actions* may be utilized by subspecialty programs from which accreditation has been withdrawn in an action separate from the core program.

Inquiries about accreditation of anesthesiology subspecialty programs should be addressed to the executive secretary of the RRC for Anesthesiology.

Program Requirements for Residency Education in the Subspecialties of Anesthesiology

These requirements apply to all of the accredited subspecialty areas and should be consulted along with the individual subspecialty Program Requirements.

I. General Information

A. A residency education program in a subspecialty of anesthesiology is an educational experience of at least 1 year designed to develop advanced knowledge and skills in a specific clinical area. All educational components of the program should be related to program goals. The program design and/or structure must be approved by the Residency Review Committee (RRC) as part of the regular review process.

Completion of an Accreditation Council for Graduate Medical Education (ACGME)-accredited anesthesiology residency, or its equivalent, is a prerequisite for entry into a subspecialty program of anesthesiology.
B. Residency education programs in the subspecialties of anesthesiology may be accredited only in an institution that either sponsors a residency education program in anesthesiology accredited by the ACGME or is related by formal agreement with the core program. Close cooperation between the subspecialty and residency program directors is required.
C. Subspecialty programs will not be approved if they have substantial negative impact on the education of the anesthesiology residents in the core program.

II. Faculty Qualifications and Responsibilities

The program director and faculty are responsible for the general administration of a program, including activities related to the recruitment and selection, supervision, counseling, evaluation and advancement of residents and the maintenance of records related to program accreditation.

Subspecialty education programs must provide a scholarly environment for acquiring the necessary cognitive and procedural clinical skills essential to the practice of the specific subspecialty. This objective can be achieved only when the program director, the supporting faculty and staff, and the administration are fully committed to the educational program. It is also imperative that appropriate resources and facilities be present. Service obligations must not compromise educational goals and objectives.

A. Qualifications of the Program Director

There must be a single program director responsible for the subspecialty program. The director must be an experienced educator and supervisor of residents in the subspecialty. He or she must be certified by the American Board of Anesthesiology or possess equivalent qualifications, and shall have had post residency experience in the subspecialty, preferably fellowship training. (See Program Requirements for Residency Education in the individual subspecialties for subspecialty certification requirements.) The program director must be licensed to practice medicine in the state where the institution that sponsors the program is located. (Certain federal programs are exempted.) The program director must be a member of the anesthesiology faculty, spend essentially all professional time in the subspecialty, and devote sufficient time to fulfill all responsibilities inherent in meeting the educational goals of the program.

B. Responsibilities of the Program Director

It is the responsibility of the subspecialty program director to support the residency education program by devoting his/her principal effort to its management and administration, as well as to teaching, research, and clinical care limited to the integrated institutions. This general responsibility includes the following specifics:

1. Preparation of a written statement outlining the educational goals of the program with respect to knowledge, skills, and other attributes of residents and for each major rotation or other program assignment. This statement must be distributed to residents and members of the teaching staff and should be readily available for review.

2. Selection of residents for appointment to the program in accordance with institutional and departmental policies and procedures.
3. Selection and supervision of the teaching staff and other program personnel at each institution participating in the program.
4. Supervision of residents through explicit written descriptions of supervisory lines of responsibility for the care of patients. Such guidelines must be communicated to all members of the program staff. Residents must be provided with prompt, reliable systems for communication and interaction with supervisory physicians.
5. Regular evaluation of residents' knowledge, skills, and overall performance, including the development of professional attitudes consistent with being a physician.
6. Implementation of fair procedures, as established by the sponsoring institution, regarding academic discipline and resident complaints or grievances.
7. Monitoring of resident stress, including mental or emotional conditions inhibiting performance or learning and drug- or alcohol-related dysfunction. Program directors and teaching staff should be sensitive to the need for timely provision of confidential counseling and psychological support services to residents. Training situations that consistently produce undesirable stress on residents must be evaluated and modified.
8. Preparation of an accurate statistical and narrative description of the program.
9. Notification of the RRC regarding major programmatic changes. Prior approval of the RRC is required for the addition or deletion of a major participating hospital and for a major change in the program's organization.

C. Faculty

There must be a sufficient number of teaching staff with documented qualifications to instruct and supervise adequately all the residents in the program. Members of the teaching staff must be able to devote sufficient time to meet their supervisory and teaching responsibilities.

All members of the teaching staff must demonstrate a strong interest in the education of residents, sound clinical and teaching abilities, support of the goals and objectives of the program, a commitment to their own continuing medical education, and participation in scholarly activities.

A member of the teaching staff of each participating institution must be designated to assume responsibility for the day-to-day activities of the program at that institution, with overall coordination by the program director.

The teaching staff must be organized and have regular documented meetings to review program goals and objectives as well as program effectiveness in achieving them. At least one resident representative should participate in these reviews.

The teaching staff should periodically evaluate the utilization of the resources available to the program, the contribution of each institution participating in the program, the financial and administrative support of the program, the volume and variety of patients available to the program for educational purposes, the performance of members of the teaching staff, and the quality of supervision of residents.

D. Other Program Personnel

Programs must be provided with the additional professional, technical, and clerical personnel needed to support the administration and educational conduct of the program.

III. Facilities and Resources

A. Space and Equipment

(See Program Requirements for Residency Education in the individual subspecialties for space and equipment requirements.)

B. Library

Residents must have ready access to a major medical library, either at the institution where the residents are located or through arrangement with convenient nearby institutions. There must be access to an on-site library or to a collection of appropriate texts and journals in each institution participating in a residency program. Access to computerized literature search facilities is necessary. On-site libraries and/or collections of texts and journals must be readily available during nights and weekends.

IV. Educational Program

The director and teaching staff must prepare and comply with written goals for the program. All educational components of the program should be related to the program goals. The program design must be approved by the RRC as part of the regular review process. A written statement of the educational objectives must be given to each resident.

A postgraduate residency must provide advanced education so that the residents can acquire special skill and knowledge in a specific subspecialty. This education should consist of a cognitive and a technical component. The cognitive component should emphasize the scholarly attributes of self-instruction, teaching, skilled clinical analysis, sound judgment, and research creativity. The technical component must provide appropriate opportunity for the residents to acquire the operative and other psychomotor skills required for the practice of the subspecialty.

A. Clinical Components

A sufficient number of patients must be available to ensure appropriate inpatient and outpatient experience for each subspecialty resident, without adversely affecting the experience of residents in the anesthesiology core program.

The total number of residents is dependent on the program's resources and its capacity to provide an excellent educational experience.

B. Didactic Components

Subspecialty conferences, including review of all current complications and deaths, seminars, and clinical and basic science instruction, must be regularly scheduled. Active participation of the subspecialty resident in the planning and the production of these meetings is essential.

C. Supervision

A resident must have the opportunity to provide consultation with faculty supervision. He or she should have clearly defined educational responsibilities for anesthesiology residents, medical students, and professional personnel. These teaching experiences should correlate basic biomedical knowledge with the clinical aspects of the subspecialty.

There must be close interaction between the core residency program in anesthesiology and the subspecialty program. Lines of responsibility for the anesthesiology residents and the subspecialty resident must be clearly defined. It is imperative that the educational program for the subspecialty resident not adversely affect the education of the anesthesiology residents, in terms of either experience or patient responsibility.

D. Duty Hours and Conditions of Work

The program director must establish an environment that is optimal both for resident education and for patient care, including the responsibility for continuity of care, while ensuring that undue stress and fatigue among residents are avoided. It is the program director's responsibility to ensure assignment of appropriate in-hospital duty hours so that residents are not subjected to excessively difficult or prolonged working hours. It is desirable that residents' work schedules be designed so that on average, excluding exceptional patient care needs, residents have at least 1 day out of 7 free of routine responsibilities and be on call in the hospital no more often than every third night.

During the on-call hours residents should be provided with adequate sleeping, lounge, and food facilities. There must be adequate backup so that patient care is not jeopardized during or following assigned periods of duty. Support services and systems must be such that the resident does not spend an inordinate amount of time in noneducational activities that can be discharged properly by other personnel.

E. Substance Abuse

The program must have a written policy specifically addressing the needs of anesthesiology and an education program regarding substance abuse.

F. Scholarly Activity

Graduate medical education must take place in an environment of inquiry and scholarship in which residents participate in the development of new knowledge, learn to evaluate research findings, and develop habits of inquiry as a continuing professional responsibility. The responsibility for establishing and maintaining an environment of inquiry and scholarship rests with the teaching staff. While not all members of a teaching staff must be investigators, the staff as a whole must demonstrate broad involvement in scholarly activity. This activity should include

1. active participation of the teaching staff in clinical discussions, rounds, and conferences in a manner that promotes a spirit of inquiry and scholarship. Scholarship implies an in-depth understanding of basic mechanisms of normal and abnormal states and the application of current knowledge to practice.
2. participation in journal clubs and research conferences.
3. active participation in regional or national professional and scientific societies, particularly through presentations at the organizations' meetings and publications in their journals.
4. participation in research, particularly in projects that are funded following peer review and/or result in publications or presentations at regional and national scientific meetings.
5. offering of guidance and technical support (eg, research design, statistical analysis) for residents involved in research.
6. provision of support for resident participation in scholarly activities.

G. Research

A subspecialty program should have an investigational component such that the residents may become familiar with the design, implementation, and interpretation of clinical research studies. Facilities should be made available for research activity. (Refer to Program Requirements for Residency Education in the individual subspecialties for additional research requirements.)

V. Evaluation

A. Residents

Subspecialty program directors must establish clearly defined procedures for regular evaluation of residents. The assessment must include cognitive, motor, and interpersonal skills as well as judgment.

The program director, with participation of members of the teaching staff, shall

1. at least semiannually evaluate the knowledge, skills, and professional growth of the residents, using appropriate criteria and procedures.
2. communicate each evaluation to the resident in a timely manner.
3. advance residents to positions of higher responsibility only on the basis of evidence of their satisfactory progressive scholarship and professional growth.
4. maintain a permanent record of evaluation for each resident and have it accessible to the resident and other authorized personnel.
5. provide a written final evaluation for each resident who completes the program. The evaluation must include a review of the resident's performance during the final period of training and should verify that the resident has demonstrated sufficient professional ability to practice competently and independently. This final evaluation should be part of the resident's permanent record maintained by the institution.

B. Faculty

Faculty must be evaluated at least annually to review teaching abilities, commitment to the educational program, clinical knowledge, and scholarly activities. Residents should participate in these evaluations.

C. Program

The educational effectiveness of a program must be evaluated in a systematic manner. In particular, the quality of the curriculum and the extent to which the educational goals have been met by residents must be assessed by the subspecialty program director, the core anesthesiology program director, and by the Institutional Review Committee on a regular basis. Written evaluations by residents should be utilized in this process.

There must be continuing quality improvement, utilization review, and evaluation.

VI. Board Certification

Questions relating to educational programs and communication for the ACGME should be directed to the Executive Director, Residency Review Committee for Anesthesiology, 515 North State Street, Suite 2000, Chicago, IL 60610. Inquiries relating to the credentials of individual applicants for certification should be directed to the American Board of Anesthesiology, 4101 Lake Boone Trail, Raleigh, NC 27607-7506.

ACGME: February 1998 Effective: July 1998

Program Requirements for Residency Education in Anesthesiology Critical Care Medicine (Anesthesiology)

In addition to the requirements described below, the statements in the Program Requirements for the anesthesiology core residency program concerning program director and faculty qualifications and responsibilities, research and scholarly activity, and evaluation mechanisms also pertain to the subspecialty programs in anesthesiology critical care medicine.

I. Introduction

A. Duration and Scope of Training

1. Anesthesiology critical care medicine (ACCM) is a subspecialty of anesthesiology devoted to the acute and long-term care of critically ill patients with multiple organ system derangements.

2. Subspecialty training in ACCM shall be a minimum of 12 months in duration beginning after satisfactory completion of a 4-year continuum in anesthesiology as required for entry into the examination system of the American Board of Anesthesiology. As such, subspecialty training in ACCM is in addition to the minimum requirements set forth in the Program Requirements for the core program in anesthesiology. At least 9 months of training in ACCM should be spent in care of critically ill patients in intensive care units (ICUs). The remaining months may be spent in meeting the objectives described below (see Section I.B).
3. Subspecialty training in ACCM should comprise 12 continuous months and there may be no more than one interruption of this period so that educational continuity may be maintained.
4. Accreditation of a subspecialty training program in ACCM will be granted only when the program is in direct association with a core residency program in anesthesiology accredited by the ACGME. Therefore, subspecialty training in ACCM can occur only in institutions where there are ACGME-accredited residency programs in anesthesiology, or in institutions related by formal agreement to the core program. In addition, there must be ACGME-accredited core residencies in general surgery and internal medicine.
5. The subspecialty program must function in conjunction with the core program in anesthesiology. The lines of responsibility between resident staffs in both the core program and the subspecialty program must be clearly delineated.
6. Subspecialty training in ACCM will occur principally in areas of the hospital commonly characterized as ICUs. Such ICUs are capable of providing acute and long-term life support of patients with multiple organ system derangements. Examples of ICUs include, but are not limited to, multidiscipline, surgical, medical, neonatal and pediatric, high-risk pregnancy, neurosurgical, trauma, and burn units.
7. There should be an institutional policy governing the educational resources committed to critical care programs assuring cooperation of all involved disciplines. Where more than one critical care program exists in an institution, it will be the responsibility of the institution to coordinate interdisciplinary requirements.

B. Objectives

1. The subspecialty program in ACCM must be structured to provide resources necessary to assure optimal patient care while providing its trainees the opportunity to develop skills in clinical care and judgment, teaching, administration, and research.
2. Exposure should be provided to a wide variety of clinical problems in adult and pediatric patients necessary for the development of broad clinical skills required for a subspecialist in CCM.

II. Personnel

A. Program Director

1. The program director of subspecialty training in ACCM must be an anesthesiologist who is certified in critical care medicine (CCM) by the American Board of Anesthesiology or who has obtained equivalent training and experience in critical care medicine. The subspecialty program director has responsibility for the teaching program in ACCM subject to the approval of the director of the core residency training program in anesthesiology.
2. The medical director of the ICU may be someone other than the subspecialty program director in ACCM. Recognizing the institutional and multidisciplinary nature of CCM, the specialty of origin of the medical director of the ICU is not as important as the provision that such an individual be certified in CCM and represent the best qualified person within the institution. However, the ACCM program director must be an associate director or co-director of the ICU(s) in which ACCM training occurs so that he/she can function in an educationally and clinically effective manner.
3. The ACCM program director must devote sufficient time to provide adequate leadership to the program and supervision for the trainees. This responsibility also includes active participation in the selection of subspecialty trainees and faculty with suitable qualifications in CCM.

B. Teaching Staff

1. There must be evidence of active participation by qualified anesthesiologists with a continuous and meaningful role in the subspecialty training program. Faculty involved in teaching subspecialty trainees in ACCM must possess expertise in the care of critically ill patients. It is recognized that such expertise will often cross specialty boundaries emphasizing the importance of collegial relationships and consultation between the CCM program director and faculty from other disciplines including, but not limited to, surgery and its subspecialties, internal medicine and its subspecialties, pediatrics, obstetrics and gynecology, pathology, and radiology. Where appropriate, supervision and teaching by faculty in these disciplines should be integrated into the teaching program for subspecialty trainees in ACCM.
2. Faculty and the CCM program director responsible for teaching subspecialty trainees in ACCM must maintain an active role in scholarly pursuits as evidenced by participation in continuing medical education at local and national meetings, as well as involvement in research as it pertains to care of critically ill patients.
3. Although the number of faculty involved in teaching trainees in ACCM will vary, it is recommended that at least three anesthesiology faculty be involved and that these be equal to two full-time equivalents, including the program director.

III. Clinical and Educational Facilities and Resources

A. An ICU must be located in a designated area within the hospital and designed specifically for care of critically ill patients.
B. Adequate numbers of specially trained nurses plus technicians with expertise in biomedical engineering and respiratory therapy must be available.
C. In order to provide sufficient range of exposure, an ICU that averages a census of at least five patients for each subspecialty trainee in ACCM is recommended.
D. Appropriate monitoring and life-support equipment must be readily available and representative of current levels of technology.
E. There should be readily available, at all times, facilities to provide laboratory measurements pertinent to care of critically ill patients with multiple organ system derangements. These include, but are not limited to, measurement of blood chemistries, blood gases and pH, culture and sensitivity, toxicology, and analysis of plasma drug concentrations.
F. Facilities for special radiologic imaging procedures and echocardiography are essential.
G. Conveniently located library facilities, and space for research and teaching conferences in CCM, are essential.

IV. Educational Program

A. The subspecialty trainee in ACCM should gain clinical experience in the following areas:
   1. Airway maintenance
   2. Mechanical ventilation of the lungs
   3. Emergency and therapeutic treatment of pneumothorax requiring placement of chest tubes

4. Emergency and therapeutic treatment requiring fiberoptic laryngotracheobronchoscopy
5. Pulmonary function tests
6. Cardiopulmonary resuscitation. The program must provide for training in advanced cardiac life support, advanced trauma life support, and pediatric advanced life support. Residents must gain certification for this training from the appropriate agency before the end of the ACCM year if they do not already possess it.
7. Placement of arterial and venous catheters
8. Emergency and therapeutic placement of artificial transvenous cardiac pacemakers
9. Pharmocologic and mechanical support of circulation
10. Monitoring central nervous system function and management of intracranial hypertension
11. Recognition and treatment of hepatic and renal dysfunction
12. Diagnosis and treatment of sepsis
13. Management of massive fluid and/or blood loss
14. Total parenteral nutrition
15. Bioengineering and monitoring
16. Interpretation of laboratory results
17. Psychiatric effects of critical illness

B. The teaching curriculum for the subspecialty trainee in ACCM should include the following areas:
1. Resuscitation
2. Cardiovascular physiology, pathology, pathophysiology, and therapy
3. Respiratory physiology, pathology, pathophysiology, and therapy
4. Renal physiology, pathology, pathophysiology, and therapy
5. Central nervous system physiology, pathology, pathophysiology, and therapy
6. Metabolic and endocrine effects of critical illness
7. Infectious disease physiology, pathology, pathophysiology, and therapy
8. Hematologic disorders secondary to critical illness
9. Gastrointestinal, genitourinary, and obstetric-gynecologic acute disorders
10. Trauma, including burns
11. Monitoring, bioengineering, biostatistics
12. Life-threatening pediatric conditions
13. Administrative and management principles and techniques
14. Transport of critically ill patients
15. Pharmacokinetics and dynamics; drug metabolism and excretion in critical illness
16. Ethical and legal aspects

C. The subspecialty training program in ACCM must provide the opportunity for active trainee participation in research projects pertinent to critical care medicine. Subspecialty trainees should be instructed in the design and interpretation of research studies, evaluation of investigation methods and interpretation of data, and should have the opportunity to develop competence in critical assessment of new therapies and of the medical literature.

D. Subspecialty trainees in ACCM should become experienced in teaching principles of critical care medicine to other resident physicians, medical students, and health care professionals. This experience should correlate basic biomedical knowledge with clinical aspects of critical care medicine, including the integration of clinical management principles applicable to patients of all age groups.

E. In preparation for roles as consultants to other specialists, the subspecialty trainee in ACCM must have the opportunity to provide consultation under the direction of faculty responsible for teaching in the ACCM program.

F. Subspecialty trainees in ACCM should gain experience in the administration of an ICU as related to appointment and training of nonphysician personnel, establishment of policies regulating functioning of the ICU, and coordination of the activities of the ICU with other in-hospital units.

G. Subspecialty conferences, including mortality and morbidity conferences, journal reviews, and research seminars, must be regularly scheduled. Active participation of the subspecialty trainee in ACCM in the planning and production of these conferences is essential. Attendance at multidisciplinary conferences is encouraged, with particular attention given to those conferences relevant to CCM.

V. Evaluation

A. Faculty responsible for teaching subspecialty trainees in ACCM must provide critical evaluations of each trainee's progress and competence to the director at the end of 6 months and 12 months of training. These evaluations should include intellectual abilities, manual skills, attitudes, and interpersonal relationships, as well as specific tasks of patient management, decision-making skills, and critical analysis of clinical situations. The subspecialty trainee in ACCM must achieve an overall satisfactory evaluation at 12 months to receive credit for training.

B. There must be written feedback of these evaluations to the subspecialty trainee.

C. Written and confidential evaluation of CCM faculty performance by the resident must take place once a year.

D. Written evaluations of patient care and subspecialty training objectives are required annually.

ACGME: February 1995 Effective: January 1996

Program Requirements for Residency Education in Anesthesiology Pain Management (Anesthesiology)

In addition to complying with the Program Requirements for Residency Education in the Subspecialties of Anesthesiology, programs must comply with the following requirements, which in some cases exceed the common requirements.

I. Scope and Duration of Training

A. Definition and Scope of the Specialty

Pain management is a discipline within the practice of medicine that specializes in the management of patients suffering from acute, chronic, and cancer pain. The management of acute and chronic pain syndromes is a complex matter involving many areas of interest and medical disciplines. Clinical and investigative efforts are vital to the progress of the specialty.

B. Duration of Training

Subspecialty training in pain management shall consist of 12 months of full-time training, beginning after satisfactory completion of a core residency program. At least 9 of the 12 months of training must be in clinical pain management. The remainder may be in clinical activities or research relevant to pain management. Assignments must not be made to activities not directly related to pain management.

II. Institutional Organization

A. Relationship to Core Program

Accreditation of a subspecialty program in pain management will be granted only when the program is in direct association with a core residency program in anesthesiology accredited by the Accreditation Council for Graduate Medical Education (ACGME). If the subspecialty program is not conducted within the institution that sponsors the core residency program, there must be an integration agreement between the core program institution and the facility in which the pain management program is conducted. Rotations outside the institution in which the pain management program is based should not exceed 4 months.

B. Appointment of Residents

Programs will be reviewed for assurance that they provide an appropriate balance between the number of residents in training and the educational resources available to them. Any proposed increase in the number of residents must receive prior approval by the RRC. Such approval will require documentation that the available clinical resources and faculty remain in compliance with the requirements.

C. Institutional Policy: Resources

Because pain management is a multidisciplinary approach to a common problem, there should be an institutional policy governing the educational resources committed to pain management that ensures cooperation of all involved disciplines.

III. Program Director/Faculty

A. Program Director

The program director must be an anesthesiologist who has been certified in pain management by the American Board of Anesthesiology or who has equivalent qualifications in pain management.

The subspecialty program director has responsibility for the teaching program in pain management subject to the approval of the director of the core residency program.

B. Medical Director

The medical director of the pain management service may be someone other than the subspecialty program director. Recognizing the institutional and multidisciplinary nature of pain management, the primary specialty of the medical director is not as important as the provision that such an individual represent the best-qualified person within the institution.

C. Faculty

Qualified physicians with expertise in pain management must have a continuous and meaningful role in the subspecialty training program. Faculty involved in teaching subspecialty residents in pain management must possess expertise in the care of patients with acute, chronic, and cancer pain problems. Such expertise frequently crosses specialty boundaries. Thus, the program is encouraged to include faculty from ABMS-recognized medical specialties other than anesthesiology. Where appropriate, supervision and teaching by faculty in these and other disciplines should be incorporated into the teaching program for subspecialty residents in pain management.

At least three anesthesiology faculty with expertise in pain management should be involved in teaching pain management residents and these should equal two or more full-time equivalents. A ratio of one full-time equivalent faculty member to two subspecialty residents shall be maintained.

IV. Facilities and Resources

A. Space and Equipment

A pain management center (clinic) must be located within a hospital/medical office complex and must be designed specifically for the management of pain patients. Space for research and teaching conferences in pain management must be available.

Appropriate monitoring and life-support equipment must be immediately available wherever invasive pain management procedures are performed.

There must be appropriate on-call facilities for male and female residents and faculty.

B. Support Services

The following functions and support must be available:
1. Appropriate laboratory facilities
2. Appropriate radiologic imaging facilities
3. Psychiatric/psychological services, including behavioral modification
4. Physical and/or occupational therapy
5. Social services
6. Medical record keeping
7. Other services as indicated (vocational, nursing, pharmacy, dietary, etc)
8. Appropriate electrodiagnostic facilities

C. Patient Population

For each subspecialty pain resident each year, there must be a minimum of 200 new patients. A minimum of 15% of the resident's experience should be spent in managing each of the three types of pain problems: acute pain, chronic pain, and cancer pain.

There must be ready access to consultation from other disciplines involved in pain management.

D. Library

There must be a departmental library with adequate material relevant to pain management. This may be supplemented but not replaced by private faculty book collections and hospital or institutional libraries.

V. The Educational Program

A. Educational Environment

An accredited program in pain management must provide education, training, and experience in an atmosphere of mutual respect between instructor and resident so that residents will be stimulated and prepared to apply acquired knowledge and talents independently.

B. Clinical Components

There should be exposure to a wide variety of clinical pain problems. Such exposure is necessary for the development of broad clinical skills and knowledge required for a specialist in pain management. Subspecialty training in pain management must include experience in the management of both inpatients and outpatients.

The resident must become familiar with the theory, benefits, indications, and practical applications of the following procedures and techniques:
1. A broad range of peripheral nerve block procedures
2. Epidural and subarachnoid injections
3. Joint and bursal sac injections
4. Cryotherapeutic techniques
5. Epidural, subarachnoid, or peripheral neurolysis
6. Electrical stimulation techniques
7. Implanted epidural and intrathecal catheters, ports, and infusion pumps
8. Acupuncture and acupressure

9. Behavioral modification
10. Physical therapy
11. Hypnosis, stress management, and relaxation techniques
12. Trigeminal ganglionectomy
13. Peripheral neurectomy and neurolysis
14. Sympathectomy techniques
15. Alternative pain therapies
16. Prevention, recognition, and management of local anesthetic overdose, including airway management and resuscitation
17. Recognition and management of therapies, side effects and complications of pharmacologic agents used in pain management.

The pain management resident must have significant experience in providing consultation.

C. Didactic Components

The pain management curriculum must include the following topics in lectures and reading:

1. Anatomy and physiology of the pain projection system
2. Epidemiology, economic impact, and sociology of pain
3. Pharmacology of opiates, non-narcotic analgesics, and nonsteroidal anti-inflammatory agents
4. Pharmacology of centrally acting drugs used in pain management
5. Measurement and assessment of pain and function
6. Principles of neural stimulation
7. Principles of diagnostic testing
8. Nerve blocks in pain management
9. Neuroablative procedures
10. Behavioral, cognitive, and supportive psychotherapeutic treatment principles, including rehabilitation and the role of team management
11. Principles and techniques of acute pain management
12. Principles and techniques of cancer pain management, including death and dying, and the ethical principles involved in hospital, hospice, and home care
13. Principles and techniques of management of other chronic pain problems
14. Principles of physical therapy, occupational therapy, and rehabilitation of the chronic pain patient
15. Principles of multidisciplinary approaches to pain management
16. Management of pain in children
17. Management of pain in the elderly
18. Principles and ethics of pain research in humans and animals
19. Organization and management of a pain management center
20. Continuing quality improvement, utilization review, and program evaluation
21. Disability assessment and rehabilitation procedures

D. Pain Center Management

Subspecialty residents in pain management must gain experience in the management of a pain center (clinic) with regard to appointment and training of nonphysician personnel, establishment of policies relating to management of pain problems, and coordination of the activities of the pain center with other inpatient and outpatient services.

E. Resident Teaching

The subspecialty resident in pain management must become experienced in teaching principles of pain management to resident physicians, medical students, and other health care professionals.

F. Conferences

Pain management conferences must be held regularly. These should include morbidity and mortality conferences, journal reviews, and research seminars. Active participation in the planning and presentation of these conferences by the pain management resident and faculty is essential. Attendance at multidisciplinary conferences is encouraged.

VI. Scholarly Activity

(Refer to the Program Requirements for Residency Education in the Subspecialties of Anesthesiology for requirements concerning scholarly activity.)

VII. Evaluation

A. Faculty responsible for teaching subspecialty residents in pain management anesthesiology must provide critical evaluations of each resident's progress and competence to the anesthesiology pain management program director at the end of 6 months and 12 months of training. These evaluations should include attitude, interpersonal relationships, fund of knowledge, manual skills, patient management, decision-making skills, and critical analysis of clinical situations. The program director or designee must inform each resident of the results of evaluations at least every 6 months during training, advise the resident on areas needing improvement, and document the communication. Subspecialty residents in pain management anesthesiology must obtain overall satisfactory evaluations at completion of 12 months of training to receive credit for training.

B. Periodic evaluation of patient care (quality assurance) is mandatory. Subspecialty residents in pain management anesthesiology should be involved in continuous quality improvement, utilization review, and risk management.

VIII. Board Certification

The record of its graduates in obtaining certification in pain management by ABMS certifying bodies represents one measure of the quality of a program. The RRC will consider this information as part of the overall evaluation of the program.

ACGME: June 1998 Effective: July 1999

Program Requirements for Residency Education in Pediatric Anesthesiology (Anesthesiology)

I. Introduction

A. Definition and Scope of the Specialty

Pediatric anesthesiology is the subspecialty of anesthesiology devoted to the preoperative, intraoperative, and postoperative anesthetic care of pediatric patients.

B. Duration and Scope of Education

Subspecialty training in pediatric anesthesiology shall be 12 months in duration, beginning after satisfactory completion of the residency program in anesthesiology as required for entry into the examination system of the American Board of Anesthesiology. Subspecialty training in pediatric anesthesiology is in addition to the minimum requirements described in the Program Requirements for the core program in anesthesiology.

The clinical training in pediatric anesthesiology must be spent in caring for pediatric patients in the operating rooms, in other anesthetizing locations, and in intensive care units. The training will include experience in providing anesthesia both for inpatient and outpatient surgical procedures and for nonoperative procedures outside the operating rooms, as well as preanesthesia preparation and postanesthesia care, pain management, and advanced life support for neonates, infants, children, and adolescents.

C. Goals and Objectives

The subspecialty program in pediatric anesthesiology must be structured to ensure optimal patient care while providing residents the opportunity to develop skills in clinical care and judgment, teaching, administration, and research. The subspecialist in pediatric anesthesiology should be proficient not only in providing anesthesia care for neonates, infants, children, and adolescents undergoing a wide variety of surgical, diagnostic, and therapeutic procedures, but also in pain management, critical perioperative care, and advanced life support. To meet these goals, the program should provide exposure to the wide variety of clinical problems in pediatric patients, as outlined in V.B., that are necessary for the development of these clinical skills.

II. Institutional Organization

A. Relationship to the Core Residency Program

Accreditation of a subspecialty program in pediatric anesthesiology will be granted only when the program is associated with a core residency program in anesthesiology that is accredited by the Accreditation Council for Graduate Medical Education (ACGME). Therefore, subspecialty training in pediatric anesthesiology can occur only in an institution in which there is an ACGME-accredited residency program in anesthesiology or in an institution related to a core program by a formal integration agreement. The director of the core anesthesiology residency program is responsible for the appointment of the director of the pediatric anesthesiology subspecialty program and determines the activities of the appointee and the duration of the appointment.

There must be close cooperation between the core program and the subspecialty training program. The division of responsibilities between residents in the core program and those in the subspecialty program must be clearly delineated.

B. Institutional Policy

There should be an institutional policy governing the educational resources committed to pediatric anesthesiology programs.

III. Faculty Qualifications and Responsibilities

A. Program Director

1. Qualifications of the Program Director
   The program director in pediatric anesthesiology must be an anesthesiologist who is certified by the American Board of Anesthesiology or who has equivalent qualifications. The program director also must be licensed to practice medicine in the state where the institution that sponsors the program is located (certain federal programs are exempted) and have an appointment in good standing to the medical staff of an institution participating in the program. He/she must have training and/or experience in providing anesthesia care for pediatric patients beyond the requirement for completion of a core anesthesiology residency. The program director in pediatric anesthesiology has responsibility for the training program subject to the approval of the program director of the core residency training program in anesthesiology. He/she must devote sufficient time to provide adequate leadership to the program and supervision for the residents. The clinical director of the pediatric anesthesiology service may be someone other than the program director.
2. Responsibilities of the Program Director
   a. Preparation, periodic review, and, if necessary, revision of a written outline of the educational goals of the program with respect to the knowledge, skills, and other attributes of residents at each level of training and for each major rotation or other program assignment. This statement must be distributed to residents and members of the teaching staff. It should be readily available for review.
   b. Selection of residents for appointment to the program in accordance with institutional and departmental policies and procedures.
   c. Selection and supervision of the teaching staff and other program personnel.
   d. Supervision of residents through explicit written descriptions of supervisory lines of responsibility for the care of patients. Such guidelines must be communicated to all members of the program staff. Residents must be provided with prompt, reliable systems for communication and interaction with supervisory physicians.
   e. Implementation of fair procedures, as established by the sponsoring institution, regarding academic discipline and resident complaints or grievances.
   f. Preparation of an accurate statistical and narrative description of the program, as requested by the Residency Review Committee (RRC).

B. Faculty

Although the number of faculty members involved in teaching residents in pediatric anesthesiology will vary, it is recommended that at least three faculty members be involved, and that these be equal to or greater than two full-time equivalents, including the program director. A ratio of no less than one full-time equivalent faculty member to one subspecialty resident shall be maintained. The RRC understands that *full-time* means that the faculty member devotes essentially all professional time to the program.

There must be evidence of active participation by qualified physicians with training and/or expertise in pediatric anesthesiology beyond the requirement for completion of a core anesthesiology residency. The faculty must possess expertise in the care of pediatric patients and must have a continuous and meaningful role in the subspecialty training program.

The program should include teaching in multidisciplinary conferences by faculty in pediatric and neonatal intensive care, pediatric medicine, and pediatric surgery.

The pediatric anesthesiology program director and faculty responsible for teaching subspecialty residents in pediatric anesthesiology must maintain an active role in scholarly pursuits pertaining to pediatric anesthesiology, as evidenced by participation in continuing medical education as well as by involvement in research as it pertains to the care of pediatric patients.

IV. Clinical and Educational Facilities and Resources

The following resources and facilities are necessary to the program:

A. Intensive care units for both newborns and older children.
B. An emergency department in which children of all ages can be effectively managed 24 hours a day.
C. Operating rooms adequately designed and equipped for the management of pediatric patients. A postanesthesia care area adequately designed and equipped for the management of pediatric patients must be located near the operating room suite.
D. Pediatric surgical patients in sufficient volume and variety to provide a broad educational experience for the program. Surgeons with special pediatric training and/or experience in general surgery, otolaryngology, neurosurgery, GU, ophthalmology, orthopedics, and plastic surgery must be available.
E. Monitoring and advanced life-support equipment representative of current levels of technology.
F. Allied health staff and other support personnel.

Program Requirements

G. Facilities that are readily available at all times to provide prompt laboratory measurements pertinent to the care of pediatric patients. These include but are not limited to measurement of blood chemistries, blood gases and pH, oxygen saturation, hematocrit/hemoglobin, and clotting function.

H. Conveniently located library facilities and space for research and teaching conferences in pediatric anesthesiology.

V. Educational Program

A. Goals and Objectives

The director and teaching staff must prepare and comply with written goals for the program. All educational components of the program should be related to the program goals. The program design must be approved by the RRC as part of the regular review process. A written statement of the educational objectives must be given to each resident.

B. Clinical Components

The subspecialty resident in pediatric anesthesiology should gain clinical experience in the following areas of care of neonates, infants, children, and adolescents:

1. Preoperative assessment of children scheduled for surgery
2. Cardiopulmonary resuscitation and advanced life support
3. Management of normal and abnormal airways
4. Mechanical ventilation
5. Temperature regulation
6. Placement of venous and arterial catheters
7. Pharmacologic support of the circulation
8. Management of both normal perioperative fluid therapy and massive fluid and/or blood loss
9. Interpretation of laboratory results
10. Management of children requiring general anesthesia for elective and emergent surgery for a wide variety of surgical conditions including neonatal surgical emergencies, cardiopulmonary bypass, solid organ transplantation, and congenital disorders
11. Techniques for administering regional anesthesia for inpatient and ambulatory surgery in children
12. Sedation or anesthesia for children outside the operating rooms, including those undergoing radiologic studies and treatment and acutely ill and severely injured children in the emergency department
13. Recognition, prevention, and treatment of pain in medical and surgical patients
14. Consultation for medical and surgical patients
15. Recognition and treatment of perioperative vital organ dysfunction
16. Diagnosis and perioperative management of congenital and acquired disorders
17. Participation in the care of critically ill infants and children in a neonatal and/or pediatric intensive care unit
18. Emergency transport of critically ill patients within the hospital and between hospitals
19. Psychological support of patients and their families

In preparation for roles as consultants to other specialists, subspecialty residents in pediatric anesthesiology should have the opportunity to provide consultation under the direction of faculty responsible for teaching in the pediatric anesthesiology program. This should include assessment of the appropriateness of a patient's preparation for surgery and recognition of when an institution's personnel, equipment, and/or facilities are not appropriate for management of the patient.

C. Didactic Components

The didactic curriculum, provided through lectures and reading, should include the following areas, with emphasis on developmental and maturational aspects as they pertain to anesthesia and life support for pediatric patients:

1. Cardiopulmonary resuscitation
2. Pharmacokinetics and pharmacodynamics and mechanisms of drug delivery
3. Cardiovascular, respiratory, renal, hepatic, and central nervous system physiology, pathophysiology, and therapy
4. Metabolic and endocrine effects of surgery and critical illness
5. Infectious disease pathophysiology and therapy
6. Coagulation abnormalities and therapy
7. Normal and abnormal physical and psychological development
8. Trauma, including burn management
9. Congenital anomalies and developmental delay
10. Medical and surgical problems common in children
11. Use and toxicity of local and general anesthetic agents
12. Airway problems common in children
13. Pain management in pediatric patients of all ages
14. Ethical and legal aspects of care
15. Transport of critically ill patients

Subspecialty conferences, including morbidity and mortality conferences, journal reviews, and research seminars, should be regularly attended. Active participation of the subspecialty resident in pediatric anesthesiology in the planning and production of these conferences is essential. However, the faculty should be the conference leaders in the majority of the sessions. Attendance by residents at multidisciplinary conferences, especially those relevant to pediatric anesthesiology, is encouraged.

D. Resident Policies

1. Duty Hours
   While the actual number of hours worked by subspecialty residents may vary, residents should have sufficient time off to avoid undue fatigue and stress. It is recommended that residents be allowed to spend, on average, at least 1 full day out of 7 away from the hospital and should be assigned on-call duty in the hospital no more frequently than, on average, every fourth night. The program director is responsible for monitoring the residents' activities to ensure adherence to this recommendation.
2. Peer Interaction
   Subspecialty residents in pediatric anesthesiology should become experienced in teaching principles of pediatric anesthesiology to other resident physicians, medical students, and other health-care professionals. This experience should correlate basic biomedical knowledge with clinical aspects of pediatric anesthesiology, including the management of patients requiring sedation outside the operating rooms as well as pain management and life support.

E. Scholarly Activities

The subspecialty training program in pediatric anesthesiology should provide the opportunity for active resident participation in research projects pertinent to pediatric anesthesia. Subspecialty residents should be instructed in the conduct of scholarly activities and the evaluation of investigative methods and interpretation of data, including statistics; they should have the opportunity to develop competence in critical assessment of new therapies and of the medical literature.

F. Additional Required Components

There should be prompt access to consultation with other disciplines, including pediatric subspecialties of neonatology, cardiology, neurology, pulmonology, radiology, critical care, emergency medicine, and pediatric subspecialties of surgical fields. To provide the necessary breadth of experience, an accredited residency training program in pediatrics is required within the institution. Residency programs or other equivalent clinical expertise in other specialties, particularly pediatric general surgery and pediatric surgical subspecialties, such as otolaryngology, GU, neurosurgery, ophthalmology, and orthopedics, and pediatric radiology, are highly desirable.

VI. Evaluation

A. Faculty responsible for teaching subspecialty residents in pediatric anesthesiology must provide critical evaluations of each resident's progress and competence to the pediatric anesthesiology program director at the end of 6 months and 12 months of training. These evaluations should include attitude, interpersonal relationships, fund of knowledge, manual skills, patient management, decision-making skills, and critical analysis of clinical situations. The program director or designee must inform each resident of the results of evaluations at least every 6 months during training, advise the resident on areas needing improvement, and document the communication. Subspecialty residents in pediatric anesthesiology must obtain overall satisfactory evaluations at completion of 12 months of training to receive credit for training.
B. There must be a regular opportunity for residents to provide written, confidential evaluation of the faculty and program.
C. Periodic evaluation of patient care (quality assurance) is mandatory. Subspecialty residents in pediatric anesthesiology should be involved in continuous quality improvement, utilization review, and risk management.
D. Periodic evaluation of subspecialty training objectives is encouraged.

ACGME: February 1997 Effective: February 1997

Program Requirements for Residency Education in Colon and Rectal Surgery

I. Introduction

A. Duration and Scope of Training

Institutions offering residencies in colon and rectal surgery must provide the necessary education to qualify the resident as a colon and rectal specialist in the care of patients, in teaching, and in research. Surgeons admitted to each residency are required to have completed a minimum of 5 years of an accredited, graded program in general surgery. Thus, the residents already should have developed a satisfactory level of clinical maturity, technical skills, and surgical judgment that will enable them to begin a residency in colon and rectal surgery for the purpose of specializing in this field of surgery. The period of training must be 1 year, and the program must comply with the Institutional Requirements for residency training.

B. Program Goals and Objectives

The director and teaching staff of a program must prepare and comply with written educational goals for the program.

C. Program Design

All educational components of a residency program should be related to program goals.

1. The program design and/or structure must be approved by the Residency Review Committee (RRC) for Colon and Rectal Surgery as part of the regular review process.
2. Participation by any institution providing more than 3 months of training must be approved by the RRC.

II. Program Personnel

The program director and the teaching staff are responsible for the general administration of a program, including those activities related to the recruitment, selection, instruction, supervision, counseling, evaluation, and advancement of residents and the maintenance of records related to program accreditation.

A. Program Director

There must be a single program director responsible for the program.

1. Qualifications of the program director:
   a. Requisite and documented clinical, educational, and administrative abilities and experience.
   b. Licensure to practice medicine in the state where the institution that sponsors the program is located. (Certain federal programs are exempted.)
   c. Certification by the American Board of Colon and Rectal Surgery or suitable equivalent qualifications.
   d. Appointment in good standing to the medical staff of an institution participating in the program.
2. Responsibilities of the program director:
   a. Full responsibility for the teaching or work done in the department or section.
   b. Preparation of a written statement outlining the educational goals of the program with respect to knowledge, skills, and other attributes of residents at each level of training and for each major rotation or other program assignment. This statement must be distributed to residents and members of the teaching staff. It should be readily available for review.

c. Selection of residents for appointment to the program in accordance with institutional and departmental policies and procedures.
d. Selection and supervision of the teaching staff and other program personnel at each institution participating in the program.
e. The supervision of residents through explicit written descriptions of supervisory lines of responsibility for the care of patients. Such guidelines must be communicated to all members of the program staff. Residents must be provided with prompt, reliable systems for communication and interaction with supervisory physicians.
f. Regular evaluation of residents' knowledge, skills, and overall performance, including the development of professional attitudes consistent with being a physician.

   The program director, with participation of members of the teaching staff, shall
   1. at least semiannually evaluate the knowledge, skills, and professional growth of the residents, using appropriate criteria and procedures.
   2. communicate each evaluation to the resident in a timely manner.
   3. advance residents to positions of higher responsibility only on the basis of evidence of their satisfactory progressive scholarship and professional growth.
   4. maintain a permanent record of evaluation for each resident and have it accessible to the resident and other authorized personnel.
g. The provision of a written final evaluation for each resident who completes the program. The evaluation must include a review of the resident's performance during the final period of training and should verify that the resident has demonstrated sufficient professional ability to practice competently and independently. This final evaluation should be part of the resident's permanent record maintained by the institution.
h. Implementation of fair procedures as established by the sponsoring institution regarding academic discipline and resident complaints or grievances.
i. Monitoring resident stress, including mental or emotional conditions inhibiting performance or learning and drug- or alcohol-related dysfunction. Program directors and teaching staff should be sensitive to the need for timely provision of confidential counseling and psychological support services to residents. Training situations that consistently produce undesirable stress on residents must be evaluated and modified.
j. Preparation of an accurate statistical and narrative description of the program, as requested by the RRC.

B. Faculty

1. There should be a minimum of two staff members, including the program director, who are certified by the American Board of Colon and Rectal Surgery or possess suitable equivalent qualifications, and who have significant teaching responsibilities. Members of the teaching staff must be able to devote sufficient time to meet their supervisory and teaching responsibilities.
2. All members must have the necessary interest and ability to perform their teaching duties adequately, have sound clinical and teaching abilities, support the goals and objectives of the program, have a commitment to their own continuing medical education, and participate in scholarly activities.
3. A member of the teaching staff of each participating institution must be designated to assume responsibility for the day-to-day activities of the program at that institution, with overall coordination by the program director.
4. The teaching staff must be organized and have regular documented meetings to review program goals and objectives as well as program effectiveness in achieving them. At least one resident representative should participate in these reviews.
5. The teaching staff should periodically evaluate the utilization of the resources available to the program, the contribution of each institution participating in the program, the financial and administrative support of the program, the volume and variety of patients available to the program for educational purposes, the performance of members of the teaching staff, and the quality of supervision of residents.

C. Other Program Personnel

Programs must be provided with the additional professional, technical, and clerical personnel needed to support the administration and educational conduct of the program.

III. Facilities and Resources

A. Residents must have ready access to a major medical library, either at the institution where the residents are located or through arrangement with convenient nearby institutions.
B. Library services should include the electronic retrieval of information from medical databases.
C. There must be access to an on-site library or to a collection of appropriate texts and journals in each institution participating in a residency program. On-site libraries and/or collections of texts and journals must be readily available during nights and weekends.

IV. Educational Program

A. The program should supply the necessary volume and variety of colon and rectal surgery to ensure adequate training of residents. If there is insufficient volume or variety in the primary institutions, arrangements should be made for an affiliation with a participating institution to correct the inadequacy. Each resident must have ample opportunity and responsibility for the care of patients with anorectal and colonic diseases.
B. The educational program also must include training in both diagnostic and therapeutic colonoscopy. The objective is to develop the necessary competence in the use of this procedure to qualify as an expert in the field. Therefore, adequate numbers of both diagnostic and therapeutic colonoscopies must be available either at the colon and rectal training program or through an appropriate institutional affiliation to satisfy this particular need.
C. An important aspect of the educational program is training in an outpatient facility to develop skills in patient evaluation, examination, office treatment, and surgical aftercare. Where feasible, such training should include work in the faculty member's office as well as in the outpatient clinic of the hospital.
D. Residents in colon and rectal surgery should be given the opportunity to obtain sufficient knowledge of those aspects of anesthesiology, radiology, and pathology that relate to colon and rectal surgery to develop overall competence as a specialist. Such training is best accomplished in cooperation with the departments of anesthesiology, radiology, and pathology.
E. Teaching contributes to the educational process, and therefore should be a regular part of the training program. The resident should assist when possible in the instruction of general surgical residents and medical students, as well as nurses and other allied health professionals. It is important to include instruction in the care of intestinal stomas, especially in institutions that do not have enterostomal therapists.
F. The responsibility for establishing and maintaining an environment of inquiry and scholarship rests with the teaching staff. While not all members of a teaching staff must be investigators,

the staff as a whole must demonstrate broad involvement in scholarly activity. This activity should include the following:
1. Active participation of the teaching staff in clinical discussions, rounds, and conferences in a manner that promotes a spirit of inquiry and scholarship. Scholarship implies an in-depth understanding of basic mechanisms of normal and abnormal states and the application of current knowledge to practice.
2. Participation in journal clubs and research conferences.
3. Active participation in regional or national professional and scientific societies, particularly through presentations at the organizations' meetings and publication in their journals.
4. Participation in research, particularly in projects that are funded following peer review and/or result in publication or presentations at regional and national scientific meetings.
5. Offering of guidance and technical support (eg, research design, statistical analysis) to residents involved in research.
6. Encouragement of trainees to undertake clinical and/or laboratory investigations, to present their research in scientific meetings, and to publish their findings in recognized medical journals.

G. Graduate education in colon and rectal surgery requires a commitment to continuity of and excellence in patient care. At the same time, patients have a right to expect an alert, responsible, and responsive physician dedicated to delivering effective and appropriate care. The program director, therefore, must ensure supervision of each resident, commensurate with that resident's knowledge, skill, and experience and with the complexity of each patient's illness. It is desirable that residents' work schedules be designed so that on the average, excluding exceptional patient care needs, residents have at least 1 day out of 7 free of resident responsibilities and be on call in the hospital no more often than every third night. The ratio of hours worked and on-call time will vary at this senior level and, therefore, necessitates flexibility.

H. The resident's activity outside the educational program should not be allowed to interfere with his or her performance in the educational process as defined in the agreement between the institution and the house officer.

I. There should be a documented semiannual evaluation of the resident's performance. Likewise, there should be opportunity for the resident to evaluate the program and the faculty.

V. Program Evaluation

The educational effectiveness of a program must be evaluated in a systematic manner. In particular, the quality of the curriculum and the extent to which the educational goals have been met by residents must be assessed. Written evaluations by residents should be utilized in this process.

VI. Other

A. One measure of the educational quality of a program is the performance of its graduates on the examination of the American Board of Colon and Rectal Surgery.

B. Those who plan to seek certification by the American Board of Colon and Rectal Surgery should communicate with the secretary of the board prior to beginning their residencies to be certain that their general surgical training is acceptable as one of the requirements for certification.

ACGME: June 1995 Effective: July 1996

Program Requirements for Residency Education in Dermatology

I. Duration and Scope of Training

A. Accredited training programs in dermatology shall be organized to provide trainees with the educational and practical experience that will enable them to deliver superior specialized care to patients with diseases of the skin, hair, nails, and mucous membranes. Such experience must be varied and broad, progressive and systematic, and of sufficient duration. Moreover, it must include instruction in the pertinent basic sciences and in all clinical areas that bear on the specialty of dermatology and training in research and teaching. Accomplishment of these objectives requires a suitable institutional environment; a cooperative and supportive administrative authority; a stable financial base; an enthusiastiç, competent, and available staff; an adequate patient population; modern, efficient equipment and space; and satisfactory liaison with other disciplines that relate to dermatology.

B. A dermatology residency may be accredited to offer either 3 or 4 years of graduate medical education.
1. A 3-year program is preceded by a broad-based clinical year of training (PGY-1) in an Accreditation Council for Graduate Medical Education (ACGME)-accredited program or similar program accredited in Canada.
2. A 4-year program must provide a broad-based clinical experience during the first year and 3 years of dermatology education in the second through fourth years of the program.
3. Approximately 75% of the resident's time during the 3 years of dermatology training must be related to the direct care of dermatologic outpatients and inpatients; this includes consultations, clinical conferences, and inpatient rounds.
4. Dermatopathology, microbiology, and other basic science lectures, seminars, and conferences are essential components of the resident's training.
5. Exceptionally, accreditation of residency programs of less than 3 years is possible, but only under the following conditions:
   a. This training must represent an unusual and highly specialized experience, in research or in a selected major area of dermatology, in an institution with extraordinary capability in such fields and with multiple accredited training programs in other disciplines.
   b. Moreover, training under such conditions will provide the trainee with only 1 year of credit to be applied against the necessary 3 years of training in dermatology. This training may not be used in lieu of the first postgraduate year or the first year of residency training in dermatology.

C. The program director and teaching staff must prepare and comply with written educational goals for the program. All educational components of a program should be related to program goals.
1. The program design and/or structure must be approved by the Residency Review Committee (RRC) as part of the regular review process.
2. Participation by any institution providing more than 6 months of training in a program must be approved by the RRC.

II. Institutional Organization

A. The sponsoring institution must ensure the financial, technical, and moral support and provide the necessary space, facilities, and supply of patients for the establishment and maintenance of an approved residency program in dermatology.

B. Adequate exposure to both outpatients and inpatients is necessary, as are opportunities to do research, to teach, and to become acquainted with administrative aspects of the specialty.
C. A cooperative relationship with other disciplines in medicine will result in the most effective implementation of these activities.
D. When the resources of two or more institutions are utilized for the clinical or basic science education of a resident in dermatology, letters of agreement must be approved by the institutional governing boards.
E. Affiliations should be avoided with institutions that
   1. Are at such a distance from the parent institution as to make resident attendance at rounds and conferences difficult, or
   2. Do not add to the educational value of the program.

III. Program Personnel

The program director and the teaching staff are responsible for the general administration of a program, including those activities related to the recruitment, selection, instruction, supervision, counseling, evaluation, and advancement of residents and the maintenance of records related to program accreditation.

A. Program Director

1. There must be a single program director responsible for the program.
2. Qualifications of the program director include:
   a. Requisite and documented clinical, educational, and administrative abilities and experience.
   b. Licensure to practice medicine in the state where the institution that sponsors the program is located. (Certain federal programs are exempted.)
   c. Certification by the American Board of Dermatology or suitable equivalent qualifications.
   d. Appointment in good standing to the medical staff of an institution participating in the program.
3. Responsibilities of the program director include:
   a. Preparation of a written statement outlining the educational goals of the program with respect to knowledge, skills, and other attributes of residents at each level of training and for each major rotation or other program assignment. This statement must be distributed to residents and members of the teaching staff. It should be readily available for review.
   b. Selection of residents for appointment to the program in accordance with institutional and departmental policies and procedures.
   c. Selection and supervision of the teaching staff and other program personnel at each institution participating in the program.
   d. The supervision of residents in accordance with explicit written descriptions of supervisory lines of responsibility for the care of patients. Such guidelines must be communicated to all members of the program staff. Residents must be provided with prompt, reliable systems for communication and interaction with supervisory physicians.
   e. Regular evaluation of residents' knowledge, skills, and overall performance, including the development of professional attitudes consistent with being a physician. The program director, with participation of members of the teaching staff, shall:
      1. At least semiannually evaluate the knowledge, skills, and professional growth of the residents, using appropriate criteria and procedures.
      2. Communicate each evaluation to the resident in a timely manner.
      3. Advance residents to positions of higher responsibility only on the basis of evidence of their satisfactory progressive scholarship and professional growth.
      4. Maintain a permanent record of evaluation for each resident and have it accessible to the resident and other authorized personnel.
   f. The provision of a written final evaluation for each resident who completes the program. The evaluation must include a review of the resident's performance during the final period of training and should verify that the resident has demonstrated sufficient professional ability to practice competently and independently. This final evaluation should be part of the resident's permanent record maintained by the institution.
   g. Implementation of fair procedures, as established by the sponsoring institution, regarding academic discipline and resident complaints or grievances.
   h. Monitoring resident stress, including mental or emotional conditions inhibiting performance or learning and drug- or alcohol-related dysfunction. Program directors and teaching staff should be sensitive to the need for timely provision of confidential counseling and psychological support services to residents. Training situations that consistently produce undesirable stress on residents must be evaluated and modified.
   i. Preparation of an accurate statistical and narrative description of the program as requested by the RRC.
   j. Internal analysis of the training program by the program director and his or her staff is essential, in addition to the regular surveys conducted by the RRC for Dermatology.
   k. The program director must notify the secretary of the RRC of any change in the program, staffing, affiliations, or facilities that might significantly alter the educational experience.
   l. At times of his or her absence, the program director must designate an interim director. If this period is for 6 months or longer, the RRC must be notified. Appointment of an interim director should not exceed 2 years, as it may have a detrimental effect on the program.
   m. A log of surgical procedures performed by residents must be kept on file and provided on request to the RRC or the site visitor. Documentation of resident evaluation, institutional and interinstitutional agreements, resident agreements, and departmental statistics should be kept on file and provided on request to the RRC or site visitor. The accurate and complete execution of application forms, progress reports, and replies to other requests from the RRC is the responsibility of the program director. The care and precision given to these responses will be taken into consideration in the assessment of the training program.
   n. The program director must ensure that residents are adequately supervised by faculty at all times. Further, resident duty and on-call assignments must be made in a manner that ensures that neither education nor quality of patient care is jeopardized by inappropriate resident stress or fatigue. Physicians must have a keen sense of personal responsibility for continuing patient care and must recognize that their obligation to patients is not automatically discharged at any given hour of the day or on any particular day of the week. In no case should a resident go off duty until the proper care and welfare of the patients have been ensured. Resident duty hours and night and weekend call must reflect the concept of responsibility for patients and provide for adequate patient care. Residents must not be required regularly to perform excessively difficult or prolonged duties. When averaged over 4 weeks, residents should spend no more than 80 hours per week in hospital duties. Residents at all levels should, on average, have the opportunity to spend at least 1 day out of 7 free of hospital duties and should be on call no more often than

every third night. There should be opportunity to rest and sleep when on call for 24 hours or more.

o. Trainees should be adequately supported to permit their undivided attention to educational and service responsibilities.

p. The program director should advise all residents planning to seek certification by the American Board of Dermatology to complete the preliminary registration form of this board and to communicate directly with the executive director of the board to be certain that they are in full compliance with the requirements for certification.

q. The program director must have a full-time commitment to the educational program and related activities.

B. Teaching Staff

1. There must be a sufficient number of teaching staff with documented qualifications to instruct and supervise adequately all the residents in the program. An instructor-to-trainee ratio of at least one-to-three is desirable, as is a minimum of two geographic full-time members of the clinical faculty, one of whom must be the training director.
2. Members of the teaching staff must be able to devote sufficient time to meet their supervisory and teaching responsibilities.
3. All members of the teaching staff must demonstrate a strong interest in the education of residents, sound clinical and teaching abilities, support of the goals and objectives of the program, a commitment to their own continuing medical education, and participation in scholarly activities.
4. A member of the teaching staff of each participating institution must be designated to assume responsibility for the day-to-day activities of the program at that institution, with overall coordination by the program director.
5. The teaching staff must be organized and have regular documented meetings to review program goals and objectives as well as program effectiveness in achieving them. At least one resident representative should participate in these reviews.
6. The teaching staff should periodically evaluate the utilization of the resources available to the program, the contribution of each institution participating in the program, the financial and administrative support of the program, the volume and variety of patients available to the program for educational purposes, the performance of members of the teaching staff, and the quality of supervision of residents.
7. Faculty from any and all clinical and basic science departments can and should be utilized to provide a complete educational experience for the trainees.

C. Other Program Personnel

Programs must be provided with the additional professional, technical, and clerical personnel needed to support the administration and educational conduct of the program.

IV. Educational Program

A. The training program shall be organized to permit the acquisition of experience and knowledge of dermatology in a graded and systematic fashion and ensure continuity of patient care.

B. Didactic training should complement and, when possible, precede or parallel the clinical activities. Such education should be organized to follow a curriculum that will ensure resident exposure to the complete range of disorders encountered by the dermatologist.

C. Appropriate clinical direction and supervision are necessary throughout the training period. As the experience and confidence of the trainees grow, increasing responsibility for patient management should be assumed; however, the authority and supervisory role of the staff at all levels of training must prevail.

D. An equivalent training experience must be ensured for all trainees.

E. Teaching methods throughout the training period should include various combinations of lectures, conferences, seminars, demonstrations, individual or group study of color transparencies and histologic slides, clinical rounds, chart and record reviews, faculty-trainee sessions in small groups and one-to-one settings, book and journal reviews, and attendance at local, regional, and national meetings.

F. Projection equipment and facilities for reviewing and taking clinical photographs should be provided.

G. A library containing the essential texts, journals, and other learning resources should be an integral part of each training area.

H. Space should also be made available for dermatology conferences, preferably dedicated for that purpose.

I. A vital part of the residency program is the structured study of the basic sciences related to dermatology, including allergy, anatomy, bacteriology, biochemistry, embryology, entomology, genetics, histology, immunology, mycology, oncology, parasitology, pathology, pharmacology, photobiology, physiology, serology, virology, and basic principles of therapy by physical agents. In addition, the structured study should include the basic medical sciences and principles that underlie dermatologic surgery and therapy by physical agents. Particular emphasis should be placed upon dermatologic microbiology, dermatopathology, and immunodermatology. There should be a well-organized course of instruction and range of experience in these three disciplines. The dermatopathology training should be directed by a physician with special qualification, or its equivalent, in dermatopathology.

J. To facilitate clinical and laboratory teaching it is essential that the department have an adequate supply of properly classified anatomic and pathologic materials, including histologic and photographic slides, and that the resident participate actively in the interpretation of histopathologic sections. Clinical laboratory facilities for microscopic analysis of biologic specimens (eg, fungal and ectoparasite scrapings, Tzanck preparations, immunofluorescence, darkfield examinations), culture for microbes (eg, fungi, bacteria, viruses), and interpretation of histologic specimens by light and electron microscopy should be conveniently available.

K. The training should be sufficient to ensure a knowledge of and competence in the performance of procedures in allergy and immunology, cryosurgery, dermatologic surgery, laser surgery, dermatopathology, clinical pathology, parasitology, patch testing, photobiology, physiotherapy, and topical and systemic pharmacotherapy and microbiology, including sexually transmitted diseases. Among these disciplines, dermatologic surgery should be given special emphasis in the organization and implementation of the training program. The surgical training should be directed by faculty who have had advanced training in dermatologic surgery. Dermatologic surgical training should include electrosurgery, cryosurgery, laser surgery, nail surgery, biopsy techniques, and excisional surgery with appropriate closures, including small flaps and grafts when indicated.

L. The practice of dermatology is concerned with both ambulatory and hospitalized patients. It is essential that an active outpatient service furnish sufficient clinical material representing the broad array of diseases seen by the dermatologist. Suitable facilities that permit the use of modern diagnostic and therapeutic techniques in the care of these patients should be provided. Inpatient facilities are also essential so that residents may have the opportunity to treat the more serious cutaneous diseases on a daily basis and observe the dermatologic manifestations of systemic disease. Dermatology staff and residents must have primary rather than consultant responsibility for patients they hospitalize with dermatologic illnesses. Properly supervised experience with appropriate follow-up in the provision of consultation to other services whose patients manifest skin diseases as secondary diagnoses is also necessary. The keeping of complete and accurate consultation records within the dermatology unit should be emphasized throughout this phase of the training. Space and equipment should be provided to permit instruction in dermatologic surgery, electrosurgery, phototherapy, cryosurgery, application of topical medicaments and dressings, physiotherapy, radiotherapy, and appropriate epicutaneous and intradermal testing, phototesting, and other diagnostic procedures.

M. During training it is necessary for trainees to gain an understanding of many diagnostic procedures and therapeutic techniques, even though they may not personally perform them. Furthermore, some of these procedures or techniques may not be available in their programs. Among these techniques are procedures such as hair transplantation, dermabrasion, Mohs micrographic surgery, and tissue augmentation. The physical modalities are especially notable, since an understanding of the basic properties of the electromagnetic spectrum is needed for the resident to become knowledgeable about the effects of various forms of this energy in the cause of disease and about its use in dermatologic diagnosis and therapy. Electron beam, x-ray, grenz ray, and laser are among these modalities. Even if some of these modalities are unavailable within a training unit, it is still an obligation of the director to ensure that the trainee has received appropriate instruction concerning the disease implication and therapeutic application of these energy sources.

N. Training must be provided in cutaneous allergy and immunology and in sexually transmitted diseases. Training should also be provided in appropriate aspects of environmental and industrial medicine, internal medicine, obstetrics and gynecology, ophthalmology, otolaryngology, pathology, pediatrics, physical medicine, preventive medicine, psychiatry, radiology, and surgery.

O. Experience in teaching dermatology to other residents, medical students, nurses, and/or allied health personnel is an important element of the residency program. In addition, trainees should, when possible, be given selected administrative responsibility commensurate with their interests, abilities, and qualifications.

V. Program Research and Scholarly Activity

A. Graduate medical education must take place in an environment of inquiry and scholarship in which residents participate in the development of new knowledge, learn to evaluate research findings, and develop habits of inquiry as a continuing professional responsibility.

B. The responsibility for establishing and maintaining an environment of inquiry and scholarship rests with the teaching staff. While not all members of a teaching staff must be investigators, the staff as a whole must demonstrate broad involvement in scholarly activity. This activity should include:
1. Active participation of the teaching staff in clinical discussions, rounds, and conferences in a manner that promotes a spirit of inquiry and scholarship. Scholarship implies an in-depth understanding of basic mechanisms of normal and abnormal states and the application of current knowledge to practice.
2. Participation in journal clubs and research conferences.
3. Active participation in regional or national professional and scientific societies, particularly through presentations at the organizations' meetings and publication in their journals.
4. Participation in research, particularly in projects that are funded following peer review and/or result in publications or presentations at regional and national scientific meetings.
5. Offering of guidance and technical support (eg, research design, statistical analysis) for residents involved in research.
6. Provision of support for resident participation in scholarly activities.

C. Residents must have ready access to a major medical library, either at the institution where the residents are located or through arrangement with convenient nearby institutions. Library services should include the electronic retrieval of information from medical databases.

D. There must be access to an on-site library or to a collection of appropriate texts and journals in each institution participating in a residency program. On-site libraries and/or collections of texts and journals must be readily available during nights and weekends.

VI. Evaluation

A. Periodic in-training evaluation of trainees should be carried out to ensure that the trainee is making satisfactory progress. Both formal examinations and performance ratings by the faculty can be utilized, and the trainee should be personally apprised of his or her strengths and weaknesses at appropriate intervals at least twice annually. Completion by the program director of resident yearly report forms, such as those requested by the American Board of Dermatology and other certifying boards, is an important part of this evaluation process.

B. The educational effectiveness of a program must be evaluated in a systematic manner. In particular, the quality of the curriculum and the extent to which the educational goals have been met by residents must be assessed. Written evaluations by residents should be utilized in this process.

C. One measure of the quality of a program is the performance of its graduates on the certifying examination of the American Board of Dermatology.

ACGME: September 1990 Effective: July 1995

Program Requirements for Residency Education in Dermatopathology (Dermatology)

I. Duration and Scope of Education

A. Dermatopathology is the subspecialty of dermatology and pathology that is concerned with the study and diagnosis of diseases of the skin and adjacent mucous membranes, cutaneous appendages, hair, nails, and subcutaneous tissues by histological, histochemical, immunological, ultrastructural, molecular, microbiological, and other related techniques.

B. Graduate medical education programs in dermatopathology must provide an organized educational experience for qualified physicians seeking to acquire the additional competence of a dermatopathologist.

C. Programs must provide organized education in all current aspects of dermatopathology, including basic science, laboratory procedures, laboratory management, quality assurance, and self-assessment.

D. The dermatopathology program must be an equal and joint function of the department of dermatology and of the department of pathology in a sponsoring institution that has an Accreditation Council for Graduate Medical Education (ACGME)-accredited residency in dermatology and an ACGME-accredited residency in anatomic pathology (AP-3) or anatomic and clinical pathology (APCP-4).

E. Dermatopathology programs must offer 12 months of education subsequent to the satisfactory completion of an ACGME-accredited residency in either dermatology or pathology.

F. For all dermatopathology residents, 50% of their education should be devoted to the study of dermatopathology, as outlined in II.A.1. For those who have completed a pathology residency, 50% of the 1-year program should be education in clinical dermatology provided by the dermatology teaching staff. For those who have completed a dermatology residency, 50% of the program should be education in anatomic pathology provided by the pathology teaching staff.

G. The director and teaching staff of the program must prepare and comply with written educational goals for the program and distribute them to applicants, residents, and members of the teaching staff. All educational components of the program should be related to these goals.

H. The program design and/or structure must be approved by the dermatopathology review committee as part of the regular review process.

I. Participation by any institution providing more than 2 months of training in the program must be approved by the subcommittee for dermatopathology.

J. The educational effectiveness of the program must be evaluated in a systematic manner. In particular, the quality of the curriculum and the extent to which the educational goals have been met by residents must be assessed. Written evaluations by residents should be utilized in this process.

II. Educational Program

A. Curriculum

1. Programs should be structured so that residents are involved in dermatopathology throughout the year. The program must include didactic instruction and practical experience in the diagnosis of skin disorders by direct inspection and by histological, histochemical, immunological, ultrastructural, molecular, microbiological, and other related techniques. Relevant aspects of mycology, bacteriology, and entomology should be included.
2. Dermatopathology residents must be given clearly defined assignments and increasing responsibility as they progress through the program.
3. The program must provide a sufficient volume and variety of dermatopathology specimens (at least 5,000 new accessions per resident per year) and other educational material for the resident to acquire the qualifications of a consultant in dermatopathology.
4. The program must provide the resident with the experience required to set up and to operate a dermatopathology laboratory and to supervise and train laboratory personnel.
5. All dermatopathology residents should participate in patient examination and autopsies appropriate to dermatopathology. Residents who are pathologists must participate in the examination of at least 1,000 dermatology patients.
6. Dermatopathology residents who are dermatologists must have exposure to autopsy and surgical pathology. This experience should emphasize contemporary diagnostic techniques and require attendance at autopsy and surgical pathology conferences, the review of slide sets of diseases relevant to dermatopathology, and participation in autopsies.

B. Educational Activities

1. Lectures, tutorials, seminars, and conferences with clinical services must be regularly scheduled and held.
2. Instruction should include the use of study sets and files of usual and unusual cases and other educational materials.

III. Program Personnel

The program director and the teaching staff are responsible for the general administration of a program, including those activities related to the recruitment, selection, instruction, supervision, counseling, evaluation, and advancement of residents and the maintenance of records related to program accreditation.

A. Program Director

1. The program director must be responsible for and have the authority to conduct the training program effectively. He or she must devote sufficient time to the program to ensure the implementation of sound administrative practices and the provision of adequate facilities, teaching staff, resident staff, and educational resource materials.
2. A program involving two or more participating institutions must have a single director with authority for the supervision and coordination of the portions of the program carried out at each institution.
3. Qualifications of the program director include:
   a. Requisite and documented clinical, educational, and administrative abilities and experience.
   b. Licensure to practice medicine in the state where the institution that sponsors the program is located. (Certain federal programs are exempted.)
   c. Certification in dermatopathology by the American Board of Dermatology or American Board of Pathology, or suitable equivalent qualifications.
   d. Appointment in good standing to the medical staff of an institution participating in the program.
4. The program director must demonstrate continuing scholarly activity.
5. Responsibilities of the program director include:
   a. Preparation of a written statement outlining the educational goals of the program with respect to knowledge, skills, and other attributes of residents at each level of training and for each major rotation or other program assignment. This statement must be distributed to residents and members of the teaching staff. It should be readily available for review.
   b. Selection of residents for appointment to the program in accordance with institutional and departmental policies and procedures.
   c. Selection, supervision, and evaluation of the teaching staff and other program personnel at each institution participating in the program.
   d. The supervision of residents in accordance with explicit written descriptions of supervisory lines of responsibility for the care of patients. Such guidelines must be communicated to all members of the program staff. Residents must be provided with prompt, reliable systems for communication and interaction with supervisory physicians.
   e. Regular evaluation of residents' knowledge, skills, and overall performance, including the development of professional attitudes consistent with being a physician. The program director, with participation of members of the teaching staff, shall:
      1. At least semiannually evaluate the knowledge, skills, and professional growth of the residents, using appropriate criteria and procedures.
      2. Communicate each evaluation to the resident in a timely manner.
      3. Advance residents to positions of higher responsibility only on the basis of evidence of their satisfactory progressive scholarship and professional growth.

4. Maintain a permanent record of evaluation for each resident and have it accessible to the resident and other authorized personnel.

f. The provision of a written final evaluation for each resident who completes the program. The evaluation must include a review of the resident's performance during the final period of training and should verify that the resident has demonstrated sufficient professional ability to practice competently and independently. This final evaluation should be part of the resident's permanent record maintained by the institution.

g. Implementation of fair procedures, as established by the sponsoring institution, regarding academic discipline and resident complaints or grievances.

h. Monitoring resident stress, including mental or emotional conditions inhibiting performance or learning and drug- or alcohol-related dysfunction. Program directors and teaching staff should be sensitive to the need for timely provision of confidential counseling and psychological support services to residents. Training situations that consistently produce undesirable stress on residents must be evaluated and modified.

i. Preparation of an accurate statistical and narrative description of the program as requested by the dermatopathology review committee.

B. Teaching Staff

1. There must be a sufficient number of teaching staff with documented qualifications in dermatopathology to instruct and supervise adequately all the residents in the program. Members of the teaching staff must be able to devote sufficient time to meet their supervisory and teaching responsibilities.
2. All members of the teaching staff must demonstrate a strong interest in the education of residents, sound clinical and teaching abilities, support of the goals and objectives of the program, a commitment to their own continuing medical education, and participation in scholarly activities.
3. A member of the teaching staff of each participating institution must be designated to assume responsibility for the day-to-day activities of the program at that institution, with overall coordination by the program director.
4. The teaching staff must be organized and have regular documented meetings to review program goals and objectives as well as program effectiveness in achieving them. At least one resident representative should participate in these reviews.
5. The teaching staff should periodically evaluate the utilization of the resources available to the program, the contribution of each institution participating in the program, the financial and administrative support of the program, the volume and variety of patients available to the program for educational purposes, the performance of members of the teaching staff, and the quality of supervision of residents.

C. Dermatopathology Residents

1. The number of positions requested must not exceed the educational resources available in a program.
2. Residents must have the opportunity to assume increasing responsibility under supervision appropriate to their experience as they progress through the program.
3. Residents should have the opportunity to become involved in dermatopathologic research and teaching during the program.
4. The program director must ensure that residents are adequately supervised by faculty at all times. Further, resident duty and on-call assignments must be made in a manner that ensures that neither education nor quality of patient care is jeopardized by resident stress or fatigue. Physicians must have a keen sense of personal responsibility for continuing patient care, and must recognize that their obligation to patients is not automatically discharged at any given hour of the day. In no case should a trainee go off duty until the proper care and welfare of the patients have been ensured. Resident duty hours and night and weekend call must reflect the concept of responsibility for patients and the provision of adequate patient care. Residents must not be required regularly to perform excessive, prolonged duties. When averaged over 4 weeks, residents should spend no more than 80 hours per week in hospital duties. Residents should, on average, have the opportunity to spend at least 1 day out of 7 free of program duties and should be on call no more often than every third night. When on call for 24 hours or more, there should be opportunity to rest and sleep.

D. Other Personnel

1. The laboratories involved in the program must be directed by qualified physicians who are licensed to practice medicine and are members in good standing of the institution's medical staff.
2. There must be a sufficient number of qualified professional, technical, and clerical personnel to support laboratory work and the educational program.

IV. Institutional Resources

A. There must be ample case material and supporting facilities to meet the training requirements in dermatopathology, dermatology, and pathology. Each dermatopathology resident should examine at least 5,000 dermatopathology specimens (ie, in-house or referred specimens in the institution's accessions file for which reports are generated).

B. There must be adequate equipment, laboratory space, office facilities, meeting rooms, classrooms, and research space to support service, teaching, and educational responsibilities.

C. The institutions and laboratories participating in the program must be appropriately accredited and/or licensed.

D. Residents must have ready access to a major medical library, either at the institution where the residents are located or through arrangement with convenient nearby institutions. Library services should include the electronic retrieval of information from medical databases. There must be access to an on-site library or to a collection of appropriate texts and journals in each institution participating in a residency program. On-site libraries and/or collections of texts and journals must be readily available during nights and weekends.

V. Research and Scholarly Activity

A. Graduate medical education must take place in an environment of inquiry and scholarship in which residents participate in the development of new knowledge, learn to evaluate research findings, and develop habits of inquiry as a continuing professional responsibility.

B. The responsibility for establishing and maintaining an environment of inquiry and scholarship rests with the teaching staff. While not all members of a teaching staff must be investigators, the staff as a whole must demonstrate broad involvement in scholarly activity. This activity should include:

1. Active participation of the teaching staff in clinical discussions, rounds, and conferences in a manner that promotes a spirit of inquiry and scholarship. Scholarship implies an in-depth understanding of basic mechanisms of normal and abnormal states and the application of current knowledge to practice.
2. Participation in journal clubs and research conferences.
3. Active participation in regional or national professional and scientific societies, particularly through presentations at the organizations' meetings and publication in their journals.

4. Participation in research, particularly in projects that are funded following peer review and/or result in publication or presentations at regional and national scientific meetings.
5. Offering of guidance and technical support (eg, research design, statistical analysis) for residents involved in research.
6. Provision of support for resident participation in scholarly activities.

VI. Evaluation

A. There must be regular, written evaluation of residents by teaching staff. Evaluations should be completed and discussed with the residents at least once every 6 months.

B. Residents should submit written evaluations of the program at least once each year for review by the director and teaching staff.

VII. Certification and Accreditation

A. The Residency Review Committees for Dermatology and Pathology are responsible for accreditation of graduate medical education programs in dermatopathology.

B. The American Board of Dermatology and American Board of Pathology are responsible for certification of individual physicians in dermatopathology. Individuals who plan to seek certification should communicate with their respective boards to obtain the latest information regarding certification.

ACGME: February 1993   Effective: July 1995

Program Requirements for Residency Education in Emergency Medicine

I. Introduction

A. General Characteristics of Accredited Programs

Residencies in emergency medicine are designed to prepare physicians for the practice of emergency medicine. These programs must teach the basic skills and knowledge that constitute the foundations of emergency medicine practice and provide progressive responsibility for and experience in the application of these principles to the management of clinical problems. Equal opportunity must be provided for the residents, under the guidance and supervision of a qualified faculty, to develop a satisfactory level of clinical maturity, judgment, and technical skill. Upon completion of the program, residents should be capable of practicing emergency medicine, incorporating new skills and knowledge during their careers, and monitoring their own physical and mental well-being and that of others in the profession.

B. Length of the Program

1. The required length of an emergency medicine residency is 36 months in a curriculum under the control of the emergency medicine program director. Accreditation by the Accreditation Council for Graduate Medical Education (ACGME) is required for all years of the educational program. The Residency Review Committee (RRC) recognizes three educational formats: PGY 1-3, PGY 2-4, and PGY 1-4. The resident must complete all years of education for which the program is accredited. [*Note:* For information concerning the transfer of residents between emergency medicine residencies with differing educational formats and advanced placement credit for training in other specialties, contact the American Board of Emergency Medicine.]
2. Programs that extend the residency beyond 36 months must present a clear educational rationale consonant with the program requirements and the objectives of the residency. The program director must obtain the approval of the sponsoring institution and the RRC prior to implementation and at each subsequent accreditation review of the program.
3. Prior to entry into the program, each resident must be notified in writing of the required length of the program. This period may not be changed for a particular resident during his or her program unless there is a significant break in his or her education or the resident needs remedial education.

C. Goals of Education

Residency programs in emergency medicine should produce physicians prepared to:

1. Provide the recognition, resuscitation, stabilization, evaluation, and care of the full range of patients who present to the emergency department.
2. Arrange appropriate follow-up or referral as required.
3. Manage the prehospital care of the acutely ill or injured patient.
4. Participate in the administration of the emergency medical services system providing prehospital care.
5. Provide appropriate patient education directed toward the prevention of illness and injury.
6. Engage in the administration and teaching of emergency medicine.
7. Understand and evaluate research methodologies and their application.

II. Institutions

The institution(s) involved in the program must provide evidence of commitment to graduate medical education, including emergency medicine. While it is recognized that the practice of emergency medicine occurs within a variety of organizational structures, the administrative and academic structure must be organized in a way that facilitates the provision of an adequate educational experience. There must be evidence of an adequate financial commitment to the program.

A. Medical School Affiliation

Medical school affiliation is desirable. When a medical school affiliation is present, there must be a written affiliation agreement or a letter of understanding documenting the duties and responsibilities of both the medical school and the program. Program core faculty should have or be able to apply for appropriate faculty appointments at the medical school.

B. Affiliation Agreements

1. When there is a cooperative educational effort involving multiple institutions, the commitment of each institution to the program must be made explicit in an affiliation agreement with each institution that conforms to ACGME Institutional Requirements Section I.C.1-5.
2. In addition, there must be a current letter of understanding between the program director and the individual responsible for each resident rotation in the program that describes:
   a. The educational objectives and the means by which they will be accomplished and evaluated.
   b. The resources and facilities in the institution(s) that will be available to each resident, including but not limited to library and medical records.
   c. The duties and responsibilities the resident will have on each rotation.
   d. The relationship that will exist between emergency medicine residents and residents and faculty in other programs.
   e. The supervision emergency medicine residents will receive on each rotation.
3. For emergency medicine rotations, the physician responsible, under the authority of the program director, for the teaching and supervision of emergency medicine residents must be identified.

C. Participating Institutions

1. The program should be based at a primary hospital (hereafter referred to as the primary clinical site). More of the didactic and clinical experiences should take place at the primary clinical site than at any other single site. Educationally justified exceptions to this requirement will be considered.
2. Programs using multiple hospitals must ensure the provision of a unified educational experience for the residents. Each affiliated institution must offer significant educational opportunities to the overall program. The reasons for including each institution must be stated. Affiliations that merely duplicate experiences otherwise available within the program are not desirable.
3. To maintain program cohesion, continuity, and critical mass, as well as to reduce stress on the residents and their families, mandated rotations to affiliated institutions that are geographically distant from the sponsoring institution are acceptable only if they offer special resources, unavailable locally, that significantly augment the overall educational experience of the program.
4. The number and geographic distribution of participating institutions must not preclude the satisfactory participation by all residents in conferences and other educational exercises.

D. Facilities and Resources

In every hospital in which the emergency department is used as a training site, the following must be provided:

1. Adequate patient care space.
2. Laboratory and diagnostic imaging results, especially those required on a STAT basis, returned on a timely basis.
3. Adequate program support space, including office space for faculty and residents.
4. Current medical library resources, including appropriate emergency medicine reference texts in the emergency department. In addition, residents must have ready access to a major medical library, either at the institution where the residents are located or through arrangement with convenient nearby institutions. Services available should include the electronic retrieval of information from medical databases.
5. Adequate and readily accessible instructional space.
6. Data information systems.
7. Security support services.

III. Personnel

The program leadership and the teaching staff are responsible for the general administration of the program, including those activities related to the recruitment, selection, instruction, supervision, counseling, evaluation, and advancement of residents and the maintenance of records related to program accreditation.

A. Head of Emergency Medicine

The head of emergency medicine shall:

1. Be a member of the program's core teaching faculty and meet the qualifications for faculty specified in paragraph III.D.2.
2. Be an experienced administrator in emergency medicine.

B. Program Director

There must be a single program director responsible for the program. The program director must function within a sound administrative organizational framework and have an effective teaching staff as essential elements of an approved residency program. Frequent changes in leadership or long periods of temporary leadership may adversely affect the accreditation status of the program. The program director shall:

1. Be licensed to practice medicine in the state where the institution that sponsors the program is located. (Certain federal programs are exempted.)
2. Be qualified and have at least 3 years' experience as a clinician, administrator, and educator in emergency medicine.
3. Be certified in emergency medicine by the American Board of Emergency Medicine or have equivalent qualifications in emergency medicine.
4. Be full time in emergency medicine, clinically active, and devote sufficient time and effort to the program to provide day-to-day continuity of leadership and to fulfill all of the responsibilities inherent in meeting the educational goals of the program.
5. Have an appointment in good standing, including clinical privileges, and work clinical shifts at the primary clinical site. He or she should be based at the primary clinical site.
6. Demonstrate active involvement in:
   a. Continuing emergency medical education
   b. State, regional, or national scientific societies
   c. Presentations and publication and other scholarly activities
7. Have at least 50% of his or her time protected from clinical service.
8. Have appropriate authority to oversee and to organize the activities of the educational program, including but not limited to:
   a. Resident appointments and assignments
   b. Supervision, direction, and administration of the educational activities

c. Evaluation of the residents, faculty, and the residency program.

C. Responsibilities of the Program Director

1. Preparation of a written statement outlining the educational goals of the program with respect to knowledge, skills, and other attributes of residents at each level of training and for each major rotation or other program assignment. This statement must be distributed to residents and members of the teaching staff. It should be readily available for review.
2. Selection of residents for appointment to the program in accordance with institutional and departmental policies and procedures.
3. Selection and supervision of the teaching staff and other program personnel at each institution participating in the program.
4. The supervision of residents through explicit written descriptions of supervisory lines of responsibility for the care of patients. Such guidelines must be communicated to all members of the program staff. Residents must be provided with prompt, reliable systems for communication and interaction with supervisory physicians.
5. Regular evaluation of residents' knowledge, skills, and overall performance, including the development of professional attitudes consistent with being a physician.
6. The provision of a written final evaluation for each resident who completes the program. The evaluation must include a review of the resident's performance during the final period of training and should verify that the resident has demonstrated sufficient professional ability to practice competently and independently. This final evaluation should be part of the resident's permanent record maintained by the institution.
7. Implementation of fair procedures, as established by the sponsoring institution, regarding academic discipline and resident complaints or grievances.
8. Monitoring resident stress, including mental or emotional conditions inhibiting performance or learning and drug- or alcohol-related dysfunction. Program directors and teaching staff should be sensitive to the need for timely provision of confidential counseling and psychological support services to residents. Training situations that consistently produce undesirable stress on residents must be evaluated and modified.
9. Preparation of an accurate statistical and narrative description of the program as requested by the RRC for Emergency Medicine.

D. Teaching Staff

1. There must be a sufficient number of teaching staff with documented qualifications to instruct and supervise adequately all the residents in the program. Members of the teaching staff must be able to devote sufficient time to meet their supervisory and teaching responsibilities.
2. All members of the teaching staff must demonstrate a strong interest in the education of residents, sound clinical and teaching abilities, support of the goals and objectives of the program, a commitment to their own continuing medical education, and participation in scholarly activities. A core physician faculty member is one who provides clinical service and teaching, devotes the majority of his or her professional efforts to the program, and has sufficient time protected from direct service responsibilities to meet the educational requirements of the program.
   a. To ensure a sufficient number of faculty to provide adequate on-line 24-hour emergency department attending staff supervision and participation in ongoing scholarly activity and research in support of the emergency medicine residents, there must be a minimum of one core physician faculty member for every three residents in the program. When the total resident complement exceeds 30, the faculty-resident ratio of one core faculty member for every three residents may be altered with appropriate educational justification.
   b. The faculty must be certified by the American Board of Emergency Medicine or have equivalent qualifications in emergency medicine. [*Note:* Board-prepared emergency physicians actively pursuing certification are considered as qualified under this requirement.]
   c. A significant number of such faculty should be residency trained in emergency medicine.
   d. The faculty should show evidence of participation in a spectrum of professional activities within the institution as well as within local, state, regional, and national associations.
   e. While not all members of a faculty need be researchers, some core physician faculty members should be engaged in research and should have protected time and adequate support services to accomplish these tasks.
   f. The core faculty should be involved in continuing scholarly activity such as publications in peer review journals, textbooks, local publications, formal lectures, and visiting professorships. Documentation of this involvement will be required and verified at the time of each periodic program review.
   g. Emergency medicine faculty members at the major clinical sites who average more than 15 hours per week in the administration and teaching (both clinical and didactic) of emergency medicine residents should have specific responsibilities defined in writing for the teaching and supervision of residents as well as for any designated administrative tasks.
3. A member of the teaching staff of each participating institution must be designated to assume responsibility for the day-to-day activities of the program at that institution, with overall coordination by the program director.
4. The teaching staff must be organized and have regular documented meetings to review program goals and objectives as well as program effectiveness in achieving them. At least one resident representative should participate in these reviews.
5. The teaching staff should periodically evaluate the utilization of the resources available to the program, the contribution of each institution participating in the program, the financial and administrative support for the program, the volume and variety of patients available to the program for educational purposes, the performance of members of the teaching staff, and the quality of supervision of residents.
6. Other individuals hired as attending staff to provide clinical care and/or resident supervision in the emergency department must meet the qualifications specified in paragraph III.D.2.b.

E. Core Faculty Development

Each program should encourage the academic growth of its faculty. Faculty development opportunities should be made available to each faculty member. A written plan for each member of the core faculty should be prepared in consultation with the faculty member for whom the plan is being developed.

F. Other Program Personnel

Programs must be provided with the additional professional, technical, and clerical personnel needed to support the administration and educational conduct of the program. Clinical support services must be provided on a 24-hour basis. The services must be adequate to meet reasonable and expected demands and must include the following services: nursing, clerical, intravenous, EKG, respiratory therapy, messenger/transporter, and phlebotomy.

IV. Educational Program

The director and teaching staff of a program must prepare and comply with written educational goals for the program. All educational components of a residency program should be related to program goals. The program design and/or structure must be approved by the RRC for Emergency Medicine as part of the regular review process.

A. Organization and Structure

1. Patient Population
   a. There must be an adequate number of patients of all ages and both sexes, with a wide variety of clinical problems to provide a patient population sufficient to meet the educational needs of emergency medicine residents and other residents who are assigned for training in emergency medicine. Except under unusual circumstances, the primary clinical site should have at least 30,000 emergency department visits annually.
   b. Pediatric experience should be at least 16% of all resident emergency department encounters or 4 months of full-time-equivalent experience dedicated to the care of infants and children. The program can balance a deficit of patients by offering dedicated rotations in the care of infants and children. The formula for achieving this balance: a 1-month rotation equals 4% of patients. Although this experience should include the critical care of infants and children, at least 50% of the 4 months should be in an emergency setting.
   c. The number of critically ill or critically injured patients treated in aggregate by the residents at the primary clinical site should be significant, constituting at least 3% or 1,200 of the emergency department patients per year (whichever is greater) who are admitted to monitored care settings, operative care, or the morgue following treatment in the emergency department. Additional critical care experience is required during off-service rotations.
   d. There shall be a policy to provide personal and consultant physicians access to the emergency department for patient care. This policy must be consistent with those for physician access to other special care areas.
2. Supervision
   a. All residents within the emergency department must be under the supervision of emergency medicine faculty in the emergency department at all times, except when residents from other services provide supervised care to patients on their service. In such circumstances, they must be supervised by emergency medicine faculty or by faculty from their services. Sufficient faculty must be present to provide supervision appropriate to the care of each patient.
   b. All residents assigned to the emergency department must have supervision commensurate with their level of training.
   c. The presence of residents from other specialties must allow sufficient opportunities for senior responsibility by emergency medicine residents.
   d. The program director should ensure that all emergency medicine residents, while on rotation on other services, are appropriately supervised and are provided with an educational experience equivalent to that of an ACGME-approved residency in that specialty.
3. Progressive Responsibility
   The program director must ensure that the degree of professional responsibility accorded to a resident is progressively increased through the course of training commensurate with skill and experience. Included should be opportunities to develop clinical and administrative judgment in the areas of patient care, teaching, administration, and leadership.
4. Number of Residents
   a. There should be a minimum of six residents per year of training to achieve a major impact in the emergency department, to ensure meaningful attendance at emergency medicine conferences, to provide for progressive responsibility, and to foster a sense of residency program and departmental identity. Exceptions to these standards will require justification based on sound educational principles and must demonstrate substantial compliance with the intent of this requirement.
   b. The program should request a number or range (minimum-maximum) of emergency medicine residents per year. The RRC will approve a range (minimum-maximum) or number of residents per year based on the educational resources of the program. [*Note:* In calculating the appropriate number and range of residents needed, the RRC will use, among other factors, the following guideline: an average of 1,500 emergency department encounters per year per emergency medicine resident.]
5. Presence of Other Residencies and Other Educational Resources
   The sponsoring institution for emergency medicine education must have a major educational commitment, as evidenced by training programs in other major specialties. The program must demonstrate the availability of other residencies or educational resources for the education of emergency medicine residents in anesthesiology, dermatology, medicine, neurology, obstetrics-gynecology, ophthalmology, orthopedics, otolaryngology, pediatrics, plastic surgery, psychiatry, radiology (including diagnostic imaging), and surgery. A lack of such resources will adversely affect the accreditation status of the program.
6. Fellowships
   Programs must notify the RRC if they sponsor any emergency medicine-related fellowships within institutions participating in the program. Documentation must be provided describing the fellowship's relationship to and impact on the residency.
   a. The appointment of other individuals, such as fellows, for special training or education must not dilute or detract from the educational opportunities of regularly appointed emergency medicine residents.
   b. Addition or integration of such individuals into an existing residency program requires a clear statement of the areas of education, clinical responsibilities, duration of training, and overall impact on the educational needs of existing emergency medicine residents.
7. Duty Hours
   a. Emergency medicine rotations
      1. As a minimum, residents shall be allowed 1 full day in 7 days away from the institution and free of any clinical or academic responsibilities.
      2. While on duty in the emergency department, residents may not work longer than 12 continuous scheduled hours. There must be at least an equivalent period of continuous time off between scheduled work periods.
      3. A resident should not work more than 60 scheduled hours per week seeing patients in the emergency department and no more than 72 duty hours per week. Duty hours comprise all assigned clinical duty time and conferences, whether spent within or outside the educational program, including all on-call hours.
   b. Other rotations
      The program director must ensure that all residents have appropriate duty hours when rotating on other clinical services, in accordance with the ACGME-approved program requirements of that specialty.
   c. Extracurricular activities
      Activities that fall outside the educational program may not be mandated, nor may they interfere with the resident's performance in the educational process as defined in the agreement between the institution and the resident.

B. Curriculum

1. The program director must provide each resident and member of the faculty in writing and in advance of the experience a comprehensive curriculum (covering the material listed in IV.B.5 and IV.B.6) specific to the educational needs of the emergency medicine resident. It shall be readily available for review. The curriculum shall include:
   a. The educational objectives for each rotation or other program assignment.
   b. Methods of implementation, including specific educational experiences used to meet each objective.
   c. Evaluation processes that are linked to the accomplishment of objectives.
   d. Feedback mechanisms.
2. Planned Educational Experiences
   Each program must offer to its residents an average of at least 5 hours per week of planned educational experiences (not including change-of-shift report) developed by the emergency medicine residency program. These educational experiences should include presentations based on the defined curriculum, morbidity and mortality conferences, journal review, administrative seminars, and research methods. They may include, but are not limited to, problem-based learning, laboratories, and computer-based instruction, as well as joint conferences cosponsored with other disciplines.
3. Emergency medicine faculty must attend and meaningfully participate in these planned educational experiences.
4. The program should ensure that residents are relieved of clinical duties to attend these planned educational experiences. Although release from some off-service rotations may not be possible, the program should require each resident to participate in at least 70% of the planned emergency medicine educational experiences offered (excluding vacations). [*Note:* Seventy percent refers to the minimum number of conferences required per week.]
   Attendance should be monitored and documented.
5. The educational program must cover:
   a. Principles of emergency care
   b. Principles of injury control and disease prevention
   c. Administrative aspects of emergency medicine
   d. Emergency medical services
   e. Physician interpersonal skills
   f. Physician wellness
   g. Medical ethics and jurisprudence
   h. Critical analysis of medical literature
6. The curriculum must also include didactic and clinical education for acute and emergency care in the following areas:
   a. Abdominal and gastrointestinal disorders
   b. Cardiovascular disorders
   c. Cutaneous disorders
   d. Endocrine, metabolic, and nutritional disorders
   e. Environmental disorders
   f. Head and neck disorders
   g. Hematologic disorders
   h. Immune system disorders
   i. Systemic infectious disorders
   j. Musculoskeletal disorders (nontraumatic)
   k. Nervous system disorders
   l. Obstetrics
   m. Pediatric disorders
   n. Psychiatric and behavioral disorders
   o. Renal disorders
   p. Thoracic-respiratory disorders
   q. Toxicology and clinical pharmacology
   r. Traumatic disorders
   s. Urogenital/gynecologic disorders
   t. Administrative aspects of emergency medicine
   u. Emergency medical services
   v. Presentations/symptoms
   w. Procedures/skills
7. The curriculum must include at least 2 months of inpatient critical care rotations, during which the residents should have decision-making experience that allows them to develop the skills and judgment necessary to manage critically ill and injured patients who present to the emergency department.
8. The program must develop a system that provides and documents efforts to teach residents the importance of patient follow-up. This should involve a representative sample of patients who are admitted to the hospital and who are discharged from the emergency department. Acceptable methods include but are not limited to the following:
   a. Written documentation of individual resident efforts (ward/ICU visits, telephone calls, and chart review)
   b. Timely provision of patient discharge summaries, operative reports, autopsy summaries, and/or consultation notes
   c. Regular case conferences (other than morbidity and mortality conference) that cover a representative sample of patient follow-ups
9. At least 50% of the training beyond the first year must take place in the emergency department. Excessive clinical time in the emergency department should not preclude adequate experience in off-service areas needed to cover the curriculum.
10. Of the total educational experience, no less than 50% should take place under the supervision of emergency medicine faculty. Such experiences can include emergency medical services, toxicology, pediatric emergency medicine, sports medicine, emergency medicine administration, and research in emergency medicine.
11. Prehospital Care
    Because prehospital care is an integral and vital part of emergency medicine, there must be a formal, structured resident experience. This should include participation in paramedic base station communications; emergency transportation and care in the field, including ground units and, if possible, air ambulance units; teaching prehospital personnel; disaster planning and drills; and quality assurance audits. If residents are required to ride on ground or in air ambulance units, they must be notified of this requirement prior to the resident selection process.
12. Resuscitations
    Each resident must have sufficient opportunities to perform invasive procedures, monitor unstable patients, and direct major resuscitations of all types on all age groups. A major resuscitation is patient care for which prolonged physician attention is needed and interventions such as defibrillation, cardiac pacing, treatment of shock, intravenous use of drugs (eg, thrombolytics, vasopressors, neuromuscular blocking agents), or invasive procedures (eg, cutdowns, central line insertion, tube thoracostomy, endotracheal intubation) are necessary for stabilization and treatment. The resident must have the opportunity to make admission recommendations and direct resuscitations.
    a. Programs must maintain a record of all major resuscitations and procedures performed by each resident. The record must document their role, ie, participant or director; the type of procedure(s); the location (ED, ICU, etc); age of patient; and admission diagnosis. Only one resident may be credited with the direction of each resuscitation and the performance of each procedure.

b. These records should be verified by the residency director and should be the basis for documenting the total number of resuscitations and procedures in the program. They should be available for review by the site visitor and the RRC.

13. Continuous Quality Improvement
Residents must actively participate in emergency department continuous quality improvement programs. There must be formal regular conferences such as mortality and morbidity conferences in which the care rendered to patients in the emergency department is critically reviewed. Efforts should be made to gain permission for postmortem examinations and to review the results of these examinations.

14. Research and Scholarly Activity
Graduate medical education must take place in an environment of inquiry and scholarship in which residents participate in the development of new knowledge, learn to evaluate research findings, and develop habits of inquiry as a continuing professional responsibility. The responsibility for establishing and maintaining an environment of inquiry and scholarship rests with the teaching staff. The staff as a whole must demonstrate broad involvement in scholarly activity. This activity should include:
a. Active participation in clinical discussions, rounds, and conferences in a manner that promotes a spirit of inquiry and scholarship. Scholarship implies an in-depth understanding of basic mechanisms of normal and abnormal states and the application of current knowledge to practice.
b. Participation in journal clubs and research conferences.
c. Active participation in regional or national professional and scientific societies, particularly through presentations at the organizations' meetings and publication in their journals.
d. Participation in research, particularly in projects that are funded following peer review and/or result in publication or presentations at regional and national scientific meetings.
e. Offering of guidance and technical support (eg, research design, statistical analysis) for residents involved in research.
f. Provision of support for resident participation in scholarly activities. The curriculum should include resident experience in scholarly activity prior to completion of the program. Some examples of suitable resident scholarly activities are the preparation of a scholarly paper such as a collective review or case report, active participation in a research project, or formulation and implementation of an original research project.
g. Residents must be taught an understanding of basic research methodologies, statistical analysis, and critical analysis of current medical literature.

15. Physician Wellness
Physical and mental well-being are critical to the emergency physician's ability to provide proper care in a stressful environment. Emergency medicine residencies should include educational programs concerning physician wellness, stress, circadian rhythms, and substance abuse.

V. Evaluation

There must be effective, ongoing evaluation of all components of the residency program. This evaluation process must relate to the educational objectives of the program and provide a mechanism to effect change.

A. Evaluation of Residents

1. At least semiannually, there must be an evaluation of the knowledge, skills, and professional growth in emergency medicine of each resident, using appropriate criteria and procedures. Documentation of management of patients with emergency conditions, to include major trauma, medical and pediatric resuscitations, and performance of emergency procedures by each resident in the program, must be kept and reviewed periodically by the program director.
2. Formal evaluation of each resident during training is required and must include oral and written examinations. In addition, there must be a mechanism for formal evaluation of the resident on each rotation. A summary of the evaluations must be communicated in writing to and should be signed by the resident. Discussions of these results between the resident and the program director or his or her designee must be held on at least a semiannual basis.
3. Residents may be advanced to positions of higher responsibility only on the basis of evidence of their satisfactory progressive scholarship and professional growth.
4. A plan to remedy deficiencies must be in writing and on file, and progress and improvement must be monitored at least every 3 months.
5. A permanent record of evaluation for each resident must be maintained and must be accessible to the resident and other authorized personnel.
6. A written final evaluation must be provided for each resident who completes the program. The evaluation must include a review of the resident's performance during the final period of training and should verify that the resident has demonstrated sufficient professional ability to practice competently and independently. This final evaluation should be part of the resident's permanent record maintained by the institution.

B. Evaluation of Faculty

1. At least annually, individual faculty members must be formally evaluated by the head of emergency medicine, who should include information from the program director and the emergency medicine residents. A mechanism for preserving resident confidentiality in the evaluation process shall be implemented.
2. Faculty evaluations should include documentation of teaching ability, clinical knowledge, administrative and interpersonal skills, and scholarly contributions. A summary of the evaluations should be communicated in writing to each faculty member.

C. Evaluation of the Program

1. At least annually, the educational effectiveness of the entire program, including the quality of the curriculum and the clinical rotations, must be evaluated by residents and faculty in a systematic manner. The extent to which the educational goals have been met by residents must be assessed. Written evaluations by residents should be used in this process. The results of these evaluations must be kept on file.
2. The RRC may take into consideration information provided by the American Board of Emergency Medicine regarding performance of the program's graduates on the certifying examinations over a period of several years.

VI. Other

A. Notice of Changes in the Program

1. The program leadership is responsible for notifying the Executive Secretary of the RRC within 30 days, in writing, of any major changes in the program that may significantly alter the educational experience for the residents, including:
a. Leadership of the department or the program;
b. Administrative structure such as an alteration in the hierarchical status of the program/department within the institution;
c. A drop in the faculty complement below the required minimum number or if one-third or more of the faculty leave within 1 year;
d. A drop below the minimum approved number of residents in the program for 2 consecutive years.

Should the RRC determine that a significant alteration of the educational resources has occurred, an immediate review of the program may be performed.

2. The program director must obtain prior approval for the following changes in the program in order for the RRC to determine if an adequate educational environment exists to support these changes:
   a. The addition or deletion of any participating institution to which a resident will rotate for 4 months or longer;
   b. The addition or deletion of any rotation of 4 months or longer;
   c. Any change in the approved resident complement of the program (Prior approval is not required for temporary changes in resident numbers due to makeup or remedial time for currently enrolled residents or to fill vacancies at the same level of education in which the vacancy occurs.);
   d. Any change in the length or educational format of the program.

   On review of a proposal for a major change in a program, the RRC may determine that a site visit is necessary.

B. Combined Programs

The RRC will review combined education program proposals only after the review and approval of the American Board of Emergency Medicine. Review by the RRC will consider only whether the residency has sufficient resources to support combined education without diluting the experience of the regularly appointed residents. The RRC does not accredit the combined education program. The proposal must be submitted to the RRC prior to the implementation of required education.

C. Certification

Residents who plan to seek certification by the American Board of Emergency Medicine should communicate with the secretary of that board for information regarding the requirements for certification.

ACGME: June 1994 Effective: July 1995

Program Requirements for Residency Education in the Subspecialties of Emergency Medicine

The following requirements pertain to programs in the subspecialties of emergency medicine. Each program must comply with the requirements listed below as well as with the specialty content found in the program requirements for the respective area.

These programs must exist in conjunction with and be an integrated part of an Accreditation Council for Graduate Medical Education (ACGME)-accredited emergency medicine residency program. Their existence should not compromise the integrity of the core program.

Residents appointed to the sports medicine programs should have completed an ACGME-accredited residency in emergency medicine, family practice, internal medicine, or pediatrics. [*Note:* Those lacking board certification in one of these areas will not be considered eligible for a Certificate of Added Qualifications from any of the corresponding specialty boards.]

I. Program Goals and Objectives

The director and teaching staff of a program must prepare and comply with written educational goals for the program.

A. Program Design

All educational components of a residency program should be related to program goals.

1. The program design and/or structure must be approved by the Residency Review Committee (RRC) for Emergency Medicine as part of the regular review process.
2. Participation by any institution providing more than 3 months of training in a program must be approved by the RRC.

B. Program Evaluation

The educational effectiveness of a program must be evaluated in a systematic manner. In particular, the quality of the curriculum and the extent to which the educational goals have been met by residents must be assessed. Written evaluations by residents should be utilized in this process.

II. Program Personnel

The program director and the teaching staff are responsible for the general administration of a program, including those activities related to the recruitment, selection, instruction, supervision, counseling, evaluation, and advancement of residents and the maintenance of records related to program accreditation.

A. Program Director

There must be a single program director responsible for the program.

1. Qualifications of the program director include:
   a. Requisite and documented clinical, educational, and administrative abilities and experience.
   b. Licensure to practice medicine in the state where the institution that sponsors the program is located. (Certain federal programs are exempted.)
   c. Certification by one of the following boards: American Board of Emergency Medicine, American Board of Family Practice, American Board of Internal Medicine, or American Board of Pediatrics, and possess a Certificate of Added Qualifications in Sports Medicine from that same board. The RRC will determine the adequacy of alternate qualifications.
   d. Appointment in good standing to the medical staff of an institution participating in the program.
2. Responsibilities of the program director include:
   a. Preparation of a written statement outlining the educational goals of the program with respect to knowledge, skills, and other attributes of residents at each level of training and for each major rotation or other program assignment. This statement must be distributed to residents and members of the teaching staff. It should be readily available for review.
   b. Selection of residents for appointment to the program in accordance with institutional and departmental policies and procedures.
   c. Selection and supervision of the teaching staff and other program personnel at each institution participating in the program.
   d. The supervision of residents through explicit written descriptions of supervisory lines of responsibility for the care of patients. Such guidelines must be communicated to all members of the program staff. Residents must be provided with prompt, reliable systems for communication and interaction with supervisory physicians.
   e. Regular evaluation of residents' knowledge, skills, and overall performance, including the development of professional attitudes consistent with being a physician.

      The program director, with participation of members of the teaching staff, shall:

1. At least semiannually evaluate the knowledge, skills, and professional growth of the residents, using appropriate criteria and procedures.
2. Communicate each evaluation to the resident in a timely manner.
3. Advance residents to positions of higher responsibility only on the basis of evidence of their satisfactory progressive scholarship and professional growth.
4. Maintain a permanent record of evaluation for each resident and have it accessible to the resident and other authorized personnel.

f. The provision of a written final evaluation for each resident who completes the program. The evaluation must include a review of the resident's performance during the final period of training and should verify that the resident has demonstrated sufficient professional ability to practice competently and independently. This final evaluation should be part of the resident's permanent record maintained by the institution.

g. Implementation of fair procedures as established by the sponsoring institution regarding academic discipline and resident complaints or grievances.

h. Monitoring resident stress, including mental or emotional conditions inhibiting performance or learning, and drug- or alcohol-related dysfunction. Program directors and teaching staff should be sensitive to the need for timely provision of confidential counseling and psychological support services to residents. Training situations that consistently produce undesirable stress on residents must be evaluated and modified.

i. Preparation of an accurate statistical and narrative description of the program as requested by a review committee.

B. Teaching Staff

1. There must be a sufficient number of teaching staff with documented qualifications to instruct and supervise adequately all the residents in the program. Members of the teaching staff must be able to devote sufficient time to meet their supervisory and teaching responsibilities.
2. All members of the teaching staff must demonstrate a strong interest in the education of residents, sound clinical and teaching abilities, support of the goals and objectives of the program, a commitment to their own continuing medical education, and participation in scholarly activities.
3. A member of the teaching staff of each participating institution must be designated to assume responsibility for the day-to-day activities of the program at that institution, with overall coordination by the program director.
4. The teaching staff must be organized and have regular documented meetings to review program goals and objectives as well as program effectiveness in achieving them. At least one resident representative should participate in these reviews.
5. The teaching staff should periodically evaluate the utilization of the resources available to the program, the contribution of each institution participating in the program, the financial and administrative support of the program, the volume and variety of patients available to the program for educational purposes, the performance of members of the teaching staff, and the quality of supervision of residents.

C. Other Program Personnel

Programs must be provided with the additional professional, technical, and clerical personnel needed to support the administration and educational conduct of the program.

III. Program Research and Scholarly Activity

Graduate medical education must take place in an environment of inquiry and scholarship in which residents participate in the development of new knowledge, learn to evaluate research findings, and develop habits of inquiry as a continuing professional responsibility.

A. Scholarly Activity

The responsibility for establishing and maintaining an environment of inquiry and scholarship rests with the teaching staff. While not all members of a teaching staff must be investigators, the staff as a whole must demonstrate broad involvement in scholarly activity. This activity should include:

1. Active participation of the teaching staff in clinical discussions, rounds, and conferences in a manner that promotes a spirit of inquiry and scholarship. Scholarship implies an in-depth understanding of basic mechanisms of normal and abnormal states and the application of current knowledge to practice.
2. Participation in journal clubs and research conferences.
3. Active participation in regional or national professional and scientific societies, particularly through presentations at the organizations' meetings and publication in their journals.
4. Participation in research, particularly in projects that are funded following peer review and/or result in publication or presentations at regional and national scientific meetings.
5. Offering of guidance and technical support (eg, research design, statistical analysis) for residents involved in research.
6. Provision of support for resident participation in scholarly activities.

B. Library

1. Residents must have ready access to a major medical library either at the institution where the residents are located or through arrangement with convenient nearby institutions.
2. Library services should include the electronic retrieval of information from medical databases.
3. There must be access to an on-site library or to a collection of appropriate texts and journals in each institution participating in a residency program. On-site libraries and/or collections of texts and journals must be readily available during nights and weekends.

ACGME: September 1994 Effective: September 1994

Program Requirements for Residency Education in Pediatric Emergency Medicine (Emergency Medicine)

In addition to complying with the Program Requirements for Residency Education in the Subspecialties of Pediatrics or Emergency Medicine, programs in pediatric emergency medicine must comply with the following requirements.

I. Introduction

The goal of a residency program in pediatric emergency medicine is to produce physicians who are clinically proficient in the practice of pediatric emergency medicine, especially in the management of the acutely ill or injured child, in the setting of an emergency department that is approved as a 911 receiving facility or its equivalent and has an emergency medical services system.

A program in pediatric emergency medicine must be administered by, and be an integral part of, an ACGME-accredited program in either emergency medicine or pediatrics and must be associated with an ACGME-accredited residency program in the corresponding discipline.

There must be written agreements between the director of the program in pediatric emergency medicine and the directors of the participating residencies in pediatrics and emergency medicine specifying the experiences that will compose this subspecialty program. These agreements should address appropriate curriculum content, supervision of the resident, amount and distribution of clinical and nonclinical time, conferences, clinical performance criteria, and mechanisms for resolving performance problems.

Prerequisite training should include satisfactory completion of an ACGME-accredited residency program in either emergency medicine or pediatrics.

II. Duration and Scope of Training

A training period of 2 years is required for all subspecialty residents. [Note: For those planning to seek certification from the American Board of Pediatrics, 3 years of training is required.] [Note: If a third year is offered, it must be described when the program is reviewed by the Residency Review Committee. Those planning to seek certification should consult with the appropriate certifying board regarding the criteria for eligibility, including duration of training.]

The educational program must be organized and conducted in a way that ensures an appropriate environment for the well-being and care of the patients and their families while providing residents the opportunity to become skilled clinicians, competent teachers, and knowledgeable investigators. The program must emphasize the fundamentals of assessment, diagnosis, and management. Residents also should be exposed to the academic debate, intensive research review, and the interaction between and among the specialties of pediatrics and emergency medicine.

III. Curriculum

The residents in pediatric emergency medicine must participate in the care of pediatric patients of all ages, from infancy through young adulthood, with a broad spectrum of illnesses and injuries of all severities. At least 12 months of the clinical experience must be obtained seeing children in an emergency department where children, ages 21 years of age or less, are treated for the full spectrum of illnesses and injuries. To provide adequate exposure for selected problems, additional experience with anesthesiologists, intensivists, neurologists, psychiatrists, pre-hospital care providers, orthopedists, surgeons, toxicologists, traumatologists who have training and experience in the care of children and adolescents, and other specialists must be available.

Specialty-specific content must include at least 4 months of training in the reciprocal specialty from which the resident enters the training program. Additional elective months of reciprocal training should be scheduled when deemed appropriate by the program director on the basis of the background of the resident and his/her progress in acquiring the essential skills of a pediatric emergency specialist.

For the emergency medicine graduate, the reciprocal time must include time spent in pediatric subspecialty and ambulatory clinics, inpatient management, neonatal management, and pediatric critical care in an ACGME-accredited residency program in pediatrics.

For the pediatric graduate, this must include 4 months in an adult emergency department that is part of an ACGME-accredited residency program in emergency medicine. One month of that experience may occur off site as approved by the ACGME-accredited program in emergency medicine, in EMS, adult trauma, or toxicology.

Additional experiences may be necessary for residents from both core specialties. For example, adolescents have unique aspects of disease and injury. Experience with blunt and penetrating trauma, and with significant gynecologic and obstetrical emergencies, as well as psychiatric emergencies of the adolescent, must be a part of a resident's training if previous experience in these areas was not adequate. These experiences should be in settings best suited for the resident's training.

The core content must include training in EMS, administration, ethics, legal issues, and procedures. It must also include but not be limited to structured opportunities to develop special competence in such areas as cardiopulmonary resuscitation; trauma; disaster and environmental medicine; transport; triage; sedation; monitoring (biomedical instrumentation); emergencies arising from toxicologic, obstetric, gynecologic, allergic/immunologic, cardiovascular, congenital, dermatologic, dental, endocrine/metabolic, gastrointestinal, hematologic/oncologic, infectious, musculoskeletal, neurologic, ophthalmic, psychosocial, and pulmonary causes; renal/genitourinary and surgical disorders; and physical and sexual abuse.

In addition to achieving an understanding of the pathophysiology, epidemiology, and management of these problems, the resident must learn how to evaluate the patient with an undifferentiated chief complaint such as abdominal pain. The resident must be taught to arrive at a diagnosis, whether it falls in areas traditionally designated medical or surgical, eg, appendicitis, ectopic pregnancy, intussusception, sickle cell anemia; to perform the evaluation rapidly in accordance with any pathophysiologic disturbances in the patient; and to proceed with an appropriate life-saving therapy, such as endotracheal intubation or thoracostomy or administration of antibiotics, before arriving at a definitive diagnosis.

The resident must learn the skills necessary to prioritize and manage the emergency care of multiple patients. Finally, the resident must have supervised experience in a range of technical/procedural skills, as they apply to pediatric patients of all ages.

The resident must be given increasing responsibilities for patient care as she or he progresses through the program. In the final year of training, the resident must be given the opportunities to demonstrate the skills appropriate to a supervisor, teacher, and a decision maker in pediatric emergencies.

There must be an emphasis on developing a compassionate understanding of the stress associated with sudden illness, injury, and death so that the resident may be responsive to the emotional needs of the patients, their families, and the staff of the emergency department. Discussion and appreciation of the many ethical issues involved in pediatric emergency medicine should be part of the educational program.

Residents should be exposed to formal sessions on organizing teaching programs, medical writing, and oral presentation. Residents should have the opportunity to develop teaching skills by conducting lectures, seminars, and clinical conferences and by preparing written reports and teaching materials. These efforts must be reviewed and evaluated by the supervising faculty in light of competency-based objectives developed by the program. The resident must receive instruction and experience in the administrative and management skills necessary to oversee a division or department.

IV. Conferences

There should be opportunities to participate in regularly scheduled, multidisciplinary conferences that include lectures, morbidity and mortality conferences, case conferences, general reviews, and research seminars. The program must include instruction in or other educational exposure to related basic sciences, including physiology, growth and development, pathophysiology, and epidemiology, and prevention of pediatric illnesses and injuries.

The program also should provide education on physician wellness and stress management.

V. Teaching Staff

There must be at least four members of the teaching staff who have experience and knowledge of the care of acute pediatric illness and injuries to provide adequate supervision of residents and to ensure the educational and research quality of the program. Two of the faculty must be certified in pediatric emergency medicine or have equivalent qualifications. For a subspecialty program that functions as an integral part of a pediatric residency program, there must be adequate exposure to faculty who are certified by the American Board of Emergency Medicine. Conversely, for a subspecialty program based in an emergency medicine residency program, there must be adequate exposure to faculty certified by the American Board of Pediatrics.

The availability of consultant and collaborative faculty in related medical and surgical disciplines, as referred to in Section III, must be ensured.

The pediatric emergency medicine faculty must have an active role in curriculum development and in the supervision and evaluation of the subspecialty residents.

VI. Patient Population

A sufficient number of patients must be available to provide adequate opportunity for subspecialty residents to acquire competence in the management of the full spectrum of acutely ill and injured children, adolescents, and young adults. The subspecialty residents must provide the initial evaluation of and treatment to all types of patients.

To meet the educational objectives of the program and to provide both the pediatric and subspecialty residents with an adequate experience to acquire competence in clinical management, there should be a minimum of 15,000 pediatric patient visits per year in the primary emergency department that is used for the program. Patient acuity and the total number of trainees will be considered in assessing the adequacy of the patient population. These must include a sufficient number of patients with major and minor trauma, airway insufficiency, ingestions, obstetric and gynecologic disorders, psychosocial disturbances, and emergent problems from all pediatric medical and surgical subspecialties.

Subspecialty residents should not serve as the only care givers for children seen in the emergency department. They should provide supervision and consultation to other residents who are assigned to the emergency department and will be caring for patients. These subspecialty residents must, however, have the opportunity to manage multiple patients at the same time, to learn the skills necessary to prioritize the evaluation and treatment of these patients. In addition, the program must provide the pediatric emergency medicine residents the opportunity to assume leadership responsibility for the pediatric emergency department.

VII. Facilities

There must be an acute care facility that receives patients via ambulance from the prehospital setting, is equipped to handle trauma, and that has a full range of services associated with residencies in pediatrics and emergency medicine. This facility should be accredited by the Joint Commission on Accreditation of Healthcare Organizations.

The emergency department must be adequately staffed, have appropriate bedside monitoring capability, and be capable of resuscitating medical and trauma patients. Facilities and equipment must meet the generally accepted standards of a modern emergency department and be available within the institution on a 24-hour-a-day basis.

The institution should have comprehensive radiologic and laboratory support systems and readily available operative suites and intensive care unit beds.

VIII. Board Certification

Residents seeking certification in the subspecialty of pediatric emergency medicine should consult their primary specialty board, ie, the American Board of Pediatrics or the American Board of Emergency Medicine, regarding the criteria for eligibility for certification in this subspecialty.

ACGME: June 1998 Effective: June 1998

Program Requirements for Residency Education in Medical Toxicology (Emergency Medicine)

I. Introduction

A. Definition and Description of the Subspecialty

1. Medical toxicology is a clinical specialty that includes the monitoring, prevention, evaluation and treatment of injury and illness due to occupational and environmental exposures, pharmaceutical agents, as well as unintentional and intentional poisoning in all age groups. A medical toxicology residency must be organized to provide residents with experience in the clinical practice of medical toxicology for all age groups and to provide a sound basis for the development of physician practitioners, educators, researchers, and administrators capable of practicing medical toxicology in academic and clinical settings.
2. Residencies in medical toxicology must teach the basic skills and knowledge that constitute the foundations of medical toxicology practice and must provide progressive responsibility for and experience in the application of these principles to the management of clinical problems. It is expected that the resident will develop a satisfactory level of clinical maturity, judgment, and technical skill that will, on completion of the program, render the resident capable of independent practice in medical toxicology.
3. Programs must provide a broad education in medical toxicology to prepare the resident to function as a specialist capable of providing comprehensive patient care.

B. Duration and Scope of Education

1. Prerequisite training for entry into a medical toxicology program should include the satisfactory completion of an ACGME-accredited residency. [Note: Candidates who do not meet this criterion should consult the American Board of Emergency Medicine, or the American Board of Preventive Medicine regarding their eligibility for subspecialty certification.]
2. The length of the educational program is 24 months. The program must be associated with an ACGME-accredited residency program in emergency medicine, or preventive medicine.
3. Prior to entry into the program, each resident must be notified in writing of the required length of the program.

II. Institutional Organization

A. Sponsoring Institution

1. The sponsoring institution must provide sufficient faculty, financial resources, and clinical, research, and library facilities to

meet the educational needs of the residents and to enable the program to comply with the requirements for accreditation. It is highly desirable that the program structure include the participation of a medical school, a school of public health, and a school of pharmacy or department of pharmacology.

2. Programs in medical toxicology should be based at a primary hospital (hereafter referred to as the primary clinical site). The majority of the didactic and clinical experiences should take place at the primary clinical site.
3. The following services must be organized and provided at the primary clinical site:
   a. An emergency service for both adult and pediatric patients, adult and pediatric inpatient facilities, and adult and pediatric intensive care facilities
   b. Renal dialysis services with 24-hour availability
   c. Toxicology laboratory services with 24-hour availability
   d. Inpatient and outpatient facilities with staff who consult the toxicology service
   e. It is desirable that hyperbaric oxygen therapy is available
4. The program must develop an institutional affiliation to provide residents with clinical experiences not provided at the primary clinical site, other than those listed in II.A.3.a-d.

B. Participating Institutions

1. All participating institutions must provide appropriate support services to ensure an adequate educational experience. This includes support personnel in all categories and physical resources to ensure that residents have sufficient time and space to carry out their clinical and educational functions.
2. The program must develop an institutional affiliation with a clinical facility to provide residents with clinical experience in critical care areas should this experience not be provided at the sponsoring institution.
   a. Approval of participating institutions will be based on the presence of sufficient opportunities for residents to manage, either as primary physicians or consultants, the entire course of critically poisoned patients in both the pediatric and adult categories.
   b. Institutional resources must be available to support the provision of clinical experience in adult and pediatric critical care areas for residents without prior experience of at least 1 month in an adult intensive care unit and 1 month in a pediatric intensive care unit.
   c. Programs using multiple participating institutions must ensure the provision of a unified educational experience for the residents. Each participating institution must offer significant educational opportunities to the overall program that do not duplicate experiences otherwise available within the program. An acceptable educational rationale must be provided for each participating institution.
   d. Participating institutions must not be geographically distant from the sponsoring institution unless special resources are provided that are not available at the primary clinical site.
   e. The number and geographic distribution of participating institutions must not preclude all residents' participation in conferences and other educational exercises.
   f. A letter of agreement with each institution participating in the program must be developed to include
      1. the educational objectives and the method to accomplish and to evaluate each objective;
      2. the resources and facilities in the institution(s) that will be available to each resident, including but not limited to library resources;
      3. the resident's duties and responsibilities and duty hours for the assignment; and
      4. the relationship that will exist between medical toxicology residents and residents and faculty in other programs.

C. Library

Residents must have ready access to a major medical library either at the institution where the residents are located or through arrangement with convenient nearby institutions. Reference material specific to the content of the subspecialty must be available in either text or electronic retrieval form.

D. Appointment of Residents

The Residency Review Committee (RRC) will approve the number of medical toxicology residents in the program. Approval will be based on the number, qualifications, and scholarly activity of the faculty; the volume and variety of the patient population available for educational purposes; and the institutional resources available to the program.

III. Faculty Qualifications and Responsibilities

A. In addition to the qualifications and responsibilities of the program director and faculty described in the Program Requirements for Residency Education in the Subspecialties of Emergency Medicine or the Program Requirements for Residency Education in Preventive Medicine, there must be a minimum of two medical toxicology faculty who each devote a minimum of 5 hours per week of direct teaching time to the residents and whose medical practice makes them available to the residents for consultations on cases.

B. The program director and faculty must be certified in medical toxicology or possess suitable equivalent qualifications as determined by the RRC.

C. Consultants from appropriate medical subspecialties including those with special expertise in disaster and mass casualty incident management, hyperbaric medicine, immunology, industrial hygiene, occupational toxicology, pulmonary medicine, biostatistics, epidemiology, public health, botany, cardiology, dermatology, gastroenterology, nephrology, ophthalmology, pathology, pharmacology, surgical subspecialty, zoology, hazardous materials and mass exposure to toxins, laboratory toxicology, forensic toxicology and environmental toxicology, and nonmedical specialties, such as botany, herpetology, and mycology should be available for consultation and academic lectures.

IV. The Educational Program

A. The director and teaching staff of a program must prepare and comply with written educational goals for the program. All educational components of a residency program should be related to program goals. The program design and/or structure must be approved by the RRC.

B. The curriculum must include the following academic and clinical content:
   1. The clinical manifestations, differential diagnosis, and management of poisoning
   2. The biochemistry of metabolic processes, the pharmacology, pharmacokinetics, and teratogenesis, toxicity, and interactions of therapeutic drugs
   3. The biochemistry of toxins, kinetics, metabolism, mechanisms of acute and chronic injury, and carcinogenesis
   4. Experimental design and statistical analysis of data as related to laboratory, clinical, and epidemiologic research
   5. Laboratory techniques in toxicology
   6. Occupational toxicology, including acute and chronic workplace exposure to intoxicants and basic concepts of the workplace and industrial hygiene

7. Prevention of poisoning, including prevention of occupational exposures by intervention methodologies, that take into account the epidemiology, environmental factors, and the role of regulation and legislation in prevention
8. Environmental toxicology, including identification of hazardous materials and the basic principles of management of large-scale environmental contamination and mass exposures
9. The function, management, and financing of poison control centers
10. Oral and written communication skills and teaching techniques
11. Principles of epidemiology and risk communication, analytical laboratory techniques, and research methodologies in toxicology

C. Clinical Experience
Residents must have a minimum of 12 months of clinical experience as the primary or consulting physician responsible for providing direct/bedside patient evaluation, management, screening, and preventive services.

Residents must be provided with experience in evaluating and managing patients with workplace and environmental exposures and must have experience in workplace evaluation, as well as in an occupational medicine or toxicology clinic.

D. Residents must have opportunities to evaluate and manage patients with acute and long-term workplace and environmental toxic exposures. Clinical training should include experience in an industrial setting or an occupational medicine clinic or access to occupational medicine patients in a referral setting. The resident should also have the opportunity to evaluate and manage intoxicated patients in both industrial and referral setting, including responsibility for providing bedside evaluation, management, screening, and preventive services for a minimum of 12 months or its full-time equivalent.

E. Regional Poison Information Center
1. The program must provide residents with educational experiences in a regional poison control center certified by the American Association of Poison Control Centers or its equivalent. It is highly desirable that the poison control center be in physical proximity to the primary clinical site.
2. Each resident must have 12 months' experience with a referral population of poisoned patients under the supervision of a physician who is certified in medical toxicology or who possesses suitable equivalent qualifications as determined by the RRC.
3. The poison control center should have at least 1,500 calls annually that require physician telephone consultation or intervention

F. Planned Educational Conferences
Each program must offer to its residents an average of at least 5 hours per week of planned educational experiences (not including change-of-shift reports). These educational experiences should include presentations based on the defined curriculum, morbidity and mortality conferences, journal review, administrative seminars, and research methods. They may include but are not limited to problem-based learning, laboratory research, and computer-based instruction, as well as joint conferences cosponsored with other disciplines.

G. Additional Educational Experiences
The program curriculum must include pharmacology, pharmacokinetics, and drug interactions. This must be accomplished by (1) an affiliation with a school of pharmacy or department of pharmacology that provides regular didactic experience and consultation to residents or (2) the presence of a Doctor of Pharmacology or PhD pharmacologist as a participating member of the teaching faculty.

H. Additional Clinical Experiences
The program should provide the opportunity for the residents to maintain their primary board skills during training, but it may not require that residents provide more than 12 hours per week of clinical practice not related to medical toxicology as a condition of the educational program.

I. Communication and Teaching Experience
Residents must have progressive experience and responsibility for the teaching of medical toxicology to health care professionals. Residents in the second year of training should participate in the teaching and supervision of first-year residents and should be responsible for regular contributions to formal didactic experiences within the training program, in other academic departments in the institution(s), and in the community. Research leading to publication should be encouraged.

V. Board Certification

Those planning to seek a subspecialty certificate from their primary board should communicate with the administrative officer of the board to ascertain the full requirements.

ACGME: June 1998 Effective: June 1998

Program Requirements for Residency Education in Sports Medicine (Emergency Medicine)

I. Introduction

In addition to complying with the requirements below, each program must comply with the Program Requirements in emergency medicine.

II. Scope and Duration of Training

An educational program in sports medicine must be organized to provide a well-supervised experience at a level sufficient for the resident to acquire the competence of a physician with added qualifications in this field. It shall be 12 months in duration.

The practice of sports medicine is the application of the physician's knowledge, skills, and attitudes to those engaged in sports and exercise. Thus, the program must provide training in the development of the clinical competencies needed to diagnose and manage medical illnesses and injuries related to sports and exercise, for example, first-degree sprains, strains, and contusions, including appropriate referrals of, for example, fractures, dislocations, and third-degree sprains. Clinical experience must include injury prevention, preparticipation evaluation, management of acute and chronic illness or injury, and rehabilitation, as applied to a broad spectrum of undifferentiated patients. There must be experience functioning as a team physician and in the promotion of physical fitness and wellness.

The program should emphasize physiology and biomechanics; principles of nutrition; pathology and pathophysiology of illness and injury; pharmacology; effects of therapeutic, performance-enhancing, and mood-altering drugs; psychological aspects of exercise, performance, and competition; ethical principles; and medical-legal aspects of exercise and sports.

III. Teaching Staff

In addition to the program director, each program must have at least one other faculty member with similar qualifications who devotes a substantial portion of professional time to the training program.

The teaching staff must include orthopedic surgeons who are engaged in the operative management of sports injuries and other conditions and who are readily available to teach and provide consultation to the residents. Teaching staff from the disciplines of nutrition, pharmacology, pathology, exercise physiology, physical therapy, behavioral science, physical medicine and rehabilitation, and clinical imaging also should be available to assist in the educational program. Coaches and athletic trainers also should be included.

IV. Facilities and Resources

The program must include the following:

A. Patient Population

A patient population that is unlimited by age or gender and is adequate in number and variety to meet the needs of the training program must be available. The program director must ensure that residents are accorded meaningful patient responsibility with the supervision of a faculty member at all facilities and sites.

B. Sports Medicine Clinic

There must be an identifiable clinic that offers continuing care to patients who seek consultation regarding sports- or exercise-related health problems. The nonsurgical trainees must be supervised by a physician who has qualifications in sports medicine and is certified by the American Board of Emergency Medicine, the American Board of Family Practice, the American Board of Internal Medicine, or the American Board of Pediatrics or who possesses suitable equivalent qualifications.

Adequate, up-to-date diagnostic imaging and rehabilitation services must be readily available and accessible to clinic patients. Consultation in medical and surgical subspecialties, physical therapy, nursing, nutrition, and pharmacy must be available. The opportunity to render continuing care and to organize recommendations from other specialties and disciplines is mandatory and will require that medical records include information pertinent to the assessment and management of patients with health problems related to sports and exercise.

C. Sporting Events/Team Sports/Mass-Participation Events

The program must have access to sporting events, team sports, and mass-participation events during which the resident can have meaningful patient responsibility.

D. Acute-Care Facility

There must be an acute-care hospital with a full range of services associated with and in proximity to the sponsoring residency. This facility must be readily accessible to patients served by the program.

V. Educational Program

The curriculum must provide the educational experiences necessary for the residents to achieve the cognitive knowledge, psychomotor skills, interpersonal skills, professional attitudes, and practical experience required of physicians in the care of patients with health problems related to sports and exercise.

Didactic as well as clinical learning opportunities must be provided as part of the required curriculum for all residents. Conferences or seminars/workshops in sports medicine should be specifically designed for the residents to augment the clinical experiences.

All educational activities must be adequately supervised, while allowing the resident to assume progressive responsibility for patient care. The clinical activities in sports medicine should represent a minimum of 50% of the time in the program. The remainder of the time should be spent in didactic, teaching, and/or research activities and in the primary care or emergency medicine ambulatory facility.

Residents must spend ½ day per week maintaining their skills in their primary specialty.

Participation in the following must be required of all residents:

A. Preparticipation Evaluation of the Athlete

The program must ensure that all sports medicine residents are involved in the development and conduct of preparticipation examination programs.

B. Acute Care

The resident must have appropriate authority and responsibility to participate meaningfully in the medical care that is provided to acute-care patients (see "Scope and Duration of Training," above). In addition, the program should arrange for residents to observe representative inpatient and outpatient operative orthopedic procedures.

C. Sports Medicine Clinic Experience

The resident must attend patients in a continuing, comprehensive manner, providing consultation for health problems related to sports and exercise. The resident shall spend at least 1 day per week for 10 months of the training period in this activity.

If patients are hospitalized, the resident should follow them during their inpatient stay and resume outpatient care following the hospitalization. Consultation with other physicians and professionals in other disciplines should be encouraged.

D. On-Site Sports Care

The resident should participate in planning and implementation of all aspects of medical care at various sporting events. The program must ensure that supervised sports medicine residents provide on-site care and management to participants in these events.

In addition, the resident must participate in the provision of comprehensive and continuing care to a sports team. Preferably, the experience should include several teams that engage in seasonal sports.

E. Mass-Participation Sports Events

The resident should participate in the planning and implementation of the provision of medical coverage for at least one mass-participation event. The program must ensure that its residents have experience that includes providing medical consultation, direct patient care, event planning, protection of participants, coordination with local EMS systems, and other medical aspects of those events.

VI. Specific Knowledge and Skills

A. Clinical

The program must provide educational experiences that enable residents to develop clinical competence in the overall field of sports medicine.

The curriculum must include but not be limited to the following content and skill areas:

1. Anatomy, physiology, and biomechanics of exercise
2. Basic nutritional principles and their application to exercise
3. Psychological aspects of exercise, performance, and competition
4. Guidelines for evaluation prior to participation in exercise and sport
5. Physical conditioning requirements for various activities
6. Special considerations related to age, gender, and disability
7. Pathology and pathophysiology of illness and injury as they relate to exercise
8. Effects of disease, eg, diabetes, cardiac conditions, arthritis, on exercise and the use of exercise in the care of medical problems

9. Prevention, evaluation, management, and rehabilitation of injuries
10. Understanding pharmacology and effects of therapeutic, performance-enhancing, and mood-altering drugs
11. Promotion of physical fitness and healthy lifestyles
12. Functioning as a team physician
13. Ethical principles as applied to exercise and sports
14. Medical-legal aspects of exercise and sports
15. Environmental effects on exercise
16. Growth and development related to exercise

B. Patient Education/Teaching

The program must provide the experiences necessary for the residents to develop and demonstrate competence in patient education regarding sports and exercise. They must have experience teaching others, eg, nurses, allied health personnel, medical students, residents, coaches, athletes, other professionals, and members of patients' families. There must also be relevant experience working in a community sports medicine network involving parents, coaches, certified athletic trainers, allied medical personnel, residents, and physicians.

ACGME: September 1994 Effective: September 1994

Program Requirements for Residency Education in Family Practice

I. Introduction

A. Duration of Training

Residencies in family practice must be 3 years in duration after graduation from medical school and must be planned so that a coherent, integrated, and progressive educational program with progressive resident responsibility is ensured.

B. Scope of Training

The programs must be specifically designed to meet the educational needs of medical school graduates intending to become family physicians and must provide experience and responsibility for the residents in those areas of medicine that will be of importance to their future practice. The goal of the family practice training program is to produce fully competent physicians capable of providing care of high quality to their patients. The presence of other programs sponsored by the residency, eg, geriatric medicine and/or sports medicine, must not result in significant dilution of the experience available to the family practice residents.

Family practice residency programs should provide opportunity for the residents to learn, in both the hospital and ambulatory settings, those procedural skills that are within the scope of family practice.

II. Institutional Organization

A. Sponsoring Institution

There must be one sponsoring institution for each residency, as mandated by the Institutional Requirements. This entity must be identified at the time of each review of the residency.

The sponsoring institution must ensure the existence and availability of those basic educational and patient care resources necessary to provide the family practice resident with meaningful involvement and responsibility in the required clinical specialties.

Since family practice programs are dependent in part on other specialties for the training of residents, the ability and commitment of the institution to fulfill these requirements must be documented. Instruction in the other specialties must be conducted by faculty with appropriate expertise. There must be agreement with specialists in other areas/services regarding the requirement that residents maintain concurrent commitment to their patients in the Family Practice Center (FPC) during these rotations.

B. Participating Institutions

When a residency relies on multiple institutions to provide curricular components, the arrangements between the program/primary site and each affiliated facility must be described in a written document that is signed by the appropriate administrators of the respective institutions. These arrangements must be specific to the family practice residency and must address the scope of the affiliation, the content and duration of the rotations involved, the duties and patient care responsibilities of the residents during these rotations and the details of the supervision and resident evaluation that will be provided. These documents should be appended to the program information forms each time there is a site visit and review of the program.

Participation by an institution that provides more than 6 of the 36 months of training in the program must be approved by the Residency Review Committee (RRC).

A member of the teaching staff of each participating institution must be designated to assume responsibility for the day-to-day activities of the program at that institution, with overall coordination by the program director.

C. Appointment of Residents

[*Note:* Applicants who have had previous graduate training may be considered for admission to family practice residencies. Credit for this other training may be given only in the amount that is compatible with the Program Requirements for Residency Education in Family Practice. Directors should consult with the American Board of Family Practice on each case prior to making a determination regarding the equivalence of such training.]

Programs should appoint only those candidates who intend to complete the full program. As a general rule, programs should appoint residents to the first year of training and those accepted into the first year of training should be assured of a position for the full 3 years, barring the development of grounds for dismissal. A family practice program should endeavor not to function as a transitional year program.

To provide adequate peer interaction a program should offer at least four positions at each level and should retain, on average, a minimum complement of 12 residents. Except for periods of transition, the program should offer the same number of positions for each of the 3 years.

In certain cases, for urban or rural areas serving underserved communities, tracks may be approved that have a smaller resident complement but with at least one resident at the second and third levels to ensure peer interaction. In such cases, programs are encouraged to arrange opportunities for the residents to interact with other residents, eg, through didactic sessions at the parent program.

The degree of resident attrition and the presence of a critical mass of residents are factors that will be considered by the RRC in the evaluation of a program.

III. Faculty Qualifications and Responsibilities

The program director and teaching staff are responsible for the general administration of the program, including those activities related to the recruitment, selection, instruction, supervision, counseling, evaluation, and advancement of residents and the maintenance of records related to program accreditation.

All members of the teaching staff must demonstrate a strong interest in the education of residents, sound clinical and teaching abilities, support of the goals and objectives of the program, a commitment to their own continuing medical education, and participation in scholarly activities.

A. Program Director

There must be a single program director responsible for the residency. Continuity of leadership over a period of years is important to the stability of a residency program. Frequent changes in leadership or long periods of temporary leadership usually have an adverse effect on an educational program and will be cause for serious concern. The RRC must be notified promptly in writing of any change in the leadership of the program.

To provide continuity of leadership and to fulfill the administrative and teaching responsibilities inherent in achieving the educational goals of the program, the director must devote sufficient time to the residency program, ie, at least 1400 hours per year exclusive of time spent in direct patient care without the presence of residents.

1. Qualifications of the Director

   The following are the requirements for the program director. An acting or interim director should be similarly qualified.

   a. Academic and professional qualifications: The director must have demonstrated ability as a teacher, clinician, and administrator; must be capable of administering the program in an effective manner; and must be actively involved in the care of patients. Prior to assuming this position, the program director must have had a minimum of 2 years full-time professional activity in family practice and should have had teaching experience in a family practice residency.
   b. Licensure: The director must be licensed to practice medicine in the state where the institution that sponsors the program is located. (Certain federal programs are exempted.)
   c. Certification requirements: The director must be currently certified by the American Board of Family Practice or have suitable equivalent qualifications. The RRC will determine the acceptability of alternate qualifications.
   d. Medical staff appointment: The director must hold an appointment in good standing to the medical staff of an institution participating in the program.

2. Responsibilities of the Director

   The program director is responsible for the following:

   a. Written educational goals: The director must prepare a written statement outlining the educational goals of the program. These must be provided in a document that outlines the specific knowledge, skills, and other attitudes expected of residents at each level of training and for each major rotation or other program assignment. The goals must be distributed to residents and teaching staff and should be available for review by the site visitor.
   b. Selection of residents: Residents for appointment to the program must be selected in accordance with institutional and departmental policies and procedures.
   c. Teaching staff and other program personnel: The director must have responsibility for selection and supervision of these staff members at each institution participating in the program.
   d. Supervision of residents: Institutional and program policies and procedures must ensure that all residents are adequately supervised in carrying out their patient care responsibilities. It is the responsibility of the program director and faculty to ensure that residents are appropriately supervised. Supervising policies of the residency should be consistent with those of the institution. They must be in writing and be distributed to all members of the program staff.

      Faculty on-call schedules must be structured to ensure that supervision is readily available to residents on duty. An appropriately qualified member of the program's faculty must be in attendance on site when the services or procedures needed exceed the capability of the most senior supervising resident or when qualified senior residents are unavailable for supervision of more junior residents.
   e. Resident evaluation: There must be regular and formal evaluation of residents with participation of the teaching staff.
   f. Discipline: The director has responsibility for the implementation of fair procedures, as established by the sponsoring institution, regarding academic discipline and resident complaints or grievances.
   g. Resident well-being: The director must monitor resident stress, including mental or emotional conditions that inhibit performance or learning, and dysfunction related to drugs or alcohol. The director and teaching staff should be sensitive to the need for timely provision of confidential counseling and psychological support service to residents. To promote physician well-being and prevent impairment, residents should be trained to balance personal and professional responsibilities in a way that can be reflected throughout their careers. Training situ-

ations that consistently produce undesirable stress on residents must be evaluated and modified.

h. Provision of accurate information: The director must submit accurate and complete information as requested by the RRC on the program information forms or in a special communication as directed by the committee.

i. Notification of change: The director must notify the RRC regarding major programmatic changes and obtain approval prior to their implementation.

B. Family Physician Faculty

The family physician faculty must be currently certified by the American Board of Family Practice or must demonstrate suitable equivalent qualifications. The RRC will determine the acceptability of alternate qualifications.

There must be at least one full-time equivalent (FTE) family physician faculty, in addition to the program director, for each six residents in the program. A full-time commitment is at least 1,400 hours per year devoted to the residency, exclusive of time spent in direct patient care without the presence of residents. Any program in operation must have at least two family physician faculty members, including the director, regardless of resident complement.

The faculty must contain teachers with the diversified interests and expertise necessary to meet the training responsibilities of the program. There must be a sufficient number of hours contributed by a critical mass of family physician faculty to prevent fragmentation of the learning experience. Where part-time faculty are utilized, there must be evidence of sufficient continuity of teaching and supervision.

The family physician faculty should have a specific time commitment to patient care to enable them to maintain their clinical skills and to serve as role models for the residents. Some of the family physician teaching staff must see patients in the FPC to serve as role models for the residents. In addition, the program must have family physician faculty with admitting privileges in the hospital(s) where the FPC patients are hospitalized.

C. Other Faculty

Physicians in the other specialties must devote sufficient time to teaching and supervising the family practice residents and providing consultation to ensure that the program's goals for their specialty areas are accomplished.

Additional teaching staff will be needed to provide training in areas such as behavioral science, nutrition, and the use of drugs and their interaction.

D. Qualifications and Development of Faculty

All of the key members of the teaching staff in the program must demonstrate suitable qualifications for their specialty areas, eg, certification by a member board of the American Board of Medical Specialties (ABMS) or equivalent qualifications for physician faculty, and appropriate credentials for the nonphysician faculty. The RRC will determine the acceptability of alternate qualifications.

There must be an explicit system to develop and maintain academic and clinical skills of the faculty and to foster their continual professional growth and development.

IV. Facilities

A program must provide the facilities required for the education of residents in sufficient proximity to the primary hospital to allow for the efficient functioning of the educational program.

A. Primary and Affiliated Hospitals

1. Multiple Hospitals

If the primary facility is unable to provide all of the required experiences, additional facilities may be used. Such arrangements will be considered acceptable only if there is no compromise in the quality of the educational program and no significant reduction in attendance of residents at teaching sessions or of camaraderie and exchange of information among residents and with the faculty. These affiliated hospitals may not be at such a distance from the primary teaching sites that they require excessive travel time or otherwise fragment the educational experience.

2. Number of Beds

It is essential that the participating hospitals, primary and affiliated, be of sufficient size and have an adequate number of occupied teaching beds to ensure a sufficient patient load and variety of problems for the education of the number of residents and other learners on the services. Inpatient facilities must also provide adequate physical, human, and educational resources for training in family practice. In determining the adequacy of the number of occupied beds in the primary and affiliated hospitals, the patient census, the types of patients, and their availability for residency education will be considered.

3. Medical Staff

The medical staff should be organized so that family physician members may participate in appropriate hospital governance activities on a basis equivalent to that of members in other specialties. Where a hospital is departmentalized, there must be a clinical department of family practice.

B. Family Practice Center

1. Introduction

The primary setting for training in the knowledge, skills, and attitudes of family practice is the model office or FPC, where each resident must provide continuing, comprehensive care to a panel of patient families. The FPC must be for the exclusive use of the residency, ie, all activities in the FPC must be residency-related and under the direction of the program director. The center must be clearly and significantly identified as an FPC.

An FPC must be in operation on the date the program begins. If a temporary center is used, it must meet the criteria specified below. If multiple centers are used for training, each must be approved by the RRC and must meet the same criteria as the primary center. All of the FPCs used in a program must provide comparable experiences.

Programs that involve training in Community or Migrant Health Centers (C/MHCs) [*Note:* See Section 330 of the Public Health Service Act.] must provide assurance that these facilities meet the criteria for an FPC, as outlined below.

2. Administration and Staffing

The program director must have administrative responsibility for and control of the FPC and its staff. The director of the FPC must report to the program director. In cases where the facility is not owned by the program, its primary hospital, or its sponsoring institution, eg, a Community Health Center, a letter of agreement must be provided that guarantees the program director's authority over and responsibility for the educational activities that take place in the facility.

The FPC must be appropriately staffed with nurses, technicians, clerks, and administrative and other health professional personnel to ensure efficiency and adequate support for patient care and educational needs.

3. Location and Access

The FPC must be close enough to the hospital to require minimal travel time. It may not be at such a distance as to require travel that interferes with the educational opportunities, efficiency, or patient care responsibility.

The facility must be designed to ensure adequate accessibility and efficient patient flow, be environmentally sensitive to patient care needs, and provide appropriate access and accommodations for the handicapped.

4. Required Areas
Each FPC must have
a. its own reception area and waiting room;
b. suitable resident work space and space for individual and small group counseling;
c. an office library, an office laboratory, and a business office;
d. two examining rooms that are large enough to accommodate the teaching and patient care activities of the program for each physician faculty member and resident when they are providing patient care; and
e. faculty offices and a conference room, if not in the FPC, then immediately adjacent to the center.

When other learners, eg, fellows, residents from other specialties, medical students, and nurses, are being trained by family physicians in the FPC, additional space may be required. Efficiency and education of the family practice residents must not be compromised by the training of other health care professionals.

5. Equipment
There must be
a. appropriate diagnostic and therapeutic equipment in the FPC to meet the basic needs of an efficient and up-to-date family practice office and an acceptable educational program for residents in family practice and
b. provision for diagnostic laboratory and imaging services so that there is prompt and convenient access by patients and residents for patient care and education.

6. Patient Access to the FPC
The FPC must be available for patient services at times commensurate with community medical standards and practice. When the center is not open, there must be a well-organized plan that ensures continuing access to the patient's personal physician or a designated family physician from the FPC.

Patients of the FPC must receive education and direction as to how they may obtain access to their physician or a substitute physician for continuity of care during the hours the center is closed. Patients should have access to printed policies and procedures of the clinic.

7. Record System
The FPC patients' records must be maintained in the FPC for easy and prompt accessibility at all times. The record system should be designed to provide information on patient care and the residents' experience. These records must be well maintained, legible, and up-to-date, and should document the patient's primary physician.

The record system must provide the data needed for patient care audit and chart review of all facets of family care, including care rendered in the FPC, in the hospital, at home, by telephone, through consultations, and by other institutions.

8. Source of Income
The fiscal operation of the FPC must reflect a balance between education and service. Service demands must not adversely affect educational objectives. A plan should be in place to ensure fiscal stability of the program.

Residents, faculty, and staff should be educated periodically on the importance of cost-effective quality health care and the importance of efficiency within the FPC.

C. Library Services

In addition to the office library in the FPC, residents must have ready access to a major medical library, either at the institution where the residents are located or through arrangement with convenient nearby institutions.

Library services should include the electronic retrieval of information from medical databases.

There must be access to an on-site library or to a collection of appropriate texts and journals in each institution participating in a residency program, and these must be readily available during nights and weekends.

D. Patient Population

A patient population of adequate size and representing a broad spectrum of problems, various ages, and both sexes should be attended in the hospital, in the FPC, at home, and in institutions for long-term care or rehabilitation. A sufficient number of inpatients must be available to provide a broad spectrum of problems in any area listed in these requirements that involves inpatient care. The disease spectrum available for resident education must be that common to the general community. These experiences must include the opportunity to attain expertise in emergency initial care of unusual or life-threatening problems.

V. The Educational Program

A. Introduction

The curricula and plans for all rotations and experiences must be developed by the family practice faculty. Other specialty faculty should be consulted for assistance as needed. All major dimensions of the curriculum should be structured educational experiences for which written goals and objectives, specific methodologies for teaching, and methods of evaluation exist.

While every residency program must have the required core curriculum as contained in this document, curriculum components may vary, with approval of the RRC, to reflect current regional practice patterns and patient care needs and may be flexible enough to utilize the strengths of the program.

Family physicians must be utilized to the fullest extent as teachers consistent with their experience, training, and current competence.

1. Program Design
The program design and/or structure must be approved by the RRC as part of the regular review process. All components of a residency program should be related to the program goals. Programs utilizing multiple sites and/or tracks must describe a core curriculum of at least 20 months that is participated in by all of the residents. If the remaining months are offered at more than one site they must be comparable in terms of their content, duration, and intensity.

Innovative and experimental educational designs and formats will be considered. For example, programs in family practice may propose utilization of a nonrotational format for providing resident education in areas usually taught in block rotations. Such proposals must demonstrate that the program provides experience equivalent to that of block rotations for its residents and must include documentation that residents will have all of the required experiences during their training, including experience with an adequate volume and mix of patients, the required continuity of care experiences, and appropriate faculty supervision.

2. Approval of Changes
Prior approval of the RRC is required for major changes in the curriculum, format, or design of the program; the addition or deletion of a major participating hospital; and/or the utilization of a new or additional FPC or the alteration of an existing center in any way that might make the facility less suitable.

On review of a proposal for major change in curriculum, facilities, or design of a program, the RRC may determine that a site visit is necessary before a decision can be made.

B. Principles of Family Practice

Continuity of care and family-oriented comprehensive care must be integral components of all programs. Residents must be taught throughout their training to demonstrate and to articulate clearly the following philosophy and concepts of family practice to patients and colleagues.

1. Continuity of Care
   The program must instruct residents in the provision of continuity of care and ensure that each resident has experience with the interrelating roles played by the physician, the patient, the patient's family, the health care system, and the community in optimizing the patient's care.

   The learning of continuity of care requires stable, protected physician-patient relationships that are structured to enhance both resident learning and patient care. This must occur primarily with a panel of patients in the FPC. Additional continuity patients, who may not be able to visit the FPC, should be enrolled and assigned as needed to provide residents with ongoing experience in home care and long-term care settings.

   The program must require that each resident maintain continuity of responsibility for his/her patients when such patients require hospitalization or consultation with other providers, both to integrate each patient's care and to optimize each resident's continuity training. The resident must maintain active involvement in management and treatment decisions.
2. Family-Oriented Comprehensive Care
   The family physician assumes responsibility for the total health care of the individual and family, taking into account social, behavioral, economic, cultural, and biologic dimensions. Therefore, a program must emphasize comprehensive, family-oriented care that must be taught in didactic and clinical settings during the entire period of residency training. Residents must have experience in all patient care contexts, including outpatient, inpatient, home, and long-term care settings.

   The resident must be given the opportunity to achieve high levels of competence in health maintenance and in disease and problem management and to develop attitudes that reflect expertise in comprehensive patient management and education.

   The program must provide the opportunity for residents to acquire knowledge and experience in the provision of longitudinal health care to families, including assisting them in coping with serious illness and loss and promoting family mechanisms to maintain wellness of its members.

   Essential elements to be integrated into the teaching of family care to residents include, for the individual patient, health assessment, health maintenance, preventive care, acute and chronic illness and injury, rehabilitation, behavioral counseling, health education, and human sexuality. Elements for the family include family structure and dynamics, genetic counseling, family development, family planning, child rearing and education, aging, end of life issues, epidemiology of illness in families, the role of family in illness care, family counseling and education, nutrition, and safety.

   The resident must be taught patterns of record keeping that incorporate a comprehensive information base, retrievable documentation of all aspects of care, and mechanisms for promotion of health maintenance and quality assessment of care.

C. Family Practice Center Experience

1. Orientation
   First-year residents must have an orientation period in the FPC to introduce the comprehensive approach to health care and to promote resident identity as a family physician.
2. Faculty Supervision
   The number of family physician faculty assigned to the FPC must be sufficient to ensure that there is always an appropriate number who, without other obligations, supervise and are immediately available on-site to the residents in the FPC whenever two or more residents are seeing patients. If there is only one resident seeing patients, the preceptor may engage in other activities in the FPC to a maximum of 50%. In addition to their availability when needed by residents, these supervisors must provide active precepting of the residents.
3. Patient Population
   Each program must document the availability of a stable patient population of sufficient number and variety to ensure comprehensiveness and continuity of experience for the residents in the FPC. Patient populations seeking only episodic care will not satisfy this requirement.

   The majority of the scheduled patient visits in the FPC should be from families for whom a resident is responsible. To achieve this, appointments must be scheduled by regular employees of the FPC or by an employee assigned specifically to scheduling family practice patients. These employees must be cognizant of the significance of the appointment policy on continuity of care and patient access to personal physicians. Wherever possible, assignment of family groups to a resident and priority scheduling with the primary provider should be considered.
4. Continuity Patient Panels
   Residents should develop and maintain a continuing physician-patient relationship with an undifferentiated panel of patients and their families throughout the 3-year period. The program must be structured to ensure that residents maintain such continuity at least throughout their second and third years of training. Residents must maintain this commitment to their panels of patients during specialty rotations. Continuity may be interrupted for a maximum of 1 month in the first year of training for remote site experiences. Limited interruptions during the second and third years may be allowed when rotations to remote sites are educationally justifiable. During each of the last 2 years of training the resident may not be away for remote site assignments longer than 2 months, and these two periods may not be consecutive. After the first remote experience, the residents must return to provide continuity care for their patient panels for at least 2 months before leaving for another remote experience.

   Each resident must be assigned to the same FPC for the number of half days specified below. A half-day session must be at least 3 hours. To gain adequate experience, each resident must see, on average, the following required minimum number of patients:
   a. First-year residents must be assigned to the FPC at least one half day per week and see a minimum of three patients per session.
   b. Second-year residents must be assigned to the FPC at least two half days per week and see a minimum of six patients per session.
   c. Third-year residents must be assigned at least three half days per week in the FPC and see a minimum of eight patients per session.

D. Focused Experiences

The program should implement a plan to ensure that residents retain their identity and commitment to the principles and philosophic attitudes of family practice throughout the training program, particularly while they rotate on other specialty services.

While the content of a rotation is more important than the time assigned to it, it is necessary to establish guidelines for the allocation of time segments to provide an objective measure of the opportunity provided for residents to achieve the cognitive knowledge, psychomotor skills, attitudinal orientation, and practical experience required of a family physician in each of the curricular elements. Concurrent time spent in the FPC may not be included when calculating the duration of the specialty rotations for which a number of required hours is specified. It is understood, however, that FPC time is included in the duration of the required rotations that are specified in months.

The following curricular areas must be included in each program.

1. Human Behavior and Mental Health
   Knowledge and skills in this area should be acquired through a program in which behavioral science and psychiatry are integrated with all disciplines throughout the resident's total educational experience. Training should be accomplished primarily in an outpatient setting through a combination of longitudinal experiences and didactic sessions. Intensive short-term experiences in facilities devoted to the care of chronically ill patients should be limited. Instruction must be provided by faculty who have the training and experience necessary to apply modern behavioral and psychiatric principles to the care of the undifferentiated patient. Family physicians, psychiatrists, and behavioral scientists should be involved in teaching this curricular component.

   There must be instruction in the following areas:
   a. Diagnosis and management of psychiatric disorders in children and adults
   b. Emotional aspects of nonpsychiatric disorders
   c. Psychopharmacology
   d. Alcoholism and other substance abuse
   e. The physician/patient relationship
   f. Patient interviewing skills
   g. Counseling skills
   h. Normal psychosocial growth and development in individuals and families
   i. Stages of stress in a family life cycle
   j. Sensitivity to gender, race, age, sexual orientation, and cultural differences in patients
   k. Family violence including child, partner, and elder abuse (physical and sexual), as well as neglect, and its effect on both victims and perpetrators
   l. Medical ethics, including patient autonomy, confidentiality, and issues concerning quality of life
   m. Factors influencing patient compliance
2. Adult Medicine
   This experience must provide the resident with the opportunity to acquire the knowledge and skills necessary for the diagnosis, treatment, and management of nonsurgical diseases of adults. This experience should enhance the resident's understanding of the pathophysiologic basis for nonsurgical diagnostic and therapeutic techniques and promote development of a disciplined, scientific approach to the practice of adult medicine. Faculty must include family physicians and may include internists or other specialists.

   There must be a minimum of 8 months of experience in adult medicine. At least 6 months should occur in the inpatient setting, on either a family practice or an internal medicine service. In all cases, experiences should progress from general to specific content areas, with graduated resident responsibilities and supervision.

   This training must include a separate defined critical care experience of at least 1 month's duration, or its equivalent, and a structured clinical experience in cardiology. The curriculum must also provide instruction in endocrinology, pulmonary diseases, hematology and oncology, gastroenterology, infectious diseases, rheumatology, nephrology, allergy and immunology, and neurology through lectures, rotations, or interaction with consultants.

   There must be education in the prevention and detection of diseases in women. Instruction on women should also cover social issues of concern to women, including domestic violence, rape, sexual abuse, and the changing role of women in our society. Residents should have the opportunity to develop an understanding of the effect of the community on women's health care, including the epidemiology of infant mortality and prevention of teenage pregnancy. Residents must have the opportunity to learn about the mental health issues of women, including problems that are seen predominantly in women, such as eating disorders and the sequelae of sexual abuse.
3. Maternity and Gynecologic Care
   a. Maternity Care
   The resident must be provided instruction in the biological and psychosocial impacts of pregnancy, delivery, and care of the newborn on a woman and her family. There must be a minimum of 2 months of experience in maternity care, including the principles and techniques of prenatal care, management of labor and delivery, and postpartum care. This must involve sufficient instruction and experience to enable residents to manage a normal pregnancy and delivery.

   The resident must be trained in the recognition and initial management of the high-risk prenatal patient, including consultation and referral. Additionally, the residents must be taught to recognize and manage complications and emergencies in pregnancy, labor, and delivery. Residents also must receive training in genetic counseling. When appropriate for the resident's future practice and patient care, the resident must be trained in the management of the high-risk prenatal patient.

   Each resident must perform a sufficient number of deliveries to ensure adequate opportunity for the achievement of competencies appropriate to family physicians. A portion of the maternity care experience must be derived from the continuity panel of patients. To accomplish the objectives of the curriculum in maternity care, residents must assume the responsibility of longitudinal provision of antenatal, natal, and postnatal care during their 3 years of training. Whenever possible, these patients should be derived from the residents' panels of patients in the FPC.

   Supervision of labor and delivery care must be immediately available. The program must have family physician faculty who are engaged in providing these services and who can supervise the residents and serve as role models for them.

   The program must make available additional training in maternity care as an elective within the 36-month curriculum. This elective experience must include high-risk maternity care, including the opportunity for residents to develop technical proficiency in appropriate operative procedures that may form a part of their future practice.

   b. Gynecological Care
   There must be a minimum of 140 hours of structured experience in the care of the gynecological system in nonpregnant women. This experience must be in addition to the routine care of continuity patients in the FPC. All residents must be provided instruction in normal growth and development; diseases of the female reproductive tract; reproductive physiology including fertility, family planning, and human sexuality; physiology of menopause; and pelvic floor dysfunction. The program also must provide adequate instruction and clinical experience in managing emergency problems of the female reproductive system. This experience should be predominantly

ambulatory, but residents must participate in the management of gynecological/surgical emergencies. The training should include some inpatient care, preoperative care, assisting in surgery, and postoperative care. The residents must have the opportunity to learn to perform appropriate procedures.

4. Care of the Surgical Patient

The program must provide instruction with special emphasis on the diagnosis and management of surgical disorders and emergencies and the appropriate and timely referral of surgical cases for specialized care.

Residents must be taught to appreciate the varieties of surgical treatments and the potential risks associated with them to enable them to give proper advice, explanation, and emotional support to patients and their families. The residents should also be taught to recognize conditions that are preferably managed on an elective basis.

The program must provide all residents with training in preoperative and postoperative care, basic surgical principles, asepsis, handling of tissue, and technical skills to assist the surgeon in the operating room. The program should provide the opportunity for residents to develop technical proficiency in those specific surgical procedures that family physicians may be called on to perform. If the residents expect to include surgery as a major aspect of their practice, additional training must be considered.

a. General Surgery

The residents must be required to participate in a structured experience in general surgery of at least 2 months, including ambulatory and operating room experience. Experiences in general surgery must be designed to provide opportunity for residents to achieve competency in the diagnosis and management of a wide variety of common surgical problems typically cared for by family physicians.

b. Surgical Subspecialties

The required experiences in surgical subspecialties may occur in a block or longitudinal format and are exclusive of time spent caring for patients in the assigned panel of FPC patients and of the learning acquired through consultations.

A minimum of 140 hours of structured experience in the care of orthopaedic disorders is required. This experience must include caring for a broad variety of acute and emergency musculoskeletal injuries and illnesses, as well as for chronic disorders. Residents must have the opportunity to develop skills in casting and splinting. The program also must provide experience in the initial evaluation and rehabilitation of adult and pediatric musculoskeletal disorders, including the appropriateness of consultation. This educational experience must include didactic conferences and clinical exposure, and should occur primarily in an outpatient setting. Supervision must be provided by faculty with demonstrated expertise in evaluation and treatment of musculoskeletal disorders.

The curriculum also must include structured experiences in the care of genitourinary disorders and disorders of the eye, ear, nose, and throat. Residents must have the opportunity under appropriate supervision to learn to perform appropriate procedures. Most of these experiences should occur in outpatient settings and must be in addition to the experiences residents have during the care of their continuity patients in the FPC.

5. Sports Medicine

The sports medicine experience must include didactic and clinical experience in the areas of preparticipation assessment, injury prevention, evaluation, management, and rehabilitation related to athletic and recreational injuries.

The orthopaedic aspects of sports medicine training may be integrated into the orthopaedic curriculum, but the time devoted to sports medicine should be in addition to the minimum requirement of 140 hours for orthopaedics.

6. Emergency Care

There must be a structured educational experience of at least a 1-month block rotation in the delivery of emergency care. Additional required or elective emergency care experiences may be in either a block or longitudinal format. There must be on-site supervision by qualified physicians whenever residents are on the service.

A sufficient volume and variety of patient visits, adequate numbers and types of support personnel, and suitable facilities must be available to ensure the residents an adequate experience in the initial management of serious illnesses and injuries.

The emergency care training should include didactic as well as clinical experiences. Residents should receive training in all standard current life support skills and procedures for both trauma and medical emergencies in patients of all ages.

7. Care of Neonates, Infants, Children, and Adolescents

There must be a structured educational experience in the care of children that is at least 4 months in duration and involves pediatric ambulatory clinic and inpatient experience with a sufficient volume of patients in each setting. This must include the newborn nursery as well as clinical experience in management of the distressed neonate who may need resuscitation, stabilization, and preparation for transport. The resident should have the opportunity to develop an understanding of the prenatal period, the growth and development of the newborn through adolescence, child rearing, and emotional problems of children and their management. In addition, the resident should be taught to recognize and manage behavioral, medical, and surgical problems of children and adolescents in home, school, ambulatory, and hospital settings.

8. Community Medicine

Residents must be taught to assess and understand the important health needs of the community in which they work. Instruction and clinical experiences in the following areas must be provided:

a. Occupational medicine, including disability assessment, employee health, and job-related injury and illness
b. Community health resources that may be utilized in the care of patients and their families, including school health services and public health (including environmental health) services
c. Disease prevention/health promotion, including appropriate strategies and behaviors such as immunizations and healthful lifestyle changes that will protect children, adults, and families from illness or injury.

9. Care of the Older Patient

Educational experience must be provided in the common and complex clinical problems of the older patient and must include the preventive aspects of health care, functional assessment, the physiological and psychological changes of senescence, the sociocultural parameters of the patient and his or her greater community, the nutritional and pathological (acute and chronic) entities of aging, and the effective utilization of all members of the health care team.

There must be experience with the older adult patient in the hospital, the FPC, a long-term care facility, and the home.

10. Care of the Skin and Associated Organs
The curriculum must include a required educational experience of at least 60 hours, most of which should be in an outpatient setting and be supplementary to the learning that results from consultations. The experience should be supervised by a physician with competence in this area.
11. Diagnostic Imaging and Nuclear Medicine
The program must provide the residents with a structured opportunity to learn the appropriate application of techniques and specialty consultations in the diagnostic imaging and nuclear medicine therapy of organs and body systems. Instruction should include the limitations and risks attendant to these techniques. The format of the instruction should be adapted to the resources available, but must include radiographic film/diagnostic imaging interpretation and nuclear medicine therapy pertinent to family practice.
12. Conferences
Conferences should be offered to cover the breadth of the specialty of family practice.

There should be a core curriculum that is based in the residency and that is specifically directed to the residents as learners. This core curriculum should be supplemented by conferences during other rotations. Residents and faculty should periodically be presenters at conferences, but residents should not be used excessively in this role. Resident and faculty attendance at conferences must be monitored and documented, and these records should be reviewed periodically by the program director and they should also be available for review by the site visitor.
13. Resident Research and Scholarly Activity
Each program must provide opportunity for residents to participate in research or other scholarly activities. Instruction in the critical evaluation of medical literature, including assessing study validity and the applicability of studies to the residents' patients, must be provided.

The participation of each resident in an active research program should be encouraged as preparation for a lifetime of self-education after the completion of formal training. Generally, this activity should be concurrent with other assignments, provided that the responsibilities of the resident are adjusted to permit a reasonable time for research activity. This experience should be designed to give the residents an awareness of the basic principles of study design, performance, analysis, and reporting, as well as of the relevance of research to patient care.

Other acceptable forms of scholarly activity include presentations at national, regional, state, or local meetings, and presentation and publication of review articles and case presentations.
14. Practice Management
There must be at least 60 hours of formal instruction in practice management in both the didactic and the practical setting. A practice management curriculum should include but not be limited to the areas of personal finance, office and personnel management, business planning, use of computers in practice, managed care, alternative practice models, professional liability, and risk management.

The FPC should be considered a primary site for teaching practice management and should serve as an example on which residents may model their future practice.
15. Electives
Electives are intended primarily to enrich the residents' training with experiences relevant to their plans for future practice or their interests as family physicians. There must be a minimum of 3 and a maximum of 6 months of appropriately supervised electives available to all residents. The choice of electives by the resident, including those for remedial purposes, must be made with the approval of the program director.

E. Resident Workload and Impairment

Each program must ensure an appropriate working environment and a duty hour schedule that are consistent with proper patient care and the educational needs of the residents. The educational goals of the program and the learning objectives of the residents must not be compromised by excessive reliance on residents to fulfill institutional service obligations.

There must be formal written policies on the following matters that demonstrate compliance with these requirements. These documents must be available to the RRC, if requested.

1. Moonlighting
It is the responsibility of the program to see that residents provide patient care in the pursuit of their education without additional remuneration based on productivity. Residency training is a full-time responsibility. The program director should monitor the effects of outside activities, including moonlighting inside or outside the participating institutions, to ensure that the quality of patient care and the resident's educational experience are not compromised.
2. Workload/Duty Hours
Resident assignments must be made in such a way as to prevent excessive patient loads, excessive new admission workups, inappropriate intensity of service or case mix, and excessive length and frequency of call contributing to excessive fatigue and sleep deprivation. The program must also ensure the following:
a. At least 1 day out of 7, averaged monthly, away from the residency program
b. On-call duty no more frequently than every third night, averaged monthly
c. Adequate backup if sudden and unexpected patient care needs create resident fatigue sufficient to jeopardize patient care during or following on-call periods

Programs must have formal mechanisms specifically designed for promotion of physician well-being and prevention of impairment. There also should be a structured and facilitated group designed for resident support that meets on a regular schedule.

F. Faculty Research and Scholarly Activity

Graduate medical education must take place in an environment of inquiry and scholarship in which residents participate in the development of new knowledge, learn to evaluate research findings, and develop habits of inquiry as a continuing professional responsibility. Scholarship implies an in-depth understanding of basic mechanisms of normal and abnormal states and the application of current knowledge to practice.

While not all members of a teaching staff must be investigators, the staff as a whole must demonstrate broad involvement in scholarly activity. This activity should include

1. Active participation in clinical discussions, rounds, and conferences in a manner that promotes a spirit of inquiry and scholarship.
2. Active participation in regional or national professional and scientific societies, particularly through presentations at the organizations' meetings and publications in their journals.
3. Participation in research, particularly in projects that are funded following peer review and/or result in publications or presentations at regional and national scientific meetings.
4. Provision of guidance and technical support (eg, research design, statistical analysis) to residents involved in research.

VI. Evaluation

A. Evaluation of Residents

There must be adequate, ongoing evaluation of the knowledge, skills, and performance of the residents. Entry evaluation assessment, interim testing, and periodic reassessment, as well as other modalities for evaluation, should be utilized. There must be a method of documenting the procedures that are performed by the residents. Such documentation must be maintained by the program, be available for review by the site visitor, and be used to provide documentation for future hospital privileges.

The faculty must provide a written evaluation of each resident after each rotation, and these must be available for review by the residents and site visitor. Written evaluation of each resident's knowledge, skills, professional growth, and performance, using appropriate criteria and procedures, must be accomplished at least semiannually and must be communicated to and discussed with the resident in a timely manner.

Residents should be advanced to positions of higher responsibility only on the basis of evidence of their satisfactory progressive scholarship and professional growth.

The program must maintain a permanent record of evaluation for each resident and have it accessible to the resident and other authorized personnel. The program director and faculty are responsible for provision of a written final evaluation for each resident who completes the program. This evaluation must include a review of the resident's performance during the final period of training and should verify that the resident has demonstrated sufficient professional ability to practice competently and independently. This final evaluation should be part of the resident's permanent record maintained by the institution.

B. Evaluation of Faculty

All teaching faculty must be formally evaluated at least annually. Documentation of faculty evaluation should include teaching ability, clinical knowledge, attitudes, and communication skills. There should be a mechanism for anonymous input by the residents.

C. Evaluation of the Program

The family practice residency must incorporate all elements of these Program Requirements. The educational effectiveness of a program must be evaluated in a systematic manner at least annually. The program should engage in self-evaluation within the context of the educational goals and objectives, the needs of the residents, teaching responsibilities of the faculty, and the availability of administrative and financial support and of adequate health care resources within the community. This evaluation should include an examination of the balance among education, research, and service. The teaching staff must hold regular, documented meetings to accomplish these reviews. At least one resident representative should participate in these reviews and written evaluations by residents and feedback from the program's graduates should be utilized in the process.

D. Evaluation of Patient Care

A mechanism must be in place to evaluate the care provided in both inpatient and outpatient settings. There should be evidence that this evaluation is used to improve education and the provision of care.

E. Evaluation of the Graduates

Each program must maintain a system of evaluation of its graduates. The residency should obtain feedback on demographic and practice profiles, licensure and board certification, the graduates' perceptions of the relevancy of training to practice, suggestions for improving the training, and ideas for new areas of curriculum. The suggested format is a written survey after 1 year and every 5 years thereafter.

The data from the evaluation of the graduates should be used as part of the program's determination of the degree to which the program's stated goals are being met.

VII. Evaluation of the Program by the RRC

The program will be evaluated by the RRC at regular intervals, at which times the RRC will judge the degree of its compliance with the Program Requirements.

One measure of the quality of a residency program is the performance of its graduates on the certifying examination of the American Board of Family Practice. In its evaluation of residency programs, the RRC will take into consideration the information provided by ABFP regarding resident performance on the certifying examinations over a period of several years.

The committee will use scores for a minimum of 3 and a maximum of 5 years and will take into consideration noticeable improvements or declines during the period considered. Poor performance will be cited if more than 10% of a program's candidates fail on the first examination over a period of consecutive years and/or the program's composite score is consistently at or below the 25th percentile in the nation.

ACGME: September 1996 Effective: July 1997

Program Requirements for Residency Education in Family Practice Geriatric Medicine and Family Practice Sports Medicine

The following generic requirements pertain to programs in Family Practice Geriatric Medicine and Family Practice Sports Medicine. Each program must comply with the requirements listed below as well as with the specialty content found in the Program Requirements for the respective area.

These programs must exist in conjunction with and be an integrated part of an Accreditation Council for Graduate Medical Education (ACGME)-accredited family practice residency program. Their existence should not compromise the integrity of the core program.

Residents who are appointed to programs in geriatric medicine must have satisfactorily completed an ACGME-accredited residency in family practice or internal medicine. Residents appointed to the sports medicine programs should have completed an ACGME-accredited residency in emergency medicine, family practice, internal medicine, or pediatrics. [*Note:* Those lacking board certification in one of these areas will not be considered eligible for a Certificate of Added Qualifications from any of the corresponding specialty boards.]

I. Program Organization

A. Program Design

The director and teaching staff of a program must prepare and comply with written educational goals for the program. All educational components of the residency program must be related to these goals and should be structured educational experiences for which a specific methodology and method of evaluation exist.

The program design and/or structure must be approved by the Residency Review Committee (RRC) as part of the regular review process.

B. Participating Institutions

Participation by any institution providing more than 3 months of training in a program must be approved by the RRC.

A member of the teaching staff of each participating institution must be designated to assume responsibility for the day-to-day activities of the program at that institution, with overall coordination by the program director.

II. Program Personnel

The program director and the teaching staff are responsible for the general administration of the program, including those activities related to the recruitment, selection, instruction, supervision, counseling, evaluation, and advancement of residents and the maintenance of records related to program accreditation.

A. Program Director

There must be a single program director responsible for the program, who is based primarily at the teaching center. The director must be fully committed to the program in order to devote sufficient time to the achievement of the educational goals and objectives. She or he must have sufficient authority to manage, control, and direct the program.

1. Qualifications
   The program director must possess the following qualifications:
   a. Requisite and documented clinical, educational, and administrative abilities and experience.
   b. Licensure to practice medicine in the state where the institution that sponsors the program is located. (Certain federal programs are exempted.)
   c. Certification by the specialty board in the discipline of the program or demonstrate suitable equivalent qualifications. For directors of programs in geriatric medicine this means certification by the American Board of Family Practice or the American Board of Internal Medicine and a Certificate of Added Qualification in Geriatric Medicine from the same board. Directors of programs in sports medicine may be certified by any of the following boards: American Board of Emergency Medicine, American Board of Family Practice, American Board of Internal Medicine, or American Board of Pediatrics, and must possess a Certificate of Added Qualification in Sports Medicine from that same board. The RRC will determine the adequacy of alternate qualifications.
   d. Appointment in good standing to the medical staff of an institution participating in the program.
2. Responsibilities
   The responsibilities of the program director include:
   a. Preparation of a written statement outlining the educational goals of the program with respect to knowledge, skills, and other attributes of residents at each level of training and for each major rotation or other program assignment. This statement must be distributed to residents and members of the teaching staff and be readily available for review.
   b. Selection of residents for appointment to the program in accordance with institutional and departmental policies and procedures.
   c. Selection and supervision of the teaching staff and other program personnel at each institution participating in the program.
   d. Supervision of residents through explicit written descriptions of supervisory lines of responsibility for the care of patients. Such guidelines must be communicated to all members of the program staff. Residents must be provided with prompt, reliable systems for communication and interaction with supervisory physicians.
   e. Preparation of an accurate statistical and narrative description of the program as requested by the RRC.

B. Teaching Staff

1. There must be a sufficient number of teaching staff with documented qualifications, ie, board certification for the physician faculty and appropriate credentials for the nonphysician teaching staff, to instruct and supervise adequately all the residents in the program. Members of the teaching staff must be able to devote sufficient time to meet their supervisory and teaching responsibilities.
2. All members of the teaching staff must demonstrate a strong interest in the education of residents, sound clinical and teaching abilities, support of the goals and objectives of the program, a commitment to their own continuing medical education, and participation in scholarly activities.

C. Other Program Personnel

Programs must be provided with the additional professional, technical, and clerical personnel needed to support the administration and educational conduct of the program.

III. Workload/Call Schedule

The schedule for the residents should allow them to make full utilization of their educational experiences without resultant counterproductive stress, fatigue, and depression. There should be adequate staff to prevent excessive patient loads and excessive length and frequency of call. On-call duty should occur no more frequently than every third night, averaged monthly, and residents must be permitted to spend a monthly average of at least 1 day out of 7 away from program duties. Formal written policies on these matters must be established and available for review.

There must be attention given to monitoring resident stress, including mental or emotional conditions inhibiting performance or learning and drug- or alcohol-related dysfunction. Program directors and teaching staff should be sensitive to the need for timely provision of confidential counseling and psychological support services to residents. Training situations that consistently produce undesirable stress on residents must be evaluated and modified.

IV. Program Research and Scholarly Activity

Graduate medical education must take place in an environment of inquiry and scholarship in which residents participate in the development of new knowledge, learn to evaluate research findings, and develop habits of inquiry as a continuing professional responsibility.

A. Teaching Staff Research/Scholarly Activity

The responsibility for establishing and maintaining an environment of inquiry and scholarship rests with the teaching staff. While not all members of a teaching staff must be investigators, the staff as a whole must demonstrate broad involvement in scholarly activity. This activity should include:

1. Active participation of the teaching staff in clinical discussions, rounds, and conferences in a manner that promotes a spirit of inquiry and scholarship. Scholarship implies an in-depth understanding of basic mechanisms of normal and abnormal states and the application of current knowledge to practice.
2. Active participation in regional or national professional and scientific societies, particularly through presentations at the organizations' meetings and publication in their journals.
3. Participation in research, particularly in projects that are funded following peer review and/or result in publication or presentations at regional and national scientific meetings.

B. Resident Research/Scholarly Activity

The residents must be exposed to and take part in research programs that provide an environment conducive to a questioning attitude and critical analysis. The program must provide support for resident participation in scholarly activities and offer guidance and technical support, eg, research design, statistical analysis, for residents involved in research. Residents must participate in journal clubs and research conferences.

C. Library

Residents must have ready access to a major medical library, either at the institution where the residents are located or through arrangement with convenient nearby institutions.

The library services should include the electronic retrieval of information from medical databases.

There must be access to an on-site library or to a collection of appropriate texts and journals in each institution participating in a residency program. On-site libraries and/or collections of texts and journals must be readily available during nights and weekends.

V. Evaluation

A. Evaluation of Residents

There must be regular evaluation of residents' knowledge, skills, and overall performance, including the development of professional attitudes consistent with being a physician. The program director, with participation of members of the teaching staff, shall

1. Evaluate the knowledge, skills, and professional growth of the residents at least semiannually, using appropriate criteria and procedures.
2. Communicate each evaluation to the resident in a timely manner.
3. Advance residents to positions of higher responsibility only on the basis of evidence of their satisfactory progressive scholarship and professional growth.
4. Maintain a permanent record of evaluation for each resident and have it accessible to the resident and other authorized personnel.
5. Provide a written final evaluation for each resident who completes the program. The evaluation must include a review of the resident's performance during the final period of training and should verify that the resident has demonstrated sufficient professional ability to practice competently and independently. This final evaluation should be part of the resident's permanent record maintained by the institution.
6. Implement fair procedures, as established by the sponsoring institution, regarding academic discipline and resident complaints or grievances.

B. Evaluation of the Teaching Staff

Formal mechanisms for annual evaluation of the teaching staff must exist and must include confidential resident participation.

C. Program Evaluation

The teaching staff must be organized and have regular documented meetings to review program goals and objectives as well as program effectiveness in achieving them. In particular, the quality of the curriculum and the extent to which the educational goals have been met by residents must be assessed. At least one resident representative should participate in these reviews, and written evaluations by residents should be utilized in this process.

There should also be periodic evaluation of the utilization of resources available to the program, the contribution of each institution participating in the program, the financial and administrative support of the program, the volume and variety of patients available to the program for educational purposes, the performance of members of the teaching staff, and the quality of supervision of residents.

One measure of the quality of a program will be the performance by its graduates on the examinations of the certifying board.

VI. Certification

Those planning to seek a Certificate of Added Qualifications from their primary board should communicate with the administrative officer of the board to ascertain the full requirements.

ACGME: September 1994 Effective: July 1995

Program Requirements for Residency Education in Family Practice Geriatric Medicine

In addition to complying with the Program Requirements for Residency Education in Family Practice Geriatric Medicine and Family Practice Sports Medicine, programs must also comply with the following requirements, which may in some cases exceed the common requirements.

I. Educational Program

An educational program in geriatric medicine must be organized to provide a well-supervised experience at a sufficient level for the resident to acquire the competence of a physician with added qualifications in the field. It shall be 12 months in duration. The program must be conducted by an accredited residency program in internal medicine or family practice.

Clinical experience must include opportunities to manage elderly patients with a wide variety of medical problems on an inpatient and outpatient basis. Residents must be given the opportunity to provide both primary care and consultation for patients in acute, ambulatory, community, and long-term care settings in order to understand the interaction of natural aging and disease as well as the techniques of assessment, therapy, and management. Additionally, residents must be given the opportunity to care for persons who are generally healthy and require primarily preventive health-care measures.

The program should include an emphasis on the physiology of aging, the pathophysiology that commonly occurs in older persons, atypical presentations of illnesses, functional assessment, cognitive status and affective assessment, and concepts of treatment and management in both the acute and long-term care settings, as well as in the community and in the home.

Attention also should be directed to the behavioral aspects of illness, socioeconomic factors, and ethical and legal considerations that may impinge on medical management.

The program must provide the opportunity for residents to maintain their basic primary skills during the course of this training. At least ½ day per week must be spent in a continuity of care experience in the resident's primary discipline.

II. Faculty and Staff

A. Program Director

The program director must be fully committed to the program in order to devote sufficient time to the achievement of the educational goals and objectives. The director must have demonstrated experience in geriatric medicine and must have demonstrated experience in education and scholarly activity and have a career commitment to academic geriatric medicine. The director must be primarily based at the teaching center.

B. Other Teaching Staff

In addition to the program director, each program must have at least one other faculty member with similar qualifications who devotes a substantial portion of professional time to the training program. For programs with more than two residents, there must be 0.5 additional faculty member for each additional resident. Some of these faculty may be part-time in geriatric medicine or drawn wholly from collaborating programs. The faculty commitment must not attenuate the quality of the core residency training program. The program must ensure that interdisciplinary relationships with the following specialties occur: physical medicine and rehabilitation, neurology, and psychiatry. Appropriate relationships with other disciplines including but not limited to general surgery, orthopedics, ophthalmology, otolaryngology, urology, gynecology, emergency medicine, dentistry, pharmacy, audiology, physical and occupational therapy, speech therapy, and nursing and social services should be maintained. Additionally, a liaison with the physician assistants, when available, should be established.

C. Geriatric Care Team

The resident must have experience with physician-directed interdisciplinary geriatric teams in an acute-care hospital, in a nursing home, that includes subacute and long-term care, in a home care setting, and in a family practice center or other outpatient settings. Essential members include a geriatrician, a nurse, and a social worker. Additional members may be included in the team as appropriate, including representatives from disciplines such as neurology, psychiatry, physical medicine and rehabilitation, physical therapy, occupational therapy and speech therapy, dentistry, pharmacy, psychology, and pastoral care. Regular team conferences must be held as dictated by the needs of the individual patient.

III. Facilities/Resources

A patient population adequate to meet the needs of the training program must be available in the facilities in which the educational experiences take place. Elderly patients of both sexes with a variety of chronic illnesses, at least some of whom have potential for rehabilitation, must be available. At all facilities utilized by the program the resident must be given opportunities to assume meaningful patient responsibility. At each setting certain activities are mandated and must be supervised and taught by the appropriate clinician. The program must include the following:

A. Acute-Care Hospital

The acute-care hospital central to the geriatric medicine program must be an integral component of a teaching center. It must have the full range of services usually ascribed to an acute-care general hospital, including intensive care units, emergency medicine, operating rooms, diagnostic laboratory and imaging services, and a pathology department.

B. Long-term Care Institution

One or more long-term care institutions, such as a skilled nursing facility or chronic care hospital, is a necessary component of the geriatric medicine program. Exposure to subacute care and rehabilitation care in the long-term care setting is desirable. The total number of beds available must be sufficient to permit a comprehensive educational experience. The institutions must be approved by the appropriate licensing agencies of the state, and the standard of facilities and care in each must be consistent with those promulgated by the Joint Commission on the Accreditation of Healthcare Organizations.

C. Long-term Noninstitutional Care

Noninstitutional care service, for example, home care, day care, residential care, or assisted living, is a major component of the geriatric medicine program. A home care program or home health agency is a necessary resource to permit residents to learn to provide care for patients who are homebound but not institutionalized. Day care or day hospital centers, life care communities, and residential care facilities for the elderly are also desirable training sites.

D. Ambulatory Care Program

The ambulatory care program must comprise a minimum of 33% of the resident's time. Each resident should evaluate approximately 1 to 3 new geriatric patients and 4 to 8 follow-up geriatric patients each week. This must include at least ½ day per week spent in a continuity of care experience. This experience must be designed to provide care in a geriatric clinic or family practice center to elderly patients who may require the services of multiple medical disciplines (including but not limited to neurology, gynecology, urology, psychiatry, podiatry, orthopedics, physical medicine and rehabilitation, dentistry, audiology, otolaryngology, and ophthalmology, as well as nursing, social work, and nutrition, among other disciplines. The opportunity to provide continuing care and to coordinate the implementation of recommendations from these medical specialties and disciplines is mandatory. In addition, experiences in relevant ambulatory specialty and subspecialty clinics (eg, geriatric psychiatry and neurology) and those that focus on geriatric syndromes (eg, falls, incontinence, osteoporosis) are highly desirable.

E. Additional Educational Environment

Peer interaction is essential for residents. To achieve this goal, an accredited training program in at least one relevant specialty other than family practice must be present at the teaching center sponsoring the training program in geriatric medicine. This may be accomplished by affiliation with another educational institution for the enrichment of the educational experience.

Involvement in other health care and community agencies is desirable. There must be a formal affiliation agreement between each long-term care facility included in the program and the sponsoring institution, in which each institution must acknowledge its responsibility to provide high-quality care, adequate resources, and administrative support for the educational mission. In addition, there must be a letter of agreement between each long-term care facility and the office of the director of the geriatric medicine program that guarantees the director appropriate authority at the long-term care institution to carry out the training program.

IV. Specific Program Content

All major dimensions of the curriculum should be structured educational experiences for which written goals and objectives, a specific methodology for teaching, and a method of evaluation exist. A written curriculum that describes the program comprehensively, including sites, educational objectives for each component, and topics to be covered in didactic sessions, should be available to residents and faculty. The curriculum must ensure the opportunity for residents to achieve the cognitive knowledge, psychomotor skills, interpersonal skills, professional attitudes, and practical experience required of a physician who specializes in the care of the aged.

Didactic as well as clinical learning opportunities must be available to the resident. Conferences or seminars/workshops in geriatric medicine should be specifically designed to augment the residents' clinical experiences. Journal club or other activities that foster interaction and develop skills in interpreting the medical literature are necessary.

All deaths of patients who receive care by residents should be reviewed and autopsies performed whenever possible.

As the residents progress through their training, they must have the opportunity to teach personnel such as nurses, allied health personnel, medical students, and residents. Appropriate experiences designed to refine educational and teaching skills of the residents and to develop the necessary administrative skills must be provided.

Appropriate faculty supervision of the residents must be provided during all of their educational experiences.

The following components must be provided:

A. Geriatric Medicine Consultation Program

This program must be formally available in the ambulatory setting, the inpatient service, and/or emergency medicine in the acute-care hospital or at an ambulatory setting administered by the primary teaching institution.

B. Long-term Care Experience

In the long-term care institutional setting each resident must have 12 months of continuing longitudinal clinical experience with an assigned panel of patients for whom the resident is the primary provider. Additional block time to provide long-term care experience is encouraged. Emphasis during the longitudinal experience should be focused on (1) the approaches to diagnosis and treatment of the acutely and chronically ill, frail elderly in a less technologically sophisticated environment than the acute-care hospital; (2) working within the limits of a decreased staff-patient ratio compared with acute-care hospitals; (3) a much greater awareness of and familiarity with subacute care physical medicine and rehabilitation; (4) the challenge of the clinical and ethical dilemmas produced by the illness of the very old; and (5) administrative aspects of long-term care.

Experience with home visits and hospice care must be included. The resident must be exposed to the organizational and administrative aspects of home health care. Continuity of care with an assigned panel of home or hospice care patients for whom the resident is the primary provider is essential.

C. Geriatric Psychiatry

Identifiable structured didactic and clinical experiences in geriatric psychiatry must be included in the program of each resident. Behavioral sciences such as psychology/social work and others must be included in the curriculum.

D. Curriculum

The training program must provide opportunities for the residents to develop clinical competence in the overall field of geriatric medicine. The curriculum of the program must exhibit, as a minimum, the following content and skill areas:

1. Current scientific knowledge of aging and longevity, including theories of aging, the physiology and natural history of aging, pathologic changes with aging, epidemiology of aging populations, and diseases of the aged.
2. Aspects of preventive medicine, including nutrition, oral health, exercise, screening, immunization, and chemoprophylaxis against disease. Instruction about and experience with community resources dedicated to these activities should be included.
3. Geriatric assessment, including medical, affective, cognitive, functional status, social support, economic, and environmental aspects related to health; activities of daily living (ADL); the instrumental activities of daily living (IADL); the appropriate use of the history; physical and mental examination; and laboratory.
4. Appropriate interdisciplinary coordination of the actions of multiple health professionals, including physicians, nurses, social workers, dieticians, and rehabilitation experts, in the assessment and implementation of treatment.
5. Topics of special interest to geriatric medicine, including but not limited to cognitive impairment, depression and related disorders, falls, incontinence, osteoporosis, fractures, sensory impairment, pressure ulcers, sleep disorders, pain, senior (elder) abuse, malnutrition, and functional impairment.
6. Diseases that are especially prominent in the elderly or that have different characteristics in the elderly, including neoplastic, cardiovascular, neurologic, musculoskeletal, metabolic, and infectious disorders.
7. Pharmacologic problems associated with aging, including changes in pharmacokinetics and pharmacodynamics, drug interactions, overmedication, appropriate prescribing, and adherence.
8. Psychosocial aspects of aging, including interpersonal and family relationships, living situations, adjustment disorders, depression, bereavement, and anxiety.
9. The economic aspects of supporting services, including Title III of the Older Americans Act, Medicare, Medicaid, capitation, and cost containment.
10. Ethical and legal issues especially pertinent to geriatric medicine, including limitation of treatment, competency, guardianship, right to refuse treatment, advance directives, wills, and durable power of attorney for medical affairs.
11. General principles of geriatric rehabilitation, including those applicable to patients with orthopedic, rheumatologic, cardiac, and neurologic impairments. These principles should include those related to the use of physical medicine modalities, exercise, functional activities, assistive devices, environmental modification, patient and family education, and psychosocial and recreational counseling.
12. Management of patients in long-term care settings, including palliative care, knowledge of the administration, regulation, and financing of long-term institutions, and the continuum from short- to long-term care.
13. Research methodologies related to geriatric medicine, including clinical epidemiology, decision analysis, and critical literature review.
14. Perioperative assessment and involvement in management.
15. Iatrogenic disorders and their prevention.
16. Communication skills with patients, families, professional colleagues, and community groups, including presenting case reports, literature searches, and research papers, when appropriate, to peers and lectures to lay audiences.
17. The pivotal role of the family in caring for many elderly and the community resources (formal support systems) required to support both patient and family.
18. Cultural aspects of aging, including knowledge about demographics, health care status of older persons of diverse ethnicities, access to health care, cross-cultural assessment, and use of an interpreter in clinical care. Issues of ethnicity in long-term care, patient education, and special issues relating to urban and rural older persons of various ethnic backgrounds should be covered.
19. Home care, including the components of a home visit, and accessing appropriate community resources to provide care in the home setting.
20. Hospice care, including pain management, symptom relief, comfort care, and end-of-life issues.

V. Certification

Those planning to seek a Certificate of Added Qualifications from the American Board of Internal Medicine or the American Board of Family Practice should communicate with the administrative officer of the board as listed in the *Graduate Medical Education Directory* to ascertain the full requirements.

ACGME: February 1998 Effective: July 1998

Program Requirements for Residency Education in Family Practice Sports Medicine

I. Introduction

In addition to complying with the Program Requirements for Residency Education in Family Practice Geriatric Medicine and Family Practice Sports Medicine, programs must also comply with the following requirements, which may in some cases exceed the common requirements.

II. Scope and Duration of Training

An educational program in sports medicine must be organized to provide a well-supervised experience at a level sufficient for the resident to acquire the competence of a physician with added qualifications in this field. It shall be 12 months in duration.

The practice of sports medicine is the application of the physician's knowledge, skills, and attitudes to those engaged in sports and exercise. Thus, the program must provide training in the development of the clinical competencies needed to diagnose and manage medical illnesses and injuries related to sports and exercise, for example, first-degree sprains, strains, and contusions, including appropriate referrals of, for example, fractures, dislocations, and third-degree sprains. Clinical experience must include injury prevention, preparticipation evaluation, management of acute and chronic illness or injury, and rehabilitation, as applied to a broad spectrum of undifferentiated patients. There must be experience functioning as a team physician and in the promotion of physical fitness and wellness.

The program should emphasize physiology and biomechanics; principles of nutrition; pathology and pathophysiology of illness and injury; pharmacology; effects of therapeutic, performance-enhancing, and mood-altering drugs; psychological aspects of exercise, performance, and competition; ethical principles; and medical-legal aspects of exercise and sports.

III. Teaching Staff

In addition to the program director, each program must have at least one other faculty member with similar qualifications who devotes a substantial portion of professional time to the training program.

The teaching staff must include orthopedic surgeons who are engaged in the operative management of sports injuries and other conditions and who are readily available to teach and provide consultation to the residents. Teaching staff from the disciplines of nutrition, pharmacology, pathology, exercise physiology, physical therapy, behavioral science, physical medicine and rehabilitation, and clinical imaging also should be available to assist in the educational program. Coaches and athletic trainers also should be included.

IV. Facilities and Resources

The program must include the following:

A. Patient Population

A patient population that is unlimited by age or gender and is adequate in number and variety to meet the needs of the training program must be available. The program director must ensure that residents are accorded meaningful patient responsibility with the supervision of a faculty member at all facilities and sites.

B. Sports Medicine Clinic

There must be an identifiable clinic that offers continuing care to patients who seek consultation regarding sports- or exercise-related health problems. The nonsurgical trainees must be supervised by a physician who has qualifications in sports medicine and is certified by the American Board of Emergency Medicine, the American Board of Family Practice, the American Board of Internal Medicine, or the American Board of Pediatrics or who possesses suitable equivalent qualifications.

Adequate, up-to-date diagnostic imaging and rehabilitation services must be readily available and accessible to clinic patients. Consultation in medical and surgical subspecialties, physical therapy, nursing, nutrition, and pharmacy must be available. The opportunity to render continuing care and to organize recommendations from other specialties and disciplines is mandatory and will require that medical records include information pertinent to the assessment and management of patients with health problems related to sports and exercise.

C. Sporting Events/Team Sports/Mass-Participation Events

The program must have access to sporting events, team sports, and mass-participation events during which the resident can have meaningful patient responsibility.

D. Acute-Care Facility

There must be an acute-care hospital with a full range of services associated with and in proximity to the sponsoring residency. This facility must be readily accessible to patients served by the program.

V. Educational Program

The curriculum must provide the educational experiences necessary for the residents to achieve the cognitive knowledge, psychomotor skills, interpersonal skills, professional attitudes, and practical experience required of physicians in the care of patients with health problems related to sports and exercise.

Didactic as well as clinical learning opportunities must be provided as part of the required curriculum for all residents. Conferences or seminars/workshops in sports medicine should be specifically designed for the residents to augment the clinical experiences.

All educational activities must be adequately supervised, while allowing the resident to assume progressive responsibility for patient care. The clinical activities in sports medicine should represent a minimum of 50% of the time in the program. The remainder of the time should be spent in didactic, teaching, and/or research activities and in the primary care or emergency medicine ambulatory facility.

Residents must spend ½ day per week maintaining their skills in their primary specialty.

Participation in the following must be required of all residents:

A. Preparticipation Evaluation of the Athlete

The program must ensure that all sports medicine residents are involved in the development and conduct of preparticipation examination programs.

B. Acute Care

The resident must have appropriate authority and responsibility to participate meaningfully in the medical care that is provided to acute-care patients (see "Scope and Duration of Training," above). In addition, the program should arrange for residents to observe representative inpatient and outpatient operative orthopedic procedures.

C. Sports Medicine Clinic Experience

The resident must attend patients in a continuing, comprehensive manner, providing consultation for health problems related to

Program Requirements

sports and exercise. The resident shall spend at least 1 day per week for 10 months of the training period in this activity.

If patients are hospitalized, the resident should follow them during their inpatient stay and resume outpatient care following the hospitalization. Consultation with other physicians and professionals in other disciplines should be encouraged.

D. On-Site Sports Care

The resident should participate in planning and implementation of all aspects of medical care at various sporting events. The program must ensure that supervised sports medicine residents provide on-site care and management to participants in these events.

In addition, the resident must participate in the provision of comprehensive and continuing care to a sports team. Preferably, the experience should include several teams that engage in seasonal sports.

E. Mass-Participation Sports Events

The resident should participate in the planning and implementation of the provision of medical coverage for at least one mass-participation event. The program must ensure that its residents have experience that includes providing medical consultation, direct patient care, event planning, protection of participants, coordination with local EMS systems, and other medical aspects of those events.

VI. Specific Knowledge and Skills

A. Clinical

The program must provide educational experiences that enable residents to develop clinical competence in the overall field of sports medicine.

The curriculum must include but not be limited to the following content and skill areas:

1. Anatomy, physiology, and biomechanics of exercise
2. Basic nutritional principles and their application to exercise
3. Psychological aspects of exercise, performance, and competition
4. Guidelines for evaluation prior to participation in exercise and sport
5. Physical conditioning requirements for various activities
6. Special considerations related to age, gender, and disability
7. Pathology and pathophysiology of illness and injury as they relate to exercise
8. Effects of disease, eg, diabetes, cardiac conditions, arthritis, on exercise and the use of exercise in the care of medical problems
9. Prevention, evaluation, management, and rehabilitation of injuries
10. Understanding pharmacology and effects of therapeutic, performance-enhancing, and mood-altering drugs
11. Promotion of physical fitness and healthy lifestyles
12. Functioning as a team physician
13. Ethical principles as applied to exercise and sports
14. Medical-legal aspects of exercise and sports
15. Environmental effects on exercise
16. Growth and development related to exercise

B. Patient Education/Teaching

The program must provide the experiences necessary for the residents to develop and demonstrate competence in patient education regarding sports and exercise. They must have experience teaching others, eg, nurses, allied health personnel, medical students, residents, coaches, athletes, other professionals, and members of patients' families. There must also be relevant experience working in a community sports medicine network involving parents, coaches, certified athletic trainers, allied medical personnel, residents, and physicians.

ACGME: September 1994 Effective: July 1995

Program Requirements for Residency Education in Internal Medicine

I. Introduction

A. Definition and Scope of Specialty

Internal medicine is the discipline encompassing the study and practice of health promotion, disease prevention, diagnosis, and treatment of men and women from adolescence to old age, during times of health and through all stages of acute and chronic illness. Intrinsic to the discipline are the application of the scientific method of problem solving, decision making, and an attitude of caring driven by humanistic and professional values.

The practice of internal medicine requires comprehensive knowledge of human biology, behavior, and spirit; an understanding of the epidemiology and pathophysiology of disease; and the mechanisms of treatment. Internal medicine requires a mastery of clinical skills in interviewing, physical examination, differential diagnosis, diagnostic testing strategies, therapeutic techniques, counseling, and disease prevention.

B. Duration and Scope of Education

1. An accredited residency program in internal medicine must provide 36 months of supervised graduate education.
2. The educational program must include core clinical experiences in general internal medicine, the subspecialties of internal medicine, and other specialties. The clinical settings in which these experiences occur must include a minimum of one-third of the time in ambulatory sites and a minimum of one-third of the time in inpatient sites. Over the 36 months of training, at least ½ day each week must be spent managing a panel of general internal medicine patients in continuity.
3. The program must include a schedule of prescribed learning experiences accomplished through teaching rounds, conferences, lectures, and discussions that ensure the residents' mastery of the knowledge, skills, and attitudes needed to practice general internal medicine or to progress into a subspecialty, research, or a teaching career in internal medicine. The training program must include a written evaluation of clinical competence, medical knowledge, skills, and professional attitudes throughout the educational experience.
4. The internal medicine component of special educational tracks must be conducted under the auspices of the Department of Internal Medicine. Although such tracks may differ in educational content, the core experience of residents must provide training in both inpatient and ambulatory general internal medicine to enable the graduates of such special tracks to function as general internists. The Residency Review Committee (RRC) evaluates special educational tracks as part of internal medicine programs in the accreditation process.

II. Institutional Organization

A. Sponsoring Institution

1. Each internal medicine residency must have a single sponsoring institution. It must
   a. provide an environment of inquiry and scholarship in which residents participate in the development of new knowledge, learn to evaluate and apply research findings, and develop habits of inquiry as a continuing professional responsibility;
   b. establish the internal medicine residency within a department of internal medicine or an administrative unit whose mission

is the advancement of internal medicine education and patient care;

c. have an affiliation with a Liaison Committee on Medical Education-accredited medical school, or demonstrate that the primary clinical site has a commitment to education and research similar to that of a medical school;

d. have affiliations with community-based institutions, if the sponsoring institution lacks sufficient diversity in faculty, facilities, and resources in the inpatient and/or ambulatory settings;

e. provide adequate faculty, resident compensation, facilities, and resources for education, clinical care, and research required for accreditation;

f. designate a single program director within the internal medicine administrative unit to lead the internal medicine residency program and its subspecialty residencies at all sites and in all special tracks or combined specialty training with internal medicine; and

g. notify the RRC promptly of
   1. major changes in leadership, governance, affiliation, or fiscal arrangements that affect the educational program and
   2. a change in the program director. The qualifications and the curriculum vitae of the new program director must be submitted to the RRC.

   The RRC may schedule a site visit when notified about either of the above changes.

2. A sponsoring institution must not place excessive reliance on residents to meet the service needs of the participating training sites. To this end, the sponsoring and participating institutions must have institutional written policies or procedures that address the following:
   a. Residents must not routinely be required to provide intravenous, phlebotomy, or messenger/transporter services.
   b. Residents' service responsibilities must be limited to patients for whom the training program bears major diagnostic and therapeutic responsibility.
   c. On inpatient rotations, residents should have continuing responsibility for most of the patients they admit.
   d. Supervision by faculty members must be provided for all patient care activities in which residents are engaged.
   e. Educational experiences must include interactions with attending physicians and other residents, as well as teaching rounds, conferences, evaluation, and formative feedback.
   f. For each rotation or major clinical assignment, the teaching ratio must not exceed a total of 8 residents or students to one teaching attending.
   g. Total required emergency medicine experience must not exceed 3 months in 3 years of training for a resident.
   h. Total required critical care experience must not exceed 6 months in 3 years of training for a resident. (*Note:* When elective experience is added in the critical care unit, it must not result in more than a total of 8 months in 3 years of training for any resident.)
   i. When averaged over any 4-week rotation or assignment, residents must not spend more than 80 hours per week in patient care duties.
   j. Residents must not be assigned on-call in-house duty more often than every third night.
   k. When averaged over any 4-week rotation or assignment, residents must have at least 1 day out of 7 free of patient care duties.
   l. During emergency medicine assignments, continuous duty must not exceed 12 hours.
   m. Emergency medicine or night float assignments must be separated by at least 8 hours of non-patient-care duties.
   n. During ambulatory assignments, a first-year resident's patient load, on average, must not exceed two new patients or more than six return patients per 1/2 day session.
   o. On inpatient rotations or assignments (*Note:* These limits may be increased by 2 in special rotations where each admission does not require a full workup, providing it is educationally justified.)
      1. a first-year resident must not be responsible for more than five new patients per admitting day.
      2. a first-year resident must not be assigned more than eight new patient admissions in a 48-hour period.
      3. a first-year resident must not be responsible for the ongoing care of more than 12 patients.
      4. when supervising more than one first-year resident, the second- or third-year resident must not be responsible for the ongoing care of more than 24 patients.
      5. the second- or third-year resident must not be responsible for admitting more than a total of 10 new patients per admitting day or more than 16 new patients in a 48-hour period, which includes the first-year resident's patients being supervised.

B. Participating Institutions

1. Participation by any institution that provides more than 6 months of the training in the program must be approved by the RRC.
2. When two or more institutions affiliate to participate in residency education, a written agreement, signed by the authorities of each institution, must document the following:
   a. Purpose and scope of the affiliation for internal medicine residency education
   b. Financial, faculty, and facility resources involved
   c. An administrative relationship between the institutions that ensures the program director's authority to accomplish the goals and objectives of the clinical and didactic curriculum at all training sites
   d. Delegation of the authority and responsibility for the day-to-day program operations at the participating institution to a key faculty member who reports to the program director
   e. Assurance that residents assigned to all training sites will attend their continuity clinics and core conferences
3. At each participating training site, the program must be provided with the necessary professional, technical, and clerical personnel needed to support the residency.

C. Residents

1. Appointment of residents
   a. The program must select residents in accordance with institutional and departmental policies and procedures. The program should demonstrate the ability to retain qualified residents by graduating at the end of the residency at least 80% of the enrolled, first-year, categorical residents.
   b. No resident who has satisfactorily completed a preliminary training year may be appointed to 1 or more additional years as a preliminary resident in that program.
   c. Before accepting a resident in transfer from another program, the program director should receive a written evaluation of the resident's past performance from the previous program director(s).
2. Resident complement

   The RRC will stipulate the maximum total number of residents that can be supported by the educational resources for the program. The program director must obtain approval from the RRC before changing the number of approved residency positions. (*Note:* The resident complement is the total number of resident positions offered in the 3-year training program. The number includes all preliminary, categorical, and special track residents. For programs that offer combined internal medicine and another specialty training, the number added to the total resident complement is half of the total complement for the full term of the combined training.)

3. Resident advancement
The program director, with participation of members of the teaching staff, must advance residents to positions of higher responsibility only on the basis of evidence of their satisfactory progressive scholarship and professional growth.

III. Program Director and Faculty Qualifications and Responsibilities

A. General Qualifications and Responsibilities

1. Qualifications
The program director and all faculty members
   a. must be licensed to practice medicine in the state where the sponsoring institution is located. (Certain federal programs are exempted.)
   b. must have an appointment in good standing to the medical staff of an institution participating in the training program.
   c. should be certified by the specialty board or present equivalent credentials or experience acceptable to the RRC.
   d. must meet professional standards of ethical behavior.
2. Responsibilities
The program director and all faculty members
   a. must have a commitment to the goals and objectives of the teaching program, including development of the residents' medical knowledge; clinical, technical, and management skills; and clinical judgment.
   b. should be able to nurture the attributes of the scholar, scientist, teacher, and humanist in residents.
   c. should be available to residents for advice and counseling.
   d. must comply with the written curriculum that describes both patient-based and educational elements of the residency.
   e. should review the written learning objectives and expectations for each rotation or assignment with residents at the beginning of the rotation or assignment.
   f. must be sensitive to the need for timely provision of confidential counseling and psychological support services to residents.
   g. must provide written and verbal feedback to residents at the end of each rotation or assignment.

B. Program Director

1. Qualifications
The program director must
   a. be an institutionally based appointee, ie, his or her home office must be at the principal clinical training institution. The program director also must bear responsibility to the sponsoring institution.
   b. have at least 5 years of participation as an active faculty member in an accredited internal medicine residency program.
   c. be certified by the American Board of Internal Medicine or present equivalent credentials acceptable to the RRC.
2. Responsibilities
The program director
   a. must dedicate the majority of his or her professional effort, ie, an average of at least 20 hours per week throughout the year, to the internal medicine training program.
   b. must be primarily responsible for the organization, implementation, and supervision of all aspects of the training program, including the selection and supervision of the faculty members and other program personnel at each institution participating in the program.
   c. must select residents for appointment to the program in accordance with institutional and departmental policies and procedures, evaluate the quality of care rendered by the residents, have the authority to ensure effective teaching, and obtain teaching commitments from other departments involved in the education of internal medicine residents.
   d. must prepare written learning objectives and expectations outlining the educational goals and objectives of the program with respect to knowledge, skills, and other attributes of residents at each level of training and for each major rotation or other program assignment.
   e. must ensure that the written learning objectives and expectations are readily available for review and are distributed to residents and faculty members.
   f. must ensure that the residency does not place excessive reliance on service as opposed to education. (*Note:* See Section II.A.2. for examples of excessive service.)
   g. must notify the RRC promptly of
      1. any change in the number of residents in the training program and
      2. major changes in the structure of the educational program.

      The RRC may schedule a site visit when notified about either of the above changes.
   h. must prepare an accurate statistical and narrative description of the program, as required by the RRC.
   i. must monitor the residents' stress, including mental or emotional conditions inhibiting performance or learning and drug- or alcohol-related dysfunction.
   j. must evaluate and modify training situations that consistently produce undesirable stress on residents.
   k. must be responsible for the general administration of the program, including those activities related to the recruitment, selection, instruction, supervision, counseling, evaluation, and advancement of residents and the maintenance of records related to program accreditation.
   l. must establish and use educational standards that determine the residents' competence in procedures and skills.
   m. should monitor any internal medicine subspecialty training programs sponsored by the institution to ensure compliance with the Accreditation Council for Graduate Medical Education (ACGME) accreditation standards.
   n. should ensure that there is a rapid and reliable system for residents to communicate with supervising attending physicians and residents.
   o. must establish a system that ensures that attending physicians are available to participate in the residents' diagnostic and management decisions in a timely manner.
   p. should outline in written policies the lines of responsibility and supervision for the care of patients on all inpatient and ambulatory settings, including all clinical sites for all members of the teaching teams and program staff.

C. Key Clinical Faculty Members

The residency program must include four institutionally based faculty members, not including the program director and chief residents.

1. Qualifications
Key clinical faculty members must
   a. be certified by the American Board of Internal Medicine or present equivalent credentials acceptable to the RRC.
   b. have documented clinical, academic, and administrative experience to ensure effective implementation of the Program Requirements.

c. be clinicians with broad knowledge of, experience with, and commitment to internal medicine, whether trained as general internists or as subspecialists.

2. Responsibilities

Key clinical faculty members

a. must dedicate the majority of their professional effort, ie, an average of at least 20 hours per week throughout the year, to the internal medicine training program.

b. should participate in prescribed faculty development programs designed to enhance their teaching effectiveness.

c. should assist in the general administration of the program, including those activities related to the recruitment, selection, instruction, supervision, counseling, evaluation, and advancement of residents and the maintenance of records related to program accreditation.

d. must assist in the preparation of a written curriculum that describes both patient-based and educational elements of the residency and outlines the goals and objectives of the program with respect to knowledge, skills, and other attributes of residents at each level of training and for each major rotation or other program assignment.

e. must demonstrate that they share with the program director a commitment to the goals and objectives of the curriculum.

f. must assist in nurturing the attributes of the scholar, scientist, teacher, and humanist in the residents.

g. must assist in monitoring resident stress, including mental or emotional conditions inhibiting performance or learning and drug- or alcohol-related dysfunction.

D. Other Faculty

1. Qualifications

a. Qualified individuals (Division Chiefs) must be certified by the American Board of Internal Medicine in their internal medicine subspecialty or present equivalent credentials acceptable to the RRC.

b. Each division chief should have a term of office to achieve the educational goals and objectives of the residency.

c. Internal medicine subspecialty support should include adequate professional and teaching staff.

d. PhD faculty members not holding an MD may be included as other teaching faculty but they may not be regarded as key clinical faculty members.

2. Responsibilities

a. Division chiefs or their designates must be appointed to be responsible for teaching activities in the recognized internal medicine subspecialties.

b. Division chiefs must organize, supervise, and implement the clinical and educational subspecialty training as specified in the curriculum.

c. Each consultative service must be headed by a qualified individual who ensures that consultants participate in the education of residents on the medical teaching services.

d. Supervisors of special educational tracks must report directly to the internal medicine program director.

IV. Facilities and Resources

Modern hospital facilities (ie, diagnostic, therapeutic, and laboratory) to fulfill the curriculum must be available and functioning. Adequate facilities, support services, and space for outpatient teaching and patient care must be available. Residents must have clinical experiences in efficient, effective ambulatory care settings.

A. Space and Equipment

There must be space and equipment for the educational program, including meeting rooms, classrooms, examination rooms, computers, visual and other educational aids, and office space for teaching staff.

B. Facilities

1. To ensure that a spectrum of cardiovascular disorders is available for resident education, cardiac catheterization facilities should be present at the site(s) where the residents see the majority of their acutely ill, hospitalized patients with a range of cardiovascular diseases. If such facilities are not present, the program must demonstrate that all residents care for patients with a similar range of cardiovascular disorders.
2. Facilities should be available to the program to ensure that residents become proficient in the effective use of current and evolving technologies, that the involved institution(s) has an appropriate patient mix, and that related educational goals and objectives are achieved. These facilities should include but not be limited to those for bronchoscopy; coagulation studies; gastrointestinal motility and endoscopy; noninvasive cardiology studies; pulmonary function studies; hemodialysis; and imaging studies including radionuclide, ultrasound, fluoroscopy, plain films, angiography, computer tomography, and magnetic resonance.
3. Internal medicine subspecialty resources should include specialized laboratory and technical facilities.
4. Residents must have sleeping, lounge, and food facilities during assigned duty hours. When residents are assigned night duty in the hospital, they must be provided with on-call facilities that are convenient and that afford privacy, safety, and a restful environment. The safety of residents at all times while on duty is essential. Residents must be instructed regarding fire protocols, electrical safety, protocols and dangers relating to hazardous materials, and assault safeguards. Security personnel must be available as necessary.
5. It is desirable that the program use community resources such as physicians' offices, neighborhood health centers, or home-care and/or managed-care facilities to broaden the base of residents' clinical experiences with ambulatory patients.

C. Medical Records

1. A medical records department that facilitates both patient care and residents' education must be available.
2. Clinical records that document both inpatient and ambulatory care must be maintained such that prompt accessibility is ensured at all times.

D. Medical Library

1. A medical library under the direction of a qualified medical librarian must be readily accessible.
2. There must be a means of access to an on-site library or to reference material in each participating institution during those times when the library is not open or staffed.
3. The library must contain a representative selection of books and journals on internal medicine.
4. At all training sites, residents should have access to a computerized literature search system and electronic medical databases.

E. Patient Population

1. Patients must be available in sufficient numbers for training purposes in general internal medicine in inpatient, ambulatory, and other settings.
2. Patients must exhibit a variety of clinical problems to provide broad experience in general internal medicine in inpatient, ambulatory, and other settings.
3. There must be patients of both sexes, with a broad range of age from adolescent to geriatric patients.
4. The clinical experience should include opportunities to have exposure to patients of a disadvantaged socioeconomic status.

F. Pathology Material

1. All deaths of patients who received care by residents must be reviewed and autopsies performed whenever possible.
2. Residents should review the gross pathological and/or histological specimens soon after autopsies are performed on their patients and should review the autopsy reports.

G. Support Services

1. Inpatient clinical support services must be available on a 24-hour basis to meet reasonable and expected demands, including intravenous services, phlebotomy services, messenger/transporter services, and laboratory and radiologic information retrieval systems that allow prompt access to results.
2. At all training sites, medical records, x-ray films, and results of diagnostic studies must be readily available.
3. Consultations from other clinical services in the hospital should be available in a timely manner. All consultations should be by or under the supervision of a qualified specialist.

V. Educational Program

A. Program Goals and Objectives (Written Curriculum)

All educational components of the residency should be related to the program's goals and objectives and set down in a written curriculum. For each rotation or major learning experience, the written curriculum

1. should include the educational purpose; teaching methods; the mix of diseases, patient characteristics, and types of clinical encounters, procedures, and services; reading lists, pathological material, and other educational resources to be used; and a method of evaluation of resident performance.
2. must include all required educational and clinical experiences specified in the Program Requirements.
3. must include the clinical experience in inpatient or outpatient settings.
4. must define the level of residents' supervision by faculty members in all patient care activities.
5. must integrate medical problems; health promotion; and cultural, socioeconomic, ethical, occupational, environmental, and behavioral issues in most rotations or major learning experiences.
6. must be approved as part of the regular review process by the RRC, along with the program design and/or structure.
7. must include teaching rounds and conferences during which residents
   a. apply knowledge of the etiology, pathogenesis, clinical presentation, and natural history of the diseases treated by internists to demonstrate skills in diagnosis, mature judgment, and resourcefulness in therapy;
   b. receive instruction and feedback to master the interviewing, communication, and interpersonal skills that are necessary to elicit and record a thorough and accurate history, establish and maintain a therapeutic physician-patient relationship, and initiate or motivate the patient to implement optimal medical management;
   c. receive instruction and feedback to develop expertise in physical examination skills that include training in bimanual female pelvic examination, PAP smears, and speculum examination of the vagina; and
   d. demonstrate the humanistic treatment of patients.
8. must indicate that residents care for patients with a wide range of clinical problems in all stages of illness.
9. should include rotations or assignments during which residents learn to work with other members of the health-care team and learn to become leaders in the organization and management of patient care.
10. should be revised by faculty members and residents to keep it current and relevant.

B. Presence of Other Residents

For each year of training, the percentage of resident-months on those inpatient services used for training internal medicine residents that can be assigned to residents other than those enrolled in internal medicine in categorical (3-year), preliminary (1-year), and special tracks (ie, primary care, combined internal medicine-specialty training) and transitional-year program residents sponsored by internal medicine must be less than 25%. (*Note:* Excluded entirely from this limitation are residents from any program who receive training in internal medicine on services to which no internal medicine residents at any level of training are concurrently assigned.)

C. Peer Interaction

1. A program must have a minimum of 12 residents enrolled and participating in the training program at all times.
2. Inpatient rotations must have first-year residents interacting with more senior internal medicine residents in the care of patients.

D. Meaningful Patient Responsibility

1. Each resident must be assigned for a minimum of 24 months to internal medicine inpatient and ambulatory rotations or assignments during which the resident has primary responsibility for patient care. These inpatient and ambulatory assignments must include development of diagnostic strategies, planning, record keeping, order or prescription writing, management, discharge summary preparation, and decision-making commensurate with residents' abilities and with appropriate supervision by the attending physician.
2. On inpatient rotations, second- or third-year residents with documented experience appropriate to the acuity, complexity, and severity of patient illness should be available at all times on-site to supervise first-year residents.
3. Residents must write all orders for patients under their care, with appropriate supervision by the attending physician. In those unusual circumstances when an attending physician or subspecialty resident writes an order on a resident's patient, the attending or subspecialty resident must communicate his or her action to the resident in a timely manner.

E. Progressive Responsibility

1. The program must ensure, with each year of training, that each resident has increasing responsibility in patient care, leadership, teaching, and administration.
2. Residents from other specialties must not supervise internal medicine residents on any internal medicine inpatient rotation.

F. Individual Responsibility

1. During rotations or assignments where meaningful patient responsibility occurs, there must be a resident schedule, including check-out and check-in procedures, so residents will learn to work in teams to ensure proper care and welfare of the patients.
2. The on-call system must include a plan for backup to ensure that patient care is not jeopardized during or following assigned periods of duty.
3. The residency is a full-time responsibility. Activities outside the training program should not interfere with the resident's educational performance.

G. Formal Teaching Program

1. Rounds
   a. Teaching rounds

Teaching rounds must be patient-based sessions in which a few cases are presented as a basis for discussion of such points as interpretation of clinical data, pathophysiology, differential diagnosis, specific management of the patient, the appropriate use of technology, and disease prevention.

1. Inpatient and ambulatory teaching rounds must be regularly scheduled and formally conducted.
2. In addition to morning report, inpatient teaching rounds must occur at least 3 days of the week for a minimum of 4 ½ hours per week.
3. Teaching rounds must include direct resident and attending interaction with the patient. The teaching sessions must include demonstration and evaluation of each resident's interview and physical examination skills.
4. Inpatient teaching rounds must include bedside teaching.

b. Management rounds by the physician of record

1. Each physician of record has the responsibility to interact at intervals with his or her patients and to communicate effectively and frequently with the resident staff participating in the care of these patients. It is desirable that this communication be achieved by the physician of record making management rounds on his or her patients at least daily with at least one member of the resident team.
2. To avoid interference with the resident's educational experience, the resident should not be required to relate to excessive numbers of physicians.
3. Although management rounds may offer many educational opportunities, they are not to be confused with or to take the place of teaching rounds. Also, management rounds by the physician of record should not interfere with resident work rounds. (*Note:* Work rounds are rounds in which a senior resident supervises a junior resident's patient care activities, without an attending physician present.) Management rounds by the physician of record are not time-specific and should be commensurate with the needs of the patient.

2. Conferences and seminars

a. Departmental conferences, seminars, and literature-review activities covering both general medicine and the internal medicine subspecialties should be conducted regularly and sufficiently often to fulfill educational goals.

b. The conference schedule must have a core conference series dealing with the major topics in general internal medicine (including issues arising in ambulatory and extended care settings) and the internal medicine subspecialties.

c. The core conference series should be repeated often enough to afford each resident an opportunity to complete the curriculum.

d. Conferences should include information from the basic medical sciences, with emphasis on the pathophysiology of disease and reviews of recent advances in clinical medicine and biomedical research.

e. Conferences correlating current pathological material, including material from autopsies, surgical specimens, and other pathology material, with the clinical course and management of patients must be held at least monthly. Faculty members and attending physicians from other disciplines should be involved.

f. Conferences should include a journal club that emphasizes a critical appraisal of the medical literature.

g. Residents and faculty members should participate in the planning, production, and presentation of conferences.

h. It is desirable that each resident attend at least 60% of those conferences designated as required by the program director.

3. Self-assessment

It is desirable that the program director have each resident use prescribed self-assessment techniques as an educational tool for monitoring his or her own progress toward the program's educational objectives. (*Note:* For example, the program director could have residents participate in in-training examinations or self-study courses.)

4. Basic sciences

a. The basic sciences should be integrated into the daily clinical activities by clearly linking the pathophysiologic process and findings to the diagnosis, treatment, and management of clinical disorders.

b. Residents should acquire an in-depth understanding of the basic mechanisms of normal and abnormal human biology and behavior and the application of current knowledge to practice.

H. Specific Patient Care Experiences

1. Experience with ambulatory patients

a. At least one-third of the residency training must be in the ambulatory care setting. (*Note:* In assessing the contribution of various clinical experiences with ambulatory patients to the 33% minimum, the following guidelines can be used: ½ day per week assigned to an ambulatory setting throughout all 3 years of training is equivalent to 10%; a 1-month block rotation is equivalent to 3%; 1 full day per week throughout a single year of training is equivalent to 7%. Examples of settings that may be counted toward this requirement are general medicine continuity clinics, subspecialty clinics, ambulatory block rotations, physicians' offices, managed health care systems, emergency medicine, "walk-in" clinics, neighborhood health clinics, and home-care visits.)

b. Residents' clinical experiences with ambulatory patients must occur in each of the 3 years of residency training.

c. The residents' clinical experiences with ambulatory patients must include first-contact, comprehensive, and continuing care covering a broad spectrum of disease.

d. No more than 2 months (6%) of emergency medicine experience will count toward the required ambulatory experience.

e. In an ambulatory setting, one faculty member must be responsible for no more than five residents.

f. On-site faculty members' primary responsibilities must include the supervision and teaching of residents. On-site supervision as well as the quality of the educational experience must be documented.

g. The patient volume in the ambulatory environment must be large enough to provide adequate numbers of new patients. In general medicine settings, patient loads should, on average, be not less than one new patient and not less than three return patients per ½-day session for each resident.

h. Residents must be able to obtain appropriate and timely consultation from other specialties for their ambulatory patients.

i. There should be services available from and collegial relationships with other health-care professionals such as nurses, social workers, and dietitians.

j. Training in ambulatory care of patients should take place in an environment similar to an office practice.

k. The residents' clinical experiences with ambulatory patients should include the opportunity to develop diagnostic and therapeutic skills and professional attitudes in the care of general internal medicine patients.

l. It is desirable that supervision be provided by physicians experienced in the broad field of general internal medicine. (*Note:* The program director may assign experienced and qualified [ie, board certified or equivalent] practitioners from other specialties [eg, family practice] to participate as teachers in the ambulatory setting.)

m. It is desirable that block rotations in the ambulatory setting in subspecialty experiences be utilized to increase the residents' ambulatory experience.
n. It is desirable that 50% of the ambulatory experience take place in a general internal medicine setting.

2. Experience with continuity ambulatory patients
   a. The residents must have continuing patient care experience (continuity clinic) in an ambulatory care setting at least ½ day each week over each of the 3 years of training. (*Note:* Preliminary year residents are excluded from this requirement.)
   b. Residents may be excused from attending their continuity clinic when they are assigned to an intensive care unit or to emergency medicine. The continuing patient care experience should not be interrupted by more than 1 month, excluding a resident's vacation.
   c. The residents' clinical experiences with ambulatory patients must provide residents the opportunity to observe and to learn the natural course of disease.
   d. During the continuity experience, arrangements should be made to minimize interruptions of the experience by residents' inpatient duties.
   e. Each resident must have the opportunity to follow patients on a long-term basis. It is desirable that such long-term observation include following patients from the ambulatory to the inpatient environment as well as from the inpatient to the ambulatory environment.
3. Experience with hospitalized patients
   a. It is desirable that 50% of the inpatient experience occur on general internal medicine services.
   b. There must be a minimum of 6 months of internal medicine teaching service assignments in the first year, and over the second and third years of training combined, a minimum of 6 months of such training.
   c. Geographic concentration of inpatients assigned to a given resident is desirable because such concentration promotes effective teaching and fosters interaction with other health personnel.
4. Emergency medicine experience
   a. Internal medicine residents assigned to emergency medicine must have first-contact responsibility for a sufficient number of unselected patients to meet the educational needs of internal medicine residents. Triage by other physicians prior to this contact is unacceptable.
   b. Internal medicine residents must be assigned to emergency medicine for at least 4 weeks of direct experience in blocks of not less than 2 weeks.
   c. Residents must have meaningful responsibility for patients, including participation in diagnosis, management, and admission decisions across the broad spectrum of medical and surgical illnesses such that the residents learn how to determine which patients require hospitalization.
   d. Internal medicine residents assigned to rotations on emergency medicine must have on-site, 24-hour, daily supervision by qualified faculty members.
   e. The rotations should be conducted in accordance with a written curriculum. Both the written curriculum and the faculty members should be acceptable to the program director in internal medicine.
   f. Consultations from other specialties should be readily available.
5. Critical care unit experience
   a. Residents must participate directly in the care of patients with various illnesses in critical care units (eg, intensive care units, cardiac care units, respiratory care units).
   b. The assignment must have supervision by trained internists with consultation by internal medicine subspecialists and other specialists.
   c. The assignment must have critical care unit teaching rounds and conferences acceptable to the program director in internal medicine.
   d. The experience must not be less than 3 months in 3 years of training for any resident.
   e. The assignment should be conducted in accordance with a written curriculum. Both the written curriculum and the faculty members should be acceptable to the program director in internal medicine.
6. Subspecialty Experience
   a. Education in the various subspecialties of internal medicine should be part of the training program and should be gained in both inpatient and ambulatory settings.
   b. Although it is not necessary that each resident be assigned to every subspecialty, it is important that each resident have exposure to the diagnostic and therapeutic methods of each of the recognized internal medicine subspecialties.
   c. At a minimum, residents should acquire knowledge sufficient to diagnose, follow, and treat patients with common disorders of the various organ systems covered by the internal medicine subspecialties and to recognize those disorders that should be referred to, or managed jointly with, the appropriate subspecialists.
7. Consultative experience
   a. Residents should have sufficient knowledge and experience to act, under supervision, as consultants to physicians in other specialties.
   b. It is desirable that the principles involved in consultation be included in the core conference series.
8. Geriatric medicine
   a. Residents must have formal instruction and regular, supervised clinical experience in geriatric medicine.
   b. The written curriculum must include experiences in the care of a broad range of elderly patients.
   c. Geriatric clinical experiences must be offered. They may occur at one or more specifically designated geriatric inpatient units, geriatric consultation services, long-term care facilities, geriatric ambulatory clinics, and/or in home-care settings.
9. Adolescent medicine
   a. Residents should be formally instructed in adolescent medicine, which may include the following topics: health promotion, family planning and human sexuality, sexually transmitted diseases (STDs), chemical dependency, sports medicine, and school health issues.
   b. Structured patient care experiences directed by faculty in advising young patients on these topics is desirable.
10. Gender-specific health care
    Residents should receive instruction in the prevention, counseling, detection, and diagnosis and treatment of diseases of women and men, as well as opportunities for clinical experience. (*Note:* This can occur in women's health clinics, obstetric or gynecologic clinics, STD clinics, general medicine clinics, urology clinics, or other specialty clinics.)
11. Experiences in other specialties
    a. Residents should have sufficient experience in neurology, psychiatry, dermatology, medical ophthalmology, otorhinolaryngology, orthopedics, and rehabilitation medicine to become familiar with those aspects of care in each specialty area that are diagnosed and managed by general internists and with

those that should be referred to, or managed jointly with, other specialists.

b. It is desirable that some of the residents' clinical experiences with ambulatory patients include these specialties.

12. Procedures and technical skills

a. Procedures

1. All residents must be instructed in indications, contraindications, complications, limitations, and interpretations of findings; they must develop technical proficiency in performing the following procedures: advanced cardiopulmonary resuscitation, access techniques to obtain venous and arterial blood, abdominal paracentesis, thoracentesis, arthrocentesis of the knee, central venous line placement, lumbar puncture, and nasogastric intubation.

2. Residents should be instructed in additional procedural skills that will be determined by the training environment, residents' practice expectations, the availability of skilled teaching faculty, and privilege delineation. These procedures may include but are not limited to arterial line placement; bone marrow aspiration; bladder catheterization; elective cardioversion; endotracheal intubation; flexible sigmoidoscopy; pulmonary artery balloon flotation catheter placement; skin biopsy (punch); temporary pacemaker placement; ambulatory electrocardiographic interpretation; treadmill exercise testing, supervision, and interpretation; fitting vaginal diaphragms; topical chemotherapy for external genital warts; endometrial biopsy; and insertion and removal of IUDs.

b. Interpretative skills

All residents should be given an opportunity to develop competency in interpretation of electrocardiograms, chest roentgenograms, Gram stains of sputum, microscopic examinations of urine, spirometry, and KOH and wet prep examinations of vaginal discharge for clue cells, candida, and trichomonas.

I. Professional Ethical Behavior

1. Physician accountability

a. The training program must have mentors, role-model clinicians, and a resident culture that demonstrates the values of professionalism, such as placing the needs of patients first, maintaining a commitment to scholarship, helping colleagues meet their responsibilities, a commitment to continued improvement, and being responsive to society's health-care needs.

b. Residents should be given the opportunity to participate in community service, professional organizations, and institutional committee activities.

2. Humanistic qualities

Physicians must have the welfare of their patients as their primary professional concern. Thus, the resident, faculty members, and program must demonstrate humanistic qualities that foster the formation of patient/physician relationships. These qualities include integrity, respect, compassion, professional responsibility, courtesy, sensitivity to patient needs for comfort and encouragement, and a professional attitude and behavior toward colleagues. The written curriculum must emphasize the importance of humanistic qualities throughout the residency.

3. Physician impairment

The residency program must instruct residents and faculty members in physician impairment, to include the recognition of, intervention in, and management of impairment such as alcohol and other substance abuse; depression; dementia; and other mental, emotional, and physical disorders in their peers, as well as the principles and methods of active intervention.

4. Professional ethics

The training program must foster a commitment to professional ethics in residents that is demonstrated by a spirit of collegiality and a high standard of moral and ethical behavior within the clinical setting in the care of patients, in the education of residents, in conducting research, and in interacting with pharmaceutical companies and funding organizations.

J. Special Educational Requirements

1. Clinical ethics

The program must include education in the principles of bioethics as applied to medical care, and the residents must participate in decision making involving ethical issues that arise in the diagnosis and management of their patients.

2. Quality assessment, quality improvement, risk management, and cost effectiveness in medicine

a. Residents should receive instruction in the social and economic impact of medical decisions on patients and society and the need to be the primary advocate for patients' needs.

b. It is desirable that all residents receive formal instruction regarding the principles, objectives, and processes of quality assessment and improvement and of risk management.

3. Preventive medicine

a. Screening for disease, disease prevention, maintenance of general health, and health promotion should be emphasized in the curriculum.

b. It is desirable that all residents receive instruction in occupational and environmental disease processes and in methods for their control.

4. Medical informatics and decision-making skills

a. Residents should receive instruction in the critical assessment of medical literature, in clinical epidemiology, in biostatistics, and in clinical decision theory.

b. Each resident should receive instruction in basic computer skills. Instruction should include an introduction to computer capabilities and medical applications, basic techniques for electronic retrieval of medical literature, computer-assisted medical instruction, and electronic information networks.

5. Law and public policy

Residents must receive instruction in the basic legal principles inherent in the practice of internal medicine, including issues of informed consent, advance medical directives, "do not resuscitate" orders, organ donation, living wills, patient advocacy, and related state laws concerning patients' rights.

6. Pain management

Each resident should receive instruction in the principles and practice of pain management, including symptom assessment and control.

7. End-of-life care

a. Each resident should receive instruction in the principles of palliative care for terminally ill patients, including the role of the health-care team. Instruction should include psychosocial, cultural, and religious issues related to death and dying.

b. It is desirable that residents participate in hospice and home care.

8. Principles of managed care

It is desirable that each resident receive instruction in the principles of managed care, including but not limited to the development and use of critical pathways and cost-efficient use of medical resources.

9. Violence

It is desirable that all residents receive instruction in the principles of recognition and management of domestic violence and of sexual, family, and elder abuse.

10. Substance use disorders

All residents should receive instruction in diagnosis and management of alcoholism and other substance abuse. The instruction should include the principles of addiction medicine and interventional techniques. Residents should have clinical experience in managing patients with alcoholism and substance abuse disorders.

11. Sports medicine and school health
It is desirable that all residents receive instruction in the areas of preparticipation sports assessment, injury prevention, evaluative management, and rehabilitation related to athletic and recreational injuries.

K. Research and Scholarly Activities

1. Faculty
The responsibility for establishing and maintaining an environment of inquiry and scholarship rests with the faculty members. While not all faculty members must be investigators, key clinical faculty members must demonstrate broad involvement in scholarly activity. Collectively, their activity must include all of the following:
   a. Active participation in clinical discussions, rounds, and conferences in a manner that promotes a spirit of inquiry and scholarship. Scholarship implies an in-depth understanding of basic mechanisms of normal and abnormal states and the application of current knowledge to practice.
   b. Participation in journal clubs that emphasize a critical appraisal of the medical literature.
   c. Active participation in regional or national professional and scientific societies.
   d. Provision of support for resident participation in scholarly activities.
   e. Regular interaction of residents with clearly identified faculty members (preferably key clinical faculty members)
      1. who participate in research conferences that emphasize the presentation of original research.
      2. who participate in research that leads to publication or to presentations at regional and national scientific meetings. (*Note:* For example, key clinical faculty member participation in original research projects subject to peer review, case reports, or single- or multi-institution clinical trials.)
      3. who offer guidance and technical support such as research design and statistical analysis to residents involved in research.
2. Residents
Prior to the completion of training, each resident
   a. must demonstrate acceptable scholarly activity such as original research, comprehensive case reports, or review of assigned clinical and research topics and
   b. should have basic science literacy and understand the fundamental principles of clinical study design and evaluation of research findings.

VI. Evaluation

A. Residents

1. Formative evaluation
   a. The program director must evaluate the clinical competence of the residents on a regular basis. The evaluation must include intellectual abilities, clinical skills, interpersonal skills and relationship building, and the development of professional attitudes consistent with being a physician. The resident must be closely observed performing specific tasks of patient management such as the interview and physical examination, choice of diagnostic studies, formulation of differential diagnosis or problem lists, development of plans for short-term and long-term medical management, communication of treatment plans, invasive procedures, and (when on inpatient services) discharge planning. A structured clinical evaluation must be conducted at least once during the first 2 years of the training program for each resident. (*Note:* For example, a mini-clinical evaluation exercise, such as that described in publications by the American Board of Internal Medicine.)
   b. Residents' humanistic qualities must be evaluated by faculty members, peers, and others during all observed clinical encounters.
   c. Chart auditing for format and quality of data entry should be done on a representative sample of resident inpatient and outpatient records (including inpatient discharge summaries) during each rotation, with feedback to the residents. The program director should ensure that the auditing of medical records is incorporated into evaluation components of the program.
   d. Records must be maintained by documentation logbook or by an equivalent method to demonstrate that residents have had experience with invasive procedures. These records must state the indications and complications and include the names of the supervising physicians. Such records must be of sufficient detail to permit use in future credentialing.
   e. Residents must be evaluated in writing and their performance reviewed with them verbally on completion of each rotation period.
   f. Formal evaluations of knowledge, skills, and professional growth of residents and required counseling by the program director or designee must occur at least semiannually.
   g. Permanent records of the evaluation and counseling process for each resident must be maintained for each resident.
   h. Such records must be available in the resident's file and must be accessible to the resident and other authorized personnel.
2. Summative evaluation
   a. The program director must prepare an evaluation (eg, the American Board of Internal Medicine's tracking form) of the clinical competence of each resident annually and at the conclusion of the resident's period of training in the program. Such evaluations stipulate the degree to which the resident has mastered each component of clinical competence (ie, clinical judgment, medical knowledge, clinical skills, humanistic qualities, professional attitudes and behavior, and provision of medical care) and has acquired proficiency in each of the various procedural skills identified in the program's curriculum. They should verify that the resident has demonstrated sufficient professional ability to practice competently and independently.
   b. A record of the evaluations must be maintained in the program files to substantiate future judgments in hospital credentialing, board certification, agency licensing, and in other bodies' actions.
   c. In the event of an adverse annual evaluation, a resident must be offered an opportunity to address a judgment of academic deficiencies or misconduct before a constituted clinical competence committee.
   d. There must be a written policy that ensures that academic due process provides fundamental fairness to the resident and protects the institution by ensuring accurate, proper, and definitive resolution of disputed evaluations.

B. Faculty Members and Program

1. Resident evaluation of faculty members and program
   a. The educational effectiveness of a program must be evaluated at least annually in a systematic manner. Specifically, the quality of the curriculum and the extent to which the educational

goals and objectives have been met by residents must be assessed. Written evaluations by residents must be utilized in developing programmatic changes.

b. The faculty must be organized and have regular documented meetings to review program goals and objectives as well as program effectiveness in achieving them.

c. At least one resident representative should participate in these reviews of the training program.

d. The faculty should at least annually evaluate the utilization of the resources available to the program, the contribution of each institution participating in the program, the financial and administrative support of the program, the volume and variety of patients available to the program for educational purposes, the performance of faculty members, and the quality of supervision of residents.

e. Provision should be made for residents to evaluate the faculty members annually. The results of the evaluations should be used for faculty-member counseling and for selecting faculty members for specific teaching assignments.

2. Certifying examination

a. A program's graduates must achieve a pass rate on the certifying examination of the American Board of Internal Medicine of at least 50% for first-time takers of the examination for the most recent defined 3-year period.

b. At least 75% of those completing their training in the program for the most recent defined 3-year period must have taken the certifying examination.

VII. Certification

Residents who plan to seek certification by the American Board of Internal Medicine should communicate with the registration section of the board regarding fulfillment of requirements for certification. Residents must be certified in internal medicine prior to seeking certification in a subspecialty.

ACGME: June 1997 Effective: July 1998

Policies and Procedures for Residency Education in the Subspecialties of Internal Medicine

1. As a general rule, subspecialty programs will be surveyed and reviewed in conjunction with the parent residency program in internal medicine. In the case of applications, or as determined by the Residency Review Committee (RRC), a subspecialty program may be surveyed and reviewed separately.
2. Subspecialty program information forms will be distributed to the director of the parent internal medicine residency program, who will coordinate the collection of information, completion of the forms, and submission of required materials to the RRC for all subspecialty programs to be reviewed.
3. The survey may be conducted by a member of the Field Staff or by a specialist selected by the RRC. The surveyor will submit a report on the internal medicine residency program as well as on each of the subspecialty programs under review.
4. Subspecialty programs will be designated as "accredited" or "nonaccredited." No other delineation of accreditation categories will be used. The accreditation status of subspecialty programs will be directly related to that of the parent internal medicine program as follows:

a. Applications for accreditation of new subspecialty programs will be considered only if the parent residency program in internal medicine carries the status of full accreditation.

b. Applications for accreditation of new subspecialty programs will not be considered if the parent residency program in internal medicine is (1) accredited on a provisional or probationary basis; or (2) involved in the process of implementing appeal procedures.

c. Application for combined subspecialty training programs such as hematology and oncology or pulmonary disease and critical care medicine will not be considered if the application is based on an existing subspecialty program accredited with warning.

d. When a subspecialty program is found not to be in substantial compliance with the *Essentials of Accredited Residencies*, the program director will be warned that accreditation will be withdrawn if the program is found not to be in substantial compliance with the *Essentials* at the time of the next scheduled review, regardless of the accreditation status of the parent internal medicine program.

e. If the parent internal medicine program is accredited on a probationary basis, or accredited on a provisional basis with a warning that adverse action will be taken if the program is not in substantial compliance with the *Essentials of Accredited Residencies* at the time of the next scheduled review, the subspecialty programs will be informed that their accreditation status is in jeopardy.

In addition, if the primary subspecialty program is accredited with a warning that an adverse action will be taken if the program is not in substantial compliance with the *Essentials of Accredited Residencies* at the time of the next scheduled review, the linked secondary subspecialty program (eg, cardiovascular disease and clinical cardiac electrophysiology) will be informed that its accreditation status is in jeopardy. Further, accreditation of the secondary subspcialty program will be administratively withdrawn if the RRC withdraws accreditation of the primary subspecialty program.

Thereafter, accreditation of the subspecialty programs will be administratively withdrawn if the RRC (1) continues accreditation of the parent residency program in internal medicine on a probationary basis beyond 2 years; (2) withdraws accreditation of the parent residency program in internal medicine.

f. Withdrawal of accreditation of the parent internal medicine residency program under circumstances other than those described above will also result in simultaneous withdrawal of all subspecialty programs.

5. In case of withholding accreditation or withdrawing accreditation of subspecialty programs, the Procedures for Proposed Adverse Actions and the Procedures for Appeal of Adverse Actions apply.

Program Requirements for Residency Education in the Subspecialties of Internal Medicine

I. General Information

A. Subspecialty training in internal medicine is a voluntary component in the continuum of the educational process; such training should take place on satisfactory completion of an accredited program in internal medicine. A minimum of 75% of residents in each subspecialty program should be graduates of an Accreditation Council for Graduate Medical Education (ACGME)-accredited internal medicine training program. (*Note:* The minimum of 75% of residents in the subspecialty of geriatric medicine should be graduates of either an ACGME-accredited internal medicine or family practice training program.)

B. To be eligible for accreditation, a subspecialty program must function as an integral part of an accredited residency program in internal medicine. There must be a reporting relationship, to ensure compliance with the ACGME accreditation standards, from the program director of the subspecialty program to the program director of the parent internal medicine residency program. The discipline must be one for which a certificate of special qualifications or a certificate of added qualifications is offered by the American Board of Internal Medicine. (The information herein applies to subspecialty disciplines in internal medicine as well as to disciplines for which a certificate of added qualifications is offered by the American Board of Internal Medicine. For editorial purposes, the term subspecialty is used throughout the document for both types of training programs.)

C. Applications for accreditation of new subspecialty programs will not be considered if the parent residency program in internal medicine is accredited on a provisional or probationary basis.

D. Sponsoring institutions must have an affiliation with a Liaison Committee on Medical Education-accredited medical school or demonstrate that the primary clinical site has a commitment to education and research similar to that of a medical school. In addition, the sponsoring institution must provide adequate faculty, resident compensation, facilities, and resources for education, clinical care, and research required for accreditation.

E. The program design and/or structure must be approved by the Residency Review Committee (RRC) as part of the regular review process.

F. Graduate education in the subspecialties of internal medicine requires a major commitment to education by the sponsoring institution. Evidence of such a commitment includes each of the following:
   1. The minimum number of resident positions in each training program must not be less than the number of accredited training years in the program.
   2. The institution must sponsor significant research in each subspecialty for which it sponsors a training program.
   3. The institution should sponsor a minimum of three accredited subspecialty programs, including three programs based at the primary training site of the parent internal medicine residency program. (*Note:* Internal medicine training programs in geriatric medicine and sports medicine are exempt.)

II. Educational Program

A. Subspecialty programs must provide advanced training to allow the resident to acquire expertise as a consultant in the subspecialty.

B. All educational components of the program should be related to the program's goals and objectives and set down in a written curriculum. The curriculum must ensure the opportunity for residents to achieve the cognitive knowledge, procedural skills, interpersonal skills, professional attitudes, humanistic qualities, and practical experience required of a subspecialist. The written curriculum should
   1. include for each rotation or major learning experience the educational purpose; teaching methods; the mix of diseases, patient characteristics, and types of clinical encounters, procedures, and services; reading lists, pathological material, and other educational resources to be used; and a method of evaluation of resident performance.
   2. include a description of all required educational and clinical experiences specified in the Program Requirements.
   3. include a description of the clinical experience in inpatient or outpatient settings.
   4. define the level of residents' supervision by faculty members in all patient care activities.
   5. integrate medical problems, health promotion, and cultural, socioeconomic, ethical, occupational, environmental, and behavioral issues in most rotations or major learning experiences.
   6. include teaching rounds and conferences.
   7. indicate that residents care for patients with a wide range of clinical problems in all stages of illness.
   8. emphasize the importance of humanistic qualities throughout the residency.
   9. document explicit methods of evaluation of residents' performance and the educational effectiveness of the program.
   10. be revised by faculty members and residents to keep it current and relevant.
   11. be approved as part of the regular review process by the RRC.

C. The program should provide residents adequate opportunity to become leaders in the organization and management of patient care.

D. The program must emphasize scholarship, self-instruction, development of critical analysis of clinical problems, and the ability to make appropriate decisions.

E. Appropriate faculty supervision of the residents must be provided during all of their educational experiences.

F. Participation by any institution providing more than 3 months of training in a program of less than 3 years in duration or more than 6 months of training in a program of 3 years in duration must be prior approved by the RRC. The principles of education enumerated in the Program Requirements for Residency Education in Internal Medicine (*Note:* Specifically, paragraphs V.E., and V.G.) and the Institutional Requirements of the *Essentials of Accredited Residencies in Graduate Medical Education* also apply to subspecialty programs. The following principles require special emphasis:
   1. Educational environment
      Refer to the Institutional Requirements of the *Essentials of Accredited Residencies in Graduate Medical Education* (I. Institutional Organization and Commitment) and the Program Requirements for Residency Education in Internal Medicine, Sections I and II.A.
   2. Duty hours
      a. When averaged over any 4-week rotation or assignment, residents must not spend more than 80 hours per week in patient care duties.
      b. Residents must not be assigned on-call in-house duty more often than every third night.
      c. When averaged over a year, excluding vacation, residents must be provided with a minimum of 48 days free of patient care duties, including home-call responsibility.
   3. Professionalism and ethical behavior
      a. Physician accountability
         1. The training program must have mentors, role-model clinicians, and a resident culture that demonstrates the values of professionalism, such as placing the needs of patients first, maintaining a commitment to scholarship, helping colleagues meet their responsibilities, establishing a commitment to continuous quality improvement, and being responsive to society's health-care needs.

2. Residents should be given the opportunity to participate in community service, professional organizations, and institutional committee activities.

b. Humanistic qualities
Physicians must have the welfare of their patients as their primary professional concern. Thus, the residents, faculty members, and program must demonstrate humanistic qualities that foster the formation of empathetic, constructive, and effective patient/physician relationships. These qualities include integrity, respect, compassion, professional responsibility, courtesy, sensitivity to patient needs for comfort and encouragement, and a professional attitude and behavior toward colleagues.

c. Physician impairment
The training program must instruct residents and faculty members in physician impairment, to include the recognition of, intervention in, and management of impairment such as alcohol and other substance abuse; depression; dementia; and other mental, emotional, and physical disorders in their peers, as well as in the principles and methods of active intervention.

d. Professional ethics
The training program must foster a commitment to professional ethics in residents that is demonstrated by a spirit of collegiality and a high standard of moral and ethical behavior within the clinical setting in the care of patients, in the education of residents, in conducting research, and in interacting with medical device and pharmaceutical companies and funding organizations.

4. Responsibility and professional relationships
Lines of responsibility must be clearly delineated for residents in subspecialty programs and for residents in internal medicine training programs. Subspecialty programs must contribute to the general internal medicine program without diluting the overall experience of the internal medicine resident. In addition, it is highly desirable that residents have a meaningful working relationship with residents in accredited programs in other disciplines. Where appropriate, qualified faculty in other disciplines should provide instruction and supervision for subspecialty residents.

G. Peer Interaction
To ensure adequate peer interaction, the total number of residents enrolled in the program must at all times be equal to or greater than the number of years of accredited training.

III. Program Director and Faculty Qualifications and Responsibilities

A. General Qualifications and Responsibilities

1. Qualifications
The program director and all key clinical faculty members
a. must be licensed to practice medicine in the state where the sponsoring institution is located. (Certain federal programs are exempted, as appropriate.)
b. must have appointments in good standing to the medical staff of an institution participating in the training program.
c. should be certified by the specialty board or present equivalent credentials acceptable to the RRC.
d. must meet professional standards of ethical behavior.

2. Responsibilities
The program director and all faculty members
a. must have a commitment to the goals and objectives of the teaching program, including development of the residents' medical knowledge; clinical, technical, and management skills; and clinical judgment.
b. should be able to nurture the attributes of the scholar, scientist, teacher, and humanist in residents.
c. must be available to residents for advice and counseling.
d. must comply with the written curriculum that describes both patient-based and educational elements of the residency.
e. should review the written learning objectives and expectations for each rotation or assignment with residents at the beginning of the rotation or assignment, when designated to a rotation or assignment.
f. must be sensitive to the need for timely provision of confidential counseling and psychological support services to residents.
g. should participate actively in the clinical practice of the subspecialty, as appropriate.
h. should participate in their own continuing education.
i. should participate in the activities of regional and national scientific societies.
j. must provide written and verbal feedback to residents at the end of each rotation or assignment, when designated as a supervisor of residents during a rotation or assignment.

B. Program Director

1. Qualifications
There must be a single program director responsible for the program. The program director must
a. be an institutionally based appointee, ie, his or her home office must be at the primary training site.
b. have at least 5 years of participation as an active faculty member in an accredited subspecialty residency program.
c. be subspecialty certified by the American Board of Internal Medicine or present equivalent credentials acceptable to the RRC.

2. Responsibilities
The program director
a. must devote an average of at least 20 hours per week throughout the year to the training program.
b. must be primarily responsible for the organization, implementation, and supervision of all aspects of the training program, including the selection and supervision of the faculty members and other program personnel at each institution participating in the program.
c. must select residents for appointment to the program in accordance with institutional and departmental policies and procedures, evaluate the quality of care rendered by the residents, have the authority to ensure effective teaching, and obtain teaching commitments from other departments involved in the education of internal medicine residents.
d. must prepare written learning objectives and expectations outlining the educational goals and objectives of the program with respect to knowledge, skills, and other attributes of residents at each level of training and for each major rotation or other program assignment.
e. must ensure that the written learning objectives and expectations are readily available for review and are distributed to residents and faculty members.
f. must ensure that the residency does not place excessive reliance on service.
g. must notify the RRC promptly of
1. any change in the total number of residents in the training program and
2. major changes in the structure of the educational program.
The RRC may schedule a site visit when notified about either of the above changes.
h. must prepare an accurate statistical and narrative description of the program, as required by the RRC.

i. must monitor the residents' stress, including mental or emotional conditions inhibiting performance or learning and drug- or alcohol-related dysfunction.
j. must evaluate and modify training situations that consistently produce undesirable stress on residents.
k. must be responsible for the general administration of the program, including those activities related to the recruitment, selection, instruction, supervision, counseling, evaluation, and advancement of residents and the maintenance of records related to program accreditation.
l. must establish and use educational standards that determine the residents' competence in procedures and skills.
m. should ensure that there is a rapid and reliable system for residents to communicate with supervising attending physicians and residents.
n. must establish a system that ensures that attending physicians are available to participate in the residents' diagnostic and management decisions in a timely manner.
o. should outline in written policies the lines of responsibility and supervision for the care of patients on all inpatient and ambulatory settings, including all clinical sites for all members of the teaching teams and program staff.

C. Key Clinical Faculty Members

The training program must include a minimum of three institutionally based key faculty members, including the program director. (*Note:* Subspecialty programs in clinical cardiac electrophysiology, interventional cardiology, internal medicine-geriatric medicine, and internal medicine-sports medicine are exempt from this requirement.) For programs with more than five residents enrolled during the accredited portion of the training program, a ratio of such faculty to residents of at least 1:1.5 must be maintained. (These minimums may be exceeded in certain subspecialties.) Each resident must have, on average, a minimum of 10 hours per week of direct clinical faculty teaching hours.

1. Qualifications
Key clinical faculty members must
a. be certified by the American Board of Internal Medicine or present equivalent credentials acceptable to the RRC.
b. have documented clinical, academic, and administrative experience to ensure effective implementation of the Program Requirements.
c. be clinicians with broad knowledge of, experience with, and commitment to the subspecialty.
2. Responsibilities
Key clinical faculty members
a. must dedicate, on average, 10 hours per week throughout the year to the training program.
b. should participate in activities designed to enhance their teaching effectiveness.
c. should assist in the general administration of the program, including those activities related to the recruitment, selection, instruction, supervision, counseling, evaluation, and advancement of residents and the maintenance of records related to program accreditation.
d. must assist in the preparation of a written curriculum that describes both patient-based and educational elements of the residency and outlines the goals and objectives of the program with respect to knowledge, skills, and other attributes of residents at each level of training and for each major rotation or other program assignment.
e. must assist in nurturing the attributes of the scholar, scientist, teacher, and humanist in the residents.
f. must assist in monitoring resident stress, including mental or emotional conditions inhibiting performance or learning and drug- or alcohol-related dysfunction.

D. Other Faculty

PhD faculty members not holding an MD may be included as other teaching faculty but they may not be regarded as key clinical faculty members.

IV. Facilities and Resources

A. The Program Requirements for Residency Education in Internal Medicine governing the provision of appropriate facilities also apply to specialty training. Unique facilities required for a particular subspecialty will be found in the Program Requirements for that subspecialty.
B. As used in this document, the primary training site shall mean the health-care facility that provides the required services, is the location of the program director's major activity, is the location where the resident spends the majority of clinical time, and is ordinarily the primary location of the core program in internal medicine.
C. Programs must be provided with the additional professional, technical, and clerical personnel needed to support the administration and educational conduct of the program. In addition, refer to the Institutional Requirements of the *Essentials of Accredited Residencies in Graduate Medical Education,* II.D.
D. A sufficient number of new and follow-up patients, including the geriatric age group, and patients of both sexes must be available to ensure adequate inpatient and ambulatory experience for each subspecialty resident without diluting the experience of the residents in the general internal medicine residency program.

V. Specific Program Content

A. Patient Care Experience

The available inpatient and ambulatory care patient population must provide experience with those illnesses that are encompassed by, and help to define, the subspecialty. Such experience should include sufficient numbers of patients over the age of 70 to provide substantial opportunities in the management of the complex physical, social, and psychological problems prevalent in elderly patients. Subspecialty programs must include the following educational components:

1. Experience with ambulatory patients
a. Consultative as well as continuing care must occur at least ½ day each week throughout the length of the training program. (*Note:* Training programs in critical care medicine are exempt from this requirement.)
b. On-site faculty members' primary responsibilities must include the supervision and teaching of residents. On-site supervision as well as the evaluation of the educational experience must be documented.
c. The patient volume in the ambulatory environment must be large enough to provide adequate numbers of new and return patients. Residents should, on average, be responsible for from one to three new patients and three to six return patients during each ½-day session.
2. Experience with continuity ambulatory patients
a. The residents should have an opportunity to follow a panel of patients with a diversity of disease.
b. The resident's clinical experiences with ambulatory patients must provide residents the opportunity to observe and to learn the course of disease.

B. Consultation Experience

Subspecialty residents must have the appropriate supervised experience to develop skills in providing consultation services on inpatient and ambulatory services, communicating with referring physicians and other members of the health-care team, and ensuring support for continuous care by the patient's primary physician.

C. Teaching Experience

The program must provide subspecialty residents with the opportunity to teach general internal medicine residents, medical students, physicians, and other professional personnel.

D. Conferences

1. Core conferences must be conducted regularly as scheduled and must be attended faculty and residents. At a minimum, these must include at least one clinical conference weekly and one basic science conference, one literature review conference (journal club), and one research conference monthly.
2. Residents must participate in formal review of gross and microscopic pathological material from patients who have been under their care.
3. Residents must participate in planning and in conducting conferences.
4. Faculty and resident attendance and participation at multidisciplinary conferences is also expected.

E. Procedures

1. Residents must develop a comprehensive understanding of indications, contraindications, limitations, complications, techniques, and interpretation of results of those diagnostic and therapeutic procedures integral to the discipline. Residents must acquire knowledge of and skill in educating patients about the technique, rationale, and complications of procedures and in obtaining procedure-specific informed consent.
2. Faculty supervision by key clinical faculty or other designated physicians of procedures performed by each resident is required until proficiency has been acquired and documented for the program director. Each program must
   a. identify key procedures.
   b. define a standard for proficiency.
   c. document achievement of proficiency.

F. Occupational Safety and Health Administration (OSHA) and Health-Care Regulations

Residents must have formal instruction in current OSHA regulations and universal precautions and protection of health-care workers.

G. Medical Informatics and Decision-Making Skills

1. Residents should receive instruction in the critical assessment of medical literature, in clinical epidemiology, in biostatistics, and in clinical decision theory.
2. Each resident should have the opportunity to learn basic computer skills, including an introduction to computer capabilities and medical applications, basic techniques for electronic retrieval of medical literature, computer-assisted medical instruction, and electronic information networks.

H. Quality Assessment, Quality Improvement, Risk Management, and Cost Effectiveness in Medicine

1. Residents should receive instruction in the social and economic impact of medical decisions on patients and society and the need to be the primary advocate for patients' needs.
2. It is desirable that all residents receive formal instruction regarding the principles, objectives, and processes of quality assessment and improvement and of risk management.

I. Clinical ethics

The program must include education in the principles of bioethics as applied to medical care, and the residents must participate in decision making involving ethical issues that arise in the diagnosis and management of their patients.

J. Educational and Counseling Skills

Residents should have instruction and experience in patient counseling skills and community education. This training should emphasize effective communication techniques for diverse populations, as well as organizational resources useful for patient and community education.

K. End-of-Life Care

1. Each resident should receive instruction in the principles of palliative care for terminally ill patients, including the role of the health-care team. Instruction should include psychosocial, cultural, and religious issues related to death and dying.
2. It is desirable that residents participate in hospice and home care.

L. Research

As part of the academic environment, an active research component must be included within each accredited subspecialty program. The program must ensure a meaningful, supervised research experience with appropriate protected time—either in blocks or concurrent with clinical rotations—for each resident, while maintaining the essential clinical experience. Evidence of recent productivity by both the program faculty and by the residents as a whole, will be required, including publication in peer-reviewed journals. Residents must learn the design and interpretation of research studies, responsible use of informed consent, and research methodology and interpretation of data. The program must provide instruction in the critical assessment of new therapies and of the medical literature. Residents should be advised and supervised by qualified faculty members in the conduct of research. (*Note:* Training programs in internal medicine-geriatric medicine are exempt from this requirement relative to research productivity by residents.)

M. Other Scholarly Activities

The resident should make presentations at lectures, medical grand rounds, journal clubs, and research and other conferences.

VI. Evaluation

A. Residents

1. Formative Evaluation
   a. Subspecialty program directors must establish procedures for evaluating and documenting the clinical and technical competence of subspecialty residents. These procedures must include observation, assessment, and substantiation of residents' comprehensive and specialized medical knowledge and provision of medical care, including advanced skills in history-taking, physical examination, clinical judgment, management, and consultation, and their ability to critically analyze clinical situations and make medical decisions. The program must also evaluate residents' technical proficiency, teaching skills, communication, humanistic qualities, professional attitudes and behavior, and commitment to scholarship as demonstrated within the clinical setting.
   b. Records must be maintained by documentation logbooks or an equivalent method to demonstrate that subspecialty residents have had adequate experience with invasive and noninvasive procedures. Records should state the indications and complications and include the name of the supervising physician. Such records must be kept in sufficient detail to permit use in future credentialing.

c. Regular and meaningful feedback to subspecialty residents about their performance is essential to their continuing growth and development as subspecialty internists. There must be regular evaluation of residents' knowledge, skills, and overall performance, including the development of professional attitudes consistent with being a physician.
d. Residents must be evaluated and their performance reviewed with them on completion of each rotation period.
e. At least semiannually, the program must provide to the resident structured feedback on performance, including appropriate counseling and other necessary remedial effort.
f. Adequate records of the evaluation and counseling process must be maintained for each resident. Such records must be available in the resident's file and must be accessible to the resident.

2. Summative Evaluation
   a. The program director must prepare a written evaluation (eg, the American Board of Internal Medicine's tracking form) of the clinical competence of each subspecialty resident annually and at the conclusion of the resident's period of training in the program. Such evaluations must stipulate the degree to which the resident has mastered each component of clinical competence (ie, clinical judgment, medical knowledge, clinical skills, humanistic qualities, professional attitudes and behavior, research and scholarship, and provision of medical care) and has acquired proficiency in each of the various procedural skills identified in the program's curriculum.

The program director must verify whether the resident has demonstrated sufficient professional ability to practice competently and independently by the end of the residency program.

   b. A record of the evaluation must be maintained in the program files to substantiate future judgments provided to hospital credentialing and privileging, board certification, and agency licensing bodies, and to support other bodies' actions.
   c. Residents must be advanced to positions of higher responsibility only on the basis of evidence of their satisfactory progressive scholarship and professional growth. In the event of an adverse annual evaluation, residents must be offered the opportunity to address judgments of academic deficiencies or misconduct before an independent, appropriately constituted clinical competence committee.
   d. There must be a written policy to ensure that academic due process provides fundamental fairness to the resident and protects the institution by ensuring accurate, proper, and definitive resolution of disputed evaluations.

B. Faculty Members and Program

1. Resident evaluation of faculty members and program
   a. The educational effectiveness of a program must be evaluated in a systematic manner. Specifically, the quality of the curriculum and the extent to which the educational goals and objectives have been met by residents must be assessed. Written evaluations by residents should be utilized in this process.
   b. The faculty must be organized and have regular documented meetings to review program goals and objectives as well as program effectiveness in achieving them.
   c. At least one resident representative must participate in these reviews of the training program.
   d. The faculty should at least annually evaluate the utilization of the resources available to the program, the contribution of each institution participating in the program, the financial and administrative support of the program, the volume and variety of patients available to the program for educational purposes, the performance of the faculty members, and the quality of supervision of residents.
   e. Provision must be made for residents to evaluate the faculty and the training program in writing at least annually. The results of such evaluations should be used for faculty counseling and for selecting faculty members for specific teaching assignments.

C. Evaluation of the Graduates

Each program must maintain a system of evaluation of its graduates. The residency should obtain feedback on demographic and practice profiles, licensure and board certification, the graduates' perceptions of the relevancy of training to practice or other career pathways, suggestions for improving the training, and ideas for new areas of curriculum. The suggested format is a written survey after 1 year and every 5 years thereafter. The data from the evaluation of the graduates should be used as part of the program's determination of the degree to which the program's stated goals are being met.

VII. Program Requirements

The Program Requirements for training programs in a specific subspecialty may exceed the minimum requirements set forth above.

ACGME: June 1998 Effective: July 1999

Program Requirements for Residency Education in Cardiovascular Disease (Internal Medicine)

I. Educational Program

A subspecialty educational program in cardiology must be organized to provide training and supervised experience in the evaluation and management of a wide variety of patients with acute and chronic cardiovascular conditions including chronic coronary heart disease, congestive heart failure, arrhythmias, acute myocardial infarction and other acute ischemic syndromes, lipid disorders, hypertension, cardiomyopathy, valvular heart disease, pulmonary heart disease, peripheral vascular disease, infections and inflammatory heart disease, and adult congenital heart disease. The training and experience must be at a sufficient level for the resident to acquire the competency of a specialist in the field. It must be 3 years in duration.

II. Key Clinical Faculty

The program must provide a minimum of four institutionally based faculty members, including the program director. In programs with a total of more than six residents enrolled, a ratio of such faculty to residents of at least 1:1.5 must be maintained.

III. Facilities and Resources

Modern facilities to accomplish the overall educational program must be available and functioning at the primary training site. These include inpatient, ambulatory care, and clinical and research laboratory resources. Specifically, there must be laboratories in which cardiac hemodynamics, angiography, percutaneous transluminal coronary angioplasty, invasive electrophysiologic studies, and other interventional procedures are performed. There must be laboratories that provide resources for electrocardiography, ambulatory electrocardiogram (ECG) recording, exercise testing, echocardiography (including Doppler and transesophageal studies), and radionuclide techniques. Other hospital resources should include facilities for assessment of peripheral vascular disease and pulmonary physiology. Critical care units must include a cardiac care unit and a cardiac surgery intensive care unit. Resources must be available for implantation of pacemakers, implantable cardioverter/defibrillator, and follow-up. There must be a cardiac catheterization laboratory and active cardiac surgery at the primary training site.

IV. Specific Program Content

The goal of the training program is to provide opportunities for the residents to develop clinical competence in the field of adult cardiovascular disease.

A. Clinical Experience

1. Special Clinical Experiences
   There must be at least 24 months of clinical training, including inpatient and special experiences. The program must provide a minimum of
   a. Four months in the cardiac catheterization laboratory
   b. Six months in noninvasive cardiac evaluations, consisting of
      1. three months of echocardiography;
      2. two months of nuclear cardiology; and
      3. one month of other noninvasive cardiac evaluations, which includes at least
         a. exercise stress testing,
         b. ECG interpretation, and
         c. ambulatory ECG recording.

   These rotations may be done in conjunction with other block rotations or concurrently with other clinical rotations.
   c. Two months devoted to electrophysiology, pacemaker follow-up and ICDs.
2. Inpatient Experience
   There must be at least 8 months of nonlaboratory clinical practice activities (eg, consultations, cardiac care units, postoperative care of cardiac surgery patients).

B. Technical and Other Skills

1. The program must provide sufficient experience for the resident to acquire skill in the performance and interpretation of
   a. history and physical examination
   b. basic and advanced cardiac life support
   c. elective cardioversion
   d. bedside right heart catheterization
   e. insertion and management of temporary pacemakers, including transvenous and transcutaneous
   f. right and left heart catheterization including coronary arteriography; residents must participate in a minimum of 100 catheterizations
   g. exercise stress testing; residents must perform a minimum of 50 ECG tests
   h. echocardiography; residents must perform and interpret a minimum of 150 studies, including transesophageal and esophageal cardiac studies
   i. pericardiocentesis
   j. programming and follow-up surveillance of permanent pacemakers and ICDs
   k. cardiovascular rehabilitation
2. The program must provide opportunities for residents to acquire experience with the performance and (where applicable) interpretation of
   a. intracardiac electrophysiologic studies
   b. intra-aortic balloon counterpulsation
   c. percutaneous transluminal coronary angioplasty and other interventional procedures
3. The program must provide sufficient experience for residents to acquire skill in the interpretation of
   a. chest x-rays
   b. a minimum of 3500 electrocardiograms
   c. a minimum of 75 ambulatory ECG recordings
   d. radionuclide studies of myocardial function and perfusion
   e. cardiovascular literature

C. Formal Instruction

The program must provide instruction in the following:
1. Basic science, including
   a. cardiovascular anatomy
   b. cardiovascular physiology
   c. cardiovascular metabolism
   d. molecular biology of the cardiovascular system
   e. cardiovascular pharmacology, including drug metabolism, adverse effects, indications, the effects on aging, relative costs of therapy, and the effects of noncardiovascular drugs upon cardiovascular function
   f. cardiovascular pathology
2. Prevention of cardiovascular disease, including
   a. epidemiology and biostatistics
   b. risk factors
   c. lipid disorders
3. Evaluation and management of patients with
   a. coronary artery disease and its manifestations and complications
   b. arrhythmias
   c. hypertension
   d. cardiomyopathy
   e. valvular heart disease
   f. pericardial disease
   g. pulmonary heart disease, including pulmonary embolism
   h. peripheral vascular disease
   i. cerebrovascular disease
   j. heart disease in pregnancy
   k. adult congenital heart disease
   l. cardiovascular trauma
4. Management of
   a. acute and chronic congestive heart failure
   b. acute myocardial infarction and other acute ischemic syndromes
   c. acute and chronic arrhythmias
   d. preoperative and postoperative patients
   e. cardiac transplant patients
   f. geriatric patients with cardiovascular disease
5. Diagnostic techniques, including
   a. magnetic resonance imaging
   b. fast computed tomography
   c. positron emission tomography

ACGME: June 1998 Effective: July 1999

Program Requirements for Residency Education in Clinical Cardiac Electrophysiology (Internal Medicine)

I. Educational Program

A. A subspecialty educational program in clinical cardiac electrophysiology (CCEP) must function as an integral component of an accredited subspecialty fellowship in cardiovascular disease and must be organized to provide training and supervised experience at a sufficient level for the resident to acquire the competency of a specialist in the field.

B. During training in CCEP, the resident's clinical experience must include opportunities to observe, diagnose, manage, and judge the effectiveness of treatment for inpatients and outpatients with palpitations, syncope, and bradyarrhythmias and with both supraventricular and ventricular tachyarrhythmias. The resident should be given opportunities to assume continuing and increasing responsibility for both acutely and chronically ill patients to learn the natural history of a wide variety of cardiac arrhythmias and how to treat them.

C. The CCEP program must be 1 year in length, following completion of an accredited cardiovascular disease residency program.

II. Key Clinical Faculty

Faculty responsible for training must be board certified in CCEP or possess equivalent qualifications. In addition, there must be a minimum of two key clinical CCEP faculty members, including the program director. In programs with a total of more than two residents enrolled, a ratio of such faculty to residents of at least 1:1 must be maintained.

III. Facilities and Resources

A. Modern facilities to accomplish the overall educational program must be available and functioning at the primary training site. Specifically, there must be a clinical cardiac electrophysiologic laboratory for invasive intracardiac electrophysiologic studies and catheter ablation and laboratories to provide the noninvasive diagnostic and therapeutic techniques detailed below.

B. The electrophysiology laboratory must contain appropriate cardiac fluoroscopic equipment, programmable stimulator, recording devices, and resuscitative equipment. An outpatient follow-up program must exist to care for patients with pacemakers and implantable cardioverters/defibrillators (ICDs). Clinical care units must include cardiac care units (CCUs), cardiac surgical intensive care units, and outpatient clinics. A cardiac surgery program must be at the primary training site.

IV. Specific Program Content

A. Clinical Experience

1. Residents must have clinical experiences with the required procedures and skills, which includes the knowledge of their indications, contraindications, risks, and limitations. Residents must be instructed in the sensitivity, specificity, and the positive and negative predictive accuracy of any test employed. They must be instructed in the appropriate techniques for evaluating patients with
   a. a variety of rhythm disorders, including but not limited to
      1. sinus node dysfunction,
      2. atrioventricular (AV) and intraventricular block, and
      3. supraventricular and ventricular tachyarrhythmias.
   b. clinical conditions such as
      1. unexplained syncope,
      2. aborted sudden cardiac death,
      3. palpitations,
      4. Wolff-Parkinson-White (WPW) syndrome, and
      5. long QT syndrome.
   c. conditions that make them candidates for nonpharmacological therapy such as ablation, surgery, and ICD implantation.
2. Clinical experiences involving
   a. consultation to physicians in other disciplines
   b. care of patients in the cardiac care unit, emergency room, or other intensive care settings.
   c. care of the patient before and after an electrophysiologic procedure.
   d. care of patients with postoperative arrhythmias.
   e. outpatient follow-up of patients treated with drugs, devices, or surgery.
   f. electrocardiography—proficiency in the interpretation of the standard 12-lead ECG, stress testing, ambulatory ECG recording, signal-averaged ECG, and telephone-transmitted ECGs.
   g. care of patients with temporary and permanent pacemakers.
   h. care of patients with ICDs.

B. Technical and Other Skills

1. To become proficient in CCEP, residents must have the opportunity to acquire a broad knowledge base of cardiac electrophysiology. There must be opportunity to develop a high level of performance in such areas as interpretation of results of noninvasive testing relevant to arrhythmia diagnoses and treatment, performance and interpretation of invasive electrophysiologic testing, performing therapeutic catheter ablation procedures, and performing or assisting in the implantation of cardioverter/defibrillators and pacemakers.
2. The program must ensure that residents have the necessary opportunities to acquire skill in the interpretation of
   a. activation sequence mapping recordings.
   b. invasive intracardiac electrophysiologic studies, including endocardial electrogram recording.
   c. relevant imaging studies, including chest radiography.
   d. tilt testing.
   e. electrocardiograms and ambulatory ECG recordings.
   f. continuous in-hospital ECG recording.
   h. signal-averaged ECG recordings.
   i. stress test ECG recordings.
   j. transtelephonic ECG readings.
3. The program must ensure that residents have the necessary opportunities to acquire skill in the performance of clinical cardiac electrophysiologic studies.
   a. The resident is expected to perform an average of three or more electrophysiology invasive diagnostic/interventional catheter procedures per week as the primary operator or as an assistant closely involved with data collection and analysis.
   b. A minimum of 150 intracardiac procedures in at least 75 patients will be required.
4. The program director of the CCEP training program will be expected to ensure the competency of the resident in the following:
   a. Electrode catheter introduction
   b. Electrode catheter positioning in atria, ventricles, coronary sinus, His bundle area, and pulmonary artery
   c. Stimulating techniques to obtain conduction times and refractory periods and to initiate and terminate tachycardias
   d. Recording techniques, including an understanding of amplifiers, filters, and signal processors
   e. Measurement and interpretation of data
5. A minimum of 75 catheter ablative procedures, including postdiagnostic testing, will be required for each resident. These cases must include a mix of AV nodal reentrant tachycardia and accessory pathway modification, atrial tachycardia and atrial flutter, AV junctional ablation and modification and ventricular tachycardia ablation.
6. Participation in a minimum of 25 initial ICD procedures, including pacemaker and ICD programming, will be required for each resident. The program must assure that the residents acquire skill in the following:
   a. Device programming
   b. Noninvasive programmed stimulation for arrhythmia induction through the device

c. Defibrillation threshold testing
d. Final prescription of antitachycardia pacing and defibrillation therapies

C. Formal Instruction

The program must provide instruction in

1. basic cardiac electrophysiology, including but not limited to genesis of arrhythmias, normal and abnormal electrophysiologic responses, autonomic influences, effects of ischemia, drugs, and other interventions.
2. clinical cardiac electrophysiology.
3. arrhythmia control device management
4. the genetic basis of pathological arrhythmias.
5. epidemiology of arrhythmias.
6. clinical trials of arrhythmia management and their impact on clinical practice.

ACGME: June 1998 Effective: July 1999

Program Requirements for Residency Education in Critical Care Medicine (Internal Medicine)

I. Educational Program

A. A subspecialty educational program in critical care medicine must be organized to provide training and supervised experience at a sufficient level for the resident to acquire competency in managing critically ill patients and in supervising critical care units.

B. Critical care medicine training programs may be 1 or 2 years in duration.
1. Programs that accept only those who have completed training in an accredited program in one of the subspecialties of internal medicine may be organized to offer a single year of training.
2. Programs organized to provide critical care medicine training in association with an accredited program in one of the subspecialties of internal medicine may fulfill training requirements by devoting 12 months to critical care out of a total of 36 months of training.
3. Otherwise, a program must provide training of 2 years in duration.

C. To provide evidence of substantial institutional support in those disciplines most relevant to critical care medicine, the sponsoring institution's primary training site should sponsor accredited subspecialty programs in cardiovascular disease, pulmonary disease, and infectious diseases and must have an accredited residency program in general surgery. The presence of training programs in these disciplines ensures the extensive educational, patient care, and research resources that are essential to the learning environment for critical care medicine residents. Furthermore, peer interaction is essential in the education of critical care medicine residents.

D. The sponsoring institution(s) must provide service for the care of patients with major trauma and must have an active open heart surgery program.

E. Institutional policies should be established to govern the educational resources committed to critical care training programs and to ensure cooperation of all involved disciplines.

II. Key Clinical Faculty

A. The program director and the critical care teaching staff must have privileges regarding the admission, treatment, and discharge of patients on the critical care unit(s).

B. The director shall have administrative responsibility for the critical care teaching program, subject to the approval of the director of the parent internal medicine training program.

C. The key clinical teaching faculty at the primary training site must include each of the following:
1. For each resident there must be no less than one key clinical faculty member.
2. There must be at least two key clinical faculty members each in nephrology, gastroenterology, pulmonary, cardiology, infectious disease, and hematology who must devote substantial effort to the education of critical care medicine residents.
3. There must be key clinical faculty members in geriatric medicine and oncology who are available to participate in the education of residents in critical care medicine.

D. Faculty members in anesthesiology, neurology, and neurosurgery who are certified by an American Board of Medical Specialties member board in their respective disciplines or who have equivalent training and experience must also participate at the primary training site in the education of residents in critical care medicine.

E. Because critical care training is multidisciplinary in nature, faculty from several related disciplines such as general surgery, thoracic surgery, pediatrics, urology, orthopedic surgery, emergency medicine, and obstetrics-gynecology must be available to participate in the training program.

F. A collegial relationship must exist between the director of the critical care training program and the teaching staff, to enhance the educational opportunities for all residents.

III. Facilities and Resources

A. Modern facilities to accomplish the educational program must be available and functioning.
1. The critical care unit(s) must be located in a designated area within the hospital and must be constructed and designed specifically for the care of critically ill patients.
2. Whether operating in separate locations or in combined facilities, the program must provide the equivalent of a medical intensive care unit (MICU), a surgical intensive care unit, and a coronary intensive care unit (CICU).
3. The MICU must be at the primary training site and should be the focus of a teaching service in which the program director in critical care medicine is responsible for the educational program.

B. Available facilities must be adequate to care for patients with acute myocardial infarction, severe trauma, shock, recent open heart surgery, recent major thoracic or abdominal surgery, and severe neurologic and neurosurgical conditions.

C. In units to which a resident is assigned, an average census of at least five patients per resident is required.

D. A sufficient number of knowledgeable personnel and the necessary equipment to care for critically ill patients must be available. Personnel must include specially trained nurses and technicians who are skilled in critical care instrumentation, respiratory function, and laboratory medicine.

E. A supporting laboratory must be available to provide complete and prompt laboratory evaluation.

F. Modern imaging services and an active emergency service must be available.

G. Nutritional support services also must be available.

IV. Specific Program Content

A. Clinical Experience

1. Ultimate integration and application of the necessary knowledge, skills, and attitudes are best experienced in the intensive care environment. The program must be structured to provide adequate and meaningful patient responsibility in critical care unit(s), at least 6 months of which must be devoted to the care of critically ill medical patients (ie, MICU/CICU or equivalent).
2. Residents must be given opportunities to assume responsibility, under appropriate supervision, for the care of patients throughout their stay in the critical care unit(s) and to monitor the subsequent course of patients throughout the remainder of their hospital stay. To assess the various aspects of critical care, the resident must also have organized opportunities to learn about former critical care patients after hospital discharge, including clinical pathological correlations when appropriate.
3. Because critical care medicine is multidisciplinary in nature, clinical experience must include opportunities to manage adult patients with a wide variety of serious illnesses and injuries requiring treatment in a critical care setting. Therefore, residents must obtain additional clinical experience with other critically ill patients, which may include surgical, shock/trauma, and neurologic/neurosurgical intensive care units; pediatric intensive care unit; burn unit; dialysis unit; anesthesia service; cardiac catheterization laboratory; high-risk pregnancy intensive care unit; and transplant unit.

B. Technical and Other Skills

1. The program must be structured to permit all critical care residents to develop the requisite procedural and technical skills, including the ability to interpret data derived from various bedside devices commonly employed to monitor patients in the critical care setting.
2. The training program must provide opportunities for residents to learn the indications, contraindications, complications, and limitations of the following critical care procedures and the technical skills necessary to perform them. This experience may ordinarily occur in a pulmonary function laboratory or respiratory care service.
   a. Establishment and maintenance of open airway in nonintubated, unconscious, paralyzed patients
   b. Pressure-cycled, volume-cycled, time-cycled, and flow-cycled mechanical ventilation
   c. Use of reservoir masks and continuous positive airway pressure masks for delivery of supplemental oxygen, humidifiers, nebulizers, and incentive spirometry
   d. Management of pneumothorax (needle insertion and drainage systems)
   e. Maintenance of circulation with
      1. Arterial puncture and blood sampling
      2. Insertion of central venous, arterial, and pulmonary artery balloon flotation catheters
      3. Basic and advanced cardiopulmonary resuscitation
      4. Cardioversion
   f. Thoracentesis
3. The training program must provide opportunities for residents to learn the indications, contraindications, limitations, and complications of the following critical care procedures and the technical skills necessary to perform them:
   a. Parenteral nutrition
   b. Monitoring/bioengineering
      1. Utilization, zeroing, and calibration of transducers
      2. Use of amplifiers and recorders
4. The program also must provide opportunities to learn the indications, contraindications, complications, and limitations of the following procedures; practical experience is recommended.
   a. Pericardiocentesis
   b. Transvenous pacemaker insertion
   c. Peritoneal dialysis
   d. Peritoneal lavage
   e. Insertion of chest tubes
   f. Percutaneous needle aspiration
   g. Intracranial pressure monitoring
5. Experience also must be provided in the analysis of data pertaining to the following:
   a. Cardiac output determinations by thermodilution and other techniques
   b. Evaluation of oliguria
   c. Management of massive transfusions
   d. Management of hemostatic defects
   e. Interpretation of antibiotic levels and sensitivities
   f. Monitoring and assessment of metabolism and nutrition
   g. Calculation of oxygen content, intrapulmonary shunt and alveolar arterial gradients
   h. Pharmacokinetics
6. Opportunities also must be available for residents to acquire those skills required to organize, administer, and direct a critical care unit and to work effectively as a member of a multidisciplinary team.

C. Formal Instruction

The training program must provide opportunities for the residents to acquire knowledge of and to develop clinical competence in the following content areas:

1. Physiology, pathophysiology, diagnosis, and therapy of disorders of the cardiovascular, respiratory, renal, gastrointestinal, genitourinary, neurologic, endocrine, hematologic, musculoskeletal, and immune systems as well as of infectious diseases
2. Electrolyte and acid-base physiology, pathophysiology, diagnosis, and therapy
3. Metabolic, nutritional, and endocrine effects of critical illnesses
4. Hematologic and coagulation disorders associated with critical illness
5. Critical obstetric and gynecologic disorders
6. Management of the immunosuppressed patient
7. Management of anaphylaxis and acute allergic reactions
8. Trauma
9. Pharmacokinetics, pharmacodynamics, and drug metabolism and excretion in critical illness
10. Use of paralytic agents
11. Ethical, economic, and legal aspects of critical illness
12. Principles and techniques of administration and management
13. Psychosocial and emotional effects of critical illnesses on patients and their families
14. Iatrogenic and nosocomial problems in critical care medicine
15. Occupational Safety and Health Administration (OSHA) regulations and universal precautions and protection of health-care workers

ACGME: June 1998 Effective: July 1999

Program Requirements for Residency Education in Endocrinology, Diabetes, and Metabolism (Internal Medicine)

I. Educational Program

A subspecialty educational program in endocrinology, diabetes, and metabolism must be organized to provide training and experience at a sufficient level for the resident to acquire the competency of a specialist in the field. It must be 2 years in duration.

II. Facilities and Resources

Modern facilities must be available and functioning. Specifically, there must be a complete biochemistry laboratory and facilities for radioimmunoassay. Available imaging services must include nuclear, ultrasonic, and radiologic facilities and expertise to conduct studies for all types of endocrine disease. There must be available endocrine surgical services and a pathology laboratory for the interpretation of surgical and cytologic specimens. There should be access to karyotyping and immunohistologic studies. In addition, there must be a close working relationship with dietary and/or nutrition services, as well as specialists in surgery, nephrology, neurology and neurosurgery, obstetrics and gynecology, ophthalmology, pediatrics, podiatry, and urology.

III. Specific Program Content

A. Clinical Experience

1. The training program must provide opportunities for the resident to develop clinical competence in the field of endocrinology, diabetes, and metabolism. Clinical experience must include opportunities to diagnose and manage inpatients and outpatients representing adolescent and adult patients of both sexes and representing variable acuity and who have a wide variety of endocrine and metabolic diseases. The program also must include opportunities to function in the role of an endocrinology consultant for patients and other physicians and services in both inpatient and outpatient settings.
2. The residents must be given opportunities to assume responsibility for and follow patients throughout the training period in both inpatient and outpatient settings to observe the evolution and natural history of these disorders, as well as the effectiveness of therapeutic interventions. To accomplish these goals, the educational program must have at least 30% of the training in endocrine subspecialty related ambulatory care settings. Residents must have experience representing variable acuity and the full spectrum of endocrine and metabolic diseases.
3. The curriculum must emphasize biochemistry and physiology, including cell and molecular biology, as they relate to endocrinology, diabetes, and metabolism. The appropriate utilization and interpretation of clinical laboratory, radionuclide, and radiologic studies for the diagnosis and treatment of endocrine and metabolic diseases must be stressed.
4. Residents must have clinical experience in a multidisciplinary diabetes education and treatment program.
5. Residents must have formal instruction, clinical experience, or opportunities to acquire expertise in the evaluation and management of the following disorders:
   a. Thyroid disorders, including
      1. hyperthyroidism and hypothyroidism
      2. nodular thyroid diseases
      3. thyroid cancer
      4. goiter, and
      5. thyroiditis, including chronic, silent, subacute, and autoimmune
   b. Hypothalamic and pituitary tumors, including
      1. pituitary tumors of all types, with particular experience in the diagnosis and management of prolactinoma, acromegaly, Cushing's disease, and clinically nonfunctioning tumors
      2. craniopharyngeoma and other space occupying and infiltrative disorders of the pituitary and hypothalamic region
      3. hypopituitarism
      4. growth hormone disorders
      5. hypothalamic insufficiency
      6. SIADH
      7. diabetes insipidus (primary and nephrogenic), and
      8. galactorrhea
   c. Type 1 and Type 2 diabetes mellitus, including
      1. patient monitoring and treatment objectives in adolescents and adults
      2. acute and chronic complications, including
         a. diabetic ketoacidosis
         b. hyperosmolar non-ketotic syndromes
         c. hypoglycemia, and
         d. microvascular and macrovascular disease, including
            i. diabetic retinopathy
            ii. diabetic nephropathy
            iii. diabetic neuropathy
            iv. dermatologic aspects of diabetes
            v. coronary heart disease
            vi. peripheral vascular disease, and
            vii. cerebral vascular disease
         e. infections in the diabetic patient
      3. gestational diabetes mellitus
      4. diabetes mellitus in the pregnant patient
      5. the surgical patient with diabetes mellitus
      6. patient education
      7. psychosocial issues
      8. genetics and genetic counseling as it relates to patients with edocrine and metabolism disorders
      9. dietary principles
   d. Hypoglycemic syndromes, including the spectrum of insulinoma and other causes
   e. The diagnosis and management of lipid and lipoprotein disorders
   f. The diagnosis and management of primary and secondary hypertension
   g. Disorders of bone and mineral metabolism, including
      1. hyperparathyroidism and other causes of hypercalcemia
      2. hypoparathyroidism and other causes of hypocalcemia
      3. metabolic bone diseases, with particular emphasis on the diagnosis and management of osteoporosis
      4. evaluation and prevention of kidney stones
      5. Paget's disease
      6. osteomalacia and disorders of vitamin D and phosphorus metabolism
      7. disorders of magnesium metabolism
   h. Disorders of the adrenal cortex and medulla including:
      1. benign and malignant adrenal tumors
      2. adrenogenital syndromes
      3. Cushing's syndrome, including drug-induced
      4. adrenal cortex hypofunction—cause and therapy.
      5. pheochromocytoma
      6. primary aldosteronism

i. Disorders of fluid, electrolyte, and acid-base metabolism, including
   1. hypernatremia and hyponatremia
   2. hyperkalemia and hypokalemia
   3. metabolic acidosis
   4. metabolic alkalosis
j. Disorders of magnesium and phosphorous metabolism
k. Endocrine aspects of psychiatric diseases
l. Endocrine aspects of aging, with particular emphasis on the care of geriatric patients with endocrine disease and diabetes and the endocrine changes associated with aging
m. Autoimmune polyglandular failure syndrome
n. Endocrine emergencies, including
   1. hypercalcemia and hypocalcemia
   2. severe hypo- and hyperthyroidism
   3. adrenal insufficiency
   4. pituitary apoplexy
o. Parenteral nutritional support
p. Nutritional disorders
   1. obesity-pathophysiology, diagnosis and management
   2. anorexia nervosa and bulimia
q. Hormone-producing neoplasms, particularly carcinoid syndromes, ectopic hormone production, islet cell tumors and multiple endocrine neoplasia syndromes
r. Female and male reproduction, including
   1. primary and secondary amenorrhea
   2. hirsutism/virilization
   3. dysfunctional uterine bleeding
   4. infertility
   5. menopause
   6. testicular tumors
   7. erectile dysfunction
   8. gynecomastia
   9. hypogonadism
s. Endocrine adaptations and maladaptations to systemic diseases, including effects on the thyroidal, adrenal, and gonadal axes.

B. Technical and Other Skills

Residents should have experience in the performance of endocrine clinical laboratory and radionuclide studies and basic laboratory techniques, including quality control, quality assurance, and proficiency standards.

Provision must be made for the residents to acquire experience and skill in the following areas:

1. The interpretation of laboratory tests; immunoassays; and radionuclide, ultrasound, radiologic, and other imaging studies for the diagnosis and treatment of endocrine and metabolic disease,
2. The effects of a variety of nonendocrine disorders on laboratory and imaging studies and performance and interpretation of stimulation and suppression tests.
3. Performance and cytologic interpretation of fine needle aspiration of the thyroid.
4. Indication and interpretation of quantitative digital radiography and other tests used in the management of osteoporosis and other metabolic bone diseases.
5. Management of adolescent and adult patients of all ages with diabetes mellitus, including but not limited to the following aspects of the disease:
   a. The utilization and interpretation of autoimmune markers of Type 1 diabetes in patient management and counseling
   b. Prescription of exercise programs
   c. Rationale for and calculation of diabetic diets
   d. Oral antidiabetic therapy
   e. The use of intravenous insulin in acute decompensated diabetes mellitus
   f. Chronic insulin administration, including the use of all varieties of insulin delivery systems
   g. Glucose monitoring devices
   h. Funduscopic examination, recognition, and appropriate referral of patients with diabetic retinopathy
   i. Foot care
   j. Psychosocial effects of diabetes mellitus on patients and their families
   k. Patient and community education

C. Formal Instruction

The formal curriculum of the program must, as a minimum, provide instruction in the following:

1. Pathogenesis and epidemiology of diabetes mellitus
2. Genetics as it relates to endocrine diseases
3. Developmental endocrinology, including growth and development, sexual differentiation, and pubertal maturation
4. Endocrine physiology and pathophysiology in systemic diseases and principles of hormone action
5. Biochemistry and physiology, including cell and molecular biology and immunology, as they relate to endocrinology and metabolism
6. Signal transduction pathways and biology of hormone receptors

ACGME: June 1998 Effective: July 1999

Program Requirements for Residency Education in Gastroenterology (Internal Medicine)

I. Educational Program

A subspecialty education program in gastroenterology must be organized to provide training and experience at a sufficient level for the resident to acquire the competency of a specialist in the field. It must be 3 years in duration.

II. Key Clinical Faculty

The program must provide a minimum of four institutionally based faculty members, including the program director. In addition, at least one key clinical faculty member should have demonstrated expertise and primary focus in hepatology.

III. Facilities and Resources

A. Modern facilities to accomplish the overall educational program must be available and functioning at the primary training site. Specifically, there must be a procedure laboratory completely equipped to provide modern capability in gastrointestinal procedures. This equipment must include an up-to-date array of complete diagnostic and therapeutic endoscopic instruments and accessories plus esophageal motility instrumentation. Facilities for parasitology testing should be provided. Supporting services including pathology, diagnostic radiology, interventional radiology, medical imaging and nuclear medicine, general surgery, and oncology also must be available.

B. Facilities for the intensive care of critically ill patients with gastrointestinal disorders must be provided, including a working relationship with surgery, oncology, pediatrics, radiology, and pathology services.

IV. Specific Program Content

A. Clinical Experience

1. The training program must provide opportunities for residents to develop clinical competence in the field of gastroenterology, including hepatology, clinical nutrition, and gastrointestinal oncology.
2. At least 18 months of the clinical experience should be in general gastroenterology, including hepatology, which should comprise approximately 30% of this experience. The additional 18 months of training must be dedicated to elective fields of training oriented to enhance competency.
3. Residents must have formal instruction, clinical experience, or opportunities to acquire expertise in the evaluation and management of the following disorders:
   a. Diseases of the esophagus
   b. Acid peptic disorders of the gastrointestinal tract
   c. Motor disorders of the gastrointestinal tract
   d. Irritable bowel syndrome
   e. Disorders of nutrient assimilation
   f. Inflammatory bowel diseases
   g. Vascular disorders of the gastrointestinal tract
   h. Gastrointestinal infections, including retroviral, mycotic, and parasitic diseases
   i. Gastrointestinal and pancreatic neoplasms
   j. Gastrointestinal diseases with an immune basis
   k. Gallstones and cholecystitis
   l. Alcoholic liver diseases
   m. Cholestatic syndromes
   n. Drug-induced hepatic injury
   o. Hepatobiliary neoplasms
   p. Chronic liver disease
   q. Gastrointestinal manifestations of HIV infections
   r. Gastrointestinal neoplastic disease
   s. Acute and chronic hepatitis
   t. Biliary and pancreatic diseases
4. Residents must have formal instruction, clinical experience, and opportunities to acquire expertise in the evaluation and management of patients with the following clinical problems:
   a. Dysphagia
   b. Abdominal pain
   c. Acute abdomen
   d. Nausea and vomiting
   e. Diarrhea
   f. Constipation
   g. Gastrointestinal bleeding
   h. Jaundice
   i. Cirrhosis and portal hypertension
   j. Malnutrition
   k. Genetic/inherited disorders
   l. Depression, neurosis, and somatization syndromes
   m. Surgical care of gastrointestinal disorders

B. Technical and Other Skills

1. The program must provide for instruction in the indications, contraindications, complications, limitations, and (where applicable) interpretation of the following diagnostic and therapeutic techniques and procedures:
   a. Imaging of the digestive system, including
      1. Ultrasound
      2. Computed tomography
      3. Magnetic resonance imaging
      4. Vascular radiography
      5. Nuclear medicine
   b. Percutaneous cholangiography
   c. Percutaneous endoscopic gastrostomy
   d. Gastric, pancreatic, and biliary secretory tests
   e. Other diagnostic and therapeutic procedures utilizing enteral intubation and bougienage
   f. Enteral and parenteral alimentation
   g. Liver transplantation
   h. Pancreatic needle biopsy
   i. ERCP, including papillotomy and biliary stent placement
2. Opportunities also must be provided for the resident to gain competence in the performance of the following procedures. A skilled preceptor must be available to teach and to supervise them. The performance of these procedures must be documented in the resident's record, giving indications, outcomes, diagnoses, and supervisor(s).
   a. Esophagogastroduodenoscopy; residents should perform a minimum of 100 supervised studies.
   b. Esophageal dilation; residents should perform a minimum of 15 supervised studies.
   c. Proctoscopy
   d. Flexible sigmoidoscopy; residents should perform a minimum of 25 supervised studies.
   e. Colonoscopy with polypectomy; residents should perform a minimum of 100 supervised colonoscopies and 20 supervised polypectomies.
   f. Percutaneous liver biopsy; residents should perform a minimum of 20 supervised studies.
   g. Percutaneous endoscopic gastrostomy; residents should perform a minimum of 10 supervised studies.
   h. Biopsy of the mucosa of esophagus, stomach, small bowel, and colon
   i. Gastrointestinal motility studies
   j. Nonvariceal hemostasis (upper and lower); residents should perform 20 supervised cases, including 10 active bleeders.
   k. Variceal hemostasis; residents should perform 15 supervised cases, including five active bleeders.
   l. Enteral and parenteral alimentation
   m. Liver biopsy

C. Formal Instruction

The program must include emphasis on the pathogenesis, manifestations, and complications of gastrointestinal disorders, including the behavioral adjustments of patients to their problems. The impact of various modes of therapy and the appropriate utilization of laboratory tests and procedures should be stressed. Additional specific content areas that must be included in the formal program (lectures, conferences, and seminars) include the following:

1. Anatomy, physiology, pharmacology, and pathology related to the gastrointestinal system, including the liver
2. The natural history of digestive diseases
3. Factors involved in nutrition and malnutrition
4. Surgical procedures employed in relation to digestive system disorders and their complications
5. Prudent, cost-effective, and judicious use of special instruments, tests, and therapy in the diagnosis and management of gastroenterologic disorders
6. Liver transplantation
7. Sedation and sedative pharmacology
8. Interpretation of abnormal liver chemistries

ACGME: June 1998 Effective: July 1999

Program Requirements

Program Requirements for Residency Education in Internal Medicine Geriatric Medicine

In addition to complying with the Program Requirements for Residency Education in the Subspecialties of Internal Medicine, programs must also comply with the following requirements, which may in some cases exceed the common requirements.

I. Educational Program

An educational program in geriatric medicine must be organized to provide a well-supervised experience at a sufficient level for the resident to acquire the competence of a physician with added qualifications in the field. It shall be 12 months in duration. The program must be conducted by an accredited residency program in internal medicine or family practice.

Clinical experience must include opportunities to manage elderly patients with a wide variety of medical problems on an inpatient and outpatient basis. Residents must be given the opportunity to provide both primary care and consultation for patients in acute, ambulatory, community, and long-term care settings in order to understand the interaction of natural aging and disease as well as the techniques of assessment, therapy, and management. Additionally, residents must be given the opportunity to care for persons who are generally healthy and require primarily preventive health-care measures.

The program should include an emphasis on the physiology of aging, the pathophysiology that commonly occurs in older persons, atypical presentations of illnesses, functional assessment, cognitive status and affective assessment, and concepts of treatment and management in both the acute and long-term care settings, as well as in the community and in the home.

Attention also should be directed to the behavioral aspects of illness, socioeconomic factors, and ethical and legal considerations that may impinge on medical management.

The program must provide the opportunity for residents to maintain their basic primary skills during the course of this training. At least ½ day per week must be spent in a continuity of care experience in the resident's primary discipline.

II. Faculty and Staff

A. Program Director

The program director must be fully committed to the program in order to devote sufficient time to the achievement of the educational goals and objectives. The director must have demonstrated experience in geriatric medicine and must have demonstrated experience in education and scholarly activity and have a career commitment to academic geriatric medicine. The director must be primarily based at the teaching center.

B. Other Teaching Staff

In addition to the program director, each program must have at least one other faculty member with similar qualifications who devotes a substantial portion of professional time to the training program. For programs with more than two residents, there must be 0.5 additional faculty member for each additional resident. Some of these faculty may be part-time in geriatric medicine or drawn wholly from collaborating programs. The faculty commitment must not attenuate the quality of the core residency training program. The program must ensure that interdisciplinary relationships with the following specialties occur: physical medicine and rehabilitation, neurology, and psychiatry. Appropriate relationships with other disciplines, including but not limited to general surgery, orthopedics, ophthalmology, otolaryngology, urology, gynecology, emergency medicine, dentistry, pharmacy, audiology, physical and occupational therapy, speech therapy, and nursing and social services should be maintained. Additionally, a liaison with the physician assistants, when available, should be established.

C. Geriatric Care Team

The resident must have experience with physician-directed interdisciplinary geriatric teams in an acute-care hospital, in a nursing home that includes subacute and long-term care, in a home care setting, and in a family practice center or other outpatient settings. Essential members include a geriatrician, a nurse, and a social worker. Additional members may be included in the team as appropriate, including representatives from disciplines such as neurology, psychiatry, physical medicine and rehabilitation, physical therapy, occupational therapy and speech therapy, dentistry, pharmacy, psychology, and pastoral care. Regular team conferences must be held as dictated by the needs of the individual patient.

III. Facilities/Resources

A patient population adequate to meet the needs of the training program must be available in the facilities in which the educational experiences take place. Elderly patients of both sexes with a variety of chronic illnesses, at least some of whom have potential for rehabilitation, must be available. At all facilities utilized by the program the resident must be given opportunities to assume meaningful patient responsibility. At each setting certain activities are mandated and must be supervised and taught by the appropriate clinician. The program must include the following:

A. Acute-Care Hospital

The acute-care hospital central to the geriatric medicine program must be an integral component of a teaching center. It must have the full range of services usually ascribed to an acute-care general hospital, including intensive care units, emergency medicine, operating rooms, diagnostic laboratory and imaging services, and a pathology department.

B. Long-term Care Institution

One or more long-term care institutions, such as a skilled nursing facility or chronic care hospital, is a necessary component of the geriatric medicine program. Exposure to subacute care and rehabilitation care in the long-term care setting is desirable. The total number of beds available must be sufficient to permit a comprehensive educational experience. The institutions must be approved by the appropriate licensing agencies of the state, and the standard of facilities and care in each must be consistent with those promulgated by the Joint Commission on the Accreditation of Healthcare Organizations.

C. Long-term Noninstitutional Care

Noninstitutional care service, for example, home care, day care, residential care, or assisted living, is a major component of the geriatric medicine program. A home care program or home health agency is a necessary resource to permit residents to learn to provide care for patients who are homebound but not institutionalized. Day care or day hospital centers, life care communities, and residential care facilities for the elderly are also desirable training sites.

D. Ambulatory Care Program

The ambulatory care program must comprise a minimum of 33% of the resident's time. Each resident should evaluate approximately 1 to 3 new geriatric patients and 4 to 8 follow-up geriatric patients each week. This must include at least ½ day per week spent in a continuity of care experience. This experience must be designed to provide care in a geriatric clinic or family practice center to elderly patients who may require the services of multiple medical disciplines (including but not limited to neurology, gynecology, urology, psychiatry, podiatry, orthopedics, physical medicine and rehabilitation, dentistry, audiology, otolaryngology, and ophthalmology, as well as nursing, social work, and nutrition, among other disciplines. The opportunity to provide continuing care and to coordinate the implementation of recommendations from these medical specialties and disciplines is mandatory. In addition, experiences in relevant ambulatory specialty and subspecialty clinics (eg, geriatric psychiatry and neurology) and those that focus on geriatric syndromes (eg, falls, incontinence, osteoporosis) are highly desirable.

E. Additional Educational Environment

Peer interaction is essential for residents. To achieve this goal, an accredited training program in at least one relevant specialty other than internal medicine must be present at the teaching center sponsoring the training program in geriatric medicine.

Involvement in other health care and community agencies is desirable. There must be a formal affiliation agreement between each long-term care facility included in the program and the sponsoring institution, in which each institution must acknowledge its responsibility to provide high-quality care, adequate resources, and administrative support for the educational mission. In addition, there must be a letter of agreement between each long-term care facility and the office of the director of the geriatric medicine program that guarantees the director appropriate authority at the long-term care institution to carry out the training program.

IV. Specific Program Content

All major dimensions of the curriculum should be structured educational experiences for which written goals and objectives, a specific methodology for teaching, and a method of evaluation exist. A written curriculum that describes the program comprehensively, including sites, educational objectives for each component, and topics to be covered in didactic sessions, should be available to residents and faculty. The curriculum must ensure the opportunity for residents to achieve the cognitive knowledge, psychomotor skills, interpersonal skills, professional attitudes, and practical experience required of a physician who specializes in the care of the aged.

Didactic as well as clinical learning opportunities must be available to the resident. Conferences or seminars/workshops in geriatric medicine should be specifically designed to augment the residents' clinical experiences. Journal club or other activities that foster interaction and develop skills in interpreting the medical literature are necessary.

All deaths of patients who receive care by residents should be reviewed and autopsies performed whenever possible.

As the residents progress through their training, they must have the opportunity to teach personnel such as nurses, allied health personnel, medical students, and residents.

Appropriate faculty supervision of the residents must be provided during all of their educational experiences.

The following components must be provided:

A. Geriatric Medicine Consultation Program

This program must be formally available in the ambulatory setting, the inpatient service, and/or emergency medicine in the acute-care hospital or at an ambulatory setting administered by the primary teaching institution.

B. Long-term Care Experience

In the long-term care institutional setting each resident must have 12 months of continuing longitudinal clinical experience with an assigned panel of patients for whom the resident is the primary provider. Additional block time to provide long-term care experience is encouraged. Emphasis during the longitudinal experience should be focused on (1) the approaches to diagnosis and treatment of the acutely and chronically ill, frail elderly in a less technologically sophisticated environment than the acute-care hospital; (2) working within the limits of a decreased staff-patient ratio compared with acute-care hospitals; (3) a much greater awareness of and familiarity with subacute care physical medicine and rehabilitation; (4) the challenge of the clinical and ethical dilemmas produced by the illness of the very old; and (5) administrative aspects of long-term care.

Experience with home visits and hospice care must be included. The resident must be exposed to the organizational and administrative aspects of home health care. Continuity of care with an assigned panel of home or hospice care patients for whom the resident is the primary provider is essential.

C. Geriatric Psychiatry

Identifiable structured didactic and clinical experiences in geriatric psychiatry must be included in the program of each resident. Behavioral sciences such as psychology/social work and others must be included in the curriculum.

D. Curriculum

The training program must provide opportunities for the residents to develop clinical competence in the overall field of geriatric medicine. The curriculum of the program must exhibit, as a minimum, the following content and skill areas:

1. Current scientific knowledge of aging and longevity, including theories of aging, the physiology and natural history of aging, pathologic changes with aging, epidemiology of aging populations, and diseases of the aged.
2. Aspects of preventive medicine, including nutrition, oral health, exercise, screening, immunization, and chemoprophylaxis against disease. Instruction about and experience with community resources dedicated to these activities should be included.
3. Geriatric assessment, including medical, affective, cognitive, functional status, social support, economic, and environmental aspects related to health; activities of daily living (ADL); the instrumental activities of daily living (IADL); the appropriate use of the history, physical and mental examination, and laboratory.
4. Appropriate interdisciplinary coordination of the actions of multiple health professionals, including physicians, nurses, social workers, dieticians, and rehabilitation experts, in the assessment and implementation of treatment.
5. Topics of special interest to geriatric medicine, including but not limited to cognitive impairment, depression and related disorders, falls, incontinence, osteoporosis, fractures, sensory impairment, pressure ulcers, sleep disorders, pain, senior (elder) abuse, malnutrition, and functional impairment.
6. Diseases that are especially prominent in the elderly or that have different characteristics in the elderly, including neoplastic, cardiovascular, neurologic, musculoskeletal, metabolic, and infectious disorders.
7. Pharmacologic problems associated with aging, including changes in pharmacokinetics and pharmacodynamics, drug interactions, overmedication, appropriate prescribing, and adherence.
8. Psychosocial aspects of aging, including interpersonal and family relationships, living situations, adjustment disorders, depression, bereavement, and anxiety.
9. The economic aspects of supporting services, including Title III of the Older Americans Act, Medicare, Medicaid, capitation, and cost containment.
10. Ethical and legal issues especially pertinent to geriatric medicine, including limitation of treatment, competency, guardianship, right to refuse treatment, advance directives, wills, and durable power of attorney for medical affairs.

11. General principles of geriatric rehabilitation, including those applicable to patients with orthopedic, rheumatologic, cardiac, and neurologic impairments. These principles should include those related to the use of physical medicine modalities, exercise, functional activities, assistive devices, environmental modification, patient and family education, and psychosocial and recreational counseling.
12. Management of patients in long-term care settings, including palliative care, knowledge of the administration, regulation, and financing of long-term institutions, and the continuum from short- to long-term care.
13. Research methodologies related to geriatric medicine, including clinical epidemiology, decision analysis, and critical literature review.
14. Perioperative assessment and involvement in management.
15. Iatrogenic disorders and their prevention.
16. Communication skills with patients, families, professional colleagues, and community groups, including presenting case reports, literature searches, and research papers, when appropriate, to peers and lectures to lay audiences.
17. The pivotal role of the family in caring for many elderly and the community resources (formal support systems) required to support both patient and family.
18. Cultural aspects of aging, including knowledge about demographics, health care status of older persons of diverse ethnicities, access to health care, cross-cultural assessment, and use of an interpreter in clinical care. Issues of ethnicity in long-term care, patient education, and special issues relating to urban and rural older persons of various ethnic backgrounds should be covered.
19. Home care, including the components of a home visit, and accessing appropriate community resources to provide care in the home setting.
20. Hospice care, including pain management, symptom relief, comfort care, and end-of-life issues.

V. Certification

Those planning to seek a Certificate of Added Qualifications from the American Board of Internal Medicine or the American Board of Family Practice should communicate with the administrative officer of the board as listed in the *Graduate Medical Education Directory* to ascertain the full requirements.

ACGME: February 1998 Effective: July 1998

Program Requirements for Residency Education in Hematology (Internal Medicine)

I. Educational Program

A subspecialty educational program in hematology must be organized to provide training and supervised experience at a sufficient level for the resident to acquire the competency of a specialist in the field. It must be 2 years in duration.

II. Faculty

See Section III, Program Requirements for Residency Education in the Subspecialties of Internal Medicine.

III. Facilities and Resources

Modern facilities to accomplish the overall educational program must be available and functioning. Specifically, the resources that must be available to the program include hematology and coagulation laboratories; advanced pathology services, including immunopathology; a blood bank; transfusion and apheresis facilities; diagnostic and therapeutic radiology services; and nuclear medicine services. The program must also participate in a multidisciplinary tumor conference that includes discussion of neoplastic blood disorders and hematologic-oncologic protocol studies. In addition, there should be a medical oncology program with which hematology residents can interact formally in an educational experience.

It is highly desirable to have the support of the nursing, rehabilitation medicine, pain management, dietetic, and social services in the care of patients with neoplastic blood disorders so that the resident may see the role of other specialties in the total care of patients with hematologic and/or neoplastic diseases.

IV. Specific Program Content

A. Clinical Experience

Clinical experience must include opportunities to observe and manage patients with a wide variety of blood diseases on both an inpatient and an outpatient basis. The resident must be given opportunities to assume continuing responsibility for acutely and chronically ill patients in order to observe the evolution of blood diseases as well as the benefits and adverse effects of therapy. Inpatient assignments should be of sufficient duration to permit continuing care of a majority of the patients throughout their hospitalization.

B.

The program must provide residents with experiences in an ambulatory care setting at least ½ day each week over the 24 months of training. In addition, the program must provide residents with continuity experiences, each at least 6 months in duration, throughout the residency program.

C. Technical and Other Skills

1. The program must provide residents with the opportunity to develop competence to work effectively as part of a multidisciplinary team.
2. The program must provide the opportunity for residents to gain competence or expertise in the performance and (where applicable) interpretation of the following:
   a. Bone marrow aspiration and biopsy, including preparation, staining, examination, and interpretation of blood smears, bone marrow aspirates, and touch preparations and interpretation of bone marrow biopsies
   b. Use of chemotherapeutic agents and biological products through all therapeutic routes
   c. Correlation of clinical information with the findings of cytology, histology, immunodiagnostic, and imaging techniques
3. The program should provide experience or observation of the following:
   a. Apheresis procedures
   b. Performance and interpretation of partial thromboplastin time, prothrombin time, platelet aggregation, and bleeding time and other standard coagulation assays
   c. Bone marrow or peripheral stem cell harvest for transplantation
   d. Fine needle aspiration and biopsy

D. Specific Program Content

The residents must have formal instruction, clinical experience, or opportunities to acquire knowledge in the following:

1. Morphology, physiology, and biochemistry of blood, marrow, lymphatic tissue, and the spleen
2. Related basic fields, including immunology, basic and clinical pharmacology and pharmacokinetics, cell and molecular biol-

ogy, tumor immunology, molecular genetics, and prenatal diagnosis
3. Basic molecular and pathophysiologic mechanisms, diagnosis, and therapy of diseases of the blood, including anemias, diseases of white blood cells and stem cells, and disorders of hemostasis and thrombosis
4. Etiology, epidemiology, natural history, diagnosis, pathology, staging, and management of neoplastic diseases of the blood, blood-forming organs, and lymphatic tissues
5. Measurement of the complete blood count, including platelets and white cell differential, using automated or manual techniques with appropriate quality control
6. Immunophenotyping, cytochemical studies, and cytogenetic and DNA analysis of neoplastic disorders of blood, blood-forming organs, and lymphatic tissues
7. Molecular mechanisms of hematopoietic and lymphopoietic malignancies, including the nature of oncogenes and their products
8. Relevant chemotherapeutic drugs, biologic products, and growth factors and their mechanisms of action, pharmacokinetics, clinical indications, and limitations
9. Multiagent chemotherapy protocols and combined modality therapy for hematopoietic and lymphopoietic malignancies
10. Management and care of indwelling venous access catheters
11. Principles and application of radiation medicine to hematopoietic and lymphopoietic malignancies
12. Management of the neutropenic and the immunocompromised patient
13. Effects of systemic disorders and drugs on the blood, blood-forming organs, and lymphatic tissues
14. Allogeneic and autologous bone marrow or peripheral blood stem cell transplantation and the nature and management of posttransplant complications
15. Tests of hemostasis and thrombosis for both congenital and acquired disorders and regulation of antithrombotic therapy
16. Treatment of patients with disorders of hemostasis and the biochemistry and pharmacology of coagulation factor replacement therapy
17. Transfusion medicine, including the evaluation of antibodies, blood compatibility, and the use of blood-component therapy and apheresis
18. Indications and application of imaging techniques in patients with blood disorders
19. Personal development, attitudes, and coping skills of physicians and other health-care professionals who care for critically ill patients
20. Pain management in patients with blood disorders
21. Rehabilitation and psychosocial aspects of clinical management of patients with hematologic disorders
22. Hospice and home care
23. Recognition and management of paraneoplastic disorders
24. Clinical epidemiology and medical statistics, including clinical study and experimental protocol design, data collection, and analysis
25. Participation in a tumor board
26. Human immunodeficiency virus-related malignancies
27. Care and management of geriatric patients with hematologic disorders

ACGME: June 1998 Effective: July 1999

Program Requirements for Residency Education in Hematology and Oncology (Internal Medicine)

I. Educational Program

A subspecialty educational program in combined hematology and oncology must be organized to provide training and supervised experience at a sufficient level for the resident to acquire the competency of a specialist in the field. It must be 3 years in duration.

II. Key Clinical Faculty

A. The combined subspecialty program faculty must include a minimum of six (three for each discipline) qualified key clinical teaching faculty members, including the program director.

B. At least two of the key clinical faculty must be certified in hematology and at least two must be certified in oncology.

C. Faculty members who are certified in infectious diseases, pulmonary diseases, endocrinology, and gastroenterology by the American Board of Internal Medicine or who have obtained equivalent training and experience must be available to participate in the education of residents in hematology/oncology. The program also must have the support of other clinical specialties, including psychiatry, neurology, dermatology, gynecology, nuclear medicine, pathology, radiation therapy, and surgical specialties.

III. Facilities and Resources

A. Modern facilities to accomplish the overall educational program must be available and functioning at the primary site. Specifically, there must be advanced pathology services, including immunopathology, resources for nuclear medicine imaging, blood banking, transfusion and apheresis facilities, coagulation laboratories, and radiation oncology facilities. A modern diagnostic radiologic service and a general surgical service and its support must be available. The program also must participate in a multidisciplinary tumor conference and cancer protocol studies.

B. It is highly desirable to have the support of oncologic nursing, rehabilitation medicine, dietetic, and social services so that the resident may see the role of other specialists in the total care of the cancer patient.

IV. Specific Program Content

A. Clinical Experience

Clinical experience must include opportunities to observe and manage both inpatients and outpatients with a wide variety of blood and neoplastic disorders. The resident must be given opportunities to assume continuing responsibility for acutely and chronically ill patients in order to observe the evolution of blood diseases and the natural history of cancer as well as the benefits and adverse effects of therapy. Inpatient assignments should be of sufficient duration to permit continuing care of a majority of the patients throughout their hospitalization. At least 18 months of the program must be devoted to clinical training.

B. Ambulatory Medicine Experience

The program must provide residents with experiences in an ambulatory care setting for at least ½ day each week over the 36 months of training. In addition, the program must provide residents with continuity experiences, each at least 6 months in duration throughout the residency program.

C. Technical and Other Skills

1. The program must provide residents with the opportunity to develop competence to work effectively as part of a multidisciplinary team.
2. The program must provide the opportunity for residents to gain competence or expertise in the performance and (where applicable) interpretation of the following:
   a. Bone marrow aspiration and biopsy, including preparation, staining, examination, and interpretation of blood smears, bone marrow aspirates, and touch preparations and interpretation of bone marrow biopsies
   b. Use of chemotherapeutic agents and biological response modifiers by all therapeutic routes
   c. Serial measurement of palpable tumor masses
   d. Assessment of tumor imaging by computed tomography, magnetic resonance, and nuclear imaging techniques
   e. Correlation of clinical information with cytology, histology, and immunodiagnostic imaging techniques
3. The program should provide experience or observation of the following:
   a. Apheresis procedures
   b. Performance and interpretation of partial thromboplastin time, prothrombin time, platelet aggregation, and bleeding time and other standard coagulation assays
   c. Bone marrow or peripheral stem cell harvest for transplantation
   d. Fine needle aspiration and biopsy

D. Specific Program Content

The residents must have formal instruction, clinical experience, or opportunities to acquire knowledge in the following:

1. Morphology, physiology, and biochemistry of blood, marrow, lymphatic tissue, and the spleen
2. Basic molecular and pathophysiologic mechanisms, diagnosis, and therapy of diseases of the blood, including anemias, diseases of white cells, and disorders of hemostasis and thrombosis
3. Etiology, epidemiology, natural history, diagnosis, pathology, staging, and management of neoplastic disorders
4. Measurement of the complete blood count, including platelets and white cell differential, using automated or manual techniques with appropriate quality control
5. Immune markers, immunophenotyping, cytochemical studies, and cytogenetic and DNA analysis of neoplastic disorders
6. Molecular mechanisms of neoplasia, including the nature of oncogenes and their products
7. Chemotherapeutic drugs, biologic products, and growth factors and their mechanisms of action, pharmacokinetics, clinical indications, and limitations, including their effects, toxicity, and interactions
8. Multiagent chemotherapy protocols and combined modality therapy in the treatment of neoplastic disorders
9. Management and care of indwelling venous access catheters
10. Principles and application of surgery and radiation therapy in the treatment of neoplastic disorders
11. Management of the neutropenic and the immunocompromised patient
12. Effects of systemic disorders, infections, solid tumors, and drugs on the blood, blood-forming organs, and lymphatic tissues
13. Allogeneic and autologous bone marrow transplantation and the nature and management of posttransplant complications
14. Indications and application of imaging techniques in patients with blood and neoplastic disorders
15. Pathophysiology and patterns of solid tumor metastases
16. Principles of multidisciplinary management of organ-specific cancers, in particular, gynecologic malignancies
17. Pain management in the cancer patient
18. Rehabilitation and psychosocial management of patients with hematologic and neoplastic disorders
19. Hospice and home care for the cancer patient
20. Recognition and management of paraneoplastic disorders
21. The etiology of cancer, including predisposing causal factors leading to neoplasia
22. Cancer prevention and screening, including competency in genetic testing and counseling as they relate to hereditary cancers and hematologic disorders for high-risk individuals
23. Participation in a tumor board
24. Tests of hemostasis and thrombosis for both congenital and acquired disorders and regulation of antithrombotic therapy
25. Treatment of patients with disorders of hemostasis and the biochemistry and pharmacology of coagulation factor replacement
26. Transfusion medicine, including the evaluation of antibodies, blood compatibility, and the use of blood component therapy and apheresis procedures
27. Personal development, attitudes, and coping skills of physicians and other health-care professionals who care for critically ill patients
28. Human immunodeficiency virus-related malignancies
29. Care and management of the geriatric patient with malignancy and hematologic disorders

ACGME: June 1998 Effective: July 1999

Program Requirements for Residency Education in Infectious Disease (Internal Medicine)

I. Educational Program

A subspecialty educational program in infectious disease must be organized to provide training and supervised experience at a sufficient level for the resident to acquire the competency of a specialist in the field. It must be 2 years in duration.

II. Facilities and Resources

Modern facilities to accomplish the overall educational program must be available and functioning at the primary training site. Specifically, there must be access to a laboratory for clinical microbiology, including diagnostic bacteriology, immunology, mycology, parasitology, and virology. Facilities for the isolation of patients with infectious diseases must be available. It is highly desirable that the training program be conducted in a setting in which training programs in surgery, obstetrics, gynecology, pediatrics, and other medical and surgical specialties and subspecialties are available.

III. Specific Program Content

A. Clinical Experience

Clinical experience must include opportunities to observe and manage adult patients with a wide variety of infectious diseases on both an inpatient and an ambulatory basis. Such opportunities must encompass longitudinal experiences in a continuum of care to observe the course of illness and the effects of therapy. Therapeutic modalities should include management of antibiotic administration in such settings as the hospital, the office, or in conjunction with home-care services. Experience with pediatric infectious diseases is encouraged.

B. Ambulatory Medicine Experience

Ambulatory care experience to provide both consultative services and continuing care in infectious disease including human immunodeficiency virus (HIV) must be included in the training program. Ambulatory training must include longitudinal care of patients with HIV infection.

C. Specific Program Content

Residents must have clinical experience or formal instruction in the prevention, evaluation, and management of the following disorders:

1. The febrile patient; specifically presenting in association with rash or as fever of unknown origin
2. Upper respiratory tract infections
3. Pleuropulmonary and bronchial infections
4. Urinary tract infections
5. Peritonitis and other intra-abdominal infections
6. Cardiovascular infections
7. Central nervous system infections
8. Skin and soft tissue infections
9. Infections related to trauma, including burns and animal and human bites
10. Gastrointestinal infections and food poisoning
11. Bone and joint infections
12. Infections of the reproductive organs
13. Sexually transmitted diseases
14. Infections of the eye
15. Viral hepatitides
16. Sepsis syndromes
17. Nosocomial infections
18. HIV infection and acquired immunodeficiency syndrome
19. Infections in the immunocompromised or neutropenic host
20. Infections in patients with acute leukemia and lymphomas
21. Infections in transplant recipients
22. Infections in solid organ transplant recipients
23. Infections in geriatric patients
24. Infections in travelers
25. Infections in parenteral drug abusers

D. Technical and Other Skills

The program must provide for practical experience or instruction in the cognitive aspects of the following:

1. Mechanisms of action and adverse reactions of antimicrobial agents; the conduct of pharmacologic studies to determine absorption and excretion of antimicrobial agents; methods of determining antimicrobial activity of a drug; techniques to determine concentration of antimicrobial agents in the blood and other body fluids; the appropriate use and management of antimicrobial agents in a variety of clinical settings, including the hospital, ambulatory practice, and the home
2. The utility of procedures for specimen collection relevant to infectious disease, including but not limited to bronchoscopy, thoracentesis, arthrocentesis, lumbar puncture, and aspiration of abscess cavities, including soft-tissue infections
3. Principles and practice of hospital infection control
4. Principles of chemoprophylaxis and immunoprophylaxis to enhance resistance
5. Mechanisms of actions of biological products, including monoclonal antibodies, cytokines, interferons, interleukins, and colony-stimulating factors, and their applications in the treatments of infectious diseases or their role in enhancing the immune response

E. Formal Instruction

Additional specific content areas that must be included in the formal program (lectures, conferences, and seminars) include

1. the factors that determine the outcome between host and parasite, including microbial virulence factors and host defense mechanisms.
2. basic concepts of immunology.
3. the epidemiology, clinical course, manifestations, diagnosis, treatment, and prevention of major infectious agents including viruses, chlamydiae, mycoplasma and ureaplasma, rickettsioses, and bacteria including spirochetes and mycobacteria, mycoses, protozoa, and helminths.
4. quality assurance and cost containment in the clinical practice of infectious diseases.

ACGME: June 1998 Effective: July 1999

Program Requirements for Residency Education in Interventional Cardiology (Internal Medicine)

I. Educational Program

A. Interventional cardiology encompasses the special knowledge and skill required of cardiologists to care for patients receiving cardiac interventional procedures. Interventional cardiology is the practice of techniques that improve coronary circulation and alleviate valvular stenosis.

B. A subspecialty educational program in interventional cardiology must function as an integral component of an accredited subspecialty residency in cardiovascular disease and must be organized to provide training and experience at a sufficient level for the resident to acquire the competency of a specialist in the field.

C. During training in interventional cardiology, the resident's clinical experience must include opportunities to diagnose, select therapies, perform interventional procedures, and manage and judge the effectiveness of treatment(s) for inpatients and outpatients with chronic coronary artery disease, acute coronary syndromes, and valvular heart disease. The resident should be given opportunities to assume continuing responsibility for both acutely and chronically ill patients to learn the natural history of these cardiac conditions.

D. The interventional cardiology program is accredited for 1 year of training. All applicants entering interventional cardiology must have completed an Accreditation Council for Graduate Medical Education (ACGME)-accredited cardiovascular disease program or its equivalent.

E. The principles enumerated in the Program Requirements for Residency Education in Internal Medicine and the General Information Section of the Program Requirements for Residency Education in the Subspecialties of Internal Medicine are also applicable to training in this subspecialty.

II. Faculty

Faculty responsible for training should be board certified in interventional cardiology or possess equivalent qualifications. There should be a minimum of two key clinically active interventional cardiology faculty members and no fewer than one key clinically active interventional cardiology faculty member per 1.5 residents. [*Note:* Clinically active is defined as a minimum of 75 interventions performed per year.] Access to faculty with expertise in cardiac surgery, radiation safety, hematology, pharmacology, congenital heart disease in adults, and research laboratories is desirable.

III. Facilities and Resources

A. Modern clinical inpatient and ambulatory care and research facilities to accomplish the overall educational goals and objectives of the program must be available and functioning.
B. There must be a cardiac catheterization laboratory at each training site wherein a minimum of 400 interventional procedures of the heart are performed per year.
   1. It must contain appropriate cardiac fluoroscopic equipment, recording devices, and resuscitative equipment.
   2. An outpatient follow-up program must exist to care for patients.
C. Clinical care units must include cardiac care units (CCUs), cardiac surgical intensive care units, and outpatient clinics.
D. Cardiac surgery must be located at the primary training site.

IV. Specific Program Content

A. Clinical Experience

1. Residents should have clinical experiences that provide the opportunity to acquire knowledge of the indications, contraindications, risks, limitations, sensitivity, specificity, predictive accuracy, and appropriate techniques for evaluating patients with a variety of cardiac disease disorders, including but not limited to
   a. chronic ischemic heart disease
   b. acute ischemic syndromes
   c. valvular heart disease
2. Residents must have the opportunity to acquire experience in the management of the bleeding complications associated with percutaneous intervention, including but not limited to
   a. bleeding after thrombolytic usage
   b. heparin usage
   c. glycoprotein IIb/IIIa inhibitor usage
3. Residents must have clinical experiences involving
   a. consultation
   b. care of patients in the cardiac care unit, emergency department, or other intensive care settings
   c. care of the patient before and after interventional procedures
   d. outpatient follow-up of patients treated with drugs, interventions, devices, or surgery
4. The program must provide sufficient experience for the residents to acquire knowledge in clinical decision making, including but not limited to
   a. the role of randomized clinical trials and registry experiences in clinical decision making
   b. the clinical importance of complete vs incomplete revascularization in a wide variety of clinical and anatomic situations
   c. strengths and limitations, both short- and long-term, of percutaneous vs surgical and medical therapy for a wide variety of clinical and anatomic situations related to cardiovascular disease
   d. strengths and limitations, both short- and long-term of differing percutaneous approaches for a wide variety of anatomic situations related to cardiovascular disease
   e. the role of emergency coronary bypass surgery in the management of complications of percutaneous intervention
   f. the use and limitations of intra-aortic balloon counterpulsation (IABP) and other hemodynamic support devices (as available)
   g. strengths and weaknesses of mechanical vs lytic approach for patients with acute myocardial infarction
   h. The use of pharamocologic agents appropriate in the postintervention management of patients
   i. strengths and limitations of both noninvasive and invasive coronary evaluation during the recovery phase after acute myocardial infarction
   j. understanding the clinical utility and limitations of valvuloplasty of both the mitral and aortic valves
   k. the assessment of plaque composition and response to intervention

B. Technical and Other Skills

1. To become proficient in interventional cardiology, residents must have the opportunity to acquire a broad-based knowledge of interventions. Toward that end, residents must have opportunities to acquire skill in the interpretation of
   a. coronary arteriograms
   b. ventriculography
   c. hemodynamics
   d. intravascular ultrasound
   e. Doppler flow and intracoronary pressure monitoring
2. Each resident must have opportunity to acquire skill in the performance of a minimum of 250 coronary interventions, to include the following: [*Note:* A single coronary intervention is defined as all coronary interventions performed during one hospitalization.]
   a. Management of mechanical complications of percutaneous intervention, including but not limited to
      1. coronary dissection
      2. thrombosis
      3. spasm
      4. perforation
      5. "slow reflow"
      6. cardiogenic shock
      7. left main trunk dissection
      8. cardiac tamponade
      9. peripheral vessel occlusion, and retained components
      10. pseudoaneurysm
   b. Femoral and brachial/radial cannulation of normal and abnormally located coronary ostia
   c. Application and usage of balloon angioplasty, stents, and other commonly used interventional devices
   d. Use of adjunctive imaging techniques such as intravascular ultrasound, angioscopy, coronary flow reserve, and pressure measurement
3. Resident experience should meet the following criteria:
   a. Participation in preprocedural planning, including the indications for the procedure and the selection of the appropriate procedure or instruments
   b. Performance of the critical technical manipulations of the procedure
   c. Substanial involvement in postprocedure care
   d. Supervision by teaching faculty responsible for the procedure
4. Residents also must have opportunities to acquire skill in the following:
   a. Use of antiarrhythmic drugs, including knowledge of pharmacokinetics and pharmacodynamics related to acute ischemic events occurring during and after interventional cardiac procedures
   b. Cardiopulmonary resuscitation
   c. Advanced cardiac life support
   d. Use of thrombolytic and antithrombolytic agents
   e. Use of vasoactive agents for epicardial and microvascular spasm

C. Formal Instruction

The program must provide instruction and opportunities to acquire knowledge in the following:
1. Role of platelets and the clotting cascade in response to vascular injury
2. Pathophysiology of restenosis
3. Strengths and limitations of various animal models used to evaluate the problem of restenosis in humans
4. Role and limitations of gene transfer and therapy for treatment of restenosis

5. Physiology of coronary flow and detection of flow-limiting conditions
6. Detailed coronary anatomy
7. Radiation physics, biology, and safety related to the use of x-ray imaging equipment
8. Critical analysis of published interventional cardiology data in laboratory and clinical research
9. Role of randomized clinical trials and registry experiences in clinical decision making

ACGME: September 1998 Effective: September 1998

Program Requirements for Residency Education in Nephrology (Internal Medicine)

I. Educational Program

A subspecialty educational program in nephrology must be organized to provide training and supervised experience at a sufficient level for the resident to acquire the competency of a specialist in the field. It must be 2 years in duration.

II. Facilities and Resources

A. Modern facilities to accomplish the overall educational program must be available and functioning at the primary training site. Specifically, there must be facilities for acute and chronic hemodialysis, continuous renal replacement therapy, acute and chronic peritoneal dialysis, and renal biopsy. The following must be available: a radiology service that can provide modern renal-related procedures, including ultrasound and computerized tomography, a diagnostic radionuclide laboratory, electron microscopy for renal biopsy material, biochemistry and serologic laboratories, a nutrition support service, and relevant social services. A meaningful working relationship must exist with other services, including surgery, urology, obstetrics, gynecology, pediatrics, psychiatry, pathology, and radiology.

B. The sponsoring institution must be approved to perform renal transplantation or have a formal written agreement with such an institution ensuring that nephrology residents receive the requisite experience with renal transplantation. The training program must have access to at least 10 new renal transplants per year per clinical resident and be responsible for the longitudinal follow-up of at least 20 patients with transplants per resident.

C. The training program should be of sufficient size to ensure adequate exposure of residents to patients with acute renal failure and a chronic dialysis patient population, including patients who utilize home dialysis treatment modalities, to ensure adequate training in chronic dialysis.

D. The training program must afford the residents the opportunity to care for patients with renal and other disorders in the intensive care unit setting.

III. Specific Program Content

A. Clinical Experience

A minimum of 12 months should be devoted to clinical experiences.

B. Specific Program Content

1. Residents must have formal instruction, clinical experience, and opportunities to acquire expertise in the prevention, evaluation, and management of the following disorders:
   a. Disorders of mineral metabolism, including nephrolithiasis and renal osteodystrophy
   b. Disorders of fluid, electrolyte, and acid-base regulation
   c. Acute renal failure
   d. Chronic renal failure and its management by conservative methods, including nutritional management of uremia
   e. End-stage renal disease
   f. Hypertensive disorders
   g. Renal disorders of pregnancy
   h. Urinary tract infections
   i. Tubulointerstitial renal diseases, including inherited diseases of transport, cystic diseases, and other congenital disorders
   j. Glomerular and vascular diseases, including the glomerulonephritides, diabetic nephropathy, and atheroembolic renal disease
   k. Disorders of drug metabolism and renal drug toxicity
   l. Genetic and inherited renal disorders
   m. Geriatric aspects of nephrology, including disorders of the aging kidney and urinary tract
2. Residents must have special experiences in renal transplantation and dialysis and extracoporeal therapy.
   a. Renal transplantation: Each resident must have a minimum of 2 months of clinical experience, preferably consecutively, on an active renal transplant service. Clinical experience must entail supervised involvement in the decision making for patients during the pre- and post-transplant care. This experience must include
      1. evaluation and selection of transplant candidates
      2. preoperative evaluation and preparation of transplant recipients and donors
      3. immediate postoperative management of transplant recipients, including administration of immunosuppressants
      4. clinical diagnosis of all forms of rejection, including laboratory, histopathologic, and imaging techniques
      5. medical management of rejection, including use of immunosuppressant drugs and other agents
      6. recognition and medical management of the surgical and nonsurgical complications of transplantations
      7. long-term follow-up of transplant recipients in the ambulatory setting
   b. Dialysis and extracorporeal therapy: Each resident should have exposure to dialysis and extracorporeal therapies during the equivalent of at least 4 months of the training program. Clinical experience must entail supervised involvement in decision making for patients undergoing these therapies. This experience must include
      1. evaluation and selection of patients for acute hemodialysis or continuous renal replacement therapies
      2. evaluation of end-stage renal disease patients for various forms of therapy and their instruction regarding treatment options
      3. drug dosage modification during dialysis and other extracorporeal therapies
      4. evaluation and management of medical complications in patients during and between dialyses and other extracorporeal therapies, including dialysis access, and an understanding of the pathogenesis and prevention of such complications
      5. long-term follow-up of patients undergoing chronic dialysis, including the dialysis prescription and modification and assessment of adequacy of dialysis
      6. an understanding of the principles and practice of peritoneal dialysis, including the establishment of peritoneal ac-

cess, the principles of dialysis catheters, and how to choose appropriate catheters
7. an understanding of the technology of peritoneal dialysis, including the use of automated cyclers
8. assessment of peritoneal dialysis efficiency, using peritoneal equilibration testing and the principles of peritoneal biopsy
9. an understanding of how to write a peritoneal dialysis prescription and how to assess peritoneal dialysis adequacy
10. the pharmacology of commonly used medications and their kinetic and dosage alteration with peritoneal dialysis
11. an understanding of the complications of peritoneal dialysis, including peritonitis and its treatment, exit site and tunnel infections and their management, hernias, plural effusions, and other less common complications and their management
12. an understanding of the special nutritional requirements of hemodialysis and peritoneal dialysis patients

C. Technical and Other Skills

1. The procedural skills in which residents must be given sufficient experience to gain expertise, including the performance of such procedures, their indications and complications, and interpretation of their results, are
   a. urinalysis
   b. percutaneous biopsy of both autologous and transplanted kidneys
   c. placement of temporary vascular access for hemodialysis and related procedures
   d. peritoneal dialysis
   e. acute and chronic hemodialysis
   f. continuous renal replacement therapy
2. The program must ensure that residents have the necessary knowledge and are familiar with the following procedures, including their indications, contraindications, complications, and interpretations of results, as well as their cost-effectiveness and application to patient care:
   a. Radiology of vascular access
   b. Balloon angioplasty of vascular access
   c. Therapeutic plasmapheresis
   d. Bone biopsy
   e. Placement of peritoneal catheters
   f. Renal ultrasound
   g. Lithotripsy

D. Formal Instruction

1. Specific content areas that must be included in the formal program (lectures, conferences, seminars, and journal clubs) include
   a. renal anatomy, physiology, and pathology
   b. pathogenesis, natural history, and management of congenital and acquired diseases of the kidney and urinary tract and renal diseases associated with systemic disorders such as diabetes, collagen-vascular diseases, and pregnancy
   c. normal mineral metabolism and its alteration in renal diseases, metabolic bone disease, and nephrolithiasis
   d. normal and abnormal blood pressure regulation
   e. clinical pharmacology, including drug metabolism and pharmacokinetics and the effects of drugs on renal structure and function
   f. nutritional aspects of renal disorders
   g. immunology, including
      1. basic principles
      2. immunologic mechanisms of renal disease
      3. fundamental aspects of diagnostic laboratory immunology relevant to renal diseases
   h. transplantation—the structured curriculum for renal transplantation must, as a minimum, include
      1. biology of transplantation rejection
      2. indications for and contraindications to renal transplantation
      3. principles of transplant recipient evaluation and selection
      4. principles of evaluation of transplant donors, both live and cadaveric, including histocompatibility testing
      5. principles of organ harvesting, preservation, and sharing
      6. psychosocial aspects of organ donation and transplantation
      7. the pathogenesis and management of urinary tract infections
      8. the pathogenesis and management of acute renal failure
      9. indications for and interpretations of radiologic tests of the kidney and urinary tract
      10. disorders of fluids and electrolytes and acid-base balance
   i. dialysis and extracorporeal therapy, including
      1. the kinetic principles of hemodialysis and peritoneal dialysis
      2. the indication for each mode of dialysis
      3. the short-term and long-term complications of each mode of dialysis and their management
      4. the principles of dialysis access (acute and chronic vascular and peritoneal), including indications, techniques, and complications
      5. urea kinetics and protein catabolic rate
      6. dialysis modes and their relation to metabolism
      7. nutritional management of dialysis patients
      8. dialysis water treatment, delivery systems, and reuse of artificial kidneys
      9. the artificial membranes used in hemodialysis and biocompatibility
      10. the psychosocial and ethical issues of dialysis
   j. geriatric medicine, including
      1. physiology and pathology of the aging kidney
      2. drug dosing and renal toxicity in elderly patients

ACGME: June 1998 Effective: July 1999

Program Requirements for Residency Education in Oncology (Internal Medicine)

I. Educational Program

A subspecialty educational program in oncology must be organized to provide training and supervised experience at a sufficient level for the resident to acquire the competency of a specialist in the field. It must be 2 years in duration.

II. Key Clinical Faculty

A. See Section III, Program Requirements for Residency Education in the Subspecialties of Internal Medicine.

B. Faculty members who are subspecialty certified by the American Board of Internal Medicine in their respective disciplines or who have obtained equivalent training and experience in infectious disease, pulmonary disease, endocrinology, gastroenterology, and hematology must be available to participate in the education of residents in oncology. The program also must have the support of other clinical specialties, including psychiatry, gynecology, nuclear medicine, pathology, neurology, neurosurgery, radiation therapy, neurology, dermatology, and surgical specialties.

III. Facilities and Resources

A. Modern facilities to accomplish the overall educational program must be available and functioning. Specifically, there must be advanced pathology services, including immunopathology resources for nuclear medicine imaging, blood banking, transfusion and apheresis facilities, and radiation oncology facilities. A modern diagnostic radiologic service, and a general surgical service and its support, must be available. The program must also participate in a multidisciplinary tumor conference and cancer protocol studies.

B. It is highly desirable to have the support of oncologic nursing, rehabilitation medicine, pain management, dietetic, and social services so that the resident may see the role of other specialties in the total care of the cancer patient.

IV. Specific Program Content

A. Clinical Experience

Clinical experience must include opportunities to observe and manage patients with a wide variety of neoplastic diseases on an inpatient and outpatient basis. The resident must be given opportunities to assume continuing responsibility for both acutely and chronically ill patients to learn the natural history of cancer as well as the effectiveness of therapeutic programs. Inpatient assignments should be of sufficient duration to permit continuing care of a majority of the patients throughout their hospitalization.

B. Ambulatory Medicine Experience

The program must provide residents with experiences in an ambulatory care setting at least ½ day each week over the 24 months of training. In addition, the program must provide residents with continuity experiences, each at least 6 months in duration, throughout the residency program.

C. Technical and Other Skills

1. The program must provide residents with the opportunity to develop the competence needed to work effectively as part of a multidisciplinary team.
2. The program must provide the opportunity for residents to gain competence or expertise in the performance and (where applicable) interpretation of the following:
   a. Serial measurement of palpable tumor masses
   b. Assessment of tumor imaging by computed tomography, magnetic resonance, and nuclear imaging techniques
   c. Bone marrow aspiration and biopsy and their interpretation
   d. Use of chemotherapeutic agents and biological products through all therapeutic routes
   e. Correlation of clinical information with the findings of cytology, histology, and immunodiagnostic techniques

D. Specific Program Content

The residents must have formal instruction, clinical experience, or opportunities to acquire knowledge in the following:

1. The etiology of cancer, including predisposing causal factors leading to neoplasia
2. Fundamental concepts of cellular and molecular biology, cytogenetics, immunology, basic and clinical pharmacology, pharmacokinetics, toxicity, and tumor immunology
3. Etiology, epidemiology, and natural history of cancer
4. Diagnosis, pathology, staging, and management of neoplastic disorders
5. Measurement of the complete blood count, including platelets and white cell differential, by means of automated or manual techniques, with appropriate quality control
6. Immune markers, immunophenotyping, cytochemical studies, and cytogenetic and DNA analysis of neoplastic disorders
7. Molecular mechanisms of neoplasia, including the nature of oncogenes and their products
8. Principles of multidisciplinary management of organ-specific cancers, in particular, gynecologic malignancy
9. Pathophysiology and patterns of tumor metastases
10. Indications and application of imaging techniques in patients with neoplastic disorders
11. Chemotherapeutic drugs, biologic products, and growth factors and their mechanisms of action, pharmacokinetics, clinical indications, and limitations, including their effects, toxicity, and interactions
12. Multiagent chemotherapeutic protocols and combined modality therapy of neoplastic disorders
13. Management and care of indwelling access catheters
14. Principles of, indications for, and limitations of surgery and radiation therapy in the treatment of cancer
15. Principles of, indications for, and complications of autologous and allogeneic bone marrow or peripheral blood stem cell transplantation and peripheral stem cell harvests, including the management of posttransplant complications
16. Fine needle aspiration biopsy
17. Concepts of supportive care, including hematologic, infectious disease, and nutritional
18. Management of the neutropenic and the immunocompromised patient
19. Pain management in the cancer patient
20. Rehabilitation and psychosocial aspects of clinical management of the cancer patient
21. Hospice and home care for the cancer patient
22. Recognition and management of paraneoplastic disorders
23. Cancer prevention and screening, including competency in genetic testing and for high-risk individuals
24. Clinical epidemiology and medical statistics, including clinical study and experimental protocol design, data collection, and analysis
25. Participation in a tumor board
26. Personal development, attitudes, and coping skills of physicians and other health-care professionals who care for critically ill patients
27. Human immunodeficiency virus-related malignancies
28. Care and management of the geriatric patient with malignancy

ACGME: June 1998 Effective: July 1999

Program Requirements for Residency Education in Pulmonary Disease (Internal Medicine)

I. Educational Program

A. A subspecialty educational program in pulmonary disease must be organized to provide training and supervised experience at a sufficient level for the resident to acquire the competency of a specialist in the field. It must be 2 years in duration, of which a minimum of 12 months must be devoted to clinical training.

B. Clinical experience must include opportunities to observe and manage inpatients and outpatients with a wide variety of pulmonary disease. The residents must be given opportunities to assume continuing responsibility for both acutely and chronically ill patients in order to learn the natural history of pulmonary disease as well as the effectiveness of therapeutic programs.

II. Facilities and Resources

A. Modern facilities to accomplish the overall educational program must be available and functioning at the primary training site. These include inpatient and ambulatory care facilities, a laboratory for pulmonary function tests and exfoliative cytology, and extensive pathology services. Appropriate space and staffing for pulmonary procedures must be available. Finally, special facilities for intensive care, postoperative care, and respiratory care services also must be provided at the primary training site.

B. There should be a close liaison with other services, including pediatrics, radiology, pathology, thoracic surgery, microbiology, laboratory medicine, occupational medicine, immunology, physical medicine, and rehabilitation. In addition, there should be a working relationship with the otolaryngology and anesthesiology services. A sleep laboratory also must be available.

III. Specific Program Content

The training program must provide the environment, patient population, and resources for residents to develop clinical competence in the field of pulmonary disease. All elements of the specific content must be provided either by clinical experience or by didactic instruction.

A. Clinical Experience

The program must provide the environment and resources for residents to acquire knowledge of and have clinical experience with a broad spectrum of pulmonary disease, including but not limited to the following:

1. Obstructive lung diseases, including asthma, bronchitis, emphysema, bronchiectasis, and cystic fibrosis
2. Pulmonary malignancy—primary and metastatic
3. Pulmonary infections, including tuberculous, fungal, and those in the immunocompromised host, eg, human immunodeficiency virus-related infections
4. Diffuse interstitial lung disease
5. Pulmonary vascular disease, including primary and secondary pulmonary hypertension and the vasculitis and pulmonary hemorrhage syndromes
6. Occupational and environmental lung diseases
7. Iatrogenic respiratory diseases, including drug-induced disease
8. Acute lung injury, including radiation, inhalation, and trauma
9. Pulmonary manifestations of systemic diseases, including collagen vascular disease and diseases that are primary in other organs
10. Respiratory failure, including the adult respiratory distress syndrome, acute and chronic respiratory failure in obstructive lung diseases, and neuromuscular respiratory drive disorders
11. Disorders of the pleura and the mediastinum
12. Genetic and developmental disorders of the respiratory system
13. Sleep disorders

B. Technical and Other Skills

1. The program must provide the environment and resources for the resident to acquire knowledge (indications, contraindications, complications, and limitations) of and competence in performing the following:
   a. Pressure-cycled, volume-cycled, time-cycled and flow-cycled mechanical ventilation
   b. Use of reservoir masks and continuous positive airway pressure masks for delivery of supplemental oxygen, humidifiers, nebulizers, and incentive spirometry
   c. Weaning and respiratory care techniques
   d. Management of pneumothorax (needle insertion and drainage system)
   e. Maintenance of circulation
      1. Arterial puncture and blood sampling
      2. Insertion of central venous, arterial, and pulmonary artery balloon flotation catheters
      3. Basic and advanced cardiopulmonary resuscitation
      4. Cardioversion
   f. Pulmonary function tests to assess respiratory mechanics, gas exchange, and respiratory drive, including spirometry, flow volume studies, lung volumes, diffusing capacity, arterial blood gas analysis, and exercise studies
   g. Diagnostic and therapeutic procedures, including thoracentesis, pleural biopsy, flexible fiber-optic bronchoscopy and related procedures, endotracheal intubation, percutaneous arterial puncture and cannulation, central venous catheterization, and pulmonary artery balloon flotation catheterization
   h. Calibration and operation of hemodynamic recording systems
   i. Ventilatory support, weaning, and respiratory care techniques
   j. Examination and interpretation of sputum, bronchopulmonary secretions, pleural fluid/tissue, and lung tissue for infectious agents, cytology, and histopathology
2. The program should provide the environment and resources for the resident to develop clinical competence in performing the following:
   a. Inhalation challenge studies
   b. Thoracostomy tube insertion and drainage
   c. Insertion of chest tubes
   d. Percutaneous needle biopsy
3. The program must provide the environment and resources for the resident to acquire knowledge of and ability to interpret the following:
   a. Imaging procedures, including
      1. chest roentgenograms
      2. computed axial tomograms
      3. radionuclide scans
      4. pulmonary angiograms
      5. other radiologic procedures
   b. Sleep studies
4. The program must provide the environment and resources for residents to develop expertise in monitoring and supervising special services, including
   a. Critical care or respiratory care units
   b. Pulmonary function laboratories
   c. Respiratory physical therapy and pulmonary rehabilitation
   d. Respiratory care techniques and services

C. Basic Sciences

The program must provide instruction in the basic sciences with particular emphasis on

1. Molecular biology
2. Pulmonary physiology
3. Pulmonary immunology

ACGME: June 1998 Effective: July 1999

Program Requirements for Residency Education in Pulmonary Disease and Critical Care Medicine (Internal Medicine)

I. Educational Program

A. A combined subspecialty program in pulmonary disease and critical care medicine must be organized to provide training and supervised experience at a sufficient level for the resident to acquire the competency of a specialist in both disciplines. Because of some degree of congruity in the knowledge base, the clinical skills, and the patient populations for each of these subspecialty areas, it is possible to compress the duration of the educational experience and still ensure these competencies. However, the combined training program must be 3 years in duration (of which a minimum of 18 months is devoted to clinical training), and all of the educational experiences and program content explicitly required for a training program in each area must be present in the combined program.

B. With respect to pulmonary disease, clinical experience must include opportunities to observe and manage inpatients and outpatients with a wide variety of pulmonary disease. The residents must be given opportunities to assume continuing responsibility for both acutely and chronically ill patients in order to learn the natural history of pulmonary disease as well as the effectiveness of therapeutic programs. There should be an educational emphasis on pulmonary physiology and its correlation with clinical disorders.

C. With respect to critical care medicine, the program must be structured to provide at least 12 months of meaningful patient care responsibility in critical care units; at least 6 of these months must be devoted to the care of critically ill medical patients (ie, MICU/CICU or equivalent).

D. To provide evidence of substantial institutional support in those disciplines most relevant to critical care medicine, the sponsoring institution's primary site should sponsor accredited subspecialty programs in cardiovascular disease and infectious disease and must have an accredited residency program in general surgery. The presence of training programs in these disciplines ensures the extensive educational, patient care, and research resources that are essential to the learning environment for critical care medicine residents. Furthermore, peer interaction is essential in the education of critical care medicine residents.

E. The sponsoring institution(s) must provide services for the care of patients with major trauma and must have an active open heart surgery program.

F. Institutional policies should be established to govern the educational resources committed to critical care training programs and to ensure cooperation of all involved disciplines.

II. Key Clinical Faculty

A. A training program must be under the direction of an internist who is certified in pulmonary disease and/or critical care medicine by the American Board of Internal Medicine or who has obtained equivalent training and experience. If the program director does not have appropriate credentials in both specialties, an appropriately credentialed full-time key clinical faculty member must be identified as responsible for the education program in the second specific area.

B. The combined subspecialty program faculty must include a minimum of six (three for each discipline) qualified key clinical teaching faculty members, including the program director. At least two of these key clinical faculty members must be certified in pulmonary disease (or possess equivalent qualifications), and at least two must be certified in critical care medicine (or possess equivalent qualifications). For programs with more than six residents enrolled, a ratio of such faculty to residents of at least 1:1 must be maintained.

At least two key clinical teaching faculty members each in nephrology, gastroenterology, cardiology, infectious disease, and hematology must devote substantial effort to the education of critical care medicine residents, and there must be key clinical faculty members in geriatric medicine and oncology who participate in the education of residents.

Faculty members in anesthesiology, neurology, and neurosurgery who are certified by an American Board of Medical Specialties member board in their respective disciplines or who have equivalent training and experience also must participate at the primary training site in the education of residents in critical care medicine.

C. The critical care teaching staff must have privileges regarding the admission, treatment, and discharge of patients on critical care units.

D. Because critical care training is multidisciplinary in nature, faculty from several related disciplines such as general surgery, thoracic surgery, urology, orthopedic surgery, and obstetrics-gynecology must be available to participate in the training program. A collegial relationship must exist between the director of the critical care training program and the teaching staff to enhance the education opportunities for all internal medicine residents and subspecialty residents.

III. Facilities and Resources

A. Modern facilities to accomplish the overall educational program must be available and functioning at the primary training site. These include inpatient and ambulatory care facilities, a laboratory for pulmonary function tests and exfoliative cytology, and extensive pathology services.

Appropriate space and staffing for pulmonary procedures must be available at the primary training site. Facilities for training in microbiology procedures, pulmonary rehabilitation, and a sleep laboratory also must be available.

B. The critical care unit(s) must be located in a designated area within the hospital and must be constructed and designed specifically for the care of critically ill patients. Whether operating in separate locations or in combined facilities, the program must provide the equivalent of a medical intensive care unit, a surgical intensive care unit, and a coronary care unit. Available facilities must be adequate to care for patients with acute myocardial infarction, severe trauma, shock, recent open heart surgery, recent major thoracic or abdominal surgery, and severe neurologic and neurosurgical conditions.

C. In units to which a resident is assigned, an average census of at least five patients per resident is required. A sufficient number of knowledgeable personnel and the necessary equipment to care for critically ill patients must be available. Personnel should include specially trained nurses and technicians who are skilled in critical care instrumentation, respiratory function, and laboratory medicine. A supporting laboratory should be available to provide complete and prompt laboratory evaluation. Modern imaging services and an active emergency service must be available. Nutritional support services also must be available.

IV. Specific Program Content

A. The training program must provide the environment, patient population, and resources for residents to develop clinical competence in the fields of pulmonary disease and critical care medicine. It must include a minimum of 6 months of clinical training specific to pulmonary disease and 6 months of clinical training specific to critical care medicine.

B. The program must provide residents with pulmonary experiences in an ambulatory care setting at least ½ day each week for 30 months of training.

C. Because critical care medicine is multidisciplinary in nature, clinical experience must include opportunities to manage adult patients with a wide variety of serious illnesses and injuries requiring treatment in a critical care setting. Therefore, residents must obtain additional clinical experience with other critically ill patients, which may include surgical, shock/trauma, and neurologic/neurosurgical intensive care units; pediatric intensive care unit; cardiac catheterization laboratory; burn unit; dialysis unit; anesthesia service; high-risk pregnancy intensive care unit; and transplant unit.

D. The resident must be given opportunities to assume responsibility, under appropriate supervision, for the care of patients throughout their stay in the critical care unit(s) and to monitor the subsequent course of patients throughout the remainder of their hospital stay. To assess the various aspects of critical care, the resident also must have organized opportunities to learn about former critical care patients after hospital discharge, including clinical pathological correlations when appropriate.

E. Opportunities also must be available for residents to acquire those skills required to organize, administer, and direct a critical care unit and to work effectively as a member of a multidisciplinary team.

F. For training in pulmonary disease, the program must provide the environment and resources for residents to acquire knowledge of and have clinical experience with a broad spectrum of pulmonary disease, including but not limited to the following:
1. Obstructive lung diseases, including asthma, bronchitis, emphysema, bronchiectasis, and cystic fibrosis
2. Pulmonary malignancy—primary and metastatic
3. Pulmonary infections, including tuberculous, fungal, and those in the immunocompromised host
4. Diffuse interstitial lung disease
5. Pulmonary vascular disease, including primary and secondary pulmonary hypertension and the vasculitis and pulmonary hemorrhage syndromes
6. Occupational and environmental lung diseases
7. Iatrogenic respiratory diseases, including drug-induced disease
8. Acute lung injury, including radiation, inhalation, and trauma
9. Pulmonary manifestations of systemic diseases, including collagen vascular diseases that are primary in other organs
10. Respiratory failure, including the adult respiratory distress syndrome, acute and chronic respiratory failure in obstructive lung diseases, and neuromuscular respiratory drive disorders
11. Disorders of the pleura and the mediastinum
12. Genetic and developmental disorders of the respiratory system
13. Sleep disorders

G. The program must provide the environment and resources for the resident to acquire knowledge (indications, contraindications, complications, and limitations) of and competence in performing the following:
1. Establishment and maintenance of open airway in nonintubated, unconscious, paralyzed patients
2. Pressure-cycled, volume-cycled, time-cycled and flow-cycled mechanical ventilation
3. Use of reservoir masks and continuous positive airway pressure masks for delivery of supplemental oxygen, humidifiers, nebulizers, and incentive spirometry
4. Weaning and respiratory care techniques
5. Management of pneumothorax (needle insertion and drainage systems)
6. Maintenance of circulation, including
   a. Arterial puncture and blood sampling
   b. Insertion of central venous, arterial, and pulmonary artery balloon flotation catheters
   c. Basic and advanced cardiopulmonary resuscitation
   d. Cardioversion
7. Pulmonary function tests to assess respiratory mechanics, gas exchange, and respiratory drive, including spirometry, flow volume studies, lung volumes, diffusing capacity, arterial blood gas analysis, and exercise studies
8. Diagnostic and therapeutic procedures, including thoracentesis, pleural biopsy, flexible fiber-optic bronchoscopy, and related procedures
9. Calibration and operation of hemodynamic recording systems
10. Ventilatory support, weaning, and respiratory care techniques
11. Examination and interpretation of sputum, bronchopulmonary secretions, pleural fluid/tissue, and lung tissue for infectious agents; cytology; and histopathology

H. The program must provide the environment and resources for the resident to acquire knowledge of and ability to interpret the following:
1. Imaging procedures, including
   a. chest roentgenograms
   b. computed axial tomograms
   c. radionuclide scans
   d. pulmonary angiograms
   e. other radiologic procedures
2. Sleep studies

I. The program must provide the environment and resources for residents to develop expertise in monitoring and supervising special services, including
1. critical and respiratory care units
2. pulmonary function laboratories
3. respiratory physical therapy and pulmonary rehabilitation services
4. respiratory care techniques and services

J. The program must provide instruction in the basic sciences with particular emphasis on
1. molecular biology
2. pulmonary physiology
3. pulmonary immunology

K. The program should provide the environment and resources for the resident to develop clinical competence in performing the following:
1. Inhalation challenge studies
2. Thoracostomy tube insertion and drainage
3. Percutaneous needle biopsy

L. In addition to the educational experience listed above, the training program must provide opportunities for the residents to acquire knowledge of and to develop clinical competence in the following content areas:
1. Physiology, pathophysiology, molecular biology, diagnosis, and therapy of disorders of the cardiovascular, respiratory, renal, gastrointestinal, genitourinary, neurologic, endocrine, hematologic, musculoskeletal, and immune systems as well as of infectious diseases

2. Electrolyte and acid-base physiology, pathophysiology, diagnosis, and therapy
3. Metabolic, nutritional, and endocrine effects of critical illnesses
4. Hematologic and coagulation disorders secondary to critical illnesses
5. Critical obstetric and gynecologic disorders
6. Management of the immunosuppressed patient
7. Management of anaphylaxis and acute allergic reactions
8. Trauma
9. Pharmacokinetics, pharmacodynamics, and drug metabolism and excretion in critical illness
10. Use of paralytic agents
11. Ethical, economic, and legal aspects of critical illness
12. Principles and techniques of administration and management
13. Psychosocial and emotional effects of critical illnesses
14. Iatrogenic and nosocomial problems in critical care medicine
15. Occupational Safety and Health Administration (OSHA) regulations and universal precautions and protection of health-care workers

M. The training program must provide opportunities for residents to learn the indications, contraindications, limitations, and complications of the following critical care procedures and the technical skills necessary to perform them:
   1. Parenteral nutrition
   2. Monitoring/bioengineering
      a. Utilization, zeroing, and calibration of transducers
      b. Use of amplifiers and recorders

N. The program also must provide opportunities to learn the indications, contraindications, limitations, and complications of the following procedures; practical experience is recommended.
   1. Pericardiocentesis
   2. Transvenous pacemaker insertion
   3. Peritoneal dialysis
   4. Peritoneal lavage
   5. Percutaneous needle aspiration and/or cutting lung biopsy
   6. Intracranial pressure monitoring

O. Experience also must be provided in the analysis of data pertaining to the following:
   1. Cardiac output determinations by thermodilution and/or other techniques
   2. Evaluation of oliguria
   3. Management of massive transfusions
   4. Management of hemostatic defects
   5. Interpretation of antibiotic levels and sensitivities
   6. Monitoring and assessment of metabolism and nutrition
   7. Calculation of oxygen content, intrapulmonary shunt, and alveolar arterial gradients
   8. Pharmacokinetics

ACGME: June 1998 Effective: July 1999

Program Requirements for Residency Education in Rheumatology (Internal Medicine)

I. Educational Program

A subspecialty educational program in rheumatology must be organized to provide training and supervised experience at a level sufficient for the resident to acquire competence in the field. It must be 2 years in duration.

II. Facilities and Resources

A. Modern facilities to accomplish the overall educational program must be available and functioning at the primary training site. These include inpatient facilities for acute and chronic care at primary, secondary, and tertiary levels; imaging facilities, including computerized tomography and magnetic resonance imaging; and a fully equipped clinical laboratory providing service on a 24-hour basis and equipped with a compensated polarized light microscope for use by residents. Rehabilitation medicine facilities and ambulatory care facilities also must be available. Resources for specialized tests used by rheumatologists must be available on the premises or by contract arrangement.

B. There must be a meaningful working relationship, including availability for teaching and consultation at the primary site, with faculty in radiology and orthopedic surgery and also with allied health professionals in physical therapy and occupational therapy.

III. Specific Program Content

A. Clinical Experience

Clinical experience as a multidisciplinary team member must include supervised opportunities to manage both inpatients and outpatients with a wide variety of rheumatic and musculoskeletal diseases and other illnesses with rheumatologic musculoskeletal manifestations.

B. Ambulatory Medicine Experience

The residents must be given opportunities to assume responsibility for and follow patients throughout the training period in both inpatient and outpatient settings to observe the evolution and natural history of these disorders, as well as the effectiveness of therapeutic interventions. To accomplish these goals, the educational program must include a minimum of 3 half-days of ambulatory care per week averaged over the 2 years of training.

C. Specific Program Content

1. The training program must provide the environment and resources for the residents to gain experience in the diagnosis and treatment of patients with
   a. diffuse connective tissue diseases
   b. rheumatoid arthritis
   c. systemic lupus erythematosus
   d. scleroderma
   e. polymyositis
   f. spondyloarthropathies
   g. vasculitis
   h. crystal-induced synovitis
   i. osteoarthritis
   j. regional musculoskeletal pain syndromes
   k. nonarticular rheumatic diseases, including fibromyalgia
   l. nonsurgical, exercise-related (sports) injury
   m. systemic diseases with rheumatic manifestations
   n. metabolic diseases of bone
   o. osteoporosis
   p. infection of joints
   q. joint surgery
   r. acute and chronic musculoskeletal pain
2. It is desirable that programs with the qualified faculty and facilities provide training in pediatric rheumatic disease.

D. Technical and Other Skills

1. The program must provide sufficient experience for the resident to acquire skill in the
   a. use of nonsteroidal anti-inflammatory drugs, disease-modifying drugs, biologic response modifiers, glucocorticoids, cytotoxic

drugs, antihyperuricemic drugs, and antibiotic therapy for septic joints.

b. examination of patients, to include a specific examination of structure and function of all joints, both axial and peripheral, as well as periarticular structure and muscle units.
c. construction of differential diagnosis for complexes of symptoms and signs related to rheumatologic diseases.
d. diagnostic aspiration and analysis by light and compensated polarized light microscopy of synovial fluid.
e. therapeutic injection of diarthrodial joints, bursae, tenosynovial structures, and entheses.

2. The program must provide sufficient experience for the resident to acquire skill in the performance or interpretation of
   a. biopsies of tissues relevant to the diagnosis of rheumatic diseases.
   b. bone and joint imaging techniques.
   c. bone density measurements.
   d. controlled clinical trials in rheumatic diseases.
   e. nailfold capillary microscopy.
   f. indications for arthroscopy.
   g. electromyography and nerve conduction studies.

E. Formal Instruction

In the study of rheumatic diseases, musculoskeletal disorders, metabolic diseases of bone, osteoporosis, and acute and chronic musculoskeletal pain, the following specific content areas as a minimum, must be included in the formal program (lectures, conferences, and seminars).

1. Anatomy, pathology, genetics, immunology, biochemistry, and physiology of connective tissue, bone, and muscle, including purine metabolism
2. The scientific basis of the methodology, indications, and interpretations of laboratory tests and imaging procedures used in diagnosis and management
3. Indications for and interpretation of electromyograms, nerve conduction studies, and muscle/nerve biopsy
4. Pharmacology and pharmacokinetics, including drug metabolism, adverse effects, interactions, and relative costs of therapy
5. Principles of physical medicine and rehabilitation in patients with rheumatologic disorders
6. Evaluation, management, and rehabilitation of exercise-related (sports) illnesses
7. Indications for surgical and orthopedic consultation
8. Geriatric and aging influences

ACGME: June 1998 Effective: July 1999

Program Requirements for Residency Education in Internal Medicine Sports Medicine

I. Introduction

In addition to complying with the requirements below, each program must comply with the Program Requirements for Residency Education in the Subspecialties of Internal Medicine.

II. Scope and Duration of Training

An educational program in sports medicine must be organized to provide a well-supervised experience at a level sufficient for the resident to acquire the competence of a physician with added qualifications in this field. It shall be 1 year in duration.

The practice of sports medicine is the application of the physician's knowledge, skills, and attitudes to those engaged in sports and exercise. Thus, the program must provide training in the development of the clinical competencies needed to diagnose and manage medical illnesses and injuries related to sports and exercise, for example, first-degree sprains, strains, and contusions, including appropriate referrals of, for example, fractures, dislocations, and third-degree sprains. Clinical experience must include injury prevention, preparticipation evaluation, management of acute and chronic illness or injury, and rehabilitation as applied to a broad spectrum of undifferentiated patients. There must be experience functioning as a team physician and in the promotion of physical fitness and wellness.

The program should emphasize physiology and biomechanics; principles of nutrition; pathology and pathophysiology of illness and injury; pharmacology; effects of therapeutic, performance-enhancing, and mood-altering drugs; psychological aspects of exercise, performance, and competition; ethical principles; and medical-legal aspects of exercise and sports.

III. Teaching Staff

In addition to the program director, each program must have at least one other faculty member with similar qualifications who devotes a substantial portion of professional time to the training program.

The teaching staff must include orthopedic surgeons who are engaged in the operative management of sports injuries and other conditions and who are readily available to teach and provide consultation to the residents. Teaching staff from the disciplines of nutrition, pharmacology, pathology, exercise physiology, physical therapy, behavioral science, physical medicine and rehabilitation, and clinical imaging also should be available to assist in the educational program. Coaches and athletic trainers also should be included.

IV. Facilities and Resources

The program must include the following:

A. Patient Population

A patient population that is unlimited by age or gender and is adequate in number and variety to meet the needs of the training program must be available. The program director must ensure that residents are accorded meaningful patient responsibility with the supervision of a faculty member at all facilities and sites.

B. Sports Medicine Clinic

There must be an identifiable clinic that offers continuing care to patients who seek consultation regarding sports- or exercise-related health problems. The nonsurgical residents must be supervised by a physician who has qualifications in sports medicine and is certified by the American Board of Emergency Medicine, the American Board of Family Practice, the American Board of Internal Medicine, or the American Board of Pediatrics or who possesses suitable equivalent qualifications.

Adequate, up-to-date diagnostic imaging and rehabilitation services must be readily available and accessible to clinic patients. Consultation in medical and surgical subspecialties, physical therapy, nursing, nutrition, and pharmacy must be available. The opportunity to render continuing care and to organize recommendations from other specialties and disciplines is mandatory and will require that medical records include information pertinent to the assessment and management of patients with health problems related to sports and exercise.

C. Sporting Events/Team Sports/Mass-Participation Events

The program must have access to sporting events, team sports, and mass-participation events during which the resident can have meaningful patient responsibility.

D. Acute-Care Facility

There must be an acute-care hospital with a full range of services associated with and in proximity to the sponsoring residency. This facility must be readily accessible to patients served by the program.

V. Educational Program

The curriculum must provide the educational experiences necessary for the residents to achieve the cognitive knowledge, psychomotor skills, interpersonal skills, professional attitudes, and practical experience required of physicians in the care of patients with health problems related to sports and exercise.

Didactic as well as clinical learning opportunities must be provided as part of the required curriculum for all residents. Conferences or seminars/workshops in sports medicine should be specifically designed for the residents to augment the clinical experiences.

All educational activities must be adequately supervised while allowing the resident to assume progressive responsibility for patient care. The clinical activities in sports medicine should represent a minimum of 50% of the time in the program. The remainder of the time should be spent in didactic, teaching, and/or research activities and in the primary care or emergency medicine ambulatory facility.

Residents must spend ½ day per week maintaining their skills in their primary specialty.

Participation in the following must be required of all residents:

A. Preparticipation Evaluation of the Athlete

The program must ensure that all sports medicine residents are involved in the development and conduct of preparticipation examination programs.

B. Acute Care

The resident must have appropriate authority and responsibility to participate meaningfully in the medical care that is provided to acute-care patients (see "Scope and Duration of Training," above). In addition, the program should arrange for residents to observe representative inpatient and outpatient operative orthopedic procedures.

C. Sports Medicine Clinic Experience

The resident must attend patients in a continuing, comprehensive manner, providing consultation for health problems related to sports and exercise. The resident shall spend at least 1 day per week for 10 months of the training period in this activity.

If patients are hospitalized, the resident should follow them during their inpatient stay and resume outpatient care following the hospitalization. Consultation with other physicians and professionals in other disciplines should be encouraged.

D. On-Site Sports Care

The resident should participate in planning and implementation of all aspects of medical care at various sporting events. The program must ensure that supervised sports medicine residents provide on-site care and management to participants in these events.

In addition, the resident must participate in the provision of comprehensive and continuing care to a sports team. Preferably, the experience should include several teams that engage in seasonal sports.

E. Mass-Participation Sports Events

The resident should participate in the planning and implementation of the provision of medical coverage for at least one mass-participation event. The program must ensure that its residents have experience that includes providing medical consultation, direct patient care, event planning, protection of participants, coordination with local EMS systems, and other medical aspects of those events.

VI. Specific Knowledge and Skills

A. Clinical

The program must provide educational experiences for the residents to develop clinical competence in the overall field of sports medicine.

The curriculum must include but not be limited to the following content and skill areas:

1. Anatomy, physiology, and biomechanics of exercise
2. Basic nutritional principles and their application to exercise
3. Psychological aspects of exercise, performance, and competition
4. Guidelines for evaluation prior to participation in exercise and sport
5. Physical conditioning requirements for various activities
6. Special considerations related to age, gender, and disability
7. Pathology and pathophysiology of illness and injury as it relates to exercise
8. Effects of disease, eg, diabetes, cardiac conditions, and arthritis, on exercise and the use of exercise in the care of medical problems
9. Prevention, evaluation, management, and rehabilitation of injuries
10. Understanding pharmacology and effects of therapeutic, performance-enhancing, and mood-altering drugs
11. Promotion of physical fitness and healthy lifestyles
12. Functioning as a team physician
13. Ethical principles as applied to exercise and sports
14. Medical-legal aspects of exercise and sports
15. Environmental effects on exercise
16. Growth and development related to exercise

B. Patient Education/Teaching

The program must provide the experiences necessary for the residents to develop and demonstrate competence in patient education regarding sports and exercise. They must have experience teaching others, eg, nurses, allied health personnel, medical students, residents, coaches, athletes, other professionals, and members of patients' families. There also must be relevant experience working in a community sports medicine network involving parents, coaches, certified athletic trainers, allied medical personnel, residents, and physicians.

ACGME: September 1994 Effective: July 1995

Program Requirements for Residency Education in Medical Genetics

I. Duration and Scope of Accredited Programs in Medical Genetics

A. Description of the Specialty

1. Clinical medical geneticists are physicians who provide comprehensive diagnostic, management, and genetic counseling services for patients with genetic, or possibly genetic, disorders. They also plan and coordinate large-scale screening programs for inborn errors of metabolism, hemoglobinopathies, chromosome abnormalities, neural tube defects, and other genetically influenced conditions.
2. Clinical medical geneticists are able to (a) diagnose and manage genetic disorders; (b) provide patient and family counseling; (c) use their knowledge of heterogeneity, variability, and natural history of genetic disorders in patient-care decision making; (d) elicit and interpret individual and family medical histories; (e) interpret clinical genetic and specialized laboratory testing information; (f) explain the causes and natural history of genetic disorders and genetic risk assessment; and (g) interact with other health-care professionals in the provision of services for patients with genetically influenced disorders.

B. Scope of Education

1. Accredited graduate medical education programs in medical genetics must provide the formal instruction and appropriately supervised clinical experience necessary for residents to develop the knowledge, skills, and attitudes essential to the practice of clinical medical genetics.
2. Programs must provide (a) opportunities for residents to become involved in research and teaching and (b) education in the basic sciences and clinical areas pertinent to medical genetics, including mendelian genetics, cytogenetics, diagnosis and treatment of inborn errors of metabolism, molecular diagnosis, syndrome identification and dysmorphology, teratology, reproductive genetics, congenital malformations, multifactorial disorders, mental retardation and developmental disabilities, genetic screening, social and ethical issues in medical genetics, genetic counseling, and quantitative human genetics.

C. Program Length

1. A clinical medical genetics residency may be accredited to provide 2 and/or 4 years of graduate medical education:
   a. Physicians who have completed a residency accredited by the Accreditation Council for Graduate Medical Education (ACGME) are eligible for appointment to a 2-year medical genetics residency.
   b. A medical genetics program director may appoint a resident to a 2-year program following 2 or more years of ACGME-accredited residency education.
   c. A 4-year program must include 2 years of pregenetics education in other ACGME-accredited residencies followed by 2 years of education in clinical medical genetics. A 4-year program must be designed prospectively by the director of the medical genetics residency and the directors of the programs to which residents will be assigned during the 2 years of pregenetics education.
2. In both 2-year and 4-year programs, the 24 months of genetics education must include at least 18 months of broad-based, clinically oriented medical genetics activities.

D. Program Goals and Objectives

1. Program Description
   a. The director and teaching staff must prepare and comply with written educational goals for the program.
   b. A written description of the educational program must be prepared and distributed to residents and teaching staff.
   c. The program description must include:
      i. A summary of the program's educational goals.
      ii. A listing and description of all required rotations and other assignments.
      iii. The goals and objectives of each rotation/assignment.
      iv. The duration of each rotation/assignment.
      v. A description of resident opportunities for teaching and research.
      vi. A description of the manner in which residents are supervised.
2. Program Design
   a. All educational components of the program should be related to program goals.
   b. The program design and/or structure must be approved by the Residency Review Committee (RRC) as part of the regular review process.
   c. Participation by any institution providing more than 3 months of training in a 2-year program or 6 months of training in a 4-year program requires prior approval by the RRC.

II. Institutional Resources

A. Graduate medical education in medical genetics must be sponsored by institutions that are able to provide sufficient faculty, administrative support, financial resources, comprehensive medical library services, research facilities, office space, support staff, and clinical facilities to meet the educational needs of residents and enable the residency to comply with accreditation requirements. Affiliations may be made with other institutions/laboratories to meet educational needs.

B. Institutions sponsoring medical genetics programs should also sponsor ACGME-accredited programs in pediatrics, internal medicine, and obstetrics/gynecology.

C. Program institutions should have a clinical cytogenetics laboratory, a clinical biochemical genetics laboratory, and a clinical molecular genetics laboratory, each of which provides an appropriate volume and variety of medical genetics-related services and has an adequate number of qualified staff. If a laboratory is not located in a program institution, a written letter of agreement from the laboratory director detailing the laboratory's contributions to the education of medical genetics residents must be prepared and kept on file by the program director.

D. Program institutions must provide a sufficient number and variety (eg, pregnant and nonpregnant, all ages) of inpatients and outpatients to permit residents to gain experience with the natural history of a wide range of genetic disorders.

III. Program Personnel

The program director and the teaching staff are responsible for the general administration of the program, including those activities related to the recruitment, selection, instruction, supervision, counseling, evaluation, and advancement of residents and the maintenance of records related to program accreditation.

A. Program Director

1. There must be a single program director who has the authority to direct the entire clinical medical genetics program and is able to devote sufficient time to fulfill the responsibilities required to meet the educational goals of the program, including the implementation of sound administrative practices and the provision of

adequate facilities, teaching staff, resident staff, support staff, and other educational resources.

2. The program director must be:
   a. A physician who has a valid license to practice medicine in the state where the institution that sponsors the program is located.
   b. Certified in Clinical Genetics by the American Board of Medical Genetics (ABMG) or possess suitable equivalent qualifications.
   c. A member in good standing of the medical staff of the institution that sponsors the program.
   d. Experienced in medical education in general and graduate medical education in genetics in particular and possess the requisite clinical, educational, and administrative abilities needed to direct a medical genetics program.
3. Responsibilities of the program director include:
   a. Preparation of a written statement outlining the educational goals of the program with respect to knowledge, skills, and other attributes of residents at each level of training and for each major rotation or other program assignment. This statement must be distributed to residents and members of the teaching staff. It should be readily available for review.
   b. Selection of residents for appointment to the program in accordance with institutional and departmental policies and procedures.
   c. Selection, supervision, and evaluation of the teaching staff and other program personnel at each institution participating in the program.
   d. The supervision of residents in accordance with explicit written descriptions of supervisory lines of responsibility for the care of patients. Such guidelines must be communicated to all members of the program staff. Residents must be provided with prompt, reliable systems for communication and interaction with supervisory physicians.
   e. Regular evaluation of residents' knowledge, skills, and overall performance, including the development of professional attitudes consistent with being a physician. The program director, with participation of members of the teaching staff, shall:
      1. At least semiannually evaluate the knowledge, skills, and professional growth of the residents, using appropriate criteria and procedures.
      2. Communicate each evaluation to the resident in a timely manner.
      3. Advance residents to positions of higher responsibility only on the basis of evidence of their satisfactory progressive scholarship and professional growth.
      4. Maintain a permanent record of evaluation for each resident and have it accessible to the resident and other authorized personnel.
   f. The provision of a written final evaluation for each resident who completes the program. The evaluation must include a review of the resident's performance during the final period of training and should verify that the resident has completed the program and demonstrated sufficient professional ability to practice competently and independently. This final evaluation should be part of the resident's permanent record maintained by the institution.
   g. Implementation of fair procedures, as established by the sponsoring institution, regarding academic discipline and resident complaints or grievances.
   h. Monitoring resident stress, including mental or emotional conditions inhibiting performance or learning, and drug- or alcohol-related dysfunction. Program directors and teaching staff should be sensitive to the need for timely provision of confidential counseling and psychological support services to residents. Training situations that consistently produce undesirable stress on residents must be evaluated and modified.
   i. Continuing involvement in scholarly activities, participation in key national scientific human genetics meetings, and contribution to medical education both locally and nationally.
   j. Communication with the RRC, including the program information that is prepared for periodic accreditation site visits and reviews. The director must also notify the committee of significant changes in the program, including:
      1. Change of program director.
      2. Major changes in institutional affiliation. Any change in formal affiliation with institutions where residents are assigned for required educational experiences requires prior approval from the RRC.
      3. An increase in the RRC-approved maximum number of residents in the program. Requests for increases in a program's resident complement require the prior approval of the RRC.
   k. Ensuring that residents are clearly informed in writing of program requirements, including the duration of the resident's course of study.
4. As continuity of the leadership of a residency is crucial to educational quality, frequent changes in the directorship and extended periods of temporary leadership have been found to have an adverse impact on programs. Therefore, institutions must develop and implement policies and procedures to ensure continuity when the program director departs, is on sabbatical, or is unable to meet his or her duties for any other reason.

B. Teaching Staff

1. There must be a sufficient number of teaching staff with documented qualifications to instruct and supervise adequately all the residents in the program. Members of the teaching staff must be able to devote sufficient time to meet their supervisory and teaching responsibilities.
2. There must be at least three members of the teaching staff (including the program director) who are certified by the ABMG (or possess equivalent qualifications) and are members of the medical staffs at program institutions. At least two of these individuals must be certified in clinical medical genetics.
3. The individual responsible for resident education in biochemical genetics must be ABMG-certified in biochemical genetics. The person responsible for resident education in molecular genetics must be ABMG-certified in molecular genetics. The individual responsible for resident education in clinical cytogenetics must be ABMG-certified in clinical cytogenetics.
4. There must be a sufficient number of teaching staff so that program faculty are readily available to residents and able to meet effectively their patient care, educational, and research responsibilities.
5. All members of the teaching staff must demonstrate a strong interest in the education of residents, sound clinical and teaching abilities, support of the goals and objectives of the program, a commitment to their own continuing medical education, and participation in scholarly activities.
6. Members of the teaching staff must regularly and actively participate in program rounds, conferences, and journal clubs.
7. Members of the teaching staff must participate in appropriate scientific societies (particularly through presentations at meetings) and pursue their own continuing education.
8. Members of the teaching staff must demonstrate an active interest in genetics research (particularly in projects that are funded following peer review and/or result in publications in peer-reviewed journals), and provide guidance and technical support

(eg, research design, statistical analysis) for residents who are involved in research or other scholarly activities.

9. A member of the teaching staff of each participating institution must be designated to assume responsibility for the day-to-day activities of the program at that institution, with overall coordination by the program director.
10. The teaching staff must be organized and have regular documented meetings to review program goals and objectives as well as program effectiveness in achieving them. At least one resident representative should participate in these reviews.
11. The teaching staff should periodically evaluate the utilization of the resources available to the program, the contribution of each institution participating in the program, the financial and administrative support of the program, the volume and variety of patients available to the program for educational purposes, the performance of members of the teaching staff, and the quality of supervision of residents.

C. Number of Residents

When reviewing a program for accreditation, the RRC will approve a maximum total number of residents to be appointed to a program. That number will be based primarily on the number, qualifications, and commitment of the teaching staff; the volume and variety of genetics patients available for educational purposes; and program facilities, finances, and organization.

D. Other Program Personnel

There must be a sufficient number of appropriately qualified patient care, administrative, technical, clerical, and other staff to support all the educational activities of the program.

IV. Program Facilities

A. Adequate space and equipment must be available to meet the educational goals of the program. In addition to space for patient care activities, this requires meeting rooms, classrooms, office space, research facilities, and facilities for record storage and retrieval.

B. Office and laboratory space must be provided for the residents for both patient-care work and participation in scholarly activities.

C. Residents must have ready access to a major medical library, either at the institution where the residents are located or through arrangement with convenient nearby institutions. The institutional library should contain standard journals and texts in genetics and related fields of medicine and provide services for the electronic retrieval of information from national medical databases to permit timely literature review.

D. Residents must have access to an on-site library or to a collection of appropriate texts and journals in each institution participating in a residency program. On-site libraries and/or collections of texts and journals must be readily available during nights and weekends.

E. Residents should have access to computer-based genetic diagnostic systems.

F. The audiovisual resources available for educational purposes should be adequate to meet the goals and objectives of the program.

V. Educational Program

The residency must be organized to provide a well-structured, integrated, and progressive educational experience in clinical medical genetics. The residents must have the opportunity to develop the abilities to diagnose genetic disorders, counsel patients, and manage the broad range of clinical problems that are encompassed within medical genetics. Because of the complex nature and multiple system involvement of genetic disorders, residents must be exposed to multidisciplinary and interdisciplinary models during the program and must become proficient at organizing teams of health-care professionals to provide the necessary resources for their patients. As medical genetics involves families and individuals of all ages, residents must be competent to work with adults and children and must have an opportunity to gain an understanding of family dynamics as they relate to issues of diagnosis, counseling, and management.

A. Clinical Components

1. Patient Population
   Residents must have the opportunity to care for a number of patients and families sufficient to permit them to develop an understanding of the wide variety of medical genetic problems, including mendelian disorders, inborn errors of metabolism, diseases of chromosome number and structure, multifactorial disorders, syndromes, congenital malformations, other birth defects, and other genetically influenced conditions. Typically, this will mean that programs will care for at least 100 different patients or families per year for each resident. These patients and families must be seen in outpatient and inpatient settings.
2. Correlation of Laboratory and Clinical Experiences
   Clinical biochemical genetic, molecular genetic, and cytogenetic laboratories must be integral components of each program, and residents must have regular opportunities to develop their abilities to understand and critically interpret laboratory data. Residents must develop an understanding of the appropriate use of laboratories during diagnosis, counseling, and management of patients with genetic disorders. Toward this end, resident education must include participation in the working conferences of laboratories as well as ongoing discussion of laboratory data during other clinical conferences.
3. Other Health Care Professionals
   Residents must have regular opportunities to work with genetic counselors, nurses, nutritionists, and other health care professionals who are involved in the provision of clinical medical genetics services.
4. Responsibilities for Patient Care
   The development of mature clinical judgment requires that residents, properly supervised, be given responsibility for patient care commensurate with their ability. This can be achieved only if the resident is involved in the decision-making process and in the continuity of patient care. Residents must be given the responsibility for direct patient care in all settings, including planning and management, both diagnostic and therapeutic, subject to review and approval by the attending physician.
   a. Supervision
      Residents must be supervised by appropriately qualified faculty at all times. Residents must be provided with rapid and reliable systems for communicating with supervising residents and attendings. Attending physicians or supervising residents with appropriate experience for the severity and complexity of the patient's condition must be available to residents at all times and must be able to respond in a timely fashion.
   b. Progressive Responsibility
      The responsibility given to residents for patient care should depend on their knowledge, skill, experience, and the complexity of the patient's counseling or medical problems. The degree of responsibility accorded to a resident, both professional and administrative, must be increased progressively. This includes responsibility in such areas as patient care, leadership, teaching, organization, and administration. The program must provide residents with experience in direct and progressively responsible patient management as they advance through the

program so that those completing the program will have developed sound clinical judgment.

c. Duty Hours and Personal Responsibility
The physician's responsibilities for continuing patient care transcend normal working hours. To fulfill this obligation, provisions for night and weekend call must be established. However, residents must not be regularly required to perform difficult or prolonged duties. Therefore, the program director must ensure assignment of reasonable in-hospital duty hours. Residents at all levels should be able to spend, on average, at least 1 full day out of 7 free of hospital duties and should be on call in the hospital no more often than every third night, except in the maintenance of continuity of care. There should be adequate opportunity to rest and to sleep when on duty for 24 hours or more. On-call rooms arranged to permit adequate rest and privacy should be available for each resident on night duty in the hospital. There should be adequate backup support if needed to maintain appropriate patient care.

B. Academic Components

1. Basic Sciences
   a. Each resident must participate formally, through lectures or other didactic sessions, in the equivalent of a 1-year graduate level course in basic, human, and medical genetics, including but not limited to population and quantitative genetics, mendelian and nonmendelian genetics, cytogenetics, biochemical genetics, and molecular genetics.
   b. Research seminars should be a part of the training experience but shall not be considered an acceptable alternative to this basic science didactic component.
2. Research and Scholarly Activity
   a. Graduate medical education must take place in an environment of inquiry and scholarship in which residents participate in the development of new knowledge, learn to evaluate research findings, and develop habits of inquiry as a continuing professional responsibility.
   b. The responsibility for establishing and maintaining an environment of inquiry and scholarship rests with the teaching staff. While not all members of the faculty must be investigators, the staff as a whole must demonstrate broad involvement in scholarly activity. This activity should include:
      1. Active participation of the teaching staff in clinical discussions, rounds, and conferences in a manner that promotes a spirit of inquiry and scholarship. Scholarship implies an in-depth understanding of basic mechanisms of normal and abnormal states and the application of current knowledge to practice.
      2. Active participation in regional or national professional and scientific societies, particularly through presentations at the organizations' meetings and publications in their journals.
      3. Participation in research, particularly in projects that are funded following peer review and/or result in publications or presentations at regional and national scientific meetings.
      4. Offering of guidance and technical support (eg, research design, statistical analysis) for residents involved in research.
      5. Provision of support and facilities for resident participation in scholarly activities. In addition to direct research involvement, residents and faculty should participate in journal clubs, research seminars, work-in-progress sessions, and reviews of intradepartmental and interdepartmental research activity.
3. Clinical Conferences
   Clinical teaching conferences must be organized by the faculty for the residents, and attendance by the residents and the faculty must be documented. These conferences must be distinct from the basic science lectures and didactic sessions. Clinical teaching conferences may include formal didactic sessions on clinical laboratory topics, medical genetics rounds, journal clubs, and follow-up conferences for genetic clinics.
4. Presence of Other Learners
   a. The presence of other learners in medical genetics and in other specialties within program institutions is essential to the maintenance of a stimulating educational environment.
   b. The appointment of other individuals for special training or education, such as fellows, residents from other specialties, and medical students, must not dilute or detract from the educational opportunities of the medical genetics residents.

VI. Evaluation

A. Evaluation of Residents

1. Regular oral and written evaluations of residents must include comment on both clinical and academic work. Evaluations of residents' patient care activities must address their abilities to carry out clinical genetic evaluations, perform appropriate clinical procedures, understand the methodologies involved in genetic laboratory tests, interpret test results, and counsel patients and families.
2. There must be formal evaluation by the faculty of each resident's knowledge, performance, and growth at least twice each year, and residents must have the opportunity to review confidential, written evaluations of their performance with the program director.

B. Evaluation of Faculty

1. Individual members of the teaching staff must be confidentially evaluated by the program director and the residents at least once each year.
2. Faculty evaluations should include comment on teaching ability, research and other scholarly activity, availability to the residents, and commitment to the training program, as well as clinical knowledge and skill.

C. Evaluation of the Program

1. The educational effectiveness of the program must be evaluated in a systematic manner. In particular, the quality of the curriculum and the extent to which the educational goals have been met by residents must be assessed.
2. There must be regular written, confidential evaluation of the program by the sponsoring institution, program director, and teaching staff.
3. At least once each year, residents and members of the teaching staff should provide the director with written evaluations of the program that give particular attention to the program's success in meeting its educational goals and objectives as well as accreditation requirements.
4. One measure of the quality of a medical genetics residency is the performance of its residents on certifying examinations of the ABMG.

VII. Certification and Accreditation

A. The RRC for Medical Genetics is responsible for accreditation of graduate medical education programs in clinical medical genetics. The ABMG is responsible for certification of individual physicians in medical genetics.
B. Questions about accreditation of residency programs should be directed to the Executive Director of the RRC.
C. Questions about certification in medical genetics should be directed to the office of the ABMG.

ACGME: June 1996 Effective: July 1997

Program Requirements for Residency Education in Neurological Surgery

I. Introduction

A. Definition of Discipline

Neurological surgery is a medical discipline that provides the operative and nonoperative management (ie, prevention, diagnosis, evaluation, treatment, critical care, and rehabilitation) of disorders that affect the central, peripheral, and autonomic nervous systems, including their supporting structures and vascular supply, and the operative and nonoperative management of pain. As such, neurological surgery encompasses the modern treatment of disorders of the brain, meninges, skull, and their blood supply, including the extracranial carotid and vertebral arteries; disorders of the pituitary gland; disorders of the spinal cord, meninges, and spine; disorders of the cranial and spinal nerves throughout their distributions; and disorders of the autonomic nervous system.

B. Duration and Scope of Education

1. The educational program must be diversified and well-balanced.
2. The training program in neurological surgery must include a minimum of 1 year of training in an Accreditation Council for Graduate Medical Education (ACGME)-accredited program in general surgery or at least 1 year of a program accredited for the acquisition of fundamental clinical skills, which must include at least 6 months of surgical disciplines other than neurological surgery. This training should be completed prior to undertaking the third year of neurological surgery training.
3. The neurological surgery training program is 60 months in duration, in addition to the year of acquisition of fundamental clinical skills, and must provide 36 months of clinical neurological surgery at the sponsoring institution or one of its approved participating institutions.
4. Twenty-one months of the total 60 months may be devoted to any of several aspects of the training program, depending on the needs of the resident. [*Note:* The program director should consult the American Board of Neurological Surgery for certification requirements concerning any training conducted outside the approved institutions of the program.] It may be spent in the study of the basic sciences, neuroradiology, neuropathology, or other appropriate subject matter related to the neurosciences as agreed upon by individual residents and the program director.
5. A block of training of 3 months minimum in an ACGME-accredited neurology training program must be arranged for all residents, unless they have previously had a minimum of 1 year of formal residency training in an accredited neurology training program.
6. There must be a 12-month period of time as senior/chief resident on the clinical service of neurological surgery in the sponsoring institution or its approved participating institutions. This is considered an essential component in each resident's planned program. The program must provide the residents with experience in direct and progressively responsible patient management as they advance through training.
   a. The senior/chief resident must have major or primary responsibility for patient management with faculty supervision.
   b. The senior/chief resident should also have administrative responsibility as designated by the program director.
7. Residents must be introduced to the practice of neurosurgery in an outpatient setting where nonemergency patients are seen by the resident for evaluation before and after surgical procedures.

A crucial element of this experience is the clear understanding by the patient that the resident is involved in making decisions concerning diagnosis and participates in operative procedures and follow-up care.

8. Prior to entry into the program, each resident must be notified in writing of the length of training. The prescribed length of training for a particular resident may not be changed without mutual agreement during his or her program unless there is a break in his or her training or the resident requires remedial training. Any training additional to the accredited residency must be based on a clear educational rationale and must not interfere with the education and training of the residents enrolled in the program.

C. Accreditation Guidelines

1. Training programs in neurological surgery are accredited by the Residency Review Committee (RRC) by authority of the ACGME. A list of accredited training programs in neurological surgery is published annually in the *Graduate Medical Education Directory*.
2. To be accredited by the ACGME an educational program in neurological surgery must be in substantial compliance with both the Program Requirements for Residency Education in Neurological Surgery and the Institutional Requirements of the *Essentials of Accredited Residencies in Graduate Medical Education*. Programs must be able to demonstrate their compliance with these requirements at the time of their site visit and subsequent review by the RRC.
3. When a change in leadership occurs within an accredited neurological surgery residency, the program must be site-visited within 18 months and reviewed by the RRC in approximately 2 years following the appointment of the new program director.

II. Institutional Organization

A. Sponsoring Institution

An educational program in neurological surgery must have one sponsoring institution within a single geographic location with primary responsibility for the entire program. Appropriate institutions include medical schools, hospitals, and medical foundations. The institution must demonstrate commitment to the program in terms of financial and academic support.

B. Participating Institutions

Participating institutions include the sponsoring institution and other integrated and/or affiliated institutions approved by the RRC for training purposes (see surgical requirements for affiliated status). Participating institutions must promote the educational goals of the program rather than simply enlarge the program and must not be added primarily for the purpose of meeting service needs.

1. An integrated institution must function as a single neurological surgery service with the sponsoring institution or, in exceptional circumstances, with an approved affiliate of the sponsoring institution. The program director must demonstrate to the RRC that the clinical service operates as a single unit in the assignment of residents and their faculty supervisors, the formulation of call and backup schedules, and in the convening of teaching conferences and related educational activities.
2. An affiliated institution functions as a separate neurological surgical service with a local training director under the direction of the program director and should be sufficiently close to the sponsoring institution to ensure peer interaction and regular attendance at joint conferences and other activities. Appropriate exceptions may be considered for special resource hospitals (eg, pediatrics, trauma, and spine).
3. Training at an additional institution, proposed for affiliated status, may be approved on a provisional basis for a maximum of 2 years, at which time such training must be either fully approved or withdrawn at the discretion of the RRC. Ordinarily, a site visit will not be necessary to confirm the permanent approval of a provisionally approved participating institution.
4. The number and distribution of participating institutions must not preclude satisfactory participation by residents in teaching and training exercises.
5. Affiliated institutions that are geographically separated from the sponsoring institution are not desirable and are acceptable only if they offer special resources that significantly augment the overall educational experience of the training program.
6. Rotations to affiliated and integrated institutions must be based on a clear statement of the value of such institutions to the teaching program as a whole.

C. Number and Quality of Residents

1. One of the measures of a training program is the quality of residents chosen and the ability of the program to ensure a steady increase in the resident's knowledge and skills.
2. The RRC will review the selection process of residents and seek evidence that the program evaluates the progression of the residents during training.
3. Where there is demonstrated excellence in providing educational experience for the residents, as determined by the RRC, a program may be authorized to enroll more than one resident per year. The ability to do so does not depend on any multiplication of the minimum requirements as established by the Program Requirements for Residency Education in Neurological Surgery. In determining the size of a resident complement, the RRC will consider:
   a. Presence of a faculty of national stature in neurological surgery.
   b. Quality of the educational program.
   c. Quality of clinical care.
   d. Total number and distribution of cases.
   e. Quality of clinical and basic research.
   f. Quality of residents trained by the program, including numbers of residents starting and finishing the program, number of graduates who take written and oral examinations of the American Board of Neurological Surgery, and the number of graduates passing these written and oral examinations.
   g. Facilities.
4. The number of residents at each year of training in a given program, except as provided below, shall not exceed the number approved by the most recent accreditation review of that program. Should a vacancy occur at any level of training in a program, the program director has the option of appointing a new resident at a level that might overlap with that of another resident in training, provided that such appointments do not adversely affect the training experience of residents already in the program. Furthermore, over a 5-year period, commencing at the time when the resident whose departure created the vacancy would have completed training, the average number of residents graduating yearly must not exceed the number approved by the RRC.

III. Faculty Qualifications and Responsibilities

The program director and the teaching staff are responsible for the general administration of a program, including those activities related to the recruitment, selection, instruction, supervision, counseling, evaluation, and advancement of residents and the maintenance of records related to program accreditation.

A. Program Director Qualifications

1. There must be a single program director responsible for the program.
2. The program director shall be a neurological surgeon who possesses and practices the necessary administrative, teaching, and clinical skills and has experience to conduct the program.
3. The program director shall be certified by the American Board of Neurological Surgery or possess suitable equivalent qualifications in neurological surgery satisfactory to the RRC.
4. The program director shall be licensed to practice medicine in the state where the institution that sponsors the program is located. (Certain federal programs are exempted.)
5. The program director shall have an appointment in good standing to the medical staff of an institution participating in the program.

B. Program Director Responsibilities

The program director must assume responsibility for all aspects of the training program and devote sufficient time to the educational program, including the following:

1. Preparation of a written statement outlining the educational goals of the program with respect to knowledge, skills, and other attributes of residents at each level of training and for each major rotation or other program assignment. This statement must be distributed to residents and members of the teaching staff. It should be readily available for review.
2. Selection of residents for appointment to the program in accordance with institutional and departmental policies and procedures.
3. Selection and supervision of the teaching staff and other program personnel at each institution participating in the program.
4. The supervision of residents through explicit written descriptions of supervisory lines of responsibility for the care of patients. Such guidelines must be communicated to all members of the program staff.
5. Regular evaluation of residents' knowledge, skills, and overall performance, including the development of professional attitudes consistent with being a physician.
6. The provision of a written final evaluation for each resident who completes the program, as specified in paragraph VI.I.
7. Implementation of fair procedures, as established by the sponsoring institution, regarding academic discipline and resident complaints or grievances.
8. Monitoring resident stress, including mental or emotional conditions inhibiting performance or learning and drug- or alcohol-related dysfunction. Program directors and teaching staff should be sensitive to the need for timely provision of confidential counseling and psychological support services to residents. Training situations that consistently produce undesirable stress on residents must be evaluated and modified.
9. Preparation of an accurate statistical and narrative description of the program as requested by the RRC for Neurological Surgery.
10. Notifying the executive secretary of the RRC in writing of any major change in the program that may significantly alter the educational experience for the residents, including:
    a. Changes in leadership of the department, such as the appointment of a permanent or acting program director and/or departmental chairman.
    b. Changes in administrative structure, such as alteration in the hierarchical status of the program/department within the institution.
11. The director of the program must obtain prior approval of the RRC for the following changes in the program to determine if an adequate educational environment exists to support these changes:
    a. The addition or deletion of any participating institution to which residents rotate
    b. The addition or deletion of any institutional rotation
    c. Any change in the resident complement of the program
    d. Any change in the format of the training program (including fellowships within the program)

Upon review of a proposal for a major change in a program, the RRC may determine that a site visit is necessary.

C. Other Teaching Faculty Qualifications and Number

1. All clinical faculty members shall possess the necessary experience and administrative, teaching, and clinical skills to conduct the program.
2. All clinical faculty members who are neurological surgeons shall be certified by, or be in the certification process of, the American Board of Neurological Surgery or possess equivalent qualifications in neurological surgery satisfactory to the RRC.
3. There must be a sufficient number of teaching staff with documented qualifications to instruct and supervise adequately all the residents in the program. Members of the teaching staff must be able to devote sufficient time to meet their supervisory and teaching responsibilities. Under most circumstances, there should be a minimum of three neurological surgeons associated with the training program.
4. All members of the teaching staff must demonstrate a strong interest in the education of residents, sound clinical and teaching abilities, support of the goals and objectives of the program, a commitment to their own continuing medical education, and participation in scholarly activities. Neurological surgery faculty participation in undergraduate medical education is highly desirable.
5. The teaching staff must be organized and have regular documented meetings to review program goals and objectives as well as program effectiveness in achieving them. At least one resident representative should participate in these reviews.
6. The teaching staff should periodically evaluate the utilization of the resources available to the program, the contribution of each institution participating in the program, the financial and administrative support of the program, the volume and variety of patients available to the program for educational purposes, the performance of members of the teaching staff, and the quality of supervision of residents.

D. Training Directors at Participating Institutions

1. The training director shall be a qualified neurological surgeon appointed by and responsible to the program director in each geographically separate institution. This individual must be responsible for the education of the residents and will also supervise the educational activities of other neurological surgeons relating to resident education in that institution. Appropriate exceptions may be considered for special resource hospitals.
2. These appointments will generally be for a 1-year period and can be renewable to ensure continuity of leadership.
3. The training director in neurological surgery at each participating institution must have major clinical responsibilities at that institution.

E. Scholarly Activity of Faculty

The responsibility for establishing and maintaining an environment of inquiry and scholarship rests with the teaching staff. While not all members of a teaching staff must be investigators, the staff as a whole must demonstrate broad involvement in scholarly activity. This activity should include:

1. Active participation of the teaching staff in clinical discussions, rounds, and conferences in a manner that promotes a spirit of inquiry and scholarship. Scholarship implies an in-depth under-

standing of basic mechanisms of normal and abnormal states and the application of current knowledge to practice.
2. Participation in journal clubs and research conferences.
3. Active participation in regional or national professional and scientific societies, particularly through presentations at the organizations' meetings and publication in their journals.
4. Participation in research, particularly in projects that are funded following peer review and/or result in publication or presentations at regional and national scientific meetings.
5. Offering of guidance and technical support (eg, research design, statistical analysis) for residents involved in research.
6. Provision of support for resident participation in scholarly activities.

F. Other Program Personnel

Programs must be provided with the additional professional, technical, and clerical personnel needed to support the administration and educational conduct of the program.

IV. Facilities and Resources

A. Inpatient Facilities

1. Inpatient facilities available for training programs in neurological surgery should be geographically identifiable and have an adequate number of beds, support personnel, and proper equipment to ensure quality education.
2. Inpatient facilities may vary from one participating institution to another but should support essential prerequisites for excellence in patient care and teaching.
3. The presence of a neurological surgery operating room with microsurgical capabilities and an intensive care unit specifically for the care of neurological surgery patients is highly desirable to a training program, as are other units for specialized neurological surgery care.
4. Similarly, neurological surgery beds should be on a unit designated for neurosurgery patients.

B. Outpatient Facilities

Residents must use outpatient facilities, clinic, and office space for training purposes in the regular preoperative evaluation and postoperative follow-up for cases for which the resident has responsibility.

C. Research Facilities

1. There should be space and support personnel for research identifiable in the neurological surgery division or department, and some activity should be ongoing in this area.
2. Clinical and/or basic research opportunities should be available to the neurological surgical resident with appropriate faculty supervision.

D. Library

1. Residents must have ready access to a major medical library, either at the institution where the residents are located or through arrangement with convenient nearby institutions.
2. Library services should include the electronic retrieval of information from medical databases.
3. There must be access to an on-site library or to a collection of appropriate texts and journals in each institution participating in a residency program. On-site libraries and/or collections of texts and journals must be readily available during nights and weekends.

V. Educational Program

The director and teaching staff of a program must prepare and comply with written educational goals for the program. All educational components of a residency program should be related to program goals. The program design and/or structure must be approved by the RRC for Neurological Surgery as part of the regular review process.

A. Clinical Components

A current, well-organized, written plan for rotation of residents among the various services and institutions involved must be maintained and must be available to the residents and faculty.

1. Patient Requirements
   There shall be sufficient patients admitted each year to ensure that the resident participates in the care of patients suffering from the full spectrum of neurosurgical diseases.
2. This participation must include substantial experience in the management (including critical care) and surgical care of adult and pediatric patients and should include disorders of the spine and of the peripheral nerves, cerebrovascular disease including extracranial vascular disease, trauma, and tumors of the nervous system.
   a. A program must demonstrate to the satisfaction of the RRC that it has both the volume of patients under neurological care and the breadth and depth of academic support to ensure that it has the capability of providing excellent neurological surgery training to residents.
   b. The former must be substantiated in part by a compilation of annual institutional operative data and resident operative data (including that from residents rotating on the service from other programs) provided in a fashion prescribed by the RRC. Under some circumstances, the program may be required to include data for a period of up to 3 years prior to the date of the submitted program information forms for accreditation or reaccreditation. The entire surgical experience of the most recently graduating resident(s) must be submitted each time the program has its periodic review.
   c. The profile of clinical experience reported to the RRC must be limited to that utilized in the resident's educational program. It also is understood that the educational requirements of the resident must be considered at all times, and assignment to a clinical service that limits or precludes educational opportunities will be adversely considered in evaluation of the program.
   d. Within the total clinical facilities available to the training program, there should be a minimum of 300 major neurological surgery procedures per year per finishing resident. It must be understood that achievement of this minimum number of clinical procedures will not ensure accreditation of a training program.
   e. The minimum number of clinical procedures (see paragraph V.A.2.d) is suggested with the understanding that the majority of the procedures must occur at the sponsoring institution.
   f. The presence within a given training program of this neurological surgery workload and the distribution of the surgical experience are equally important. For instance, the cases should be appropriately distributed among cranial, extracranial, spinal, and peripheral nerve surgical procedures and should represent a well-balanced spectrum of neurological surgery in both adults and children. This spectrum should include craniotomies for trauma, verified neoplasms, aneurysms, and vascular malformations; extracranial carotid and vertebral artery surgery; transsphenoidal and stereotaxic surgery; and spinal procedures of a sufficient number and complexity using modern techniques that encompass a variety of disorders (such as trauma, neoplasia, infection, and degenerative disorders).
   g. No affiliated hospital unit in the training program should be a component of a training program unless there are a minimum of 100 major neurological surgery procedures per year distributed appropriately among the spectrum of cases as described in paragraph f, above. Again, exception may be made if a hospi-

tal offers special clinical resources, eg, stereotaxic surgery, trauma, or pediatric neurological surgery, that significantly augment the resources of the training program as a whole.

3. Residents must have opportunities to evaluate patients referred for elective surgery in an outpatient environment. Under appropriate supervision, this experience should include obtaining a complete history, conducting an examination, ordering (if necessary) and interpreting diagnostic studies, and arriving independently at a diagnosis and plan of management. Consonant with their skills and level of experience, residents should be actively involved in preoperative decision-making and subsequent operative procedures under the supervision of the attending physician who has ultimate responsibility for the patient. Residents should similarly be actively involved in postsurgical care and follow-up evaluation of their patients to develop skills in assessing postoperative recovery, recognizing and treating complications, communicating with referring physicians, and developing the physician-patient relationship. Preoperative interview and examination of patients already scheduled for a surgical procedure will not satisfy these requirements.

B. Didactic Components

There must be a well-coordinated schedule of teaching conferences, rounds, and other educational activities in which both the neurological surgery faculty and the residents participate. Conferences must be coordinated among institutions in a training program to facilitate attendance by a majority of staff and residents.

C. Resident Policies

1. Supervision
The program director must ensure, direct, and document proper supervision of residents at all times. Residents must be provided with prompt, reliable systems for communication and interaction with supervisory physicians. Attending physicians or supervising residents with appropriate experience for the severity and complexity of the patient's condition must be available at all times on site. The responsibility or independence given to residents in patient care should depend on their knowledge, manual skill, experience, and the complexity of the patient's illness and the risk of the operations.
2. Progressive Responsibility
Resident participation in and responsibility for operative procedures embracing the entire neurosurgical spectrum should increase progressively throughout the training period.
3. Continuity of Care
Graduate training in neurological surgery requires a commitment to continuity of patient care, as practiced by qualified neurological surgeons. This continuity of care must take precedence—without regard to the time of day, day of the week, number of hours already worked, or on-call schedules. At the same time, patients have a right to expect a healthy, alert, responsible, and responsive physician dedicated to delivering effective and appropriate care.
4. Duty Hours
   a. The program director must establish an environment that is optimal for both resident education and patient care, while assuring that undue stress and fatigue among residents are avoided. It is his or her responsibility to ensure assignment of appropriate in-hospital duty hours so that residents are not required to perform excessively difficult or prolonged duties regularly. It is desirable that residents' work schedules be designed so that, on average, excluding exceptional patient care needs, residents have at least 1 day out of 7 free of routine responsibilities and be on-call in the hospital no more often than every third night. Different rotations may require different working hours and patterns. There must be adequate backup so that patient care is not jeopardized during or following assigned periods of duty.
   b. A distinction must be made between on-call time in the hospital and on-call availability at home vis-a-vis actual hours worked. The ratio of hours worked and on-call time will vary, particularly at the senior levels, and therefore necessitates flexibility.
   c. During these hours residents must be provided with adequate sleeping, lounge, and food facilities. Support services must be such that the resident does not spend an inordinate amount of time in noneducational activities that can be discharged properly by other personnel.
5. Extracurricular Activities
Residency training in neurological surgery is a full-time responsibility; activities outside the educational program must not interfere with the residents' performance in the educational process, as determined by the program director, and must not interfere with the residents' opportunities for rest, relaxation, and study.

D. Other Required Educational Components

Graduate medical education must take place in an environment of inquiry and scholarship in which residents participate in the development of new knowledge, learn to evaluate research findings, and develop habits of inquiry as a continuing professional responsibility.

1. Educational experience in neuroradiology and neuropathology must be an integral part of the training program designed for the education of the neurological surgery residents. Such experience should be under the direction of qualified neuroradiologists and neuropathologists.
2. The program must provide opportunities for experience and instruction in the basic neurosciences.
3. The residents should participate in scholarly activities such as ongoing clinical and/or basic research projects with which appropriate faculty are involved.
4. Resident participation in undergraduate medical education is highly desirable.
5. Related Disciplines
   a. Recognizing the nature of the specialty of neurological surgery, it is unlikely that a program can mount an adequate educational experience for neurological surgery residents without approved training programs in related fields. Clinically oriented training programs in the sponsoring institution of the neurological surgery program should include accredited training programs in neurology, general surgery, internal medicine, pediatrics, and radiology.
   b. There should be clinical resources for the education of neurological surgery residents in anesthesiology, endocrinology, ophthalmology, orthopedics, otolaryngology, pathology, and psychiatry. A lack of such resources will adversely affect the accreditation status of the neurological surgery program.
6. Appointment of Fellows
   a. The appointment of other individuals for special training or education, such as fellows, must not dilute or detract from the educational opportunities of regularly appointed residents.
   b. Programs must notify the RRC when they sponsor or participate in any clinical fellowships within institutions participating in the program before the commencement of such training and at each subsequent review of the program. Documentation must be provided describing the fellowship's relationship to and impact on the residency.
   c. If fellows so appointed will, in the judgment of the RRC, detract from the education of the regularly appointed residents, the accreditation status of the program may be adversely affected.

VI. Evaluation

The educational effectiveness of a program must be evaluated in a systematic manner. In particular, the quality of the curriculum and the extent to which the educational goals have been met by residents must be assessed. Written evaluations by residents should be utilized in this process.

A. The program director is responsible for the annual collection, compilation, and retention of the number and types of neurological surgery operative procedures performed in all institutions and facilities utilized in the clinical education of residents. This information must be provided on request in the format and form specified by the RRC.

B. Annually, the program director must ensure the compilation of a comprehensive record of the number and type of operative procedures performed by each resident completing the program. This record must include all of the procedures in which the neurological surgery resident was either surgeon or assistant and must be signed by both the resident and the program director as a statement of its accuracy. This information must be provided upon request in the format specified by the RRC. These records must be accurately maintained by the program director.

C. The knowledge, skills, professional growth, and progress of each resident, including professional conduct, must be evaluated by the program director in consultation with the teaching staff in a semiannual, written review. These evaluations must be provided to and discussed with each resident in a timely manner. Appropriate criteria and procedures must be used.

D. Residents must be advanced to positions of higher responsibility only on the basis of evidence of their satisfactory progressive scholarship and professional growth.

E. The program must maintain a permanent record of evaluation for each resident and have it accessible to the resident and other authorized personnel.

F. At least annually, all individual faculty members must be formally evaluated by the program director of neurological surgery as well as by the residents. A mechanism for sharing the results of such evaluations with the faculty that preserves individual resident confidentiality must be employed.

G. At least annually, the program rotations and conferences must be evaluated by both residents and faculty. The results of these evaluations should be kept on file.

H. The thoroughness of resident, faculty, and program evaluations, as well as the accurate and timely provision of program-related information to the RRC, will be monitored in the overall review of the residency program.

I. The program director must provide a written final evaluation for each resident who completes the program. The evaluation must include a review of the resident's performance during the final period of training and should verify that the resident has demonstrated sufficient professional ability to practice competently and independently. This final evaluation should be part of the resident's permanent record maintained by the institution.

VII. Board Certification

A. Performance on Examination

One measure of the quality of a program is the participation in and performance of its graduates on the examinations of the American Board of Neurological Surgery. The number of residents completing training and taking and passing the certification examinations will be part of the RRC's evaluation of the program.

B. Certification Requirements

Residents who seek certification by the American Board of Neurological Surgery should communicate with the secretary of the board to be sure that the requirements for certification have been fulfilled. The current address of this office is published in each edition of the *Graduate Medical Education Directory*. Requests regarding evaluation of educational programs in neurological surgery and all related program inquiries should be addressed to the Executive Secretary of the Residency Review Committee for Neurological Surgery, 515 N State St/Ste 2000, Chicago, IL 60610.

ACGME: June 1994 Effective: July 1995

Program Requirements for Residency Education in Neurology

[*Note:* This material constitutes the Program Requirements for Residency Education in Neurology. The reader is referred to the Institutional Requirements for Residency Education and to the Program Requirements for Residency Education in Child Neurology. The reader is also referred to the publications of the Accreditation Council for Graduate Medical Education (ACGME) that outline the composition and function of all Residency Review Committees (RRCs); indicate the actions that any RRC may take, as well as the actions that the ACGME may take; and describe the appeals procedure, types of programs, and the relationships between the RRCs, their parent organizations, and the ACGME.

Requests to have a program accredited to train residents in neurology (or related inquiries regarding residency programs) should be addressed to Executive Director, Residency Review Committee for Neurology, 515 N State St, Suite 2000, Chicago, IL 60610. All inquiries as to whether a physician is qualified to be examined for certification in neurology should be addressed to Executive Vice President, American Board of Psychiatry and Neurology (ABPN), 500 Lake Cook Rd, Suite 335, Deerfield, IL 60015.]

I. Introduction

A. Definition

Neurology is a medical specialty concerned with the diagnosis and treatment of all categories of disease involving the central, peripheral and autonomic nervous systems, including their coverings, blood vessels, and all effector tissue, such as muscle. For these diseases, the neurologist is often the principal care physician and may render all levels of care commensurate with his or her training.

B. Duration and Scope of Training

A complete neurology residency is 48 months. Approved residencies in neurology must provide at least 36 months of this education. The program meeting these requirements may be of two types:

1. Those that provide 4 years of residency training, the first year of which training (accredited by the ACGME) must include a broad clinical experience in general internal medicine. This year must include at least one of the following: (a) 8 months in internal medicine with primary responsibility in patient care or (b) 6 months in internal medicine with primary responsibility in patient care and a period of at least 2 months total time in pediatrics or emergency medicine or both. Residents must spend no more than 2 months in neurology during this year.
2. Those that provide 3 years of residency training but accept only residents who have had an initial first year of graduate training in an ACGME-accredited program. This first year must meet the minimum requirements as noted in B.1. above.

C. Goals and Objectives for Residency Education

The purpose of the training program is to prepare the physician for the independent practice of clinical neurology. This training must be based on supervised clinical work with increasing responsibility for outpatients and inpatients. It must have a foundation of organized instruction in the basic neurosciences.

D. Program Design

1. All educational components of a residency program must be related to program goals. The program design and structure must be approved by the RRC for Neurology as part of the regular review process.
2. Programs that cosponsor combined training in neurology and another specialty must so inform the RRC. Residents in such training must be informed of the necessary requirements of the specialty boards in question.

II. Administration and Organization

A. Participating Institutions

Participation by any institution providing 6 months or more of training in a program of 3 or more years must be approved by the RRC.

B. Appointment of Residents

1. The exact number of residents that may be appointed to a given program is not specifically designated. However, the number of residents appointed to the program must be commensurate with the educational resources specifically available to the residents in terms of faculty, the number and variety of patient diagnoses, and the availability of basic science and research education.
2. The program director will establish the maximum number of resident positions that can be supported by the educational resources for the program, subject to the approval of the RRC. The program director must report any increase or decrease in the resident complement (at the beginning of the academic year), and any resulting change in the structure of the program, to the RRC. (The resident complement is the total number of resident positions offered in the training program. The number includes all PG-1 and categorical positions and ½ of the positions for combined training in neurology and another specialty.)
3. All additional trainees in the program other than regularly appointed residents must be identified and designated as such and must not compromise resident education.

Programs that fail to recruit any new residents for 2 consecutive years may be subject to adverse action because of inactivity in the educational program.

C. Leave and Vacation Policy

Each program must have an equitable leave and vacation policy for residents, in accordance with overall institutional policy.

III. Faculty Qualifications and Responsibilities

The director and teaching staff of a program must prepare and comply with written educational goals for the program. The program director and the teaching staff are responsible for the general administration of a program, including those activities related to the recruitment, selection, instruction, supervision, counseling, evaluation, and advancement of residents, and the maintenance of records related to program accreditation.

A. Program Director

There must be a single program director responsible for the program.

1. Qualifications of the program director include:
   a. requisite and documented clinical, educational, and administrative abilities and experience
   b. licensure to practice medicine in the state where the institution that sponsors the program is located (Certain federal programs are exempted.)
   c. certification by the American Board of Psychiatry and Neurology (ABPN) or suitable equivalent qualifications
   d. appointment in good standing to the medical staff of an institution participating in the program
2. Responsibilities of the program director include:
   a. devotion of sufficient time to provide leadership to the program and supervision of the residents.
   b. monitoring the content and ensuring the quality of the program.
   c. preparation of a written statement outlining the educational goals and objectives of the program with respect to knowledge,

skills and other attributes of residents at each level of training and for each major rotation or other program assignment. These goals and objectives must be consistent with and linked to the program's overall goals and objectives, to the educational experiences in the curriculum (both didactic and clinical), and to the Program Requirements. This statement must be distributed to residents and members of the teaching staff as they begin the program. It should be readily available for review. The program director also must develop criteria to use in the assessment of the extent to which the program's goals and objectives are met.

d. selection of residents for appointment to the program in accordance with institutional and departmental policies and procedures.

e. selection and supervision of the teaching staff and other program personnel at each institution participating in the program.

f. supervision of residents through explicit written descriptions of supervisory lines of responsibility for the care of patients. Such guidelines must be communicated to all members of the program staff. Residents must be provided with prompt, reliable systems for communication and interaction with supervisory physicians.

g. regular evaluation of residents' knowledge, skills, and overall performance, including the development of professional attitudes and ethical behavior consistent with being a capable neurologist. The program director, with participation of members of the teaching staff, shall
   1. at least semiannually evaluate the knowledge, skills, and professional growth of the residents, using appropriate criteria and procedures.
   2. communicate each evaluation to the resident in a timely manner.
   3. advance residents to positions of higher responsibility only on the basis of evidence of their satisfactory progressive scholarship and professional growth.
   4. maintain a permanent record of evaluation for each resident and have it accessible to the resident and other authorized personnel.

h. provision of a written final evaluation for each resident who completes the program. The evaluation must include a review of the resident's performance during the final period of training and should verify that the resident has demonstrated sufficient professional ability to practice competently and independently. This final evaluation must be part of the resident's permanent record maintained by the institution.

i. implementation of fair procedures as established by the sponsoring institution regarding academic discipline and resident complaints or grievances.

j. monitoring resident stress, including mental or emotional conditions inhibiting performance or learning and drug- or alcohol-related dysfunction. Program directors and teaching staff must be sensitive to the need for timely provision of confidential counseling and psychological support services to residents. Training situations that consistently produce undesirable stress on residents must be evaluated and modified.

k. preparation of an accurate statistical and narrative description of the program, as requested by the RRC.

l. notification in writing to the Executive Director of the RRC within 60 days of any major change in the program that may significantly alter the educational experience for the residents, including but not limited to
   1. changes in the program directorship or the departmental leadership and
   2. changes in administrative structure, such as a change in the hierarchical status of the program and/or department within the institution.

Notification of a change in the program directorship must include a copy of the new director's curriculum vitae, including details of his or her experience and qualifications in graduate medical education.

B. Teaching Staff

1. Besides the program director, there must be a minimum of five neurology faculty, in addition to child neurology faculty, fully committed to the residency program, who devote sufficient time to the program to ensure basic and clinical education for the residents. Within the department or section of neurology, a faculty-to-resident ratio of at least 1:1 in the total program is required. The program director may be counted as one of the faculty in determining the ratio.
2. Neurologists with teaching responsibilities must be certified by the ABPN or have equivalent qualifications.
3. There must be faculty who have diverse interests and skills in an appropriate range of teaching and research; who ensure adequate clinical opportunities for residents; and who provide continued instruction through seminars, conferences, and teaching rounds.
4. The program must have a sufficient number of qualified faculty involved in the teaching of residents in each of the component institutions of the program.
5. Faculty with special expertise in all the disciplines related to neurology, including neuro-ophthalmology, neuromuscular disease, cerebrovascular disease, epilepsy, movement disorders, critical care, clinical neurophysiology, behavioral neurology, neuroimmunology, infectious disease, neuro-otology, neuroimaging, neuro-oncology, pain management, neurogenetics, child neurology, the neurology of aging, and psychiatry must be available on a regular basis to neurology residents.
6. All members of the teaching staff must demonstrate a strong interest in the education of residents, sound clinical and teaching abilities, support of the goals and objectives of the program, and a commitment to their own continuing medical education.
7. The teaching staff must actively pursue scholarly activity in the neurosciences and encourage residents to engage in scholarly activity.
8. A member of the teaching staff of each participating institution must be designated to assume responsibility for the day-to-day activities of the program at that institution, with overall coordination by the program director.
9. The teaching staff must be organized and have regular documented meetings to review program goals and objectives as well as program effectiveness in achieving them. At least one resident representative must participate in these reviews.
10. The teaching staff must periodically evaluate the utilization of the resources available to the program, the contribution of each institution participating in the program, the financial and administrative support of the program, the volume and variety of patients available to the program for educational purposes, the performance of members of the teaching staff, and the quality of supervision of residents.

C. Other Program Personnel

Programs must be provided with the additional professional, technical, and clerical personnel needed to support the administration and educational conduct of the program.

IV. Facilities and Resources

A. Patient Population

It is the program director's responsibility to ensure that the number of patients is appropriate. They must be diversified as to age and sex, short-term and long-term neurologic problems, and inpatients and outpatients. Neurology residents must have management responsibility for patients with neurological disorders. Neurology residents must be involved in the management of patients with neurological disorders who require emergency and intensive care.

B. Facilities

There must be adequate inpatient and outpatient facilities, examining areas, conference rooms, and research laboratories. There must be adequate space for offices for faculty members. Space for study, chart work, and dictation must be available for the residents. There must be adequate contemporary clinical laboratory facilities that report rapidly the results of necessary laboratory evaluations, including clinical-pathological, electrophysiological, imaging, and other studies needed by neurological services. Adequate chart and record-keeping systems must be in use for patient treatment.

C. Library

Residents must have access to an adequate medical library. Library services must include the electronic retrieval of information from medical databases. There must be access to an on-site library or to a collection of appropriate texts and journals in each institution participating in a residency program. On-site libraries, collections of texts and journals, and electronic retrieval of information from medical databases must be readily available during nights and weekends.

V. Educational Program

A. Basic Curriculum

1. Patient care, teaching, and research must be present in every training program. Patient care responsibilities must ensure a balance between patient care and education that achieves for the trainee an optimal educational experience consistent with the best medical care. Patient care responsibilities must include inpatient, outpatient, and consultation experiences.
2. The program must include a minimum of 18 months (full-time equivalent) of clinical adult neurology with management responsibility for patient care. This must include at least 6 months (full-time equivalent) of outpatient experience in clinical adult neurology. The outpatient experience also must include a resident longitudinal/continuity clinic with attendance by each resident one-half day weekly throughout the program. (The resident may be excused from this clinic when a rotation site is more than 1 hour travel time from the clinic site.)
3. Residents in neurology must have experience with neurological disorders in children under the supervision of a child neurologist with ABPN certification or suitable equivalent qualifications. This must consist of a minimum of 3 months (full-time equivalent) in clinical child neurology with management responsibility in patient care.

B. Teaching Rounds

Clinical teaching rounds must be supervised by faculty. They must occur at least 5 days per week. Residents must present cases and their diagnostic and therapeutic plans.

C. Clinical Teaching

1. The resident must have instruction and practical experience in obtaining an orderly and detailed history from the patient, in conducting a thorough general and neurological examination, and in organizing and recording data. The training must include the indications for and limitations of clinical neurodiagnostic tests and their interpretation. The resident must learn to correlate the information derived from these neurodiagnostic studies with the clinical history and examination in formulating a differential diagnosis and management plan.
2. Residents must participate in the evaluation of and decision making for patients with disorders of the nervous system requiring surgical management. The existence of a neurosurgical service with close interaction with the neurology service is essential.
3. The residents must participate in the management of patients with psychiatric disorders. They must learn about the psychological aspects of the patient-physician relationship and the importance of personal, social, and cultural factors in disease processes and their clinical expression. Residents must learn the principles of psychopathology, psychiatric diagnosis, and therapy and the indications for and complications of drugs used in psychiatry.
4. Residents must learn the basic principles of rehabilitation for neurological disorders.
5. The resident must participate in the management of patients with acute neurological disorders in an intensive care unit and an emergency department.
6. The resident must receive instruction in the principles of bioethics and in the provision of appropriate and cost-effective evaluation and treatment for patients with neurologic disorders.
7. The resident must receive instruction in appropriate and compassionate methods of end-of-life palliative care, including adequate pain relief and psychosocial support and counseling for patients and family members about these issues.

D. Progressive Responsibility

Programs must provide opportunities for increasing responsibility and professional maturation of residents. Early clinical assignments must be based on direct patient responsibility for a limited number of patients. Subsequent assignments must place the resident in a position of taking increased responsibility for patients. Night call is essential in accomplishing these goals. Adequate faculty supervision is essential throughout the program. Neurological training must include assignment on a consultation service to the medical, surgical, obstetric and gynecologic, pediatric, rehabilitation medicine, and psychiatry services.

E. Basic and Related Science

Residents must learn the basic sciences on which clinical neurology is founded, including neuroanatomy, neuropathology, neurophysiology, neuroimaging, neuropsychology, neural development, neurochemistry, neuropharmacology, molecular biology, genetics, immunology, and epidemiology and statistics. Concentrated training in one or more of these areas, accomplished with a full-time equivalent experience of at least 2 months total, is required for each resident. Specific goals and objectives must be developed for this experience.

F. Electives

Resident assignments need not be identical for each resident, and elective time should accommodate individual resident interests and previous training. Elective time should be a minimum of 3 months.

G. Seminars and Conferences

Residents must regularly attend seminars and conferences in the following disciplines: neuropathology, neuroradiology, neuro-ophthalmology, neuromuscular disease, cerebrovascular disease, epilepsy, movement disorders, critical care, clinical neurophysiology, behavioral neurology, neuroimmunology, infectious disease, neuro-otology, neuroimaging, neuro-oncology, pain management, neurogenetics, rehabilitation, child neurology, the neurology of aging, and general neurology. There must be gross and microscopic pathology conferences and clinical pathological conferences. The resident must have increasing responsibility for the planning and supervision of the conferences.

The resident must learn about major developments in both the basic and clinical sciences relating to neurology. Residents must attend periodic seminars, journal clubs, lectures in basic science, didactic courses, and meetings of local and national neurological societies.

H. Educational Policies

The program must provide for the following:

1. Residents must be allowed to spend an average of at least 1 full day out of 7 away from the hospital.
2. Residents must provide on-call duty in the hospital, but no more frequently than an average of every third night.
3. There must be adequate physician coverage if unexpected patient care needs create resident fatigue sufficient to jeopardize patient care during or following on-call periods.

I. Resident Participation in Research

Graduate medical education must take place in an environment of inquiry and scholarship in which residents participate in the development of new knowledge, learn to evaluate research findings, and develop habits of inquiry as a continuing professional responsibility. The responsibility for establishing and maintaining an environment of inquiry and scholarship rests with the teaching staff. While not all members of a teaching staff must be investigators, training must be conducted by neurology departments in centers in which there is active research in both clinical and basic neuroscience. This activity must include:

1. active participation of the teaching staff in clinical discussions, rounds, and conferences in a manner that promotes a spirit of inquiry and scholarship. Scholarship implies an in-depth understanding of basic mechanisms of normal and abnormal states and the application of current knowledge to practice.
2. participation in research, particularly in projects that are funded following peer review and result in publications or presentations at regional and national scientific meetings.
3. offering of guidance and technical support (eg, research design, statistical analysis) for residents involved in research.
4. provision of support for research opportunities for residents.

J. Resident Responsibility for Teaching

Teaching of other residents, medical students, nurses, and other health care personnel, formally and informally, are required aspects of the resident's education in neurology.

VI. Evaluation

A. Resident Evaluation (See also Section III.A.2.)

The program must have an evaluation system that provides information about each resident's educational progress and the extent to which each resident has accomplished the program's learning and performance objectives.

1. Formative Evaluation
   a. Resident performance must be monitored and feedback provided on an ongoing basis.
   b. A written evaluation of the resident's attainment of objectives specific to the rotation must be made after each rotation and reviewed with the resident so that areas of weakness and strength can be communicated to the resident.
   c. The program director or his or her designee must meet with each resident semiannually in a formal feedback session to discuss the resident's standing in relation to specific learning and performance objectives. Plans to correct any deficiencies must be discussed. Each resident must be an active participant in formulating plans for his or her development. Evaluation data should be used to advise the resident and to make decisions regarding the progression in the resident's level of responsibility.
2. Final Evaluation
   At the conclusion of the resident's period of training in the program, the program director must prepare a detailed, written evaluation of the resident's performance in relation to the program's learning and performance objectives and discuss this evaluation with the resident.
3. Records
   a. A written record of the contents of the semiannual review session must be prepared and filed in the resident's permanent record. The written record of the evaluation and the review must be signed by the resident. The resident must have the opportunity to append a written response to the written record of the evaluation and review.
   b. Each resident's permanent record must include the written evaluations completed for each defined educational experience, the written records from the semiannual reviews, results of formal assessments, and the resident's final evaluation. Written descriptions of any deficiencies and problem areas, plans for correcting the deficiencies, disciplinary actions, and commendations, where appropriate, should be included.

B. Program Evaluation

The educational effectiveness of a program must be evaluated in a systematic manner. In particular, the quality of the curriculum and the extent to which the educational goals have been met by residents must be assessed. Written evaluations by residents must be utilized in this process.

1. Evaluations of residents' attainment of the program's learning and performance objectives must be used as the basis for program evaluation. Comparisons of these data against the program's own criteria, performance criteria set by the RRC, and attainment levels of residents at comparable levels of training should be performed as a primary means of assessing attainment of goals and objectives. In this context, a suitable in-service examination, such as the RITE examination, must be used.
2. Residents must evaluate the program at least annually.

C. Board Certification

One measure of the quality of a training program is the proportion of its residents who take the examinations of the ABPN and the proportion who pass those examinations. This information must be used in the evaluation of the educational effectiveness of the program. A program will be judged deficient by the RRC if during the most recent 5-year period fewer than 60% of its graduates who take the examinations pass either the written (Part I) or oral (Part II) examination on the first try.

ACGME: February 1998 Effective: January 1999

Policies and Procedures for Residency Education in the Subspecialties of Neurology

1. The initial application for a subspecialty program will not require a site visit, but will require submission of all application materials and information and must be signed by the director of the subspecialty program and the director of the core program in neurology. (Applications for programs in child neurology must be

cosigned by the directors of the accredited programs in both pediatrics and neurology.) The Residency Review Committee (RRC) for Neurology will take initial action based on a "paper review" of the program, namely, a review without a site visit.

2. Subsequent review of subspecialty programs will be in conjunction with the survey and review of the core program in neurology. The subspecialty program director will complete a separate set of forms for review of the subspecialty program. In special cases determined by the RRC, a subspecialty program may be surveyed and reviewed separately. The RRC will also entertain interim requests and, on occasion, ask for interim progress reports.
3. The RRC will designate programs as being accredited or not accredited. No further delineation of accreditation categories will be utilized. The accreditation of a program will be directly tied to that of the core. If the core program (either neurology or pediatrics for child neurology programs) is subsequently accredited on a probationary basis, this is simultaneously a warning to the related subspecialty program that accreditation is in jeopardy. Withdrawal of accreditation of the core program (either neurology or pediatrics for child neurology programs) will result in a simultaneous loss of accreditation of the subspecialty program.
4. If the core program (either neurology or pediatrics for child neurology programs) remains in good standing, but the RRC judges the subspecialty program to be in noncompliance with the applicable program requirements, a warning will be issued. If these areas of noncompliance are not corrected, accreditation may be withdrawn from the subspecialty program. The Procedures for Proposed Adverse Actions and the Procedures for Appeal of Adverse Actions may be utilized by programs from which accreditation has been withdrawn in an action separate from withdrawal of accreditation of a core program.
5. Inquiries about accreditation of subspecialty programs should be directed to the Executive Secretary of the RRC for Neurology.

Program Requirements for Residency Education in Child Neurology (Neurology)

[*Note:* This material constitutes the Program Requirements for Residency Education in Child Neurology. The reader should refer as well to the Program Requirements for Residency Education in Neurology for information on requirements for core programs, to which programs in child neurology must be attached. The reader is also referred to the Institutional Requirements of the Essentials of Accredited Residencies in Graduate Medical Education and to other publications of the Accreditation Council for Graduate Medical Education (ACGME), which outline the composition and function of all Residency Review Committees (RRCs); indicate the actions that any RRC may take, as well as the actions that the ACGME may take; and describe the appeals procedure, types of programs, and the relationships among the RRCs, their parent organizations, and the ACGME.

Requests to have a program accredited to train residents in child neurology (or related inquiries regarding residency programs) should be addressed to Executive Director, RRC for Neurology, 515 N State St, Suite 2000, Chicago, IL 60610. All inquiries concerning prerequisite training or whether a physician is qualified to be examined for certification in neurology with special qualification in child neurology should be addressed to Executive Vice President, American Board of Psychiatry and Neurology (ABPN), 500 Lake Cook Rd/Ste 335, Deerfield, IL 60015.]

I. Introduction

A. Duration and Scope of Training

Training in child neurology shall encompass a total of 3 years. One year of training must be in clinical adult neurology. One year of training shall be referred to as flexible, and the resident must learn the principles of neurophysiology, neuropathology, neuroradiology, neuro-ophthalmology, psychiatry, rehabilitation, neurological surgery, neurodevelopment, and the basic neurosciences. One year of training shall be in clinical child neurology.

B. Prerequisite Training

The training can be initiated following one of three options: (1) 2 years of residency training in pediatrics in an ACGME-accredited program; (2) one PG-1 year (as described in the Program Requirements for Residency Education in Neurology, Section I.A.1) and 1 year of residency training in pediatrics; or (3) 1 year of pediatrics plus 1 year of basic neuroscience training. The program director must review and determine the acceptability of these initial 2 years of training.

C. Goals and Objectives for Residency Training

The purpose of the training program is to prepare the physician for the independent practice of clinical child neurology. This training must be based on supervised clinical work with increasing responsibility for outpatients and inpatients. It must have a foundation of organized instruction in the basic neurosciences.

D. Program Design

All educational components of a residency program should be related to program goals. The program design and/or structure must be approved by the RRC for Neurology as part of the regular review process.

II. Administration and Organization

A. Relation to Core Programs

The 3 years of training in child neurology must take place in a center in which there are accredited residency programs in both pediatrics and neurology and with the approval and support of the program directors of both of these departments.

B. Participating Institutions

Participation by any institution providing 6 months or more of training in a program must be approved by the RRC.

C. Appointment of Residents

The exact number of residents that may be appointed to a given program is not specifically designated. However, the number of residents appointed to the program must be commensurate with the educational resources specifically available to the residents in terms of faculty, the number and variety of patient diagnoses, and the availability of basic science and research education.

All additional trainees in the program other than regularly appointed residents must be identified and designated as such and must not compromise resident education.

D. Leave and Vacation Policy

Each program must have an equitable leave and vacation policy for residents, in accordance with overall institutional policy.

III. Faculty Qualifications and Responsibilities

The director and teaching staff of a program must prepare and comply with written educational goals for the program. The program director and the teaching staff are responsible for the general administration of a program, including those activities related to the recruitment, selection, instruction, supervision, counseling, evaluation, and advancement of residents, and the maintenance of records related to program accreditation.

A. Program Director

There must be a single program director responsible for the program.

1. Qualifications of the program director include:
   a. requisite and documented clinical, educational, and administrative abilities and experience.
   b. licensure to practice medicine in the state where the institution that sponsors the program is located. (Certain federal programs are exempted.)
   c. certification by the ABPN with Special Qualification in Child Neurology or suitable equivalent qualifications.
   d. appointment in good standing to the medical staff of an institution participating in the program.
2. Responsibilities of the program director include:
   a. devotion of sufficient time and full commitment to provide leadership to the program and supervision of the residents.
   b. monitoring the content and ensuring the quality of the program.
   c. preparation of a written statement outlining the educational goals and objectives of the program with respect to knowledge, skills, and other attributes of residents at each level of training and for each major rotation or other program assignment. These goals and objectives must be consistent with and linked to the program's overall goals and objectives, the educational experiences in the curriculum (both didactic and clinical), and the Program Requirements. This statement must be distributed to residents and members of the teaching staff as they begin the program. It should be readily available for review. The program director also must develop criteria to use in the assessment of the extent to which the program's goals and objectives are met.
   d. selection of residents for appointment to the program in accordance with institutional and departmental policies and procedures.
   e. selection and supervision of the teaching staff and other program personnel at each institution participating in the program.
   f. supervision of residents through explicit written descriptions of supervisory lines of responsibility for the care of patients. Such guidelines must be communicated to all members of the program staff. Residents must be provided with prompt, reliable systems for communication and interaction with supervisory physicians.
   g. regular evaluation of residents' knowledge, skills, and overall performance, including the development of professional attitudes consistent with being a physician. The program director, with participation of members of the teaching staff, shall
      1. at least semiannually evaluate the knowledge, skills, and professional growth of the residents, using appropriate criteria and procedures.
      2. communicate each evaluation to the resident in a timely manner.
      3. advance residents to positions of higher responsibility only on the basis of evidence of their satisfactory progressive scholarship and professional growth.
      4. maintain a permanent record of evaluation for each resident and have it accessible to the resident and other authorized personnel.
   h. provision of a written final evaluation for each resident who completes the program. The evaluation must include a review of the resident's performance during the final period of training and should verify that the resident has demonstrated sufficient professional ability to practice competently and independently. This final evaluation should be part of the resident's permanent record maintained by the institution.
   i. implementation of fair procedures, as established by the sponsoring institution, regarding academic discipline and resident complaints or grievances.
   j. monitoring resident stress, including mental or emotional conditions inhibiting performance or learning and drug- or alcohol-related dysfunction. Program directors and teaching staff should be sensitive to the need for timely provision of confidential counseling and psychological support services to residents. Training situations that consistently produce undesirable stress on residents must be evaluated and modified.
   k. preparation of an accurate statistical and narrative description of the program as requested by the RRC.
   l. notification in writing of the Executive Director of the RRC within 60 days of any major change in the program that may significantly alter the educational experience for the residents, including but not limited to
      1. changes in the program directorship or the departmental leadership and
      2. changes in administrative structure, such as a change in the hierarchical status of the program and/or department within the institution.

      Notification of a change in the program directorship must include a copy of the new director's curriculum vitae, including details of his or her experience and qualifications in graduate medical education.

B. Teaching Staff

1. In addition to the program director, the program providing training in child neurology must have at least two child neurology faculty, in addition to the adult neurology faculty, fully committed to the residency program who devote sufficient time to the training program to ensure adequate clinical training of the child neurology residents. Within the section of child neurology, a faculty-to-resident ratio of at least 1:1 in the total program is required. The program director may be counted as one of the faculty in determining the ratio.
2. Neurologists with teaching responsibilities must be certified by the ABPN in Neurology with Special Qualification in Child Neurology or possess equivalent qualifications.
3. There must be enough faculty with diverse interests and skills to make the breadth of teaching and research appropriate to a program meeting these program requirements; to ensure adequate clinical opportunities for residents; and to provide continued instruction through seminars, conferences, and teaching rounds.
4. The program must have a sufficient number of qualified staff involved in the teaching of residents in each of the component institutions of the program.
5. Faculty with special expertise in the disciplines related to child neurology, including cognitive development, neuro-ophthalmology, neuromuscular disease, epilepsy, movement disorders, critical care, clinical neurophysiology, neuroimmunology, infectious disease, neuro-otology, neuroimaging, neurogenetics, neuro-oncology, and pain management, must be available to child neurology residents.
6. All members of the teaching staff must demonstrate a strong interest in the education of residents, sound clinical and teaching abilities, support of the goals and objectives of the program, a commitment to their own continuing medical education, and participation in scholarly activities.
7. The staff must actively pursue scholarly activity in the neurosciences and encourage residents to engage in scholarly activity.

8. A member of the teaching staff of each participating institution must be designated to assume responsibility for the day-to-day activities of the program at that institution, with overall coordination by the program director.
9. The teaching staff must be organized and have regular documented meetings to review program goals and objectives as well as program effectiveness in achieving them. At least one resident representative should participate in these reviews.
10. The teaching staff should periodically evaluate the utilization of the resources available to the program, the contribution of each institution participating in the program, the financial and administrative support of the program, the volume and variety of patients available to the program for educational purposes, the performance of members of the teaching staff, and the quality of supervision of residents.

C. Other Program Personnel

Programs must be provided with the additional professional, technical, and clerical personnel needed to support the administration and educational conduct of the program.

IV. Facilities and Resources

A. Patient Population

During the year of training in clinical child neurology, the resident must work in the outpatient clinic and on the inpatient service on a regular basis. The number and type of patients must be appropriate. The patient population must be diversified as to age and sex, short-term and long-term neurologic problems, and inpatients and outpatients. Child neurology residents must have management responsibility for hospitalized patients with neurological disorders. Neurology residents must be involved in the management of patients with neurological disorders who require emergency and intensive care.

B. Facilities

1. The department or division of child neurology shall be part of the department of pediatrics and/or the department of neurology.
2. There must be adequate inpatient and outpatient facilities, examining areas, conference rooms, and research laboratories. There must be adequate space for offices for faculty members. Space for study, chart work, and dictation must be available for the residents. There must be adequate contemporary clinical laboratory facilities that report rapidly the results of necessary laboratory evaluations, including clinical-pathological, electrophysiological, imaging, and other studies needed by neurological services. Adequate chart and record-keeping systems must be in use for patient treatment.

C. Library

Residents must have access to an adequate medical library. Library services must include the electronic retrieval of information from medical databases. There must be access to an on-site library or to a collection of appropriate texts and journals in each institution participating in a residency program. On-site libraries, collections of texts and journals, and electronic retrieval of information from medical databases must be readily available during nights and weekends.

V. Educational Program

A. Basic Curriculum

1. Patient care, teaching, and research must be present in every training program. Patient care responsibilities must ensure a balance between patient care and education that achieves for the trainee an optimal educational experience consistent with the best medical care. Patient care responsibilities must include inpatient, outpatient, and consultation experiences.
2. In the program there must be a minimum of 12 months (full-time equivalent) of clinical child neurology with management responsibility for patient care. This must include at least 4 months (full-time equivalent) of outpatient experience in clinical child neurology. The outpatient experience also must include a resident longitudinal/continuity clinic with attendance by each resident at least ½ day weekly throughout the program. (The resident may be excused from this clinic when a rotation site is more than 1 hour travel time from the clinic site.)

B. Teaching Rounds

Clinical teaching rounds must be supervised and directed by the faculty of the child neurology department or division. They must occur at least 5 days per week. The resident in child neurology must present cases and their diagnostic and therapeutic plans.

C. Clinical Teaching

1. The resident must have instruction and practical experience in obtaining an orderly and detailed history from the patient, in conducting a thorough general and neurological examination, and in organizing and recording data. The training must include the indications for neurodiagnostic tests and their interpretation. The resident must learn to correlate the information derived from these neurodiagnostic studies with the clinical history and examination in formulating a differential diagnosis and management plan.
2. Residents must participate in the evaluation of and decision making for patients with disorders of the nervous system requiring surgical management. This experience must be part of the clinical child neurology experience. The existence of a neurosurgical service with close interaction with the neurology service is essential.
3. The residents must participate in the management of children and adolescents with psychiatric disorders. They must learn about the psychological aspects of the patient-physician relationship and the importance of personal, social, and cultural factors in disease processes and their clinical expression. Residents must become familiar with the principles of psychopathology, psychiatric diagnosis and therapy, and the indications for and complications of drugs used in psychiatry. This must be accomplished by at least a 1-month experience (full-time equivalent) under the supervision of a qualified child and adolescent psychiatrist.
4. Residents must learn the basic principles of rehabilitation for neurological disorders, including pediatric neurological disorders.
5. The resident must participate in the management of pediatric patients with acute neurological disorders in an intensive care unit and an emergency department.
6. The resident must receive instruction in the principles of bioethics and in the provision of appropriate and cost-effective evaluation and treatment for children with neurologic disorders.
7. The resident must receive instruction in appropriate and compassionate methods of terminal palliative care, including adequate pain relief, and psychosocial support and counseling for patients and family members about these issues.

D. Progressive Responsibility

Programs must provide opportunities for increasing responsibility and professional maturity of residents. Early clinical assignments must be based on direct patient responsibility for a limited number of patients. Subsequent assignments must place the resident in a position of taking increased responsibility for patients and in a liaison relationship with staff and referring physicians. Night call is essential in accomplishing this goal. Adequate faculty supervision is essential throughout the program. Neurological training must include assignment on a consultation service to the medical, surgical, and psychiatric services.

E. Basic and Related Science

Residents must learn the basic sciences on which clinical child neurology is founded, including neuroanatomy, neural and behavioral development, neuropathology, neurophysiology, neuroimaging, neuropsychology, neurochemistry, neuropharmacology, molecular biology, genetics, immunology, and epidemiology and statistics. Concentrated training in one or more of these areas, accomplished with a full-time equivalent experience of at least 2 months total, is required for each resident. Specific goals and objectives must be developed for this experience.

F. Electives

Resident assignments need not be identical for each resident. Elective time should accommodate individual resident interests and previous training. Elective time should be a minimum of 3 months.

G. Seminars and Conferences

1. Residents must regularly attend seminars and conferences in the following disciplines: neuropathology, clinical neurophysiology, neuroradiology, neuro-ophthalmology, cognitive development, neuromuscular disease, epilepsy, movement disorders, critical care, neuroimmunology, infectious disease, neuro-otology, neuroimaging, neurogenetics, neuro-oncology, pain management, and general and child neurology. There must be gross and microscopic pathology conferences and clinical pathological conferences. The resident must have increasing responsibility for the planning and supervision of the conferences.
2. The resident must learn about major developments in both the basic and clinical sciences relating to child neurology. Residents must attend periodic seminars, journal clubs, lectures, didactic courses, and meetings of local and national neurological societies.

H. Educational Policies

The program must provide for the following:

1. Residents must be allowed to spend an average of at least 1 full day out of 7 away from the hospital.
2. Residents must provide on-call duty in the hospital, but no more frequently than an average of every third night.
3. There must be adequate physician coverage if unexpected patient care needs create resident fatigue sufficient to jeopardize patient care during or following on-call periods.

I. Resident Participation in Research

Graduate medical education must take place in an environment of inquiry and scholarship in which residents participate in the development of new knowledge, learn to evaluate research findings, and develop habits of inquiry as a continuing professional responsibility. The responsibility for establishing and maintaining an environment of inquiry and scholarship rests with the teaching staff. While not all members of a teaching staff must be investigators, the staff as a whole must demonstrate broad involvement in scholarly activity, and child neurology training must be conducted in centers where there is active research activity both in clinical and basic neuroscience fields. This activity must include:

1. active participation of the teaching staff in clinical discussions, rounds, and conferences in a manner that promotes a spirit of inquiry and scholarship. Scholarship implies an in-depth understanding of basic mechanisms of normal and abnormal states and the application of current knowledge to practice.
2. participation in journal clubs and research conferences.
3. active participation in regional or national professional and scientific societies, particularly through presentations at the organizations' meetings and publication in their journals.
4. participation in research, particularly in projects that are funded following peer review and result in publications or presentations at regional and national scientific meetings.
5. offering of guidance and technical support (eg, research design, statistical analysis) for residents involved in research.
6. provision of support and encouragement for resident participation in scholarly activities.

J. Resident Responsibility for Teaching

Teaching of other residents, medical students, nurses, and other health care personnel, formally and informally, are required aspects of the resident's education in neurology.

VI. Evaluation

A. Resident Evaluation (See also Section III.A.2.)

The program must have an evaluation system that provides information about each resident's educational progress and the extent to which each resident has accomplished the program's learning and performance objectives.

1. Formative Evaluation
   a. Resident performance must be monitored and feedback provided on an ongoing basis.
   b. A written evaluation of the resident's attainment of objectives specific to the rotation must be made after each rotation and reviewed with the resident so that areas of weakness and strength can be communicated to the resident. This evaluation must incorporate evaluations obtained from faculty in the department of neurology during the resident's rotation on the adult clinical service and flexible year experiences, together with evaluations obtained from other faculty in the department or division of child neurology.
   c. The program director or his or her designee must meet with each resident semiannually in a formal feedback session to discuss the resident's standing in relation to specific learning and performance objectives. Plans to correct any deficiencies must be discussed. Each resident must be an active participant in formulating plans for his or her development. Evaluation data should be used to advise the resident and to make decisions regarding the progression in the resident's level of responsibility.
2. Final Evaluation
   At the conclusion of the resident's period of training in the program, the program director must prepare a detailed, written evaluation of the resident's performance in relation to the program's learning and performance objectives and discuss this evaluation with the resident.
3. Records
   a. A written record of the contents of the semiannual review session must be prepared and filed in the resident's permanent record. The written record of the evaluation and the review must be signed by the resident. The resident must have the opportunity to append a written response to the written record of the evaluation and review.
   b. Each resident's permanent record must include the written evaluations completed for each defined educational experience, the written records from the semiannual reviews, results of formal assessments, and the resident's final evaluation. Written descriptions of any deficiencies and problem areas, plans for correcting the deficiencies, disciplinary actions, and commendations, where appropriate, should be included.

B. Program Evaluation

The educational effectiveness of a program must be evaluated in a systematic manner. In particular, the quality of the curriculum and the extent to which the educational goals have been met by residents must be assessed. Written evaluations by residents must be utilized in this process.

1. Evaluations of residents' attainment of the program's learning and performance objectives must be used as the basis for program evaluation. Comparisons of these data against the program's own criteria, performance criteria set by the RRC, and attainment levels of residents at comparable levels of training should be performed as a primary means of assessing attainment of goals and objectives.
2. The residents must have an opportunity to evaluate the program in writing at least annually.

C. Board Certification

One measure of the quality of a training program is the proportion of its graduates who take the examinations of the ABPN and their performance on those examinations.

ACGME: February 1998 Effective: January 1999

Program Requirements for Residency Education in Clinical Neurophysiology (Neurology)

I. Introduction

A. Definition

Clinical neurophysiology is an area of medicine in which selected neurologic disorders involving central, peripheral, and autonomic nervous systems and muscles are assessed, monitored, and treated using a combination of clinical evaluation and electrophysiological testing. A derangement of the normal physiology of the nervous system underlies these selected disorders, and an assessment of the electrophysiological abnormalities is an integral part of the evaluation process.

Clinical neurophysiology requires a detailed knowledge of the normal physiology of the nervous system, the altered abnormal electrophysiology, and the disease states involved. Clinical neurophysiology is not confined to diagnostic techniques, but includes the application of electrical, magnetic, and mechanical methods to the evaluation and treatment of a wide range of diseases including the epilepsies, demyelinating disorders of the nervous system, stroke, Parkinson's disease and other movement disorders, sleep disorders, traumatic disorders, congenital and genetic disorders, intracranial mass lesions, and degenerative diseases. Another application of increasing importance is the use of intraoperative monitoring to guide surgical interventions.

B. Duration and Scope of Training

Training in neurophysiology shall encompass a total of 1 year, which must be preceded by the completion of a residency program in neurology, child neurology, general psychiatry, or physical medicine and rehabilitation accredited in the United States. The training must be separate and distinct from all training required for certification in neurology, child neurology, general psychiatry, or physical medicine and rehabilitation. The 1 year in clinical neurophysiology should be in a program that provides training in the broad area of clinical neurophysiology. The training should cover this broad area and include extensive experience in one or more of the following: evoked potential studies, motor and sensory nerve conduction studies, diagnostic electromyography, single fiber electromyography, electrodiagnostic movement disorder assessment, electroencephalography, testing of motor and sensory reflexes, polysomnography, and testing of autonomic function.

C. Objective

The objective of the total training outlined above is to provide the resident with the opportunity to develop the expertise necessary to evaluate and manage patients using the procedures and techniques of clinical neurophysiology.

D. Program Design

All educational components of a residency program should be related to program goals.

1. The program design and/or structure must be approved by the RRC for Neurology as part of the regular review process.
2. Participation by any institution providing 2 months or more of training in a program must be approved by the RRC.

II. Personnel

The director and teaching staff of a program must prepare and comply with written educational goals for the program. The program director and the teaching staff are responsible for the general administration of a program, including those activities related to the recruitment, selection, instruction, supervision, counseling, evaluation, and advancement of residents and the maintenance of records related to program accreditation.

A. Program Director

There must be a single program director responsible for the program.

1. Qualifications of the program director include:
   a. Requisite and documented clinical, educational, and administrative abilities and experience.
   b. Licensure to practice medicine in the state where the institution that sponsors the program is located. (Certain federal programs are exempted.)
   c. Certification by the American Board of Psychiatry and Neurology (ABPN) with Special Qualification in Clinical Neurophysiology or suitable equivalent qualifications, as determined by the RRC.
   d. Appointment in good standing to the medical staff of an institution participating in the program.
2. Responsibilities of the program director include:
   a. Devotion of sufficient time to provide leadership to the program and supervision of the residents in the program. (It is highly desirable that the director be a full-time faculty member.)
   b. Monitoring the content and ensuring the quality of the program.
   c. Preparation of a written statement outlining the educational goals of the program with respect to knowledge, skills, and other attributes of residents at each level of training and for each major rotation or other program assignment. This statement must be distributed to residents and members of the teaching staff. It should be readily available for review.
   d. Selection of residents for appointment to the program in accordance with institutional and departmental policies and procedures.
   e. Selection and supervision of the teaching staff and other program personnel at each institution participating in the program.
   f. The supervision of residents through explicit written descriptions of supervisory lines of responsibility for the care of patients. Such guidelines must be communicated to all members of the program staff. Residents must be provided with prompt, reliable systems for communication and interaction with supervisory physicians.

g. Regular evaluation of residents' knowledge, skills, and overall performance, including the development of professional attitudes consistent with being a physician.

The program director, with participation of members of the teaching staff, shall:

1. At least semiannually evaluate the knowledge, skills, and professional growth of the residents, using appropriate criteria and procedures.
2. Communicate each evaluation to the resident in a timely manner.
3. Advance residents to positions of higher responsibility only on the basis of evidence of their satisfactory progressive scholarship and professional growth.
4. Maintain a permanent record of evaluation for each resident and have it accessible to the resident and other authorized personnel.

h. The provision of a written final evaluation for each resident who completes the program. The evaluation must include a review of the resident's performance during the final period of training and should verify that the resident has demonstrated sufficient professional ability to practice competently and independently. This final evaluation should be part of the resident's permanent record maintained by the institution.

i. Implementation of fair procedures, as established by the sponsoring institution, regarding academic discipline and resident complaints or grievances.

j. Monitoring resident stress, including mental or emotional conditions inhibiting performance or learning and drug- or alcohol-related dysfunction. Program directors and teaching staff should be sensitive to the need for timely provision of confidential counseling and psychological support services to residents. Training situations that consistently produce undesirable stress on residents must be evaluated and modified.

k. Preparation of an accurate statistical and narrative description of the program, as requested by the RRC.

B. Teaching Staff

1. There must be a sufficient number of teaching staff with documented qualifications to instruct and supervise adequately all the residents in the program. Members of the teaching staff must be able to devote sufficient time to meet their supervisory and teaching responsibilities. The program providing training in clinical neurophysiology must have at least two faculty neurologists, including the director, who have completed training in this subspecialty. It is desirable that they be full-time members of the Department of Neurology.
2. Each of these members of the teaching staff should be certified by the ABPN with ABPN-added qualifications in clinical neurophysiology or possess suitable equivalent qualifications.
3. Expertise in the areas of electroencephalography, evoked potentials, nerve conduction studies, and electromyography must be represented among the director and the faculty. The RRC recognizes that expertise in clinical neurophysiology is available from physicians who are board certified in many medical specialties, particularly physical medicine and rehabilitation, anesthesia, internal medicine, and psychiatry, and actively encourages multidisciplinary cooperation in the training of residents.
4. The faculty shall devote sufficient time to the training program to ensure adequate clinical training of the resident in clinical neurophysiology and will be primarily involved in direction of the resident during the 1-year training.
5. All members of the teaching staff must demonstrate a strong interest in the education of residents, sound clinical and teaching abilities, support of the goals and objectives of the program, a commitment to their own continuing medical education, and participation in scholarly activities.
6. A member of the teaching staff of each participating institution must be designated to assume responsibility for the day-to-day activities of the program at that institution, with overall coordination by the program director.
7. The teaching staff must be organized and have regular documented meetings to review program goals and objectives as well as program effectiveness in achieving them. At least one resident representative should participate in these reviews.
8. The teaching staff should periodically evaluate the utilization of the resources available to the program, the contribution of each institution participating in the program, the financial and administrative support of the program, the volume and variety of patients available to the program for educational purposes, the performance of members of the teaching staff, and the quality of supervision of residents.

C. Other Teaching Staff

In addition, faculty with suitable training and experience from other disciplines may be included in the teaching program.

D. Other Program Personnel

Programs must be provided with the additional professional, technical, and clerical personnel needed to support the administration and educational conduct of the program.

E. Residents

Programs that fail to recruit any new residents for 2 consecutive years will be subject to adverse action.

III. Clinical and Educational Facilities and Resources

A. Facilities

The section of clinical neurophysiology shall be within the Department or Division of Neurology and have facilities adequate for the educational program.

B. Library

1. Residents must have ready access to a major medical library, either at the institution where the residents are located or through arrangement with convenient nearby institutions.
2. Library services should include the electronic retrieval of information from medical databases.
3. There must be access to an on-site library or to a collection of appropriate texts and journals in each institution participating in a residency program. On-site libraries and/or collections of texts and journals must be readily available during nights and weekends.

IV. Educational Programs

A. Curriculum

The training program is largely a clinical experience in which the resident develops and executes a plan of evaluation and treatment, including the appropriate technical skills to deal with patients with various neurological disorders.

B. Seminars and Conferences

The section of clinical neurophysiology shall conduct formal lectures and teaching conferences, including but not limited to electroencephalography, polysomnography, electromyography, nerve conduction studies, auditory evoked potentials, visual evoked potentials, somatosensory evoked potentials, motor evoked potentials, autonomic function studies, and monitoring of neural function during surgery. These must include clinical applications for and relevance to underlying disease. The clinical neurophysiology resident

Program Requirements

must participate actively on a weekly basis in the primary teaching conferences directed by the Department of Neurology in which the section resides. Participation in clinical conferences dealing with epilepsy and neuromuscular disorders is of particular importance. The resident in clinical neurophysiology must have the opportunity to develop competencies in these areas.

C. Teaching and Supervision

Supervisory faculty and staff must be available on a full-time basis. The resident in clinical neurophysiology should take an active role in the teaching and training of neurology residents in the Department of Neurology in which the section resides.

D. Clinical and Basic Science Teaching

1. Clinical Science

The resident must have instruction and practical experience to permit him or her to develop diagnostic, procedural, technical, and interventional skills essential to the performance of clinical neurophysiology. The clinical experience must include opportunities to observe, evaluate, and manage patients of all ages with a wide variety of disorders of the nervous system and muscles, as well as to learn the effectiveness of the procedures. It should provide for basic and advanced training and education, as well as professional development. Clinical experience must include inpatient care, outpatient care, and support services in the fields of pathology, radiology, and engineering. Examples of clinical problems that should be included in the experience of the resident for the development of knowledge and skills specific to clinical neurophysiology include but are not limited to epilepsy, neuromuscular diseases, trauma and its sequelae, congenital and developmental disorders, sleep disorders, infections, metabolic disorders, neoplasia, vascular disorders, and degenerative diseases. There should be experience in the development and execution of a plan of evaluation and treatment, including the appropriate technical skills to deal with patients with the above disorders. The opportunity should include experience in clinical diagnosis and accumulation/interpretation of laboratory data relevant to the above disorders as part of outpatient and hospitalized patient diagnostic evaluations. Additional, similar experience during intraoperative and paraoperative monitoring is desirable.

Experience should include training in each of the following:

a. Visual evoked potentials, auditory evoked potentials, somatosensory evoked potentials
b. Motor and sensory nerve conduction studies
c. Diagnostic electromyography and single fiber electromyography
d. Electrodiagnostic movement disorder assessment
e. Electroencephalography
f. Testing of motor and sensory reflexes
g. Testing of autonomic function
h. Polysomnography

The resident's experience should include independent studies of a sufficient number of patients to achieve competence in the assessment of patients with a wide range of clinical disorders.

2. Basic Science

Residents must be provided with an advanced and extensive background in those basic sciences on which clinical neurophysiology is founded. These include neurophysiology, neuroanatomy, neuropharmacology, and neuropathology. Didactic lectures and seminars in all or some of the basic sciences are necessary to provide an overall review and understanding of the field as it relates to clinical neurophysiology. A particularly good way for the resident to review the basic sciences is to participate in the teaching and laboratory supervision of the neuroscience courses that are offered in medical schools.

E. Resident/Patient Ratio

The number of patients must be adequate to provide a sound educational program. It is the program director's responsibility to ensure that the number of patients is appropriate. Patients must be diversified as to age, sex, short-term and long-term neurological problems, and inpatients and outpatients. The patients available to the resident must not interfere with the training of residents in the core neurology training program.

F. Faculty/Resident Ratio

In general, there should be enough faculty with diverse interests and skills to make the breadth of training appropriate to a program meeting these program requirements; to ensure adequate clinical experience for residents; and to provide continued interaction (eg, through seminars, conferences, clinical supervision) among residents and faculty.

G. Diagnostic Skills

Clinical assignments should include progressively increasing responsibility for patient care with direct supervision by the appropriate faculty member or staff. Adequate faculty supervision is essential throughout the program.

H. Subspecialty Experience

While a wide range of clinical experience is mandatory, each resident should have extensive experience in one or more areas of clinical neurophysiology. Clinical assignments need not be identical for each resident. Subspecialty experience should accommodate individual interests.

I. Resident Evaluation

Resident evaluation by staff should be made at regular intervals so that areas of weakness and strength can be communicated to the resident. Records shall be maintained documenting resident experience and performance. Periodic review of the resident's performance is essential for planning his or her subsequent educational program. The evaluation will include judging the fund of knowledge, basic clinical competence, general skills in the primary specialty, and specific technical skills required for clinical neurophysiology. The summary and final evaluation of the resident in clinical neurophysiology should be prepared by the program director of the clinical neurophysiology training program and should reflect the periodic evaluation of all the faculty. Each resident should be required to be proficient in the technical skills determined to be necessary for a clinical neurophysiologist and any related standards relevant to neurology. The educational effectiveness of a program must be evaluated in a systematic manner. In particular, the quality of the curriculum and the extent to which the educational goals have been met by residents must be assessed. Written evaluations by residents should be utilized in this process.

J. Resident Participation in Research

The responsibility for establishing and maintaining an environment of inquiry and scholarship rests with the teaching staff. While not all members of a teaching staff must be investigators, the staff as a whole must demonstrate broad involvement in scholarly activity, and clinical neurophysiology training must be conducted in centers where there is research in clinical neurophysiology. The program should include opportunities for the resident to participate in clinical and basic research projects relating to the field of clinical neurophysiology. This activity should include:

1. Active participation of the teaching staff in clinical discussions, rounds, and conferences in a manner that promotes a spirit of inquiry and scholarship. Scholarship implies an in-depth understanding of basic mechanisms of normal and abnormal states and the application of current knowledge to practice.
2. Participation in journal clubs and research conferences.

3. Active participation in regional or national professional and scientific societies, particularly through presentations at the organizations' meetings and publication in their journals.
4. Participation in research, particularly in projects that are funded following peer review and/or result in publication or presentations at regional and national scientific meetings.
5. Offering of guidance and technical support (eg, research design, statistical analysis) for residents involved in research.
6. Provision of support and encouragement for resident participation in scholarly activities.

K. Resident Responsibility

The resident's education in clinical neurophysiology is reinforced by teaching the discipline to other residents in neurology and other disciplines, medical students, nurses, and other health-care personnel. Residents must be given this opportunity.

L. Resident Duty Hours

To ensure an appropriate educational environment and prevent an excessive patient load, the program should provide for the following:

1. Residents should be allowed to spend an average of at least 1 full day out of 7 away from the hospital.
2. Residents should be assigned on-call duty in the hospital no more frequently than an average of every third night.
3. There should be adequate physician coverage if unexpected patient care needs create resident fatigue sufficient to jeopardize patient care during or following on-call periods.

V. Other

A. Relation to Core Program

The 1 year of training in clinical neurophysiology must take place in a center in which there is an accredited residency program in neurology and with the written approval and support of the director of the neurology program.

B. Use of Board Examinations

One measure of the quality of a training program is the proportion of its graduates who take the examination for added qualifications in clinical neurophysiology provided by the American Board of Psychiatry and Neurology, as well as their performance on those examinations.

C. Evaluation of the Program

The provisions of the Institutional Requirements for residency training of the Accreditation Council for Graduate Medical Education must also be met for approval of training in clinical neurophysiology.

ACGME: September 1994 Effective: September 1994

Program Requirements for Residency Education in Nuclear Medicine

I. Introduction

A. Definition and Scope of the Specialty

Nuclear medicine is the clinical and laboratory medical specialty that employs the measured nuclear properties of radioactive and stable nuclides for diagnosis, therapy, and research and to evaluate metabolic, physiologic, and pathologic conditions of the body.

B. Duration and Scope of Education

1. Length of program. The length of the nuclear medicine residency program is 2 years, following 1 year of preparatory clinical residency training (see below).
2. Admission prerequisites. The length of the nuclear medicine residency program is 2 years. However, a minimum of 3 years of graduate medical education is necessary to train a physician in the field of nuclear medicine. Before entering a nuclear medicine residency, residents must satisfactorily complete 1 year of training in an ACGME-accredited program that provides broad clinical education, with primary emphasis on the patient and the patient's clinical problems. Residents should have a sufficiently broad knowledge of medicine to obtain a pertinent history, perform an appropriate physical examination, and arrive at a differential diagnosis.
3. Specific description of program format. Residencies in nuclear medicine must teach the basic skills and clinical competence that constitute the foundations of nuclear medicine practice and must provide progressive responsibility for and experience in the application of these principles to the management of clinical problems. Clinical experience must include the opportunity to recommend and plan, conduct, supervise, interpret, and dictate reports for nuclear medicine procedures that are appropriate for the existing clinical problem or condition.

C. Broad Description of Training Objectives and Goals

The program must be structured so that the resident's clinical responsibilities increase progressively during training. At the completion of the training program, residents should be proficient in all areas of clinical nuclear medicine and be able to function independently as nuclear medicine consultants, plan and perform appropriate nuclear medicine procedures, interpret the test results, and formulate a diagnosis and an appropriate differential diagnosis. They should be qualified to recommend therapy or further studies. If radionuclide therapy is indicated, they should be capable of assuming responsibility for patient care. It is expected that residents will develop a satisfactory level of clinical maturity, judgment, and technical skill that will, on completion of the program, render them capable of the independent practice of nuclear medicine.

The director and teaching staff of a program shall prepare and comply with written educational goals for the program. All educational components of a residency program should be related to program goals. The program design and/or structure must be approved by the Residency Review Committee (RRC) for Nuclear Medicine as part of the regular review process and must be distributed to residents on commencement of their training.

II. Institutional Organization

Graduate medical education must take place in an environment of inquiry and scholarship in which residents participate in the development of new knowledge, learn to evaluate research findings, and develop habits of inquiry as a continuing professional responsibility.

A. Sponsoring Institution

A residency program in nuclear medicine must have a single sponsoring institution. The sponsoring institution must provide sufficient faculty, financial resources, and clinical, research, and library facilities to meet the educational needs of the residents and to enable the program to comply with the requirements for accreditation.

B. Participating Institutions

Limited outside rotations may be utilized to supplement training in a branch of nuclear medicine, eg, position emission tomography (PET) and radionuclide therapy, if there is insufficient patient volume in the sponsoring institution. When the resources of another institution are utilized, letters of affiliation must be approved by the institutional governing boards. Affiliated institutions should not be so distant as to make it difficult for residents to travel between institutions for participation in clinical responsibilities or didactic activities. Assignments at affiliated institutions must not be made primarily to meet service needs. A member of the teaching staff of each participating institution must be designated to assume responsibility for day-to-day activities of the program at that institution, with overall coordination by the program director.

Participation by any institution providing 3 months or more of training in the program must be approved by the RRC for Nuclear Medicine, according to criteria similar to those applied to the primary institution. A maximum of 6 months of the 2-year nuclear medicine program may be spent outside the parent institution and integrated institutions on rotation to affiliated sites. [*Note:* An affiliation may be said to exist where there is a formal agreement between an accredited program and another institution to make facilities, clinical experience, supervision, and teaching sessions available to residents of the program who will rotate through the affiliated hospital. Rotations to affiliates are restricted, as noted above.

An integrated relationship is one in which the program director (a) appoints the members of the teaching staff and makes recommendations for the appointment of the chief of service at the integrated institution, (b) determines all rotations and assignments at the integrated institution, and (c) is responsible for the overall conduct of the educational program in the integrated institution. The amount of time spent in integrated institutions is not restricted.]

C. Appointment of Residents

Programs must demonstrate the ability to recruit and retain qualified residents. Residents must be selected for appointment to the program in accordance with institutional and departmental policies and procedures. Residents should be appointed only when their documented prior experience and attitudes demonstrate the presence of abilities necessary to master successfully the clinical knowledge and skills required of all program graduates. All residents must have demonstrated understanding and facility in using the English language. Residents should be reappointed only when their clinical judgment, medical knowledge, history-taking, professional attitudes, moral and ethical behavior, and clinical performance are documented to be entirely satisfactory.

The total number of residents enrolled in the program must not exceed the faculty, patient, and facility resources available to support an appropriate educational program.

The RRC may withdraw accreditation from a program, regardless of its current accreditation status, if the program has been inactive for at least 2 years.

III. Faculty Qualifications and Responsibilities

A. Program Director

1. Qualifications of the Program Director
   There must be a single program director responsible for the program. The strength of the program is directly related to the professional competence and leadership qualities of the program director, whose term of appointment must be sufficient to ensure continuity for the program. The qualifications of the program director include
   a. documented clinical, educational, and administrative abilities and experience;
   b. certification by the American Board of Nuclear Medicine or equivalent credentials and experience acceptable to the RRC for Nuclear Medicine;
   c. broad knowledge of, experience with, and commitment to general nuclear medicine, along with sufficient academic and administrative experience to ensure effective implementation of these Program Requirements and sufficient experience participating as an active faculty member in an accredited residency program;
   d. compliance with professional standards of ethical behavior;
   e. a strong interest in the education of residents, sound clinical and teaching abilities, support of the goals and objectives of the program, a commitment to his or her own continuing medical education, and participation in scholarly activities; and
   f. appointment in good standing to the medical staff of an institution participating in the program and licensure to practice in the state where the sponsoring institution is located. (Certain federal programs are exempted.)

   A complete curriculum vitae of the program director shall be filed with the executive director of the RRC at the time of appointment and updated with each review of the program by the RRC.
2. Responsibilities of the Program Director
   The program director is responsible for the general administration of a program, including those activities related to the recruitment, selection, instruction, supervision, counseling, evaluation, and advancement of residents and the maintenance of records related to program accreditation.
   Specific responsibilities include
   a. preparation of a written statement outlining the educational goals of the program with respect to knowledge, skills, and other attributes of residents at each level of training and for each major rotation or other program assignment. This statement must be distributed to residents and members of the teaching staff. It should be readily available for review.
   b. selection of residents for appointment to the program in accordance with institutional and departmental policies and procedures.
   c. selection and supervision of the teaching staff and other program personnel at each institution participating in the program.
   d. supervision of residents through explicit written descriptions of supervisory lines of responsibility for the care of patients. Such guidelines must be communicated to all members of the program staff. Residents must be provided with prompt, reliable systems for communication and interaction with supervisory physicians. (See also Section V.C.1, "Resident Policies," on supervision of residents.)
   e. regular evaluation of residents' knowledge, skills, and overall performance, including the development of professional attitudes consistent with being a physician.
   f. implementation of fair personnel procedures, as established by the sponsoring institution, regarding academic discipline and resident complaints or grievances.

g. provision of notice to the RRC of any changes, as they occur, that might significantly alter the educational experience, such as a change in program director, key faculty members, institutional affiliation, or in the number of residency positions offered.
h. preparation of an accurate statistical and narrative description of the program, as requested by the RRC.

B. Faculty

1. Number of Faculty Required
The number of nuclear medicine faculty and the size of the technologist staff must be large enough to carry out the workload of the facility as well as the responsibilities of the teaching program. The ratio of faculty to residents shall be sufficient to ensure adequate clinical supervision of residents at all times and to provide teaching of the clinical and basic sciences.
2. Certification Requirements
The medical faculty who participate in the program must be certified by the American Board of Nuclear Medicine or possess equivalent credentials and/or experience acceptable to the RRC for Nuclear Medicine. Basic science faculty should possess equivalent qualifications in their fields of interest, including credentials or experience acceptable to the RRC for Nuclear Medicine.
3. Academic and Professional Qualifications
All members of the faculty must demonstrate a strong interest in the education of residents, sound clinical and teaching abilities, support of the goals and objectives of the program, and a commitment to their own continuing medical education. Faculty members should participate actively in the educational program and be willing to devote the necessary time and effort. The faculty must be able to nurture the attributes of the scholar, teacher, and humanist and must be available to residents for advice and counseling.
4. Scholarly Activities
While not all faculty members must be investigators, the faculty as a whole must demonstrate involvement in research or other scholarly activities, including
   a. participation in clinical discussions, rounds, and conferences in a manner that promotes a spirit of inquiry, scholarship, and learning;
   b. participation in journal clubs and research conferences;
   c. participation in research, particularly in projects that result in publication in scientific, peer-reviewed journals or recognized educational publications or in presentations at regional and national scientific meetings;
   d. participation in regional or national professional and scientific societies, particularly through presentations at meetings and publication in such societies' journals;
   e. offering of guidance and technical support such as research design and statistical analysis for residents involved in research or other scholarly activities.

The faculty as a whole must have demonstrated ongoing participation in such activities during the past 5 years.

The faculty must be organized and have regular, documented meetings to review program goals and objectives as well as program effectiveness in achieving them. At least one resident representative should participate in these reviews.

C. Other Program Personnel

Programs must be provided with the additional professional, technical, and clerical personnel needed to support the administration and educational conduct of the program.

IV. Facilities and Resources

A. Patient Population and Procedures

The institution sponsoring a residency program in nuclear medicine should be of sufficient size and composition to provide an adequate volume and variety of patients for resident training.

B. Space and Equipment

The program must provide adequate space, equipment, and other pertinent facilities to ensure an effective educational experience for residents in nuclear medicine and must possess the modern facilities and equipment required to practice nuclear medicine.

C. Other Specialties

A nuclear medicine residency program requires the support of services in other specialties, notably medicine, surgery, radiology, pediatrics, and pathology. Training resources should be such that the total number of residents in the institution is large enough to permit peer interaction and intellectual exchange with residents in the nuclear medicine program.

D. Library

Residents must have ready access to a major medical library with a representative selection of books and journals related to nuclear medicine, either at the institution where the residents are located or through arrangement with convenient nearby institutions. Library services should include the electronic retrieval of information from medical databases. There must be access to an on-site library or to a collection of appropriate texts and journals in each institution participating in a residency program. On-site libraries and/or collections of texts and journals must be readily available during nights and weekends.

V. Educational Program

A. Clinical Components

1. Curriculum Content
The residency program in nuclear medicine should include the diagnostic, therapeutic, and investigational uses of radionuclides. It should be of sufficient breadth to ensure that all residents become thoroughly acquainted with current nuclear medicine diagnostic and therapeutic applications. The training experience should ensure ample opportunity to attain sequentially increasing competence in selecting the most appropriate nuclear medicine studies for the patient, performing these studies in the technically correct manner, interpreting the information obtained, correlating this information with other diagnostic studies, and treating and following up the patient who receives radionuclide therapy. Under adequate faculty supervision, the resident should participate directly in the performance of imaging studies, nonimaging measurements and assays, and therapeutic procedures.

   Residents must be provided structured opportunities to (a) learn the indications, contraindications, complications, and limitations of specific procedures; (b) develop technical proficiency in performing these procedures; and (c) learn to interpret the results of these procedures. The program must provide adequate opportunity for residents to participate in and personally perform and analyze a broad range of common clinical nuclear medicine procedures. This must include experience in the following:
   a. Myocardial perfusion imaging procedures performed with radioactive perfusion agents in association with treadmill and pharmacologic stress (planar and tomographic). Specific applications should include patient monitoring, with special emphasis on electrocardiographic interpretation, cardiopulmonary resuscitation during interventional stress tests with radiopharmaceuticals or exercise, pharmacology of cardioactive

drugs, and hands-on experience for performance of the stress procedure (exercise or pharmacologic agents) for a minimum of 50 patients. Program directors must be able to document the experience of residents in this area.

b. Pulmonary perfusion and ventilation procedures performed with radiolabeled particles or macroaggregates and radioactive gas or aerosols.

c. Radionuclide ventriculography performed with ECG gating for evaluation of ventricular performance. The experience should include first pass and equilibrium studies and calculation of ventricular performance parameters, eg, ejection fraction and regional wall motion assessment.

d. Whole body imaging procedures for detection of musculoskeletal disease performed with radiolabeled bone tracers; cancer detection and staging performed with monoclonal antibodies, receptor binding radiolabeled agents, or radioactive gallium; and abscess and focal inflammatory disease detection performed with labeled leukocytes or radiogallium.

e. Genitourinary tract imaging, including renal perfusion and function procedures, clearance methods, renal scintigraphy with pharmacologic interventions and renal transplant evaluation, and scrotal and testicular imaging.

f. Therapeutic administration of radiopharmaceuticals, to include patient selection and understanding and calculation of the administered dose. Specific applications should include radioiodine in hyperthyroidism and thyroid carcinoma, and may include radiophosphorus (soluble) in polycythemia vera and other myeloproliferative disorders, radiocolloids for therapy, radionuclides for painful bone disease, and radioligand therapy. Program directors must be able to document the experience of residents in this area, for example, by resident logbooks.

g. Single-photon tomographic imaging procedures (SPECT) with a variety of radiopharmaceuticals and single and multihead tomographic imaging systems.

h. Where available, imaging procedures using positron-emitting radionuclides, medical cyclotron operation for production of PET radionuclides such as fluorine 18-labeled fluorodeoxyglucose (FDG), and PET radiochemistry synthesis.

In addition, each resident must be given the experience to participate in being on-call and assuming the responsibility for providing consultative activities for procedures performed on an emergency basis.

2. Patient Population Requirements

While the number of procedures may vary from one training program to another, a well-designed program will ensure resident involvement in at least 4,000 common nuclear medicine imaging procedures annually, a wide variety of nonimaging procedures to include in vivo kinetic and body composition procedures, and at least 15 radionuclide therapeutic procedures annually. Imaging procedures should be distributed over the entire spectrum of nuclear medicine practice, including the pediatric age group. An approximate minimum of 100 pediatric nuclear medicine cases should be available annually. Resident rotations to hospitals with a large pediatric caseload should be considered if the number of pediatric studies in the primary institution is fewer than 200 averaged over 2 years. The program director must be able to document the experience of residents in the performance of cardiovascular nuclear medicine procedures and therapeutic nuclear medicine procedures.

The program must provide the residents with experience in direct and progressively responsible patient management as they advance through training. This training must culminate in sufficient independent responsibility for clinical decision making to ensure that the graduating resident has achieved the ability to function independently and in a proficient manner in all nuclear medicine consultative areas.

B. Didactic Components

1. Basic Science Content

Study of the basic sciences that constitute the foundation for clinical nuclear medicine must be part of the resident's education. This is most effectively accomplished through a combination of formal didactic lectures and discussion of these topics in conferences. The program director must develop a formal didactic schedule that indicates the specific date and time of each lecture, the topic of the lecture, the faculty individual presenting the lecture, and the duration of the lecture. This schedule must incorporate each of the elements of basic science detailed below, and the program director must provide written documentation of this schedule as part of the information submitted to the RRC for its review of the program. The schedule must be current for each academic year. Visiting faculty and residents may provide some of the lectures.

The training program must provide didactic instruction in the following areas:

a. Physics: structure of matter, modes of radioactive decay, particle and photon emissions, and interactions of radiation with matter

b. Instrumentation: principles of instrumentation used in detection, measurement, and imaging of radioactivity with special emphasis on gamma cameras, including single photon and PET devices, and associated electronic instrumentation and computers employed in image production and display

c. Mathematics, statistics, and computer sciences: probability distributions; medical decision making; basic aspects of computer structure, function, programming, and processing; applications of mathematics to tracer kinetics; compartmental modeling; and quantification of physiologic processes

d. Radiation biology and protection: biological effects of ionizing radiation, means of reducing radiation exposure, calculation of the radiation dose, evaluation of radiation overexposure, medical management of persons overexposed to ionizing radiation, management and disposal of radioactive substances, and establishment of radiation safety programs in accordance with federal and state regulations

e. Radiopharmaceuticals: reactor, cyclotron, and generator production of radionuclides; radiochemistry; pharmacokinetics; and formulation of radiopharmaceuticals

An aggregate of at least 200 hours should be devoted to basic science instruction, ie, formal lectures and formal labs, over the 2-year training period, with an appropriate balance of time allocated to the major subject areas, which must include physical science and instrumentation, 100 hours; radiobiology and radiation protection, 30 hours; mathematics, 20 hours; radiopharmaceutical chemistry, 30 hours; and computer science, 20 hours. Instruction in the basic sciences should not be limited to only didactic sessions. The resident's activities also should include laboratory experience and regular contact with basic scientists in their clinical adjunctive roles.

2. Didactic Clinical Content

There must be didactic instruction in both diagnostic imaging and nonimaging nuclear medicine applications and therapeutic applications. The instruction must be well organized, thoughtfully integrated, and carried out on a regularly scheduled basis. The program director must develop a formal didactic schedule that indicates the specific date and time of each lecture, the topic of the lecture, the faculty individual presenting the lecture, and the duration of the lecture. This schedule must incorporate each of the elements of the clinical specialty detailed below, and the program director must provide written documentation of this schedule to the RRC for its review of the program. Visiting faculty and residents may provide some of the lectures. The schedule must be current for each academic year.

Instruction must include the following areas:

a. Diagnostic use of radiopharmaceuticals: clinical indications, technical performance, and interpretation of in vivo imaging of the body organs and systems, using external detectors and scintillation cameras, including single photon tomography and PET
b. Exercise and pharmacologic stress testing: to include the pharmacology of cardioactive drugs; physiologic gating techniques; patient monitoring during interventional procedures; management of cardiac emergencies, including electrocardiographic interpretation and cardiopulmonary life support; and correlation of nuclear medicine procedures with other pertinent imaging modalities such as angiography, computed tomography, bone density measurement, ultrasonography, and magnetic resonance imaging.
c. Nonimaging studies: training and experience in the application of a variety of nonimaging procedures, including instruction in the principles of immunology; radioimmunoassay and receptor assay technology; preparation of radiolabeled antibodies; radiopharmaceutical absorption, excretion, and dilution studies; cellular kinetics; measurement of organ function; and body composition studies
d. Therapeutic uses of unsealed radiopharmaceuticals: patient selection and management, including dose administration and dosimetry, radiation toxicity, and radiation protection considerations in the treatment of metastatic cancer and bone pain, primary neoplasms, solid tumors, and malignant effusions; and the treatment of hematologic, endocrine, and metabolic disorders
e. Quality management and improvement: principles of quality management and performance improvement, efficacy assessment, and compliance with other regulations of the Nuclear Regulatory Commission and the Joint Commission on the Accreditation of Healthcare Organizations

3. Conferences and Seminars

All residents must participate in regularly scheduled clinical nuclear medicine conferences and seminars and interdisciplinary conferences, in which the resident is responsible for presenting case materials and discussing the relevant theoretical and practical issues. There should be active resident participation in well-structured seminars and journal clubs that review the pertinent literature with respect to current clinical problems and that include discussion of additional topics to supplement the didactic curriculum.

a. Clinical interpretation conference

All residents must participate in regularly scheduled, usually daily, procedure interpretation and review conferences. The program must provide the resident with the opportunity to gain progressively independent responsibility for review, technical approval and acceptance, and interpretation and dictation of consultative reports on completed nuclear medicine procedures.

b. Teaching files

Teaching case files involving diagnostic and therapeutic nuclear medicine procedures should cover the full spectrum of clinical applications; they should be indexed, coded with correlative and follow-up data, and readily accessible for resident use. There must be a mechanism for maintaining case records and treatment results to facilitate patient follow-up and to provide teaching material.

Electronic availability of teaching files is acceptable as an enhancement of on-site teaching case files.

C. Resident Policies

1. Supervision

All patient care services provided by residents must be supervised by appropriately qualified faculty. The program director must ensure, direct, and document proper supervision of residents at all times. Residents must be provided with rapid, reliable systems for communicating with supervising residents and attendings. Attending physicians or supervising residents with appropriate experience for the severity and complexity of the procedure and the patient's condition must be present at all times for the procedure. The resident must review with a nuclear medicine faculty member all patient studies that the resident has dictated.

2. Duty Hours and Work Conditions

The practice of nuclear medicine requires 24-hour physician availability. Duty hours and night and weekend call for residents must reflect the concept of responsibility for patients and must provide for adequate patient care. Residents must not be required to regularly perform unduly prolonged duties. However, in no case should the resident go off duty until the proper care and welfare of the patient have been ensured. All residents should have the opportunity to spend an average of at least 1 full day out of 7 free of hospital duties and should be assigned on-call duty in the hospital no more frequently than, on average, every third night. It is the responsibility of the program director to ensure assignment of reasonable in-hospital and on-call duty hours.

Resident stress, including mental or emotional conditions inhibiting performance or learning and drug- or alcohol-related dysfunction, should be monitored. Program directors and teaching faculty should be sensitive to the need for timely provision of confidential counseling and psychological support services to residents. Training situations that consistently produce undesirable stress on residents must be evaluated and modified.

3. Other

The residents also must be provided basic life-support training, and advanced cardiac life-support training is recommended.

D. Scholarly Activity

Graduate medical education must take place in an environment of inquiry and scholarship in which residents participate in the development of new knowledge, learn to evaluate research findings, and develop habits of inquiry as a continuing professional responsibility. The responsibility for establishing and maintaining an environment of inquiry and scholarship rests with the teaching staff. The resident must demonstrate broad involvement in research and scholarly activity. This activity may include

a. active participation in regional or national professional and scientific societies, through presentations at the organizations' meetings and publication in their journals.
b. participation in research, particularly in projects that are funded following peer review and/or result in publications or presentations at regional and national scientific meetings.

VI. Evaluation

A. Resident Evaluation

Resident evaluation should be carried out at least every 6 months and should concern itself with intellectual abilities, technical skills, attitudes, and interpersonal relationships. Observation of the resident performing specific tasks such as image interpretation, taking a history and performing a physical examination, choosing diagnostic studies, formulating patient management, and communicating effectively should be included. There must be provision for appropriate and timely feedback of the content of these evaluations to the resident. Residents should be advanced to positions of higher responsibility only on the basis of evidence of their satisfactory progressive scholarship and professional growth. The program must maintain a permanent record of the evaluation and counseling process for each resident. Such records must be accessible to the resident and other authorized personnel.

The program director must provide a written final evaluation for each resident who completes the program. The evaluation must include a review of the resident's performance during the final period of training and should verify that the resident has demonstrated sufficient professional ability to practice competently and independently. This final evaluation should be part of the resident's permanent record maintained by the institution.

B. Program Evaluation

The educational effectiveness of a program must be evaluated in a systematic manner. In particular, the quality of the curriculum and the extent to which the educational goals have been met by the program must be assessed. Written evaluations by residents must be utilized in this process. Residents should be given the opportunity to provide confidential written evaluations of the faculty and program at least annually. The teaching staff also should evaluate periodically the utilization of the resources available to the program, the contribution of each institution participating in the program, the financial and administrative support of the program, the volume and variety of patients available to the program for educational purposes, the performance of members of the teaching staff, and the quality of supervision of residents.

VII. Board Certification

Residents who plan to seek certification by the American Board of Nuclear Medicine should communicate with the office of that board regarding the requirements for certification.

ACGME: February 1998 Effective: January 1999

Program Requirements for Residency Education in Obstetrics and Gynecology

I. Introduction

A. Program Goals

A residency program in obstetrics-gynecology must constitute a structured educational experience, planned in continuity with undergraduate and continuing medical education, in the health care area encompassed by this specialty. While such residency programs contain a patient-service component, they must be designed to provide education as a first priority and not function primarily to provide hospital service.

An educational program in obstetrics-gynecology must provide an opportunity for resident physicians to achieve the knowledge, skills, and attitudes essential to the practice of obstetrics and gynecology and must also be geared toward the development of competence in the provision of ambulatory primary health care for women. The program must provide opportunity for increasing responsibility, appropriate supervision, formal instruction, critical evaluation, and counseling for the resident.

B. Program Design

All educational components of a residency program should be related to program goals.

1. The program design and/or structure must be approved by the Residency Review Committee (RRC) for Obstetrics-Gynecology as part of the regular review process.
2. Participation by any institution providing 6 months or more of training in a program of 3 or more years must be approved by the RRC.

II. Institutional Organization

A. Administration

The administration of the sponsoring institution must demonstrate a commitment to educational and scholarly activities by meeting all provisions of the Institutional Requirements of the *Essentials for Accredited Residencies in Graduate Medical Education* for approval of a residency program.

B. Participating Institutions

The RRC for Obstetrics-Gynecology uses the following categories for the purpose of monitoring the structure of residencies. In all cases, where more than one institution is involved, a formal written agreement must be developed between the responsible administrative bodies of those institutions.

1. Independent—An independent program is conducted within a single educational institution under a single program director. Extramural rotations for a total of no more than 6 months are permitted under the regulations applied to all programs (see II.B.3).
2. Integrated—An integrated program is conducted within multiple educational institutions but under a single program director. Each educational institution involved in an integrated program must provide the same quality of education and level of supervision required of an independent program and must formally acknowledge the authority of the program director and the role that the institution will play in the overall program. Residents may rotate at any level, including the final year of the program. The program director must have authority over the educational program in each hospital, including the teaching appointments and assignments of all faculty and all residents, and must ensure the adequacy of the educational experience for each resident. Ad-

ditional extramural rotations for a total of no more than 6 months are permitted under the regulations applied to all programs (see II.B.3). If a program includes rotations for a total of more than 6 months for any resident at institutions other than those included in the integrated program, that program becomes an affiliated program.

3. Affiliated—An affiliated program is one in which any resident spends a total of more than 6 months in extramural rotations outside the parent institution (or institutions, in the case of integrated programs).

   Extramural rotations may be arranged by the program director of either an independent or an integrated program to enhance the educational experience of the residents. Only under exceptional circumstances, and with prior written approval of the RRC, may they be included in the final senior resident year. Residents are appointed by their parent program and assigned by it to the affiliated hospitals, where they spend no more than 18 months in obstetrics-gynecology and primary care educational experiences. Two types of extramural rotations may be considered:

   a. If the total time of extramural rotation from the parent program by any resident during the entire residency exceeds 6 months, the program is considered to be an affiliated program, and the entire program must receive prior approval by the RRC.
   b. Rotations for a total of less than 6 months will not require that the program be designated as an affiliated program, and these rotations may be arranged by the program director without prior RRC approval.

C. Resident Numbers

1. The number of residents that can be adequately and responsibly educated depends on several interrelated factors. Clinical involvement alone does not constitute an educational experience. The provision of adequate supervision, education, individual evaluation, and administrative support is critical. With this, it is of utmost importance that each resident have sufficient independent operative and clinical responsibilities to prepare for practice in the specialty.
2. The maximum number of residents in a program is linked to the number that can be accommodated within the framework of these requirements. One of the most important considerations is the clinical experience available to give each resident adequate primary responsibility. Because this usually centers on the senior resident year, the maximum number of residents in a program depends on how many senior residents the program can educate. Usually the maximum number of residents in a program is the number of senior residents the program can accommodate multiplied by three or four, depending on the length of the program.
3. The minimum number of residents in an accreditable program is two per year. Accreditation is granted on the basis of a balance between the educational resources and the number of residents in the program. Appointment of residents in excess of the approved number may adversely affect the quality of the total experience of each resident. Therefore, changes in the educational resources should be reported to the RRC, and proposed increases in the number of residents must first be approved in writing by the RRC.
4. All requests for a change in the number of residents must demonstrate a distinct and substantial improvement in the educational opportunities for all residents in the program. Such requests must be based not only on the availability of an adequate patient population but also on adequate resources for supervision, education, and evaluation. A request for a change in the number of residents must describe the predicted impact on the total experience of each of the senior residents under the new circumstances. The request will be considered incomplete if it lists only expansion in beds, hospitals, or overall clinical experience and does not address the question of the expansion of faculty and administrative support necessary to teach, supervise, and evaluate the additional residents. Conversely, a reduction in beds or hospitals, or other changes in the program that may lead to an anticipated decrease in total experience for the residents, must be promptly called to the attention of the RRC to determine if a reduction in the number of resident positions in a given graduate medical program is necessary.

III. Faculty Qualifications and Responsibilities

The director and teaching staff of a program must prepare and comply with written educational goals for the program. The program director and the teaching staff are responsible for the general administration of a program, including those activities related to the recruitment, selection, instruction, supervision, counseling, evaluation, and advancement of residents and the maintenance of records related to program accreditation.

A. Program Director

There must be a single program director responsible for the program.

1. Qualifications of the program director
   a. The program director must be qualified and experienced as a clinician, administrator, and educator in obstetrics and gynecology and must have experience in and commitment to ambulatory primary health care for women. There must be a minimum of 5 years' experience (postresidency/fellowship) in such activities. The program director must be certified by the American Board of Obstetrics and Gynecology or must possess suitable equivalent qualifications.
   b. The program director must have licensure to practice medicine in the state where the institution that sponsors the program is located. (Certain federal programs are exempted.)
   c. The program director must have appointment in good standing to the medical staff of an institution participating in the program.
2. Responsibilities of the program director
   a. The program director must devote sufficient time and effort to the program to provide day-to-day continuity of leadership and to fulfill all of the responsibilities inherent in meeting the educational goals of the program.
   b. The program director must function within a sound administrative organizational framework and have an effective teaching staff as essential elements of an approved residency program. Continuity of leadership over a period of years is important to the stability of a residency program. Frequent changes in leadership or long periods of temporary leadership usually have an adverse effect on an educational program.
   c. The program director should demonstrate active involvement in (1) clinical practice, (2) continuing obstetrics/gynecology education, (3) regional or national scientific societies, (4) presentations and publications, and (5) scholarly activities.
   d. The program director must have appropriate authority to oversee and to organize the activities of the educational program. The responsibilities of this position should include but not be limited to the following:
      1. Resident appointments and assignments;
      2. Supervision, direction, and administration of the educational activities; and
      3. Evaluation of the house staff, faculty, and residency program.
   e. The program director must provide a clearly defined assignment of responsibilities for resident education, including

preparation of a written statement outlining the educational goals of the program with respect to knowledge, skills, and other attributes of residents at each level of training and for each major rotation or other program assignment. This statement must be distributed to residents and members of the teaching staff. It should be readily available for review.

f. The program director must provide for the selection of residents for appointment to the program in accordance with institutional and departmental policies and procedures.

g. The program director must provide for the selection and supervision of the teaching staff and other program personnel at each institution participating in the program.

h. The program director must provide for the supervision of residents through explicit written descriptions of supervisory lines of responsibility for the care of patients. Such guidelines must be communicated to all members of the program staff. Residents must be provided with prompt, reliable systems for communication and interaction with supervisory physicians.

i. The program director must provide for the regular evaluation of residents' knowledge, skills, and overall performance, including the development of professional attitudes consistent with being a physician.

The program director, with participation of members of the teaching staff, shall

1. at least semiannually evaluate the knowledge, skills, and professional growth of the residents, using appropriate criteria and procedures.
2. communicate each evaluation to the resident in a timely manner.
3. advance residents to positions of higher responsibility only on the basis of evidence of their satisfactory progressive scholarship and professional growth.
4. maintain a permanent record of evaluation for each resident and have it accessible to the resident and other authorized personnel.

j. The program director must verify that residents have satisfactorily completed the program and provide a written final evaluation for each resident who completes the program. The evaluation must include a review of the resident's performance during the final period of training and should verify that the resident has demonstrated sufficient professional ability to practice competently and independently. This final evaluation should be part of the resident's permanent record maintained by the institution.

k. The program director must provide for implementation of fair procedures as established by the sponsoring institution regarding academic discipline and resident complaints or grievances.

l. The program director must provide for monitoring resident stress, including mental or emotional conditions inhibiting performance or learning and drug- or alcohol-related dysfunction. Program directors and teaching staff should be sensitive to the need for timely provision of confidential counseling and psychological support services to residents. Training situations that consistently produce undesirable stress on residents must be evaluated and modified.

m. The program leadership is responsible for notifying the executive secretary of the RRC, in writing, within 30 days of any major change in the program that may significantly alter the educational experience for the residents, including

1. changes in leadership of the department or the program;
2. changes in administrative structure, such as an alteration in the hierarchical status of the program/department within the institution; and
3. substantial changes in volume and/or variety of the patient population.

n. The program director is responsible for communicating to the RRC any change in the use of rotations to participating institutions (including additions or deletions of institutions) and any significant change in the number of patient cases available at the sponsoring and/or participating institutions, if residency education would be adversely affected. The program director must describe the effect of these changes and the corrective action taken to address them.

o. The program director must obtain prior approval for the following changes in the program so the RRC may determine if an adequate educational environment exists to support these changes:

1. The addition or deletion of any participating institution to which residents rotate for 6 months or longer
2. The addition or deletion of any rotation of 6 months or longer
3. Any change in the approved resident complement of the program
4. Any change in the length or major change in the educational format of the program

On review of a proposal for a major change in a program, the RRC may determine that a site visit is necessary.

B. Faculty

1. An obstetrics-gynecology education program must have a sufficient and appropriate number of attending staff with professional ability, enthusiasm, dedication, and a sense of responsibility for teaching residents. Members of the teaching staff must be able to devote sufficient time to meet their supervisory and teaching responsibilities. It would be well for the staff to regard these attributes as a prerequisite to active faculty membership and promotion. The faculty complement should include appropriately educated generalist faculty. The quality of teaching and supervision by the faculty must be reviewed at least annually by the program director and through written feedback provided to individual faculty members. When deficiencies occur, corrective action should be undertaken. Regular and protected input into this evaluation by the residents must be an integral component of such reviews.
2. All members of the teaching staff must demonstrate a strong interest in the education of residents, sound clinical and teaching abilities, support of the goals and objectives of the program, a commitment to their own continuing medical education, and participation in scholarly activities.
3. A member of the teaching staff of each participating institution must be designated to assume responsibility for the day-to-day activities of the program at that institution, with overall coordination by the program director.
4. The teaching staff must be organized and have regular documented meetings to review program goals and objectives as well as program effectiveness in achieving them. At least one resident representative should participate in these reviews.
5. The teaching staff should periodically evaluate the utilization of the resources available to the program, the contribution of each institution participating in the program, the financial and administrative support of the program, the volume and variety of patients available to the program for educational purposes, the performance of members of the teaching staff, and the quality of supervision of residents.

C. Other Program Personnel

Programs must be provided with the additional professional, technical, and clerical personnel needed to support the administration and educational conduct of the program.

IV. Facilities and Resources

A. Outpatient Facilities

Appropriate facilities and equipment including patient medical and laboratory data retrieval capabilities to manage patients in a timely fashion must be provided so that efficient and effective education in the ambulatory care aspects of the discipline can be accomplished.

B. Inpatient Facilities

Appropriate facilities and equipment including patient medical and laboratory data retrieval capabilities must be provided to achieve the educational objectives, including the management of critically ill patients and those undergoing obstetric or gynecologic operative procedures.

C. Medical Records

The fundamentals of good medical history taking and thoughtful, meticulous physical examination must be taught. Information gained by these procedures must be carefully recorded in the medical record. A reliable measure of the quality of a program is the quality of hospital records. These records should include daily appropriate progress notes by residents, together with a discharge summary. The hospital should maintain a records room with adequate cross indexing and ready reference for study of patients' charts. Periodic summaries of department statistics are essential for the evaluation of results and usually will be requested at the time a program is reviewed by the RRC.

D. Medical Library

The medical library is an important resource to the obstetrics-gynecology education program. The library may be sponsored by the hospital or the department, but it must be readily accessible to staff and residents, both during the day and in the evening, including weekends. In addition, there must be access to an on-site library or to a collection of appropriate texts and journals in each institution participating in the residency program. The textbooks should be kept up-to-date, and there should be an ample supply of current journals devoted to obstetrics-gynecology and related subjects. When a comprehensive library is not available in the hospital, an active reference system should be provided through ready access to larger medical libraries. Programs must provide instruction in retrieval and assessment of medical literature, and library services should include the electronic retrieval of information from medical databases.

E. Resident Facilities and Support Services

Adequate facilities for residents to carry out their patient care and personal educational responsibilities are required. These include adequate on-call, lounge, and food facilities for residents while on duty and on call. Also required are clinical support services such as pathology and radiology, including laboratory and radiologic information retrieval systems that allow rapid access to results, intravenous (IV) services, phlebotomy services, and messenger/transporter services in sufficient number to meet reasonable demands at all times.

F. Other Graduate Medical Education Programs

The program must exist in an educational environment that includes at least two other relevant graduate medical education programs such as internal medicine, pediatrics, surgery, or family practice. The program director must obtain teaching commitments from the other departments involved in the education of obstetrics-gynecology residents.

V. The Educational Program

A. General

1. Organization and Structure
   a. Resident education in obstetrics-gynecology must include 4 years of accredited, clinically oriented graduate medical education, of which 3 years must be focused on reproductive health care and ambulatory primary health care for women, including health maintenance, disease prevention, diagnosis, treatment, consultation, and referral. Residency programs may, with prior RRC approval, contain more residents in the first year than the number approved for subsequent years or may have no residents in the first year.
   b. The RRC has the responsibility for the review of all graduate medical education programs in obstetrics-gynecology seeking accreditation. If a program includes sponsorship of a first-graduate-year experience, then the RRC has the responsibility for review of that first graduate year.
   c. A program director, under suitable circumstances, may elect to credit a resident with a period of graduate education in obstetrics and gynecology gained by the resident before entering the program. The period of education must have been of 4 or more months in duration and must have been received in a hospital conducting a currently accredited residency in obstetrics-gynecology. This period may then be used to provide time, within the 36 months of obstetrics-gynecology, for appropriate electives on other clinical services. It may not be used to shorten the total length of the residency program.
   d. The majority of residents are preparing for a practice that provides reproductive health care and ambulatory primary and preventive health care for women, and residency programs may vary as to when and how these requirements are met. The ambulatory primary care component of residency, with the exception of the continuity clinics, may be obtained in an approved family medicine or internal medicine graduate medical education program prior to entering an obstetrics and gynecology residency.
   e. Growth in knowledge and experience in the primary and preventive care role is best provided to residents by maximizing their participation in an ambulatory environment designed to enable continuity of care over an extended period of time. It is required that continuity clinics be provided and be attended by residents throughout 3 years of the residency.
   f. Specific educational experiences for the primary and preventive care role should occupy the equivalent of at least 6 months of the 4 years of residency and may be addressed in any of the 4 years of residency. The emphasis should be on ambulatory care of the patient, which requires both knowledge and skills in the areas of health maintenance, disease prevention, risk assessment, counseling, and the use of consultants and community resources. These experiences should be evident in the residents' exposure to continuity of care, general gynecology, general obstetrics, prevention or control of disease (eg, sexually transmitted disease), substance abuse, or prevention of pregnancy. In addition to rotations in obstetrics-gynecology, general medical management experience should also be obtained during rotations in internal medicine and/or family practice, emergency medicine, and geriatric medicine. The individual's role and experience in these rotations should be equivalent to those of residents on these services and relevant to the health care of women. Experiences should be strongly oriented toward ambulatory care and must include at a mini-

mum a 4-month rotation in general medicine or family practice medicine and a 1-month rotation in emergency medicine. In addition, residents must have a structured experience in geriatric medicine that is the equivalent of at least 1 month of a block rotation.

g. The patient population on which the educational program is based should be sufficient in size and composition so that the broad spectrum of experiences necessary to meet the educational objectives will be provided.

h. The ambulatory care experiences of residents preparing for their roles as providers of primary and preventive care require the same attention, supervision, and guidance as those experiences in specialty clinics. It is essential to provide a closely supervised experience by appropriately educated generalist faculty that assures patients of continuity of care by an individual resident. Increasing responsibility should be given to the resident under the supervision of a qualified, on-site, attending staff/faculty member. Residents should develop and maintain a continuing physician-patient relationship with a panel of patients, at least ½ day per week, throughout at least 3 of the 4 years of education. The use of remote sites or institutions or clinical services must not interrupt continuity of care clinics for longer than 2 months each year. Residents should be provided opportunity on at least a weekly basis to return to the parent institution for their continuity clinic experience. Alternatively, if the geographic proximity of the remote site or institution permits, the continuity clinic experience may take place at that location.

2. Content of Curriculum

a. The resident's ability to personally evaluate a patient's complaint, provide an accurate examination, employ appropriate diagnostic tests, arrive at a correct diagnosis, and recommend the appropriate treatment is of paramount importance.

b. Formal teaching activities in obstetrics-gynecology should be structured and regularly scheduled. They generally should consist of patient rounds, case conferences, journal clubs, and coverage of appropriate basic sciences pertinent to the specialty. In cross-disciplinary conferences such as perinatology, physicians from appropriate specialties should be invited to participate.

c. Wise judgment regarding the need for a surgical procedure and recognition and management of complications are as important as the technical aspects of residency education. The program must, therefore, ensure that residents' clinical experience emphasizes appropriate involvement in the process that leads to selection of the surgical option, the preoperative assessment, and the postoperative care of the patients for whom they share surgical responsibility. Continuity of care of these patients must be documented. A residency program in obstetrics-gynecology must be able to provide substantial, diverse, and appropriate surgical experience after residents have mastered the basic skills.

d. The program must provide a structured didactic and clinical educational experience in all methods of family planning. Topics must include all reversible methods of contraception, including natural methods, as well as sterilization. This must include experience in management of complications as well as training in the performance of these procedures. This education can be provided outside the institution, in an appropriate facility, under the supervision of appropriately educated faculty.

e. No program or resident with a religious or moral objection shall be required to provide training in or to perform induced abortions. Otherwise, access to experience with induced abortion must be part of residency education. This education can be provided outside the institution. Experience with management of complications of abortion must be provided to all residents. If a residency program has a religious, moral, or legal restriction that prohibits the residents from performing abortions within the institution, the program must ensure that the residents receive satisfactory education and experience in managing the complications of abortion. Furthermore, such residency programs (1) must not impede residents in the programs who do not have religious or moral objections from receiving education and experience in performing abortions at another institution and (2) must publicize such policy to all applicants to those residency programs.

f. Because an increasing percentage of women seeking their medical care from obstetrician-gynecologists are postmenopausal, there must be appropriate didactic instruction and sufficient clinical experience in the management of the problems of women in the postreproductive age.

3. Educational Objectives

a. To be accredited, every program must have a written statement of the educational objectives for the residents in that program, and a list of those objectives must be given to each resident. One example of such objectives is set forth in the current "Educational Objectives for Residents in Obstetrics and Gynecology," produced under the auspices of the Council on Residency Education in Obstetrics and Gynecology (CREOG). Directors of programs must be able to document that they are reviewing the implementation of the educational objectives and that the residents are indeed accomplishing what is anticipated of them. Any program that does not establish a system that clearly demonstrates that each resident has or has not successfully accomplished each of the items indicated in the program's statement of educational aims and objectives cannot be considered an adequate program.

b. It is neither essential nor desirable that all educational programs or individual resident experiences be identical in structure or function. Variations that provide creative solutions and opportunities or allow greater efficiency in the educational program may be implemented with the prior written approval of the RRC. It is, however, mandatory that each residency program provide quality education and experience for each of the residents completing the program.

4. Patient Responsibility/Supervision

a. Supervision of residents in obstetrics and gynecology is required to ensure proper (1) education, (2) quality of care, (3) patient safety, and (4) fulfillment of responsibility of the attending physicians to their patients. These considerations must be integrated with the goal of independent competence in the full range of obstetrics and gynecology at the completion of residency. This implies a graduated and increasing level of independent resident action. Each program director must balance quality assurance for patient care, resident education, and independent resident action. The level of resident supervision should be commensurate with the amount of independent function that is designated at each resident level. Residents, as well as faculty, may provide supervision.

b. On an obstetrics and gynecology service, adequate supervision requires the 24-hour presence of faculty in the hospital except when residents are not assigned in-house call responsibilities. Faculty must be immediately available to the resident if clinical activity is taking place in the operating rooms and/or labor and delivery areas. Faculty must be within easy walking distance of patient care units. Clinical services provided in ambulatory (office) locations require on-site supervision. Open and generously used lines of two-way communication are important and should be encouraged.

c. If the program director judges that the size and nature of the patient population does not require the 24-hour presence of residents and faculty, this situation must be carefully defined and reviewed and should include information about the nature of the hospital, the patient population, the nature of attending staff, and the geographic and climatic situations. Exceptions require prior written approval from the RRC.

d. Supervision of residents is a responsibility of the program director and teaching staff. It is the responsibility of the institution sponsoring a residency program to establish oversight to ensure that programs meet the supervisory provisions of these Program Requirements.

5. Graded Responsibility

Complete management of a patient's care under adequate supervision should be considered the highest level of residency education. There are, however, circumstances under which the resident may not assume complete management:

a. When the program director or his/her designee does not believe the resident's expertise or understanding is adequate to ensure the best care of the patient

b. When the attending physician is unable to delegate the necessary degree of responsibility

c. When the resident, for religious or moral reasons, does not wish to participate in proposed procedures

An essential feature of resident education is that a significant number of staff support the principle of delegation of complete management under supervision.

Increasing responsibility must progress in an orderly fashion, culminating in a senior resident year. The senior resident year consists of 12 months of clinical experience in the last year of the resident's program. Elective time in the senior resident year requires the prior approval of the RRC. The senior resident must have sufficient independent operating experience to become technically competent and have enough total responsibility for management of patients to ensure proficiency in the diagnostic and treatment skills that are required of a specialist in obstetrics-gynecology in office and hospital practice.

6. Duty Hours and Personal Responsibilities

On-call requirements are essential for an optimal educational environment and to ensure continuity of patient care. The number of residents and faculty should be adequate to prevent excessive frequency and length of on-call duty. The scheduling of on-call duty should consider that clinical events in obstetrics and gynecology do take place at any time; that both safe, effective patient care and a good learning environment require adequate periods of rest; and that the residency program appointment is the resident's full-time compensated occupation. The frequency of on-call duty for residents should be, on the average, no more often than every third night. Residents should be allowed to spend, on the average, at least 1 full day out of 7 away from program duties. The program director must also ensure adequate backup if sudden and unexpected patient care needs create resident fatigue sufficient to jeopardize patient care during or following on-call periods.

B. Specific Educational Experiences

Resident education must include but not necessarily be limited to the following:

1. Obstetrics
   a. The full range of obstetrics, including high-risk obstetrics and medical and surgical complications of pregnancy
   b. Genetics, including the performance of genetic amniocentesis and patient counseling
   c. Learning and performing operative vaginal deliveries, including the use of obstetric forceps and/or the vacuum extractor
   d. Performing vaginal breech and vaginal multifetal deliveries
   e. Performing vaginal births after previous cesarean delivery
   f. Obstetric anesthesia (Residents must learn the principles of general and conduction anesthesia, together with the management and the complications of these techniques.)
   g. Experience in the management of critically ill patients
   h. Immediate care of the newborn (Every resident must have experience in resuscitation of the human newborn, including tracheal intubation. The principles of general neonatal complications must be learned as well.)
   i. The full range of commonly employed obstetrical diagnostic procedures, including ultrasonography and other relevant imaging techniques
   j. The emotional and psychosocial impact of pregnancy on an individual and her family, in a variety of circumstances
   k. The counseling of women regarding nutrition, exercise, health maintenance, high-risk behaviors, and preparation for pregnancy and childbirth
   l. Obstetric pathology
2. Gynecology
   a. The full range of medical and surgical gynecology for all age groups
   b. Diagnosis and management of pelvic floor dysfunction, including experience with the various operations for its correction
   c. Diagnosis and medical and surgical management of urinary incontinence
   d. Oncology, including prevention, diagnosis, and treatment
   e. Diagnosis and nonsurgical management of breast disease, including fine-needle aspiration
   f. Reproductive endocrinology and infertility
   g. Clinical skills in family planning
   h. Psychosomatic and psychosexual counseling
   i. The full range of commonly employed gynecologic diagnostic procedures, including ultrasonography and other relevant imaging techniques
   j. Experience in the management of critically ill patients
   k. Counseling and educating patients about the normal physiology of the reproductive tract and about high-risk behaviors that may compromise reproductive function
   l. Gynecologic pathology
3. Primary and Preventive Care
   a. Comprehensive history taking, including medical, nutritional, sexual, family, genetic, and social behavior data, and the ability to assess health risks
   b. Complete physical examination
   c. Appropriate use of laboratory studies and diagnostic techniques
   d. Patient education and counseling
   e. Screening appropriate to patients of various ages and risk factors
   f. Immunizations needed at specific ages and under specific circumstances
   g. Diagnosis and treatment of the common nonreproductive illnesses affecting women
   h. Management of the health care of patients in a continuous manner through all the reproductive and postreproductive years
   i. Appropriate use of community resources and other physicians through consultation when necessary
   j. Appropriate awareness and knowledge of the behavioral and societal factors that influence health among women of differing socioeconomic and cultural backgrounds

k. Behavioral medicine and psychosocial problems, including domestic violence, sexual assault, and substance abuse
l. Emergency care
m. Ambulatory primary care problems of the geriatric patient
n. Basics of epidemiology, statistics, data collection and management, and use of medical literature and assessment of its value
o. Ethics and medical jurisprudence
p. Community medicine
q. Health care systems
r. Information processing and decision making

C. Other Residents and Trainees

1. The number of residents from other graduate medical education programs in any specialty who are assigned to the obstetrics-gynecology residency should not be so large as to compromise the educational resources of the obstetrics-gynecology residency.
2. For those residency programs associated with postresidency fellowships, the education of fellows must not compromise the experience of residents.

D. Research

The quality of the educational experience within a department of obstetrics and gynecology is enhanced by an active research environment. It is highly desirable that every program encourage each resident to be involved in a research project.

E. Scholarly Environment

Documentation of scholarly activity on the part of the program and the faculty must be submitted at the time of program review. The responsibility for establishing and maintaining an environment of inquiry and scholarship rests with the teaching staff. While not all members of a teaching staff must be investigators, the staff as a whole must demonstrate broad, ongoing involvement in scholarly activity. This activity should include the following:

1. Active participation of the teaching staff in clinical discussions, rounds, and conferences in a manner that promotes a spirit of inquiry and scholarship (Scholarship implies an in-depth understanding of basic mechanisms of normal and abnormal states and the application of current knowledge to practice.)
2. Participation in journal clubs and research conferences
3. Participation in regional or national professional societies
4. Presentation and/or publication of studies
5. Participation in research, particularly in projects that are funded following peer review and/or result in publication or presentations at regional and national scientific meetings
6. Offering of guidance and technical support (eg, research design, statistical analysis) for residents involved in research
7. Provision of support for resident participation in scholarly activities

VI. Evaluation

A. Resident Performance

1. The program director must establish methods of periodically and systematically evaluating and documenting the level of performance, experience, and technical skills of the residents. One example of an acceptable mechanism helpful in evaluating cognitive knowledge is the CREOG in-training examination. On at least a semiannual basis, program directors or their designees must inform the residents of their individual progress, emphasizing strong points and offering guidance with regard to correcting deficiencies. These evaluations, as well as a list of skills that the resident has mastered, must be documented and available (without revealing the specific resident's identity) at the time the program is reviewed for approval.
2. Physicians must have the welfare of their patients as their primary professional concern. The resident must therefore demonstrate those humanistic qualities that foster the formation of appropriate patient/physician relationships. These include integrity, respect, compassion, professional responsibility, sensitivity to the patient's needs for comfort and encouragement, and an appropriate professional attitude and behavior toward colleagues. These attributes should be emphasized throughout the curriculum and must be evaluated.

B. Evaluation and Program Review

1. The educational effectiveness of a program must be evaluated in a systematic manner. In particular, the quality of the curriculum and the extent to which the educational goals have been met by residents must be assessed. Written evaluations by residents should be utilized in this process.
2. For the purpose of program review, accurate and complete documentation of each individual resident's experience for each year of the program is mandatory. These records should indicate the level of participation of the resident and skills achieved. The program director must review the record of operative experience with individual residents at least semiannually for breadth and depth of experience as well as for evidence of continuing growth in technical achievements. These cumulative data will be reviewed in detail at the time of survey for program approval or continued program approval. For the purposes of these records, there is no distinction between private and service patients.
3. Annually, the program director must collect, compile, and retain the numbers and types of operative procedures performed by residents in the program, together with information describing the total resident experience in each institution and facility utilized in the clinical education of residents. This information must be provided in the format and form specified by the RRC.
4. One significant measure of the quality of a program is the performance of its graduates on the examinations of the American Board of Obstetrics and Gynecology.

VII. Board Certification

Program directors must notify residents who plan to seek certification by the American Board of Obstetrics and Gynecology that they should communicate with the executive director of the board to obtain the latest information regarding current requirements for certification.

ACGME: September 1995 Effective: January 1996

Program Requirements for Residency Education in Ophthalmology

I. Introduction

A. The Program Requirements for Residency Education in Ophthalmology set forth the educational prerequisites for residents and the minimum components that a residency training program in ophthalmology must possess, including the duration of training, institutional support and administration, faculty, educational program, patient resources, and facilities.

B. Residency training programs in ophthalmology should be organized to provide a stable, well-coordinated, progressive educational experience for the resident rather than simply to provide health care to patients.

II. Prerequisites

All applicants entering ophthalmology training programs must have taken a postgraduate clinical year (PGY-1) in a program accredited by the Accreditation Council for Graduate Medical Education (ACGME) or the Royal College of Physicians and Surgeons of Canada. The PGY-1 year must comprise training in which the resident has primary responsibility for patient care in fields such as internal medicine, neurology, pediatrics, surgery, family practice, or emergency medicine. As a minimum, 6 months of this year must be a broad experience in direct patient care.

III. Program Goals and Duration

A. Program Goals and Design

1. The director and teaching staff of a program must prepare and comply with written educational goals for the program. All educational components of a residency program should be related to program goals.
2. The program design and/or structure must be approved by the Residency Review Committee (RRC) as part of the regular review process.

B. Duration of Training

1. The length of training in ophthalmology must be at least 36 calendar months, including appropriate short periods for vacation, special assignments, or exceptional individual circumstances approved by the program director.
2. Any program that extends the length of training beyond 36 calendar months must present an educational rationale that is consonant with the program requirements and the objectives for residency training. Approval for the extended curriculum must be obtained prior to implementation and at each subsequent review. Prior to entry into the program, each resident must be notified in writing of the required curriculum length.
3. The length of time of residency training for a particular resident may be extended by the program director if a resident progresses at a slower pace than provided by the standard rotations. If the extension is only 6 months or less, the program director must notify the RRC of the extension and must describe the proposed curriculum for that resident and the measures taken to minimize the impact on other residents. (See below, IV.C.4.b.)

IV. Institutional Support and Program Administration

A. General

1. There must be a single program director responsible for the program.
2. The institution must ensure that the program director is given sufficient authority, financial support, and facilities by the governing body of the sponsoring institution to permit him or her to organize and supervise the following activities of the training program: resident selection and evaluation, instructional program, patient management, research, and initiation of recommendations for staff recruitment.

B. Qualifications of the Program Director

1. The program director must be a qualified ophthalmologist, who either is certified by the American Board of Ophthalmology or is judged by the RRC to possess suitable equivalent qualifications. The term of appointment of the program director must be adequate to ensure stability and continuity of the program.
2. The program director must be licensed to practice medicine in the state where the institution that sponsors the program is located. (Certain federal programs are exempted.)
3. The program director must have an appointment in good standing to the medical staff of an institution participating in the program.
4. The program director who serves as administrator, educator, and research coordinator must devote sufficient time to the administration and conduct of the residency training program so that the educational experience for the residents is satisfactory. The RRC for Ophthalmology will evaluate the overall effectiveness of the program director as an administrator, educator, and research coordinator.

C. Responsibilities of the Program Director

1. The program director must prepare a written statement outlining the educational goals of the program with respect to knowledge, skills, and other attributes of residents at each level of training and for each major rotation or other program assignment. This statement must be distributed to residents and members of the teaching staff. It should be readily available for review.
2. The program director, with the support of the institution, must develop and maintain current documentation of institutional or interinstitutional agreements, resident selection and agreements, patient care statistics, faculty evaluations, and assessment of resident performance. This documentation must be provided to the RRC as indicated in the Program Information Forms supplied by the committee secretary.
3. The program director is responsible for notifying the executive secretary of the RRC of any changes in program director and/or departmental chairman as well as of a formal affiliation with another institution.
4. The program director is required to have prior approval of the RRC for the following changes:
   a. A required rotation of 4 months or more to any institution other than the parent.
   b. The number of resident positions in the training program, both total number and the number at any level. If the change in resident complement results from the extension of training of a current resident, as described in III.B.3 above, and is not greater than 6 months, only prior notification of the RRC is required.
   c. The number of years of training.

   The appropriate educational justification and documentation must accompany all of these requests so that the RRC may evaluate whether the quality of the program and the resources available are adequate to support the requested change.
5. To ensure proper supervision, the program director must prepare explicit, written descriptions of lines of responsibility for the care of patients and make these clear to all members of teaching teams. Residents must be provided with rapid, reliable systems for communication with and appropriate involvement of supervi-

sory physicians in a manner appropriate for quality patient care and educational programs.

6. The program director must ensure the implementation of fair procedures as established by the sponsoring institution regarding academic discipline and resident complaints or grievances.
7. The program director must monitor resident stress, including mental or emotional conditions inhibiting performance or learning and drug- or alcohol-related dysfunction. Program directors and teaching staff should be sensitive to the need for timely provision of confidential counseling and psychological support services to residents. Training situations that consistently produce undesirable stress on residents must be evaluated and modified.

V. Minimum Resident Complement

The RRC recognizes the importance of interaction among residents themselves as well as between faculty and residents in the conduct of conferences and patient care. A critical mass or minimum number of residents is essential to provide an opportunity for meaningful interaction throughout the training period. Each program must be structured to have a minimum of two residents in each year of training.

VI. Teaching Faculty

A. The faculty must be highly qualified and possess appropriate clinical and teaching skills. The faculty must devote adequate time to the education of residents. The faculty must have a broad range of subspecialty expertise. Such expertise will usually be acquired by subspecialty fellowship training.

B. Faculty members should be certified by the American Board of Ophthalmology or possess suitable equivalent qualifications.

C. There must be sufficient faculty in the program to provide a minimum of one full-time equivalent faculty person for every three residents in the program.

D. All members of the teaching staff must demonstrate a strong interest in the education of residents, sound clinical and teaching abilities, support of the goals and objectives of the program, a commitment to their own continuing medical education, and participation in scholarly activities.

E. The teaching staff must be organized and have regular documented meetings to review program goals and objectives as well as program effectiveness in achieving them. At least one resident representative should participate in these reviews.

F. The teaching staff should periodically evaluate the utilization of the resources available to the program, the contribution of each institution participating in the program, the financial and administrative support of the program, the volume and variety of patients available to the program for educational purposes, the performance of members of the teaching staff, and the quality of supervision of residents.

VII. Other Program Personnel

Programs must be provided with the additional professional, technical, and clerical personnel needed to support the administration and educational conduct of the program.

VIII. Program Research and Scholarly Activity

Graduate medical education must take place in an environment of inquiry and scholarship in which residents participate in the development of new knowledge, learn to evaluate research findings, and develop habits of inquiry as a continuing professional responsibility.

Scholarly Activity

The responsibility for establishing and maintaining an environment of inquiry and scholarship rests with the teaching staff. While not all members of a teaching staff must be investigators, the staff as a whole must demonstrate broad involvement in scholarly activity. This activity should include:

1. Active participation of the teaching staff in clinical discussions, rounds, and conferences in a manner that promotes a spirit of inquiry and scholarship. Scholarship implies an in-depth understanding of basic mechanisms of normal and abnormal states and the application of current knowledge to practice.
2. Participation in journal clubs and research conferences.
3. Active participation in regional or national professional and scientific societies, particularly through presentations at the organizations' meetings and publication in their journals.
4. Participation in research, particularly in projects that are funded following peer review and/or result in publication or presentations at regional and national scientific meetings.
5. Offering of guidance and technical support (eg, research design, statistical analysis) for residents involved in research.
6. Provision of support for resident participation in scholarly activities.

IX. Participating Institutions

A residency program in ophthalmology must have a designated parent institution where the majority of the required clinical and didactic educational experiences occur and are coordinated by the program director. Affiliations with other institutions may sometimes be desirable to provide complementary educational experiences for the residents. Programs that depend on rotations to hospitals other than the parent institution must submit documentation that the following criteria are being fulfilled:

A. Purpose

There must be a clear statement in the narrative section of the Program Information Forms regarding the purpose of each participating institution, indicating how they enhance the total program and how they are coordinated with the other components of the overall educational experience.

B. Local Director

There must be a designated local director of the program at each participating institution. The program director must appoint or be consulted in the appointment of the local program director, and this arrangement must be documented in writing by the appropriate individuals at each institution. There must be evidence of ongoing coordination of the various components of the overall program, which would include planning of the rotations, evaluation of residents, and evaluation of each institution by the residents.

C. Physical Facilities

The program director should ensure that the physical facilities of each participating institution, including outpatient clinic, inpatient facilities, operating rooms, and their respective equipment, meet the program requirements.

D. Educational Experiences

1. The program director is ultimately responsible for the schedule and composition of the residents' rotations at each participating institution, as well as for the extent of faculty supervision on the clinical services and in the operating room.
2. The program director is ultimately responsible for the content and quality of didactic lectures and conferences and must ensure that these are coordinated with the overall educational activities of the program. Sample schedules must be submitted along with those from the parent institution.
3. If a participating institution is sufficiently remote from the parent institution to prevent regular attendance by residents at the didactic and clinical conferences at the parent institution or if the rotation otherwise prevents such attendance, the program direc-

tor must demonstrate that each resident is exposed to a formal educational experience that fulfills the program requirements.

4. Formal teaching case presentations should be included at each participating institution to ensure optimal utilization of patients for teaching purposes; alternatively, cases should be brought from participating institutions to the parent institution for presentation if formal teaching case presentations are held only there.
5. The program director must ensure that all residents have equivalent educational experiences.
6. Rotations to foreign countries shall not be used to meet minimum educational standards.

X. Educational Program

The program director is responsible for the structure and content of the educational program and must provide the RRC with a statement of objectives, methods of implementation, and procedures for assessment of the program by the faculty and the residents. The educational experience must be designed and supervised by the program director. The educational program should include:

A. Didactic Instruction in the Basic and Clinical Sciences

Residents should be educated in basic and clinical sciences through lectures and/or regularly scheduled discussions relevant to the practice of ophthalmology. Regularly scheduled required lectures or seminars should be held at the parent institution. The didactic curriculum must encompass a minimum of 360 hours of instruction for residents during the 36-month training program, at least 240 of which must be intramural. The program director is responsible for documenting resident attendance at conferences.

B. Case Presentations and Clinical Conferences

A minimum of 8 hours per month should be devoted to regularly scheduled formal teaching case presentations and clinical conferences attended by several faculty and a majority of residents.

C. Pathology

The training experience in ocular pathology should comprise continuing intramural lectures, clinicopathological conferences, and a minimum of 50 hours of laboratory experience in gross and microscopic examination of pathological specimens. This latter experience with a qualified pathologist may take place intramurally or extramurally at a laboratory considered by the RRC to be capable of providing such training. If utilized, this extramural effort should occur during the 36 months of residency training, preferably early in the program, and would not be construed to be a substitute for the continuing intramural program. A short exposure to ophthalmic pathology at a remote course may supplement this training but will not be considered as a substitute for the pathology requirement.

D. Clinical Experiences

The volume and variety of clinical ophthalmological problems in children and adults must be sufficient to afford each resident a graduated supervised experience with the entire spectrum of ophthalmic diseases so that the resident may develop diagnostic, therapeutic, and manual skills and judgment as to their appropriate use.

1. Outpatient Experience
   During the course of training residents should be responsible for the care of an adequate number of outpatients who represent a broad range of ophthalmic diseases. There must be appropriate faculty supervision of the residents in all outpatient visits. Appropriate faculty supervision occurs when the faculty is readily available to residents for consultation or assistance when requested.
   a. Each resident should participate in a minimum of 3,000 outpatient visits in which the resident performs a substantial portion of the examination and has responsibility for the care of the patient.
   b. There should be direct faculty supervision of the residents in at least 1,000 outpatient visits. Direct faculty supervision occurs when teaching staff also examine the patient with the resident and discuss the management of the patient with the resident before the patient leaves the clinic.
   c. A minimum of 1,500 outpatients should be refracted by each resident.
2. Surgical Experience
   a. Residents must perform and assist at sufficient surgery to become skilled as general ophthalmic surgeons. That is, each resident must have major technical and patient care responsibilities in the surgery (including laser surgery) of cataract, strabismus, cornea, glaucoma, retina/vitreous, oculoplastic, and trauma to provide an adequate base for a general ophthalmic practice.
   b. The program director is responsible for documenting the surgical experiences of each resident, to include the number of cases in each category where the resident has served as the primary surgeon or the assistant surgeon. This documentation must be provided to the RRC on its Program Information Forms, and individual resident logs must be available at the time of the site visit.
3. Systemic Disease Consultation Experience
   Each resident should care for a minimum of 150 patients seen in consultation during the course of 3 years of training. The types of cases seen should cover a wide spectrum of ophthalmic diseases and ophthalmic manifestations of systemic diseases.

E. Duty Hours and Personal Responsibility

Duty hours and night and weekend call for residents must reflect the concept of responsibility for patients and provide for adequate patient care. Residents must not be required regularly to perform excessively difficult or prolonged duties. When averaged over 4 weeks, residents should spend no more than 80 hours per week in patient care activities. Residents at all levels should, on average, have the opportunity to spend at least 1 day out of 7 free of patient care activities and should, on average, have patient care activities no more often than every third night.

F. Fellowship Program

If the residency training program is conducted in conjunction with fellowship training programs for teaching advanced competence in specialized areas of ophthalmology, such fellowship programs must not adversely affect the experience of residents in the core training program.

XI. Facilities

A. Clinic

The outpatient area of each participating institution must have a minimum of one fully equipped examining lane for each resident in the clinic. There must be access to current diagnostic equipment. This should encompass equipment designed for ophthalmic photography (including fluorescein angiography), perimetry, ultrasonography, keratometry, retinal electrophysiology, and microbiology, as well as other appropriate equipment.

B. Operating Room Facilities

The surgical facilities at each participating institution in which residents are trained in surgery must include at least one operating room fully equipped for ophthalmic surgery, including an operating microscope.

C. Inpatient Facilities

There must be inpatient facilities with access to sufficient space and beds for good patient care. An eye examination room with a slit lamp should be easily accessible.

D. Library

1. Residents must have ready access to a major medical library, either at the institution where the residents are located or through arrangement with convenient nearby institutions.
2. Library services should include the electronic retrieval of information from medical databases.
3. There must be readily available an on-site library or a collection of ophthalmological and general medical texts, journals, films, records, and tapes in each institution participating in a residency program. On-site libraries and/or collections of texts and journals must be readily available during nights and weekends.

XII. Evaluation

A. Program and Faculty Evaluation

The educational effectiveness of a program must be evaluated in a systematic manner. In particular, the quality of the curriculum and the extent to which the educational goals have been met by residents must be assessed.

Teaching faculty must be evaluated on a regular basis. Documentation of faculty evaluation should include teaching ability and commitment as well as clinical knowledge.

Written evaluations by residents, through a mechanism that ensures anonymity, should be utilized in the evaluation of both the program and the faculty.

B. Resident Evaluation

There must be regular evaluation of residents' knowledge, skills, and overall performance, including the development of professional attitudes consistent with being a physician.

The program director, with participation of members of the teaching staff, shall:

1. At least semiannually evaluate the knowledge, skills, and professional growth of the residents, using appropriate criteria and procedures.
2. Communicate each evaluation to the resident in a timely manner.
3. Advance residents to positions of higher responsibility only on the basis of evidence of their satisfactory progressive scholarship and professional growth.
4. Maintain a permanent record of evaluation for each resident and have it accessible to the resident and other authorized personnel.

C. Final Evaluation

The program director must provide a written final evaluation for each resident who completes the program. The evaluation must include a review of the resident's performance during the final period of training and should verify that the resident has demonstrated sufficient professional ability to practice competently and independently. This final evaluation should be part of the resident's permanent record maintained by the institution.

XIII. Other

A. Use of Board Examinations

In its review and evaluation of training programs the RRC for Ophthalmology may use the pass rate on the examinations of the American Board of Ophthalmology for residents completing a particular program as one measure of the quality of that training program.

B. Institutional Requirements

Training programs in ophthalmology should comply with all of the provisions of the Institutional Requirements.

C. Certification

Residents who plan to seek certification by the American Board of Ophthalmology should communicate with the executive director of the board regarding specific requirements for certification.

ACGME: February 1993 Effective: July 1995

Program Requirements for Residency Education in Orthopaedic Surgery

I. Introduction

A. Definition and Scope of the Specialty

Orthopaedic surgery is the medical specialty that includes the study and prevention of musculoskeletal diseases, disorders, and injuries and their treatment by medical, surgical, and physical methods.

B. Definition and Scope of Education

1. Until July 1, 2000, an orthopaedic residency may be accredited to offer either 4 or 5 years of graduate medical education. After July 1, 2000, orthopaedic residencies will be accredited to offer 5 years of graduate medical education.
2. A 4-year program must be preceded by a year of education in an Accreditation Council for Graduate Medical Education (ACGME)-accredited residency in a general medical specialty such as general surgery, internal medicine, or pediatrics. No more than 3 months of orthopaedic surgery education should be offered during that year.
3. In a 5-year program the orthopaedic residency director is responsible for the design, implementation, and oversight of a PGY-1 year that will prepare residents for specialty education in orthopaedic surgery. This year must include resident participation in clinical and didactic activities that will give them the opportunity to
   a. develop the knowledge, attitudes, and skills needed to formulate principles and assess, plan and initiate treatment of adult and pediatric patients with surgical and/or medical problems;
   b. be involved in the care of patients with surgical and medical emergencies, multiple organ system trauma, soft tissue wounds, nervous system injuries and diseases, peripheral vascular injuries and diseases, and rheumatologic and other medical diseases;
   c. gain experience in the care of critically ill surgical and medical patients;
   d. participate in the pre-, intra-, and post-operative care of surgical patients; and
   e. develop an understanding of surgical anesthesia, including anesthetic risks and the management of intraoperative anesthetic complications.
4. In order to meet these goals the PGY-1 year must include
   a. A minimum of 6 months of structured education in surgery, to include multisystem trauma, plastic surgery/burn care, intensive care, and vascular surgery;
   b. A minimum of 1 month of structured education in at least three of the following: emergency medicine, medical/cardiac intensive care, internal medicine, neurology, neurological surgery, rheumatology, anesthesiology, musculoskeletal imaging, and rehabilitation; and
   c. A maximum of 3 months of orthopaedic surgery.
5. The program director is also responsible for the design, implementation, and oversight of PGY-2 through PGY-5 years that
   a. must include at least 3 years of rotations on orthopaedic services.
   b. may include rotations on related services such as plastic surgery, physical medicine and rehabilitation, rheumatology, or neurological surgery.

C. The director and teaching staff of a program must prepare and comply with written educational goals for the program. All educational components of a residency program should be related to program goals.

1. The program design and/or structure must be approved by the Residency Review Committee (RRC) as part of the regular review process.
2. Participation by any institution providing more than 6 months of training in a program requires prior approval by the RRC.

D. The educational effectiveness of a program must be evaluated in a systematic manner. In particular, the quality of the curriculum and the extent to which the educational goals have been met by residents must be assessed. Written evaluations by residents should be utilized in this process.

II. Institutional Organization

A. Sponsoring Institution

1. An orthopaedic residency must have a single sponsoring institution and one primary site where most of the residents' basic science and research education is provided.
   a. Residents' clinical education at the primary site should include extensive experience in patient care. Preoperative evaluation and postoperative follow-up, as well as evaluation and treatment of patients not requiring surgery, must be included.
   b. Basic science education and the principal clinical conferences should be provided at the primary site. Supplemental conferences may also be provided at other locations, but the program's didactic activities should be provided at the program's primary site.
2. The governing body of the sponsoring institution must provide support for the program director in teaching, recruiting staff, selecting residents, assigning residents to an appropriate workload, and dismissing residents whose performance is unsatisfactory and must encourage continuity in the program directorship.
3. In communities where the didactic programs of several residencies are combined, the staff of each accredited program must actively and consistently participate in the combined effort.
4. To provide an adequate interdisciplinary educational experience, the institution that sponsors the orthopaedic program should also participate in ACGME-accredited programs in general surgery, internal medicine, and pediatrics.

B. Participating Institutions

1. When the resources of two or more institutions are utilized for the clinical or basic science education of orthopaedic residents, an affiliation agreement specifying the contribution of each institution to the orthopaedic surgery residency must be approved by institutional governing boards.
2. A program involving more than two institutions must clearly demonstrate the educational need for each institution's participation in the program. Clinical responsibility alone does not constitute a suitable educational experience.
3. Affiliations should be avoided with institutions that are at such a distance from the sponsoring institution as to make resident participation in program conferences and rounds difficult, unless the participating institution provides comparable activities.
4. The program director must have the responsibility and authority to coordinate program activities at all participating institutions and must maintain a file of written descriptions of the educational activities provided at each institution involved in the program.

III. Faculty Qualifications and Responsibilities

The program director and the teaching staff are responsible for the general administration of a program, including those activities related to the recruitment, selection, instruction, supervision, counseling, evaluation, and advancement of residents and the maintenance of records related to program accreditation.

A. Program Director

There must be a single program director responsible for the program. The program director should be the chief administrator of the department, division, or section of orthopaedic surgery.

1. Qualifications of the Program Director
   a. Requisite and documented clinical, educational, and administrative abilities and experience.
   b. Licensure to practice medicine in the state where the institution that sponsors the program is located. (Certain federal programs are exempted.)
   c. Certification by the American Board of Orthopaedic Surgery or suitable equivalent qualifications.
   d. Appointment in good standing to the medical staff of an institution participating in the program.
2. Responsibilities of the Program Director
   a. Preparing a written statement outlining the educational goals of the program with respect to knowledge, skills, and other attributes of residents at each level of training and for each major rotation or other program assignment. This statement must be distributed to residents and members of the teaching staff. It should be readily available for review.
   b. Selecting residents for appointment to the program in accordance with institutional and departmental policies and procedures.
   c. Selecting, supervising, and evaluating the teaching staff and other program personnel at each institution participating in the program.
   d. Supervising residents in accordance with explicit written descriptions of supervisory lines of responsibility for the care of patients. Such guidelines must be communicated to all members of the program staff. Residents must be provided with prompt, reliable systems for communication and interaction with supervisory physicians.
   e. Regularly evaluating residents' knowledge, skills, and overall performance, including the development of professional attitudes consistent with being a physician. The program director, with participation of members of the teaching staff, shall
      1. at least semiannually evaluate the knowledge, skills, and professional growth of the residents, using appropriate criteria and procedures.
      2. communicate each evaluation to the resident in a timely manner.
      3. advance residents to positions of higher responsibility only on the basis of evidence of their satisfactory progressive scholarship and professional growth.
      4. maintain a permanent record of evaluation for each resident and have it accessible to the resident and other authorized personnel.
   f. Providing a written final evaluation for each resident who completes the program. The evaluation must include a review of the resident's performance during the final period of training and should verify that the resident has demonstrated sufficient professional ability to practice competently and independently. This final evaluation should be part of the resident's permanent record maintained by the institution.
   g. Implementing fair procedures as established by the sponsoring institution regarding academic discipline and resident complaints or grievances.
   h. Monitoring each resident's performance and progress in the development of the cognitive and interpersonal skills, ethics, manual abilities, and affective qualities needed by an orthopaedic surgeon.
   i. Monitoring resident stress, including mental or emotional conditions inhibiting performance or learning and drug- or alcohol-related dysfunction. Program directors and teaching staff should be sensitive to the need for timely provision of confidential counseling and psychological support services to residents. Training situations that consistently produce undesirable stress on residents must be evaluated and modified.
   j. Preparing an accurate statistical and narrative description of the program as requested by the RRC.
   k. Ensuring the provision of adequate facilities, teaching staff, resident staff, teaching beds, educational resource materials, outpatient facilities, and research facilities.
   l. Ensuring that resident performance is not impaired by excessive fatigue, whether caused by program duties or other activities. It is desirable that residents' work schedules be designed so that, on average, excluding exceptional patient care needs, residents have at least 1 day out of 7 free of routine responsibilities and be on call in the hospital no more often than every third night. The ratio of hours worked to on-call time will vary, particularly at the senior levels, and therefore necessitates flexibility.
   m. In institutions that offer postgraduate fellowships and/or other educational experiences, ensuring that these activities do not compromise resident education.
   n. Maintaining a file of current, written institutional and interinstitutional agreements, resident agreements, patient care statistics, the operative experience of individual residents, policies on duty hours and supervision, and regular assessments of resident performance. These documents must be provided on request to the RRC or to the site visitor.
   o. Notifying the secretary of the RRC of any change that may significantly alter the educational experience. Examples of such changes are
      1. change of program director.
      2. major changes in institutional affiliation. Any change in formal affiliation with an institution where a resident spends 6 months or longer requires prior approval by the RRC.
      3. extension of a resident's educational period. A program director may retain a resident longer than the duration for which the program is accredited in orthopaedic surgery so that the resident may achieve sufficient competence in the specialty. The RRC must be notified of such retention.
      4. change in number of residents. Any change in the number of residents at any level of training or a change in the total number of residents must receive prior approval of the RRC.

B. Teaching Staff

1. There must be a sufficient number of teaching staff with documented qualifications to instruct and supervise adequately all the residents in the program. Members of the teaching staff must be able to devote sufficient time to meet their supervisory and teaching responsibilities.
   a. All programs must have at least three faculty who devote at least 20 hours each week to the program.
   b. There must be at least one full-time faculty equivalent (one FTE equals 45 hours per week devoted to the residency) for every four residents in the program (excluding residents in nonorthopaedic education).
2. All members of the teaching staff must demonstrate a strong interest in the education of residents, sound clinical and teaching abilities, support of the goals and objectives of the program, a commitment to their own continuing medical education, and participation in scholarly activities.
3. A member of the teaching staff of each participating institution must be designated to assume responsibility for the day-to-day ac-

tivities of the program at that institution, with overall coordination by the program director.

4. The teaching staff must be organized and have regular documented meetings to review program goals and objectives as well as program effectiveness in achieving them. At least one resident representative should participate in these reviews.
5. At least once a year the teaching staff should evaluate the utilization of the resources available to the program, the contribution of each institution participating in the program, the financial and administrative support of the program, the volume and variety of patients available to the program for educational purposes, the performance of members of the teaching staff, and the quality of supervision of residents.
6. At least once a year the teaching staff must evaluate the educational effectiveness of the program. In particular, the quality of the curriculum and the extent to which educational goals have been met by residents must be assessed. Written evaluations of the program by residents should be utilized in the process.
7. It is the responsibility of the teaching staff to
    a. ensure that the structure and content of the residency program reflect an education-to-service ratio that identifies the resident as a student and provide adequate experience in preoperative and postoperative, as well as intraoperative, patient management. This responsibility must include direct supervision appropriate to a resident's competence and level of training in all patient care settings, including operative, inpatient, outpatient, and emergency, and participation in patient care conferences and other educational activities.
    b. participate in appropriate scientific societies, pursue their own continuing education, and demonstrate an active interest in related research.
    c. evidence ethical medical practice.

C. Other Personnel

Programs must be provided with the additional professional, technical, and clerical personnel needed to support the administration and educational conduct of the program.

D. Residents

When reviewing a program for accreditation, the RRC will approve a maximum total number of residents to be educated in the program and the maximum that may be educated at each level of the program. Those numbers will be based primarily on the number, qualifications, and commitment of the faculty; the volume and variety of the patient population available for educational purposes; the quality of the educational offering; and the totality of institutional resources. It is important that the resident complement be sufficient in number to sustain an educational environment.

IV. Educational Program

A. Clinical Resources

Clinical problems must be of sufficient variety and volume to afford the residents adequate experience in the diagnosis and management of adult and pediatric orthopaedic disorders. The residents' clinical experience must include adult orthopaedics, including joint reconstruction; pediatric orthopaedics, including pediatric trauma; trauma, including multisystem trauma; surgery of the spine, including disk surgery, spinal trauma, and spinal deformities; hand surgery; foot surgery in adults and children; athletic injuries, including arthroscopy; metastatic disease; and orthopaedic rehabilitation, including amputations and postamputation care.

B. Related Areas of Instruction

Resident education must include orthopaedic oncology, rehabilitation of neurologic injury and disease, spinal cord injury rehabilitation, orthotics and prosthetics, and the ethics of medical practice.

C. Continuity of Care

All residents must have the opportunity to develop competence in the preadmission care, hospital care, operative care, and follow-up care (including rehabilitation) of patients.

D. Nonoperative Outpatient Experience

Residents must have adequate experience in nonoperative outpatient diagnosis and care, including all orthopaedic anatomic areas and patients of all age groups.

E. Progressive Responsibility

Residents must have the opportunity to assume increasing responsibility for patient care, under direct faculty supervision (as appropriate for a resident's ability and experience), as they progress through a program. Inpatient and outpatient experience with all age groups is necessary.

F. Teaching Rounds and Conferences

Faculty and residents must attend and participate in regularly scheduled and held teaching rounds, lectures, and conferences. Treatment indications, clinical outcomes, complications, morbidity, and mortality must be critically reviewed and discussed on a regular basis. Subjects of mutual interest and the changing practice of medicine should be discussed at interdisciplinary conferences. On average, there must be at least 4 hours of formal teaching activities each week.

G. Basic Medical Sciences

Basic science education must include substantial instruction in anatomy, biomechanics, pathology, and physiology. The basic science program must also include resident education in embryology, immunology, pharmacology, biochemistry, and microbiology.

1. Instruction in anatomy must include study and dissection of anatomic specimens by the residents and lectures or other formal sessions.
2. Instruction in pathology must include organized instruction in correlative pathology in which gross and microscopic pathology are related to clinical and roentgenographic findings.
3. Instruction in biomechanics should be presented in seminars or conferences emphasizing principles, terminology, and application to orthopaedics.
4. Organized instruction in the basic medical sciences must be integrated into the daily clinical activities by clearly linking the pathophysiologic process and findings to the diagnosis, treatment, and management of clinical disorders.
5. Organized instruction in the appropriate use and interpretation of radiographic and other imaging techniques must be provided for all residents.

H. Basic Motor Skills

Instruction in basic motor skills must include experience in the proper use of surgical instruments and operative techniques. Evaluation of new or experimental techniques and/or materials should be emphasized. The application of basic motor skills must be integrated into daily clinical activities, especially in the operating room.

I. Research and Scholarly Activity

1. Graduate medical education must take place in an environment of inquiry and scholarship in which residents participate in the development of new knowledge, learn to evaluate research findings, and develop habits of inquiry as a continuing professional responsibility.

2. The responsibility for establishing and maintaining an environment of inquiry and scholarship rests with the teaching staff. While not all members of a teaching staff must be investigators, the staff as a whole must demonstrate broad involvement in scholarly activity. This activity should include
   a. active participation of the teaching staff in clinical discussions, rounds, and conferences in a manner that promotes a spirit of inquiry and scholarship. Scholarship implies an in-depth understanding of basic mechanisms of normal and abnormal states and the application of current knowledge to practice.
   b. participation in journal clubs and research conferences.
   c. active participation in regional or national professional and scientific societies, particularly through presentations at the organizations' meetings and publications in their journals.
   d. participation in research, particularly in projects that are funded following peer review and/or result in publications or presentations at regional and national scientific meetings.
   e. offering of guidance and technical support (eg, research design, statistical analysis) for residents involved in research.
   f. provision of support for resident participation in scholarly activities.
3. To develop the abilities to critically evaluate medical literature, research, and other scholarly activity, resident education must include instruction in experimental design, hypothesis testing, and other current research methods, as well as participation in clinical or basic research.
4. Space, equipment, faculty expertise and supervision, conferences, support personnel, time, and funding must be provided for research in the program.
5. Program directors must maintain a current record of research activity by residents and faculty.
6. Library Resources
   a. Residents must have ready access to a major medical library, either at the institution where the residents are located or through arrangement with convenient nearby institutions.
   b. Library resources must include current and past orthopaedic periodicals and reference books that are readily accessible to all orthopaedic residents in the program.
   c. Library services should include the electronic retrieval of information from medical databases.
   d. There must be access to an on-site library or to a collection of appropriate texts and journals in each institution participating in a residency program. On-site libraries and/or collections of texts and journals must be readily available during nights and weekends.

V. Other

A. Examinations

One measure of the quality of a program is the performance of its graduates on examinations for certification by the American Board of Orthopaedic Surgery. Program graduates should take the examination, and at least 75% of those who take the exam for the first time should pass.

B. Change of Program Director

Programs that have acting directors for more than 1 year will be subject to review, which may include a site visit.

C. Board Certification

Residents should contact the American Board of Orthopaedic Surgery for information regarding certification.

ACGME: September 1997 Effective: July 1998

Program Requirements for Residency Education in Adult Reconstructive Orthopaedics (Orthopaedic Surgery)

I. Introduction

A. Adult reconstructive orthopaedics is a subspecialty of orthopaedic surgery that includes the in-depth study, prevention, and reconstructive treatment of musculoskeletal diseases, disorders, and sequelae of injuries by medical, physical, and surgical methods. An educational program in adult reconstructive orthopaedics may include the care of arthritis and related disorders in many anatomic regions or be limited to areas such as the hip, knee, shoulder, elbow, or ankle and foot. The program must be organized to provide sufficient experience for fellows to acquire the competency of a specialist in the field.

B. Postgraduate fellowship education in orthopaedic surgery is a component in the continuum of the educational process, and such education will take place after completion of an accredited residency. Graduate medical education programs in the subspecialties of orthopaedic surgery will be accredited to offer 12 months of education.

C. Postgraduate fellowship programs in the subspecialties of orthopaedic surgery may be accredited in institutions that sponsor accredited residency programs in orthopaedic surgery or that are affiliated with an Accreditation Council for Graduate Medical Education (ACGME)-accredited orthopaedic surgery residency. Requests for exceptions to this policy will be reviewed on a case-by-case basis.

D. When orthopaedic residents and fellows are being educated in the same institution, the residency director and the director of the fellowship must jointly prepare and approve a written agreement specifying the educational relationship between the residency and fellowship programs, the roles of the residency and fellowship directors in determining the educational program of residents and fellows, and the roles of the residents and fellows in patient care.

E. The director and teaching staff of a program must prepare and comply with written educational goals for the program. All educational components of a program should be related to program goals.
   1. The program design and/or structure must be approved by the Residency Review Committee (RRC) as part of the regular review process.
   2. Participation by any institution providing more than 2 months of training must be approved by the RRC.

II. Institutional Resources and Organization

A. Programs must provide an intellectual environment for acquiring the knowledge, skills, clinical judgment, and attitudes essential to the practice of adult reconstructive orthopaedics. This objective can be achieved only when the program director, the supporting faculty and staff, and the administration are fully committed to the educational program and when appropriate resources and facilities are present. Effective graduate education is not achieved when the educational program functions primarily to meet service commitments.

B. A sufficient number of new and follow-up patients must be available to ensure adequate inpatient and outpatient experience for each fellow without adversely diluting the educational experience of the orthopaedic surgery residents or the educational experience of residents in other specialties.

C. There must be close monitoring of the interface between residency and fellowship education. It is imperative that orthopaedic fellowship education not interfere with the education of residents. Lines of responsibility for the orthopaedic resident and the fellow must be clearly defined. In addition, the fellow should maintain a close working relationship with orthopaedic residents and other fellows in orthopaedic surgery and in other disciplines.

D. Facilities to support the overall educational program must be available and functioning. These include outpatient, inpatient, imaging, laboratory, rehabilitation, and research resources. Operating rooms must be state of the art and contain modern equipment for reconstructive surgery.

E. There should be broad support from other clinical specialties, including radiology, laboratory medicine, rheumatology, endocrinology, infectious disease, pathology, and rehabilitation.

III. Program Personnel

The program director and the teaching staff are responsible for the general administration of a program, including those activities related to the recruitment, selection, instruction, supervision, counseling, evaluation, and advancement of residents and the maintenance of records related to program accreditation.

A. Program Director

The director of the subspecialty program and the director of the affiliated orthopaedic surgery program, in conjunction with the administration of the institution, will be responsible for ensuring that adequate facilities and other necessary resources are available to provide an education of high quality.

There must be a single program director responsible for the program.

1. Qualifications of the program director include:
   a. Requisite and documented clinical, educational, and administrative abilities and experience.
   b. Licensure to practice medicine in the state where the institution that sponsors the program is located. (Certain federal programs are exempted.)
   c. Certification by the American Board of Orthopaedic Surgery or suitable equivalent qualifications.
   d. Appointment in good standing to the medical staff of an institution participating in the program.
2. Responsibilities of the program director include:
   a. Preparation of a written statement outlining the educational goals of the program with respect to knowledge, skills, and other attributes of residents at each level of training and for each major rotation or other program assignment. This statement must be distributed to residents and members of the teaching staff. It should be readily available for review.
   b. Selection of residents for appointment to the program in accordance with institutional and departmental policies and procedures.
   c. Selection and supervision of the teaching staff and other program personnel at each institution participating in the program.
   d. The supervision of residents in accordance with explicit written descriptions of supervisory lines of responsibility for the care of patients. Such guidelines must be communicated to all members of the program staff. Residents must be provided with prompt, reliable systems for communication and interaction with supervisory physicians.
   e. Regular evaluation of residents' knowledge, skills, and overall performance, including the development of professional attitudes consistent with being a physician. The program director, with participation of members of the teaching staff, shall:
      1. At least semiannually evaluate the knowledge, skills, and professional growth of the residents, using appropriate criteria and procedures.
      2. Communicate each evaluation to the resident in a timely manner.
      3. Advance residents to positions of higher responsibility only on the basis of evidence of their satisfactory progressive scholarship and professional growth.
      4. Maintain a permanent record of evaluation for each resident and have it accessible to the resident and other authorized personnel.
   f. The provision of a written final evaluation for each resident who completes the program. The evaluation must include a review of the resident's performance during the final period of training and should verify that the resident has demonstrated sufficient professional ability to practice competently and independently. This final evaluation should be part of the resident's permanent record maintained by the institution.
   g. Fellowship directors must ensure that trainees are given reasonable duty and call assignments. It is desirable that fellows' work schedules be designed so that on average, excluding exceptional patient care needs, fellows have at least 1 day out of 7 free of routine responsibilities and be on call in the hospital no more often than every third night. Scheduling will necessitate flexibility, as fellows are at the postgraduate level, so the ratio of hours worked and on-call time may vary.
   h. Implementation of fair procedures, as established by the sponsoring institution, regarding academic discipline and resident complaints or grievances.
   i. Monitoring resident stress, including mental or emotional conditions inhibiting performance or learning and drug- or alcohol-related dysfunction. Program directors and teaching staff should be sensitive to the need for timely provision of confidential counseling and psychological support services to residents. Training situations that consistently produce undesirable stress on residents must be evaluated and modified.
   j. Preparation of an accurate statistical and narrative description of the program as requested by the RRC.

B. Teaching Staff

1. There must be a sufficient number of teaching staff with documented qualifications to instruct and supervise adequately all the residents in the program.
2. Members of the teaching staff must be able to devote sufficient time to meet their supervisory and teaching responsibilities.
3. All members of the teaching staff must demonstrate a strong interest in the education of residents, sound clinical and teaching abilities, support of the goals and objectives of the program, a commitment to their own continuing medical education, and participation in scholarly activities.
4. A member of the teaching staff of each participating institution must be designated to assume responsibility for the day-to-day activities of the program at that institution, with overall coordination by the program director.
5. The teaching staff must be organized and have regular documented meetings to review program goals and objectives as well as program effectiveness in achieving them. At least one resident representative should participate in these reviews.
6. The teaching staff should periodically evaluate the utilization of the resources available to the program, the contribution of each institution participating in the program, the financial and administrative support of the program, the volume and variety of patients available to the program for educational purposes, the

performance of members of the teaching staff, and the quality of supervision of residents.

C. Other Program Personnel

Programs must be provided with the additional professional, technical, and clerical personnel needed to support the administration and educational conduct of the program.

IV. Educational Program

A. The fellowship must provide sufficiently advanced education to allow the fellow to acquire the expertise of a specialist in adult reconstructive orthopaedics. This education must consist of academic and technical components.
  1. The academic component must emphasize a scholarly approach to clinical problem-solving, self-directed study, teaching, development of analytic skills and surgical judgment, and research.
  2. The technical component should ensure the ability of the fellow to perform skillfully the procedures required for practice of the subspecialty.

B. The program must offer supervised training in the operative and other technical skills integral to adult reconstructive orthopaedics. Instruction and experience must be sufficient for the fellow to understand the indications, risks, and limitations of the commonly performed procedures in the subspecialty.

C. Fellows must have the opportunity to provide consultation with faculty supervision and should have clearly defined educational responsibilities for residents, medical students, and allied health personnel. These teaching experiences should correlate basic biomedical knowledge with the clinical aspects of the subspecialty.

D. Clinical experience must include opportunities to observe and to manage patients with a variety of problems involving orthopaedic reconstruction on both an inpatient and outpatient basis, and the breadth of patient experience should include the evaluation and care of individuals through a wide range of ages, both sexes, and involve acute, subacute, and chronic conditions.

E. The educational curriculum must include opportunities for fellows to study anatomy, physiology, biomechanics, pathology, microbiology, pharmacology, and immunology as they relate to adult reconstructive orthopaedics.

F. The program must have regularly scheduled and held subspecialty conferences with active faculty and fellow participation.

G. The program must emphasize the diagnosis of clinical disorders of the bones, joints, and soft tissues; the pathogenesis of these disorders; the treatment modalities available for managing these disorders; and the results and complications of such treatment. Fellows must assume a major role in the continuing care of patients and have progressive responsibility in patient assessment, preoperative evaluation, operative experience, and postoperative management and rehabilitation.

H. The fellow must keep a record of the diagnosis and procedure for each operation in which he or she is an operating surgeon or first assistant. This must be kept on file and available for review.

I. The fellowship program must provide sufficient training to permit fellows to develop clinical competence in the field of adult reconstructive orthopaedics. Reconstructive principles may be broadly based or taught in a context of specific anatomic regions. Examples of knowledge and skills that are desirable include but are not limited to the following:
  1. The basic sciences related to adult reconstructive orthopaedics.
  2. The natural history of joint diseases.
  3. Prudent use of diagnostic laboratory tests.
  4. Interpretation of the radiographic and various imaging modality examination of the musculoskeletal system with an appreciation of the risk and information expected of the procedures.
  5. Development of a treatment plan to manage patients with traumatic, congenital and developmental, infectious, metabolic, degenerative, and rheumatologic disorders.
  6. Development of operative skills in reconstructive orthopaedics, including soft-tissue procedures, osteotomy, bone grafting, excisional arthroplasty, arthrodesis, and prosthetic arthroplasty.
  7. Recognition and management of complications of treatment.
  8. Assessment of the effectiveness of treatment methods.
  9. Sufficient familiarity with current research methods to enable the fellow to critically analyze research reports and to design and implement clinical or basic research in the field of adult reconstructive orthopaedics.
  10. Acquisition of teaching skills in adult reconstructive orthopaedics.

V. Program Research and Scholarly Activity

Graduate medical education must take place in an environment of inquiry and scholarship in which residents participate in the development of new knowledge, learn to evaluate research findings, and develop habits of inquiry as a continuing professional responsibility.

A. The responsibility for establishing and maintaining an environment of inquiry and scholarship rests with the teaching staff. While not all members of a teaching staff must be investigators, the staff as a whole must demonstrate broad involvement in scholarly activity. This activity should include:
  1. Active participation of the teaching staff in clinical discussions, rounds, and conferences in a manner that promotes a spirit of inquiry and scholarship. Scholarship implies an in-depth understanding of basic mechanisms of normal and abnormal states and the application of current knowledge to practice.
  2. Participation in journal clubs and research conferences.
  3. Active participation in regional or national professional and scientific societies, particularly through presentations at the organizations' meetings and publication in their journals.
  4. Participation in research, particularly in projects that are funded following peer review and/or result in publication or presentations at regional and national scientific meetings.
  5. Offering of guidance and technical support (eg, research design, statistical analysis) for residents involved in research.
  6. Provision of support for resident participation in scholarly activities.

B. Fellows must participate in basic and/or clinical research.
  1. Fellows must learn to design, implement, and interpret research studies under supervision by qualified faculty.
  2. The program must provide time and facilities for research activities by fellows.

VI. Library

1. Residents must have ready access to a major medical library, either at the institution where the residents are located or through arrangement with convenient nearby institutions.
2. Library services should include the electronic retrieval of information from medical databases.
3. There must be access to an on-site library or to a collection of appropriate texts and journals in each institution participating in a residency program. On-site libraries and/or collections of texts and journals must be readily available during nights and weekends.

VII. Evaluation

A. Program directors must have a clearly defined method for regular periodic assessment of the performance of the fellow. The assessment must include cognitive, motor, and interpersonal skills; attitudinal traits; and surgical judgment. There must be at least semiannual communication of this information to the fellow and to the director of the residency program in orthopaedic surgery.

B. The educational effectiveness of a program must be evaluated in a systematic manner. In particular, the quality of the curriculum and the extent to which the educational goals have been met by residents must be assessed. Written evaluations by residents should be utilized in this process.

ACGME: September 1989 Effective: July 1995

Program Requirements for Residency Education in Foot and Ankle Orthopaedics (Orthopaedic Surgery)

I. Introduction

A. Foot and ankle orthopaedics is a subspecialty of orthopaedic surgery that includes the in-depth study, prevention, and treatment of musculoskeletal diseases, disorders, and sequelae of injuries in this anatomic region by medical, physical, and surgical methods.

B. Programs in foot and ankle orthopaedics will be accredited to offer 1 year of postresidency education to individuals who have completed an Accreditation Council for Graduate Medical Education (ACGME)-accredited orthopaedic surgery residency.

C. Postgraduate fellowship education in orthopaedic surgery is a component in the continuum of the educational process, and such education will take place after completion of an accredited residency.

D. Postgraduate fellowship programs in the subspecialties of orthopaedic surgery may be accredited in institutions that sponsor accredited residency programs in orthopaedic surgery or that are affiliated with an ACGME-accredited orthopaedic surgery residency. Requests for exceptions to this policy will be reviewed on a case-by-case basis.

E. The director and teaching staff of a program must prepare and comply with written educational goals for the program. All educational components of a residency program should be related to program goals.

1. The program design and/or structure must be approved by the Residency Review Committee (RRC) as part of the regular review process.
2. Participation by any institution providing more than 2 months of training in a program must be approved by the RRC.

F. When orthopaedic residents and fellows are being educated in the same institution, the residency director and the director of the fellowship must jointly prepare and approve a written agreement specifying the educational relationship between the residency and fellowship programs, the roles of the residency and fellowship directors in determining the educational program of residents and fellows, and the roles of the residents and fellows in patient care.

II. Institutional Resources and Organization

A. Adequate facilities to support the overall educational program must be available and functioning. These include outpatient, inpatient, imaging, laboratory, rehabilitation, and research resources. Operating rooms must be adequately equipped for reconstructive surgery.

B. A sufficient number of new and follow-up patients must be available to ensure adequate inpatient and outpatient experience for each fellow without adversely diluting the educational experience of the orthopaedic surgery residents or the educational experience of residents in other specialties.

C. There should be broad support from other clinical subspecialties, including radiology, pathology, rheumatology, endocrinology, laboratory medicine, infectious disease, rehabilitation, and prosthetics and orthotics.

D. Programs must provide an intellectual environment for acquiring the knowledge, skills, clinical judgment, and attitudes essential to the practice of foot and ankle orthopaedics. This objective can be achieved only when the program director, the supporting faculty and staff, and the administration are fully committed to the educational program and when appropriate resources and facilities are present. Effective graduate education is not achieved when the educational program functions primarily to meet service commitments.

E. There must be close monitoring of the interface between residency and fellowship education. It is imperative that orthopaedic fellowship education not interfere with the education of residents. Lines of responsibility for the orthopaedic resident and the fellow must be clearly defined. In addition, the fellow should maintain a close working relationship with orthopaedic residents and other fellows in orthopaedic surgery and in other disciplines.

III. Program Personnel

The program director and the teaching staff are responsible for the general administration of a program, including those activities related to the recruitment, selection, instruction, supervision, counseling, evaluation, and advancement of residents and the maintenance of records related to program accreditation.

A. Program Director

The director of the subspecialty program and the director of the affiliated orthopaedic surgery program, in conjunction with the administration of the institution, will be responsible for ensuring that adequate facilities and other necessary resources are available to provide an education of high quality.

There must be a single program director responsible for the program.

1. Qualifications of the program director include:
   a. Requisite and documented clinical, educational, and administrative abilities and experience.
   b. Licensure to practice medicine in the state where the institution that sponsors the program is located. (Certain federal programs are exempted.)
   c. Certification by the American Board of Orthopaedic Surgery or suitable equivalent qualifications.
   d. Appointment in good standing to the medical staff of an institution participating in the program.
2. Responsibilities of the program director include:
   a. Preparation of a written statement outlining the educational goals of the program with respect to knowledge, skills, and other attributes of residents at each level of training and for each major rotation or other program assignment. This statement must be distributed to residents and members of the teaching staff. It should be readily available for review.

b. Selection of residents for appointment to the program in accordance with institutional and departmental policies and procedures.
c. Selection and supervision of the teaching staff and other program personnel at each institution participating in the program.
d. The supervision of residents in accordance with explicit written descriptions of supervisory lines of responsibility for the care of patients. Such guidelines must be communicated to all members of the program staff. Residents must be provided with prompt, reliable systems for communication and interaction with supervisory physicians.
e. Regular evaluation of residents' knowledge, skills, and overall performance, including the development of professional attitudes consistent with being a physician. The program director, with participation of members of the teaching staff, shall:
    1. At least semiannually evaluate the knowledge, skills, and professional growth of the residents, using appropriate criteria and procedures.
    2. Communicate each evaluation to the resident in a timely manner.
    3. Advance residents to positions of higher responsibility only on the basis of evidence of their satisfactory progressive scholarship and professional growth.
    4. Maintain a permanent record of evaluation for each resident and have it accessible to the resident and other authorized personnel.
f. The provision of a written final evaluation for each resident who completes the program. The evaluation must include a review of the resident's performance during the final period of training and should verify that the resident has demonstrated sufficient professional ability to practice competently and independently. This final evaluation should be part of the resident's permanent record maintained by the institution.
g. Fellowship directors must ensure that trainees are given reasonable duty and call assignments. It is desirable that fellows' work schedules be designed so that on average, excluding exceptional patient care needs, fellows have at least 1 day out of 7 free of routine responsibilities and be on call in the hospital no more often than every third night. Scheduling will necessitate flexibility, as fellows are at the postgraduate level, so the ratio of hours worked and on-call time may vary.
h. Implementation of fair procedures, as established by the sponsoring institution, regarding academic discipline and resident complaints or grievances.
i. Monitoring resident stress, including mental or emotional conditions inhibiting performance or learning and drug- or alcohol-related dysfunction. Program directors and teaching staff should be sensitive to the need for timely provision of confidential counseling and psychological support services to residents. Training situations that consistently produce undesirable stress on residents must be evaluated and modified.
j. Preparation of an accurate statistical and narrative description of the program as requested by the RRC.

B. Teaching Staff

1. There must be a sufficient number of teaching staff with documented qualifications to instruct and supervise adequately all the residents in the program. In addition to the program director, there must be at least one other orthopaedist who actively participates in the academic and clinical components of the program and regularly provides supervision and instruction of residents.
2. Members of the teaching staff must be able to devote sufficient time to meet their supervisory and teaching responsibilities.
3. All members of the teaching staff must demonstrate a strong interest in the education of residents, sound clinical and teaching abilities, support of the goals and objectives of the program, a commitment to their own continuing medical education, and participation in scholarly activities.
4. A member of the teaching staff of each participating institution must be designated to assume responsibility for the day-to-day activities of the program at that institution, with overall coordination by the program director.
5. The teaching staff must be organized and have regular documented meetings to review program goals and objectives as well as program effectiveness in achieving them. At least one resident representative should participate in these reviews.
6. The teaching staff should periodically evaluate the utilization of the resources available to the program, the contribution of each institution participating in the program, the financial and administrative support of the program, the volume and variety of patients available to the program for educational purposes, the performance of members of the teaching staff, and the quality of supervision of residents.

C. Other Program Personnel

Programs must be provided with the additional professional, technical, and clerical personnel needed to support the administration and educational conduct of the program.

IV. Educational Program

A. The educational program in foot and ankle orthopaedics may include the orthopaedic management and appropriate referral for the care of related disorders (eg, rheumatoid arthritis, neuromuscular disorders, and diabetes), as well as those disorders of the leg that may directly or indirectly affect the foot and ankle (eg, compartment syndrome, neuromuscular disease, malalignment of the leg, bone instability).
B. The educational program must be organized to provide advanced experience for residents to acquire the competency of a specialist in the field. Clinical experience must include opportunities to observe and to manage patients with a variety of problems involving orthopaedic repair of the foot and ankle on both an inpatient and an outpatient basis. The breadth of patient experience should include the evaluation and care of individuals through a wide range of ages and both sexes, and should involve acute, subacute, and chronic conditions.
C. A postgraduate fellowship program must provide sufficiently advanced education to allow the fellow to acquire special expertise in foot and ankle orthopaedics. This education must consist of academic and technical components. The academic component must emphasize a scholarly approach to clinical problem solving, self-directed study, teaching, development of analytic skills and surgical judgment, and research. The technical component should ensure the ability of the fellow to perform skillfully the procedures required for practice of foot and ankle orthopaedics.
D. Programs must provide supervised training in the operative and other technical skills integral to foot and ankle orthopaedics. Instruction and experience must be sufficient for the fellow to understand the indications, risks, and limitations of the commonly performed procedures in foot and ankle orthopaedics.
E. The educational curriculum must include the study of anatomy, physiology, biomechanics and gait, pathology, microbiology, pharmacology, and immunology as they relate to foot and ankle orthopaedics.
F. The program must have regularly held and attended subspecialty conferences, including at least one weekly teaching conference and a monthly morbidity-mortality conference, with active fac-

ulty and resident participation. A monthly journal club covering appropriate topics in foot and ankle surgery should be held.

G. The program must emphasize the diagnosis of clinical disorders of the bones, joints, and soft tissues of the foot and ankle. The pathogenesis of these disorders, the treatment modalities available, and the results and complications of such treatment should be emphasized.

H. Residents must assume a major role in the continuing care of patients and have progressive responsibility for patient assessment, decisions regarding treatment, preoperative evaluation, operative experience, nonoperative management, postoperative management, rehabilitation, long-term follow-up, and other outpatient care.

I. A fellow must have the opportunity to provide consultation with faculty supervision and should have clearly defined educational responsibilities for residents, medical students, and allied health personnel. These teaching experiences should correlate basic biomedical knowledge with the clinical aspects of foot and ankle orthopaedics.

J. Residents must keep a record of the diagnosis and procedure for each operation for which he or she is an operating room surgeon or first assistant. This must be kept on file and available for review.

K. The program must provide sufficient education to permit residents to develop clinical competence in the field of foot and ankle orthopaedics. Examples of knowledge and skills that are essential include but are not limited to:

1. The basic sciences related to foot and ankle orthopaedics.
2. The natural history of disease and disorders of the foot and ankle, including an understanding of the deformed, injured, or diseased pediatric foot.
3. Prudent use of diagnostic laboratory tests.
4. Interpretation of the radiographic examination of the musculoskeletal system, particularly the foot and ankle, with an understanding of the risk and information expected of these procedures.
5. Development of a treatment plan to manage patients with traumatic, congenital and developmental, infectious, metabolic, degenerative, neurologic, and rheumatologic disorders.
6. An understanding of the importance of the timing of orthopaedic procedures in the overall context of foot and ankle injuries.
7. Prevention and treatment methods for the management of bony and soft-tissue injuries of the foot and ankle, including the indications for various types of internal and external fixation devices and their applications to foot and ankle trauma.
8. Development of operative skills in reconstructive orthopaedics such as soft-tissue procedures, osteotomies, bone grafting, excisional arthroplasty, arthrodesis, and prosthetic arthroplasty.
9. Understanding of the dysvascular and neurologically impaired foot, including the neuropathic foot, and the indications for various amputation procedures of the foot and ankle.
10. Recognition and management of complications of treatment.
11. Assessment of the efficacy of treatment methods.
12. Sufficient familiarity with current research methods to enable the resident to critically analyze research reports and to design and implement clinical or basic research in the field of foot and ankle orthopaedics.
13. Recuperative and rehabilitation techniques including the use of physical and occupational therapy designed to return the patient to normal activities and work.
14. Understanding of prosthetics and orthotics pertaining to disorders of the foot, gait, and amputation.
15. Development of teaching skills, lecture techniques, and instructional materials in foot and ankle orthopaedics.

V. Program Research and Scholarly Activity

A. Graduate medical education must take place in an environment of inquiry and scholarship in which residents participate in the development of new knowledge, learn to evaluate research findings, and develop habits of inquiry as a continuing professional responsibility.

B. The responsibility for establishing and maintaining an environment of inquiry and scholarship rests with the teaching staff. While not all members of a teaching staff must be investigators, the staff as a whole must demonstrate broad involvement in scholarly activity. This activity should include:

1. Active participation of the teaching staff in clinical discussions, rounds, and conferences in a manner that promotes a spirit of inquiry and scholarship. Scholarship implies an in-depth understanding of basic mechanisms of normal and abnormal states and the application of current knowledge to practice.
2. Participation in journal clubs and research conferences.
3. Active participation in regional or national professional and scientific societies, particularly through presentations at the organizations' meetings and publication in their journals.
4. Participation in research, particularly in projects that are funded following peer review and/or result in publication or presentations at regional and national scientific meetings.
5. Offering of guidance and technical support (eg, research design, statistical analysis) for residents involved in research.
6. Provision of support for resident participation in scholarly activities.

C. All residents must participate in clinical or basic research, and this should culminate in the development and publication and/or presentation of an appropriate paper.

D. Fellows must learn to design, implement, and interpret research studies under supervision by qualified faculty, and the program must provide time and facilities for research activities by faculty and fellows.

VI. Library

1. Residents must have ready access to a major medical library, either at the institution where the residents are located or through arrangement with convenient nearby institutions.
2. Library services should include the electronic retrieval of information from medical databases.
3. There must be access to an on-site library or to a collection of appropriate texts and journals in each institution participating in a residency program. On-site libraries and/or collections of texts and journals must be readily available during nights and weekends.

VII. Evaluation

A. The educational effectiveness of a program must be evaluated in a systematic manner. In particular, the quality of the curriculum and the extent to which the educational goals have been met by residents must be assessed.

B. The program, the educational process, and its faculty, in respect to academic performance, should be evaluated at least every 2 or 3 years to see if goals and objectives are being met.

C. This review process must include direct observation and discussion of case management with the resident.

D. In order to ensure that residents meet the academic and clinical goals of the program, evaluation procedures must include:

1. Formal testing of residents' cognitive capabilities.

2. Systematic evaluation and documentation of residents' clinical abilities.
3. Evaluation of residents' interpersonal skills and attitudinal traits.

E. Formal review of residents by the program director and members of the teaching staff must include:
1. Written evaluation of the knowledge, skills, and professional growth of the residents, using appropriate criteria and procedures, at least once every 6 months.
2. Timely communication and review of the written evaluation to the resident.

F. Programs must maintain a permanent record of evaluation for each resident and have it accessible to the resident and other authorized personnel.

ACGME: September 1994 Effective: July 1995

Program Requirements for Residency Education in Hand Surgery (Orthopaedic Surgery)

I. Introduction

A. Definition of the Specialty

Hand surgery is a surgical subspecialty that deals with congenital and acquired defects of the hand and wrist that compromise the function of the hand. A hand surgery educational program is designed to educate physicians in the art and science of hand surgery and to develop a competent hand surgeon who is capable of independent function. The educational program should provide experience in the repair, resection, and reconstruction of defects of form and function of the hand; in the design, construction, and transfer of flaps and the transplantation of tissues, including microsurgery of multiple tissues; in replantation of upper extremity parts; in surgical and ancillary methods of treatment of tumors; in management of complex wounds; and in the use of alloplastic materials.

B. Scope of Education

1. Prerequisite resident education must be completed in a general surgery, orthopaedic surgery, or plastic surgery program accredited by the Accreditation Council for Graduate Medical Education (ACGME) or the Royal College of Physicians and Surgeons of Canada.
2. The length of the educational program is 1 year.

II. Institutional Organization

A. Sponsoring Institution

The educational program should have one sponsoring institution that has primary responsibility for the entire program. The sponsoring institution should provide sufficient faculty; financial resources; and clinical, research, and library facilities to meet the educational needs of the residents and to permit the program to comply with the requirements for accreditation.

B. Participating Institutions

1. When multiple institutions participate in the educational program, the commitment of each participating institution must be documented in a written agreement that complies with the ACGME Institutional Requirements.
2. Assignments to participating institutions must be based on an appropriate educational rationale. Assignments that dilute the education of residents or that do not provide proper supervision and coordination of educational activities should not be established or maintained.
3. Assignments to participating institutions that are geographically distant from the sponsoring institution are not desirable. To be justifiable, such assignments must offer special resources or opportunities not otherwise available to the program.
4. The number and location of participating institutions must not preclude the participation of residents and faculty in the educational activities of the hand surgery course of study.

C. Appointment of Residents

1. The total number of residents must be approved in advance by the Residency Review Committee (RRC). The number of residents shall be based primarily on the number, qualifications, and commitment of the faculty; the volume and variety of the patient population available for educational purposes; and the institutional resources committed to resident education.
2. Programs may not graduate more hand surgery residents in any given year than the number of residents approved by the RRC.
3. Any increase, including a temporary increase in resident complement, must receive prior approval of the RRC. Requests for changes in the approved resident complement of a program must include a strong educational rationale.

III. Faculty Qualifications and Responsibilities

The program director and the faculty are responsible for the general administration of a program, including those activities related to the recruitment, selection, instruction, supervision, counseling, evaluation, and advancement of residents and the maintenance of records related to program accreditation.

A. Program Director

A single program director must be responsible for the program.

1. Qualifications of the program director
   a. Requisite and documented clinical, educational, and administrative abilities and experience.
   b. Licensure to practice medicine in the state where the institution that sponsors the program is located.
   c. Certification by the appropriate ABMS Board or suitable equivalent qualifications in the appropriate specialty and a certificate of added qualifications in hand surgery or suitable equivalent qualifications in hand surgery. The RRC will determine the acceptability of equivalent qualifications.
   d. Appointment in good standing to the medical staff of an institution participating in the program.
   e. Frequent changes in leadership or long periods of temporary leadership are undesirable and may adversely affect the accreditation status of the program.
2. Responsibilities of the program director
   a. Prepare a written statement outlining the educational goals of the program with respect to knowledge, skills, and other attributes of hand surgery residents at each level of education and for each assignment. This statement must be distributed to hand surgery residents and members of the faculty. It should be readily available for review.
   b. Select residents for appointment to the program according to institutional and departmental policies and procedures.
   c. Select and supervise the faculty and other program personnel at each participating institution.
   d. Supervise residents through explicit written descriptions of supervisory lines of responsibility for the care of patients. Such guidelines must be communicated to all members of the faculty. Residents must be provided with prompt, reliable systems for communication and interaction with supervising physicians.

e. Regularly evaluate residents' knowledge, skills, and overall performance. The program director, with participation of the faculty, must
   1. at least quarterly, evaluate the progress of each hand surgery resident in writing, using appropriate criteria and procedures;
   2. communicate each evaluation to the resident in a timely manner;
   3. advance residents to positions of higher responsibility only on evidence of their satisfactory progressive scholarship and growth;
   4. maintain a permanent record of evaluation for each resident and have it accessible to the resident and other authorized personnel; and
   5. provide a final written evaluation to each hand surgery resident who completes the program. The evaluation must include a review of the resident's performance during the final period of education and should verify that the resident has demonstrated sufficient professional ability to practice competently and independently. Each evaluation should be signed by the resident and program director and be maintained on file by the program director for at least 5 years following completion of the program.
f. Implement fair procedures, as established by the sponsoring institution, regarding academic discipline and resident complaints or grievances.
g. Monitor resident stress, including mental or emotional conditions inhibiting performance or learning and drug- or alcohol-related dysfunction. Program directors and faculty should be sensitive to the need for timely provision of counseling and psychological support services to residents. Educational situations that consistently produce undesirable stress on residents must be evaluated and modified.
h. Prepare an accurate statistical and narrative description of the program, as requested by the RRC.
i. Ensure that each resident is provided with a sufficient educational program, including a sufficient volume and variety of operative experience and progressive surgical responsibility.
j. Annually collect, compile, and retain the number and types of hand surgery operative procedures performed in all institutions used for resident education. These data must be provided in the form and format specified by the RRC.
k. Annually collect, compile, and retain a comprehensive record of the operative procedures performed by each hand surgery resident completing the program. This information must be provided in the form and format specified by the RRC. This record must be signed by the hand surgery resident and the program director, attesting to its accuracy.
l. Advise applicants of the prerequisite requirements of the appropriate specialty board.
m. Document the satisfactory completion of prerequisite education before the resident begins the hand surgery program.
n. Notify the executive director of the RRC in writing of any major change in the program that significantly alters the educational experience for the residents, including
   1. changes in program leadership, to include any change in appointment of the program director, section or division head, or department chair, and
   2. changes in administrative structure that affect the status of the parent department in the institution.
o. Obtain prior RRC approval for the following changes in the program:
   1. the addition or deletion of any participating institution to which residents are assigned for a total of 2 months or longer;
   2. any change in the approved resident complement of the program; and
   3. any change in the length or format of the program.

B. Faculty

1. The hand surgery faculty must be certified by the one of the sponsoring boards, or possess suitable equivalent qualifications and be certified in hand surgery or possess suitable equivalent qualifications. The majority of the faculty must possess certificates of added qualifications in hand surgery. The RRC will determine the acceptability of equivalent qualifications.
2. There must be a sufficient number of qualified faculty to adequately instruct and supervise hand surgery residents to ensure optimal patient care and resident education. The faculty must be able to devote sufficient time to the program to meet their supervisory and teaching responsibilities.
3. The faculty must demonstrate a strong interest in the education of residents, sound clinical and teaching abilities, support of the goals and objectives of the program, a commitment to their own continuing medical education, and participation in scholarly activities.
4. A faculty member at each participating institution must be designated to assume responsibility for the day-to-day activities of the program at that institution, with overall coordination by the program director.
5. The faculty must be organized and have regular documented meetings to review program goals and objectives and program effectiveness in achieving these goals. The hand surgery resident should participate in these reviews.
6. The faculty should, at least annually, evaluate the utilization of the resources available to the program, the contribution of each institution participating in the program, the financial and administrative support of the program, the volume and variety of patients available to the program for educational purposes, the performance of the faculty, and the quality of resident supervision.

C. Scholarly Activity

Graduate medical education must take place in an environment of inquiry and scholarship in which residents participate in the development of new knowledge, learn to evaluate research findings, and develop habits of inquiry as a continuing professional responsibility. The responsibility for establishing and maintaining an environment of inquiry and scholarship rests with the faculty. While not all members of the faculty must be research investigators, the faculty as a whole must demonstrate broad involvement in scholarly activity. Scholarship is defined as an in-depth understanding of basic mechanisms of normal and abnormal states and the application of current knowledge to practice. This activity should include

1. participation in clinical discussions, rounds, and conferences in a manner that promotes a spirit of inquiry and scholarship;
2. participation in journal clubs and research conferences;
3. active participation in regional or national professional and scientific societies, particularly through presentations at the organizations' meetings and publication in their journals;
4. participation in research, particularly in projects funded following peer review and/or that result in publications or presentations at regional and national scientific meetings;
5. offering of guidance and technical support (eg, research design, statistical analysis) for residents involved in research; and
6. provision of support for resident participation in scholarly activities.

D. Other Program Personnel

Programs must be provided with the additional professional, technical, and clerical personnel needed to support the administration and educational conduct of the program.

IV. Facilities and Resources

A. Inpatient Facilities

1. Inpatient facilities should have a sufficient number of beds, support personnel, and proper equipment to ensure quality patient care and education.
2. Operating suite and diagnostic and treatment facilities must contain technologically current equipment.

B. Outpatient Facilities

Appropriately equipped outpatient facilities including support staff, operating suites, and clinic and office space must be available for resident participation in the preoperative evaluation, treatment, and postoperative follow-up of patients for whom the resident has responsibility.

C. Library Facilities

1. The residents must have ready access to a major medical library, either at the institution where the residents are located or through arrangement with convenient nearby institutions.
2. Library services should include the electronic retrieval of information from medical databases.

V. The Educational Program

A. Program Design

1. The program director and faculty must prepare and implement written educational goals for the program.
2. The program design and/or structure must be approved by the RRC as part of the regular review process.

B. Clinical Component

1. Residents must be provided with education in surgical design, surgical diagnosis, embryology, surgical and artistic anatomy, surgical physiology and pathology, pharmacology, wound healing, microbiology, adjunctive oncological therapy, biomechanics, rehabilitation, and surgical instrumentation.
2. A sufficient number and variety of adult and pediatric hand surgery patients must be available for resident education.
3. Generally equivalent and sufficient distribution of operative procedures among the residents in all categories of hand surgery must be demonstrated.
4. Residents should be provided with graduated and progressive patient management responsibility.
5. Because judgment and technical capability to achieve satisfactory surgical results are mandatory qualities for the hand surgeon, education should be provided in the following areas:
   a. Skin repair, including grafts and flaps, multiple tissue flaps, free microscopic tissue transfers, and insertion of tissue expanders
   b. Fingertip injuries
   c. Tendon repair, including flexor tendon repair and graft, implantation of tendon spacer, extensor tendon repair, and tenolysis/tenodesis
   d. Tendon transfer and tendon balancing
   e. Nerve repair, including major and digital, graft, neurolysis, surgical treatment of neuroma, transpositions, and nerve decompressions
   f. Management of fractures and dislocations, including phalangeal or metacarpal with and without internal fixation; wrist, radius, and ulna with and without internal fixation; and injuries to joint ligaments
   g. Bone grafts
   h. Joint and tendon sheath repairs, including release of contracture, synovectomy, arthroplasty with and without implant, arthrodesis, trigger finger release, and stiff joints that result from rheumatoid or other injury
   i. Pollicization or ray transfer
   j. Foot to hand transfer
   k. Tumors, benign and malignant
   l. Dupuytren's contracture
   m. Replantation, revascularization
   n. Amputations
   o. Fasciotomy, deep incision and drainage for infection, and wound débridement
   p. Congenital deformities, including syndactyly and others
   q. Management of upper extremity vascular disorders and insufficiencies
   r. Foreign body, implant removal
   s. Thermal injuries
   t. Arthroscopy
   u. Upper extremity pain management

C. Didactic Components

1. A comprehensive, organized course of study must be offered, to include educational conferences that are well defined, documented, and regularly held. At minimum, the program must provide a didactic component for clinical education referencing section V.B.1 of these Program Requirements for Residency Education in Hand Surgery.
2. The written course of study should reflect careful planning, with evidence of a cyclical presentation of core specialty knowledge supplemented by the addition of current information, including practice management, ethics, and medicolegal topics as they relate to hand surgery.

Conferences must include basic science subjects related to clinical surgery of the hand, such as anatomy, physiology, pathology, genetics, microbiology, and pharmacology. A periodic review of the morbidity and mortality experience of the service must be included.

3. A list of the conferences should be maintained and available for review at the time of the site visit.
4. Conferences should be attended by both the residents and the faculty, and such attendance should be documented.
5. Conferences should be organized by the faculty to ensure that sufficient educational experience is provided. Hand surgery residents assigned to participating institutions other than the sponsoring institution should attend the hand surgery conferences at those sites.
6. Residents should make presentations at conferences and actively participate in conference discussions. Adequate time for resident preparation should be permitted to maximize the educational experience.
7. Hand surgery residents should be encouraged to pursue clinical or basic science research interests.

D. Supervision

1. All patient care services must be supervised by qualified hand surgery faculty. The program director must ensure, direct, and document proper supervision of residents at all times.
2. Residents must be provided with rapid, reliable systems for communicating with faculty at all times.
3. Hand surgery residents may function as intermediate supervisors when documented prior experience makes it appropriate, but faculty supervision must be available.

E. Duty Hours
1. It is desirable that residents' work schedules be designed so that on the average, excluding exceptional patient care needs, residents have at least 1 day out of 7 free of routine responsibilities and be on call in the hospital no more often than every third night. The ratio of hours worked to on-call time will vary, particularly at senior levels, and flexibility will be necessary.
2. There must be adequate backup so that patient care is not jeopardized during or following assigned periods of duty.
3. Sufficient support services must be provided to ensure that residents are not required to spend excessive time in noneducational activities that can be discharged properly by other personnel.
4. The hand surgery residency is a full-time responsibility. Activities outside the educational program must not interfere with resident performance in the educational program as determined by the program director and must not interfere with resident opportunity for rest, relaxation, and study.

F. Appointment of Other Residents
1. The appointment of other residents for hand surgery education must not dilute or detract from the educational opportunities of hand surgery residents.
2. The appointment of other residents to the hand surgery service requires a clear statement of the areas of education, clinical responsibilities, and duration of the education. This statement must be supplied to the RRC at the time the program is reviewed.
3. If such residents so appointed will, in the judgment of the RRC, detract from the education of the hand surgery residents, the accreditation status of the program may be adversely affected.

VI. Evaluation
A. Resident Evaluation
The program director and faculty are responsible for regularly evaluating the residents' knowledge, skills, and overall performance, including the development of professional attitudes consistent with being a physician.

B. Faculty Evaluation
1. At least annually, all individual faculty members must be formally evaluated by the program director. Hand surgery residents should be provided with the opportunity to evaluate faculty.
2. A mechanism for sharing the results of such evaluations with the faculty that preserves resident confidentiality in the evaluation process must be employed.
3. The program should demonstrate that such evaluations are used in improving the program.

C. Program Evaluation
1. The educational effectiveness of a program must be evaluated at least annually. In particular, the quality of the curriculum and the extent to which the educational goals have been met by residents must be assessed. Written evaluations by hand surgery residents should be utilized in this process.
2. One measure of the quality of a program is the performance of its graduates on the examination for the certificate of added qualifications in hand surgery given by one of the sponsoring boards. The RRC may consider this information as part of the overall evaluation of the program.

VII. Board Certification
Residents who plan to seek hand surgery certification as administered by the American Board of Orthopaedic Surgery should communicate with the executive director of the board to ascertain the current requirements for acceptance as a candidate for certification.

ACGME: September 1997 Effective: July 1998

Program Requirements for Residency Education in Musculoskeletal Oncology (Orthopaedic Surgery)

I. Introduction
A. Postgraduate fellowship education in orthopaedic surgery is a component in the continuum of the educational process, and such education will take place after completion of an accredited residency. Graduate medical education programs in the subspecialties of orthopaedic surgery will be accredited to offer 12 months of education.

B. Postgraduate fellowship programs in the subspecialties of orthopaedic surgery may be accredited in institutions that sponsor accredited residency programs in orthopaedic surgery or that are affiliated with an Accreditation Council for Graduate Medical Education (ACGME)-accredited orthopaedic surgery residency. Requests for exceptions to this policy will be reviewed on a case-by-case basis.

C. When orthopaedic residents and fellows are being educated in the same institution, the residency director and the director of the fellowship must jointly prepare and approve a written agreement specifying the educational relationship between the residency and fellowship programs, the roles of the residency and fellowship directors in determining the educational program of residents and fellows, and the roles of the residents and fellows in patient care.

D. The director and teaching staff of a program must prepare and comply with written educational goals for the program. All educational components of a program should be related to program goals.
1. The program design and/or structure must be approved by the Residency Review Committee (RRC) as part of the regular review process.
2. Participation by any institution providing more than 2 months of training must be approved by the RRC.

II. Institutional Resources and Organization
A. Programs must provide an intellectual environment for acquiring the knowledge, skills, clinical judgment, and attitudes essential to the practice of musculoskeletal oncology. This objective can be achieved only when the program director, the supporting faculty and staff, and the administration are fully committed to the educational program and when appropriate resources and facilities are present. Effective graduate education is not achieved when the educational program functions primarily to meet service commitments.

B. A sufficient number of new and follow-up patients must be available to ensure adequate inpatient and outpatient experience for each fellow without adversely diluting the educational experience of the orthopaedic surgery residents or the educational experience of residents in other specialties.

C. There must be close monitoring of the interface between residency and fellowship education. It is imperative that orthopaedic fellowship education not interfere with the education of residents. Lines of responsibility for the orthopaedic resident and the fellow must be clearly defined. In addition, the fellow should maintain a close working relationship with orthopaedic residents and other fellows in orthopaedic surgery and in other disciplines.

D. There should be broad support from other clinical specialties, including diagnostic and therapeutic radiology, pediatrics, nuclear medicine, pathology, surgery and its subspecialties, and medical oncology. Support of oncologic nursing, rehabilitation, nutrition, dietetic, and social services, as well as physical and occupational rehabilitation, is desirable.

E. Modern facilities to accomplish the overall educational program must be available and functioning. These include inpatient ambulatory care and laboratory resources. Specifically, there should be advanced pathology services, including electron microscopy and immunopathology; resources for nuclear medical imaging, musculoskeletal angiography, and computed tomographic scanning; and sufficient facilities for qualitative correlative studies.

F. The fellow must have day-to-day access to pathologists and to radiologists with recognized expertise in musculoskeletal pathology and radiology.

G. On-site radiation and medical oncology facilities and a modern diagnostic radiologic service are necessary.

H. It is desirable that there be other clinical subspecialties of orthopaedic surgery and general surgery to which the orthopaedic oncology fellow may relate formally, as well as special facilities for musculoskeletal pathology.

I. There must be a minimum of 200 new cases of benign and malignant tumors with an appropriate mix of primary and metastatic lesions to afford the fellow adequate educational experience in musculoskeletal oncology. This experience must include the care of both inpatients and outpatients.

J. The program should include access to computer facilities and a teaching collection of slides, x-rays, and specimens that are appropriately indexed for easy retrieval.

III. Program Personnel

The program director and the teaching staff are responsible for the general administration of a program, including those activities related to the recruitment, selection, instruction, supervision, counseling, evaluation, and advancement of residents and the maintenance of records related to program accreditation.

A. Program Director

The director of the subspecialty program and the director of the affiliated orthopaedic surgery program, in conjunction with the administration of the institution, will be responsible for ensuring that adequate facilities and other necessary resources are available to provide an education of high quality.

There must be a single program director responsible for the program.

1. Qualifications of the program director include:
   a. Requisite and documented clinical, educational, and administrative abilities and experience.
   b. Licensure to practice medicine in the state where the institution that sponsors the program is located. (Certain federal programs are exempted.)
   c. Certification by the American Board of Orthopaedic Surgery or suitable equivalent qualifications.
   d. Appointment in good standing to the medical staff of an institution participating in the program.
2. Responsibilities of the program director include:
   a. Preparation of a written statement outlining the educational goals of the program with respect to knowledge, skills, and other attributes of residents at each level of training and for each major rotation or other program assignment. This statement must be distributed to residents and members of the teaching staff. It should be readily available for review.
   b. Selection of residents for appointment to the program in accordance with institutional and departmental policies and procedures.
   c. Selection and supervision of the teaching staff and other program personnel at each institution participating in the program.
   d. The supervision of residents in accordance with explicit written descriptions of supervisory lines of responsibility for the care of patients. Such guidelines must be communicated to all members of the program staff. Residents must be provided with prompt, reliable systems for communication and interaction with supervisory physicians.
   e. Regular evaluation of residents' knowledge, skills, and overall performance, including the development of professional attitudes consistent with being a physician. The program director, with participation of members of the teaching staff, shall:
      1. At least semiannually evaluate the knowledge, skills, and professional growth of the residents, using appropriate criteria and procedures.
      2. Communicate each evaluation to the resident in a timely manner.
      3. Advance residents to positions of higher responsibility only on the basis of evidence of their satisfactory progressive scholarship and professional growth.
      4. Maintain a permanent record of evaluation for each resident and have it accessible to the resident and other authorized personnel.
   f. The provision of a written final evaluation for each resident who completes the program. The evaluation must include a review of the resident's performance during the final period of training and should verify that the resident has demonstrated sufficient professional ability to practice competently and independently. This final evaluation should be part of the resident's permanent record maintained by the institution.
   g. Fellowship directors must ensure that trainees are given reasonable duty and call assignments. It is desirable that fellows' work schedules be designed so that on average, excluding exceptional patient care needs, fellows have at least 1 day out of 7 free of routine responsibilities and be on call in the hospital no more often than every third night. Scheduling will necessitate flexibility, as fellows are at the postgraduate level, so the ratio of hours worked and on-call time may vary.
   h. Implementation of fair procedures, as established by the sponsoring institution, regarding academic discipline and resident complaints or grievances.
   i. Monitoring resident stress, including mental or emotional conditions inhibiting performance or learning and drug- or alcohol-related dysfunction. Program directors and teaching staff should be sensitive to the need for timely provision of confidential counseling and psychological support services to residents. Training situations that consistently produce undesirable stress on residents must be evaluated and modified.
   j. Preparation of an accurate statistical and narrative description of the program as requested by the RRC.

B. Teaching Staff

1. There must be a sufficient number of teaching staff with documented qualifications to instruct and supervise adequately all the residents in the program.
2. Members of the teaching staff must be able to devote sufficient time to meet their supervisory and teaching responsibilities.
3. All members of the teaching staff must demonstrate a strong interest in the education of residents, sound clinical and teaching

abilities, support of the goals and objectives of the program, a commitment to their own continuing medical education, and participation in scholarly activities.

4. A member of the teaching staff of each participating institution must be designated to assume responsibility for the day-to-day activities of the program at that institution, with overall coordination by the program director.
5. The teaching staff must be organized and have regular documented meetings to review program goals and objectives as well as program effectiveness in achieving them. At least one resident representative should participate in these reviews.
6. The teaching staff should periodically evaluate the utilization of the resources available to the program, the contribution of each institution participating in the program, the financial and administrative support of the program, the volume and variety of patients available to the program for educational purposes, the performance of members of the teaching staff, and the quality of supervision of residents.

C. Other Program Personnel

Programs must be provided with the additional professional, technical, and clerical personnel needed to support the administration and educational conduct of the program.

IV. Educational Program

A. The fellowship must provide sufficiently advanced education to allow the fellow to acquire the expertise of a specialist in musculoskeletal oncology. This education must consist of academic and technical components.
   1. The academic component must emphasize a scholarly approach to clinical problem solving, self-directed study, teaching, development of analytic skills and surgical judgment, and research.
   2. The technical component should ensure the ability of the fellow to perform skillfully the procedures required for practice of the subspecialty.

B. The program must offer supervised training in the operative and other technical skills integral to musculoskeletal oncology. Instruction and experience must be sufficient for the fellow to understand the indications, risks, and limitations of the commonly performed procedures in the subspecialty.

C. Fellows must have the opportunity to provide consultation with faculty supervision and should have clearly defined educational responsibilities for residents, medical students, and allied health personnel. These teaching experiences should correlate basic biomedical knowledge with the clinical aspects of the subspecialty.

D. The educational program in musculoskeletal oncology must be organized to provide experience at a sufficient level for the fellow to acquire the competency of a specialist in the field. Clinical experience must include opportunities to observe and to manage patients with a wide variety of clinical orthopaedic oncologic problems on both an inpatient and an outpatient basis.

E. The fellow must be given an opportunity to assume continuing responsibility for both acutely and chronically ill patients to learn the natural history of musculoskeletal neoplasia as well as the effectiveness of therapeutic programs.

F. There should be a weekly multidisciplinary tumor conference involving radiation and medical oncologists, a weekly pathology conference, and ongoing prospective protocol studies.

G. The educational curriculum must include sufficient material to ensure that the fellow acquires basic knowledge in surgical oncology, radiation therapy, and chemotherapy.

H. The program must provide training to develop clinical competence in the overall field of musculoskeletal oncology. Examples of knowledge and skill that are desirable include but are not limited to the following:
   1. The natural history of musculoskeletal neoplasia
   2. Knowledge of musculoskeletal surgical pathology
   3. Management of treatment protocols
   4. Knowledge of the indications for and limitations of surgery, radiation therapy, and chemotherapy in the treatment of musculoskeletal neoplasms
   5. Knowledge of the methodology and techniques to perform creditable clinical and/or basic research in musculoskeletal oncology
   6. Acquisition of teaching skills in musculoskeletal pathology and oncology

V. Program Research and Scholarly Activity

A. Graduate medical education must take place in an environment of inquiry and scholarship in which residents participate in the development of new knowledge, learn to evaluate research findings, and develop habits of inquiry as a continuing professional responsibility.

B. The responsibility for establishing and maintaining an environment of inquiry and scholarship rests with the teaching staff. While not all members of a teaching staff must be investigators, the staff as a whole must demonstrate broad involvement in scholarly activity. This activity should include:
   1. Active participation of the teaching staff in clinical discussions, rounds, and conferences in a manner that promotes a spirit of inquiry and scholarship. Scholarship implies an in-depth understanding of basic mechanisms of normal and abnormal states and the application of current knowledge to practice.
   2. Participation in journal clubs and research conferences.
   3. Active participation in regional or national professional and scientific societies, particularly through presentations at the organizations' meetings and publication in their journals.
   4. Participation in research, particularly in projects that are funded following peer review and/or result in publication or presentations at regional and national scientific meetings.
   5. Offering of guidance and technical support (eg, research design, statistical analysis) for residents involved in research.
   6. Provision of support for resident participation in scholarly activities.

C. Fellows must participate in basic and/or clinical research.
   1. Fellows must learn to design, implement, and interpret research studies under supervision by qualified faculty.
   2. The program must provide time and facilities for research activities by fellows.

VI. Library

1. Residents must have ready access to a major medical library, either at the institution where the residents are located or through arrangement with convenient nearby institutions.
2. Library services should include the electronic retrieval of information from medical databases.
3. There must be access to an on-site library or to a collection of appropriate texts and journals in each institution participating in a residency program. On-site libraries and/or collections of texts and journals must be readily available during nights and weekends.

VII. Evaluation

A. Program directors must have a clearly defined method for regular periodic assessment of the performance of the fellow. The assessment must include cognitive, motor, and interpersonal skills; attitudinal traits; and surgical judgment. There must be at least semiannual communication of this information to the fellow and to the director of the residency program in orthopaedic surgery.

B. The educational effectiveness of a program must be evaluated in a systematic manner. In particular, the quality of the curriculum and the extent to which the educational goals have been met by residents must be assessed. Written evaluations by residents should be utilized in this process.

ACGME: June 1986 Effective: July 1995

Program Requirements for Residency Education in Orthopaedic Sports Medicine (Orthopaedic Surgery)

I. Introduction

A. Postgraduate fellowship education in orthopaedic surgery is a component in the continuum of the educational process, and such education will take place after completion of an accredited residency. Graduate medical education programs in the subspecialties of orthopaedic surgery will be accredited to offer 12 months of education.

B. Postgraduate fellowship programs in the subspecialties of orthopaedic surgery may be accredited in institutions that sponsor accredited residency programs in orthopaedic surgery or that are affiliated with an Accreditation Council for Graduate Medical Education (ACGME)-accredited orthopaedic surgery residency. Requests for exceptions to this policy will be reviewed on a case-by-case basis.

C. When orthopaedic residents and fellows are being educated in the same institution, the residency director and the director of the fellowship must jointly prepare and approve a written agreement specifying the educational relationship between the residency and fellowship programs, the roles of the residency and fellowship directors in determining the educational program of residents and fellows, and the roles of the residents and fellows in patient care.

D. The director and teaching staff of a program must prepare and comply with written educational goals for the program. All educational components of a program should be related to program goals.
   1. The program design and/or structure must be approved by the Residency Review Committee (RRC) as part of the regular review process.
   2. Participation by any institution providing more than 2 months of training must be approved by the RRC.

II. Institutional Resources and Organization

A. Programs must provide an intellectual environment for acquiring the knowledge, skills, clinical judgment, and attitudes essential to the practice of orthopaedic sports medicine. This objective can be achieved only when the program director, the supporting faculty and staff, and the administration are fully committed to the educational program and when appropriate resources and facilities are present. Effective graduate education is not achieved when the educational program functions primarily to meet service commitments.

B. A sufficient number of new and follow-up patients must be available to ensure adequate inpatient and outpatient experience for each fellow without adversely diluting the educational experience of the orthopaedic surgery residents or the educational experience of residents in other specialties.

C. There must be close monitoring of the interface between residency and fellowship education. It is imperative that orthopaedic fellowship education not interfere with the education of residents. Lines of responsibility for the orthopaedic resident and the fellow must be clearly defined. In addition, the fellow should maintain a close working relationship with orthopaedic residents and other fellows in orthopaedic surgery and in other disciplines.

D. Facilities to accomplish the clinical and educational objectives of the specialty must be available and functioning for both inpatients and outpatients.
   1. The physical therapy and the athletic training departments must be completely equipped with the modern therapeutic modalities used in the treatment of the injured athlete.
   2. The operating room facilities must contain modern equipment, including arthroscopes, adjunctive equipment for arthroscopy, and necessary radiologic equipment.

E. The educational program must be conducted in a setting that will allow interaction with the disciplines of radiology, physical therapy, internal medicine, and such other specialties ordinarily encountered in sports medicine.

III. Program Personnel

The program director and the teaching staff are responsible for the general administration of a program, including those activities related to the recruitment, selection, instruction, supervision, counseling, evaluation, and advancement of residents and the maintenance of records related to program accreditation.

A. Program Director

The director of the subspecialty program and the director of the affiliated orthopaedic surgery program, in conjunction with the administration of the institution, will be responsible for ensuring that adequate facilities and other necessary resources are available to provide an education of high quality.

There must be a single program director responsible for the program.

1. Qualifications of the program director include:
   a. Requisite and documented clinical, educational, and administrative abilities and experience.
   b. Licensure to practice medicine in the state where the institution that sponsors the program is located. (Certain federal programs are exempted.)
   c. Certification by the American Board of Orthopaedic Surgery or suitable equivalent qualifications.
   d. Appointment in good standing to the medical staff of an institution participating in the program.
2. Responsibilities of the program director include:
   a. Preparation of a written statement outlining the educational goals of the program with respect to knowledge, skills, and other attributes of residents at each level of training and for each major rotation or other program assignment. This statement must be distributed to residents and members of the teaching staff. It should be readily available for review.
   b. Selection of residents for appointment to the program in accordance with institutional and departmental policies and procedures.
   c. Selection and supervision of the teaching staff and other program personnel at each institution participating in the program.
   d. The supervision of residents in accordance with explicit written descriptions of supervisory lines of responsibility for the care of patients. Such guidelines must be communicated to all members of the program staff. Residents must be provided

with prompt, reliable systems for communication and interaction with supervisory physicians.

e. Regular evaluation of residents' knowledge, skills, and overall performance, including the development of professional attitudes consistent with being a physician. The program director, with participation of members of the teaching staff, shall:
   1. At least semiannually evaluate the knowledge, skills, and professional growth of the residents, using appropriate criteria and procedures.
   2. Communicate each evaluation to the resident in a timely manner.
   3. Advance residents to positions of higher responsibility only on the basis of evidence of their satisfactory progressive scholarship and professional growth.
   4. Maintain a permanent record of evaluation for each resident and have it accessible to the resident and other authorized personnel.

f. The provision of a written final evaluation for each resident who completes the program. The evaluation must include a review of the resident's performance during the final period of training and should verify that the resident has demonstrated sufficient professional ability to practice competently and independently. This final evaluation should be part of the resident's permanent record maintained by the institution.

g. Fellowship directors must ensure that trainees are given reasonable duty and call assignments. It is desirable that fellows' work schedules be designed so that on average, excluding exceptional patient care needs, fellows have at least 1 day out of 7 free of routine responsibilities and be on call in the hospital no more often than every third night. Scheduling will necessitate flexibility, as fellows are at the postgraduate level, so the ratio of hours worked and on-call time may vary.

h. Implementation of fair procedures as established by the sponsoring institution regarding academic discipline and resident complaints or grievances.

i. Monitoring resident stress, including mental or emotional conditions inhibiting performance or learning and drug- or alcohol-related dysfunction. Program directors and teaching staff should be sensitive to the need for timely provision of confidential counseling and psychological support services to residents. Training situations that consistently produce undesirable stress on residents must be evaluated and modified.

j. Preparation of an accurate statistical and narrative description of the program as requested by the RRC.

B. Teaching Staff

1. There must be a sufficient number of teaching staff with documented qualifications to instruct and supervise adequately all the residents in the program.
2. Members of the teaching staff must be able to devote sufficient time to meet their supervisory and teaching responsibilities.
3. All members of the teaching staff must demonstrate a strong interest in the education of residents, sound clinical and teaching abilities, support of the goals and objectives of the program, a commitment to their own continuing medical education, and participation in scholarly activities.
4. A member of the teaching staff of each participating institution must be designated to assume responsibility for the day-to-day activities of the program at that institution, with overall coordination by the program director.
5. The teaching staff must be organized and have regular documented meetings to review program goals and objectives as well as program effectiveness in achieving them. At least one resident representative should participate in these reviews.
6. The teaching staff should periodically evaluate the utilization of the resources available to the program, the contribution of each institution participating in the program, the financial and administrative support of the program, the volume and variety of patients available to the program for educational purposes, the performance of members of the teaching staff, and the quality of supervision of residents.

C. Other Program Personnel

Programs must be provided with the additional professional, technical, and clerical personnel needed to support the administration and educational conduct of the program.

IV. Educational Program

A. The fellowship must provide sufficiently advanced education to allow the fellow to acquire the expertise of a specialist in orthopaedic sports medicine. This education must consist of academic and technical components.
   1. The academic component must emphasize a scholarly approach to clinical problem solving, self-directed study, teaching, development of analytic skills and surgical judgment, and research.
   2. The technical component should ensure the ability of the fellow to perform skillfully the procedures required for practice of the subspecialty.

B. The program must offer supervised training in the operative and other technical skills integral to orthopaedic sports medicine. Instruction and experience must be sufficient for the fellow to understand the indications, risks, and limitations of the commonly performed procedures in the subspecialty.

C. Fellows must have the opportunity to provide consultation with faculty supervision and should have clearly defined educational responsibilities for residents, medical students, and allied health personnel. These teaching experiences should correlate basic biomedical knowledge with the clinical aspects of the subspecialty.

D. Clinical experience must include inpatient and outpatient opportunities to observe, manage, operate, and follow patients with a wide variety of sports medicine problems.

E. The program must be structured to provide the fellow with an opportunity to assume continuing responsibility with appropriate supervision for patients with acute and chronic injuries and to observe the natural course of athletic injuries and the effects of various therapeutic modalities on their outcome.

F. The program should provide the fellow with the opportunity to work with athletic teams and/or athletic organizations.

G. The program must emphasize the pathology and biomechanics of athletic injuries and the effects of injury on the athlete, including both physical and psychological manifestations. Appropriate utilization of laboratory tests, physical modalities, and operative procedures for the diagnosis and treatment of athletic injuries must be stressed.

H. The program must provide the fellow with specific experience with athletic trainers and physical therapists and with related experience in writing appropriate prescriptions and in monitoring patient progress.

I. The program must provide sufficient opportunity for the fellow to gain knowledge and skill in a number of areas that include but are not limited to:
   1. Taking a history and performing an appropriate physical examination for orthopaedic sports injuries.
   2. Exposure to patients with typical histories and physical findings of chronic orthopaedic sports injuries and the management of those injuries.

3. Differentiating between those sports injuries that require immediate surgical treatment and those that can be treated nonoperatively.
4. Recognizing those sports injuries for which a minor delay in treatment would not be deleterious to the patient.
5. Acute care of orthopaedic and other acute sports medicine injuries that may occur during athletic competition and how to deal with those injuries on the athletic field.
6. How to order and interpret radiologic examinations that are used for diagnosis of sports injuries, including specific views, tomograms, bone scans, arthrograms, computerized axial tomography scans, and magnetic resonance imaging.
7. Therapeutic modalities offered in the department of physical therapy, how to use them, and how to judge the appropriateness and efficacy of a treatment plan.
8. Diagnostic and operative arthroscopy.
9. Nonorthopaedic problems that occur in sports medicine and how to deal with those problems or how to refer them appropriately.
10. The psychological effect of injuries on athletes and how to deal with them or how to select consultants to assist in their management.
11. Sports equipment, particularly protective devices intended to allow the athlete to continue to compete, including helmets, protective pads, knee braces, foot orthotics, and others not specifically named.

V. Program Research and Scholarly Activity

A. Graduate medical education must take place in an environment of inquiry and scholarship in which residents participate in the development of new knowledge, learn to evaluate research findings, and develop habits of inquiry as a continuing professional responsibility.

B. The responsibility for establishing and maintaining an environment of inquiry and scholarship rests with the teaching staff. While not all members of a teaching staff must be investigators, the staff as a whole must demonstrate broad involvement in scholarly activity. This activity should include:

1. Active participation of the teaching staff in clinical discussions, rounds, and conferences in a manner that promotes a spirit of inquiry and scholarship. Scholarship implies an in-depth understanding of basic mechanisms of normal and abnormal states and the application of current knowledge to practice.
2. Participation in journal clubs and research conferences.
3. Active participation in regional or national professional and scientific societies, particularly through presentations at the organizations' meetings and publication in their journals.
4. Participation in research, particularly in projects that are funded following peer review and/or result in publication or presentations at regional and national scientific meetings.
5. Offering of guidance and technical support (eg, research design, statistical analysis) for residents involved in research.
6. Provision of support for resident participation in scholarly activities.

C. Fellows must participate in basic and/or clinical research.

1. Fellows must learn to design, implement, and interpret research studies under supervision by qualified faculty.
2. The program must provide time and facilities for research activities by fellows.

VI. Library

1. Residents must have ready access to a major medical library, either at the institution where the residents are located or through arrangement with convenient nearby institutions.
2. Library services should include the electronic retrieval of information from medical databases.
3. There must be access to an on-site library or to a collection of appropriate texts and journals in each institution participating in a residency program. On-site libraries and/or collections of texts and journals must be readily available during nights and weekends.

VII. Evaluation

A. Program directors must have a clearly defined method for regular periodic assessment of the performance of the fellow. The assessment must include cognitive, motor, and interpersonal skills; attitudinal traits; and surgical judgment. There must be at least semiannual communication of this information to the fellow and to the director of the residency program in orthopaedic surgery.

B. The educational effectiveness of a program must be evaluated in a systematic manner. In particular, the quality of the curriculum and the extent to which the educational goals have been met by residents must be assessed. Written evaluations by residents should be utilized in this process.

ACGME: June 1986 Effective: July 1995

Program Requirements for Residency Education in Orthopaedic Surgery of the Spine (Orthopaedic Surgery)

I. Introduction

A. Subspecialty training in orthopaedic spine surgery includes the in-depth study, prevention, and treatment of spinal column diseases, disorders, and injuries by medical, physical, and surgical methods. The educational program of a fellowship in orthopaedic surgery of the spine must be organized to provide sufficient experience for a fellow to acquire the competency of a specialist in the field.

B. Postgraduate fellowship education in orthopaedic surgery is a component in the continuum of the educational process, and such education will take place after completion of an accredited residency. Graduate medical education programs in the subspecialties of orthopaedic surgery will be accredited to offer 12 months of education.

C. Postgraduate fellowship programs in the subspecialties of orthopaedic surgery may be accredited in institutions that sponsor accredited residency programs in orthopaedic surgery or that are affiliated with an Accreditation Council for Graduate Medical Education (ACGME)-accredited orthopaedic surgery residency. Requests for exceptions to this policy will be reviewed on a case-by-case basis.

D. When orthopaedic residents and fellows are being educated in the same institution, the residency director and the director of the fellowship must jointly prepare and approve a written agreement specifying the educational relationship between the residency and fellowship programs, the roles of the residency and fellowship directors in determining the educational program of residents and fellows, and the roles of the residents and fellows in patient care.

E. The director and teaching staff of a program must prepare and comply with written educational goals for the program. All educational components of a program should be related to program goals.

1. The program design and/or structure must be approved by the Residency Review Committee (RRC) as part of the regular review process.
2. Participation by any institution providing more than 2 months of training must be approved by the RRC.

II. Institutional Resources and Organization

A. Programs must provide an intellectual environment for acquiring the knowledge, skills, clinical judgment, and attitudes essential to the practice of spine surgery. This objective can be achieved only when the program director, the supporting faculty and staff, and the administration are fully committed to the educational program and when appropriate resources and facilities are present. Effective graduate education is not achieved when the educational program functions primarily to meet service commitments.

B. A sufficient number of new and follow-up patients must be available to ensure adequate inpatient and outpatient experience for each fellow without adversely diluting the educational experience of the orthopaedic surgery residents or the educational experience of residents in other specialties.

C. There must be close monitoring of the interface between residency and fellowship education. It is imperative that orthopaedic fellowship education not interfere with the education of residents. Lines of responsibility for the orthopaedic resident and the fellow must be clearly defined. In addition, the fellow should maintain a close working relationship with orthopaedic residents and other fellows in orthopaedic surgery and in other disciplines.

D. Facilities and equipment to support the overall educational program must be readily available and functioning. These include outpatient, inpatient, imaging, laboratory, rehabilitation, and research resources. Operating rooms must be state of the art and contain modern equipment for surgery of the spine.

E. Institutions sponsoring programs in orthopaedic surgery of the spine should also have an ACGME-accredited residency in neurological surgery. The educational program must involve close cooperation with neurological surgery and should maintain close collegial relationships with related clinical specialties including but not limited to physical medicine and rehabilitation, neurology, radiology, pathology, laboratory medicine, anesthesiology, and infectious disease. Exceptions to this standard will be considered on a case-by-case basis and will require justification based on sound educational principles, as well as demonstration of substantial compliance with the intent of this requirement.

III. Program Personnel

The program director and the teaching staff are responsible for the general administration of a program, including those activities related to the recruitment, selection, instruction, supervision, counseling, evaluation, and advancement of residents and the maintenance of records related to program accreditation.

A. Program Director

The director of the subspecialty program and the director of the affiliated orthopaedic surgery program, in conjunction with the administration of the institution, will be responsible for ensuring that adequate facilities and other necessary resources are available to provide an education of high quality.

There must be a single program director responsible for the program.

1. Qualifications of the program director include:
   a. Requisite and documented clinical, educational, and administrative abilities and experience.
   b. Licensure to practice medicine in the state where the institution that sponsors the program is located. (Certain federal programs are exempted.)
   c. Certification by the American Board of Orthopaedic Surgery or suitable equivalent qualifications.
   d. Appointment in good standing to the medical staff of an institution participating in the program.
2. Responsibilities of the program director include:
   a. Preparation of a written statement outlining the educational goals of the program with respect to knowledge, skills, and other attributes of residents at each level of training and for each major rotation or other program assignment. This statement must be distributed to residents and members of the teaching staff. It should be readily available for review.
   b. Selection of residents for appointment to the program in accordance with institutional and departmental policies and procedures.
   c. Selection and supervision of the teaching staff and other program personnel at each institution participating in the program.
   d. The supervision of residents in accordance with explicit written descriptions of supervisory lines of responsibility for the care of patients. Such guidelines must be communicated to all members of the program staff. Residents must be provided with prompt, reliable systems for communication and interaction with supervisory physicians.
   e. Regular evaluation of residents' knowledge, skills, and overall performance, including the development of professional attitudes consistent with being a physician. The program director, with participation of members of the teaching staff, shall:
      1. At least semiannually evaluate the knowledge, skills, and professional growth of the residents, using appropriate criteria and procedures.
      2. Communicate each evaluation to the resident in a timely manner.
      3. Advance residents to positions of higher responsibility only on the basis of evidence of their satisfactory progressive scholarship and professional growth.
      4. Maintain a permanent record of evaluation for each resident and have it accessible to the resident and other authorized personnel.
   f. The provision of a written final evaluation for each resident who completes the program. The evaluation must include a review of the resident's performance during the final period of training and should verify that the resident has demonstrated sufficient professional ability to practice competently and independently. This final evaluation should be part of the resident's permanent record maintained by the institution.
   g. Fellowship directors must ensure that trainees are given reasonable duty and call assignments. It is desirable that fellows' work schedules be designed so that on average, excluding exceptional patient care needs, fellows have at least 1 day out of 7 free of routine responsibilities and be on call in the hospital no more often than every third night. Scheduling will necessitate flexibility, as fellows are at the postgraduate level, so the ratio of hours worked and on-call time may vary.
   h. Implementation of fair procedures, as established by the sponsoring institution, regarding academic discipline and resident complaints or grievances.
   i. Monitoring resident stress, including mental or emotional conditions inhibiting performance or learning and drug- or alcohol-related dysfunction. Program directors and teaching staff should be sensitive to the need for timely provision of confidential counseling and psychological support services to residents.

Training situations that consistently produce undesirable stress on residents must be evaluated and modified.

j. Preparation of an accurate statistical and narrative description of the program as requested by the RRC.

B. Teaching Staff

1. There must be a sufficient number of teaching staff with documented qualifications to instruct and supervise adequately all the residents in the program.
2. Members of the teaching staff must be able to devote sufficient time to meet their supervisory and teaching responsibilities.
3. All members of the teaching staff must demonstrate a strong interest in the education of residents, sound clinical and teaching abilities, support of the goals and objectives of the program, a commitment to their own continuing medical education, and participation in scholarly activities.
4. A member of the teaching staff of each participating institution must be designated to assume responsibility for the day-to-day activities of the program at that institution, with overall coordination by the program director.
5. The teaching staff must be organized and have regular documented meetings to review program goals and objectives as well as program effectiveness in achieving them. At least one resident representative should participate in these reviews.
6. The teaching staff should periodically evaluate the utilization of the resources available to the program, the contribution of each institution participating in the program, the financial and administrative support of the program, the volume and variety of patients available to the program for educational purposes, the performance of members of the teaching staff, and the quality of supervision of residents.

C. Other Program Personnel

Programs must be provided with the additional professional, technical, and clerical personnel needed to support the administration and educational conduct of the program.

IV. Educational Program

A. The fellowship must provide sufficiently advanced education to allow the fellow to acquire the expertise of a specialist in orthopaedic surgery of the spine. This education must consist of academic and technical components.
   1. The academic component must emphasize a scholarly approach to clinical problem solving, self-directed study, teaching, development of analytic skills and surgical judgment, and research.
   2. The technical component should ensure the ability of the fellow to perform skillfully the procedures required for practice of the subspecialty.

B. The program must offer supervised training in the operative and other technical skills integral to orthopaedic surgery of the spine. Instruction and experience must be sufficient for the fellow to understand the indications, risks, and limitations of the commonly performed procedures in the subspecialty.

C. Fellows must have the opportunity to provide consultation with faculty supervision and should have clearly defined educational responsibilities for residents, medical students, and allied health personnel. These teaching experiences should correlate basic biomedical knowledge with the clinical aspects of the subspecialty.

D. The fellows' clinical experience must include opportunities to observe and manage patients on both an inpatient and an outpatient basis as well as for the evaluation and care of individuals through a wide range of ages and of both sexes, and with a wide variety of problems in various spinal regions.

E. The educational curriculum must include anatomy, physiology, biomechanics, microbiology, pathology, and other sciences as they relate to orthopaedic surgery of the spine.

F. The program must have regularly scheduled and held subspecialty conferences with active faculty and fellow participation.

G. The program must emphasize the diagnosis of clinical disorders of the spine, the pathogenesis of these disorders, the operative and nonoperative treatment modalities available for managing these disorders, and the results and complications of such treatment.

H. The educational program will not include experience in the treatment of intradural pathology. When spinal disease or injury and neurological deficit coexist, the educational program will ensure appropriate interdisciplinary cooperation with neurological surgery and rehabilitation medicine. The program structure must ensure that the fellow plays a major role and has progressive responsibility in the assessment, preoperative evaluation, surgical care, and postoperative management and rehabilitation of patients. There must be an opportunity for continuing evaluation of treated patients.

I. Fellows must maintain a record of the diagnosis and procedure for each operation in which they are an operating surgeon or first assistant that is available for review by the RRC and its site visitors.

J. Fellows must have the opportunity to develop clinical competence in the field of orthopaedic surgery of the spine. Principles may be broadly based or taught in a context of specific anatomic regions. Examples of knowledge and skills that are essential include but are not limited to:
   1. The basic sciences related to the musculoskeletal system.
   2. The natural history of spinal degeneration.
   3. The ability to assess clinically the neurologic function of the spinal cord and nerve roots.
   4. Prudent use of diagnostic laboratory tests (including electrophysiologic monitoring).
   5. Indications for and interpretation of imaging studies of the spine, including an appreciation of the risk and information expected of the procedures.
   6. Development of a treatment plan to manage patients with traumatic, congenital, developmental, infectious, metabolic, degenerative, and rheumatologic disorders of the spine.
   7. Development of operative skills for the management of patients with orthopaedic disorders of the spine.
   8. Recognition and management of complications of treatment (including appropriate consultations with subspecialists).
   9. Assessment of the effectiveness of diagnostic and treatment methods.
   10. Familiarity with currently used research methods.
   11. Acquisition of teaching skills in evaluation and care of spinal problems.

V. Program Research and Scholarly Activity

A. Graduate medical education must take place in an environment of inquiry and scholarship, in which residents participate in the development of new knowledge, learn to evaluate research findings, and develop habits of inquiry as a continuing professional responsibility.

B. The responsibility for establishing and maintaining an environment of inquiry and scholarship rests with the teaching staff. While not all members of a teaching staff must be investigators, the staff as a whole must demonstrate broad involvement in scholarly activity. This activity should include:
   1. Active participation of the teaching staff in clinical discussions, rounds, and conferences in a manner that promotes a spirit of inquiry and scholarship. Scholarship implies an in-depth un-

derstanding of basic mechanisms of normal and abnormal states and the application of current knowledge to practice.
2. Participation in journal clubs and research conferences.
3. Active participation in regional or national professional and scientific societies, particularly through presentations at the organizations' meetings and publication in their journals.
4. Participation in research, particularly in projects that are funded following peer review and/or result in publications or presentations at regional and national scientific meetings.
5. Offering of guidance and technical support (eg, research design, statistical analysis) for residents involved in research.
6. Provision of support for resident participation in scholarly activities.

C. Fellows must participate in basic and/or clinical research.
1. Fellows must learn to design, implement, and interpret research studies under supervision by qualified faculty.
2. The program must provide time and facilities for research activities by fellows.

VI. Library

1. Residents must have ready access to a major medical library, either at the institution where the residents are located or through arrangement with convenient nearby institutions.
2. Library services should include the electronic retrieval of information from medical databases.
3. There must be access to an on-site library or to a collection of appropriate texts and journals in each institution participating in a residency program. On-site libraries and/or collections of texts and journals must be readily available during nights and weekends.

VII. Evaluation

A. Program directors must have a clearly defined method for regular periodic assessment of the performance of the fellow. The assessment must include cognitive, motor, and interpersonal skills; attitudinal traits; and surgical judgment. There must be at least semiannual communication of this information to the fellow and to the director of the residency program in orthopaedic surgery.

B. The educational effectiveness of a program must be evaluated in a systematic manner. In particular, the quality of the curriculum and the extent to which the educational goals have been met by residents must be assessed. Written evaluations by residents should be utilized in this process.

ACGME: February 1991 Effective: July 1995

Program Requirements for Residency Education in Orthopaedic Trauma (Orthopaedic Surgery)

I. Introduction

A. Orthopaedic trauma is a subspecialty of orthopaedic surgery that includes the in-depth study and treatment of injuries to the locomotor system and their sequelae. An educational program in orthopaedic trauma must be organized to provide sufficient experience for fellows to acquire the competency of a specialist in the field.

B. Postgraduate fellowship education in orthopaedic surgery is a component in the continuum of the educational process, and such education will take place after completion of an accredited residency. Graduate medical education programs in the subspecialties of orthopaedic surgery will be accredited to offer 12 months of education.

C. Postgraduate fellowship programs in the subspecialties of orthopaedic surgery may be accredited in institutions that sponsor accredited residency programs in orthopaedic surgery or that are affiliated with an Accreditation Council for Graduate Medical Education (ACGME)-accredited orthopaedic surgery residency. Requests for exceptions to this policy will be reviewed on a case-by-case basis.

D. When orthopaedic residents and fellows are being educated in the same institution, the residency director and the director of the fellowship must jointly prepare and approve a written agreement specifying the educational relationship between the residency and fellowship programs, the roles of the residency and fellowship directors in determining the educational program of residents and fellows, and the roles of the residents and fellows in patient care.

E. The director and teaching staff of a program must prepare and comply with written educational goals for the program. All educational components of a program should be related to program goals.
1. The program design and/or structure must be approved by the Residency Review Committee (RRC) as part of the regular review process.
2. Participation by any institution providing more than 2 months of training must be approved by the RRC.

II. Institutional Resources and Organization

A. Programs must provide an intellectual environment for acquiring the knowledge, skills, clinical judgment, and attitudes essential to the practice of orthopaedic trauma. This objective can be achieved only when the program director, the supporting faculty and staff, and the administration are fully committed to the educational program and when appropriate resources and facilities are present. Effective graduate education is not achieved when the educational program functions primarily to meet service commitments.

B. A sufficient number of new and follow-up patients must be available to ensure adequate inpatient and outpatient experience for each fellow without adversely diluting the educational experience of the orthopaedic surgery residents or the educational experience of residents in other specialties.

C. There must be close monitoring of the interface between residency and fellowship education. It is imperative that orthopaedic fellowship education not interfere with the education of residents. Lines of responsibility for the orthopaedic resident and the fellow must be clearly defined. In addition, the fellow should maintain a close working relationship with orthopaedic residents and other fellows in orthopaedic surgery and in other disciplines.

D. Modern facilities to support the overall educational program must be available and functioning. The primary hospital in which the fellow works must be a Level I or II trauma center or equivalent with 24-hour full services, acute and emergency surgery, and at least 50 cases of major trauma each year. It must have a modern operating room facility, image intensification, compatible fracture table, orthopaedic implants in stock, and ideally, a special room dedicated to acute and emergency surgery.

E. There must be access to records and x-rays of orthopaedic trauma cases for at least 5 years following patient discharge with computerized or some other efficient coding system. There should be photographic records and photography support readily available.

F. There must be broad support and cooperation from other clinical services, particularly emergency medicine, general surgery, neurosurgery, anesthesia, intensive care, and radiology (including computed tomography and angiography available on an emergency basis). Plastic surgery, urology, otolaryngology, ophthalmology, and pulmonary medical specialists also should be available to provide emergency consultation.

III. Program Personnel

The program director and the teaching staff are responsible for the general administration of a program, including those activities related to the recruitment, selection, instruction, supervision, counseling, evaluation, and advancement of residents and the maintenance of records related to program accreditation.

A. Program Director

The director of the subspecialty program and the director of the affiliated orthopaedic surgery program, in conjunction with the administration of the institution, will be responsible for ensuring that adequate facilities and other necessary resources are available to provide an education of high quality.

There must be a single program director responsible for the program.

1. Qualifications of the program director include:
   a. Requisite and documented clinical, educational, and administrative abilities and experience.
   b. Licensure to practice medicine in the state where the institution that sponsors the program is located. (Certain federal programs are exempted.)
   c. Certification by the American Board of Orthopaedic Surgery or suitable equivalent qualifications.
   d. Appointment in good standing to the medical staff of an institution participating in the program.
2. Responsibilities of the program director include:
   a. Preparation of a written statement outlining the educational goals of the program with respect to knowledge, skills, and other attributes of residents at each level of training and for each major rotation or other program assignment. This statement must be distributed to residents and members of the teaching staff. It should be readily available for review.
   b. Selection of residents for appointment to the program in accordance with institutional and departmental policies and procedures.
   c. Selection and supervision of the teaching staff and other program personnel at each institution participating in the program.
   d. The supervision of residents in accordance with explicit written descriptions of supervisory lines of responsibility for the care of patients. Such guidelines must be communicated to all members of the program staff. Residents must be provided with prompt, reliable systems for communication and interaction with supervisory physicians.
   e. Regular evaluation of residents' knowledge, skills, and overall performance, including the development of professional attitudes consistent with being a physician. The program director, with participation of members of the teaching staff, shall:
      1. At least semiannually evaluate the knowledge, skills, and professional growth of the residents, using appropriate criteria and procedures.
      2. Communicate each evaluation to the resident in a timely manner.
      3. Advance residents to positions of higher responsibility only on the basis of evidence of their satisfactory progressive scholarship and professional growth.
      4. Maintain a permanent record of evaluation for each resident and have it accessible to the resident and other authorized personnel.
   f. The provision of a written final evaluation for each resident who completes the program. The evaluation must include a review of the resident's performance during the final period of training and should verify that the resident has demonstrated sufficient professional ability to practice competently and independently. This final evaluation should be part of the resident's permanent record maintained by the institution.
   g. Fellowship directors must ensure that trainees are given reasonable duty and call assignments. It is desirable that fellows' work schedules be designed so that on average, excluding exceptional patient care needs, fellows have at least 1 day out of 7 free of routine responsibilities and be on call in the hospital no more often than every third night. Scheduling will necessitate flexibility, as fellows are at the postgraduate level, so the ratio of hours worked and on-call time may vary.
   h. Implementation of fair procedures, as established by the sponsoring institution, regarding academic discipline and resident complaints or grievances.
   i. Monitoring resident stress, including mental or emotional conditions inhibiting performance or learning and drug- or alcohol-related dysfunction. Program directors and teaching staff should be sensitive to the need for timely provision of confidential counseling and psychological support services to residents. Training situations that consistently produce undesirable stress on residents must be evaluated and modified.
   j. Preparation of an accurate statistical and narrative description of the program as requested by the RRC.

B. Teaching Staff

1. There must be a sufficient number of teaching staff with documented qualifications to instruct and supervise adequately all the residents in the program.
2. Members of the teaching staff must be able to devote sufficient time to meet their supervisory and teaching responsibilities.
3. All members of the teaching staff must demonstrate a strong interest in the education of residents, sound clinical and teaching abilities, support of the goals and objectives of the program, a commitment to their own continuing medical education, and participation in scholarly activities.
4. A member of the teaching staff of each participating institution must be designated to assume responsibility for the day-to-day activities of the program at that institution, with overall coordination by the program director.
5. The teaching staff must be organized and have regular documented meetings to review program goals and objectives as well as program effectiveness in achieving them. At least one resident representative should participate in these reviews.
6. The teaching staff should periodically evaluate the utilization of the resources available to the program, the contribution of each institution participating in the program, the financial and administrative support of the program, the volume and variety of patients available to the program for educational purposes, the performance of members of the teaching staff, and the quality of supervision of residents.

C. Other Program Personnel

Programs must be provided with the additional professional, technical, and clerical personnel needed to support the administration and educational conduct of the program.

IV. Educational Program

A. The fellowship must provide sufficiently advanced education to allow the fellow to acquire the expertise of a specialist in orthopaedic trauma. This education must consist of academic and technical components.
   1. The academic component must emphasize a scholarly approach to clinical problem solving, self-directed study, teaching, development of analytic skills and surgical judgment, and research.
   2. The technical component should ensure the ability of the fellow to perform skillfully the procedures required for practice of the subspecialty.

B. The program must offer supervised training in the operative and other technical skills integral to the treatment of orthopaedic trauma. Instruction and experience must be sufficient for the fellow to understand the indications, risks, and limitations of the commonly performed procedures in the subspecialty.

C. Fellows must have the opportunity to provide consultation with faculty supervision and should have clearly defined educational responsibilities for residents, medical students, and allied health personnel. These teaching experiences should correlate basic biomedical knowledge with the clinical aspects of the subspecialty.

D. Clinical experience must include opportunities to observe and to manage patients with a wide variety of problems in orthopaedic trauma, and the breadth of patient experience should include the evaluation and care of individuals of a wide range of ages and both sexes. Generally, care of these patients involves several specialties and a cooperative effort in trauma centers.

E. The educational curriculum must include opportunities for fellows to study anatomy, physiology, biomechanics, pathology, microbiology, pharmacology, and immunology as they relate to orthopaedic trauma.

F. The program must hold regularly scheduled subspecialty conferences, including at least one weekly teaching conference, a monthly morbidity/mortality conference, and a monthly conference with other trauma services, with active faculty and fellow participation.

G. The program must emphasize the diagnosis of clinical orthopaedic trauma problems, the mechanism of injury, the treatment modalities available, and the results and complications of such treatment. Fellows must have the opportunity to assume a major role in the continuity of care of patients and have progressive responsibility for patient assessment, preoperative planning, operative experience, postoperative intensive care, other postoperative management, rehabilitation, and other outpatient care of patients.

H. The fellow must keep a record of the diagnosis and procedure for each operation in which he/she is an operating surgeon or first assistant. This must be kept on file and available for review.

I. The fellowship program must provide sufficient training to permit fellows to develop clinical competence in the field of orthopaedic trauma, and in resuscitation as applied to the patient with polytrauma. Examples of knowledge and skills that are desirable include but are not limited to the following:
   1. The basic sciences related to orthopaedic trauma.
   2. An understanding of the integration of the orthopaedic traumatologist in a trauma team and an appreciation of the importance of the timing of orthopaedic procedures in the overall care of the severely injured patient.
   3. Indications for various types of internal and external fixation devices and their applications in multiple trauma situations, both in the axial and appendicular skeletons.
   4. Prophylactic and treatment protocols for severe soft-tissue injuries and secondary organ failures in polytrauma.
   5. Indications for early or immediate amputation rather than salvage attempts in severely injured limbs.
   6. Pathophysiology of severe musculoskeletal trauma and secondary organ failure.
   7. Psychiatric and psychologic implications of severe musculoskeletal trauma for the patient and family members.
   8. Recuperative and rehabilitation techniques and use of physical and occupational therapy designed to return the patient to normal activities and work.
   9. Sufficient familiarity with current research methods to enable the fellow to critically analyze research reports and to design and implement clinical or basic research in the field of musculoskeletal trauma.
   10. Teaching skills and lecture techniques and materials in orthopaedic traumatology.
   11. Overall, the fellow must develop medical, surgical and psychosociological skills in the management of the severely injured patient.

V. Program Research and Scholarly Activity

A. Graduate medical education must take place in an environment of inquiry and scholarship in which residents participate in the development of new knowledge, learn to evaluate research findings, and develop habits of inquiry as a continuing professional responsibility.

B. The responsibility for establishing and maintaining an environment of inquiry and scholarship rests with the teaching staff. While not all members of a teaching staff must be investigators, the staff as a whole must demonstrate broad involvement in scholarly activity. This activity should include:
   1. Active participation of the teaching staff in clinical discussions, rounds, and conferences in a manner that promotes a spirit of inquiry and scholarship. Scholarship implies an in-depth understanding of basic mechanisms of normal and abnormal states and the application of current knowledge to practice.
   2. Participation in journal clubs and research conferences.
   3. Active participation in regional or national professional and scientific societies, particularly through presentations at the organizations' meetings and publication in their journals.
   4. Participation in research, particularly in projects that are funded following peer review and/or result in publication or presentations at regional and national scientific meetings.
   5. Offering of guidance and technical support (eg, research design, statistical analysis) for residents involved in research.
   6. Provision of support for resident participation in scholarly activities.

C. Fellows must participate in basic and/or clinical research.
   1. Fellows must learn to design, implement, and interpret research studies under supervision by qualified faculty.
   2. The program must provide time and facilities for research activities by fellows.

VI. Library

1. Residents must have ready access to a major medical library, either at the institution where the residents are located or through arrangement with convenient nearby institutions.
2. Library services should include the electronic retrieval of information from medical databases.
3. There must be access to an on-site library or to a collection of appropriate texts and journals in each institution participating in a residency program. On-site libraries and/or collections of

texts and journals must be readily available during nights and weekends.

VII. Evaluation

A. Program directors must have a clearly defined method for regular periodic assessment of the performance of the fellow. The assessment must include cognitive, motor, and interpersonal skills; attitudinal traits; and surgical judgment. There must be at least semiannual communication of this information to the fellow and to the director of the residency program in orthopaedic surgery.

B. The educational effectiveness of a program must be evaluated in a systematic manner. In particular, the quality of the curriculum and the extent to which the educational goals have been met by residents must be assessed. Written evaluations by residents should be utilized in this process.

ACGME: September 1989 Effective: July 1995

Program Requirements for Residency Education in Pediatric Orthopaedics (Orthopaedic Surgery)

I. Introduction

A. Postgraduate fellowship education in orthopaedic surgery is a component in the continuum of the educational process, and such education will take place after completion of an accredited residency. Graduate medical education programs in the subspecialties of orthopaedic surgery will be accredited to offer 12 months of education.

B. Postgraduate fellowship programs in the subspecialties of orthopaedic surgery may be accredited in institutions that sponsor accredited residency programs in orthopaedic surgery or that are affiliated with an Accreditation Council for Graduate Medical Education (ACGME)-accredited orthopaedic surgery residency. Requests for exceptions to this policy will be reviewed on a case-by-case basis.

C. When orthopaedic residents and fellows are being educated in the same institution, the residency director and the director of the fellowship must jointly prepare and approve a written agreement specifying the educational relationship between the residency and fellowship programs, the roles of the residency and fellowship directors in determining the educational program of residents and fellows, and the roles of the residents and fellows in patient care.

D. The director and teaching staff of a program must prepare and comply with written educational goals for the program. All educational components of a program should be related to program goals.
   1. The program design and/or structure must be approved by the Residency Review Committee (RRC) as part of the regular review process.
   2. Participation by any institution providing more than 2 months of training must be approved by the RRC.

II. Institutional Resources and Organization

A. Programs must provide an intellectual environment for acquiring the knowledge, skills, clinical judgment, and attitudes essential to the practice of pediatric orthopaedics. This objective can be achieved only when the program director, the supporting faculty and staff, and the administration are fully committed to the educational program and when appropriate resources and facilities are present. Effective graduate education is not achieved when the educational program functions primarily to meet service commitments.

B. A sufficient number of new and follow-up patients must be available to ensure adequate inpatient and outpatient experience for each fellow without adversely diluting the educational experience of the orthopaedic surgery residents or the educational experience of residents in other specialties.

C. There must be close monitoring of the interface between residency and fellowship education. It is imperative that orthopaedic fellowship education not interfere with the education of residents. Lines of responsibility for the orthopaedic resident and the fellow must be clearly defined. In addition, the fellow should maintain a close working relationship with orthopaedic residents and other fellows in orthopaedic surgery and in other disciplines.

D. Inpatient, ambulatory care, and laboratory facilities must be available and functioning.

E. The program must be conducted in a setting in which comprehensive surgical, medical, and pediatric consultation services are available.

III. Program Personnel

The program director and the teaching staff are responsible for the general administration of a program, including those activities related to the recruitment, selection, instruction, supervision, counseling, evaluation, and advancement of residents and the maintenance of records related to program accreditation.

A. Program Director

The director of the subspecialty program and the director of the affiliated orthopaedic surgery program, in conjunction with the administration of the institution, will be responsible for ensuring that adequate facilities and other necessary resources are available to provide an education of high quality.

There must be a single program director responsible for the program.

1. Qualifications of the program director include:
   a. Requisite and documented clinical, educational, and administrative abilities and experience.
   b. Licensure to practice medicine in the state where the institution that sponsors the program is located. (Certain federal programs are exempted).
   c. Certification by the American Board of Orthopaedic Surgery or suitable equivalent qualifications.
   d. Appointment in good standing to the medical staff of an institution participating in the program.
2. Responsibilities of the program director include:
   a. Preparation of a written statement outlining the educational goals of the program with respect to knowledge, skills, and other attributes of residents at each level of training and for each major rotation or other program assignment. This statement must be distributed to residents and members of the teaching staff. It should be readily available for review.
   b. Selection of residents for appointment to the program in accordance with institutional and departmental policies and procedures.
   c. Selection and supervision of the teaching staff and other program personnel at each institution participating in the program.
   d. The supervision of residents in accordance with explicit written descriptions of supervisory lines of responsibility for the care of patients. Such guidelines must be communicated to all members of the program staff. Residents must be provided with prompt, reliable systems for communication and interaction with supervisory physicians.

e. Regular evaluation of residents' knowledge, skills, and overall performance, including the development of professional attitudes consistent with being a physician. The program director, with participation of members of the teaching staff, shall:
   1. At least semiannually evaluate the knowledge, skills, and professional growth of the residents, using appropriate criteria and procedures.
   2. Communicate each evaluation to the resident in a timely manner.
   3. Advance residents to positions of higher responsibility only on the basis of evidence of their satisfactory progressive scholarship and professional growth.
   4. Maintain a permanent record of evaluation for each resident and have it accessible to the resident and other authorized personnel.

f. The provision of a written final evaluation for each resident who completes the program. The evaluation must include a review of the resident's performance during the final period of training and should verify that the resident has demonstrated sufficient professional ability to practice competently and independently. This final evaluation should be part of the resident's permanent record maintained by the institution.

g. Fellowship directors must ensure that trainees are given reasonable duty and call assignments. It is desirable that fellows' work schedules be designed so that on average, excluding exceptional patient care needs, fellows have at least 1 day out of 7 free of routine responsibilities and be on call in the hospital no more often than every third night. Scheduling will necessitate flexibility, as fellows are at the postgraduate level, so the ratio of hours worked and on-call time may vary.

h. Implementation of fair procedures, as established by the sponsoring institution, regarding academic discipline and resident complaints or grievances.

i. Monitoring resident stress, including mental or emotional conditions inhibiting performance or learning and drug- or alcohol-related dysfunction. Program directors and teaching staff should be sensitive to the need for timely provision of confidential counseling and psychological support services to residents. Training situations that consistently produce undesirable stress on residents must be evaluated and modified.

j. Preparation of an accurate statistical and narrative description of the program as requested by the RRC.

B. Teaching Staff

1. There must be a sufficient number of teaching staff with documented qualifications to instruct and supervise adequately all the residents in the program.
2. Members of the teaching staff must be able to devote sufficient time to meet their supervisory and teaching responsibilities.
3. All members of the teaching staff must demonstrate a strong interest in the education of residents, sound clinical and teaching abilities, support of the goals and objectives of the program, a commitment to their own continuing medical education, and participation in scholarly activities.
4. A member of the teaching staff of each participating institution must be designated to assume responsibility for the day-to-day activities of the program at that institution, with overall coordination by the program director.
5. The teaching staff must be organized and have regular documented meetings to review program goals and objectives as well as program effectiveness in achieving them. At least one resident representative should participate in these reviews.
6. The teaching staff should periodically evaluate the utilization of the resources available to the program, the contribution of each institution participating in the program, the financial and administrative support of the program, the volume and variety of patients available to the program for educational purposes, the performance of members of the teaching staff, and the quality of supervision of residents.

C. Other Program Personnel

Programs must be provided with the additional professional, technical, and clerical personnel needed to support the administration and educational conduct of the program.

IV. Educational Program

A. The fellowship must provide sufficiently advanced education to allow the fellow to acquire the expertise of a specialist in pediatric orthopaedics. This education must consist of academic and technical components.
   1. The academic component must emphasize a scholarly approach to clinical problem solving, self-directed study, teaching, development of analytic skills and surgical judgment, and research.
   2. The technical component should ensure the ability of the fellow to perform skillfully the procedures required for practice of the subspecialty.

B. The program must offer supervised training in the operative and other technical skills integral to pediatric orthopaedics. Instruction and experience must be sufficient for the fellow to understand the indications, risks, and limitations of the commonly performed procedures in the subspecialty.

C. Fellows must have the opportunity to provide consultation with faculty supervision and should have clearly defined educational responsibilities for residents, medical students, and allied health personnel. These teaching experiences should correlate basic biomedical knowledge with the clinical aspects of the subspecialty.

D. The fellows' clinical experience should include observation and treatment of both inpatients and outpatients with a wide variety of orthopaedic disorders.

E. Fellows must have the opportunity to assume continuous responsibility for both acutely and chronically ill patients so as to learn the natural history of pediatric orthopaedic disorders as well as the effectiveness of treatment programs and the impact of growth on these disorders.

F. The program should emphasize normal physiologic mechanisms and the pathogenesis and complications of pediatric orthopaedic disorders.

G. Utilization of appropriate laboratory procedures and allied medical personnel should be stressed.

H. The knowledge and skills the program must cover include but are not limited to:
   1. Prudent and judicious use of diagnostic tests.
   2. Use of data resources and the need for and interpretation of data.
   3. Interpretation of radiologic examination of the musculoskeletal system, including vascular studies and the modalities of nuclear medicine (and other advanced techniques) with an appreciation of the risk and expected yield of the procedures.
   4. Understanding of the roles of physical and occupational therapists, orthotists, and prosthetists in the rehabilitation and ongoing management of pediatric orthopaedic disorders.
   5. Performance of pediatric orthopaedic surgical procedures.

V. Program Research and Scholarly Activity

A. Graduate medical education must take place in an environment of inquiry and scholarship in which residents participate in the development of new knowledge, learn to evaluate research findings, and develop habits of inquiry as a continuing professional responsibility.

B. The responsibility for establishing and maintaining an environment of inquiry and scholarship rests with the teaching staff. While not all members of a teaching staff must be investigators, the staff as a whole must demonstrate broad involvement in scholarly activity. This activity should include:
   1. Active participation of the teaching staff in clinical discussions, rounds, and conferences in a manner that promotes a spirit of inquiry and scholarship. Scholarship implies an in-depth understanding of basic mechanisms of normal and abnormal states and the application of current knowledge to practice.
   2. Participation in journal clubs and research conferences.
   3. Active participation in regional or national professional and scientific societies, particularly through presentations at the organizations' meetings and publication in their journals.
   4. Participation in research, particularly in projects that are funded following peer review and/or result in publication or presentations at regional and national scientific meetings.
   5. Offering of guidance and technical support (eg, research design, statistical analysis) for residents involved in research.
   6. Provision of support for resident participation in scholarly activities.

C. Fellows must participate in basic and/or clinical research.
   1. Fellows must learn to design, implement, and interpret research studies under supervision by qualified faculty.
   2. The program must provide time and facilities for research activities by fellows.

VI. Library

1. Residents must have ready access to a major medical library, either at the institution where the residents are located or through arrangement with convenient nearby institutions.
2. Library services should include the electronic retrieval of information from medical databases.
3. There must be access to an on-site library or to a collection of appropriate texts and journals in each institution participating in a residency program. On-site libraries and/or collections of texts and journals must be readily available during nights and weekends.

VII. Evaluation

A. Program directors must have a clearly defined method for regular periodic assessment of the performance of the fellow. The assessment must include cognitive, motor, and interpersonal skills; attitudinal traits; and surgical judgment. There must be at least semiannual communication of this information to the fellow and to the director of the residency program in orthopaedic surgery.

B. The educational effectiveness of a program must be evaluated in a systematic manner. In particular, the quality of the curriculum and the extent to which the educational goals have been met by residents must be assessed. Written evaluations by residents should be utilized in this process.

ACGME: June 1985 Effective: July 1995

Program Requirements for Residency Education in Otolaryngology

I. Introduction

A. Definition and Scope of the Specialty

Residency programs in otolaryngology-head and neck surgery are designed to provide residents with education in the comprehensive medical and surgical care of patients with diseases and disorders that affect the ears, the upper respiratory and upper alimentary systems and related structures, and the head and neck. The educational program should include the core knowledge, skills, and understanding of the basic medical sciences relevant to the head and neck; the upper respiratory and upper alimentary systems; the communication sciences, including the knowledge of audiology and speech pathology and audiologic and speech rehabilitation; and the chemical senses and allergy, endocrinology, and neurology as they relate to the head and neck area. The educational program also should include the clinical aspects of diagnosis and the medical and/or surgical therapy for: prevention of diseases, neoplasms, deformities, disorders and/or injuries of the ears, the upper respiratory and upper alimentary systems, the face, the jaws, and other head and neck systems; head and neck oncology; and facial plastic and reconstructive surgery.

Following completion of the educational program, residents should be prepared to care for patients of all ages with medical and surgical disorders of the ears, the upper respiratory and upper alimentary systems and related structures, and the head and neck; to carry out diagnostic evaluations of patients with otolaryngology disorders; and to carry out the surgical and nonsurgical management of otolaryngology disorders, including rehabilitation and referral to subspecialists when appropriate.

B. Duration and Scope of Education

1. Residency programs in otolaryngology-head and neck surgery must be of 5 years' duration, which must include 1 year of general surgery and 4 years of progressive education in the specialty. Experience in the basic surgical sciences should precede the otolaryngology-head and neck surgery education. The final year of the 4 years of otolaryngology education must be a chief resident experience and must be spent within institutions approved as part of the program.
2. Prior to admission, the program must notify each resident in writing of the required length of the educational program. The required length of the educational program for a particular resident may not be changed without mutual agreement during his or her program unless there is a significant break in his or her training or the resident requires remedial education.
3. While it is not essential that all programs have the same curriculum or offer a uniform sequence of experience, all accredited programs should adequately cover the entire scope of the discipline with interdisciplinary interaction as appropriate.
4. The program should provide a comprehensive educational experience in bronchoesophagology, endocrinology, facial plastic and reconstructive surgery, head and neck surgery, immunology, laryngology, otology, otolaryngic allergy, neurology, neurotology, pediatric otolaryngology, and rhinology. The program must provide sufficient clinical and operative experience to enable the residents, on completion of their education, to practice this specialty in a scientific, a knowledgeable, and an independent manner.

II. Institutional Organization

A. Sponsoring Institution

The sponsoring institution must provide sufficient faculty, financial resources, support space, clinical and research facilities, and library materials to meet the educational needs of the residents and to enable the program to comply with the requirements for accreditation. The governing body of the sponsoring institution must grant the program director sufficient authority, financial support, and access to facilities to organize and supervise the following activities: resident selection and evaluation; the didactic and clinical components of the program, including patient management and scholarly activity; and staff recruitment and evaluation. There must be sufficient operative time available to ensure an adequate resident surgical experience.

B. Participating Institutions

1. A program need not be confined to a single hospital. However, in programs involving two or more hospitals, the sponsoring institution must organize the program to provide residents with a progressive educational experience.
2. Each participating institution must offer significant educational opportunities to the program. Resident education at each participating institution must comply with the Program Requirements for Otolaryngology. Assignments that dilute the education of residents or that do not provide proper supervision and coordination of educational activities should not be established or maintained.
3. There must be a qualified otolaryngologist-head and neck surgeon appointed by and responsible to the program director in each geographically separate institution. This individual must be responsible for the education of the residents and also will supervise the educational activities of the other faculty relating to resident education in that institution. The program director at each participating institution must have major clinical responsibilities at that institution.
4. The educational program may not include assignments to any nonapproved participating institutions for more than a total of 3 months without prior approval of the Residency Review Committee (RRC).

C. Appointment of Residents

1. The total number of residents and the number of residents per year must be approved in advance by the RRC. The number of residents will be based on the number, qualifications, and commitment of the faculty; the volume and variety of the patient population available for educational purposes; and the totality of institutional resources committed to resident education.
2. Programs may not graduate more residents in any given year than the number of residents approved by the RRC, except in cases where a resident's educational program is extended because the program director has determined the need for additional education to meet minimum requirements for competency. The program director must request approval in writing from the RRC to extend a resident's educational program. Any increase in the number of residents at any year of the program or in the total number of residents must receive prior approval of the RRC. Any request for change in the approved resident complement must include a strong educational rationale.
3. A vacancy in a resident complement, if filled, must be at the same level in which the vacancy occurs, unless otherwise approved by the RRC.

   Violations of these requirements will result in an adverse accreditation action.

D. Appointment of Subspecialty Residents

1. The appointment of subspecialty residents for special training or education must not dilute or detract from the educational opportunities of regularly appointed otolaryngology residents.
2. Any program with subspecialty residents must submit a clear statement of the areas of education, clinical responsibilities, and duration of the educational program. This statement must be supplied to the RRC at the time the program is site visited.
3. If subspecialty residents will, in the judgment of the RRC, detract from the education of the regularly appointed otolaryngology residents, the accreditation status of the program may be adversely affected.

III. Faculty Qualifications and Responsibilities

The program director and the faculty are responsible for the general administration of the program, including those activities related to the recruitment, selection, instruction, supervision, counseling, evaluation, and advancement of residents and the maintenance of records related to program accreditation.

A. Program Director

There must be a single program director responsible for the program.

1. Qualifications of the program director
   a. Requisite and documented clinical, educational, and administrative abilities and experience
   b. Licensure to practice medicine in the state where the institution that sponsors the program is located (Certain federal programs are exempted.)
   c. Certification by the American Board of Otolaryngology or suitable equivalent qualifications in otolaryngology-head and neck surgery
   d. Appointment in good standing to the medical staff of an institution participating in the program
2. Responsibilities of the program director
   a. Preparing a written statement outlining the educational goals of the program with respect to knowledge, skills, and other attributes of residents at each level of training and for each major rotation or other program assignment. This statement must be distributed to residents and faculty and should be readily available for review.
   b. Devoting sufficient time to the program to provide continuity of leadership and to fulfill all of the responsibilities inherent in meeting the educational goals of the program. Continuity of leadership over a period of years is important to the stability of a residency program. Frequent changes in leadership or long periods of temporary leadership usually have an adverse effect on an educational program and will be cause for serious concern.
   c. Developing a sound administrative organizational framework and an effective faculty as essential elements of an approved residency program.
   d. Active involvement in clinical practice, continuing medical education, regional or national scientific societies, presentations and publications, and research.
   e. Overseeing and organizing the activities of the educational program. The responsibilities of this position should include but not be limited to
      1. selection of residents for appointment to the program according to institutional and departmental policies and procedures;
      2. supervision, direction, and administration of the educational activities;
      3. evaluation of the residents, faculty, and residency program;

4. selection and supervision of the faculty and other program personnel at each institution participating in the program, to include the appointment of program directors at participating institutions.

f. Supervising residents through explicit written descriptions of supervisory lines of responsibility for the care of patients. Such guidelines must be communicated to all members of the program staff. Residents must be provided with prompt, reliable systems for communication and interaction with supervisory physicians.

g. Regularly evaluating residents' knowledge, skills, and overall performance, including the development of professional attitudes consistent with being a physician.

h. Implementing fair procedures, as established by the sponsoring institution, regarding academic discipline and resident complaints or grievances.

i. Monitoring resident stress, including mental or emotional conditions inhibiting performance or learning, and drug- or alcohol-related dysfunction. The program director and faculty should be sensitive to the need for timely provision of confidential counseling and psychological support services to residents. Situations that consistently produce undesirable stress on residents must be evaluated and modified.

j. Preparing an accurate statistical and narrative description of the program as requested by the RRC.

k. Promptly notifying the executive director of the RRC in writing of any major change in the program that may significantly alter the educational experience for the residents, including
  1. changes in leadership of the department, such as the appointment of a permanent or acting program director and/or department chair;
  2. changes in administrative structure, such as an alteration in the status of the program within the institution.

l. Obtaining prior approval of the RRC for the following changes in the program to determine if an adequate educational environment exists to support these changes:
  1. The addition of any institution to which residents rotate for more than 3 months
  2. Any change in the approved resident complement of the program
  3. Any change in the length or format of the educational program

  On review of a proposal for a major change in a program, the RRC may determine that a site visit is necessary.

B. Faculty

1. There must be a sufficient number of faculty with documented qualifications to instruct and supervise adequately all residents in the program. Members of the faculty must be able to devote sufficient time to meet their supervisory and teaching responsibilities.
2. The faculty is responsible for ensuring that the structure and content of the residency program reflect an appropriate education-to-service ratio. The resident should be recognized as a student and provided with a sufficient experience in nonoperative management and the preoperative, intraoperative, and postoperative patient care of patients with otolaryngology disorders. This responsibility must include on-site supervision of the resident in operative, inpatient, outpatient, and emergency cases and participation in patient care conferences and other educational exercises.
3. It is desirable that there be at least two other members of the faculty with qualifications similar to those of the program director.
4. All members of the faculty must demonstrate a strong interest in the education of residents, sound clinical and teaching abilities, and support for the goals and objectives of the educational program. The faculty must be willing to devote the necessary time and effort to the educational program and be engaged in scholarly activities, including
   a. participation and presentation of their work at regional or national scientific societies;
   b. participation in their own continuing medical education;
   c. participation in clinical and/or basic research;
   d. publication in refereed journals, monographs, or books.

   A faculty that does not exhibit such characteristics will be the cause of concern to the RRC as to its adequacy and suitability for conducting a program of graduate education in otolaryngology-head and neck surgery.
5. There must be clear documentation of adequate faculty commitment to the residency program. One measure of this commitment is the extent to which faculty permit residents to participate in the management of faculty members' private patients.
6. A faculty member from each participating institution must be designated to assume responsibility for the day-to-day activities of the program at that institution, with overall coordination by the program director.
7. The faculty must be organized and have regular documented meetings at least annually to review program goals and objectives and program effectiveness in achieving them. At least one resident representative should participate in these reviews.
8. The faculty should evaluate at least annually the utilization of the resources available to the program, the contribution of each institution participating in the program, the financial and administrative support of the program, the volume and variety of patients available to the program for educational purposes, the performance of members of the faculty, and the quality of supervision of residents.

C. Other Program Personnel

Programs must be provided with the additional professional, technical, and clerical personnel needed to support the administration and educational conduct of the program.

IV. Facilities and Resources

There must be adequate space and equipment for the educational program, including meeting rooms; classrooms with audiovisual and other educational aids; office space for staff; pertinent library materials and current information technology readily available for clinical care; and diagnostic, therapeutic, and research facilities.

A. Within each institution, beds sufficient for the needs of the service must be provided.

B. Residents must have access to outpatient facilities, clinics, and office space for education in the regular preoperative evaluation and postoperative follow-up of cases for which the resident has responsibility.

C. Technologically current equipment considered necessary for diagnosis and treatment must be available.

D. A patient information system that facilitates both quality patient care and education must be available.
  1. The patient information system should be supervised by qualified staff.
  2. The patient information system should be maintained to ensure easy and prompt access at all times.
  3. The patient information system should be organized to permit the collection and evaluation of selected material from clinical records for investigative and review purposes.

E. Residents should be provided with adequate office, sleeping, lounge, and food facilities during assigned duty hours. Adequate clerical support services also must be provided.

F. Library
1. Residents must have ready access to a major medical library, either at the institution where the residents are located or through arrangement with convenient nearby institutions.
2. Library services should include the electronic retrieval of information from medical databases.
3. There must be access to an on-site library or to a collection of appropriate texts and journals in each institution participating in the residency program. On-site libraries and/or collections of texts and journals must be readily available during nights and weekends.

V. The Educational Program

A. Program Goals and Objectives

The program director and faculty must prepare and implement written educational goals for the program.

1. Program Design
All educational components of a residency program should be related to program goals. The program design and/or structure must be approved by the RRC as part of the regular review process.
2. The program must have a comprehensive, well-organized, and effective curriculum, including the cyclical presentation of core specialty knowledge supplemented by the addition of current information. There must be evidence that the teaching is conducted in a variety of educational settings such as clinics, classrooms, operating rooms, bedsides, and laboratories, employing accepted educational principles.

B. Specialty Content

The broad scope of the specialty of otolaryngology-head and neck surgery requires that the program provide surgical and medical education in the following areas:

1. Morphology, physiology, pharmacology, pathology, microbiology, biochemistry, genetics, and immunology relevant to the head and neck; the upper respiratory and upper alimentary systems; the communication sciences, including knowledge of audiology and speech-language pathology; the chemical senses and allergy, endocrinology, and neurology as they relate to the head and neck; and voice sciences as they relate to laryngology
2. Diagnosis and diagnostic methods: audiologic and vestibular assessments, techniques in voice assessment, electrophysiologic techniques, and other related laboratory procedures for diagnosing diseases and disorders of the ears, the upper respiratory and upper alimentary systems, and the head and neck
3. Therapeutic and diagnostic radiology: the interpretation of medical imaging techniques relevant to the head and neck and the thorax, including studies of the temporal bone, skull, nose, paranasal sinuses, salivary and thyroid glands, larynx, neck, lungs, and esophagus
4. Diagnostic evaluation and management of congenital anomalies, allergy, trauma, and diseases affecting the regions and systems mentioned above
5. Management of congenital, inflammatory, endocrine, neoplastic, degenerative, and traumatic states, including operative intervention and preoperative and postoperative care of the following major categories:
   a. General otolaryngology
   b. Head and neck surgery
   c. Plastic and reconstructive surgery
   d. Otology
   e. Endoscopy
6. Habilitation and rehabilitation techniques and procedures including respiration, deglutition, chemoreception, balance, speech, and hearing
7. Diagnostic and therapeutic techniques involving the application and utilization of lasers and flexible and rigid perioral endoscopy
8. Ethical, socioeconomic, and medicolegal issues affecting graduate medical education and how to apply cost-effective measures in the provision of patient care
9. Current information technology and clinical outcomes analysis and their impact on quality patient care

C. Surgical Experience

1. The sponsoring and participating institutions approved for the program must have a sufficient number and variety of adult and pediatric medical and surgical patients who are available for resident education.
2. While not all residents are expected to have operative experience in all surgical specialty procedures, the surgical procedures performed by the residents must be sufficient in number and variety to provide education in the entire scope of the specialty. There must be adequate distribution and sufficient complexity within the principal categories of the specialty.
3. Generally equivalent and adequate distribution of categories and procedures among the residents must be demonstrated. Significantly unequal experience in volume and/or complexity of cases managed by the residents will be considered serious noncompliance with these requirements. In some instances, the quality of care may require that case management be conducted with other specialties (eg, hypophysectomy, cerebellopontine tumor).
4. Documentation of each individual resident's operative experience must be provided. The cumulative operative experience of each resident must be reviewed at least semiannually by the program director as a part of his or her responsibility for evaluation of the balanced progress of individual residents. The program director is responsible for compiling accurate information regarding the institutional operative records and the individual resident operative reports annually at the end of each academic year and for submitting these records for review as requested by the RRC.

D. Resident Policies

1. Supervision
All cases must be adequately supervised by appropriately qualified faculty. The program director must ensure, direct, and document proper supervision of residents at all times. Residents must be provided with rapid, reliable systems for communicating with supervising residents and faculty. Faculty or supervising residents with experience appropriate to the severity and complexity of a patient's condition must be available at all times on site. The responsibility or independence given to residents in patient care should depend on each resident's knowledge, manual skill, and experience and on the complexity of a patient's illness and the risk of the operation(s).
2. Duty hours
The physician's responsibilities for continuing patient care transcend normal working hours. To fulfill this obligation, provisions for night and weekend call should be established. However, residents should not be required regularly to perform excessively difficult or prolonged duties. The program director must ensure assignment of reasonable in-hospital duty hours. Residents at all levels should have the opportunity to spend, on average, at least 1 full day out of 7 free of hospital duties and should be on call in the hospital no more often than every third night, except in the maintenance of continuity of care. There should be adequate opportunity to rest and to sleep when on duty for 24 hours or more. On-call rooms arranged to permit adequate rest and privacy

should be available for each resident on night duty in the hospital. There should be adequate backup support if needed to maintain appropriate patient care.

3. Graded responsibility
The program must provide the residents with experience in direct and progressively responsible patient management as they advance through the educational program. This education must culminate in sufficient independent responsibility for clinical decision making to reflect that the graduating resident has developed sound clinical judgment and possesses the ability to formulate and carry out appropriate management plans.

E. Research and Scholarly Activities

1. Graduate medical education must take place in an environment of inquiry and scholarship in which residents participate in the development of new knowledge, learn to evaluate research findings, and develop habits of inquiry as a continuing professional responsibility. Research offers an important opportunity for the application of the basic sciences to clinical problems and is an important part of the preparation of the resident for a lifetime of self-education after the completion of formal residency education.
2. The educational program should provide a structured research experience for the residents, sufficient to result in an understanding of the basic principles of study design, performance, analysis, and reporting. The research experience may be clinical or basic in nature and should reflect careful advice and planning with the faculty. Facilities and protected time for research by the residents should be provided, with guidance and supervision by qualified faculty.
3. The responsibility for establishing and maintaining an environment of inquiry and scholarship rests with the faculty. While not all members of the faculty must be investigators, the faculty as a whole must demonstrate broad involvement in scholarly activity. This activity should include
   a. participation of the faculty in clinical discussions, rounds, and conferences in a manner that promotes a spirit of inquiry and scholarship. Scholarship implies an in-depth understanding of basic mechanisms of normal and abnormal states and the application of current knowledge to practice.
   b. participation in journal clubs and research conferences.
   c. participation in regional or national professional and scientific societies, particularly through presentations at the organizations' meetings and publication in their journals.
   d. participation in research, particularly in projects that are funded following peer review and/or result in publications or presentations at regional and national scientific meetings.
   e. offering of guidance and technical support (eg, research design, statistical analysis) for residents involved in research.
   f. provision of support for resident participation in scholarly activities.

F. Outpatient Experience

1. There must be a well-organized and well-supervised outpatient service. This service must operate in relation to an inpatient service used in the program. Residents must have the opportunity to see patients, establish provisional diagnoses, and initiate preliminary treatment plans. An opportunity for follow-up care must be provided so that the results of surgical care may be evaluated by the responsible residents. These activities must be carried out under appropriate faculty supervision.
2. If residents participate in preoperative and postoperative care in a private office, the program director must ensure that the resident functions with an appropriate degree of responsibility with adequate supervision. Experience should be provided in office practice procedures and management.
3. Residents must have experience in the emergency care of critically ill and injured patients with otolaryngology-head and neck conditions.

G. Conferences

1. Basic Science
There must be a structured educational experience in basic science. Ordinarily, this should be provided within the participating institutions of the residency program. Any program that provides the requisite basic science experience outside the approved participating institutions must demonstrate that the educational experience provided meets these designated criteria. Faculty must participate in basic science education, resident attendance must be monitored, education must be evaluated, and content must be integrated into the educational program. The basic science education should meet the following requirements:
   a. Basic science education should include instruction in anatomy, biochemistry, cell biology, embryology, immunology, molecular genetics, pathology, pharmacology, physiology, and other basic sciences related to the head and neck.
   b. Sufficient resources, including space, equipment, personnel, and funding for instruction and study of the basic sciences should be available to permit satisfactory correlation between basic science knowledge and clinical application.
   c. Resident instruction in anatomy should include study and dissection of cadaver anatomic specimens, including the temporal bone, with appropriate lectures and other formal sessions.
   d. Resident instruction in pathology should include formal instruction in correlative pathology in which gross and microscopic pathology relating to the head and neck area are included. The resident should study and discuss with the pathology service tissues removed at operations and autopsy material. It is desirable to have residents assigned to the Department of Pathology.
2. Clinical Conferences
Clinical conferences must be held regularly and should be attended by all residents and faculty. Grand rounds, mortality and morbidity conferences, tumor conferences, and conferences on other pertinent topics must be included in the educational program. Interdisciplinary conferences are encouraged.

VI. Evaluation

A. Resident Evaluation

1. The program must develop mechanisms by which the residents can demonstrate the acquisition of fundamental knowledge and clinical skills before progression to the level of supervised, semi-independent patient management and operative care.
2. Each resident's performance and progress in the cognitive, judgmental, interpersonal, and manual skills should be continuously monitored. Residents who fail to demonstrate appropriate industry, competence, responsibility, learning abilities, and ethics should be successively counseled and, after due process, dismissed if remediation has not occurred.
3. It is essential that the residents participate in existing national examinations. The annual otolaryngology examination of the American Academy of Otolaryngology-Head and Neck Surgery is one example of an objective test that can be used by the program. An analysis of the results of these testing programs should guide the faculty in assessing the strengths and weaknesses of individual residents and the program. The program director should also monitor the performance of program graduates on the examinations of the American Board of Otolaryngology.

4. The program director, with participation of faculty, shall
   a. at least semiannually provide formal written evaluations of the knowledge, skills, and professional growth of the residents, using appropriate criteria and procedures.
   b. communicate each evaluation to the resident in a timely manner.
   c. advance residents to positions of higher responsibility only on the basis of evidence of their satisfactory progressive scholarship and professional growth.
   d. maintain a permanent record of evaluation for each resident and have it accessible to the resident and other authorized personnel.
   e. provide a written final evaluation for each resident who completes the program. The evaluation must include a review of the resident's performance during the final period for education and should verify that the resident has demonstrated sufficient professional ability to practice competently and independently. This final evaluation should be part of the resident's permanent record maintained by the institution.

B. Faculty Evaluation

Faculty also must be evaluated on an annual basis. Documentation of faculty evaluation should include teaching ability and commitment, clinical knowledge, and scholarly contributions. Residents should participate in this evaluation.

C. Program Evaluation

1. The educational effectiveness of a program must be evaluated in a systematic manner at least annually. In particular, the quality of the curriculum and the extent to which the educational goals have been met by residents must be assessed. Written and confidential evaluations by residents must be utilized in this process.
2. There should be documented evidence of periodic self-evaluation of the program in relation to the educational goals, the needs of the residents, and the teaching responsibilities of the faculty. This evaluation must include an assessment of the balance between the educational and service components of the residency.
3. One measure of the quality of a residency program is the performance of its graduates on the certifying examinations of the American Board of Otolaryngology. In its evaluation of residency programs, the RRC will take into consideration the information provided by the American Board of Otolaryngology regarding resident performance on the certifying examination.

VII. Board Certification

Residents who plan to seek certification by the American Board of Otolaryngology should communicate with the executive vice president of the board to ascertain the current requirements for acceptance as a candidate for certification.

ACGME: June 1996 Effective: July 1997

Program Requirements for Residency Education in Otology-Neurotology (Otolaryngology)

I. Introduction

A. Definition and Description of the Specialty

The otology-neurotology lateral skull base surgery program will provide advanced education in the diagnosis and management of disorders of the temporal bone, lateral skull base, and related structures. Surgery of the lateral skull base that involves the mesial aspect of the dura or intradural structure requires the joint effort of an otology-neurotology and neurological surgery team. A 24-month educational program will ensure that concentrated time is available for the otology-neurotology resident to develop advanced diagnostic expertise and advanced medical and surgical management skills not afforded in the basic otolaryngology residency program; ie, for the care of diseases and disorders of the petrous apex, infratemporal fossa, internal auditory canals, cranial nerves (eg, vestibular nerve section and joint otology-neurotology resection of intradural VIII nerve tumors), and lateral skull base, including the occipital bone, sphenoid bone, and temporal bone. This advanced education is required so that the neurotology resident may develop expertise with extradural skull base approaches in collaboration with neurological surgery. The postoperative care of these lateral skull base surgery patients requires the joint management of both neurological surgery and otology-neurotology. The advanced education is also necessary to gain expertise in the joint collaborative management of patients undergoing lateral skull base surgery. In addition, the program will permit exposure to new research opportunities and time to explore new research ideas.

B. Duration and Scope of Education

1. Admission to a program is contingent on completion of a residency program in otolaryngology accredited by the Accreditation Council for Graduate Medical Education (ACGME).
2. The duration of the program is 24 months, all of which must be spent in participating institutions approved by the Residency Review Committee (RRC). The otology-neurotology program must be associated with an ACGME-accredited otolaryngology program. Resident experiences in related specialties such as physical medicine and rehabilitation, neurology, neurological surgery, neuroradiology, and neuropathology must be offered by the sponsoring institution.
3. One otology-neurotology resident should be enrolled each year. A program without a resident for 2 successive years will be administratively withdrawn. The RRC will develop an annual resident reporting system to ensure that ACGME procedures are followed in this respect.

C. Program Goals and Objectives

The program course of study must be comprehensive and well organized and must provide each resident with opportunities for progressive management responsibility in both inpatient and outpatient environments. The goals and objectives of the program must include the following experiences:

1. The program must include increasing responsibility in both inpatient and outpatient environments. Direct surgical experience with all procedures must be documented. The experience must include neurotology and lateral skull base surgery techniques with intracranial exposures performed jointly with neurosurgery.
2. Program faculty must be responsible to the patient and the otology-neurotology resident so that when an otologist-neurotologist plans an operation in which the dura may be entered, neurological consultation will be obtained to determine the appropriateness and planning of a joint surgical effort by both otology-neurotology and neurosurgery.
3. The refinement of diagnostic expertise and the development of medical and surgical management strategies, including intracranial exposure, and postoperative care necessary to treat congenital, inflammatory, neoplastic, idiopathic, and traumatic diseases of the petrous apex, internal auditory canal, cerebellopontine angle, cranial nerves, and lateral skull base, including the occipital bone, temporal bone, and craniovertebral junction.

4. Because advanced otology-neurotology is multidisciplinary in nature and because interactions with peers from related disciplines contribute to the quality of education, the faculty from related disciplines such as neurology, neurological surgery, audiology, neuro-ophthalmology, neuroradiology, and neuropathology should participate in the program to enhance the educational opportunities for the otology-neurotology residents. Close interaction with physical medicine and rehabilitation in the aspect of otologic-neurologic rehabilitation is highly desirable.
5. In addition to combined educational conferences with the other disciplines listed in C.4 above, cooperative efforts in the diagnostic area with neurological surgeons, surgical team approaches to operative therapy with neurosurgeons, and combined approaches to rehabilitative efforts with physical medicine and rehabilitation must be emphasized. The program faculty must be responsible to the patient and the otology-neurotology resident so that when an otologist-neurotologist plans an operation in which the dura may be entered, it is expected that neurosurgical consultation will be obtained to determine the appropriateness and planning of a joint effort by otology-neurotology and neurosurgery.
6. The otology-neurotology resident must be provided with experience in the habilitation and rehabilitation of the vertiginous patient and the treatment of intracranial and intratemporal facial nerve disorders.
7. Participation in a multidisciplinary surgical team that manages disorders of the temporal bone, cerebellopontine angle, lateral skull base, and related structures is required. Members of the team should include audiologists, electrophysiologists, head and neck surgeons, neurologists, neuroradiologists, neurological surgeons, neuro-ophthalmologists, neuropathologists, neurotologists, and physiatrists.

II. Institutional Organization

A. Sponsoring Institution

1. A single sponsoring institution must sponsor the otology-neurology program, as stated in the Institutional Requirements.
2. The sponsoring institution must provide sufficient faculty, financial resources, and clinical and research support. Other educational resources, such as a temporal bone dissection laboratory; testing facilities for complete auditory and vestibular evaluation that include facilities for intracranial nerve monitoring; and other appropriate diagnostic, therapeutic, and research facilities to meet the educational needs of the otology-neurotology residents, are required.
3. Service commitments must not compromise the achievement of the program's educational goals and objectives.

B. Participating Institutions

1. If the resources of two or more institutions are used, interinstitutional agreements must be developed by the institutional governing boards, as referenced in the Institutional Requirements.
2. The RRC must approve the addition and deletion of all participating institutions prospectively. Such approval will be based on a clear educational rationale and the value of the institution to the program as a whole.

C. Library

1. Residents must have ready access to a major medical library, either at the institution where the residents are located or through arrangements with convenient nearby institutions.
2. Library services should include the electronic retrieval of information from medical databases.
3. There must be access to an onsite library or to a collection of appropriate texts and journals in each institution participating in the educational program.

D. Appointment of Residents

1. The RRC will approve a total number of otology-neurotology residents in the program for each year. The number of residents will be based on the number, qualifications, and commitment of the faculty; the volume and variety of the patient population available for educational purposes; and the institutional resources committed to the educational program.
2. A program may not graduate more residents in any given year than are approved by the RRC unless prior approval has been received.

III. Program Personnel

The program director and faculty are responsible for the general administration of the program, including those activities related to the recruitment, selection, instruction, supervision, counseling, evaluation, and advancement of residents and the maintenance of records related to program accreditation.

A. Program Director

1. Qualifications
   a. A single program director with the requisite and documented clinical and educational experience must be responsible for the program. The program director must be licensed to practice medicine in the state where the institution that sponsors the program is located and must be appointed in good standing to the medical staff of an institution participating in the program.
   b. The program director must be certified by the American Board of Otolaryngology and be certified in the subspecialty or possess suitable equivalent qualifications, as determined by the RRC.
   c. The program director must have administrative responsibility for the otology-neurotology program and should possess the skills of administrator, clinician, teacher, and researcher. The program director must devote sufficient time to the program to ensure continuity of leadership and to fulfill all of the responsibilities inherent in meeting the educational goals of the program. Frequent changes of leadership or long periods of temporary leadership will be cause for serious concern. The executive secretary should be notified promptly of any change in program leadership.
2. Responsibilities
   a. Development of a sound administrative and organizational framework, to include an effective faculty as an essential element of the program.
   b. Maintenance of the record of otology-neurotology operative cases performed by the service and for each otology-neurotology resident. These records must be reviewed annually by the program director with the resident as a part of the director's responsibility for evaluation of the balanced progress of each resident and of the total program. These data must be submitted to the RRC at the time of the program review.
   c. Preparation of a written statement outlining the educational goals of the program with respect to the knowledge, skills, and other attributes of otology-neurotology residents at each level of education and for each major rotation or other program assignment. This statement must be distributed to residents and members of the faculty and must be readily available for review.
   d. Selection of residents for appointment to the program in accordance with institutional and departmental policies and procedures.
   e. Selection and supervision of faculty and other personnel at each institution participating in the program.

f. Supervision of residents through explicit written descriptions of supervisory lines of responsibility for the care of patients. Such guidelines must be communicated to all members of the program faculty. Residents must be provided with prompt, reliable systems for communication and interaction with supervising physicians.
g. Implementation of fair procedures, as established by the sponsoring institution, regarding academic discipline and resident complaints or grievances.
h. Monitoring resident stress, including mental or emotional conditions inhibiting performance or learning and drug- or alcohol-related dysfunction. Program directors and faculty should be sensitive to the need for timely provision of confidential counseling and psychological support services to residents. Educational situations that consistently produce undesirable stress on residents must be evaluated and modified.
i. Preparation of an accurate statistical and narrative description of the program, as requested by the RRC.

B. Faculty

1. There must be one otology-neurotology faculty member in addition to the program director who is certified by the American Board of Otolaryngology with additional appropriate professional qualifications in otology-neurotology or other equivalent qualifications, as determined by the RRC.
2. Members of the faculty must be able to devote sufficient time to meet their supervisory and teaching responsibilities.
3. The faculty must demonstrate a strong interest in the education of residents, sound clinical and teaching abilities, support for the goals and objectives of the program, a commitment to their own continuing education, and participation in scholarly activities. One measure of this commitment is the extent to which faculty members permit otology-neurotology residents to participate in the management of patients in their care.
4. The faculty must be organized and have regular documented meetings to review program goals and objectives and program effectiveness in achieving them. At least one resident should participate in these reviews.
5. The faculty should periodically evaluate the use of resources available to the program, the contribution of each participating institution, the financial and administrative support for the program, the volume and variety of patients available to the program for educational purposes, the performance of members of the faculty, and the quality of resident supervision.
6. The faculty must demonstrate involvement in scholarly activities, including
   a. participation in their own continuing education;
   b. participation in regional and national scientific societies;
   c. presentation and publication of scientific studies;
   d. active participation in research as it pertains to otology-neurotology;
   e. offering of guidance and technical support, eg, research design and statistical analysis, for residents involved in research; and
   f. active participation in clinical discussions, rounds, and conferences in a manner that promotes the spirit of inquiry and scholarship.
7. Because otology-neurotology is multidisciplinary in nature and because interaction with peers from related disciplines contributes to the quality of education, faculty from related disciplines such as audiology, neuro-ophthalmology, neurological surgery, neurology, physical medicine and rehabilitation, psychiatry, and radiology should participate in the program to enhance the residents' educational opportunities. These faculty members should have recognized expertise in otology-neurotology.

C. Other Program Personnel

Programs must be provided with the additional professional, technical, and clerical personnel needed to support the administration and educational conduct of the program.

IV. The Educational Program

The educational program must provide an intellectual environment for acquiring the knowledge, skills, clinical judgment, and attitudes that are essential for the practice of the specialty. This objective can be achieved only when the program leadership, the faculty, and the sponsoring institution are committed to the educational program and when appropriate resources and facilities are available.

A. General

1. The program director is responsible for developing a structured curriculum with written, defined goals and objectives. Clinical, basic science, and research conferences and seminars and critical literature review activities about the subspecialty must be conducted regularly and as scheduled. The otology-neurotology residents must participate in planning and in conducting conferences. Both the faculty and otology-neurotology residents must attend and participate in multidisciplinary conferences.
2. The otology-neurotology residents must be provided with the opportunity to develop skills in providing consultation, in communication with colleagues and referring physicians, and in teaching medical students, physicians, and other professional personnel.
3. Lines of responsibility must be clearly delineated between otology-neurotology residents and otolaryngology residents in the areas of training, clinical responsibilities, and duration of training. Such information must be supplied to the RRC at the time of the review and survey.
4. The same resident duty hours and supervision requirements apply to these subspecialty residents as documented in the core Program Requirements for Residency Education in Otolaryngology.

B. Course of Study

1. Academic
   The academic component should provide supplemental education in the basic sciences related to otology-neurotology, including allergy and immunology, audiology and rehabilitative audiology, genetics, neuroanatomy, neurophysiology, neuropathology, neuropharmacology, neuro-ophthalmology, physical medicine and rehabilitation, temporal bone histopathology, and vestibular pathophysiology. The course of study must reflect the following content areas:
   a. Neurophysiology, neuropathophysiology, diagnosis, and therapy of advanced otologic-neurotologic disorders, including advanced audiologic and vestibular testing; evaluation of cranial nerves and related structures; interpretation of imaging techniques of the temporal bone and lateral skull base; and electrophysiologic monitoring of cranial nerves VII, VIII, X, XI, and XII
   b. Vestibular rehabilitation
   c. Auditory and speech rehabilitation of the hearing impaired, included cochlear implants
   d. Management and rehabilitation of extradural cranial nerve defects and those defined in the definition and description of the specialty (Section I.A)
   e. Didactic and laboratory experience teaching advanced surgical techniques to deal with diseases and disorders of the auditory and vestibular systems; extradural skull base, including the sphenoid bone; temporal bone; and reconstructive techniques for repair of deficits in these areas

C. Clinical

1. Programs must provide structured clinical opportunities for residents to develop advanced skills in otology-neurotology and lateral skull base surgery, including exposure to intracranial approaches.
2. A sufficient volume and variety of cases must be available to ensure adequate inpatient and outpatient experience for each otology-neurotology resident.
3. Each otology-neurotology resident must prepare documentation of surgical experience as both assistant surgeon and surgeon in the surgical revision procedures for the treatment of chronic otitis media; disorders of the vestibular system; otosclerosis; profound hearing loss; facial nerve disorders; and congenital inflammatory, neoplastic, idiopathic, and traumatic disorders of the extradural petrous bone and apex, occipital bone, sphenoid bone, and related structures.
4. The diagnosis and medical and surgical management of congenital, traumatic, inflammatory, degenerative, neoplastic, and idiopathic diseases and other disease states of the temporal bone, occipital bone, sphenoid bone, craniovertebral junction, and related structures are required experiences.
5. Audiometric testing including auditory brainstem responses and otacoustic emissions, vestibular testing, facial nerve testing, electrophysiologic monitoring strategies, and neuroradiologic procedures used to evaluate the temporal bone, skull base, and related structures are required experiences.
6. Rehabilitation techniques and procedures concerning the vestibular disorders, cranial nerve neuropathies, assistive listening devices and hearing aids, and cochlear implants must be provided.

D. Research and Scholarly Activity

1. Graduate medical education must take place in an environment of inquiry and scholarship in which otology-neurotology residents participate in the development of new knowledge, learn to evaluate research findings, and develop habits of inquiry as a continuing professional responsibility. The responsibility for establishing and maintaining an environment of inquiry and scholarship rests with the faculty.
2. The course of study must include research methodology, not to exceed 6 months, with protected time for the pursuit of scholarly activities and research. The otology-neurotology resident should study epidemiology, statistical methods, experimental design, and manuscript preparation, including literature searches and the use of computerized databases.
3. It is highly desirable that the resident prepare and submit at minimum one paper for publication in a peer-reviewed journal. While the specific content will be related to the particular expertise, interest, and capability of the program faculty and institutional resources, the general goal of the research experience should be maintained.

V. Evaluation

A. Resident Evaluation

The program director with participation of the faculty must

1. evaluate each resident in writing at least semiannually, using appropriate criteria and procedures. The evaluation must be confidential and must include observation, assessment, and substantiation of the resident's acquired body of knowledge, skills in physical examination and patient communication, technical proficiency, professional attitudes, humanistic qualities as demonstrated in the clinical setting, consultation skills, patient management, decision making, and critical analysis of clinical situations.
2. communicate each evaluation to the resident in a timely manner and provide feedback on his or her performance, including appropriate counseling and necessary remedial effort.
3. advance residents to positions of higher responsibility based on evidence of satisfactory progressive scholarship and professional growth.
4. maintain a permanent record of evaluation for each resident and have it accessible to the resident and other authorized personnel.
5. provide a final written evaluation for each resident graduating from the program that includes a review of resident performance during the program. This evaluation should verify that the resident has demonstrated sufficient professional ability to practice competently and independently. The final record should be part of the resident's permanent record maintained at the institution.
6. maintain the record of surgical operative procedures performed by the resident during the educational program. These records must be submitted to the program director and kept in a permanent file for review as requested.

B. Faculty Evaluation

All faculty must be evaluated on a regular basis. This evaluation should include teaching ability and commitment to the educational program, clinical knowledge, and scholarly contributions. Residents should participate in this evaluation.

C. Program Evaluation

There should be documented evidence of periodic self-evaluation of the program in relation to the educational goals, the needs of the otology-neurotology residents, and the extent to which the goals of resident education have been met. Confidential written evaluations by residents should be included in this process.

ACGME: June 1995 Effective: June 1995

Program Requirements for Residency Education in Pediatric Otolaryngology (Otolaryngology)

I. Introduction

A. Definition of the Subspecialty

Pediatric otolaryngology is a subspecialty within otolaryngology-head and neck surgery defined by both the age of the patient served and the knowledge and skill of the physician providing medical and surgical care. The pediatric otolaryngologist has special expertise in the management of infants and children with complex problems generally referred to tertiary care pediatric institutions with a multidisciplinary team of full-time hospital-based medical specialists. A pediatric otolaryngology educational program will be based in a tertiary care pediatric institution where the care of children can be readily coordinated with other subspecialists, thus allowing sufficient exposure and broad experience in the management of uncommon and complex otolaryngology disorders in children. A pediatric otolaryngology educational program must provide the following experiences for the pediatric otolaryngology residents: the diagnosis and care of congenital and acquired conditions involving the aerodigestive tract, nose and paranasal sinuses, the ear, diseases and disorders of the laryngotracheal complex and the head and neck; expertise in the diagnosis, treatment, and management of childhood disorders of voice, speech, language, and hearing; and a knowledge of genetics. The program should provide opportunities for the pediatric otolaryngologist to function as an advocate for the child and facilitate patient management in the home, school, or institutional setting.

B. Duration and Scope of Education

1. Admission to a pediatric otolaryngology program is contingent on completion of an Accreditation Council for Graduate Medical Education (ACGME) accredited residency program in otolaryngology.
2. The duration of a pediatric otolaryngology program is 24 months, all of which must be spent in participating institutions approved by the Residency Review Committee (RRC). The pediatric otolaryngology program must be associated with an ACGME-accredited otolaryngology program.
3. One pediatric otolaryngology resident should be enrolled each year. A program without a resident for 2 successive years will be administratively withdrawn. The RRC will develop an annual resident reporting system to ensure that the ACGME procedures are followed in this respect.

C. Program Goals and Objectives

The overall goal for residency education is to provide the pediatric otolaryngology resident with diagnostic and surgical skills for the care of ear, nose, throat, head and neck, and bronchoesophageal disorders of children that are uncommon and complex. Specific objectives include

1. an in-depth study of the embryology, developmental anatomy and physiology, microbiology, oncology, and psychology of the infant and child as related to the head and neck;
2. an understanding of the differences among the medical management of infant, childhood, and adult diseases of the head and neck;
3. provision for a sufficient number and variety of pediatric otolaryngology surgical procedures in the scope of the specialty with emphasis on those procedures infrequently encountered in the general practice of otolaryngology;
4. an appreciation for the inherent complexities of interacting with children and their families compared with adult patients; and
5. the ability to teach otoscopic and other diagnostic skills to pediatricians and other primary care physicians.

II. Institutional Organization

A. Sponsoring Institution

1. A pediatric otolaryngology educational program must be sponsored by a single sponsoring institution, as stated in the Institutional Requirements. In addition, the program must be based within a pediatric tertiary care institution that provides sufficient exposure and broad experience in the management of uncommon and complex otolaryngology disorders of children. The RRC will develop an annual resident reporting system to ensure that ACGME procedures are followed in this respect.
2. The sponsoring institution must provide sufficient faculty, clinical material, research and other educational resources to meet the needs of the pediatric otolaryngology residents.
3. Service commitments must not compromise the achievement of educational goals and objectives.

B. Participating Institutions

1. If the resources of two or more institutions are used, interinstitutional agreements must be developed by the institutional governing boards, as referenced in the Institutional Requirements.
2. The RRC must approve the addition or deletion of all participating institutions prospectively. Such approval will be based on a clear educational rationale and the value of the institution to the program.

C. Appointment of Residents

1. The RRC will approve a total number of pediatric otolaryngology residents in the program for each year. The number will be based on the number, qualifications, and commitment of the faculty; the volume and variety of the patient population available for educational purposes; and the institutional resources committed to the program.
2. The program may not graduate more residents in any year than are approved by the RRC unless prior approval has been received.

III. Program Personnel

The program director and faculty are responsible for the general administration of the program, including those activities related to the recruitment, selection, instruction, supervision, counseling, evaluation, and advancement of residents and the maintenance of records related to program accreditation.

A. Program Director

1. Qualifications
   a. There must be a single program director responsible for the program with requisite and documented clinical, educational, and administrative abilities and experience. The program director must be licensed to practice medicine in the state where the institution that sponsors the program is located and must be appointed in good standing to the medical staff of an institution participating in the program.
   b. The program director must be certified by the American Board of Otolaryngology and be certified in the subspecialty or possess suitable equivalent qualifications as determined by the RRC for Otolaryngology.
   c. The program director must have administrative responsibility for the pediatric otolaryngology program and should possess the skills of administrator, clinician, teacher, and researcher. The program director must devote sufficient time to the program to ensure continuity of leadership and to fulfill all the responsibilities inherent in meeting the educational goals of the program. The executive secretary should be notified promptly of any change in program leadership.
2. Responsibilities
   a. Development of a sound administrative and organizational framework that includes an effective faculty as an essential element of the program. Continuity of leadership is essential to the program's stability. Frequent changes in leadership or long periods of temporary leadership will be cause for serious concern. The executive secretary should be notified promptly of any change in program leadership.
   b. Maintenance of a record of pediatric otolaryngology operative cases performed by the service and a record of operative experience for each pediatric otolaryngology resident. These records must be reviewed at least semiannually by the program director as a part of his or her responsibility for evaluation of the balanced progress of each individual resident and of the total program. These data must be submitted to the RRC at the time of each program review.
   c. Preparation of a written statement outlining the educational goals of the program with respect to the knowledge, skills, and other attributes of residents at each level of education and for each major rotation or other program assignment. This statement must be distributed to residents and members of the faculty and be readily available for review.
   d. Selection of residents for appointment to the program in accordance with institutional and departmental policies and procedures.
   e. Selection and supervision of faculty and other personnel at each institution participating in the program.

f. Supervision of residents through explicit written descriptions of supervisory lines of responsibility for the care of patients. Such guidelines must be communicated to all members of the faculty. Residents must be provided with prompt, reliable systems for communication and interaction with supervising physicians.
g. Implementation of fair procedures as established by the sponsoring institution regarding academic discipline and resident complaints or grievances.
h. Monitoring resident stress, including mental or emotional conditions inhibiting performance or learning and drug- or alcohol-related dysfunction. Program directors and faculty should be sensitive to the need for timely provision of confidential counseling and psychological support services to residents. Situations that consistently produce undesirable stress on residents must be evaluated and modified.
i. Preparation of an accurate statistical and narrative description of the program, as requested by the RRC.

B. Faculty

1. There must be one pediatric otolaryngology faculty member in addition to the program director who is certified by the American Board of Otolaryngology with additional appropriate professional qualifications in pediatric otolaryngology or other equivalent qualifications, as determined by the RRC.
2. There must be a sufficient number of faculty with documented qualifications to instruct and supervise adequately all pediatric otolaryngology residents in the program. Members of the faculty must be able to devote sufficient time to meet their supervisory and teaching responsibilities.
3. Because the care of pediatric otolaryngology patients may be multidisciplinary in nature, additional peers from pediatrics and other related pediatric disciplines should participate in the program to enhance the residents' educational opportunities. Examples of related faculty may include anesthesiology; medical genetics; radiology; neonatology; pediatric neurology; audiology, speech, voice, and hearing specialists; plastic surgery; and pathology.
4. The faculty must demonstrate a strong interest in the education of residents, sound clinical and teaching abilities, support for the goals and objectives of the program, a commitment to their own continuing medical education, and participation in scholarly activities. One measure of this commitment is the extent to which faculty members permit pediatric residents to participate in the management of patients under their care.
5. The faculty must be organized and have regular documented meetings to review program goals and objectives and program effectiveness in achieving them. At least one pediatric otolaryngology resident should participate in these reviews.
6. The faculty should periodically evaluate the utilization of resources available to the program, the contribution of each participating institution, the financial and administrative support for the program, the volume and variety of patients available to the program for educational purposes, the performance of members of the faculty, and the quality of resident supervision.
7. The faculty must demonstrate involvement in scholarly activities, to include
   a. participation in their own continuing education;
   b. participation in regional and national scientific societies;
   c. presentation and publication of scientific studies;
   d. active participation in research as it pertains to pediatric otolaryngology;
   e. offering of guidance and technical support (eg, research design, statistical analysis) for residents involved in research; and
   f. active participation in clinical discussions, rounds, and conferences to promote a spirit of inquiry and scholarship.

C. Other Program Personnel

Programs must be provided with the additional professional, technical, and clerical personnel needed to support the administration and educational conduct of the program.

IV. The Educational Program

The educational program must provide an intellectual environment for acquiring the knowledge, skills, clinical judgment, and attitudes that are essential for the practice of the subspecialty.

This objective can be achieved only when the program leadership, the faculty, and the sponsoring institution are committed to the educational program and when appropriate resources and facilities are available.

A. General

1. The program director is responsible for developing a structured curriculum with written, defined goals and objectives. Clinical, basic science, and research conferences and seminars and journal club activities pertaining to the subspecialty must be conducted regularly. The pediatric otolaryngology resident must participate in planning and conducting the conferences. Both the faculty and the resident must attend and participate in multidisciplinary conferences.
2. The pediatric otolaryngology resident must be provided with opportunities to develop skills in providing consultation, in communicating with colleagues and referring physicians, and in teaching medical students, residents, physicians, and other professional personnel.
3. Lines of responsibility must be clearly defined between pediatric otolaryngology and otolaryngology residents in the areas of education, clinical responsibilities, and duration of education. Such information must be supplied to the RRC at the time of the survey and review.
4. The same resident duty hours and supervision requirements apply to these subspecialty residents as those documented in the Program Requirements for Residency Education in Otolaryngology.

B. Clinical

1. Outpatient Experiences
   a. There must be adequate outpatient experiences to provide a sufficient number of visits for the evaluation of patients with varied types of disorders to provide the residents with wide experience in diagnosis and outpatient management of patients with otolaryngology disorders. Residents are required to attend a minimum of two clinic sessions per week.
   b. Experience in the ambulatory care setting should include evaluation of children with common disorders and experience with the diagnosis and management of children with congenital abnormalities of the head and neck, hearing impairment, inherited disorders and developmental abnormalities, swallowing disorders, and sinus disease.
   c. In addition, multispecialty, interdisciplinary team experience should be provided to include, for example, a craniofacial and/or cleft palate team.
2. Inpatient
   a. An adequate inpatient facility must be available to provide a broad range of pediatric consultative experience.
   b. Pediatric intensive care facilities must be available for resident experience.
   c. There must be a sufficient number and variety of surgical cases to provide the pediatric otolaryngology resident with operative experience in all aspects of pediatric otolaryngology. The surgical case load should include experience in the following areas:

laryngobronchoesophagology, head and neck surgery, laryngotracheal surgery, otologic surgery, surgery of the nose and paranasal sinuses, surgery for congenital abnormalities of the head and neck, and surgery for benign and malignant head and neck disorders.

3. Diagnostic
   a. Complete diagnostic facilities for infants and children with otolaryngologic disorders must be available to provide the resident with the opportunity to interpret the results of diagnostic studies.
   b. The diagnostic studies for complete audiologic, voice, speech, language, and developmental assessments must be available. In addition, state-of-the-art diagnostic, therapeutic, and laboratory facilities must be provided.

C. Research and Scholarly Activity

1. Graduate medical education must take place in an environment of inquiry and scholarship in which pediatric otolaryngology residents participate in the development of new knowledge, learn to evaluate research findings, and develop habits of inquiry as a continuing professional responsibility. The responsibility for establishing and maintaining an environment of inquiry and scholarship rests with the faculty.
2. The course of study must include research methodology, not to exceed 6 months, with protected time for the pursuit of scholarly activities and research. The pediatric otolaryngology resident should study epidemiology, statistical methods, experimental design, and manuscript preparation, including literature searches and the use of computerized databases. It is highly desirable that the resident prepare and submit one paper for publication in a peer-reviewed journal.

D. Library

1. Residents must have ready access to a major medical library, either at the institution where the residents are located or through arrangements with convenient nearby institutions.
2. Library services should include the electronic retrieval of information from medical databases.
3. There must be access to an onsite library or to collections of appropriate texts and journals in each institution participating in the educational program.

V. Evaluation

A. Resident Evaluation

The program director, with faculty participation, must

1. evaluate residents in writing at least semiannually regarding the knowledge, skills, and professional growth using appropriate criteria and procedures. The procedures must be confidential and must include observation, assessment, and substantiation of the resident's acquired body of knowledge, skills in physical examination and patient communication, technical proficiency, professional attitudes, and humanistic qualities demonstrated in the clinical setting, consultation skills, patient management, decision making, and critical analysis of clinical situations.
2. communicate each evaluation to the resident in a timely manner and provide feedback on his or her performance, including appropriate counseling and necessary remedial effort.
3. advance residents to positions of higher responsibility based on evidence of satisfactory progressive scholarship and professional growth.
4. maintain a permanent record of evaluation for each resident and have it accessible to the resident and other authorized personnel.
5. provide a final written evaluation for each resident graduating from the program that includes a review of the resident's performance during the program. This evaluation should verify that the resident has demonstrated sufficient professional ability to practice competently and independently. This final evaluation should be part of the resident's permanent record at the institution.
6. maintain the list of all surgical operative procedures performed by the resident during the educational program. These data must be submitted to the program director and kept in a permanent file for review by the RRC at the time of the site visit and review.

B. Faculty Evaluation

All faculty must be evaluated on a regular basis. This evaluation should include teaching ability and commitment to the educational program, clinical knowledge, and scholarly contributions. Residents should participate in this evaluation.

C. Program Evaluation

There should be documented evidence of periodic self-evaluation of the program in relation to the educational goals, the needs of the pediatric otolaryngology residents, and the extent to which the goals of resident education have been met. Confidential written evaluations by residents should be included in this process.

ACGME: June 1995 Effective: June 1995

Program Requirements

Residency Education in Pathology

Graduate medical education programs in pathology are accredited in the following categories:

APCP-4	Four-year programs in anatomic and clinical pathology
AP-3	Three-year programs in anatomic pathology
CP-3	Three-year programs in clinical pathology
BB-1	One-year programs in blood banking/transfusion medicine
PCH-1	One-year programs in chemical pathology
PCP-1	One-year programs in cytopathology
DP-1	One-year programs in dermatopathology
FP-1	One-year programs in forensic pathology
HMP-1	One-year programs in hematology
IMP-1	One-year programs in immunopathology
MM-1	One-year programs in medical microbiology
NP-2	Two-year programs in neuropathology
PP-1	One-year programs in pediatric pathology
SP	Training in selective pathology

Programs in the SP category are ordinarily approved in highly specialized hospitals of acknowledged excellence that, because of the limitations of their clinical material, cannot provide general training in all aspects of anatomic and/or clinical pathology.

Accredited programs in all categories must meet institutional requirements as well as the applicable program requirements.

Program Requirements for Residency Education in Pathology–Anatomic and Clinical

I. Duration and Scope of Training

A. Graduate medical education programs in anatomic and/or clinical pathology must provide an organized educational experience for qualified physicians seeking to acquire the basic competence of a pathologist.

B. Programs must offer residents the opportunity to acquire a broad understanding of anatomic and/or clinical pathology, the techniques and methods of those disciplines, and the consultative role of the pathologist in patient-care decision making.

C. APCP-4 programs are accredited to offer 4 years of education/training in anatomic and clinical pathology, 3 years of training in anatomic pathology (AP-3), and 3 years of training in clinical pathology (CP-3.)

D. APCP-4 programs must include 18 months of formal education in anatomic pathology and 18 months of formal education in clinical pathology. The remaining 12 months of training may be a continuation of structured anatomic pathology or clinical pathology education or may be devoted to a specialized facet of pathology. AP-3 and CP-3 programs must include 24 months of anatomic pathology or clinical pathology education. The remaining 12 months of training may be a continuation of structured anatomic pathology or clinical pathology education or may be devoted to a specialized facet of pathology. The education must occur in the Department of Pathology under the direction of the program director or designated member of the teaching staff. The program director must clearly define, as part of the program description, the available opportunities whereby residents may accomplish the additional 12 months of pathology education. The program director must approve all such opportunities and monitor their progress.

II. Institutional Support of Graduate Medical Education

A. Institutions involved in residency programs must be in compliance with the Institutional Requirements of the Essentials of Accredited Residencies in Graduate Medical Education. Institutional commitment to graduate medical education is a critical influence on a residency and will be carefully evaluated when pathology programs are reviewed.

B. When the resources of two or more institutions are utilized in a program, valid letters of agreement from the appropriate institutional representatives detailing the educational role of each institution must be kept on file by the director of the residency program.

C. As other residency programs facilitate peer interchange and augment the breadth of the educational experience, institutions providing graduate medical education in anatomic and/or clinical pathology should also sponsor at least three additional accredited residency programs. Programs in internal medicine, family practice, obstetrics and gynecology, general surgery, pediatrics, and radiology are considered to be most complementary to pathology education. Requests for exceptions to this requirement will be considered on a case-by-case basis.

D. Resident assignments away from the primary institution in a program should not prevent regular resident participation in rounds and conferences, either at the parent institution or in equivalent conferences at participating institutions.

III. Program Goals and Objectives

A. The director and teaching staff of a program must prepare and comply with written educational goals for the program.

B. All educational components of a residency program should be related to program goals.
   1. The program design and/or structure must be approved by the Residency Review Committee (RRC) as part of the regular review process.
   2. Participation by an institution providing more than 6 months of training in a program must be approved by the RRC.

C. There must be a program statement, available for review by applicants, residents, and the RRC, describing the program and each rotation, assignment, or other experience.
   1. The program statement must include:
      a. A description of the program's educational goals and philosophy.
      b. A listing and description of all required rotations, including their duration.
      c. A listing and description of elective rotations, the year(s) of the program in which they are available, and their duration.
      d. A description of resident opportunities for teaching and research.
      e. A description of the manner in which residents and the program are evaluated and how such evaluations are used.
      f. A description of the manner in which residents are supervised.
   2. The description of rotations, assignments, or other experiences must include:
      a. The goals and objectives of the experience.
      b. The duration of the experience.
      c. The duties and responsibilities of residents at each year of training.
      d. The teaching staff responsible for the supervision and instruction of the residents during the experience.
      e. The manner in which residents are supervised and evaluated during the experience.

IV. Curriculum

A. Education in anatomic pathology must include autopsy and surgical pathology, cytopathology, pediatric pathology, dermatopathology, forensic pathology, immunopathology, histochemistry, neuropathology, ultrastructural pathology, cytogenetics, molecular biology, and other advanced diagnostic techniques as they become available.
B. Education in clinical pathology must include microbiology (including bacteriology, mycology, parasitology, and virology), immunopathology, blood banking/transfusion medicine, chemical pathology, cytogenetics, hematology, coagulation, toxicology, medical microscopy (including urinalysis), molecular biologic techniques, and other advanced diagnostic techniques as they become available.
C. Programs must provide instruction and experience in the major aspects of the administration of a hospital laboratory, including resident participation in interpretation of laboratory data as part of patient-care decision making, conferences, rounds, patient-care consultation, management and direction of the laboratory, quality assurance, data processing, teaching, and scholarly activity.
D. The educational experiences detailed above may be provided through separate, exclusive rotations, by rotations that combine more than one area, or by other means; but in any case, all rotations and other assignments must conform to the educational goals and objectives of the program.

V. Program Personnel

The program director and the teaching staff are responsible for the general administration of a program, including those activities related to the recruitment, selection, instruction, supervision, counseling, evaluation, and advancement of residents and the maintenance of records related to program accreditation.

A. Program Director

1. The program director is responsible for, and must have the authority to conduct, the entire program and must devote sufficient time to fulfill the responsibilities inherent in meeting the educational goals of the program, including the implementation of sound administrative practices and the provision of adequate facilities, teaching staff, resident staff, and educational resource materials.
2. A program involving two or more institutions must have a single director with the responsibility and authority for the supervision and coordination of the portions of the program carried out at each institution.
3. Continuity of leadership over a period of years is important to the stability of a residency program. Frequent changes in the directorship or long periods of temporary leadership are cause for serious concern by the RRC.
4. The program director must demonstrate a continuing involvement in scholarly activity.
5. Qualifications of the program director include:
   a. Requisite and documented clinical, educational, and administrative abilities and experience.
   b. Licensure to practice medicine in the state where the institution that sponsors the program is located. (Certain federal programs are exempted.)
   c. Certification by the American Board of Pathology (in anatomic and clinical pathology, anatomic pathology, or clinical pathology) or suitable equivalent qualifications.
   d. Appointment in good standing to the medical staff of an institution participating in the program.
6. Responsibilities of the program director include:
   a. Preparation of a written statement outlining the educational goals of the program with respect to knowledge, skills, and other attributes of residents at each level of training and for each major rotation or other program assignment. This statement must be distributed to residents and members of the teaching staff. It should be readily available for review.
   b. Selection of residents for appointment to the program in accordance with institutional and departmental policies and procedures.
   c. Selection and supervision of the teaching staff and other program personnel at each institution participating in the program.
   d. The supervision of residents in accordance with explicit written descriptions of supervisory lines of responsibility for the care of patients. Such guidelines must be communicated to all members of the program staff. Residents must be provided with prompt, reliable systems for communication and interaction with supervisory physicians.
   e. Regular evaluation of residents' knowledge, skills, and overall performance, including the development of professional attitudes consistent with being a physician.
   f. The program director, with participation of members of the teaching staff, shall:
      1. At least semiannually evaluate the knowledge, skills, and professional growth of the residents, using appropriate criteria and procedures.
      2. Communicate each evaluation to the resident in a timely manner.
      3. Advance residents to positions of higher responsibility only on the basis of evidence of their satisfactory progressive scholarship and professional growth.
      4. Maintain a permanent record of evaluation for each resident and have it accessible to the resident and other authorized personnel.
   g. The provision of a written final evaluation for each resident who completes the program. The evaluation must include a review of the resident's performance during the final period of training and should verify that the resident has demonstrated sufficient professional ability to practice competently and independently. This final evaluation should be part of the resident's permanent record maintained by the institution.
   h. Implementation of fair procedures, as established by the sponsoring institution, regarding academic discipline and resident complaints or grievances.
   i. Monitoring resident stress, including mental or emotional conditions inhibiting performance or learning and drug- or alcohol-related dysfunction. Program directors and teaching staff should be sensitive to the need for timely provision of confidential counseling and psychological support services to residents. Training situations that consistently produce undesirable stress on residents must be evaluated and modified.
   j. Preparation of an accurate statistical and narrative description of the program as requested by a review committee.

B. Teaching Staff

1. There must be a sufficient number of teaching staff with documented qualifications to instruct and supervise adequately all the residents in the program. Members of the teaching staff must be able to devote sufficient time to meet their supervisory and teaching responsibilities.
2. All members of the teaching staff must demonstrate a strong interest in the education of residents, sound clinical and teaching abilities, support of the goals and objectives of the program, a commitment to their own continuing medical education, and participation in scholarly activities.

3. A member of the teaching staff of each participating institution must be designated to assume responsibility for the day-to-day activities of the program at that institution, with overall coordination by the program director.
4. The teaching staff must be organized and have regular documented meetings to review program goals and objectives as well as program effectiveness in achieving them. At least one resident representative should participate in these reviews.
5. The teaching staff should periodically evaluate the utilization of the resources available to the program, the contribution of each institution participating in the program, the financial and administrative support of the program, the volume and variety of patients available to the program for educational purposes, the performance of members of the teaching staff, and the quality of supervision of residents.

C. Number of Residents

1. The number of resident positions requested must not exceed the educational resources available in a program.
2. When reviewing a program for accreditation, the RRC will approve a maximum number of residents to be trained in the program at any one time. Any increase in that number requires prior written approval of the RRC.
3. Programs must maintain a number of residents sufficient to promote an intellectually stimulating educational environment. There should be at least two residents enrolled in each year of a program. A lesser number is cause for concern by the RRC.

D. Appointment of Fellows

1. The appointment of other individuals for special training or education, such as fellows, must not dilute or detract from the educational opportunities of the regularly appointed residents.
2. The appointment of fellows by a program director requires a clear statement of the areas of training, responsibilities, and duration of the fellowship. This statement must be provided to the RRC at the time the program is reviewed.

E. Other Personnel

1. The laboratories providing patient-care services must be accredited by the appropriate organizations and must be directed by a qualified physician who is licensed to practice medicine and is a member of the medical staff.
2. The number and qualifications of medical technologists and other support personnel must be adequate for the volume of work in the laboratory and the educational activities of the institution.
3. Programs must be provided with the additional professional, technical, and clerical personnel needed to support the administration and educational conduct of the program.

VI. Program Facilities

A. Adequate space and equipment must be available for the conduct of the program, including equipment for the performance of all the functions described above, meeting rooms, classrooms, and office and research space for staff.

B. Office and laboratory space must be provided for the residents for both patient-care work and participation in scholarly activities.

C. The patient material of the department must be indexed in such a way as to permit appropriate retrieval.

D. Residents must have ready access to a major medical library, either at the institution where the residents are located or through arrangement with convenient nearby institutions. The services provided by the library should include the electronic retrieval of information from medical databases.

E. There must be access to an on-site library or to a collection of appropriate texts and journals in each institution participating in a residency program. On-site libraries and/or collections of texts and journals must be readily available during nights and weekends.

F. The audiovisual resources available for educational purposes should be adequate to meet the goals and objectives of the program.

VII. Educational Program

A. Resources for Anatomic Pathology

1. The volume and variety of material available in the program for anatomic pathology education must be sufficient to ensure that residents have a broad exposure to both common conditions and unusual entities, develop proficiency in diagnosis and problem solving, and develop the necessary technical skills to perform the functions of an anatomic pathologist.
2. While the quality of an educational program is not based on volume of teaching material alone, programs should have sufficient volume and variety of material available for educational purposes to ensure the opportunity for:
   a. The performance of at least 75 autopsies per resident during the program. It is highly desirable that this experience include forensic and stillborn autopsies.
   b. The examination and signing out of at least 2,000 surgical pathology specimens per resident during the program. This material must be from an adequate mix of cases to ensure exposure to both common and uncommon conditions.
   c. The examination of at least 1,500 cytologic specimens per resident during the program. This material must include a variety of both exfoliative and aspiration specimens.
   d. The performance of at least 200 operating room consultations (frozen sections) per resident during the program.

B. Resources for Clinical Pathology

1. The volume and variety of material available in the program for training in clinical pathology should be sufficient to ensure that residents have a broad exposure to both common conditions and unusual entities, develop proficiency in diagnosis and problem solving, and develop the necessary technical skills to perform the functions of a clinical pathologist.
2. The number and variety of tests performed in the laboratories utilized in the program should be sufficient to give residents experience in the range of tests typically available in a general hospital. Further, resident experience should be augmented through the use of seminar and course materials and laboratory indices of unusual cases.
3. While the quality of an educational program is not based on the volume of teaching material alone, programs should have a laboratory workload of at least 500,000 weighted workload units (according to the standards of the workload recording program of the College of American Pathologists or equivalent) per resident during the program. Further, this material must include an adequate variety of clinical pathology procedures.
4. A sufficient number of supervisory personnel and medical technologists, as well as modern equipment, must be available in each of the laboratories utilized in the program.

C. Seminars, Conferences, and Rounds

1. There must be regularly scheduled seminars and conferences devoted to the basic and applied medical sciences and clinical correlation conferences.
2. Clinical correlation conferences (eg, a pediatric mortality conference) should be held with clinical services such as internal medicine, surgery, gynecology, radiology, pediatrics, and their subspecialties.

3. There must be departmental conferences for detailed discussion of difficult and unusual cases in which both faculty and residents participate.
4. Residents must participate in the regular, formal clinical, and teaching rounds corresponding to the laboratory services to which they are assigned. For example, infectious disease service rounds should be attended during an assignment in microbiology.

D. Consultation

1. Both faculty and residents must be regularly involved in consultative activity.
2. Patient-care consultations should be both intra- and interdepartmental.

E. Teaching

1. Residents should participate in the education of medical students and other residents.
2. The effectiveness of residents as teachers should be monitored and evaluated by the program director and teaching staff.

VIII. Evaluation

A. There must be regular, formal, written evaluation of residents by the teaching staff. Evaluations should be completed at least once every 6 months and after rotations outside the primary institutions or to specialty experiences. Evaluations should be discussed with the residents by the program director or appropriate designee at least once each year.

B. The educational effectiveness of a program must be evaluated in a systematic manner. In particular, the quality of the curriculum and the extent to which the educational goals have been met by residents must be assessed. As part of this process, residents should provide periodic written evaluations of the program and teaching staff.

IX. Research and Scholarly Activity

A. Graduate medical education must take place in an environment of inquiry and scholarship in which residents participate in the development of new knowledge, learn to evaluate research findings, and develop habits of inquiry as a continuing professional responsibility.

B. The responsibility for establishing and maintaining an environment of inquiry and scholarship rests with the teaching staff. While not all members of a teaching staff must be investigators, the staff as a whole must demonstrate broad involvement in scholarly activity. This activity should include:

1. Active participation of the teaching staff in clinical discussions, rounds, and conferences in a manner that promotes a spirit of inquiry and scholarship. Scholarship implies an in-depth understanding of basic mechanisms of normal and abnormal states and the application of current knowledge to practice.
2. Participation in journal clubs and research conferences.
3. Active participation in regional or national professional and scientific societies, particularly through presentations at the organizations' meetings and publication in their journals.
4. Participation in research, particularly in projects that are funded following peer review and/or result in publications or presentations at regional and national scientific meetings.
5. Offering of guidance and technical support (eg, research design, statistical analysis) for residents involved in research.
6. Provision of support for resident participation in scholarly activities.

X. Resident Research

A. Throughout their time in the program, residents should be exposed to and encouraged to participate in clinical or laboratory research, research seminars, work-in-progress sessions, and organized reviews of intradepartmental research.

B. Resident involvement in research may be related to methods development, clinical or basic research, or literature surveys, but in all cases the program should provide an environment that promotes research or scholarly activity by residents.

XI. Resident Responsibility

A. Residents must be considered integral members of the staff of the Department of Pathology and must have the opportunity to participate in discussion of matters related to management of the department.

B. There must be periods of time when decision making in the laboratory is the direct responsibility of residents, under appropriate supervision.

C. Duty hours and night and weekend call for residents must reflect the fact that responsibilities for continuing patient care are not automatically discharged at any given hour of the day or any particular day of the week. However, the program director must ensure that residents are given reasonable duty and call assignments. All residents should, on the average, have the opportunity to spend at least 1 full day out of 7 free from hospital duties and should be on call no more often than every third night. Backup support should be provided for residents when their patient care responsibilities are especially difficult or prolonged.

XII. Residency Review Committee

A. When a program is scheduled for review by the RRC, the accuracy of the program information forms required by the committee is the responsibility of the program director. Action by the RRC will be deferred or an adverse action considered if the forms are not completed as requested.

B. The RRC must be provided written notification of major changes in a program, including changes in leadership, within 90 days. Prior approval of the committee is required for the addition or deletion of a major participating institution, a major change in the design of the program, or an increase or decrease in the approved number of residents in the program.

XIII. Certification and Accreditation

A. The RRC for Pathology is responsible for accreditation of graduate medical education programs in pathology. The American Board of Pathology is responsible for certification of individual physicians in pathology.

B. Questions about accreditation of residency programs should be directed to the executive director of the RRC.

C. Individuals who plan to seek certification by the American Board of Pathology should communicate with the executive vice president of the board to obtain the latest information regarding certification.

ACGME: June 1989 Effective: July 1995

Program Requirements for Residency Education in Blood Banking/Transfusion Medicine (Pathology)

I. Definition, Duration, and Scope of Education

A. Blood banking/transfusion medicine is the practice of laboratory and clinical medicine concerned with all aspects of blood transfusion, including the scientific basis of transfusion, selection and recruitment of blood donors, utilization and quality control, preparation of blood components, pretransfusion testing, transfusion of blood components, adverse effects of blood transfusion, autoimmunity, transplantation, histocompatibility, therapeutic apheresis and phlebotomy, blood substitutes, medicolegal considerations of transfusion, paternity analysis, management aspects of blood services, and the history of blood transfusion. Blood banking/transfusion medicine requires a strong foundation in clinical pathology as well as clinical medicine.

B. Graduate medical education programs in blood banking/transfusion medicine must provide an organized educational experience for qualified physicians seeking to acquire additional competence in blood banking/transfusion medicine.

C. Programs will be accredited to offer 1 year of organized education in all aspects of blood banking/transfusion medicine.

II. Program Goals and Objectives

A. The director and teaching staff of a program must prepare and comply with written educational goals for the program.

B. All educational components of a residency program should be related to program goals.

1. The program design and/or structure must be approved by the Residency Review Committee (RRC) as part of the regular review process.
2. Participation by any institution providing more than 2 months of training must be approved by the RRC.

III. Educational Program

A. Curriculum

1. The program must be structured to give residents clearly defined graduated responsibilities and delegated authority. Written goals and objectives for the educational program must be clearly defined.
2. There must be sufficient opportunity for the resident to develop comprehensive knowledge of the technical aspects of blood banking and immunohematology. There must be an opportunity to acquire knowledge and skills in new technologies as they become available.
3. Clinical aspects of transfusion medicine must be emphasized throughout the program. Residents must participate in ongoing clinical consultations regarding all aspects of blood transfusion and have opportunity to develop competence in providing services to patients and other physicians.

B. Educational Activities

1. Lectures, tutorials, seminars, and conferences must be regularly scheduled and held, with active participation of clinical services. The residents must have the opportunity to attend regional or national meetings.
2. Instruction should include studies illustrating usual and unusual cases.

IV. Personnel

The program director and the teaching staff are responsible for the general administration of a program, including those activities related to the recruitment, selection, instruction, supervision, counseling, evaluation, and advancement of residents and the maintenance of records related to program accreditation.

A. Program Director

1. A program involving two or more institutions must have a single director with authority for the supervision and coordination of the portions of the program carried out at each institution.
2. Qualifications of the program director include:
   a. Requisite and documented clinical, educational, and administrative abilities and experience.
   b. Licensure to practice medicine in the state where the institution that sponsors the program is located. (Certain federal programs are exempted.)
   c. Certification by the American Board of Pathology in Blood Banking/Transfusion Medicine or suitable equivalent qualifications.
   d. Appointment in good standing to the medical staff of an institution participating in the program.
3. Responsibilities of the program director include:
   a. Preparation of a written statement outlining the educational goals of the program with respect to knowledge, skills, and other attributes of residents at each level of training and for each major rotation or other program assignment. This statement must be distributed to residents and members of the teaching staff. It should be readily available for review.
   b. Selection of residents for appointment to the program in accordance with institutional and departmental policies and procedures.
   c. Selection, supervision, and evaluation of the teaching staff and other program personnel at each institution participating in the program.
   d. The supervision of residents through explicit written descriptions of supervisory lines of responsibility for the care of patients. Such guidelines must be communicated to all members of the program staff. Residents must be provided with prompt, reliable systems for communication and interaction with supervisory physicians.
   e. Regular evaluation of residents' knowledge, skills, and overall performance, including the development of professional attitudes consistent with being a physician.
      The program director, with participation of members of the teaching staff, shall:
      1. At least semiannually evaluate the knowledge, skills, and professional growth of the residents, using appropriate criteria and procedures.
      2. Communicate each evaluation to the resident in a timely manner.
      3. Advance residents to positions of higher responsibility only on the basis of evidence of their satisfactory progressive scholarship and professional growth.
      4. Maintain a permanent record of evaluation for each resident and have it accessible to the resident and other authorized personnel.
   f. The provision of a written final evaluation for each resident who completes the program. The evaluation must include a review of the resident's performance during the final period of training and should verify that the resident has demonstrated sufficient professional ability to practice competently and independently. This final evaluation should be part of the resident's permanent record maintained by the institution.

g. Implementation of fair procedures, as established by the sponsoring institution, regarding academic discipline and resident complaints or grievances.
h. Monitoring resident stress, including mental or emotional conditions inhibiting performance or learning and drug- or alcohol-related dysfunction. Program directors and teaching staff should be sensitive to the need for timely provision of confidential counseling and psychological support services to residents. Training situations that consistently produce undesirable stress on residents must be evaluated and modified.
i. Preparation of an accurate statistical and narrative description of the program as requested by the RRC.
j. The program director must be responsible for and have the authority to conduct the training program effectively. He or she must devote sufficient time to fulfill the responsibilities inherent in meeting the educational goals of the program, including implementation of sound administrative practices and evaluation procedures and the provision of adequate facilities, teaching staff, resident staff, and educational resource materials.
k. The program director must demonstrate a continuing record of scholarly activity.
l. The program director must ensure that residents are given reasonable duty and call assignments.

B. Teaching Staff

1. There must be a sufficient number of teaching staff with documented qualifications to instruct and supervise adequately all the residents in the program. Members of the teaching staff must be able to devote sufficient time to meet their supervisory and teaching responsibilities.
2. All members of the teaching staff must demonstrate a strong interest in the education of residents, sound clinical and teaching abilities, support of the goals and objectives of the program, a commitment to their own continuing medical education, and participation in scholarly activities.
3. A member of the teaching staff of each participating institution must be designated to assume responsibility for the day-to-day activities of the program at that institution, with overall coordination by the program director.
4. The teaching staff must be organized and have regular documented meetings to review program goals and objectives as well as program effectiveness in achieving them. At least one resident representative should participate in these reviews.
5. The teaching staff should periodically evaluate the utilization of the resources available to the program, the contribution of each institution participating in the program, the financial and administrative support of the program, the volume and variety of patients available to the program for educational purposes, the performance of members of the teaching staff, and the quality of supervision of residents.

C. Residents

1. The resident should have completed training in anatomic and clinical pathology or in clinical pathology, or be certified by a primary medical specialty board of the American Board of Medical Specialties.
2. The number of resident positions requested must be consistent with the educational resources available in the program.
3. Residents must have the opportunity to assume increasing responsibilities as they progress through the program.
4. Residents should have the opportunity to become involved in basic scientific or clinical research and teaching during the program.
5. It is desirable that residents' work schedules be designed so that on the average, excluding exceptional patient care needs, residents have at least 1 day out of 7 free of routine responsibilities and be on-call in the hospital no more often than every third night. The ratio of hours worked and on-call time will vary, particularly at the senior levels, and therefore necessitate flexibility.

D. Other Personnel

1. The laboratories and clinical services involved in the program must be directed by qualified physicians who are licensed to practice medicine and are members in good standing of the institution's medical staff.
2. Programs must be provided with the additional professional, technical, and clerical personnel needed to support the administration and educational conduct of the program.

V. Program Research and Scholarly Activity

A. Graduate medical education must take place in an environment of inquiry and scholarship in which residents participate in the development of new knowledge, learn to evaluate research findings, and develop habits of inquiry as a continuing professional responsibility.

B. The responsibility for establishing and maintaining an environment of inquiry and scholarship rests with the teaching staff. While not all members of a teaching staff must be investigators, the staff as a whole must demonstrate broad involvement in scholarly activity. This activity should include:
1. Active participation of the teaching staff in clinical discussions, rounds, and conferences in a manner that promotes a spirit of inquiry and scholarship. Scholarship implies an in-depth understanding of basic mechanisms of normal and abnormal states and the application of current knowledge to practice.
2. Participation in journal clubs and research conferences.
3. Active participation in regional or national professional and scientific societies, particularly through presentations at the organizations' meetings and publication in their journals.
4. Participation in research, particularly in projects that are funded following peer review and/or result in publications or presentations at regional and national scientific meetings.
5. Offering of guidance and technical support (eg, research design, statistical analysis) for residents involved in research.
6. Provision of support for resident participation in scholarly activities.

VI. Library

1. Residents must have ready access to a major medical library, either at the institution where the residents are located or through arrangement with convenient nearby institutions.
2. Library services should include the electronic retrieval of information from medical databases.
3. There must be access to an on-site library or to a collection of appropriate texts and journals in each institution participating in a residency program. On-site libraries and/or collections of texts and journals must be readily available during nights and weekends.

VII. Institutional Resources

A. The program must have a sufficient number and variety of patients to offer training in the widest range of blood banking/transfusion medicine. There must be a mechanism for the retrieval and review of cases. There must be effective mechanisms to facilitate clinical correlation with laboratory findings.

B. There must be adequate equipment, laboratory facilities, offices, meeting rooms, classrooms, and space to support service, teaching, educational, and research activities.

Program Requirements

C. The institutions, laboratories, and clinical services participating in the program must be appropriately accredited and/or licensed.

VIII. Evaluation

A. There must be regular, formal, and written evaluations of the residents by the teaching staff. Evaluations should be completed and discussed with the residents at least once every 6 months.

B. The educational effectiveness of a program must be evaluated in a systematic manner. In particular, the quality of the curriculum and the extent to which the educational goals have been met by residents must be assessed. Residents should submit formal, written evaluations of the program and faculty at least once each year for review by the director and the teaching staff.

IX. Administrative Structure

Each blood banking/transfusion medicine program should be administratively attached to an Accreditation Council for Graduate Medical Education-accredited residency in anatomic and/or clinical pathology when feasible.

X. Certification and Accreditation

A. The RRC for Pathology is responsible for accreditation of graduate medical education programs in blood banking/transfusion medicine. The American Board of Pathology is responsible for certification of individual physicians in pathology and blood banking/transfusion medicine.

B. Questions about accreditation of residency programs should be directed to the executive director of the RRC.

C. Individuals who plan to seek certification from the American Board of Pathology in blood banking/transfusion medicine should communicate with the executive vice president of the board to obtain current information regarding certification.

ACGME: February 1993 Effective: July 1995

Program Requirements for Residency Education in Chemical Pathology (Pathology)

I. Introduction

A. The minimum training program in chemical pathology shall be 1 year in addition to the completion of acceptable residency training in an Accreditation Council for Graduate Medical Education (ACGME)-accredited program of anatomic and/or clinical pathology, as outlined in the *Graduate Medical Education Directory*, or equivalent postgraduate training and experience.

B. The director and teaching staff of a program must prepare and comply with written educational goals for the program.

C. All educational components of a residency program should be related to program goals.

1. The program design and/or structure must be approved by the Residency Review Committee (RRC) as part of the regular review process.
2. Participation by any institution providing more than 2 months of training in a program must be approved by the RRC.

D. The educational effectiveness of a program must be evaluated in a systematic manner. In particular, the quality of the curriculum and the extent to which the educational goals have been met by residents must be assessed. Written evaluations by residents should be utilized in this process.

II. Program Personnel

The program director and the teaching staff are responsible for the general administration of a program, including those activities related to the recruitment, selection, instruction, supervision, counseling, evaluation, and advancement of residents and the maintenance of records related to program accreditation.

A. Program Director

1. There must be a single program director responsible for the program.
2. Qualifications of the program director include:
   a. Requisite and documented clinical, educational, and administrative abilities and experience.
   b. Licensure to practice medicine in the state where the institution that sponsors the program is located. (Certain federal programs are exempted.)
   c. Certification by the American Board of Pathology in Chemical Pathology or suitable equivalent qualifications.
   d. Appointment in good standing to the medical staff of an institution participating in the program.
3. Responsibilities of the program director include:
   a. Preparation of a written statement outlining the educational goals of the program with respect to knowledge, skills, and other attributes of residents at each level of training and for each major rotation or other program assignment. This statement must be distributed to residents and members of the teaching staff. It should be readily available for review.
   b. Selection of residents for appointment to the program in accordance with institutional and departmental policies and procedures.
   c. Selection and supervision of the teaching staff and other program personnel at each institution participating in the program.
   d. The supervision of residents through explicit written descriptions of supervisory lines of responsibility for the care of patients. Such guidelines must be communicated to all members of the program staff. Residents must be provided with prompt, reliable systems for communication and interaction with supervisory physicians.
   e. Regular evaluation of residents' knowledge, skills, and overall performance, including the development of professional attitudes consistent with being a physician.

   The program director, with participation of members of the teaching staff, shall:

   1. At least semiannually evaluate the knowledge, skills, and professional growth of the residents, using appropriate criteria and procedures.
   2. Communicate each evaluation to the resident in a timely manner.
   3. Advance residents to positions of higher responsibility only on the basis of evidence of their satisfactory progressive scholarship and professional growth.
   4. Maintain a permanent record of evaluation for each resident and have it accessible to the resident and other authorized personnel.
   5. The provision of a written final evaluation for each resident who completes the program. The evaluation must include a review of the resident's performance during the final period of training and should verify that the resident has demonstrated sufficient professional ability to practice competently and independently. This final evaluation should be part of the resident's permanent record maintained by the institution.

f. Implementation of fair procedures, as established by the sponsoring institution, regarding academic discipline and resident complaints or grievances.
g. Monitoring resident stress, including mental or emotional conditions inhibiting performance or learning and drug- or alcohol-related dysfunction. Program directors and teaching staff should be sensitive to the need for timely provision of confidential counseling and psychological support services to residents. Training situations that consistently produce undesirable stress on residents must be evaluated and modified.
h. Preparation of an accurate statistical and narrative description of the program as requested by the RRC.

B. Teaching Staff

1. There must be a sufficient number of teaching staff with documented qualifications to instruct and supervise adequately all the residents in the program. Members of the teaching staff must be able to devote sufficient time to meet their supervisory and teaching responsibilities.
2. All members of the teaching staff must demonstrate a strong interest in the education of residents, sound clinical and teaching abilities, support of the goals and objectives of the program, a commitment to their own continuing medical education, and participation in scholarly activities.
3. A member of the teaching staff of each participating institution must be designated to assume responsibility for the day-to-day activities of the program at that institution, with overall coordination by the program director.
4. The teaching staff must be organized and have regular documented meetings to review program goals and objectives as well as program effectiveness in achieving them. At least one resident representative should participate in these reviews.
5. The teaching staff should periodically evaluate the utilization of the resources available to the program, the contribution of each institution participating in the program, the financial and administrative support of the program, the volume and variety of patients available to the program for educational purposes, the performance of members of the teaching staff, and the quality of supervision of residents.

C. Other Program Personnel

Programs must be provided with the additional professional, technical, and clerical personnel needed to support the administration and educational conduct of the program.

III. Educational Program

A. The program must provide opportunities for residents to become expert in the development, operation, and quality control of a chemical pathology laboratory and in the clinical interpretation of laboratory results; and to become a consultant in these areas to physicians and patients.
B. The analytical repertoire of the laboratory must be distributed satisfactorily within the various categories and subdivisions of chemical pathology to provide experience at a sufficient level for the resident to acquire the competency of a specialist in chemical pathology.
C. Clinical training in relation to chemical pathology, including the use and interpretation of chemical analyses in clinical diagnosis and management, must be an integral part of the training program.
D. The training program must provide opportunities for residents to develop knowledge and skills relating to (1) analytical chemical pathology, both basic and applied; (2) instrumentation; (3) administration and management of a chemical pathology laboratory; and (4) data processing. It is further expected that the resident will engage in research activities during the period of training.

IV. Institutional Organization and Resources

A. The training institution should be of sufficient size to provide the program with the necessary volume and variety of clinical material in chemical pathology.
B. The laboratory must have office and bench space sufficient to provide for both laboratory personnel and residents. The facilities should be well equipped with modern instrumentation in all major areas of analytical work.
C. The training program should be administratively attached to an ACGME-accredited program whenever feasible.

V. Program Research and Scholarly Activity

A. Graduate medical education must take place in an environment of inquiry and scholarship in which residents participate in the development of new knowledge, learn to evaluate research findings, and develop habits of inquiry as a continuing professional responsibility.
B. The responsibility for establishing and maintaining an environment of inquiry and scholarship rests with the teaching staff. While not all members of a teaching staff must be investigators, the staff as a whole must demonstrate broad involvement in scholarly activity. This activity should include:
   1. Active participation of the teaching staff in clinical discussions, rounds, and conferences in a manner that promotes a spirit of inquiry and scholarship. Scholarship implies an in-depth understanding of basic mechanisms of normal and abnormal states and the application of current knowledge to practice.
   2. Participation in journal clubs and research conferences.
   3. Active participation in regional or national professional and scientific societies, particularly through presentations at the organizations' meetings and publication in their journals.
   4. Participation in research, particularly in projects that are funded following peer review and/or result in publication or presentations at regional and national scientific meetings.
   5. Offering of guidance and technical support (eg, research design, statistical analysis) for residents involved in research.
   6. Provision of support for resident participation in scholarly activities.
C. Residents must have ready access to a major medical library, either at the institution where the residents are located or through arrangement with convenient nearby institutions.
   1. Library services should include the electronic retrieval of information from medical databases.
   2. There must be access to an on-site library or to a collection of appropriate texts and journals in each institution participating in a residency program. On-site libraries and/or collections of texts and journals must be readily available during nights and weekends.

ACGME: November 1983 Effective: July 1995

Program Requirements for Residency Education in Cytopathology (Pathology)

I. Definition, Duration, and Scope of Education

A. Cytopathology is the practice of pathology concerned with the study and diagnosis of human disease manifested in cells. Cytology requires a strong foundation in anatomic pathology.

B. Graduate medical education programs in cytopathology must provide an organized educational experience for qualified physicians seeking to acquire the competence of a cytopathologist.

C. Programs will be accredited to offer 1 year of organized education in all current aspects of cytopathology, including laboratory procedures, laboratory management, quality assurance, self-assessment, diagnostic and patient care decision making, and the scientific basis of cytopathology.

II. Program Goals and Objectives

A. The director and teaching staff of a program must prepare and comply with written educational goals for the program.

B. All educational components of a residency program should be related to program goals.

1. The program design and/or structure must be approved by the Residency Review Committee (RRC) as part of the regular review process.
2. Participation by any institution providing more than 2 months of training in a program must be approved by the RRC.

III. Educational Program

A. Curriculum

1. The program must be structured to give residents clearly defined graduated responsibilities and delegated authority. Written goals and objectives for the educational program must be clearly defined.
2. There must be ample opportunity for residents to develop knowledge and skills in the techniques of screening, specimen collection, cytopreparation, fine needle aspiration, flow cytometric and image analysis, in situ hybridization, hormone receptor assessment, and other new immunological and molecular techniques as they become applicable to the study of cells.
3. Diagnosis, pathogenesis, clinical correlation, consultative skills, and prognostic significance must be emphasized throughout the program.
4. Residents must be instructed and involved in correlating cytologic and histopathologic specimens.

B. Educational Activities

1. Lectures, tutorials, seminars, and conferences with clinical services must be regularly scheduled and held.
2. Instruction should include the use of study sets of usual and unusual cases and other educational materials.

IV. Program Personnel

The program director and the teaching staff are responsible for the general administration of a program, including those activities related to the recruitment, selection, instruction, supervision, counseling, evaluation, and advancement of residents and the maintenance of records related to program accreditation.

A. Program Director

A program involving two or more institutions must have a single director with authority for the supervision and coordination of the portions of the program carried out at each institution.

1. Qualifications of the program director include:
   a. Requisite and documented clinical, educational, and administrative abilities and experience.
   b. Licensure to practice medicine in the state where the institution that sponsors the program is located. (Certain federal programs are exempted.)
   c. Certification by the American Board of Pathology in Cytopathology or suitable equivalent qualifications.
   d. Appointment in good standing to the medical staff of an institution participating in the program.
2. Responsibilities of the program director include:
   a. Conducting the training program effectively. He or she must devote sufficient time to fulfill the responsibilities inherent in meeting the educational goals of the program, including the implementation of sound administrative practices and evaluation procedures and the provision of adequate facilities, teaching staff, resident staff, and educational resource materials.
   b. Ensuring that residents are given reasonable duty and call assignments.
   c. Preparation of a written statement outlining the educational goals of the program with respect to knowledge, skills, and other attributes of residents at each level of training and for each major rotation or other program assignment. This statement must be distributed to residents and members of the teaching staff. It should be readily available for review.
   d. Selection of residents for appointment to the program in accordance with institutional and departmental policies and procedures.
   e. Selection and supervision of the teaching staff and other program personnel at each institution participating in the program.
   f. The supervision of residents through explicit written descriptions of supervisory lines of responsibility for the care of patients. Such guidelines must be communicated to all members of the program staff. Residents must be provided with prompt, reliable systems for communication and interaction with supervisory physicians.
   g. Regular evaluation of residents' knowledge, skills, and overall performance, including the development of professional attitudes consistent with being a physician. The program director, with participation of members of the teaching staff, shall:
      1. At least semiannually evaluate the knowledge, skills, and professional growth of the residents, using appropriate criteria and procedures.
      2. Communicate each evaluation to the resident in a timely manner.
      3. Advance residents to positions of higher responsibility only on the basis of evidence of their satisfactory progressive scholarship and professional growth.
      4. Maintain a permanent record of evaluation for each resident and have it accessible to the resident and other authorized personnel.
      5. The provision of a written final evaluation for each resident who completes the program. The evaluation must include a review of the resident's performance during the final period of training and should verify that the resident has demonstrated sufficient professional ability to practice competently and independently. This final evaluation should be

part of the resident's permanent record maintained by the institution.

h. Implementation of fair procedures, as established by the sponsoring institution, regarding academic discipline and resident complaints or grievances.

i. Monitoring resident stress, including mental or emotional conditions inhibiting performance or learning and drug- or alcohol-related dysfunction. Program directors and teaching staff should be sensitive to the need for timely provision of confidential counseling and psychological support services to residents. Training situations that consistently produce undesirable stress on residents must be evaluated and modified.

j. Preparation of an accurate statistical and narrative description of the program as requested by the RRC.

B. Teaching Staff

1. There must be a sufficient number of teaching staff with documented qualifications to instruct and supervise adequately all the residents in the program. Members of the teaching staff must be able to devote sufficient time to meet their supervisory and teaching responsibilities.
2. All members of the teaching staff must demonstrate a strong interest in the education of residents, sound clinical and teaching abilities, support of the goals and objectives of the program, a commitment to their own continuing medical education, and participation in scholarly activities.
3. A member of the teaching staff of each participating institution must be designated to assume responsibility for the day-to-day activities of the program at that institution, with overall coordination by the program director.
4. The teaching staff must be organized and have regular documented meetings to review program goals and objectives as well as program effectiveness in achieving them. At least one resident representative should participate in these reviews.
5. The teaching staff should periodically evaluate the utilization of the resources available to the program, the contribution of each institution participating in the program, the financial and administrative support of the program, the volume and variety of patients available to the program for educational purposes, the performance of members of the teaching staff, and the quality of supervision of residents.

C. Residents

1. Prior to enrollment in a cytopathology program, residents should have completed training in:
   a. Anatomic and clinical pathology or
   b. Anatomic pathology.
2. The number of resident positions requested must be consistent with the educational resources available in the program.
3. Residents must have the opportunity to assume increasing responsibility as they progress through the program.
4. Residents should have the opportunity to become involved in cytopathologic research and teaching during the program.
5. Residents' performance must not be impaired by fatigue, whether caused by program duties or other activities. On average, residents should have the opportunity to spend at least 1 full day out of 7 free from hospital duties and should be on call no more often than every third night.

D. Other Personnel

1. The laboratories involved in the program must be directed by qualified physicians who are licensed to practice medicine and are members in good standing of the institution's medical staff.
2. Programs must be provided with the additional professional, technical, and clerical personnel needed to support the administration and educational conduct of the program.

V. Institutional Resources and Organization

A. The program must have access to a large volume and variety of cytopathology material. The material and files must be indexed to permit appropriate retrieval. There must be mechanisms to facilitate correlation with anatomic material.

B. There must be adequate equipment, laboratory facilities, offices, meeting rooms, classrooms, and space to support service, teaching, educational, and research activities.

C. The institutions and laboratories participating in the program must be appropriately accredited and/or licensed.

D. A cytopathology program should be administratively attached to an Accreditation Council for Graduate Medical Education (ACGME)-accredited residency in anatomic and clinical pathology or anatomic pathology when feasible.

VI. Program Research and Scholarly Activity

A. Graduate medical education must take place in an environment of inquiry and scholarship in which residents participate in the development of new knowledge, learn to evaluate research findings, and develop habits of inquiry as a continuing professional responsibility.

B. The responsibility for establishing and maintaining an environment of inquiry and scholarship rests with the teaching staff. While not all members of a teaching staff must be investigators, the staff as a whole must demonstrate broad involvement in scholarly activity. This activity should include:

1. Active participation of the teaching staff in clinical discussions, rounds, and conferences in a manner that promotes a spirit of inquiry and scholarship. Scholarship implies an in-depth understanding of basic mechanisms of normal and abnormal states and the application of current knowledge to practice.
2. Participation in journal clubs and research conferences.
3. Active participation in regional or national professional and scientific societies, particularly through presentations at the organizations' meetings and publication in their journals.
4. Participation in research, particularly in projects that are funded following peer review and/or result in publication or presentations at regional and national scientific meetings.
5. Offering of guidance and technical support (eg, research design, statistical analysis) for residents involved in research.
6. Provision of support for resident participation in scholarly activities.

C. Residents must have ready access to a major medical library, either at the institution where the residents are located or through arrangement with convenient nearby institutions.

1. Library services should include the electronic retrieval of information from medical databases.
2. There must be access to an on-site library or to a collection of appropriate texts and journals in each institution participating in a residency program. On-site libraries and/or collections of texts and journals must be readily available during nights and weekends.

VII. Evaluation

A. There must be regular, formal, written evaluation of residents by teaching staff. Evaluations should be completed and discussed with the residents at least once every 6 months.

B. The educational effectiveness of a program must be evaluated in a systematic manner. In particular, the quality of the curriculum and the extent to which the educational goals have been met by residents must be assessed. Residents should submit formal, written evaluations of the program at least once each year for review by the director and the teaching staff.

VIII. Certification and Accreditation

A. The RRC for Pathology is responsible for accreditation of graduate medical education programs in pathology. The American Board of Pathology is responsible for certification of individual physicians in pathology.
B. Questions about accreditation of residency programs should be directed to the Executive Secretary of the RRC.
C. Individuals who plan to seek certification by the American Board of Pathology should communicate with the executive vice president of the board.

ACGME: June 1991 Effective: July 1995

Program Requirements for Residency Education in Dermatopathology (Pathology)

I. Duration and Scope of Education

A. Dermatopathology is the subspecialty of dermatology and pathology that is concerned with the study and diagnosis of diseases of the skin and adjacent mucous membranes, cutaneous appendages, hair, nails, and subcutaneous tissues by histological, histochemical, immunological, ultrastructural, molecular, microbiological, and other related techniques.
B. Graduate medical education programs in dermatopathology must provide an organized educational experience for qualified physicians seeking to acquire the additional competence of a dermatopathologist.
C. Programs must provide organized education in all current aspects of dermatopathology, including basic science, laboratory procedures, laboratory management, quality assurance, and self-assessment.
D. The dermatopathology program must be an equal and joint function of the Department of Dermatology and of the Department of Pathology in a sponsoring institution that has an Accreditation Council for Graduate Medical Education (ACGME)-accredited residency in Dermatology and an ACGME-accredited residency in Anatomic Pathology (AP-3) or Anatomic and Clinical Pathology (APCP-4).
E. Dermatopathology programs must offer 12 months of education subsequent to the satisfactory completion of an ACGME-accredited residency in either dermatology or pathology.
F. For all dermatopathology residents, 50% of their education should be devoted to the study of dermatopathology, as outlined in II.A.1. For those who have completed a pathology residency, 50% of the 1-year program should be education in clinical dermatology provided by the dermatology teaching staff. For those who have completed a dermatology residency, 50% of the program should be education in anatomic pathology provided by the pathology teaching staff.
G. The director and teaching staff of the program must prepare and comply with written educational goals for the program and distribute them to applicants, residents, and members of the teaching staff. All educational components of the program should be related to these goals.
H. The program design and/or structure must be approved by the dermatopathology review committee as part of the regular review process.
I. Participation by any institution providing more than 2 months of training in the program must be approved by the subcommittee for dermatopathology.
J. The educational effectiveness of the program must be evaluated in a systematic manner. In particular, the quality of the curriculum and the extent to which the educational goals have been met by residents must be assessed. Written evaluations by residents should be utilized in this process.

II. Educational Program

A. Curriculum

1. Programs should be structured so that residents are involved in dermatopathology throughout the year. The program must include didactic instruction and practical experience in the diagnosis of skin disorders by direct inspection and by histological, histochemical, immunological, ultrastructural, molecular, microbiological, and other related techniques. Relevant aspects of mycology, bacteriology, and entomology should be included.
2. Dermatopathology residents must be given clearly defined assignments and increasing responsibility as they progress through the program.
3. The program must provide a sufficient volume and variety of dermatopathology specimens (at least 5,000 new accessions per resident per year) and other educational material for the resident to acquire the qualifications of a consultant in dermatopathology.
4. The program must provide the resident with the experience required to set up and to operate a dermatopathology laboratory and to supervise and train laboratory personnel.
5. All dermatopathology residents should participate in patient examination and autopsies appropriate to dermatopathology. Residents who are pathologists must participate in the examination of at least 1,000 dermatopathology patients.
6. Dermatopathology residents who are dermatologists must have exposure to autopsy and surgical pathology. This experience should emphasize contemporary diagnostic techniques (including the use of a wide variety of monoclonal antibodies) and require attendance at autopsy and surgical pathology conferences, the review of slide sets of diseases relevant to dermatopathology, and participation in autopsies.

B. Educational Activities

1. Lectures, tutorials, seminars, and conferences with clinical services must be regularly scheduled and held.
2. Instruction should include the use of study sets and files of usual and unusual cases and other educational materials.

III. Program Personnel

The program director and the teaching staff are responsible for the general administration of a program, including those activities related to the recruitment, selection, instruction, supervision, counseling, evaluation, and advancement of residents and the maintenance of records related to program accreditation.

A. Program Director

1. The program director must be responsible for and have the authority to conduct the training program effectively. He or she must devote sufficient time to the program to ensure the implementation of sound administrative practices and the provision of adequate facilities, teaching staff, resident staff, and educational resource materials.
2. A program involving two or more participating institutions must have a single director with authority for the supervision and coordination of the portions of the program carried out at each institution.
3. Qualifications of the program director include:
   a. Requisite and documented clinical, educational, and administrative abilities and experience.

b. Licensure to practice medicine in the state where the institution that sponsors the program is located. (Certain federal programs are exempted.)
c. Certification in dermatopathology by the American Board of Dermatology or American Board of Pathology or suitable equivalent qualifications.
d. Appointment in good standing to the medical staff of an institution participating in the program.

4. The program director must demonstrate continuing scholarly activity.
5. Responsibilities of the program director include:
   a. Preparation of a written statement outlining the educational goals of the program with respect to knowledge, skills, and other attributes of residents at each level of training and for each major rotation or other program assignment. This statement must be distributed to residents and members of the teaching staff. It should be readily available for review.
   b. Selection of residents for appointment to the program in accordance with institutional and departmental policies and procedures.
   c. Selection, supervision, and evaluation of the teaching staff and other program personnel at each institution participating in the program.
   d. The supervision of residents in accordance with explicit written descriptions of supervisory lines of responsibility for the care of patients. Such guidelines must be communicated to all members of the program staff. Residents must be provided with prompt, reliable systems for communication and interaction with supervisory physicians.
   e. Regular evaluation of residents' knowledge, skills, and overall performance, including the development of professional attitudes consistent with being a physician. The program director, with participation of members of the teaching staff, shall:
      1. At least semiannually evaluate the knowledge, skills, and professional growth of the residents, using appropriate criteria and procedures.
      2. Communicate each evaluation to the resident in a timely manner.
      3. Advance residents to positions of higher responsibility only on the basis of evidence of their satisfactory progressive scholarship and professional growth.
      4. Maintain a permanent record of evaluation for each resident and have it accessible to the resident and other authorized personnel.
   f. The provision of a written final evaluation for each resident who completes the program. The evaluation must include a review of the resident's performance during the final period of training and should verify that the resident has demonstrated sufficient professional ability to practice competently and independently. This final evaluation should be part of the resident's permanent record maintained by the institution.
   g. Implementation of fair procedures, as established by the sponsoring institution, regarding academic discipline and resident complaints or grievances.
   h. Monitoring resident stress, including mental or emotional conditions inhibiting performance or learning and drug- or alcohol-related dysfunction. Program directors and teaching staff should be sensitive to the need for timely provision of confidential counseling and psychological support services to residents. Training situations that consistently produce undesirable stress on residents must be evaluated and modified.
   i. Preparation of an accurate statistical and narrative description of the program as requested by the dermatopathology review committee.

B. Teaching Staff

1. There must be a sufficient number of teaching staff with documented qualifications in dermatopathology to instruct and supervise adequately all the residents in the program. Members of the teaching staff must be able to devote sufficient time to meet their supervisory and teaching responsibilities.
2. All members of the teaching staff must demonstrate a strong interest in the education of residents, sound clinical and teaching abilities, support of the goals and objectives of the program, a commitment to their own continuing medical education, and participation in scholarly activities.
3. A member of the teaching staff of each participating institution must be designated to assume responsibility for the day-to-day activities of the program at that institution, with overall coordination by the program director.
4. The teaching staff must be organized and have regular documented meetings to review program goals and objectives as well as program effectiveness in achieving them. At least one resident representative should participate in these reviews.
5. The teaching staff should periodically evaluate the utilization of the resources available to the program, the contribution of each institution participating in the program, the financial and administrative support of the program, the volume and variety of patients available to the program for educational purposes, the performance of members of the teaching staff, and the quality of supervision of residents.

C. Dermatopathology Residents

1. The number of positions requested must not exceed the educational resources available in a program.
2. Residents must have the opportunity to assume increasing responsibility under supervision appropriate to their experience as they progress through the program.
3. Residents should have the opportunity to become involved in dermatopathologic research and teaching during the program.
4. The program director must ensure that residents are adequately supervised by faculty at all times. Further, resident duty and on-call assignments must be made in a manner that ensures that neither education nor quality of patient care is jeopardized by resident stress or fatigue. Physicians must have a keen sense of personal responsibility for continuing patient care, and must recognize that their obligation to patients is not automatically discharged at any given hour of the day. In no case should a trainee go off duty until the proper care and welfare of the patients have been ensured. Resident duty hours and night and weekend call must reflect the concept of responsibility for patients and the provision of adequate patient care. Residents must not be required regularly to perform excessive, prolonged duties. When averaged over 4 weeks, residents should spend no more than 80 hours per week in hospital duties. Residents should, on average, have the opportunity to spend at least 1 day out of 7 free of program duties and should be on call no more often than every third night. When on call for 24 hours or more, there should be opportunity to rest and sleep.

D. Other Personnel

1. The laboratories involved in the program must be directed by qualified physicians who are licensed to practice medicine and are members in good standing of the institution's medical staff.
2. There must be a sufficient number of qualified professional, technical, and clerical personnel to support laboratory work and the educational program.

IV. Institutional Resources

A. There must be ample case material and supporting facilities to meet the training requirements in dermatopathology, dermatology, and pathology. Each dermatopathology resident should examine at least 5,000 dermatopathology specimens (ie, in-house or referred specimens in the institution's accessions file for which reports are generated).

B. There must be adequate equipment, laboratory space, office facilities, meeting rooms, classrooms, and research space to support service, teaching, and educational responsibilities.

C. The institutions and laboratories participating in the program must be appropriately accredited and/or licensed.

D. Residents must have ready access to a major medical library, either at the institution where the residents are located or through arrangement with convenient nearby institutions. Library services should include the electronic retrieval of information from medical databases. There must be access to an on-site library or to a collection of appropriate texts and journals in each institution participating in a residency program. On-site libraries and/or collections of texts and journals must be readily available during nights and weekends.

V. Research and Scholarly Activity

A. Graduate medical education must take place in an environment of inquiry and scholarship in which residents participate in the development of new knowledge, learn to evaluate research findings, and develop habits of inquiry as a continuing professional responsibility.

B. The responsibility for establishing and maintaining an environment of inquiry and scholarship rests with the teaching staff. While not all members of a teaching staff must be investigators, the staff as a whole must demonstrate broad involvement in scholarly activity. This activity should include:
   1. Active participation of the teaching staff in clinical discussions, rounds, and conferences in a manner that promotes a spirit of inquiry and scholarship. Scholarship implies an in-depth understanding of basic mechanisms of normal and abnormal states and the application of current knowledge to practice.
   2. Participation in journal clubs and research conferences.
   3. Active participation in regional or national professional and scientific societies, particularly through presentations at the organizations' meetings and publication in their journals.
   4. Participation in research, particularly in projects that are funded following peer review and/or result in publication or presentations at regional and national scientific meetings.
   5. Offering of guidance and technical support (eg, research design, statistical analysis) for residents involved in research.
   6. Provision of support for resident participation in scholarly activities.

VI. Evaluation

A. There must be regular, written evaluation of residents by teaching staff. Evaluations should be completed and discussed with the residents at least once every 6 months.

B. Residents should submit written evaluations of the program at least once each year for review by the director and teaching staff.

VII. Certification and Accreditation

A. The Residency Review Committees for Dermatology and Pathology are responsible for accreditation of graduate medical education programs in dermatopathology.

B. The American Board of Dermatology and American Board of Pathology are responsible for certification of individual physicians in dermatopathology. Individuals who plan to seek certification should communicate with their respective boards to obtain the latest information regarding certification.

ACGME: February 1993 Effective: July 1995

Program Requirements for Residency Education in Forensic Pathology (Pathology)

I. Introduction

A. The program shall be for a period of 1 year and must be directed by a pathologist who is certified by the American Board of Pathology in Forensic Pathology or has equivalent qualifications.

B. The director and teaching staff of a program must prepare and comply with written educational goals for the program.

C. All educational components of a residency program should be related to program goals.
   1. The program design and/or structure must be approved by the Residency Review Committee (RRC) as part of the regular review process.
   2. Participation by any institution providing more than 2 months of training in a program must be approved by the RRC.

D. The educational effectiveness of a program must be evaluated in a systematic manner. In particular, the quality of the curriculum and the extent to which the educational goals have been met by residents must be assessed. Written evaluations by residents should be utilized in this process.

II. Program Personnel

The program director and the teaching staff are responsible for the general administration of a program, including those activities related to the recruitment, selection, instruction, supervision, counseling, evaluation, and advancement of residents and the maintenance of records related to program accreditation.

A. Program Director

1. There must be a single program director responsible for the program.
2. Qualifications of the program director include:
   a. Requisite and documented clinical, educational, and administrative abilities and experience.
   b. Licensure to practice medicine in the state where the institution that sponsors the program is located. (Certain federal programs are exempted.)
   c. Certification by the American Board of Pathology in Forensic Pathology or suitable equivalent qualifications.
   d. Appointment in good standing to the medical staff of an institution participating in the program.
3. Responsibilities of the program director include:
   a. Preparation of a written statement outlining the educational goals of the program with respect to knowledge, skills, and other attributes of residents at each level of training and for each major rotation or other program assignment. This statement must be distributed to residents and members of the teaching staff. It should be readily available for review.
   b. Selection of residents for appointment to the program in accordance with institutional and departmental policies and procedures.
   c. Selection and supervision of the teaching staff and other program personnel at each institution participating in the program.

d. The supervision of residents through explicit written descriptions of supervisory lines of responsibility for the care of patients. Such guidelines must be communicated to all members of the program staff. Residents must be provided with prompt, reliable systems for communication and interaction with supervisory physicians.
e. Regular evaluation of residents' knowledge, skills, and overall performance, including the development of professional attitudes consistent with being a physician.
   The program director, with participation of members of the teaching staff, shall:
   1. At least semiannually evaluate the knowledge, skills, and professional growth of the residents, using appropriate criteria and procedures.
   2. Communicate each evaluation to the resident in a timely manner.
   3. Advance residents to positions of higher responsibility only on the basis of evidence of their satisfactory progressive scholarship and professional growth.
   4. Maintain a permanent record of evaluation for each resident and have it accessible to the resident and other authorized personnel.
f. The provision of a written final evaluation for each resident who completes the program. The evaluation must include a review of the resident's performance during the final period of training and should verify that the resident has demonstrated sufficient professional ability to practice competently and independently. This final evaluation should be part of the resident's permanent record maintained by the institution.
g. Implementation of fair procedures, as established by the sponsoring institution, regarding academic discipline and resident complaints or grievances.
h. Monitoring resident stress, including mental or emotional conditions inhibiting performance or learning and drug- or alcohol-related dysfunction. Program directors and teaching staff should be sensitive to the need for timely provision of confidential counseling and psychological support services to residents. Training situations that consistently produce undesirable stress on residents must be evaluated and modified.
i. Preparation of an accurate statistical and narrative description of the program as requested by the RRC.

B. Teaching Staff

1. There must be a sufficient number of teaching staff with documented qualifications to instruct and supervise adequately all the residents in the program. Members of the teaching staff must be able to devote sufficient time to meet their supervisory and teaching responsibilities.
   a. The teaching staff must include at least two forensic pathologists (including the program director).
   b. Programs that offer training for two or more residents must have a senior staff of qualified forensic pathologists that numbers at least one more than the number of residency positions.
2. All members of the teaching staff must demonstrate a strong interest in the education of residents, sound clinical and teaching abilities, support of the goals and objectives of the program, a commitment to their own continuing medical education, and participation in scholarly activities.
3. A member of the teaching staff of each participating institution must be designated to assume responsibility for the day-to-day activities of the program at that institution, with overall coordination by the program director.
4. The teaching staff must be organized and have regular documented meetings to review program goals and objectives as well as program effectiveness in achieving them. At least one resident representative should participate in these reviews.
5. The teaching staff should periodically evaluate the utilization of the resources available to the program, the contribution of each institution participating in the program, the financial and administrative support of the program, the volume and variety of patients available to the program for educational purposes, the performance of members of the teaching staff, and the quality of supervision of residents.

C. Other Program Personnel

Programs must be provided with the additional professional, technical, and clerical personnel needed to support the administration and educational conduct of the program.

III. Educational Program

A. A resident should perform 250 to 350 autopsies in a year of approved training and should have experience in scene investigations, including examination of the body before it has been disturbed.
B. The resident should have responsibility for the performance of autopsies in cases that are likely to result in criminal prosecution or civil litigation, and it is highly desirable for residents to have opportunities to participate in the legal follow-up of cases if such occurs during the course of their year of training.
C. It is highly desirable for residents to accompany staff pathologists when they testify in court and give depositions.
D. During the year of approved training, the resident must have a period of approximately 4 to 8 weeks devoted exclusively to laboratory experience in toxicology, physical anthropology, and components of the crime laboratory such as firearms, serology, and trace evidence.

IV. Institutional Resources

A. Approximately 500 medicolegal autopsies should be conducted in an approved program each year. Of these, 100 or more should be in cases in which death is due to the immediate (within 24 hours) and direct effects of physical or chemical injury.
B. The institution or office should conduct approximately 300 additional autopsies for each additional residency position requested.
C. Adequate facilities and competent personnel shall be available and properly utilized for the conduct of all bacteriologic, biochemical, toxicology, firearms, trace evidence, physical anthropology, odontology, and other scientific studies as may be needed to ensure complete postmortem investigation. When such support services are not housed at the medicolegal facility, they should be available and accessible to the resident at suitable laboratories.
D. If the resident is to spend parts of the training program at other laboratories or institutions, such training must be adequately supervised by qualified personnel.

V. Program Research and Scholarly Activity

A. Graduate medical education must take place in an environment of inquiry and scholarship in which residents participate in the development of new knowledge, learn to evaluate research findings, and develop habits of inquiry as a continuing professional responsibility.
B. The responsibility for establishing and maintaining an environment of inquiry and scholarship rests with the teaching staff. While not all members of a teaching staff must be investigators, the staff as a whole must demonstrate broad involvement in scholarly activity. This activity should include:
   1. Active participation of the teaching staff in clinical discussions, rounds, and conferences in a manner that promotes a spirit of

inquiry and scholarship. Scholarship implies an in-depth understanding of basic mechanisms of normal and abnormal states and the application of current knowledge to practice.
2. Participation in journal clubs and research conferences.
3. Active participation in regional or national professional and scientific societies, particularly through presentations at the organizations' meetings and publication in their journals.
4. Participation in research, particularly in projects that are funded following peer review and/or result in publication or presentations at regional and national scientific meetings.
5. Offering of guidance and technical support (eg, research design, statistical analysis) for residents involved in research.
6. Provision of support for resident participation in scholarly activities.

C. Residents must have ready access to a major medical library, either at the institution where the residents are located or through arrangement with convenient nearby institutions.
1. Library services should include the electronic retrieval of information from medical databases.
2. There must be access to an on-site library or to a collection of appropriate texts and journals in each institution participating in a residency program. On-site libraries and/or collections of texts and journals must be readily available during nights and weekends.

VI. Evaluation

A. There must be regular, formal, written evaluation of residents by teaching staff. Evaluations should be completed and discussed with the residents at least once every 6 months.

B. The educational effectiveness of a program must be evaluated in a systematic manner. In particular, the quality of the curriculum and the extent to which the educational goals have been met by residents must be assessed. Residents should submit formal, written evaluations of the program at least once each year for review by the director and the teaching staff.

VII. Certification and Accreditation

A. The RRC for Pathology is responsible for accreditation of graduate medical education programs in pathology. The American Board of Pathology is responsible for certification of individual physicians in pathology.

B. Questions about accreditation of residency programs should be directed to the executive director of the RRC.

C. Individuals who plan to seek certification by the American Board of Pathology should communicate with the executive vice president of the board.

ACGME: February 1986 Effective: July 1995

Program Requirements for Residency Education in Hematology (Pathology)

I. Definition, Duration, and Scope of Education

A. Hematology is the practice of pathology concerned with the study and diagnosis of human diseases involving the hematopoietic tissues and cells. Hematology requires a strong foundation in pathology.

B. Graduate medical education programs in hematology must provide an organized educational program for qualified physicians seeking to acquire additional competence in hematology and should be associated with an active program in clinical hematology of both adults and children.

C. Programs will be accredited to offer 1 year of organized training in all current aspects of hematology, including clinical laboratory procedures, laboratory management, database management, quality assurance, self-assessment, clinical consultation, and the scientific basis of hematology.

II. Program Goals and Objectives

A. The director and teaching staff of a program must prepare and comply with written educational goals for the program.

B. All educational components of a residency program should be related to program goals.
1. The program design and/or structure must be approved by the Residency Review Committee (RRC) as part of the regular review process.
2. Participation by any institution providing more than 2 months of training in a program must be approved by the RRC.

III. Educational Program

A. Curriculum

1. The program must be structured to give hematology residents clearly defined graduated responsibilities and delegated authority. Written goals and objectives for the educational program must be clearly defined.
2. There must be ample opportunity for the residents to develop knowledge and skills in the techniques of specimen collection and preparation for routine hematologic testing, bone marrow aspiration, biopsy and interpretation, lymph node interpretation, coagulation testing, cell analysis systems, and the applications of advanced technology, including in situ hybridization, image analysis, immunocytochemistry, cytogenetics, and molecular probe diagnosis, to hematologic problems. Adult and pediatric diagnostic material must be available.
3. Diagnosis, pathogenesis, clinical correlation, and prognostic significance of hematologic disease must be emphasized throughout the program.
4. Residents must be given increasing responsibilities for services to patients and other physicians as they progress through the program.
5. Residents must be instructed in methods of correlating data from cytological, histopathological, and clinical pathology assessments of hematologic disease.

B. Educational Activities

1. Lectures, tutorials, seminars, rounds, and conferences with clinical services must be regularly scheduled and held.
2. Instruction should include the use of study sets of usual and unusual cases, performance of tests under supervision, and interpretation of results with generation of narrative reports.

IV. Program Personnel

The program director and the teaching staff are responsible for the general administration of a program, including those activities related to the recruitment, selection, instruction, supervision, counseling, evaluation, and advancement of residents and the maintenance of records related to program accreditation.

A. Program Director

A program involving two or more institutions must have a single director with authority for the supervision and coordination of the portions of the program carried out at each institution.
1. Qualifications of the program director include:
   a. Requisite and documented clinical, educational, and administrative abilities and experience.

b. Licensure to practice medicine in the state where the institution that sponsors the program is located. (Certain federal programs are exempted.)
c. Certification by the American Board of Pathology in Hematology or suitable equivalent qualifications.
d. Appointment in good standing to the medical staff of an institution participating in the program.

2. Responsibilities of the program director include:
   a. Conducting the training program effectively. He or she must devote sufficient time to fulfill the responsibilities inherent in meeting the educational goals of the program, including the implementation of sound administrative practices, evaluation procedures, and the provision of adequate facilities, teaching staff, resident staff, and educational resource materials.
   b. Ensuring that residents are given reasonable duty and call assignments.
   c. Preparation of a written statement outlining the educational goals of the program with respect to knowledge, skills, and other attributes of residents at each level of training and for each major rotation or other program assignment. This statement must be distributed to residents and members of the teaching staff. It should be readily available for review.
   d. Selection of residents for appointment to the program in accordance with institutional and departmental policies and procedures.
   e. Selection and supervision of the teaching staff and other program personnel at each institution participating in the program.
   f. The supervision of residents through explicit written descriptions of supervisory lines of responsibility for the care of patients. Such guidelines must be communicated to all members of the program staff. Residents must be provided with prompt, reliable systems for communication and interaction with supervisory physicians.
   g. Regular evaluation of residents' knowledge, skills, and overall performance, including the development of professional attitudes consistent with being a physician. The program director, with participation of members of the teaching staff, shall:
      1. At least semiannually evaluate the knowledge, skills, and professional growth of the residents, using appropriate criteria and procedures.
      2. Communicate each evaluation to the resident in a timely manner.
      3. Advance residents to positions of higher responsibility only on the basis of evidence of their satisfactory progressive scholarship and professional growth.
      4. Maintain a permanent record of evaluation for each resident and have it accessible to the resident and other authorized personnel.
   h. The provision of a written final evaluation for each resident who completes the program. The evaluation must include a review of the resident's performance during the final period of training and should verify that the resident has demonstrated sufficient professional ability to practice competently and independently. This final evaluation should be part of the resident's permanent record maintained by the institution.
   i. Implementation of fair procedures, as established by the sponsoring institution, regarding academic discipline and resident complaints or grievances.
   j. Monitoring resident stress, including mental or emotional conditions inhibiting performance or learning and drug- or alcohol-related dysfunction. Program directors and teaching staff should be sensitive to the need for timely provision of confidential counseling and psychological support services to residents. Training situations that consistently produce undesirable stress on residents must be evaluated and modified.
   k. Preparation of an accurate statistical and narrative description of the program as requested by the RRC.

B. Teaching Staff

1. There must be a sufficient number of teaching staff with documented qualifications to instruct and supervise adequately all the residents in the program. Members of the teaching staff must be able to devote sufficient time to meet their supervisory and teaching responsibilities.
2. All members of the teaching staff must demonstrate a strong interest in the education of residents, sound clinical and teaching abilities, support of the goals and objectives of the program, a commitment to their own continuing medical education, and participation in scholarly activities.
3. A member of the teaching staff of each participating institution must be designated to assume responsibility for the day-to-day activities of the program at that institution, with overall coordination by the program director.
4. The teaching staff must be organized and have regular documented meetings to review program goals and objectives as well as program effectiveness in achieving them. At least one resident representative should participate in these reviews.
5. The teaching staff should periodically evaluate the utilization of the resources available to the program, the contribution of each institution participating in the program, the financial and administrative support of the program, the volume and variety of patients available to the program for educational purposes, the performance of members of the teaching staff, and the quality of supervision of residents.

C. Residents

1. The resident should have completed training in anatomic and clinical pathology, anatomic pathology or clinical pathology, or primary certification in another primary medical specialty board of the American Board of Medical Specialties.
2. The number of resident positions requested must be consistent with the educational resources available in a program.
3. Residents must have the opportunity to assume increasing responsibility as they progress through the program.
4. Residents should have the opportunity to become involved in hematology research and teaching during the program.
5. It is desirable that residents' work schedules be designed so that on the average, excluding exceptional patient care needs, residents have 1 day out of 7 free of routine responsibilities and be on call in the hospital no more often than every third night. The ratio of hours worked and on-call time will vary, particularly at the senior levels, and therefore necessitate flexibility.

D. Other Personnel

1. The laboratories involved in the program must be directed by qualified physicians who are licensed to practice medicine and are members in good standing of the institution's medical staff.
2. Programs must be provided with the additional professional, technical, and clerical personnel needed to support the administration and educational conduct of the program. There must be a sufficient number of qualified and credentialed technical, clerical, and other personnel to support laboratory work and the educational program.

V. Institutional Resources

A. The program must have access to the number and variety of patients needed to provide education in hematology. The material and files must be indexed to permit appropriate retrieval. There must be mechanisms to facilitate correlation with anatomical material.

B. There must be adequate equipment, laboratory facilities, offices, meeting rooms, classrooms, and space to support service, teaching, educational, and research activities.
C. The institutions and laboratories participating in the program must be appropriately accredited and/or licensed.

VI. Program Research and Scholarly Activity

A. Graduate medical education must take place in an environment of inquiry and scholarship in which residents participate in the development of new knowledge, learn to evaluate research findings, and develop habits of inquiry as a continuing professional responsibility.
B. The responsibility for establishing and maintaining an environment of inquiry and scholarship rests with the teaching staff. While not all members of a teaching staff must be investigators, the staff as a whole must demonstrate broad involvement in scholarly activity. This activity should include:
   1. Active participation of the teaching staff in clinical discussions, rounds, and conferences in a manner that promotes a spirit of inquiry and scholarship. Scholarship implies an in-depth understanding of basic mechanisms of normal and abnormal states and the application of current knowledge to practice.
   2. Participation in journal clubs and research conferences.
   3. Active participation in regional or national professional and scientific societies, particularly through presentations at the organizations' meetings and publication in their journals.
   4. Participation in research, particularly in projects that are funded following peer review and/or result in publication or presentations at regional and national scientific meetings.
   5. Offering of guidance and technical support (eg, research design, statistical analysis) for residents involved in research.
   6. Provision of support for resident participation in scholarly activities.
C. Residents must have ready access to a major medical library, either at the institution where the residents are located or through arrangement with convenient nearby institutions.
   1. Library services should include the electronic retrieval of information from medical databases.
   2. There must be access to an on-site library or to a collection of appropriate texts and journals in each institution participating in a residency program. On-site libraries and/or collections of texts and journals must be readily available during nights and weekends.

VII. Evaluation

A. There must be regular, formal, written evaluations of residents by teaching staff. Evaluations should be completed and discussed with the residents at least once every 6 months.
B. The educational effectiveness of a program must be evaluated in a systematic manner. In particular, the quality of the curriculum and the extent to which the educational goals have been met by residents must be assessed. Residents should submit formal, written evaluations of the program and faculty at least once each year for review by the director and the teaching staff.

VIII. Administrative Structure

A hematology program should be administratively attached to an Accreditation Council for Graduate Medical Education-accredited residency in anatomic and/or clinical pathology.

IX. Certification and Accreditation

A. The RRC for Pathology is responsible for accreditation of graduate medical education programs in hematology. The American Board of Pathology is responsible for certification of individual physicians in hematology.
B. Questions about accreditation of residency programs should be directed to the executive director of the RRC.
C. Individuals who plan to seek certification from the American Board of Pathology should communicate with the executive vice president of the board to obtain the latest information regarding certification.

ACGME: February 1993 Effective: July 1995

Program Requirements for Residency Education in Immunopathology (Pathology)

I. Introduction

A. Educational programs in immunopathology must be 1 year in length and must provide a structured educational experience in all current aspects of the discipline, including basic science, diagnostic laboratory procedures, laboratory management, and patient care consultation. Programs must be designed to teach residents to integrate immunopathologic data into medical consultations with clinicians in the diagnosis and management of patients with immunologic disease.
B. The director and teaching staff of a program must prepare and comply with written educational goals for the program.
C. All educational components of a residency program should be related to program goals.
   1. The program design and/or structure must be approved by the Residency Review Committee (RRC) as part of the regular review process.
   2. Participation by any institution providing more than 2 months of training during the program must be approved by the RRC.

II. Program Personnel

The program director and the teaching staff are responsible for the general administration of a program, including those activities related to the recruitment, selection, instruction, supervision, counseling, evaluation, and advancement of residents and the maintenance of records related to program accreditation.

A. Program Director

A program involving two or more institutions must have a single director, whose primary professional activity must be in immunopathology, with authority for the supervision and coordination of the portions of the program carried out at each institution.

1. Qualifications of the program director include:
   a. Requisite and documented clinical, educational, and administrative abilities and experience.
   b. Licensure to practice medicine in the state where the institution that sponsors the program is located. (Certain federal programs are exempted.)
   c. Certification by the American Board of Pathology in Immunopathology or suitable equivalent qualifications.
   d. Appointment in good standing to the medical staff of an institution participating in the program.
2. Responsibilities of the program director include:

a. Conducting the training program effectively. He or she must devote sufficient time to fulfill the responsibilities inherent in meeting the educational goals of the program, including the implementation of sound administrative practices, evaluation procedures and the provision of adequate facilities, teaching staff, resident staff, and educational resource materials.
b. Preparation of a written statement outlining the educational goals of the program with respect to knowledge, skills, and other attributes of residents at each level of training and for each major rotation or other program assignment. This statement must be distributed to residents and members of the teaching staff. It should be readily available for review.
c. Selection of residents for appointment to the program in accordance with institutional and departmental policies and procedures.
d. Selection and supervision of the teaching staff and other program personnel at each institution participating in the program.
e. The supervision of residents through explicit written descriptions of supervisory lines of responsibility for the care of patients. Such guidelines must be communicated to all members of the program staff. Residents must be provided with prompt, reliable systems for communication and interaction with supervisory physicians.
f. Regular evaluation of residents' knowledge, skills, and overall performance, including the development of professional attitudes consistent with being a physician. The program director, with participation of members of the teaching staff, shall:
   1. At least semiannually evaluate the knowledge, skills, and professional growth of the residents, using appropriate criteria and procedures.
   2. Communicate each evaluation to the resident in a timely manner.
   3. Advance residents to positions of higher responsibility only on the basis of evidence of their satisfactory progressive scholarship and professional growth.
   4. Maintain a permanent record of evaluation for each resident and have it accessible to the resident and other authorized personnel.
g. The provision of a written final evaluation for each resident who completes the program. The evaluation must include a review of the resident's performance during the final period of training and should verify that the resident has demonstrated sufficient professional ability to practice competently and independently. This final evaluation should be part of the resident's permanent record maintained by the institution.
h. Implementation of fair procedures, as established by the sponsoring institution, regarding academic discipline and resident complaints or grievances.
i. Monitoring resident stress, including mental or emotional conditions inhibiting performance or learning and drug- or alcohol-related dysfunction. Program directors and teaching staff should be sensitive to the need for timely provision of confidential counseling and psychological support services to residents. Training situations that consistently produce undesirable stress on residents must be evaluated and modified.
j. Preparation of an accurate statistical and narrative description of the program as requested by the RRC.

B. Teaching Staff

1. There must be a sufficient number of teaching staff with documented qualifications to instruct and supervise adequately all the residents in the program. Members of the teaching staff must be able to devote sufficient time to meet their supervisory and teaching responsibilities.
2. All members of the teaching staff must demonstrate a strong interest in the education of residents, sound clinical and teaching abilities, support of the goals and objectives of the program, a commitment to their own continuing medical education, and participation in scholarly activities.
3. A member of the teaching staff of each participating institution must be designated to assume responsibility for the day-to-day activities of the program at that institution, with overall coordination by the program director.
4. The teaching staff must be organized and have regular documented meetings to review program goals and objectives as well as program effectiveness in achieving them. At least one resident representative should participate in these reviews.
5. The teaching staff should periodically evaluate the utilization of the resources available to the program, the contribution of each institution participating in the program, the financial and administrative support of the program, the volume and variety of patients available to the program for educational purposes, the performance of members of the teaching staff, and the quality of supervision of residents.

C. Residents

1. The number of residents in a program must conform to the resources available for educational purposes, and all programs should have at least two residents.
2. Programs that fail to recruit new residents for 2 consecutive years will be subject to review and possible adverse accreditation action.

D. Other Personnel

Programs must be provided with the additional professional, technical, and clerical personnel needed to support the administration and educational conduct of the program.

III. Institutional Resources

A. Space, Equipment, Support Services

Administrative, financial, and library services, as well as technical personnel, laboratory space and equipment, and resident office space must be available to adequately support training in immunopathologic methods.

B. Patient Population

A sufficient volume and variety of adult and pediatric patients must be available for educational purposes to provide residents a broad exposure to consultations regarding congenital and acquired immunologic disease.

IV. Educational Program

A. Curriculum

1. Educational goals and objectives must be clearly defined for the program and must be evident in the curriculum.
2. All rotations, including external rotations, and other major educational activities must explicitly contribute to the objectives of the program and effectively address graded responsibility, resident evaluation and counseling, and the roles of the faculty and the resident.
3. Residents must be given a systematic introduction to modern and traditional immunopathologic methods, including but not limited to immunohistochemistry of neoplasia and infection; diagnostic surgical pathology of immunologically related diseases in the endocrine, cutaneous, urinary, intestinal, respiratory, renal, skeletal, lymphoid, and nervous systems; immunopathologic techniques in the management of organ transplantation; serum autoantibody and leukocyte marker techniques; normal and abnormal serum proteins; histocompatibility-locus antigens; leuko-

cyte function; leukocyte identification; tumor antigens; relevant molecular and genetic techniques; and immunotherapy.

4. Residents must gain experience as consultants in clinical decision making in conjunction with professionals from related disciplines and in the cost-effective use of immunopathologic techniques.
5. Indexes of classic and unusual cases as well as materials from local and national courses and seminars that augment knowledge of diseases not frequently encountered must be available to the program for educational purposes.

B. Teaching Conferences

There must be regularly scheduled inter- and intradepartmental conferences and educational meetings that provide for progressive resident participation. Both staff and residents must attend and participate on a regular basis. The schedule must be comprehensive in scope and must treat both clinical and research subjects.

V. Program Research and Scholarly Activity

A. Graduate medical education must take place in an environment of inquiry and scholarship in which residents participate in the development of new knowledge, learn to evaluate research findings, and develop habits of inquiry as a continuing professional responsibility.

B. The responsibility for establishing and maintaining an environment of inquiry and scholarship rests with the teaching staff. While not all members of a teaching staff must be investigators, the staff as a whole must demonstrate broad involvement in scholarly activity. This activity should include:

1. Active participation of the teaching staff in clinical discussions, rounds, and conferences in a manner that promotes a spirit of inquiry and scholarship. Scholarship implies an in-depth understanding of basic mechanisms of normal and abnormal states and the application of current knowledge to practice.
2. Participation in journal clubs and research conferences.
3. Active participation in regional or national professional and scientific societies, particularly through presentations at the organizations' meetings and publication in their journals.
4. Participation in research, particularly in projects that are funded following peer review and/or result in publication or presentations at regional and national scientific meetings.
5. Offering of guidance and technical support (eg, research design, statistical analysis) for residents involved in research.
6. Provision of support for resident participation in scholarly activities.

C. Residents must have ready access to a major medical library, either at the institution where the residents are located or through arrangement with convenient nearby institutions.

1. Library services should include the electronic retrieval of information from medical databases.
2. There must be access to an on-site library or to a collection of appropriate texts and journals in each institution participating in a residency program. On-site libraries and/or collections of texts and journals must be readily available during nights and weekends.

VI. Administrative Structure

Immunopathology programs should be administratively attached to an Accreditation Council for Graduate Medical Education-accredited anatomic and clinical pathology program wherever possible.

VII. Evaluation

A. Residents should be provided with a summary of the assessment of their performance and professional growth on completion of each rotation or other major educational assignment.

B. The educational effectiveness of a program must be evaluated in a systematic manner. In particular, the quality of the curriculum and the extent to which the educational goals have been met by residents must be assessed. Written evaluations by residents should be utilized in this process.

VIII. Certification

Residents who plan to seek certification by the American Board of Pathology should communicate with the executive vice president of the board regarding certification matters.

ACGME: February 1988 Effective: July 1995

Program Requirements for Residency Education in Medical Microbiology (Pathology)

I. Introduction

A. The minimum training period in medical microbiology shall be 1 year in addition to the completion of acceptable residency training in an Accreditation Council for Graduate Medical Education (ACGME)-accredited program of anatomic and/or clinical pathology, as outlined in the *Graduate Medical Education Directory*, or equivalent postgraduate training and experience.

B. The director and teaching staff of a program must prepare and comply with written educational goals for the program.

C. All educational components of a residency program should be related to program goals.

1. The program design and/or structure must be approved by the Residency Review Committee (RRC) as part of the regular review process.
2. Participation by any institution providing more than 2 months of training in a program must be approved by the RRC.

D. The educational effectiveness of a program must be evaluated in a systematic manner. In particular, the quality of the curriculum and the extent to which the educational goals have been met by residents must be assessed. Written evaluations by residents should be utilized in this process.

II. Program Personnel

The program director and the teaching staff are responsible for the general administration of a program, including those activities related to the recruitment, selection, instruction, supervision, counseling, evaluation, and advancement of residents and the maintenance of records related to program accreditation.

A. Program Director

1. There must be a single program director responsible for the program.
2. Qualifications of the program director include:
   a. Requisite and documented clinical, educational, and administrative abilities and experience.
   b. Licensure to practice medicine in the state where the institution that sponsors the program is located. (Certain federal programs are exempted.)
   c. Certification by the American Board of Pathology in Medical Microbiology or suitable equivalent qualifications.
   d. Appointment in good standing to the medical staff of an institution participating in the program.
3. Responsibilities of the program director include:
   a. Preparation of a written statement outlining the educational goals of the program with respect to knowledge, skills, and

other attributes of residents at each level of training and for each major rotation or other program assignment. This statement must be distributed to residents and members of the teaching staff. It should be readily available for review.

b. Selection of residents for appointment to the program in accordance with institutional and departmental policies and procedures.

c. Selection and supervision of the teaching staff and other program personnel at each institution participating in the program.

d. The supervision of residents through explicit written descriptions of supervisory lines of responsibility for the care of patients. Such guidelines must be communicated to all members of the program staff. Residents must be provided with prompt, reliable systems for communication and interaction with supervisory physicians.

e. Regular evaluation of residents' knowledge, skills, and overall performance, including the development of professional attitudes consistent with being a physician.

The program director, with participation of members of the teaching staff, shall:

1. At least semiannually evaluate the knowledge, skills, and professional growth of the residents, using appropriate criteria and procedures.
2. Communicate each evaluation to the resident in a timely manner.
3. Advance residents to positions of higher responsibility only on the basis of evidence of their satisfactory progressive scholarship and professional growth.
4. Maintain a permanent record of evaluation for each resident and have it accessible to the resident and other authorized personnel.

f. The provision of a written final evaluation for each resident who completes the program. The evaluation must include a review of the resident's performance during the final period of training and should verify that the resident has demonstrated sufficient professional ability to practice competently and independently. This final evaluation should be part of the resident's permanent record maintained by the institution.

g. Implementation of fair procedures, as established by the sponsoring institution, regarding academic discipline and resident complaints or grievances.

h. Monitoring resident stress, including mental or emotional conditions inhibiting performance or learning and drug- or alcohol-related dysfunction. Program directors and teaching staff should be sensitive to the need for timely provision of confidential counseling and psychological support services to residents. Training situations that consistently produce undesirable stress on residents must be evaluated and modified.

i. Preparation of an accurate statistical and narrative description of the program as requested by the RRC.

B. Teaching Staff

1. There must be a sufficient number of teaching staff with documented qualifications to instruct and supervise adequately all the residents in the program. Members of the teaching staff must be able to devote sufficient time to meet their supervisory and teaching responsibilities.
2. All members of the teaching staff must demonstrate a strong interest in the education of residents, sound clinical and teaching abilities, support of the goals and objectives of the program, a commitment to their own continuing medical education, and participation in scholarly activities.
3. A member of the teaching staff of each participating institution must be designated to assume responsibility for the day-to-day activities of the program at that institution, with overall coordination by the program director.
4. The teaching staff must be organized and have regular documented meetings to review program goals and objectives as well as program effectiveness in achieving them. At least one resident representative should participate in these reviews.
5. The teaching staff should periodically evaluate the utilization of the resources available to the program, the contribution of each institution participating in the program, the financial and administrative support of the program, the volume and variety of patients available to the program for educational purposes, the performance of members of the teaching staff, and the quality of supervision of residents.

C. Other Program Personnel

Programs must be provided with the additional professional, technical, and clerical personnel needed to support the administration and educational conduct of the program.

III. Educational Program

A. The training program in medical microbiology must be designed to provide a broad knowledge in the discipline through didactic instruction and a personal participation in microbiologic techniques and methodology, as well as in the reporting and interpretation of laboratory results, principles of laboratory management, teaching, and investigation.

B. The training program must provide opportunities for residents to develop knowledge and skills relating to preparation and examination of cultures, identification of microorganisms, and performance of diagnostic immunologic procedures, supplemented with stock cultures of infrequently encountered and medically important microorganism microscope slides, photographs, and seminar material.

C. Knowledge of specimen collection, transport, and processing; microscopic examination of specimens; histopathologic and clinical correlation of microbiologic data; activity and pharmacokinetics of antimicrobial agents; antibiotic assay; antimicrobial susceptibility testing; and interpretation of findings are important educational objectives.

D. Residents must develop knowledge and skills related to principles of disinfection and sterilization, hospital infection control, infection control committee functions and responsibilities, microbiologic safety, quality control, workload accounting, budgeting, personnel supervision, and hospital and public health epidemiology.

E. Educational experiences should include opportunities to observe patients, both adults and children, with a wide variety of infectious diseases through interaction with physicians from other clinical services.

F. The program should provide regular administrative meetings, seminars, and conferences in medical microbiology, pathology, and the clinical and epidemiologic aspects of infectious diseases.

G. Instruction should include but not be limited to training in medical bacteriology, mycobacteriology, mycology, virology, parasitology, and immunology.

IV. Institutional Organization and Resources

A. The training program should provide the necessary clinical material and analytical capability in medical microbiology to provide experience at a sufficient level for the resident to acquire the competency of a specialist in medical microbiology.

B. Access to reference laboratories should be available for training in specialized procedures not available in the laboratory.

C. The laboratory should have adequate modern facilities, policies and procedures, equipment, and personnel for the performance of all laboratory aspects of medical microbiology, epidemiology, and infectious diseases.

D. The training program should be administratively attached to an ACGME-accredited program whenever feasible.

V. Program Research and Scholarly Activity

A. Graduate medical education must take place in an environment of inquiry and scholarship in which residents participate in the development of new knowledge, learn to evaluate research findings, and develop habits of inquiry as a continuing professional responsibility.

B. The responsibility for establishing and maintaining an environment of inquiry and scholarship rests with the teaching staff. While not all members of a teaching staff must be investigators, the staff as a whole must demonstrate broad involvement in scholarly activity. This activity should include:

1. Active participation of the teaching staff in clinical discussions, rounds, and conferences in a manner that promotes a spirit of inquiry and scholarship. Scholarship implies an in-depth understanding of basic mechanisms of normal and abnormal states and the application of current knowledge to practice.
2. Participation in journal clubs and research conferences.
3. Active participation in regional or national professional and scientific societies, particularly through presentations at the organizations' meetings and publication in their journals.
4. Participation in research, particularly in projects that are funded following peer review and/or result in publication or presentations at regional and national scientific meetings.
5. Offering of guidance and technical support (eg, research design, statistical analysis) for residents involved in research.
6. Provision of support for resident participation in scholarly activities.

C. Residents must have ready access to a major medical library, either at the institution where the residents are located or through arrangement with convenient nearby institutions.

1. Library services should include the electronic retrieval of information from medical databases.
2. There must be access to an on-site library or to a collection of appropriate texts and journals in each institution participating in a residency program. On-site libraries and/or collections of texts and journals must be readily available during nights and weekends.

ACGME: November 1983 Effective: July 1995

Program Requirements for Residency Education in Neuropathology (Pathology)

I. Introduction

A. The educational program must be 2 years in length and provide a structured educational experience in all current aspects of the discipline, including basic science, laboratory management, and patient care consultation.

B. The director and teaching staff of the program must prepare and comply with written educational goals for the program.

C. All educational components of the residency program should be related to program goals.

1. The program design and/or structure must be approved by the Residency Review Committee (RRC) as part of the regular review process.
2. Participation by any institution providing more than 2 months of training in the program must be approved by the RRC.

II. Program Personnel

The program director and the teaching staff are responsible for the general administration of the program, including those activities related to the recruitment, selection, instruction, supervision, counseling, evaluation, and advancement of residents, and the maintenance of records related to program accreditation.

A. Program Director

There must be a single program director, whose primary professional responsibility must be neuropathology.

1. Qualifications of the program director
   a. Requisite and documented clinical, educational, and administrative abilities and experience.
   b. Licensure to practice medicine in the state where the institution that sponsors the program is located. (Certain federal programs are exempted.)
   c. Certification by the American Board of Pathology in neuropathology or suitable equivalent qualifications.
   d. Appointment in good standing to the medical staff of an institution participating in the program.
2. Responsibilities of the program director
   a. Preparation of a written statement outlining the educational goals of the program with respect to knowledge, skills, and other attributes of residents at each level of training and for each major rotation or other program assignment. This statement must be distributed to residents and members of the teaching staff. It should be readily available for review.
   b. Selection of residents for appointment to the program in accordance with institutional and departmental policies and procedures.
   c. Selection and supervision of the teaching staff and other program personnel at each institution participating in the program.
   d. Supervision of residents through explicit written descriptions of supervisory lines of responsibility for the care of patients. Such guidelines must be communicated to all members of the program staff. Residents must be provided with prompt, reliable systems for communication and interaction with supervisory physicians.
   e. Regular evaluation of residents' knowledge, skills, and overall performance, including the development of professional attitudes consistent with being a physician.
3. The program director, with participation of members of the teaching staff, shall
   a. at least semiannually evaluate the knowledge, skills, and professional growth of the residents, using appropriate criteria and procedures.
   b. communicate each evaluation to the resident in a timely manner.
   c. advance residents to positions of higher responsibility only on the basis of evidence of their satisfactory progressive scholarship and professional growth.
   d. maintain a permanent record of evaluation for each resident and have it accessible to the resident and other authorized personnel.
   e. The provision of a written final evaluation for each resident who completes the program. The evaluation must include a review of the resident's performance during the final period of training and should verify that the resident has demonstrated sufficient professional ability to practice competently and independently. This final evaluation should be part of the resident's permanent record maintained by the institution.

f. implement fair procedures, as established by the sponsoring institution, regarding academic discipline and resident complaints or grievances.
g. monitor resident stress, including mental or emotional conditions inhibiting performance or learning and drug- or alcohol-related dysfunction. Program directors and teaching staff should be sensitive to the need for timely provision of confidential counseling and psychological support services to residents. Training situations that consistently produce undesirable stress on residents must be evaluated and modified.
h. prepare an accurate statistical and narrative description of the program as requested by a review committee.

4. The program director must have the authority to organize and oversee the program and ensure that an appropriate educational environment is maintained.

B. Teaching Staff

1. There must be a sufficient number of teaching staff with documented qualifications to instruct and supervise adequately all the residents in the program. Members of the teaching staff must be able to devote sufficient time to meet their supervisory and teaching responsibilities.
2. All members of the teaching staff must demonstrate a strong interest in the education of residents, sound clinical and teaching abilities, support of the goals and objectives of the program, a commitment to their own continuing medical education, and participation in scholarly activities.
3. A member of the teaching staff of each participating institution must be designated to assume responsibility for the day-to-day activities of the program at that institution, with overall coordination by the program director.
4. The teaching staff must be organized and have regular documented meetings to review program goals and objectives as well as program effectiveness in achieving them. At least one resident representative should participate in these reviews.
5. The teaching staff should periodically evaluate the utilization of the resources available to the program, the contribution of each institution participating in the program, the financial and administrative support of the program, the volume and variety of patients available to the program for educational purposes, the performance of members of the teaching staff, and the quality of supervision of residents.

C. Number of Residents

The number of residents must conform to the neuropathologic resources available for educational purposes. Programs that fail to recruit new residents in 2 consecutive years will be subject to review and possible adverse accreditation action.

D. Other Program Personnel

Programs must be provided with the additional professional, technical, and clerical personnel needed to support the administration and educational conduct of the program.

III. The Educational Program

A. Residents must actively participate in the evaluation of a comprehensive body of pathological lesions of the central nervous system, peripheral nervous system, and neuromuscular systems.
B. Residents should regularly participate in basic neuroscience activities, teaching conferences in neuropathology, and joint conferences with the pathology department and clinical services involved in the diagnosis and management of neurological disorders.
C. Programs must be designed to teach neuropathology residents to integrate neuropathologic information into medical consultations with clinicians in the diagnosis and management of patients.

IV. Institutional Resources and Organization

A. The neuropathology program must be based in institutions where each year
1. at least 200 necropsies that include examination of the nervous system are performed; and
2. there are at least 100 neurosurgical specimens from the brain, spinal cord, pituitary gland, and eyes (including neoplastic, degenerative, infectious, and immune disorders) of significance in the treatment and management of pediatric and adult patients.

B. The neuropathology program should ensure that sufficient material is available for each trainee to examine at least 50 neuromuscular biopsy specimens and to study neoplasms and related lesions of peripheral nerves and the sympathetic and parasympathetic nervous systems.
C. Appropriate laboratory space, facilities, and personnel should be available for the conduct of special neuropathologic procedures, including but not limited to ultrastructural, histochemical, immunopathologic, and molecular-biologic techniques.
D. Indexes of usual and unusual cases, course and seminar materials, microscopic slide collections augmented by photographs, and museum specimens sufficient for the study of conditions and diseases not frequently encountered in routine necropsy and surgical specimens should be readily available to the program for educational purposes.
E. Neuropathology programs should be administratively attached to an Accreditation Council for Graduate Medical Education-accredited anatomic and clinical pathology (APCP) program.

V. Program Research and Scholarly Activity

A. Graduate medical education must take place in an environment of inquiry and scholarship in which residents participate in the development of new knowledge, learn to evaluate research findings, and develop habits of inquiry as a continuing professional responsibility.
B. The responsibility for establishing and maintaining an environment of inquiry and scholarship rests with the teaching staff. While not all members of a teaching staff must be investigators, the staff as a whole must demonstrate broad involvement in scholarly activity. This activity should include the following
1. Active participation of the teaching staff in clinical discussions, rounds and conferences in a manner that promotes a spirit of inquiry and scholarship. Scholarship implies an in-depth understanding of basic mechanisms of normal and abnormal states and the application of current knowledge to practice.
2. Participation in journal clubs and research conferences.
3. Active participation in regional or national professional and scientific societies, particularly through presentations at the organizations' meetings and publications in their journals.
4. Participation in research, particularly in projects that are funded following peer review and/or result in publications or presentations at regional and national scientific meetings.
5. Offering of guidance and technical support (eg, research design, statistical analysis) for residents involved in research.
6. Provision of support for resident participation in scholarly activities.

C. Residents must have ready access to a major medical library either at the institution where the residents are located or through arrangement with convenient nearby institutions.
1. Library services should include the electronic retrieval of information from medical databases.

Program Requirements

2. There must be access to an on-site library or to a collection of appropriate texts and journals in each institution participating in a residency program. On-site libraries and/or collections of texts and journals must be readily available during nights and weekends.

VI. Evaluation

A. Residents should be provided with a summary of the assessment of their performance and professional growth following each rotation or other major educational assignment.

B. The educational effectiveness of a program must be evaluated in a systematic manner. In particular, the quality of the curriculum and the extent to which the educational goals have been met by residents must be assessed. Neuropathology residents should evaluate the program, the faculty, and the facilities in writing at least once each academic year.

VII. Certification

Residents who plan to seek certification by the American Board of Pathology should communicate with the executive vice president of the board regarding certification matters.

ACGME: September 1997 Effective: July 1998

Program Requirements for Residency Education in Pediatric Pathology (Pathology)

I. Definition, Duration, and Scope of Education

A. Pediatric pathology is that practice of pathology concerned with the study and diagnosis of human disease manifested in the embryo, fetus, infant, child, and adolescent. Pediatric pathology requires a strong foundation in pathology and its clinical interpretation.

B. Graduate medical education programs in pediatric pathology must provide an organized educational experience for qualified physicians seeking to acquire advanced competence in the diagnosis of childhood diseases.

C. Programs will be accredited to offer 1 year of organized education in pediatric pathology, which must include formal education in diagnostic pediatric pathology and management and quality assessment issues germane to the pediatric laboratory environment.

D. The director and teaching staff of a program must prepare and comply with written educational goals for the program.

E. All educational components of a residency program should be related to program goals.

1. The program design and/or structure must be approved by the Residency Review Committee (RRC) as part of the regular review process.
2. Participation by any institution providing more than 2 months of training during the program must be approved by the RRC.

II. Educational Program

A. Curriculum

1. The program must be structured to give residents clearly defined graduated responsibilities and delegated authority. The descriptions of rotations, assignments, or other experiences must include:
   a. The goals and objectives of the experience.
   b. The duration of the experience.
   c. The duties and responsibilities of residents at each year of training.
   d. The teaching staff responsible for the supervision and instruction of the residents during the experience.
   e. The manner in which residents are supervised during the experience.
2. There must be a program statement available for review by applicants, residents, and staff. The program statement must include:
   a. A description of the program's educational goals and philosophy.
   b. A listing and description of all required rotations, including their duration.
   c. A listing and description of elective rotations and their duration.
   d. A description of resident opportunities for teaching and research, including the manner in which such research is funded.
   e. A description of the manner in which residents and the program are evaluated and how such evaluations are used.
3. The education in pediatric pathology must include general and systemic aspects of autopsy and surgical pathology (including embryo-fetal, perinatal, and placental pathology as well as pediatric aspects of dermatopathology, gynecological and obstetrical pathology, forensic pathology, and neuropathology), immunopathologic and histochemical techniques, cytopathology, ultrastructural pathology, cytogenetics, molecular biologic techniques including diagnostic techniques for metabolic diseases, and other advanced diagnostic techniques as they relate to pediatric pathology.
4. Programs must provide instruction and experience in the major aspects of a hospital laboratory as it relates to diagnosis in pediatric pathology, including resident participation in interpretation of laboratory data as part of pediatric patient-care consultation, conferences, rounds, laboratory management, quality assurance, data processing, teaching, and scholarly activity.

B. Educational Activities

1. The educational experiences detailed above may be provided through separate, exclusive rotations or by rotations that combine more than one area or by other means.
2. Lectures, tutorials, seminars, and conferences with clinical services including pediatric surgery, pediatric hematology, pediatric oncology, medical microbiology, medical genetics, pediatric radiology, obstetrics, and pediatrics must be regularly scheduled and held.
3. Instruction should include the use of study sets of usual and unusual cases and other educational materials.

III. Program Personnel

The program director and the teaching staff are responsible for the general administration of a program, including those activities related to the recruitment, selection, instruction, supervision, counseling, evaluation, and advancement of residents and the maintenance of records related to program accreditation.

A. Program Director

A program involving two or more institutions must have a single director who has the authority for the supervision and coordination of the portions of the program carried out at each institution.

1. Qualifications of the program director include:
   a. Requisite and documented clinical, educational, and administrative abilities and experience.
   b. Licensure to practice medicine in the state where the institution that sponsors the program is located. (Certain federal programs are exempted.)

c. Certification by the American Board of Pathology in Pediatric Pathology or suitable equivalent qualifications.
d. Appointment in good standing to the medical staff of an institution participating in the program.

2. Responsibilities of the program director include:
a. Conducting the training program effectively. He or she must devote sufficient time to fulfilling the responsibilities inherent in meeting the educational goals of the program, including the implementation of sound administrative practices, evaluation procedures and the provision of adequate facilities, teaching staff, resident staff, and educational resource materials.
b. Preparation of a written statement outlining the educational goals of the program with respect to knowledge, skills, and other attributes of residents at each level of training and for each major rotation or other program assignment. This statement must be distributed to residents and members of the teaching staff. It should be readily available for review.
c. Selection of residents for appointment to the program in accordance with institutional and departmental policies and procedures.
d. Selection and supervision of the teaching staff and other program personnel at each institution participating in the program.
e. The supervision of residents through explicit written descriptions of supervisory lines of responsibility for the care of patients. Such guidelines must be communicated to all members of the program staff. Residents must be provided with prompt, reliable systems for communication and interaction with supervisory physicians.
f. Regular evaluation of residents' knowledge, skills, and overall performance, including the development of professional attitudes consistent with being a physician. The program director, with participation of members of the teaching staff, shall:
   1. At least semiannually evaluate the knowledge, skills, and professional growth of the residents, using appropriate criteria and procedures.
   2. Communicate each evaluation to the resident in a timely manner.
   3. Advance residents to positions of higher responsibility only on the basis of evidence of their satisfactory progressive scholarship and professional growth.
   4. Maintain a permanent record of evaluation for each resident and have it accessible to the resident and other authorized personnel.
g. The provision of a written final evaluation for each resident who completes the program. The evaluation must include a review of the resident's performance during the final period of training and should verify that the resident has demonstrated sufficient professional ability to practice competently and independently. This final evaluation should be part of the resident's permanent record maintained by the institution.
h. Implementation of fair procedures, as established by the sponsoring institution, regarding academic discipline and resident complaints or grievances.
i. Monitoring resident stress, including mental or emotional conditions inhibiting performance or learning and drug- or alcohol-related dysfunction. Program directors and teaching staff should be sensitive to the need for timely provision of confidential counseling and psychological support services to residents. Training situations that consistently produce undesirable stress on residents must be evaluated and modified.
j. Preparation of an accurate statistical and narrative description of the program as requested by the RRC.
k. Ensuring that residents are given reasonable duty and call assignments.

B. Teaching Staff

1. There must be a sufficient number of teaching staff with documented qualifications to instruct and supervise adequately all the residents in the program. Members of the teaching staff must be able to devote sufficient time to meet their supervisory and teaching responsibilities.
2. All members of the teaching staff must demonstrate a strong interest in the education of residents, sound clinical and teaching abilities, support of the goals and objectives of the program, a commitment to their own continuing medical education, and participation in scholarly activities.
3. A member of the teaching staff of each participating institution must be designated to assume responsibility for the day-to-day activities of the program at that institution, with overall coordination by the program director.
4. The teaching staff must be organized and have regular documented meetings to review program goals and objectives as well as program effectiveness in achieving them. At least one resident representative should participate in these reviews.
5. The teaching staff should periodically evaluate the utilization of the resources available to the program, the contribution of each institution participating in the program, the financial and administrative support of the program, the volume and variety of patients available to the program for educational purposes, the performance of members of the teaching staff, and the quality of supervision of residents.

C. Residents

1. Residents should have completed at least 2 years of training in residencies in anatomic and clinical pathology prior to appointment to a pediatric pathology program.
2. The number of resident positions requested must be consistent with the educational resources available in a program.
3. Residents must have the opportunity to assume increasing responsibility as they progress through the program.
4. The number of residents should be sufficient to promote an intellectually stimulating educational environment. Typically, there should be at least one resident enrolled in each year of a program.
5. Resident performance must not be impaired by fatigue, whether caused by program duties or other activities. On average, residents should have the opportunity to spend at least 1 full day out of 7 free from hospital duties and should be on call no more often than every third night.
6. The appointment of other individuals for special training or education must not dilute or detract from the educational opportunities of the regularly appointed residents in pediatric pathology.

D. Other Personnel

1. The laboratories involved in the program must be directed by qualified physicians who are licensed to practice medicine and are members in good standing of the institution's medical staff.
2. Programs must be provided with the additional professional, technical, and clerical personnel needed to support the administration and educational conduct of the program.

IV. Institutional Resources

A. The program must have access to an adequate volume and variety of pediatric pathology material. The material and files must be indexed to permit appropriate retrieval. There must be mechanisms to facilitate correlation with anatomical material.

B. There must be adequate equipment, laboratory facilities, offices, meeting rooms, classrooms, and space to support service, teaching, educational, and research activities.
C. The institutions and laboratories participating in the program must be appropriately accredited and/or licensed.
D. Each pediatric pathology program should be administratively attached to an Accreditation Council for Graduate Medical Education-accredited residency in anatomic and clinical pathology or anatomic pathology when feasible.
E. To facilitate peer interchange and augment the breadth of the educational experiences, institutions providing programs in pediatric pathology must be affiliated with accredited specialty training programs in pediatrics, obstetrics, surgery, and radiology.
F. While the quality of an educational program is not based on the volume of teaching material alone, programs must have sufficient volume and variety of materials available for educational purposes to ensure the opportunity for:
  1. The participation in at least 40 pediatric autopsies per resident during the program. This experience must include general pediatric, metabolic, forensic, perinatal, and stillborn autopsies. It is highly desirable that this experience also include embryofetal autopsies.
  2. Examination of at least 2,000 pediatric surgical pathology specimens per resident during the program. This material must be from an adequate mix of cases, including obstetrics-related materials (placentas and abortions) and cytology.
  3. The performance of at least 50 intraoperative consultations (frozen sections, smears) per resident during the program.
  4. The number and variety of laboratory tests utilized in the program should be sufficient to give each resident experience in the range of laboratory examinations typically available and useful in the diagnoses and following of both common and unusual pediatric diagnostic problems, including metabolic, prenatal, genetic, neoplastic, and other diseases of the pediatric population.

V. Program Research and Scholarly Activity

A. Graduate medical education must take place in an environment of inquiry and scholarship in which residents participate in the development of new knowledge, learn to evaluate research findings, and develop habits of inquiry as a continuing professional responsibility.
B. The responsibility for establishing and maintaining an environment of inquiry and scholarship rests with the teaching staff. While not all members of a teaching staff must be investigators, the staff as a whole must demonstrate broad involvement in scholarly activity. This activity should include:
  1. Active participation of the teaching staff in clinical discussions, rounds, and conferences in a manner that promotes a spirit of inquiry and scholarship. Scholarship implies an in-depth understanding of basic mechanisms of normal and abnormal states and the application of current knowledge to practice.
  2. Participation in journal clubs and research conferences.
  3. Active participation in regional or national professional and scientific societies, particularly through presentations at the organizations' meetings and publication in their journals.
  4. Participation in research, particularly in projects that are funded following peer review and/or result in publications or presentations at regional and national scientific meetings.
  5. Offering of guidance and technical support (eg, research design, statistical analysis) for residents involved in research.
  6. Provision of support for resident participation in scholarly activities.

C. Residents must have ready access to a major medical library, either at the institution where the residents are located or through arrangement with convenient nearby institutions.
  1. Library services should include the electronic retrieval of information from medical databases.
  2. There must be access to an on-site library or to a collection of appropriate texts and journals in each institution participating in a residency program. On-site libraries and/or collections of texts and journals must be readily available during nights and weekends.

VI. Evaluation

A. There must be regular, formal, written evaluation of residents by teaching staff. Evaluations should be completed and discussed with the residents at least once every 6 months.
B. The educational effectiveness of a program must be evaluated in a systematic manner. In particular, the quality of the curriculum and the extent to which the educational goals have been met by residents must be assessed. Residents should submit confidential, written evaluations of the program and teaching staff at least once each year.

VII. Certification and Accreditation

A. The RRC for Pathology is responsible for accreditation of graduate medical education programs in pathology. The American Board of Pathology is responsible for certification of individual physicians in pathology.
B. Questions about accreditation of residency programs should be directed to the executive secretary of the RRC.
C. Individuals who plan to seek certification from the American Board of Pathology should communicate with the executive vice president of the board to obtain the latest information regarding certification.

ACGME: June 1994 Effective: July 1995

Program Requirements for Residency Education in Pediatrics

I. Introduction

A. Scope of Training

Programs must provide residents with a broad exposure to the health care of children and substantial experience in the management of diverse pathologic conditions. This must include experience in child health supervision and those conditions commonly encountered in primary care practice. It must also include experience with a wide range of acute and chronic medical conditions of pediatrics in both the inpatient and ambulatory settings.

Preventive health care, ethical issues, and discussions of the cost of diagnostic tests, procedures, and therapies should be a part of all rotations.

Throughout the 3 years of training, emphasis must be placed on enhancement of residents' competence in the medical interview, physical examination, and communication and interpersonal skills.

B. Duration and Levels of Training

Programs must provide a progressive educational experience with increasing patient care responsibility over a 3-year period. The first year (PL-1) should include an introduction to the basic experiences on which the rest of the training will be based. During the last 24 months of training the program must require at least 5 months of supervising the activities of more junior residents within the approved educational settings. The supervisory responsibilities must involve both inpatient and outpatient experience.

C. Goal of the Residency

The goal of residency training in pediatrics is to provide educational experiences that prepare residents to be competent general pediatricians able to provide comprehensive, coordinated care to a broad range of pediatric patients. The residents' educational experiences must emphasize the competencies and skills needed to practice general pediatrics of high quality in the community. In addition, residents must become sufficiently familiar with the fields of subspecialty pediatrics to enable them to participate as team members in the care of patients with chronic and complex disorders.

Residents must be given the opportunity to function with other members of the health care team in both inpatient and ambulatory settings to become proficient as leaders in the organization and management of patient care.

II. Institutional Organization

A. Sponsoring Institution

There must be one sponsoring institution for each residency, as mandated by the Institutional Requirements. This entity must be identified at the time of each review of the residency.

B. Participating Institutions

1. Single or Multiple Institutions
   An accredited program may be independent or may occur in two or more institutions that develop formal agreements and conjoint responsibilities to provide complementary facilities, teaching staff, and teaching sessions. When affiliated institutions are utilized and a single program director assumes responsibility for the entire residency, including the appointment of all residents and teaching staff, the affiliated institution is designated as integrated. Within a single program some participating hospitals may qualify as integrated, while others are merely affiliated.
2. Agreements with Participating Institutions

When a residency program relies on other institutions to provide some components of the curriculum, the arrangement between the institutions must be designed to meet the educational needs of the residents and must be described in a written document that is signed by the appropriate persons from the respective institutions. These agreements must relate specifically to the residency program in pediatrics and must be current at the time of the site visit. Copies of these written arrangements, specifying administrative, organizational, and educational relationships, must be submitted with the program information forms at the time of each evaluation by the Residency Review Committee (RRC). These must address the following:

a. The nature and scope of the affiliation or integration as it pertains to the residency;
b. The resources in the affiliated or integrated institutions that will be available to the pediatric residents and whether space is ensured in the desired rotations;
c. The specific content of the rotations;
d. The duties and responsibilities the pediatric residents will have at the affiliated or integrated institution, including the degree of responsibility for patient care and whether supervisory experience is involved;
e. The relationship that will exist between the residents of this program and the staff and residents at the affiliated or integrated institution;
f. The names and qualifications of the staff with major teaching commitment for these proposed rotations, particularly in the subspecialty areas; and
g. the method of evaluation of residents by teaching staff at the affiliated or integrated institution and how this is communicated to the program director.

C. Appointment of Residents

The development of a satisfactory program requires careful selection of applicants for appointment to the residency. When appointing residents, the program director must adhere to the criteria for resident eligibility that are specified in the Institutional Requirements. To determine the appropriate level of training for a resident who is transferring from another ACGME-accredited pediatrics program, the program director must receive written verification of the previous educational experiences in a pediatric residency and a statement regarding the performance evaluation of the transferring resident prior to accepting that resident into the program. The program director is also required to provide verification of training, if requested to do so, for any residents who may leave the program prior to completion of training.

III. Faculty Qualifications and Responsibilities

The chief of pediatrics/department chair must have overall responsibility for all educational programs that are carried on within the Department of Pediatrics, including those in the subspecialties. All program descriptions submitted to the RRC from this department must bear this person's signature, in addition to that of the program director, indicating that the chief/chair has reviewed and approved the materials submitted.

The program director and teaching staff are responsible for the general administration of a program, including those activities related to the recruitment, selection, instruction, supervision, counseling, evaluation, and advancement of residents and the maintenance of records related to program accreditation.

A. Program Director

There must be a single program director responsible for the program. The RRC must be notified immediately in writing of a change in leadership of the program. Continuity of leadership over a period of years is important for the stability of a residency program. Frequent changes in leadership or long periods of temporary leadership usually have an adverse effect on an educational program and will be cause for serious concern.

1. Qualifications
   a. Experience/Ability: The director of the residency program must have demonstrated ability as a clinician, medical educator, and administrator and have an understanding of, and commitment to, general pediatric education.
   b. Licensure: The director must be licensed to practice medicine in the state where the institution that sponsors the program is located. (Certain federal programs are exempted.)
   c. Board Certification: The director must be currently certified by the American Board of Pediatrics or must possess suitable equivalent qualifications. The adequacy of alternate qualifications will be determined by the RRC.
   d. Medical Staff Appointment: The director must hold an appointment in good standing to the medical staff of an institution participating in the residency.
2. Responsibilities
   The program director must devote sufficient time to the residency program to provide continuity of leadership and to fulfill the administrative and teaching responsibilities inherent in achieving the educational goals of the program.
   The responsibilities of the director include the following:
   a. Preparation of a written statement outlining the educational goals of the program with respect to knowledge, skills, and other attributes of residents at each level of training and for each major rotation or other program assignment, and distribution of the statement to residents and members of the teaching staff.
   b. Selection of residents for appointment to the program in accordance with institutional and departmental policies and procedures.
   c. Selection and supervision of the teaching staff and other program personnel at each institution participating in the program.
   d. Supervision of residents.
   e. Regular evaluation of residents' knowledge, skills, and overall performance, including the development of professional attitudes consistent with being a physician.
   f. Implementation of fair procedures as established by the sponsoring institution regarding academic discipline and resident complaints or grievances.
   g. Monitoring resident stress, including mental or emotional conditions inhibiting performance or learning and drug- or alcohol-related dysfunction. Training situations that consistently produce undesirable stress on residents must be evaluated and modified. The director should be sensitive to the need for timely provision of confidential counseling and psychological support services to residents.
   h. Program directors are required to provide accurate and complete statistical and narrative information as requested by the RRC for these evaluations.
   i. Notification of the RRC of major changes in the program.

B. Faculty

The teaching staff must have sufficient background and expertise to ensure that the educational goals, objectives, and/or curricular content can be met. They must be actively involved in the establishment of educational goals and objectives for the resident experiences in which they participate and in the evaluation of both the residents and the program.

1. Sufficient Numbers and Diversity
   There must be a sufficient number of pediatric teaching staff who function as general pediatrician and subspecialist role models for the residents and who contribute adequate time to the program to meet the educational needs of the residents.
   Within the primary hospital and/or integrated participating hospitals there must be teaching staff with expertise in the area of general pediatrics who will serve as teachers, researchers, and role models for general pediatrics. Hospital-based as well as community-based general pediatricians should participate actively in the program as leaders of formal teaching sessions, as outpatient preceptors, and as attending physicians on the general inpatient services. The number of general pediatricians actively involved in the teaching program must be sufficient to enable each resident to establish close working relationships that foster role-modeling. Where teaching staff participate on a part-time basis, there must be evidence of sufficient involvement and continuity in teaching. These physicians should have a continuing time commitment to direct patient care to maintain their clinical skills.
   There must be teaching staff with training and/or experience in behavioral and developmental pediatrics, as well as teaching staff with training and/or experience in adolescent medicine. Within the primary hospital and/or integrated participating hospitals, there also must be teaching staff in at least four of the pediatric subspecialties listed in Section V.C.3 from which the four required 1-month rotations must be chosen. These subspecialists must function as integral parts of the clinical and didactic components of the program in both outpatient and inpatient settings.
   A surgeon having significant experience with pediatric patients must play a major role in the residents' education with respect to surgical diagnoses and preoperative and postoperative care. A pathologist and a radiologist who have significant experience with pediatric problems and who interact regularly with the pediatric residents are essential.
2. Commitment to Education
   The faculty must demonstrate a commitment to the education of residents, sound clinical and teaching abilities, support of the goals and objectives of the program, a commitment to their own continuing medical education, and participation in scholarly activities. A measure of the commitment of the teaching staff to the program is the degree to which patients under their care are available for resident education.
3. Participating Institutions
   Where multiple hospitals participate, a member of the teaching staff of each participating institution must be designated to assume responsibility for the day-to-day activities of the program at that institution, with overall coordination by the program director.
4. Qualifications
   All of the physician teaching staff must be currently board-certified and have achieved subspecialty certification where appropriate or must possess suitable equivalent qualifications. Each time the program is evaluated by the RRC it is the responsibility of the program director to provide evidence of equivalent qualifications for teaching staff who lack board certification. The RRC will judge the adequacy of alternate qualifications.

C. Other Program Personnel

Teaching by other health professionals such as nurses, pharmacists, social workers, child life specialists, physical and occupational therapists, speech and hearing pathologists, respiratory therapists, psychologists, and nutritionists is highly desirable.

D. Support Staff

Additional professional, technical, and clerical personnel needed to support the administration and educational conduct of the program must be provided.

IV. Facilities and Resources

A. Inpatient and Outpatient Facilities

The inpatient and outpatient facilities must be adequate in size and variety and must have the appropriate equipment necessary for a broad educational experience in pediatrics.

There must be an appropriately equipped and staffed emergency facility for the care of pediatric patients. The program must also have an intensive care facility that is appropriately equipped and staffed for the care of a sufficient number of seriously ill pediatric patients to provide adequate experience for the number of residents in the program.

B. Medical Library

Residents must have ready access to a major medical library, either at the institution where they are located or through arrangement with convenient nearby institutions. These library services should include the electronic retrieval of information from medical databases. There must also be access to an on-site library or to a collection of appropriate texts and journals in each institution participating in a residency program. On-site libraries and/or collections of texts and journals must be readily available during nights and weekends.

C. Patient Population

Programs must provide residents with patient care experience in both inpatient and outpatient settings. A sufficient number, variety, and complexity of patients, ranging in age from infancy through young adulthood, must be present. A deficient or excessive patient load may jeopardize the accreditation status of the program.

V. Educational Program

A. Curriculum, Goals, and Objectives

Each program must describe a core curriculum that complies with the RRC's requirements and is participated in by all residents. Programs that utilize multiple hospitals or that offer more than one track must provide evidence of a unified educational experience for each resident. Where multiple tracks exist within one program, each track must comply with the requirements, and residents in all tracks must have a minimum of 18 months of training in common. The provisions of the Institutional Requirements also must be met for accreditation.

Written goals and objectives and a method of evaluation must exist for each curricular component. The residency curriculum must be a structured educational experience that reflects an appropriate balance between clinical and didactic elements. The curriculum should be competency-based and focus on skill attainment and skill maintenance. It should emphasize attitudes and skills necessary for lifelong learning.

1. Resident Assignments

   Assignments to affiliated institutions must be designed to fulfill the educational goals and objectives of the program and must not be made primarily to meet service needs.

   While no limit is placed on the duration of rotations to institutions that are integrated with the primary hospital's pediatric program, rotations to participating institutions that are not integrated with the primary hospital may not exceed a total of 9 months during the 3 years of training. No more than 3 months of these outside rotations may be in institutions that do not have their own pediatric residencies.

   Rotations to other programs should enrich but not replace core experiences. When residents rotate to an institution that has its own accredited pediatric residency, the rotating residents must be fully absorbed into the prevailing pattern of instruction and patient care at the same level as the pediatric residents of that affiliated institution.

   Residency programs that offer training to residents from other pediatric residencies must provide instruction and experience equivalent to that given to their own residents. They should enter into agreement with other programs only if they are prepared to absorb those residents into the prevailing pattern of education and patient care.

2. Approval of Changes

   The program design or format must be approved by the RRC as part of the regular review process. Major changes in the content or format of a program that are proposed between regular reviews and/or the addition or deletion of a participating institution that provides 6 months or more of training require RRC approval before implementation. The RRC may determine that a site visit is required before a decision is made on such proposals.

B. General Pediatrics

In keeping with the commitment to general pediatrics, a minimum of 50% of clinical training should be devoted to ambulatory experiences. This may include all assignments in the continuity practice, emergency and acute care, and community-based experiences, as well as the ambulatory portion of normal/term newborn, subspecialty, behavior/development, and adolescent experiences.

1. Inpatient Experience

   General inpatient pediatrics must constitute at least 5 months of a resident's overall experience, exclusive of intensive care rotations. It must be structured to provide the resident with a concentrated exposure and continuity of involvement to ensure a primary role in patient care. The inpatient care experience must be designed to develop resident competency in managing patients with diverse illnesses of such complexity and severity as to require in-hospital care but not care in a critical care unit. This can be achieved most effectively through block rotations. An experience that is integrated with other educational activities will be considered acceptable if the program can demonstrate that the educational goals and objectives are met and that the primary role of the resident in the ongoing care of patients is ensured.

   The experience must be structured to enable residents to develop

   a. an understanding of which patients require in-hospital care and why, including medical, psychosocial, and environmental considerations;
   b. skills in determining which patients can be managed in a general inpatient setting and which require higher levels of care and expertise in a critical care unit;
   c. skills and competence in the evaluation, diagnosis, management, and appropriate disposition of pediatric patients in the hospital setting;
   d. skills in working with an organized inpatient health care team, including nursing, child life therapy, social services, physical therapy, occupational therapy, and discharge planning; and
   e. skills in the appropriate utilization of consultants and selection of studies in the care of pediatric patients in the hospital setting.

   The program must ensure that each resident has the opportunity for independent evaluation and development of a differential diagnosis, planning diagnostic studies, formulating and implementing therapeutic options, and planning for discharge of patients under their care. It is not an appropriate educational experience if the above are all accomplished by attending physicians without the pediatric inpatient resident's involvement.

The resident must be given progressive responsibility under close faculty supervision within a team that fosters peer and supervisory interchange. The availability of consultative resources appropriate to the patient base must be ensured, while allowing the resident to participate in the full spectrum of patient care from admission through discharge.

Regularly scheduled teaching/attending rounds that include all patients for whom the resident is responsible must be conducted by qualified teachers who are immediately available for consultation and who are supported by consultants in subspecialty areas appropriate to the patient population. Rounds should be targeted to the knowledge and skills required of a general pediatrician in an inpatient setting and should emphasize the appropriate utilization of subspecialist colleagues. The correlation of basic pathophysiologic principles with the disease process should be stressed. Rounds that focus on the educational objectives of inpatient care must be held at least three times per week and may not be replaced by rounds that are primarily work-oriented.

The patient load for residents at all levels of training should allow time for close and effective management and detailed study of patients, yet should challenge the resident with diverse and complex problems at increasing levels of responsibility. A first-year resident should be responsible for approximately 6 to 10 inpatients, depending on the average length of stay and the nature and severity of the illness. Second- and third-year residents may be involved in the care of more patients in a supervisory capacity, but this number should not exceed 30 in most situations.

The patient population available for resident education on the inpatient service must be of sufficient number, age distribution, and variety of complex and diverse pathology to assure the residents of adequate experience with infants, children, and adolescents who have acute and chronic illnesses, as well as with those with life-threatening conditions. Although there is increasing emphasis on outpatient care for a broad spectrum of pediatric illness, resident experience that is limited to the ambulatory setting will not be considered adequate for patient groups that require inpatient care as part of their ongoing treatment.

The comprehensive curriculum should include but not be limited to the following core content and should emphasize the pathophysiologic correlates of the clinical situations:

a. Interviewing techniques with specific emphasis on behavioral, psychosocial, environmental, and family unit correlates of disease
b. Physical examination, both general and system-specific, as a tool in initial diagnosis and subsequent patient monitoring
c. Utilization of appropriate members of the health care team to ensure comprehensive yet cost-effective care of the patient and the family
d. Diagnosis and management of acute episodic medical illness including but not limited to meningitis, sepsis, dehydration, pneumonia, diarrhea, renal failure, seizure, coma, hypotension, hypertension, and respiratory illnesses
e. Diagnosis and management of acute problems associated with chronic diseases including but not limited to diabetic ketoacidosis, status asthmaticus, status epilepticus, oncologic therapy and complications, congenital heart disease, cystic fibrosis, chronic renal disease, gastrointestinal disorders, hepatic failure, metabolic disorders, and neurologic disorders
f. Pediatric aspects of the management of surgical patients, both preoperatively and postoperatively, including interaction with the surgical team
g. Principles of discharge planning to ensure efficient transition and continuity of care

Residents on the inpatient service must be supervised by pediatric faculty who have extensive experience in and knowledge of the care of pediatric patients with illnesses of sufficient severity to warrant hospitalization. The utilization of general pediatricians in this role is encouraged, provided that consultative services from pediatric subspecialists and other specialists appropriate to the patient population are readily available.

2. Emergency and Acute Illness Experience (See also Section V.G.2, paragraph 7)

The experience in emergency and acute illness must constitute a minimum of 4 months.

Two of these months should be in emergency medicine; at least 1 of these months must be a block rotation in an emergency department that serves as the receiving point for EMS transport and ambulance traffic and is the access point for seriously injured and acutely ill pediatric patients in the service area. This may be either a pediatric emergency department or a combined pediatric/adult emergency department. Assignment to an acute care center or walk-in clinic to which patients are triaged from the emergency department will not fulfill this requirement.

The remaining required experience may be in the emergency department or, if patients are available in sufficient numbers, in another setting where acutely ill pediatric patients are seen. Optional sites may include walk-in clinics, acute care centers, and/or community-based primary care practice settings. Preferably, this experience would be as a block rotation, but integration into other longitudinal experiences is acceptable if the required duration and the educational goals and objectives can be met and appropriate supervision ensured.

The experience must be designed to develop resident competence in managing unselected and unscheduled patients with acute illness and injury of varying degrees of severity, from very minor to life-threatening.

Specific objectives of this experience must include but not be limited to development skills in the following:

a. Evaluation and care of patients with acute illnesses or injuries of varying degrees of severity
b. Resuscitation, stabilization, and triage of patients after initial evaluation
c. Interaction with other professionals involved in emergency care in the emergency department, including the trauma team; emergency physicians; specialists in surgery, anesthesia, radiology, and relevant pediatric and surgical subspecialties; dentists; and others as appropriate
d. Participation with the emergency medical system in the provision of prehospital care for acutely ill or injured patients, including access to appropriate transport systems and triage

The program director must ensure that the pediatric residents have first-contact evaluation of pediatric patients and continuous on-site supervision. It is not a sufficient educational experience if the pediatric resident functions only on a consultative basis or deals only with a preselected patient population. Residents in these settings must have on-site supervision by members of the pediatric teaching staff or by other attending staff who have extensive experience in and knowledge of the care of acute pediatric illnesses and injuries.

The resident should have the opportunity to work on a multidisciplinary clinical team to learn the role of the general pediatrician in such a setting. A system for patient outcome feedback to the resident should be established. The resident's performance must be evaluated on a regular basis by staff directly involved in the acute and emergency care experience, and appropriate feedback must be provided to the resident and to the program director.

Although they may be called on to care for some adult patients to ensure adequate volume and diversity, the pediatric residents' major responsibility must be for an appropriate range of pediatric patients. Programs that share the emergency and acute illness patient base with other training programs, such as emergency medicine, pediatric emergency medicine, and family practice, must document that a sufficient and appropriately diverse pediatric patient population is available to the pediatric residency program.

The comprehensive experience for all residents should include but not be limited to the following disorders and should emphasize the pathophysiologic correlates of the clinical situations:

a. Acute major and minor medical problems such as respiratory infection, respiratory failure, cardiopulmonary arrest (including sudden infant death syndrome, or SIDS), dehydration, coma, seizures, diabetic ketoacidosis, asthma, skin disorders, pyelonephritis, sepsis, shock, fever, and childhood exanthems
b. Acute major and minor surgical problems such as appendicitis, bowel obstruction, burns, foreign body inhalation and ingestion, abscess drainage, and head trauma
c. Poisonings and ingestion
d. Physical and sexual abuse
e. Minor trauma (including splinting, casting, and suturing)
f. Major trauma (including active participation with the trauma team)
g. Participation in prehospital management and transport
h. Acute psychiatric, behavioral, and psychosocial problems
i. Admission or discharge planning, including communication with the personal physician

3. Continuity Experience

The program must provide adequate continuity experience for all residents to allow them the opportunity to develop an understanding of and appreciation for the longitudinal nature of general pediatric care, including aspects of physical and emotional growth and development, health promotion/disease prevention, management of chronic and acute medical conditions, family and environmental impacts, and practice management. Residents must assume responsibility for the continuing care of a group of patients throughout their training. Inherent in the principle of continuity of care is that patients are seen on a regular and continuing basis, rather than on a single occasion. Isolated block experiences will not satisfy this requirement.

The continuity of care experience must include participation in a setting that is structured and designed to emulate the practice of general pediatrics and that is conducive to efficient processing and management of patients. This setting may be an office-based practice, an institutional-based continuity clinic, or a community-based center. Ideally, residents should participate in the care of their patients through any hospitalization, assess them during acute illnesses, and be available to facilitate other services, such as school-related evaluations and specialty referrals.

Residents must devote at least ½ day per week to their continuity experience throughout the 3 years, and an additional one-half day session per week is suggested. This experience must receive priority over other responsibilities, and may be interrupted only for vacations and outside rotations located at too great a distance to allow residents to return. The periods of interruption may not exceed 2 months in any 1 year or 3 consecutive months at any time.

The program must ensure that residents are exposed to a continuity patient population sufficient in number and of adequate variety to meet the educational objectives. It must include well patients as well as those with complex and chronic problems. Patients initially managed in the normal newborn nursery, emergency department, inpatient service, intensive care unit (pediatric and neonatal), subspecialty clinics, and other sites may be enrolled in the residents' panels. Guidelines for numbers of continuity panel patients seen per half-day experience are three to six patients per resident in the PL-1 year, four to eight patients in the PL-2 year, and five to ten patients in the PL-3 year. Acceptable minimum numbers for each resident's patient panel are approximately 50 patients for each PL-1 resident and approximately 100 patients for each PL-2 and PL-3 resident.

The curriculum should emphasize the generalist approach to common office-based pediatric issues including anticipatory guidance from birth through young adulthood, developmental and behavioral issues, and immunization practices and health promotion, as well as the care of children with chronic conditions. The resident must learn to serve as the coordinator of comprehensive primary care for children with complex and multiple health-related problems and to function as part of a health care team. Subspecialty consultants and allied health personnel must be available to residents in the care of their continuity patients.

The number of teaching staff in the continuity clinic must be sufficient to ensure an appropriate educational experience for all residents present. Teaching staff who serve as attendings in the continuity clinic must have expertise in the area of general pediatrics and be able to function as role models in general pediatrics. They must be actively involved in direct patient care to maintain their expertise and credibility. These and other competing responsibilities, however, must not compromise their availability for supervision and consultation with the residents.

Record maintenance must be designed to allow verification of the adequacy of each resident's experience.

4. Normal/Term Newborn Experience

There must be the equivalent of at least 1 month in the care of normal/term newborns. This may not be part of a neonatal intensive care unit (NICU) rotation but it may be combined with another experience over a longer period of time if an equivalent duration is demonstrated and the educational goals of both experiences can be met. Preferably, this rotation should take place in the first year of training to provide an experience on which more advanced training will be based, and it should be supervised primarily by general pediatric faculty. This experience should include longitudinal follow-up of selected infants discharged from the nursery. The experience should also include at least the following:

a. Recognition and appropriate intervention for high-risk infants
b. Distinguishing well from ill infants
c. Performance of physical examination on newborn infants, which includes assessment of gestational age and the appropriateness of intrauterine growth
d. Identification of common anomalies, birth defects, and syndromes, including counseling the parents
e. Provision of routine newborn care
f. Recognition and treatment of common physiologic deviations in the newborn
g. Identification and management of infants of mothers with substance abuse and/or sexually transmitted diseases (STDs) or other infections
h. Routine newborn screening and appropriate follow-up of infants with positive test results
i. Preventive measures including immunization schedules and safety issues, such as counseling parents on the importance of infant safety seats and knowledge of normal infant nutrition,

including breast feeding, as well as knowledge of normal newborn growth and development
j. Discharge planning
5. Community Experiences
There must be structured educational experiences that prepare residents for the role of advocate for the health of children within the community. These should include both didactic and experiential components that may be integrated into other parts of the curriculum, eg, continuity, adolescent behavior/development, or they may be designed as distinct longitudinal or block rotations.

Residents must be supervised by pediatricians and other health professionals experienced in the relevant content areas. The curriculum should include but not be limited to the following subjects:
a. Community-oriented care with focus on the health needs of all children within a community, particularly underserved populations
b. The multicultural dimensions of health care
c. Environmental toxicants and their effect on child health
d. The role of the pediatrician within school and day care settings
e. The role of the pediatrician in the legislative process
f. The role of the pediatrician in disease and injury prevention
g. The role of the pediatrician in the regional emergency medical system for children

These experiences should utilize settings within the community, such as
a. community-based primary care practice settings;
b. community health resources and organizations, including governmental and voluntary agencies, eg, local and state public health departments, services for children with disabilities, Head Start;
c. schools and day-care settings, including elementary school through college;
d. home-care services for children with special health care needs; and
e. facilities for incarcerated youth.
6. Behavioral/Developmental Pediatrics
The program must provide all residents with an adequate experience in behavioral/developmental pediatrics to ensure that the resident recognizes normal and abnormal behavior and understands child development from infancy through young adulthood. The program must educate the residents in the intrinsic and extrinsic factors that influence behavior to enable them to differentiate behavior that can and should be managed by the general pediatrician from behavior that warrants referral to other specialists. Clinical and didactic components of behavioral, psychosocial, and developmental pediatrics should be integrated into the general educational program and into each patient encounter, when possible.

The experience must be supervised by faculty with training and/or experience in the behavioral/developmental aspects of pediatrics.

The experience must include, as a minimum, a 1-month block rotation to ensure a focused experience in behavioral/developmental pediatrics. The program also must provide an integrated experience that incorporates behavioral developmental issues into ambulatory and inpatient experiences throughout the 3 years, eg, inpatient unit, community setting, continuity clinic, and subspecialty rotations. The program must include formal instruction in at least the following components to enable the residents to develop appropriate skills:
a. Normal and abnormal child behavior and development, including cognitive, language, motor, social, and emotional components
b. Family structure, adoption, and foster care
c. Interviewing parents and children
d. Psychosocial and developmental screening techniques
e. Behavioral counseling and referral
f. Management strategies for children with developmental disabilities or special needs
g. Needs of children at risk, eg, those in poverty, from fragmented families, or victims of child abuse/neglect
h. Impact of chronic diseases, terminal conditions, and death on patients and their families

C. Subspecialty Education

Education in the various subspecialties of pediatrics must be a vital part of the training of general pediatricians. Although it is not possible for each resident to rotate through every subspecialty, it is required that all residents be exposed to the specialized knowledge and methods of the major pediatric subspecialties through longitudinal experiences on the general inpatient and intensive care services and in outpatient settings. Residents should be taught when to seek consultation, when to refer to the subspecialist, and how to manage chronic illness as a team member with the subspecialist.

The curriculum must be designed to teach each resident the knowledge and skills appropriate for a general pediatrician, including the management of psychosocial problems affecting children with complex chronic disorders and their families. The experiences should include appropriate reading assignments and subspecialty conferences and familiarizing the residents with the techniques and skills used by the subspecialist.

All subspecialty rotations must have an adequate number, variety, and complexity of patients to provide each resident with an appropriately broad experience in the subspecialty. Outpatient experiences should be integrated into all subspecialty rotations to provide an opportunity for residents to develop the skills needed to manage patients with complex illnesses in a primary care practice.

The resident must be given appropriate patient care responsibilities with an opportunity to evaluate and formulate management plans for subspecialty patients. In the outpatient subspecialty clinics and with appropriate supervision by a subspecialist, the resident should function as the physician of first contact. Experiences in which the resident is solely an observer will not fulfill this requirement.

Subspecialty faculty must be directly involved in the supervision of residents and be readily available for consultation on a continuing basis. The supervision must be provided by pediatricians who are currently certified by the appropriate subboard of the American Board of Pediatrics or by other specialists who care for pediatric patients and who are certified by a specialty board approved by the American Board of Medical Specialties. In the absence of such certification, documentation of suitable equivalent qualifications must be provided. The acceptability of alternate qualifications will be determined by the RRC.
1. Intensive Care Experience (NICU and PICU)
The intensive care experiences must provide the opportunity for residents to deal with the special needs of critically ill patients and their families. Intensive care experience must be for a minimum of 4 and a maximum of 6 months and must include at least 3 block months of neonatal intensive care (Level II or III) and 1 block month of pediatric intensive care. Night and weekend responsibilities in the NICU, when the residents are on other rotations, will be included in the allowable maximum period of intensive care experience, with 200 hours being considered the equivalent of 1 month.

Programs with 4 block months of neonatal intensive care experience may allow an additional 200 hours of night and weekend responsibilities while the residents are on other rotations. Programs with 3 block months may have 400 hours of additional call. Programs with 5 block months may have no additional NICU call.

The curricula in neonatal and pediatric intensive care must be structured to familiarize the resident with the special multidisciplinary and multiorgan implications of fluid, electrolyte, and metabolic disorders; trauma, nutrition, and cardiorespiratory management; infection control; and recognition and management of congenital anomalies in pediatric patients. It also must be designed to teach the following:

a. Recognition and management of isolated and multiorgan system failure and assessment of its reversibility
b. Understanding of the variations in organ system dysfunction by age of patient
c. Integration of clinical assessment and laboratory data to formulate management and therapeutic plans for critically ill patients
d. Invasive and noninvasive techniques for monitoring and supporting pulmonary, cardiovascular, cerebral, and metabolic functions
e. Participation in decision making in the admitting, discharge, and transfer of patients in the intensive care units
f. Resuscitation, stabilization, and transportation of patients to the ICUs and within the hospital
g. Understanding of the appropriate roles of the generalist pediatrician and the intensivist/neonatologist in these settings
h. Participation in preoperative and postoperative management of surgical patients, including understanding the appropriate roles of the general pediatric practitioner and the intensivist in this setting
i. Participation, during the neonatal intensive care experience, in perinatal diagnostic and management discussions
j. Resuscitation and care of newborns in the delivery room
k. Evaluation and management, during the pediatric intensive care experience, of patients following traumatic injury

2. Adolescent Medicine

The program must provide all residents with experience in adolescent medicine that will enable them to recognize normal and abnormal growth and development in adolescent patients. This experience must be supervised by faculty having training and/or experience in adolescent medicine.

The experience must include, as a minimum, a 1-month block rotation to ensure a focused experience in the area of adolescent medicine. The program must also provide the resident with an integrated experience that incorporates adolescent issues into ambulatory and inpatient experiences throughout the 3 years, eg, inpatient unit, community settings, continuity clinic, or subspecialty rotations.

It must include instruction and experience in at least the following:

a. Normal pubertal growth and development and the associated physiologic and anatomic changes
b. Health promotion, disease prevention, and anticipatory guidance of adolescents
c. Common adolescent health problems, including chronic illness, sports-related issues, motor vehicle safety, and the effects of violence in conflict resolution
d. Interviewing the adolescent patient with attention to confidentiality, consent, and cultural background
e. Psychosocial issues, such as peer and family relations, depression, eating disorders, substance abuse, suicide, and school performance
f. Male and female reproductive health, including sexuality, pregnancy, contraception, and STDs

3. Additional Required Subspecialty Experience

Excluding the adolescent medicine and intensive care experiences, the time committed by any resident to subspecialty rotations must be a minimum of 6 months. During the 3 years of training no more than 3 block months, or its equivalent, may be spent by a resident in any one of the subspecialties in the lists below. Subspecialty research electives that involve no clinical activities need not be included in the calculation of a resident's subspecialty months.

The program must require that each resident complete a minimum of four different 1-month block rotations taken from the following list of pediatric subspecialties:

Allergy/Immunology	Infectious Disease
Cardiology	Nephrology
Endocrinology/Metabolism	Neurology
Gastroenterology	Pulmonology
Genetics	Rheumatology
Hematology/Oncology	

At least two of the four subspecialty rotations must be taken at the primary teaching site and/or integrated hospitals. Two of these subspecialties may be combined over a 2-month block if the outpatient and inpatient experiences of the two disciplines can be successfully integrated.

Additional subspecialty experiences needed to comply with the minimum requirements may be scheduled either as block assignments or as part of rotations in the outpatient department or inpatient services. The daytime equivalent of a block month is 140 hours. These may be selected from the list above or from the following list:

Child Psychiatry	Otolaryngology
Dermatology	Pediatric Radiology
Ophthalmology	Pediatric Surgery
Orthopaedics and Sports Medicine	

Two subspecialty areas from this second list may be combined over a 1- or 2-month period to provide a more effective educational experience.

D. Additional Curricular Requirements

Departmental conferences, seminars, teaching rounds, and other structured educational experiences must be conducted on a regular basis sufficiently often to fulfill educational goals. Reasonable requirements for resident attendance should be established, and resident and staff attendance should be monitored and documented. In addition to providing instruction in topics relevant to general pediatrics and to the subspecialty disciplines, there must be a structured curriculum in each of the following areas:

1. Medical ethics, including but not limited to the ethical principles of medical practice and the ethical aspects of
   a. the relationship of the physician to patients, eg, initiating and discontinuing the treatment relationship, confidentiality, consent, and issues of life-sustaining treatments
   b. the relationship of the physician to other physicians and to society, eg, the impaired physician, peer review, conflicts of interest, resource allocation, institutional ethics committees, and ethical issues in research.
2. Quality assessment, quality improvement, risk management, and cost effectiveness in medicine
3. Health care organization, financing, and practice management, with instruction in

a. the organization and financing of health care services for children at the local, state, and national levels, including an understanding of the role of the pediatrician in the legislative process
b. the organization and financing of office practice, including personnel and business management, scheduling, billing and coding procedures, and maintenance of an appropriate patient record system.
4. Medical information sciences, emphasizing the skills necessary to prepare the resident for continued self-learning and including instruction in
a. basic computer skills, techniques for electronic retrieval of the medical literature, and the use of electronic information networks
b. the critical evaluation of the medical literature, study design, and the applicability of clinical studies to patient care
c. clinical decision theory and its application to clinical practice.

E. Development of Procedural Skills

The program must teach residents, in both hospital and ambulatory settings, those procedural skills appropriate for a general pediatrician. These educational experiences should be graduated so that residents build and maintain skills throughout the training program.

1. Each program must provide sufficient training in and monitor resident development of at least the following skills:
a. Basic and advanced life support
b. Endotracheal intubation
c. Placement of intraosseous and intravenous lines
d. Arterial puncture
e. Venipuncture
f. Umbilical artery and vein catheter placement
g. Lumbar puncture
h. Bladder catheterization
i. Thoracentesis
j. Chest tube placement
k. Gynecologic evaluation of prepubertal and postpubertal females
l. Wound care and suturing of lacerations
m. Subcutaneous, intradermal, and intramuscular injections
n. Developmental screening test.

Each program must have a formal system for documenting resident experience and for monitoring resident compliance with the documentation process. Documentation of skills, eg, procedure logs, must be maintained by the program in the resident files. Supervision and documentation of skills must be by faculty or others with documented competence in the procedures. Residents should be informed about the procedures they are expected to learn and must receive feedback on their proficiency as part of the evaluation process.

2. In addition, programs should provide exposure to the following procedures or skills:
a. Circumcision
b. Conscious sedation
c. Tympanometry and audiometry interpretation
d. Vision screening
e. Hearing screening
f. Simple removal of foreign bodies, eg, from ears or nose
g. Inhalation medications
h. Incision and drainage of superficial abscesses
i. Suprapubic tap
j. Reduction and splinting of simple dislocations
k. Pain management.

All residents should maintain certification in pediatric (PALS) and neonatal advanced cardiac life support or in equivalent lifesaving systems.

F. Elective Experiences

Electives are intended to enrich the educational experience of residents in conformity with their needs, interests, and/or future professional plans. Electives must be well-constructed, purposeful, and effective learning experiences, with written goals and objectives. The choice of electives must be made with the advice and approval of the program director.

G. Resident Policies

1. Supervision of Residents

The supervision of residents must be accomplished through explicit written descriptions of supervisory lines of responsibility for the care of patients. Such guidelines must be communicated to all members of the program staff. Residents must be provided with prompt, reliable systems for communication and interaction with supervisory physicians. On-call schedules for teaching staff must be structured to ensure that supervision is readily available to residents on duty.

Residents must be supervised by teaching staff in a way that will allow them to assume progressively increasing responsibility for patient care according to their level of training, their ability, and their experience. The level of responsibility accorded to each resident must be determined by the teaching staff.

2. Duty Hours and Conditions of Work

Residency training is a full-time responsibility. The program director should monitor the effects of outside activities, including moonlighting in or outside the primary hospital, to ensure that the quality of patient care and the educational experience, as outlined in the agreement between the institution and the residents, is not compromised. Formal written policies on outside professional activities must be provided to the residents and should be available to the RRC, if requested.

Clinical duties must not be so pressing or consuming that they preclude ample time for educational activities, other important phases of the training program, or personal needs.

It is equally important that the residents have a keen sense of personal responsibility for patient care. Residents should be taught that their obligation to patients is not automatically discharged at any given hour of the day or any particular day of the week. The resident should not be relieved of duty until the proper care and welfare of the patients have been ensured by the presence of a suitable professional replacement.

On-call duty should occur with a monthly average of every third to fourth night for inpatient rotations requiring call. Call may be less frequent for outpatient or elective rotations. The call expected is in-house call for services with acutely ill patients, ie, inpatient and intensive care. Call on other rotations or electives may be in-house or by phone. There should also be a resident backup call schedule or alternate plan to provide coverage in the event that the assigned resident is unable to fulfill the assignment.

Call-free rotations should not occur on regular inpatient services where such a schedule would compromise the concept of continuity of care and interfere with the educational experience, eg, teaching rounds. Call-free rotations should not exceed 4 months during the 3 years of training.

The purposes of night call are to provide patient care, assume clinical responsibility, teach and supervise, and accumulate clinical experience including skill maintenance. Night and weekend duties must be sufficient to permit implementation of the concept of continuity of patient care.

The schedule should be designed to provide a monthly average of at least 1 day out of 7 without assigned duties in the program. Emergency department shifts should not exceed 12 hours, with consecutive shifts separated by at least 8 hours. Night float rotations must not occur so frequently in the program as to interfere with the educational experience for the residents.

3. Resident Complement/Peer Interchange
Because peer interchange is a very important component of the learning process, each program is expected to recruit and retain a sufficient number of qualified residents to fulfill the need for peer interaction among those training in pediatrics. The number of residents from other specialties or programs who rotate on the pediatric service must not dilute the experience and peer interaction of the pediatric residents.

There must be a sufficient number of residents at each level to provide appropriate peer interaction including frequent and meaningful discussion during all phases of the training program, eg, neonatal, outpatient, inpatient, and emergency services. Residents at more than one level of training must interact in the care of inpatients. To achieve this, a program should offer a minimum total of 12 resident positions, ie, four at each level, exclusive of subspecialty residents. Except for periods of transition, the same number of positions should be offered in each of the 3 years of training. The RRC will consider the presence of residents from combined pediatrics programs, eg, medicine/pediatrics or pediatrics/emergency medicine, when it evaluates the adequacy of the resident complement and of peer interaction. An inability to recruit the required minimum number of residents and/or a high rate of resident attrition from a program over a period of years will be a cause of concern to the RRC.

H. Scholarly Activity

The responsibility for establishing and maintaining an environment of inquiry and scholarship rests with the teaching staff. Scholarship implies an in-depth understanding of basic mechanisms of normal and abnormal states and the application of current knowledge to practice. While not all members of a teaching staff must be investigators, the staff as a whole must demonstrate broad involvement in scholarly activity, which should include the following:

1. Active participation of the teaching staff in clinical discussions, rounds, and conferences in a manner that promotes a spirit of inquiry and scholarship;
2. Active participation in regional or national professional and scientific societies, particularly through presentations at the organizations' meetings and publications in their journals;
3. Participation in research, particularly in projects that are funded following peer review and/or result in publications or presentations at regional and national scientific meetings;
4. Provision of guidance and technical support for residents involved in research, eg, research design, statistical analysis; and
5. Provision of support for resident participation in scholarly activities.

There should be evidence of clinical investigation and research that is designed to provide an environment of inquiry and scholarship in which the residents participate in the development of new knowledge, learn to evaluate research findings, and develop habits of inquiry as a continuing professional responsibility. This must include

1. a journal club and research conferences in which members of the teaching faculty participate and
2. opportunity to participate in scholarly activities, which may include clinical investigation and/or basic research.

VI. Evaluation

The program director is responsible for developing and implementing formal mechanisms for evaluation, as described below.

A. Evaluation of Residents

The program must have formal mechanisms for monitoring and documenting each resident's acquisition of fundamental knowledge and clinical skills and his or her overall performance prior to progression to the level of supervised semi-independent patient management. The supervising faculty must evaluate each resident in writing at the completion of each rotation. The resident should be evaluated on the acquisition of knowledge, skills, and attitudes, and should receive formal feedback about these evaluations at least twice a year. The program should advance residents to positions of higher responsibility only on the basis of evidence of satisfactory performance, progressive scholarship, and professional growth.

Written documentation of regular periodic evaluation of each resident must be maintained and must be available for review by the site visitor. Evaluations must include noncognitive areas such as interpersonal and communication skills, attitudes, and professional behavior, as well as moral and ethical characteristics.

Program directors are required to keep accurate documentation of the general and subspecialty experience of each resident in the program and to submit this information to the RRC if it is requested. The exact nature of the general and subspecialty experiences of residents at other institutions and evaluation of their performance must be documented in the residents' files.

It is essential that residents participate in existing national examinations. The annual In-Training Examination of the American Board of Pediatrics is one example of an objective test that can be utilized by the programs. An analysis of the results of these testing programs should be used by the faculty to identify the cognitive strengths and weaknesses of individual residents and weaknesses in the teaching program and to develop remedial activity, if warranted.

The program director and faculty are responsible for provision of a written final evaluation for each resident who completes the program. The evaluation must include a review of the resident's performance during the final period of training and should verify that the resident has demonstrated sufficient professional ability to practice competently and independently. This final evaluation should be part of the resident's permanent record that is maintained by the institution.

B. Evaluation of Faculty

Teaching faculty must be evaluated at least annually. Documentation of faculty evaluation should include teaching ability and commitment as well as clinical knowledge. There must be a formal mechanism by which residents participate in this evaluation in a confidential manner.

C. Evaluation of the Program

The teaching staff must be organized and have regular, documented meetings to review program goals and objectives, the program's effectiveness in achieving them, and the needs of the residents. At least one resident representative should participate in these reviews. In particular, the quality of the curriculum and the extent to which the educational goals have been met by residents must be addressed.

This evaluation should include an assessment of the balance between the educational and service components of the residency. In addition, the utilization of the resources available to the program, the contribution of each institution participating in the program, the financial and administrative support of the program, the volume and variety of patients available to the program for educational purposes, and the quality of supervision of the residents should be evaluated. Written evaluation by residents should be utilized in the process.

As part of the evaluation of the effectiveness of the program, the director must monitor the performance by the program's graduates on the certifying examination of the American Board of Pediatrics. Information gained from the results should be used to improve the program.

VII. Board Certification

One measure of the quality of a residency program is the performance of its graduates on the certifying examinations of the American Board of Pediatrics. In its evaluation of residency programs, the RRC will take into consideration the information provided by the American Board of Pediatrics regarding resident performance on the certifying examinations during the most recent 3 to 5 years. A program will be judged deficient if, over a period of years, the rate of those passing the examination on their first attempt is less than 50% and/or if fewer than 75% of those completing the program take the certifying examination.

Residents who plan to seek certification by the American Board of Pediatrics should communicate with the president of the board to obtain the latest information regarding certification.

ACGME: February 1996 Effective: February 1997

Program Requirements for Residency Education in the Subspecialties of Pediatrics

I. Introduction

Each subspecialty program must be organized and conducted in a way that ensures an appropriate environment for the well-being and care of the patients, provides residents with adequate training in the diagnosis and management of these subspecialty patients, and develops scholarship on the part of those residents. [*Note:* Those in accredited subspecialty programs are called residents or subspecialty residents. The term fellow is not used.]

These subspecialty programs must exist in conjunction with and be an integrated part of an Accreditation Council for Graduate Medical Education (ACGME)-accredited pediatric residency program. Their existence should not compromise the integrity of the core program.

Prerequisite training for entry into a pediatric subspecialty program should include the satisfactory completion of an ACGME-accredited pediatric residency or other suitable training. [*Note:* Candidates who do not meet this criterion should consult the American Board of Pediatrics or other appropriate board regarding their eligibility for subspecialty certification.]

The director and teaching staff of a program must prepare and comply with written educational goals for the program, and all educational components of a program should be related to these goals.

The program design and/or structure must be approved by the Residency Review Committee (RRC) as part of the regular review process. Participation by any institution providing more than 6 months of training in the program must be approved by the RRC.

II. Duration and Scope of Training

Pediatric subspecialty programs must provide 2 years of training, which must include progressive clinical, technical, and consultative experiences that will enable the resident to acquire expertise as a consultant in the subspecialty. [*Note:* If a third year is offered, it must be described when the program is reviewed by the RRC. Those planning to seek certification by the subboard should consult the American Board of Pediatrics regarding the criteria for eligibility, including length of training.] A program must emphasize scholarship, self-instruction, development of critical analysis of clinical problems, and the ability to make appropriate decisions. There should be progressive acquisition of skills in investigative efforts related to the subspecialty.

III. Service Duties

Service commitments must neither compromise the educational goals and objectives nor preclude adequate time for personal needs. The call schedule should not be more frequent than every third night, averaged monthly, and the overall schedule should be designed to provide a monthly average of at least 1 day out of 7 without assigned duties in the program.

The program director and teaching staff must monitor resident stress, including mental or emotional conditions inhibiting performance or learning and drug- or alcohol-related dysfunction, and should be sensitive to the need for timely provision of confidential counseling and psychological support services to residents. Training situations that consistently produce undesirable stress on residents must be evaluated and modified.

IV. Program Leadership and Teaching Staff

The program director and the teaching staff are responsible for the general administration of a program, including those activities related to the recruitment, selection, instruction, supervision, counseling, evaluation, and advancement of residents and the maintenance of records related to program accreditation.

A. Program Director

There must be a single program director responsible for the program. This director must be fully committed to the program in order to devote sufficient time to the achievement of the educational goals and objectives and must be based at the primary teaching site. The RRC must be notified promptly of a change in the leadership of the program.

1. Qualifications
   The director must possess the following qualifications:
   a. Requisite and documented clinical, educational, investigative, and administrative abilities and experience.
   b. Licensure to practice medicine in the state where the institution that sponsors the program is located. (Certain federal programs are exempted.)
   c. Certification by the relevant subboard of the American Board of Pediatrics or acceptable equivalent credentials. The adequacy of alternate qualifications will be judged by the RRC.
   d. Appointment in good standing to the medical staff of an institution participating in the program.
2. Responsibilities
   The responsibilities of the program director include the following:
   a. Preparation of a written statement outlining the educational goals of the program with respect to knowledge, skills, and other attributes of the subspecialty residents at each level of training and for each major rotation or other program assignment. This statement must be distributed to residents and members of the teaching staff. It should be readily available for review.
   b. Selection of residents for appointment to the program in accordance with institutional and departmental policies and procedures.
   c. Selection and supervision of the teaching staff and other program personnel at each institution participating in the program.
   d. The supervision of residents through explicit written descriptions of supervisory lines of responsibility for the care of patients. Such guidelines must be communicated to all members of the program staff. Residents must be provided with prompt,

reliable systems for communication and interaction with supervisory physicians.

Supervision of subspecialty residents must be provided by members of the teaching staff who are skilled in medical education as well as in the care of patients and who can devote adequate time to both of these endeavors. The supervising faculty must include teaching staff who are active and competent in their respective subspecialty disciplines and who are available to ensure proper education and to intervene in patient care as appropriate.

e. Implementation of fair procedures, as established by the sponsoring institution, regarding academic discipline and resident complaints or grievances.

B. Teaching Staff

1. In addition to the program director, there must be at least one other member of the teaching staff who is similarly qualified in the subspecialty to ensure continuity of the educational program.
2. A member of the teaching staff of each participating institution must be designated to assume responsibility for the day-to-day activities of the program at that institution, with overall coordination by the program director.
3. All members of the teaching staff must demonstrate a strong interest in the education of residents, sound clinical and teaching abilities, support of the goals and objectives of the program, a commitment to their own continuing medical education, and participation in scholarly activities.
4. Appropriate consultant faculty must be available to provide the residents with a defined educational experience in related disciplines, as delineated in the Program Requirements for each subspecialty.

C. Other Program Personnel

Programs must be provided with the additional professional, technical, and clerical personnel needed to support the administration and educational conduct of the program.

V. Scholarly Activity and Research

As part of the academic environment, an active research component must be included within each accredited subspecialty program. The responsibility for establishing and maintaining an environment of inquiry and scholarship rests with the teaching staff. Recent productivity by the program and by the residents will be assessed.

Participation of the teaching staff in clinical discussions, rounds, and conferences in a manner that promotes a spirit of inquiry and scholarship must be demonstrated. Scholarship implies an in-depth understanding of basic mechanisms of normal and abnormal states and the application of current knowledge to practice.

There must be adequate resources for scholarly activity, including research and critical analysis. Adequate laboratory space, equipment, and computer services for data analysis and statistical consultative services must be available to both the faculty and the residents.

A. Faculty Research/Scholarly Activity

The teaching staff must provide evidence of a commitment to and productivity in research in the pediatric subspecialty area. This research must be ongoing in clinical and/or basic aspects of the pediatric subspecialty field.

The RRC will consider the following as indicative of the commitment of the teaching staff to research:

1. Projects that are funded by agencies requiring peer review
2. Publication in peer-reviewed journals
3. Presentations at national or regional scientific meetings
4. Research protocols that have been approved by the local Institutional Review Board

B. Research Program for Subspecialty Residents

Within the institution there must be provision of support for resident participation in scholarly activities. The subspecialty resident must be exposed to and take part in research projects that are conducive to a questioning attitude, to protocol development, and to critical analysis of new therapies and medical literature. Research experience should begin in the first year and continue for the entire period of training to allow adequate time for the development of research skills and to bring a project to completion.

Residents must help design, conduct, evaluate, and prepare for publication a clinical or laboratory research project in the subspecialty area. They also should be required to conduct research seminars and prepare a written report of their research activities.

Instruction in related basic sciences and associated disciplines such as research design, biostatistics, and epidemiology must be offered through courses, workshops, and seminars.

C. Medical Education

Subspecialty residents should be actively involved in the education of house staff and medical students. They should understand the appropriate role of the pediatric generalist in subspecialty care and participate in the residency and continuing education activities. This should include a knowledge of curricular design and an active involvement in conferences, lectures, and clinical experiences for general pediatric residents.

Residents should have experience and guidance in the critical evaluation of pertinent medical literature and in medical writing and oral presentations. They should have the opportunity to develop teaching skills by giving lectures, conducting seminars and clinical conferences, and preparing teaching materials. These efforts should be reviewed and evaluated by supervising faculty.

VI. Patient Population

Adequate numbers of pediatric subspecialty inpatients and outpatients, both new and follow-up, must be available to provide a broad experience for the residents. These should range in age from infancy through young adulthood, where appropriate. There is a critical balance among the number and variety of patients, the number of preceptors, and the number of residents in the program.

VII. Library Facilities

Residents must have access to an on-site library or to a collection of appropriate texts and journals in each institution participating in a program.

The training program must provide access to facilities for the residents to engage in scholarly activities, including conference rooms, medical library, and research laboratories. The library should be available day and night and should have an ample supply of current pediatric subspecialty textbooks and journals. Access to computerized literature search facilities is necessary.

VIII. Evaluation

There must be an ongoing mechanism for the assessment of resident performance, faculty performance, patient care, and program objectives.

A. Evaluation of Residents

The program must have formal mechanisms by which the knowledge, skills, and professional growth of the residents are evaluated at least semiannually. This assessment must specify how the acquisition of requisite skills for subspecialty competence is accomplished. A written record of these evaluations must be maintained, must be formally reviewed with the residents, and must be accessible to authorized personnel. Residents should be advanced to positions of higher responsibility only on the basis of evidence of their satisfactory progressive scholarship and professional growth.

The program director must provide a written final evaluation for each resident who completes the program. This evaluation must include a review of the resident's performance during the final period of training and should verify that the resident has demonstrated sufficient professional ability to practice in this pediatric subspecialty competently and independently. This final evaluation should be part of the resident's permanent record maintained by the institution.

B. Evaluation of Faculty

Teaching faculty must be evaluated on a regular basis. Documentation of faculty evaluation must include teaching ability and commitment, as well as clinical knowledge and participation in scholarly activity. There must be a formal mechanism by which residents in both the core and subspecialty programs participate in this evaluation.

C. Evaluation of the Program

There must be documented evidence of periodic review and evaluation of the program in relation to the educational goals, the needs of the residents, and the clinical and research responsibilities of the faculty. At least one resident representative should participate in these reviews.

The teaching staff should periodically evaluate the utilization of the resources available to the program, the contribution of each institution participating in the program, the financial and administrative support of the program, the volume and variety of patients available to the program for educational purposes, the performance of members of the teaching staff, and the quality of supervision of residents.

The educational effectiveness of a program must be evaluated in a systematic manner. In particular, the quality of the curriculum and the extent to which the educational goals have been met by residents must be assessed. Written evaluations by residents should be utilized in this process.

Information gained from these evaluations should be used to implement improvements in the program.

IX. Evaluation by the RRC

Each program will be evaluated by the RRC at regular intervals, usually in conjunction with a review of the core program to which the subspecialty program is attached. Prior approval of the RRC should be obtained before implementation of major changes in the program during the interval between regular reviews.

Program directors are responsible for submitting complete and accurate information on the program to the RRC. Upon review of this information, the committee will judge the degree of compliance with the published standards.

In addition to complying with the requirements outlined in this document, each program must comply with the program requirements for the respective subspecialty, which may exceed the minimum requirements set forth above.

One measure of the quality of a training program is the performance of its graduates on the certifying examination of the subboard. In its evaluation of these programs the RRC will take into consideration the information provided by the American Board of Pediatrics.

ACGME: September 1991 Effective: July 1995

Program Requirements for Residency Education in Adolescent Medicine (Pediatrics)

Introduction

In addition to complying with the Program Requirements for Residency Education in the Subspecialties of Pediatrics, programs in adolescent medicine also must comply with the following requirements.

I. Scope and Duration of Training

Programs in adolescent medicine must provide training in and include an appropriate balance among clinical, didactic, and research activities. They must provide education in the broad and diverse knowledge base of this multidisciplinary field that focuses on the unique physical, psychological, and social characteristics of adolescents, their health-care problems and needs.

Adolescence links childhood with the adult years, covering the period from the start of puberty to early adulthood, programs in adolescent medicine must, therefore, integrate the relevant areas of pediatrics and the pediatric subspecialties with family practice, general internal medicine, psychiatry, obstetrics/gynecology, sports medicine, dermatology, and surgery and with related fields such as clinical pharmacology/toxicology, law, psychology, social work, education, nutrition, juvenile justice, sociology, and public health.

II. Faculty

Appropriate physician and nonphysician faculty in numbers sufficient for the size of the program must be available to provide ongoing teaching and supervision of the subspecialty residents. In addition to the program director, there must be at least one other physician who possesses appropriate qualifications in adolescent medicine, as described in the Program Requirements for Residency Education in the Subspecialties of Pediatrics.

In addition to the full range of pediatric subspecialists, consultant faculty in the following areas must be available to the program:

A. Child/adolescent psychiatry
B. Child neurology
C. Obstetrics/gynecology
D. General surgery
E. Orthopedic surgery
F. Sports medicine
G. Dermatology

In addition, personnel from the following categories should be available:

A. Psychology
B. Social work
C. Public and private school systems
D. Education
E. Public health
F. Chemical dependency
G. Nutrition
H. Clinical pharmacology

III. Facilities/Training Sites

The facilities and settings used by the program must be adequate for the program to accomplish the educational goals, and must include access to the following:

A. An inpatient medical service
B. An outpatient service
C. Clinical consultation

D. Additional clinical settings should include a school-based clinic, a summer camp, a crisis center, juvenile justice facilities, a college health program and a community health center, psychiatric, drug and alcohol facilities, and a family plan program.

IV. Curriculum

A. Core Knowledge Areas

The program must provide adequate instruction and clinical experience for all of the adolescent medicine residents to enable them to gain sufficient knowledge of and skill in the following:

1. Physical, physiologic, and psychosocial changes associated with pubertal maturation and its disorders
2. Organ-specific conditions frequently encountered during the teenage years
3. The effects of adolescence on preexisting conditions
4. Mental illnesses of adolescence (including psychopharmacology and psychophysiologic disorders)
5. Family dynamics, conflicts, and problems
6. Adolescent parenthood
7. Disorders of cognition, learning, attention, and education
8. Social and emotional development of the adolescent, including cultural/ethnic diversity
9. Chronic handicapping conditions
10. Disorders of the endocrine system and metabolism
11. Sexuality, including sexual identity, development, and sexual health problems
12. Sexually transmitted diseases (prevention and treatment)
13. Reproductive health issues of males and females (eg, menstrual disorders, gynecomastia, contraception, pregnancy, fertility)
14. Nutrition, including normal needs, health problems and deficiencies, and nutritional needs of special populations
15. Health promotion, disease prevention, screening, and immunizations
16. Infectious diseases, including epidemiology, microbiology, and treatment
17. Pharmacology and toxicity
18. Substance abuse, including alcohol and tobacco
19. Eating disorders, eg, obesity, anorexia nervosa, and bulimia
20. Social/environmental morbidities including physical and sexual abuse, risk-taking behaviors, injuries, sexual assault, and violence
21. Juvenile justice
22. Sports medicine
23. Legal and ethical issues including advocacy
24. Interviewing/short-term counseling skills for teens and their parents
25. Public health issues including demographics, social epidemiology, population-based interventions, and adolescent health promotion
26. Financing adolescent health care in public, private, and academic managed care environments

B. Clinical and Continuity Experience

The program must provide on-site clinical supervision of the subspecialty residents in a manner that allows them to assume graded responsibility for both the provision of clinical services and the supervision of other learners during the years of training.

The subspecialty resident must be given the opportunity to assume continuing responsibility for both acute and chronic health problems of adolescents in both inpatient and outpatient settings and to provide direct and consultative care to adolescents of various ages and socioeconomic and racial backgrounds in a variety of hospital and community settings. It is essential that the adolescent medicine resident have an outpatient continuity experience to include at least ½ day per week in an adolescent medicine setting.

C. Didactic Sessions

Conferences must emphasize the core knowledge and skill areas enumerated above. In addition, clinical conferences must include discussion of the basic clinical sciences. Health education, current health-care legislation, biomedical ethics, and preventive measures should also be addressed. Faculty must be available to provide instruction in interdisciplinary patient management and case conferences.

D. Administrative Instruction

Adolescent medicine residents must be exposed to formal sessions on the organization and leadership of, and membership in, a comprehensive health-care team. This must include utilization of the services of all relevant health-care professionals, including those in social services, nursing, education, mental health, and community resources.

The subspecialty resident must be provided with instruction and experience in the administrative aspects of an adolescent health care program, eg, knowledge of staffing needs, program management, continuous quality improvement, the organization and financing of health-care services, preparation of grant proposals, and planning for program development in a variety of settings.

ACGME: September 1997 Effective: September 1997

Program Requirements for Residency Education in Neonatal-Perinatal Medicine (Pediatrics)

In addition to complying with the Program Requirements for Residency Education in the Subspecialties of Pediatrics, programs must comply with the following requirements, which may in some cases exceed the common requirements.

I. Scope of Training

The purpose of the training program in neonatal-perinatal medicine is to provide residents with the background to understand the physiology of the normal neonate and the pathophysiology of the sick infant and to diagnose and manage problems of the newborn. To ensure an appropriate educational environment, training programs in neonatal-perinatal medicine must exist in conjunction with an accredited obstetrical residency program as well as with an accredited program in pediatrics.

The training program must emphasize the fundamentals of clinical diagnosis and management of problems seen in the continuum of the development of the fetus through prenatal, intrapartum, and neonatal periods, including follow-up. Each resident must participate in the long-term follow-up of high-risk infants and must have the opportunity to learn to identify the high-risk pregnancy, to evaluate fetal well-being and maturation, and to become familiar with the aberrant factors that may develop during the intrapartum period. The resident must have the opportunity to develop special competence in the management of critically ill newborn infants, including techniques of neonatal resuscitation, venous and arterial access, endotracheal intubation, preparation for transport, ventilatory support, continuous monitoring, temperature control, nutritional support, and general principles of critical care. The residents should have the opportunity to develop an appreciation of the social implications of disorders of the fetus and newborn infant.

The program should also provide opportunity for residents to teach and assume some departmental administrative responsibilities.

II. Patient Population

An adequate number of infants with a variety of neonatal disorders must be available so that each neonatal-perinatal resident may acquire competency in the management of the critically ill infant and in the technical aspects of care. The obstetrical and neonatal-perinatal programs must be closely associated, and there should be a sufficient number and variety of high-risk obstetrical patients to ensure that the residents become knowledgeable in identifying high-risk pregnancies and evaluating fetal well-being and maturation.

The number of infants requiring ventilatory assistance must be sufficient to provide each resident with the opportunity to become skilled in the management of these infants. Similarly, there should be an adequate number of infants requiring major surgery, including cardiac surgery, to afford the resident the opportunity to become skilled in the preoperative and postoperative management of these infants.

Residents must follow discharged infants in sufficient numbers to become skilled in the evaluation and management of such infants, as well as to become aware of the socioeconomic impact and the psychosocial stress that such infants may place on a family.

III. Laboratory Techniques

Residents must be instructed in laboratory techniques essential to the care of the high-risk infant. Experience in tabulating and evaluating institutional and regional fetal and neonatal morbidity and mortality should be provided. There also should be experience and instruction in techniques of collation and critical interpretation of data pertaining to immediate outcome and sequelae of various disease entities such as hyaline membrane disease, asphyxia, neonatal sepsis, blood group incompatibilities and congenital anomalies. This experience should be closely related to the evaluations of various modalities of therapy used in these disorders.

IV. Basic Sciences and Conferences

The program must include instruction in related basic sciences. Seminars, conferences, courses, and appropriate laboratory experiences must be offered in the basic disciplines related to pregnancy, the fetus, and the newborn. Examples of these are maternal physiological, biochemical, and pharmacological influences on the fetus; fetal physiology; fetal development; placental function (placental circulation, gas exchange, growth); physiological and biochemical adaptation to birth; physiology, biochemistry, pharmacology, and pathology relevant to diseases of the newborn; psychology of pregnancy and maternal-infant interaction; breast feeding and lactation; growth and nutrition; genetics; epidemiology; and biostatistics.

Residents should participate in regularly scheduled multidisciplinary conferences, such as sessions that review perinatal mortality, morbidity, and patient care, as well as in case conferences and current literature and research conferences.

V. Teaching Staff

Essential staff for the training program are

1. A minimum of three neonatologists to provide adequate supervision and to ensure the educational and research quality of the program.
2. A pediatric cardiologist as a consultant and teacher.
3. A surgeon skilled in pediatric surgery as a consultant and teacher.
4. A cardiovascular surgeon skilled in pediatric cardiovascular surgery as a consultant and teacher.
5. An obstetrician with special competence in fetal-maternal medicine.
6. A pediatrician skilled in neurodevelopment as a consultant and teacher.

Appropriate consultant faculty must be available to provide the residents with a defined educational experience in related disciplines, including other pediatric subspecialties, fetal-maternal medicine, pediatric surgery, radiology, anesthesiology, pathology, social service, and nursing.

Staff from other disciplines should be readily available. These should include but not be limited to neurology, ultrasonography, genetics, infectious disease, neurosurgery, ophthalmology, urology, orthopedics, and otorhinolaryngology.

The following staff also are recommended: a bioengineer, an ultrasonographer well versed in perinatal ultrasonic techniques, and a statistician and/or epidemiologist.

Nursing staffs must be sufficient to meet appropriate standards of care. This implies leadership by nurses skilled in neonatal and obstetrical intensive care. Medical social workers, qualified in maternal-child health, also must be available.

VI. Facilities and Laboratories

Because neonatal intensive care is an integral part of the institution in which the training program is housed, it is essential that the following facilities be available within that institution or in another readily available institution that ensures access to them on a 24-hour-a-day basis:

1. Microchemical laboratory
2. Blood gas laboratory
3. Perinatal diagnostic laboratory
4. Radiology and ultrasound imaging facilities
5. Diagnostic bacteriology and virology laboratory
6. Hematology laboratory
7. Blood bank
8. Electrocardiographic and electroencephalographic laboratories
9. Computed tomography and/or magnetic resonance imaging facilities

In addition to these essential diagnostic facilities, the following should be available within a reasonable period of time at the primary teaching site or nearby:

1. Screening laboratory for inborn errors of metabolism
2. Clinical toxicology laboratory
3. Nuclear medicine facilities
4. Cytogenetics laboratory

ACGME: September 1991 Effective: July 1995

Program Requirements for Residency Education in Pediatric Cardiology (Pediatrics)

In addition to complying with the Program Requirements for Residency Education in the Subspecialties of Pediatrics, programs must comply with the following requirements, which may in some cases exceed the common requirements.

I. Scope and Duration of Training

An accredited program in pediatric cardiology must provide 3 years of training.

The purpose of a training program in pediatric cardiology is to provide subspecialty residents with the foundation for understanding normal and abnormal cardiovascular conditions. Graduate training in pediatric cardiology should provide for properly balanced, well-organized, and progressive responsibility for care and study of patients on inpatient services, in intensive care units, and in ambulatory centers. The program must prepare the residents to provide optimal care and consultation for children with cardiovascular disease. Clinical training must be broad and include inpatient and outpatient experience, with the opportunity to observe heart disease in adults, particularly congenital and rheumatic disease. This responsibility must encompass age groups from the fetus and newborn through the young adult. The resident must be exposed to pathologic conditions ranging from mild to those requiring extensive or continued intensive care. There must be experience with a broad spectrum of congenital and acquired heart disease, both surgical and medical, and chronic as well as acute or emergency situations.

There must be opportunities to participate in and learn the fundamentals of administration of a pediatric cardiology program, including organization of clinics, organization and function of the cardiac team, and interaction with support agencies in the community such as government programs, third-party insurance companies, school nurses, public health nurses, and others.

The resident also must be provided experience in organizational responsibilities of a pediatric cardiologist in the community. This should include the functioning of a cardiac catheterization laboratory and a hospital-based pediatric cardiology service.

Residents must become familiar with preventive cardiology and with the psychosocial, ethical, and legal aspects of pediatric cardiology.

II. Clinical Experience

Programs in pediatric cardiology must include but not be limited to training in the following fundamental skills:

A. Noninvasive Techniques

Clinical diagnosis with special emphasis on auscultation and physical examination, roentgenology, electrocardiography, 2-D and M-mode echocardiography, Doppler ultrasound, exercise testing, Holter monitoring, and any other laboratory tests or imaging methods that may become established to facilitate diagnosis and management.

B. Invasive Techniques

Experience and instruction in the techniques and understanding of the value and limitations of diagnostic cardiac catheterization, selective angiocardiography, electrophysiology, and therapeutic catheter techniques.

C. Resuscitation Techniques

Experience and instruction in the techniques and understanding of the value and limitations of pericardiocentesis, thoracentesis, cardiopulmonary resuscitation, cardioversion, and temporary pacing.

D. Cardiac Catheterizations

The residents must be taught the use of relevant electronic equipment, recording devices, and angiographic equipment necessary to perform cardiac catheterization. In addition, the program must instruct the residents in the fundamentals of radiation safety. Accredited training programs should have a minimum yearly pediatric caseload of approximately 100 cardiac catheterizations and 75 operations employing extracorporeal circulation. Of these, approximately 30 catheterizations and approximately 24 open-heart surgical procedures should be performed on patients less than 1 year of age.

Experience with preoperative and postoperative care of patients having cardiac surgery, both by closed and open methods, in close cooperation with the cardiothoracic surgical staff, is required. Residents must have sufficient exposure to or instruction in current surgical techniques, methods of cardiopulmonary bypass, and hypothermia to develop adequate understanding of them. The resident should be instructed in the management of postoperative patients and postoperative complications, both immediate and delayed. Opportunity for long-term follow-up observations of both preoperative and postoperative patients must be provided.

The resident should participate in consultations or conferences in which the medical and surgical staffs evaluate the results of surgery and the patient's cardiac status prior to discharge from the hospital. The resident should have the opportunity to arrange for follow-up visits and send information to the referring physician to assist him or her in the future management of the patient.

In addition, the program must provide the resident with education in and exposure to rheumatic fever, collagen diseases, infective endocarditis, and other infections and metabolic conditions. Residents should be instructed in the etiologic and risk factors in hypertensive and atherosclerotic heart disease, including hyperlipidemic states, and should gain experience in the prevention, diagnosis, and management of patients with these cardiovascular problems.

There must be a regularly scheduled pediatric cardiology clinic, which must be supervised by one or more members of the cardiology staff. Time and space in this clinic must be available for residents to provide continuity and follow-up care for all patients under their care.

Clinical data, including inpatients, outpatients, and patients undergoing catheterization and/or surgery, should be cross-indexed and kept in such a manner as to allow rapid evaluation and analysis of the assembled information, including age, diagnosis, outcome, etc.

III. Basic Sciences and Conferences

The program should offer courses, seminars, workshops, or laboratory experience to provide appropriate background in basic and fundamental disciplines related to the heart and cardiovascular system, such as anatomy, physiology, biochemistry, embryology, pathology, pharmacology, genetics, nutrition, bioelectronics, and biostatistics.

The resident must receive instruction in cardiovascular pathology. Specimens demonstrating the various types of congenital cardiovascular anomalies should be classified and readily available for study. Conferences involving current pathological material must be held and closely correlated with clinical experience; such conferences should have clinicians, surgeons, anesthesiologists, roentgenologists, and pathologists in attendance.

There must be structured education in embryology and anatomy of the normal heart and vascular system as well as potential deviations from normal. Normal and abnormal cardiovascular and cardiopulmonary physiology and metabolism should be taught, as well as fundamentals of cardiovascular pharmacology, including mechanisms of drug action, therapeutic indications, and side effects.

Conferences must be held on a regular basis in the areas of clinical diagnosis and therapy, including quality assurance evaluation, cardiovascular research, and clinical morphologic correlations. Conferences with other disciplines such as physiology, pharmacology, neonatology, cardiovascular radiology, cardiothoracic surgery, and adult cardiology are encouraged.

IV. Teaching Staff

A general pediatric staff with a broad range of subspecialty interests is essential to teach complete care of infants, children, adolescents, and young adults with cardiac problems. Members of the pediatric cardiology training staff must be board-certified in the subspecialty or possess suitable equivalent qualifications. Residents must also be assured of access to medical cardiologists and basic scientists actively engaged in cardiovascular research. Special staff expertise is desirable in electrophysiology, exercise physiology, invasive and interventional cardiac catheterization procedures, intensive care, preventive cardiology, and echo-Doppler (including fetal). A ratio of two pediatric cardiology training staff members to each resident is desirable.

The physician in charge of the catheterization procedures must be certified by the subboard of Pediatric Cardiology or possess suitable equivalent qualifications and must be able to carry out the technical aspects of the procedures and correlate the results of the study with clinical information in reaching sound anatomic, hemodynamic, and electrophysiologic conclusions. A second physician should be available to the catheterization lab in the event that additional help is needed or a complication develops.

In addition, an anesthesiologist and a cardiothoracic surgeon, all having expertise in the pediatric cardiovascular aspects of their specialties, should be immediately available for consultation, assistance, and emergency surgical procedures. Additional personnel, adequately trained in pediatric cardiovascular techniques, should be available.

Staff from other disciplines, including cardiovascular radiology, cardiothoracic surgery, adult cardiology, anesthesiology, neonatology, pulmonary disease, pathology, hematology, nephrology, gastroenterology, and genetics, should be readily available.

Residents should be taught to work with and utilize the special skills of pediatric cardiovascular nurses, intensive care nurses, catheterization laboratory technicians, operating room personnel, social workers, and psychologists.

V. Facilities and Equipment

It is desirable that all facilities be located at the same institution. Where a facility is shared by several institutions in the interest of cost and efficiency, the program director may arrange for a resident to rotate to that facility.

A. Catheterization Laboratory

To provide a comprehensive experience for the resident, the catheterization laboratory should be located within a facility completely equipped to take care of patients. A program utilizing a catheterization laboratory located in a facility that cannot meet this criterion will be expected to provide evidence that the educational experience is not compromised in this regard.

Up-to-date equipment in the catheterization laboratory must include facilities for diagnostic biplanar cineangiocardiography and blood gas analyses and should include equipment for electrophysiological studies and interventional cardiology. A method for recording catheterization laboratory complications must be used and records kept of all complications. Resuscitation equipment must be available for all pediatric patients.

B. Inpatient Service

An active inpatient pediatric cardiology service is essential. It should provide all the diagnostic and treatment services characteristic of a comprehensive children's facility. Patients admitted to the inpatient service should be under the direct or indirect supervision of the training program staff and available to the residents.

C. Support Facilities

The following facilities should be available on a 24-hour basis:

1. General x-ray diagnostic facilities and nuclear cardiology
2. A graphics laboratory with facilities for recording the standard electrocardiogram and 2-D and Doppler echocardiograms
3. Laboratories to do routine analyses of blood and urine; to determine blood gas values, blood chemistries, and blood clotting studies; and to cross-match blood
4. An operating room designed and equipped for cardiopulmonary extracorporeal circulation with appropriate monitoring devices, defibrillators, and cardiac pacing devices
5. A blood bank equipped to meet the demands of cardiac surgery, which must be closely affiliated with the center
6. An intensive care unit in each center in which patients with heart disease are cared for under the supervision of the training program staff and are available to the residents and in which there are preoperative and postoperative patients with heart disease, as well as appropriate personnel and equipment to allow provision of the special and constant care needed by these patients

ACGME: February 1992 Effective: July 1995

Program Requirements for Residency Education in Pediatric Critical Care Medicine (Pediatrics)

In addition to complying with the Program Requirements for Residency Education in the Subspecialties of Pediatrics, programs must comply with the following requirements, which may in some cases exceed the common requirements.

I. Scope of Training

The purpose of the training program in pediatric critical care medicine is to provide subspecialty residents with a foundation for understanding the pathophysiology of acute, life-threatening disease, as well as the physiology of advanced life support; to prepare them for the care of critically ill pediatric patients; and to enable them to contribute to this pediatric subspecialty.

If there is more than one program in critical care medicine in the institution, there should be an institutional policy governing the educational resources committed to these programs and ensuring cooperation of all involved disciplines.

These programs must be organized and conducted in a manner that assures optimum patient care while providing residents with the opportunity to become skilled clinicians, competent teachers, and knowledgeable investigators familiar with and capable of administering a critical care unit.

To achieve this, the program must emphasize the fundamentals of clinical diagnosis, patient assessment, and clinical management. The subspecialty residents in pediatric critical care medicine must participate in the care of pediatric patients of all ages, from the infant to the young adult, and they must have the opportunity to acquire the knowledge and skills to diagnose and manage patients with acute life-threatening problems. This will include but not be limited to the opportunity to develop special competence in such areas as cardiopulmonary resuscitation; stabilization for transport; trauma; triage; ventilatory, circulatory, and neurologic support; management of renal and hepatic failure, poisoning, and complicated hematological, infectious, and immune problems; continuous monitoring; and nutritional support. The residents should have some of their clinical experience in other critical care settings, such as with anesthesiologists, in a medical intensive care unit (ICU), in a neonatal ICU, and in a surgical ICU.

There must be emphasis on developing a compassionate understanding of critical illness and death, so that the resident may be responsive to the emotional needs of the patients, their families, and the critical care staff.

Interpretation of laboratory studies essential to the care of the critically ill pediatric patient must be included in the curriculum. The program must teach pharmacologic principles and provide opportunity for the subspecialty residents to apply them to the critically ill patient. Instruction in biomedical instrumentation must be offered to familiarize the resident with current technology. The curriculum should include instruction in collation and critical interpretation of patient care data. The resident in pediatric critical care medicine must function as a teacher and assume some administrative responsibilities. Though clinical training in pediatric critical care medicine must include direct patient care responsibilities, a graduated experience should propel the resident toward supervisory and teaching roles.

II. Conferences/Basic Science

There should be opportunities to participate in regularly scheduled, multidisciplinary conferences such as sessions reviewing morbidity and mortality, case conferences, journal review, and research conferences.

The training program must include instruction in (or other educational exposure to) related basic sciences, including pathology, physiology, microbiology, nutrition/metabolism, biomedical instrumentation, and biostatistics.

III. Faculty

Appropriate consultant and collaborating faculty in related disciplines must be available at the facility housing the residency program. This must include specialists in the various pediatric subspecialties and surgeons having special expertise with pediatric patients. The faculty must also include specialists in cardiovascular surgery, neurosurgery, radiology, anesthesiology, orthopedics, otolaryngology, neurology, psychiatry, nephrology, pathology, social services, and nursing who have sufficient experience with pediatric patients to qualify them to play a part in the residents' education.

Essential physician staff for the training program are

1. At least two pediatric intensivists, to provide adequate supervision of residents and to ensure the educational and research quality of the program
2. A pediatric cardiologist as a consultant and teacher who must be certified by the appropriate subspecialty board or have equivalent credentials
3. A pediatric pulmonologist as a consultant and teacher who must be certified by the appropriate subspecialty committee or have equivalent credentials
4. A neonatologist as a consultant and teacher who must be certified by the appropriate subspecialty board or have equivalent credentials
5. An anesthesiologist with pediatric expertise as a consultant and teacher; there should be in-house, 24-hour anesthesiology coverage
6. A pediatric infectious disease specialist

All of the members of the physician teaching staff should be currently certified by the appropriate specialty board and should be certified by the relevant subboard of the American Board of Pediatrics, where appropriate. Where this is not the case, evidence of suitable equivalent qualifications must be provided. The Residency Review Committee will determine the acceptability of equivalent qualifications.

The following other staff are essential to the program to contribute to the resident's understanding of the broad impact of pediatric intensive care:

1. A respiratory therapy staff adequate to meet the clinical needs of patients and the educational needs of the resident in pediatric critical care
2. A skilled nursing staff capable of providing pediatric intensive care to the patients and contributing to the resident's understanding of the bedside nursing procedures involved in caring for these patients
3. Pediatric social workers and support staff to meet the needs of ICU patients and their families

The following staff are recommended:

1. A bioengineer
2. A statistician and/or epidemiologist
3. An ethicist

IV. Patient Population

An adequate number of pediatric ICU patients must be available for the subspecialty resident in pediatric critical care to acquire competence in the management of critically ill infants, children, adolescents, and young adults, including preoperative and postoperative care of the surgical patient. In the case of a patient on the surgical service, the pediatric resident should collaboratively participate with the surgeon who is managing the care of the patient. To meet the educational objectives of the program, the average daily census in the ICU should be at least four patients per resident assigned to the pediatric critical care service.

The number of patients requiring mechanical ventilation must be sufficient to provide each resident with the opportunity to become skilled in their management. There must be available to the teaching program an adequate number of patients in the pediatric age groups requiring major surgery, including cardiac and neurosurgery, to ensure that the subspecialty resident participates in the intensive care of these patients.

V. Facilities

A. Facilities and equipment must meet the generally accepted standards of modern intensive care units and must be available within the institution on a 24-hour-a-day basis. These include but are not limited to the following:
   1. Microchemistry laboratory
   2. Blood gas laboratory
   3. Hematology laboratory
   4. Blood bank
   5. Diagnostic bacteriology and virology laboratories
   6. Radiology facilities with portable capabilities for bedside use
   7. Facilities for special radiographic imaging including computerized axial tomography and radionuclide scanning
   8. Electrocardiographic laboratory with portable capabilities for bedside use
   9. Echocardiography laboratory with portable facilities
   10. Electrocardiographic laboratory with portable capabilities for bedside use
   11. Cardiac catheterization facility

B. In addition to these essential diagnostic and support facilities, the following are considered highly desirable and should be available:
   1. Clinical toxicology laboratory
   2. Laboratory that can screen for inborn errors of metabolism

ACGME: February 1991 Effective: July 1995

Program Requirements For Residency Education in Pediatric Emergency Medicine (Pediatrics)

In addition to complying with the Program Requirements for Residency Education in the Subspecialties of Pediatrics or Emergency Medicine, programs in pediatric emergency medicine must comply with the following requirements.

I. Introduction

The goal of a residency program in pediatric emergency medicine is to produce physicians who are clinically proficient in the practice of pediatric emergency medicine, especially in the management of the acutely ill or injured child, in the setting of an emergency department that is approved as a 911 receiving facility or its equivalent and has an emergency medical services system.

A program in pediatric emergency medicine must be administered by, and be an integral part of, an ACGME-accredited program in either emergency medicine or pediatrics and must be associated with an ACGME-accredited residency program in the corresponding discipline.

There must be written agreements between the director of the program in pediatric emergency medicine and the directors of the participating residencies in pediatrics and emergency medicine specifying the experiences that will compose this subspecialty program. These agreements should address appropriate curriculum content, supervision of the resident, amount and distribution of clinical and nonclinical time, conferences, clinical performance criteria, and mechanisms for resolving performance problems.

Prerequisite training should include satisfactory completion of an ACGME-accredited residency program in either emergency medicine or pediatrics.

II. Duration and Scope of Training

A training period of 2 years is required for all subspecialty residents. [*Note:* For those planning to seek certification from the American Board of Pediatrics, 3 years of training is required.] [*Note:* If a third year is offered, it must be described when the program is reviewed by the Residency Review Committee. Those planning to seek certification should consult with the appropriate certifying board regarding the criteria for eligibility, including duration of training.]

The educational program must be organized and conducted in a way that ensures an appropriate environment for the well-being and care of the patients and their families while providing residents the opportunity to become skilled clinicians, competent teachers, and knowledgeable investigators. The program must emphasize the fundamentals of assessment, diagnosis, and management. Residents also should be exposed to the academic debate, intensive research review, and the interaction between and among the specialties of pediatrics and emergency medicine.

III. Curriculum

The residents in pediatric emergency medicine must participate in the care of pediatric patients of all ages, from infancy through young adulthood, with a broad spectrum of illnesses and injuries of all severities. At least 12 months of the clinical experience must be obtained seeing children in an emergency department where children, ages 21 years of age or less, are treated for the full spectrum of illnesses and injuries. To provide adequate exposure for selected problems, additional experience with anesthesiologists, intensivists, neurologists, psychiatrists, pre-hospital care providers, orthopedists, surgeons, toxicologists, traumatologists, who have training and experience in the care of children and adolescents, and other specialists must be available.

Specialty-specific content must include at least 4 months of training in the reciprocal specialty from which the resident enters the training program. Additional elective months of reciprocal training should be scheduled when deemed appropriate by the program director on the basis of the background of the resident and his/her progress in acquiring the essential skills of a pediatric emergency specialist.

For the emergency medicine graduate, the reciprocal time must include time spent in pediatric subspecialty and ambulatory clinics, inpatient management, neonatal management, and pediatric critical care in an ACGME-accredited residency program in pediatrics.

For the pediatric graduate, this must include 4 months in an adult emergency department that is part of an ACGME-accredited residency program in emergency medicine. One month of that experience may occur off site as approved by the ACGME-accredited program in emergency medicine, in EMS, adult trauma, or toxicology.

Additional experiences may be necessary for residents from both core specialties. For example, adolescents have unique aspects of disease and injury. Experience with blunt and penetrating trauma, and with significant gynecologic and obstetrical emergencies, as well as psychiatric emergencies of the adolescent, must be a part of a resident's training if previous experience in these areas was not adequate. These experiences should be in settings best suited for the resident's training.

The core content must include training in EMS, administration, ethics, legal issues, and procedures. It must also include but not be limited to structured opportunities to develop special competence in such areas as cardiopulmonary resuscitation; trauma; disaster and environmental medicine; transport; triage; sedation; monitoring (biomedical instrumentation); emergencies arising from toxicologic, obstetric, gynecologic, allergic/immunologic, cardiovascular, congenital, dermatologic, dental, endocrine/metabolic, gastrointestinal, hematologic/oncologic, infectious, musculoskeletal, neurologic, ophthalmic, psychosocial, and pulmonary causes; renal/genitourinary and surgical disorders; and physical and sexual abuse.

In addition to achieving an understanding of the pathophysiology, epidemiology, and management of these problems, the resident must learn how to evaluate the patient with an undifferentiated chief complaint such as abdominal pain. The resident must be taught to arrive at a diagnosis, whether it falls in areas traditionally designated medical or surgical, eg, appendicitis, ectopic pregnancy, intussusception, sickle cell anemia; to perform the evaluation rapidly in accordance with any pathophysiologic disturbances in the patient; and to proceed with an appropriate life-saving therapy, such as endotracheal intubation or thoracostomy or administration of antibiotics, before arriving at a definitive diagnosis.

The resident must learn the skills necessary to prioritize and manage the emergency care of multiple patients. Finally, the resident must have supervised experience in a range of technical/procedural skills, as they apply to pediatric patients of all ages.

The resident must be given increasing responsibilities for patient care as she or he progresses through the program. In the final year of training, the resident must be given the opportunities to demonstrate the skills appropriate to a supervisor, teacher, and a decision maker in pediatric emergencies.

There must be an emphasis on developing a compassionate understanding of the stress associated with sudden illness, injury, and death so that the resident may be responsive to the emotional needs of the patients, their families, and the staff of the emergency department. Discussion and appreciation of the many ethical issues involved in pediatric emergency medicine should be part of the educational program.

Residents should be exposed to formal sessions on organizing teaching programs, medical writing, and oral presentation. Residents should have the opportunity to develop teaching skills by conducting lectures, seminars, and clinical conferences and by preparing written reports and teaching materials. These efforts must be reviewed and evaluated by the supervising faculty in light of competency based objectives developed by the program. The resident must receive instruction and experience in the administrative and management skills necessary to oversee a division or department.

IV. Conferences

There should be opportunities to participate in regularly scheduled, multidisciplinary conferences that include lectures, morbidity and mortality conferences, case conferences, general reviews, and research seminars. The program must include instruction in or other educational exposure to related basic sciences, including physiology, growth and development, pathophysiology, and epidemiology, and prevention of pediatric illnesses and injuries.

The program also should provide education on physician wellness and stress management.

V. Teaching Staff

There must be at least four members of the teaching staff who have experience and knowledge of the care of acute pediatric illness and injuries to provide adequate supervision of residents and to ensure the educational and research quality of the program. Two of the faculty must be certified in pediatric emergency medicine or have equivalent qualifications. For a subspecialty program that functions as an integral part of a pediatric residency program, there must be adequate exposure to faculty who are certified by the American Board of Emergency Medicine. Conversely, for a subspecialty program based in an emergency medicine residency program, there must be adequate exposure to faculty certified by the American Board of Pediatrics.

The availability of consultant and collaborative faculty in related medical and surgical disciplines, as referred to in Section III, must be ensured.

The pediatric emergency medicine faculty must have an active role in curriculum development and in the supervision and evaluation of the subspecialty residents.

VI. Patient Population

A sufficient number of patients must be available to provide adequate opportunity for subspecialty residents to acquire competence in the management of the full spectrum of acutely ill and injured children, adolescents, and young adults. The subspecialty residents must provide the initial evaluation of and treatment to all types of patients.

To meet the educational objectives of the program and to provide both the pediatric and subspecialty residents with an adequate experience to acquire competence in clinical management, there should be a minimum of 15,000 pediatric patient visits per year in the primary emergency department that is used for the program. Patient acuity and the total number of trainees will be considered in assessing the adequacy of the patient population. These must include a sufficient number of patients with major and minor trauma, airway insufficiency, ingestions, obstetric and gynecologic disorders, psychosocial disturbances, and emergent problems from all pediatric medical and surgical subspecialties.

Subspecialty residents should not serve as the only care givers for children seen in the emergency department. They should provide supervision and consultation to other residents who are assigned to the emergency department and will be caring for patients. These subspecialty residents must, however, have the opportunity to manage multiple patients at the same time, to learn the skills necessary to prioritize the evaluation and treatment of these patients. In addition, the program must provide the pediatric emergency medicine residents the opportunity to assume leadership responsibility for the pediatric emergency department.

VII. Facilities

There must be an acute care facility that receives patients via ambulance from the prehospital setting, is equipped to handle trauma, and that has a full range of services associated with residencies in pediatrics and emergency medicine. This facility should be accredited by the Joint Commission on Accreditation of Healthcare Organizations.

The emergency department must be adequately staffed, have appropriate bedside monitoring capability, and be capable of resuscitating medical and trauma patients. Facilities and equipment must meet the generally accepted standards of a modern emergency department and be available within the institution on a 24-hour-a-day basis.

The institution should have comprehensive radiologic and laboratory support systems and readily available operative suites and intensive care unit beds.

VIII. Board Certification

Residents seeking certification in the subspecialty of pediatric emergency medicine should consult their primary specialty board, ie, the American Board of Pediatrics or the American Board of Emergency Medicine, regarding the criteria for eligibility for certification in this subspecialty.

ACGME: June 1998 Effective: June 1998

Program Requirements for Residency Education in Pediatric Endocrinology (Pediatrics)

In addition to complying with the Program Requirements for Residency Education in the Subspecialties of Pediatrics, programs must comply with the following requirements, which may in some cases exceed the common requirements.

I. Scope of Training

The purpose of the training program must be to provide the residents with the background to diagnose and manage endocrine diseases and to understand the physiology of hormonal regulation in childhood, adolescence, and young adulthood.

The program must emphasize fundamentals of clinical diagnosis with special emphasis on history taking and physical examination. An opportunity must be available for the residents to learn about the pertinent aspects of genetics. Particular emphasis should be placed on the areas of counseling and biochemical genetics, cytogenetics, and their phenotypic expression.

II. Patient Population

Adequate numbers of patients, representing a wide variety and complexity of endocrine disorders and ranging in age from newborn to young adult, must be available to the training program. It is important that residents have a continuing responsibility for the care of patients in the outpatient clinic throughout their training.

The clinical experience must include patients in but not limited to the following categories:

1. Short stature, including constitutional delay
2. Disorders of anterior pituitary hormone physiology, including growth hormone deficiency
3. Disorders of posterior pituitary hormone physiology, including diabetes insipidus
4. Disorders of hypothalamic regulation of hormonal secretion
5. Disorders of thyroid hormone physiology; secretion and synthesis
6. Diagnosis and management of thyroid nodules and neoplasms
7. Disorders of the adrenal gland physiology; secretion and metabolism
8. Disorders of androgen and estrogen metabolism
9. Disorders of sexual differentiation and development
10. Disorders of calcium, phosphorus, and vitamin D metabolism
11. Disorders of parathyroid gland physiology
12. Disorders of fluid and electrolyte metabolism
13. Disorders of carbohydrate metabolism, including diabetes mellitus and hypoglycemia

It is particularly important that the resident have continuing responsibility for care of patients with diabetes mellitus and other chronic endocrine disorders. The clinical program must provide sufficient experience in the management of outpatients with diabetes mellitus as well as experience with the hospitalized diabetic. The residents must be involved in the care of adolescents to gain knowledge of normal and abnormal pubertal and hormonal alterations occurring during this phase of life. The residents must be involved in an endocrine clinic that meets at least weekly.

III. Laboratory Experience

The residents must be exposed to the proper use of laboratory techniques for measurement of hormones in body fluids; particular emphasis should be placed on recognition of the limitations and pitfalls of interpretation of laboratory results. They should be instructed in the normal variations that occur in laboratory data at different ages. Formal rotations through such laboratories should be included. Residents should be provided with a background that will enable them to utilize current diagnostic procedures of endocrinology involving radiology and nuclear medicine.

IV. Basic Science/Conferences

The training program must include instruction in related basic sciences. These include (1) endocrine physiology and biochemistry; (2) embryology of endocrine and related systems with emphasis on sexual differentiation; (3) genetics, including laboratory methods, cytogenetics, and enzymology; and (4) aspects of immunology pertinent to understanding endocrine disease and the use of immunoassays.

In addition, regular conferences reviewing patient management must be scheduled with required attendance.

V. Teaching Staff

Appropriate consultant faculty and staff must be available to provide the resident with a defined educational experience in related disciplines, including surgery, obstetrics/gynecology, internal medicine, psychiatry, neurology, radiology, nuclear medicine, genetics, pathology, nutrition, psychosocial support, and diabetes education.

VI. Facilities and Support Services

Facilities should include (1) space in an ambulatory setting for optimal evaluation and care of patients and (2) an inpatient area with a full array of pediatric and related services staffed by pediatric residents and faculty. Full support services must include radiology, laboratory, nuclear medicine, pathology, nutrition, and social services.

ACGME: September 1991 Effective: July 1995

Program Requirements for Residency Education in Pediatric Gastroenterology (Pediatrics)

In addition to complying with the Program Requirements for Residency Education in the Subspecialties of Pediatrics, programs must comply with the following requirements, which may in some cases exceed the common requirements.

I. Introduction

The principal goal of a training program should be the development of competent subspecialists. The program must provide the resident in gastroenterology with the background and experience to diagnose and manage patients with acute and chronic diseases of the digestive system (esophagus, stomach, intestines, liver, and pancreas), including those that are life-threatening, and to conduct research in this specialized field. The resident must be guided in developing clinical judgment and skills and in acquiring medical knowledge, humanistic qualities, and professional attitudes and behaviors that are appropriate for the pediatric gastroenterologist.

II. Duration and Scope of Training

A. Length of Training

A period of 2 years of progressive educational experience is required, which includes the development of procedural skills, responsibility for patient care, and participation in research.

Any program that extends training beyond the minimum requirements must present a clear educational rationale consonant with the Program Requirements and objectives for residency training. The program director must obtain approval of the Residency Review Committee prior to implementation and at each subsequent review of the program. Prior to entry into the program, each resident must be notified in writing of the required length of training.

The educational program must be organized and conducted in a way that ensures an appropriate environment for the well-being and care of the patients and their families.

B. Breadth of Experience

The program must emphasize developmental gastrointestinal physiology in infants, children, adolescents, and young adults and the correlation of pathophysiology with clinical disorders to develop the residents' competence in the clinical diagnosis and medical management of patients with these disorders. There must be training in the selection, performance, and evaluation of procedures necessary for morphological, physiological, immunological, microbiological, and psychosocial assessment of gastrointestinal diseases.

Residents must have clinical experience in the use of a variety of diagnostic tests and therapeutic procedures, eg, the use of imaging techniques such as computed tomography and magnetic resonance imaging, as well as conventional x-rays (contrast studies), ultrasound and hepatobiliary scans, tests of digestive system function, and assessment of nutritional status and pancreatic function.

C. Procedures

Residents must receive training in the following procedures:

- Colonoscopy
- Diagnostic upper panendoscopy
- Establishment and maintenance of patients with enteral and parenteral nutrition (include nutritional assessment)
- Flexible and rigid sigmoidoscopy

Paracentesis
Percutaneous liver biopsy
Rectal biopsy
Small bowel biopsy

In addition, residents should have training in the following:

Anorectal manometry
Breath hydrogen analysis
Dilatation of esophagus
Endoscopic retrograde cholangiopancreatography (ERCP)
Therapeutic upper pandendoscopy (sclerosis of esophageal varices)
Colonoscopy with polypectomy
Esophageal manometry
Pancreatic stimulation test
Esophageal pH monitoring
Placement of percutaneous gastrostomy

The program must have formal mechanisms for monitoring each resident's development of skills in the performance of these procedures and for including this in the regular evaluations.

D. Didactic and Laboratory Experience

The program should offer instruction, through courses, workshops, seminars, and laboratory experience, to provide an appropriate background for residents in the basic and fundamental disciplines related to the digestive system, such as embryology, physiology, pharmacology, nutrition, pathology, biochemistry, molecular biology, immunopathology, and genetics. Training in the evaluation of the psychosocial aspects of chronic gastrointestinal disease as they affect the child and competence in counseling chronically ill patients and their families should be components of the training program. Health education, biomedical ethics, and preventive measures for digestive disease also should be emphasized.

E. Administrative Experience

The residents must receive instruction and experience in the operational aspects of a pediatric gastroenterology facility, eg, staffing needs, unit management, and planning for program development.

III. Patient Population

The clinical component must involve broadly based experience with an appropriate range of pediatric patients having gastrointestinal problems. The patient population available to the program must have sufficiently varied and complex diseases and a volume sufficiently great to ensure that the residents have the opportunity to become clinically competent in the management of common as well as uncommon gastrointestinal, hepatobiliary, and pancreatic diseases in patients ranging from infancy through young adulthood.

Residents must have ongoing responsibility for the continuing care of patients with chronic gastrointestinal problems and must have sufficient opportunities to provide consultation on a wide variety of patients to become familiar with the gastrointestinal manifestations of a broad spectrum of pediatric illnesses.

This clinical experience must involve the management of patients with gastrointestinal disorders, including but not limited to the following categories:

A. Signs and Symptoms

1. Vomiting (including gastroesophageal reflux)
2. Acute and chronic abdominal pain
3. Acute and chronic diarrhea
4. Constipation (including Hirschsprung's disease)
5. Gastrointestinal bleeding

B. Diseases/Disorders

1. Growth failure and malnutrition (including an understanding of nutritional assessment and parenteral nutrition)
2. Malabsorption (celiac disease, cystic fibrosis, pancreatic insufficiency, etc)
3. Gastrointestinal allergy
4. Peptic ulcer disease
5. Jaundice
6. Liver failure (including evaluation and follow-up care of the patient requiring liver transplantation)
7. Digestive tract anomalies
8. Chronic inflammatory bowel disease
9. Functional bowel disorders
10. Evolution of gastrointestinal problems in the immune-compromised host
11. Other gastrointestinal disorders, such as gastrointestinal infections, motility disorders, infectious and metabolic liver diseases, and pancreatitis

IV. Facilities and Support Services

The following must be available to the program:

A. Space in an ambulatory setting for optimal evaluation and care of outpatients
B. An inpatient area with a full array of pediatric and related services (including surgery and psychiatry) staffed by pediatric residents and faculty
C. Full support services, including radiology, laboratory, nuclear medicine, pathology, and nutrition
D. Pediatric intensive care unit
E. Neonatal intensive care unit
F. Access to gastrointestinal function laboratory capable of measuring intestinal absorptive function, esophageal physiology pancreatic function, and nutritional parameters in pediatric patients
G. Flexible endoscopy facilities

V. Faculty

A. Specialty Consultants

In addition to the minimum of two pediatric gastroenterologists (see Program Requirements for Residency Education in the Subspecialties of Pediatrics), consultant and collaborative faculty in the following related pediatric disciplines must be readily available to the program: neonatology, hematology, immunology, genetics, and infectious disease, as well as specialists in pediatric surgery, pediatric anesthesiology, pediatric pathology, pediatric radiology, and child psychiatry and/or psychology.

B. Other Personnel

A nutritionist or registered dietitian with special skills in pediatrics must be available. Also, a nurse specialist or physician extender in pediatric gastroenterology should be available to the program.

ACGME: February 1993 Effective: July 1995

Program Requirements for Residency Education in Pediatric Hematology/Oncology (Pediatrics)

In addition to complying with the Program Requirements for Residency Education in the Subspecialties of Pediatrics, programs must also comply with the following requirements, which may in some cases exceed the common requirements.

I. Scope of Training

A program in pediatric hematology/oncology must provide the educational environment for the resident to develop an understanding of the pathophysiology of pediatric hematologic and oncologic disorders and to develop competence in the clinical diagnosis and management of these disorders. There must be training in the selection, performance, and evaluation of procedures necessary for appropriate assessment of these disorders.

The program must emphasize the fundamentals of clinical diagnosis, with special emphasis on history taking and physical examination, and must provide sufficient clinical experience with both inpatients and outpatients having hematologic and oncologic disorders to allow residents to develop skill in diagnosing and managing both common and unusual problems.

The clinical experience must involve patients who have a broad variety of hematologic-oncologic problems, and should include but not be limited to the following categories:

1. Leukemias, both acute and chronic
2. Solid tumors of organs, soft tissue, bone, and central nervous system
3. Lymphomas
4. Bone marrow failure
5. Hemoglobinopathies, including the thalassemia syndromes
6. Inherited and acquired disorders of the red-cell membrane and of red-cell metabolism
7. Autoimmune hemolytic anemia
8. Nutritional anemia
9. Inherited and acquired disorders of white blood cells
10. Platelet disorders, including ITP and acquired and inherited platelet function defects
11. Hemophilia, von Willebrand's disease, and other inherited and acquired coagulopathies
12. Hematologic disorders of the newborn
13. Transfusion medicine and use of blood products
14. Congenital and acquired immunodeficiencies

The resident must also have experience with bone marrow transplantation and its complications, including graft versus host disease.

The resident must become familiar with all aspects of chemotherapy, surgical therapy, and radiotherapy, including treatment protocols and management of complications, diagnosis and treatment of infections in the compromised host, appropriate use of transfusion of the various blood components, plasmapheresis, and bone marrow transplantation. The program should provide the resident with experience as a member of a multidisciplinary team for patients with cancer and chronic life-threatening hematologic disorders.

The resident should be instructed in the methods of physiologic support of the cancer patient, including parenteral nutrition, control of nausea, and management of pain. The pediatric oncology component of the program must include education in the staging and classification of tumors, the application of multimodal therapy, how to function as a member of the oncology team, the epidemiology and etiology of childhood cancer, how to make appropriate observations, and how to keep accurate patient data.

The resident should participate in the activities of the tumor board and in the provision of comprehensive care to the child with cancer and should have experience in support of the patient, family, and staff in dealing with terminal illness. Residents should be guided in the development of skills in communication and counseling.

II. Patient Population

Adequate numbers of patients with hematologic and oncologic disorders, ranging in age from newborn through young adult, must be available to the training program. Residents must have continuing responsibility for the care of patients with malignant disease and chronic hematologic problems. A program having fewer than 40 teaching patients with newly diagnosed oncologic disease each year must specifically demonstrate that it is able to provide the breadth of experience required for a training program. There should be opportunity for the residents to provide consultation for a sufficient variety of patients to become familiar with the hematologic manifestations of a broad spectrum of pediatric illnesses.

III. Laboratory Experience and Related Services

The residents must be exposed to the proper use of laboratory techniques for diagnosis. There should be particular emphasis on recognition of the limitations of the various methods and the pitfalls in interpretation of laboratory results. Residents should be instructed in the normal variations in laboratory data that occur at different ages and the influence of medications, toxins, and systemic disease on hematologic values.

The residents should be provided with a background that will enable them to utilize the current diagnostic procedures of hematology and oncology. These include (a) the performance and interpretation of bone marrow aspiration and biopsy, (b) lumbar puncture with evaluation of cerebrospinal fluid, (c) microscopic interpretation of peripheral blood films, and (d) interpretation of all hematologic laboratory diagnostic tests. Appropriate educational experiences in the laboratories, including blood bank and tissue pathology, should be included.

The principal training institution should have available the diagnostic services of radiology, nuclear medicine, computerized tomography, sonography, angiography, clinical chemistry, microbiology, immunology, and genetics.

IV. Basic Sciences/Conferences

The training program should provide instruction in the related basic sciences, including the structure and function of hemoglobin and iron metabolism, the phagocytic system, splenic function, cell kinetics, immunology, coagulation, genetics, the principles of radiation therapy, the characteristics of malignant cells, tissue typing, blood groups, pharmacology of chemotherapeutic agents, microbiology and anti-infective agents in the compromised host, and nutrition.

V. Teaching Staff

At least three pediatric hematologists/oncologists must be based at the primary teaching site and must devote sufficient time to the program to ensure adequate teaching and to provide critical evaluation of the progress and competence of the residents. Appropriate consultant faculty must be available to provide the resident with a definitive educational experience in related disciplines, including pediatric surgery and surgical specialties, radiation oncology, diagnostic radiology, gynecology, infectious disease, pathology, psychiatry, clinical psychology, immunology, cardiology, neurology, endocrinology, gastroenterology, genetics, nutrition, pain control, and physical medicine and rehabilitation.

VI. Facilities

Space in an ambulatory setting must be provided for optimal evaluation and care of patients, including facilities for outpatient chemotherapy and transfusions. An inpatient area with full array of pediatric and related services staffed by pediatric residents and faculty must also be present. Full support must include radiology, laboratory, pathology, intensive care, respiratory therapy, physical therapy, nutrition, social services, psychiatry, and psychology.

The program must also have access to specialized laboratories capable of assaying red-cell enzymes, identifying unusual hemoglobins, performing human lymphocyte antigen typing, immunophenotyping of leukemic blast cells, cytogenetic analysis, and identifying complex congenital and/or acquired hemostatic abnormalities.

ACGME: September 1991 Effective July 1995

Program Requirements for Residency Education in Pediatric Infectious Diseases (Pediatrics)

I. Introduction

In addition to complying with the Program Requirements for Residency Education in the Subspecialties of Pediatrics, programs in pediatric infectious diseases also must comply with the following requirements.

II. Scope of Training

The purpose of a training program in pediatric infectious diseases is to provide subspecialty residents with the background and experience that will enable them to provide optimal care and consultation to pediatric patients with infectious diseases. To achieve this, the training must include properly balanced, well-organized, and progressive clinical, technical, teaching, research, and consultative experiences. The educational program also must encompass basic concepts in immunology, epidemiology, and infection control as they relate to patient care and training in the prevention of infectious diseases.

III. Faculty

Supervision of subspecialty residents must be provided by members of the teaching staff who are skilled in medical education as well as in care of patients and who can devote adequate time to both of these endeavors. The supervising faculty must include teaching staff who are active and competent in pediatric infectious diseases and who are available to ensure proper education and to intervene in patient care as appropriate. Clinical supervision must be on a 24-hour-a-day, 7-day-a-week basis with as much continuity as is feasible.

Consultant faculty in related disciplines must also be available at the institution where the training occurs, including:

1. Allergy-immunology
2. Pediatric cardiology
3. Pediatric critical care
4. Dermatology
5. Pediatric gastroenterology
6. Genetics
7. Pediatric hematology-oncology
8. Microbiology
9. Neonatology
10. Pediatric nephrology
11. Pediatric neurology
12. Pathology
13. Pediatric pulmonology
14. Pediatric radiology
15. Pediatric surgery/surgery subspecialties

Consultants in nutrition, and clinical pharmacology also should be available.

IV. Facilities/Resources

Facilities and resources available to the program for the required clinical experiences must include at least the following:

A. Outpatient and Inpatient

The following facilities must be available at the primary teaching site:

1. An ambulatory facility for appropriate evaluation and care of patients from the newborn period to early adulthood
2. An inpatient facility with full pediatric (including adolescent) and related services that are staffed by pediatric residents and faculty and that includes
   a. facilities for isolation of patients with infectious diseases;
   b. pediatric and neonatal intensive care units; and
   c. complete support services including radiology, hematology, nuclear medicine, and pathology.

B. Laboratories

There must be clinical microbiology laboratories that include areas of diagnostic bacteriology, mycology, parasitology, virology, and immunology, all of which incorporate rapid diagnostic tests.

C. Other

There must be an infection control program with a physician leader (with knowledge of epidemiology of pediatric infectious diseases), written protocols for prevention of infection and its spread, an active surveillance system, and an interventional plan for outbreak control.

V. Educational Program

A. Curriculum

The program must have a well-developed, formally structured curriculum that is designed to

1. provide subspecialty residents with the information and experience necessary to diagnose and manage pediatric patients with a wide variety of acute and chronic infectious diseases, including disorders of host defense;
2. prepare the subspecialty resident to understand and deal with the principles of disease control, prevention of nosocomial infections, and immunization programs;
3. teach basic epidemiologic and biostatistical methods and their application to clinical research and patient care;
4. teach the subspecialty resident the functions and appropriate utilization of diagnostic microbiology, immunology, virology, mycology, and parasitology laboratories;
5. prepare the subspecialty residents to conduct research in the broad area of pediatric infectious diseases; and
6. ensure acquisition of appropriate teaching skills that can be used in the area of pediatric infectious diseases.

The educational program must include training in

1. the appropriate use of antimicrobial agents in a variety of clinical settings, their mechanisms of action, and their potential adverse reactions;
2. microbiological and immunologic factors that determine the outcome of the interaction between host and microbe, ie, the host-parasite relationship;
3. the effects of underlying disease states and immunosuppressive therapies on host response to infectious agents;
4. mechanisms of enhancement of resistance by active or passive immunization and immunomodulating agents;
5. pharmacologic mechanisms that affect absorption, metabolism, excretion, and interaction of antimicrobial agents;
6. methods of determining activity of antimicrobial agents and techniques to determine their concentrations in blood and other body fluids;
7. indications for procedures for specimen collection relevant to infectious diseases, including but not limited to bronchoscopy, thoracentesis, arthrocentesis, lumbar puncture, and aspiration of abscess cavities and soft tissues;

8. culture techniques for and/or methods of identification in tissues and fluids of bacteria, mycobacteria, fungi, viruses, rickettsiae, chlamydiae, and parasites;
9. the sensitivity, specificity, efficacy, benefits, and risks of contemporary technologies, such as those for rapid microbiologic diagnosis and for diagnostic imaging;
10. the principles and practice of hospital epidemiology and infection control;
11. quality improvement, clinical outcomes analysis, and cost containment in the clinical practice of infectious diseases;
12. the understanding of adverse events attributed to specific immunizations and immunomodulators;
13. ethical and medicolegal issues pertinent to pediatric infectious diseases; and
14. recognition of social and emotional issues pertinent to pediatric infectious diseases.

B. Clinical Experience

Clinical experience in the application and interpretation of diagnostic tests and indications, risks, and interpretation of the results of therapeutic procedures must be provided for all subspecialty residents in the program. This must involve experience with outpatients and inpatients having infectious diseases due to bacteria, fungi, viruses, parasites, rickettsiae, and chlamydiae that include at least the following categories:

1. Nonspecific systemic infections
2. Upper respiratory tract infections
3. Lower respiratory tract infections
4. Central nervous system infections
5. Urinary tract infections
6. Cardiovascular infections
7. Bone and joint infections
8. Skin/soft tissue/muscle infections
9. Gastrointestinal tract/intra-abdominal infections
10. Lymphoreticular infections
11. Hepatic/biliary infections
12. Ocular infections
13. Reproductive tract infections
14. Sexually transmitted diseases
15. Foreign-body and catheter-related infections

C. Patient Population

An adequate number and variety of patients with infectious diseases, ranging in age from newborn through young adulthood, must be available to the educational program and to each subspecialty resident. This patient population must include inpatients, outpatients, and patients with chronic diseases.

The program must ensure that each subspecialty resident provides consultation for an appropriate variety of patients in order to become familiar with the manifestations of a broad spectrum of infectious diseases. Such experiences must encompass longitudinal care, which provides the opportunity for observation of the course of illness and the benefits and risks of therapy.

The clinical population must include but not be limited to patients with the following conditions:

1. Primary immunodeficiency
2. Prematurity, low birth weight infants
3. Both congenital and acquired barrier defects
4. HIV disease
5 Immunosuppression secondary to malignancies and to chemotherapeutic or immunosuppressive agents
6. Malnutrition
7. Cystic fibrosis
8. Burns
9. Postoperative state following surgical procedures

ACGME: June 1996 Effective: June 1996

Program Requirements for Residency Education in Pediatric Nephrology (Pediatrics)

In addition to complying with the Program Requirements for Residency Education in the Subspecialties of Pediatrics, programs must comply with the following requirements, which may in some cases exceed the common requirements.

I. Scope of Training

The purpose of the training program is to provide residents with the capability and experience to diagnose and manage renal diseases and to understand the physiology of fluid and electrolyte regulation.

The training program must be designed to develop the physician's competence in the clinical diagnosis, pathophysiology, and medical treatment of disorders of the kidneys; urologic abnormalities; hypertension; and disorders of body fluid physiology in newborns, infants, children, adolescents, and young adults. Longitudinal experience must be provided in the therapy of acute renal failure and end-stage renal disease, including hemodialysis, continuous arteriovenous hemofiltration, peritoneal dialysis, and renal transplantation. Training and experience in the selection, performance, and evaluation of procedures, including renal biopsy, necessary for morphologic and physiologic assessment of renal disease, must be included.

There also should be training in the evaluation of psychosocial aspects of life-threatening and chronic diseases as they affect the patient and the family, and in counseling both acutely and chronically ill patients and their families.

The resident also should be provided with instruction and experience in the operational aspects of a pediatric nephrology service, including the dialysis facility. Knowledge of staffing needs, unit management, preparation of grants and proposals, quality assurance programs, appropriate communication with referring physicians, and planning for program development should be acquired during the training.

II. Patient Population

Adequate numbers of patients with a wide variety and complexity of renal disorders must be available to the training program. It is important that residents have a continuing responsibility for the care of outpatients throughout their training.

The clinical experience must involve but not be limited to patients in the following categories:

1. Congenital anomalies of the genitourinary tract
2. Hypertension
3. Renal disorders in systemic disease
4. Renal infections
5. Acute renal failure
6. Chronic renal failure
7. Renal transplantation
8. Neoplasms of the kidney
9. Fluid and electrolyte disorders
10. Acute and chronic glomerular diseases
11. Renal tubular disorders
12. Nephrolithiasis

III. Basic Sciences/Conferences

The program must offer instruction through courses, workshops, seminars, and laboratory experience to provide appropriate background for residents in diagnostic techniques and in the basic and fundamental disciplines related to the kidney. These should include embryology, physiology, pharmacology, pathology, immunopathology, genetics, biochemistry, cell biology, molecular biology, parenteral nutrition, magnetic resonance imaging, computed tomography, ultrasound, and nuclear medicine.

IV. Teaching Staff

Appropriate consultant faculty must be available to provide the resident with a definitive educational experience in related disciplines, including but not limited to urology, surgery, pathology, radiology, immunology, infectious disease, neonatology, hematology-oncology, and organ transplantation.

V. Facilities and Support Services

The facilities available must be sufficient to provide continuing contact with patients in both inpatient and outpatient settings. Transplantation and dialysis are essential components of the program.

In addition, certain ancillary support services and facilities must be available. These include urology, radiology, pathology, psychiatry and/or psychology, nuclear medicine, clinical laboratory, nutritional support services, nursing services, and social services.

ACGME: September 1991 Effective July 1995

Program Requirements for Residency Education in Pediatric Pulmonology (Pediatrics)

In addition to complying with the Program Requirements for Residency Education in the Subspecialties of Pediatrics, programs must comply with the following requirements, which may in some cases exceed the common requirements.

I. Scope of Training

The purpose of the training program is to provide the resident with the background to diagnose and manage pediatric patients with acute and chronic respiratory disorders, including those that are life-threatening, and to prepare the resident to conduct research in this special field. The program should emphasize normal pulmonary physiology in pediatric patients and correlation of pathophysiology with clinical disorders. It must require research and provide opportunity for the development of teaching skills on the part of the residents. This educational program must be organized and conducted in a way that ensures an appropriate environment for the well-being and care of the patients and their families.

The training program must be designed to develop the physician's competence in the clinical diagnosis, pathophysiology, and medical treatment of respiratory disorders in infants, children, adolescents, and young adults. There must be training in the selection, performance, and evaluation of procedures necessary for morphologic and physiologic assessment of pulmonary diseases.

The clinical component must be broadly based, with experience in a variety of pediatric pulmonary problems. The patient population must be sufficiently varied and frequently encountered to ensure that the pediatric pulmonology resident has the opportunity to become clinically competent in its management.

Clinical experience in the interpretation of a variety of diagnostic tests and the performance of therapeutic procedures must be available to the resident. Examples are the interpretation of new imaging techniques in relation to conventional x-rays and lung scans, tests of pulmonary function, evaluation of host defense mechanisms, and assessment of nonrespiratory functions of the lungs. The resident must have the opportunity to become proficient in bronchoscopy, thoracentesis, and physical and respiratory therapy. Training must include experience in respiratory intensive care procedures, eg, tracheal intubation, mechanical ventilation, cardio-pulmonary resuscitation, and must provide the opportunity for residents to develop an understanding of how a patient's critical respiratory problems affect other critical organ systems.

The program must offer instruction through courses, workshops, seminars, and laboratory experience to provide an appropriate experience for residents in the basic and fundamental disciplines related to the lung, such as embryology, physiology, pharmacology, pathology, allergy and immunology, immunopathology, and genetics. Training must be provided in the evaluation of the psychosocial aspects of chronic pulmonary disease as they affect the pediatric patient and his or her family. Opportunity also must be provided for residents to develop competence in counseling chronically ill patients and their families. Health education and preventive measures related to pulmonary disease also should be emphasized.

The resident in pediatric pulmonology should be exposed to formal sessions on organizing teaching programs, on medical writing, and on oral presentation. The resident must have the opportunity to develop teaching skills by conducting lectures, seminars, and clinical conferences and by preparing written reports and teaching material. These efforts must be reviewed and evaluated by the supervising faculty.

The resident must be provided with instruction and experience in operational aspects of a pediatric pulmonology facility. Knowledge of staffing needs, unit management, grant proposals, and planning for program development must be acquired.

II. Patient Population and Facilities

A. Patient Population

An adequate number and variety of patients with pulmonary disorders, who range in age from newborn through young adulthood, must be available. It is particularly important that residents have continuing responsibility for the care of patients with chronic pulmonary problems. There should be sufficient opportunity for the resident to provide consultation on a variety of patients to become familiar with the pulmonary manifestations of a broad spectrum of pediatric illnesses.

The clinical experience must involve patients having a broad variety of pediatric pulmonary problems, including but not limited to the following categories:

1. Asthma and allergic disorders affecting the pulmonary system
2. Bronchopulmonary dysplasia
3. Cystic fibrosis
4. Lower respiratory tract infections
5. Newborn respiratory diseases
6. Pulmonary intensive care of infants and children
7. Disorders of control of breathing, eg, apnea
8. Airway appliances and chronic ventilatory assistance
9. Aspiration syndromes
10. Anomalies of the respiratory system
11. Chronic suppurative lung disease
12. Evolution of pulmonary problems in the compromised airway
13. Other respiratory diseases, such as collagen vascular disease, hemosiderosis, fibrosing alveolitis, and acute lung injuries
14. Multiple trauma, to include carbon monoxide poisoning, respiratory distress associated with head trauma, and rib fracture

B. Facilities Must Include:

1. Space in an ambulatory setting for optimal evaluation and care of patients

2. An inpatient area with full pediatric and related services staffed by pediatric residents and faculty
3. Full support services, including radiology, laboratory, nuclear medicine, and pathology
4. Pediatric intensive care unit
5. Neonatal intensive care unit
6. Pediatric pulmonary function laboratory capable of measuring lung volumes, including body plethysmography, flows, gas exchange, and bronchoprovocation studies
7. Invasive and noninvasive pediatric cardiac laboratories
8. An inpatient unit capable of meeting the needs of young adults with cystic fibrosis, including consultative evaluation by internists where appropriate
9. Flexible bronchoscopy capability
10. Adequate resources for research, including statistical consultation, laboratory space, and computer services

III. Faculty

In addition to the program director, there must be at least one other similarly qualified faculty member in pediatric pulmonology to ensure continuity of the educational program and to provide adequate supervision of the residents and the required academic and research components of their training.

Consultant faculty in related disciplines must also be available at the institution where the training takes place. These must include faculty with special expertise in the following areas:

1. Pediatric cardiology
2. Pediatric critical care
3. Neonatology
4. Pediatric surgery
5. Allergy/immunology
6. Pediatric otolaryngology
7. Pediatric infectious disease
8. Pediatric radiology
9. Pediatric anesthesiology
10. Pediatric pathology

These essential members of the teaching staff should be certified by the appropriate subboard of the American Board of Pediatrics or must possess suitable equivalent qualifications. The Residency Review Committee will determine the acceptability of such equivalent qualifications. In addition, consultants should be available in the following areas:

1. Genetics
2. Pediatric gastroenterology
3. Pediatric neurology
4. Developmental pediatrics
5. Nutrition

IV. Other Personnel

The following staff are essential:

1. A pediatric respiratory therapy staff sufficient to meet the clinical needs of patients and the teaching of parents and to contribute to the education of the resident
2. Nurses experienced in pediatric pulmonology
3. Pediatric social workers
4. Pediatric nutritionists

ACGME: September 1991 Effective: July 1995

Program Requirements for Residency Education in Pediatric Rheumatology (Pediatrics)

In addition to complying with the Program Requirements for Residency Education in the Subspecialties of Pediatrics, programs in pediatric rheumatology must comply with the following specialty requirements, which may in some cases exceed the generic requirements.

I. Scope and Duration of Training

A. Length of Training

An accredited program in pediatric rheumatology must provide 3 years of training to allow sufficient time for the subspecialty residents to develop expertise in the long-term continuity of care that is required for the patients and to understand the natural history of the diseases. Continuity of care for a panel of patients throughout the 3 years is required.

B. Breadth of Experience

The purpose of a program in pediatric rheumatology is to provide subspecialty residents in pediatric rheumatology with the background to diagnose and manage patients with acute and chronic rheumatic diseases, including those that are life-threatening, and to help them develop investigative skills related to this specialized field, as is specified in the Program Requirements for Residency Education in the Subspecialties of Pediatrics.

The program must provide subspecialty residents with a thorough knowledge of normal growth and development as well as a broad understanding of all aspects of child health care, both of which are prerequisites for the proper management of pediatric patients with rheumatic diseases. The program should ensure the availability of all facilities and personnel necessary for the complete care of infant, child, adolescent, and young adult patients with rheumatic diseases. A patient population of sufficient size must be available to ensure training of both the general pediatric residents and the rheumatology residents.

The program must ensure that each subspecialty resident has the opportunity to provide continuing responsibility for both acute and chronic rheumatic diseases in order to observe the natural history of the disease process and effectiveness of therapeutic programs. Continuing responsibility for the care of patients with chronic rheumatic diseases is of particular importance.

II. Clinical Experience

The clinical component of the program must provide broadly based experience with a variety of rheumatic diseases and must be designed to develop the subspecialty resident's understanding of the pathophysiology of various rheumatic diseases and competence in the clinical diagnoses and medical management of these disorders. There must be training in the selection, performance, and evaluation of procedures necessary for pathologic, physiologic, immunologic, microbiologic, and psychosocial assessment of rheumatic diseases.

A. Diagnostic Tests and Procedures

Clinical experience in the indication for and interpretation of diagnostic tests and therapeutic procedures must be available to each subspecialty resident, eg, arthroscopy, the use of imaging techniques such as magnetic resonance imaging of the joints, nuclear imaging, contrast studies such as angiogram, ultrasound, and slitlamp examination of the eye.

The program must provide sufficient training to the residents to enable them to become proficient in the performance of the following:

1. Aspiration and injection of joints and interpretations of analysis of joint fluid
2. Prescription of physical therapy, occupational therapy, splints, and other therapeutic modalities
3. Interpretation of various imaging techniques used in the diagnosis and the care of rheumatology patients
4. Evaluation for surgical intervention, including participation in both preoperative and postoperative patient management
5. Interpretation of various laboratory tests as they relate to rheumatic disorders
6. Understanding of indications for and interpretations of electromyographic (EMG) and nerve conduction studies and of muscle and nerve biopsies.

The program must have mechanisms to document the proficiency of each subspecialty resident in the performance of these tasks.

There should be sufficient opportunity for the subspecialty resident to provide consultation on a wide variety of patients with rheumatic complaints common in the spectrum of other childhood diseases.

B. Patient Population

The patient population must be sufficiently varied and the volume sufficiently large to ensure the subspecialty resident the opportunity to become clinically competent in the management of common as well as uncommon rheumatic disorders. The patient population must be characterized by ample diversity of rheumatic diseases including but not limited to the following categories:

1. Acute rheumatic fever
2. Juvenile rheumatoid arthritis
3. Kawasaki disease
4. Lyme disease
5. Systemic lupus erythematosus
6. Scleroderma
7. Dermatomyositis/polymyositis
8. Henoch-Schönlein purpura
9. Other vasculitic disorders
10. Nonarticular rheumatic diseases including reflex neurovascular dystrophy and fibromyalgia
11. Skeletal dysplasias and metabolic bone diseases
12. Infections of bones and joints
13. Neonates with consequences of maternal rheumatic diseases or medications for rheumatic diseases
14. Spondyloarthropathies, psoriasis, and other HLA B27-related disorders
15. Malignancies of bone and muscle
16. Disorders of collagen and connective tissue
17. Rheumatic aspects in a child who is immunocompromised (congenital or acquired)
18. Rheumatic aspects of systemic diseases such as endocrine, metabolic, and gastrointestinal diseases
19. Sports injuries (exercise-related syndromes)
20. Secondary osteoarthritis, osteochondritis, avascular necrosis
21. Osteochondritis syndromes, such as Osgood-Schlatter disease and Legg-Perthes syndrome.

III. Basic Sciences and Conferences

The program must emphasize anatomy, physiology, biochemistry, genetics, and molecular biology of the musculoskeletal system in the developing child and the young adult.

A. Didactic and Laboratory Experience

The program should offer instruction in the form of courses, workshops, seminars, and laboratory experience, to provide an appropriate background for subspecialty residents in the basic and fundamental disciplines related to the musculoskeletal system, eg, anatomy, biochemistry, embryology, genetics, immunopathology, molecular biology, pathology, pharmacology, and physiology. Instruction and experience in rehabilitative and psychosocial aspects of chronic rheumatic diseases as they affect the child are essential. Experience in counseling chronically ill patients and their families must be a component of the training program. Health education, current health care legislation, biomedical ethics, and preventive measures also should be emphasized.

B. Health Care Team

The subspecialty residents must be exposed to formal sessions on organization and leadership of a comprehensive health care team and the utilization of the services of all relevant allied health professionals, including those in social services, rehabilitation, education, and mental health. There also must be education in the use of community resources in the care of children with rheumatic diseases.

C. Administrative Experience

The subspecialty resident must be provided with instruction and experience in the operational aspects of the rheumatology program, including staffing needs, unit management, working with team members, preparation of grant proposals, and planning for program development.

IV. Teaching Staff

A. Core Faculty

There must be at least two pediatric rheumatologists in the program to ensure adequate time for the administrative, clinical, and research activities involved in educating the subspecialty residents.

B. Specialty Consultants

Consultant and collaborative faculty in related disciplines, particularly pediatric orthopedics, must be available at the institution where training takes place. There must be pediatric subspecialists available in cardiology, gastroenterology, hematology/oncology, immunology, infectious disease, and nephrology, as well as specialists who have expertise with pediatric patients in at least the following areas: anesthesiology, clinical genetics, dermatology, neurology, ophthalmology, pathology, physical medicine and rehabilitation, and radiology. Collaboration with basic science departments and with adult rheumatology programs is encouraged.

C. Other Personnel

Staff from allied health disciplines, including registered physical and occupational therapists, must be available. The presence of a nurse specialist, a pediatric social worker, and a nutritionist is highly recommended.

V. Facilities, Equipment, and Support Services

A. Outpatient and Inpatient Areas

There must be adequate space in an ambulatory setting for optimum care and evaluation of patients. An inpatient area staffed by pediatric residents and faculty and with prompt availability of pediatric and related services must be present.

B. Support Services

In addition, there must be full support services, including radiology, laboratory, nuclear medicine, and pathology, as well as access to a pediatric rehabilitation program and to a clinical immunology laboratory.

ACGME: June 1995 Effective: June 1995

Program Requirements for Residency Education in Pediatric Sports Medicine (Pediatrics)

I. Introduction

In addition to complying with the requirements below, each program must comply with the Program Requirements for Residency Education in the Subspecialties of Pediatrics.

II. Scope and Duration of Training

An educational program in sports medicine must be organized to provide a well-supervised experience at a level sufficient for the resident to acquire the competence of a physician with added qualifications in this field. It shall be 12 months in duration.

The practice of sports medicine is the application of the physician's knowledge, skills, and attitudes to those engaged in sports and exercise. Thus, the program must provide training in the development of the clinical competencies needed to diagnose and manage medical illnesses and injuries related to sports and exercise, for example, first-degree sprains, strains, and contusions, including appropriate referrals of, for example, fractures, dislocations, and third-degree sprains. Clinical experience must include injury prevention, preparticipation evaluation, management of acute and chronic illness or injury, and rehabilitation as applied to a broad spectrum of undifferentiated patients. There must be experience functioning as a team physician and in the promotion of physical fitness and wellness.

The program should emphasize physiology and biomechanics; principles of nutrition; pathology and pathophysiology of illness and injury; pharmacology; effects of therapeutic, performance-enhancing, and mood-altering drugs; psychological aspects of exercise, performance, and competition; ethical principles; and medical-legal aspects of exercise and sports.

III. Teaching Staff

In addition to the program director, each program must have at least one other faculty member with similar qualifications who devotes a substantial portion of professional time to the training program.

The teaching staff must include orthopedic surgeons who are engaged in the operative management of sports injuries and other conditions and who are readily available to teach and provide consultation to the residents. Teaching staff from the disciplines of nutrition, pharmacology, pathology, exercise physiology, physical therapy, behavioral science, physical medicine and rehabilitation, and clinical imaging also should be available to assist in the educational program. Coaches and athletic trainers should also be included.

IV. Facilities and Resources

The program must include the following:

A. Patient Population

A patient population, unlimited by age or gender and adequate in number and variety to meet the needs of the training program, must be available. The program director must ensure that residents are accorded meaningful patient responsibility with the supervision of a faculty member at all facilities and sites.

B. Sports Medicine Clinic

There must be an identifiable clinic that offers continuing care to patients who seek consultation regarding sports- or exercise-related health problems. Nonsurgical residents must be supervised by a physician who has qualifications in sports medicine and is certified by the American Board of Emergency Medicine, the American Board of Family Practice, the American Board of Internal Medicine, or the American Board of Pediatrics or who possesses suitable equivalent qualifications.

Adequate up-to-date diagnostic imaging and rehabilitation services must be readily available and accessible to clinic patients. Consultation in medical and surgical subspecialties, physical therapy, nursing, nutrition, and pharmacology must be available. The opportunity to render continuing care and to organize recommendations from other specialties and disciplines is mandatory and will require that medical records include information pertinent to the assessment and management of patients with health problems related to sports and exercise.

C. Sporting Events/Team Sports/Mass-Participation Events

The program must have access to sporting events, team sports, and mass-participation events during which the resident can have meaningful patient responsibility.

D. Acute-Care Facility

There must be an acute-care hospital, with a full range of services, associated with and in proximity to the sponsoring residency. This facility must be readily accessible to patients served by the program.

V. Educational Program

The curriculum must provide the educational experiences necessary for the residents to achieve the cognitive knowledge, psychomotor skills, interpersonal skills, professional attitudes, and practical experience required of physicians in the care of patients with health problems related to sports and exercise.

Didactic as well as clinical learning opportunities must be provided as part of the required curriculum for all residents. Conferences or seminars/workshops in sports medicine should be specifically designed for the residents to augment the clinical experiences.

All educational activities must be adequately supervised, while allowing the resident to assume progressive responsibility for patient care. The clinical activities in sports medicine should represent a minimum of 50% of the time in the program. The remainder of the time should be spent in didactic, teaching, and/or research activities and the primary care or emergency medicine ambulatory facility.

Residents must spend ½ day per week maintaining their skills in their primary specialty.

Participation in the following must be required of all residents:

A. Preparticipation Evaluation of the Athlete

The program must ensure that all sports medicine residents are involved in the development and conduct of preparticipation examination programs.

B. Acute Care

The resident must have appropriate authority and responsibility to participate meaningfully in the medical care that is provided to acute-care patients (see "Scope and Duration of Training," above). In addition, the program should arrange for residents to observe representative inpatient and outpatient operative orthopedic procedures.

C. Sports Medicine Clinic Experience

The resident must attend patients in a continuing, comprehensive manner, providing consultation for health problems related to sports and exercise. The resident shall spend at least 1 day per week for 10 months of the training period in this activity.

If patients are hospitalized, the resident should follow them during their inpatient stay and resume outpatient care following the hospitalization. Consultation with other physicians and professionals in other disciplines should be encouraged.

D. On-Site Sports Care

The resident should participate in planning and implementation of all aspects of medical care at various sporting events. The program must ensure that supervised sports medicine residents provide on-site care and management to participants in these events.

In addition, the resident must participate in the provision of comprehensive and continuing care to a sports team. Preferably, the experience should include several teams that engage in seasonal sports.

E. Mass-Participation Sports Events

The resident should participate in the planning and implementation of the provision of medical coverage for at least one mass-participation event. The program must ensure that its residents have experience that includes providing medical consultation, direct patient care, event planning, protection of participants, coordination with local emergency medical systems, and other medical aspects of those events.

VI. Specific Knowledge and Skills

A. Clinical

The program must provide educational experiences for the residents to develop clinical competence in the overall field of sports medicine.

The curriculum must include but not be limited to the following content and skill areas:

1. Anatomy, physiology, and biomechanics of exercise
2. Basic nutritional principles and their application to exercise
3. Psychological aspects of exercise, performance, and competition
4. Guidelines for evaluation prior to participation in exercise and sport
5. Physical conditioning requirements for various activities
6. Special considerations related to age, gender, and disability
7. Pathology and pathophysiology of illness and injury as they relate to exercise
8. Effects of disease, eg, diabetes, cardiac conditions, arthritis, on exercise and the use of exercise in the care of medical problems
9. Prevention, evaluation, management, and rehabilitation of injuries
10. Understanding pharmacology and effects of therapeutic, performance-enhancing, and mood-altering drugs
11. Promotion of physical fitness and healthy lifestyles
12. Functioning as a team physician
13. Ethical principles as applied to exercise and sports
14. Medical-legal aspects of exercise and sports
15. Environmental effects on exercise
16. Growth and development related to exercise

B. Patient Education/Teaching

The program must provide the experiences necessary for the residents to develop and demonstrate competence in patient education regarding sports and exercise. They must have experience teaching others, eg, nurses, allied health personnel, medical students, residents, coaches, athletes, other professionals, and members of patients' families. There must also be relevant experience working in a community sports medicine network involving parents, coaches, certified athletic trainers, allied medical personnel, residents, and physicians.

ACGME: September 1994 Effective: July 1995

Program Requirements for Residency Education in Physical Medicine and Rehabilitation

I. Introduction

A. Definition of Physical Medicine and Rehabilitation

Physical medicine and rehabilitation, also referred to as *physiatry*, is a medical specialty concerned with diagnosing, evaluating, and treating patients with limited function as a consequence of diseases, injuries, impairments, and/or disabilities. Emphasis is placed on maximal restoration of the physical, psychological, social, and vocational functions of the person; on the maintenance of health and the prevention of secondary complications of disability; and on alleviation of pain. Physiatrists have special training in therapeutic exercise and physical modalities; prosthetics, orthotics, and the use of other durable medical equipment; gait analysis; diagnostic and therapeutic injections; electrodiagnostic studies; and rehabilitation management.

B. Program Design and Evaluation

The director and teaching staff of a program must prepare and comply with written educational goals for the program.

1. Program Design

   All educational components of a residency program should be related to program goals.

   a. The program design and/or structure must be approved by the Residency Review Committee (RRC) for Physical Medicine and Rehabilitation as part of the regular review process.

   b. Participation by any institution providing 6 months or more of training in a program of 3 or more years must be approved by the RRC.

2. Program Evaluation

   The educational effectiveness of a program must be evaluated in a systematic manner. In particular, the quality of the curriculum and the extent to which the educational goals have been met by residents must be assessed. Written evaluations by residents should be utilized in this process.

C. Duration of Training

1. a. Four years of graduate medical education is necessary to train a physician contemplating specialization in this field, and 3 of these years must be physical medicine and rehabilitation training. Of these 3 years no more than 6 months can be elective.

   b. One year of the 4 years of training is to develop fundamental clinical skills. This year of training in fundamental clinical skills must consist of an accredited Transitional Year or include 6 months or more in accredited training in family practice, internal medicine, pediatrics, or surgery, or any combination of these patient care experiences. The remaining months of this year may include any combination of accredited specialties or subspecialties.

   Accredited training in any of the specialties or subspecialties selected must be for a period of at least 4 weeks. No more than 8 weeks may be in nondirect patient care experiences. This training must take place within the first 2 years of the 4-year training program.

2. Training programs may choose either to provide 3 years of physical medicine and rehabilitation training and appoint residents at the PG-2 level contingent on satisfactory completion of 1 year's accredited training in fundamental clinical skills or to provide 4 years of training to include these fundamental clinical skills.

3. A training program of 3 years' duration is responsible for the 36 months of physical medicine and rehabilitation training and responsible for ensuring that residents appointed at the PG-2 level have received satisfactory training in fundamental clinical skills. A training program of 4 years' duration is responsible for the quality of the integrated educational experience for the entire training program, including training in fundamental clinical skills.

D. Objectives for Residency Training

1. An approved residency in physical medicine and rehabilitation must document that it provides an educational experience of such quality and excellence as to offer its graduates the opportunity for attainment of those competencies necessary for entry-level independent practice of this specialty. This must include knowledge about the diagnosis, pathogenesis, treatment, prevention, and rehabilitation of those neuromusculoskeletal, cardiovascular, pulmonary, and other system disorders common to this specialty in patients of both sexes and all ages. The training program must provide the opportunity for the graduate to develop the attitudes and psychomotor skills required to
   a. modify history-taking technique to include data critical to the recognition of functional abilities and physical and psychosocial impairments that may create functional disabilities;
   b. perform the general and specific physiatric examinations, including electromyography, nerve conduction studies, and other procedures common to the practice of physical medicine and rehabilitation;
   c. make sound clinical judgments; and
   d. design and monitor rehabilitation treatment programs to minimize and prevent impairment and maximize functional abilities.
2. The training program must provide the opportunity for the graduate to coordinate effectively and efficiently an interdisciplinary team of allied rehabilitation professionals for the maximum benefit of the patient by
   a. an understanding of each allied health professional's role,
   b. the ability to write adequately detailed prescriptions based on functional goals for physiatric management, and
   c. the development of management and leadership skills.
3. Additionally, the training program must stress the importance of self-evaluation, continuing medical education, and continued professional development after graduation. The training program must provide the opportunity for the resident to develop the necessary written and verbal communication skills essential to the efficient practice of physiatry.
4. The organization and philosophy of the residency program must provide the opportunity for development of the clinical competence of the resident. The curiosity and creativity of all residents must be stimulated. Their critical appraisal of current literature must be encouraged.
5. All provisions of the Institutional Requirements must also be met for accreditation.

II. Administration and Organization

A. Physical medicine and rehabilitation should be organized as an identifiable specialty within the sponsoring institution.

B. Institutions sponsoring or participating in residency training in physical medicine and rehabilitation should be appropriately accredited by the Joint Commission on Accreditation of Healthcare Organizations for rehabilitation or the Commission on Accreditation of Rehabilitation Facilities. If the institution is not so accredited, reasons why accreditation was not sought or was denied must be explained.

C. Number of residents: To ensure the stimulating educational atmosphere that a peer group provides, residents should be enrolled in a training program at all times. All training programs should have at least two residents per year in each year of training, with an approximately equal distribution of these residents. In addition, each training program should provide educational experiences that bring together all of the residents of the training program at frequent and regular intervals. Failure to recruit any new residents for 2 consecutive years will result in RRC review and possible adverse action.

III. Faculty Qualifications and Responsibilities

A. Program Director

1. Qualifications of the program director
   a. To achieve and maintain high quality of the training program, the program director must have the professional ability, enthusiasm, and sense of responsibility for this mission. The director must have the authority and time needed to fulfill administrative and teaching responsibilities so as to achieve the educational goals of the training program and to participate with other institutional program directors in maintaining the quality of all training programs.
   b. The program director must devote sufficient time to provide adequate leadership to the training program, implementation of the *Essentials,* and supervision for residents. To maintain training program continuity, the program director should have adequate tenure of office and be assigned over a period of years. Changes of program directorship must be reported *immediately* to the RRC for review of approval status.
   c. The program director must have licensure to practice medicine in the state where the institution that sponsors the program is located. (Certain federal programs are exempted.)
   d. The program director must be experienced and qualified as a teacher, clinician, and administrator and be certified by the American Board of Physical Medicine and Rehabilitation or possess suitable equivalent qualifications as a physiatrist.
2. Responsibilities of the program director
   a. The program director is responsible for the accuracy and timeliness of the information on the program information forms and other communications with the RRC.
   b. The program director must provide for the preparation of a written statement outlining the educational goals of the program with respect to knowledge, skills, and other attributes of residents at each level of training and for each major rotation or other program assignment. This statement must be distributed to residents and members of the teaching staff. It should be readily available for review.
   c. The program director must provide for the selection of residents for appointment to the program in accordance with institutional and departmental policies and procedures.
   d. The program director must provide for the selection and supervision of the teaching staff and other program personnel at each institution participating in the program.
   e. The program director must provide for the supervision of residents through explicit written descriptions of supervisory lines of responsibility for the care of patients. Such guidelines must be communicated to all members of the program staff. Residents must be provided with prompt, reliable systems for communication and interaction with supervisory physicians.
   f. The program director must provide for the regular evaluation of residents' knowledge, skills, and overall performance, including the development of professional attitudes consistent with being a physician.

      The program director, with participation of members of the teaching staff, shall

1. at least semiannually evaluate the knowledge, skills, and professional growth of the residents, using appropriate criteria and procedures.
2. communicate each evaluation to the resident in a timely manner.
3. advance residents to positions of higher responsibility only on the basis of evidence of their satisfactory progressive scholarship and professional growth.
4. maintain a permanent record of evaluation for each resident and have it accessible to the resident and other authorized personnel.

g. The program director must provide for a written final evaluation for each resident who completes the program. The evaluation must include a review of the resident's performance during the final period of training and should verify that the resident has demonstrated sufficient professional ability to practice competently and independently. This final evaluation should be part of the resident's permanent record maintained by the institution.

h. The program director must provide for the implementation of fair procedures as established by the sponsoring institution regarding academic discipline and resident complaints or grievances.

i. The program director must provide for monitoring resident stress, including mental or emotional conditions inhibiting performance or learning and drug- or alcohol-related dysfunction. Program directors and teaching staff should be sensitive to the need for timely provision of confidential counseling and psychological support services to residents. Training situations that consistently produce undesirable stress on residents must be evaluated and modified.

j. The program director must provide for the preparation of an accurate statistical and narrative description of the program as requested by the RRC.

B. Faculty

1. There must be a sufficient number of medical staff who are highly competent clinicians and motivated to teach residents. There should be a minimum of three full-time equivalent faculty members, including the program director, with a ratio of at least one full-time equivalent physiatric faculty member for every three PG-2 through PG-4 residents.
2. The faculty must be certified by the American Board of Physical Medicine and Rehabilitation or possess suitable equivalent qualifications. Nonphysiatric medical faculty must be appropriately certified or possess suitable equivalent qualifications. These teachers must participate regularly and systematically in the training program, both clinical and didactic, and must be readily available to the residents for consultations and during clinical crises. Part-time faculty should have specific, regular teaching responsibilities.
3. The faculty as a whole must set examples for residents, make reasonable scholarly contributions, provide quality clinical care, participate in research, and contribute to the professional literature.
4. A member of the teaching staff of each participating institution must be designated to assume responsibility for the day-to-day activities of the program at that institution, with overall coordination by the program director.
5. The teaching staff must be organized and have regular documented meetings to review program goals and objectives as well as program effectiveness in achieving them. At least one resident representative should participate in these reviews.
6. The teaching staff should periodically evaluate the utilization of the resources available to the program, the contribution of each institution participating in the program, the financial and administrative support of the program, the volume and variety of patients available to the program for educational purposes, the performance of members of the teaching staff, and the quality of supervision of residents.

C. Professional Staff

Professional staff who are appropriately credentialed in the disciplines of nursing, occupational therapy, orthotics and prosthetics, physical therapy, psychology, rehabilitation nursing, social service, speech-language pathology, recreational services, and vocational counseling should be integrated into both the didactic and clinical experience of the resident whenever relevant.

D. Other Program Personnel

Programs must be provided with the additional professional, technical, and clerical personnel needed to support the administration and educational conduct of the program.

IV. Facilities and Resources

A. It is necessary to have beds assigned to the physical medicine and rehabilitation service, grouped in one or more geographic areas. A minimum census of eight physical medicine and rehabilitation inpatients should be available for each resident while assigned full-time to an inpatient rehabilitation service.

B. There must be adequate equipment and space available to carry out a comprehensive training program in physical medicine and rehabilitation. There must be specific equipment for physical medicine interventions, and residents must have actual experience with this equipment. Equipment must be suitable for all age groups, with special attention to modified equipment for pediatric and geriatric patients. These include diathermies, ultrasound, radiant and conductive heat sources, other thermotherapy and hydrotherapy devices, ultraviolet, exercise equipment, ambulatory aids, wheelchairs, special devices for the impaired driver, electrodiagnostic and EMG equipment, cystometric equipment and urodynamic laboratory instruments, and simple splinting apparatuses. The occupational therapy area must be adequately equipped to give the residents experience in activities of daily living and in the evaluation and training in the use of devices to improve skills in activities of daily living. Psychometric and vocational and social evaluation facilities and test instruments must be adequate to expose the resident to the broad spectrum of their prescription and of their use and interpretation in the common practice of rehabilitation medicine. Adequate office space should be available for the faculty and residents to participate in both clinical examination of patients and self-study.

C. The sponsoring institution should provide an adequate, available professional library with suitable basic textbooks and journals pertinent to general medicine and surgery as well as to the specialty of physical medicine and rehabilitation. Loan arrangements with other main or lending libraries should be available. There also must be access to an on-site library or collection of appropriate texts and journals in each institution participating in the residency program. Library services should include the electronic retrieval of information from medical databases. On-site libraries and/or collections of texts and journals must be readily available to residents during evening hours and weekends. Some scholarly experience that demands the use of library reference facilities should be a part of the residency program.

D. Basic teaching aids such as slide projectors and videotape facilities are essential. Reasonable access to audiovisual areas on nights and weekends for residents and staff must be available.

Adequate space must be available for seminars, lectures, and other teaching experiences. There must be facilities for team conferences and specialty care clinics, such as orthotics, prosthetics, children's handicaps, and the like.

E. Peer Interaction

Facilities must be accessible to persons with disabilities.

V. Educational Program

A. Clinical Components

1. The clinical portion of the curriculum must include a sufficient variety, depth, and number of clinical experiences. However, clinical activities must not compromise the educational requirements of the training program.
2. The training program must include a significant amount of time spent in primary responsibility for the direct patient care management of hospitalized patients on the physical medicine and rehabilitation service. Residents must devote at least one-third of their residency experience to the care of these hospitalized patients with need for physical medicine and rehabilitation. They must spend at least one-third of their training in the care of outpatients, including a significant experience in the care of musculoskeletal problems.
3. Clinical experiences should allow for progressive responsibility with lesser degrees of supervision as the resident advances and demonstrates additional competencies. The program director must establish written guidelines for appropriate supervision of junior residents by senior residents and of all residents by attending physicians, with attention to the acuity, complexity, and severity of patient illness. Supervision must include faculty review of a clearly written patient history and physical examination and a meaningful continuous record of the patient's illness, background, and management strategies, as well as lucid presentations of the case summary.
4. Provision must be made for residents personally to review pertinent laboratory, roentgenographic, and other imaging materials for the patient. Opportunity to observe directly and participate in the various therapies in the treatment areas must occur regularly throughout the residency program, including proper use and function of equipment and tests.
5. Residents must have the opportunity to observe and gain fundamental understanding of orthotics and prosthetics, including fitting and manufacturing, through documented arrangements made with appropriate orthotic-prosthetic facilities.
6. Residents should have the opportunity to observe and gain fundamental understanding of the types of patients served, referral patterns, and services available in the continuum of rehabilitation care in community rehabilitation facilities. These include subacute units and skilled nursing facilities, sheltered workshops and other vocational facilities, schools for persons with multiple handicaps including deafness and blindness, independent living facilities for individuals with severe physical impairments, day hospitals and home health care services, and community reentry services. Some introduction to these options for care should be made by on-site visits to some of these facilities as well as by didactic lectures. Residents should be encouraged to interact with health care consumer groups and organizations.
7. The clinical curriculum must be written and implemented for the comprehensive development of measurable competencies for each resident in the following areas:
    a. History and physical examination pertinent to physical medicine and rehabilitation
    b. Assessment of neurological, musculoskeletal, and cardiovascular-pulmonary systems
    c. Determining impairment and disability
    d. Data gathering and interpreting of psychosocial and vocational factors
    e. Performance of electromyography, nerve conduction, and somatosensory evoked potential studies and other electrodiagnostic studies (In general, involvement in approximately 200 electrodiagnostic consultations per resident, under appropriate supervision, represents an adequate number.)
    f. Physiatric therapeutic and diagnostic injection techniques
    g. Prescriptions for orthotics, prosthetics, wheelchairs and ambulatory devices, special beds, and other assistive devices
    h. Written prescriptions with specific details appropriate to the patient for therapeutic modalities, therapeutic exercises, and testing performed by physical therapists, occupational therapists, and speech-language pathologists (It is necessary to provide for an understanding and coordination of psychologic and vocational interventions and tests.)
    i. Familiarity with the safety and maintenance, as well as the actual use, of medical equipment common to the various therapy areas and laboratories
    j. A formal experience in evaluation and application of cardiac and pulmonary rehabilitation as they relate to physiatric responsibilities
    k. The rehabilitation of children
    l. Collaboration with other medical professionals and members of the allied health team, including management techniques consistent with the resident's team leadership role and the treatment program management role of the physiatrist
    m. Geriatric rehabilitation
    n. Injury, illness, and disability prevention
8. The resident must have opportunities for progressive responsibility in diagnosing, assessing, and managing the conditions commonly encountered by the physiatrist in the rehabilitative management of at least the following:
    a. Acute musculoskeletal pain syndromes, including sports and occupational injuries
    b. Chronic pain management
    c. Congenital or acquired myopathies, peripheral neuropathies, and motor neuron and motor system diseases
    d. Rehabilitative care of traumatic brain injury
    e. Hereditary, developmental, and acquired central nervous system disorders, including cerebral palsy, stroke, myelomeningocele, and multiple sclerosis
    f. Rehabilitative care of spinal cord trauma and diseases, including management of bladder and bowel dysfunction and pressure ulcer prevention and treatment
    g. Rehabilitative care of amputations for both congenital and acquired conditions in patients of all ages
    h. Sexual dysfunction common to the physically impaired
    i. Postfracture care and rehabilitation of postoperative joint arthroplasty
    j. Pulmonary, cardiac, oncologic, and other common medical conditions seen in patients with physical disabilities
    k. Diseases, impairments, and functional limitations seen in the geriatric population
    l. Rheumatologic disorders treated by the physiatrist
    m. Medical conditions or complications commonly seen and managed in the physiatric patient
    n. Medical conditioning, reconditioning and fitness
    o. Soft-tissue disorders, such as burns and ulcers, and wound care

B. Didactic and Formal Components

1. Formal education should have a high priority. Didactic instruction must be well organized, thoughtfully integrated, based on sound educational principles, and carried out on a regularly scheduled basis. In a progressive fashion, it must expose residents to topics

appropriate to their level of training. Systematically organized formal instruction (prepared lectures, seminars, assigned reading, etc) must be an essential part of the residency. Staff meetings, clinical case conferences, journal clubs, and lectures by visitors are desirable adjuncts but must not be used as a substitute for an organized didactic curriculum. Active participation by the faculty in the didactic program is required.

2. The curriculum must include adequate and systematic training in basic sciences relevant to physical medicine and rehabilitation, such as anatomy, physiology, pathology, and pathophysiology of the neuromusculoskeletal, cardiovascular, and pulmonary systems; kinesiology; functional anatomy; physics; electronics; fundamental research design and methodologies; and instrumentation related to the field, which should pertain to physiologic responses to the various physical modalities and therapeutic exercises and the procedures commonly employed by physiatry. This training should be correlated with clinical training but should, when appropriate, involve basic science faculty. An accessible anatomy laboratory for dissection is highly desirable.
3. The training program must provide adequate and supervised experience in administration, unit management, cost containment activities, quality improvement, ethics, and teaching.
4. Bedside teaching rounds on hospitalized patients on the physical medicine and rehabilitation service must be made by residents with faculty at least five times per week.

C. Educational Policies

1. The clinical care of patients is the core of an adequate residency program, because the chief objective of residency training is the development of clinical competence in its graduates. The attainment of this chief objective must not be attenuated by participation of the resident in other activities.

   Physicians must have a keen sense of personal responsibility for continuing patient care and must recognize that their obligations to patients are not automatically discharged at any given time of the day or any particular day of the week. Duty hours and weekend call for residents reflect the concept of responsibility for patients and provide for adequate patient care. It is the responsibility of the program director, however, to ensure and monitor assignment of reasonable inpatient and outpatient duty hours to ensure that the resident is not subjected regularly to excessively difficult or unduly prolonged duties. Residents at all levels, on the average, should have the opportunity to spend 1 full day out of 7 free of inpatient and outpatient care duties and, on average, should be on night call no more often than every third night. The resident must be provided with adequate support, such as sleeping and food facilities, during duty hours.

   Satisfactory performance in the residency program is the resident's primary responsibility. Activities outside the educational program must be monitored proactively to ensure that they do not interfere with the resident's ability to perform in the educational process. It is the program director's responsibility to have and to implement written guidelines that address all of the above issues.
2. Each training program must have a written statement of educational objectives for the residents in that program. The program director must be able to document the implementation and achievement of these objectives.

D. Research and Scholarly Activity

1. The responsibility for establishing and maintaining an environment of inquiry and scholarship rests with the teaching staff. While not all members of a teaching staff must be investigators, the staff as a whole must demonstrate broad involvement in scholarly activity. This activity should include
   a. active participation of the teaching staff in clinical discussions, rounds, and conferences in a manner that promotes a spirit of inquiry and scholarship. Scholarship implies an in-depth understanding of basic mechanisms of normal and abnormal states and the application of current knowledge to practice.
   b. participation in journal clubs and research conferences.
   c. active participation in regional or national professional and scientific societies, particularly through presentations at the organizations' meetings and publication in their journals.
   d. participation in research, particularly in projects that are funded following peer review and/or result in publication or presentations at regional and national scientific meetings.
   e. offering of guidance and technical support (eg, research design, statistical analysis) for residents involved in research.
   f. provision of support for resident participation in scholarly activities.
2. Residents should have the opportunity to participate in structured, supervised research training. It is desirable that each resident produce a peer-reviewed publication during the residency program. A program director may elect to offer a special research or academic track for selected residents. This may take the form of an elective or research rotation, not to exceed 6 months, within the 36 months of physical medicine and rehabilitation residency training.

E. Peer Interaction

Physical medicine and rehabilitation residents must have interaction with residents from other specialties and/or medical students to provide opportunities for peer interaction and teaching.

VI. Evaluation

A. There must be a documented, confidential, organized, and formal system for resident evaluation by faculty members at least every 6 months and annual in-service examinations, post-rotation evaluations, or external examinations such as those provided by the American Academy of Physical Medicine and Rehabilitation. Residents must meet with the program director or designee at least twice a year for formal review and feedback and have access to their evaluation folders. The residents' rights must be protected by due process procedures. Residents must be aware of their rights and of the institution's obligations and rights.

B. A formal system must exist to identify special competencies and weaknesses of faculty and to make appropriate teaching, clinical, and research assignments. Residents must have an effective, formal, written, confidential, and anonymous mechanism for faculty and rotation evaluation. Such evaluations must be reviewed at least annually by the program director. Where indicated, substantive efforts should be made to correct faculty weaknesses.

C. A formal system to identify strengths and weaknesses of the training program must exist. Residents must have an effective, formal mechanism for evaluation of the residency program. Such evaluations must be reviewed by the program director at least annually. Other types of evaluation (sponsoring institution's internal reviews, in-service examinations, performance on board examinations, etc) also should be utilized. Where indicated, substantive efforts should be made to correct residency program weakness.

VII. Board Certification

Residents who plan to seek certification by the American Board of Physical Medicine and Rehabilitation should communicate with the executive director of the board. The program director must complete a final evaluation for the American Board of Physical Medicine and Rehabilitation concerning the resident's admissibility to the certifying examination.

One measure of the quality of a residency program is the performance of its residents on the examinations of the American Board of Physical Medicine and Rehabilitation.

ACGME: February 1995 Effective: January 1996

Policies and Procedures for Residency Education in the Subspecialties of Physical Medicine and Rehabilitation

A. The initial application for a subspecialty program will not require an on-site survey, but will require submission of all application materials and information signed by the director of the subspecialty program and the director of the accredited sponsoring program in a relevant core specialty such as anesthesiology, emergency medicine, family practice, internal medicine, neurological surgery, neurology, orthopedic surgery, pediatrics, physical medicine and rehabilitation, plastic surgery, surgery, or urology. The Residency Review Committee for Physical Medicine and Rehabilitation (RRC) will take initial action based on a "paper review" of the program, namely, a review without survey.

B. Subsequent review of subspecialty programs will be in conjunction with the survey and review of the core program. A separate set of forms will have to be completed by the subspecialty program director. In special cases determined by the RRC, the subspecialty program will be surveyed and reviewed separately. The RRC will also entertain interim requests and, on occasion, ask for interim progress reports.

C. The Residency Review Committee will designate programs as being accredited or not accredited. No further delineation of accreditation categories will be utilized. The accreditation of a program will be directly tied to that of the core. If the core program is subsequently accredited on a probationary basis, this is simultaneously a warning to the related subspecialty program that accreditation is in jeopardy. Withdrawal of accreditation of the core program will result in a simultaneous loss of accreditation of the subspecialty program.

D. If the core program remains in good standing but the RRC judges the subspecialty program to be in noncompliance with the applicable program requirements, a warning will be issued. If these areas of noncompliance are not corrected, accreditation may be withdrawn from the subspecialty program. The *Procedures for Proposed Adverse Actions* and the *Procedures for Appeal of Adverse Actions* may be utilized by programs from which the accreditation has been withdrawn in an action separate from withdrawal of accreditation of the core program.

E. Inquiries about accreditation of subspecialty programs should be directed to the Executive Secretary of the Residency Review Committee for Physical Medicine and Rehabilitation.

Program Requirements for Residency Education in Spinal Cord Injury Medicine (Physical Medicine and Rehabilitation)

I. Introduction

A. Definition

1. Spinal Cord Injury Medicine (SCIM) addresses the prevention, diagnosis, treatment, and management of traumatic spinal cord injury (SCI) and nontraumatic myelopathies, including the prevention, diagnosis, and treatment of related medical, physical, psychosocial, and vocational disabilities and complications during the lifetime of the patient.
2. The management of persons with spinal cord dysfunction (SCD) requires a team and interspecialty approach, with contributions from several medical and surgical specialties as well as other health care professionals. The specialist in SCIM should serve as the team leader after the patient is medically and surgically stabilized. When the spinal disability is secondary to an active process or a chronic degenerative disorder, the management of the patient's primary disease is the responsibility of a physician in the appropriate discipline.

B. Duration and Scope of Education

1. Training in SCIM shall be 12 months in duration beginning after satisfactory completion of an approved residency program in a specialty relevant to SCIM, such as anesthesiology, emergency medicine, family practice, internal medicine, neurological surgery, neurology, orthopedic surgery, pediatrics, physical medicine and rehabilitation, plastic surgery, surgery, or urology.
2. The program must provide for individuals to acquire, within the interdisciplinary SCI team, knowledge of emergency care and knowledge and skills in the following areas:
   a. post-initial care,
   b. initial and ongoing medical rehabilitation,
   c. discharge planning,
   d. lifelong care, and
   e. scholarly activity in support of these skills.
3. Any program that extends training beyond the 12-month minimum requirement must present a clear educational rationale consonant with the program requirements and objectives for subspecialty training. The program director must obtain approval of the Residency Review Committee (RRC) prior to implementation and at each subsequent review of the program. Prior to entry in the program, each resident must be notified in writing of the required length of training.

C. Program Goals and Objectives

The director and teaching staff of a program must prepare and comply with written educational goals for the program.

1. Goals: An approved subspecialty program must be designed to provide an educational experience to ensure that its graduates possess the advanced knowledge and competencies necessary to practice this subspecialty.
2. Objectives: The program must provide the resident opportunities to develop a unique set of attitudes, knowledge, and psychomotor skills because SCD affects multiple organ systems of the body and its treatment involves many specialty areas of expertise. The resident must be given the opportunity to gain knowledge of
   a. the impact of SCD on the various organ systems,

b. the natural history, pharmacologic management, and evolution of organ system functioning after SCD and the interaction among the various organ systems,
c. the impact of aging and long-standing injury on organ system decline,
d. the prevention and treatment of secondary complications of SCD, and
e. the maximal functions possible, based on the characteristics and level of SCD and how to achieve them.

The resident must be given the opportunity to become proficient in:

a. coordination in the postinitial care setting of the impact and timing of treatment of each organ system's dysfunction so that an optimum treatment effect can be obtained,
b. planning of the most efficient and effective treatment approaches for acquisition of skills and knowledge by the patient in order to acquire the highest level of functioning, and
c. promotion of patient education about all aspects of SCD in order to promote patient independence and patient recognition of illness.

The program must prepare the person trained as an SCIM specialist to implement, over the course of the individual patient's lifetime, a health maintenance and disease prevention program with early recognition and effective treatment of complications related to SCD, and must promote awareness of the impact of aging on SCD.

D. Program Design

All educational components of a residency program should be related to program goals.

1. The program design and/or structure must be approved by the appropriate review committee as part of the regular review process.
2. Participation by any institution providing more than 3 months of training must be approved by the RRC.

II. Institutional Organization

A. Sponsoring Institution

1. The institution sponsoring the SCIM program must be a center for care of persons with SCD or affiliated with such a center. Affiliation with an accredited medical school is desirable. The institution should be accredited by the Joint Commission on Accreditation of Healthcare Organizations-Rehabilitation Section or the Commission on Accreditation of Rehabilitation Facilities.
2. Accreditation of a subspecialty program in SCIM will be granted only when the program is administratively attached to an ACGME-accredited residency program in a relevant specialty.
3. There must be close cooperation between the core residency training program and the subspecialty program. The lines of responsibility between resident staffs in the core program and the subspecialty program must be clearly delineated.
4. The sponsoring institution should exercise the necessary administrative management of the training program.
5. There should be an institutional policy, reviewed at the time of regular institutional or internal review, governing the educational resources committed to the SCIM program assuring cooperation of all involved disciplines.
6. The institution must provide for financial resources including, but not limited to, salaries, fringe benefits, and opportunities for continuing medical education for residents.

B. Participating Institutions

It is highly desirable for participating institutions to be in the same geographic location and conveniently and safely accessible to residents.

C. Appointment of Residents

1. The program shall establish written policies and procedures regarding selection and appointment of residents. The resident complement should be appropriate to the available clinical and educational resources. It is highly desirable to have at least one resident in the program at all times.
2. The program shall have and implement written policies and procedures, based on the educational resources available, for determining the number of resident positions.
3. The program shall have and implement written policies and procedures, based on the educational resources available, regarding changes in resident complement or filling vacant positions.
4. The applicant must be licensed for unrestricted practice in a state or province of the United States or Canada.

III. Faculty Qualifications and Responsibilities

The program director and the teaching staff are responsible for the general administration of a program, including those activities related to the recruitment, selection, instruction, supervision, counseling, evaluation, and advancement of residents and the maintenance of records related to program accreditation.

A. Program Director

There must be a single program director responsible for the program.

1. Qualifications of the program director include:
   a. Documented qualifications as a clinician, administrator, and educator in the field of SCIM.
   b. Board certification in a specialty or subspecialty related to the care of persons with SCD and subspecialty certification in SCIM or suitable equivalent qualifications.
   c. Licensure to practice medicine in the state where the institution that sponsors the program is located. (Certain federal programs are exempted.)
   d. Appointment in good standing to the medical staff of an institution participating in the program.
2. Responsibilities of the program director include:
   a. Sufficient time devoted to provide continuous leadership to the program as well as supervision of the residents.
   b. Active participation in research and scholarly activities in SCIM.
   c. Preparation of a written statement outlining the educational goals of the program with respect to knowledge, skills, and other attributes of residents at each level of training and for each major rotation or other program assignment. This statement must be distributed to residents and members of the teaching staff. It should be readily available for review.
   d. Selection of residents for appointment to and assignment in the program in accordance with institutional and departmental policies and procedures.
   e. Selection and supervision of the teaching staff and other program personnel at each institution participating in the program. The program director should assign faculty and perform annual evaluations of their performance.
   f. The supervision of residents through explicit written descriptions of supervisory lines of responsibility for the care of patients. Such guidelines must be communicated to all members of the program staff. Residents must be provided with prompt, reliable systems for communication and interaction with supervisory physicians.
   g. Regular evaluation of residents' knowledge, skills, and overall performance, including the development of professional attitudes consistent with being a physician.

   The program director, with participation of members of the teaching staff, shall:

1. At least semiannually evaluate the knowledge, skills, and professional growth of the residents, using appropriate criteria and procedures.
2. Communicate each evaluation to the resident in a timely manner.
3. Advance residents to positions of higher responsibility only on the basis of evidence of their satisfactory progressive scholarship and professional growth.
4. Maintain a permanent record of evaluation for each resident and have it accessible to the resident and other authorized personnel.

h. The provision of a written final evaluation for each resident who completes the program. The evaluation must include a review of the resident's performance during the final period of training and should verify that the resident has demonstrated sufficient professional ability to practice competently and independently. This final evaluation should be part of the resident's permanent record maintained by the institution.

i. Implementation of fair procedures as established by the sponsoring institution regarding academic discipline and resident complaints or grievances.

j. Monitoring resident stress, including mental or emotional conditions inhibiting performance or learning and drug- or alcohol-related dysfunction. Program directors and teaching staff should be sensitive to the need for timely provision of confidential counseling and psychological support services to residents. Training situations that consistently produce undesirable stress on residents must be evaluated and modified.

k. Preparation of an accurate statistical and narrative description of the program as requested by the RRC. Adequate data collection and analysis is necessary for overall program evaluation and total quality management. The program director should gather, analyze, and maintain data regarding resident and faculty performance.

l. Gathering and analyzing initial, discharge, and follow-up data regarding the functional outcomes of persons served.

m. Notification to the RRC of major programmatic changes. The RRC must be notified immediately of any change in program directorship.

B. Number and Qualifications of Faculty

1. There must be a sufficient number of teaching staff with documented qualifications to instruct and supervise adequately all the residents in the program. Members of the teaching staff must be able to devote sufficient time to meet their supervisory and teaching responsibilities. In addition to the program director, there must be at least one other faculty member with expertise in SCIM who is dedicated to the program.
2. All members of the teaching staff must demonstrate a strong interest in the education of residents, sound clinical and teaching abilities in the field of SCIM, support of the goals and objectives of the program, a commitment to their own continuing medical education, and participation in scholarly activities. The faculty should actively participate in teaching, research, and scholarly activity in the field of SCIM.
3. The faculty should be board-certified in a specialty or subspecialty related to the care of persons with SCD or possess suitable equivalent qualifications.
4. A member of the teaching staff of each participating institution must be designated to assume responsibility for the day-to-day activities of the program at that institution, with overall coordination by the program director.
5. The teaching staff must be organized and have regular documented meetings to review program goals and objectives as well as program effectiveness in achieving them. At least one resident representative should participate in these reviews.
6. The teaching staff should periodically evaluate the utilization of the resources available to the program, the contribution of each institution participating in the program, the financial and administrative support of the program, the volume and variety of patients available to the program for educational purposes, the performance of members of the teaching staff, and the quality of supervision of residents.

C. Other Program Personnel

Programs must be provided the additional professional, technical, and clerical personnel needed to support the administration and educational conduct of the program.

IV. Facilities and Resources

A. Institutional Facilities

Education in SCIM should include experience in both inpatient and outpatient facilities. The sponsoring and participating institutions must operate or have access to a service delivery system dedicated to the care of persons with SCD. Necessary resources include:

1. an emergency department that treats patients with SCI,
2. an accredited acute care hospital,
3. a dedicated inpatient rehabilitation unit,
4. a designated outpatient clinic for persons with SCD, and
5. availability of home care and independent living programs.

B. Specific Facilities and Resources

1. The sponsoring institution must have available the equipment, diagnostic imaging devices, electrodiagnostic devices, laboratory services, a urodynamic laboratory, and clinical facilities necessary to provide appropriate care to persons with SCD. Medical library facilities and facilities for teaching experiences must be available, along with a medical records system that allows for efficient case retrieval.
2. The sponsoring institutions must have available specialty consultant services in anesthesia, emergency medicine, family practice, internal medicine (including the relevant subspecialties), neurological surgery, neurology, orthopedic surgery, pathology, pediatrics, physical medicine and rehabilitation, plastic surgery, psychiatry, radiology, surgery, and urology. Other health care professionals are essential to the care of persons with SCD.

C. Library

1. Residents must have ready access to a major medical library either at the institution where the residents are located or through arrangement with convenient nearby institutions.
2. Library services should include the electronic retrieval of information from medical databases.
3. There must be access to an on-site library or to a collection of appropriate texts and journals in each institution participating in a residency program. On-site libraries and/or collections of texts and journals must be readily available during nights and weekends.

D. Patient Population

The patient population must be of sufficient size and diversity of age so as to provide the resident with the opportunity to care for an adequate number of persons with new SCD, to care for persons readmitted to the hospital with intercurrent illness, and to care for appropriate numbers of outpatients. There should be a minimum census of eight patients per resident.

V. Educational Program

A. Clinical Components

1. The clinical portion of the curriculum must include a sufficient variety, depth, and volume of clinical experiences. The educational program should take into consideration the resident's documented past educational and patient care experiences. The training program must provide for the resident to spend a significant amount of time in responsibility for the direct care of hospitalized as well as nonhospitalized patients. Residents must devote at least one-third of their clinical experience to the care of hospitalized patients and at least one-third to nonhospitalized patients.
2. The educational program must be designed for the resident to attain the following knowledge and competencies within the interspecialty and interdisciplinary care team:
   a. Initial Care
      1. Understand the organization and interdisciplinary practices of the Emergency Medical Services system relating to the prehospital and initial Emergency Department care of the spinal cord injured as well as concomitant and associated injuries. This is not meant to interfere with the independent decision making of the attending physician during the initial care.
      2. Understand the techniques of appropriate spinal immobilization in order to protect patients from additional neurological damage.
      3. Understand the supportive role of SCIM to neurological surgery, orthopedic surgery, emergency medicine, and other appropriate physicians in the initial care.
      4. Understand the management of the abnormalities and complications in other body systems resulting from SCI, especially the following: pulmonary, genitourinary, endocrine, metabolic, vascular, cardiac, gastrointestinal, musculoskeletal, and integumentary.

   b. Post-Initial Care
      1. Understand how the stability of the spine is evaluated and know the various options for treatment of fractures/dislocations at all vertebral levels.
      2. Understand the optimal coordination of services of the various physicians and other health professionals in the prevention and treatment of complications in each organ system.
      3. Develop the skills to initiate and direct appropriate rehabilitation programming in the early hospital phase of treatment.
      4. Understand the relationship between the extent and level of SCI on the ultimate residual functional capacity and be able to inform and counsel the patient, the family, and other health specialists on a timely basis about the impact of the disability.
      5. Understand special needs and problems that children and adolescents with SCI may have in areas such as behavior, bladder and bowel and skin care, growth and development, immunizations, mobility, nutrition, pediatrics, self-care, recreation, and schooling through lectures and adequate clinical assignments under the integrated services of pediatricians and specialists in SCIM. Also understand the special needs of parents and others in relating to and assisting with these problems.

   c. Initial and Ongoing Medical Rehabilitation
      1. Coordinate the transition from postinitial care to rehabilitation and assume primary management responsibility.
      2. Establish short- and long-term rehabilitation goals and coordinate the implementation of the rehabilitation program to meet such goals.
      3. Monitor the evolution of neural dysfunction to recognize conditions that may require additional evaluation, consultation, or modification of treatment.
      4. After postinitial care, in conjunction with the interspecialty SCI team, participate in the management of SCI following either operative or nonoperative stabilization, including activity restrictions and appropriate orthotic support.
      5. Understand the collaborative role of integral members of the SCI care team.
      6. Recognize, diagnose, and coordinate treatment for respiratory complications such as tracheostomies, airway obstruction, atelectasis, pneumonia, tracheal stenosis, and mechanical methods of respiration including both fixed and portable equipment. The resident should be able to manage patients with high quadriplegia and respirator-dependent patients in weaning the patient from the respirator and in evaluating indications and contraindications of phrenic nerve pacing, motorized wheelchairs, portable respirators, environmental control systems, home modifications, etc.
      7. Recognize, diagnose, and treat orthostatic hypotension and other cardiovascular abnormalities during initial mobilization of the patient.
      8. Evaluate and manage skin problems utilizing various techniques of prevention, such as the proper use of specialized beds, other surfaces, cushions, wheelchairs, etc, to manage pressure ulcers effectively; and, in consultation with surgical colleagues, determine the indications for various surgical procedures including resection of bone and the development of flaps and other techniques for soft tissue coverage. The resident should also develop an understanding of the preoperative and postoperative management of these patients.
      9. With appropriate consultation, identify the risk of infection and coordinate treatment and infection control, including the judicious use of antimicrobials.
      10. Coordinate and implement management of the neurogenic bowel.
      11. Understand management of the neurogenic bladder and that the role of the urologist in the diagnosis and management of bladder dysfunction, urinary tract infection, urinary calculi, sexual dysfunction, obstructive uropathy with or without stones, infertility, and problems of ejaculation is pivotal and should be utilized early in the care of these patients.
      12. Diagnose and treat, with appropriate consultation, complications such as deep vein thrombosis, pulmonary embolus, autonomic hyperreflexia, substance abuse, pain, spasticity, depression, and the sequelae of associated illnesses and pre-existing diseases.
      13. Recognize pharmacologic alterations associated with SCI, including changes in pharmacokinetics, pharmacodynamics, drug interactions, over-medication, and compliance.
      14. Diagnose and manage the psychological dysfunction associated with SCI.
      15. Perform a functional assessment based on neurological, musculoskeletal, and cardiopulmonary examinations and psychosocial and prevocational evaluations.
      16. Determine functional goals for self-care, mobility, and vocational and avocational activities based on the level and completeness of the lesion.

17. If appropriate, prescribe motor retraining and conditioning activities, orthoses, and the adaptive equipment needed to meet the rehabilitation goals.
18. Anticipate the approximate length of stay, cost of hospitalization, equipment needs, etc, with the involvement of the patient, the patient's support persons, and appropriate agencies.
19. Identify the indications for and the use of clinical neurophysiologic testing to assess the extent of neuropraxia, denervation, reinnervation, phrenic nerve function, and spinal cord function.
20. Identify the indications and use of functional electrical stimulation (FES) as applied to the management of spinal cord impairment.
21. Understand the kinesiology of upper extremity function and the use of muscle substitution patterns in retraining; the value, indications, and contraindications of tendon and muscle transfers and other operative procedures that would enhance function.
22. Within the interdisciplinary and interspecialty SCI teams, understand the concepts of muscle and tendon transfers and other operative procedures that enhance extremity function and manage the postoperative retraining, when indicated.
23. Understand group process and team dynamics, and coordinate the activities of the interdisciplinary team through daily rounds, staff conferences, and patient and family educational and training sessions to maximize the goals established by the patient and team.
24. Understand the training and capabilities of rehabilitation nurses, social workers, psychologists, physical therapists, occupational therapists, prosthetists, orthotists, speech/language pathologists, and recreational and vocational counselors; recognize the professional role and contributions of the various allied health professions individually and collectively; encourage their full participation in patient care management while maintaining medical responsibility; and appreciate that a team effort, with as much continuity as practical, will produce a more satisfying outcome and experience for the patient, family, and team members.
25. Conduct a problem-oriented conference and set goals with the participation of the allied health staff.

d. Discharge Planning
1. Determine when the rehabilitation goals have been achieved, finalize the discharge plan, and arrange for the appropriate level of care to match the patient's needs.
2. Participate in family meetings/discharge planning conferences, with focus on community integration and adjustment to disability.
3. Organize and conduct programs of patient and family education.
4. In concert with appropriate disciplines and other team members, manage the psychological effects of the impairment to prevent their interference with the reintegration and re-entry to the community.
5. Use the full range of community resources to facilitate the transition to the community.
6. Understand the needs for personal care attendants, architectural modifications, and community follow-up care.

e. Follow-Up Phase—Sustaining Care
1. Recognize, diagnose, and treat intercurrent disease in conjunction with the proper consultants. There should be special emphasis on the prevention and management of these diseases in patients at various levels of SCI.
2. Diagnose and coordinate the treatment of the complications associated with chronic SCI, including pressure sores, spasticity, pain, urinary calculi, urinary tract infection, fractures, post-traumatic syringomyelia, and progressive respiratory decline.
3. Set up a program of regular follow-up, evaluation, and preventive health care to keep the person at his/her maximum health and rehabilitation status, and coordinate this care with the patient's personal community physician.
4. Direct to, or establish the patient in, a program of vocational rehabilitation, if appropriate.
5. Appreciate that the ultimate goal is to return and maintain the person with SCI as a satisfied and productive member of society.
6. Understand the prevention and management of complications associated with long-standing disability, the effects of aging with a disability, and the provision of long-term follow-up services.
7. Coordinate and manage an SCI home care program.
8. Develop and maintain as needed a professional relationship with primary care physicians and be available to assist or, when asked to, temporarily provide primary care for needed follow-up examination and for complex issues of SCI care.
9. In all phases of care, understand and define the ethical and legal issues especially pertinent to spinal cord injury, including diminished competence and the right to refuse treatment.

3. The program should be designed so that the resident has an opportunity to follow individual patients longitudinally as well as the ability to encounter a wide variety of patient problems.
4. The program should be designed so that the resident has an opportunity to develop a management style compatible with the interdisciplinary team process.

B. Didactic Components

1. Basic science content. There should be a didactic curriculum taught by faculty and a self-directed learning program to address the theoretical and clinical principles that form the fundamentals for care of patients with SCD. Pathophysiology, discussion and knowledge of clinical manifestations, and management principles should constitute the major topics for study.
2. Specialty content. Specialists in anesthesiology, emergency medicine, internal medicine (including the relevant subspecialties), neurology, neurosurgery, orthopedic surgery, pediatrics, physical medicine and rehabilitation, plastic surgery, psychiatry, surgery, and urology should take an active role in the didactic curriculum, providing instruction in the areas of their practices relevant to SCD.
3. Conferences
   a. Required conferences should include case-oriented multidisciplinary conferences, journal clubs, and quality management seminars relevant to clinical care on the spinal cord program.
   b. Conferences must be of sufficient quality and frequency to provide in-depth coverage of the major topics in SCIM over 1 year.
   c. There must be documentation of staff and resident attendance.
   d. Educational activities must be carried out under the direct supervision of faculty members.

C. Resident Policies

1. Supervision
   a. The level of supervision of the residents should be determined by the program director based on formal and informal evaluations.

b. The program director should assign a member of the faculty as supervisor to each resident. Written objectives for each clinical rotation must be provided to the resident.

c. The supervisor is responsible for the educational experience according to the written plan developed at the beginning of the training. The supervisor must meet regularly with the program director and resident for appropriate monitoring and feedback.

2. Duty hours. While the actual number of hours worked by a subspecialty resident may vary, the resident should have sufficient off-duty time to avoid undue fatigue and stress. The resident should be allowed to spend, on average, at least 1 full day out of 7 away from the hospital, and should be assigned on-call duty in the hospital no more frequently than an average of every third night. The program director is responsible for monitoring according to written policies on-duty assignments as well as activities outside the program.
3. Graded responsibility. Clinical experiences should allow for progressive responsibility with lesser degrees of supervision as the resident advances and demonstrates additional competencies. The program should be flexible but sufficiently structured to allow for such graded responsibility.
4. Peer interaction. The resident must have opportunity to meet and share experience with residents in the core program and in other specialties. It is desirable for the resident to interact with peers in primary care and relevant subspecialties. Residents should have the opportunity to teach other residents, medical students, and other health care professionals.
5. Presence of other learners/fellows. Rotation to the SCIM program by residents from other specialties or subspecialties as well as medical students is desirable.

D. Other Program Components

1. Research and scholarly activity. Graduate medical education must take place in an environment of inquiry and scholarship in which residents participate in the development of new knowledge, learn to evaluate research findings, and develop habits of inquiry as a continuing professional responsibility. The responsibility for establishing and maintaining an environment of inquiry and scholarship rests with the teaching staff. While not all members of a teaching staff must be investigators, the staff as a whole must demonstrate broad involvement in scholarly activity. This activity should include:
   a. Active participation of the teaching staff in clinical discussions, rounds, and conferences in a manner that promotes a spirit of inquiry and scholarship. Scholarship implies an in-depth understanding of basic mechanisms of normal and abnormal states and the application of current knowledge to practice.
   b. Participation in journal clubs and research conferences.
   c. Active participation in regional or national professional and scientific societies, particularly through presentations at the organizations' meetings and publication in their journals.
   d. Participation in research, particularly in projects that are funded following peer review and/or result in publication or presentations at regional and national scientific meetings.
   e. Offering of guidance and technical support (eg, research design, statistical analysis) for residents involved in research.
   f. Provision of support for resident participation in scholarly activities. The resident should have assigned time to conduct research or other scholarly activities. The goal for the resident should be at least one scientific presentation, abstract, or publication.
2. Management. Within the interspecialty and interdisciplinary SCIM care team, the resident should be taught and should understand and apply principles of organizational and group behavior, leadership and management styles, evaluation and modification of performance, labor-management issues, cost accounting and containment, and quality assurance techniques. The resident should gain an understanding and some proficiency in the areas of budget planning and presentation, preparation of management briefings, information systems, and external reviews such as the Joint Commission for the Accreditation of Healthcare Organizations and the Commission on Accreditation of Rehabilitation Facilities.
3. Teaching by the resident. The resident should have the opportunity to:
   a. Teach local medical communities and the general public about prevention of SCI;
   b. teach prehospital personnel and other health care providers how to stabilize patients with SCI and institute a rational protocol for their prehospital care;
   c. teach other hospital personnel and health care providers, patients, and patient support systems about the rehabilitation needs and long-term care of patients with SCI;
   d. teach medical students, medical residents, and other health professionals;
   e. understand and utilize learning theory, including assessment of learning needs, development of objectives and curriculum plans, effective use of audiovisual and other teaching materials, and evaluation of teaching outcomes;
   f. provide instruction to patients and families; and
   g. participate in educational activities within the interspecialty and interdisciplinary SCIM care team.

VI. Evaluation

Evaluation is an essential component of the program. The program director and faculty must have a plan that addresses the evaluation of residents, faculty, and the program. Well-designed evaluation combined with feedback improves the program and focuses the learning process.

A. Residents:

1. Policy and Principles
   a. Evaluation should be based on the program objectives and on the objectives of the resident's individualized program.
   b. Evaluation must be carried out semi-annually and should be followed by extensive feedback to the resident. Remedial objectives may be established.
2. The following areas should be evaluated:
   a. acquisition of described competencies,
   b. problem-solving skills,
   c. interpersonal relationship skills,
   d. ability to access, retrieve, and critically evaluate the literature,
   e. information management,
   f. quality and cost-effectiveness measures of patient care, and
   g. research and other scholarly accomplishments.

B. Faculty and Program

1. Faculty evaluation by residents should be on a semi-annual basis.
2. Areas to be evaluated are:
   a. clinical skills and competencies,
   b. teaching skills,
   c. scholarly activity,
   d. leadership skills, and
   e. interpersonal skills.
3. The educational effectiveness of the program must be evaluated annually and in a systematic manner. In particular, the quality of the curriculum and the extent to which the educational goals have been met by the residents must be assessed. Written evaluations by residents should be utilized in this process. Resident satisfaction at the completion of training should also be assessed.

4. One measure of the quality of a program is the performance of its residents on the examinations of the American Board of Physical Medicine and Rehabilitation for special qualifications in SCIM.

VII. Board Certification

Residents who plan to seek certification by the American Board of Physical Medicine and Rehabilitation in Spinal Cord Injury Medicine should communicate with the executive director of the ABPMR to ascertain the current requirements for acceptance as a candidate for certification.

ACGME: February 1996 Effective: February 1996

Program Requirements for Residency Education in Plastic Surgery

I. Introduction

A. Definition of the Specialty

Training in the specialty of plastic surgery deals with the resection, repair, replacement, and reconstruction of defects of form and function of the integument and its underlying anatomic systems, including the craniofacial structures, the oropharynx, the trunk, the extremities, the breast, and the perineum. It includes aesthetic (cosmetic) surgery of structures with undesirable form. Special knowledge and skill in the design and transfer of flaps, in the transplantation of tissues, and in the replantation of structures are vital to these ends, as is skill in excisional surgery, in management of complex wounds, and in the use of alloplastic materials. Residency training in plastic surgery is designed to educate and train physicians broadly in the art and science of plastic and reconstructive surgery and to develop a competent and responsible plastic surgeon with high moral and ethical character capable of functioning as an independent surgeon. A variety of educational plans will produce the desired result.

B. Scope of Training (Including Prerequisites)

1. All prerequisite residency training must be taken within programs accredited by the following organizations: the Accreditation Council for Graduate Medical Education (ACGME), the Royal College of Physicians and Surgeons of Canada, or the American Dental Association.
2. The curriculum for residency training in plastic surgery is 2 years. A program may be accredited for more than 2 years (such as in the integrated model or the independent model using a 3-year format) when it is demonstrated that there is a clear educational rationale, consonant with the Program Requirements for Residency Education in Plastic Surgery and the objectives for residency training, that cannot be met in a 2-year curriculum or when the program director has delineated a program with special goals that exceed those defined in the program requirements.
3. Training Models: the Residency Review Committee (RRC) for Plastic Surgery recognizes two training models, independent and integrated.
   a. Independent Model
   In the independent model of training, residents complete 2 or 3 years of concentrated plastic surgery training, with no less than 12 months of senior/chief responsibility, after successful completion of one of the following prerequisite curricula:
      1. A minimum of 3 years of clinical training with progressive responsibility in the same program in general surgery. Transitional year or rotating internships may not be used to fulfill this requirement.
      2. A complete neurological surgery, orthopedic surgery, otolaryngology, or urology residency.
      3. Satisfactory completion of a residency program in oral and maxillofacial surgery approved by the American Dental Association (ADA) is an alternate pathway for prerequisite training prior to a plastic surgery residency. This pathway is available only to those individuals holding a DMD/MD or DDS/MD degree. Training must also include a minimum of 24 months of progressive responsibility on surgical rotations under the direction of the general surgery program director after receipt of the MD degree. Rotations in general surgery during medical school, prior to receiving the MD degree,

will not be considered as fulfilling any part of the 24-month minimum requirement.

b. Integrated Model
In the integrated model, residents complete 5 or 6 years of ACGME-accredited plastic surgery training following receipt of an MD or DO degree from an institution accredited by the Liaison Committee on Medical Education (LCME) or the American Osteopathic Association.
  1. The integrated curriculum must contain no less than 5 years of clinical surgical training under the authority and direction of the plastic surgery program director.
  2. Of these 5 or 6 years, no less than 24 months must be concentrated plastic surgery training with no less than 12 months of senior/chief responsibility on the clinical service of plastic surgery.
  3. Additional clinical experiences appropriate to the training of a plastic surgeon should be provided in anesthesiology, burn management, critical care medicine, emergency medicine, cardiothoracic surgery, general surgery, neurological surgery, oncologic surgery, orthopedic surgery, otolaryngology, pediatric surgery, trauma management, and vascular surgery.
  4. Accreditation by the ACGME is required for all years of the training program.
  5. The program director must obtain the approval of the sponsoring institution and the RRC for the length of training prior to implementation and at each subsequent review of the program.
  6. Prior to entry into the program, each resident must be notified in writing of the required length of training. The required length of training for a particular resident may not be changed without mutual agreement during his or her program unless there is a break in his or her training or the resident requires remedial training. All such changes must have prior approval of the RRC.
  7. Residents must complete the length of training for which they have enrolled (ie, although residents may transfer from one program to another, they may not change from one model of training to another without RRC prior approval).
  8. Experience beyond the approved residency that may be required by the American Board of Plastic Surgery or other certifying body (eg, a period of time in independent practice) is not reviewed by the RRC.

II. Institutional Organization

A. Sponsoring Institutions

An educational program in plastic surgery must have one sponsoring institution within a single geographic location with primary responsibility for the entire program. Appropriate institutions include medical schools, hospitals, and medical foundations. The sponsoring institution must provide sufficient faculty, financial resources, and academic support to enable the program to comply with the requirements for accreditation. This support must include sufficient operating time to ensure adequate resident surgical experience.

B. Participating Institutions

When there is a cooperative educational effort involving multiple institutions, the commitment of each institution to the program must be documented in an affiliation agreement that conforms to ACGME Institutional Requirements I.C.

1. Participating institutions include the sponsoring institution and other affiliated institutions approved by the RRC for clinical training.
2. Participating institutions must promote the educational goals of the program rather than simply enlarging the program, and they must not be added primarily for the purpose of meeting service needs.
3. Programs using multiple hospitals must ensure the provision of a unified educational experience for the residents. Affiliations that merely duplicate experiences otherwise available within the program are not acceptable.
4. Participating institutions that are geographically distant from the sponsoring institution are not desirable. These are acceptable only if they offer special resources, which are unavailable locally, that significantly augment the overall educational experience of the residents.
5. The number and distribution of participating institutions must not preclude the satisfactory participation of residents and faculty in conferences and other educational activities of the program.

C. Appointment of Residents

1. The RRC will approve a total number of residents to be trained in the program by training year. The number will be based primarily upon the number, qualifications, and commitment of the faculty; the volume and variety of the patient population available for educational purposes; the totality of institutional resources committed to resident education; and the state of the program's compliance with the Institutional and Program Requirements at the time of the most recent accreditation review of the program.
2. Programs may not enroll more residents at any level of training than the number of residents approved by the RRC for that year of training, except when a resident's training is extended because the program director has determined the need for additional training to meet the minimum requirements for competency. In this circumstance, the program director must notify the RRC in writing of the decision to extend a resident's training. Otherwise, any increase (including temporary increases) in the number of residents at any level of training or increase in the total number of residents must receive prior approval of the RRC. Requests for changes in the approved resident complement of a program must include a strong educational rationale. Requests based primarily on service considerations will not be approved.
3. Vacancies
   a. In an independent training model, a vacancy in resident complement, if filled, must be at the same level in which the vacancy occurs, unless otherwise approved by the RRC.
   b. In an integrated training model, the program director may appoint a new resident at a level that overlaps that of another resident in the program, provided that (1) each appointment does not adversely affect the training experience of residents already in the program and (2) commencing at the time when the resident whose departure created the vacancy would have completed training, the average number of residents graduating yearly will not exceed the number approved by the RRC over the accredited length of the program.

III. Faculty Qualifications and Responsibilities

The program director and the teaching staff are responsible for the general administration of a program, including those activities related to the recruitment, selection, instruction, supervision, counseling, evaluation, and advancement of residents and the maintenance of records related to program accreditation.

A. Program Director

There must be a single program director responsible for the program.

1. Qualifications of the program director include:

a. An experienced, clinically active, competent teacher, clinician, and administrator.
b. Licensure to practice medicine in the state where the institution that sponsors the program is located. (Certain federal programs are exempted.)
c. Certification by the American Board of Plastic Surgery or suitable equivalent qualifications in plastic surgery, as determined by the RRC.
d. Appointment in good standing to the medical staff of an institution participating in the program.
e. Frequent changes in leadership or long periods of temporary leadership are undesirable and may adversely affect the accreditation status of the program.

2. Responsibilities of the program director include:
a. Familiarity with the current Institutional Requirements and Program Requirements approved by the ACGME. These requirements must be met for approval of a program.
b. Preparation of a written statement outlining the educational goals of the program with respect to knowledge, skills, and other attributes of residents at each level of training and for each major rotation or other program assignment. This statement must be distributed to residents and members of the teaching staff. It should be readily available for review.
c. Prompt notification of the executive secretary of the RRC in writing of any major change in the program that may significantly alter the educational experience for the residents, including:
   1. Changes in leadership of a section, division, or department of plastic surgery, such as appointment as a permanent or acting program director, section head, division head or chief, or department chairman.
   2. Changes in administrative structure that affect the status of the program/division or department of plastic surgery within the institution.
d. Obtaining prior approval of the RRC for the following changes in the program to determine if an adequate educational environment exists to support these changes. On review of a proposal for a major change in a program, the RRC may determine that a site visit is necessary.
   1. The addition or deletion of any participating institution to which residents rotate for 3 months or longer (including individual rotations of less than 3 months, which taken collectively total 3 months or longer)
   2. The addition or deletion of any rotation for 3 months or longer
   3. Any change in the approved resident complement of the program
   4. Any change in the length or format of the training program
e. Developing, maintaining, and communicating written guidelines specifically delineating the supervisory responsibilities of the faculty and attending staff in each hospital or facility utilized by the training program, to include promulgation of regular call schedules for the attending and resident staffs.
f. Ensuring that the educational environment, the volume and variety of patient population, and the concept of progressive surgical responsibility are scrupulously followed.
g. Selecting residents for appointment to the program in accordance with institutional and departmental policies and procedures.
h. Selecting and supervising the teaching staff and other program personnel at each institution participating in the program.
i. Annually collecting, compiling, and retaining records of the number and types of plastic surgery operative procedures performed in all institutions and facilities utilized in the clinical education of residents. This information must be provided as requested in the format and form specified by the RRC.
j. Annually compiling a comprehensive record of the number and type of operative procedures performed by each resident completing the program. This record must include all of the procedures in which the plastic surgery resident was either surgeon or assistant during that year and must be signed by both the resident and the program director as a statement of its accuracy. This information must be provided as requested in the format and form specified by the RRC. These records must be maintained by the program director.
k. Having documentation on file of the satisfactory completion of prerequisite training before the candidate begins plastic surgery training.
l. Verifying the credentials of a transferring resident prior to accepting the resident into the program. Verification should include documentation of all rotations for which the transferring resident has been given credit by the previous program director. The program director who accepts a transferring resident should modify the individual's course of study as needed to ensure that the resident completes all training requirements prior to graduation.
m. Regularly evaluating the residents and the program, as noted in Section VI of these Program Requirements.
n. Advising resident applicants of the prerequisite requirements of the American Board of Plastic Surgery.
o. Implementing fair procedures, as established by the sponsoring institution, regarding academic discipline and resident complaints or grievances.
p. Monitoring resident stress, including mental or emotional conditions inhibiting performance or learning and drug- or alcohol-related dysfunction. Program directors and teaching staff should be sensitive to the need for timely provision of confidential counseling and psychological support services to residents. Training situations that consistently produce undesirable stress on residents must be evaluated and modified.
q. Preparing an accurate statistical and narrative description of the program as requested by the RRC.

B. Number and Qualifications of Faculty

1. There must be sufficient numbers of qualified faculty and/or attending staff available at all times at each of the participating institutions to supervise and instruct residents to ensure optimal patient care and resident education.
2. The faculty of plastic surgeons must be certified by the American Board of Plastic Surgery or possess suitable equivalent qualifications in plastic surgery, as determined by the RRC.
3. The faculty and attending staff should possess qualifications that contribute to the training program, including high moral and ethical standards, and should demonstrate an appropriate commitment in time and energy to fulfill the teaching assignments.
4. There must be evidence of scholarly activity among the plastic surgery faculty. Such evidence should include a high order of teaching skills, participation in clinical and/or basic research, involvement in plastic surgery and/or other medical scientific organizations and their meetings, and publication in refereed journals, monographs, and books.
5. A member of the faculty of each participating institution must be designated to assume responsibility for the day-to-day activities of the program at that institution, with overall coordination by the program director.
6. The faculty must be organized and have regular documented meetings to review program goals and objectives as well as program effectiveness in achieving them. At least one resident representative should participate in these reviews.

7. The faculty should periodically evaluate the utilization of the resources available to the program, the contribution of each institution participating in the program, the financial and administrative support of the program, the volume and variety of patients available to the program for educational purposes, the performance of members of the faculty, and the quality of supervision of residents.

C. Program Research and Scholarly Activity

Graduate medical education must take place in an environment of inquiry and scholarship in which residents participate in the development of new knowledge, learn to evaluate research findings, and develop habits of inquiry as a continuing professional responsibility.

The responsibility for establishing and maintaining an environment of inquiry and scholarship rests with the teaching staff. While not all members of a teaching staff must be investigators, the staff as a whole must demonstrate broad involvement in scholarly activity. This activity should include:

1. Active participation of the teaching staff in clinical discussions, rounds, and conferences in a manner that promotes a spirit of inquiry and scholarship. Scholarship implies an in-depth understanding of basic mechanisms of normal and abnormal states and the application of current knowledge to practice.
2. Participation in journal clubs and research conferences.
3. Active participation in regional or national professional and scientific societies, particularly through presentations at the organizations' meetings and publication in their journals.
4. Participation in research, particularly in projects that are funded following peer review and/or result in publication or presentations at regional and national scientific meetings.
5. Offering of guidance and technical support (eg, research design, statistical analysis) for residents involved in research.
6. Provision of support for resident participation in scholarly activities.

D. Other Program Personnel

Programs must be provided with the additional professional, technical, and clerical personnel needed to support the administration and educational conduct of the program.

IV. Facilities and Resources

A. Inpatient Facilities

1. Although inpatient facilities may vary from one participating institution to another, the plastic surgery inpatient service should have an adequate number of beds, support personnel, and proper equipment to ensure quality patient care and education.
2. Operating suites as well as diagnostic and treatment facilities must contain technologically current equipment.

B. Outpatient Facilities

Appropriately equipped outpatient facilities, including operating suites, clinics, and office space, must be available for resident participation in the regular preoperative evaluation, treatment, and postoperative follow-up of patients for whom the resident has responsibility.

C. Library Facilities

1. Residents must have ready access to a major medical library, either at the institution where the residents are located or through arrangement with convenient nearby institutions.
2. Library services should include the electronic retrieval of information from medical databases.
3. There must be access to an on-site library or to a collection of appropriate texts and journals in each institution participating in a residency program. On-site libraries and/or collections of texts and journals must be readily available during nights and weekends.

D. Other Facilities and Resources

Within the participating institutions of the program, the following must be adequate and readily available:

1. Laboratory services
2. Diagnostic imaging
3. Medical library resources, including current texts and journals relevant to the practice of plastic surgery, that are accessible to residents on a 24-hour basis
4. Adequate space and resources for conferences, including appropriate audiovisual equipment
5. Data information systems sufficient to support research activities and enable the program to meet its record-keeping and data-reporting needs
6. Sufficient technical and clerical support personnel to meet the needs of the educational program

V. Educational Program

A. Program Goals and Objectives

The director and faculty of a program must prepare and comply with written educational goals for the program.

1. Program Design
   All educational components of a residency program should be related to program goals.
   a. The program design and/or structure must be approved by the appropriate review committee as part of the regular review process.
   b. Participation by an institution providing more than 3 months of training must be approved by the RRC.
2. Program Evaluation
   The educational effectiveness of a program must be evaluated in a systematic manner. In particular, the quality of the curriculum and the extent to which the educational goals have been met by residents must be assessed. Written evaluations by residents should be utilized in this process.

B. Clinical Components

Knowledge of surgical design, surgical diagnosis, embryology, surgical and artistic anatomy, surgical physiology and pharmacology, wound healing, surgical pathology and microbiology, adjunctive oncological therapy, biomechanics, rehabilitation, and surgical instrumentation is fundamental to this specialty. The judgment and technical capability for achieving satisfactory surgical results are mandatory qualities for the plastic surgeon.

1. Specific training should be provided in the following areas:
   a. Congenital defects of the head and neck, including clefts of the lip and palate, and craniofacial surgery
   b. Neoplasms of the head and neck, including the oropharynx, and training in appropriate endoscopy
   c. Craniomaxillofacial trauma, including fractures
   d. Aesthetic (cosmetic) surgery of the head and neck, trunk, and extremities
   e. Plastic surgery of the breast
   f. Surgery of the hand/upper extremities
   g. Plastic surgery of the lower extremities
   h. Plastic surgery of congenital and acquired defects of the trunk and genitalia
   i. Burn management, acute and reconstructive
   j. Microsurgical techniques applicable to plastic surgery
   k. Reconstruction by tissue transfer, including flaps and grafts
   l. Surgery of benign and malignant lesions of the skin and soft tissues

2. There must be a well-organized and well-supervised outpatient clinic. This clinic must operate in relation to an inpatient service used in the program.
   a. Residents must have the opportunity to see patients, establish provisional diagnoses, and initiate preliminary plans prior to the patients' treatment.
   b. An opportunity for follow-up care must be provided so that the results of surgical care may be evaluated by the responsible residents.
   c. These activities must be carried out under appropriate faculty supervision. If residents participate in preoperative and postoperative care in a private office, the program director must ensure that the resident functions with an appropriate degree of responsibility with adequate supervision.
   d. Adequate experience should be provided in office practice procedures and management.
3. The institutions in the program must have an adequate number and variety of adult and pediatric surgical patients available for resident education. Experience in all 12 categories of surgical experience is important and must not be limited by excessive clinical responsibility in any one or several categories or by excessive nonclinical activities.
4. Generally equivalent and adequate distribution of categories and cases among the residents must be demonstrated.
5. Resident experience in patient management should demonstrate graduated and progressive responsibility.
6. Senior plastic surgery residents may be expected to serve as intermediate supervisors when documented prior experience makes it appropriate, but they must always have supervision available from faculty or staff.

C. Didactic Components

The scope of plastic surgery is so broad that a well-organized, comprehensive, and effective educational curriculum is necessary to ensure that all residents experience training in all the various areas of the specialty, including pertinent related basic science applications. The written curriculum should reflect careful planning of all years of the program, with evidence that the cyclical presentation of core specialty knowledge is being supplemented by the addition of current information, including practice management, ethics, and medical-legal topics as related to plastic surgery.

1. Conferences should be organized by the faculty and held to allow discussion of topics selected to broaden knowledge in the wide field of plastic surgery and to evaluate current information.
2. Conferences should embrace the scope of plastic surgery training as outlined in sections I.A and V.B.1.a-l of these Program Requirements.
3. Teaching conferences must include basic science subjects, such as anatomy, physiology, pathology, embryology, radiation biology, genetics, microbiology, and pharmacology.
4. There should be regular, documented attendance of plastic surgery conferences by residents and staff. Residents on off-service rotations should attend the conferences of that rotation.
5. Periodic review of the morbidity and mortality experiences of the service must be documented.
6. Participation in and presentation of educational material at conferences is expected of residents. Adequate time for preparation should be permitted, both to maximize the educational experience for the residents and to emphasize the importance of the experience.

D. Resident Policies

1. Supervision
   It is incumbent on the program director to ensure that there is adequate supervision for all resident patient care and educational activities.
2. Working Conditions and Environment
   a. The program director must establish an environment that is optimal both for resident education and for patient care, while ensuring that undue stress and fatigue among residents are avoided. It is his or her responsibility to ensure assignment of appropriate in-hospital duty hours so that residents are not required to perform excessively difficult or prolonged duties regularly.
   b. It is desirable that residents' work schedules be designed so that on average, excluding exceptional patient care needs, residents have at least 1 day out of 7 free of routine responsibilities and be on call in the hospital no more often than every third night.
   c. During these on-call hours, residents should be provided with adequate sleeping, lounge, and food facilities.
   d. There must be adequate backup so that patient care is not jeopardized during or following assigned periods of duty.
   e. Annual vacation time shall be additional time off.
   f. Support services must be such that residents do not spend an inordinate amount of time in noneducational activities that can be discharged properly by other personnel.
   g. Different rotations may require different working hours and patterns. A distinction must be made between on-call time in the hospital and on-call availability at home vis-a-vis actual hours worked. The ratio of hours worked and on-call time will vary, particularly at the senior levels, and therefore necessitates flexibility.
3. Residency training in plastic surgery is a full-time responsibility; activities outside the educational program must not interfere with the residents' performance in the educational process as determined by the program director and must not interfere with the residents' opportunities for rest, relaxation, and study.
4. Appointment of Individuals for Special Training
   a. The appointment of other individuals for special training or education must not detract from the educational opportunities of the residents. The appointment of such individuals must be reported to the RRC.
   b. Addition of such individuals by a program director and/or institution requires a clear statement of the areas of training, clinical responsibilities, duration of the training, and the impact of these individuals on the training of the residents, regardless of the level of training of the resident. This statement is to be supplied to the RRC at the time the program is reviewed.
   c. If individuals so appointed, in the judgment of the RRC, detract from the education of the residents, the accreditation status of the program may be adversely affected.

E. Other Required Components

1. Training must take place in an environment of inquiry and scholarship. Residents must be taught to understand and apply the scientific method to clinical medicine through scholarly activity. Residents should have genuine opportunities to engage in scholarly activities such as participation in ongoing clinical and/or basic research projects with which appropriate faculty are involved, preparation of reports for publication (eg, case reports, summaries of current scientific knowledge, or reviews of recent developments in plastic surgery), and participation in scientific meetings.
2. Recognizing the comprehensive nature of the specialty of plastic surgery, there should be clinical resources for the education of

plastic surgery residents in anesthesiology, burn management, emergency medicine, cardiothoracic surgery, general surgery, neurological surgery, orthopedic surgery, otolaryngology, pediatric surgery, surgical critical care, surgical oncology, trauma management, and vascular surgery.

VI. Evaluation

A. Evaluation of Residents

Residents should be evaluated at the completion of each rotation by the faculty member who is responsible for the resident's supervision and training. The progress of each resident, including personality characteristics and ethics, knowledge, skills, and professional growth, must be evaluated by the program director in consultation with the faculty in a semiannual, written review using appropriate criteria and procedures. The semiannual review should accomplish the following:

1. The evaluations must document any efficiencies to be corrected prior to completion of the residency program.
2. The evaluations must be communicated in a timely manner to the individual resident in a confidential conference with the program director, with a discussion of remedial steps, if any. The review and comments should be signed by the resident and program director and be maintained on file by the program director for at least 5 years following the resident's completion of the program.
3. The record of evaluations for each resident must be maintained and must be accessible to the resident and other authorized personnel.
4. A final written evaluation for each resident who completes the program must be provided. The evaluation must include a review of the resident's performance during the final period of training and should verify that the resident has demonstrated sufficient professional ability to practice competently and independently. This final evaluation should be part of the resident's permanent record maintained by the institution.
5. There must be a written basis for annual advancement of a resident and written procedures for redress of grievances and for due process.

B. Faculty Evaluation

1. At least annually, all individual faculty members must be formally evaluated by the program director as well as by the residents. A mechanism for sharing the results of such evaluations with the faculty that preserves resident confidentiality in the evaluation process must be employed.
2. The program should demonstrate that such evaluations are used in improving the program.

C. Internal Evaluation

There should be provisions for annual internal evaluation of the educational, research, and clinical aspects of the program. Residents should participate in this evaluation. A written summary of these evaluations should be made available at the time of the periodic survey and review of the program.

VII. Board Certification

A. One measure of the quality of a program is the performance of its graduates with respect to the American Board of Plastic Surgery certification process. Graduates of ACGME-approved programs are expected to complete this process successfully. A program will be judged deficient if during the most recent 5-year period more than 50% of its graduates fail either the qualifying or the certifying examination on the first try.

B. Residents who plan to seek certification by the American Board of Plastic Surgery should communicate with the secretary of the board to obtain current information regarding certification prior to beginning their training.

ACGME: February 1994 Effective: July 1995

Program Requirements for Residency Education in the Subspecialties of Plastic Surgery

General Information

A. A postgraduate fellowship is a prescribed post-plastic surgery residency educational experience of at least 1 year devoted to the enhancement of knowledge and skills in a defined area of plastic surgery. Postgraduate fellowship programs of graduate education in the subspecialties of plastic surgery may be accredited only in institutions that sponsor accredited residency programs in plastic surgery, or that are related by formal agreement to such institutions or programs. Accordingly, subspecialty programs will be considered for accreditation only if they function in direct association with a residency program in plastic surgery accredited by the Accreditation Council for Graduate Medical Education.

B. Postgraduate fellowship education in plastic surgery is a component in the continuum of the educational process; therefore, such education will take place only after completion of an accredited residency in plastic surgery, except under very unusual circumstances and with the prior approval of the Residency Review Committee.

C. Postgraduate fellowship programs will be considered for accreditation only in subspecialty areas that meet the requirements for accreditation as established by the Accreditation Council for Graduate Medical Education.

D. The essentials enumerated in the Program Requirements for Residency Education in Plastic Surgery are also applicable to the postgraduate fellowships. In conformity with the Program Requirements, programs must provide an intellectual environment for acquiring the knowledge, skills, clinical judgment, and attitudes that are essential to the practice of the specific subspecialty. This objective can be achieved only when the program director, the supporting faculty and staff, and the administration are fully committed to the educational program and when appropriate resources and facilities are present. Effective graduate education is not achieved when the educational program functions primarily to meet service commitments.

The following items, adapted from the Program Requirements for Residency Education in Plastic Surgery, merit emphasis:

1. The postgraduate fellowship program director must be qualified to supervise and to educate fellows appropriately in the specific subspecialty and must be certified by the American Board of Plastic Surgery or possess equivalent qualifications. The program director will be responsible for ensuring that adequate facilities and other necessary resources are available to provide an education of high quality. There should be a sufficient number of qualified faculty to provide the educational experience and to evaluate the progress and performance of the fellow. As with residency program directors in plastic surgery, it is essential that postgraduate fellowship program directors devote sufficient time and effort to the postgraduate fellowship program and related activities. It is desirable that the postgraduate fellowship program be appointed on a full-time basis.

Program Requirements

2. A postgraduate fellowship must provide sufficiently advanced education to allow the fellow to acquire special skill and knowledge in a specific subspecialty. This education should consist of academic and technical components. The academic component should emphasize scholarship, self-instruction, teaching, development of analytic skills and surgical judgment, and research creativity. The technical component should ensure the ability of the fellow to perform skillfully the procedures required for the practice of the subspecialty.

E. Programs will be evaluated according to the following postgraduate fellowship prerequisites:
1. A sufficient number of new and follow-up patients must be present to ensure appropriate inpatient and outpatient experience for each fellow.
2. Subspecialty conferences, seminars, and literature review activities of high quality and of sufficient number must be regularly scheduled. Active participation of the fellow in the planning and the production of these meetings is essential.
3. A fellow must have the opportunity to provide consultation with faculty supervision and should have clearly defined educational responsibilities for residents, medical students, and allied health personnel. These teaching experiences should correlate basic biomedical knowledge with the clinical aspects of the subspecialty.
4. There must be close interaction between the parent residency program in plastic surgery and the postgraduate fellowship programs. Lines of responsibility for the plastic surgery resident and the fellow must be clearly defined. In addition, the fellow should maintain a defined interaction with residents and fellows in other disciplines.
5. A postgraduate fellowship program should have an investigational component. A fellow must learn to design, to carry out, and to interpret research studies. Supervised participation in research projects should occur. Time and facilities must be available to research activity.
6. A postgraduate fellowship must offer supervised training in the operative procedures and in the technical skills integral to the subspecialty discipline involved. Instruction and experience must be sufficient for the fellow to acquire an understanding of the common procedures of the subspecialty and their indications, risks, and limitations.

F. Postgraduate fellowship program directors must have a clearly defined method for regular periodic assessment of the performance of the fellow. The assessment must include cognitive, motor, and interpersonal skills and surgical judgment. There must be provision for regular communication of this information to the fellow and to the residency program director.

G. The following policies and procedures pertain to the accreditation of postgraduate fellowship programs:
1. Program information forms to be used for accreditation of a postgraduate fellowship will be distributed to the director of the plastic surgery residency program. It will be the responsibility of the residency program director to collect information from directors of the postgraduate fellowship programs that are to be reviewed for accreditation. A site visitor will review the entire institutional program in plastic surgery, including the postgraduate fellowship programs being considered for accreditation. The statistical and narrative reports for all components of the program will be forwarded to the Residency Review Committee for Plastic Surgery (RRC-PS). The RRC-PS will review the institutional program in its entirety and will determine the accreditation of the plastic surgery residency program and the postgraduate fellowship programs.
2. Postgraduate fellowship programs will be accredited only if the residency program in plastic surgery is accredited. The accreditation status of postgraduate fellowship programs may equal but not exceed the accreditation status of the parent plastic surgery residency program. A plastic surgery residency program may achieve and retain accreditation whether or not the affiliated postgraduate fellowship programs are accredited. Loss of accreditation of the plastic surgery residency program will result in loss of accreditation of all postgraduate fellowship programs related to that residency.
3. The review cycle for postgraduate fellowship programs will be coordinated with the review cycle for the plastic surgery residency program with provision for separate review of a postgraduate fellowship program when major changes occur.
4. Progress reports may be used to obtain additional information regarding postgraduate fellowship program progress and development.

ACGME: February 1986 Effective: July 1995

Program Requirements for Residency Education in Craniofacial Surgery (Plastic Surgery)

I. Introduction

A. Definition of the Specialty

1. Craniofacial surgery is a subspecialty of plastic surgery that includes the in-depth study and reconstructive treatment of disorders of the soft and hard tissues of the face and cranial areas, such as congenital anomalies and posttraumatic and other acquired conditions. Although craniofacial surgery includes combined intracranial and extracranial surgery, the broad scope of the subspecialty is applicable to other procedures in the craniofacial region. Surgeons trained in craniofacial surgery should be able to manage any hard- or soft-tissue reconstruction problem of the craniofacial region.
2. The team approach to many problems may be appropriate, resulting in the integration of other specialties into the craniofacial team. In addition to plastic surgery, these specialties should include neurological surgery, ophthalmology, otolaryngology, oral surgery, and orthodontics.
3. The primary goals of a craniofacial surgery educational program are to provide a broad education in the art and science of the specialty and sufficient experience for surgeons to acquire competency as specialists in the field.

B. Duration and Scope of Education

1. The length of the educational program in craniofacial surgery is 1 year. Before entry into the program, each prospective craniofacial surgery resident must be notified in writing of the length of the program.
2. Admission to a craniofacial surgery educational program is open to those who have satisfactorily completed an accredited plastic surgery residency program or to other appropriately qualified surgeons.
3. The craniofacial surgery educational program must be associated with an accredited program in plastic surgery. The educational relationship should demonstrate the use of shared resources to in-

clude, for example, faculty, educational conferences, patient management, and other institutional resources.

C. Program Goals and Objectives

1. Although educational programs in craniofacial surgery may differ in format and objectives, each program must demonstrate that residents are provided with the opportunity to obtain the knowledge, skills, clinical judgment, and attitudes essential to the practice of craniofacial surgery.
2. The craniofacial surgery resident must be provided with progressive senior surgical responsibility in the four essential phases of total patient care: preoperative evaluation, therapeutic decision making, operative experience, and postoperative management.
3. The craniofacial surgery resident must be provided with sufficient knowledge of the sciences of embryology, anatomy, physiology, and pathology as these relate to the diagnosis and treatment of diseases of the craniofacial areas. Education in the diagnosis and management of disease and deformity involving the jaws, teeth, and occlusion also must be included in the program.

II. Institutional Organization

A. Sponsoring Institution

1. There must be one institution responsible for the conduct of the educational program as required by the Institutional Requirements.
2. The sponsoring institution must provide sufficient resources to meet the educational needs of the residents and to enable the program to comply with the requirements for accreditation.
3. A sufficient number of patients must be available to ensure inpatient and outpatient experiences for each craniofacial surgery resident without diluting the educational experience for regularly enrolled plastic surgery residents or residents in other specialties.

B. Participating Institutions

1. If the resources of two or more institutions are required to support the program, interinstitutional agreements must be developed by the sponsoring and participating institutions as required by the Institutional Requirements.
2. Participation by any institution that provides 2 months or more of the educational program must be approved prospectively by the Residency Review Committee (RRC) for Plastic Surgery.
3. Assignments to participating institutions must be based on a clear educational rationale and should provide special clinical resources not otherwise available to the program.

C. Library

1. Residents must have ready access to a major medical library, either at the institution where the residents are located or through arrangement with convenient nearby institutions.
2. Library services should include the electronic retrieval of information from medical databases.
3. There must be access to an on-site library or to a collection of appropriate texts and journals at each institution participating in the program. On-site libraries and/or collections of texts and journals must be readily available during nights and weekends.

D. Appointment of Residents

1. The RRC will approve a total number of residents in the program per year, based on the number and qualifications of the faculty, the volume and variety of patients available for educational purposes, and the institutional resources committed to the program. The minimum faculty/resident ratio is 1:1.
2. The program may not graduate more residents in any given year than are approved by the RRC unless prior approval has been obtained.

III. Faculty Qualifications and Responsibilities

The program director and faculty are responsible for the general administration of the program, including activities related to the recruitment, selection, instruction, supervision, counseling, evaluation, and advancement of residents and the maintenance of records related to program accreditation.

A. Program Director

There must be one program director responsible for the program.

1. Qualifications of the program director
   a. Requisite and documented clinical, educational, and administrative abilities and experience in craniofacial surgery
   b. Licensure to practice medicine in the state where the sponsoring institution is located
   c. Certification in plastic surgery and appropriate qualifications in craniofacial surgery, or possession of suitable equivalent qualifications
   d. Appointment in good standing to the medical staff of an institution participating in the program
2. Responsibilities of the program director
   a. Preparation of a written statement outlining the educational goals of the program with respect to the knowledge, skills, and other attributes of residents at each level of education and for each major clinical assignment. This statement must be distributed to residents and members of the faculty. It should be readily available for review.
   b. Selection of residents for appointment to the program in accordance with institutional and departmental policies and procedures.
   c. Selection and supervision of faculty and other program personnel at each institution participating in the program.
   d. Supervision of residents through explicit written description of supervisory lines of responsibility for the care of patients. Such guidelines must be communicated to all members of the program. Residents must be provided with prompt, reliable systems for communication and interaction with supervisory physicians.
   e. Regular evaluation of the resident's knowledge, skills, and overall performance, including the development of professional attitudes consistent with being a physician.
   f. The program director, with participation of the faculty, shall
      1. at least semiannually evaluate the knowledge, skills, and professional growth of the craniofacial surgery residents, using appropriate criteria and procedures;
      2. communicate each evaluation to the resident in a timely manner;
      3. advance residents to positions of higher responsibility only on the basis of evidence of their satisfactory progressive scholarship and professional growth;
      4. maintain a permanent record of evaluation for each resident and have it accessible to the resident and other authorized personnel; and
      5. provide a final written evaluation for each resident who completes the program. The evaluation must include a review of the resident's performance during the final period of education and should verify that the resident has demonstrated sufficient professional ability to practice competently and independently. The final evaluation should be part of the resident's permanent record maintained by the institution.
   g. Implement fair procedures, as established by the sponsoring institution, regarding academic discipline and resident complaints or grievances.
   h. Monitor resident stress, including mental or emotional conditions inhibiting performance or learning and drug- or alcohol-related dysfunction. The program director and faculty should

be sensitive to the need for timely provision of confidential counseling and psychological support services for residents.

Educational situations that consistently produce undesirable stress on residents must be evaluated and modified.

i. Prepare an accurate statistical and narrative description of the program as requested by the RRC.

j. Notify the Executive Director of the RRC for Plastic Surgery of any changes that might substantially alter the educational experience, eg, a change in program director or changes in participating institutions.

B. Faculty

1. There must be a sufficient number of faculty with documented qualifications in craniofacial surgery to instruct and supervise adequately all residents in the program. Members of the faculty must be able to devote sufficient time to meet their supervisory and teaching responsibilities.
2. All members of the faculty must demonstrate a strong interest in the education of residents, sound clinical and teaching abilities, support for the goals and objectives of the program, a commitment to their own continuing medical education, and participation in scholarly activities.
3. A member of the faculty of each participating institution must be designated to assume responsibility for the day-to-day activities of the program at that institution, with overall coordination by the program director.
4. The faculty must be organized and have regular, documented meetings to review program goals and objectives and program effectiveness in achieving them. At least one resident representative should participate in these reviews.
5. The faculty should periodically evaluate the utilization of the resources available to the program, the contribution of each institution participating in the program, the financial and administrative support for the program, the volume and variety of patients available to the program for educational purposes, the didactic course of study, the performance of the faculty, and the quality of resident supervision.

C. Other Program Personnel

The program must be provided with the professional, technical, and clerical personnel to support the administration and educational conduct of the program.

IV. The Educational Program

The program director and the faculty are responsible for providing the intellectual environment necessary for acquiring the knowledge, skills, clinical judgment, and attitudes that are essential for the practice of the specialty. These objectives can be achieved only when the program leadership, the faculty, and the sponsoring institution are committed to the educational program and when appropriate resources and facilities are available.

A. General

1. The program director and faculty must prepare and comply with written educational goals for the program. All educational components of the program must be related to program goals and objectives.
2. The program design and structure must be approved by the RRC as part of the review process.
3. Clinical, basic science, and research conferences; monthly morbidity and mortality sessions; and other conferences focused specifically on craniofacial surgery must be conducted regularly and as scheduled. The topic and subject matter of these conferences must be linked to the goals and objectives for the course of study.
4. Written lines of responsibility describing the relationship between craniofacial surgery residents and plastic surgery residents regarding their clinical responsibilities must be supplied to the RRC at the time of the review.

B. Academic and Clinical Components

The educational program should include the areas outlined below.

1. Basic science
   a. Normal and abnormal embryology and fetal development of the head and neck with special emphasis on the development of the cranium, the maxillary and mandibular complex, the mechanisms of clefting, and the development of the temporomandibular joint and surrounding musculature
   b. Normal growth and development of the cranium and face with special attention to dental development and occlusion and to the consequences of congenital anomalies, trauma, surgery, and radiation
   c. Dental radiographs, cephalometric analysis, and study models; construction of splints and their use in craniofacial and maxillofacial surgery
   d. Interpretation of sophisticated diagnostic imaging modalities used in craniofacial surgery, such as computed tomography, magnetic resonance imaging, and arteriography
   e. Standards of beauty and normalcy as they relate to the face and an understanding of the relationship of cephalometric values to soft-tissue features
   f. Bone healing, including primary healing, malunion, nonunion, osteomyelitis, and the physiology and methods of bone grafting
   g. Use of alloplastic materials used for reconstruction
   h. Congenital, developmental, and secondary deformities of the head and face, including the embryology, pathogenesis, anatomy, natural history, and course of the disease following treatment
2. Congenital anomalies and disorders

   The foundation of this subspecialty is the treatment of congenital craniofacial anomalies. Because such treatment can be applied to a variety of acquired deformities, the program must include in-depth training, education, and participation in the diagnosis, planning, operative treatment, and postoperative care of craniofacial problems including but not necessarily limited to
   a. craniosynostosis;
   b. congenital and developmental deformities of the face that may be related to craniosynostosis, including midface hypoplasia and facial asymmetries;
   c. syndromal malformations of the face such as Treacher Collins, hemifacial microsomia;
   d. congenital orbital dysmorphologies including orbitofacial clefts and hypertelorism;
   e. facial cleft deformities;
   f. atrophic and hypertrophic disorders such as Romberg's disease, bone dysplasia;
   g. craniofacial manifestations of systemic disorders such as neurofibromatosis and vascular malformations and lymphatic disorders;
   h. posttraumatic complex skull and facial deformities;
   i. congenital and acquired disorders of the facial skeleton and occlusal relationships; and
   j. craniofacial concepts in the exposure and/or reconstruction in cranial base oncologic surgery.
3. Clinical activities

   The clinical education should include active participation in an integrated craniofacial team with sufficient patient volume to provide an exposure to diverse craniofacial problems. In addition to plastic surgery, the craniofacial team should include neurological surgery, ophthalmology, otolaryngology, dentistry, and orthodontics. Clinical activities should include

a. education, training, and participation in the surgical methods of craniofacial surgery, including rigid fixation of skull facial bones and training in the fabrication of dental splints;
b. preoperative assessment and decision making regarding methods and timing of intervention in craniofacial disorders;
c. management of craniofacial patients from the preoperative through the postoperative stages; and
d. knowledge of critical care in the postoperative management of craniofacial patients.

4. Education and experience in the following areas is desirable:
a. Diagnostic methods and treatment techniques of temporomandibular joint disorders
b. Aesthetic contour deformities such as masseteric hypertrophy, frontal cranial remodeling
c. Elective orthognathic surgery for orthodontic problems
d. Surgical correction of congenital clefts of the lip and palate with emphasis on both primary and late repairs and revisions
e. Reconstructive management of defects after ablative surgery for malignancy about the maxillofacial region, including pedicle and free flap surgery and bone grafting techniques

C. Operative Experience

1. A program of graduate education in craniofacial surgery must provide a sufficient number and variety of surgical experiences to ensure that residents receive sufficient exposure to a wide range of diseases and injuries to the soft and hard tissues of the craniofacial region.
2. The resident must be allowed senior responsibility as the operating surgeon while performing critical portions of the surgery in the operative management of a range of common craniofacial surgery procedures.
3. The craniofacial surgery resident is not a substitute for faculty and should not act on a regular basis as a teaching assistant to the chief resident in plastic surgery. If the craniofacial surgery resident and the plastic surgery resident share operative experience, only one surgeon may receive credit as surgeon for the experience.

D. Resident Policies

1. Supervision
All patient care services must be supervised by appropriately qualified faculty. The program director must ensure, direct, and document proper supervision of residents at all times. Residents must be provided with rapid, reliable systems for communicating with other residents and faculty. The level and appropriateness of resident supervision must be based on the severity and complexity of the patient's condition.
2. Duty hours and conditions of work
The resident's work schedule should be designed so that on the average, excluding exceptional patient care needs, residents have at least 1 day out of 7 free of routine responsibilities, and be on call in the hospital no more often that every third night. The ratio of hours worked to on-call time will vary and necessitate flexibility.

E. Program Research and Scholarly Activity

Graduate medical education must take place in an environment of inquiry and scholarship in which residents participate in the development of new knowledge, learn to evaluate research findings, and develop habits of inquiry as a continuing professional responsibility.

1. The responsibility for establishing and maintaining an environment of inquiry and scholarship rests with the faculty. While not all members of the faculty may be investigators, the faculty as a whole must demonstrate broad involvement in scholarly activity.
2. The types of activities should include
a. participation in clinical discussion, rounds, and conferences in a manner that promotes a spirit of inquiry and scholarship. Scholarship implies an in-depth understanding of basic mechanisms of normal and abnormal states and the application of current knowledge to practice.
b. participation in journal clubs and conferences.
c. participation in regional and national professional and scientific societies, particularly through presentations at the organizations' meetings and publications in peer-reviewed journals.
d. participation in research, particularly in projects funded following peer review and/or that result in publications or presentations at regional and national scientific meetings.
e. offering of guidance and technical support, for example, research design or statistical analysis, for residents involved in research.
f. provision of support for resident participation in scholarly activities.

V. Evaluation

A. Resident Evaluation

1. Semiannual written evaluation of each resident is required as defined in section III.A.2.f.
2. The resident operative experience must be submitted yearly to the RRC to permit evaluation of each resident's experience.

B. Faculty Evaluation

All faculty must be evaluated annually to review teaching abilities, commitment to the educational program, clinical knowledge, and scholarly activities. Residents should participate in faculty evaluation.

C. Program Evaluation

The educational effectiveness of the program must be evaluated in a systematic manner. In particular, the quality of the curriculum and the extent to which the educational goals have been met by residents must be assessed. Confidential written evaluations by residents should be used in this process.

ACGME: September 1997 Effective: September 1997

Program Requirements for Residency Education in Hand Surgery (Plastic Surgery)

I. Introduction

A. Definition of the Specialty

Hand surgery is a surgical subspecialty that deals with congenital and acquired defects of the hand and wrist that compromise the function of the hand. A hand surgery educational program is designed to educate physicians in the art and science of hand surgery and to develop a competent hand surgeon who is capable of independent function. The educational program should provide experience in the repair, resection, and reconstruction of defects of form and function of the hand; in the design, construction, and transfer of flaps and the transplantation of tissues, including microsurgery of multiple tissues; in replantation of upper extremity parts; in surgical and ancillary methods of treatment of tumors; in management of complex wounds; and in the use of alloplastic materials.

B. Scope of Education

1. Prerequisite resident education must be completed in a general surgery, orthopaedic surgery, or plastic surgery program accred-

ited by the Accreditation Council for Graduate Medical Education (ACGME) or the Royal College of Physicians and Surgeons of Canada.
2. The length of the educational program is 1 year.

II. Institutional Organization

A. Sponsoring Institution

The educational program should have one sponsoring institution that has primary responsibility for the entire program. The sponsoring institution should provide sufficient faculty; financial resources; and clinical, research, and library facilities to meet the educational needs of the residents and to permit the program to comply with the requirements for accreditation.

B. Participating Institutions

1. When multiple institutions participate in the educational program, the commitment of each participating institution must be documented in a written agreement that complies with the ACGME Institutional Requirements.
2. Assignments to participating institutions must be based on an appropriate educational rationale. Assignments that dilute the education of residents or that do not provide proper supervision and coordination of educational activities should not be established or maintained.
3. Assignments to participating institutions that are geographically distant from the sponsoring institution are not desirable. To be justifiable, such assignments must offer special resources or opportunities not otherwise available to the program.
4. The number and location of participating institutions must not preclude the participation of residents and faculty in the educational activities of the hand surgery course of study.

C. Appointment of Residents

1. The total number of residents must be approved in advance by the Residency Review Committee (RRC). The number of residents shall be based primarily on the number, qualifications, and commitment of the faculty; the volume and variety of the patient population available for educational purposes; and the institutional resources committed to resident education.
2. Programs may not graduate more hand surgery residents in any given year than the number of residents approved by the RRC.
3. Any increase, including a temporary increase in resident complement, must receive prior approval of the RRC. Requests for changes in the approved resident complement of a program must include a strong educational rationale.

III. Faculty Qualifications and Responsibilities

The program director and the faculty are responsible for the general administration of a program, including those activities related to the recruitment, selection, instruction, supervision, counseling, evaluation, and advancement of residents and the maintenance of records related to program accreditation.

A. Program Director

A single program director must be responsible for the program.

1. Qualifications of the program director
   a. Requisite and documented clinical, educational, and administrative abilities and experience.
   b. Licensure to practice medicine in the state where the institution that sponsors the program in located.
   c. Certification by the appropriate ABMS Board or suitable equivalent qualifications in the appropriate specialty and a certificate of added qualifications in hand surgery or suitable equivalent qualifications in hand surgery. The RRC will determine the acceptability of equivalent qualifications.
   d. Appointment in good standing to the medical staff of an institution participating in the program.
   e. Frequent changes in leadership or long periods of temporary leadership are undesirable and may adversely affect the accreditation status of the program.
2. Responsibilities of the program director
   a. Prepare a written statement outlining the educational goals of the program with respect to knowledge, skills, and other attributes of hand surgery residents at each level of education and for each assignment. This statement must be distributed to hand surgery residents and members of the faculty. It should be readily available for review.
   b. Select residents for appointment to the program according to institutional and departmental policies and procedures.
   c. Select and supervise the faculty and other program personnel at each participating institution.
   d. Supervise residents through explicit written descriptions of supervisory lines of responsibility for the care of patients. Such guidelines must be communicated to all members of the faculty. Residents must be provided with prompt, reliable systems for communication and interaction with supervising physicians.
   e. Regularly evaluate residents' knowledge, skills, and overall performance. The program director, with participation of the faculty, must
      1. at least quarterly, evaluate the progress of each hand surgery resident in writing, using appropriate criteria and procedures;
      2. communicate each evaluation to the resident in a timely manner;
      3. advance residents to positions of higher responsibility only on evidence of their satisfactory progressive scholarship and growth;
      4. maintain a permanent record of evaluation for each resident and have it accessible to the resident and other authorized personnel; and
      5. provide a final written evaluation to each hand surgery resident who completes the program. The evaluation must include a review of the resident's performance during the final period of education and should verify that the resident has demonstrated sufficient professional ability to practice competently and independently. Each evaluation should be signed by the resident and program director and be maintained on file by the program director for at least 5 years following completion of the program.
   f. Implement fair procedures, as established by the sponsoring institution, regarding academic discipline and resident complaints or grievances.
   g. Monitor resident stress, including mental or emotional conditions inhibiting performance or learning and drug- or alcohol-related dysfunction. Program directors and faculty should be sensitive to the need for timely provision of counseling and psychological support services to residents. Educational situations that consistently produce undesirable stress on residents must be evaluated and modified.
   h. Prepare an accurate statistical and narrative description of the program, as requested by the RRC.
   i. Ensure that each resident is provided with a sufficient educational program, including a sufficient volume and variety of operative experience and progressive surgical responsibility.
   j. Annually collect, compile, and retain the number and types of hand surgery operative procedures performed in all institutions used for resident education. These data must be provided in the form and format specified by the RRC.

k. Annually collect, compile, and retain a comprehensive record of the operative procedures performed by each hand surgery resident completing the program. This information must be provided in the form and format specified by the RRC. This record must be signed by the hand surgery resident and the program director, attesting to its accuracy.
l. Advise applicants of the prerequisite requirements of the appropriate specialty board.
m. Document the satisfactory completion of prerequisite education before the resident begins the hand surgery program.
n. Notify the executive director of the RRC in writing of any major change in the program that significantly alters the educational experience for the residents, including
   1. changes in program leadership, to include any change in appointment of the program director, section or division head, or department chair, and
   2. changes in administrative structure that affect the status of the parent department in the institution.
o. Obtain prior RRC approval for the following changes in the program:
   1. the addition or deletion of any participating institution to which residents are assigned for a total of 2 months or longer;
   2. any change in the approved resident complement of the program; and
   3. any change in the length or format of the program.

B. Faculty

1. The hand surgery faculty must be certified by the one of the sponsoring boards, or possess suitable equivalent qualifications and be certified in hand surgery or possess suitable equivalent qualifications. The majority of the faculty must possess certificates of added qualifications in hand surgery. The RRC will determine the acceptability of equivalent qualifications.
2. There must be a sufficient number of qualified faculty to adequately instruct and supervise hand surgery residents to ensure optimal patient care and resident education. The faculty must be able to devote sufficient time to the program to meet their supervisory and teaching responsibilities.
3. The faculty must demonstrate a strong interest in the education of residents, sound clinical and teaching abilities, support of the goals and objectives of the program, a commitment to their own continuing medical education, and participation in scholarly activities.
4. A faculty member at each participating institution must be designated to assume responsibility for the day-to-day activities of the program at that institution, with overall coordination by the program director.
5. The faculty must be organized and have regular documented meetings to review program goals and objectives and program effectiveness in achieving these goals. The hand surgery resident should participate in these reviews.
6. The faculty should, at least annually, evaluate the utilization of the resources available to the program, the contribution of each institution participating in the program, the financial and administrative support of the program, the volume and variety of patients available to the program for educational purposes, the performance of the faculty, and the quality of resident supervision.

C. Scholarly Activity

Graduate medical education must take place in an environment of inquiry and scholarship in which residents participate in the development of new knowledge, learn to evaluate research findings, and develop habits of inquiry as a continuing professional responsibility. The responsibility for establishing and maintaining an environment of inquiry and scholarship rests with the faculty. While not all members of the faculty must be research investigators, the faculty as a whole must demonstrate broad involvement in scholarly activity. Scholarship is defined as an in-depth understanding of basic mechanisms of normal and abnormal states and the application of current knowledge to practice. This activity should include

1. participation in clinical discussions, rounds, and conferences in a manner that promotes a spirit of inquiry and scholarship;
2. participation in journal clubs and research conferences;
3. active participation in regional or national professional and scientific societies, particularly through presentations at the organizations' meetings and publication in their journals;
4. participation in research, particularly in projects funded following peer review and/or that result in publications or presentations at regional and national scientific meetings;
5. offering of guidance and technical support (eg, research design, statistical analysis) for residents involved in research; and
6. provision of support for resident participation in scholarly activities.

D. Other Program Personnel

Programs must be provided with the additional professional, technical, and clerical personnel needed to support the administration and educational conduct of the program.

IV. Facilities and Resources

A. Inpatient Facilities

1. Inpatient facilities should have a sufficient number of beds, support personnel, and proper equipment to ensure quality patient care and education.
2. Operating suite and diagnostic and treatment facilities must contain technologically current equipment.

B. Outpatient Facilities

Appropriately equipped outpatient facilities including support staff, operating suites, and clinic and office space must be available for resident participation in the preoperative evaluation, treatment, and postoperative follow-up of patients for whom the resident has responsibility.

C. Library Facilities

1. The residents must have ready access to a major medical library, either at the institution where the residents are located or through arrangement with convenient nearby institutions.
2. Library services should include the electronic retrieval of information from medical databases.

V. The Educational Program

A. Program Design

1. The program director and faculty must prepare and implement written educational goals for the program.
2. The program design and/or structure must be approved by the RRC as part of the regular review process.

B. Clinical Component

1. Residents must be provided with education in surgical design, surgical diagnosis, embryology, surgical and artistic anatomy, surgical physiology and pathology, pharmacology, wound healing, microbiology, adjunctive oncological therapy, biomechanics, rehabilitation, and surgical instrumentation.
2. A sufficient number and variety of adult and pediatric hand surgery patients must be available for resident education.

3. Generally equivalent and sufficient distribution of operative procedures among the residents in all categories of hand surgery must be demonstrated.
4. Residents should be provided with graduated and progressive patient management responsibility.
5. Because judgment and technical capability to achieve satisfactory surgical results are mandatory qualities for the hand surgeon, education should be provided in the following areas:
   a. Skin repair, including grafts and flaps, multiple tissue flaps, free microscopic tissue transfers, and insertion of tissue expanders
   b. Fingertip injuries
   c. Tendon repair, including flexor tendon repair and graft, implantation of tendon spacer, extensor tendon repair, and tenolysis/tenodesis
   d. Tendon transfer and tendon balancing
   e. Nerve repair, including major and digital, graft, neurolysis, surgical treatment of neuroma, transpositions, and nerve decompressions
   f. Management of fractures and dislocations, including phalangeal or metacarpal with and without internal fixation; wrist, radius, and ulna with and without internal fixation; and injuries to joint ligaments
   g. Bone grafts
   h. Joint and tendon sheath repairs, including release of contracture, synovectomy, arthroplasty with and without implant, arthrodesis, trigger finger release, and stiff joints that result from rheumatoid or other injury
   i. Pollicization or ray transfer
   j. Foot to hand transfer
   k. Tumors, benign and malignant
   l. Dupuytren's contracture
   m. Replantation, revascularization
   n. Amputations
   o. Fasciotomy, deep incision and drainage for infection, and wound débridement
   p. Congenital deformities, including syndactyly and others
   q. Management of upper extremity vascular disorders and insufficiencies
   r. Foreign body, implant removal
   s. Thermal injuries
   t. Arthroscopy
   u. Upper extremity pain management

C. Didactic Components

1. A comprehensive, organized course of study must be offered, to include educational conferences that are well defined, documented, and regularly held. At minimum, the program must provide a didactic component for clinical education referencing section V.B.1 of these Program Requirements for Residency Education in Hand Surgery.
2. The written course of study should reflect careful planning, with evidence of a cyclical presentation of core specialty knowledge supplemented by the addition of current information, including practice management, ethics, and medicolegal topics as they relate to hand surgery.

   Conferences must include basic science subjects related to clinical surgery of the hand, such as anatomy, physiology, pathology, genetics, microbiology, and pharmacology. A periodic review of the morbidity and mortality experience of the service must be included.
3. A list of the conferences should be maintained and available for review at the time of the site visit.
4. Conferences should be attended by both the residents and the faculty, and such attendance should be documented.
5. Conferences should be organized by the faculty to ensure that sufficient educational experience is provided. Hand surgery residents assigned to participating institutions other than the sponsoring institution should attend the hand surgery conferences at those sites.
6. Residents should make presentations at conferences and actively participate in conference discussions. Adequate time for resident preparation should be permitted to maximize the educational experience.
7. Hand surgery residents should be encouraged to pursue clinical or basic science research interests.

D. Supervision

1. All patient care services must be supervised by qualified hand surgery faculty. The program director must ensure, direct, and document proper supervision of residents at all times.
2. Residents must be provided with rapid, reliable systems for communicating with faculty at all times.
3. Hand surgery residents may function as intermediate supervisors when documented prior experience makes it appropriate, but faculty supervision must be available.

E. Duty Hours

1. It is desirable that residents' work schedules be designed so that on the average, excluding exceptional patient care needs, residents have at least 1 day out of 7 free of routine responsibilities and be on call in the hospital no more often than every third night. The ratio of hours worked to on-call time will vary, particularly at senior levels, and flexibility will be necessary.
2. There must be adequate backup so that patient care is not jeopardized during or following assigned periods of duty.
3. Sufficient support services must be provided to ensure that residents are not required to spend excessive time in noneducational activities that can be discharged properly by other personnel.
4. The hand surgery residency is a full-time responsibility. Activities outside the educational program must not interfere with resident performance in the educational program as determined by the program director and must not interfere with resident opportunity for rest, relaxation, and study.

F. Appointment of Other Residents

1. The appointment of other residents for hand surgery education must not dilute or detract from the educational opportunities of hand surgery residents.
2. The appointment of other residents to the hand surgery service requires a clear statement of the areas of education, clinical responsibilities, and duration of the education. This statement must be supplied to the RRC at the time the program is reviewed.
3. If such residents so appointed will, in the judgment of the RRC, detract from the education of the hand surgery residents, the accreditation status of the program may be adversely affected.

VI. Evaluation

A. Resident Evaluation

The program director and faculty are responsible for regularly evaluating the residents' knowledge, skills, and overall performance, including the development of professional attitudes consistent with being a physician.

B. Faculty Evaluation

1. At least annually, all individual faculty members must be formally evaluated by the program director. Hand surgery residents should be provided with the opportunity to evaluate faculty.
2. A mechanism for sharing the results of such evaluations with the faculty that preserves resident confidentiality in the evaluation process must be employed.

3. The program should demonstrate that such evaluations are used in improving the program.

C. Program Evaluation

1. The educational effectiveness of a program must be evaluated at least annually. In particular, the quality of the curriculum and the extent to which the educational goals have been met by residents must be assessed. Written evaluations by hand surgery residents should be utilized in this process.
2. One measure of the quality of a program is the performance of its graduates on the examination for the certificate of added qualifications in hand surgery given by one of the sponsoring boards. The RRC may consider this information as part of the overall evaluation of the program.

VII. Board Certification

Residents who plan to seek hand surgery certification as administered by the American Board of Plastic Surgery should communicate with the secretary of the board to ascertain the current requirements for acceptance as a candidate for certification.

ACGME: September 1997 Effective: July 1998

Program Requirements for Residency Education in Preventive Medicine

This document is divided into four sections: the Common Program Requirements, Program Requirements for Public Health and General Preventive Medicine, Program Requirements for Occupational Medicine, and Program Requirements for Aerospace Medicine. The Common Program Requirements describe the essentials common to the specialty. Sections 2-4 contain the essentials for each of the areas of specialization. Each program must comply with the Common Program Requirements in addition to the essentials for the specific area of specialization.

Common Program Requirements

I. Introduction

A. Definition

The primary foci of preventive medicine are the study of disease processes as they occur in communities and defined population groups and the stimulation of practices with respect to the community and the individual that will advance health by promoting health-enhancing environments and behaviors, preventing disease and injury, making possible early diagnosis and treatment, and fostering habilitation and rehabilitation of persons with disabilities.

B. Basic Components

Preventive medicine has certain common basic components, whatever the area of specialization. A given component may be of major importance in some fields of practice and of lesser importance in others, but basic competence is essential in each. These components are the

1. application of biostatistical principles and methodology;
2. recognition of epidemiological principles and methodology;
3. planning, administration, and evaluation of health and medical programs and the evaluation of outcomes of health behavior and medical care;
4. recognition, assessment, and control of environmental hazards to health, including those of occupational environments;
5. recognition of the social, cultural, and behavioral factors in medicine;
6. application and evaluation of primary, secondary, and tertiary prevention; and
7. assessment of population and individual health needs.

C. Program Phases

1. To impart the knowledge and develop the skills necessary to achieve the stated objectives, graduate education in preventive medicine must include three phases: the clinical, the academic, and the practicum. Each of these phases must be no less than 1 year in duration, except the academic phase, as described in section IV.A.3 of the Common Program Requirements.
2. A program may be accredited for one, two, or three phases. A clinical phase will not be accredited by the Residency Review Committee (RRC) for Preventive Medicine if that phase has been accredited by another specialty.

II. Faculty Qualifications and Responsibilities

The program director and the faculty are responsible for the general administration of the program, including those activities related to the recruitment, selection, instruction, supervision, counseling, evaluation, and advancement of residents and the maintenance of records related to program accreditation.

A. Program Director

1. Qualifications
   a. The entire residency program should be under the supervision of one physician who is certified by the American Board of Preventive Medicine in the appropriate field of preventive medicine or who possesses suitable equivalent qualifications. The RRC will determine the acceptability of equivalent qualifications. For example, knowledge and experience of at least 3 years in the field of preventive medicine after completion of residency education may be considered as suitable equivalent qualifications.
   b. The program director must be able to devote sufficient time and effort to the program to ensure its educational quality. At all times, there must be continuity and direction in the education and supervision of residents.
   c. Other qualifications include:
      1. requisite and documented clinical, educational, and administrative abilities and experience.
      2. licensure to practice medicine in the state where the institution that sponsors the program is located. (Certain federal programs are exempted.)
      3. appointment in good standing to the medical staff of an institution participating in the program.
2. Responsibilities
   Responsibilities of the program director include the following:
   a. Counseling residents in the academic phase in the selection of assignments, services, or elective courses that will help provide the skills and knowledge needed in the resident's practicum experiences and area of specialization in preventive medicine. The program director must provide information that describes the program's accreditation status to each applicant and resident.
   b. Preparing a written statement outlining the educational goals of the program with respect to knowledge, skills, and other attributes of residents at each level of training and for each major rotation or other program assignment. This statement must be distributed to residents and members of the faculty. It should be readily available for review.
   c. Selecting residents for appointment to the program in accordance with institutional and departmental policies and procedures.
   d. Selecting and supervising the faculty and other program personnel at each institution participating in the program.
   e. Supervising residents through explicit written descriptions of supervisory lines of responsibility for the care of patients. Such guidelines must be communicated to all members of the program. Residents must be provided with prompt, reliable systems for communication and interaction with supervisory physicians.
   f. Regularly evaluating residents' knowledge, skills, and overall performance, including the development of professional attitudes consistent with being a physician.
   g. Implementing fair procedures, as established by the sponsoring institution, regarding academic discipline and resident complaints or grievances.
   h. Monitoring resident stress, including mental or emotional conditions inhibiting performance or learning and drug- or alcohol-related dysfunction. Program directors and faculty should be sensitive to the need for timely provision of confidential counseling and psychological support services to residents. Educational situations that consistently produce undesirable stress on residents must be evaluated and modified.
   i. Preparing an accurate statistical and narrative description of the program as requested by the RRC.
   j. Notifying the RRC regarding major program changes.

B. Faculty

1. There must be a sufficient number of faculty with documented qualifications to instruct and supervise adequately all residents in the program. Faculty members must be able to devote sufficient time to meet their supervisory and teaching responsibilities.
2. All members of the faculty must demonstrate a strong interest in the education of residents, sound clinical and teaching abilities, support for the goals and objectives of the program, a commitment to their own continuing medical education, and participation in scholarly activities.
3. A faculty member at each participating institution must be designated to assume responsibility for the day-to-day activities of the program at that institution, with overall coordination by the program director.
4. The faculty must be organized and have regular, documented meetings to review program goals and objectives and program effectiveness in achieving them. At least one resident representative should participate in these reviews.
5. The faculty should periodically evaluate the utilization of the resources available to the program, the contribution of each institution participating in the program, the financial and administrative support of the program, the volume and variety of patients available to the program for educational purposes, the performance of members of the faculty, and the quality of supervision of residents.

C. Other Program Personnel

Programs must be provided with the additional professional, technical, and clerical personnel needed to support the administration and educational conduct of the program.

D. Residency Advisory Committee

There must be a residency advisory committee (RAC), comprising members expert in the field, that must evaluate and advise on the content, conduct, and effectiveness of the educational program and make appropriate recommendations.

1. A substantial number of RAC members must be persons other than the primary faculty or staff of the sponsoring institution.
2. The program director must be an ex-officio member and must not chair the RAC.
3. The chair of the RAC must be a physician.
4. Residents in the program should be represented on the RAC.
5. The RAC must meet with the frequency required to discharge these responsibilities, but not less than semiannually, and should report at least annually to the head of the sponsoring institution.
6. Formal minutes of the RAC meetings must be kept and must be submitted to the RRC with the annual report.
7. The residents must provide the chair of the RAC with their annual evaluation of the program.

III. Facilities and Resources

A. General Support

The sponsoring institution must maintain adequate facilities, including office and laboratory space and access to computer facilities. A basic collection of reference texts and periodicals in preventive medicine and public health must be maintained. Support services, including secretarial services, should be provided. Residents must be provided with adequate office facilities during assigned duty hours. All residents should be provided funds for travel to designated professional meetings.

B. Participating Institutions

Individual parts of the program may be offered at participating institutions. Agreements between the sponsoring and the participating institutions must be defined.

1. New or updated affiliation agreements must be included with the annual report.
2. The program must have all active agreements available for review at the site visit.
3. The program director is responsible for reviewing the agreements annually and for supplying updates as needed to ensure currency.
4. The reciprocal commitments of the residency program and the participating institutions must be explicit in a written agreement or contract indicating
   a. the educational objectives;
   b. the scope of the experience, with placement locations noted;
   c. the resources, including space, support services, and clinical facilities, that will be available to the residents;
   d. the duties and responsibilities of the residents;
   e. the relationship that will exist between residents and faculty of the residency program and the participating institution; and
   f. the supervisory relationship and identified supervisor who shall be qualified by certification or equivalent experience, as determined by the program director. There must be active participation by the residents at the participating institution, and resident supervision on-site must be performed by a physician or appropriately qualified health professional.

C. Library

1. Residents must have ready access to a major medical library, either at the institution where the residents are located or through arrangement with convenient nearby institutions.
2. Library services should include the electronic retrieval of information from a medical database.
3. There must be access to an on-site library or to a collection of appropriate texts and journals in each institution participating in a residency program. On-site libraries and/or collections of texts and journals must be readily available during nights and weekends.

IV. The Educational Program

A. Required Program Phases

1. General Information
   a. The RRC will consider accreditation for programs that offer (1) the clinical, academic, and practicum phases; (2) the academic and practicum phases; or (3) the practicum phase alone.
   b. Programs based in nonacademic institutions that offer only a practicum year must have formal affiliation with a school of public health, a medical school offering an MPH or equivalent degree, or another program's accredited academic phase.
   c. Programs that offer only the academic and practicum phases or only the practicum phase are to accept only residents who have completed education in an accredited clinical phase.
   d. If the clinical phase is not taken as part of the preventive medicine residency program, the resident should meet the clinical phase requirement with a year in an accredited program in one of the recognized direct primary patient care specialties, eg, family practice, pediatrics, internal medicine, and obstetrics and gynecology, or in a transitional year program.
2. Clinical Phase
   The clinical phase constitutes a graduate year of clinical education and experience in direct patient care. It must provide broad experience in direct patient care, including ambulatory and inpatient hospital experience, eg, family practice, pediatrics, internal medicine, and obstetrics and gynecology, or in a transitional year, and it must be completed prior to the start of the practicum phase. If the preventive medicine residency program offers a clinical year, it must meet the following requirements for accreditation:
   a. In addition to the preventive medicine residency, there must be at least one Accreditation Council for Graduate Medical Education (ACGME)-accredited primary care residency at the same institution.
   b. Other departments participating in the clinical year education shall be identified and have delineated roles. The qualifications of the participating faculty should be equivalent to those of the faculty in the accredited primary care residency.
   c. The curriculum should include at least 3 months of hospital experience in internal medicine. In addition, there should be a balanced program of outpatient and inpatient care, including pediatrics, obstetrics and gynecology, and emergency medicine to provide a broad range of exposure to other types of patients. Elective assignments should be determined by the needs of the individual resident and/or the requirements of the specialty program. A clinical year consisting exclusively of a series of outpatient clinic rotations will not be considered as offering an adequate breadth of education.
   d. All participating institutions must be accredited by the Joint Commission on Accreditation of Healthcare Organizations (JCAHO) or an equivalent organization.
3. Academic Phase
   The academic phase consists of a course of study leading to the MPH or equivalent degree in an institution accredited by a nationally recognized accrediting agency. The course of study requires a minimum of 1 full academic year or its equivalent, as determined by the RRC. The resident who is in a degree-granting institution must meet all requirements for the degree. When no degree is granted, a postbaccalaureate curriculum of equivalent content, depth, and rigor may be acceptable, provided the curriculum is approved by an appropriate body, such as the graduate school or academic senate of an institution accredited by a nationally recognized accrediting agency. In such a case, the written notification of approval must be supplied to the RRC.
   a. Required Course Work
   The required course work shall include biostatistics, epidemiology, health services organization and administration, environmental and occupational health, and social and behavioral influences on health.
   b. Research Activities
   Adequate opportunities should be available for the resident to participate in research activities appropriate to the chosen field of education.
4. Practicum Phase
   The practicum phase is a year of continued learning and supervised application of the knowledge, skills, and attitudes of preventive medicine in the field.
   a. Duration
   The practicum phase shall be the equivalent of 12 full months' duration. Programs that offer a combined 2-year academic/practicum program must provide the RRC with a clearly delineated schedule showing that adequate time is available to complete both the academic and practicum components of the program. Academic work shall precede or be concurrent with activities of the practicum phase that apply the principles embodied in the academic program.
   b. Content
   The practicum phase shall offer both didactic and applied components that shall be provided in settings in which there are

well-organized programs appropriate to the particular field of preventive medicine. There shall be provision for the supervised application of the knowledge, skills, and attitudes of preventive medicine gained in the academic phase and in the didactic component of the practicum phase. The resident must assume progressive responsibility during this phase of the educational program.

c. Prerequisites
Programs accredited to offer only the practicum year can permit the resident to begin the practicum year only if the resident has
1. satisfactorily completed a course of study leading to an MPH or equivalent degree, as specified in these Common Program Requirements IV. A. 3., or
2. made substantive progress in a course of study demonstrated by completion of the required course work specified in these Common Program Requirements IV. A. 3. a.

B. Program Goals and Objectives

1. The program director and faculty must prepare and comply with written educational goals for the program. All educational components of a residency program shall be related to program goals.
2. The program design and/or structure must be approved by the RRC as part of the regular review process.
3. Participation by any institution providing more than 2 months of education in a 1-year program; 4 months of education in a 2-year program, or 6 months of education in a 3-year program must be approved by the RRC.

C. Duty Hours

Resident duty hours in a clinical setting must be scheduled and monitored to avoid excessive stress and fatigue. Residents must have a keen sense of personal responsibility for continuing patient care, and must recognize that their obligations to patients are not automatically discharged at any given hour of the day or any particular day of the week. In no case should residents go off duty until the proper care and welfare of patients have been ensured. Duty hours and night and weekend call for residents must reflect the concept of responsibility for patients and provide for adequate patient care. Residents must not be required regularly to perform excessively difficult or prolonged duties. When averaged over 4 weeks, residents should spend no more than 80 hours per week in all duties. Residents at all levels should, on average, have the opportunity to spend at least 1 day out of 7 free of hospital duties and should be on call no more often than every third night. There should be adequate opportunity to rest and sleep when on call for 24 hours or more. There should be adequate backup so that patient care is not jeopardized during or following assigned periods of duty.

D. Program Research and Scholarly Activity

Graduate medical education must take place in an environment of inquiry and scholarship in which residents participate in the development of new knowledge, learn to evaluate research findings, and develop habits of inquiry as a continuing professional responsibility. The responsibility for establishing and maintaining this environment of inquiry and scholarship rests with the faculty. While not all members of a faculty must be investigators, the faculty as a whole must demonstrate broad involvement in scholarly activity. This activity should include

1. participation of the faculty in clinical discussions, rounds, and conferences in a manner that promotes a spirit of inquiry and scholarship. Scholarship infers an in-depth understanding of basic mechanisms of normal and abnormal states and the application of current knowledge to practice.
2. participation in journal clubs and research conferences.
3. participation in regional or national professional and scientific societies, particularly through presentation at the organizations' meetings and publications in their journals.
4. participation in research, particularly in projects funded following peer review that result in publications or presentations at regional and national scientific meetings.
5. offering of guidance and technical support (eg, research design, statistical analysis) to residents involved in research.
6. provision of support for resident participation in scholarly activities.

V. Evaluation

A. Resident Evaluation

The program director, with participation of the faculty, must at least semiannually evaluate the knowledge, skills, and professional growth of residents, using appropriate criteria and procedures. The evaluations must be communicated to residents formally and in a timely manner. Where appropriate, interim evaluation is encouraged. Residents should be advanced to positions of higher responsibility only on the basis of evidence of their satisfactory progressive scholarship and professional growth.

1. The resident's supervisor in the clinical and practicum phases shall provide a written evaluation to the program director and the resident on completion of the rotation.
2. The evaluations for each resident must be kept available for review by the individual resident and by the reviewer at the time of the survey.
3. The program director and faculty must certify that residents completing the program have fulfilled all established requirements based on the above evaluations. The final evaluation should be part of each resident's permanent record maintained by the institution, and must be accessible to the resident and other authorized personnel. The evaluation must include a review of the resident's performance during the final period of education and should verify that the resident has demonstrated sufficient professional responsibility to practice competently and independently.
4. Each program must develop and use specific performance measures. A variety of acceptable techniques for performance assessment may be used. A record must be maintained of the instruments and processes used for assessment.
5. Evaluation of residents in the academic phase is the responsibility of the sponsoring institution and must include a transcript or equivalent document provided to each resident. All academic activities should be coordinated with the individual resident's program director.

B. Program Evaluation

1. Except in the year when accreditation occurs, an annual report must be submitted to the RRC. The program director must describe each individual resident's activities and any significant change in program staffing, affiliations, or facilities for the year covered by the report. Minutes of the RAC meetings and new or updated interinstitutional agreements must be furnished with the report. The annual report forms will be furnished to the program directors by the executive director of the RRC.
2. The educational effectiveness of a program must be evaluated in a systematic manner. In particular, the quality of the curriculum and the extent to which the educational goals have been met by residents must be assessed at least annually. Residents must have the opportunity to provide written confidential evaluations of the adequacy, quality, and appropriateness of each component of the educational program. This evaluation must be provided to the chair of the RAC annually. A record must be maintained of

the internal assessments of the program by the program director, faculty, and residents.

3. The RRC may consider the performance of graduates on the examinations of the American Board of Preventive Medicine as one measure of the quality of the educational program.

VI. Other

Residents should contact the executive director of the American Board of Preventive Medicine for information regarding Board Certification.

Public Health and General Preventive Medicine

I. Introduction

A. Scope of the Specialty

Public health and general preventive medicine is the area of specialization in preventive medicine that deals with health promotion and disease prevention in communities and in defined populations. Practitioners in this field are found in governmental and voluntary health agencies, academic and health care institutions, group practice settings, and health service research organizations. Many of these specialists deal with public health practice, the direction and management of health care institutions and delivery systems, the community's health, and the health status and demographics of population groups. Some of these specialists provide prevention interventions for individual patients, while others are involved in the health status of both groups and individuals.

B. General Objectives

The achievement of knowledge and skills in the component functions of preventive medicine will enable the graduate practitioner to

1. perform epidemiological investigations of acute and chronic diseases and injuries;
2. use appropriate statistical techniques in the design of studies and interpretation of findings relative to disease interventions performed on individuals and in monitoring and experimental protocols;
3. plan, administer, and evaluate programs to promote health and prevent disease in medical practice settings and in public health agencies;
4. design, perform, and evaluate clinical trials;
5. apply clinical interventions in the general population;
6. assess health risk factors in individual persons and groups and prescribe appropriate interventions;
7. assess and ameliorate the impact of environmental and occupational risk factors on individual persons and on groups;
8. assess the clinical and public health program needs of populations, eg, workers, communities, military groups;
9. achieve maximum advantage through collaboration with other members of the health promotion and preventive medicine team;
10. develop budgeting and personnel management skills; and
11. develop research skills in other areas appropriate to health promotion and disease prevention.

II. Sponsoring and Participating Institutions

The facilities in which education is provided need not conform to a rigid pattern. The sponsoring institution may be an educational institution, a research center, or an operating health agency. These relationships must be documented by written agreements, as specified in the Common Program Requirements for Residency Education in Preventive Medicine.

A. If the sponsoring institution is an educational or research institution, it should have resources for developing a comprehensive graduate program in preventive medicine. In the case of a sponsoring institution that is not a public health agency, affiliation must be negotiated with a health department or other health agencies or organizations to ensure appropriate didactic and research opportunities.

B. If the sponsoring institution is a health agency, it should offer a comprehensive experience in community or public health. The program may include communicable and chronic disease control, health care administration, health protection and promotion, maternal and child health, environmental health and sanitation, and mental health. To ensure an appropriate didactic component, including the gathering and analyzing of data, affiliations must be negotiated with a medical school or school of public health and that relationship documented in a written agreement, as specified in the Common Program Requirements.

C. In addition to the sponsoring institution, a practicum may be given in a participating institution that is chosen to meet a particular need of a resident.

III. Facilities

A. The resources and structure of a participating institution should be well established and should serve a population or provide research and educational programs sufficiently comprehensive to ensure appropriate experience in public health and general preventive medicine.

B. The competence and interest of the professional and supervisory staff in residency education should be ensured to the satisfaction of the RRC.

IV. Required Phases

A. Clinical Phase

The clinical phase is described in the Common Program Requirements. If the resident has already chosen an area of special emphasis, the clinical phase should be designed to strengthen skills in that area.

B. Academic Phase

The academic phase is described in the Common Program Requirements. Program directors must counsel residents on course work that should be taken as electives. Electives should be chosen according to the area of specialization and interest of the resident and the Program Requirements.

C. Practicum Phase

1. The purpose of the practicum phase is to give the resident experience in practicing general preventive medicine and public health in established programs under the guidance of skilled practitioners. The scope of that experience must be broad enough to ensure an appreciation for and ability to cope with a range of preventive medical problems in different settings. Additionally, the education must provide opportunity for concentrated experience in an area of special emphasis.
2. This phase shall be the equivalent of 12 months duration. Programs that offer a combined 2-year academic/practicum program must provide the RRC with a clearly delineated schedule showing that adequate time is available to complete both the academic and the practicum phases.
3. Didactic education must be documented and must offer a broad range of topics such as the medical aspects of health promotion, disease prevention and surveillance, toxic exposure, health economics, clinical issues in prevention, management techniques, and current epidemiological issues.

4. Residency programs are encouraged to make experiences in occupational medicine available to their residents.
5. The program should include studies that offer each resident an opportunity to participate in data gathering and analysis procedures.
6. The program must provide at least a 1-month experience in a public health agency, and this must be documented for each resident.
7. The adequacy of highly fragmented assignments may require special documentation.
8. Because the practitioners of public health and preventive medicine will need management skills, the program should include experience in budgeting, fiscal control, personnel practice, and administrative techniques, including automated record keeping and computer applications in the management of health services.
9. Special attention should be given to the political process, governmental structure, and health policy. It is highly desirable that observation or participation in legislative and regulatory procedures as well as public relations be included.

Occupational Medicine

I. Introduction

Occupational medicine is the area of specialization in preventive medicine that focuses on the relationships among the health of workers; the ability to perform work; the arrangements of work; and the physical, chemical, and social environments of the workplace. Practitioners in this field recognize that work and the environment in which work is performed can have favorable or adverse effects on the health of workers as well as on that of other populations, that the nature or circumstances of work can be arranged to protect worker health, and that health and well-being in the workplace are promoted when workers' physical attributes or limitations are accommodated in job placement.

The principal concerns of occupational medicine are

A. *the workers*: The appraisal, maintenance, restoration, and improvement of health through the application of the principles of preventive medicine, medical care, rehabilitation, and environmental medicine; the matching of health or physical attributes of workers with the requirements of jobs.

B. *the workplace*: The appraisal and design of work and the workplace for the purpose of controlling within safe limits exposures to potentially injurious substances or conditions, evaluating hazards or toxic materials in the workplace, and arranging work so that it conforms to the physiological requirements of workers.

C. *information management*: The collection, collation, storage, and analysis of health data to facilitate epidemiological study of health phenomena related to work or to health-enhancing activities; to disseminate health-relevant information to workers, regulatory agencies, customers, and others who may benefit from such information; and to protect against inappropriate release of confidential medical information.

D. *administration*: The application of social, economic, and management principles to organize, implement, and assess activities designed to promote the health and well-being of workers and to enhance the capability to deal with relevant regulatory, legal, and industrial relations organizations.

II. Educational Program

A. Phases

1. Clinical Phase
The clinical phase is described in the Common Program Requirements for Residency Education in Preventive Medicine.
2. Academic Phase
The requirements of the academic phase are described in the Common Program Requirements. The academic phase shall include the required courses listed in those Common Program Requirements as well as topics selected from the list of didactic components referenced in section II.B.1. of these Program Requirements.
3. Practicum Phase
The practicum phase shall prepare the resident for the comprehensive practice of occupational medicine and shall afford opportunities for the resident to deal with clinical, scientific, social, legal, and administrative issues from the perspectives of workers and their representatives, employers, and regulatory or legal authorities.
   a. There shall be opportunities for the planned and supervised application of the knowledge and skills acquired in the prior phases of residency education. Residents shall have sufficient continuity of service in practicum activities to foster the assumption of authentic clinical and administrative responsibility and the development of mature judgment and resourcefulness.
   b. For at least 4 months the resident shall engage in supervised practice within the real world of work. Through interaction with occupational health personnel, workers, human resources and industrial relations personnel, line supervisors, worker representatives, and the medical community, the resident must gain experience in the clinical and administrative aspects of direct worker care and job assignment, medical screening and surveillance, health conservation and promotion, environmental assessment, employee assistance, and relevant regulatory compliance.

      Appropriate practicum opportunities may be found in a variety of settings in which a comprehensive program of occupational medicine and related health and administrative services exists. Suitable sites may include heavy and light manufacturing; the utilities, services, and transportation sectors; and clinics that provide comprehensive services to workers and employers.

      Although diagnostic and referral clinics organized primarily for the diagnosis and assessment of occupational disease can have a vital role in the education of residents, they do not afford the broad practicum opportunities specified above. This experience need not be obtained at a single site, nor must the experience be received in a single 4-month block; however, sufficient sustained attendance at each facility must occur to permit the assumption of significant clinical and administrative responsibility.
   c. A 4-month equivalent based on distributed time totaling 4 months may be acceptable, provided that less-than-full-time attendance does not compromise the assumption of responsibility. The program director must document the distributed time totaling 4 months to the satisfaction of the RRC. The adequacy of highly fragmented assignments may require special documentation.

      Assignments that do not afford opportunity for the development of responsibility are not acceptable.
   d. Extensive time commitments to the care of minor employee complaints or to service functions characterized by highly repetitive or standardized procedures do not contribute to professional growth and must not be permitted to dilute the educational value of the practicum experience.
   e. Because the team approach is an important aspect of occupational medicine practice, residents must have assignments that require collaborative work not only with industrial hygienists, nurses, and safety personnel, but also with counselors or others concerned with psychosocial issues.

f. Residents are encouraged to engage in research during the practicum phase with the advice and supervision of the teaching faculty. However, the practicum must be primarily an educational experience that prepares the resident for the comprehensive practice of occupational medicine. The commitment of time to the development of new knowledge, however valuable, must not impair achievement of the fundamental objectives of the practicum by diluting the educational experience, diminishing peer interaction, or impeding the assumption of progressive clinical and administrative responsibility.

B. Required Components

The following components are required. They may be addressed in more than one phase of the program.

1. Didactic Component

   A didactic component must be provided in the practicum phase. This component shall include structured lectures, journal clubs, symposia, etc, that focus on the following topics:

   a. Environmental physiology, including responses to heat, pressure, noise, and other physical stresses
   b. Occupational disease, including diagnosis, differential diagnosis, prevention, and treatment
   c. Toxicology, including basic principles, clinical applications, and risk assessment
   d. Industrial hygiene, including instrumentation, data interpretation, and basic environmental control measures
   e. Safety, including behavioral factors in accident causation and control and medical support of accident investigations
   f. Ergonomics
   g. Determination of fitness to work, placement of workers, adaptations of work to accommodate handicaps
   h. Employee assistance programs, including substance abuse and rehabilitation
   i. Health education and health promotion; lifestyle risk factors as they are affected by the occupational environment
   j. Occupational health data management and analysis
   k. Management and administrative aspects of an occupational health program
   l. Clinical preventive activities to improve the health of workers and their families

2. Clinical Component

   The clinical component shall include but not be limited to each of the following topics:

   a. Clinical care of workers in the prevention, diagnosis, treatment, and rehabilitation of work-related disorders
   b. Evaluation of the fitness of workers for normal or modified job assignments in a wide variety of work environments and the assessment of impairment and disability
   c. Counseling and education of workers and supervisors with respect to work or environmental hazards, health-related habits of living, and the arrangements of work

3. Administrative Component

   The administrative component shall provide the resident with opportunities for management responsibilities and shall include but not be limited to each of the following topics:

   a. The planning, administration, supervision, and evaluation of a broad program for the protection and promotion of the health and safety of workers in the work setting, including health risk assessment, accident evaluation, and risk reduction
   b. Application of administrative and scientific principles to achieve compliance with regulatory requirements and the requirements of workers' compensation plans
   c. Acquisition, collation, storage, and analysis of health and environmental data

Aerospace Medicine

I. Introduction

Aerospace medicine is the area of specialization in preventive medicine that focuses on the health of a population group consisting of the operating crews and passengers of air and space vehicles together with the support personnel who are required to operate such vehicles. Segments of this population often work and live in remote, isolated, and sometimes closed environments under conditions of physical and psychological stress rarely encountered in terrestrial life. Education in this field must, therefore, address the diagnosis, prevention, and treatment of disorders associated with these unique environments and with the adaptive systems designed to enhance performance and support life under such conditions.

II. Educational Program

In addition to the Common Program Requirements for Residency Education in Preventive Medicine, the phases of a residency in aerospace medicine shall contain the following:

A. Clinical Phase

The clinical phase is described in the Common Program Requirements. Residency education in this area of specialization should emphasize neuropsychiatry, ophthalmology, cardiopulmonary diagnosis, and emergency medicine. It is desirable that this year of clinical education be accomplished in a hospital or medical complex in which patients with aerospace medical problems are frequently encountered. Progressive patient responsibility should be assigned to residents. Supplemental clinical education in the areas mentioned above shall be provided during the practicum year, as described in section C below.

B. Academic Phase

The requirements of the academic phase are described in the Common Program Requirements. Additional academic requirements for aerospace medicine are normally integrated into the course of study leading to a postbaccalaureate degree. In addition to the course work required in the Common Program Requirements, course work should emphasize environmental physiology and toxicology with respect to the biological effects of altered pressure, temperature, atmospheric chemistry, and ionizing radiation. Facilities should be available for laboratory or clinical investigation of problems with direct application to the specialty, and supervised participation by the resident in a formal research project should be encouraged. Because of the paramount role of clinical care in an aerospace medicine practice, it is desirable that the academic faculty be either part of or formally affiliated with an accredited school of medicine.

C. Practicum Phase

This year of supervised application should be accomplished in an institutional setting where operational aeromedical problems are routinely encountered and aerospace life support systems are under active study and development. Aircraft accident investigation and aircraft certification regulations must be included. Laboratory facilities should be equipped to provide simulated environments in which the effects of and adaptation to extreme conditions of temperature, barometric pressure, acceleration, weightlessness, and psychological stress can be studied. A flight training program should be available both to familiarize the resident with basic aeronautical skills and to serve as a source of clinical material for the supervised management of common clinical problems encountered among flight personnel.

ACGME: June 1996 Effective: July 1997

Program Requirements for Residency Education in Medical Toxicology (Preventive Medicine)

I. Introduction

A. Definition and Description of the Subspecialty

1. Medical toxicology is a clinical specialty that includes the monitoring, prevention, evaluation and treatment of injury and illness due to occupational and environmental exposures, pharmaceutical agents, as well as unintentional and intentional poisoning in all age groups. A medical toxicology residency must be organized to provide residents with experience in the clinical practice of medical toxicology for all age groups and to provide a sound basis for the development of physician practitioners, educators, researchers, and administrators capable of practicing medical toxicology in academic and clinical settings.
2. Residencies in medical toxicology must teach the basic skills and knowledge that constitute the foundations of medical toxicology practice and must provide progressive responsibility for and experience in the application of these principles to the management of clinical problems. It is expected that the resident will develop a satisfactory level of clinical maturity, judgment, and technical skill that will, on completion of the program, render the resident capable of independent practice in medical toxicology.
3. Programs must provide a broad education in medical toxicology to prepare the resident to function as a specialist capable of providing comprehensive patient care.

B. Duration and Scope of Education

1. Prerequisite training for entry into a medical toxicology program should include the satisfactory completion of an ACGME-accredited residency. [*Note:* Candidates who do not meet this criterion should consult the American Board of Emergency Medicine, or the American Board of Preventive Medicine regarding their eligibility for subspecialty certification.]
2. The length of the educational program is 24 months. The program must be associated with an ACGME-accredited residency program in emergency medicine, or preventive medicine.
3. Prior to entry into the program, each resident must be notified in writing of the required length of the program.

II. Institutional Organization

A. Sponsoring Institution

1. The sponsoring institution must provide sufficient faculty, financial resources, and clinical, research, and library facilities to meet the educational needs of the residents and to enable the program to comply with the requirements for accreditation. It is highly desirable that the program structure include the participation of a medical school, a school of public health, and a school of pharmacy or department of pharmacology.
2. Programs in medical toxicology should be based at a primary hospital (hereafter referred to as the primary clinical site). The majority of the didactic and clinical experiences should take place at the primary clinical site.
3. The following services must be organized and provided at the primary clinical site:
   a. An emergency service for both adult and pediatric patients, adult and pediatric inpatient facilities, and adult and pediatric intensive care facilities
   b. Renal dialysis services with 24-hour availability
   c. Toxicology laboratory services with 24-hour availability
   d. Inpatient and outpatient facilities with staff who consult the toxicology service
   e. It is desirable that hyperbaric oxygen therapy is available
4. The program must develop an institutional affiliation to provide residents with clinical experiences not provided at the primary clinical site, other than those listed in II.A.3.a-d.

B. Participating Institutions

1. All participating institutions must provide appropriate support services to ensure an adequate educational experience. This includes support personnel in all categories and physical resources to ensure that residents have sufficient time and space to carry out their clinical and educational functions.
2. The program must develop an institutional affiliation with a clinical facility to provide residents with clinical experience in critical care areas should this experience not be provided at the sponsoring institution.
   a. Approval of participating institutions will be based on the presence of sufficient opportunities for residents to manage, either as primary physicians or consultants, the entire course of critically poisoned patients in both the pediatric and adult categories.
   b. Institutional resources must be available to support the provision of clinical experience in adult and pediatric critical care areas for residents without prior experience of at least 1 month in an adult intensive care unit and 1 month in a pediatric intensive care unit.
   c. Programs using multiple participating institutions must ensure the provision of a unified educational experience for the residents. Each participating institution must offer significant educational opportunities to the overall program that do not duplicate experiences otherwise available within the program. An acceptable educational rationale must be provided for each participating institution.
   d. Participating institutions must not be geographically distant from the sponsoring institution unless special resources are provided that are not available at the primary clinical site.
   e. The number and geographic distribution of participating institutions must not preclude all residents' participation in conferences and other educational exercises.
   f. A letter of agreement with each institution participating in the program must be developed to include
      1. the educational objectives and the method to accomplish and to evaluate each objective;
      2. the resources and facilities in the institution(s) that will be available to each resident, including but not limited to library resources;
      3. the resident's duties and responsibilities and duty hours for the assignment; and
      4. the relationship that will exist between medical toxicology residents and residents and faculty in other programs.

C. Library

Residents must have ready access to a major medical library either at the institution where the residents are located or through arrangement with convenient nearby institutions. Reference material specific to the content of the subspecialty must be available in either text or electronic retrieval form.

D. Appointment of Residents

The Residency Review Committee (RRC) will approve the number of medical toxicology residents in the program. Approval will be based on the number, qualifications, and scholarly activity of the faculty; the volume and variety of the patient population available for educational purposes; and the institutional resources available to the program.

III. Faculty Qualifications and Responsibilities

A. In addition to the qualifications and responsibilities of the program director and faculty described in the Program Requirements for Residency Education in the Subspecialties of Emergency Medicine or the Program Requirements for Residency Education in Preventive Medicine, there must be a minimum of two medical toxicology faculty who each devote a minimum of 5 hours per week of direct teaching time to the residents and whose medical practice makes them available to the residents for consultations on cases.

B. The program director and faculty must be certified in medical toxicology or possess suitable equivalent qualifications as determined by the RRC.

C. Consultants from appropriate medical subspecialties including those with special expertise in disaster and mass casualty incident management, hyperbaric medicine, immunology, industrial hygiene, occupational toxicology, pulmonary medicine, biostatistics, epidemiology, public health, botany, cardiology, dermatology, gastroenterology, nephrology, ophthalmology, pathology, pharmacology, surgical subspecialty, zoology, hazardous materials and mass exposure to toxins, laboratory toxicology, forensic toxicology and environmental toxicology, and nonmedical specialties, such as botany, herpetology, and mycology should be available for consultation and academic lectures.

IV. The Educational Program

A. The director and teaching staff of a program must prepare and comply with written educational goals for the program. All educational components of a residency program should be related to program goals. The program design and/or structure must be approved by the RRC.

B. The curriculum must include the following academic and clinical content:

1. The clinical manifestations, differential diagnosis, and management of poisoning
2. The biochemistry of metabolic processes, the pharmacology, pharmacokinetics, and teratogenesis, toxicity, and interactions of therapeutic drugs
3. The biochemistry of toxins, kinetics, metabolism, mechanisms of acute and chronic injury, and carcinogenesis
4. Experimental design and statistical analysis of data as related to laboratory, clinical, and epidemiologic research
5. Laboratory techniques in toxicology
6. Occupational toxicology, including acute and chronic workplace exposure to intoxicants and basic concepts of the workplace and industrial hygiene
7. Prevention of poisoning, including prevention of occupational exposures by intervention methodologies, that take into account the epidemiology, environmental factors, and the role of regulation and legislation in prevention
8. Environmental toxicology, including identification of hazardous materials and the basic principles of management of large-scale environmental contamination and mass exposures
9. The function, management, and financing of poison control centers
10. Oral and written communication skills and teaching techniques
11. Principles of epidemiology and risk communication, analytical laboratory techniques, and research methodologies in toxicology

C. Clinical Experience
Residents must have a minimum of 12 months of clinical experience as the primary or consulting physician responsible for providing direct/bedside patient evaluation, management, screening, and preventive services.

Residents must be provided with experience in evaluating and managing patients with workplace and environmental exposures and must have experience in workplace evaluation, as well as in an occupational medicine or toxicology clinic.

D. Residents must have opportunities to evaluate and manage patients with acute and long-term workplace and environmental toxic exposures. Clinical training should include experience in an industrial setting or an occupational medicine clinic or access to occupational medicine patients in a referral setting. The resident should also have the opportunity to evaluate and manage intoxicated patients in both industrial and referral setting, including responsibility for providing bedside evaluation, management, screening, and preventive services for a minimum of 12 months or its full-time equivalent.

E. Regional Poison Information Center

1. The program must provide residents with educational experiences in a regional poison control center certified by the American Association of Poison Control Centers or its equivalent. It is highly desirable that the poison control center be in physical proximity to the primary clinical site.
2. Each resident must have 12 months' experience with a referral population of poisoned patients under the supervision of a physician who is certified in medical toxicology or who possesses suitable equivalent qualifications as determined by the RRC.
3. The poison control center should have at least 1,500 calls annually that require physician telephone consultation or intervention.

F. Planned Educational Conferences
Each program must offer to its residents an average of at least 5 hours per week of planned educational experiences (not including change-of-shift reports). These educational experiences should include presentations based on the defined curriculum, morbidity and mortality conferences, journal review, administrative seminars, and research methods. They may include but are not limited to problem-based learning, laboratory research, and computer-based instruction, as well as joint conferences cosponsored with other disciplines.

G. Additional Educational Experiences
The program curriculum must include pharmacology, pharmacokinetics, and drug interactions. This must be accomplished by (1) an affiliation with a school of pharmacy or department of pharmacology that provides regular didactic experience and consultation to residents or (2) the presence of a Doctor of Pharmacology or PhD pharmacologist as a participating member of the teaching faculty.

H. Additional Clinical Experiences
The program should provide the opportunity for the residents to maintain their primary board skills during training, but it may not require that residents provide more than 12 hours per week of clinical practice not related to medical toxicology as a condition of the educational program.

I. Communication and Teaching Experience
Residents must have progressive experience and responsibility for the teaching of medical toxicology to health care professionals. Residents in the second year of training should participate in the teaching and supervision of first-year residents and should be responsible for regular contributions to formal didactic experiences within the training program, in other academic departments in the institution(s), and in the community. Research leading to publication should be encouraged.

V. Board Certification

Those planning to seek a subspecialty certificate from their primary board should communicate with the administrative officer of the board to ascertain the full requirements.

ACGME: June 1998 Effective: June 1998

Program Requirements for Residency Education in Psychiatry

I. Introduction

A. Description of the Specialty

An approved residency program in psychiatry must provide an educational experience designed to ensure that its graduates will possess sound clinical judgment, requisite skills, and a high order of knowledge about the diagnosis, treatment, and prevention of all psychiatric disorders and the common medical and neurological disorders that relate to the practice of psychiatry. While residents cannot be expected to achieve the highest possible degree of expertise in all of the diagnostic and treatment procedures used in psychiatry in 4 years of training, those individuals who satisfactorily complete residency programs in psychiatry must be competent to render effective professional care to patients. Furthermore, they must have a keen awareness of their own strengths and limitations and of the necessity for continuing their own professional development.

B. Duration and Scope of Education

1. Admission Requirements

   Physicians may enter psychiatry programs at either the first-year or second-year postgraduate level. Physicians may enter programs at the second-year postgraduate level only after successful completion of one of the following:

   a. A broad-based clinical year of accredited training in the United States or Canada in programs in internal medicine, family practice, or pediatrics;

   b. An Accreditation Council for Graduate Medical Education (ACGME)-accredited transitional year program;

   c. One year of an ACGME-accredited residency in a clinical specialty requiring comprehensive and continuous patient care.

2. Length of the Program

   a. A complete psychiatry residency is 48 months. Twelve of those months may be spent in an ACGME-approved child and adolescent psychiatry residency. Accreditation by the ACGME is required for all years of the training program. Programs may not permit residents to use vacation time or other benefit time to advance the date of graduation from training. Although residency is best completed on a full-time basis, part-time training at no less than half time is permissible to accommodate residents with personal commitments (eg, child care).

   b. Any program that alters the length of training beyond these minimum requirements must present a clear educational rationale consonant with the program requirements and objectives for residency training. The program director must obtain the approval of the sponsoring institution and the Residency Review Committee (RRC) prior to implementation and at each subsequent review of the program.

   c. Prior to entry into the program, each resident must be notified in writing of the required length of training for which the program is accredited. The required length of training for a particular resident may not be changed without mutual agreement during his or her program, unless there is a break in his or her training or the resident requires remedial training.

   d. Programs should meet all of the Program Requirements for Residency Education in Psychiatry. Under rare and unusual circumstances, programs of either 1 year's or 2 years' duration may be approved, even though they do not meet all of the above requirements for psychiatry. Such 1- or 2-year programs will be approved only if they provide some highly specialized educational and/or research programs. Also, such programs will be approved only if they ensure that residents will complete the didactic and clinical requirements outlined in the program requirements.

3. Program Format by Year of Training
   a. First Year of Training
      A psychiatric first postgraduate year must include at least 4 months in internal medicine, family practice, and/or pediatrics. This training must be in a clinical setting that provides comprehensive and continuous patient care.
      1. Neurology rotations may not be used to fulfill this 4-month requirement.
      2. One month, but no more, of this requirement can be fulfilled by an emergency medicine rotation, as long as the experience is predominantly with medical evaluation and treatment, as opposed to surgical procedures.
      3. For residents transferring into a program, there must be documentation in the training record that they have met this requirement in either current or prior training.
      4. A psychiatric first postgraduate year should not include more than 6 months in psychiatry and must not include more than 8 months in psychiatry.
      5. A minimum of 2 months of neurology, or its full-time equivalent on a part-time basis, is required prior to completion of training. It is highly desirable that this experience occur during a psychiatric first postgraduate year.
      6. It is highly desirable that the Department of Psychiatry maintain contact with residents during the first postgraduate year while they are on services other than psychiatry.
   b. The Second Through Fourth Years of Training
      Although some of the training described below may be offered in the first postgraduate year, all must be completed prior to graduation from the program.
      1. The program must have an explicitly described educational curriculum covering the broad spectrum of clinical psychiatry as outlined in V.B.1.a-o.
      2. The formal didactic instruction must include regularly scheduled lectures, teaching rounds, seminars, clinical conferences, and required reading assignments covering the topics identified in Section V.
      3. There must be an educationally sound balance among time spent in direct patient care, clinical and didactic teaching, and supervision. Formal educational activity shall have high priority in the allotment of the resident's time and energies. Service needs and clinical responsibilities must not prevent the resident from obtaining the requisite didactic educational activities and formal instruction.

II. Institutional Organization

A. Sponsoring Organization

1. Programs should be conducted under the sponsorship of an institution that meets the Institutional Requirements that apply to residency programs in all specialties, as outlined in the *Essentials of Accredited Residencies.*
2. The administration of the sponsoring institution(s) should be understanding of and sympathetic to the attainment of educational goals and should evidence the willingness and ability to support these goals philosophically and financially. The latter includes a commitment by the institution and by the program that embraces appropriate compensation for faculty and residents, adequate offices and educational facilities, and support services, as well as opportunities for research.
3. It is important that each affiliated institution offer significant educational opportunities to the overall program. The reasons for including each institution within the program must be stated. The number and distribution of participating training sites must not preclude satisfactory participation by residents in teaching and training exercises. Geographic proximity will be one factor in evaluating program cohesion, continuity, and "critical mass." Affiliated training sites will be evaluated on the basis of whether they contribute to a well-integrated educational program with respect to both didactic and clinical experiences.

B. Selection and Appointment of Residents

1. The program director is responsible for maintaining a process for selecting resident physicians who are personally and professionally suited for training in psychiatry. It is highly desirable that each program have a residency selection committee to advise the program director.
2. The program should document the procedures used to select residents. Application records should contain complete information from medical schools and graduate medical education programs. A documented procedure should be in place for evaluating the credentials, clinical training experiences, past performance, and professional integrity of residents transferring from one program to another, including from an adult to a child and adolescent psychiatry program. This procedure must include solicitation and documentation of relevant information from the training directors of the previous programs participated in by the transferring resident. This documentation must specify all clinical and didactic experiences for which the resident has been given credit. Those residents selected at the second postgraduate year or above must have satisfied the training objectives cited above for reaching that level of training.
3. The residency program director must accept only those applicants whose qualifications for residency include sufficient command of English to facilitate accurate, unimpeded communication with patients and teachers.
4. A transferring resident's educational program must be sufficiently individualized so that he or she will have met all the educational and clinical experiences of the program, as accredited, prior to graduation.
5. The RRC will determine the size of the program's permanent resident complement based on the program's clinical and academic resources.
6. To promote an educationally sound, intellectually stimulating atmosphere and effective graded responsibility, programs must maintain a critical mass of at least three residents at each level of training. Programs that fall below this prescribed critical mass will be reviewed, and if this deficiency is not corrected, they will be subject to negative action.
7. Programs in which the number of residents exceed the resources of patient population, faculty, or facilities for adequate training will be found deficient on the basis of size.
8. Any permanent change in the number of approved positions requires prior approval by the RRC. (Programs seeking interim approval of a permanent increase in the number of approved resident positions should contact the executive secretary of the RRC.) Prior approval is not required for temporary changes in resident numbers due to makeup or remedial time for currently enrolled residents or to fill vacancies. Approval of permanent increases will require documentation that didactic and clinical training, including supervision, will not be compromised.

III. Faculty Qualifications and Responsibilities

The program director and the teaching staff are responsible for the general administration of a program, including those activities related to the recruitment, selection, instruction, supervision, counseling, evaluation, and advancement of residents and the maintenance of records related to program accreditation.

A. Program Director

There must be a single program director responsible for the program. Each residency program must be under the direction of an experienced, fully trained, and qualified psychiatrist whose major responsibility is to maintain an excellent educational program. The residency program director must possess the necessary administrative, teaching, and clinical skills and experience to conduct the program. Continuity of leadership over a period of years is important to the stability of a residency program. Frequent changes in leadership or long periods of temporary leadership usually have a negative effect on an educational program and may adversely affect the accreditation status of the program. The program director must:

1. Be licensed to practice medicine in the state where the institution that sponsors the program is located. (Certain federal programs are exempted.)
2. Be certified by the American Board of Psychiatry and Neurology or possess equivalent qualifications in psychiatry satisfactory to the RRC.
3. Have an appointment in good standing to the medical staff of an institution participating in the program.
4. Devote at least one-half of his or her time to the administration and operation of the educational program, including didactic, supervisory, and clinical teaching activities. Programs with multiple institutions, many residents, and/or a large clinical population will require additional time.

B. Responsibilities of the Program Director

1. The program director must have appropriate authority to oversee and to organize the activities of the educational program. The responsibilities of this position should include but not be limited to the following:
   a. Resident appointments and assignments in accordance with institutional and departmental policies and procedures.
   b. Supervision, direction, and administration of the educational activities.
   c. Coordination of training in each geographically separate institution.
   d. Selection and supervision of the teaching staff and other program personnel at each institution participating in the program.
   e. The supervision of residents through explicit written descriptions of supervisory lines of responsibility for the care of patients. Such guidelines must be communicated to all members of the program staff.
   f. Regular evaluation of residents' knowledge, skills, and overall performance, including the development of professional attitudes consistent with being a physician.
   g. Provision of a written final evaluation for each resident who completes the program, as specified in Section VI.A.7.
   h. Preparation of a written statement outlining the educational goals of the program with respect to knowledge, skills, and other attributes of residents at each level of training and for each major rotation or other program assignment. This statement must be distributed to applicants, residents, and members of the teaching staff. It should be readily available for review.
   i. Provision of written information to applicants and residents regarding financial compensation, liability coverage, and the policies regarding vacations, sick leave, and parental leave, as well as other special leaves.
   j. Implementation of fair procedures, as established by the sponsoring institution, regarding academic discipline and resident complaints or grievances.
   k. Monitoring resident stress, including mental or emotional conditions inhibiting performance or learning and drug- or alcohol-related dysfunction. Program directors and teaching staff should be sensitive to the need for timely provision of confidential counseling and psychological support services to residents. Training situations that consistently produce undesirable stress on residents must be evaluated and modified.
   l. Maintenance of a permanent record of evaluation for each resident and having it accessible to the resident and other authorized personnel. These will be made available on review of the program.
   m. Preparation of an accurate statistical and narrative description of the program as requested by the RRC for Psychiatry.
   n. Notification in writing of the executive secretary of the RRC within 60 days of any major change in the program that may significantly alter the educational experience for the residents, including:
      1. Changes in leadership of the department or the program.
      2. Changes in administrative structure, such as an alteration in the hierarchical status of the program/department within the institution.
      3. Changes in the resident complement that would bring the number of residents below the required critical mass of three residents per year for 2 consecutive years.
2. The program director must obtain prior approval for the following changes in the program for the RRC to determine if an adequate educational environment exists to support these changes:
   a. The addition of any participating institution to which residents rotate for 6 months or longer.
   b. The addition or deletion of any rotation of 6 months or longer.
   c. Any increase in the approved number of resident positions in the program.
   d. Any change in the total length of the program.

   On review of such proposals or important changes in a program, the RRC may determine that a site visit is necessary.

C. Education Policy Committee

The director of the residency program should have an educational policy committee composed of members of the psychiatry program teaching staff that includes representation from the residents as well as a member of the teaching staff from each ACGME-approved subspecialty residency that may be affiliated with the psychiatry residency. There should be a written description of the committee, including its responsibility to the sponsoring department or institution and to the program director. This committee should participate actively in:

1. Planning, developing, implementing, and evaluating all significant features of the residency program, including the selection of residents (unless there is a separate residency selection committee)
2. Determining curriculum goals and objectives
3. Evaluating both the teaching staff and residents

D. Number and Qualifications of the Faculty

All members of the teaching staff must demonstrate a strong interest in the education of residents, sound clinical and teaching abilities, support of the goals and objectives of the program, commitment to their own continuing medical education, and participation in scholarly activities.

1. There must be a sufficient number of teaching staff to instruct and supervise adequately all the residents in the program. Members of the teaching staff must be able to devote sufficient time to meet their supervisory and teaching responsibilities. The residency must be staffed by a sufficiently wide variety and appropriate number of capable psychiatrists and other mental health professionals with documented qualifications to achieve the goals and objectives of the training program.

2. The faculty psychiatrists should be certified by the American Board of Psychiatry and Neurology or have equivalent qualifications in psychiatry satisfactory to the RRC.
3. A written record of the educational responsibilities of all staff and faculty members (whether full-time or part-time) who participate directly in the education of residents is essential. That record should include the qualifications and experience of the faculty member and the nature, as well as the frequency, duration, and site, of the teaching activity.
4. There must be evidence of scholarly activity among the faculty psychiatrists. Scholarly activity is defined as professional activities that serve to enhance the profession or professional knowledge. While not all members of a faculty need be investigators, scholarly activities should be present on a continuous basis. There should also be evidence of participation in a spectrum of academic and professional activities within the institution as well as within local and national associations. Such evidence should include:
   a. Documentation of teaching excellence
   b. Participation in clinical and/or basic research
   c. Involvement in relevant medical scientific organizations and their meetings
   d. Publication in refereed journals, monographs, and books
5. The faculty must participate regularly and systematically in the training program and be readily available for consultation whenever a resident is faced with a major therapeutic or diagnostic problem.
6. The faculty psychiatrists should actively participate in the planning, organization, and presentation of conferences as well as clinical teaching and supervision.
7. A member of the teaching staff of each participating institution must be designated to assume responsibility for the day-to-day activities of the program at that institution, with overall coordination by the program director.
8. The teaching staff must be organized and have regular documented meetings to review program goals and objectives as well as program effectiveness in achieving them. At least one resident representative should participate in these reviews.
9. The teaching staff should periodically evaluate the utilization of the resources available to the program, the contribution of each institution participating in the program, the financial and administrative support of the program, the volume and variety of patients available to the program for educational purposes, the performance of members of the teaching staff, and the quality of supervision of residents.

E. Other Program Personnel

Programs must be provided with the additional professional, technical, and clerical personnel needed to support the administration and educational conduct of the program.

IV. Program Facilities and Resources

A. Clinical Facilities and Resources

1. All programs must have adequate patient populations for each mode of required training and, minimally, must include organized clinical services in inpatient, outpatient, emergency, consultation-liaison, and child and adolescent psychiatry.
2. Training programs must have available to them adequate inpatient and outpatient facilities, clinics, agencies, and other suitable placements where the residents can meet the educational objectives of the program. The program should specify the facilities in which the goals and objectives are to be implemented.
3. All residents must have available offices adequate in size and decor to allow them to interview patients and accomplish their duties in a professional manner. The facility must also provide adequate and specifically designated areas in which residents can perform basic physical examinations and other necessary diagnostic procedures.

B. Other Educational Resources

1. The administration of the facility must provide ample space and equipment for educational activities. There must be adequate space and equipment specifically designated for seminars, lectures, and other teaching exercises.
2. The program must have available audiovisual equipment and teaching material such as films, audio cassettes, and videotapes, as well as the capability to record and play back videotapes.
3. Residents must have ready access to a major medical library, either at the institution where the residents are located or through arrangement with convenient nearby institutions. Library services should include the electronic retrieval of information from medical databases.
4. There must be access to an on-site library or to a collection of appropriate texts and journals in each institution participating in a residency program. On-site libraries and/or collections of texts and journals must be readily available during nights and weekends.
   This library should provide:
   a. A substantial number of current basic textbooks in psychiatry, neurology, and general medicine
   b. A number of the major journals in psychiatry, neurology, and medicine sufficient for an excellent educational program
   c. The capability to obtain textbooks and journals on loan from major medical libraries
   d. Capability to perform MEDLINE or other medical information searches (or ready access to a library that has this capacity).
5. Each clinical service must have a mechanism that ensures that charts are appropriately maintained and readily accessible for regular review for supervisory and educational purposes. Randomly selected charts will be reviewed at the time of survey.

V. Educational Program

The director and teaching staff of a program must prepare and comply with written educational goals for the program. All educational components of a residency program should be related to program goals. The program design and/or structure must be approved by the RRC for Psychiatry as part of the regular review process.

A. Objectives of Training

1. First Year
   The training obtained during the first postgraduate year should provide residents with medical skills most relevant to psychiatric practice. These include being able to
   a. Undertake the initial clinical and laboratory studies of patients presenting with a broad range of common medical and surgical disorders
   b. Diagnose common medical and surgical disorders and formulate appropriate initial treatment plans
   c. Provide limited, but appropriate, continuous care of patients with medical illnesses and make appropriate referrals
   d. Be especially conversant with medical disorders displaying symptoms likely to be regarded as psychiatric and with psychiatric disorders displaying symptoms likely to be regarded as medical
   e. Be especially cognizant of the nature of the interactions between psychiatric treatments and medical and surgical treatments

f. Relate to patients and their families, as well as other members of the health-care team with compassion, respect, and professional integrity

2. Second Through Fourth Years

The program must provide a well-planned, high-quality curriculum that includes specific, assessable objectives for program components as well as criteria for graduation. These must be written and provided to each resident and faculty member. Residents must be taught to conceptualize all illnesses in terms of biological, psychological, and sociocultural factors that determine normal and disordered behavior. They must be educated to gather and organize data, integrate these data with a comprehensive formulation of the problem to support a well-reasoned differential diagnosis, formulate a treatment plan, and implement treatment and follow-up. The program must provide residents with sufficient opportunities to develop professionalism, knowledge, clinical skills, and professional principles.

a. The didactic curriculum should include:
   1. Critical appraisals of the major theories and viewpoints in psychiatry, together with a thorough grounding in the generally accepted facts
   2. Presentation of the biological, psychological, sociocultural, economic, ethnic, gender, religious/spiritual, sexual orientation, and family factors that significantly influence physical and psychological development in infancy, childhood, adolescence, and adulthood
   3. Presentation of the etiologies, prevalence, diagnosis, treatment, and prevention of all of the psychiatric conditions in the current standard diagnostic statistical manual, to include the biological, psychological, sociocultural, and iatrogenic factors that affect the long-term course and treatment of psychiatric illness
   4. Comprehension of the diagnosis and treatment of neurologic disorders commonly encountered in psychiatric patients, such as neoplasms, dementia, headaches, head trauma, infectious diseases, movement disorders, multiple sclerosis, Parkinson's disease, seizure disorders, and stroke and related disorders
   5. The use, reliability, and validity of the generally accepted diagnostic techniques, including physical examination of the patient, laboratory testing, imaging, neurophysiologic testing, and psychological testing
   6. The financing and regulation of psychiatric practice, including information about the structure of governmental and private organizations that influence mental health care
   7. Medical ethics as applied to psychiatric practice
   8. The history of psychiatry and its relationship to the evolution of modern medicine
   9. The legal aspects of psychiatric practice
   10. When and how to refer
   11. Research methods in the clinical and behavioral sciences related to psychiatry

b. Clinical training should provide sufficient experiences in:
   1. The elements of clinical diagnosis with all age groups (of both sexes and including some ethnic minorities), such as interviewing; clear and accurate history taking; physical, neurological, and mental status examination; and complete and systematic recording of findings
   2. Relating history and clinical findings to the relevant biological, psychological, and social issues associated with etiology and treatment
   3. Formulating a differential diagnosis and treatment plan for all conditions in the current standard nomenclature, taking into consideration all relevant data
   4. The major types of therapy, including short- and long-term individual psychotherapy, psychodynamic psychotherapy, family therapy, group therapy, cognitive and behavior therapy, crisis intervention, pharmacological and other somatic therapies, and drug and alcohol detoxification
   5. Providing continuous care for a variety of patients from different age groups, seen regularly and frequently for an extended time, in a variety of treatment modalities
   6. Psychiatric consultation in a variety of medical, surgical, and community settings
   7. Providing care and treatment for the chronically mentally ill with appropriate psychopharmacologic, psychotherapeutic, and social rehabilitative interventions
   8. Psychiatric administration, especially leadership of interdisciplinary teams
   9. Providing psychiatric care to patients who are receiving treatment from nonmedical therapists and coordinating such treatment
   10. Knowledge of the indications for and limitations of the more common psychological tests
   11. Critically appraising the professional and scientific literature
   12. Ability to teach psychiatry to students in the health professions

B. Curriculum

1. Clinical Experience

Carefully supervised clinical care of patients is the core of an adequate program. The clinical services must be so organized that residents have major responsibility for the care of a significant proportion of all patients assigned to them and that they have sufficient and high-quality supervision. The number of patients for whom residents have primary responsibility at any one time must be small enough to permit residents to provide each patient with appropriate treatment and to have sufficient time for other aspects of their educational program. At the same time, the total number must be large enough to provide an adequate depth and variety of clinical experiences.

The amount and type of patient care responsibility a resident assumes must increase as the resident advances in training. Each resident must have major responsibility for the diagnosis and treatment of a reasonable number and adequate variety of patients with both acute and chronic illnesses representing the major psychotic and nonpsychotic categories of psychiatric illness. Adequate experience must also be ensured in the diagnosis and management of the medical and neurological disorders encountered in psychiatric practice. Each resident must have supervised experience in the evaluation and treatment of patients of both sexes, of various ages from childhood to old age, and from a variety of ethnic, racial, social, and economic backgrounds.

It is desirable that residents have didactic learning and supervised experiences in the delivery of psychiatric services in the public sector (such as community mental health centers and public hospitals and agencies) and in managed-care health systems. The clinical experiences are to be designed to develop the requisite skills as outlined in Section V.A.2.b, above. Specific clinical experiences must include:

a. Neurology. Supervised clinical experience in the diagnosis and treatment of neurological patients. This 2-month experience (or its equivalent if done on a part-time basis) may occur on either an inpatient and/or an outpatient basis. The training must provide opportunities to conduct initial evaluations, to participate in the subsequent diagnostic process, and to follow patients during the treatment and/or evolution of their neurological illness. The training in neurology should provide sufficient didactic and clinical experience to develop expertise in the diagnosis of those neurological conditions that might reasonably be expected to be encountered in psychiatric practice and that must be considered in the differential diagnosis of psychiatric conditions.

b. Inpatient. Significant responsibility for the assessment, diagnosis, and treatment of an appropriate number and variety of general adult psychiatric inpatients for a period of not less than 9 months but no more than 18 months (or its full-time equivalent if done on a part-time basis) in 4 years of training. In general, it is highly desirable that the minimum general, adult inpatient experience be 12 months in duration, although it is recognized that in some settings other training opportunities might lead to the absolute minimum of 9 months. Inpatient rotations on specialized clinical services such as substance abuse, geriatrics, research units, day and/or partial hospitalization, and child and adolescent psychiatry will not be included in assessing the required minimum 9-month inpatient experiences for residency training, unless the rotation on such specialized units is comparable in breadth, depth, and experience to training on general inpatient units. Those rotations not fulfilling the above requirement will be included in assessing the maximum allowable 18-month inpatient experience.

c. Outpatient. An organized, continuous, supervised clinical experience in the assessment, diagnosis, and treatment of outpatients of at least 1 year (or its full-time equivalent if done on a part-time basis) that emphasizes a developmental and biopsychosocial approach to outpatient treatment. This must include experience with a wide variety of disorders, patients, and treatment modalities, with experience in both brief and long-term care of patients, using individual psychotherapy (including psychodynamic, cognitive, behavioral, biological, and social rehabilitation approaches to outpatient treatment). Long-term psychotherapy experience must include a sufficient number of patients seen at least weekly for at least 1 year, under supervision. Other long-term treatment experiences should include patients with differing disorders and chronicity and should include some patients who are chronically mentally ill.

d. Child and adolescent psychiatry. An organized clinical experience under the supervision of qualified child and adolescent psychiatrists in the evaluation, diagnosis, and treatment of children, adolescents, and their families. Such experiences should be no less than 2 months full-time equivalent and involve a sufficient number and variety of patients, by both age and psychopathology, treated with a variety of interventional modalities. Residents should have experiences in determining the developmental status and needs for intervention with the children of some of their adult patients and in consulting with these patients regarding the referral of their children for psychiatric services. Residents must have patient care responsibility under the supervision of qualified child and adolescent psychiatrists. While adolescent inpatient units may be used to satisfy a portion of this requirement, rotations to student health services may not.

e. Consultation/liaison. Supervised psychiatric consultation/liaison responsibility of a minimum of 2 months full-time equivalent, involving patients on other medical and surgical services. While on-call experiences may be a part of this training, such experiences alone will not be sufficient to constitute adequate training in consultation/liaison psychiatry.

f. Emergency psychiatry. Supervised responsibility on an organized, 24-hour psychiatric emergency service that is responsible for evaluation, crisis management, and triage of psychiatric patients. Instruction and experience should be provided in learning crisis intervention techniques, including the evaluation and management of suicidal patients. A psychiatric emergency service that is a part of or interfaces with other medical emergency services is desirable because of the opportunities for collaboration and educational exchange with colleagues in other specialties. There must be organized instruction and supervised clinical experience in emergency psychiatry that lead to the development of knowledge and skills in the emergency evaluation, crisis management, and triage of patients. This should include the assessment and management of patients who are a danger to themselves or others, the evaluation and reduction of risk to caregivers, and knowledge of relevant issues in forensic psychiatry. There should be sufficient continued contact with patients to enable the resident to evaluate the effectiveness of clinical interventions. While on-call experiences may be a part of this training, such experiences alone will not be sufficient to constitute adequate training in emergency psychiatry.

g. Community psychiatry. Supervised responsibility in community-based mental health activities. This should include consultation with at least one community agency.

h. Geriatric psychiatry. Supervised clinical management of geriatric patients with a variety of psychiatric disorders, including familiarity with long-term care in a variety of settings.

i. Addiction psychiatry. Supervised clinical management of patients with alcoholism and drug abuse, including detoxification and long-term management in inpatient and/or outpatient settings and familiarity with self-help groups.

j. Forensic psychiatry. Supervised experience in evaluation of patients with forensic problems under the supervision of a psychiatrist.

k. Supervised clinical experience in the evaluation and treatment of couples, families, and groups.

l. Techniques for evaluation and management of danger (of the patient dangerous to self and others) should be taught in every aspect of patient care.

m. Psychological testing. Supervised experience with the more common psychological test procedures, including neuropsychological assessment, in a sufficient number of cases to give the resident an understanding of the clinical usefulness of these procedures and of the correlation of psychological test findings with clinical data. Under the guidance of a qualified clinical supervisor, residents should have experience with the interpretation of the psychological tests most commonly used, and some of this experience should be with their own patients.

n. Supervised experience in utilization review and total quality management.

o. Supervised, active collaboration with psychologists, psychiatric nurses, social workers, and other professional and paraprofessional mental health personnel in the treatment of patients.

2. Didactic Components

The didactic and clinical curriculum must be of sufficient breadth and depth to provide residents with a thorough and well-balanced presentation of the generally accepted theories, schools of thought, and major diagnostic and therapeutic procedures in the field of psychiatry.

a. The curriculum must include a significant number of interdisciplinary clinical conferences and didactic seminars for residents in which psychiatric faculty members collaborate with neurologists, internists, and colleagues from other medical specialties and mental health disciplines.

b. Didactic instruction must be systematically organized, thoughtfully integrated, and based on sound educational principles, and must include prepared lectures, seminars, and assigned readings that are carried out on a regularly scheduled basis. In a progressive fashion, it should expose residents to topics appropriate to their level of training as outlined in Section V.A.2, above. Staff meetings, clinical case conferences, journal clubs, and lectures by visitors are desirable adjuncts, but they must not be used as substitutes for an organized didactic curriculum.

c. The curriculum must include adequate and systematic instruction in neurobiology, psychopharmacology, and other clinical sciences relevant to psychiatry; child and adult development; major psychological theories, including learning theory and psychodynamic theory; and appropriate material from social and behavioral sciences such as sociology and anthropology. The curriculum should address development, psychopathology, and topics relevant to treatment employed with psychiatric illness, including the chronically mentally ill.

d. The residency program should provide its residents with instruction about American culture and subcultures, particularly those found in the patient community associated with the training program. This instruction should include such issues as sex, race, ethnicity, religion/spirituality, and sexual orientation. Many physicians may not be sufficiently familiar with attitudes, values, and social norms prevalent among various groups of contemporary Americans. Therefore, the curriculum should contain enough instruction about these issues to enable residents to render competent care to patients from various cultural backgrounds. This instruction must be especially comprehensive in those programs with residents whose cultural backgrounds are significantly different from those of their patients.

e. Didactic exercises should include resident presentation and discussion of clinical case material at conferences attended by faculty and fellow residents. This training should involve experiences in formulating and discussing the theoretical and practical issues involved in the diagnosis and management of the cases presented.

3. Supervision
Clinical training must include adequate, regularly scheduled, individual supervision. Each resident must have at least 2 hours of individual supervision weekly, in addition to teaching conferences and rounds, in the PG-2 through PG-4 years of training. Residents must be provided with prompt, reliable systems for communication and interaction with supervisory physicians.

4. Clinical Records
Clinical records must reflect the residents' ability to:
a. Record an adequate history and mental status, physical, and neurological examinations
b. Organize a comprehensive differential diagnosis
c. Proceed with appropriate laboratory and other diagnostic procedures
d. Develop and implement an appropriate treatment plan accompanied by regular and relevant progress notes
e. Prepare an adequate discharge summary and plan

C. Resident Policies

1. The program should not allow on-call schedules and activities outside the residency to interfere with education, performance, or clinical responsibility. The program should ensure:
a. One day out of 7 free of program duties;
b. On average, on-call duty no more than every third night;
c. Adequate backup if patient care needs create resident fatigue sufficient to jeopardize patient care or resident welfare during or following on-call periods.
2. Each resident must be given a copy of the *Essentials of Accredited Residencies* at the beginning of training.
3. Readily available procedures for assisting the resident to obtain appropriate help for significant personal or professional problems should be in place.

D. Other Required Components

1. Scholarly Activity of the Residents and Faculty
Graduate medical education must take place in an environment of inquiry and scholarship in which residents participate in the development of new knowledge, learn to evaluate research findings, and develop habits of inquiry as a continuing professional responsibility. The following components of a scholarly environment should be present:
a. The program must promote an atmosphere of scholarly inquiry, including the provision of access to ongoing research activity in psychiatry. Residents must be taught the design and interpretation of research studies, including the responsible use of informed consent, research methodology, and interpretation of data. The program must teach expertise in the critical assessment of new therapies and developments as described in the literature. Residents must be advised and supervised by faculty members qualified in the conduct of research. Programs must have a plan to foster the development of skills for those residents interested in conducting psychiatric research. This plan should include opportunities for conducting research under the supervision of a mentor and training in the principles and methods of research.
b. Active participation of the teaching staff in clinical discussions, rounds, and conferences in a manner that promotes a spirit of inquiry and scholarship. Scholarship implies an in-depth understanding of basic mechanisms of normal and abnormal states and the application of current knowledge to practice.
c. Participation in journal clubs and research conferences.
d. Active participation in regional or national professional and scientific societies, particularly through presentations at the organizations' meetings and publication in their journals.
e. Participation in research, particularly in projects that are funded following peer review and/or result in publication or presentations at regional and national scientific meetings.
f. Offering of guidance and technical support (eg, research design, statistical analysis) for residents involved in research.
g. Provision of support for resident participation in scholarly activities.

2. Progressive Responsibility
Under supervision, resident clinical experience in patient management should demonstrate graduated and progressive responsibility.

3. Teaching Opportunities
An important part of the education of the resident is the development of teaching skills. Residents should have ample opportunity to teach students in the health professions.

4. Electives
All programs should provide residents an opportunity to pursue individually chosen electives.

5. Resident Logs
There must be a record maintained of specific cases treated by residents, in a manner that does not identify patients but that illustrates each resident's clinical experience in the program. This record must demonstrate that each resident has met the educational requirements of the program with regard to variety of patients, diagnoses, and treatment modalities. In the case of

transferring residents, the records should include the experiences in the prior as well as the current program. This record should be reviewed periodically with the program director or a designee, and be made available to the surveyor of the program.

VI. Internal Evaluation

The educational effectiveness of a program must be evaluated in a systematic manner. In particular, the quality of the curriculum and the extent to which the educational goals have been met by residents must be assessed. Written evaluations by residents should be utilized in this process.

A. Evaluation of Residents

All programs should state specifically and as clearly as possible the objectives and competencies required for successful completion of the program. These objectives and criteria should be made available to residency applicants.

1. Regular, systematic, documented evaluation of the knowledge, skills, and professional growth of each resident, using appropriate criteria and procedures, must be maintained, including complete records of evaluations containing explicit statements on the resident's progress toward meeting educational objectives and his or her major strengths and weaknesses. Each evaluation should be communicated to the resident in a timely manner.
2. The program must provide opportunity for and document regularly scheduled meetings between the resident and the program director or designated faculty members. These meetings should be of sufficient frequency, length, and depth to ensure that the residents are continually aware of the quality of their progress toward attainment of professional expertise. These evaluation sessions should be held at least semiannually and preferably more frequently. The program should give residents opportunities to assess the program and the faculty in a manner that ensures resident confidentiality. Provision should be made for remediation in cases of unsatifactory performance.
3. The program must formally examine the cognitive knowledge of each resident at least annually in the PG-2 through PG-4 years, and conduct an organized examination of clinical skills at least twice during the 4 years of training.
4. Residents should be advanced to positions of higher responsibility only on the basis of evidence of their satisfactory progressive scholarship and professional growth.
5. A written set of due-process procedures must be in place for resolving problems that occur when a resident's performance fails to meet required standards. These procedures must conform to those policies and procedures adopted by the sponsoring institution for the provision of due process to all residents training in sponsored programs and must include the criteria for any adverse action, such as placing a resident on probation, or for terminating a resident whose performance is unsatisfactory. The procedures should be fair to the resident, to patients under care, and to the training program. A copy should be provided to residents at the beginning of training.
6. On any resident's departure from a program (including by graduation), the program director must prepare a letter describing the nature and length of the rotations for which the resident has been given credit. If a resident departs the program without receiving full credit for all educational experiences, the reasons for withholding credit must be specified in the letter. The resident must be given the letter, and a copy must be retained in the resident's permanent file.
7. When a resident leaves the program (including by graduation), the program director will affirm in the training record that there is no documented evidence of unethical behavior, of unprofessional behavior, or of serious question of clinical competence. Where there is such evidence, it will be comprehensively recorded, along with the responses of the resident. The evaluation should verify that the resident has demonstrated sufficient professional ability to practice competently and independently. This final evaluation should be part of the resident's permanent record maintained by the institution.

B. Program Evaluation

1. Participation in and performance of graduates on examinations for certification by the American Board of Psychiatry and Neurology may be one measure of the quality of a program used by the RRC in its evaluation of each program. Therefore, it is highly desirable that programs use such information as one measure of their quality control.
2. Programs must demonstrate that they have an ongoing mechanism to evaluate the effectiveness of their didactic and clinical teaching.

VII. Inquiries Concerning Accreditation and Certification

A. All inquiries concerning the accreditation of psychiatry residencies should be addressed to Executive Secretary, Residency Review Committee for Psychiatry, 515 N State St/Ste 2000, Chicago, IL 60610.

B. All inquiries as to whether a physician is qualified to be admitted for examination for certification in psychiatry should be addressed to Executive Vice President, American Board of Psychiatry and Neurology, 500 Lake Cook Rd/Ste 335, Deerfield, IL 60015.

ACGME: June 1994 Effective: July 1995

Program Requirements for Residency Education in Addiction Psychiatry (Psychiatry)

I. Introduction

A. Definition of the Subspecialty

Addiction psychiatry is the psychiatric subspecialty that focuses on the prevention, evaluation, and treatment of substance abuse and dependence as well as related education and research efforts. In addition, the addiction psychiatrist will be fully trained in the techniques required in the treatment of the larger group of patients with the dual diagnosis of addictive disorders and other psychiatric disorders. Subspecialty training in addiction psychiatry is a component in the continuum of the educational process in psychiatry, taking place on satisfactory completion of an Accreditation Council for Graduate Medical Education (ACGME)-accredited psychiatry residency.

B. Duration and Scope of Education

1. The training period in addiction psychiatry must be 12 months. Any program that extends training beyond these minimum requirements must present a clear educational rationale consonant with the Program Requirements and objectives for residency training in addiction psychiatry.
2. The addiction psychiatry resident must have satisfactorily completed an ACGME-accredited psychiatry residency prior to entering the program.
3. Training in addiction psychiatry that occurred during the general residency training will not be credited toward this 1-year requirement.

4. Training is best accomplished on a full-time basis. If it is undertaken on a part-time basis, the 12-month program must be completed within a 2-year period.
5. Prior to entry, each addiction psychiatry resident must be notified in writing of the required length of training for which the program is accredited. The required length of training for a particular individual may not be changed without mutual agreement during his or her program unless there is a break in his or her training or the individual requires remedial training.

C. Educational Goals and Objectives

1. The program must offer advanced training such that the knowledge, skills, clinical judgment, and attitudes essential to the practice of addiction psychiatry at the consultant level are provided.
2. Clinical experience must include the opportunity to evaluate and follow a variety of patients of both sexes, including adolescents and adult and geriatric age groups spanning a broad range of diagnoses, as enumerated in Program Requirements V.A.1.a-d. Residents must provide both primary and consultative care in both inpatient (including intensive care) and outpatient settings for patients whose conditions encompass a wide variety of types of substance abuse. Where the primary site of training is devoted to the care of patients with only a particular form of substance abuse, appropriate affiliations must be arranged to ensure that adequate exposure to a sufficient number and variety of substance-abusing patients is provided.
3. Programs must be based on a structured written curriculum with well-defined goals and objectives. Clinical, basic science, and research conferences, as well as seminars and critical literature review activities pertaining to substance abuse, must be conducted regularly and as scheduled. The curriculum must include sufficient didactic content so that the graduates will have comprehensive understanding of the pharmacology of all commonly abused substances, as well as the actions of pharmacological agents used to treat these conditions. Clinical experience and didactics should be integrated to provide appropriate progressive learning.
4. Training must focus on the biopsychosocial and functional concepts of diagnosis and treatment as applied to inpatient, outpatient, and other community settings. Iatrogenic aspects of illness, as well as sociocultural, ethnic, economic, ethical, and legal considerations that may affect or interact with the psychiatric care of these patients, must be included in the program.
5. The program should present the epidemiology of substance abuse, such as social, cultural, and familial factors affecting the availability and use of addicting substances.

II. Institutional Organization

A. The program must be administratively attached to and sponsored by a core residency program in psychiatry that holds full accreditation from the ACGME. Ongoing general psychiatry programs that have been comprehensively reorganized and reaccredited on a provisional basis may be exempted from this requirement. The program must function in close relationship to the psychiatry residency.

B. The presence of residents in addiction psychiatry must not dilute or otherwise detract from the didactic or clinical experience available to general psychiatry residents. The Residency Review Committee (RRC) shall approve the size of the resident complement. Any permanent changes in resident complement will require prior approval by the RRC.

C. The program must take place in facilities approved by the appropriate state licensing agencies and, where appropriate, by the Joint Commission on Accreditation of Healthcare Organizations.

D. There shall be a clear educational rationale for the inclusion of each participating institution. The number of and distance between participating institutions shall not impair training and participation in conferences and other organized educational aspects of the program.

E. There must be current, written affiliation agreements between the sponsoring institution of the addiction psychiatry program and each of the participating institutions that conform to institutional requirements I.C.1-5. There should be an additional agreement between the addiction psychiatry program director and the individual responsible for addiction psychiatry education in each participating institution that specifies:

1. The addiction psychiatry program goals and objectives and the means by which they will be accomplished.
2. The resources and facilities in the institution(s) that will be available to addiction psychiatry residents.
3. Information on professional liability insurance, fringe benefits, and vacations.
4. The duties and responsibilities the addiction psychiatry residents will have in each institution.
5. The relationship that will exist between addiction psychiatry residents and the residents and faculty in other programs, as appropriate.
6. The supervision each addiction psychiatry resident will receive from the faculty in each institution.
7. The provision of due process to all parties in the event of a dispute, disciplinary action, or termination.

III. Faculty and Staff

The program director and the teaching staff are responsible for the general administration of a program, including those activities related to the recruitment, selection, instruction, supervision, counseling, evaluation, and advancement of residents and the maintenance of records related to program accreditation.

A. Program Director

There must be a single program director responsible for the program. The program director should be an active clinician and must devote sufficient time to the program to ensure achievement of the educational goals and objectives. The program director should be primarily based at the main program teaching site.

1. Program Director Qualifications
   The program director must be:
   a. Certified by the American Board of Psychiatry and Neurology (ABPN) with Added Qualifications in Addiction Psychiatry or have equivalent qualifications in addiction psychiatry satisfactory to the RRC.
   b. Appropriately qualified by training and experience in psychiatric education and administration to direct and supervise the program.
   c. Licensed to practice medicine in the state where the institution that sponsors the program is located. (Certain federal programs are exempted.)
   d. Appointed in good standing to the medical staff of an institution participating in the program.
   e. Participate in scholarly activities appropriate to the subspecialty, such as local, regional, and national specialty societies; research; presentations; and publication.
2. Program Director Responsibilities
   The program director will be the person who has primary responsibility for the administration of the program. Frequent changes in leadership or long periods of temporary leadership are undesirable and may adversely affect the accreditation status of the program. The program director shall be responsible for:
   a. Preparing a written statement outlining the educational goals of the program with respect to knowledge, skills, and other attributes of residents at each level of training and for each ma-

jor rotation or other program assignment. This statement must be distributed to residents and members of the teaching staff. It should be readily available for review.

b. Supervising the recruitment, selection, and appointment process for applicants, including compliance with appropriate credentialing policies and procedures in accordance with institutional and departmental policies and procedures. The director must receive documentation from the prior general psychiatry program to verify satisfactory completion of all educational and ethical requirements for graduation before appointment to the program.

c. Ensuring the provision of written descriptions of departmental policies regarding salary and benefits, due process, sickness and other leaves, call responsibilities, and vacation time to all residents on appointment to the program. All residents must be provided with written descriptions of the malpractice coverage provided for each clinical assignment.

d. Monitoring the progress of each addiction psychiatry resident, including the maintenance of a training record that documents completion of all required components of the program as well as evaluations of residents' clinical and didactic work by supervisors and teachers. This record shall include a patient log for each addiction psychiatry resident, which shall document that each resident has completed all clinical experiences required by the program requirements and the educational objectives of the program.

e. Supervising residents through explicit written descriptions of supervisory lines of responsibility for the care of patients. Such guidelines must be communicated to all members of the program staff.

f. Regularly evaluating, with participation of members of the teaching staff, the residents' knowledge, skills, and overall performance, including the development of professional attitudes consistent with being a physician.

g. Selecting and supervising the teaching staff and other program personnel at each institution participating in the program.

h. Monitoring the quality of all didactic and clinical experiences, including the collection and review of periodic written confidential evaluations by residents of all such experiences and supervision.

i. Maintaining all other training records, including those related to appointment; departmental processes regarding due process, sickness, and other leaves; call responsibilities; and vacation time.

j. Providing a written final evaluation that documents the satisfactory completion of all program requirements for each resident who completes the program. The evaluation must include a review of the resident's performance during the final period of training and should verify that the resident has demonstrated sufficient professional ability to practice competently and independently. This final evaluation should be part of the resident's permanent record maintained by the institution.

k. Monitoring resident stress, including mental or emotional conditions inhibiting performance or learning and drug- or alcohol-related dysfunction. Program directors and teaching staff should be sensitive to the need for timely provision of confidential counseling and psychological support services to residents. Training situations that consistently produce undesirable stress on residents must be evaluated and modified.

l. Implementating fair procedures, as established by the sponsoring institution, regarding academic discipline and resident complaints or grievances.

m. Notifying the RRC promptly of any major changes in the program or its leadership. Participation by any institution providing more than 3 months of training must be approved by the RRC.

n. Preparing timely, accurate program information forms and related materials in preparation for review by the RRC.

o. Reporting to the RRC by September 1 of each year the name of each resident in the program.

B. Number and Qualifications of the Physician Faculty

All members of the teaching staff must demonstrate a strong interest in the education of residents, sound clinical and teaching abilities, support of the goals and objectives of the program, a commitment to their own continuing medical education, and participation in scholarly activities.

1. There must be a sufficient number of physician faculty members with documented qualifications to maintain a quality didactic and clinical educational program and to ensure adequate instruction and supervision of all residents in the program. In addition to the program director, there must be at least one other faculty member certified by the ABPN with Added Qualifications in Addiction Psychiatry or its equivalent. Programs with large patient populations, multiple institutions, and large resident complements will be expected to have additional faculty appropriate to their size and structure.
2. These individuals must be additionally qualified by experience in addiction psychiatry to provide the expertise needed to fulfill the didactic, clinical, and research goals of the program.
3. The faculty must devote sufficient time to the educational program in addiction psychiatry to ensure fulfillment of its goals and objectives and to meet their supervisory and teaching responsibilities.
4. The responsibility for establishing and maintaining an environment of inquiry and scholarship rests with the teaching staff. While not all members of a teaching staff must be investigators, the staff as a whole must demonstrate broad involvement in scholarly activity. This activity should include:
   a. Active participation of the teaching staff in clinical discussions, rounds, and conferences in a manner that promotes a spirit of inquiry and scholarship. Scholarship implies an in-depth understanding of basic mechanisms of normal and abnormal states and the application of current knowledge to practice.
   b. Participation in journal clubs and research conferences.
   c. Active participation in regional or national professional and scientific societies, particularly through presentations at the organizations' meetings and publication in their journals.
   d. Participation in research, particularly in projects that are funded following peer review and/or result in publication or presentations at regional and national scientific meetings.
   e. Offering of guidance and technical support (eg, research design, statistical analysis) for residents involved in research.
   f. Provision of support for resident participation in scholarly activities.
5. The teaching staff must be organized and have regular documented meetings to review program goals and objectives as well as program effectiveness in achieving them. At least one resident representative should participate in these reviews.
6. The director of addiction psychiatry training at each participating institution shall be appointed by or with the concurrence of the addiction psychiatry program director to assume responsibility for the day-to-day activities of the program at that institution, with overall coordination by the program director.

C. Multidisciplinary Team Exposure

Addiction psychiatry residents must be provided with meaningful patient care experiences as part of an interdisciplinary care team. The resident should work in settings that include representatives from clinical disciplines such as social work, psychology, psychiatric nursing, therapeutic activities, pharmacology, and nutrition, as well as clinicians in anesthesia (including pain management), emergency medicine, family practice, geriatrics, internal medicine, neurology, obstetrics-gynecology, surgical specialties, and pediatric/adolescent medicine as appropriate for the care of the patient. In addition, residents should work with others such as substance abuse counselors and, where appropriate, with teachers.

D. Other Program Personnel

Programs must be provided with the additional professional, technical, and clerical personnel needed to support the administration and educational conduct of the program.

IV. Facilities and Resources

All elements of the program must be located in designated facilities based on written affiliation agreements between the participating institutions and the administration of the program.

A. Inpatient Care Facility

The department sponsoring the program must be a part of, or affiliated with, at least one acute-care general hospital with a full range of services, including medical and surgical services, intensive care units, emergency department, diagnostic laboratory, and imaging services. If the acute-care hospital is specialized and does not itself have the full spectrum of services described above, the program must document that it has access for training purposes to other affiliated acute-care facilities that have the services not present at the specialized facility.

B. Partial Hospitalization and Day Treatment Center

Programs must have access to a partial hospitalization or other day-care program. Such programs may be located in community-based institutions or within the sponsoring department of psychiatry in its acute-care hospital. Exposure to self-help and other community programs (such as 12-step programs widely used by substance-abusing patients) must be provided.

C. Ambulatory Care Service

The program must provide experience in a multidisciplinary ambulatory care facility such as a methadone maintenance clinic, an alcohol treatment clinic, or other specialized outpatient program.

D. Library

Residents must have ready access to a major medical library, either at the institution where the residents are located or through arrangement with convenient nearby institutions.

1. Library services should include the electronic retrieval of information from medical databases.
2. There must be access to an on-site library or to a collection of appropriate texts and journals in each institution participating in a residency program. On-site libraries and/or collections of texts and journals must be readily available during nights and weekends.

E. Ancillary Support Services

At all participating facilities, there must be appropriate support services to ensure an adequate educational experience. This includes support personnel in all categories and physical resources to ensure that residents have sufficient time and space to carry out their clinical and educational functions.

F. Patient Population

The number and variety of new and follow-up patients spanning the life cycle from adolescence to old age must be sufficient to ensure an adequate outpatient and inpatient experience, as specified in I.C.2 and V.A.1-7. The spectrum of patients should include diverse socioeconomic, educational, and cultural backgrounds.

G. Additional Educational Environment

The program must provide opportunities for the residents to render continuing care and to exercise leadership responsibilities in organizing recommendations from the treatment team, including the integration of recommendations from consulting medical specialists and other professionals in allied disciplines.

H. Faculty Supervision

Residents must be supervised in the performance of procedures integral to the specialty of addiction psychiatry. Supervision must include observation, assessment, and substantiation of the residents' knowledge and skills in clinical evaluation, technical proficiency, and professional attitudes. Residents must be provided with prompt, reliable systems for communication and interaction with supervisory physicians.

V. Educational Program

The director and teaching staff of a program must prepare and comply with written educational goals for the program. All educational components of a residency program should be related to program goals. The program design and/or structure must be approved by the RRC for Psychiatry as part of the regular review process. The training program must provide opportunities for residents to develop advanced clinical knowledge and skills in the field of addiction psychiatry. These objectives will be accomplished by a combination of supervised clinical experience and formal didactic conferences. The curriculum must ensure the opportunity for residents to achieve the cognitive knowledge, interpersonal skills, professional attitudes, and practical experience required of an addiction psychiatrist providing acute and chronic care for the substance-abusing patient. All major dimensions of the curriculum must be structured educational experiences guided by written goals and objectives as well as by specified teaching and evaluation methods. The goals and objectives of each major component of the curriculum must be provided to the residents in writing on entering the program.

A. Clinical Experiences

The training program must include the following clinical components:

1. Evaluation, consultation, and treatment of
   a. Patients with primary alcohol and/or drug abuse and their families.
   b. Medical and surgical patients in the emergency department, intensive care units, and general wards of the hospital with acute and chronic drug and/or alcohol abuse and dependency, including acute intoxication and overdose.
   c. Psychiatric inpatients and outpatients with chemical dependencies and comorbid psychopathology, to include a broad range of psychiatric diagnoses, such as affective disorders, psychotic disorders, organic disorders, personality disorders, and anxiety disorders, as well as patients suffering from medical conditions commonly associated with substance abuse such as hepatitis and acquired immune deficiency syndrome.
   d. Medication-dependent patients with chronic medical disorders.
2. Exposure to the following substance-abuse problems:
   a. Alcohol
   b. Opioids
   c. Cocaine and other stimulants

d. Marijuana and hallucinogens
e. Benzodiazepines
f. Other drugs of abuse, including sedative/hypnotics and nicotine
g. Miscellaneous/unusual, eg, khat, nutmeg, designer drugs, organic solvents

3. Resident treatment of a minimum of five addicted outpatients with a variety of diagnoses requiring individual treatment for at least 6 months.
4. Rotations should provide residents with experience in evaluating acute and chronic substance-abusing patients in inpatient and outpatient settings. There should be an identifiable structured educational experience in neuropsychiatry relevant to the practice of addiction psychiatry that includes both didactic and clinical training methods. The curriculum should emphasize functional assessment, signs and symptoms of neuropsychiatric impairment associated with substance abuse, and the identification of physical illnesses and iatrogenic factors that can alter mental status, behavior, and management.
5. The program must provide specific experience in consultation to acute and chronic, medically ill substance-abusing patients being treated on medical, emergency, intensive care, and/or surgical services of a general hospital. Supervision of addiction psychiatry residents in their clinical evaluation of such patients, as well as in their consultative role, is essential. The program should provide residents with the opportunity to function at the level of a specialist consultant to physicians in the primary care specialties and to intensive care specialists.
6. Experience in working with multidisciplinary teams as a consultant and as a team leader.
7. Experience in working with patients who are concurrently participating in self-help programs.

B. Curriculum Content

The field of addiction psychiatry requires knowledge of neurology, pharmacology, psychiatry, general medicine, and psychology, as well as an understanding of the interaction of these disciplines. Programs must include both direct experience in clinical care and formal conferences. Instruction and experience must include the performance of the mental status examination, a neuropsychiatric evaluation instrument such as the Mini-Mental Status examination, community and environmental assessment, family and caregiver assessment, medical assessment, and physical and psychological functional assessments. These skills compose the basis for formal assessment of the addicted patient using a synthesis of clinical findings, historical and current information, and data from laboratory and other special studies. Residents must acquire knowledge and skills in the following areas:

1. Knowledge of the signs and symptoms of the use and abuse of all of the major categories of drugs enumerated in V.A.2.a-g, as well as knowledge of the types of treatment required for each.
2. Knowledge of the signs of withdrawal from these major categories of drugs and knowledge and experience with the range of options for treatment of the withdrawal syndromes and the complications commonly associated with such withdrawal.
3. Knowledge of the signs and symptoms of overdose, the medical and psychiatric sequelae of overdose, and experience in providing proper treatment of overdose.
4. Management of detoxification and acute hospital treatment of the chronic user of the major categories of drugs. Experience in working collaboratively with specialists in the emergency department and intensive care units in the diagnosis and management of acute overdose symptoms.
5. Knowledge of the signs and symptoms of the social and psychological problems as well as the medical and psychiatric disorders that often accompany the chronic use and abuse of the major categories of drugs.
6. Experience in the use of psychoactive medications in the treatment of psychiatric disorders often accompanying the major categories of substance abuse.
7. Experience in the use of techniques required for confrontation of and intervention with a chronic drug abuser and in dealing with the defense mechanisms that cause the patient to resist entry into treatment.
8. Experience in the use of the various psychotherapeutic modalities involved in the ongoing management of the chronic drug-abusing patient, including individual psychotherapies, couples therapy, family therapy, cognitive-behavioral therapy, and group therapy.
9. Experience in working collaboratively with other mental health providers and allied health professionals, including nurses, social workers, psychologists, nurse practitioners, counselors, pharmacists, and others who participate in the care of substance-abusing patients.
10. Knowledge and understanding of the special problems of the pregnant drug abuser and of the babies born to substance-abusing mothers.
11. Knowledge of family systems and dynamics relevant to the etiology, diagnosis, and treatment of substance abuse disorders.
12. Knowledge of the genetic vulnerabilities, risk and protective factors, epidemiology, and prevention of substance-abuse disorders.
13. Familiarity with the major medical journals and professional-scientific organizations dealing with research on the understanding and treatment of substance abuse.
14. Critical analysis of research reports, as presented in journal clubs and seminars.
15. Experience in teaching and supervising student clinicians in the care of substance-abusing patients.
16. Understanding of the current economic aspects of providing psychiatric and other health-care services to the addicted patient.
17. Knowledge of quality assurance measures and cost effectiveness of various treatment modalities for substance-abusing patients.

C. Conferences

Conferences in addiction psychiatry, such as grand rounds, case conferences, reading seminars, and journal clubs, should be specifically designed to complement the clinical experiences. Regular attendance by residents and faculty should be documented.

D. Policies Regarding Residents, Supervision, and Participation

1. The program director must ensure, direct, and document proper supervision of all addiction psychiatry residents at all times by appropriately qualified faculty. The responsibility and independence allowed residents in patient contact should depend on their knowledge, skill, experience, and the complexity of the clinical problem. Residents must be provided with rapid, reliable methods for communicating with supervising physicians. Each resident must have a minimum of 2 hours of individual supervision of clinical activities weekly.
2. The program should carefully monitor and document any clinical activity outside the program that could potentially interfere with educational performance or clinical responsibility. The program must carefully monitor all on-call schedules and hours within the program to ensure a balanced and appropriate educational and clinical experience. This monitoring should ensure
   a. one full day out of 7 free of program-related duties.
   b. on average, on-call duty no more than every third night.
   c. adequate backup if patient care needs create resident fatigue sufficient to jeopardize patient care or resident welfare during or following on-call periods.

d. adequate faculty backup if residents encounter complex clinical situations while on call.
3. At all program facilities, residents must be afforded responsibilities commensurate with their postgraduate status and experience level in the provision of patient care.

E. Other Program Components

1. Scholarly Activity
Graduate medical education must take place in an environment of inquiry and scholarship in which residents participate in the development of new knowledge, learn to evaluate research findings, and develop habits of inquiry as a continuing professional responsibility. As part of the academic environment, an active scholarly component must be included within the addiction psychiatry program. Faculty members should participate actively in basic, clinical, and/or health services research.
The program should provide each resident with a meaningful, individually supervised opportunity to participate in research or scholarly activity.
2. Presence of Other Training Programs
The addiction psychiatry program should provide peer interaction between its residents and those of other medical specialties. To achieve this goal, an ACGME-accredited training program in at least one nonpsychiatric specialty should be present within the participating institutions of the program, such as neurology, internal medicine, or family practice. Peer interaction among the programs should occur in the course of clinical and/or didactic work, but is most satisfactory when organized around joint patient evaluation and/or care.
3. Resident Teaching Experiences
The program should provide appropriate experiences designed to develop the administrative and teaching skills of the addiction psychiatry residents. As the residents progress through the program, they should have the opportunity to teach personnel such as other residents, medical students, nurses, and other allied health professionals.

VI. Evaluation

A. Evaluation of Residents

There must be at least quarterly written evaluations of the residents by all supervisors and the directors of clinical components of training. These must be discussed with the residents and placed in the training record. The program director shall:

1. At least semiannually evaluate the knowledge, skills, and professional growth of the residents, using appropriate criteria and procedures.
2. Communicate each evaluation to the resident in a timely manner.
3. Advance residents to positions of higher responsibility only on the basis of evidence of their satisfactory progressive scholarship and professional growth.
4. Maintain a permanent record of evaluation for each resident and have it accessible to the resident and other authorized personnel.

B. Faculty Evaluation

There must be in place a mechanism for the written confidential evaluation of all supervisors by addiction psychiatry residents, as well as of the didactic and clinical elements of the educational program.

C. Program Evaluation

1. The educational effectiveness of a program must be evaluated in a systematic manner. In particular, the quality of the curriculum and the extent to which the educational goals have been met by residents must be assessed. The teaching staff should periodically evaluate the utilization of the resources available to the program, the contribution of each institution participating in the program, the financial and administrative support of the program, the volume and variety of patients available to the program for educational purposes, the performance of members of the teaching staff, and the quality of supervision of residents.
2. Written evaluations by residents should be utilized in this process.
3. One measure of the quality of the program will be participation in and performance of its graduates on the Added Qualifications certifying examination conducted by the ABPN.

VII. Certification

Those individuals planning to seek Added Qualifications certification through the ABPN should communicate with the administrative officer of the ABPN prior to beginning training to ascertain its requirements.

ACGME: September 1994 Effective: July 1995

Program Requirements for Residency Education in Child and Adolescent Psychiatry (Psychiatry)

I. Introduction

Scope of Training

Child and adolescent psychiatry is a specialty of medical practice within psychiatry. The goal of residency training in child and adolescent psychiatry is to produce specialists in the delivery of skilled and comprehensive medical care of children and adolescents suffering from psychiatric disorders. The child and adolescent psychiatrist must have a thorough understanding of the development and prevention of psychopathology as it appears from infancy through adulthood. He or she should also have the skills to serve as an effective consultant to primary care physicians and to community agencies and institutions serving children and adolescents.

Approved residencies in child and adolescent psychiatry must offer well-supervised and well-balanced clinical experiences with inpatients, outpatients, and consultees and must also provide a formal educational experience. The residency must provide a combination of didactic and clinical work that is both broad enough to ensure knowledge of the full spectrum of disorders of childhood and adolescence and yet intensive enough to ensure thorough diagnostic, treatment, and consultative skills. Diagnostic and therapeutic experiences must be provided in sufficient numbers and depth with preschool, grade school, and adolescent patients of both sexes and their families for the resident to understand the disorders and situations studied.

II. Program Length and Prerequisites

A. In addition to the postgraduate first year and a minimum of 2 years of accredited training in general psychiatry, 2 years' training in an Accreditation Council for Graduate Medical Education-accredited child and adolescent psychiatry program is required.
B. To achieve greater flexibility in the sequence of residency training and to assist in recruitment, the 2-year child and adolescent psychiatry training experience may be initiated at any point beyond the PGY-1 level in the psychiatry residency sequence. Training is best done full-time, and it must be done in no more than two blocks. If done in two blocks, the blocks must not be more than 5 years apart, and the shorter block must not be less than 6 months long. At the discretion of the program director, 1 year of training credit may be given for 2 years at half-time; 2 years of

training credit may be given for 3 years at two-thirds time or 4 years at half-time.

C. In general, training in child and adolescent psychiatry obtained as part of the curriculum for general psychiatry training may not count toward residency training in child and adolescent psychiatry. However, certain clinical experiences, including but not limited to pediatric neurology, forensic consultation, and pediatric consultation/liaison, may be designed to fulfill the Program Requirements in general psychiatry and child and adolescent psychiatry if approved by both program directors. The program director must document areas for which credit is given in both programs. These experiences may not be used to reduce the total length of time devoted to training in either general or child and adolescent psychiatry.

D. Prior to entry into the program, each resident must be notified in writing of the required length of training for which the program is accredited. The required length of training for a particular resident may not be changed during his or her program without mutual agreement, unless there is an interruption in his or her training or the resident requires remedial training.

III. Institutional Organization

A. Institutional Support

The administration of the sponsoring institution(s) should understand the educational goals and should evidence its willingness and ability to support these goals philosophically and financially.

B. Affiliation Agreements

1. In programs where more than one clinical site is used for the training of residents, there must be affiliation agreements between the sponsor of the child and adolescent psychiatry residency and each participating institution that conform to Institutional Requirements I.C.1-5.
2. In addition, each training program accredited for child and adolescent psychiatry must have a formal educational affiliation agreement with a psychiatry residency program that is accredited for at least 3 years of training. The written agreement of such affiliation must be signed by the residency directors of both programs, and copies must be filed with the Residency Review Committee (RRC).

C. Participating Institutions

It is important that each affiliated institution offer significant educational opportunities to the overall program. The number and distribution of participating training sites must not preclude satisfactory participation by residents in teaching and training exercises. Geographic proximity will be one factor in evaluating program cohesion, continuity, and "critical mass." Affiliated training sites will be evaluated on the basis of whether they contribute to a well-integrated educational program with respect to both didactic and clinical experiences.

D. Appointment of Residents

1. The program should document the procedures used to select residents in accordance with institutional and departmental policies and procedures. Application records should document information from graduate medical education programs. A documented procedure should be in place for checking the credentials, the clinical training experiences, and the past performance and professional integrity of residents transferring from one program to another, including from an adult to a child and adolescent psychiatry program. This procedure must include solicitation and documentation of relevant information from the training directors of the previous programs participated in by the transferring resident.
2. The residency program director must accept only those applicants whose qualifications for residency include sufficient command of English to permit accurate, unimpeded communication.
3. A program must have at least two residents in each of the 2 years of training. Peer interaction and the need for group discussion in seminars and conferences are crucial.
4. The number of residents from other graduate medical education programs and mental health disciplines who participate in the child and adolescent psychiatry educational curriculum should not be so large as to compromise the educational resources of the child and adolescent psychiatry residency.

IV. Faculty Qualifications and Responsibilities

There must be a single program director responsible for the program. The program director and the teaching staff are responsible for the general administration of a program, including those activities related to the recruitment, selection, instruction, supervision, counseling, evaluation, and advancement of residents and the maintenance of records related to program accreditation.

A. Program Director Qualifications

1. Qualifications of the Program Director include:
   a. The residency program in child and adolescent psychiatry must be under the direction of a fully trained child and adolescent psychiatrist with documented clinical, educational, and administrative abilities and experience, who is certified in child and adolescent psychiatry by the American Board of Psychiatry and Neurology (ABPN) or who possesses suitable equivalent qualifications as determined by the RRC.
   b. The program director must be licensed to practice medicine in the state where the institution that sponsors the program is located. (Certain federal programs are exempted.)
   c. The program director must be appointed to and in good standing with the medical staff of an institution participating in the program.
2. Responsibilities of the Program Director
   The program director is responsible for selecting residents, planning the curriculum, evaluating individual resident progress, and maintaining records of these endeavors. The program director shall provide residents with the goals of training, their responsibilities, and the evaluation procedures. Responsibilities of the program director include:
   a. Devotion of at least half-time to the training program, including teaching activities.
   b. Preparation of a written statement outlining the educational goals of the program with respect to knowledge, skills, and other attributes of residents at each level of training and for each major rotation or other program assignment. This statement must be distributed to applicants, residents, and members of the teaching staff. It should be readily available for review.
   c. Selection of residents for appointment to the program in accordance with institutional and departmental policies and procedures.
   d. Selection and supervision of the teaching staff and other program personnel at each institution participating in the program in consultation with the chair or division chief.
   e. The supervision of residents through explicit written descriptions of supervisory lines of responsibility for the care of patients. Such guidelines must be communicated to all members of the program staff.
   f. Regular evaluation, with participation of members of the teaching staff, of residents' knowledge, skills, and overall performance, including the development of professional attitudes consistent with being a physician as specified in Section VI.

g. The provision of a written final evaluation for each resident who completes the program and maintenance of a permanent record of evaluation for each resident that is accessible to the resident and other authorized personnel.
h. Implementation of fair procedures, as established by the sponsoring institution, regarding academic discipline and resident complaints or grievances.
i. Monitoring resident stress, including mental or emotional conditions inhibiting performance or learning and drug- or alcohol-related dysfunction. Program directors and teaching staff should be sensitive to the need for timely provision of confidential counseling and psychological support services to residents. Training situations that consistently produce undesirable stress on residents must be evaluated and modified.
j. Evaluation of faculty teaching and supervision in writing.
k. Providing applicants with written descriptions of the clinical rotations and educational program. Written information must be provided regarding financial compensation, liability coverage, and the policies regarding vacations, sick leave, and family leave, as well as other special leaves.
l. Preparation of an accurate statistical and narrative description of the program as requested by the RRC for Psychiatry.
m. Notification requirements—the program leadership is responsible for notifying the executive secretary of the RRC in writing within 30 days of any major change in the program that may significantly alter the educational experience for the residents, including:
   1. Changes in leadership of the department or the program.
   2. Changes in administrative structure, such as an alteration in the status of the program/department within the institution.
   3. Any year there is a reduction in the critical mass of residents below two for each year of training.
   4. A reduction in the number of faculty below three full-time-equivalent positions in more than 1 year.
n. Prior approval requirements—the program director must obtain prior approval for the following changes in the RRC program to determine if an adequate educational environment exists to support these changes and if the program's clinical and academic resources are adequate to support these changes:
   1. The addition or deletion of any training site to which residents are assigned half-time or more for 6 months or longer for the full-time equivalent of at least 4 months.
   2. Any increase in the approved resident complement of the program.

B. Number and Qualifications of the Faculty

1. The residency must be staffed by an appropriate number of capable, qualified psychiatrists and other mental health professionals with sufficient breadth and depth of documented qualifications to instruct and supervise adequately all the residents in the program. Members of the teaching staff must be able to devote sufficient time to meet their supervisory and teaching responsibilities. The faculty must include a total of at least three full-time-equivalent, fully trained child and adolescent psychiatrists who devote substantial time to the residency program.
2. The psychiatric faculty should be certified by the ABPN or have equivalent qualifications in psychiatry satisfactory to or determined by the RRC for Psychiatry.
3. Psychiatric faculty must participate regularly and systematically in the training program. All members of the teaching staff must demonstrate a strong interest in the education of residents, sound clinical and teaching abilities, support of the goals and objectives of the program, a commitment to their own continuing medical education, and participation in scholarly activities.
4. A member of the teaching staff of each participating institution must be designated to assume responsibility for the day-to-day activities of the program at that institution, with overall coordination by the program director.
5. The teaching staff must be organized and have regular documented meetings to review program goals and objectives as well as program effectiveness in achieving them. At least one resident representative should participate in these reviews.

C. Other Program Personnel

Programs must be provided with the additional professional, technical, and clerical personnel needed to support the administration and educational conduct of the program.

V. Facilities and Resources

A. Training programs must have adequate facilities and affiliations to meet the educational objectives of the program. Adequate office space with readily accessible play materials must be available for each resident to see patients.
B. Special space for physical and neurological examinations, as well as the appropriate medical equipment, must be readily available in the training facility.
C. There must be adequate space and equipment specifically designated for seminars, lectures, and other educational activities. The program must have available such basic teaching aids as one-way mirrors and audiovisual equipment.
D. The sponsoring institution must provide residents with ready access to a library that contains a substantial number of current basic textbooks and major journals in psychiatry, child and adolescent psychiatry, neurologic pediatrics, and general medicine, sufficient for an excellent educational program. The library must be capable of obtaining textbooks and journals on loan from major medical libraries and of carrying out MEDLINE and other medical information searches (or accessing a library that has this capacity), and it must be reasonably available to residents on weekends and during evening hours.

VI. Educational Program

A. Goals

The director and teaching staff of a program must prepare and comply with written educational goals for the program. All educational components of a residency program should be related to program goals. There must be sufficient, stable leadership, faculty, clinical facilities, and affiliations to provide a consistent educational experience. The program design and/or structure must be approved by the RRC as part of the regular review process.

B. Curriculum

An approved program must have an explicitly described and distributed educational curriculum composed of formal didactic instruction and a program of graduated learning and supervised experience through the 2 years. The latter is to be marked by graduated and increased clinical responsibility for the diagnosis and treatment of preschool and grade-school children, adolescents, and their families.

Educational quality must have the highest priority in the allotment of the residents' time and energy. The clinical responsibilities of residents must not infringe unduly upon didactic activities.

C. Clinical Experience

1. Each resident must have responsibility for the evaluation and treatment of a sufficient number and adequate variety of patients representing the full spectrum of psychiatric illnesses in

children and adolescents. The number of patients for which residents have primary responsibility at any one time must permit them to provide each patient with appropriate treatment and to have sufficient time for other aspects of their educational program. The depth and variety of clinical experiences must be adequate.

2. Clinical records, recorded by the child and adolescent psychiatry residents, should document an adequate individual and family history, mental status, physical and neurological examinations when appropriate, supplementary medical and psychological data, and integration of these data into a formulation, differential diagnosis, and comprehensive treatment plan.
3. Opportunities for the development of both conceptual understanding of and clinical skills in the major types of therapy with children and adolescents, including short- and long-term individual psychotherapy, psychodynamic psychotherapy, family therapy, crisis intervention, and pharmacological therapies, must be provided. There must be opportunities for residents to be involved in providing continuous care for a variety of patients from different age groups, seen regularly and frequently for an extended time, in a variety of treatment modalities. Residents should have some experience with continuity of patient care across clinical programs providing different levels of care. Work with outpatients must include work with some child and adolescent patients for at least a year's duration.
4. Residents must receive training so that they have an opportunity to evaluate and to treat patients from various cultural backgrounds and socioeconomic levels.
5. Training must include supervised, active collaboration with other professional mental health personnel (ie, psychologists, psychiatric nurses, social workers) in the evaluation and treatment of patients.
6. There must be teaching about the appropriate uses and limitations of psychological tests. Residents should have the opportunity to observe some of their patients being tested.
7. There must be teaching and clinical experience in pediatric neurology, mental retardation, and other developmental disorders.
8. Residents should have experiences in the management of psychiatric emergencies and acute disturbances in children and adolescents.
9. Experience with 24-hour responsibility in working with acutely and severely disturbed children or young adolescents is an essential part of training. This experience must occur in settings with an organized treatment program, such as inpatient units, residential treatment facilities, partial hospitalization programs, and/or day treatment programs. This experience must be the full-time equivalent of not less than 4 nor more than 10 months.
10. Residents must have experience as consultants in situations in which they do not primarily engage in treatment but use their specialized knowledge and skills to assist others to function better in their roles. Training and experience in consultation to facilities serving children, adolescents, and their families should include:
    a. Supervised consultation experience with an adequate number of pediatric patients in outpatient and/or inpatient medical facilities
    b. Supervised formal observation and/or consultation experiences in schools
    c. Training and experience in legal issues relevant to child and adolescent psychiatry, including forensic consultation experience and court testimony
11. Administrative experiences, in which residents function in positions of leadership, are essential.

D. Didactic Curriculum

Didactic instruction must be well organized, thoughtfully integrated, based on sound educational principles, and carried out on a regularly scheduled basis. Systematically organized formal instruction (prepared lectures, seminars, assigned reading, etc) must be integral to the residency. Staff meetings, clinical case conferences, journal clubs, and lectures by visitors are desirable adjuncts, but must not be used as substitutes for an organized didactic curriculum.

1. Emphasis on developmental considerations is the hallmark of training in child and adolescent psychiatry. The teaching of developmental knowledge and the integration of biopsychosocial data into a comprehensive formulation of clinical problems are essential. Teaching about normal development should include observation of and interaction with normal children.
2. The didactic and clinical curriculum must be of sufficient breadth and depth to provide residents with a thorough and well-balanced presentation of the generally accepted theories; schools of thought; and major diagnostic, therapeutic, and preventive procedures in the field of child and adolescent psychiatry.
3. The curriculum must include adequate and systematic instruction in basic biological, psychological, and clinical sciences relevant to psychiatry; in psychodynamic theory; and in the application of developmental psychological theories relevant to the understanding of psychopathology. It must provide teaching about the full gamut of psychopathology in children and adolescents, including the etiologies, epidemiology, diagnosis, treatment, and prevention of all of the psychiatric conditions that affect children and adolescents.
4. There must be teaching in ethical aspects of child and adolescent psychiatric practice.
5. The opportunity for residents to be involved in research must be available.
6. The curriculum must include an adequate number of interdisciplinary clinical conferences and didactic seminars for residents, in which faculty psychiatrists collaborate in teaching with colleagues from other medical specialties and mental health disciplines.

E. Other Required Components

1. Scholarly Activity

   Graduate medical education must take place in an environment of inquiry and scholarship in which residents participate in the development of new knowledge, learn to evaluate research findings, and develop habits of inquiry as a continuing professional responsibility. The responsibility for establishing and maintaining an environment of inquiry and scholarship rests with the teaching staff. While not all members of a teaching staff must be investigators, the staff as a whole must demonstrate broad involvement in scholarly activity. This activity should include:
    a. Active participation of the teaching staff in clinical discussions, rounds, and conferences in a manner that promotes a spirit of inquiry and scholarship. Scholarship implies an in-depth understanding of basic mechanisms of normal and abnormal states and the application of current knowledge to practice.
    b. Participation in journal clubs and research conferences.
    c. Active participation in regional or national professional and scientific societies, particularly through presentations at the organizations' meetings and publication in their journals.
    d. Participation in research, particularly in projects that are funded following peer review and/or result in publications or presentations at regional and national scientific meetings.
    e. Offering of guidance and technical support (eg, research design, statistical analysis) for residents involved in research.

f. Provision of support for resident participation in scholarly activities.

2. Teaching Opportunities
Opportunities for residents to teach community groups, medical students, and/or other residents should be available.

F. Resident Policies

1. Supervision
Each resident must have at least 2 hours of individual supervision weekly, in addition to teaching conferences and rounds. Residents must be provided with prompt, reliable systems for communication and interaction with supervisory physicians.
2. Duty Hours
The program should carefully monitor any professional activity outside the residency and ensure that it does not interfere with education, performance, or clinical responsibility. The program should carefully monitor all on-call schedules and hours within and outside residency to prevent undue interference with education, performance, or clinical responsibility. The monitoring should ensure:
a. On average, 1 full day out of 7 free of program duties.
b. On average, on-call duty no more than every third night.
c. Adequate backup if patient care needs create resident fatigue sufficient to jeopardize patient care or resident welfare during or following on-call periods.

VII. Internal Evaluation

The program will maintain records of all evaluations required in this section and these will be made available on review of the program.

A. Evaluation of Residents

1. The program must provide opportunity for and document regularly scheduled meetings between the resident and the program director or designated faculty members. These meetings should be of sufficient frequency, length, and depth to ensure that the residents are continually aware of the quality of their progress toward attainment of program goals. At least semiannually, the program director must evaluate the knowledge, skills, and professional growth of the residents, using appropriate criteria and procedures. Provision should be made for remediation in cases of unsatisfactory performance.
2. Each evaluation must be communicated to the resident in a timely manner.
3. Residents must be advanced to positions of higher responsibility only on the basis of evidence of their satisfactory progressive scholarship and professional growth.
4. In addition to periodic assessments, an annual evaluation procedure is required that must include a written examination of the knowledge base as well as a formal documented clinical skills examination.
5. Evaluation must include a review of the resident's performance during the final period of training and should verify that the resident has demonstrated sufficient professional ability to practice competently and independently. At the time of the resident's graduation, the program director will affirm in the training record that there is no documented evidence of unethical behavior, unprofessional behavior, or clinical incompetence. Where there is such evidence, it must be comprehensively recorded, along with the responses of the resident. This final evaluation should be part of the resident's permanent record maintained by the institution.
6. A written set of due-process procedures must be in place for resolving problems that occur if a resident's performance fails to meet required standards. These must include the criteria for any adverse action, such as placing a resident on probation, or for terminating a resident whose performance is unsatisfactory. The procedures should be fair to the resident, patients under care, and the training program. A copy should be provided to the residents at the beginning of training.

B. Faculty Evaluation

The program director is responsible for the evaluation of faculty teaching and supervision, which must include an annual written assessment of faculty members by the residents.

C. Program Evaluation

The educational effectiveness of a program must be evaluated in a systematic manner. In particular, the quality of the curriculum and the extent to which the educational goals have been met by residents must be assessed. Written evaluations by residents should be utilized in this process. The teaching staff should periodically evaluate the utilization of the resources available to the program, the contribution of each institution participating in the program, the financial and administrative support of the program, the volume and variety of patients available to the program for educational purposes, the performance of members of the teaching staff, and the quality of supervision of residents.

ACGME: June 1994 Effective: July 1995

Program Requirements For Residency Education in Forensic Psychiatry (Psychiatry)

I. Introduction

A. Definition of the Subspecialty

Forensic psychiatry is the psychiatric subspecialty that focuses on interrelationships between psychiatry and the law (including civil, criminal, and administrative law), including (1) the psychiatric evaluation of individuals involved with the legal system; (2) the specialized psychiatric treatment required by those who have been incarcerated in jails, prisons, or special forensic psychiatric hospitals; (3) active involvement in the area of legal regulation of general psychiatric practice; and (4) related education and research efforts. Subspecialty training in forensic psychiatry is a component in the continuum of the educational process in psychiatry, taking place on satisfactory completion of a psychiatry residency accredited by the Accreditation Council for Graduate Medical Education (ACGME).

B. Duration and Scope of Education

1. The training period in forensic psychiatry must be 12 months.
2. Training in forensic psychiatry that occurs during the general residency training will not be credited toward this 1-year requirement.
3. Training is best accomplished on a full-time basis. If it is undertaken on a part-time basis, the 12-month program must be completed within a 2-year period.
4. Prior to entry, each forensic psychiatry resident must be notified in writing of the required length of training for which the program is accredited and the requirements for satisfactory completion of the program. Neither the required length of training for a particular individual nor the graduation requirements may be changed without mutual agreement during his or her program unless there is a break in his or her training or the individual requires remedial training.

C. Educational Goals and Objectives

1. The program must offer advanced training that affords sufficient opportunities for the resident to develop the knowledge, skills, clinical judgment, and attitudes essential to the practice of forensic psychiatry.
2. Clinical experience must include experiences in the following three areas: (a) forensic evaluation of a variety of subjects of both genders, including adolescent, adult, and geriatric age groups, spanning a broad range of mental disorders and circumstances, including both civil and criminal contexts; (b) consultation to general psychiatric services on issues related to the legal regulation of psychiatric practice, such as civil commitment, confidentiality, refusal of treatment, decision-making competence, guardianship, etc; (c) treatment of persons involved in the criminal justice system. Appropriate affiliations must be arranged to ensure that adequate exposure to a sufficient number and variety of experiences is provided.
3. Programs must be based on a structured written curriculum with well-defined goals and objectives. Clinical case conferences and seminars dealing with topics such as law, ethics, the relevant basic and social sciences, and research must be conducted regularly and as scheduled. The curriculum must include sufficient didactic content so that graduates will be knowledgeable about the content outlined in V.A.2.a-d.
4. Training must focus on the social and legal context for forensic work, both civil and criminal. Instruction should take into account the sociocultural, ethnic, economic, and ethical considerations that affect mentally ill persons who come into contact with the legal system.

II. Institutional Organization

A. Sponsoring Institution

1. The sponsoring institution must provide sufficient faculty, financial resources, and clinical, research, and library facilities to meet the educational needs of the residents and to enable the program to comply with the requirements for accreditation.
2. The program must be administratively attached to and sponsored by a residency program in psychiatry that is accredited by the ACGME. Applications for the accreditation of new forensic psychiatry programs will be considered only if the sponsoring psychiatry residency carries the status of full accreditation. Exception may be made for existing psychiatry programs that have been comprehensively reorganized and reaccredited as provisional programs. The program must function in close relationship with the psychiatry residency.
3. The presence of residents in forensic psychiatry must not dilute or otherwise detract from the didactic or clinical experience available to general psychiatry residents.

   The RRC shall approve the size of the resident complement. Any changes in resident complement require prior approval by the RRC.

B. Participating Institutions

1. The program should take place in facilities recognized, accredited, and/or licensed by the appropriate state and/or federal licensing agencies, the courts, and, where appropriate, by the Joint Commission on Accreditation of Healthcare Organizations. When participating facilities are not so recognized, accredited, and/or licensed, the program must provide a rationale and explanation for participation.
2. There must be a clear educational rationale for the inclusion of each participating institution. The number of and distance between participating institutions should not be so great as to interfere with training and participation in conferences and other organized educational aspects of the program.
3. There must be written affiliation agreements specific to the provision of training in forensic psychiatry between the institution sponsoring the program and each of the participating institutions. These agreements should specify the following for each participating institution:
   a. The program goals and objectives and the means by which they will be accomplished.
   b. The resources and facilities in the institution that will be available to residents.
   c. Information on professional liability insurance, fringe benefits, and vacations.
   d. The duties and responsibilities that forensic psychiatry residents will have in the institution.
   e. The relationship that will exist between forensic psychiatry residents and the residents, trainees, and faculty in other programs, as appropriate.
   f. The type of supervision each forensic psychiatry resident will receive from the faculty in the institution.
   g. The provision of fair procedures to all parties in the event of a dispute, disciplinary action, or termination.

C. Appointment of Residents

The development of a satisfactory program requires careful selection of applicants for appointment to the subspecialty residency. The program director must adhere to the criteria for resident eligibility that are specified in the institutional requirements. An excessively high rate of resident attrition from a program will be a cause of concern to the RRC.

III. Faculty and Staff

A. Program Director

The program director and the teaching staff are responsible for the general administration of the program, including those activities related to the recruitment, selection, instruction, supervision, counseling, evaluation, and advancement of residents and the maintenance of records related to program accreditation.

1. Qualifications of the Program Director
   a. Documented clinical, educational, and administrative abilities and experience.
   b. Licensure to practice medicine in the state where the institution that sponsors the program is located. (Certain federal programs are exempted.)
   c. Certification by the American Board of Psychiatry and Neurology (ABPN) with Added Qualifications in Forensic Psychiatry or equivalent qualifications in forensic psychiatry satisfactory to the RRC.
   d. Appointment in good standing to the medical staff of an institution participating in the program.
   e. The program director should be an active practitioner and must devote sufficient time to the program to ensure achievement of the educational goals and objectives.
   f. Participation in scholarly activities appropriate to the subspecialty, such as local, regional, and national specialty societies; research; presentations; and publication.
2. Responsibilities of the Program Director

   The program director has primary responsibility for the administration of the program. Frequent changes in leadership or long periods of temporary leadership are undesirable and may adversely affect the accreditation status of the program. Responsibilities of the program director include
   a. preparation of a written statement outlining the educational goals of the program with respect to knowledge, skills, and

other attributes of residents at each level of training and for each major rotation or other program assignment. This statement must be distributed to residents and members of the teaching staff on beginning that aspect of training and must include the requirements for satisfactory completion of the program. It should be readily available for review.

b. selection of residents for appointment to the program in accordance with institutional and departmental policies and procedures. The director must receive documentation from the general psychiatry program completed by an applicant to verify satisfactory completion of all educational and ethical requirements for graduation before the applicant is appointed to the program. Agreements with applicants made prior to the completion of the general residency must be contingent on this requirement.

c. selection and supervision of the teaching staff and other program personnel at each institution participating in the program.

d. the supervision of residents through explicit written descriptions of supervisory lines of responsibility for the care of patients. Such guidelines must be communicated to all members of the program staff. Residents must be provided with prompt, reliable systems for communication and interaction with supervisory physicians.

e. monitoring the progress of each subspecialty resident, including the maintenance of a training record that documents completion of all required components of the program and requirements for satisfactory completion of the program as well as evaluations of residents' clinical and didactic work by supervisors and teachers. This record shall include a patient log for each subspecialty resident that shall document that each resident has completed all clinical experiences required by the Program Requirements and the educational objectives of the program.

f. regular evaluation of residents' knowledge, skills, and overall performance, including the development of professional attitudes consistent with being a physician.

g. The program director, with participation of members of the teaching staff, must
   1. at least semiannually evaluate the knowledge, skills, and professional growth of each resident, using appropriate criteria and procedures.
   2. communicate each evaluation to the resident in a timely manner.
   3. advance residents to positions of higher responsibility only on the basis of evidence of their satisfactory progressive scholarship and professional growth.
   4. maintain a permanent record of evaluation for each resident and have it accessible to the resident and other authorized personnel.
   5. monitor the quality of didactic and clinical experiences, including the collection and review of periodic written evaluations by residents of all such experiences and supervision.
   6. ensure the provision of written descriptions of departmental policies regarding salary and benefits, due process, sickness and other leaves, call responsibilities, and vacation time to all residents on their appointment to the program. All residents must be provided with written descriptions of the malpractice coverage provided for each clinical assignment.
   7. prepare an accurate statistical and narrative description of the program as requested by a review committee.
   8. implement fair procedures, as established by the sponsoring institution, regarding academic discipline and resident complaints or grievances.
   9. monitor resident stress, including mental or emotional conditions inhibiting performance or learning and drug- or alcohol-related dysfunction. Program directors and teaching staff should be sensitive to the need for timely provision of confidential counseling and psychological support services to residents. Training situations that consistently produce undesirable stress on residents must be evaluated and modified.
   10. notify the RRC promptly of any major changes in the program or its leadership.
   11. prepare timely, accurate program information forms and related materials in preparation for review by the RRC.
   12. report the name of each resident in the program to the RRC by September 1 of each year.

B. Number and Qualifications of the Physician Faculty

1. There must be a sufficient number of qualified physician faculty members to maintain high-quality didactic and clinical educational programs. In addition to the program director, there must be a least one other faculty member certified by the ABPN with Added Qualification in Forensic Psychiatry or its equivalent and at least one certified child and adolescent psychiatrist. Programs with large patient populations, multiple institutions, and large resident complements will be expected to have additional faculty appropriate to their size and structure.
2. Faculty must be additionally qualified by experience in forensic psychiatry to provide the expertise needed to fulfill the didactic, clinical, and research goals of the program.
3. The faculty must devote sufficient time to the educational program in forensic psychiatry to ensure fulfillment of its goals and objectives.
4. A member of the teaching staff of each participating institution must be designated to assume responsibility for the day-to-day activities of the program at that institution, with overall coordination by the program director. The director of forensic psychiatry training at each participating institution shall be appointed by or with the concurrence of the forensic psychiatry program director.
5. The teaching staff must be organized and have regular documented meetings to review program goals and objectives as well as program effectiveness in achieving them. At least one resident representative should participate in these reviews.
6. The teaching staff should periodically evaluate the utilization of the resources available to the program, the contribution of each institution participating in the program, the financial and administrative support of the program, the volume and variety of patients available to the program for educational purposes, the performance of members of the teaching staff, and the quality of supervision of residents.

C. Other Faculty and Program Personnel

1. In addition to the faculty psychiatrists, the faculty must include a lawyer and a forensic psychologist. It is desirable that there be other appropriate nonmedical professionals in the faculty such as judges, social workers, criminologists, and others. The number of these faculty members must be sufficient for the size of the program.
2. Programs must be provided with the additional professional, technical, and clerical personnel needed to support the administration and educational conduct of the program.

IV. Facilities and Resources

A. Requirements for Facilities

All elements of the program must be located in designated facilities based on written affiliation agreements and must include experiences in the following three venues:

1. Facilities in which forensic psychiatric evaluations are performed on subjects with a broad variety of psychiatric disorders, where residents can learn evaluation techniques. These may include court clinics, inpatient forensic units, outpatient forensic clinics, and private practices.
2. Facilities that provide general psychiatric services to patients with a broad variety of psychiatric disorders, where residents can learn consultation regarding legal issues in psychiatric practice. These may include inpatient and outpatient facilities or may be specialized facilities that provide psychiatric care to correctional populations.
3. Facilities that treat persons in the correctional system, where residents can learn about the specialized treatment issues raised by these populations and settings. These may include prisons, jails, hospital-based correctional units, halfway facilities, rehabilitation programs, community probation programs, and forensic clinics.

Appropriate support services to ensure an adequate educational experience at all participating institutions must be available, including support personnel and a physically safe environment in which residents may carry out their clinical and educational functions.

B. Library

1. Residents must have ready access to a major medical library, either at the institution where the residents are located or through arrangement with convenient nearby institutions.
2. Library services should include the electronic retrieval of information from medical databases.
3. There must be access to an on-site library or to a collection of appropriate texts and journals in each institution participating in a residency program. On-site libraries and/or collections of texts and journals must be readily available during nights and weekends.
4. There must be an adequate number of texts and journals in psychiatry and law. Access for residents to a law library or a comprehensive legal on-line service must be available.

V. Educational Program

The training program must provide opportunities for residents to acquire advanced clinical knowledge and skills in the field of forensic psychiatry. These objectives will be accomplished by a combination of supervised clinical experiences and formal didactic conferences. The curriculum must assure residents the opportunity to acquire the cognitive knowledge, interpersonal skills, professional attitudes, and practical experience required of a psychiatrist with added qualifications in forensic psychiatry. All major dimensions of the curriculum must be structured educational experiences guided by written goals and objectives as well as by specified teaching and evaluation methods. The goals and objectives of each major component of the curriculum must be provided to residents in writing when they enter the program.

A. Components of the Educational Program

1. Forensic experiences
   a. Clinical experiences must provide residents with sufficient opportunity for the psychiatric evaluation of individuals involving
      1. criminal behavior,
      2. criminal responsibility and competency to stand trial,
      3. sexual misconduct, and
      4. dangerousness.

   b. Residents also must have experience in the review of written records, including clinical and legal documents, and in the preparation of written reports and/or testimony in a diversity of cases, for example:
      1. aiding the court in the sentencing of criminal offenders;
      2. domestic relations cases;
      3. personal injury cases;
      4. allegations of sexual abuse; and
      5. other cases involving the ethical issues and legal regulation of psychiatry, ie, involuntary hospitalization, confidentiality, right to treatment, right to refuse treatment, informed consent, and professional liability.

   c. Residents must have supervised experience in testifying in court or in mock trial simulations.

   d. Residents must have supervised training in the relevance of legal documents, police reports, court testimony, polygraphs, hypnosis, narcoanalysis, psychological and neuropsychological testing, brain-imaging techniques, and other procedures relevant to assessments and treatment in forensic psychiatry.

   e. Consultative experiences must provide residents with an opportunity to consult with general psychiatric clinicians regarding legal issues that arise in psychiatric practice. This can occur in inpatient or outpatient settings and should include patients from diverse socioeconomic, educational, ethnic, and cultural backgrounds, with a variety of diagnoses. At a minimum, residents should have the opportunity to consult with clinicians regarding civil commitment and dangerousness, confidentiality, decision-making competence, guardianship, and refusal of treatment.

   f. Clinical placement must provide residents with experience in the evaluation and management of acutely and chronically ill patients in correctional systems such as prisons, jails, and community programs. There also must be experience in working with other professionals and personnel in both forensic and community settings. A sufficient number and variety of patients, ranging from adolescence to old age and of diverse backgrounds, should be provided to ensure an adequate experience. Residents must have at least 6 months' experience in the management of at least two patients in the correctional system.

   g. Direct clinical work with children under the age of 14 years should be limited to residents who have previously completed ACGME-approved training in child and adolescent psychiatry.

2. Didactic curriculum

   The didactic curriculum must include the following components:

   a. A psychiatric curriculum that includes the
      1. history of forensic psychiatry;
      2. roles and responsibilities of forensic psychiatrists;
      3. assessment of competency to stand trial, criminal responsibility, amnesia, testamentary capacity, and civil competency;
      4. issues involved in the assessment of dangerousness;
      5. assessment of the accused sexual offender;
      6. evaluation and treatment of incarcerated individuals;
      7. ethical, administrative, and legal issues in forensic psychiatry;
      8. legal regulation of psychiatric practice;
      9. writing of a forensic report;
      10. eyewitness testimony of children; and
      11. ethics of genetic counseling.

   b. A law curriculum that covers issues in the legal system related to forensic psychiatry, such as
      1. fundamentals of law, statutes, and administrative regulations;

2. the structure of federal and state court systems;
3. use of a law library;
4. theory and practice of sentencing of the convicted offender;
5. basic civil procedure;
6. basic criminal procedure;
7. jurisdiction;
8. responsibility;
9. tort law;
10. children's rights;
11. family law; and
12. confessions of minors.

c. A civil law curriculum that includes issues such as
1. conservators and guardianships;
2. child custody determinations;
3. parental competence and termination of parental rights;
4. child abuse/neglect;
5. psychiatric disability determinations;
6. testamentary capacity;
7. psychiatric malpractice;
8. personal injury litigation;
9. abandonment law; and
10. developmental disability law, ie, individualized educational needs and the right to the least restrictive environment for education.

d. A criminal law curriculum that includes issues such as
1. competence to stand trial;
2. competence to enter a plea;
3. testimonial capacity;
4. voluntariness of confessions;
5. insanity defense(s);
6. diminished capacity;
7. evaluations in aid of sentencing;
8. safe release of persons acquitted by reason of insanity; and
9. competence to be executed.

e. Conferences in forensic psychiatry, such as grand rounds, case conferences, readings seminars, and journal clubs, should be specifically designed to augment the clinical experiences. Regular attendance by the residents and the faculty should be documented.

B. Policies Regarding Supervision, Duty Hours, and Progressive Responsibility

1. The program director must ensure, direct, and document proper supervision of all forensic psychiatry residents by appropriately qualified faculty. The responsibility and independence allowed residents in patient contact should depend on their knowledge, skill, and experience and the complexity of the clinical problem. Residents must be provided with rapid, reliable methods for communicating with supervising physicians. Each resident must have a minimum of 2 hours of individual supervision of clinical activities weekly.
2. The program director should carefully monitor and document any clinical activity outside the program that could potentially interfere with educational performance or clinical responsibility. The program director must carefully monitor all on-call schedules and duty hours within the program to ensure a balanced and appropriate educational and clinical experience. This monitoring should ensure
a. One full day out of every 7 free of program-related duties;
b. on average, on-call duty no more than every third night;
c. adequate backup if patient care needs create resident fatigue sufficient to jeopardize patient care or resident welfare during or following on-call periods; and
d. adequate faculty backup if residents encounter complex clinical situations while on call.
3. Residents must be supervised in the performance of procedures integral to the specialty of forensic psychiatry. Supervision must include observation, assessment, and substantiation of the residents' knowledge and skills in clinical evaluation, technical proficiency, and professional attitudes.
4. At all program facilities, residents must be afforded responsibilities commensurate with their postgraduate status and experience level in the provision of patient care.

C. Scholarly Activity

Graduate medical education must take place in an environment of inquiry and scholarship in which residents participate in the development of new knowledge, learn to evaluate research findings, and develop habits of inquiry as a continuing professional responsibility. The responsibility for establishing and maintaining an environment of inquiry and scholarship rests with the teaching staff. While not all members of a teaching staff must be investigators, the staff as a whole must demonstrate broad involvement in scholarly activity. This activity should include

1. active participation of the teaching staff in clinical discussions, rounds, and conferences in a manner that promotes a spirit of inquiry and scholarship. Scholarship implies an in-depth understanding of basic mechanisms of normal and abnormal states and the application of current knowledge to practice.
2. participation in journal clubs and research conferences.
3. active participation in regional or national professional and scientific societies, particularly through presentations at the organizations' meetings and publication in their journals.
4. participation in research, particularly in projects that are funded following peer review and/or that result in publication or presentations at regional and national scientific meetings.
5. offering of guidance and technical support (eg, research design, statistical analysis) to residents involved in research.

As part of the academic environment, an active scholarly component should be included within the forensic psychiatry program. Faculty members should participate actively in scholarly medical activities and research related to the field of forensic psychiatry. The program should offer a meaningful, individually supervised scholarly experience for each resident.

D. Other Program Components

1. Presence of Other Training Programs
The forensic psychiatry program should provide peer interaction between its residents and those of other specialties. To achieve this goal, an accredited training program in at least one nonpsychiatric medical specialty should be present within the program's participating institutions. In addition, peer interaction with students in the fields of law, social work, etc, is highly desirable. Peer interaction among the programs should occur in the course of clinical and/or didactic work, but it is most satisfactory when organized around joint patient evaluation and/or care.
2. Resident Administrative and Teaching Experiences
The program should provide appropriate experience designed to develop the administrative and teaching skills of forensic psychiatry residents. As residents progress through the program, they should have the opportunity to teach personnel such as other residents, mental health professionals, and students.

VI. Evaluation

A. Evaluation of Residents

There must be at least quarterly written evaluations of the residents by all supervisors and the directors of clinical components of training. These must be discussed with the residents and placed in the training record.

B. Faculty Evaluation

There must be in place a mechanism for the written evaluation by forensic psychiatry residents of all supervisors, as well as of the didactic and clinical elements of the educational program.

C. Program Evaluation

1. The educational effectiveness of a program must be evaluated in a systematic manner. In particular, the quality of the curriculum and the extent to which the educational goals have been met by residents must be assessed. The teaching staff should periodically evaluate the utilization of the resources available to the program, the contribution of each institution participating in the program, the financial and administrative support of the program, the volume and variety of patients available to the program for educational purposes, the performance of members of the teaching staff, and the quality of supervision of residents.
2. Written evaluations by residents should be utilized in this process.
3. One measure of the quality of the program will be participation in and performance of its graduates on the Added Qualifications certifying examination conducted by the ABPN.

VII. Certification

Those individuals planning to seek Added Qualifications certification through the ABPN should communicate with the administrative officer of the ABPN prior to beginning training to ascertain the board's requirements if there are any questions about them.

ACGME: February 1996 Effective: February 1996

Program Requirements for Residency Education in Geriatric Psychiatry (Psychiatry)

I. Introduction

A. Definition of the Subspecialty

Geriatric psychiatry is that area of psychiatry that focuses on prevention, diagnosis, evaluation, and treatment of mental disorders and disturbances seen in older adult patients. An educational program in geriatric psychiatry must be organized to provide professional knowledge and a well-supervised clinical experience.

B. Duration and Scope of Education

1. The training period in geriatric psychiatry must be 12 months. Any program that extends the length of the program beyond 12 months must present an educational rationale consistent with the program requirements and the objectives for resident education.
2. The geriatric psychiatry resident must have satisfactorily completed an Accreditation Council for Graduate Medical Education (ACGME)-accredited psychiatry residency prior to entering the program.
3. Training in geriatric psychiatry that occurred during general residency training will not be counted toward meeting this requirement.
4. Training is best accomplished on a full-time basis. If it is undertaken on a part-time basis, the 12-month program must be completed within a 2-year period.
5. Prior to entry into the program, each geriatric psychiatry resident must be notified in writing of the required length of training for which the program is accredited. The required length of training for a particular individual may not be changed without mutual agreement during his or her program unless there is a break in his or her training or the individual requires remedial training.

C. Educational Goals and Objectives

1. Geriatric psychiatry programs must provide advanced training for the resident to function as a consultant in the subspecialty. Programs must emphasize scholarship, self-instruction, development of critical analysis of clinical problems, and the ability to make appropriate decisions.
2. Clinical experience must include opportunities to assess and manage elderly inpatients and ambulatory patients of both sexes with a wide variety of psychiatric problems. Geriatric psychiatry residents must be given the opportunity to provide both primary and consultative care for patients in both inpatient and outpatient settings to understand the interaction of normal aging and disease as well as to gain mastery in assessment, therapy, and management.
3. The program must include training in the biological and psychosocial aspects of normal aging; the psychiatric impact of acute and chronic physical illnesses; and the biological and psychosocial aspects of the pathology of primary psychiatric disturbances beginning in or continuing into older age.
4. There must be a focus on multidimensional biopsychosocial concepts of treatment and management as applied both in inpatient facilities (acute and long-term care) and in the community or home settings. There must also be emphasis on the medical and iatrogenic aspects of illness as well as on sociocultural, ethnic, economic, ethical, and legal considerations that may affect psychiatric management.

II. Institutional Organization

A. The program must be administratively attached to and sponsored by a core residency program in psychiatry that holds full accreditation from the ACGME. Ongoing general psychiatry programs that have been comprehensively reorganized and reaccredited on a provisional basis may be exempted from this requirement. The program must function as an integral part of the psychiatry residency.

B. The presence of residents in geriatric psychiatry must not dilute or otherwise detract from the didactic or clinical experience available to general psychiatry residents. The Residency Review Committee (RRC) shall approve the size of the geriatric psychiatry resident complement. Any changes in this complement will require prior approval by the RRC.

C. The training program must take place in facilities that are approved by the appropriate state licensing agencies and, where appropriate, by the Joint Commission on Accreditation of Healthcare Organizations.

D. There shall be a clear educational rationale for the inclusion of each participating institution.

E. There must be current, written affiliation agreements between the sponsoring institution of the geriatric psychiatry program and each of its participating institutions. These agreements must comply with Institutional Requirements Section I.C.1-5. There should be an additional agreement between the geriatric psychiatry program director and the individual responsible for geriatric psychiatry education in each participating institution that specifies:

1. The geriatric psychiatry program goals and objectives for each rotation in the participating institution and the means by which they will be accomplished.
2. The resources and facilities in the institution(s) that will be available to each geriatric psychiatry resident.
3. Information on professional liability insurance, fringe benefits, and vacations, to be provided by each institution.

4. The duties and responsibilities the geriatric psychiatry resident will have in each institution.
5. The relationship that will exist between geriatric psychiatry residents and the residents and faculties in other programs, as appropriate.
6. The supervision each geriatric psychiatry resident will receive by the faculty in each institution.

III. Faculty and Staff

The program director and the teaching staff are responsible for the general administration of a program, including those activities related to the recruitment, selection, instruction, supervision, counseling, evaluation, and advancement of residents and the maintenance of records related to program accreditation.

A. Program Director

There must be a single program director responsible for the program. The program director should be an active clinician and must devote sufficient time to the program to ensure achievement of the educational goals and objectives. The program director should be primarily based at the main program teaching site.

1. Qualifications of the Program Director
   The program director must be:
   a. Certified by the American Board of Psychiatry and Neurology (ABPN) with Added Qualifications in Geriatric Psychiatry or have equivalent qualifications in geriatric psychiatry.
   b. Appropriately qualified by training and experience in psychiatric education and administration to direct and supervise the program.
   c. Licensed to practice medicine in the state where the institution that sponsors the program is located. (Certain federal programs are exempted.)
   d. Appointed in good standing to the medical staff of an institution participating in the program.
   e. Participating in scholarly activities appropriate to the profession, such as local, regional, and national specialty societies; research; presentations; and publications.
2. Program Director Responsibilities
   The program director will be the person who has primary responsibility for the administration of the program. The program director shall be responsible for:
   a. Preparing a written statement outlining the educational goals of the program with respect to knowledge, skills, and other attributes of residents at each level of training and for each major rotation or other program assignment. This statement must be distributed to residents and members of the teaching staff. It should be readily available for review.
   b. Supervising the recruitment and appointment process for applicants, including compliance with appropriate credentialing policies and procedures in accordance with institutional and departmental policies and procedures. No applicant who has completed a general psychiatry residency in another program shall be appointed without written communication from the prior program director that verifies satisfactory completion of all educational and ethical requirements for graduation.
   c. Monitoring the progress of each geriatric psychiatry resident, including the maintenance of a training record that documents completion of all required components of the program as well as the evaluations of performance by supervisors and teachers. This record shall include a patient log for each geriatric psychiatry resident that shall document that each resident has completed all clinical experiences required by the program requirements and the educational objectives of the program.
   d. Supervising residents through explicit written descriptions of supervisory lines of responsibility for the care of patients. Such guidelines must be communicated to all members of the program staff.
   e. Regularly evaluating, with the participation of members of the teaching staff, the residents' knowledge, skills, and overall performance, including the development of professional attitudes consistent with being a physician.
   f. Selecting and supervising the teaching staff and other program personnel at each institution participating in the program.
   g. Monitoring the quality of all didactic and clinical experiences, including the collection and review of periodic written evaluation by the resident of all such experiences and supervision.
   h. Maintaining all other training records, including those related to appointment, the departmental processes regarding due process, sickness and other leaves, call responsibilities, and vacation time.
   i. Providing to each geriatric psychiatry resident the written goals and objectives for each component of the program at the beginning of that aspect of training.
   j. Ensuring that residents are provided written descriptions of the departmental policies regarding due process, sickness and other leaves, call responsibilities, and vacation time on appointment to the program. All residents must be provided with written descriptions of the professional liability coverage provided for each clinical assignment.
   k. Providing a written final evaluation that documents the satisfactory completion of all program requirements for each resident who completes the program. The evaluation must include a review of the resident's performance during the final period of training and should verify that the resident has demonstrated sufficient professional ability to practice competently and independently. This final evaluation should be part of the resident's permanent record maintained by the institution.
   l. Monitoring resident stress, including mental or emotional conditions inhibiting performance or learning and drug- or alcohol-related dysfunction. Program directors and teaching staff should be sensitive to the need for timely provision of confidential counseling and psychological support services to residents. Training situations that consistently produce undesirable stress on residents must be evaluated and modified.
   m. Implementing fair procedures, as established by the sponsoring institution, regarding academic discipline and resident complaints or grievances.
   n. Notifying the RRC promptly of any major changes in the program or its leadership. Participation by any institution providing more than 3 months of training must be approved by the RRC.
   o. Preparing timely, accurate program information forms and related materials in preparation for review by the RRC.
   p. Reporting to the RRC by September of each year the name of each geriatric psychiatry resident in the program.

B. Number and Qualifications of the Physician Faculty

All members of the teaching staff must demonstrate a strong interest in the education of residents, sound clinical and teaching abilities, support of the goals and objectives of the program, a commitment to their own continuing medical education, and participation in scholarly activities.

1. There must be a sufficient number of qualified physician faculty members with documented qualifications to maintain a quality didactic and clinical educational program and to ensure the adequate instruction and supervision of all residents in the program. In addition to the program director, there must be at least one

other faculty member who is certified by the ABPN with Added Qualifications in Geriatric Psychiatry (or its equivalent).

2. These individuals must be additionally qualified by experience in geriatric psychiatry to provide the expertise needed to fulfill the didactic, clinical, and research goals of the program.
3. The faculty must devote sufficient time to the educational program in geriatric psychiatry to ensure fulfillment of its goals and objectives and to meet their supervisory and teaching responsibilities.
4. The responsibility for establishing and maintaining an environment of inquiry and scholarship rests with the teaching staff. While not all members of a teaching staff must be investigators, the staff as a whole must demonstrate broad involvement in scholarly activity. This activity should include:
   a. Active participation of the teaching staff in clinical discussions, rounds, and conferences in a manner that promotes a spirit of inquiry and scholarship. Scholarship implies an in-depth understanding of basic mechanisms of normal and abnormal states and the application of current knowledge to practice.
   b. Participation in journal clubs and research conferences.
   c. Active participation in regional or national professional and scientific societies, particularly through presentations at the organizations' meetings and publication in their journals.
   d. Participation in research, particularly in projects that are funded following peer review and/or result in publications or presentations at regional and national scientific meetings.
   e. Offering of guidance and technical support (eg, research design, statistical analysis) for residents involved in research.
   f. Provision of support for resident participation in scholarly activities.
5. The teaching staff must be organized and have regular documented meetings to review program goals and objectives as well as program effectiveness in achieving them. At least one resident representative should participate in these reviews.
6. The director of geriatric training at each participating institution shall be appointed by or with the concurrence of the geriatric psychiatry program director to assume responsibility for the day-to-day activities of the program at that institution, with overall coordination by the program director.

C. Geriatric Care Team

Geriatric psychiatry residents must be provided with meaningful patient care experiences as part of an interdisciplinary care team.

1. In addition to geriatric psychiatry, the geriatric care team should include representatives from related clinical disciplines such as psychology, social work, psychiatric nursing, activity or occupational therapy, physical therapy, pharmacology, and nutrition.
2. A variety of individuals representing disciplines within medicine, such as family practice and internal medicine (including their geriatric subspecialties), neurology, and physical medicine and rehabilitation, should be available for participation on the geriatric care team as needed for patient care and teaching purposes.
3. It is highly desirable that geriatric psychiatry residents have access to professionals representing allied disciplines (such as ethics, law, and pastoral care) as needed for patient care and teaching purposes.
4. Geriatric psychiatry residents should be provided with opportunities to participate as members of medical geriatric teams in institutions where such teams are present.

D. Other Program Personnel

Programs must be provided with the additional professional, technical, and clerical personnel needed to support the administration and educational conduct of the program.

IV. Facilities and Resources

A. Acute-Care Hospital

The psychiatry department sponsoring the program must be a part of or affiliated with at least one acute-care general hospital that has the full range of services usually ascribed to such a facility, including both medical and surgical services, intensive care units, emergency department, diagnostic laboratory and imaging services, and pathology department. If the acute-care hospital is specialized (eg, in geriatric or psychiatric care) and does not itself have the full spectrum of services described above, the program must document that it has access for training purposes to other affiliated acute-care facilities that have the remaining general services not present at the specialized facility.

B. Long-Term-Care Facility

Inclusion of at least one long-term-care facility is an essential component of the geriatric psychiatry program. Such facilities may be either discrete institutions separate from an acute-care hospital or formally designated units or services within an acute-care hospital. Suitable training sites include both nonpsychiatric facilities (such as a nursing facility or chronic care hospital) and psychiatric facilities.

C. Ambulatory-Care Service

The ambulatory-care service must be designed to render care in a multidisciplinary environment such as a geriatric clinic, psychiatric outpatient department, or community mental health center where nonpsychiatric medical specialists are also available.

D. Ancillary Support Services

At all participating facilities, there must be sufficient administrative support to ensure adequate teaching facilities, appropriate office space, support personnel, and teaching resources.

E. Library

Residents must have ready access to a major medical library, either at the institution where the residents are located or through arrangement with convenient nearby institutions.

1. Library services should include the electronic retrieval of information from medical databases.
2. There must be access to an on-site library or to a collection of appropriate texts and journals in each institution participating in a residency program. On-site libraries and/or collections of texts and journals must be readily available during nights and weekends.

F. Patient Population

There must be sufficient number and variety of patients in all institutions where training takes place to accomplish the educational goals. This should include not only the spectrum of psychiatric diagnoses but also experience with a diversity of patients by sex and socioeconomic, educational, and cultural backgrounds.

G. Additional Educational Environment

The program must provide opportunities for the geriatric psychiatry resident to render continuing care and to exercise leadership responsibilities in organizing recommendations from the mental health team and in integrating recommendations and input from primary care physicians, consulting medical specialists, and representatives of other allied disciplines.

V. Educational Program

The director and teaching staff of a program must prepare and comply with written educational goals for the program. All educational components of a residency program should be related to program goals. The program design and/or structure must be approved by the RRC for Psychiatry as part of the regular review process. The training program must provide opportunities for the residents to develop advanced clinical knowledge and skills in the overall field of geriatric psychiatry. These objectives will be accomplished by a combination of supervised clinical experiences and formal didactic conferences.

The curriculum must ensure the opportunity for geriatric psychiatry residents to achieve the cognitive knowledge, interpersonal skills, professional attitudes, and practical experience required of a geriatric psychiatrist in the care of the aged. Didactic as well as clinical learning opportunities must be available to the resident. All major dimensions of the curriculum must be structured educational experiences that are guided by written goals and objectives as well as by specified teaching and evaluation methods. The goals and objectives of each major component of the curriculum should be provided to the residents in writing on entering the program.

A. Clinical Experiences

The training program must include the following clinical components:

1. Geriatric Psychiatry Consultation Experience
Attaining skills as a consultant is an essential part of training. Consultation experiences should be formally available on the nonpsychiatric services of an acute-care hospital. They should include consultation to inpatient, outpatient, and emergency services. There should also be consultative experience in long-term-care facilities. Familiarity with the organizational and administrative aspects of home health-care services should be provided. Exposure to outreach services and crisis intervention services in both community and home settings should be provided.
2. Long-term-care Experience
All geriatric psychiatry residents should have the opportunity to follow and treat a sufficient number of long-term-care patients at a senior level of responsibility. This experience should be of sufficient duration for the resident to understand the problems and learn the skills associated with long-term management and treatment. Emphasis during this experience should be placed on approaches to consultation, diagnosis, and treatment of the acutely and chronically ill elderly in a diversity of care settings, both medical and psychiatric, including those with less technologically sophisticated environments. Training should include instruction on the use of group and activity therapies; on the psychosocial impact of institutionalization; on teaching nonmental health professionals about mental health in the aged; on the bioethical dilemmas encountered when treating illness in the very old; and on working within facilities that may have limitations, such as a decreased staff-patient ratio.
3. Other Medical Specialty Experience
There should be an identifiable, structured educational experience in neurology, physical medicine and rehabilitation, and geriatric medicine or geriatric family practice relative to the practice of psychiatry that includes both didactic and clinical training methods. The curriculum should address functional assessment, altered signs and symptoms of physical illness that occur in the elderly, and the identification of physical illnesses and iatrogenic factors that can alter mental status and behavior.

B. Specialty Content

The program curriculum must address, as a minimum, the following content and skill areas:

1. The current scientific understanding of aging and longevity, including theories of aging, epidemiology and natural history of aging, and diseases of the aged. This includes specific knowledge of the effects of biologic aging on human physiology, with emphasis on altered pharmacokinetics, pharmacodynamics, and sensory acuity in the elderly and on the differences and gradations between normal and abnormal age changes, with particular reference to such areas as memory and cognition, affective stability, personality and behavioral patterns, and sexuality. There must be an understanding of successful and maladaptive responses to stressors frequently encountered in older adults, such as retirement, widowhood, role changes, interpersonal and health status losses, financial reverses, environmental relocations, and increased dependency.
2. The relevance of cultural and ethnic differences and the special problems of disadvantaged minority groups, as these bear on distinguishing and treating abnormal and maladaptive clinical changes as well as the use of psychosocial support services.
3. The epidemiology, diagnosis, and treatment of all major psychiatric disorders seen in the elderly. Such disorders, seen alone and in combination, typically include but are not limited to affective disorders, dementia, delirium, late-onset psychoses, medical presentations of psychiatric disorders, iatrogenesis, adjustment disorders, anxiety disorders, sleep disorders, sexual disorders, substance abuse disorders, personality disorders, and continuation of psychiatric illnesses that began earlier in life.
4. The performance of mental status examination, community and environmental assessment, family and caregiver assessment, medical assessment, and physical functional assessment. Such skills form the basis for formal multidimensional geriatric assessment, using the appropriate synthesis of clinical findings and historical as well as current information acquired from the patient and/or relevant others (such as family members, caregivers, and other health-care professionals). The multidimensional assessment is essential to short-term and long-term diagnostic and treatment planning; as such, training must be provided in formulating the various assessments into an appropriate and coherent treatment plan.
5. The formal and informal administrative leadership of the mental health-care team, including skills in communicating treatment plans to the patient and the family.
6. The selection and use of clinical laboratory tests; radiologic and other imaging procedures; and polysomnographic, electrophysiologic, and neuropsychologic tests, as well as making appropriate referrals to and consultations with other health-care specialists.
7. The initiation and flexible guidance of treatment, with the need for ongoing monitoring of changes in mental and physical health status and medical regimens. Residents should be taught to recognize and manage psychiatric comorbid disorders (eg, dementia and depression), as well as the management of other disturbances often seen in the elderly, such as agitation, wandering, changes in sleep patterns, and aggressiveness.
8. The recognition of the stressful impact of psychiatric illness on caregivers. Attention should be placed on the appropriate guidance of and protection of caregivers, as well as the assessment of their ability to function.
9. Recognition and assessment of direct or indirect elder abuse.
10. The appropriate use of community or home health services, respite care, and the need for institutional long-term care.
11. The management of the care of elderly persons with emotional or behavioral disorders, including the awareness of appropriate modifications in techniques and goals in applying the various psychotherapies (with individual, group, and family focuses) and behavioral strategies.
12. The indications, side effects, and therapeutic limitations of psychoactive drugs and the pharmacologic alterations associated with aging, including changes in pharmacokinetics, pharmacodynamics, drug interactions, overmedication, and problems with

compliance. Attention should be given to the psychiatric manifestations of iatrogenic influences such as the multiple medications frequently taken by the elderly.

13. The use of nonpharmacologic approaches, with particular reference to applications and limitations of behavioral therapeutic strategies, physical restraints, and the appropriate use and application of electroconvulsive therapy in the elderly.
14. The appropriate use of psychodynamic understanding of developmental problems, conflict, and adjustment difficulties in the elderly that may complicate the clinical presentation and influence the doctor-patient relationship or treatment planning.
15. The ethical and legal issues especially pertinent to geriatric psychiatry, including competence, guardianship, right to refuse treatment, wills, informed consent, patient abuse, and the withholding of medical treatments.
16. The current economic aspects of supporting services, including but not limited to Title III of the Older Americans Act, Medicare, Medicaid, and cost containment.
17. The research methodologies related to geriatric psychiatry, including biostatistics, clinical epidemiology, medical information sciences, decision analysis, critical literature review, and research design (including cross-sectional and longitudinal methods).

C. Conferences

Conferences in geriatric psychiatry, such as grand rounds, case conferences, readings seminars, and journal clubs, should be specifically designed to augment the clinical experiences. Regular attendance by the residents and the faculty should be documented.

D. Resident Policies

1. The program director must ensure, direct, and document proper supervision of all geriatric psychiatry residents at all times by appropriately qualified faculty. The responsibility or independence given to residents in patient care should depend on their knowledge, skill, experience, and the complexity of the patient's illness. Residents must be provided with rapid, reliable methods for communicating with supervising physicians. Each resident shall have a minimum of 2 hours of individual supervision of clinical activities weekly.
2. The program should carefully monitor any activity outside the program that interferes with education, performance, or clinical responsibility. The program should carefully monitor all on-call schedules and hours within and outside the program to prevent interference with education, performance, or clinical responsibility. The monitoring should ensure:
   a. One full day out of 7 free of program duties.
   b. On average, on-call duty no more than every third night.
   c. Adequate backup if patient care needs create resident fatigue sufficient to jeopardize patient care or resident welfare during or following on-call periods.
3. At all program facilities, the geriatric psychiatry residents must be given responsibilities commensurate with their postgraduate status and appropriate to their skill and experience in the provision of patient care. Residents must actively participate in a physician-directed geriatric team on both inpatient and outpatient services.

E. Other Program Components

1. Scholarly Activity
   Graduate medical education must take place in an environment of inquiry and scholarship, in which residents participate in the development of new knowledge, learn to evaluate research findings, and develop habits of inquiry as a continuing professional responsibility. As part of the academic environment, an active scholarly component must be included within the geriatric psychiatry program. Faculty members should participate actively in basic, clinical, and/or health services research. The program should provide each resident with a meaningful, individually supervised opportunity to participate in research or scholarly activity.
2. Presence of Other Training Programs
   The program should provide peer interaction between its geriatric psychiatry residents and those of other medical specialties. To achieve this goal, there should be an ACGME-accredited training program in at least one relevant nonpsychiatric specialty, such as neurology, internal medicine, family practice, or physical medicine and rehabilitation, within the participating institutions of the geriatric psychiatry program. Peer interaction among the programs should occur in the course of clinical and/or didactic work but is most satisfactory when organized around joint patient evaluation and/or care.
3. Resident Teaching Experiences
   The program should provide appropriate experiences designed to develop the administrative and teaching skills of the geriatric psychiatry residents. As the geriatric psychiatry residents progress through the program, they should have the opportunity to teach personnel such as other residents, medical students, nurses, and allied health professionals.

VI. Evaluation

A. Evaluation of Residents

There must be at least quarterly evaluation of the geriatric psychiatry residents by all supervisors and the directors of clinical components of training. These evaluations must be discussed with the resident and placed in the training record. The program director shall:

1. At least semiannually evaluate the knowledge, skills, and professional growth of the residents, using appropriate criteria and procedures.
2. Communicate each evaluation to the resident in a timely manner.
3. Advance residents to positions of higher responsibility only on the basis of evidence of their satisfactory progressive scholarship and professional growth.
4. Maintain a permanent record of evaluation for each resident and have it accessible to the resident and other authorized personnel.

B. Faculty Evaluation

Geriatric psychiatry residents must also be provided with a mechanism for the written evaluation of all supervisors and of the didactic and clinical components of the educational program.

C. Program Evaluation

1. The educational effectiveness of a program must be evaluated in a systematic manner. In particular, the quality of the curriculum and the extent to which the educational goals have been met by residents must be assessed. The teaching staff should periodically evaluate the utilization of the resources available to the program, the contribution of each institution participating in the program, the financial and administrative support of the program, the volume and variety of patients available to the program for educational purposes, the performance of members of the teaching staff, and the quality of supervision of residents.
2. Written evaluations by residents should be utilized in this process.
3. One measure of the quality of the program will be the participation in and performance of its graduates on the Added Qualifications certifying examination conducted by the ABPN.

VII. Certification

Those individuals planning to seek Added Qualifications certification through the ABPN should communicate with the administrative officer of the ABPN prior to beginning training to ascertain the requirements.

ACGME: June 1994 Effective: July 1995

Program Requirements for Residency Education in Diagnostic Radiology

I. Introduction

A. Definition and Scope

Diagnostic radiology encompasses a variety of diagnostic and image-guided therapeutic techniques, including all aspects of radiological diagnosis, nuclear radiology, diagnostic ultrasound, magnetic resonance, computed tomography, interventional procedures, and the use of other forms of radiant energy. The residency program in diagnostic radiology shall offer a quality graduate medical educational experience of adequate scope and depth in all of these associated diagnostic disciplines.

B. Duration and Scope of Education

Resident education in diagnostic radiology must include 5 years of clinically oriented graduate medical education, of which 4 years must be in diagnostic radiology. The clinical year must consist of Accreditation Council for Graduate Medical Education (ACGME) or equivalent accredited training in internal medicine, pediatrics, surgery or surgical specialties, obstetrics and gynecology, neurology, family practice, emergency medicine, or any combination of these, or an ACGME or equivalent accredited transitional year.

If the clinical year is offered by the institution of the core residency, and it is not itself an ACGME-accredited year, the program director will be responsible for assuring the quality of the year. The clinical year should be completed within the first 24 months of training.

The diagnostic radiology program shall offer a minimum of 4 years of graduate medical education (including vacation and meeting time) in diagnostic radiology, of which at least 42 months of training must be in the parent or integrated institution(s). [*Note:* Time spent attending the AFIP course is excluded.] The minimum period of training in nuclear radiology shall be 6 months. The maximum period of training in any subspecialty area shall be 12 months.

II. Institutional Organization

All educational components of a residency program should be related to program goals. The program design and structure must be approved by the Residency Review Committee (RRC) as part of the regular review process.

A. Sponsoring Institution

The residency program in diagnostic radiology must have one parent institution with primary responsibility for the entire program. When any institution(s) other than the parent is utilized for the clinical or basic science education of a resident in diagnostic radiology, letters of agreement must be provided by the appropriate institutional authority.

The institution must demonstrate commitment to the program in terms of financial and academic support, including the timely appointment of a permanent department chair.

B. Participating Institutions

Institutions may participate on an affiliated or an integrated basis. An accredited program may be independent or may occur in two or more institutions that develop formal agreements and conjoint responsibilities to provide complementary facilities, teaching staff, and teaching sessions. When another institution is utilized and a single program director assumes responsibility for the entire residency, including the appointment of all residents and teaching staff, that institution is designated as integrated. Within a single program some participating hospitals may qualify as integrated, while others are merely affiliated. Rotations to affiliated institutions may not exceed 6 months during the 4 years of training. [*Note:* Time spent attending the AFIP course is excluded.] Rotations to integrated institutions are not limited in duration. Participation by any affiliated institution providing more than 3 months of training must be approved by the RRC. Prior approval of the RRC must be obtained for participation of an institution on an integrated basis, regardless of the duration of the rotations.

The purpose of another institution's participation and the educational contribution to the total training program shall be defined. Service responsibility alone at a participating institution does not constitute a suitable educational experience. Affiliation shall be avoided with institutions that are at such a distance from the parent institution as to make resident attendance at rounds and conferences impractical, unless there is a comparable educational experience at the affiliated institution.

C. Appointment of Residents

Peer contact and discussion are as important to the learning process as contact with teaching faculty. The number of diagnostic radiology residents in the program must be sufficient to provide for frequent and meaningful discussion with peers as well as to provide appropriate coverage for adequate patient care. Appointment of a minimum of eight residents with, on average, two appointed each year, is required for an efficient learning environment. Prior approval by the RRC is required for an increase in the number of residents.

The complement of residents must be commensurate with the total capacity of the program to offer an adequate educational experience in diagnostic radiology. A reasonable volume is no less than 7,000 radiologic examinations per year per resident. The number of examinations in each of the subspecialty areas must be of sufficient volume to ensure adequate training experience.

III. Faculty Qualifications and Responsibilities

The program director and teaching faculty are responsible for the general administration of a program, including those activities related to the recruitment, selection, instruction, supervision, counseling, evaluation, and advancement of residents and the maintenance of records related to program accreditation.

A. Program Director

1. Qualifications of the Program Director
   a. There must be a single program director responsible for the program. The program director must be a faculty member who is a diagnostic radiologist and must contribute sufficient time to the program to fulfill all the responsibilities inherent in meeting the educational goals of the program. The program director must have appropriate authority to organize and fulfill administrative and teaching responsibilities to achieve the educational goals.
   b. The program director must be licensed to practice medicine in the state where the institution that sponsors the program is located. (Certain federal programs are exempted.)
   c. The program director shall be certified by the American Board of Radiology or possess suitable equivalent qualifications, as determined by the RRC.
   d. The program director also must hold an appointment in good standing to the medical staff of an institution participating in the program. A complete curriculum vitae of the program director shall be filed with the Executive Director of the RRC at the time of appointment and updated with each review of the program by the RRC.
   e. The program director should have sufficient academic and administrative experience to ensure effective implementation of these Program Requirements and should have at least 3 years of participation as an active faculty member in an accredited residency program.
2. Responsibilities of the Program Director

The program director shall be responsible for the total training in diagnostic radiology, which includes the instruction and supervision of residents. The program director shall be responsible for evaluation of the teaching faculty in concert with the department chair.

The program director is responsible for promptly notifying the Executive Director of the RRC in writing of any major changes in the program, including changes in leadership. Prior approval of the RRC is required for the addition or deletion of a major participating hospital, for an increase in the number of residents in the program, and for a major change in the format of the program. On review of a proposal for major change in a program, the RRC may determine that a site visit is necessary.

The program director is also responsible for the following:

a. Preparation of a written statement outlining the curriculum and educational goals and objectives of the program with respect to knowledge, skills, and other attributes of residents at each level of training and for each major rotation or other program assignment. This statement must be distributed to residents and members of the teaching faculty. It should be readily available for review.
b. Selection of residents for appointment to the program in accordance with institutional and departmental policies and procedures
c. Selection and supervision of resident rotations, teaching faculty from the department professional staff, and other program personnel at each institution participating in the program
d. Supervision of residents through explicit written descriptions of supervisory lines of responsibility for the care of patients. Such guidelines must be communicated to all members of the program faculty. Residents must be provided with prompt, reliable systems for communication and interaction with supervisory physicians.
e. Implementation of fair procedures, as established by the sponsoring institution, regarding academic discipline and resident complaints or grievances
f. Preparation of an accurate statistical and narrative description of the program as requested by the RRC
g. Monitoring of resident stress, including mental or emotional conditions and drug- or alcohol-related dysfunction, inhibiting performance or learning. The program director and teaching faculty should be sensitive to the need for timely provision of confidential counseling and psychological support services to residents. Training situations that consistently produce undesirable stress on residents must be evaluated and modified.

B. Faculty

1. All members of the teaching faculty must demonstrate a strong interest in the education of residents, sound clinical and teaching abilities, support of the goals and objectives of the program, a commitment to their own continuing medical education, and participation in scholarly activities. There must be a sufficient number of teaching faculty. At a minimum, there must be one full-time equivalent physician faculty member at the parent and integrated institutions for every resident in training in the program. The teaching faculty must be qualified in those areas in which they are assigned to instruct and supervise residents, and

they must contribute sufficient time to the program to provide adequate instruction and supervision.

2. Didactic and clinical teaching must be provided by faculty with documented interests and expertise in the subspecialty involved. The teaching faculty responsible for the training in each designated subspecialty area must demonstrate a commitment to the subspecialty. Such commitment may be demonstrated by any of the following: (1) fellowship training or 3 years of subspecialty practice, (2) membership in a subspecialty society, (3) publications and presentations in the subspecialty, (4) annual CME credits in the subspecialty.
3. At least one faculty member must be designated to have primary responsibility for the educational content of each of the nine subspecialty areas. This individual must practice at least 50% of his/her time in the department. The nine subspecialty areas are neuroradiology, musculoskeletal radiology, vascular and interventional radiology, chest radiology, breast imaging, abdominal radiology, pediatric radiology, ultrasonography (including obstetrical and vascular ultrasound), and nuclear radiology. No faculty member can have primary responsibility for the educational content of more than one subspecialty area, although faculty can have clinical responsibility and/or teaching responsibilities in several subspecialty areas. A pediatric radiologist may have a primary appointment at another institution and still be the designated faculty member supervising pediatric radiologic education.
4. A member of the teaching faculty of each participating institution must be designated to assume responsibility for the day-to-day activities of the program at that institution, with overall coordination by the program director.
5. The teaching faculty must be organized and have regular documented meetings to review program goals and objectives as well as program effectiveness in achieving them. At least one resident representative should participate in these reviews. The faculty should evaluate the utilization of the resources available to the program, the contribution of each institution participating in the program, the financial and administrative support of the program, the volume and variety of patients available to the program for educational purposes, the performance of members of the teaching faculty, and the quality of supervision of residents.

C. Other Program Personnel

Programs must be provided with the additional professional, technical, and clerical personnel needed to support the administration and educational conduct of the program.

IV. Facilities and Resources

A. The program must provide not only adequate space, equipment, and other pertinent facilities to ensure an effective educational experience for residents in diagnostic radiology but also the modern facilities and equipment required in all of the subspecialty rotations.

B. There must be 24-hour access to an on-site departmental library or to a collection of journals, references, and resource materials pertinent to progressive levels of education in diagnostic radiology and associated fields in each institution participating in a residency program. On-site libraries and/or collections of texts and journals must include standard diagnostic radiology and radiological subspecialty textbooks and major radiology journals.

C. Residents must have ready access to a major medical library, either at the institution where the residents are located or through arrangement with convenient nearby institutions. The institutional library must have facilities for electronic retrieval of information from medical databases and on-line literature searches.

D. Service commitments must not compromise the achievement of the program's educational goals and objectives.

V. The Educational Program

A. Clinical Components

The program in diagnostic radiology must provide a sufficient volume and variety of patients to ensure that residents gain experience in the full range of radiologic examinations, procedures, and interpretations. A reasonable volume is no less than 75,000 total radiologic examinations at the parent or integrated program, and no less than 7,000 radiologic examinations per year per resident. The number of examinations in each of the subspecialty areas must be of sufficient volume to ensure adequate training experience. If volume in any subspecialty area is less than acceptable, a plan must be developed to increase trainee exposure. The presence of residents and subspecialty residents from outside institutions for limited rotations should not dilute the educational experience of the core program residents.

The clinical training must provide for progressive, supervised responsibility for patient care and must ensure that the supervised resident performs those procedures commonly accepted in all aspects of diagnostic radiology. The training must include progressive study and experience in all of the diagnostic radiologic subspecialties. The training program should ensure sufficient time to gain experience in neuroradiology, musculoskeletal radiology, vascular and interventional radiology, chest radiology, breast imaging, abdominal radiology, pediatric radiology, ultrasonography (including obstetrical and vascular ultrasound), and nuclear radiology.

Additionally, each resident must have documented supervised experience in interventional procedures, for example, image-guided biopsies, drainage procedures, noncoronary angioplasty, embolization and infusion procedures, and percutaneous introduction techniques.

The program director must require that residents maintain a record (electronic or written) in which they document the performance, interpretation, and complications of vascular, interventional, and invasive procedures. The record must be reviewed by the program director or faculty designee on a yearly basis.

Training and experience are required in plain film interpretation, computed tomography, magnetic resonance imaging, ultrasonography, angiography, and nuclear radiology examinations related to cardiovascular disease. The program also must provide instruction in cardiac anatomy, physiology, and pathology, including the coronary arteries, as essential to the interpretation of cardiac imaging studies. This training must include both the adult and the pediatric age group.

Radiologic education in different organ systems must provide the opportunity for residents to develop adequate knowledge regarding normal and pathologic physiology, including the biologic and pharmacologic actions of materials administered to patients in diagnostic studies.

Each resident must have basic life-support training, and advanced cardiac life-support training is recommended.

B. Didactic Components

The education in diagnostic radiology must occur in an environment that encourages the interchange of knowledge and experience among residents in the program and with residents in other major clinical specialties located in those institutions participating in the program.

Diagnostic radiologic physics, radiation biology, radiation protection, and pathology are required elements of the curriculum. In view of the importance of understanding pathology as a basis for radiologic diagnosis, emphasis should be placed on its study. Radiologic/pathologic conferences are required for those residents who do not participate in formalized extramural pathology teaching programs.

Computer applications in radiology, practice management, and health systems and quality improvement are also required curriculum components.

Teaching files (electronic or film) of cases related to all aspects of diagnostic radiology must be available for use by residents. Aggregates of these files should contain a minimum of 1,000 cases that are actively maintained and continually enhanced with new cases. The American College of Radiology learning file or its equivalent should be available to residents; this only partially meets the teaching file requirements.

Conferences and teaching rounds must be correlated and provide for progressive resident participation. There should be intradepartmental conferences as well as interdepartmental conferences of appropriate frequency with each major clinical department in which both residents and faculty participate on a regular basis.

C. Resident Policies

1. Supervision
The responsibility or independence given to residents should depend on their knowledge, manual skill, and experience. Faculty supervision must be available at all sites of training.
The resident in the first year of training in the diagnostic radiology program must have a minimum of 6 months of training in diagnostic radiology prior to independent in-house on-call responsibilities. Residents must always have faculty backup when taking night or weekend call. All radiologic images must be reviewed and all reports must be signed by faculty.
2. Duty Hours and Conditions of Work
Duty hours and night and weekend call for residents must reflect the concept of responsibility for adequate patient care. However, residents must not be required regularly to perform excessively difficult or prolonged duties. It is recommended that residents should be allowed to spend at least 1 full day out of 7 away from the hospital and should be assigned on-call duty in the hospital no more than, on average, every third night. It is the responsibility of the program director to monitor resident assignments to ensure adherence to this recommendation.

D. Other Required Components

1. Scholarly Activity
Graduate medical education must take place in an environment of inquiry and scholarship in which residents participate in the development of new knowledge, learn to evaluate research findings, and develop habits of inquiry as a continuing professional responsibility. The responsibility for establishing and maintaining an environment of inquiry and scholarship rests with the teaching faculty. While not all members of a teaching faculty must be investigators, the faculty as a whole must demonstrate broad involvement in scholarly activity. This activity should include the following:
   a. Active participation of the teaching faculty in clinical discussions, rounds, and conferences in a manner that promotes a spirit of inquiry and scholarship. Scholarship implies an in-depth understanding of basic mechanisms of normal and abnormal states and the application of current knowledge to practice.
   b. Participation in journal clubs and research conferences
   c. Active participation in regional or national professional and scientific societies, particularly through presentations at the organizations' meetings and publication in their journals
   d. Participation in continuing medical education programs
   e. Participation in research, particularly in projects that are funded following peer review and/or result in publication or presentations at regional and national scientific meetings
   f. Offering of guidance and technical support (eg, research design, statistical analysis) for residents involved in scholarly activities
2. Resident Research
During their training, all residents should be encouraged to engage in an investigative project under faculty supervision. This may take the form of laboratory research, clinical research, or the retrospective analysis of data from patients, and results of such projects shall be suitable for publication or presentation at local, regional, or national scientific meetings.

VI. Evaluation

A. Resident Evaluation

The program director is responsible for regular evaluation of residents' knowledge, skills, and overall performance, including the development of professional attitudes consistent with being a physician. Evaluations of each resident's progress and competence should be conducted preferably at the end of each rotation, but not less than four times yearly. The evaluation must concern itself with intellectual abilities, attitudes and character skills, and clinical and technical competence. The program director or the program director's designee must meet with all the residents at least semiannually to discuss these evaluations and provide feedback on performance. More frequent reviews of performance for residents experiencing difficulties or receiving unfavorable evaluations are required. There must be provision for appropriate and timely feedback of the content of all evaluations to the resident. Residents should be advanced to positions of higher responsibility only on the basis of their satisfactory progressive scholarship and professional growth. The program must maintain a permanent record of the evaluation and counseling process for each resident. Such records must be accessible to the resident and other authorized personnel.

There must be a written final evaluation for each resident who completes the program. The evaluation must include a review of the resident's performance during the final period of training and should verify that the resident has demonstrated sufficient professional ability to practice competently and independently. The final evaluation should be part of the resident's permanent record maintained by the institution.

B. Faculty and Program Evaluation

The program must provide the opportunity for residents to provide written confidential evaluation of the faculty and the program at least annually. Each faculty member must review his or her evaluations.

The educational effectiveness of a program must be evaluated in a systematic manner. In particular, the quality of the curriculum and the extent to which the educational goals have been met by residents must be assessed. Anonymous written evaluations by residents should be utilized in this process.

VII. Board Certification

The RRC will consider the performance of a program's graduates on the examinations of the American Board of Radiology as one measure of the quality of the training program. During the most recent 5-year period, at least 50% of its graduates should pass without condition the written and oral examinations on the first attempt.

Residents who plan to seek certification by the American Board of Radiology should communicate with the Executive Director of the Board to be certain of all requirements, including duration of training, for admission to the examination process.

ACGME: June 1998 Effective: July 1999

Policies and Procedures for Residency Education in the Subspecialties of Diagnostic Radiology

Subspecialty programs must be administratively linked to an accredited core residency program in diagnostic radiology. (The only exception is pediatric radiology, as discussed below.) An application for accreditation of a new subspecialty program will be considered only if the core program has full accreditation. An application will not be accepted for review if the core program in diagnostic radiology is accredited on a provisional or a probationary basis, or if it has been accredited with a warning that adverse action will be taken if it is not in substantial compliance with the *Essentials of Accredited Residencies in Graduate Medical Education* at the time of the next review.

A subspecialty program in pediatric radiology may not necessarily be administratively linked to an accredited core residency program in diagnostic radiology if the pediatric radiology program is conducted in a children's hospital. In such a case, the subspecialty program may be considered free-standing and, therefore, not required to be under the sponsorship of a diagnostic radiology residency program.

An on-site survey of the proposed program is required for the initial review by the Residency Review Committee. Accreditation will be granted on the basis of the application and the written report from the on-site survey of the proposed program. Following the initial approval, the subspecialty program will be surveyed and reviewed in conjunction with the core diagnostic radiology program.

Subspecialty programs will be designated as "accredited" or "nonaccredited." No other delineation of accreditation categories will be used. The accreditation status of the subspecialty program will be directly related to that of the core diagnostic radiology program, as follows:

Subspecialty programs may be cited for deficiencies and advised that either the deficiencies must be corrected by the specified time or accreditation will be withdrawn regardless of the accreditation status of the associated diagnostic radiology program.

If the associated diagnostic radiology program is accredited on a probationary basis, or accredited with a warning that adverse action will be taken, the subspecialty program will be informed that its accreditation status is also in jeopardy. Thereafter, accreditation of the subspecialty programs will be withdrawn if the Residency Review Committee finds that the sponsoring institution(s) is (are) not making satisfactory progress in addressing the adverse accreditation status of the core diagnostic radiology program.

Withdrawal of accreditation of the core diagnostic radiology residency program will result in simultaneous withdrawal of accreditation of the subspecialty program.

In the case of withholding of accreditation or withdrawing accreditation of subspecialty programs, the *Procedures for Proposed Adverse Actions* and the *Procedures for Appeal of Adverse Actions* apply.

Program Requirements for Residency Education in the Subspecialties of Diagnostic Radiology

These requirements apply to all of the accredited subspecialty areas and should be consulted with the individual subspecialty Program Requirements.

I. General Information

A. A residency education program in a subspecialty of diagnostic radiology is an educational experience of at least 1 year designed to develop advanced knowledge and skills in a specific clinical area. All educational components of the program should be related to program goals. The program design and/or structure must be approved by the Residency Review Committee (RRC) as part of the regular review process.

Completion of an Accreditation Council for Graduate Medical Education (ACGME)-accredited diagnostic radiology residency or its equivalent is a prerequisite for entry into a subspecialty program of diagnostic radiology.

B. Residency education programs in the subspecialties of diagnostic radiology may be accredited only in institutions that either sponsor a residency education program in diagnostic radiology accredited by the ACGME or are integrated by formal agreement into such programs. (See Program Requirements for Residency Education in Pediatric Radiology for exceptions to this requirement.) Close cooperation between the subspecialty and residency program directors is required.

C. Rotations to affiliated institutions can be approved for a period not exceeding 25% of the total program; adequate educational justification for such rotations must be provided to the RRC prior to implementation. The definitions governing affiliated and integrated institutions in the Program Requirements for Residency Education in Diagnostic Radiology also apply to the subspecialty programs of diagnostic radiology.

D. Subspecialty programs will not be approved if they have substantial negative impact on the education of the diagnostic radiology residents in the core program.

II. Faculty Qualifications and Responsibilities

The program director and faculty are responsible for the general administration of a program, including activities related to the recruitment and selection, supervision, counseling, evaluation, and advancement of residents and the maintenance of records related to program accreditation.

Subspecialty education programs must provide a scholarly environment for acquiring the necessary cognitive and procedural clinical skills essential to the practice of the specific subspecialty. This objective can be achieved only when the program director, the supporting faculty and staff, and the administration are fully committed to the educational program. It is also imperative that appropriate resources and facilities be present. Service obligations must not compromise educational goals and objectives.

A. Qualifications of the Program Director

There must be a single program director responsible for the subspecialty program. The director must be an experienced educator and supervisor of residents in the subspecialty. He or she must be certified by the American Board of Radiology in diagnostic radiology or radiology or possess equivalent qualifications, and shall have had postresidency experience in the subspecialty, preferably fellowship training. (See Program Requirements for Residency Education in the individual subspecialties for subspecialty certification requirements.) The program director must be licensed to practice medicine in the state where the institution that sponsors the program is located. (Certain federal programs are exempted.) The program director must be a member of the radiology faculty, spend essentially all professional time in the subspecialty, and devote sufficient time to fulfill all responsibilities inherent in meeting the educational goals of the program.

B. Responsibilities of the Program Director

It is the responsibility of the subspecialty program director to support the residency education program by devoting his/her principal effort to its management and administration, as well as to teaching, research, and clinical care limited to the integrated institutions. This general responsibility includes the following specifics:

1. Preparation of a written statement outlining the educational goals of the program with respect to knowledge, skills, and other attributes of residents and for each major rotation or other program assignment. This statement must be distributed to residents and members of the teaching staff and should be readily available for review.
2. Selection of residents for appointment to the program in accordance with institutional and departmental policies and procedures.
3. Selection and supervision of the teaching staff and other program personnel at each institution participating in the program.
4. Supervision of residents through explicit written descriptions of supervisory lines of responsibility for the care of patients. Such guidelines must be communicated to all members of the program staff. Residents must be provided with prompt, reliable systems for communication and interaction with supervisory physicians.
5. Regular evaluation of residents' knowledge, skills, and overall performance, including the development of professional attitudes consistent with being a physician.
6. Implementation of fair procedures, as established by the sponsoring institution, regarding academic discipline and resident complaints or grievances.
7. Monitoring of resident stress, including mental or emotional conditions inhibiting performance or learning and drug- or alcohol-related dysfunction. Program directors and teaching staff should be sensitive to the need for timely provision of confidential counseling and psychological support services to residents. Training situations that consistently produce undesirable stress on residents must be evaluated and modified.
8. Preparation of an accurate statistical and narrative description of the program.
9. Notification of the RRC regarding major programmatic changes. Prior approval of the RRC is required for the addition or deletion of a major participating hospital, for an increase in the number of residents in the program, and for a major change in the program's organization.

C. Faculty

There must be a sufficient number of teaching staff with documented qualifications to instruct and supervise adequately all the residents in the program. Members of the teaching staff must be able to devote sufficient time to meet their supervisory and teaching responsibilities.

All members of the teaching staff must demonstrate a strong interest in the education of residents, sound clinical and teaching abilities, support of the goals and objectives of the program, a commitment to their own continuing medical education, and participation in scholarly activities.

A member of the teaching staff of each participating institution must be designated to assume responsibility for the day-to-day activities of the program at that institution, with overall coordination by the program director.

The teaching staff must be organized and have regular documented meetings to review program goals and objectives as well as program effectiveness in achieving them. At least one resident representative should participate in these reviews.

The teaching staff should periodically evaluate the utilization of the resources available to the program, the contribution of each institution participating in the program, the financial and administrative support of the program, the volume and variety of patients available to the program for educational purposes, the performance of members of the teaching staff, and the quality of supervision of residents.

D. Other Program Personnel

Programs must be provided with the additional professional, technical, and clerical personnel needed to support the administration and educational conduct of the program.

III. Facilities and Resources

A. Space and Equipment

(See Program Requirements for Residency Education in the individual subspecialties for space and equipment requirements.)

B. Library

Residents must have ready access to a major medical library, either at the institution where the residents are located or through arrangement with convenient nearby institutions. There must be access to an on-site library or to a collection of appropriate texts and journals in each institution participating in a residency program. Access to computerized literature search facilities is necessary. On-site libraries and/or collections of texts and journals must be readily available during nights and weekends.

IV. Educational Program

The director and teaching staff must prepare and comply with written goals for the program. All educational components of the program should be related to the program goals. The program design must be approved by the RRC as part of the regular review process. A written statement of the educational objectives must be given to each resident.

A postgraduate residency must provide advanced education so that the residents can acquire special skill and knowledge in a specific subspecialty. This education should consist of a cognitive and a technical component. The cognitive component should emphasize the scholarly attributes of self-instruction, teaching, skilled clinical analysis, sound judgment, and research creativity. The technical component must provide appropriate opportunity for the residents to acquire the operative and other psychomotor skills required for the practice of the subspecialty.

A. Clinical Components

A sufficient number of patients must be available to ensure appropriate inpatient and outpatient experience for each subspecialty resident without adversely affecting the experience of residents in the diagnostic radiology core program.

The total number of residents is dependent on the program's resources and its capacity to provide an excellent educational experience.

B. Didactic Components

Subspecialty conferences, including review of all current complications and deaths, seminars, and clinical and basic science instruction, must be regularly scheduled. Active participation of the subspecialty resident in the planning and the production of these meetings is essential.

C. Supervision

A resident must have the opportunity to provide consultation with faculty supervision. He or she should have clearly defined educational responsibilities for diagnostic radiology residents, medical students, and professional personnel. These teaching experiences should correlate basic biomedical knowledge with the clinical aspects of the subspecialty.

There must be close interaction between the core residency program in diagnostic radiology and the subspecialty program. Lines of responsibility for the diagnostic radiology residents and the subspecialty resident must be clearly defined. It is imperative that the educational program for the subspecialty resident not adversely affect the education of the diagnostic radiology residents, in terms of either experience or patient responsibility.

D. Duty Hours and Conditions of Work

The program director must establish an environment that is optimal both for resident education and for patient care, including the responsibility for continuity of care, while ensuring that undue stress and fatigue among residents are avoided. It is the program director's responsibility to ensure assignment of appropriate in-hospital duty hours so that residents are not subjected to excessively difficult or prolonged working hours. It is desirable that residents' work schedules be designed so that on average, excluding exceptional patient care needs, residents have at least 1 day out of 7 free of routine responsibilities and be on call in the hospital no more often than every third night.

During the on-call hours residents should be provided with adequate sleeping, lounge, and food facilities. There must be adequate backup so that patient care is not jeopardized during or following assigned periods of duty. Support services and systems must be such that the resident does not spend an inordinate amount of time in noneducational activities that can be discharged properly by other personnel.

E. Scholarly Activity

Graduate medical education must take place in an environment of inquiry and scholarship in which residents participate in the development of new knowledge, learn to evaluate research findings, and develop habits of inquiry as a continuing professional responsibility. The responsibility for establishing and maintaining an environment of inquiry and scholarship rests with the teaching staff. While not all members of a teaching staff must be investigators, the staff as a whole must demonstrate broad involvement in scholarly activity. This activity should include

1. active participation of the teaching staff in clinical discussions, rounds, and conferences in a manner that promotes a spirit of inquiry and scholarship. Scholarship implies an in-depth understanding of basic mechanisms of normal and abnormal states and the application of current knowledge to practice.
2. participation in journal clubs and research conferences.
3. active participation in regional or national professional and scientific societies, particularly through presentations at the organizations' meetings and publications in their journals.
4. participation in research, particularly in projects that are funded following peer review and/or result in publications or presentations at regional and national scientific meetings.
5. offering of guidance and technical support (eg, research design, statistical analysis) for residents involved in research.
6. provision of support for resident participation in scholarly activities.

F. Research

A subspecialty program should have an investigational component such that the residents may become familiar with the design, implementation, and interpretation of clinical research studies. Facilities should be made available for research activity. (See Program Requirements for the individual subspecialties for further requirements.)

V. Evaluation

A. Residents

Subspecialty program directors must establish clearly defined procedures for regular evaluation of residents' knowledge, skills, and overall performance, including the development of professional attitudes consistent with being a physician. The assessment must include cognitive, motor, and interpersonal skills as well as judgment.

The program director, with participation of members of the teaching staff, shall

1. at least semiannually evaluate the knowledge, skills, and professional growth of the residents, using appropriate criteria and procedures.
2. communicate each evaluation to the resident in a timely manner.
3. advance residents to positions of higher responsibility only on the basis of evidence of their satisfactory progressive scholarship and professional growth.
4. maintain a permanent record of evaluation for each resident and have it accessible to the resident and other authorized personnel.
5. provide a written final evaluation for each resident who completes the program. The evaluation must include a review of the resident's performance during the final period of training and should verify that the resident has demonstrated sufficient professional ability to practice competently and independently. This final evaluation should be part of the resident's permanent record maintained by the institution.

B. Faculty

Faculty must be evaluated at least annually to review teaching abilities, commitment to the educational program, clinical knowledge, and scholarly activities. Residents should participate in these evaluations.

C. Program

The educational effectiveness of a program must be evaluated in a systematic manner. In particular, the quality of the curriculum and the extent to which the educational goals have been met by residents must be assessed by the subspecialty program director, the core diagnostic radiology program director, and the Institutional Review Committee on a regular basis. Written evaluations by residents should be utilized in this process.

VI. Board Certification

Residents who plan to seek certification by the American Board of Radiology should communicate with the Executive Director of the Board to ascertain the current requirements for acceptance as a candidate for subspecialty certification.

ACGME: February 1994 Effective: January 1995

Program Requirements for Residency Education in Abdominal Radiology (Radiology-Diagnostic)

In addition to complying with the Program Requirements for Residency Education in the Subspecialties of Diagnostic Radiology, programs must comply with the following requirements, which in some cases may exceed the common requirements.

I. Scope and Duration of Training

A. Definition and Scope of the Specialty

Abdominal radiology constitutes the application and interpretation of conventional radiology, computed tomography, ultrasonography, magnetic resonance (MR) imaging, nuclear medicine, fluoroscopy, and interventional methods customarily included within the specialty of diagnostic radiology as they apply to diseases involving the gastrointestinal tract, the genitourinary tract, and the intraperitoneal and extraperitoneal abdominal organs.

The program must be organized to enhance substantially the residents' knowledge of the application of all forms of diagnostic imaging and interventional techniques to the unique clinical pathophysiologic problems encountered in diseases affecting the gastrointestinal and genitourinary systems. The program should include education in normal and pathologic anatomy and physiology of gastrointestinal and genitourinary disease and be structured to develop expertise in the appropriate application of all forms of diagnostic imaging and interventions to problems of the abdomen and pelvis.

B. Duration of Training

The program shall offer 1 year of graduate medical education in abdominal radiology. This year of training must follow successful completion of an ACGME-accredited program in diagnostic radiology or its equivalent.

II. Faculty Qualifications and Responsibilities

The director of the program in abdominal radiology must be an experienced educator and supervisor of residents in abdominal radiology. The program director must be certified by the American Board of Radiology in radiology or diagnostic radiology, or possess equivalent qualifications, and shall have had postresidency experience in abdominal radiology, preferably fellowship training.

The faculty should include, in addition to the program director, at least one other full-time radiologist specializing in abdominal radiology. At a minimum, the program faculty must have two full-time equivalent faculty members dedicated to the program. Although it is desirable that abdominal radiologists supervise special imaging such as computed tomography, ultrasonography, and magnetic resonance imaging, in instances where they are not expert in a special imaging technique, other radiologists who are specialists in those areas must be part-time members of the abdominal radiology faculty. The faculty must provide didactic teaching and supervision of the residents' performance and interpretation of all abdominal imaging procedures.

(See Program Requirements for the Subspecialties of Diagnostic Radiology for additional program director and faculty requirements.)

The total number of residents in the program must be commensurate with the capacity of the program to offer an adequate educational experience in abdominal radiology. The minimum number of residents need not be greater than one, but at least two residents is desirable. To ensure adequate supervision and evaluation of the residents' academic progress, the faculty/resident ratio should not be less than one faculty member to each resident.

III. Facilities and Resources

A. Space and Equipment

Modern imaging equipment and adequate space must be available to accomplish the overall educational program in abdominal radiology. There must be state-of-the-art equipment for conventional radiography, digital fluoroscopy, computed tomography, ultrasonography, nuclear medicine, and magnetic resonance imaging. Laboratory and pathology services must be adequate to support the educational experience in abdominal radiology. Adequate areas for display of images, interpretation of images, and consultation with clinicians must be available.

B. Library

Ancillary teaching resources must include access to a medical library. A variety of textbooks, journals, and other teaching materials in abdominal radiology and related medical and surgical fields must be available. A subspecialty teaching file and in-house file must be actively developed and available for use by residents. The ACR teaching files in gastrointestinal and genitourinary radiology only partially meet this requirement.

IV. Educational Program

A. Clinical Components

The program must provide both clinical and didactic experiences that encompass the full breadth of diseases and their pathophysiology, including coverage of uncommon problems involving the gastrointestinal tract, genitourinary tract, and abdomen, including but not limited to the liver and biliary system, pancreas, stomach, esophagus, small bowel, colon, spleen, kidneys, adrenal glands, bladder, male and female reproductive systems, and lymphatic system.

The program must provide an adequate volume and variety of imaging studies and interventional procedures and must provide instruction in their indications, appropriate utilization, risks, and alternatives. The resident must have the opportunity to perform the abdominal imaging studies, including urethrography; urography; cystography; hysterosalpingography; computed tomography; ultrasonography; MR imaging; and plain radiographic and fluoroscopic studies of the hollow gastrointestinal tract.

The resident also must gain experience in performing guided biopsies of intraperitoneal and retroperitoneal structures and aspiration and drainage of abscesses. The resident must be familiar with the indications and complications of percutaneous nephrostomy, and transhepatic cholangiography and obtain experience in providing fluoroscopic guidance for the dilation of gastrointestinal, biliary, pancreatic, and ureteric duct strictures. Interpretation of endoscopic retrograde cholangiopancreatography (ERCP) and operative cholangiography must be taught. The program also should provide opportunity, through conferences and individual consultation, for the residents to integrate invasive procedures, where indicated, into optimal care plans for patients, even though formal responsibility for performing the procedures may not be part of the program.

The program must provide instruction in the indications for, as well as the complications of, certain procedures, such as visceral angiography, tumor embolization, radionuclide scintigraphy, lithotripsy, gastrostomy, nephrostomy, and cholecystostomy.

Graded responsibility or independence given to residents should depend on their knowledge, technical skill, and experience. Attending faculty must be available to perform and/or supervise procedures as required.

B. Didactic Components

A major goal of the didactic portion of the training program should be to provide the resident with understanding of the pathophysiology of diseases that affect the gastrointestinal and genitourinary tracts. Diagnostic skill and understanding of uncommon problems in abdominal disease, as well as of the indications, risks, limitations, alternatives, and appropriate utilization of imaging and interventional procedures, should be part of the body of knowledge imparted.

Education must be available in the basic radiologic sciences, eg, diagnostic radiologic physics, radiation biology, and the pharmacology of radiographic contrast materials.

There must be intradepartmental conferences, as well as conferences with related clinical departments, in which residents in abdominal radiology participate on a regular basis. These should include one or more weekly departmental conferences in abdominal radiology and at least one monthly interdepartmental clinical conference.

Residents must be given the opportunity to present the radiologic aspects of cases in combined clinical conferences related to allied disciplines. They also should prepare clinically and/or pathologically proven cases for inclusion in an ongoing teaching file. There must be daily image interpretation sessions that require that residents reach their own diagnostic conclusions, which then are reviewed and critiqued by faculty. Diagnostic reports generated by residents should be closely reviewed for content, level of confidence, grammar, and style.

Residents should be encouraged to attend and participate in regional conferences. They should attend at least one national meeting or postgraduate course in abdominal radiology during the year of fellowship training.

C. Additional Required Components

There should be an ACGME-accredited residency or subspecialty training program available in general surgery, gastroenterology, oncology, urology, gynecology, and pathology; at a minimum there must be Board-certified (or equivalent) specialists in these areas to provide appropriate patient populations and educational resources in the institution. These specialists may serve as additional faculty.

D. Scholarly Activities

The training program should have a research component that offers an opportunity for residents to learn the fundamentals of design, performance, and interpretation of research studies, as well as how to evaluate investigative methods. Particular attention should be given to developing competence in critical assessment of new imaging modalities and of the radiologic literature, and residents will be expected to participate actively in research projects. The program must provide sufficient office space, supplies, and secretarial support to enable residents to conduct research projects as well as perform literature searches, manuscript preparation, statistical analysis, and photography.

VI. Evaluation

(See Program Requirements for the Subspecialties of Diagnostic Radiology for evaluation requirements.)

ACGME: June 1998 Effective: June 1998

Program Requirements for Residency Education in Musculoskeletal Radiology (Radiology-Diagnostic)

In addition to complying with the Program Requirements for Residency Education in the Subspecialties of Diagnostic Radiology, programs must comply with the following requirements, which in some cases may exceed the common requirements.

I. Scope and Duration of Training

A. Definition and Scope of the Subspecialty

The musculoskeletal radiology training program constitutes a closely supervised experience in the application and interpretation of all imaging examinations and procedures as they relate to the analysis of disorders of the musculoskeletal system, including bones, joints, and soft tissues. The imaging methods and procedures include, but are not necessarily limited to, routine radiography, computed tomography, ultrasonography, radionuclide scintigraphy, magnetic resonance, arthrography, and image-guided percutaneous biopsy techniques. The objective of training in musculoskeletal radiology is to provide an organized, comprehensive, supervised, and progressively responsible full-time educational experience in the selection, interpretation, and performance of these examinations and procedures. A further objective is to provide the resident an opportunity to develop skills necessary for clinical and/or basic research in the subspecialty of musculoskeletal radiology.

B. Duration of Training

The program shall offer 1 year of graduate medical education in musculoskeletal radiology.

Completion of an Accreditation Council for Graduate Medical Education (ACGME)-accredited program in diagnostic radiology or its equivalent must precede the period of training in musculoskeletal radiology.

II. Faculty Qualifications and Responsibilities

The program director must be certified in diagnostic radiology or radiology by the American Board of Radiology or possess equivalent qualifications.

In addition to the program director, the program must include at least one person experienced in musculoskeletal radiology who has a substantial commitment to the training program. If necessary, other radiologists with expertise in certain imaging methods or procedures may function at least as part-time members of the training program. To ensure adequate supervision of the residents, there must be at least one full-time faculty person available for each two residents in the program.

III. Facilities and Resources

A. Space and Equipment

Modern facilities and equipment and adequate space must be available to ensure an adequate educational experience for the resident. Access to routine radiographic, computed tomographic, scintigraphic, magnetic resonance, and ultrasound equipment must be provided. Adequate space for film display, film interpretation, and consultation with referring physicians must be available, and adequate office space, office supplies, and secretarial help for the conduct of research projects should be provided for musculoskeletal radiology faculty and residents. Assistance with literature searches, editing, statistical tabulation, and photography should be provided.

B. Library

The training program must provide ancillary teaching resources including access to a medical library with a sufficient number of textbooks and journals related to musculoskeletal diseases and electronic literature search capabilities. A musculoskeletal radiology/pathology teaching file must be developed and available for use by the residents. The American College of Radiology teaching file will only partially meet this requirement.

IV. Educational Program

A. Clinical Components

Residents in musculoskeletal radiology must be provided access to a variety of patients encompassing the entire range of disorders of the musculoskeletal system, including articular, degenerative, metabolic, hematopoietic, infectious, traumatic, vascular, congenital, and neoplastic diseases. The imaging methods and procedures available for training should include routine radiography, computed tomography, ultrasonography, radionuclide scintigraphy, magnetic resonance, arthrography, and image-guided percutaneous biopsy techniques.

The program curriculum must provide clinical experience and didactic sessions encompassing the entire spectrum of musculoskeletal diseases. This must include both the axial and the appendicular skeletons of both adult and pediatric patients. The resident must interpret, under appropriate supervision, diagnostic examinations that include routine radiography, computed tomography, and magnetic resonance. Furthermore, the resident must perform and interpret arthrograms. The program must provide experience with image-guided percutaneous biopsy procedures and exposure to ultrasonography, bone densitometry, and radionuclide scintigraphy as they relate to diseases of the musculoskeletal system. A log must be kept by each resident documenting the types of arthrographic and biopsy procedures that she or he performs. With regard to invasive procedures, residents are to be given graduated responsibility as competence increases; such responsibility should include preprocedural and postprocedural patient care. Emphasis is placed on close coordination and cooperation with referring physicians, including orthopedic surgeons, rheumatologists, and emergency department specialists, and on establishment of proper imaging protocols to ensure that excessive or inappropriate examinations are not ordered and performed. Access to both inpatients and outpatients is required.

B. Didactic Components

There must be didactic conferences and teaching sessions that provide coverage of musculoskeletal concepts related to anatomy, physiology, pathology, orthopedic surgery, and rheumatology. Attendance at and participation in department conferences such as daily film interpretation sessions are required. Regularly scheduled interdepartmental conferences in, for example, orthopedic surgery, neurosurgery, and other appropriate surgical specialties; pathology; rheumatology; and oncology are also necessary components of the program. In addition, the training experience should include radiology oriented conferences with medical students and graduate medical staff. The resident also should be encouraged to attend at least one national meeting or postgraduate course dealing with musculoskeletal radiology during his/her fellowship year.

Although the precise responsibility of the resident will vary from one clinical conference to another, opportunities must exist for active participation in the formulation of a diagnosis and/or the generation of an imaging protocol; such participation is to be used as a means by which the program director and other faculty members judge the resident's progress.

C. Resident Participation in Research

The training period in musculoskeletal radiology should provide sufficient research opportunities for the resident. He or she should be able to participate in the design, performance, and interpretation of research studies and have the opportunity to develop competence in critical assessment of investigative techniques. Completion of at least one clinical or basic research investigation during the period of training is encouraged. Laboratory facilities to support research projects should be available in the institution.

D. Interchange With Residents in Other Specialties

The presence of accredited training programs in orthopedic surgery and rheumatology is highly desirable.

Shared experiences with residents in orthopedic surgery, rheumatology, pathology, and other appropriate specialties, including surgical subspecialties, are strongly encouraged. When appropriate, supervision and teaching by faculty expert in these additional disciplines should be available.

V. Evaluation

(See Program Requirements for Residency Education in the Subspecialties of Diagnostic Radiology for details concerning evaluation requirements.)

ACGME: February 1996 Effective: February 1996

Program Requirements for Residency Education in Neuroradiology (Radiology-Diagnostic)

In addition to complying with the Program Requirements for Residency Education in the Subspecialties of Diagnostic Radiology, programs must comply with the following requirements, which may in some cases exceed the common requirements.

I. Scope and Duration of Training

A. Definition and Scope of the Subspecialty

The body of knowledge and practice of neuroradiology comprises both imaging and interventional procedures related to the brain, spine and spinal cord, head, neck, and organs of special sense in adults and children. Special training and skills are required to enable the neuroradiologist to function as an expert diagnostic and therapeutic consultant and practitioner. The objective of training in this subspecialty of radiology is to provide residents with an organized, comprehensive and highly supervised full-time educational experience in the selection, interpretation, and performance of these examinations and procedures and to provide them with opportunities and skills for research in the field of neuroradiology.

B. Duration of Training

The program shall offer 1 year of graduate medical education in neuroradiology. This year of training must follow successful completion of an Accreditation Council for Graduate Medical Education (ACGME)-accredited program in diagnostic radiology or its equivalent.

II. Faculty Qualifications and Responsibilities

The program director shall have had appropriate postresidency experience in neuroradiology, preferably fellowship training.

At a minimum, the neuroradiology faculty must include, in addition to the program director, one or more neuroradiologists whose total time commitment to neuroradiology is at least one half-time equivalent and who are able to devote adequate time to the program. Their expertise may be limited to a segment of neuroradiology or a related discipline, eg, interventional neuroradiology, pediatric neuroradiology, or head and neck radiology. The faculty must provide didactic teaching and supervision of the residents' performance and interpretations of neuroradiologic procedures.

The minimum number of residents need not be greater than one, but two residents are desirable. To ensure adequate supervision and evaluation of a resident's academic progress, the faculty/resident ratio should not be less than one full-time faculty person for every two residents.

III. Facilities and Resources

A. Space and Equipment

The following equipment, which should be "state of the art," should be available: magnetic resonance (MR) imager, computed tomography (CT) scanner, film-screen and digital subtraction angiography (DSA) equipment, a radiographic-fluoroscopic room(s) with tilt table suitable for performing myelography, and conventional radiographic and tomographic equipment. The examination rooms should be equipped for monitoring so that examinations may be performed in high-risk patients. Adjacent to or within examination rooms there should be facilities for storing the catheters, gowns, embolic materials, contrast material, and other supplies needed for the conduct of neuroradiological procedures. A room should be available near the angiographic room for sterilization and preparation of catheters, instrument trays, and other reusable supplies. There must be adequate space within the department to house these facilities.

Adequate areas for film display, interpretation of films, and consultation with clinicians must be available. There must be adequate office space and support space for neuroradiology faculty/staff and residents.

The program should provide office space, office supplies, and secretarial help for the conduct of research projects. Assistance with literature searches, editing, statistical tabulation, and photography should be provided.

B. Laboratory

The institution should provide laboratory facilities to support research projects. It is highly desirable to have an animal facility with radiographic-fluoroscopic equipment, particularly that which might be used for invasive diagnostic and therapeutic neuroradiologic procedures.

C. Library

There should be ready access to a library of general medical texts and periodicals. In particular, there should be periodicals and texts in the fields of neuroradiology, diagnostic radiology, head and neck radiology, neurology, neurosurgery, neuroanatomy, and orthopedic surgery. It is desirable that computerized literature search facilities also be available.

IV. Educational Program

A. Curriculum

The program must offer the opportunity for residents to perform, consult, conduct, and interpret, under close supervision, invasive as well as noninvasive procedures in neuroradiology. The procedures shall include cerebral angiography, myelography, CT, MR imaging, ultrasound of the central nervous system and vessels, and plain film radiography related to the brain, head, neck, and spine. It is also desirable that there be exposure to positron emission tomography (PET) and magnetic resonance spectroscopy. With regard to invasive procedures, residents must be given graduated responsibility in the performance of the procedures as competence increases. Responsibility for these procedures should include preprocedural and postprocedural patient care.

B. Clinical Components

Clinical and educational experience in the basic clinical neurosciences, eg, neurosurgery, neurology, neuropathology, neuro-otolaryngology, and neuro-ophthalmology, and in the basic radiological sciences, eg, radiation and MR physics, radiation biology, and the pharmacology of radiographic contrast materials, must be provided. It is expected that there will be strong clinical services in neurological surgery and neurology in the institution sponsoring the neuroradiology program. The majority of the time in the program should be spent in clinical training in neuroradiology.

The program in neuroradiology must provide a sufficient volume and variety of patients with neurological, neurosurgical, neuro-ophthalmologic, neuro-otorhinolaryngologic, spinal, and other pertinent disorders so that residents gain adequate experience in the full gamut of neuroradiologic examinations, procedures, and interpretations. The program must provide an adequate volume and variety of invasive procedures, eg, neuroangiography, myelography, DSA, and therapeutic embolization, and noninvasive neuroradiologic examinations, eg, CT, MR, and plain film studies. The program director should require residents to maintain documentation of the invasive cases in which they have been the performing radiologist and should review the logs with them at least once in the course of the training year. Clinical experience may be supplemented by training through affiliations with other institutions.

C. Didactic Components

There shall be intradepartmental conferences as well as conferences with related clinical departments in which residents and residents participate on a regular basis. These should include one or more weekly departmental conferences in neuroradiology, as well as institutional conferences in clinical neurosciences that are held at least monthly. Residents should be encouraged to attend and participate in local extramural conferences and should attend at least one national meeting or postgraduate course in neuroradiology while in training.

Residents should be encouraged to present the radiological aspects of cases that are discussed in clinical conferences related to the allied disciplines, such as neurosurgery and the neurological sciences. They should also prepare clinically or pathologically proved cases for inclusion in the teaching file.

There should be daily "film reading" conferences that should require residents to reach their own diagnostic conclusions, which should then be reviewed and criticized by faculty/staff. These conferences need not be limited to clinically current cases, but may be based on cases that are already within the teaching file. Diagnostic reports generated by residents should be closely reviewed for content, level of confidence, grammar, and style.

D. Resident Participation in Research

Residents should be encouraged to undertake investigative study of either a clinical or basic science nature. At least one project of such merit that it could be submitted for publication should be encouraged.

E. Interchange With Residents in Other Specialties and Students

Residents should be encouraged to participate in the research projects of residents and staff persons in other specialties. They should attend clinical conferences in other specialties and serve as consultants to these conferences. It is desirable that they participate in the clinical teaching of medical students and also in the preclinical curriculum in subjects such as anatomy and physiology.

V. Evaluation

(See Program Requirements for Residency Education in the Subspecialties of Diagnostic Radiology for details concerning evaluation requirements.)

ACGME: February 1990 Effective: July 1995

Program Requirements for Residency Education in Nuclear Radiology (Radiology-Diagnostic)

In addition to complying with the Program Requirements for Residency Education in the Subspecialties of Diagnostic Radiology, programs must comply with the following requirements, which may in some cases exceed the common requirements.

I. Scope and Duration of Training

A. Definition and Scope of the Specialty

Nuclear radiology is defined as a clinical subspecialty of radiology involving imaging by external detection of radionuclides and/or biodistribution by external detection of radionuclides in the body for diagnosis of disease. Residency training programs in nuclear radiology must provide advanced training in the medical uses of radionuclides for in vivo imaging.

A training program in nuclear radiology will be accredited only in those institutions that have an accredited training program in diagnostic radiology.

A program in nuclear radiology will be reviewed and accredited in conjunction with the review and accreditation of the residency program in diagnostic radiology.

B. Duration of Training

The program shall offer 1 year of graduate medical education in nuclear radiology. The year of training must follow successful completion of an Accreditation Council for Graduate Medical Education (ACGME)-accredited residency program in diagnostic radiology or its equivalent.

II. Institutional Organization

Those aspects of institutional support that pertain to residencies in diagnostic radiology shall also apply to programs in nuclear radiology, eg, administrative support, facilities, and clinical resources.

III. Faculty Qualifications and Responsibilities

The program director is responsible for the instructional program and for supervision of residents. The program director shall be certified by the American Board of Radiology with Special Competence in Nuclear Radiology or by the American Board of Nuclear Medicine or possess suitable equivalent qualifications. It is desirable that faculty members be certified in boards appropriate to those areas in which they are assigned to instruct and supervise residents. They must contribute sufficient time to the program to provide adequate instruction and supervision.

A faculty (nuclear medicine physician)-to-resident ratio of 1:2 should adequately provide for teaching and supervisory responsibilities.

IV. Facilities and Resources

State-of-the-art nuclear imaging equipment should be available for instructional purposes.

V. Educational Program

The educational program must provide for well-balanced and progressive resident participation through examination of a diverse patient population, with continuous teaching and an active research effort in nuclear radiology.

A. Clinical Component

1. The training program shall include graduated study, experience, and responsibility in all facets of nuclear radiological diagnosis, medical nuclear and diagnostic radiological physics, radiobiology, health physics and protection, nuclear medical instrumentation, radiopharmaceutical chemistry and instrumentation, clinical applications of nuclear radiology, and pathology.
2. The program must provide adequate opportunity for a resident to participate in and personally perform a broad range of nuclear radiological procedures.

B. Didactic Components

1. Formal instruction in diagnostic radiological and medical nuclear physics, radiobiology, and radiopharmaceutical chemistry is required.
2. Appropriate emphasis must be placed on the educational value of teaching rounds and conferences. In addition, there should be frequent interdepartmental teaching conferences.

C. Research

The program should provide an environment in which a resident is encouraged to engage in investigative work with appropriate faculty supervision. Documentation of this environment should be made in the application and indicated by papers published by residents and/or clinical faculty.

D. Teaching File

A teaching file of images referable to all aspects of nuclear radiology must be available for use by residents. This file should be indexed, coded, and currently maintained.

VI. Evaluation

(See Program Requirements for Residency Education in the Subspecialties of Diagnostic Radiology for details concerning evaluation requirements.)

ACGME: September 1996 Effective: July 1997

Program Requirements for Residency Education in Pediatric Radiology (Radiology-Diagnostic)

In addition to complying with the Program Requirements for Residency Education in the Subspecialties of Diagnostic Radiology, programs must comply with the following requirements, which may in some cases exceed the common requirements.

I. Scope and Duration of Training

A. Definition and Scope of the Specialty

The training program in the subspecialty of pediatric radiology constitutes a supervised experience in the pediatric applications and interpretation of radiography, computed tomography, ultrasonography, angiography, interventional techniques, nuclear radiology, magnetic resonance, and any other imaging modality customarily included within the specialty of diagnostic radiology.

The program should be structured to enhance substantially the resident's knowledge of the applications of all forms of diagnostic imaging to the unique clinical/pathophysiologic problems of the newborn, infant, child, and adolescent. The fundamentals of radiobiology, radiological physics, and radiation protection as they relate to the infant, child, and adolescent should be reviewed during the pediatric radiology training experience. The program must provide residents direct and progressively responsible experience in pediatric imaging as they advance through training. This training must culminate in sufficiently independent responsibility for clinical decision making such that the program is assured that the graduating resident has achieved the ability to execute sound clinical judgment.

B. Duration of Training

The program shall offer 1 year of graduate medical education in pediatric radiology. Completion of an Accreditation Council for Graduate Medical Education (ACGME)-accredited program in diagnostic radiology or its equivalent must precede advanced training in pediatric radiology.

C. Objectives and Goals

The educational program in pediatric radiology shall meet training objectives so that on completion of the program the resident is able to

1. understand the developmental and acquired disease processes of the newborn, infant, child, and adolescent, which are basic to the practice of pediatric and adolescent medicine.
2. perform and interpret radiological and imaging studies of the pediatric patient.
3. supervise and teach the elements of radiography and radiology as they pertain to infants and children.
4. understand how to design and perform research (clinical, biomedical, educational, health services).

II. Institutional Organization

A program of pediatric radiology training should function whenever feasible in direct association and/or affiliation with an ACGME accredited program in diagnostic radiology. Pediatric radiology programs may be conducted in either a children's hospital or a general hospital.

III. Faculty Qualifications and Responsibilities

A. Program Director

The program director must have sufficient academic and administrative experience to ensure effective implementation of these program requirements and should have had at least 5 years of participation as an active faculty member in an accredited pediatric radiology program. The program director must be certified by the American Board of Radiology in radiology or diagnostic radiology or possess equivalent qualifications. The program director must have received the Certificate of Added Qualifications in Pediatric Radiology granted by the American Board of Radiology or possess equivalent qualifications. The director must devote sufficient time to the program to fulfill all of the responsibilities inherent in meeting the educational goals of the program. The program director is responsible for establishing the curriculum as well as procedures for evaluation of the resident's competency. Periodic evaluation of the resident with feedback is required. The program director shall select and supervise the trainees and shall select pediatric radiology program faculty members.

B. Faculty

There should be sufficient qualified professional personnel to constitute a teaching faculty. The faculty should comprise no fewer than three experienced radiologists, including the program director, who work full-time in pediatric radiology and its related subspecialty areas and are able to devote adequate time to the program. The minimum faculty requirement may be met by the program director and two other full-time equivalent (ie, a total of three or more individuals) faculty members. Although it is desirable that pediatric radiologists supervise special imaging (ie, angiography, interventional radiology, nuclear radiology, computed tomography, magnetic resonance), in instances where they are not expert in an imaging technique, other radiologists who are specialists in that imaging method should be part-time members of the pediatric radiology faculty. Because such radiologists are usually not broadly experienced in the discipline and practice of pediatric radiology, pediatric radiologists should participate in the interpretation and correlation of the findings of these special imaging examinations.

A ratio of at least two pediatric radiologists for every resident is essential to provide adequate opportunity for teaching and supervision.

IV. Facilities and Resources

A. Space and Equipment

Modern facilities and equipment in adequate space must be available and functioning to accomplish the overall educational program in pediatric radiology. Diagnostic imaging modalities shall include radiography, computed tomography, ultrasonography, radionuclide scintigraphy, angiography, and magnetic resonance imaging. The department must have a minimum of one radiographic/fluoroscopic room, one ultrasound unit, one angiographic room, one computed tomography (CT) scanner, one magnetic resonance (MR) imaging unit, and one nuclear radiology gamma camera. All equipment must be up-to-date. There must be justification for continued use of any equipment that is more than 10 years of age.

In general hospitals that treat patients of all ages, pediatric radiology often is a section of the radiology department; similarly, special imaging services of such departments are separate sections. In such cases, there should be recognition within the special imaging sections of the particular needs of the pediatric radiology program. There should be low-dose roentgenographic/fluoroscopic facilities specifically for children. The availability of all special imaging services for pediatric radiology residents is essential.

Laboratory and pathology services must be adequate to permit residents to enhance their educational experience during the diagnostic imaging and care of patients and to obtain timely correlation with diagnostic imaging studies.

B. Inpatient and Outpatient Services

The hospital must have sufficient inpatient and outpatient services in general and subspecialty pediatrics to ensure a broad, in-depth exposure to pediatrics. The pediatric clinical services must be part of the teaching program and should require diagnostic imaging input for many of their patients.

C. Library

Learning resources should include access to an institutional and/or departmental library with current journals and textbooks sufficient to cover the specialty of pediatrics and pediatric subspecialties, radiology, and related fields. The library must contain journals and current textbooks on all aspects of pediatric radiology. The institutional library must have a librarian and facilities for electronic database searches. Moreover, the methods of performing such electronic database searches must be taught to residents. A pediatric radiology teaching file must be available for use by pediatric radiology residents. This teaching file should contain a minimum of 500 cases that are indexed, coded, actively maintained, and continually enhanced with new cases. Availability of the American College of Radiology pediatric learning file or its equivalent is desirable; this only partially meets the teaching file requirements.

D. Patient Population

There should be an ACGME-accredited residency in pediatrics, as well as pediatric medical and surgical subspecialty programs, to provide an appropriate patient population and educational resources in the institution. In addition to full-time pediatricians, there should be one or more pediatric surgeons, one or more pediatric pathologists, as well as a broad range of pediatric medical and surgical subspecialists.

The institution's pediatric population must include patients with a diversity of pediatric illnesses from which broad experience can be gained. The number of pediatric radiology residents in a program at any given time should reflect the patient census to ensure each trainee of an adequate experience. The program must have sufficient volume and variety of patients to assure that residents gain experience in the full range of pediatric radiological examinations, procedures, and interpretations. A reasonable experience is no less than 15,000 pediatric radiological examinations per year per resident.

V. Educational Program

A. Curriculum

The training should consist of didactic and clinical experiences that encompass the scope of pediatric radiology from the neonate to the adolescent. Every organ system should be studied in the contexts of growth and development, congenital malformations, diseases peculiar to infants and children, and diseases beginning in childhood but causing substantial residual impairment in adulthood. The didactic component should promote scholarship, self-instruction, self-evaluation, teaching, and research activity. It should foster the development of analytic skills and judgment. The clinical component should facilitate skillful technical performance of low radiation dose procedures on all organ systems that are examined in the practice of pediatric radiology. The pediatric imaging experience should include both inpatient and outpatient studies.

Residents must have graded responsibility and supervision in the performance of procedures and the perfection of technical and interpretive skills. It is essential that the pediatric radiology trainee be instructed in common pediatric imaging technical procedures and their indications, limitations, judicious utilization, and risks, including radiation dose considerations. The pediatric radiology resident must also be instructed in the risks and benefits of pediatric sedation; this includes an understanding of the physician's role in the monitoring and management of pediatric patients during and after sedation for diagnostic and therapeutic procedures. Where the program is conducted in a general hospital, the pediatric radiology trainee must have training in imaging examinations of pediatric patients. The scope of a 1-year training program in pediatric radiology shall include all diagnostic imaging applicable to the pediatric patient. The 1-year training program should include no more than 4 weeks' vacation. The curriculum must include the central nervous, musculoskeletal, cardiopulmonary, gastrointestinal, and genitourinary systems. In each organ system, the effective and appropriate use of imaging modalities, including ultrasound, CT, MR, nuclear radiology, and vascular/interventional radiology, should be taught. The resident is responsible for following the imaging workup of the patient and must be substantially involved in the performance and interpretation of examinations that utilize various modalities. Correlation of radiological findings with the clinical management and outcome of the pediatric patient is essential.

B. Clinical Component

The pediatric radiology training program should provide a minimum number of procedures available per year per resident as follows:

- 300 fluoroscopic procedures
- 300 ultrasound examinations
- 200 body imaging (CT/MR) examinations

The number of these procedures available for the pediatric radiology resident should not have an adverse impact on the education of the diagnostic radiology residents in the same institution.

The pediatric radiology resident must have at least 3 weeks of experience in each of the following specialized areas, pediatric neuroradiology, vascular/interventional radiology, and nuclear radiology. This experience may be obtained through a combination of lectures, conferences, seminars, and involvement as the primary or secondary operator and by observing procedures. Supervised instruction should be provided by physicians with special expertise in those disciplines. It is acceptable to supplement the pediatric experience with adult patients in some specialties, such as vascular and interventional radiology, to enhance teaching. The program must require that residents maintain a logbook and document their training in nuclear radiology, neuroradiology, and vascular/interventional radiology. The logbook should include the patient name, medical record number, and procedure(s) performed. The minimum numbers of procedures per resident performed in these specialized areas of pediatric radiology are as follows:

- 50 pediatric nuclear radiology studies
- 200 neuroimaging studies
- 25 vascular/interventional studies

Residents in pediatric radiology should serve as pediatric radiologic consultants with the supervision and mentoring of faculty pediatric radiologists. The teaching experience should include pediatric- and radiological-oriented conferences with medical students, residents, medical staff, and health care professionals.

C. Didactic Component

Study of clinical and basic sciences as they relate to radiology and pediatrics shall be a part of the didactic program. Subspecialty conferences, seminars, and academic review activities in pediatric radiology must be regularly scheduled. It is essential that the resident participate in the planning and presenting of conferences. In addition to conferences, study is integrated with the performance and interpretation of roentgenographic and other imaging examinations.

Residents must attend a minimum of 3 departmental conferences per week dedicated to pediatric radiology and participate in 3 or more interdepartmental conferences or rounds per week. When attending the conferences of other specialties, for example, tumor board, morbidity and mortality, and surgery conferences, the pediatric residents should present the radiographic portions of the conferences. The resident must be involved in daily radiology working conferences (daily conferences reviewing radiographs of intensive care units, other inpatient teams, etc). In the course of the 12-month program residents should attend and participate in at least 20 teaching conferences, such as grand rounds, sponsored by pediatric subspecialty departments. A journal club or research club must meet monthly.

D. Resident Policies

1. Supervision
   The responsibility or independence given to residents should depend on their knowledge, skills, and experience. Additional personnel must be available within an appropriate time interval to perform or to supervise procedures.
2. Duty Hours and Conditions of Work
   Duty hours and night and weekend call for trainees must reflect responsibility for patients and provide for adequate patient care. Residents must not be required regularly to perform excessively difficult or prolonged duties. It is the responsibility of the program director to ensure assignment of reasonable in-hospital duty hours. Residents who are taking night or weekend call must always have assigned faculty who are available for on-call coverage.

E. Other Required Components

1. Resident Participation in Research
   The training program in pediatric radiology should have a research component that will offer the resident an opportunity to learn the fundamentals of design, performance, interpretation of research studies, and evaluation of investigative methods. Train-

ees should develop competence in critical assessment of imaging research, patient outcome data, and the scientific literature.

The resident should participate in clinical, basic biomedical, or health services research projects and submit at least one scientific paper or exhibit to a regional or national meeting. The resident should participate in the quality improvement program of the department.

2. Appointment of Other Residents
The training program should have close interaction with a diagnostic radiology residency. Shared experience with residents in general pediatrics and in the pediatric-related subspecialties, ie, surgery, pathology, and cardiology, is strongly encouraged; where appropriate, supervision and teaching by expert faculty in these disciplines should occur.

The resident must also be involved in teaching conferences for medical students, radiology residents, other residents rotating on the pediatric radiology service, and other health professional training programs.

The subspecialty program in pediatric radiology must not have an adverse impact, such as by dilution of the available clinical material, on the education of the diagnostic radiology residents in the same institution.

VI. Evaluation

The RRC will consider as one measure of a program's quality the performance of its graduates on the examination of the American Board of Radiology for the Certificate of Added Qualifications in Pediatric Radiology. All program graduates should take the examination. (See Program Requirements for Residency Education in the Subspecialties of Diagnostic Radiology for additional evaluation requirements.)

ACGME: September 1997 Effective: July 1998

Program Requirements for Residency Education in Vascular and Interventional Radiology (Radiology-Diagnostic)

In addition to complying with the Program Requirements for Residency Education in the Subspecialties of Diagnostic Radiology, programs must comply with the following requirements, which in some cases exceed the common requirements.

I. Scope and Duration of Training

A. Definition and Scope of the Specialty

The unique clinical and invasive nature of practice in vascular and interventional radiology requires special training and skills. The educational program in the subspecialty of vascular and interventional radiology must be organized to provide comprehensive, full-time training and experience in the evaluation and management of patients requiring imaging guided diagnostic vascular and interventional procedures and a supervised experience in performance of imaging guided diagnostic methods of treating disease. Vascular and interventional procedures are guided by a number of imaging modalities including fluoroscopy, angiography, computed tomography, ultrasonography, magnetic resonance imaging, radionuclide scintigraphy, and other modalities included within the specialty of radiology. The training program must be structured to enhance substantially the resident's knowledge of the application of all forms of imaging to the performance and interpretation of vascular and interventional procedures.

The program in vascular and interventional radiology must be structured to enhance the resident's knowledge of the signs and symptoms of disorders amenable to diagnosis and/or treatment by percutaneous techniques. The significance of the symptoms must be understood, as well as the pathophysiology and natural history of the disorders. Residents must know the indications for and contraindications to vascular and interventional procedures and understand the medical and surgical alternatives to those procedures. The vascular and interventional radiologist must have a complete understanding of imaging methods used to guide percutaneous procedures. The resident must become skilled in the technical aspects of percutaneous procedures. The fundamentals of radiation physics, radiation biology, and radiation protection should all be reviewed during the vascular and interventional training experience. In addition, training should provide opportunities for research into new technologies and evaluation of the clinical outcomes of interventional radiology.

B. Duration of Training

The program shall offer 1 year of graduate medical education in vascular and interventional radiology. This year of training must follow successful completion of an ACGME-accredited program in diagnostic radiology or its equivalent.

C. Faculty/Resident Numbers

The minimum number of residents is one. To ensure an adequate educational experience as well as adequate supervision and evaluation of a resident's academic progress the faculty-to-resident ratio must not be less than one full-time faculty person for every resident.

II. Program Director/Faculty

A. Program Director

The program director must be certified by the American Board of Radiology in diagnostic radiology or radiology and have a Certificate of Added Qualifications in Vascular and Interventional Radiology from the American Board of Radiology or possess equivalent qualifications.

B. Faculty

There should be sufficient qualified professional personnel to constitute a teaching faculty. The faculty should comprise at least two full-time vascular and interventional radiologists, including the program director. While the expertise of any one faculty member may be limited to a particular aspect of vascular and interventional radiology, the training program must provide experience that includes all aspects of vascular and nonvascular interventional radiology. The faculty must provide didactic teaching and direct supervision of residents' performance in the clinical patient management, procedural, interpretative, and consultative aspects of vascular and interventional radiology. The faculty must demonstrate a commitment to the subspecialty of vascular interventional radiology. Such commitment includes membership in professional societies, publications in the field, and/or a minimum of 30 hours of CME Category I credit per year.

(See Program Requirements for Residency Education in the Subspecialties of Diagnostic Radiology for additional program director and faculty requirements.)

III. Facilities and Resources

A. Space and Equipment

Modern imaging/procedure rooms and equipment in adequate space must be available to permit the performance of all vascular and interventional radiologic procedures. Imaging modalities in the department should include fluoroscopy, angiography, computed tomography, ultrasonography, magnetic resonance imaging, and radionuclide scintigraphy. Fluoroscopic equipment should be high resolution and have digital display with postprocedure image processing capability. Rooms in which vascular and interventional procedures are performed must be equipped with physiologic monitoring and resuscitative equipment. Suitable recovery and patient holding areas should be available. Adjacent to or within procedure rooms, there should be facilities for storing catheters, guide wires, contrast materials, embolic agents, and other supplies. There must be adequate space and facilities for image display, image interpretation, and consultation with other clinicians. There must be adequate office space and support space for vascular and interventional radiology faculty or staff and residents.

B. Patient Population

The institution's patient population must have a diversity of illnesses from which a broad experience in vascular and interventional radiology can be obtained. There also must be an adequate variety and number of interventional procedures for each resident. Each resident must document his/her direct participation in a minimum of 500 vascular and interventional procedures that cover the entire range of the specialty. The procedures should be recorded in a personal case log that should be reviewed periodically with the program director. Clinical experience may be supplemented by training affiliations to other institutions.

C. Library

Teaching resources must include a medical library with access to a variety of textbooks and journals in radiology, vascular and interventional radiology, and related fields. A coded vascular and interventional radiology teaching film file is desirable. The resident should have access to computerized literature search facilities.

D. Support Services

Pathology and medical laboratory services and consultation must be regularly and conveniently available to meet the needs of patients, as determined by the medical staff. Services should be available each day throughout the entire 24 hours. At least one qualified medical technologist must be on duty or available at all times. Diagnostic laboratories for the noninvasive assessment of peripheral vascular disease also must be available. Nursing support should be readily available, particularly if conscious sedation might be administered.

E. Research Facilities

The institution should provide laboratory and ancillary facilities to support research projects. These laboratory facilities and research opportunities may be made available to vascular and interventional radiology residents through cooperative arrangements with other departments or institutions.

IV. The Educational Program

A. Clinical Components

The training program curriculum must include didactic and clinical experiences that encompass the full clinical spectrum of vascular and interventional radiology. Residents must have the opportunity to carry out all of the following under close, graded responsibility and supervision: clinical preprocedure evaluation of patients, interpretation of preliminary diagnostic studies, consultation with clinicians on other services, performance of vascular and interventional procedures, generation of procedural reports, and delivery of both short- and long-term follow-up care. The continuity of care must be of sufficient duration to enable the resident to obtain appropriate feedback regarding the management of patients under his/her care.

Both vascular and nonvascular interventional procedures, excluding the intracerebral vascular system, must be included in the training program. Examples of vascular procedures include but are not limited to arteriography, venography, lymphography, angioplasty and related percutaneous revascularization procedures, embolotherapy, transcatheter infusion therapy, intravascular foreign body removal, and percutaneous placement of endovascular prostheses such as stent grafts and inferior vena cava filters and insertion of vascular access devices and catheters. Examples of nonvascular procedures include, but are not limited to, percutaneous imaging-guided biopsy; percutaneous gastrostomy; percutaneous nephrostomy; ureteral stenting and other transcatheter genitourinary procedures for diagnosis and for treatment of lithiasis, obstruction, and fistula; percutaneous transhepatic and transcholecystic biliary procedures; percutaneous drainage for diagnosis and treatment of infections and other fluid collections; and miscellaneous percutaneous imaging-guided procedures such as ablation of neoplasms and cysts. Residents must have specific clinical time dedicated to the performance and interpretation of vascular ultrasound studies, magnetic resonance angiograms, and CT angiograms.

The responsibility or independence given to residents must depend on an assessment of their knowledge, manual skill, and experience. In supervising residents during vascular and interventional procedures, faculty members should reinforce the understanding gained during residency training of x-ray generators, image intensifiers, film, screen-film combinations, film changers, film processing, ultrasonography, computed tomography, and other imaging modalities. Residents must be provided with instruction in the use of needles, catheters, and guide wires and must be directly supervised and given graduated responsibility in the performance of procedures as competence increases. A thorough understanding of the clinical indications, risks, interpretation, and limitations of vascular and interventional procedures is essential to the practice of vascular and interventional radiology. Residents must be instructed in these areas. Residents should also be instructed in proper use and interpretation of laboratory tests and in methods that are adjunctive to vascular and interventional procedures, such as use of physiologic monitoring devices, noninvasive vascular testing, and noninvasive vascular imaging. There should be specific instruction in the clinical aspects of patient assessment, patient treatment, planning, and patient management related to vascular and interventional radiology. There also should be instruction in the use of analgesics, antibiotics, and other drugs commonly employed in conjunction with these procedures. The residents must be thoroughly familiar with all aspects of administering and monitoring sedation of the conscious patient. They also must have advanced cardiac life support training.

Residents should serve as consultants under the supervision of staff vascular and interventional radiologists. Direct interactions of residents with patients must be closely observed to ensure that appropriate standards of care and concern for patient welfare are strictly maintained. Communication, consultation, and coordination of care with the referring clinical staff and clinical services must be maintained and documented with appropriate notes in the medical record. Reports for the medical record generated by residents should be closely reviewed by faculty for accuracy of content, grammar, style, and level of confidence. The vascular/interventional residents should also assist and train diagnostic radiology residents in the performance and interpretation of procedures.

B. Didactic Components

There shall be scheduled intradepartmental conferences as well as conferences with related clinical departments in which residents participate on a regular basis. These should include one or more specific weekly departmental conferences and at least one interdisciplinary conference per week at which attendance is required. In particular, interdepartmental conferences with the surgical specialties should be an important teaching component. The resident's teaching experience should include conferences with medical students, graduate medical staff, and allied health personnel. Scheduled presentations by the resident during these conferences should be encouraged.

Clinical and basic sciences as they relate to radiology and vascular and interventional radiology should be part of the didactic program. This should include but not be limited to the anatomy, physiology, and pathophysiology of the hematological, circulatory, respiratory, gastrointestinal, genitourinary, and musculoskeletal systems. Relevant pharmacology, patient evaluation and management skills, and diagnostic techniques also should be addressed.

There must be documented regular review of all mortality and morbidity related to the performance of interventional procedures. Residents must participate actively in this review, which should be held not less than monthly. Residents should be encouraged to attend and participate in local extramural conferences and should attend at least one national meeting or postgraduate course in interventional radiology while in training. Participation in local or national vascular and interventional radiology societies should be encouraged. Residents should be encouraged to present the radiologic aspects of cases that are discussed in multidisciplinary conferences. They also should prepare clinically or pathologically proven cases for inclusion in the teaching file.

C. Other Required Components

1. Resident participation in research
   The residents should learn the fundamentals of experimental design, performance, and interpretation of results. They should participate in clinical, basic biomedical, or health services research projects and should be encouraged to undertake at least one project as principal investigator. They should submit at least one scientific paper or exhibit to a regional or national meeting. The opportunity also must be provided for residents to develop their competence in critical assessment of new imaging modalities and of new procedures in vascular and interventional radiology.
2. Scholarly activity (See Program Requirements for Residency Education in the Subspecialties of Diagnostic Radiology for details concerning scholarly activity requirements.)
3. Duty hours and conditions of work (See Program Requirements for Residency Education in the Subspecialties of Diagnostic Radiology for details concerning duty hour requirements.)

V. Evaluation

(See Program Requirements for Residency Education in the Subspecialties of Diagnostic Radiology for details concerning evaluation requirements.)

VI. Board Certification

The Residency Review Committee will consider as one measure of a program's quality the performance of its graduates on the examination of the American Board of Radiology for the Certificate of Added Qualifications in Vascular Interventional Radiology. All program graduates should take the examination.

ACGME: June 1998 Effective: July 1999

Program Requirements for Residency Education in Radiation Oncology

I. Introduction

A. Definition of the Specialty

Radiation oncology is that branch of clinical medicine that utilizes ionizing radiation to treat patients with cancer and occasionally with diseases other than cancer. Radiation oncologists are an integral part of the multidisciplinary management of the cancer patient and must collaborate closely with physicians in related disciplines and be familiar with their role in the management of the patient.

B. Program Goals and Objectives

The objective of the residency program is to educate and train physicians to be skillful in the practice of radiation oncology and to be caring and compassionate in the treatment of patients. To accomplish this goal, adequate structure, facilities, faculty, patient resources, and educational environment must be provided.

The director and teaching staff of a program must prepare and comply with written educational goals for the residency program. All educational components of the program should be related to program goals. The program design and/or structure must be approved by the Residency Review Committee (RRC) for Radiation Oncology as part of the regular review process.

C. Length and Scope of Training

Resident education in radiation oncology must include 5 years of accredited clinically oriented graduate medical education. The first year of postgraduate clinical training must be spent in a medicine, family practice, surgery, pediatrics, or a transitional year program. This clinical experience must then be followed by 4 years focused in radiation oncology.

No fewer than 36 months of the 4-year program must be spent in the clinical core curriculum of radiation oncology. In addition, the program must provide a 2-month rotation or its equivalent in hematology/medical oncology and exposure to oncologic pathology, either by its integration into the conference schedules and tumor boards or by a 1-month rotation in oncologic pathology. The remaining months must allow for in-depth experience in individually selected areas applicable to clinical radiation oncology, as described in Section V.A.2, "Clinical Curriculum." A research component, either clinical or basic laboratory research, is desirable.

II. Institution

A. Sponsoring Institution

The administration of the institution sponsoring the program in radiation oncology must provide funding for space, equipment, staff, nonprofessional personnel, and residents. It must assist the program director in teaching and recruiting faculty, as well as in selecting, evaluating, and dismissing residents whose performance is unsatisfactory.

B. Other Accredited Residencies

Education in radiation oncology must occur in an environment that encourages the exchange of knowledge and experience among residents both in the program and in other oncology specialties within the sponsoring institution. There should be other Accreditation Council for Graduate Medical Education (ACGME)-accredited residency programs, including internal medicine and general surgery, in the institution.

C. Participating Institutions: Affiliation and Integration

Extramural educational experience may be used to complement the training program, but the preponderance of the educational experience must take place in the parent institution. If residents are to be sent to another institution to obtain experience lacking in the parent institution, the program director must obtain prior approval from the RRC when the outside rotation totals more than 3 months.

Institutions may participate on an affiliated or integrated basis. The program may establish an *affiliated* relationship with another institution for the purpose of limited rotations. Affiliated institutions must provide additional resources and experience and must not be added primarily for the purpose of meeting service needs. Rotations to affiliated institutions may not exceed 6 months over the course of the program.

An institution is considered *integrated* when the program director (a) appoints the members of the faculty and is involved in the appointment of the chief of service at the integrated institution, (b) determines all rotations and assignments of residents, and (c) is responsible for the overall conduct of the educational program in the integrated institution. There must be a written agreement between the parent institution and the integrated institution stating that these provisions are in effect. Rotations to integrated institutions are not limited in duration.

In seeking approval from the RRC for either an affiliated or integrated arrangement with another institution, the program director must explain the reasons for the rotation, must specify the number and types of patients and procedures available to the residents, and must provide a signed agreement approved by the institutional governing boards. Arrangements for rotations should not be made with institutions that do not add to the educational value of the program or that are at such a distance from the parent institution as to make resident attendance at rounds and conferences difficult. The RRC will not approve rotations to an institution where the resident acts only as an observer or where clinical experience is so diluted by the presence of other rotating residents as not to be meaningful. Clinical responsibility alone does not constitute a suitable educational experience.

D. Resident Complement

The RRC recognizes the importance of peer interaction among residents themselves, as well as of interactions between faculty and residents in the conduct of conferences and patient care. A minimum number of residents is essential to provide an opportunity for meaningful interaction throughout the training period. Each program must be structured to have a minimum of four residents. The RRC will accredit a program for a maximum number of residents commensurate with the total capacity of the program, to offer an appropriate educational experience in radiation oncology. There should be not more than 1.5 residents for every staff radiation oncologist during any resident's training in clinical radiation oncology. If a program director wants to increase the number of residents in a program beyond the authorized number, prior approval must be obtained from the RRC. Requests based primarily on service considerations will not be approved.

E. Other Trainees

The residents' experience must not be significantly diminished by the presence of other trainees, such as fellows and postgraduate trainees or residents rotating from another accredited residency program.

III. Program Personnel

The program director and the teaching staff are responsible for the general administration of a program, including those activities related to the recruitment, selection, instruction, supervision, counseling, evaluation, and advancement of residents, and the maintenance of records related to program accreditation.

A. Program Director

1. Qualifications: There must be a single program director responsible for the program.
   The program director must be a highly qualified radiation oncologist with substantial experience in education in radiation oncology, who must demonstrate the ability to organize and direct the teaching program, maintain a quality teaching staff, and provide a significant commitment of time and effort to the residency program. He or she must be currently certified by the American Board of Radiology in Radiation Oncology or possess suitable equivalent qualifications. The program director must be licensed to practice medicine in the state where the institution that sponsors the program is located (certain federal programs are exempted), and also must hold an appointment in good standing to the medical staff of an institution participating in the program. A complete curriculum vitae of the program director shall be filed with the executive secretary of the RRC at the time of appointment and updated with each review of the program by the RRC.
2. Responsibilities: The program director is responsible for the structure and content of the educational program and must document the provision of training in clinical radiation oncology, treatment planning, radiation physics, and radiobiology. The director also is responsible for the following:
   a. Arrangement for provision of adequate facilities and clinical and educational resources.
   b. Preparation of a written statement outlining the educational goals of the program with respect to knowledge, skills, and other attributes of residents at each level of training and for each major rotation or other program assignment. This statement must be distributed to residents and members of the teaching staff. It should be readily available for review.
   c. Prompt notification to the executive secretary of the RRC, in writing, of any changes as they occur that might significantly alter the educational experience, such as a change in program director, faculty, the number of residency positions offered, institutional affiliation, or equipment.
   d. Selection of residents for appointment to the program in accordance with institutional and departmental policies and procedures.
   e. Selection and supervision of the teaching staff and other program personnel at each institution participating in the program.
   f. Supervision of residents through explicit written descriptions of supervisory lines of responsibility for the care of patients. Such guidelines must be communicated to all members of the program staff. Residents must be provided with prompt, reliable systems for communication and interaction with supervisory physicians.
   g. Monitoring resident stress, including mental or emotional conditions inhibiting performance or learning and drug- or alcohol-related dysfunction. Program directors and teaching staff should be sensitive to the need for timely provision of confidential counseling and psychological support services to residents. Training situations that consistently produce undesirable stress on residents must be evaluated and modified.
   h. Regular evaluation of residents' knowledge, skills, and overall performance, including the development of professional attitudes consistent with being a physician.
   i. Implementation of fair procedures, as established by the sponsoring institution, regarding academic discipline and resident complaints or grievances.

Program Requirements

j. Preparation of an accurate statistical and narrative description of the program as requested by the RRC.

B. Teaching Staff

The program must provide a minimum of four radiation oncologists who devote essentially all of their professional time to the program for the teaching of clinical radiation oncology. In addition, the faculty must include one full-time radiation biologist or basic scientist, who must be on-site, for the teaching of radiation biology and one full-time medical physicist, who must also be on-site, for the teaching of radiation physics. The radiation oncologists and the medical physicist must be certified by the American Board of Radiology or possess suitable equivalent qualifications.

Graduate medical education must take place in an environment of inquiry and scholarship in which residents participate in the development of new knowledge, learn to evaluate research findings, and develop habits of inquiry as a continuing professional responsibility. The responsibility for establishing and maintaining an environment of inquiry and scholarship rests with the teaching staff. While not all members of a teaching staff must be investigators, the staff as a whole must demonstrate broad involvement in scholarly activity. This activity should include

1. active participation of the teaching staff in clinical discussions, rounds, conferences, and didactic lectures in a manner that promotes a spirit of inquiry and scholarship.
2. participation in journal clubs and research conferences.
3. active participation in regional or national professional and scientific societies, particularly through presentations at the organizations' meetings and publication in their journals.
4. participation in research, particularly in projects that are peer reviewed and/or result in publication or presentations at regional and national scientific meetings.
5. providing guidance and technical support (eg, research design, statistical analysis) for residents involved in research or scholarly activities.

The curriculum vitae of each faculty member must document his or her qualifications to teach and supervise residents in training. The faculty must be committed to the teaching of the residents and document the time and effort they devote to the educational program. They must supervise the residents and provide the opportunity for the residents to gradually accept more responsibility for patient care as training progresses. Members of the teaching staff must be able to devote sufficient time to meet their supervisory and teaching responsibilities. A faculty that does not meet the stated qualifications or fails to devote itself to the teaching of residents shall be considered unsuitable for conducting a program of graduate education in radiation oncology.

A member of the teaching staff of each participating institution must be designated to assume responsibility for the day-to-day activities of the program at that institution, with overall coordination by the program director.

The teaching staff must be organized and have regular documented meetings to review program goals and objectives as well as program effectiveness in achieving them. At least one resident representative should participate in these reviews.

C. Other Program Personnel

Programs must be provided with the additional professional, technical, and clerical personnel needed to support the administration and educational conduct of the program.

IV. Facilities and Resources

A. Facilities

A training program in radiation oncology must have adequate space and equipment to train residents in state-of-the-art radiation oncology. There must be two or more megavoltage machines, a machine with a broad range of electron beam capabilities, a dedicated therapy simulator, computerized treatment planning, a mold room and/or machine shop for the construction of treatment aids, and equipment to do interstitial and intracavitary brachytherapy. Access to kilovoltage capability is desirable.

B. Other Services

Adequate medical services must be available in the specialties of hematology/medical oncology, surgical oncology and its subspecialties, gynecologic oncology, and pediatric oncology. There must be access to current imaging techniques, nuclear medicine, pathology, a clinical laboratory, and a tumor registry.

C. Library Resources

A sufficient variety of journals, reference books, and resource materials pertinent to radiation oncology and associated fields in oncology and basic sciences must be provided in a radiation oncology library and must be immediately accessible at all times, including nights and weekends, for resident study. In addition, residents must have access to a general medical library. The sponsoring institution must provide residents with ready access to a computerized search system and rapid access to national databases in medicine to permit timely literature review.

V. Educational Program

A. Clinical Components

1. Clinical Resources

   To ensure adequate numbers and variety of patients for resident training, at least 600 patients must be irradiated yearly in the parent institution or integrated program, and the number of patients seen by each resident must be no fewer than 150 per year, or a minimum of 450 during the clinical radiation oncology rotations. A resident should not treat more than 250 patients per year.

2. Clinical Curriculum

   The program must provide the resident with the opportunity to gain in-depth knowledge of clinical radiation oncology, including the indications for irradiation and special therapeutic considerations unique to each site and stage of disease. The resident must be trained in standard radiation techniques as well as in the use of treatment aids and treatment planning to optimize the distribution of the radiation dose. The principles of normal tissue tolerance to radiation and tumor dose-response must be taught. The use of combined modality therapy and altered fractionation schemes should also be part of the clinical curriculum.

   The clinical core curriculum shall include experience with gastrointestinal, gynecologic, genitourinary, reticuloendothelial, breast, soft tissue and bone, skin, head and neck, lung, pediatric, and central nervous system tumors. In addition, the curriculum must provide instruction in the physics, biology, and clinical applicability of the following areas: radiosurgery, intraoperative radiation therapy, conformal therapy, three-dimensional treatment planning, radioimmunotherapy, total body irradiation as used in bone-marrow transplantation, total skin irradiation, high-dose-rate brachytherapy, hyperthermia, plaque therapy, particle therapy, and any others that may be developed, as they apply to the core curriculum.

   The resident also must be trained in the use of external beam modalities, including superficial irradiation; megavoltage irradiation, such as Cobalt 60 and low- and high-energy x-rays; electron beam; simulation to localize anatomy; and computerized treatment planning. The faculty must ensure that the resident personally performs technical procedures, including treatment setups as well as intracavitary and interstitial placement of radiation sources, and that the resident keeps a detailed log of these procedures.

It is required that a resident perform no fewer than five interstitial implants and ten intracavitary implants and assist in an additional five interstitial and ten intracavitary implants during the course of training.

Follow-up of the irradiated patients by the resident on an inpatient or outpatient basis is a required part of resident training and must be demonstrated by the program to ensure that residents have the opportunity to learn about the problems of recurrent and disseminated tumors and of late aftereffects and complications of radiation therapy.

3. Resident Logs
The program director must submit at the RRC's request the residents' logs of patients irradiated, procedures performed and observed, and modalities used. The program director should review the logs with all residents at least twice yearly.
4. Duty Hours
While the actual number of hours worked by residents may vary, residents must have sufficient off-duty time to avoid undue fatigue and stress. It is required that residents be allowed to spend, on average, at least 1 full day out of 7 away from the hospital and not be assigned on-call duty in the hospital more frequently than every third night. The program director is responsible for monitoring on-duty assignments for residents to ensure adherence to this recommendation.

B. Didactic Components

1. Conferences
Conferences and teaching rounds must provide for progressive resident participation. There must be adequate frequency of conferences, with attendance by residents, radiation oncologists, and other staff documented by the program director. Adequate conference room and audiovisual facilities must be provided.

The clinical and basic sciences must be taught through regularly scheduled lectures, case presentations, conferences, and discussions relevant to the practice of radiation oncology. The training program must provide curricula for the teaching of basic sciences essential to training in radiation oncology, including radiation biology and medical physics. The curriculum in medical physics must include didactic lectures and laboratory demonstrations of radiation safety procedures, calibration of radiation therapy machines, the use of the computer for treatment planning, the construction of treatment aids, and the safe handling of sealed and unsealed radionuclides. The radiation biology curriculum must include didactic lectures on all aspects of radiation effects on normal and neoplastic tissues. The program also must familiarize the resident with medical statistics, through an organized program of lectures or conferences, and oncologic pathology, with special emphasis on neoplasia and radiation effects.

There must be didactic instruction in the potential value and limitations of other oncologic disciplines, such as medical oncology, surgical oncology, gynecologic oncology, hematologic oncology, pediatric oncology, and the various surgical subspecialties that play a role in the management of the patient. This will be accomplished by attendance at multidisciplinary and departmental conferences.

There must be intradepartmental clinical oncology conferences, including new patient conferences, weekly chart reviews, problem case conferences, morbidity and mortality, physics, dosimetry, radiation biology, and journal review.

2. Resident Investigative Project
During their training, residents will be required to engage in an investigative project under faculty supervision. This may take the form of laboratory research, clinical research, or the retrospective analysis of data from treated patients, and results of such projects shall be suitable for publication or presentation at local, regional, or national scientific meetings.

VI. Evaluation

1. Resident Evaluation: Evaluation of each resident's progress and competence must be conducted at least twice yearly. The evaluations must include an assessment of intellectual abilities, attitudes, and interpersonal relationships as well as clinical competence, decision-making, and clinical management skills. There must be provision for appropriate and timely feedback of the content of these evaluations to the resident. Residents should be advanced to positions of higher responsibility only on the basis of evidence of their satisfactory progressive scholarship and professional growth. The program must maintain a permanent record of the evaluation and counseling process for each resident. Such records must be accessible to the resident and other authorized personnel.

The program director must provide a written final evaluation for each resident who completes the program. The evaluation must include a review of the resident's performance during the final period of training and should verify that the resident has demonstrated sufficient professional ability to practice competently and independently. This final evaluation should be part of the resident's permanent record maintained by the institution.

2. Program Evaluation: The educational effectiveness of a program must be evaluated in a systematic manner. In particular, the quality of the curriculum and the extent to which the educational goals have been met by residents must be assessed. Residents should have the opportunity at least annually to evaluate the faculty and the program. Written evaluations by residents should be utilized in the program evaluation process.

The teaching staff should periodically evaluate the utilization of the resources available to the program, the contribution of each institution participating in the program, the financial and administrative support of the program, the volume and variety of patients available to the program for educational purposes, the performance of members of the teaching staff, and the quality of supervision of residents.

One measure of the quality of a program is the performance of its graduates on examinations given by the American Board of Radiology. The RRC will consider this information as part of the overall evaluation of the program.

VII. Certification

Residents who plan to seek certification by the American Board of Radiology should communicate with the office of the board regarding the full requirements for certification.

ACGME: September 1995 Effective: July 1996

Program Requirements for Residency Education in General Surgery

I. Introduction

A. Definition and Scope of the Specialty

The training of surgeons for the practice of general surgery encompasses education in basic sciences, training in cognitive and technical skills, development of clinical knowledge and maturity, and acquisition of surgical judgment.

1. The program must provide the opportunity for residents to learn in depth the fundamentals of basic science as applied to clinical surgery. These include but are not limited to the elements of wound healing, hemostasis, hematologic disorders, oncology, shock, circulatory physiology, surgical microbiology, respiratory physiology, gastrointestinal physiology, genitourinary physiology, surgical endocrinology, surgical nutrition, fluid and electrolyte balance, metabolic response to injury including burns, musculoskeletal biomechanics and physiology, immunobiology and transplantation, applied surgical anatomy, and surgical pathology.
2. The program must provide experience in preoperative, operative, and postoperative care for patients in all areas that constitute the principal components of general surgery: specifically, diseases of the head and neck, breast, skin and soft tissues, alimentary tract, abdomen, vascular system, endocrine system, the comprehensive management of trauma and emergency operations, and surgical critical care. Additional components that must also be encompassed in the teaching program, as described in I.C.5, are cardiothoracic surgery, pediatric surgery, plastic surgery, burn management, transplant surgery, endoscopy, urology, gynecology, neurosurgery, orthopedics, and anesthesiology.
3. The goal of a surgical residency program is to prepare the resident to function as a qualified practitioner of surgery at the high level of performance expected of a board-certified specialist; the educational components of the program, therefore, must be of the highest priority. Residents must be provided adequate time and sufficient facilities for study and be assured of a rotation schedule that provides an equivalent educational opportunity for each resident. While every residency carries with it a commitment of service to patients in the institution, the service responsibilities must support and not detract from the educational activities.

B. Program Goals and Design

1. The director and teaching staff of a program must prepare and comply with written educational goals for the program. All educational components of a residency program should be related to these goals.
2. The program design and/or structure must be approved by the review committee as part of the regular review process.

C. Duration and Scope of Education

Five years of graduate training in surgery after graduation from medical school is the minimum amount of time required for acquisition of necessary knowledge, technical skill, and judgment. Any program that extends training beyond these minimum requirements must present a clear educational rationale consonant with the Program Requirements and objectives for residency training. The program director must obtain approval of the Residency Review Committee (RRC) prior to implementation and at each subsequent review of the program. Prior to entry in the program each resident must be notified in writing of the required length of training. All years must be in an accredited program under the guidance of the program director in surgery, regardless of rotations to other disciplines.

Following are the components of an acceptable program.

1. The program must consist of at least 5 years, of which
   a. not more than 12 months may be devoted to education in a single surgical discipline other than the principal components of surgery;
   b. not more than 6 months in total may be allocated to nonsurgical clinical disciplines such as internal medicine, pediatrics, gastroenterology, anesthesiology, or surgical pathology;
   c. at least 3½ years must be clinical surgery, with experience in endoscopy, surgical intensive care, and emergency care included under this category;
   d. Three of the clinical surgery years must be concerned with the principal components of general surgery as listed in I.A.2.
2. The program must commit the chief clinical year to the principal components of general surgery at the parent or integrated institution(s). The majority of the 12 months of the chief year must be served in the final year of the program. However, to take advantage of a unique educational opportunity in a program during a resident's final year, a portion of the chief year may be served in the next to the last year, provided it is not earlier than the fourth clinical year and has been approved in advance by the Residency Review Committee for Surgery.
   a. In the chief year, not more than 4 months may be devoted exclusively to any one principal component of general surgery.
   b. In the chief year, residents must rotate only on services devoted to the principal components of general surgery, but they may have primary responsibility for surgical specialty cases if patients are on a general surgical service.
   c. In the chief year, with prior approval of the RRC, a rotation on a pediatric surgical service may be acceptable under the following conditions:
      1. The resident's experience in the principal components of general surgery is adequate.
      2. The resident is responsible for the preoperative, operative, and postoperative care of the pediatric surgical patient.
      3. The volume and complexity of cases are appropriate for a chief resident.
3. The program must provide opportunity for each resident to perform a variety of rigid and flexible endoscopic procedures, particularly proctosigmoidoscopy, colonoscopy, esophagogastroduodenoscopy, laparoscopy, and operative choledochoscopy, as well as provide experience in other relevant diagnostic and therapeutic techniques including laryngoscopy, bronchoscopy, and fine-needle aspiration.

   The program should also provide opportunity for the resident to become familiar with the appropriate use of evolving diagnostic and therapeutic methods, such as laser applications, investigations and manipulations of the distal common bile duct (including sphincterotomy), stereotactic breast biopsy, physiologic testing and evaluation of the gastrointestinal tract, non-invasive diagnostic evaluation of the vascular system, and invasive vascular interventional techniques. Residents should also have the opportunity to become familiar with ultrasonography of the head and neck, breast, abdomen (including laparoscopic intra-abdominal), and endorectal ultrasound.
4. The program must provide sufficient experience in an emergency room and in intensive care units to enable residents to manage patients with severe and complex illnesses and with major injuries requiring critical care.
5. The program must enable the resident to acquire an understanding of the principles of and to have personal clinical experience in the surgical specialties, including

a. preoperative, operative, and postoperative care in cardiothoracic surgery, pediatric surgery, plastic surgery, and transplant surgery;
b. participation in the overall management of patients with common problems in urology, gynecology, neurological surgery, orthopedics, burns, and anesthesiology.

These experiences may be provided either by a rotation through that specialty or through patient care activities, which must be documented by means of an operative log, record, or registry. At the time of program review, a listing of the goals and objectives that each program maintains for each surgical specialty should be available, as well as a description of the process through which these goals are to be achieved for each resident.

6. The program must provide the opportunity for surgical residents to manage, on the surgical services, patients who may or may not require surgical intervention (eg, patients with pancreatitis, portal hypertension, multiple trauma, immunosuppression) and to acquire skill in such nonoperative management.
7. The program must provide teaching in critical thinking, design of experiments, and evaluation of data as well as in technological advances that relate to surgery and the care of patients with surgical diseases.
8. The program must encourage participation by the residents in clinical and/or laboratory research.

II. Institutional Organization

A. Requirements for Sponsoring Institution

1. Inasmuch as general surgery is a discipline of great breadth and is often consultative in nature, the program should be conducted in institutions accredited by the Joint Commission on Accreditation of Healthcare Organizations or its equivalent and classified as general hospitals. These institutions, by definition, must include facilities and staff for a variety of services, including radiology and pathology.
2. There must be at least one additional residency program, in internal medicine or pediatrics or family practice, whose residents rotate through the same integrated institutions as the surgical residents.

B. Participating Institutions

An institution that cannot provide sufficient resources and clinical experience within its own facilities may make arrangements with other institutions through formal written agreements to provide additional resources and experience. All such agreements are subject to approval by the RRC, either as indicated below in item II.B.3 or at the time of program review.

1. Institutions may be *affiliated* with the parent institution through an Affiliation Agreement, which must cover the areas specified in the Institutional Requirements. Affiliated institutions must promote the educational goals of the program rather than simply enlarge the program and must not be added primarily for the purpose of meeting service needs.
2. Institutions may be *integrated* with the parent institution through an Integration Agreement that must specify—in addition to the Institutional Requirements—that the program director of the parent institution (1) appoint the members of the teaching staff at the integrated institution, (2) appoint the chief or director of the teaching service in the integrated institution, (3) appoint all residents in the program, and (4) determine all rotations and assignments of both residents and members of the teaching staff. As a general rule, institutions integrated with parent hospitals must be in close geographic proximity to allow all residents to attend joint conferences, basic science lectures, and morbidity and mortality reviews on a regular documented basis in a central location. If the institutions are geographically so remote that joint conferences cannot be held, an equivalent educational program of lectures and conferences in the integrated institution must be fully documented.
3. Prior approval must be obtained from the RRC (1) for a portion of the final year to be spent at an affiliated institution, (2) for *affiliations* with rotations of 6 months or more as well as for all integrations, and (3) for more than 1 year total to be spent away from the integrated institution(s).

C. Number of Approved Residency Positions

1. The number of positions in the training program must be approved by the RRC; this number will include all residents who are appointed for a full academic year in the training program. Any request for changes in the resident complement must be justified in terms of the educational goals of the program.
2. Residency positions shall be allocated to one of three groups: categorical, designated preliminary, and nondesignated preliminary. *Categorical residents* are those accepted into the residency program who intend to complete the full general surgical training, normally 5 clinical years, assuming satisfactory performance. *Designated preliminary residents* are those accepted for 1, 2, or 3 years prior to continuing their education in another surgical or nonsurgical specialty or subspecialty program with which there are established written agreements of preacceptance of the residents. *Nondesignated preliminary residents* are those accepted into the general surgical program, normally for 1, 2, or, rarely, 3 years, who at the time of matching have not determined their further residency training.
3. a. At each level the number of categorical PGY1, PGY2, and PGY3 positions shall not exceed the number of approved chief residency positions. Modest variations, not to exceed a 10% increase in the total number of categorical PGY1, PGY2, and PGY3 residents, may be permitted on a temporary basis only.
   b. The number of designated preliminary positions shall not be specifically limited, as long as the total number of residents does not exceed the educational capacity of the surgical program.
   c. The number of nondesignated preliminary residents in the PGY1, PGY2, and PGY3 years combined shall not exceed 150% of the number of categorical chief residents. Evidence of continuation in graduate medical education must be provided for these residents. Exceptions to this number of nondesignated preliminary residents will require not only adequate documentation of continuing in graduate medical education in another program but also clear evidence of educational benefit to the overall program.

A modest increase from the approved number of nondesignated preliminary PGY1, PGY2, and PGY3 positions is permitted on a temporary (1-year) basis only. A modest increase is understood by the RRC as within a 10% variation in the total number of PGY1, PGY2, and PGY3 positions.

III. Teaching Staff

The establishment of an inquiring and scholarly environment in the parent and integrated institution(s) is the primary responsibility of the teaching staff in a general surgery training program. Only in such a milieu can residents develop the facility for critical analysis and further growth potential necessary to a lifetime of self-education after the completion of formal residency training. The teaching staff responsible for the direction and execution of the program must be well qualified to create and maintain such an environment and be of sufficient diversity of interest that the many facets of surgery are represented.

A. Program Director

There must be a single program director responsible for the program.

1. Qualifications of the program director
   a. Documented qualification in surgery, requisite administrative abilities and experience, and dedication to surgical education and scholarship, as evidenced by his or her curriculum vitae.
   b. Licensure to practice medicine in the state where the institution that sponsors the program is located. (Certain federal programs are exempted.)
   c. Certification by the American Board of Surgery or suitable equivalent qualifications, as determined by the RRC.
   d. Appointment in good standing to the medical staff of the parent or one of the integrated institutions participating in the program.
   e. Appointment, as a normal rule, for at least the duration of the program plus 1 year, that is, a minimum of 6 years. Persons appointed or elected for short durations or in an honorary capacity cannot serve as program directors.
2. Responsibilities of the program director
   The program director's responsibility is to support the residency training program by devoting his or her principal effort to its management and administration, as well as to teaching, research, and clinical care limited to the parent or integrated institution(s). Therefore, the program director shall
   a. prepare a written statement outlining the educational goals of the program with respect to knowledge, skills, and other attributes of residents at each level of training and for each major rotation or other program assignment. This statement must be distributed to residents and members of the teaching staff. It should be readily available for review.
   b. designate other well-qualified surgeons to assist in the supervision of the resident staff so that, in addition to the program director, for each approved chief residency position there is at least one geographic full-time teaching staff member whose major function is to support the residency program. These key staff members must be appointed for a period long enough to ensure adequate continuity in the supervision of the resident staff.
   c. be responsible for rotations and staff appointments of attending surgeons on the teaching services in the parent and in all integrated institutions.
   d. select residents for appointment to the program in accordance with institutional and departmental policies and procedures, make resident assignments, and be responsible for the proper conduct of the educational activities; namely, for their supervision, direction, and administration in all participating institutions.
   e. provide residents with explicit written descriptions of supervisory lines of responsibility for the care of patients. Such guidelines must be communicated to all members of the program staff. Residents must be provided with prompt, reliable systems for communication and interaction with supervisory physicians.
   f. implement fair procedures, as established by the sponsoring institution, regarding academic discipline and resident complaints or grievances.
   g. monitor resident stress, including mental or emotional conditions inhibiting performance or learning and drug- or alcohol-related dysfunction. Program directors and teaching staff should be sensitive to the need for timely provision of confidential counseling and psychological support services to residents. Training situations that consistently produce undesirable stress on residents must be evaluated and modified.
   h. provide complete and accurate program information forms and resident operative records to the RRC so that an appropriate assessment of the program can be made.

B. Other Teaching Staff

1. There must be a sufficient number of teaching staff with documented qualifications to instruct and supervise adequately all the residents in the program. Surgeons with teaching responsibilities should be certified by the American Board of Surgery or possess suitable equivalent qualifications, as determined by the RRC. Members of the teaching staff must be able to devote sufficient time to meet their supervisory and teaching responsibilities.
2. The teaching staff must include members with diverse expertise to meet the needs of the training program. All members of the staff must demonstrate a strong interest in the education of residents, sound clinical and teaching abilities, support of the goals and objectives of the program, a commitment to their own continuing medical education, and participation in scholarly activities.
3. A member of the teaching staff of each participating institution must be designated to assume responsibility for the day-to-day activities of the program at that institution, with overall coordination by the program director.
4. The teaching staff must be organized and have regular documented meetings to review program goals and objectives as well as program effectiveness in achieving them. At least one resident representative should participate in these reviews.
5. The teaching staff should periodically evaluate the utilization of the resources available to the program, the contribution of each institution participating in the program, the financial and administrative support of the program, the volume and variety of patients available to the program for educational purposes, the performance of members of the teaching staff, and the quality of supervision of residents.

C. Other Program Personnel

Programs must be provided with the additional professional, technical, and clerical personnel needed to support the administration and educational conduct of the program.

IV. Facilities and Resources

Library

1. Residents must have ready access to a major medical library, either at the institution where the residents are located or through arrangement with convenient nearby institutions.
2. Library services should include the electronic retrieval of information from medical databases.
3. There must be access to an on-site library or to a collection of appropriate texts and journals in each institution participating in a residency program. On-site libraries and/or collections of texts and journals must be readily available during nights and weekends.

V. The Educational Program

A. Volume and Complexity of Operative Experience

Operative skill is essential for the surgeon and can be acquired only through personal experience and training. The program must provide for sufficient operative experience to train qualified surgeons, taking into account individual capability and rate of progress.

1. The volume and variety of the operative experience of each resident for the entire training program must be such as to ensure
   a. a balanced experience in each of the principal components of general surgery, namely, head and neck; breast; skin and soft tissues; alimentary tract; abdomen; vascular system; endocrine

system; the comprehensive management of trauma, burns, and emergency surgery; and surgical critical care.

b. a sufficient number and distribution of complex cases, as determined by the RRC, for the achievement of adequate operative skill and surgical judgment.

2. The program director must ensure that the operative experience of residents in the same program is comparable. While the overall number of major operations to be performed by each resident is not specified, an acceptable range is from 500 to 1,000 major cases over all 5 years, with from 150 to 300 major cases in the chief year.

   Operative experience of any one resident in excess of 450 cases for the chief year or 1,500 cases for all years must be justified by the program director.
3. When previous personal operative experience justifies a teaching role, residents should act as teaching assistants and list such cases for the fourth and fifth years only.
4. A resident is considered to be the surgeon when he or she can document a significant role in the following aspects of management: determination or confirmation of the diagnosis, provision of preoperative care, selection and accomplishment of the appropriate operative procedure, direction of the postoperative care, and accomplishment of sufficient follow-up to be acquainted with both the course of the disease and the outcome of its treatment. Participation in the operation only, without preoperative and postoperative care, is inadequate.

B. Supervision

The attending physician has both an ethical and a legal responsibility for the overall care of the individual patient and for the supervision of the resident involved in the care of that patient. Although senior residents require less direction than junior residents, even the most senior must be supervised. A chain of command that emphasizes graded authority and increasing responsibility as experience is gained must be established. Judgments on this delegation of responsibility must be made by the attending surgeon who is ultimately responsible for the patient's care; such judgments shall be based on the attending surgeon's direct observation and knowledge of each resident's skills and ability.

To ensure the fulfillment of these responsibilities, the following principles of supervision must be operative within a training program:

1. Supervision of residents must be specified in the bylaws, policies, procedures, rules, and/or regulations of the department, which must not be less demanding than those of the institution.
2. Evidence that adequate supervision exists within a program must be provided to the site visitor at the time of program review in the form of signed notes in the patient charts and/or other such records, as well as through personal interviews of residents.
3. Proper supervision must not conflict with progressively more independent decision making on the part of the resident; thus, the degree of supervision may vary with the clinical circumstances and the training level of the resident. However, to exercise their responsibilities properly, members of the teaching staff always must be immediately available for consultation and support.

C. Outpatient Responsibilities

To be adequate, a program must document both inpatient and outpatient activities. Outpatient activities constitute an essential component of adequate experience in continuity of patient care. These activities should be conducted in such a way that the resident has an opportunity to examine patients preoperatively, has ample opportunity to consult with the attending surgeon regarding operative care, and has an opportunity to participate in the operation and in the immediate postoperative care until release from the facility. To participate in posthospital care, the resident has the responsibility for seeing patients personally in an outpatient setting and consulting with the attending surgeon regarding follow-up care.

D. Educational Conferences

Educational conferences must be adequate in quality and quantity to provide a review of clinical surgery as well as of advances in surgery.

The conferences should be scheduled to permit the residents to attend on a regular basis. Participation by both residents and teaching staff must be documented.

The following types of conferences must exist within a program:

1. Weekly review of all current complications and deaths, including radiological and pathological correlation of surgical specimens and autopsies
2. A course or a structured series of conferences to ensure coverage of the basic and clinical sciences fundamental to surgery in general; sole reliance on textbook review is inadequate
3. Regular organized clinical teaching, such as ward rounds and clinical conferences

E. Special Trainees

At the time of each program survey, or at other times on request of the RRC, the program must provide to the RRC a report on all special trainees of any training programs, both approved and unapproved, in the parent and integrated institutions that might affect the experience of the residents in the core program in general surgery. Examples of such programs include fellowships or residencies in vascular surgery, oncologic surgery, head and neck surgery, critical care, trauma, endoscopy, gastroenterology, transplantation, pediatric surgery, and endocrine surgery that provide clinical experience to trainees outside the general surgery residency program. The report must describe in detail the relationship of the special trainee(s) to the residents in the general surgery program. A program in which the experience of general surgery residents is adversely affected by the presence of other trainees will be subject to adverse action by the RRC.

In particular, the following are noted:

1. A special trainee may not supervise chief residents.
2. A chief resident and a special trainee may not have primary responsibility for the same patients.

F. Working Environment and Hours

Graduate education in surgery requires a commitment to continuity of patient care. This continuity of care must take precedence—without regard to the time of day, day of the week, number of hours already worked, or on-call schedules. At the same time, patients have a right to expect a healthy, alert, responsible, and responsive physician dedicated to delivering effective and appropriate care.

The program director must establish an environment that is optimal both for resident education and for patient care, while ensuring that undue stress and fatigue among residents are avoided. It is his or her responsibility to ensure assignment of appropriate in-hospital duty hours so that residents are not required to perform excessively difficult or prolonged duties regularly. It is desirable that residents' work schedules be designed so that on average, excluding exceptional patient care needs, residents have at least 1 day out of 7 free of routine responsibilities and be on call in the hospital no more often than every third night. During these on-call hours residents should be provided with adequate sleeping, lounge, and food facilities. There must be adequate backup so that patient care is not jeopardized during or following assigned periods of duty. Support services must be such that residents do not spend an inordinate amount of time in noneducational activities that can be discharged properly by other personnel.

Different specialties and different rotations may require different working hours and patterns. A distinction must be made between on-call time in the hospital and on-call availability at home and their relation to actual hours worked. The ratio of hours worked to on-call time will vary particularly at the senior levels and therefore necessitates flexibility.

Residency training in surgery is a full-time responsibility; activities outside the educational program must not interfere with the resident's performance in the educational process, as determined by the program director, nor must they interfere with the residents' opportunities for rest, relaxation, and study.

G. Scholarly Environment

The quality of the educational environment of the parent and integrated institutions is of paramount importance to the program. Staff activity at affiliated institutions cannot account or substitute for the educational environment of the parent and integrated institutions. Adequate documentation of scholarly activity on the part of the program director and the teaching staff at the parent and integrated institutions must be submitted at the time of the program review. Documentation of scholarly activity is based on

1. participation in continuing surgical education;
2. participation in regional or national surgical scientific societies;
3. presentation and publication of scientific studies; and
4. demonstration of an active interest in research as it pertains to their own special surgical interests. The RRC will consider documented involvement in the following as indications of the commitment of the staff to research:
   a. Projects that are funded following peer review,
   b. Publications in peer-reviewed journals,
   c. Presentations at national and regional scientific meetings, and
   d. Research protocols that have been approved by appropriate institutional committees or other organizations.

While not all members of a teaching staff can be investigators, clinical and/or basic science research must be ongoing in the department of surgery of the parent and integrated institution(s). Research on the part of residents is not a substitute for the involvement of the program director and teaching staff. The staff as a whole must document active involvement in all phases of scholarly activity as defined above if they are to be considered adequate to conduct a program of graduate education in surgery.

VI. Evaluation

A. Programs of graduate education in surgery must be so constructed that there is a clear demonstration by the resident of acquisition of a solid foundation of fundamental surgical knowledge prior to progression in the program to the level of independent but supervised patient management and operative care. An objective test mechanism is required as a component of the process of demonstration of this cognitive capability. While each program may utilize its own test instruments, the American Board of Surgery In-Training Examination (ABSITE) is considered a most desirable example. However, results of the in-training examination should not be used as the only criterion of resident performance.

In addition to measuring the cognitive capability of the resident, the program must also have a system by which to measure the level of the resident's clinical qualifications as he or she progresses through the program. Any program that does not establish a system of trainee evaluation that clearly documents the progress of each resident in meeting the cognitive and clinical goals of the program will not be considered acceptable.

B. Including the evaluation processes indicated in the previous paragraph (VI.A), the overall performance of each resident must be evaluated by the teaching staff at least every 6 months.

1. A documented record of that evaluation must be prepared and maintained for subsequent review. This permanent record of evaluation for each resident is to be accessible to the resident and other authorized personnel.
2. All evaluations must be reviewed at least every 6 months with trainees.

C. A written final evaluation for each resident who completes the program must be provided. The evaluation must include a review of the resident's performance during the final period of training and should verify that the resident has demonstrated sufficient professional ability to practice competently and independently. This final evaluation should be part of the resident's permanent record maintained by the institution.

D. The educational effectiveness of a program must be evaluated in a systematic manner. In particular, the quality of the curriculum and the extent to which the educational goals have been met by residents must be assessed. Written evaluations by residents of the teaching staff and the program should be utilized in this process.

E. A program must strive for the highest possible quality of educational experience for the residents; it will be judged on this basis. One measure of the quality of a program is the performance of its graduates with respect to the American Board of Surgery certification process. Graduates of ACGME-approved programs are expected to complete this process successfully. At a minimum, for the most recent 5-year period, 60% of the graduates must pass the qualifying and certifying examinations on the first try.

ACGME: February 1998 Effective: January 1999

Program Requirements for Residency Education in the Subspecialties of General Surgery

I. General Information

A. A residency education program in a subspecialty of general surgery is an educational experience of at least 1 year designed to develop advanced knowledge and skills in a specific clinical area. All educational components of the program should be related to program goals. The program design and/or structure must be approved by the Residency Review Committee (RRC) as part of the regular review process.

Subspecialty education is a component in the continuum of the education process and must be in addition to the requirements for complete residency education in general surgery. Ordinarily the subspecialty education will follow completion of an accredited general surgery residency program.

B. Residency education programs in the subspecialties of general surgery may be accredited only in institutions that either sponsor a residency education program in general surgery or pediatric surgery accredited by the Accreditation Council for Graduate Medical Education (ACGME) or are integrated by formal agreement into such programs. The subspecialty programs will be approved only as an administratively integrated part of the approved core program in general surgery. Rotations to affiliated institutions can be approved for a period not exceeding 25% of the total program; adequate educational justification for such rotations must be provided to the RRC prior to implementation.

The description and regulations governing affiliated and integrated institutions in the Program Requirements for Residency

Education in General Surgery also apply to the subspecialty programs of surgery.

C. Subspecialty programs will not be approved if they have substantial negative impact on the education of the general surgery residents in the core program.

II. Program Director and Teaching Staff

Subspecialty education programs must provide a scholarly environment for acquiring the necessary cognitive and procedural clinical skills essential to the practice of the specific subspecialty. This objective can be achieved only when the program director, the supporting faculty and staff, and the administration are fully committed to the educational program. It is also imperative that appropriate resources and facilities be present. Service obligations must not compromise educational goals and objectives.

A. Program Director

There must be a single program director responsible for the program.

1. Qualifications of the Program Director:
   The subspecialty program director must be a surgeon who is qualified to supervise and to educate residents appropriately in the specific subspecialty.
   a. The director must either be certified in the subspecialty by the American Board of Surgery or possess equivalent qualifications, as determined by the RRC.
   b. The director must have an appointment in good standing to the medical staff of an institution participating in the program.
   c. The director must be licensed to practice medicine in the state where the institution that sponsors the program is located. (Certain federal programs are exempted.)
2. Responsibilities of the Program Director:
   It is the responsibility of the subspecialty program director to support the residency education program by devoting his/her principal effort to its management and administration, as well as to teaching, research, and clinical care limited to the integrated institutions. This general responsibility includes the following specifics:
   a. Preparation of a written statement outlining the educational goals of the program with respect to knowledge, skills, and other attributes of residents at each level of training and for each major rotation or other program assignment. This statement must be distributed to residents and members of the teaching staff. It should be readily available for review.
   b. Selection of residents for appointment to the program in accordance with institutional and departmental policies and procedures.
   c. Selection and supervision of the teaching staff and other program personnel at each institution participating in the program.
   d. The supervision of residents through explicit written descriptions of supervisory lines of responsibility for the care of patients. Such guidelines must be communicated to all members of the program staff. Residents must be provided with prompt, reliable systems for communication and interaction with supervisory physicians.
   e. Implementation of fair procedures as established by the sponsoring institution regarding academic discipline and resident complaints or grievances.
   f. Monitoring resident stress, including mental or emotional conditions inhibiting performance or learning, and drug- or alcohol-related dysfunction. Program directors and teaching staff should be sensitive to the need for timely provision of confidential counseling and psychological support services to residents. Training situations that consistently produce undesirable stress on residents must be evaluated and modified.
   g. Preparation of an accurate statistical and narrative description of the program

B. Teaching Staff

1. There must be a sufficient number of teaching staff with documented qualifications to instruct and supervise adequately all the residents in the program. Members of the teaching staff must be able to devote sufficient time to meet their supervisory and teaching responsibilities.
2. All members of the teaching staff must demonstrate a strong interest in the education of residents, sound clinical and teaching abilities, support of the goals and objectives of the program, a commitment to their own continuing medical education, and participation in scholarly activities.
3. A member of the teaching staff of each participating institution must be designated to assume responsibility for the day-to-day activities of the program at that institution, with overall coordination by the program director.
4. The teaching staff must be organized and have regular documented meetings to review program goals and objectives as well as program effectiveness in achieving them. At least one resident representative should participate in these reviews.
5. The teaching staff should periodically evaluate the utilization of the resources available to the program, the contribution of each institution participating in the program, the financial and administrative support of the program, the volume and variety of patients available to the program for educational purposes, the performance of members of the teaching staff, and the quality of supervision of residents.

C. Other Program Personnel

Programs must be provided the additional professional, technical, and clerical personnel needed to support the administration and educational conduct of the program.

III. Educational Principles

The principles of education enumerated in the Program Requirements for Residency Education in General Surgery are also applicable to the subspecialty programs.

A. The program directors for both the subspecialty and the core programs, as well as the institution itself, are responsible for ensuring that adequate facilities and resources are available to achieve the educational objectives.

B. A postgraduate residency must provide advanced education so that the residents can acquire special skill and knowledge in a specific subspecialty. This education should consist of a cognitive and a technical component. The cognitive component should emphasize the scholarly attributes of self-instruction, teaching, skilled clinical analysis, sound surgical judgment, and research creativity. The technical component must provide appropriate opportunity for the residents to acquire the operative and other psychomotor skills required for the practice of the subspecialty.

C. The program director must establish an environment that is optimal both for resident education and for patient care, including the responsibility for continuity of care, while assuring that undue stress and fatigue among residents are avoided. It is the program director's responsibility to ensure assignment of appropriate in-hospital duty hours so that residents are not subjected to excessively difficult or prolonged working hours. It is desirable that residents' work schedules be designed so that on average, excluding exceptional patient care needs, residents have at least 1 day out of 7 free of routine responsibilities and be on call in the hospital no more often than every third night. Different specialties and different rotations may require different working hours and patterns. A distinction must be made between on-call time in the hospital and on-call availability at home vis-a-vis actual hours worked. The ratio of hours worked and on-call time will vary, particularly at the senior levels, and therefore necessitates flexibility.

D. During the on-call hours residents should be provided with adequate sleeping, lounge, and food facilities. There must be adequate backup so that patient care is not jeopardized during or following assigned periods of duty. Support services and systems must be such that the resident does not spend an inordinate amount of time in noneducational activities that can be discharged properly by other personnel.

IV. Educational Components

Subspecialty programs must include the following educational components:

A. A sufficient number of patients must be available to assure appropriate inpatient and outpatient experience for each subspecialty resident, without adversely affecting the experience of residents in the general surgery core program. There must be adequate responsibility for continuity of care, to include prehospital and posthospital experience.

B. Subspecialty conferences, including review of all current complications and deaths; seminars; and clinical and basic science instruction must be regularly scheduled. Active participation of the subspecialty resident in the planning and the production of these meetings is essential.

C. A resident must have the opportunity to provide consultation with faculty supervision. He or she should have clearly defined educational responsibilities for other residents, medical students, and professional personnel. These teaching experiences should correlate basic biomedical knowledge with the clinical aspects of the subspecialty.

D. There must be close interaction between the core residency program in general surgery and the subspecialty program. Lines of responsibility for the general surgery residents and the subspecialty resident must be clearly defined. It is imperative that the educational program for the subspecialty resident not adversely affect the education of the general surgery residents, either in terms of operative experience or patient responsibility. In particular, the following are noted:

1. A subspecialty surgical resident may be a teaching assistant for residents other than general surgery chief residents.
2. Unless explicitly allowed by the Program Requirements for Residency Education in the specific subspecialty of general surgery, a chief resident in general surgery and a subspecialty resident may not have primary responsibility for the same patients.

The subspecialty resident should maintain a close working relationship with residents and fellows in general surgery and in other disciplines such as radiology, pathology, medicine, and pediatrics.

E. A subspecialty program must offer supervised training to assure the acquisition of the necessary preoperative, operative, and postoperative skills integral to the subspecialty discipline. Instruction and experience must be sufficient for the residents to acquire an understanding of the common procedures of the subspecialty, their indications, risks, and limitations.

F. Adequate and appropriate supervision of subspecialty residents must be provided at all times in accord with their level of experience and expertise.

V. Program Research and Scholarly Activity

Graduate medical education must take place in an environment of inquiry and scholarship in which residents participate in the development of new knowledge, learn to evaluate research findings, and develop habits of inquiry as a continuing professional responsibility.

A. Scholarly Activity

The responsibility for establishing and maintaining an environment of inquiry and scholarship rests with the teaching staff. While not all members of a teaching staff must be investigators, the staff as a whole must demonstrate broad involvement in scholarly activity. This activity should include:

1. Active participation of the teaching staff in clinical discussions, rounds, and conferences in a manner that promotes a spirit of inquiry and scholarship. Scholarship implies an in-depth understanding of basic mechanisms of normal and abnormal states and the application of current knowledge to practice.
2. Participation in journal clubs and research conferences.
3. Active participation in regional or national professional and scientific societies, particularly through presentations at the organization's meetings and publications in their journals.
4. Participation in research, particularly in projects that are funded following peer review and/or result in publications or presentations at regional and national scientific meetings.
5. Offering of guidance and technical support (eg, research design, statistical analysis) for residents involved in research.
6. Provision of support for resident participation in scholarly activities.

B. Research

A subspecialty program should have an investigational component such that the residents may become familiar with the design, implementation, and interpretation of clinical research studies. Facilities should be made available for research activity.

C. Library

1. Residents must have ready access to a major medical library either at the institution where the residents are located or through arrangement with convenient nearby institutions.
2. Library services should include the electronic retrieval of information from medical databases.
3. There must be access to an on-site library or to a collection of appropriate texts and journals in each institution participating in a residency program. On-site libraries and/or collections of texts and journals must be readily available during nights and weekends.

VI. Evaluation

A. Residents

Subspecialty program directors must establish clearly defined procedures for regular evaluation of residents' knowledge, skills, and overall performance, including the development of professional attitudes consistent with being a physician. The assessment must include cognitive, motor, and interpersonal skills as well as surgical judgment.

The program director, with participation of members of the teaching staff, shall:

1. At least semiannually evaluate the knowledge, skills, and professional growth of the residents, using appropriate criteria and procedures.
2. Communicate each evaluation to the resident in a timely manner.
3. Advance residents to positions of higher responsibility only on the basis of evidence of their satisfactory progressive scholarship and professional growth.

4. Maintain a permanent record of evaluation for each resident and have it accessible to the resident and other authorized personnel.

The provision of a written final evaluation is required for each resident who completes the program. The evaluation must include a review of the resident's performance during the final period of training and should verify that the resident has demonstrated sufficient professional ability to practice competently and independently. This final evaluation should be part of the resident's permanent record maintained by the institution.

B. Program Director

The subspecialty program director should be evaluated annually by the director of the core general surgery program regarding teaching, scholarly activities including research productivity, patient care activities, and administrative capabilities.

C. Program

The educational effectiveness of a program must be evaluated in a systematic manner. In particular, the quality of the curriculum and the extent to which the educational goals have been met by residents must be assessed by the program director, the core General Surgery program director, and by the Institutional Review Committee on a regular basis. Written evaluations by residents should be utilized in this process.

D. Efficacy of the Program

An important measure of the efficacy of the program is the performance of its graduates on the certification examinations offered by the American Board of Surgery. It is expected that 60% or more of the graduates of the program will become certified on their first attempt.

ACGME: September 1996 Effective: July 1997

Program Requirements for Residency Education in Surgical Critical Care (Surgery-General)

I. Introduction

A. Definition and Scope of the Specialty

1. Surgical critical care deals with complex surgical and medical problems in critically ill surgical patients. Institutions sponsoring graduate educational programs in surgical critical care must provide the educational, clinical, and administrative resources to allow residents to develop advanced proficiency in the management of critically ill surgical patients, to develop the qualifications necessary to supervise surgical critical care units, and to conduct scholarly activities in surgical critical care. The educational program must be an integral part of and enhance an accredited core program in general surgery.
2. Completion of at least 3 clinical years in an accredited graduate educational program in the disciplines of general surgery, neurosurgery, urology, or obstetrics and gynecology is a prerequisite. A subspecialty educational program in surgical critical care is in addition to the requirements for critical care education set forth in the Program Requirements for these core programs. There should be an institutional policy governing the educational resources committed to critical care programs and ensuring cooperation of all involved disciplines.
3. Residents in one of the surgical disciplines listed in Section I.A.2 who enter the program prior to completing a residency must have a categorical residency position in their specialty available to them on satisfactory completion of the critical care fellowship.

B. Duration and Scope of Training

1. Graduate education in surgical critical care shall be 12 months, of which 2 months may be elective rotations. These 12 months must be devoted to advanced educational and clinical activities related to the care of critically ill patients and to the administration of critical care units.
2. A surgical critical care program must include primary educational activities in a surgical critical care unit with pediatric and/or adult patients, located in an institution that has been approved by the Residency Review Committee (RRC) for surgery as an integrated institution (as defined in the Program Requirements for Residency Education in General Surgery) with a core general surgery or pediatric surgery residency program.

   Training may take place in various settings that provide for the care of critically ill adult and/or pediatric surgical patients, including those with general surgical conditions such as trauma, burns, and surgical oncology; with cardiothoracic, neurosurgical, and high risk pregnancy conditions; and with organ transplantation.
3. In some instances residents may devote up to 25% of their time to direct operative care of critically ill patients. During such operative care, the critical care resident and chief resident in general surgery may not share primary responsibility for the same patient. However, in the nonoperative management of critically ill surgical patients the surgical critical care residents and general surgery residents may interact as long as they share primary responsibility in patient management decisions. The final decision and responsibility rests with the supervising attending surgeon.

C. Objectives

1. The completion of an accredited surgical residency training program qualifies the surgeon to manage critically ill surgical patients. Therefore, the surgical critical care program must enable the resident to acquire an advanced body of knowledge and level of skill in the management of critically ill surgical patients in order to assume a leadership role in teaching and in research in surgical critical care. This advanced body of knowledge and level of skill must include the mastery of (1) the use of advanced technology and instrumentation to monitor the physiologic status of children or adults of both sexes, including those in the neonatal, pediatric, child-bearing, or advanced years; (2) organizational and administrative aspects of a critical care unit; and (3) ethical, economic, and legal issues as they pertain to critical care.
2. In addition, individuals completing a training program in surgical critical care will be expected to be able to
   a. teach the specialty of surgical critical care.
   b. undertake investigations into the various areas of surgical critical care, such as new instrumentation, identification of important physiologic parameters, evaluation of pharmacologic agents in critically ill patients, or health outcomes and/or health policy issues related to surgical critical care.
   c. administer a surgical critical care unit and appoint, train, and supervise specialized personnel, establish policy and procedures for the unit, and coordinate the activities of the unit with other administrative units within the hospital.

II. Faculty Qualification and Responsibilities

A. Program Director

1. The critical care training program must be under the direction of a surgeon who is certified in surgical critical care by the American Board of Surgery or who has equivalent surgical training as

well as the appropriate qualifications and documented experience in surgical critical care.

2. The program director of the critical care program must be the director or codirector of one or more of the critical care units in which the clinical aspects of the critical care program take place, and he or she must be personally involved in clinical supervision and teaching of general surgery and surgical critical care residents in that unit.
3. The program director shall have administrative responsibility for the surgical critical care educational program and shall appoint all residents and teaching staff to the program and determine their duties.

B. Faculty

1. In the teaching environment of the surgical critical care unit, it is recognized that the teaching staff in surgery, medicine, pediatrics, obstetrics and gynecology, anesthesiology, and other disciplines may all be involved in the care of specific patients. Therefore, a collegial relationship must exist between the surgical director of the critical care educational program and the teaching staff to enhance the educational opportunities for all residents and trainees.
2. The teaching staff must be specifically qualified in the care of critically ill surgical patients and must provide the program director with regular evaluations of the residents. At least one surgeon qualified in surgical critical care must be appointed to the teaching staff for every surgical critical care resident enrolled in the program.
3. The teaching staff must have real and demonstrated interest in teaching and set an example for residents by documented engagement in scholarly pursuits, to include (1) participation in their own continuing education in surgical critical care, (2) participation in regional and national surgical scientific societies, and (3) demonstration of an active interest in research as it pertains to critical care problems.

III. Facilities and Resources

A. The surgical critical care program must function in a unit that has sufficient numbers of knowledgeable personnel and the necessary equipment to care for critically ill surgical patients.

B. Personnel should include specially trained nurses and technicians who are skilled in critical care instrumentation, respiratory function, and laboratory medicine.

C. The critical care unit must be located in a designated area within the hospital, constructed and designed specifically for the care of critically ill patients.

D. Equipment and personnel in the critical care unit should be centrally concentrated to provide efficient and expeditious operation.

E. There should be a supporting laboratory available to provide complete and prompt laboratory evaluation.

F. The objectives of a surgical critical care program can be achieved only when the program is based within an institution that has an accredited residency program in general surgery. It is desirable for the institution to have accredited residencies in the surgical specialties and in disciplines that particularly relate to surgery, such as internal medicine, radiology, pathology, and anesthesiology.

G. An adequate hospital library must be readily available to provide easy access to information for patient care or scholarly pursuits.

H. Conveniently located and adequate space for conferences and study is essential.

I. The average daily census for each surgical critical care unit to which the residents are assigned shall permit a resident-to-patient ratio of one resident to five patients. The qualified surgical faculty-to-critical care resident ratio shall be at least one to one. These ratios are sufficient to provide an adequate clinical and supervisory base. When more than one critical care program exists in an institution, it will be the responsibility of the institution to coordinate interdisciplinary requirements and to ensure that each resident meets the Program Requirements for Residency Education in Critical Care in their primary discipline (eg, medicine, anesthesiology, etc).

J. To provide sufficient breadth in patient exposure, a critical care program that averages a daily census of at least 10 patients is required.

K. The record-keeping system must maintain the records of patients in the critical care unit as retrievable parts of the hospital chart, so they can be available for evaluation.

IV. The Educational Program

A. Curriculum Overview

The program must provide the opportunity for residents to acquire advanced knowledge of the following aspects of critical care, particularly as they relate to the management of patients with hemodynamic instability, multiple system organ failure, and complex coexisting medical problems:

1. Cardiorespiratory resuscitation
2. Physiology, pathophysiology, diagnosis, and therapy of disorders of the cardiovascular, respiratory, gastrointestinal, genitourinary, neurologic, endocrine, musculoskeletal, and immune systems, as well as of infectious diseases
3. Metabolic, nutritional, and endocrine effects of critical illness
4. Hematologic and coagulation disorders
5. Critical obstetric and gynecologic disorders
6. Trauma, thermal, electrical, and radiation injuries
7. Inhalation and immersion injuries
8. Monitoring and medical instrumentation
9. Critical pediatric surgical conditions
10. Pharmacokinetics and dynamics of drug metabolism and excretion in critical illness
11. Ethical and legal aspects of surgical critical care
12. Principles and techniques of administration and management
13. Biostatistics and experimental design

B. Critical Care Skills

The program must provide supervised training that will enable the resident to gain competence in the performance and application of the following critical care skills:

1. Respiratory: airway management, including endoscopy and management of respiratory systems
2. Circulatory: invasive and noninvasive monitoring techniques, including transesophageal and precordial cardiac ultrasound and application of transvenous pacemakers; computations of cardiac output and of systemic and pulmonary vascular resistance; monitoring electrocardiograms and management of cardiac assist devices
3. Neurological: the performance of complete neurological examinations; use of intracranial pressure monitoring techniques and of the electroencephalogram to evaluate cerebral function; application of hypothermia in the management of cerebral trauma
4. Renal: the evaluation of renal function; peritoneal dialysis and hemofiltration; knowledge of the indications and complications of hemodialysis
5. Gastrointestinal: utilization of gastrointestinal intubation and endoscopic techniques in the management of the critically ill patient; application of enteral feedings; management of stomas, fistulas, and percutaneous catheter devices
6. Hematologic: application of autotransfusion; assessment of coagulation status; appropriate use of component therapy

7. Infectious disease: classification of infections and application of isolation techniques, pharmacokinetics, drug interactions, and management of antibiotic therapy during organ failure; nosocomial infections; indications for applications of hyperbaric oxygen therapy
8. Nutritional: application of parenteral and enteral nutrition; monitoring and assessing metabolism and nutrition
9. Monitoring/bioengineering: use and calibration of transducers, amplifiers, and recorders
10. Miscellaneous: use of special beds for specific injuries; employment of pneumatic antishock garments, traction, and fixation devices

V. Documentation of Experience

The program must document to the site visitor that residents in the surgical critical care program have had direct involvement in the management of a broad spectrum of critically ill surgical patients. In addition, each resident must submit an operative log of the number and type of operative experiences while a surgical critical care resident.

VI. Other Information

In addition to these requirements specific to surgical critical care, the Program Requirements for Residency Education in the Subspecialties of General Surgery also apply to all surgical critical care programs.

ACGME: September 1996 Effective: July 1997

Program Requirements for Residency Education in Hand Surgery (Surgery-General)

I. Introduction

A. Definition of the Specialty

Hand surgery is a surgical subspecialty that deals with congenital and acquired defects of the hand and wrist that compromise the function of the hand. A hand surgery educational program is designed to educate physicians in the art and science of hand surgery and to develop a competent hand surgeon who is capable of independent function. The educational program should provide experience in the repair, resection, and reconstruction of defects of form and function of the hand; in the design, construction, and transfer of flaps and the transplantation of tissues, including microsurgery of multiple tissues; in replantation of upper extremity parts; in surgical and ancillary methods of treatment of tumors; in management of complex wounds; and in the use of alloplastic materials.

B. Scope of Education

1. Prerequisite resident education must be completed in a general surgery, orthopaedic surgery, or plastic surgery program accredited by the Accreditation Council for Graduate Medical Education (ACGME) or the Royal College of Physicians and Surgeons of Canada.
2. The length of the educational program is 1 year.

II. Institutional Organization

A. Sponsoring Institution

The educational program should have one sponsoring institution that has primary responsibility for the entire program. The sponsoring institution should provide sufficient faculty; financial resources; and clinical, research, and library facilities to meet the educational needs of the residents and to permit the program to comply with the requirements for accreditation.

B. Participating Institutions

1. When multiple institutions participate in the educational program, the commitment of each participating institution must be documented in a written agreement that complies with the ACGME Institutional Requirements.
2. Assignments to participating institutions must be based on an appropriate educational rationale. Assignments that dilute the education of residents or that do not provide proper supervision and coordination of educational activities should not be established or maintained.
3. Assignments to participating institutions that are geographically distant from the sponsoring institution are not desirable. To be justifiable, such assignments must offer special resources or opportunities not otherwise available to the program.
4. The number and location of participating institutions must not preclude the participation of residents and faculty in the educational activities of the hand surgery course of study.

C. Appointment of Residents

1. The total number of residents must be approved in advance by the Residency Review Committee (RRC). The number of residents shall be based primarily on the number, qualifications, and commitment of the faculty; the volume and variety of the patient population available for educational purposes; and the institutional resources committed to resident education.
2. Programs may not graduate more hand surgery residents in any given year than the number of residents approved by the RRC.
3. Any increase, including a temporary increase in resident complement, must receive prior approval of the RRC. Requests for changes in the approved resident complement of a program must include a strong educational rationale.

III. Faculty Qualifications and Responsibilities

The program director and the faculty are responsible for the general administration of a program, including those activities related to the recruitment, selection, instruction, supervision, counseling, evaluation, and advancement of residents and the maintenance of records related to program accreditation.

A. Program Director

A single program director must be responsible for the program.

1. Qualifications of the program director
   a. Requisite and documented clinical, educational, and administrative abilities and experience.
   b. Licensure to practice medicine in the state where the institution that sponsors the program is located.
   c. Certification by the appropriate ABMS Board or suitable equivalent qualifications in the appropriate specialty and a certificate of added qualifications in hand surgery or suitable equivalent qualifications in hand surgery. The RRC will determine the acceptability of equivalent qualifications.
   d. Appointment in good standing to the medical staff of an institution participating in the program.
   e. Frequent changes in leadership or long periods of temporary leadership are undesirable and may adversely affect the accreditation status of the program.
2. Responsibilities of the program director
   a. Prepare a written statement outlining the educational goals of the program with respect to knowledge, skills, and other attributes of hand surgery residents at each level of education and for each assignment. This statement must be distributed

Program Requirements

to hand surgery residents and members of the faculty. It should be readily available for review.

b. Select residents for appointment to the program according to institutional and departmental policies and procedures.
c. Select and supervise the faculty and other program personnel at each participating institution.
d. Supervise residents through explicit written descriptions of supervisory lines of responsibility for the care of patients. Such guidelines must be communicated to all members of the faculty. Residents must be provided with prompt, reliable systems for communication and interaction with supervising physicians.
e. Regularly evaluate residents' knowledge, skills, and overall performance. The program director, with participation of the faculty, must
   1. at least quarterly, evaluate the progress of each hand surgery resident in writing, using appropriate criteria and procedures;
   2. communicate each evaluation to the resident in a timely manner;
   3. advance residents to positions of higher responsibility only on evidence of their satisfactory progressive scholarship and growth;
   4. maintain a permanent record of evaluation for each resident and have it accessible to the resident and other authorized personnel; and
   5. provide a final written evaluation to each hand surgery resident who completes the program. The evaluation must include a review of the resident's performance during the final period of education and should verify that the resident has demonstrated sufficient professional ability to practice competently and independently. Each evaluation should be signed by the resident and program director and be maintained on file by the program director for at least 5 years following completion of the program.
f. Implement fair procedures, as established by the sponsoring institution, regarding academic discipline and resident complaints or grievances.
g. Monitor resident stress, including mental or emotional conditions inhibiting performance or learning and drug- or alcohol-related dysfunction. Program directors and faculty should be sensitive to the need for timely provision of counseling and psychological support services to residents. Educational situations that consistently produce undesirable stress on residents must be evaluated and modified.
h. Prepare an accurate statistical and narrative description of the program, as requested by the RRC.
i. Ensure that each resident is provided with a sufficient educational program, including a sufficient volume and variety of operative experience and progressive surgical responsibility.
j. Annually collect, compile, and retain the number and types of hand surgery operative procedures performed in all institutions used for resident education. These data must be provided in the form and format specified by the RRC.
k. Annually collect, compile, and retain a comprehensive record of the operative procedures performed by each hand surgery resident completing the program. This information must be provided in the form and format specified by the RRC. This record must be signed by the hand surgery resident and the program director, attesting to its accuracy.
l. Advise applicants of the prerequisite requirements of the appropriate specialty board.
m. Document the satisfactory completion of prerequisite education before the resident begins the hand surgery program.
n. Notify the executive director of the RRC in writing of any major change in the program that significantly alters the educational experience for the residents, including
   1. changes in program leadership, to include any change in appointment of the program director, section or division head, or department chair, and
   2. changes in administrative structure that affect the status of the parent department in the institution.
o. Obtain prior RRC approval for the following changes in the program:
   1. the addition or deletion of any participating institution to which residents are assigned for a total of 2 months or longer;
   2. any change in the approved resident complement of the program; and
   3. any change in the length or format of the program.

B. Faculty

1. The hand surgery faculty must be certified by the one of the sponsoring boards, or possess suitable equivalent qualifications and be certified in hand surgery or possess suitable equivalent qualifications. The majority of the faculty must possess certificates of added qualifications in hand surgery. The RRC will determine the acceptability of equivalent qualifications.
2. There must be a sufficient number of qualified faculty to adequately instruct and supervise hand surgery residents to ensure optimal patient care and resident education. The faculty must be able to devote sufficient time to the program to meet their supervisory and teaching responsibilities.
3. The faculty must demonstrate a strong interest in the education of residents, sound clinical and teaching abilities, support of the goals and objectives of the program, a commitment to their own continuing medical education, and participation in scholarly activities.
4. A faculty member at each participating institution must be designated to assume responsibility for the day-to-day activities of the program at that institution, with overall coordination by the program director.
5. The faculty must be organized and have regular documented meetings to review program goals and objectives and program effectiveness in achieving these goals. The hand surgery resident should participate in these reviews.
6. The faculty should, at least annually, evaluate the utilization of the resources available to the program, the contribution of each institution participating in the program, the financial and administrative support of the program, the volume and variety of patients available to the program for educational purposes, the performance of the faculty, and the quality of resident supervision.

C. Scholarly Activity

Graduate medical education must take place in an environment of inquiry and scholarship in which residents participate in the development of new knowledge, learn to evaluate research findings, and develop habits of inquiry as a continuing professional responsibility. The responsibility for establishing and maintaining an environment of inquiry and scholarship rests with the faculty. While not all members of the faculty must be research investigators, the faculty as a whole must demonstrate broad involvement in scholarly activity. Scholarship is defined as an in-depth understanding of basic mechanisms of normal and abnormal states and the application of current knowledge to practice. This activity should include

1. participation in clinical discussions, rounds, and conferences in a manner that promotes a spirit of inquiry and scholarship;
2. participation in journal clubs and research conferences;

3. active participation in regional or national professional and scientific societies, particularly through presentations at the organizations' meetings and publication in their journals;
4. participation in research, particularly in projects funded following peer review and/or that result in publications or presentations at regional and national scientific meetings;
5. offering of guidance and technical support (eg, research design, statistical analysis) for residents involved in research; and
6. provision of support for resident participation in scholarly activities.

D. Other Program Personnel

Programs must be provided with the additional professional, technical, and clerical personnel needed to support the administration and educational conduct of the program.

IV. Facilities and Resources

A. Inpatient Facilities

1. Inpatient facilities should have a sufficient number of beds, support personnel, and proper equipment to ensure quality patient care and education.
2. Operating suite and diagnostic and treatment facilities must contain technologically current equipment.

B. Outpatient Facilities

Appropriately equipped outpatient facilities including support staff, operating suites, and clinic and office space must be available for resident participation in the preoperative evaluation, treatment, and postoperative follow-up of patients for whom the resident has responsibility.

C. Library Facilities

1. The residents must have ready access to a major medical library, either at the institution where the residents are located or through arrangement with convenient nearby institutions.
2. Library services should include the electronic retrieval of information from medical databases.

V. The Educational Program

A. Program Design

1. The program director and faculty must prepare and implement written educational goals for the program.
2. The program design and/or structure must be approved by the RRC as part of the regular review process.

B. Clinical Component

1. Residents must be provided with education in surgical design, surgical diagnosis, embryology, surgical and artistic anatomy, surgical physiology and pathology, pharmacology, wound healing, microbiology, adjunctive oncological therapy, biomechanics, rehabilitation, and surgical instrumentation.
2. A sufficient number and variety of adult and pediatric hand surgery patients must be available for resident education.
3. Generally equivalent and sufficient distribution of operative procedures among the residents in all categories of hand surgery must be demonstrated.
4. Residents should be provided with graduated and progressive patient management responsibility.
5. Because judgment and technical capability to achieve satisfactory surgical results are mandatory qualities for the hand surgeon, education should be provided in the following areas:
   a. Skin repair, including grafts and flaps, multiple tissue flaps, free microscopic tissue transfers, and insertion of tissue expanders
   b. Fingertip injuries
   c. Tendon repair, including flexor tendon repair and graft, implantation of tendon spacer, extensor tendon repair, and tenolysis/tenodesis
   d. Tendon transfer and tendon balancing
   e. Nerve repair, including major and digital, graft, neurolysis, surgical treatment of neuroma, transpositions, and nerve decompressions
   f. Management of fractures and dislocations, including phalangeal or metacarpal with and without internal fixation; wrist, radius, and ulna with and without internal fixation; and injuries to joint ligaments
   g. Bone grafts
   h. Joint and tendon sheath repairs, including release of contracture, synovectomy, arthroplasty with and without implant, arthrodesis, trigger finger release, and stiff joints that result from rheumatoid or other injury
   i. Pollicization or ray transfer
   j. Foot to hand transfer
   k. Tumors, benign and malignant
   l. Dupuytren's contracture
   m. Replantation, revascularization
   n. Amputations
   o. Fasciotomy, deep incision and drainage for infection, and wound débridement
   p. Congenital deformities, including syndactyly and others
   q. Management of upper extremity vascular disorders and insufficiencies
   r. Foreign body, implant removal
   s. Thermal injuries
   t. Arthroscopy
   u. Upper extremity pain management

C. Didactic Components

1. A comprehensive, organized course of study must be offered, to include educational conferences that are well defined, documented, and regularly held. At minimum, the program must provide a didactic component for clinical education referencing section V.B.1 of these Program Requirements for Residency Education in Hand Surgery.
2. The written course of study should reflect careful planning, with evidence of a cyclical presentation of core specialty knowledge supplemented by the addition of current information, including practice management, ethics, and medicolegal topics as they relate to hand surgery. Conferences must include basic science subjects related to clinical surgery of the hand, such as anatomy, physiology, pathology, genetics, microbiology, and pharmacology. A periodic review of the morbidity and mortality experience of the service must be included.
3. A list of the conferences should be maintained and available for review at the time of the site visit.
4. Conferences should be attended by both the residents and the faculty, and such attendance should be documented.
5. Conferences should be organized by the faculty to ensure that sufficient educational experience is provided. Hand surgery residents assigned to participating institutions other than the sponsoring institution should attend the hand surgery conferences at those sites.
6. Residents should make presentations at conferences and actively participate in conference discussions. Adequate time for resident preparation should be permitted to maximize the educational experience.
7. Hand surgery residents should be encouraged to pursue clinical or basic science research interests.

D. Supervision

1. All patient care services must be supervised by qualified hand surgery faculty. The program director must ensure, direct, and document proper supervision of residents at all times.
2. Residents must be provided with rapid, reliable systems for communicating with faculty at all times.
3. Hand surgery residents may function as intermediate supervisors when documented prior experience makes it appropriate, but faculty supervision must be available.

E. Duty Hours

1. It is desirable that residents' work schedules be designed so that on the average, excluding exceptional patient care needs, residents have at least 1 day out of 7 free of routine responsibilities and be on call in the hospital no more often than every third night. The ratio of hours worked to on-call time will vary, particularly at senior levels, and flexibility will be necessary.
2. There must be adequate backup so that patient care is not jeopardized during or following assigned periods of duty.
3. Sufficient support services must be provided to ensure that residents are not required to spend excessive time in noneducational activities that can be discharged properly by other personnel.
4. The hand surgery residency is a full-time responsibility. Activities outside the educational program must not interfere with resident performance in the educational program as determined by the program director and must not interfere with resident opportunity for rest, relaxation, and study.

F. Appointment of Other Residents

1. The appointment of other residents for hand surgery education must not dilute or detract from the educational opportunities of hand surgery residents.
2. The appointment of other residents to the hand surgery service requires a clear statement of the areas of education, clinical responsibilities, and duration of the education. This statement must be supplied to the RRC at the time the program is reviewed.
3. If such residents so appointed will, in the judgment of the RRC, detract from the education of the hand surgery residents, the accreditation status of the program may be adversely affected.

VI. Evaluation

A. Resident Evaluation

The program director and faculty are responsible for regularly evaluating the residents' knowledge, skills, and overall performance, including the development of professional attitudes consistent with being a physician.

B. Faculty Evaluation

1. At least annually, all individual faculty members must be formally evaluated by the program director. Hand surgery residents should be provided with the opportunity to evaluate faculty.
2. A mechanism for sharing the results of such evaluations with the faculty that preserves resident confidentiality in the evaluation process must be employed.
3. The program should demonstrate that such evaluations are used in improving the program.

C. Program Evaluation

1. The educational effectiveness of a program must be evaluated at least annually. In particular, the quality of the curriculum and the extent to which the educational goals have been met by residents must be assessed. Written evaluations by hand surgery residents should be utilized in this process.
2. One measure of the quality of a program is the performance of its graduates on the examination for the certificate of added qualifications in hand surgery given by the American Board of Surgery. The RRC may consider this information as part of the overall evaluation of the program.

VII. Board Certification

Residents who plan to seek hand surgery certification as administered by the American Board of Surgery should communicate with the secretary of the board to ascertain the current requirements for acceptance as a candidate for certification.

ACGME: September 1997 Effective July 1998

Program Requirements for Residency Education in Pediatric Surgery (Surgery-General)

I. General Characteristics of Accredited Programs

A residency program in pediatric surgery must provide a structured curriculum and adequate clinical experience in the fundamental areas of surgery related to infants and children. The goal is to prepare residents to function as qualified practitioners of pediatric surgery at the high level of performance expected of board-certified specialists. The educational components of the program, therefore, must be of the highest priority. Residents must be provided adequate time and sufficient facilities for study. While every program carries a commitment of service to patients, the service responsibilities must support and not detract from the educational activities.

II. Teaching Staff

The staff responsible for the organization and performance of the pediatric surgical program must be well qualified and diversified, so as to represent the many facets of pediatric surgery.

A. Program Director

The program director must be dedicated to and actively engaged in surgical education and must be responsible for the proper conduct of the educational activities of the program. The program director must:

1. Be institutionally based and be appointed for at least the duration of the program plus 1 year
2. Be qualified in surgery, certified by the American Board of Surgery, and hold a current Certificate of Special Qualifications in Pediatric Surgery or have equivalent qualifications
3. Be responsible for rotations and staff appointments of attending surgeons on the teaching services
4. Make resident appointments and assignments and be responsible for the proper conduct of the educational activities, particularly for the supervision and direction of the residents
5. Provide complete and accurate program information forms and resident operative records to the Residency Review Committee (RRC) so that an appropriate assessment of the program can be made.

B. Other Teaching Staff

1. The teaching staff must include, at a minimum, one other pediatric surgeon who possesses the qualifications listed for the program director in II.A.2.
2. The key staff members must be appointed for a period long enough to ensure continuity in the supervision of the program. They must be formally organized and meet regularly.
3. It is essential that the members of the teaching staff provide exemplary models to the trainees by their dedication to patient care and education. Participation and productivity in scholarly

pursuits by the teaching staff is a required attribute of an accredited program.

III. Institution

In addition to the essentials outlined in the Institutional Requirements, institutions with an approved training program in pediatric surgery must have the following characteristics:

A. There shall be inpatient pediatric surgical admissions adequate to provide educational experience for the program. Intensive care units for both infants and older children are essential.

B. Pediatric surgical outpatient care sessions must meet on a regular basis. They shall include initial evaluation of ambulatory patients with surgical conditions as well as both short-term and ongoing follow-up management of these patients.

C. An emergency department in which infants and children can be efficiently managed 24 hours a day is essential. The pediatric surgical staff will ordinarily serve as consultants for this department. The pediatric surgical service must direct the care of all patients with traumatic or thermal injuries involving multiple organ systems.

D. To provide the necessary breadth of experience, an accredited residency training program in pediatrics is required within the primary institution. Residency programs or other equivalent clinical expertise in other specialties, particularly radiology and pathology, are highly desirable.

E. The department of radiology must have one or more staff with training, interest, competence, and experience in the radiologic evaluation of infants and children. The department should be staffed and organized to permit efficient and complete evaluation of patients 24 hours a day. The department should be furnished and equipped to provide up-to-date imaging capability, including such procedures as ultrasonography and computerized scanning. Facilities for nuclear medicine, magnetic resonance imaging, and interventional radiography should be available within the institution.

F. The department of pathology should have one or more staff with special training, interest, competence, and experience in pediatric pathology. The department should provide efficient and expert surgical pathology service, and surgical pathology consultation must be available at all times. The department of pathology must participate in the pediatric surgical educational program, including the conduct of appropriate conferences at which the current surgical pathology material is presented and discussed. These conferences must be attended by both staff and residents of the pediatric surgical service.

G. Within the department of anesthesiology there must be anesthesiologists with special training, interest, competence, and experience in the anesthesia of infants and children. The number of such anesthesiologists must be consistent with the volume of surgical cases in the pediatric age group.

H. The institutional library must contain a representative and authoritative collection of books and journals on pediatric surgery, pediatrics, general surgery, other surgical specialties, radiology, and the basic sciences. The library shall be managed and supervised by a well-qualified medical librarian. The Index Medicus must be part of the library, and access to computerized literature search facilities is highly desirable.

IV. Duration of Training

A. Before beginning a residency in pediatric surgery, each resident must have satisfactorily completed a program in general surgery accredited by the Accreditation Council for Graduate Medical Education (ACGME) or the Royal College of Physicians and Surgeons of Canada. He or she must be admissible to examination by the American Board of Surgery (or its equivalent) or be certified by that board.

B. The residency program in pediatric surgery must be accredited for 2 years, 18 months of which must be devoted to clinical pediatric surgery. The remaining required 6 months may be devoted to related clinical disciplines designed to enhance the educational experience or may be devoted to scholarly activities. The last 12 months of the clinical training must be at the chief pediatric surgical resident level with a high degree of responsibility for patient management, including semi-independent operative experience under appropriate supervision.

V. Scope and Content of Program

A. The program must provide both clinical experience and education in the fundamental areas of surgery related to infants and children.

1. Residents must be given responsibility for surgical management so that they may attain detailed knowledge of congenital, neoplastic, infectious, and other acquired conditions of the gastrointestinal system and other abdominal organs; of the blood and vascular system; of the integument; of the diaphragm and thorax, exclusive of the heart; of the endocrine glands; of the gonads and reproductive organs; and of the head and neck.
2. In addition, an opportunity for similar experience in traumatic conditions of the abdomen, chest, head and neck, and extremities must be provided. Particularly, the resident must have sufficient experience to become expert in the management of children who have sustained injuries to multiple organs. The resident also must have sufficient opportunity to manage on the surgical service patients who may or may not require surgical intervention and to acquire skill in such nonoperative management.
3. The resident also should have sufficient exposure in endoscopy to become competent in endoscopy of the airway and gastrointestinal tract, including laryngoscopy, bronchoscopy, esophagoscopy, and gastroduodenoscopy. Experiences in lower intestinal endoscopy, laparoscopy, and cystoscopy are desirable.
4. The resident must gain adequate understanding of the principles and operative experience in the management of the more common problems in urologic surgery.
5. The resident must have the opportunity to gain adequate knowledge of the basic principles of cardiothoracic surgery, gynecology, neurologic surgery, orthopedics, otorhinolaryngology, anesthesia, vascular surgery, transplant surgery, and the management of burns. While rotations on these services are highly desirable, the program may enable the resident to acquire an understanding of the principles of these subspecialties by a structured curriculum that adequately deals with these surgical areas.
6. The resident must gain experience and competence in the complete care of the critically ill infant or child, including the following: (a) cardiopulmonary resuscitation, (b) management of patients on respirators, (c) invasive monitoring techniques and interpretation, (d) nutritional assessment and management, and (e) competence in the recognition and management of clotting and coagulation disorders.

B. The program must provide a course or structured series of conferences to ensure coverage of the basic and clinical sciences fundamental to pediatric surgery, to include but not be limited to embryology; genetics; wound healing; hemostasis and blood disorders; immunobiology; transplantation; and physiology and pathology of the circulatory, respiratory, gastrointestinal, genitourinary, and endocrine systems. Similarly, the program must provide appropriate education in fluid and electrolyte balance, nutrition, infection, metabolic response to injury, and anesthesiology.

C. The program must incorporate structured educational activities on a regular basis, to include:
   1. Teaching rounds with bedside teaching conducted by the surgical staff.
   2. Staff supervision of surgical procedures performed by the resident.
   3. Regular teaching conferences, held at least twice monthly, to include pediatric surgical grand rounds, morbidity and mortality conferences, and radiology conferences.
   4. Other relevant multidisciplinary conferences, including surgical pathology and tumor conferences.
   5. During the senior year, the residents are to be given the opportunity for personally organizing the more formal of the pediatric surgical conferences, including pediatric surgical grand rounds and the mortality and morbidity conferences. They also shall be directly responsible for a significant share of the presentations and discussions at these conferences.

D. The residents must participate in outpatient activities as an integral component of the program. In the surgical outpatient facility, the residents must have the opportunity to evaluate patients, make appropriate provisional diagnoses, initiate diagnostic procedures, and form preliminary treatment plans. In addition and of particular importance, the residents must have the opportunity for outpatient follow-up care of surgical patients. This care shall include not only the short-term evaluation and progress of patients who have had recent surgical problems or procedures but also the opportunity to see patients on a long-term basis, particularly those who have had operations for major congenital anomalies or neoplasms. An effective mechanism for follow-up must be provided for all patients, whether seen in clinics or private office settings. The program must document a satisfactory mechanism for follow-up care by the residents.

E. To meet the requirements of direct and responsible patient management, it is essential that those patients whose primary problem is surgical be on the pediatric surgical service and be directly managed by the surgical staff. Appropriate consultation with specialists such as neonatologists and intensivists is strongly encouraged. It is emphasized, however, that newborns with surgical conditions, as well as surgical patients requiring intensive care, must be on the pediatric surgical service where the care is the responsibility of the surgical staff.

F. Residents should have significant teaching responsibilities for more junior house officers and medical students assigned to the service and should also share in the development and the presentation of the formal teaching conferences. The resident's effectiveness as a teacher shall be a part of his or her overall evaluation.

G. Residents may be given the opportunity to engage in scholarly activities.

H. Rotations not to exceed 3 months may be spent at outside institutions at the discretion of the program director during the first year of training. Rotations outside the parent institution exceeding 3 months may be made only with prior approval of the RRC for Surgery. In no circumstance may outside rotations exceed a total of 6 months of the 24-month training period.

VI. Patient Volume

To be approved for training in pediatric surgery, an institution must provide an adequate number and variety of pediatric surgical patients.

A. The general pediatric surgical service should perform a minimum of 900 operations per year.

B. The chief resident must be provided with a broad and varied experience; each is expected to be responsible for at least 250 pediatric surgical operations under supervision during this year.

C. The operative experience of the residents must include a sufficient number of neonatal cases to ensure the opportunity to acquire adequate experience, knowledge, and competence in the conditions falling under this category; there also should be an adequate number of major solid tumor procedures.

D. When previous personal operative experience justifies a teaching role, residents may act as teaching assistants and list such cases in the appropriate manner.

VII. Evaluation

A. The performance of each house officer must be evaluated by the teaching staff at least every 6 months; it is required that input from other departments or services involved in the training of the residents be included in this evaluation. Records documenting the 6-month evaluations must be maintained.

B. Prior to advancement to the senior or chief resident level of supervised and semi-independent patient management and operative experience, a resident must clearly demonstrate acquisition of basic knowledge in pediatric surgery. An objective test for this purpose is required. While each program may utilize its own testing mechanism, an excellent instrument is the annual In-Training Examination in Pediatric Surgery. In addition to measuring the cognitive capability of the resident, the program also must have a system by which to measure the level of the resident's clinical qualifications as he or she progresses through the program. The program must establish a system of evaluation that clearly documents the progress of each resident in meeting the cognitive and clinical goals of the program.

C. A program will be judged on the quality of educational experience provided to the residents. One measure of the quality of a program is the performance of its graduates with respect to the American Board of Surgery examinations for Certification of Special Qualification in Pediatric Surgery. Graduates of ACGME-approved programs are expected to complete this process successfully. A program will be judged deficient unless during the most recent 5-year period at least 50% of its graduates pass the qualifying and certifying examinations on the first try.

VIII. Special Information

In addition to these requirements specific to pediatric surgery, the Program Requirements for Residency Education in the Subspecialties of General Surgery also apply to all pediatric surgery programs.

All questions concerning the examination for Certification of Special Qualifications in Pediatric Surgery should be addressed to the Secretary, American Board of Surgery, Inc.

ACGME: June 1993 Effective: July 1995

Program Requirements for Residency Education in General Vascular Surgery (Surgery-General)

I. General Characteristics of Approved Programs

Graduate training programs in general vascular surgery should be designed to provide the educational resources appropriate for the development of proficiency in the diagnosis and treatment of diseases of the arterial, venous, and lymphatic circulatory systems, exclusive of those components intrinsic to the heart, thoracic aorta, and intracranial vessels. The foregoing definition describes what is hereinafter referred to as the vascular system. The training objectives are most appropriately achieved through a structured program that is properly supervised and accredited.

II. Types of Programs

A. Appropriate education and training in general vascular surgery may be attained through two types of programs. Provision should be made, however, to ensure that in either type of program the general surgery residents' experience in vascular surgery, which is one of the principal components of general surgery, is not adversely affected, in terms of either operative experience or patient responsibility. The two types of programs are:
   1. A general vascular surgery residency that follows the completion of an accredited residency program in general surgery and/or thoracic surgery.
   2. A general vascular surgery residency that is a component of an accredited cardiothoracic surgery program, in which patient material is adequate to fulfill the requirements of both areas of training. This specialized training in general vascular surgery is in addition to the requirement of 7 years for completion of the programs in general surgery and thoracic surgery.

B. An application for a general vascular surgery residency will not be accepted if the core program in either general surgery or thoracic surgery is not provisionally or fully approved. There should be only one general vascular surgery program per sponsoring institution.

III. Duration and Scope of Training

A. The general vascular surgery program must be of sufficient duration to allow the resident to acquire an advanced level of skill in the diagnosis and treatment of vascular diseases. The program shall not be less than 12 months in duration and shall be exclusively devoted to general vascular surgery. It shall be in addition to the training required for certification in either general surgery or thoracic surgery. Any program that extends clinical training beyond these minimum requirements must present a clear educational rationale consonant with the program requirements and objectives for residency training. The program director must obtain approval of the Residency Review Committee prior to implementation and at each subsequent review of the program. Prior to entry into the program, each resident must be notified in writing of the required length of training.

B. The program must provide instruction and require the resident to become knowledgeable in the fundamental sciences, including anatomy, embryology, physiology, and pathology, as they relate to the diagnosis and treatment of vascular lesions.

C. Familiarity with special diagnostic techniques is of great importance in the management of vascular lesions. It is essential that the resident have an acquaintance with the methods and techniques of angiography and competence in the interpretation of angiographic findings. The resident should have experience in the application, interpretation, and limitations of noninvasive vascular diagnostic techniques.

D. The resident must be provided with progressive senior surgical responsibilities in the four phases of total patient care, consisting of patient evaluation, therapeutic decisions, operative experience, and postoperative management. The focus of the program is clinical education; research, laboratory, and nonvascular clinical assignments should be related to this focus.

IV. Organization and Staff

A. To provide an effective training program, a general vascular surgery service must be organized as an identifiable unit, even though it is within the framework of a larger administrative entity such as a department of surgery or general surgery or thoracic surgery. It is highly desirable that all patients with vascular disease who are available for teaching purposes be admitted to this unit so that the patients may be centralized and utilized most efficiently for teaching.

The general vascular surgery program must be under the direction of a vascular or cardiovascular surgeon certified by the American Board of Surgery and/or Thoracic Surgery, or possessing equivalent qualifications, and dedicated to the teaching of general vascular surgery. The director of the general vascular surgery program must have continuous responsibility and authority for administrative and teaching policies of the service.

B. Privileges on the general vascular surgery teaching service should be granted to surgeons only with the understanding that their patients are to be available for coordinated graduate education of residents. All members of the staff of the general vascular surgery unit must be highly qualified in general vascular surgery, dedicated to teaching, and must devote the necessary time and effort to the educational program. They should also engage in scholarly activities.

V. Patient Population

The institution, department, or service accredited to conduct a program of graduate education in general vascular surgery must be able to provide a sufficient number and variety of vascular surgery patients to ensure that residents have an adequate exposure to a wide spectrum of lesions of the vascular system so that they may acquire a high level of skill in their diagnosis and management. There must be a scheduled conference, at least twice monthly, to review current morbidity and mortality.

VI. Operative Experience

The resident must be afforded the opportunity to have chief or senior resident responsibility in the operative management of a wide range of patients who require the commonly employed reconstructive and nonreconstructive vascular procedures within the scope of general vascular surgery. Chief or senior resident operative experience is defined as activity in the course of which the resident functions as the operating surgeon or performs the critical technical portions of the operation. The resident should perform a minimum of 70 major vascular reconstructive procedures that reflect an adequate representation of current trends in the spectrum of surgical care of vascular diseases.

It is the responsibility of the program directors in both general surgery and general vascular surgery to ensure that the allocation of patients to the vascular surgery resident(s) does not have substantial negative impact on the training of the general surgery residents.

VII. Other Requirements

In addition to these requirements specific to vascular surgery, the Program Requirements for Residency Education in the Subspecialties of General Surgery also apply to all vascular surgery programs.

ACGME: September 1991 Effective: July 1995

Program Requirements for Residency Education in Thoracic Surgery

I. Introduction

A. Definition of Thoracic Surgery

Thoracic surgery encompasses the operative and perioperative care as well as critical care of patients with pathologic conditions within the chest. Included is the surgical care of coronary artery disease; cancers of the lung, esophagus, and chest wall; abnormalities of the great vessels and heart valves; congenital anomalies of the chest and heart; tumors of the mediastinum; and diseases of the diaphragm. The management of the airway and injuries of the chest is within the scope of the specialty.

B. Program Goals and Design

1. The director and teaching staff of a program must prepare and comply with written educational goals for the program. All educational components of a residency program should be related to these goals.
2. The program design and/or structure must be approved by the Residency Review Committee (RRC) as part of the regular review process.

C. Objective of Thoracic Surgery Training

The objective of a residency training program in thoracic surgery is to provide the trainee with factual knowledge and technical skills in the preoperative evaluation, operative management, and postoperative care of patients with pathologic conditions involving thoracic structures to prepare the trainee to function as a qualified practitioner of thoracic and cardiovascular surgery at the high level of performance expected of a certified specialist.

D. Compliance With the Institutional and Program Requirements

For a residency program in thoracic surgery to be accredited, compliance is required with both the Institutional Requirements and the Program Requirements, as stated in the *Essentials of Accredited Residencies*.

II. General Characteristics of Accredited Programs

A. Core Knowledge and Skills

A thoracic surgery residency is a graduate education program designed to give the resident a broad clinical experience in pulmonary, esophageal, mediastinal, chest wall, diaphragmatic, and cardiovascular disorders in all age groups. On completion of the program, the residents are expected to be clinically proficient in these areas as well as knowledgeable in the use of cardiac and respiratory support devices.

B. Additional Required Skills

Although operative experience constitutes the most important aspect of the program, the training should include the opportunity to correlate the pathologic and diagnostic aspects of cardiothoracic disorders. The resident is required to be skilled in important diagnostic procedures such as bronchoscopy and esophagoscopy and to be able to interpret all appropriate imaging studies (ultrasound, computed tomography, roentgenographic, radionuclide), cardiac catheterization, pulmonary function, and esophageal function studies. The resident must have the opportunity under supervision to:

1. Provide preoperative management, including the selection and timing of operative intervention and the selection of appropriate operative procedures.
2. Provide and be responsible for the postoperative management of thoracic and cardiovascular patients.
3. Provide and be responsible for the critical care of patients with thoracic and cardiovascular surgical disorders, including trauma patients, whether or not operative intervention is required.

C. Duration and Scope of Training

1. Duration of Training
   a. Two years of clinical experience on clearly defined thoracic surgical services is the minimum amount of time required in thoracic surgery for the acquisition of the necessary knowledge, judgment, and technical skills. Laboratory investigation is not permitted as a portion of this minimum time. An interruption of the required years of clinical experience should not exceed 2 years.
   b. Any program that extends training beyond these minimum requirements must present a clear educational rationale consonant with the program requirements and objectives for residency training. The program director must obtain approval of the RRC prior to implementation and at each subsequent review of the program. Prior to entry into the program, each resident must be notified in writing of the required length of training.
   c. Specific rotations in nonsurgical areas such as cardiac catheterization and/or esophageal or pulmonary function may not exceed a total of 3 months during the clinical program and may not occur in the final year.
2. Scope of Training
   a. The resident must complete a general surgery residency program accredited by either the Accreditation Council for Graduate Medical Education (ACGME) or the Royal College of Physicians and Surgeons of Canada before beginning training in thoracic surgery.
   b. Residents must be provided with progressively increasing responsibility. The final year of thoracic surgical training must be served in the integrated institutions of the program, except with prior approval of the RRC. During the final year the resident must assume senior responsibility for the preoperative, intraoperative, and postoperative care of patients with thoracic and cardiovascular disease.
   c. The RRC recognizes the importance of interaction among trainees themselves, as well as between teaching staff and trainees in the conduct of conferences and patient care. A number of residents is essential to provide an opportunity for meaningful interaction throughout the training period. Each program must be structured to have a minimum of two thoracic surgery residents in training.

III. Institutional Responsibilities

A. Institutional Commitment

1. Sponsoring Institution
   An educational program in thoracic surgery must have one sponsoring institution with primary responsibility for the entire program. The sponsoring institution must provide evidence of commitment to graduate medical education, including thoracic surgery, and must assume responsibility for the educational validity of all components of the program.
2. Participating Institutions
   When there is a cooperative residency program involving multiple institutions, the commitment of each institution to the program must be made explicit and should be embodied in current letters/contracts of affiliation or integration.

a. Affiliated Institutions
The formal written agreement must cover:
1. The scope of the affiliation
2. The resources and facilities in all participating institutions that will be available to the residents
3. The duties and responsibilities the resident will have in the participating institutions
4. The relationship that will exist between the thoracic surgery residents and the residents and faculty in other programs in the participating institutions
5. The supervision the residents will receive by faculty in each institution

b. Integrated Institutions
The formal written agreement must specify, in addition to the points under III.A.2.a, that the program director of the parent institution:
1. Appoints the members of the teaching staff at the integrated institution
2. Appoints the chief or director of the teaching service in the integrated institution
3. Appoints all residents in the program
4. Determines all rotations and assignments of both residents and members of the teaching staff

Participating institutions and their teaching staffs must ensure that all educational experiences and resources offered are consistent with the goals of the program and meet the standards set forth herein. When several institutions participate in sponsoring a program, the program director has the primary responsibility for developing mechanisms to coordinate the overall educational mission to facilitate the accomplishment of the program's goals and be in substantial compliance with the requirements. A program in which any participating institution does not allow appropriate supervision or coordination of educational experiences is not acceptable.

B. Institutional Resources and Facilities

1. Institutional Resources
Institutions must assume responsibility for ensuring an administrative and academic structure that provides for management of educational and financial resources dedicated to the needs of the program, such as appointment of teaching faculty and residents, and for adequate program planning and evaluation.
2. Facilities
Facilities must be appropriate and sufficient for the effective accomplishment of the educational mission of each program. In every institution used as a training site for thoracic surgery, there must be adequate space for patient care, program support, and research; trained medical and paramedical personnel; laboratory and imaging support; and medical library resources.
3. Supporting Disciplines
a. Recognizing the nature of the specialty of thoracic surgery, it is important that thoracic surgery residents have the opportunity to interact with residents in other related specialties in all of the participating institutions.
b. To ensure a cohesive educational environment, the program director must cooperate with the leadership of related disciplines and actively foster the training of thoracic surgery residents in those disciplines. Program directors, teaching staff, and residents in thoracic surgery must work together to provide an operating system whereby the goals and requirements of the training programs can be met.

IV. Teaching and Resident Staff

The program director and the teaching staff are responsible for the general administration of a program, including those activities related to the recruitment, selection, instruction, supervision, counseling, evaluation, and advancement of residents and the maintenance of records related to program accreditation.

A. Program Director

There must be a single program director responsible for the program.
1. Qualifications of the Program Director
a. Requisite and documented clinical, educational, and administrative abilities and experience.
b. Licensure to practice medicine in the state where the institution that sponsors the program is located. (Certain federal programs are exempted.)
c. Certification by the American Board of Thoracic Surgery (ABTS) or suitable equivalent qualifications, as determined by the RRC.
d. Appointment in good standing to the medical staff of an institution participating in the program.
2. Responsibilities of the Program Director
The program director must have appropriate authority and adequate stability as well as give sufficient time to organize and to fulfill administrative and teaching responsibilities. A stable educational environment cannot be maintained without continuity in program leadership.
The responsibilities include:
a. Preparation of a written statement outlining the educational goals of the program with respect to knowledge, skills, and other attributes of residents at each level of training and for each major rotation or other program assignment. This statement must be distributed to residents and members of the teaching staff. It should be readily available for review.
b. Selection of residents for appointment to the program in accordance with institutional and departmental policies and procedures. In selecting from among qualified applicants for first-year thoracic surgery resident positions, the thoracic surgery program should participate in the Thoracic Surgery Matching Program.
c. Selection and supervision of the teaching staff and other program personnel at each institution participating in the program. Opportunities for development of the teaching staff should be made available to each member of the staff and should include development of skills in teaching, research, and scientific writing.
d. The supervision of residents through explicit written descriptions of supervisory lines of responsibility for the care of patients. Such guidelines must be communicated to all members of the program staff. Residents must be provided with prompt, reliable systems for communication and interaction with supervisory physicians.
e. Implementation of fair procedures, as established by the sponsoring institution, regarding academic discipline and resident complaints or grievances.
f. Monitoring resident stress, including mental or emotional conditions inhibiting performance or learning and drug- or alcohol-related dysfunction. Program directors and teaching staff should be sensitive to the need for timely provision of confidential counseling and psychological support services to residents. Training situations that consistently produce undesirable stress on residents must be evaluated and modified.
g. Ensuring assignment of reasonable in-hospital duty hours so that residents are not required regularly to perform excessively prolonged periods of duty. It is desirable that residents' work schedules be designed so that on average, excluding exceptional patient care needs, residents have at least 1 day out of 7 free of routine responsibilities and be on call in the hospi-

Program Requirements

tal no more often than every third night. Since training in thoracic surgery is at senior levels, the ratio of hours worked and on-call time varies considerably and necessitates flexibility.

h. Notification of the executive secretary of the RRC in writing of any program change that may significantly alter the educational experience for the residents. This will include a change in
   1. program director and/or department chairman and/or
   2. formal affiliation with another institution.
i. Requesting prior approval from the RRC for the following changes so that the committee may determine that there is adequate educational justification and that an adequate educational environment exists to support these changes:
   1. Formal integration with another institution
   2. A required rotation to any institution other than those already participating in the program in which the duration is 4 months or longer or a foreign rotation of any duration
   3. The number of resident positions offered
   4. The number of years of training required in the program
j. It is essential that the program director provide complete and accurate program information forms to the RRC so that an adequate assessment of the program can be made. A comprehensive and accurate evaluation of the program is not possible without the detailed information requested. The program director is also responsible for the accuracy of the residents' records of their surgical experience and for making these records available to the RRC on request. Program directors should pay particular attention to consistency in the reporting of "Operative Experience Reports" for the institutions, the residents, and any other fellows/special trainees appointed to the program. In the evaluation of the program, it is essential that the statistics in all reports cover the same period of time for comparison purposes, ie, the institution's report must be consistent with the residents' reports and those of fellows/special trainees. Failure to furnish the required information in the program information forms may jeopardize the accreditation of the program.

B. Teaching Staff

1. There must be a sufficient number of teaching staff with documented qualifications to instruct and supervise adequately all the residents in the program. Physicians with teaching responsibilities should be board-certified in thoracic surgery or possess suitable equivalent qualifications, as determined by the RRC. Members of the teaching staff must be able to devote sufficient time to meet their supervisory and teaching responsibilities.
2. All members of the teaching staff must demonstrate a strong interest in the education of residents, sound clinical and teaching abilities, support of the goals and objectives of the program, a commitment to their own continuing medical education, and participation in scholarly activities.
3. There should be at least one designated cardiothoracic faculty member responsible for coordinating multidisciplinary clinical conferences and organizing instruction and research in general thoracic surgery.
4. A member of the teaching staff of each participating institution must be designated to assume responsibility for the day-to-day activities of the program at that institution, with overall coordination by the program director.
5. The teaching staff must be organized and have regular documented meetings to review program goals and objectives as well as program effectiveness in achieving them. At least one resident representative should participate in these reviews.
6. The teaching staff should periodically evaluate the utilization of the resources available to the program, the contribution of each institution participating in the program, the financial and administrative support of the program, the volume and variety of patients available to the program for educational purposes, the performance of members of the teaching staff, and the quality of supervision of residents.

C. Other Program Personnel

Programs must be provided with the additional professional, technical, and clerical personnel needed to support the administration and educational conduct of the program.

D. Scholarly Environment

Graduate medical education must take place in an environment of inquiry and scholarship in which residents participate in the development of new knowledge, learn to evaluate research findings, and develop habits of inquiry as a continuing professional responsibility. Adequate documentation of scholarly activity on the part of the program director and the teaching staff at the sponsoring and integrated institutions must be submitted at the time of the program review. Documentation of scholarly activity is based on:

1. Participation in continuing surgical education;
2. Participation in regional or national surgical scientific societies;
3. Presentation and publication of scientific studies;
4. Demonstration of an active interest in research as it pertains to their own special surgical interests. The RRC will consider documented involvement in the following as indications of the commitment of the staff to research:
   a. Projects that are funded following peer review
   b. Publication in peer-reviewed journals
   c. Presentations at national and regional scientific meetings
   d. Research protocols that have been approved by appropriate institutional committees or other organizations

E. Residents

1. Resident Selection
   Residents who are eligible to enter graduate medical education programs accredited by the ACGME must meet the qualifications stipulated in the institutional requirements.
2. Resident Responsibilities
   The hallmark of surgical care has long been the commitment of surgeons to be available for their patients throughout the surgical experience. In residency training a commitment to continuity of care involves the development of a keen sense of personal responsibility for patient care that is not automatically discharged at any given hour. Duty hours and night and weekend call for residents must reflect this concept of longitudinal responsibility for patients by providing for adequate continuity of patient care. At the same time, duty assignments must not regularly be of such excessive length and frequency that they cause undue fatigue and sleep deprivation.

V. Educational Program

A. Surgical Volume

1. Minimum Standards
   Guidelines for the minimum operative experience of each resident are as follows:
   a. An annual average of 125 major operations from those listed on the program information forms.
   b. An adequate distribution of categories and complexity of procedures such that each resident is ensured a balanced and equivalent operative experience.
   c. The categories of procedures must include but are not limited to the following: lungs, pleura, chest wall, esophagus, mediastinum, diaphragm, thoracic aorta and great vessels, congenital heart anomalies, valvular heart diseases, and myocardial

revascularization. Residents should also have experience in cardiac pacemaker implantation, mediastinoscopy, pleuroscopy, and flexible and rigid esophagoscopy and bronchoscopy.

2. Resident Credit for Operative Experience
Operative experience should meet the following criteria:
   a. The resident participated in the diagnosis, preoperative planning, and selection of the operation for the patient.
   b. The resident performed those technical manipulations that constituted the essential parts of the patient's operation.
   c. The resident was substantially involved in postoperative care.
   d. The resident was supervised by responsible teaching staff.

B. Supervision

Programs in thoracic surgery require that residents be directly involved in providing care under supervision in all institutions that accept responsibility for the quality of the educational program. There must be procedures established by the program director that ensure that all residents are supervised during their operative and clinical training.

Program directors and residents should note that the ABTS may have its own specific guidelines for adequate operative experience.

C. Rotations

1. Rotation Plan
The program director is responsible for providing an organized written plan and a block diagram for the rotations of residents among the various services and institutions in the program so that continuity in the care of patients can be achieved. The residents' rotations should be carefully structured so that graded levels of responsibilities can be maintained, all residents receive a balanced training and experience in the program, and the requirements stipulated under Section II.C.2, "Scope of Training, can be met.
2. Rotation Objectives
The objectives of each rotation should be well defined in the curriculum. A number of abbreviated rotations among several participating institutions to meet minimum requirements is discouraged. Simultaneous assignment to more than one institution must be avoided.

D. Number of Residents and Other Trainees

1. Evaluation of Resident Complement
As part of its review process, the RRC evaluates the number of residents participating in each program. The program director must ensure that there are adequate facilities, qualified teaching staff, and an adequate clinical volume and distribution of surgical cases for the number of residents participating in a given program.
2. Appointment of Other Trainees
The appointment of other trainees to the program and their operative experience must be reported to the RRC so that the committee can determine whether the educational experience of the residents already in training is compromised. Dilution of the residents' experience by other appointees may be deemed substantial noncompliance with this requirement.

E. Conferences

The program director is responsible for providing separate and regularly scheduled teaching conferences, mortality and morbidity conferences, rounds, and other educational activities in which both the thoracic surgery teaching staff and the residents attend and participate. Such experiences should be under the direction of qualified thoracic surgeons and other teaching staff in related disciplines. Records of attendance must be kept and be available for review by the site visitor.

F. Patient Care Responsibilities

The educational mission of each program must not be compromised by an excessive reliance on residents to fulfill institutional service obligations. In addition, excellence in patient care must not be compromised or jeopardized by needs of the educational program.

G. Outpatient Responsibilities

Outpatient activities constitute an essential component for providing adequate experience in continuity of patient care. These activities should be conducted in such a way that the resident has an opportunity to examine the patient preoperatively, has ample opportunity to consult with the attending surgeon regarding operative care, and has an opportunity to participate in the operation and in the postoperative care. To participate in posthospital care, the resident has the responsibility for seeing the patient personally in an outpatient setting and/or, as a minimum in some cases, consulting with the attending surgeon regarding the follow-up care rendered to the patient in the doctor's office.

The policies and procedures governing prehospital and posthospital involvement of the residents must be documented. Evidence of the elements of this process, in the form of notes on the patient's chart as well as other records, must be available to the site visitor at the time of program review.

H. Library

1. Residents must have ready access to a major medical library, either at the institution where the residents are located or through arrangement with convenient nearby institutions.
2. Library services should include the electronic retrieval of information from medical databases.
3. There must be access to an on-site library or to a collection of appropriate texts and journals in each institution participating in a residency program. On-site libraries and/or collections of texts and journals must be readily available during nights and weekends.

I. Autopsies

Permission for performing an autopsy should be sought in all deaths. Autopsy material must be appropriately reviewed by teaching staff and residents.

VI. Evaluation

A. The educational effectiveness of a program must be evaluated in a systematic manner. In particular, the quality of the curriculum and the extent to which the educational goals have been met by residents must be assessed. Written evaluations by residents of the teaching staff and the program should be utilized in this process.

B. Regular evaluation of residents' knowledge, skills, and overall performance, including the development of professional attitudes consistent with being a thoracic surgeon, should be documented.

The program director, with participation of members of the teaching staff, shall:

1. At least semiannually evaluate the knowledge, skills, and professional growth of the residents, using appropriate criteria and procedures.
2. Communicate each evaluation to the resident in a timely manner.
3. Advance residents to positions of higher responsibility only on the basis of evidence of their satisfactory progressive scholarship and professional growth.
4. Maintain a permanent record of evaluation for each resident and have it accessible to the resident and other authorized personnel.

C. A written final evaluation for each resident who completes the program must be provided. The evaluation must include a review of the resident's performance during the final period of training and should verify that the resident has demonstrated sufficient professional ability to practice competently and independently. This final evaluation should be part of the resident's permanent record maintained by the institution.

D. One measure of the quality of a program may be the percentage of program graduates who take the certification examination of the ABTS and their performance on that examination.

Application forms may be obtained by writing to Executive Secretary, Residency Review Committee for Thoracic Surgery, 515 N State St/Ste 2000, Chicago, IL 60610.

ACGME: September 1992 Effective: July 1995

Program Requirements for Residency Education in Urology

I. Introduction

A. Definition of the Specialty

Urology is the medical and surgical specialty involving disorders of the genitourinary tract, including the adrenal gland. Specialists in this discipline must demonstrate knowledge, skill, and understanding of the basic medical sciences relevant to the genitourinary tract and adrenal gland. Residency education in this specialty is designed to educate physicians in the clinical aspects of diagnosis, medical and surgical therapy, and the prevention and reconstruction of urologic diseases, neoplasms, deformities, disorders, and injuries.

B. Scope of Education

1. Five years of postgraduate education are required. Twelve months must be spent in general surgery in an Accreditation Council for Graduate Medical Education (ACGME)-accredited program, and 36 months must be spent in clinical urology. Six months of the remaining 12 months must be spent in general surgery, urology, or in other clinical disciplines relevant to urology. The following educational formats are possible:
   a. Two years of surgery and 3 years of clinical urology
   b. Two years of surgery, 6 months of research, and 3½ years of clinical urology
   c. One year of surgery and 4 years of clinical urology.

   The final 12 months of the urology educational program must be spent as a chief resident with appropriate clinical responsibility under supervision in institutions that are an approved part of the program.
2. Any program that extends the urology educational program beyond 3 years must present a clear educational rationale consonant with the Program Requirements and objectives for residency education.

   The program director must obtain approval of the Residency Review Committee (RRC) prior to implementation and at each subsequent review of the program.
3. Accreditation by the ACGME is required for all years of the educational program. To be considered a graduate of the program, residents must complete the full length of the educational program for which the specific program is accredited.
4. Prior to admission, the program must notify each resident in writing of the required length of the educational program. The required length of the educational program for a particular resident may not be changed without mutual agreement with the resident during his or her program unless there is a significant break in his or her educational program or the resident requires remedial education. All changes to the length of the educational program for any resident must have prior approval of the RRC.

II. Institutional Organization

Institutions involved in the education of urology residents must provide opportunities for resident education, including scholarly activities and relevant clinical experience, across the full range of urologic disease in both children and adults.

A. Sponsoring Institution

The educational program must have a single sponsoring institution that has primary responsibility for the entire program. The institution must demonstrate commitment to the program in terms of financial and academic support.

B. Participating Institutions

1. There must be an appropriately executed interinstitutional agreement that conforms to the Institutional Requirements for the sponsoring institution and each participating institution.
2. The number of participating institutions must not preclude satisfactory participation by residents in educational activities. The committee considers four participating institutions as optimal to promote educational and peer activities.
3. Assignments to participating institutions must be based on an appropriate educational rationale. Assignments that dilute the education of residents or that do not provide proper supervision and coordination of educational activities must not be established or maintained.
4. Assignments to institutions distant from the sponsoring institution are not desirable. To be justifiable, they must offer special resources or opportunities otherwise not available to the program.
5. A single resident should not be assigned to a participating institution unless special resources or opportunities are offered at that institution that are not available otherwise in the educational program. Residents must be included in program educational activities during the assignment.
6. The primary teaching faculty must have major clinical responsibilities in their respective institutions. Residents must have rapid access at all times to the faculty responsible for patients in the institution where the resident is assigned.

C. Appointment of Residents

1. The total number of residents and the number of residents per year must be approved in advance by the RRC. The number of residents will be based primarily on the number, qualifications, and commitment of the faculty; the volume and variety of the patient population available for educational purposes; and the institutional resources committed to resident education.
2. Programs may not graduate more residents in any given year than the number of residents approved by the RRC. Any change in the number of residents by year or any change in the total number of residents must receive prior approval of the RRC. Requests for changes in the resident complement of a program must include a strong educational rationale.
3. A vacancy in a resident complement, if filled, must be at the same level in which the vacancy occurs, unless otherwise approved by the RRC.

III. Faculty Qualifications and Responsibilities

The program director and the faculty are responsible for the general administration of a program, including those activities related to the recruitment, selection, instruction, supervision, counseling, evaluation, and advancement of residents and the maintenance of records related to program accreditation.

A. Program Director

There must be a single program director responsible for the program.

1. Qualifications of the program director
   a. Requisite and documented clinical, educational, and administrative abilities and experience
   b. Licensure to practice medicine in the state where the institution that sponsors the program is located (Certain federal programs are exempted)
   c. Certification by the American Board of Urology or suitable equivalent qualifications
   d. Appointment in good standing to the medical staff of an institution participating in the program
   e. Based geographic full-time at the sponsoring institution unless otherwise approved by the RRC
2. Responsibilities of the program director
   a. Devoting sufficient time and effort to the program to provide day-to-day continuity of leadership and to fulfill all of the responsibilities inherent in meeting the educational goals of the program.
   b. Developing a sound organizational framework and an effective teaching staff as essential elements of an approved residency program. Continuity of leadership is important to the stability of a residency program. Frequent changes in leadership or long periods of temporary leadership will be cause for serious concern.
   c. Engaging in scholarly activities such as active involvement in continuing medical education in urology; active participation in regional or national scientific societies, presentations, and publications; and active interest in research.
   d. Ensuring that residents have access to a balanced and comprehensive surgical experience and that the progress of each resident is regularly evaluated.
   e. Preparing a written statement outlining the educational goals of the program with respect to knowledge, skills, and other attributes of residents at each level of education and for each major rotation or other program assignment. This statement must be distributed to residents and members of the faculty. It should be readily available for review.
   f. Maintaining an annual log, in the form and format provided by the RRC, of procedures performed by the urology service within each participating institution to which residents rotate for clinical experience.
   g. Compiling annually an accurate statistical and narrative description of the program as requested by the RRC. This log must include a comprehensive record of the number and types of operative procedures performed by each resident completing the program and all of the procedures in which the resident was either surgeon or assistant surgeon, and it must be signed by both the resident and the program director as a statement of its accuracy. The log must include ambulatory or outpatient procedures performed by the resident in office practice or ambulatory facilities. This information must be provided in the format and form specified by the RRC.
   h. Supervising residents through explicit written descriptions of supervisory lines of responsibility for the care of patients. Such guidelines must be communicated to all members of the program staff. Residents must be provided with prompt, reliable systems for communication and interaction with supervisory physicians.
   i. Evaluating regularly residents' knowledge, skills, and overall performance, including the development of professional attitudes consistent with being a physician.
   j. Implementing fair procedures, as established by the sponsoring institution, regarding academic discipline and resident complaints or grievances.
   k. Monitoring resident stress, including mental or emotional conditions inhibiting performance or learning and drug- or alcohol-related dysfunction. Program directors and the faculty should be sensitive to the need for timely provision of confidential counseling and psychological support services to residents. Educational situations that consistently produce undesirable stress on residents must be evaluated and modified.
   l. Having appropriate authority to oversee and to organize the activities of the educational program. The responsibilities of this position should include but not be limited to

1. resident selection, appointment, and assignment in accordance with institutional and departmental policies and procedures;
2. supervision, direction, and administration of the educational activities at all participating institutions;
3. evaluation of the faculty, other staff, and the residency program;
4. appointment of local training directors and other personnel in participating institutions.

m. Notifying the RRC Executive Director in writing of any major change in the program that may significantly alter the educational experience or environment for the residents, including
1. changes in department leadership such as the appointment of the program director and/or department chair;
2. changes in administrative structure, such as an alteration in the hierarchical status of the program/department within the institution.

n. Obtaining prior approval of the RRC for the following changes in the program to determine if an adequate educational environment exists to support these changes:
1. The addition or deletion of any participating institution to which residents rotate
2. Any change in the approved resident complement of the program
3. Any change in the length or format of the educational program

On review of a proposal for a major change in a program, the RRC may determine that a site visit is necessary.

B. Faculty Qualifications

1. Besides the program director, there must be a minimum of two clinical urology faculty committed fully to the educational objectives of the residency program who devote sufficient time to the supervision and teaching of the residents. A faculty-to-resident ratio of at least 1:2 in the total program is required. The program director may be counted as one of the faculty in determining the ratio. The program director must notify the RRC if the number of clinical urology faculty members drops below 2, or if the ratio falls below 1:2 and remains below that level longer than 1 year.
2. Urologists with teaching responsibilities must be certified or in the process of certification by the American Board of Urology or have equivalent qualifications.
3. All members of the faculty must demonstrate a strong interest in the education of residents and sound clinical and teaching abilities, support the goals and objectives of the educational program, have a commitment to their own continuing medical education, and participate in scholarly activities. Members of the faculty must devote sufficient time to meet their supervisory and teaching responsibilities.
4. One measure of adequate faculty commitment to the residency program is the extent to which faculty members permit residents to participate in all aspects of the management of patients under the faculty members' care.
5. Faculty involved in teaching should have clearly defined responsibilities including but not limited to supervision of residents, teaching, administration, and/or research. The amount of time dedicated to the educational program should be specified.
6. The faculty must be organized and have regular documented meetings at least annually to review program goals and objectives and program effectiveness in achieving them. At least one resident representative should participate in these reviews.
7. The faculty should evaluate at least annually the availability of resources for the program, the contribution of each institution participating in the program, the financial and administrative support of the program, the volume and variety of patients available to the program for educational purposes, the performance of members of the faculty, and the quality of supervision of residents.
8. To provide the greatest depth of knowledge in a variety of subjects, it is highly desirable that the faculty possess special knowledge in several different urological domains such as pediatric urology; female urology; renal transplantation; renal vascular disease; oncology; infertility, impotence, and endocrinology; stone disease; and urodynamics.

C. Other Program Personnel

Programs must be provided with the additional professional, technical, and clerical personnel needed to support the administration and educational conduct of the program.

D. Directors at Participating Institutions

1. There must be a qualified urologist appointed by and responsible to the program director in each geographically separate institution. This urologist must be responsible for the education of the residents and must supervise the educational activities of the urology faculty in that institution.
2. These appointments should be for a 1-year period and should be renewable to ensure continuity of leadership.
3. The urology director at each participating institution must have the majority of his or her clinical responsibilities based at that institution.

IV. Facilities and Resources

There must be adequate space and equipment for the educational program, including meeting rooms; classrooms with audiovisual and other educational aids; office space for staff; pertinent library materials; and diagnostic, therapeutic, and research facilities.

A. Within each institution, bed space sufficient for the needs of the urology service must be provided.

B. Technologically current diagnostic and treatment facilities providing cystoscopy, imaging with biopsy, imaging with percutaneous access to the kidney, ultrasound with biopsy, endourology, laser, and urodynamics equipment must be present. The use of video imaging for educational purposes is desirable.

C. An extracorporeal shock wave lithotripsy facility must be available for resident education in the treatment of urinary calculi.

D. Residents must have access to outpatient facilities, clinic, and office space for preoperative evaluation and postoperative follow-up for cases for which the resident has responsibility.

E. A medical records department that facilitates both quality patient care and education must be available. Clinical records must be maintained to ensure easy and prompt access at all times.

F. Residents must be provided with adequate office, sleeping, lounge, and food facilities during assigned duty hours. Adequate clerical support services also must be provided.

G. Institutions should provide adequate resources for research, such as statistical consultation and computer services. Research laboratories, while not mandatory for accreditation, should be available.

H. There must be access to an on-site library or to a collection of appropriate texts and journals in each institution that participates in a residency program. On-site libraries and/or collections of texts and journals must be readily available during nights and weekends. Library services should include the electronic retrieval of information from medical databases.

V. The Educational Program

A. Program design

1. The program director and faculty must prepare and implement written educational goals for the program.

2. The program design and/or structure must be approved by the RRC as a part of the regular review process.

B. Conferences

1. A comprehensive, organized course of study must be developed to include educational conferences that are well-defined, documented, and regularly scheduled. The conferences must include a combined morbidity and mortality conference for all participating hospitals, urological imaging, urological pathology, journal review, and other subjects having educational value in the basic and clinical domains of urology. The domains of urology are andrology, infertility, impotence, sexuality; calculus disease, endourology, extracorporeal shock wave lithotripsy; female urology; infectious disease; neurourology; obstructive disease; oncology; pediatric urology; psychological disorders; renovascular disease; surgery of the adrenal; renal transplantation; trauma; and urodynamics.
2. A list of the conferences must be maintained and available for review at the time of the site visit. The list should include the names of those attending, the subjects discussed, and the principal speaker.
3. Conferences should be well attended by both residents and faculty, and such attendance must be documented.
4. A faculty member should supervise each conference to ensure that a worthwhile educational experience is provided.

C. Clinical Component

1. A sufficient number and variety of adult and pediatric patients with urologic disease must be available for resident education. Resident experience with medical and surgical patients must extend beyond common urological problems to include all of the urology domains and areas pertinent to urology as a medical discipline.
2. Generally equivalent and adequate distribution of operative procedures among the residents must be demonstrated. Significantly unequal experience in volume and/or complexity of operative procedures among the residents demonstrates noncompliance with these requirements.
3. All patients on the urology service must be reviewed by the faculty on regular teaching rounds with the residents according to a predetermined schedule.

D. Graded Responsibility

1. The program must provide the residents with experience in direct and progressively responsible patient management as they advance through the program. The educational program must culminate in sufficiently independent responsibility for clinical decision making to ensure that the graduating resident has developed sound clinical judgment and possesses the ability to carry out appropriate management plans.
2. The level of resident responsibility should be increased progressively with each year of education. This includes responsibility in such areas as patient care, leadership, teaching, organization, and administration. Appropriately qualified senior residents may supervise or act as consultants to junior residents.
3. The resident should have responsibility under supervision for the total care of the patient, including initial evaluation, establishment of diagnosis, selection of appropriate therapy, implementation of therapy, and management of complications. The resident must participate in the continuity of patient care through preoperative and postoperative clinics and inpatient contact.
4. When residents participate in preoperative and postoperative care in a clinic or private office setting, the program director must ensure that the resident functions with an appropriate degree of responsibility under adequate supervision.

E. Supervision

1. The program director must ensure, direct, and document proper supervision of residents at all times. A supervising urologist must be responsible for each patient. The supervising urologist should see the patient, discuss the case with the resident, and write or countersign notes.
2. Residents must be provided with rapid, reliable systems for communicating with supervising residents and faculty. Supervising physicians or supervising residents with appropriate experience for the severity and complexity of the patient's condition must be available at all times on site. The responsibility or independence given to residents in patient care should depend on each resident's knowledge, manual skill, experience, the complexity of the patient's illness, and the risk of the operation.

F. Duty Hours

1. Physicians must have a keen sense of personal responsibility for continuing patient care and must recognize that their obligation to patients is not automatically discharged at any given hour of the day or any particular day of the week. Duty hours and night and weekend call for residents must reflect the concept of responsibility for patients and provide for adequate patient care. However, residents must not be required regularly to perform excessively difficult or prolonged duties. It is the responsibility of the program director to ensure assignment of reasonable in hospital duty hours.
2. Residents at all levels should, on average, have the opportunity to spend at least 1 full day out of 7 free of scheduled hospital duties and should be on call in the hospital no more often than every third night, except in the maintenance of continuity of care.
3. There should be adequate opportunity to rest and to sleep when on call for 24 hours or more. On-call rooms arranged to permit adequate rest and privacy must be available for each resident on night duty in the hospital.
4. There should be adequate backup support if the volume of patient care required jeopardizes the quality of patient care during or following assigned periods of duty.
5. Residency is a full-time responsibility. Activities outside the educational program must not interfere with the resident's performance in the educational process as defined in the agreement between the institution and the resident.

G. Scholarly activity

The faculty and residents should be involved in activities that keep them abreast of current developments in medicine and that enable them to explore new directions in the science of urology. Because research also offers an important opportunity for the application of the basic sciences to clinical problems, it is an essential part of the preparation of the resident for a lifetime of self-education after the completion of the formal residency program.

1. Faculty scholarly activities

   The responsibility for establishing and maintaining an environment of inquiry and scholarship rests with the faculty. While not all members of the faculty must be investigators, the faculty as a whole must demonstrate broad involvement in scholarly activity. This activity should include

   a. participation of the faculty in clinical discussions, rounds, and conferences in a manner that promotes a spirit of inquiry and scholarship. Scholarship implies an in-depth understanding of basic mechanisms of normal and abnormal states and the application of current knowledge to practice.
   b. participation in journal clubs and research conferences.
   c. participation in regional or national professional and scientific societies, particularly through presentations at the organizations' meetings and publication in their journals.

Program Requirements

   d. participation in research, particularly in projects that are funded following peer review and/or result in publication or presentations at regional and national scientific meetings.
   e. offering guidance and technical support to residents involved in research.
   f. provision of support for resident participation in scholarly activities.
2. Resident scholarly activities
   a. The residents must be provided with research exposure sufficient to result in an understanding of the basic principles of study design, performance, analysis, and reporting, including statistics and epidemiology. The research exposure may be clinical or basic in nature and should reflect careful advice and planning with the faculty.
   b. The residents should be exposed to developments outside their own program by resident attendance at regional or national meetings and other educational conferences or by visits to the program from recognized authorities from other institutions. A listing of these activities should be made available at the time of review.

H. Related Disciplines

Because clinical problems often involve multidisciplinary care, consultative support from other disciplines must be available. The disciplines of internal medicine, surgery, pediatrics, obstetrics and gynecology, pathology, and radiology should be available to facilitate an appropriate educational environment.

I. Appointment of Subspecialty Residents

1. The appointment of subspecialty residents for special education must not dilute or detract from the educational opportunities of regularly appointed urology residents.
2. Any program with subspecialty residents must submit a clear statement of the areas of education, clinical responsibilities, and duration of the educational program. This statement must be supplied to the RRC at the time of the site visit. A log detailing the operative experience of the subspecialty resident must be submitted with the urology residents' logs at the time of the site visit.
3. If subspecialty residents detract from the education of the urology residents, the accreditation status of the program may be affected adversely.

VI. Evaluation

A. Resident Evaluation

1. The program should develop mechanisms for residents to demonstrate the acquisition of fundamental knowledge, attitudes, and skills necessary for current urologic practice. Each program must develop and use specific performance measures such as inservice examinations. At the conclusion of the educational program, residents should be qualified to provide competent care.
2. Written evaluations of resident performance are required at least semiannually and must be reviewed formally and communicated in a timely manner to the resident. Subsequent analysis of these evaluations should guide the program director and faculty in judging the strengths and weaknesses of individual residents.
3. Residents must be advanced to positions of higher responsibility based on evidence of their satisfactory progressive scholarship and professional growth.
4. A permanent record of evaluation for each resident must be maintained and must be accessible to the resident and other authorized personnel.
5. Each resident must be provided with a written final evaluation. This evaluation must include a review of the resident's performance during the final period of education and should verify that the resident has demonstrated the ability to practice competently and independently. This final evaluation should be part of the resident's permanent record maintained by the institution.

B. Faculty Evaluation

The teaching ability, commitment, clinical knowledge, and scholarly activities of faculty require review and confidential evaluation at least annually. A summary of the review must be communicated directly to each faculty member by the program director. Confidential resident evaluation must be a part of this review.

C. Program Evaluation

1. The educational effectiveness of the program must be evaluated in a systematic manner. In particular, the quality of the curriculum and the extent to which educational goals have been met by residents must be assessed. Written confidential evaluations by residents should be utilized in this process.
2. Programs must conduct and document evidence of periodic evaluations of the entire program at all participating institutions, to include
   a. evidence of satisfactory attainment of educational goals,
   b. attention to the needs of the residents, especially regarding the balance between educational and service components of the program,
   c. adequate performance of teaching responsibilities by the faculty,
   d. performance of residents on examinations such as the inservice examination and the American Board of Urology Qualifying (Part I) and Certifying (Part II) Examinations.
3. One measure of the quality of a program is the performance of its graduates on the examinations given by the American Board of Urology. The RRC may consider this information as part of the overall evaluation of the program.

VII. Board Certification

Residents who plan to seek certification by the American Board of Urology should communicate with the executive secretary of the board to be certain of the requirements for acceptance as a candidate for certification.

ACGME: June 1996 Effective: July 1997

Program Requirements for Residency Education in Pediatric Urology (Urology)

I. Scope of Education

A. Subspecialty education in pediatric urology involves all aspects of congenital anomalies, childhood-acquired urologic problems such as tumors and trauma, and overlapping problems of adolescence. The subspecialty education in pediatric urology must provide an experience of sufficient level for the pediatric urology resident to acquire advanced skills in the management of congenital anomalies and pediatric urologic problems.

B. Duration of Education
To be accredited, pediatric urology programs must contain 1 continuous clinical year taken subsequent to the completion of an accredited residency in urology.

II. Institutional Organization

A pediatric urology educational program can be provided only in conjunction with an Accreditation Council for Graduate Medical

Education (ACGME)-accredited urology residency program. The institution sponsoring the pediatric urology program must provide a sufficient volume and variety of pediatric urology experience to meet the needs of the pediatric urology resident without compromising the quality of resident education in general urology. The pediatric urology program must be centered at a children's hospital or a medical center with pediatric medical, surgical, and radiologic subspecialties. The sponsoring institution of the pediatric urology program may seek a complementary affiliation with other institutions that offer significant educational opportunities to the residency program.

III. Faculty Qualifications and Responsibilities

The program director and faculty are responsible for the general administration of the program, including those activities related to the recruitment, selection, instruction, supervision, counseling, evaluation, and advancement of residents and the maintenance of records related to program accreditation.

A. Program Director

There must be a single program director responsible for the program. The program director should be based at the institution where the education occurs and must be dedicated to, and actively engaged in, pediatric urology education.

1. Qualifications of the program director
   a. Requisite and documented clinical, educational, and administrative abilities and experience in all aspects of pediatric urology
   b. Licensure to practice medicine in the state where the institution that sponsors the program is located (Certain federal programs are exempted.)
   c. Certification by the American Board of Urology or suitable equivalent qualifications and qualifications and experience in the practice of pediatric urology
   d. Appointment in good standing to the medical staff of an institution participating in the program
2. Responsibilities of the program director
   a. Preparation of a written statement outlining the educational goals of the program with respect to knowledge, skills, and other attributes of residents at each level of training and for each major rotation or other program assignment. This statement must be distributed to residents and faculty members. It should be readily available for review.
   b. Selection of residents for appointment to the program in accordance with institutional and departmental policies and procedures.
   c. Selection and supervision of the faculty and other program personnel at each institution participating in the program.
   d. The supervision of residents through explicit written descriptions of supervisory lines of responsibility for the care of patients. Such guidelines must be communicated to all members of the program staff. Residents must be provided with prompt, reliable systems for communication and interaction with supervisory physicians.
   e. Regular evaluation of residents' knowledge, skills, and overall performance, including the development of professional attitudes consistent with being a physician.
   f. Implementation of fair procedures as established by the sponsoring institution regarding academic discipline and resident complaints or grievances.
   g. Monitoring resident stress, including mental or emotional conditions inhibiting performance or learning and drug- or alcohol-related dysfunction. Program directors and faculty should be sensitive to the need for timely provision of confidential counseling and psychological support services to residents. Educational situations that consistently produce undesirable stress on residents must be evaluated and modified.
   h. Preparation of an accurate statistical and narrative description of the program as requested by the review committee.

B. Faculty

1. There must be a sufficient number of faculty with documented qualifications to instruct and supervise adequately all pediatric urology residents in the program. Members of the faculty must be able to devote sufficient time to meet their supervisory and teaching responsibilities.
2. All members of the faculty must demonstrate a strong interest in the education of residents, sound clinical and teaching abilities, support of the goals and objectives of the program, a commitment to their own continuing medical education, and participation in scholarly activities.
3. A member of the faculty of each participating institution must be designated to assume responsibility for the day-to-day activities of the program at that institution, with overall coordination by the program director.
4. The faculty must be organized and have regular documented meetings to review program goals and objectives as well as program effectiveness in achieving them. At least one resident representative should participate in these reviews.
5. The faculty should evaluate at least annually the utilization of the resources available to the program, the contribution of each institution participating in the program, the financial and administrative support of the program, the volume and variety of patients available to the program for educational purposes, the performance of members of the faculty, and the quality of supervision of residents.

C. Other Program Personnel

Programs must be provided with the additional professional, technical, and clerical personnel needed to support the administration and educational conduct of the program.

IV. Facilities and Resources

A. To be considered for accreditation, the institution should have the following resources available for resident education: a broad spectrum of urologic diseases; a sufficient volume and broad variety of pediatric urology surgical procedures consisting of 200 major, 200 intermediate, and 100 minor procedures per year; and 2,000 pediatric urologic outpatient visits per year, including urology subspecialty clinics. Representative examples of these classifications include: Minor: circumcision, meatotomy, diagnostic endoscopy, percutaneous aspiration or tube insertion; Intermediate: therapeutic endoscopy, inguinal surgery >2 years, distal hypospadias (no urethroplasty), diagnostic laparoscopy; Major: all abdominal surgery, flank surgery, hypospadias, laparoscopic surgery, valve ablation, inguinal surgery <2 years.

B. Diagnostic facilities should include body imaging equipment suitable for the care of pediatric patients.

C. Program research and scholarly activity

Graduate medical education must take place in an environment of inquiry and scholarship in which residents participate in the development of new knowledge, learn to evaluate research findings, and develop habits of inquiry as a continuing professional responsibility.

1. Scholarly activity

   The responsibility for establishing and maintaining an environment of inquiry and scholarship rests with the faculty. While not all members of a faculty must be investigators, the staff as a whole must demonstrate broad involvement in scholarly activity. This activity should include

a. active participation of the faculty in clinical discussions, rounds, and conferences in a manner that promotes a spirit of inquiry and scholarship. Scholarship implies an in-depth understanding of basic mechanisms of normal and abnormal states and the application of current knowledge to practice.
b. participation in journal clubs and research conferences.
c. active participation in regional or national professional and scientific societies, particularly through presentations at the organizations' meetings and publications in their journals.
d. participation in research, particularly in projects that are funded following peer review and/or result in publications or presentations at regional and national scientific meetings.
e. offering of guidance and technical support (eg, research design, statistical analysis) for residents involved in research.
f. Provision of support for resident participation in scholarly activities.

2. Library
   a. Residents must have ready access to a major medical library, either at the institution where the residents are located or through arrangement with convenient nearby institutions.
   b. Library services should include the electronic retrieval of information from medical databases.
   c. There must be access to an on-site library or to a collection of appropriate texts and journals in each institution participating in a residency program. On-site libraries and/or collections of texts and journals must be readily available during nights and weekends.

V. Educational Program

The director and faculty of a program must prepare and comply with written educational goals for the program.

A. Program Design

All educational components of the program should be related to program goals.

1. The program design and/or structure must be approved by the appropriate review committee as part of the regular review process.
2. Participation by any institution providing more than 2 months of education in the program must be approved by the residency review committee.

B. Program Course of Study

The educational program must provide sufficient clinical experience for the residents to develop clinical competence in pediatric urology. The clinical component of the program must include the following experience in:

1. The surgical aspects of pediatric urology. Such experience must be documented in an accurate, comprehensive, operative log maintained by the resident and reviewed by the program director quarterly. All operative procedures in which the pediatric urology resident acts as surgeon or teaching assistant should be separately documented.
2. Inpatient consultation and outpatient management of pediatric urologic disease, with graded responsibility for patient care, which must be similarly documented and maintained.
3. Body imaging modalities used in the care of pediatric patients.
4. Performance and evaluation of urodynamic studies must be included.
5. Multidisciplinary management of patients with urologic tumors.
6. Multidisciplinary management of patients with urologic trauma.
7. Multidisciplinary management of nephrological disease.
8. Neonatal and intensive care unit treatment for all pediatric ages.
9. Multidisciplinary management of myelomeningocele and other neuropathic bladder entities.
10. Multidisciplinary management of patients with problems relating to sexual development and medical aspects of intersex states.
11. Performance of genetic counseling for renal and genital anomalies.
12. Pediatric infectious disease and its treatment.

C. Pediatric Urology Resident Duty Hours

The same resident duty hours and supervision requirements apply to pediatric urology residents as provided in the Program Requirements for Residency Education in Urology.

VI. Evaluation

The pediatric urology program must have an ongoing assessment of the following components of the educational program: resident performance, faculty performance, and program objectives.

A. Pediatric Urology Resident Evaluation

The program director, with participation of members of the faculty, shall

1. at least semiannually evaluate the knowledge, skills, and professional growth of the residents, using appropriate criteria and procedures.
2. communicate each evaluation to the resident in a timely manner.
3. advance residents to positions of higher responsibility only on the basis of evidence of their satisfactory progressive scholarship and professional growth.
4. maintain a permanent record of evaluation for each resident and have it accessible to the resident and other authorized personnel.
5. provide a written final evaluation for each resident who completes the program. The evaluation must include a review of the resident's performance during the final period of training and should verify that the resident has demonstrated sufficient professional ability to practice competently and independently. This final evaluation should be part of the resident's permanent record maintained by the institution.

B. Program and Faculty Evaluation

The educational effectiveness of the program and faculty must be evaluated in a systematic manner. In particular, the quality of the curriculum and the extent to which the educational goals have been met by residents must be assessed. Confidential, written evaluations by residents should be utilized in this process.

VII. Board Certification

Individuals should communicate with the Executive Secretary of the American Board of Urology regarding the status of requirements for certification.

ACGME: September 1998 Effective: January 1999

Program Requirements for the Transitional Year

I. Purpose of a Transitional Year

The transitional year must be designed to fulfill the educational needs of medical school graduates who:

A. Have chosen a career specialty for which the respective program in graduate medical education has, as a prerequisite, 1 year of fundamental clinical education, which may also contain certain specific experiences for development of desired skills; or

B. Have not yet made a career choice or specialty selection and desire a broad-based year to assist them in making that decision; or

C. Are planning to serve in organizations such as the public health service or on active duty in the military as general medical officers or primary flight/undersea medicine physicians prior to completing a program in graduate medical education; or

D. Have at least 1 year of fundamental clinical education prior to entering a career path that does not require broad clinical skill, such as administrative medicine or nonclinical research.

The objective of the transitional year is to provide a well-balanced program of graduate medical education in multiple clinical disciplines designed to facilitate the choice of and/or preparation for a specific specialty. The transitional year is not meant to be a complete graduate education program in preparation for the practice of medicine.

The sponsoring institution and the transitional year program must demonstrate substantial compliance with both the Institutional Requirements of the *Essentials of Accredited Residencies* and the Program Requirements that follow.

II. Administration

A. Sponsorship

1. The transitional year program must be offered by an institution and its affiliate(s) conducting two or more Accreditation Council for Graduate Medical Education (ACGME)-accredited residency programs, which must participate in the education of transitional year residents. One of these accredited residency programs must be identified as the sponsoring program. Other disciplines may serve as participants in the transitional year.
2. Each of the accredited sponsors must exist in the parent institution and its affiliate(s) offering the transitional year. The sponsors and participating disciplines must represent a component of the transitional year program.
3. Programs that do not regularly provide educational experiences for the transitional year residents should not be designated as participating disciplines.
4. One of the accredited sponsors must provide experiences for the transitional year residents to develop fundamental clinical skills. Those disciplines considered to provide these experiences are family practice, internal medicine, obstetrics/gynecology, pediatrics, and general surgery.
5. The sponsoring programs and participating disciplines must provide written goals and objectives for the areas of knowledge and skills to be developed by the transitional year resident and demonstrate a commitment to meeting those goals and objectives through the provision of quality teaching and allocation of adequate educational resources. These goals and objectives must be distributed to the residents and be readily available for review.

B. Program Director

1. There must be a single program director responsible for the program. The process by which the program director of the transitional year program is appointed must be consistent with the policies for the appointment of other program directors in the sponsoring institution.
2. The program director's tenure should be of sufficient duration to assure continuity of the educational program. The program director should be appointed for a minimum of 3 years.
3. The program director must be a physician with demonstrated and documented clinical, educational, and administrative abilities and experience in graduate medical education. The qualifications of the program director must include:
   a. The ability to devote the time required for program development, implementation, administration, and supervision
   b. Certification by a specialty board or suitable equivalent qualifications
   c. Licensure to practice medicine in the state where the institution that sponsors the program is located. (Certain federal programs are exempt.)
   d. Appointment in good standing to the medical staff of an institution participating in the program.
4. The program director must coordinate the educational experiences within the separate categorical programs and participating disciplines. Sufficient authority must be delegated to the program director by the sponsoring institution to facilitate effective organization and management.
5. The responsibilities of the program director must include the following:
   a. To select the residents for appointment to the program in accordance with institutional policies and procedures.
   b. To select and supervise the teaching staff and other program personnel at each institution participating in the program.
   c. To arrange and implement educational programs in fundamental clinical skills.
   d. To counsel transitional year residents in the development of a curriculum appropriate to their individual learning needs and career goals.
   e. To apply to the transitional year residents those institutional policies that apply to all other residents in the institution.
   f. To develop and implement systems for periodic evaluation of (1) the quality of the educational experience and program performance, (2) resident performance, (3) resident assessment of the program's educational components including the faculty, and (4) faculty performance.
   g. To advance residents to positions of higher responsiblity only on the basis of evidence of their satisfactory progressive scholarship and professional growth.
   h. To maintain records of (1) all residents appointed to the transitional year program; (2) the transitional year objectives, curriculum content offered by the program, and the curriculum undertaken by each resident; (3) the performance evaluations; (4) the residents' subsequent training or other professional activities until they enter a categorical program or determine a career path. Tracking of residents must be done for at least 1 year and need not exceed 5 consecutive years.
   i. To implement fair procedures, as established by the sponsoring institution, regarding academic discipline and resident complaints or grievances.
   j. To monitor resident stress, including mental or emotional conditions inhibiting performance or learning and drug- or alcohol-related dysfunction. Program directors and teaching staff should be sensitive to the need for timely provision of confidential counseling and psychological support services to residents. Training situations that consistently produce undesirable stress on residents must be evaluated and modified.
   k. To prepare statistical, narrative, and progress reports, as requested by the Transitional Year Review Committee.

l. To prepare for and participate in Transitional Year Review Committee surveys and to participate in Residency Review Committee surveys of the sponsoring programs.
m. To inform the Transitional Year Review Committee of the appointment of a new program director when such changes occur.

C. Institutional Coordination Committee

1. An institutional coordination committee must be appointed and have major responsibility for conducting and monitoring the activities of the transitional year program. It should be convened by the parent institution at least four times a year. This committee should be composed of but not limited to the transitional year program director, the program directors (or designees) of disciplines regularly included in the curriculum, and the chief executive officer(s) (or designee[s] in hospital administration) of the parent institution.
2. The responsibilities of the committee must include the following:
a. To recommend to the governing body of the sponsoring institution policies that establish the educational content of the transitional year and the allocation of resources for the effective conduct of the program.
b. To ensure that the quality of medical care provided by transitional year residents is equivalent to that expected of first-year residents in other ACGME-accredited programs within the institution.
c. To monitor the impact of the transitional year program on the categorical residents' programs to ensure that there is no compromise of the educational resources. This includes monitoring the adequacy of the number of patients, variety of illnesses, educational materials, teaching/attending physicians, and financial support.
d. To review at least twice a year the transitional year residents' performance evaluations and their assessment of the components of the transitional year, to include the faculty.
e. To ensure within acceptable standards of medical care that the educational opportunities provided transitional year residents are equivalent to those provided first-year residents in the categorical programs in which the transitional year residents participate.
f. To ensure that the quality of education provided by the nonaccredited components of the program is reasonably comparable to that provided to the first-year residents in accredited programs.
g. To approve the curriculum of each transitional year resident, which has been planned with the transitional year program director in accordance with the individual needs of the residents and the Program Requirements for the Transitional Year.
h. To ensure that the transitional year program undergoes a periodic internal review in accordance with the general institutional requirements.
i. To maintain records documenting the committee's activities for each of the above requirements and to have copies of these records available for transmission to the Transitional Year Review Committee.

III. Faculty

Qualifications/Responsibilities

1. The faculty of the transitional year program must be the same persons or have qualifications equivalent to those of the faculty of the participating categorical programs.
2. There must be a sufficient number of teaching staff with documented qualifications to instruct and supervise adequately all the residents in the program. Members of the teaching staff must be able to devote sufficient time to meet their supervisory and teaching responsibilities.
3. All members of the teaching staff must demonstrate a strong interest in the education of residents, sound clinical and teaching abilities, support of the goals and objectives of the program, a commitment to their own continuing medical education, and participation in scholarly activities.
4. A member of the teaching staff of each participating institution must be designated to assume responsibility for the day-to-day activities of the rotation at that institution, with overall coordination by the program director.
5. There must be active participation of the teaching staff in clinical discussions, rounds, and conferences in a manner that promotes a spirit of inquiry and scholarship. Scholarship implies an in-depth understanding of basic mechanisms of normal and abnormal states and the application of current knowledge to practice.
6. The faculty providing educational experiences in the disciplines not accredited by ACGME must have credentials within their respective specialties similar in professional status to the other transitional year faculty.
7. The teaching and supervision of transitional year residents must be the same as that provided residents in categorical programs.

IV. Curriculum

A. Duration and Content

1. The duration of the transitional year program must be 1 year (12 calendar months).
2. At least 6 months of each resident's curriculum must be provided by disciplines offering fundamental clinical skills as defined above.
3. Other rotations should be a minimum of 1 month or 4 weeks in duration to ensure a reasonable continuity of education and patient care.
4. The curriculum should include emphasis not only on clinical problems but also on discussion of moral, ethical, legal, social, and economic issues.

B. Skill Development

1. During the rotations in disciplines offering fundamental clinical skills, the transitional year residents should develop the skills necessary to obtain a medical history; perform a complete physical examination; define a patient's problems; develop a rational plan for diagnosis; and implement therapy based on the etiology, pathogenesis, and clinical manifestations of various diseases.
2. Educational experiences must ensure development not only of cognitive and procedural/technical skills, but also of humane qualities that enhance interactions between the physician, the patients, and the patients' families.

C. Electives

The transitional year residents should have no fewer than 2 months of electives. Elective rotations should be determined by the needs of the individual resident and/or the requirements of the future residency program chosen.

D. Emergency Medicine

1. The transitional year residents must have a 1-month rotation in emergency medicine under the supervision of qualified teaching staff within the sponsoring or an affiliated institution.
2. The transitional year residents should have experience in the diagnosis and management of all types of patients treated in an institution's emergency department.

E. Ambulatory Care

1. The transitional year residents should have at least 1 month of experience in ambulatory care other than that acquired in the

emergency department. This experience may consist of a 1-month block of time or be divided into lesser periods of time on different services to approximate 1 month.

2. Outpatient experience must be obtained within the ambulatory programs of the sponsoring or affiliated institutions.

F. Conferences/Rounds

All disciplines participating in the transitional year program must involve the transitional year residents in their departmental programs, such as seminars, conferences, and grand rounds.

G. Service vs Educational Objectives

The transitional year program must be designed to meet the educational needs of the residents. Service obligations of the sponsoring institution must be secondary to the transitional year educational objectives.

H. Number of Residents

1. Program applications will be reviewed for assurance that there is an appropriate balance between the number of transitional year residents in training and the educational resources available to them.
2. Any proposed change in the number of transitional year residents must receive prior approval by the Transitional Year Review Committee. Programs that fail consistently to fill the designated number of approved positions may be asked to reduce the number offered.

I. Support Facilities/Departments

1. Pathology, radiology, and nuclear medicine facilities must exist in the parent and affiliated institutions. These entities must be directed by qualified physicians who are committed to medical education and to providing competent instruction to the transitional year residents when patients require these diagnostic and/or therapeutic modalities.
2. During working and on-call hours, the transitional year residents must be provided with adequate sleeping, lounge, and food facilities. There should be adequate backup so that patient care is not jeopardized during or following assigned periods of duty. Support services must be such that the transitional year residents do not spend an inordinate amount of time in noneducational activities that can be discharged properly by other personnel. Ancillary support services, facilities, and personnel must contribute to the transitional year program in accordance with the Institutional Requirements of the *Essentials of Accredited Residencies*.
3. Transitional year residents must be provided with rapid, reliable systems for communicating with supervising residents and attendings.
4. Residents must have ready access to a major medical library, either at the institution where the residents are located or through arrangement with convenient nearby institutions. Library services should include the electronic retrieval of information from medical databases. There must be access to an on-site library or to a collection of appropriate texts and journals in each institution participating in a residency program. On-site libraries and/or collections of texts and journals must be readily available during nights and weekends.

V. Resident Supervision and Working Environment

A. Supervision

1. The transitional year program director and the faculty of the disciplines participating in the transitional year must ensure, direct, and document proper supervision of the residents in the program at all times.
2. At least 6 months of each transitional year resident's rotations must be on clinical services where he or she works directly with more-senior residents in ACGME-accredited programs. On services where senior residents are not present, there must be effective supervision by faculty and evaluation systems in place.
3. Attending physicians or senior residents with experience appropriate for the severity and complexity of a patient's condition must be available at all times on site.
4. The responsibility or independence given to the transitional year residents by the supervising physician for the care of patients should depend on the residents' knowledge, manual skill, experience, and the complexity of the patients' illnesses and the risk of any procedures that residents perform.

B. Hours

1. Graduate training requires a commitment to continuity of patient care. This continuity of care takes precedence without regard to the time of day, day of the week, number of hours already worked, or on-call schedules.
2. The transitional year program director and the faculty of the disciplines participating in the transitional year must establish an environment that is optimal both for resident education and for patient care, while ensuring that undue stress and fatigue among residents are avoided. It is the responsibility of the transitional year program director and faculty to ensure that in-hospital duty hours shall correspond to the program requirements of the categorical programs to which the transitional year resident is assigned so that residents are not required to perform excessively difficult or prolonged duties regularly.
3. A distinction must be made between on-call time in the hospital and on-call availability at home vis-a-vis actual hours worked. The ratio of hours worked to on-call time may vary with each rotation, and therefore precludes a mandated pattern of established hours.

VI. Assessment

Performance Evaluations

1. The transitional year program director must receive a performance evaluation of each transitional year resident by the participating discipline on each resident's completion of a rotation in that discipline. These evaluations must include an assessment of the resident's knowledge, skills, and professional growth using appropriate criteria and procedures.
2. At least twice a year, the transitional year residents must be apprised individually by the program director of their evaluations. These evaluations must be communicated to the resident in a timely manner.
3. The program director must provide a written final evaluation for each resident who completes the program. The evaluation must include a review of the resident's performance during the final period of training and should verify that the resident has demonstrated sufficient professional ability to advance into a categorical program.
4. The transitional year residents must provide written evaluations of the adequacy, quality, and appropriateness of each component of their educational program, including an evaluation of the faculty members.
5. The program director must maintain a permanent record of evaluations, as noted in this section, for each resident and have it accessible to the resident and other authorized personnel. These records must be made available for inspection during the process of accreditation of the program.

VII. Completion of Training

A. Institutional Certificates

Institutional certificates to be awarded at the conclusion of training in the transitional year program must clearly indicate that the experience was that of a Transitional Year.

B. Continuation of Residency Training

If more than 20% of the transitional year residents, when averaged over 5 years, enter clinical practice without further training, such will be considered as evidence that a program is ineffective in achieving its essential objectives and may be cause for an adverse accreditation action.

ACGME: June 1991 Effective: July 1995

Section III

Accredited Graduate Medical Education Programs

Introduction

This section of the *Directory* contains a list of graduate medical education (GME) programs accredited by the Accreditation Council for Graduate Medical Education (ACGME).

Programs are listed by specialty under the state and city of the sponsoring institution (refer to sample, below). Listed under the program title is the institution that sponsors the residency program, followed by the major participating institution(s), which are recognized by at least one ACGME residency review committee as providing a major portion of required GME. Hospitals and other institutions that provide rotations of less than one-sixth of the program length or less than a total of 6 months are not listed in the *Directory*.

Listings contain the program director's name, address, telephone and fax numbers, and e-mail address, as well as the program Internet web site, a new feature for this year's edition. Additional information on each program includes the ACGME-accredited length of the program, the program size (the total number of *filled and unfilled* positions for 1999-2000 as reported by the program), and the number of graduate year one (GY1) positions (ie, positions that do not require prior GME), if any. (*Note:* The published program length reflects the length approved by the Residency Review Committee. The program may require or offer additional years; these data are included in FREIDA Online.) The program identification number appears at the bottom of each listing; the first three digits of this number indicate the specialty/subspecialty code (see "Specialties/Subspecialties with ACGME Program Requirements," p 363) and the next two the state code.

Sample Listing

Title of the Program

Sponsor: The program's sponsoring institution
The program's major participating institution(s)
Program Director:
Name
Program co-director name (if any)
Address
City, state, zip code
Telephone number, fax number
E-mail address
Internet address
Accred Length: Program length *Program Size:* for 1998-1999
(*GY1:* first-year size of programs that do not require prior GME)
Program ID: 000-00-00-000

Data Accuracy

Much of the data listed in the following pages is collected by the AMA through its Annual Survey of Graduate Medical Education Programs; 98.5% of programs provided updated information during the 1998 survey cycle. Listings of programs that did not respond to the survey may show inaccurate or outdated information. *Programs interested in providing updated information should contact the AMA at 312 464-4635.*

Preventive Medicine Programs

The preventive medicine programs listed in Section III include programs that offer areas of specialization in aerospace medicine, occupational medicine, public health, and general preventive medicine. Refer to the identifying text with each program to determine the area of specialization.

Transitional Year Programs

Transitional Year programs are available for physicians seeking broad clinical experience before entering GME in their chosen field or for physicians who have not yet decided on a medical specialty.

Combined Specialty Programs

Combined specialty programs (listed in Appendix A) have been approved by each respective specialty board; resident physicians completing these programs are eligible for board certification. Neither the ACGME nor the Residency Review Committees accredit combined programs; they accredit each specialty program separately. Information in the combined program list was provided by specialty boards and through the AMA Annual Survey of Graduate Medical Education Programs. Applicants to combined specialty programs are encouraged to review requirements for admission to the certification process of each board in Appendix B of this *Directory.*

Restricted-entry GME Programs

US Armed Services Graduate Medical Education Programs

In most cases, *only persons enrolled in the US Armed Services are eligible for appointment to residency positions at US Army, Navy, and Air Force hospitals and teaching institutions.* These programs are identified in Section III with the text, *US Armed Services Program.* For further information, consult Section I, "Graduate Medical Education Information."

Centers for Disease Control and Prevention GME Programs

GME programs at the Centers for Disease Control and Prevention (CDC) are usually open only to CDC physicians.

Programs on Probation

The *Directory* may include programs that are on probation. For information on a program's current accreditation status, contact the ACGME, 515 N State St/Ste 2000, Chicago, IL 60610; 312 464-4920; 312 464-4098 Fax; http://www.acgme.org.

Sources for Additional Information

Most programs start in June or July, but several begin in January or at other times. (*Note:* For a list of these programs, consult the *Graduate Medical Education Directory Supplement, 1999-2000.*) For this or other information about a particular program, candidates can also contact program directors or refer to FREIDA Online (Fellowship and Residency Electronic Interactive Database Access), an Internet database available through the AMA home page (http://www.ama-assn.org/freida).

Graduates of medical schools not accredited by the Liaison Committee on Medical Education should carefully read Section I before applying to a program.

Specialties/Subspecialties with ACGME Program Requirements

Code	Abbr.	Accred Length(s)	GY1*	# of Programs	Specialty/Subspecialty
020	AI	2	N	77	Allergy and Immunology
025	ALI	1	N	11	Clinical and Laboratory Immunology
040	AN	3 4	S	134	Anesthesiology
042	PAN	1	N	15	Pediatric Anesthesiology
045	CCA	1	N	55	Critical Care Medicine
048	APM	1	N	97	Pain Management
060	CRS	1	N	33	Colon and Rectal Surgery
080	D	3 4	S	102	Dermatology
100	DMP	1	N	39	Dermatopathology
110	EM	3 4	S	121	Emergency Medicine
114	PE	2	N		Pediatric Emergency Medicine
116	ESM	1	N	1	Sports Medicine
118	ETX	2	N		Medical Toxicology
120	FP	3	Y	498	Family Practice
125	FPG	1	N	20	Geriatric Medicine
127	FSM	1	N	42	Sports Medicine
130	MG	2 4	S	40	Medical Genetics
140	IM	3	Y	408	Internal Medicine
141	CD	3	N	186	Cardiovascular Disease
142	CCM	1 2	N	40	Critical Care Medicine
143	END	2	N	122	Endocrinology, Diabetes, and Metabolism
144	GE	2	N	165	Gastroenterology
145	HEM	2	N	32	Hematology
146	ID	2	N	138	Infectious Disease
147	ON	2	N	41	Oncology
148	NEP	2	N	127	Nephrology
149	PUD	2	N	48	Pulmonary Disease
150	RHU	2	N	106	Rheumatology
152	IC	1	N		Interventional Cardiology
151	IMG	2	N	92	Geriatric Medicine
154	ICE	1	N	70	Clinical Cardiac Electrophysiology
155	HO	3	N	105	Hematology and Oncology
156	PCC	3	N	109	Pulmonary Disease and Critical Care Medicine
157	ISM	1	N	1	Sports Medicine
160	NS	5	S	95	Neurological Surgery
180	N	3 4	S	117	Neurology
185	CHN	3	N	70	Child Neurology
187	CN	1	N	68	Clinical Neurophysiology
200	NM	2	N	71	Nuclear Medicine
220	OBG	4	Y	262	Obstetrics and Gynecology
240	OPH	3 4	N	127	Ophthalmology
260	ORS	4 5	S	157	Orthopaedic Surgery
261	OAR	1	N	11	Adult Reconstructive Orthopaedics
262	OFA	1	N	1	Foot and Ankle Orthopaedics
263	HSO	1	N	52	Hand Surgery
265	OP	1	N	28	Pediatric Orthopaedics
267	OSS	1	N	14	Orthopaedic Surgery of the Spine
268	OSM	1	N	57	Orthopaedic Sports Medicine
269	OTR	1	N	4	Orthopaedic Trauma
270	OMO	1	N	7	Musculoskeletal Oncology
280	OTO	4	N	104	Otolaryngology
286	NO	2	N	5	Otology-Neurotology
288	PDO	2	N	4	Pediatric Otolaryngology
300	PTH	4	Y	165	Pathology—Anatomic and Clinical
301	SP	1	N	10	Selective Pathology
305	BBK	1	N	48	Blood Banking/Transfusion Medicine
306	PCH	1	N	4	Chemical Pathology
307	PCP	1	N	75	Cytopathology
310	FOP	1	N	42	Forensic Pathology
311	HMP	1	N	59	Hematology
313	PIP	1 2	N	7	Immunopathology
314	MM	1	N	9	Medical Microbiology
315	NP	2	N	44	Neuropathology
316	PP	1	N	25	Pediatric Pathology
320	PD	3	Y	209	Pediatrics
321	ADL	3	N	10	Adolescent Medicine
323	CCP	3	N	61	Pediatric Critical Care Medicine
324	PEM	2	N		Pediatric Emergency Medicine
325	PDC	3	N	46	Pediatric Cardiology
326	PDE	3	N	61	Pediatric Endocrinology
327	PHO	3	N	64	Pediatric Hematology/Oncology
328	PN	3	N	45	Pediatric Nephrology
329	NPM	3	N	99	Neonatal-Perinatal Medicine
330	PDP	3	N	47	Pediatric Pulmonology
331	PPR	3	N	18	Pediatric Rheumatology
332	PG	3	N	48	Pediatric Gastroenterology
333	PSM	1	N		Pediatric Sports Medicine
335	PDI	3	N	55	Pediatric Infectious Diseases
340	PM	3 4	S	82	Physical Medicine and Rehabilitation
345	SCI	1	N	6	Spinal Cord Injury Medicine
360	PS	2 3 5 6	S	93	Plastic Surgery
361	CFS	1	N		Craniofacial Surgery
363	HSP	1	N	16	Hand Surgery
380	GPM	1 2 3	S	90	Preventive Medicine
399	PTX	2	N		Medical Toxicology
400	P	4	Y	186	Psychiatry
401	ADP	1	N	34	Addiction Psychiatry
405	CHP	2	N	117	Child and Adolescent Psychiatry
406	PFP	1	N	21	Forensic Psychiatry
407	PYG	1	N	49	Geriatric Psychiatry
420	DR	4	S	197	Radiology-Diagnostic
421	AR	1	N		Abdominal Radiology
423	RNR	1	N	86	Neuroradiology
424	PDR	1	N	43	Pediatric Radiology
425	NR	1	N	28	Nuclear Radiology
426	MSR	1	N	7	Musculoskeletal Radiology
427	VIR	1	N	89	Vascular and Interventional Radiology
430	RO	4	N	77	Radiation Oncology
440	GS	5	Y	261	Surgery-General
442	CCS	1	N	60	Surgical Critical Care
443	HSS	1	N	2	Hand Surgery
445	PDS	2	N	32	Pediatric Surgery
450	VS	1	N	82	Vascular Surgery
460	TS	2 3	N	89	Thoracic Surgery
480	U	3 4	N	121	Urology
485	UP	1	N	11	Pediatric Urology
999	TY	1	Y	148	Transitional Year
				7,607	**Total**

* Y = GY1 positions available
N = No GY1 positions available
S = Some programs offer GY1 positions

Programs

Addiction Psychiatry (Psychiatry)

Colorado

Denver

University of Colorado Program
Sponsor: University of Colorado Health Sciences Center
Veterans Affairs Medical Center (Denver)
Program Director:
Jonathan I Ritvo, MD
Denver Health Med Ctr
777 Bannock St/MC 0490
Denver, CO 80204-4507
Tel: 303 436-6660 *Fax:* 303 436-5184
E-mail: addiction@dhha.org
Accred Length: 1 Year *Program Size:* 2
Program ID: 401-07-21-006

Connecticut

Farmington

Institute of Living/University of Connecticut Program
Sponsor: University of Connecticut School of Medicine
Hartford Hospital
Program Director:
Henry R Kranzler, MD
Univ of Connecticut Health Ctr
263 Farmington Ave (MC2103)
Farmington, CT 06030
Tel: 860 679-1283 *Fax:* 860 679-1316
E-mail: kranzler@psychiatry.uchc.edu
Accred Length: 1 Year *Program Size:* 2
Program ID: 401-08-21-021

New Haven

Yale-New Haven Medical Center Program
Sponsor: Yale-New Haven Hospital
Connecticut Mental Health Center
Veterans Affairs Medical Center (West Haven)
Program Director:
Richard Schottenfeld, MD
34 Park St
New Haven, CT 06519
Tel: 203 974-7349 *Fax:* 203 974-7606
E-mail: richard.schottenfeld?@yale.edu
Accred Length: 1 Year *Program Size:* 6
Program ID: 401-08-21-016

Florida

Miami

University of Miami-Jackson Memorial Medical Center Program
Sponsor: University of Miami-Jackson Memorial Medical Center
Mount Sinai Medical Center of Greater Miami
Program Director:
Lauren Williams, MD
Univ of Miami-Jackson Memorial Med Ctr
1400 NW 10th Ave/Ste 307
Miami, FL 33136
Tel: 305 243-4644 *Fax:* 305 243-2599
Accred Length: 1 Year *Program Size:* 2
Program ID: 401-11-21-029

Tampa

University of South Florida Program
Sponsor: University of South Florida College of Medicine
James A Haley Veterans Hospital
Program Director:
Elie Francis, MD
Univ of South Florida Coll of Med
13000 Bruce B Downs Blvd
Tampa, FL 33612
Tel: 813 972-7665
Accred Length: 1 Year *Program Size:* 0
Program ID: 401-11-21-034

Hawaii

Honolulu

University of Hawaii Program
Sponsor: University of Hawaii John A Burns School of Medicine
Hawaii State Hospital
Queen's Medical Center
Program Director:
Jon Streltzer, MD
1356 Lusitana St/4th Fl
Honolulu, HI 96813
Tel: 803 586-2900
Accred Length: 1 Year *Program Size:* 0
Program ID: 401-14-21-033

Illinois

Chicago

McGaw Medical Center of Northwestern University Program
Sponsor: Northwestern University Medical School
Veterans Affairs Lakeside Medical Center (Chicago)
Program Director:
John E Franklin, MD
Northwestern Univ
303 E Superior St/Ste 552
Chicago, IL 60611
Tel: 312 908-2107 *Fax:* 312 908-4840
E-mail: jef@wu.edu
Accred Length: 1 Year *Program Size:* 1
Program ID: 401-16-21-009

University of Illinois College of Medicine at Chicago Program
Sponsor: University of Illinois College of Medicine at Chicago
University of Illinois Hospital and Clinics
Program Director:
Norman S Miller, MD
Dept of Psychiatry (M/C 913)
912 S Wood St
Chicago, IL 60612
Tel: 312 996-7712 *Fax:* 312 996-4358
E-mail: nsm@psych.uic.edu
Accred Length: 1 Year *Program Size:* 1
Program ID: 401-16-21-012

Indiana

Indianapolis

Indiana University School of Medicine Program
Sponsor: Indiana University School of Medicine
Richard L Roudebush Veterans Affairs Medical Center
William N Wishard Memorial Hospital
Program Director:
Alan D Schmetzer, PhD
1001 W 10th St
Indianapolis, IN 46202
Tel: 317 630-8801
Accred Length: 1 Year *Program Size:* 0
Program ID: 401-17-21-030

Kentucky

Lexington

University of Kentucky Medical Center Program
Sponsor: University of Kentucky Hospital
Charter Ridge Hospital
Veterans Affairs Medical Center (Lexington)
Program Director:
Lon R Hays, MD
Univ of Kentucky Med Ctr
Dept of Psychiatry
Kentucky Clinic/Wing B
Lexington, KY 40536-0284
Tel: 606 323-6021, ext 234 *Fax:* 606 323-1194
Accred Length: 1 Year *Program Size:* 1
Program ID: 401-20-21-001

Louisiana

New Orleans

Tulane University Program
Sponsor: Tulane University School of Medicine
DePaul/Tulane Behavioral Health Center
Veterans Affairs Medical Center-LSU Service (New Orleans)
Program Director:
Jose M Pena, MD
Tulane Univ Med Ctr
Tidewater Bldg
1440 Canal St/TB 53
New Orleans, LA 70112
Tel: 504 588-5405 *Fax:* 504 587-4270
Accred Length: 1 Year *Program Size:* 2
Program ID: 401-21-21-027

Maryland

Baltimore

University of Maryland Program
Sponsor: University of Maryland Medical System
Veterans Affairs Medical Center (Baltimore)
Walter P Carter Mental Health Center
Program Director:
Joseph G Liberto, MD
701 W Pratt St
Baltimore, MD 21201
Tel: 410 328-6969 *Fax:* 410 328-3311
Accred Length: 1 Year *Program Size:* 4
Program ID: 401-23-21-002

Massachusetts

Boston

Boston University Medical Center Program
Sponsor: Boston Medical Center
Veterans Affairs Medical Center (Boston)
Program Director:
John A Renner, MD
VA Outpatient Clinic
251 Causeway St
Boston, MA 02114
Tel: 617 248-1030 *Fax:* 617 248-1496
E-mail: renner.john@boston.va.gov
Accred Length: 2 Years *Program Size:* 2
Program ID: 401-24-21-019

Michigan

Ann Arbor

University of Michigan Program
Sponsor: University of Michigan Hospitals
Veterans Affairs Medical Center (Ann Arbor)
Program Director:
Kirk J Brower, MD
Univ of Michigan Alcohol Research Ctr
400 E Eisenhower Pkwy/Ste A
Ann Arbor, MI 48108
Tel: 734 930-0201, ext 33 *Fax:* 734 930-0727
E-mail: kbrower@umich.edu
Internet:
http://www.med.umich.edu/psych/education/fellowship/addiction.html
Accred Length: 1 Year *Program Size:* 2
Program ID: 401-25-21-022

Minnesota

Minneapolis

University of Minnesota Program
Sponsor: University of Minnesota Medical School
Fairview-University Medical Center
Veterans Affairs Medical Center (Minneapolis)
Program Director:
James A Halikas, MD
Box 393
420 Delaware St SE
Minneapolis, MN 55455
Tel: 612 626-6361 *Fax:* 612 626-5185
Accred Length: 1 Year *Program Size:* 3
Program ID: 401-26-21-003

Rochester

Mayo Graduate School of Medicine (Rochester) Program
Sponsor: Mayo Graduate School of Medicine-Mayo Foundation
St Mary's Hospital of Rochester
Program Director:
Joyce Tinsley, MD
Mayo Graduate Sch of Med
200 First St SW
Rochester, MN 55905
Tel: 507 284-2649
Accred Length: 1 Year *Program Size:* 0
Program ID: 401-26-21-031

Nebraska

Omaha

Creighton University/University of Nebraska Program
Sponsor: Creighton University School of Medicine
St Joseph Center for Mental Health
Veterans Affairs Medical Center (Omaha)
Program Director:
Ernest Haffke, MD
Omaha VA Med Ctr
4101 Woolworth Ave
Omaha, NE 68105-1873
Tel: 402 449-0679 *Fax:* 402 449-0677
E-mail: haffke,ernest@omaha.va.gov
Accred Length: 1 Year *Program Size:* 2
Program ID: 401-30-21-025

New Hampshire

Lebanon

Dartmouth-Hitchcock Medical Center Program
Sponsor: Mary Hitchcock Memorial Hospital
Veterans Affairs Medical Center (White River Junction)
Program Director:
Donald A West, MD
Dartmouth-Hitchcock Med Ctr
1 Medical Center Dr
Lebanon, NH 03756
Tel: 603 650-5805 *Fax:* 603 650-7503
E-mail: donald.west@dartmouth.edu
Accred Length: 1 Year *Program Size:* 1
Program ID: 401-32-21-024

New York

Bronx

Albert Einstein College of Medicine at Bronx-Lebanon Hospital Center Program
Sponsor: Bronx-Lebanon Hospital Center
Program Director:
John Osei-Tutu, MD
Bronx-Lebanon Hospital Ctr
1276 Fulton Ave
Bronx, NY 10456
Tel: 718 901-6133 *Fax:* 718 901-6356
E-mail: oseitutu@erols.com
Accred Length: 1 Year *Program Size:* 3
Program ID: 401-35-31-017

Albert Einstein College of Medicine Program
Sponsor: Albert Einstein College of Medicine of Yeshiva University
Jacobi Medical Center
North Central Bronx Hospital
Program Director:
Michelle Rottenstein, MD
Albert Einstein Coll of Med
260 E 161st St/T Level
Bronx, NY 10451
Tel: 718 993-3397 *Fax:* 718 993-2460
E-mail: rottenst@aecom.yu.edu
Accred Length: 1 Year *Program Size:* 1
Program ID: 401-35-21-023

Manhasset

North Shore University Hospital/NYU School of Medicine Program
Sponsor: North Shore University Hospital
St John's Episcopal Hospital-South Shore
Program Director:
Robert Hirsch, MD
300 Community Dr
Manhasset, NY 11030
Tel: 516 562-3010 *Fax:* 516 562-3996
Accred Length: 1 Year *Program Size:* 2
Program ID: 401-35-31-007

New York

Albert Einstein College of Medicine at Beth Israel Medical Center Program
Sponsor: Beth Israel Medical Center
Program Director:
Richard N Rosenthal, MD
Beth Israel Med Ctr
1st Ave at 16th St/9 Fierman
New York, NY 10003
Tel: 212 420-2421 *Fax:* 212 420-3442
E-mail: rrosenthal@bethisraelny.org
Accred Length: 1 Year *Program Size:* 2
Program ID: 401-35-21-010

New York and Presbyterian Hospital (Columbia Campus) Program
Sponsor: New York and Presbyterian Hospital
New York and Presbyterian Hospital (Columbia Campus)
New York State Psychiatric Institute
Program Director:
Frances Levin, MD
New York and Presbyterian Hospital
722 W 168th St
New York, NY 10032
Tel: 212 543-5896
Accred Length: 1 Year *Program Size:* 0
Program ID: 401-35-21-032

New York and Presbyterian Hospital (Cornell Campus) Program
Sponsor: New York and Presbyterian Hospital
New York and Presbyterian Hospital (Cornell Campus)
New York and Presbyterian Hospital-Payne Whitney Clinic
Program Director:
Robert B Millman, MD
New York and Presbyterian Hospital
411 E 69th St
New York, NY 10021
Tel: 212 746-1248 *Fax:* 212 746-8544
Accred Length: 1 Year *Program Size:* 0
Program ID: 401-35-11-018

Programs

New York University Medical Center Program
Sponsor: New York University Medical Center
Bellevue Hospital Center
Program Director:
Marc Galanter, MD
New York Univ Med Ctr
550 First Ave
NB 20N31
New York, NY 10016
Tel: 212 263-6960
Accred Length: 2 Years *Program Size:* 5
Program ID: 401-35-21-004

North Carolina

Durham

Duke University Program
Sponsor: Duke University Medical Center
John Umstead Hospital
Veterans Affairs Medical Center (Durham)
Program Director:
Roy Stein, MD
Psychiatry Service (116A), VA Med Ctr
508 Fulton St
Durham, NC 27705
Tel: 919 286-0411, ext 7483 *Fax:* 919 416-5831
E-mail: roy.stein@duke.edu
Accred Length: 1 Year *Program Size:* 2
Program ID: 401-36-21-035

Ohio

Cincinnati

University Hospital/University of Cincinnati College of Medicine Program
Sponsor: University Hospital Inc
Veterans Affairs Medical Center (Cincinnati)
Program Director:
R Jeffrey Goldsmith, MD
Univ of Cincinnati Med Ctr
231 Bethesda Ave/Mail Location #559
Cincinnati, OH 45267-0559
Tel: 513 558-5190 *Fax:* 513 558-3477
E-mail: goldsmith.richard_j@cincinnati.va.gov.
Internet: http://www.uc.edu/~liang
Accred Length: 1 Year *Program Size:* 1
Program ID: 401-38-21-013

Pennsylvania

Philadelphia

University of Pennsylvania Program
Sponsor: Hospital of the University of Pennsylvania
Veterans Affairs Medical Center (Philadelphia)
Program Director:
Charles P O'Brien, MD PhD
Hospital of Univ of Pennsylvania
Dept of Psych/Addiction Med
3900 Chestnut St
Philadelphia, PA 19104-6178
Tel: 215 222-3200, ext 140 *Fax:* 215 386-6770
E-mail: obrien@research.trc.upenn.edu
Accred Length: 1 Year *Program Size:* 4
Program ID: 401-41-21-011

Pittsburgh

St Francis Medical Center Program
Sponsor: St Francis Medical Center
Program Director:
Wesley E Sowers, MD
St Francis Med Ctr
Medical Education
400 45th St
Pittsburgh, PA 15201
Tel: 412 622-4511
E-mail: sowers@sfhs.edu
Accred Length: 1 Year *Program Size:* 2
Program ID: 401-41-21-026

South Carolina

Charleston

Medical University of South Carolina Program
Sponsor: Medical University of South Carolina College of Medicine
MUSC Medical Center
Program Director:
Kathleen T Brady, MD
171 Ashley Ave
Charleston, SC 29425
Tel: 803 792-5215 *Fax:* 803 792-7353
Accred Length: 1 Year *Program Size:* 2
Program ID: 401-45-21-014

Tennessee

Nashville

Vanderbilt University Program
Sponsor: Vanderbilt University Medical Center
Psychiatric Hospital at Vanderbilt
Program Director:
Paul W Ragan, MD
A-2205 Med Ctr North
21st Ave S and Garland Ave
Nashville, TN 37232-2647
Tel: 615 343-7920 *Fax:* 615 343-8639
E-mail: paul.ragan@mcmail
Accred Length: 1 Year *Program Size:* 2
Program ID: 401-47-21-015

Texas

Dallas

University of Texas Southwestern Medical School Program
Sponsor: University of Texas Southwestern Medical School
Veterans Affairs Medical Center (Dallas)
Program Director:
Bryon H Adinoff, MD
VA North Texas Health Care System
4500 Lancaster Rd
VA Med Ctr
Dallas, TX 75216
Tel: 214 857-0835 *Fax:* 214 857-0902
E-mail: bryadinoff@aol.com
Accred Length: 1 Year *Program Size:* 2
Program ID: 401-48-21-028

San Antonio

University of Texas Health Science Center at San Antonio Program
Sponsor: University of Texas Medical School at San Antonio
Audie L Murphy Memorial Veterans Hospital (San Antonio)
Program Director:
John T Pichot, MD
Univ of Texas Health Science Ctr
7703 Floyd Curl Dr
San Antonio, TX 78284-7790
Tel: 210 567-5430 *Fax:* 210 567-6941
E-mail: pichot@swbell.net
Internet: http://psych68.uthscsa.edu
Accred Length: 1 Year *Program Size:* 2
Program ID: 401-48-21-008

Washington

Seattle

University of Washington Program
Sponsor: University of Washington School of Medicine
Veterans Affairs Medical Center (Seattle)
Program Director:
Andrew L Saxon, MD
VA Puget Sound Health Care System
1660 S Columbian Way
Addictions Treatment Ctr
Seattle, WA 98108
Tel: 206 764-2782 *Fax:* 206 764-2293
E-mail: asaxon@u.washington.edu
Accred Length: 1 Year *Program Size:* 3
Program ID: 401-54-21-005

Adolescent Medicine (Pediatrics)

California

Los Angeles

Children's Hospital of Los Angeles Program
Sponsor: Children's Hospital of Los Angeles
Program Director:
Richard MacKenzie, MD
Children's Hospital of Los Angeles
PO Box 54700/Mailstop #2
Los Angeles, CA 90054-0700
Tel: 323 669-2112 *Fax:* 323 913-3691
Accred Length: 3 Years *Program Size:* 4
Program ID: 321-05-21-018

Indiana

Indianapolis

Indiana University School of Medicine Program
Sponsor: Indiana University School of Medicine
Clarian Methodist Hospital of Indiana
Clarian Riley Hospital for Children
William N Wishard Memorial Hospital
Program Director:
Donald P Orr, MD
Indiana Univ Med Ctr
702 Barnhill Dr/1740 North
Indianapolis, IN 46202
Tel: 317 274-8812 *Fax:* 317 274-0133
Accred Length: 3 Years *Program Size:* 6
Program ID: 321-17-21-006

Maryland

Baltimore

Johns Hopkins University Program
Sponsor: Johns Hopkins University School of Medicine
Johns Hopkins Hospital
Program Director:
Alain Joffe, MD
Johns Hopkins Hospital
600 N Wolfe St/Park 307
Baltimore, MD 21287-2530
Tel: 410 955-2910 *Fax:* 410 955-4079
Accred Length: 3 Years *Program Size:* 3
Program ID: 321-23-21-007

Massachusetts

Boston

Children's Hospital/Boston Medical Center Program
Sponsor: Children's Hospital
Program Director:
S Jean Emans, MD
Children's Hospital
300 Longwood Ave
Boston, MA 02115
Tel: 617 355-7170 *Fax:* 617 730-0442
Accred Length: 3 Years *Program Size:* 6
Program ID: 321-24-21-002

New York

Bronx

Albert Einstein College of Medicine Program
Sponsor: Albert Einstein College of Medicine of Yeshiva University
Montefiore Medical Center-Henry and Lucy Moses Division
Program Director:
Elizabeth M Alderman, MD
Montefiore Med Ctr
Div of Adolescent Medicine
111 E 210th St-NW674
Bronx, NY 10467
Tel: 718 920-6614 *Fax:* 718 920-5289
Accred Length: 3 Years *Program Size:* 3
Program ID: 321-35-21-008

Manhasset

North Shore University Hospital/NYU School of Medicine Program
Sponsor: North Shore University Hospital
Program Director:
Martin Fisher, MD
North Shore Univ Hospital
300 Community Dr
Manhasset, NY 11030
Tel: 516 622-5075 *Fax:* 516 622-5074
Accred Length: 3 Years *Program Size:* 2
Program ID: 321-35-21-010

New Hyde Park

Albert Einstein College of Medicine at Long Island Jewish Medical Center Program
Sponsor: Long Island Jewish Medical Center
Schneider Children's Hosp (Long Island Jewish Med Ctr)
Program Director:
I Ronald Shenker, MD
Schneider Children's Hospital
410 Lakeville Rd
Ste 108
New Hyde Park, NY 11040
Tel: 516 465-3270 *Fax:* 516 465-5299
Accred Length: 3 Years *Program Size:* 2
Program ID: 321-35-31-011

Rochester

University of Rochester Program
Sponsor: Strong Memorial Hospital of the University of Rochester
Rochester General Hospital
Program Director:
Richard E Kreipe, MD
Strong Memorial Hospital-Univ of Rochester
601 Elmwood Ave/Box 690
Rochester, NY 14642
Tel: 716 275-7844 *Fax:* 716 242-9733
E-mail: richard_kreipe@urmc.rochester.edu
Accred Length: 3 Years *Program Size:* 6
Program ID: 321-35-12-013

Ohio

Cincinnati

Children's Hospital Medical Center/University of Cincinnati College of Medicine Program
Sponsor: Children's Hospital Medical Center
Program Director:
Frank M Biro, MD
Children's Hospital Med Ctr
Div of Adolescent Medicine
3333 Burnet Ave
Cincinnati, OH 45229-2899
Tel: 513 636-8587 *Fax:* 513 636-7844
Accred Length: 3 Years *Program Size:* 3
Program ID: 321-38-21-014

Pennsylvania

Philadelphia

Children's Hospital of Philadelphia Program
Sponsor: Children's Hospital of Philadelphia
Hospital of the University of Pennsylvania
Program Director:
Donald F Schwarz, MD
Children's Hospital of Philadelphia
Div of General Pediatrics
Philadelphia, PA 19104-4399
Tel: 215 590-1462 *Fax:* 215 590-3050
Accred Length: 3 Years *Program Size:* 2
Program ID: 321-41-21-015

Adult Reconstructive Orthopaedics (Orthopaedic Surgery)

California

Stanford

Stanford University Program
Sponsor: Stanford University Hospital
Program Director:
David J Schurman, MD
300 Pasteur Dr/R-144
Stanford, CA 94305-5341
Tel: 650 723-7806 *Fax:* 650 723-6396
E-mail: diane.starrett@forslythe.stanford.edu
Accred Length: 1 Year *Program Size:* 1
Program ID: 261-05-21-016

Florida

Gainesville

University of Florida Program
Sponsor: University of Florida College of Medicine
Shands Hospital at the University of Florida
Program Director:
Scott Myers, MD
Univ of Florida
PO Box 100246/HSC
Gainesville, FL 32610-0246
Tel: 352 392-4251 *Fax:* 352 392-8637
Internet: http://www.med.ufl.edu/ortho
Accred Length: 1 Year *Program Size:* 1
Program ID: 261-11-21-004

Illinois

Chicago

University of Chicago Program
Sponsor: Louis A Weiss Memorial Hospital
Program Director:
Henry A Finn, MD MD
Univ of Chicago-Bone and Joint Replacement Ctr
4646 N Marine Dr
Chicago, IL 60640
Tel: 773 564-5888 *Fax:* 773 564-5886
Accred Length: 1 Year *Program Size:* 1
Program ID: 261-16-21-012

Michigan

Detroit

Wayne State University/Detroit Medical Center Program
Sponsor: Wayne State University/Detroit Medical Center
Detroit Receiving Hospital and University Health Center
Hutzel Hospital
Program Director:
Jeffrey W Mast, MD
4707 St Antoine
Rm 207
Detroit, MI 48201
Tel: 810 573-3131 *Fax:* 810 573-3135
Accred Length: 1 Year *Program Size:* 1
Program ID: 261-25-21-013

Minnesota

Rochester

Mayo Graduate School of Medicine (Rochester) Program
Sponsor: Mayo Graduate School of Medicine-Mayo Foundation
Mayo Clinic (Rochester)
Rochester Methodist Hospital
Program Director:
Miguel E Cabanela, MD
Application Processing Ctr
Mayo Graduate Sch of Med
200 First St SW/Siebens 5
Rochester, MN 55905
Tel: 507 284-4331 *Fax:* 507 284-0999
E-mail: mgsm.surgical.specialties@mayo.edu
Internet: http://www.mayo.edu/
Accred Length: 1 Year *Program Size:* 3
Program ID: 261-26-21-015

New York

New York

Albert Einstein College of Medicine at Beth Israel Medical Center Program
Sponsor: Beth Israel Medical Center
Program Director:
John N Insall, MD
170 E End Ave
New York, NY 10128
Tel: 212 870-9760 *Fax:* 212 535-2703
Internet: http://isk-institute.com
Accred Length: 1 Year *Program Size:* 4
Program ID: 261-35-21-020

New York and Presbyterian Hospital (Columbia Campus) Program
Sponsor: New York and Presbyterian Hospital
New York and Presbyterian Hospital (Columbia Campus)
Program Director:
Louis U Bigliani, MD
Columbia Presbyterian Med Ctr
Dept of Ortho Surgery/Shoulder Service
622 W 168th St/11-1131
New York, NY 10032
Tel: 212 305-5564 *Fax:* 212 305-4040
E-mail: reidyca@pegasus.cpmc.columbia.edu
Internet:
http://cpmcnet.columbia.edu/dept/ortho/shoulder/welcome/html
Accred Length: 1 Year *Program Size:* 2
Program ID: 261-35-21-010

Pennsylvania

Philadelphia

Thomas Jefferson University Program
Sponsor: Thomas Jefferson University Hospital
Pennsylvania Hospital (UPHS)
Program Director:
Richard H Rothman, MD PhD
Thomas Jefferson Univ Hospital
925 Chestnut St
Rm 0566
Philadelphia, PA 19107
Tel: 215 503-0566 *Fax:* 215 923-3794
Accred Length: 1 Year *Program Size:* 2
Program ID: 261-41-31-008

University of Pennsylvania Program
Sponsor: Hospital of the University of Pennsylvania
Crozer-Keystone Health System
Program Director:
Paul A Lotke, MD
Univ of Pennsylvania Sch of Med
3400 Spruce St
Philadelphia, PA 19104
Tel: 215 349-8729 *Fax:* 215 349-5928
E-mail: lotkepa@mailmed.upenn.edu
Accred Length: 1 Year *Program Size:* 1
Program ID: 261-41-21-001

Texas

San Antonio

University of Texas Health Science Center at San Antonio Program
Sponsor: University of Texas Medical School at San Antonio
Audie L Murphy Memorial Veterans Hospital (San Antonio)
University Hospital-South Texas Medical Center
Program Director:
Charles A Rockwood, MD
Univ of Texas Health Science Ctr
Dept of Orthopaedics
7703 Floyd Curl Dr
San Antonio, TX 78284-7774
Tel: 210 567-5125 *Fax:* 210 567-5167
E-mail: orthopresprg@uthscsa.edu
Internet: http://www.mabrey.uthscsa.edu
Accred Length: 1 Year *Program Size:* 1
Program ID: 261-48-21-007

Virginia

Charlottesville

University of Virginia Program
Sponsor: University of Virginia Medical Center
Program Director:
Gwo-Jaw Wang, MD
Univ of Virginia Health Sciences Ctr
Dept of Ortho Surgery
HSC Box 159
Charlottesville, VA 22908
Tel: 804 924-2935 *Fax:* 804 924-5613
E-mail: bjl7e@virginia.edu
Internet:
http://www.med.va.edu/medicine/clinical/orthopaedics
Accred Length: 1 Year *Program Size:* 1
Program ID: 261-51-21-009

Allergy and Immunology

Alabama

Birmingham

University of Alabama Medical Center Program
Sponsor: University of Alabama Hospital
Program Director:
Max D Cooper, MD
Univ of Alabama
Rm 263
Birmingham, AL 35294
Tel: 205 975-7203 *Fax:* 205 975-7218
Accred Length: 2 Years *Program Size:* 2
Program ID: 020-01-21-109

California

La Jolla

Scripps Clinic/Scripps Green Hospital Program
Sponsor: Scripps Clinic
Scripps Green Hospital
Program Director:
Bruce L Zuraw, MD
Sandra C Christiansen, MD
Dept of Grad Med Educ/403C
Scripps Clinic-Green Hospital
10666 N Torrey Pines Rd
La Jolla, CA 92037-1093
Tel: 619 554-8582 *Fax:* 619 554-6310
E-mail: gme@scripps.edu
Internet: http://scrippsclinic.com/edu
Accred Length: 2 Years *Program Size:* 3
Program ID: 020-05-31-002

Los Angeles

Southern California Kaiser Permanente Medical Care (Los Angeles) Program
Sponsor: Southern California Kaiser Permanente Medical Group
Kaiser Foundation Hospital (Los Angeles)
Program Director:
Michael Kaplan, MD
Kaiser Foundation Hospital
1515 Vermont/5th Fl
Los Angeles, CA 90027
Tel: 323 783-4647 *Fax:* 323 783-4646
Accred Length: 2 Years *Program Size:* 2
Program ID: 020-05-12-003

UCLA Medical Center Program
Sponsor: UCLA School of Medicine
UCLA Medical Center
Program Director:
E Richard Stiehm, MD
Andrew Saxon, MD
UCLA Children's Hospital
Div of Ped Allergy
10833 Le Conte Ave/22-387 MDCC
Los Angeles, CA 90095-1752
Tel: 310 825-6481 *Fax:* 310 206-5843
E-mail: estiehm@pediatrics.medsch.ucla.edu
Accred Length: 2 Years *Program Size:* 3
Program ID: 020-05-11-038

University of Southern California Program
Sponsor: Los Angeles County-USC Medical Center
Program Director:
Craig Jones, MD
Los Angeles County-USC Med Ctr
1801 E Marengo
Rm 1G1
Los Angeles, CA 90033
Tel: 323 226-3813 *Fax:* 323 226-5049
Accred Length: 2 Years *Program Size:* 2
Program ID: 020-05-21-065

VA Greater Los Angeles Healthcare System Program
Sponsor: VA Greater Los Angeles Healthcare System
Children's Hospital of Los Angeles
Program Director:
William B Klaustermeyer, MD
West Los Angeles VA Med Ctr
11301 Wilshire Blvd/111R
Los Angeles, CA 90073
Tel: 310 268-3011 *Fax:* 310 268-4922
Accred Length: 2 Years *Program Size:* 2
Program ID: 020-05-21-096

Orange

University of California (Irvine) Program
Sponsor: University of California (Irvine) Medical Center
Veterans Affairs Medical Center (Long Beach)
Program Director:
Sudhir Gupta, MD
Univ of California
C240 Medical Sciences I
Irvine, CA 92697-4069
Tel: 949 824-5818 *Fax:* 949 824-4362
E-mail: sgupta@uci.edu
Accred Length: 2 Years *Program Size:* 2
Program ID: 020-05-21-064

Sacramento

University of California (Davis) Program
Sponsor: University of California (Davis) Medical Center
Program Director:
Suzanne S Teuber, MD
Univ of California Davis Sch of Med
Div of Rheum/Allergy/Clin Immun
One Shields Ave/TB 192
Davis, CA 95616-8660
Tel: 530 752-2884 *Fax:* 530 754-6047
E-mail: ssteuber@ucdavis.edu
Accred Length: 2 Years *Program Size:* 3
Program ID: 020-05-21-048

San Diego

University of California (San Diego) Program
Sponsor: University of California (San Diego) Medical Center
Program Director:
Diana L Marquardt, MD
Univ of California San Diego Med Ctr
Div of Allergy/Immunology
9500 Gilman Dr
La Jolla, CA 92093-0635
Tel: 619 534-2033 *Fax:* 619 534-2110
Accred Length: 2 Years *Program Size:* 1
Program ID: 020-05-21-066

San Francisco

University of California (San Francisco)/Stanford University Program
Sponsor: University of California (San Francisco) Medical Center
Lucile Salter Packard Children's Hospital at Stanford
Stanford University Hospital
Program Director:
Richard S Shames, MD
Stanford Univ Med Ctr
Div of Allergy/Immunology
Rm G309 Stanford Univ Med Ctr
Stanford, CA 94305-5208
Tel: 650 723-5227 *Fax:* 650 498-5560
E-mail: maribel.ortiz@stanford.edu
Internet: http://www-med.stanford.edu/scholl/pediatrics/asthma_center/index.html
Accred Length: 2 Years *Program Size:* 3
Program ID: 020-05-21-116

Torrance

Los Angeles County-Harbor-UCLA Medical Center Program
Sponsor: Los Angeles County-Harbor-UCLA Medical Center
Program Director:
Gildon N Beall, MD
Los Angeles County-Harbor-UCLA Med Ctr
1000 W Carson St
Torrance, CA 90509-2910
Tel: 310 222-2365 *Fax:* 310 533-0447
Accred Length: 2 Years *Program Size:* 3
Program ID: 020-05-21-102

Colorado

Denver

University of Colorado Program A
Sponsor: University of Colorado Health Sciences Center
National Jewish Ctr for Immunology and Respiratory Medicine
Program Director:
Andrew H Liu, MD
National Jewish Med and Research Ctr
Dept of Pediatrics
1400 Jackson St
Denver, CO 80206-2762
Tel: 303 398-1245 *Fax:* 303 270-2182
E-mail: liua@njc.org
Internet: http://www.njc.org
Accred Length: 2 Years *Program Size:* 5
Program ID: 020-07-31-010

University of Colorado Program B
Sponsor: University of Colorado Health Sciences Center
National Jewish Ctr for Immunology and Respiratory Medicine
Program Director:
Lanny J Rosenwasser, MD
Stephen C Dreskin, MD
National Jewish Ctr for Immunology and Resp Med
1400 Jackson St
Denver, CO 80206
Tel: 303 398-1656 *Fax:* 303 398-1806
E-mail: rosenwasserl@njc.org
Accred Length: 2 Years *Program Size:* 3
Program ID: 020-07-31-086

Connecticut

New Haven

Yale-New Haven Medical Center Program

Sponsor: Yale-New Haven Hospital

Program Director:
Philip W Askenase, MD
Fred S Kantor, MD
Yale Univ Sch of Med
Sect for Allergy/Clin Immunology
333 Cedar St/LCI 904
New Haven, CT 06520-8013
Tel: 203 785-4142 *Fax:* 203 785-3229
E-mail: askanase.lab@quickmail.yale.edu
Internet: http://www.info.med.yale.edu/intmed/
Accred Length: 2 Years *Program Size:* 3
Program ID: 020-08-21-099

District of Columbia

Washington

Children's National Medical Center Program

Sponsor: Children's National Medical Center

Program Director:
R Michael Sly, MD
Dept of Pediatrics
111 Michigan Ave NW
Washington, DC 20010-2970
Tel: 202 884-2033 *Fax:* 202 884-3461
Accred Length: 2 Years *Program Size:* 2
Program ID: 020-10-11-039

Walter Reed Army Medical Center Program

Sponsor: Walter Reed Army Medical Center

Program Director:
Col Renata J Engler, MD
Michael A O'Connell , MD
Walter Reed Army Med Ctr
Allergy/Immunology Dept
6825 16th St NW
Washington, DC 20307-5001
Tel: 202 782-6850 *Fax:* 202 782-7093
E-mail: col_renata_engler@wramc1-amedd.army.mil
Accred Length: 2 Years *Program Size:* 6
Program ID: 020-10-11-087
US Armed Services Program

Florida

St Petersburg

University of South Florida (All Children's) Program

Sponsor: University of South Florida College of Medicine
All Children's Hospital

Program Director:
Robert A Good, MD
Sami L Bahna, MD
All Children's Hospital
801 Sixth St S
St Petersburg, FL 33701-4899
Tel: 727 892-4470 *Fax:* 727 892-8542
E-mail: goodr@allkids.org
Accred Length: 2 Years *Program Size:* 7
Program ID: 020-11-21-106

Tampa

University of South Florida Program

Sponsor: University of South Florida College of Medicine
James A Haley Veterans Hospital

Program Director:
Richard F Lockey, MD
Univ of South Florida Coll of Med
VA Hospital, Div of Allergy/Immun
13000 Bruce B Downs Blvd (111D)
Tampa, FL 33612
Tel: 813 972-7631 *Fax:* 813 972-7623
Internet: http://www.med.usf.edu/intmed/allergy/
Accred Length: 2 Years *Program Size:* 2
Program ID: 020-11-21-093

Georgia

Atlanta

Emory University Program

Sponsor: Emory University School of Medicine
Egleston Children's Hospital at Emory University
Emory University Hospital
Grady Memorial Hospital

Program Director:
Timothy J Sullivan, MD
Keith M Phillips, MD
Emory Clinic
4th Fl
1365 Clifton Rd NE
Atlanta, GA 30322
Tel: 404 778-4867 *Fax:* 404 778-4147
Accred Length: 2 Years *Program Size:* 4
Program ID: 020-12-21-101

Augusta

Medical College of Georgia Program

Sponsor: Medical College of Georgia Hospital and Clinics

Program Director:
Betty B Wray, MD
Chester T Stafford, MD
Med Coll of Georgia
Dept of Peds/Med
BG-230
Augusta, GA 30912-3790
Tel: 706 721-3531 *Fax:* 706 721-2527
E-mail: bettyw@mail.mcg.edu
Accred Length: 2 Years *Program Size:* 4
Program ID: 020-12-21-013

Illinois

Chicago

McGaw Medical Center of Northwestern University Program

Sponsor: Northwestern University Medical School
Children's Memorial Medical Center
Northwestern Memorial Hospital

Program Director:
Paul A Greenberger, MD
Northwestern Univ Med Sch
Div of Allergy/Immunology
303 E Chicago Ave/S207
Chicago, IL 60611-3008
Tel: 312 909-8171 *Fax:* 312 908-0205
E-mail: p-greenberger@nwu.edu
Internet: http://www.medicine.nwu.edu/allergy
Accred Length: 2 Years *Program Size:* 8
Program ID: 020-16-31-016

Rush-Presbyterian-St Luke's Medical Center Program

Sponsor: Rush-Presbyterian-St Luke's Medical Center
Cook County Hospital

Program Director:
Anita Gewurz, MD
Rush-Presbyterian-St Luke's Med Ctr
1725 W Harrison St/Ste 207
Chicago, IL 60612
Tel: 312 942-6296 *Fax:* 312 563-2201
E-mail: agewurz@rush.edu
Internet: http://www.rush.edu/med/allergy
Accred Length: 2 Years *Program Size:* 5
Program ID: 020-16-21-108

Iowa

Iowa City

University of Iowa Hospitals and Clinics Program B

Sponsor: University of Iowa Hospitals and Clinics

Program Director:
Zuhair K Ballas, MD
Univ of Iowa Hospitals and Clinics
Dept of Int Med
200 Hawkins Dr
Iowa City, IA 52242-1081
Tel: 319 356-3697 *Fax:* 319 356-8280
E-mail: ballasz@uiowa.edu
Accred Length: 2 Years *Program Size:* 4
Program ID: 020-18-21-081

Kansas

Kansas City

University of Kansas Medical Center Program

Sponsor: University of Kansas School of Medicine
University of Kansas Medical Center

Program Director:
Daniel J Stechschulte, MD
Univ of Kansas Med Ctr
Rm 4035 Wescoe
3901 Rainbow Blvd
Kansas City, KS 66160-7317
Tel: 913 588-6008 *Fax:* 913 588-3987
E-mail: dstechsc@kumc.edu
Accred Length: 2 Years *Program Size:* 2
Program ID: 020-19-21-117

Louisiana

New Orleans

Louisiana State University Program

Sponsor: Louisiana State University School of Medicine
Childrens Hospital
Medical Center of Louisiana at New Orleans

Program Director:
Prem Kumar, MD
Ricardo U Sorensen, MD
Sect of Allergy/Immunology
Louisiana State Univ Med Ctr
1542 Tulane Ave
New Orleans, LA 70112-2822
Tel: 504 568-4580 *Fax:* 504 568-3899
Accred Length: 2 Years *Program Size:* 4
Program ID: 020-21-21-070

Tulane University Program
Sponsor: Tulane University School of Medicine
Louisiana State University Medical College Campus
Medical Center of Louisiana at New Orleans
Tulane University Hospital and Clinics
Veterans Affairs Medical Center (New Orleans)
Veterans Affairs Medical Center-LSU Service (New Orleans)
Program Director:
Manuel Lopez, MD
Tulane Med Ctr
1700 Perdido St
Box SL57
New Orleans, LA 70112
Tel: 504 588-5578 *Fax:* 504 584-3686
E-mail: malopez@mailhost.tcs.tulane.edu
Accred Length: 2 Years *Program Size:* 4
Program ID: 020-21-31-017

Shreveport

Louisiana State University (Shreveport) Program
Sponsor: Louisiana State University Hospital-Shreveport
Tulane University Hospital and Clinics
Program Director:
Bettina C Hilman, MD
Louisiana State Univ Med Ctr Hospital
Med Educ Dept
PO Box 33932
Shreveport, LA 71130-3932
Tel: 318 675-6094 *Fax:* 318 675-7668
E-mail: bhilma@lsumc.edu
Accred Length: 2 Years *Program Size:* 3
Program ID: 020-21-21-060

Maryland

Baltimore

Johns Hopkins University Program
Sponsor: Johns Hopkins University School of Medicine
Johns Hopkins Bayview Medical Center
Johns Hopkins Hospital
Program Director:
N Franklin Adkinson Jr, MD
Peyton A Eggleston, MD
Johns Hopkins Asthma and Allergy Ctr
5501 Hopkins Bayview Cir
Baltimore, MD 21224-6801
Tel: 410 550-2337 *Fax:* 410 550-2055
E-mail: fadkinso@welchlink.welch.jhu.edu
Accred Length: 2 Years *Program Size:* 8
Program ID: 020-23-21-094

Bethesda

National Institutes of Health Clinical Center Program
Sponsor: NIH Warren Grant Magnuson Clinical Center
Program Director:
Dean D Metcalfe, MD
NIAID/Laboratory Allergic Diseases
Bldg 10/Rm 11C205
10 Center Dr/MSC 1881
Bethesda, MD 20892-1881
Tel: 301 496-2165 *Fax:* 301 480-8384
E-mail: dean metcalfe@nih.gov
Accred Length: 2 Years *Program Size:* 9
Program ID: 020-23-21-090

Massachusetts

Boston

Boston University Medical Center Program
Sponsor: Boston Medical Center
Veterans Affairs Medical Center (Boston)
Program Director:
Helen M Hollingsworth, MD
Boston Med Ctr
80 E Concord St/Rm R304
Boston, MA 02118
Tel: 617 638-4933 *Fax:* 617 638-5298
E-mail: hollings@bupula.bu.edu
Accred Length: 2 Years *Program Size:* 3
Program ID: 020-24-21-112

Brigham and Women's Hospital Program
Sponsor: Brigham and Women's Hospital
Program Director:
Dirk K Greineder, MD PhD
K Frank Austen, MD
Brigham and Women's Hospital
Smith Bldg/Rm 638
One Jimmy Fund Way
Boston, MA 02115
Tel: 617 525-1300 *Fax:* 617 525-1310
E-mail: mcfisher@warren.med.harvard.edu
Accred Length: 2 Years *Program Size:* 4
Program ID: 020-24-21-031

Children's Hospital Program
Sponsor: Children's Hospital
Program Director:
Raif S Geha, MD
Lynda C Schneider, MD
Children's Hospital
300 Longwood Ave
Boston, MA 02115-5747
Tel: 617 355-7602 *Fax:* 617 355-8205
E-mail: geha@al.tch.harvard.edu
Internet: http://web1.tch.harvard.edu/allergy/
Accred Length: 2 Years *Program Size:* 9
Program ID: 020-24-21-061

Massachusetts General Hospital Program
Sponsor: Massachusetts General Hospital
Program Director:
Johnson T Wong, MD
Immunology/Allergy Unit
100 Blossom St/Cox 5
Boston, MA 02114
Tel: 617 726-3850 *Fax:* 617 726-2365
Internet: http://www.mgh.harvard.edu/
Accred Length: 2 Years *Program Size:* 2
Program ID: 020-24-21-051

Michigan

Ann Arbor

University of Michigan Program
Sponsor: University of Michigan Hospitals
Program Director:
James R Baker Jr, MD
William R Solomon, MD
Univ of Michigan Hospitals
Div of Allergy/Immunology
3918 Taubman Ctr
Ann Arbor, MI 48109-0380
Tel: 734 647-2777 *Fax:* 734 936-2990
E-mail: jbakerjr@umich.edu
Accred Length: 2 Years *Program Size:* 4
Program ID: 020-25-21-045

Detroit

Henry Ford Hospital Program
Sponsor: Henry Ford Hospital
Program Director:
John A Anderson, MD
Henry Ford Hospital
2799 W Grand Blvd
Detroit, MI 48202
Tel: 313 876-2662 *Fax:* 313 876-2094
Accred Length: 2 Years *Program Size:* 3
Program ID: 020-25-11-032

Wayne State University/Detroit Medical Center Program
Sponsor: Wayne State University/Detroit Medical Center
Children's Hospital of Michigan
Detroit Receiving Hospital and University Health Center
Veterans Affairs Medical Center (Detroit)
Program Director:
Michael Simon, MD
VA Med Ctr 111F
4646 John R St
Detroit, MI 48201
Tel: 313 576-1000, ext 3796 *Fax:* 313 576-1122
E-mail: simon.michael_r@allen-park.va.gov
Accred Length: 2 Years *Program Size:* 3
Program ID: 020-25-21-071

Minnesota

Minneapolis

University of Minnesota Program
Sponsor: University of Minnesota Medical School
Fairview-University Medical Center
Program Director:
Malcolm N Blumenthal, MD
Univ of Minnesota
C378 Mayo Bldg/Box 434
420 Delaware St SE
Minneapolis, MN 55455
Tel: 612 624-5456 *Fax:* 612 624-9188
E-mail: blume001@maroon.tc.umn.edu
Internet: http://www.dept.med.umn.edu/medicine/
Accred Length: 2 Years *Program Size:* 1
Program ID: 020-26-21-091

Rochester

Mayo Graduate School of Medicine (Rochester) Program A
Sponsor: Mayo Graduate School of Medicine-Mayo Foundation
Mayo Clinic (Rochester)
Rochester Methodist Hospital
Program Director:
James T Li, MD
Mayo Graduate Sch of Med
Application Processing Ctr
200 First St SW
Rochester, MN 55905
Tel: 507 284-3126 *Fax:* 507 284-0999
E-mail: mgsm.intmed.specialties@mayo.edu
Internet: http://www.mayo.edu/
Accred Length: 2 Years *Program Size:* 3
Program ID: 020-26-11-018

Mayo Graduate School of Medicine (Rochester) Program B
Sponsor: Mayo Graduate School of Medicine-Mayo Foundation
Mayo Clinic (Rochester)
St Mary's Hospital of Rochester
Program Director:
Martin I Sachs, DO PhD
Mayo Graduate Sch of Med
Siebens 5th Fl
Application Processing Ctr
Rochester, MN 55905
Tel: 507 284-2922 *Fax:* 507 284-0564
E-mail: mgsm.intmed.specialties@mayo.edu
Internet: http://www.mayo.edu/
Accred Length: 2 Years *Program Size:* 1
Program ID: 020-26-21-057

Mayo Graduate School of Medicine (Rochester) Program
Sponsor: Mayo Graduate School of Medicine-Mayo Foundation
Program Director:
James T Li, MD
200 First Street, SW
Rochester, MN 55095
Tel: 507 284-4966 *Fax:* 507 284-0902
Accred Length: 2 Years *Program Size:* 0
Program ID: 020-26-21-115

Missouri

Kansas City

University of Missouri at Kansas City Program
Sponsor: University of Missouri-Kansas City School of Medicine
Children's Mercy Hospital
Truman Medical Center-West
Program Director:
Jay M Portnoy, MD
Children's Mercy Hospital
Sect of Allergy Asthma Immunology
2401 Gillham Rd
Kansas City, MO 64108
Tel: 816 234-3097 *Fax:* 816 346-1301
E-mail: jportnoy@cmh.edu
Internet: http://www.cmh.edu/allergy
Accred Length: 2 Years *Program Size:* 3
Program ID: 020-28-21-114

St Louis

St Louis University School of Medicine Program
Sponsor: St Louis University School of Medicine
SSM Cardinal Glennon Children's Hospital
St Louis University School of Medicine
Program Director:
Mark S Dykewicz, MD
Alan P Knutsen, MD
St Louis Univ Sch of Med
1402 S Grand Blvd
R209
St Louis, MO 63104-1028
Tel: 314 577-8456 *Fax:* 314 577-8459
E-mail: dykewicz@slu.edu
Internet:
http://www.slu.edu/colleges/med/graduatemed/allergy
Accred Length: 2 Years *Program Size:* 3
Program ID: 020-28-21-019

Washington University/B-JH/SLCH Consortium Program
Sponsor: Washington University/B-JH/SLCH Consortium
Barnes-Jewish Hospital
St Louis Children's Hospital
Program Director:
Daniel L Hamilos, MD
Jonathan Gitlin, MD
Washington Univ Sch of Med
660 S Euclid Ave/Box 8122
St Louis, MO 63110
Tel: 314 454-7377 *Fax:* 314 454-5140
E-mail: dhamilos@imgate.wustl.edu
Internet: http://www:internalmed.wustl.edu
Accred Length: 2 Years *Program Size:* 7
Program ID: 020-28-21-095

Nebraska

Omaha

Creighton University Program
Sponsor: Creighton University School of Medicine
Ehrling Bergquist Hospital
Tenet St Joseph Hospital at Creighton Univ Medical Center
Program Director:
Robert G Townley, MD
Creighton Univ
Allergic Disease Ctr
2500 California Plaza
Omaha, NE 68178
Tel: 402 280-2940 *Fax:* 402 280-1843
E-mail: diva@creighton.edu
Internet: http://www.medicine.creighton.edu/allergy/fellowshipdesc.html
Accred Length: 2 Years *Program Size:* 2
Program ID: 020-30-21-088

New Jersey

Newark

UMDNJ-New Jersey Medical School Program
Sponsor: UMDNJ-New Jersey Medical School
UMDNJ-University Hospital
Veterans Affairs Medical Center (East Orange)
Program Director:
Leonard Bielory, MD
James Oleske, MD MPH
UMDNJ-New Jersey Med Sch
Allergy/Immunology Dept
90 Bergen St/DOC 4700
Newark, NJ 07103-2499
Tel: 973 972-2762 *Fax:* 973 972-2769
Accred Length: 2 Years *Program Size:* 5
Program ID: 020-33-11-040

New York

Bronx

Albert Einstein College of Medicine Program
Sponsor: Albert Einstein College of Medicine of Yeshiva University
Jacobi Medical Center
Montefiore Medical Center-Weiler Hospital
Program Director:
Arye Rubinstein, MD
Albert Einstein Coll of Med
1300 Morris Park Ave
Mazer Bldg/Rm 200
Bronx, NY 10461
Tel: 718 430-2319 *Fax:* 718 430-8982
E-mail: rubinste@aecom.yu.edu
Accred Length: 2 Years *Program Size:* 3
Program ID: 020-35-21-054

Brooklyn

Long Island College Hospital Program
Sponsor: Long Island College Hospital
Program Director:
Arlene T Schneider, MD
Long Island College Hospital
339 Hicks St
Brooklyn, NY 11201
Tel: 718 780-4674 *Fax:* 718 780-1493
Accred Length: 2 Years *Program Size:* 2
Program ID: 020-35-11-041

SUNY Health Science Center at Brooklyn Program
Sponsor: SUNY Health Science Center at Brooklyn
Kings County Hospital Center
University Hospital-SUNY Health Science Center at Brooklyn
Program Director:
Alan S Josephson, MD
SUNY Health Science Ctr-Brooklyn
Dept of Med
450 Clarkson Ave/Box 50
Brooklyn, NY 11203-2098
Tel: 718 270-2156 *Fax:* 718 270-1831
E-mail: ajosephson@aol.com
Accred Length: 2 Years *Program Size:* 3
Subspecialties: ALI
Program ID: 020-35-21-092

Buffalo

SUNY at Buffalo Graduate Medical-Dental Education Consortium Program
Sponsor: SUNY at Buffalo Grad Medical-Dental Education Consortium
CGF Health System (Buffalo General Hospital)
CGF Health System (Children's Hospital of Buffalo)
Program Director:
Mark Ballow, MD
Stanley Schwartz, MD
Children's Hospital
219 Bryant St
Buffalo, NY 14222-2099
Tel: 716 878-7105 *Fax:* 716 888-3841
E-mail: ballow@acsu.buffalo.edu
Accred Length: 2 Years *Program Size:* 4
Program ID: 020-35-21-053

East Meadow

Nassau County Medical Center Program
Sponsor: Nassau County Medical Center
North Shore University Hospital
Program Director:
Marianne Frieri, MD PhD
Savita Pahwa, MD
Nassau County Med Ctr
Div of Clinical Immunopathology
2201 Hempstead Trnpk
East Meadow, NY 11554-5400
Tel: 516 572-3214 *Fax:* 516 572-5614
Accred Length: 2 Years *Program Size:* 4
Program ID: 020-35-11-020

New Hyde Park

Albert Einstein College of Medicine at Long Island Jewish Medical Center Program
Sponsor: Long Island Jewish Medical Center
Schneider Children's Hosp (Long Island Jewish Med Ctr)
Program Director:
Vincent R Bonagura, MD
Long Island Jewish Med Ctr
270-05 76th Ave
New Hyde Park, NY 11040-1432
Tel: 718 470-3300 *Fax:* 718 347-0859
E-mail: bonagura@lij.com
Internet: http://www.lij.edu
Accred Length: 2 Years *Program Size:* 3
Program ID: 020-35-21-105

New York

Mount Sinai School of Medicine Program
Sponsor: Mount Sinai School of Medicine
Mount Sinai Medical Center
Program Director:
Lloyd F Mayer, MD
Charlotte Cunningham-Rundles, MD
Mount Sinai Med Ctr
1425 Madison Ave
Rm 11-20 East Bldg
New York, NY 10029-6574
Tel: 212 241-5992 *Fax:* 212 987-5593
E-mail: lmayer@smtplink.mssm.edu
Accred Length: 2 Years *Program Size:* 3
Program ID: 020-35-21-083

New York and Presbyterian Hospital (Columbia Campus) Program
Sponsor: New York and Presbyterian Hospital
New York and Presbyterian Hospital (Columbia Campus)
Program Director:
William J Davis, MD
Vincent Butler Jr, MD
Columbia Univ Coll of Physicians and Surgeons
630 W 168th St
New York, NY 10032
Tel: 212 305-2300 *Fax:* 212 305-4538
Accred Length: 2 Years *Program Size:* 1
Program ID: 020-35-21-082

New York and Presbyterian Hospital (Cornell Campus) Program
Sponsor: New York and Presbyterian Hospital
New York and Presbyterian Hospital (Cornell Campus)
Program Director:
David J Valacer, MD
Irwin Rappaport, MD
New York Hospital
525 E 68th St
Rm J116
New York, NY 10021
Tel: 212 746-3313 *Fax:* 212 746-3988
Accred Length: 2 Years *Program Size:* 2
Program ID: 020-35-21-046

New York and Presbyterian Hospital (Cornell Campus) Program
Sponsor: New York and Presbyterian Hospital
New York and Presbyterian Hospital (Cornell Campus)
Program Director:
Kendall Smith, MD
Cornell Univ Med Coll
Allergy/Immunology Dept
525 E 68th St/Box 41
New York, NY 10021-0021
Tel: 212 746-4464 *Fax:* 212 746-8167
Accred Length: 2 Years *Program Size:* 2
Program ID: 020-35-21-084

Rochester

University of Rochester Program
Sponsor: Strong Memorial Hospital of the University of Rochester
Program Director:
Stephen I Rosenfeld, MD
Univ of Rochester Med Ctr
601 Elmwood Ave/Box 695
Rochester, NY 14642-8695
Tel: 716 275-2891 *Fax:* 716 273-1070
Internet: http://www.urmc.rochester.edu/smd/air
Accred Length: 2 Years *Program Size:* 2
Program ID: 020-35-11-043

Stony Brook

SUNY at Stony Brook Program
Sponsor: University Hospital-SUNY at Stony Brook
Program Director:
Raymond J Dattwyler, MD
Div of Allergy/Clin Immunology
SUNY Health Sciences Ctr
T16 Rm 040
Stony Brook, NY 11794-8161
Tel: 516 444-3808 *Fax:* 516 444-3475
E-mail: bdagnelli@mail.som.sunysb.edu
Accred Length: 2 Years *Program Size:* 2
Program ID: 020-35-21-089

North Carolina

Durham

Duke University Program
Sponsor: Duke University Medical Center
Program Director:
Rebecca H Buckley, MD
Barton F Haynes, MD
Duke Univ Med Ctr
Div of Ped Allergy/Immunology
Box 2898
Durham, NC 27710
Tel: 919 684-2922 *Fax:* 919 681-7979
E-mail: buckl003@mc.duke.edu
Accred Length: 2 Years *Program Size:* 6
Program ID: 020-36-21-022

Greenville

East Carolina University Program
Sponsor: East Carolina University School of Medicine
Pitt County Memorial Hospital
Program Director:
W James Metzger, MD
East Carolina Univ Sch of Med
Dept of Med/Brody 3E-129
Greenville, NC 27858-4354
Tel: 252 816-3144 *Fax:* 252 816-3481
E-mail: metzger@brody.med.ecu.edu
Accred Length: 2 Years *Program Size:* 2
Program ID: 020-36-21-107

Winston-Salem

Wake Forest University School of Medicine Program
Sponsor: Wake Forest University Baptist Medical Center
Program Director:
John W Georgitis, MD
Wake Forest Univ Baptist Med Ctr
Medical Center Blvd
Winston-Salem, NC 27157
Tel: 336 716-0512 *Fax:* 336 716-7100
E-mail: jgeorgit@bgsm.edu
Accred Length: 2 Years *Program Size:* 2
Program ID: 020-36-11-047

Ohio

Cincinnati

University Hospital/University of Cincinnati College of Medicine Program
Sponsor: University Hospital Inc
Children's Hospital Medical Center
Veterans Affairs Medical Center (Cincinnati)
Program Director:
Amal H Assa'ad, MD
David I Bernstein, MD
Children's Hospital Med Ctr
3333 Burnet Ave
Cincinnati, OH 45229-2899
Tel: 513 636-6771 *Fax:* 513 636-4615
E-mail: assa0@chmcc.org
Accred Length: 2 Years *Program Size:* 4
Program ID: 020-38-21-113

Cleveland

Cleveland Clinic Foundation Program
Sponsor: Cleveland Clinic Foundation
Program Director:
Alton L Melton Jr, MD
Cleveland Clinic Foundation
Dept of Allergy/A72
9500 Euclid Ave
Cleveland, OH 44195-5242
Tel: 216 444-5690 *Fax:* 216 444-1162
E-mail: meded@cestmp.ccf.org
Internet: http://www.ccf.org
Accred Length: 2 Years *Program Size:* 4
Program ID: 020-38-21-104

Pennsylvania

Philadelphia

Children's Hospital of Philadelphia Program
Sponsor: Children's Hospital of Philadelphia
Hospital of the University of Pennsylvania
Program Director:
Nicholas A Pawlowski, MD
Children's Hospital
34th St and Civic Center Blvd
5th Fl Wood Ctr
Philadelphia, PA 19104-4399
Tel: 215 590-2017, ext 1997 *Fax:* 215 590-2025
E-mail: pawlowski@email.chop.edu
Accred Length: 2 Years *Program Size:* 1
Program ID: 020-41-21-074

Thomas Jefferson University Program
Sponsor: Thomas Jefferson University Hospital
Program Director:
Stephen J McGeady, MD
Jefferson Univ
841 Chestnut St
3rd Fl
Philadelphia, PA 19107-5541
Tel: 215 955-6504 *Fax:* 215 923-5816
Accred Length: 2 Years *Program Size:* 4
Program ID: 020-41-11-034

University of Pennsylvania Program
Sponsor: Hospital of the University of Pennsylvania
Program Director:
Arnold Levinson, MD
Univ of Pennsylvania Sch of Med
726 Clinical Research Bldg
415 Curie Blvd
Philadelphia, PA 19104-6144
Tel: 215 898-4592 *Fax:* 215 898-0189
E-mail: frog@mail.med.upenn.edu
Accred Length: 2 Years *Program Size:* 6
Program ID: 020-41-21-075

Pittsburgh

University Health Center of Pittsburgh Program
Sponsor: University Health Center of Pittsburgh
Children's Hospital of Pittsburgh
Program Director:
David P Skoner, MD
Children's Hospital
3705 Fifth Ave
4B 320
Pittsburgh, PA 15213-2583
Tel: 412 692-6850 *Fax:* 412 692-8499
E-mail: jaskom@caplink.chp.edu
Accred Length: 2 Years *Program Size:* 2
Program ID: 020-41-21-076

Tennessee

Memphis

University of Tennessee Program
Sponsor: University of Tennessee College of Medicine
Baptist Memorial Hospital
LeBonheur Children's Medical Center
St Jude Children's Research Hospital
University of Tennessee Medical Center (UT Bowld Hospital)
Veterans Affairs Medical Center (Memphis)
Program Director:
Tai June Yoo, MD PhD
Michael Blaiss, MD
Univ of Tennessee Coll of Med
Div of Allerg/Immunology
956 Court Ave/Rm H300
Memphis, TN 38163
Tel: 901 448-6663 *Fax:* 901 448-5735
E-mail: tyoo@utmeml.utmem.edu
Accred Length: 2 Years *Program Size:* 4
Program ID: 020-47-21-025

Nashville

Vanderbilt University Program
Sponsor: Vanderbilt University Medical Center
Program Director:
Samuel R Marney Jr, MD
Vanderbilt Univ
1500 21st Ave S/Ste 3500 VAV
Nashville, TN 37212-8112
Tel: 615 322-7424 *Fax:* 615 343-0623
E-mail: samuel.m arney@mcmail.vanderbilt.edu
Accred Length: 2 Years *Program Size:* 4
Program ID: 020-47-21-097

Texas

Dallas

University of Texas Southwestern Medical School Program
Sponsor: University of Texas Southwestern Medical School
Children's Medical Center of Dallas
Dallas County Hospital District-Parkland Memorial Hospital
Zale-Lipshy University Hospital
Program Director:
David A Khan, MD
Univ of Texas Southwestern Med Ctr
5323 Harry Hines Blvd
Dallas, TX 75235-8859
Tel: 214 648-3004 *Fax:* 214 648-9100
E-mail: dkhan@mednet.swmed.edu
Accred Length: 2 Years *Program Size:* 4
Program ID: 020-48-21-085

Galveston

University of Texas Medical Branch Hospitals Program
Sponsor: University of Texas Medical Branch Hospitals
Program Director:
Rafeul Alam, MD PhD
Univ of Texas Med Branch Hospitals
301 University Blvd
CSB 409
Galveston, TX 77555-0762
Tel: 409 772-3410 *Fax:* 409 772-5841
E-mail: ralam@utmb.edu
Internet:
http://www.intmed.utmb.edu/division/allergy/allergy.html
Accred Length: 2 Years *Program Size:* 2
Program ID: 020-48-11-026

Houston

Baylor College of Medicine Program
Sponsor: Baylor College of Medicine
Methodist Hospital
Texas Children's Hospital
Program Director:
William T Shearer, MD PhD
David P Huston, MD
Baylor Coll of Med
Dept of Ped/Allergy-Immunology
One Baylor Plaza
Houston, TX 77030
Tel: 713 770-1319 *Fax:* 713 770-1260
E-mail: tmccumber@msmail.is5.tch.tmc.edu
Accred Length: 2 Years *Program Size:* 10
Program ID: 020-48-21-063

Lackland AFB

San Antonio Uniformed Services Health Education Consortium Program
Sponsor: San Antonio Uniformed Services Health Education Consortium
Wilford Hall Medical Center (AETC)
Program Director:
Theodore M Freeman, MD
Wilford Hall Med Ctr/MMIA
2200 Bergquist Dr/Ste 1
Lackland AFB
San Antonio, TX 78236-5300
Tel: 210 292-5717 *Fax:* 210 292-7033
E-mail: freeman_t@whmc-lafb.af.mil
Accred Length: 2 Years *Program Size:* 4
Program ID: 020-48-21-077
US Armed Services Program

Virginia

Charlottesville

University of Virginia Program
Sponsor: University of Virginia Medical Center
Program Director:
Lisa M Wheatley, MD MD
Thomas A Platts-Mills Jr, MD PhD
Univ of Virginia
Allergy/Immunology Dept
Box 225
Charlottesville, VA 22908
Tel: 804 924-2227 *Fax:* 804 924-5779
Accred Length: 2 Years *Program Size:* 4
Program ID: 020-51-21-100

Richmond

Medical College of Virginia/Virginia Commonwealth University Program
Sponsor: Medical College of Virginia/Virginia Commonwealth University
Medical College of Virginia Hospitals
Program Director:
Lawrence B Schwartz, MD PhD
Med Coll of Virginia
Div of Rheum/Allergy/Immun
PO Box 980263
Richmond, VA 23298-0263
Tel: 804 828-9685 *Fax:* 804 828-0283
E-mail: lschwartz@hsc.vcu.edu
Internet: http://www.views.vcu.edu/internal-medicine/
Accred Length: 2 Years *Program Size:* 2
Subspecialties: ALI
Program ID: 020-51-21-056

Washington

Seattle

University of Washington Program
Sponsor: University of Washington School of Medicine
Children's Hospital and Medical Center
University of Washington Medical Center
Program Director:
William R Henderson Jr, MD
Clifton T Furukawa, MD
Univ of Washington Med Ctr
Dept of Med/Box 356523
1959 NE Pacific St
Seattle, WA 98195-6523
Tel: 206 543-3780 *Fax:* 206 685-9318
E-mail: joangb@u.washington.edu
Accred Length: 2 Years *Program Size:* 3
Program ID: 020-54-21-078

Wisconsin

Madison

University of Wisconsin Program

Sponsor: University of Wisconsin Hospital and Clinics
William S Middleton Veterans Hospital

Program Director:
Robert F Lemanske Jr, MD
Univ of Wisconsin Hospital and Clinics
600 Highland Ave/Rm H4-432
Madison, WI 53792-4108
Tel: 608 263-6174 *Fax:* 608 263-3104
E-mail: rfl@medicine.wisc.edu
Internet: http://www.medicine.wisc.edu/sections/allergy/
Accred Length: 2 Years *Program Size:* 5
Program ID: 020-56-21-028

Milwaukee

Medical College of Wisconsin Program

Sponsor: Medical College of Wisconsin Affiliated Hospitals Inc
Children's Hospital of Wisconsin
Clement J Zablocki Veterans Affairs Medical Center
Froedtert Memorial Lutheran Hospital

Program Director:
Kevin J Kelly, MD
Jordan N Fink, MD
Children's Hospital
9000 W Wisconsin Ave
PO Box 1997
Milwaukee, WI 53201
Tel: 414 266-6840 *Fax:* 414 266-6437
Accred Length: 2 Years *Program Size:* 2
Program ID: 020-56-31-037

Anesthesiology

Alabama

Birmingham

University of Alabama Medical Center Program

Sponsor: University of Alabama Hospital
Carraway Methodist Medical Center
Children's Hospital of Alabama
Cooper Green Hospital
Veterans Affairs Medical Center (Birmingham)

Program Director:
David H Chestnut, MD
Univ of Alabama, Dept of Anesth
Jefferson Tower 964
619 S 19th St
Birmingham, AL 35233-6810
Tel: 205 934-6525 *Fax:* 205 975-5963
E-mail: aboudreaux@ms.jt.anes.uab.edu
Internet: http://www.anes.uab.edu
Accred Length: 3 Years *Program Size:* 48
Subspecialties: APM
Program ID: 040-01-21-010

Arizona

Tucson

University of Arizona Program

Sponsor: University of Arizona College of Medicine
Maricopa Medical Center
University Medical Center
Veterans Affairs Medical Center (Tucson)

Program Director:
Steven J Barker, PhD MD
Univ of Arizona Health Sciences Ctr
PO Box 245114
1501 N Campbell Ave
Tucson, AZ 85724-5114
Tel: 520 626-7141 *Fax:* 520 626-6943
E-mail: marthena@u.arizona.edu
Internet: http://www.ahsc.arizona.edu/anesth/
Accred Length: 4 Years *Program Size:* 26
Subspecialties: APM, CCA
Program ID: 040-03-21-012

Arkansas

Little Rock

University of Arkansas for Medical Sciences Program

Sponsor: University of Arkansas College of Medicine
Arkansas Children's Hospital
John L McClellan Memorial Veterans Hospital
University Hospital of Arkansas

Program Director:
Michael L Schmitz, MD
Univ of Arkansas for Med Sciences
4301 W Markham St
Slot 515
Little Rock, AR 72205-7199
Tel: 501 320-2933 *Fax:* 501 320-2939
E-mail: mahnkenestherm@exchange.uams.edu
Internet: http://www.uams.edu
Accred Length: 3 Years *Program Size:* 31 (*GY1:* 7)
Subspecialties: PAN
Program ID: 040-04-21-013

California

Loma Linda

Loma Linda University Program

Sponsor: Loma Linda University Medical Center

Program Director:
Wayne K Jacobsen, MD
Loma Linda Univ Med Ctr
Dept of Anesthesia/Rm 2539
Loma Linda, CA 92354
Tel: 909 824-4475 *Fax:* 909 824-4143
Accred Length: 3 Years *Program Size:* 36
Subspecialties: APM
Program ID: 040-05-21-016

Los Angeles

Charles R Drew University Program

Sponsor: Charles R Drew University of Medicine and Science
LAC-King/Drew Medical Center

Program Director:
Calvin L Johnson, MD
Martin Luther King Jr-Drew Med Ctr
12021 S Wilmington Ave
Los Angeles, CA 90059
Tel: 310 668-4683 *Fax:* 310 764-5906
Accred Length: 4 Years *Program Size:* 10 (*GY1:* 0)
Program ID: 040-05-21-019

UCLA Medical Center Program

Sponsor: UCLA School of Medicine
Cedars-Sinai Medical Center
UCLA Medical Center
VA Greater Los Angeles Healthcare System

Program Director:
Patricia A Kapur, MD
UCLA Sch of Med
Dept of Anesthesiology
Box 951778
Los Angeles, CA 90095-1778
Tel: 310 825-3316 *Fax:* 310 267-1790
E-mail: cdb@anes.ucla.edu
Internet: http://www.anes.ucla.edu
Accred Length: 3 Years *Program Size:* 57
Subspecialties: APM
Program ID: 040-05-21-020

University of Southern California Program

Sponsor: Los Angeles County-USC Medical Center

Program Director:
Ronald L Katz, MD
Los Angeles County-USC Med Ctr
1200 N State St/Rm 14-901
Los Angeles, CA 90033
Tel: 323 226-4597 *Fax:* 323 226-2794
E-mail: merit@hsc.edu
Internet:
http://www.usc.edu/hsc/medicine/anesthesiology
Accred Length: 4 Years *Program Size:* 55
Program ID: 040-05-21-018

Programs

Orange

University of California (Irvine) Program
Sponsor: University of California (Irvine) Medical Center
San Bernardino County Medical Center
Veterans Affairs Medical Center (Long Beach)
Program Director:
Elizabeth C Behringer, MD
Univ of California Irvine Med Ctr
101 The City Dr S/Bldg 53 Rm 227
Orange, CA 92868
Tel: 714 456-7568 *Fax:* 714 456-7702
E-mail: ebehring@uci.edu
Internet: http://www.com.uci.edu
Accred Length: 3 Years *Program Size:* 28
Subspecialties: APM, CCA
Program ID: 040-05-21-015

Sacramento

University of California (Davis) Program
Sponsor: University of California (Davis) Medical Center
Program Director:
Peter G Moore, MD PhD
Univ of California Davis Med Ctr
PSSB Ste 1200
4150 V St
Sacramento, CA 95817
Tel: 916 734-5169 *Fax:* 916 734-7980
E-mail: smgaskins@ucdavis.edu
Internet: http://www.anesthesiology.ucdmc.ucdavis.edu/
Accred Length: 3 Years *Program Size:* 24
Subspecialties: APM
Program ID: 040-05-21-014

San Diego

Naval Medical Center (San Diego) Program
Sponsor: Naval Medical Center (San Diego)
Program Director:
David Leivers, MD
Naval Med Ctr
Dept of Anesthesia
San Diego, CA 92134-5000
Tel: 619 532-8941 *Fax:* 619 532-8945
E-mail: dleivers@snd10.med.navy.mil.
Accred Length: 3 Years *Program Size:* 17
Program ID: 040-05-21-006
US Armed Services Program

University of California (San Diego) Program
Sponsor: University of California (San Diego) Medical Center
Children's Hospital and Health Center
Veterans Affairs Medical Center (San Diego)
Program Director:
John C Drummond, MD
UCSD Med Ctr
200 W Arbor Dr
San Diego, CA 92103-8770
Tel: 619 543-5297 *Fax:* 619 543-5424
Internet: http://anes-lxin.ucsd.edu/
Accred Length: 4 Years *Program Size:* 25
Subspecialties: APM
Program ID: 040-05-21-022

San Francisco

University of California (San Francisco) Program
Sponsor: University of California (San Francisco) School of Medicine
Mount Zion Medical Center of the University of California
San Francisco General Hospital Medical Center
University of California (San Francisco) Medical Center
Program Director:
Ronald D Miller, MD
513 Parnassus Ave
Rm S-436/Box 0648
San Francisco, CA 94143-0648
Tel: 415 476-3235 *Fax:* 415 502-5375
E-mail: janet_molinari@quickmail.ucsf.edu
Internet: http://anesthesia.ucsf.edu/anesthweb
Accred Length: 4 Years *Program Size:* 66
Subspecialties: APM, CCA
Program ID: 040-05-21-023

Stanford

Stanford University Program
Sponsor: Stanford University Hospital
Santa Clara Valley Medical Center
Veterans Affairs Palo Alto Health Care System
Program Director:
Donald R Stanski, MD
Stanford Univ Med Ctr
300 Pasteur Dr/Rm H3580
Stanford, CA 94305-5117
Tel: 650 723-7377 *Fax:* 650 725-8544
Internet:
http://www.-leland.stanford.edu/dept/anesthesia
Accred Length: 3 Years *Program Size:* 47
Subspecialties: APM, CCA, PAN
Program ID: 040-05-21-025

Torrance

Los Angeles County-Harbor-UCLA Medical Center Program
Sponsor: Los Angeles County-Harbor-UCLA Medical Center
Program Director:
Elaine C Yang, MD
Los Angeles County-Harbor-UCLA Med Ctr
Box 10
1000 W Carson St
Torrance, CA 90509-2910
Tel: 310 222-3472 *Fax:* 310 782-1467
Accred Length: 4 Years *Program Size:* 12
Program ID: 040-05-11-026

Colorado

Denver

University of Colorado Program
Sponsor: University of Colorado Health Sciences Center
Denver Health and Hospitals
Veterans Affairs Medical Center (Denver)
Program Director:
Charles P Gibbs, MD
Univ of Colorado Health Sciences Ctr
Dept of Anesth/B113
4200 E Ninth Ave
Denver, CO 80262
Tel: 303 394-8275 *Fax:* 303 270-8329
E-mail: jhratterree@ski.uhcolorado.edu
Internet: http://www.uchsc.edu/sm/anesth
Accred Length: 3 Years *Program Size:* 36
Subspecialties: APM, PAN
Program ID: 040-07-21-028

Connecticut

Farmington

University of Connecticut Program
Sponsor: University of Connecticut School of Medicine
Connecticut Children's Medical Center
Hartford Hospital
St Francis Hospital and Medical Center
Univ of Connecticut Health Center/John Dempsey Hospital
Program Director:
Richard B Lilly, MD
Univ of Connecticut Sch of Med
263 Farmington Ave
Farmington, CT 06030-2015
Tel: 860 679-3597 *Fax:* 860 679-1275
Internet:
http://www.resprog.uchc.edu/md/anesthesiology/home.html
Accred Length: 3 Years *Program Size:* 24
Program ID: 040-08-21-172

New Haven

Yale-New Haven Medical Center Program
Sponsor: Yale-New Haven Hospital
Veterans Affairs Medical Center (West Haven)
Program Director:
Abraham L Mandel, MD
Yale-New Haven Med Ctr, Dept of Anesth
PO Box 3333
New Haven, CT 06501-8110
Tel: 203 785-2802 *Fax:* 203 785-6664
Internet: http://info.med.yale.edu/anesthes/
Accred Length: 3 Years *Program Size:* 50
Subspecialties: APM, CCA, PAN
Program ID: 040-08-21-030

District of Columbia

Washington

George Washington University Program
Sponsor: George Washington University School of Medicine
George Washington University Hospital (UHS)
Program Director:
Michael J Berrigan, PhD MD
George Washington Univ Med Ctr
901 23rd St NW
Washington, DC 20037
Tel: 202 994-3134 *Fax:* 202 994-5620
E-mail: berrigan@gwis2.circ.gwu.edu
Internet: http://www.gwumc.edu
Accred Length: 3 Years *Program Size:* 21
Subspecialties: CCA, PAN
Program ID: 040-10-21-033

Georgetown University Program
Sponsor: Georgetown University Medical Center
Program Director:
David E Lees, MD
Georgetown Univ Hospital
3800 Reservoir Rd NW
Washington, DC 20007
Tel: 202 687-8556 *Fax:* 202 687-8854
E-mail: leesd@gunet.georgetown.edu
Internet:
http://www.dm1.georgetown.edu/depts/anesthesia/residency
Accred Length: 4 Years *Program Size:* 13
Subspecialties: APM
Program ID: 040-10-21-032

Howard University Program
Sponsor: Howard University Hospital
Program Director:
Melville Q Wyche Jr, MD
Howard Univ Hospital
2041 Georgia Ave NW/Ste B105
Washington, DC 20060
Tel: 202 865-6711 *Fax:* 202 865-6713
Accred Length: 4 Years *Program Size:* 19 (*GY1:* 2)
Program ID: 040-10-11-034

Florida

Gainesville

University of Florida Program
Sponsor: University of Florida College of Medicine
Shands Hospital at the University of Florida
Veterans Affairs Medical Center (Gainesville)
Program Director:
Nikolaus Gravenstein, MD
Univ of Florida
Dept of Anesthesiology
1600 SW Archer Rd
Gainesville, FL 32610-0254
Tel: 352 395-0077 *Fax:* 352 395-6922
E-mail: mahla@anest2.anest.ufl.edu
Internet: http://www.anest.ufl.edu
Accred Length: 4 Years *Program Size:* 68 (*GY1:* 12)
Subspecialties: APM, CCA, PAN
Program ID: 040-11-21-035

Miami

University of Miami-Jackson Memorial Medical Center Program
Sponsor: University of Miami-Jackson Memorial Medical Center
Miami Children's Hospital
Mount Sinai Medical Center of Greater Miami
Veterans Affairs Medical Center (Miami)
Program Director:
N W Brian Craythorne, MD
Univ of Miami Sch of Med
PO Box 016370
R370
Miami, FL 33101
Tel: 305 585-6970 *Fax:* 305 545-6753
E-mail: lpatton@umdas.med.miami.edu
Internet: http://umdas.med.miami.edu
Accred Length: 4 Years *Program Size:* 104 (*GY1:* 10)
Subspecialties: APM, CCA, PAN
Program ID: 040-11-21-036

Tampa

University of South Florida Program
Sponsor: University of South Florida College of Medicine
H Lee Moffitt Cancer Center
Tampa General Healthcare
Program Director:
John B Downs, MD
Univ of South Florida Med Ctr
MDC 59
12901 Bruce B Downs Blvd
Tampa, FL 33612-4799
Tel: 813 251-7082 *Fax:* 813 251-7418
E-mail: casanova@com1.med.usf.edu
Internet:
http://www.med.usf.edu/anesthesiology/index.html
Accred Length: 4 Years *Program Size:* 52 (*GY1:* 10)
Subspecialties: APM, CCA
Program ID: 040-11-21-178

Georgia

Atlanta

Emory University Program
Sponsor: Emory University School of Medicine
Egleston Children's Hospital at Emory University
Emory University Hospital
Grady Memorial Hospital
Program Director:
John L Waller, MD
Emory Univ Sch of Med
Dept of Anesthesiology
1364 Clifton Rd NE
Atlanta, GA 30322
Tel: 404 778-3378 *Fax:* 404 778-5405
E-mail: barbara_jones@emory.org
Internet:
http://www.cc.emory.edu/whsc/med/anesthesiology/index.html
Accred Length: 3 Years *Program Size:* 42
Subspecialties: APM, CCA
Program ID: 040-12-21-037

Augusta

Medical College of Georgia Program
Sponsor: Medical College of Georgia Hospital and Clinics
Veterans Affairs Medical Center (Augusta)
Program Director:
Robert S Crumrine, MD
Med Coll of Georgia
Dept of Anesthesiology
1120 15th St/BIW-2144
Augusta, GA 30912-2700
Tel: 706 721-4544 *Fax:* 706 721-7753
E-mail: sdawkins@mail.mcg.edu
Accred Length: 4 Years *Program Size:* 16 (*GY1:* 4)
Subspecialties: APM
Program ID: 040-12-11-038

Illinois

Chicago

Cook County Hospital Program
Sponsor: Cook County Hospital
Program Director:
Alon P Winnie, MD
Cook County Hospital
Dept of Anesthesiology
1835 W Harrison St
Chicago, IL 60612-9985
Tel: 312 633-6176 *Fax:* 312 633-5773
Internet: http://www.cookcountyhospital.edu
Accred Length: 4 Years *Program Size:* 28 (*GY1:* 7)
Program ID: 040-16-12-039

Illinois Masonic Medical Center Program
Sponsor: Illinois Masonic Medical Center
Program Director:
M Ramez Salem, MD
Illinois Masonic Med Ctr
Dept of Anesthesiology
836 W Wellington Ave
Chicago, IL 60657-5193
Tel: 773 296-7035 *Fax:* 773 296-5088
E-mail: dmartin@immc.org
Internet: http://www.immc.org
Accred Length: 4 Years *Program Size:* 26
Program ID: 040-16-21-040

McGaw Medical Center of Northwestern University Program
Sponsor: Northwestern University Medical School
Children's Memorial Medical Center
Evanston Hospital
Northwestern Memorial Hospital
Veterans Affairs Lakeside Medical Center (Chicago)
Program Director:
Barry A Shapiro, MD
Northwestern Univ Med Sch
303 E Superior St/Ste 360
Chicago, IL 60611-3053
Tel: 312 908-8254 *Fax:* 312 908-3233
Internet: http://www.careermd.com1
Accred Length: 4 Years *Program Size:* 39
Subspecialties: APM, CCA
Program ID: 040-16-21-042

Rush-Presbyterian-St Luke's Medical Center Program
Sponsor: Rush-Presbyterian-St Luke's Medical Center
Program Director:
Anthony D Ivankovich, MD
1653 W Congress Pkwy
Chicago, IL 60612
Tel: 312 942-6504 *Fax:* 312 942-8858
Accred Length: 4 Years *Program Size:* 49 (*GY1:* 12)
Subspecialties: APM
Program ID: 040-16-21-043

University of Chicago Program
Sponsor: University of Chicago Hospitals
Program Director:
Michael F Roizen, MD
Univ of Chicago
5841 S Maryland Ave/MC4028
Chicago, IL 60637-1470
Tel: 773 702-6700 *Fax:* 773 834-0063
E-mail: webmaster@dacc.bsd.uchicago.edu
Internet: http://www.webmaster@dacc.bsd.uchicago.edu
Accred Length: 4 Years *Program Size:* 52 (*GY1:* 7)
Subspecialties: APM
Program ID: 040-16-11-044

University of Illinois College of Medicine at Chicago Program
Sponsor: University of Illinois College of Medicine at Chicago
Michael Reese Hospital and Medical Center
University of Illinois Hospital and Clinics
Program Director:
Ronald F Albrecht, MD
Univ of Illinois-Chicago Coll of Med
Dept of Anesth (M/C 515)
1740 W Taylor St
Chicago, IL 60612-7239
Tel: 312 996-4021 *Fax:* 312 996-4019
E-mail: mouse@uic.edu
Accred Length: 4 Years *Program Size:* 77 (*GY1:* 18)
Subspecialties: APM
Program ID: 040-16-11-041

Maywood

Loyola University Program
Sponsor: Loyola University Medical Center
Edward J Hines Jr Veterans Affairs Hospital
Program Director:
Stephen Slogoff, MD
Loyola Univ Med Ctr
Dept of Anesthesiology
2160 S First Ave
Maywood, IL 60153
Tel: 708 216-9169 *Fax:* 708 216-1249
E-mail: sslogof@luc.edu
Accred Length: 4 Years *Program Size:* 18 (*GY1:* 2)
Subspecialties: APM
Program ID: 040-16-11-046

Programs

Indiana

Indianapolis

Indiana University School of Medicine Program

Sponsor: Indiana University School of Medicine
Clarian IU Hospital
Clarian Riley Hospital for Children
Richard L Roudebush Veterans Affairs Medical Center
William N Wishard Memorial Hospital

Program Director:
Robert K Stoelting, MD
Indiana Univ Sch of Med
1120 South Dr/FH 204
Indianapolis, IN 46202-5115
Tel: 317 274-0269 *Fax:* 317 274-0256
E-mail: robert_stoelting@anesthesia.iupui.edu
Internet: http://www.iupui.edu/~anesth/index.html
Accred Length: 4 Years *Program Size:* 67
Subspecialties: APM
Program ID: 040-17-21-048

Iowa

Iowa City

University of Iowa Hospitals and Clinics Program

Sponsor: University of Iowa Hospitals and Clinics
Veterans Affairs Medical Center (Iowa City)

Program Director:
David L Brown, MD
Univ of Iowa Hospitals and Clinics
Dept of Anesthesia
200 Hawkins Dr
Iowa City, IA 52242-1009
Tel: 319 356-2633 *Fax:* 319 356-2940
E-mail: david-brown@uiowa.edu
Internet: http://www.anesth.uiowa.edu
Accred Length: 4 Years *Program Size:* 48 (*GY1:* 12)
Subspecialties: APM, CCA
Program ID: 040-18-21-049

Kansas

Kansas City

University of Kansas Medical Center Program

Sponsor: University of Kansas School of Medicine
University of Kansas Medical Center

Program Director:
Kirk T Benson, MD
Univ of Kansas Med Ctr
3901 Rainbow Blvd
Kansas City, KS 66160-7415
Tel: 913 588-3304 *Fax:* 913 588-3365
E-mail: pcampbell@kumc.edu
Internet: http://www.kumc.edu/anes
Accred Length: 3 Years *Program Size:* 15
Program ID: 040-19-11-050

Wichita

University of Kansas (Wichita) Program

Sponsor: University of Kansas School of Medicine (Wichita)
Columbia Wesley Medical Center
Via Christi Regional Medical Center
Via Christi Regional Medical Center-St Joseph

Program Director:
Byran L Black, MD
Dept of Anesthesiology
929 N St Francis/Rm 8074
Wichita, KS 67214-3882
Tel: 316 268-6147 *Fax:* 316 291-7759
E-mail: anesthe1@kumc.edu
Internet: http://www.kumc.edu/wichita/dept/anes/
Accred Length: 4 Years *Program Size:* 7 (*GY1:* 3)
Program ID: 040-19-22-051

Kentucky

Lexington

University of Kentucky Medical Center Program

Sponsor: University of Kentucky Hospital

Program Director:
William O Witt, MD
Univ of Kentucky-Albert B Chandler Med Ctr
800 Rose St/Rm N 202
Lexington, KY 40536-0293
Tel: 606 323-5956, ext 123 *Fax:* 606 323-1080
Internet: http://www.anes.uky.edu
Accred Length: 4 Years *Program Size:* 32
Subspecialties: APM
Program ID: 040-20-21-052

Louisville

University of Louisville Program

Sponsor: University of Louisville School of Medicine
Kosair Children's Hospital (Alliant Health System)
University of Louisville Hospital
Veterans Affairs Medical Center (Louisville)

Program Director:
Benjamin M Rigor, MD
Univ of Louisville Sch of Med
Dept of Anesthesiology
545 S Jackson St/Ste 100
Louisville, KY 40202-3617
Tel: 502 852-5851 *Fax:* 502 852-6056
Internet: http://www.louisville.edu/medschool/anesth/
Accred Length: 4 Years *Program Size:* 23
Program ID: 040-20-21-053

Louisiana

New Orleans

Alton Ochsner Medical Foundation Program

Sponsor: Alton Ochsner Medical Foundation

Program Director:
James R Douglas Jr, MD PhD
Alton Ochsner Med Foundation
Dept of Grad Med Educ
1516 Jefferson Hwy
New Orleans, LA 70121
Tel: 504 842-3260 *Fax:* 504 842-3193
E-mail: dlambert@ochsner.org
Internet: http://www.oschner.org
Accred Length: 4 Years *Program Size:* 13 (*GY1:* 3)
Program ID: 040-21-12-055

Tulane University Program

Sponsor: Tulane University School of Medicine
Medical Center of Louisiana at New Orleans
Tulane University Hospital and Clinics

Program Director:
Melvin C Gitlin, MD
Tulane Univ Sch of Med
1430 Tulane Ave
New Orleans, LA 70112-2699
Tel: 504 588-5904 *Fax:* 504 584-3501
Internet: http://www.tmc.tulane.edu/anes
Accred Length: 4 Years *Program Size:* 30
Program ID: 040-21-31-168

Shreveport

Louisiana State University (Shreveport) Program

Sponsor: Louisiana State University Hospital-Shreveport

Program Director:
Randall C Cork, MD PhD
Louisiana State Univ Med Ctr Hospital
1501 Kings Hwy
PO Box 33932
Shreveport, LA 71130-3932
Tel: 318 675-5300 *Fax:* 318 675-6681
E-mail: mharri6@lsumc.edu
Internet: http://www.anesthesia.lsumc.edu
Accred Length: 3 Years *Program Size:* 14
Subspecialties: APM
Program ID: 040-21-11-056

Maine

Portland

Maine Medical Center Program

Sponsor: Maine Medical Center

Program Director:
Kenneth L Raessler, MD
Maine Med Ctr
22 Bramhall St
Portland, ME 04102-3175
Tel: 207 871-2526 *Fax:* 207 871-6236
Accred Length: 4 Years *Program Size:* 11 (*GY1:* 2)
Program ID: 040-22-11-057

Maryland

Baltimore

Johns Hopkins University Program

Sponsor: Johns Hopkins University School of Medicine
Johns Hopkins Bayview Medical Center
Johns Hopkins Hospital

Program Director:
Edward D Miller Jr, MD
Dept of Anes/Critical Care Med
Johns Hopkins Hospital
600 N Wolfe St/Blalock 1415
Baltimore, MD 21287-4963
Tel: 410 955-7609 *Fax:* 410 955-5607
E-mail: jkirsch@welchlink.welch.jhu.edu
Internet: http://www.med.jhu.edu/anesthesiology
Accred Length: 4 Years *Program Size:* 66
Subspecialties: APM, CCA, PAN
Program ID: 040-23-21-058

University of Maryland Program
Sponsor: University of Maryland Medical System
Program Director:
Jane Matjasko, MD
Univ of Maryland
Dept of Anesthesiology
22 S Greene St/Box 253
Baltimore, MD 21201
Tel: 410 328-6120 *Fax:* 410 328-5531
Internet: http://anesthesia.ummc.ab.umd.edu
Accred Length: 3 Years *Program Size:* 21
Subspecialties: APM, CCA
Program ID: 040-23-11-059

Bethesda

National Capital Consortium Program
Sponsor: National Capital Consortium
National Naval Medical Center (Bethesda)
Walter Reed Army Medical Center
Program Director:
Alvin R Manalaysay, MD
National Naval Med Ctr
8901 Wisconsin Ave
Bethesda, MD 20889
Tel: 301 295-4455 *Fax:* 301 295-5063
E-mail: bth0plm@bth12.med.navy.mil
Accred Length: 3 Years *Program Size:* 36
Program ID: 040-10-21-190
US Armed Services Program

Massachusetts

Boston

Beth Israel Deaconess Medical Center Program
Sponsor: Beth Israel Deaconess Medical Center
Program Director:
Leonard S Bushnell, MD
Beth Israel Deaconess Med Ctr
Dept of Anes/Critical Care
330 Brookline Ave
Boston, MA 02215
Tel: 617 754-2713 *Fax:* 617 667-5013
Internet:
http://www.harvard.med.edu/programs/anesthesia/bih
Accred Length: 4 Years *Program Size:* 47
Subspecialties: APM, CCA
Program ID: 040-24-11-060

Boston University Medical Center Program
Sponsor: Boston Medical Center
Program Director:
Keith P Lewis, MD MBA
Boston Med Ctr
Anesthesiology Dept
One Boston Medical Center Pl
Boston, MA 02118-2393
Tel: 617 638-6950 *Fax:* 617 638-6959
Internet: http://www.bmc.org/anesthesia
Accred Length: 3 Years *Program Size:* 14
Program ID: 040-24-21-062

Brigham and Women's Hospital Program
Sponsor: Brigham and Women's Hospital
Program Director:
Simon Gelman, MD PhD
Brigham and Women's Hospital
Attn: Eileen Stanford, Registrar
75 Francis St
Boston, MA 02115
Tel: 617 732-8210 *Fax:* 617 730-9534
E-mail: eileen@zeus.bwh.harvard.edu
Internet: http://zeus.bwh.harvard.edu
Accred Length: 4 Years *Program Size:* 80
Subspecialties: APM, CCA
Program ID: 040-24-21-066

Massachusetts General Hospital Program
Sponsor: Massachusetts General Hospital
Program Director:
Warren M Zapol, MD
Massachusetts General Hospital
Dept of Anesthesia/Critical Care
Fruit St
Boston, MA 02114
Tel: 617 726-3030 *Fax:* 617 726-3032
Internet: http://www.mghdacc.com
Accred Length: 3 Years *Program Size:* 66
Subspecialties: APM, CCA
Program ID: 040-24-31-064

New England Medical Center Hospitals Program
Sponsor: New England Medical Center Hospitals
Program Director:
W Heinrich Wurm, MD
New England Med Ctr
750 Washington St
NEMC Box 298
Boston, MA 02111
Tel: 617 636-6044 *Fax:* 617 636-8384
E-mail: ralph.yarnell@es.nemc.org
Internet: http://www.nemc.org/anes/anesres.htm
Accred Length: 3 Years *Program Size:* 12
Subspecialties: APM, PAN
Program ID: 040-24-21-065

St Elizabeth's Medical Center of Boston Program
Sponsor: St Elizabeth's Medical Center of Boston
Program Director:
David J Cullen, MD MS
St Elizabeth's Med Ctr
736 Cambridge St
CMP2A
Boston, MA 02135-2997
Tel: 617 789-2777 *Fax:* 617 254-6384
E-mail: ppatters@semc.org
Internet: http://www.semc.org
Accred Length: 4 Years *Program Size:* 30
Program ID: 040-24-21-067

Springfield

Baystate Medical Center Program
Sponsor: Baystate Medical Center
Program Director:
Prasad R Kilaru, MD
Dept of Anesthesiology
759 Chestnut St
Springfield, MA 01199
Tel: 413 794-4326 *Fax:* 413 794-5349
E-mail: kristen.kolb@bhs.org
Internet: http://www.baystatehealth.com
Accred Length: 4 Years *Program Size:* 27 (*GYI:* 6)
Subspecialties: APM
Program ID: 040-24-12-069

Worcester

University of Massachusetts Program
Sponsor: University of Massachusetts Medical School
UMass Memorial Health Care (University Campus)
Program Director:
Philomena M Verghese, MD
Univ of Massachusetts Med Sch
Dept of Anesthesiology
55 Lake Ave N
Worcester, MA 01655
Tel: 508 856-3821 *Fax:* 508 856-5911
Accred Length: 4 Years *Program Size:* 18
Subspecialties: APM, CCA
Program ID: 040-24-31-070

Michigan

Ann Arbor

University of Michigan Program
Sponsor: University of Michigan Hospitals
Program Director:
Kevin K Tremper, PhD MD
1G323 UH 0048
1500 E Medical Center Dr
Ann Arbor, MI 48109-0048
Tel: 313 936-4280 *Fax:* 313 936-9091
Internet: http://www.anes.med.umich.edu/
Accred Length: 4 Years *Program Size:* 59
Subspecialties: APM, CCA, PAN
Program ID: 040-25-21-071

Detroit

Henry Ford Hospital Program
Sponsor: Henry Ford Hospital
Program Director:
Fathy S Gabriel, MD BS
Henry Ford Hospital
Dept of Anesthesiology
2799 W Grand Blvd
Detroit, MI 48202
Tel: 313 876-7648 *Fax:* 313 556-9867
Accred Length: 4 Years *Program Size:* 18 (*GYI:* 6)
Subspecialties: APM, CCA
Program ID: 040-25-21-185

Wayne State University/Detroit Medical Center Program
Sponsor: Wayne State University/Detroit Medical Center
Program Director:
H Michael Marsh, MD
Sinai Hospital
6767 W Outer Dr
Detroit, MI 48235
Tel: 313 493-5335 *Fax:* 313 493-5112
Accred Length: 4 Years *Program Size:* 22 (*GYI:* 9)
Subspecialties: CCA
Program ID: 040-25-31-073

Minnesota

Minneapolis

University of Minnesota Program

Sponsor: University of Minnesota Medical School
Fairview-University Medical Center
Hennepin County Medical Center

Program Director:
Richard J Palahniuk, MD
Univ of Minnesota Hospital and Clinics
420 Delaware St SE
Box 294 UMHC
Minneapolis, MN 55455-0392
Tel: 612 624-9990 *Fax:* 612 626-2363
E-mail: palah001@maroon.tc.umn.edu
Internet: http://www.umn.edu/anesthes/anes_hp.thml
Accred Length: 4 Years *Program Size:* 22 (*GY1:* 4)
Program ID: 040-26-31-075

Rochester

Mayo Graduate School of Medicine (Rochester) Program

Sponsor: Mayo Graduate School of Medicine-Mayo Foundation
Mayo Clinic (Jacksonville)
Mayo Clinic (Rochester)
Mayo Clinic (Scottsdale)
Rochester Methodist Hospital
Scottsdale Healthcare-Shea
St Luke's Hospital
St Mary's Hospital of Rochester

Program Director:
Duane K Rorie, MD PhD
Application Processing Ctr
Mayo Graduate Sch of Med
200 First St SW
Rochester, MN 55905
Tel: 507 255-6219 *Fax:* 507 255-2939
E-mail: mgsm.roch.mn.anesthesiology@mayo.edu
Internet: http://www.mayo.edu/
Accred Length: 4 Years *Program Size:* 64 (*GY1:* 7)
Subspecialties: APM, CCA
Program ID: 040-26-21-076

Mississippi

Jackson

University of Mississippi Medical Center Program

Sponsor: University of Mississippi School of Medicine
University Hospital

Program Director:
John H Eichhorn, MD
Univ of Mississippi Med Ctr
Dept of Anesthesiology
2500 N State St
Jackson, MS 39216-4505
Tel: 601 984-5900 *Fax:* 601 984-5912
E-mail: cgriffin@anesthesia.umsmed.edu
Accred Length: 4 Years *Program Size:* 27 (*GY1:* 7)
Program ID: 040-27-11-077

Missouri

Columbia

University of Missouri-Columbia Program

Sponsor: University of Missouri-Columbia School of Medicine
University Hospitals and Clinics

Program Director:
Noel W Lawson, MD
Univ of Missouri-Columbia
Anesthesiology/DC00500
One Hospital Dr
Columbia, MO 65212
Tel: 573 882-2568 *Fax:* 573 882-2226
Internet: http://www.missouri.edu/~anespp
Accred Length: 4 Years *Program Size:* 12 (*GY1:* 4)
Program ID: 040-28-11-078

Kansas City

University of Missouri at Kansas City Program

Sponsor: University of Missouri-Kansas City School of Medicine
Saint Luke's Hospital
Truman Medical Center-West

Program Director:
Eugene E Fibuch, MD
St Luke's Hospital
44th and Wornall Rd
Kansas City, MO 64111
Tel: 816 932-5132 *Fax:* 816 932-5179
E-mail: lyoung@saint-lukes.org
Internet: http://www.umkc.edu/
Accred Length: 4 Years *Program Size:* 24 (*GY1:* 6)
Program ID: 040-28-12-080

St Louis

St Louis University School of Medicine Program

Sponsor: St Louis University School of Medicine
SSM Cardinal Glennon Children's Hospital
St Louis University School of Medicine

Program Director:
Lawrence J Baudendistel, MD PhD
St Louis Univ Sch of Med
3635 Vista Ave
PO Box 15250
St Louis, MO 63110-0250
Tel: 314 577-8750 *Fax:* 314 268-5102
E-mail: elmorejr@slucare1.sluh.edu
Internet: http://www.anesthesia.sluh.edu
Accred Length: 4 Years *Program Size:* 33
Program ID: 040-28-21-166

Washington University/B-JH/SLCH Consortium Program

Sponsor: Washington University/B-JH/SLCH Consortium
Barnes-Jewish Hospital

Program Director:
James M Shear, MD
Washington Univ Sch of Med
660 S Euclid Ave/Box 8054
St Louis, MO 63110
Tel: 800 329-5971 *Fax:* 314 362-1185
Internet: http://www.anest.wuslt.edu
Accred Length: 3 Years *Program Size:* 24
Subspecialties: APM, CCA
Program ID: 040-28-11-081

Nebraska

Omaha

University of Nebraska Program

Sponsor: University of Nebraska Medical Center

Program Director:
John H Tinker, MD
Univ of Nebraska Med Ctr
Dept of Anesthesiology
984455 Nebraska Med Ctr
Omaha, NE 68198-4455
Tel: 402 559-7405 *Fax:* 402 559-7372
E-mail: jchapin@unmc.edu
Internet: http://www.unmc.edu/gme/anesth-web.htm
Accred Length: 3 Years *Program Size:* 22
Subspecialties: APM
Program ID: 040-30-11-082

New Hampshire

Lebanon

Dartmouth-Hitchcock Medical Center Program

Sponsor: Mary Hitchcock Memorial Hospital

Program Director:
D David Glass, MD
Dartmouth-Hitchcock Med Ctr
One Medical Center Dr
Lebanon, NH 03756
Tel: 603 650-6177 *Fax:* 603 650-8980
E-mail: lisa.wirth@hitchcock.org
Internet:
http://www.hitchcock.org./pages/anes/deptofanes.html
Accred Length: 4 Years *Program Size:* 18
Subspecialties: APM, CCA
Program ID: 040-32-11-083

New Jersey

Livingston

St Barnabas Medical Center Program

Sponsor: St Barnabas Medical Center

Program Director:
Norman J Zeig, MD
St Barnabas Med Ctr
Dept of Anesthesiology
94 Old Short Hills Rd/1002
Livingston, NJ 07039
Tel: 973 322-5512 *Fax:* 973 322-8165
E-mail: nzeig@sbhcs.com
Accred Length: 4 Years *Program Size:* 9
Program ID: 040-33-12-085

Newark

UMDNJ-New Jersey Medical School Program

Sponsor: UMDNJ-New Jersey Medical School
UMDNJ-University Hospital

Program Director:
Philip Liu, MD
UMDNJ-New Jersey Med Sch
185 S Orange Ave/MSB E-538
Newark, NJ 07103-2714
Tel: 973 972-5006 *Fax:* 973 972-4172
E-mail: liuph@umdnj.edu
Internet: http://www.umdnj.edu/anesnweb/title.htm
Accred Length: 4 Years *Program Size:* 33 (*GY1:* 9)
Subspecialties: APM
Program ID: 040-33-21-087

Paterson

St Joseph's Hospital and Medical Center Program
Sponsor: St Joseph's Hospital and Medical Center
St Elizabeth Hospital
Program Director:
Anna Stanec, MD
St Joseph's Hospital and Med Ctr
703 Main St
Paterson, NJ 07503
Tel: 973 754-2323 *Fax:* 973 977-9455
Accred Length: 4 Years *Program Size:* 19 (*GY1:* 1)
Program ID: 040-33-21-089

Piscataway

UMDNJ-Robert Wood Johnson Medical School Program
Sponsor: UMDNJ-Robert Wood Johnson Medical School
Robert Wood Johnson University Hospital
Program Director:
Sanford L Klein, MD DDS
UMDNJ-Robert Wood Johnson Med Sch
Dept of Anesthesia CAB/Ste 3100
125 Paterson St
New Brunswick, NJ 08901-1977
Tel: 732 235-7827 *Fax:* 732 235-6131
E-mail: sklein@umdnj.edu
Internet: http://www2.umdnj.edu/anes web /watch fire. htm.
Accred Length: 4 Years *Program Size:* 24 (*GY1:* 6)
Subspecialties: APM, CCA
Program ID: 040-33-21-180

New Mexico

Albuquerque

University of New Mexico Program
Sponsor: University of New Mexico School of Medicine
Veterans Affairs Medical Center (Albuquerque)
Program Director:
Stephen E Abram, MD
Univ of New Mexico Sch of Med
2701 Frontier Blvd NE
Suge Bldg/Rm 110
Albuquerque, NM 87131
Tel: 505 272-2610 *Fax:* 505 272-1300
E-mail: jfabian@salud.unm.edu
Internet:
http://macbeth.unm.edu/som/gme/anesthesiology.html
Accred Length: 4 Years *Program Size:* 24 (*GY1:* 6)
Subspecialties: APM, PAN
Program ID: 040-34-21-183

New York

Albany

Albany Medical Center Program
Sponsor: Albany Medical Center
Program Director:
Kevin Roberts, MD MD
Albany Med Ctr Hospital
Dept of Anesth(131)
47 New Scotland Ave
Albany, NY 12208-3478
Tel: 518 262-4302 *Fax:* 518 262-4736
E-mail: kushniv@mail.amc.edu
Internet: http://www.albanyanesth.com
Accred Length: 4 Years *Program Size:* 16
Subspecialties: APM, CCA
Program ID: 040-35-21-167

Bronx

Albert Einstein College of Medicine Program
Sponsor: Albert Einstein College of Medicine of Yeshiva University
Jacobi Medical Center
Montefiore Medical Center-Henry and Lucy Moses Division
Montefiore Medical Center-Weiler Hospital
Program Director:
Albert J Saubermann, MD
Albert Einstein Coll of Med
Montefiore Med Ctr
111 E 210th St
Bronx, NY 10467
Tel: 718 920-4383 *Fax:* 718 881-2245
E-mail: asauberm@montefiore.org
Accred Length: 3 Years *Program Size:* 45
Subspecialties: APM, CCA
Program ID: 040-35-21-181

Brooklyn

Brookdale University Hospital Medical Center Program
Sponsor: Brookdale University Hospital Medical Center
Program Director:
Adel R Abadir, MD
Brookdale Univ Hospital and Med Ctr
1 Brookdale Plaza/Rm 727 CHC
Brooklyn, NY 11212
Tel: 718 240-5356 *Fax:* 718 240-5367
Accred Length: 4 Years *Program Size:* 33 (*GY1:* 0)
Subspecialties: APM
Program ID: 040-35-31-097

Maimonides Medical Center Program
Sponsor: Maimonides Medical Center
Coney Island Hospital
Program Director:
Ketan Shevde, MD
Dept of Anesthesiology
4802 Tenth Ave
Brooklyn, NY 11219
Tel: 718 283-8301 *Fax:* 718 283-8377
E-mail: ksheve@maimonidesmed.org
Accred Length: 3 Years *Program Size:* 21
Program ID: 040-35-11-101

New York Methodist Hospital Program
Sponsor: New York Methodist Hospital
Program Director:
Joseph Schianodicola, MD
New York Methodist Hospital
506 Sixth St
Brooklyn, NY 11215
Tel: 718 780-3279 *Fax:* 718 780-3281
Accred Length: 4 Years *Program Size:* 13
Program ID: 040-35-11-102

SUNY Health Science Center at Brooklyn Program
Sponsor: SUNY Health Science Center at Brooklyn
Kings County Hospital Center
Long Island College Hospital
University Hospital-SUNY Health Science Center at Brooklyn
Program Director:
James E Cottrell, MD
SUNY Health Science Ctr-Brooklyn
450 Clarkson Ave
Box 6
Brooklyn, NY 11203-2098
Tel: 718 270-3070 *Fax:* 718 270-3066
E-mail: auci@hscbklyn.edu
Accred Length: 4 Years *Program Size:* 63
Subspecialties: APM, CCA
Program ID: 040-35-21-110

Buffalo

SUNY at Buffalo Graduate Medical-Dental Education Consortium Program
Sponsor: SUNY at Buffalo Grad Medical-Dental Education Consortium
CGF Health System (Buffalo General Hospital)
CGF Health System (Children's Hospital of Buffalo)
CGF Health System (Millard Fillmore Hospitals)
Erie County Medical Center
Roswell Park Cancer Institute
Veterans Affairs Medical Center (Buffalo)
Program Director:
Jared C Barlow, MD PhD
Hamlin House/2nd Fl
100 High St
Buffalo, NY 14203
Tel: 716 859-4525 *Fax:* 716 859-4529
Accred Length: 4 Years *Program Size:* 28
Subspecialties: APM, CCA
Program ID: 040-35-21-093

East Meadow

Nassau County Medical Center Program
Sponsor: Nassau County Medical Center
Program Director:
Kenneth J Freese, MD
Nassau County Med Ctr
2201 Hempstead Trnpk
East Meadow, NY 11554-5400
Tel: 516 572-6803 *Fax:* 516 572-5019
E-mail: anesthes@ncmc.co.nassau.ny.us
Accred Length: 3 Years *Program Size:* 15
Program ID: 040-35-11-094

New York

Albert Einstein College of Medicine at Beth Israel Medical Center Program
Sponsor: Beth Israel Medical Center
Program Director:
Isaac Azar, MD
Beth Israel Med Ctr
First Ave at 16th St
New York, NY 10003
Tel: 212 420-2385, ext 2385 *Fax:* 212 420-2364
Accred Length: 4 Years *Program Size:* 12
Program ID: 040-35-11-096

Mount Sinai School of Medicine Program
Sponsor: Mount Sinai School of Medicine
Elmhurst Hospital Center-Mount Sinai Services
Mount Sinai Medical Center
Program Director:
Paul L Goldiner, MD
Dept of Anesthesiology/Box 1010
Mount Sinai Med Ctr
One Gustave L Levy Pl
New York, NY 10029-6574
Tel: 212 241-8392 *Fax:* 212 876-3906
E-mail: adam_levine@smtplink.mssm.edu
Internet: http://www.mssm.edu/anesthesia
Accred Length: 3 Years *Program Size:* 42
Subspecialties: APM, CCA
Program ID: 040-35-21-104

New York and Presbyterian Hospital (Columbia Campus) Program
Sponsor: New York and Presbyterian Hospital
New York and Presbyterian Hospital (Columbia Campus)
Program Director:
Margaret Wood, MD
New York Presbyterian Hospital
Columbia-Presbyterian Campus
622 W 168 St
New York, NY 10032-3784
Tel: 212 305-3117 *Fax:* 212 305-3296
E-mail: crb4@columbia.edu
Internet:
http://cpmcnet.columbia.edu/dept/anesthesiology
Accred Length: 3 Years *Program Size:* 36
Subspecialties: CCA
Program ID: 040-35-11-107

New York and Presbyterian Hospital (Cornell Campus) Program
Sponsor: New York and Presbyterian Hospital
Memorial Sloan-Kettering Cancer Center
New York and Presbyterian Hospital (Cornell Campus)
Program Director:
John J Savarese, MD
New York Presbyterian Hospital-Cornell Campus
525 E 68th St
New York, NY 10021
Tel: 212 746-2941 *Fax:* 212 746-8713
E-mail: aishapir@mail.med.cornell.edu
Internet: http://www.anestres.edu.med
Accred Length: 4 Years *Program Size:* 44 (*GY1:* 13)
Subspecialties: APM, CCA
Program ID: 040-35-21-098

New York Medical College at St Vincent's Hospital and Medical Center of New York Program
Sponsor: New York Medical College
St Vincent's Hospital and Medical Center of New York
Program Director:
George G Neuman, MD
St Vincent's Hospital and Med Ctr
153 W 11th St/NR Rm 408
New York, NY 10011
Tel: 212 604-7566 *Fax:* 212 604-2637
Accred Length: 4 Years *Program Size:* 21 (*GY1:* 7)
Subspecialties: APM
Program ID: 040-35-12-109

New York University Medical Center Program
Sponsor: New York University Medical Center
Bellevue Hospital Center
Veterans Affairs Medical Center (Manhattan)
Program Director:
Herman Turndorf, MD
Dept of Anesthesiology
550 First Ave/Rm IRM-625
New York, NY 10016
Tel: 212 263-6343 *Fax:* 212 263-7254
Internet: http://www.mcan15.med.nyu.edu
Accred Length: 3 Years *Program Size:* 51
Subspecialties: APM, CCA
Program ID: 040-35-21-106

St Luke's-Roosevelt Hospital Center Program
Sponsor: St Luke's-Roosevelt Hospital Center
St Luke's-Roosevelt Hospital Center-St Luke's Division
Program Director:
Daniel M Thys, MD
St Luke's-Roosevelt Hospital Ctr
1111 Amsterdam Ave
New York, NY 10025
Tel: 212 523-2500 *Fax:* 212 523-3930
E-mail: dmt3@columbia.edu
Internet: http://www.docnet.org/dept/anesthesia/
Accred Length: 3 Years *Program Size:* 30
Subspecialties: APM
Program ID: 040-35-11-108

Rochester

University of Rochester Program
Sponsor: Strong Memorial Hospital of the University of Rochester
Program Director:
Denham S Ward, MD PhD
Univ of Rochester Med Ctr
Dept of Anesth/Box 604
601 Elmwood Ave
Rochester, NY 14642
Tel: 716 275-1384 *Fax:* 716 244-7271
Internet: http://www.anes.rochester.edu
Accred Length: 4 Years *Program Size:* 32
Subspecialties: APM, CCA
Program ID: 040-35-11-111

Stony Brook

SUNY at Stony Brook Program
Sponsor: University Hospital-SUNY at Stony Brook
Program Director:
Paul J Poppers, MD
Dept of Anesthesiology
HSC L-4 060
Stony Brook, NY 11794-8480
Tel: 516 444-2975 *Fax:* 516 444-2907
Accred Length: 3 Years *Program Size:* 24 (*GY1:* 8)
Subspecialties: APM
Program ID: 040-35-21-170

Syracuse

SUNY Health Science Center at Syracuse Program
Sponsor: University Hospital-SUNY Health Science Center at Syracuse
Crouse Hospital
Veterans Affairs Medical Center (Syracuse)
Program Director:
Enrico M Camporesi, MD
SUNY Health Science Ctr, Dept of Anesthesiology
750 E Adams St
Syracuse, NY 13210
Tel: 315 464-4720 *Fax:* 315 464-4905
Internet: http://eja.anes.hscsyr.edu/anes/home.html
Accred Length: 3 Years *Program Size:* 28
Subspecialties: APM, CCA
Program ID: 040-35-21-113

Valhalla

New York Medical College at Westchester Medical Center Program
Sponsor: New York Medical College
Metropolitan Hospital Center
Sound Shore Medical Center of Westchester
Westchester Medical Center
Program Director:
Elizabeth A M Frost, MD
New York Med Coll
Macy West Pavilion/Rm 2395
Valhalla, NY 10595
Tel: 914 493-7692 *Fax:* 914 285-7927
E-mail: elizabeth_frost@nymc.edu
Internet: http://www.nymc.edu
Accred Length: 3 Years *Program Size:* 28
Subspecialties: APM
Program ID: 040-35-21-105

North Carolina

Chapel Hill

University of North Carolina Hospitals Program
Sponsor: University of North Carolina Hospitals
Program Director:
Philip G Boysen, MD
Univ of North Carolina Sch of Med
223 Burnett-Womack Bldg/CB7010
Chapel Hill, NC 27599-7010
Tel: 919 966-5136 *Fax:* 919 966-4873
E-mail: boysen@aims.unc.edu
Internet:
http://www.aims.unc.edu/dept/anesthesiology.html
Accred Length: 4 Years *Program Size:* 31 (*GY1:* 9)
Subspecialties: APM, CCA
Program ID: 040-36-21-114

Durham

Duke University Program
Sponsor: Duke University Medical Center
Program Director:
J G Reves, MD
Duke Univ Med Ctr
Box 3094
Durham, NC 27710
Tel: 919 681-2924 *Fax:* 919 681-7893
E-mail: lineb001@mc.duke.edu
Internet: http://anesthesia.mc.duke.edu
Accred Length: 4 Years *Program Size:* 26
Subspecialties: APM, CCA
Program ID: 040-36-31-115

Winston-Salem

Wake Forest University School of Medicine Program
Sponsor: Wake Forest University Baptist Medical Center
Program Director:
Raymond C Roy, MD
300 S Hawthorne Rd
Winston-Salem, NC 27103
Tel: 336 716-4497 *Fax:* 336 716-3394
E-mail: mpegram@wfubmd.edu
Internet: http://www.wfubme.edu.com
Accred Length: 4 Years *Program Size:* 41 (*GY1:* 8)
Subspecialties: APM, CCA
Program ID: 040-36-21-116

Ohio

Cincinnati

University Hospital/University of Cincinnati College of Medicine Program

Sponsor: University Hospital Inc
Children's Hospital Medical Center

Program Director:
Phillip O Bridenbaugh, MD
Univ of Cincinnati
PO Box 670531
231 Bethesda Ave
Cincinnati, OH 45267-0531
Tel: 513 558-6356 *Fax:* 513 558-0995
E-mail: fischecg@email.uc.edu
Internet: http://www.med.uc.edu/htdocs/medicine/anesthesia/index.htm
Accred Length: 4 Years *Program Size:* 20 (*GY1:* 2)
Subspecialties: APM, PAN
Program ID: 040-38-21-118

Cleveland

Case Western Reserve University (MetroHealth) Program

Sponsor: MetroHealth Medical Center

Program Director:
Tejbir S Sidhu, MD
MetroHealth Med Ctr
2500 MetroHealth Dr
Cleveland, OH 44109-1998
Tel: 216 778-4801 *Fax:* 216 778-5378
E-mail: tsidhu@mhnet.mhmc.org
Accred Length: 4 Years *Program Size:* 14 (*GY1:* 2)
Program ID: 040-38-21-174

Case Western Reserve University Program

Sponsor: University Hospitals of Cleveland
Veterans Affairs Medical Center (Cleveland)

Program Director:
Helmut F Cascorbi, MD PhD
Univ Hospitals of Cleveland
Dept of Anesthesiology
11100 Euclid Ave
Cleveland, OH 44106-5007
Tel: 216 844-7330 *Fax:* 216 844-3781
E-mail: christine.cimaglia@uhhs.com
Internet: http://www.anesth.com
Accred Length: 4 Years *Program Size:* 20 (*GY1:* 3)
Subspecialties: APM, CCA, PAN
Program ID: 040-38-21-119

Cleveland Clinic Foundation Program

Sponsor: Cleveland Clinic Foundation

Program Director:
F George Estafanous, MD
Cleveland Clinic Foundation
Dept of Anesthesiology
9500 Euclid Ave
Cleveland, OH 44195-5242
Tel: 216 444-5690 *Fax:* 216 444-1162
E-mail: meded@cestmp.ccf.org
Internet: http://www.ccf.org
Accred Length: 4 Years *Program Size:* 80 (*GY1:* 12)
Subspecialties: APM, CCA
Program ID: 040-38-22-120

Meridia Huron Hospital Program

Sponsor: Meridia Huron Hospital

Program Director:
John G Poulos, MD
Meridia Huron Hospital
Dept of Anesthesiology
13951 Terracve Rd
Cleveland, OH 44112
Tel: 216 761-4280 *Fax:* 216 761-7980
Accred Length: 3 Years *Program Size:* 12
Program ID: 040-38-22-122

Columbus

Ohio State University Program

Sponsor: Ohio State University Medical Center

Program Director:
Ronald L Harter, MD
Ohio State Univ Med Ctr
N-416 Doan Hall
410 W Tenth Ave
Columbus, OH 43210-1228
Tel: 614 293-8487 *Fax:* 614 293-8153
Internet: http://www.med.ohio-state.edu/anes
Accred Length: 3 Years *Program Size:* 21
Subspecialties: CCA
Program ID: 040-38-11-123

Toledo

Medical College of Ohio Program

Sponsor: Medical College of Ohio
Flower Hospital
Medical College of Ohio Hospital
Toledo Hospital

Program Director:
Marc A Huntoon, MD
Med Coll of Ohio Hospital
Dept of Anesthesiology
3000 Arlington Ave
Toledo, OH 43614-2598
Tel: 419 383-3556 *Fax:* 419 383-3550
Accred Length: 4 Years *Program Size:* 16 (*GY1:* 3)
Subspecialties: APM
Program ID: 040-38-21-125

Oklahoma

Oklahoma City

University of Oklahoma Health Sciences Center Program

Sponsor: University of Oklahoma College of Medicine
Children's Hospital of Oklahoma
University Hospital
Veterans Affairs Medical Center (Oklahoma City)

Program Director:
Robin J Elwood, MD
Univ of Oklahoma Coll of Med
Dept of Anesthesiology
PO Box 53188
Oklahoma City, OK 73152
Tel: 405 271-4803, ext 55117 *Fax:* 405 271-1216
E-mail: robin-elwood@ouhsc.edu
Internet: http://w3.ouhsc.edu/anesthesiology/
Accred Length: 4 Years *Program Size:* 25 (*GY1:* 8)
Subspecialties: APM
Program ID: 040-39-21-128

Oregon

Portland

Oregon Health Sciences University Program

Sponsor: Oregon Health Sciences University Hospital

Program Director:
Harry G Kingston, MB BCh MBA
Oregon Health Sciences Univ
3181 SW Sam Jackson Park Rd/UHS-2
Portland, OR 97201-3098
Tel: 503 494-7641 *Fax:* 503 494-4588
E-mail: altonr@ohsu.edu
Internet: http://www.ohsu.edu
Accred Length: 3 Years *Program Size:* 18
Subspecialties: APM
Program ID: 040-40-21-129

Pennsylvania

Hershey

Penn State Geisinger Health System/Milton S Hershey Medical Center Program

Sponsor: Penn State Geisinger Health System
Milton S Hershey Medical Center

Program Director:
Philip D Lumb, MB BS
Milton S Hershey Med Ctr
Dept of Anesthesia/H187
500 University Dr/PO Box 850
Hershey, PA 17033
Tel: 800 206-7718 *Fax:* 717 531-6221
Internet: http://www.anes.hmc.psu.edu
Accred Length: 4 Years *Program Size:* 19 (*GY1:* 6)
Subspecialties: APM, CCA
Program ID: 040-41-11-130

Philadelphia

MCP Hahnemann University Program

Sponsor: MCP Hahnemann University
Hahnemann University Hospital

Program Director:
Alan J Schwartz, MD MS Ed
Hahnemann Univ Hospital
Broad and Vine Sts
MS 310
Philadelphia, PA 19102-1192
Tel: 215 762-7922 *Fax:* 215 762-8656
Accred Length: 3 Years *Program Size:* 15
Program ID: 040-41-21-133

Temple University Program

Sponsor: Temple University Hospital

Program Director:
Lydia A Conlay, MD PhD MBA
Dept of Anesthesiology
Temple Univ Hospital
3401 N Broad St
Philadelphia, PA 19140
Tel: 215 707-3326 *Fax:* 215 707-8028
E-mail: anesres.blue.temple.edu
Internet: http://www.temple.edu/anes
Accred Length: 3 Years *Program Size:* 18
Subspecialties: APM, CCA
Program ID: 040-41-31-136

Thomas Jefferson University Program
Sponsor: Thomas Jefferson University Hospital

Program Director:
Joseph L Seltzer, MD
Thomas Jefferson Univ Hospital
Dept of Anesthesiology
111 S 11th St/8490-G
Philadelphia, PA 19107
Tel: 215 955-6161 *Fax:* 215 923-5507
Internet: http://www.jeffline.tju.edu/cwis/dept/anesthesiology/index.html
Accred Length: 3 Years *Program Size:* 36
Subspecialties: APM
Program ID: 040-41-21-137

University of Pennsylvania Program
Sponsor: Hospital of the University of Pennsylvania
Children's Hospital of Philadelphia
Veterans Affairs Medical Center (Philadelphia)

Program Director:
David E Longnecker, MD
Hospital of Univ of Pennsylvania
Dept of Anesthesia
3400 Spruce St
Philadelphia, PA 19104-4283
Tel: 215 662-3738 *Fax:* 215 349-5341
E-mail: apfeifer@mail.med.upenn.edu
Internet: http://www.med.upenn.edu/~dripps/
Accred Length: 4 Years *Program Size:* 45
Subspecialties: APM, CCA
Program ID: 040-41-21-134

Pittsburgh

Allegheny General Hospital Program
Sponsor: Allegheny General Hospital

Program Director:
Glenn P Gravlee, MD
Allegheny General Hospital
Dept of Anesthesiology
320 E North Ave
Pittsburgh, PA 15212-9986
Tel: 412 359-3155 *Fax:* 412 359-3483
E-mail: bdavis@aherf.edu
Internet: http://www.wizard.asri.edu/aghanes/brochues/contact.html
Accred Length: 3 Years *Program Size:* 18
Subspecialties: APM
Program ID: 040-41-11-138

Mercy Hospital of Pittsburgh Program
Sponsor: Mercy Hospital of Pittsburgh

Program Director:
William D Hetrick, MD
Mercy Hospital of Pittsburgh
Dept of Anesthesiology
1400 Locust St
Pittsburgh, PA 15219-5166
Tel: 412 232-8009 *Fax:* 412 232-7960
E-mail: anesthesiology.residency@mercy.pmhs.org
Internet: http://www.mercy-meded.com
Accred Length: 4 Years *Program Size:* 13
Subspecialties: CCA
Program ID: 040-41-12-140

University Health Center of Pittsburgh Program
Sponsor: University Health Center of Pittsburgh
Presbyterian University Hospital/UPMC

Program Director:
Leonard L Firestone, MD
Univ Health Ctr of Pittsburgh
3471 Fifth Ave/Ste 910 LSK
Pittsburgh, PA 15213
Tel: 412 692-4503 *Fax:* 412 692-4515
Internet: http://www.anes.upmc.edu
Accred Length: 3 Years *Program Size:* 20
Subspecialties: APM, CCA, PAN
Program ID: 040-41-21-139

Western Pennsylvania Hospital Program
Sponsor: Western Pennsylvania Hospital

Program Director:
Scott D Brinkmeyer, DO
Western Pennsylvania Hospital
Anesthesiology Dept
4800 Friendship Ave
Pittsburgh, PA 15224
Tel: 412 578-5323 *Fax:* 412 578-4981
Internet: http://www.westpennhospital.com/resident/anes.htm
Accred Length: 3 Years *Program Size:* 18
Program ID: 040-41-32-141

Puerto Rico

San Juan

University of Puerto Rico Program
Sponsor: University of Puerto Rico School of Medicine
San Juan City Hospital
University Hospital
Veterans Affairs Medical Center (San Juan)

Program Director:
Armando Lopez-Tristani, MD
Univ of Puerto Rico Sch of Med, Dept of Anesth
PO Box 365067
San Juan, PR 00936-5067
Tel: 787 758-0640 *Fax:* 787 758-1327
E-mail: arm_lopez@rcmaca.upr.clu.edu
Internet: http://home.coqui.net/jasantos
Accred Length: 4 Years *Program Size:* 23 (*GY1:* 6)
Program ID: 040-42-21-142

South Carolina

Charleston

Medical University of South Carolina Program
Sponsor: Medical University of South Carolina College of Medicine
MUSC Medical Center
Ralph H Johnson Dept of Veterans Affairs Med Center

Program Director:
Joanne M Conroy, MD
Med Univ of South Carolina
Dept of Anesthesiology
171 Ashley Ave
Charleston, SC 29425-2207
Tel: 803 792-2322 *Fax:* 803 792-2726
E-mail: conroyj@musc.edu
Internet: http://www.musc.edu/ane/index.htm
Accred Length: 4 Years *Program Size:* 25 (*GY1:* 7)
Subspecialties: APM
Program ID: 040-45-22-143

Tennessee

Knoxville

University of Tennessee Medical Center at Knoxville Program
Sponsor: University of Tennessee Graduate School of Medicine
University of Tennessee Memorial Hospital

Program Director:
Steve A Morris, MD
Univ of Tennessee Med Ctr
Graduate Sch of Med
1924 Alcoa Hwy
Knoxville, TN 37920-6999
Tel: 423 544-9220
Internet: http://www.mc.utk.edu
Accred Length: 3 Years *Program Size:* 24
Subspecialties: CCA
Program ID: 040-47-11-144

Memphis

University of Tennessee Program
Sponsor: University of Tennessee College of Medicine
Regional Medical Center at Memphis
University of Tennessee Medical Center (UT Bowld Hospital)

Program Director:
John Zanella Jr, MD PhD
Univ of Tennessee
Dept of Anesthesiology
800 Madison Ave
Memphis, TN 38163
Tel: 901 448-5664 *Fax:* 901 448-5540
E-mail: bplants@utmeml.utmem.edu
Internet: http://www.utmgopher.utmem.edu/anes/anesthesiology.html
Accred Length: 3 Years *Program Size:* 12
Program ID: 040-47-21-145

Nashville

Vanderbilt University Program
Sponsor: Vanderbilt University Medical Center

Program Director:
Charles Beattie, PhD MD
Vanderbilt Univ Hospital
1313 21st Ave S/504 Oxford House
Nashville, TN 37232-4125
Tel: 615 343-9419 *Fax:* 615 343-6272
E-mail: chas.beattie@mcmail.vanderbilt.edu
Internet: http://www.anesthesiology.mc.vanderbilt.edu
Accred Length: 4 Years *Program Size:* 44 (*GY1:* 8)
Subspecialties: APM, CCA
Program ID: 040-47-11-146

Texas

Dallas

University of Texas Southwestern Medical School Program
Sponsor: University of Texas Southwestern Medical School
Dallas County Hospital District-Parkland Memorial Hospital
Program Director:
Dennis F Landers, MD PhD
Univ of Texas Southwestern Med Ctr
5323 Harry Hines Blvd
Dallas, TX 75235-9068
Tel: 214 648-5460 *Fax:* 214 648-5461
Internet:
http://www.swmed.edu/home_pages/anesth/depanes.html
Accred Length: 4 Years *Program Size:* 48
Subspecialties: APM
Program ID: 040-48-21-147

El Paso

Texas Tech University (El Paso) Program
Sponsor: Texas Tech University Health Sciences Center at El Paso
R E Thomason General Hospital
Program Director:
Swapna M Chaudhuri, MD PhD
Texas Tech Univ Health Sciences Ctr
Dept of Anesthesiology
4800 Alberta Ave
El Paso, TX 79905-2400
Tel: 915 545-6573 *Fax:* 915 545-6521
E-mail: aneesev@ttuhsc.edu.
Internet: http://www.ttuhsc.edu
Accred Length: 3 Years *Program Size:* 9
Program ID: 040-48-21-187

Galveston

University of Texas Medical Branch Hospitals Program
Sponsor: University of Texas Medical Branch Hospitals
Program Director:
Donald S Prough, MD
Univ of Texas Med Branch
Dept of Anesthesiology
301 University Blvd
Galveston, TX 77555-0591
Tel: 409 772-1221 *Fax:* 409 772-1224
E-mail: cbreish@utmb.edu
Internet: http://www.utmb.edu
Accred Length: 4 Years *Program Size:* 49 (*GY1:* 12)
Subspecialties: CCA
Program ID: 040-48-11-149

Houston

Baylor College of Medicine Program
Sponsor: Baylor College of Medicine
Harris County Hospital District-Ben Taub General Hospital
Methodist Hospital
Veterans Affairs Medical Center (Houston)
Program Director:
William F Childres, MD
Baylor Coll of Med
Dept of Anesthesiology
6550 Fannin St/Smith Tower 1003
Houston, TX 77030
Tel: 713 798-5117 *Fax:* 713 798-7345
E-mail: chilton@bcm.tmc.edu
Internet: http://www.bcm.tmc.edu/anesth
Accred Length: 4 Years *Program Size:* 42 (*GY1:* 6)
Subspecialties: APM
Program ID: 040-48-31-150

University of Texas at Houston Program
Sponsor: University of Texas Medical School at Houston
Memorial Hermann Healthcare System
Program Director:
Jeffrey Katz, MD
Univ of Texas Health Science Ctr
6431 Fannin St/MSB 5020
Houston, TX 77030
Tel: 713 500-6200, ext 6270 *Fax:* 713 500-6201
Internet: http://www.-anes.uth.tmc.edu
Accred Length: 4 Years *Program Size:* 68 (*GY1:* 10)
Subspecialties: APM, CCA
Program ID: 040-48-31-152

Lackland AFB

San Antonio Uniformed Services Health Education Consortium Program
Sponsor: San Antonio Uniformed Services Health Education Consortium
Brooke Army Medical Center
Wilford Hall Medical Center (AETC)
Program Director:
Lt Col Thomas E Grissom, MD
Brooke Army Med Ctr
Attn: Medical Education (P Bolt)
3851 Roger Brooke Dr
Fort Sam Houston, TX 78234-6200
Tel: 210 916-2222 *Fax:* 210 916-5187
Accred Length: 3 Years *Program Size:* 30
Program ID: 040-48-21-091
US Armed Services Program

Lubbock

Texas Tech University (Lubbock) Program
Sponsor: Texas Tech University Health Sciences Center at Lubbock
University Medical Center
Program Director:
Gabor B Racz, MD
Texas Tech Univ Health Sciences Ctr
3601 4th St/Rm 1C282
Lubbock, TX 79430
Tel: 806 743-2981 *Fax:* 806 743-2984
E-mail: aneblc@ttuhsc.edu
Internet: http://www.anes001.ttuhsc.edu/
Accred Length: 4 Years *Program Size:* 15 (*GY1:* 3)
Subspecialties: APM
Program ID: 040-48-11-153

San Antonio

University of Texas Health Science Center at San Antonio Program
Sponsor: University of Texas Medical School at San Antonio
Audie L Murphy Memorial Veterans Hospital (San Antonio)
University Hospital-South Texas Medical Center
Program Director:
R Brian Smith, MD
Univ of Texas Health Science Ctr
Dept of Anesthesiology
7703 Floyd Curl Dr
San Antonio, TX 78284-7838
Tel: 210 567-4507 *Fax:* 210 567-6135
E-mail: amf@aries.uthscsa.edu
Internet: http://www.anesthes.uthscsa.edu
Accred Length: 4 Years *Program Size:* 30
Subspecialties: APM
Program ID: 040-48-21-155

Temple

Texas A&M College of Medicine-Scott and White Program
Sponsor: Scott and White Memorial Hospital
Central Texas Veterans Affairs Healthcare System
Program Director:
Charles H McLeskey, MD
Texas A&M-Scott and White
Dept of Anesthesiology
2401 S 31st St
Temple, TX 76508
Tel: 254 724-5306 *Fax:* 254 724-5369
E-mail: gmebjh@swmail.sw.org
Internet: http://www.sw.org/gme/anesth/anesth.htm
Accred Length: 4 Years *Program Size:* 24 (*GY1:* 6)
Program ID: 040-48-21-156

Utah

Salt Lake City

University of Utah Program
Sponsor: University of Utah Medical Center
Program Director:
Christopher M Viscomi, MD
Univ of Utah Med Ctr
50 N Medical Dr
Salt Lake City, UT 84132
Tel: 801 581-6393 *Fax:* 801 581-4367
Internet: http://carf.med.utah.edu:8002
Accred Length: 3 Years *Program Size:* 30
Subspecialties: APM
Program ID: 040-49-31-157

Vermont

Burlington

University of Vermont Program
Sponsor: Fletcher Allen Health Care
Program Director:
Howard M Schapiro, MD
Dept of Anesthesia
Fletcher Allen Health Care
111 Colchester Ave
Burlington, VT 05401
Tel: 802 656-2415 *Fax:* 802 656-5324
E-mail: howard.schapiro@vtmednet.org
Internet: http://www.uvm.edu
Accred Length: 3 Years *Program Size:* 15
Subspecialties: APM
Program ID: 040-50-11-158

Virginia

Charlottesville

University of Virginia Program
Sponsor: University of Virginia Medical Center
Program Director:
Roger A Johns, MD MD
Univ of Virginia Med Ctr
PO Box 10010
Charlottesville, VA 22906-0010
Tel: 804 982-4307 *Fax:* 804 982-0019
E-mail: raj2d@virginia.edu
Internet:
http://www.med.virginia.edu:80/som-cl/anesth/index.html
Accred Length: 4 Years *Program Size:* 46 (*GY1:* 10)
Subspecialties: APM, CCA
Program ID: 040-51-11-159

Programs

Portsmouth

Naval Medical Center (Portsmouth) Program
Sponsor: Naval Medical Center (Portsmouth)
Program Director:
Capt William L Little Jr, DO
Dept of Anesthesiology
Naval Med Ctr
620 John Paul Jones Cir
Portsmouth, VA 23708-5000
Tel: 757 398-5129 *Fax:* 757 398-7907
Accred Length: 3 Years *Program Size:* 12
Subspecialties: APM
Program ID: 040-51-21-008
US Armed Services Program

Richmond

Medical College of Virginia/Virginia Commonwealth University Program
Sponsor: Medical College of Virginia/Virginia Commonwealth University
Hunter Holmes McGuire VA Medical Center (Richmond)
Medical College of Virginia Hospitals
Program Director:
Wayne K Marshall, MD
Med Coll of Virginia Campus/VCU
PO Box 980459
Richmond, VA 23298-0459
Tel: 804 828-0733 *Fax:* 804 828-8682
E-mail: jdunaway@hsc.edu.vcu
Internet: http://www.views.vcv.edu/~aneweb
Accred Length: 4 Years *Program Size:* 28 (*GY1:* 4)
Subspecialties: APM
Program ID: 040-51-11-160

Washington

Seattle

University of Washington Program
Sponsor: University of Washington School of Medicine
Harborview Medical Center
University of Washington Medical Center
Program Director:
Frederick W Cheney, MD
Dept of Anesthesiology
Univ of Washington
1959 NE Pacific St/Box 356540
Seattle, WA 98195-6540
Tel: 206 543-2773 *Fax:* 206 543-2958
E-mail: lfg@u.washington.edu
Internet:
http://weber.u.washington.edu/anesth/index.html
Accred Length: 3 Years *Program Size:* 54
Subspecialties: APM
Program ID: 040-54-21-161

Virginia Mason Medical Center Program
Sponsor: Virginia Mason Medical Center
Program Director:
Stephen M Rupp, MD
Virginia Mason Med Ctr
Grad Med Educ/H8-GME
925 Seneca St
Seattle, WA 98111
Tel: 206 583-6079
Internet: http://www.vmmc.org
Accred Length: 4 Years *Program Size:* 25 (*GY1:* 6)
Subspecialties: APM
Program ID: 040-54-12-162

West Virginia

Morgantown

West Virginia University Program
Sponsor: West Virginia University Hospitals
Program Director:
Robert E Johnstone, MD
West Virginia Univ Sch of Med
Dept of Anesthesiology
Box 9134/3618 Health Sciences Ctr
Morgantown, WV 26506-9134
Tel: 304 598-4122 *Fax:* 304 598-4037
E-mail: kofke@jazz.wvnet.edu or turnerr@rcbhsc.wvu.edu
Internet: http://www.hsc.wvu.edu/som/anesth/index.html
Accred Length: 4 Years *Program Size:* 22
Subspecialties: APM
Program ID: 040-55-11-163

Wisconsin

Madison

University of Wisconsin Program
Sponsor: University of Wisconsin Hospital and Clinics
William S Middleton Veterans Hospital
Program Director:
Susan L Goelzer, MD
Univ of Wisconsin Hospital and Clinics
600 Highland Ave/Rm B6-319
Madison, WI 53792-3272
Tel: 608 263-8114 *Fax:* 608 263-0575
E-mail: info@anesthesia.wisc.edu
Internet: http://www.anesthesia.wisc.edu
Accred Length: 4 Years *Program Size:* 32 (*GY1:* 8)
Subspecialties: CCA
Program ID: 040-56-21-164

Milwaukee

Medical College of Wisconsin Program
Sponsor: Medical College of Wisconsin Affiliated Hospitals Inc
Clement J Zablocki Veterans Affairs Medical Center
Froedtert Memorial Lutheran Hospital
Program Director:
John P Kampine, MD PhD
Med Coll of Wisconsin
Dept of Anesthesiology
9200 W Wisconsin Ave
Milwaukee, WI 53226
Tel: 414 257-6269 *Fax:* 414 257-8047
E-mail: jpk@mcw.edu
Internet: http://www.mcw.edu/anesthesia
Accred Length: 4 Years *Program Size:* 59
Subspecialties: APM, CCA
Program ID: 040-56-21-165

Blood Banking/Transfusion Medicine (Pathology)

Alabama

Birmingham

University of Alabama Medical Center Program
Sponsor: University of Alabama Hospital
American Red Cross Blood Services-Alabama Region
Program Director:
Shu T Huang, MD
Univ of Alabama-Birmingham
619 S 19th St
West Pavilion P230
Birmingham, AL 35233-7331
Tel: 205 934-6421 *Fax:* 205 975-4468
E-mail: huang@path.uab.edu
Internet: http://path.uab.edu
Accred Length: 1 Year *Program Size:* 1
Program ID: 305-01-21-041

California

Long Beach

Long Beach Memorial Medical Center/American Red Cross Blood and Tissue Services Program
Sponsor: Long Beach Memorial Medical Center
American Red Cross Blood Services-South Calif Region
Program Director:
Emanuel Ferro, MD
George Garratty, MD PhD
Long Beach Memorial Med Ctr
2801 Atlantic Ave
Long Beach, CA 90801-1428
Tel: 562 933-0829 *Fax:* 562 933-0791
Accred Length: 1 Year *Program Size:* 0
Program ID: 305-05-21-014

Los Angeles

Cedars-Sinai Medical Center Program
Sponsor: Cedars-Sinai Medical Center
Program Director:
Dennis Goldfinger, MD
Div of Transfusion Med
Dept of Path/Lab Med
8700 Beverly Blvd
Los Angeles, CA 90048
Tel: 310 855-5418 *Fax:* 310 659-2306
Accred Length: 1 Year *Program Size:* 1
Program ID: 305-05-21-015

UCLA Medical Center Program
Sponsor: UCLA School of Medicine
American Red Cross Blood Services-South Calif Region
UCLA Medical Center
University of Louisville Hospital
Program Director:
Lawrence D Petz, MD
UCLA Med Ctr
Rm A6-238 CHS
10833 Le Conte Ave
Los Angeles, CA 90095-1713
Tel: 310 825-9916 *Fax:* 310 206-3707
Accred Length: 1 Year *Program Size:* 1
Program ID: 305-05-11-049

University of Southern California Program
Sponsor: Los Angeles County-USC Medical Center
Program Director:
Ira A Shulman, MD
Los Angeles County-USC Med Ctr
1200 N State St/Box 778
Los Angeles, CA 90033
Tel: 323 226-5993 *Fax:* 323 226-5742
E-mail: ishulman@hsc.usc.edu
Accred Length: 1 Year *Program Size:* 1
Program ID: 305-05-21-016

San Francisco

Blood Centers of the Pacific Program
Sponsor: Blood Centers of the Pacific
University of California (San Francisco) Medical Center
Program Director:
Herbert A Perkins, MD
Blood Ctrs of the Pacific
270 Masonic Ave
San Francisco, CA 94118
Tel: 415 567-6400, ext 652 *Fax:* 415 921-6184
E-mail: hperkins@pacbell.net
Accred Length: 1 Year *Program Size:* 2
Program ID: 305-05-21-017

Torrance

Los Angeles County-Harbor-UCLA Medical Center Program
Sponsor: Los Angeles County-Harbor-UCLA Medical Center
Program Director:
Priscilla I Figueroa, MD MD
Harbor-UCLA Med Ctr
1000 W Carson St/Box 12
Torrance, CA 90509-2910
Tel: 310 222-2250 *Fax:* 310 222-6485
Accred Length: 1 Year *Program Size:* 1
Program ID: 305-05-21-067

Connecticut

Farmington

University of Connecticut Program
Sponsor: University of Connecticut School of Medicine
Connecticut Red Cross Blood Services
Hartford Hospital
St Francis Hospital and Medical Center
Univ of Connecticut Health Center/John Dempsey Hospital
Program Director:
Ritchard G Cable, MD
American Red Cross Blood Services
209 Farmington Ave
Farmington, CT 06032
Tel: 860 678-2770 *Fax:* 860 676-8093
Accred Length: 1 Year *Program Size:* 1
Program ID: 305-08-21-025

Hartford

Hartford Hospital Program
Sponsor: Hartford Hospital
Program Director:
Herbert Silver, MD
Hartford Hospital
80 Seymour St
PO Box 5037
Hartford, CT 06102-5037
Tel: 860 545-2634 *Fax:* 860 545-3655
E-mail: hsilver@harthosp.org
Accred Length: 1 Year *Program Size:* 1
Program ID: 305-08-21-070

New Haven

Yale-New Haven Medical Center Program
Sponsor: Yale-New Haven Hospital
Connecticut Red Cross Blood Services
Program Director:
Edward L Snyder, MD
Blood Bank/Laboratory Med 459-CB
Yale-New Haven Hospital
20 York St
New Haven, CT 06504
Tel: 203 785-2441 *Fax:* 203 737-2748
E-mail: edward.snyder@yale.edu
Internet:
http://info.med.yale.edu/labmed/bloodbank.html
Accred Length: 1 Year *Program Size:* 1
Program ID: 305-08-21-052

District of Columbia

Washington

Georgetown University Program
Sponsor: Georgetown University Medical Center
Program Director:
S Gerald Sandler, MD
Georgetown Univ Med Ctr
Blood Donor Service/Rm M-1306
3800 Reservoir Rd NW
Washington, DC 20007
Tel: 202 687-8520 *Fax:* 202 784-2440
Accred Length: 1 Year *Program Size:* 1
Program ID: 305-10-21-057

Florida

Tampa

Florida Blood Services Program
Sponsor: Florida Blood Services
Program Director:
German F Leparc, MD
Florida Blood Services
PO Box 2125
Tampa, FL 33601-2125
Tel: 813 903-1161 *Fax:* 813 903-1177
E-mail: gleparc@fbsblood.org
Internet: http://www.fbsblood.org
Accred Length: 1 Year *Program Size:* 1
Program ID: 305-11-21-031

Georgia

Atlanta

Emory University Program
Sponsor: Emory University School of Medicine
Program Director:
Christopher D Hillyer, MD
Pathology Education Office
H-189 Emory Univ Hospital
1364 Clifton Rd NE
Atlanta, GA 30322-8110
Tel: 404 727-5914 *Fax:* 404 727-2519
E-mail: chillye@emory.edu
Internet: http://www.emory.edu.pathology/residency/
Accred Length: 1 Year *Program Size:* 1
Program ID: 305-12-31-056

Augusta

Medical College of Georgia Program
Sponsor: Medical College of Georgia Hospital and Clinics
Program Director:
Lloyd O Cook, MD
Med Coll of Georgia
Blood Bank
1120 15th St
Augusta, GA 30912-3620
Tel: 706 721-2731, ext 2731 *Fax:* 706 721-6333
E-mail: gendel.lcook@mail.mcg.edu
Accred Length: 1 Year *Program Size:* 1
Program ID: 305-12-21-053

Illinois

Chicago

University of Chicago Program
Sponsor: University of Chicago Hospitals
Program Director:
Beverly W Baron, MD
Univ of Chicago Hospitals
Blood Bank MC0007
5841 S Maryland Ave
Chicago, IL 60637
Tel: 773 702-1439 *Fax:* 773 702-4543
E-mail: bbaron@mcis.bsd.uchicago.edu
Accred Length: 1 Year *Program Size:* 1
Program ID: 305-16-21-054

Maywood

Loyola University Program
Sponsor: Loyola University Medical Center
Program Director:
Simone Silberman, MD
Loyola Univ Med Ctr
2160 S First Ave
Bldg 103/Rm 01777
Maywood, IL 60153
Tel: 708 327-2580 *Fax:* 708 327-2620
E-mail: ssilber@luc.edu
Accred Length: 1 Year *Program Size:* 1
Program ID: 305-16-21-075

Indiana

Indianapolis

Indiana University School of Medicine Program
Sponsor: Indiana University School of Medicine
Central Indiana Regional Blood Center
Clarian IU Hospital
Program Director:
Leo J McCarthy, MD
Indiana Univ Med Ctr
Transfusion Med/Rm 4435
550 N University Blvd
Indianapolis, IN 46202-5283
Tel: 317 274-8189 *Fax:* 317 274-2166
E-mail: lmmcarth@iupui.edu
Internet: http://www.pathology.iupui.edu
Accred Length: 1 Year *Program Size:* 1
Program ID: 305-17-21-058

Iowa

Iowa City

University of Iowa Hospitals and Clinics Program

Sponsor: University of Iowa Hospitals and Clinics

Program Director:
Ronald G Strauss, MD
Univ of Iowa Hospitals and Clinics
Dept of Pathology
200 Hawkins Dr
Iowa City, IA 52242-1009
Tel: 319 335-8150 *Fax:* 319 335-6555
E-mail: ronald-strauss@uiowa.edu
Internet: http://www.medicine.uiowa.edu/pathology/path_folder/ education/tm.html
Accred Length: 1 Year *Program Size:* 2
Program ID: 305-18-21-039

Kentucky

Louisville

American Red Cross Blood Services-Louisville Region Program

Sponsor: American Red Cross Blood Services (Louisville Region)
Kosair Children's Hospital (Alliant Health System)
Norton Hospital (Alliant Health System)
University of Louisville Hospital

Program Director:
William B Lockwood, MD PhD
American Red Cross Blood Services-River Valley Region
520 E Chestnut St
PO Box 3168
Louisville, KY 40201-3168
Tel: 502 540-7050 *Fax:* 502 540-7194
Accred Length: 1 Year *Program Size:* 1
Program ID: 305-20-21-059

Louisiana

New Orleans

Louisiana State University Program

Sponsor: Louisiana State University School of Medicine
Medical Center of Louisiana at New Orleans
The Blood Center

Program Director:
Yuan-Shiang Kao, MD
Louisiana State Univ Med Ctr
1901 Perdido St
New Orleans, LA 70112-1393
Tel: 504 568-6031 *Fax:* 504 568-6037
Accred Length: 1 Year *Program Size:* 1
Program ID: 305-21-21-063

Maryland

Baltimore

Johns Hopkins University Program

Sponsor: Johns Hopkins University School of Medicine
American Red Cross Blood Services
Johns Hopkins Hospital

Program Director:
Paul M Ness, MD
Johns Hopkins Hospital
600 N Wolfe St
Baltimore, MD 21287-6667
Tel: 410 955-6583 *Fax:* 410 955-0618
Accred Length: 1 Year *Program Size:* 2
Program ID: 305-23-21-026

Bethesda

National Institutes of Health Clinical Center Program

Sponsor: NIH Warren Grant Magnuson Clinical Center

Program Director:
Cathy Conry-Cantilena, MD
NIH Clinical Ctr, Dept of Transfusion Med
10 Center Dr/MSC 1184
Bldg 10/Rm 1c711
Bethesda, MD 20892-1184
Tel: 301 496-4506, ext 293 *Fax:* 301 402-1360
E-mail: cathyc@cc.nih.gov
Accred Length: 1 Year *Program Size:* 4
Program ID: 305-23-21-001

Massachusetts

Boston

Beth Israel Deaconess Medical Center (West Campus) Program

Sponsor: Beth Israel Deaconess Medical Center

Program Director:
Lynne Uhl, MD
Beth Israel Deaconess Med Ctr
330 Brookline Ave
Boston, MA 02215
Tel: 617 667-3648 *Fax:* 617 667-4533
E-mail: luhl@caregroup.harvard.edu
Accred Length: 1 Year *Program Size:* 1
Program ID: 305-24-31-069

Brigham and Women's Hospital Program

Sponsor: Brigham and Women's Hospital
Children's Hospital
Massachusetts General Hospital

Program Director:
W Hallowell Churchill, MD
75 Francis St
Boston, MA 02115
Tel: 617 732-6623 *Fax:* 617 277-9013
E-mail: whchurchil@bics.bwh.harvard.edu
Accred Length: 1 Year *Program Size:* 1
Program ID: 305-24-31-073

Massachusetts General Hospital Program

Sponsor: Massachusetts General Hospital

Program Director:
Christopher P Stowell, MD PhD
55 Fruit St
GRJ-212
Boston, MA 02114
Tel: 617 726-2815 *Fax:* 617 726-6832
E-mail: cstowell@partners.org
Accred Length: 1 Year *Program Size:* 1
Program ID: 305-24-21-064

Springfield

Baystate Medical Center Program

Sponsor: Baystate Medical Center

Program Director:
Chester Andrzejewski, MD
Baystate Med Ctr
Dept of Pathology
759 Chestnut St
Springfield, MA 01199
Tel: 413 794-5085 *Fax:* 413 794-5893
E-mail: csullivan@bhs.org
Internet: http://www.baystatehealth.com
Accred Length: 1 Year *Program Size:* 1
Program ID: 305-24-21-072

Michigan

Royal Oak

William Beaumont Hospital Program

Sponsor: William Beaumont Hospital
American Red Cross Blood Serv-Southeastern Michigan Region

Program Director:
A Bradley Eisenbrey, MD PhD
Bruce Newman, MD
William Beaumont Hospital
3601 W 13 Mile Rd
Royal Oak, MI 48072-6769
Tel: 248 551-8013
E-mail: beisenbrey@beaumont.edu
Internet: http://www.beaumont.edu/html/gme
Accred Length: 1 Year *Program Size:* 1
Program ID: 305-25-32-012

Minnesota

Minneapolis

University of Minnesota Program

Sponsor: University of Minnesota Medical School
American Red Cross Blood Services-St Paul Region
Fairview-University Medical Center
Memorial Blood Centers of Minnesota
Veterans Affairs Medical Center (Minneapolis)

Program Director:
Jeffrey McCullough, MD
Box 609/Mayo Bldg
Univ of Minnesota
420 Delaware St SE
Minneapolis, MN 55455
Tel: 612 626-3272 *Fax:* 612 625-0617
Accred Length: 1 Year *Program Size:* 3
Program ID: 305-26-21-013

Rochester

Mayo Graduate School of Medicine (Rochester) Program

Sponsor: Mayo Graduate School of Medicine-Mayo Foundation
Mayo Clinic (Rochester)

Program Director:
Alvaro A Pineda, MD
Application Processing Ctr
Mayo Graduate Sch of Med
200 First St SW
Rochester, MN 55905
Tel: 507 284-1196 *Fax:* 507 284-1599
E-mail: mgsm.medlab.specialties@mayo.edu
Internet: http://www.mayo.edu/
Accred Length: 1 Year *Program Size:* 1
Program ID: 305-26-21-005

Missouri

St Louis

Washington University/B-JH/SLCH Consortium Program

Sponsor: Washington University/B-JH/SLCH Consortium
Barnes-Jewish Hospital
Barnes-Jewish Hospital (North Campus)

Program Director:
Douglas M Lublin, MD PhD
Barnes-Jewish Hospital
One Barnes Hospital Plaza
St Louis, MO 63110
Tel: 314 362-8849 *Fax:* 314 362-3016
E-mail: lublin@labmed.wustl.edu
Internet: http://www.medinfo.wustl.edu/~labmed
Accred Length: 1 Year *Program Size:* 2
Program ID: 305-28-22-006

New York

New York

New York Blood Center Program

Sponsor: New York Blood Center
Memorial Sloan-Kettering Cancer Center
Mount Sinai Medical Center
New York University Medical Center
Westchester Medical Center

Program Director:
Celso Bianco, MD
New York Blood Ctr
310 E 67th St
New York, NY 10021-6295
Tel: 212 570-3101 *Fax:* 212 794-1957
E-mail: cbianco@nybc.org
Accred Length: 1 Year *Program Size:* 3
Program ID: 305-35-21-019

Stony Brook

SUNY at Stony Brook Program

Sponsor: University Hospital-SUNY at Stony Brook
New York Blood Center

Program Director:
Dennis K Galanakis, MD
SUNY-Stony Brook Health Science Ctr
Basic Science Tower 9/Rm 140
Stony Brook, NY 11794-8691
Tel: 516 444-2626 *Fax:* 516 444-3137
E-mail: dgalanakis@path.som.sunysb.edu
Accred Length: 1 Year *Program Size:* 1
Program ID: 305-35-21-051

Syracuse

SUNY Health Science Center at Syracuse/American Red Cross Blood Services Program

Sponsor: University Hospital-SUNY Health Science Center at Syracuse
American Red Cross Blood Services-Syracuse Region
Crouse Hospital

Program Director:
John B Henry, MD
SUNY Health Science Ctr-Syracuse
750 E Adams St
Syracuse, NY 13210
Tel: 315 464-7186 *Fax:* 315 464-7187
E-mail: henryjb@vax.cs.hscsyr.edu
Accred Length: 1 Year *Program Size:* 1
Program ID: 305-35-21-034

North Carolina

Chapel Hill

University of North Carolina Hospitals Program

Sponsor: University of North Carolina Hospitals

Program Director:
Mark E Brecher, MD
Univ of North Carolina Hospitals
1021 East Wing/Transfusion Med
101 Manning Dr
Chapel Hill, NC 27514
Tel: 919 966-8465 *Fax:* 919 966-5013
E-mail: brecher@med.unc.edu
Internet: http://www.pathology.med.unc.edu
Accred Length: 1 Year *Program Size:* 1
Program ID: 305-36-21-020

Ohio

Cincinnati

Hoxworth Blood Center/University of Cincinnati College of Medicine Program

Sponsor: Hoxworth Blood Center

Program Director:
Thomas F Zuck, MD
Hoxworth Blood Ctr-Univ of Cincinnati
3130 Highland Ave
PO Box 670055
Cincinnati, OH 45267-0055
Tel: 513 558-1200 *Fax:* 513 558-1300
Accred Length: 1 Year *Program Size:* 3
Program ID: 305-38-21-027

Cleveland

American Red Cross Northern Ohio Region Program

Sponsor: American Red Cross Northern Ohio Region
Cleveland Clinic Foundation
University Hospitals of Cleveland

Program Director:
John P Miller, MD PhD
American Red Cross Blood Serv-Northern Ohio Region
3747 Euclid Ave
Cleveland, OH 44115-2501
Tel: 216 431-3056 *Fax:* 216 391-3505
E-mail: millerjo@usa.redcross.org
Accred Length: 1 Year *Program Size:* 1
Program ID: 305-38-21-071

Columbus

Ohio State University Program

Sponsor: Ohio State University Medical Center
American Red Cross Central Ohio Region

Program Director:
Larry C Lasky, MD
Ohio State Univ Med Ctr
E-312 Doan Hall
410 W Tenth Ave
Columbus, OH 43210
Tel: 614 293-3020 *Fax:* 614 293-7273
E-mail: lasky.4@osu.edu
Internet: http://www.pathology.med.ohio-state.edu
Accred Length: 1 Year *Program Size:* 1
Program ID: 305-38-31-061

Oklahoma

Oklahoma City

University of Oklahoma Health Sciences Center Program

Sponsor: University of Oklahoma College of Medicine
Children's Hospital of Oklahoma
University Hospital
Veterans Affairs Medical Center (Oklahoma City)

Program Director:
Lesley A Kresie, MD
Univ of Oklahoma Health Sciences Ctr
Dept of Pathology/BMSB 451
940 Stanton L Young
Oklahoma City, OK 73104
Tel: 405 271-2422 *Fax:* 405 271-2568
E-mail: dianne-wright@ouhsc.edu
Accred Length: 1 Year *Program Size:* 1
Program ID: 305-39-21-076

Pennsylvania

Philadelphia

Thomas Jefferson University Program

Sponsor: Thomas Jefferson University Hospital
American Red Cross Blood Services-Penn-Jersey Region

Program Director:
Samir K Ballas, MD
Thomas Jefferson Univ Hospital
1015 Walnut St/Curtis Bldg
Philadelphia, PA 19107
Tel: 215 955-8485 *Fax:* 215 923-7859
Accred Length: 1 Year *Program Size:* 1
Program ID: 305-41-21-037

University of Pennsylvania Program

Sponsor: Hospital of the University of Pennsylvania

Program Director:
Leslie E Silberstein, MD
Hospital of Univ of Pennsylvania
Blood Bank/6079 Founders Pavilion
3400 Spruce St
Philadelphia, PA 19104-4283
Tel: 215 662-3427 *Fax:* 215 662-6891
Accred Length: 1 Year *Program Size:* 1
Program ID: 305-41-21-007

Pittsburgh

Central Blood Bank Program

Sponsor: Central Blood Bank
Allegheny General Hospital
Children's Hospital of Pittsburgh
Presbyterian University Hospital/UPMC

Program Director:
Darrell J Triulzi, MD
Inst for Transfusion Med
3636 Blvd of the Allies
Pittsburgh, PA 15213
Tel: 412 209-7304 *Fax:* 412 209-7325
E-mail: darrell_j._triulzi@itxm.org
Internet: http://www.itxm.org
Accred Length: 1 Year *Program Size:* 1
Program ID: 305-41-21-065

Texas

Dallas

University of Texas Southwestern Medical School Program
Sponsor: University of Texas Southwestern Medical School
Program Director:
Laurie J Sutor, MD
Univ of Texas Southwestern Med Ctr
5323 Harry Hines Blvd
Dallas, TX 75235-9073
Tel: 214 648-7884 *Fax:* 214 648-8037
E-mail: lsutor@carter.bloodcare.org
Internet: http://athcuric1.swmed.edu
Accred Length: 1 Year *Program Size:* 1
Program ID: 305-48-31-068

Houston

University of Texas M D Anderson Cancer Center Program
Sponsor: University of Texas M D Anderson Cancer Center
Harris County Hospital District-Ben Taub General Hospital
Program Director:
Harald E Fischer, MD
Office of Education-165
Univ of Texas MD Anderson Cancer Ctr
1515 Holcombe Blvd
Houston, TX 77030
Tel: 713 792-2644 *Fax:* 713 794-1410
E-mail: hfischer@mdanderson.org
Accred Length: 1 Year *Program Size:* 2
Program ID: 305-48-21-044

San Antonio

University of Texas Health Science Center at San Antonio Program
Sponsor: University of Texas Medical School at San Antonio
University Hospital-South Texas Medical Center
Program Director:
Chantal R Harrison, MD
Univ of Texas Health Science Ctr
Dept of Path/Blood Banking
7703 Floyd Curl Dr
San Antonio, TX 78284-7750
Tel: 210 567-4090 *Fax:* 210 567-2367
E-mail: harrisonc@uthscsa.edu
Internet: http://pathologyweb.uthscsa.edu/residency.html
Accred Length: 1 Year *Program Size:* 2
Program ID: 305-48-21-045

Virginia

Charlottesville

University of Virginia Program
Sponsor: University of Virginia Medical Center
Program Director:
Pamela Clark, MD JD
Univ of Virginia
Box 286
Charlottesville, VA 22908
Tel: 804 982-0145 *Fax:* 804 982-0140
E-mail: pc4b@virginia.edu
Accred Length: 1 Year *Program Size:* 1
Program ID: 305-51-21-074

Washington

Seattle

Puget Sound Blood Center Program
Sponsor: Puget Sound Blood Center
Program Director:
Alexander P Reiner, MD
Puget Sound Blood Ctr
921 Terry Ave
Seattle, WA 98104-1256
Tel: 206 292-1888 *Fax:* 206 343-5043
E-mail: apreiner@u.washington.edu
Internet: http://www.psbc.org
Accred Length: 1 Year *Program Size:* 4
Program ID: 305-54-21-066

Wisconsin

Madison

University of Wisconsin Program
Sponsor: University of Wisconsin Hospital and Clinics
American Red Cross Blood Services-Badger Region
Program Director:
James S Malter, MD
Alice J Hibbard, MD
Univ of Wisconsin Hospital and Clinics
B4/263 Clinical Science Ctr
600 Highland Ave
Madison, WI 53792-2472
Tel: 608 263-1559 *Fax:* 608 263-1568
E-mail: js.malter@usmsg.hosp.wisc.edu
Internet: http://www.biostat.wisc.edu/path/transfu.html
Accred Length: 1 Year *Program Size:* 1
Program ID: 305-56-21-048

Milwaukee

Medical College of Wisconsin Program
Sponsor: Medical College of Wisconsin Affiliated Hospitals Inc
Blood Center of Southeastern Wisconsin
Froedtert Memorial Lutheran Hospital
Program Director:
Jerome L Gottschall, MD
Blood Ctr of Southeastern Wisconsin
638 N 18th St
PO Box 2178
Milwaukee, WI 53201-2178
Tel: 414 937-6231 *Fax:* 414 933-6803
E-mail: jlgottschall@bcsew.edu
Accred Length: 1 Year *Program Size:* 1
Program ID: 305-56-21-023

Cardiovascular Disease (Internal Medicine)

Alabama

Birmingham

University of Alabama Medical Center Program
Sponsor: University of Alabama Hospital
Program Director:
Vera A Bittner, MD
Univ of Alabama, Div of Cardiovascular Dis
306 Lyons Harrison Research Bldg
701 S 19th St
Birmingham, AL 35294-0007
Tel: 205 934-0820 *Fax:* 205 975-8568
E-mail: vbittner@cardio.dom.uab.edu
Accred Length: 3 Years *Program Size:* 14
Program ID: 141-01-21-151

Mobile

University of South Alabama Program
Sponsor: University of South Alabama Medical Center
Program Director:
Vaskar Mukerji, MD
Univ of South Alabama Med Ctr
2451 Fillingim St
10th Fl/Ste D
Mobile, AL 36617
Tel: 334 471-7923 *Fax:* 334 470-5888
Accred Length: 3 Years *Program Size:* 4
Program ID: 141-01-11-060

Arizona

Phoenix

Good Samaritan Regional Medical Center Program
Sponsor: Good Samaritan Regional Medical Center
Carl T Hayden Veterans Affairs Medical Center (Phoenix)
Program Director:
Kenneth B Desser, MD
Good Samaritan Regional Med Ctr
Cardiology Fellowship
1111 E McDowell Rd/WT4
Phoenix, AZ 85006
Tel: 602 239-6743 *Fax:* 602 239-5094
Accred Length: 3 Years *Program Size:* 7
Program ID: 141-03-21-039

Tucson

University of Arizona Program
Sponsor: University of Arizona College of Medicine
University Medical Center
Veterans Affairs Medical Center (Tucson)
Program Director:
Gordon A Ewy, MD
William R Roeske, MD
Univ of Arizona Health Sciences Ctr
1501 N Campbell Ave
Tucson, AZ 85724
Tel: 520 626-6221 *Fax:* 520 626-0967
Accred Length: 3 Years *Program Size:* 5
Program ID: 141-03-21-131

Arkansas

Little Rock

University of Arkansas for Medical Sciences Program

Sponsor: University of Arkansas College of Medicine
John L McClellan Memorial Veterans Hospital
University Hospital of Arkansas

Program Director:
Joel D Talley, MD
Univ of Arkansas for Med Sciences
Div of Cardiology
4301 W Markham/Slot 532
Little Rock, AR 72205-7199
Tel: 501 686-5880 *Fax:* 501 686-8319
E-mail: jtalley@medlan.uams.edu
Internet: http://www.uams.edu
Accred Length: 3 Years *Program Size:* 9
Program ID: 141-04-21-132

California

La Jolla

Scripps Clinic/Scripps Green Hospital Program

Sponsor: Scripps Clinic
Scripps Green Hospital

Program Director:
Guy P Curtis, MD PhD
Dept of Grad Med Educ/403C
Scripps Clinic and Research Foundation
10666 N Torrey Pines Rd
La Jolla, CA 92037-1093
Tel: 619 554-8582 *Fax:* 619 554-6310
E-mail: gme@scripps.edu
Internet: http://scrippsclinic.com
Accred Length: 3 Years *Program Size:* 4
Program ID: 141-05-21-086

Loma Linda

Loma Linda University Program

Sponsor: Loma Linda University Medical Center
Jerry L Pettis Memorial Veterans Hospital

Program Director:
Paulo A Ribeiro, MD PhD
Loma Linda Univ Med Ctr
Cardiology Sect
PO Box 2000
Loma Linda, CA 92354
Tel: 909 824-4652 *Fax:* 909 558-0390
Accred Length: 3 Years *Program Size:* 6
Program ID: 141-05-21-153

Los Angeles

Cedars-Sinai Medical Center Program

Sponsor: Cedars-Sinai Medical Center

Program Director:
Prediman K Shah, MD
Cedars-Sinai Med Ctr
8700 Beverly Blvd
Los Angeles, CA 90048-1865
Tel: 310 855-3884 *Fax:* 310 967-0144
Internet: http://www.csmc.edu
Accred Length: 3 Years *Program Size:* 9
Program ID: 141-05-11-134

Southern California Kaiser Permanente Medical Care (Los Angeles) Program

Sponsor: Southern California Kaiser Permanente Medical Group
Kaiser Foundation Hospital (Los Angeles)
St Vincent Medical Center

Program Director:
Michael Jorgensen, MD
Dept of Cardiology
1526 N Edgemont St
Los Angeles, CA 90027
Tel: 323 783-4516
Accred Length: 3 Years *Program Size:* 9
Program ID: 141-05-12-041

UCLA Medical Center Program

Sponsor: UCLA School of Medicine
UCLA Medical Center

Program Director:
Gregg C Fonarow, MD
Ctr for Health Sciences/Rm 47-123
10833 Le Conte Ave
Los Angeles, CA 90095-1679
Tel: 310 794-9736 *Fax:* 310 206-9133
E-mail: slafranc@medicine.medsch.ucla.edu
Internet: http://www.med.ucla.edu
Accred Length: 3 Years *Program Size:* 11
Program ID: 141-05-11-155

University of Southern California Program

Sponsor: Los Angeles County-USC Medical Center

Program Director:
David P Faxon, MD
Univ of Southern California Med Ctr
Ambulatory Health Ctr
1355 San Pablo St/Rm 117
Los Angeles, CA 90033-1026
Tel: 323 442-5480 *Fax:* 323 442-5481
E-mail: uscheart@hsc.usc.edu
Accred Length: 3 Years *Program Size:* 12
Program ID: 141-05-21-061

VA Greater Los Angeles Healthcare System Program

Sponsor: VA Greater Los Angeles Healthcare System
Olive View-UCLA Medical Center

Program Director:
Bramah N Singh, MD PhD
West Los Angeles VA Med Ctr
Div of Cardiology (W111E)
11301 Wilshire Blvd
Los Angeles, CA 90073
Tel: 310 268-3643, ext 41473 *Fax:* 310 268-4288
Accred Length: 3 Years *Program Size:* 10
Program ID: 141-05-31-073

Orange

University of California (Irvine) Program

Sponsor: University of California (Irvine) Medical Center
Long Beach Memorial Medical Center
Veterans Affairs Medical Center (Long Beach)

Program Director:
Julius M Gardin, MD
Univ of California Irvine Med Ctr
Div of Cardiology
101 City Dr S/Rte 81 Bl 53
Orange, CA 92868-3298
Tel: 714 456-6545 *Fax:* 714 456-8895
E-mail: jmgardin@uci.edu
Accred Length: 3 Years *Program Size:* 10
Program ID: 141-05-21-180

Sacramento

University of California (Davis) Program

Sponsor: University of California (Davis) Medical Center

Program Director:
Lawrence Laslett, MD
2315 Stockton Blvd
Sacramento, CA 95817
Tel: 916 734-3764 *Fax:* 916 734-8394
Internet:
http://www.ucdmc.ucdavis.edu/medser/cardiology/index.html
Accred Length: 3 Years *Program Size:* 9
Program ID: 141-05-21-111

San Diego

Naval Medical Center (San Diego) Program

Sponsor: Naval Medical Center (San Diego)

Program Director:
Cdr Peter E Linz, MD
Naval Med Ctr
Cardiology Div
34800 Bob Wilson Dr
San Diego, CA 92134-5000
Tel: 619 532-7403 *Fax:* 619 532-9863
Accred Length: 3 Years *Program Size:* 11
Program ID: 141-05-12-181
US Armed Services Program

University of California (San Diego) Program

Sponsor: University of California (San Diego) Medical Center
Scripps Mercy Hospital
Veterans Affairs Medical Center (San Diego)

Program Director:
Wilbur Lew, MD
UCSD Med Ctr
Div of Cardiology
200 W Arbor Dr
San Diego, CA 92103-8411
Tel: 619 543-3406 *Fax:* 619 543-3305
Accred Length: 3 Years *Program Size:* 9
Program ID: 141-05-21-209

San Francisco

California Pacific Medical Center Program

Sponsor: California Pacific Medical Center
California Pacific Medical Center

Program Director:
Andrew Rosenblatt, MD
CPMC/Div of Cardiology
2333 Buchanan St/#2367
San Francisco, CA 94115
Tel: 415 923-3236 *Fax:* 415 885-8664
Internet: http://www.cpmc.org
Accred Length: 3 Years *Program Size:* 6
Program ID: 141-05-12-183

St Mary's Hospital and Medical Center Program

Sponsor: St Mary's Hospital and Medical Center
University of California (San Francisco) Medical Center

Program Director:
Richard Podolin, MD
St Marys Hospital and Med Ctr
450 Stanyan St
San Francisco, CA 94117-1079
Tel: 415 750-5507 *Fax:* 415 750-5948
Accred Length: 3 Years *Program Size:* 3
Program ID: 141-05-22-233

University of California (San Francisco) Program
Sponsor: University of California (San Francisco) School of Medicine
San Francisco General Hospital Medical Center
University of California (San Francisco) Medical Center
Veterans Affairs Medical Center (San Francisco)
Program Director:
William W Parmley, MD
Dept of Med
1186 Moffitt Hospital
505 Parnassus Ave/Box 0124
San Francisco, CA 94143-0124
Tel: 415 502-1115 *Fax:* 415 502-8627
E-mail: parmley@medicine.ucsf.edu
Internet: http://www.cardio.his.ucsf.edu/
Accred Length: 3 Years *Program Size:* 16
Program ID: 141-05-21-184

Stanford

Stanford University Program
Sponsor: Stanford University Hospital
Veterans Affairs Palo Alto Health Care System
Program Director:
Edwin L Alderman, MD
Stanford Univ, Cardiovascular Med Div
CVRC-261
Stanford, CA 94305-5406
Tel: 650 723-6008 *Fax:* 650 725-1599
Accred Length: 3 Years *Program Size:* 23
Program ID: 141-05-21-025

Torrance

Los Angeles County-Harbor-UCLA Medical Center Program
Sponsor: Los Angeles County-Harbor-UCLA Medical Center
Program Director:
Kenneth A Narahara, MD
Harbor-UCLA Med Ctr
Div of Cardiology
1000 W Carson St/RB2
Torrance, CA 90509
Tel: 310 222-2515 *Fax:* 310 787-0448
Accred Length: 3 Years *Program Size:* 12
Program ID: 141-05-11-210

Colorado

Denver

University of Colorado Program
Sponsor: University of Colorado Health Sciences Center
Denver Health and Hospitals
Veterans Affairs Medical Center (Denver)
Program Director:
Edward P Havranek, MD
Div of Cardiology
Univ of Colorado Health Sciences Ctr
4200 E Ninth Ave/Box B-130
Denver, CO 80262
Tel: 303 315-4398 *Fax:* 303 315-5082
E-mail: ehavrane@dhha.org
Accred Length: 3 Years *Program Size:* 18
Program ID: 141-07-21-074

Connecticut

Bridgeport

Yale University (Bridgeport) Program
Sponsor: Bridgeport Hospital
Program Director:
Craig A McPherson, MD
Bridgeport Hospital
267 Grant St
Bridgeport, CT 06610
Tel: 203 384-3842 *Fax:* 203 384-3664
E-mail: pcmcph@bpthosp.org
Accred Length: 3 Years *Program Size:* 4
Program ID: 141-08-11-211

Farmington

University of Connecticut Program 1
Sponsor: University of Connecticut School of Medicine
Mount Sinai Hospital
St Francis Hospital and Medical Center
Univ of Connecticut Health Center/John Dempsey Hospital
Program Director:
Peter Schulman, MD
Univ of Connecticut Health Ctr
263 Farmington Ave
Farmington, CT 06030-2202
Tel: 860 679-2771 *Fax:* 860 679-3346
E-mail: bournival@nso1.uchc.edu
Internet: http://www.uchc.edu
Accred Length: 3 Years *Program Size:* 8
Program ID: 141-08-31-001

University of Connecticut Program 2
Sponsor: University of Connecticut School of Medicine
Hartford Hospital
Univ of Connecticut Health Center/John Dempsey Hospital
Program Director:
Gary V Heller, MD PhD
80 Seymour St
Hartford, CT 06102-5037
Tel: 860 545-2880 *Fax:* 860 545-3168
E-mail: aalvara@harthosp.org
Accred Length: 3 Years *Program Size:* 9
Program ID: 141-08-31-253

New Haven

Yale-New Haven Medical Center Program
Sponsor: Yale-New Haven Hospital
Veterans Affairs Medical Center (West Haven)
Program Director:
Lawrence H Young, MD
Yale Univ Sch of Med
Sect of Cardiovascular Med
333 Cedar St/PO Box 208017 3FMP
New Haven, CT 06520-8017
Tel: 203 785-4102 *Fax:* 203 785-7144
Internet: http://www.cardio.med.yale.edu
Accred Length: 3 Years *Program Size:* 15
Program ID: 141-08-21-026

District of Columbia

Washington

George Washington University Program
Sponsor: George Washington University School of Medicine
George Washington University Hospital (UHS)
Program Director:
Conor F Lundergan, MD
George Washington Univ Hospital
Div of Cardiology
Ste 4-414
Washington, DC 20037
Tel: 202 994-6113 *Fax:* 202 994-3673
E-mail: clundergan@aol.com
Accred Length: 3 Years *Program Size:* 6
Program ID: 141-10-21-136

Georgetown University Program
Sponsor: Georgetown University Medical Center
Veterans Affairs Medical Center (Washington, DC)
Program Director:
Allen J Solomon, MD
Georgetown Univ Hospital
Div of Cardiology (M4222)
3800 Reservoir Rd NW
Washington, DC 20007-2197
Tel: 202 687-4034 *Fax:* 202 687-7797
E-mail: steelewe@gunet.georgetown.edu
Accred Length: 3 Years *Program Size:* 12
Program ID: 141-10-21-107

Howard University Program
Sponsor: Howard University Hospital
District of Columbia General Hospital
Program Director:
Charles L Curry, MD
Howard Univ Hospital
2041 Georgia Ave NW
Ste 6C-03
Washington, DC 20060
Tel: 202 865-6791 *Fax:* 202 865-4449
Accred Length: 3 Years *Program Size:* 9
Program ID: 141-10-21-158

Walter Reed Army Medical Center Program
Sponsor: Walter Reed Army Medical Center
National Naval Medical Center (Bethesda)
Program Director:
Lee W Jordan, MD
Walter Reed Army Med Ctr
6825 16th St NW
Washington, DC 20307-5001
Tel: 202 782-9870 *Fax:* 202 782-3813
Accred Length: 3 Years *Program Size:* 18
Program ID: 141-10-11-159
US Armed Services Program

Washington Hospital Center Program
Sponsor: Washington Hospital Center
Program Director:
Joseph Lindsay Jr, MD
Washington Hospital Ctr
110 Irving St NW
Washington, DC 20010-2975
Tel: 202 877-7597 *Fax:* 202 877-2247
E-mail: jml2@mhg.edu
Accred Length: 3 Years *Program Size:* 6
Program ID: 141-10-11-160

Florida

Gainesville

University of Florida Program
Sponsor: University of Florida College of Medicine
Shands Hospital at the University of Florida
Veterans Affairs Medical Center (Gainesville)

Program Director:
Jamie B Conti, MD
Univ of Florida, Dept of Med
PO Box 100277
1600 SW Archer Rd
Gainesville, FL 32610-0277
Tel: 352 392-5691 *Fax:* 352 846-0314
Accred Length: 3 Years *Program Size:* 9
Program ID: 141-11-21-045

Jacksonville

University of Florida Health Science Center/Jacksonville Program
Sponsor: University of Florida College of Medicine at Jacksonville
University Medical Center (UFHSC/J)

Program Director:
Daniel S Goldman, MD
Univ of Florida Health Science Ctr-Jacksonville
655 W 8th St
Jacksonville, FL 32209
Tel: 904 549-3065 *Fax:* 904 549-3102
Accred Length: 3 Years *Program Size:* 9
Program ID: 141-11-21-027

Miami

University of Miami-Jackson Memorial Medical Center Program
Sponsor: University of Miami-Jackson Memorial Medical Center
Veterans Affairs Medical Center (Miami)

Program Director:
Robert J Myerburg, MD
Univ of Miami Sch of Med
Div of Cardiology (D-39)
PO Box 016960
Miami, FL 33101-6960
Tel: 305 585-5523 *Fax:* 305 585-7089
E-mail: rmyerbur@mednet.med.miamiedu
Accred Length: 3 Years *Program Size:* 16
Program ID: 141-11-21-212

Miami Beach

Mount Sinai Medical Center of Greater Miami Program
Sponsor: Mount Sinai Medical Center of Greater Miami

Program Director:
Gervasio A Lamas, MD
Mount Sinai Med Ctr of Greater Miami
Div of Cardiology
4300 Alton Rd
Miami Beach, FL 33140
Tel: 305 674-2260 *Fax:* 305 674-2146
E-mail: glamas@msmc.com
Internet: http://www.mountsinaimiami.org
Accred Length: 3 Years *Program Size:* 12
Program ID: 141-11-12-076

Tampa

University of South Florida Program
Sponsor: University of South Florida College of Medicine
James A Haley Veterans Hospital
Tampa General Healthcare

Program Director:
Hector L Fontanet, MD
Harbourside Med Tower
4 Columbia Dr/Ste 630
Tampa, FL 33606
Tel: 813 974-2880 *Fax:* 813 254-4701
Internet:
http://www.med.usf.edu/intmed/cardiology/index.html
Accred Length: 3 Years *Program Size:* 9
Program ID: 141-11-21-046

Georgia

Atlanta

Emory University Program
Sponsor: Emory University School of Medicine
Crawford Long Hospital of Emory University
Emory University Hospital
Grady Memorial Hospital
Veterans Affairs Medical Center (Atlanta)

Program Director:
W Robert Taylor, MD PhD
Emory Univ Sch of Med
1639 Pierce Dr/WMB Ste 319
Atlanta, GA 30322
Tel: 404 727-4724 *Fax:* 404 727-3330
E-mail: cardiology@emory.edu
Internet: http://www.cc.emory.edu/cardiology/
Accred Length: 3 Years *Program Size:* 37
Program ID: 141-12-21-161

Augusta

Medical College of Georgia Program
Sponsor: Medical College of Georgia Hospital and Clinics
Veterans Affairs Medical Center (Augusta)

Program Director:
Louis Michael Prisant, MD
Med Coll of Georgia
BBR-6515A, Sect of Cardiology
1120 15th St
Augusta, GA 30912-3105
Tel: 706 721-2736 *Fax:* 706 721-2785
E-mail: mprisant@mail.mcg.edu
Accred Length: 3 Years *Program Size:* 9
Program ID: 141-12-21-004

Illinois

Chicago

Cook County Hospital Program
Sponsor: Cook County Hospital

Program Director:
Russell F Kelly, MD
Cook County Hospital
Div of Adult Cardiology
1825 W Harrison St
Chicago, IL 60612
Tel: 312 633-7862 *Fax:* 312 633-7270
Accred Length: 3 Years *Program Size:* 9
Program ID: 141-16-12-047

Illinois Masonic Medical Center/Rush Medical College Program
Sponsor: Illinois Masonic Medical Center

Program Director:
Peter J Stecy, MD
Illinois Masonic Med Ctr
Sect of Cardiology
836 W Wellington Ave
Chicago, IL 60657-5193
Tel: 773 296-7044 *Fax:* 773 296-5940
Internet: http://www.immc.org
Accred Length: 3 Years *Program Size:* 9
Program ID: 141-16-11-220

McGaw Medical Center of Northwestern University Program
Sponsor: Northwestern University Medical School
Northwestern Memorial Hospital
Veterans Affairs Lakeside Medical Center (Chicago)

Program Director:
George Gubernikoff, MD
Northwestern Univ Med Sch
250 E Superior St
Wesley 520
Chicago, IL 60611
Tel: 312 908-4954 *Fax:* 312 908-8133
E-mail: g-gubernikoff@nwu.edu
Internet: http://www.medicine.nwu.edu/cardio/
Accred Length: 3 Years *Program Size:* 11
Program ID: 141-16-21-090

Rush-Presbyterian-St Luke's Medical Center Program
Sponsor: Rush-Presbyterian-St Luke's Medical Center
MacNeal Memorial Hospital

Program Director:
Joseph E Parrillo, MD
Rush-Presbyterian-St Luke's Med Ctr
1653 W Congress Pkwy
Chicago, IL 60612-3864
Tel: 312 942-2998 *Fax:* 312 942-5829
E-mail: jparrill@rush.edu
Accred Length: 3 Years *Program Size:* 21
Program ID: 141-16-11-162

University of Chicago Program
Sponsor: University of Chicago Hospitals

Program Director:
Roberto M Lang, MD
Univ of Chicago
5841 S Maryland Ave
MC6088
Chicago, IL 60637
Tel: 773 702-5211 *Fax:* 773 702-2681
E-mail: amurphy@medicine.bsd.uchicago.edu
Internet:
http://card-mac14.bsd.uchicago.edu/levin/cardiology.html
Accred Length: 3 Years *Program Size:* 14
Program ID: 141-16-11-077

University of Illinois College of Medicine at Chicago Program 1
Sponsor: University of Illinois College of Medicine at Chicago
University of Illinois Hospital and Clinics
Veterans Affairs West Side Medical Center

Program Director:
George T Kondos, MD
Univ of Illinois-Chicago
Sect of Cardiology M/C 787
840 S Wood St/9th Fl
Chicago, IL 60612
Tel: 312 996-6730 *Fax:* 312 413-1616
E-mail: gtkondos@uic.edu
Accred Length: 3 Years *Program Size:* 10
Program ID: 141-16-21-163

University of Illinois College of Medicine at Chicago/Michael Reese Hospital Program

Sponsor: University of Illinois College of Medicine at Chicago
Michael Reese Hospital and Medical Center

Program Director:
Pablo Denes, MD
Michael Reese Hospital and Med Ctr
2929 S Ellis Ave
Chicago, IL 60616
Tel: 312 791-3160 *Fax:* 312 791-8006
Internet: http://www.michaelreese.com
Accred Length: 3 Years *Program Size:* 9
Program ID: 141-16-21-028

Maywood

Loyola University Program

Sponsor: Loyola University Medical Center
Edward J Hines Jr Veterans Affairs Hospital

Program Director:
Ronald R Schreiber, MD
Henry S Loeb, MD
Loyola Univ Med Ctr
EMS Bldg 110 Rm 6231
2160 S First Ave
Maywood, IL 60153
Tel: 708 327-2747 *Fax:* 708 327-2771
Accred Length: 3 Years *Program Size:* 20
Program ID: 141-16-21-005

North Chicago

Finch University of Health Sciences/Chicago Medical School Program

Sponsor: Finch University of Health Sciences/Chicago Medical School
Mount Sinai Hospital Medical Center of Chicago
Veterans Affairs Medical Center (North Chicago)

Program Director:
Jeffrey B Lakier, MD
Finch Univ of Health Sciences-Chicago Med Sch
Dept of Med
3333 Green Bay Rd
North Chicago, IL 60064-3095
Tel: 847 578-3227 *Fax:* 847 578-8647
E-mail: serdarc@mis.finchcms.edu
Internet: http://www.finchcms.edu
Accred Length: 3 Years *Program Size:* 7
Program ID: 141-16-21-062

Oak Lawn

University of Illinois College of Medicine at Chicago/Christ Hospital Program

Sponsor: University of Illinois College of Medicine at Chicago
Christ Hospital and Medical Center

Program Director:
Marc A Silver, MD
Christ Hospital-Univ of Illinois
4440 W 95th St/Ste 428S
Oak Lawn, IL 60453
Tel: 708 346-8000 *Fax:* 708 346-4097
E-mail: dropsy1@.com
Internet: http://www.advocate.health.com
Accred Length: 3 Years *Program Size:* 8
Program ID: 141-16-21-091

Park Ridge

Lutheran General Hospital Program

Sponsor: Lutheran General Hospital

Program Director:
Jeffrey B Lakier, MD
Lutheran General Hospital
1775 W Dempster St
Park Ridge, IL 60068-1174
Tel: 847 723-7997 *Fax:* 847 723-2131
E-mail: jeffrey.lakier-md@advocatehealth.com
Accred Length: 3 Years *Program Size:* 9
Program ID: 141-16-21-255

Indiana

Indianapolis

Indiana University School of Medicine Program

Sponsor: Indiana University School of Medicine
Clarian IU Hospital

Program Director:
Eric S Williams, MD
Indiana Univ Med Ctr
Krannert Inst of Cardiology
1111 W 10th St
Indianapolis, IN 46202-4800
Tel: 317 630-7716 *Fax:* 317 630-8009
E-mail: mehamilt@iupui.edu
Accred Length: 3 Years *Program Size:* 12
Program ID: 141-17-21-185

Iowa

Iowa City

University of Iowa Hospitals and Clinics Program

Sponsor: University of Iowa Hospitals and Clinics

Program Director:
Joseph A Hill, MD
Univ of Iowa Hospitals and Clinics
4207 RCP
200 Hawkins Dr
Iowa City, IA 52242-1009
Tel: 319 354-9829 *Fax:* 319 353-6343
E-mail: joseph-hill@uiowa.edu
Accred Length: 3 Years *Program Size:* 7
Program ID: 141-18-21-112

Kansas

Kansas City

University of Kansas Medical Center Program

Sponsor: University of Kansas School of Medicine
University of Kansas Medical Center

Program Director:
Steven B Gollub, MD
Univ of Kansas Med Ctr
Cardiovascular Div
3901 Rainbow Blvd
Kansas City, KS 66160-7378
Tel: 913 588-6015 *Fax:* 913 588-6010
Accred Length: 3 Years *Program Size:* 6
Program ID: 141-19-21-137

Kentucky

Lexington

University of Kentucky Medical Center Program

Sponsor: University of Kentucky Hospital
Veterans Affairs Medical Center (Lexington)

Program Director:
Santosh G Menon, MD
Univ Hospital-Albert B Chandler Med Ctr
Div of Cardiovascular Med
740 S Limestone/L543
Lexington, KY 40536-0284
Tel: 606 323-5479 *Fax:* 606 323-6475
E-mail: sgmenon@pop.uky.edu
Accred Length: 3 Years *Program Size:* 10
Program ID: 141-20-21-213

Louisville

University of Louisville Program

Sponsor: University of Louisville School of Medicine
University of Louisville Hospital
Veterans Affairs Medical Center (Louisville)

Program Director:
Stephen G Wagner, MD
Univ of Louisville Sch of Med
ACB/3rd Fl/Cardiology
530 S Jackson St
Louisville, KY 40292
Tel: 502 852-7959 *Fax:* 502 852-7147
Accred Length: 3 Years *Program Size:* 14
Program ID: 141-20-31-215

Louisiana

New Orleans

Alton Ochsner Medical Foundation Program

Sponsor: Alton Ochsner Medical Foundation

Program Director:
Tyrone Collins, MD
Alton Ochsner Med Foundation
Dept of Grad Med Educ
1516 Jefferson Hwy
New Orleans, LA 70121
Tel: 504 842-3260 *Fax:* 504 842-3193
E-mail: dlambert@ochsner.org
Internet: http://www.ochsner.org
Accred Length: 3 Years *Program Size:* 16
Program ID: 141-21-22-123

Louisiana State University Program

Sponsor: Louisiana State University School of Medicine
Medical Center of Louisiana at New Orleans

Program Director:
Luke Glancy, MD MD
2021 Perdido St
New Orleans, LA 70112
Tel: 504 568-5845 *Fax:* 504 599-0525
Accred Length: 3 Years *Program Size:* 12
Program ID: 141-21-21-246

Tulane University Program

Sponsor: Tulane University School of Medicine
Medical Center of Louisiana at New Orleans
Tulane University Hospital and Clinics
Veterans Affairs Medical Center (New Orleans)
Veterans Affairs Medical Center-LSU Service (New Orleans)

Program Director:
Dwight Stapleton, MD
Tulane Univ Sch of Med
Sect of Cardiology
1430 Tulane Ave/SL-48
New Orleans, LA 70112-2699
Tel: 504 585-6139 *Fax:* 504 587-4237
E-mail: deidwell@tmc.tulane.edu
Accred Length: 3 Years *Program Size:* 14
Program ID: 141-21-21-130

Shreveport

Louisiana State University (Shreveport) Program

Sponsor: Louisiana State University Hospital-Shreveport
Overton Brooks Veterans Affairs Medical Center

Program Director:
Frank M Sheridan, MD
Louisiana State Univ Med Ctr
Cardiology Sect
1501 Kings Hwy/PO Box 33932
Shreveport, LA 71130-3932
Tel: 318 675-5940 *Fax:* 318 675-5686
E-mail: fsheri@lsumc.edu
Accred Length: 3 Years *Program Size:* 10
Program ID: 141-21-21-078

Maine

Portland

Maine Medical Center Program

Sponsor: Maine Medical Center

Program Director:
Costas T Lambrew, MD
Maine Med Ctr
22 Bramhall St
Portland, ME 04102
Tel: 207 871-2413 *Fax:* 207 871-6038
E-mail: lambrc@mail.mmc.org
Internet: http://www.mmc.org
Accred Length: 3 Years *Program Size:* 7
Program ID: 141-22-11-092

Maryland

Baltimore

Johns Hopkins University Program

Sponsor: Johns Hopkins University School of Medicine
Johns Hopkins Hospital

Program Director:
Lewis C Becker, MD
Johns Hopkins Hospital
600 N Wolfe St/Halsted 500
Baltimore, MD 21287
Tel: 410 955-5997 *Fax:* 410 955-0852
E-mail: lbecker@welchlink.welch.jhu.edu
Accred Length: 3 Years *Program Size:* 26
Program ID: 141-23-11-093

University of Maryland Program

Sponsor: University of Maryland Medical System
Veterans Affairs Medical Center (Baltimore)

Program Director:
Gary D Plotnick, MD
Univ of Maryland Med System
Div of Cardiology
22 S Greene St/Gudelsky Bldg
Baltimore, MD 21201-1595
Tel: 410 328-4394 *Fax:* 410 328-1498
E-mail: mbileck@heart.ab.umd.edu
Accred Length: 3 Years *Program Size:* 10
Program ID: 141-23-21-049

Massachusetts

Boston

Beth Israel Deaconess Medical Center (East Campus) Program

Sponsor: Beth Israel Deaconess Medical Center

Program Director:
James P Morgan, MD PhD
Beth Israel Deaconess Med Ctr
330 Brookline Ave
Boston, MA 02215
Tel: 617 667-2191 *Fax:* 617 667-4833
E-mail: jmorgan@bidmc.harvard.edu
Internet: http://www.bidmc.harvard.edu/cardiology
Accred Length: 3 Years *Program Size:* 27
Program ID: 141-24-21-006

Boston University Medical Center Program

Sponsor: Boston Medical Center
Veterans Affairs Medical Center (Boston)

Program Director:
Wilson S Colucci, MD
Boston Med Ctr
Sect of Cardiology
88 E Newton St
Boston, MA 02118
Tel: 617 638-8706 *Fax:* 617 638-8712
Accred Length: 3 Years *Program Size:* 20
Program ID: 141-24-21-187

Brigham and Women's Hospital Program 1

Sponsor: Brigham and Women's Hospital

Program Director:
Sharon C Reimold, MD
Brigham and Women's Hospital
Dept of Med
75 Francis St
Boston, MA 02115
Tel: 617 732-5500, ext 3451 *Fax:* 617 277-4981
E-mail: screimold@bics.bwh.harvard.edu
Internet: http://www.heartdoc.org
Accred Length: 3 Years *Program Size:* 21
Program ID: 141-24-21-007

Brigham and Women's Hospital Program 2

Sponsor: Brigham and Women's Hospital

Program Director:
Thomas B Graboys, MD
Lown Cardiovascular Ctr
21 Longwood Ave
Brookline, MA 02146
Tel: 617 732-1318 *Fax:* 617 734-5763
E-mail: tbgraboys@bics.bwh.harvard.edu
Internet: http://www.healthnet.org/lown
Accred Length: 3 Years *Program Size:* 5
Program ID: 141-24-21-008

Massachusetts General Hospital Program

Sponsor: Massachusetts General Hospital

Program Director:
Peter Yurchak, MD
Massachusetts General Hospital
Cardiac Unit
55 Fruit St
Boston, MA 02114
Tel: 617 726-2898 *Fax:* 617 726-3062
Accred Length: 3 Years *Program Size:* 19
Program ID: 141-24-11-079

New England Medical Center Hospitals Program

Sponsor: New England Medical Center Hospitals

Program Director:
Marvin A Konstam, MD
750 Washington St
NEMC #108
Boston, MA 02111
Tel: 617 636-5911 *Fax:* 617 636-7667
Accred Length: 3 Years *Program Size:* 13
Program ID: 141-24-21-010

St Elizabeth's Medical Center of Boston Program

Sponsor: St Elizabeth's Medical Center of Boston

Program Director:
Bernard D Kosowsky, MD
St Elizabeth's Med Ctr
736 Cambridge St
Boston, MA 02135
Tel: 617 789-2000 *Fax:* 617 789-5029
Internet: http://www.semc.org
Accred Length: 3 Years *Program Size:* 11
Program ID: 141-24-21-063

Burlington

Lahey Clinic Program

Sponsor: Lahey Clinic

Program Director:
Sherif B Labib, MD
Lahey Clinic
41 Mall Rd
Burlington, MA 01805
Tel: 781 744-8002 *Fax:* 781 744-5261
E-mail: lauren.manganaro@lahey.org
Accred Length: 3 Years *Program Size:* 6
Program ID: 141-24-21-222

Springfield

Baystate Medical Center Program

Sponsor: Baystate Medical Center

Program Director:
James B Kirchhoffer, MD
Baystate Med Ctr
Div of Cardiology
759 Chestnut St
Springfield, MA 01199
Tel: 413 794-4490 *Fax:* 413 794-0198
Accred Length: 3 Years *Program Size:* 10
Program ID: 141-24-11-095

Worcester

St Vincent Hospital Program

Sponsor: St Vincent Hospital
UMass Memorial Health Care (University Campus)

Program Director:
David H Spodick, MD
St Vincent Hospital
25 Winthrop St
Worcester, MA 01604
Tel: 508 798-6162
Accred Length: 3 Years *Program Size:* 8
Program ID: 141-24-21-239

Programs

University of Massachusetts Program
Sponsor: University of Massachusetts Medical School
UMass Memorial Health Care (University Campus)
Program Director:
Gerard Aurigemma, MD
Univ of Massachusetts Med Sch
Cardiovascular Div
55 Lake Ave N
Worcester, MA 01655
Tel: 508 856-3064 *Fax:* 508 856-4571
E-mail: jackie.jolie@banyan.ummed.edu
Internet:
http://www.ummed.edu/dept/cardiovascular_med/
Accred Length: 3 Years *Program Size:* 14
Program ID: 141-24-21-011

Michigan

Ann Arbor

University of Michigan Program
Sponsor: University of Michigan Hospitals
Veterans Affairs Medical Center (Ann Arbor)
Program Director:
Mark R Starling, MD
Univ of Michigan Hospitals
1500 E Medical Center Dr
3910 Taubman
Ann Arbor, MI 48109-0366
Tel: 734 761-7978 *Fax:* 734 769-7381
E-mail: mrstar@umich.edu
Accred Length: 3 Years *Program Size:* 24
Program ID: 141-25-21-096

Detroit

Henry Ford Hospital Program
Sponsor: Henry Ford Hospital
Program Director:
Howard S Rosman, MD
Henry Ford Hospital
Int Med/Cardiovascular Dis
2799 W Grand Blvd
Detroit, MI 48202
Tel: 313 916-2871 *Fax:* 313 556-8205
Accred Length: 3 Years *Program Size:* 15
Program ID: 141-25-11-164

St John Hospital and Medical Center Program
Sponsor: St John Hospital and Medical Center
Program Director:
Theodore L Schreiber, MD
St John Hospital and Med Ctr
Dept of Med Educ
22101 Moross Rd
Detroit, MI 48236
Tel: 313 343-7837 *Fax:* 313 343-7556
E-mail: sue.moynihan@stjohn.org
Internet: http://www.stjohn.org
Accred Length: 3 Years *Program Size:* 6
Program ID: 141-25-31-258

Wayne State University/Detroit Medical Center Program
Sponsor: Wayne State University/Detroit Medical Center
Detroit Receiving Hospital and University Health Center
Harper Hospital
Veterans Affairs Medical Center (Detroit)
Program Director:
Paul E Ruble, MD
Harper Hospital, Div of Cardiology
3990 John R St
8 Webber Core
Detroit, MI 48201
Tel: 313 745-2635 *Fax:* 313 993-0243
Accred Length: 3 Years *Program Size:* 12
Program ID: 141-25-21-057

East Lansing

Michigan State University Program
Sponsor: Michigan State University College of Human Medicine
Sparrow Hospital
Program Director:
George S Abela, MD
Michigan State Univ
B206 Clinical Ctr
East Lansing, MI 48824-1313
Tel: 517 353-4830
Accred Length: 3 Years *Program Size:* 6
Program ID: 141-25-11-259

Royal Oak

William Beaumont Hospital Program
Sponsor: William Beaumont Hospital
Program Director:
Pamela Marcovitz, MD
William Beaumont Hospital
3601 W 13 Mile Rd
Royal Oak, MI 48073-6769
Tel: 248 551-5482 *Fax:* 248 551-4199
Internet: http://www.beaumont.edu/html/gme
Accred Length: 3 Years *Program Size:* 12
Program ID: 141-25-12-216

Southfield

Providence Hospital and Medical Centers Program
Sponsor: Providence Hospital and Medical Centers
Program Director:
Wolf F C Duvernoy, MD
Providence Hospital
Med Educ
16001 W Nine Mile Rd
Southfield, MI 48075-4818
Tel: 248 424-3216 *Fax:* 248 424-5324
Accred Length: 3 Years *Program Size:* 6
Program ID: 141-25-11-214

Minnesota

Minneapolis

University of Minnesota Program
Sponsor: University of Minnesota Medical School
Fairview-University Medical Center
Regions Hospital
Veterans Affairs Medical Center (Minneapolis)
Program Director:
Harold L Kennedy, MD MPH
Univ of Minnesota
Cardiovascular Training
420 Delaware St SE
Minneapolis, MN 55455
Tel: 612 625-9100 *Fax:* 612 626-4411
E-mail: heart.card.umn.edukenne045@tc.umn.edu
Accred Length: 3 Years *Program Size:* 12
Program ID: 141-26-21-139

Rochester

Mayo Graduate School of Medicine (Rochester) Program
Sponsor: Mayo Graduate School of Medicine-Mayo Foundation
Mayo Clinic (Rochester)
Rochester Methodist Hospital
St Mary's Hospital of Rochester
Program Director:
Guy S Reeder, MD
Application Processing Ctr
Siebens 5th Fl
Mayo Graduate Sch of Med
Rochester, MN 55905
Tel: 507 284-3126 *Fax:* 507 284-0999
E-mail: mgsm.intmed.specialties@mayo.edu
Internet: http://www.mayo.edu/
Accred Length: 3 Years *Program Size:* 24
Program ID: 141-26-21-066

Mississippi

Jackson

University of Mississippi Medical Center Program
Sponsor: University of Mississippi School of Medicine
University Hospital
Veterans Affairs Medical Center (Jackson)
Program Director:
Thomas N Skelton, MD
Div of Cardiovascular Diseases
Univ Med Ctr
2500 N State St
Jackson, MS 39216-4505
Tel: 601 984-5630 *Fax:* 601 984-5638
E-mail: tskelton@medicine.umsmed.edu
Internet: http://www.umsmed.edu
Accred Length: 3 Years *Program Size:* 7
Program ID: 141-27-21-097

Missouri

Columbia

University of Missouri-Columbia Program
Sponsor: University of Missouri-Columbia School of Medicine
Harry S Truman Memorial Veterans Hospital
University Hospitals and Clinics
Program Director:
Karl T Weber, MD
Univ of Missouri-Columbia
#30 Hadley Hall
One Hospital Dr
Columbia, MO 65212
Tel: 573 882-7272 *Fax:* 573 884-4641
Accred Length: 3 Years *Program Size:* 15
Program ID: 141-28-21-098

Kansas City

University of Missouri at Kansas City Program

Sponsor: University of Missouri-Kansas City School of Medicine
Saint Luke's Hospital
Truman Medical Center-West

Program Director:
Alan D Forker, MD
Dept of Med
2301 Holmes
Kansas City, MO 64108
Tel: 816 556-4073 *Fax:* 816 881-6224
Accred Length: 3 Years *Program Size:* 6
Program ID: 141-28-31-140

St Louis

St Louis University School of Medicine Program

Sponsor: St Louis University School of Medicine
St Louis University School of Medicine
Veterans Affairs Medical Center (St Louis)

Program Director:
Bernard R Chaitman, MD
St Louis Univ Sch of Med
Div of Cardiology
3635 Vista Ave
St Louis, MO 63110-0250
Tel: 314 577-8890 *Fax:* 314 268-5172
E-mail: chaitman@sluvca.slu.edu
Internet: http://www.slu.edu/departments/medicine
Accred Length: 3 Years *Program Size:* 16
Program ID: 141-28-21-108

Washington University/B-JH/SLCH Consortium (South Campus) Program

Sponsor: Washington University/B-JH/SLCH Consortium
Barnes-Jewish Hospital
Barnes-Jewish Hospital (North Campus)

Program Director:
Benico Barzilai, MD
Washington Univ Sch of Med
Campus Box 8086
660 S Euclid Ave
St Louis, MO 63110
Tel: 314 362-8902 *Fax:* 314 362-9982
E-mail: bbarzila@imgate.wustl.edu
Accred Length: 3 Years *Program Size:* 31
Program ID: 141-28-21-188

Nebraska

Omaha

Creighton University Program

Sponsor: Creighton University School of Medicine
Tenet St Joseph Hospital at Creighton Univ Medical Center

Program Director:
Aryan N Mooss, MD
Creighton Univ Cardiac Ctr
3006 Webster St
Omaha, NE 68131-2044
Tel: 402 280-4626 *Fax:* 402 280-5182
Internet: http://www.creighton.edu
Accred Length: 3 Years *Program Size:* 9
Program ID: 141-30-21-190

University of Nebraska Program

Sponsor: University of Nebraska Medical Center
Veterans Affairs Medical Center (Omaha)

Program Director:
Arthur R Easley Jr, MD
Univ of Nebraska Med Ctr
600 S 42nd St
Box 982265
Omaha, NE 68198-2265
Tel: 402 559-5151 *Fax:* 402 559-8355
E-mail: aeasley@unmc.edu
Internet: http://www.unmc.edu/gme/programs.htm
Accred Length: 3 Years *Program Size:* 6
Program ID: 141-30-21-191

New Hampshire

Lebanon

Dartmouth-Hitchcock Medical Center Program

Sponsor: Mary Hitchcock Memorial Hospital

Program Director:
Edward Catherwood, MD
Dartmouth-Hitchcock Med Ctr
One Medical Center Dr
Lebanon, NH 03756
Tel: 603 650-6009 *Fax:* 603 650-6164
E-mail: edward,catherwood@hitchcock.org
Accred Length: 3 Years *Program Size:* 9
Program ID: 141-32-21-178

New Jersey

Camden

UMDNJ-Robert Wood Johnson Medical School (Camden) Program

Sponsor: Cooper Hospital-University Medical Center

Program Director:
Toby R Engel, MD
Cooper Hospital-Univ Med Ctr
One Cooper Plaza
Cardiology Dept
Camden, NJ 08103-1489
Tel: 609 342-2567 *Fax:* 609 968-8300
E-mail: engel-toby@cooperhealth.edu
Accred Length: 3 Years *Program Size:* 7
Program ID: 141-33-21-240

Jersey City

Mount Sinai School of Medicine (Jersey City) Program

Sponsor: Mount Sinai School of Medicine
Jersey City Medical Center

Program Director:
Feridoun Rezai, MD
Jersey City Med Ctr
50 Baldwin Ave
Jersey City, NJ 07304
Tel: 201 915-2448 *Fax:* 201 915-2443
Accred Length: 3 Years *Program Size:* 0
Program ID: 141-33-21-203

Newark

UMDNJ-New Jersey Medical School Program

Sponsor: UMDNJ-New Jersey Medical School
Hackensack University Medical Center
UMDNJ-University Hospital
Veterans Affairs Medical Center (East Orange)

Program Director:
Edward M Dwyer, MD
UMDNJ-New Jersey Med Sch
185 S Orange Ave
Newark, NJ 07103-2714
Tel: 973 972-4731 *Fax:* 973 972-2243
E-mail: dwyerem@umdnj.edu
Accred Length: 3 Years *Program Size:* 8
Program ID: 141-33-21-237

Piscataway

UMDNJ-Robert Wood Johnson Medical School Program

Sponsor: UMDNJ-Robert Wood Johnson Medical School
Deborah Heart and Lung Center
Robert Wood Johnson University Hospital

Program Director:
Abel E Moreyra, MD
UMDNJ-Robert Wood Johnson Med Sch
One Robert Wood Johnson Pl/CN 19
New Brunswick, NJ 08903-0019
Tel: 732 235-7855 *Fax:* 732 246-8722
E-mail: moreyrae@umdnj.edu
Internet: http://www2.umdnj.edu/:ucgweb
Accred Length: 3 Years *Program Size:* 10
Program ID: 141-33-21-029

South Orange

Seton Hall University School of Graduate Medical Education Program

Sponsor: Seton Hall University School of Graduate Medical Education
St Joseph's Hospital and Medical Center
St Michael's Medical Center (Cathedral Hlth Srvcs Inc)

Program Director:
Rita M Watson, MD
St Elizabeth Hospital
225 Williamson St
Elizabeth, NJ 07207
Tel: 908 527-5041 *Fax:* 908 527-5346
Accred Length: 3 Years *Program Size:* 9
Program ID: 141-33-11-223

New Mexico

Albuquerque

University of New Mexico Program

Sponsor: University of New Mexico School of Medicine
Lovelace Medical Center
University Hospital
Veterans Affairs Medical Center (Albuquerque)

Program Director:
Michael H Crawford, MD
Univ of New Mexico Sch of Med
Div of Cardiology/ACC 5th Fl
2211 Lomas Blvd NE
Albuquerque, NM 87131-5271
Tel: 505 272-6020 *Fax:* 505 272-4356
E-mail: nwhalen@salud.unm.edu
Internet:
http://macbeth.unm.edu/som/gme/cardiology.html
Accred Length: 3 Years *Program Size:* 9
Program ID: 141-34-21-165

New York

Albany

Albany Medical Center Program

Sponsor: Albany Medical Center
Veterans Affairs Medical Center (Albany)

Program Director:
Theodore L Biddle, MD
Albany Med Coll
47 New Scotland Ave/A-44
Albany, NY 12208-3479
Tel: 518 262-5076 *Fax:* 518 262-5082
Accred Length: 3 Years *Program Size:* 7
Program ID: 141-35-31-030

Bronx

Albert Einstein College of Medicine Program

Sponsor: Albert Einstein College of Medicine of Yeshiva University
Montefiore Medical Center-Henry and Lucy Moses Division
Montefiore Medical Center-Weiler Hospital

Program Director:
Jamshid Shirani, MD
Albert Einstein Coll of Med-Montefiore Med Ctr
1300 Morris Park Ave
Forchheimer Bldg/Rm G42
Bronx, NY 10461
Tel: 718 430-3315 *Fax:* 718 430-8989
E-mail: shirani@aecom.yu.edu
Accred Length: 3 Years *Program Size:* 20
Program ID: 141-35-21-124

Bronx-Lebanon Hospital Center Program

Sponsor: Bronx-Lebanon Hospital Center

Program Director:
Edward J Brown Jr, MD
Bronx-Lebanon Hospital Ctr
1650 Grand Concourse
Bronx, NY 10457
Tel: 718 518-5222 *Fax:* 718 518-5585
Accred Length: 3 Years *Program Size:* 6
Program ID: 141-35-11-125

Brooklyn

Brooklyn Hospital Center Program

Sponsor: Brooklyn Hospital Center

Program Director:
Kenneth Ong, MD
Brooklyn Hospital Ctr
121 DeKalb Ave
Brooklyn, NY 11201
Tel: 718 250-8265 *Fax:* 718 250-6216
Accred Length: 3 Years *Program Size:* 8
Program ID: 141-35-12-166

Coney Island Hospital Program

Sponsor: Coney Island Hospital

Program Director:
Mohandas Shenoy, MD
Coney Island Hospital
2601 Ocean Pkwy
Brooklyn, NY 11235
Tel: 718 616-3543 *Fax:* 718 616-3797
Accred Length: 3 Years *Program Size:* 9
Program ID: 141-35-11-207

Interfaith Medical Center Program

Sponsor: Interfaith Medical Center
Maimonides Medical Center
St Luke's-Roosevelt Hospital Center

Program Director:
Sanford Leff, MD
Interfaith Med Ctr
555 Prospect Pl
Brooklyn, NY 11238
Tel: 718 935-7511 *Fax:* 718 935-7514
Accred Length: 3 Years *Program Size:* 3
Program ID: 141-35-21-224

Long Island College Hospital Program

Sponsor: Long Island College Hospital
Woodhull Medical and Mental Health Center

Program Director:
Balendu C Vasavada, MD
Long Island Coll Hospital, Dept of Cardiology
340 Henry St
Brooklyn, NY 11201
Tel: 718 833-3692 *Fax:* 718 780-1619
Accred Length: 3 Years *Program Size:* 8
Program ID: 141-35-11-032

Maimonides Medical Center Program

Sponsor: Maimonides Medical Center

Program Director:
Jacob Shani, MD
Maimonides Med Ctr
Cardiology Div
4802 Tenth Ave
Brooklyn, NY 11219
Tel: 718 283-7489 *Fax:* 718 283-8956
Accred Length: 3 Years *Program Size:* 12
Program ID: 141-35-11-192

SUNY Health Science Center at Brooklyn Program

Sponsor: SUNY Health Science Center at Brooklyn
Brookdale University Hospital Medical Center
Kings County Hospital Center
University Hospital-SUNY Health Science Center at Brooklyn
Veterans Affairs Medical Center (Brooklyn)

Program Director:
Luther T Clark, MD
SUNY Health Science Ctr-Brooklyn
450 Clarkson Ave
Box 1199
Brooklyn, NY 11203-2098
Tel: 718 270-1568 *Fax:* 718 270-2917
Accred Length: 3 Years *Program Size:* 18
Program ID: 141-35-21-013

Buffalo

SUNY at Buffalo Graduate Medical-Dental Education Consortium Program

Sponsor: SUNY at Buffalo Grad Medical-Dental Education Consortium
CGF Health System (Buffalo General Hospital)
CGF Health System (Millard Fillmore Hospitals)
Erie County Medical Center
Veterans Affairs Medical Center (Buffalo)

Program Director:
Avery K Ellis, MD PhD
SUNY-Buffalo
3495 Bailey Ave
Buffalo, NY 14215
Tel: 716 862-3638 *Fax:* 716 862-4727
E-mail: ellis.avery k@buffalo.va.gov
Internet: http://members.aol.com/ubcardio
Accred Length: 3 Years *Program Size:* 9
Program ID: 141-35-31-051

East Meadow

SUNY at Stony Brook (East Meadow) Program

Sponsor: Nassau County Medical Center
Winthrop-University Hospital

Program Director:
Arnold R Conrad, MD
Nassau County Med Ctr
2201 Hempstead Trnpk
East Meadow, NY 11554
Tel: 516 572-8784, ext 3030 *Fax:* 516 572-3172
Accred Length: 3 Years *Program Size:* 4
Program ID: 141-35-21-113

Elmhurst

Mount Sinai School of Medicine (Elmhurst) Program

Sponsor: Mount Sinai School of Medicine
Elmhurst Hospital Center-Mount Sinai Services

Program Director:
John E Madias, MD
Elmhurst Hospital Ctr
79-01 Broadway
Elmhurst, NY 11373
Tel: 718 334-5005 *Fax:* 718 334-5990
Accred Length: 3 Years *Program Size:* 6
Program ID: 141-35-11-141

Jamaica

Catholic Medical Center of Brooklyn and Queens Program

Sponsor: Catholic Medical Center of Brooklyn and Queens Inc
Catholic Medical Center (Mary Immaculate Hospital)
Catholic Medical Center (St John's Queens Hospital)
Long Island Jewish Medical Center

Program Director:
Bernard H Boal, MD
Catholic Med Ctr of Brooklyn and Queens
88-25 153rd St
Jamaica, NY 11432
Tel: 718 657-7208 *Fax:* 718 558-7010
E-mail: selkparr@aol.com
Accred Length: 3 Years *Program Size:* 6
Program ID: 141-35-22-059

Manhasset

North Shore University Hospital/NYU School of Medicine Program

Sponsor: North Shore University Hospital

Program Director:
Stanley Katz, MD
North Shore Univ Hospital
Div of Cardiology
Manhasset, NY 11030
Tel: 516 562-4100 *Fax:* 516 562-2352
Accred Length: 3 Years *Program Size:* 12
Program ID: 141-35-21-201

Mineola

Winthrop-University Hospital Program

Sponsor: Winthrop-University Hospital

Program Director:
Jason M Lazar, MD
Winthrop-Univ Hospital
259 First St
Mineola, NY 11501
Tel: 516 663-4481 *Fax:* 516 663-2054
Accred Length: 3 Years *Program Size:* 7
Program ID: 141-35-11-100

New Hyde Park

Albert Einstein College of Medicine at Long Island Jewish Medical Center Program

Sponsor: Long Island Jewish Medical Center

Program Director:
Ira L Weg, MD
Long Island Jewish Med Ctr
270-05 76th Ave
New Hyde Park, NY 11040
Tel: 718 470-7331 *Fax:* 718 343-9762
Internet: http://www.lij.edu
Accred Length: 3 Years *Program Size:* 9
Program ID: 141-35-21-167

New York

Albert Einstein College of Medicine at Beth Israel Medical Center Program

Sponsor: Beth Israel Medical Center

Program Director:
Steven F Horowitz, MD
Div of Cardiology
Beth Israel Med Ctr
16th St at First Ave
New York, NY 10003
Tel: 212 420-4560 *Fax:* 212 420-2406
Accred Length: 3 Years *Program Size:* 12
Program ID: 141-35-11-080

Harlem Hospital Center Program

Sponsor: Harlem Hospital Center

Program Director:
Eric J Vanderbush, MD
Harlem Hospital Ctr
506 Lenox Ave
Rm 15101
New York, NY 10037
Tel: 212 939-4701 *Fax:* 212 939-4706
E-mail: eric@mail.eclipse.net
Accred Length: 3 Years *Program Size:* 7
Program ID: 141-35-11-206

Lenox Hill Hospital Program

Sponsor: Lenox Hill Hospital

Program Director:
Neil L Coplan, MD
Lenox Hill Hospital
100 E 77th St
New York, NY 10021
Tel: 212 434-2170 *Fax:* 212 434-2111
Accred Length: 3 Years *Program Size:* 9
Program ID: 141-35-11-231

Mount Sinai School of Medicine (Cabrini) Program

Sponsor: Mount Sinai School of Medicine
Cabrini Medical Center
Mount Sinai Medical Center

Program Director:
Philip Varriale, MD
Cabrini Med Ctr
227 E 19th St
New York, NY 10003
Tel: 212 995-6124 *Fax:* 212 995-6912
Accred Length: 3 Years *Program Size:* 3
Program ID: 141-35-31-114

Mount Sinai School of Medicine Program 1

Sponsor: Mount Sinai School of Medicine
Mount Sinai Medical Center
Veterans Affairs Medical Center (Bronx)

Program Director:
Mark B Taubman, MD
Mount Sinai Med Ctr
Div of Cardiology/Box 1269
One Gustave L Levy Pl
New York, NY 10029
Tel: 212 241-0047 *Fax:* 212 369-3269
E-mail: m_taubman@smtplink.mssm.edu
Internet: http://www.mssm.edu
Accred Length: 3 Years *Program Size:* 15
Program ID: 141-35-31-193

New York and Presbyterian Hospital (Columbia Campus) Program

Sponsor: New York and Presbyterian Hospital
New York and Presbyterian Hospital (Columbia Campus)

Program Director:
Paul J Cannon, MD
New York Presbyterian Hospital
622 W 168th St
New York, NY 10032
Tel: 212 305-9052 *Fax:* 212 305-4648
E-mail: pjc4@columbia.edu
Internet: http://cpmcnet.columbia.edu/dept/cardiology/
Accred Length: 3 Years *Program Size:* 13
Program ID: 141-35-11-081

New York and Presbyterian Hospital (Cornell Campus) Program

Sponsor: New York and Presbyterian Hospital
New York and Presbyterian Hospital (Cornell Campus)

Program Director:
Stephen Scheidt, MD
New York Hospital-Cornell Med Ctr
525 E 68th St
New York, NY 10021
Tel: 212 746-2148
Accred Length: 3 Years *Program Size:* 20
Program ID: 141-35-21-202

New York Medical College at St Vincent's Hospital and Medical Center of New York Program

Sponsor: New York Medical College
St Vincent's Hospital and Medical Center of New York

Program Director:
James T Mazzara, MD
St Vincent's Hospital and Med Ctr
153 W 11th St
New York, NY 10011
Tel: 212 604-2224 *Fax:* 212 604-3843
Internet: http://svh.nymc.edu
Accred Length: 3 Years *Program Size:* 8
Program ID: 141-35-11-033

New York University Medical Center (Veterans) Program

Sponsor: New York University Medical Center
Bellevue Hospital Center
Veterans Affairs Medical Center (Manhattan)

Program Director:
Steven Sedlis, MD
VA Med Ctr
423 E 23rd St
New York, NY 10010
Tel: 212 951-3335
Accred Length: 3 Years *Program Size:* 4
Program ID: 141-35-21-144

New York University Medical Center Program

Sponsor: New York University Medical Center
Bellevue Hospital Center

Program Director:
Richard I Levin, MD
New York Univ Med Ctr
550 First Ave
New York, NY 10016
Tel: 212 263-6554 *Fax:* 212 263-7060
E-mail: richard.levin@med.nyu.edu
Internet: http://www.med.nyu.edu/medicine/cardio.htm
Accred Length: 3 Years *Program Size:* 13
Program ID: 141-35-21-143

St Luke's-Roosevelt Hospital Center Program

Sponsor: St Luke's-Roosevelt Hospital Center
St Luke's-Roosevelt Hospital Center-St Luke's Division

Program Director:
Jonathan S Steinberg, MD
St Luke's-Roosevelt Hospital Ctr
Div of Cardiology
1111 Amsterdam Ave
New York, NY 10025
Tel: 212 523-4007 *Fax:* 212 523-3915
Accred Length: 3 Years *Program Size:* 9
Program ID: 141-35-21-251

Rochester

University of Rochester Program

Sponsor: Strong Memorial Hospital of the University of Rochester
Rochester General Hospital

Program Director:
Richard M Pomerantz, MD
Strong Memorial Hospital
Cardiology/Box 679
601 Elmwood Ave
Rochester, NY 14642-8679
Tel: 716 275-7736 *Fax:* 716 473-1573
Internet: http://www.urmc.rochester.edu/smd/cardio/
Accred Length: 3 Years *Program Size:* 9
Program ID: 141-35-11-232

Staten Island

New York Medical College (Richmond) Program

Sponsor: New York Medical College
Sisters of Charity Medical Center-St Vincent's Campus

Program Director:
Richard S Grodman, MD
Sisters of Charity Med Ctr-St Vincent's Campus
355 Bard Ave
Staten Island, NY 10310-1699
Tel: 718 876-4642 *Fax:* 718 876-2755
Accred Length: 3 Years *Program Size:* 6
Program ID: 141-35-11-170

Stony Brook

SUNY at Stony Brook Program

Sponsor: University Hospital-SUNY at Stony Brook
Veterans Affairs Medical Center (Northport)

Program Director:
Peter F Cohn, MD
Div of Cardiology
SUNY-Stony Brook
Health Sciences Ctr/T-17-020
Stony Brook, NY 11794-8171
Tel: 516 444-1060 *Fax:* 516 444-1054
Accred Length: 3 Years *Program Size:* 9
Program ID: 141-35-21-014

Syracuse

SUNY Health Science Center at Syracuse Program

Sponsor: University Hospital-SUNY Health Science Center at Syracuse
Veterans Affairs Medical Center (Syracuse)

Program Director:
Harold Smulyan, MD
Dept of Med
SUNY Health Science Ctr
750 E Adams St
Syracuse, NY 13210
Tel: 315 464-9572 *Fax:* 315 464-9571
Accred Length: 3 Years *Program Size:* 9
Program ID: 141-35-21-128

Valhalla

New York Medical College at Westchester Medical Center Program

Sponsor: New York Medical College
Westchester Medical Center

Program Director:
Melvin B Weiss, MD
Westchester Med Ctr
Div of Cardiology
Valhalla, NY 10595
Tel: 914 493-8816 *Fax:* 914 493-5726
Accred Length: 3 Years *Program Size:* 11
Program ID: 141-35-11-015

North Carolina

Chapel Hill

University of North Carolina Hospitals Program

Sponsor: University of North Carolina Hospitals

Program Director:
Park W Willis IV, MD
Univ of North Carolina Sch of Med
CB 7075 349 Burnett-Womack Bldg
Chapel Hill, NC 27599-7075
Tel: 919 966-5205 *Fax:* 919 966-1743
E-mail: hodges.cards@mhs.unc.edu
Internet: http://www.med.unc.edu/medicine/cardiolo
Accred Length: 3 Years *Program Size:* 11
Program ID: 141-36-21-171

Durham

Duke University Program

Sponsor: Duke University Medical Center
Veterans Affairs Medical Center (Durham)

Program Director:
Thomas M Bashore, MD
Duke Univ Med Ctr
Box 3012
Durham, NC 27710
Tel: 919 684-2407 *Fax:* 919 681-7917
E-mail: basho001@mc.duke.edu
Internet:
http://www.taylor.mc.duke.edu/card/training.html
Accred Length: 3 Years *Program Size:* 36
Program ID: 141-36-21-172

Greenville

East Carolina University Program

Sponsor: East Carolina University School of Medicine
Pitt County Memorial Hospital

Program Director:
Harry J DeAntonio, DO
Pitt County Memorial Hospital
East Carolina Univ Sch of Med
Dept of Med/Cardiology PCMH-TA 378
Greenville, NC 27858-4354
Tel: 919 816-5569 *Fax:* 919 816-5884
E-mail: sauls@brody.med.ecu.edu
Accred Length: 3 Years *Program Size:* 6
Program ID: 141-36-11-245

Winston-Salem

Wake Forest University School of Medicine Program

Sponsor: Wake Forest University Baptist Medical Center

Program Director:
Robert J Applegate, MD
Wake Forest Univ Sch of Med
Sect on Cardiology
Medical Center Blvd
Winston-Salem, NC 27157-1045
Tel: 336 716-2718 *Fax:* 336 716-5324
Accred Length: 3 Years *Program Size:* 16
Program ID: 141-36-21-016

Ohio

Cincinnati

University Hospital/University of Cincinnati College of Medicine Program

Sponsor: University Hospital Inc
Veterans Affairs Medical Center (Cincinnati)

Program Director:
Charles R Hattemer Sr, MD
Univ of Cincinnati
231 Bethesda Ave/ML 542
Cincinnati, OH 45267-0542
Tel: 513 558-4721 *Fax:* 513 558-3116
Internet: http://www.med.uc.edu/cardiology
Accred Length: 3 Years *Program Size:* 9
Program ID: 141-38-21-102

Cleveland

Case Western Reserve University (MetroHealth) Program

Sponsor: MetroHealth Medical Center
Mount Sinai Medical Center of Cleveland

Program Director:
Lee A Biblo, MD
MetroHealth Med Ctr
Div of Cardiology
2500 MetroHealth Dr
Cleveland, OH 44109-1998
Tel: 216 778-2748 *Fax:* 216 778-3927
E-mail: lbiblo@metrohealth.org
Accred Length: 3 Years *Program Size:* 7
Program ID: 141-38-11-196

Case Western Reserve University Program

Sponsor: University Hospitals of Cleveland
Veterans Affairs Medical Center (Cleveland)

Program Director:
Frank V Brozovich, MD
Case Western Reserve Univ-Univ Hospitals of Cleveland
Div of Cardiology
11100 Euclid Ave
Cleveland, OH 44106-5038
Tel: 216 844-7603 *Fax:* 216 844-8954
E-mail: cvfellow@po.cwru.edu
Internet: http://www.cwru.edu/med/cardiology.html
Accred Length: 3 Years *Program Size:* 11
Program ID: 141-38-21-194

Cleveland Clinic Foundation Program

Sponsor: Cleveland Clinic Foundation

Program Director:
Brian Griffin, MD
Cleveland Clinic Foundation
Dept of Cardiovascular Disease/F25
9500 Euclid Ave
Cleveland, OH 44195-5242
Tel: 216 444-5690 *Fax:* 216 444-1162
E-mail: meded@cestmp.ccf.org
Internet: http://www.ccf.org
Accred Length: 3 Years *Program Size:* 36
Program ID: 141-38-12-197

Columbus

Ohio State University Program

Sponsor: Ohio State University Medical Center

Program Director:
Albert J Kolibash Jr, MD
Ohio State Univ Hospitals
1654 Upham Dr
601 Means Hall
Columbus, OH 43210-1228
Tel: 614 293-8962 *Fax:* 614 293-5614
Accred Length: 3 Years *Program Size:* 6
Program ID: 141-38-11-179

Dayton

Wright State University Program

Sponsor: Wright State University School of Medicine
Good Samaritan Hospital and Health Center
Veterans Affairs Medical Center (Dayton)

Program Director:
Mohsen Sakhaii, MD
Good Samaritan Hospital
2222 Philadelphia Dr
Dayton, OH 45406
Tel: 513 278-6251, ext 3311 *Fax:* 513 276-8253
Accred Length: 3 Years *Program Size:* 6
Program ID: 141-38-21-217

Toledo

Medical College of Ohio Program

Sponsor: Medical College of Ohio
Medical College of Ohio Hospital

Program Director:
Joseph Abruzzo, MD
Med Coll of Ohio
Dept of Med
3120 Glendale Ave
Toledo, OH 43614
Tel: 419 383-3697 *Fax:* 419 383-3041
E-mail: cariologyao@gemini.mco.edu
Internet:
http://www.mco.edu/medicine/fellowship/index.html
Accred Length: 3 Years *Program Size:* 5
Program ID: 141-38-21-068

Oklahoma

Oklahoma City

University of Oklahoma Health Sciences Center Program

Sponsor: University of Oklahoma College of Medicine
University Hospital
Veterans Affairs Medical Center (Oklahoma City)

Program Director:
C A Sivaram, MD
Univ of Oklahoma Health Sciences Ctr
PO Box 26901
VAMC-111B
Oklahoma City, OK 73190
Tel: 405 270-4742, ext 3268 *Fax:* 405 270-1576
E-mail: chittur_sivaram@uokhsc.edu
Accred Length: 3 Years *Program Size:* 11
Program ID: 141-39-21-103

Oregon

Portland

Oregon Health Sciences University Program

Sponsor: Oregon Health Sciences University Hospital
Veterans Affairs Medical Center (Portland)

Program Director:
Edward S Murphy, MD
Oregon Health Sciences Univ
Div of Cardiology
3181 SW Sam Jackson Park Rd/UHN62
Portland, OR 97201-3098
Tel: 503 494-8750 *Fax:* 503 494-8550
Accred Length: 3 Years *Program Size:* 8
Program ID: 141-40-31-198

Pennsylvania

Danville

Penn State Geisinger Health System/Geisinger Medical Center Program

Sponsor: Penn State Geisinger Health System
Geisinger Medical Center

Program Director:
John M Costello, MD
Geisinger Med Ctr
100 N Academy Ave
Danville, PA 17822-2013
Tel: 717 271-6423 *Fax:* 717 271-8795
E-mail: ckrebs@psghs.edu
Accred Length: 3 Years *Program Size:* 8
Program ID: 141-41-11-173

Hershey

Penn State Geisinger Health System/Milton S Hershey Medical Center Program

Sponsor: Penn State Geisinger Health System
Milton S Hershey Medical Center

Program Director:
Joseph A Gascho, MD
Div of Cardiology
Milton S Hershey Med Ctr
PO Box 850/H047
Hershey, PA 17033
Tel: 717 531-8407 *Fax:* 717 531-7969
Accred Length: 3 Years *Program Size:* 11
Program ID: 141-41-11-017

Philadelphia

Albert Einstein Medical Center Program

Sponsor: Albert Einstein Medical Center

Program Director:
Larry Jacobs, MD
Albert Einstein Med Ctr
5401 Old York Rd
Klein Bldg/Ste 363
Philadelphia, PA 19141
Tel: 215 456-7266 *Fax:* 215 455-1933
E-mail: kotlerm@aehn2.einstein.edu
Internet: http://www.einstein.edu
Accred Length: 3 Years *Program Size:* 11
Program ID: 141-41-11-082

Episcopal Hospital Program

Sponsor: Episcopal Hospital (TUHS)

Program Director:
Gerardo Voci, MD PhD
Episcopal Hospital
100 E Lehigh Ave
MAB Ste 305
Philadelphia, PA 19125-1098
Tel: 215 427-6216 *Fax:* 215 427-7358
Accred Length: 3 Years *Program Size:* 10
Program ID: 141-41-11-052

Graduate Hospital Program

Sponsor: Graduate Hospital

Program Director:
Thomas Kreulen, MD
Graduate Hospital
Pepper Pavilion/Ste101
Philadelphia, PA 19146-1497
Tel: 215 893-2495 *Fax:* 215 893-2648
E-mail: kreulen@ix.netcom.com
Accred Length: 3 Years *Program Size:* 9
Program ID: 141-41-11-174

MCP Hahnemann University Program

Sponsor: MCP Hahnemann University
Hahnemann University Hospital
Medical College of Pennsylvania Hospital

Program Director:
William G Kussmaul III, MD
Hahnemann Univ Hosp
Dept of Cardiology
Broad and Vine Sts/MS 119
Philadelphia, PA 19102
Tel: 215 762-7093 *Fax:* 215 762-3196
Accred Length: 3 Years *Program Size:* 35
Program ID: 141-41-21-145

Temple University Program

Sponsor: Temple University Hospital

Program Director:
Alfred E Buxton, MD
Temple Univ Hospital
Cardiology Section
3401 N Broad St
Philadelphia, PA 19140
Tel: 215 707-3346 *Fax:* 215 707-3946
E-mail: abuxton@nimbus.ocis.temple.edu
Accred Length: 3 Years *Program Size:* 9
Program ID: 141-41-21-036

Thomas Jefferson University Program

Sponsor: Thomas Jefferson University Hospital

Program Director:
Arnold J Greenspon, MD
Thomas Jefferson Univ Hospital
1025 Walnut St/Ste 403
Philadelphia, PA 19107
Tel: 215 955-1976 *Fax:* 215 923-2539
E-mail: greenspl@jeflin.tju.edu
Accred Length: 3 Years *Program Size:* 14
Program ID: 141-41-21-037

University of Pennsylvania Program

Sponsor: Hospital of the University of Pennsylvania

Program Director:
Martin G St John Sutton, MD
Hospital of Univ of Pennsylvania
Cardiovascular Div/9 Gates
3400 Spruce St
Philadelphia, PA 19104-4283
Tel: 215 662-3990 *Fax:* 215 349-8190
E-mail: rghall@mail.med.upenn.edu
Accred Length: 3 Years *Program Size:* 22
Program ID: 141-41-21-023

Pittsburgh

Allegheny General Hospital Program

Sponsor: Allegheny General Hospital

Program Director:
Christopher M Kramer, MD
Allegheny General Hospital
Div of Cardiology
320 E North Ave
Pittsburgh, PA 15212-9986
Tel: 412 359-8700 *Fax:* 412 359-8964
Accred Length: 3 Years *Program Size:* 12
Program ID: 141-41-11-053

Shadyside Hospital/UPMC Program

Sponsor: Shadyside Hospital/UPMC

Program Director:
Robert J Ruffner, MD
UPMC Shadyside
Med Educ Dept
5230 Centre Ave
Pittsburgh, PA 15232
Tel: 412 623-2296 *Fax:* 412 683-0191
Internet: http://ssh.edu
Accred Length: 3 Years *Program Size:* 9
Program ID: 141-41-22-069

University Health Center of Pittsburgh Program

Sponsor: University Health Center of Pittsburgh
Presbyterian University Hospital/UPMC
Veterans Affairs Medical Center (Pittsburgh)

Program Director:
James A Shaver, MD
Presbyterian Univ Hospital
S-555 Scaife Hall
200 Lothrop St
Pittsburgh, PA 15213
Tel: 412 383-8750 *Fax:* 412 383-8857
E-mail: shaverja@msx.upmc.edu
Internet: http://www.upmc.edu/cardiology
Accred Length: 3 Years *Program Size:* 15
Program ID: 141-41-21-054

Western Pennsylvania Hospital Program

Sponsor: Western Pennsylvania Hospital

Program Director:
Alan H Gradman, MD
Western Pennsylvania Hospital
4800 Friendship Ave
Ste 3411/N Tower
Pittsburgh, PA 15224
Tel: 412 578-6934 *Fax:* 412 578-4471
E-mail: gradmanmd@aol.com
Accred Length: 3 Years *Program Size:* 6
Program ID: 141-41-11-083

Wynnewood

Lankenau Hospital Program
Sponsor: Lankenau Hospital
Program Director:
James F Burke, MD
Lankenau Hospital
100 Lancaster Ave
Medical Office Bldg East/Ste 558
Wynnewood, PA 19096
Tel: 610 645-2682 *Fax:* 610 896-0643
Accred Length: 3 Years *Program Size:* 9
Program ID: 141-41-11-035

Puerto Rico

Ponce

Hospital de Damas Program
Sponsor: Hospital de Damas
Hospital San Lucas
Program Director:
Felix M Cortes, MD
Hospital de Damas
2213 Ponce By Pass
Ponce, PR 00731-7779
Tel: 787 840-8686, ext 6123
Accred Length: 3 Years *Program Size:* 6
Program ID: 141-42-11-117

Rio Piedras

San Juan City Hospital Program
Sponsor: San Juan City Hospital
University of Puerto Rico School of Medicine
Program Director:
Jorge E Lugo-Rodriguez, MD
San Juan City Hospital
PO Box 70344
CMMS #68
San Juan, PR 00936
Tel: 787 766-2222, ext 2401 *Fax:* 787 756-7796
Accred Length: 3 Years *Program Size:* 6
Program ID: 141-42-11-118

San Juan

University of Puerto Rico Program
Sponsor: University of Puerto Rico School of Medicine
University Hospital
Program Director:
Mario R Garcia-Palmieri, MD
Univ Hospital
Box 365067
San Juan, PR 00936-5067
Tel: 787 767-8499 *Fax:* 787 754-1739
Accred Length: 3 Years *Program Size:* 9
Program ID: 141-42-21-148

Veterans Affairs Medical and Regional Office Center Program
Sponsor: Veterans Affairs Medical Center (San Juan)
Program Director:
Edgardo Hernandez-Lopez, MD
Cardiology Sect
VA Med Ctr
One Veterans Plaza
San Juan, PR 00927-5800
Tel: 787 766-6520 *Fax:* 787 766-6021
Accred Length: 3 Years *Program Size:* 5
Program ID: 141-42-31-147

Rhode Island

Providence

Brown University Program 2
Sponsor: Rhode Island Hospital
Memorial Hospital of Rhode Island
Miriam Hospital
Veterans Affairs Medical Center (Providence)
Program Director:
Peter L Tilkemeier, MD
Miriam Hospital
164 Smmit Ave
Providence, RI 02906
Tel: 401 793-4104 *Fax:* 401 793-4049
E-mail: peter_tilkemeier@brown.edu
Internet:
http://biomedcs.biomed.brown.edu/catmed/cardio_fellows
Accred Length: 3 Years *Program Size:* 12
Program ID: 141-43-21-260

Brown University Program
Sponsor: Rhode Island Hospital
Program Director:
Lynne L Johnson, MD
Div of Cardiology
Rhode Island Hospital
593 Eddy St
Providence, RI 02903
Tel: 401 277-5891 *Fax:* 401 444-5124
E-mail: lynne_johnson@brown.edu
Accred Length: 3 Years *Program Size:* 8
Program ID: 141-43-11-149

South Carolina

Charleston

Medical University of South Carolina Program
Sponsor: Medical University of South Carolina College of Medicine
MUSC Medical Center
Program Director:
Bruce W Usher, MD
Med Univ of South Carolina
Cardiology Div
MUSC 600 Complex Ste 816
Charleston, SC 29425-2221
Tel: 803 792-4411 *Fax:* 803 792-7771
Accred Length: 3 Years *Program Size:* 12
Program ID: 141-45-21-129

Columbia

Palmetto Health Alliance/University of South Carolina School of Medicine Program
Sponsor: Palmetto Health Alliance
Palmetto Richland Memorial Hospital
William Jennings Bryan Dorn Veterans Hospital
Program Director:
Nowamagbe A Omoigui, MD MPH
Palmetto Richland Memorial Hospital
Two Medical Park Rd/Ste 501
Columbia, SC 29203
Tel: 803 540-1100 *Fax:* 803 540-1110
E-mail: nowa@richmed.medpark.sc.edu
Internet: http://www.med.sc.edu/heart
Accred Length: 3 Years *Program Size:* 6
Program ID: 141-45-21-110

Tennessee

Johnson City

East Tennessee State University Program
Sponsor: James H Quillen College of Medicine
Johnson City Medical Center Hospital
Veterans Affairs Medical Center (Mountain Home)
Program Director:
David S Sheps, MD
East Tennessee State Univ
Dept of Internal Med
PO Box 70622
Johnson City, TN 37614-0622
Tel: 423 232-4884 *Fax:* 423 439-6387
Accred Length: 3 Years *Program Size:* 8
Program ID: 141-47-21-104

Memphis

University of Tennessee Program
Sponsor: University of Tennessee College of Medicine
Regional Medical Center at Memphis
Veterans Affairs Medical Center (Memphis)
Program Director:
Jay M Sullivan, MD
Dept of Med
956 Court Ave/Rm D334
Memphis, TN 38163
Tel: 901 448-5759 *Fax:* 901 448-8084
E-mail: jmsu@meditech.vowld.utmem.edu
Accred Length: 3 Years *Program Size:* 7
Program ID: 141-47-21-175

Nashville

Vanderbilt University Program
Sponsor: Vanderbilt University Medical Center
Program Director:
Douglas E Vaughan, MD
Vanderbilt Univ Sch of Med
Div of Cardiology
315 MRBII
Nashville, TN 37232-6300
Tel: 615 936-1720 *Fax:* 615 936-1872
Accred Length: 3 Years *Program Size:* 12
Program ID: 141-47-31-018

Texas

Dallas

Baylor University Medical Center Program
Sponsor: Baylor University Medical Center
Program Director:
Peter J Wells, MD
Baylor Univ Med Ctr
Dept of Int Med
3500 Gaston Ave
Dallas, TX 75246
Tel: 214 820-6202 *Fax:* 214 820-6385
Internet:
http://www.bhcs.com/bumc/medicaleducation/residencies.htm
Accred Length: 3 Years *Program Size:* 6
Program ID: 141-48-31-176

University of Texas Southwestern Medical School Program
Sponsor: University of Texas Southwestern Medical School
Dallas County Hospital District-Parkland Memorial Hospital
Veterans Affairs Medical Center (Dallas)
Program Director:
Thomas C Andrews, MD
Univ of Texas Southwestern Med Ctr
Cardiology Div CS7102
5323 Harry Hines Blvd
Dallas, TX 75235-9047
Tel: 214 648-6893 *Fax:* 214 648-6783
Internet: http://www.swmed.edu/home_pages/cardiology/
Accred Length: 3 Years *Program Size:* 14
Program ID: 141-48-21-119

Fort Sam Houston

San Antonio Uniformed Services Health Education Consortium (BAMC) Program
Sponsor: San Antonio Uniformed Services Health Education Consortium
Brooke Army Medical Center
Program Director:
Karl C Stajduhar, MD
Brooke Army Med Ctr
Cardiology Service
3851 Roger Brooke Dr/Bldg 3600
Fort Sam Houston, TX 78234-6200
Tel: 210 916-3305 *Fax:* 210 916-3051
Accred Length: 3 Years *Program Size:* 20
Program ID: 141-48-12-177
US Armed Services Program

Galveston

University of Texas Medical Branch Hospitals Program
Sponsor: University of Texas Medical Branch Hospitals
Program Director:
Marschall S Runge, MD PhD
Univ of Texas Med Branch
301 University Blvd
Galveston, TX 77555-0553
Tel: 409 772-1533 *Fax:* 409 772-4982
Accred Length: 3 Years *Program Size:* 14
Program ID: 141-48-21-070

Houston

Baylor College of Medicine Program 1
Sponsor: Baylor College of Medicine
Harris County Hospital District-Ben Taub General Hospital
Methodist Hospital
Veterans Affairs Medical Center (Houston)
Program Director:
Robert Roberts, MD
Baylor Coll of Med
Sect of Cardiology
6550 Fannin St/MS SM677
Houston, TX 77030
Tel: 713 790-4871 *Fax:* 713 790-4348
E-mail: rroberts@bcm.tmc.edu
Internet: http://www.bmc.tmc.edu
Accred Length: 3 Years *Program Size:* 32
Program ID: 141-48-21-106

Baylor College of Medicine Program 2
Sponsor: Baylor College of Medicine
St Luke's Episcopal Hospital
Program Director:
Robert J Hall, MD
St Luke's Episcopal Hospital
6720 Bertner Ave/Rm P332
Mail Code 1-133
Houston, TX 77030
Tel: 713 794-6676 *Fax:* 713 791-8374
Accred Length: 3 Years *Program Size:* 18
Program ID: 141-48-21-120

University of Texas at Houston Program
Sponsor: University of Texas Medical School at Houston
Lyndon B Johnson General Hospital
Memorial Hermann Healthcare System
Program Director:
Francisco Fuentes, MD
UTMSH, Div of Cardiology
6431 Fannin St
PO Box 20708
Houston, TX 77025
Tel: 713 500-6577 *Fax:* 713 500-6556
E-mail: ralvarez@med.uth.tmc.edu
Accred Length: 3 Years *Program Size:* 17
Program ID: 141-48-31-019

Lubbock

Texas Tech University (Lubbock) Program
Sponsor: Texas Tech University Health Sciences Center at Lubbock
University Medical Center
Program Director:
Leigh Ann Jenkins, MD
Texas Tech Univ Health Sciences Ctr
Cardiology Div
3601 Fourth St
Lubbock, TX 79430
Tel: 806 743-3155 *Fax:* 806 743-3148
Accred Length: 3 Years *Program Size:* 6
Program ID: 141-48-21-121

San Antonio

University of Texas Health Science Center at San Antonio Program
Sponsor: University of Texas Medical School at San Antonio
Audie L Murphy Memorial Veterans Hospital (San Antonio)
University Hospital-South Texas Medical Center
Program Director:
Sumanth D Prabhu, MD
Univ of Texas Health Science Ctr
Div of Cardiology
7703 Floyd Curl Dr
San Antonio, TX 78284-7872
Tel: 210 567-4602 *Fax:* 210 567-6960
E-mail: prabhu@uthscsa.edu
Internet: http://amplatz.uthscsa.edu
Accred Length: 3 Years *Program Size:* 10
Program ID: 141-48-21-084

Temple

Texas A&M College of Medicine-Scott and White Program
Sponsor: Scott and White Memorial Hospital
Program Director:
D Scott Gantt, DO
Texas A&M-Scott & White
Grad Med Education
2401 S 31st St
Temple, TX 76508-0001
Tel: 254 724-9290 *Fax:* 254 724-8425
E-mail: jlsmith@swmail.sw.org
Internet: http://www.sw.org
Accred Length: 3 Years *Program Size:* 6
Program ID: 141-48-21-020

Utah

Salt Lake City

University of Utah Program
Sponsor: University of Utah Medical Center
Veterans Affairs Medical Center (Salt Lake City)
Program Director:
Jay W Mason, MD
Univ of Utah Health Sciences Ctr
Cardiology Div
50 N Medical Dr
Salt Lake City, UT 84132-1001
Tel: 801 581-7715 *Fax:* 801 581-7735
E-mail: jay.mason@hsc.utah.edu
Accred Length: 3 Years *Program Size:* 11
Program ID: 141-49-21-199

Vermont

Burlington

University of Vermont Program
Sponsor: Fletcher Allen Health Care
Program Director:
Mark Capeless, MD
Cardiology Dept
Med Ctr Hospital of Vermont
Burlington, VT 05401
Tel: 802 656-3734 *Fax:* 802 656-3637
Accred Length: 3 Years *Program Size:* 9
Program ID: 141-50-21-200

Virginia

Charlottesville

University of Virginia Program
Sponsor: University of Virginia Medical Center
Program Director:
David E Haines, MD
Univ of Virginia Health Sciences Ctr
Box 158/Cardiovascular Div
Charlottesville, VA 22908
Tel: 804 924-2675 *Fax:* 804 243-2625
E-mail: aguenther@virginia.edu
Internet: http://www.virginia.edu/docs/heart
Accred Length: 3 Years *Program Size:* 15
Program ID: 141-51-21-021

Richmond

Medical College of Virginia/Virginia Commonwealth University Program
Sponsor: Medical College of Virginia/Virginia Commonwealth University
Medical College of Virginia Hospitals
Program Director:
Anthony J Minisi, MD
Med Coll of Virginia, Div of Cardiology
PO Box 980128
Richmond, VA 23298-0128
Tel: 804 828-9989 *Fax:* 804 828-3544
Accred Length: 3 Years *Program Size:* 14
Program ID: 141-51-21-022

Washington

Seattle

University of Washington Program
Sponsor: University of Washington School of Medicine
University of Washington Medical Center
Veterans Affairs Medical Center (Seattle)
Program Director:
Catherine M Otto, MD
Univ of Washington
Box 356422
1959 NE Pacific St
Seattle, WA 98195
Tel: 206 685-1397 *Fax:* 206 685-9394
E-mail: uwcard@u.washington.edu
Accred Length: 3 Years *Program Size:* 14
Program ID: 141-54-21-105

Tacoma

Madigan Army Medical Center Program
Sponsor: Madigan Army Medical Center
Program Director:
Alice M Mascette, MD
Cardiology Service
Madigan Army Med Ctr
Tacoma, WA 98431
Tel: 253 968-1090 *Fax:* 253 968-0100
Accred Length: 3 Years *Program Size:* 3
Program ID: 141-54-21-252
US Armed Services Program

West Virginia

Huntington

Marshall University School of Medicine Program
Sponsor: Marshall University School of Medicine
Cabell Huntington Hospital
St Mary's Hospital
Veterans Affairs Medical Center (Huntington)
Program Director:
Paulette S Wehner, MD
Marshall Univ Sch of Med
Dept of Med
1600 Medical Center Dr/Ste G-500
Huntington, WV 25701-3655
Tel: 304 691-1084 *Fax:* 304 691-1693
Accred Length: 3 Years *Program Size:* 9
Program ID: 141-55-21-038

Morgantown

West Virginia University Program
Sponsor: West Virginia University Hospitals
Program Director:
Abnash C Jain, MD
West Virginia Univ
2203 Health Science Ctr South
Morgantown, WV 26506-9157
Tel: 304 293-4096 *Fax:* 304 293-7828
E-mail: acjain@wvnvm.wvnet.edu
Accred Length: 3 Years *Program Size:* 6
Program ID: 141-55-11-219

Wisconsin

Madison

University of Wisconsin Program
Sponsor: University of Wisconsin Hospital and Clinics
William S Middleton Veterans Hospital
Program Director:
Ford Ballantyne III, MD
Univ of Wisconsin Hospital and Clinics
600 Highland Ave/Rm H6-349
Madison, WI 53792-3248
Tel: 608 263-0891 *Fax:* 608 263-0405
E-mail: paf@medicine.wisc.edu
Internet:
http://www.medicine.wisc.edu/sections/cardiology/cardio_fellow.html
Accred Length: 3 Years *Program Size:* 12
Program ID: 141-56-21-150

Milwaukee

Aurora Health Care Program
Sponsor: Aurora Health Care
Sinai Samaritan Medical Center
Program Director:
Dianne L Zwicke, MD
Sinai Samaritan Med Ctr
PO Box 342
945 N 12th St
Milwaukee, WI 53201-0342
Tel: 414 219-3317 *Fax:* 414 219-7809
Accred Length: 3 Years *Program Size:* 9
Program ID: 141-56-21-072

Medical College of Wisconsin Program
Sponsor: Medical College of Wisconsin Affiliated Hospitals Inc
Clement J Zablocki Veterans Affairs Medical Center
Froedtert Memorial Lutheran Hospital
Program Director:
John C Wynsen, MD
Med Coll of Wisconsin
Cardiovascular Med
9200 W Wisconsin Ave
Milwaukee, WI 53226-8110
Tel: 414 456-6761 *Fax:* 414 456-6203
Accred Length: 3 Years *Program Size:* 9
Program ID: 141-56-31-056

Chemical Pathology (Pathology)

Michigan

Ann Arbor

University of Michigan Program
Sponsor: University of Michigan Hospitals
Program Director:
Anthony A Killeen, MD
1301 Catherine St
Ann Arbor, MI 48109-0602
Tel: 734 936-1873 *Fax:* 734 936-2756
E-mail: ekilleen@umich.edu
Accred Length: 1 Year *Program Size:* 0
Program ID: 306-25-21-010

Royal Oak

William Beaumont Hospital Program
Sponsor: William Beaumont Hospital
Program Director:
Elizabeth Sykes, MB BS
William Beaumont Hospital
3601 W 13 Mile Rd
Royal Oak, MI 48073
Tel: 248 551-8022 *Fax:* 248 551-3694
E-mail: esykes@beaumont.edu
Internet: http://www.beaumont.edu/html/gme
Accred Length: 1 Year *Program Size:* 1
Program ID: 306-25-21-008

Texas

Houston

University of Texas M D Anderson Cancer Center Program
Sponsor: University of Texas M D Anderson Cancer Center
Program Director:
Frank J Liu, MD
Univ of Texas-MD Anderson Cancer Ctr
Lab Med/Box 37
1515 Holcombe Blvd
Houston, TX 77030
Tel: 713 792-4749 *Fax:* 713 792-4793
E-mail: fjl@notes.mdacc.tmc.edu
Accred Length: 1 Year *Program Size:* 1
Program ID: 306-48-21-004

Virginia

Richmond

Medical College of Virginia/Virginia Commonwealth University Program
Sponsor: Medical College of Virginia/Virginia Commonwealth University
Medical College of Virginia Hospitals
Program Director:
Richard A McPherson, MD
Greg Miller, PhD
Med Coll of Virginia
Dept of Pathology
PO Box 980258
Richmond, VA 23298-0258
Tel: 804 828-5389 *Fax:* 804 828-6156
Accred Length: 1 Year *Program Size:* 1
Program ID: 306-51-21-002

Child and Adolescent Psychiatry (Psychiatry)

Alabama

Birmingham

University of Alabama Medical Center Program
Sponsor: University of Alabama Hospital
Children's Hospital of Alabama
Program Director:
Lee I Ascherman, MD
Dept of Child/Adolescent Psych
Smolian Bldg/3rd Fl
1700 7th Ave S
Birmingham, AL 35294-0018
Tel: 205 975-8204 *Fax:* 205 934-4659
E-mail: lascher@smopsy1.his.uab.edu
Accred Length: 2 Years *Program Size:* 6
Program ID: 405-01-21-172

Arizona

Tucson

University of Arizona Program
Sponsor: University of Arizona College of Medicine
University Medical Center
Program Director:
Patrick M Burke, MD PhD
Arizona Health Sciences Ctr
1501 N Campbell Ave
PO Box 245002
Tucson, AZ 85724-5002
Tel: 520 626-6473 *Fax:* 520 626-2004
E-mail: burke@u.arizona.edu
Internet: http://www.medicine.arizona edu/psychiatry/
Accred Length: 2 Years *Program Size:* 4
Program ID: 405-03-21-142

Arkansas

Little Rock

University of Arkansas for Medical Sciences Program
Sponsor: University of Arkansas College of Medicine
Arkansas Children's Hospital
Arkansas State Hospital-Little Rock Hospital
University Hospital of Arkansas
Program Director:
Andre Derdeyn, MD
Univ of Arkansas for Med Sciences
Arkansas Children's Hospital
1120 Marshall St/Slot 654
Little Rock, AR 72202-3591
Tel: 501 320-4670 *Fax:* 501 320-1592
E-mail: derdeynandrep@exchange.uam.edu
Accred Length: 2 Years *Program Size:* 4
Program ID: 405-04-21-146

California

Los Angeles

Cedars-Sinai Medical Center Program
Sponsor: Cedars-Sinai Medical Center
Program Director:
Roxy Szeftel, MD
Cedars-Sinai Med Ctr
8730 Alden Dr/E-201
Los Angeles, CA 90048-0750
Tel: 310 855-3564 *Fax:* 310 967-0114
E-mail: roxy.szeftel@cshs.org
Internet: http://www.csmc.edu
Accred Length: 2 Years *Program Size:* 6
Program ID: 405-05-11-008

UCLA Medical Center Program
Sponsor: UCLA School of Medicine
UCLA Neuropsychiatric Hospital
Program Director:
Bonnie Zima, MD
UCLA Neuropsychiatric Inst
Attn: Sandra Lipschultz, Admin
760 Westwood Plaza/Rm C8-852
Los Angeles, CA 90024-1759
Tel: 310 825-0548 *Fax:* 310 825-0340
E-mail: sandrajl@npih.medsch.ucla.edu
Internet: http://www.mentalhealth.ucla.edu/trainees
Accred Length: 2 Years *Program Size:* 12
Program ID: 405-05-12-012

University of Southern California Program
Sponsor: Los Angeles County-USC Medical Center
Program Director:
Sidney Russak, MD PhD
Los Angeles County-USC Psychiatric Hospital
1937 Hospital Pl
Graduate Hall/Rm 155
Los Angeles, CA 90033
Tel: 213 226-5288 *Fax:* 213 226-5822
Accred Length: 2 Years *Program Size:* 14
Program ID: 405-05-11-010

Orange

University of California (Irvine) Program
Sponsor: University of California (Irvine) Medical Center
Program Director:
Kenneth Steinhoff, MD
Univ of California Irvine Med Ctr
Neuropsychiatric Ctr/Bldg 3 Rte 88
101 City Dr S
Orange, CA 92668
Tel: 714 456-5823 *Fax:* 714 586-1484
E-mail: ksteinho@uci.edu
Accred Length: 2 Years *Program Size:* 4
Program ID: 405-05-11-007

Sacramento

University of California (Davis) Program
Sponsor: University of California (Davis) Medical Center
Program Director:
Emily Harris, MD
Univ of California Davis Med Ctr
2315 Stockton Blvd
Sacramento, CA 95817
Tel: 916 734-2614 *Fax:* 916 451-9946
E-mail: esharris@ucdavis.edu
Internet:
http://www.neuroscience.ucdavis.edu/psychiatry
Accred Length: 2 Years *Program Size:* 6
Program ID: 405-05-11-005

San Diego

University of California (San Diego) Program
Sponsor: University of California (San Diego) Medical Center
Children's Hospital and Health Center
Program Director:
Ellen K Heyneman, MD
UCSD Med Ctr
3030 Children's Way
Ste 103
San Diego, CA 92123-4226
Tel: 619 495-4939 *Fax:* 619 627-0710
E-mail: eheyneman@ucsd.edu
Accred Length: 2 Years *Program Size:* 6
Program ID: 405-05-21-014

San Francisco

University of California (San Francisco) Program
Sponsor: University of California (San Francisco) School of Medicine
University of California (San Francisco) Medical Center
Program Director:
Graeme Hanson, MD
Univ of California San Francisco
401 Parnassus Ave
Box CAS-0984
San Francisco, CA 94143-0984
Tel: 415 476-7233 *Fax:* 415 476-7163
E-mail: graemeh@lppi.ucsf.edu
Internet: http://itsa.ucsf.edu/~lppi
Accred Length: 2 Years *Program Size:* 8
Program ID: 405-05-21-018

Stanford

Stanford University Program
Sponsor: Stanford University Hospital
Program Director:
Hans Steiner, MD
Stanford Univ Sch of Med
Div of Child Psychiatry
401 Quarry Rd/Rm C107B
Stanford, CA 94305-5719
Tel: 650 725-0957 *Fax:* 650 723-5531
E-mail: marsha@leland.stanford.edu
Internet:
http://www-cap.stanford.edu/training/index.html
Accred Length: 2 Years *Program Size:* 6
Program ID: 405-05-21-019

Torrance

Los Angeles County-Harbor-UCLA Medical Center Program
Sponsor: Los Angeles County-Harbor-UCLA Medical Center
College Hospital
Program Director:
Zev Nathan, MD PhD
Los Angeles County-Harbor-UCLA Med Ctr
1000 W Carson St/Box 498
PO Box 2910
Torrance, CA 90509-2910
Tel: 310 222-1615 *Fax:* 310 328-7217
E-mail: z_nathan@humc.edu
Accred Length: 2 Years *Program Size:* 6
Program ID: 405-05-21-020

Colorado

Denver

University of Colorado Program
Sponsor: University of Colorado Health Sciences Center
Program Director:
Donald W Bechtold, MD
Univ of Colorado Sch of Med
Campus Box B148
4200 E Ninth Ave
Denver, CO 80262
Tel: 303 315-7748 *Fax:* 303 315-4048
E-mail: dbechtold@crete.uchsc.edu
Accred Length: 2 Years *Program Size:* 10
Program ID: 405-07-11-021

Connecticut

Farmington

Institute of Living/University of Connecticut Program
Sponsor: University of Connecticut School of Medicine
Connecticut Children's Medical Center
Institute of Living
Mount Sinai Hospital
Univ of Connecticut Health Center/John Dempsey Hospital
Program Director:
Lisa Namerow, MD
Institute of Living
400 Washington St
Hartford, CT 06106
Tel: 860 545-7183
Accred Length: 2 Years *Program Size:* 6
Program ID: 405-08-21-022

New Haven

Yale-New Haven Medical Center Program
Sponsor: Yale-New Haven Hospital
Riverview Hospital for Children
Program Director:
Dorothy E Stubbe, MD
Yale Univ Child Study Ctr
PO Box 207900
230 S Frontage Rd
New Haven, CT 06520-7900
Tel: 203 785-2516 *Fax:* 203 785-7400
Accred Length: 2 Years *Program Size:* 12
Program ID: 405-08-11-023

District of Columbia

Washington

Children's National Medical Center Program
Sponsor: Children's National Medical Center
Program Director:
Kenneth E Towbin, MD
Children's Hospital National Med Ctr
Dept of Psychiatry
111 Michigan Ave NW
Washington, DC 20010-2970
Tel: 202 884-5420 *Fax:* 202 745-4112
Accred Length: 2 Years *Program Size:* 8
Program ID: 405-10-21-024

Florida

Gainesville

University of Florida Program
Sponsor: University of Florida College of Medicine
Shands Hospital at the University of Florida
University Medical Center (UFHSC/J)
Program Director:
Regina Bussing, MD
Div of Child/Adolescent Psych
PO Box 100234/UFHSC
1600 SW Archer Rd
Gainesville, FL 32610-0234
Tel: 352 392-3641 *Fax:* 352 392-4588
Accred Length: 2 Years *Program Size:* 8
Program ID: 405-11-11-026

Miami

University of Miami-Jackson Memorial Medical Center Program
Sponsor: University of Miami-Jackson Memorial Medical Center
University of Miami Hospital and Clinics
Program Director:
Jon A Shaw, MD
Univ of Miami Sch of Med
Dept of Psychiatry D-29
PO Box 016960
Miami, FL 33101
Tel: 305 585-6862 *Fax:* 305 325-8355
Accred Length: 2 Years *Program Size:* 11
Program ID: 405-11-21-027

Tampa

University of South Florida Program
Sponsor: University of South Florida College of Medicine
Tampa General Healthcare
TGH University Psychiatry Center
Program Director:
Kailie R Shaw, MD
Univ of South Florida
3515 E Fletcher Ave
Tampa, FL 33613
Tel: 813 974-2388 *Fax:* 813 974-3223
E-mail: kshaw@com1.med.usf.edu.
Internet: http://www.med.usf.edu.psych.psychome.html
Accred Length: 2 Years *Program Size:* 4
Program ID: 405-11-21-140

Georgia

Atlanta

Emory University Program
Sponsor: Emory University School of Medicine
Egleston Children's Hospital at Emory University
Georgia Mental Health Institute
Grady Memorial Hospital
Program Director:
Arden D Dingle, MD
Emory Univ Sch of Med
Briarcliff Childrens Unit 8
1256 Briarcliff Rd NE
Atlanta, GA 30306
Tel: 404 894-6303 *Fax:* 404 894-5847
E-mail: adingle@emory.edu
Accred Length: 2 Years *Program Size:* 8
Program ID: 405-12-21-028

Augusta

Medical College of Georgia Program
Sponsor: Medical College of Georgia Hospital and Clinics
Dwight David Eisenhower Army Medical Center
Georgia Regional Hospital at Augusta
Program Director:
Allan M Josephson, MD
Med Coll of Georgia
Dept of Psychiatry
1515 Pope Ave
Augusta, GA 30912-3800
Tel: 706 721-6699 *Fax:* 706 721-1793
E-mail: ajosephs@mail.mcg.edu
Accred Length: 2 Years *Program Size:* 8
Program ID: 405-12-21-148

Hawaii

Honolulu

Tripler Army Medical Center Program
Sponsor: Tripler Army Medical Center
Kahi Mohala Hospital
Program Director:
Wayne B Batzer, MD
Tripler Army Med Ctr, Child/Adolescent Psych Service
MCHK-PSC
1 Jarrett White Rd
Tripler AMC, HI 96859-5000
Tel: 808 433-6418 *Fax:* 808 433-4591
E-mail:
ltc_wayne_batzer@smtplink.tamc.amedd.army.mil
Internet: http://www.tamc.amedd.army.mil
Accred Length: 2 Years *Program Size:* 5
Program ID: 405-14-21-143
US Armed Services Program

University of Hawaii Program
Sponsor: University of Hawaii John A Burns School of Medicine
Kahi Mohala Hospital
Kapiolani Medical Center for Women and Children
Program Director:
Alayne Yates, MD
Univ of Hawaii
1319 Punahou St/Rm 635
Honolulu, HI 96826
Tel: 808 983-8375 *Fax:* 808 942-5725
E-mail: yatesa@jabsom.biomed.hawaii.edu
Accred Length: 2 Years *Program Size:* 6
Program ID: 405-14-31-029

Illinois

Chicago

McGaw Medical Center of Northwestern University Program
Sponsor: Northwestern University Medical School
Children's Memorial Medical Center
Northwestern Memorial Hospital
Program Director:
Carrie E Sylvester, MD MPH
2300 Children's Plaza/Box 10
Chicago, IL 60614-3394
Tel: 773 880-4833 *Fax:* 773 880-4066
E-mail: c-sylvester@nwu.edu
Internet: http://www.childmmc.edu/hmhweb/cmhdepts/psychweb/psychresprogram.html
Accred Length: 2 Years *Program Size:* 8
Program ID: 405-16-31-032

Rush-Presbyterian-St Luke's Medical Center Program
Sponsor: Rush-Presbyterian-St Luke's Medical Center
Program Director:
Reneé D Mehlinger, MD
Rush-Presbyterian-St Luke's Med Ctr
Sect of Child Psychiatry
1720 W Polk St
Chicago, IL 60612-4393
Tel: 312 942-2185 *Fax:* 312 942-3186
E-mail: rmehlin1@rush.edu
Internet: http://www.rush.edu
Accred Length: 2 Years *Program Size:* 4
Program ID: 405-16-21-153

University of Chicago Program
Sponsor: University of Chicago Hospitals
HCA Chicago Lakeshore Hospital
Program Director:
Kathleen M Kelley, MD
Univ of Chicago Hospitals
5841 S Maryland Ave/MC3077
Chicago, IL 60637-1470
Tel: 773 702-0529 *Fax:* 773 702-4297
E-mail: education@yoda.bsd.uchicago.edu
Accred Length: 2 Years *Program Size:* 6
Program ID: 405-16-21-034

University of Illinois College of Medicine at Chicago Program
Sponsor: University of Illinois College of Medicine at Chicago
Program Director:
Geri Fox, MD
Univ of Illinois Chicago-Inst for Juvenile Research
907 S Wolcott Ave (M/C 747)
Chicago, IL 60612-7347
Tel: 312 996-7721 *Fax:* 312 996-9534
E-mail: foxg@uic.edu
Internet: http://www.psych.uic.edu/ijr.html
Accred Length: 2 Years *Program Size:* 8
Program ID: 405-16-21-030

Indiana

Indianapolis

Indiana University School of Medicine Program
Sponsor: Indiana University School of Medicine
Clarian Riley Hospital for Children
Larue D Carter Memorial Hospital
William N Wishard Memorial Hospital
Program Director:
David Dunn, MD
Riley Hospital for Children
702 Barnhill Dr
Rm 3701
Indianapolis, IN 46202-5200
Tel: 317 274-8162 *Fax:* 317 278-0609
E-mail: jraetz@iupui.edu
Accred Length: 2 Years *Program Size:* 8
Program ID: 405-17-21-038

Iowa

Iowa City

University of Iowa Hospitals and Clinics Program
Sponsor: University of Iowa Hospitals and Clinics
Program Director:
Beth C Cizadlo, MD
Univ of Iowa Hospitals and Clinics
Dept of Psychiatry
200 Hawkins Dr
Iowa City, IA 52242-1057
Tel: 319 353-6042 *Fax:* 319 356-2587
E-mail: beth-cizadlo@uiowa.edu
Internet: http://www.uihc.uiowa.edu/pubinfo/psychl.htm
Accred Length: 2 Years *Program Size:* 6
Program ID: 405-18-11-039

Kansas

Kansas City

University of Kansas Medical Center Program
Sponsor: University of Kansas School of Medicine
University of Kansas Medical Center
Program Director:
David J Ermer, MD
Univ of Kansas Med Ctr
Dept of Child Psychiatry
3901 Rainbow Blvd
Kansas City, KS 66160-7341
Tel: 913 588-6475 *Fax:* 913 588-1305
Accred Length: 2 Years *Program Size:* 4
Program ID: 405-19-11-040

Topeka

Menninger School of Psychiatry Program
Sponsor: Menninger Clinic
C F Menninger Memorial Hospital
Program Director:
Kirby K Pope, MD
Children's Hospital-Menninger Foundation
PO Box 829
Topeka, KS 66601-0829
Tel: 785 350-5893 *Fax:* 785 350-5392
E-mail: reppat@menninger.edu
Internet: http://www.menninger.edu
Accred Length: 2 Years *Program Size:* 8
Program ID: 405-19-22-041

Kentucky

Lexington

University of Kentucky Medical Center Program
Sponsor: University of Kentucky Hospital
Charter Ridge Hospital
Program Director:
Debra A Katz, MD
Univ of Kentucky Med Ctr
Dept of Psychiatry
Kentucky Clinic/Wing B
Lexington, KY 40536-0284
Tel: 606 323-6021, ext 272 *Fax:* 606 323-1194
E-mail: dkatz0@pop.uky.edu
Accred Length: 2 Years *Program Size:* 4
Program ID: 405-20-21-042

Louisville

University of Louisville Program
Sponsor: University of Louisville School of Medicine
Child Psychiatric Services (Bingham Child Guidance Clinic)
Kosair Children's Hospital (Alliant Health System)
Program Director:
Mohammad Shafii, MD
Div of Child/Adolescent Psych
Bingham Child Guidance Ctr
200 E Chestnut St
Louisville, KY 40202
Tel: 502 852-7548 *Fax:* 502 852-1055
E-mail: arwill01@homer.louisville.edu
Internet: http://www.louisville.edu/~arwill01/
Accred Length: 2 Years *Program Size:* 4
Program ID: 405-20-21-043

Louisiana

New Orleans

Louisiana State University Program
Sponsor: Louisiana State University School of Medicine
Medical Center of Louisiana at New Orleans
Program Director:
Humberto Quintana, MD
Louisiana State Univ Med Ctr
Dept of Psychiatry
1542 Tulane Ave
New Orleans, LA 70112-2822
Tel: 504 568-3031 *Fax:* 504 568-8647
E-mail: jconst1@lsumc.edu
Accred Length: 2 Years *Program Size:* 6
Program ID: 405-21-21-159

Tulane University Program
Sponsor: Tulane University School of Medicine
Tulane University Hospital and Clinics
Program Director:
Betty A Muller, MD
Tulane Univ Sch of Med
Dept of Psych/Neurology
1430 Tulane Ave
New Orleans, LA 70112
Tel: 504 588-5405 *Fax:* 504 587-4264
E-mail: bmuller@mailhost.tcs.tulane.edu
Internet: http://www1.omi.tulane.edu/departments/psych_neuro/psnra01.htm
Accred Length: 2 Years *Program Size:* 6
Program ID: 405-21-21-045

Maine

Portland

Maine Medical Center Program
Sponsor: Maine Medical Center
Jackson Brook Institute
Program Director:
Andrew Hinkens, MD MPH
Maine Med Ctr
22 Bramhall St
Portland, ME 04102
Tel: 207 871-2733 *Fax:* 207 871-6783
E-mail: hinkea@mail.mmc.org
Internet: http://www.mmc.org/psych
Accred Length: 2 Years *Program Size:* 4
Program ID: 405-22-11-046

Maryland

Baltimore

Johns Hopkins University Program
Sponsor: Johns Hopkins University School of Medicine
Johns Hopkins Hospital
Program Director:
Emily J Frosch, MD
Johns Hopkins Hospital
CMSC 338
600 N Wolfe St
Baltimore, MD 21287-3325
Tel: 410 955-4298 *Fax:* 410 955-8691
E-mail: efrosch@jhmi.edu
Internet:
http://www.med.jhu.edu/jhhpsychiatry/master.htm
Accred Length: 2 Years *Program Size:* 12
Program ID: 405-23-11-047

University of Maryland Program
Sponsor: University of Maryland Medical System
Sheppard and Enoch Pratt Hospital
Program Director:
Richard Sarles, MD
Div of Child/Adolescent Psych
Inst of Psychiatry and Human Behavior
701 W Pratt St/Rm 422
Baltimore, MD 21201-1549
Tel: 410 328-3522 *Fax:* 410 328-0202
E-mail: rsarles@umpsy.ab.umd.edu
Accred Length: 2 Years *Program Size:* 10
Program ID: 405-23-21-048

Bethesda

National Capital Consortium Program
Sponsor: National Capital Consortium
Walter Reed Army Medical Center
Program Director:
Stephen J Cozza, MD
Dept of Psychiatry
Borden Pavilion/Bldg 6
Walter Reed Army Med Ctr
Washington, DC 20307-5001
Tel: 202 782-5961 *Fax:* 202 782-8387
Accred Length: 2 Years *Program Size:* 8
Program ID: 405-10-12-002
US Armed Services Program

Massachusetts

Boston

Boston University Medical Center Program
Sponsor: Boston Medical Center
Somerville Hospital
Program Director:
Glenn Saxe, MD
Dowling 1 North
818 Harrison Ave
Boston, MA 02118
Tel: 617 414-5490 *Fax:* 617 414-5520
Accred Length: 2 Years *Program Size:* 3
Program ID: 405-24-21-052

Children's Hospital/Judge Baker Guidance Center Program
Sponsor: Children's Hospital
Judge Baker Guidance Center
Massachusetts Mental Health Center
Program Director:
Stuart J Goldman, MD
Children's Hospital-Harvard Med Sch
Dept of Psychiatry
300 Longwood Ave
Boston, MA 02115-5737
Tel: 617 355-6745 *Fax:* 617 264-9681
E-mail: goldmans@a1.tch.harvard.edu
Accred Length: 2 Years *Program Size:* 10
Program ID: 405-24-21-053

Harvard Medical School Program
Sponsor: Massachusetts General Hospital
McLean Hospital
Program Director:
Eugene V Beresin, MD
Massachusetts General Hospital
55 Fruit St
Bulfinch 449
Boston, MA 02114
Tel: 617 726-1620 *Fax:* 617 726-8479
E-mail: beresine@a1.mgh.harvard.edu
Internet: http://www.mgh.harvard.edu/
Accred Length: 2 Years *Program Size:* 12
Program ID: 405-24-21-167

New England Medical Center Hospitals Program
Sponsor: New England Medical Center Hospitals
Program Director:
Joseph J Jankowski, MD
New England Med Ctr
750 Washington St/Box 39
Boston, MA 02111
Tel: 617 636-1635 *Fax:* 617 636-4852
Internet: http://www.nemc.org/psych/training.htm
Accred Length: 2 Years *Program Size:* 8
Program ID: 405-24-21-056

Cambridge

Cambridge Hospital/Cambridge Health Alliance Program
Sponsor: Cambridge Hospital/Cambridge Health Alliance
New England Memorial Hospital
Program Director:
Timothy F Dugan, MD
Cambridge Hospital-Cambridge Health Alliance
Dept of Psychiatry
1493 Cambridge St
Cambridge, MA 02139
Tel: 617 498-1183 *Fax:* 617 498-1204
Accred Length: 2 Years *Program Size:* 10
Program ID: 405-24-21-057

Worcester

University of Massachusetts Program
Sponsor: University of Massachusetts Medical School
UMass Memorial Health Care (University Campus)
Program Director:
W Peter Metz, MD
Univ of Massachusetts Med Sch
55 Lake Ave N/7th Fl
Worcester, MA 01655
Tel: 508 856-4094 *Fax:* 508 856-6426
E-mail: peter.metz@banyan.ummed.edu
Accred Length: 2 Years *Program Size:* 4
Program ID: 405-24-21-156

Michigan

Ann Arbor

University of Michigan Program
Sponsor: University of Michigan Hospitals

Program Director:
James E Dillon, MD
Child and Adolescent Psychiatric Hospital
1500 E Medical Center Dr
3881TC/0390
Ann Arbor, MI 48109-0390
Tel: 734 936-6335 *Fax:* 734 936-8907
E-mail: dillonj@umich.edu
Internet: http://www.psych.umich.edu/web/cd/
Accred Length: 2 Years *Program Size:* 12
Program ID: 405-25-11-060

Detroit

Wayne State University/Detroit Medical Center Program
Sponsor: Wayne State University/Detroit Medical Center
Hawthorn Center Hospital

Program Director:
Beth Ann Brooks, MD
Univ Psychiatric Ctr-Central Campus
101 E Alexandrine
Detroit, MI 48201
Tel: 313 577-5986 *Fax:* 313 577-6031
E-mail: babrooks@med.wayne.edu
Internet: http://psychiatry1.med.wayne.edu
Accred Length: 2 Years *Program Size:* 12
Program ID: 405-25-21-173

Minnesota

Minneapolis

University of Minnesota Program
Sponsor: University of Minnesota Medical School
Fairview-University Medical Center

Program Director:
Jonathan B Jensen, MD
William F Clark, MD
Univ of Minnesota Med Sch
Box 95 UMHC
420 Delaware St SE
Minneapolis, MN 55455
Tel: 612 626-3691 *Fax:* 612 626-5591
E-mail: haran001@tc.umn.edu
Accred Length: 2 Years *Program Size:* 6
Program ID: 405-26-11-066

Rochester

Mayo Graduate School of Medicine (Rochester) Program
Sponsor: Mayo Graduate School of Medicine-Mayo Foundation
Mayo Clinic (Rochester)
Rochester Methodist Hospital
St Mary's Hospital of Rochester

Program Director:
John J Huxsahl, MD
Mayo Graduate Sch of Med
200 First St SW
Rochester, MN 55905
Tel: 507 284-1043 *Fax:* 507 284-4157
E-mail: mgsm.medlab.specialties@mayo.edu
Internet: http://www.mayo.edu/
Accred Length: 2 Years *Program Size:* 6
Program ID: 405-26-21-067

Mississippi

Jackson

University of Mississippi Medical Center Program
Sponsor: University of Mississippi School of Medicine
University Hospital

Program Director:
Cynthia L Undesser, MD
2500 N State St
Jackson, MS 39216
Tel: 601 984-5820 *Fax:* 601 984-5857
Accred Length: 2 Years *Program Size:* 4
Program ID: 405-27-21-176

Missouri

Columbia

University of Missouri-Columbia Program
Sponsor: University of Missouri-Columbia School of Medicine
Charter Hospital of Columbia
Mid-Missouri Mental Health Center
Royal Oaks Hospital
University Hospitals and Clinics

Program Director:
Thomas D Eppright, MD
Univ of Missouri-Columbia
1 Hospital Dr/DCO67.00
Columbia, MO 65212
Tel: 573 882-8907 *Fax:* 573 884-5396
E-mail: statet@brain.missouri.edu
Internet: http://www.hsc.missouri.edu/~dmhs/psychneur/
Accred Length: 2 Years *Program Size:* 6
Program ID: 405-28-21-068

St Louis

St Louis University School of Medicine Program
Sponsor: St Louis University School of Medicine
SSM Cardinal Glennon Children's Hospital

Program Director:
Linda Bock, MD
St Louis Univ Sch of Med
Child/Adolescent Psych
1221 S Grand Blvd
St Louis, MO 63104-1094
Tel: 314 577-8724 *Fax:* 314 664-7248
Internet: http://www.slu.edu/colleges/med/depar
Accred Length: 2 Years *Program Size:* 4
Program ID: 405-28-21-157

Washington University/B-JH/SLCH Consortium Program
Sponsor: Washington University/B-JH/SLCH Consortium
Barnes-Jewish Hospital
Barnes-Jewish Hospital (North Campus)
St Louis Children's Hospital

Program Director:
Joan L Luby, MD
Washington Univ Sch of Med
Box 8134
4940 Children's Pl
St Louis, MO 63110
Tel: 314 286-2730 *Fax:* 314 286-2732
E-mail: lubyj@psychiatry.wustl.edu
Accred Length: 2 Years *Program Size:* 6
Program ID: 405-28-21-070

Nebraska

Omaha

Creighton University/University of Nebraska Program
Sponsor: Creighton University School of Medicine
St Joseph Center for Mental Health

Program Director:
Shashi K Bhatia, MD
Creighton-Nebraska, Dept of Psychiatry
3528 Dodge St
Omaha, NE 68131
Tel: 402 595-1067 *Fax:* 402 595-2752
E-mail: sbhatia@mail.unmc.edu
Accred Length: 2 Years *Program Size:* 6
Program ID: 405-30-31-071

New Hampshire

Lebanon

Dartmouth-Hitchcock Medical Center Program
Sponsor: Mary Hitchcock Memorial Hospital
Brattleboro Retreat

Program Director:
Robert J Racusin, MD
Dartmouth-Hitchcock Med Ctr
Dept of Psychiatry
One Medical Center Dr
Lebanon, NH 03756
Tel: 603 650-5835 *Fax:* 603 650-5842
E-mail: robert.j.racusin@dartmouth.edu
Internet: http://www.hitchcock.org
Accred Length: 2 Years *Program Size:* 6
Program ID: 405-32-21-073

New Jersey

Newark

UMDNJ-New Jersey Medical School Program
Sponsor: UMDNJ-New Jersey Medical School
UMDNJ-Community Mental Health Center at Newark
UMDNJ-University Hospital

Program Director:
Adrian Sondheimer, MD
UMDNJ-New Jersey Med Sch
UBHC B-60C
215 S Orange Ave
Newark, NJ 07103-2700
Tel: 973 972-4284 *Fax:* 973 972-6976
Accred Length: 2 Years *Program Size:* 4
Program ID: 405-33-21-150

Piscataway

UMDNJ-Robert Wood Johnson Medical School Program
Sponsor: UMDNJ-Robert Wood Johnson Medical School
Robert Wood Johnson University Hospital
UMDNJ-Community Behavioral HealthCare at Piscataway

Program Director:
Myron Gessner, MD
UMDNJ-Robert Wood Johnson Med Sch
671 Hoes Ln/UBHC/C-206
Piscataway, NJ 08854-5633
Tel: 732 235-4433 *Fax:* 732 235-4821
Accred Length: 2 Years *Program Size:* 6
Program ID: 405-33-21-074

New Mexico

Albuquerque

University of New Mexico Program

Sponsor: University of New Mexico School of Medicine
University Hospital

Program Director:
Claudia K Berenson, MD
Univ of New Mexico Sch of Med
2400 Tucker NE
Albuquerque, NM 87131-5326
Tel: 505 272-5002 *Fax:* 505 272-4639
E-mail: cberenso@cph.unm.edu
Internet: http://hsc.unm.edu/som/psychiatry/index.htm
Accred Length: 2 Years *Program Size:* 8
Program ID: 405-34-21-144

New York

Bronx

Albert Einstein College of Medicine at Bronx-Lebanon Hospital Center Program

Sponsor: Bronx-Lebanon Hospital Center

Program Director:
Arthur Gillman, MD
Bronx-Lebanon Hospital Ctr
1844 Webster Ave
Bronx, NY 10457
Tel: 718 901-6831 *Fax:* 718 901-6880
E-mail: aegillman@pol.net
Accred Length: 2 Years *Program Size:* 4
Program ID: 405-35-21-177

Albert Einstein College of Medicine Program

Sponsor: Albert Einstein College of Medicine of Yeshiva University
Bronx Children's Psychiatric Center
Jacobi Medical Center
Montefiore Medical Center-Henry and Lucy Moses Division

Program Director:
Harvey Kranzler, MD
Montefiore Med Ctr
Dept of Psychiatry
3317 Rochambeau Ave
Bronx, NY 10467
Tel: 718 920-7970 *Fax:* 718 798-3810
Accred Length: 2 Years *Program Size:* 8
Program ID: 405-35-21-077

Brooklyn

Brookdale University Hospital Medical Center Program

Sponsor: Brookdale University Hospital Medical Center

Program Director:
Jerome Pollack, MD
Brookdale Hospital and Med Ctr
Linden Blvd at Brookdale Plaza
Brooklyn, NY 11212
Tel: 718 240-5997 *Fax:* 718 240-5042
Accred Length: 2 Years *Program Size:* 6
Program ID: 405-35-31-078

SUNY Health Science Center at Brooklyn Program

Sponsor: SUNY Health Science Center at Brooklyn
Kings County Hospital Center
University Hospital-SUNY Health Science Center at Brooklyn

Program Director:
Lenore Engel, MD
SUNY Health Science Ctr-Brooklyn
Child/Adolescent Psych
450 Clarkson Ave/Box 1203
Brooklyn, NY 11203
Tel: 718 270-1430 *Fax:* 718 245-2517
Accred Length: 2 Years *Program Size:* 6
Program ID: 405-35-21-094

Buffalo

SUNY at Buffalo Graduate Medical-Dental Education Consortium Program

Sponsor: SUNY at Buffalo Grad Medical-Dental Education Consortium
CGF Health System (Children's Hospital of Buffalo)
SUNY at Buffalo School of Medicine
Western New York Children's Psychiatric Center

Program Director:
David L Kaye, MD
Children's Hospital
219 Bryant St
Buffalo, NY 14222
Tel: 716 878-1200 *Fax:* 716 888-3999
E-mail: dlkaye@acsu.buffalo.edu
Accred Length: 2 Years *Program Size:* 6
Program ID: 405-35-21-161

Elmhurst

Mount Sinai School of Medicine (Elmhurst) Program

Sponsor: Mount Sinai School of Medicine
Elmhurst Hospital Center-Mount Sinai Services

Program Director:
Dimitrios Padouvas, MD
Elmhurst Hospital Ctr-Mount Sinai Services
79-01 Broadway
Elmhurst, NY 11373
Tel: 718 334-1331 *Fax:* 718 334-3557
Accred Length: 2 Years *Program Size:* 5
Program ID: 405-35-11-079

Manhasset

North Shore University Hospital/NYU School of Medicine Program

Sponsor: North Shore University Hospital

Program Director:
Victor M Fornari, MD
North Shore Univ Hospital
Dept of Psychiatry
400 Community Dr
Manhasset, NY 11030
Tel: 516 562-3005 *Fax:* 516 562-4786
E-mail: vfornari@nshs.edu
Accred Length: 2 Years *Program Size:* 6
Program ID: 405-35-11-076

New Hyde Park

Albert Einstein College of Medicine at Long Island Jewish Medical Center Program

Sponsor: Long Island Jewish Medical Center
Schneider Children's Hosp (Long Island Jewish Med Ctr)

Program Director:
Richard R Pleak, MD
Long Island Jewish Med Ctr
Schneider Children's Hospital
269-01 76th Ave/Ste 441
New Hyde Park, NY 11040
Tel: 718 470-3550 *Fax:* 718 470-0524
Internet: http://www.lij.edu/lij-homepage-ns.html
Accred Length: 2 Years *Program Size:* 10
Program ID: 405-35-11-082

New York

Harlem Hospital Center Program

Sponsor: Harlem Hospital Center
Rockland Children's Psychiatric Center

Program Director:
Sady Sultan, MD
Harlem Hospital Ctr
506 Lenox Ave
New York, NY 10032
Tel: 212 939-3065 *Fax:* 212 939-3064
Accred Length: 2 Years *Program Size:* 6
Program ID: 405-35-21-081

Mount Sinai School of Medicine Program

Sponsor: Mount Sinai School of Medicine
Mount Sinai Medical Center

Program Director:
Henry P Schwartz, MD
Mount Sinai Hospital
One Gustave L Levy Pl
Box 1230
New York, NY 10029
Tel: 212 824-7055 *Fax:* 212 348-8436
E-mail: jeffrey-newcorn@smtplink.mssm.edu
Accred Length: 2 Years *Program Size:* 4
Program ID: 405-35-11-085

New York and Presbyterian Hospital (Columbia Campus) Program

Sponsor: New York and Presbyterian Hospital
New York and Presbyterian Hospital (Columbia Campus)
New York State Psychiatric Institute

Program Director:
Clarice J Kestenbaum, MD
New York State Psychiatric Inst
722 W 168th St
Box 60
New York, NY 10032
Tel: 212 543-5583 *Fax:* 212 543-6093
E-mail: kapigian@child.cpmc.columbia.edu
Internet: http://www.nyspi.cpmc.columbia.edu
Accred Length: 2 Years *Program Size:* 14
Program ID: 405-35-11-080

New York and Presbyterian Hospital (Cornell Campus) Program

Sponsor: New York and Presbyterian Hospital
New York and Presbyterian Hospital (Cornell Campus)
New York and Presbyterian Hospital-Payne Whitney Clinic

Program Director:
Theodore Shapiro, MD
New York Hospital
525 E 68th St
Box 147
New York, NY 10021
Tel: 212 821-0724 *Fax:* 212 821-0792
Accred Length: 2 Years *Program Size:* 6
Program ID: 405-35-11-086

New York Medical College (Metropolitan) Program
Sponsor: New York Medical College
Metropolitan Hospital Center
Program Director:
Yvette G Janssen, MD
Rm 4M14B Psychiatric Pavillion
1901 First Ave
New York, NY 10029
Tel: 212 423-7060 *Fax:* 212 423-7434
Accred Length: 2 Years *Program Size:* 4
Program ID: 405-35-11-087

New York Medical College at St Vincent's Hospital and Medical Center of New York Program
Sponsor: New York Medical College
St Vincent's Hospital and Medical Center of New York
Program Director:
A Reese Abright, MD
St Vincent's Hospital and Med Ctr
203 W 12th St/O'Toole 606
New York, NY 10011
Tel: 212 604-8213 *Fax:* 212 604-8794
Internet: http://svh.nymc.edu
Accred Length: 2 Years *Program Size:* 6
Program ID: 405-35-22-092

New York University Medical Center Program
Sponsor: New York University Medical Center
Bellevue Hospital Center
Program Director:
Wayne Hugo Green, MD
Bellevue Hospital
462 First Ave
NB 21-S-6
New York, NY 10016
Tel: 212 263-6244 *Fax:* 212 263-0202
Accred Length: 2 Years *Program Size:* 10
Program ID: 405-35-21-088

St Luke's-Roosevelt Hospital Center Program
Sponsor: St Luke's-Roosevelt Hospital Center
St Luke's-Roosevelt Hospital Center-Roosevelt Division
St Luke's-Roosevelt Hospital Center-St Luke's Division
Program Director:
Raul R Silva, MD
St Luke's-Roosevelt Hospital Ctr
411 W 114th St/Ste 3A
New York, NY 10025
Tel: 212 523-3069, ext 3069 *Fax:* 212 523-3064
Internet: http://www.docnet.org/dept/psych
Accred Length: 2 Years *Program Size:* 6
Program ID: 405-35-31-166

Rochester

University of Rochester Program
Sponsor: Strong Memorial Hospital of the University of Rochester
Rochester Psychiatric Center
Program Director:
Stephen W Munson, MD
Univ of Rochester Med Ctr
300 Crittenden Blvd
Rochester, NY 14642-8409
Tel: 716 275-3137 *Fax:* 716 273-1076
E-mail: louise_haskins@urmc.rochester.edu
Internet: http://www.urmc.rochester.edu/smh/psych.html
Accred Length: 2 Years *Program Size:* 5
Program ID: 405-35-11-095

Stony Brook

SUNY at Stony Brook Program
Sponsor: University Hospital-SUNY at Stony Brook
Program Director:
Judith A Crowell, MD
SUNY-Stony Brook
Div of Child Psychiatry
Health Sciences Ctr/T-10
Stony Brook, NY 11794-8101
Tel: 516 632-8840 *Fax:* 516 632-8953
Accred Length: 2 Years *Program Size:* 5
Program ID: 405-35-21-158

Valhalla

New York Medical College at Westchester Medical Center Program
Sponsor: New York Medical College
Westchester Medical Center
Program Director:
Klaus Schreiber, MD
New York Med Coll-Westchester Med Ctr
Div of Child/Adolescent Psych
Behavioral Health Ctr/Rm B102
Valhalla, NY 10595
Tel: 914 493-1829 *Fax:* 914 493-7152
E-mail: klaus_schreiber@nymc.edu
Accred Length: 2 Years *Program Size:* 6
Program ID: 405-35-21-097

White Plains

New York and Presbyterian Hospital (Cornell Campus)/Westchester Program
Sponsor: New York and Presbyterian Hospital
New York and Presbyterian Hospital-Westchester Division
Program Director:
Paulina F Kernberg, MD
New York Presbyterian Hospital-Westchester Div
21 Bloomingdale Rd
White Plains, NY 10605-1504
Tel: 914 997-5951 *Fax:* 914 682-6988
E-mail: pkernber%westnyh@nyh.med.cornell.edu
Accred Length: 2 Years *Program Size:* 6
Program ID: 405-35-21-098

North Carolina

Chapel Hill

University of North Carolina Hospitals Program
Sponsor: University of North Carolina Hospitals
Dorothea Dix Hospital
Program Director:
Albert J Naftel, MD
Univ of North Carolina
CB7160/Rm 10602 Neurosciences Hospital
Chapel Hill, NC 27599-7160
Tel: 919 966-2127 *Fax:* 919 966-2220
Internet: http://www.psychiatry.unc.edu
Accred Length: 2 Years *Program Size:* 10
Program ID: 405-36-21-100

Durham

Duke University Program
Sponsor: Duke University Medical Center
John Umstead Hospital
Program Director:
Charles Keith, MD
Div of Child/Adolescent Psych
Box 2906
Duke Univ Med Ctr
Durham, NC 27710
Tel: 919 684-3044 *Fax:* 919 286-6069
Accred Length: 2 Years *Program Size:* 8
Program ID: 405-36-31-101

Greenville

East Carolina University Program
Sponsor: East Carolina University School of Medicine
Cherry Hospital
Pitt County Memorial Hospital
Pitt County Mental Health Center
Program Director:
Kaye L McGinty, MD
East Carolina Univ Sch of Med
Dept of Psychiatry/Brody Bldg 4E
600 Moye Blvd
Greenville, NC 27858-4354
Tel: 919 816-2673 *Fax:* 919 816-3815
E-mail: kmcginty@brody.med.ecu.edu
Accred Length: 2 Years *Program Size:* 4
Program ID: 405-36-21-162

Winston-Salem

Wake Forest University School of Medicine Program
Sponsor: Wake Forest University Baptist Medical Center
Program Director:
Guy D Palmes, MD
Dept of Psychiatry/Behav Med
Medical Center Blvd
Winston-Salem, NC 27157-1087
Tel: 336 716-2240 *Fax:* 336 716-6830
Internet: http://www.wfubmc.edu/psychiatry/
Accred Length: 2 Years *Program Size:* 4
Program ID: 405-36-31-163

Ohio

Cincinnati

University Hospital/University of Cincinnati College of Medicine Program
Sponsor: University Hospital Inc
Children's Hospital Medical Center
Program Director:
Michael T Sorter, MD
Univ of Cincinnati Med Ctr
231 Bethesda Ave/ML 0559
Cincinnati, OH 45267-0559
Tel: 513 558-5190 *Fax:* 513 558-3477
E-mail: sortmi@chmcc.org
Internet: http://www.chmcc.org/departments/47/
Accred Length: 2 Years *Program Size:* 5
Program ID: 405-38-21-102

Cleveland

Case Western Reserve University Program
Sponsor: University Hospitals of Cleveland

Program Director:
Robert L Findling, MD
Case Western Reserve Univ
Div of Child/Adolescent Psychiatry
11100 Euclid Ave/Mail Stop 5080
Cleveland, OH 44106
Tel: 216 844-1707 *Fax:* 216 844-5883
E-mail: rlf5@po.cwru.edu
Accred Length: 2 Years *Program Size:* 6
Program ID: 405-38-11-103

Cleveland Clinic Foundation Program
Sponsor: Cleveland Clinic Foundation

Program Director:
John P Glazer, MD
Sect of Child/Adolescent Psych
Dept of Psychiatry/P57
9500 Euclid Ave
Cleveland, OH 44195
Tel: 216 444-0477 *Fax:* 216 444-9054
E-mail: glazerj@cesmtp.ccf.org
Internet: http://www.ccf.org
Accred Length: 2 Years *Program Size:* 6
Program ID: 405-38-21-171

Columbus

Ohio State University Program
Sponsor: Ohio State University Medical Center

Program Director:
Craig Williams, MD
Ohio State Univ
1670 Upham Dr/Ste 560
Columbus, OH 43210-1250
Tel: 614 293-8230 *Fax:* 614 293-4200
Accred Length: 2 Years *Program Size:* 4
Program ID: 405-38-21-104

Dayton

Wright State University Program
Sponsor: Wright State University School of Medicine
Children's Medical Center
Franciscan Medical Center-Dayton Campus
Good Samaritan Hospital and Health Center

Program Director:
William M Klykylo, MD
Div of Child/Adolescent Psych
Wright State Univ Sch of Med
PO Box 927
Dayton, OH 45401-0927
Tel: 937 276-8325, ext 5 *Fax:* 937 275-2817
E-mail: wklykylo@desire.wright.edu
Internet: http://www.med.wright.edu/som/resident/psych/child.htm
Accred Length: 2 Years *Program Size:* 4
Program ID: 405-38-21-169

Toledo

Medical College of Ohio Program
Sponsor: Medical College of Ohio

Program Director:
Wun Jung Kim, MD MPH
Med Coll of Ohio Hospital
Kobacker Ctr
3130 Glendale Ave
Toledo, OH 43614-5810
Tel: 419 383-5494 *Fax:* 419 383-3098
E-mail: fgrindle@gemini.mco.edu or wjkim@mco.edu
Internet: http://www.mco.edu/depts/psych
Accred Length: 2 Years *Program Size:* 4
Program ID: 405-38-11-105

Oklahoma

Oklahoma City

University of Oklahoma Health Sciences Center Program
Sponsor: University of Oklahoma College of Medicine
Children's Hospital of Oklahoma

Program Director:
James R Allen, MD MPH
Univ of Oklahoma Health Sciences Ctr
PO Box 26901/3WP3070
Oklahoma City, OK 73190-3048
Tel: 405 271-4219 *Fax:* 405 271-3808
Accred Length: 2 Years *Program Size:* 4
Program ID: 405-39-11-106

Oregon

Portland

Oregon Health Sciences University Program
Sponsor: Oregon Health Sciences University Hospital

Program Director:
Nancy C Winters, MD
Oregon Health Sciences Univ
3181 SW Sam Jackson Park Rd/DC7P
Portland, OR 97201-3098
Tel: 503 418-5775 *Fax:* 503 418-5774
E-mail: winterna@ohsu.edu
Accred Length: 2 Years *Program Size:* 10
Program ID: 405-40-21-107

Pennsylvania

Hershey

Penn State Geisinger Health System/Milton S Hershey Medical Center Program
Sponsor: Penn State Geisinger Health System
Milton S Hershey Medical Center

Program Director:
H Allen Handford Sr, MD MD
500 University Dr/PO Box 850
Hershey, PA 17033-0850
Tel: 717 531-8515 *Fax:* 717 531-6491
E-mail: tms2@psu.edu
Accred Length: 2 Years *Program Size:* 6
Program ID: 405-41-21-147

Philadelphia

MCP Hahnemann University Program
Sponsor: MCP Hahnemann University
Hahnemann University Hospital
Medical College of Pennsylvania Hospital

Program Director:
William A Sonis, MD
Eastern Pennsylvania Psychiatric Inst
Henry Ave and Abbotsford Rd
Philadelphia, PA 19129
Tel: 215 842-4429 *Fax:* 215 843-8207
E-mail: sonis@auhs.edu
Accred Length: 2 Years *Program Size:* 14
Program ID: 405-41-21-110

Philadelphia Child Guidance Center Program
Sponsor: Philadelphia Child Guidance Center

Program Director:
Judith W Dogin, MD
Children's Hospital of Philadelphia
34th St and Civic Center Blvd
Philadelphia, PA 19104-4322
Tel: 215 590-7567 *Fax:* 215 590-7540
E-mail: dogin@email.chop.edu
Accred Length: 2 Years *Program Size:* 10
Program ID: 405-41-11-111

Thomas Jefferson University Program
Sponsor: Thomas Jefferson University Hospital

Program Director:
Harris Rabinovich, MD
Thomas Jefferson Univ Hospital
1201 Chestnut St/#1512
Philadelphia, PA 19107
Tel: 215 955-7663 *Fax:* 215 568-2329
Accred Length: 2 Years *Program Size:* 5
Program ID: 405-41-11-113

Pittsburgh

Allegheny General Hospital Program
Sponsor: Allegheny General Hospital

Program Director:
Judith A Cohen, MD
Allegheny General Hospital
320 E North Ave
Pittsburgh, PA 15212-4772
Tel: 412 330-4321 *Fax:* 412 330-4319
E-mail: jcohen1@aherf.edu
Accred Length: 2 Years *Program Size:* 4
Program ID: 405-41-21-174

University Health Center of Pittsburgh Program
Sponsor: University Health Center of Pittsburgh
Presbyterian University Hospital/UPMC
Western Psychiatric Institute and Clinic/UPMC

Program Director:
Viveca A Meyer, MD
Western Psychiatric Inst and Clinic
3811 O'Hara St
Pittsburgh, PA 15213-2593
Tel: 412 624-2876 *Fax:* 412 624-0319
E-mail: meyerva@msx.upmc.edu
Internet: http://www.wpic.pitt.edu
Accred Length: 2 Years *Program Size:* 10
Program ID: 405-41-31-114

Puerto Rico

San Juan

University of Puerto Rico Program
Sponsor: University of Puerto Rico School of Medicine
University Hospital

Program Director:
Ricardo M Velas Fossas, MD
Univ of Puerto Rico
Dept of Psychiatry
GPO Box 5067
San Juan, PR 00936
Tel: 787 757-1800, ext 635 *Fax:* 787 769-3735
Accred Length: 2 Years *Program Size:* 4
Program ID: 405-42-21-116

Rhode Island

Providence

Brown University Program

Sponsor: Rhode Island Hospital
Emma Pendleton Bradley Hospital
Program Director:
Henrietta L Leonard, MD
Rhode Island Hospital, Dept of Child/Family Psych
593 Eddy St
Providence, RI 02903
Tel: 401 444-3762 *Fax:* 401 444-8879
Accred Length: 2 Years *Program Size:* 10
Program ID: 405-43-21-117

South Carolina

Charleston

Medical University of South Carolina Program

Sponsor: Medical University of South Carolina College of Medicine
MUSC Medical Center
Program Director:
Lisa D Hand, MD
2 North Inst of Psychiatry
67 President St
PO Box 250861
Charleston, SC 29425-0742
Tel: 843 792-0135 *Fax:* 843 792-5598
E-mail: handld@musc.edu
Internet: http://www.musc.edu/psychiatry
Accred Length: 2 Years *Program Size:* 10
Program ID: 405-45-21-118

Columbia

Palmetto Health Alliance/University of South Carolina School of Medicine Program

Sponsor: Palmetto Health Alliance
William S Hall Psychiatric Institute
Program Director:
Margaret Shugart, MD
William S Hall Psychiatric Inst
1800 Colonial Dr
PO Box 202
Columbia, SC 29202
Tel: 803 734-7267 *Fax:* 803 734-7894
Internet: http://www.ceb.sc.edu
Accred Length: 2 Years *Program Size:* 8
Program ID: 405-45-21-119

South Dakota

Sioux Falls

University of South Dakota Program

Sponsor: University of South Dakota School of Medicine
Sioux Valley Hospital
Program Director:
Jessica Oesterheld, MD
Dept of Psychiatry
Univ of South Dakota Sch of Med
800 E 21st St
Sioux Falls, SD 57101
Tel: 605 367-5950 *Fax:* 605 367-5598
E-mail: joesterhj@dakota.net
Accred Length: 2 Years *Program Size:* 4
Program ID: 405-46-21-164

Tennessee

Memphis

University of Tennessee Program

Sponsor: University of Tennessee College of Medicine
LeBonheur Children's Medical Center
St Joseph Hospital
University of Tennessee Medical Center (UT Bowld Hospital)
Program Director:
David Pruitt, MD
Univ of Tennessee
711 Jefferson/Ste 137
Memphis, TN 38163
Tel: 901 448-5944 *Fax:* 901 448-6913
Accred Length: 2 Years *Program Size:* 4
Program ID: 405-47-21-120

Nashville

Vanderbilt University Program

Sponsor: Vanderbilt University Medical Center
Psychiatric Hospital at Vanderbilt
Program Director:
Catherine Fuchs, MD
Vanderbilt Univ Med Ctr
Div of Child/Adolescent Psychiatry
1601 23rd Ave S/Ste 303
Nashville, TN 37212-8645
Tel: 615 327-7019 *Fax:* 615 327-7136
Accred Length: 2 Years *Program Size:* 6
Program ID: 405-47-21-121

Texas

Austin

Austin State Hospital Program

Sponsor: Austin State Hospital
Brackenridge Hospital
Program Director:
Beverly J Sutton, MD
Austin Psychiatric Residency Program
Austin State Hospital
4110 Guadalupe
Austin, TX 78751-4296
Tel: 512 419-2116 *Fax:* 512 419-2163
E-mail: beverly.sutton@mhmr.state.tx.us
Accred Length: 2 Years *Program Size:* 6
Program ID: 405-48-12-122

Dallas

University of Texas Southwestern Medical School Program

Sponsor: University of Texas Southwestern Medical School
Children's Medical Center of Dallas
Dallas County Hospital District-Parkland Memorial Hospital
Program Director:
Gail S Alexander, MD
Univ of Texas Southwestern Med Ctr
5323 Harry Hines Blvd
Dallas, TX 75235-8589
Tel: 214 648-5302 *Fax:* 214 648-5229
E-mail: ggarre@mednet.swmed.edu
Accred Length: 2 Years *Program Size:* 9
Program ID: 405-48-21-123

Galveston

University of Texas Medical Branch Hospitals Program

Sponsor: University of Texas Medical Branch Hospitals
Program Director:
Christopher R Thomas, MD
Div of Child/Adolescent Psych
Univ of Texas Med Branch
301 University Blvd
Galveston, TX 77555-0425
Tel: 409 772-1055 *Fax:* 409 772-2885
E-mail: crthomas@utmb.edu
Internet: http://www.psy.utmb.edu
Accred Length: 2 Years *Program Size:* 8
Program ID: 405-48-11-124

Houston

Baylor College of Medicine Program

Sponsor: Baylor College of Medicine
Texas Children's Hospital
Program Director:
Florence F Eddins, MD
Baylor Coll of Med
Dept of Psych/Behav Science
One Baylor Plaza/Rm 109-D
Houston, TX 77030
Tel: 713 798-4768 *Fax:* 713 796-9718
Accred Length: 2 Years *Program Size:* 8
Program ID: 405-48-21-125

University of Texas at Houston Program

Sponsor: University of Texas Medical School at Houston
University of Texas Mental Sciences Institute
Program Director:
Ann Saunders, MD
Univ of Texas Health Sciences Ctr
1300 Moursund/Rm 179
Houston, TX 77030
Tel: 713 794-1460 *Fax:* 713 500-2669
Accred Length: 2 Years *Program Size:* 6
Program ID: 405-48-21-139

San Antonio

University of Texas Health Science Center at San Antonio Program

Sponsor: University of Texas Medical School at San Antonio
Child Guidance Center of San Antonio
Southwest Neuropsychiatric Institute
Program Director:
Kenneth L Matthews, MD
Univ of Texas Health Science Ctr
7703 Floyd Curl Dr
San Antonio, TX 78284-7792
Tel: 210 567-5430 *Fax:* 210 567-6941
E-mail: matthewsk@uthscsa.edu
Internet: http://psych68.uthscsa.edu
Accred Length: 2 Years *Program Size:* 7
Program ID: 405-48-21-126

Temple

Texas A&M College of Medicine-Scott and White Program

Sponsor: Scott and White Memorial Hospital
Cedar Crest Residential Treatment Center
Darnall Army Community Hospital
Program Director:
Helen Zaphiris, MD
2401 S 31st St
Temple, TX 76508
Tel: 254 724-1768 *Fax:* 254 724-1747
E-mail: psych@bellnet.tamu.edu
Internet: http://www.sw.org
Accred Length: 2 Years *Program Size:* 2
Program ID: 405-48-21-175

Utah

Salt Lake City

University of Utah Program
Sponsor: University of Utah Medical Center
Children's Center
Primary Children's Medical Center
Valley Mental Health
Program Director:
Frances L Burger, MD
Univ of Utah Sch of Med
Dept of Psychiatry
50 N Medical Dr
Salt Lake City, UT 84132
Tel: 801 581-3936 *Fax:* 801 581-5604
E-mail: laura.hart@hsc.utah.edu
Accred Length: 2 Years *Program Size:* 6
Program ID: 405-49-21-127

Virginia

Charlottesville

University of Virginia Program
Sponsor: University of Virginia Medical Center
De Jarnette Center
Program Director:
Roger C Burket, MD
Univ of Virginia Health Sciences Ctr
Div of Child/Family Psych
1 Boar's Head Ln
Charlottesville, VA 22903
Tel: 804 243-6950 *Fax:* 804 243-6970
Accred Length: 2 Years *Program Size:* 4
Program ID: 405-51-11-130

Richmond

Medical College of Virginia/Virginia Commonwealth University Program
Sponsor: Medical College of Virginia/Virginia Commonwealth University
MCV-Virginia Treatment Center for Children
Medical College of Virginia Hospitals
Program Director:
Aradhana A Sood, MD
Med Coll of Virginia
PO Box 980489
Richmond, VA 23298-0489
Tel: 804 828-4058 *Fax:* 804 828-3504
E-mail: bsood@gems.vcu.edu
Accred Length: 2 Years *Program Size:* 6
Program ID: 405-51-11-131

Washington

Seattle

University of Washington Program
Sponsor: University of Washington School of Medicine
Children's Hospital and Medical Center
Sacred Heart Medical Center
University of Washington Medical Center
Program Director:
Christopher K Varley, MD
Children's Hospital and Regional Med Ctr
PO Box 5371
4800 Sand Point Way NE
Seattle, WA 98105-0371
Tel: 206 368-4957 *Fax:* 206 368-4969
E-mail: cvarley@u.washington.edu
Accred Length: 2 Years *Program Size:* 8
Program ID: 405-54-21-132

West Virginia

Charleston

West Virginia University (Charleston Division) Program
Sponsor: Charleston Area Medical Center
Program Director:
Peter R Edelman, MD
Child and Adolescent Psych
Robert C Byrd Health Sciences Ctr
PO Box 1547
Charleston, WV 25326
Tel: 304 341-1500, ext 1528 *Fax:* 304 341-1522
E-mail: pete edelman@camcare.com
Accred Length: 2 Years *Program Size:* 4
Program ID: 405-55-21-170

Wisconsin

Madison

University of Wisconsin Program
Sponsor: University of Wisconsin Hospital and Clinics
HCA Parkway Hospital
Mendota Mental Health Institute
Program Director:
Hugh F Johnston, MD
Wisconsin Psychiatric Inst and Clinics
Dept of Psychiatry
6001 Research Park Blvd
Madison, WI 53719-1176
Tel: 608 263-6084 *Fax:* 608 263-0265
E-mail: hfjohnst@facstaff.wisc.edu
Accred Length: 2 Years *Program Size:* 4
Program ID: 405-56-21-134

Milwaukee

Medical College of Wisconsin Program
Sponsor: Medical College of Wisconsin Affiliated Hospitals Inc
Children's Hospital of Wisconsin
Milwaukee Psychiatric Hospital-Dewey Center
Program Director:
Anthony D Meyer, MD
Milwaukee Psychiatric Hospital
1220 Dewey Ave
Wauwatosa, WI 53213
Tel: 414 454-6609 *Fax:* 414 454-6604
Accred Length: 2 Years *Program Size:* 5
Program ID: 405-56-21-135

Child Neurology (Neurology)

Alabama

Birmingham

University of Alabama Medical Center Program
Sponsor: University of Alabama Hospital
Children's Hospital of Alabama
Program Director:
Alan K Percy, MD
Univ of Alabama
1600 7th Ave S
Ste 516-ACC
Birmingham, AL 35233
Tel: 205 939-9588 *Fax:* 205 939-6184
E-mail: apercy@peds.uab.edu
Accred Length: 3 Years *Program Size:* 3
Program ID: 185-01-21-008

Arizona

Phoenix

St Joseph's Hospital and Medical Center Program
Sponsor: St Joseph's Hospital and Medical Center
Program Director:
Stanley D Johnsen, MD
Barrow Neurological Inst
St Joseph's Hospital and Med Ctr
PO Box 2071
Phoenix, AZ 85001-2071
Tel: 602 406-3196 *Fax:* 602 406-4104
Internet: http://www.chw.edu/mha/mha.mtml
Accred Length: 3 Years *Program Size:* 3
Program ID: 185-03-21-024

Arkansas

Little Rock

University of Arkansas for Medical Sciences Program
Sponsor: University of Arkansas College of Medicine
Arkansas Children's Hospital
John L McClellan Memorial Veterans Hospital
Program Director:
May L Griebel, MD
Univ of Arkansas Coll of Med
800 Marshall St
Little Rock, AR 72202
Tel: 501 320-1850 *Fax:* 501 320-6269
Accred Length: 3 Years *Program Size:* 0
Program ID: 185-04-21-085

California

Loma Linda

Loma Linda University Program

Sponsor: Loma Linda University Medical Center

Program Director:
Stephen Ashwal, MD
Loma Linda Univ Med Ctr
11234 Anderson St/Rm A1120G Coleman
Loma Linda, CA 92354
Tel: 909 824-0800, ext 42212 *Fax:* 909 824-4184
Accred Length: 3 Years *Program Size:* 1
Program ID: 185-05-21-075

Los Angeles

UCLA Medical Center Program

Sponsor: UCLA School of Medicine
UCLA Medical Center

Program Director:
W Donald Shields, MD
UCLA Sch of Med
Div of Ped Neurology
PO Box 951752
Los Angeles, CA 90095-1752
Tel: 310 825-6196 *Fax:* 310 825-5834
E-mail: wdshields@pediatrics.medsch.ucla.edu
Accred Length: 3 Years *Program Size:* 3
Program ID: 185-05-21-062

University of Southern California Program

Sponsor: Los Angeles County-USC Medical Center
Children's Hospital of Los Angeles

Program Director:
Wendy G Mitchell, MD
Univ of Southern California Sch of Med
Children's Hospital Los Angeles
4650 Sunset Blvd
Los Angeles, CA 90027
Tel: 323 669-2498 *Fax:* 323 667-2019
E-mail: wmitchell@chlais.usc.edu
Accred Length: 3 Years *Program Size:* 3
Program ID: 185-05-21-065

Orange

University of California (Irvine) Program

Sponsor: University of California (Irvine) Medical Center

Program Director:
Ira T Lott, MD
Univ of California Irvine Med Ctr
101 City Dr S/Rte 81
Bldg 2 Zot Code 4482
Orange, CA 92868-3298
Tel: 714 456-5333 *Fax:* 714 456-7658
E-mail: itlott@uci.edu
Accred Length: 3 Years *Program Size:* 3
Program ID: 185-05-21-006

San Diego

University of California (San Diego) Program

Sponsor: University of California (San Diego) Medical Center
Children's Hospital and Health Center
Veterans Affairs Medical Center (San Diego)

Program Director:
Doris A Trauner, MD
UCSD Med Ctr
9500 Gilman Dr (MC0935)
La Jolla, CA 92093
Tel: 619 587-4004 *Fax:* 619 587-8050
E-mail: dtrauner@ucsd.edu
Accred Length: 3 Years *Program Size:* 1
Program ID: 185-05-21-020

San Francisco

University of California (San Francisco) Program

Sponsor: University of California (San Francisco) School of Medicine
San Francisco General Hospital Medical Center
University of California (San Francisco) Medical Center
Veterans Affairs Medical Center (San Francisco)

Program Director:
Donna M Ferreiro, BS MD
Univ of California San Francisco Med Ctr
Dept of Neurology
Box 0114/C-214
San Francisco, CA 94143-0114
Tel: 415 502-1099 *Fax:* 415 502-5821
E-mail: dmf@itsa.ucsf.edu
Accred Length: 3 Years *Program Size:* 4
Program ID: 185-05-21-069

Stanford

Stanford University Program

Sponsor: Stanford University Hospital
Santa Clara Valley Medical Center
Veterans Affairs Palo Alto Health Care System

Program Director:
Jin S Hahn, MD
Stanford Univ Med Ctr
Dept of Ped Neurology
300 Pasteur Dr/Rm H-3160
Stanford, CA 94305-5235
Tel: 650 723-6841 *Fax:* 650 725-7459
E-mail: jhahn@stanford.edu
Internet: http://www.stanford.edu/group/neurology
Accred Length: 3 Years *Program Size:* 3
Program ID: 185-05-21-061

Torrance

Los Angeles County-Harbor-UCLA Medical Center Program

Sponsor: Los Angeles County-Harbor-UCLA Medical Center

Program Director:
Kenneth R Huff, MD
Harbor-UCLA Med Ctr
Dept of Pediatrics Box 468
1000 W Carson St
Torrance, CA 90509
Tel: 310 222-4168 *Fax:* 310 212-7440
E-mail: huff@harbor2.humc.edu
Accred Length: 3 Years *Program Size:* 3
Program ID: 185-05-21-017

Colorado

Denver

University of Colorado Program

Sponsor: University of Colorado Health Sciences Center
Children's Hospital
Denver Health and Hospitals

Program Director:
Alan R Seay, MD
Univ of Colorado Sch of Med
Children's Hospital
1056 E 19th Ave/Box B155
Denver, CO 80218
Tel: 303 861-6895 *Fax:* 303 861-3984
Accred Length: 3 Years *Program Size:* 4
Program ID: 185-07-21-023

Connecticut

New Haven

Yale-New Haven Medical Center Program

Sponsor: Yale-New Haven Hospital
Veterans Affairs Medical Center (West Haven)

Program Director:
Bennett A Shaywitz, MD
333 Cedar St
New Haven, CT 06520-8064
Tel: 203 785-4641 *Fax:* 203 785-6369
E-mail: bennett.shaywitz@yale.edu
Accred Length: 3 Years *Program Size:* 0
Program ID: 185-08-21-077

District of Columbia

Washington

George Washington University Program

Sponsor: Children's National Medical Center
George Washington University Hospital (UHS)

Program Director:
Roger J Packer, MD
Children's National Med Ctr
111 Michigan Ave NW/Ste W-4 800
Washington, DC 20010
Tel: 202 884-2120, ext 2652 *Fax:* 202 884-5226
E-mail: rpacker@cnmc.org
Accred Length: 3 Years *Program Size:* 3
Program ID: 185-10-21-048

Florida

Gainesville

University of Florida Program

Sponsor: University of Florida College of Medicine
Shands Hospital at the University of Florida

Program Director:
Bernard L Maria, MD MBA
Univ of Florida
Div of Ped Neurology
JHMHC/Box J296
Gainesville, FL 32610
Tel: 352 392-8183 *Fax:* 352 392-9802
E-mail: maria@ufbi.ufl.edu
Accred Length: 3 Years *Program Size:* 1
Program ID: 185-11-21-087

Miami

University of Miami-Jackson Memorial Medical Center Program

Sponsor: University of Miami-Jackson Memorial Medical Center

Program Director:
Richard G Curless, MD
Univ of Miami-Jackson Memorial Med Ctr
Mailman Ctr D 820
PO Box 016960
Miami, FL 33101
Tel: 305 243-7257 *Fax:* 305 243-7260
E-mail: rcurless@mednet.med.miami.edu
Accred Length: 3 Years *Program Size:* 5
Program ID: 185-11-21-005

Georgia

Atlanta

Emory University Program

Sponsor: Emory University School of Medicine
Egleston Children's Hospital at Emory University
Grady Memorial Hospital

Program Director:
John T Sladky, MD
Emory Univ Sch of Med
Div of Ped Neurology
2040 Ridgewood Dr NE
Atlanta, GA 30322
Tel: 404 727-5756 *Fax:* 404 727-1981
Accred Length: 3 Years *Program Size:* 1
Program ID: 185-12-21-058

Augusta

Medical College of Georgia Program

Sponsor: Medical College of Georgia Hospital and Clinics
University Hospital
Veterans Affairs Medical Center (Augusta)

Program Director:
James E Carroll, MD
Sect of Child Neurology
CJ 2103
Med Coll of Georgia
Augusta, GA 30912-3255
Tel: 706 721-3376 *Fax:* 706 721-3377
E-mail: carroll@neuro.mcg.edu
Accred Length: 3 Years *Program Size:* 3
Program ID: 185-12-21-019

Illinois

Chicago

McGaw Medical Center of Northwestern University Program

Sponsor: Northwestern University Medical School
Children's Memorial Medical Center
Northwestern Memorial Hospital

Program Director:
Charles N Swisher, MD
Children's Memorial Hospital
2300 Children's Plaza
Chicago, IL 60614
Tel: 773 880-3886 *Fax:* 773 880-3374
Accred Length: 3 Years *Program Size:* 3
Program ID: 185-16-21-021

University of Chicago Program

Sponsor: University of Chicago Hospitals

Program Director:
Peter R Huttenlocher, MD
Univ of Chicago
Pediatrics/Neurology
5841 S Maryland Ave/MC3055
Chicago, IL 60637-1470
Tel: 773 702-6487 *Fax:* 773 702-4786
E-mail: phutten@peds.bsd.uchicago.edu
Accred Length: 3 Years *Program Size:* 2
Program ID: 185-16-21-001

Maywood

Loyola University Program

Sponsor: Loyola University Medical Center
Edward J Hines Jr Veterans Affairs Hospital

Program Director:
Kenneth Silver, MD
Loyola Univ-Stritch Sch of Med
Dept of Neurology
2160 S First Ave
Maywood, IL 60153
Tel: 708 216-3407 *Fax:* 708 216-5617
E-mail: ksilver@.it.luc.edu
Internet: http://www.lumc.edu/neurology
Accred Length: 3 Years *Program Size:* 1
Program ID: 185-16-21-045

Indiana

Indianapolis

Indiana University School of Medicine Program

Sponsor: Indiana University School of Medicine
Clarian Riley Hospital for Children

Program Director:
Bhuwan P Garg, MD
Indiana Univ Med Ctr
Dept of Neurology
702 Barnhill Dr/RI 1757
Indianapolis, IN 46202-5200
Tel: 317 274-8747 *Fax:* 317 274-3622
E-mail: bpgarg@indyvax.iupui.edu
Internet: http://www.medlib.iupui.edu/neuro/
Accred Length: 3 Years *Program Size:* 3
Program ID: 185-17-21-050

Louisiana

New Orleans

Louisiana State University Program

Sponsor: Louisiana State University School of Medicine
Childrens Hospital
Medical Center of Louisiana at New Orleans

Program Director:
Ann Henderson-Tilton, MD
Dept of Neurology
Louisiana State Univ Med Ctr
1542 Tulane Ave
New Orleans, LA 70112-2822
Tel: 504 568-4081 *Fax:* 504 568-7130
Internet: http://www.lsumc.edu/campus/neur/neurology/lsuneuro.htm
Accred Length: 3 Years *Program Size:* 3
Program ID: 185-21-21-022

Tulane University Program

Sponsor: Tulane University School of Medicine
Childrens Hospital
Medical Center of Louisiana at New Orleans
Tulane University Hospital and Clinics

Program Director:
Deborah A Lee, MD PhD
Tulane Univ Sch of Med
1430 Tulane Ave
Dept of Neurology TB-52
New Orleans, LA 70112-2699
Tel: 504 588-2241 *Fax:* 504 584-3695
E-mail: neuro@mailhost.tcs.tulane.edu
Accred Length: 3 Years *Program Size:* 1
Program ID: 185-21-21-064

Maryland

Baltimore

Johns Hopkins University Program

Sponsor: Johns Hopkins University School of Medicine
Johns Hopkins Hospital

Program Director:
Harvey S Singer, MD
Johns Hopkins Univ Sch of Med
Harvey 811
600 N Wolfe St
Baltimore, MD 21287-8811
Tel: 410 955-7212 *Fax:* 410 614-2297
E-mail: hsinger@welchlink.welch.jhu.edu
Internet:
http://hopkins.med.jhu.edu/healthcarepros/neuro/neuroped/htm
Accred Length: 3 Years *Program Size:* 5
Program ID: 185-23-21-027

Bethesda

National Capital Consortium Program

Sponsor: National Capital Consortium
Walter Reed Army Medical Center

Program Director:
Michael H Mitchell, MD
Child Neurology Service
Walter Reed Army Med Ctr
6825 16th St NW
Washington, DC 20307-5001
Tel: 202 782-6864 *Fax:* 202 782-0740
Accred Length: 3 Years *Program Size:* 2
Program ID: 185-10-11-010
US Armed Services Program

Massachusetts

Boston

Beth Israel Deaconess Medical Center/Harvard Medical School Program

Sponsor: Children's Hospital
Beth Israel Deaconess Medical Center
Brigham and Women's Hospital

Program Director:
Robert Rust, MD
Children's Hospital
Dept of Neurology
300 Longwood Ave
Boston, MA 02115
Tel: 617 355-6386 *Fax:* 617 730-0416
E-mail: trapilo@a1.tch.harvard.edu
Internet:
http://web1.tch.harvard.edu/neurology/childres.html
Accred Length: 3 Years *Program Size:* 9
Program ID: 185-24-21-051

Massachusetts General Hospital Program

Sponsor: Massachusetts General Hospital

Program Director:
Elizabeth C Dooling, MD
Massachusetts General Hospital
32 Fruit St/VBK 731
Boston, MA 02114
Tel: 617 726-3877 *Fax:* 617 724-7860
Accred Length: 3 Years *Program Size:* 3
Program ID: 185-24-31-067

Tufts University Program
Sponsor: New England Medical Center Hospitals
Program Director:
N Paul Rosman, MD
New England Med Ctr
NEMC #330
750 Washington St
Boston, MA 02111
Tel: 617 636-6096 *Fax:* 617 636-8375
E-mail: paul.rosman@es.nemc.org
Accred Length: 3 Years *Program Size:* 6
Program ID: 185-24-21-028

Worcester

University of Massachusetts Program
Sponsor: University of Massachusetts Medical School
UMass Memorial Health Care (University Campus)
Program Director:
Israel F Abroms, MD
Univ of Massachusetts Med Sch
55 Lake Ave N
Worcester, MA 01655
Tel: 508 856-3247 *Fax:* 508 856-4287
Accred Length: 3 Years *Program Size:* 1
Program ID: 185-24-21-029

Michigan

Ann Arbor

University of Michigan Program
Sponsor: University of Michigan Hospitals
Program Director:
Faye S Silverstein, MD
Univ of Michigan Hospitals
Ped Neurology
MSRB III/Box 0646 Rm 8301
Ann Arbor, MI 48109-0646
Tel: 734 763-4097 *Fax:* 734 764-4279
E-mail: fsilvers@umich.edu
Accred Length: 3 Years *Program Size:* 3
Program ID: 185-25-21-030

Detroit

Wayne State University/Detroit Medical Center Program
Sponsor: Wayne State University/Detroit Medical Center
Children's Hospital of Michigan
Harper Hospital
Program Director:
Susan L Smietana, DO
Children's Hospital of Michigan
Dept of Neurology
3901 Beaubien Blvd
Detroit, MI 48201
Tel: 313 745-5906 *Fax:* 313 745-0955
E-mail: ssmietan@med.wayne.edu
Internet: http://www.phymac.med.wayne.edu/departments/neurology/dept.html
Accred Length: 3 Years *Program Size:* 4
Program ID: 185-25-21-052

Minnesota

Minneapolis

University of Minnesota Program
Sponsor: University of Minnesota Medical School
Fairview-University Medical Center
Hennepin County Medical Center
Regions Hospital
Program Director:
Lawrence A Lockman, MD
Univ of Minnesota
Pediatric Neurology/Box 486
420 Delaware St SE
Minneapolis, MN 55455
Tel: 612 625-7466 *Fax:* 612 624-7681
E-mail: lockm001@maroon.tc.umn.edu
Accred Length: 3 Years *Program Size:* 1
Program ID: 185-26-21-016

Rochester

Mayo Graduate School of Medicine (Rochester) Program
Sponsor: Mayo Graduate School of Medicine-Mayo Foundation
Mayo Clinic (Rochester)
Rochester Methodist Hospital
St Mary's Hospital of Rochester
Program Director:
Jeffrey R Buchhalter, MD PhD
Application Processing Ctr
Mayo Graduate Sch of Med
200 First St SW
Rochester, MN 55905
Tel: 507 284-3373 *Fax:* 507 284-0999
E-mail: mgsm.roch.mn.neurology@mayo.edu
Internet: http://www.mayo.edu/
Accred Length: 3 Years *Program Size:* 3
Program ID: 185-26-21-053

Mississippi

Jackson

University of Mississippi Medical Center Program
Sponsor: University of Mississippi School of Medicine
University Hospital
Program Director:
S Robert Snodgrass, MD
Dept of Ped Neurology
Univ of Mississippi Med Ctr
2500 N State St
Jackson, MS 39216-4505
Tel: 601 984-5275 *Fax:* 601 984-5981
E-mail: sr67s@umsmed.edu
Accred Length: 3 Years *Program Size:* 3
Program ID: 185-27-21-031

Missouri

St Louis

St Louis University School of Medicine Program
Sponsor: St Louis University School of Medicine
SSM Cardinal Glennon Children's Hospital
St Louis University School of Medicine
Program Director:
Suresh Kotagal, MD
St Louis Univ Sch of Med-Cardinal Glennon Child Hospital
1465 S Grand Blvd
St Louis, MO 63104-1095
Tel: 314 268-4105 *Fax:* 314 268-6411
E-mail: suresh@slucare1.sluh.edu
Internet:
http://medschool.slu.edu/departments/neurology
Accred Length: 3 Years *Program Size:* 2
Program ID: 185-28-21-033

Washington University/B-JH/SLCH Consortium Program
Sponsor: Washington University/B-JH/SLCH Consortium
Barnes-Jewish Hospital
St Louis Children's Hospital
Program Director:
Steven M Rothman, MD
St Louis Children's Hospital
One Children's Pl/Ste 12E25
St Louis, MO 63110-1077
Tel: 314 454-6042 *Fax:* 314 454-2523
E-mail: rothman@kids.wustl.edu
Internet: http://www.neuro.wustl.edu
Accred Length: 3 Years *Program Size:* 6
Program ID: 185-28-21-034

New Jersey

Newark

UMDNJ-New Jersey Medical School Program
Sponsor: UMDNJ-New Jersey Medical School
UMDNJ-University Hospital
Veterans Affairs Medical Center (East Orange)
Program Director:
M Richard Koenigsberger, MD
UMDNJ-New Jersey Med Sch
185 S Orange Ave
Newark, NJ 07103
Tel: 973 972-5204 *Fax:* 973 972-2369
E-mail: koenigmr@njms.edu
Accred Length: 3 Years *Program Size:* 3
Program ID: 185-33-21-011

New Mexico

Albuquerque

University of New Mexico Program
Sponsor: University of New Mexico School of Medicine
University Hospital
Program Director:
Leslie A Morrison, MD
Dept of Neurology
Univ of New Mexico Sch of Med
915 Camino de Salud NE
Albuquerque, NM 87131-5281
Tel: 505 272-3342 *Fax:* 505 272-6692
E-mail: lmorrison@salud.unm.edu
Internet: http://www.salud.unm..edu/neuro/
Accred Length: 3 Years *Program Size:* 1
Program ID: 185-34-21-083

New York

Bronx

Albert Einstein College of Medicine Program

Sponsor: Albert Einstein College of Medicine of Yeshiva University
Jacobi Medical Center
Montefiore Medical Center-Henry and Lucy Moses Division
Montefiore Medical Center-Weiler Hospital

Program Director:
Solomon L Moshe, MD
Albert Einstein Coll of Med
Kennedy Ctr/Rm 316
1410 Pelham Pkwy S
Bronx, NY 10461
Tel: 718 430-2447 *Fax:* 718 430-8899
E-mail: moshe@aecom.yu.edu
Accred Length: 3 Years *Program Size:* 5
Program ID: 185-35-21-002

Brooklyn

SUNY Health Science Center at Brooklyn Program

Sponsor: SUNY Health Science Center at Brooklyn
Kings County Hospital Center
University Hospital-SUNY Health Science Center at Brooklyn

Program Director:
Romaine Schubert, MD
SUNY Health Science Ctr-Brooklyn
450 Clarkson Ave/Box 118
Brooklyn, NY 11203-2098
Tel: 718 270-2042 *Fax:* 718 270-3748
E-mail: rschubert@earthlink.net
Internet: http://www.hscbklyn.edu/suny/depts/pedneur/default.html
Accred Length: 3 Years *Program Size:* 5
Program ID: 185-35-21-054

Buffalo

SUNY at Buffalo Graduate Medical-Dental Education Consortium Program

Sponsor: SUNY at Buffalo Grad Medical-Dental Education Consortium
CGF Health System (Children's Hospital of Buffalo)
Erie County Medical Center
Veterans Affairs Medical Center (Buffalo)

Program Director:
Thomas J Langan, MD
Dept of Child Neurology
219 Bryant St
Buffalo, NY 14222
Tel: 716 878-7848 *Fax:* 716 878-7326
E-mail: mecohen@acsu.buffalo.edu
Accred Length: 3 Years *Program Size:* 2
Program ID: 185-35-21-035

East Meadow

Nassau County Medical Center Program

Sponsor: Nassau County Medical Center

Program Director:
Satish Kadakia, MD
Nassau County Med Ctr
2201 Hempstead Trnpk
East Meadow, NY 11554-5400
Tel: 516 572-3107 *Fax:* 516 572-5715
Internet: http://www.ncmc.co.nassau.ny.us
Accred Length: 3 Years *Program Size:* 3
Program ID: 185-35-21-036

New Hyde Park

Albert Einstein College of Medicine at Long Island Jewish Medical Center Program

Sponsor: Long Island Jewish Medical Center
Schneider Children's Hosp (Long Island Jewish Med Ctr)

Program Director:
Lydia Eviatar, MD
Schneider Childrens Hospital
Ped Neurology
269-01 76th Ave
New Hyde Park, NY 11040
Tel: 718 470-3450 *Fax:* 718 343-5826
Internet: http://www.lij.edu
Accred Length: 3 Years *Program Size:* 6
Program ID: 185-35-21-055

New York

Mount Sinai School of Medicine Program

Sponsor: Mount Sinai School of Medicine
Mount Sinai Medical Center

Program Director:
Alan M Aron, MD
Mount Sinai Sch of Med
One Gustave L Levy Pl
New York, NY 10029
Tel: 212 831-4393 *Fax:* 212 426-7627
Accred Length: 3 Years *Program Size:* 2
Program ID: 185-35-21-046

New York and Presbyterian Hospital (Columbia Campus) Program

Sponsor: New York and Presbyterian Hospital
New York and Presbyterian Hospital (Columbia Campus)

Program Director:
Darryl C De Vivo, MD
Columbia-Presbyterian Hospital
710 W 168th St
New York, NY 10032
Tel: 212 305-5244 *Fax:* 212 305-7036
E-mail: dcd1@columbia.edu
Accred Length: 3 Years *Program Size:* 6
Program ID: 185-35-21-059

New York and Presbyterian Hospital (Cornell Campus) Program

Sponsor: New York and Presbyterian Hospital
New York and Presbyterian Hospital (Cornell Campus)

Program Director:
Abe Chutorian, MD
Div of Ped Neurology
525 E 68th St
New York, NY 10021
Tel: 212 746-3278 *Fax:* 212 746-8137
Accred Length: 3 Years *Program Size:* 3
Program ID: 185-35-21-015

New York University Medical Center Program

Sponsor: New York University Medical Center
Bellevue Hospital Center

Program Director:
Ruth Nass, MD
New York Univ Med Ctr
550 First Ave
New York, NY 10016
Tel: 212 263-7753 *Fax:* 212 263-7721
Accred Length: 3 Years *Program Size:* 5
Program ID: 185-35-21-057

Rochester

University of Rochester Program

Sponsor: Strong Memorial Hospital of the University of Rochester

Program Director:
Leon G Epstein, MD
Univ of Rochester Med Ctr
Child Neurology/Rm 4-3259
601 Elmwood Ave/Box 631
Rochester, NY 14642-8677
Tel: 716 275-4783, ext 4783 *Fax:* 716 275-3683
E-mail: lepstein@mail.neurology.rochester.edu
Internet: http://www.urmc.rochester.edu/smd/neuro
Accred Length: 3 Years *Program Size:* 3
Program ID: 185-35-21-013

Stony Brook

SUNY at Stony Brook Program

Sponsor: University Hospital-SUNY at Stony Brook

Program Director:
Nicholas J Lenn, MD PhD
SUNY-Stony Brook
Dept of Neurology
HSC T12/020
Stony Brook, NY 11794-8121
Tel: 516 444-7878 *Fax:* 516 444-1474
E-mail: dboehle@neuro.som.sunysb.edu
Internet:
http://www.informatics.s...edu/neurology/index.html.
Accred Length: 3 Years *Program Size:* 3
Program ID: 185-35-21-081

North Carolina

Chapel Hill

University of North Carolina Hospitals Program

Sponsor: University of North Carolina Hospitals

Program Director:
Robert S Greenwood, MD
Univ of North Carolina Sch of Med
751 Burnett-Womack Bldg/CB7025
Chapel Hill, NC 27599-7025
Tel: 919 966-2528 *Fax:* 919 966-2922
E-mail: greenwor@med.unc.edu
Internet: http://www.med.unc/nrkunits/2depts/neurology
Accred Length: 3 Years *Program Size:* 3
Program ID: 185-36-21-003

Durham

Duke University Program

Sponsor: Duke University Medical Center

Program Director:
Darrell V Lewis Jr, MD
Duke Univ Med Ctr
Div of Ped Neurology
Durham, NC 27710
Tel: 919 684-3219 *Fax:* 919 681-8943
Accred Length: 3 Years *Program Size:* 3
Program ID: 185-36-21-080

Winston-Salem

Wake Forest University School of Medicine Program
Sponsor: Wake Forest University Baptist Medical Center
Program Director:
Cesar C Santos, MD
Wake Forest Univ Sch of Med
Medical Center Blvd
Winston-Salem, NC 27157-1078
Tel: 336 716-2151 *Fax:* 336 716-9489
E-mail: csantos@wfubmc.edu
Internet: http://www.bgsm.edu/bgsm/neurology/neu
Accred Length: 3 Years *Program Size:* 3
Program ID: 185-36-21-037

Ohio

Cincinnati

Children's Hospital Medical Center/University of Cincinnati College of Medicine Program
Sponsor: Children's Hospital Medical Center
University Hospital Inc
Program Director:
Antonius J deGrauw, MD PhD
Children's Hospital Med Ctr
3333 Burnet Ave
Cincinnati, OH 45229-3039
Tel: 513 636-4222, ext 8681 *Fax:* 513 636-3980
E-mail: neuro@chmcc.org
Internet: http://www.chmcc.org
Accred Length: 3 Years *Program Size:* 6
Program ID: 185-38-21-038

Cleveland

Cleveland Clinic Foundation Program
Sponsor: Cleveland Clinic Foundation
Program Director:
A David Rothner, MD
Cleveland Clinic Foundation
Dept of Child Neurology/S90
9500 Euclid Ave
Cleveland, OH 44195-5242
Tel: 216 444-2435 *Fax:* 216 444-0236
E-mail: tripepl@cesmtp.ccf.org
Internet: http://www.ccf.org
Accred Length: 3 Years *Program Size:* 6
Program ID: 185-38-21-004

Oklahoma

Oklahoma City

University of Oklahoma Health Sciences Center Program
Sponsor: University of Oklahoma College of Medicine
Children's Hospital of Oklahoma
University Hospital
Veterans Affairs Medical Center (Oklahoma City)
Program Director:
Charles T Gay, MD
Univ of Oklahoma Health Sciences Ctr
711 Stanton L Young Blvd/Ste 215
Oklahoma City, OK 73104-5023
Tel: 405 271-4113 *Fax:* 405 271-5723
E-mail: charles-gay@ouhsc.edu
Internet: http://w3.ouhsc.edu/neuro
Accred Length: 3 Years *Program Size:* 3
Program ID: 185-39-21-086

Pennsylvania

Philadelphia

Children's Hospital of Philadelphia Program
Sponsor: Children's Hospital of Philadelphia
Hospital of the University of Pennsylvania
Program Director:
Donald P Younkin, MD
Children's Hospital of Philadelphia
Div of Neurology
34th St and Civic Center Blvd
Philadelphia, PA 19104-9786
Tel: 215 590-1719 *Fax:* 215 590-1771
E-mail: younkin@email.chop.edu
Accred Length: 3 Years *Program Size:* 6
Program ID: 185-41-21-041

St Christopher's Hospital for Children Program
Sponsor: St Christopher's Hospital for Children
Program Director:
Joseph J Melvin, DO JD
St Christopher's Hospital for Children
Erie Ave at Front St
Philadelphia, PA 19134-1095
Tel: 215 427-5470 *Fax:* 215 427-4393
E-mail: melvinj@wpo.auhs.edu
Accred Length: 3 Years *Program Size:* 1
Program ID: 185-41-21-040

Pittsburgh

University Health Center of Pittsburgh Program
Sponsor: University Health Center of Pittsburgh
Children's Hospital of Pittsburgh
Presbyterian University Hospital/UPMC
Program Director:
Michael J Painter, MD
Children's Hospital
3705 Fifth Ave
Pittsburgh, PA 15213
Tel: 412 692-6182 *Fax:* 412 692-6787
Internet: http://www.chp.edu
Accred Length: 3 Years *Program Size:* 4
Program ID: 185-41-21-012

Rhode Island

Providence

Brown University Program
Sponsor: Rhode Island Hospital
Program Director:
Generoso G Gascon, MD
Rhode Island Hospital
110 Lockwood St/Ste 342
Providence, RI 02903
Tel: 401 444-4345 *Fax:* 401 444-3236
E-mail: generoso_gascon@brown.edu
Accred Length: 3 Years *Program Size:* 3
Program ID: 185-43-21-074

Tennessee

Memphis

University of Tennessee Program
Sponsor: University of Tennessee College of Medicine
Baptist Memorial Hospital
LeBonheur Children's Medical Center
Regional Medical Center at Memphis
Veterans Affairs Medical Center (Memphis)
Program Director:
Douglas F Rose, MD
Univ of Tennessee Coll of Med
777 Washington Ave/Ste 350
Memphis, TN 38105
Tel: 901 572-4538, ext 9015 *Fax:* 901 572-4587
Accred Length: 3 Years *Program Size:* 1
Program ID: 185-47-21-079

Nashville

Vanderbilt University Program
Sponsor: Vanderbilt University Medical Center
Program Director:
Gerald M Fenichel, MD
Dept of Neurology
2100 Pierce Ave
Nashville, TN 37212
Tel: 615 936-2024 *Fax:* 615 936-0223
E-mail: gerald.fenichel@mcmail.vanderbilt.edu
Accred Length: 3 Years *Program Size:* 3
Program ID: 185-47-21-042

Texas

Dallas

University of Texas Southwestern Medical School Program
Sponsor: University of Texas Southwestern Medical School
Children's Medical Center of Dallas
Dallas County Hospital District-Parkland Memorial Hospital
Texas Scottish Rite Hospital for Children
Program Director:
Anthony R Riela, MD
Children's Med Ctr
1935 Motor St
Dallas, TX 75235
Tel: 214 640-8403 *Fax:* 214 640-7671
E-mail: ariela@mednet.swmed.edu
Internet: http://www.swmed.edu
Accred Length: 3 Years *Program Size:* 7
Program ID: 185-48-21-043

Houston

Baylor College of Medicine Program
Sponsor: Baylor College of Medicine
Texas Children's Hospital
Program Director:
Marvin A Fishman, MD
Texas Children's Hospital
Ped Neurology
6621 Fannin St/MC 3-3311
Houston, TX 77030
Tel: 713 770-3964 *Fax:* 713 796-2340
E-mail: mfishman@bcm.tmc.edu
Internet: http://www.bcm.tmc.edu/neurol
Accred Length: 3 Years *Program Size:* 6
Program ID: 185-48-21-018

University of Texas at Houston Program
Sponsor: University of Texas Medical School at Houston
Memorial Hermann Healthcare System
Shriners Hospitals for Children (Houston)
University of Texas M D Anderson Cancer Center
Program Director:
Ian J Butler, MD
Univ of Texas-Houston Med Sch
Div of Child Neurology
6431 Fannin St/7044/MSB
Houston, TX 77030-1501
Tel: 713 500-7100, ext 7113 *Fax:* 713 500-7019
E-mail: mcandela@neuro.med.uth.tmc.edu
Internet: http://neurology.uth.tmc.edu/index.htm
Accred Length: 3 Years *Program Size:* 1
Program ID: 185-48-31-078

Utah

Salt Lake City

University of Utah Program
Sponsor: University of Utah Medical Center
Primary Children's Medical Center
Program Director:
Francis Filloux, MD
Primary Children's Med Ctr
Div of Child Neurology
100 N Medical Dr
Salt Lake City, UT 84113-1100
Tel: 801 588-3385 *Fax:* 801 588-3392
E-mail: fran.filloux@hsc.utah.edu
Internet: http://www.ped.med.utah.edu
Accred Length: 3 Years *Program Size:* 3
Program ID: 185-49-21-044

Virginia

Richmond

Medical College of Virginia/Virginia Commonwealth University Program
Sponsor: Medical College of Virginia/Virginia Commonwealth University
Medical College of Virginia Hospitals
Program Director:
Edwin C Myer, MD
Virginia Commonwealth Univ-Med Coll of Virginia
PO Box 980211
Richmond, VA 23298-0211
Tel: 804 828-0442 *Fax:* 804 828-6690
E-mail: ecmyer@hsc.vcu.edu
Internet: http://www.nsc.vcu.edu
Accred Length: 3 Years *Program Size:* 3
Program ID: 185-51-21-060

Washington

Seattle

University of Washington Program
Sponsor: University of Washington School of Medicine
Children's Hospital and Medical Center
Harborview Medical Center
University of Washington Medical Center
Program Director:
Harvey Sarnat, MD MD
Children's Hospital and Med Ctr
4800 Sand Point Way NE
CH-49/Box 359300
Seattle, WA 98105-0371
Tel: 206 526-2078 *Fax:* 206 528-2649
Accred Length: 3 Years *Program Size:* 3
Program ID: 185-54-21-047

West Virginia

Morgantown

West Virginia University Program
Sponsor: West Virginia University Hospitals
Program Director:
John Bodensteiner, MD
Dept of Neurology
RC Byrd Health Science Ctr-West Virginia Univ
PO Box 9180
Morgantown, WV 26506-9180
Tel: 304 293-2341 *Fax:* 304 293-3352
E-mail: mgarlick@wvuhsc1.hsc.wvu.edu
Internet: http://www.hsc.wvu.edu
Accred Length: 3 Years *Program Size:* 1
Program ID: 185-55-11-068

Wisconsin

Milwaukee

Medical College of Wisconsin Program
Sponsor: Medical College of Wisconsin Affiliated Hospitals Inc
Children's Hospital of Wisconsin
Clement J Zablocki Veterans Affairs Medical Center
Froedtert Memorial Lutheran Hospital
Program Director:
Edward Kovnar, MD
Med Coll of Wisconsin, Div of Child Neurology
9200 W Wisconsin Ave
Milwaukee, WI 53226
Tel: 414 266-4090 *Fax:* 414 266-8676
E-mail: ekovnar@mcw.edu
Accred Length: 3 Years *Program Size:* 3
Program ID: 185-56-21-070

Clinical and Laboratory Immunology (Allergy and Immunology)

California

Orange

University of California (Irvine) Program
Sponsor: University of California (Irvine) Medical Center
University of California (Irvine) College of Medicine
Program Director:
Sudhir Gupta, MD PhD
Univ of California
Div of Immunology
C240 Med Sci 1
Irvine, CA 92697-4069
Tel: 949 824-5818 *Fax:* 949 824-4362
E-mail: sgupta@uci.edu
Accred Length: 1 Year *Program Size:* 1
Program ID: 025-05-21-016

Colorado

Denver

University of Colorado Program
Sponsor: University of Colorado Health Sciences Center
Immunological Associates of Denver
National Jewish Ctr for Immunology and Respiratory Medicine
Program Director:
Lanny J Rosenwasser, MD
Div of Allergy/Clin Immunology
1400 Jackson St
Denver, CO 80206
Tel: 303 398-1656 *Fax:* 303 398-1806
E-mail: rosenwasserl@njc.org
Accred Length: 1 Year *Program Size:* 1
Program ID: 025-07-21-005

District of Columbia

Washington

Walter Reed Army Medical Center Program
Sponsor: Walter Reed Army Medical Center
NIH Warren Grant Magnuson Clinical Center
Program Director:
Michael A O'Connell, MD
Walter Reed Army Med Ctr
Allergy/Immunology Services I-J
6900 Georgia Ave NW
Washington, DC 20307-5001
Tel: 202 782-6850 *Fax:* 202 782-7093
E-mail: ltc_michael_o'connell@wramc1-amedd.army.mil
Accred Length: 1 Year *Program Size:* 1
Program ID: 025-10-21-006
US Armed Services Program

Florida

St Petersburg

University of South Florida (All Children's) Program

Sponsor: University of South Florida College of Medicine
All Children's Hospital

Program Director:
Robert A Good, MD
Noorbibi K Day, PhD
All Children's Hospital
801 Sixth St S
St Petersburg, FL 33701
Tel: 727 892-4470 *Fax:* 727 892-8536
E-mail: dayn@allkids.org
Accred Length: 1 Year *Program Size:* 2
Program ID: 025-11-31-010

Tampa

University of South Florida Program

Sponsor: University of South Florida College of Medicine
All Children's Hospital
James A Haley Veterans Hospital
Tampa General Healthcare

Program Director:
Dennis K Ledford, MD
Univ of South Florida Coll of Med
Div of Allergy/Immunology, VAMC
13000 Bruce B Downs Blvd (111D)
Tampa, FL 33612
Tel: 813 972-7631 *Fax:* 813 972-7623
E-mail: dledford@com1.med.usf.edu
Internet: http://www.med.usf.edu/intmed/allergy/
Accred Length: 1 Year *Program Size:* 1
Program ID: 025-11-21-001

Maryland

Bethesda

National Institutes of Health Clinical Center Program

Sponsor: NIH Warren Grant Magnuson Clinical Center
Walter Reed Army Medical Center

Program Director:
Thomas A Fleisher, MD
Bldg 10/Rm 2C410
National Institutes of Health
Bethesda, MD 20892-1508
Tel: 301 496-5668 *Fax:* 301 402-1612
Internet: http://www.helix.uih.gov:8001/oe
Accred Length: 1 Year *Program Size:* 1
Program ID: 025-23-21-007

New York

Brooklyn

SUNY Health Science Center at Brooklyn Program

Sponsor: SUNY Health Science Center at Brooklyn
Kings County Hospital Center
University Hospital-SUNY Health Science Center at Brooklyn

Program Director:
Alan S Josephson, MD
Div of Allergy/Clin Immunology
SUNY Health Science Ctr-Brooklyn
450 Clarkson Ave/Box 50
Brooklyn, NY 11203-2098
Tel: 718 270-2156 *Fax:* 718 270-1831
E-mail: ajosephson@aol.com
Accred Length: 1 Year *Program Size:* 1
Program ID: 025-35-31-018

East Meadow

Nassau County Medical Center Program

Sponsor: Nassau County Medical Center
North Shore University Hospital

Program Director:
Marianne Frieri, MD PhD
Savita Pahwa, MD
Div of Clin Immunopathology
Nassau County Med Ctr
2201 Hempstead Trnpk
East Meadow, NY 11554-5400
Tel: 516 572-3214 *Fax:* 516 572-5614
Accred Length: 1 Year *Program Size:* 1
Program ID: 025-35-21-015

Texas

Houston

Baylor College of Medicine Program

Sponsor: Baylor College of Medicine
Methodist Hospital
Texas Children's Hospital

Program Director:
David P Huston, MD
William T Shearer, MD PhD
Baylor Coll of Med
One Baylor Plaza
FBRN B567
Houston, TX 77030-3498
Tel: 713 790-5310 *Fax:* 713 793-1445
E-mail: dhuston@bcm.tmc.edu
Internet: http://www.bcm.tmc.edu/medicine/residency/
Accred Length: 1 Year *Program Size:* 1
Program ID: 025-48-21-012

Lackland AFB

San Antonio Uniformed Services Health Education Consortium Program

Sponsor: San Antonio Uniformed Services Health Education Consortium
Wilford Hall Medical Center (AETC)

Program Director:
Theodore H Freeman, MD
Wilford Hall Med Ctr/MMIA
2200 Bergquist Dr/Ste 1
Lackland AFB, TX 78236-5300
Tel: 210 292-5717 *Fax:* 210 292-7033
Accred Length: 1 Year *Program Size:* 1
Program ID: 025-48-31-017
US Armed Services Program

Virginia

Richmond

Medical College of Virginia/Virginia Commonwealth University Program

Sponsor: Medical College of Virginia/Virginia Commonwealth University
Medical College of Virginia Hospitals

Program Director:
P Franklin Mullinax, MD
Med Coll of Virginia
PO Box 980263
Richmond, VA 23298-0263
Tel: 804 828-9685 *Fax:* 804 828-0283
E-mail: pfmullinax@gems.vcu.edu
Internet: http://www.views.vcu.edu/internal-medicine
Accred Length: 1 Year *Program Size:* 1
Program ID: 025-51-21-021

Clinical Cardiac Electrophysiology (Internal Medicine)

California

Los Angeles

Cedars-Sinai Medical Center Program
Sponsor: Cedars-Sinai Medical Center
Program Director:
Peng-Sheng Chen, MD
Cedars-Sinai Med Ctr
Div of Cardiology/Rm 5342
8700 Beverly Blvd
Los Angeles, CA 90048-1865
Tel: 310 855-4851 *Fax:* 310 289-0780
E-mail: chenp@csmc.edu
Internet: http://www.csmc.edu/cards
Accred Length: 1 Year *Program Size:* 2
Program ID: 154-05-21-002

University of Southern California Program
Sponsor: Los Angeles County-USC Medical Center
USC University Hospital
Program Director:
Koonlawee Nademanee, MD
Univ of Southern California
1355 San Pablo St/AHC-117
Los Angeles, CA 90033-4581
Tel: 323 442-8922 *Fax:* 323 442-5227
E-mail: nademane@hsc.usc.edu
Accred Length: 1 Year *Program Size:* 1
Program ID: 154-05-12-005

VA Greater Los Angeles Healthcare System Program
Sponsor: VA Greater Los Angeles Healthcare System
Program Director:
Philip Sager, MD
West Los Angeles VA Med Ctr
11301 Wilshire Blvd
Los Angeles, CA 90073
Tel: 310 268-3643 *Fax:* 310 268-4288
Accred Length: 1 Year *Program Size:* 1
Program ID: 154-05-13-006

San Diego

University of California (San Diego) Program
Sponsor: University of California (San Diego) Medical Center
Program Director:
Gregory K Feld, MD
200 W Arbor Dr
San Diego, CA 92103-8411
Tel: 619 543-5428 *Fax:* 619 543-7418
E-mail: gfeld@ucsd.edu
Accred Length: 1 Year *Program Size:* 2
Program ID: 154-05-22-007

San Francisco

University of California (San Francisco) Program
Sponsor: University of California (San Francisco) School of Medicine
University of California (San Francisco) Medical Center
Program Director:
Michael D Lesh, MD
Univ of California San Francisco
MU E Tower
513 Parnassus Ave/S-224
San Francisco, CA 94143-1354
Tel: 415 476-5709 *Fax:* 415 476-6260
E-mail: lesh@ep4.ucsf.edu
Accred Length: 1 Year *Program Size:* 6
Program ID: 154-05-23-008

Stanford

Stanford University Program
Sponsor: Stanford University Hospital
Santa Teresa Community Hospital
Veterans Affairs Palo Alto Health Care System
Program Director:
Ruey J Sung, MD
Stanford Univ Med Ctr
H-2146
300 Pasteur Dr
Stanford, CA 94305-5233
Tel: 650 725-4931 *Fax:* 650 725-7568
Accred Length: 1 Year *Program Size:* 4
Program ID: 154-05-32-009

Torrance

Los Angeles County-Harbor-UCLA Medical Center Program
Sponsor: Los Angeles County-Harbor-UCLA Medical Center
Program Director:
Anil K Bhandari, MD
Los Angeles County-Harbor-UCLA Med Ctr
Int Med/Cardiac Electrophys
1225 Wilshire Blvd
Los Angeles, CA 90017
Tel: 213 977-2239 *Fax:* 213 977-2209
Accred Length: 1 Year *Program Size:* 2
Program ID: 154-05-31-003

Colorado

Denver

University of Colorado Program
Sponsor: University of Colorado Health Sciences Center
Program Director:
Michael J Reiter, MD
Univ of Colorado Health Sciences Ctr
4200 E 9th Ave
Denver, CO 80262
Tel: 303 315-7558 *Fax:* 303 372-8028
Accred Length: 1 Year *Program Size:* 5
Program ID: 154-07-21-010

District of Columbia

Washington

George Washington University Program
Sponsor: George Washington University School of Medicine
George Washington University Hospital (UHS)
Veterans Affairs Medical Center (Washington, DC)
Program Director:
Sung W Lee, MD
George Washington Univ
ACC Ste 4-421
2150 Pennsylvania Ave NW
Washington, DC 20037
Tel: 202 994-6113 *Fax:* 202 994-3673
E-mail: domswl@gwumc.edu
Accred Length: 1 Year *Program Size:* 1
Program ID: 154-10-31-012

Georgetown University Program
Sponsor: Georgetown University Medical Center
Veterans Affairs Medical Center (Washington, DC)
Program Director:
Cynthia M Tracy, MD
Georgetown Univ Med Ctr
Med/EP Fellowship (c/o W Steele 5 PHC)
3800 Reservoir Rd NW
Washington, DC 20007
Tel: 202 687-4034 *Fax:* 202 687-7797
E-mail: steelewe@gunet.georgetown.edu
Accred Length: 1 Year *Program Size:* 2
Program ID: 154-10-21-011

Florida

Gainesville

University of Florida Program
Sponsor: University of Florida College of Medicine
Shands Hospital at the University of Florida
Veterans Affairs Medical Center (Gainesville)
Program Director:
Anne B Curtis, MD
Univ of Florida
Box 100277
Gainesville, FL 32610-2610
Tel: 352 392-2469 *Fax:* 352 846-0314
E-mail: curtis@medicine.ufl.edu
Accred Length: 1 Year *Program Size:* 2
Program ID: 154-11-21-081

Miami

University of Miami-Jackson Memorial Medical Center Program
Sponsor: University of Miami-Jackson Memorial Medical Center
Program Director:
Alberto Interian Jr, MD
Univ of Miami Sch of Med
Jackson Memorial Hospital
PO Box 016960
Miami, FL 33101
Tel: 305 585-5532 *Fax:* 305 585-5090
Accred Length: 1 Year *Program Size:* 2
Program ID: 154-11-21-014

Georgia

Atlanta

Emory University Program

Sponsor: Emory University School of Medicine
Crawford Long Hospital of Emory University

Program Director:
Jonathan J Langberg, MD
Emory Univ Hospital
1364 Clifton Rd NE
Ste F-414
Atlanta, GA 30322
Tel: 404 712-4942 *Fax:* 404 712-4374
E-mail: jlangbe@emory.edu
Internet: http://www.heartweb.eushc.org
Accred Length: 1 Year *Program Size:* 2
Program ID: 154-12-21-015

Illinois

Chicago

Illinois Masonic Medical Center/Rush Medical College Program

Sponsor: Illinois Masonic Medical Center

Program Director:
Richard F Kehoe, MD
Illinois Masonic Med Ctr
Cardiac Arrhythmia Consultants
3000 N Halsted St/Ste 803
Chicago, IL 60657
Tel: 773 296-7135 *Fax:* 773 296-7982
Internet: http://www.immc.org
Accred Length: 1 Year *Program Size:* 2
Program ID: 154-16-21-016

McGaw Medical Center of Northwestern University Program

Sponsor: Northwestern University Medical School
Northwestern Memorial Hospital

Program Director:
Alan Kadish, MD
Northwestern Memorial Hospital
250 E Superior/Ste 520
Chicago, IL 60611
Tel: 312 908-4753 *Fax:* 312 908-6003
E-mail: a-kadish@nwu.edu
Accred Length: 1 Year *Program Size:* 1
Program ID: 154-16-31-017

Rush-Presbyterian-St Luke's Medical Center Program

Sponsor: Rush-Presbyterian-St Luke's Medical Center

Program Director:
Richard G Trohman, MD PhD
1653 W Congress Pkwy
Chicago, IL 60612-0612
Tel: 312 942-6858 *Fax:* 312 942-5862
Accred Length: 1 Year *Program Size:* 2
Program ID: 154-16-11-018

University of Chicago Program

Sponsor: University of Chicago Hospitals

Program Director:
David J Wilber, MD
5841 S Maryland Ave
MC 9064
Chicago, IL 60637-0637
Tel: 773 702-5988 *Fax:* 773 702-4666
Accred Length: 1 Year *Program Size:* 2
Program ID: 154-16-12-019

Maywood

Loyola University Program

Sponsor: Loyola University Medical Center

Program Director:
Brian Olshansky, MD
Loyola Univ Med Ctr
2160 S First Ave
Bldg 107/Rm 1847
Maywood, IL 60153
Tel: 708 216-9449 *Fax:* 708 216-6829
E-mail: internet:bolshan@luc.edu
Accred Length: 1 Year *Program Size:* 1
Program ID: 154-16-13-020

Indiana

Indianapolis

Indiana University School of Medicine Program

Sponsor: Indiana University School of Medicine
Richard L Roudebush Veterans Affairs Medical Center

Program Director:
John M Miller, MD
Krannert Inst of Cardiology
1111 W 10th St
Indianapolis, IN 46202-4800
Tel: 317 630-6668 *Fax:* 317 630-2555
E-mail: jmiller6@iupui.edu
Accred Length: 1 Year *Program Size:* 2
Program ID: 154-17-21-021

Iowa

Iowa City

University of Iowa Hospitals and Clinics Program

Sponsor: University of Iowa Hospitals and Clinics
Veterans Affairs Medical Center (Iowa City)

Program Director:
James B Martins, MD
Univ of Iowa Hospitals and Clinics
Dept of Int Med/E 318-3 GH
200 Hawkins Dr
Iowa City, IA 52242
Tel: 319 356-2740 *Fax:* 319 356-6343
E-mail: james-martins@uiowa.edu
Accred Length: 1 Year *Program Size:* 1
Program ID: 154-18-21-022

Kentucky

Louisville

University of Louisville Program

Sponsor: University of Louisville School of Medicine
Jewish Hospital
University of Louisville Hospital
Veterans Affairs Medical Center (Louisville)

Program Director:
Igor Singer, MD
Univ of Louisville, Div of Cardiology
530 S Jackson St
Ambulatory Care Bldg 3rd Fl
Louisville, KY 40292
Tel: 502 852-7956
E-mail: iosing01@athena.louisville.edu
Accred Length: 1 Year *Program Size:* 1
Program ID: 154-20-21-023

Maryland

Baltimore

Johns Hopkins University Program

Sponsor: Johns Hopkins University School of Medicine
Johns Hopkins Hospital

Program Director:
Hugh Calkins, MD
Carnegie 592
600 N Wolfe St
Baltimore, MD 21287-0409
Tel: 410 955-7405 *Fax:* 410 614-1345
E-mail: hcalkins@welchlink.welch.jhu.edu
Accred Length: 1 Year *Program Size:* 4
Program ID: 154-23-21-024

University of Maryland Program

Sponsor: University of Maryland Medical System
Veterans Affairs Medical Center (Baltimore)

Program Director:
Michael R Gold, MD PhD
Univ of Maryland Hospital
22 S Greene St/Ste N3W77
Baltimore, MD 21201
Tel: 410 328-6056 *Fax:* 410 328-2062
E-mail: mgold@medicine.ab.umd.edu
Accred Length: 1 Year *Program Size:* 2
Program ID: 154-23-31-025

Massachusetts

Boston

Beth Israel Deaconess Medical Center (East Campus) Program

Sponsor: Beth Israel Deaconess Medical Center

Program Director:
Mark E Josephson, MD
Beth Israel Deaconess Med Ctr
330 Brookline Ave
Boston, MA 02215
Tel: 617 667-4387 *Fax:* 617 667-4833
E-mail: mjoseph2@bidmc.harvard.edu
Internet: http://www.bidmc.harvard.edu/cardiology
Accred Length: 1 Year *Program Size:* 2
Program ID: 154-24-21-026

Brigham and Women's Hospital Program

Sponsor: Brigham and Women's Hospital
Brockton-West Roxbury Veterans Affairs Medical Center

Program Director:
William G Stevenson, MD
75 Francis St
Boston, MA 02115
Tel: 617 732-7517 *Fax:* 617 277-4981
E-mail: wgstevenso@bics.bwh.harvard.edu
Accred Length: 1 Year *Program Size:* 3
Program ID: 154-24-11-028

Massachusetts General Hospital Program

Sponsor: Massachusetts General Hospital

Program Director:
Jeremy N Ruskin, MD
32 Fruit St
Boston, MA 02114
Tel: 617 726-8514 *Fax:* 617 726-3852
E-mail: ruskin.jeremy@mgh.harvard.edu
Internet: http://www.mgh.harvard.edu
Accred Length: 1 Year *Program Size:* 3
Program ID: 154-24-12-029

New England Medical Center Hospitals Program
Sponsor: New England Medical Center Hospitals
Program Director:
N A Mark Estes III, MD
750 Washington St/Box 197
Boston, MA 02111
Tel: 617 636-6156 *Fax:* 617 636-5913
Accred Length: 1 Year *Program Size:* 2
Program ID: 154-24-13-030

Burlington

Lahey Clinic Program
Sponsor: Lahey Clinic
Program Director:
David T Martin, MD
Lahey Clinic Med Ctr
41 Mall Rd
Burlington, MA 01805
Tel: 781 744-8863 *Fax:* 781 744-5261
E-mail: david.t.martin@lahey.org
Internet: http://www.lahey.org
Accred Length: 1 Year *Program Size:* 1
Program ID: 154-24-23-032

Springfield

Baystate Medical Center Program
Sponsor: Baystate Medical Center
Program Director:
James B Kirchhoffer, MD
Baystate Med Ctr
Cardiology Service/Springfield 4
759 Chestnut St
Springfield, MA 01199
Tel: 413 794-4490 *Fax:* 413 794-0198
Accred Length: 1 Year *Program Size:* 1
Program ID: 154-24-32-033

Worcester

University of Massachusetts Program
Sponsor: University of Massachusetts Medical School
UMass Memorial Health Care (University Campus)
Program Director:
Robert S Mittleman, MD MS
Univ of Massachusetts Med Sch
Div of Cardiology
55 Lake Ave N
Worcester, MA 01655
Tel: 508 856-6149 *Fax:* 508 856-4571
E-mail: rmittlem@umassmed.ummed.edu
Accred Length: 1 Year *Program Size:* 1
Program ID: 154-24-33-034

Michigan

Ann Arbor

University of Michigan Program
Sponsor: University of Michigan Hospitals
Oakwood Hospital
Program Director:
Fred Morady, MD
1500 E Medical Center Dr
Rm BIF245
Ann Arbor, MI 48109-0022
Tel: 734 936-4025 *Fax:* 734 936-7641
E-mail: fmorady@umich.edu
Accred Length: 1 Year *Program Size:* 4
Program ID: 154-25-21-035

Detroit

Wayne State University/Detroit Medical Center Program
Sponsor: Wayne State University/Detroit Medical Center
Sinai Hospital
St John Hospital and Medical Center
Program Director:
Russell T Steinman, MD
Sinai Hospital
Dept of Medicine
6767 W Outer Dr
Detroit, MI 48235
Tel: 313 493-5780 *Fax:* 313 493-6892
Accred Length: 1 Year *Program Size:* 0
Program ID: 154-25-31-036

Minnesota

Minneapolis

University of Minnesota Program
Sponsor: University of Minnesota Medical School
Fairview-University Medical Center
Program Director:
David G Benditt, MD
Box 508 UMHC
420 Delaware St SE
Minneapolis, MN 55455
Tel: 612 625-4401 *Fax:* 612 624-4937
Accred Length: 1 Year *Program Size:* 1
Program ID: 154-26-21-037

Rochester

Mayo Graduate School of Medicine (Rochester) Program
Sponsor: Mayo Graduate School of Medicine-Mayo Foundation
St Mary's Hospital of Rochester
Program Director:
Stephen C Hammill, MD
Application Processing Ctr
Mayo Graduate Sch of Med
200 First St SW
Rochester, MN 55905
Tel: 507 284-3126 *Fax:* 507 284-0999
E-mail: mgsm.intmed.specialties@mayo.edu
Internet: http://www.mayo.edu/
Accred Length: 1 Year *Program Size:* 3
Program ID: 154-26-31-038

Missouri

Kansas City

University of Missouri at Kansas City Program
Sponsor: University of Missouri-Kansas City School of Medicine
Saint Luke's Hospital
Program Director:
David M Steinhaus, MD
Cardiovascular Consultants PC
4330 Wornall Rd/Ste 2000
Kansas City, MO 64111
Tel: 816 931-1883 *Fax:* 816 531-7408
Accred Length: 1 Year *Program Size:* 1
Program ID: 154-28-21-039

St Louis

Washington University/B-JH/SLCH Consortium (South Campus) Program
Sponsor: Washington University/B-JH/SLCH Consortium
Barnes-Jewish Hospital
Barnes-Jewish Hospital (North Campus)
Program Director:
Bruce D Lindsay, MD
Washington Univ Sch of Med
660 S Euclid Ave/Box 8086
St Louis, MO 63110-3110
Tel: 314 362-1045 *Fax:* 314 362-0057
E-mail: blindsay@im.wustl.edu
Accred Length: 1 Year *Program Size:* 4
Program ID: 154-28-31-040

New Hampshire

Lebanon

Dartmouth-Hitchcock Medical Center Program
Sponsor: Mary Hitchcock Memorial Hospital
Program Director:
Mark L Greenberg, MD
Dartmouth-Hitchcock Med Ctr
1 Medical Center Dr
Lebanon, NH 03756
Tel: 603 650-7837 *Fax:* 603 650-6164
E-mail: mark.greenberg@hitchcock.org
Accred Length: 1 Year *Program Size:* 1
Program ID: 154-32-21-041

New York

Bronx

Albert Einstein College of Medicine Program
Sponsor: Albert Einstein College of Medicine of Yeshiva University
Montefiore Medical Center-Henry and Lucy Moses Division
Program Director:
John D Fisher, MD
Montefiore Med Ctr
111 E 210th St
Bronx, NY 10467
Tel: 718 920-4116 *Fax:* 718 920-6798
Accred Length: 1 Year *Program Size:* 1
Program ID: 154-35-21-042

Brooklyn

SUNY Health Science Center at Brooklyn Program
Sponsor: SUNY Health Science Center at Brooklyn
Program Director:
Nabil El-Sherif, MD
450 Clarkson Ave/Box 1199
Brooklyn, NY 11203-2098
Tel: 718 270-4147 *Fax:* 718 270-4106
Accred Length: 1 Year *Program Size:* 2
Program ID: 154-35-31-043

Manhasset

North Shore University Hospital/NYU School of Medicine Program

Sponsor: North Shore University Hospital

Program Director:
Ram L Jadonath, MD
North Shore Univ Hospital
Cardiology/EPS
300 Community Dr
Manhasset, NY 11030
Tel: 516 562-2300 *Fax:* 516 562-2352
Internet: http://www.nshs.edu
Accred Length: 1 Year *Program Size:* 1
Program ID: 154-35-11-044

New Hyde Park

Albert Einstein College of Medicine at Long Island Jewish Medical Center Program

Sponsor: Long Island Jewish Medical Center

Program Director:
Steven Evans, MD
Long Island Jewish Med Ctr
Rm 2135
New Hyde Park, NY 11042
Tel: 718 470-7333 *Fax:* 718 470-1821
Internet: http://www.lij.edu
Accred Length: 1 Year *Program Size:* 1
Program ID: 154-35-13-046

New York

Mount Sinai School of Medicine Program

Sponsor: Mount Sinai School of Medicine
Mount Sinai Medical Center

Program Director:
Anthony J Gomes, MD
Mount Sinai Med Ctr
One Gustave L Levy Pl
Box 1030
New York, NY 10029
Tel: 212 241-7272 *Fax:* 212 534-2776
Accred Length: 1 Year *Program Size:* 1
Program ID: 154-35-22-047

New York and Presbyterian Hospital (Columbia Campus) Program

Sponsor: New York and Presbyterian Hospital
New York and Presbyterian Hospital (Columbia Campus)

Program Director:
James Reiffel, MD
161 Fort Washington Ave/Rm 349
New York, NY 10032
Tel: 212 305-5206 *Fax:* 212 305-1386
Accred Length: 1 Year *Program Size:* 1
Program ID: 154-35-33-050

New York and Presbyterian Hospital (Cornell Campus) Program

Sponsor: New York and Presbyterian Hospital
New York and Presbyterian Hospital (Cornell Campus)

Program Director:
Bruce B Lerman, MD
New York Hospital-Cornell Med Ctr
525 E 68th St/Starr 4
New York, NY 10021
Tel: 212 746-2169 *Fax:* 212 746-6951
E-mail: blerman@mail.med.cornell.edu
Accred Length: 1 Year *Program Size:* 2
Program ID: 154-35-23-048

New York University Medical Center Program

Sponsor: New York University Medical Center
Bellevue Hospital Center

Program Director:
Larry A Chinitz, MD
New York Univ Med Ctr
560 First Ave
New York, NY 10016
Tel: 212 263-5656 *Fax:* 212 263-8534
Accred Length: 1 Year *Program Size:* 1
Program ID: 154-35-32-049

St Luke's-Roosevelt Hospital Center Program

Sponsor: St Luke's-Roosevelt Hospital Center
St Luke's-Roosevelt Hospital Center-St Luke's Division

Program Director:
Jonathan Steinberg, MD
1111 Amsterdam Ave
New York, NY 10025
Tel: 212 523-4007 *Fax:* 212 523-3915
E-mail: jss7@columbia.edu
Internet: http://www.arrhythmia.com
Accred Length: 1 Year *Program Size:* 2
Program ID: 154-35-42-051

Rochester

University of Rochester Program

Sponsor: Strong Memorial Hospital of the University of Rochester

Program Director:
James P Daubert, MD
Strong Memorial Hospital
601 Elmwood Ave/Box 679
Rochester, NY 14642-8679
Tel: 716 275-7736 *Fax:* 716 473-1573
Accred Length: 1 Year *Program Size:* 2
Program ID: 154-35-43-052

North Carolina

Chapel Hill

University of North Carolina Hospitals Program

Sponsor: University of North Carolina Hospitals

Program Director:
William E Sanders Jr, MD
Univ of North Carolina Hospitals
CB7075 Burnett-Womack Bldg
Chapel Hill, NC 27599-7075
Tel: 919 966-6455 *Fax:* 919 966-4366
Accred Length: 1 Year *Program Size:* 1
Program ID: 154-36-21-053

Durham

Duke University Program

Sponsor: Duke University Medical Center

Program Director:
J Marcus Wharton, MD
Box 3816
Duke Univ
Durham, NC 27710
Tel: 919 681-6478 *Fax:* 919 681-8980
E-mail: whart002@mc.duke.edu
Internet: http://www.mc.duke.edu
Accred Length: 1 Year *Program Size:* 3
Program ID: 154-36-31-054

Winston-Salem

Wake Forest University School of Medicine Program

Sponsor: Wake Forest University Baptist Medical Center

Program Director:
David M Fitzgerald, MD
Wake Forest Univ Sch of Med
Dept of Int Med/Cardiology
Winston-Salem, NC 27157-1046
Tel: 336 716-4838 *Fax:* 336 716-7771
Accred Length: 1 Year *Program Size:* 4
Program ID: 154-36-11-055

Ohio

Cleveland

Case Western Reserve University Program

Sponsor: University Hospitals of Cleveland
Veterans Affairs Medical Center (Cleveland)

Program Director:
Albert L Waldo, MD
Univ Hospitals of Cleveland
11100 Euclid Ave
Cleveland, OH 44106-5038
Tel: 216 844-7690 *Fax:* 216 844-7196
E-mail: alw2@po.cwru.edu
Internet: http://www.cwru.edu/med/cardiology.html
Accred Length: 1 Year *Program Size:* 3
Program ID: 154-38-21-056

Cleveland Clinic Foundation Program

Sponsor: Cleveland Clinic Foundation

Program Director:
Gregory A Kidwell, MD
Dept of Cardiology/F15
9500 Euclid Ave
Cleveland, OH 44195
Tel: 216 444-4293
E-mail: meded@cesmtp.ccf.org
Internet: http://www.ccf.org
Accred Length: 1 Year *Program Size:* 2
Program ID: 154-38-21-083

Oklahoma

Oklahoma City

University of Oklahoma Health Sciences Center Program

Sponsor: University of Oklahoma College of Medicine
University Hospital
Veterans Affairs Medical Center (Oklahoma City)

Program Director:
Warren M Jackman, MD
Univ of Oklahoma Health Sciences Ctr
5SP300/PO Box 26901
920 S L Young Blvd/WP3120
Oklahoma City, OK 73104
Tel: 405 271-8764 *Fax:* 405 271-2619
Accred Length: 1 Year *Program Size:* 3
Program ID: 154-39-21-059

Oregon

Portland

Oregon Health Sciences University Program

Sponsor: Oregon Health Sciences University Hospital
Veterans Affairs Medical Center (Portland)

Program Director:
John H McAnulty, MD
3181 SW Sam Jackson Park Rd/UHN62
Portland, OR 97201
Tel: 503 494-2375 *Fax:* 503 494-8550
Accred Length: 1 Year *Program Size:* 2
Program ID: 154-40-21-060

Pennsylvania

Hershey

Penn State Geisinger Health System/Milton S Hershey Medical Center Program

Sponsor: Penn State Geisinger Health System
Milton S Hershey Medical Center

Program Director:
Jerry C Luck, MD
500 University Dr
PO Box 850
Hershey, PA 17033
Tel: 717 531-8407 *Fax:* 717 531-7969
Accred Length: 1 Year *Program Size:* 0
Program ID: 154-41-21-084

Philadelphia

MCP Hahnemann University Program

Sponsor: MCP Hahnemann University
Hahnemann University Hospital
Medical College of Pennsylvania Hospital

Program Director:
Francis E Marchlinski, MD
MCP Hahnemann Univ Hospital
3300 Henry Ave
Ste 803
Philadelphia, PA 19129
Tel: 215 842-6408 *Fax:* 215 991-4881
Accred Length: 1 Year *Program Size:* 5
Program ID: 154-41-31-062

Temple University Program

Sponsor: Temple University Hospital

Program Director:
Alfred E Buxton, MD
Cardiac Electrophysiology Program
903 Parkinson Pavilion/TUH
3401 N Broad St
Philadelphia, PA 19140
Tel: 215 707-4724 *Fax:* 215 707-7718
E-mail: abuxton@nimbus.ocis.temple.edu
Accred Length: 1 Year *Program Size:* 2
Program ID: 154-41-12-064

University of Pennsylvania Program

Sponsor: Hospital of the University of Pennsylvania
Veterans Affairs Medical Center (Philadelphia)

Program Director:
Michael Hanna, MD
Cardiovascular Section
3400 Spruce St
9 Founders
Philadelphia, PA 19104
Tel: 215 662-6800 *Fax:* 215 662-2879
E-mail: mhanna@mail.med.upenn.edu
Accred Length: 1 Year *Program Size:* 2
Program ID: 154-41-22-065

Pittsburgh

University Health Center of Pittsburgh Program

Sponsor: University Health Center of Pittsburgh

Program Director:
Raul Weiss, MD
Univ of Pittsburgh Med Ctr
200 Lothrop St/Rm B535
Pittsburgh, PA 15213-2582
Tel: 412 647-6272 *Fax:* 412 647-7979
E-mail: weissr@msx.upmc.edu
Accred Length: 1 Year *Program Size:* 2
Program ID: 154-41-22-066

Wynnewood

Lankenau Hospital Program

Sponsor: Lankenau Hospital

Program Director:
Roger A Marinchak, MD
Lankenau Hospital
100 Lancaster Ave
Ste 558/Medical Office Bldg East
Wynnewood, PA 19096
Tel: 610 645-2682 *Fax:* 610 896-0643
E-mail: jrbbn@aol.com
Accred Length: 1 Year *Program Size:* 1
Program ID: 154-41-23-067

Tennessee

Nashville

Vanderbilt University Program

Sponsor: Vanderbilt University Medical Center
Metropolitan Nashville General Hospital
Veterans Affairs Medical Center (Nashville)

Program Director:
Mark E Anderson, MD PhD
Vanderbilt Univ
315 Med Research Bldg II
Nashville, TN 37232-6300
Tel: 615 936-1720 *Fax:* 615 936-1872
E-mail: mark.anderson@mcmail.vanderbilt.edu
Accred Length: 1 Year *Program Size:* 1
Program ID: 154-47-21-069

Texas

Dallas

University of Texas Southwestern Medical School Program

Sponsor: University of Texas Southwestern Medical School
Dallas County Hospital District-Parkland Memorial Hospital
Veterans Affairs Medical Center (Dallas)

Program Director:
Richard L Page, MD
5323 Harry Hines Blvd
Dallas, TX 75235-9047
Tel: 214 590-5055 *Fax:* 214 590-5032
E-mail: rpage@parknet.pmh.org
Internet: http://www.swmed.edu/home_pages/cardiology/
Accred Length: 1 Year *Program Size:* 2
Program ID: 154-48-21-070

Houston

Baylor College of Medicine (St Luke's) Program

Sponsor: Baylor College of Medicine
St Luke's Episcopal Hospital

Program Director:
Ali Massumkhani, MD
St Luke's Episcopal Hospital
6720 Bertner (1-133)
Houston, TX 77030
Tel: 713 794-6676 *Fax:* 713 791-8374
Accred Length: 1 Year *Program Size:* 1
Program ID: 154-48-13-073

Baylor College of Medicine Program

Sponsor: Baylor College of Medicine
Harris County Hospital District-Ben Taub General Hospital
Methodist Hospital
Veterans Affairs Medical Center (Houston)

Program Director:
Dennis W Zhu, MD
Baylor Coll of Med
6550 Fannin St/MS SM1246
Houston, TX 77030
Tel: 713 790-6490 *Fax:* 713 790-6195
E-mail: dzhu@bcm.tmc.edu
Internet: http://www.bmc.tmc.edu
Accred Length: 1 Year *Program Size:* 1
Program ID: 154-48-11-072

University of Texas at Houston Program

Sponsor: University of Texas Medical School at Houston
Memorial Hermann Healthcare System

Program Director:
Anne Hamilton Dougherty, MD
Univ of Texas Med Sch
6431 Fannin St/MSB 1246
Houston, TX 77030
Tel: 713 500-6590 *Fax:* 713 500-6556
Accred Length: 1 Year *Program Size:* 4
Program ID: 154-48-21-082

Utah

Salt Lake City

University of Utah Program

Sponsor: University of Utah Medical Center
Veterans Affairs Medical Center (Salt Lake City)

Program Director:
Roger A Freedman, MD
Univ of Utah Med Ctr
50 N Medical Dr
Salt Lake City, UT 84132
Tel: 801 581-7715 *Fax:* 801 581-7735
E-mail: roger.freedman@hsc.utah.edu
Accred Length: 1 Year *Program Size:* 1
Program ID: 154-49-21-075

Virginia

Charlottesville

University of Virginia Program
Sponsor: University of Virginia Medical Center
Program Director:
John P DiMarco, MD PhD
Univ of Virginia
Dept of Int Med
Box 158
Charlottesville, VA 22908
Tel: 804 924-2031 *Fax:* 804 924-2581
E-mail: jdimarco@virginia.edu
Accred Length: 1 Year *Program Size:* 1
Program ID: 154-51-21-076

Richmond

Medical College of Virginia/Virginia Commonwealth University Program
Sponsor: Medical College of Virginia/Virginia Commonwealth University
Hunter Holmes McGuire VA Medical Center (Richmond)
Medical College of Virginia Hospitals
Program Director:
Kenneth A Ellenbogen, MD
Med Coll of Virginia
PO Box 980053
Richmond, VA 23298-0053
Tel: 804 828-7565 *Fax:* 804 828-6082
E-mail: kellenbogen@pol.net
Internet: http://www.views.vcu.edu.eps
Accred Length: 1 Year *Program Size:* 3
Program ID: 154-51-31-077

Washington

Seattle

University of Washington Program
Sponsor: University of Washington School of Medicine
University of Washington Medical Center
Program Director:
Peter J Kudenchuk, MD
Univ of Washington
Div of Cardiology/Box 356422
Seattle, WA 98195
Tel: 206 685-4176 *Fax:* 206 616-1022
Accred Length: 1 Year *Program Size:* 1
Program ID: 154-54-21-078

Wisconsin

Milwaukee

Aurora Health Care Program
Sponsor: Aurora Health Care
Sinai Samaritan Medical Center
St Luke's Medical Center
Program Director:
Mohammad R Jazayeri, MD
Aurora Health Care-Sinai Samaritan Med Ctr
945 N 12th St
PO Box 342
Milwaukee, WI 53201-0342
Tel: 414 219-7686 *Fax:* 414 219-6211
Accred Length: 1 Year *Program Size:* 2
Program ID: 154-56-21-079

Clinical Neurophysiology (Neurology)

Alabama

Birmingham

University of Alabama Medical Center Program
Sponsor: University of Alabama Hospital
Veterans Affairs Medical Center (Birmingham)
Program Director:
Shin J Oh, MD
Univ of Alabama at Birmingham
UAB Station
Birmingham, AL 35294
Tel: 205 934-2120 *Fax:* 205 975-6758
E-mail: sjoh@email.neuro.uab.edu
Accred Length: 1 Year *Program Size:* 4
Program ID: 187-01-21-038

Arizona

Phoenix

St Joseph Hospital and Medical Center Program
Sponsor: St Joseph's Hospital and Medical Center
Program Director:
Jau-Shin Lou, MD
St Joseph's Hospital and Med Ctr
350 W Thomas Rd
Phoenix, AZ 85013
Tel: 602 406-6315 *Fax:* 602 406-7187
Accred Length: 1 Year *Program Size:* 0
Program ID: 187-03-21-094

California

Los Angeles

UCLA Medical Center Program
Sponsor: UCLA School of Medicine
Olive View-UCLA Medical Center
UCLA Medical Center
Program Director:
Marc R Nuwer, MD PhD
710 Westwood Plaza
Reed Bldg 1-194
Los Angeles, CA 90095
Tel: 310 206-3093 *Fax:* 310 206-8461
E-mail: mrn@ucla.edu
Accred Length: 1 Year *Program Size:* 5
Program ID: 187-05-21-004

Sacramento

University of California (Davis) Program
Sponsor: University of California (Davis) Medical Center
David Grant Medical Center
Program Director:
Masud Seyal, MD
2315 Stockton Blvd/Rm 5308
Sacramento, CA 95817
Tel: 916 736-2976 *Fax:* 916 452-2739
Accred Length: 1 Year *Program Size:* 1
Program ID: 187-05-31-005

San Francisco

University of California (San Francisco) Program
Sponsor: University of California (San Francisco) School of Medicine
San Francisco General Hospital Medical Center
University of California (San Francisco) Medical Center
Program Director:
Michael J Aminoff, MD
505 Parnassus Ave
San Francisco, CA 94143-0114
Tel: 415 476-1986 *Fax:* 415 476-3518
E-mail: aminoff@itsa.ucsf.edu
Accred Length: 1 Year *Program Size:* 2
Program ID: 187-05-11-006

Stanford

Stanford University Program
Sponsor: Stanford University Hospital
California Pacific Medical Center (California Campus)
Lucile Salter Packard Children's Hospital at Stanford
Program Director:
Les Dorfman, MD
Neurology H-3160
300 Pasteur Dr
Stanford, CA 94305-5235
Tel: 650 723-6888 *Fax:* 650 725-7459
Accred Length: 1 Year *Program Size:* 5
Program ID: 187-05-21-022

Torrance

Los Angeles County-Harbor-UCLA Medical Center Program
Sponsor: Los Angeles County-Harbor-UCLA Medical Center
Program Director:
Hugh B McIntyre, MD PhD
Harbor-UCLA Med Ctr
1000 W Carson St
Torrance, CA 90509
Tel: 310 222-3897 *Fax:* 310 533-8905
E-mail: hbmcintyre@pol.net
Accred Length: 1 Year *Program Size:* 2
Program ID: 187-05-21-068

Connecticut

New Haven

Yale-New Haven Medical Center Program
Sponsor: Yale-New Haven Hospital
Veterans Affairs Medical Center (West Haven)
Program Director:
Jonathan M Goldstein, MD
Dept of Neurology LCI-702
333 Cedar St
New Haven, CT 06510
Tel: 203 688-2495 *Fax:* 203 785-5694
E-mail: jonathan.goldstein@yale.edu
Internet:
http://www.info.med.yale.edu/neurol/cneurophysiol/clinnp.html
Accred Length: 1 Year *Program Size:* 1
Program ID: 187-08-21-058

Programs

Florida

Gainesville

University of Florida Program
Sponsor: University of Florida College of Medicine
Shands Hospital at the University of Florida
Veterans Affairs Medical Center (Gainesville)
Program Director:
Robin L Gilmore, MD
Univ of Florida
Box 100236 UFHSC
Gainesville, FL 32610-0236
Tel: 352 392-3491 *Fax:* 352 392-6893
E-mail: gilmore@medicine.ufl.edu
Accred Length: 1 Year *Program Size:* 2
Program ID: 187-11-21-025

Georgia

Augusta

Medical College of Georgia Program
Sponsor: Medical College of Georgia Hospital and Clinics
Program Director:
Michael H Rivner, MD
Med Coll of Georgia
EMG Lab BP3117
1120 15th St
Augusta, GA 30912-3200
Tel: 706 721-2681 *Fax:* 706 721-6757
E-mail: mrivner@neuro.mcg.edu
Internet: http://www.neuro.mcg.edu
Accred Length: 1 Year *Program Size:* 2
Program ID: 187-12-21-070

Illinois

Chicago

McGaw Medical Center of Northwestern University Program
Sponsor: Northwestern University Medical School
Children's Memorial Medical Center
Northwestern Memorial Hospital
Program Director:
Albert Ehle, MD
710 N Lakeshore Dr/11th Fl
Chicago, IL 60611
Tel: 312 908-3300 *Fax:* 312 908-6637
Accred Length: 1 Year *Program Size:* 1
Program ID: 187-16-21-041

Rush-Presbyterian-St Luke's Medical Center Program
Sponsor: Rush-Presbyterian-St Luke's Medical Center
Program Director:
Matthew N Meriggioli, MD
Sect of Neuromuscular Disorders
1725 W Harrison St/Ste 1106-1118
Chicago, IL 60612
Tel: 312 942-6121 *Fax:* 312 942-2380
E-mail: mmeriggi@neuro.rpslmc.edu
Accred Length: 1 Year *Program Size:* 5
Program ID: 187-16-21-026

University of Chicago Program
Sponsor: University of Chicago Hospitals
Program Director:
Jean-Paul C Spire, MD
5841 S Maryland Ave
Chicago, IL 60637
Tel: 773 702-1780 *Fax:* 773 702-7998
E-mail: eegs@midway.uchicago.edu
Internet: http://drugs.bsd.uchicago.edu/~neurowww
Accred Length: 1 Year *Program Size:* 3
Program ID: 187-16-21-086

University of Illinois College of Medicine at Chicago Program
Sponsor: University of Illinois College of Medicine at Chicago
Program Director:
John R Hughes, MD PhD
912 S Wood St (M/C 796)
Chicago, IL 60612
Tel: 312 996-4169 *Fax:* 312 413-1388
E-mail: jhughes@uic.edu
Accred Length: 1 Year *Program Size:* 1
Program ID: 187-16-21-001

Maywood

Loyola University Program
Sponsor: Loyola University Medical Center
Edward J Hines Jr Veterans Affairs Hospital
Program Director:
Gastone G Celesia, MD
Loyola Univ Med Ctr
2160 S First Ave
Maywood, IL 60153
Tel: 708 216-3405 *Fax:* 708 216-5617
E-mail: gcelesi@luc.edu
Internet: http://www.umc.edu/neurology
Accred Length: 1 Year *Program Size:* 1
Program ID: 187-16-21-051

Springfield

Southern Illinois University Program
Sponsor: Southern Illinois University School of Medicine
Memorial Medical Center
St John's Hospital
Program Director:
Dean K Naritoku, MD
Southern Illinois Univ Sch of Med
PO Box 19637
Springfield, IL 62794-9637
Tel: 217 782-0168 *Fax:* 217 524-4539
Internet: http://www.siumed.edu/neuro
Accred Length: 1 Year *Program Size:* 1
Program ID: 187-16-31-008

Indiana

Indianapolis

Indiana University School of Medicine Program
Sponsor: Indiana University School of Medicine
Clarian IU Hospital
Clarian Riley Hospital for Children
Program Director:
Omkar N Markand, MD
EEG/Epilepsy Sect UH 1711
550 N University Blvd
Indianapolis, IN 46202-5200
Tel: 317 274-0181 *Fax:* 317 274-1472
E-mail: omarkand@iumc.iupui.edu
Accred Length: 1 Year *Program Size:* 3
Program ID: 187-17-21-003

Iowa

Iowa City

University of Iowa Hospitals and Clinics Program
Sponsor: University of Iowa Hospitals and Clinics
Program Director:
Gwendolyn C Ford, MD
Univ of Iowa Hospitals and Clinics
Dept of Neurology 0181 RCP
200 Hawkins Dr
Iowa City, IA 52242
Tel: 319 356-3059 *Fax:* 319 356-1209
E-mail: gwendolyn-ford@uiowa.edu
Accred Length: 1 Year *Program Size:* 1
Program ID: 187-18-21-054

Louisiana

New Orleans

Louisiana State University Program
Sponsor: Louisiana State University School of Medicine
Childrens Hospital
Medical Center of Louisiana at New Orleans
Program Director:
Bruce J Fisch, MD
Louisiana State Univ Med Ctr
Dept of Neurology
1542 Tulane Ave
New Orleans, LA 70112-2822
Tel: 504 568-4081 *Fax:* 504 568-7130
E-mail: bfisch@lsumc.edu
Internet:
http://www.lsumc.edu/campus/neur/neurology/lsuneuro.htm
Accred Length: 1 Year *Program Size:* 4
Program ID: 187-21-21-078

Maryland

Baltimore

Johns Hopkins University Program
Sponsor: Johns Hopkins University School of Medicine
Program Director:
Vinay Chaudhry, MD
600 N Wolfe St
Meyer 6-119
Baltimore, MD 21287
Tel: 410 955-9167 *Fax:* 410 614-8337
E-mail: vchaudh@jhmi.edu
Accred Length: 1 Year *Program Size:* 4
Program ID: 187-23-21-027

University of Maryland Program
Sponsor: University of Maryland Medical System
Program Director:
Elizabeth Barry, MD
Univ of Maryland Sch of Med
22 S Greene St/N4W46
Baltimore, MD 21201
Tel: 410 328-6266 *Fax:* 410 328-0697
Accred Length: 1 Year *Program Size:* 2
Program ID: 187-23-21-016

Bethesda

National Capital Consortium (Bethesda) Program

Sponsor: National Capital Consortium
National Naval Medical Center (Bethesda)
Children's National Medical Center
NIH Warren Grant Magnuson Clinical Center

Program Director:
Susumu Sato, MD
Office of Clinical Dir/NINDS
10 Ctr Dr/Bldg 10/Rm 5C101
Bethesda, MD 20892-1404
Tel: 301 496-5121 *Fax:* 301 402-8796
Internet: http://www.intra.nindo.nih.gov/ocd/index.html
Accred Length: 1 Year *Program Size:* 2
Program ID: 187-10-31-028
US Armed Services Program

National Capital Consortium Program

Sponsor: National Capital Consortium
Walter Reed Army Medical Center

Program Director:
Bahman Jabbari, MD
Dept of Neurology
Walter Reed Army Med Ctr
6825 16th St NW
Washington, DC 20307-5001
Tel: 202 782-8677 *Fax:* 202 782-5014
Accred Length: 1 Year *Program Size:* 1
Program ID: 187-10-31-024
US Armed Services Program

Massachusetts

Boston

Beth Israel Deaconess Medical Center/Harvard Medical School Program

Sponsor: Children's Hospital

Program Director:
Gregory L Holmes, MD
300 Longwood Ave
Clinical Neurophysiology Lab
Hunnewell 2
Boston, MA 02115
Tel: 617 355-8461 *Fax:* 617 355-6814
E-mail: holmesg@a1.tch.harvard.edu
Accred Length: 1 Year *Program Size:* 5
Program ID: 187-24-21-071

Worcester

University of Massachusetts Program

Sponsor: University of Massachusetts Medical School
UMass Memorial Health Care (University Campus)

Program Director:
David A Chad, MD
Univ of Massachusetts Med Sch
Dept of Neurology
55 Lake Ave N
Worcester, MA 01655
Tel: 508 856-3083 *Fax:* 508 856-6778
Accred Length: 1 Year *Program Size:* 1
Program ID: 187-24-21-009

Michigan

Ann Arbor

University of Michigan Program

Sponsor: University of Michigan Hospitals

Program Director:
Michael S Aldrich, MD
1500 E Medical Center Dr
UH8D8820/0117
Ann Arbor, MI 48109-0117
Tel: 734 647-9064 *Fax:* 734 647-9065
E-mail: maldrich@umich.edu
Accred Length: 1 Year *Program Size:* 7
Program ID: 187-25-21-010

Detroit

Henry Ford Hospital Program

Sponsor: Henry Ford Hospital

Program Director:
Bashiruddin K Ahmad, MD
Henry Ford Hospital
2799 W Grand Blvd
Detroit, MI 48202-2689
Tel: 313 876-3822 *Fax:* 313 876-2187
E-mail: ahmad@neuro.hfh..edu
Accred Length: 1 Year *Program Size:* 4
Program ID: 187-25-21-057

Wayne State University/Detroit Medical Center Program

Sponsor: Wayne State University/Detroit Medical Center
Children's Hospital of Michigan
Detroit Receiving Hospital and University Health Center

Program Director:
James F Selwa, MD
Neurology 6E-UHC
4201 St Antoine
Detroit, MI 48201
Tel: 313 745-8328 *Fax:* 313 993-0643
E-mail: jselwamd@dmc.org
Accred Length: 1 Year *Program Size:* 4
Program ID: 187-25-21-042

Minnesota

Minneapolis

University of Minnesota Program

Sponsor: University of Minnesota Medical School
Fairview-University Medical Center
Hennepin County Medical Center
Veterans Affairs Medical Center (Minneapolis)

Program Director:
John W Day, MD
Box 295 Mayo Bldg
Univ of Minnesota
Minneapolis, MN 55455-0392
Tel: 612 625-6180 *Fax:* 612 625-7950
Accred Length: 1 Year *Program Size:* 2
Program ID: 187-26-21-030

Rochester

Mayo Graduate School of Medicine (Rochester) Program

Sponsor: Mayo Graduate School of Medicine-Mayo Foundation
Mayo Clinic (Rochester)
Rochester Methodist Hospital
St Mary's Hospital of Rochester

Program Director:
Barbara F Westmoreland, MD
Application Processing Ctr
Mayo Graduate Sch of Med
200 First St SW
Rochester, MN 55905
Tel: 507 284-3255 *Fax:* 507 284-8686
E-mail: mgsm.roch.mn.neurology@mayo.edu
Internet: http://www.mayo.edu/
Accred Length: 1 Year *Program Size:* 5
Program ID: 187-26-21-011

Mississippi

Jackson

University of Mississippi Medical Center Program

Sponsor: University of Mississippi School of Medicine

Program Director:
A Arturo Leis, MD
Neurology EEG/EMG
2500 N State St
Jackson, MS 39216-4505
Tel: 601 984-4765 *Fax:* 601 984-4895
E-mail: aleis@neurology.umsmed.edu
Accred Length: 1 Year *Program Size:* 2
Program ID: 187-27-21-043

Missouri

St Louis

St Louis University School of Medicine Program

Sponsor: St Louis University School of Medicine
SSM Cardinal Glennon Children's Hospital
St Louis University School of Medicine
Veterans Affairs Medical Center (St Louis)

Program Director:
Ghazala Hayat, MD
St Louis Univ Sch of Med
Dept of Neurology
3635 Vista Ave
St Louis, MO 63110
Tel: 314 577-8026 *Fax:* 314 268-5101
E-mail: hayatg@slucare1.sluh.edu
Accred Length: 1 Year *Program Size:* 2
Program ID: 187-28-21-031

Washington University/B-JH/SLCH Consortium Program

Sponsor: Washington University/B-JH/SLCH Consortium
Barnes-Jewish Hospital
St Louis Children's Hospital

Program Director:
John W Miller, MD PhD
660 S Euclid Ave/Box 8111
St Louis, MO 63110
Tel: 314 362-7845 *Fax:* 314 362-0296
E-mail: millerjw@neuro.wush.edu
Accred Length: 1 Year *Program Size:* 0
Program ID: 187-28-21-072

New Mexico

Albuquerque

University of New Mexico Program

Sponsor: University of New Mexico School of Medicine
Veterans Affairs Medical Center (Albuquerque)

Program Director:
Jerry J Shih, MD
2211 Lomas Blvd NE
Albuquerque, NM 87131-5281
Tel: 505 272-3342 *Fax:* 505 272-6692
E-mail: jshih@salud.unm.edu
Internet: http://www.salud.unm.edu/neuro
Accred Length: 1 Year *Program Size:* 1
Program ID: 187-34-21-061

New York

Bronx

Albert Einstein College of Medicine Program

Sponsor: Albert Einstein College of Medicine of Yeshiva University
Montefiore Medical Center-Henry and Lucy Moses Division

Program Director:
Solomon L Moshe, MD
Montefiore Med Ctr
111 E 210th St
Bronx, NY 10467
Tel: 718 920-8417 *Fax:* 718 881-0838
Accred Length: 1 Year *Program Size:* 3
Program ID: 187-35-21-012

Brooklyn

SUNY Health Science Center at Brooklyn Program

Sponsor: SUNY Health Science Center at Brooklyn
Kings County Hospital Center
Long Island College Hospital
University Hospital-SUNY Health Science Center at Brooklyn

Program Director:
Larry S Bernardo, MD PhD
SUNY Health Science Ctr
450 Clarkson Ave/Box 118
Brooklyn, NY 11203
Tel: 718 270-2035 *Fax:* 718 270-3840
E-mail: lbernardo@netmail.hscbklyn.edu
Accred Length: 1 Year *Program Size:* 1
Program ID: 187-35-21-062

Buffalo

SUNY at Buffalo Graduate Medical-Dental Education Consortium Program

Sponsor: SUNY at Buffalo Grad Medical-Dental Education Consortium
CGF Health System (Buffalo General Hospital)
CGF Health System (Children's Hospital of Buffalo)
CGF Health System (Millard Fillmore Hospitals)
Erie County Medical Center
Veterans Affairs Medical Center (Buffalo)

Program Director:
Edward J Fine, MD
219 Bryant St
Buffalo, NY 14222
Tel: 716 834-9200 *Fax:* 716 878-7326
E-mail: efine@acsu.buffalo.edu
Accred Length: 1 Year *Program Size:* 1
Program ID: 187-35-21-032

New York

New York and Presbyterian Hospital (Columbia Campus) Program

Sponsor: New York and Presbyterian Hospital
New York and Presbyterian Hospital (Columbia Campus)

Program Director:
Ronald G Emerson, MD
Neurological Inst
710 W 168th St
New York, NY 10032
Tel: 212 305-2121 *Fax:* 212 305-1315
E-mail: rge2@columbia.edu
Accred Length: 1 Year *Program Size:* 4
Program ID: 187-35-31-033

New York and Presbyterian Hospital (Cornell Campus) Program

Sponsor: New York and Presbyterian Hospital
Hospital for Special Surgery
New York and Presbyterian Hospital (Cornell Campus)

Program Director:
Jonathan D Victor, MD PhD
Cornell Univ Med Coll
1300 York Ave
New York, NY 10021
Tel: 212 746-2343 *Fax:* 212 746-8984
E-mail: jdvicto@med.cornell.edu
Internet:
http://neuro.med.cornell.edu/nyh-cmc/n-cliniclab.html
Accred Length: 1 Year *Program Size:* 2
Program ID: 187-35-11-034

New York University Medical Center Program

Sponsor: New York University Medical Center

Program Director:
Aleksandar Beric, MD
Hospital for Joint Diseases
301 E 17th St
New York, NY 10003
Tel: 212 598-6194 *Fax:* 212 598-6009
E-mail: berica@mcns09.med.nyu.edu
Accred Length: 1 Year *Program Size:* 5
Program ID: 187-35-31-063

Rochester

University of Rochester Program

Sponsor: Strong Memorial Hospital of the University of Rochester

Program Director:
Eric Logigian, MD
Univ of Rochester Med Ctr
601 Elmwood Ave
Box 673
Rochester, NY 14642
Tel: 716 275-4568 *Fax:* 716 473-6622
E-mail: elogigian@mail.neurology.rochester.edu
Accred Length: 1 Year *Program Size:* 2
Program ID: 187-35-21-045

Stony Brook

SUNY at Stony Brook Program

Sponsor: University Hospital-SUNY at Stony Brook
Veterans Affairs Medical Center (Northport)

Program Director:
Mary R Andriola, MD
Health Science Ctr
SUNY-Stony Brook/T12-020
Stony Brook, NY 11794-8121
Tel: 516 444-1450 *Fax:* 516 444-1474
E-mail: mandriol@neuro.som.sunysb.edu
Internet:
http://www.informatics.s...edu/neurology/index.html
Accred Length: 1 Year *Program Size:* 2
Program ID: 187-35-11-064

Syracuse

SUNY Health Science Center at Syracuse Program

Sponsor: University Hospital-SUNY Health Science Center at Syracuse
Veterans Affairs Medical Center (Syracuse)

Program Director:
Jeremy M Shefner, MD
750 E Adams St
Syracuse, NY 13210
Tel: 315 464-5358 *Fax:* 315 464-5006
E-mail: shefnerj@vax.cs.hscsyr.edu
Accred Length: 1 Year *Program Size:* 2
Program ID: 187-35-21-085

North Carolina

Durham

Duke University Program

Sponsor: Duke University Medical Center
Veterans Affairs Medical Center (Durham)

Program Director:
Rodney A Radtke, MD
Box 3678
Duke Univ
Durham, NC 27710
Tel: 919 681-3448 *Fax:* 919 684-8955
E-mail: radtk002@mcduke.duke .edu
Accred Length: 1 Year *Program Size:* 2
Program ID: 187-36-21-088

Ohio

Cincinnati

University Hospital/University of Cincinnati College of Medicine Program

Sponsor: University Hospital Inc
Children's Hospital Medical Center
Veterans Affairs Medical Center (Cincinnati)

Program Director:
Michael Privitera, MD
Univ of Cincinnati Med Ctr
231 Bethesda Ave/ML 0525
Cincinnati, OH 45267-0525
Tel: 513 558-5440 *Fax:* 513 558-4305
E-mail: michael.privitera@uc.edu
Internet:
http://www.med.uc.edu/htdocs/medicine/departme/neuro/neuro3.htm
Accred Length: 1 Year *Program Size:* 1
Program ID: 187-38-21-083

Cleveland

Case Western Reserve University Program

Sponsor: University Hospitals of Cleveland
Veterans Affairs Medical Center (Cleveland)

Program Director:
Bashar Katirji, MD
11100 Euclid Ave
Cleveland, OH 44106
Tel: 216 844-4854 *Fax:* 216 844-7624
Accred Length: 1 Year *Program Size:* 2
Program ID: 187-38-21-046

Cleveland Clinic Foundation Program
Sponsor: Cleveland Clinic Foundation

Program Director:
Kerry H Levin, MD
Cleveland Clinic Foundation
Dept of Neurology/S90
9500 Euclid Ave
Cleveland, OH 44195
Tel: 216 444-8370 *Fax:* 216 445-4653
E-mail: levink@cesmtp.ccf.org
Internet: http://www.ccf.org
Accred Length: 1 Year *Program Size:* 10
Program ID: 187-38-31-047

Pennsylvania

Hershey

Penn State Geisinger Health System/Milton S Hershey Medical Center Program
Sponsor: Penn State Geisinger Health System
Milton S Hershey Medical Center

Program Director:
Zachary Simmons, MD
500 University Dr
Hershey, PA 17033
Tel: 717 531-8692 *Fax:* 717 531-4694
E-mail: zsimmons@psghs.edu.psghs.edu
Accred Length: 1 Year *Program Size:* 1
Program ID: 187-41-21-035

Philadelphia

MCP Hahnemann University (Graduate) Program
Sponsor: MCP Hahnemann University
Graduate Hospital
Hahnemann University Hospital
Medical College of Pennsylvania Hospital
St Christopher's Hospital for Children

Program Director:
Albert J Tahmoush, MD
Ste 900 Pepper Pavilion
1800 Lombard St
Philadelphia, PA 19146
Tel: 215 893-2449 *Fax:* 215 893-7644
Accred Length: 1 Year *Program Size:* 0
Program ID: 187-41-31-089

MCP Hahnemann University Program
Sponsor: MCP Hahnemann University
Hahnemann University Hospital
Medical College of Pennsylvania Hospital

Program Director:
Mercedes P Jacobson, MD
Med Coll of Pennsylvania Hospital
Dept of Neurology
3300 Henry Ave
Philadelphia, PA 19129
Tel: 215 842-7706 *Fax:* 215 848-2035
E-mail: jacobson@auhs.edu
Internet: http://www.auhs.edu
Accred Length: 1 Year *Program Size:* 3
Program ID: 187-41-21-048

Temple University Program
Sponsor: Temple University Hospital
St Christopher's Hospital for Children

Program Director:
Joseph F Hulihan, MD
Rm 558 Parkinson Pavilion
3401 N Broad St
Philadelphia, PA 19140
Tel: 215 707-3040 *Fax:* 215 707-8235
Accred Length: 1 Year *Program Size:* 0
Program ID: 187-41-31-049

Thomas Jefferson University Program
Sponsor: Thomas Jefferson University Hospital

Program Director:
Leopold J Streletz, MD
Jefferson Med Coll
Dept of Neurology/Ste 310C
1025 Walnut St
Philadelphia, PA 19107
Tel: 215 955-7571 *Fax:* 215 923-6792
E-mail: joayn.hill@mail.edu.tju
Accred Length: 1 Year *Program Size:* 2
Program ID: 187-41-31-036

University of Pennsylvania Program
Sponsor: Hospital of the University of Pennsylvania
Children's Hospital of Philadelphia

Program Director:
Shawn J Bird, MD
Univ of Pennsylvania
Dept of Neurology
3400 Spruce St
Philadelphia, PA 19104-4283
Tel: 215 662-6551 *Fax:* 215 349-5579
E-mail: sbird@mail.med.upenn.edu
Internet: http://www.med.upenn.edu/neuro
Accred Length: 1 Year *Program Size:* 1
Program ID: 187-41-21-087

Pittsburgh

University Health Center at Pittsburgh Program
Sponsor: University Health Center of Pittsburgh
Children's Hospital of Pittsburgh
Western Psychiatric Institute and Clinic/UPMC

Program Director:
Richard P Brenner, MD
Western Psychiatric Inst and Clinic
3811 O'Hara St
Pittsburgh, PA 15213
Tel: 412 624-2369 *Fax:* 412 624-3388
E-mail: rpb@med.pitt.edu
Accred Length: 1 Year *Program Size:* 2
Program ID: 187-41-21-065

Rhode Island

Providence

Brown University Program
Sponsor: Rhode Island Hospital

Program Director:
James M Gilchrist, MD
593 Eddy St/APC 689
Providence, RI 02903
Tel: 401 444-8761 *Fax:* 401 444-5929
Accred Length: 1 Year *Program Size:* 3
Program ID: 187-43-21-015

South Carolina

Charleston

Medical University of South Carolina Program
Sponsor: Medical University of South Carolina College of Medicine
MUSC Medical Center

Program Director:
David A Griesemer, MD
Dept of Neurology
600 MUSC Complex/Ste 309
Charleston, SC 29425
Tel: 803 792-3224 *Fax:* 803 792-8626
E-mail: grieseda@musc.edu
Accred Length: 1 Year *Program Size:* 3
Program ID: 187-45-21-020

Tennessee

Memphis

University of Tennessee Program
Sponsor: University of Tennessee College of Medicine
LeBonheur Children's Medical Center
Methodist Hospitals of Memphis-Central

Program Director:
Michael Jacewicz, MD
855 Monroe Ave/Rm 415
Memphis, TN 38163
Tel: 901 448-6661 *Fax:* 901 448-7440
E-mail: hham@utmem1.utmem.edu
Accred Length: 1 Year *Program Size:* 1
Program ID: 187-47-21-084

Nashville

Vanderbilt University Program
Sponsor: Vanderbilt University Medical Center

Program Director:
Bassel Abou-Khalil, MD
2100 Pierce Ave/Ste 336
Nashville, TN 37212
Tel: 615 936-2027 *Fax:* 615 936-0223
Accred Length: 1 Year *Program Size:* 2
Program ID: 187-47-21-073

Texas

Dallas

University of Texas Southwestern Medical School Program
Sponsor: University of Texas Southwestern Medical School
Dallas County Hospital District-Parkland Memorial Hospital
Veterans Affairs Medical Center (Dallas)

Program Director:
Richard J Barohn, MD
Univ of Texas Southwestern Med Ctr
5323 Harry Hines Blvd
Dallas, TX 75235-8897
Tel: 214 648-6419 *Fax:* 214 648-9311
E-mail: cbeise@mednet.swmed.edu
Accred Length: 1 Year *Program Size:* 7
Program ID: 187-48-21-074

Houston

Baylor College of Medicine Program
Sponsor: Baylor College of Medicine
Methodist Hospital
Texas Children's Hospital
Program Director:
Eli M Mizrahi, MD
Baylor Coll of Med
Sect of Neurophysiology
One Baylor Plaza
Houston, TX 77030
Tel: 713 790-3109 *Fax:* 713 793-1574
Accred Length: 1 Year *Program Size:* 2
Program ID: 187-48-21-037

University of Texas at Houston Program
Sponsor: University of Texas Medical School at Houston
Memorial Hermann Healthcare System
Program Director:
Francine Vriesendorp, MD
Univ of Texas-Houston Med Sch
Dept of Neurology
6431 Fannin St/7044/MSB
Houston, TX 77030-1501
Tel: 713 500-7100, ext 7024 *Fax:* 713 500-7019
E-mail: jhaas@neuro.med.uth.tmc.edu
Internet: http://www.neurology.uth.tmc.edu/index.htm
Accred Length: 1 Year *Program Size:* 2
Program ID: 187-48-21-066

San Antonio

University of Texas Health Science Center at San Antonio Program
Sponsor: University of Texas Medical School at San Antonio
Audie L Murphy Memorial Veterans Hospital (San Antonio)
University Hospital-South Texas Medical Center
Wilford Hall Medical Center (AETC)
Program Director:
Carlayne E Jackson, MD
Univ of Texas Health Science Ctr
Dept of Med/Neurology
7703 Floyd Curl Dr
San Antonio, TX 78284-7883
Tel: 210 567-1945 *Fax:* 210 567-1948
E-mail: jacksonce@uthscsa.edu
Accred Length: 1 Year *Program Size:* 2
Program ID: 187-48-31-077

Utah

Salt Lake City

University of Utah Program
Sponsor: University of Utah Medical Center
Primary Children's Medical Center
Program Director:
Mark B Bromberg, MD PhD
Univ of Utah Med Ctr
50 N Medical Dr/Rm 3R152
Salt Lake City, UT 84132
Tel: 801 581-6873 *Fax:* 801 585-2054
E-mail: mbromberg@hsc.utah.edu
Accred Length: 1 Year *Program Size:* 3
Program ID: 187-49-21-075

Vermont

Burlington

University of Vermont Program
Sponsor: Fletcher Allen Health Care
Program Director:
Keith J Nagle, MD
Clinical Neurophysiology Lab
Fletcher Allen Health Care
111 Colchester Ave/Brown 301
Burlington, VT 05401
Tel: 802 656-2788 *Fax:* 802 656-5679
E-mail: keith.nagle@vtmednet.org
Accred Length: 1 Year *Program Size:* 1
Program ID: 187-50-21-081

Virginia

Charlottesville

University of Virginia Program
Sponsor: University of Virginia Medical Center
Program Director:
Lawrence H Phillips II, MD
Univ of Virginia
Dept of Neurology
Box 394
Charlottesville, VA 22908
Tel: 804 924-5361 *Fax:* 804 982-1850
E-mail: lhp3n@virginia.edu
Internet:
http://www.med.virginia.edu/medicine/clinical/neurology/
Accred Length: 1 Year *Program Size:* 3
Program ID: 187-51-21-050

Richmond

Medical College of Virginia/Virginia Commonwealth University Program
Sponsor: Medical College of Virginia/Virginia Commonwealth University
Hunter Holmes McGuire VA Medical Center (Richmond)
Medical College of Virginia Hospitals
Program Director:
Robert T Leshner, MD
Med Coll of Virginia
PO Box 980599
Richmond, VA 23298-0599
Tel: 804 828-9350 *Fax:* 804 828-4459
E-mail: rleshner@gems.vcu.edu
Accred Length: 1 Year *Program Size:* 4
Program ID: 187-51-31-053

West Virginia

Morgantown

West Virginia University Program
Sponsor: West Virginia University Hospitals
Program Director:
Laurie Gutmann, MD
West Virginia Univ Health Sciences Ctr
Dept of Neurology
PO Box 9180
Morgantown, WV 26506-9180
Tel: 304 293-3527 *Fax:* 304 293-3352
E-mail: madamsmi@wvu.edu or
mgarlick@wvuhsc1.hsc.wvu.edu
Internet: http://www.hsc.wvu.edu
Accred Length: 1 Year *Program Size:* 1
Program ID: 187-55-21-002

Wisconsin

Milwaukee

Medical College of Wisconsin Program
Sponsor: Medical College of Wisconsin Affiliated Hospitals Inc
Children's Hospital of Wisconsin
Clement J Zablocki Veterans Affairs Medical Center
Froedtert Memorial Lutheran Hospital
Program Director:
Safwan S Jaradeh, MD
Med Coll of Wisconsin
9200 W Wisconsin Ave
Milwaukee, WI 53226
Tel: 414 454-5202 *Fax:* 414 259-0469
E-mail: sjaradeh@mcw.edu
Accred Length: 1 Year *Program Size:* 1
Program ID: 187-56-21-067

Colon and Rectal Surgery

California

Los Angeles

University of Southern California Program
Sponsor: Los Angeles County-USC Medical Center
Kenneth Norris Jr Cancer Hospital and Research Institute
Program Director:
Robert W Beart Jr, MD
Univ of Southern California
Div of Colon/Rectal Surgery
1450 San Pablo St/Ste 5400
Los Angeles, CA 90033-4612
Tel: 323 442-5751 *Fax:* 323 442-5756
Internet:
http://www.surgery.usc.edu/divisions/cr/index.html
Accred Length: 1 Year *Program Size:* 2
Program ID: 060-05-21-042

Connecticut

Hartford

St Francis Hospital and Medical Center Program
Sponsor: St Francis Hospital and Medical Center
Program Director:
David A Cherry, MD
Colon and Rectal Surgeons of Greater Hartford
6 Northwestern Dr/Ste 305
Bloomfield, CT 06002-6002
Tel: 860 242-8591 *Fax:* 860 242-2511
Accred Length: 1 Year *Program Size:* 1
Program ID: 060-08-21-032

District of Columbia

Washington

Washington Hospital Center Program
Sponsor: Washington Hospital Center
Program Director:
Lee E Smith, MD
110 Irving St NW
Ste 3B-31
Washington, DC 20010
Tel: 202 877-8484 *Fax:* 202 877-8483
Accred Length: 1 Year *Program Size:* 1
Program ID: 060-10-21-045

Florida

Fort Lauderdale

Cleveland Clinic Foundation (Florida) Program
Sponsor: Cleveland Clinic Foundation
Cleveland Clinic Hospital
Cleveland Clinic Florida
Program Director:
Steven D Wexner, MD
Cleveland Clinic Florida
3000 W Cypress Creek Rd
Fort Lauderdale, FL 33309-1743
Tel: 954 978-5238 *Fax:* 954 978-5757
E-mail: warrenk@cestmp.ccf.org
Internet: http://www.ccf.org/ed/ccfed.htm
Accred Length: 1 Year *Program Size:* 3
Program ID: 060-11-21-038

Orlando

Orlando Regional Healthcare System Program
Sponsor: Orlando Regional Medical Center
Florida Hospital
Program Director:
Sergio W Larach, MD
Orlando Regional Healthcare System
86 W Underwood St/Ste 201
Orlando, FL 32806
Tel: 407 422-3790 *Fax:* 407 425-4358
E-mail: crcorlando@aol.com
Internet: http://www.orhs-surged.org
Accred Length: 1 Year *Program Size:* 2
Program ID: 060-11-21-037

Illinois

Chicago

Cook County Hospital Program
Sponsor: Cook County Hospital
Program Director:
Charles P Orsay, MD MS
Cook County Hospital
1825 W Harrison St/M-4
Chicago, IL 60612
Tel: 312 633-6202 *Fax:* 312 633-3058
E-mail: corsay@pol.net
Accred Length: 1 Year *Program Size:* 2
Program ID: 060-16-12-001

Urbana

Carle Foundation Hospital Program
Sponsor: Carle Foundation Hospital
Program Director:
Lyn E Tangen, MD
Carle Foundation Hospital
611 W Park St/PVC-4
Urbana, IL 61801
Tel: 217 383-3022, ext 34637 *Fax:* 217 383-3121
Accred Length: 1 Year *Program Size:* 2
Program ID: 060-16-11-002

Louisiana

New Orleans

Alton Ochsner Medical Foundation Program
Sponsor: Alton Ochsner Medical Foundation
Program Director:
Terry C Hicks, MD
Alton Ochsner Med Foundation
Dept of Grad Med Educ
1514 Jefferson Hwy
New Orleans, LA 70121
Tel: 504 842-3260 *Fax:* 504 842-3193
E-mail: dlambert@ochsner.org
Internet: http://www.ochsner.org
Accred Length: 1 Year *Program Size:* 2
Program ID: 060-21-12-003

Shreveport

Louisiana State University (Shreveport) Program
Sponsor: Louisiana State University Hospital-Shreveport
Schumpert Medical Center
Program Director:
H Whitney Boggs Jr, MD
Dept of Colon/Rectal Surgery
1801 Fairfield Ave/Ste 401
Shreveport, LA 71101-4474
Tel: 318 424-8373 *Fax:* 318 222-1542
Accred Length: 1 Year *Program Size:* 1
Program ID: 060-21-21-004

Maryland

Baltimore

Greater Baltimore Medical Center Program
Sponsor: Greater Baltimore Medical Center
Program Director:
Alan V Abrams, MD
Greater Baltimore Med Ctr
6569 N Charles St/Ste 502
Baltimore, MD 21204
Tel: 410 494-1191 *Fax:* 410 296-1739
E-mail: aabrams@gbmc.org
Accred Length: 1 Year *Program Size:* 1
Program ID: 060-23-12-005

Massachusetts

Burlington

Lahey Clinic Program
Sponsor: Lahey Clinic
Program Director:
John J Murray, MD
Lahey Clinic
41 Mall Rd
Burlington, MA 01805
Tel: 781 744-8971 *Fax:* 781 744-2945
Internet: http://www.lahey.org
Accred Length: 1 Year *Program Size:* 2
Program ID: 060-24-12-007

Michigan

Detroit

Henry Ford Hospital Program
Sponsor: Henry Ford Hospital
Program Director:
Eric J Szilagy, MD
Henry Ford Hospital
2799 W Grand Blvd
Detroit, MI 48202-8202
Tel: 313 916-2498 *Fax:* 313 664-2932
E-mail: eszilag1@hfhs.org
Internet: http://www.mich.com/~hfhcrs
Accred Length: 1 Year *Program Size:* 1
Program ID: 060-25-31-043

Grand Rapids

Spectrum Health-East Campus Program
Sponsor: Spectrum Health-East Campus
Program Director:
Martin A Luchtefeld, MD
Ferguson Clinic
75 Sheldon Blvd SE
Grand Rapids, MI 49503
Tel: 616 356-4100 *Fax:* 616 356-4040
Accred Length: 1 Year *Program Size:* 2
Program ID: 060-25-12-009

Royal Oak

William Beaumont Hospital Program
Sponsor: William Beaumont Hospital
Program Director:
Donald C Barkel, MD
William Beaumont Hospital
3601 W 13 Mile Rd
Royal Oak, MI 48073
Tel: 248 551-0403 *Fax:* 248 551-8880
E-mail: jgibson@beaumont.edu
Internet: http://www.beaumont.edu/html/gme
Accred Length: 1 Year *Program Size:* 1
Program ID: 060-25-12-010

Minnesota

Minneapolis

University of Minnesota Program
Sponsor: University of Minnesota Medical School
Abbott-Northwestern Hospital
Fairview-University Medical Center
United Hospital
Veterans Affairs Medical Center (Minneapolis)
Program Director:
Ann C Lowry, MD
Dept of Colon/Rectal Surgery
2550 University Ave W/Rm 313N
St Paul, MN 55114-1084
Tel: 651 641-1707 *Fax:* 651 641-1720
E-mail: alowry@wavefront.com
Accred Length: 1 Year *Program Size:* 4
Program ID: 060-26-21-011

Rochester

Mayo Graduate School of Medicine (Rochester) Program
Sponsor: Mayo Graduate School of Medicine-Mayo Foundation
Mayo Clinic (Rochester)
Rochester Methodist Hospital
St Mary's Hospital of Rochester
Program Director:
Richard M Devine, MD
Dept of Colon/Rectal Surgery
200 First St SW
Rochester, MN 55905
Tel: 507 284-5366 *Fax:* 507 284-1794
Internet: http://www.mayo.edu/
Accred Length: 1 Year *Program Size:* 3
Program ID: 060-26-21-012

Missouri

St Louis

St Louis University School of Medicine Program
Sponsor: St Louis University School of Medicine
St John's Mercy Medical Center
St Louis University School of Medicine
Program Director:
Walter E Longo, MD
St Louis Univ Sch of Med
3635 Vista Ave
PO Box 15250
St Louis, MO 63110-0250
Tel: 314 577-8317 *Fax:* 314 268-5466
E-mail: surgweb@slu.edu
Internet:
http://www.slu.edu/colleges/med/departments/surgery/
Accred Length: 1 Year *Program Size:* 1
Program ID: 060-28-21-039

Washington University/B-JH/SLCH Consortium Program
Sponsor: Washington University/B-JH/SLCH Consortium
Barnes-Jewish Hospital (North Campus)
Program Director:
James W Fleshman Jr, MD
Barnes Jewish Hospital-North Campus
3rd Fl KHB/Campus Box 8109
216 S Kingshighway Blvd
St Louis, MO 63110
Tel: 314 454-7177 *Fax:* 314 454-5249
E-mail: fleshmanj@msnotes.wustl.edu
Internet: http://www.surgery.wustl.edu
Accred Length: 1 Year *Program Size:* 2
Program ID: 060-28-21-025

Nebraska

Omaha

Creighton University Program
Sponsor: Creighton University School of Medicine
Tenet St Joseph Hospital at Creighton Univ Medical Center
Program Director:
Alan G Thorson, MD
Dept of Surgery
601 N 30th St/Ste 3520
Omaha, NE 68131-2137
Tel: 402 280-4533 *Fax:* 402 280-4534
E-mail: agtcr@creighton.edu
Accred Length: 1 Year *Program Size:* 1
Program ID: 060-30-21-035

New Jersey

Piscataway

UMDNJ-Robert Wood Johnson Medical School Program
Sponsor: UMDNJ-Robert Wood Johnson Medical School
JFK Medical Center
Muhlenberg Regional Medical Center
Program Director:
Theodore E Eisenstat, MD
Associated Colon and Rectal Surgeons
1010 Park Ave
Plainfield, NJ 07060
Tel: 908 756-6640 *Fax:* 908 549-8204
Accred Length: 1 Year *Program Size:* 3
Program ID: 060-33-12-013

New York

Buffalo

SUNY at Buffalo Graduate Medical-Dental Education Consortium Program
Sponsor: SUNY at Buffalo Grad Medical-Dental Education Consortium
CGF Health System (Buffalo General Hospital)
Program Director:
Amarjit Singh, MD
SUNY-Buffalo
85 High St
Buffalo, NY 14203
Tel: 716 856-1200 *Fax:* 716 856-2930
Accred Length: 1 Year *Program Size:* 1
Program ID: 060-35-12-014

New York

Mount Sinai School of Medicine Program
Sponsor: Mount Sinai School of Medicine
Mount Sinai Medical Center
Program Director:
Jeffrey W Milsom, MD
Mount Sinai Med Ctr
5 E 98th St
Box 1259
New York, NY 10029
Tel: 212 241-9289 *Fax:* 212 534-2654
Accred Length: 1 Year *Program Size:* 1
Program ID: 060-35-21-046

St Luke's-Roosevelt Hospital Center Program
Sponsor: St Luke's-Roosevelt Hospital Center
St Luke's-Roosevelt Hospital Center-Roosevelt Division
Program Director:
Lester Gottesman, MD
St Luke's-Roosevelt Hospital Ctr
Dept of Colon and Rectal Surgery
1000 Tenth Ave/Ste 2B
New York, NY 10019
Tel: 212 523-7780 *Fax:* 212 523-6495
E-mail: lg40@columbia.edu
Accred Length: 1 Year *Program Size:* 1
Program ID: 060-35-21-034

Ohio

Cleveland

Cleveland Clinic Foundation Program

Sponsor: Cleveland Clinic Foundation

Program Director:
Scott Strong, MD
Cleveland Clinic Foundation
Dept of Colorectal Surgery/A111
9500 Euclid Ave
Cleveland, OH 44195-5242
Tel: 216 444-5690 *Fax:* 216 444-1162
E-mail: meded@cesmtp.ccf.org
Internet: http://www.ccf.org
Accred Length: 1 Year *Program Size:* 4
Program ID: 060-38-12-016

Columbus

Grant Medical Center (OhioHealth) Program

Sponsor: Grant Medical Center (OhioHealth)

Program Director:
Pedro S Aguilar, MD
Grant Med Ctr
Medical Education Dept
111 S Grant Ave
Columbus, OH 43215-4632
Tel: 614 566-9041 *Fax:* 614 566-8073
Accred Length: 1 Year *Program Size:* 2
Program ID: 060-38-12-017

Pennsylvania

Allentown

Lehigh Valley Hospital/Pennsylvania State University Program

Sponsor: Lehigh Valley Hospital

Program Director:
Robert D Riether, MD
Lehigh Valley Hospital
Cedar Crest and I78/PO Box 689
Allentown, PA 18105-1556
Tel: 610 402-8966 *Fax:* 610 402-1667
E-mail: colonres@lvhhn.org
Internet:
http://www.lvhhn.org/academic/residency/colon/home.html
Accred Length: 1 Year *Program Size:* 2
Program ID: 060-41-21-029

Erie

St Vincent Health Center Program

Sponsor: St Vincent Health Center

Program Director:
John C Reilly, MD
St Vincent Health Ctr
Graduate Medical Education
2314 Sassafras St/Ste 200
Erie, PA 16502
Tel: 814 452-5100
Accred Length: 1 Year *Program Size:* 2
Program ID: 060-41-12-019

Philadelphia

Thomas Jefferson University Program

Sponsor: Thomas Jefferson University Hospital

Program Director:
Jan Rakinic, MD
Thomas Jefferson Univ Hospital
1100 Walnut St/Ste 702
Philadelphia, PA 19107
Tel: 215 955-5875 *Fax:* 215 955-2404
Internet: http://jeffline.tju.edu/cwis/dept/colosurg
Accred Length: 1 Year *Program Size:* 1
Program ID: 060-41-21-031

Texas

Dallas

Baylor University Medical Center Program

Sponsor: Baylor University Medical Center

Program Director:
R D Dignan, MD
Baylor Univ Med Ctr
3600 Gaston Ave
Ste 1209/LB164
Dallas, TX 75246-1812
Tel: 214 824-2573 *Fax:* 214 824-2575
Internet: http://www.bhcs.com/bumc/medicaleducation/residencies.htm
Accred Length: 1 Year *Program Size:* 2
Program ID: 060-48-21-021

Presbyterian Hospital of Dallas Program

Sponsor: Presbyterian Hospital of Dallas
Dallas County Hospital District-Parkland Memorial Hospital

Program Director:
Clifford L Simmang, MD
Univ of Texas Southwestern Med Ctr, Dept of Surgery
5323 Harry Hines Blvd
Dallas, TX 75235-9156
Tel: 214 648-3013 *Fax:* 214 648-2301
E-mail: csimma@mednet.swmed.edu
Accred Length: 1 Year *Program Size:* 1
Program ID: 060-48-21-022

Houston

University of Texas at Houston Program

Sponsor: University of Texas Medical School at Houston
Memorial Hermann Healthcare System

Program Director:
H Randolph Bailey, MD
Univ of Texas Health Science Ctr
6550 Fannin Smith Tower/Ste 2307
Houston, TX 77030-2723
Tel: 713 790-9250 *Fax:* 713 790-9251
E-mail: hrbailey@utsurg.med.uth.tmc.edu
Accred Length: 1 Year *Program Size:* 4
Program ID: 060-48-21-023

San Antonio

University of Texas Health Sciences Center at San Antonio Program

Sponsor: University of Texas Medical School at San Antonio
University Hospital-South Texas Medical Center

Program Director:
Jaime L Mayoral, MD
Dept of General Surgery
8711 Village Dr/Ste 320
San Antonio, TX 78217
Tel: 210 655-0844 *Fax:* 210 655-5705
Accred Length: 1 Year *Program Size:* 1
Program ID: 060-48-21-044

Washington

Seattle

Northwest Colon and Rectal Clinic Program

Sponsor: Northwest Colon and Rectal Clinic, PS
Northwest Hospital
Swedish Medical Center-Seattle

Program Director:
Richard P Billingham, MD
1101 Madison/Ste 500
Seattle, WA 98104
Tel: 206 386-6600 *Fax:* 206 386-2452
E-mail: rbham@u.washington.edu
Accred Length: 1 Year *Program Size:* 1
Program ID: 060-54-21-040

Critical Care Medicine (Anesthesiology)

Arizona

Tucson

University of Arizona Program
Sponsor: University of Arizona College of Medicine
Maricopa Medical Center
University Medical Center
Program Director:
Charles W Otto, MD
Arizona Health Sciences Ctr
PO Box 245114
1501 N Campbell Ave
Tucson, AZ 85724-5114
Tel: 520 626-7141 *Fax:* 520 626-6943
Internet: http://www.ahsc.arizona.edu/anesth
Accred Length: 1 Year *Program Size:* 2
Program ID: 045-03-21-046

California

Orange

University of California (Irvine) Program
Sponsor: University of California (Irvine) Medical Center
Veterans Affairs Medical Center (Long Beach)
Program Director:
Elizabeth C Behringer, MD
Long Beach VA Med Ctr
5901 E Seventh St (139)
Long Beach, CA 90822
Tel: 562 494-5412 *Fax:* 562 494-5991
E-mail: ebehring@uci.edu
Accred Length: 1 Year *Program Size:* 2
Program ID: 045-05-21-011

San Francisco

University of California (San Francisco) Program
Sponsor: University of California (San Francisco) School of Medicine
San Francisco General Hospital Medical Center
University of California (San Francisco) Medical Center
Program Director:
Neal H Cohen, MD MPH MS
Univ of California San Francisco
505 Parnassus Ave/M-917
Box 0624
San Francisco, CA 94143-0624
Tel: 415 476-1116 *Fax:* 415 476-0722
E-mail: neal_cohen@quickmail.ucsf.edu
Accred Length: 1 Year *Program Size:* 8
Program ID: 045-05-21-021

Stanford

Stanford University Program
Sponsor: Stanford University Hospital
Program Director:
Myer H Rosenthal, MD
Stanford Univ Sch of Med
Dept of Anesthesiology
300 Pasteur Dr
Stanford, CA 94305-5115
Tel: 650 723-7662 *Fax:* 650 725-8544
E-mail: mhr@leland.stanford.edu
Accred Length: 1 Year *Program Size:* 5
Program ID: 045-05-21-002

Connecticut

Farmington

University of Connecticut Program
Sponsor: University of Connecticut School of Medicine
Hartford Hospital
Univ of Connecticut Health Center/John Dempsey Hospital
Program Director:
Thomas C Mort, MD
Critical Care Med/Anesthesia
Hartford Hospital-Univ of Connecticut Sch of Med
80 Seymour St
Hartford, CT 06115
Tel: 860 545-5022
E-mail: tmort@harthosp.org
Accred Length: 1 Year *Program Size:* 1
Program ID: 045-08-21-035

New Haven

Yale-New Haven Medical Center Program
Sponsor: Yale-New Haven Hospital
Program Director:
Stanley H Rosenbaum, MD
PO Box 208051
333 Cedar St
New Haven, CT 06520-8051
Tel: 203 785-2802 *Fax:* 203 785-6664
Internet: http://gasnet.med.yale.edu/local/yale
Accred Length: 1 Year *Program Size:* 1
Program ID: 045-08-21-058

District of Columbia

Washington

George Washington University Program
Sponsor: George Washington University School of Medicine
George Washington University Hospital (UHS)
Program Director:
Christopher D Junker, MD
George Washington Univ Med Ctr
901 23rd St NW
Washington, DC 20037
Tel: 202 994-3134 *Fax:* 202 994-5620
E-mail: junker@gwis2.circ.gwu.edu
Accred Length: 1 Year *Program Size:* 2
Program ID: 045-10-21-039

Florida

Gainesville

University of Florida Program
Sponsor: University of Florida College of Medicine
Shands Hospital at the University of Florida
Veterans Affairs Medical Center (Gainesville)
Program Director:
T James Gallagher, MD
Univ of Florida
Box 100254 JHMHC
Gainesville, FL 32610-0254
Tel: 352 395-0463 *Fax:* 352 338-9861
Accred Length: 1 Year *Program Size:* 3
Program ID: 045-11-21-009

Miami

University of Miami-Jackson Memorial Medical Center Program
Sponsor: University of Miami-Jackson Memorial Medical Center
Program Director:
Albert J Varon, MD
Univ of Miami-Jackson Memorial Med Ctr
Div of Trauma Anes/Critical Care
PO Box 016370 (M820)
Miami, FL 33101
Tel: 305 585-6970 *Fax:* 305 545-6501
Internet: http://umdas.med.miami.edu
Accred Length: 1 Year *Program Size:* 3
Program ID: 045-11-21-004

Tampa

University of South Florida Program
Sponsor: University of South Florida College of Medicine
Tampa General Healthcare
Veterans Affairs Medical Center (Bay Pines)
Program Director:
Roy D Cane, MB BCh
Univ of South Florida
12901 Bruce B Downs Blvd/MDC59
Tampa, FL 33612
Tel: 813 251-7438 *Fax:* 813 251-7418
E-mail: rcane@com1.med.usf.edu
Internet:
http://www.med.usf.edu/anesthesiology/index.html
Accred Length: 1 Year *Program Size:* 4
Program ID: 045-11-21-050

Georgia

Atlanta

Emory University Program
Sponsor: Emory University School of Medicine
Crawford Long Hospital of Emory University
Grady Memorial Hospital
Program Director:
James G Ramsay, MD
Emory Univ Sch of Med
Dept of Anesthesiology
1364 Clifton Rd NE
Atlanta, GA 30322
Tel: 404 778-5874 *Fax:* 404 778-5194
E-mail: james_ramsay@emory.org
Internet:
http://www.cc.emory.edu/whsc/med/anesthesiology/index.html
Accred Length: 1 Year *Program Size:* 2
Program ID: 045-12-21-059

Illinois

Chicago

McGaw Medical Center of Northwestern University Program

Sponsor: Northwestern University Medical School
Northwestern Memorial Hospital
Veterans Affairs Lakeside Medical Center (Chicago)

Program Director:
William T Peruzzi, MD
Northwestern Memorial Hospital
250 E Superior St
Ste 678
Chicago, IL 60611-3053
Tel: 312 908-2537 *Fax:* 312 908-1700
E-mail: wperuzzi@nmff.nwu.edu
Accred Length: 1 Year *Program Size:* 3
Program ID: 045-16-21-014

Iowa

Iowa City

University of Iowa Hospitals and Clinics Program

Sponsor: University of Iowa Hospitals and Clinics

Program Director:
J Steven Hata, MD
Univ of Iowa Hospitals and Clinics
Dept of Anesthesia
200 Hawkins Dr
Iowa City, IA 52242-1009
Tel: 319 353-7303 *Fax:* 319 356-1120
E-mail: steven-hata@uiowa.edu
Internet:
http://www.anesth.uiowa.edu/anesthesia/home.htm
Accred Length: 1 Year *Program Size:* 4
Program ID: 045-18-21-003

Maryland

Baltimore

Johns Hopkins University Program

Sponsor: Johns Hopkins University School of Medicine
Johns Hopkins Hospital

Program Director:
Todd Dorman, MD
Meyer 299A
600 N Wolfe St
Baltimore, MD 21287-7294
Tel: 410 955-9080 *Fax:* 410 955-8978
E-mail: tdorman@jhmi.edu
Internet:
http://hopkins.med.jhu.edu/healthcarepros/ccm/ccf.html
Accred Length: 1 Year *Program Size:* 7
Program ID: 045-23-21-034

University of Maryland Program

Sponsor: University of Maryland Medical System

Program Director:
Mary J Njoku, MD
Univ of Maryland
22 S Greene St/Box 253
Baltimore, MD 21201-1595
Tel: 410 328-1239 *Fax:* 410 328-0546
E-mail: mjohnson@anesth.ab.umd.edu
Internet: http://anesthesia.ummc.ab.umd.edu
Accred Length: 1 Year *Program Size:* 3
Program ID: 045-23-21-029

Bethesda

National Capital Consortium Program

Sponsor: National Capital Consortium
Walter Reed Army Medical Center

Program Director:
Marianne C Reis, MD
Walter Reed Army Med Ctr
Critical Care Med Service
6825 16th St NW
Washington, DC 20307-5001
Tel: 202 782-3891 *Fax:* 202 782-5043
Accred Length: 1 Year *Program Size:* 2
Program ID: 045-10-21-042
US Armed Services Program

Massachusetts

Boston

Beth Israel Deaconess Medical Center (East Campus) Program

Sponsor: Beth Israel Deaconess Medical Center
Children's Hospital

Program Director:
Alan Lisbon, MD
Beth Israel Deaconess Med Ctr
Dept of Anes/Critical Care RS-951
330 Brookline Ave
Boston, MA 02215
Tel: 617 667-5298 *Fax:* 617 667-5003
E-mail: alisbon@bih.harvard.edu
Internet:
http://www.med.harvard.edu/programs/anesthesia/bih
Accred Length: 1 Year *Program Size:* 2
Program ID: 045-24-11-001

Massachusetts General Hospital Program

Sponsor: Massachusetts General Hospital

Program Director:
William E Hurford, MD
Massachusetts General Hospital
Dept of Anes/Critical Care
Fruit St
Boston, MA 02114
Tel: 617 726-2859 *Fax:* 617 724-8511
E-mail: hurford@etherdome.mgh.harvard.edu
Internet: http://www.mghdacc.com
Accred Length: 1 Year *Program Size:* 5
Program ID: 045-24-31-015

Springfield

Baystate Medical Center Program

Sponsor: Baystate Medical Center

Program Director:
Thomas L Higgins, MD
Baystate Med Ctr
759 Chestnut St
Springfield, MA 01199
Tel: 413 794-5439 *Fax:* 413 794-5389
E-mail: thomas.higgins@bhs.org
Internet: http://www.baystatehealth.com
Accred Length: 1 Year *Program Size:* 2
Program ID: 045-24-21-063

Worcester

University of Massachusetts Program

Sponsor: University of Massachusetts Medical School
UMass Memorial Health Care (University Campus)
Worcester City Hospital

Program Director:
Stephen O Heard, MD
Univ of Massachusetts Med Sch
Dept of Anesthesia
55 Lake Ave N
Worcester, MA 01655
Tel: 508 856-5581 *Fax:* 508 856-4060
E-mail: stephen.heard@banyan.ummed.edu
Accred Length: 1 Year *Program Size:* 2
Program ID: 045-24-31-017

Michigan

Ann Arbor

University of Michigan Program

Sponsor: University of Michigan Hospitals

Program Director:
Jeremy Lieberman, MD
1500 E Medical Center Dr
Ann Arbor, MI 48109-0048
Tel: 734 936-4280 *Fax:* 734 936-9091
Accred Length: 1 Year *Program Size:* 2
Program ID: 045-25-21-060

Detroit

Wayne State University/Detroit Medical Center (Sinai Hospital) Program

Sponsor: Wayne State University/Detroit Medical Center

Program Director:
William Pavlik, MD
Sinai Hospital
6767 W Outer Dr
Detroit, MI 48235-2899
Tel: 313 493-5760 *Fax:* 313 493-5112
Accred Length: 1 Year *Program Size:* 1
Program ID: 045-25-31-019

Minnesota

Minneapolis

University of Minnesota Program

Sponsor: University of Minnesota Medical School
Fairview-University Medical Center
Regions Hospital
Veterans Affairs Medical Center (Minneapolis)

Program Director:
Ian Hasinoff, MD
Box 294
420 Delaware St SE
Minneapolis, MN 55455
Tel: 612 624-9990 *Fax:* 612 626-2363
E-mail: hasin002@gold.tc.umn.edu
Internet:
http://www1.umn.edu/anesthes/critcare/critical-care.html
Accred Length: 1 Year *Program Size:* 1
Program ID: 045-26-21-061

Rochester

Mayo Graduate School of Medicine (Rochester) Program
Sponsor: Mayo Graduate School of Medicine-Mayo Foundation
Mayo Clinic (Rochester)
Program Director:
Martin L DeRuyter, MD
Application Processing Ctr
Mayo Graduate Sch of Med
200 First St SW/Siebens 5
Rochester, MN 55905
Tel: 507 284-4331 *Fax:* 507 284-0999
E-mail: mgsm.roch.mnanesthesiology@mayo.edu
Internet: http://www.mayo.edu/
Accred Length: 1 Year *Program Size:* 6
Program ID: 045-26-21-024

Missouri

St Louis

Washington University/B-JH/SLCH Consortium Program
Sponsor: Washington University/B-JH/SLCH Consortium
Barnes-Jewish Hospital
Program Director:
Walter A Boyle III, MD
Washington Univ Sch of Med
600 S Euclid Ave
Campus Box 8054
St Louis, MO 63110
Tel: 314 747-3581 *Fax:* 314 747-1710
E-mail: boylew@notes.wustl.edu
Accred Length: 1 Year *Program Size:* 4
Program ID: 045-28-21-056

New Hampshire

Lebanon

Dartmouth-Hitchcock Medical Center Program
Sponsor: Mary Hitchcock Memorial Hospital
Program Director:
Athos J Rassias, MD
Dartmouth-Hitchcock Med Ctr
One Medical Center Dr
Lebanon, NH 03756-0001
Tel: 603 650-5000, ext 4642 *Fax:* 603 650-4360
E-mail: athos.j.rassias@hitchcock.org
Accred Length: 1 Year *Program Size:* 3
Program ID: 045-32-21-030

New Jersey

Camden

UMDNJ-Robert Wood Johnson Medical School (Camden) Program
Sponsor: Cooper Hospital-University Medical Center
Program Director:
W Eric Scott, MD
1 Cooper Plaza/Dorrance Ste 222
Camden, NJ 08103
Tel: 609 342-2408 *Fax:* 609 968-8253
E-mail: scottwe@umdnj.edu
Internet: http://www.umdnj.edu
Accred Length: 1 Year *Program Size:* 1
Program ID: 045-33-21-041

New York

Albany

Albany Medical Center Program
Sponsor: Albany Medical Center
Program Director:
Kevin W Roberts, MD MD
Albany Med Ctr Hospital
Dept of Anesth(131)
43 New Scotland Ave
Albany, NY 12208-3478
Tel: 518 262-4302 *Fax:* 518 262-4736
E-mail: kushniv@mail.amc.edu
Accred Length: 1 Year *Program Size:* 1
Program ID: 045-35-21-044

Bronx

Albert Einstein College of Medicine Program
Sponsor: Albert Einstein College of Medicine of Yeshiva University
Montefiore Medical Center-Henry and Lucy Moses Division
Program Director:
Christopher W Bryan-Brown, MD
Montefiore Med Ctr
Dept of Anesthesiology
111 E 210th St
Bronx, NY 10467
Tel: 718 920-4175 *Fax:* 718 881-2245
E-mail: cwildonbb@aol.com
Accred Length: 1 Year *Program Size:* 2
Program ID: 045-35-21-026

Brooklyn

SUNY Health Science Center at Brooklyn Program
Sponsor: SUNY Health Science Center at Brooklyn
Kings County Hospital Center
Long Island College Hospital
University Hospital-SUNY Health Science Center at Brooklyn
Program Director:
Ashraf Boutros, MD
SUNY Health Science Ctr-Brooklyn
Dept of Anes/Critical Care
450 Clarkson Ave/Box 6
Brooklyn, NY 11203
Tel: 718 270-3269 *Fax:* 718 270-3298
Accred Length: 1 Year *Program Size:* 2
Program ID: 045-35-11-054

Buffalo

SUNY at Buffalo Graduate Medical-Dental Education Consortium Program
Sponsor: SUNY at Buffalo Grad Medical-Dental Education Consortium
CGF Health System (Buffalo General Hospital)
CGF Health System (Children's Hospital of Buffalo)
Erie County Medical Center
Roswell Park Cancer Institute
Veterans Affairs Medical Center (Buffalo)
Program Director:
Carlos J Kurek, MD
VA Med Ctr
Dept of Anesthesiology
3495 Bailey Ave
Buffalo, NY 14215
Tel: 716 834-9200 *Fax:* 716 862-3395
E-mail: kurek.carlos.j@buffalo.va.gov
Internet: http://www.wings.buffalo.edu/smbs/anest
Accred Length: 1 Year *Program Size:* 2
Program ID: 045-35-21-051

New York

Mount Sinai School of Medicine Program
Sponsor: Mount Sinai School of Medicine
Elmhurst Hospital Center-Mount Sinai Services
Mount Sinai Medical Center
Program Director:
Andrew B Leibowitz, MD
Mount Sinai Hospital
Surgical ICU (Box 1264)
One Gustave L Levy Pl
New York, NY 10029-6574
Tel: 212 241-8867 *Fax:* 212 860-3669
E-mail: aleibow @smtplink.mssm.edu
Accred Length: 1 Year *Program Size:* 2
Program ID: 045-35-21-020

New York and Presbyterian Hospital (Columbia Campus) Program
Sponsor: New York and Presbyterian Hospital
New York and Presbyterian Hospital (Columbia Campus)
Program Director:
Robert N Sladen, MD
Presbyterian Hospital
Dept of Anes/Critical Care
622 W 168th St
New York, NY 10032-3784
Tel: 212 305-8633 *Fax:* 212 305-9482
E-mail: rs543@columbia.edu
Accred Length: 1 Year *Program Size:* 3
Program ID: 045-35-11-007

New York and Presbyterian Hospital (Cornell Campus) Program
Sponsor: Memorial Sloan-Kettering Cancer Center
New York and Presbyterian Hospital (Cornell Campus)
Program Director:
Roger S Wilson, MD
Memorial Sloan-Kettering Cancer Ctr
1275 York Ave/Rm
New York, NY 10021
Tel: 212 639-6848 *Fax:* 212 772-8646
E-mail: wilsonr@mskcc.org
Accred Length: 1 Year *Program Size:* 2
Program ID: 045-35-21-006

New York University Medical Center Program
Sponsor: New York University Medical Center
Bellevue Hospital Center
Program Director:
Brian S Kaufman, MD
550 First Ave
New York, NY 10016
Tel: 212 263-5072 *Fax:* 212 263-7254
Accred Length: 1 Year *Program Size:* 3
Program ID: 045-35-21-016

Rochester

University of Rochester Program
Sponsor: Strong Memorial Hospital of the University of Rochester
Genesee Hospital
Rochester General Hospital
Program Director:
Niels Lund, MD PhD
Univ of Rochester Med Ctr
Dept of Anesth/Box 604
601 Elmwood Ave
Rochester, NY 14642
Tel: 716 275-2141 *Fax:* 716 244-7271
Accred Length: 1 Year *Program Size:* 6
Program ID: 045-35-11-022

Syracuse

SUNY Health Science Center at Syracuse Program
Sponsor: University Hospital-SUNY Health Science Center at Syracuse
Program Director:
Michael F Mascia, MD MPH
SUNY Health Science Ctr-Syracuse
Dept of Anes/Critical Care Med
750 E Adams St
Syracuse, NY 13210
Tel: 315 464-4890 *Fax:* 315 464-4866
Accred Length: 1 Year *Program Size:* 2
Program ID: 045-35-31-053

North Carolina

Chapel Hill

University of North Carolina Hospitals Program
Sponsor: University of North Carolina Hospitals
Program Director:
Philip G Boysen, MD
Univ of North Carolina, Dept of Anesthesiology
223 Burnett-Womack Bldg/CB7010
Chapel Hill, NC 27599-7010
Tel: 919 966-5136 *Fax:* 919 966-4873
E-mail: boysen@aims.unc.edu
Internet: http://www.aims.unc.edu
Accred Length: 1 Year *Program Size:* 1
Program ID: 045-36-21-062

Durham

Duke University Program
Sponsor: Duke University Medical Center
Veterans Affairs Medical Center (Durham)
Program Director:
Christopher C Young, MD
Duke Univ
Dept of Anes/Critical Care
PO Box 3094
Durham, NC 27710
Tel: 919 681-6656 *Fax:* 919 681-7893
E-mail: carr0001@mc.duke.edu
Internet: http://anesthsia.mc.duke.edu/duke2.htm
Accred Length: 1 Year *Program Size:* 3
Program ID: 045-36-21-052

Winston-Salem

Wake Forest University School of Medicine Program
Sponsor: Wake Forest University Baptist Medical Center
Program Director:
Richard C Prielipp, MD
Wake Forest Univ Sch of Med
Medical Center Blvd
Winston-Salem, NC 27157-1009
Tel: 336 716-4498 *Fax:* 336 716-8190
Internet: http://www.anes.wfubmc.edu
Accred Length: 1 Year *Program Size:* 4
Program ID: 045-36-21-023

Ohio

Cleveland

Case Western Reserve University Program
Sponsor: University Hospitals of Cleveland
Program Director:
Howard S Nearman, MD
Univ Hospitals of Cleveland
11100 Euclid Ave
Cleveland, OH 44106-5007
Tel: 216 844-7333 *Fax:* 216 844-3781
Accred Length: 1 Year *Program Size:* 2
Program ID: 045-38-21-012

Cleveland Clinic Foundation Program
Sponsor: Cleveland Clinic Foundation
Program Director:
Marc J Popovich, MD
Cleveland Clinic Foundation
Dept of Critical Care Med/E3
9500 Euclid Ave
Cleveland, OH 44195
Tel: 216 444-5690 *Fax:* 216 444-1162
E-mail: meded@cesmtp.ccf.org
Internet: http://www.ccf.org
Accred Length: 1 Year *Program Size:* 6
Program ID: 045-38-21-031

Columbus

Ohio State University Program
Sponsor: Ohio State University Medical Center
Arthur G James Cancer Hospital and Research Institute
Children's Hospital
Program Director:
Thomas E Reilley, DO
N-416 Doan Hall
410 W Tenth Ave
Columbus, OH 43210
Tel: 614 293-8487 *Fax:* 614 293-8153
Accred Length: 1 Year *Program Size:* 3
Program ID: 045-38-21-049

Pennsylvania

Hershey

Penn State Geisinger Health System/Milton S Hershey Medical Center Program
Sponsor: Penn State Geisinger Health System
Milton S Hershey Medical Center
Program Director:
John K Stene, MD
Milton S Hershey Med Ctr
Dept of Anesthesia/H187
PO Box 850
Hershey, PA 17033-0850
Tel: 800 206-7718 *Fax:* 717 531-6221
Internet: http://www.anes.hmc.psu.edu
Accred Length: 1 Year *Program Size:* 1
Program ID: 045-41-21-038

Philadelphia

Temple University Program
Sponsor: Temple University Hospital
Fox Chase Cancer Center
St Christopher's Hospital for Children
Program Director:
Rodger E Barnette, MD
Temple Univ Hospital
Critical Care Program
3401 N Broad St
Philadelphia, PA 19140
Tel: 215 707-3326 *Fax:* 215 707-8028
E-mail: rodger@vm.temple.edu
Accred Length: 1 Year *Program Size:* 2
Program ID: 045-41-21-047

University of Pennsylvania Program
Sponsor: Hospital of the University of Pennsylvania
Children's Hospital of Philadelphia
Program Director:
Clifford S Deutschman, MD
Andrew T Costarino Jr, MD
Hospital of Univ of Pennsylvania
Dept of Anesthesia
3400 Spruce St
Philadelphia, PA 19104
Tel: 215 662-3719 *Fax:* 215 349-5341
E-mail: apfeifer@mail.med.upenn.edu
Accred Length: 1 Year *Program Size:* 2
Program ID: 045-41-21-005

Pittsburgh

University Health Center of Pittsburgh Program
Sponsor: University Health Center of Pittsburgh
Presbyterian University Hospital/UPMC
Program Director:
Ake Grenvik, MD
Univ Health Ctr of Pittsburgh
Critical Care Med
655 Scaife Hall
Pittsburgh, PA 15261
Tel: 412 647-3135 *Fax:* 412 647-8060
E-mail: mcctp@smtp.anes.upmc.edu
Internet: http://www.anes.upmc.edu/mcctp/
Accred Length: 1 Year *Program Size:* 4
Program ID: 045-41-21-028

Tennessee

Knoxville

University of Tennessee Medical Center at Knoxville Program
Sponsor: University of Tennessee Graduate School of Medicine
University of Tennessee Memorial Hospital
Program Director:
Steve A Morris, MD
Univ of Tennessee Med Ctr
Dept of Anesthesiology
1924 Alcoa Hwy/U-109
Knoxville, TN 37920-6999
Tel: 423 544-9220
Internet: http://www.mc.utk.edu
Accred Length: 1 Year *Program Size:* 1
Program ID: 045-47-21-045

Nashville

Vanderbilt University Program
Sponsor: Vanderbilt University Medical Center

Program Director:
Kevin P Clarkson, MD
Vanderbilt Univ Med Ctr
1313 21st Ave S/504 Oxford House
Nashville, TN 37232-4125
Tel: 615 936-2800 *Fax:* 615 343-6272
E-mail: kevin.clarkson@mcmail.vanderbilt.edu
Internet: http://www.anesthesiology.mc.vanderbilt.edu
Accred Length: 1 Year *Program Size:* 2
Program ID: 045-47-21-057

Texas

Galveston

University of Texas Medical Branch Hospitals Program
Sponsor: University of Texas Medical Branch Hospitals

Program Director:
Mali Mathru, MD
Univ of Texas Med Branch
Dept of Anesthesiology
301 University Blvd
Galveston, TX 77555-0591
Tel: 409 747-5781 *Fax:* 409 747-4314
E-mail: cjb@utmb.edu
Internet: http://www.utmb.edu
Accred Length: 1 Year *Program Size:* 2
Program ID: 045-48-21-048

Houston

University of Texas at Houston Program
Sponsor: University of Texas Medical School at Houston
Memorial Hermann Healthcare System

Program Director:
Joseph L Nates, MD
Univ of Texas Med Sch
Dept of Anesthesiology
6431 Fannin St/5020 MSB
Houston, TX 77030
Tel: 713 500-6183 *Fax:* 713 500-6201
E-mail: jnates@anes1.med.uth.tmc.edu
Internet: http://www-anes.uth.tmc.edu
Accred Length: 1 Year *Program Size:* 2
Program ID: 045-48-21-032

Lackland AFB

San Antonio Uniformed Services Health Education Consortium (WHMC) Program
Sponsor: San Antonio Uniformed Services Health Education Consortium
Wilford Hall Medical Center (AETC)
Brooke Army Medical Center

Program Director:
Kenneth S Papier, DO
59th MDW/PSSA
2200 Bergquist Dr/Ste 1
San Antonio, TX 78236-5300
Tel: 210 292-5558 *Fax:* 210 292-7986
E-mail: papier@pol.net
Accred Length: 1 Year *Program Size:* 3
Program ID: 045-48-21-033
US Armed Services Program

Virginia

Charlottesville

University of Virginia Program
Sponsor: University of Virginia Medical Center

Program Director:
Charles G Durbin Jr, MD
Univ of Virginia Health Service
Box 10010
Charlottesville, VA 22906-0010
Tel: 804 924-2283 *Fax:* 804 982-0019
E-mail: cgd8v@virginia.edu
Internet:
http://www.med.virginia.edu/som-cl/anesth/index.html
Accred Length: 1 Year *Program Size:* 2
Program ID: 045-51-11-027

Wisconsin

Madison

University of Wisconsin Program
Sponsor: University of Wisconsin Hospital and Clinics
William S Middleton Veterans Hospital

Program Director:
Douglas B Coursin, MD
Univ of Wisconsin Clinical Sciences Ctr
Dept of Anesth B6/319
600 Highland Ave
Madison, WI 53792-3272
Tel: 608 263-8114 *Fax:* 608 263-0575
E-mail: info@anesthesia.wisc.edu
Internet: http://www.anesthesia.wisc.edu
Accred Length: 1 Year *Program Size:* 2
Program ID: 045-56-21-008

Milwaukee

Medical College of Wisconsin Program
Sponsor: Medical College of Wisconsin Affiliated Hospitals Inc
Froedtert Memorial Lutheran Hospital

Program Director:
Eugene Y Cheng, MD
Med Coll of Wisconsin
Anesthesiology Dept
9200 W Wisconsin Ave
Milwaukee, WI 53226
Tel: 414 259-2715 *Fax:* 414 259-1522
E-mail: eycheng@mcw.edu
Internet:
http://www.mcw.edu/my_html/dp-anesthesiology.html
Accred Length: 1 Year *Program Size:* 2
Program ID: 045-56-21-025

Critical Care Medicine (Internal Medicine)

California

Los Angeles

Cedars-Sinai Medical Center Program
Sponsor: Cedars-Sinai Medical Center

Program Director:
Lawrence S Maldonado, MD
Michael I Lewis, MD
Cedars-Sinai Med Ctr
8700 Beverly Blvd/Rm B114
Los Angeles, CA 90048-1865
Tel: 310 855-4658 *Fax:* 310 657-6175
E-mail: lawrence.maldonado@cshs.org
Accred Length: 2 Years *Program Size:* 2
Program ID: 142-05-11-005

UCLA Medical Center Program
Sponsor: UCLA School of Medicine
UCLA Medical Center

Program Director:
Paul E Bellamy, MD
UCLA Sch of Med, Dept of Med
37-131 CHS
10833 Le Conte Ave
Los Angeles, CA 90095-1690
Tel: 310 285-5988
Accred Length: 2 Years *Program Size:* 6
Program ID: 142-05-11-007

San Francisco

University of California (San Francisco) Program
Sponsor: University of California (San Francisco) School of Medicine
University of California (San Francisco) Medical Center

Program Director:
Michael A Matthay, MD
John M Luce, MD
Univ of California
Cardiovascular Research Inst
505 Parnassus Ave/M-917
San Francisco, CA 94143-0624
Tel: 415 476-2807 *Fax:* 415 476-0722
E-mail: mmatt@itsa.ucsf.edu
Accred Length: 2 Years *Program Size:* 2
Program ID: 142-05-21-011

Stanford

Stanford University Program
Sponsor: Stanford University Hospital

Program Director:
Norman W Rizk, MD
Stanford Univ Med Ctr
Div of Pulm/Critical Care Med H3142
300 Pasteur Dr
Stanford, CA 94305-5236
Tel: 650 723-7377 *Fax:* 650 725-5489
Accred Length: 2 Years *Program Size:* 7
Program ID: 142-05-21-013

District of Columbia

Washington

George Washington University Program 1
Sponsor: George Washington University School of Medicine
George Washington University Hospital (UHS)
Program Director:
Michael Seneff, MD
George Washington Univ Med Ctr
901 23rd St NW
Washington, DC 20037
Tel: 202 994-3837 *Fax:* 202 994-4800
E-mail: anemgs@gwumc.edu
Accred Length: 2 Years *Program Size:* 2
Program ID: 142-10-21-103

Walter Reed Army Medical Center Program
Sponsor: Walter Reed Army Medical Center
Program Director:
Thomas M Fitzpatrick, MD PhD
Critical Care Med Service
Walter Reed Army Med Ctr
6825 16th St NW
Washington, DC 20307-5001
Tel: 202 782-2063 *Fax:* 202 782-5043
E-mail: ltc_thomas_fitzpatrick@wramc1-amedd.army.mil
Accred Length: 2 Years *Program Size:* 3
Program ID: 142-10-21-125
US Armed Services Program

Florida

Miami

University of Miami-Jackson Memorial Medical Center Program
Sponsor: University of Miami-Jackson Memorial Medical Center
Mount Sinai Medical Center of Greater Miami
Veterans Affairs Medical Center (Miami)
Program Director:
Roland M H Schein, MD
VA Med Ctr
Critical Care Med (111)
1201 NW 16th St
Miami, FL 33125
Tel: 305 324-3153 *Fax:* 305 324-3366
E-mail: rschein@mednet.med.miami.edu
Accred Length: 2 Years *Program Size:* 2
Program ID: 142-11-21-020

Illinois

Chicago

Rush-Presbyterian-St Luke's Medical Center Program
Sponsor: Rush-Presbyterian-St Luke's Medical Center
Program Director:
R Phillip Dellinger, MD
Rush-Presbyterian-St Luke's Med Ctr
1653 W Congress Pkwy
Chicago, IL 60612
Tel: 312 942-2998 *Fax:* 312 942-5829
E-mail: pdelli@rush.edu
Accred Length: 2 Years *Program Size:* 4
Program ID: 142-16-11-027

University of Chicago Program
Sponsor: University of Chicago Hospitals
Program Director:
Gregory Schmidt, MD
Dept of Med
5841 S Maryland Ave
MC 6026
Chicago, IL 60637
Tel: 773 702-1454 *Fax:* 773 702-4754
Accred Length: 2 Years *Program Size:* 3
Program ID: 142-16-11-024

North Chicago

Finch University of Health Sciences/Chicago Medical School Program
Sponsor: Finch University of Health Sciences/Chicago Medical School
Cook County Hospital
Mount Sinai Hospital Medical Center of Chicago
Veterans Affairs Medical Center (North Chicago)
Program Director:
Eric Gluck, MD
Finch Univ of Health Sciences-Chicago Med Sch
Dept of Med
3333 Green Bay Rd
North Chicago, IL 60064-3095
Tel: 847 688-1900 *Fax:* 847 578-3868
Accred Length: 2 Years *Program Size:* 6
Program ID: 142-16-21-026

Louisiana

New Orleans

Tulane University Program
Sponsor: Tulane University School of Medicine
Tulane University Hospital and Clinics
Veterans Affairs Medical Center-LSU Service (New Orleans)
Program Director:
Kevin L Kovitz, MD
Tulane Med Ctr
1430 Tulane Ave
Box SL9
New Orleans, LA 70112-2699
Tel: 504 588-2250 *Fax:* 504 587-2144
E-mail: ijeffer@tmcpop.tmc.tulane.edu
Accred Length: 1 Year *Program Size:* 9
Program ID: 142-21-21-153

Shreveport

Louisiana State University (Shreveport) Program
Sponsor: Louisiana State University Hospital-Shreveport
Overton Brooks Veterans Affairs Medical Center
Program Director:
Steven A Conrad, MD PhD
Louisiana State Univ Med Ctr
Dept of Med Educ
1501 Kings Hwy/PO Box 33932
Shreveport, LA 71130-3932
Tel: 318 675-6885 *Fax:* 318 675-6878
E-mail: sconrad@lsumc.edu
Internet: http://www.ccm.lsumc.edu
Accred Length: 2 Years *Program Size:* 4
Program ID: 142-21-21-032

Maryland

Bethesda

National Institutes of Health Clinical Center Program
Sponsor: NIH Warren Grant Magnuson Clinical Center
Washington Hospital Center
Program Director:
Frederick P Ognibene, MD
National Insts of Health
10 Center Dr
Bldg 10 Rm 7D43
Bethesda, MD 20892-1662
Tel: 301 496-9320 *Fax:* 301 402-1213
E-mail: fognibene@cc.nih.gov
Accred Length: 2 Years *Program Size:* 15
Program ID: 142-23-21-128

Massachusetts

Worcester

University of Massachusetts Program
Sponsor: University of Massachusetts Medical School
UMass Memorial Health Care (University Campus)
Program Director:
Nicholas A Smyrnios, MD
Univ of Massachusetts Med Sch
55 Lake Ave N
Worcester, MA 01655
Tel: 508 856-3122
E-mail: nicholas.smyrnios@banyan.ummed.edu
Accred Length: 2 Years *Program Size:* 2
Program ID: 142-24-21-035

Michigan

Detroit

Wayne State University/Detroit Medical Center Program
Sponsor: Wayne State University/Detroit Medical Center
Detroit Receiving Hospital and University Health Center
Harper Hospital
Program Director:
Joseph J Bander, MD
Harper Hospital
Pulmonary/Critical Care Div V534
3990 John R
Detroit, MI 48201
Tel: 313 745-8107 *Fax:* 313 745-8846
E-mail: jbander@oncgate.roc.wayne.edu
Internet: http://www.intmed.wayne.edu
Accred Length: 2 Years *Program Size:* 12
Program ID: 142-25-21-043

Minnesota

Minneapolis

Hennepin County Medical Center Program

Sponsor: Hennepin County Medical Center
Methodist Hospital

Program Director:
James W Leatherman, MD
Hennepin County Med Ctr
701 Park Ave S
Minneapolis, MN 55415
Tel: 612 347-2625 *Fax:* 612 904-4299
Accred Length: 2 Years *Program Size:* 3
Program ID: 142-26-21-118

Rochester

Mayo Graduate School of Medicine (Rochester) Program

Sponsor: Mayo Graduate School of Medicine-Mayo Foundation
Mayo Clinic (Rochester)
Rochester Methodist Hospital
St Mary's Hospital of Rochester

Program Director:
William F Dunn, MD
Mayo Graduate Sch of Med
Application Processing Ctr
Siebens 5th Fl
Rochester, MN 55905
Tel: 507 284-3126 *Fax:* 507 284-0999
E-mail: mgsm.intmed.specialties@mayo.edu
Internet: http://www.mayo.edu/
Accred Length: 2 Years *Program Size:* 5
Program ID: 142-26-21-100

Missouri

St Louis

St Louis University School of Medicine Program

Sponsor: St Louis University School of Medicine
St John's Mercy Medical Center
St Louis University School of Medicine

Program Director:
Robert W Taylor, MD
St John's Mercy Med Ctr
621 S New Ballas Rd/Ste 5007B
St Louis, MO 63141
Tel: 314 569-6486 *Fax:* 314 995-4155
E-mail: rwtaylor@inlink.com
Accred Length: 2 Years *Program Size:* 10
Program ID: 142-28-21-048

New Hampshire

Lebanon

Dartmouth-Hitchcock Medical Center Program

Sponsor: Mary Hitchcock Memorial Hospital

Program Director:
Athos J Rassias, MD
Dartmouth-Hitchcock Med Ctr
One Medical Center Dr
Lebanon, NH 03756
Tel: 603 650-5000, ext 4642 *Fax:* 603 650-4360
E-mail: athos.j.rassias@hitchcock.org
Accred Length: 2 Years *Program Size:* 6
Program ID: 142-32-21-140

New Jersey

Camden

UMDNJ-Robert Wood Johnson Medical School (Camden) Program

Sponsor: Cooper Hospital-University Medical Center

Program Director:
David R Gerber, DO
Cooper Hospital-Univ Med Ctr
Three Cooper Plaza/Ste 312
Camden, NJ 08103
Tel: 609 342-2406 *Fax:* 609 541-3968
E-mail: gerberdr@umdnj.edu
Internet: http://www.umdnj.edu
Accred Length: 2 Years *Program Size:* 3
Program ID: 142-33-21-051

South Orange

Seton Hall University School of Graduate Medical Education Program

Sponsor: Seton Hall University School of Graduate Medical Education
JFK Medical Center
St Michael's Medical Center (Cathedral Hlth Srvcs Inc)

Program Director:
Marc R Adelman, MD
St Michael's Med Ctr
306 Martin Luther King Blvd
Newark, NJ 07102
Tel: 201 877-5090 *Fax:* 201 877-2737
Accred Length: 2 Years *Program Size:* 3
Program ID: 142-33-11-050

New Mexico

Albuquerque

University of New Mexico Program

Sponsor: University of New Mexico School of Medicine
University Hospital
Veterans Affairs Medical Center (Albuquerque)

Program Director:
Howard Levy, MD PhD
Univ of New Mexico, Dept of Med
5th Fl Ambulatory Care Ctr
2211 Lomas Blvd NE
Albuquerque, NM 87131-5271
Tel: 505 272-4751 *Fax:* 505 272-8700
E-mail: howard_levy@somasf.unm.edu
Internet: http://macbeth.unm.edu/som/gme
Accred Length: 1 Year *Program Size:* 2
Program ID: 142-34-21-053

New York

Bronx

Albert Einstein College of Medicine Program

Sponsor: Albert Einstein College of Medicine of Yeshiva University
Jacobi Medical Center
Montefiore Medical Center-Henry and Lucy Moses Division

Program Director:
Vladimir Kvetan, MD
Montefiore Med Ctr
Div of Critical Care Med
111 E 210th St
Bronx, NY 10467
Tel: 718 920-5440 *Fax:* 718 652-2464
E-mail: vkvetan@aol.com
Accred Length: 2 Years *Program Size:* 8
Program ID: 142-35-21-067

Brooklyn

Maimonides Medical Center Program

Sponsor: Maimonides Medical Center

Program Director:
Sidney Tessler, MD
Maimonides Med Ctr
4802 Tenth Ave
Brooklyn, NY 11219
Tel: 718 435-9700 *Fax:* 718 283-7884
E-mail: stessler@maimonidesmed.org
Accred Length: 2 Years *Program Size:* 4
Program ID: 142-35-11-056

SUNY Health Science Center at Brooklyn Program

Sponsor: SUNY Health Science Center at Brooklyn
Kings County Hospital Center
St John's Episcopal Hospital-South Shore
University Hospital-SUNY Health Science Center at Brooklyn
Veterans Affairs Medical Center (Brooklyn)

Program Director:
Linda S Efferen, MD
SUNY Health Science Ctr-Brooklyn
450 Clarkson Ave/Box 19
Brooklyn, NY 11203-2098
Tel: 718 270-1770 *Fax:* 718 270-1733
Accred Length: 2 Years *Program Size:* 4
Program ID: 142-35-21-065

New York

Mount Sinai School of Medicine Program

Sponsor: Mount Sinai School of Medicine
Englewood Hospital and Medical Center
Mount Sinai Medical Center
Veterans Affairs Medical Center (Bronx)

Program Director:
John M Oropello, MD
Ernest Benjamin, MD
Mount Sinai Med Ctr
Surgical ICU (Box 1264)
One Gustave L Levy Pl
New York, NY 10029-6574
Tel: 212 241-7331 *Fax:* 212 860-3669
E-mail: joropel@smtplink.mssm.edu
Accred Length: 2 Years *Program Size:* 12
Program ID: 142-35-31-060

New York and Presbyterian Hospital (Columbia Campus) Program
Sponsor: New York and Presbyterian Hospital
New York and Presbyterian Hospital (Columbia Campus)
Program Director:
Randolph P Cole, MD
Presbyterian Hospital in the City of New York
630 W 168th St/Box 91
PH 8 Center
New York, NY 10032
Tel: 212 305-9817 *Fax:* 212 305-8464
Internet:
http://cpmcnet.columbia.edu/dept/pulmonary/fellowship.html
Accred Length: 1 Year *Program Size:* 3
Program ID: 142-35-11-148

New York and Presbyterian Hospital (Cornell Campus) Program
Sponsor: Memorial Sloan-Kettering Cancer Center
Program Director:
Jeffrey S Groeger, MD
Memorial Sloan-Kettering Cancer Ctr
1275 York Ave/Rm M210B
New York, NY 10021
Tel: 212 639-8114 *Fax:* 212 794-4333
E-mail: groegerj@mskcc.org
Accred Length: 2 Years *Program Size:* 6
Program ID: 142-35-21-064

New York Medical College at St Vincent's Hospital and Medical Center of New York Program
Sponsor: New York Medical College
St Vincent's Hospital and Medical Center of New York
Program Director:
Mark E Astiz, MD
St Vincent's Hospital and Med Ctr
Dept of Med
153 W 11th St
New York, NY 10011
Tel: 212 604-2004 *Fax:* 212 604-8061
Internet: http://svh.nymc.edu
Accred Length: 2 Years *Program Size:* 5
Program ID: 142-35-11-058

Rochester

University of Rochester Program
Sponsor: Strong Memorial Hospital of the University of Rochester
Genesee Hospital
Program Director:
Michael J Apostolakos, MD
Strong Memorial Hospital
Pulmonary/Critical Care Unit
601 Elmwood Ave/Box #692
Rochester, NY 14642
Tel: 716 275-2050 *Fax:* 716 273-1126
E-mail: michael_apostolakos@urmc.rochester.edu
Accred Length: 2 Years *Program Size:* 2
Program ID: 142-35-21-141

North Carolina

Winston-Salem

Wake Forest University School of Medicine Program
Sponsor: Wake Forest University Baptist Medical Center
Program Director:
David L Bowton, MD
Wake Forest Univ Sch of Med
Critical Care Med
Medical Center Blvd
Winston Salem, NC 27157-1009
Tel: 336 716-6533 *Fax:* 336 716-8190
E-mail: dbowton@wfubmc.edu
Internet: http://www.wfubmc.edu
Accred Length: 2 Years *Program Size:* 4
Program ID: 142-36-21-069

Pennsylvania

Hershey

Penn State Geisinger Health System/Milton S Hershey Medical Center Program
Sponsor: Penn State Geisinger Health System
Milton S Hershey Medical Center
Program Director:
Rebecca Bascom, MD MPH
Penn State Geisinger Health System
MC H041
PO Box 850
Hershey, PA 17033-0850
Tel: 717 531-6525 *Fax:* 717 531-5785
Accred Length: 1 Year *Program Size:* 6
Program ID: 142-41-11-079

Pittsburgh

University Health Center of Pittsburgh Program
Sponsor: University Health Center of Pittsburgh
Presbyterian University Hospital/UPMC
Veterans Affairs Medical Center (Pittsburgh)
Program Director:
Paul L Rogers, MD
Univ Health Center of Pittsburgh
3550 Terrace St
655 Scaife Hall
Pittsburgh, PA 15261
Tel: 412 647-3135 *Fax:* 412 647-8060
E-mail: rogers@smtp.anes.upmc.edu
Internet: http://www.anes.upmc.edu/mcctp
Accred Length: 2 Years *Program Size:* 24
Program ID: 142-41-21-114

Rhode Island

Providence

Brown University (Miriam) Program
Sponsor: Miriam Hospital
Rhode Island Hospital
Program Director:
Paul C Yodice, MD
Miriam Hospital
Div of Critical Care Med/Rm 223
164 Summit Ave
Providence, RI 02906
Tel: 401 793-4501, ext 34501 *Fax:* 401 793-4511
E-mail: paul_yodice@brown.edu
Accred Length: 1 Year *Program Size:* 3
Program ID: 142-43-11-083

Brown University Program
Sponsor: Rhode Island Hospital
Roger Williams Medical Center
Veterans Affairs Medical Center (Providence)
Program Director:
Sidney S Braman, MD
Rhode Island Hospital
593 Eddy St
Providence, RI 02903
Tel: 401 444-8410 *Fax:* 401 444-5914
Accred Length: 1 Year *Program Size:* 4
Program ID: 142-43-11-082

Tennessee

Memphis

University of Tennessee Program
Sponsor: University of Tennessee College of Medicine
Regional Medical Center at Memphis
Veterans Affairs Medical Center (Memphis)
Program Director:
A Stacey Headley, MD
Univ of Tennessee
956 Court Ave/Rm H314
Memphis, TN 38163
Tel: 901 448-5757 *Fax:* 901 448-7726
Accred Length: 1 Year *Program Size:* 2
Program ID: 142-47-21-123

Texas

Fort Sam Houston

San Antonio Uniformed Services Health Education Consortium (BAMC) Program
Sponsor: San Antonio Uniformed Services Health Education Consortium
Brooke Army Medical Center
Program Director:
Lt Col David P Ciceri, MD
Brooke Army Med Ctr
Critical Care Med Service
3851 Roger Brooke Dr
Fort Sam Houston, TX 78234-6200
Tel: 210 916-5250 *Fax:* 210 916-1602
E-mail: dpaulc@earthlink.net
Accred Length: 2 Years *Program Size:* 4
Program ID: 142-48-12-087
US Armed Services Program

Houston

Baylor College of Medicine Program
Sponsor: Baylor College of Medicine
Methodist Hospital
Program Director:
Al Davies, MD
Baylor Coll of Med-Methodist Hospital
6550 Fannin St/Ste 1233
Houston, TX 77030
Tel: 713 790-2238 *Fax:* 713 790-3648
E-mail: adavies@bcm.tmc.edu
Internet: http://www.bcm.tmc.edu/medicine/pulmonary
Accred Length: 2 Years *Program Size:* 6
Program ID: 142-48-21-091

Virginia

Charlottesville

University of Virginia Program
Sponsor: University of Virginia Medical Center
Program Director:
Jonathon D Truwit, MD
Univ of Virginia Health Systems
Box 546
Charlottesville, VA 22908-0001
Tel: 804 924-5270 *Fax:* 804 924-9682
E-mail: truwit@virginia.edu
Accred Length: 2 Years *Program Size:* 2
Program ID: 142-51-21-107

Washington

Seattle

University of Washington Program
Sponsor: University of Washington School of Medicine
University of Washington Medical Center
Program Director:
Leonard D Hudson, MD
Harborview Med Ctr
325 Ninth Ave
Box 359762
Seattle, WA 98104
Tel: 206 731-8483 *Fax:* 206 731-8584
E-mail: kathleen@colossus.pulmcc.washington.edu
Internet: http://weber.u.washington.edu/~pulmcc
Accred Length: 2 Years *Program Size:* 0
Program ID: 142-54-21-094

Cytopathology (Pathology)

Alabama

Birmingham

University of Alabama Medical Center Program
Sponsor: University of Alabama Hospital
Veterans Affairs Medical Center (Birmingham)
Program Director:
William H Rodgers, PhD MD
Kracke Bldg/Rm 532A
1922 7th Ave S
Birmingham, AL 35233-1924
Tel: 205 975-8898 *Fax:* 205 975-7284
E-mail: wrodgers@path.uab.edu
Internet: http://www.uab.edu
Accred Length: 1 Year *Program Size:* 1
Program ID: 307-01-21-041

Arkansas

Little Rock

University of Arkansas for Medical Sciences Program
Sponsor: University of Arkansas College of Medicine
John L McClellan Memorial Veterans Hospital
Program Director:
Ricardo H Bardales, MD
Univ of Arkansas for Med Sciences
4301 W Markham St/Slot 517
Little Rock, AR 72205-7199
Tel: 501 686-5171 *Fax:* 501 686-5874
E-mail: bardalesricardoh@exchange.uams.edu
Accred Length: 1 Year *Program Size:* 1
Program ID: 307-04-21-034

California

Los Angeles

UCLA Medical Center Program
Sponsor: UCLA School of Medicine
UCLA Medical Center
Program Director:
Roberta K Nieberg, MD
UCLA Med Ctr
A3-231N
Los Angeles, CA 90095
Tel: 310 825-9670 *Fax:* 310 206-5178
E-mail: rnieberg@pathology.medsch.ucla.edu
Internet: http://www.pathnet.medsch.ucla.edu
Accred Length: 1 Year *Program Size:* 1
Program ID: 307-05-21-013

University of Southern California Program
Sponsor: Los Angeles County-USC Medical Center
Program Director:
Sue E Martin, MD PhD
1441 Eastlake Ave
Topping Tower Rm 2420
Los Angeles, CA 90033-0804
Tel: 323 865-3270 *Fax:* 323 865-0077
Accred Length: 1 Year *Program Size:* 3
Program ID: 307-05-21-063

San Francisco

University of California (San Francisco) Program
Sponsor: University of California (San Francisco) School of Medicine
San Francisco General Hospital Medical Center
Program Director:
Britt-Marie Ljung, MD
Univ of California San Francisco
2356 Sutter St/7th Fl
San Francisco, CA 94143
Tel: 415 885-7220 *Fax:* 415 567-5584
E-mail: bml@itsa.ucsf.edu
Internet: http://www.pangloss.ucsf.edu/af/docs
Accred Length: 1 Year *Program Size:* 2
Program ID: 307-05-21-075

Connecticut

Hartford

Hartford Hospital Program
Sponsor: Hartford Hospital
Program Director:
Mark E Ludwig, MD
Hartford Hospital
Dept of Pathology
80 Seymour St
Hartford, CT 06102-5037
Tel: 860 545-2866 *Fax:* 860 522-0045
Accred Length: 1 Year *Program Size:* 2
Program ID: 307-08-21-053

New Haven

Yale-New Haven Medical Center Program
Sponsor: Yale-New Haven Hospital
Program Director:
David L Rimm, MD PhD
600 York St
New Haven, CT 06504
Tel: 203 737-4204 *Fax:* 203 737-5089
E-mail: david.rimm@yale.edu
Internet:
http://info.med.yale.edu/pathol/cytology/cytol.htm
Accred Length: 1 Year *Program Size:* 1
Program ID: 307-08-21-078

District of Columbia

Washington

George Washington University Program
Sponsor: George Washington University School of Medicine
George Washington University Hospital (UHS)
Program Director:
Mary K Sidawy, MD
George Washington Univ Med Ctr
2300 Eye St NW
Ross Hall/Rm 502
Washington, DC 20037
Tel: 202 994-3391
Internet: http://www.gwumc.edu/dept/path
Accred Length: 1 Year *Program Size:* 1
Program ID: 307-10-21-005

Georgetown University Program
Sponsor: Georgetown University Medical Center
Program Director:
David F Garvin, MD
Elizabeth Montgomery, MD
3900 Reservoir Rd NW
Washington, DC 20007
Tel: 202 687-2904 *Fax:* 202 687-8935
Accred Length: 1 Year *Program Size:* 1
Program ID: 307-10-21-073

Florida

Gainesville

University of Florida Program
Sponsor: University of Florida College of Medicine
Shands Hospital at the University of Florida
Veterans Affairs Medical Center (Gainesville)
Program Director:
Edward J Wilkinson, MD
Univ of Florida Coll of Med
Dept of Pathology
PO Box 100275
Gainesville, FL 32610-0275
Tel: 352 395-0238 *Fax:* 352 395-0437
E-mail: wilkinso.pathology@mail.health.ufl.edu
Internet: http://www.med.ufl.edu/path/homepage
Accred Length: 1 Year *Program Size:* 1
Program ID: 307-11-21-047

Jacksonville

University of Florida Health Science Center/Jacksonville Program
Sponsor: University of Florida College of Medicine at Jacksonville
University Medical Center (UFHSC/J)
Program Director:
Shahla Masood, MD
Univ of Florida Health Science Ctr-Jacksonville
Dept of Pathology
655 W Eighth St
Jacksonville, FL 32209-6511
Tel: 904 549-4387 *Fax:* 904 549-4060
E-mail: sm.umc5@mail.health.ufl.edu
Internet: http://www.ufhscj.edu/path/index.html
Accred Length: 1 Year *Program Size:* 2
Program ID: 307-11-21-014

Miami

University of Miami-Jackson Memorial Medical Center Program
Sponsor: University of Miami-Jackson Memorial Medical Center
Program Director:
Parvin Ganjei Azar, MD
Univ of Miami-Jackson Memorial Med Ctr
Div of Cytopathology
PO Box 016960 (R-1)
Miami, FL 33101
Tel: 305 585-6055 *Fax:* 305 585-2598
Accred Length: 1 Year *Program Size:* 1
Program ID: 307-11-21-024

Tampa

University of South Florida Program
Sponsor: University of South Florida College of Medicine
H Lee Moffitt Cancer Center
Program Director:
Santo V Nicosia, MD
12901 Bruce B Downs Blvd
MDC Box 11
Tampa, FL 33612-4799
Tel: 813 974-3133
E-mail: snicosia@com1.med.usf.edu
Accred Length: 1 Year *Program Size:* 1
Program ID: 307-11-21-068

Georgia

Atlanta

Emory University Program
Sponsor: Emory University School of Medicine
Egleston Children's Hospital at Emory University
Emory University Hospital
Grady Memorial Hospital
Program Director:
Melinda M Lewis, MD
Pathology Education Office
Emory Univ Hospital/Rm H-189
1364 Clifton Rd NE
Atlanta, GA 30322-8110
Tel: 404 727-7328 *Fax:* 404 727-2519
E-mail: aboyett@.emory.edu
Internet: http://www.emory.edu/pathology/residency/
Accred Length: 1 Year *Program Size:* 2
Program ID: 307-12-21-058

Illinois

Chicago

McGaw Medical Center of Northwestern University Program
Sponsor: Northwestern University Medical School
Northwestern Memorial Hospital
Veterans Affairs Lakeside Medical Center (Chicago)
Program Director:
Carlos Bedrossian, MD
Dept of Cytopathology
303 E Superior St
Passavant Pavilion/Rm 226A
Chicago, IL 60611
Tel: 312 908-1191 *Fax:* 312 908-8950
E-mail: c-bedrossian@nwu.edu
Accred Length: 1 Year *Program Size:* 2
Program ID: 307-16-21-037

University of Chicago Program
Sponsor: University of Chicago Hospitals
Program Director:
Richard M DeMay, MD
5841 S Maryland Ave/MC 2050
MARP 212
Chicago, IL 60637
Tel: 773 702-9121 *Fax:* 773 702-6570
Accred Length: 1 Year *Program Size:* 1
Program ID: 307-16-21-061

University of Illinois College of Medicine at Chicago Program
Sponsor: University of Illinois College of Medicine at Chicago
University of Illinois Hospital and Clinics
Program Director:
Leopoldo T Gerardo, MD
Dept of Pathology (M/C 847)
1819 W Polk St/Rm 446
Chicago, IL 60612
Tel: 312 996-9288
Accred Length: 1 Year *Program Size:* 26
Program ID: 307-16-21-050

Maywood

Loyola University Program
Sponsor: Loyola University Medical Center
Edward J Hines Jr Veterans Affairs Hospital
Program Director:
Suzanne M Selvaggi, MD
Loyola Univ Med Ctr
2160 S First Ave
Maywood, IL 60153
Tel: 708 327-2600 *Fax:* 708 327-2620
E-mail: sselvag@luc.edu
Accred Length: 1 Year *Program Size:* 2
Program ID: 307-16-21-001

Indiana

Indianapolis

Indiana University School of Medicine Program
Sponsor: Indiana University School of Medicine
Clarian IU Hospital
Clarian Riley Hospital for Children
Richard L Roudebush Veterans Affairs Medical Center
William N Wishard Memorial Hospital
Program Director:
Liang-Che Tao, MD
Indiana Univ Hospital
Div of Cytopathology
550 N University Blvd/Rm 3465
Indianapolis, IN 46202-5280
Tel: 317 274-2361 *Fax:* 317 274-5346
E-mail: ltao@iupui.edu
Internet: http://www.pathology.iupui.edu/tao.html
Accred Length: 1 Year *Program Size:* 2
Program ID: 307-17-21-002

Iowa

Iowa City

University of Iowa Hospitals and Clinics Program
Sponsor: University of Iowa Hospitals and Clinics
Veterans Affairs Medical Center (Iowa City)
Program Director:
Timothy G Timmerman, MD
Univ of Iowa Hospitals and Clinics
Dept of Pathology
200 Hawkins Dr/5243 RCP
Iowa City, IA 52242-1009
Tel: 319 356-4510 *Fax:* 319 356-8470
E-mail: timothy-timmerman@uiowa.edu
Accred Length: 1 Year *Program Size:* 2
Program ID: 307-18-21-025

Kansas

Kansas City

University of Kansas Medical Center Program

Sponsor: University of Kansas School of Medicine
University of Kansas Medical Center

Program Director:
Patricia A Thomas, MD
3901 Rainbow Blvd
Kansas City, KS 66160
Tel: 913 588-1744 *Fax:* 913 588-1160
E-mail: pthomas@kumc.edu
Accred Length: 1 Year *Program Size:* 3
Program ID: 307-19-21-079

Kentucky

Lexington

University of Kentucky Medical Center Program

Sponsor: University of Kentucky Hospital
Veterans Affairs Medical Center (Lexington)

Program Director:
Diane Davis Davey, MD
Univ of Kentucky Med Ctr
Pathology/Ste MS117
Lexington, KY 40536-0084
Tel: 606 257-5357, ext 232 *Fax:* 606 323-2094
E-mail: ddavey@pop.uky.edu
Internet:
http://www.uky.edu/medicine/departments/pathology/pathology.html
Accred Length: 1 Year *Program Size:* 1
Program ID: 307-20-21-008

Louisville

University of Louisville Program

Sponsor: University of Louisville School of Medicine

Program Director:
Sidney Murphree, MD
Univ of Louisville Sch of Med
Dept of Pathology
512 S Hancock St/Carmichael Bldg Rm 201
Louisville, KY 40202
Tel: 502 852-8203, ext 8203 *Fax:* 502 852-8299
E-mail: msdixo01@gwise.louisville.edu
Accred Length: 1 Year *Program Size:* 1
Program ID: 307-20-21-036

Louisiana

New Orleans

Louisiana State University Program

Sponsor: Louisiana State University School of Medicine
Medical Center of Louisiana at New Orleans

Program Director:
Lester Vial Jr, MD
Louisiana State Univ Sch of Med
Dept of Pathology Box P5-1
1901 Perdido St
New Orleans, LA 70112-1393
Tel: 504 568-6049 *Fax:* 504 568-6037
Accred Length: 1 Year *Program Size:* 1
Program ID: 307-21-21-051

Tulane University Program

Sponsor: Tulane University School of Medicine
Medical Center of Louisiana at New Orleans

Program Director:
Nina Dhurander, MD
1430 Tulane Ave
New Orleans, LA 70112-2699
Tel: 504 588-5224 *Fax:* 504 587-7389
Accred Length: 1 Year *Program Size:* 1
Program ID: 307-21-21-080

Shreveport

Louisiana State University (Shreveport) Program

Sponsor: Louisiana State University Hospital-Shreveport

Program Director:
Elba A Turbat-Herrera, MD
1501 S Kings Hwy
PO Box 33932
Shreveport, LA 71130-3932
Tel: 318 675-5862 *Fax:* 318 675-7662
E-mail: eturba@lsumc.edu
Accred Length: 1 Year *Program Size:* 2
Program ID: 307-21-21-074

Maryland

Baltimore

Johns Hopkins University Program

Sponsor: Johns Hopkins University School of Medicine
Armed Forces Institute of Pathology
Johns Hopkins Hospital

Program Director:
Dorothy Rosenthal, MD BS
Johns Hopkins Med Insts
600 N Wolfe St
Pathology 406
Baltimore, MD 21287-6940
Tel: 410 955-1180 *Fax:* 410 614-9556
E-mail: drosenth@pathlan.path.jhu.edu
Internet: http://www.pathology.jhu.edu/cytoweb
Accred Length: 1 Year *Program Size:* 3
Program ID: 307-23-21-065

Bethesda

National Capital Consortium Program

Sponsor: National Capital Consortium
National Naval Medical Center (Bethesda)
National Cancer Institute

Program Director:
Michael Henry, MD
National Naval Med Ctr
Lab Dept Bldg 9
8901 Wisconsin Ave
Bethesda, MD 20889-5600
Tel: 301 295-5774 *Fax:* 301 295-1415
Accred Length: 1 Year *Program Size:* 1
Program ID: 307-10-21-033
US Armed Services Program

National Institutes of Health Clinical Center Program

Sponsor: NIH Warren Grant Magnuson Clinical Center
National Naval Medical Center (Bethesda)

Program Director:
Andrea Abati, MD
NIH National Cancer Inst
9000 Rockville Pike
Bldg 10/Rm 2A19
Bethesda, MD 20892
Tel: 301 496-6355 *Fax:* 301 402-2585
Accred Length: 1 Year *Program Size:* 1
Program ID: 307-23-21-032

Massachusetts

Boston

Beth Israel Deaconess Medical Center Program

Sponsor: Beth Israel Deaconess Medical Center

Program Director:
Helen H Wang, MD PhD
Dept of Pathology
Beth Israel Deaconess Med Ctr-East Campus
330 Brookline Ave
Boston, MA 02215
Tel: 617 667-7284 *Fax:* 617 667-7120
Accred Length: 1 Year *Program Size:* 2
Program ID: 307-24-21-030

Boston University Medical Center Program

Sponsor: Boston Medical Center

Program Director:
Antonio de las Morenas, MD
Boston Med Ctr, Mallory Inst of Pathology
784 Massachusetts Ave
Boston, MA 02118
Tel: 617 414-5059 *Fax:* 617 414-5315
Accred Length: 1 Year *Program Size:* 2
Program ID: 307-24-21-003

Brigham and Women's Hospital Program

Sponsor: Brigham and Women's Hospital

Program Director:
Edmund S Cibas, MD
Brigham and Women's Hospital
Dept of Pathology
75 Francis St
Boston, MA 02115
Tel: 617 732-6797 *Fax:* 617 739-6192
E-mail: escibas@bics.bwh.harvard.edu
Accred Length: 1 Year *Program Size:* 2
Program ID: 307-24-21-029

Massachusetts General Hospital Program

Sponsor: Massachusetts General Hospital

Program Director:
Debra A Bell, MD
Massachusetts General Hospital
Fruit St
Boston, MA 02114
Tel: 617 726-3977 *Fax:* 617 726-7474
Accred Length: 1 Year *Program Size:* 1
Program ID: 307-24-21-016

Springfield

Baystate Medical Center Program

Sponsor: Baystate Medical Center

Program Director:
Martin Bur, MD
Baystate Med Ctr
Dept of Pathology
759 Chestnut St
Springfield, MA 01199
Tel: 413 794-5085 *Fax:* 413 794-5893
E-mail: csullivan@bhs.org
Internet: http://www.baystatehealth.com
Accred Length: 1 Year *Program Size:* 1
Program ID: 307-24-21-071

Michigan

Ann Arbor

University of Michigan Program

Sponsor: University of Michigan Hospitals

Program Director:
Claire W Michael, MD
Univ Hospital
1500 E Medical Center Dr
Rm 2G332/0054
Ann Arbor, MI 48109-0054
Tel: 734 936-6770 *Fax:* 734 763-4095
E-mail: clairemi@umich.edu
Accred Length: 1 Year *Program Size:* 1
Program ID: 307-25-31-019

Detroit

Henry Ford Hospital Program

Sponsor: Henry Ford Hospital

Program Director:
Sudha R Kini, MD
Henry Ford Hospital
Div of Cytopathology
2799 W Grand Blvd
Detroit, MI 48202
Tel: 313 916-2352 *Fax:* 313 916-2385
Accred Length: 1 Year *Program Size:* 2
Program ID: 307-25-21-020

Wayne State University/Detroit Medical Center Program

Sponsor: Wayne State University/Detroit Medical Center
Harper Hospital
Hutzel Hospital

Program Director:
Latha R Pisharodi, MD
Pathology Dept, Detroit Med Ctr-Hutzel Hospital
4707 St Antonio Blvd
Detroit, MI 48201
Tel: 313 745-0834 *Fax:* 313 993-8894
E-mail: pisharod@kci.wayne.edu
Accred Length: 1 Year *Program Size:* 2
Program ID: 307-25-21-046

Royal Oak

William Beaumont Hospital Program

Sponsor: William Beaumont Hospital

Program Director:
Tomi Jo Kuntzman, DO
William Beaumont Hospital
Dept of Anatomic Pathology
3601 W 13 Mile Rd
Royal Oak, MI 48073
Tel: 248 551-1256 *Fax:* 248 551-1257
Internet: http://www.beaumont.edu/html/gme
Accred Length: 1 Year *Program Size:* 1
Program ID: 307-25-21-015

Mississippi

Jackson

University of Mississippi Medical Center Program

Sponsor: University of Mississippi School of Medicine
Veterans Affairs Medical Center (Jackson)

Program Director:
Luciano B Lemos, MD
Univ of Mississippi Med Ctr
2500 N State St
Jackson, MS 39216-4505
Tel: 601 984-1550 *Fax:* 601 984-1531
E-mail: llemos@pathology.umsmed.edu
Accred Length: 1 Year *Program Size:* 1
Program ID: 307-27-21-057

Missouri

St Louis

St Louis University School of Medicine Program

Sponsor: St Louis University School of Medicine
St Louis University School of Medicine
Veterans Affairs Medical Center (St Louis)

Program Director:
Brian Collins, MD
St Louis Univ Sch of Med
Dept of Pathology
1402 S Grand Blvd
St Louis, MO 63104
Tel: 314 577-8782 *Fax:* 314 268-5120
E-mail: collinbt@slu.edu
Internet:
http://www.slu.edu/colleges/med/departments/path/edu/medical/
Accred Length: 1 Year *Program Size:* 1
Program ID: 307-28-21-040

Washington University/B-JH/SLCH Consortium Program

Sponsor: Washington University/B-JH/SLCH Consortium
Barnes-Jewish Hospital
Barnes-Jewish Hospital (North Campus)
St Louis Children's Hospital

Program Director:
Rosa M Davila, MD
Barnes-Jewish Hospital
One Barnes Hospital Plaza
Peters Bldg/Ste 300
St Louis, MO 63110
Tel: 314 362-0101 *Fax:* 314 747-2040
E-mail: davila@path.wustl.edu
Accred Length: 1 Year *Program Size:* 1
Program ID: 307-28-21-062

New York

Bronx

Albert Einstein College of Medicine Program

Sponsor: Albert Einstein College of Medicine of Yeshiva University
Montefiore Medical Center-Henry and Lucy Moses Division

Program Director:
Leopold G Koss, MD
Montefiore Med Ctr
Central Bldg/Rm 313
111 E 210th St
Bronx, NY 10467-2490
Tel: 718 920-5185 *Fax:* 718 515-9841
E-mail: steinber@aecom.yu.edu
Internet: http://www.aecom.yu.edu
Accred Length: 1 Year *Program Size:* 2
Program ID: 307-35-31-027

New Hyde Park

Albert Einstein College of Medicine at Long Island Jewish Medical Center Program

Sponsor: Long Island Jewish Medical Center

Program Director:
Patricia G Wasserman, MD
Long Island Jewish Med Ctr
Dept of Pathology/Rm B67
270-05 76th Ave
New Hyde Park, NY 11040
Tel: 718 470-7709 *Fax:* 718 347-9171
Internet: http://www.lij.edu
Accred Length: 1 Year *Program Size:* 1
Program ID: 307-35-21-066

New York

Memorial Sloan-Kettering Cancer Center Program

Sponsor: Memorial Sloan-Kettering Cancer Center

Program Director:
Maureen F Zakowski, MD
Memorial Sloan-Kettering Cancer Ctr
Cytology Service
1275 York Ave
New York, NY 10021
Tel: 212 639-5900 *Fax:* 212 639-6318
E-mail: zakowskm@mskcc.org
Accred Length: 1 Year *Program Size:* 2
Program ID: 307-35-21-006

Mount Sinai School of Medicine Program

Sponsor: Mount Sinai School of Medicine
Mount Sinai Medical Center
Queens Hospital Center

Program Director:
David E Burstein, MD
Mount Sinai Med Ctr, Div of Cytopathology
One Gustave L Levy Pl
Annenberg 15-64
New York, NY 10029
Tel: 212 241-0463 *Fax:* 212 534-7491
Accred Length: 1 Year *Program Size:* 2
Program ID: 307-35-31-048

New York and Presbyterian Hospital (Cornell Campus) Program

Sponsor: New York and Presbyterian Hospital
New York and Presbyterian Hospital (Cornell Campus)

Program Director:
Daniel M Knowles, MD
New York Hospital-Cornell Med Ctr
Papanicolaou Cytology Lab F766
525 E 68th St
New York, NY 10021
Tel: 212 746-4528 *Fax:* 212 746-8359
Internet: http://www.nycornell.org/pathology/
Accred Length: 1 Year *Program Size:* 1
Program ID: 307-35-21-042

New York University Medical Center Program

Sponsor: New York University Medical Center
Bellevue Hospital Center

Program Director:
Jerry Waisman, MD
New York Univ Med Ctr
550 First Ave/Skirball Bldg 7S
New York, NY 10016
Tel: 212 263-5475 *Fax:* 212 263-5509
Accred Length: 1 Year *Program Size:* 2
Program ID: 307-35-21-070

Rochester

University of Rochester Program

Sponsor: Strong Memorial Hospital of the University of Rochester

Program Director:
Lisa A Teot, MD
601 Elmwood Ave/Box 626
Rochester, NY 14642
Tel: 716 275-1602 *Fax:* 716 442-1766
Accred Length: 1 Year *Program Size:* 1
Program ID: 307-35-21-031

Syracuse

SUNY Health Science Center at Syracuse Program

Sponsor: University Hospital-SUNY Health Science Center at Syracuse

Program Director:
Kamal K Khurana, MD MD
SUNY Health Science Ctr-Syracuse
Path/Cytopathology
750 E Adams St
Syracuse, NY 13210
Tel: 315 464-4270 *Fax:* 315 464-4267
Accred Length: 1 Year *Program Size:* 1
Program ID: 307-35-21-022

Valhalla

New York Medical College at Westchester Medical Center Program

Sponsor: New York Medical College
Westchester Medical Center

Program Director:
Muhammad B Zaman, MD
New York Med Coll
Basic Sciences Bldg/Rm 413
Valhalla, NY 10595
Tel: 914 594-4148 *Fax:* 914 594-4163
Accred Length: 1 Year *Program Size:* 1
Program ID: 307-35-31-007

North Carolina

Chapel Hill

University of North Carolina Hospitals Program

Sponsor: University of North Carolina Hospitals

Program Director:
Susan J Maygarden, MD
Univ of North Carolina Sch of Med
CB7525 Brinkhous-Bullitt Bldg
Chapel Hill, NC 27599-7525
Tel: 919 966-2339 *Fax:* 919 966-6417
Internet:
http://www.pathology.med.unc.edu/path/welcome.htm
Accred Length: 1 Year *Program Size:* 1
Program ID: 307-36-21-044

Durham

Duke University Program

Sponsor: Duke University Medical Center

Program Director:
Sandra H Bigner, MD
Duke Univ Med Ctr
Box 3712
Durham, NC 27710
Tel: 919 684-2486 *Fax:* 919 684-6306
Accred Length: 1 Year *Program Size:* 1
Program ID: 307-36-21-039

Greenville

East Carolina University Program

Sponsor: East Carolina University School of Medicine
Pitt County Memorial Hospital

Program Director:
James L Finley, MD
East Carolina Univ Sch of Med
Dept of Cytology
Brody 7-S10
Greenville, NC 27858-4354
Tel: 252 816-4951 *Fax:* 252 816-8200
Accred Length: 1 Year *Program Size:* 1
Program ID: 307-36-21-021

Ohio

Akron

Summa Health System (Akron City Hospital)/NEOUCOM Program

Sponsor: Summa Health System
Akron City Hospital (Summa Health System)
Children's Hospital Medical Center of Akron

Program Director:
Sheila Kashkari, MD
Summa Health System
Dept of Cytopathology
525 E Market St
Akron, OH 44309
Tel: 330 375-4967 *Fax:* 330 375-4874
Internet: http://www.summahealth.org/edu/
Accred Length: 1 Year *Program Size:* 1
Program ID: 307-38-21-045

Cincinnati

University Hospital/University of Cincinnati College of Medicine Program

Sponsor: University Hospital Inc

Program Director:
Jose L Mira, MD
Univ of Cincinnati
231 Bethesda Ave
PO Box 670529
Cincinnati, OH 45267-0529
Tel: 513 558-7113 *Fax:* 513 558-2289
E-mail: dana.brindley@uc.edu
Internet:
http://www.med.uc.edu/departme/pathdept/web/resident/respage.htm
Accred Length: 1 Year *Program Size:* 1
Program ID: 307-38-21-035

Cleveland

Case Western Reserve University (MetroHealth) Program

Sponsor: MetroHealth Medical Center

Program Director:
Amer Khiyami, MD
MetroHealth Med Ctr
Div of Cytopathology
2500 MetroHealth Dr
Cleveland, OH 44109-1998
Tel: 216 778-5181 *Fax:* 216 778-5701
Internet: http://www.pathology.metrohealth.org
Accred Length: 1 Year *Program Size:* 1
Program ID: 307-38-21-038

Case Western Reserve University Program

Sponsor: University Hospitals of Cleveland

Program Director:
Fadi W Abdul-Karim, MD
Univ Hospitals of Cleveland
Dept of Pathology
11100 Euclid Ave
Cleveland, OH 44106
Tel: 216 844-1807 *Fax:* 216 844-1810
Internet: http://www.uhhs.com/to
teach/pathology/index.html
Accred Length: 1 Year *Program Size:* 1
Program ID: 307-38-21-072

Columbus

Ohio State University Program

Sponsor: Ohio State University Medical Center

Program Director:
Sedigheh Keyhani-Rofagha, MD
Ohio State Univ Med Ctr
S-305 Rhodes Hall
410 W 10th Ave
Columbus, OH 43210
Tel: 614 293-3880 *Fax:* 614 293-7273
E-mail: keyhani-1@medctr.osu.edu
Internet: http://www.pathology.med.ohio-state.edu
Accred Length: 1 Year *Program Size:* 1
Program ID: 307-38-31-077

Pennsylvania

Danville

Penn State Geisinger Health System/Geisinger Medical Center Program

Sponsor: Penn State Geisinger Health System
Geisinger Medical Center

Program Director:
Steven C Meschter, MD
Geisinger Med Ctr
100 N Academy Ave
Danville, PA 17822-0131
Tel: 717 271-6338 *Fax:* 717 271-6105
E-mail: smeschter@psghs.edu
Accred Length: 1 Year *Program Size:* 1
Program ID: 307-41-21-059

Philadelphia

MCP Hahnemann University Program

Sponsor: MCP Hahnemann University
Hahnemann University Hospital
Medical College of Pennsylvania Hospital

Program Director:
Lorenzo Galindo, MD
Hahnemann Univ Hospital
Dept of Cytopathology
Broad and Vine Sts/MS 435
Philadelphia, PA 19102
Tel: 215 842-7074 *Fax:* 215 843-0590
Accred Length: 1 Year *Program Size:* 3
Program ID: 307-41-21-028

Thomas Jefferson University Program

Sponsor: Thomas Jefferson University Hospital

Program Director:
Marluce Bibbo, MD
260 A Main Bldg
121 S 10th St
Philadelphia, PA 19107
Tel: 215 955-1197 *Fax:* 215 923-7591
Accred Length: 1 Year *Program Size:* 1
Program ID: 307-41-31-009

University of Pennsylvania Program

Sponsor: Hospital of the University of Pennsylvania

Program Director:
Prabodh K Gupta, MD
Univ of Pennsylvania Med Ctr
6th Fl/Founders Pavilion
3400 Spruce St
Philadelphia, PA 19104-4283
Tel: 215 662-3238 *Fax:* 215 349-8994
E-mail: prabodh_gupta@path1a.med.upenn.edu
Accred Length: 1 Year *Program Size:* 5
Program ID: 307-41-21-004

Pittsburgh

Allegheny General Hospital Program

Sponsor: Allegheny General Hospital

Program Director:
Stephen S Raab, MD
Allegheny General Hospital
Dept of Lab Med
320 E North Ave
Pittsburgh, PA 15212
Tel: 412 359-6886
Accred Length: 1 Year *Program Size:* 1
Program ID: 307-41-21-076

University Health Center of Pittsburgh Program

Sponsor: University Health Center of Pittsburgh
Magee-Women's Hospital
Presbyterian University Hospital/UPMC

Program Director:
Manju Nath, MD
Dept of Pathology
Magee-Women's Hospital
300 Halket St
Pittsburgh, PA 15213
Tel: 412 641-4651 *Fax:* 412 641-1675
E-mail: mnath@mail.magee.edu
Accred Length: 1 Year *Program Size:* 2
Program ID: 307-41-31-049

Wynnewood

Lankenau Hospital Program

Sponsor: Lankenau Hospital

Program Director:
Vaidehi Kannan, MD
Lankenau Hospital
100 Lancaster Ave
Wynnewood, PA 19096
Tel: 610 645-2623 *Fax:* 610 645-8470
Accred Length: 1 Year *Program Size:* 2
Program ID: 307-41-21-010

South Carolina

Charleston

Medical University of South Carolina Program

Sponsor: Medical University of South Carolina College of Medicine

Program Director:
Mary M B Wilson, MD
Div of Cytopathology
165 Ashley Ave/Ste 309
PO Box 250908
Charleston, SC 29425-0555
Tel: 843 792-3121 *Fax:* 843 792-0555
E-mail: wilsonmb@musc.edu
Accred Length: 1 Year *Program Size:* 3
Program ID: 307-45-21-012

Texas

Dallas

University of Texas Southwestern Medical School Program

Sponsor: University of Texas Southwestern Medical School
Dallas County Hospital District-Parkland Memorial Hospital

Program Director:
Raheela Ashfaq, MD
Univ of Texas Southwestern Med Ctr
5323 Harry Hines Blvd
Dallas, TX 75235-9072
Tel: 214 590-8743 *Fax:* 214 590-2721
Internet: http://www.swmed.edu
Accred Length: 1 Year *Program Size:* 1
Program ID: 307-48-21-060

Houston

Baylor College of Medicine Program

Sponsor: Baylor College of Medicine
Harris County Hospital District-Ben Taub General Hospital
Methodist Hospital
Veterans Affairs Medical Center (Houston)

Program Director:
Ibrahim Ramzy, MD
Baylor Coll of Med
Div of Cytopathology
One Baylor Plaza
Houston, TX 77030-3498
Tel: 713 790-4508 *Fax:* 713 793-1603
E-mail: iramzy@bcm.tmc.edu
Internet: http://www.bcm.tmc.edu/pathology
Accred Length: 1 Year *Program Size:* 4
Program ID: 307-48-21-023

University of Texas M D Anderson Cancer Center Program

Sponsor: University of Texas M D Anderson Cancer Center

Program Director:
Gregg Staerkel, MD
Univ of Texas-MD Anderson Cancer Ctr
1515 Holcombe Blvd/Box 53
Houston, TX 77030-4095
Tel: 713 794-5625 *Fax:* 713 794-5664
E-mail: jknight@notes.mdacc.tmc.edu
Accred Length: 1 Year *Program Size:* 5
Program ID: 307-48-21-054

Lackland AFB

San Antonio Uniformed Services Health Education Consortium Program

Sponsor: San Antonio Uniformed Services Health Education Consortium

Program Director:
Prabha H Solanki, MD
2200 Bergquist Dr/Ste 1
Lackland AFB, TX 78236-5300
Tel: 210 292-5507 *Fax:* 210 292-7484
Accred Length: 1 Year *Program Size:* 2
Program ID: 307-48-21-011
US Armed Services Program

San Antonio

University of Texas Health Science Center at San Antonio Program

Sponsor: University of Texas Medical School at San Antonio
Audie L Murphy Memorial Veterans Hospital (San Antonio)
University Hospital-South Texas Medical Center

Program Director:
Philip T Valente, MD
Univ of Texas Health Science Ctr
Dept of Cytopathology
7703 Floyd Curl Dr
San Antonio, TX 78284-7750
Tel: 210 567-4134 *Fax:* 210 567-2478
Internet: http://pathologyweb.uthscsa.edu/residency.html
Accred Length: 1 Year *Program Size:* 1
Program ID: 307-48-11-018

Programs

Vermont

Burlington

University of Vermont Program
Sponsor: Fletcher Allen Health Care
Program Director:
Matthew Zarka, MD
Fletcher Allen Health Care-Univ of Vermont
111 Colchester Ave
Burlington, VT 05401
Tel: 802 656-3921 *Fax:* 802 656-3632
E-mail: matthew.zarka@vtmednet.org
Accred Length: 1 Year *Program Size:* 1
Program ID: 307-50-21-056

Virginia

Charlottesville

University of Virginia Program
Sponsor: University of Virginia Medical Center
Program Director:
Henry F Frierson Jr, MD
Univ of Virginia Health Sciences Ctr
Dept of Pathology
Box 214
Charlottesville, VA 22908
Tel: 804 982-4404 *Fax:* 804 924-8767
E-mail: hff@virginia.edu
Accred Length: 1 Year *Program Size:* 2
Program ID: 307-51-21-069

Richmond

Medical College of Virginia/Virginia Commonwealth University Program
Sponsor: Medical College of Virginia/Virginia Commonwealth University
Medical College of Virginia Hospitals
Program Director:
Celeste N Powers, MD PhD
Med Coll of Virginia, Dept of Pathology
PO Box 980115
Richmond, VA 23298-0115
Tel: 804 828-9738 *Fax:* 804 828-8733
E-mail: powersc@hsc.vcu.edu
Accred Length: 1 Year *Program Size:* 2
Program ID: 307-51-21-055

Wisconsin

Madison

University of Wisconsin Program
Sponsor: University of Wisconsin Hospital and Clinics
Program Director:
Daniel F Kurtycz, BS MD
Univ of Wisconsin
State Laboratory of Hygiene
465 Henry Mall
Madison, WI 53706-1578
Tel: 608 262-1297 *Fax:* 608 265-6294
E-mail: dkurtycz@facstaff.wisc.edu
Internet: http://www.biostat.wisc.edu/path/cyto.html
Accred Length: 1 Year *Program Size:* 1
Program ID: 307-56-21-052

Dermatology

Alabama

Birmingham

University of Alabama Medical Center Program
Sponsor: University of Alabama Hospital
Veterans Affairs Medical Center (Birmingham)
Program Director:
Craig A Elmets, MD
Univ of Alabama Sch of Med, Dept of Dermatology
703 S 19th St/Rm 239
Univ Station SDB-76
Birmingham, AL 35294-0007
Tel: 205 975-6415 *Fax:* 205 934-5766
E-mail: medd011@uabdpo.dpo.uab.edu
Accred Length: 3 Years *Program Size:* 6
Program ID: 080-01-21-010

Arizona

Tucson

University of Arizona Program
Sponsor: University of Arizona College of Medicine
University Medical Center
Veterans Affairs Medical Center (Tucson)
Program Director:
Ronald C Hansen, MD
Univ of Arizona Health Sciences Ctr
1501 N Campbell Ave
PO Box 245038
Tucson, AZ 85724-5038
Tel: 520 626-7783 *Fax:* 520 626-4299
E-mail: pcasilla@u.arizona.edu
Accred Length: 3 Years *Program Size:* 5
Program ID: 080-03-21-012

Arkansas

Little Rock

University of Arkansas for Medical Sciences Program
Sponsor: University of Arkansas College of Medicine
John L McClellan Memorial Veterans Hospital
University Hospital of Arkansas
Program Director:
Thomas D Horn, MD
Univ of Arkansas Coll of Med
4301 W Markham St/Slot 576
Little Rock, AR 72205
Tel: 501 686-5110 *Fax:* 501 686-7264
Accred Length: 3 Years *Program Size:* 7
Program ID: 080-04-21-013

California

Loma Linda

Loma Linda University Program
Sponsor: Loma Linda University Medical Center
Jerry L Pettis Memorial Veterans Hospital
Program Director:
Nancy Anderson, MD
Loma Linda Univ Med Ctr
Dermatology/FMO Ste 2600
11370 Anderson St
Loma Linda, CA 92354
Tel: 909 796-4842 *Fax:* 909 478-6448
Accred Length: 3 Years *Program Size:* 3
Program ID: 080-05-21-111

Los Angeles

Charles R Drew University Program
Sponsor: Charles R Drew University of Medicine and Science
LAC-King/Drew Medical Center
Program Director:
A Paul Kelly, MD
Martin Luther King Jr-Drew Med Ctr
12021 S Wilmington Ave
Rm 4016
Los Angeles, CA 90059
Tel: 310 668-4578 *Fax:* 310 639-3842
E-mail: apkelly@cdrewu.edu
Accred Length: 3 Years *Program Size:* 6
Program ID: 080-05-12-016

UCLA Medical Center Program
Sponsor: UCLA School of Medicine
UCLA Medical Center
VA Greater Los Angeles Healthcare System
Program Director:
Robert L Modlin, MD
UCLA Sch of Med
Div of Dermatology
CHS 52-121
Los Angeles, CA 90095-1750
Tel: 310 825-7375 *Fax:* 310 825-5791
E-mail: troth@medicine.medsch.ucla.edu
Accred Length: 3 Years *Program Size:* 9
Program ID: 080-05-21-017

University of Southern California Program
Sponsor: Los Angeles County-USC Medical Center
Program Director:
Arnold W Gurevitch, MD
Los Angeles County-USC Med Ctr
1200 N State St/Rm 8440
Los Angeles, CA 90033
Tel: 213 226-3373 *Fax:* 213 226-2654
Accred Length: 3 Years *Program Size:* 9
Program ID: 080-05-11-015

Orange

University of California (Irvine) Program
Sponsor: University of California (Irvine) Medical Center
Veterans Affairs Medical Center (Long Beach)
Program Director:
Gary Cole, MD
Dermatology Service (110)
VA Med Ctr
5901 E Seventh St
Long Beach, CA 90822
Tel: 562 494-5458 *Fax:* 562 494-5742
E-mail: gwcole@edu.uci
Internet: http://www.med.uci.edu/~derm/
Accred Length: 3 Years *Program Size:* 9
Subspecialties: DMP
Program ID: 080-05-21-014

Sacramento

University of California (Davis) Program
Sponsor: University of California (Davis) Medical Center
Program Director:
Monica A Lawry, MD
Univ of California Davis
Dept of Dermatology
4860 Y St/Ste 3400
Sacramento, CA 95817
Tel: 916 734-6795 *Fax:* 916 734-6793
Accred Length: 3 Years *Program Size:* 6
Program ID: 080-05-21-101

San Diego

Naval Medical Center (San Diego) Program
Sponsor: Naval Medical Center (San Diego)
Program Director:
Terry L Barrett, MD
Naval Med Ctr
Dept of Dermatology
34800 Bob Wilson Dr
San Diego, CA 92134-5000
Tel: 619 532-9666 *Fax:* 619 532-9458
E-mail: tbarrett@snd10.med.navy.mil
Accred Length: 3 Years *Program Size:* 15
Program ID: 080-05-31-006
US Armed Services Program

University of California (San Diego) Program
Sponsor: University of California (San Diego) Medical Center
Veterans Affairs Medical Center (San Diego)
Program Director:
Constance Nagi, MD
UCSD Med Ctr
Div of Dermatology/8420
200 W Arbor Dr
San Diego, CA 92103-8420
Tel: 619 543-5580 *Fax:* 619 543-2144
Accred Length: 3 Years *Program Size:* 6
Program ID: 080-05-21-018

San Francisco

University of California (San Francisco) Program
Sponsor: University of California (San Francisco) School of Medicine
San Francisco General Hospital Medical Center
University of California (San Francisco) Medical Center
Veterans Affairs Medical Center (San Francisco)
Program Director:
Timothy G Berger, MD
Univ of California San Francisco
Dermatology Units, UCSF Box 0316
1701 Divisadero St/3rd Fl
San Francisco, CA 94143-0316
Tel: 415 353-7879 *Fax:* 415 353-7850
E-mail: tgberger@orca.ucsf.edu
Internet: http://www.dermatology.ucsf.edu
Accred Length: 3 Years *Program Size:* 11
Program ID: 080-05-21-019

Stanford

Stanford University Program
Sponsor: Stanford University Hospital
Santa Clara Valley Medical Center
Veterans Affairs Palo Alto Health Care System
Program Director:
Susan M Swetter, MD
900 Blake Wilbur Dr/Rm W0069
Stanford, CA 94305-5334
Tel: 650 723-7893 *Fax:* 650 723-7796
E-mail: emeea@stanford.edu
Internet: http://www-leland.stanford.edu/dept/derm/
Accred Length: 3 Years *Program Size:* 13
Program ID: 080-05-21-020

Colorado

Denver

University of Colorado Program
Sponsor: University of Colorado Health Sciences Center
Denver Health and Hospitals
Veterans Affairs Medical Center (Denver)
Program Director:
James E Fitzpatrick, MD
Univ of Colorado Health Sciences Ctr
Box B-153
4200 E Ninth Ave
Denver, CO 80262
Tel: 303 315-7738 *Fax:* 303 315-8272
Internet: http://www.uchsc.edu/sm/derma/
Accred Length: 3 Years *Program Size:* 6
Program ID: 080-07-21-022

Connecticut

New Haven

Yale-New Haven Medical Center Program
Sponsor: Yale-New Haven Hospital
Veterans Affairs Medical Center (West Haven)
Program Director:
Jean L Bolognia, MD
Yale Univ
333 Cedar St
New Haven, CT 06520
Tel: 203 785-4092 *Fax:* 203 785-7637
E-mail: donna.carroll@yale.edu
Internet: http://www.info.med.yale.edu.dermatology
Accred Length: 3 Years *Program Size:* 7
Program ID: 080-08-21-023

District of Columbia

Washington

George Washington University Program
Sponsor: George Washington University School of Medicine
George Washington University Hospital (UHS)
Program Director:
Brenda J Berberian, MD
George Washington Univ Hospital Med Ctr
2150 Pennsylvania Ave NW
Ste 6-A
Washington, DC 20037
Tel: 202 994-3093 *Fax:* 202 994-8036
Accred Length: 3 Years *Program Size:* 3
Subspecialties: DMP
Program ID: 080-10-21-024

Howard University Program
Sponsor: Howard University Hospital
Children's National Medical Center
Veterans Affairs Medical Center (Washington, DC)
Program Director:
Rebat M Halder, MD
Howard Univ Hospital
Dept of Dermatology
2041 Georgia Ave NW
Washington, DC 20060-0060
Tel: 202 865-6725 *Fax:* 202 865-1757
Accred Length: 3 Years *Program Size:* 5
Program ID: 080-10-21-025

Washington Hospital Center Program
Sponsor: Washington Hospital Center
Program Director:
Thomas P Nigra, MD
Washington Hospital Ctr
110 Irving St NW/2B-44
Washington, DC 20010-2975
Tel: 202 877-6654 *Fax:* 202 877-3288
Accred Length: 3 Years *Program Size:* 6
Program ID: 080-10-21-106

Florida

Gainesville

University of Florida Program
Sponsor: University of Florida College of Medicine
Shands Hospital at the University of Florida
Veterans Affairs Medical Center (Gainesville)
Program Director:
Franklin P Flowers, MD
Univ of Florida
Div of Dermatology
Box 100277 JHMHC
Gainesville, FL 32610
Tel: 352 392-4984 *Fax:* 352 392-5376
Accred Length: 3 Years *Program Size:* 6
Program ID: 080-11-21-115

Miami

University of Miami-Jackson Memorial Medical Center Program
Sponsor: University of Miami-Jackson Memorial Medical Center
Mount Sinai Medical Center of Greater Miami
Veterans Affairs Medical Center (Miami)
Program Director:
William H Eaglstein, MD
Univ of Miami Sch of Med
Dept of Dermatology
PO Box 016250 (R-250)
Miami, FL 33101-6250
Tel: 305 243-6734 *Fax:* 305 243-6191
Accred Length: 3 Years *Program Size:* 20
Subspecialties: DMP
Program ID: 080-11-21-026

Tampa

University of South Florida Program

Sponsor: University of South Florida College of Medicine
H Lee Moffitt Cancer Center
James A Haley Veterans Hospital
Tampa General Healthcare
Veterans Affairs Medical Center (Bay Pines)

Program Director:
Neil A Fenske, MD
Univ of South Florida Coll of Med
12901 Bruce B Downs Blvd (MDC 19)
Tampa, FL 33612-4799
Tel: 813 974-2854 *Fax:* 813 974-4272
E-mail: blane@com1.med.usf.edu
Accred Length: 3 Years *Program Size:* 9
Program ID: 080-11-21-096

Georgia

Atlanta

Emory University Program

Sponsor: Emory University School of Medicine
Emory University Hospital
Grady Memorial Hospital
Veterans Affairs Medical Center (Atlanta)

Program Director:
Cheryl A Armstrong, MD
Emory Univ Sch of Med
Dept of Dermatology
5001 Woodruff Memorial Bldg
Atlanta, GA 30322
Tel: 404 727-5872 *Fax:* 404 727-5878
Accred Length: 3 Years *Program Size:* 13
Program ID: 080-12-21-028

Augusta

Medical College of Georgia Program

Sponsor: Medical College of Georgia Hospital and Clinics
Veterans Affairs Medical Center (Augusta)

Program Director:
Jack L Lesher Jr, MD
Med Coll of Georgia, Sect of Dermatology
1004 Chafee Ave
Augusta, GA 30912
Tel: 706 721-6231 *Fax:* 706 721-6220
E-mail: jlesher@mail.mcg.edu
Internet: http://www.jlesher@mail.mcg.edu
Accred Length: 3 Years *Program Size:* 8
Program ID: 080-12-11-029

Illinois

Chicago

Cook County Hospital Program

Sponsor: Cook County Hospital

Program Director:
Darryl M Bronson, MD
Cook County Hospital
Administration Bldg/Rm 519
1900 W Polk St
Chicago, IL 60612-9985
Tel: 312 633-8734 *Fax:* 312 633-3347
Accred Length: 3 Years *Program Size:* 9
Program ID: 080-16-12-030

McGaw Medical Center of Northwestern University Program

Sponsor: Northwestern University Medical School
Children's Memorial Medical Center
Northwestern Memorial Hospital
Veterans Affairs Lakeside Medical Center (Chicago)

Program Director:
Brian Cook, MD MBA
Dept of Dermatology
303 E Chicago Ave
Chicago, IL 60611
Tel: 312 908-8173 *Fax:* 312 908-0664
Accred Length: 3 Years *Program Size:* 3
Program ID: 080-16-21-031

Rush-Presbyterian-St Luke's Medical Center Program

Sponsor: Rush-Presbyterian-St Luke's Medical Center

Program Director:
Michael D Tharp, MD
Rush-Presbyterian-St Luke's Med Ctr
Dept of Dermatology
1653 W Congress Pkwy
Chicago, IL 60612-3865
Tel: 312 942-6096 *Fax:* 312 942-7778
E-mail: derm@rush.edu
Accred Length: 3 Years *Program Size:* 4
Program ID: 080-16-11-032

University of Chicago Program

Sponsor: University of Chicago Hospitals

Program Director:
James C Shaw, MD
Sect of Dermatology
MC5067
5841 S Maryland Ave
Chicago, IL 60637-1470
Tel: 773 702-6559 *Fax:* 773 702-8398
Accred Length: 3 Years *Program Size:* 6
Program ID: 080-16-11-033

University of Illinois College of Medicine at Chicago Program

Sponsor: University of Illinois College of Medicine at Chicago
Edward J Hines Jr Veterans Affairs Hospital
University of Illinois Hospital and Clinics
Veterans Affairs West Side Medical Center

Program Director:
Virginia C Fiedler, MD
Univ of Illinois-Chicago
808 S Wood St (M/C 624)
Chicago, IL 60612-7307
Tel: 312 996-6966 *Fax:* 312 996-1188
E-mail: vfiedler@uic.edu
Internet: http://www.uic.edu/depts/mcde/derm.html
Accred Length: 3 Years *Program Size:* 9
Program ID: 080-16-21-034

Springfield

Southern Illinois University Program

Sponsor: Southern Illinois University School of Medicine
Memorial Medical Center
St John's Hospital

Program Director:
Lucinda S Buescher, MD
Southern Illinois Univ Sch of Med
PO Box 19230
Springfield, IL 62794-1414
Tel: 217 785-3821, ext 2110 *Fax:* 217 524-4485
E-mail: jhicks@siumed.edu
Accred Length: 3 Years *Program Size:* 6
Program ID: 080-16-21-118

Indiana

Indianapolis

Indiana University School of Medicine Program

Sponsor: Indiana University School of Medicine
Clarian IU Hospital
Clarian Riley Hospital for Children
Richard L Roudebush Veterans Affairs Medical Center
William N Wishard Memorial Hospital

Program Director:
Evan R Farmer, MD
Indiana Univ Med Ctr
550 N University Blvd/Ste 3240
Indianapolis, IN 46202-5267
Tel: 317 274-7741 *Fax:* 317 274-7051
E-mail: efarmer@iupui.edu
Internet: http://www.iupui.edu/it/derm/tocderm.html
Accred Length: 3 Years *Program Size:* 6
Program ID: 080-17-21-035

Iowa

Iowa City

University of Iowa Hospitals and Clinics Program

Sponsor: University of Iowa Hospitals and Clinics

Program Director:
Richard D Sontheimer, MD
Univ of Iowa Hospitals and Clinics
BT-2045-1
200 Hawkins Dr
Iowa City, IA 52242-1090
Tel: 319 356-3609 *Fax:* 319 356-8317
Internet: http://tray.dermatology.uiowa.edu/home.html
Accred Length: 3 Years *Program Size:* 13
Program ID: 080-18-21-036

Kansas

Kansas City

University of Kansas Medical Center Program

Sponsor: University of Kansas School of Medicine
University of Kansas Medical Center

Program Director:
Donald V Belsito, MD
Univ of Kansas Med Ctr
Dermatology Div
3901 Rainbow Blvd
Kansas City, KS 66160-7319
Tel: 913 588-3840 *Fax:* 913 588-4060
E-mail: cboxmeyer@kumc.edu
Internet: http://eagle.cc.ukans.edu/~kvo038/index.htm
Accred Length: 3 Years *Program Size:* 6
Program ID: 080-19-11-037

Kentucky

Louisville

University of Louisville Program

Sponsor: University of Louisville School of Medicine
University of Louisville Hospital
Veterans Affairs Medical Center (Louisville)

Program Director:
Jeffrey P Callen, MD
Univ of Louisville Health Science Ctr
Div of Dermatology
310 E Broadway
Louisville, KY 40292
Tel: 502 852-7287 *Fax:* 502 583-3028
E-mail: jpcall01@ulkyvm.louisville.edu
Accred Length: 3 Years *Program Size:* 6
Program ID: 080-20-21-038

Louisiana

New Orleans

Louisiana State University Program

Sponsor: Louisiana State University School of Medicine
Medical Center of Louisiana at New Orleans
Overton Brooks Veterans Affairs Medical Center

Program Director:
Lee T Nesbitt Jr, MD
Louisiana State Univ Sch of Med
1542 Tulane Ave/Rm 634
New Orleans, LA 70112-2822
Tel: 504 568-7110 *Fax:* 504 568-2170
E-mail: lnesbi@lsumc.edu
Internet:
http://www.medschool.lsumc.edu/departments/asp/derm.asp
Accred Length: 3 Years *Program Size:* 15
Program ID: 080-21-21-109

Tulane University Program

Sponsor: Tulane University School of Medicine
Medical Center of Louisiana at New Orleans
Tulane University Hospital and Clinics

Program Director:
Larry E Millikan, MD
Tulane Univ Med Ctr
1430 Tulane Ave/SL-73
New Orleans, LA 70112-2699
Tel: 504 588-5114 *Fax:* 504 587-7382
E-mail: larry.millikan@tulane.edu
Internet:
http://www.mcl.tulane.edu/departments/dermatology/dermatology.html
Accred Length: 3 Years *Program Size:* 11
Program ID: 080-21-21-108

Maryland

Baltimore

Johns Hopkins University Program

Sponsor: Johns Hopkins University School of Medicine
Johns Hopkins Bayview Medical Center
Johns Hopkins Hospital

Program Director:
Francisco Tausk, MD
Johns Hopkins Med Institutions-JHOC
601 N Caroline St/Rm 6062
Baltimore, MD 21287-0900
Tel: 410 614-4198 *Fax:* 410 955-0123
E-mail: ftausk@welchlink.welch.jhu.edu
Accred Length: 3 Years *Program Size:* 8
Program ID: 080-23-21-040

University of Maryland Program

Sponsor: University of Maryland Medical System
Veterans Affairs Medical Center (Baltimore)

Program Director:
Mark H Lowitt, MD
Univ of Maryland Med System
405 W Redwood St/6th Fl
Baltimore, MD 21201
Tel: 410 328-5766 *Fax:* 410 328-0098
E-mail: mlowitt@umaryland.edu
Internet: http://som1.ab.umd.edu/smderm/
Accred Length: 3 Years *Program Size:* 4
Program ID: 080-23-21-041

Bethesda

National Capital Consortium Program

Sponsor: National Capital Consortium
National Naval Medical Center (Bethesda)
Walter Reed Army Medical Center

Program Director:
Paul M Benson, MD
Walter Reed Army Med Ctr
Dermatology Service/Rm 1J
Washington, DC 20307-5001
Tel: 202 782-9484 *Fax:* 202 782-9118
Accred Length: 3 Years *Program Size:* 15
Program ID: 080-10-21-123
US Armed Services Program

National Institutes of Health Clinical Center Program

Sponsor: NIH Warren Grant Magnuson Clinical Center

Program Director:
Stephen I Katz, MD PhD
Bldg 10/Rm 12N238
10 Center Dr/MSC 1908
Bethesda, MD 20892
Tel: 301 496-2481 *Fax:* 301 496-5370
Accred Length: 1 Year *Program Size:* 4
Program ID: 080-23-12-008

Massachusetts

Boston

Boston University Medical Center/Tufts University Program

Sponsor: Boston Medical Center
New England Medical Center Hospitals
Veterans Affairs Medical Center (Boston)

Program Director:
Barbara A Gilchrest, MD
David S Feingold, MD
Boston Univ Sch of Med
Dept of Dermatology/J-100
715 Albany St
Boston, MA 02118
Tel: 617 638-5500, ext 5538 *Fax:* 617 638-5515
Accred Length: 3 Years *Program Size:* 15
Program ID: 080-24-21-044

Harvard Medical School Program

Sponsor: Massachusetts General Hospital
Beth Israel Deaconess Medical Center
Brigham and Women's Hospital
Cambridge Hospital/Cambridge Health Alliance
Children's Hospital
Lahey Clinic

Program Director:
John A Parrish, MD
Massachusetts General Hospital
Dept of Dermatology
55 Fruit St/Wel-224
Boston, MA 02114
Tel: 617 726-1684 *Fax:* 617 724-9595
E-mail: kovacevd@ai.mgh.harvard.edu
Accred Length: 3 Years *Program Size:* 15
Program ID: 080-24-31-043

Worcester

University of Massachusetts Program

Sponsor: University of Massachusetts Medical School
UMass Memorial Health Care (University Campus)

Program Director:
Thomas G Cropley, MD
Univ of Massachusetts Med Ctr
Div of Dermatology
55 Lake Ave N
Worcester, MA 01655
Tel: 508 856-2156 *Fax:* 508 856-2085
Accred Length: 3 Years *Program Size:* 3
Program ID: 080-24-21-114

Michigan

Ann Arbor

University of Michigan Program

Sponsor: University of Michigan Hospitals
Veterans Affairs Medical Center (Ann Arbor)

Program Director:
Charles N Ellis, MD
Univ of Michigan Med Ctr
Dermatology Residency
1500 E Medical Center Dr/1910 TC
Ann Arbor, MI 48109-0314
Tel: 734 936-6674 *Fax:* 734 936-6395
E-mail: res-appl@mailgw.derm.med.umich.edu
Internet: http://www.med.umich.edu/derm
Accred Length: 3 Years *Program Size:* 16
Program ID: 080-25-31-045

Detroit

Henry Ford Hospital Program

Sponsor: Henry Ford Hospital

Program Director:
Henry W Lim, MD
Henry Ford Hospital
Dept of Dermatology
2799 W Grand Blvd
Detroit, MI 48202
Tel: 313 916-2960 *Fax:* 313 916-2093
E-mail: hlm1@hfhs.or9
Accred Length: 3 Years *Program Size:* 18
Program ID: 080-25-12-046

Wayne State University/Detroit Medical Center Program

Sponsor: Wayne State University/Detroit Medical Center
Children's Hospital of Michigan
Detroit Receiving Hospital and University Health Center
Harper Hospital
Veterans Affairs Medical Center (Detroit)

Program Director:
Ken Hashimoto, MD
Wayne State Univ-Detroit Med Ctr
4201 St Antoine
5E Univ Health Ctr
Detroit, MI 48201
Tel: 313 577-5061 *Fax:* 313 577-8866
Accred Length: 3 Years *Program Size:* 10
Program ID: 080-25-21-047

Minnesota

Minneapolis

University of Minnesota Program

Sponsor: University of Minnesota Medical School
Fairview-University Medical Center
Hennepin County Medical Center
Regions Hospital
Veterans Affairs Medical Center (Minneapolis)

Program Director:
Whitney D Tope, MD
Univ of Minnesota
Dept of Dermatology, Mayo Box 284
420 Delaware St SE
Minneapolis, MN 55455
Tel: 612 626-2419 *Fax:* 612 625-3238
E-mail: ehre0001@tc.umn.edu
Internet: http://www.dept.med.umn.edu/dermatology
Accred Length: 3 Years *Program Size:* 15
Program ID: 080-26-31-048

Rochester

Mayo Graduate School of Medicine (Rochester) Program

Sponsor: Mayo Graduate School of Medicine-Mayo Foundation
Mayo Clinic (Rochester)
Rochester Methodist Hospital
St Mary's Hospital of Rochester

Program Director:
Arnold L Schroeter, MD
Mayo Graduate Sch of Med
Application Processing Ctr
Siebens 5th Fl
Rochester, MN 55905
Tel: 507 284-3108 *Fax:* 507 284-0999
E-mail: mgsm.medlab.specialties@mayo.edu
Internet: http://www.mayo.edu/
Accred Length: 3 Years *Program Size:* 18
Program ID: 080-26-21-049

Missouri

Columbia

University of Missouri-Columbia Program

Sponsor: University of Missouri-Columbia School of Medicine
Harry S Truman Memorial Veterans Hospital
University Hospitals and Clinics

Program Director:
Karen E Zanol, MD
Univ of Missouri-Columbia
One Hospital Dr
Rm M173 HSC
Columbia, MO 65212
Tel: 573 882-8578 *Fax:* 573 884-5947
E-mail: karen_zanol@mailsvr.hsc.missouri.edu
Internet:
http://www.hsc.missouri.edu/internal_medicine/
Accred Length: 3 Years *Program Size:* 8
Program ID: 080-28-21-050

St Louis

St Louis University School of Medicine Program

Sponsor: St Louis University School of Medicine
St Louis University School of Medicine

Program Director:
George T Nahass, MD
St Louis Univ Sch of Med
Dept of Dermatology
1402 S Grand Blvd
St Louis, MO 63104
Tel: 314 268-5215 *Fax:* 314 268-5131
E-mail: nahassgt@wpogate.slu.edu
Accred Length: 3 Years *Program Size:* 6
Program ID: 080-28-21-116

Washington University/B-JH/SLCH Consortium Program

Sponsor: Washington University/B-JH/SLCH Consortium
Barnes-Jewish Hospital

Program Director:
Arthur Z Eisen, MD
Washington Univ Sch of Med
Div of Dermatology
660 S Euclid Ave/Box 8123
St Louis, MO 63110
Tel: 314 362-8180
Internet: http://www.dermatology.wustl.edu
Accred Length: 3 Years *Program Size:* 15
Program ID: 080-28-21-051

New Hampshire

Lebanon

Dartmouth-Hitchcock Medical Center Program

Sponsor: Mary Hitchcock Memorial Hospital
Veterans Affairs Medical Center (White River Junction)

Program Director:
Daniel W Collison, MD
Dartmouth-Hitchcock Med Ctr
One Medical Center Dr
Lebanon, NH 03756
Tel: 603 650-5180 *Fax:* 603 650-6499
E-mail: dhmcderm@dartmouth.edu
Internet: http://www.hitchcock.org
Accred Length: 3 Years *Program Size:* 6
Program ID: 080-32-21-053

New Jersey

Camden

UMDNJ-Robert Wood Johnson Medical School Program

Sponsor: Cooper Hospital-University Medical Center

Program Director:
Warren R Heymann, MD
Cooper Hospital-Univ Med Ctr
Div of Dermatology
3 Cooper Plaza/Ste 220
Camden, NJ 08103
Tel: 609 342-2014 *Fax:* 609 966-0735
Accred Length: 3 Years *Program Size:* 3
Program ID: 080-33-21-117

Newark

UMDNJ-New Jersey Medical School Program

Sponsor: UMDNJ-New Jersey Medical School
UMDNJ-University Hospital
Veterans Affairs Medical Center (East Orange)

Program Director:
Robert A Schwartz, MD MPH
UMDNJ-New Jersey Med Sch
185 S Orange Ave
Newark, NJ 07103-2714
Tel: 973 972-6255 *Fax:* 973 972-7092
Accred Length: 3 Years *Program Size:* 5
Program ID: 080-33-21-107

New Mexico

Albuquerque

University of New Mexico Program

Sponsor: University of New Mexico School of Medicine
University Hospital
Veterans Affairs Medical Center (Albuquerque)

Program Director:
R Steven Padilla, MD
Univ of New Mexico Sch of Med
4775 Indian School Rd NE/Ste 100
Albuquerque, NM 87110
Tel: 505 272-6000 *Fax:* 505 272-6003
E-mail: kwerblow@salud.unm.edu
Accred Length: 3 Years *Program Size:* 4
Program ID: 080-34-21-054

New York

Albany

Albany Medical Center Program

Sponsor: Albany Medical Center

Program Director:
George Murakawa, MD PhD
Albany Med Coll
Div of Dermatology/MC-7
47 New Scotland Ave
Albany, NY 12208
Tel: 518 262-6252 *Fax:* 518 262-6251
E-mail: bj_best@ccgateway.amc.edu
Accred Length: 3 Years *Program Size:* 4
Subspecialties: DMP
Program ID: 080-35-31-119

Bronx

Albert Einstein College of Medicine Program
Sponsor: Albert Einstein College of Medicine of Yeshiva University
Beth Israel Medical Center
Jacobi Medical Center
Montefiore Medical Center-Henry and Lucy Moses Division
Montefiore Medical Center-Weiler Hospital

Program Director:
Michael Fisher, MD
1300 Morris Park Ave
Bronx, NY 10461
Tel: 718 918-4273 *Fax:* 718 918-7158
Accred Length: 3 Years *Program Size:* 11
Program ID: 080-35-31-058

Brooklyn

SUNY Health Science Center at Brooklyn Program
Sponsor: SUNY Health Science Center at Brooklyn
Kings County Hospital Center
University Hospital-SUNY Health Science Center at Brooklyn
Veterans Affairs Medical Center (Brooklyn)

Program Director:
Alan R Shalita, MD
SUNY Health Science Ctr-Brooklyn
450 Clarkson Ave/Box 46
Brooklyn, NY 11203
Tel: 718 270-1229 *Fax:* 718 270-2794
Accred Length: 3 Years *Program Size:* 13
Program ID: 080-35-21-065

Buffalo

SUNY at Buffalo Graduate Medical-Dental Education Consortium Program
Sponsor: SUNY at Buffalo Grad Medical-Dental Education Consortium
CGF Health System (Buffalo General Hospital)
CGF Health System (Children's Hospital of Buffalo)
Erie County Medical Center
Roswell Park Cancer Institute
Veterans Affairs Medical Center (Buffalo)

Program Director:
Stephanie H Pincus, MD
SUNY-Buffalo
100 High St/Ste C319
Buffalo, NY 14203
Tel: 716 859-1566 *Fax:* 716 859-1569
Accred Length: 3 Years *Program Size:* 7
Program ID: 080-35-21-057

New York

Mount Sinai School of Medicine Program
Sponsor: Mount Sinai School of Medicine
Elmhurst Hospital Center-Mount Sinai Services
Mount Sinai Medical Center
Veterans Affairs Medical Center (Bronx)

Program Director:
Mark Lebwohl, MD
Mount Sinai Med Ctr
One Gustave Levy Pl/Box 1047
New York, NY 10029-6594
Tel: 212 824-7130 *Fax:* 212 348-7434
E-mail: gay_megherian@smtplink.mssm.edu
Accred Length: 3 Years *Program Size:* 8
Subspecialties: DMP
Program ID: 080-35-21-061

New York and Presbyterian Hospital (Columbia Campus) Program
Sponsor: New York and Presbyterian Hospital
New York and Presbyterian Hospital (Columbia Campus)

Program Director:
David R Bickers, MD
New York Presbyterian Hospital (Columbia Campus)
161 Ft Washington Ave
New York, NY 10032
Tel: 212 305-5317 *Fax:* 212 305-4571
Accred Length: 3 Years *Program Size:* 8
Program ID: 080-35-21-104

New York and Presbyterian Hospital (Cornell Campus) Program
Sponsor: New York and Presbyterian Hospital
Lincoln Medical and Mental Health Center
New York and Presbyterian Hospital (Cornell Campus)

Program Director:
Richard D Granstein, MD
New York Hospital-Cornell Med Ctr
525 E 68th St/Rm F-340
New York, NY 10021
Tel: 212 746-7274 *Fax:* 212 746-8656
E-mail: rdgranst@mail.med.cornell.edu
Accred Length: 3 Years *Program Size:* 12
Program ID: 080-35-21-062

New York University Medical Center Program
Sponsor: New York University Medical Center
Bellevue Hospital Center
Veterans Affairs Medical Center (Manhattan)

Program Director:
Irwin M Freedberg, MD
New York Univ Med Ctr
550 First Ave
New York, NY 10016
Tel: 212 263-5245 *Fax:* 212 263-8752
E-mail: irwin.freedberg@med.nyu.edu
Internet: http://www.med.nyu.edu/derm/homepage.htm
Accred Length: 3 Years *Program Size:* 19
Program ID: 080-35-21-064

St Luke's - Roosevelt Hospital Center Program
Sponsor: St Luke's-Roosevelt Hospital Center
St Luke's-Roosevelt Hospital Center-Roosevelt Division
St Luke's-Roosevelt Hospital Center-St Luke's Division

Program Director:
Vincent A Deleo, MD
St Luke's Roosevelt Hospital Ctr
1090 Amsterdam Ave
Ste 11B
New York, NY 10025
Tel: 212 388-3814 *Fax:* 212 388-3808
Accred Length: 3 Years *Program Size:* 5
Program ID: 080-35-21-124

Rochester

University of Rochester Program
Sponsor: Strong Memorial Hospital of the University of Rochester

Program Director:
Marc D Brown, MD
Univ of Rochester Med Ctr
601 Elmwood Ave
Rochester, NY 14642
Tel: 716 275-0193 *Fax:* 716 461-3509
E-mail: marylou_williams@urmc.rochester.edu
Internet: http://www.urmc.rochester.edu/smp/derm
Accred Length: 3 Years *Program Size:* 6
Program ID: 080-35-21-102

Stony Brook

SUNY at Stony Brook Program
Sponsor: University Hospital-SUNY at Stony Brook
Veterans Affairs Medical Center (Northport)

Program Director:
Richard A Clark, MD
SUNY-Stony Brook
Dept of Dermatology
Health Science Ctr/T-16-060
Stony Brook, NY 11794-8165
Tel: 516 444-3843 *Fax:* 516 444-3844
Accred Length: 3 Years *Program Size:* 6
Program ID: 080-35-21-113

Valhalla

New York Medical College at Westchester Medical Center Program
Sponsor: New York Medical College
Bayley Seton Hospital
Lincoln Medical and Mental Health Center
Metropolitan Hospital Center
Our Lady of Mercy Medical Center
Westchester Medical Center

Program Director:
Bijan Safai, MD
New York Med Coll
Dept of Dermatology
Vosburgh Pavillion/Rm 217
Valhalla, NY 10595-8110
Tel: 914 594-4566 *Fax:* 914 594-4019
E-mail: safai@aol.com
Accred Length: 3 Years *Program Size:* 11
Program ID: 080-35-21-063

North Carolina

Chapel Hill

University of North Carolina Hospitals Program
Sponsor: University of North Carolina Hospitals

Program Director:
Robert A Briggaman, MD
Univ of North Carolina Sch of Med
Dept of Dermatology/CB7287
Ste 3100 Thurston-Bowles Bldgs
Chapel Hill, NC 27599-7287
Tel: 919 966-0785 *Fax:* 919 966-3898
E-mail: mjowebb@med.unc.edu
Internet: http://www.med.unc.edu/derm/
Accred Length: 3 Years *Program Size:* 10
Program ID: 080-36-11-066

Durham

Duke University Program
Sponsor: Duke University Medical Center
Veterans Affairs Medical Center (Durham)

Program Director:
Sarah Myers, MD
Duke Univ Med Ctr
PO Box 3852
Durham, NC 27710
Tel: 919 684-6185 *Fax:* 919 681-8073
E-mail: myers011@mc.duke.edu
Accred Length: 3 Years *Program Size:* 10
Program ID: 080-36-21-067

Winston-Salem

Wake Forest University School of Medicine Program
Sponsor: Wake Forest University Baptist Medical Center
Program Director:
Joseph L Jorizzo, MD
Wake Forest Univ Sch of Med
Dept of Dermatology
Medical Center Blvd
Winston-Salem, NC 27157-1071
Tel: 910 716-2768 *Fax:* 910 716-7732
E-mail: jjorizzo@wfubmc.edu
Accred Length: 3 Years *Program Size:* 9
Program ID: 080-36-21-110

Ohio

Cincinnati

University Hospital/University of Cincinnati College of Medicine Program
Sponsor: University Hospital Inc
Program Director:
Diya Mutasim, MD
Dept of Dermatology
Univ of Cincinnati Coll of Med
PO Box 670592
Cincinnati, OH 45267-0592
Tel: 513 558-6242 *Fax:* 513 558-0198
E-mail: griggsjm@email.uc.edu
Internet:
http://www.med.uc.edu/dermatology/dermatol.htm
Accred Length: 3 Years *Program Size:* 9 (*GY1:* 2)
Program ID: 080-38-21-068

Cleveland

Case Western Reserve University Program
Sponsor: University Hospitals of Cleveland
MetroHealth Medical Center
Veterans Affairs Medical Center (Cleveland)
Program Director:
Bryan R Davis, MD
11100 Euclid Ave
Cleveland, OH 44106
Tel: 216 844-5794 *Fax:* 216 844-8993
Internet:
http://www.uhhs.com/toteach/dermatology/training.html
Accred Length: 3 Years *Program Size:* 12
Program ID: 080-38-21-120

Cleveland Clinic Foundation Program
Sponsor: Cleveland Clinic Foundation
Program Director:
Charles Camisa, MD
Cleveland Clinic Foundation
Dept of Dermatology/A61
9500 Euclid Ave
Cleveland, OH 44195-5242
Tel: 216 444-5690 *Fax:* 216 444-1162
E-mail: meded@cestmp.ccf.org
Internet: http://www.ccf.org
Accred Length: 4 Years *Program Size:* 13 (*GY1:* 3)
Program ID: 080-38-12-070

Columbus

Ohio State University Program
Sponsor: Ohio State University Medical Center
Program Director:
Arthur E Pellegrini, MD
Ohio State Univ
4731 Univ Hospitals Clinic
456 W Tenth Ave
Columbus, OH 43210-1282
Tel: 614 293-8111 *Fax:* 614 293-8090
Accred Length: 3 Years *Program Size:* 6
Program ID: 080-38-11-072

Dayton

Wright State University Program
Sponsor: Wright State University School of Medicine
Children's Medical Center
Franciscan Medical Center-Dayton Campus
Veterans Affairs Medical Center (Dayton)
Wright-Patterson Medical Center
Program Director:
Julian J Trevino, MD
Wright State Univ Sch of Med
Sect of Dermatology
PO Box 927
Dayton, OH 45401-0927
Tel: 937 262-0214 *Fax:* 937 262-0211
Internet:
http://www.med.wright.edu/som/academic/dermlgy.html
Accred Length: 3 Years *Program Size:* 6
Program ID: 080-38-21-073

Oklahoma

Oklahoma City

University of Oklahoma Health Sciences Center Program
Sponsor: University of Oklahoma College of Medicine
Children's Hospital of Oklahoma
University Hospital
Veterans Affairs Medical Center (Oklahoma City)
Program Director:
Dennis A Weigand, MD
Univ of Oklahoma Health Sciences Ctr
619 NE 13th St
Oklahoma City, OK 73104
Tel: 405 271-6600 *Fax:* 405 236-5618
E-mail: warren-churchill@ouhsc.edu
Accred Length: 3 Years *Program Size:* 6
Program ID: 080-39-21-074

Oregon

Portland

Oregon Health Sciences University Program
Sponsor: Oregon Health Sciences University Hospital
Veterans Affairs Medical Center (Portland)
Program Director:
Neil Swanson, MD
Oregon Health Sciences Univ
3181 SW Sam Jackson Park Rd
Mail Stop L-468
Portland, OR 97201-3098
Tel: 503 494-1375 *Fax:* 503 494-8513
E-mail: dermatol@ohsu.edu
Accred Length: 3 Years *Program Size:* 9
Program ID: 080-40-21-075

Pennsylvania

Danville

Penn State Geisinger Health System/Geisinger Medical Center Program
Sponsor: Penn State Geisinger Health System
Geisinger Medical Center
Program Director:
Michele S Maroon, MD
Geisinger Med Ctr
Dept of Dermatology
100 N Academy Ave
Danville, PA 17822
Tel: 717 271-8010
E-mail: ckrebs@psghs.edu
Accred Length: 3 Years *Program Size:* 6
Program ID: 080-41-12-076

Hershey

Penn State Geisinger Health System/Milton S Hershey Medical Center Program
Sponsor: Penn State Geisinger Health System
Milton S Hershey Medical Center
Program Director:
James G Marks Jr, MD
Milton S Hershey Med Ctr
500 University Dr/PO Box 850
Sect of Dermatology HU14
Hershey, PA 17033-0850
Tel: 717 531-8307 *Fax:* 717 531-6516
E-mail: jmarks@med.hmc.psghs.edu
Internet: http://www.hmc.psu.edu.derm
Accred Length: 3 Years *Program Size:* 6
Program ID: 080-41-21-103

Philadelphia

MCP Hahnemann University Program
Sponsor: MCP Hahnemann University
Hahnemann University Hospital
Program Director:
Gary R Kantor, MD
Hahnemann Univ Hospital
Dept of Dermatology/MS401
Broad and Vine Sts
Philadelphia, PA 19102-1192
Tel: 215 762-8252 *Fax:* 215 299-5178
Accred Length: 3 Years *Program Size:* 9
Subspecialties: DMP
Program ID: 080-41-21-077

Thomas Jefferson University Program
Sponsor: Thomas Jefferson University Hospital
Program Director:
Jouni Uitto, MD PhD
Jefferson Med Coll
Bluemle Life Sciences Bldg/Ste 450
233 S 10th St
Philadelphia, PA 19107
Tel: 215 503-5785 *Fax:* 215 503-5788
E-mail: jouni.uitto@mail.tju.edu
Accred Length: 3 Years *Program Size:* 11
Program ID: 080-41-11-079

University of Pennsylvania Program
Sponsor: Hospital of the University of Pennsylvania
Children's Hospital of Philadelphia
Graduate Hospital
Pennsylvania Hospital (UPHS)
Veterans Affairs Medical Center (Philadelphia)
Program Director:
William D James, MD
Hospital of Univ of Pennsylvania
211B Clinical Research Bldg
415 Curie Blvd
Philadelphia, PA 19104-4283
Tel: 215 898-3240 *Fax:* 215 573-2033
E-mail: hookerj@mail.med.upenn.edu
Internet: http://www.med.upenn.edu/dermatol/
Accred Length: 3 Years *Program Size:* 10
Program ID: 080-41-21-080

Pittsburgh

University Health Center of Pittsburgh Program
Sponsor: University Health Center of Pittsburgh
Children's Hospital of Pittsburgh
Presbyterian University Hospital/UPMC
Veterans Affairs Medical Center (Pittsburgh)
Program Director:
Brian V Jegasothy, MD
Univ Dermatology Assoc
3601 Fifth Ave
Pittsburgh, PA 15213
Tel: 412 648-3250 *Fax:* 412 648-8117
Accred Length: 3 Years *Program Size:* 9
Program ID: 080-41-11-081

Puerto Rico

San Juan

University of Puerto Rico Program
Sponsor: University of Puerto Rico School of Medicine
San Juan City Hospital
University Hospital
Program Director:
Jorge L Sanchez, MD
Univ of Puerto Rico Med Sciences Campus
Dept of Dermatology
PO Box 365067
San Juan, PR 00936-5067
Tel: 787 765-7950 *Fax:* 787 767-0467
E-mail: rcm_dermatol@rcmac.upr.clu.edu
Accred Length: 3 Years *Program Size:* 6
Program ID: 080-42-21-082

Rhode Island

Providence

Brown University Program
Sponsor: Rhode Island Hospital
Memorial Hospital of Rhode Island
Veterans Affairs Medical Center (Providence)
Program Director:
Charles J McDonald, MD
Rhode Island Hospital
APC Bldg 10th Fl
593 Eddy St
Providence, RI 02903
Tel: 401 444-7816 *Fax:* 401 444-7105
Internet:
http://www.biomedcs.biomed.brown.edu/dermatology/
brownderm_home_page.html
Accred Length: 3 Years *Program Size:* 10
Program ID: 080-43-21-122

Roger Williams Medical Center Program
Sponsor: Roger Williams Medical Center
Veterans Affairs Medical Center (Providence)
Program Director:
Vincent Falanga, MD
Roger Williams Med Ctr
825 Chalkstone Ave
Providence, RI 02908
Tel: 401 456-2033 *Fax:* 401 456-6719
Accred Length: 3 Years *Program Size:* 6
Program ID: 080-43-21-083

South Carolina

Charleston

Medical University of South Carolina Program
Sponsor: Medical University of South Carolina College of Medicine
MUSC Medical Center
Ralph H Johnson Dept of Veterans Affairs Med Center
Program Director:
John C Maize, MD
Med Univ of South Carolina
171 Ashley Ave
Charleston, SC 29425-2215
Tel: 843 792-5858 *Fax:* 843 792-9157
E-mail: maizejc@musc.edu
Accred Length: 3 Years *Program Size:* 7
Program ID: 080-45-21-099

Tennessee

Memphis

University of Tennessee Program
Sponsor: University of Tennessee College of Medicine
Baptist Memorial Hospital
Regional Medical Center at Memphis
University of Tennessee Medical Center (UT Bowld Hospital)
Veterans Affairs Medical Center (Memphis)
Program Director:
E William Rosenberg, MD
Univ of Tennessee
956 Court Ave/Rm E332
Memphis, TN 38163
Tel: 901 448-5795 *Fax:* 901 448-8284
Accred Length: 3 Years *Program Size:* 6
Program ID: 080-47-21-084

Nashville

Vanderbilt University Program
Sponsor: Vanderbilt University Medical Center
Metropolitan Nashville General Hospital
St Thomas Hospital
Veterans Affairs Medical Center (Nashville)
Program Director:
Lloyd E King Jr, MD PhD
Vanderbilt Univ Sch of Med
3900 Vanderbilt Clinic
22nd Ave S
Nashville, TN 37232-5227
Tel: 615 343-3958 *Fax:* 615 343-3947
E-mail: lloyd.king@mcmail.vanderbilt.edu
Accred Length: 3 Years *Program Size:* 8
Program ID: 080-47-21-098

Texas

Dallas

University of Texas Southwestern Medical School Program
Sponsor: University of Texas Southwestern Medical School
Children's Medical Center of Dallas
Dallas County Hospital District-Parkland Memorial Hospital
Veterans Affairs Medical Center (Dallas)
Zale-Lipshy University Hospital
Program Director:
Ponciano D Cruz Jr, MD
Univ of Texas Southwestern Med Ctr
5323 Harry Hines Blvd
Dallas, TX 75235-9069
Tel: 214 648-8806 *Fax:* 214 648-9292
E-mail: jurquh@mednet.swmed.edu
Internet: http://www.swmed.edu/home_pages/derma/
Accred Length: 3 Years *Program Size:* 12
Program ID: 080-48-21-085

Galveston

University of Texas Medical Branch Hospitals Program
Sponsor: University of Texas Medical Branch Hospitals
Program Director:
Edgar B Smith, MD
Univ of Texas Med Branch Hospitals
Dept of Dermatology
301 University Blvd
Galveston, TX 77555-0783
Tel: 409 772-1911 *Fax:* 409 772-1943
E-mail: ebsmith@utmb.edu
Accred Length: 3 Years *Program Size:* 7
Program ID: 080-48-11-086

Houston

Baylor College of Medicine Program
Sponsor: Baylor College of Medicine
Harris County Hospital District-Ben Taub General Hospital
Methodist Hospital
Veterans Affairs Medical Center (Houston)
Program Director:
John E Wolf Jr, MD
Baylor Coll of Med
One Baylor Plaza (F840)
Houston, TX 77030-3498
Tel: 713 798-4046 *Fax:* 713 798-6923
E-mail: jwolf@bcm.tmc.edu
Internet: http://www.bmc.tmc.edu/dermamtology
Accred Length: 3 Years *Program Size:* 10
Program ID: 080-48-21-087

University of Texas at Houston Program
Sponsor: University of Texas Medical School at Houston
Lyndon B Johnson General Hospital
Memorial Hermann Healthcare System
University of Texas M D Anderson Cancer Center
Program Director:
Robert E Jordon, MD
Univ of Texas-Houston Med Sch
Dept of Dermatology
6431 Fannin St/MSB 1204
Houston, TX 77030
Tel: 713 500-7163 *Fax:* 713 500-7168
E-mail: imorales@utmmg.med.uth.tmc.edu
Accred Length: 3 Years *Program Size:* 9
Program ID: 080-48-21-100

Lackland AFB

San Antonio Uniformed Services Health Education Consortium Program
Sponsor: San Antonio Uniformed Services Health Education Consortium
Program Director:
James H Keeling, MD
Brooke Army Med Ctr
3851 Roger Brooke Dr
Fort Sam Houston, TX 78234-6200
Tel: 210 916-2120 *Fax:* 210 916-3103
Accred Length: 3 Years *Program Size:* 18
Program ID: 080-48-21-121
US Armed Services Program

Lubbock

Texas Tech University (Lubbock) Program
Sponsor: Texas Tech University Health Sciences Center at Lubbock
University Medical Center
Program Director:
Ronald P Rapini, MD
Texas Tech Univ Health Sciences Ctr
Dept of Dermatology
3601 Fourth St
Lubbock, TX 79430
Tel: 806 743-2456, ext 228 *Fax:* 806 743-1105
E-mail: derrpr@ttuhsc.edu
Internet:
http://www.ttuhsc.edu/pages/derm/der4/index.htm
Accred Length: 3 Years *Program Size:* 6
Program ID: 080-48-21-105

San Antonio

University of Texas Health Science Center at San Antonio Program
Sponsor: University of Texas Medical School at San Antonio
Audie L Murphy Memorial Veterans Hospital (San Antonio)
University Hospital-South Texas Medical Center
Program Director:
Ronald E Grimwood Jr, MD
Univ of Texas Health Science Ctr
Div of Dermatology
7703 Floyd Curl Dr
San Antonio, TX 78284-7876
Tel: 210 567-4885 *Fax:* 210 567-6679
E-mail: grimwood@uthscsa.edu
Accred Length: 3 Years *Program Size:* 3
Program ID: 080-48-22-088

Utah

Salt Lake City

University of Utah Program
Sponsor: University of Utah Medical Center
Primary Children's Medical Center
Veterans Affairs Medical Center (Salt Lake City)
Program Director:
Marta J Petersen, MD
Univ of Utah Sch of Med
Dept of Dermatology
50 N Medical Dr
Salt Lake City, UT 84132
Tel: 801 581-7837 *Fax:* 801 581-6484
E-mail: petersen@derm.med.utah.edu
Accred Length: 3 Years *Program Size:* 5
Program ID: 080-49-21-112

Virginia

Charlottesville

University of Virginia Program
Sponsor: University of Virginia Medical Center
Program Director:
Kenneth E Greer, MD
Univ of Virginia
Dept of Dermatology/Box 134
Charlottesville, VA 22908
Tel: 804 924-5115 *Fax:* 804 924-5936
Internet: http://www.med.virginia.edu~kk3p/
Accred Length: 3 Years *Program Size:* 6
Program ID: 080-51-11-089

Richmond

Medical College of Virginia/Virginia Commonwealth University Program
Sponsor: Medical College of Virginia/Virginia Commonwealth University
Hunter Holmes McGuire VA Medical Center (Richmond)
Medical College of Virginia Hospitals
Program Director:
Julia R Nunley, MD
Med Coll of Virginia
PO Box 980164
Richmond, VA 23298-0164
Tel: 804 828-9595, ext 207 *Fax:* 804 828-9596
Accred Length: 3 Years *Program Size:* 6
Program ID: 080-51-21-090

Washington

Seattle

University of Washington Program
Sponsor: University of Washington School of Medicine
University of Washington Medical Center
Program Director:
Gregory J Raugi, MD PhD
Univ of Washington Med Ctr
Div of Dermatology/Box 356524
Seattle, WA 98195-6524
Tel: 206 543-5290 *Fax:* 206 543-2489
E-mail: skin@u.washington.edu
Internet: http://weber.u.washington.edu/~medweb
Accred Length: 3 Years *Program Size:* 8
Program ID: 080-54-31-091

West Virginia

Morgantown

West Virginia University Program
Sponsor: West Virginia University Hospitals
Program Director:
William A Welton, MD
West Virginia Univ
PO Box 9158/Health Sciences Ctr N
Morgantown, WV 26506
Tel: 304 293-6618 *Fax:* 304 293-2710
Accred Length: 3 Years *Program Size:* 3
Subspecialties: DMP
Program ID: 080-55-11-092

Wisconsin

Madison

University of Wisconsin Program
Sponsor: University of Wisconsin Hospital and Clinics
Marshfield Clinic-St Joseph's Hospital
William S Middleton Veterans Hospital
Program Director:
Derek J Cripps, MD
Univ Station Clinics
2880 University Ave
PO Box 5902
Madison, WI 53705
Tel: 608 263-6230 *Fax:* 608 263-4993
Internet: http://www.medicine.wisc.edu
Accred Length: 3 Years *Program Size:* 5
Program ID: 080-56-21-093

Milwaukee

Medical College of Wisconsin Program
Sponsor: Medical College of Wisconsin Affiliated Hospitals Inc
Clement J Zablocki Veterans Affairs Medical Center
Froedtert Memorial Lutheran Hospital
Program Director:
Janet A Fairley, MD
Matthew G Fleming, MD
Med Coll of Wisconsin-Froedtert West Clinic
Dept of Dermatology
9200 W Wisconsin Ave
Milwaukee, WI 53226
Tel: 414 454-5300 *Fax:* 414 258-8085
E-mail: jfairley@mcw.edu
Internet: http://www.mcw.edu/derm
Accred Length: 3 Years *Program Size:* 10
Program ID: 080-56-21-095

Dermatopathology (Dermatology and Pathology)

Alabama

Birmingham

University of Alabama Medical Center Program
Sponsor: University of Alabama Hospital
Birmingham Baptist Medical Center-Montclair
Veterans Affairs Medical Center (Birmingham)
Program Director:
Emily F Omura, MD
Univ of Alabama
1922 7th Ave S
Kracke Bldg/Rm 101
Birmingham, AL 35294-0007
Tel: 205 934-3352 *Fax:* 205 975-6504
E-mail: gramer@uab.edu
Accred Length: 1 Year *Program Size:* 1
Program ID: 100-01-21-024

Arkansas

Little Rock

University of Arkansas for Medical Sciences Program
Sponsor: University of Arkansas College of Medicine
John L McClellan Memorial Veterans Hospital
University Hospital of Arkansas
Program Director:
Bruce R Smoller, MD
4301 W Markham
Slot 517
Little Rock, AR 72205
Tel: 501 686-5170
E-mail: smollerbr@exchange.uams.edu
Accred Length: 1 Year *Program Size:* 1
Program ID: 100-04-21-062

California

Orange

University of California (Irvine) Program
Sponsor: University of California (Irvine) Medical Center
Veterans Affairs Medical Center (Long Beach)
Program Director:
Ronald J Barr, MD
Dermatopathology Laboratory
Bldg 52/Rte 98
101 City Dr S
Orange, CA 92868
Tel: 714 456-5557 *Fax:* 714 456-8859
Accred Length: 1 Year *Program Size:* 1
Program ID: 100-05-21-053

San Francisco

University of California (San Francisco) Program
Sponsor: University of California (San Francisco) School of Medicine
Program Director:
Philip E LeBoit, MD
Univ of California San Francisco
Dermatopathology Sect
1701 Divisadero St/Ste 350
San Francisco, CA 94115
Tel: 415 353-7550 *Fax:* 415 353-7553
E-mail: philipl@itsa.ucsf.edu
Accred Length: 1 Year *Program Size:* 1
Program ID: 100-05-21-035

Stanford

Stanford University Program
Sponsor: Stanford University Hospital
Program Director:
Sabine Kohler, MD
Stanford Univ Med Ctr
300 Pasteur Dr
Stanford, CA 94305
Tel: 650 723-6736 *Fax:* 650 725-6902
E-mail: skohler@pathology.stanford.edu
Accred Length: 1 Year *Program Size:* 2
Program ID: 100-05-21-041

Connecticut

New Haven

Yale-New Haven Medical Center Program
Sponsor: Yale-New Haven Hospital
Program Director:
Earl J Glusac Jr, MD
Yale Univ Sch of Med
333 Cedar St/LMP 5034
New Haven, CT 06520-8059
Tel: 203 785-7668, ext 3218
Accred Length: 1 Year *Program Size:* 1
Program ID: 100-08-21-045

District of Columbia

Washington

Armed Forces Institute of Pathology Program
Sponsor: Armed Forces Institute of Pathology
Walter Reed Army Medical Center
Program Director:
George P Lupton, MD
Armed Forces Inst of Pathology
Dept of Dermatopathology
6825 16th St NW
Washington, DC 20306-6000
Tel: 202 782-2125 *Fax:* 202 782-3075
Accred Length: 1 Year *Program Size:* 2
Program ID: 100-10-21-019
US Armed Services Program

Florida

Miami

University of Miami-Jackson Memorial Medical Center Program
Sponsor: University of Miami-Jackson Memorial Medical Center
Program Director:
George W Elgart, MD
Univ of Miami-Jackson Memorial Med Ctr
1444 NW 9th Ave/3rd Fl
Miami, FL 33136
Tel: 305 243-6272 *Fax:* 305 243-4628
Accred Length: 1 Year *Program Size:* 1
Program ID: 100-11-21-059

Georgia

Atlanta

Emory University Program
Sponsor: Emory University School of Medicine
Emory University Hospital
Grady Memorial Hospital
Veterans Affairs Medical Center (Atlanta)
Program Director:
Alvin R Solomon, MD
Woodruff Memorial Bldg/Rm 5001
1440 Clifton Rd NE
Atlanta, GA 30322
Tel: 404 727-5872 *Fax:* 404 727-5878
E-mail: asolomo@emory.edu
Accred Length: 1 Year *Program Size:* 2
Program ID: 100-12-21-044

Illinois

Chicago

University of Chicago Program
Sponsor: University of Chicago Hospitals
Michael Reese Hospital and Medical Center
Program Director:
Keyoumars Soltani, MD
Univ of Chicago Med Ctr
Dept of Dermatopathology
5841 S Maryland Ave/MC5067
Chicago, IL 60637-1470
Tel: 773 702-6558 *Fax:* 773 702-8398
Accred Length: 1 Year *Program Size:* 1
Program ID: 100-16-31-001

Indiana

Indianapolis

Indiana University School of Medicine Program

Sponsor: Indiana University School of Medicine
Clarian IU Hospital
Clarian Riley Hospital for Children
Richard L Roudebush Veterans Affairs Medical Center
William N Wishard Memorial Hospital

Program Director:
Antoinette F Hood, MD
Indiana Univ Sch of Med
550 N University Blvd/Rm 3274
Indianapolis, IN 46202
Tel: 317 274-4212 *Fax:* 317 278-1310
E-mail: ahood@.iupui.edu
Internet: http://www.pathology.iupui.edu
Accred Length: 1 Year *Program Size:* 1
Program ID: 100-17-21-020

Louisiana

New Orleans

Tulane University Program

Sponsor: Tulane University School of Medicine
Medical Center of Louisiana at New Orleans

Program Director:
Richard Marshall, MD
Tulane Univ Med Ctr
Dept of Pathology, SL-79
1430 Tulane Ave
New Orleans, LA 70112
Tel: 504 588-5224 *Fax:* 504 587-7389
Accred Length: 1 Year *Program Size:* 1
Program ID: 100-21-21-052

Maryland

Baltimore

Johns Hopkins University Program

Sponsor: Johns Hopkins University School of Medicine
Johns Hopkins Bayview Medical Center
Johns Hopkins Hospital

Program Director:
Raymond L Barnhill, MD
Johns Hopkins Med Institutions
Div of Dermatopathology
600 N Wolfe St/Blalock 907
Baltimore, MD 21287-9977
Tel: 410 955-3484 *Fax:* 410 955-2445
Accred Length: 1 Year *Program Size:* 2
Program ID: 100-23-21-026

Massachusetts

Boston

Boston University Medical Center Program

Sponsor: Boston Medical Center
Mallory Institute of Pathology
New England Medical Center Hospitals

Program Director:
Jag Bhawan, MD
Boston Univ Sch of Med
Dept of Dermatology/Rm J-308
609 Albany St
Boston, MA 02118-2515
Tel: 617 638-5570 *Fax:* 617 638-5575
E-mail: ddorfer@acs.bu.edu
Internet: http://skinpathlab.com
Accred Length: 1 Year *Program Size:* 2
Program ID: 100-24-21-033

Harvard Medical School Program

Sponsor: Massachusetts General Hospital
Beth Israel Deaconess Medical Center
Brigham and Women's Hospital

Program Director:
Lyn M Duncan, MD
Dermatopathology Unit Warren Bldg
55 Fruit St/Rm 827
Boston, MA 02114-2696
Tel: 617 726-8890 *Fax:* 617 726-1866
E-mail: duncan@helix.mgh.harvard.edu
Accred Length: 1 Year *Program Size:* 3
Program ID: 100-24-31-002

Minnesota

Rochester

Mayo Graduate School of Medicine (Rochester) Program

Sponsor: Mayo Graduate School of Medicine-Mayo Foundation
Mayo Clinic (Rochester)
Rochester Methodist Hospital
St Mary's Hospital of Rochester

Program Director:
Lawrence E Gibson, MD
Mayo Graduate Sch of Med
Application Processing Ctr
Siebens 5th Fl
Rochester, MN 55905
Tel: 507 284-3108 *Fax:* 507 284-0999
E-mail: mgsm.medlab.specialties@mayo.edu
Internet: http://www.mayo.edu/
Accred Length: 1 Year *Program Size:* 1
Program ID: 100-26-21-004

Missouri

St Louis

Washington University/B-JH/SLCH Consortium Program

Sponsor: Washington University/B-JH/SLCH Consortium
Barnes-Jewish Hospital

Program Director:
Louis P Dehner, MD
Mark R Wick, MD
Barnes-Jewish Hospital
Div of Anatomical Pathology
One Barnes-Jewish Hospital Plaza
St Louis, MO 63110
Tel: 314 362-0104 *Fax:* 314 362-0327
Accred Length: 1 Year *Program Size:* 1
Program ID: 100-28-21-036

New Jersey

Newark

UMDNJ-New Jersey Medical School Program

Sponsor: UMDNJ-New Jersey Medical School
UMDNJ-University Hospital

Program Director:
W Clark Lambert, MD PhD
UMDNJ-New Jersey Med Sch
185 S Orange Ave
Medical Science Bldg/Rm H-576
Newark, NJ 07103-2714
Tel: 973 972-6255 *Fax:* 973 972-7092
Accred Length: 1 Year *Program Size:* 1
Program ID: 100-33-21-034

New York

Albany

Albany Medical Center Program

Sponsor: Albany Medical Center

Program Director:
John Andrew Carlson, MD
Albany Med Coll
47 New Scotland Ave
Albany, NY 12208
Tel: 518 262-6252 *Fax:* 518 262-6251
E-mail: ebrisson@ccgateway.amc.edu
Accred Length: 1 Year *Program Size:* 1
Program ID: 100-35-21-060

New York

Mount Sinai School of Medicine Program

Sponsor: Mount Sinai School of Medicine
Mount Sinai Medical Center

Program Director:
Robert G Phelps, MD
Mount Sinai Sch of Med
Dept of Pathology
One Gustave L Levy Pl/Box 1194
New York, NY 10029-6574
Tel: 212 241-6064 *Fax:* 212 534-7491
E-mail: robert_phelps@smtplink.mssm.edu
Internet: http://academic.mssm.edu/path
Accred Length: 1 Year *Program Size:* 1
Program ID: 100-35-21-056

New York and Presbyterian Hospital (Cornell Campus) Program
Sponsor: New York and Presbyterian Hospital
Memorial Sloan-Kettering Cancer Center
New York and Presbyterian Hospital (Cornell Campus)
Rockefeller University Hospital

Program Director:
N Scott McNutt, MD
New York Hospital
Div of Dermatopathology/F-309
525 E 68th St
New York, NY 10021-4897
Tel: 212 746-6434 *Fax:* 212 746-8570
Internet: http://www.nycornell.org/pathology/
Accred Length: 1 Year *Program Size:* 1
Program ID: 100-35-21-027

New York University Medical Center Program
Sponsor: New York University Medical Center
Bellevue Hospital Center
Veterans Affairs Medical Center (Manhattan)

Program Director:
Hideko Kamino, MD
New York Univ Med Ctr
530 First Ave/Ste 7J
New York, NY 10016
Tel: 212 263-7250 *Fax:* 212 684-2991
Accred Length: 1 Year *Program Size:* 4
Program ID: 100-35-21-005

North Carolina

Durham

Duke University Program
Sponsor: Duke University Medical Center
Veterans Affairs Medical Center (Durham)

Program Director:
Christopher R Shea, MD
Duke Univ Med Ctr
Box 3712
Durham, NC 27710
Tel: 919 681-6462 *Fax:* 919 684-4445
E-mail: shea0002@mc.duke.edu
Accred Length: 1 Year *Program Size:* 1
Program ID: 100-36-21-006

Winston-Salem

Wake Forest University School of Medicine Program
Sponsor: Wake Forest University Baptist Medical Center

Program Director:
Wain L White, MD
Bowman Gray Sch of Med
Medical Center Blvd
Winston-Salem, NC 27157-1072
Tel: 336 716-2636 *Fax:* 336 716-7595
E-mail: wwhite@wfubmc.edu
Accred Length: 1 Year *Program Size:* 1
Program ID: 100-36-21-039

Ohio

Cleveland

Cleveland Clinic Foundation Program
Sponsor: Cleveland Clinic Foundation

Program Director:
Wilma F Bergfeld, MD
Cleveland Clinic Foundation
Dept of Dermatopathology/A61
9500 Euclid Ave
Cleveland, OH 44195
Tel: 216 444-5722 *Fax:* 216 444-1162
E-mail: bergfew@cestmp.ccf.org
Internet: http://www.ccf.org
Accred Length: 1 Year *Program Size:* 1
Program ID: 100-38-12-009

Columbus

Ohio State University Program
Sponsor: Ohio State University Medical Center

Program Director:
Arthur E Pellegrini, MD
Ohio State Univ Med Ctr
4731 Univ Hospitals Clinic
456 W 10th Ave
Columbus, OH 43210
Tel: 614 293-8163 *Fax:* 614 293-8090
Accred Length: 1 Year *Program Size:* 1
Program ID: 100-38-21-046

Oklahoma

Oklahoma City

University of Oklahoma Health Sciences Center Program
Sponsor: University of Oklahoma College of Medicine
Children's Hospital of Oklahoma
University Hospital
Veterans Affairs Medical Center (Oklahoma City)

Program Director:
Dennis A Weigand, MD
Univ of Oklahoma Health Sciences Ctr
Dept of Dermatopathology
619 NE 13th St
Oklahoma City, OK 73104
Tel: 405 271-6600 *Fax:* 405 236-5618
Accred Length: 1 Year *Program Size:* 0
Program ID: 100-39-21-010

Pennsylvania

Philadelphia

MCP Hahnemann University Program
Sponsor: MCP Hahnemann University
Hahnemann University Hospital

Program Director:
Gary R Kantor, MD
MCP Hahnemann Univ Hospital
Dept of Dermatology/10th Fl
219 N Broad St
Philadelphia, PA 19107
Tel: 215 299-5190 *Fax:* 215 299-5195
Accred Length: 1 Year *Program Size:* 1
Program ID: 100-41-21-047

Thomas Jefferson University Program
Sponsor: Thomas Jefferson University Hospital

Program Director:
A Bernard Ackerman, MD
Thomas Jefferson Univ
Dermatopathology
130 S 9th St/Ste 1410
Philadelphia, PA 19107
Tel: 215 955-6123 *Fax:* 215 923-3412
E-mail: lmckenna@inst-dermpath.com
Internet: http://www.inst-dermpath.com
Accred Length: 1 Year *Program Size:* 7
Program ID: 100-41-21-055

University of Pennsylvania Program
Sponsor: Hospital of the University of Pennsylvania

Program Director:
Rosalie Elenitsas, MD
Univ of Pennsylvania
217 Clinical Research Bldg
415 Curie Blvd
Philadelphia, PA 19104-4218
Tel: 215 898-3241 *Fax:* 215 898-0201
E-mail: cblument@mail.med.upenn.edu
Accred Length: 1 Year *Program Size:* 2
Program ID: 100-41-11-012

Pittsburgh

University Health Center of Pittsburgh Program
Sponsor: University Health Center of Pittsburgh
Presbyterian University Hospital/UPMC

Program Director:
Brian V Jegasothh, MD
E Leon Barnes, MD
145 Lothrop Hall
190 Lothrop St
Pittsburgh, PA 15213
Tel: 412 648-3261 *Fax:* 412 648-8117
E-mail: rumba@ai.esd.upmc.edu
Accred Length: 1 Year *Program Size:* 1
Program ID: 100-41-21-028

Rhode Island

Providence

Roger Williams Medical Center Program
Sponsor: Roger Williams Medical Center

Program Director:
Caroline S Wilkel, MD
Roger Williams Med Ctr
825 Chalkstone Ave
Providence, RI 02908
Tel: 401 456-2162 *Fax:* 401 456-2131
Accred Length: 1 Year *Program Size:* 1
Program ID: 100-43-21-031

South Carolina

Charleston

Medical University of South Carolina Program
Sponsor: Medical University of South Carolina College of Medicine
MUSC Medical Center
Program Director:
John C Maize, MD
Med Univ Hospital
171 Ashley Ave
Charleston, SC 29425-2215
Tel: 843 792-5858 *Fax:* 843 792-9157
E-mail: maizejc@musc.edu
Accred Length: 1 Year *Program Size:* 2
Program ID: 100-45-21-023

Tennessee

Memphis

University of Tennessee Program
Sponsor: University of Tennessee College of Medicine
Baptist Memorial Hospital
Veterans Affairs Medical Center (Memphis)
Program Director:
George F Bale, MD
Pathology Group of the Mid South
6046 Kinght Arnould Rd
Memphis, TN 38115
Tel: 901 542-6800 *Fax:* 901 542-6871
Accred Length: 1 Year *Program Size:* 1
Program ID: 100-47-21-040

Texas

Dallas

University of Texas Southwestern Medical School Program
Sponsor: University of Texas Southwestern Medical School
Dallas County Hospital District-Parkland Memorial Hospital
Program Director:
Clay J Cockerell, MD
2330 Butler St/Ste 115
Dallas, TX 75235-7800
Tel: 214 638-2222 *Fax:* 214 630-5210
E-mail: ccockerell@skincancer.com
Internet: http://www.skincancer.com
Accred Length: 1 Year *Program Size:* 3
Program ID: 100-48-21-013

Galveston

University of Texas Medical Branch Hospitals Program
Sponsor: University of Texas Medical Branch Hospitals
Program Director:
Ramon L Sanchez, MD
Univ of Texas Med Branch Hospitals
Dept of Dermatology
4112 McCullogh Bldg
Galveston, TX 77555-0783
Tel: 409 772-1911 *Fax:* 409 772-1943
E-mail: rlsanchez@utmb.edu
Accred Length: 1 Year *Program Size:* 1
Program ID: 100-48-21-048

Houston

Baylor College of Medicine Program
Sponsor: Baylor College of Medicine
Harris County Hospital District-Ben Taub General Hospital
Methodist Hospital
Program Director:
Mary R Schwartz, MD
Baylor Coll of Med
Dept of Pathology
One Baylor Plaza
Houston, TX 77030
Tel: 713 798-4661 *Fax:* 713 798-5838
E-mail: melindaf@bcm.tmc.edu
Internet: http://www.bcm.tmc.edu/pathology
Accred Length: 1 Year *Program Size:* 2
Program ID: 100-48-21-057

Virginia

Charlottesville

University of Virginia Program
Sponsor: University of Virginia Medical Center
Program Director:
James W Patterson, MD
Univ of Virginia Hospital
Box 214/Old Medical School Bldg
University Ave
Charlottesville, VA 22908
Tel: 804 982-4402 *Fax:* 804 924-0217
E-mail: jwp9e@virginia.edu
Accred Length: 1 Year *Program Size:* 2
Program ID: 100-51-21-061

West Virginia

Morgantown

West Virginia University Program
Sponsor: West Virginia University Hospitals
Program Director:
William A Welton, MD
West Virginia Univ Hospital
Health Science Ctr-N
Rm 4089/Box 9158
Morgantown, WV 26506
Tel: 304 293-6618 *Fax:* 304 293-2710
Accred Length: 1 Year *Program Size:* 1
Program ID: 100-55-21-049

Emergency Medicine

Arizona

Phoenix

Maricopa Medical Center Program
Sponsor: Maricopa Medical Center
Program Director:
Paul A Blackburn, DO
Maricopa Med Ctr
Dept of Emergency Med
2601 E Roosevelt St
Phoenix, AZ 85008
Tel: 602 267-5808 *Fax:* 602 267-5907
E-mail: nkissling@medicine.maricopa.gov
Internet:
http://www.maricopa.gov/medcenter/ed/edhome.html
Accred Length: 3 Years *Program Size:* 33 (*GY1:* 8)
Program ID: 110-03-21-082

Tucson

University of Arizona Program
Sponsor: University of Arizona College of Medicine
University Medical Center
Program Director:
Samuel M Keim, MD
Univ of Arizona Health Sciences Ctr
Sect of Emergency Med
PO Box 245057
Tucson, AZ 85724-5057
Tel: 520 626-7233 *Fax:* 520 626-2480
E-mail: donna@aemrc.arizona.edu
Internet:
http://www.ahsc.arizona.edu/emresidn/emhome.htm
Accred Length: 3 Years *Program Size:* 30 (*GY1:* 10)
Program ID: 110-03-12-056

Arkansas

Little Rock

University of Arkansas for Medical Sciences Program
Sponsor: University of Arkansas College of Medicine
University Hospital of Arkansas
Program Director:
Martin J Carey, MB ChB MPH
Univ of Arkansas Med Sciences
4301 W Markham St/Slot 584
Little Rock, AR 72205-7199
Tel: 501 686-5515 *Fax:* 501 686-8586
E-mail: careymartinj@exchange.uams.edu
Internet: http://www.uams.edu/ems/hompg4.htm
Accred Length: 3 Years *Program Size:* 24 (*GY1:* 8)
Program ID: 110-04-21-071

California

Bakersfield

Kern Medical Center Program

Sponsor: Kern Medical Center

Program Director:
Mitesh B Patel, MD
Kern Med Ctr
Dept of Emergency Med
1830 Flower St
Bakersfield, CA 93305
Tel: 805 326-2160 *Fax:* 805 326-2165
E-mail: kmcemed@lightspeed.net.
Internet: http://www.kmcemed.edu
Accred Length: 3 Years *Program Size:* 21
Program ID: 110-05-12-001

Fresno

University of California (San Francisco)/Fresno Program

Sponsor: UCSF-Fresno Medical Education Program
University Medical Center

Program Director:
Herbert G Bivins, MD
Univ Med Ctr
445 S Cedar Ave
Fresno, CA 93702-2907
Tel: 209 459-5105 *Fax:* 209 459-3844
E-mail: darmijo@chsnet.com
Internet: http://www.ucsfresno.edu/em
Accred Length: 3 Years *Program Size:* 18
Program ID: 110-05-12-002

Loma Linda

Loma Linda University Program

Sponsor: Loma Linda University Medical Center
Riverside County Regional Medical Center

Program Director:
Steven M Green, MD
Loma Linda Univ Med Ctr
Dept of Emergency Med A108
11234 Anderson St
Loma Linda, CA 92354
Tel: 909 824-4085 *Fax:* 909 478-4121
E-mail: khaimson@ahs.llumc.edu
Internet: http://www.llu.edu/llumc/emergency/
Accred Length: 4 Years *Program Size:* 30 (*GY1:* 10)
Program ID: 110-05-12-068

Los Angeles

Charles R Drew University Program

Sponsor: Charles R Drew University of Medicine and Science
LAC-King/Drew Medical Center

Program Director:
Eugene Hardin, MD
Martin Luther King Jr-Drew Med Ctr
12021 S Wilmington Ave/Rm 1034
Los Angeles, CA 90059
Tel: 310 668-4510 *Fax:* 310 632-6591
Internet: http://members.aol.com/leon salem/mlker
Accred Length: 3 Years *Program Size:* 42 (*GY1:* 14)
Program ID: 110-05-12-004

UCLA Medical Center/Olive View-UCLA Medical Center Program

Sponsor: UCLA School of Medicine
Olive View-UCLA Medical Center
UCLA Medical Center

Program Director:
Scott R Votey, MD
UCLA Emergency Medicine Ctr
924 Westwood Blvd/Ste 300
Los Angeles, CA 90024-1777
Tel: 310 794-0585 *Fax:* 310 794-0599
E-mail: svotey@ucla.edu
Internet: http://www.pacificocean.com/uclaem
Accred Length: 3 Years *Program Size:* 36
Program ID: 110-05-12-003

University of Southern California Program

Sponsor: Los Angeles County-USC Medical Center

Program Director:
William K Mallon, MD
Los Angeles County-USC Med Ctr
1200 N State St/Box 789
Los Angeles, CA 90033-1084
Tel: 323 226-6675 *Fax:* 323 226-6454
Internet: http://www.usc.edu/hsc/medicine/emergmed
Accred Length: 4 Years *Program Size:* 54 (*GY1:* 18)
Program ID: 110-05-12-005

Oakland

Alameda County Medical Center Program

Sponsor: Alameda County Medical Center

Program Director:
Barry C Simon, MD
Alameda County Med Ctr-Highland Hospital
Dept of Emergency Med
1411 E 31st St
Oakland, CA 94602-1018
Tel: 510 437-4564 *Fax:* 510 437-8322
E-mail: apply@hghed.com
Internet: http://www.hghed.com
Accred Length: 4 Years *Program Size:* 38 (*GY1:* 10)
Subspecialties: TY
Program ID: 110-05-12-006

Orange

University of California (Irvine) Program

Sponsor: University of California (Irvine) Medical Center
Long Beach Memorial Medical Center

Program Director:
Mark I Langdorf, MD MPH
Univ of California Irvine Med Ctr
Dept of Emergency Med
101 City Dr S/Rte 128
Orange, CA 92868-3298
Tel: 714 456-5239 *Fax:* 714 456-5390
E-mail: milangdo@uci.edu
Internet: http://www.com.uci.edu
Accred Length: 3 Years *Program Size:* 18 (*GY1:* 6)
Program ID: 110-05-21-078

Sacramento

University of California (Davis) Program

Sponsor: University of California (Davis) Medical Center
Kaiser Foundation Hospital (South Sacramento)

Program Director:
Edward A Panacek, MD
2315 Stockton Blvd
PSSB Ste 2100
Sacramento, CA 95817
Tel: 916 734-8571 *Fax:* 916 734-7950
E-mail: emres@ucdmc.ucdavis.edu
Internet: http://www.emergency.ucdmc.ucdavis.edu/
Accred Length: 3 Years *Program Size:* 28 (*GY1:* 9)
Program ID: 110-05-21-097

San Diego

Naval Medical Center (San Diego) Program

Sponsor: Naval Medical Center (San Diego)

Program Director:
Paul D Pearigen, MD
Naval Med Ctr
Dept of Emergency Med/Ste 118
San Diego, CA 92134-5000
Tel: 619 532-8229 *Fax:* 619 532-5307
E-mail: pearigen@snd10.med.navy.mil
Accred Length: 3 Years *Program Size:* 25
Program ID: 110-05-12-067
US Armed Services Program

University of California (San Diego) Program

Sponsor: University of California (San Diego) Medical Center

Program Director:
Peter Rosen, MD
UCSD Med Ctr
Dept of Emergency Med
200 W Arbor Dr
San Diego, CA 92103-8819
Tel: 619 543-6236 *Fax:* 619 543-7598
E-mail: kmrichardson@ucsd.edu
Internet: http://www.medicine.ucsd.edu/emergencymed/
Accred Length: 3 Years *Program Size:* 19
Program ID: 110-05-21-080

Stanford

Stanford University Hospital/Kaiser Permanente Medical Center Program

Sponsor: Stanford University Hospital
Kaiser Permanente Medical Center (Santa Clara)

Program Director:
Rebecca Smith-Coggins, MD
Stanford Univ Med Ctr
Dept of Emergency Med
300 Pasteur Dr/MSOB-X300
Stanford, CA 94305
Tel: 650 723-9215 *Fax:* 650 723-0121
E-mail: em.residency@forsythe.stanford.edu
Internet: http://www.stanford.edu/dept/emed
Accred Length: 3 Years *Program Size:* 26 (*GY1:* 8)
Program ID: 110-05-21-098

Torrance

Los Angeles County-Harbor-UCLA Medical Center Program

Sponsor: Los Angeles County-Harbor-UCLA Medical Center

Program Director:
Howard A Bessen, MD
Los Angeles County-Harbor-UCLA Med Ctr
1000 W Carson St/Box 21
PO Box 2910
Torrance, CA 90509-2910
Tel: 310 222-3500 *Fax:* 310 782-1763
E-mail: bessen@emedharbor.edu
Internet: http://www.emedharbor.edu
Accred Length: 3 Years *Program Size:* 39 (*GY1:* 13)
Program ID: 110-05-12-008

Colorado

Denver

Denver Health Medical Center Program

Sponsor: Denver Health and Hospitals

Program Director:
Lee W Shockley, MD
Denver Health Med Ctr
Mailcode 0108
777 Bannock St
Denver, CO 80204-4507
Tel: 303 436-7147 *Fax:* 303 436-7541
E-mail: dghems@aol.com
Internet: http://www.dghems.org
Accred Length: 3 Years *Program Size:* 40
Program ID: 110-07-12-009

Connecticut

Farmington

University of Connecticut Program

Sponsor: University of Connecticut School of Medicine
Hartford Hospital
St Francis Hospital and Medical Center

Program Director:
Susan Dufel, MD
Univ of Connecticut Med Ctr (JDH)
Dept of Traumatology/Emergency Med
263 Farmington Ave
Farmington, CT 06030-1930
Tel: 860 679-4988 *Fax:* 860 679-3489
E-mail: nelson@nso.uchc.edu
Internet:
http://www.resprog.uchc.edu/md/emergency/home.html
Accred Length: 3 Years *Program Size:* 30 (*GY1:* 10)
Program ID: 110-08-21-120

New Haven

Yale-New Haven Medical Center Program

Sponsor: Yale-New Haven Hospital
Bridgeport Hospital

Program Director:
Scott Jolin, MD
Sect of Emergency Med
464 Congress Ave
New Haven, CT 06519-1313
Tel: 203 785-5174 *Fax:* 203 785-4580
Accred Length: 4 Years *Program Size:* 40 (*GY1:* 10)
Program ID: 110-08-21-139

Delaware

Wilmington

Christiana Care Health Services Program

Sponsor: Christiana Care Health Services Inc

Program Director:
Robert E O'Connor, MD MPH
Med Ctr of Delaware Residency Programs
PO Box 6001
Newark, DE 19718
Tel: 302 733-4176 *Fax:* 302 733-1595
E-mail: emed.residencyj@med.gen.de.us
Internet: http://www.christianacare.org/residency/emed
Accred Length: 3 Years *Program Size:* 36 (*GY1:* 12)
Program ID: 110-09-12-057

District of Columbia

Washington

George Washington University Program

Sponsor: George Washington University School of Medicine
Alexandria Hospital
Fairfax Hospital
George Washington University Hospital (UHS)

Program Director:
James L Scott, MD
George Washington Univ
Dept of Emergency Med
2140 Pennsylvania Ave NW
Washington, DC 20037
Tel: 202 994-3921 *Fax:* 202 994-3924
E-mail: emdlag@gwumc.edu
Internet: http://www.gwemed.edu
Accred Length: 3 Years *Program Size:* 24
Program ID: 110-10-12-011

Howard University Program

Sponsor: Howard University Hospital
District of Columbia General Hospital
Fairfax Hospital
Prince George's Hospital Center

Program Director:
Michelle G Ervin, MD
Howard Univ Hospital
Dept of Emergency Med
2041 Georgia Ave NW
Washington, DC 20060
Tel: 202 865-1121 *Fax:* 202 865-4492
E-mail: mgrant-ervin@fac.howard.edu
Accred Length: 3 Years *Program Size:* 30 (*GY1:* 10)
Program ID: 110-10-12-010

Florida

Jacksonville

University of Florida Health Science Center/Jacksonville Program

Sponsor: University of Florida College of Medicine at Jacksonville
University Medical Center (UFHSC/J)

Program Director:
David C Seaberg, MD
Univ of Florida Health Science Ctr-Jacksonville
Div of Emergency Med
655 W Eighth St/Shell Bldg
Jacksonville, FL 32209-6561
Tel: 904 549-4106 *Fax:* 904 549-4508
E-mail: seaberg@ems.umc.ufl.edu
Internet: http://ora.umc.ufl.edu/emergencymedicine/
Accred Length: 3 Years *Program Size:* 39 (*GY1:* 13)
Program ID: 110-11-12-058

Orlando

Orlando Regional Healthcare System Program

Sponsor: Orlando Regional Medical Center

Program Director:
Jay L Falk, MD
Orlando Regional Med Ctr
Dept of Emergency Med
1414 Kuhl Ave
Orlando, FL 32806-2134
Tel: 407 237-6329 *Fax:* 407 649-3083
E-mail: jayf@orhs.org
Internet: http://www.orhs.org
Accred Length: 3 Years *Program Size:* 30 (*GY1:* 10)
Program ID: 110-11-21-072

Georgia

Atlanta

Emory University Program

Sponsor: Emory University School of Medicine
Crawford Long Hospital of Emory University
Grady Memorial Hospital

Program Director:
Katherine Helpern, MD
Emory Univ Sch of Med
Dept of Emergency Med
69 Butler St SE
Atlanta, GA 30303-3219
Tel: 404 616-6673 *Fax:* 404 659-6012
E-mail: emres@emory.edu
Internet: http://www.emory.edu/em/
Accred Length: 3 Years *Program Size:* 48 (*GY1:* 16)
Program ID: 110-12-12-012

Augusta

Medical College of Georgia Program

Sponsor: Medical College of Georgia Hospital and Clinics
University Hospital

Program Director:
Richard Schwartz, MD
Med Coll of Georgia
Dept of Emergency Med
1120 15th St/Box 8158
Augusta, GA 30912-4007
Tel: 706 721-2613 *Fax:* 706 721-7718
Internet: http://www.mcg.edu
Accred Length: 3 Years *Program Size:* 22
Program ID: 110-12-21-090

Illinois

Chicago

Cook County Hospital Program

Sponsor: Cook County Hospital

Program Director:
Constance S Greene, MD
Cook County Hospital
Dept of Emergency Med
1900 W Polk St/10th Fl
Chicago, IL 60612
Tel: 312 633-3226 *Fax:* 312 633-8189
E-mail: vrichmond@ccbh.org
Internet:
http://www.rush.edu/departments/emergencymedicine
Accred Length: 3 Years *Program Size:* 54 (*GY1:* 18)
Program ID: 110-16-21-083

McGaw Medical Center of Northwestern University Program

Sponsor: Northwestern University Medical School
Evanston Hospital
Northwestern Memorial Hospital

Program Director:
Edward A Michelson, MD
216 E Superior/Rm 100
Chicago, IL 60611
Tel: 312 908-4415 *Fax:* 312 908-6004
E-mail: emedres@nwu.edu
Internet: http://www.medicine/nwu.edu/emergency
Accred Length: 4 Years *Program Size:* 29 (*GY1:* 7)
Program ID: 110-16-12-015

Resurrection Medical Center Program

Sponsor: Resurrection Medical Center
Michael Reese Hospital and Medical Center

Program Director:
Teresita M Hogan, MD
Resurrection Med Ctr
Dept of Emergency Med
7435 W Talcott Ave
Chicago, IL 60631-3746
Tel: 773 792-7921 *Fax:* 773 594-7805
E-mail: thogan@reshealthcare.org
Internet: http://www.reshealth.org
Accred Length: 3 Years *Program Size:* 36 (*GY1:* 12)
Program ID: 110-16-31-146

University of Chicago Program

Sponsor: University of Chicago Hospitals
Lutheran General Hospital

Program Director:
David S Howes, MD
Univ of Chicago Hospitals
5841 S Maryland Ave/MC5068
Chicago, IL 60637-1470
Tel: 773 702-9500 *Fax:* 773 702-3135
E-mail: btorres@medicine.bsd.uchicago.edu
Internet: http://www2.uchicago.edu/med-em
Accred Length: 3 Years *Program Size:* 36 (*GY1:* 12)
Program ID: 110-16-12-014

University of Illinois College of Medicine at Chicago Metropolitan Group Hospitals Program

Sponsor: University of Illinois College of Medicine at Chicago
Illinois Masonic Medical Center
Mercy Hospital and Medical Center
University of Illinois Hospital and Clinics

Program Director:
Timothy Erickson, MD
Univ of Illinois-Chicago
1819 W Polk St
Rm 618 CMW-M/C 724
Chicago, IL 60612-7354
Tel: 312 413-7393 *Fax:* 312 413-0289
E-mail: jstrange@uic.edu
Internet: http://www.er.uic.edu
Accred Length: 3 Years *Program Size:* 36 (*GY1:* 12)
Program ID: 110-16-12-016

Oak Lawn

Christ Hospital and Medical Center Program

Sponsor: Christ Hospital and Medical Center

Program Director:
Robert C Harwood, MD
Christ Hospital and Med Ctr
Dept of Emergency Med
4440 W 95th St
Oak Lawn, IL 60453
Tel: 708 346-5375 *Fax:* 708 346-1028
Accred Length: 3 Years *Program Size:* 27 (*GY1:* 9)
Program ID: 110-16-12-017

Peoria

University of Illinois College of Medicine at Peoria Program

Sponsor: University of Illinois College of Medicine at Peoria
St Francis Medical Center

Program Director:
Marc D Squillante, DO
OSF St Francis Med Ctr
Emergency Dept
530 NE Glen Oak Ave
Peoria, IL 61637
Tel: 309 655-6710 *Fax:* 309 655-2602
E-mail: glendah@uic.edu
Internet:
http://www.uicomp.uic.edu/html/erres/emergres.html
Accred Length: 3 Years *Program Size:* 24 (*GY1:* 8)
Program ID: 110-16-12-069

Indiana

Indianapolis

Indiana University School of Medicine Program

Sponsor: Indiana University School of Medicine
Clarian Methodist Hospital of Indiana

Program Director:
Carey D Chisholm, MD
Methodist Hospital of Indiana
I-65 at 21st St
PO Box 1367
Indianapolis, IN 46206-1367
Tel: 317 929-5975 *Fax:* 317 929-2306
E-mail: cchisholm@clarian.com
Internet: http://www.iupui.edu/~emergmed/
Accred Length: 3 Years *Program Size:* 33 (*GY1:* 11)
Program ID: 110-17-12-018

Kentucky

Lexington

University of Kentucky Medical Center Program

Sponsor: University of Kentucky Hospital

Program Director:
C Keith Stone, MD
Univ of Kentucky
800 Rose St/Rm M-53
Lexington, KY 40536-0298
Tel: 606 323-5083 *Fax:* 606 323-0236
E-mail: ckston1@pop.uky.edu
Internet:
http://www.uky.edu/medicine/departments/emergency_med/resident.html
Accred Length: 3 Years *Program Size:* 18 (*GY1:* 6)
Program ID: 110-20-21-129

Louisville

University of Louisville Program

Sponsor: University of Louisville School of Medicine
Kosair Children's Hospital (Alliant Health System)
Norton Hospital (Alliant Health System)
University of Louisville Hospital

Program Director:
Salvator J Vicario, MD
Royce D Coleman, MD
Univ of Louisville Hospital
530 S Jackson St
Louisville, KY 40202
Tel: 502 852-5689 *Fax:* 502 852-0066
E-mail: sssapp01@ulkyvm.louisville.edu
Internet: http://www.louiville.edu/~emergmed/
Accred Length: 3 Years *Program Size:* 27 (*GY1:* 9)
Program ID: 110-20-12-020

Louisiana

Baton Rouge

Louisiana State University (Baton Rouge) Program

Sponsor: Earl K Long Medical Center
Baton Rouge General Medical Center

Program Director:
Cris V Mandry, MD
Earl K Long Med Ctr
5825 Airline Hwy
Baton Rouge, LA 70805-2498
Tel: 225 358-3940 *Fax:* 225 358-3939
Accred Length: 3 Years *Program Size:* 36 (*GY1:* 12)
Program ID: 110-21-21-117

New Orleans

Louisiana State University Program

Sponsor: Louisiana State University School of Medicine
Medical Center of Louisiana at New Orleans

Program Director:
Peter M DeBlieux, MD
Charity Hospital
1532 Tulane Ave/Rm 1351
New Orleans, LA 70112-2822
Tel: 504 568-3930 *Fax:* 504 568-5383
E-mail: lindahill@worldnet.att.net
Internet:
http://www.lsumc.edu/campus/emed/lsumchomepage.htm
Accred Length: 4 Years *Program Size:* 53 (*GY1:* 15)
Program ID: 110-21-12-021

Maine

Portland

Maine Medical Center Program

Sponsor: Maine Medical Center

Program Director:
Mark W Fourre, MD
Maine Med Ctr
Dept of Emergency Med
22 Bramhall St
Portland, ME 04102-3175
Tel: 207 772-8850, ext 320 *Fax:* 207 772-4036
E-mail: kanej@mail.mmc.org
Internet: http://www.mmc.org/mmcem
Accred Length: 3 Years *Program Size:* 18 (*GY1:* 6)
Program ID: 110-22-21-142

Maryland

Baltimore

Johns Hopkins University Program

Sponsor: Johns Hopkins University School of Medicine
Johns Hopkins Bayview Medical Center
Johns Hopkins Hospital

Program Director:
Gabor D Kelen, MD
Johns Hopkins Hospital
600 N Wolfe St
Marburg B186
Baltimore, MD 21287-2080
Tel: 410 955-8191 *Fax:* 410 955-0141
Accred Length: 3 Years *Program Size:* 36 (*GY1:* 12)
Program ID: 110-23-12-022

University of Maryland Program

Sponsor: University of Maryland Medical System
Mercy Medical Center

Program Director:
Brian D Euerle, MD
Univ of Maryland Med Ctr
419 W Redwood St/Ste 280
Baltimore, MD 21201
Tel: 410 328-8025 *Fax:* 410 328-8028
E-mail: emera@surgery1.ab.umd.edu
Internet:
http://www.umm.edu/center/training/residency.html
Accred Length: 3 Years *Program Size:* 30 (*GY1:* 10)
Program ID: 110-23-21-101

Massachusetts

Boston

Boston University Medical Center Program

Sponsor: Boston Medical Center

Program Director:
Andrew S Ulrich, MD
Boston Med Ctr
Dept of Emergency Med
818 Harrison Ave/Dowling 1
Boston, MA 02118
Tel: 617 534-3452 *Fax:* 617 534-7759
E-mail: aulrich@bu.edu
Internet: http://med-www.bu.edu/emed/home.html
Accred Length: 3 Years *Program Size:* 34
Program ID: 110-24-21-084

Harvard Medical School Program

Sponsor: Brigham and Women's Hospital
Massachusetts General Hospital

Program Director:
Richard Wolfe, MD
Brigham and Women's Hospital
75 Francis St
PBB-G
Boston, MA 02115
Tel: 617 732-8070 *Fax:* 617 264-6848
E-mail: rewolfe@bics.bwh.harvard.edu
Internet: http://www.emergency.mgh.harvard.edu
Accred Length: 4 Years *Program Size:* 49 (*GY1:* 13)
Program ID: 110-24-21-150

Springfield

Baystate Medical Center Program

Sponsor: Baystate Medical Center

Program Director:
Stephen J Playe, MD
Baystate Med Ctr
Dept of Emergency Med
759 Chestnut St
Springfield, MA 01199
Tel: 413 794-5999 *Fax:* 413 794-8070
Accred Length: 3 Years *Program Size:* 18 (*GY1:* 6)
Program ID: 110-24-21-116

Worcester

University of Massachusetts Program

Sponsor: University of Massachusetts Medical School
St Vincent Hospital
UMass Memorial Health Care (Memorial Campus)
UMass Memorial Health Care (University Campus)

Program Director:
Francis P Renzi, MD
Univ of Massachusetts Med Sch
55 Lake Ave N/H1-712
Worcester, MA 01655
Tel: 508 856-4101 *Fax:* 508 856-6902
E-mail: fran.renzi@banyan@ummed.edu
Accred Length: 3 Years *Program Size:* 36 (*GY1:* 12)
Program ID: 110-24-21-074

Michigan

Ann Arbor

University of Michigan Program

Sponsor: University of Michigan Hospitals
St Joseph Mercy Health System

Program Director:
Steven C Dronen, MD
Michael G Mikhail, MD
Univ of Michigan Med Ctr
Dept of Emergency Med
TC B1354 Box 0303
Ann Arbor, MI 48109-0303
Tel: 734 763-7919 *Fax:* 734 936-9414
Internet: http://www.med.umich.edu/surg/em
Accred Length: 4 Years *Program Size:* 33 (*GY1:* 10)
Program ID: 110-25-21-106

Detroit

Henry Ford Hospital Program

Sponsor: Henry Ford Hospital

Program Director:
Christopher A Lewandowski, MD
Henry Ford Hospital
Emergency Med Program/ECFP-1
2799 W Grand Blvd
Detroit, MI 48202-2608
Tel: 313 916-1552 *Fax:* 313 916-7437
Internet: http://www.henryfordhealth.org
Accred Length: 3 Years *Program Size:* 39 (*GY1:* 13)
Program ID: 110-25-12-025

St John Hospital and Medical Center Program

Sponsor: St John Hospital and Medical Center

Program Director:
Don Michael Benson, DO
St John Hospital and Med Ctr
Dept of Med Educ
22101 Moross Rd
Detroit, MI 48236-2172
Tel: 313 343-3875 *Fax:* 313 343-7840
E-mail: sue.moynihan@stjohn.org
Internet: http://www.stjohn.org
Accred Length: 3 Years *Program Size:* 24 (*GY1:* 8)
Program ID: 110-25-21-132

Wayne State University/Detroit Medical Center (Grace Hospital) Program

Sponsor: Wayne State University/Detroit Medical Center
Grace Hospital

Program Director:
Terry Kowalenko, MD
Grace Hospital
6071 W Outer Dr
Detroit, MI 48235-2679
Tel: 313 966-1020 *Fax:* 313 966-1024
E-mail: tkowelen@med.wayne.edu
Accred Length: 3 Years *Program Size:* 24 (*GY1:* 8)
Program ID: 110-25-12-059

Wayne State University/Detroit Medical Center Program

Sponsor: Wayne State University/Detroit Medical Center
Children's Hospital of Michigan
Detroit Receiving Hospital and University Health Center

Program Director:
Robert P Wahl, MD
Emergency Med Dept
8D Univ Health Ctr
4201 St Antoine
Detroit, MI 48201-2194
Tel: 313 993-2530 *Fax:* 313 993-7703
E-mail: rwahl@med.wayne.edu
Internet: http://www.med.wayne.edu/er/
Accred Length: 3 Years *Program Size:* 36 (*GY1:* 12)
Program ID: 110-25-12-024

Grand Rapids

Spectrum Health-Downtown Campus/Michigan State University Program

Sponsor: Spectrum Health-Downtown Campus

Program Director:
Gwendolyn L Hoffman, MD
Spectrum Health-Downtown Campus
100 Michigan Ave NE/MC49
Grand Rapids, MI 49503
Tel: 616 391-1973 *Fax:* 616 391-3674
E-mail: marte.bergman@spectrum-health.org
Internet: http://www.shdem.com/residency
Accred Length: 3 Years *Program Size:* 27 (*GY1:* 9)
Program ID: 110-25-12-026

Kalamazoo

Kalamazoo Center for Medical Studies/Michigan State University Program

Sponsor: Kalamazoo Center for Medical Studies
Borgess Medical Center
Bronson Methodist Hospital

Program Director:
David T Overton, MD
Michigan State Univ-Kalamazoo Ctr for Med Studies
Dept of Emergency Med
1000 Oakland Dr
Kalamazoo, MI 49008-1284
Tel: 616 337-6600 *Fax:* 616 337-6475
E-mail: brzezinski@kcms.msu.edu
Internet: http://www.kcms.msu.edu
Accred Length: 3 Years *Program Size:* 30 (*GY1:* 10)
Program ID: 110-25-21-124

Lansing

Sparrow Hospital/Michigan State University Program

Sponsor: Sparrow Hospital
Michigan Capital Medical Center

Program Director:
Earl J Reisdorff, MD
Michigan State Univ-Lansing
PO Box 30480
1215 S Michigan Ave
Lansing, MI 48909
Tel: 517 483-2583 *Fax:* 517 483-2763
Internet: http://www.chm.msu.edu/emr/emlansing.html
Accred Length: 3 Years *Program Size:* 30 (*GY1:* 10)
Program ID: 110-25-12-027

Royal Oak

William Beaumont Hospital Program

Sponsor: William Beaumont Hospital
William Beaumont Hospital-Troy

Program Director:
Keith C Wilkinson, MD
William Beaumont Hospital
3601 W 13 Mile Rd
Royal Oak, MI 48073
Tel: 248 551-2015 *Fax:* 248 551-2017
E-mail: kcwilkinson@beaumont.edu
Internet: http://www.beaumont.edu/html/gme
Accred Length: 3 Years *Program Size:* 30 (*GY1:* 10)
Subspecialties: TY
Program ID: 110-25-12-065

Saginaw

Saginaw Cooperative Hospitals/Michigan State University Program

Sponsor: Saginaw Cooperative Hospitals Inc
Covenant Medical Center
Saginaw General Hospital
St Mary's Medical Center

Program Director:
Robert W Wolford, MD
Saginaw Cooperative Hospitals
1000 Houghton Ave
Saginaw, MI 48602
Tel: 517 771-6817 *Fax:* 517 754-2741
Internet: http://www.chm.msu.edu:/saginaw/index.html
Accred Length: 3 Years *Program Size:* 16 (*GY1:* 8)
Program ID: 110-25-11-138

Minnesota

Minneapolis

Hennepin County Medical Center Program

Sponsor: Hennepin County Medical Center

Program Director:
Douglas D Brunette, MD
Hennepin County Med Ctr
Emergency Med/#825
701 Park Ave S
Minneapolis, MN 55415
Tel: 612 347-5683 *Fax:* 612 904-4241
E-mail: doug.brunette@co.hennepin.mn.us
Internet: http://www.hcmcem.com
Accred Length: 3 Years *Program Size:* 30 (*GY1:* 10)
Program ID: 110-26-12-028

St Paul

HealthPartners Institute for Medical Education Program

Sponsor: HealthPartners Institute for Medical Education
Regions Hospital

Program Director:
Robert K Knopp, MD
Regions Hospital
Dept of Emergency Med
640 Jackson St
St Paul, MN 55101-2595
Tel: 651 221-1290 *Fax:* 651 221-8756
E-mail: kris.m.alfonso@healthpartners.com
Internet:
http://www.healthpartners.com/regions/em/index.html
Accred Length: 3 Years *Program Size:* 24 (*GY1:* 8)
Program ID: 110-26-21-144

Mississippi

Jackson

University of Mississippi Medical Center Program

Sponsor: University of Mississippi School of Medicine
University Hospital

Program Director:
Robert L Galli, MD
Univ of Mississippi Med Ctr
Dept of Emergency Med
2500 N State St
Jackson, MS 39216-4505
Tel: 601 984-5570 *Fax:* 601 984-5583
Accred Length: 3 Years *Program Size:* 22
Program ID: 110-27-21-073

Missouri

Kansas City

University of Missouri at Kansas City Program

Sponsor: University of Missouri-Kansas City School of Medicine
Truman Medical Center-West

Program Director:
Joseph A Salomone III, MD
Truman Med Ctr
Dept of Emergency Med
2301 Holmes St
Kansas City, MO 64108
Tel: 816 556-3127 *Fax:* 816 881-6282
E-mail: jlross@cctr.umkc.edu
Internet:
http://www.research.med.umkc.edu/residency/em
Accred Length: 3 Years *Program Size:* 27 (*GY1:* 9)
Program ID: 110-28-12-029

St Louis

Washington University/B-JH/SLCH Consortium Program

Sponsor: Washington University/B-JH/SLCH Consortium
Barnes-Jewish Hospital
Barnes-Jewish Hospital (North Campus)
St Louis Children's Hospital

Program Director:
Dane M Chapman, MD PhD
Washington Univ
660 S Euclid Ave
Campus Box 8072
St Louis, MO 63110-1093
Tel: 314 362-9177 *Fax:* 314 362-0478
E-mail: dchapman@imgate.wustl.edu
Internet:
http://www.internalmed.wustl.edu/divisions.emer_med/emer_med.htm
Accred Length: 4 Years *Program Size:* 48 (*GY1:* 12)
Program ID: 110-28-21-154

New Jersey

Camden

UMDNJ-Robert Wood Johnson Medical School (Camden) Program

Sponsor: Cooper Hospital-University Medical Center

Program Director:
Sarah A Stahmer, MD
Dept of Emergency Med
One Cooper Plaza
Camden, NJ 08103
Tel: 609 342-2351 *Fax:* 609 968-8272
Internet: http://www.umdnj.edu/emedweb
Accred Length: 3 Years *Program Size:* 18 (*GY1:* 6)
Program ID: 110-33-21-118

Morristown

Morristown Memorial Hospital Program

Sponsor: Morristown Memorial Hospital

Program Director:
Mark Mandell, MD
Morristown Memorial Hospital
100 Madison Ave
PO Box 1956
Morristown, NJ 07962-1956
Tel: 973 971-5044 *Fax:* 973 290-7202
E-mail: mark.mandell @mmh.ahsys.org
Internet: http://www.embbs.com/mmh
Accred Length: 3 Years *Program Size:* 18 (*GY1:* 6)
Program ID: 110-33-12-060

Newark

Newark Beth Israel Medical Center Program
Sponsor: Newark Beth Israel Medical Center
St Barnabas Medical Center
Program Director:
Ioliene Boenau, MD
Newark Beth Israel Med Ctr
201 Lyons Ave
Newark, NJ 07112
Tel: 973 926-6671 *Fax:* 973 282-0562
E-mail: jjohnson@bethi.com
Accred Length: 3 Years *Program Size:* 30 (*GY1:* 10)
Program ID: 110-33-21-158

New Mexico

Albuquerque

University of New Mexico Program
Sponsor: University of New Mexico School of Medicine
Presbyterian Healthcare Services
University Hospital
Program Director:
Judith C Brillman, MD
Univ of New Mexico Sch of Med
Dept of Emergency Med
2211 Lomas Blvd NE/Ambulatory Care Ctr 4 West
Albuquerque, NM 87131-5246
Tel: 505 272-5062 *Fax:* 505 272-6503
E-mail: jbrillman@salud.unm.edu
Internet: http://hsc.unm.edu/som/emerdmed/index.html
Accred Length: 3 Years *Program Size:* 24 (*GY1:* 8)
Program ID: 110-34-21-075

New York

Albany

Albany Medical Center Program
Sponsor: Albany Medical Center
Program Director:
Joel Bartfield, MD
Albany Med Coll
Dept of Emergency Med/MC-139
47 New Scotland Ave
Albany, NY 12208-3479
Tel: 518 262-3773 *Fax:* 518 262-3236
E-mail: joel_bartfield@ccgateway.amc.edu
Internet:
http://www.amc.edu/html/emergency_medicine_residency.html
Accred Length: 3 Years *Program Size:* 21 (*GY1:* 7)
Program ID: 110-35-21-086

Bronx

Albert Einstein College of Medicine Program
Sponsor: Albert Einstein College of Medicine of Yeshiva University
Jacobi Medical Center
Program Director:
Adrienne Birnbaum, MD
1W20 Jacobi Hospital
Pelham Pkwy and Eastchester Rd
Bronx, NY 10461
Tel: 718 918-5812 *Fax:* 718 918-7459
E-mail: jacobi-em@mindspring.com
Internet: http://www.jacobi-em.com
Accred Length: 3 Years *Program Size:* 51
Program ID: 110-35-12-030

Lincoln Medical and Mental Health Center Program
Sponsor: Lincoln Medical and Mental Health Center
Our Lady of Mercy Medical Center
Program Director:
Joel Gernsheimer, MD
Lincoln Med and Mental Health Ctr
234 E 149th St
Bronx, NY 10451
Tel: 718 579-6011 *Fax:* 718 579-4822
Accred Length: 3 Years *Program Size:* 29
Program ID: 110-35-12-053

Brooklyn

Brooklyn Hospital Center Program
Sponsor: Brooklyn Hospital Center
Program Director:
Lisandro Irizarry, MD
Brooklyn Hospital Ctr
121 Dekalb Ave
Brooklyn, NY 11201
Tel: 718 250-6889 *Fax:* 718 250-6528
Internet: http://www.bklyned.com
Accred Length: 4 Years *Program Size:* 24 (*GY1:* 6)
Program ID: 110-35-21-093

New York Methodist Hospital Program
Sponsor: New York Methodist Hospital
Program Director:
Theodore J Gaeta, DO
New York Methodist Hospital
506 Sixth St
Brooklyn, NY 11215-9008
Tel: 718 780-5040 *Fax:* 718 780-3153
E-mail: nymhemr@aol.com
Internet: http://www.nymhemr.com
Accred Length: 3 Years *Program Size:* 24 (*GY1:* 8)
Program ID: 110-35-21-147

SUNY Health Science Center at Brooklyn Program
Sponsor: SUNY Health Science Center at Brooklyn
Kings County Hospital Center
University Hospital-SUNY Health Science Center at Brooklyn
Program Director:
Michael Lucchesi, MD
SUNY Health Science Ctr-Brooklyn
Dept of Emergency Med
450 Clarkson Ave/Box 1228
Brooklyn, NY 11203
Tel: 718 245-2973 *Fax:* 718 245-4799
E-mail: sunybklynem@msn.com
Accred Length: 4 Years *Program Size:* 52 (*GY1:* 13)
Program ID: 110-35-31-135

Buffalo

SUNY at Buffalo Graduate Medical-Dental Education Consortium Program
Sponsor: SUNY at Buffalo Grad Medical-Dental Education Consortium
CGF Health System (Buffalo General Hospital)
CGF Health System (Millard Fillmore Hospitals)
Erie County Medical Center
Program Director:
Richard S Krause, MD
Buffalo General Hospital
Dept of Emergency Med
100 High St
Buffalo, NY 14203-1154
Tel: 716 859-1993 *Fax:* 716 859-1555
E-mail: sunyabem@bgh.edu
Accred Length: 3 Years *Program Size:* 28 (*GY1:* 9)
Program ID: 110-35-31-127

Manhasset

North Shore University Hospital/NYU School of Medicine Program
Sponsor: North Shore University Hospital
Program Director:
Joseph LaMantia, MD
North Shore Univ Hospital
Dept of Emergency Med
300 Community Dr
Manhasset, NY 11030
Tel: 516 562-2925 *Fax:* 516 562-3680
E-mail: lamantia@nshs.edu
Internet: http://www.nsuh-emergency.edu
Accred Length: 3 Years *Program Size:* 24 (*GY1:* 8)
Program ID: 110-35-21-141

New Hyde Park

Albert Einstein College of Medicine at Long Island Jewish Medical Center Program
Sponsor: Long Island Jewish Medical Center
Jacobi Medical Center
Program Director:
Stacy Nunberg, MD
Long Island Jewish Med Ctr
270-05 76th Ave
New Hyde Park, NY 11040
Tel: 718 470-7873 *Fax:* 718 470-9113
E-mail: foti@lij.edu
Internet: http://www.lij.edu
Accred Length: 3 Years *Program Size:* 25
Program ID: 110-35-12-062

New York

Albert Einstein College of Medicine at Beth Israel Medical Center Program
Sponsor: Beth Israel Medical Center
Program Director:
Kai M Sturmann, MD
Beth Israel Med Ctr
Dept of Emergency Med
First Ave at 16th St
New York, NY 10003-3881
Tel: 212 420-3948 *Fax:* 212 420-2863
E-mail: emergmedres@bethisraelny.org
Internet: http://www.bethisraelny.org
Accred Length: 3 Years *Program Size:* 24 (*GY1:* 8)
Program ID: 110-35-11-149

Mount Sinai School of Medicine Program
Sponsor: Mount Sinai School of Medicine
Elmhurst Hospital Center-Mount Sinai Services
Mount Sinai Medical Center
Program Director:
Lynne D Richardson, MD
Mount Sinai Sch of Med
Dept of Emergency Med
One Gustave L Levy Pl/Box 1149
New York, NY 10029
Tel: 212 241-3870 *Fax:* 212 426-1946
E-mail: lynne_richardson@smtplink.mssm.edu
Internet: http://academic.mssm.edu/emergmed
Accred Length: 3 Years *Program Size:* 28 (*GY1:* 8)
Program ID: 110-35-21-087

New York Medical College (Metropolitan) Program
Sponsor: New York Medical College
Metropolitan Hospital Center
St Vincent's Hospital and Medical Center of New York
Program Director:
Monica Parraga, MD
Metropolitan Hospital Ctr
Dept of Emergency Med
1901 First Ave
New York, NY 10029
Tel: 212 423-6011, ext 6011 *Fax:* 212 423-6383
Accred Length: 3 Years *Program Size:* 24 (*GY1:* 9)
Program ID: 110-35-12-031

New York University Medical Center Program
Sponsor: New York University Medical Center
Bellevue Hospital Center
Program Director:
Wallace A Carter Jr, MD
Bellevue Hospital Ctr
Emergency Dept
27th St and First Ave
New York, NY 10016
Tel: 212 562-4317 *Fax:* 212 263-6826
E-mail: hoffma01@popmail.med.nyu.edu
Internet: http://www.med.nyu.edu
Accred Length: 4 Years *Program Size:* 52 (*GY1:* 13)
Program ID: 110-35-21-092

St Luke's-Roosevelt Hospital Center Program
Sponsor: St Luke's-Roosevelt Hospital Center
St Luke's-Roosevelt Hospital Center-Roosevelt Division
St Luke's-Roosevelt Hospital Center-St Luke's Division
Program Director:
Marc Borenstein, MD
St Luke's-Roosevelt Hospital Ctr
Dept of Emergency Med
1000 Tenth Ave
New York, NY 10019-1105
Tel: 212 523-8158 *Fax:* 212 523-8000
E-mail: mborenstein@slrhc.org
Internet:
http://www.wehealny/professionals/residency/slr_em.html
Accred Length: 3 Years *Program Size:* 26 (*GY1:* 8)
Program ID: 110-35-21-109

Rochester

University of Rochester Program
Sponsor: Strong Memorial Hospital of the University of Rochester
Program Director:
Linda L Spillane, MD
Strong Memorial Hospital
Dept of Emergency Med
601 Elmwood Ave/Box 4-9200
Rochester, NY 14642
Tel: 716 273-4124 *Fax:* 716 473-3516
E-mail: linda_spillane@urmc.rochester.edu
Internet:
http://www.urmc.rochester.edu/smd/emergmed/residency.html
Accred Length: 3 Years *Program Size:* 22 (*GY1:* 7)
Program ID: 110-35-21-131

Stony Brook

SUNY at Stony Brook Program
Sponsor: University Hospital-SUNY at Stony Brook
Program Director:
Frederick M Schiavone, MD
SUNY-Stony Brook
Univ Med Ctr/Level 4-515
Stony Brook, NY 11794-7400
Tel: 516 444-3880 *Fax:* 516 444-3919
E-mail: fschiavone@epo.hsc.sunysb.edu
Internet: http://www.uhmc.sunysb.edu.emed/index.htm
Accred Length: 3 Years *Program Size:* 21 (*GY1:* 7)
Program ID: 110-35-21-091

Syracuse

SUNY Health Science Center at Syracuse Program
Sponsor: University Hospital-SUNY Health Science Center at Syracuse
St Joseph's Hospital Health Center
Program Director:
Gary A Johnson, MD
Univ Hospital
Dept of Emergency Med
750 E Adams St
Syracuse, NY 13210
Tel: 315 464-4363 *Fax:* 315 464-6229
E-mail: resapp@mailbox.hscsyr.edu
Internet: http://www.hscyr.edu
Accred Length: 3 Years *Program Size:* 23 (*GY1:* 8)
Subspecialties: TY
Program ID: 110-35-21-121

North Carolina

Chapel Hill

University of North Carolina Hospitals Program
Sponsor: University of North Carolina Hospitals
Wake Medical Center
Program Director:
Judith E Tintinalli, MD MS
Univ of North Carolina Sch of Med
Dept of Emergency Med/CB #7594
Chapel Hill, NC 27599-7594
Tel: 919 966-5643
E-mail: lbiggs@med.unc.edu
Internet: http://www.med.unc.edu/emergmed/
Accred Length: 3 Years *Program Size:* 18 (*GY1:* 6)
Program ID: 110-36-21-130

Charlotte

Carolinas Medical Center Program
Sponsor: Carolinas Medical Center
Program Director:
Robert E Schneider, MD
Carolinas Med Ctr
PO Box 32861
Charlotte, NC 28232-2861
Tel: 704 355-3658 *Fax:* 704 355-7047
E-mail: lklotz@carolinas.org
Internet: http://www.carolinas.org/emergency
Accred Length: 3 Years *Program Size:* 30 (*GY1:* 10)
Program ID: 110-36-12-032

Greenville

East Carolina University Program
Sponsor: East Carolina University School of Medicine
Pitt County Memorial Hospital
Program Director:
Charles K Brown, MD
East Carolina Univ Sch of Med
Dept of Emergency Med
600 Moye Blvd
Greenville, NC 27858-4354
Tel: 252 816-4184 *Fax:* 252 816-5014
E-mail: ckbrown@brody.med.ecu.edu
Internet:
http://www.med.ecu.edu/htdocs/emer_med/index.htm
Accred Length: 3 Years *Program Size:* 30 (*GY1:* 10)
Program ID: 110-36-12-063

Winston-Salem

Wake Forest University School of Medicine Program
Sponsor: Wake Forest University Baptist Medical Center
Program Director:
Earl Schwartz, MD
Wake Forest Univ Baptist Med Ctr
Medical Center Blvd
Winston-Salem, NC 27157-1089
Tel: 336 716-4625 *Fax:* 336 716-5438
E-mail: emedres@wfubmc.edu
Internet: http://www.wfubmc.edu/em/
Accred Length: 3 Years *Program Size:* 25 (*GY1:* 8)
Program ID: 110-36-12-033

Ohio

Akron

Akron General Medical Center/NEOUCOM Program
Sponsor: Akron General Medical Center
Program Director:
John C Bradford, DO
Akron General Med Ctr
400 Wabash Ave
Akron, OH 44307
Tel: 330 384-6326 *Fax:* 330 384-1529
E-mail: meded@agmc.org
Internet: http://agmc.org
Accred Length: 3 Years *Program Size:* 18 (*GY1:* 6)
Program ID: 110-38-12-035

Summa Health System (Akron City Hospital)/NEOUCOM Program
Sponsor: Summa Health System
Akron City Hospital (Summa Health System)
Program Director:
Michael Beeson, MD MBA
Summa Health System
Med Educ/Mary Yanik
525 E Market St
Akron, OH 44309
Tel: 800 322-0517
Internet: http://www.summahealth.org/edu
Accred Length: 3 Years *Program Size:* 24 (*GY1:* 8)
Subspecialties: TY
Program ID: 110-38-12-034

Cincinnati

University Hospital/University of Cincinnati College of Medicine Program

Sponsor: University Hospital Inc

Program Director:
W Brian Gibler, MD
Univ of Cincinnati Med Ctr
231 Bethesda Ave/PO Box 670769
Cincinnati, OH 45267-0769
Tel: 513 558-8114 *Fax:* 513 558-5791
E-mail: rose.alden@uc.edu
Internet: http://www.emermed.uc.edu
Accred Length: 4 Years *Program Size:* 40 (*GY1:* 10)
Program ID: 110-38-12-036

Cleveland

Case Western Reserve University (MetroHealth) Program

Sponsor: MetroHealth Medical Center
Cleveland Clinic Foundation

Program Director:
Rita K Cydulka, MD
MetroHealth Med Ctr
2500 MetroHealth Dr/Rm S1-206
Cleveland, OH 44109-1998
Tel: 216 778-5088 *Fax:* 216 778-5349
E-mail: emresidency@metrohealth.org
Internet: http://www.metrohealth.org
Accred Length: 3 Years *Program Size:* 33 (*GY1:* 11)
Program ID: 110-38-21-110

Mount Sinai Medical Center of Cleveland Program

Sponsor: Mount Sinai Medical Center of Cleveland

Program Director:
Joyce M Mitchell-Savinsky, MD
Mount Sinai Med Ctr
One Mt Sinai Dr
Cleveland, OH 44106-4198
Tel: 216 421-4022 *Fax:* 216 421-6901
E-mail: msmcclved@stratos.net
Accred Length: 3 Years *Program Size:* 19 (*GY1:* 6)
Program ID: 110-38-12-037

Columbus

Ohio State University Program

Sponsor: Ohio State University Medical Center
Riverside Methodist Hospitals (OhioHealth)

Program Director:
Daniel R Martin, MD
Ohio State Univ Med Ctr
016 Prior Health Sciences Library
376 W 10th Ave
Columbus, OH 43210-1252
Tel: 614 293-8305 *Fax:* 614 293-3124
E-mail: martin.23@osu.edu
Internet: http://www-em.med.ohio-state.edu
Accred Length: 3 Years *Program Size:* 24 (*GY1:* 8)
Program ID: 110-38-12-038

Dayton

Wright State University Program

Sponsor: Wright State University School of Medicine
Good Samaritan Hospital and Health Center
Kettering Medical Center
Wright-Patterson Medical Center

Program Director:
Jonathan Singer, MD
Dept of Emergency Med
3525 Southern Blvd
Kettering, OH 45429
Tel: 937 296-7839 *Fax:* 937 296-4287
E-mail: wsuemed@erinet.com
Internet:
http://www.med.wright.edu/som/resident/emed/emhome.htm
Accred Length: 3 Years *Program Size:* 36 (*GY1:* 12)
Program ID: 110-38-12-039

Toledo

St Vincent Mercy Medical Center/Toledo Hospital Program

Sponsor: St Vincent Mercy Medical Center
Toledo Hospital

Program Director:
Randall W King, MD
St Vincent Mercy Med Ctr
2213 Cherry St
Toledo, OH 43608
Tel: 419 251-4723, ext 4723 *Fax:* 419 251-2698
E-mail: kathy_ansted@mail.svmc.org
Internet: http://www.svmmc.emres.mhsnr.org
Accred Length: 3 Years *Program Size:* 38 (*GY1:* 12)
Program ID: 110-38-12-040

Oklahoma

Oklahoma City

University of Oklahoma Health Sciences Center Program

Sponsor: University of Oklahoma College of Medicine
Children's Hospital of Oklahoma
Columbia Presbyterian Hospital
Integris Baptist Medical Center
St Anthony Hospital
University Hospital

Program Director:
James S Walker, DO
Univ of Oklahoma Coll of Med
PO Box 26307
Rm EB #319
Oklahoma City, OK 73126
Tel: 405 271-5135 *Fax:* 405 271-7007
E-mail: jswalker@ionet.net
Internet: http://www.uokhsc.edu
Accred Length: 4 Years *Program Size:* 24 (*GY1:* 6)
Program ID: 110-39-12-041

Oregon

Portland

Oregon Health Sciences University Program

Sponsor: Oregon Health Sciences University Hospital

Program Director:
Harold A Thomas, MD
Oregon Health Sciences Univ/UHN 52
3181 SW Sam Jackson Park Rd
Portland, OR 97201-3098
Tel: 503 494-7010 *Fax:* 503 494-4997
E-mail: shiolas@ohsu.edu
Internet: http://www.ohsu.edu/som-emergmed
Accred Length: 3 Years *Program Size:* 21 (*GY1:* 7)
Program ID: 110-40-12-042

Pennsylvania

Bethlehem

St Luke's Hospital Program

Sponsor: St Luke's Hospital

Program Director:
Michael B Heller, MD
St Luke's Hospital
Emergency Med Residency
801 Ostrum St
Bethlehem, PA 18015
Tel: 610 954-4903 *Fax:* 610 954-2153
E-mail: em-residency@slhn.org
Internet: http://www.slhn-lehighvalley.org
Accred Length: 3 Years *Program Size:* 18 (*GY1:* 6)
Program ID: 110-41-21-111

Danville

Penn State Geisinger Health System/Geisinger Medical Center Program

Sponsor: Penn State Geisinger Health System
Geisinger Medical Center

Program Director:
Douglas F Kupas, MD
Geisinger Med Ctr
Dept of Emergency Med
100 N Academy Ave
Danville, PA 17821
Tel: 717 271-8001 *Fax:* 717 271-6507
E-mail: ckrebs@psghs.edu
Accred Length: 3 Years *Program Size:* 21 (*GY1:* 7)
Program ID: 110-41-12-043

Philadelphia

Albert Einstein Medical Center Program

Sponsor: Albert Einstein Medical Center

Program Director:
John W Becher, DO
Albert Einstein Med Ctr
5501 Old York Rd
Korman B-9
Philadelphia, PA 19141
Tel: 215 456-6336 *Fax:* 215 456-8502
E-mail: becherj@aehn2.einstein.edu
Accred Length: 4 Years *Program Size:* 46 (*GY1:* 12)
Program ID: 110-41-21-122

MCP Hahnemann University Program
Sponsor: MCP Hahnemann University
Hahnemann University Hospital
Medical College of Pennsylvania Hospital
Mercy Hospital of Philadelphia
Program Director:
Robert M McNamara, MD
MCP Hahneman Sch of Med
3300 Henry Ave
Philadelphia, PA 19129
Tel: 215 842-6548 *Fax:* 215 843-5121
E-mail: ekelly@auhs.edu
Internet: http://www.pond.com/~slithey/mcp.htm
Accred Length: 3 Years *Program Size:* 50 (*GY1:* 16)
Program ID: 110-41-12-045

Temple University Program
Sponsor: Temple University Hospital
Program Director:
David Brian Levy, DO
3401 N Broad St
Philadelphia, PA 19140
Tel: 215 707-7529 *Fax:* 215 707-3494
E-mail: owleddoc@aol.com
Accred Length: 3 Years *Program Size:* 24
Program ID: 110-41-21-155

Thomas Jefferson University Program
Sponsor: Thomas Jefferson University Hospital
Methodist Hospital
Program Director:
Mark L Zwanger, MD
Thomas Jefferson Univ Hospital
Div of Emer Med/239 Thompson Bldg
11th and Walnut Sts
Philadelphia, PA 19107
Tel: 215 955-6844 *Fax:* 215 923-6225
E-mail: em.residency@mail.tju.edu
Internet:
http://jeffline.tju.edu/cwis/dept/emerg-med/main.htm
Accred Length: 3 Years *Program Size:* 36 (*GY1:* 12)
Program ID: 110-41-12-064

University of Pennsylvania Program
Sponsor: Hospital of the University of Pennsylvania
Program Director:
Suzanne M Shepherd, MD
Hospital of Univ of Pennsylvania
3400 Spruce St
Ground Fl Silverstein
Philadelphia, PA 19104-4283
Tel: 215 662-6305 *Fax:* 215 662-3953
E-mail: eminfo@mail.med.upenn.edu
Internet: http://www.med.upenn.edu/~em/
Accred Length: 4 Years *Program Size:* 24 (*GY1:* 9)
Program ID: 110-41-21-148

Pittsburgh

Allegheny General Hospital Program
Sponsor: Allegheny General Hospital
Program Director:
Dennis P Hanlon, MD
Allegheny General Hospital
Dept of Emergency Med
320 E North Ave
Pittsburgh, PA 15212-9986
Tel: 412 359-4905 *Fax:* 412 359-4963
Accred Length: 3 Years *Program Size:* 24 (*GY1:* 8)
Program ID: 110-41-12-054

University Health Center of Pittsburgh Program
Sponsor: University Health Center of Pittsburgh
Mercy Hospital of Pittsburgh
Presbyterian University Hospital/UPMC
Western Pennsylvania Hospital
Program Director:
Allan B Wolfson, MD
Univ Health Ctr of Pittsburgh
230 McKee Pl/Ste 500
Pittsburgh, PA 15213-4901
Tel: 412 578-3180 *Fax:* 412 578-3241
E-mail: emres@pop.pitt.edu
Internet: http://www.pitt.edu/~emergres/
Accred Length: 3 Years *Program Size:* 36 (*GY1:* 12)
Program ID: 110-41-12-055

York

York Hospital Program
Sponsor: York Hospital
Program Director:
David A Kramer, MD
York Hospital
1001 S George St
York, PA 17405
Tel: 717 851-3070 *Fax:* 717 851-3469
E-mail: ed_wtucker@yorkhospital.edu
Internet: http://www.yorkhealth.org
Accred Length: 3 Years *Program Size:* 30 (*GY1:* 10)
Program ID: 110-41-21-089

Puerto Rico

San Juan

University of Puerto Rico Program
Sponsor: University of Puerto Rico School of Medicine
Dr Federico Trilla - Carolina Regional Hospital
Program Director:
Juan A Gonzalez-Sanchez, MD
Univ of Puerto Rico Sch of Med
GPO Box 365067
San Juan, PR 00936
Tel: 787 758-2525, ext 2066 *Fax:* 787 754-4105
E-mail: juan_gonzalez@compuserve.com
Accred Length: 3 Years *Program Size:* 25
Program ID: 110-42-12-046

Rhode Island

Providence

Brown University Program
Sponsor: Rhode Island Hospital
Program Director:
Daniel L Savitt, MD
Rhode Island Hospital
Samuels Bldg/2nd Fl
593 Eddy St
Providence, RI 02903
Tel: 401 444-4247 *Fax:* 401 444-6662
E-mail: daniel_savitt@brown.edu
Internet:
http://www.brown.edu/administration/emergency_medicine/index.html
Accred Length: 4 Years *Program Size:* 46 (*GY1:* 12)
Program ID: 110-43-21-114

South Carolina

Columbia

Palmetto Health Alliance Program
Sponsor: Palmetto Health Alliance
Palmetto Richland Memorial Hospital
Program Director:
Joseph S Myslinski, MD
Palmetto Richland Memorial Hospital
Dept of Emergency Med
5 Richland Medical Pk Dr
Columbia, SC 29203-6897
Tel: 803 434-3790 *Fax:* 803 434-3946
E-mail: em.residency@rmh.edu
Internet: http://www.palmettorichland.edu
Accred Length: 3 Years *Program Size:* 25 (*GY1:* 8)
Program ID: 110-45-12-047

Tennessee

Nashville

Vanderbilt University Program
Sponsor: Vanderbilt University Medical Center
Program Director:
Keith D Wrenn, MD
Vanderbilt Univ Med Ctr
1313 21st Ave S/Ste 703
Oxford House
Nashville, TN 37232-4700
Tel: 615 343-4836 *Fax:* 615 936-1316
E-mail: keith.wrenn@mcmail.vanderbilt.edu
Internet:
http://www.mc.vanderbilt.edu/vumcdept/emergency/
Accred Length: 3 Years *Program Size:* 28 (*GY1:* 8)
Program ID: 110-47-21-113

Texas

Dallas

University of Texas Southwestern Medical School Program
Sponsor: University of Texas Southwestern Medical School
Dallas County Hospital District-Parkland Memorial Hospital
Program Director:
Michael P Wainscott, MD
Div of Emergency Med
5323 Harry Hines Blvd
Dallas, TX 75235-8579
Tel: 214 590-1352 *Fax:* 214 590-4079
E-mail: michael.wainscott@email.swmed.edu
Internet: http://www.swmed.edu/home_pages.emrp
Accred Length: 3 Years *Program Size:* 48 (*GY1:* 16)
Program ID: 110-48-21-153

El Paso

Texas Tech University (El Paso) Program
Sponsor: Texas Tech University Health Sciences Center at El Paso
R E Thomason General Hospital
Program Director:
John M MacKay, MD
Texas Tech Univ Health Sciences Ctr
Dept of Emergency Med
6090 Surety Dr/#412
El Paso, TX 79905-2060
Tel: 915 771-6482 *Fax:* 915 774-4905
E-mail: emmemle@ttuhsc.edu
Internet: http://www.ttuhsc.edu/pages/emme/emme.htm
Accred Length: 3 Years *Program Size:* 23 (*GYI:* 8)
Program ID: 110-48-12-070

Fort Hood

Darnall Army Community Hospital Program
Sponsor: Darnall Army Community Hospital
Program Director:
Benjamin P Harrison, MD
Darnall Army Community Hospital
Emergency Med Program
36000 Darnall Loop
Fort Hood, TX 76544-4752
Tel: 254 288-8302 *Fax:* 254 286-7055
Accred Length: 3 Years *Program Size:* 22 (*GYI:* 7)
Program ID: 110-48-12-048
US Armed Services Program

Houston

University of Texas at Houston Program
Sponsor: University of Texas Medical School at Houston
Lyndon B Johnson General Hospital
Memorial Hermann Healthcare System
Program Director:
Ginger W Wilhelm, MD
Univ of Texas-Houston
Div of Emergency Med
PO Box 20708
Houston, TX 77225
Tel: 713 500-7882 *Fax:* 713 500-0758
E-mail: smiller@em.med.uth.tmc.edu
Internet:
http://oac.hsc.uth.tmc.edu/uth_orgs/emer_med/
Accred Length: 3 Years *Program Size:* 24 (*GYI:* 8)
Program ID: 110-48-21-096

Lackland AFB

San Antonio Uniformed Services Health Education Consortium Program
Sponsor: San Antonio Uniformed Services Health Education Consortium
Program Director:
James A Morgan, DO
Brooke Army Med Ctr
Dept of Emergency Med
3851 Roger Brooke Dr
Fort Sam Houston, TX 78234-6200
Tel: 210 916-1006 *Fax:* 210 916-2265
Accred Length: 3 Years *Program Size:* 42
Program ID: 110-48-21-085
US Armed Services Program

Temple

Texas A&M College of Medicine-Scott and White Program
Sponsor: Scott and White Memorial Hospital
Program Director:
Marco Coppola, DO
Texas A&M-Scott and White
Dept of Emergency Med
2401 S 31st St
Temple, TX 76508-0001
Tel: 800 299-4463, ext 45815 *Fax:* 254 724-1044
E-mail: emresi@bellnet.tamu.edu
Internet: http://www.sw.org/gme
Accred Length: 3 Years *Program Size:* 18 (*GYI:* 6)
Program ID: 110-48-21-102

Virginia

Charlottesville

University of Virginia Program
Sponsor: University of Virginia Medical Center
Program Director:
Andrew T Guertler, MD
Dept of Emergency Med
Univ of Virginia Health Science Ctr
PO Box 10014
Charlottesville, VA 22906-0014
Tel: 804 982-1800 *Fax:* 804 982-4118
Internet:
http://www.med.virginia.edu/medicine/clinical/emergency/residency/emr.htm
Accred Length: 3 Years *Program Size:* 24 (*GYI:* 8)
Program ID: 110-51-21-125

Norfolk

Eastern Virginia Medical School Program
Sponsor: Eastern Virginia Medical School
Sentara Norfolk General Hospital
Program Director:
Francis L Counselman, MD
Dept of Emergency Med
Raleigh Bldg/Rm 206
600 Gresham Dr
Norfolk, VA 23507
Tel: 757 668-3397 *Fax:* 757 668-2885
E-mail: evms@pilot.infi.net
Internet: http://www.evms.edu
Accred Length: 3 Years *Program Size:* 24 (*GYI:* 8)
Program ID: 110-51-12-050

Portsmouth

Naval Medical Center (Portsmouth) Program
Sponsor: Naval Medical Center (Portsmouth)
DePaul Medical Center
Program Director:
Kevin J Knoop, MD
Naval Hospital
Dept of Emergency Med
Portsmouth, VA 23708-5000
Tel: 757 953-7794 *Fax:* 757 953-6907
E-mail: pnh1kjk@pnh10.med.navy.mil
Accred Length: 3 Years *Program Size:* 24
Program ID: 110-51-21-105
US Armed Services Program

Washington

Tacoma

Madigan Army Medical Center Program
Sponsor: Madigan Army Medical Center
Program Director:
Matthew M Rice, MD
Madigan Army Med Ctr, Dept of Emergency Med
Bldg 9040
Fitzsimmons Dr
Tacoma, WA 98431-5000
Tel: 253 968-1260 *Fax:* 253 968-2550
Internet: http://weber.u.washington.edu/~muwemres/
Accred Length: 3 Years *Program Size:* 31
Program ID: 110-54-12-051
US Armed Services Program

West Virginia

Morgantown

West Virginia University Program
Sponsor: West Virginia University Hospitals
Program Director:
Rosanna Sikora, MD
Robert C Byrd Health Sciences Ctr
Dept of Emergency Med
PO Box 9149
Morgantown, WV 26506-9149
Tel: 304 293-7215 *Fax:* 304 293-6702
E-mail: rsikora@wvuem1.hsc.wvu.edu
Internet: http://www.hsc.wvu.edu/som/em/ed.htm
Accred Length: 3 Years *Program Size:* 18 (*GYI:* 6)
Program ID: 110-55-21-128

Wisconsin

Milwaukee

Medical College of Wisconsin Program
Sponsor: Medical College of Wisconsin Affiliated Hospitals Inc
Froedtert Memorial Lutheran Hospital
Program Director:
Gary L Swart, MD
Dept of Emergency Med
Froedtert Memorial Lutheran Hospital
9200 W Wisconsin Ave
Milwaukee, WI 53226
Tel: 414 257-5388 *Fax:* 414 257-8040
E-mail: fmlhem@post.its.mcw.edu
Internet: http://www.mcw.edu/emr
Accred Length: 3 Years *Program Size:* 23
Program ID: 110-56-12-052

Endocrinology, Diabetes, and Metabolism (Internal Medicine)

Alabama

Birmingham

University of Alabama Medical Center Program
Sponsor: University of Alabama Hospital
Program Director:
Jeffrey E Kudlow, MD
Univ of Alabama Med Ctr
Univ Station
1808 7th Ave S/BDB 756
Birmingham, AL 35294
Tel: 205 934-4116 *Fax:* 205 934-4389
E-mail: kudlow@endo.dom.uab.edu
Accred Length: 2 Years *Program Size:* 2
Program ID: 143-01-21-103

Arizona

Phoenix

Good Samaritan Regional Medical Center Program
Sponsor: Good Samaritan Regional Medical Center
Carl T Hayden Veterans Affairs Medical Center (Phoenix)
Maricopa Medical Center
Program Director:
James V Felicetta, MD
Carl T Hayden VA Med Ctr
Med Service (111)
650 E Indian School Rd
Phoenix, AZ 85012
Tel: 602 222-6436 *Fax:* 602 222-6494
Accred Length: 2 Years *Program Size:* 6
Program ID: 143-03-21-169

Tucson

University of Arizona Program
Sponsor: University of Arizona College of Medicine
University Medical Center
Veterans Affairs Medical Center (Tucson)
Program Director:
David G Johnson, MD
Univ of Arizona, Dept of Med
1501 N Campbell Ave
Tucson, AZ 85724
Tel: 520 626-6376 *Fax:* 520 626-8110
E-mail: djohnson@u.arizona.edu
Accred Length: 2 Years *Program Size:* 2
Program ID: 143-03-21-090

Arkansas

Little Rock

University of Arkansas for Medical Sciences Program
Sponsor: University of Arkansas College of Medicine
John L McClellan Memorial Veterans Hospital
University Hospital of Arkansas
Program Director:
Debra L Simmons, MD
Univ of Arkansas for Med Sciences
4301 W Markham St/Slot 587
Little Rock, AR 72205-7199
Tel: 501 686-5130 *Fax:* 501 686-8148
E-mail: simmonsdebral@exchange.uams.edu
Accred Length: 2 Years *Program Size:* 4
Program ID: 143-04-21-165

California

La Jolla

Scripps Clinic/Scripps Green Hospital Program
Sponsor: Scripps Clinic
Scripps Green Hospital
Program Director:
George Dailey III, MD
Dept of Grad Med Educ/403C
Scripps Clinic-Green Hospital
10666 N Torrey Pines Rd
La Jolla, CA 92037-1093
Tel: 619 554-8582 *Fax:* 619 554-6310
E-mail: gme@scripps.edu
Internet: http://scrippsclinic.com
Accred Length: 2 Years *Program Size:* 2
Program ID: 143-05-21-057

Los Angeles

Cedars-Sinai Medical Center Program
Sponsor: Cedars-Sinai Medical Center
Program Director:
Philip S Barnett, MD PhD
Cedars Sinai Med Ctr
8700 Beverly Blvd
Becker Bldg 131
Los Angeles, CA 90048
Tel: 310 855-4774 *Fax:* 310 967-0119
E-mail: barnettp@cshs.org
Accred Length: 2 Years *Program Size:* 2
Program ID: 143-05-11-092

Charles R Drew University Program
Sponsor: Charles R Drew University of Medicine and Science
LAC-King/Drew Medical Center
LAC-Rancho Los Amigos Medical Center
Program Director:
Shalender Bhasin, MD
1621 E 120th St/MP02
Los Angeles, CA 90059
Tel: 213 563-9353 *Fax:* 213 563-9352
E-mail: sbhasin@ucla.edu
Accred Length: 2 Years *Program Size:* 6
Program ID: 143-05-21-173

UCLA Medical Center Program
Sponsor: UCLA School of Medicine
UCLA Medical Center
VA Greater Los Angeles Healthcare System
Program Director:
Andre Van Herle, MD
UCLA Med Ctr, Dept of Med/Endocrinology
900 Veteran Ave
24-130 Warren Hall
Los Angeles, CA 90095-1736
Tel: 310 825-5874 *Fax:* 310 794-7654
E-mail: avanherl@med1.medsch.ucla.edu
Accred Length: 2 Years *Program Size:* 6
Program ID: 143-05-11-105

University of Southern California Program
Sponsor: Los Angeles County-USC Medical Center
USC University Hospital
Program Director:
Jonathan S LoPresti, MD PhD
Univ of Southern California Sch of Med
1975 Zonal Ave
Unit I-Rm 6602
Los Angeles, CA 90033
Tel: 213 226-4632 *Fax:* 213 226-2796
Accred Length: 2 Years *Program Size:* 5
Program ID: 143-05-21-041

VA Greater Los Angeles Healthcare System Program
Sponsor: VA Greater Los Angeles Healthcare System
Program Director:
Jerome M Hershman, MD
West Los Angeles VA Med Ctr
11301 Wilshire Blvd/111D
Los Angeles, CA 90073
Tel: 310 268-4879 *Fax:* 310 268-4288
E-mail: jhershmn@ucla.edu
Accred Length: 2 Years *Program Size:* 3
Program ID: 143-05-31-049

Orange

University of California (Irvine) Program
Sponsor: University of California (Irvine) Medical Center
Veterans Affairs Medical Center (Long Beach)
Program Director:
Ellis R Levin, MD
Univ of California Irvine Med Ctr
VA Med Ctr
5901 E Seventh St (11-111I)
Long Beach, CA 90822
Tel: 562 494-5748 *Fax:* 562 494-5515
E-mail: elevin@pop.long-beach.va.gov
Accred Length: 2 Years *Program Size:* 2
Program ID: 143-05-21-122

Sacramento

University of California (Davis) Program
Sponsor: University of California (Davis) Medical Center
Program Director:
Mahmoud M Benbarka, MD
Univ of California Davis Med Ctr
4150 V St/PSSB Ste G400
Sacramento, CA 95817
Tel: 916 734-3739 *Fax:* 916 734-7953
Accred Length: 2 Years *Program Size:* 2
Program ID: 143-05-21-078

San Diego

University of California (San Diego) Program
Sponsor: University of California (San Diego) Medical Center
Veterans Affairs Medical Center (San Diego)
Program Director:
Steven Edelman, MD
Patricia Wu, MD
225 Dickinson St
San Diego, CA 92103
Tel: 619 534-0343 *Fax:* 619 642-6242
Accred Length: 2 Years *Program Size:* 8
Program ID: 143-05-21-139

San Francisco

University of California (San Francisco) Program
Sponsor: University of California (San Francisco) School of Medicine
San Francisco General Hospital Medical Center
University of California (San Francisco) Medical Center
Veterans Affairs Medical Center (San Francisco)
Program Director:
Dolores M Shoback, MD
VA Med Ctr (111-N)
Univ of California San Francisco
4150 Clement St
San Francisco, CA 94121
Tel: 415 750-2089 *Fax:* 415 750-6929
Accred Length: 2 Years *Program Size:* 10
Program ID: 143-05-21-124

Stanford

Stanford University Program
Sponsor: Stanford University Hospital
Santa Clara Valley Medical Center
Veterans Affairs Palo Alto Health Care System
Program Director:
Fredric B Kraemer, MD
Div of Endocrinology/S 005
Stanford Univ Med Ctr
300 Pasteur Dr
Stanford, CA 94305-5103
Tel: 650 723-6054 *Fax:* 650 725-7085
E-mail: joyce.loewy@forsythe.stanford.edu
Accred Length: 2 Years *Program Size:* 4
Program ID: 143-05-21-022

Torrance

Los Angeles County-Harbor-UCLA Medical Center Program
Sponsor: Los Angeles County-Harbor-UCLA Medical Center
Program Director:
Ronald S Swerdloff, MD
Los Angeles County-Harbor-UCLA Med Ctr
1000 W Carson St/Box 446
Torrance, CA 90509-2910
Tel: 310 222-1867 *Fax:* 310 533-0627
E-mail: endocrine@harbor2.humc.edu
Accred Length: 2 Years *Program Size:* 2
Program ID: 143-05-11-140

Colorado

Denver

University of Colorado Program
Sponsor: University of Colorado Health Sciences Center
Denver Health and Hospitals
Veterans Affairs Medical Center (Denver)
Program Director:
E Chester Ridgway, MD
Univ of Colorado Health Sciences Ctr
Div of Endo/Metab/Diabetes
4200 E Ninth Ave/B151
Denver, CO 80262
Tel: 303 315-8443 *Fax:* 303 315-4525
Accred Length: 2 Years *Program Size:* 8
Program ID: 143-07-21-050

Connecticut

Farmington

University of Connecticut Program
Sponsor: University of Connecticut School of Medicine
Hartford Hospital
St Francis Hospital and Medical Center
Univ of Connecticut Health Center/John Dempsey Hospital
Program Director:
Kamal C Shoukri, MD
Carl D Malchoff, MD PhD
Univ of Connecticut Health Ctr
263 Farmington Ave
Farmington, CT 06030
Tel: 860 679-2129 *Fax:* 860 679-1258
Accred Length: 2 Years *Program Size:* 3
Program ID: 143-08-31-001

New Haven

Yale-New Haven Medical Center Program
Sponsor: Yale-New Haven Hospital
Veterans Affairs Medical Center (West Haven)
Program Director:
Robert S Sherwin, MD
Yale Univ Sch of Med, Dept of Med
Box 208020 Fitkin 1
New Haven, CT 06520-8020
Tel: 203 737-5071 *Fax:* 203 737-5558
E-mail: phyllis_strumpf@qm.yale.edu
Accred Length: 2 Years *Program Size:* 6
Program ID: 143-08-21-023

District of Columbia

Washington

George Washington University Program
Sponsor: George Washington University School of Medicine
George Washington University Hospital (UHS)
Veterans Affairs Medical Center (Washington, DC)
Program Director:
Kenneth L Becker, MD PhD
George Washington Univ Med Ctr
2150 Pennsylvania Ave NW
Washington, DC 20037
Tel: 202 994-0326 *Fax:* 202 994-9953
E-mail: klb1@erols.com
Accred Length: 2 Years *Program Size:* 4
Program ID: 143-10-21-093

Georgetown University Program
Sponsor: Georgetown University Medical Center
Program Director:
Joseph G Verbalis, MD
Georgetown Univ Med Ctr
Div of Endocrinology/Metabolism
4000 Reservoir Rd NW/232 Bldg D
Washington, DC 20007-2145
Tel: 202 687-2818 *Fax:* 202 687-2040
Accred Length: 2 Years *Program Size:* 3
Program ID: 143-10-21-072

Howard University Program
Sponsor: Howard University Hospital
District of Columbia General Hospital
Program Director:
Gail Nunlee-Bland, MD
Howard Univ Hospital
2041 Georgia Ave NW
Washington, DC 20060
Tel: 202 865-6620 *Fax:* 202 865-4607
Accred Length: 2 Years *Program Size:* 2
Program ID: 143-10-21-107

Florida

Gainesville

University of Florida Program
Sponsor: University of Florida College of Medicine
Shands Hospital at the University of Florida
Veterans Affairs Medical Center (Gainesville)
Program Director:
Maria Grant, MD
Univ of Florida Coll of Med
PO Box 100226
1600 SW Archer Rd
Gainesville, FL 32610
Tel: 352 392-2726 *Fax:* 352 846-2231
E-mail: ccg.med@shands.ufl.edu
Accred Length: 2 Years *Program Size:* 2
Program ID: 143-11-21-033

Jacksonville

University of Florida Health Science Center/Jacksonville Program
Sponsor: University of Florida College of Medicine at Jacksonville
University Medical Center (UFHSC/J)
Program Director:
Julie A Bauer, MD
Univ of Florida Health Science Ctr-Jacksonville
653-1 W 8th St
Jacksonville, FL 32209
Tel: 904 549-3071 *Fax:* 904 549-3087
Internet: http://www.ufhscj.edu
Accred Length: 2 Years *Program Size:* 2
Program ID: 143-11-21-024

Miami

University of Miami-Jackson Memorial Medical Center Program
Sponsor: University of Miami-Jackson Memorial Medical Center
Veterans Affairs Medical Center (Miami)
Program Director:
Peter J Gkonos, MD
Univ of Miami Sch of Med
Div of Endocrinology
PO Box 016960 (D-503)
Miami, FL 33101
Tel: 305 324-3388 *Fax:* 305 324-3365
E-mail: vroos@mednet.med.miami.edu
Accred Length: 2 Years *Program Size:* 3
Program ID: 143-11-21-141

Tampa

University of South Florida Program
Sponsor: University of South Florida College of Medicine
James A Haley Veterans Hospital
Tampa General Healthcare
Program Director:
Robert V Farese, MD
Univ of South Florida Coll of Med
12901 Bruce B Downs Blvd
MDC Box 19
Tampa, FL 33612
Tel: 813 972-7662 *Fax:* 813 972-7623
E-mail: rfarese@com1.med.usf.edu
Accred Length: 2 Years *Program Size:* 2
Program ID: 143-11-21-034

Georgia

Atlanta

Emory University Program
Sponsor: Emory University School of Medicine
Emory University Hospital
Grady Memorial Hospital
Veterans Affairs Medical Center (Atlanta)
Program Director:
Lawrence C Phillips, MD
Emory Univ Sch of Med
Div of Endocrinology
1639 Pierce Dr NE/Rm 1301 WMRB
Atlanta, GA 30322
Tel: 404 727-1391 *Fax:* 404 727-1300
Accred Length: 2 Years *Program Size:* 4
Program ID: 143-12-21-109

Augusta

Medical College of Georgia Program
Sponsor: Medical College of Georgia Hospital and Clinics
Veterans Affairs Medical Center (Augusta)
Program Director:
Roberto A Calle, MD MD
Med Coll of Georgia
Dept of Med
1467 Harper St/HB-5025
Augusta, GA 30912
Tel: 706 721-2131 *Fax:* 706 721-6892
Accred Length: 2 Years *Program Size:* 2
Program ID: 143-12-21-002

Illinois

Chicago

Cook County Hospital Program
Sponsor: Cook County Hospital
Program Director:
C R Kannan, MD
Cook County Hospital
Div of Endocrinology
1825 W Harrison
Chicago, IL 60612
Tel: 312 633-8971 *Fax:* 312 633-7101
Accred Length: 2 Years *Program Size:* 2
Program ID: 143-16-12-035

McGaw Medical Center of Northwestern University Program
Sponsor: Northwestern University Medical School
Northwestern Memorial Hospital
Veterans Affairs Lakeside Medical Center (Chicago)
Program Director:
Larry Jameson, MD PhD
Northwestern Univ Med Sch
303 E Chicago Ave
Tarry 15-701
Chicago, IL 60611-3008
Tel: 312 908-8023 *Fax:* 312 908-9032
E-mail: ljameson@nwu.edu
Internet: http://www.medicine.nwu.edu/cemmindex.html
Accred Length: 2 Years *Program Size:* 4
Program ID: 143-16-21-060

University of Chicago Program
Sponsor: University of Chicago Hospitals
Program Director:
Kenneth S Polonsky, MD
Univ of Chicago
5841 S Maryland Ave
MC1027
Chicago, IL 60637
Tel: 773 702-6217 *Fax:* 773 702-9194
Internet: http://endocrinology.uchicago.edu
Accred Length: 2 Years *Program Size:* 7
Program ID: 143-16-21-157

University of Illinois College of Medicine at Chicago Program
Sponsor: University of Illinois College of Medicine at Chicago
Christ Hospital and Medical Center
Michael Reese Hospital and Medical Center
University of Illinois Hospital and Clinics
Veterans Affairs West Side Medical Center
Program Director:
Elena Barengolts, MD
Sect of Endocrinology (M/C 640)
1819 W Polk St
Chicago, IL 60612
Tel: 312 996-6060 *Fax:* 312 413-0437
E-mail: eibareng@uic.edu
Accred Length: 2 Years *Program Size:* 5
Program ID: 143-16-21-170

Maywood

Loyola University Program
Sponsor: Loyola University Medical Center
Edward J Hines Jr Veterans Affairs Hospital
Program Director:
Nicholas V Emanuele, MD
Div of Endocrinology/Metabolism
Loyola Univ Med Ctr
2160 S First Ave/Bldg 117 Rm 11
Maywood, IL 60153
Tel: 708 216-6200 *Fax:* 708 216-4113
E-mail: nemanue@luc.edu
Accred Length: 2 Years *Program Size:* 2
Program ID: 143-16-21-003

North Chicago

Finch University of Health Sciences/Chicago Medical School Program
Sponsor: Finch University of Health Sciences/Chicago Medical School
Mount Sinai Hospital Medical Center of Chicago
Veterans Affairs Medical Center (North Chicago)
Program Director:
Sant P Singh, MD
Univ of Health Sciences-Chicago Med Sch
Dept of Med
3333 Green Bay Rd
North Chicago, IL 60064-3095
Tel: 847 578-3227 *Fax:* 847 578-8647
E-mail: singhs@finchcms.edu
Accred Length: 2 Years *Program Size:* 2
Program ID: 143-16-21-042

Springfield

Southern Illinois University Program
Sponsor: Southern Illinois University School of Medicine
Memorial Medical Center
St John's Hospital
Program Director:
Romesh Khardori, MD MB
Southern Illinois Univ Sch of Med
801 N Rutledge/MS 1618
PO Box 19230
Springfield, IL 62794-9230
Tel: 217 782-0166 *Fax:* 217 524-9125
Accred Length: 2 Years *Program Size:* 2
Program ID: 143-16-21-164

Indiana

Indianapolis

Indiana University School of Medicine Program
Sponsor: Indiana University School of Medicine
Clarian IU Hospital
Richard L Roudebush Veterans Affairs Medical Center
William N Wishard Memorial Hospital
Program Director:
Marian S Kirkman, MD
Indiana Univ Sch of Med
541 N Clinical Dr/CL 459
Indianapolis, IN 46202-5111
Tel: 317 274-1339 *Fax:* 317 278-0658
E-mail: ekurtz@iupui.edu
Internet: http://www.iupui.edu/it/medschl/home.html
Accred Length: 2 Years *Program Size:* 5
Program ID: 143-17-21-125

Iowa

Iowa City

University of Iowa Hospitals and Clinics Program
Sponsor: University of Iowa Hospitals and Clinics
Program Director:
Robert Bar, MD
Univ of Iowa Hospitals and Clinics
Dept of Int Med/Endocrinology
200 Hawkins Dr
Iowa City, IA 52242-1009
Tel: 319 338-0581, ext 7625 *Fax:* 319 339-7025
Accred Length: 2 Years *Program Size:* 3
Program ID: 143-18-21-079

Kentucky

Louisville

University of Louisville Program

Sponsor: University of Louisville School of Medicine
Jewish Hospital
Norton Hospital (Alliant Health System)
University of Louisville Hospital
Veterans Affairs Medical Center (Louisville)

Program Director:
Vasti L Broadstone, MD
Univ of Louisville
Div of Endocrinology
530 S Jackson St
Louisville, KY 40292
Tel: 502 852-5237 *Fax:* 502 852-4978
Accred Length: 2 Years *Program Size:* 2
Program ID: 143-20-31-073

Louisiana

New Orleans

Alton Ochsner Medical Foundation Program

Sponsor: Alton Ochsner Medical Foundation

Program Director:
Alan L Burshell, MD
Alton Ochsner Med Foundation
Dept of Grad Med Educ
1516 Jefferson Hwy
New Orleans, LA 70121
Tel: 504 842-3260 *Fax:* 504 842-3193
E-mail: lblonde@ochsner.org
Internet: http://www.ochsner.org
Accred Length: 2 Years *Program Size:* 2
Program ID: 143-21-22-118

Louisiana State University Program

Sponsor: Louisiana State University School of Medicine
Medical Center of Louisiana at New Orleans

Program Director:
Frank Svec, MD PhD
Louisiana State Univ Med Ctr
Endocrinology/Box T4M-5
1542 Tulane Ave
New Orleans, LA 70112-2822
Tel: 504 568-6446 *Fax:* 504 568-4159
Accred Length: 2 Years *Program Size:* 2
Program ID: 143-21-21-051

Tulane University Program

Sponsor: Tulane University School of Medicine
Medical Center of Louisiana at New Orleans
Tulane University Hospital and Clinics

Program Director:
Ramona Granda-Ayala, MD
Tulane Univ Med Ctr
1430 Tulane Ave/SL53
New Orleans, LA 70112-2699
Tel: 504 584-1851 *Fax:* 504 585-4028
E-mail: lripley@tmcpop.tmc.tulane.edu
Accred Length: 2 Years *Program Size:* 3
Program ID: 143-21-21-089

Shreveport

Louisiana State University (Shreveport) Program

Sponsor: Louisiana State University Hospital-Shreveport

Program Director:
Steven Levine, MD
Louisiana State Univ Med Ctr Hospital
Dept of Med/Endocrinology
1501 Kings Hwy/PO Box 33932
Shreveport, LA 71130-3932
Tel: 318 675-5984 *Fax:* 318 675-7176
E-mail: slevin@lsumc.edu
Accred Length: 2 Years *Program Size:* 2
Program ID: 143-21-21-074

Maine

Portland

Maine Medical Center Program

Sponsor: Maine Medical Center

Program Director:
Daniel S Oppenheim, MD PhD
Maine Med Ctr
Div of Endocrinology
100 US Route 1/Unit 116
Scarborough, ME 04074-9308
Tel: 207 885-7700 *Fax:* 207 885-7701
Accred Length: 2 Years *Program Size:* 1
Program ID: 143-22-21-155

Maryland

Baltimore

Johns Hopkins University Program

Sponsor: Johns Hopkins University School of Medicine
Johns Hopkins Hospital

Program Director:
Paul W Ladenson, MD
Johns Hopkins Univ Sch of Med
Div of Endocrinology/Metabolism
600 N Wolfe St/Blalock 904
Baltimore, MD 21287-4904
Tel: 410 955-3663 *Fax:* 410 955-8172
E-mail: ladenson@welchlink.welch.jhu.edu
Accred Length: 2 Years *Program Size:* 6
Program ID: 143-23-11-061

University of Maryland Program

Sponsor: University of Maryland Medical System
Veterans Affairs Medical Center (Baltimore)

Program Director:
John F Wilber, MD
Univ of Maryland Med System
Div of Endocrinology/Rm N3W50
22 S Greene St
Baltimore, MD 21201-1595
Tel: 410 328-2515 *Fax:* 410 328-1623
E-mail: jwilber@medicine.ab.umd.edu
Accred Length: 2 Years *Program Size:* 4
Program ID: 143-23-21-036

Bethesda

National Institutes of Health Clinical Center Program

Sponsor: NIH Warren Grant Magnuson Clinical Center

Program Director:
Monica C Skarulls, MD
Bldg 10 Rm 85-235B
National Institutes of Health
10 Center Dr
Bethesda, MD 20892-1770
Tel: 301 496-6087 *Fax:* 301 480-4517
E-mail: monica_skarulls@nih.gov
Internet: http://www.nih.gov:8001/oe
Accred Length: 2 Years *Program Size:* 14
Program ID: 143-23-21-161

National Naval Medical Center (Bethesda) Program

Sponsor: National Naval Medical Center (Bethesda)
Walter Reed Army Medical Center

Program Director:
K M M Shakir, MD MD
National Naval Med Ctr
Endocrinology/Metabolism Div
Bethesda, MD 20889-5600
Tel: 301 295-5165 *Fax:* 301 295-1939
Accred Length: 2 Years *Program Size:* 8
Program ID: 143-23-11-126
US Armed Services Program

Massachusetts

Boston

Beth Israel Deaconess Medical Center (East Campus) Program

Sponsor: Beth Israel Deaconess Medical Center

Program Director:
Jeffrey S Flier, MD
Beth Israel Deaconess Med Ctr
Research N 325 Endocrine Div
330 Brookline Ave
Boston, MA 02215
Tel: 617 667-3249 *Fax:* 617 667-2927
E-mail: jflier@bidmc.harvard.edu
Accred Length: 2 Years *Program Size:* 5
Program ID: 143-24-21-004

Beth Israel Deaconess Medical Center (West Campus) Program

Sponsor: Beth Israel Deaconess Medical Center
Joslin Diabetes Center

Program Director:
Edward S Horton, MD
New England Deaconess Hospital
Joslin Diabetes Ctr
One Joslin Pl
Boston, MA 02215
Tel: 617 732-2501 *Fax:* 617 732-2574
E-mail: ehorton@joslin.harvard.edu.
Accred Length: 2 Years *Program Size:* 4
Program ID: 143-24-21-111

Boston University Medical Center Program

Sponsor: Boston Medical Center

Program Director:
Alan O Malabanan, MD
Boston Univ Sch of Med
715 Albany St/M-1013
Boston, MA 02118
Tel: 617 534-5320 *Fax:* 617 534-7208
E-mail: malaplan@bu.edu
Accred Length: 2 Years *Program Size:* 2
Program ID: 143-24-21-127

Brigham and Women's Hospital Program

Sponsor: Brigham and Women's Hospital
Brockton-West Roxbury Veterans Affairs Medical Center

Program Director:
Gordon H Williams, MD
Brigham and Women's Hospital
Endocrine/Hypertension Div
221 Longwood Ave
Boston, MA 02115
Tel: 617 732-5661 *Fax:* 617 732-5764
Accred Length: 2 Years *Program Size:* 6
Program ID: 143-24-21-005

Massachusetts General Hospital Program

Sponsor: Massachusetts General Hospital

Program Director:
Anne Klibanski, MD
Massachusetts General Hospital
Endocrine Program WEL 501
Fruit St
Boston, MA 02114
Tel: 617 724-7777 *Fax:* 617 726-7543
E-mail: minyard@helix.mgh.harvard.edu
Accred Length: 2 Years *Program Size:* 9
Program ID: 143-24-11-052

New England Medical Center Hospitals Program

Sponsor: New England Medical Center Hospitals

Program Director:
Ronald M Lechan, MD PhD
New England Med Ctr
Div of Endo/Diabetes/Metabolism
750 Washington St/Box 268
Boston, MA 02111
Tel: 617 636-5689 *Fax:* 617 636-4719
E-mail: ron.lechan@es.nemc.org
Internet: http://www.nemc.org
Accred Length: 2 Years *Program Size:* 5
Program ID: 143-24-21-006

Burlington

Lahey Clinic Program

Sponsor: Lahey Clinic
Joslin Diabetes Center

Program Director:
Mary Beth Hodge, MD
Lahey Clinic
41 Mall Rd
Burlington, MA 01805
Tel: 781 744-8493 *Fax:* 781 744-5348
E-mail: marybeth.hodge@lahey.org
Internet: http://www.lahey.org
Accred Length: 2 Years *Program Size:* 2
Program ID: 143-24-21-119

Springfield

Baystate Medical Center Program

Sponsor: Baystate Medical Center

Program Director:
Mary Pat Roy, MD
Baystate Med Ctr
Endocrine/Metabolic/Diabetes Div
759 Chestnut St
Springfield, MA 01199
Tel: 413 794-0207 *Fax:* 413 794-9329
E-mail: marypat.roy@bhs.org
Internet: http://www.baystatehealth.com
Accred Length: 2 Years *Program Size:* 2
Program ID: 143-24-11-062

Worcester

University of Massachusetts Program

Sponsor: University of Massachusetts Medical School
UMass Memorial Health Care (University Campus)

Program Director:
Neil Aronin, MD
Univ of Massachusetts Med Sch
Div of Endocrinology
55 Lake Ave N
Worcester, MA 01655
Tel: 508 856-3115 *Fax:* 508 856-6950
E-mail: chasemer@massmed.org
Accred Length: 2 Years *Program Size:* 5
Program ID: 143-24-21-007

Michigan

Ann Arbor

University of Michigan Program

Sponsor: University of Michigan Hospitals
Veterans Affairs Medical Center (Ann Arbor)

Program Director:
Robert Lash, MD
Univ of Michigan Hospitals
3920 Taubman Ctr/Box 0354
1500 E Medical Center Dr
Ann Arbor, MI 48109-0354
Tel: 734 936-8279 *Fax:* 734 936-9240
E-mail: rwlash@medmail.umich.edu
Accred Length: 2 Years *Program Size:* 8
Program ID: 143-25-21-063

Detroit

Henry Ford Hospital Program

Sponsor: Henry Ford Hospital

Program Director:
Max Wisgerhof, MD
Henry Ford Hospital
2799 W Grand Blvd
Detroit, MI 48202
Tel: 313 876-3468 *Fax:* 313 556-8343
Accred Length: 2 Years *Program Size:* 4
Program ID: 143-25-11-112

Wayne State University/Detroit Medical Center Program

Sponsor: Wayne State University/Detroit Medical Center
Detroit Receiving Hospital and University Health Center
Harper Hospital
Veterans Affairs Medical Center (Detroit)

Program Director:
James R Sowers, MD
Endocrinology
Univ Health Ctr-4H
4201 St Antoine
Detroit, MI 48201
Tel: 313 745-4008 *Fax:* 313 993-0903
E-mail: rbufkin@oncgate.roc.wayne.edu
Accred Length: 2 Years *Program Size:* 5
Program ID: 143-25-21-040

Minnesota

Minneapolis

University of Minnesota Program

Sponsor: University of Minnesota Medical School
Fairview-University Medical Center
Veterans Affairs Medical Center (Minneapolis)

Program Director:
Cary N Mariash, MD
Fairview-Univ Med Ctr
Endocrinology/Diabetes Box 101
420 Delaware St SE
MInneapolis, MN 55455
Tel: 612 626-1960 *Fax:* 612 626-3133
E-mail: med-endo@tc.umn.edu
Internet:
http://www.dept.med.umn.edu/medicine/div/dem.htm
Accred Length: 2 Years *Program Size:* 6
Program ID: 143-26-21-096

Rochester

Mayo Graduate School of Medicine (Rochester) Program

Sponsor: Mayo Graduate School of Medicine-Mayo Foundation
Mayo Clinic (Rochester)
Rochester Methodist Hospital
St Mary's Hospital of Rochester

Program Director:
John C Morris III, MD
Application Processing Ctr
Siebens 5th Fl
Mayo Graduate Sch of Med
Rochester, MN 55905
Tel: 507 284-3126 *Fax:* 507 284-0999
E-mail: mgsm.intmed.specialties@mayo.edu
Internet: http://www.mayo.edu/
Accred Length: 2 Years *Program Size:* 9
Program ID: 143-26-21-043

Mississippi

Jackson

University of Mississippi Medical Center Program

Sponsor: University of Mississippi School of Medicine
University Hospital
Veterans Affairs Medical Center (Jackson)

Program Director:
Donald A McClain, MD PhD
2500 N State St
Jackson, MS 39216-4505
Tel: 601 984-5525 *Fax:* 601 984-5769
E-mail: dmcclain@medicine.umsmed.edu
Accred Length: 2 Years *Program Size:* 1
Program ID: 143-27-21-171

Missouri

Columbia

University of Missouri-Columbia Program

Sponsor: University of Missouri-Columbia School of Medicine
Harry S Truman Memorial Veterans Hospital
University Hospitals and Clinics

Program Director:
George T Griffing, MD
D111 Cosmopolitan Int Diabetes Ctr
Univ of Missouri Hospitals and Clinics
1 Hospital Dr
Columbia, MO 65212-0001
Tel: 573 882-2265 *Fax:* 573 884-4609
E-mail: dklachko@pol.net
Accred Length: 2 Years *Program Size:* 3
Program ID: 143-28-21-064

St Louis

St Louis University School of Medicine Program

Sponsor: St Louis University School of Medicine
St Louis University School of Medicine

Program Director:
Arshag D Mooradian, MD
St Louis Univ Sch of Med
1402 S Grand Blvd
St Louis, MO 63104-1096
Tel: 314 577-8458 *Fax:* 314 773-4567
Accred Length: 2 Years *Program Size:* 2
Program ID: 143-28-21-080

Washington University/B-JH/SLCH Consortium (South Campus) Program

Sponsor: Washington University/B-JH/SLCH Consortium
Barnes-Jewish Hospital
Barnes-Jewish Hospital (North Campus)

Program Director:
Philip E Cryer, MD
Barnes-Jewish Hospital
Metabolism Box 8127
One Barnes Hospital Plaza
St Louis, MO 63110
Tel: 314 362-7617 *Fax:* 314 362-7989
E-mail: pcryer@imgate.wustl.edu
Accred Length: 2 Years *Program Size:* 9
Program ID: 143-28-21-159

Nebraska

Omaha

University of Nebraska Program

Sponsor: University of Nebraska Medical Center
Creighton University School of Medicine

Program Director:
Jennifer L Larsen, MD
Univ of Nebraska Med Ctr
Div of Diabetes/Endo/Metabolism
983020 Nebraska Med Ctr
Omaha, NE 68198-3020
Tel: 402 559-4837 *Fax:* 402 559-9504
E-mail: jlarsen@unmc.edu
Accred Length: 2 Years *Program Size:* 3
Program ID: 143-30-21-160

New Jersey

Newark

UMDNJ-New Jersey Medical School Program

Sponsor: UMDNJ-New Jersey Medical School
UMDNJ-University Hospital
Veterans Affairs Medical Center (East Orange)

Program Director:
Marvin A Kirschner, MD
UMDNJ-New Jersey Med Sch
185 S Orange Ave
MSB I-588
Newark, NJ 07103
Tel: 973 972-6170 *Fax:* 973 972-5185
E-mail: kirschma@umdnj.edu
Accred Length: 2 Years *Program Size:* 2
Program ID: 143-33-21-148

Piscataway

UMDNJ-Robert Wood Johnson Medical School Program

Sponsor: UMDNJ-Robert Wood Johnson Medical School
Robert Wood Johnson University Hospital
St Peter's University Hospital

Program Director:
Louis F Amorosa, MD
UMDNJ-Robert Wood Johnson Med School
Div of Endocrinology/MEB 384
PO Box 19
New Brunswick, NJ 08903-0019
Tel: 732 235-7751 *Fax:* 732 235-7096
Accred Length: 2 Years *Program Size:* 2
Program ID: 143-33-21-026

New Mexico

Albuquerque

University of New Mexico Program

Sponsor: University of New Mexico School of Medicine
University Hospital
Veterans Affairs Medical Center (Albuquerque)

Program Director:
R Philip Eaton, MD
Univ of New Mexico Sch of Med
Dept of Med
ACC/5th Fl
Albuquerque, NM 87131-5191
Tel: 505 272-4658 *Fax:* 505 272-5155
E-mail: rpeaton@salud.unm.edu
Accred Length: 2 Years *Program Size:* 2
Program ID: 143-34-21-113

New York

Albany

Albany Medical Center Program

Sponsor: Albany Medical Center

Program Director:
Matthew C Leinung, MD
Albany Med Ctr
47 New Scotland Ave/Mail Code 141
Albany, NY 12208
Tel: 518 262-5185 *Fax:* 518 262-6303
E-mail: matthew_leinung@ccgateway.amc.edu
Accred Length: 2 Years *Program Size:* 2
Program ID: 143-35-31-027

Bronx

Albert Einstein College of Medicine Program

Sponsor: Albert Einstein College of Medicine of Yeshiva University
Jacobi Medical Center
Montefiore Medical Center-Henry and Lucy Moses Division
Montefiore Medical Center-Weiler Hospital
North Central Bronx Hospital

Program Director:
Martin I Surks, MD
Montefiore Med Ctr
111 E 210th St
Bronx, NY 10467
Tel: 718 920-4331 *Fax:* 718 920-5202
E-mail: surks@aecom.yu.edu
Accred Length: 2 Years *Program Size:* 4
Program ID: 143-35-21-097

Brooklyn

Interfaith Medical Center Program

Sponsor: Interfaith Medical Center
Coney Island Hospital

Program Director:
Maria Fernandez-Renedo, MD
Interfaith Med Ctr
555 Prospect Pl
Brooklyn, NY 11238
Tel: 718 935-7852 *Fax:* 718 935-7323
Accred Length: 2 Years *Program Size:* 2
Program ID: 143-35-21-143

SUNY Health Science Center at Brooklyn Program

Sponsor: SUNY Health Science Center at Brooklyn
Kings County Hospital Center
University Hospital-SUNY Health Science Center at Brooklyn
Veterans Affairs Medical Center (Brooklyn)

Program Director:
Harold E Lebovitz, MD
SUNY-Brooklyn
450 Clarkson Ave/Box 1205
Brooklyn, NY 11203
Tel: 718 270-1698 *Fax:* 718 270-1699
Accred Length: 2 Years *Program Size:* 4
Program ID: 143-35-21-010

Buffalo

SUNY at Buffalo Graduate Medical-Dental Education Consortium Program

Sponsor: SUNY at Buffalo Grad Medical-Dental Education Consortium
Erie County Medical Center
Veterans Affairs Medical Center (Buffalo)

Program Director:
Paresh Dandona, MD
3 Gates Cir
Buffalo, NY 14209
Tel: 716 887-4523 *Fax:* 716 887-4773
E-mail: pmaher@mfhs.edu
Accred Length: 2 Years *Program Size:* 3
Program ID: 143-35-31-008

East Meadow

SUNY at Stony Brook (East Meadow) Program
Sponsor: Nassau County Medical Center
Program Director:
W N Kromholz, MD
Nassau County Med Ctr
2201 Hempstead Trnpk
East Meadow, NY 11554-5400
Tel: 516 572-6504 *Fax:* 516 572-5609
E-mail: kromholz@ncmc.co.nassau.ny.us
Accred Length: 2 Years *Program Size:* 2
Program ID: 143-35-21-081

Mineola

Winthrop-University Hospital Program
Sponsor: Winthrop-University Hospital
Program Director:
John F Aloia, MD
Winthrop-Univ Hospital
222 Station Plaza N/Ste #350
Mineola, NY 11501
Tel: 516 663-2540 *Fax:* 516 663-4780
E-mail: jaloia@winthrop.org
Internet: http://www.winthrop.org
Accred Length: 2 Years *Program Size:* 4
Program ID: 143-35-11-065

New Hyde Park

Albert Einstein College of Medicine at Long Island Jewish Medical Center Program
Sponsor: Long Island Jewish Medical Center
Queens Hospital Center
Program Director:
Bruce S Schneider, MD
Long Island Jewish Med Ctr
270-05 76th Ave
New Hyde Park, NY 11040
Tel: 718 470-7241 *Fax:* 718 470-0827
Internet: http://www.lij.edu/lij-homepage-ns.html
Accred Length: 2 Years *Program Size:* 0
Program ID: 143-35-21-114

New York

Albert Einstein College of Medicine at Beth Israel Medical Center Program
Sponsor: Beth Israel Medical Center
Program Director:
Barnett Zumoff, MD
Beth Israel Med Ctr
First Ave at 16th St
New York, NY 10003
Tel: 212 420-4008 *Fax:* 212 420-2224
E-mail: bzumoff@bethisraelny.org
Accred Length: 2 Years *Program Size:* 2
Program ID: 143-35-11-009

Mount Sinai School of Medicine Program
Sponsor: Mount Sinai School of Medicine
Mount Sinai Medical Center
Veterans Affairs Medical Center (Bronx)
Program Director:
Terry F Davies, MD
Mount Sinai Med Ctr
One Gustave L Levy Pl/Box 1055
New York, NY 10029-6574
Tel: 212 241-6091 *Fax:* 212 241-4218
E-mail: tdavies@smtplink.mssm.edu
Internet:
http://www.mssm.edu/medicine/endocrinology/home-page.html
Accred Length: 2 Years *Program Size:* 6
Program ID: 143-35-31-130

New York and Presbyterian Hospital (Columbia Campus) Program
Sponsor: New York and Presbyterian Hospital
New York and Presbyterian Hospital (Columbia Campus)
Program Director:
John P Bilezikian, MD
Presbyterian Hospital
622 W 168th St/PH 8 W
New York, NY 10032
Tel: 212 305-6238 *Fax:* 212 305-6486
E-mail: bilezik@medicine1.cpmc.columbia.edu
Accred Length: 2 Years *Program Size:* 7
Program ID: 143-35-11-053

New York and Presbyterian Hospital (Cornell Campus) Program
Sponsor: New York and Presbyterian Hospital
New York and Presbyterian Hospital (Cornell Campus)
Program Director:
Julianne Imperato-McGinley, MD
New York Hospital-Cornell Med Ctr
525 E 68th St/Rm F-263
New York, NY 10021
Tel: 212 746-4745 *Fax:* 212 746-8922
E-mail: mhsu@cumc.cornell.edu
Internet:
http://www.nycornell.org/medicine/edm/index.html
Accred Length: 2 Years *Program Size:* 4
Program ID: 143-35-21-136

New York Medical College at St Vincent's Hospital and Medical Center of New York Program
Sponsor: New York Medical College
St Vincent's Hospital and Medical Center of New York
Cabrini Medical Center
The Rogosin Institute
Program Director:
Iven S Young, MD
St Vincent's Hospital and Med Ctr
153 W 11th St/MP 7-D
New York, NY 10011
Tel: 212 604-8918 *Fax:* 212 604-3844
Internet: http://svh.nymc.edu
Accred Length: 2 Years *Program Size:* 2
Program ID: 143-35-21-162

New York University Medical Center Program
Sponsor: New York University Medical Center
Bellevue Hospital Center
Veterans Affairs Medical Center (Manhattan)
Program Director:
Herbert H Samuels, MD
New York Univ Med Ctr
Div of Clinical/Molecular Endocrinology
550 First Ave
New York, NY 10016
Tel: 212 263-6279 *Fax:* 212 263-7701
Accred Length: 2 Years *Program Size:* 6
Program ID: 143-35-21-098

St Luke's-Roosevelt Hospital Center Program
Sponsor: St Luke's-Roosevelt Hospital Center
St Luke's-Roosevelt Hospital Center-St Luke's Division
Program Director:
F Xavier Pi-Sunyer, MD
St Luke's-Roosevelt Hospital Ctr-St Luke's Div
Div of Endocrinology
1111 Amsterdam Ave
New York, NY 10025
Tel: 212 523-4161 *Fax:* 212 523-4830
E-mail: fxp1@columbia.edu
Accred Length: 2 Years *Program Size:* 2
Program ID: 143-35-21-086

Rochester

University of Rochester Program
Sponsor: Strong Memorial Hospital of the University of Rochester
Genesee Hospital
Rochester General Hospital
St Mary's Hospital (Unity Health System)
Program Director:
Laurence S Jacobs, MD
Strong Memorial Hospital
601 Elmwood Ave
PO Box 693
Rochester, NY 14642-8693
Tel: 716 275-2901 *Fax:* 716 256-2789
E-mail: larry_jacobs@urmc.rochester.edu
Accred Length: 2 Years *Program Size:* 3
Program ID: 143-35-11-145

Stony Brook

SUNY at Stony Brook Program
Sponsor: University Hospital-SUNY at Stony Brook
Veterans Affairs Medical Center (Northport)
Program Director:
Harold E Carlson, MD
SUNY-Stony Brook
Div of Endocrinology
Health Science Ctr T15-060
Stony Brook, NY 11794-8154
Tel: 516 444-1038 *Fax:* 516 444-3410
E-mail: hcarlson@mail.som.sunysb.edu
Accred Length: 2 Years *Program Size:* 4
Program ID: 143-35-21-011

Syracuse

SUNY Health Science Center at Syracuse Program
Sponsor: University Hospital-SUNY Health Science Center at Syracuse
Veterans Affairs Medical Center (Syracuse)
Program Director:
Ruth S Weinstock, MD PhD
SUNY Health Science Ctr
Dept of Med
750 E Adams St
Syracuse, NY 13210
Tel: 315 464-5740 *Fax:* 315 464-5718
E-mail: weinstor@vax.cs.hscsyr.edu
Accred Length: 2 Years *Program Size:* 2
Program ID: 143-35-21-087

Valhalla

New York Medical College at Westchester Medical Center Program
Sponsor: New York Medical College
Sound Shore Medical Center of Westchester
Westchester Medical Center
Program Director:
A Louis Southren, MD
New York Med Coll-Westchester Med Ctr
Div of Endocrinology/Metabolism
Munger Pavillion Rm 622
Valhalla, NY 10595
Tel: 914 493-7578
Accred Length: 2 Years *Program Size:* 2
Program ID: 143-35-21-172

North Carolina

Chapel Hill

University of North Carolina Hospitals Program

Sponsor: University of North Carolina Hospitals

Program Director:
David R Clemmons, MD
Univ of North Carolina Sch of Med
MacNider Bldg/CB #7170
Chapel Hill, NC 27599-7170
Tel: 919 966-4735 *Fax:* 919 966-6025
Accred Length: 2 Years *Program Size:* 4
Program ID: 143-36-21-115

Durham

Duke University Program

Sponsor: Duke University Medical Center
Veterans Affairs Medical Center (Durham)

Program Director:
Marc Drezner, MD
Duke Univ Med Ctr
Box 3285
Durham, NC 27710
Tel: 919 684-5197 *Fax:* 919 681-8926
E-mail: drezn001@mc.duke.edu
Accred Length: 2 Years *Program Size:* 6
Program ID: 143-36-21-116

Winston-Salem

Wake Forest University School of Medicine Program

Sponsor: Wake Forest University Baptist Medical Center

Program Director:
K Patrick Ober, MD
North Carolina Baptist Hospital
Medical Center Blvd
Winston-Salem, NC 27157-1047
Tel: 336 716-4658 *Fax:* 336 716-5895
E-mail: kpober@wfubmc.edu
Accred Length: 2 Years *Program Size:* 3
Program ID: 143-36-21-013

Ohio

Cincinnati

University Hospital/University of Cincinnati College of Medicine Program

Sponsor: University Hospital Inc
Veterans Affairs Medical Center (Cincinnati)

Program Director:
James A Fagin, MD
Univ of Cincinnati
PO Box 670547
Cincinnati, OH 45267-0547
Tel: 513 558-4444 *Fax:* 513 558-8581
E-mail: jeannie.wilson@uc.edu
Accred Length: 2 Years *Program Size:* 2
Program ID: 143-38-21-066

Cleveland

Case Western Reserve University Program

Sponsor: University Hospitals of Cleveland
Veterans Affairs Medical Center (Cleveland)

Program Director:
Baha M Arafah, MD
Sch of Med/BRB 433
10900 Euclid Ave
Cleveland, OH 44106-4951
Tel: 216 368-6129 *Fax:* 216 368-5824
Accred Length: 2 Years *Program Size:* 3
Program ID: 143-38-21-131

Cleveland Clinic Foundation Program

Sponsor: Cleveland Clinic Foundation

Program Director:
S Sethu Reddy, MD
Cleveland Clinic Foundation
Dept of Endocrinology/A30
9500 Euclid Ave
Cleveland, OH 44195-5242
Tel: 216 444-5690 *Fax:* 216 444-1162
E-mail: meded@cestmp.ccf.org
Internet: http://www.ccf.org
Accred Length: 2 Years *Program Size:* 4
Program ID: 143-38-12-132

Columbus

Ohio State University Program

Sponsor: Ohio State University Medical Center

Program Director:
Daryl A Cottrell, MD
Ohio State Univ Med Ctr
485 McCampbell Hall
1581 Dodd Dr
Columbus, OH 43210-1228
Tel: 614 292-5201 *Fax:* 614 292-1550
Accred Length: 2 Years *Program Size:* 2
Program ID: 143-38-11-121

Oklahoma

Oklahoma City

University of Oklahoma Health Sciences Center Program

Sponsor: University of Oklahoma College of Medicine
University Hospital
Veterans Affairs Medical Center (Oklahoma City)

Program Director:
David C Kem, MD
Univ of Oklahoma Coll of Med
PO Box 26901
WP-1345
Oklahoma City, OK 73190
Tel: 405 271-5963 *Fax:* 405 271-7522
E-mail: david-kem@uokhsc.edu
Accred Length: 2 Years *Program Size:* 2
Program ID: 143-39-21-067

Oregon

Portland

Oregon Health Sciences University Program

Sponsor: Oregon Health Sciences University Hospital
Veterans Affairs Medical Center (Portland)

Program Director:
Peter S Rotwein, MD
Oregon Health Sciences Univ (NRC3)
3181 SW Sam Jackson Park Rd
Portland, OR 97201-3098
Tel: 503 494-7328 *Fax:* 503 494-7368
E-mail: endocrin@ohsu.edu
Accred Length: 2 Years *Program Size:* 6
Program ID: 143-40-31-147

Pennsylvania

Hershey

Penn State Geisinger Health System/Milton S Hershey Medical Center Program

Sponsor: Penn State Geisinger Health System
Milton S Hershey Medical Center

Program Director:
Andrea Manni, MD
Milton S Hershey Med Ctr
PO Box 850/H044
500 University Dr
Hershey, PA 17033-0850
Tel: 717 531-8395 *Fax:* 717 531-5726
Accred Length: 2 Years *Program Size:* 3
Program ID: 143-41-11-015

Philadelphia

MCP Hahnemann University Program

Sponsor: MCP Hahnemann University
Medical College of Pennsylvania Hospital
Veterans Affairs Medical Center (Philadelphia)

Program Director:
Stefan Hasinski, MD
MCP Hahnemann Univ Hospital
230 N Broad St
MS 426
Philadelphia, PA 19102
Tel: 215 762-8114 *Fax:* 215 246-5913
Accred Length: 2 Years *Program Size:* 4
Program ID: 143-41-21-099

Thomas Jefferson University Program

Sponsor: Thomas Jefferson University Hospital

Program Director:
Barry J Goldstein, MD PhD
Jefferson Med Coll
Div of Endocrinology
1020 Locust St/Rm 349
Philadelphia, PA 19107-6799
Tel: 215 503-1272 *Fax:* 215 923-7932
Accred Length: 2 Years *Program Size:* 2
Program ID: 143-41-21-166

University of Pennsylvania Program

Sponsor: Hospital of the University of Pennsylvania

Program Director:
Susan J Mandel, MD MPH
611 Clinical Research Bldg
415 Curie Blvd
Philadelphia, PA 19104
Tel: 215 898-0210 *Fax:* 215 898-5408
E-mail: geniene@mail.med.upenn.edu
Accred Length: 2 Years *Program Size:* 4
Program ID: 143-41-21-021

Pittsburgh

University Health Center of Pittsburgh Program
Sponsor: University Health Center of Pittsburgh
Presbyterian University Hospital/UPMC
Veterans Affairs Medical Center (Pittsburgh)
Program Director:
Frederick R DeRubertis, MD
Univ Health Ctr of Pittsburgh
Terrace St
E1140 Biomedical Science Tower
Pittsburgh, PA 15261
Tel: 412 688-6000, ext 4693 *Fax:* 412 688-6947
E-mail: derubertis.frederick.r@va.gov
Internet: http://www.upmc.edu/endodocs
Accred Length: 2 Years *Program Size:* 8
Program ID: 143-41-21-037

Puerto Rico

Rio Piedras

San Juan City Hospital Program
Sponsor: San Juan City Hospital
Program Director:
Gildred E Colon, MD
San Juan Municipal Hospital, Dept of Med
Box 21405
Puerto Rico Med Ctr
San Juan, PR 00928
Tel: 809 765-5147 *Fax:* 809 763-1778
Accred Length: 2 Years *Program Size:* 1
Program ID: 143-42-11-082

San Juan

University of Puerto Rico Program
Sponsor: University of Puerto Rico School of Medicine
University Hospital
Program Director:
Francisco Aguilo, MD
Univ Hospital-Puerto Rico Med Ctr
Box 5067
San Juan, PR 00935
Tel: 787 754-3633 *Fax:* 787 754-3592
Accred Length: 2 Years *Program Size:* 16
Program ID: 143-42-21-100

Rhode Island

Providence

Brown University Program
Sponsor: Rhode Island Hospital
Roger Williams Medical Center
Veterans Affairs Medical Center (Providence)
Program Director:
Ivor Jackson, MD
Brown Univ
Box G-RIH
Providence, RI 02912
Tel: 401 444-4170 *Fax:* 401 444-4921
E-mail: ivor_jackson@brown.edu
Accred Length: 2 Years *Program Size:* 4
Program ID: 143-43-11-101

South Carolina

Charleston

Medical University of South Carolina Program
Sponsor: Medical University of South Carolina College of Medicine
MUSC Medical Center
Ralph H Johnson Dept of Veterans Affairs Med Center
Program Director:
Ronald K Mayfield, MD
Med Univ of South Carolina
171 Ashley Ave
Charleston, SC 29425-2222
Tel: 803 792-2529 *Fax:* 803 792-4114
Internet:
http://www.musc.edu/endocrinology/training.htm
Accred Length: 2 Years *Program Size:* 4
Program ID: 143-45-21-088

Columbia

Palmetto Health Alliance/University of South Carolina School of Medicine Program
Sponsor: Palmetto Health Alliance
Palmetto Richland Memorial Hospital
William Jennings Bryan Dorn Veterans Hospital
Program Director:
Tu Lin, MD
Univ of South Carolina Sch of Med
Medical Library Bldg/#316
Columbia, SC 29208
Tel: 803 733-3112 *Fax:* 803 733-1547
Accred Length: 2 Years *Program Size:* 2
Program ID: 143-45-21-077

Tennessee

Memphis

University of Tennessee Program
Sponsor: University of Tennessee College of Medicine
Baptist Memorial Hospital
Regional Medical Center at Memphis
Veterans Affairs Medical Center (Memphis)
Program Director:
Abbas E Kitabchi, PhD MD
Univ of Tennessee
951 Court Ave/Rm 335-M
Memphis, TN 38163
Tel: 901 448-5802 *Fax:* 901 448-4340
Accred Length: 2 Years *Program Size:* 4
Program ID: 143-47-21-117

Nashville

Vanderbilt University Program
Sponsor: Vanderbilt University Medical Center
Program Director:
James M May, MD
Div of Endocrinology/Diabetes
Vanderbilt Univ Sch of Med
2220 Pierce Ave/715 Medical Research Bldg II
Nashville, TN 37232-6303
Tel: 615 936-1653 *Fax:* 615 936-1667
E-mail: james.may@mcmail.vanderbilt.edu
Accred Length: 2 Years *Program Size:* 7
Program ID: 143-47-31-016

Texas

Dallas

University of Texas Southwestern Medical School Program
Sponsor: University of Texas Southwestern Medical School
Children's Medical Center of Dallas
Dallas County Hospital District-Parkland Memorial Hospital
Veterans Affairs Medical Center (Dallas)
Program Director:
James E Griffin, MD
Univ of Texas Southwestern Med Ctr
5323 Harry Hines Blvd
Dallas, TX 75235-8857
Tel: 214 648-3494 *Fax:* 214 648-8917
E-mail: jgrif2@mednet.swmed.edu
Internet:
http://www.swmed.edu:80/home_pages/endocrine/index.html
Accred Length: 2 Years *Program Size:* 7
Program ID: 143-48-21-083

Galveston

University of Texas Medical Branch Hospitals Program
Sponsor: University of Texas Medical Branch Hospitals
Program Director:
Randall J Urban, MD
Univ of Texas Med Branch
8.138 MRB/1060
Galveston, TX 77555-1060
Tel: 409 772-1176 *Fax:* 409 772-8709
E-mail: rurban@utmb.edu
Internet:
http://www.intmed.utmb.edu/subspec/endofell.htm
Accred Length: 2 Years *Program Size:* 2
Program ID: 143-48-21-163

Houston

Baylor College of Medicine Program
Sponsor: Baylor College of Medicine
Harris County Hospital District-Ben Taub General Hospital
Methodist Hospital
University of Texas M D Anderson Cancer Center
Veterans Affairs Medical Center (Houston)
Program Director:
Glenn R Cunningham, MD
Baylor Coll of Med
Texas Med Ctr
One Baylor Plaza/Rm 537-E
Houston, TX 77030-3498
Tel: 713 798-6053 *Fax:* 713 798-4585
E-mail: pamelal@bcm.tmc.edu
Accred Length: 2 Years *Program Size:* 9
Program ID: 143-48-21-070

University of Texas at Houston Program
Sponsor: University of Texas Medical School at Houston
Lyndon B Johnson General Hospital
Memorial Hermann Healthcare System
Program Director:
Philip Orlander, MD
Univ of Texas-Houston Med Sch
Int Med/Endocrinology
PO Box 20708
Houston, TX 77225-0708
Tel: 713 500-6646 *Fax:* 713 500-6647
E-mail: orlander@heart.med.uth.tmc.edu
Accred Length: 2 Years *Program Size:* 2
Program ID: 143-48-31-017

Lackland AFB

San Antonio Uniformed Services Health Education Consortium (WHMC) Program
Sponsor: San Antonio Uniformed Services Health Education Consortium
Wilford Hall Medical Center (AETC)
Program Director:
Sharon G Harris, MD
59th Medical Wing (AETC)
Endocrinology Flight/MMIE
2200 Bergquist Dr/Ste 1
Lackland AFB, TX 78236-5300
Tel: 210 292-6475 *Fax:* 210 292-7868
Accred Length: 2 Years *Program Size:* 2
Program ID: 143-48-12-048
US Armed Services Program

San Antonio

University of Texas Health Science Center at San Antonio Program
Sponsor: University of Texas Medical School at San Antonio
Audie L Murphy Memorial Veterans Hospital (San Antonio)
University Hospital-South Texas Medical Center
Program Director:
Jan M Bruder, MD
Univ of Texas Health Science Ctr-San Antonio
Div of Endocrinology/Metabolism
7703 Floyd Curl Dr
San Antonio, TX 78284-7877
Tel: 210 567-4900 *Fax:* 210 567-6693
Accred Length: 2 Years *Program Size:* 3
Program ID: 143-48-21-055

Vermont

Burlington

University of Vermont Program
Sponsor: Fletcher Allen Health Care
Program Director:
John L Leahy, MD
Univ of Vermont Coll of Med
Dept of Med
Given C-331
Burlington, VT 05405-0068
Tel: 802 656-2530 *Fax:* 802 656-8031
E-mail: jleahy@zoo.uvm.edu
Accred Length: 2 Years *Program Size:* 1
Program ID: 143-50-21-134

Virginia

Charlottesville

University of Virginia Program
Sponsor: University of Virginia Medical Center
Program Director:
Alan C Dalkin, MD
Univ of Virginia Health Sciences Ctr
Div of Endocrinology
Box 511
Charlottesville, VA 22908
Tel: 804 982-3683 *Fax:* 804 982-0088
E-mail: acd6v@virginia.edu
Accred Length: 2 Years *Program Size:* 5
Program ID: 143-51-21-019

Richmond

Medical College of Virginia/Virginia Commonwealth University Program
Sponsor: Medical College of Virginia/Virginia Commonwealth University
Hunter Holmes McGuire VA Medical Center (Richmond)
Medical College of Virginia Hospitals
Program Director:
John E Nestler, MD
Med Coll of Virginia
PO Box 980111
Richmond, VA 23298-0111
Tel: 804 828-9695 *Fax:* 804 828-8389
E-mail: nestler@hsc.vcu.edu
Internet:
http://views.vcu.edu/internal-medicine/divisions/endocrin/endocrinology_metabolism.html
Accred Length: 2 Years *Program Size:* 3
Program ID: 143-51-21-020

Washington

Seattle

University of Washington Program
Sponsor: University of Washington School of Medicine
Harborview Medical Center
University of Washington Medical Center
Veterans Affairs Medical Center (Seattle)
Program Director:
John D Brunzell, MD
Div of Metab/Endocrin/Nutrition
Univ of Washington
Box 356426
Seattle, WA 98195-6426
Tel: 206 548-4700 *Fax:* 206 548-2890
E-mail: brunzell@u.washington.edu
Internet: http://weber.u.washington.edu/~metab
Accred Length: 2 Years *Program Size:* 12
Program ID: 143-54-21-071

West Virginia

Huntington

Marshall University School of Medicine Program
Sponsor: Marshall University School of Medicine
Cabell Huntington Hospital
St Mary's Hospital
Veterans Affairs Medical Center (Huntington)
Program Director:
Bruce S Chertow, MD
Marshall Univ Sch of Med
Dept of Med
1600 Medical Center Dr/Ste G500
Huntington, WV 25701-3655
Tel: 304 691-1095 *Fax:* 304 691-1693
E-mail: chertow@marshall.edu
Accred Length: 2 Years *Program Size:* 2
Program ID: 143-55-21-031

Wisconsin

Madison

University of Wisconsin Program
Sponsor: University of Wisconsin Hospital and Clinics
William S Middleton Veterans Hospital
Program Director:
Yoram Shenker, MD
Univ of Wisconsin Hospital and Clinics
H4/568 CSC
600 Highland Ave
Madison, WI 53792-5148
Tel: 608 263-9221 *Fax:* 608 263-9983
E-mail: yshenker@facstaff.wisc.edu
Accred Length: 2 Years *Program Size:* 3
Program ID: 143-56-21-102

Milwaukee

Medical College of Wisconsin Program
Sponsor: Medical College of Wisconsin Affiliated Hospitals Inc
Clement J Zablocki Veterans Affairs Medical Center
Froedtert Memorial Lutheran Hospital
Program Director:
Albert L Jochen, MD
Med Coll of Wisconsin
Froedtert Memorial Lutheran Hospital
9200 W Wisconsin Ave
Milwaukee, WI 53226
Tel: 414 456-6810 *Fax:* 414 456-6210
E-mail: vdodge@mcw.edu
Accred Length: 2 Years *Program Size:* 2
Program ID: 143-56-31-039

Family Practice

Alabama

Anniston

Northeast Alabama Regional Medical Center Program
Sponsor: Northeast Alabama Regional Medical Center
Program Director:
C Neal Canup, MD
Anniston Family Practice Program
PO Box 2208
400 E 10th St
Anniston, AL 36207
Tel: 205 231-8877 *Fax:* 205 231-8689
E-mail: mhall@hvps.com
Internet: http://www.rmccares.org
Accred Length: 3 Years *Program Size:* 4 (*GY1:* 4)
Program ID: 120-01-21-636

Birmingham

Carraway Methodist Medical Center Program
Sponsor: Carraway Methodist Medical Center
Program Director:
Marshall N Boone Jr, MD PhD
Carraway Methodist Med Ctr
Dept of Family Med
3001 27th St N
Birmingham, AL 35207
Tel: 205 502-5809 *Fax:* 205 502-5586
E-mail: fpres@mail.carraway.com
Internet: http://www.carraway.org
Accred Length: 3 Years *Program Size:* 12 (*GY1:* 4)
Program ID: 120-01-31-019

Medical Center East Program
Sponsor: Medical Center East
Program Director:
Marion H Sims, MD
Family Practice Ctr
2152 Old Springville Rd
Birmingham, AL 35215
Tel: 205 853-2223 *Fax:* 205 815-3928
Accred Length: 3 Years *Program Size:* 15 (*GY1:* 5)
Program ID: 120-01-31-020

University of Alabama Medical Center Program
Sponsor: University of Alabama Hospital
Program Director:
Cynthia M Moore-Sledge, MD
Univ of Alabama
Dept of Family/Com Med
930 S 20th St
Birmingham, AL 35294-2042
Tel: 205 934-3863 *Fax:* 205 934-7802
E-mail: fammedres@fms.uab.edu
Accred Length: 3 Years *Program Size:* 18 (*GY1:* 6)
Program ID: 120-01-21-021

Huntsville

University of Alabama Medical Center (Huntsville) Program
Sponsor: University of Alabama School of Medicine
Huntsville Hospital
Program Director:
Michael M Linder, MD
Univ of Alabama Sch of Med-Huntsville
Dept of Family Practice
201 Governors Dr
Huntsville, AL 35801
Tel: 205 551-4632 *Fax:* 205 551-4633
E-mail: edwardsh@email.uah.edu
Accred Length: 3 Years *Program Size:* 36 (*GY1:* 12)
Subspecialties: FSM
Program ID: 120-01-11-023

Mobile

University of South Alabama Program
Sponsor: University of South Alabama Medical Center
Program Director:
Perry Dickinson, MD
Univ of South Alabama
Dept of Fam Prac/Com Med
1504 Springhill Ave
Mobile, AL 36604
Tel: 334 434-3484 *Fax:* 334 434-3495
E-mail: fpres@jaguar1.usouthal.edu
Internet: http://www.southalabama.edu/famprac
Accred Length: 3 Years *Program Size:* 23 (*GY1:* 8)
Program ID: 120-01-11-024

Montgomery

Baptist Outreach Services (Montgomery) Program
Sponsor: Baptist Outreach Services
Baptist Medical Center
Program Director:
Samuel Saliba, MD
Baptist Health
4371 Narrow Lane Rd
Ste 100
Montgomery, AL 36116-2952
Tel: 334 613-3699 *Fax:* 334 613-3685
E-mail: montfammed@bmcmont.hbocvan.com
Internet: http://www.fam-medmontgomery.org
Accred Length: 3 Years *Program Size:* 11 (*GY1:* 6)
Program ID: 120-01-21-624

Selma

University of Alabama Medical Center (Selma Dallas County) Program
Sponsor: Four Rivers Medical Center
Vaughan Regional Medical Center
Program Director:
Boyd L Bailey, MD
UAB-Selma Family Medicine Ctr
429 Lauderdale St
Selma, AL 36701
Tel: 334 875-4184 *Fax:* 334 874-0027
E-mail: sfm@tomnet.com
Accred Length: 3 Years *Program Size:* 15 (*GY1:* 5)
Program ID: 120-01-21-026

Tuscaloosa

University of Alabama Medical Center (Tuscaloosa) Program
Sponsor: University of Alabama College of Community Health Sciences
DCH Regional Medical Center
Program Director:
Marc A Armstrong, MD
Univ of Alabama Sch of Med-Tuscaloosa
Family Practice Program
Box 870377
Tuscaloosa, AL 35487-0377
Tel: 205 348-1373 *Fax:* 205 348-2695
E-mail: uatfprp@cchs.ua.edu
Internet: http://bama.ua.edu/~fpres
Accred Length: 3 Years *Program Size:* 37 (*GY1:* 12)
Program ID: 120-01-21-027

Alaska

Anchorage

Providence Hospital Program
Sponsor: Providence Hospital
Program Director:
Harold Johnston, MD
3546 LaTouche St
Anchorage, AK 99508
Tel: 907 561-4500 *Fax:* 907 561-4806
Internet: http://www.alaska.net/~akfpr
Accred Length: 3 Years *Program Size:* 24 (*GY1:* 8)
Program ID: 120-02-21-596

Arizona

Phoenix

Good Samaritan Regional Medical Center Program
Sponsor: Good Samaritan Regional Medical Center
Program Director:
Jeffrey D Wolfrey, MD
GSRMC Family Practice Residency
1300 N 12th St/#605
Phoenix, AZ 85006
Tel: 602 239-2668 *Fax:* 602 239-2067
E-mail: lorilog@samaritan.edu
Internet: http://www.samaritan.edu
Accred Length: 3 Years *Program Size:* 26 (*GY1:* 8)
Program ID: 120-03-12-028

Maricopa Medical Center Program
Sponsor: Maricopa Medical Center
Program Director:
Armaity V Austin, MD MPH
Dept of Family/Community Med
Maricopa Med Ctr
2601 E Roosevelt St
Phoenix, AZ 85008
Tel: 602 267-5426 *Fax:* 602 267-5196
Internet: http://www.maricopa.gov/medcenter/mmc.html
Accred Length: 3 Years *Program Size:* 18 (*GY1:* 6)
Program ID: 120-03-21-563

Phoenix Baptist Hospital and Medical Center Program
Sponsor: Phoenix Baptist Hospital and Medical Center
Program Director:
Christopher P Shearer, MD
Phoenix Baptist Family Med Ctr
2000 W Bethany Home Rd
Phoenix, AZ 85015
Tel: 602 246-5521 *Fax:* 602 246-5945
E-mail: pbhfmc01@swlink.net
Internet: http://www.baptistresidency.org
Accred Length: 3 Years *Program Size:* 23 (*GY1:* 8)
Program ID: 120-03-21-029

St Joseph's Hospital and Medical Center Program
Sponsor: St Joseph's Hospital and Medical Center
Program Director:
Paul Steinberg, MD
St Joseph's Hospital and Med Ctr
350 W Thomas Rd
PO Box 2071
Phoenix, AZ 85001-2071
Tel: 602 406-3152 *Fax:* 602 406-4122
E-mail: psteinb@mha.chw.edu
Internet:
http://www.mha.chw.edu/mha/research/meded.html
Accred Length: 3 Years *Program Size:* 24 (*GY1:* 8)
Subspecialties: FPG
Program ID: 120-03-12-030

Scottsdale

Mayo Graduate School of Medicine (Scottsdale) Program
Sponsor: Mayo Graduate School of Medicine-Mayo Foundation
Scottsdale Healthcare-Shea
Program Director:
Susan S Wilder, MD
13737 N 92nd St
Scottsdale, AZ 85260
Tel: 602 860-4800, ext 4868 *Fax:* 602 860-4820
Internet: http://www.mayo.edu
Accred Length: 3 Years *Program Size:* 18 (*GY1:* 6)
Program ID: 120-03-21-570

Scottsdale Healthcare-Osborn Program
Sponsor: Scottsdale Healthcare Hospitals
Maricopa Medical Center
Program Director:
Robert J Creager, MD
Family Practice Residency
7301 E Second St/Ste 210
Scottsdale, AZ 85251
Tel: 602 675-4890 *Fax:* 602 675-6801
E-mail: fpres@shc.org
Internet: http://www.shc.org/fpres
Accred Length: 3 Years *Program Size:* 24 (*GY1:* 8)
Program ID: 120-03-32-031

Tucson

University of Arizona Program
Sponsor: University of Arizona College of Medicine
University Medical Center
Program Director:
Victoria E Murrain, DO
Dept of Family/Com Med
1450 N Cherry Ave
Tucson, AZ 85719-4296
Tel: 520 626-7816 *Fax:* 520 626-6134
E-mail: rmn@u.arizona.edu
Internet:
http://www.ahsc.arizona.edu/~fcm/famresid.html
Accred Length: 3 Years *Program Size:* 24 (*GY1:* 8)
Subspecialties: FPG
Program ID: 120-03-12-032

Arkansas

El Dorado

University of Arkansas for Medical Sciences AHEC (South Arkansas) Program
Sponsor: UAMS-Area Health Education Centers
Area Health Education Center (South Arkansas)
Medical Center of South Arkansas
Program Director:
Rodney M Dixon, MD
Area Health Education Ctr-South Arkansas
460 W Oak/3rd Fl E
El Dorado, AR 71730
Tel: 501 862-2489, ext 342 2 *Fax:* 501 862-6353
E-mail: odonohoes@ahecsa.uams.edu or abdellage@ahecsa.uams.edu
Internet: http://www.uams.edu/ahec/ahec22.htm
Accred Length: 3 Years *Program Size:* 17 (*GY1:* 5)
Program ID: 120-04-21-405

Fayetteville

University of Arkansas for Medical Sciences AHEC (Northwest) Program
Sponsor: UAMS-Area Health Education Centers
Area Health Education Center (Northwest)
Washington Regional Medical Center
Program Director:
F Allen Martin, MD
Univ of Arkansas Med Sch-AHEC Northwest
2907 E Joyce
Fayetteville, AR 72703
Tel: 501 521-0263 *Fax:* 501 521-8723
E-mail: nwarfpr@ahecnw.uams.edu
Internet: http://www.ahecnw.uams.edu
Accred Length: 3 Years *Program Size:* 27 (*GY1:* 9)
Program ID: 120-04-21-033

Fort Smith

University of Arkansas for Medical Sciences AHEC (Fort Smith) Program
Sponsor: UAMS-Area Health Education Centers
Sparks Regional Medical Center
Program Director:
Jimmy D Acklin, MD
AHEC-Fort Smith Family Practice Residency Program
612 S 12th St
Fort Smith, AR 72901
Tel: 501 785-2431 *Fax:* 501 785-0732
E-mail: cmizell@ahecfs.uams.edu
Internet: http://www.ahecfsweb.uams.edu
Accred Length: 3 Years *Program Size:* 21 (*GY1:* 8)
Program ID: 120-04-21-034

Jonesboro

University of Arkansas for Medical Sciences AHEC (Northeast) Program
Sponsor: UAMS-Area Health Education Centers
St Bernards Regional Medical Center
Program Director:
Joe Stallings, MD
AHEC Northeast
Family Practice Program
223 E Jackson
Jonesboro, AR 72401
Tel: 870 972-0063, ext 30 *Fax:* 870 930-2914
E-mail: doris@ahecne.uams.edu
Internet: http://www.ahecne.uams.edu
Accred Length: 3 Years *Program Size:* 19 (*GY1:* 6)
Program ID: 120-04-21-406

Little Rock

University of Arkansas for Medical Sciences Program
Sponsor: University of Arkansas College of Medicine
John L McClellan Memorial Veterans Hospital
University Hospital of Arkansas
Program Director:
David A Nelsen Jr, MD
4301 W Markham/Slot 530
Little Rock, AR 72205-7199
Tel: 501 686-6610 *Fax:* 501 686-8421
Accred Length: 3 Years *Program Size:* 21 (*GY1:* 7)
Program ID: 120-04-21-035

Pine Bluff

University of Arkansas for Medical Sciences AHEC (Pine Bluff) Program
Sponsor: UAMS-Area Health Education Centers
Jefferson Regional Medical Center
Program Director:
Herbert F Fendley, MD
AHEC-Pine Bluff
Dept of Family Practice
4010 Mulberry
Pine Bluff, AR 71603
Tel: 870 541-6010 *Fax:* 870 541-6034
E-mail: resdirector@ahecpb.uams.edu
Internet: http://www.uams.edu/ahec/ahec21.htm
Accred Length: 3 Years *Program Size:* 30 (*GY1:* 10)
Program ID: 120-04-11-037

California

Anaheim

Southern California Kaiser Permanente Medical Care (Anaheim) Program
Sponsor: Southern California Kaiser Permanente Medical Group
Kaiser Foundation Hospitals (Anaheim)
Program Director:
Timothy A Munzing, MD
Kaiser Permanente Med Care
393 E Walnut St
Pasadena, CA 91188-8013
Tel: 800 541-7946 *Fax:* 714 967-4767
E-mail: scal.oc-residents@kp.org
Internet: http://www.kpscal.org
Accred Length: 3 Years *Program Size:* 19 (*GY1:* 6)
Program ID: 120-05-31-515

Bakersfield

Kern Medical Center Program
Sponsor: Kern Medical Center
Program Director:
Navin M Amin, MD
Kern Med Ctr
Dept of Family Med
1830 Flower St
Bakersfield, CA 93305-4197
Tel: 805 326-2191 *Fax:* 805 326-2181
E-mail: masengae@kernmedctr.com
Internet: http://frontpage.lightspeed.net/kmc-fp
Accred Length: 3 Years *Program Size:* 16 (*GY1:* 6)
Program ID: 120-05-11-038

Camp Pendleton

Naval Hospital (Camp Pendleton) Program

Sponsor: Naval Hospital (Camp Pendleton)

Program Director:
William L Roberts, MD
Dept of Family Practice
Naval Hospital
Box 555191
Camp Pendleton, CA 92055-5191
Tel: 760 725-0406 *Fax:* 760 725-1101
E-mail: pen1wjm@pen10.med.navy.mil
Accred Length: 3 Years *Program Size:* 36 (*GY1:* 12)
Program ID: 120-05-12-014
US Armed Services Program

Chula Vista

Scripps Memorial Hospital (Chula Vista) Program

Sponsor: Scripps Memorial Hospital-Chula Vista

Program Director:
Marianne McKennett, MD
1637 Third Ave
Chula Vista, CA 91911
Tel: 619 422-0354, ext 990 *Fax:* 619 425-5072
E-mail: scrippsfp@chw.edu
Accred Length: 3 Years *Program Size:* 6 (*GY1:* 6)
Program ID: 120-05-21-632

Fontana

Southern California Kaiser Permanente Medical Care (Fontana) Program

Sponsor: Southern California Kaiser Permanente Medical Group
Kaiser Foundation Hospital (Fontana)

Program Director:
Janis F Neuman, MD
Kaiser Permanente Med Care
393 E Walnut St
Pasadena, CA 91188-8013
Tel: 909 427-5083 *Fax:* 909 427-5619
Internet: http://ca.kaiserpermanente.org/
Accred Length: 3 Years *Program Size:* 27 (*GY1:* 9)
Subspecialties: FSM
Program ID: 120-05-12-040

Fresno

University of California (San Francisco)/Fresno Program

Sponsor: UCSF-Fresno Medical Education Program
University Medical Center

Program Director:
John Zweifler, MD MPH
Family Practice Dept
University Med Ctr
445 S Cedar Ave
Fresno, CA 93702
Tel: 209 459-5705 *Fax:* 209 459-4443
E-mail: zweifler@medisun.ucsfresno.edu
Internet: http://www.ucsfresno.edu/family
Accred Length: 3 Years *Program Size:* 39 (*GY1:* 13)
Program ID: 120-05-21-041

Glendale

Glendale Adventist Medical Center Program

Sponsor: Glendale Adventist Medical Center
White Memorial Medical Center

Program Director:
Janet Cunningham, MD
Glendale Adventist Med Ctr
Dept of Family Practice
801 S Chevy Chase Dr/#201
Glendale, CA 91205
Tel: 818 500-5594 *Fax:* 818 500-5550
E-mail: gamcfprp@ni.net
Accred Length: 3 Years *Program Size:* 24 (*GY1:* 8)
Program ID: 120-05-21-372

La Mesa

Sharp HealthCare (La Mesa) Program

Sponsor: Sharp HealthCare
Grossmont Hospital
Sharp Chula Vista Medical Center

Program Director:
Joseph F Leonard, MD
Grossmont Hospital
5555 Grossmont Ctr Dr
La Mesa, CA 91942
Tel: 619 644-4166, ext 3220 *Fax:* 619 644-4167
E-mail: jamipiearson@sharp.com
Internet: http://www.fprsharp.com
Accred Length: 3 Years *Program Size:* 30 (*GY1:* 10)
Subspecialties: FSM
Program ID: 120-05-21-539

Loma Linda

Loma Linda University Program

Sponsor: Loma Linda University Community Hospital

Program Director:
Dennis deLeon, MD
Loma Linda Univ Community Med Ctr
25455 Barton Rd/Rm 209-B
Loma Linda, CA 92354
Tel: 909 558-6688 *Fax:* 909 558-6656
E-mail: sreile@ccmail.llu.edu
Internet: http://www.llu.edu/llumc/family
Accred Length: 3 Years *Program Size:* 18 (*GY1:* 6)
Program ID: 120-05-21-471

Long Beach

Long Beach Memorial Medical Center Program

Sponsor: Long Beach Memorial Medical Center

Program Director:
Susan Y Melvin, DO
Long Beach Memorial Med Ctr
Memorial Family Med Program
450 E Spring St/#1
Long Beach, CA 90806-1625
Tel: 562 933-0063 *Fax:* 562 933-0079
E-mail: kambrose@memnet.org
Accred Length: 3 Years *Program Size:* 24 (*GY1:* 8)
Program ID: 120-05-21-044

Los Angeles

Charles R Drew University Program

Sponsor: Charles R Drew University of Medicine and Science
LAC-King/Drew Medical Center

Program Director:
Zakaria Boshra, MD
King-Drew Med Ctr
Dept of Family Med
1621 E 120th St/I&R Bldg Rm 2-110
Los Angeles, CA 90059
Tel: 310 668-4965 *Fax:* 310 763-8557
E-mail: dorothy_bush@dhs.co.la.ca.us
Accred Length: 3 Years *Program Size:* 21 (*GY1:* 7)
Program ID: 120-05-11-048

Southern California Kaiser Permanente Medical Care (Los Angeles) Program

Sponsor: Southern California Kaiser Permanente Medical Group
Kaiser Foundation Hospital (Los Angeles)

Program Director:
Jimmy H Hara, MD
Kaiser Foundation Hospital
4747 Sunset Blvd
Los Angeles, CA 90027
Tel: 323 783-8700
Internet: http://www.kpscal.org
Accred Length: 3 Years *Program Size:* 24 (*GY1:* 8)
Subspecialties: FPG
Program ID: 120-05-11-047

UCLA Medical Center Program

Sponsor: UCLA School of Medicine
Olive View-UCLA Medical Center
UCLA Medical Center

Program Director:
Martin A Quan, MD
UCLA Family Health Ctr
200 UCLA Med Plaza/Ste 220
Los Angeles, CA 90095-1628
Tel: 310 206-8718 *Fax:* 310 825-6826
Internet: http://www.medsch.ucla.edu/som/fammed
Accred Length: 3 Years *Program Size:* 24 (*GY1:* 8)
Subspecialties: FSM
Program ID: 120-05-11-049

University of Southern California (North Hollywood) Program

Sponsor: University of Southern California School of Medicine
Medical Center of North Hollywood
USC University Hospital

Program Director:
Tracey Lee Norton, DO
1420 San Pablo St
Los Angeles, CA 90033
Tel: 213 342-1313 *Fax:* 213 342-3070
E-mail: ranville@hsc.usc.edu
Internet: http://www.usc.edu/hsc/medicine/family_med
Accred Length: 3 Years *Program Size:* 30 (*GY1:* 10)
Program ID: 120-05-21-622

University of Southern California/California Medical Center (Los Angeles) Program

Sponsor: California Hospital Medical Center

Program Director:
Maureen P Strohm, MD
Univ of Southern California-California Hospital Med Ctr
1401 S Grand Blvd
Los Angeles, CA 90015
Tel: 213 742-5754 *Fax:* 213 742-5409
E-mail: famprac@chmc.unihealth.org
Internet: http://www.usc.edu
Accred Length: 3 Years *Program Size:* 21 (*GY1:* 7)
Program ID: 120-05-21-458

Programs

White Memorial Medical Center Program
Sponsor: White Memorial Medical Center
Program Director:
Luis Samaniego, MD
1720 Cesar Chavez Ave
Los Angeles, CA 90033
Tel: 323 260-5789 *Fax:* 323 881-8641
E-mail: tinatanner@msn.com
Internet: http://www.whitememorial.com
Accred Length: 3 Years *Program Size:* 21 (*GY1:* 7)
Program ID: 120-05-21-480

Martinez

Contra Costa County Health Services Program
Sponsor: Contra Costa Regional Medical Center
Program Director:
Jeff Smith, MD
Contra Costa Health Services Program
2500 Alhambra Ave
Martinez, CA 94553-3191
Tel: 925 370-5117 *Fax:* 925 370-5142
Accred Length: 3 Years *Program Size:* 27 (*GY1:* 9)
Program ID: 120-05-31-050

Merced

Sutter/Merced Community Medical Center Program
Sponsor: Sutter Merced Medical Center
Program Director:
David Araujo, MD
Sutter Merced Med Ctr
Dept of Family Practice
315 E 13th St
Merced, CA 95340
Tel: 209 385-7172 *Fax:* 209 385-7893
E-mail: mercedfp@elite.net
Internet: http://www.faccommed.ucdmc.ucdavis.edu
Accred Length: 3 Years *Program Size:* 18 (*GY1:* 6)
Program ID: 120-05-21-459

Modesto

Stanislaus County Health Services Program
Sponsor: Stanislaus County Health Services
Doctors Medical Center
Program Director:
John C Payne, MD
Stanislaus County Family Practice Program
PO Box 4138
Modesto, CA 95352
Tel: 209 576-3528 *Fax:* 209 576-3597
E-mail: kathy.garcia@tenethealth.com
Accred Length: 3 Years *Program Size:* 27 (*GY1:* 9)
Program ID: 120-05-11-052

Moreno Valley

Riverside County Regional Medical Center Program
Sponsor: Riverside County Regional Medical Center
Program Director:
Asma B Jafri, MD
Riverside County Regional Med Ctr
Family Practice Program
26520 Cactus Ave
Moreno Valley, CA 92555
Tel: 909 486-5610 *Fax:* 909 486-5620
E-mail: rghfp@co.riverside.ca.us
Internet:
http://www.geocities.com/yosemite/2088/index.htm
Accred Length: 3 Years *Program Size:* 27 (*GY1:* 9)
Program ID: 120-05-21-421

Northridge

Northridge Hospital Medical Center Program
Sponsor: Northridge Hospital Medical Center
Program Director:
Myron C Greengold, MD
Northridge Family Practice Residency
18406 Roscoe Blvd
Northridge, CA 91325
Tel: 818 993-4054 *Fax:* 818 993-1917
E-mail: nfp@deepfocus.com
Internet:
http://www.deepfocus.com/northridgefamilypractice
Accred Length: 3 Years *Program Size:* 20 (*GY1:* 7)
Program ID: 120-05-11-053

Orange

University of California (Irvine) Program
Sponsor: University of California (Irvine) Medical Center
Western Medical Center
Program Director:
Thomas C Bent, MD
Univ of California Irvine Med Ctr
Dept of Family Med
101 City Dr S/Bldg 200 Rt 81 Rm 512
Orange, CA 92868-3298
Tel: 714 456-6502 *Fax:* 714 456-7984
E-mail: apalega@uci.edu
Accred Length: 3 Years *Program Size:* 36 (*GY1:* 12)
Program ID: 120-05-21-042

Pomona

Pomona Valley Hospital Medical Center Program
Sponsor: Pomona Valley Hospital Medical Center
Program Director:
James E Cruz, MD
1770 N Orange Grove/Ste 201
Pomona, CA 91767
Tel: 909 469-9490 *Fax:* 909 865-2982
E-mail: pomfprp@earthlink.net
Internet: http://www.1.primenet.com/~fprp/
Accred Length: 3 Years *Program Size:* 16 (*GY1:* 6)
Program ID: 120-05-21-610

Redding

University of California (Davis)/Redding Program
Sponsor: Mercy Medical Center
University of California (Davis) Medical Center
Program Director:
Ronald W Sand, MD
Shasta-Cascade Family Practice Residency
2175 Rosaline Ave
PO Box 496009
Redding, CA 96049-6009
Tel: 916 225-6090 *Fax:* 916 225-6093
E-mail: tdailey@chw.edu
Internet: http://www.mercy.org
Accred Length: 3 Years *Program Size:* 24 (*GY1:* 8)
Program ID: 120-05-31-054

Riverside

Southern California Kaiser Permanente Medical Care (Riverside) Program
Sponsor: Southern California Kaiser Permanente Medical Group
Kaiser Foundation Hospital (Riverside)
Program Director:
Walter C Morgan, MD
Kaiser Permanente Med Ctr
393 E Walnut St
Pasadena, CA 91188-8013
Tel: 800 541-7946 *Fax:* 818 405-2675
Accred Length: 3 Years *Program Size:* 18 (*GY1:* 6)
Program ID: 120-05-21-509

Sacramento

Methodist Hospital of Sacramento Program
Sponsor: Methodist Hospital of Sacramento
University of California (Davis) Medical Center
Program Director:
Amir R Sweha, MD MD
Methodist Hospital
Family Practice Program
7500 Hospital Dr
Sacramento, CA 95823
Tel: 916 423-6009 *Fax:* 916 688-0225
Internet: http://www.calweb.com/~mhsfpres
Accred Length: 3 Years *Program Size:* 18 (*GY1:* 6)
Program ID: 120-05-21-564

Sutter Health Program
Sponsor: Sutter Health
Sutter Davis Hospital
Sutter General Hospital
Sutter Memorial Hospital
Program Director:
William R Gillanders, MD
1201 Alhambra Blvd/Ste 340
Sacramento, CA 95816
Tel: 916 731-7866 *Fax:* 916 731-7867
E-mail: sutterfprp@aol.com
Internet: http://www.sutterheatlh.org
Accred Length: 3 Years *Program Size:* 18 (*GY1:* 6)
Program ID: 120-05-31-556

University of California (Davis) Program
Sponsor: University of California (Davis) Medical Center
Program Director:
James Nuovo, MD '
Univ of California Davis Med Ctr
Lawrence J Ellison Ambulatory Care Ctr
4860 Y St/Ste 2300
Sacramento, CA 95817
Tel: 916 734-3432 *Fax:* 916 734-5641
E-mail: jim.nuovo@ucdmc.ucdavis.edu
Internet: http://famcommed.ucdmc.ucdavis.edu
Accred Length: 3 Years *Program Size:* 39 (*GY1:* 13)
Program ID: 120-05-11-039

Salinas

Natividad Medical Center Program
Sponsor: Natividad Medical Center
Program Director:
Richard E Brunader, MD
Natividad Med Ctr
PO Box 81611
1330 Natividad Rd
Salinas, CA 93912-1611
Tel: 408 755-4201 *Fax:* 408 755-6315
E-mail: nmcfpres@moco.monterey.ca.us
Internet: http://www.natividad.com/res
Accred Length: 3 Years *Program Size:* 21 (*GY1:* 7)
Program ID: 120-05-21-056

San Bernardino

San Bernardino County Medical Center Program

Sponsor: San Bernardino County Medical Center

Program Director:
Andre V Blaylock, MD
San Bernardino County Med Ctr
Dept of Family Med
780 E Gilbert St
San Bernardino, CA 92415-0935
Tel: 909 387-7882 *Fax:* 909 387-0407
E-mail: fammed@co.san-bernardino.ca.us
Internet:
http://www.co.san-bernardino.ca.us/cmc/fammed/residency/htm
Accred Length: 3 Years *Program Size:* 54 (*GYI:* 18)
Program ID: 120-05-11-057

San Diego

University of California (San Diego) Program

Sponsor: University of California (San Diego) Medical Center

Program Director:
William A Norcross, MD
UCSD Family Medicine Residency Program
PO Box 3027
200 W Arbor Dr/#8809
San Diego, CA 92163-1027
Tel: 619 543-5776 *Fax:* 619 543-5996
E-mail: mdixon@ucsd.edu
Internet: http://www.ucsd.edu/famres
Accred Length: 3 Years *Program Size:* 24 (*GYI:* 8)
Subspecialties: FSM
Program ID: 120-05-21-058

San Francisco

University of California (San Francisco) Program

Sponsor: University of California (San Francisco) School of Medicine
San Francisco General Hospital Medical Center

Program Director:
Peter Sommers, MD
San Francisco General Hospital-Community Health Network
Bldg 80/Ward 83
1001 Potrero Ave
San Francisco, CA 94110
Tel: 415 206-8610 *Fax:* 415 476-3454
E-mail: ucsffp@itsa.ucsf.edu
Internet: http://itsa.ucsf.edu/~sfghfp/
Accred Length: 3 Years *Program Size:* 39 (*GYI:* 13)
Program ID: 120-05-11-059

San Jose

San Jose Medical Center Program

Sponsor: San Jose Medical Center

Program Director:
Robert M Norman, MD
San Jose Med Ctr
25 N 14th St/Ste 1060
San Jose, CA 95112
Tel: 408 977-4507 *Fax:* 408 977-4456
Accred Length: 3 Years *Program Size:* 18 (*GYI:* 6)
Subspecialties: FSM
Program ID: 120-05-22-061

Santa Monica

Santa Monica-UCLA Medical Center Program

Sponsor: Santa Monica-UCLA Medical Center

Program Director:
Denise K Sur, MD
Santa Monica-UCLA Med Ctr
Dept of Family Practice
1255 15th St
Santa Monica, CA 90404
Tel: 310 319-4709 *Fax:* 310 393-5659
E-mail: dchalme@mednet.ucla.edu
Internet: http://www.mednet.ucla.edu/healthnet/santamonica/residency
Accred Length: 3 Years *Program Size:* 24 (*GYI:* 8)
Program ID: 120-05-11-064

Santa Rosa

University of California (San Francisco)/Santa Rosa Program

Sponsor: Sutter Medical Center of Santa Rosa

Program Director:
Marshall K Kubota, MD
Sutter Med Ctr of Santa Rosa
Dept of Family Practice
3324 Chanate Rd
Santa Rosa, CA 95404
Tel: 707 576-4070 *Fax:* 707 576-4087
E-mail: fp_srosa@ix.netcom.com
Internet: http://www.fpresidencysantarosa.org
Accred Length: 3 Years *Program Size:* 33 (*GYI:* 10)
Program ID: 120-05-11-065

Stockton

San Joaquin General Hospital Program

Sponsor: San Joaquin General Hospital

Program Director:
Dale Bishop, MD
San Joaquin General Hospital
Dept of Family Practice
PO Box 1020
Stockton, CA 95201
Tel: 209 468-6835 *Fax:* 209 468-6747
E-mail: sjgh@softcom.net
Accred Length: 3 Years *Program Size:* 21 (*GYI:* 7)
Program ID: 120-05-31-066

Torrance

Los Angeles County-Harbor-UCLA Medical Center Program

Sponsor: Los Angeles County-Harbor-UCLA Medical Center

Program Director:
Daniel B Castro, MD MPH
Harbor-UCLA Med Ctr
1001 W Carson St/Ste E
Torrance, CA 90502
Tel: 310 222-5205 *Fax:* 310 782-0752
E-mail: harborfp@aol.com
Internet:
http://members.aol.com/harborfp/fammed/index.htm
Accred Length: 3 Years *Program Size:* 40 (*GYI:* 12)
Program ID: 120-05-21-478

Travis AFB

David Grant Medical Center Program

Sponsor: David Grant Medical Center

Program Director:
Lt Col Brian V Reamy, MD
60th Med Operations Sqd/SGOL
101 Bodin Cir
Travis AFB, CA 94535-1800
Tel: 707 423-3735 *Fax:* 707 423-3501
E-mail: brian.reamy@60mdg.travis.af.mil
Accred Length: 3 Years *Program Size:* 31 (*GYI:* 10)
Program ID: 120-05-11-001
US Armed Services Program

Ventura

Ventura County Medical Center Program

Sponsor: Ventura County Medical Center

Program Director:
Lanyard K Dial, MD
Ventura County Med Ctr
Med Educ Dept
3291 Loma Vista Rd
Ventura, CA 93003
Tel: 805 652-6228 *Fax:* 805 652-6606
Accred Length: 3 Years *Program Size:* 39 (*GYI:* 13)
Program ID: 120-05-11-068

Whittier

University of Southern California Program

Sponsor: Presbyterian Intercommunity Hospital
Los Angeles County-USC Medical Center

Program Director:
Ana G Bejinez Eastman, MD
Presbyterian Intercommunity Hospital
12401 Washington Blvd
Whittier, CA 90602
Tel: 562 698-0811, ext 2786 *Fax:* 562 698-0010
E-mail: uscpih@linkonline.net
Internet: http://www.usc.edu/hsc/med/family_med
Accred Length: 3 Years *Program Size:* 23 (*GYI:* 6)
Program ID: 120-05-21-352

Woodland Hills

Southern California Kaiser Permanente Medical Care (Woodland Hills) Program

Sponsor: Southern California Kaiser Permanente Medical Group
Kaiser Foundation Hospital (Woodland Hills)

Program Director:
Jeffrey Safer, MD
Kaiser Permanente
5601 De Soto Ave
Woodland Hills, CA 91365-4084
Tel: 818 719-3973 *Fax:* 818 719-3784
E-mail: jilly.l.ducatman@kp.org
Internet: http://www.kpscal.org
Accred Length: 3 Years *Program Size:* 18 (*GYI:* 6)
Program ID: 120-05-21-514

Colorado

Denver

Exempla St Joseph Hospital Program

Sponsor: Exempla St Joseph Hospital
Program Director:
Martin Kiernan, MD
Exempla-St Joseph Hospital-Family Practice Ctr
2005 Franklin St
Midtown II/Ste 200
Denver, CO 80205
Tel: 303 764-2005 *Fax:* 303 764-2040
E-mail: kiernanm@exempla.org
Internet: http://www.saintjosephdenver.org
Accred Length: 3 Years *Program Size:* 24 (*GY1:* 8)
Program ID: 120-07-12-070

St Anthony Hospital Program

Sponsor: St Anthony Hospital Central
St Anthony Hospital North
Program Director:
Timothy E Dudley, MD
St Anthony Central Hospital
4231 W 16th Ave/Kuhlman Bldg
Denver, CO 80204
Tel: 303 629-3890 *Fax:* 303 595-6656
E-mail: veras@csn.net
Internet: http://www.sni.net/~veras/
Accred Length: 3 Years *Program Size:* 36 (*GY1:* 12)
Program ID: 120-07-12-069

University of Colorado (Denver Health and Hospital) Program

Sponsor: University of Colorado Health Sciences Center
Denver Health and Hospitals
Program Director:
Conry M Colleen, MD
Lucy Loomis, MD MPH
Denver Health and Hospitals
Dept of Family Med
777 Bannock St/MC1914
Denver, CO 80204
Tel: 303 436-6471 *Fax:* 303 436-5772
E-mail: lloomis@dhha.org
Accred Length: 3 Years *Program Size:* 4 (*GY1:* 2)
Program ID: 120-07-21-621

University of Colorado (University Hospital) Program

Sponsor: University of Colorado Health Sciences Center
University Hospital
Program Director:
Colleen Conry, MD
University Hospital
5250 Leetsdale Dr
Ste 302
Denver, CO 80246-1452
Tel: 303 388-0965, ext 601 *Fax:* 303 388-1168
E-mail: regina.garrison@uhcolorado.edu
Internet: http://atlas.uchsc.edu
Accred Length: 3 Years *Program Size:* 12 (*GY1:* 4)
Program ID: 120-07-21-619

University of Colorado at Columbia Rose Medical Center Program

Sponsor: University of Colorado Health Sciences Center
Denver Health and Hospitals
Rose Medical Center
Program Director:
Richard Nicholas, MD
Univ of Colorado Health Sciences Ctr
Rose Family Med Program
2149 S Holly St
Denver, CO 80222
Tel: 303 584-7913 *Fax:* 303 584-0300
E-mail: nicholar@rfmr.com
Internet: http://www.rfmr.com
Accred Length: 3 Years *Program Size:* 21 (*GY1:* 6)
Subspecialties: FP
Program ID: 120-07-21-071

University of Colorado Rural Program

Sponsor: University of Colorado Health Sciences Center
Avista Hospital
Denver Health and Hospitals
Rose Medical Center
Veterans Affairs Medical Center (Denver)
Program Director:
Colleen Conry, MD
UCHSC, Dept of Family Med
1180 Clermont St
Denver, CO 80220
Tel: 303 315-9711 *Fax:* 303 315-9748
E-mail: colleen.conry@uhcolorado.edu
Internet: http://hypoxia.uchsc.edu:8080/rose.res
Accred Length: 3 Years *Program Size:* 4 (*GY1:* 0)
Program ID: 120-07-21-537

Englewood

University of Colorado at Columbia Swedish Medical Center Program

Sponsor: University of Colorado Health Sciences Center
Swedish Medical Center
Program Director:
Richard J Drexelius, MD
Residency Administration
191 E Orchard Rd/#200
Littleton, CO 80121
Tel: 303 795-5494 *Fax:* 303 795-2912
Internet: http://www.sfmr.com
Accred Length: 3 Years *Program Size:* 18 (*GY1:* 6)
Program ID: 120-07-21-544

Fort Collins

Fort Collins Family Medicine Program

Sponsor: Poudre Valley Hospital
Program Director:
Roger P Bermingham, MD
Fort Collins Family Medicine Program
1025 Pennock Pl
Fort Collins, CO 80524-3250
Tel: 970 495-8803 *Fax:* 970 495-8891
Accred Length: 3 Years *Program Size:* 18 (*GY1:* 6)
Program ID: 120-07-31-072

Grand Junction

St Mary's Hospital and Medical Center Program

Sponsor: St Mary's Hospital and Medical Center
Program Director:
Daniel R Dill, MD
St Mary's Family Practice Program
1160 Patterson Rd
Grand Junction, CO 81506
Tel: 970 244-2195 *Fax:* 970 244-7522
E-mail: eharris@stmarygj.com
Internet: http://www.stmarygj.com
Accred Length: 3 Years *Program Size:* 18 (*GY1:* 6)
Program ID: 120-07-31-073

St Mary's Hospital and Medical Center Rural Program

Sponsor: St Mary's Hospital and Medical Center
Program Director:
Daniel R Dill, MD
St Mary's Family Practice Program
1160 Patterson Rd
Grand Junction, CO 81506
Tel: 970 244-2800 *Fax:* 970 244-7522
E-mail: eharris@stmarygj.com
Internet: http://www.stmarygj.com
Accred Length: 3 Years *Program Size:* 3 (*GY1:* 1)
Program ID: 120-07-21-597

Greeley

North Colorado Medical Center Program

Sponsor: North Colorado Medical Center
Program Director:
Mark E Wallace, MD MPH
North Colorado Med Ctr
1600 23rd Ave
Greeley, CO 80631
Tel: 800 336-6236 *Fax:* 970 346-2828
Internet: http://www.ncfm.edu
Accred Length: 3 Years *Program Size:* 21 (*GY1:* 7)
Program ID: 120-07-11-074

North Colorado Medical Center Rural Program

Sponsor: North Colorado Medical Center
Wray Community District Hospital
Program Director:
Mark Wallace, MD
North Colorado Med Ctr
1600 23rd Ave
Greeley, CO 80631
Tel: 800 336-6236 *Fax:* 970 346-2828
Internet: http://www.ncfm.edu
Accred Length: 3 Years *Program Size:* 31 (*GY1:* 8)
Program ID: 120-07-31-524

Pueblo

Southern Colorado Family Medicine Program

Sponsor: Centura Health St Mary-Corwin Medical Center
Program Director:
Charles H Raye, MD
Southern Colorado Family Med
1008 Minnequa Ave
Pueblo, CO 81004
Tel: 719 560-5870 *Fax:* 719 560-4730
E-mail: nhamilto@centura.org
Internet: http://s-co-familymed.com
Accred Length: 3 Years *Program Size:* 24 (*GY1:* 8)
Program ID: 120-07-21-075

Connecticut

Hartford

University of Connecticut Program

Sponsor: University of Connecticut School of Medicine
St Francis Hospital and Medical Center
Program Director:
Maria E Pharr, MD
Asylum Hill Family Practice Ctr
99 Woodland St
Hartford, CT 06105-1207
Tel: 860 714-6527 *Fax:* 860 714-8079
E-mail: wwiggles@stfranciscare.org
Accred Length: 3 Years *Program Size:* 18 (*GY1:* 6)
Program ID: 120-08-21-076

Middletown

Middlesex Hospital Program

Sponsor: Middlesex Hospital

Program Director:
Michael A Stehney, MD MPH
Family Practice Residency Program
Middlesex Hospital
90 S Main St
Middletown, CT 06457-8110
Tel: 860 344-6305 *Fax:* 860 344-6650
E-mail: family_practice@midhosp.chime.org
Internet: http://www.midhosp.org
Accred Length: 3 Years *Program Size:* 24 *(GY1:* 8)
Program ID: 120-08-21-077

Stamford

Stamford Hospital/Columbia University College of Physicians and Surgeons Program

Sponsor: Stamford Hospital

Program Director:
Joseph Connelly, MD
St Joseph Med Ctr
128 Strawberry Hill Ave
Stamford, CT 06904-1222
Tel: 203 353-2270 *Fax:* 203 353-2303
E-mail: joseph_connelly@stamhosp.chime.org
Accred Length: 3 Years *Program Size:* 15 *(GY1:* 5)
Program ID: 120-08-11-078

Delaware

Wilmington

Christiana Care Health Services Program

Sponsor: Christiana Care Health Services Inc

Program Director:
Daniel L De Pietropaolo, MD
Med Ctr of Delaware
Family Med Ctr
1401 Foulk Rd
Wilmington, DE 19803-2754
Tel: 302 477-3320 *Fax:* 302 477-3311
E-mail: fpres@mcd.gen.de.us
Internet: http://www.christianacare.org/residency/
Accred Length: 3 Years *Program Size:* 25 *(GY1:* 8)
Subspecialties: FSM, TY
Program ID: 120-09-11-079

Temple University (Wilmington) Program

Sponsor: St Francis Hospital

Program Director:
Kim L Carpenter, MD
Med Services Bldg Level II
7th and Clayton Sts
Wilmington, DE 19805
Tel: 302 575-8041 *Fax:* 302 575-8005
E-mail: francis@fwd.org
Internet: http://www.dca.net/~stfweb/fprp/
Accred Length: 3 Years *Program Size:* 18 *(GY1:* 6)
Program ID: 120-09-21-415

District of Columbia

Washington

George Washington University Program

Sponsor: George Washington University School of Medicine
Holy Cross Hospital of Silver Spring

Program Director:
Joyce Evans, MD
George Washington-Holy Cross Family Practice
255 Rockville Pike
Ste 101A
Rockville, MD 20850-4166
Tel: 301 738-3290 *Fax:* 301 738-3293
E-mail: gwfamily@gwis2.circ.gwu.edu
Internet:
http://www.gwumc.edu/dept/dhcs/meded/reside/fpr
Accred Length: 3 Years *Program Size:* 19 *(GY1:* 6)
Program ID: 120-10-21-555

Georgetown University/Providence Hospital Program

Sponsor: Providence Hospital

Program Director:
Robert J Carr, MD
Georgetown Univ-Providence Hospital
Family Practice Program
1150 Varnum St NE
Washington, DC 20017
Tel: 301 699-7707 *Fax:* 301 779-9001
E-mail: wallacab@gucfm.georgetown.edu
Internet:
http://www.gucfm.cfm.georgetown.edu/fpres.html
Accred Length: 3 Years *Program Size:* 21 *(GY1:* 7)
Subspecialties: FPG
Program ID: 120-10-21-080

Howard University Program

Sponsor: Howard University Hospital

Program Director:
Thomas Gaiter, MD
Dept of Com Health/Fam Pract
2041 Georgia Ave NW
Tower Bldg/Ste #3400
Washington, DC 20060
Tel: 202 865-1452 *Fax:* 202 865-3637
Accred Length: 3 Years *Program Size:* 18 *(GY1:* 6)
Program ID: 120-10-21-081

Florida

Clearwater

University of South Florida at Morton Plant Mease Health Care Program

Sponsor: University of South Florida College of Medicine
Morton Plant Hospital

Program Director:
Bruce Flareau, MD
Morton Plant Hospital
323 Jeffords St/MS 21
Clearwater, FL 33756
Tel: 813 518-2011 *Fax:* 813 461-8029
E-mail: emorroni@com1.med.usf.edu
Internet: http://mpmhealth.com
Accred Length: 3 Years *Program Size:* 14 *(GY1:* 8)
Program ID: 120-11-21-625

Daytona Beach

Halifax Medical Center Program

Sponsor: Halifax Medical Center

Program Director:
Richard T Branoff, MD
Halifax Med Ctr
PO Box 2830
303 N Clyde Morris Blvd
Daytona Beach, FL 32120-2830
Tel: 904 254-4167 *Fax:* 904 258-4867
Internet: http://www.halifax.org
Accred Length: 3 Years *Program Size:* 24 *(GY1:* 8)
Program ID: 120-11-11-083

Eglin AFB

Headquarters Air Force Development Test Center (AFMC) Program

Sponsor: Headquarters Air Force Development Test Center (AFMC)

Program Director:
Charles W Mackett III, MD
96th Med Group (AFMC)/SGOL
307 Boatner Rd/Ste 114
Eglin AFB, FL 32542-1282
Tel: 850 883-8288 *Fax:* 850 883-8192
E-mail: mackett@eglin.af.mil
Accred Length: 3 Years *Program Size:* 24 *(GY1:* 8)
Program ID: 120-11-12-003
US Armed Services Program

Fort Lauderdale

University of Florida/North Broward Hospital District Program

Sponsor: University of Florida College of Medicine
Broward General Medical Center
Coral Springs Medical Center

Program Director:
Bridget M Silva, MD
Dept of Family Practice
Coral Springs Med Ctr
3000 Coral Hills Dr
Coral Springs, FL 33065
Tel: 954 344-4269 *Fax:* 954 344-3187
E-mail: u-f-nbhd@bridge.net
Internet: http://www.netrox.net/~u-f-nbhd
Accred Length: 3 Years *Program Size:* 18 *(GY1:* 6)
Program ID: 120-11-31-549

Gainesville

University of Florida Program

Sponsor: University of Florida College of Medicine
Alachua General Hospital
Shands Hospital at the University of Florida

Program Director:
Karen L Hall, MD
Univ of Florida-Shands/AGH Family Practice
625 SW Fourth Ave
PO Box 147001
Gainesville, FL 32614
Tel: 352 392-4541 *Fax:* 352 392-7766
E-mail: zinkel@fpmg.health.ufl.edu
Internet: http://www.med.ufl.edu/chfm/fprp/brochure
Accred Length: 3 Years *Program Size:* 26 *(GY1:* 9)
Program ID: 120-11-21-084

Jacksonville

Mayo Graduate School of Medicine (Jacksonville) Program

Sponsor: Mayo Graduate School of Medicine-Mayo Foundation
Mayo Clinic (Jacksonville)
St Luke's Hospital

Program Director:
Sandra L Argenio, MD
4500 San Pablo Rd
Jacksonville, FL 32224
Tel: 904 296-4078 *Fax:* 904 296-3892
E-mail: mgsm.jack.fl.familymed@mayo.edu
Internet: http://www.mayo.edu/
Accred Length: 3 Years *Program Size:* 18 (*GY1:* 6)
Program ID: 120-11-21-545

Naval Hospital (Jacksonville) Program

Sponsor: Naval Hospital (Jacksonville)

Program Director:
Robert F Raspa, MD
Naval Hospital
Dept of Family Practice
2080 Child St
Jacksonville, FL 32214-5227
Tel: 904 777-7762 *Fax:* 904 542-7836
E-mail: jak0cah@jak10.med.navy.mil
Accred Length: 3 Years *Program Size:* 39 (*GY1:* 13)
Program ID: 120-11-21-015
US Armed Services Program

St Vincent's Medical Center Program

Sponsor: St Vincent's Medical Center

Program Director:
Frank J Kuczler Jr, MD
St Vincent's Med Ctr
2708 St Johns Ave
Jacksonville, FL 32205
Tel: 904 308-7374 *Fax:* 904 308-2998
E-mail: gnelson@jax-inter.net
Internet: http://www.baptist-stvincents.com
Accred Length: 3 Years *Program Size:* 30 (*GY1:* 10)
Program ID: 120-11-11-085

University of Florida Health Science Center/Jacksonville Program

Sponsor: University of Florida College of Medicine at Jacksonville
University Medical Center (UFHSC/J)

Program Director:
Marcia W Funderburk, MD
Family Practice Dept
Univ of Florida-Jacksonville
1255-B Lila St
Jacksonville, FL 32208
Tel: 904 549-5840 *Fax:* 904 549-5825
E-mail: funderbu@ufpc.umc.ufl.edu
Internet: http://chfmj.umc.ufl.edu
Accred Length: 3 Years *Program Size:* 30 (*GY1:* 10)
Program ID: 120-11-21-456

Miami

University of Miami-Jackson Memorial Medical Center Program

Sponsor: University of Miami-Jackson Memorial Medical Center

Program Director:
Enrique S Fernandez, MD
Univ of Miami-Jackson Memorial Med Ctr
Family Practice Program
PO Box 016700-R700
Miami, FL 33101
Tel: 305 243-2951 *Fax:* 305 243-2905
Accred Length: 3 Years *Program Size:* 24 (*GY1:* 8)
Program ID: 120-11-21-087

Orlando

Florida Hospital Program

Sponsor: Florida Hospital

Program Director:
Richard L Milholm, MD
Florida Hospital
2501 N Orange Ave/#235
Orlando, FL 32804-4641
Tel: 407 897-1514 *Fax:* 407 897-1885
E-mail: norma_hill@mail.flhmis.net
Internet:
http://www.flhosp.org/residency/familypractice/index.html
Accred Length: 3 Years *Program Size:* 48 (*GY1:* 16)
Program ID: 120-11-11-088

Pensacola

Naval Hospital (Pensacola) Program

Sponsor: Naval Hospital (Pensacola)

Program Director:
Thomas J Kersch, MD
Naval Hospital
Code 55
6000 Hwy 98 W
Pensacola, FL 32512-0003
Tel: 850 505-6472 *Fax:* 850 505-6501
E-mail: psa1bah@psa10.med.navy.mil
Accred Length: 3 Years *Program Size:* 32 (*GY1:* 12)
Program ID: 120-11-12-016
US Armed Services Program

St Petersburg

Bayfront Medical Center Program

Sponsor: Bayfront Medical Center

Program Director:
Corey H Evans, MD
Bayfront Med Ctr
700 6th St S
St Petersburg, FL 33701-4891
Tel: 813 893-6156 *Fax:* 813 553-7340
E-mail: fpweb@bayfront.org
Internet: http://www.bayfront.org
Accred Length: 3 Years *Program Size:* 27 (*GY1:* 9)
Program ID: 120-11-11-090

Tallahassee

Tallahassee Family Practice Program

Sponsor: Tallahassee Memorial Regional Medical Center

Program Director:
John R Purvis, MD
Family Practice Residency Program
1301 Hodges Dr
Tallahassee, FL 32308-4676
Tel: 850 681-5714 *Fax:* 850 841-6403
E-mail: fprp@mail.tmh.org
Internet: http://www.tmh.org
Accred Length: 3 Years *Program Size:* 30 (*GY1:* 10)
Program ID: 120-11-11-086

Georgia

Albany

Phoebe Putney Memorial Hospital Program

Sponsor: Phoebe Putney Memorial Hospital

Program Director:
Paul S Williamson, MD
Southwest Georgia Family Practice Residency
2336 Dawson Rd
Albany, GA 31701-2442
Tel: 912 888-8890 *Fax:* 912 888-8815
Accred Length: 3 Years *Program Size:* 18 (*GY1:* 6)
Program ID: 120-12-21-525

Atlanta

Emory University Program

Sponsor: Emory University School of Medicine
Crawford Long Hospital of Emory University
Grady Memorial Hospital

Program Director:
Lawrence L Golusinski, MD
Emory Univ Sch of Med
478 Peachtree St NE/Ste 818
Atlanta, GA 30308
Tel: 404 686-8213 *Fax:* 404 686-4366
E-mail: emoryfpr@fpm.eushc.org
Accred Length: 3 Years *Program Size:* 31 (*GY1:* 10)
Program ID: 120-12-21-562

Georgia Baptist Medical Center Program

Sponsor: Georgia Baptist Medical Center

Program Director:
Frank R Don Diego, MD
Georgia Baptist Family Practice Program
1000 Corporate Ctr Dr/Ste 200
Morrow, GA 30260
Tel: 770 968-6460 *Fax:* 770 968-6465
Accred Length: 3 Years *Program Size:* 18 (*GY1:* 6)
Program ID: 120-12-21-536

Morehouse School of Medicine Program

Sponsor: Morehouse School of Medicine
Southwest Community Hospital and Medical Center

Program Director:
Harry S Strothers III, MD
Michelle Nichols, MD
Southwest Professional Bldg
505 Fairburn Rd SW
Atlanta, GA 30331-2099
Tel: 404 756-1230 *Fax:* 404 756-1229
Accred Length: 3 Years *Program Size:* 15 (*GY1:* 5)
Program ID: 120-12-21-439

Augusta

Medical College of Georgia Program

Sponsor: Medical College of Georgia Hospital and Clinics

Program Director:
Paul D Forney, MD
Med Coll of Georgia
Dept of Family Med/HB3020
1120 Fifteenth St
Augusta, GA 30912-3500
Tel: 800 729-3157 *Fax:* 706 721-7518
E-mail: jhammon@mail.mcg.edu
Internet: http://www.mcg.edu/resident/fm/index/html
Accred Length: 3 Years *Program Size:* 24 (*GY1:* 8)
Program ID: 120-12-21-091

Columbus

The Medical Center Program

Sponsor: The Medical Center Inc

Program Director:
John R Bucholtz, DO
Med Ctr, Dept of Family Med
1900 Tenth Ave
Ste 100
Columbus, GA 31902
Tel: 706 571-1430 *Fax:* 706 660-2895
Accred Length: 3 Years *Program Size:* 36 (*GY1:* 12)
Program ID: 120-12-11-092

Fort Benning

Martin Army Community Hospital Program

Sponsor: Martin Army Community Hospital

Program Director:
Lt Col Jeffrey R Rifkin, MD
Martin Army Community Hospital
Dept of Family Pract/Com Med
Attn: MCXB-FRT
Fort Benning, GA 31905-6100
Tel: 706 544-1556 *Fax:* 706 544-3234
E-mail: etta_dudley@smtplink.benning.amedd.army.mil
Internet:
http://-benning.army.mil/fbhome/mach/fpres.htm
Accred Length: 3 Years *Program Size:* 27 (*GY1:* 7)
Program ID: 120-12-11-008
US Armed Services Program

Fort Gordon

Dwight David Eisenhower Army Medical Center Program

Sponsor: Dwight David Eisenhower Army Medical Center

Program Director:
Brian K Unwin, MD
Dwight David Eisenhower Army Med Ctr
Dept of Family/Com Med
Fort Gordon, GA 30905-5650
Tel: 706 787-9358 *Fax:* 706 787-9356
Accred Length: 3 Years *Program Size:* 24 (*GY1:* 6)
Program ID: 120-12-21-009
US Armed Services Program

Macon

Mercer University School of Medicine Program

Sponsor: Medical Center of Central Georgia

Program Director:
Fred S Girton, MD
Med Ctr of Central Georgia
3780 Eisenhower Pkwy
Macon, GA 31206
Tel: 912 784-3587 *Fax:* 912 784-3550
E-mail: fp.residency@mail.mccg.org
Accred Length: 3 Years *Program Size:* 24 (*GY1:* 8)
Program ID: 120-12-12-093

Rome

Floyd Medical Center Program

Sponsor: Floyd Medical Center

Program Director:
Mallory G Smith, MD
Dept of Family Practice
Floyd Med Ctr
2 Professional Ct
Rome, GA 30165-2832
Tel: 706 295-5644 *Fax:* 706 236-2174
E-mail: romefp@floydmed.org
Internet: http://gain.mercer.edu./floyd/contents.htm
Accred Length: 3 Years *Program Size:* 21 (*GY1:* 7)
Program ID: 120-12-31-094

Savannah

Memorial Medical Center Program

Sponsor: Memorial Medical Center

Program Director:
Keith E Ellis, MD
Memorial Med Ctr
PO Box 23089
Savannah, GA 31403-3089
Tel: 912 350-8837 *Fax:* 912 350-5118
Internet: http://www.memorialmed.com
Accred Length: 3 Years *Program Size:* 18 (*GY1:* 6)
Program ID: 120-12-11-095

Waycross

Medical College of Georgia (Okefenokee Satilla) Program

Sponsor: Medical College of Georgia Hospital and Clinics
Satilla Regional Medical Center

Program Director:
Paul D Forney, MD
Satilla Regional Med Ctr
410 Darling Ave
PO Box 139
Waycross, GA 31502
Tel: 912 287-4168 *Fax:* 912 284-2450
E-mail: kathiej@accessatc.net
Internet: http://www.satilla.org
Accred Length: 3 Years *Program Size:* 6 (*GY1:* 2)
Program ID: 120-12-21-637

Hawaii

Honolulu

Tripler Army Medical Center Program

Sponsor: Tripler Army Medical Center

Program Director:
Mary Wyman, MD
Dept of Family Pract/Community Med
Attn: MCHK-FMR
1 Jarrett White Rd
Tripler AMC, HI 96859-5000
Tel: 808 433-3313 *Fax:* 808 433-1153
E-mail: mary_j.wyman@tamc.chcs.amedd.army.mil
Internet: http://www.tamc.amedd.army.mil
Accred Length: 3 Years *Program Size:* 18 (*GY1:* 6)
Program ID: 120-14-21-502
US Armed Services Program

Wahiawa

University of Hawaii Program

Sponsor: University of Hawaii John A Burns School of Medicine
Wahiawa General Hospital

Program Director:
Neal A Palafox, MD
Physician Ctr at Mililani
95-390 Kuahelani Ave
Mililani, HI 96786
Tel: 808 627-3230 *Fax:* 808 627-3265
E-mail: wabinga@jabsom.biomed.hawaii.ea
Accred Length: 3 Years *Program Size:* 18 (*GY1:* 6)
Program ID: 120-14-21-541

Idaho

Boise

Family Practice Residency of Idaho Program

Sponsor: Family Practice Residency of Idaho
St Alphonsus Regional Medical Center
St Luke's Regional Medical Center

Program Director:
Todd K Swanson, MD
FPRI
777 N Raymond St
Boise, ID 83704
Tel: 208 367-6042 *Fax:* 208 322-7018
E-mail: meliblak@mailstn.sarmc.org
Internet: http://www.sarmc.org/residency
Accred Length: 3 Years *Program Size:* 28 (*GY1:* 9)
Program ID: 120-15-11-097

Family Practice Residency of Idaho Rural Program

Sponsor: Family Practice Residency of Idaho
St Luke's Regional Medical Center

Program Director:
Todd Swanson, MD
FPRI
777 N Raymond St
Boise, ID 83704
Tel: 208 367-6042 *Fax:* 208 322-7018
E-mail: meliblak@mailstn.sarmc.org
Internet: http://www.sarmc.org/residency
Accred Length: 3 Years *Program Size:* 3 (*GY1:* 1)
Subspecialties: FP
Program ID: 120-15-21-588

Pocatello

Idaho State University Program

Sponsor: Idaho State University
Bannock Regional Medical Center
Pocatello Regional Medical Center

Program Director:
Jonathan Cree, MD BS
Idaho State Univ
Dept of Family Med
Campus Box 8357
Pocatello, ID 83209-8357
Tel: 208 236-4508 *Fax:* 208 236-4818
Internet: http://www.clinic.isu.edu/fammed.html
Accred Length: 3 Years *Program Size:* 12 (*GY1:* 4)
Program ID: 120-15-21-521

Illinois

Aurora

Rush Medical College/Copley Memorial Hospital Program

Sponsor: Rush-Presbyterian-St Luke's Medical Center
Copley Memorial Hospital

Program Director:
Edward C Foley, MD MPH
Rush-Copley Family Practice Ctr
2020 Ogden Ave/Ste 325
Aurora, IL 60504
Tel: 630 978-6207 *Fax:* 630 375-2812
Accred Length: 3 Years *Program Size:* 12 (*GY1:* 4)
Program ID: 120-16-21-604

Belleville

St Louis University School of Medicine (Belleville) Program

Sponsor: St Louis University School of Medicine
St Elizabeth's Hospital
375th Medical Group

Program Director:
Michael P Temporal, MD
St Louis Univ Sch of Med-Belleville Program
180 S Third St/Ste 400
Belleville, IL 62220-1914
Tel: 618 233-7880, ext 1405 *Fax:* 618 233-3265
Internet: http://medschool.slu.edu/fpp
Accred Length: 3 Years *Program Size:* 42 (*GY1:* 14)
Program ID: 120-16-21-427

Berwyn

MacNeal Memorial Hospital Program

Sponsor: MacNeal Memorial Hospital

Program Director:
Penny Tenzer, MD
MacNeal Memorial Hospital
Dept of Family Practice
3231 S Euclid Ave
Berwyn, IL 60402
Tel: 708 783-3425 *Fax:* 708 783-3656
Internet: http://www.macneal.com/fpresidency
Accred Length: 3 Years *Program Size:* 32 (*GY1:* 12)
Program ID: 120-16-11-098

Carbondale

Southern Illinois University (Carbondale) Program

Sponsor: Southern Illinois University School of Medicine
Memorial Hospital of Carbondale

Program Director:
Penelope K Tippy, MD
Southern Illinois Univ Family Practice Ctr
305 W Jackson/Ste 200
Carbondale, IL 62901-6815
Tel: 618 536-6621, ext 221 *Fax:* 618 453-1102
E-mail: cnull@siu.edu
Internet: http://www.siumed.edu/fammed/carb.html
Accred Length: 3 Years *Program Size:* 18 (*GY1:* 6)
Program ID: 120-16-11-099

Chicago

Catholic Health Partners Program

Sponsor: Catholic Health Partners
St Joseph Health Centers and Hospital

Program Director:
Roger A Nosal, MD PhD
2900 N Lake Shore Dr
Chicago, IL 60657-6274
Tel: 773 665-3300 *Fax:* 773 665-3228
E-mail: stjfmed@cath-health.org
Internet: http://www.cath-health.org
Accred Length: 3 Years *Program Size:* 18 (*GY1:* 6)
Program ID: 120-16-11-103

Cook County Hospital Program

Sponsor: Cook County Hospital

Program Director:
Janice L Benson, MD
Dept of Family Practice
13th Fl Administration Bldg
1900 W Polk St
Chicago, IL 60612
Tel: 312 633-8587 *Fax:* 312 633-8454
E-mail: cchfpres@enteract.com.
Accred Length: 3 Years *Program Size:* 42 (*GY1:* 14)
Program ID: 120-16-11-100

Jackson Park Hospital Program

Sponsor: Jackson Park Hospital

Program Director:
Lakshmi P Dodda, MD
Jackson Park Hospital Family Practice Ctr
7501 Stony Island Ave
Chicago, IL 60649
Tel: 773 947-7310 *Fax:* 773 947-2487
E-mail: jpheras@flash.net
Internet: http://www.flash.net/~jphosp.
Accred Length: 3 Years *Program Size:* 13 (*GY1:* 7)
Program ID: 120-16-12-363

Loyola University Medical Center/Provident Hospital of Cook County Program

Sponsor: Loyola University Medical Center
Provident Hospital of Cook Country

Program Director:
Crystal Cash, MD
Provident Hospital of Cook County
Dept of Family Med
500 E 51st St
Chicago, IL 60615
Tel: 773 572-2673 *Fax:* 773 572-2677
Accred Length: 3 Years *Program Size:* 12 (*GY1:* 4)
Program ID: 120-16-21-612

Mount Sinai Hospital Medical Center of Chicago Program

Sponsor: Mount Sinai Hospital Medical Center of Chicago

Program Director:
Augustine Wong, MD
Mount Sinai Hospital Med Ctr
California Ave at 15th St/Rm L1026
Chicago, IL 60608
Tel: 773 257-6097 *Fax:* 773 257-6045
Accred Length: 3 Years *Program Size:* 19 (*GY1:* 6)
Program ID: 120-16-31-618

Resurrection Medical Center Program

Sponsor: Resurrection Medical Center

Program Director:
Robert L Buckley, MD
Family Practice Ctr
7447 W Talcott
Ste 182
Chicago, IL 60631
Tel: 773 792-5155 *Fax:* 773 594-7975
E-mail: rbuckley@reshealthcare.org
Internet: http://www.reshealth.org
Accred Length: 3 Years *Program Size:* 18 (*GY1:* 6)
Program ID: 120-16-11-102

Rush-Presbyterian-St Luke's Medical Center/Illinois Masonic Medical Center Program

Sponsor: Rush-Presbyterian-St Luke's Medical Center
Illinois Masonic Medical Center

Program Director:
Susan Vanderberg-Dent, MD
Rush-Illinois Masonic Family Practice Residency
1653 W Congress Pkwy
Chicago, IL 60612
Tel: 773 296-5290 *Fax:* 773 296-8020
E-mail: jsameshi@immc.org
Accred Length: 3 Years *Program Size:* 21 (*GY1:* 7)
Program ID: 120-16-21-543

St Elizabeth's Hospital Program

Sponsor: St Elizabeth's Hospital

Program Director:
James E Lang, MD
St Elizabeth's Hospital
1431 N Western Ave/Ste 406
Chicago, IL 60622
Tel: 312 633-5842 *Fax:* 312 633-5936
E-mail: stefprp@ancilla.org
Accred Length: 3 Years *Program Size:* 18 (*GY1:* 6)
Program ID: 120-16-21-428

St Mary of Nazareth Hospital Center Program

Sponsor: St Mary of Nazareth Hospital Center

Program Director:
Adolfo M Llano, MD
St Mary of Nazareth Hospital Ctr
Family Practice Program
2233 W Division St
Chicago, IL 60622-3043
Tel: 312 770-2060 *Fax:* 312 770-3264
Accred Length: 3 Years *Program Size:* 24 (*GY1:* 8)
Program ID: 120-16-11-104

Swedish Covenant Hospital Program

Sponsor: Swedish Covenant Hospital

Program Director:
Walten I Baba, MD PhD
Swedish Covenant Hospital
5145 N California Ave
Chicago, IL 60625-3642
Tel: 773 989-3808
E-mail: slasater@schosp.org or rarregui@schosp.org
Accred Length: 3 Years *Program Size:* 19 (*GY1:* 7)
Program ID: 120-16-31-106

University of Illinois College of Medicine at Chicago Program

Sponsor: University of Illinois College of Medicine at Chicago
University of Illinois Hospital and Clinics

Program Director:
Jeffrey C Rubin, MD
Univ of Illinois-Chicago Coll of Med
Dept of Family Med
1919 W Taylor St (M/C 663)
Chicago, IL 60612-7248
Tel: 312 996-8209 *Fax:* 312 996-2579
E-mail: davidgs@uic.edu
Internet: http://www.uic.edu/depts/mcfp/resident.html
Accred Length: 3 Years *Program Size:* 21 (*GY1:* 8)
Program ID: 120-16-21-488

University of Illinois College of Medicine at Chicago/Ravenswood Hospital Program

Sponsor: University of Illinois College of Medicine at Chicago
Ravenswood Hospital Medical Center

Program Director:
Margaret Wiedmann, MD
Ravenswood Hospital Med Ctr
4550 N Winchester Ave
Chicago, IL 60640-5205
Tel: 773 878-4300, ext 1248 *Fax:* 773 279-3982
E-mail: ravenswoodfpr@rhmc.com
Internet: http://www.advocatehealth.com
Accred Length: 3 Years *Program Size:* 15 (*GY1:* 5)
Program ID: 120-16-21-467

Decatur

Southern Illinois University (Decatur) Program

Sponsor: Southern Illinois University School of Medicine
Decatur Memorial Hospital
St Mary's Hospital

Program Director:
John G Bradley, MD
SIU-Decatur Family Practice Program
250 W Kenwood Ave
Decatur, IL 62526
Tel: 217 876-5850 *Fax:* 217 876-5822
E-mail: mtohill@somsclinics.siumed.edu
Internet: http://www.siumed.edu./dfpc
Accred Length: 3 Years *Program Size:* 18 (*GY1:* 6)
Program ID: 120-16-21-354

Evanston

St Francis Hospital of Evanston Program
Sponsor: St Francis Hospital of Evanston
Program Director:
Barbara J Moront, MD
St Francis Family Practice Residency
Lincolnwood Health Ctr
7126 N Lincoln Ave
Lincolnwood, IL 60646
Tel: 847 316-5961 *Fax:* 847 316-5395
E-mail: bmorontpd@hotmail.com
Internet: http://www.reshealth.org
Accred Length: 3 Years *Program Size:* 18 (*GY1:* 6)
Program ID: 120-16-21-599

Hinsdale

Hinsdale Hospital Program
Sponsor: Hinsdale Hospital
Program Director:
Gerald A Lofthouse, MD
Hinsdale Hospital-Hinsdale Family Practice
135 N Oak St
Hinsdale, IL 60521-3829
Tel: 630 856-8950 *Fax:* 630 856-8923
E-mail: hfpr@megsinet.net
Internet: http://ahsmidwest.org
Accred Length: 3 Years *Program Size:* 29 (*GY1:* 9)
Program ID: 120-16-21-109

Joliet

Provena St Joseph Medical Center Program
Sponsor: Provena St Joseph Medical Center
Program Director:
Jeffrey D Tiemstra, MD
Provena St Joseph Family Practice Residency
24024 W Brancaster Dr
Naperville, IL 60564-8044
Tel: 630 904-1220 *Fax:* 630 904-0967
E-mail: tiemstra@aol.com
Accred Length: 3 Years *Program Size:* 12 (*GY1:* 4)
Program ID: 120-16-21-647

Kewanee

University of Illinois College of Medicine at Peoria Rural Program
Sponsor: University of Illinois College of Medicine at Peoria
Kewanee Hospital
Methodist Medical Center of Illinois
Program Director:
Thomas B Golemon, MD
Methodist Family Med Ctr
815 Main St/Ste C
Peoria, IL 61602
Tel: 800 336-2380 *Fax:* 309 672-4790
E-mail: cbutenhoff@mmci.org
Internet: http://www.uicomp.uic.edu/
Accred Length: 3 Years *Program Size:* 31 (*GY1:* 11)
Program ID: 120-16-21-629

LaGrange

La Grange Memorial Hospital Program
Sponsor: La Grange Memorial Hospital
Program Director:
William J Nelson, MD
LaGrange Memorial Hospital
Community Family Practice Ctr
1323 Memorial Dr/Ste 214
LaGrange, IL 60525-2601
Tel: 708 482-1561 *Fax:* 708 352-3867
E-mail: mykaelmoss@interaccess.com
Accred Length: 3 Years *Program Size:* 21 (*GY1:* 7)
Program ID: 120-16-11-110

Oak Lawn

University of Illinois College of Medicine at Chicago/Christ Hospital Program
Sponsor: University of Illinois College of Medicine at Chicago
Christ Hospital and Medical Center
Program Director:
Kevin M Sherin, MD
Univ of Illinois-Christ Hospital
4400 W 95th St/Ste 207
Oak Lawn, IL 60453
Tel: 708 346-5324 *Fax:* 708 346-2003
E-mail: ksherin@uic.edu
Internet: http://www.uic.edu/orgs/uiccfp
Accred Length: 3 Years *Program Size:* 30 (*GY1:* 10)
Program ID: 120-16-21-364

Oak Park

West Suburban Hospital Medical Center Program
Sponsor: West Suburban Hospital Medical Center
Program Director:
Katherine A Walsh, MD
West Suburban Family Practice Program
7411 W Lake St
River Forest, IL 60305
Tel: 708 488-2367 *Fax:* 708 763-2162
Accred Length: 3 Years *Program Size:* 36 (*GY1:* 12)
Subspecialties: TY
Program ID: 120-16-31-112

Park Ridge

Lutheran General Hospital Program
Sponsor: Lutheran General Hospital
Program Director:
Ronald A Ferguson, MD MBA
Lutheran General Hospital
1775 W Dempster St
Park Ridge, IL 60068
Tel: 847 723-7969 *Fax:* 847 723-5615
E-mail: marie.markovich@advocatehealth.com
Internet: http://www.lghfpres.com
Accred Length: 3 Years *Program Size:* 24 (*GY1:* 8)
Subspecialties: FSM
Program ID: 120-16-11-107

Peoria

University of Illinois College of Medicine at Peoria Program
Sponsor: University of Illinois College of Medicine at Peoria
Methodist Medical Center of Illinois
Program Director:
Thomas B Golemon, MD
Methodist Family Med Ctr
815 Main St
Ste C
Peoria, IL 61602
Tel: 800 336-2380 *Fax:* 309 672-4790
E-mail: cbutenhoff@mmci.org
Internet: http://www.uicomp.uic.edu/
Accred Length: 3 Years *Program Size:* 30 (*GY1:* 10)
Program ID: 120-16-11-113

Quincy

Southern Illinois University (Quincy) Program
Sponsor: Southern Illinois University School of Medicine
Blessing Hospital
Program Director:
Jerry Kruse, MD
Quincy Family Practice Ctr
2325 Elm
Quincy, IL 62301
Tel: 217 224-9484 *Fax:* 217 224-7950
Internet: http://www.quincyfp.org
Accred Length: 3 Years *Program Size:* 16 (*GY1:* 5)
Program ID: 120-16-21-365

Rockford

University of Illinois College of Medicine at Rockford Program
Sponsor: University of Illinois College of Medicine at Rockford
Swedish American Health System
Program Director:
Peter J MacDonald, MD
L P Johnson Family Health Ctr
1221 E State St
Rockford, IL 61104-2232
Tel: 815 972-1037 *Fax:* 815 972-1092
E-mail: pjmacd@uic.edu
Internet: http://www.rockford.uic.edu/fprp.htm
Accred Length: 3 Years *Program Size:* 27 (*GY1:* 9)
Program ID: 120-16-31-115

Springfield

Southern Illinois University Program
Sponsor: Southern Illinois University School of Medicine
Memorial Medical Center
St John's Hospital
Program Director:
Janet Albers, MD
Dept of Family/Community Med
PO Box 19230
Springfield, IL 62794-1613
Tel: 217 757-0317 *Fax:* 217 757-8155
Internet: http://www.mhs1(cecelia fox)@attmail.com
Accred Length: 3 Years *Program Size:* 24 (*GY1:* 8)
Program ID: 120-16-21-117

Urbana

Carle Foundation Hospital Program
Sponsor: Carle Foundation Hospital
Program Director:
Timothy S Meneely, DO
602 W University Ave
South Clinic 2
Urbana, IL 61801
Tel: 217 383-3302 *Fax:* 217 383-3121
E-mail: timothy.meneely@carle.com
Internet: http://www.carle.com/residency/fp/index.htm
Accred Length: 3 Years *Program Size:* 12 (*GY1:* 4)
Program ID: 120-16-21-492

Indiana

Beech Grove

St Francis Hospital and Health Centers Program
Sponsor: St Francis Hospital and Health Centers
Program Director:
Richard D Feldman, MD
Family Practice Ctr
1500 Albany St/Ste 807
Beech Grove, IN 46107
Tel: 317 783-8923 *Fax:* 317 782-6916
Accred Length: 3 Years *Program Size:* 18 (*GY1:* 6)
Program ID: 120-17-11-125

Evansville

Deaconess Hospital Program
Sponsor: Deaconess Hospital
Program Director:
Kim A Volz, MD
Deaconess Family Practice Residency
Wallace M Adye Ctr
515 Read St
Evansville, IN 47710-1700
Tel: 812 426-6068 *Fax:* 812 426-3071
E-mail: deacfp@dynasty.net
Internet: http://www.deaconess.com
Accred Length: 3 Years *Program Size:* 18 (*GY1:* 6)
Program ID: 120-17-21-119

St Mary's Medical Center Program
Sponsor: St Mary's Medical Center
Program Director:
Thimjon Ferguson, MD
St Mary's Med Ctr
3700 Washington Ave
Evansville, IN 47750
Tel: 812 485-4173 *Fax:* 812 485-7968
E-mail: dmoehlen@stm2.smmcevv.com
Internet: http://www.stmarys.org
Accred Length: 3 Years *Program Size:* 20 (*GY1:* 6)
Program ID: 120-17-21-120

Fort Wayne

Fort Wayne Medical Education Program
Sponsor: Fort Wayne Medical Education Program
Lutheran Hospital of Indiana
Parkview Memorial Hospital
St Joseph's Medical Center
Program Director:
Frederic L Jackson, DO MPH
Fort Wayne Med Education Program
2448 Lake Ave
Fort Wayne, IN 46805
Tel: 219 422-6573 *Fax:* 219 423-6621
E-mail: fjackson@fwmep.edu
Internet: http://www.fwmep.edu
Accred Length: 3 Years *Program Size:* 30 (*GY1:* 10)
Program ID: 120-17-21-121

Gary

Methodist Hospitals Program
Sponsor: Methodist Hospitals
Program Director:
David E Ross, MD
600 Grant St
Gary, IN 46402
Tel: 219 886-4636 *Fax:* 219 886-4106
Accred Length: 3 Years *Program Size:* 12 (*GY1:* 4)
Program ID: 120-17-21-493

Indianapolis

Community Hospitals of Indianapolis Program
Sponsor: Community Hospitals of Indianapolis
Program Director:
Robin H Ledyard, MD
Community Hospitals of Indianapolis
10122 E 10th St/Ste 100
Indianapolis, IN 46229-2601
Tel: 317 355-5913 *Fax:* 317 898-9760
Accred Length: 3 Years *Program Size:* 23 (*GY1:* 7)
Program ID: 120-17-11-123

Indiana University School of Medicine Program
Sponsor: Indiana University School of Medicine
Clarian Methodist Hospital of Indiana
Program Director:
J Christopher Shank, MD
Clarian Methodist Hospital
1520 N Senate Ave
Indianapolis, IN 46202-2213
Tel: 317 929-8188 *Fax:* 317 929-6722
E-mail: mbishop@clarian.com
Internet: http://www.iupui.edu/~famprac/
Accred Length: 3 Years *Program Size:* 30 (*GY1:* 9)
Subspecialties: FSM
Program ID: 120-17-11-126

St Vincent Hospital and Health Care Center Program
Sponsor: St Vincent Hospital and Health Care Center
Program Director:
Judith A Monroe, MD
St Vincent Family Medicine Program
8220 Naab Rd/Ste 200
Indianapolis, IN 46260
Tel: 317 338-7600 *Fax:* 317 338-7606
E-mail: dmeastma@stvincent.org
Internet: http://www.stvincent.org
Accred Length: 3 Years *Program Size:* 24 (*GY1:* 8)
Subspecialties: TY
Program ID: 120-17-11-127

Muncie

Ball Memorial Hospital Program
Sponsor: Ball Memorial Hospital
Program Director:
Stewart C Brown, MD
Ball Memorial Hospital
2300 W Gilbert St
Muncie, IN 47303
Tel: 765 747-3376 *Fax:* 765 741-1983
Internet: http://www.ballhospital.org
Accred Length: 3 Years *Program Size:* 24 (*GY1:* 8)
Program ID: 120-17-11-128

South Bend

Memorial Hospital of South Bend Program
Sponsor: Memorial Hospital of South Bend
Program Director:
Robert J Riley, MD
Memorial Family Practice
714 N Michigan St
South Bend, IN 46601-1035
Tel: 219 284-7913 *Fax:* 219 284-6819
E-mail: memorialofsb@prodigy.net
Internet: http://www.qualityoflife.org/fpc.htm
Accred Length: 3 Years *Program Size:* 27 (*GY1:* 9)
Subspecialties: FSM
Program ID: 120-17-11-129

St Joseph's Medical Center of South Bend Program
Sponsor: St Joseph's Regional Medical Center of South Bend
Program Director:
Martin Wieschhaus, MD
St Joseph's Med Ctr of South Bend
801 E LaSalle St/PO Box 1935
South Bend, IN 46634
Tel: 219 237-7637 *Fax:* 219 239-6088
E-mail: mastaghp@sjcg.org
Internet: http://www.sjmed.com
Accred Length: 3 Years *Program Size:* 26 (*GY1:* 8)
Subspecialties: FSM
Program ID: 120-17-11-130

Terre Haute

Union Hospital Program
Sponsor: Union Hospital
Program Director:
Randall L Stevens, MD
Union Hospital, Dept of Family Practice
1513 N 6-1/2 St
Terre Haute, IN 47807
Tel: 812 238-7632 *Fax:* 812 238-7003
Accred Length: 3 Years *Program Size:* 18 (*GY1:* 6)
Program ID: 120-17-11-131

Iowa

Cedar Rapids

Cedar Rapids Medical Education Foundation Program
Sponsor: Cedar Rapids Medical Education Foundation
Mercy Medical Center
St Luke's Methodist Hospital
Program Director:
Gordon H Baustian, MD
Cedar Rapids Med Educ Foundation
1026 A Ave NE
PO Box 3026
Cedar Rapids, IA 52406-3026
Tel: 319 369-7393 *Fax:* 319 369-8351
E-mail: crmef@crstlukes.com
Internet: http://crmef.mercycare.org
Accred Length: 3 Years *Program Size:* 21 (*GY1:* 7)
Program ID: 120-18-22-132

Davenport

Genesis Medical Education Foundation Program
Sponsor: Genesis Medical Education Foundation
Genesis Medical Center
Program Director:
Monte L Skaufle, MD
Quad Cities Genesis Family Practice Program
1345 W Central Pk
Davenport, IA 52804-1844
Tel: 319 421-4450 *Fax:* 319 421-4449
E-mail: rwarhank@revealed.net
Internet: http://www.home.revealed.net/rwarhank/
Accred Length: 3 Years *Program Size:* 18 (*GY1:* 6)
Program ID: 120-18-21-133

Des Moines

Broadlawns Medical Center Program
Sponsor: Broadlawns Medical Center
Program Director:
Larry D Beaty, MD
Broadlawns Med Ctr
1801 Hickman Rd
Des Moines, IA 50314
Tel: 515 282-2565 *Fax:* 515 282-2332
E-mail: lbeaty@broadlawns.org
Internet: http://broadlawns.org
Accred Length: 3 Years *Program Size:* 30 (*GY1:* 10)
Program ID: 120-18-11-134

Iowa Lutheran Hospital Program
Sponsor: Iowa Lutheran Hospital
Program Director:
David A McInnes, MD
Iowa Lutheran Hospital
Family Practice Program
840 E University Ave
Des Moines, IA 50316-2396
Tel: 515 265-1050 *Fax:* 515 265-6884
Internet:
http://www.ihsdesmoines.org/familypractice.html
Accred Length: 3 Years *Program Size:* 16 (*GY1:* 8)
Program ID: 120-18-31-135

Mayo Graduate School of Medicine (Des Moines) Program
Sponsor: Mayo Graduate School of Medicine-Mayo Foundation
Mercy Hospital Medical Center
Program Director:
Charles H Korte, MD
Mercy Med Ctr
250 Laurel St
Des Moines, IA 50314
Tel: 515 643-4610 *Fax:* 515 643-4662
E-mail: mgsdm.medlab.specialties@mayo.edu
Internet: http://www.mercydesmoines.org
Accred Length: 3 Years *Program Size:* 24 (*GY1:* 8)
Program ID: 120-18-21-598

Iowa City

University of Iowa Hospitals and Clinics Program
Sponsor: University of Iowa Hospitals and Clinics
Mercy Hospital
Program Director:
Robert E Garrett, MD
Dept of Family Practice
01110-D PFP
Iowa City, IA 52242
Tel: 319 384-7507 *Fax:* 319 384-7822
E-mail: robert-garrett@uiowa.edu
Internet: http://www.uiowa.edu/~famprac/index.html
Accred Length: 3 Years *Program Size:* 24 (*GY1:* 8)
Program ID: 120-18-11-136

Mason City

North Iowa Mercy Health Center Program
Sponsor: North Iowa Mercy Health Center
Program Director:
Michael L Sparacino, DO
Family Practice Ctr
1000 4th St SW
Mason City, IA 50401-2999
Tel: 515 422-7779 *Fax:* 515 422-7125
E-mail: sparacim@mercyhealth.com
Internet: http://www.netins.net/showcase/nimres
Accred Length: 3 Years *Program Size:* 18 (*GY1:* 6)
Program ID: 120-18-21-373

Sioux City

Siouxland Medical Education Foundation Program
Sponsor: St Luke's Regional Medical Center
Marian Health Center
Program Director:
Michael J Jung, MD
Siouxland Med Education Foundation
2501 Pierce St
Sioux City, IA 51104
Tel: 712 294-5018 *Fax:* 712 294-5091
E-mail: leonards@mail.stlukes.org
Accred Length: 3 Years *Program Size:* 18 (*GY1:* 6)
Program ID: 120-18-21-137

Waterloo

Northeast Iowa Medical Education Foundation Program
Sponsor: Northeast Iowa Medical Education Foundation
Allen Memorial Hospital
Covenant Medical Center
Program Director:
John E Sutherland, MD
Northeast Iowa Family Practice Residency Program
2055 Kimball Ave
Waterloo, IA 50702-5047
Tel: 800 211-9283 *Fax:* 319 272-2527
E-mail: neifpr@sbt.net
Accred Length: 3 Years *Program Size:* 18 (*GY1:* 6)
Program ID: 120-18-21-138

Kansas

Kansas City

University of Kansas Medical Center (Hays) Rural Program
Sponsor: University of Kansas School of Medicine
Hays Medical Center
University of Kansas Medical Center
Program Director:
Mark C Meyer, MD
Univ of Kansas Med Ctr
Dept of Family Practice
3901 Rainbow Blvd
Kansas City, KS 66160-7370
Tel: 913 588-1902 *Fax:* 913 588-1951
E-mail: cplotycia@kumc.edu
Accred Length: 3 Years *Program Size:* 1 (*GY1:* 0)
Program ID: 120-19-31-554

University of Kansas Medical Center (Junction City) Rural Program
Sponsor: University of Kansas School of Medicine
Geary Community Hospital
University of Kansas Medical Center
Program Director:
Mark C Meyer, MD
Univ of Kansas Med Ctr
Dept of Family Med
3901 Rainbow Blvd
Kansas City, KS 66160-7370
Tel: 913 588-1902 *Fax:* 913 588-1951
E-mail: cplotyci@kumc.edu
Internet: http://www.kumc.edu/fammed
Accred Length: 3 Years *Program Size:* 3 (*GY1:* 1)
Program ID: 120-19-21-553

University of Kansas Medical Center Program
Sponsor: University of Kansas School of Medicine
University of Kansas Medical Center
Program Director:
Mark C Meyer, MD
Univ of Kansas Med Ctr
Dept of Family Med
39th and Rainbow Blvd
Kansas City, KS 66160-7370
Tel: 913 588-1902 *Fax:* 913 588-1951
E-mail: cplotyci@kumc.edu
Internet: http://www.kumc.edu/fammed
Accred Length: 3 Years *Program Size:* 48 (*GY1:* 16)
Subspecialties: FP
Program ID: 120-19-11-139

Salina

University of Kansas (Wichita)/Salina Program
Sponsor: University of Kansas School of Medicine (Wichita)
Salina Regional Health Center
Program Director:
Charles Allred, MD
Smoky Hill Family Practice Ctr
Salina Health Education Foundation
501 S Santa Fe/Ste 200
Salina, KS 67401
Tel: 913 825-7251 *Fax:* 913 825-1605
E-mail: smokyhil@kumc.edu
Internet:
http://www.kumc.edu/wichita/dept/fcm/smoky.html
Accred Length: 3 Years *Program Size:* 12 (*GY1:* 4)
Program ID: 120-19-21-366

Topeka

Kansas Medical Education Foundation Program
Sponsor: Kansas Medical Education Foundation
St Francis Hospital and Medical Center
Stormont-Vail Regional Health Center
Program Director:
Karen E Bruce, MD
3520 SW 6th St
Topeka, KS 66606-2806
Tel: 913 234-0880 *Fax:* 913 234-4150
E-mail: kbruce@cjnetworks.com
Internet: http://www.fmrp.org
Accred Length: 3 Years *Program Size:* 12 (*GY1:* 4)
Program ID: 120-19-21-534

Wichita

University of Kansas (Wichita) Program

Sponsor: University of Kansas School of Medicine (Wichita)
Via Christi Regional Medical Center
Via Christi Regional Medical Center-St Joseph

Program Director:
Richard H Leu, MD
Via Christi Regional Med Ctr
925 N Emporia
Wichita, KS 67214
Tel: 316 268-5996 *Fax:* 316 291-7869
Accred Length: 3 Years *Program Size:* 54 (*GY1:* 18)
Program ID: 120-19-21-630

University of Kansas (Wichita)/Wesley Program

Sponsor: University of Kansas School of Medicine (Wichita)
Columbia Wesley Medical Center

Program Director:
Carol A Johnson, MD
UKSM-W Family Practice Program
Wesley Med Ctr
3340 E Central
Wichita, KS 67208-3104
Tel: 316 688-3976
E-mail: kreed@kumc.edu
Internet:
http://www.kumc.edu/wichita/dept/fcm/wesley.html
Accred Length: 3 Years *Program Size:* 27 (*GY1:* 9)
Program ID: 120-19-11-142

Kentucky

Edgewood

St Elizabeth Medical Center Program

Sponsor: St Elizabeth Medical Center

Program Director:
Donald J Swikert, MD
St Elizabeth Family Practice Ctr
413 S Loop Rd
Edgewood, KY 41017
Tel: 606 344-3841 *Fax:* 606 344-3920
E-mail: kmward1@aol.com
Accred Length: 3 Years *Program Size:* 24 (*GY1:* 8)
Program ID: 120-20-11-143

Glasgow

University of Louisville (Glasgow) Program

Sponsor: University of Louisville School of Medicine
T J Samspon Community Hospital

Program Director:
Peter A Rives, MD
T J Samson Family Practice Ctr
1330 N Race St
Glasgow, KY 42141
Tel: 502 651-6791 *Fax:* 502 651-3182
E-mail: nlv@scrtc.blue.net
Internet: http://www.glasgow-uofl.org
Accred Length: 3 Years *Program Size:* 9 (*GY1:* 4)
Program ID: 120-20-21-613

Hazard

University of Kentucky Medical Center Rural Program

Sponsor: University of Kentucky College of Medicine
ARH Regional Medical Center
University of Kentucky Hospital

Program Director:
Joseph A Florence, MD
East Kentucky Family Practice Residency
100 Airport Gardens Rd
Ste 7
Hazard, KY 41701-9500
Tel: 606 439-3557, ext 244 *Fax:* 606 436-8833
E-mail: jaf@pop.uky.edu
Internet: http://www2.mccs.uky.edu/ruralhealth
Accred Length: 3 Years *Program Size:* 12 (*GY1:* 4)
Program ID: 120-20-21-512

Lexington

University of Kentucky Medical Center Program

Sponsor: University of Kentucky Hospital

Program Director:
Mark Scott, MD
Univ of Kentucky Coll of Med
Dept of Family Practice
Kentucky Clinic
Lexington, KY 40536-0284
Tel: 606 323-6711 *Fax:* 606 323-6661
Internet: http://www.family.gws.uky.edu/fp/fam_pr.htm
Accred Length: 3 Years *Program Size:* 24 (*GY1:* 8)
Program ID: 120-20-21-144

Louisville

University of Louisville Program

Sponsor: University of Louisville School of Medicine
Jewish Hospital
University of Louisville Hospital

Program Director:
Stephen F Wheeler, MD MD
Univ of Louisville Sch of Med
201 Abraham Flexner Way/Ste 690
Louisville, KY 40292
Tel: 502 852-5499 *Fax:* 502 587-4031
E-mail: mmshie01@med.louisville.edu
Internet: http://www.louisville.edu
Accred Length: 3 Years *Program Size:* 24 (*GY1:* 8)
Program ID: 120-20-21-145

Madisonville

Trover Clinic Foundation Program

Sponsor: Trover Clinic Foundation
Regional Medical Center of Hopkins County

Program Director:
Robert L Wood, MD
Trover Foundation
Family Practice Residency
435 N Kentucky Ave/Ste D
Madisonville, KY 42431
Tel: 502 824-3705 *Fax:* 502 824-3732
E-mail: famdoc@wko.com
Accred Length: 3 Years *Program Size:* 24 (*GY1:* 8)
Program ID: 120-20-31-146

Louisiana

Alexandria

Louisiana State University (Shreveport)/Rapides Program

Sponsor: Louisiana State University Hospital-Shreveport
Rapides Regional Medical Center

Program Director:
Dennis LaRavia, MD
Louisiana State Univ Med Ctr-Shreveport
Dept of Family Practice
821 Elliott St
Alexandria, LA 71301
Tel: 318 441-1063 *Fax:* 318 441-1066
E-mail: lsufamilymed@centuryinter.net
Accred Length: 3 Years *Program Size:* 17 (*GY1:* 8)
Program ID: 120-21-31-566

Baton Rouge

Baton Rouge General Medical Center Program

Sponsor: Baton Rouge General Medical Center

Program Director:
Robert Chasuk, MD
Family Health Ctr
3801 North Blvd
Baton Rouge, LA 70806
Tel: 504 387-7899 *Fax:* 504 381-2579
E-mail: #fmrp@generalhealth.org
Internet: http://www.generalhealth.org
Accred Length: 3 Years *Program Size:* 24 (*GY1:* 8)
Program ID: 120-21-21-560

Louisiana State University (Baton Rouge) Program

Sponsor: Earl K Long Medical Center

Program Director:
John T Howe, MD
Dept of Family Practice
5825 Airline Hwy
Baton Rouge, LA 70805
Tel: 504 358-1383 *Fax:* 504 358-1211
E-mail: mgrege@mail.ekl.lsumc.edu
Accred Length: 3 Years *Program Size:* 18 (*GY1:* 6)
Program ID: 120-21-21-400

Homer

Louisiana State University Medical Center (Shreveport) Rural Program

Sponsor: Louisiana State University Hospital-Shreveport
Homer Memorial Hospital

Program Director:
Michael B Harper, MD
Dept of Family Practice
Louisiana State Univ Med Ctr
PO Box 33932
Shreveport, LA 71130-3932
Tel: 318 675-5815 *Fax:* 318 675-7950
E-mail: mharpe@lsumc.edu
Accred Length: 3 Years *Program Size:* 6 (*GY1:* 2)
Program ID: 120-21-11-567

Kenner

Louisiana State University (Kenner) Program

Sponsor: Louisiana State University School of Medicine
Kenner Regional Medical Center
Medical Center of Louisiana at New Orleans

Program Director:
Roger J Zoorob, MD MPH
Louisiana State Univ Sch of Med-New Orleans
Dept of Fam Med-Kenner Program
1542 Tulane Ave/Ste 123
New Orleans, LA 70112
Tel: 504 471-2750 *Fax:* 504 471-2764
E-mail: rzooro@lsumc.edu
Internet: http://www.lsumc.edu
Accred Length: 3 Years *Program Size:* 18 (*GY1:* 6)
Program ID: 120-21-21-641

Lafayette

Louisiana State University (Lafayette) Program

Sponsor: University Medical Center (Lafayette)

Program Director:
Albert C Rees, MD
Univ Med Ctr
2390 W Congress St
Lafayette, LA 70506-4016
Tel: 318 261-6690 *Fax:* 318 261-6662
E-mail: arees@umc.lhca.state.la.us
Internet: http://155.58.21.21
Accred Length: 3 Years *Program Size:* 24 (*GY1:* 8)
Program ID: 120-21-11-149

Lake Charles

Louisiana State University (Shreveport)/Lake Charles Program

Sponsor: Louisiana State University Hospital-Shreveport
Lake Charles Memorial Hospital

Program Director:
Alan LeBato, MD
Lake Charles Memorial Hospital
Family Practice Clinic
1525 Oak Park Blvd
Lake Charles, LA 70601
Tel: 318 494-2023 *Fax:* 318 494-6750
E-mail: lsumc@lcmh.com
Internet: http://www.lcmh.com/lsumc-s.htm
Accred Length: 3 Years *Program Size:* 18 (*GY1:* 6)
Program ID: 120-21-21-594

Metairie

East Jefferson General Hospital Program

Sponsor: East Jefferson General Hospital

Program Director:
David W Euans, MD
East Jefferson General Hospital
Family Practice Program
4228 Houma Blvd/Ste 230
Metairie, LA 70006
Tel: 504 883-3722 *Fax:* 504 883-3723
E-mail: jthornhi@ejhospital.com
Accred Length: 3 Years *Program Size:* 18 (*GY1:* 6)
Program ID: 120-21-21-631

Monroe

Louisiana State University (Shreveport)/Monroe Program

Sponsor: E A Conway Medical Center

Program Director:
Donald N Givler Jr, MD
E A Conway Med Ctr
PO Box 1881
Monroe, LA 71210-1881
Tel: 318 330-7650 *Fax:* 318 330-7613
E-mail: eac-residency@lsumc.edu
Internet:
http://www.conway.lsumc.edu/resident/homepage.htm
Accred Length: 3 Years *Program Size:* 24 (*GY1:* 8)
Program ID: 120-21-21-440

New Orleans

Alton Ochsner Medical Foundation Program

Sponsor: Alton Ochsner Medical Foundation
Leonard J Chabert Medical Center

Program Director:
William R Brandon, MD
Ochsner Clinic
Dept of Family Practice
5701 Deer Park Blvd
New Orleans, LA 70127
Tel: 504 243-6024 *Fax:* 504 243-6052
E-mail: wbrandon@ochsner.org
Internet: http://www.ochsner.org
Accred Length: 3 Years *Program Size:* 12 (*GY1:* 4)
Program ID: 120-21-21-505

Shreveport

Louisiana State University (Shreveport) Program

Sponsor: Louisiana State University Hospital-Shreveport
Schumpert Medical Center

Program Director:
Michael B Harper, MD
Louisiana State Univ Med Ctr Hospital
Med Educ/Family Practice
1501 Kings Hwy/PO Box 33932
Shreveport, LA 71130-3932
Tel: 318 675-5815 *Fax:* 318 675-7950
E-mail: mharpe@lsumc.edu
Accred Length: 3 Years *Program Size:* 26 (*GY1:* 10)
Program ID: 120-21-21-150

Maine

Augusta

Maine-Dartmouth Family Practice Program

Sponsor: MaineGeneral Medical Center
Maine General Medical Center

Program Director:
Daniel K Onion, MD MPH
Maine-Dartmouth Family Practice Residency
15 E Chestnut St
Augusta, ME 04330-5796
Tel: 207 626-1894 *Fax:* 207 626-1902
E-mail: mdfpr@dartmouth.edu
Internet: http://www.dartmouth.edu/dms/mdfpr
Accred Length: 3 Years *Program Size:* 27 (*GY1:* 9)
Program ID: 120-22-22-151

Bangor

Eastern Maine Medical Center Program

Sponsor: Eastern Maine Medical Center

Program Director:
James A Raczek, MD
EMMC Family Practice Program
895 Union St
Ste 12
Bangor, ME 04401-0667
Tel: 207 973-7973, ext 7949 *Fax:* 207 973-7684
E-mail: emmcfprp@emh.org
Internet: http://www.emh.org/fprp
Accred Length: 3 Years *Program Size:* 27 (*GY1:* 9)
Program ID: 120-22-12-152

Lewiston

Central Maine Medical Center Program

Sponsor: Central Maine Medical Center

Program Director:
Timothy J Pollard, MD
76 High St
Lewiston, ME 04240-7681
Tel: 207 795-2803 *Fax:* 207 795-2190
E-mail: cmmcfpr@cmhc.org
Internet: http://www.cmmc.org
Accred Length: 3 Years *Program Size:* 18 (*GY1:* 6)
Program ID: 120-22-11-153

Portland

Maine Medical Center Program

Sponsor: Maine Medical Center

Program Director:
Ann K Skelton, MD
Maine Med Ctr
22 Bramhall St
Portland, ME 04102
Tel: 207 871-2875 *Fax:* 207 871-6055
Internet: http://www.mmc.org/mmcfp
Accred Length: 3 Years *Program Size:* 23 (*GY1:* 7)
Program ID: 120-22-31-154

Maryland

Andrews AFB

National Capital Consortium Program

Sponsor: National Capital Consortium
Malcolm Grow Medical Center (SGE)

Program Director:
William S Sykora, MD
Stonehouse E Stephen, MD
89 MDG/SGOEF
1075 W Perimeter Rd
Andrews AFB, MD 20762
Tel: 301 981-3956 *Fax:* 301 981-3011
E-mail: sykorw@mgmc.af.mil
Internet: http://usafsg.satx.disa.mil/~mgmcfp
Accred Length: 3 Years *Program Size:* 30 (*GY1:* 10)
Program ID: 120-23-21-002
US Armed Services Program

Baltimore

Franklin Square Hospital Center Program
Sponsor: Franklin Square Hospital Center
Program Director:
William D Hakkarinen, MD
Franklin Square Hospital Ctr
Dept of Family Practice
9000 Franklin Square Dr
Baltimore, MD 21237-3998
Tel: 410 682-7304 *Fax:* 410 682-8298
E-mail: williamh@helix.org
Internet: http://www.helixhealth.com
Accred Length: 3 Years *Program Size:* 24 (*GY1:* 8)
Program ID: 120-23-12-155

University of Maryland Program
Sponsor: University of Maryland Medical System
Union Memorial Hospital
Program Director:
Kevin S Ferentz, MD
Univ of Maryland
Univ Family Med
29 S Paca St/Lower Level
Baltimore, MD 21201
Tel: 410 328-5012 *Fax:* 410 328-0639
E-mail: sdiggs@schmed01.ab.umd.edu
Internet: http://www.umm.edu
Accred Length: 3 Years *Program Size:* 39 (*GY1:* 13)
Program ID: 120-23-21-156

Cheverly

Prince George's Hospital Center Program
Sponsor: Prince George's Hospital Center
Program Director:
A Clark Holmes, MD
Prince George's Hospital Ctr
Family Health Ctr
3001 Hospital Dr
Cheverly, MD 20785
Tel: 301 618-3433 *Fax:* 301 618-3943
Accred Length: 3 Years *Program Size:* 6 (*GY1:* 0)
Program ID: 120-23-31-157

Massachusetts

Beverly

Beverly Hospital Program
Sponsor: Beverly Hospital
Program Director:
Mark B Mengel, MD MPH
Beverly Hospital
75 Lindall St
Danvers, MA 01923
Tel: 508 762-4797 *Fax:* 508 762-6455
E-mail: mmengel@nhs-healthlink.org
Internet: http://www.nhs.healthlink.org
Accred Length: 3 Years *Program Size:* 18 (*GY1:* 6)
Program ID: 120-24-21-531

Boston

Boston University Medical Center Program
Sponsor: Boston Medical Center
Program Director:
Brian Jack, MD
Dowling 5 South
One Boston Medical Center Pl
Boston, MA 02118
Tel: 617 414-4465 *Fax:* 617 414-3345
E-mail: brian.jack@bmc.org
Accred Length: 3 Years *Program Size:* 8 (*GY1:* 6)
Program ID: 120-24-21-644

Fitchburg

University of Massachusetts (Fitchburg) Program
Sponsor: University of Massachusetts Medical School
Health Alliance Hospital-Leominster
Program Director:
Peter C McConarty, MD
Fitchburg Family Practice Program
275 Nichols Rd/4th Fl
Fitchburg, MA 01420
Tel: 978 665-5925 *Fax:* 978 665-5922
Internet:
http://www.family.medicine@banyan@ummed.edu
Accred Length: 3 Years *Program Size:* 18 (*GY1:* 6)
Program ID: 120-24-31-159

Lawrence

Greater Lawrence Family Health Center Program
Sponsor: Greater Lawrence Family Health Center Inc
Lawrence General Hospital
Program Director:
Scott C Early, MD
Lawrence Family Practice Residency
34 Haverhill St
Lawrence, MA 01841
Tel: 978 725-7410 *Fax:* 978 687-2106
E-mail: residency@glfhc.org
Internet: http://www.lawrencefpr.org
Accred Length: 3 Years *Program Size:* 24 (*GY1:* 8)
Program ID: 120-24-21-528

Malden

Malden Hospital Program
Sponsor: Malden Hospital
Program Director:
Joseph W Gravel Jr, MD
Peter F Jeffries, MD
Malden Hospital
Dept of Family Practice
100 Hospital Rd
Malden, MA 02148-3951
Tel: 781 397-6017 *Fax:* 781 397-6055
Internet: http://tmhfprp@shore.net
Accred Length: 3 Years *Program Size:* 18 (*GY1:* 6)
Subspecialties: TY
Program ID: 120-24-21-506

Worcester

University of Massachusetts Program
Sponsor: University of Massachusetts Medical School
St Vincent Hospital
UMass Memorial Health Care (Memorial Campus)
UMass Memorial Health Care (University Campus)
Program Director:
Vance Brown, MD
Benedict Bldg/A3-232
55 Lake Ave N
Worcester, MA 01655
Tel: 508 856-3011 *Fax:* 508 856-6400
Internet: http://www.ummed.edu
Accred Length: 3 Years *Program Size:* 45 (*GY1:* 15)
Program ID: 120-24-21-160

Michigan

Ann Arbor

St Joseph Mercy Hospital Program
Sponsor: St Joseph Mercy Health System
Program Director:
Eric Skye, MD
St Joseph Mercy Hospital
5333 McAuley Dr/RHB-4001
PO Box 995
Ann Arbor, MI 48106
Tel: 734 712-5015 *Fax:* 734 712-8777
Accred Length: 3 Years *Program Size:* 0
Program ID: 120-25-21-642

University of Michigan Program
Sponsor: University of Michigan Hospitals
Chelsea Community Hospital
Program Director:
John M O'Brien, MD
Univ of Michigan Hospitals
Dept of Family Med
1018 Fuller St
Ann Arbor, MI 48109-0708
Tel: 734 998-9173 *Fax:* 734 998-7335
Internet: http://www.med.umich.edu/fpc
Accred Length: 3 Years *Program Size:* 30 (*GY1:* 10)
Subspecialties: FSM
Program ID: 120-25-21-425

Dearborn

Oakwood Hospital Program
Sponsor: Oakwood Hospital
Program Director:
Michael J Worzniak, MD
Oakwood Healthcare System
18101 Oakwood Blvd
PO Box 2500
Dearborn, MI 48123-2500
Tel: 313 593-7798 *Fax:* 313 436-2071
Internet: http://www.oakwood.org
Accred Length: 3 Years *Program Size:* 24 (*GY1:* 8)
Subspecialties: TY
Program ID: 120-25-21-161

Detroit

Henry Ford Hospital Program
Sponsor: Henry Ford Hospital
Henry Ford Cottage Hospital
Samaritan Health Center-Mercy Hospital
Program Director:
Christine Jerpbak, MD
Henry Ford Hospital
Dept of Family Practice
One Ford Pl/Rm 2C
Detroit, MI 48202
Tel: 313 874-5373 *Fax:* 313 874-5381
E-mail: ddehrin1@hfhs.org
Accred Length: 3 Years *Program Size:* 36 (*GY1:* 12)
Program ID: 120-25-21-484

St John Hospital and Medical Center Program
Sponsor: St John Hospital and Medical Center
Program Director:
Aaron R Ellis, MD
St John Hospital and Med Ctr
Dept of Med Educ
22101 Moross Rd
Detroit, MI 48236
Tel: 313 343-3875 *Fax:* 313 343-7840
E-mail: sue.moynihan@stjohn.org
Internet: http://www.stjohn.org
Accred Length: 3 Years *Program Size:* 24 (*GY1:* 8)
Program ID: 120-25-11-163

Wayne State University/Detroit Medical Center Program
Sponsor: Wayne State University/Detroit Medical Center
Grace Hospital
Huron Valley-Sinai Hospital
Program Director:
Bruce R Deschere, MD
WSU Family Practice Residency Program
26454 Woodward
Royal Oak, MI 48034
Tel: 248 543-9915 *Fax:* 248 543-4246
E-mail: mlipman@med.wayne.edu
Internet: http://www.med.wayne.edu
Accred Length: 3 Years *Program Size:* 45 (*GY1:* 15)
Program ID: 120-25-21-164

Flint

McLaren Regional Medical Center Program
Sponsor: McLaren Regional Medical Center
Program Director:
Paul Lazar, MD
McLaren Family Practice
401 S Ballenger Hwy
Flint, MI 48532-3685
Tel: 810 733-9635 *Fax:* 810 733-9690
Accred Length: 3 Years *Program Size:* 18 (*GY1:* 6)
Program ID: 120-25-21-573

Grand Blanc

Genesys Regional Medical Center Program
Sponsor: Genesys Regional Medical Center
Program Director:
William K Stetson, MD
Genesys Regional Med Ctr
One Genesys Pkwy
Grand Blanc, MI 48439-1477
Tel: 810 606-5980 *Fax:* 810 606-5990
Internet:
http://msufame.msu.edu/family_practice/genframe.htm
Accred Length: 3 Years *Program Size:* 39 (*GY1:* 13)
Program ID: 120-25-31-166

Grand Rapids

St Mary's Health Services/Spectrum Health-Downtown Campus Program
Sponsor: St Mary's Health Services
Spectrum Health-Downtown Campus
Program Director:
Susan L Radecky, MD
Grand Rapids Family Practice Residency
200 Jefferson Ave SE
Grand Rapids, MI 49503
Tel: 616 752-6741 *Fax:* 616 732-3033
E-mail: mederaf@iserv.net
Internet: http://pilot.msu.edu/user/martinr3/grfpr_0.htm
Accred Length: 3 Years *Program Size:* 30 (*GY1:* 10)
Program ID: 120-25-21-167

Grosse Pointe

Bon Secours Hospital Program
Sponsor: Bon Secours Hospital
Program Director:
Peter Rodin, DO
Bon Secours Hospital
468 Cadieux Rd
Grosse Pointe, MI 48230
Tel: 313 343-1490 *Fax:* 313 343-1611
Accred Length: 3 Years *Program Size:* 18 (*GY1:* 6)
Program ID: 120-25-21-168

Kalamazoo

Kalamazoo Center for Medical Studies/Michigan State University Program
Sponsor: Kalamazoo Center for Medical Studies
Borgess Medical Center
Bronson Methodist Hospital
Program Director:
Robert W Reinhardt, MD
Michigan State Univ-Kalamazoo Ctr for Med Studies
Dept of Family Practice
1000 Oakland Dr
Kalamazoo, MI 49008-1284
Tel: 616 337-6550 *Fax:* 616 337-6565
E-mail: famprac@kcms.msu.edu
Internet: http://www.kcms.msu.edu
Accred Length: 3 Years *Program Size:* 21 (*GY1:* 8)
Subspecialties: FSM, TY
Program ID: 120-25-21-169

Lansing

Sparrow Hospital Program
Sponsor: Sparrow Hospital
Program Director:
George F Smith, MD
Sparrow-MSU Family Practice Program
Ste 245-C Sparrow Professional Bldg
PO Box 30480
Lansing, MI 48909
Tel: 517 364-5772 *Fax:* 517 364-5764
E-mail: dmlafave@aol.com
Accred Length: 3 Years *Program Size:* 40 (*GY1:* 12)
Program ID: 120-25-21-170

Marquette

Marquette General Hospital Program
Sponsor: Marquette General Hospital
Program Director:
John L Lehtinen, MD
Marquette General Hospital
Family Care Doctors
1414 W Fair Ave/Ste 36
Marquette, MI 49855
Tel: 906 225-3867 *Fax:* 906 225-7667
E-mail: residency@mgh.org
Internet: http://www.mgh.org/
Accred Length: 3 Years *Program Size:* 18 (*GY1:* 6)
Program ID: 120-25-21-370

Midland

MidMichigan Regional Medical Center Program
Sponsor: MidMichigan Regional Medical Center
Program Director:
William Dery, MD
MidMichigan Regional Med Ctr
Office of Med Educ
4005 Orchard Dr
Midland, MI 48670
Tel: 517 839-3320 *Fax:* 517 839-3344
E-mail: fpresidency@midmichigan.org
Internet: http://www.midmichigan.org
Accred Length: 3 Years *Program Size:* 18 (*GY1:* 6)
Program ID: 120-25-31-171

Pontiac

North Oakland Medical Center Program
Sponsor: North Oakland Medical Center
Program Director:
Anthony N Vettraino Jr, MD
North Oakland Med Ctrs
Family Practice Ctr
461 W Huron
Pontiac, MI 48341
Tel: 248 857-6700
E-mail: nomcfamprac@psinet.com
Accred Length: 3 Years *Program Size:* 18 (*GY1:* 6)
Program ID: 120-25-12-172

Royal Oak

William Beaumont Hospital Program
Sponsor: William Beaumont Hospital
William Beaumont Hospital-Troy
Program Director:
Paul W Misch, MD
William Beaumont Hospital
44201 Dequindre Rd
Troy, MI 48098
Tel: 248 828-5345 *Fax:* 248 828-6085
E-mail: pmisch@beaumont.edu
Internet: http://www.beaumont.edu/html/gme
Accred Length: 3 Years *Program Size:* 18 (*GY1:* 6)
Program ID: 120-25-21-374

Saginaw

Saginaw Cooperative Hospitals Program
Sponsor: Saginaw Cooperative Hospitals Inc
Covenant Medical Center
Saginaw General Hospital
Program Director:
Thomas J Zuber, MD
Saginaw Cooperative Hospitals
1000 Houghton Ave
Saginaw, MI 48602
Tel: 517 771-6901 *Fax:* 517 771-6941
E-mail: pruitt@pilot.msu.edu
Internet:
http://www.chm.msu.edu:80/saginaw/index.html
Accred Length: 3 Years *Program Size:* 24 (*GY1:* 8)
Program ID: 120-25-31-174

South Haven

Kalamazoo Center for Medical Studies/Michigan State University Rural Program
Sponsor: Kalamazoo Center for Medical Studies
South Haven Community Hospital
Borgess Medical Center
Bronson Methodist Hospital
Program Director:
Robert Reinhardt, MD
1000 Oakland Dr
Kalamazoo, MI 49008
Tel: 616 337-6554 *Fax:* 616 337-6565
E-mail: dickson@kcms.msu.edu
Internet: http://www.kcms.msu.edu
Accred Length: 3 Years *Program Size:* 4 (*GY1:* 2)
Program ID: 120-25-21-638

Southfield

Providence Hospital and Medical Centers Program

Sponsor: Providence Hospital and Medical Centers

Program Director:
Gary G Otsuji, MD
Providence Family Practice Ctr/5th Fl PMB
22250 Providence Dr
Southfield, MI 48075-4818
Tel: 248 424-3447 *Fax:* 248 424-8277
E-mail: gotsugi@ic.net
Internet: http://ic.net/piepwin/4b.htm
Accred Length: 3 Years *Program Size:* 33 (*GY1:* 11)
Subspecialties: FSM
Program ID: 120-25-21-175

Traverse City

Munson Medical Center Program

Sponsor: Munson Medical Center

Program Director:
Daniel M Webster, MD
Munson Family Practice Residency
Grad Med Educ Office
1400 Medical Campus Dr
Traverse City, MI 49684
Tel: 616 935-8070 *Fax:* 616 935-8098
Accred Length: 3 Years *Program Size:* 15 (*GY1:* 5)
Program ID: 120-25-21-602

Minnesota

Duluth

Duluth Graduate Medical Education Council Program

Sponsor: St Luke's Hospital
St Mary's Medical Center

Program Director:
Thomas W Day, MD
Duluth Family Practice Residency Program
330 N Eighth Ave E
Duluth, MN 55805
Tel: 218 725-2601 *Fax:* 218 725-2620
E-mail: jlonetto@d.umn.edu
Internet: http://www.d.umn.edu/medweb/mwdfpr/
Accred Length: 3 Years *Program Size:* 30 (*GY1:* 10)
Program ID: 120-26-21-176

Maplewood

University of Minnesota/St John's Hospital Program

Sponsor: University of Minnesota Medical School
St John's Hospital

Program Director:
David C Current, MD
Univ Family Physicians-Phalen Village
1414 Maryland Ave E
St Paul, MN 55106
Tel: 651 772-3461 *Fax:* 651 772-2605
E-mail: residency@famprac.umn.edu
Internet: http://www.med.umn.edu/fp
Accred Length: 3 Years *Program Size:* 18 (*GY1:* 6)
Program ID: 120-26-11-652

Minneapolis

Hennepin County Medical Center Program

Sponsor: Hennepin County Medical Center

Program Director:
Patricia Cole, MD
Family Med Ctr
5 W Lake St
Minneapolis, MN 55408
Tel: 612 827-9777 *Fax:* 612 827-9734
E-mail: mindy.chatelle@co.hennepin.mn.us
Internet: http://www.hcmc.org
Accred Length: 3 Years *Program Size:* 39 (*GY1:* 12)
Subspecialties: FSM
Program ID: 120-26-11-177

University of Minnesota (Waseca-Mankato) Program

Sponsor: University of Minnesota Medical School
Immanuel-St Joseph's Hospital
St John's Hospital

Program Director:
James W Jessen, MD
Univ of Minnesota
Dept of Family Practice
501 N State St
Waseca, MN 56093-2899
Tel: 507 837-4143 *Fax:* 507 837-4179
E-mail: wnowak@famprac.umn.edu
Internet: http://www.med.umn.edu/fp/index.htm
Accred Length: 3 Years *Program Size:* 18 (*GY1:* 6)
Program ID: 120-26-21-568

University of Minnesota-Health System Minnesota Program

Sponsor: University of Minnesota Medical School
Methodist Hospital

Program Director:
Kenneth N Kephart, MD
HealthSystem Minnesota-Univ of Minnesota
Creekside Family Physicians
6600 Excelsior/Ste 160
St Louis Park, MN 55426
Tel: 612 938-0794 *Fax:* 612 938-3135
E-mail: hsmrsdnt@hsmnet.com
Internet: http://www.med.umn.edu/fp/
Accred Length: 3 Years *Program Size:* 19 (*GY1:* 6)
Program ID: 120-26-21-617

University of Minnesota/Fairview-University Medical Center Program

Sponsor: University of Minnesota Medical School
Fairview-University Medical Center

Program Director:
Gregory J Gepner, MD
Smiley's Clinic
2615 E Franklin Ave
Minneapolis, MN 55406
Tel: 612 333-0770 *Fax:* 612 333-1986
E-mail: residency@famprac.umn.edu
Internet: http://www.med.umn.edu/fp
Accred Length: 3 Years *Program Size:* 32 (*GY1:* 10)
Program ID: 120-26-21-650

Robbinsdale

University of Minnesota/North Memorial Health Care Program

Sponsor: University of Minnesota Medical School
North Memorial Health Care

Program Director:
Mark R Bixby, MD
1020 W Broadway
Minneapolis, MN 55411
Tel: 612 521-4721 *Fax:* 612 521-4725
E-mail: residency@famprac.umn.edu
Internet: http://www.med.umn.edu/fp
Accred Length: 3 Years *Program Size:* 33 (*GY1:* 10)
Program ID: 120-26-31-651

Rochester

Mayo Graduate School of Medicine (Rochester) Program

Sponsor: Mayo Graduate School of Medicine-Mayo Foundation
Mayo Clinic (Rochester)
Rochester Methodist Hospital
St Mary's Hospital of Rochester

Program Director:
Matthew E Bernard, MD
Application Processing Ctr
Mayo Graduate Sch of Med
200 First St SW
Rochester, MN 55905
Tel: 507 266-0251 *Fax:* 507 284-5067
E-mail: mgsm.medlab.specialties@mayo.edu
Internet: http://www.mayo.edu/
Accred Length: 3 Years *Program Size:* 24 (*GY1:* 8)
Program ID: 120-26-21-179

St Cloud

Mayo Graduate School of Medicine (St Cloud) Program

Sponsor: Mayo Graduate School of Medicine-Mayo Foundation
St Cloud Hospital

Program Director:
George Schoephoerster, MD
Family Practice Ctr
1520 Whitney Ct/Ste 200
St Cloud, MN 56303
Tel: 320 240-3182 *Fax:* 320 240-3165
Internet: http://www.mayo.edu/mgsm/rschmfp.htm
Accred Length: 3 Years *Program Size:* 12 (*GY1:* 4)
Program ID: 120-26-21-586

St Paul

Allina Health System Program

Sponsor: Allina Health System
United Hospital
Children's Health Care (St Paul)

Program Director:
Kathleen M Macken, MD
United Family Medicine Program
545 W Seventh St
St Paul, MN 55102
Tel: 651 293-0069 *Fax:* 651 293-5889
E-mail: jgray@allina.com
Accred Length: 3 Years *Program Size:* 18 (*GY1:* 6)
Program ID: 120-26-21-526

HealthPartners Institute for Medical Education Program

Sponsor: HealthPartners Institute for Medical Education
Regions Hospital

Program Director:
Gwen W Halaas, MD MBA
HealthPartners Family Medicine Program
Regions Hospital
640 Jackson St
St Paul, MN 55101-2595
Tel: 612 221-3540 *Fax:* 612 221-4360
E-mail: dee.m.st_george@healthpartners.com
Accred Length: 3 Years *Program Size:* 36 (*GY1:* 12)
Program ID: 120-26-11-180

University of Minnesota/HealthEast St Joseph's Hospital Program

Sponsor: University of Minnesota Medical School
Healtheast St Joseph's Hospital

Program Director:
James S Van Vooren, MD
Univ Family Physicians-Bethesda Clinic
580 Rice St
St Paul, MN 55103
Tel: 612 227-1804 *Fax:* 612 227-6551
E-mail: residency@famprac.umn.edu
Internet: http://www.med.umn.edu/fp
Accred Length: 3 Years *Program Size:* 30 (*GY1:* 8)
Program ID: 120-26-12-653

Mississippi

Jackson

University of Mississippi Medical Center Program

Sponsor: University of Mississippi School of Medicine
University Hospital

Program Director:
Diane K Beebe, MD
Univ Hospital
Dept of Family Med
2500 N State St
Jackson, MS 39216-4505
Tel: 601 984-5426 *Fax:* 601 984-6835
E-mail: brousard@fiona.usmed.edu
Accred Length: 3 Years *Program Size:* 33 (*GY1:* 10)
Program ID: 120-27-21-181

Tupelo

North Mississippi Medical Center (Tupelo) Program

Sponsor: North Mississippi Medical Center
University of Mississippi School of Medicine

Program Director:
Edward Hill, MD
North Mississippi Med Ctr
1680 S Green St
Tupelo, MS 38801
Tel: 601 791-2261 *Fax:* 601 791-2263
E-mail: jconwill@nmhs.net
Internet: http://www.nmhs.net
Accred Length: 3 Years *Program Size:* 18 (*GY1:* 6)
Program ID: 120-27-21-558

Missouri

Columbia

University of Missouri-Columbia Program

Sponsor: University of Missouri-Columbia School of Medicine
University Hospitals and Clinics

Program Director:
Erika N Ringdahl, MD
Univ of Missouri-Columbia
Dept of Family/Com Med
One Hospital Dr/DC032.00
Columbia, MO 65212
Tel: 573 882-9099 *Fax:* 573 882-9096
E-mail: resident@health.missouri.edu
Internet: http://www.fcm.missouri.edu
Accred Length: 3 Years *Program Size:* 36 (*GY1:* 12)
Subspecialties: FPG
Program ID: 120-28-11-182

Kansas City

Baptist Medical Center Program

Sponsor: Baptist Medical Center

Program Director:
Lawrence A Rues, MD
Goppert Family Care Ctr
6601 Rockhill Rd
Kansas City, MO 64131
Tel: 816 276-7650 *Fax:* 816 276-7090
E-mail: bagould@healthmidwest.org
Internet: http://www.bmc-goppert.com
Accred Length: 3 Years *Program Size:* 24 (*GY1:* 8)
Program ID: 120-28-21-183

Trinity Lutheran Hospital Program

Sponsor: Trinity Lutheran Hospital

Program Director:
Scott W Thompson, MD
Trinity Lutheran Hospital
2900 Baltimore/Ste 400
Kansas City, MO 64108
Tel: 816 751-5000 *Fax:* 816 751-4499
E-mail: tlhfmc@unicom.net
Internet: http://www.trinityfp-kc.org
Accred Length: 3 Years *Program Size:* 24 (*GY1:* 8)
Program ID: 120-28-21-451

University of Missouri at Kansas City Program

Sponsor: University of Missouri-Kansas City School of Medicine
Truman Medical Center-East
Truman Medical Center-West

Program Director:
Walter A Forred, MD
Truman Med Ctr
7900 Lee's Summit Rd
Kansas City, MO 64139-1246
Tel: 816 373-6228 *Fax:* 816 478-7534
E-mail: umkcfprp@qni.com
Internet: http://www.qni.com/~umkcfprp
Accred Length: 3 Years *Program Size:* 36 (*GY1:* 12)
Subspecialties: FPG
Program ID: 120-28-21-422

Springfield

Cox Medical Centers Program

Sponsor: Cox Medical Center North
Cox Medical Center South

Program Director:
Larry W Halverson, MD
Cox Health Systems
1423 N Jefferson/Ste A100
Springfield, MO 65802
Tel: 417 269-8787 *Fax:* 417 269-8750
E-mail: vgreenw@coxnet.org
Internet: http://www.coxnet.org/fpr
Accred Length: 3 Years *Program Size:* 24 (*GY1:* 8)
Program ID: 120-28-21-476

St Louis

Deaconess Hospital Program

Sponsor: Deaconess Hospital

Program Director:
David C Campbell, MD
Deaconess Hospital
6125 Clayton Ave/Ste 201
St Louis, MO 63139
Tel: 314 768-3204 *Fax:* 314 768-3015
E-mail: docdav19@mail.idt.net
Accred Length: 3 Years *Program Size:* 27 (*GY1:* 9)
Program ID: 120-28-21-479

St John's Mercy Medical Center Program

Sponsor: St John's Mercy Medical Center

Program Director:
Peter G Danis, MD
St John's Mercy Med Ctr
615 S New Ballas Rd
St Louis, MO 63141-8277
Tel: 314 569-6012 *Fax:* 314 995-4127
Internet: http://www.mercy-fammed.com
Accred Length: 3 Years *Program Size:* 21 (*GY1:* 7)
Program ID: 120-28-21-186

Montana

Billings

Montana Family Practice Residency Program

Sponsor: Montana Family Practice Residency
Deaconess Medical Center

Program Director:
Roxanne Fahrenwald, MD
123 S 27th St/Ste B
Billings, MT 59101
Tel: 406 247-3306 *Fax:* 406 247-3307
E-mail: info@mfpr.fammed.washington.edu
Accred Length: 3 Years *Program Size:* 15 (*GY1:* 5)
Program ID: 120-29-21-590

Glasgow

Montana Family Practice Residency Rural Program

Sponsor: Montana Family Practice Residency
Frances Mahon Deaconess Hospital
Deaconess Medical Center

Program Director:
Roxanne Fahrenwald, MD
Montana Family Practice Residency
123 S 27th St/Ste B
Billings, MT 59101
Tel: 406 247-3306 *Fax:* 406 247-3307
E-mail: info@mfpr.fammed.washington.edu
Accred Length: 3 Years *Program Size:* 3 (*GY1:* 1)
Program ID: 120-29-31-591

Nebraska

Lincoln

Lincoln Medical Education Foundation Program

Sponsor: Lincoln Medical Education Foundation
BryanLGH Medical Center East
BryanLGH Medical Center West
St Elizabeth Community Health Center

Program Director:
Bruce E Gfeller, MD
Lincoln Family Practice Program
4600 Valley Rd/Ste 210
Lincoln, NE 68510
Tel: 402 483-4591 *Fax:* 402 483-5079
E-mail: lincfamprac@medlinc.com
Accred Length: 3 Years *Program Size:* 24 (*GY1:* 8)
Program ID: 120-30-31-187

Omaha

Clarkson Regional Health Service Program

Sponsor: Clarkson Regional Health Service

Program Director:
Richard H Hurd, MD
Clarkson Family Medicine
4200 Douglas St
Omaha, NE 68131-2700
Tel: 402 552-2050 *Fax:* 402 552-2186
E-mail: mmiller@clarkhosp.nhsnet.org
Accred Length: 3 Years *Program Size:* 18 (*GY1:* 6)
Program ID: 120-30-21-498

Creighton University Program

Sponsor: Creighton University School of Medicine
Tenet St Joseph Hospital at Creighton Univ Medical Center

Program Director:
Donald R Frey, MD
Creighton Family Practice
601 N 30th St/Ste 6720
Omaha, NE 68131-2179
Tel: 402 280-4111
Internet:
http://www.medicine.creighton.edu/medschool/family/default.htm
Accred Length: 3 Years *Program Size:* 26 (*GY1:* 8)
Program ID: 120-30-31-188

University of Nebraska Program

Sponsor: University of Nebraska Medical Center
Ehrling Bergquist Hospital
Methodist Hospital

Program Director:
James H Stageman Jr, MD
Dept of Family Med
Univ of Nebraska Med Ctr
600 S 42nd St
Omaha, NE 68198-3075
Tel: 402 559-7249 *Fax:* 402 559-6501
E-mail: unmcfp@mail.unmc.edu
Internet: http://www.unmc.edu/familymed
Accred Length: 3 Years *Program Size:* 44 (*GY1:* 12)
Program ID: 120-30-21-189

University of Nebraska Rural Program

Sponsor: University of Nebraska Medical Center
Good Samaritan Hospital (Kearney)
Great Plains Regional Medical Center
Regional West Medical Center
St Francis Medical Center (Grand Island)

Program Director:
Jeffrey D Harrison, MD
Dept of Family Med
Univ of Nebraska Med Ctr
983075 Nebraska Med Ctr
Omaha, NE 68198-3075
Tel: 402 559-8252 *Fax:* 402 559-6501
E-mail: unmcfpr@mail.unmc.edu
Internet: http://www.unmc.edu/familymed
Accred Length: 3 Years *Program Size:* 24 (*GY1:* 8)
Program ID: 120-30-21-517

Nevada

Las Vegas

University of Nevada (Las Vegas) Program

Sponsor: University of Nevada School of Medicine
University Medical Center of Southern Nevada

Program Director:
Roy Henderson, MD MPH
Univ of Nevada Sch of Med
Dept of Family/Com Med
6375 W Charleston Blvd (M/S A100)
Las Vegas, NV 89146
Tel: 702 877-4974, ext 210 *Fax:* 702 877-6876
E-mail: mraetz@med.unr.edu
Internet: http://www.unr.edu/med
Accred Length: 3 Years *Program Size:* 13 (*GY1:* 4)
Program ID: 120-31-21-481

Reno

University of Nevada (Reno) Program

Sponsor: University of Nevada School of Medicine
Ioannis A Lougaris Veterans Affairs Medical Center
Washoe Medical Center

Program Director:
Robert B Bannister, DO
Univ of Nevada Sch of Med
Dept of Family/Com Med
Brigham Bldg (316)
Reno, NV 89557-0046
Tel: 702 784-6180 *Fax:* 702 784-4473
E-mail: kselbach@med.unr.edu
Internet:
http://www.unr.edu/med/residency/northfp.html
Accred Length: 3 Years *Program Size:* 18 (*GY1:* 6)
Program ID: 120-31-21-482

New Hampshire

Concord

Concord Hospital Program

Sponsor: Concord Hospital

Program Director:
Daniel F Eubank, MD
New Hampshire Dartmouth Family Practice Residency-Concord
250 Pleasant St
Concord, NH 03301
Tel: 603 225-2711, ext 2936 *Fax:* 603 228-7173
Accred Length: 3 Years *Program Size:* 12 (*GY1:* 4)
Program ID: 120-32-31-557

Lebanon

Dartmouth-Hitchcock Medical Center Program

Sponsor: Mary Hitchcock Memorial Hospital
Concord Hospital

Program Director:
Patricia T Glowa, MD
Two Buck Rd/Ste 3
Hanover, NH 03755
Tel: 603 650-4070 *Fax:* 603 650-4090
Accred Length: 3 Years *Program Size:* 12 (*GY1:* 4)
Program ID: 120-32-21-551

New Jersey

Edison

JFK Medical Center Program

Sponsor: JFK Medical Center

Program Director:
Robin O Winter, MD
JFK Med Ctr
Family Practice Ctr
65 James St
Edison, NJ 08818
Tel: 732 321-7493 *Fax:* 732 906-4986
E-mail: famprac@jfk.hbocvan.com
Internet: http://www.jfkhs.org/rfamprac.htm
Accred Length: 3 Years *Program Size:* 21 (*GY1:* 7)
Program ID: 120-33-11-190

Flemington

Hunterdon Medical Center Program

Sponsor: Hunterdon Medical Center

Program Director:
Stanley M Kozakowski, MD
Hunterdon Med Ctr
2100 Wescott Dr
Flemington, NJ 08822
Tel: 908 788-6160 *Fax:* 908 788-2538
E-mail: kozakost@umdnj.edu
Internet: http://www.hunterfpr.org
Accred Length: 3 Years *Program Size:* 18 (*GY1:* 6)
Program ID: 120-33-11-191

Hoboken

St Mary Hospital Program

Sponsor: St Mary Hospital

Program Director:
Abbie Jacobs, MD
St Mary Hospital
308 Willow Ave
Hoboken, NJ 07030
Tel: 201 418-3126 *Fax:* 201 418-3148
Accred Length: 3 Years *Program Size:* 27 (*GY1:* 9)
Program ID: 120-33-11-192

Montclair

Mountainside Hospital Program

Sponsor: Mountainside Hospital

Program Director:
Sofia H Anthony, MD
Mountainside Family Practice Associates
799 Bloomfield Ave
Verona, NJ 07044-1374
Tel: 973 746-7050 *Fax:* 973 509-4477
E-mail: santhonymd@pol.net
Accred Length: 3 Years *Program Size:* 18 (*GY1:* 6)
Program ID: 120-33-11-193

Mount Holly

Memorial Hospital of Burlington County Program

Sponsor: Memorial Hospital of Burlington County
Program Director:
Mark A Van Kooy, MD
Memorial Hospital of Burlington County
Dept of Family Practice
175 Madison Ave
Mount Holly, NJ 08060
Tel: 609 261-7019 *Fax:* 609 261-9225
E-mail: mvankooy@mhbc.org
Internet: http://www.memorial-nj.org/famprac
Accred Length: 3 Years *Program Size:* 18 (*GY1:* 6)
Program ID: 120-33-21-444

Paterson

St Joseph's Hospital and Medical Center Program

Sponsor: St Joseph's Hospital and Medical Center
Program Director:
John DeGhetto Jr, DO
St Joseph's-Mt Sinai Family Medicine Program
716 Broad St/2nd Fl
Clifton, NJ 07013-1642
Tel: 973 754-4120 *Fax:* 973 754-4190
E-mail: sjfm@sjhmc.org
Internet: http://www.sjhmc.org
Accred Length: 3 Years *Program Size:* 18 (*GY1:* 6)
Program ID: 120-33-21-449

Phillipsburg

Warren Hospital Program

Sponsor: Warren Hospital
Program Director:
John C Brogan, MD
Warren Hospital, Dept of Family Practice
410 Coventry Dr
Phillipsburg, NJ 08865
Tel: 908 859-6785, ext 9216 *Fax:* 908 454-9889
E-mail: cfp@fast.net
Accred Length: 3 Years *Program Size:* 21 (*GY1:* 7)
Program ID: 120-33-21-436

Piscataway

UMDNJ-Robert Wood Johnson Medical School Program

Sponsor: UMDNJ-Robert Wood Johnson Medical School
St Peter's University Hospital
Program Director:
Laura Micek-Galinat, MD MPH
UMDNJ-Robert Wood Johnson Med Sch
Dept of Family Med
One Robert Wood Johnson Pl/PO Box 19
New Brunswick, NJ 08903-0019
Tel: 732 235-7664 *Fax:* 732 235-6095
E-mail: bundybs@umdnj.edu
Internet: http://www2.umdnj.edu/fmedweb/sp_rwj/
Accred Length: 3 Years *Program Size:* 30 (*GY1:* 10)
Subspecialties: FPG, FSM
Program ID: 120-33-21-419

Somerville

Somerset Medical Center Program

Sponsor: Somerset Medical Center
Program Director:
Melodee S Lasky, MD
Somerset Family Practice Residency Program
110 Rehill Ave
Somerville, NJ 08876
Tel: 908 685-2900 *Fax:* 908 704-0083
E-mail: kschmidt@somerset-healthcare.com
Internet: http://www.smchealthwise.com
Accred Length: 3 Years *Program Size:* 21 (*GY1:* 7)
Program ID: 120-33-11-194

Summit

Overlook Hospital Program

Sponsor: Overlook Hospital
Program Director:
Susan T Kaye, MD
Overlook Hospital
99 Beauvoir Ave
PO Box 220
Summit, NJ 07902-0220
Tel: 908 522-2907 *Fax:* 908 522-0804
E-mail: peggy.nadzan@oh.ahsys.org
Accred Length: 3 Years *Program Size:* 21 (*GY1:* 7)
Program ID: 120-33-11-195

Trenton

Capital Health System-Fuld Campus/Robert Wood Johnson Medical School Program

Sponsor: Capital Health System-Fuld Campus
Program Director:
Martha H Lansing, MD
UMDNJ-RWJ Family Practice Residency-Capital Health System
666 Plainsboro Rd
Ste 355
Plainsboro, NJ 08536-3209
Tel: 609 275-8674 *Fax:* 609 275-1933
E-mail: fprhfmc@bellatlantic.net
Internet: http://www2.umdnj.edu/fmedweb/
Accred Length: 3 Years *Program Size:* 12 (*GY1:* 4)
Program ID: 120-33-21-559

Voorhees

West Jersey Health System Program

Sponsor: West Jersey Hospital-Voorhees
Program Director:
Mary A Willard, MD
West Jersey Health System
Tatem-Brown Family Practice Ctr
One Carnie Blvd
Voorhees, NJ 08043
Tel: 609 795-7075 *Fax:* 609 325-3705
E-mail: wjfpres@wjhs.org
Internet: http://www.wjhs.org/residency
Accred Length: 3 Years *Program Size:* 19 (*GY1:* 6)
Program ID: 120-33-11-196

Woodbury

Underwood-Memorial Hospital Program

Sponsor: Underwood-Memorial Hospital
Program Director:
Stephen Colameco, MD
Family Practice Ctr
Underwood-Memorial Hospital
35 Oak St
Woodbury, NJ 08096
Tel: 609 853-2056 *Fax:* 609 848-2879
Accred Length: 3 Years *Program Size:* 12 (*GY1:* 4)
Program ID: 120-33-21-445

New Mexico

Albuquerque

University of New Mexico (Santa Fe) Rural Program

Sponsor: University of New Mexico School of Medicine
University Hospital
Program Director:
Mario Pacheco, MD
PO Box 5395
1035 Alto St
Santa Fe, NM 87502-5395
Tel: 505 982-4425 *Fax:* 505 982-8440
E-mail: deborah.weiss@stvin.org
Accred Length: 3 Years *Program Size:* 6 (*GY1:* 2)
Program ID: 120-34-21-595

University of New Mexico Program

Sponsor: University of New Mexico School of Medicine
University Hospital
Program Director:
Martha Cole McGrew, MD
Univ of New Mexico
Dept of Family/Community Med
2400 Tucker Ave NE
Albuquerque, NM 87131-5266
Tel: 505 272-4918 *Fax:* 505 272-1348
E-mail: mmcgrew@salud.unm.edu
Internet: http://somasf.unm.edu/gme
Accred Length: 3 Years *Program Size:* 44 (*GY1:* 20)
Program ID: 120-34-21-197

Las Cruces

University of New Mexico (Las Cruces) Rural Program

Sponsor: Memorial Medical Center, Inc
University Hospital
Program Director:
Mark A Knox, MD
Memorial Med Ctr
2450 S Telshor Blvd
Las Cruces, NM 88011
Tel: 505 521-5374 *Fax:* 505 521-5568
Accred Length: 3 Years *Program Size:* 12 (*GY1:* 4)
Program ID: 120-34-21-577

Roswell

University of New Mexico (Roswell) Rural Program

Sponsor: University of New Mexico School of Medicine
Eastern New Mexico Medical Center
University Hospital
Program Director:
Karen Vaillant, MD
Eastern New Mexico Med Ctr
603 W Country Club Rd
Roswell, NM 88201
Tel: 505 627-4175 *Fax:* 505 624-5603
E-mail: enmfprp@dfn.com
Accred Length: 3 Years *Program Size:* 7 (*GY1:* 2)
Program ID: 120-34-21-608

Programs

New York

Albany

Albany Medical Center Program

Sponsor: Albany Medical Center
St Peter's Hospital

Program Director:
Neil C Mitnick, DO
Dept of Family Practice
1 Clara Barton Dr/A-21
Albany, NY 12208-3495
Tel: 518 462-5041 *Fax:* 518 262-5192
E-mail: neil_mitnick@ccgateway.amc.edu
Internet: http://www.amc.edu
Accred Length: 3 Years *Program Size:* 24 (*GY1:* 8)
Program ID: 120-35-21-198

Bay Shore

Southside Hospital Program

Sponsor: Southside Hospital

Program Director:
Richard J Bonanno, MD
Southside Hospital
301 E Main St
Bay Shore, NY 11706-8458
Tel: 516 968-3295 *Fax:* 516 968-3210
Accred Length: 3 Years *Program Size:* 27 (*GY1:* 9)
Program ID: 120-35-21-199

Binghamton

Wilson Memorial Regional Medical Center (United Health Services) Program

Sponsor: Wilson Memorial Regional Medical Center (United Health Svs)

Program Director:
Richard R Terry, DO
33-57 Harrison St
Johnson City, NY 13790
Tel: 607 763-5334 *Fax:* 607 763-5415
E-mail: linda_kinsey@uhs.org
Internet: http://www.hscsyr.edu/~wilsonfp/index.htm
Accred Length: 3 Years *Program Size:* 27 (*GY1:* 9)
Subspecialties: TY
Program ID: 120-35-11-203

Bronx

Albert Einstein College of Medicine Program

Sponsor: Albert Einstein College of Medicine of Yeshiva University
Montefiore Medical Center-Henry and Lucy Moses Division

Program Director:
Victoria Gorski, MD
Albert Einstein Coll of Med
3544 Jerome Ave
Bronx, NY 10467
Tel: 718 920-5521 *Fax:* 718 515-5416
E-mail: algonzal@montefiore.org
Internet: http://www.raccoon. aecom.yu.edu
Accred Length: 3 Years *Program Size:* 30 (*GY1:* 10)
Program ID: 120-35-21-209

Bronx-Lebanon Hospital Center Program

Sponsor: Bronx-Lebanon Hospital Center

Program Director:
Margaret Rosenberg, MD
Bronx-Lebanon Hospital Family Practice Ctr
1265 Franklin Ave/3rd Fl
Bronx, NY 10456
Tel: 718 901-8749 *Fax:* 718 901-8704
E-mail: blres@interactive.net
Accred Length: 3 Years *Program Size:* 30 (*GY1:* 10)
Program ID: 120-35-21-465

Brooklyn

Brooklyn Hospital Center Program

Sponsor: Brooklyn Hospital Center

Program Director:
Maritza De La Rosa, MD
Brooklyn Hospital Ctr
Dept of Family Practice
121 DeKalb Ave
Brooklyn, NY 11201-9973
Tel: 718 250-8621 *Fax:* 718 250-8878
E-mail: famp@tbh.org
Internet: http://www.tbh.org
Accred Length: 3 Years *Program Size:* 12 (*GY1:* 4)
Program ID: 120-35-21-530

Lutheran Medical Center Program

Sponsor: Lutheran Medical Center

Program Director:
Claudia Lyon, DO
Lutheran Med Ctr
Med Educ Office
150 55th St
Brooklyn, NY 11220-2574
Tel: 718 630-7350 *Fax:* 718 492-2776
E-mail: fplmc.ny@ibm.net
Internet: http://www.lmcmc.com
Accred Length: 3 Years *Program Size:* 33 (*GY1:* 11)
Program ID: 120-35-11-207

SUNY Health Science Center at Brooklyn Program

Sponsor: SUNY Health Science Center at Brooklyn
Kings County Hospital Center
University Hospital-SUNY Health Science Center at Brooklyn

Program Director:
Gwyneth A Davis, MD
Dept of Family Practice
450 Clarkson Ave/Box 67
Brooklyn, NY 11203-2098
Tel: 718 270-2560 *Fax:* 718 270-2125
E-mail: gjichetti@netmail.hscbklyn.edu
Internet: http://www.aafp.org/residencies259html
Accred Length: 3 Years *Program Size:* 25 (*GY1:* 9)
Program ID: 120-35-21-210

Wyckoff Heights Medical Center Program

Sponsor: Wyckoff Heights Medical Center

Program Director:
Andreas Cohrssen, MD
Wyckoff Heights Med Ctr
374 Stockholm St
Brooklyn, NY 11237
Tel: 718 963-7587 *Fax:* 718 963-6575
Accred Length: 3 Years *Program Size:* 13 (*GY1:* 4)
Program ID: 120-35-21-507

Buffalo

SUNY at Buffalo Graduate Medical-Dental Education Consortium Program

Sponsor: SUNY at Buffalo Grad Medical-Dental Education Consortium
CGF Health System (Buffalo General Hospital)
CGF Health System (Millard Fillmore Hospitals)
Erie County Medical Center

Program Director:
Daniel Morelli, MD
SUNY-Buffalo
Dept of Family Med
462 Grider St
Buffalo, NY 14215
Tel: 716 898-5972 *Fax:* 716 898-4750
E-mail: jgkrause@acsu.buffalo.edu
Internet: http://www.wings.buffalo.edu/smbs/fammed
Accred Length: 3 Years *Program Size:* 47 (*GY1:* 16)
Program ID: 120-35-21-489

SUNY at Buffalo Graduate Medical-Dental Education Consortium Rural Program

Sponsor: SUNY at Buffalo Grad Medical-Dental Education Consortium
CGF Health System (Buffalo General Hospital)
Olean General Hospital

Program Director:
Daniel Morelli, MD
SUNY-Buffalo
Dept of Family Med
462 Grider St
Buffalo, NY 14215
Tel: 716 898-5972 *Fax:* 716 898-4750
Internet: http://www.llwings.buffalo.edu/smbs/fam-med/
Accred Length: 3 Years *Program Size:* 6 (*GY1:* 2)
Program ID: 120-35-21-516

Glen Cove

North Shore University Hospital at Glen Cove Program

Sponsor: North Shore University Hospital at Glen Cove

Program Director:
George F Dunn, MD
North Shore Univ Hospital-Glen Cove
101 St Andrews Ln
Glen Cove, NY 11542
Tel: 516 674-7637 *Fax:* 516 674-7639
E-mail: gcfpprog@nshs.edu
Accred Length: 3 Years *Program Size:* 21 (*GY1:* 7)
Program ID: 120-35-11-202

Jamaica

Catholic Medical Center of Brooklyn and Queens Program

Sponsor: Catholic Medical Center of Brooklyn and Queens Inc
Catholic Medical Center (Mary Immaculate Hospital)

Program Director:
Joseph G Lurio, MD
Catholic Med Ctr of Brooklyn and Queens
Dept of Family Pract/Community Med
88-25 153rd St/Ste 2-L
Jamaica, NY 11432
Tel: 718 558-7195, ext 106 *Fax:* 718 558-7205
E-mail: family.practice@cmcny.com
Accred Length: 3 Years *Program Size:* 18 (*GY1:* 6)
Program ID: 120-35-21-420

Jamaica Hospital Program

Sponsor: Jamaica Hospital

Program Director:
Alan R Roth, DO
Jamaica Hospital Med Ctr
Dept of Family Med
8900 Van Wyck Expwy
Jamaica, NY 11418
Tel: 718 206-6914 *Fax:* 718 206-8716
E-mail: alandocr@aol.com
Internet: http://www.jhfamprac.org
Accred Length: 3 Years *Program Size:* 24 (*GY1:* 8)
Program ID: 120-35-11-206

Kingston

Mid-Hudson Family Health Institute Program

Sponsor: Mid-Hudson Family Health Institute
Benedictine Hospital
Kingston Hospital
Program Director:
Mark Josefski, MD
Mid-Hudson Family Practice Residency Program
Kingston Hospital
396 Broadway
Kingston, NY 12401
Tel: 914 338-5344 *Fax:* 914 338-0307
Accred Length: 3 Years *Program Size:* 18 (*GY1:* 6)
Program ID: 120-35-21-204

New York

Albert Einstein College of Medicine at Beth Israel Medical Center Program

Sponsor: Beth Israel Medical Center
The Institute for Urban Family Health
Program Director:
Richard O'Keefe, MD
Beth Israel Med Ctr
Inst for Urban Family Health
16 E 16th St
New York, NY 10003
Tel: 212 206-5255, ext 5214 *Fax:* 212 206-5251
Internet: http://www.institute2000.org
Accred Length: 3 Years *Program Size:* 27 (*GY1:* 8)
Program ID: 120-35-32-538

New York and Presbyterian Hospital (Columbia Campus) Program

Sponsor: New York and Presbyterian Hospital
New York and Presbyterian Hospital (Columbia Campus)
Program Director:
Christopher Wang, MD MPH
Columbia Presbyterian Med Ctr
Family Health Ctr
64 Nagle Ave
New York, NY 10040-1406
Tel: 212 567-2291 *Fax:* 212 567-1945
E-mail: cpmcfam@cpmc3.cis.columbia.edu
Internet: http://cpmcnet.columbia.edu.dept/family
Accred Length: 3 Years *Program Size:* 18 (*GY1:* 6)
Program ID: 120-35-21-581

Niagara Falls

SUNY at Buffalo Graduate Medical-Dental Education Consortium (Niagara Falls) Program

Sponsor: SUNY at Buffalo Grad Medical-Dental Education Consortium
Niagara Falls Memorial Medical Center
Program Director:
Jerome C Andres, MD
Niagara Falls Memorial Med Ctr
Dept of Family Practice
501 Tenth St
Niagara Falls, NY 14301
Tel: 716 278-4618 *Fax:* 716 285-8992
Accred Length: 3 Years *Program Size:* 10 (*GY1:* 3)
Program ID: 120-35-12-211

Oceanside

South Nassau Communities Hospital Program

Sponsor: South Nassau Communities Hospital
Program Director:
Scott D Kirsch, MD
South Nassau Communities Hospital
2445 Oceanside Rd
Oceanside, NY 11572
Tel: 516 763-3909 *Fax:* 516 763-3475
E-mail: fammed@mindspring.com
Accred Length: 3 Years *Program Size:* 24 (*GY1:* 8)
Program ID: 120-35-11-212

Poughkeepsie

Mount Sinai School of Medicine (Poughkeepsie) Program

Sponsor: Mount Sinai School of Medicine
St Francis Hospital
Vassar Brothers Hospital
Program Director:
Margaret Rodriquez, MD
Hudson Valley Family Practice Residency
4 Jefferson Plaza
Poughkeepsie, NY 12601-4025
Tel: 914 431-8123 *Fax:* 914 485-3740
Accred Length: 3 Years *Program Size:* 18 (*GY1:* 6)
Program ID: 120-35-21-483

Rochester

University of Rochester/Highland Hospital of Rochester Program

Sponsor: Highland Hospital of Rochester
Rochester General Hospital
Strong Memorial Hospital of the University of Rochester
Program Director:
Jeffrey J Harp, MD
Jacob W Holler Family Med Ctr
885 South Ave
Rochester, NY 14620-2399
Tel: 716 442-7470, ext 219 *Fax:* 716 442-8319
E-mail: fmres@urmc.rochester.edu
Internet: http://www.urmc.rochester.edu/smd/fammed/
Accred Length: 3 Years *Program Size:* 33 (*GY1:* 10)
Program ID: 120-35-21-214

University of Rochester/Highland Hospital of Rochester Rural Program

Sponsor: Highland Hospital of Rochester
Frederick Ferris Thompson Systems
Geneva General Hospital
Soldiers and Sailors Memorial Hospital of Yates County
Program Director:
Jeffrey J Harp, MD
885 South Ave
Rochester, NY 14620
Tel: 716 442-7470, ext 7175 *Fax:* 716 442-8319
E-mail: ruralres@netacc.net
Internet:
http://www.urmc.rochester.edu/smd/fammed/index.html
Accred Length: 3 Years *Program Size:* 6 (*GY1:* 2)
Program ID: 120-35-31-535

Schenectady

St Clare's Hospital of Schenectady Program

Sponsor: St Clare's Hospital of Schenectady
Program Director:
Gary R Dunkerley, MD
St Clare's Hospital
Cushing Ctr
624 McClellan St
Schenectady, NY 12304
Tel: 518 347-5293, ext 5293 *Fax:* 518 347-5007
E-mail: dunkerley@stclares.org
Internet: http://www.stclares.org
Accred Length: 3 Years *Program Size:* 29 (*GY1:* 9)
Program ID: 120-35-12-215

Stony Brook

SUNY at Stony Brook Program

Sponsor: University Hospital-SUNY at Stony Brook
Program Director:
Donna Meltzer, MD
SUNY-Stony Brook
Dept of Family Med
Level 4/Rm 050
Stony Brook, NY 11794-8461
Tel: 516 444-2300
Internet: http://www.fammed.sunysb.edu
Accred Length: 3 Years *Program Size:* 27 (*GY1:* 9)
Program ID: 120-35-21-408

Syracuse

SUNY Health Science Center at Syracuse/Crouse Hospital Program

Sponsor: Crouse Hospital
Program Director:
Peter M Nalin, MD
Lafayette Family Medicine Residency
2394 Rte 11
Lafayette, NY 13084
Tel: 315 677-9469 *Fax:* 315 677-3945
E-mail: cimfmres@vax.cs.hscsyr.edu
Internet: http://www.crouse.org/partners
Accred Length: 3 Years *Program Size:* 18 (*GY1:* 6)
Program ID: 120-35-21-571

SUNY Health Science Center at Syracuse/St Joseph's Hospital Health Center Program

Sponsor: St Joseph's Hospital Health Center
Program Director:
James B Tucker, MD
St Joseph's Hospital Health Ctr
301 Prospect Ave
Syracuse, NY 13203
Tel: 315 448-5537 *Fax:* 315 448-6313
E-mail: louisa45@sjhsyr.org
Internet: http://www.sjhsyr.org/fampract
Accred Length: 3 Years *Program Size:* 39 (*GY1:* 13)
Program ID: 120-35-21-216

Utica

Bassett Healthcare (Utica) Program

Sponsor: Bassett Healthcare
St Elizabeth Medical Center

Program Director:
Carol A Stewart, MD
Family Practice Center
120 Hobart St
Utica, NY 13501
Tel: 800 848-8344 *Fax:* 315 734-3572
E-mail: bassedfp@telenet.net
Internet:
http://www.cooperstown.net/bassett/bh/meded/familymed.html
Accred Length: 3 Years *Program Size:* 26 (*GY1:* 8)
Program ID: 120-35-11-217

Yonkers

New York Medical College at St Joseph's Medical Center Program

Sponsor: New York Medical College
St Joseph's Medical Center

Program Director:
Joseph L Halbach, MD
St Joseph's Med Ctr
127 S Broadway
Yonkers, NY 10701-4080
Tel: 914 378-7586 *Fax:* 914 378-1071
E-mail: stjosfp@chcn.org
Internet: http://www.saintjosephs.org
Accred Length: 3 Years *Program Size:* 30 (*GY1:* 10)
Program ID: 120-35-11-218

North Carolina

Asheville

Mountain Area Health Education Center Program

Sponsor: Mountain Area Health Education Center
Memorial Mission Hospital

Program Director:
Stephen D Hulkower, MD
MAHEC Family Practice Program
118 W T Weaver Blvd
Asheville, NC 28804-3415
Tel: 828 258-0670 *Fax:* 828 257-4738
Internet: http://www.mtn.ncahec.org
Accred Length: 3 Years *Program Size:* 24 (*GY1:* 8)
Program ID: 120-36-11-219

Chapel Hill

University of North Carolina Hospitals Program

Sponsor: University of North Carolina Hospitals
Wake Medical Center

Program Director:
Clark R Denniston, MD
Univ of North Carolina Sch of Med
Dept of Family Med/CB7595
Manning Dr
Chapel Hill, NC 27599-7595
Tel: 919 966-2716 *Fax:* 919 966-6125
E-mail: uncfpr@med.unc.edu
Internet: http://www.fammed.unc.edu
Accred Length: 3 Years *Program Size:* 24 (*GY1:* 8)
Program ID: 120-36-31-220

Charlotte

Carolinas Medical Center Program

Sponsor: Carolinas Medical Center

Program Director:
Mary N Hall, MD
Dept of Family Practice
Carolinas Med Ctr
PO Box 32861/CMC-Myers Park
Charlotte, NC 28232-2861
Tel: 704 355-3172 *Fax:* 704 446-1221
E-mail: fprp@carolinas.org
Internet: http://www.carolinas.org
Accred Length: 3 Years *Program Size:* 28 (*GY1:* 8)
Program ID: 120-36-11-221

Concord

Northeast Medical Center Program

Sponsor: Northeast Medical Center

Program Director:
L Allen Dobson Jr, MD
Northeast Med Ctr
315 Medical Park Dr/#203
Concord, NC 28025
Tel: 704 783-1044 *Fax:* 704 783-1077
E-mail: kleatherman@northeastmedical.org
Internet: http://www.cfmrp.org
Accred Length: 3 Years *Program Size:* 24 (*GY1:* 8)
Program ID: 120-36-21-580

Durham

Duke University Program

Sponsor: Duke University Medical Center
Durham Regional Hospital

Program Director:
Margaret Gradison, MD
Duke Univ Med Ctr
Dept of Family Practice
Box 3886
Durham, NC 27710
Tel: 919 681-3064 *Fax:* 919 681-6560
E-mail: fmrperas@mc.duke.edu
Internet: http://cfm.mc.duke.edu/resident/
Accred Length: 3 Years *Program Size:* 24 (*GY1:* 8)
Program ID: 120-36-21-222

Fayetteville

Duke University/Southern Regional Area Health Education Center Program

Sponsor: Southern Regional Health Education Center
Cape Fear Valley Medical Center

Program Director:
Lenard D Salzberg, MD
Southern Regional AHEC Family Med Program
1601 Owen Dr
Fayetteville, NC 28304-3482
Tel: 910 678-7259 *Fax:* 910 678-0115
E-mail: crussell@med.unc.edu
Internet: http://www2.mc.duke.edu/srahec
Accred Length: 3 Years *Program Size:* 20 (*GY1:* 6)
Program ID: 120-36-31-223

Fort Bragg

Womack Army Medical Center Program

Sponsor: Womack Army Medical Center

Program Director:
David B Sproat, MD MSA
Dept of Family Med
2500 Normandy Dr
Fort Bragg, NC 28307-5000
Tel: 910 432-9704 *Fax:* 910 432-7732
E-mail: drdave5523@aol.com
Internet: http://www.bragg.army.mil/Fampract/index.htm
Accred Length: 3 Years *Program Size:* 33 (*GY1:* 9)
Program ID: 120-36-21-011
US Armed Services Program

Greensboro

Moses H Cone Memorial Hospital Program

Sponsor: Moses H Cone Memorial Hospital

Program Director:
Karl B Fields, MD
Moses H Cone Memorial Hospital
Family Practice Ctr
1125 N Church St
Greensboro, NC 27401-1007
Tel: 336 832-8132 *Fax:* 336 832-7078
E-mail: susan.rice@mosescone.com
Internet: http://www.med.unc.edu/gahec/
Accred Length: 3 Years *Program Size:* 26 (*GY1:* 8)
Subspecialties: FSM
Program ID: 120-36-11-224

Greenville

East Carolina University Program

Sponsor: East Carolina University School of Medicine
Pitt County Memorial Hospital

Program Director:
George S Poehlman, MD MPH
East Carolina Univ Sch of Med
Dept of Family Med
Family Practice Ctr
Greenville, NC 27858-4354
Tel: 252 816-4616 *Fax:* 252 816-4614
E-mail: poehlman@brody.med.ecu.edu
Internet: http://www.med.ecu.edu/fammed/residenc.htm
Accred Length: 3 Years *Program Size:* 36 (*GY1:* 12)
Subspecialties: FPG
Program ID: 120-36-11-225

East Carolina University Rural Program

Sponsor: East Carolina University School of Medicine
Martin General Hospital
Pitt County Memorial Hospital
Roanoke-Chowan Hospital
Sampson County Memorial Hospital

Program Director:
Dana E King, MD
Dept of Family Med
East Carolina Univ Sch of Med
Family Practice Ctr
Greenville, NC 27858-4354
Tel: 252 816-5517 *Fax:* 252 816-4614
E-mail: dking@brody.med.ecu.edu
Internet: http://www.med.ecu.edu/fammed/fmhome.htm
Accred Length: 3 Years *Program Size:* 18 (*GY1:* 6)
Program ID: 120-36-21-533

Hendersonville

Mountain Area Health Education Center Rural Program
Sponsor: Mountain Area Health Education Center
Margaret R Pardee Memorial Hospital
Memorial Mission Hospital
Program Director:
Wail Malaty, MD
Hendersonville Family Practice Program
604 Connor Ave
Hendersonville, NC 28791-3404
Tel: 828 696-1255 *Fax:* 828 696-1257
E-mail: janets@shamu.mtn.nchacec.org
Internet: http://www.mtn.ncahec.org
Accred Length: 3 Years *Program Size:* 6 (*GY1:* 2)
Program ID: 120-36-21-575

Monroe

Carolinas Medical Center Rural Program
Sponsor: Carolinas Medical Center
Union Regional Medical Center
Program Director:
J Lewis Sigmon Jr, MD
CORPCE-Carolinas Med Ctr
PO Box 32861
Charlotte, NC 28232-2861
Tel: 704 355-8233 *Fax:* 704 355-8380
E-mail: rrpfp@carolinas.org
Internet: http://www.carolinas.org
Accred Length: 3 Years *Program Size:* 6 (*GY1:* 2)
Program ID: 120-36-21-634

Wilmington

New Hanover Regional Medical Center Program
Sponsor: New Hanover Regional Medical Center
Program Director:
James G Lenhart, MD
New Hanover Regional Med Ctr
Coastal Family Med Ctr
2523 Delaney Ave
Wilmington, NC 28403
Tel: 910 343-1122 *Fax:* 910 343-1999
E-mail: nhrmcfm@med.unc.edu
Internet: http://www.med.unc.edu/coahec/
Accred Length: 3 Years *Program Size:* 13 (*GY1:* 4)
Program ID: 120-36-21-611

Winston-Salem

Wake Forest University School of Medicine Program
Sponsor: Wake Forest University Baptist Medical Center
Forsyth Memorial Hospital
Program Director:
Mark Knudson, MD
Wake Forest Univ Baptist Med Ctr
Dept of Family/Community Med
Medical Center Blvd
Winston-Salem, NC 27157
Tel: 336 716-2832 *Fax:* 336 716-9126
E-mail: dgant@wfubmc.edu
Internet: http://www.bgsm.edu/fam_med/
Accred Length: 3 Years *Program Size:* 30 (*GY1:* 10)
Subspecialties: FSM
Program ID: 120-36-31-226

North Dakota

Bismarck

University of North Dakota (Bismarck) Program
Sponsor: Univ of North Dakota School of Medicine & Health Sciences
Medcenter One Inc
St Alexius Medical Center
Program Director:
Guy P Tangedahl, MD
515 E Broadway
Bismarck, ND 58501
Tel: 701 328-9950 *Fax:* 701 328-9957
Internet: http://www.med.und.nodak.edu
Accred Length: 3 Years *Program Size:* 15 (*GY1:* 5)
Program ID: 120-37-21-227

Fargo

University of North Dakota (Fargo) Program
Sponsor: Univ of North Dakota School of Medicine & Health Sciences
MeritCare Hospital
Dakota Hospital
Program Director:
John R Baird, MD
Univ of North Dakota-Fargo
Family Practice Residency
306 4th St N
Fargo, ND 58102-4820
Tel: 701 239-2297 *Fax:* 701 239-7134
E-mail: jbaird@medicine.nodak.edu
Internet:
http://www.med.und.nodak.edu/depts/fpcfar/home.htm
Accred Length: 3 Years *Program Size:* 15 (*GY1:* 5)
Program ID: 120-37-21-228

Grand Forks

University of North Dakota (Grand Forks) Program
Sponsor: Univ of North Dakota School of Medicine & Health Sciences
Altru Health System Hospital
Program Director:
Larry Halvorson, MD
Family Practice Ctr/Ste 100
1300 S Columbia Rd
Grand Forks, ND 58201-4012
Tel: 701 780-6810 *Fax:* 701 780-6817
E-mail: larryh@mail.med.und.nodak.edu
Internet:
http://www.med.und.nodak.edu/depts/fpc/res_pgm.htm
Accred Length: 3 Years *Program Size:* 18 (*GY1:* 6)
Program ID: 120-37-31-229

Minot

University of North Dakota (Minot) Program
Sponsor: Univ of North Dakota School of Medicine & Health Sciences
UniMed Medical Center
Trinity Medical Center
Program Director:
C Milton Smith, MD
Pat W Mitchel, MD
Univ of North Dakota
Minot Ctr for Family Medicine
123 First St SW
Minot, ND 58701
Tel: 701 858-6700, ext 6750 *Fax:* 701 858-6749
E-mail: karenru@mail.med.und.nodak.edu
Internet: http://www.minot8.med.und.nodak.edu/
Accred Length: 3 Years *Program Size:* 18 (*GY1:* 6)
Program ID: 120-37-31-230

Ohio

Akron

Akron General Medical Center/NEOUCOM Program
Sponsor: Akron General Medical Center
Program Director:
Margaret P Panzner, MD
Akron General Med Ctr
400 Wabash Ave
Akron, OH 44307
Tel: 330 384-7671 *Fax:* 330 384-6852
E-mail: meded@agmc.org
Internet: http://agmc.org
Accred Length: 3 Years *Program Size:* 15 (*GY1:* 5)
Program ID: 120-38-31-232

Summa Health System (Akron City Hospital)/NEOUCOM Program
Sponsor: Summa Health System
Akron City Hospital (Summa Health System)
Program Director:
Richard M Hines, MD
Summa Health System
Med Educ/Mary Yanik
525 E Market St
Akron, OH 44304
Tel: 800 322-0517
Internet: http://www.summahealth.org/edu/
Accred Length: 3 Years *Program Size:* 24 (*GY1:* 8)
Program ID: 120-38-21-231

Barberton

Barberton Citizens Hospital/NEOUCOM Program
Sponsor: Barberton Citizens Hospital
Program Director:
Anthony J Costa, MD
Barberton Citizens Hospital
155 Fifth St NE
Barberton, OH 44203
Tel: 330 745-5008 *Fax:* 330 848-7829
Internet: http://www.barbhosp.com
Accred Length: 3 Years *Program Size:* 18 (*GY1:* 6)
Program ID: 120-38-21-437

Bellefontaine

Ohio State University Rural Program

Sponsor: Ohio State University Medical Center
Mary Rutan Hospital

Program Director:
Randall L Longenecker, MD
OSU-Oakhill Rural Family Practice Program
4879 US Rte 68 South
West Liberty, OH 43357
Tel: 937 599-1411 *Fax:* 937 465-9945
E-mail: rll.mrfp@logan.net
Internet: http://www.fammed.ohio-state.edu
Accred Length: 3 Years *Program Size:* 6 (*GY1:* 2)
Program ID: 120-38-21-640

Canton

Aultman Hospital/NEOUCOM Program

Sponsor: Aultman Hospital

Program Director:
Susan Mercer, MD
Family Practice Ctr-Aultman Hospital
2600 Seventh St SW
Canton, OH 44710
Tel: 330 438-6250 *Fax:* 330 580-5509
E-mail: smercer@aultman.com
Internet: http://www.aultmanresidencies.com
Accred Length: 3 Years *Program Size:* 21 (*GY1:* 7)
Program ID: 120-38-11-234

Cincinnati

Bethesda Hospital Program

Sponsor: Bethesda Hospital Inc

Program Director:
Toby Acheson, MD
Bethesda Hospital
4411 Montgomery Rd/Ste 206
Cincinnati, OH 45212
Tel: 513 631-0750 *Fax:* 513 631-0796
E-mail: bethesda@one.net
Internet: http://www.trihealth.com
Accred Length: 3 Years *Program Size:* 18 (*GY1:* 6)
Program ID: 120-38-21-474

University Hospital/University of Cincinnati College of Medicine Program

Sponsor: University Hospital Inc
Franciscan Hospital-Mount Airy Campus

Program Director:
Jeffery E Heck, MD
Univ of Cincinnati Med Ctr
Dept of Family Med
2446 Kipling Ave
Cincinnati, OH 45239-6695
Tel: 513 853-4350 *Fax:* 513 541-3902
E-mail: mullensf@fmmail.uc.edu
Internet: http://www.familymedicine.uc.edu
Accred Length: 3 Years *Program Size:* 36 (*GY1:* 12)
Subspecialties: FPG
Program ID: 120-38-21-235

Cleveland

Case Western Reserve University (MetroHealth) Program

Sponsor: MetroHealth Medical Center

Program Director:
Christine Alexander, MD MD
MetroHealth Med Ctr
Dept of Family Practice
2500 MetroHealth Dr
Cleveland, OH 44109-1998
Tel: 216 778-5031 *Fax:* 216 778-8225
E-mail: fpres@metrohealth.org
Accred Length: 3 Years *Program Size:* 18 (*GY1:* 6)
Program ID: 120-38-11-237

Case Western Reserve University Program

Sponsor: University Hospitals of Cleveland
Mount Sinai Medical Center of Cleveland

Program Director:
Michael Rowane, DO
Univ Hospitals of Cleveland
Dept of Family Practice
11100 Euclid Ave/Bolwell 1200
Cleveland, OH 44106-5036
Tel: 216 844-3791 *Fax:* 216 844-3799
Internet: http://www.uhhs.com/toteach/
Accred Length: 3 Years *Program Size:* 23 (*GY1:* 7)
Program ID: 120-38-11-236

Fairview Health System Program

Sponsor: Fairview Health System
Fairview Health System (Fairview General Hospital)

Program Director:
Stephen P Flynn, MD MPH
Fairview Hospital
Center for Family Med
18200 Lorain Ave
Cleveland, OH 44111-5628
Tel: 216 476-7084 *Fax:* 216 476-7604
E-mail: kgaughan@apk.net
Internet: http://www.webcom.com/fairres
Accred Length: 3 Years *Program Size:* 20 (*GY1:* 6)
Subspecialties: FSM
Program ID: 120-38-11-238

Columbus

Grant Medical Center (OhioHealth) Program

Sponsor: Grant Medical Center (OhioHealth)

Program Director:
Robert Skully, MD
Grant Med Ctr, Med Education Dept
111 S Grant Ave
Columbus, OH 43215
Tel: 614 566-9290 *Fax:* 614 566-8073
E-mail: fbass@ohiohealth.com
Internet: http://www.ohiohealth.com.gmeded.htm
Accred Length: 3 Years *Program Size:* 39 (*GY1:* 13)
Subspecialties: FSM
Program ID: 120-38-31-239

Mount Carmel Health Program

Sponsor: Mount Carmel Medical Center

Program Director:
John G O'Handley, MD
Mount Carmel Health System
1335 Dublin Rd/Ste 110E
Columbus, OH 43215
Tel: 614 234-0373 *Fax:* 614 234-0392
E-mail: gscherer@mchs.com
Internet: http://mchsresidency.org
Accred Length: 3 Years *Program Size:* 22 (*GY1:* 7)
Program ID: 120-38-32-240

Ohio State University Program

Sponsor: Ohio State University Medical Center
Park Medical Center

Program Director:
Victor Trianfo Jr, DO
Ohio State Univ
2231 N High St/Rm 205
Columbus, OH 43210-1228
Tel: 614 688-3908 *Fax:* 614 688-3698
E-mail: trianfo-1@medctr.osu.edu
Internet: http://www.fammed.ohio-state.edu
Accred Length: 3 Years *Program Size:* 31 (*GY1:* 9)
Subspecialties: FSM
Program ID: 120-38-21-241

Riverside Methodist Hospitals (OhioHealth) Program

Sponsor: Riverside Methodist Hospitals (OhioHealth)

Program Director:
Edward T Bope, MD
Riverside Methodist Hospital
Riverside Family Practice Ctr
697 Thomas Ln
Columbus, OH 43214
Tel: 614 566-4398 *Fax:* 614 566-6843
Internet: http://www.ohiohealth.com
Accred Length: 3 Years *Program Size:* 18 (*GY1:* 6)
Program ID: 120-38-21-242

Dayton

Franciscan Medical Center (Dayton) Program

Sponsor: Franciscan Medical Center-Dayton Campus

Program Director:
Anthony E Foley, MD
Franciscan Med Ctr
St Elizabeth Family Practice Residency
One Franciscan Way
Dayton, OH 45408-1498
Tel: 937 229-6495 *Fax:* 937 229-7288
Accred Length: 3 Years *Program Size:* 36 (*GY1:* 12)
Subspecialties: FSM
Program ID: 120-38-11-245

Good Samaritan Hospital and Health Center Program

Sponsor: Good Samaritan Hospital and Health Center

Program Director:
Michael F Bosworth, DO
2345 Philadelphia Dr
Dayton, OH 45406-1816
Tel: 937 276-4141 *Fax:* 937 277-7249
E-mail: family_practice@shp-dayton.org
Internet: http://www.ketthealth.com/fme/dcfpr.htm
Accred Length: 3 Years *Program Size:* 24 (*GY1:* 8)
Program ID: 120-38-31-243

Miami Valley Hospital Program

Sponsor: Miami Valley Hospital

Program Director:
Theodore E Wymyslo, MD
Miami Valley Hospital
101 Wyoming St
Dayton, OH 45409-2793
Tel: 937 208-2427 *Fax:* 937 341-8349
E-mail: mvhfpr@mvh.org
Accred Length: 3 Years *Program Size:* 21 (*GY1:* 7)
Program ID: 120-38-31-244

Sylvania

Flower Hospital Program

Sponsor: Flower Hospital
Toledo Hospital

Program Director:
Crystal R Goveia, MD
Flower Hospital Family Physicians Assoc
5300 Harroun Rd
Ste 304
Sylvania, OH 43560
Tel: 419 824-1100, ext 1371 *Fax:* 419 824-1771
E-mail: farah.dharamshi@promedica.org
Internet: http://www.flower.org/fpr/
Accred Length: 3 Years *Program Size:* 18 (*GY1:* 6)
Program ID: 120-38-11-246

Toledo

Medical College of Ohio Program

Sponsor: Medical College of Ohio
Medical College of Ohio Hospital
St Vincent Mercy Medical Center
Program Director:
Allan J Wilke, MD
Dept of Family Med
Med Coll of Ohio
1015 Garden Lake Pkwy
Toledo, OH 43614-2798
Tel: 419 383-5523 *Fax:* 419 382-7876
E-mail: rcalhoun@mco.edu
Internet:
http://www.mco.edu:80/depts/familymed/index.html
Accred Length: 3 Years *Program Size:* 16 (*GY1:* 4)
Program ID: 120-38-31-247

Mercy Health Partners Program

Sponsor: St Vincent Mercy Medical Center
Program Director:
Archie W Bedell, MD PhD
2127 Jefferson Ave
Toledo, OH 43624
Tel: 419 251-1859 *Fax:* 419 242-9806
E-mail: mercyfp@primenet.com
Internet: http://www.primenet.com/~mercyfp
Accred Length: 3 Years *Program Size:* 18 (*GY1:* 6)
Program ID: 120-38-31-249

Toledo Hospital Program

Sponsor: Toledo Hospital
Program Director:
William J Geiger, MD
Toledo Hospital Family Practice Residency
2051 W Central Ave
Toledo, OH 43606
Tel: 800 860-2051 *Fax:* 419 479-6952
E-mail: tthfpr@promedica.org
Internet: http://www.promedica.org/tth/fpr/index.htm
Accred Length: 3 Years *Program Size:* 18 (*GY1:* 6)
Subspecialties: FSM
Program ID: 120-38-21-250

Wilmington

Clinton Memorial Hospital Program

Sponsor: Clinton Memorial Hospital
Program Director:
Keith B Holten, MD
Clinton Memorial Hospital
825 W Locust St
Wilmington, OH 45177
Tel: 937 383-3382 *Fax:* 937 383-0610
E-mail: cmh-familypracticeresidency@in-touch.net
Internet: http://www.cmhregional.com
Accred Length: 3 Years *Program Size:* 12 (*GY1:* 4)
Program ID: 120-38-21-626

Youngstown

St Elizabeth Health Center/NEOUCOM Program

Sponsor: St Elizabeth Health Center
Program Director:
Mark H Belfer, DO
St Elizabeth Health Ctr-Family Health Ctr
1053 Belmont Ave
Youngstown, OH 44504
Tel: 330 744-0301 *Fax:* 330 480-2948
E-mail: rosey_hilland@hmis.org
Accred Length: 3 Years *Program Size:* 13 (*GY1:* 4)
Program ID: 120-38-11-251

Western Reserve Care System/NEOUCOM Program

Sponsor: Western Reserve Care System
Forum Health-Northside Medical Center
Southside Medical Center
Program Director:
James C Dewar, MD
Western Reserve Care System
Family Practice Ctr
500 Gypsy Ln
Youngstown, OH 44501
Tel: 330 740-3983 *Fax:* 330 740-5678
E-mail: mevanchick@onecom.com
Internet: http://www.wrhc.org
Accred Length: 3 Years *Program Size:* 12 (*GY1:* 4)
Program ID: 120-38-11-359

Oklahoma

Enid

University of Oklahoma/Garfield County Medical Society Rural Program

Sponsor: Bass Memorial Baptist Hospital
St Mary's Mercy Hospital
University Hospital
Program Director:
J Michael Pontious, MD
Enid Family Med Clinic
620 S Madison/Ste 304
Enid, OK 73701-7266
Tel: 405 242-1300 *Fax:* 405 233-3721
E-mail: mike-pontious@uokhsc.edu
Internet: http://www.fammed.uokhsc.edu/enid/enid.htm
Accred Length: 3 Years *Program Size:* 12 (*GY1:* 4)
Program ID: 120-39-11-253

Oklahoma City

Great Plains Medical Foundation Program

Sponsor: Great Plains Medical Foundation
Integris Baptist Medical Center
Program Director:
Neal Clemenson, MD
Great Plains Family Practice Program
3500 NW 56/#100
Oklahoma City, OK 73112-4518
Tel: 405 951-2623 *Fax:* 405 951-2824
E-mail: grtplain@integris-health.com
Internet: http://www.greatplains-fp.com
Accred Length: 3 Years *Program Size:* 15 (*GY1:* 5)
Program ID: 120-39-21-585

St Anthony Hospital Program

Sponsor: St Anthony Hospital
Program Director:
Richard L Boothe II, MD
St Anthony Hospital
608 NW Ninth St/Ste 1000
Oklahoma City, OK 73102
Tel: 405 272-7494 *Fax:* 405 272-6985
Internet: http://www.saintafpr.com
Accred Length: 3 Years *Program Size:* 17 (*GY1:* 6)
Program ID: 120-39-21-513

University of Oklahoma Health Sciences Center Program

Sponsor: University of Oklahoma College of Medicine
University Hospital
Program Director:
John P Zubialde, MD
Univ of Oklahoma Health Sciences Ctr
900 NE 10th St
Oklahoma City, OK 73104
Tel: 405 271-2230 *Fax:* 405 271-4366
E-mail: fam-med-okc@ouhsc.edu
Internet: http://www.fammed.ouhsc.edu
Accred Length: 3 Years *Program Size:* 36 (*GY1:* 12)
Subspecialties: FSM
Program ID: 120-39-21-254

Tulsa

In His Image at Hillcrest Medical Center Program

Sponsor: In His Image Inc
Hillcrest Medical Center
Program Director:
John R Crouch Jr, MD
7600 S Lewis Ave
Tulsa, OK 74136
Tel: 918 493-7816 *Fax:* 918 493-7888
E-mail: admin@inhisimage.org
Internet: http://www.inhisimage.org
Accred Length: 3 Years *Program Size:* 30 (*GY1:* 10)
Program ID: 120-39-21-499

University of Oklahoma College of Medicine-Tulsa Program

Sponsor: University of Oklahoma College of Medicine-Tulsa
Hillcrest Medical Center
St Francis Hospital
St John Medical Center
Program Director:
Loui D Elfrink, MD
Univ of Oklahoma Coll of Med-Tulsa
Dept of Family Med
9920 E 21st St
Tulsa, OK 74129
Tel: 918 663-6885 *Fax:* 918 663-6893
E-mail: debbie-phillips@ouhsc.edu
Internet:
http://www.tulsa.ouhscc.edu/family/residency.htm
Accred Length: 3 Years *Program Size:* 36 (*GY1:* 12)
Program ID: 120-39-21-256

University of Oklahoma College of Medicine-Tulsa Rural Program

Sponsor: University of Oklahoma College of Medicine-Tulsa
St John Medical Center
Program Director:
W Michael Woods, MD
Univ of Oklahoma Coll of Med-Tulsa
400 Wyandotte
PO Box 420
Ramona, OK 74061
Tel: 918 536-2104
E-mail: mwoods@fullnet.net
Internet: http://www.fullnet.net/np/ourural/
Accred Length: 3 Years *Program Size:* 6 (*GY1:* 2)
Program ID: 120-39-21-600

Programs

Oregon

Klamath Falls

Oregon Health Sciences University (Cascades East) Program

Sponsor: Oregon Health Sciences University Hospital
Merle West Medical Center
St Charles Medical Center
Program Director:
James F Calvert Jr, MD
Cascades East Family Practice
2800 Daggett St
Klamath Falls, OR 97601
Tel: 541 885-0325 *Fax:* 541 885-2643
E-mail: resident.cefp@mwmc.org
Internet:
http://www.ohsu.edu/som-fammed/cerespgm.htm
Accred Length: 3 Years *Program Size:* 18 (*GY1:* 6)
Program ID: 120-40-21-540

Portland

Oregon Health Sciences University Program

Sponsor: Oregon Health Sciences University Hospital
Program Director:
Eric Walsh, MD
Oregon Health Sciences Univ
Dept of Family Med/FP
3181 SW Sam Jackson Park Rd
Portland, OR 97201-3098
Tel: 503 494-6600 *Fax:* 503 494-7659
E-mail: fournies@ohsu.edu
Internet:
http://www.ohsu.edu/som-fammed/residpgm.htm
Accred Length: 3 Years *Program Size:* 36 (*GY1:* 12)
Subspecialties: FP
Program ID: 120-40-21-371

Pennsylvania

Abington

Abington Memorial Hospital Program

Sponsor: Abington Memorial Hospital
Program Director:
Gerald J Hansen III, MD
Abington Memorial Hospital
Abington Family Medicine
817 Old York Rd
Jenkintown, PA 19046-1623
Tel: 215 576-2729 *Fax:* 215 884-7344
E-mail: fpresamh@shrsys.hslc.org
Internet: http://www.amh.org
Accred Length: 3 Years *Program Size:* 20 (*GY1:* 7)
Program ID: 120-41-11-258

Allentown

Lehigh Valley Hospital/Pennsylvania State University Program

Sponsor: Lehigh Valley Hospital
Program Director:
William L Miller, MD
Lehigh Valley Hospital
17th and Chew Sts
PO Box 7017
Allentown, PA 18105-7017
Tel: 610 402-4970 *Fax:* 610 402-4952
E-mail: familypractice@lvhhn.org
Internet:
http://www.lvhhn.org/academic/residency/family/home.html
Accred Length: 3 Years *Program Size:* 18 (*GY1:* 6)
Program ID: 120-41-21-572

Temple University (Allentown) Program

Sponsor: Sacred Heart Hospital
Program Director:
Christian F Sorensen, MD
Sacred Heart Hospital
Fourth and Chew Sts
Allentown, PA 18102-3490
Tel: 610 776-4888 *Fax:* 610 776-5176
Internet: http://www.shh.org
Accred Length: 3 Years *Program Size:* 21 (*GY1:* 7)
Program ID: 120-41-21-259

Altoona

Altoona Hospital Program

Sponsor: Altoona Hospital
Program Director:
Elissa J Palmer, MD
Allegheny Family Physicians-Altoona Hospital
501 Howard Ave/Ste F2
Altoona, PA 16601-4882
Tel: 814 946-2020 *Fax:* 814 946-7864
Internet: http://www.altoonahosp.org/afpmain.htp
Accred Length: 3 Years *Program Size:* 18 (*GY1:* 6)
Program ID: 120-41-11-260

Beaver

The Medical Center (Beaver, PA) Program

Sponsor: The Medical Center (Beaver PA)
Program Director:
James P McKenna, MD
Family Practice Ctr
918 Third Ave
Beaver Falls, PA 15010
Tel: 724 843-6007 *Fax:* 724 847-7840
E-mail: rapplications@vhsnet.org
Accred Length: 3 Years *Program Size:* 18 (*GY1:* 6)
Program ID: 120-41-21-409

Bethlehem

St Luke's Hospital Program

Sponsor: St Luke's Hospital
Program Director:
James L Martin, MD
St Luke's Family Practice Residency
2830 Easton Ave
Bethlehem, PA 18017-4204
Tel: 610 954-3550 *Fax:* 610 954-3560
E-mail: fpresidency@slhn.org
Internet:
http://slhn-lehighvalley.org/services/resident/famres.htm
Accred Length: 3 Years *Program Size:* 18 (*GY1:* 6)
Program ID: 120-41-21-603

Bryn Mawr

Bryn Mawr Hospital Program

Sponsor: Bryn Mawr Hospital
Program Director:
Gerard F Klinzing, MD
Bryn Mawr Hospital
Med Educ Dept
130 S Bryn Mawr Ave
Bryn Mawr, PA 19010-3157
Tel: 610 526-3066 *Fax:* 610 526-3683
E-mail: klinzingg@mlhs.org
Accred Length: 3 Years *Program Size:* 18 (*GY1:* 6)
Program ID: 120-41-31-261

Danville

Penn State Geisinger Health System/Geisinger Medical Center Program

Sponsor: Penn State Geisinger Health System
Geisinger Medical Center
Program Director:
Mark Burd, MD
Geisinger Med Ctr
100 N Academy Ave
Danville, PA 17822
Tel: 717 271-6114 *Fax:* 717 271-5269
E-mail: ckrebs@psghs.edu
Accred Length: 3 Years *Program Size:* 19 (*GY1:* 6)
Program ID: 120-41-11-262

Erie

Hamot Medical Center Program

Sponsor: Hamot Medical Center
Program Director:
Mark J Levine, MD
Hamot Family Practice Residency
104 E Second St
Erie, PA 16507
Tel: 814 877-6187 *Fax:* 814 877-6741
E-mail: kathy.hull@hamot.org
Internet: http://www.hamot.org
Accred Length: 3 Years *Program Size:* 18 (*GY1:* 6)
Program ID: 120-41-11-263

St Vincent Health Center Program

Sponsor: St Vincent Health Center
Program Director:
Gary J Silko, MD MS
2314 Sassafras St/Ste 200
Erie, PA 16502
Tel: 814 452-5100 *Fax:* 814 452-5097
E-mail: gsilko@svhs.org
Accred Length: 3 Years *Program Size:* 21 (*GY1:* 7)
Program ID: 120-41-11-264

Harrisburg

PinnacleHealth Hospitals Program

Sponsor: PinnacleHealth System-Harrisburg Hospital
Program Director:
Ellen G Smith, MD
PinnacleHealth-Harrisburg Hospital
Dept of Family Practice
205 S Front St/PO Box 8700
Harrisburg, PA 17105-8700
Tel: 717 231-8650 *Fax:* 717 782-5702
E-mail: esmith@pinnaclehealth.org
Internet: http://www.pinnaclehealth.org/harrisburg.html
Accred Length: 3 Years *Program Size:* 27 (*GY1:* 9)
Program ID: 120-41-11-265

Johnstown

Conemaugh Valley Memorial Hospital Program

Sponsor: Conemaugh Valley Memorial Hospital
Program Director:
Orlando F Mills, MD MPH
Conemaugh Health System-Memorial Med Ctr
Family Med Ctr
1086 Franklin St
Johnstown, PA 15905-4398
Tel: 814 534-9364, ext 9364 *Fax:* 814 534-3136
E-mail: omills@conemaugh.org
Internet: http://www.jfmc.com
Accred Length: 3 Years *Program Size:* 18 (*GY1:* 6)
Program ID: 120-41-11-269

Lancaster

Lancaster General Hospital Program

Sponsor: Lancaster General Hospital

Program Director:
Nikitas J Zervanos, MD
Lancaster General Hospital
555 N Duke St/PO Box 3555
Lancaster, PA 17604-3555
Tel: 717 290-4940 *Fax:* 717 290-4149
E-mail: njzervan@lha.org
Internet: http://www.lha.org_residency.html
Accred Length: 3 Years *Program Size:* 39 (*GY1:* 13)
Program ID: 120-41-12-270

Latrobe

Thomas Jefferson University (Latrobe) Program

Sponsor: Latrobe Area Hospital

Program Director:
John G Bertolino, MD MPH
Latrobe Area Hospital
Family Practice Program
121 W 2nd Ave
Latrobe, PA 15650-1096
Tel: 724 537-1485
E-mail: lahpad@lah.com
Internet: http://www.lah.com
Accred Length: 3 Years *Program Size:* 17 (*GY1:* 6)
Program ID: 120-41-11-277

Lebanon

Penn State Geisinger Health System/Good Samaritan Hospital Program

Sponsor: Penn State Geisinger Health System
Good Samaritan Hospital
Milton S Hershey Medical Center

Program Director:
Edward G Paul, MD
Penn State Univ-Good Samaritan Hospital
PO Box 1520
Lebanon, PA 17042-1520
Tel: 717 270-1949 *Fax:* 717 270-1958
E-mail: fpr@gshleb.com
Internet: http://gshleb.com/fppprog.html
Accred Length: 3 Years *Program Size:* 18 (*GY1:* 6)
Program ID: 120-41-21-504

McKeesport

McKeesport Hospital/UPMC Program

Sponsor: McKeesport Hospital/UPMC

Program Director:
Robert J Grealish, MD
UPMC McKeesport
1500 Fifth Ave
McKeesport, PA 15132-2483
Tel: 412 664-2131 *Fax:* 412 664-2720
E-mail: kramersb@msx.upmc.edu
Internet: http://www.mckeehosp.org
Accred Length: 3 Years *Program Size:* 18 (*GY1:* 6)
Program ID: 120-41-12-271

Meadville

Meadville Medical Center Program

Sponsor: Meadville Medical Center

Program Director:
Ronald A Kellogg, MD
Family Medicine Meadville
765 Liberty St
Ste 105
Meadville, PA 16335
Tel: 814 333-5461 *Fax:* 814 333-5025
E-mail: mmcfpr@mmchs.org
Internet: http://practicelink.com
Accred Length: 3 Years *Program Size:* 4 (*GY1:* 4)
Program ID: 120-41-21-645

Monroeville (Pittsburgh)

Allegheny University Hospitals-Forbes Regional Program

Sponsor: Allegheny University Hospitals-Forbes Regional

Program Director:
Martin I Seltman, MD
Forbes Health System
500 Finley St
Pittsburgh, PA 15206
Tel: 412 858-2768 *Fax:* 412 858-2765
E-mail: mtomina@aherf.edu
Internet: http://www.pgh.aherf.edu/forbesfp/
Accred Length: 3 Years *Program Size:* 18 (*GY1:* 6)
Program ID: 120-41-22-278

Norristown

Montgomery Hospital Program

Sponsor: Montgomery Hospital

Program Director:
Louis D Mancano III, MD
Montgomery Family Practice Program
1330 Powell St/Ste 409
Norristown, PA 19401
Tel: 610 277-0964 *Fax:* 610 270-2184
E-mail: mfpc@earthlink.net
Internet: http://home.earthlink.net/~mfpc
Accred Length: 3 Years *Program Size:* 18 (*GY1:* 6)
Program ID: 120-41-11-272

Philadelphia

Chestnut Hill Hospital Program

Sponsor: Chestnut Hill Hospital

Program Director:
Marc W McKenna, MD
Chestnut Hill Hospital
Family Practice Ctr
8815 Germantown Ave/5th Fl
Philadelphia, PA 19118
Tel: 215 248-8145 *Fax:* 215 248-8852
E-mail: bosca@chh.org
Internet: http://www.chh.org
Accred Length: 3 Years *Program Size:* 18 (*GY1:* 6)
Program ID: 120-41-31-275

MCP Hahnemann University Program

Sponsor: MCP Hahnemann University
Medical College of Pennsylvania Hospital
Warminster Hospital

Program Director:
Judy L Gerard-Ciminera, MD
Hahnemann Univ Hospitals-Bucks County
Dept of Family Practice
225 Newtown Rd
Warminster, PA 18974
Tel: 215 441-7560 *Fax:* 215 441-7585
E-mail: fpres@auhs.edu
Accred Length: 3 Years *Program Size:* 12 (*GY1:* 4)
Program ID: 120-41-31-576

Thomas Jefferson University Program

Sponsor: Thomas Jefferson University Hospital

Program Director:
Janice E Nevin, MD MPH
Thomas Jefferson Univ Hospital
1015 Walnut St/Rm 401
Philadelphia, PA 19107
Tel: 215 955-2352 *Fax:* 215 923-6256
Accred Length: 3 Years *Program Size:* 26 (*GY1:* 8)
Subspecialties: FPG, FSM
Program ID: 120-41-21-276

University of Pennsylvania Program

Sponsor: Hospital of the University of Pennsylvania
Presbyterian Medical Center (UPHS)

Program Director:
Judith A Fisher, MD
Univ of Pennsylvania
6th Fl Mutch Bldg/Dept of Fam Practice
39th and Market Sts
Philadelphia, PA 19104
Tel: 215 662-8949 *Fax:* 215 243-3290
E-mail: tcs@mail.med.upenn.edu
Internet:
http://www.med.upenn.edu/fampract/residency.html
Accred Length: 3 Years *Program Size:* 18 (*GY1:* 6)
Program ID: 120-41-21-633

Pittsburgh

Mercy Hospital of Pittsburgh Program

Sponsor: Mercy Hospital of Pittsburgh

Program Director:
Michael J Essig, MD MD
Mercy Hospital of Pittsburgh
Dept of Family Practice
1400 Locust St
Pittsburgh, PA 15219-5166
Tel: 412 323-5609 *Fax:* 412 323-5685
E-mail: family.practice.residency@mercy.pmhs.org
Internet: http://www.mercy-meded.com
Accred Length: 3 Years *Program Size:* 19 (*GY1:* 6)
Program ID: 120-41-11-578

Shadyside Hospital/UPMC Program

Sponsor: Shadyside Hospital/UPMC

Program Director:
David A Blandino, MD
UPMC Shadyside
Dept of Family Practice
5230 Centre Ave
Pittsburgh, PA 15232
Tel: 412 623-2236 *Fax:* 412 623-3012
E-mail: davidb@ssh.edu
Internet: http://ssh.edu
Accred Length: 3 Years *Program Size:* 27 (*GY1:* 9)
Subspecialties: FSM, TY
Program ID: 120-41-12-280

University of Pittsburgh Medical Center (St Margaret) Program

Sponsor: University of Pittsburgh Medical Center (St Margaret)

Program Director:
Ted C Schaffer, MD
UPMC St Margaret
815 Freeport Rd
Pittsburgh, PA 15215-3384
Tel: 412 784-4232 *Fax:* 412 784-5274
E-mail: smhfpr@fyi.net
Accred Length: 3 Years *Program Size:* 36 (*GY1:* 12)
Subspecialties: FPG, FSM
Program ID: 120-41-12-279

Western Pennsylvania Hospital Program
Sponsor: Western Pennsylvania Hospital
Program Director:
Marian R Block, MD
Western Pennsylvania Hospital
Family Practice Program
4800 Friendship Ave/Ste N221
Pittsburgh, PA 15224
Tel: 412 578-1649 *Fax:* 412 688-7711
E-mail: wphfprp@yahoo.com
Internet:
http://www.westpennhospital.com/resident/family.htm
Accred Length: 3 Years *Program Size:* 18 (*GY1:* 6)
Program ID: 120-41-12-579

Reading

Reading Hospital and Medical Center Program
Sponsor: Reading Hospital and Medical Center
Program Director:
D Michael Baxter, MD
Reading Hospital and Med Ctr
Family Med Program
301 S Seventh Ave/Ste 2120
Reading, PA 19612-6052
Tel: 610 378-6855 *Fax:* 610 378-6390
E-mail: fmres@readinghospital.org
Internet:
http://www.readinghospital.org/familymed/familymed.asp
Accred Length: 3 Years *Program Size:* 18 (*GY1:* 6)
Program ID: 120-41-12-281

St Joseph Medical Center Program
Sponsor: St Joseph Medical Center
Program Director:
Margaret M Wilkins, DO
145 N 6th St
2nd Floor
Reading, PA 19604
Tel: 610 378-2080 *Fax:* 610 378-2434
E-mail: sjmcfprp@enter.net
Internet: http://www.enter.net/~sjmcfprp
Accred Length: 3 Years *Program Size:* 18 (*GY1:* 5)
Program ID: 120-41-11-282

Sayre

Guthrie Healthcare System Program
Sponsor: Guthrie Healthcare System
Robert Packer Hospital
Program Director:
Franklyn D Dornfest, MD
Guthrie Family Practice Residency
1st Level-Guthrie Clinic
Guthrie Sq
Sayre, PA 18840
Tel: 570 882-3292 *Fax:* 570 882-2807
E-mail: fampract@inet.guthrie.org
Internet: http://www.guthrie.org/family.htm
Accred Length: 3 Years *Program Size:* 12 (*GY1:* 4)
Program ID: 120-41-21-518

Upland

Crozer-Keystone Health System Program
Sponsor: Crozer-Chester Medical Center
Crozer-Keystone Health System
Program Director:
John A Zapp, MD
Crozer-Keystone Fam Practice Residency
1260 E Woodland Ave/Ste 200
Springfield, PA 19064-3988
Tel: 610 690-4480 *Fax:* 610 328-9391
E-mail: jzapp@crozer.org
Internet: http://www.hslc.org/ccm/ccm.html
Accred Length: 3 Years *Program Size:* 21 (*GY1:* 7)
Subspecialties: FSM
Program ID: 120-41-21-477

Washington

Washington Hospital Program
Sponsor: Washington Hospital
Program Director:
Paul T Cullen, MD
Washington Hospital
Family Practice Ctr
95 Leonard Ave
Washington, PA 15301
Tel: 724 223-3548 *Fax:* 724 229-2178
Internet: http://www.welnet.org
Accred Length: 3 Years *Program Size:* 24 (*GY1:* 8)
Program ID: 120-41-12-283

Wilkes-Barre

United Health and Hospital Services Program
Sponsor: Wyoming Valley Health Care System
WVHCS-Hospital
Program Director:
Richard B English, MD
Wyoming Valley Family Practice Residency
2 Sharpe St/Caller 3500
Kingston, PA 18704-0350
Tel: 717 552-8900 *Fax:* 717 552-8958
Internet: http://wvfprp.com
Accred Length: 3 Years *Program Size:* 18 (*GY1:* 6)
Program ID: 120-41-21-284

Williamsport

Williamsport Hospital and Medical Center Program
Sponsor: Williamsport Hospital and Medical Center
Program Director:
David N Ambrose, MD
Williamsport Hospital
Family Practice Program
699 Rural Ave
Williamsport, PA 17701-3198
Tel: 717 321-2340 *Fax:* 717 321-2359
E-mail: wmsptfp@shscares.org
Internet: http://www.shscares.org/famlprac/index.htm
Accred Length: 3 Years *Program Size:* 21 (*GY1:* 7)
Program ID: 120-41-31-285

York

York Hospital Program
Sponsor: York Hospital
Program Director:
Richard W Sloan, MD RPh
York Hospital
1001 S George St
York, PA 17405
Tel: 717 851-3038 *Fax:* 717 851-5852
E-mail: fp_rsloan@yorkhospital.edu
Internet: http://www.yorkhealth.org
Accred Length: 3 Years *Program Size:* 24 (*GY1:* 8)
Subspecialties: TY
Program ID: 120-41-11-286

Puerto Rico

Bayamon

Hospital San Pablo Program
Sponsor: Hospital San Pablo
Program Director:
Felix Betancourt-Bojos, MD
Hospital San Pablo
PO Box 236
Bayamon, PR 00960
Tel: 787 740-4747, ext 396 *Fax:* 787 740-5775
Accred Length: 3 Years *Program Size:* 15 (*GY1:* 5)
Program ID: 120-42-21-448

Universidad Central del Caribe Program
Sponsor: University Hospital Ramon Ruiz Arnau
Program Director:
Harry E Mercado, MD
Univ Central del Caribe
Dept of Family Med
Call Box 60327
Bayamon, PR 00960-6032
Tel: 787 740-4343 *Fax:* 787 740-4343
E-mail: reinforma@caribe.net
Accred Length: 3 Years *Program Size:* 20 (*GY1:* 6)
Program ID: 120-42-21-510

Caguas

University of Puerto Rico Program
Sponsor: University of Puerto Rico School of Medicine
Caguas Regional Hospital
Program Director:
Paquita L Moya-Huff, MD
Gurabo Community Health Ctr
Box 1277
Gurabo, PR 00778
Tel: 787 737-6690 *Fax:* 787 737-6624
Accred Length: 3 Years *Program Size:* 30 (*GY1:* 10)
Subspecialties: FPG
Program ID: 120-42-21-287

Manati

Dr Alejandro Otero Lopez Hospital Program
Sponsor: Hospital Dr Alejandro Otero Lopez
Program Director:
Enid M Mateo-Reyes, MD
Dr Alejandro Otero Lopez Hospital
PO Box 1142
Manati, PR 00674
Tel: 787 854-3700 *Fax:* 787 884-6403
Accred Length: 3 Years *Program Size:* 18 (*GY1:* 6)
Program ID: 120-42-21-501

Mayaguez

Bella Vista Hospital Program
Sponsor: Bella Vista Hospital
Program Director:
Eliasin Munoz, MD
Laura Mata, MD
Bella Vista Hospital
PO Box 1750
Mayaguez, PR 00681
Tel: 787 834-2350, ext 6214 *Fax:* 787 831-6315
E-mail: bvfamilymedicine@hotmail.com
Accred Length: 3 Years *Program Size:* 8 (*GY1:* 4)
Program ID: 120-42-21-620

Ponce

Dr Pila Hospital/Ponce School of Medicine Program
Sponsor: Dr Pila Hospital
Ponce University Hospital
Program Director:
Muneca I Rivera, MD
Dr Pila Hospital-Ponce Sch of Med
PO Box 1910
Ponce, PR 00733-1910
Tel: 787 844-6405, ext 236 *Fax:* 787 844-6400
E-mail: imfdepon@caribe.net
Accred Length: 3 Years *Program Size:* 12 (*GY1:* 4)
Program ID: 120-42-21-466

Rhode Island

Pawtucket

Brown University Program
Sponsor: Memorial Hospital of Rhode Island
Program Director:
John B Murphy, MD
Memorial Hospital of Rhode Island-Brown Univ
111 Brewster St
Pawtucket, RI 02860
Tel: 401 729-2236 *Fax:* 401 729-2923
E-mail: john_murphy@mhri.org
Internet:
http://biomed.brown.edu/medicine_department/familymedicine/home.html
Accred Length: 3 Years *Program Size:* 39 (*GY1:* 13)
Program ID: 120-43-21-288

South Carolina

Anderson

Anderson Area Medical Center Program
Sponsor: Anderson Area Medical Center
Program Director:
James R Buehler, MD
Dept of Family Practice
600 N Fant St
Anderson, SC 29621
Tel: 864 224-8100, ext 1916 *Fax:* 864 260-3702
E-mail: andersonfp@anmed.com
Accred Length: 3 Years *Program Size:* 28 (*GY1:* 9)
Program ID: 120-45-11-289

Charleston

Medical University of South Carolina Program
Sponsor: Medical University of South Carolina College of Medicine
Program Director:
Peter J Carek, MD MS
Med Univ of South Carolina
Dept of Family Med
295 Calhoun St/PO Box 250192
Charleston, SC 29425
Tel: 843 824-9566, ext 244 *Fax:* 843 569-2243
E-mail: fammedres@musc.edu
Internet: http://www.musc.edu/dfm/homepage.htm
Accred Length: 3 Years *Program Size:* 36 (*GY1:* 12)
Program ID: 120-45-21-290

Columbia

Palmetto Health Alliance/University of South Carolina School of Medicine Program
Sponsor: Palmetto Health Alliance
Palmetto Richland Memorial Hospital
Program Director:
John J Lammie, MD
Palmetto Richland Memorial Hospital
Dept of Family Practice
Six Richland Memorial Hospital
Columbia, SC 29203
Tel: 803 434-6116 *Fax:* 803 434-7529
E-mail: jlammiefpgw.rmh.edu
Internet: http://www.prevmed.sc.edu/fp.htm
Accred Length: 3 Years *Program Size:* 36 (*GY1:* 12)
Subspecialties: FSM
Program ID: 120-45-11-291

Florence

McLeod Regional Medical Center Program
Sponsor: McLeod Regional Medical Center
Program Director:
William H Hester, MD
McLeod Family Med Ctr
555 E Cheves St
Florence, SC 29506-2617
Tel: 843 667-2812 *Fax:* 843 667-2829
E-mail: dbacon@mcleodregional.org
Internet: http://www.mcleodregional.org
Accred Length: 3 Years *Program Size:* 26 (*GY1:* 8)
Program ID: 120-45-21-375

Greenville

Greenville Hospital System Program
Sponsor: Greenville Hospital System
Program Director:
Palmira S Snape, MD
Ctr for Family Medicine
877 W Faris Rd
Greenville, SC 29605
Tel: 864 455-7831 *Fax:* 864 455-9015
E-mail: cfm@.ghs.org
Accred Length: 3 Years *Program Size:* 30 (*GY1:* 10)
Program ID: 120-45-11-292

Greenwood

Greenwood Family Practice Program
Sponsor: Self Memorial Hospital
Program Director:
Stoney A Abercrombie, MD
Family Practice Program
160 Academy Ave
Greenwood, SC 29646
Tel: 864 227-4869 *Fax:* 864 227-4883
E-mail: sabercrombie@emeraldis.com
Internet: http://www.emeraldis.com/greenwoodfp
Accred Length: 3 Years *Program Size:* 27 (*GY1:* 9)
Program ID: 120-45-21-376

Spartanburg

Spartanburg Regional Healthcare System Program
Sponsor: Spartanburg Regional Healthcare System
Program Director:
Otis L Baughman III, MD
Spartanburg Family Medicine Program
853 N Church St/Ste 510
Spartanburg, SC 29303
Tel: 864 560-1558 *Fax:* 864 560-1565
E-mail: sfmr@bigfoot.com
Internet: http://www.spartfam.org
Accred Length: 3 Years *Program Size:* 36 (*GY1:* 12)
Program ID: 120-45-11-293

South Dakota

Rapid City

Rapid City Regional Hospital Program
Sponsor: Rapid City Regional Hospital
Program Director:
Douglas A Bright, MD
Rapid City Regional Hospital
502 E Monroe St
Rapid City, SD 57701
Tel: 605 341-8828 *Fax:* 605 399-4244
E-mail: tbrcrhfp@rapidnet.com
Internet: http://www.rcrhfpr.org
Accred Length: 3 Years *Program Size:* 18 (*GY1:* 6)
Program ID: 120-46-21-547

Sioux Falls

University of South Dakota Program
Sponsor: University of South Dakota School of Medicine
Avera McKennan Hospital
Sioux Valley Hospital
Program Director:
Earl D Kemp, MD
Ctr for Family Medicine
2300 S Dakota Ave
Sioux Falls, SD 57105
Tel: 605 339-1783 *Fax:* 605 335-1006
E-mail: edkemp@iw.net
Internet: http://www.iw.net/sffpr
Accred Length: 3 Years *Program Size:* 27 (*GY1:* 8)
Subspecialties: TY
Program ID: 120-46-11-294

Tennessee

Bristol

East Tennessee State University (Bristol) Program
Sponsor: James H Quillen College of Medicine
Bristol Regional Medical Center
Program Director:
Raymond H Feierabend Jr, MD
Bristol Family Practice Ctr
100 Bristol College Dr
Bristol, TN 37620
Tel: 423 989-4069 *Fax:* 423 989-4057
E-mail: bfpc@etsu.edu
Internet: http://www.etsu-tn.edu/
Accred Length: 3 Years *Program Size:* 24 (*GY1:* 8)
Program ID: 120-47-31-296

Chattanooga

East Tennessee State University (Chattanooga) Program

Sponsor: James H Quillen College of Medicine
Memorial Hospital

Program Director:
Thomas A Cable, MD
Memorial Hospital
2525 de Sales Ave
Chattanooga, TN 37404-3322
Tel: 423 495-6377 *Fax:* 423 698-2329
E-mail: tom_cable@memorial.org
Accred Length: 3 Years *Program Size:* 18 (*GY1:* 6)
Program ID: 120-47-11-587

University of Tennessee College of Medicine at Chattanooga Program

Sponsor: University of Tennessee College of Medicine-Chattanooga Unit
Erlanger Medical Center

Program Director:
J Mack Worthington, MD
Univ of Tennessee Coll of Med
Dept of Family Med
1100 E Third St
Chattanooga, TN 37403
Tel: 423 778-2957 *Fax:* 423 778-2959
E-mail: utfammed@erlanger.org
Internet: http://www.erlanger.org/utcom/famprac.html
Accred Length: 3 Years *Program Size:* 24 (*GY1:* 8)
Program ID: 120-47-31-584

Jackson

University of Tennessee (Jackson) Program

Sponsor: University of Tennessee College of Medicine
Jackson-Madison County General Hospital

Program Director:
David E Roberts, MD
Dept of Family Med
294 Summar Dr
Jackson, TN 38301-3983
Tel: 901 423-1932, ext 227 *Fax:* 901 423-4919
E-mail: deroberts@utmem.edu
Internet: http://206.240.216.21/jackson.html
Accred Length: 3 Years *Program Size:* 24 (*GY1:* 8)
Program ID: 120-47-21-299

Johnson City

East Tennessee State University Program

Sponsor: James H Quillen College of Medicine
Johnson City Medical Center Hospital
Veterans Affairs Medical Center (Mountain Home)

Program Director:
Daniel J David, MD
East Tennessee State Univ
Dept of Family Med
917 W Walnut St
Johnson City, TN 37604
Tel: 423 439-6463 *Fax:* 423 439-7118
E-mail: fammed@etsu.edu
Internet: http://www.etsu.edu/fammed
Accred Length: 3 Years *Program Size:* 21 (*GY1:* 7)
Program ID: 120-47-21-410

Kingsport

East Tennessee State University (Kingsport) Program

Sponsor: James H Quillen College of Medicine
Wellmont Health System-Holston Valley

Program Director:
Reid B Blackwelder, MD
201 Cassel Dr
Kingsport, TN 37660
Tel: 423 245-9635 *Fax:* 423 245-9634
Internet: http://www.etsu-tn.edu/~fammed
Accred Length: 3 Years *Program Size:* 24 (*GY1:* 8)
Program ID: 120-47-31-297

Knoxville

University of Tennessee Medical Center at Knoxville Program

Sponsor: University of Tennessee Graduate School of Medicine
University of Tennessee Memorial Hospital

Program Director:
Gregory H Blake, MD MPH
Univ of Tennessee Grad Sch of Med
1924 Alcoa Hwy/U-67
Knoxville, TN 37920-6999
Tel: 423 544-9352 *Fax:* 423 544-6532
E-mail: utfprp@mc.utmck.edu
Internet: http://www.mc.utk.edu
Accred Length: 3 Years *Program Size:* 30 (*GY1:* 10)
Subspecialties: FSM
Program ID: 120-47-11-298

Memphis

University of Tennessee (Healthplex) Program

Sponsor: University of Tennessee College of Medicine
Baptist Memorial Hospital

Program Director:
J Sloan Manning, MD
Healthplex Family Practice
1121 Union Ave
Memphis, TN 38104
Tel: 901 448-7368 *Fax:* 901 448-1860
Internet: http://132.192.48.70healthplex.html
Accred Length: 3 Years *Program Size:* 36 (*GY1:* 12)
Program ID: 120-47-21-462

University of Tennessee Program

Sponsor: University of Tennessee College of Medicine
St Francis Hospital
University of Tennessee Medical Center (UT Bowld Hospital)

Program Director:
Michael A Murphy, MD
St Francis Family Practice Clinic
1301 Primacy Pkwy
Memphis, TN 38119
Tel: 901 761-2997 *Fax:* 901 763-3649
E-mail: utsffpr@utmem1.utmem.edu
Internet: http://132.192.48.70/st.francis.html
Accred Length: 3 Years *Program Size:* 24 (*GY1:* 8)
Program ID: 120-47-21-453

Nashville

Meharry Medical College Program

Sponsor: Meharry Medical College
Alvin C York Veterans Affairs Medical Center
Metropolitan Nashville General Hospital

Program Director:
Harold V Nevels, MD
Meharry Med Coll
1005 D B Todd Jr Blvd
Nashville, TN 37208
Tel: 615 327-6572 *Fax:* 615 327-5834
Accred Length: 3 Years *Program Size:* 19 (*GY1:* 6)
Program ID: 120-47-21-463

Texas

Amarillo

Texas Tech University (Amarillo) Program

Sponsor: Texas Tech University Health Sciences Center at Amarillo
Northwest Texas Health Care System
St Anthony's Hospital

Program Director:
Barton E Freeman, MD
Texas Tech Univ Health Sciences Ctr
1400 Wallace Blvd
Amarillo, TX 79106
Tel: 806 354-5462 *Fax:* 806 351-3791
E-mail: pat@cortex.ama.ttuhsc.edu
Internet: http://www.ama.ttuhsc.edu
Accred Length: 3 Years *Program Size:* 18 (*GY1:* 6)
Program ID: 120-48-21-511

Austin

CTMF of Seton Healthcare Network Program

Sponsor: CTMF of Seton Healthcare Network
Brackenridge Hospital

Program Director:
Cynthia C Brinson, MD
Central Texas Med Foundation
Dept of Family Med
4614 N I H-35
Austin, TX 78751
Tel: 512 458-9176 *Fax:* 512 458-1783
Accred Length: 3 Years *Program Size:* 21 (*GY1:* 7)
Program ID: 120-48-11-302

Baytown

San Jacinto Methodist Hospital Program

Sponsor: San Jacinto Methodist Hospital

Program Director:
Clare Hawkins, MD
Family Practice Center
4301 Garth Rd/Ste 400
Baytown, TX 77521
Tel: 713 420-8400 *Fax:* 713 420-8480
E-mail: sjfprp@tmh.tmc.edu
Internet:
http://www.methodisthealth.com/sanjacinto/residency
Accred Length: 3 Years *Program Size:* 24 (*GY1:* 8)
Program ID: 120-48-21-432

Bryan

Family Practice Foundation of Brazos Valley Program

Sponsor: Family Practice Foundation of the Brazos Valley
St Joseph Regional Health Center

Program Director:
Dallas E Coate, MD
Family Practice Residency-Brazos Valley
1301 Memorial Dr/#210
Bryan, TX 77802
Tel: 409 862-4465 *Fax:* 409 774-6603
E-mail: coate@tamu.edu
Internet: http://www.fpresidency-brazos.org
Accred Length: 3 Years *Program Size:* 18 (*GY1:* 6)
Program ID: 120-48-31-605

Conroe

University of Texas Medical Branch Hospitals (Conroe) Program

Sponsor: University of Texas Medical Branch Hospitals
Conroe Regional Medical Center

Program Director:
Joseph G Ewing, MD
Family Practice Ctr
701 E Davis St/Ste C
Conroe, TX 77301-3018
Tel: 409 539-5161 *Fax:* 409 539-3635
E-mail: conroe@lcc.net
Internet: http://129.109.37.53/
Accred Length: 3 Years *Program Size:* 21 (*GY1:* 7)
Program ID: 120-48-21-454

Corpus Christi

Spohn Memorial Hospital Program

Sponsor: Spohn Memorial Hospital

Program Director:
Rick D Edwards, MD
Spohn Memorial Hospital
2606 Hospital Blvd
Corpus Christi, TX 78405
Tel: 512 902-4499 *Fax:* 512 902-4588
E-mail: ccfprp@worldnet.att.net
Internet: http://home.att.net/~ccfprp
Accred Length: 3 Years *Program Size:* 36 (*GY1:* 12)
Program ID: 120-48-22-303

Dallas

St Paul Medical Center/University of Texas Southwestern Medical Center Program

Sponsor: St Paul Medical Center
Dallas County Hospital District-Parkland Memorial Hospital

Program Director:
Phillip H Disraeli, MD
Inwood Rd at I-35
5909 Harry Hines Blvd
Dallas, TX 75235
Tel: 972 789-1787 *Fax:* 972 960-8299
E-mail: phillipdisraeli@hmhs.com
Internet: http://www.texashealth.org/spfamprac/
Accred Length: 3 Years *Program Size:* 12 (*GY1:* 4)
Program ID: 120-48-21-361

University of Texas Southwestern Medical Center (Methodist) Program

Sponsor: Methodist Hospitals of Dallas
Charlton Methodist Hospital
Dallas County Hospital District-Parkland Memorial Hospital

Program Director:
Luis C Palacios, MD
Methodist Hospitals of Dallas
3400 W Wheatland Rd
Dallas, TX 75237-3498
Tel: 214 947-5420 *Fax:* 214 947-5425
E-mail: helenmalone@mhdcme.org
Internet: http://www.mhdcme.org
Accred Length: 3 Years *Program Size:* 20 (*GY1:* 8)
Subspecialties: FSM
Program ID: 120-48-21-433

University of Texas Southwestern Medical School (Parkland Memorial) Program

Sponsor: University of Texas Southwestern Medical School
Dallas County Hospital District-Parkland Memorial Hospital

Program Director:
Robert D Frey, MD
Univ of Texas Southwestern Med Ctr
5323 Harry Hines Blvd
Dallas, TX 75235-9165
Tel: 214 648-3085 *Fax:* 214 648-1085
E-mail: mhanso@mednet.swmed.edu
Internet: http://www.swmed.edu/home_pages/famprac
Accred Length: 3 Years *Program Size:* 18 (*GY1:* 6)
Program ID: 120-48-21-601

El Paso

Texas Tech University (El Paso) Program

Sponsor: Texas Tech University Health Sciences Center at El Paso
R E Thomason General Hospital

Program Director:
Mary C Spalding, MD
Texas Tech Family Med
10060 Rushing
El Paso, TX 79924-3803
Tel: 915 757-3178 *Fax:* 915 751-4378
Internet:
http://www.ttuhsc.edu/pages/fammed/tthscfp.html
Accred Length: 3 Years *Program Size:* 25 (*GY1:* 8)
Program ID: 120-48-11-309

Fort Worth

University of Texas Southwestern Medical School (Fort Worth) Program

Sponsor: John Peter Smith Hospital (Tarrant County Hospital District)

Program Director:
Joane Baumer, MD
John Peter Smith Hospital
Dept of Family Practice
1500 S Main St
Fort Worth, TX 76104-4940
Tel: 817 927-1200 *Fax:* 817 927-1691
E-mail: bamckeon@aol.com
Internet: http://www.jpshealthnet.org
Accred Length: 3 Years *Program Size:* 72 (*GY1:* 24)
Program ID: 120-48-31-304

Galveston

University of Texas Medical Branch Hospitals Program

Sponsor: University of Texas Medical Branch Hospitals

Program Director:
Angela J Shepherd, MD
Univ of Texas Med Branch
Dept of Family Med
301 University Blvd
Galveston, TX 77555-1123
Tel: 409 772-3123 *Fax:* 409 747-8582
E-mail: tgeronda@utmb.edu
Internet: http://www.fammed1.utmb.edu
Accred Length: 3 Years *Program Size:* 42 (*GY1:* 14)
Program ID: 120-48-21-305

Garland

Baylor Medical Center at Garland Program

Sponsor: Baylor Medical Center at Garland
Family Healthcare Medical Education Center at Garland

Program Director:
C Tim Lambert, MD
Garland Family Practice Program
3262 Medical Plaza Dr/Ste 111
Garland, TX 75044
Tel: 972 495-4955 *Fax:* 972 496-9239
E-mail: fp.resident@baylordallas.edu
Accred Length: 3 Years *Program Size:* 18 (*GY1:* 6)
Program ID: 120-48-21-574

Harlingen

Valley Baptist Medical Center Program

Sponsor: Valley Baptist Medical Center

Program Director:
Bruce A Leibert, MD
2222 Benwood St
Harlingen, TX 78850
Tel: 956 389-2448 *Fax:* 956 389-2498
Accred Length: 3 Years *Program Size:* 12 (*GY1:* 4)
Program ID: 120-48-21-593

Houston

Baylor College of Medicine Program

Sponsor: Baylor College of Medicine
AMI Park Plaza Hospital
Harris County Hospital District-Ben Taub General Hospital
St Luke's Episcopal Hospital

Program Director:
James B Schindler, MD MPH
Baylor Family Practice Ctr
5510 Greenbriar Dr
Houston, TX 77005-2646
Tel: 713 798-7791 *Fax:* 713 798-7789
E-mail: jbschin@bcm.tmc.edu
Internet: http://www.bcm.tmc.edu/familymed/
Accred Length: 3 Years *Program Size:* 36 (*GY1:* 12)
Program ID: 120-48-11-306

Memorial Hermann Hospital System Program

Sponsor: Memorial Herman Hospital System

Program Director:
George O Zenner Jr, MD
Memorial Family Practice Residency Program
7737 Southwest Frwy #420
Houston, TX 77074
Tel: 713 776-5684 *Fax:* 713 776-5935
E-mail: memfpadmit@mhcs.org
Internet: http://www.mhcs.org/residency/index.html
Accred Length: 3 Years *Program Size:* 48 (*GY1:* 16)
Program ID: 120-48-21-307

St Joseph Hospital Program
Sponsor: St Joseph Hospital
Program Director:
Mark A Koch, MD
St Joseph Hospital
1315 St Joseph Pkwy/Ste 1400
Houston, TX 77002
Tel: 713 756-4129 *Fax:* 713 657-7391
E-mail: louis_johnston@stjoe.sch.org
Internet: http://www.stjosephfp.com
Accred Length: 3 Years *Program Size:* 24 (*GY1:* 8)
Program ID: 120-48-21-565

University of Texas at Houston Program
Sponsor: University of Texas Medical School at Houston
Lyndon B Johnson General Hospital
Memorial Hermann Healthcare System
Program Director:
Rebecca H Gladu, MD
Univ of Texas Med Sch
6431 Fannin St/Rm 2104
Houston, TX 77030
Tel: 713 500-7610 *Fax:* 713 500-7619
E-mail: dheidemann@fpcm.med.uth.tmc.edu
Internet: http://www.uth.tmc.edu/schools/med/fam_prac/
Accred Length: 3 Years *Program Size:* 35 (*GY1:* 11)
Program ID: 120-48-21-490

Lubbock

Texas Tech University (Lubbock) Program
Sponsor: Texas Tech University Health Sciences Center at Lubbock
St Mary of the Plains Hospital
University Medical Center
Program Director:
Roger M Ragain, MD
Texas Tech Univ Health Sciences Ctr
Dept of Family Med
3601 Fourth St
Lubbock, TX 79430
Tel: 806 743-2770 *Fax:* 806 743-3955
E-mail: fmprmr@ttuhsc.edu
Internet:
http://www.ttuhsc.edu/pages/fammed/deptpage.html
Accred Length: 3 Years *Program Size:* 27 (*GY1:* 9)
Program ID: 120-48-21-310

McAllen

University of Texas at San Antonio (McAllen) Program
Sponsor: University of Texas Medical School at San Antonio
McAllen Medical Center
Program Director:
Juan J Trevino, MD
McAllen Med Ctr
205 E Toronto
McAllen, TX 78503
Tel: 956 687-6155, ext 42 *Fax:* 956 618-0451
E-mail: bakers0@hiline
Accred Length: 3 Years *Program Size:* 24 (*GY1:* 8)
Program ID: 120-48-11-311

Odessa

Texas Tech University (Odessa) Program
Sponsor: Texas Tech University Health Sciences Center at Odessa
Medical Center Hospital
Program Director:
Leonard W Morgan, MD
Texas Tech Univ Health Sciences Ctr
800 W Fourth St
Odessa, TX 79763-4362
Tel: 915 335-5311 *Fax:* 915 335-5316
E-mail: fmpolah@tthsc8.odessa.ttuhsc.edu
Internet: http://www.ttuhsc.edu
Accred Length: 3 Years *Program Size:* 18 (*GY1:* 6)
Program ID: 120-48-21-457

Port Arthur

University of Texas Medical Branch (Port Arthur) Program
Sponsor: University of Texas Medical Branch Hospitals
St Mary Hospital
Program Director:
James J Hrachovy, MD
3535 Gates Blvd
Ste 100
Port Arthur, TX 77642
Tel: 409 989-5147 *Fax:* 409 983-6519
E-mail: teddip@exp.net
Accred Length: 3 Years *Program Size:* 30 (*GY1:* 10)
Program ID: 120-48-21-424

San Antonio

Santa Rosa Health Care Program
Sponsor: Santa Rosa Health Care Corporation
Northeastern Baptist Hospital
Program Director:
James C Martin, MD
Santa Rosa Family Practice Program
519 W Houston St
San Antonio, TX 78207-3198
Tel: 210 704-2535 *Fax:* 210 704-2545
E-mail: sharon_winnek@srhcc.org
Internet: http://198.8.16.3/1**fampract.html
Accred Length: 3 Years *Program Size:* 18 (*GY1:* 6)
Program ID: 120-48-21-616

University of Texas Health Science Center at San Antonio Program
Sponsor: University of Texas Medical School at San Antonio
Audie L Murphy Memorial Veterans Hospital (San Antonio)
University Health Center-Downtown
University Hospital-South Texas Medical Center
Program Director:
Joshua Freeman, MD
Univ of Texas Health Science Ctr
Dept of Family Practice
7703 Floyd Curl Dr
San Antonio, TX 78284-7795
Tel: 210 358-3920 *Fax:* 210 220-3763
Internet: http://macorb.uthscsa.edu/famprac
Accred Length: 3 Years *Program Size:* 36 (*GY1:* 12)
Subspecialties: FSM
Program ID: 120-48-21-312

Temple

Texas A&M College of Medicine-Scott and White Program
Sponsor: Scott and White Memorial Hospital
Program Director:
Steven L Smith, MD
Texas A&M-Scott and White
Grad Med Educ
2401 S 31st St
Temple, TX 76508-0001
Tel: 254 771-8403 *Fax:* 254 771-8493
E-mail: fammedresi@bellnet.tamu.edu
Internet: http://www.sw.org
Accred Length: 3 Years *Program Size:* 24 (*GY1:* 8)
Program ID: 120-48-21-469

Texarkana

University of Arkansas for Medical Sciences AHEC (Southwest) Program
Sponsor: UAMS-Area Health Education Centers
Health Care Center
Wadley Regional Medical Center (Texarkana TX)
Program Director:
George M Finley, MD
Univ of Arkansas Med Sch-AHEC Southwest
300 E 6th St
Texarkana, AR 71854
Tel: 870 779-6042 *Fax:* 870 779-6093
E-mail: n_scales@ahecsw.uams.edu
Accred Length: 3 Years *Program Size:* 22 (*GY1:* 8)
Program ID: 120-04-21-527

Tyler

University of Texas Health Center at Tyler Program
Sponsor: University of Texas Health Center at Tyler
Mother Frances Hospital Regional Health Care Center
Program Director:
Richard M Viken, MD
Univ of Texas Health Ctr-Tyler
Family Practice Dept
11937 US Hwy 271 N
Tyler, TX 75708-3154
Tel: 903 877-7204 *Fax:* 903 877-7778
E-mail: kdennis@uthct.edu
Internet: http://www.uthct.edu
Accred Length: 3 Years *Program Size:* 22 (*GY1:* 7)
Program ID: 120-48-21-464

Waco

McLennan County Medical Education and Research Foundation Program
Sponsor: McLennan County Medical Education and Research Foundation
Hillcrest Baptist Medical Center
Providence Health Center
Program Director:
Roland A Goertz, MD
Family Practice Ctr
1600 Providence Dr
Waco, TX 76707
Tel: 254 750-8201 *Fax:* 254 750-8326
Accred Length: 3 Years *Program Size:* 36 (*GY1:* 12)
Program ID: 120-48-11-313

Wichita Falls

North Central Texas Medical Foundation Program
Sponsor: North Central Texas Medical Foundation
Bethania Regional Health Care Center
United Regional Health Care System
Program Director:
D Clifford Burross, MD
North Central Texas Med Foundation
1301 Third St/Ste 200
Wichita Falls, TX 76301-2213
Tel: 940 767-5145 *Fax:* 940 767-3027
E-mail: wfallsfp@wf.net
Internet: http://www.wf.net/~wfallsfp
Accred Length: 3 Years *Program Size:* 24 (*GY1:* 8)
Program ID: 120-48-21-435

Utah

Ogden

McKay-Dee Hospital Center Program
Sponsor: McKay-Dee Hospital Center
Program Director:
Richard C Arbogast, MD
McKay-Dee Family Practice Program
3955 Harrison Blvd
Ogden, UT 84403
Tel: 801 398-2749 *Fax:* 801 398-5970
E-mail: pomkres@ihc.com
Internet: http://www.ihc.com/mckay-dee/fpres
Accred Length: 3 Years *Program Size:* 18 (*GY1:* 6)
Program ID: 120-49-21-495

Provo

Utah Valley Regional Medical Center Program
Sponsor: Utah Valley Regional Medical Center
Program Director:
Michael J Beller, MD
Utah Valley Family Practice Residency
1134 N 500 West
Provo, UT 84605-0390
Tel: 801 371-7940 *Fax:* 801 371-7927
E-mail: uvdmcelr@ihc.com
Internet: http://www.ihc.com/uvrmc/fpres
Accred Length: 3 Years *Program Size:* 14 (*GY1:* 6)
Program ID: 120-49-21-583

Salt Lake City

St Mark's Health Care Foundation Program
Sponsor: St Mark's Health Care Foundation
St Mark's Hospital
Program Director:
John W Robinson, MD
6947 S 900 E
Midvale, UT 84047
Tel: 801 566-7204 *Fax:* 801 561-1324
E-mail: info@columbia-utah.com
Internet: http://www.columbia-utah.com/residency
Accred Length: 3 Years *Program Size:* 12 (*GY1:* 4)
Program ID: 120-49-21-529

University of Utah Program
Sponsor: University of Utah Medical Center
Salt Lake Regional Medical Center
Program Director:
Stephen D Ratcliffe, MD
Univ of Utah Sch of Med
Family/Prev Med
50 N Medical Dr/Rm 1C26
Salt Lake City, UT 84132
Tel: 801 581-7234 *Fax:* 801 581-2771
E-mail: fpresidency@dfpm.utah.edu
Internet: http://www.med.utah.edu/dfpm/fpresidency/
Accred Length: 3 Years *Program Size:* 36 (*GY1:* 12)
Program ID: 120-49-21-315

Vermont

Burlington

University of Vermont Program
Sponsor: Fletcher Allen Health Care
Program Director:
Thomas C Peterson, MD
Univ of Vermont Coll of Med
Milton Family Practice
28 Centre Dr
Milton, VT 05468
Tel: 802 893-0136 *Fax:* 802 893-2410
E-mail: gail.coletti@vtmednet.org
Internet: http://www.vtmednet.orgfamprac/uvmfp.htm
Accred Length: 3 Years *Program Size:* 18 (*GY1:* 6)
Program ID: 120-50-21-316

Virginia

Blackstone

Medical College of Virginia/Virginia Commonwealth University (Blackstone) Program
Sponsor: Medical College of Virginia/Virginia Commonwealth University
Blackstone Family Practice Center
Medical College of Virginia Hospitals
Program Director:
Benjamin H McIlwaine, MD
Blackstone Family Practice Ctr
920 S Main St
Blackstone, VA 23824
Tel: 804 292-7261 *Fax:* 804 298-0908
E-mail: bhmcilwa@hsc.vcu.edu
Internet: http://www.bfpc.org
Accred Length: 3 Years *Program Size:* 18 (*GY1:* 6)
Program ID: 120-51-11-321

Charlottesville

University of Virginia Program
Sponsor: University of Virginia Medical Center
Program Director:
Steven A Meixel, MD
Univ of Virginia Health Sciences Ctr
Dept of Family Med
PO Box 414
Charlottesville, VA 22908
Tel: 804 924-5348 *Fax:* 804 982-4306
E-mail: mw6r@virginia.edu
Internet:
http://www.med.virginia.edu/som-cl/familymed/home.html
Accred Length: 3 Years *Program Size:* 24 (*GY1:* 8)
Program ID: 120-51-11-317

Falls Church

Medical College of Virginia/Virginia Commonwealth University (Falls Church) Program
Sponsor: Medical College of Virginia/Virginia Commonwealth University
Fairfax Hospital
Program Director:
Samuel M Jones, MD
Fairfax Family Practice Ctr
3650 Joseph Siewick Dr/4th Fl
Fairfax, VA 22033
Tel: 703 391-2020, ext 174 *Fax:* 703 391-1211
E-mail: ffpcres@erols.com
Internet: http://views.vcu.edu/~fapweb/
Accred Length: 3 Years *Program Size:* 24 (*GY1:* 8)
Program ID: 120-51-11-322

Fort Belvoir

DeWitt Army Community Hospital Program
Sponsor: DeWitt Army Community Hospital
Program Director:
Thomas M Howard, MD
DeWitt Army Community Hospital
Family Health Ctr of Fort Belvoir
9501 Farrel Rd/Ste GC11
Fort Belvoir, VA 22060-5141
Tel: 703 805-0045 *Fax:* 703 805-0284
Accred Length: 3 Years *Program Size:* 18 (*GY1:* 6)
Program ID: 120-51-12-012
US Armed Services Program

Lynchburg

Centra Health Program
Sponsor: Centra Health Inc
Program Director:
Dean Gianakos, MD
Lynchburg Family Practice Residency
2097 Langhorne Rd
Lynchburg, VA 24501
Tel: 804 947-5210 *Fax:* 804 947-5213
E-mail: dean.gianakos@centrahealth.com
Internet: http://www.centrahealth.com
Accred Length: 3 Years *Program Size:* 12 (*GY1:* 4)
Program ID: 120-51-21-318

Newport News

Riverside Regional Medical Center Program
Sponsor: Riverside Regional Medical Center
Program Director:
Charles O Frazier, MD
Riverside Family Practice Ctr
316 Main St/3rd Fl
Newport News, VA 23601
Tel: 757 594-3878 *Fax:* 757 591-9021
E-mail: ruth@visi.net
Internet: http://views.vcu.edu/views/fap/rs
Accred Length: 3 Years *Program Size:* 36 (*GY1:* 12)
Program ID: 120-51-31-323

Norfolk

Eastern Virginia Medical School Program

Sponsor: Eastern Virginia Medical School
Sentara Norfolk General Hospital

Program Director:
Thooma Grant, MD
Ghent Family Practice Ctr
721 Fairfax Ave
Norfolk, VA 23507
Tel: 757 446-5983 *Fax:* 757 446-5196
Internet: http://www.evms.edu/fcm/gfp/
Accred Length: 3 Years *Program Size:* 18 (*GY1:* 6)
Program ID: 120-51-21-319

Portsmouth

Eastern Virginia Medical School Program

Sponsor: Eastern Virginia Medical School
Portsmouth General Hospital
Maryview Hospital

Program Director:
Anne Lockett, MD
Portsmouth Family Med
2700 London Blvd
Portsmouth, VA 23707-3647
Tel: 804 446-7400 *Fax:* 804 393-4869
E-mail: v-m@fammed.evms.edu
Internet: http://www.evms.edu/fcm/pfm/pfm.html
Accred Length: 3 Years *Program Size:* 18 (*GY1:* 6)
Program ID: 120-51-21-442

Richmond

Medical College of Virginia/Virginia Commonwealth University (Chesterfield) Program

Sponsor: Medical College of Virginia/Virginia Commonwealth University
Columbia-HCA Chippenham Medical Center
Columbia-HCA Johnston-Willis Hospital

Program Director:
W Jefferson McCarter, MD
Chesterfield Family Practice Ctr
2500 Pocoshock Pl
Richmond, VA 23235
Tel: 804 276-9305
E-mail: cfpcres@erols.com
Internet: http://www.chesterfieldfp.com
Accred Length: 3 Years *Program Size:* 24 (*GY1:* 8)
Program ID: 120-51-11-320

Medical College of Virginia/Virginia Commonwealth University Program

Sponsor: Medical College of Virginia/Virginia Commonwealth University
Medical College of Virginia Hospitals

Program Director:
Michael J Petrizzi, MD
Hanover Family Physicians
9376 Atlee Station Rd
Mechanicsville, VA 23116
Tel: 804 730-4810, ext 142 *Fax:* 804 730-3375
E-mail: hanoverfp@aol.com
Accred Length: 3 Years *Program Size:* 18 (*GY1:* 6)
Program ID: 120-51-21-485

Roanoke

Carilion Health System Program

Sponsor: Carilion Health System
Carilion Roanoke Community Hospital
Carilion Roanoke Memorial Hospital

Program Director:
J A Hagy, MD
Carilion Health System
Family Practice Residency Program
1314 Peters Creek Rd
Roanoke, VA 24017-2500
Tel: 540 562-5702 *Fax:* 540 562-4258
E-mail: psnidow@carilion.com
Internet: http://www.carilion.com/residency
Accred Length: 3 Years *Program Size:* 36 (*GY1:* 12)
Program ID: 120-51-11-325

Winchester

MCV/VCU-Valley Health System Program

Sponsor: Valley Health System

Program Director:
Andrew A White, MD
1840 Amherst St
Winchester, VA 22601
Tel: 540 545-4120 *Fax:* 540 545-4125
E-mail: tsimance@valleyhealthlink.com
Accred Length: 3 Years *Program Size:* 12 (*GY1:* 4)
Program ID: 120-51-21-627

Washington

Bremerton

Naval Hospital (Bremerton) Program

Sponsor: Naval Hospital (Bremerton)

Program Director:
Capt Jeffrey H Brodie, MD
Puget Sound Family Med Residency
HPO1 Boone Rd
Bremerton, WA 98312-1898
Tel: 360 475-4345 *Fax:* 360 475-4512
E-mail: 1mendiola@pnw.med.navy.mil
Internet: http://www.nh_bremerton.med.navy.mil/
Accred Length: 3 Years *Program Size:* 18 (*GY1:* 6)
Program ID: 120-54-21-494
US Armed Services Program

Olympia

St Peter Hospital Program

Sponsor: St Peter Hospital

Program Director:
Keith Frey, MD
Providence-St Peter Hospital
Family Practice Program
525 Lilly Rd NE/PBP09
Olympia, WA 98506-5166
Tel: 360 493-4020 *Fax:* 360 493-5524
E-mail: rossf@psph.providence.org
Internet: http://www.providence.org/swsa
Accred Length: 3 Years *Program Size:* 18 (*GY1:* 6)
Program ID: 120-54-21-497

Renton

Valley Medical Center Program

Sponsor: Valley Medical Center

Program Director:
Andrew B Oliveira, MD
Valley Med Ctr FPR
Valley Professional Ctr North
3915 Talbot Rd S/Ste 401
Renton, WA 98055
Tel: 425 656-4287 *Fax:* 425 656-5395
E-mail: jeanb@vmc.fammed.washington.edu
Internet:
http://www.valleymed.org/fampracticeframe.htm
Accred Length: 3 Years *Program Size:* 24 (*GY1:* 8)
Program ID: 120-54-21-470

Seattle

Group Health Cooperative of Puget Sound Program

Sponsor: Group Health Cooperative of Puget Sound
Virginia Mason Medical Center

Program Director:
Fred Heidrich, MD
Group Health Cooperative of Puget Sound
200 15th Ave E/CWB100
Seattle, WA 98112
Tel: 206 326-3585 *Fax:* 206 326-3543
Internet: http://www.ghcorg/fpr
Accred Length: 3 Years *Program Size:* 15 (*GY1:* 5)
Program ID: 120-54-21-327

Providence Seattle Medical Center Program

Sponsor: Providence Seattle Medical Center

Program Director:
Samuel W Cullison, MD
Medalia Family Med Ctr
550 16th Ave/Ste 100
Seattle, WA 98122
Tel: 206 320-2233 *Fax:* 206 320-8173
E-mail: lmcsherr@pmfmc.fammed.washington.edu
Internet:
http://www.fammed.washington.edu/network/providence
Accred Length: 3 Years *Program Size:* 30 (*GY1:* 10)
Program ID: 120-54-21-328

Swedish Medical Center-Seattle Program

Sponsor: Swedish Medical Center-Seattle

Program Director:
Joseph N Scardapane, MD
Swedish Med Ctr-Seattle
1401 Madison/#100
Seattle, WA 98104-1338
Tel: 206 386-6054 *Fax:* 206 386-6113
E-mail: sfmscard@u.washington.edu
Internet:
http://www.weber.u.washington.edu/~mtuggy/sfm/webpage1.htm
Accred Length: 3 Years *Program Size:* 30 (*GY1:* 10)
Program ID: 120-54-31-326

University of Washington Program

Sponsor: University of Washington School of Medicine
University of Washington Medical Center

Program Director:
David P Losh, MD
Univ of Washington Med Ctr
Dept of Family Practice
4245 Roosevelt Way NE/Box 354775
Seattle, WA 98105
Tel: 206 548-2883 *Fax:* 206 548-5769
E-mail: residency@fammed.washington.edu
Internet: http://www.fammed.washington.edu/residency/
Accred Length: 3 Years *Program Size:* 25 (*GY1:* 8)
Program ID: 120-54-31-329

Spokane

Inland Empire Hospital Services Association Program
Sponsor: Inland Empire Hospital Services Association
Deaconess Medical Center
Sacred Heart Medical Center
Program Director:
Gary R Newkirk, MD
Inland Empire Hospital Services Assoc
Family Med Spokane
104 W 5th/Ste 200W
Spokane, WA 99201-4839
Tel: 509 624-2313 *Fax:* 509 459-0686
E-mail: info@fms.fammed.washington.edu
Internet: http://www.inhs.org.spokanemed/famed.htm
Accred Length: 3 Years *Program Size:* 21 (*GY1:* 7)
Subspecialties: FP, TY
Program ID: 120-54-21-330

Inland Empire Hospital Services Association Rural Program
Sponsor: Inland Empire Hospital Services Association
Klickitat Valley Hospital
Mid-Valley Hospital
Mount Carmel Hospital
Program Director:
Gary R Newkirk, MD
Inland Empire Hospital Services Assoc Rural Program
104 W 5th/Ste 200W
Spokane, WA 99201-4839
Tel: 509 624-2313 *Fax:* 509 459-0686
E-mail: info@fms.fammed.washington.edu
Internet: http://www.inhs.org/spokanemed/famed.html
Accred Length: 3 Years *Program Size:* 5 (*GY1:* 2)
Program ID: 120-54-21-552

Tacoma

Madigan Army Medical Center Program
Sponsor: Madigan Army Medical Center
Program Director:
Guy P Runkle, MD MA
Madigan Army Med Ctr
Attn: MCHJ-FP (Lt Col Runkle)
Tacoma, WA 98431
Tel: 253 968-1340 *Fax:* 253 968-2608
Internet: http://192.138.33.222/famprac/mamcfp.htm
Accred Length: 3 Years *Program Size:* 18 (*GY1:* 6)
Program ID: 120-54-21-013
US Armed Services Program

Multicare Medical Center Program
Sponsor: MultiCare Medical Center
Mary Bridge Children's Hospital and Health Center
Tacoma General Hospital
Program Director:
Judith A Pauwels, MD
Tacoma Family Med
521 Martin Luther King Jr Way
Tacoma, WA 98405-4272
Tel: 253 552-2945 *Fax:* 253 552-2938
E-mail: lquanrud@multicare.com
Internet:
http://www.fammed.washington.edu/network/htm
Accred Length: 3 Years *Program Size:* 28 (*GY1:* 8)
Program ID: 120-54-31-331

Vancouver

Southwest Washington Medical Center Program
Sponsor: Southwest Washington Medical Center
Program Director:
David R Ruiz, MD
Family Med of Southwest Washington
PO Box 1600
Vancouver, WA 98668-1600
Tel: 360 260-7560 *Fax:* 360 260-7587
E-mail: nmoyer@swmedctr.com
Internet: http://resnet.fammed.washington.edu/~fmsw
Accred Length: 3 Years *Program Size:* 19 (*GY1:* 6)
Program ID: 120-54-21-546

Yakima

Yakima Valley Memorial Hospital/Providence Yakima Medical Center Program
Sponsor: Yakima Valley Memorial Hospital
Providence Yakima Medical Center
Program Director:
Michael W Maples, MD
Central Washington Family Med
1806 W Lincoln Ave
Yakima, WA 98902
Tel: 509 452-4946 *Fax:* 509 457-3989
E-mail: info@cwfm.fammed.washington.edu
Internet: http://www.cwfm.org
Accred Length: 3 Years *Program Size:* 18 (*GY1:* 6)
Program ID: 120-54-21-522

West Virginia

Charleston

West Virginia University (Charleston Division) Program
Sponsor: Charleston Area Medical Center
Thomas Memorial Hospital
Program Director:
Jeffrey V Ashley, MD
Dept of Family Med
1201 Washington St E/#108
Charleston, WV 25301
Tel: 304 347-4620 *Fax:* 304 347-4621
E-mail: family.medicine@camcare.com
Internet: http://www.camcare.com
Accred Length: 3 Years *Program Size:* 24 (*GY1:* 8)
Program ID: 120-55-11-337

Clarksburg

United Hospital Center Program
Sponsor: United Hospital Center
Program Director:
Eric Radcliffe, MD
United Hospital Ctr
One Hospital Plaza
PO Box 2308
Clarksburg, WV 26302-2308
Tel: 304 624-2224 *Fax:* 304 624-2787
Accred Length: 3 Years *Program Size:* 24 (*GY1:* 8)
Program ID: 120-55-22-334

Huntington

Marshall University School of Medicine Program
Sponsor: Marshall University School of Medicine
Cabell Huntington Hospital
Program Director:
Stephen M Petrany, MD
Marshall Univ Sch of Med
Dept of Family Med
1600 Medical Center Dr/Ste 1500
Huntington, WV 25701-3655
Tel: 304 691-1165 *Fax:* 304 691-1153
E-mail: badkins@marshall.edu
Internet: http://meb.marshall.edu/fch
Accred Length: 3 Years *Program Size:* 24 (*GY1:* 8)
Program ID: 120-55-21-335

Morgantown

West Virginia University Program
Sponsor: West Virginia University Hospitals
Program Director:
James G Arbogast, MD
West Virginia Univ
Robert C Byrd Health Sciences Ctr
PO Box 9152
Morgantown, WV 26506-9152
Tel: 304 293-1728 *Fax:* 304 293-8788
E-mail: wvfmdoc@wvnvm.wvnet.edu
Internet: http://wvnvm.wvnet.edu/~wvfmdoc
Accred Length: 3 Years *Program Size:* 18 (*GY1:* 6)
Program ID: 120-55-11-336

West Virginia University Rural Program
Sponsor: West Virginia University Hospitals
City Hospital
Program Director:
Konrad C Nau, MD
Harpers Ferry Family Med Ctr
PO Box 550
1399 Washington St
Harpers Ferry, WV 25425
Tel: 304 535-6362 *Fax:* 304 535-6618
E-mail: pope.joanna@consult.hsc.wvu.edu
Internet: http://wvnvm.wvnet.edu/~wvfmdoc/rural.htm
Accred Length: 3 Years *Program Size:* 12 (*GY1:* 4)
Program ID: 120-55-21-569

Wheeling

Wheeling Hospital Program
Sponsor: Wheeling Hospital
Program Director:
Terry L Elliott, MD
Family Health Ctr
40 Medical Park/Ste 401
Wheeling, WV 26003-8110
Tel: 304 243-3880 *Fax:* 304 243-3895
E-mail: fmlyhlth@wheelinghosp.com
Accred Length: 3 Years *Program Size:* 18 (*GY1:* 6)
Program ID: 120-55-22-338

Wisconsin

Antigo

University of Wisconsin Rural Program

Sponsor: University of Wisconsin Medical School
Langlade Memorial Hospital
Wausau Hospital
Program Director:
Hilary Scully, MD
995 Campus Dr
Wausau, WI 54401
Tel: 715 675-3391 *Fax:* 715 675-4253
E-mail: hscully@wausau.fammed.wisc.edu
Internet: http://www.fammed.wisc.edu
Accred Length: 3 Years *Program Size:* 2 (*GY1:* 1)
Program ID: 120-56-21-635

Appleton

University of Wisconsin (Appleton) Program

Sponsor: University of Wisconsin Medical School
Appleton Medical Center
St Elizabeth Hospital
Program Director:
Lee M Vogel, MD
Fox Valley Family Practice Residency
229 S Morrison St
Appleton, WI 54911-5760
Tel: 414 738-8413 *Fax:* 414 832-2635
Internet: http://www.fammed.wisc.edu
Accred Length: 3 Years *Program Size:* 18 (*GY1:* 6)
Program ID: 120-56-31-368

Baraboo

University of Wisconsin (Baraboo) Rural Program

Sponsor: University of Wisconsin Medical School
St Clare Hospital and Health Services
St Marys Hospital Medical Center
Program Director:
James R Damos, MD
777 S Mills St
Madison, WI 53715-1896
Tel: 608 845-9531 *Fax:* 608 845-8684
E-mail: jdamos@verona.fammed.wisc.edu
Internet: http://www.fammed.wisc.edu
Accred Length: 3 Years *Program Size:* 2 (*GY1:* 0)
Program ID: 120-56-21-609

Eau Claire

University of Wisconsin (Eau Claire) Program

Sponsor: University of Wisconsin Medical School
Luther Hospital
Sacred Heart Hospital
Program Director:
Richard R McClaflin, MD
Eau Claire Family Med Program
807 S Farwell St
Eau Claire, WI 54701
Tel: 715 839-5177 *Fax:* 715 839-4733
E-mail: rsuechti@eauclair.fammed.wisc.edu
Internet: http://www.fammed.wisc.edu
Accred Length: 3 Years *Program Size:* 21 (*GY1:* 7)
Program ID: 120-56-31-342

Janesville

Mercy Health System Program

Sponsor: Mercy Health System
Program Director:
Giovino M James, MD
Mercy Health System Family Practice Program
849 Kellogg Ave
Janesville, WI 53546-9978
Tel: 800 236-6877 *Fax:* 608 755-7873
E-mail: respro@mhsjvinet.org
Internet:
http://www.mercyhealthsystem.org/resident.htm
Accred Length: 3 Years *Program Size:* 18 (*GY1:* 6)
Program ID: 120-56-21-503

La Crosse

Franciscan Skemp Healthcare Program

Sponsor: Franciscan Skemp Healthcare-La Crosse Campus
Program Director:
Thomas J Grau, MD
La Crosse-Mayo Family Practice Residency
815 S 10th St
La Crosse, WI 54601
Tel: 608 785-0940, ext 2890 *Fax:* 608 791-9408
E-mail: grau.thomas@mayo.edu
Accred Length: 3 Years *Program Size:* 18 (*GY1:* 6)
Program ID: 120-56-11-339

Franciscan Skemp Healthcare Rural Program

Sponsor: Franciscan Skemp Healthcare-La Crosse Campus
Lutheran Hospital-La Crosse
Mile Bluff Medical Center (Mauston)
Program Director:
Thomas J Grau, MD
Franciscan Skemp Healthcare
815 S 10th St
La Crosse, WI 54601
Tel: 608 785-0940, ext 2890 *Fax:* 608 791-9408
E-mail: grau.thomas@mayo.edu
Accred Length: 3 Years *Program Size:* 6 (*GY1:* 3)
Program ID: 120-56-21-628

Madison

University of Wisconsin Program

Sponsor: University of Wisconsin Medical School
St Marys Hospital Medical Center
University of Wisconsin Hospital and Clinics
Program Director:
Louis A Sanner, MD
Dept of Family Med
777 S Mills St
Madison, WI 53715-1896
Tel: 608 265-4668 *Fax:* 608 263-5813
E-mail: flease@fammed.wisc.edu
Internet: http://www.fammed.wisc.edu
Accred Length: 3 Years *Program Size:* 42 (*GY1:* 14)
Program ID: 120-56-11-343

Menomonie

University of Wisconsin (Menomonie) Rural Program

Sponsor: University of Wisconsin Medical School
Myrtle Werth Medical Center
Luther Hospital
Sacred Heart Hospital
Program Director:
Richard R McClaflin, MD
David Eitrheim, MD
Eau Claire Family Medicine Clinic
807 S Farwell St
Eau Claire, WI 54701
Tel: 715 839-5177 *Fax:* 715 839-4733
Internet: http://www.fammed.wisc.edu
Accred Length: 3 Years *Program Size:* 1 (*GY1:* 1)
Program ID: 120-56-21-615

Milwaukee

Aurora Health Care Program

Sponsor: Aurora Health Care
St Luke's Medical Center
Program Director:
Dennis J Baumgardner, MD
Health Science Bldg E/Ste 175
St Luke's Family Practice Ctr
2801 W Kinnickinnic River Pkwy
Milwaukee, WI 53215-3660
Tel: 414 649-7909 *Fax:* 414 649-3361
E-mail: fpslmc@execpc.com
Internet: http://www.aurorahealthcare.com
Accred Length: 3 Years *Program Size:* 30 (*GY1:* 10)
Program ID: 120-56-21-348

Medical College of Wisconsin (Columbia) Program

Sponsor: Medical College of Wisconsin Affiliated Hospitals Inc
Columbia Hospital
Program Director:
Russell G Robertson, MD
Columbia Family Care Ctr
210 W Capitol Dr
Milwaukee, WI 53212
Tel: 414 961-1810 *Fax:* 414 967-2124
Accred Length: 3 Years *Program Size:* 28 (*GY1:* 8)
Program ID: 120-56-21-496

Medical College of Wisconsin (Froedtert Memorial) Program

Sponsor: Medical College of Wisconsin Affiliated Hospitals Inc
Froedtert Memorial Lutheran Hospital
Program Director:
B Clair Eliason, MD
Dept of Family/Community Med
1000 N 92nd St
Milwaukee, WI 53226
Tel: 414 456-4728 *Fax:* 414 456-6522
E-mail: beliason@mcw.edu
Accred Length: 3 Years *Program Size:* 0
Program ID: 120-56-31-639

Medical College of Wisconsin (St Mary's) Program

Sponsor: Medical College of Wisconsin Affiliated Hospitals Inc
St Mary's Hospital of Milwaukee
Program Director:
Loren A Leshan, MD
St Mary's Hospital Family Practice Ctr
2320 N Lake Dr
Milwaukee, WI 53211
Tel: 414 291-1602 *Fax:* 414 291-1613
E-mail: chrish@post.its.mcw.edu
Accred Length: 3 Years *Program Size:* 24 (*GY1:* 8)
Subspecialties: FSM
Program ID: 120-56-21-344

Medical College of Wisconsin (St Michael) Program

Sponsor: Medical College of Wisconsin Affiliated Hospitals Inc
St Michael Hospital

Program Director:
David S Smith, MD
St Michael Hospital
2400 W Villard Ave
Milwaukee, WI 53209
Tel: 414 527-8348 *Fax:* 414 527-8046
E-mail: stmikefp@mcw.edu
Internet: http://www.family.mcw.edu
Accred Length: 3 Years *Program Size:* 24 (*GY1:* 8)
Program ID: 120-56-31-349

Racine

Medical College of Wisconsin (Racine) Program

Sponsor: Medical College of Wisconsin Affiliated Hospitals Inc
St Mary's Medical Center
All Saints Healthcare System, Inc.

Program Director:
Len Scarpinato, DO
Racine Family Practice Program
PO Box 548
Racine, WI 53401-0548
Tel: 414 638-5656 *Fax:* 414 638-5657
Accred Length: 3 Years *Program Size:* 18 (*GY1:* 6)
Program ID: 120-56-21-438

Waukesha

Medical College of Wisconsin (Waukesha) Program

Sponsor: Medical College of Wisconsin Affiliated Hospitals Inc
Waukesha Memorial Hospital

Program Director:
Richard B Lewan, MD
Waukesha Family Practice Program
210 NW Barstow St/Ste 201
Waukesha, WI 53188
Tel: 414 548-6907 *Fax:* 414 548-3820
E-mail: wfprp@phci.org
Internet: http://execpc.com/~chriswd
Accred Length: 3 Years *Program Size:* 18 (*GY1:* 6)
Program ID: 120-56-21-345

Wausau

University of Wisconsin (Wausau) Program

Sponsor: University of Wisconsin Medical School
Wausau Hospital

Program Director:
Kevin J O'Connell, MD
Wausau Family Practice Ctr
995 Campus Dr
Wausau, WI 54401-1898
Tel: 715 675-3391 *Fax:* 715 675-4253
E-mail: koconnel@wausau.fammed.wisc.edu
Internet: http://www.fammed.wisc.edu
Accred Length: 3 Years *Program Size:* 19 (*GY1:* 7)
Program ID: 120-56-21-350

Wyoming

Casper

University of Wyoming (Casper) Program

Sponsor: University of Wyoming College of Health Sciences
Wyoming Medical Center

Program Director:
Joe K Schoeber, MD
Univ of Wyoming
Dept of Family Practice
1522 East A St
Casper, WY 82601
Tel: 307 266-3076 *Fax:* 307 235-6202
E-mail: uwfpcas@uwyo.edu
Internet: http://www.uwyo.edu/hs/casfamprac/
Accred Length: 3 Years *Program Size:* 24 (*GY1:* 8)
Program ID: 120-57-12-351

Cheyenne

University of Wyoming (Cheyenne) Program

Sponsor: University of Wyoming College of Health Sciences
United Medical Center
Veterans Affairs Center

Program Director:
Scott T Henderson, MD MA
Univ of Wyoming
Family Practice Program-Cheyenne
821 E 18th St
Cheyenne, WY 82001-4775
Tel: 307 777-7911 *Fax:* 307 638-3616
E-mail: uwcheyfp@uwyo.edu
Internet: http://www.uwyo.edu/chyfamprac/cheyfpr.htm
Accred Length: 3 Years *Program Size:* 18 (*GY1:* 6)
Program ID: 120-57-12-369

Foot and Ankle Orthopaedics (Orthopaedic Surgery)

New York

New York

Hospital for Joint Diseases Orthopaedic Institute Program

Sponsor: Hospital for Joint Diseases Orthopaedic Institute

Program Director:
Donna J Astion, MD
Hospital for Joint Diseases
301 E 17th St
New York, NY 10003
Tel: 212 598-6497 *Fax:* 212 598-6581
Internet: http://www.hjd.edu
Accred Length: 1 Year *Program Size:* 1
Program ID: 262-35-21-001

Forensic Pathology (Pathology)

Alabama

Birmingham

University of Alabama Medical Center Program

Sponsor: University of Alabama Hospital
Jefferson County Coroner/Medical Examiner's Office

Program Director:
Robert M Brissie, MD
Jefferson County Coroner-Med Examiner Office
1515 6th Ave S
Birmingham, AL 35233
Tel: 205 930-3603 *Fax:* 205 930-3595
E-mail: brissie@path.uab.edu
Internet: http://www.path.uab.edu
Accred Length: 1 Year *Program Size:* 1
Program ID: 310-01-21-049

Arkansas

Little Rock

University of Arkansas for Medical Sciences Program

Sponsor: University of Arkansas College of Medicine
Arkansas State Crime Laboratory

Program Director:
William Q Sturner, MD
Arkansas State Crime Lab-Med Examiners Office
3 Natural Resources Dr
PO Box 8500
Little Rock, AR 72215
Tel: 501 227-5936 *Fax:* 501 221-1653
Accred Length: 1 Year *Program Size:* 1
Program ID: 310-04-21-070

California

Los Angeles

County of Los Angeles-Department of Coroner Program

Sponsor: County of Los Angeles-Department of Coroner

Program Director:
Lakshmanan Sathyavagiswaran, MD
Christopher Rogers, MD
Dept of Coroner
1104 N Mission Rd
Los Angeles, CA 90033
Tel: 323 343-0522 *Fax:* 323 225-2235
Accred Length: 1 Year *Program Size:* 6
Program ID: 310-05-12-002

Sacramento

Northern California Forensic Pathology Program

Sponsor: North California Forensic Pathology
University of California (Davis) Medical Center

Program Director:
Gregory D Reiber, MD
Northern California Forensic Pathology
2443 Fair Oaks Blvd/Ste 311
Sacramento, CA 95825
Tel: 916 482-6237 *Fax:* 916 737-6506
E-mail: vicdoe@inreach.com
Accred Length: 1 Year *Program Size:* 1
Program ID: 310-05-21-065

San Bernardino

San Bernardino County Coroner's Office Program

Sponsor: San Bernardino County Coroner's Office

Program Director:
Frank P Sheridan, MD
San Bernardino County Coroner's Office
175 S Lena Rd
San Bernardino, CA 92415-0037
Tel: 909 387-2561 *Fax:* 909 387-2989
Accred Length: 1 Year *Program Size:* 1
Program ID: 310-05-21-062

San Diego

San Diego County Medical Examiner Program

Sponsor: San Diego County Medical Examiner

Program Director:
Brian D Blackbourne, MD
San Diego Med Examiner Office
5555 Overland Ave/Bldg 14
San Diego, CA 92123
Tel: 619 694-2895 *Fax:* 619 495-5956
E-mail: bblackmx@co.san-diego.ca.us
Accred Length: 1 Year *Program Size:* 1
Program ID: 310-05-21-059

District of Columbia

Washington

Armed Forces Institute of Pathology Program

Sponsor: Armed Forces Institute of Pathology

Program Director:
Jerry D Spencer, MD JD
AFIP-OAFME
1413 Research Blvd/Bldg 102
Rockville, MD 20850-6000
Tel: 301 319-0000 *Fax:* 301 319-0635
E-mail: afipcme@afip.osd.mil
Internet: http://www.afip.mil
Accred Length: 1 Year *Program Size:* 4
Program ID: 310-10-32-001
US Armed Services Program

Florida

Fort Lauderdale

Broward County Medical Examiner's Office Program

Sponsor: Broward County Medical Examiner's Office

Program Director:
Joshua A Perper, MD MS
Office of District Med Examiner
5301 SW 31st Ave
Fort Lauderdale, FL 33312-6199
Tel: 954 964-0218 *Fax:* 954 964-0212
E-mail: jperper@co.broward.fl.usa
Accred Length: 1 Year *Program Size:* 1
Program ID: 310-11-21-056

Miami

University of Miami-Dade County Medical Examiner's Office Program

Sponsor: Metropolitan Dade County Office of Medical Examiner

Program Director:
Roger E Mittleman, MD
Univ of Miami-Miami-Dade County Med Examiner
Number One on Bob Hope Rd
Miami, FL 33136-1133
Tel: 305 545-2425 *Fax:* 305 545-2412
Accred Length: 1 Year *Program Size:* 4
Program ID: 310-11-21-055

Orlando

Florida Medical Examiner's Office, District Nine Program

Sponsor: Office of the Medical Examiner, District Nine

Program Director:
William R Anderson, MD
Office of Med Examiner District 9
1401 Lucerne Terr
Orlando, FL 32806
Tel: 407 836-9400 *Fax:* 407 836-9450
Accred Length: 1 Year *Program Size:* 1
Program ID: 310-11-21-064

Tampa

University of South Florida Program

Sponsor: University of South Florida College of Medicine
Hillsborough County Medical Examiner Department

Program Director:
Vernard I Adams, MD
401 S Morgan St
Tampa, FL 33602-5441
Tel: 813 272-5342 *Fax:* 813 272-6268
Accred Length: 1 Year *Program Size:* 1
Program ID: 310-11-31-066

Georgia

Atlanta

Emory University Program

Sponsor: Emory University School of Medicine
Fulton County Medical Examiner's Office
Grady Memorial Hospital

Program Director:
Randy L Hanzlick, MD
Fulton County Med Examiner's Office
50 Coca-Cola Place SE
Atlanta, GA 30303
Tel: 404 730-4400 *Fax:* 404 730-4405
E-mail: rxh5@cdc.gov
Accred Length: 1 Year *Program Size:* 2
Program ID: 310-12-21-052

Illinois

Chicago

Office of the Medical Examiner of Cook County Program

Sponsor: Office of the Medical Examiner of Cook County

Program Director:
Edmund R Donoghue, MD
Office of the Medical Examiner of Cook County
2121 W Harrison St
Chicago, IL 60612-3705
Tel: 312 997-4500 *Fax:* 312 997-4516
Accred Length: 1 Year *Program Size:* 2
Program ID: 310-16-21-035

Indiana

Indianapolis

Indiana University School of Medicine Program

Sponsor: Indiana University School of Medicine

Program Director:
John E Pless, MD
Indiana Univ Sch of Med
635 Barnhill Dr/Rm 128
Indianapolis, IN 46202-5120
Tel: 317 274-2973 *Fax:* 317 278-0221
E-mail: jpless@iupui.edu
Internet: http://www.pathology.iupui.edu/pless.html
Accred Length: 1 Year *Program Size:* 1
Program ID: 310-17-21-076

Kentucky

Louisville

University of Louisville Program

Sponsor: University of Louisville School of Medicine
Office of Chief Medical Examiner
University of Louisville Hospital

Program Director:
Tracey C Handy, MD
Office of Med Examiner
Urban County Government Ctr
810 Barret Ave
Louisville, KY 40204
Tel: 502 852-5587 *Fax:* 502 852-1767
E-mail: litlwichtc@aol.com
Accred Length: 1 Year *Program Size:* 1
Program ID: 310-20-21-048

Louisiana

New Orleans

Louisiana State University Program

Sponsor: Louisiana State University School of Medicine
Parish of Orleans Coroner's Office

Program Director:
Alvaro T Hunt, MD
LSU Med Ctr
1901 Perdido St
New Orleans, LA 70112
Tel: 504 568-6055
Accred Length: 1 Year *Program Size:* 1
Program ID: 310-21-21-079

Maryland

Baltimore

Office of the Chief Medical Examiner/State of Maryland Program

Sponsor: Office of the Chief Medical Examiner

Program Director:
John E Smialek, MD
Office of Chief Med Examiner
111 Penn St
Baltimore, MD 21201
Tel: 410 333-3225 *Fax:* 410 333-3063
Accred Length: 1 Year *Program Size:* 3
Program ID: 310-23-11-012

Massachusetts

Boston

Boston University Medical Center Program

Sponsor: Boston Medical Center
Office of the Chief Medical Examiner

Program Director:
Stanton C Kessler, MD
Boston Med Ctr-Office Chief Med Examiner
720 Albany St
Boston, MA 02118
Tel: 617 267-6767, ext 245 *Fax:* 617 266-6763
Internet: http://www1.shore.net/~ocmema/index.html
Accred Length: 1 Year *Program Size:* 3
Program ID: 310-24-21-061

Michigan

Detroit

Wayne County Medical Examiner's Office Program

Sponsor: Wayne County Medical Examiner's Office

Program Director:
Sawait Kanluen, MD
1300 E Warren Ave
Detroit, MI 48207-1051
Tel: 313 833-2504 *Fax:* 313 833-2534
Accred Length: 1 Year *Program Size:* 2
Program ID: 310-25-11-013

Minnesota

Minneapolis

Hennepin County Medical Examiner Program

Sponsor: Hennepin County Medical Examiner

Program Director:
Garry F Peterson, MD JD
730 S 7th St
Minneapolis, MN 55415-1798
Tel: 612 347-2125 *Fax:* 612 904-4323
E-mail: garry.peterson@co.hennepin.mn.us
Accred Length: 1 Year *Program Size:* 1
Program ID: 310-26-12-014

Missouri

St Louis

St Louis University School of Medicine Program

Sponsor: St Louis University School of Medicine
St Louis County Medical Examiner's Office

Program Director:
Michael Graham, MD
St Louis Univ Sch of Med
Forensic Pathology
3556 Caroline St/Rm C305
St Louis, MO 63104
Tel: 314 577-8298 *Fax:* 314 268-5124
E-mail: grahamma@slu.edu
Accred Length: 1 Year *Program Size:* 1
Program ID: 310-28-21-075

New Mexico

Albuquerque

University of New Mexico Program

Sponsor: University of New Mexico School of Medicine
Office of the Medical Investigator

Program Director:
Ross E Zumwalt, MD
Office of the Medical Investigator
Univ of New Mexico
Health Sciences Ctr
Albuquerque, NM 87131-5091
Tel: 505 272-3053 *Fax:* 505 272-0727
E-mail: rzumwalt@quincy.unm.edu
Internet: http://www.unm.edu/~snunez/index.html
Accred Length: 1 Year *Program Size:* 3
Program ID: 310-34-21-015

New York

East Meadow

Nassau County Medical Examiner's Office Program

Sponsor: Nassau County Medical Examiner's Office

Program Director:
Leslie Lukash, MD
Nassau County Med Examiner
PO Box 160
East Meadow, NY 11554-0160
Tel: 516 572-5150 *Fax:* 516 572-5099
Accred Length: 1 Year *Program Size:* 1
Program ID: 310-35-31-016

New York

Office of the Chief Medical Examiner-City of New York Program

Sponsor: Office of Chief Medical Examiner-City of New York

Program Director:
Charles S Hirsch, MD
Mark Flomenbaum, MD PhD
Office of Chief Med Examiner
520 First Ave
New York, NY 10016
Tel: 212 447-2034 *Fax:* 212 447-2744
Accred Length: 1 Year *Program Size:* 5
Program ID: 310-35-21-063

Rochester

Monroe County Medical Examiners Office Program
Sponsor: Monroe County Medical Examiners Office
Program Director:
Nicholas T Forbes, MD
Monroe County Med Examiners Office
740 E Henrietta Rd
Rochester, NY 14623
Tel: 716 274-7970 *Fax:* 716 274-7979
Accred Length: 1 Year *Program Size:* 1
Program ID: 310-35-31-069

North Carolina

Chapel Hill

University of North Carolina Hospitals Program
Sponsor: University of North Carolina Hospitals
Office of the Chief Medical Examiner
Program Director:
Karen E Chancellor, MD
Office of Chief Med Examiner
CB7850
Chapel Hill, NC 27599-7580
Tel: 919 966-2253 *Fax:* 919 962-6263
E-mail: kchance@ocme.unc.edu
Internet: http://www.ocme.unc.edu
Accred Length: 1 Year *Program Size:* 2
Program ID: 310-36-21-019

Ohio

Cincinnati

Hamilton County Coroner's Office Program
Sponsor: Hamilton County Coroner's Office
Program Director:
Robert R Pfalzgraf, MD
Hamilton County Coroner's Office
3159 Eden Ave
Cincinnati, OH 45219
Tel: 513 221-4524 *Fax:* 513 221-0307
Accred Length: 1 Year *Program Size:* 1
Program ID: 310-38-21-073

Cleveland

Cuyahoga County Coroner's Office Program
Sponsor: Cuyahoga County Coroner's Office
Program Director:
Elizabeth K Balraj, MD
Cuyahoga County Coroner's Office
2121 Adelbert Rd
Cleveland, OH 44106
Tel: 216 721-5610 *Fax:* 216 721-2559
E-mail: ekb@po.cwru.edu
Accred Length: 1 Year *Program Size:* 3
Program ID: 310-38-11-021

Dayton

Office of the Montgomery County Coroner Program
Sponsor: Office of the Montgomery County Coroner
Program Director:
Jeffrey S Nine, MD
Montgomery County Coroner's Office
361 W Third St
Dayton, OH 45402
Tel: 937 225-4156, ext 2133 *Fax:* 937 496-7916
E-mail: jnine@ccl.co.montgomery.oh.us
Internet: http://www.siscom.net/~mcco
Accred Length: 1 Year *Program Size:* 1
Program ID: 310-38-21-067

Oklahoma

Oklahoma City

Office of the Chief Medical Examiner Program
Sponsor: Office of the Chief Medical Examiner-State of Oklahoma
Program Director:
Fred B Jordan, MD
Office of Chief Medical Examiner
901 N Stonewall
Oklahoma City, OK 73117
Tel: 405 239-7141 *Fax:* 405 239-2430
Accred Length: 1 Year *Program Size:* 1
Program ID: 310-39-11-022

Pennsylvania

Philadelphia

MCP Hahnemann University Program
Sponsor: MCP Hahnemann University
Hahnemann University Hospital
Medical College of Pennsylvania Hospital
Office of the Medical Examiner
Program Director:
Haresh Mirchandani, MD
Ian C Hood, MB ChB
Office of Med Examiner
321 University Ave
Philadelphia, PA 19104
Tel: 215 685-7470 *Fax:* 215 685-9075
Accred Length: 1 Year *Program Size:* 3
Program ID: 310-41-12-023

Pittsburgh

Allegheny County Coroner's Office Program
Sponsor: Allegheny County Coroner's Office
Program Director:
Abdulrezzak Shakir, MD
Allegheny County Coroner's Office
542 Fourth Ave
Pittsburgh, PA 15219-2186
Tel: 412 350-4800 *Fax:* 412 350-4899
Accred Length: 1 Year *Program Size:* 1
Program ID: 310-41-21-024

Puerto Rico

San Juan

Institute of Forensic Sciences of Puerto Rico Program
Sponsor: Institute of Forensic Sciences of Puerto Rico
Program Director:
Maria S Conte Miller, MD
Inst of Forensic Sciences
Call Box 11878
Caparra Heights Station
San Juan, PR 00922-1878
Tel: 787 765-0615, ext 325 *Fax:* 787 759-7315
E-mail: lyalvarez@prtc.net
Accred Length: 1 Year *Program Size:* 1
Program ID: 310-42-21-072

South Carolina

Charleston

Medical University of South Carolina Program
Sponsor: Medical University of South Carolina College of Medicine
MUSC Medical Center
Program Director:
Kimberly A Collins, MD
Dept of Pathology/Lab Med
Med Univ of South Carolina
165 Ashley Ave/Ste 309
Charleston, SC 29425
Tel: 803 792-3500 *Fax:* 803 792-3537
Accred Length: 1 Year *Program Size:* 1
Program ID: 310-45-21-026

Tennessee

Memphis

University of Tennessee Program
Sponsor: University of Tennessee College of Medicine
Program Director:
Jerry T Francisco, MD
Univ of Tennessee
Dept of Pathology
1060 Madison
Memphis, TN 38103-8163
Tel: 901 448-6320 *Fax:* 901 544-7211
E-mail: jfranisco@utmem1.utmem.edu
Accred Length: 1 Year *Program Size:* 1
Program ID: 310-47-21-027

Texas

Dallas

Southwestern Institute of Forensic Sciences Program
Sponsor: Southwestern Institute of Forensic Sciences
Program Director:
Jeffrey J Barnard, MD
Southwestern Inst of Forensic Sciences
PO Box 35728
5230 Medical Center Dr
Dallas, TX 75235-0728
Tel: 214 920-5900 *Fax:* 214 920-5908
Accred Length: 1 Year *Program Size:* 2
Program ID: 310-48-11-028

Houston

Harris County Medical Examiner Department Program
Sponsor: Harris County Medical Examiner Department
Program Director:
Joye M Carter, MD
1885 Old Spanish Trail
Houston, TX 77054-2098
Tel: 713 796-6789 *Fax:* 713 796-6828
E-mail: joye_carter@meo.co.harris.tx.us
Accred Length: 1 Year *Program Size:* 2
Program ID: 310-48-21-080

San Antonio

Bexar County Forensic Science Center Program
Sponsor: Bexar County Forensic Science Center
Program Director:
Vincent J M Di Maio, MD
Bexar County Med Examiner's Office
7337 Louis Pasteur
San Antonio, TX 78229
Tel: 210 335-4053 *Fax:* 210 335-4052
E-mail: dimaio@co.bexar.tx.us
Accred Length: 1 Year *Program Size:* 1
Program ID: 310-48-21-044

Utah

Salt Lake City

State of Utah Office of the Medical Examiner Program
Sponsor: State of Utah Department of Health
St Louis University School of Medicine
Program Director:
Todd C Grey, MD
State of Utah Office of Med Examiner
48 N Medical Dr
Salt Lake City, UT 84113
Tel: 801 584-8410 *Fax:* 801 584-8435
E-mail: hldels.tgrey@state.ut.us
Accred Length: 1 Year *Program Size:* 0
Program ID: 310-49-21-074

Virginia

Richmond

Medical College of Virginia/Virginia Commonwealth University Program
Sponsor: Medical College of Virginia/Virginia Commonwealth University
Medical College of Virginia Hospitals
Program Director:
Marcella F Fierro, MD
Dept of Legal Med
400 E Jackson St
Richmond, VA 23219-3694
Tel: 804 786-1033 *Fax:* 804 371-8595
E-mail: mfierro@vdhstate.va.us
Internet: http://vdhsrv15/medexam
Accred Length: 1 Year *Program Size:* 2
Program ID: 310-51-21-030

Washington

Seattle

King County Medical Examiner's Office Program
Sponsor: King County Medical Examiner's Office
Program Director:
Richard C Harruff, Md PhD
HMC/Box 359792
325 Ninth Ave
Seattle, WA 98104-2499
Tel: 206 731-3232 *Fax:* 206 731-8555
Internet: http://www.metrokc.gov/health/med_ex/
Accred Length: 1 Year *Program Size:* 2
Program ID: 310-54-21-031

Wisconsin

Milwaukee

Milwaukee County Medical Examiner's Office Program
Sponsor: Milwaukee County Medical Examiner's Office
Program Director:
John R Teggatz, MD
Milwaukee County Med Examiner's Office
933 W Highland Ave
Milwaukee, WI 53233
Tel: 414 223-1200, ext 1217 *Fax:* 414 223-1237
Accred Length: 1 Year *Program Size:* 2
Program ID: 310-56-21-053

Forensic Psychiatry (Psychiatry)

California

Los Angeles

University of Southern California Program
Sponsor: Los Angeles County-USC Medical Center
Program Director:
Tim Botello, MD MPH
1937 N Hospital Pl
PO Box 86125
Los Angeles, CA 90086-0125
Tel: 323 226-4942 *Fax:* 323 226-2777
Accred Length: 1 Year *Program Size:* 5
Program ID: 406-05-31-002

Sylmar

UCLA San Fernando Valley Program
Sponsor: Olive View-UCLA Medical Center
Atascadero State Hospital
Program Director:
Neena Sachinvala, MD
14445 Olive View Dr
Sylmar, CA 91342
Tel: 818 364-3432 *Fax:* 818 364-4577
Accred Length: 1 Year *Program Size:* 4
Program ID: 406-05-11-003

Colorado

Denver

University of Colorado Program
Sponsor: University of Colorado Health Sciences Center
Colorado Mental Health Institute at Pueblo
Program Director:
Robert D Miller, MD
Campus Box C-249-27
4200 E 9th Ave
Denver, CO 80262
Tel: 303 315-5248 *Fax:* 303 315-3781
Accred Length: 1 Year *Program Size:* 0
Program ID: 406-07-21-004

Connecticut

New Haven

Yale-New Haven Medical Center Program
Sponsor: Yale-New Haven Hospital
Connecticut Mental Health Center
Program Director:
Howard V Zonana, MD
34 Park St
New Haven, CT 06519
Tel: 203 789-7421 *Fax:* 203 974-7178
E-mail: howard.zonana@yale.edu
Accred Length: 1 Year *Program Size:* 2
Program ID: 406-08-21-005

Programs

Florida

Gainesville

University of Florida Program

Sponsor: University of Florida College of Medicine

Program Director:
Richard A Greer, MD
Univ of Florida
PO Box 100256
Gainesville, FL 32610-0256
Tel: 352 392-3284 *Fax:* 352 392-0887
E-mail: rgreen352@aol.com
Accred Length: 1 Year *Program Size:* 0
Program ID: 406-11-21-007

Georgia

Atlanta

Emory University Program

Sponsor: Emory University School of Medicine
Grady Memorial Hospital

Program Director:
Peter Ash, MD
Emory Univ Psychiatry and Law Service
Grady Memorial Hosp/Box 26238
80 Butler St SE
Atlanta, GA 30335-3801
Tel: 404 616-5492 *Fax:* 404 616-3241
E-mail: pash01@emory.edu
Internet:
http://userwww.service.emory.edu/~pash01/fellow.html
Accred Length: 1 Year *Program Size:* 2
Program ID: 406-12-21-008

Illinois

Chicago

Rush-Presbyterian-St Luke's Medical Center Program

Sponsor: Rush-Presbyterian-St Luke's Medical Center

Program Director:
Jonathan R Kelly, MD
Isaac Ray Ctr
1725 W Harrison St/Ste 110
Chicago, IL 60612
Tel: 312 942-5588 *Fax:* 312 829-1476
E-mail: astpier1@rush.edu
Internet: http://www.isaacraycenter.com
Accred Length: 1 Year *Program Size:* 2
Program ID: 406-16-21-009

Louisiana

New Orleans

Louisiana State University Program

Sponsor: Louisiana State University School of Medicine
Medical Center of Louisiana at New Orleans

Program Director:
Debra K DePrato, MD
Louisiana State Univ Sch of Med
1542 Tulane Ave
New Orleans, LA 70112
Tel: 504 568-6339 *Fax:* 504 568-6465
Accred Length: 1 Year *Program Size:* 0
Program ID: 406-21-21-024

Tulane University Program

Sponsor: Tulane University School of Medicine
Tulane University Hospital and Clinics

Program Director:
John W Thompson, MD
Dept of Psychiatry/Neurology TB 53
1440 Canal St
New Orleans, LA 70112
Tel: 504 588-2201 *Fax:* 504 587-7457
Accred Length: 1 Year *Program Size:* 2
Program ID: 406-21-21-010

Maryland

Baltimore

University of Maryland Program

Sponsor: University of Maryland School of Medicine
Clifton T Perkins Hospital Center

Program Director:
Christiane Tellefsen, MD
Clifton T Perkins Hospital Ctr
8450 Dorsey Run Rd
PO Box 1000
Jessup, MD 20794-1000
Tel: 410 724-3149 *Fax:* 410 724-3009
E-mail: ctellefsen@aol.com
Internet: http://members.aol.com/cvole 36425/
Accred Length: 1 Year *Program Size:* 3
Program ID: 406-23-21-011

Massachusetts

Boston

Massachusetts General Hospital/Mclean Hospital Program

Sponsor: Massachusetts General Hospital

Program Director:
Ronald Schouten, MD
Massachusetts General Hospital
60 Staniford St
Boston, MA 02114
Tel: 617 726-5195 *Fax:* 617 724-2808
E-mail: rschouten@partners.org
Accred Length: 1 Year *Program Size:* 1
Program ID: 406-24-21-012

Worcester

University of Massachusetts Program

Sponsor: University of Massachusetts Medical School
UMass Memorial Health Care (University Campus)

Program Director:
Kenneth Appelbaum, MD
55 Lake Ave N
Worcester, MA 01655
Tel: 508 856-6762 *Fax:* 508 856-6426
E-mail: kenneth.appelbaum@banyan.ummed.edu
Internet:
http://www.ummed.edu/dept/psychiatry/resprog.html
Accred Length: 1 Year *Program Size:* 3
Program ID: 406-24-31-013

Michigan

Ann Arbor

University of Michigan Program

Sponsor: Center for Forensic Psychiatry
University of Michigan Hospitals

Program Director:
Stephen C Cook, MD
3501 Willis Rd/PO Box 2060
Ann Arbor, MI 48106-2060
Tel: 313 429-2531, ext 352 *Fax:* 313 429-0485
E-mail: cooks2@state.mi.us
Accred Length: 1 Year *Program Size:* 3
Program ID: 406-25-21-014

New York

Bronx

Albert Einstein College of Medicine Program

Sponsor: Albert Einstein College of Medicine of Yeshiva University
Bronx Psychiatric Center

Program Director:
Merrill Rotter, MD
1500 Waters Pl
Bronx, NY 10461
Tel: 718 931-0600, ext 3103 *Fax:* 718 931-4789
Accred Length: 1 Year *Program Size:* 2
Program ID: 406-35-21-015

New York

New York University Medical Center Program

Sponsor: New York University Medical Center
Bellevue Hospital Center

Program Director:
Henry C Weinstein, MD
New York Univ Med Ctr
550 First Ave
New York, NY 10016
Tel: 212 263-6242 *Fax:* 212 876-2002
Accred Length: 1 Year *Program Size:* 3
Program ID: 406-35-31-016

Rochester

University of Rochester Program

Sponsor: Strong Memorial Hospital of the University of Rochester
Rochester Psychiatric Center
St Mary's Hospital (Unity Health System)

Program Director:
J Richard Ciccone, MD
300 Crittenden Blvd
Rochester, NY 14642
Tel: 716 275-4986 *Fax:* 716 244-4734
E-mail: jrce@uhura.cc.rochester.edu
Internet: http://www.urmc.rochester.edu/smd/psych
Accred Length: 1 Year *Program Size:* 2
Program ID: 406-35-11-017

North Carolina

Butner

Duke University Program
Sponsor: Duke University Medical Center
Federal Correctional Institution-Butner
Program Director:
Sally Johnson, MD
Duke Univ
FCI-Butner/PO Box 1000
Butner, NC 27509-1000
Tel: 919 575-4541, ext 3650 *Fax:* 919 575-2017
Accred Length: 1 Year *Program Size:* 2
Program ID: 406-36-21-018

Ohio

Cleveland

Case Western Reserve University Program
Sponsor: University Hospitals of Cleveland
Program Director:
Phillip J Resnick, MD
Univ Hospitals of Cleveland
11100 Euclid Ave
Cleveland, OH 44106
Tel: 216 844-3415 *Fax:* 216 844-1703
E-mail: pxr5@po.cwru.edu
Accred Length: 1 Year *Program Size:* 3
Program ID: 406-38-21-019

South Carolina

Columbia

Palmetto Health Alliance/University of South Carolina School of Medicine Program
Sponsor: Palmetto Health Alliance
William S Hall Psychiatric Institute
Program Director:
Donna Schwartz-Watts, MD
USC Sch of Med
3555 Harden St
Ste 104-A
Columbia, SC 29203
Tel: 803 434-4250 *Fax:* 803 434-4277
E-mail: donnasw@npsy.ceb.sc.edu
Accred Length: 1 Year *Program Size:* 2
Program ID: 406-45-21-020

Washington

Tacoma

University of Washington Program
Sponsor: University of Washington School of Medicine
Western State Hospital
Program Director:
Bruce C Gage, MD
9601 Steilacoom Blvd
Tacoma, WA 98498-7213
Tel: 253 756-3921 *Fax:* 253 756-3987
E-mail: gage@u.washington.edu
Accred Length: 1 Year *Program Size:* 1
Program ID: 406-54-21-022

Wisconsin

Milwaukee

Medical College of Wisconsin Program
Sponsor: Medical College of Wisconsin Affiliated Hospitals Inc
Mendota Mental Health Institute
Milwaukee County Mental Health Complex
Program Director:
Joseph B Layde, MD JD
Med Coll of Wisconsin, Dept of Psychiatry
8701 Watertown Plank Rd
Milwaukee, WI 53226
Tel: 414 257-5995 *Fax:* 414 257-7228
E-mail: jlayde@mcw.edu
Internet: http://www.aapl.org/fellow.htm#mcw
Accred Length: 1 Year *Program Size:* 2
Program ID: 406-56-21-023

Gastroenterology (Internal Medicine)

Alabama

Birmingham

University of Alabama Medical Center Program
Sponsor: University of Alabama Hospital
Program Director:
Charles M Wilcox, MD
Univ of Alabama Hospitals
Univ Station
Birmingham, AL 35294
Tel: 205 934-6060 *Fax:* 205 934-8493
Accred Length: 2 Years *Program Size:* 2
Program ID: 144-01-21-127

Mobile

University of South Alabama Program
Sponsor: University of South Alabama Medical Center
USA Knollwood Park Hospital
Program Director:
Jack A DiPalma, MD
Univ of South Alabama Med Ctr
2451 Fillingim St
Mobile, AL 36617
Tel: 334 471-7905 *Fax:* 334 471-6901
Internet: http://gastro@usouthal.campus.mci.net
Accred Length: 2 Years *Program Size:* 5
Program ID: 144-01-21-213

Arizona

Tucson

University of Arizona Program
Sponsor: University of Arizona College of Medicine
Carl T Hayden Veterans Affairs Medical Center (Phoenix)
Good Samaritan Regional Medical Center
University Medical Center
Veterans Affairs Medical Center (Tucson)
Program Director:
Richard E Sampliner, MD
Univ of Arizona Health Sciences Ctr
PO Box 245028
1501 N Campbell Ave
Tucson, AZ 85724
Tel: 520 626-6119 *Fax:* 520 626-0826
Internet:
http://www.medicine.arizona.edu/gastroenterology/
Accred Length: 2 Years *Program Size:* 3
Program ID: 144-03-21-110

Arkansas

Little Rock

University of Arkansas for Medical Sciences Program

Sponsor: University of Arkansas College of Medicine
John L McClellan Memorial Veterans Hospital
University Hospital of Arkansas

Program Director:
Jean-Pierre Raufman, MD
Univ of Arkansas for Med Sciences
4301 W Markham St/Slot 567
Little Rock, AR 72205
Tel: 501 686-6217 *Fax:* 501 686-6248
E-mail: raufmanjeanpierre@exchange.uams.edu
Internet: http://www.uams.edu
Accred Length: 2 Years *Program Size:* 6
Program ID: 144-04-21-111

California

La Jolla

Scripps Clinic/Scripps Green Hospital Program

Sponsor: Scripps Clinic
Scripps Green Hospital

Program Director:
Vance D Rodgers, MD
Div of Gastroenterology/203N
Scripps Clinic-Green Hospital
10666 N Torrey Pines Rd
La Jolla, CA 92037-1093
Tel: 619 554-8877 *Fax:* 619 554-4544
E-mail: vr@scripps.edu
Internet: http://scrippsclinic.com
Accred Length: 2 Years *Program Size:* 3
Program ID: 144-05-21-073

Loma Linda

Loma Linda University Program

Sponsor: Loma Linda University Medical Center
Jerry L Pettis Memorial Veterans Hospital

Program Director:
Terence D Lewis, MB BS
Loma Linda Univ Med Ctr
Dept of Med
Rm 1556
Loma Linda, CA 92354
Tel: 909 824-4905 *Fax:* 909 478-4490
Accred Length: 2 Years *Program Size:* 4
Program ID: 144-05-21-087

Los Angeles

Charles R Drew University Program

Sponsor: Charles R Drew University of Medicine and Science
LAC-King/Drew Medical Center

Program Director:
Ioannis Giannikopoulos, MD
LAC/King-Drew Med Ctr
Div of Gastroenterology MP 11
12021 S Wilmington Ave
Los Angeles, CA 90059
Tel: 213 563-5924 *Fax:* 213 357-3422
Accred Length: 2 Years *Program Size:* 4
Program ID: 144-05-21-221

Southern California Kaiser Permanente Medical Care (Los Angeles) Program

Sponsor: Southern California Kaiser Permanente Medical Group
Kaiser Foundation Hospital (Los Angeles)

Program Director:
Karl T Esrason, MD
Donald Gerety, MD
Kaiser Foundation Hospital
1526 N Edgemont St/7th Fl
Los Angeles, CA 90027
Tel: 323 783-6830 *Fax:* 323 783-3832
Accred Length: 2 Years *Program Size:* 3
Program ID: 144-05-12-037

UCLA Medical Center Program

Sponsor: UCLA School of Medicine
Cedars-Sinai Medical Center
Los Angeles County-Harbor-UCLA Medical Center
Olive View-UCLA Medical Center
UCLA Medical Center
VA Greater Los Angeles Healthcare System

Program Director:
Jonathan D Kaunitz, MD
West Los Angeles VA Med Ctr
CURE (115/115)
11301 Wilshire Blvd
Los Angeles, CA 90073-1736
Tel: 310 312-9284 *Fax:* 310 268-4963
E-mail: sromano@med1.medsch.ucla.edu
Accred Length: 2 Years *Program Size:* 19
Program ID: 144-05-11-130

University of Southern California Program

Sponsor: Los Angeles County-USC Medical Center

Program Director:
Neil Kaplowitz, MD
Univ of Southern California Sch of Med
2011 Zonal Ave/HMR 101
Los Angeles, CA 90033
Tel: 323 442-5576 *Fax:* 323 442-5567
E-mail: kaplowit@hsc.usc.edu
Accred Length: 2 Years *Program Size:* 11
Program ID: 144-05-21-053

Orange

University of California (Irvine) Program

Sponsor: University of California (Irvine) Medical Center
Long Beach Memorial Medical Center
Veterans Affairs Medical Center (Long Beach)

Program Director:
Hooshang Meshkinpour, MD
Univ of California Irvine, Dept of Med/Gastro
101 The City Dr
Bldg 53 Rt 81
Orange, CA 92868
Tel: 714 456-5140 *Fax:* 714 456-7753
Accred Length: 2 Years *Program Size:* 8
Program ID: 144-05-21-151

Sacramento

University of California (Davis) Program

Sponsor: University of California (Davis) Medical Center
Kaiser Foundation Hospital (Sacramento)

Program Director:
Joseph Leung, MD
Univ of California Davis Med Ctr
Div of Gastroenterology
4150 V St/Ste 3500
Sacramento, CA 95817
Tel: 916 734-3751 *Fax:* 916 734-7908
Accred Length: 2 Years *Program Size:* 6
Program ID: 144-05-21-094

San Diego

Naval Medical Center (San Diego) Program

Sponsor: Naval Medical Center (San Diego)

Program Director:
Cdr Oscar Sven Brann, MD
Dept of Navy
Naval Hospital
San Diego, CA 92134-5000
Tel: 619 532-9725 *Fax:* 619 532-9620
E-mail: obrann@snd.10.med.navy.mil
Accred Length: 2 Years *Program Size:* 3
Program ID: 144-05-12-152
US Armed Services Program

University of California (San Diego) Program

Sponsor: University of California (San Diego) Medical Center
Veterans Affairs Medical Center (San Diego)

Program Director:
C Richard Boland, MD
Univ of California San Diego
4028 Basic Science Bldg
9500 Gilman Dr
La Jolla, CA 92093-0688
Tel: 619 822-0304 *Fax:* 619 822-0301
E-mail: crboland@ucsd.edu
Internet: http://www.medicine.ucsd.edu/gastro
Accred Length: 2 Years *Program Size:* 6
Program ID: 144-05-21-174

San Francisco

California Pacific Medical Center Program

Sponsor: California Pacific Medical Center
California Pacific Medical Center

Program Director:
Michael Verhille, MD
California Pacific Med Ctr
2351 Clay St/#362
San Francisco, CA 94115
Tel: 800 743-7707 *Fax:* 415 775-7437
Internet: http://www.cpmc.org
Accred Length: 2 Years *Program Size:* 2
Program ID: 144-05-12-153

University of California (San Francisco) Program

Sponsor: University of California (San Francisco) School of Medicine
San Francisco General Hospital Medical Center
University of California (San Francisco) Medical Center
Veterans Affairs Medical Center (San Francisco)

Program Director:
Montgomery Bissell, MD
Div of Gastroenterology
513 Parnassus Ave/S-375
San Francisco, CA 94143-0538
Tel: 415 476-2777 *Fax:* 415 476-0659
E-mail: dmbiss@itsa.ucsf.edu
Internet: http://gi.ucsf.edu
Accred Length: 2 Years *Program Size:* 12
Program ID: 144-05-21-154

Stanford

Stanford University Program
Sponsor: Stanford University Hospital
Santa Clara Valley Medical Center
Veterans Affairs Palo Alto Health Care System
Program Director:
Harry B Greenberg, MD
Stanford Univ Med Ctr
Gastroenterology P-304
300 Pasteur Dr
Stanford, CA 94305-5487
Tel: 650 498-6080 *Fax:* 650 852-3259
Internet: http://www.leland.stanford.edu/group/gastrol
Accred Length: 2 Years *Program Size:* 10
Program ID: 144-05-21-022

Colorado

Denver

University of Colorado Program
Sponsor: University of Colorado Health Sciences Center
Denver Health and Hospitals
Veterans Affairs Medical Center (Denver)
Program Director:
Dennis Ahnen, MD
Univ of Colorado Health Sciences Ctr
4200 E Ninth Ave
Campus Box B-158
Denver, CO 80262
Tel: 303 315-2537 *Fax:* 303 315-5711
E-mail: dennis.ahnen@uchsc.edu
Accred Length: 2 Years *Program Size:* 9
Program ID: 144-07-21-065

Connecticut

Bridgeport

Yale University (Bridgeport) Program
Sponsor: Bridgeport Hospital
Program Director:
Ingram M Roberts, MD
Bridgeport Hospital
267 Grant St
Div of Gastroenterology
Bridgeport, CT 06602
Tel: 203 384-3175 *Fax:* 203 384-4294
E-mail: pirobe@bpthosp.org
Accred Length: 2 Years *Program Size:* 3
Program ID: 144-08-11-190

Farmington

University of Connecticut Program
Sponsor: University of Connecticut School of Medicine
Hartford Hospital
New Britain General Hospital
St Francis Hospital and Medical Center
Univ of Connecticut Health Center/John Dempsey Hospital
Program Director:
George Y Wu, MD PhD
Univ of Connecticut Sch of Med
Rm AM-044
263 Farmington Ave
Farmington, CT 06030-1845
Tel: 860 679-3158 *Fax:* 860 679-3159
E-mail: wu@nso.uchc.edu
Accred Length: 2 Years *Program Size:* 6
Program ID: 144-08-31-001

New Haven

Yale-New Haven Medical Center Program
Sponsor: Yale-New Haven Hospital
Veterans Affairs Medical Center (West Haven)
Program Director:
Fred S Gorelick, MD
Yale-New Haven Med Ctr, Dept of Med
PO Box 208019
333 Cedar St
New Haven, CT 06520-8019
Tel: 203 785-4138 *Fax:* 203 785-7273
E-mail: fred.gorelick@yale.edu
Internet: http://www.info.med.yale.edu/intmed/digdis
Accred Length: 2 Years *Program Size:* 12
Program ID: 144-08-21-023

Norwalk

Norwalk Hospital Program
Sponsor: Norwalk Hospital
Program Director:
Joan Culpepper-Morgan, MD
Norwalk Hospital
Sect of Gastroenterology
Maple St
Norwalk, CT 06856
Tel: 203 852-2372 *Fax:* 203 852-2075
E-mail: joan.culpepper-morgan@norwalkhealth.org
Internet: http://www.norwalkhosp.org
Accred Length: 2 Years *Program Size:* 3
Program ID: 144-08-31-002

District of Columbia

Washington

George Washington University Program
Sponsor: George Washington University School of Medicine
George Washington University Hospital (UHS)
Program Director:
Hans Fromm, MD
George Washington Univ Hospital
2150 Pennsylvania Ave NW/Rm 3-412
Washington, DC 20037
Tel: 202 994-4418 *Fax:* 202 994-7955
E-mail: domhxf@gwumc.edu
Accred Length: 2 Years *Program Size:* 2
Program ID: 144-10-21-114

Georgetown University Program
Sponsor: Georgetown University Medical Center
District of Columbia General Hospital
NIH Warren Grant Magnuson Clinical Center
Veterans Affairs Medical Center (Washington, DC)
Program Director:
Stanley B Benjamin, MD
Georgetown Univ Med Ctr
GI Fellowships (Med 5 PHC)
3800 Reservoir Rd NW
Washington, DC 20007-2197
Tel: 202 687-4034 *Fax:* 202 687-7797
E-mail: steelewe@gunet.georgetown.edu
Accred Length: 2 Years *Program Size:* 11
Program ID: 144-10-21-088

Howard University Program
Sponsor: Howard University Hospital
District of Columbia General Hospital
Program Director:
Victor F Scott, MD
Howard Univ Hospital
Div of Gastroenterology
2041 Georgia Ave NW/Ste 5100
Washington, DC 20060
Tel: 202 865-6632 *Fax:* 202 865-7268
E-mail: vscott@fac.howard.edu
Accred Length: 2 Years *Program Size:* 4
Program ID: 144-10-21-133

Washington Hospital Center Program
Sponsor: Washington Hospital Center
Program Director:
Leonard Wartofsky, MD
Frank Kim, MD
Washington Hospital Ctr
Sect of Gastroenterology/1B-39
110 Irving St NW
Washington, DC 20010
Tel: 202 877-7108 *Fax:* 202 877-8163
Internet: http://www.mhg.edu/gme/
Accred Length: 2 Years *Program Size:* 3
Program ID: 144-10-21-212

Florida

Gainesville

University of Florida Program
Sponsor: University of Florida College of Medicine
Shands Hospital at the University of Florida
Veterans Affairs Medical Center (Gainesville)
Program Director:
Phillip P Toskes, MD
Univ of Florida Coll of Med
J Hillis Miller Med Ctr/J-277
1600 SW Archer Rd
Gainesville, FL 32610
Tel: 352 392-2877 *Fax:* 352 392-3618
Accred Length: 2 Years *Program Size:* 7
Program ID: 144-11-21-039

Jacksonville

Mayo Graduate School of Medicine (Jacksonville) Program
Sponsor: Mayo Graduate School of Medicine-Mayo Foundation
Mayo Clinic (Jacksonville)
St Luke's Hospital
Program Director:
Mark E Stark, MD
Mayo Clinic Jacksonville
4500 San Pablo Rd
Jacksonville, FL 32224
Tel: 904 953-3863 *Fax:* 904 953-7260
E-mail: stark.mark@mayo.edu
Accred Length: 2 Years *Program Size:* 3
Program ID: 144-11-21-222

University of Florida Health Science Center/Jacksonville Program

Sponsor: University of Florida College of Medicine at Jacksonville
University Medical Center (UFHSC/J)

Program Director:
Louis Lambiase, MD
Univ of Florida Health Science Ctr-Jacksonville
653 W Eighth St
Jacksonville, FL 32209-6511
Tel: 904 549-3980 *Fax:* 904 549-3403
E-mail: jaffront@umc.ufl.edu
Internet: http://www.ufhscj.edu
Accred Length: 2 Years *Program Size:* 6
Program ID: 144-11-21-024

Miami

University of Miami-Jackson Memorial Medical Center Program

Sponsor: University of Miami-Jackson Memorial Medical Center
Mount Sinai Medical Center of Greater Miami
Veterans Affairs Medical Center (Miami)

Program Director:
Arvey I Rogers, MD
Univ of Miami-Jackson Memorial Med Ctr
PO Box 016960 (D-49)
Miami, FL 33101
Tel: 305 585-5120 *Fax:* 305 325-9476
Accred Length: 2 Years *Program Size:* 11
Program ID: 144-11-21-176

Tampa

University of South Florida Program

Sponsor: University of South Florida College of Medicine
James A Haley Veterans Hospital
Tampa General Healthcare

Program Director:
H Juergen Nord, MD
Univ of South Florida Coll of Med
12901 Bruce B Downs Blvd
MDC Box 19
Tampa, FL 33612-4799
Tel: 813 974-2034 *Fax:* 813 974-5333
E-mail: jpenders@com1.med.usf.edu
Accred Length: 2 Years *Program Size:* 7
Program ID: 144-11-21-040

Georgia

Atlanta

Emory University Program

Sponsor: Emory University School of Medicine
Emory University Hospital
Grady Memorial Hospital
Veterans Affairs Medical Center (Atlanta)

Program Director:
Steve Goldschmid, MD
Emory Univ Sch of Med
Div of Digestive Diseases
1639 Pierce Dr NE/Rm 2101 WMB
Atlanta, GA 30322-0463
Tel: 404 727-5638 *Fax:* 404 727-5767
Internet: http://www.emory.edu/whsc/med/gi
Accred Length: 2 Years *Program Size:* 9
Program ID: 144-12-21-136

Augusta

Medical College of Georgia Program

Sponsor: Medical College of Georgia Hospital and Clinics
Veterans Affairs Medical Center (Augusta)

Program Director:
Robert R Schade, MD
Med Coll of Georgia
Sect of Gastroenterology-BBR2536
1120 15th St
Augusta, GA 30912-3120
Tel: 706 721-2238 *Fax:* 706 721-0331
E-mail: deptmed.rschade@mail.mcg.edu
Accred Length: 2 Years *Program Size:* 5
Program ID: 144-12-21-003

Illinois

Chicago

Cook County Hospital Program

Sponsor: Cook County Hospital

Program Director:
Bashar M Attar, MD
Cook County Hospital
1825 W Harrison St
Chicago, IL 60612
Tel: 312 633-7213 *Fax:* 312 633-7604
Accred Length: 2 Years *Program Size:* 8
Program ID: 144-16-12-041

McGaw Medical Center of Northwestern University Program

Sponsor: Northwestern University Medical School
Northwestern Memorial Hospital
Veterans Affairs Lakeside Medical Center (Chicago)

Program Director:
Robert Craig, MD
320 E Superior St/Searle 10-541
Chicago, IL 60611
Tel: 312 908-7280 *Fax:* 312 908-9620
E-mail: r-craig@nwu.edu
Internet: http://www.medicine.nwu.edu/gastro/
Accred Length: 2 Years *Program Size:* 6
Program ID: 144-16-21-074

Rush-Presbyterian-St Luke's Medical Center Program

Sponsor: Rush-Presbyterian-St Luke's Medical Center

Program Director:
Seymour M Sabesin, MD
Rush-Presbyterian-St Luke's Med Ctr
1725 W Harrison St/Ste 206
Chicago, IL 60612
Tel: 312 942-8914 *Fax:* 312 942-9943
Accred Length: 2 Years *Program Size:* 6
Program ID: 144-16-11-137

University of Chicago Program

Sponsor: University of Chicago Hospitals

Program Director:
Eli D Ehrenpreis, MD
Univ of Chicago
5841 S Maryland Ave/MC4076
Chicago, IL 60637-1470
Tel: 773 702-6950 *Fax:* 773 702-2182
Accred Length: 2 Years *Program Size:* 9
Program ID: 144-16-11-067

University of Illinois College of Medicine at Chicago Program

Sponsor: University of Illinois College of Medicine at Chicago
Michael Reese Hospital and Medical Center
Mount Sinai Hospital Medical Center of Chicago
St Francis Hospital of Evanston
University of Illinois Hospital and Clinics
Veterans Affairs West Side Medical Center

Program Director:
Richard V Benya, MD
Univ of Illinois-Chicago
Digestive/Liver Diseases
840 S Wood St (M/C 787)
Chicago, IL 60612-7323
Tel: 312 996-6651 *Fax:* 312 996-5103
E-mail: prandle@uic.edu
Internet: http://www.uic.edu/com/dom/gastro
Accred Length: 2 Years *Program Size:* 8
Program ID: 144-16-21-138

Maywood

Loyola University Program

Sponsor: Loyola University Medical Center
Edward J Hines Jr Veterans Affairs Hospital

Program Director:
Mark T DeMeo, MD
Loyola Univ
2160 S First Ave
Rm 25/Bldg 117
Maywood, IL 60153
Tel: 708 216-6801 *Fax:* 708 216-4113
E-mail: mtdemeo@wpo.it.luc.edu
Accred Length: 2 Years *Program Size:* 9
Program ID: 144-16-21-004

Park Ridge

Lutheran General Hospital Program

Sponsor: Lutheran General Hospital

Program Director:
Hymie Kavin, MD
Lutheran General Hospital
1775 W Dempster St
6 South
Park Ridge, IL 60068-1174
Tel: 847 723-6464 *Fax:* 847 723-5615
Accred Length: 2 Years *Program Size:* 2
Program ID: 144-16-21-214

Springfield

Southern Illinois University Program

Sponsor: Southern Illinois University School of Medicine
Memorial Medical Center
St John's Hospital

Program Director:
Fernando Castro-Pavia, MD
Memorial Med Ctr
800 N Rutledge
Rm D123
Springfield, IL 62781
Tel: 217 782-0173 *Fax:* 217 788-5459
Internet: http://www.siumed.edu
Accred Length: 2 Years *Program Size:* 3
Program ID: 144-16-21-208

Indiana

Indianapolis

Indiana University School of Medicine Program

Sponsor: Indiana University School of Medicine
Clarian IU Hospital
Richard L Roudebush Veterans Affairs Medical Center
William N Wishard Memorial Hospital

Program Director:
John O'Brien, MD
Indiana Univ Med Ctr
Div of Gastro/Hepatology
550 N University Blvd/UH 2300
Indianapolis, IN 46202
Tel: 317 274-3332 *Fax:* 317 278-0164
E-mail: jjobrien@iupui.edu
Internet: http://medicine.iupui.edu
Accred Length: 2 Years *Program Size:* 6
Program ID: 144-17-21-155

Iowa

Iowa City

University of Iowa Hospitals and Clinics Program

Sponsor: University of Iowa Hospitals and Clinics

Program Director:
Joel Weinstock, MD
Univ of Iowa Hospitals and Clinics
Dept of Int Med
200 Hawkins Dr/Rm 4607 JCP
Iowa City, IA 52242-1081
Tel: 319 356-3127 *Fax:* 319 353-6399
Accred Length: 2 Years *Program Size:* 4
Program ID: 144-18-21-095

Kansas

Kansas City

University of Kansas Medical Center Program

Sponsor: University of Kansas School of Medicine
University of Kansas Medical Center

Program Director:
Richard W McCallum, MD
Univ of Kansas Med Ctr
Gastroenterology Div
3901 Rainbow Blvd
Kansas City, KS 66160-7350
Tel: 913 588-6003 *Fax:* 913 588-3975
E-mail: rmccallum@kumc.edu
Accred Length: 2 Years *Program Size:* 9
Program ID: 144-19-21-115

Kentucky

Lexington

University of Kentucky Medical Center Program

Sponsor: University of Kentucky Hospital
Veterans Affairs Medical Center (Lexington)

Program Director:
Nicholas Nickl, MD
Univ of Kentucky Med Ctr
Lexington, KY 40536-0293
Tel: 606 323-5575 *Fax:* 606 257-8860
Accred Length: 2 Years *Program Size:* 2
Program ID: 144-20-21-177

Louisville

University of Louisville Program

Sponsor: University of Louisville School of Medicine
Jewish Hospital
Norton Hospital (Alliant Health System)
University of Louisville Hospital
Veterans Affairs Medical Center (Louisville)

Program Director:
Richard A Wright, MD
Ambulatory Care Building
550 S Jackson St
Louisville, KY 40292
Tel: 502 588-6991 *Fax:* 502 852-0846
E-mail: rawrig02@ulkyvm.louisville.edu
Internet:
http://www.louisville.edu/medschool/medicine/gastro
Accred Length: 2 Years *Program Size:* 6
Program ID: 144-20-31-089

Louisiana

New Orleans

Alton Ochsner Medical Foundation Program

Sponsor: Alton Ochsner Medical Foundation

Program Director:
Robert P Perrillo, MD
Alton Ochsner Med Foundation
Dept of Grad Med Educ
1516 Jefferson Hwy
New Orleans, LA 70121
Tel: 504 842-3260 *Fax:* 504 842-3193
E-mail: dlambert@ochsner.org
Internet: http://www.ochsner.org/gastro
Accred Length: 2 Years *Program Size:* 6
Program ID: 144-21-22-149

Louisiana State University Program

Sponsor: Louisiana State University School of Medicine
Medical Center of Louisiana at New Orleans
Memorial Medical Center

Program Director:
Luis Balart, MD
Louisiana State Univ Med Ctr
1542 Tulane Ave
New Orleans, LA 70112
Tel: 504 568-8841 *Fax:* 504 568-2127
Accred Length: 2 Years *Program Size:* 3
Program ID: 144-21-21-139

Tulane University Program

Sponsor: Tulane University School of Medicine
Medical Center of Louisiana at New Orleans
Tulane University Hospital and Clinics
Veterans Affairs Medical Center-LSU Service (New Orleans)

Program Director:
Roy C Orlando, MD
Tulane Univ Med Ctr
Gastro/Hepatology SL35
1430 Tulane Ave
New Orleans, LA 70112-2699
Tel: 504 588-5329 *Fax:* 504 587-2188
E-mail: rorland@tmcpop.tmc.tulane.edu
Accred Length: 2 Years *Program Size:* 6
Program ID: 144-21-21-108

Shreveport

Louisiana State University (Shreveport) Program

Sponsor: Louisiana State University Hospital-Shreveport
Overton Brooks Veterans Affairs Medical Center

Program Director:
Paul A Jordan, MD
Louisiana State Univ Med Ctr Hospital
Med Educ Dept (Gastro)
1501 Kings Hwy/PO Box 33932
Shreveport, LA 71130-3932
Tel: 318 675-5982 *Fax:* 318 675-5957
Accred Length: 2 Years *Program Size:* 6
Program ID: 144-21-21-203

Maryland

Baltimore

Johns Hopkins University Bayview Medical Center Program

Sponsor: Johns Hopkins University School of Medicine
Johns Hopkins Bayview Medical Center

Program Director:
Lawrence J Cheskin, MD
Johns Hopkins Bayview Med Ctr
4940 Eastern Ave
Baltimore, MD 21224
Tel: 410 550-0794 *Fax:* 410 558-9346
E-mail: cheskin@jhmi.edu
Accred Length: 2 Years *Program Size:* 4
Program ID: 144-23-11-140

Johns Hopkins University Program

Sponsor: Johns Hopkins University School of Medicine
Johns Hopkins Hospital

Program Director:
Francis M Giardiello, MD
Gastroenterology/Hepatology
1830 E Monument St
Rm 431
Baltimore, MD 21205
Tel: 410 955-2635 *Fax:* 410 614-8337
Accred Length: 2 Years *Program Size:* 9
Program ID: 144-23-11-075

University of Maryland Program

Sponsor: University of Maryland Medical System

Program Director:
Stephen P James, MD
Univ of Maryland Med Ctr
22 S Greene St/Rm N3W62
Baltimore, MD 21201-1595
Tel: 410 328-8728 *Fax:* 410 328-8315
E-mail: sjames@medicine.ab.umd.edu
Accred Length: 2 Years *Program Size:* 8
Program ID: 144-23-21-042

Bethesda

National Naval Medical Center (Bethesda) Program

Sponsor: National Naval Medical Center (Bethesda)

Program Director:
James W Kikendall, MD
National Naval Med Ctr
Div of Gastroenterology
8901 Wisconsin Ave
Bethesda, MD 20889-5600
Tel: 202 782-5263 *Fax:* 202 782-4416
Accred Length: 2 Years *Program Size:* 9
Program ID: 144-23-11-156
US Armed Services Program

Massachusetts

Boston

Beth Israel Deaconess Medical Center (East Campus) Program

Sponsor: Beth Israel Deaconess Medical Center

Program Director:
Jay Thomas Lamont, MD
Beth Israel Deaconess Med Ctr-East Campus
Dana 601
330 Brookline Ave
Boston, MA 02215
Tel: 617 667-8377 *Fax:* 617 975-5071
Accred Length: 2 Years *Program Size:* 8
Program ID: 144-24-21-005

Beth Israel Deaconess Medical Center (West Campus) Program

Sponsor: Beth Israel Deaconess Medical Center

Program Director:
Myron Falchunk, MD
Deaconess Hospital
110 Francis St/Ste 8E
Boston, MA 02215
Tel: 617 734-5552 *Fax:* 617 739-6813
Accred Length: 2 Years *Program Size:* 0
Program ID: 144-24-21-184

Boston University Medical Center Program

Sponsor: Boston Medical Center
Veterans Affairs Medical Center (Boston)

Program Director:
M Michael Wolfe, MD
Boston Med Ctr
88 E Newton St
Evans 201
Boston, MA 02118
Tel: 617 638-8330 *Fax:* 617 638-7785
Accred Length: 2 Years *Program Size:* 6
Program ID: 144-24-21-157

Brigham and Women's Hospital Program

Sponsor: Brigham and Women's Hospital
Brockton-West Roxbury Veterans Affairs Medical Center

Program Director:
Richard S Blumberg, MD MD
Brigham and Women's Hospital
Gastroenterology Div
75 Francis St
Boston, MA 02115-6195
Tel: 617 732-5824 *Fax:* 617 264-5185
E-mail: blumberg@bustoff.bwh.harvard.edu
Accred Length: 2 Years *Program Size:* 12
Program ID: 144-24-21-006

Massachusetts General Hospital Program

Sponsor: Massachusetts General Hospital

Program Director:
Daniel K Podolsky, MD
Massachusetts General Hospital
55 Fruit St/GRJ 719
Boston, MA 02114-2696
Tel: 617 726-7411 *Fax:* 617 724-2136
E-mail: podolsky.daniel@mgh.harvard.edu
Internet: http://www.mgh.harvard.edu
Accred Length: 2 Years *Program Size:* 9
Program ID: 144-24-11-068

New England Medical Center Hospitals Program

Sponsor: New England Medical Center Hospitals

Program Director:
Young-Mee Lee, MD
New England Med Ctr
750 Washington St/Box 233
Boston, MA 02111
Tel: 617 636-9140 *Fax:* 617 636-4207
Accred Length: 2 Years *Program Size:* 4
Program ID: 144-24-21-007

St Elizabeth's Medical Center of Boston Program

Sponsor: St Elizabeth's Medical Center of Boston
Faulkner Hospital
Lemuel Shattuck Hospital

Program Director:
David R Cave, MD
Dept of Gastroenterology
736 Cambridge St
Boston, MA 02130
Tel: 617 789-2423 *Fax:* 617 789-2427
E-mail: drcave@pol.met
Accred Length: 2 Years *Program Size:* 5
Program ID: 144-24-21-057

Burlington

Lahey Clinic Program

Sponsor: Lahey Clinic
Beth Israel Deaconess Medical Center

Program Director:
Gale S Fiarman, MD
Richard P MacDermott, MD
Lahey Clinic
41 Mall Rd
Burlington, MA 01805
Tel: 781 744-8767 *Fax:* 781 744-5276
E-mail: elaine.miscovitch@lahey.org
Internet: http://www.lahey.org/
Accred Length: 2 Years *Program Size:* 6
Program ID: 144-24-21-141

Worcester

University of Massachusetts Program

Sponsor: University of Massachusetts Medical School
St Vincent Hospital
UMass Memorial Health Care (University Campus)

Program Director:
Herbert L Bonkovsky, MD
Univ of Massachusetts Med Sch
Div of Digestive Disease
55 Lake Ave N
Worcester, MA 01655
Tel: 508 856-3068 *Fax:* 508 856-3981
Internet: http://www.ummed.edu/dept/gastro
Accred Length: 2 Years *Program Size:* 6
Program ID: 144-24-21-008

Michigan

Ann Arbor

University of Michigan Program

Sponsor: University of Michigan Hospitals
Veterans Affairs Medical Center (Ann Arbor)

Program Director:
Chung Owyang, MD
Gastroenterology Div
Univ of Michigan Health Systems
3912 Taubman Ctr/Box 0362
Ann Arbor, MI 48109-0362
Tel: 313 936-6591 *Fax:* 313 936-7966
E-mail: forests@umich.edu
Accred Length: 2 Years *Program Size:* 13
Program ID: 144-25-21-077

Detroit

Henry Ford Hospital Program

Sponsor: Henry Ford Hospital

Program Director:
Surinder K Batra, MD
Henry Ford Hospital
Int Med/Gastroenterology
2799 W Grand Blvd
Detroit, MI 48202
Tel: 313 876-2408 *Fax:* 313 876-1633
Accred Length: 2 Years *Program Size:* 9
Program ID: 144-25-11-142

Wayne State University/Detroit Medical Center Program

Sponsor: Wayne State University/Detroit Medical Center
Detroit Receiving Hospital and University Health Center
Harper Hospital
Veterans Affairs Medical Center (Detroit)

Program Director:
Joseph L Kinzie, MD
Harper Hospital
3990 John R St
Detroit, MI 48201
Tel: 313 745-8601 *Fax:* 313 745-8843
Accred Length: 2 Years *Program Size:* 7
Program ID: 144-25-21-049

East Lansing

Michigan State University Program

Sponsor: Michigan State University College of Human Medicine

Program Director:
James E Mayle, MD
Dept of Med, B220 Life Sciences Bldg
Michigan State Univ
East Lansing, MI 48824-1317
Tel: 517 353-4811 *Fax:* 517 353-5436
Accred Length: 2 Years *Program Size:* 0
Program ID: 144-25-21-078

Royal Oak

William Beaumont Hospital Program

Sponsor: William Beaumont Hospital

Program Director:
Michael C Duffy, MD
William Beaumont Hospital
3601 W 13 Mile Rd
Royal Oak, MI 48073-6769
Tel: 248 551-5134 *Fax:* 248 551-8800
E-mail: adavid@beaumont.edu
Internet: http://www.beaumont.edu/html/gme
Accred Length: 2 Years *Program Size:* 3
Program ID: 144-25-12-180

Southfield

Providence Hospital and Medical Centers Program
Sponsor: Providence Hospital and Medical Centers
Program Director:
Eugene Gelzayd, MD
Providence Hospital
16001 W Nine Mile Rd
Southfield, MI 48075-4818
Tel: 248 424-3216 *Fax:* 248 424-5324
Accred Length: 2 Years *Program Size:* 2
Program ID: 144-25-11-178

Minnesota

Minneapolis

University of Minnesota Program
Sponsor: University of Minnesota Medical School
Fairview-University Medical Center
Veterans Affairs Medical Center (Minneapolis)
Program Director:
Roger L Gebhard, MD
VA Medical Center
One Veterans Dr
Box 111-D
Minneapolis, MN 55417-2399
Tel: 612 725-2034, ext 4100 *Fax:* 612 725-2248
Accred Length: 2 Years *Program Size:* 6
Program ID: 144-26-21-117

Rochester

Mayo Graduate School of Medicine (Rochester) Program
Sponsor: Mayo Graduate School of Medicine-Mayo Foundation
Mayo Clinic (Rochester)
Rochester Methodist Hospital
St Mary's Hospital of Rochester
Program Director:
John J Poterucha, MD
Application Processing Ctr
Siebens 5th Fl
Mayo Graduate Sch of Med
Rochester, MN 55905
Tel: 507 284-3126 *Fax:* 507 284-0999
Internet: http://www.mayo.edu/
Accred Length: 2 Years *Program Size:* 16
Program ID: 144-26-21-058

Mississippi

Jackson

University of Mississippi Medical Center Program
Sponsor: University of Mississippi School of Medicine
University Hospital
Veterans Affairs Medical Center (Jackson)
Program Director:
Makau Lee, MD
Univ of Mississippi Med Ctr
2500 N State St
Jackson, MS 39216
Tel: 601 984-4540 *Fax:* 601 984-4548
Accred Length: 2 Years *Program Size:* 6
Program ID: 144-27-21-079

Missouri

Columbia

University of Missouri-Columbia Program
Sponsor: University of Missouri-Columbia School of Medicine
Harry S Truman Memorial Veterans Hospital
University Hospitals and Clinics
Program Director:
Paul King, MD
MA 421 Health Sciences Ctr
Univ of Missouri Hospital
One Hospital Dr
Columbia, MO 65212
Tel: 573 882-1013 *Fax:* 573 884-4595
Internet:
http://www.hsc.missouri.edu/internal_medicine/gastro/
Accred Length: 2 Years *Program Size:* 5
Program ID: 144-28-21-080

Kansas City

University of Missouri at Kansas City Program
Sponsor: University of Missouri-Kansas City School of Medicine
Truman Medical Center-West
Program Director:
Stella G Quiason, MD
Univ of Missouri-Kansas City
2411 Holmes St
Kansas City, MO 64108
Tel: 816 276-1980 *Fax:* 816 556-3913
Accred Length: 2 Years *Program Size:* 3
Program ID: 144-28-31-118

St Louis

St Louis University School of Medicine Program
Sponsor: St Louis University School of Medicine
St Louis University School of Medicine
St Mary's Health Center
Veterans Affairs Medical Center (St Louis)
Program Director:
Bruce R Bacon, MD
St Louis Univ Sch of Med
3635 Vista Ave
PO Box 15250
St Louis, MO 63110-0250
Tel: 314 577-8764 *Fax:* 314 577-8125
E-mail: baconbr@wpogate.slu.edu
Internet:
http://www.slu.edu/departments/medicine/resid/resid/html
Accred Length: 2 Years *Program Size:* 9
Program ID: 144-28-21-182

Washington University/B-JH/SLCH Consortium (South Campus) Program
Sponsor: Washington University/B-JH/SLCH Consortium
Barnes-Jewish Hospital
Program Director:
Nicholas O Davidson, MD
Gastroenterology Div
Washington Univ
660 S Euclid Ave/Box 8124
St Louis, MO 63110
Tel: 314 362-8940 *Fax:* 314 362-8959
E-mail: nod@imgate.wustl.edu
Accred Length: 2 Years *Program Size:* 12
Program ID: 144-28-21-158

Nebraska

Omaha

University of Nebraska Program
Sponsor: University of Nebraska Medical Center
Veterans Affairs Medical Center (Omaha)
Program Director:
Renee L Young, MD
Univ of Nebraska Med Ctr
982000 Nebraska Med Ctr
Omaha, NE 68198-2000
Tel: 402 559-4356 *Fax:* 402 559-9004
E-mail: rlyoung@mail.unmc.edu
Internet: http://www.unmc.edu/gme/gi.htm
Accred Length: 2 Years *Program Size:* 5
Program ID: 144-30-21-160

New Hampshire

Lebanon

Dartmouth-Hitchcock Medical Center Program
Sponsor: Mary Hitchcock Memorial Hospital
Veterans Affairs Medical Center (White River Junction)
Program Director:
Richard I Rothstein, MD
Dartmouth-Hitchcock Med Ctr
One Medical Center Dr
Lebanon, NH 03756-0001
Tel: 603 650-5261 *Fax:* 603 650-5225
Accred Length: 2 Years *Program Size:* 3
Program ID: 144-32-21-150

New Jersey

Camden

UMDNJ-Robert Wood Johnson Medical School (Camden) Program
Sponsor: Cooper Hospital-University Medical Center
Program Director:
Steven R Peikin, MD
401 Haddon Ave
Camden, NJ 08103
Tel: 609 757-7732 *Fax:* 609 968-9564
Accred Length: 2 Years *Program Size:* 3
Program ID: 144-33-21-050

Newark

UMDNJ-New Jersey Medical School Program
Sponsor: UMDNJ-New Jersey Medical School
UMDNJ-University Hospital
Veterans Affairs Medical Center (East Orange)
Program Director:
Gerald Salen, MD
UMDNJ-New Jersey Med Sch
185 S Orange Ave
MSB H538
Newark, NJ 07103-2714
Tel: 973 972-5252 *Fax:* 973 972-3144
E-mail: saleng@umdnj.edu
Accred Length: 2 Years *Program Size:* 7
Program ID: 144-33-21-200

Piscataway

UMDNJ-Robert Wood Johnson Medical School Program

Sponsor: UMDNJ-Robert Wood Johnson Medical School
Robert Wood Johnson University Hospital
Veterans Affairs Medical Center (Lyons)
Program Director:
Kiron M Das, MD PhD
UMDNJ-Robert Wood Johnson Med Sch
Dept of Med
One Robert Wood Johnson Pl/CN 19
New Brunswick, NJ 08903-0019
Tel: 732 235-7784 *Fax:* 732 235-7792
Accred Length: 2 Years *Program Size:* 4
Program ID: 144-33-21-026

South Orange

Seton Hall University School of Graduate Medical Education Program

Sponsor: Seton Hall University School of Graduate Medical Education
St Joseph's Hospital and Medical Center
Program Director:
Walid Baddoura, MD
St Joseph's Hospital and Med Ctr
703 Main St
Paterson, NJ 07503
Tel: 973 754-2390 *Fax:* 973 754-2382
Accred Length: 2 Years *Program Size:* 5
Program ID: 144-33-21-051

New Mexico

Albuquerque

University of New Mexico Program

Sponsor: University of New Mexico School of Medicine
Lovelace Medical Center
University Hospital
Veterans Affairs Medical Center (Albuquerque)
Program Director:
Denis M McCarthy, MD
Univ of New Mexico Sch of Med
Dept of Med/Gastro
2211 Lomas Blvd NE/ACC-5
Albuquerque, NM 87131-5271
Tel: 505 272-4755 *Fax:* 505 272-4628
Accred Length: 2 Years *Program Size:* 5
Program ID: 144-34-21-143

New York

Albany

Albany Medical Center Program

Sponsor: Albany Medical Center
Program Director:
John B Rodgers, MD
Albany Med Coll
47 New Scotland Ave/MC-48
Albany, NY 12208-3479
Tel: 518 262-5276 *Fax:* 518 262-6470
Accred Length: 2 Years *Program Size:* 2
Program ID: 144-35-31-027

Bronx

Albert Einstein College of Medicine Program

Sponsor: Albert Einstein College of Medicine of Yeshiva University
Jacobi Medical Center
Montefiore Medical Center-Henry and Lucy Moses Division
North Central Bronx Hospital
Program Director:
Leslie H Bernstein, MD
Montefiore Med Ctr
Div of Gastroenterology
111 E 210th St
Bronx, NY 10467-2490
Tel: 718 920-4846 *Fax:* 718 798-6408
E-mail: lesbern@aecom.yu.edu
Accred Length: 2 Years *Program Size:* 9
Program ID: 144-35-21-102

Bronx-Lebanon Hospital Center Program

Sponsor: Bronx-Lebanon Hospital Center
Program Director:
Alan A Bloom, MD
Bronx-Lebanon Hospital Ctr
1650 Grand Concourse
Bronx, NY 10457
Tel: 718 518-5550 *Fax:* 718 518-5111
E-mail: alan@bloom.net
Accred Length: 2 Years *Program Size:* 6
Program ID: 144-35-11-103

New York Medical College (Our Lady of Mercy) Program

Sponsor: New York Medical College
Our Lady of Mercy Medical Center
Program Director:
C S Pitchumoni, MD
Our Lady of Mercy Med Ctr
Dept of Med
600 E 233rd St
Bronx, NY 10466
Tel: 718 920-9692 *Fax:* 718 920-9036
E-mail: olmmcmeded@aol.com
Accred Length: 2 Years *Program Size:* 3
Program ID: 144-35-21-043

Brooklyn

Brooklyn Hospital Center Program

Sponsor: Brooklyn Hospital Center
Program Director:
Maurice A Cerulli, MD
Brooklyn Hospital Ctr
121 DeKalb Ave
Brooklyn, NY 11201
Tel: 718 250-6945 *Fax:* 718 250-6489
Accred Length: 2 Years *Program Size:* 4
Program ID: 144-35-12-185

Interfaith Medical Center Program

Sponsor: Interfaith Medical Center
Memorial Sloan-Kettering Cancer Center
Program Director:
Franklin Marsh, MD
Interfaith Med Ctr
555 Prospect Pl
Brooklyn, NY 11238
Tel: 718 935-7325 *Fax:* 718 935-7588
Accred Length: 2 Years *Program Size:* 3
Program ID: 144-35-21-186

Long Island College Hospital Program

Sponsor: Long Island College Hospital
Woodhull Medical and Mental Health Center
Program Director:
Irwin M Grosman, MD
Long Island College Hospital
339 Hicks St
Brooklyn, NY 11201
Tel: 718 780-1738 *Fax:* 718 780-1391
Accred Length: 2 Years *Program Size:* 4
Program ID: 144-35-11-069

Maimonides Medical Center Program

Sponsor: Maimonides Medical Center
Program Director:
Eliot H Zimbalist, MD
Maimonides Med Ctr
4802 Tenth Ave
Brooklyn, NY 11219
Tel: 718 283-7476 *Fax:* 718 283-8630
Accred Length: 2 Years *Program Size:* 3
Program ID: 144-35-11-162

SUNY Health Science Center at Brooklyn Program

Sponsor: SUNY Health Science Center at Brooklyn
Brookdale University Hospital Medical Center
Kings County Hospital Center
St John's Episcopal Hospital-South Shore
Staten Island University Hospital
University Hospital-SUNY Health Science Center at Brooklyn
Veterans Affairs Medical Center (Brooklyn)
Program Director:
Eugene W Straus, MD
SUNY-Brooklyn
450 Clarkson Ave
Brooklyn, NY 11203
Tel: 718 270-1112 *Fax:* 718 270-3107
Accred Length: 2 Years *Program Size:* 15
Program ID: 144-35-21-011

Buffalo

SUNY at Buffalo Graduate Medical-Dental Education Consortium Program

Sponsor: SUNY at Buffalo Grad Medical-Dental Education Consortium
CGF Health System (Buffalo General Hospital)
Erie County Medical Center
Roswell Park Cancer Institute
Veterans Affairs Medical Center (Buffalo)
Program Director:
M P Lance, MD
Div of Gastroenterology
Buffalo General Hospital
100 High St
Buffalo, NY 14203
Tel: 716 859-2508 *Fax:* 716 859-2009
E-mail: plance@acsu.buffalo.edu
Internet:
http://www.smbs.buffalo.edu/med/gastro/index.html
Accred Length: 2 Years *Program Size:* 7
Program ID: 144-35-31-009

East Meadow

SUNY at Stony Brook (East Meadow) Program

Sponsor: Nassau County Medical Center

Program Director:
Crescens P Pellecchia, MD
Nassau County Med Ctr
Div of Gastroenterology
2201 Hempstead Trnpk
East Meadow, NY 11554-5400
Tel: 516 572-6573 *Fax:* 516 572-5609
Accred Length: 2 Years *Program Size:* 3
Program ID: 144-35-21-090

Elmhurst

Mount Sinai School of Medicine (Elmhurst) Program

Sponsor: Mount Sinai School of Medicine
Elmhurst Hospital Center-Mount Sinai Services
Mount Sinai Medical Center

Program Director:
Vivek V Gumaste, MD
Elmhurst Hospital Ctr
Dept of Int Med
79-01 Broadway
Elmhurst, NY 11373
Tel: 718 334-2288
Accred Length: 2 Years *Program Size:* 3
Program ID: 144-35-11-119

Flushing

New York Hospital Medical Center of Queens/Cornell University Medical College Program

Sponsor: New York Hospital Medical Center of Queens

Program Director:
George T Martin, MD
New York Hospital Med Ctr of Queens
56-45 Main St
Flushing, NY 11355-2966
Tel: 718 670-1070 *Fax:* 718 461-2943
E-mail: gtmartin%queens@nyh.med.cornell.edu
Internet: http://www.nyhq.org
Accred Length: 2 Years *Program Size:* 3
Program ID: 144-35-11-091

Manhasset

North Shore University Hospital/NYU School of Medicine Program

Sponsor: North Shore University Hospital

Program Director:
Gerard Mullin, MD
North Shore Univ Hospital
Dept of Med
300 Community Dr
Manhasset, NY 11030
Tel: 516 562-4281 *Fax:* 516 562-2683
E-mail: gerard@nshs.edu
Accred Length: 2 Years *Program Size:* 3
Program ID: 144-35-21-170

Mineola

Winthrop-University Hospital Program

Sponsor: Winthrop-University Hospital

Program Director:
Robert Burakoff, MD
Winthrop-Univ Hospital
222 Station Plaza N/Ste 429
Mineola, NY 11501-3893
Tel: 516 663-2527 *Fax:* 516 663-4617
E-mail: rburakof@winthrop.org
Accred Length: 2 Years *Program Size:* 3
Program ID: 144-35-11-109

New Hyde Park

Albert Einstein College of Medicine at Long Island Jewish Medical Center Program

Sponsor: Long Island Jewish Medical Center
Queens Hospital Center

Program Director:
Simmy Bank, MD
Long Island Jewish Med Ctr
270-05 76th Ave
New Hyde Park, NY 11040
Tel: 718 470-4692 *Fax:* 718 343-0128
Internet: http://www.lij.edu
Accred Length: 2 Years *Program Size:* 4
Program ID: 144-35-21-144

New York

Albert Einstein College of Medicine at Beth Israel Medical Center Program

Sponsor: Beth Israel Medical Center

Program Director:
Alvin M Gelb, MD
Beth Israel Med Ctr
Dept of Gastroenterology
First Ave at 16th St
New York, NY 10003
Tel: 212 420-4015 *Fax:* 212 420-4373
E-mail: agelb@bethisrael.org
Internet: http://www.bethisraelny.org.
Accred Length: 2 Years *Program Size:* 3
Program ID: 144-35-11-010

Harlem Hospital Center Program

Sponsor: Harlem Hospital Center

Program Director:
Lisa A Ozick, MD
Harlem Hospital Ctr
506 Lenox Ave
New York, NY 10037
Tel: 212 939-1430 *Fax:* 212 939-1432
E-mail: lao3@columbia.edu
Accred Length: 2 Years *Program Size:* 3
Program ID: 144-35-11-172

Lenox Hill Hospital Program

Sponsor: Lenox Hill Hospital

Program Director:
Burton I Korelitz, MD
Lenox Hill Hospital
100 E 77th St
New York, NY 10021-1883
Tel: 212 434-2140 *Fax:* 212 434-2446
Accred Length: 2 Years *Program Size:* 3
Program ID: 144-35-11-194

Mount Sinai School of Medicine (Cabrini) Program

Sponsor: Mount Sinai School of Medicine
Cabrini Medical Center

Program Director:
Herbert Dyrzska, MD
Cabrini Med Ctr
227 E 19th St
New York, NY 10003
Tel: 212 995-6934 *Fax:* 212 979-3442
Accred Length: 2 Years *Program Size:* 2
Program ID: 144-35-31-098

Mount Sinai School of Medicine Program

Sponsor: Mount Sinai School of Medicine
Elmhurst Hospital Center-Mount Sinai Services
Mount Sinai Medical Center
Queens Hospital Center
Veterans Affairs Medical Center (Bronx)

Program Director:
David B Sachar, MD
Mount Sinai Hospital
One Gustave L Levy Pl
Box 1069
New York, NY 10029-6574
Tel: 212 241-6749 *Fax:* 212 987-5584
E-mail: sharon_nieman@smtplink.mssm.edu
Accred Length: 2 Years *Program Size:* 13
Program ID: 144-35-31-163

New York and Presbyterian Hospital (Columbia Campus) Program

Sponsor: New York and Presbyterian Hospital
New York and Presbyterian Hospital (Columbia Campus)

Program Director:
Michael Field, MD
Columbia-Presbyterian Med Ctr
PS 10-508
630 W 168th St
New York, NY 10032
Tel: 212 305-8156 *Fax:* 212 305-6443
E-mail: mf9@columbia.edu
Internet: http://www.cpmcnet.columbia.edu/dept/gi
Accred Length: 2 Years *Program Size:* 8
Program ID: 144-35-11-070

New York and Presbyterian Hospital (Cornell Campus) Program 2

Sponsor: Memorial Sloan-Kettering Cancer Center

Program Director:
Robert C Kurtz, MD
Memorial Sloan-Kettering Cancer Ctr
1275 York Ave
New York, NY 10021
Tel: 212 639-8286 *Fax:* 212 639-2766
E-mail: kurtzr@mskcc.org
Internet: http://www.mskcc.org
Accred Length: 2 Years *Program Size:* 6
Program ID: 144-35-21-179

New York and Presbyterian Hospital (Cornell Campus) Program

Sponsor: New York and Presbyterian Hospital
New York and Presbyterian Hospital (Cornell Campus)
New York Methodist Hospital

Program Director:
Suzanne Rose, MD
New York Hospital
520 E 70th St
Ste J-314
New York, NY 10021
Tel: 212 746-4404 *Fax:* 212 746-8696
Accred Length: 2 Years *Program Size:* 4
Program ID: 144-35-21-171

New York Medical College at St Vincent's Hospital and Medical Center of New York Program

Sponsor: New York Medical College
St Vincent's Hospital and Medical Center of New York

Program Director:
James Robilotti, MD
St Vincent's Hospital and Med Ctr
153 W 11th St
New York, NY 10011
Tel: 212 604-8325 *Fax:* 212 604-8446
Internet: http://svh.nymc.edu
Accred Length: 2 Years *Program Size:* 4
Program ID: 144-35-11-029

New York University Medical Center Program
Sponsor: New York University Medical Center
Bellevue Hospital Center
Program Director:
Arthur Lindner, MD
Robert Raicht, MD
New York Univ Med Ctr
550 First Ave
New York, NY 10016
Tel: 212 263-7270 *Fax:* 212 263-0205
Accred Length: 2 Years *Program Size:* 6
Program ID: 144-35-21-120

St Luke's-Roosevelt Hospital Center Program
Sponsor: St Luke's-Roosevelt Hospital Center
St Luke's-Roosevelt Hospital Center-Roosevelt Division
St Luke's-Roosevelt Hospital Center-St Luke's Division
Program Director:
Peter R Holt, MD
St Luke's-Roosevelt Hospital Ctr
1111 Amsterdam Ave
New York, NY 10025
Tel: 212 523-3680 *Fax:* 212 523-3683
Accred Length: 2 Years *Program Size:* 6
Program ID: 144-35-21-105

Rochester

University of Rochester Program
Sponsor: Strong Memorial Hospital of the University of Rochester
Genesee Hospital
St Mary's Hospital (Unity Health System)
Program Director:
William Y Chey, MD MS MD
Strong Memorial Hospital
601 Elmwood Ave
PO Box 646
Rochester, NY 14642
Tel: 716 275-4713 *Fax:* 716 271-7868
E-mail: williamy_chey@urmc.rochester.edu
Accred Length: 2 Years *Program Size:* 5
Program ID: 144-35-21-220

Stony Brook

SUNY at Stony Brook Program
Sponsor: University Hospital-SUNY at Stony Brook
Veterans Affairs Medical Center (Northport)
Program Director:
Edward H Cheng, MD
Health Science Ctr
Div of Gastro/Hepatology
T-17/Rm 060
Stony Brook, NY 11794-8173
Tel: 516 444-2119 *Fax:* 516 444-8886
E-mail: cheng.edward@northport.va.gov
Accred Length: 2 Years *Program Size:* 5
Program ID: 144-35-21-012

Syracuse

SUNY Health Science Center at Syracuse Program
Sponsor: University Hospital-SUNY Health Science Center at Syracuse
Veterans Affairs Medical Center (Syracuse)
Program Director:
Philip G Holtzapple, MD
Dept of Med
SUNY Health Science Ctr
750 E Adams St
Syracuse, NY 13210
Tel: 315 464-5804 *Fax:* 315 464-5797
E-mail: holtzapp@vax.cs.hscsyr.edu
Accred Length: 2 Years *Program Size:* 3
Program ID: 144-35-21-106

Valhalla

New York Medical College at Westchester Medical Center Program
Sponsor: New York Medical College
Lincoln Medical and Mental Health Center
Metropolitan Hospital Center
Westchester Medical Center
Program Director:
Edward Lebovics, MD
New York Med Coll
Div of Gastro/Hepatobiliary Diseases
Munger Pavilion/Rm 206
Valhalla, NY 10595
Tel: 914 493-7337 *Fax:* 914 594-4317
Internet: http://www.nymc.edu
Accred Length: 2 Years *Program Size:* 7
Program ID: 144-35-11-013

North Carolina

Chapel Hill

University of North Carolina Hospitals Program
Sponsor: University of North Carolina Hospitals
Program Director:
Kim L Isaacs, MD PhD
Univ of North Carolina Sch of Med
326 Burnette-Womack Bldg/CB7080
Chapel Hill, NC 27599-7080
Tel: 919 966-2511 *Fax:* 919 966-6842
E-mail: klisaacs@med.unc.edu
Accred Length: 2 Years *Program Size:* 9
Program ID: 144-36-21-145

Durham

Duke University Program
Sponsor: Duke University Medical Center
Veterans Affairs Medical Center (Durham)
Program Director:
Rodger A Liddle, MD
Duke Univ Med Ctr
Int Med/Gastroenterology
Box 3913
Durham, NC 27710
Tel: 919 684-5066 *Fax:* 919 684-8857
Accred Length: 2 Years *Program Size:* 10
Program ID: 144-36-21-146

Greenville

East Carolina University Program
Sponsor: East Carolina University School of Medicine
Pitt County Memorial Hospital
Program Director:
Balbir S Minhas, MD MD
East Carolina Univ Sch of Med
Dept of Med/Gastroenterology
PCMH-TA 308
Greenville, NC 28590
Tel: 252 816-4652 *Fax:* 252 816-8426
E-mail: mddamone@ecuvm1.cis.ecu.edu
Internet: http://www.med.ecu.edu/medicine/gi
Accred Length: 2 Years *Program Size:* 2
Program ID: 144-36-21-219

Winston-Salem

Wake Forest University School of Medicine Program
Sponsor: Wake Forest University Baptist Medical Center
Program Director:
Richard B Weinberg, MD
Wake Forest Univ Sch of Med
Medical Center Blvd
Winston-Salem, NC 27157-1048
Tel: 910 716-4612 *Fax:* 910 716-6376
Accred Length: 2 Years *Program Size:* 4
Program ID: 144-36-21-014

Ohio

Cincinnati

University Hospital/University of Cincinnati College of Medicine Program
Sponsor: University Hospital Inc
Veterans Affairs Medical Center (Cincinnati)
Program Director:
Kenneth E Sherman, MD PhD
Univ of Cincinnati Coll of Med
231 Bethesda Ave
ML 0595
Cincinnati, OH 45267-0595
Tel: 513 558-5244 *Fax:* 513 558-1744
E-mail: kenneth.sherman@uc.edu
Internet:
http://www.med.uc.edu/departme/digest/uc1.htm
Accred Length: 2 Years *Program Size:* 5
Program ID: 144-38-21-081

Cleveland

Case Western Reserve University (MetroHealth) Program
Sponsor: MetroHealth Medical Center
Program Director:
Kevin D Mullen, MD
MetroHealth Med Ctr
2500 MetroHealth Dr
Cleveland, OH 44109-1998
Tel: 216 778-5736 *Fax:* 216 778-4873
E-mail: kdm@po.cwru.edu
Accred Length: 2 Years *Program Size:* 6
Program ID: 144-38-11-165

Case Western Reserve University Program
Sponsor: University Hospitals of Cleveland
Veterans Affairs Medical Center (Cleveland)
Program Director:
Gregory Cooper, MD
Univ Hospitals of Cleveland
Div of Gastroenterology
11100 Euclid Ave
Cleveland, OH 44106-5066
Tel: 216 844-5386 *Fax:* 216 844-8011
E-mail: gxc12@po.cwru.edu
Accred Length: 2 Years *Program Size:* 6
Program ID: 144-38-21-164

Cleveland Clinic Foundation Program
Sponsor: Cleveland Clinic Foundation

Program Director:
John J Vargo, MD
Dept of Gastroenterology/S40
Cleveland Clinic Foundation
9500 Euclid Ave
Cleveland, OH 44195-5242
Tel: 216 444-5690 *Fax:* 216 444-1162
E-mail: meded@cestmp.ccf.org
Internet: http://www.ccf.org
Accred Length: 2 Years *Program Size:* 8
Program ID: 144-38-12-166

Columbus

Ohio State University Program
Sponsor: Ohio State University Medical Center

Program Director:
Sheryl A Pfeil, MD
Ohio State Univ Hospital
Div of Gastroenterology
410 W Tenth Ave N213 Doan Hall
Columbus, OH 43210
Tel: 614 293-4262 *Fax:* 614 293-8518
E-mail: pfeil.4@osu.edu
Accred Length: 2 Years *Program Size:* 5
Program ID: 144-38-11-092

Dayton

Wright State University Program
Sponsor: Wright State University School of Medicine
Veterans Affairs Medical Center (Dayton)
Wright-Patterson Medical Center

Program Director:
N Gopalswamy, MD
Wright State Univ Sch of Med
Dept of Med
4100 W Third St (111W)
Dayton, OH 45428
Tel: 937 262-0201 *Fax:* 937 267-5310
E-mail: sbush@discover.wright.edu
Accred Length: 2 Years *Program Size:* 3
Program ID: 144-38-21-099

Oklahoma

Oklahoma City

University of Oklahoma Health Sciences Center Program
Sponsor: University of Oklahoma College of Medicine
University Hospital
Veterans Affairs Medical Center (Oklahoma City)

Program Director:
Richard F Harty, MD
Digestive Dis/Nutrition Sect
Univ of Oklahoma Health Sciences Ctr
UH7NP526 Box 26307
Oklahoma City, OK 73126-0307
Tel: 405 271-5428 *Fax:* 405 271-5803
E-mail: richard-harty@ouhsc.edu
Accred Length: 2 Years *Program Size:* 4
Program ID: 144-39-21-082

Oregon

Portland

Oregon Health Sciences University Program
Sponsor: Oregon Health Sciences University Hospital
Veterans Affairs Medical Center (Portland)

Program Director:
Kenneth D Flora, MD
Oregon Health Sciences Univ
Div of Gastroenterology/PV-310
Portland, OR 97201-3098
Tel: 503 494-8577 *Fax:* 503 494-7556
E-mail: florak@ohsu.edu
Accred Length: 2 Years *Program Size:* 6
Program ID: 144-40-31-167

Pennsylvania

Danville

Penn State Geisinger Health System/Geisinger Medical Center Program
Sponsor: Penn State Geisinger Health System
Geisinger Medical Center

Program Director:
Michael Komar, MD
Geisinger Med Ctr
Dept of Gastro/Nutrition
100 N Academy Ave
Danville, PA 17822-2111
Tel: 717 271-6405 *Fax:* 717 271-6852
E-mail: ckrebs@psghs.edu
Accred Length: 2 Years *Program Size:* 3
Program ID: 144-41-21-211

Hershey

Penn State Geisinger Health System/Milton S Hershey Medical Center Program
Sponsor: Penn State Geisinger Health System
Milton S Hershey Medical Center
Veterans Affairs Medical Center (Lebanon)

Program Director:
Ann Ouyang, MD
Milton S Hershey Med Ctr-Penn State Geisinger Health System
Gastroenterology/MC H045
PO Box 850
Hershey, PA 17033-0850
Tel: 717 531-8741 *Fax:* 717 531-6770
Accred Length: 2 Years *Program Size:* 5
Program ID: 144-41-11-015

Philadelphia

Albert Einstein Medical Center Program
Sponsor: Albert Einstein Medical Center

Program Director:
Gary M Levine, MD
Div of Gastroenterology
5501 Old York Rd
Klein PO Box 350
Philadelphia, PA 19141
Tel: 215 456-8210 *Fax:* 215 455-1933
Accred Length: 2 Years *Program Size:* 3
Program ID: 144-41-31-218

Graduate Hospital Program
Sponsor: Graduate Hospital

Program Director:
Steven A Edmundowicz, MD
One Graduate Plaza
Philadelphia, PA 19146
Tel: 215 893-6168 *Fax:* 215 893-6154
E-mail: dkatzka@mem.po.com
Accred Length: 2 Years *Program Size:* 6
Program ID: 144-41-11-187

MCP Hahnemann University Program
Sponsor: MCP Hahnemann University
Episcopal Hospital (TUHS)
Medical College of Pennsylvania Hospital

Program Director:
James C Reynolds, MD
MCP Hahnemann Univ
Broad and Vine Sts
MS 131
Philadelphia, PA 19102
Tel: 215 762-8101 *Fax:* 215 246-5432
Accred Length: 2 Years *Program Size:* 4
Program ID: 144-41-21-122

Temple University Program
Sponsor: Temple University Hospital

Program Director:
Robert S Fisher, MD
Temple Univ Hospital
3401 N Broad St
Philadelphia, PA 19140
Tel: 215 707-3433 *Fax:* 215 707-2684
E-mail: krevsky@vm.temple.edu
Internet: http://www.temple.edu/gisection
Accred Length: 2 Years *Program Size:* 7
Program ID: 144-41-21-033

Thomas Jefferson University Program
Sponsor: Thomas Jefferson University Hospital

Program Director:
Anthony J DiMarino Jr, MD
Div of Gastroenterology
132 S 10th St
480 Main Bldg
Philadelphia, PA 19107
Tel: 215 955-8900 *Fax:* 215 955-0872
Internet: http://jeffline.tsu.edu/cwis/dept/gi
Accred Length: 2 Years *Program Size:* 9
Program ID: 144-41-21-034

University of Pennsylvania Program
Sponsor: Hospital of the University of Pennsylvania
Presbyterian Medical Center (UPHS)

Program Director:
Anil K Rustgi, MD
Univ of Pennsylvania Health System
GI Div, 3 Ravdin HUP
3400 Spruce St
Philadelphia, PA 19104-6144
Tel: 215 898-0154 *Fax:* 215 812-1320
E-mail: anil2@mail-med.upenn.edu
Internet: http://www.med.upenn.edu/~gicenter
Accred Length: 2 Years *Program Size:* 12
Program ID: 144-41-21-021

Pittsburgh

Allegheny General Hospital Program
Sponsor: Allegheny General Hospital

Program Director:
Rad M Agrawal, MD
Allegheny General Hospital
Div of Gastroenterology
320 E North Ave
Pittsburgh, PA 15212-4772
Tel: 412 359-3846 *Fax:* 412 359-3484
Accred Length: 2 Years *Program Size:* 6
Program ID: 144-41-11-045

Programs

Shadyside Hospital/UPMC Program
Sponsor: Shadyside Hospital/UPMC

Program Director:
Farhad Ismail-Beigi, MD
UPMC Shadyside
Med Educ
5230 Centre Ave
Pittsburgh, PA 15232
Tel: 412 623-2296 *Fax:* 412 683-0191
Internet: http://ssh.edu
Accred Length: 2 Years *Program Size:* 3
Program ID: 144-41-22-035

University Health Center of Pittsburgh Program
Sponsor: University Health Center of Pittsburgh
Presbyterian University Hospital/UPMC
Veterans Affairs Medical Center (Pittsburgh)

Program Director:
Arnold Wald, MD
Presbyterian Univ Hospital
Div of GI/Hepatology
Mezzanine Level/C-Wing
Pittsburgh, PA 15213-2582
Tel: 412 648-9241 *Fax:* 412 648-9378
E-mail: wald@med1.dept-med.pitt.edu
Accred Length: 2 Years *Program Size:* 10
Program ID: 144-41-21-060

Western Pennsylvania Hospital Program
Sponsor: Western Pennsylvania Hospital

Program Director:
Robert J Kania, MD
Western Pennsylvania Hospital
Dept of Med
4800 Friendship Ave
Pittsburgh, PA 15224
Tel: 412 578-5272 *Fax:* 412 578-6804
E-mail: intermedwph@yahoo.com
Internet: http://www.pitt.edu/~westpenn/westpenn.html
Accred Length: 2 Years *Program Size:* 3
Program ID: 144-41-11-046

Wynnewood

Lankenau Hospital Program
Sponsor: Lankenau Hospital

Program Director:
Giancarlo Mercogliano, MD
Lankenau Hospital
252 Lankenau Medical Bldg East
100 Lancaster Ave W of City Line
Wynnewood, PA 19096
Tel: 610 896-7360 *Fax:* 610 896-5207
Accred Length: 2 Years *Program Size:* 3
Program ID: 144-41-11-032

Puerto Rico

Ponce

Hospital de Damas Program
Sponsor: Hospital de Damas
Ponce University Hospital

Program Director:
Alvaro Reymunde, MD
Hospital de Damas
Dept de Educacion Medica
2213 Ponce By Pass
Ponce, PR 00731-7779
Tel: 787 840-8686, ext 7369
Accred Length: 2 Years *Program Size:* 3
Program ID: 144-42-11-206

San Juan

University of Puerto Rico Program
Sponsor: University of Puerto Rico School of Medicine
University Hospital
Veterans Affairs Medical Center (San Juan)

Program Director:
Esther A Torres, MD
Univ of Puerto Rico Sch of Med
Dept of Med
PO Box 365067
San Juan, PR 00936-5067
Tel: 787 751-6034 *Fax:* 787 754-1739
E-mail: etorres@pol.net
Accred Length: 2 Years *Program Size:* 6
Program ID: 144-42-21-124

Rhode Island

Providence

Brown University Program
Sponsor: Rhode Island Hospital
Roger Williams Medical Center
Veterans Affairs Medical Center (Providence)

Program Director:
Jose Behar, MD
Rhode Island Hospital
GI Unit APC 421
593 Eddy St
Providence, RI 02903
Tel: 401 444-5031 *Fax:* 401 444-6194
Accred Length: 2 Years *Program Size:* 6
Program ID: 144-43-11-125

South Carolina

Charleston

Medical University of South Carolina Program
Sponsor: Medical University of South Carolina College of Medicine
MUSC Medical Center
Ralph H Johnson Dept of Veterans Affairs Med Center

Program Director:
Frederick A Wilson, MD
Div of Gastroenterology 916 CSB
Med Univ of South Carolina
171 Ashley Ave
Charleston, SC 29425-2223
Tel: 803 792-2301 *Fax:* 803 792-8395
Accred Length: 2 Years *Program Size:* 6
Program ID: 144-45-21-107

Columbia

Palmetto Health Alliance/University of South Carolina School of Medicine Program
Sponsor: Palmetto Health Alliance
Palmetto Richland Memorial Hospital
William Jennings Bryan Dorn Veterans Hospital

Program Director:
Rajeev Vasudeva, MD
Div of Digestive Dis/Nutrition
2 Richland Medical Pk/Ste 502
Columbia, SC 29203
Tel: 803 540-1000, ext 1012 *Fax:* 803 540-1050
E-mail: rvasude@richmed.medpark.sc.edu
Accred Length: 2 Years *Program Size:* 5
Program ID: 144-45-21-093

Tennessee

Johnson City

East Tennessee State University Program
Sponsor: James H Quillen College of Medicine
Johnson City Medical Center Hospital
Veterans Affairs Medical Center (Mountain Home)

Program Director:
Thomas Borthwick, MD
East Tennessee State Univ
Dept of Int Med
Box 70622
Johnson City, TN 37614-0622
Tel: 423 929-7111
Accred Length: 2 Years *Program Size:* 2
Program ID: 144-47-21-084

Memphis

University of Tennessee Program
Sponsor: University of Tennessee College of Medicine
Regional Medical Center at Memphis
Veterans Affairs Medical Center (Memphis)

Program Director:
Christopher R Marino, MD
Univ of Tennessee
951 Court Ave
Rm 555/Dobbs
Memphis, TN 38163
Tel: 901 448-5813 *Fax:* 901 448-7091
E-mail: mwilliams@utmem1.utmem.edu
Internet: http://utmggi1.utmem.edu/gi_fellowship.html
Accred Length: 2 Years *Program Size:* 6
Program ID: 144-47-21-188

Nashville

Vanderbilt University Program
Sponsor: Vanderbilt University Medical Center
St Thomas Hospital
Veterans Affairs Medical Center (Nashville)

Program Director:
Raymond N DuBois, MD
Vanderbilt Univ
23rd and Garland
MCN C-2104
Nashville, TN 37232-2279
Tel: 615 343-4747 *Fax:* 615 343-6229
Internet: http://www.mc.vanderbilt.edu
Accred Length: 2 Years *Program Size:* 7
Program ID: 144-47-31-016

Texas

Dallas

Baylor University Medical Center Program
Sponsor: Baylor University Medical Center

Program Director:
Lawrence R Schiller, MD
Baylor Univ Med Ctr
3500 Gaston Ave
Dallas, TX 75246
Tel: 214 820-2671 *Fax:* 214 818-8179
E-mail: lrsmd@aol.com
Accred Length: 2 Years *Program Size:* 4
Program ID: 144-48-31-148

University of Texas Southwestern Medical School Program

Sponsor: University of Texas Southwestern Medical School
Dallas County Hospital District-Parkland Memorial Hospital
Veterans Affairs Medical Center (Dallas)
Program Director:
Walter L Peterson, MD
Univ of Texas Southwestern Med Ctr
Dallas VA Med Ctr (111B1)
4500 S Lancaster Rd
Dallas, TX 75216-7191
Tel: 214 371-2464 *Fax:* 214 857-1571
E-mail: enright.julie@dallas.va.gov
Accred Length: 2 Years *Program Size:* 10
Program ID: 144-48-21-100

Galveston

University of Texas Medical Branch Hospitals Program

Sponsor: University of Texas Medical Branch Hospitals
Program Director:
Roger D Soloway, MD
4106 John McCullough Bldg G64
Univ of Texas Med Branch
301 University Blvd
Galveston, TX 77555-0764
Tel: 409 772-1501 *Fax:* 409 772-4789
E-mail: rsoloway@utmb.edu
Internet: http://www.utmb.edu
Accred Length: 2 Years *Program Size:* 9
Program ID: 144-48-21-062

Houston

Baylor College of Medicine Program

Sponsor: Baylor College of Medicine
Harris County Hospital District-Ben Taub General Hospital
Methodist Hospital
Veterans Affairs Medical Center (Houston)
Program Director:
Richard W Goodgame, MD
Baylor Coll of Med
Med-Gastroenterology
One Baylor Plaza/Rm 525D
Houston, TX 77030
Tel: 713 798-6679 *Fax:* 713 797-1849
E-mail: goodgame@bcm.tmc.edu
Internet: http://www.bcm.tmc.edu/gastro/
Accred Length: 2 Years *Program Size:* 8
Program ID: 144-48-21-085

University of Texas at Houston Program

Sponsor: University of Texas Medical School at Houston
Lyndon B Johnson General Hospital
Memorial Hermann Healthcare System
University of Texas M D Anderson Cancer Center
Program Director:
Joseph H Sellin, MD
Univ of Texas Med Sch, Dept of Med
PO Box 20708
Houston, TX 77025
Tel: 713 500-6677 *Fax:* 713 500-6699
E-mail: jsellin@heart.med.uth.tmc.edu
Accred Length: 2 Years *Program Size:* 8
Program ID: 144-48-31-017

Lackland AFB

San Antonio Uniformed Services Health Education Consortium (BAMC) Program

Sponsor: San Antonio Uniformed Services Health Education Consortium
Brooke Army Medical Center
Program Director:
Shailesh C Kadakia, MD
Brooke Army Med Ctr
Attn: Medical Education (P Bolt)
3851 Roger Brooke Dr
Fort Sam Houston, TX 78219-6200
Tel: 210 916-4578 *Fax:* 210 916-3195
E-mail: col shailesh kadakia@medcen1111_bamc
Accred Length: 2 Years *Program Size:* 9
Program ID: 144-48-12-147
US Armed Services Program

San Antonio Uniformed Services Health Education Consortium (WHMC) Program

Sponsor: San Antonio Uniformed Services Health Education Consortium
Wilford Hall Medical Center (AETC)
Program Director:
Shailesh C Kadakia, MD
59th Med Wing/MMIG
Attn: Col Kadakia
2200 Bergquist Dr/Ste 1
Lackland AFB, TX 78236-5300
Tel: 210 292-6470 *Fax:* 210 292-7660
E-mail:
col_shailesh_kadakia@bamc.smtplink.amedd.army.mil
Accred Length: 2 Years *Program Size:* 18
Program ID: 144-48-12-063
US Armed Services Program

Lubbock

Texas Tech University (Lubbock) Program

Sponsor: Texas Tech University Health Sciences Center at Lubbock
University Medical Center
Program Director:
David S Hodges, MD
Texas Tech Univ Health Sciences Ctr
Div of Gastroenterology
3601 Fourth St
Lubbock, TX 79430
Tel: 806 743-3155 *Fax:* 806 743-3148
E-mail: meddsh@ttuhsc.edu
Accred Length: 2 Years *Program Size:* 3
Program ID: 144-48-21-195

San Antonio

University of Texas Health Science Center at San Antonio Program

Sponsor: University of Texas Medical School at San Antonio
Audie L Murphy Memorial Veterans Hospital (San Antonio)
University Hospital-South Texas Medical Center
Program Director:
Charles E Brady, MD
Univ of Texas Health Science Ctr
Div of Gastro/Nutrition
7703 Floyd Curl Dr
San Antonio, TX 78284-7878
Tel: 210 691-6514 *Fax:* 210 567-1976
E-mail: mundym@uthscsa.edu
Accred Length: 2 Years *Program Size:* 6
Program ID: 144-48-21-072

Temple

Texas A&M College of Medicine-Scott and White Program

Sponsor: Scott and White Memorial Hospital
Program Director:
Richard A Erickson, MD
Texas A&M-Scott and White
Div of Gastroenterology
2401 S 31st St
Temple, TX 76508
Tel: 800 299-4463, ext 47633 *Fax:* 254 724-9280
E-mail: blculp@swmail.sw.org
Accred Length: 2 Years *Program Size:* 6
Program ID: 144-48-21-018

Utah

Salt Lake City

University of Utah Program

Sponsor: University of Utah Medical Center
Veterans Affairs Medical Center (Salt Lake City)
Program Director:
Randall W Burt, MD
Univ of Utah Sch of Med
50 N Medical Dr/Rm 4R118
Salt Lake City, UT 84132
Tel: 801 581-7802 *Fax:* 801 581-7476
Accred Length: 2 Years *Program Size:* 5
Program ID: 144-49-21-168

Vermont

Burlington

University of Vermont Program

Sponsor: Fletcher Allen Health Care
Program Director:
Nicholas Ferrentino, MD
Division of Gastroenterology + Hepatology
UVM College of Medicine
Burgess 414
Burlington, VT 05401
Tel: 802 656-2554 *Fax:* 802 656-4928
E-mail: nicholas.ferrentino@vtmednet.org
Accred Length: 2 Years *Program Size:* 3
Program ID: 144-50-21-169

Virginia

Charlottesville

University of Virginia Program

Sponsor: University of Virginia Medical Center
Veterans Affairs Medical Center (Salem)
Program Director:
Fabio Cominelli, MD PhD
Mark Worthington, MD
Univ of Virginia Health Sciences Ctr
Div of Gastro/Hepatology
PO Box 10013
Charlottesville, VA 22906-0013
Tel: 804 243-6400 *Fax:* 804 243-6405
E-mail: fc4q@virginia.edu
Internet: http://maz6rpc.med.virginia.edu/gi/default.htm
Accred Length: 2 Years *Program Size:* 10
Program ID: 144-51-21-019

Richmond

Medical College of Virginia/Virginia Commonwealth University Program
Sponsor: Medical College of Virginia/Virginia Commonwealth University
Medical College of Virginia Hospitals
Program Director:
Z Reno Vlahcevic, MD
Med Coll of Virginia, Dept of Med
Virginia Commonwealth Univ
1101 E Marshall St/PO Box 980711
Richmond, VA 23298-0711
Tel: 804 828-5396 *Fax:* 804 828-7430
E-mail: zviahcevic@gems.vcu.edu
Internet:
http://views.vcu.edu/internal-medicine/divisions/gastroenterology/gastro.html
Accred Length: 2 Years *Program Size:* 7
Program ID: 144-51-21-020

Washington

Seattle

University of Washington Program
Sponsor: University of Washington School of Medicine
University of Washington Medical Center
Program Director:
Sum P Lee, MD PhD
Univ of Washington Sch of Med
Div of Gastroenterology
1959 NE Pacific St/Box 356424
Seattle, WA 98195
Tel: 206 616-4602 *Fax:* 206 685-8684
E-mail: splee@u.washington.edu
Internet: http://weber.u.washington.edu/~gastro/
Accred Length: 2 Years *Program Size:* 10
Program ID: 144-54-21-086

Wisconsin

Madison

University of Wisconsin Program
Sponsor: University of Wisconsin Hospital and Clinics
William S Middleton Veterans Hospital
Program Director:
Ward A Olsen, MD
Univ of Wisconsin Hospital and Clinics
600 Highland Ave/Rm H6-516
Madison, WI 53792-5124
Tel: 608 263-7322 *Fax:* 608 265-5677
E-mail: waolsen@vms2.macc.wisc.edu
Internet: http://www.medicine.wisc.edu/sections/gastro/
Accred Length: 2 Years *Program Size:* 5
Program ID: 144-56-21-126

Milwaukee

Aurora Health Care Program
Sponsor: Aurora Health Care
Sinai Samaritan Medical Center
Program Director:
Vincents Dindzans, MD
Sinai Samaritan Med Ctr
PO Box 342
945 N 12th St
Milwaukee, WI 53201-0342
Tel: 414 219-7695 *Fax:* 414 219-7108
Accred Length: 2 Years *Program Size:* 3
Program ID: 144-56-21-210

Medical College of Wisconsin Program
Sponsor: Medical College of Wisconsin Affiliated Hospitals Inc
Clement J Zablocki Veterans Affairs Medical Center
Froedtert Memorial Lutheran Hospital
St Joseph's Hospital
Program Director:
Konrad H Soergel, MD
Medical College of Wisconsin
9200 W Wisconsin Ave
Milwaukee, WI 53226-3596
Tel: 414 456-6835 *Fax:* 414 456-6214
Accred Length: 2 Years *Program Size:* 6
Program ID: 144-56-31-048

Geriatric Medicine (Family Practice)

Arizona

Phoenix

St Joseph's Hospital and Medical Center Program
Sponsor: St Joseph's Hospital and Medical Center
Program Director:
Walter J Nieri, MD
Boswell Memorial Hospital/Rm D135
10401 W Thunderbird Blvd
Sun City, AZ 85351
Tel: 602 876-5601 *Fax:* 602 815-2981
E-mail: wnieri@mail.sunhealth.org
Internet: http://www.chw.edu/mha/mha.html
Accred Length: 1 Year *Program Size:* 4
Program ID: 125-03-21-029

California

Los Angeles

Southern California Kaiser Permanente Medical Care (Los Angeles) Program
Sponsor: Southern California Kaiser Permanente Medical Group
Kaiser Foundation Hospital (Los Angeles)
Program Director:
Kreighton L Chan, MD
Kaiser Foundation Hospital
Geriatrics Department
4733 Sunset Blvd/Mezz
Los Angeles, CA 90027
Tel: 323 783-4516 *Fax:* 323 783-4771
Accred Length: 1 Year *Program Size:* 4
Program ID: 125-05-21-025

San Bernardino

San Bernardino County Medical Center Program
Sponsor: San Bernardino County Medical Center
Program Director:
John F Randolph, MD
Dept of Community Med
Krikes Family Health Ctr
780 E Gilbert St
San Bernardino, CA 92415-0935
Tel: 909 387-7905 *Fax:* 909 387-8057
E-mail: frandolph@pol.net
Accred Length: 1 Year *Program Size:* 4
Program ID: 125-05-21-033

District of Columbia

Washington

Georgetown University/Providence Hospital Program

Sponsor: Georgetown University Medical Center
Providence Hospital
Program Director:
Henry M Wieman, MD
Georgetown Univ Sch of Med-Providence Hospital
1150 Varnum St NE
Washington, DC 20017
Tel: 301 699-7707, ext 34 *Fax:* 301 779-9001
E-mail: hwieman@erols.com
Accred Length: 1 Year *Program Size:* 2
Program ID: 125-10-21-028

Florida

Orlando

Florida Hospital Program

Sponsor: Florida Hospital
Program Director:
David George Pocock, MD
2501 N Orange Ave/Ste 235
Orlando, FL 32804
Tel: 407 897-1514 *Fax:* 407 897-1885
Accred Length: 1 Year *Program Size:* 1
Program ID: 125-11-21-032

Indiana

Muncie

Ball Memorial Hospital Program

Sponsor: Ball Memorial Hospital
Program Director:
Anthony R Dowell, MD
Ball Memorial Hospital
Geriatric Med
2401 W University Ave
Muncie, IN 47303
Tel: 765 751-1356 *Fax:* 765 751-1451
E-mail: klamb@cami3.com
Internet: http://www.ballhospital.org/
Accred Length: 1 Year *Program Size:* 4
Program ID: 125-17-21-030

Iowa

Iowa City

University of Iowa Hospitals and Clinics Program

Sponsor: University of Iowa Hospitals and Clinics
Program Director:
Gerald J Jogerst, MD
Univ of Iowa Hospitals and Clinics
200 Hawkins Dr
Iowa City, IA 52242-1097
Tel: 319 384-7500 *Fax:* 319 384-7822
Accred Length: 1 Year *Program Size:* 0
Program ID: 125-18-21-034

Kentucky

Louisville

University of Louisville Program

Sponsor: University of Louisville School of Medicine
University of Louisville Hospital
Program Director:
Steven H Smoger, MD
530 S Jackson St
Louisville, KY 40202
Tel: 502 852-7945 *Fax:* 502 852-8980
Internet: http://www.louisville.edu
Accred Length: 1 Year *Program Size:* 2
Program ID: 125-20-21-035

Michigan

Lansing

Sparrow Hospital Program

Sponsor: Sparrow Hospital
St Lawrence Hospital and HealthCare Services
Program Director:
John W Jones, MD
Geriatric Assessment Ctr
St Lawrence Hospital
1210 W Saginaw
Lansing, MI 48915-1999
Tel: 517 377-0330 *Fax:* 517 377-0436
Accred Length: 1 Year *Program Size:* 2
Program ID: 125-25-31-021

Minnesota

Minneapolis

University of Minnesota/HealthEast St Joseph's Hospital Program

Sponsor: University of Minnesota Medical School
Fairview-University Medical Center
Regions Hospital
Veterans Affairs Medical Center (Minneapolis)
Program Director:
Stanley L Smith, MD MPH
Dept of Family Practice
825 Washington Ave SE/Box 25
Minneapolis, MN 55414-3034
Tel: 612 627-4299 *Fax:* 612 627-4314
Internet: http://www.med.umn.edu/fp
Accred Length: 1 Year *Program Size:* 8
Program ID: 125-26-21-020

Missouri

Columbia

University of Missouri-Columbia Program

Sponsor: University of Missouri-Columbia School of Medicine
Harry S Truman Memorial Veterans Hospital
University Hospitals and Clinics
Program Director:
David R Mehr, MD MS
Univ of Missouri-Columbia Sch of Med
Dept of Family/Com Med
M228 Med Sciences Bldg
Columbia, MO 65212
Tel: 573 882-2190 *Fax:* 573 884-6172
E-mail: mehrd@health.missouri.edu
Accred Length: 1 Year *Program Size:* 2
Program ID: 125-28-21-026

Kansas City

University of Missouri at Kansas City Program

Sponsor: University of Missouri-Kansas City School of Medicine
Truman Medical Center-East
Program Director:
Jon F Dedon, MD
Univ of Missouri-Kansas City
Truman Med Ctr-East
7900 Lee's Summit Rd
Kansas City, MO 64139
Tel: 816 373-6228 *Fax:* 816 478-7534
E-mail: umkcfprp@qni.com
Internet: http://www.qni.com/~umkcfprp
Accred Length: 1 Year *Program Size:* 4
Program ID: 125-28-31-027

New Jersey

Piscataway

UMDNJ-Robert Wood Johnson Medical School Program

Sponsor: UMDNJ-Robert Wood Johnson Medical School
St Peter's University Hospital
Program Director:
David F Howarth, MD MPH
UMDNJ-Robert Wood Johnson Med Sch
Dept of Family Med
One Robert Wood Johnson Pl
New Brunswick, NJ 08903-0019
Tel: 732 235-7669 *Fax:* 732 246-8084
Internet: http://www2.umdnj.edu/fmedweb/grfellow.htm
Accred Length: 1 Year *Program Size:* 5
Program ID: 125-33-21-009

North Carolina

Greenville

East Carolina University Program

Sponsor: East Carolina University School of Medicine
Pitt County Memorial Hospital
Program Director:
Kenneth K Steinweg, MD
East Carolina Univ Sch of Med
Div of Geriatrics
Greenville, NC 27858-4354
Tel: 252 816-2597 *Fax:* 252 816-3040
E-mail: ksteinweg@brody.med.ecu.edu
Internet: http://www.med.ecu.edu/fammed/fellowsh.htm
Accred Length: 1 Year *Program Size:* 4
Program ID: 125-36-11-011

Ohio

Cincinnati

University Hospital/University of Cincinnati College of Medicine Program
Sponsor: University Hospital Inc
Christ Hospital
Drake Center
Franciscan Hospital-Mount Airy Campus
Program Director:
Gregg A Warshaw, MD
Univ Hospital-Univ of Cincinnati Coll of Med
Dept of Family Med
PO Box 670504
Cincinnati, OH 45267-0504
Tel: 513 584-0650 *Fax:* 513 584-2809
Accred Length: 1 Year *Program Size:* 4
Program ID: 125-38-21-012

Cleveland

Case Western Reserve University (MetroHealth) Program
Sponsor: MetroHealth Medical Center
Program Director:
James W Campbell, MD
2500 MetroHealth Dr
Cleveland, OH 44109-1998
Tel: 216 778-5223 *Fax:* 216 778-8225
E-mail: jcampbell@metrohealth.org
Accred Length: 1 Year *Program Size:* 3
Program ID: 125-38-21-031

Pennsylvania

Philadelphia

Thomas Jefferson University Program
Sponsor: Thomas Jefferson University Hospital
Program Director:
Karen D Novielli, MD
Thomas Jefferson Univ Hospital
1015 Walnut St/Ste 401
Philadelphia, PA 19107-5587
Tel: 215 955-2361 *Fax:* 215 923-6256
E-mail: novielli1@jeflin.tju.edu
Accred Length: 1 Year *Program Size:* 4
Program ID: 125-41-21-015

Pittsburgh

University of Pittsburgh Medical Center (St Margaret) Program
Sponsor: University of Pittsburgh Medical Center (St Margaret)
Program Director:
Karen A Powers, MD
UPMC St Margaret Hospital
Dept of Gerontology
815 Freeport Rd
Pittsburgh, PA 15215
Tel: 412 784-5070 *Fax:* 412 784-5077
Accred Length: 1 Year *Program Size:* 2
Program ID: 125-41-12-016

Puerto Rico

Caguas

University of Puerto Rico Program
Sponsor: University of Puerto Rico School of Medicine
Caguas Regional Hospital
Program Director:
Rafael Vega, MD
Univ of Puerto Rico
Dept of Family Med
GPO Box 1277
Gurabo, PR 00778
Tel: 787 737-1222 *Fax:* 787 737-1220
Accred Length: 1 Year *Program Size:* 4
Program ID: 125-42-21-017

Virginia

Newport News

Riverside Regional Medical Center Program
Sponsor: Riverside Regional Medical Center
Program Director:
Sharon Petitjean, MD
316 Main St/3rd Fl
Newport News, VA 23601
Tel: 757 594-3878 *Fax:* 757 591-9021
E-mail: ruth.mccormick@rivhs.com
Accred Length: 1 Year *Program Size:* 1
Program ID: 125-51-21-037

Geriatric Medicine (Internal Medicine)

Alabama

Birmingham

University of Alabama Medical Center Program
Sponsor: University of Alabama Hospital
Veterans Affairs Medical Center (Birmingham)
Program Director:
Richard V Sims, MD
Community Health Services Bldg (CHSB-19)
933 S 19th St/Ste 219E
Birmingham, AL 35294-2041
Tel: 205 934-9632 *Fax:* 205 975-7099
E-mail: rsims@aging.dom.uab.edu
Internet: http://www.aging.uab.edu
Accred Length: 2 Years *Program Size:* 4
Program ID: 151-01-21-001

Arizona

Phoenix

Good Samaritan Regional Medical Center Program
Sponsor: Good Samaritan Regional Medical Center
Carl T Hayden Veterans Affairs Medical Center (Phoenix)
Program Director:
Paul C Rousseau, MD
VA Med Ctr
650 E Indian School Rd
Phoenix, AZ 85012
Tel: 602 277-5551, ext 2615 *Fax:* 602 222-6514
E-mail: rousseau.paul@phoenix.va.gov
Accred Length: 2 Years *Program Size:* 2
Program ID: 151-03-21-102

Tucson

University of Arizona Program
Sponsor: University of Arizona College of Medicine
University Medical Center
Veterans Affairs Medical Center (Tucson)
Program Director:
John T Boyer, MD
Univ of Arizona-Ctr on Aging
1821 E Elm St
Tucson, AZ 85719
Tel: 520 626-6854 *Fax:* 520 626-2019
Accred Length: 2 Years *Program Size:* 4
Program ID: 151-03-21-122

Arkansas

Little Rock

University of Arkansas for Medical Sciences Program

Sponsor: University of Arkansas College of Medicine
John L McClellan Memorial Veterans Hospital
University Hospital of Arkansas

Program Director:
Cathey S Powers, MD
Univ of Arkansas for Med Sciences
4301 W Markham St/Slot 748
Little Rock, AR 72205
Tel: 501 686-6097 *Fax:* 501 686-5884
E-mail: cooperchristinam@exchange.uams.edu
Accred Length: 2 Years *Program Size:* 8
Program ID: 151-04-21-003

California

Los Angeles

Charles R Drew University Program

Sponsor: Charles R Drew University of Medicine and Science
LAC-King/Drew Medical Center

Program Director:
Arnel M Joaquin, MD
Div of Geriatrics
Charles R Drew Univ
1731 E 120th St
Los Angeles, CA 90059
Tel: 323 563-4822 *Fax:* 323 563-9393
E-mail: ajoaquin@cdrewu.edu
Accred Length: 2 Years *Program Size:* 4
Program ID: 151-05-11-108

UCLA Medical Center Program

Sponsor: UCLA School of Medicine
UCLA Medical Center
VA Greater Los Angeles Healthcare System

Program Director:
Bruce A Ferrell, MD
UCLA Med Ctr
Div of Geriatrics
10945 Le Conte Ave/Ste 2339
Los Angeles, CA 90095
Tel: 310 312-0531 *Fax:* 310 312-0546
E-mail: rneal@ucla.edu
Accred Length: 2 Years *Program Size:* 12
Program ID: 151-05-21-005

University of Southern California Program

Sponsor: Los Angeles County-USC Medical Center

Program Director:
Loren H Lipson, MD
AHC140
1355 San Pablo St
Los Angeles, CA 90033
Tel: 213 342-2960 *Fax:* 213 225-9283
Accred Length: 2 Years *Program Size:* 0
Program ID: 151-05-21-114

Orange

University of California (Irvine) Program

Sponsor: University of California (Irvine) Medical Center
Kaiser Foundation Hospitals (Anaheim)
Long Beach Memorial Medical Center

Program Director:
Laura A Mosqueda, MD
Univ of California Irvine Med Ctr
101 The City Dr South
Rte 81/Bldg 53 Rm 204D
Orange, CA 92868-3297
Tel: 714 456-5530 *Fax:* 714 456-7933
E-mail: mosqueda@uci.edu
Accred Length: 2 Years *Program Size:* 2
Program ID: 151-05-21-086

Sacramento

University of California (Davis) Program

Sponsor: University of California (Davis) Medical Center

Program Director:
Calvin Hirsch, MD
Univ of California Davis Med Ctr
Div of General Med-PSSB2400
4150 V St
Sacramento, CA 95817
Tel: 916 734-7004 *Fax:* 916 734-2732
E-mail: chhirsch@ucdavis.edu
Accred Length: 2 Years *Program Size:* 3
Program ID: 151-05-21-006

San Diego

University of California (San Diego) Program

Sponsor: University of California (San Diego) Medical Center
Veterans Affairs Medical Center (San Diego)

Program Director:
Joe W Ramsdell, MD
UCSD Med Ctr
200 W Arbor Dr
San Diego, CA 92103-8415
Tel: 619 543-5589 *Fax:* 619 543-3383
E-mail: vkrikes@ucsd.edu
Accred Length: 2 Years *Program Size:* 3
Program ID: 151-05-21-046

San Francisco

University of California (San Francisco)/Mount Zion Program

Sponsor: University of California (San Francisco) School of Medicine
Mount Zion Medical Center of the University of California

Program Director:
C Seth Landefeld, MD
VA Med Ctr
4150 Clement St (111G)
San Francisco, CA 94121
Tel: 415 750-6625 *Fax:* 415 750-6641
E-mail: sethl@medicine.ucsf.edu
Accred Length: 2 Years *Program Size:* 8
Program ID: 151-05-31-007

Stanford

Stanford University Program

Sponsor: Stanford University Hospital
Veterans Affairs Palo Alto Health Care System

Program Director:
Peter Pompei, MD
VA Palo Alto Health Care System
3801 Miranda Ave
GRECC 182-B
Palo Alto, CA 94304-1290
Tel: 415 858-3933 *Fax:* 415 855-9437
E-mail: pompei@leland.stanford.edu
Accred Length: 2 Years *Program Size:* 4
Program ID: 151-05-21-053

Colorado

Denver

University of Colorado Program

Sponsor: University of Colorado Health Sciences Center
Veterans Affairs Medical Center (Denver)

Program Director:
Laurence J Robbins, MD
VA Med Ctr
Geriatrics Sect (111D)
1055 Clermont St
Denver, CO 80220
Tel: 303 393-2822 *Fax:* 303 393-5128
E-mail: laurence.robbins@med.va.gov
Accred Length: 2 Years *Program Size:* 4
Program ID: 151-07-21-073

Connecticut

Farmington

University of Connecticut Program

Sponsor: University of Connecticut School of Medicine
Univ of Connecticut Health Center/John Dempsey Hospital

Program Director:
Gail M Sullivan, MD MPH
Univ of Connecticut Health Ctr
Ctr on Aging/MC-5215
Farmington, CT 06030-5215
Tel: 860 679-3956 *Fax:* 860 679-1307
E-mail: gsullivan@nso1.uchc.edu
Accred Length: 2 Years *Program Size:* 9
Program ID: 151-08-31-008

New Haven

Yale-New Haven Medical Center Program

Sponsor: Yale-New Haven Hospital
Veterans Affairs Medical Center (West Haven)

Program Director:
Sharon K Inouye, MD MPH
Yale Univ Sch of Med
20 York St/TMP-15
New Haven, CT 06504
Tel: 203 688-7302 *Fax:* 203 688-4209
E-mail: bonanno@gwpo.ynhh.com
Accred Length: 2 Years *Program Size:* 4
Program ID: 151-08-21-054

District of Columbia

Washington

George Washington University Program

Sponsor: George Washington University School of Medicine
George Washington University Hospital (UHS)
Program Director:
Elizabeth L Cobbs, MD
George Washington Univ Med Ctr
Div of Aging Studies/Services
2150 Pennsylvania Ave NW
Washington, DC 20037
Tel: 202 994-8292 *Fax:* 202 994-8531
E-mail: hcsjlj@gwumc.edu
Accred Length: 2 Years *Program Size:* 5
Program ID: 151-10-21-055

Florida

Gainesville

University of Florida Program

Sponsor: University of Florida College of Medicine
Shands Hospital at the University of Florida
Veterans Affairs Medical Center (Gainesville)
Program Director:
David T Lowenthal, MD
GRECC
VA Med Ctr/VA 182
Gainesville, FL 32608
Tel: 352 376-1611 *Fax:* 352 374-6412
Accred Length: 2 Years *Program Size:* 4
Program ID: 151-11-21-009

Miami

University of Miami-Jackson Memorial Medical Center Program

Sponsor: University of Miami-Jackson Memorial Medical Center
Miami Jewish Home and Hospital for the Aged
Mount Sinai Medical Center of Greater Miami
Veterans Affairs Medical Center (Miami)
Program Director:
Michael A Silverman, MD
Miami VA Med Ctr (11GRC)
1201 NW 16th St
Miami, FL 33125
Tel: 305 324-3388 *Fax:* 305 324-3365
Accred Length: 2 Years *Program Size:* 6
Program ID: 151-11-21-010

Tampa

University of South Florida Program

Sponsor: University of South Florida College of Medicine
James A Haley Veterans Hospital
Tampa General Healthcare
Program Director:
Ronald S Schonwetter, MD MD
Univ of South Florida Coll of Med
12901 Bruce B Downs Blvd
Box 19
Tampa, FL 33612
Tel: 813 974-2460 *Fax:* 813 974-2580
E-mail: gerimed@com1.med.usf.edu
Internet:
http://www.med.usf.edu/intmed/geriatrics/index.html
Accred Length: 2 Years *Program Size:* 4
Program ID: 151-11-21-011

Georgia

Atlanta

Emory University Program

Sponsor: Emory University School of Medicine
Veterans Affairs Medical Center (Atlanta)
Wesley Woods Geriatric Hospital
Program Director:
Joseph G Ouslander, MD
Emory Univ Sch of Med
Wesley Woods Geriatric Ctr
1841 Clifton Rd NE
Atlanta, GA 30329
Tel: 404 728-6295 *Fax:* 404 728-6245
E-mail: jouslan@emory.edu
Internet: http://www.emory.edu/med_ger/startup.html
Accred Length: 2 Years *Program Size:* 7
Program ID: 151-12-21-100

Hawaii

Honolulu

University of Hawaii Program

Sponsor: University of Hawaii John A Burns School of Medicine
Kaiser Foundation Hospital (Moanalua)
Kuakini Medical Center
Program Director:
Patricia L Blanchette, MD MPH
John A Burns Sch of Med
347 N Kuakini St/HPM 9
Honolulu, HI 96817
Tel: 808 523-8461 *Fax:* 808 528-1897
E-mail: blanchet@hhp2.hawaii-health.com
Accred Length: 2 Years *Program Size:* 11
Program ID: 151-14-21-047

Illinois

Chicago

McGaw Medical Center of Northwestern University Program

Sponsor: Northwestern University Medical School
Northwestern Memorial Hospital
Veterans Affairs Lakeside Medical Center (Chicago)
Program Director:
Janice B Schwartz, MD
Div of Geriatric Med
303 E Superior St
Jennings 209
Chicago, IL 60611
Tel: 312 908-3235 *Fax:* 312 908-6591
E-mail: jbs157@nwu.edu
Accred Length: 2 Years *Program Size:* 3
Program ID: 151-16-21-079

Rush-Presbyterian-St Luke's Medical Center Program

Sponsor: Rush-Presbyterian-St Luke's Medical Center
Program Director:
Martin Gorbien, MD
Rush-Presbyterian-St Luke's Med Ctr
710 S Paulina Ave
Chicago, IL 60612-3872
Tel: 312 942-3600 *Fax:* 312 942-3601
E-mail: mgorbien@rush.edu
Accred Length: 2 Years *Program Size:* 4
Program ID: 151-16-11-081

University of Chicago Program

Sponsor: University of Chicago Hospitals
Program Director:
Mark A Rudberg, MD
Univ of Chicago
5841 S Maryland Ave
MC6098
Chicago, IL 60637-1470
Tel: 773 702-3564 *Fax:* 773 702-3538
E-mail: mrudberg@medicine.bsd.uchicago.edu
Accred Length: 2 Years *Program Size:* 4
Program ID: 151-16-11-012

University of Illinois College of Medicine at Chicago Program

Sponsor: University of Illinois College of Medicine at Chicago
University of Illinois Hospital and Clinics
Veterans Affairs West Side Medical Center
Program Director:
David O Staats, MD
Univ of Illinois Hospital
840 S Wood St (M/C 787)
Chicago, IL 60612
Tel: 312 996-4750 *Fax:* 312 413-2693
E-mail: davido@uic.edu
Accred Length: 2 Years *Program Size:* 7
Program ID: 151-16-21-091

Maywood

Loyola University Program

Sponsor: Loyola University Medical Center
Edward J Hines Jr Veterans Affairs Hospital
La Grange Memorial Hospital
Program Director:
Ileana Soneru, MD
Hines VA Hospital
Geriatrics/Extended Care (181)
Bldg 1/Rm C-124D
Hines, IL 60141-5000
Tel: 708 216-2592 *Fax:* 708 216-2163
Accred Length: 2 Years *Program Size:* 8
Program ID: 151-16-21-013

Park Ridge

Lutheran General Hospital Program

Sponsor: Lutheran General Hospital
Program Director:
Herbert C Sier, MD
Div of Geriatrics
Lutheran General Hospital
1775 W Dempster St
Park Ridge, IL 60068
Tel: 847 723-1680 *Fax:* 847 696-3391
Accred Length: 2 Years *Program Size:* 4
Program ID: 151-16-21-120

Indiana

Indianapolis

Indiana University School of Medicine Program

Sponsor: Indiana University School of Medicine
Richard L Roudebush Veterans Affairs Medical Center
William N Wishard Memorial Hospital

Program Director:
Jeffrey C Darnell, MD
Indiana Univ Sch of Med
WD/OPW Bldg M200
1001 W 10th St
Indianapolis, IN 46202-2859
Tel: 317 630-6906 *Fax:* 317 630-2667
E-mail: gwestmor@iupui.edu
Internet: http://medicine.iupu.edu/fellow.html#geriatric
Accred Length: 2 Years *Program Size:* 1
Program ID: 151-17-21-016

Kansas

Kansas City

University of Kansas Medical Center Program

Sponsor: University of Kansas School of Medicine
University of Kansas Medical Center

Program Director:
Stephanie A Studenski, MD
Univ of Kansas Med Ctr
Ctr on Aging
3901 Rainbow Blvd
Kansas City, KS 66160-7117
Tel: 913 588-1265 *Fax:* 913 588-3162
E-mail: sstudens@kumc.edu
Internet: http://www2.kumc.edu/coa/index.htm
Accred Length: 2 Years *Program Size:* 6
Program ID: 151-19-21-056

Kentucky

Lexington

University of Kentucky Medical Center Program

Sponsor: University of Kentucky Hospital

Program Director:
Timothy S Caudill, MD MPH
Univ of Kentucky, Dept of Int Med
K512 Kentucky Clinic UKMC
Lexington, KY 40536
Tel: 606 257-5499 *Fax:* 606 257-2605
E-mail: tscaud1@pop.uky.edu
Accred Length: 2 Years *Program Size:* 2
Program ID: 151-20-21-087

Louisiana

New Orleans

Tulane University Program

Sponsor: Tulane University School of Medicine
Veterans Affairs Medical Center-LSU Service (New Orleans)

Program Director:
Neil Nusbaum, MD JD
VA Med Ctr (COS8)
1601 Perdido St
New Orleans, LA 70112-1262
Tel: 504 589-5907 *Fax:* 504 619-4072
E-mail: nusbaum.neil@new-orleans.med.va.gov
Accred Length: 2 Years *Program Size:* 4
Program ID: 151-21-21-115

Maryland

Baltimore

Johns Hopkins University Program

Sponsor: Johns Hopkins University School of Medicine
Johns Hopkins Bayview Medical Center
Johns Hopkins Hospital

Program Director:
Richard Bennett, MD
Johns Hopkins Geriatrics Ctr
5505 Hopkins Bayview Cir
Baltimore, MD 21224-2780
Tel: 410 550-0781 *Fax:* 410 550-1069
E-mail: rbennett@jhmi.edu
Internet:
http://www.jhbmc.jhu.edu/geriat/trainprg/trainprg01.html
Accred Length: 2 Years *Program Size:* 10
Program ID: 151-23-11-018

Union Memorial Hospital Program

Sponsor: Union Memorial Hospital

Program Director:
F Michael Gloth III, MD
Union Memorial Hospital
201 E University Pkwy
Ste 415
Baltimore, MD 21218-2895
Tel: 410 554-2923 *Fax:* 410 554-6794
Internet:
http://www.helixhealth.com/resident/union/gerinfo.htm
Accred Length: 2 Years *Program Size:* 4
Program ID: 151-23-21-116

University of Maryland Program

Sponsor: University of Maryland Medical System
Veterans Affairs Medical Center (Baltimore)

Program Director:
Conrad May, MD
Baltimore VA Med Ctr
Geriatrics Service (18)
10 N Greene St
Baltimore, MD 21201-1542
Tel: 410 605-7185 *Fax:* 410 605-7913
E-mail: bireland@umaryland.edu
Internet: http://www.grecc.ab.umd.edu
Accred Length: 2 Years *Program Size:* 4
Program ID: 151-23-21-104

Massachusetts

Boston

Beth Israel Deaconess Medical Center (East Campus) Program

Sponsor: Beth Israel Deaconess Medical Center
Brockton-West Roxbury Veterans Affairs Medical Center

Program Director:
Muriel R Gillick, MD
Hebrew Rehabilitation Ctr for Aged
1200 Centre St
Boston, MA 02131
Tel: 617 325-8000, ext 8577 *Fax:* 617 363-8929
E-mail: gillick@mail.hrca.harvard.edu
Accred Length: 2 Years *Program Size:* 12
Program ID: 151-24-21-019

Boston University Medical Center Program

Sponsor: Boston Medical Center
Edith Nourse Rogers Memorial Veterans Hospital
Jewish Memorial Hospital

Program Director:
Sharon Levine, MD
Boston Med Ctr
88 E Newton St/F-4
Boston, MA 02118
Tel: 617 638-6155 *Fax:* 617 638-8387
E-mail: sharon.levine@bmc.org
Accred Length: 2 Years *Program Size:* 3
Program ID: 151-24-31-020

Michigan

Ann Arbor

University of Michigan Program

Sponsor: University of Michigan Hospitals
Veterans Affairs Medical Center (Ann Arbor)

Program Director:
Jeffrey B Halter, MD
1500 E Medical Center Dr
Rm 1111 CCGCB
Ann Arbor, MI 48109-0926
Tel: 734 763-4002 *Fax:* 734 763-2064
E-mail: zpine@umich.edu
Accred Length: 2 Years *Program Size:* 8
Program ID: 151-25-21-024

Detroit

Wayne State University/Detroit Medical Center Program

Sponsor: Wayne State University/Detroit Medical Center
Veterans Affairs Medical Center (Detroit)

Program Director:
Joel Steinberg, MD
Geriatric Med Fellowship
4201 St Antoine
Detroit, MI 48201
Tel: 313 577-5025 *Fax:* 313 577-0157
Accred Length: 2 Years *Program Size:* 6
Program ID: 151-25-21-111

Royal Oak

William Beaumont Hospital Program

Sponsor: William Beaumont Hospital

Program Director:
Michael E Maddens, MD
3535 W 13 Mile Rd
Ste 105
Royal Oak, MI 48073
Tel: 248 551-0622 *Fax:* 248 551-1244
Internet: http://www.beaumont.edu/html/gme
Accred Length: 2 Years *Program Size:* 4
Program ID: 151-25-31-117

Minnesota

Rochester

Mayo Graduate School of Medicine (Rochester) Program

Sponsor: Mayo Graduate School of Medicine-Mayo Foundation
Mayo Clinic (Rochester)
Rochester Methodist Hospital
St Mary's Hospital of Rochester

Program Director:
Darryl S Chutka, MD
Application Processing Ctr
Mayo Graduate Sch of Med
200 First St SW
Rochester, MN 55905
Tel: 507 284-3126 *Fax:* 507 284-0999
E-mail: mgsm.intmed.specialties@mayo.edu
Internet: http://www.mayo.edu/
Accred Length: 2 Years *Program Size:* 3
Program ID: 151-26-21-085

Missouri

St Louis

St Louis University School of Medicine Program

Sponsor: St Louis University School of Medicine
St Louis University School of Medicine
Veterans Affairs Medical Center (St Louis)

Program Director:
David W Bentley, MD
St Louis Univ Sch of Med
Rm M238
1402 S Grand Blvd
St Louis, MO 63104
Tel: 314 577-8462 *Fax:* 314 771-8575
Internet: http://www.slu.edu
Accred Length: 2 Years *Program Size:* 9
Program ID: 151-28-21-095

Washington University/B-JH/SLCH Consortium (South Campus) Program

Sponsor: Washington University/B-JH/SLCH Consortium
Barnes-Jewish Hospital
Barnes-Jewish Hospital (North Campus)

Program Director:
David B Carr, MD
4488 Forest Park Blvd/Ste 201
St Louis, MO 63108-2293
Tel: 314 286-2700 *Fax:* 314 286-2701
E-mail: dcarr@imgate.wustl.edu
Accred Length: 2 Years *Program Size:* 2
Program ID: 151-28-21-027

Nebraska

Omaha

University of Nebraska Program

Sponsor: University of Nebraska Medical Center

Program Director:
Jane F Potter, MD
Univ of Nebraska Med Ctr
Univ Geriatric Ctr
985620 Nebraska Med Ctr
Omaha, NE 68198-5620
Tel: 402 559-7512 *Fax:* 402 559-8228
E-mail: bwilson@mail.unmc.edu
Internet: http://www.unmc.edu.gme/geriatrics.html
Accred Length: 2 Years *Program Size:* 3
Program ID: 151-30-21-028

New Jersey

Newark

UMDNJ-New Jersey Medical School Program

Sponsor: UMDNJ-New Jersey Medical School
Bergen Regional Medical Center
Hackensack University Medical Center
Newark Beth Israel Medical Center
UMDNJ-University Hospital

Program Director:
Knight Steel, MD
Homecare Inst
Hackensack Univ Med Ctr
30 Prospect Ave
Hackensack, NJ 07601
Tel: 201 996-2503 *Fax:* 201 883-0870
E-mail: 103106.1164@compuserve.com
Accred Length: 2 Years *Program Size:* 3
Program ID: 151-33-21-103

New Mexico

Albuquerque

University of New Mexico Program

Sponsor: University of New Mexico School of Medicine
University Hospital
Veterans Affairs Medical Center (Albuquerque)

Program Director:
Robert D Lindeman, MD
Dept of Int Med ACC-5
2211 Lomas Blvd NE
Albuquerque, NM 87131-5271
Tel: 505 272-6082 *Fax:* 505 272-4628
E-mail: rlindeman@salud.unm.edu
Accred Length: 2 Years *Program Size:* 4
Program ID: 151-34-21-093

New York

Albany

Albany Medical Center Program

Sponsor: Albany Medical Center

Program Director:
Dean A Thompson, MD
VA Healthcare Network Upstate New York-Albany
Geriatrics and Extended Care
113 Holland Ave
Albany, NY 12208-3473
Tel: 518 462-3311, ext 3167 *Fax:* 518 432-1320
E-mail: thompson.dean_at@albany.vagov
Internet:
http://www.va.gov/visns/visn02/cslines/gecline/gecline.html%0
Accred Length: 2 Years *Program Size:* 3
Program ID: 151-35-31-058

Bronx

Albert Einstein College of Medicine Program

Sponsor: Albert Einstein College of Medicine of Yeshiva University
Montefiore Medical Center-Henry and Lucy Moses Division

Program Director:
Laurie G Jacobs, MD
Montefiore Med Ctr
Div of Geriatric Med
111 E 210th St
Bronx, NY 10467
Tel: 718 920-6721 *Fax:* 718 655-9672
E-mail: ljacobs@aecom.yu.edu
Accred Length: 2 Years *Program Size:* 4
Program ID: 151-35-21-083

New York Medical College (Our Lady of Mercy) Program

Sponsor: New York Medical College
Our Lady of Mercy Medical Center

Program Director:
T S Dharmarajan, MD
New York Med Coll
600 E 233rd St
Bronx, NY 10466
Tel: 718 920-9168 *Fax:* 718 920-9036
Accred Length: 2 Years *Program Size:* 8
Program ID: 151-35-11-107

Brooklyn

Maimonides Medical Center Program

Sponsor: Maimonides Medical Center

Program Director:
Robert D Kennedy, MD
Maimonides Med Ctr
4802 Tenth Ave
Brooklyn, NY 11219
Tel: 718 283-8549 *Fax:* 718 283-8498
E-mail: rkennedy@maimonidesmed.org
Accred Length: 2 Years *Program Size:* 4
Program ID: 151-35-11-126

New York Methodist Hospital Program

Sponsor: New York Methodist Hospital

Program Director:
Thayyullathil Bharathan, MD
New York Methodist Hospital
506 Sixth St
Brooklyn, NY 11215
Tel: 718 780-5246 *Fax:* 718 780-3259
Accred Length: 2 Years *Program Size:* 2
Program ID: 151-35-21-121

Buffalo

SUNY at Buffalo Graduate Medical-Dental Education Consortium Program

Sponsor: SUNY at Buffalo Grad Medical-Dental Education Consortium
Veterans Affairs Medical Center (Buffalo)

Program Director:
Bruce Naughton, MD
Div of Geriatrics
Deaconess Ctr
1001 Humboldt Pkwy
Buffalo, NY 14208
Tel: 716 887-8195 *Fax:* 716 887-8244
Accred Length: 2 Years *Program Size:* 3
Program ID: 151-35-31-030

Flushing

New York Flushing Hospital Medical Center Program

Sponsor: New York Flushing Hospital Medical Center
New York Hospital Medical Center of Queens

Program Director:
Anthony T Vela, MD
New York Flushing Hospital
4500 Parsons Blvd
Flushing, NY 11355
Tel: 718 670-5590 *Fax:* 718 670-5666
Accred Length: 2 Years *Program Size:* 4
Program ID: 151-35-21-123

Jamaica

Catholic Medical Center of Brooklyn and Queens Program

Sponsor: Catholic Medical Center of Brooklyn and Queens Inc
Catholic Medical Center (Mary Immaculate Hospital)
Catholic Medical Center (St John's Queens Hospital)

Program Director:
Dharamjit N Kumar, MD
Catholic Med Ctr of Brooklyn and Queens
88-25 153th St
Jamaica, NY 11432
Tel: 718 558-2891 *Fax:* 718 558-2476
E-mail: dkumar@cmcny.com
Accred Length: 2 Years *Program Size:* 4
Program ID: 151-35-31-124

Manhasset

North Shore University Hospital/NYU School of Medicine Program

Sponsor: North Shore University Hospital

Program Director:
Howard J Guzik, MD
North Shore Univ Hospital
300 Community Dr
Manhasset, NY 11030
Tel: 516 562-8005 *Fax:* 516 562-8064
Accred Length: 2 Years *Program Size:* 4
Program ID: 151-35-21-084

Mineola

Winthrop-University Hospital Program

Sponsor: Winthrop-University Hospital

Program Director:
Lucy O Macina, MD
Winthrop-Univ Hospital
222 Station Plaza N
Rm 518
Mineola, NY 11501
Tel: 516 663-2588 *Fax:* 516 663-4644
Accred Length: 2 Years *Program Size:* 4
Program ID: 151-35-21-088

New Hyde Park

Albert Einstein College of Medicine at Long Island Jewish Medical Center Program

Sponsor: Long Island Jewish Medical Center

Program Director:
Conn J Foley, MD
Parker Jewish Inst for Health Care and Rehab
271-11 76th Ave
New Hyde Park, NY 11040-1433
Tel: 718 289-2100, ext 2277 *Fax:* 718 289-2345
E-mail: cfoley@parkerinstitute.org
Internet: http://www.lij.edu/lij-homepage-ns.html
Accred Length: 2 Years *Program Size:* 8
Program ID: 151-35-21-031

New York

Mount Sinai School of Medicine Program

Sponsor: Mount Sinai School of Medicine
Mount Sinai Medical Center

Program Director:
Rosanne M Leipzig, MD PhD
Dept of Geriatrics/Adult Develop/Box 1070
Mount Sinai Med Ctr
One Gustave L Levy Pl
New York, NY 10029
Tel: 212 241-4274 *Fax:* 212 987-0793
Accred Length: 2 Years *Program Size:* 12
Program ID: 151-35-31-062

New York and Presbyterian Hospital (Cornell Campus) Program

Sponsor: New York and Presbyterian Hospital
New York and Presbyterian Hospital (Cornell Campus)

Program Director:
Mark Lachs, MD MPH
Ronald Adelman, MD
New York and Presbyterian Hospital (Cornell Campus)
525 E 68th St
Box 46
New York, NY 10021
Tel: 212 746-1677 *Fax:* 212 746-4808
Accred Length: 2 Years *Program Size:* 4
Program ID: 151-35-12-127

New York Medical College at St Vincent's Hospital and Medical Center of New York Program

Sponsor: New York Medical College
St Vincent's Hospital and Medical Center of New York

Program Director:
Judith Ahronheim, MD
St Vincent's Hospital and Med Ctr
Dept of Med
153 W 11th St/NR 12-11
New York, NY 10011
Tel: 212 604-2127 *Fax:* 212 604-2128
Internet: http://svh.nymc.edu
Accred Length: 2 Years *Program Size:* 2
Program ID: 151-35-21-090

New York University Medical Center Program

Sponsor: New York University Medical Center
Bellevue Hospital Center
Hospital for Joint Diseases Orthopaedic Institute

Program Director:
Michael L Freedman, MD
Bellevue Hospital Ctr
Rm 2-N-69
First Ave and 27th St
New York, NY 10016
Tel: 212 562-6380
Accred Length: 2 Years *Program Size:* 6
Program ID: 151-35-21-101

Rochester

University of Rochester Program

Sponsor: Strong Memorial Hospital of the University of Rochester
Monroe Community Hospital

Program Director:
Paul R Katz, MD
Monroe Community Hospital
435 E Henrietta Rd
Rochester, NY 14620
Tel: 716 760-6352 *Fax:* 716 760-6376
E-mail: katz1@frontiernet.net
Accred Length: 2 Years *Program Size:* 6
Program ID: 151-35-31-105

Staten Island

Staten Island University Hospital Program

Sponsor: Staten Island University Hospital

Program Director:
Vincent Calamia, MD
Staten Island Univ Hospital
Div of Geriatric Med
475 Seaview Ave/MAP 2nd Fl
Staten Island, NY 10305
Tel: 718 226-6346 *Fax:* 718 226-6282
Accred Length: 2 Years *Program Size:* 4
Program ID: 151-35-21-110

Stony Brook

SUNY at Stony Brook Program

Sponsor: University Hospital-SUNY at Stony Brook
Veterans Affairs Medical Center (Northport)

Program Director:
Suzanne D Fields, MD
Dept of Med
SUNY-Stony Brook
HSC T-16-080
Stony Brook, NY 11794-8163
Tel: 516 444-7840 *Fax:* 516 444-6004
E-mail: sfields@epo.som.sunysb.edu
Accred Length: 2 Years *Program Size:* 5
Program ID: 151-35-22-109

Syracuse

SUNY Health Science Center at Syracuse Program

Sponsor: University Hospital-SUNY Health Science Center at Syracuse

Program Director:
Sharon A Brangman, MD
SUNY Health Science Ctr-Syracuse
750 E Adams St
Syracuse, NY 13210
Tel: 315 464-5167 *Fax:* 315 464-5771
Accred Length: 2 Years *Program Size:* 3
Program ID: 151-35-21-097

Valhalla

New York Medical College at Westchester Medical Center Program

Sponsor: New York Medical College
Westchester Medical Center

Program Director:
Krishan Gupta, MD
New York Med Coll
Munger Pavilion/Rm B06A
Valhalla, NY 10595
Tel: 914 493-7729 *Fax:* 914 493-7727
Accred Length: 2 Years *Program Size:* 2
Program ID: 151-35-11-032

North Carolina

Chapel Hill

University of North Carolina Hospitals Program

Sponsor: University of North Carolina Hospitals

Program Director:
Jan Busby-Whitehead, MD
Univ of North Carolina Sch of Med
Program on Aging
141 MacNider Bldg CB #7550
Chapel Hill, NC 27599-7550
Tel: 919 966-5945 *Fax:* 919 962-0467
E-mail: mairgold@med.unc.edu
Internet: http://www.med.unc.edu/aging/
Accred Length: 2 Years *Program Size:* 2
Program ID: 151-36-21-059

Durham

Duke University Program

Sponsor: Duke University Medical Center
Veterans Affairs Medical Center (Durham)

Program Director:
Harvey J Cohen, MD
Duke Univ Med Ctr
Box 3003
Durham, NC 27710
Tel: 919 660-7502 *Fax:* 919 684-8569
E-mail: cohen015@mc.duke.edu
Accred Length: 2 Years *Program Size:* 8
Program ID: 151-36-21-033

Winston-Salem

Wake Forest University School of Medicine Program

Sponsor: Wake Forest University Baptist Medical Center

Program Director:
Paul E McGann, MD MS
J Paul Sticht Ctr on Aging
Medical Center Blvd
Ground Fl Admin Ste
Winston-Salem, NC 27157-1051
Tel: 336 713-8549 *Fax:* 336 713-8588
Accred Length: 2 Years *Program Size:* 10
Program ID: 151-36-21-034

Ohio

Cleveland

Case Western Reserve University Program

Sponsor: University Hospitals of Cleveland
Veterans Affairs Medical Center (Cleveland)

Program Director:
Jerome Kowal, MD
12200 Fairhill Rd
Cleveland, OH 44120
Tel: 216 844-6370 *Fax:* 216 844-6492
E-mail: jxk9@po.cwru.edu
Internet: http://www.cwru.edu/orgs/gerimed/index.html
Accred Length: 2 Years *Program Size:* 7
Program ID: 151-38-21-035

Cleveland Clinic Foundation Program

Sponsor: Cleveland Clinic Foundation

Program Director:
Robert M Palmer, MD
Cleveland Clinic Foundation
Dept of Geriatric Med/A91
9500 Euclid Ave
Cleveland, OH 44195-5242
Tel: 216 444-5690 *Fax:* 216 444-1162
E-mail: meded@cesmtp.ccf.org
Internet: http://www.ccf.org
Accred Length: 2 Years *Program Size:* 2
Program ID: 151-38-12-037

Oklahoma

Oklahoma City

University of Oklahoma Health Sciences Center Program

Sponsor: University of Oklahoma College of Medicine
University Hospital
Veterans Affairs Medical Center (Oklahoma City)

Program Director:
Marie A Bernard, MD
Univ of Oklahoma Health Sciences Ctr
PO Box 26901/VAMC-11G
Oklahoma City, OK 73190
Tel: 405 270-0501, ext 5957 *Fax:* 405 270-5195
E-mail: marie-bernard@uokhsc.edu
Accred Length: 2 Years *Program Size:* 4
Program ID: 151-39-21-112

Oregon

Portland

Oregon Health Sciences University Program

Sponsor: Oregon Health Sciences University Hospital
Veterans Affairs Medical Center (Portland)

Program Director:
Nora Tobin, MD
VA Med Ctr
Medical Service (P3-Geri)
PO Box 1034
Portland, OR 97207
Tel: 503 273-5015 *Fax:* 503 721-7807
E-mail: tobin.nora@portland.va.gov
Accred Length: 2 Years *Program Size:* 4
Program ID: 151-40-31-038

Pennsylvania

Philadelphia

Albert Einstein Medical Center Program

Sponsor: Albert Einstein Medical Center

Program Director:
Todd H Goldberg, MD
Albert Einstein Med Ctr
Div of Geriatric Med
5501 Old York Rd
Philadelphia, PA 19141
Tel: 215 456-8608 *Fax:* 215 456-7512
E-mail: goldbert@aehn2.einstein.edu
Internet: http://www.einstein.edu/phl/1202a.html
Accred Length: 2 Years *Program Size:* 4
Program ID: 151-41-11-078

MCP Hahnemann University Program

Sponsor: MCP Hahnemann University
Medical College of Pennsylvania Hospital

Program Director:
Mary T Hofmann, MD
Med Coll of Pennsylvania Hospital
3300 Henry Ave
Philadelphia, PA 19129
Tel: 215 842-7377 *Fax:* 215 848-7169
Accred Length: 2 Years *Program Size:* 3
Program ID: 151-41-21-098

Temple University Program

Sponsor: Temple University Hospital

Program Director:
Karen G Kelly, MD
Philadelphia Geriatric Ctr
5301 Old York Rd
Philadelphia, PA 19141-2996
Tel: 215 456-2099 *Fax:* 215 456-2883
Internet: http://www.pgc.org
Accred Length: 2 Years *Program Size:* 8
Program ID: 151-41-21-118

University of Pennsylvania Program

Sponsor: Hospital of the University of Pennsylvania
Veterans Affairs Medical Center (Philadelphia)

Program Director:
Edna P Schwab, MD MD
Hospital of Univ of Pennsylvania
Dept of Med/Box 708
3400 Spruce St
Philadelphia, PA 19104
Tel: 215 662-4411 *Fax:* 215 662-4438
E-mail: eschwab@mail.med.upenn.edu
Internet: http://www.med.upenn.edu/aging/fellprog
Accred Length: 2 Years *Program Size:* 4
Program ID: 151-41-21-060

Pittsburgh

Shadyside Hospital/UPMC Program

Sponsor: Shadyside Hospital/UPMC

Program Director:
David C Martin, MD
UPMC Shadyside
5230 Centre Ave
Pittsburgh, PA 15232
Tel: 412 623-2700 *Fax:* 412 623-1235
E-mail: davidm@ssh.edu
Internet: http://ssh.edu
Accred Length: 2 Years *Program Size:* 4
Program ID: 151-41-21-082

University Health Center of Pittsburgh Program

Sponsor: University Health Center of Pittsburgh
Presbyterian University Hospital/UPMC
Veterans Affairs Medical Center (Pittsburgh)

Program Director:
Evelyn C Granieri, MD
Univ of Pittsburgh Sch of Med
Div of Geriatric Med
3520 Fifth Ave/Ste 300
Pittsburgh, PA 15213
Tel: 412 624-4052 *Fax:* 412 383-1972
E-mail: ghturner@juno.com
Accred Length: 2 Years *Program Size:* 6
Program ID: 151-41-21-077

Puerto Rico

San Juan

University of Puerto Rico Program

Sponsor: University of Puerto Rico School of Medicine
Dr Federico Trilla - Carolina Regional Hospital
University Hospital
Veterans Affairs Medical Center (San Juan)

Program Director:
Ivonne Jimenez-Velaquez, MD
Univ of Puerto Rico Sch of Med
Box 365067
San Juan, PR 00936-5067
Tel: 787 751-6034 *Fax:* 787 754-1739
Accred Length: 2 Years *Program Size:* 4
Program ID: 151-42-21-089

South Carolina

Columbia

Palmetto Health Alliance/University of South Carolina School of Medicine Program

Sponsor: Palmetto Health Alliance
Palmetto Richland Memorial Hospital

Program Director:
G Paul Eleazer, MD
Palmetto Richland Memorial Hospital
15 Richland Medical Pk/Ste 203
Columbia, SC 29203
Tel: 803 434-4039 *Fax:* 803 434-3773
E-mail: 75013.1666@compuserve.com
Internet: http://www.rmh.edu
Accred Length: 2 Years *Program Size:* 3
Program ID: 151-45-21-119

Tennessee

Nashville

Vanderbilt University Program

Sponsor: Vanderbilt University Medical Center

Program Director:
Sarah White, MD
Senior Care Service
7155 Vanderbilt Med Ctr East
Nashville, TN 37232
Tel: 615 936-3274 *Fax:* 615 936-3156
Accred Length: 1 Year *Program Size:* 2
Program ID: 151-47-21-125

Texas

Galveston

University of Texas Medical Branch Hospitals Program

Sponsor: University of Texas Medical Branch Hospitals

Program Director:
John E Carlson, MD
Univ of Texas Med Branch
Div of Geriatrics
301 University Blvd
Galveston, TX 77555-0460
Tel: 409 772-1987 *Fax:* 409 772-6931
E-mail: jcarlson@utmb.edu
Accred Length: 2 Years *Program Size:* 4
Program ID: 151-48-21-106

Houston

Baylor College of Medicine Program

Sponsor: Baylor College of Medicine
Veterans Affairs Medical Center (Houston)

Program Director:
George E Taffet, MD
Baylor Coll of Med
Huffington Ctr on Aging
One Baylor Plaza/M320
Houston, TX 77030-3498
Tel: 713 798-5804 *Fax:* 713 798-6688
E-mail: tmarchand@bcm.tmc.edu
Internet: http://www.hcoa.org/
Accred Length: 2 Years *Program Size:* 7
Program ID: 151-48-31-040

San Antonio

University of Texas Health Science Center at San Antonio Program

Sponsor: University of Texas Medical School at San Antonio
Audie L Murphy Memorial Veterans Hospital (San Antonio)
University Hospital-South Texas Medical Center

Program Director:
Laura K Chiodo, MD MPH
Univ of Texas Health Science Ctr-San Antonio
Div of Geriatrics/Gerontology
7703 Floyd Curl Dr
San Antonio, TX 78284-7875
Tel: 210 617-5311 *Fax:* 210 617-5312
E-mail: chiodo@uthscsa.edu
Accred Length: 2 Years *Program Size:* 6
Program ID: 151-48-21-075

Utah

Salt Lake City

University of Utah Program

Sponsor: University of Utah Medical Center
Veterans Affairs Medical Center (Salt Lake City)

Program Director:
Laurence J Meyer, MD PhD
GRECC-Salt Lake City VA Med Ctr
500 Foothill Blvd
Salt Lake City, UT 84148
Tel: 801 584-2522 *Fax:* 801 585-3884
E-mail: meyer@med.utah.edu
Internet: http://www.grecc.med.utah.edu
Accred Length: 2 Years *Program Size:* 4
Program ID: 151-49-21-052

Virginia

Charlottesville

University of Virginia Program

Sponsor: University of Virginia Medical Center

Program Director:
Diane G Snustad, MD
Univ of Virginia Hospitals
Dept of Int Med
Box 426
Charlottesville, VA 22908
Tel: 804 924-1212 *Fax:* 804 295-6311
E-mail: dgs6t@virginia.edu
Accred Length: 2 Years *Program Size:* 2
Program ID: 151-51-21-042

Richmond

Medical College of Virginia/Virginia Commonwealth University Program

Sponsor: Medical College of Virginia/Virginia Commonwealth University
Hunter Holmes McGuire VA Medical Center (Richmond)
Medical College of Virginia Hospitals

Program Director:
Angela Gentili, MD
Geriatric/Extended Care Service Line (181C)
VA Med Ctr
1201 Broad Rock Blvd
Richmond, VA 23249
Tel: 804 675-5000, ext 4740 *Fax:* 804 675-5130
E-mail: gentili.angela@richmond.va.gov
Accred Length: 2 Years *Program Size:* 4
Program ID: 151-51-21-043

Washington

Seattle

University of Washington Program 1

Sponsor: University of Washington School of Medicine
Harborview Medical Center
Veterans Affairs Medical Center (Seattle)

Program Director:
Itamar B Abrass, MD
Harborview Med Ctr
Box 359755 Rm HH565
325 Ninth Ave
Seattle, WA 98104-2499
Tel: 206 731-3089 *Fax:* 206 731-8753
E-mail: itamar@u.washington.edu
Internet: http://weber.u.washington.edu/~geront/
Accred Length: 2 Years *Program Size:* 5
Program ID: 151-54-21-044

Tacoma

Madigan Army Medical Center Program

Sponsor: Madigan Army Medical Center
VA Puget Sound Health Care System-American Lake Div

Program Director:
Sharon Falzgraf, MD
Madigan Army Med Ctr
Dept of Med
Tacoma, WA 98431-5000
Tel: 253 582-8440, ext 6085 *Fax:* 253 589-4017
Accred Length: 2 Years *Program Size:* 4
Program ID: 151-54-12-074
US Armed Services Program

Wisconsin

Madison

University of Wisconsin Program

Sponsor: University of Wisconsin Hospital and Clinics
William S Middleton Veterans Hospital

Program Director:
Steven R Barczi, MD
Wm S Middleton Memorial VA Hospital
GRECC
2500 Overlook Terrace
Madison, WI 53705
Tel: 608 262-7000 *Fax:* 608 262-7648
E-mail: steven.barczi@med.va.gov
Accred Length: 2 Years *Program Size:* 4
Program ID: 151-56-21-049

Milwaukee

Aurora Health Care Program
Sponsor: Aurora Health Care
Sinai Samaritan Medical Center
Program Director:
Ashok Choithani, MD
Sinai Samaritan Med Ctr
945 N 12th St
PO Box 342
Milwaukee, WI 53201-0342
Tel: 414 219-7312 *Fax:* 414 219-6078
Accred Length: 2 Years *Program Size:* 3
Program ID: 151-56-21-076

Medical College of Wisconsin Program
Sponsor: Medical College of Wisconsin Affiliated Hospitals Inc
Clement J Zablocki Veterans Affairs Medical Center
Program Director:
Edith A Burns, MD
Med Coll of Wisconsin
Div of Geriatrics/PC-00G
5000 W National Ave
Milwaukee, WI 53295
Tel: 414 384-2000, ext 2775 *Fax:* 414 382-5319
Accred Length: 2 Years *Program Size:* 2
Program ID: 151-56-31-048

Geriatric Psychiatry (Psychiatry)

Alabama

Birmingham

University of Alabama Medical Center Program
Sponsor: University of Alabama Hospital
Veterans Affairs Medical Center (Birmingham)
Program Director:
Terri S Steele, MD
Univ of Alabama Sch of Med
1713 6th Ave S/CPM 249
Birmingham, AL 35294-0018
Tel: 205 934-6054 *Fax:* 205 975-7829
Accred Length: 1 Year *Program Size:* 1
Program ID: 407-01-21-040

California

Los Angeles

UCLA Medical Center Program
Sponsor: UCLA School of Medicine
UCLA Neuropsychiatric Hospital
VA Greater Los Angeles Healthcare System
Program Director:
Gary W Small, MD
UCLA Neuropsychiatric Inst
Attn: Sandra Lipschultz, Admin
760 Westwood Plaza/Rm C8-852
Los Angeles, CA 90024-1759
Tel: 310 825-0548 *Fax:* 310 825-0340
E-mail: sandrajl@npih.medsch.ucla.edu
Internet: http://www.mentalhealth.ucla.edu/trainees
Accred Length: 1 Year *Program Size:* 5
Program ID: 407-05-21-001

San Diego

University of California (San Diego) Program
Sponsor: University of California (San Diego) Medical Center
Veterans Affairs Medical Center (San Diego)
Program Director:
Dilip V Jeste, MD
Univ of California San Diego
VA San Diego Healthcare System
3350 La Jolla Village Dr (116A-1)
San Diego, CA 92161
Tel: 619 534-4020 *Fax:* 619 552-7404
E-mail: behernan@ucsd.edu
Accred Length: 1 Year *Program Size:* 3
Program ID: 407-05-31-002

Stanford

Stanford University Program
Sponsor: Stanford University Hospital
Program Director:
Jared Tinklenberg, MD
Stanford Univ
Academic Affairs Office
401 Quarry Rd/Rm 2109
Stanford, CA 94305-5723
Tel: 650 725-5591 *Fax:* 650 725-5594
E-mail: fae.sloss@leland.stanford.edu
Accred Length: 1 Year *Program Size:* 1
Program ID: 407-05-11-003

Connecticut

New Haven

Yale-New Haven Medical Center Program
Sponsor: Yale-New Haven Hospital
Veterans Affairs Medical Center (West Haven)
Program Director:
J Craig Nelson, MD
Yale-New Haven Hospital
20 York St/EP-01-835C
New Haven, CT 06504
Tel: 203 688-2157
Accred Length: 1 Year *Program Size:* 0
Program ID: 407-08-21-052

Florida

Gainesville

University of Florida Program
Sponsor: University of Florida College of Medicine
Shands Hospital at the University of Florida
Veterans Affairs Medical Center (Gainesville)
Program Director:
Michael J Tueth, MD
Univ of Florida Health Science Ctr
PO Box 100256
Gainesville, FL 32610
Tel: 352 374-6014 *Fax:* 352 379-4170
Accred Length: 1 Year *Program Size:* 2
Program ID: 407-11-21-041

Miami

University of Miami-Jackson Memorial Medical Center Program
Sponsor: University of Miami-Jackson Memorial Medical Center
Miami Jewish Home and Hospital for the Aged
Mount Sinai Medical Center of Greater Miami
Veterans Affairs Medical Center (Miami)
Program Director:
Maria D Llorente, MD
Miami VA Med Ctr
Dept of Psychiatry/Behav Sci
1201 NW 16th St/#116A
Miami, FL 33125
Tel: 305 674-2194 *Fax:* 305 324-3413
E-mail: mdll@compuserve.com
Accred Length: 1 Year *Program Size:* 5
Program ID: 407-11-21-004

Tampa

University of South Florida Program
Sponsor: University of South Florida College of Medicine
James A Haley Veterans Hospital
TGH University Psychiatry Center
Program Director:
B Ashok Raj, MD
Univ of South Florida Psychiatry Ctr
3515 E Fletcher Ave
Tampa, FL 33613
Tel: 813 974-4354 *Fax:* 813 974-3223
E-mail: araj@com1.med.usf.edu
Internet: http://www.med.usf.edu/psych/psychome
Accred Length: 1 Year *Program Size:* 3
Program ID: 407-11-31-005

Georgia

Atlanta

Emory University Program

Sponsor: Emory University School of Medicine
Emory University Hospital
Wesley Woods Geriatric Hospital
Program Director:
Larry E Tune, MD
Dept of Psychiatry
Emory Clinic-Wesley Woods
1842 Clifton Rd
Atlanta, GA 30329
Tel: 404 728-4969 *Fax:* 404 728-4963
E-mail: ltune@emory.edu
Accred Length: 1 Year *Program Size:* 2
Program ID: 407-12-21-006

Hawaii

Honolulu

University of Hawaii Program

Sponsor: University of Hawaii John A Burns School of Medicine
Hawaii State Hospital
VA Regional Office-Outpatient Clinic (Honolulu)
Program Director:
Iqbal Ahmed, MD
Univ of Hawaii, Dept of Psychiatry
1356 Lusitana St/4th Fl
Honolulu, HI 96813
Tel: 808 586-2900 *Fax:* 808 586-2940
Accred Length: 1 Year *Program Size:* 2
Program ID: 407-14-21-007

Illinois

Chicago

McGaw Medical Center of Northwestern University Program

Sponsor: Northwestern University Medical School
Northwestern Memorial Hospital
Program Director:
Sanford I Finkel, MD
Dept of Geriatric Psychiatry
McGaw Med Ctr
303 E Ohio St/#550
Chicago, IL 60611
Tel: 312 908-9841 *Fax:* 312 908-6276
E-mail: s-finkel@nwu.edu
Accred Length: 1 Year *Program Size:* 2
Program ID: 407-16-21-008

Indiana

Indianapolis

Indiana University School of Medicine Program

Sponsor: Indiana University School of Medicine
Clarian IU Hospital
Clarian Methodist Hospital of Indiana
William N Wishard Memorial Hospital
Program Director:
Hugh C Hendrie, MB ChB
Indiana Univ Sch of Med
541 N Clinical Dr/Rm 298
Indianapolis, IN 46202-5111
Tel: 317 274-4012 *Fax:* 317 274-1248
E-mail: hhendri@iupui.edu
Internet: http://www.iupui.edu/~psych
Accred Length: 1 Year *Program Size:* 2
Program ID: 407-17-21-009

Kansas

Wichita

University of Kansas (Wichita) Program

Sponsor: University of Kansas School of Medicine (Wichita)
Via Christi Regional Medical Center
Via Christi Regional Medical Center-St Joseph
Program Director:
George Dyck, MD
1010 N Kansas
Wichita, KS 67214-3199
Tel: 316 261-2647 *Fax:* 316 291-1874
E-mail: gdyck@kumc.edu
Internet: http://www.kumc.edu/wickita/dept/index.html
Accred Length: 1 Year *Program Size:* 2
Program ID: 407-19-21-010

Louisiana

New Orleans

Louisiana State University Program

Sponsor: Louisiana State University School of Medicine
Touro Infirmary
Program Director:
Kenneth M Sakauye, MD
Louisiana State Univ Sch of Med
1542 Tulane Ave
New Orleans, LA 70112-2822
Tel: 504 568-6001, ext 2126 *Fax:* 504 568-8647
E-mail: ksakau@aol.com
Accred Length: 1 Year *Program Size:* 2
Program ID: 407-21-21-011

Maryland

Baltimore

Johns Hopkins University Program

Sponsor: Johns Hopkins University School of Medicine
Johns Hopkins Hospital
Program Director:
Peter V Rabins, MD
Johns Hopkins Univ
Meyer 279/Johns Hopkins Hospital
600 N Wolfe St
Baltimore, MD 21287-7279
Tel: 410 955-6736 *Fax:* 410 614-1094
E-mail: pvrabins@welchlink.welch.jhu.edu
Accred Length: 1 Year *Program Size:* 1
Program ID: 407-23-21-012

University of Maryland Program

Sponsor: University of Maryland Medical System
Veterans Affairs Medical Center (Baltimore)
Program Director:
Paul E Ruskin, MD
Psychiatry Service (116A)
Baltimore VA
10 N Greene St
Baltimore, MD 21201
Tel: 410 605-7354 *Fax:* 410 605-7918
E-mail: ruskin.paul@baltimore.va.gov
Accred Length: 1 Year *Program Size:* 3
Program ID: 407-23-31-013

Massachusetts

Belmont

McLean Hospital Program

Sponsor: McLean Hospital
Program Director:
Sumer Verma, MD
Dept of Psychiatry
McLean Hospital
115 Mill St
Belmont, MA 02178
Tel: 617 855-3293 *Fax:* 617 855-3246
E-mail: skverma@aol.com
Accred Length: 1 Year *Program Size:* 1
Program ID: 407-24-21-014

Michigan

Ann Arbor

University of Michigan Program

Sponsor: University of Michigan Hospitals
Veterans Affairs Medical Center (Ann Arbor)
Program Director:
Alan M Mellow, MD
1500 E Medical Center Dr
Ann Arbor, MI 48109-0704
Tel: 734 761-7024 *Fax:* 734 769-7410
Accred Length: 2 Years *Program Size:* 2
Program ID: 407-25-21-015

Detroit

Wayne State University/Lafayette Clinic Program

Sponsor: Wayne State University/Detroit Medical Center
Walter P Reuther Psychiatric Hospital
Program Director:
Antoun C Manganas, MD
UPC-Central Campus
101 E Alexandrine
Detroit, MI 48201
Tel: 313 577-5267, ext 201 *Fax:* 313 577-2233
E-mail: ab3847@wayne.edu
Accred Length: 1 Year *Program Size:* 3
Program ID: 407-25-31-016

Minnesota

Minneapolis

University of Minnesota Program

Sponsor: University of Minnesota Medical School
Veterans Affairs Medical Center (Minneapolis)
Program Director:
Gabe J Maletta, MD PhD
VA Med Ctr (11M)
One Veterans Dr
Minneapolis, MN 55417
Tel: 612 725-2052 *Fax:* 612 727-5958
E-mail: maletta.gabe@minneapolis.va.gov
Accred Length: 1 Year *Program Size:* 1
Program ID: 407-26-21-017

Missouri

St Louis

St Louis University School of Medicine Program

Sponsor: St Louis University School of Medicine
St Louis University School of Medicine
Program Director:
George T Grossberg, MD
St Louis Univ Sch of Med
David P Wohl Sr Memorial Inst
1221 S Grand Blvd
St Louis, MO 63104
Tel: 314 577-8720 *Fax:* 314 268-5186
E-mail: grossbgt@wpogate.slu.edu
Internet: http://www.slu.edu
Accred Length: 1 Year *Program Size:* 3
Program ID: 407-28-21-018

Nebraska

Omaha

Creighton University/University of Nebraska Program

Sponsor: Creighton University School of Medicine
University of Nebraska Medical Center
Program Director:
William H Roccaforte, MD
Dept of Psychiatry
Univ of Nebraska Med Ctr
600 S 42nd St/PO Box 985575
Omaha, NE 68198-5575
Tel: 402 559-5012 *Fax:* 402 559-9945
Internet: http://www.unmc.edu/cme/gmehome.htm
Accred Length: 1 Year *Program Size:* 2
Program ID: 407-30-21-019

New Hampshire

Lebanon

Dartmouth Hitchcock Medical Center Program

Sponsor: Mary Hitchcock Memorial Hospital
New Hampshire Hospital
Program Director:
Thomas E Oxman, MD
Dept of Psychiatry
Dartmouth Hitchcock Med Ctr
One Medical Center Dr
Lebanon, NH 03756-0001
Tel: 603 650-6147 *Fax:* 603 650-5842
E-mail: thomas.oxman@dartmouth.edu
Accred Length: 1 Year *Program Size:* 2
Program ID: 407-32-21-020

New Jersey

Piscataway

UMDNJ-Robert Wood Johnson Medical School Program

Sponsor: UMDNJ-Robert Wood Johnson Medical School
Medical Center at Princeton
Robert Wood Johnson University Hospital
Program Director:
Peter M Aupperle, MD MPH
COPSA, Div of Geriatric Psych
UMDNJ-Robert Wood Johnson Med Sch
667 Hoes Ln/PO Box 1392
Piscataway, NJ 08855-1392
Tel: 732 235-5730 *Fax:* 732 235-4920
E-mail: aupperpm@umdnj.edu
Internet:
http://www.rwja.umdnj.edu/~coyne/residency.htm
Accred Length: 1 Year *Program Size:* 3
Program ID: 407-33-21-021

New York

Binghamton

New York and Presbyterian Hospital (Columbia Campus) Program

Sponsor: New York and Presbyterian Hospital
Binghamton Psychiatric Center
New York and Presbyterian Hospital (Columbia Campus)
Program Director:
D Peter Birkett, MD
100 Haven Ave/Tower #3-30F
New York, NY 10032
Tel: 212 781-0600 *Fax:* 212 795-7696
Accred Length: 1 Year *Program Size:* 3
Program ID: 407-35-21-042

Bronx

Albert Einstein College of Medicine Program

Sponsor: Albert Einstein College of Medicine of Yeshiva University
Bronx Psychiatric Center
Montefiore Medical Center-Henry and Lucy Moses Division
Program Director:
Gary J Kennedy, MD
Montefiore Med Ctr
Dept of Psychiatry
111 E 210th St
Bronx, NY 10467
Tel: 718 920-4236 *Fax:* 718 920-6538
E-mail: gkennedy@aecom.yu.edu
Accred Length: 1 Year *Program Size:* 5
Program ID: 407-35-21-022

Brooklyn

SUNY Health Science Center at Brooklyn Program

Sponsor: SUNY Health Science Center at Brooklyn
Kingsboro Psychiatric Center
University Hospital-SUNY Health Science Center at Brooklyn
Program Director:
Carl I Cohen, MD
SUNY Health Science Ctr-Brooklyn
450 Clarkson Ave
Brooklyn, NY 11203
Tel: 718 270-2907 *Fax:* 718 270-4104
E-mail: cohen_c@hscbklyn.edu
Accred Length: 1 Year *Program Size:* 4
Program ID: 407-35-31-023

New Hyde Park

Albert Einstein College of Medicine at Long Island Jewish Medical Center Program

Sponsor: Long Island Jewish Medical Center
Central Islip Psychiatric Center
Hillside Hospital (Long Island Jewish Medical Center)
St John's Episcopal Hospital-South Shore
Program Director:
Blaine S Greenwald, MD
Albert Einstein Coll of Med-Hillside Hospital
Long Island Jewish Med Ctr
75-59 263rd St
Glen Oaks, NY 11004
Tel: 718 470-8159 *Fax:* 718 470-9784
E-mail: greenwal@lij.edu
Internet: http://www.lij.edu
Accred Length: 1 Year *Program Size:* 6
Program ID: 407-35-11-024

New York

Albert Einstein College of Medicine at Beth Israel Medical Center Program

Sponsor: Beth Israel Medical Center
Program Director:
J Paul Teusink, MD
Beth Israel Med Ctr
Dept of Psychiatry
1st Ave at 16th St
New York, NY 10003-3896
Tel: 212 420-4680 *Fax:* 212 844-7659
Accred Length: 1 Year *Program Size:* 2
Program ID: 407-35-12-025

New York Medical College at St Vincent's Hospital and Medical Center of New York Program

Sponsor: New York Medical College
St Vincent's Hospital and Medical Center of New York

Program Director:
David Cordon, MD
St Vincent's Hospital
203 W 12th St/Rm 603
New York, NY 10011
Tel: 212 604-1525 *Fax:* 212 604-8794
Accred Length: 1 Year *Program Size:* 4
Program ID: 407-35-23-028

New York University Medical Center Program

Sponsor: New York University Medical Center
Bellevue Hospital Center
Goldwater Memorial Hospital
Manhattan Psychiatric Center

Program Director:
Jeffrey R Foster, MD
New York Univ Med Ctr
Dept of Psychiatry
550 First Ave
New York, NY 10016
Tel: 212 686-9668 *Fax:* 212 263-8135
Accred Length: 1 Year *Program Size:* 2
Program ID: 407-35-22-027

Rochester

University of Rochester Program

Sponsor: Strong Memorial Hospital of the University of Rochester

Program Director:
Katherine Duffy, MD
Univ of Rochester Med Ctr
Dept of Psychiatry
300 Crittenden Blvd
Rochester, NY 14642-8409
Tel: 716 275-6737 *Fax:* 716 273-1082
E-mail: katherine_duffy@urmc.rochester.edu
Internet: http://www.urmc.rochester.edu/smh/psych
Accred Length: 1 Year *Program Size:* 1
Program ID: 407-35-32-029

White Plains

New York and Presbyterian Hospital (Cornell Campus)/Westchester Program

Sponsor: New York and Presbyterian Hospital
New York and Presbyterian Hospital-Westchester Division

Program Director:
George Alexopoulos, MD
Cornell Univ Med Coll
Dept of Psychiatry
21 Bloomingdale Rd
White Plains, NY 10605
Tel: 914 997-5767 *Fax:* 914 997-5958
Accred Length: 1 Year *Program Size:* 2
Program ID: 407-35-21-030

North Carolina

Durham

Duke University Program

Sponsor: Duke University Medical Center
John Umstead Hospital
Veterans Affairs Medical Center (Durham)

Program Director:
Keith G Meador, MD MPH
DUMC-3837
Durham, NC 27710
Tel: 919 681-5171 *Fax:* 919 684-2290
Accred Length: 1 Year *Program Size:* 2
Program ID: 407-36-21-047

Ohio

Cincinnati

University Hospital/University of Cincinnati College of Medicine Program

Sponsor: University Hospital Inc

Program Director:
John W Kasckow, MD PhD
Univ of Cincinnati
231 Bethesda Ave/ML 559
Cincinnati, OH 45267-0559
Tel: 513 558-5118 *Fax:* 513 558-4805
E-mail: kasckowj@uc.campus.mci.net
Internet: http://www.uc.edu
Accred Length: 1 Year *Program Size:* 2
Program ID: 407-38-21-038

Cleveland

Case Western Reserve University Program

Sponsor: University Hospitals of Cleveland

Program Director:
Mahmoud A Parsa, MD
Univ Hospitals of Cleveland
11100 Euclid Ave/HPV5080
Cleveland, OH 44106
Tel: 216 844-1447 *Fax:* 216 844-1703
Accred Length: 1 Year *Program Size:* 2
Program ID: 407-38-21-045

Oregon

Portland

Oregon Health Sciences University Program

Sponsor: Oregon Health Sciences University Hospital
Oregon State Hospital
Veterans Affairs Medical Center (Portland)

Program Director:
Linda K Ganzini, MD
Oregon Health Sciences Univ
Mental Health Div/P-7-1DMH
PO Box 1034
Portland, OR 97207-9823
Tel: 503 220-8262, ext 56492 *Fax:* 503 721-1053
E-mail: ganzinil@0hsu.edu
Accred Length: 1 Year *Program Size:* 2
Program ID: 407-40-21-031

Pennsylvania

Hershey

Penn State Geisinger Health System/Milton S Hershey Medical Center Program

Sponsor: Penn State Geisinger Health System
Milton S Hershey Medical Center

Program Director:
Paul A Kettl, MD
Milton S Hershey Med Ctr, Dept of Psychiatry
Pennsylvania State Univ
500 University Dr
Hershey, PA 17033
Tel: 717 531-7237 *Fax:* 717 531-8868
Accred Length: 1 Year *Program Size:* 2
Program ID: 407-41-21-032

Philadelphia

Albert Einstein Medical Center Program

Sponsor: Albert Einstein Medical Center
Belmont Center for Comprehensive Treatment

Program Director:
Kenneth I Rosenstein, MD
4200 Monument Rd
Philadelphia, PA 19131
Tel: 215 677-9415 *Fax:* 215 677-3457
Accred Length: 1 Year *Program Size:* 3
Program ID: 407-41-21-044

University of Pennsylvania Program

Sponsor: Hospital of the University of Pennsylvania
Friends Hospital

Program Director:
Joel E Streim, MD
Ralston-Penn Ctr
Sect of Geriatric Psychiatry
3615 Chestnut St
Philadelphia, PA 19104-2676
Tel: 215 662-7426 *Fax:* 215 662-6093
Accred Length: 1 Year *Program Size:* 2
Program ID: 407-41-31-033

Pittsburgh

University Health Center of Pittsburgh Program

Sponsor: University Health Center of Pittsburgh
Western Psychiatric Institute and Clinic/UPMC

Program Director:
Jules Rosen, MD
Univ of Pittsburgh Med Ctr
Dept of Geriatric Psychiatry
3811 O'Hara St/Rm 827
Pittsburgh, PA 15213-2593
Tel: 412 624-8189 *Fax:* 412 624-2698
E-mail: rosenji@msx.upmc.edu
Accred Length: 1 Year *Program Size:* 4
Program ID: 407-41-11-034

Programs

Rhode Island

Providence

Brown University Program
Sponsor: Butler Hospital
Eleanor Slater Hospital
Miriam Hospital
Program Director:
Robert Kohn, MD
Brown Univ, Dept of Psych/Human Behavior
Butler Hospital
345 Blackstone Blvd
Providence, RI 02906-9980
Tel: 401 455-6277 *Fax:* 401 455-6293
E-mail: robert_kohn@brown.edu
Internet: http://www.brown.edu/departments/psychiatry/
Accred Length: 2 Years *Program Size:* 3
Program ID: 407-43-21-048

South Carolina

Charleston

Medical University of South Carolina Program
Sponsor: Medical University of South Carolina College of Medicine
Ralph H Johnson Dept of Veterans Affairs Med Center
Program Director:
Jacobo E Mintzer, MD
Med Univ of South Carolina Inst of Psychiatry
PH 141-H
67 President St
Charleston, SC 29425
Tel: 843 792-6895 *Fax:* 843 792-7374
Accred Length: 1 Year *Program Size:* 2
Program ID: 407-45-21-035

Tennessee

Johnson City

East Tennessee State University Program
Sponsor: James H Quillen College of Medicine
Bristol Regional Medical Center
Veterans Affairs Medical Center (Mountain Home)
Program Director:
Robert Kuwik, MD
James H Quillen Coll of Med
116A Bldg 37
Mountain Home, TN 37684
Tel: 423 926-1171 *Fax:* 423 461-7929
Accred Length: 1 Year *Program Size:* 0
Program ID: 407-47-21-050

Nashville

Vanderbilt University Program
Sponsor: Vanderbilt University Medical Center
Program Director:
Richard A Margolin, MD
1500 21st Ave S/Ste 2000
Nashville, TN 37212
Tel: 615 322-0325 *Fax:* 615 343-9038
Accred Length: 1 Year *Program Size:* 1
Program ID: 407-47-21-046

Texas

Dallas

University of Texas Southwestern Medical School Program
Sponsor: University of Texas Southwestern Medical School
Dallas County Hospital District-Parkland Memorial Hospital
Dallas County Mental Health and Mental Retardation Center
Presbyterian Hospital of Dallas
Program Director:
Myron F Weiner, MD
Univ of Texas Southwestern Med Ctr
Dept of Psychiatry
5323 Harry Hines Blvd/F5400
Dallas, TX 75235-9070
Tel: 214 648-3400 *Fax:* 214 648-7980
E-mail: mweine@mednet.swmed.edu
Accred Length: 1 Year *Program Size:* 3
Program ID: 407-48-21-036

Virginia

Charlottesville

University of Virginia Program
Sponsor: University of Virginia Medical Center
Program Director:
Suzanne Holroyd, MD
Univ of Virginia Health Sciences Ctr
Box 623
Charlottesville, VA 22908
Tel: 804 924-2241 *Fax:* 804 924-5149
Accred Length: 1 Year *Program Size:* 1
Program ID: 407-51-21-043

Washington

Seattle

University of Washington Program
Sponsor: University of Washington School of Medicine
Harborview Medical Center
University of Washington Medical Center
Program Director:
Richard Veith, MD
Dept of Psych/Behavioral Sciences (Box 356560)
Univ of Washington Sch of Med
1959 NE Pacific
Seattle, WA 98195
Tel: 206 543-3750 *Fax:* 206 543-9520
E-mail: rcv@u.washington.edu
Accred Length: 1 Year *Program Size:* 3
Program ID: 407-54-21-037

Wisconsin

Madison

University of Wisconsin Program
Sponsor: University of Wisconsin Hospital and Clinics
Mendota Mental Health Institute
William S Middleton Veterans Hospital
Program Director:
Timothy Howell, MD
Dept of Psychiatry/Med
2500 Overlook Terr
Madison, WI 53705
Tel: 608 262-7084 *Fax:* 608 262-7095
E-mail: howell.timothy@madison.va.gov
Accred Length: 1 Year *Program Size:* 2
Program ID: 407-56-21-039

Hand Surgery (General Surgery)

Kentucky

Louisville

University of Louisville Program

Sponsor: University of Louisville School of Medicine
Jewish Hospital
Program Director:
Thomas W Wolff, MD
225 Abraham Flexner Way
One Medical Center Plaza/Ste 850
Louisville, KY 40202
Tel: 502 562-0312 *Fax:* 502 562-0326
Internet: http://www.thepoint.net/~cmki/index.htm
Accred Length: 1 Year *Program Size:* 8
Program ID: 443-20-21-003

Maryland

Baltimore

Union Memorial Hospital Program

Sponsor: Union Memorial Hospital
Program Director:
E F Shaw Wilgis, MD
Union Memorial Hospital
National Ctr for Treatment of Hand and Upper Extremity
3333 N Calvert St
Baltimore, MD 21218-2895
Tel: 410 554-6593 *Fax:* 410 554-2979
Accred Length: 1 Year *Program Size:* 3
Program ID: 443-23-21-001

Hand Surgery (Orthopaedic Surgery)

Alabama

Birmingham

University of Alabama Medical Center Program

Sponsor: University of Alabama Hospital
Program Director:
Donald H Lee, MD
Univ of Alabama
1813 6th Ave S
MEB 505
Birmingham, AL 35294-3295
Tel: 205 975-2663 *Fax:* 205 975-9626
E-mail: janet.mcdaniel@ortho.uab.edu
Internet: http://www.ortho.uab.edu
Accred Length: 1 Year *Program Size:* 3
Program ID: 263-01-20-018

Arizona

Phoenix

Maricopa Medical Center Program

Sponsor: Maricopa Medical Center
Hand Surgery Associates
Program Director:
Robert L Wilson, MD
Hand Surgery Associates
2610 N Third St
Phoenix, AZ 85008
Tel: 602 264-3541
Internet: http://www.maricopa.gov/medcenter/mmc.html
Accred Length: 1 Year *Program Size:* 3
Program ID: 263-03-21-044

Arkansas

Little Rock

University of Arkansas for Medical Sciences Program

Sponsor: University of Arkansas College of Medicine
Arkansas Children's Hospital
John L McClellan Memorial Veterans Hospital
Program Director:
Harris Gellman, MD
Dept of Orthopaedic Surgery
4301 W Markham St/Slot 531
Little Rock, AR 72205
Tel: 501 686-5590 *Fax:* 501 686-7824
E-mail: gellmanharris@exchange.uams.edu
Accred Length: 1 Year *Program Size:* 1
Program ID: 263-04-21-064

California

Loma Linda

Loma Linda University Program

Sponsor: Loma Linda University Medical Center
San Bernardino County Medical Center
Program Director:
Virchel E Wood, MD
Loma Linda Univ Med Ctr
11234 Anderson St
Rm A519
Loma Linda, CA 92354
Tel: 909 824-4413, ext 42859 *Fax:* 909 824-4820
Accred Length: 1 Year *Program Size:* 3
Program ID: 263-05-21-006

Los Angeles

UCLA Medical Center Program

Sponsor: UCLA School of Medicine
UCLA Medical Center
VA Greater Los Angeles Healthcare System
Program Director:
Neil Ford Jones, MD
UCLA Sch of Med
Dept of Ortho Surgery
Medical Education Sect
Los Angeles, CA 90095-6902
Tel: 310 825-6986 *Fax:* 310 825-1311
E-mail: jderenne@mednet.ucla.edu
Internet: http://149.142.183.2
Accred Length: 1 Year *Program Size:* 2
Program ID: 263-05-21-014

University of Southern California Program

Sponsor: Los Angeles County-USC Medical Center
Joseph H Boyes Foundation
Program Director:
Stephen B Schnall, MD
Los Angeles County-USC Med Ctr
Dept of Ortho Surgery
1200 N State St/G-8 Rm 3900
Los Angeles, CA 90033
Tel: 323 442-3336
Accred Length: 1 Year *Program Size:* 2
Program ID: 263-05-21-039

Sacramento

University of California (Davis) Program

Sponsor: University of California (Davis) Medical Center
Program Director:
Robert M Szabo, MD MPH
Univ of California Davis Med Ctr
Dept of Orthopaedics
4860 Y St/Ste 3800
Sacramento, CA 95817-1419
Tel: 916 734-3678 *Fax:* 916 734-7904
E-mail: tammy.brau@ucdmc.ucdavis.edu
Accred Length: 1 Year *Program Size:* 1
Program ID: 263-05-21-023

San Diego

University of California (San Diego) Program
Sponsor: University of California (San Diego) Medical Center
Veterans Affairs Medical Center (San Diego)
Program Director:
Reid A Abrams, MD
UCSD Med Ctr
200 W Arbor Dr/8894
San Diego, CA 92103-8894
Tel: 619 543-5555 *Fax:* 619 543-2540
Internet: http://www.medicine.ucsd.edu/ortho
Accred Length: 1 Year *Program Size:* 1
Program ID: 263-05-31-024

San Francisco

California Pacific Medical Center Program
Sponsor: California Pacific Medical Center
California Pacific Medical Center
San Francisco SurgiCentre
Program Director:
Leonard Gordon, MD
California Pacific Med Ctr
Hand and Microsurgery Med Group
2300 California St/Ste 300
San Francisco, CA 94115
Tel: 415 923-0992 *Fax:* 415 923-1036
Accred Length: 1 Year *Program Size:* 1
Program ID: 263-05-21-040

University of California (San Francisco) Program
Sponsor: University of California (San Francisco) School of Medicine
San Francisco General Hospital Medical Center
Program Director:
Edward Diao, MD
Univ of California San Francisco
500 Parnassus Ave/Rm MU320W
Box 0728
San Francisco, CA 94143-0728
Tel: 415 476-1167 *Fax:* 415 502-5265
E-mail: diaoe@orthosurg.ucsf.edu
Accred Length: 1 Year *Program Size:* 1
Program ID: 263-05-21-019

Stanford

Stanford University Program
Sponsor: Stanford University Hospital
Lucile Salter Packard Children's Hospital at Stanford
Veterans Affairs Palo Alto Health Care System
Program Director:
Amy L Ladd, MD
900 Blake Wilbur Dr
Palo Alto, CA 94304
Tel: 650 723-6796 *Fax:* 650 723-6786
Accred Length: 1 Year *Program Size:* 1
Program ID: 263-05-31-054

Connecticut

Farmington

University of Connecticut Program
Sponsor: University of Connecticut School of Medicine
Hartford Hospital
Univ of Connecticut Health Center/John Dempsey Hospital
Program Director:
H Kirk Watson, MD
Connecticut Combined Hand Surgery Service
85 Seymour St/Ste 816
Hartford, CT 06106
Tel: 860 527-7161 *Fax:* 860 728-3227
Accred Length: 1 Year *Program Size:* 2
Program ID: 263-08-21-030

New Haven

Yale-New Haven Medical Center Program
Sponsor: Yale-New Haven Hospital
Program Director:
Scott W Wolfe, MD
Yale Univ
PO Box 208071
New Haven, CT 06520-8071
Tel: 203 737-5661 *Fax:* 203 785-7132
E-mail: scott.wolfe@yale.edu
Internet: http://info.med.yale.edu/ortho/hand.phtml
Accred Length: 1 Year *Program Size:* 1
Program ID: 263-08-21-061

District of Columbia

Washington

Walter Reed Army Medical Center Program
Sponsor: Walter Reed Army Medical Center
Georgetown University Medical Center
Union Memorial Hospital
Program Director:
Col Allan C Smith, MD
Walter Reed Army Med Ctr
6825 16th St NW
Washington, DC 20307-5001
Tel: 202 782-7804 *Fax:* 202 782-6845
Accred Length: 1 Year *Program Size:* 2
Program ID: 263-10-21-056
US Armed Services Program

Florida

Gainesville

University of Florida Program
Sponsor: University of Florida College of Medicine
Shands Hospital at the University of Florida
Program Director:
Paul C Dell, MD
Univ of Florida
Hampton Oaks
PO Box 100241
Gainesville, FL 32610-0241
Tel: 352 395-0644 *Fax:* 352 395-0657
E-mail: paul@ortho.ufl.edu
Accred Length: 1 Year *Program Size:* 2
Program ID: 263-11-21-011

Miami

University of Miami-Jackson Memorial Medical Center Program
Sponsor: University of Miami-Jackson Memorial Medical Center
Veterans Affairs Medical Center (Miami)
Program Director:
Elizabeth A Ouellette, MD
Univ of Miami Sch of Med
Dept of Ortho/Rehab
PO Box 016960 (D-27)
Miami, FL 33101
Tel: 305 585-7152 *Fax:* 305 324-7658
E-mail: eouellet@mednet.med.miami.edu
Accred Length: 1 Year *Program Size:* 1
Program ID: 263-11-21-013

Illinois

Chicago

University of Chicago Program
Sponsor: University of Chicago Hospitals
Program Director:
Daniel P Mass, MD
Univ of Chicago Med Ctr
Hand Surgery Service
5841 S Maryland Ave/MC6032
Chicago, IL 60637-1470
Tel: 773 702-6306 *Fax:* 773 702-4378
E-mail: dmass@surgery.bsd.uchicago.edu
Accred Length: 1 Year *Program Size:* 1
Program ID: 263-16-21-035

Indiana

Indianapolis

Indiana University School of Medicine Program
Sponsor: Indiana University School of Medicine
Clarian IU Hospital
Indiana Hand Center
St Vincent Hospital and Health Care Center
Program Director:
Alexander D Mih, MD
Indiana Hand Ctr
8501 Harcourt Rd
PO Box 80434
Indianapolis, IN 46280-0434
Tel: 317 875-9105, ext 334 *Fax:* 317 875-8638
Accred Length: 1 Year *Program Size:* 6
Program ID: 263-17-21-041

Iowa

Iowa City

University of Iowa Hospitals and Clinics Program
Sponsor: University of Iowa Hospitals and Clinics
Program Director:
Curtis M Steyers, MD
Univ of Iowa Hospitals and Clinics
Dept of Ortho Surgery
200 Hawkins Dr
Iowa City, IA 52242-1009
Tel: 319 356-3943
E-mail: curtis-steyers@uiowa.edu
Accred Length: 1 Year *Program Size:* 1
Program ID: 263-18-21-009

Massachusetts

Boston

Harvard Medical School (Massachusetts General) Program

Sponsor: Massachusetts General Hospital
Program Director:
Jesse B Jupiter, MD
Massachusetts General Hospital
Dept of Hand Surgery Serv/ACC527
15 Parkman St
Boston, MA 02114
Tel: 617 726-5100 *Fax:* 617 724-8532
E-mail: jupiter.jesse@mgh.harvard.edu
Accred Length: 1 Year *Program Size:* 2
Program ID: 263-24-21-057

Harvard Medical School Program

Sponsor: Brigham and Women's Hospital
Beth Israel Deaconess Medical Center
Brockton-West Roxbury Veterans Affairs Medical Center
Children's Hospital
Program Director:
Barry P Simmons, MD
Brigham and Women's Hospital
Dept of Ortho Surgery
75 Francis St
Boston, MA 02215-6195
Tel: 617 732-5378 *Fax:* 617 732-6937
E-mail: simmons@ortho.bwh.harvard.edu
Accred Length: 1 Year *Program Size:* 2
Program ID: 263-24-21-034

Tufts University Program

Sponsor: New England Medical Center Hospitals
New England Baptist Hospital
Newton-Wellesley Hospital
Program Director:
Leonard K Ruby, MD
New England Med Ctr
750 Washington St/Box 26
Boston, MA 02111
Tel: 617 636-5155 *Fax:* 617 636-5178
E-mail: leonard.ruby@es.nemc.org
Accred Length: 1 Year *Program Size:* 2
Program ID: 263-24-21-029

Michigan

Grand Rapids

Spectrum Health-East Campus Program

Sponsor: Spectrum Health-East Campus
Program Director:
Alfred B Swanson, MD
Spectrum Health East Campus
Dept of Ortho Surgery
1840 Wealthy St SE/Rm 3E-69
Grand Rapids, MI 49506
Tel: 616 774-7426 *Fax:* 616 774-5337
Accred Length: 1 Year *Program Size:* 1
Program ID: 263-25-21-058

Minnesota

Minneapolis

University of Minnesota Program

Sponsor: University of Minnesota Medical School
Fairview-University Medical Center
Gillette Children's Speciality Healthcare
Methodist Hospital
Program Director:
Matthew D Putnam, MD
420 Delaware St SE/Box 492
Minneapolis, MN 55455
Tel: 612 625-2157 *Fax:* 612 626-6032
E-mail: putna002@maroon.tc.umn.edu
Accred Length: 1 Year *Program Size:* 2
Program ID: 263-26-21-037

Rochester

Mayo Graduate School of Medicine (Rochester) Program

Sponsor: Mayo Graduate School of Medicine-Mayo Foundation
Mayo Clinic (Rochester)
Rochester Methodist Hospital
St Mary's Hospital of Rochester
Program Director:
Robert D Beckenbaugh, MD
Mayo Graduate Sch of Med
Application Processing Ctr
200 First St SW
Rochester, MN 55905
Tel: 507 284-4331 *Fax:* 507 284-0999
E-mail: mgsm.surgical.specialties@mayo.edu
Internet: http://www.mayo.edu/
Accred Length: 1 Year *Program Size:* 3
Program ID: 263-26-21-007

Mississippi

Jackson

University of Mississippi Medical Center Program

Sponsor: University of Mississippi School of Medicine
University Hospital
Veterans Affairs Medical Center (Jackson)
Program Director:
Alan E Freeland, MD
Michael F Angel, MD
Univ of Mississippi Med Ctr
Dept of Ortho Surgery
2500 N State St
Jackson, MS 39216-4505
Tel: 601 984-5155 *Fax:* 601 984-5151
E-mail: jmuzzi@orthopedics.umsmed.edu
Accred Length: 1 Year *Program Size:* 1
Program ID: 263-27-21-032

Missouri

St Louis

Washington University/B-JH/SLCH Consortium Program

Sponsor: Washington University/B-JH/SLCH Consortium
Program Director:
Richard H Gelberman, MD
Washington Univ, Dept of Orthopaedic Surgery
Ste 11300 West Pavilion
1 Barnes-Jewish Hospital Plaza
St Louis, MO 63110
Tel: 314 747-2543 *Fax:* 314 747-2597
E-mail: orthsurg@msnotes.wustl.edu
Internet: http://www.ortho.wustl.edu
Accred Length: 1 Year *Program Size:* 2
Program ID: 263-28-21-003

New Mexico

Albuquerque

University of New Mexico Program

Sponsor: University of New Mexico School of Medicine
University Hospital
Program Director:
Moheb S Moneim, MD
Univ of New Mexico Health Sciences Ctr
Dept of Orthopaedics/Hand Fellowship
ACC 2 West
Albuquerque, NM 87131-5296
Tel: 505 272-4107 *Fax:* 505 272-3581
E-mail: mmoneim@salud.unm.edu
Internet: http://www.unm.edu/~ortho
Accred Length: 1 Year *Program Size:* 2
Program ID: 263-34-21-027

New York

Buffalo

SUNY at Buffalo Graduate Medical-Dental Education Consortium Program

Sponsor: SUNY at Buffalo Grad Medical-Dental Education Consortium
CGF Health System (Millard Fillmore Hospitals)
Erie County Medical Center
Program Director:
Clayton A Peimer, MD
Hand Ctr of WNY
Millard Fillmore Hospital
3 Gates Cir
Buffalo, NY 14209
Tel: 716 887-4040 *Fax:* 716 887-5090
Accred Length: 1 Year *Program Size:* 3
Program ID: 263-35-21-012

New York

Hospital for Joint Diseases Orthopaedic Institute Program

Sponsor: Hospital for Joint Diseases Orthopaedic Institute
Program Director:
Martin A Posner, MD
Hospital for Joint Diseases
Dept of Hand Service
301 E 17th St
New York, NY 10003
Tel: 212 598-6497 *Fax:* 212 598-6581
Accred Length: 1 Year *Program Size:* 2
Program ID: 263-35-21-047

Programs

Hospital for Special Surgery/Cornell Medical Center Program

Sponsor: Hospital for Special Surgery
New York and Presbyterian Hospital (Cornell Campus)
St Luke's-Roosevelt Hospital Center

Program Director:
Robert N Hotchkiss, MD
Hospital for Special Surgery
535 E 70th St
New York, NY 10021
Tel: 212 606-1466
Internet: http://www.hss.edu
Accred Length: 1 Year *Program Size:* 3
Program ID: 263-35-21-017

New York and Presbyterian Hospital (Columbia Campus) Program

Sponsor: New York and Presbyterian Hospital
New York and Presbyterian Hospital (Columbia Campus)

Program Director:
Melvin P Rosenwasser, MD
New York Orthopaedic Hospital
161 Fort Washington Ave/Rm 251
New York, NY 10032
Tel: 212 305-8036 *Fax:* 212 305-7314
E-mail: rosenwas@pegasus.cpmc.columbia.edu
Internet:
http://www.cpmcnet.columbia.edu/dept/ortho/hand/html
Accred Length: 1 Year *Program Size:* 1
Program ID: 263-35-31-008

New York University Medical Center Program

Sponsor: New York University Medical Center
Bellevue Hospital Center
Veterans Affairs Medical Center (Manhattan)

Program Director:
Keith B Raskin Jr, MD
New York Univ Med Ctr-Hospital for Joint Diseases
317 E 34th St
New York, NY 10016
Tel: 212 683-4263
Accred Length: 1 Year *Program Size:* 3
Program ID: 263-35-21-063

St Luke's-Roosevelt Hospital Center Program

Sponsor: St Luke's-Roosevelt Hospital Center
St Luke's-Roosevelt Hospital Center-Roosevelt Division

Program Director:
Steven Z Glickel, MD
St Luke's-Roosevelt Hospital Ctr
CV Starr Hand Surgery Ctr
1000 Tenth Ave
New York, NY 10019
Tel: 212 523-7590 *Fax:* 212 523-7592
Accred Length: 1 Year *Program Size:* 2
Program ID: 263-35-21-055

Rochester

University of Rochester Program

Sponsor: Strong Memorial Hospital of the University of Rochester

Program Director:
Richard I Burton, MD
R Christie Wray, MD
Univ of Rochester Med Ctr
601 Elmwood Ave
Box 665
Rochester, NY 14642
Tel: 716 275-5168 *Fax:* 716 756-4721
E-mail: kyick@orthomail.ortho.rochester.edu
Internet:
http://www.urme.rochester.edu/smd/ortho/orthohome.html
Accred Length: 1 Year *Program Size:* 1
Program ID: 263-35-21-010

Stony Brook

SUNY at Stony Brook Program

Sponsor: University Hospital-SUNY at Stony Brook

Program Director:
Lawrence C Hurst, MD
SUNY-Stony Brook
Div of Hand Surgery
HSC T-18
Stony Brook, NY 11794-8181
Tel: 516 444-3145 *Fax:* 516 444-7671
Accred Length: 1 Year *Program Size:* 1
Program ID: 263-35-31-026

Syracuse

SUNY Health Science Center at Syracuse Program

Sponsor: University Hospital-SUNY Health Science Center at Syracuse
Crouse Hospital

Program Director:
Andrew K Palmer, MD
SUNY Health Science Ctr
Hand Surgery Serv
550 Harrison Ctr
Syracuse, NY 13202
Tel: 315 472-2015 *Fax:* 315 472-2980
E-mail: shortw@vax.cs.hscsyr.edu
Internet:
http://www.ec.hscsyr.edu:8001/worksinprogress/orthopedics/ortho.html
Accred Length: 1 Year *Program Size:* 2
Program ID: 263-35-21-021

North Carolina

Durham

Duke University Program

Sponsor: Duke University Medical Center

Program Director:
James R Urbaniak, MD
Duke Univ Med Ctr
PO Box 2912
Durham, NC 27710
Tel: 919 684-3170 *Fax:* 919 684-8280
Accred Length: 1 Year *Program Size:* 3
Program ID: 263-36-21-022

Winston-Salem

Wake Forest University School of Medicine Program

Sponsor: Wake Forest University Baptist Medical Center

Program Director:
L Andrew Koman, MD
North Carolina Baptist Hospital
Box 1070
Medical Center Blvd
Winston-Salem, NC 27157-1070
Tel: 336 716-3946 *Fax:* 336 716-6286
E-mail: hermance@wfubmc..edu
Internet: http://www.wfubmc.edu/ortho
Accred Length: 1 Year *Program Size:* 1
Program ID: 263-36-21-060

Ohio

Cincinnati

University Hospital/University of Cincinnati College of Medicine Program

Sponsor: University Hospital Inc
Bethesda Hospital Inc

Program Director:
Peter J Stern, MD
Mary S Stern Hand Surgery Foundation
2800 Winslow Ave/Ste 401
Cincinnati, OH 45206
Tel: 513 961-4263 *Fax:* 513 961-1503
Accred Length: 1 Year *Program Size:* 2
Program ID: 263-38-21-015

Cleveland

Cleveland Combined Hand Fellowship Program

Sponsor: Cleveland Clinic Foundation
MetroHealth Medical Center
University Hospitals of Cleveland

Program Director:
James E Culver, MD
Cleveland Combined Hand Fellowship
PO Box 1969-169
Cleveland, OH 44106
Tel: 216 444-2615 *Fax:* 216 445-3694
E-mail: meded@cesmtp.ccf.org
Internet: http://www.ccf.org
Accred Length: 1 Year *Program Size:* 3
Program ID: 263-38-21-045

Columbus

Ohio State University Program

Sponsor: Ohio State University Medical Center
Children's Hospital
Riverside Methodist Hospitals (OhioHealth)

Program Director:
Carl Richard Coleman, MD
Riverside Methodist Hospital
Med Educ Dept
3535 Olentangy River Rd
Columbus, OH 43214
Tel: 614 566-5762 *Fax:* 614 566-6852
Internet: http://www.ohiohealth.com
Accred Length: 1 Year *Program Size:* 0
Program ID: 263-38-21-005

Oklahoma

Oklahoma City

Integris Baptist Medical Center Program

Sponsor: Integris Baptist Medical Center
Columbia Presbyterian Hospital

Program Director:
Ghazi M Rayan, MD
Physicians Bldg D/Ste 700
3366 NW Expressway
Oklahoma City, OK 73112
Tel: 405 945-4888 *Fax:* 405 945-4887
Accred Length: 1 Year *Program Size:* 1
Program ID: 263-39-21-049

Pennsylvania

Philadelphia

Thomas Jefferson University Program

Sponsor: Thomas Jefferson University Hospital

Program Director:
Lee Osterman, MD
Div of Hand Surgery
Philadelphia Hand Ctr/PC
700 S Henderson Rd/Ste 200
King of Prussia, PA 19406
Tel: 610 768-4467 *Fax:* 610 768-4469
Internet: http://www.handcenters.com
Accred Length: 1 Year *Program Size:* 4
Program ID: 263-41-21-001

University of Pennsylvania Program

Sponsor: Hospital of the University of Pennsylvania
Children's Hospital of Philadelphia
Mercy Fitzgerald Hospital

Program Director:
David R Steinberg, MD
Hospital of the Univ of Pennsylvania
3400 Spruce St/2 Silverstein
Philadelphia, PA 19104-4283
Tel: 215 662-3350 *Fax:* 215 349-5890
Accred Length: 1 Year *Program Size:* 2
Program ID: 263-41-21-004

Pittsburgh

Allegheny General Hospital Program

Sponsor: Allegheny General Hospital

Program Director:
Joseph E Imbriglia, MD
Allegheny General Hospital
Dept of Ortho Surgery
320 E North Ave
Pittsburgh, PA 15212
Tel: 412 359-6501 *Fax:* 412 359-6265
E-mail: lhays@aherf.edu
Accred Length: 1 Year *Program Size:* 3
Program ID: 263-41-21-031

University Health Center of Pittsburgh Program

Sponsor: University Health Center of Pittsburgh
Children's Hospital of Pittsburgh
Veterans Affairs Medical Center (Pittsburgh)

Program Director:
Dean G Sotereanos, MD
Dept of Ortho Surgery
Liliane Kaufmann Bldg/Ste 1010
3471 Fifth Ave
Pittsburgh, PA 15213-3221
Tel: 412 605-3209 *Fax:* 412 687-3724
E-mail: kneiderm@uoi.upmc.edu
Internet: http://www.orthonet.upmc.edu
Accred Length: 1 Year *Program Size:* 1
Program ID: 263-41-21-051

Tennessee

Memphis

University of Tennessee Program

Sponsor: University of Tennessee College of Medicine
University of Tennessee-Campbell Clinic

Program Director:
Phillip E Wright II, MD
Univ of Tennessee-Campbell Clinic
Dept of Ortho/Hand Surgery
910 Madison Ave/Ste 500
Memphis, TN 38104-3403
Tel: 901 729-3136 *Fax:* 901 759-3278
Accred Length: 1 Year *Program Size:* 0
Program ID: 263-47-21-046

Texas

Houston

Baylor College of Medicine Program

Sponsor: Baylor College of Medicine
Harris County Hospital District-Ben Taub General Hospital
Methodist Hospital
Veterans Affairs Medical Center (Houston)

Program Director:
David H Hildreth, MD
Baylor Coll of Med
Dept of Ortho Surgery
6550 Fannin St/Ste 2625
Houston, TX 77030
Tel: 713 986-7390 *Fax:* 713 986-7391
Accred Length: 1 Year *Program Size:* 2
Program ID: 263-48-31-002

San Antonio

University of Texas Health Science Center at San Antonio Program

Sponsor: University of Texas Medical School at San Antonio
St Luke's Baptist Hospital
University Hospital-South Texas Medical Center

Program Director:
David P Green, MD
Hand Ctr of San Antonio
9150 Huebner Rd/#290
San Antonio, TX 78240
Tel: 210 558-7025, ext 121 *Fax:* 210 558-4664
Internet: http://www.handcentersa.com
Accred Length: 1 Year *Program Size:* 4
Program ID: 263-48-21-025

Utah

Salt Lake City

University of Utah Program

Sponsor: University of Utah Medical Center

Program Director:
Douglas T Hutchinson, MD
Univ of Utah Med Ctr
50 N Medical Dr/Rm 3B165
Salt Lake City, UT 84132-0001
Tel: 801 581-7601 *Fax:* 801 581-6178
E-mail: dhutchinson@ortho.med.ut.edu
Accred Length: 1 Year *Program Size:* 2
Program ID: 263-49-21-048

Washington

Seattle

University of Washington Program

Sponsor: University of Washington School of Medicine
Harborview Medical Center
University of Washington Medical Center

Program Director:
Thomas Trumble, MD
Univ of Washington Med Ctr
Dept of Orthopaedics
Box 356600
Seattle, WA 98195
Tel: 206 543-3690 *Fax:* 206 685-3139
Internet: http://weber.u.washington.edu/~trumble/
Accred Length: 1 Year *Program Size:* 3
Program ID: 263-54-21-033

Hand Surgery (Plastic Surgery)

California

Los Angeles

University of Southern California Program
Sponsor: Los Angeles County-USC Medical Center
Southern California Orthopedic Institute
Program Director:
Randolph Sherman, MD
Univ of Southern California
Plastic/Reconstructive Surgery
1450 San Pablo St/Ste 2000
Los Angeles, CA 90033
Tel: 323 442-6482 *Fax:* 323 442-6481
E-mail: randys@hsc.usc.edu
Accred Length: 1 Year *Program Size:* 2
Program ID: 363-05-21-014

San Francisco

University of California (San Francisco) Program
Sponsor: University of California (San Francisco) School of Medicine
Davies Medical Center
University of California (San Francisco) Medical Center
Program Director:
Harry J Buncke, MD
Microsurgical Replant/Transplant Dept
CPMGI Davies Campus
45 Castro St/Ste 140
San Francisco, CA 94114
Tel: 415 565-6136 *Fax:* 415 864-1654
E-mail: pps@buncke.org
Internet: http://www.summit.stanford.edu/buncke
Accred Length: 1 Year *Program Size:* 2
Program ID: 363-05-31-017

Connecticut

New Haven

Yale-New Haven Medical Center Program
Sponsor: Yale-New Haven Hospital
Hospital of St Raphael
Veterans Affairs Medical Center (West Haven)
Program Director:
J Grant Thomson, MD
333 Cedar St
PO Box 208041
New Haven, CT 06520
Tel: 203 737-5130 *Fax:* 203 785-5714
Accred Length: 1 Year *Program Size:* 1
Program ID: 363-08-21-024

Florida

Tampa

University of South Florida Program
Sponsor: University of South Florida College of Medicine
James A Haley Veterans Hospital
Shriners Hospitals for Children (Tampa)
Tampa General Healthcare
Program Director:
Robert Belsole, MD
Univ of South Florida
4 Columbia Dr/#730
Tampa, FL 33606
Tel: 813 259-0857 *Fax:* 813 259-0885
E-mail: rbelsole@com1.med.usf.edu
Accred Length: 1 Year *Program Size:* 2
Program ID: 363-11-21-022

Illinois

Springfield

Southern Illinois University Program
Sponsor: Southern Illinois University School of Medicine
Memorial Medical Center
St John's Hospital
Program Director:
Richard E Brown, MD
501 N 1st St
PO Box 19248
Springfield, IL 62794-9248
Tel: 217 789-7480 *Fax:* 217 789-9716
Accred Length: 1 Year *Program Size:* 1
Program ID: 363-16-21-023

Massachusetts

Boston

Harvard Medical School Program 1
Sponsor: Massachusetts General Hospital
Program Director:
W P Andrew Lee, MD
Massachusetts General Hospital
15 Parkman St/Ste 453
Boston, MA 02114
Tel: 617 724-0400 *Fax:* 617 726-2824
E-mail: lee.wpa@mgh.harvard.edu
Accred Length: 1 Year *Program Size:* 1
Program ID: 363-24-21-001

Harvard Medical School Program 2
Sponsor: Beth Israel Deaconess Medical Center
Cambridge Hospital/Cambridge Health Alliance
Program Director:
Joseph Upton, MD
830 Boylston St/Ste 212
Chestnut Hill, MA 02467
Tel: 617 739-1972 *Fax:* 617 739-6624
Accred Length: 1 Year *Program Size:* 1
Program ID: 363-24-31-012

Michigan

Detroit

Wayne State University/Detroit Medical Center Program
Sponsor: Wayne State University/Detroit Medical Center
Harper Hospital
Program Director:
Mehul M Mehta, MD
Wayne State Univ-Detroit Med Ctr
3990 John R St
Detroit, MI 48201
Tel: 313 831-4800 *Fax:* 313 831-3578
Accred Length: 1 Year *Program Size:* 2
Program ID: 363-25-21-020

Missouri

St Louis

Washington University/B-JH/SLCH Consortium Program
Sponsor: Washington University/B-JH/SLCH Consortium
Barnes-Jewish Hospital
Program Director:
Susan E Mackinnon, MD
Washington Univ
One Barnes-Jewish Hospital Plaza/Ste 17424
St Louis, MO 63110
Tel: 314 362-4585 *Fax:* 314 362-4536
E-mail: woltmanr@msnotes.wustl.edu
Accred Length: 1 Year *Program Size:* 2
Program ID: 363-28-21-005

New York

New York

New York University Medical Center Program
Sponsor: New York University Medical Center
Bellevue Hospital Center
Mount Sinai Medical Center
Program Director:
Robert W Beasley, MD
Inst of Reconstructive Plastic Surgery
New York Univ Med Ctr
550 First Ave
New York, NY 10016
Tel: 212 685-3834 *Fax:* 212 545-1388
Accred Length: 1 Year *Program Size:* 2
Program ID: 363-35-21-010

Oregon

Portland

Oregon Health Sciences University Program
Sponsor: Oregon Health Sciences University Hospital
Shriners Hospitals for Children (Portland)
Veterans Affairs Medical Center (Portland)
Program Director:
Alan E Seyfer, MD
Oregon Heatlh Sciences Univ
3181 SW Sam Jackson Park Rd/L352A
Portland, OR 97201
Tel: 503 494-7824 *Fax:* 503 494-0441
E-mail: seyfera@ohsu.edu
Internet: http://www.ohsu.edu/som/plasticsurg
Accred Length: 1 Year *Program Size:* 1
Program ID: 363-40-21-018

Pennsylvania

Pittsburgh

University Health Center of Pittsburgh Program
Sponsor: University Health Center of Pittsburgh
Presbyterian University Hospital/UPMC
Program Director:
N Ake Nystrom, MD PhD
Univ of Pittsburgh
Div of Plastic Surgery
660 Scaife Hall
Pittsburgh, PA 15261
Tel: 412 648-4460 *Fax:* 412 648-1987
E-mail: nystrom@pittsurg.nb.upmc.edu
Accred Length: 1 Year *Program Size:* 1
Program ID: 363-41-21-016

Texas

Dallas

University of Texas Southwestern Medical School Program
Sponsor: University of Texas Southwestern Medical School
Dallas County Hospital District-Parkland Memorial Hospital
Texas Scottish Rite Hospital for Children
Program Director:
Harry H Orenstein, MD
Univ of Texas Southwestern Med Ctr
Dept of Plastic Surgery
5323 Harry Hines Blvd
Dallas, TX 75235-9132
Tel: 214 648-3661 *Fax:* 214 648-6776
Internet: http://www.swmed.edu/home_pages/plastsurg
Accred Length: 1 Year *Program Size:* 1
Program ID: 363-48-21-004

Houston

Baylor College of Medicine Program
Sponsor: Baylor College of Medicine
Harris County Hospital District-Ben Taub General Hospital
St Luke's Episcopal Hospital
Texas Children's Hospital
Veterans Affairs Medical Center (Houston)
Program Director:
Fred B Kessler, MD
Baylor Coll of Med
Div of Plastic Surgery
6560 Fannin/Ste 800
Houston, TX 77030
Tel: 713 798-8555 *Fax:* 713 798-3806
E-mail: mateo@bcm.tmc.edu
Accred Length: 1 Year *Program Size:* 2
Program ID: 363-48-31-008

Virginia

Charlottesville

University of Virginia Program
Sponsor: University of Virginia Medical Center
Program Director:
David B Drake, MD
Univ of Virginia Health Sciences Ctr
Dept of Plastic Surgery
PO Box 376
Charlottesville, VA 22908
Tel: 804 924-1234 *Fax:* 804 924-1333
Accred Length: 1 Year *Program Size:* 1
Program ID: 363-51-21-013

Wisconsin

Milwaukee

Medical College of Wisconsin Program
Sponsor: Medical College of Wisconsin Affiliated Hospitals Inc
Children's Hospital of Wisconsin
Froedtert Memorial Lutheran Hospital
Program Director:
Hani S Matloub, MD
Med Coll of Wisconsin Clinics-Froedtert East
Dept of Plastic Surgery
9200 W Wisconsin Ave
Milwaukee, WI 53226-3596
Tel: 414 454-5447 *Fax:* 414 259-0901
E-mail: cromellp@mcw.edu
Accred Length: 1 Year *Program Size:* 1
Program ID: 363-56-21-007

Hematology (Internal Medicine)

Arkansas

Little Rock

University of Arkansas for Medical Sciences Program
Sponsor: University of Arkansas College of Medicine
John L McClellan Memorial Veterans Hospital
University Hospital of Arkansas
Program Director:
Susan C Guba, MD
Clive S Zent, MD MD
Univ of Arkansas for Med Sciences
4301 W Markham St/Slot 508
Little Rock, AR 72205-7199
Tel: 501 686-8511 *Fax:* 501 686-7861
Accred Length: 2 Years *Program Size:* 6
Program ID: 145-04-21-096

California

La Jolla

Scripps Clinic/Scripps Green Hospital Program
Sponsor: Scripps Clinic
Scripps Green Hospital
Program Director:
Michael P Kosty, MD
Scripps Clinic-Green Hospital
Dept of Grad Med Educ
10666 N Torrey Pines Rd/403C
La Jolla, CA 92037-1093
Tel: 619 554-8582 *Fax:* 619 554-6310
E-mail: gme@scripps.edu
Internet: http://www.scrippsclinic.com
Accred Length: 2 Years *Program Size:* 4
Program ID: 145-05-21-062

Los Angeles

UCLA Medical Center Program
Sponsor: UCLA School of Medicine
UCLA Medical Center
VA Greater Los Angeles Healthcare System
Program Director:
Robert A Figlin, MD
UCLA Med Ctr
Dept of Med/Hem-Onc
10833 Le Conte Ave
Los Angeles, CA 90095-1736
Tel: 310 825-5788 *Fax:* 310 206-5414
E-mail: rfiglin@med1.medsch.ucla.edu
Accred Length: 2 Years *Program Size:* 17
Program ID: 145-05-11-112

University of Southern California Program
Sponsor: Los Angeles County-USC Medical Center
Program Director:
Alexandra Levine, MD
Univ of Southern California Sch of Med
Norris Cancer Hospital
1441 Eastlake Ave/MS 34
Los Angeles, CA 90033
Tel: 323 865-3913 *Fax:* 323 865-0060
E-mail: hornor@hsc.usc.edu
Accred Length: 2 Years *Program Size:* 6
Program ID: 145-05-21-046

Orange

University of California (Irvine) Program

Sponsor: University of California (Irvine) Medical Center
Long Beach Memorial Medical Center
Veterans Affairs Medical Center (Long Beach)

Program Director:
Randall F Holcombe, MD
Dept of Med/Hem-Onc
101 City Dr S
Bldg 23 Rm 244 Rte 81
Orange, CA 92868-3298
Tel: 714 456-5153 *Fax:* 714 456-2242
E-mail: rholcomb@uci.edu
Accred Length: 2 Years *Program Size:* 7
Program ID: 145-05-21-130

Stanford

Stanford University Program

Sponsor: Stanford University Hospital
Veterans Affairs Palo Alto Health Care System

Program Director:
Stanley L Schrier, MD
Stanford Univ Med Ctr
Div of Hematology/Rm S161
300 Pasteur Dr
Stanford, CA 94305-5112
Tel: 650 723-5007 *Fax:* 650 723-1269
Accred Length: 2 Years *Program Size:* 9
Program ID: 145-05-21-020

Connecticut

New Haven

Yale-New Haven Medical Center Program

Sponsor: Yale-New Haven Hospital

Program Director:
Bernard Forget, MD
Yale Univ Sch of Med
Hematology Sect/WWW 403
333 Cedar St
New Haven, CT 06520-8021
Tel: 203 785-4144 *Fax:* 203 785-7232
E-mail: bernard.forget@yale.edu
Accred Length: 2 Years *Program Size:* 6
Program ID: 145-08-21-021

District of Columbia

Washington

Georgetown University Program

Sponsor: Georgetown University Medical Center

Program Director:
Carl E Freter, MD PhD
Georgetown Univ Med Ctr
Div of Hematology/Oncology LCC
3800 Reservoir Rd NW/P Corr B
Washington, DC 20007-2197
Tel: 202 687-1686 *Fax:* 202 687-4429
E-mail: hussc@gunet.georgetown.edu
Accred Length: 2 Years *Program Size:* 8
Program ID: 145-10-21-078

Howard University Program

Sponsor: Howard University Hospital
District of Columbia General Hospital

Program Director:
Elliott Perlin, MD
Howard Univ Hospital
2041 Georgia Ave NW/Ste 5146
Washington, DC 20060
Tel: 202 865-1511 *Fax:* 202 865-6180
Accred Length: 2 Years *Program Size:* 2
Program ID: 145-10-21-114

Kansas

Kansas City

University of Kansas Medical Center Program

Sponsor: University of Kansas School of Medicine
University of Kansas Medical Center

Program Director:
David C Bodensteiner, MD
Univ of Kansas Med Ctr
Hematology Div/1417 Bell
3901 Rainbow Blvd
Kansas City, KS 66160-7233
Tel: 913 588-6077 *Fax:* 913 588-3996
Accred Length: 2 Years *Program Size:* 5
Program ID: 145-19-21-100

Louisiana

New Orleans

Louisiana State University Program

Sponsor: Louisiana State University School of Medicine
Medical Center of Louisiana at New Orleans

Program Director:
Robert Veith, MD
Louisiana State Univ Med Ctr
1542 Tulane Ave
New Orleans, LA 70112
Tel: 504 568-5843 *Fax:* 504 568-3694
E-mail: rveth@lsumc.edu
Accred Length: 2 Years *Program Size:* 4
Program ID: 145-21-21-173

Maryland

Baltimore

Johns Hopkins University Program

Sponsor: Johns Hopkins University School of Medicine
Johns Hopkins Hospital

Program Director:
Chi V Dang, MD PhD
Johns Hopkins Univ Sch of Med
Dept of Med
Baltimore, MD 21205-2196
Tel: 410 955-9175 *Fax:* 410 955-0185
E-mail: cvdang@welchlink.welch.jhu.edu
Internet:
http://ww2.med.jhu.edu/hematology/first_page.html
Accred Length: 2 Years *Program Size:* 2
Program ID: 145-23-11-064

Bethesda

National Institutes of Health Clinical Center Program

Sponsor: NIH Warren Grant Magnuson Clinical Center

Program Director:
Cynthia E Dunbar, MD
Hematology Branch/NHLBI
9000 Rockville Pike
Bldg 10/Rm 7C103
Bethesda, MD 20892-1652
Tel: 301 496-5093 *Fax:* 301 496-8396
E-mail: dunbar@gwgate.nhlbi.nih.gov
Accred Length: 2 Years *Program Size:* 11
Program ID: 145-23-21-177

Michigan

Detroit

Wayne State University/Detroit Medical Center Program

Sponsor: Wayne State University/Detroit Medical Center
Harper Hospital

Program Director:
Neil Lachant, MD
Harper Hospital/4 Brush S
Div of Hemotology/Oncology
3990 John R St
Detroit, MI 48201
Tel: 313 745-8853 *Fax:* 313 993-0307
E-mail: lachantn@karmanos.org
Internet: http://www.karmanos.org
Accred Length: 2 Years *Program Size:* 4
Program ID: 145-25-21-186

New Jersey

South Orange

Seton Hall University School of Graduate Medical Education Program

Sponsor: Seton Hall University School of Graduate Medical Education
St Joseph's Hospital and Medical Center
St Michael's Medical Center (Cathedral Hlth Srvcs Inc)

Program Director:
Arnold Rubin, MD
St Joseph's Hospital and Med Ctr
703 Main St
Paterson, NJ 07503
Tel: 973 754-2432 *Fax:* 973 754-2444
Accred Length: 2 Years *Program Size:* 4
Program ID: 145-33-11-138

New York

Albany

Albany Medical Center Program

Sponsor: Albany Medical Center

Program Director:
Peter T Burkart, MD
Albany Med Coll
Div of Hematology/Oncology (A-52)
47 New Scotland Ave
Albany, NY 12208
Tel: 518 262-5355 *Fax:* 518 262-5975
Accred Length: 2 Years *Program Size:* 2
Program ID: 145-35-31-026

Bronx

Albert Einstein College of Medicine Program

Sponsor: Albert Einstein College of Medicine of Yeshiva University
Jacobi Medical Center
Montefiore Medical Center-Henry and Lucy Moses Division
North Central Bronx Hospital

Program Director:
Shirley P Levine, MD
Montefiore Med Ctr
111 E 210th St
Bronx, NY 10467
Tel: 718 920-7388 *Fax:* 718 881-2666
Accred Length: 2 Years *Program Size:* 4
Program ID: 145-35-21-089

Brooklyn

Brooklyn Hospital Center Program

Sponsor: Brooklyn Hospital Center
Woodhull Medical and Mental Health Center

Program Director:
Perry Cook, MD
Brooklyn Hospital Ctr
121 Dekalb Ave
Brooklyn, NY 11201
Tel: 718 250-6960 *Fax:* 718 250-6492
E-mail: percook@earthlink.net
Accred Length: 2 Years *Program Size:* 3
Program ID: 145-35-12-161

Coney Island Hospital Program

Sponsor: Coney Island Hospital

Program Director:
Joel M Schwartz, MD
Coney Island Hospital
2601 Ocean Pkwy/Rm 9N8
Brooklyn, NY 11235
Tel: 718 616-3183 *Fax:* 718 616-3182
Accred Length: 2 Years *Program Size:* 3
Program ID: 145-35-11-149

New York Methodist Hospital Program

Sponsor: New York Methodist Hospital

Program Director:
Muthuswamy Krishnamurthy, MD
New York Methodist Hospital
506 Sixth St
Brooklyn, NY 11215
Tel: 718 780-5246 *Fax:* 718 780-3259
Accred Length: 2 Years *Program Size:* 4
Program ID: 145-35-11-122

Buffalo

SUNY at Buffalo Graduate Medical-Dental Education Consortium Program

Sponsor: SUNY at Buffalo Grad Medical-Dental Education Consortium
CGF Health System (Buffalo General Hospital)
Erie County Medical Center
Veterans Affairs Medical Center (Buffalo)

Program Director:
Gerald L Logue, MD
Erie County Med Ctr
Dept of Medicine
462 Grider St
Buffalo, NY 14215
Tel: 716 898-3941 *Fax:* 716 898-3279
Accred Length: 2 Years *Program Size:* 6
Program ID: 145-35-31-008

East Meadow

SUNY at Stony Brook (East Meadow) Program

Sponsor: Nassau County Medical Center

Program Director:
Stephen Feffer, MD
Nassau County Med Ctr
2201 Hempstead Trnpk
East Meadow, NY 11554-5400
Tel: 516 572-4713 *Fax:* 516 572-5609
Accred Length: 2 Years *Program Size:* 2
Program ID: 145-35-21-084

New York

New York University Medical Center Program

Sponsor: New York University Medical Center
Bellevue Hospital Center
Veterans Affairs Medical Center (Manhattan)

Program Director:
Simon Karpatkin, MD
New York Univ Med Ctr
550 First Ave
New York, NY 10016
Tel: 212 263-5609 *Fax:* 212 263-0695
E-mail: simon.karpatkin@mcfpo.med.nyu.edu
Internet: http://www.med.nyu.edu/medicine/hem2.htm2
Accred Length: 2 Years *Program Size:* 8
Program ID: 145-35-21-104

St Luke's-Roosevelt Hospital Center Program

Sponsor: St Luke's-Roosevelt Hospital Center
St Luke's-Roosevelt Hospital Center-Roosevelt Division
St Luke's-Roosevelt Hospital Center-St Luke's Division

Program Director:
Arthur Karanas, MD
St Luke's-Roosevelt Hospital Ctr
1000 Tenth Ave
Ste 3B-20
New York, NY 10019
Tel: 212 523-7281 *Fax:* 212 523-6677
Accred Length: 2 Years *Program Size:* 5
Program ID: 145-35-11-091

Pennsylvania

Philadelphia

Thomas Jefferson University Program

Sponsor: Thomas Jefferson University Hospital

Program Director:
Barbara A Konkle, MD
Thomas Jefferson Univ
Cardeza Foundation, Div of Hematology
1015 Walnut St/Rm 705
Philadelphia, PA 19107-5099
Tel: 215 955-7786 *Fax:* 215 955-2366
E-mail: barbara.konkle@mail.tju.edu
Accred Length: 2 Years *Program Size:* 12
Program ID: 145-41-21-031

Pittsburgh

University Health Center of Pittsburgh Program

Sponsor: University Health Center of Pittsburgh
Presbyterian University Hospital/UPMC
Veterans Affairs Medical Center (Pittsburgh)

Program Director:
Robert R Redner, MD
Univ of Pittsburgh
Med Oncology, 7 Main North
200 Lothrop St
Pittsburgh, PA 15213
Tel: 412 648-6686 *Fax:* 412 692-2757
E-mail: manndj@msx.upmc.edu
Accred Length: 2 Years *Program Size:* 12
Program ID: 145-41-21-040

Puerto Rico

Rio Piedras

San Juan City Hospital Program

Sponsor: San Juan City Hospital
University Hospital Ramon Ruiz Arnau
Veterans Affairs Medical Center (San Juan)

Program Director:
Luis Baez, MD
San Juan Municipal Hospital, Dept of Med
PO Box 21405
Rio Piedras, PR 00928
Tel: 787 758-7348 *Fax:* 787 758-7348
Accred Length: 2 Years *Program Size:* 4
Program ID: 145-42-11-086

Tennessee

Memphis

University of Tennessee Program

Sponsor: University of Tennessee College of Medicine
Baptist Memorial Hospital
Regional Medical Center at Memphis
Veterans Affairs Medical Center (Memphis)

Program Director:
Harvey B Niell, MD
Dept of Med
3 N Dunlap/Rm 326
Memphis, TN 38163
Tel: 901 448-5717 *Fax:* 901 448-5033
Accred Length: 2 Years *Program Size:* 4
Program ID: 145-47-21-125

Texas

Houston

Baylor College of Medicine Program

Sponsor: Baylor College of Medicine
Harris County Hospital District-Ben Taub General Hospital
Methodist Hospital
Veterans Affairs Medical Center (Houston)

Program Director:
Lawrence Rice, MD
Baylor Coll of Med
Texas Med Ctr
6550 Fannin St/MS 9023
Houston, TX 77030
Tel: 713 790-2157 *Fax:* 713 790-0828
Accred Length: 2 Years *Program Size:* 3
Program ID: 145-48-21-076

University of Texas at Houston Program
Sponsor: University of Texas Medical School at Houston
Lyndon B Johnson General Hospital
Memorial Hermann Healthcare System
University of Texas M D Anderson Cancer Center
Program Director:
Perumal Thiagarajan, MD
Univ of Texas Med Sch
6431 Fannin St/Rm 5284
Houston, TX 77030
Tel: 713 500-6800 *Fax:* 713 500-6810
E-mail: perumal@heart.med.uth.tmc.edu
Accred Length: 2 Years *Program Size:* 2
Program ID: 145-48-31-016

Washington

Seattle

University of Washington Program
Sponsor: University of Washington School of Medicine
University of Washington Medical Center
Program Director:
John M Harlan, MD
Univ Med Ctr
1959 NE Pacific St
Box 357710
Seattle, WA 98195-7710
Tel: 206 685-7866 *Fax:* 206 543-3560
E-mail: jharlan@u.washington.edu
Internet: http://weber.u.washington.edu/~hemat/
Accred Length: 2 Years *Program Size:* 10
Program ID: 145-54-21-077

Wisconsin

Madison

University of Wisconsin Program
Sponsor: University of Wisconsin Hospital and Clinics
William S Middleton Veterans Hospital
Program Director:
Eliot C Williams, MD PhD
Univ of Wisconsin Hospital and Clinics
600 Highland Ave/Rm H4-534
Madison, WI 53792-5156
Tel: 608 263-1836 *Fax:* 608 262-1982
E-mail: williams@medicine.wisc.edu
Internet: http://www.medicine.wisc.edu
Accred Length: 2 Years *Program Size:* 2
Program ID: 145-56-21-109

Hematology (Pathology)

Alabama

Birmingham

University of Alabama Medical Center Program
Sponsor: University of Alabama Hospital
Program Director:
Catherine M Listinsky, MD
Vishnu Reddy, MD
619 S 19th St
Birmingham, AL 35233
Tel: 205 975-8880 *Fax:* 205 975-7284
E-mail: clistinsky@path.uab.edu
Accred Length: 1 Year *Program Size:* 1
Program ID: 311-01-21-056

Arkansas

Little Rock

University of Arkansas for Medical Sciences Program
Sponsor: University of Arkansas College of Medicine
John L McClellan Memorial Veterans Hospital
University Hospital of Arkansas
Program Director:
James T Flick, MD PhD
Univ of Arkansas Med Ctr
Dept of Pathology
4301 W Markham St
Little Rock, AR 72205
Tel: 501 686-7015 *Fax:* 501 296-1053
Accred Length: 1 Year *Program Size:* 1
Program ID: 311-04-21-038

California

Duarte

City of Hope National Medical Center Program
Sponsor: City of Hope National Medical Center
Program Director:
Daniel A Arber, MD
City of Hope National Med Ctr
Anatomic Pathology
1500 E Duarte Rd
Duarte, CA 91010
Tel: 626 359-8111, ext 2456 *Fax:* 626 301-8145
E-mail: darber@coh.org
Internet: http://www.coh.org
Accred Length: 1 Year *Program Size:* 2
Program ID: 311-05-21-040

Los Angeles

Cedars-Sinai Medical Center Program
Sponsor: Cedars-Sinai Medical Center
Program Director:
Stephen Lee, MD
Div of Hematology/Immunology
8700 Beverly Blvd
Rm 4533
Los Angeles, CA 90048
Tel: 310 855-5471 *Fax:* 310 659-2306
Accred Length: 1 Year *Program Size:* 2
Program ID: 311-05-21-016

UCLA Medical Center Program
Sponsor: UCLA School of Medicine
UCLA Medical Center
Program Director:
Faramarz Naeim, MD
UCLA Dept of Pathology
A2-179 Ctr for Health Sciences
Los Angeles, CA 90095-1713
Tel: 310 825-4275 *Fax:* 310 206-3900
E-mail: fnaeim@pathology.medsch.ucla.edu
Internet: http://www.pathnet.medsch.ucla.edu
Accred Length: 1 Year *Program Size:* 1
Program ID: 311-05-21-062

University of Southern California Program
Sponsor: Los Angeles County-USC Medical Center
Program Director:
Russel K Brynes, MD
Bhart N Nathwani, MD
Los Angeles County-USC Med Ctr
Dept of Pathology
1200 N State St/Rm 2426
Los Angeles, CA 90033
Tel: 323 226-7020 *Fax:* 323 226-2686
Accred Length: 1 Year *Program Size:* 1
Program ID: 311-05-21-017

Sacramento

University of California (Davis) Program
Sponsor: University of California (Davis) Medical Center
Program Director:
Edward C Larkin, MD
Univ of California Davis Med Ctr
4625 Second Ave
Sacramento, CA 95817-2283
Tel: 916 734-2370 *Fax:* 916 734-0299
E-mail: elarkin@clb.ucdmc.ucdavis.edu
Internet: http://www.pathology.ucdmc.ucdavis.edu
Accred Length: 1 Year *Program Size:* 1
Program ID: 311-05-21-009

San Francisco

University of California (San Francisco) Program
Sponsor: University of California (San Francisco) School of Medicine
University of California (San Francisco) Medical Center
Program Director:
Susan K Atwater, MD
Univ of California San Francisco
505 Parnassus Ave
Rm M524D
San Francisco, CA 94143-0010
Tel: 415 476-2094 *Fax:* 415 476-3303
E-mail: atwater@pangloss.ucsf.edu
Accred Length: 1 Year *Program Size:* 1
Program ID: 311-05-21-053

Stanford

Stanford University Program
Sponsor: Stanford University Hospital
Program Director:
Joanne Cornbleet, MD
Clinical Laboratories H1524
300 Pasteur Dr
Stanford, CA 94305-5627
Tel: 650 723-5946 *Fax:* 650 723-3147
E-mail: jcornbleet@pathology.stanford.edu
Accred Length: 1 Year *Program Size:* 2
Program ID: 311-05-21-073

Connecticut

Hartford

Hartford Hospital Program
Sponsor: Hartford Hospital
Program Director:
William N Rezuke, MD
Hartford Hospital, Div of Hematology
80 Seymour St
PO Box 5037
Hartford, CT 06102-5037
Tel: 860 545-2008 *Fax:* 860 545-5206
E-mail: wrezuke@harthosp.org
Accred Length: 1 Year *Program Size:* 2
Program ID: 311-08-11-021

Florida

Gainesville

University of Florida Program
Sponsor: University of Florida College of Medicine
Shands Hospital at the University of Florida
Program Director:
Raul C Braylan, MD
Univ of Florida
PO Box 100275
Gainesville, FL 32610-0275
Tel: 352 392-3477 *Fax:* 352 392-4693
E-mail: braylan@ufl.edu
Accred Length: 1 Year *Program Size:* 1
Program ID: 311-11-21-051

Georgia

Atlanta

Emory University Program
Sponsor: Emory University School of Medicine
Emory University Hospital
Program Director:
Diane C Farhi, MD
Educ Office/Dept of Pathology
H-189 Emory Univ Hospital
1364 Clifton Rd NE
Atlanta, GA 30322-8110
Tel: 404 727-4283 *Fax:* 404 727-2519
E-mail: dfarhi@emory. edu
Internet: http://www.emory.edu/pathology/residency/
Accred Length: 1 Year *Program Size:* 1
Program ID: 311-12-21-027

Illinois

Chicago

McGaw Medical Center of Northwestern University Program
Sponsor: Northwestern University Medical School
Northwestern Memorial Hospital
Program Director:
LoAnn Peterson, MD
Northwestern Memorial Hospital
250 E Superior St
Wesley Pavilion/Rm 393
Chicago, IL 60611
Tel: 312 908-2687 *Fax:* 312 908-1403
E-mail: loannc@nwu.edu
Accred Length: 1 Year *Program Size:* 1
Program ID: 311-16-21-058

University of Chicago Program
Sponsor: University of Chicago Hospitals
Program Director:
James W Vardiman, MD
Univ of Chicago Hospitals
Dept of Pathology
5841 S Maryland Ave/MC0008
Chicago, IL 60637
Tel: 773 702-6196 *Fax:* 773 702-1200
Accred Length: 1 Year *Program Size:* 1
Program ID: 311-16-21-037

University of Illinois College of Medicine at Chicago Program
Sponsor: University of Illinois College of Medicine at Chicago
Program Director:
Basil A Bradlow, MD
Div of Clinical Pathology (M/C 750)
Univ of Illinois Coll of Med
840 S Wood St
Chicago, IL 60612
Tel: 312 413-0285 *Fax:* 312 413-0156
E-mail: bbradlow@uic.edu
Accred Length: 1 Year *Program Size:* 1
Program ID: 311-16-21-041

Maywood

Loyola University Program
Sponsor: Loyola University Medical Center
Edward J Hines Jr Veterans Affairs Hospital
Program Director:
Serhan Alkan, MD
Loyola Univ Med Ctr
2160 S First Ave
Maywood, IL 60153
Tel: 708 327-2610 *Fax:* 708 327-2620
E-mail: salkan@luc.edu
Accred Length: 1 Year *Program Size:* 2
Program ID: 311-16-21-018

Indiana

Indianapolis

Indiana University School of Medicine Program
Sponsor: Indiana University School of Medicine
Clarian IU Hospital
Clarian Riley Hospital for Children
Program Director:
Richard S Neiman, MD
Riley Hospital for Children
Div of Hematopathology/Rm 0969
702 Barnhill Dr
Indianapolis, IN 46202-5200
Tel: 317 274-7250 *Fax:* 317 274-0149
E-mail: rneiman@indyunix.iupui.edu
Accred Length: 1 Year *Program Size:* 1
Program ID: 311-17-21-045

Iowa

Iowa City

University of Iowa Hospitals and Clinics Program
Sponsor: University of Iowa Hospitals and Clinics
Program Director:
Fred R Dick, MD
Univ of Iowa Hospitals and Clinics
Dept of Pathology/6227 RCP
200 Hawkins Dr
Iowa City, IA 52242-1009
Tel: 319 356-2991 *Fax:* 319 356-2243
E-mail: fred-dick@uiowa.edu
Accred Length: 1 Year *Program Size:* 2
Program ID: 311-18-21-023

Louisiana

New Orleans

Tulane University Program
Sponsor: Tulane University School of Medicine
Alton Ochsner Medical Foundation
Program Director:
John R Krause, MD
1430 Tulane Ave
New Orleans, LA 70112-2699
Tel: 504 588-5224 *Fax:* 504 587-7389
Accred Length: 1 Year *Program Size:* 1
Program ID: 311-21-31-076

Maryland

Baltimore

Johns Hopkins University Program
Sponsor: Johns Hopkins University School of Medicine
Johns Hopkins Hospital
Program Director:
Michael J Borowitz, MD PhD
Johns Hopkins Hospital
600 N. Wolfe St
Carnegie 422
Baltimore, MD 21287-6417
Tel: 410 614-2888 *Fax:* 410 614-2904
E-mail: mborowit@pathlan.path.jhu.edu
Internet: http://pathology.jhu.edu
Accred Length: 1 Year *Program Size:* 1
Program ID: 311-23-21-072

Programs

University of Maryland Program
Sponsor: University of Maryland Medical System
National Cancer Institute
Program Director:
Sanford A Stass II, MD
Univ of Maryland Med System
22 S Greene St/NBW43
Baltimore, MD 21201-1595
Tel: 410 328-5555 *Fax:* 410 328-5508
Accred Length: 1 Year *Program Size:* 1
Program ID: 311-23-21-059

Massachusetts

Boston

Beth Israel Deaconess Medical Center (East Campus) Program
Sponsor: Beth Israel Deaconess Medical Center
Program Director:
Marshall E Kadin, MD
Beth Israel Deaconess Med Ctr
Dept of Pathology
330 Brookline Ave
Boston, MA 02215
Tel: 617 667-3648, ext 5886 *Fax:* 617 667-4533
E-mail: mkadin@bih.harvard.edu
Accred Length: 1 Year *Program Size:* 3
Program ID: 311-24-21-036

Boston University Medical Center Program
Sponsor: Boston Medical Center
Program Director:
Carl J O'Hara, MD
784 Massachusetts Ave
Boston, MA 02118
Tel: 617 414-5182 *Fax:* 617 414-5315
Accred Length: 1 Year *Program Size:* 1
Program ID: 311-24-21-077

Brigham and Women's Hospital Program
Sponsor: Brigham and Women's Hospital
Program Director:
Geraldine S Pinkus, MD
Brigham and Women's Hospital
Div of Hematopathology
75 Francis St
Boston, MA 02115
Tel: 617 732-7519 *Fax:* 617 713-3044
Accred Length: 1 Year *Program Size:* 2
Program ID: 311-24-21-048

Michigan

Ann Arbor

University of Michigan Program
Sponsor: University of Michigan Hospitals
Program Director:
Bertram Schnitzer, MD
Univ of Michigan Med Sch
M5242B Med Science I
1301 Catherine Rd
Ann Arbor, MI 48109-0602
Tel: 734 936-1874 *Fax:* 734 936-2756
E-mail: raven@umich.edu
Accred Length: 1 Year *Program Size:* 1
Program ID: 311-25-21-026

Royal Oak

William Beaumont Hospital Program
Sponsor: William Beaumont Hospital
Program Director:
Joan C Mattson, MD
William Beaumont Hospital
3601 W 13 Mile Rd
Royal Oak, MI 48073-6769
Tel: 248 551-2935 *Fax:* 248 551-8057
Internet: http://www.beaumont.edu/html/gme
Accred Length: 1 Year *Program Size:* 2
Program ID: 311-25-21-033

Minnesota

Rochester

Mayo Graduate School of Medicine (Rochester) Program
Sponsor: Mayo Graduate School of Medicine-Mayo Foundation
Mayo Clinic (Rochester)
Program Director:
Paul J Kurtin, MD
Application Processing Ctr
Mayo Graduate Sch of Med
200 First St SW
Rochester, MN 55905
Tel: 507 284-3108 *Fax:* 507 284-0999
E-mail: mgsm.medlab.specialties@mayo.edu
Internet: http://www.mayo.edu/
Accred Length: 1 Year *Program Size:* 1
Program ID: 311-26-21-029

Missouri

St Louis

St Louis University School of Medicine Program
Sponsor: St Louis University School of Medicine
St Louis University School of Medicine
Program Director:
Cherie H Dunphy, MD
St Louis Univ Sch of Med
1402 S Grand Blvd
St Louis, MO 63104
Tel: 314 577-8481 *Fax:* 314 268-5132
Accred Length: 1 Year *Program Size:* 1
Program ID: 311-28-21-074

Washington University/B-JH/SLCH Consortium Program
Sponsor: Washington University/B-JH/SLCH Consortium
Barnes-Jewish Hospital
Program Director:
Mary M Zutter, MD
Barnes-Jewish Hospital
One Barnes-Jewish Hospital Plaza
St Louis, MO 63110
Tel: 314 362-0114 *Fax:* 314 361-4909
Accred Length: 1 Year *Program Size:* 1
Program ID: 311-28-21-050

Nebraska

Omaha

University of Nebraska Program
Sponsor: University of Nebraska Medical Center
Program Director:
Dennis D Weisenburger, MD
Univ of Nebraska Med Ctr
Dept of Path/Microbiology
983135 Nebraska Med Ctr
Omaha, NE 68198-3135
Tel: 402 559-7689 *Fax:* 402 559-6018
E-mail: dweisenb@unmc.edu
Internet: http://www.unmc.edu/gme/gmehome.htm
Accred Length: 1 Year *Program Size:* 2
Program ID: 311-30-21-010

New Jersey

Piscataway

UMDNJ-Robert Wood Johnson Medical School Program
Sponsor: UMDNJ-Robert Wood Johnson Medical School
Robert Wood Johnson University Hospital
Program Director:
Lauri A Goodell, MD
Dept of Pathology/MEB212
UMDNJ-Robert Wood Johnson Med Sch
New Brunswick, NJ 08903-0019
Tel: 908 937-8593
Accred Length: 1 Year *Program Size:* 1
Program ID: 311-33-21-025

New Mexico

Albuquerque

University of New Mexico Program
Sponsor: University of New Mexico School of Medicine
University Hospital
Program Director:
Cheryl L Willman, MD
Univ of New Mexico Sch of Med
Cancer Research Facility Rm 101
2325 Camino de Salud NE
Albuquerque, NM 87131-5636
Tel: 505 272-5622 *Fax:* 505 272-8047
E-mail: cwillman@unm.edu
Accred Length: 1 Year *Program Size:* 2
Program ID: 311-34-21-013

New York

Albany

Albany Medical Center Program
Sponsor: Albany Medical Center
Veterans Affairs Medical Center (Albany)
Program Director:
Tipu Nazeer, MD
Albany Med Ctr
Dept of Pathology/A-81
47 New Scotland Ave
Albany, NY 12208
Tel: 518 262-6019 *Fax:* 518 262-3663
E-mail: tipu_nazeer@cgateway.amc.edu
Accred Length: 1 Year *Program Size:* 1
Program ID: 311-35-31-031

Bronx

Albert Einstein College of Medicine Program
Sponsor: Albert Einstein College of Medicine of Yeshiva University
Montefiore Medical Center-Weiler Hospital
Program Director:
Howard Ratech, MD
Albert Einstein Coll of Med
110 E 210th St
Bronx, NY 10467
Tel: 718 920-7782 *Fax:* 718 920-7611
E-mail: ratech@aecom.yu.edu
Accred Length: 1 Year *Program Size:* 1
Program ID: 311-35-31-068

New York

Albert Einstein College of Medicine at Beth Israel Medical Center Program
Sponsor: Beth Israel Medical Center
Program Director:
Carl Teplitz, MD
Dept of Diagnostic Path/Lab Med
Beth Israel Med Ctr
First Ave at 16th St
New York, NY 10003
Tel: 212 420-4030 *Fax:* 212 420-3449
Accred Length: 1 Year *Program Size:* 0
Program ID: 311-35-21-006

New York University Medical Center Program
Sponsor: New York University Medical Center
Bellevue Hospital Center
Program Director:
Giorgio Inghirami, MD
New York Univ Med Ctr
Dept of Hematopathology
550 First Ave
New York, NY 10016
Tel: 212 263-5967 *Fax:* 212 263-7712
Accred Length: 1 Year *Program Size:* 1
Program ID: 311-35-21-060

Syracuse

SUNY Health Science Center at Syracuse Program
Sponsor: University Hospital-SUNY Health Science Center at Syracuse
Program Director:
Robert E Hutchison, MD
SUNY Health Science Ctr-Syracuse
750 E Adams St
Syracuse, NY 13210
Tel: 315 464-6772 *Fax:* 315 464-7322
Accred Length: 1 Year *Program Size:* 1
Program ID: 311-35-21-030

North Carolina

Chapel Hill

University of North Carolina Hospitals Program
Sponsor: University of North Carolina Hospitals
Program Director:
Georgette A Dent, MD
Univ of North Carolina Hospitals
Dept of Path Laboratory Med/CB#7525
101 Manning Dr
Chapel Hill, NC 27599-7525
Tel: 919 966-2318 *Fax:* 919 966-6407
E-mail: georgette_dent@med.unc.edu
Internet: http://www.pathology.med.unc./path/fellowsp/hemepath.htm
Accred Length: 1 Year *Program Size:* 1
Program ID: 311-36-21-032

Charlotte

Carolinas Medical Center Program
Sponsor: Carolinas Medical Center
Program Director:
Peter M Banks, MD
Carolinas Med Ctr
1000 Blythe Blvd
Charlotte, NC 28232
Tel: 704 355-2251 *Fax:* 704 355-2156
E-mail: banks pds@aol.com
Accred Length: 1 Year *Program Size:* 1
Program ID: 311-36-21-066

Durham

Duke University Program
Sponsor: Duke University Medical Center
Veterans Affairs Medical Center (Durham)
Program Director:
Karen P Mann, MD PhD
Duke Univ Med Ctr
Box 3712
Durham, NC 27710
Tel: 919 684-2952 *Fax:* 919 681-8932
E-mail: mann0002@mc.duke.edu
Accred Length: 1 Year *Program Size:* 1
Program ID: 311-36-21-055

Ohio

Cincinnati

University Hospital/University of Cincinnati College of Medicine Program
Sponsor: University Hospital Inc
Program Director:
Harold R Schumacher, MD
Univ of Cincinnati Med Ctr
PO Box 670529
231 Bethesda Ave
Cincinnati, OH 45267-0529
Tel: 513 558-3118 *Fax:* 513 558-4176
E-mail: schumah@uc.edu
Internet:
http://www.med.uc.edu/departme/pathdept/web/division/main.htm
Accred Length: 1 Year *Program Size:* 1
Program ID: 311-38-21-042

Cleveland

Case Western Reserve University Program
Sponsor: University Hospitals of Cleveland
Program Director:
Howard Meyerson, MD
Univ Hospitals of Cleveland
Dept of Pathology
11100 Euclid Ave
Cleveland, OH 44106-5077
Tel: 216 844-1839 *Fax:* 216 844-5601
Accred Length: 1 Year *Program Size:* 1
Program ID: 311-38-21-011

Cleveland Clinic Foundation Program
Sponsor: Cleveland Clinic Foundation
Program Director:
Michael L Miller, DO
Cleveland Clinic Foundation
Dept of Laboratory Hematology/L40
9500 Euclid Ave
Cleveland, OH 44195
Tel: 216 444-8095
E-mail: meded@cesmtp.ccf.org
Internet: http://www.ccf.org
Accred Length: 1 Year *Program Size:* 1
Program ID: 311-38-21-065

Columbus

Ohio State University Program
Sponsor: Ohio State University Medical Center
Program Director:
John T Brandt, MD
Ohio State Univ Med Ctr
E-310 Doan Hall
410 W Tenth Ave
Columbus, OH 43210
Tel: 614 293-2458 *Fax:* 614 293-7273
Accred Length: 1 Year *Program Size:* 1
Program ID: 311-38-21-052

Pennsylvania

Philadelphia

Temple University Program
Sponsor: Temple University Hospital
St Christopher's Hospital for Children
Program Director:
Patti Cohen, MD
3401 N Broad St
Philadelphia, PA 19140
Tel: 215 707-3238 *Fax:* 215 707-2053
Accred Length: 1 Year *Program Size:* 1
Program ID: 311-41-21-063

University of Pennsylvania Program
Sponsor: Hospital of the University of Pennsylvania
Program Director:
Mariusz A Wasik, MD
Univ of Pennsylvania
3400 Spruce St
7 Founders Pavillion
Philadelphia, PA 19104
Tel: 215 662-3467 *Fax:* 215 349-5910
Accred Length: 1 Year *Program Size:* 1
Program ID: 311-41-21-069

Pittsburgh

Allegheny General Hospital Program
Sponsor: Allegheny General Hospital

Program Director:
Karl R Fox, MD
Allegheny General Hospital
Div of Clinical Pathology
320 E North Ave
Pittsburgh, PA 15212-9986
Tel: 412 359-3541 *Fax:* 412 359-3860
Accred Length: 1 Year *Program Size:* 1
Program ID: 311-41-21-035

University Health Center of Pittsburgh Program
Sponsor: University Health Center of Pittsburgh
Children's Hospital of Pittsburgh
Presbyterian University Hospital/UPMC

Program Director:
Steven H Swerdlow, MD
UPMC Health System
UPMC-Presbyterian Rm C606.1
200 Lothrop St
Pittsburgh, PA 15213-2582
Tel: 412 647-5191 *Fax:* 412 647-4008
E-mail: swerdlowsh@msx.upmc.edu
Accred Length: 1 Year *Program Size:* 1
Program ID: 311-41-21-014

South Carolina

Charleston

Medical University of South Carolina Program
Sponsor: Medical University of South Carolina College of Medicine
MUSC Medical Center

Program Director:
John Lazarchick, MD
Med Univ of South Carolina
171 Ashley Ave
Charleston, SC 29425
Tel: 843 792-2933
E-mail: lazarj@musc.edu
Accred Length: 1 Year *Program Size:* 1
Program ID: 311-45-21-057

Tennessee

Nashville

Vanderbilt University Program
Sponsor: Vanderbilt University Medical Center
Veterans Affairs Medical Center (Nashville)

Program Director:
John B Cousar, MD
Vanderbilt Univ, Div of Hematopathology
4800B TVC
23rd and Pierce Ave
Nashville, TN 37232-5310
Tel: 615 322-0146, ext 20146 *Fax:* 615 343-8420
E-mail: john.cousar@mcmail.vanderbilt.edu
Accred Length: 1 Year *Program Size:* 2
Program ID: 311-47-21-070

Texas

Dallas

University of Texas Southwestern Medical School Program
Sponsor: University of Texas Southwestern Medical School
Children's Medical Center of Dallas
Dallas County Hospital District-Parkland Memorial Hospital

Program Director:
Robert W McKenna, MD
5323 Harry Hines Blvd
Dallas, TX 75235-9072
Tel: 214 648-4004 *Fax:* 214 648-4070
Internet: http://www.swmed.edu
Accred Length: 1 Year *Program Size:* 2
Program ID: 311-48-21-064

Houston

Baylor College of Medicine Program
Sponsor: Baylor College of Medicine
Harris County Hospital District-Ben Taub General Hospital
Methodist Hospital
Texas Children's Hospital

Program Director:
Abdus Saleem, MD
Methodist Hospital, Dept of Pathology
6565 Fannin St/MS205
Houston, TX 77030
Tel: 713 790-2439 *Fax:* 713 793-1473
E-mail: melindaf@bcm.tmc.edu
Internet: http://www.bcm.tmc.edu/pathology
Accred Length: 1 Year *Program Size:* 1
Program ID: 311-48-21-012

University of Texas M D Anderson Cancer Center Program
Sponsor: University of Texas M D Anderson Cancer Center

Program Director:
Maher Albitar, MD
Univ of Texas-MD Anderson Cancer Ctr
1515 Holcombe Blvd
Houston, TX 77030
Tel: 713 794-1292 *Fax:* 713 794-1800
E-mail: malbitar@mdac.tmc.edu
Accred Length: 1 Year *Program Size:* 3
Program ID: 311-48-21-019

San Antonio

University of Texas Health Science Center at San Antonio Program
Sponsor: University of Texas Medical School at San Antonio
Audie L Murphy Memorial Veterans Hospital (San Antonio)
University Hospital-South Texas Medical Center

Program Director:
Fiona E Craig, MD
Univ of Texas Health Science Ctr
Dept of Path/Hematology
7703 Floyd Curl Dr
San Antonio, TX 78284-7750
Tel: 210 567-6731 *Fax:* 210 567-6729
E-mail: craigf@uthscsa.edu
Internet: http://pathologyweb.uthscsa.edu/residency.html
Accred Length: 1 Year *Program Size:* 2
Program ID: 311-48-21-020

Temple

Texas A&M College of Medicine-Scott and White Program
Sponsor: Scott and White Memorial Hospital
Central Texas Veterans Affairs Healthcare System

Program Director:
Edward S Rappaport, MD
Texas A&M-Scott and White
Grad Med Educ
2401 S 31st St
Temple, TX 76508
Tel: 800 299-4463 *Fax:* 817 724-4391
E-mail: dhinson@swmail.sw.org
Internet: http://www.swinfo.tamu.edu
Accred Length: 1 Year *Program Size:* 1
Program ID: 311-48-21-044

Utah

Salt Lake City

University of Utah Program
Sponsor: University of Utah Medical Center

Program Director:
Carl R Kjeldsberg, MD
Univ of Utah Sch of Med
Dept of Pathology
50 N Medical Dr
Salt Lake City, UT 84132
Tel: 801 581-5854 *Fax:* 801 581-4517
Accred Length: 1 Year *Program Size:* 4
Program ID: 311-49-21-024

Washington

Seattle

University of Washington Program
Sponsor: University of Washington School of Medicine
Children's Hospital and Medical Center

Program Director:
Daniel E Sabath, MD PhD
Univ of Washington
Dept of Laboratory Med
Box 357110
Seattle, WA 98195-7110
Tel: 206 548-6833 *Fax:* 206 548-6189
E-mail: dsabath@u.washington.edu
Internet:
http://www.labmed.washington.edu/division/hematology/hpfellowship.html
Accred Length: 1 Year *Program Size:* 2
Program ID: 311-54-21-067

Wisconsin

Madison

University of Wisconsin Program
Sponsor: University of Wisconsin Hospital and Clinics

Program Director:
Patrick J Buckley, MD PhD
Univ Hospital and Clinics
B4/243 CSC
600 Highland Ave
Madison, WI 53792-2472
Tel: 608 262-7158 *Fax:* 608 263-1568
E-mail: pj.buckley@hosp.wisc.edu
Internet: http://www.biostat.wisc.edu/path/hemato.html
Accred Length: 1 Year *Program Size:* 1
Program ID: 311-56-21-061

Milwaukee

Medical College of Wisconsin Program
Sponsor: Medical College of Wisconsin Affiliated Hospitals Inc
Froedtert Memorial Lutheran Hospital
Program Director:
Michael Whittaker, MD
9200 W Wisconsin Ave
Milwaukee, WI 53226-0509
Tel: 414 257-6209 *Fax:* 414 257-7815
Accred Length: 1 Year *Program Size:* 1
Program ID: 311-56-21-071

Hematology and Oncology (Internal Medicine)

Alabama

Birmingham

University of Alabama Medical Center Program
Sponsor: University of Alabama Hospital
Program Director:
Brian K Adler, MD
Univ of Alabama-Birmingham
Univ Station/WTI 520
Birmingham, AL 35294-3300
Tel: 205 934-9591 *Fax:* 205 934-9573
Internet: http://info.dom.uab.edu/hemonc
Accred Length: 3 Years *Program Size:* 12
Program ID: 155-01-21-001

Mobile

University of South Alabama Program
Sponsor: University of South Alabama Medical Center
Program Director:
Marcel E Conrad, MD
USA Cancer Ctr 414
Univ of South Alabama
2451 Fillingrim St
Mobile, AL 36688
Tel: 334 460-7194 *Fax:* 334 460-7637
Accred Length: 3 Years *Program Size:* 3
Program ID: 155-01-31-002

Arizona

Tucson

University of Arizona Program
Sponsor: University of Arizona College of Medicine
University Medical Center
Veterans Affairs Medical Center (Tucson)
Program Director:
Frederick R Ahmann, MD
Arizona Cancer Ctr
1515 N Campbell Ave
Tucson, AZ 85724
Tel: 520 626-8096 *Fax:* 520 626-2284
Internet: http://www.azcc.arizona.edu
Accred Length: 3 Years *Program Size:* 6
Program ID: 155-03-21-003

California

Los Angeles

Cedars-Sinai Medical Center Program
Sponsor: Cedars-Sinai Medical Center
Olive View-UCLA Medical Center
Program Director:
H Phillip Koeffler, MD
Cedars-Sinai Med Ctr
Div of Hematology/Oncology
8700 Beverly Blvd/B-213
Los Angeles, CA 90048-1865
Tel: 310 855-4502 *Fax:* 310 659-9741
E-mail: parkd@cshs.org
Accred Length: 3 Years *Program Size:* 2
Program ID: 155-05-21-004

VA Greater Los Angeles Healthcare System (Sepulveda) Program
Sponsor: VA Greater Los Angeles Healthcare System
Cedars-Sinai Medical Center
Olive View-UCLA Medical Center
Program Director:
Nancy R Feldman, MD
VA Med Ctr, Attn: Bonnie Hummicutt
16111 Plummer St/111T
Sepulveda, CA 91343
Tel: 818 895-9395 *Fax:* 818 895-9516
Accred Length: 3 Years *Program Size:* 6
Program ID: 155-05-13-008

Sacramento

University of California (Davis) Program
Sponsor: University of California (Davis) Medical Center
Kaiser Foundation Hospital (Sacramento)
Program Director:
Theodore Wun, MD
Univ of California Davis Cancer Ctr
4501 X St
Sacramento, CA 95817
Tel: 916 734-3772 *Fax:* 916 734-7946
E-mail: linda.glasson@ucdmc.ucdavis.edu
Internet: http://cancer.ucdmc.ucdavis.edu
Accred Length: 3 Years *Program Size:* 8
Program ID: 155-05-31-005

San Diego

University of California (San Diego) Program
Sponsor: University of California (San Diego) Medical Center
Veterans Affairs Medical Center (San Diego)
Program Director:
Elaine A Muchmore, MD
VA San Diego Healthcare System
Hematology/Oncology (111E)
3350 La Jolla Village Dr
San Diego, CA 92161
Tel: 619 552-8585, ext 7631 *Fax:* 619 552-7537
E-mail: vahemonc@popmail.ucsd.edu
Accred Length: 3 Years *Program Size:* 7
Program ID: 155-05-12-007

San Francisco

University of California (San Francisco) Program

Sponsor: University of California (San Francisco) School of Medicine
San Francisco General Hospital Medical Center
University of California (San Francisco) Medical Center
Veterans Affairs Medical Center (San Francisco)

Program Director:
Patricia A Cornett, MD
505 Parnassus Ave/Rm M1282
Box 1270
San Francisco, CA 94143-1270
Tel: 415 476-9492 *Fax:* 415 476-0624
E-mail: hemonc_fellowship@quickmail.ucsf.edu
Accred Length: 3 Years *Program Size:* 12
Program ID: 155-05-21-113

Torrance

Los Angeles County-Harbor-UCLA Medical Center Program 1

Sponsor: Los Angeles County-Harbor-UCLA Medical Center

Program Director:
Jerome B Block, MD
Los Angeles County-Harbor-UCLA Med Ctr
1000 W Carson St
Torrance, CA 90509
Tel: 310 222-2444 *Fax:* 310 782-0486
Accred Length: 3 Years *Program Size:* 5
Program ID: 155-05-31-093

Los Angeles County-Harbor-UCLA Medical Center Program 2

Sponsor: Los Angeles County-Harbor-UCLA Medical Center
City of Hope National Medical Center

Program Director:
Kouichi R Tanaka, MD
Los Angeles County-Harbor-UCLA Med Ctr
1000 W Carson St/Box-400
Torrance, CA 90509-2910
Tel: 310 222-3695 *Fax:* 310 328-1308
Accred Length: 3 Years *Program Size:* 6
Program ID: 155-05-21-087

Colorado

Denver

University of Colorado Program

Sponsor: University of Colorado Health Sciences Center
Denver Health and Hospitals
Rose Medical Center
Veterans Affairs Medical Center (Denver)

Program Director:
Catherine E Klein, MD
1055 Clermont/IIB
Denver, CO 80220
Tel: 303 315-8802 *Fax:* 303 393-3177
E-mail: cklein@calvin.uchsc.edu
Accred Length: 3 Years *Program Size:* 3
Program ID: 155-07-21-096

Connecticut

Farmington

University of Connecticut Program

Sponsor: University of Connecticut School of Medicine
Hartford Hospital
St Francis Hospital and Medical Center
Univ of Connecticut Health Center/John Dempsey Hospital

Program Director:
Robert D Bona, MD
Dept of Med
Univ of Connecticut Health Ctr
Farmington, CT 06030
Tel: 860 679-2255 *Fax:* 860 679-4451
E-mail: bona@up.uchc.edu
Accred Length: 3 Years *Program Size:* 4
Program ID: 155-08-21-009

District of Columbia

Washington

George Washington University Program

Sponsor: George Washington University School of Medicine
George Washington University Hospital (UHS)
Veterans Affairs Medical Center (Washington, DC)

Program Director:
Imad A Tabbara, MD
George Washington Univ
2150 Pennsylvania Ave NW
Ste 3-428
Washington, DC 20037
Tel: 202 994-3556 *Fax:* 202 994-4524
E-mail: itabbara@gwis2.circ.gwu.edu
Accred Length: 3 Years *Program Size:* 5
Program ID: 155-10-21-074

Washington Hospital Center Program

Sponsor: Washington Hospital Center
Veterans Affairs Medical Center (Washington, DC)

Program Director:
Dennis A Priebat, MD
Washington Hospital Ctr
110 Irving St NW
Ste C-2151
Washington, DC 20010
Tel: 202 877-6998 *Fax:* 202 877-8909
E-mail: dap3@mhg.edu
Accred Length: 3 Years *Program Size:* 6
Program ID: 155-10-31-011

Florida

Gainesville

University of Florida Program

Sponsor: University of Florida College of Medicine
Shands Hospital at the University of Florida
Veterans Affairs Medical Center (Gainesville)

Program Director:
James W Lynch Jr, MD
Univ of Florida
Box 100277 JHMHC
Gainesville, FL 32610-0277
Tel: 352 392-3000 *Fax:* 352 392-8530
Accred Length: 3 Years *Program Size:* 6
Program ID: 155-11-21-104

Jacksonville

Mayo Graduate School of Medicine (Jacksonville) Program

Sponsor: Mayo Graduate School of Medicine-Mayo Foundation
Mayo Clinic (Jacksonville)
St Luke's Hospital

Program Director:
Gerardo Colon-Otero, MD
Mayo Clinic Jacksonville
4500 San Pablo Rd
Jacksonville, FL 32224
Tel: 904 953-2000 *Fax:* 904 953-2315
E-mail: mgsm.jack.fl.internalmed@mayo.edu
Internet: http://www.mayo.edu/
Accred Length: 3 Years *Program Size:* 3
Program ID: 155-11-31-108

Miami

University of Miami-Jackson Memorial Medical Center Program

Sponsor: University of Miami-Jackson Memorial Medical Center
Veterans Affairs Medical Center (Miami)

Program Director:
Pasquale Benedetto, MD
Sylvester Cancer Ctr
1475 NW 12th Ave (D8 4)
Miami, FL 33136
Tel: 305 243-4929 *Fax:* 305 243-9161
E-mail: pbenedet@mednet.med.miani.edu
Accred Length: 3 Years *Program Size:* 11
Program ID: 155-11-21-012

Tampa

University of South Florida Program

Sponsor: University of South Florida College of Medicine
H Lee Moffitt Cancer Center
James A Haley Veterans Hospital
Tampa General Healthcare

Program Director:
Kenneth Zuckerman, MD
Div of Med Oncology/Hematology
H Lee Moffitt Cancer Ctr
12902 Magnolia Dr/Ste 3157
Tampa, FL 33612
Tel: 813 972-8477 *Fax:* 813 972-8468
E-mail: zuckerman@moffitt.usf.edu
Accred Length: 3 Years *Program Size:* 12
Program ID: 155-11-31-013

Georgia

Atlanta

Emory University Program

Sponsor: Emory University School of Medicine
Emory University Hospital
Grady Memorial Hospital

Program Director:
Laurence Harker, MD
Emory Univ Hem/Onc
1639 Pierce Dr/Rm1003
Atlanta, GA 30322
Tel: 404 727-7016 *Fax:* 404 727-3404
E-mail: lharker@emory.edu
Internet: http://www.emory.edu/whsc/med/hemonc/
Accred Length: 3 Years *Program Size:* 11
Program ID: 155-12-21-014

Augusta

Medical College of Georgia Program

Sponsor: Medical College of Georgia Hospital and Clinics
Veterans Affairs Medical Center (Augusta)

Program Director:
Abdullah Kutlar, MD
Med Coll of Georgia
Sect of Hem/Oncology
1120 15th St
Augusta, GA 30912-3125
Tel: 706 721-2505 *Fax:* 706 721-8302
Accred Length: 3 Years *Program Size:* 3
Program ID: 155-12-31-015

Illinois

Chicago

Cook County Hospital Program

Sponsor: Cook County Hospital

Program Director:
Gail M Shiomoto, MD
Cook County Hospital
1835 W Harrison St
Chicago, IL 60612
Tel: 312 633-7117, ext 6594 *Fax:* 312 633-8131
Accred Length: 3 Years *Program Size:* 4
Program ID: 155-16-21-106

McGaw Medical Center of Northwestern University Program

Sponsor: Northwestern University Medical School
Northwestern Memorial Hospital
Veterans Affairs Lakeside Medical Center (Chicago)

Program Director:
William J Gradishar, MD
233 E Erie/Ste 700
Chicago, IL 60611-2906
Tel: 312 908-9412 *Fax:* 312 908-4844
E-mail: w-gradishar@nwu.edu
Internet: http://www.medicine.nwu.edu/hem-onc/
Accred Length: 3 Years *Program Size:* 9
Program ID: 155-16-21-016

Rush-Presbyterian-St Luke's Medical Center Program

Sponsor: Rush-Presbyterian-St Luke's Medical Center

Program Director:
Anastasio Raptis, MD PhD
Rush-Presbyterian-St Luke's Med Ctr
1653 W Congress Pkwy
Chicago, IL 60612-3833
Tel: 312 942-6534 *Fax:* 312 733-1590
E-mail: araptis@rush.edu
Internet: http://www.rush.edu/
Accred Length: 3 Years *Program Size:* 5
Program ID: 155-16-21-085

University of Chicago Program

Sponsor: University of Chicago Hospitals

Program Director:
Olufunmilay I Olopade, MB BS
Univ of Chicago Hospitals
5841 S Maryland Ave
Box 420
Chicago, IL 60637-1470
Tel: 773 702-4400 *Fax:* 773 702-0963
E-mail: fiolopad@mcis.bsd.uchicago.edu
Accred Length: 3 Years *Program Size:* 15
Program ID: 155-16-21-079

University of Illinois College of Medicine at Chicago Program

Sponsor: University of Illinois College of Medicine at Chicago
University of Illinois Hospital and Clinics
Veterans Affairs West Side Medical Center

Program Director:
Steven M Devine, MD
Univ of Illinois-Chicago
840 S Wood St (M/C 787)
Chicago, IL 60612
Tel: 312 413-9288 *Fax:* 312 413-7963
E-mail: sdevine@uic.edu
Accred Length: 3 Years *Program Size:* 11
Program ID: 155-16-31-017

University of Illinois College of Medicine at Chicago/Michael Reese Hospital Program

Sponsor: University of Illinois College of Medicine at Chicago
Michael Reese Hospital and Medical Center

Program Director:
Margaret Telfer, MD
2816 S Ellis
RC-1200
Chicago, IL 60616
Tel: 312 791-2123 *Fax:* 312 791-2024
Accred Length: 3 Years *Program Size:* 2
Program ID: 155-16-11-018

Maywood

Loyola University Program

Sponsor: Loyola University Medical Center
Edward J Hines Jr Veterans Affairs Hospital
MacNeal Memorial Hospital

Program Director:
Kenneth C Micetch, MD
Div of Hematology/Oncology
Cardinal Bernardin Cancer Ctr
2160 S First Ave
Maywood, IL 60153
Tel: 708 327-3144 *Fax:* 708 327-3220
E-mail: kmiceti@luc.edu
Internet: http://www.luc.edu
Accred Length: 3 Years *Program Size:* 7
Program ID: 155-16-21-110

Indiana

Indianapolis

Indiana University School of Medicine Program

Sponsor: Indiana University School of Medicine
Clarian IU Hospital

Program Director:
Lawrence H Einhorn, MD
University Hospital/Rm 1730
550 N University Blvd
Indianapolis, IN 46223-5265
Tel: 317 274-0920 *Fax:* 317 274-0396
E-mail: larry_einhorn@iucc.iupui.edu
Accred Length: 3 Years *Program Size:* 9
Program ID: 155-17-21-020

Iowa

Iowa City

University of Iowa Hospitals and Clinics Program

Sponsor: University of Iowa Hospitals and Clinics

Program Director:
George Weiner, MD
Univ of Iowa Hospitals and Clinics
Hematology/Oncology
200 Hawkins Dr
Iowa City, IA 52242
Tel: 319 356-2810
E-mail: george-weiner@uiowa.edu
Internet:
http://www.indy.radiology.uiowa.edu/welcome/uihc/uihcmeddepts/cancercntr/html/hemoncfellowship.html
Accred Length: 3 Years *Program Size:* 8
Program ID: 155-18-21-021

Kentucky

Lexington

University of Kentucky Medical Center Program

Sponsor: University of Kentucky Hospital
Veterans Affairs Medical Center (Lexington)

Program Director:
Rita K Munn, MD
Univ of Kentucky-Markey Cancer Ctr
Lexington, KY 40536
Tel: 606 323-8043 *Fax:* 606 257-7715
Accred Length: 3 Years *Program Size:* 5
Program ID: 155-20-21-103

Louisville

University of Louisville Program

Sponsor: University of Louisville School of Medicine
James Graham Brown Medical Center
University of Louisville Hospital
Veterans Affairs Medical Center (Louisville)

Program Director:
Fred J Hendler, MD PhD
Univ of Louisville, Div of Hematology/Oncology
Brown Cancer Ctr
529 S Jackson St
Louisville, KY 40292
Tel: 502 852-6930 *Fax:* 502 852-4707
E-mail: fjhend01@ulkyvm.louisville.edu
Accred Length: 3 Years *Program Size:* 4
Program ID: 155-20-21-022

Louisiana

New Orleans

Tulane University Program

Sponsor: Tulane University School of Medicine
Medical Center of Louisiana at New Orleans
Tulane University Hospital and Clinics
Veterans Affairs Medical Center-LSU Service (New Orleans)

Program Director:
German Beltran, MD
1430 Tulane Ave/SL78
New Orleans, LA 70112-2699
Tel: 504 588-5482 *Fax:* 504 588-5483
E-mail: gbeltran@tmcpop.tmc.tulane.edu
Accred Length: 3 Years *Program Size:* 6
Program ID: 155-21-21-023

Shreveport

Louisiana State University (Shreveport) Program
Sponsor: Louisiana State University Hospital-Shreveport
Program Director:
Glenn M Mills, MD
1501 S Kings Hwy
PO Box 33932
Shreveport, LA 71132-3932
Tel: 318 675-5970 *Fax:* 318 675-5944
E-mail: gmills@lsumc.edu
Internet: http://www.cancercenter.lsumc.edu
Accred Length: 3 Years *Program Size:* 6
Program ID: 155-21-31-024

Maryland

Baltimore

University of Maryland Program
Sponsor: University of Maryland Medical System
Program Director:
Judith E Karp, MD
Univ of Maryland
22 S Greene St
Baltimore, MD 21201
Tel: 410 328-7394 *Fax:* 410 328-6896
E-mail: jkarp@umcc01.umcc.ab.umd.edu
Accred Length: 3 Years *Program Size:* 7
Program ID: 155-23-21-025

Bethesda

National Naval Medical Center (Bethesda) Program
Sponsor: National Naval Medical Center (Bethesda)
Walter Reed Army Medical Center
Program Director:
Lou Drehl, MD
National Naval Med Ctr
Dept of Med
8901 Wisconsin Ave
Bethesda, MD 20889-5600
Tel: 301 435-5332 *Fax:* 301 480-9926
Accred Length: 3 Years *Program Size:* 12
Program ID: 155-23-21-088
US Armed Services Program

Massachusetts

Boston

Beth Israel Deaconess Medical Center (East Campus) Program
Sponsor: Beth Israel Deaconess Medical Center
Program Director:
Reed E Drews, MD
Beth Israel Deaconess Med Ctr-East Campus
330 Brookline Ave
Boston, MA 02215
Tel: 617 667-2131 *Fax:* 617 667-3915
E-mail: rdrews@bidmc.harvard.edu
Internet: http://www.cancercenter.bidmc.harvard.edu
Accred Length: 3 Years *Program Size:* 19
Program ID: 155-24-21-026

Beth Israel Deaconess Medical Center (West Campus) Program
Sponsor: Beth Israel Deaconess Medical Center
Program Director:
Keith Stuart, MD
Deaconess Hospital
110 Francis St/Ste 4A
Boston, MA 02215
Tel: 617 632-8646 *Fax:* 617 566-8043
Accred Length: 3 Years *Program Size:* 1
Program ID: 155-24-11-028

Boston University Medical Center Program
Sponsor: Boston Medical Center
Veterans Affairs Medical Center (Boston)
Program Director:
Kevan L Hartshorn, MD
Hematology/Oncology Sect
80 E Concord St/Rm E-556
Boston, MA 02118
Tel: 617 638-7002 *Fax:* 617 638-7530
E-mail: ajasperse@med-med1.bu.edu
Accred Length: 3 Years *Program Size:* 9
Program ID: 155-24-31-027

Brigham and Women's Hospital Program
Sponsor: Brigham and Women's Hospital
Massachusetts General Hospital
Program Director:
Robert J Mayer, MD
Dana-Farber Cancer Inst
44 Binney St
Boston, MA 02115
Tel: 617 632-3474 *Fax:* 617 632-2260
E-mail: carol_stearns@dfci.harvard.edu
Accred Length: 3 Years *Program Size:* 42
Program ID: 155-24-21-073

New England Medical Center Hospitals Program
Sponsor: New England Medical Center Hospitals
Program Director:
John K Erban, MD
New England Med Ctr
750 Washington St
Box 542
Boston, MA 02111
Tel: 617 636-5147 *Fax:* 617 636-0342
E-mail: john.erban@es.nemc.org
Internet: http://www.nemc.org/hemonc
Accred Length: 3 Years *Program Size:* 15
Program ID: 155-24-12-029

St Elizabeth's Medical Center of Boston Program
Sponsor: St Elizabeth's Medical Center of Boston
Program Director:
Paul J Hesketh, MD
St Elizabeth's Med Ctr
736 Cambridge St
Boston, MA 02135
Tel: 617 789-2317 *Fax:* 617 789-2959
Accred Length: 3 Years *Program Size:* 7
Program ID: 155-24-21-124

Springfield

Baystate Medical Center Program
Sponsor: Baystate Medical Center
Program Director:
Grace Makari-Judson, MD
Baystate Med Ctr
759 Chestnut St
Springfield, MA 01199
Tel: 413 787-5768 *Fax:* 413 784-3613
Accred Length: 3 Years *Program Size:* 3
Program ID: 155-24-13-030

Worcester

University of Massachusetts Program
Sponsor: University of Massachusetts Medical School
UMass Memorial Health Care (University Campus)
Program Director:
Robert Emmons, MD
Univ of Massachusetts Med Sch
55 Lake Ave N
Worcester, MA 01655
Tel: 508 856-6884 *Fax:* 508 856-6715
E-mail: robert.emmons@ummed.edu
Accred Length: 3 Years *Program Size:* 4
Program ID: 155-24-21-075

Michigan

Ann Arbor

University of Michigan Program
Sponsor: University of Michigan Hospitals
Veterans Affairs Medical Center (Ann Arbor)
Program Director:
Scott D Gitlin, MD
Univ of Michigan
1150 W Medical Center Dr
5301 MSRB III/Box 0640
Ann Arbor, MI 48109-0640
Tel: 734 647-8921 *Fax:* 734 647-8792
E-mail: sgitlin@umich.edu
Internet:
http://www.med.umich.edu/intmed/hemeonc/hoinfos.itm
Accred Length: 3 Years *Program Size:* 12
Program ID: 155-25-21-098

Detroit

Henry Ford Hospital Program
Sponsor: Henry Ford Hospital
Program Director:
Robert Chapman, MD
Leslie J Bricker, MD
Henry Ford Hospital
2799 W Grand Blvd/K-13
Detroit, MI 48202
Tel: 313 876-1850 *Fax:* 313 876-7911
Accred Length: 3 Years *Program Size:* 3
Program ID: 155-25-21-031

East Lansing

Michigan State University Program
Sponsor: Michigan State University College of Human Medicine
Michigan Capital Medical Center
Sparrow Hospital
St Lawrence Hospital and HealthCare Services
Program Director:
Kenneth A Schwartz, MD
Michigan State Univ Coll of Human Med
Dept of Medicine
B-226 Life Sciences Bldg
East Lansing, MI 48824-1317
Tel: 517 353-3728 *Fax:* 517 353-5436
Accred Length: 3 Years *Program Size:* 6
Program ID: 155-25-21-126

Minnesota

Minneapolis

University of Minnesota Program

Sponsor: University of Minnesota Medical School
Fairview-University Medical Center

Program Director:
Linda J Burns, MD
Gerard Johnson, MD
Univ of Minnesota
Box 286 UMHC
Harvard St at East River Rd
Minneapolis, MN 55455
Tel: 612 626-0400 *Fax:* 612 626-1441
E-mail: stockoll@tc.umn.edu
Internet: http://www.dept.med.umn.edu
Accred Length: 3 Years *Program Size:* 14
Program ID: 155-26-21-032

Rochester

Mayo Graduate School of Medicine (Rochester) Program

Sponsor: Mayo Graduate School of Medicine-Mayo Foundation
Mayo Clinic (Rochester)
Rochester Methodist Hospital
St Mary's Hospital of Rochester

Program Director:
Joseph Rubin, MD
Application Processing Ctr
Mayo Graduate Sch of Med
200 First St SW/Siebens 5
Rochester, MN 55905
Tel: 507 284-3126 *Fax:* 507 284-0999
E-mail: mgsm.intmed.specialties@mayo.edu
Internet: http://www.mayo.edu/
Accred Length: 3 Years *Program Size:* 20
Program ID: 155-26-31-033

Mississippi

Jackson

University of Mississippi Medical Center Program

Sponsor: University of Mississippi School of Medicine
University Hospital
Veterans Affairs Medical Center (Jackson)

Program Director:
Stephanie L Elkins, MD
Univ of Mississippi Med Ctr
2500 N State St
Jackson, MS 39216-4505
Tel: 601 984-5615 *Fax:* 601 984-5689
Accred Length: 3 Years *Program Size:* 9
Program ID: 155-27-21-114

Missouri

Columbia

University of Missouri-Columbia Program

Sponsor: University of Missouri-Columbia School of Medicine
Ellis Fischel Cancer Center
Harry S Truman Memorial Veterans Hospital
University Hospitals and Clinics

Program Director:
Michael C Perry, MD
Univ of Missouri Health Sciences Ctr
Ellis Fischell Cancer Ctr
115 Business Loop 70 West
Columbia, MO 65203-3299
Tel: 573 882-6964 *Fax:* 573 884-6051
E-mail: mperry@efcc.missouri.edu
Accred Length: 3 Years *Program Size:* 6
Program ID: 155-28-21-083

Kansas City

University of Missouri at Kansas City Program

Sponsor: University of Missouri-Kansas City School of Medicine
Truman Medical Center-West

Program Director:
Loretta S Loftus, MD
Univ of Missouri-Kansas City Sch of Med
2411 Holmes St
Kansas City, MO 64108
Tel: 816 235-1863 *Fax:* 816 235-5277
E-mail: lloftus@cctr.umkc.edu
Accred Length: 3 Years *Program Size:* 3
Program ID: 155-28-21-034

St Louis

St Louis University School of Medicine Program

Sponsor: St Louis University School of Medicine
St Louis University School of Medicine

Program Director:
Paul J Petruska, MD
St Louis Univ Sch of Med
Div of Hematology/Oncology
3635 Vista Ave/PO Box 15250
St Louis, MO 63110-0250
Tel: 314 577-8854 *Fax:* 314 773-1167
E-mail: haasebh@wpogate.slu.edu
Accred Length: 3 Years *Program Size:* 6
Program ID: 155-28-11-036

Washington University/B-JH/SLCH Consortium (South Campus) Program

Sponsor: Washington University/B-JH/SLCH Consortium
Barnes-Jewish Hospital

Program Director:
Stuart Kornfeld, MD
Joanne Mortimer, MD
Washington Univ Sch of Med
660 S Euclid Ave/Campus Box 8125
St Louis, MO 63110
Tel: 314 362-8803 *Fax:* 314 362-8826
E-mail: skornfel@im.wustl.edu
Accred Length: 3 Years *Program Size:* 12
Program ID: 155-28-31-035

Nebraska

Omaha

University of Nebraska Program

Sponsor: University of Nebraska Medical Center
Veterans Affairs Medical Center (Omaha)

Program Director:
Philip J Bierman, MD
Univ of Nebraska Med Ctr
Dept of Oncology/Hematology
983330 Nebraska Med Ctr
Omaha, NE 68198-3330
Tel: 402 559-6210 *Fax:* 402 559-6520
E-mail: pjbierma@mail.unmc.edu
Accred Length: 3 Years *Program Size:* 11
Program ID: 155-30-21-037

New Hampshire

Lebanon

Dartmouth-Hitchcock Medical Center Program

Sponsor: Mary Hitchcock Memorial Hospital
Veterans Affairs Medical Center (White River Junction)

Program Director:
Thomas H Davis, MD
Dartmouth-Hitchcock Med Ctr
One Medical Center Dr
Lebanon, NH 03756
Tel: 603 650-5516 *Fax:* 603 650-7791
E-mail: thomas.h.davis@hitchcock.org
Internet:
http://www.dartmouth.edu/~hemonic/index.htm
Accred Length: 3 Years *Program Size:* 6
Program ID: 155-32-21-038

New Jersey

Camden

UMDNJ-Robert Wood Johnson Medical School (Camden) Program

Sponsor: Cooper Hospital-University Medical Center

Program Director:
Alexandre Hageboutros, MD
Cooper Hospital-Univ Med Ctr
Three Cooper Plaza/Ste 220
Camden, NJ 08103
Tel: 609 963-3572 *Fax:* 609 338-9211
E-mail: hagebout@umdnj.edu
Accred Length: 3 Years *Program Size:* 3
Program ID: 155-33-21-039

Piscataway

UMDNJ-Robert Wood Johnson Medical School Program

Sponsor: UMDNJ-Robert Wood Johnson Medical School
Medical Center at Princeton
Robert Wood Johnson University Hospital
St Peter's University Hospital

Program Director:
Parvin Saidi, MD
UMDNJ-Robert Wood Johnson Med Sch, Dept of Med
One Robert Wood Johnson Pl
New Brunswick, NJ 08903
Tel: 732 235-7679 *Fax:* 732 235-7115
Accred Length: 3 Years *Program Size:* 9
Program ID: 155-33-21-040

New Mexico

Albuquerque

University of New Mexico Program
Sponsor: University of New Mexico School of Medicine
University Hospital
Program Director:
Larry K Kvols, MD
Univ of New Mexico
Cancer Research and Treatment Ctr
900 Camino de Salud NE
Albuquerque, NM 87131-5636
Tel: 505 272-5837 *Fax:* 505 272-2841
Internet: http://medlab1.unm.edu/index.html/gme.
Accred Length: 3 Years *Program Size:* 3
Program ID: 155-34-21-115

New York

Brooklyn

Brookdale University Hospital Medical Center Program
Sponsor: Brookdale University Hospital Medical Center
Program Director:
Mark Levin, MD
Brookdale Univ Hospital and Med Ctr
One Brookdale Plaza
Brooklyn, NY 11212
Tel: 718 240-6147 *Fax:* 718 240-6634
E-mail: mlvmd@aol.com
Internet: http://www.brookdale.org
Accred Length: 3 Years *Program Size:* 5
Program ID: 155-35-21-041

Long Island College Hospital Program
Sponsor: Long Island College Hospital
Woodhull Medical and Mental Health Center
Program Director:
Michael Geraghty, MD
339 Hicks St
Brooklyn, NY 11201
Tel: 718 780-1524 *Fax:* 718 780-1594
Accred Length: 3 Years *Program Size:* 3
Program ID: 155-35-11-089

Maimonides Medical Center Program
Sponsor: Maimonides Medical Center
Program Director:
Ismat U Nawabi, MD
6323 Seventh Ave
Brooklyn, NY 11220
Tel: 718 283-6900 *Fax:* 718 283-6930
Accred Length: 3 Years *Program Size:* 3
Program ID: 155-35-31-042

SUNY Health Science Center at Brooklyn Program
Sponsor: SUNY Health Science Center at Brooklyn
Kings County Hospital Center
University Hospital-SUNY Health Science Center at Brooklyn
Veterans Affairs Medical Center (Brooklyn)
Program Director:
Sheldon Rothenberg, MD
SUNY Health Science Ctr-Brooklyn
450 Clarkson Ave/Box 20
Brooklyn, NY 11203
Tel: 718 270-2785 *Fax:* 718 270-1578
E-mail: rothes28@hscbklyn.edu
Accred Length: 3 Years *Program Size:* 10
Program ID: 155-35-11-043

Manhasset

North Shore University Hospital/NYU School of Medicine Program
Sponsor: North Shore University Hospital
Program Director:
Philip Schulman, MD
North Shore Univ Hospital
300 Community Dr
Manhasset, NY 11030
Tel: 516 562-8955 *Fax:* 516 562-8950
Accred Length: 3 Years *Program Size:* 9
Program ID: 155-35-31-116

Mineola

Winthrop-University Hospital Program
Sponsor: Winthrop-University Hospital
Program Director:
Harry Staszewski, MD
Winthrop-Univ Hospital
222 Station Plaza N
Ste 300
Mineola, NY 11501
Tel: 516 663-2310 *Fax:* 516 663-4613
E-mail: hstaszew@winthrop.org
Accred Length: 3 Years *Program Size:* 4
Program ID: 155-35-13-045

New Hyde Park

Albert Einstein College of Medicine at Long Island Jewish Medical Center Program
Sponsor: Long Island Jewish Medical Center
Program Director:
Dilip V Patel, MD
270-05 76th Ave
New Hyde Park, NY 11042
Tel: 718 470-8931 *Fax:* 718 470-0169
E-mail: patel@lij.edu
Internet: http://www.lij.edu/lij-homepage-ns.html
Accred Length: 3 Years *Program Size:* 6
Program ID: 155-35-22-046

New York

Albert Einstein College of Medicine at Beth Israel Medical Center Program
Sponsor: Beth Israel Medical Center
Program Director:
Ralph Zalusky, MD
Beth Israel Med Ctr
First Ave at 16th St
New York, NY 10003
Tel: 212 420-4185 *Fax:* 212 420-4385
E-mail: rzalusky@bethisraelny.org
Internet:
http://www.bethisraelny.org/professional/residency
Accred Length: 3 Years *Program Size:* 3
Program ID: 155-35-23-047

Lenox Hill Hospital Program
Sponsor: Lenox Hill Hospital
Program Director:
Colette Spaccavento, MD
Keith R Brunckhorst, MD
Lenox Hill Hospital
Sect of Hem/Onc
100 E 77th St
New York, NY 10021-1883
Tel: 212 434-2155, ext 5188 *Fax:* 212 434-3413
Accred Length: 3 Years *Program Size:* 4
Program ID: 155-35-33-049

Mount Sinai School of Medicine (Cabrini) Program
Sponsor: Mount Sinai School of Medicine
Cabrini Medical Center
Program Director:
Ariel Distenfeld, MD
Cabrini Med Ctr
227 E 19th St
New York, NY 10003
Tel: 212 995-6082 *Fax:* 212 979-3529
Internet: http://www.cabrininy.org
Accred Length: 3 Years *Program Size:* 4
Program ID: 155-35-32-048

Mount Sinai School of Medicine Program
Sponsor: Mount Sinai School of Medicine
Elmhurst Hospital Center-Mount Sinai Services
Mount Sinai Medical Center
Veterans Affairs Medical Center (Bronx)
Program Director:
Peter C Harpel, MD
Mount Sinai Med Ctr
One Gustave L Levy Pl
Box 1079
New York, NY 10029-6574
Tel: 212 241-0546 *Fax:* 212 996-1029
Accred Length: 3 Years *Program Size:* 9
Program ID: 155-35-21-050

New York and Presbyterian Hospital (Columbia Campus) Program
Sponsor: New York and Presbyterian Hospital
Harlem Hospital Center
New York and Presbyterian Hospital (Columbia Campus)
Program Director:
Karen H Antman, MD
Columbia Univ
MHB 6N 435
177 Fort Washington Ave
New York, NY 10032
Tel: 212 305-8602 *Fax:* 212 305-3035
E-mail: kha4@columbia.edu
Internet: http://www.ccc.columbia.edu
Accred Length: 3 Years *Program Size:* 12
Program ID: 155-35-11-052

New York and Presbyterian Hospital (Cornell Campus) Program 2
Sponsor: Memorial Sloan-Kettering Cancer Center
Program Director:
Dean Bajorin, MD
Memorial Sloan-Kettering Cancer Ctr
1275 York Ave/Box 8
New York, NY 10021
Tel: 212 639-5809 *Fax:* 212 639-2283
Internet: http://www.mskcc.org
Accred Length: 3 Years *Program Size:* 45
Program ID: 155-35-21-084

New York and Presbyterian Hospital (Cornell Campus) Program
Sponsor: New York and Presbyterian Hospital
New York and Presbyterian Hospital (Cornell Campus)
Program Director:
Ronit Simantov, MD
New York Presbyterian Hospital
525 E 68th St
New York, NY 10021
Tel: 212 746-2060 *Fax:* 212 746-8866
Accred Length: 3 Years *Program Size:* 9
Program ID: 155-35-31-051

New York Medical College at St Vincent's Hospital and Medical Center of New York Program

Sponsor: New York Medical College
St Vincent's Hospital and Medical Center of New York

Program Director:
Alan B Astrow, MD
St Vincent's Hospital and Med Ctr
153 W 11th St
New York, NY 10011
Tel: 212 604-2427 *Fax:* 212 604-6082
E-mail: aastrow@svccc.salick.com
Internet: http://svh.nymc.edu
Accred Length: 3 Years *Program Size:* 3
Program ID: 155-35-12-053

Rochester

University of Rochester Program

Sponsor: Strong Memorial Hospital of the University of Rochester

Program Director:
Karen L Kaplan, MD
Deepak Sahasrabudhe, MD
601 Elmwood
Box 704
Rochester, NY 14642
Tel: 716 275-3761 *Fax:* 716 473-4314
E-mail: karen_kaplan@urmc.rochester.edu
Accred Length: 3 Years *Program Size:* 7
Program ID: 155-35-21-100

Stony Brook

SUNY at Stony Brook Program

Sponsor: University Hospital-SUNY at Stony Brook
Veterans Affairs Medical Center (Northport)

Program Director:
Wadie F Bahou, MD
T-15 Rm 040 Health Science Ctr
Hematology Div
SUNY-Stony Brook
Stony Brook, NY 11794-8151
Tel: 516 444-2059 *Fax:* 516 444-7530
E-mail: wbahou@mail.som.sunysb.edu
Internet:
http://www.informatics.sunysb.edu/internalmed/hematol/hemhm.html
Accred Length: 3 Years *Program Size:* 6
Program ID: 155-35-13-054

Syracuse

SUNY Health Science Center at Syracuse Program

Sponsor: University Hospital-SUNY Health Science Center at Syracuse
Veterans Affairs Medical Center (Syracuse)

Program Director:
Jonathan Wright, MD
SUNY Health Science Ctr-Syracuse
750 E Adams St
Syracuse, NY 13210
Tel: 315 464-4353 *Fax:* 315 464-8280
Accred Length: 3 Years *Program Size:* 4
Program ID: 155-35-31-086

Valhalla

New York Medical College at Westchester Medical Center Program

Sponsor: New York Medical College
Westchester Medical Center

Program Director:
Robert G Lerner, MD
Westchester Med Ctr
Dept of Med
Munger Pavillion
Valhalla, NY 10595
Tel: 914 594-4415 *Fax:* 914 594-4432
E-mail: lerner@nymc.edu
Accred Length: 3 Years *Program Size:* 7
Program ID: 155-35-31-101

North Carolina

Chapel Hill

University of North Carolina Hospitals Program

Sponsor: University of North Carolina Hospitals

Program Director:
Mark A Socinski, MD
3009 Old Clinic Bldg 226H
Chapel Hill, NC 27599-7305
Tel: 919 966-4431 *Fax:* 919 966-6735
Accred Length: 3 Years *Program Size:* 9
Program ID: 155-36-21-055

Durham

Duke University Program

Sponsor: Duke University Medical Center

Program Director:
Marilyn Telen, MD
Duke Univ Med Ctr
Box 2615
Durham, NC 27710
Tel: 919 684-5378 *Fax:* 919 681-7688
E-mail: telen002@mc.duke.edu
Accred Length: 3 Years *Program Size:* 16
Program ID: 155-36-31-056

Winston-Salem

Wake Forest University School of Medicine Program

Sponsor: Wake Forest University Baptist Medical Center

Program Director:
John Owen, MD MBA
Wake Forest Univ Sch of Med
Medical Center Blvd
Winston-Salem, NC 27157-1082
Tel: 910 716-0457 *Fax:* 910 716-5687
E-mail: mhdavis@bgsm.edu
Internet: http://www.bgsm.edu/research/cancer.html
Accred Length: 3 Years *Program Size:* 11
Program ID: 155-36-21-076

Ohio

Cincinnati

University Hospital/University of Cincinnati College of Medicine Program

Sponsor: University Hospital Inc
Veterans Affairs Medical Center (Cincinnati)

Program Director:
John C Winkelmann, MD
231 Bethesda Ave
Pavilion K/Rm 308
PO Box 670508
Cincinnati, OH 45267-0508
Tel: 513 584-2195 *Fax:* 513 584-6703
E-mail: winkeljc@ucmail.uc.edu
Accred Length: 3 Years *Program Size:* 5
Program ID: 155-38-21-102

Cleveland

Case Western Reserve University Program

Sponsor: University Hospitals of Cleveland
Veterans Affairs Medical Center (Cleveland)

Program Director:
Jack O Hensold, MD
10900 Euclid Ave (BRB 333)
Cleveland, OH 44106-4937
Tel: 216 368-1175 *Fax:* 216 368-1166
E-mail: joh2@po.cwru.edu
Accred Length: 3 Years *Program Size:* 8
Program ID: 155-38-21-117

Cleveland Clinic Foundation Program

Sponsor: Cleveland Clinic Foundation

Program Director:
Robert J Pelley, MD
Cleveland Clinic Foundation
Dept of Hematology/Oncology/T40
9500 Euclid Ave
Cleveland, OH 44195-5242
Tel: 216 444-5690 *Fax:* 216 444-1162
E-mail: meded@cestmp.ccf.org
Internet: http://www.ccf.org
Accred Length: 3 Years *Program Size:* 12
Program ID: 155-38-21-057

Columbus

Ohio State University Program

Sponsor: Ohio State University Medical Center
Arthur G James Cancer Hospital and Research Institute

Program Director:
Michael A Caligiuri, MD
Ohio State Univ
Div of Hematology/Oncology
320 W Tenth Ave/Starling-Loving Hall
Columbus, OH 43210-1228
Tel: 614 293-8858 *Fax:* 614 293-4372
E-mail: caligiuri.1@osu.edu
Accred Length: 3 Years *Program Size:* 14
Program ID: 155-38-31-058

Dayton

Wright State University Program
Sponsor: Wright State University School of Medicine
Good Samaritan Hospital and Health Center
Veterans Affairs Medical Center (Dayton)
Program Director:
Michael A Baumann, MD
Div of Hematology/Oncology
4100 W Third St
Dayton, OH 45428
Tel: 513 262-0203 *Fax:* 513 267-5310
E-mail: baumann.michael@dayton.va.gov
Accred Length: 3 Years *Program Size:* 3
Program ID: 155-38-11-059

Oklahoma

Oklahoma City

University of Oklahoma Health Sciences Center Program
Sponsor: University of Oklahoma College of Medicine
University Hospital
Veterans Affairs Medical Center (Oklahoma City)
Program Director:
James N George, MD
Univ of Oklahoma Health Sciences Ctr
PO Box 26901/UH-EB-271
Oklahoma City, OK 73190
Tel: 405 271-4222 *Fax:* 405 271-6444
E-mail: jim-george@uokhsc.edu
Accred Length: 3 Years *Program Size:* 3
Program ID: 155-39-21-060

Oregon

Portland

Oregon Health Sciences University Program
Sponsor: Oregon Health Sciences University Hospital
Veterans Affairs Medical Center (Portland)
Program Director:
Craig R Nichols, MD
3181 SW Sam Jackson Park Rd/L580
Portland, OR 97201
Tel: 503 494-8534 *Fax:* 503 494-4285
E-mail: nicholsc@ohsu.edu
Internet: http://www.ohsu.edu/som-hemonc
Accred Length: 3 Years *Program Size:* 6
Program ID: 155-40-21-118

Pennsylvania

Hershey

Penn State Geisinger Health System/Milton S Hershey Medical Center Program
Sponsor: Penn State Geisinger Health System
Milton S Hershey Medical Center
Program Director:
Harold A Harvey, MD
Sect of Hematology/Oncology
PO Box 850/MC H046
Milton S Hershey Med Ctr
Hershey, PA 17033-0850
Tel: 717 531-5059 *Fax:* 717 531-8274
E-mail: mfmoore@psghs.edu
Internet: http://www.hmc.psu.edu
Accred Length: 3 Years *Program Size:* 6
Program ID: 155-41-21-061

Philadelphia

MCP Hahnemann University Program
Sponsor: MCP Hahnemann University
Hahnemann University Hospital
Medical College of Pennsylvania Hospital
Program Director:
Michael J Styler, MD
Hahnemann Univ Hospital
Broad and Vine Sts
Philadelphia, PA 19102
Tel: 215 762-8547 *Fax:* 215 762-8857
E-mail: styler@auhs.edu
Accred Length: 3 Years *Program Size:* 10
Program ID: 155-41-31-062

Temple University Program
Sponsor: Temple University Hospital
Fox Chase Cancer Center
Program Director:
Russell J Schilder, MD
Temple Univ Hospital
Dept of Medicine
3401 N Broad St
Philadelphia, PA 19140
Tel: 215 707-2847 *Fax:* 215 707-2746
Accred Length: 3 Years *Program Size:* 12
Program ID: 155-41-21-091

University of Pennsylvania Program
Sponsor: Hospital of the University of Pennsylvania
Program Director:
Dupont Guerry, MD
Univ of Pennsylvania
510 Maloney
36th and Spruce St
Philadelphia, PA 19104-4283
Tel: 215 662-4139 *Fax:* 215 349-5866
E-mail: mereditd@mail.med.upenn.edu
Internet: http://www.med.upenn.edu/"hematol"
Accred Length: 3 Years *Program Size:* 18
Program ID: 155-41-21-081

Wynnewood

Lankenau Hospital Program
Sponsor: Lankenau Hospital
Program Director:
Paul B Gilman, MD
Lankenau Hospital Cancer Ctr
100 Lancaster Ave
Wynnewood, PA 19096
Tel: 610 645-2494 *Fax:* 610 645-4456
Accred Length: 3 Years *Program Size:* 3
Program ID: 155-41-31-077

Puerto Rico

San Juan

University of Puerto Rico Program
Sponsor: University of Puerto Rico School of Medicine
University Hospital
Program Director:
Enrique O Velez-Garcia, MD
Univ Hospital
PO Box 365067
San Juan, PR 00936-5067
Tel: 787 754-3896 *Fax:* 787 756-5866
Accred Length: 3 Years *Program Size:* 3
Program ID: 155-42-21-080

Rhode Island

Providence

Roger Williams Medical Center Program
Sponsor: Roger Williams Medical Center
Emma Pendleton Bradley Hospital
Memorial Hospital of Rhode Island
Veterans Affairs Medical Center (Providence)
Program Director:
Alan Weitberg, MD
Roger Williams Med Ctr
825 Chalkstone Ave
Providence, RI 02908
Tel: 401 456-2000
Accred Length: 3 Years *Program Size:* 2
Program ID: 155-43-21-120

South Carolina

Charleston

Medical University of South Carolina Program
Sponsor: Medical University of South Carolina College of Medicine
MUSC Medical Center
Ralph H Johnson Dept of Veterans Affairs Med Center
Program Director:
Lawrence B Afrin, MD
Med Univ of South Carolina
Hematology/Oncology Div
96 Jonathan Lucas St/Ste 903
Charleston, SC 29425
Tel: 843 792-4271 *Fax:* 843 792-0644
E-mail: cassidyt@musc.edu
Internet: http://www.musc.edu/medcenter/hollings.html
Accred Length: 3 Years *Program Size:* 9
Program ID: 155-45-21-063

Tennessee

Nashville

Vanderbilt University Program
Sponsor: Vanderbilt University Medical Center
St Thomas Hospital
Veterans Affairs Medical Center (Nashville)
Program Director:
Kenneth R Hande, MD
Div of Hematology/Oncology
1956 Vanderbilt Clinic
Nashville, TN 37232-5536
Tel: 615 322-4967 *Fax:* 615 343-7602
Accred Length: 3 Years *Program Size:* 12
Program ID: 155-47-31-065

Texas

Dallas

University of Texas Southwestern Medical School Program

Sponsor: University of Texas Southwestern Medical School
Dallas County Hospital District-Parkland Memorial Hospital
Veterans Affairs Medical Center (Dallas)
Program Director:
Cynthia J Rutherford, MB ChB
Eugene P Frenkel, MD
Univ of Texas Southwestern Med Sch
5323 Harry Hines Blvd
Dallas, TX 75235-8852
Tel: 214 648-2647 *Fax:* 214 648-2792
E-mail: levia.brazzle@email.swmed.edu
Accred Length: 3 Years *Program Size:* 10
Program ID: 155-48-21-066

Fort Sam Houston

San Antonio Uniformed Services Health Education Consortium (BAMC) Program

Sponsor: San Antonio Uniformed Services Health Education Consortium
Brooke Army Medical Center
Program Director:
Rickey C Myhand, MD
Brooke Army Med Ctr
Hem-Onc Service
3851 Roger Brooke Dr
Fort Sam Houston, TX 78234-6200
Tel: 210 916-0504 *Fax:* 210 916-3099
Accred Length: 3 Years *Program Size:* 15
Program ID: 155-48-31-067
US Armed Services Program

San Antonio

University of Texas Health Science Center at San Antonio Program

Sponsor: University of Texas Medical School at San Antonio
Audie L Murphy Memorial Veterans Hospital (San Antonio)
St Luke's Baptist Hospital
University Hospital-South Texas Medical Center
Program Director:
Kevin Harris, MD
Univ of Texas Health Science Ctr
Med/Oncology
7703 Floyd Curl Dr
San Antonio, TX 78284
Tel: 210 617-5186 *Fax:* 210 567-4822
Accred Length: 3 Years *Program Size:* 12
Program ID: 155-48-21-099

Utah

Salt Lake City

University of Utah Program

Sponsor: University of Utah Medical Center
Program Director:
John H Ward, MD
Univ of Utah Sch of Med
50 N Medical Dr
Salt Lake City, UT 84132
Tel: 801 581-6734 *Fax:* 801 585-5469
E-mail: john.ward@hsc.utah.edu
Internet: http://medstat.med.utah.edu/hematology/
Accred Length: 3 Years *Program Size:* 8
Program ID: 155-49-21-082

Vermont

Burlington

University of Vermont Program

Sponsor: Fletcher Allen Health Care
Program Director:
Richard F Branda, MD
Fletcher Allen Health Care
MCHV Campus Patrick 534
111 Colchester Ave
Burlington, VT 05401-1429
Tel: 802 656-3827 *Fax:* 802 656-5946
Accred Length: 3 Years *Program Size:* 3
Program ID: 155-50-21-069

Virginia

Charlottesville

University of Virginia Program

Sponsor: University of Virginia Medical Center
Program Director:
Kerry L Kilbridge, MD
Univ of Virginia Health Sciences Ctr
Dept of Int Med
Box 502
Charlottesville, VA 22908
Tel: 804 982-4194 *Fax:* 804 243-6086
E-mail: mn8t@virginia.edu
Accred Length: 3 Years *Program Size:* 6
Program ID: 155-51-31-078

Richmond

Medical College of Virginia/Virginia Commonwealth University Program

Sponsor: Medical College of Virginia/Virginia Commonwealth University
Hunter Holmes McGuire VA Medical Center (Richmond)
Medical College of Virginia Hospitals
Program Director:
Emmanuel N Dessypris, MD
McGuire VA Med Ctr
1201 Broad Rock Blvd (111K)
Richmond, VA 23249
Tel: 804 675-5446 *Fax:* 804 675-5447
E-mail: edessypris@hsc.vcu.edu
Accred Length: 3 Years *Program Size:* 4
Program ID: 155-51-21-070

West Virginia

Morgantown

West Virginia University Program

Sponsor: West Virginia University Hospitals
Program Director:
Edward B Crowell Jr, MD
Robert C Byrd Health Sciences Ctr
Dept of Med
PO Box 9162
Morgantown, WV 26506-9162
Tel: 304 293-4229 *Fax:* 304 293-2519
E-mail: ecrowell@wvu.edu
Accred Length: 3 Years *Program Size:* 6
Program ID: 155-55-21-109

Wisconsin

Milwaukee

Medical College of Wisconsin Program

Sponsor: Medical College of Wisconsin Affiliated Hospitals Inc
Clement J Zablocki Veterans Affairs Medical Center
Froedtert Memorial Lutheran Hospital
Program Director:
Paul Ritch, MD
Med Coll of Wisconsin
9200 W Wisconsin Ave
Div of Hem/Oncology-Froedtert East Clinics
Milwaukee, WI 53226-3596
Tel: 414 805-4600 *Fax:* 414 805-4606
E-mail: pritch@mcw.edu
Internet: http://www.mcw.edu/hemonc
Accred Length: 3 Years *Program Size:* 2
Program ID: 155-56-21-119

Immunopathology (Pathology)

Florida

Miami

University of Miami-Jackson Memorial Medical Center Program
Sponsor: University of Miami-Jackson Memorial Medical Center
Program Director:
Phillip Ruiz, MD PhD
Univ of Miami Sch of Med
Dept of Pathology (D-33)
PO Box 016960
Miami, FL 33101
Tel: 305 585-7344 *Fax:* 305 324-0149
E-mail: pruiz@mednet.med.miami.edu
Accred Length: 1 Year *Program Size:* 1
Program ID: 313-11-21-017

Iowa

Iowa City

University of Iowa Hospitals and Clinics Program
Sponsor: University of Iowa Hospitals and Clinics
Program Director:
James A Goeken, MD
Univ of Iowa Hospitals and Clinics
Dept of Pathology
200 Hawkins Dr
Iowa City, IA 52242-1009
Tel: 319 356-1966 *Fax:* 319 356-8470
E-mail: james-goeken@uiowa.edu
Accred Length: 2 Years *Program Size:* 2
Program ID: 313-18-21-005

Maryland

Baltimore

Johns Hopkins University Program
Sponsor: Johns Hopkins University School of Medicine
Johns Hopkins Hospital
Program Director:
William M Baldwin, MD PhD
Johns Hopkins Univ
Ross 664D
720 Rutland Ave
Baltimore, MD 21205-2196
Tel: 410 614-2053 *Fax:* 410 614-3548
E-mail: wbaldwin@welchlink.welch.jhu.edu
Internet: http://www.pathology.jhu.edu
Accred Length: 2 Years *Program Size:* 2
Program ID: 313-23-11-008

Massachusetts

Boston

Massachusetts General Hospital Program
Sponsor: Massachusetts General Hospital
Brigham and Women's Hospital
Program Director:
Atul K Bhan, MD
Massachusetts General Hospital
Dept of Pathology
100 Blossom St/Cox 5
Boston, MA 02114
Tel: 617 726-2588 *Fax:* 617 726-2365
E-mail: abhan@partners.org
Accred Length: 1 Year *Program Size:* 2
Program ID: 313-24-21-019

New York

Bronx

Bronx-Lebanon Hospital Center Program
Sponsor: Bronx-Lebanon Hospital Center
Program Director:
Young J Choi, MD
Bronx-Lebanon Hospital Ctr
1650 Grand Concourse
Bronx, NY 10457
Tel: 718 518-5148 *Fax:* 212 716-8242
Accred Length: 2 Years *Program Size:* 2
Program ID: 313-35-12-003

North Carolina

Chapel Hill

University of North Carolina Hospitals Program
Sponsor: University of North Carolina Hospitals
Program Director:
Georgette A Dent, MD
Dept of Laboratories
Univ of North Carolina Hospitals
101 Manning Dr
Chapel Hill, NC 27514
Tel: 919 966-2318 *Fax:* 919 966-6407
E-mail: gadent@med.unc.edu
Accred Length: 1 Year *Program Size:* 1
Program ID: 313-36-21-015

Texas

Dallas

University of Texas Southwestern Medical School Program
Sponsor: University of Texas Southwestern Medical School
Dallas County Hospital District-Parkland Memorial Hospital
Program Director:
Mohammad Q Ansari, MD
Univ of Texas Southwestern Med Ctr
5323 Harry Hines Blvd
Dallas, TX 75235-9072
Tel: 214 648-9153 *Fax:* 214 648-4070
Accred Length: 2 Years *Program Size:* 1
Program ID: 313-48-21-014

Infectious Disease (Internal Medicine)

Alabama

Birmingham

University of Alabama Medical Center Program
Sponsor: University of Alabama Hospital
Program Director:
William E Dismukes, MD
Univ of Alabama, Div of Infectious Dis
Tinsley Harrison Tower 229
1900 University Blvd
Birmingham, AL 35294-0006
Tel: 205 934-5191 *Fax:* 205 934-5155
E-mail: wdismukes@uabid.dom.uab.edu
Internet: http://info.dom.uab.edu/id
Accred Length: 2 Years *Program Size:* 8
Program ID: 146-01-21-121

Mobile

University of South Alabama Program
Sponsor: University of South Alabama Medical Center
Program Director:
Keith M Ramsey, MD
Univ of South Alabama
Div of Infectious Diseases
307 University Blvd/CC-CB 472
Mobile, AL 36688-0002
Tel: 334 460-7220 *Fax:* 334 460-6981
E-mail: kramsey@usamail.usouthal.edu
Accred Length: 2 Years *Program Size:* 2
Program ID: 146-01-11-089

Arkansas

Little Rock

University of Arkansas for Medical Sciences Program
Sponsor: University of Arkansas College of Medicine
John L McClellan Memorial Veterans Hospital
University Hospital of Arkansas
Program Director:
Robert W Bradsher Jr, MD
Univ of Arkansas for Med Sciences
4301 W Markham St/Slot 639
Little Rock, AR 72205
Tel: 501 686-5585 *Fax:* 501 686-8188
E-mail: mccalliebrendal@exchange.uams.edu
Internet: http://www.uams.edu/dim/infect.htm
Accred Length: 2 Years *Program Size:* 1
Program ID: 146-04-21-107

California

Los Angeles

Charles R Drew University Program

Sponsor: Charles R Drew University of Medicine and Science
LAC-King/Drew Medical Center
Program Director:
Vinod K Dhawan, MD
Charles R Drew Univ of Med and Science
12021 S Wilmington Ave
Los Angeles, CA 90059
Tel: 310 668-3439 *Fax:* 310 763-8929
Accred Length: 2 Years *Program Size:* 2
Program ID: 146-05-11-123

Southern California Kaiser Permanente Medical Care (Los Angeles) Program

Sponsor: Southern California Kaiser Permanente Medical Group
Kaiser Foundation Hospital (Los Angeles)
Program Director:
Joel Ruskin, MD
Kaiser Foundation Hospital
1505 Edgemont/2nd Fl
Los Angeles, CA 90027
Tel: 323 783-4559 *Fax:* 323 783-4514
E-mail: joel.x.ruskin@kp.org
Accred Length: 2 Years *Program Size:* 2
Program ID: 146-05-12-032

UCLA Medical Center Program

Sponsor: UCLA School of Medicine
UCLA Medical Center
Program Director:
David A Pegues, MD
UCLA Sch of Med
Ctr for Health Sciences
Div of Infectious Dis
Los Angeles, CA 90095-1688
Tel: 310 825-7225
Accred Length: 2 Years *Program Size:* 4
Program ID: 146-05-11-124

University of Southern California Program

Sponsor: Los Angeles County-USC Medical Center
LAC-Rancho Los Amigos Medical Center
Program Director:
John M Leedom, MD
Los Angeles County-USC Med Ctr
1200 N State St/Rm 6442
Los Angeles, CA 90033
Tel: 213 226-7504 *Fax:* 213 226-7726
E-mail: jsaito@hsc.usc.edu or jmleedom@hsc.usc.edu
Accred Length: 2 Years *Program Size:* 5
Program ID: 146-05-21-042

VA Greater Los Angeles Healthcare System Program

Sponsor: VA Greater Los Angeles Healthcare System
Cedars-Sinai Medical Center
Olive View-UCLA Medical Center
Program Director:
Matthew B Goetz, MD
West Los Angeles VA Med Ctr
Infectious Diseases Sect (111F)
11301 Wilshire Blvd
Los Angeles, CA 90073
Tel: 310 268-3015 *Fax:* 310 268-4928
E-mail: matthew.goetz.@med.va.gov
Accred Length: 2 Years *Program Size:* 8
Program ID: 146-05-21-195

Orange

University of California (Irvine) Program

Sponsor: University of California (Irvine) Medical Center
Veterans Affairs Medical Center (Long Beach)
Program Director:
Jeremiah G Tilles, MD
Univ of California Irvine Med Ctr
101 City Dr S/Bldg 53/Rt 81
Orange, CA 92668
Tel: 714 456-5134 *Fax:* 714 456-8325
E-mail: jgtilles@uci.edu
Accred Length: 2 Years *Program Size:* 4
Program ID: 146-05-21-141

Sacramento

University of California (Davis) Program

Sponsor: University of California (Davis) Medical Center
David Grant Medical Center
Program Director:
Stuart H Cohen, MD
Univ of California Davis Med Ctr
2315 Stockton Blvd
Sacramento, CA 95817-2282
Tel: 916 734-3741 *Fax:* 916 734-7766
E-mail: stcohen@ucdavis.edu
Internet:
http://internalmedicine.ucdmc.ucdavis.edu/infdis/
Accred Length: 2 Years *Program Size:* 3
Program ID: 146-05-21-095

San Diego

Naval Medical Center (San Diego) Program

Sponsor: Naval Medical Center (San Diego)
Program Director:
Mark R Wallace, MD
Naval Med Ctr
34800 Bob Wilson Dr
San Diego, CA 92134-5000
Tel: 619 532-7475 *Fax:* 619 532-7478
E-mail: mwallace@sndlo.med.navy.mil
Accred Length: 2 Years *Program Size:* 4
Program ID: 146-05-12-142
US Armed Services Program

University of California (San Diego) Program

Sponsor: University of California (San Diego) Medical Center
Veterans Affairs Medical Center (San Diego)
Program Director:
Joshua Fierer, MD
VA Med Ctr
3350 La Jolla Village Dr
San Diego, CA 92161
Tel: 619 552-7446 *Fax:* 619 552-4398
E-mail: jfierer@ucsd.edu
Accred Length: 2 Years *Program Size:* 5
Program ID: 146-05-21-163

San Francisco

University of California (San Francisco) Program

Sponsor: University of California (San Francisco) School of Medicine
San Francisco General Hospital Medical Center
University of California (San Francisco) Medical Center
Veterans Affairs Medical Center (San Francisco)
Program Director:
Richard M Locksley, MD
Dept of Infectious Diseases
Box 0654/Rm C443
Univ of California San Francisco Med Ctr
San Francisco, CA 94143-0654
Tel: 415 476-9362 *Fax:* 415 476-9364
E-mail: locksley@medicine.west.edu
Accred Length: 2 Years *Program Size:* 12
Program ID: 146-05-21-144

University of California (San Francisco)/Mount Zion Program

Sponsor: University of California (San Francisco) School of Medicine
Mount Zion Medical Center of the University of California
Program Director:
W Lawrence Drew, MD PhD
Univ of California San Francisco-Mount Zion Med Ctr
1600 Divisadero St
San Francisco, CA 94115
Tel: 415 885-7315 *Fax:* 415 885-7522
Accred Length: 2 Years *Program Size:* 0
Program ID: 146-05-31-143

Stanford

Stanford University Program

Sponsor: Stanford University Hospital
Santa Clara Valley Medical Center
Veterans Affairs Palo Alto Health Care System
Program Director:
Jeffery S Loutit, MD
Stanford Univ Hospital
Div of Inf Dis/Rm S-156
300 Pasteur Dr
Stanford, CA 94305-5107
Tel: 650 725-6542 *Fax:* 650 498-7011
Accred Length: 2 Years *Program Size:* 13
Program ID: 146-05-21-023

Torrance

Los Angeles County-Harbor-UCLA Medical Center Program

Sponsor: Los Angeles County-Harbor-UCLA Medical Center
Program Director:
John E Edwards Jr, MD
Los Angeles County-Harbor-UCLA Med Ctr
Div of Adult Infectious Diseases
1000 W Carson St/Bldg RB2
Torrance, CA 90509
Tel: 310 222-3813 *Fax:* 310 782-2016
E-mail: edwards@humc.edu
Internet: http://www.afp76.humc.edu/id
Accred Length: 2 Years *Program Size:* 2
Program ID: 146-05-11-164

Colorado

Denver

University of Colorado Program

Sponsor: University of Colorado Health Sciences Center
Denver Health and Hospitals
Veterans Affairs Medical Center (Denver)

Program Director:
Nancy E Madinger, MD
Univ of Colorado Health Sciences Ctr
Div of Infectious Diseases
4200 E Ninth Ave/Box B-168
Denver, CO 80262
Tel: 303 315-7233 *Fax:* 303 315-8681
E-mail: madinger_n@defiance.uchsc.edu
Accred Length: 2 Years *Program Size:* 8
Program ID: 146-07-21-050

Connecticut

Farmington

University of Connecticut Program 1

Sponsor: University of Connecticut School of Medicine
Mount Sinai Hospital
Univ of Connecticut Health Center/John Dempsey Hospital

Program Director:
John D Shanley, MD
Univ of Connecticut Health Ctr
Div of Infectious Diseases
263 Farmington Ave
Farmington, CT 06030-3212
Tel: 860 679-4700 *Fax:* 860 679-4701
E-mail: klein@nso1.uchc.edu
Accred Length: 2 Years *Program Size:* 4
Program ID: 146-08-31-001

University of Connecticut Program 2

Sponsor: University of Connecticut School of Medicine
Hartford Hospital
Univ of Connecticut Health Center/John Dempsey Hospital

Program Director:
Brian Cooper, MD
Univ of Connecticut Sch of Med
80 Seymour St
Hartford, CT 06102-5037
Tel: 860 524-2878 *Fax:* 860 545-4256
Accred Length: 2 Years *Program Size:* 0
Program ID: 146-08-31-183

New Haven

Yale-New Haven Medical Center Program

Sponsor: Yale-New Haven Hospital
Veterans Affairs Medical Center (West Haven)

Program Director:
Vincent J Quagliarello, MD
Yale Univ Sch of Med
Infectious Disease Sect
333 Cedar St/PO Box 208022 LCI808
New Haven, CT 06520-8022
Tel: 203 785-4140 *Fax:* 203 785-3864
E-mail: vincent.quagliarello@yale.edu
Internet: http://www.info.med.yale.edu/intmed/infdis/
Accred Length: 2 Years *Program Size:* 9
Program ID: 146-08-21-024

District of Columbia

Washington

George Washington University Program

Sponsor: George Washington University School of Medicine
George Washington University Hospital (UHS)

Program Director:
Gary L Simon, MD PhD
George Washington Univ Med Ctr
Div of Infectious Diseases
2150 Pennsylvania Ave NW
Washington, DC 20037
Tel: 202 994-4717 *Fax:* 202 994-3949
E-mail: domgls@gwumc.edu
Accred Length: 2 Years *Program Size:* 2
Program ID: 146-10-21-109

Georgetown University Program

Sponsor: Georgetown University Medical Center

Program Director:
Princy N Kumar, MD
Georgetown Univ Hospital
Inf Diseases (#110 Kober-Cogan)
3800 Reservoir Rd NW
Washington, DC 20007
Tel: 202 687-6845 *Fax:* 202 687-6476
Accred Length: 2 Years *Program Size:* 3
Program ID: 146-10-21-090

Howard University Program

Sponsor: Howard University Hospital

Program Director:
Vinod R Mody, MD
Howard Univ Hospital
2041 Georgia Ave NW/Rm 5C02
Washington, DC 20060
Tel: 202 865-1872 *Fax:* 202 865-4607
Accred Length: 2 Years *Program Size:* 2
Program ID: 146-10-21-091

Walter Reed Army Medical Center Program

Sponsor: Walter Reed Army Medical Center
National Naval Medical Center (Bethesda)

Program Director:
Robert A Gasser Jr, MD
Walter Reed Army Med Ctr
6825 16th St NW
Washington, DC 20307-5001
Tel: 202 782-1663 *Fax:* 202 782-3765
E-mail: col_robert_gasser_at_wrair3__washdc@wrsmtp-ccmail.army.mil
Internet: http://www.wramc.amedd.army.mil/departments/medicine/infdis/id_felw.htm
Accred Length: 2 Years *Program Size:* 11
Program ID: 146-10-11-127
US Armed Services Program

Washington Hospital Center Program

Sponsor: Washington Hospital Center
Veterans Affairs Medical Center (Washington, DC)

Program Director:
Daniel Lucey, MD
Washington Hospital Ctr
Sect of Infectious Diseases
110 Irving St NW/Rm 2A-56
Washington, DC 20010-2975
Tel: 202 877-7164 *Fax:* 202 877-6130
Accred Length: 2 Years *Program Size:* 5
Program ID: 146-10-11-179

Florida

Gainesville

University of Florida Program

Sponsor: University of Florida College of Medicine
Shands Hospital at the University of Florida
Veterans Affairs Medical Center (Gainesville)

Program Director:
Frederick S Southwick, MD
Univ of Florida
1600 SW Archer Rd/ARB R2-124
Box 100277 JHMHC
Gainesville, FL 32610-0227
Tel: 352 392-4058 *Fax:* 352 392-6481
E-mail: southfs@medmac.ufl.edu
Accred Length: 2 Years *Program Size:* 4
Program ID: 146-11-21-033

Jacksonville

University of Florida Health Science Center/Jacksonville Program

Sponsor: University of Florida College of Medicine at Jacksonville
University Medical Center (UFHSC/J)
Baptist Medical Center (UFHSC/J)

Program Director:
Alexander G Vandevelde, MD
Univ of Florida Health Science Ctr-Jacksonville
Dept of Int Med (ID)
655 W Eighth St
Jacksonville, FL 32209-6597
Tel: 904 549-3077 *Fax:* 904 549-3087
Internet: http://www.ufhscj.edu
Accred Length: 2 Years *Program Size:* 2
Program ID: 146-11-21-186

Miami

University of Miami-Jackson Memorial Medical Center Program

Sponsor: University of Miami-Jackson Memorial Medical Center
Mount Sinai Medical Center of Greater Miami
Veterans Affairs Medical Center (Miami)

Program Director:
Thomas A Hoffman, MD
Univ of Miami-Jackson Memorial Med Ctr
PO Box 016960 (R-63)
Miami, FL 33101
Tel: 305 243-7618 *Fax:* 305 243-7621
Accred Length: 2 Years *Program Size:* 7
Program ID: 146-11-21-165

Tampa

University of South Florida Program

Sponsor: University of South Florida College of Medicine
H Lee Moffitt Cancer Center
James A Haley Veterans Hospital
Tampa General Healthcare

Program Director:
John T Sinnott, MD
Univ of South Florida Coll of Med
Div of Infectious Disease/MDC#19
12901 Bruce B Downs Blvd
Tampa, FL 33612-4799
Tel: 813 251-7670 *Fax:* 813 251-7605
E-mail: jsinnott@com1.med.usf.edu
Internet: http://www.med.usf.edu/intmed/index.html
Accred Length: 2 Years *Program Size:* 6
Program ID: 146-11-21-034

Georgia

Atlanta

Emory University Program
Sponsor: Emory University School of Medicine
Emory University Hospital
Grady Memorial Hospital
Program Director:
David Stephens, MD
Emory Univ Sch of Med, Infectious Diseases
69 Butler St SE
Atlanta, GA 30303
Tel: 404 616-3600 *Fax:* 404 880-9305
E-mail: dstep01@emory.edu
Internet: http://www.emory.edu/med_inf/idweb.html
Accred Length: 2 Years *Program Size:* 11
Program ID: 146-12-21-129

Augusta

Medical College of Georgia Program
Sponsor: Medical College of Georgia Hospital and Clinics
Veterans Affairs Medical Center (Augusta)
Program Director:
J Peter Rissing, MD
Med Coll of Georgia
Infectious Disease Sect
1120 15th St
Augusta, GA 30912-3130
Tel: 706 721-2236 *Fax:* 706 721-2000
E-mail: prissing@mail.mcg.edu
Accred Length: 2 Years *Program Size:* 2
Program ID: 146-12-21-003

Illinois

Chicago

McGaw Medical Center of Northwestern University Program
Sponsor: Northwestern University Medical School
Northwestern Memorial Hospital
Veterans Affairs Lakeside Medical Center (Chicago)
Program Director:
John P Phair, MD
Northwestern Univ Med Sch
680 N Lake Shore Dr/Ste 1106
Chicago, IL 60611
Tel: 312 908-9137 *Fax:* 312 908-5820
E-mail: s-perez@nwu.edu
Accred Length: 2 Years *Program Size:* 4
Program ID: 146-16-21-059

Rush-Presbyterian-St Luke's Medical Center Program
Sponsor: Rush-Presbyterian-St Luke's Medical Center
Cook County Hospital
Program Director:
Gordon M Trenholme, MD
Rush-Presbyterian-St Luke's Med Ctr
Sect of Infectious Diseases
600 S Paulina/Ste 143 AAC
Chicago, IL 60612
Tel: 312 942-5865 *Fax:* 312 942-2184
E-mail: gtrenhol@rush.edu
Accred Length: 2 Years *Program Size:* 10
Program ID: 146-16-11-130

University of Illinois College of Medicine at Chicago Program
Sponsor: University of Illinois College of Medicine at Chicago
Michael Reese Hospital and Medical Center
University of Chicago Hospitals
University of Illinois Hospital and Clinics
Veterans Affairs West Side Medical Center
Program Director:
David L Pitrak, MD
Univ of Illinois-Univ of Chicago
Joint Infectious Disease Fellowship
820 S Wood St (M/C 735)
Chicago, IL 60612
Tel: 312 996-6732 *Fax:* 312 413-1657
E-mail: pitrak,david@chicago-west.va.gov
Accred Length: 2 Years *Program Size:* 8
Program ID: 146-16-21-131

Maywood

Loyola University Program
Sponsor: Loyola University Medical Center
Edward J Hines Jr Veterans Affairs Hospital
Program Director:
Nigar Kirmani, MD PhD
Dept of Med/Rm 7604
2160 S First Ave
Maywood, IL 60153
Tel: 708 216-3232 *Fax:* 708 216-8198
Internet: http://www.meddean.luc.edu/lumen/deptwebs/medicine/medres/medres.htm
Accred Length: 2 Years *Program Size:* 2
Program ID: 146-16-21-004

North Chicago

Finch University of Health Sciences/Chicago Medical School Program
Sponsor: Finch University of Health Sciences/Chicago Medical School
Mount Sinai Hospital Medical Center of Chicago
Veterans Affairs Medical Center (North Chicago)
Program Director:
Walid Khayr, MD
Finch Univ of Health Sciences-Chicago Med Sch
Dept of Med
3333 Green Bay Rd
North Chicago, IL 60064-3095
Tel: 847 578-3227 *Fax:* 847 578-8647
Accred Length: 2 Years *Program Size:* 3
Program ID: 146-16-21-044

Springfield

Southern Illinois University Program
Sponsor: Southern Illinois University School of Medicine
Memorial Medical Center
St John's Hospital
Program Director:
Nancy Khardori, MD
Div of Infectious Diseases
Southern Illinois Univ Sch of Med
PO Box 19230
Springfield, IL 62794-9636
Tel: 217 782-9148 *Fax:* 217 788-5504
E-mail: nwalker@siumed.edu
Accred Length: 2 Years *Program Size:* 2
Program ID: 146-16-21-180

Indiana

Indianapolis

Indiana University School of Medicine Program
Sponsor: Indiana University School of Medicine
Program Director:
Michael Frank, MD
Indiana Univ Sch of Med
Emerson Hall/Rm 435
545 Barnhill Dr
Indianapolis, IN 46202-5124
Tel: 317 274-8113 *Fax:* 317 274-1587
E-mail: mifrank@iupui.edu
Accred Length: 2 Years *Program Size:* 5
Program ID: 146-17-21-146

Iowa

Iowa City

University of Iowa Hospitals and Clinics Program
Sponsor: University of Iowa Hospitals and Clinics
Program Director:
Bradley E Britigan, MD
Univ of Iowa Hospitals and Clinics
Dept of Int Med
200 Hawkins Dr
Iowa City, IA 52242-1009
Tel: 319 356-3674 *Fax:* 319 356-4600
Accred Length: 2 Years *Program Size:* 6
Program ID: 146-18-21-096

Kansas

Kansas City

University of Kansas Medical Center Program
Sponsor: University of Kansas School of Medicine
University of Kansas Medical Center
Program Director:
Elliot Goldstein, MD
Univ of Kansas Med Ctr
Infectious Diseases Div
3901 Rainbow Blvd
Kansas City, KS 66160-7354
Tel: 913 588-6035 *Fax:* 913 588-6024
E-mail: egoldste@kumc.edu
Accred Length: 2 Years *Program Size:* 3
Program ID: 146-19-21-110

Kentucky

Lexington

University of Kentucky Medical Center Program
Sponsor: University of Kentucky Hospital
Veterans Affairs Medical Center (Lexington)
Program Director:
Claire Pomeroy, MD
Univ of Kentucky Hospital
800 Rose St
Lexington, KY 40536-0084
Tel: 606 323-6326 *Fax:* 606 323-1020
Accred Length: 2 Years *Program Size:* 2
Program ID: 146-20-21-196

Louisville

University of Louisville Program
Sponsor: University of Louisville School of Medicine
University of Louisville Hospital
Veterans Affairs Medical Center (Louisville)
Program Director:
Julio A Ramirez, MD
Univ of Louisville
Div of Infectious Diseases
MDR Bldg 6th Fl
Louisville, KY 40292
Tel: 502 558-5131 *Fax:* 502 852-1147
E-mail: jarami01@ulkyvm.louisville.edu
Accred Length: 2 Years *Program Size:* 3
Program ID: 146-20-31-092

Louisiana

New Orleans

Alton Ochsner Medical Foundation Program
Sponsor: Alton Ochsner Medical Foundation
Program Director:
Joseph R Dalovisio, MD
Alton Ochsner Med Foundation
Dept of Grad Med Educ
1516 Jefferson Hwy
New Orleans, LA 70121
Tel: 504 842-3260 *Fax:* 504 842-3193
E-mail: dlambert@ochsner.org
Internet: http://www.ochsner.org
Accred Length: 2 Years *Program Size:* 2
Program ID: 146-21-22-100

Louisiana State University Program
Sponsor: Louisiana State University School of Medicine
Medical Center of Louisiana at New Orleans
Program Director:
Julio E Figueroa Jr, MD
Louisiana State Univ Med Ctr
1542 Tulane Ave
New Orleans, LA 70112-2822
Tel: 504 568-5031 *Fax:* 504 568-6752
E-mail: jfigue@lsumc.edu
Internet: http://www.lsumc.edu
Accred Length: 2 Years *Program Size:* 6
Program ID: 146-21-21-051

Tulane University Program
Sponsor: Tulane University School of Medicine
Medical Center of Louisiana at New Orleans
Veterans Affairs Medical Center-LSU Service (New Orleans)
Program Director:
Newton E Hyslop Jr, MD
Tulane Univ Sch of Med
1430 Tulane Ave/SL-87
New Orleans, LA 70112-2699
Tel: 504 587-7316 *Fax:* 504 584-3644
E-mail: infdis@mailhost.tcs.tulane.edu
Internet: http://www.tulane.edu/~tmcid/index.htm
Accred Length: 2 Years *Program Size:* 4
Program ID: 146-21-21-105

Shreveport

Louisiana State University (Shreveport) Program
Sponsor: Louisiana State University Hospital-Shreveport
Overton Brooks Veterans Affairs Medical Center
Program Director:
John W King, MD
Louisiana State Univ Med Ctr
Med Educ/Infectious Diseases
PO Box 33932
Shreveport, LA 71130-3932
Tel: 318 675-5904 *Fax:* 318 675-5907
Accred Length: 2 Years *Program Size:* 2
Program ID: 146-21-21-052

Maine

Portland

Maine Medical Center Program
Sponsor: Maine Medical Center
Program Director:
Robert P Smith, MD MPH
Maine Med Ctr
22 Bramhall St
Portland, ME 04102
Tel: 207 871-2099 *Fax:* 207 871-6116
E-mail: smithr.data@mmc.org
Internet: http://www.mmc.org
Accred Length: 2 Years *Program Size:* 2
Program ID: 146-22-21-182

Maryland

Baltimore

Johns Hopkins University Program
Sponsor: Johns Hopkins University School of Medicine
Johns Hopkins Hospital
Program Director:
Cynthia L Sears, MD
Johns Hopkins Univ Sch of Med
1830 E Monument St
Rm 455
Baltimore, MD 21205
Tel: 410 614-3269 *Fax:* 410 955-7889
E-mail: csears@welchlink.welch.jhu.edu
Internet: http://hopkins-id.edu
Accred Length: 2 Years *Program Size:* 11
Program ID: 146-23-11-060

University of Maryland Program
Sponsor: University of Maryland Medical System
Veterans Affairs Medical Center (Baltimore)
Program Director:
John W Warren, MD
Univ of Maryland
10 S Pine St/Rm 9-00
Baltimore, MD 21201
Tel: 410 706-7560 *Fax:* 410 706-8700
E-mail: lhorne@umppa1.ab.umd.edu
Accred Length: 2 Years *Program Size:* 8
Program ID: 146-23-21-036

Bethesda

National Institutes of Health Clinical Center Program
Sponsor: NIH Warren Grant Magnuson Clinical Center
Program Director:
John E Bennett, MD
Bldg 10/Rm 11-C-304
National Institutes of Health
10 Center Dr/MSC 1882
Bethesda, MD 20892-1882
Tel: 301 496-3461 *Fax:* 301 480-0050
E-mail: jb46y@nih.gov
Internet:
http://www.helix.nih.gov:8001/oe/clinical/clin14.html
Accred Length: 2 Years *Program Size:* 8
Program ID: 146-23-21-184

Massachusetts

Boston

Beth Israel Deaconess Medical Center (West Campus) Program
Sponsor: Beth Israel Deaconess Medical Center
Program Director:
Tamar F Barlam, MD
Beth Israel Deaconess Med Ctr
One Deaconess Rd
Kennedy-6
Boston, MA 02215
Tel: 617 632-0760 *Fax:* 617 632-0766
E-mail: tbarlam@bidmc.harvard.edu
Accred Length: 2 Years *Program Size:* 15
Program ID: 146-24-21-132

Boston University Medical Center Program
Sponsor: Boston Medical Center
Veterans Affairs Medical Center (Boston)
Program Director:
Brant Viner, MD
ENC-E336
Boston Med Ctr
88 E Newton St
Boston, MA 02118-2393
Tel: 617 638-7909 *Fax:* 617 638-8070
Accred Length: 2 Years *Program Size:* 8
Program ID: 146-24-21-148

Massachusetts General Hospital Program
Sponsor: Massachusetts General Hospital
Brigham and Women's Hospital
Program Director:
David C Hooper, MD
MGH-BWH Combined Harvard Program
J504 Massachusetts General Hospital
55 Fruit St
Boston, MA 02114-2696
Tel: 617 726-3812 *Fax:* 617 726-7416
E-mail: dhooper@partners.org
Accred Length: 2 Years *Program Size:* 18
Program ID: 146-24-21-021

New England Medical Center Hospitals Program
Sponsor: New England Medical Center Hospitals
Program Director:
Gerald T Keusch, MD
New England Med Ctr
750 Washington St/Box 041
Boston, MA 02111
Tel: 617 636-7001 *Fax:* 617 636-5292
E-mail: gerald.keusch@es.nemc.org
Accred Length: 2 Years *Program Size:* 7
Program ID: 146-24-21-006

Springfield

Baystate Medical Center Program
Sponsor: Baystate Medical Center
Program Director:
Richard B Brown, MD
Baystate Med Ctr
Infectious Disease Div
759 Chestnut St
Springfield, MA 01199
Tel: 413 794-5376 *Fax:* 413 794-4199
E-mail: richard.brown@bhs.org
Internet: http://www.baystatehealth.com
Accred Length: 2 Years *Program Size:* 2
Program ID: 146-24-11-061

Worcester

University of Massachusetts Program
Sponsor: University of Massachusetts Medical School
UMass Memorial Health Care (University Campus)
Program Director:
Richard T Ellison, MD
Univ of Massachusetts Med Sch
Div of Infectious Disease
55 Lake Ave N
Worcester, MA 01655
Tel: 508 856-3158 *Fax:* 508 856-5981
E-mail: kathy.scalley@banyan.ummed.edu
Internet: http://www.ummed.edu/dept/idi
Accred Length: 2 Years *Program Size:* 5
Program ID: 146-24-21-007

Michigan

Ann Arbor

University of Michigan Program
Sponsor: University of Michigan Hospitals
Veterans Affairs Medical Center (Ann Arbor)
Program Director:
Cary Engleberg, MD
Univ of Michigan Health System
1500 E Medical Center Dr
3116 Taubman Ctr
Ann Arbor, MI 48109-0378
Tel: 734 936-5205 *Fax:* 734 936-2737
E-mail: cengleb@umich.edu
Internet: http://www.med.umich.edu/intmed/infectious/
Accred Length: 2 Years *Program Size:* 5
Program ID: 146-25-21-062

Detroit

Henry Ford Hospital Program
Sponsor: Henry Ford Hospital
Program Director:
Douglas L Mayers, MD
Henry Ford Hospital
Div of Infectious Disease
2799 W Grand Blvd
Detroit, MI 48202
Tel: 313 916-2573 *Fax:* 313 916-2993
E-mail: pmcfarll1@hfhs.org
Accred Length: 2 Years *Program Size:* 6
Program ID: 146-25-11-133

St John Hospital and Medical Center Program
Sponsor: St John Hospital and Medical Center
Program Director:
Riad Khatib, MD
St John Hospital and Med Ctr
Dept of Med Educ
22101 Moross Rd
Detroit, MI 48236
Tel: 313 343-3875 *Fax:* 313 343-7840
E-mail: sue.moynihan@stjohn.org
Internet: http://www.stjohn.org
Accred Length: 2 Years *Program Size:* 3
Program ID: 146-25-21-191

Wayne State University/Detroit Medical Center Program
Sponsor: Wayne State University/Detroit Medical Center
Detroit Receiving Hospital and University Health Center
Harper Hospital
Veterans Affairs Medical Center (Detroit)
Program Director:
Pranatharthi H Chandrasekar, MD
Division of Infectious Diseases
4201 St Antoine
Rm 5Q-14
Detroit, MI 48201
Tel: 313 745-9649 *Fax:* 313 993-0302
E-mail: pchandrasekar@oncgate.roc.wayne.edu
Accred Length: 2 Years *Program Size:* 6
Program ID: 146-25-21-040

Royal Oak

William Beaumont Hospital Program
Sponsor: William Beaumont Hospital
Program Director:
Jeffrey D Band, MD
William Beaumont Hospital
3601 W 13 Mile Rd
Royal Oak, MI 48073-6769
Tel: 248 551-4041 *Fax:* 248 551-1110
E-mail: jband@beaumont.edu
Internet: http://www.beaumont.edu/html/gme
Accred Length: 2 Years *Program Size:* 3
Program ID: 146-25-12-102

Minnesota

Minneapolis

University of Minnesota Program
Sponsor: University of Minnesota Medical School
Fairview-University Medical Center
Hennepin County Medical Center
Veterans Affairs Medical Center (Minneapolis)
Program Director:
Edward N Janoff, MD
Infectious Disease Sect II I F
VA Med Ctr/Univ of Minnesota 1
1 Veterans Dr
Minneapolis, MN 55417
Tel: 612 775-2000, ext 4185 *Fax:* 612 727-5659
E-mail: janof001@tc.uhn.edu
Accred Length: 2 Years *Program Size:* 3
Program ID: 146-26-21-112

Rochester

Mayo Graduate School of Medicine (Rochester) Program
Sponsor: Mayo Graduate School of Medicine-Mayo Foundation
Mayo Clinic (Rochester)
Rochester Methodist Hospital
St Mary's Hospital of Rochester
Program Director:
Michael R Keating, MD
Application Processing Ctr
Mayo Graduate Sch of Med
200 First St SW/Siebens 5
Rochester, MN 55905
Tel: 507 284-3126 *Fax:* 507 284-0999
E-mail: keating.michael@mayo.edu
Internet: http://www.mayo.edu/mgsm/rid.htm
Accred Length: 2 Years *Program Size:* 9
Program ID: 146-26-21-045

Mississippi

Jackson

University of Mississippi Medical Center Program
Sponsor: University of Mississippi School of Medicine
University Hospital
Veterans Affairs Medical Center (Jackson)
Program Director:
Stanley W Chapman, MD
Univ of Mississippi Med Ctr
2500 N State St/N502
Jackson, MS 39216-4505
Tel: 601 984-5560 *Fax:* 601 984-5565
Accred Length: 2 Years *Program Size:* 2
Program ID: 146-27-21-063

Missouri

Columbia

University of Missouri-Columbia Program
Sponsor: University of Missouri-Columbia School of Medicine
Harry S Truman Memorial Veterans Hospital
University Hospitals and Clinics
Program Director:
E Dale Everett, MD
Univ of Missouri Health Sciences Ctr
MA425 Med Science Bldg
Columbia, MO 65212
Tel: 573 882-3107 *Fax:* 573 884-3996
E-mail: dale_everett@muccmail.missouri.edu
Internet: http://www.hsc.missouri.edu/internal-medicine/
Accred Length: 2 Years *Program Size:* 2
Program ID: 146-28-21-064

Kansas City

University of Missouri at Kansas City Program

Sponsor: University of Missouri-Kansas City School of Medicine
Saint Luke's Hospital
Truman Medical Center-West

Program Director:
David Bamberger, MD
Univ of Missouri
2411 Holmes St
Kansas City, MO 64108-2792
Tel: 816 235-1942 *Fax:* 816 881-6209
E-mail: dbamberger@cctr.umkc.edu
Internet: http://www.med.umkc.edu
Accred Length: 2 Years *Program Size:* 2
Program ID: 146-28-31-113

St Louis

St Louis University School of Medicine Program

Sponsor: St Louis University School of Medicine
St Louis University School of Medicine
Veterans Affairs Medical Center (St Louis)

Program Director:
Robert B Belshe, MD
St Louis Univ Sch of Med
Div of Infectious Diseases
3635 Vista Ave/FDT-8N
St Louis, MO 63110-0250
Tel: 314 577-8648 *Fax:* 314 771-3816
E-mail: prices@wpogate.slu.edu
Internet:
http://slu.edu/colleges/med/graduatemed/residencies/infectiousdiseases
Accred Length: 2 Years *Program Size:* 4
Program ID: 146-28-21-177

Washington University/B-JH/SLCH Consortium (South Campus) Program

Sponsor: Washington University/B-JH/SLCH Consortium
Barnes-Jewish Hospital

Program Director:
William G Powderly, MD
Washington Univ Sch of Med
Infectious Diseases Div
660 S Euclid Ave/Box 8051
St Louis, MO 63110
Tel: 314 747-0160
E-mail: wpowderl@imgate.wustl.edu
Internet: http://www.id.wustl.edu
Accred Length: 2 Years *Program Size:* 10
Program ID: 146-28-21-149

Nebraska

Omaha

Creighton University Program

Sponsor: Creighton University School of Medicine
Tenet St Joseph Hospital at Creighton Univ Medical Center
University of Nebraska Medical Center
Veterans Affairs Medical Center (Omaha)

Program Director:
Gary L Gorby, MD
VA Med Ctr
4101 Woolworth Ave (111D)
Omaha, NE 68105-1873
Tel: 402 449-0650 *Fax:* 402 977-5601
E-mail: gorby@omaha.va.gov
Accred Length: 2 Years *Program Size:* 3
Program ID: 146-30-21-151

New Hampshire

Lebanon

Dartmouth-Hitchcock Medical Center Program

Sponsor: Mary Hitchcock Memorial Hospital
Veterans Affairs Medical Center (White River Junction)

Program Director:
Jeffrey Parsonnet, MD
Dartmouth-Hitchcock Med Ctr
One Medical Center Dr
Lebanon, NH 03756
Tel: 603 650-8840 *Fax:* 603 650-6199
E-mail: jeffrey.parsonnet@hitchcock.org
Accred Length: 2 Years *Program Size:* 3
Program ID: 146-32-21-187

New Jersey

Camden

UMDNJ-Robert Wood Johnson Medical School (Camden) Program

Sponsor: Cooper Hospital-University Medical Center

Program Director:
Carl W Norden, MD
Cooper Hospital-Univ Med Ctr
Educ and Research Bldg/Rm 270
401 Haddon Ave
Camden, NJ 08103
Tel: 609 757-7767 *Fax:* 609 757-7803
Accred Length: 2 Years *Program Size:* 2
Program ID: 146-33-21-173

Newark

UMDNJ-New Jersey Medical School Program

Sponsor: UMDNJ-New Jersey Medical School
Hackensack University Medical Center
UMDNJ-University Hospital
Veterans Affairs Medical Center (East Orange)

Program Director:
Robert H Eng, MD
Dept of Infectious Diseases
185 S Orange Ave
MSB Rm I-510
Newark, NJ 07103-2757
Tel: 973 972-7598 *Fax:* 973 972-7790
E-mail: eng.robert@east-orange va.gov
Accred Length: 2 Years *Program Size:* 5
Program ID: 146-33-21-172

Piscataway

UMDNJ-Robert Wood Johnson Medical School Program

Sponsor: UMDNJ-Robert Wood Johnson Medical School
Jersey Shore Medical Center
Robert Wood Johnson University Hospital

Program Director:
Joseph F John, MD
Dept of Med/MEB Rm 362
One Robert Wood Johnson Pl
New Brunswick, NJ 08903-0019
Tel: 732 235-7710 *Fax:* 732 235-7951
E-mail: john@umdnj.edu
Internet: http://www.umdnj.edu
Accred Length: 2 Years *Program Size:* 5
Program ID: 146-33-21-026

South Orange

Seton Hall University School of Graduate Medical Education Program

Sponsor: Seton Hall University School of Graduate Medical Education
St Joseph's Hospital and Medical Center
St Michael's Medical Center (Cathedral Hlth Srvcs Inc)

Program Director:
Stephen M Smith, MD
Seton Hall Sch of Grad Med Education
St Michael's Med Ctr
268 Dr Martin Luther King Jr Blvd
Newark, NJ 07102
Tel: 201 877-2711 *Fax:* 201 877-2661
E-mail: ssmith1824@aol.com
Accred Length: 2 Years *Program Size:* 7
Program ID: 146-33-11-152

New Mexico

Albuquerque

University of New Mexico Program

Sponsor: University of New Mexico School of Medicine
University Hospital
Veterans Affairs Medical Center (Albuquerque)

Program Director:
Gregory Mertz, MD
Div of Infectious Diseases
Univ of New Mexico Health Sciences Ctr
Albuquerque, NM 87131-5271
Tel: 505 272-5666 *Fax:* 505 272-8441
E-mail: gmertz@salud.unm.edu
Accred Length: 2 Years *Program Size:* 4
Program ID: 146-34-21-134

New York

Albany

Albany Medical Center Program

Sponsor: Albany Medical Center
Veterans Affairs Medical Center (Albany)

Program Director:
Michael H Miller, MD
Albany Med Coll
Infectious Disease Div/A-49
47 New Scotland Ave
Albany, NY 12208
Tel: 518 262-5343 *Fax:* 518 262-6727
Accred Length: 2 Years *Program Size:* 2
Program ID: 146-35-31-027

Bronx

Albert Einstein College of Medicine Program

Sponsor: Albert Einstein College of Medicine of Yeshiva University
Jacobi Medical Center
Montefiore Medical Center-Henry and Lucy Moses Division

Program Director:
Neal H Steigbigel, MD
Montefiore Med Ctr
Div of Infectious Diseases
111 E 210th St
Bronx, NY 10467-2490
Tel: 718 920-5439 *Fax:* 718 920-2746
Accred Length: 2 Years *Program Size:* 15
Program ID: 146-35-21-101

Brooklyn

Maimonides Medical Center Program
Sponsor: Maimonides Medical Center

Program Director:
Edward Chapnick, MD
Maimonides Med Ctr
4802 Tenth Ave
Brooklyn, NY 11219
Tel: 718 283-7492 *Fax:* 718 283-8813
E-mail: echapnick@maimonidesmed.org
Accred Length: 2 Years *Program Size:* 2
Program ID: 146-35-11-171

SUNY Health Science Center at Brooklyn Program
Sponsor: SUNY Health Science Center at Brooklyn
Kings County Hospital Center
University Hospital-SUNY Health Science Center at Brooklyn
Veterans Affairs Medical Center (Brooklyn)

Program Director:
William M McCormack, MD
SUNY Health Science Ctr
450 Clarkson Ave/Box 56
Brooklyn, NY 11203
Tel: 718 270-1432 *Fax:* 718 270-4123
Accred Length: 2 Years *Program Size:* 8
Program ID: 146-35-21-011

Buffalo

SUNY at Buffalo Graduate Medical-Dental Education Consortium Program
Sponsor: SUNY at Buffalo Grad Medical-Dental Education Consortium
Erie County Medical Center
Veterans Affairs Medical Center (Buffalo)

Program Director:
Timothy F Murphy, MD
VA Med Ctr (151)
3495 Bailey Ave
Buffalo, NY 14215
Tel: 716 862-3303 *Fax:* 716 862-3419
E-mail: murphyt@acsu.buffalo.edu
Accred Length: 2 Years *Program Size:* 2
Program ID: 146-35-31-009

East Meadow

SUNY at Stony Brook (East Meadow) Program
Sponsor: Nassau County Medical Center

Program Director:
Getachew Feleke, MD
Div of Infectious Diseases/DCB1024
Nassau County Med Ctr
2201 Hempstead Trnpk
East Meadow, NY 11554-5400
Tel: 516 572-6506 *Fax:* 516 572-5648
Accred Length: 2 Years *Program Size:* 2
Program ID: 146-35-21-093

Flushing

New York Hospital Medical Center of Queens/Cornell University Medical College Program
Sponsor: New York Hospital Medical Center of Queens

Program Director:
James J Rahal, MD
New York Hospital Med Ctr of Queens
56-45 Main St
Flushing, NY 11355
Tel: 718 670-1924 *Fax:* 718 353-9819
Accred Length: 2 Years *Program Size:* 3
Program ID: 146-35-21-178

Jamaica

Catholic Medical Center of Brooklyn and Queens Program
Sponsor: Catholic Medical Center of Brooklyn and Queens Inc
Catholic Medical Center (Mary Immaculate Hospital)
Catholic Medical Center (St John's Queens Hospital)

Program Director:
Aaron E Glatt, MD
Catholic Med Ctr of Brooklyn and Queens
88-25 153rd St/Ste 3-S
Jamaica, NY 11432
Tel: 718 558-7291 *Fax:* 718 558-6165
E-mail: aglatt@pol.net
Accred Length: 2 Years *Program Size:* 5
Program ID: 146-35-22-041

Manhasset

North Shore University Hospital/NYU School of Medicine Program
Sponsor: North Shore University Hospital

Program Director:
David H Shepp, MD
North Shore Univ Hospital
Div of Infectious Diseases
300 Community Dr
Manhasset, NY 11030
Tel: 516 562-4280 *Fax:* 516 562-2626
E-mail: dshepp@nshs.edu
Internet: http://www.nshs.edu
Accred Length: 2 Years *Program Size:* 2
Program ID: 146-35-21-160

Mineola

Winthrop-University Hospital Program
Sponsor: Winthrop-University Hospital

Program Director:
Burke A Cunha, MD
Winthrop-Univ Hospital
222 Station Plaza North
Ste 432
Mineola, NY 11501
Tel: 516 663-2505 *Fax:* 516 663-2753
Accred Length: 2 Years *Program Size:* 3
Program ID: 146-35-11-065

New Hyde Park

Albert Einstein College of Medicine at Long Island Jewish Medical Center Program
Sponsor: Long Island Jewish Medical Center

Program Director:
Carol Singer, MD
Long Island Jewish Med Ctr
270-05 76th Ave
3rd Fl/Oncology Bldg Rm 333
New Hyde Park, NY 11040
Tel: 718 470-7290 *Fax:* 718 470-9859
Internet: http://www.lij.edu/lij-homepage-ns.html
Accred Length: 2 Years *Program Size:* 3
Program ID: 146-35-21-135

New York

Albert Einstein College of Medicine at Beth Israel Medical Center Program
Sponsor: Beth Israel Medical Center

Program Director:
Robert L Yarrish, MD
Beth Israel Med Ctr
Div of Infectious Diseases
First Ave at 16th St
New York, NY 10003
Tel: 212 420-4005 *Fax:* 212 420-4498
Accred Length: 2 Years *Program Size:* 4
Program ID: 146-35-11-010

Harlem Hospital Center Program
Sponsor: Harlem Hospital Center

Program Director:
Wafaa El-Sadr, MD
Harlem Hospital Ctr
506 Lenox Ave
New York, NY 10037
Tel: 212 939-2940 *Fax:* 212 939-2968
E-mail: wme1@columbia.edu
Accred Length: 2 Years *Program Size:* 4
Program ID: 146-35-11-162

Mount Sinai School of Medicine (Cabrini) Program
Sponsor: Mount Sinai School of Medicine
Cabrini Medical Center

Program Director:
Michael P Mullen, MD
Cabrini Med Ctr
227 E 19th St
New York, NY 10003
Tel: 212 995-6871 *Fax:* 212 979-3484
Accred Length: 2 Years *Program Size:* 3
Program ID: 146-35-31-097

Mount Sinai School of Medicine Program
Sponsor: Mount Sinai School of Medicine
Elmhurst Hospital Center-Mount Sinai Services
Mount Sinai Medical Center

Program Director:
Mary E Klotman, MD
Mount Sinai Med Ctr
One Gustave L Levy Pl
Box 1090
New York, NY 10029-6574
Tel: 212 241-6741 *Fax:* 212 534-3240
E-mail: m_klotman@smtplink.mssm.edu
Internet: http://www.mssm.edu
Accred Length: 2 Years *Program Size:* 4
Program ID: 146-35-31-153

New York and Presbyterian Hospital (Columbia Campus) Program
Sponsor: New York and Presbyterian Hospital
New York and Presbyterian Hospital (Columbia Campus)

Program Director:
Glenda J Garvey, MD
Presbyterian Hospital
622 W 168th St
New York, NY 10032-3702
Tel: 212 305-3395 *Fax:* 212 305-7290
Accred Length: 2 Years *Program Size:* 4
Program ID: 146-35-11-054

Programs

New York and Presbyterian Hospital (Cornell Campus) Program 2
Sponsor: Memorial Sloan-Kettering Cancer Center
Program Director:
Kent Sepkowitz, MD
Memorial Sloan-Kettering Cancer Ctr
1275 York Ave/Box 288
New York, NY 10021-6007
Tel: 212 639-2441 *Fax:* 212 639-4386
E-mail: sepkowik@mskcc.org
Accred Length: 2 Years *Program Size:* 4
Program ID: 146-35-21-167

New York and Presbyterian Hospital (Cornell Campus) Program
Sponsor: New York and Presbyterian Hospital
New York and Presbyterian Hospital (Cornell Campus)
Program Director:
Warren D Johnson Jr, MD
New York Hospital
525 E 68th St
Rm A-421
New York, NY 10021
Tel: 212 746-6320 *Fax:* 212 746-8675
E-mail: wdjohnso@mail.med.cornell.edu
Accred Length: 2 Years *Program Size:* 6
Program ID: 146-35-21-161

New York Medical College at St Vincent's Hospital and Medical Center of New York Program
Sponsor: New York Medical College
St Vincent's Hospital and Medical Center of New York
Program Director:
Glenn S Turett, MD
St Vincent's Hospital and Med Ctr
153 W 11th St
New York, NY 10011
Tel: 212 604-8328 *Fax:* 212 604-2738
Internet: http://svh.nymc.edu
Accred Length: 2 Years *Program Size:* 2
Program ID: 146-35-11-174

New York University Medical Center Program
Sponsor: New York University Medical Center
Bellevue Hospital Center
Veterans Affairs Medical Center (Manhattan)
Program Director:
H Sherwood Lawrence, MD
Dept of Int Med
New York Univ Med Ctr
550 First Ave
New York, NY 10016
Tel: 212 263-6400 *Fax:* 212 263-7369
Internet:
http://www.med.nyu.edu/medicine/infecdis.html
Accred Length: 2 Years *Program Size:* 6
Program ID: 146-35-21-114

St Luke's-Roosevelt Hospital Center Program
Sponsor: St Luke's-Roosevelt Hospital Center
St Luke's-Roosevelt Hospital Center-St Luke's Division
Program Director:
Michael Lange, MD
St Luke's-Roosevelt Hospital Ctr
1000 Tenth Ave
New York, NY 10019-1196
Tel: 212 523-6568 *Fax:* 212 523-6724
Accred Length: 2 Years *Program Size:* 3
Program ID: 146-35-21-103

Rochester

University of Rochester Program
Sponsor: Strong Memorial Hospital of the University of Rochester
Program Director:
Paul S Graman, MD
Infectious Diseases Unit
Univ of Rochester Med Ctr
601 Elmwood Ave/Box 689
Rochester, NY 14642
Tel: 716 275-5871 *Fax:* 716 442-9328
E-mail: paul_graman@urmc.rochester.edu
Internet:
http://www.urmc.rochester.edu/smd/infdis/id.htm
Accred Length: 2 Years *Program Size:* 4
Program ID: 146-35-11-170

Stony Brook

SUNY at Stony Brook Program
Sponsor: University Hospital-SUNY at Stony Brook
Veterans Affairs Medical Center (Northport)
Program Director:
William H Greene, MD
Health Sciences Ctr
HSC T-15 080
SUNY-Stony Brook
Stony Brook, NY 11794-8153
Tel: 516 444-1660 *Fax:* 516 444-7518
E-mail: wgreene@mail.som.sunysb.edu
Internet: http://www.uhmc.sunysb.edu/som/resident.html
Accred Length: 2 Years *Program Size:* 4
Program ID: 146-35-21-012

Syracuse

SUNY Health Science Center at Syracuse Program
Sponsor: University Hospital-SUNY Health Science Center at Syracuse
Crouse Hospital
Veterans Affairs Medical Center (Syracuse)
Program Director:
Donald C Blair, MD
Dept of Med
SUNY Health Science Ctr
750 E Adams St
Syracuse, NY 13210
Tel: 315 464-5533 *Fax:* 315 464-5579
Accred Length: 2 Years *Program Size:* 2
Program ID: 146-35-21-140

Valhalla

New York Medical College at Westchester Medical Center Program
Sponsor: New York Medical College
Metropolitan Hospital Center
Westchester Medical Center
Program Director:
Gary P Wormser, MD
New York Med Coll-Westchester County Med Ctr
Div of Infectious Diseases
Macy Pavilion Rm 209 SE
Valhalla, NY 10595
Tel: 914 285-8865 *Fax:* 914 285-7289
Accred Length: 2 Years *Program Size:* 3
Program ID: 146-35-11-013

North Carolina

Chapel Hill

University of North Carolina Hospitals Program
Sponsor: University of North Carolina Hospitals
Program Director:
Myron S Cohen, MD
Univ of North Carolina Sch of Med
547 Burnett-Womack Bldg/CB7030
Chapel Hill, NC 27599-7030
Tel: 919 966-2536 *Fax:* 919 966-6714
E-mail: mscohen@med.unc.edu
Accred Length: 2 Years *Program Size:* 8
Program ID: 146-36-21-136

Durham

Duke University Program
Sponsor: Duke University Medical Center
Veterans Affairs Medical Center (Durham)
Program Director:
John D Hamilton, MD
Duke Univ Med Ctr
Box 3867
Durham, NC 27710-7599
Tel: 919 684-2660 *Fax:* 919 684-8902
Accred Length: 2 Years *Program Size:* 9
Program ID: 146-36-21-137

Winston-Salem

Wake Forest University School of Medicine Program
Sponsor: Wake Forest University Baptist Medical Center
Program Director:
Robert J Sherertz, MD
Wake Forest Univ Sch of Med
Medical Center Blvd
Winston-Salem, NC 27157-1042
Tel: 336 716-4584 *Fax:* 336 716-3825
E-mail: sherert@wfubmc.edu
Internet: http://www.bgsm.edu
Accred Length: 2 Years *Program Size:* 3
Program ID: 146-36-21-014

Ohio

Cincinnati

University Hospital/University of Cincinnati College of Medicine Program
Sponsor: University Hospital Inc
Veterans Affairs Medical Center (Cincinnati)
Program Director:
George S Deepe, MD
Univ of Cincinnati
PO Box 670560
Cincinnati, OH 45267-0560
Tel: 513 558-4704 *Fax:* 513 558-2089
E-mail: buchanj@ucmail.uc.edu
Accred Length: 2 Years *Program Size:* 2
Program ID: 146-38-21-066

Cleveland

Case Western Reserve University Program
Sponsor: University Hospitals of Cleveland
MetroHealth Medical Center
Veterans Affairs Medical Center (Cleveland)
Program Director:
Robert A Salata, MD
Div of Infectious Diseases
Univ Hospitals of Cleveland
11100 Euclid Ave
Cleveland, OH 44106-5083
Tel: 216 844-3287 *Fax:* 216 844-1632
E-mail: ras7@po.cwru.edu
Internet: http://www.uhhs.com
Accred Length: 2 Years *Program Size:* 8
Program ID: 146-38-21-154

Cleveland Clinic Foundation Program
Sponsor: Cleveland Clinic Foundation
Program Director:
Carlos M Isada, MD
Cleveland Clinic Foundation
Dept of Infectious Disease/S32
9500 Euclid Ave
Cleveland, OH 44195-5242
Tel: 216 444-2762 *Fax:* 216 445-9446
E-mail: meded@cesmtp.ccf.org
Internet: http://www.ccf.org
Accred Length: 2 Years *Program Size:* 6
Program ID: 146-38-12-156

Columbus

Ohio State University Program
Sponsor: Ohio State University Medical Center
Program Director:
Susan L Koletar, MD
Ohio State Univ Hospitals
N-1135 Doan Hall
410 W Tenth Ave
Columbus, OH 43210-1228
Tel: 614 293-8745 *Fax:* 614 293-4556
E-mail: koletar.1@osu.edu
Accred Length: 2 Years *Program Size:* 4
Program ID: 146-38-11-094

Dayton

Wright State University Program
Sponsor: Wright State University School of Medicine
Good Samaritan Hospital and Health Center
Miami Valley Hospital
Veterans Affairs Medical Center (Dayton)
Program Director:
Jack M Bernstein, MD
Wright State Univ Sch of Med
4100 W Third St (111W)
Dayton, OH 45428
Tel: 937 262-0201 *Fax:* 937 267-5310
E-mail: bernstein@wsu-id.dayton.oh.us
Internet:
http://www.med.wright.edu/som/academic/internalmed/infectious.html
Accred Length: 2 Years *Program Size:* 2
Program ID: 146-38-31-189

Toledo

Medical College of Ohio Program
Sponsor: Medical College of Ohio
Program Director:
Haig Donabedian, MD
Med Coll of Ohio
Dept of Med
3120 Glendale Ave
Toledo, OH 43614
Tel: 419 383-4328 *Fax:* 419 383-6244
E-mail: hdonabedian@magnum.mco.edu
Accred Length: 2 Years *Program Size:* 4
Program ID: 146-38-21-015

Oklahoma

Oklahoma City

University of Oklahoma Health Sciences Center Program
Sponsor: University of Oklahoma College of Medicine
University Hospital
Veterans Affairs Medical Center (Oklahoma City)
Program Director:
Ronald A Greenfield, MD
Univ of Oklahoma Coll of Med
PO Box 26901
VAMC-111C
Oklahoma City, OK 73190
Tel: 405 270-0501, ext 3284 *Fax:* 405 297-5934
E-mail: ron-greenfield@uokhsc.edu
Accred Length: 2 Years *Program Size:* 2
Program ID: 146-39-21-067

Pennsylvania

Hershey

Penn State Geisinger Health System/Milton S Hershey Medical Center Program
Sponsor: Penn State Geisinger Health System
Milton S Hershey Medical Center
Program Director:
John N Goldman, MD
Univ Hospital-Milton S Hershey Med Ctr
PO Box 850
500 University Dr
Hershey, PA 17033-0850
Tel: 717 531-8881 *Fax:* 717 531-4633
E-mail: jgoldman@med.hmc.psghs.edu
Accred Length: 2 Years *Program Size:* 1
Program ID: 146-41-11-016

Philadelphia

MCP Hahnemann University Program
Sponsor: MCP Hahnemann University
Hahnemann University Hospital
Medical College of Pennsylvania Hospital
Program Director:
Abdolghader Molavi, MD
Broad and Vine Sts
MS 461
Philadelphia, PA 19102-1192
Tel: 215 762-6555 *Fax:* 215 762-3031
E-mail: molavi@auhs.edu
Accred Length: 2 Years *Program Size:* 5
Program ID: 146-41-21-046

Temple University Program
Sponsor: Temple University Hospital
Program Director:
Bennett Lorber, MD
Temple Univ Hospital, Dept of Med
3401 N Broad St
Philadelphia, PA 19140
Tel: 215 707-3807 *Fax:* 215 707-4414
E-mail: tomfeke@astro.temple.edu
Internet: http://www.temple.edu/id
Accred Length: 2 Years *Program Size:* 4
Program ID: 146-41-21-029

Thomas Jefferson University Program
Sponsor: Thomas Jefferson University Hospital
Pennsylvania Hospital (UPHS)
Program Director:
Timothy J Babinchak, MD
Jefferson Med Coll
1015 Chestnut St/Rm 610
Philadelphia, PA 19107
Tel: 215 955-0571 *Fax:* 215 955-9362
Accred Length: 2 Years *Program Size:* 4
Program ID: 146-41-21-056

University of Pennsylvania Program
Sponsor: Hospital of the University of Pennsylvania
Pennsylvania Hospital (UPHS)
Veterans Affairs Medical Center (Philadelphia)
Program Director:
Harvey M Friedman, MD
536 Johnson Pavilion
Univ of Pennsylvania
Philadelphia, PA 19104-6073
Tel: 215 662-3557 *Fax:* 215 349-5111
E-mail: hfriedma@mail.med.upenn.edu
Accred Length: 2 Years *Program Size:* 5
Program ID: 146-41-21-022

Pittsburgh

University Health Center of Pittsburgh Program
Sponsor: University Health Center of Pittsburgh
Presbyterian University Hospital/UPMC
Veterans Affairs Medical Center (Pittsburgh)
Program Director:
David J Tweardy, MD
Univ of Pittsburgh Med Ctr
Div of Inf Dis/501 Kaufmann Bldg
200 Lothrop St
Pittsburgh, PA 15213-2582
Tel: 412 648-6401 *Fax:* 412 648-6399
E-mail: tweardy+@pitt.edu
Accred Length: 2 Years *Program Size:* 5
Program ID: 146-41-21-037

Puerto Rico

San Juan

University of Puerto Rico Program
Sponsor: University of Puerto Rico School of Medicine
University Hospital
Veterans Affairs Medical Center (San Juan)
Program Director:
Carlos H Ramirez-Ronda, MD
Univ Hospital
Dept of Infectious Diseases
PO Box 363606
San Juan, PR 00936-3606
Tel: 787 766-6513 *Fax:* 787 754-2266
Accred Length: 2 Years *Program Size:* 4
Program ID: 146-42-21-118

Veterans Affairs Medical and Regional Office Center Program
Sponsor: Veterans Affairs Medical Center (San Juan)
Program Director:
Carlos H Ramirez-Ronda, MD
VA Med and Regional Office Ctr
One Veterans Plaza (111)
San Juan, PR 00927-5800
Tel: 787 758-6900 *Fax:* 787 771-3601
Accred Length: 2 Years *Program Size:* 4
Program ID: 146-42-31-117

Rhode Island

Providence

Roger Williams Medical Center Program
Sponsor: Roger Williams Medical Center
Memorial Hospital of Rhode Island
Miriam Hospital
Rhode Island Hospital
Veterans Affairs Medical Center (Providence)
Program Director:
Stephen H Zinner, MD
Roger Williams Med Ctr
825 Chalkstone Ave
Providence, RI 02908
Tel: 401 456-2074 *Fax:* 401 456-6839
Accred Length: 2 Years *Program Size:* 5
Program ID: 146-43-31-038

South Carolina

Charleston

Medical University of South Carolina Program
Sponsor: Medical University of South Carolina College of Medicine
MUSC Medical Center
Ralph H Johnson Dept of Veterans Affairs Med Center
Program Director:
Joseph R Cantey, MD
Med Univ of South Carolina
Infectious Diseases Div
100 Doughty St/PO Box 250752
Charleston, SC 29425
Tel: 803 792-4541 *Fax:* 803 792-6680
E-mail: canteyjr@musc.edu
Internet: http://www.musc.edu/muscid/fellowship.html
Accred Length: 2 Years *Program Size:* 5
Program ID: 146-45-21-104

Tennessee

Johnson City

East Tennessee State University Program
Sponsor: James H Quillen College of Medicine
Johnson City Medical Center Hospital
Veterans Affairs Medical Center (Mountain Home)
Program Director:
Felix A Sarubbi, MD
East Tennessee State Univ
PO Box 70622
Johnson City, TN 37614-0622
Tel: 423 439-6380 *Fax:* 423 232-6932
E-mail: vasquez.jose@mtn home.va.gov
Accred Length: 2 Years *Program Size:* 2
Program ID: 146-47-21-047

Memphis

University of Tennessee Program
Sponsor: University of Tennessee College of Medicine
Regional Medical Center at Memphis
Veterans Affairs Medical Center (Memphis)
Program Director:
James B Dale, MD
Michael S Bronze, MD
Univ of Tennessee
Dept of Med
956 Court Ave/H308
Memphis, TN 38163
Tel: 901 577-7207 *Fax:* 901 448-8231
E-mail: james.dale@med.va.gov
Accred Length: 2 Years *Program Size:* 2
Program ID: 146-47-21-138

Nashville

Vanderbilt University Program
Sponsor: Vanderbilt University Medical Center
St Thomas Hospital
Veterans Affairs Medical Center (Nashville)
Program Director:
Ban Mishou Allos, MD
Vanderbilt Univ Sch of Med
A-3310 Medical Center North
1161 21st Ave S
Nashville, TN 37232-2605
Tel: 615 322-2035 *Fax:* 615 343-6160
E-mail: ban.mishu.allos@mcmail.vanderbilt.edu
Accred Length: 2 Years *Program Size:* 12
Program ID: 146-47-31-017

Texas

Dallas

University of Texas Southwestern Medical School Program
Sponsor: University of Texas Southwestern Medical School
Dallas County Hospital District-Parkland Memorial Hospital
Veterans Affairs Medical Center (Dallas)
Program Director:
Justin D Radolf, MD
Univ of Texas Southwestern Med Ctr
5323 Harry Hines Blvd
Dallas, TX 75235-9113
Tel: 214 648-3480 *Fax:* 214 648-9478
E-mail: justin.radolf@email.swmed.edu
Accred Length: 2 Years *Program Size:* 5
Program ID: 146-48-21-098

Fort Sam Houston

San Antonio Uniformed Services Health Education Consortium (BAMC) Program
Sponsor: San Antonio Uniformed Services Health Education Consortium
Brooke Army Medical Center
Program Director:
Matthew J Dolan, MD
59 MDW/MMII
Wilford Hall Med Ctr (AETC)
2200 Bergquist Dr/Ste 1
Lackland AFB, TX 78236-5300
Tel: 210 292-7444 *Fax:* 210 292-3740
E-mail: dolan@whmc-lafb.af.mil
Accred Length: 2 Years *Program Size:* 8
Program ID: 146-48-12-139
US Armed Services Program

Galveston

University of Texas Medical Branch Hospitals Program
Sponsor: University of Texas Medical Branch Hospitals
Program Director:
C Glen Mayhall, MD
Div of Infectious Diseases/0835
Univ of Texas Med Branch
301 University Blvd
Galveston, TX 77555-0835
Tel: 409 747-0236 *Fax:* 409 772-6527
E-mail: cmayhall@utmb.edu
Internet: http://stem.utmb.edu/id/
Accred Length: 2 Years *Program Size:* 6
Program ID: 146-48-21-048

Houston

Baylor College of Medicine Program
Sponsor: Baylor College of Medicine
Harris County Hospital District-Ben Taub General Hospital
Methodist Hospital
St Luke's Episcopal Hospital
Veterans Affairs Medical Center (Houston)
Program Director:
Daniel Musher, MD
Infectious Diseases Sect
Rm 4B-370
VA Hospital
Houston, TX 77030
Tel: 713 794-7386 *Fax:* 713 794-7045
Accred Length: 2 Years *Program Size:* 4
Program ID: 146-48-21-070

University of Texas at Houston Program
Sponsor: University of Texas Medical School at Houston
Lyndon B Johnson General Hospital
Memorial Hermann Healthcare System
University of Texas M D Anderson Cancer Center
Program Director:
Robert M Rakita, MD
Univ of Texas Med Sch
6431 Fannin St/JFB 1.728
Houston, TX 77030
Tel: 713 500-6767 *Fax:* 713 500-5495
E-mail: jncox@heart.med.uth.tmc.edu
Internet:
http://www.uth.tmc.edu/schools/med/imed/infect/index.htm
Accred Length: 2 Years *Program Size:* 11
Program ID: 146-48-31-018

Lackland AFB

San Antonio Uniformed Services Health Education Consortium (WHMC) Program
Sponsor: San Antonio Uniformed Services Health Education Consortium
Wilford Hall Medical Center (AETC)
Brooke Army Medical Center
Program Director:
Matthew J Dolan, MD
Wilford Hall Med Ctr
759 MDOS/MMII
2200 Bergquist Dr/Ste 1
Lackland AFB, TX 78236-5300
Tel: 210 292-7444 *Fax:* 210 292-3740
E-mail: dolan@whmc.af.mil
Accred Length: 2 Years *Program Size:* 8
Program ID: 146-48-12-049
US Armed Services Program

San Antonio

University of Texas Health Science Center at San Antonio Program
Sponsor: University of Texas Medical School at San Antonio
Audie L Murphy Memorial Veterans Hospital (San Antonio)
University Hospital-South Texas Medical Center
Program Director:
Tom Patterson, MD
Univ of Texas Health Science Ctr
7703 Floyd Curl Dr
San Antonio, TX 78284-7881
Tel: 210 567-4823 *Fax:* 210 567-4670
Accred Length: 2 Years *Program Size:* 4
Program ID: 146-48-21-057

Utah

Salt Lake City

University of Utah Program
Sponsor: University of Utah Medical Center
Veterans Affairs Medical Center (Salt Lake City)
Program Director:
Harry Rosado Santos, MD
Div of Infectious Diseases
Univ of Utah Sch of Med
50 N Medical Dr/Rm 4B319
Salt Lake City, UT 84132
Tel: 801 581-8812 *Fax:* 801 585-3377
E-mail: harry.rosado@hsc.utah.edu
Internet: http://www.int.med.utah.edu
Accred Length: 2 Years *Program Size:* 4
Program ID: 146-49-21-158

Vermont

Burlington

University of Vermont Program
Sponsor: Fletcher Allen Health Care
Program Director:
Christopher Grace, MD
Fletcher Allen Health Care
Brown 325
Burlington, VT 05401
Tel: 802 656-4836 *Fax:* 802 656-5322
E-mail: christopher.grace@vtmednet.org
Accred Length: 2 Years *Program Size:* 2
Program ID: 146-50-21-194

Virginia

Charlottesville

University of Virginia Program
Sponsor: University of Virginia Medical Center
Program Director:
William A Petri Jr, MD PhD
Univ of Virginia Health Sciences Ctr
Box 385
Div of Infectious Disease
Charlottesville, VA 22908
Tel: 804 924-5942 *Fax:* 804 982-0002
Internet:
http://www.med.virginia.edu/som-cl/internal/id/fellowship.html
Accred Length: 2 Years *Program Size:* 6
Program ID: 146-51-21-019

Richmond

Medical College of Virginia/Virginia Commonwealth University Program
Sponsor: Medical College of Virginia/Virginia Commonwealth University
Hunter Holmes McGuire VA Medical Center (Richmond)
Medical College of Virginia Hospitals
Program Director:
Gordon L Archer, MD
Med Coll of Virginia-Virginia Commonwealth Univ
PO Box 980049
1101 E Marshall St/Rm 7-082A
Richmond, VA 23298-0049
Tel: 804 828-9711 *Fax:* 804 828-3097
E-mail: garcher@hsc.vcu.edu
Internet: http://www.cbil.vcu.edu/som
Accred Length: 2 Years *Program Size:* 4
Program ID: 146-51-21-020

Washington

Seattle

University of Washington Program
Sponsor: University of Washington School of Medicine
University of Washington Medical Center
Program Director:
Walter E Stamm, MD
Univ of Washington
Div of Allergy/Infectious Dis
1959 NE Pacific St
Seattle, WA 98195-6523
Tel: 206 616-4170 *Fax:* 206 616-4898
E-mail: wes@u.washington.edu
Internet: http://www.weber.washington.edu/~daid
Accred Length: 2 Years *Program Size:* 16
Program ID: 146-54-21-071

West Virginia

Morgantown

West Virginia University Program
Sponsor: West Virginia University Hospitals
Program Director:
Rashida Khakoo, MD
West Virginia Univ Hospital
Dept of Med/Infectious Dis
PO Box 9163
Morgantown, WV 26506-9163
Tel: 304 293-3306 *Fax:* 304 293-8677
E-mail: rkhakoo2@wvu.edu
Accred Length: 2 Years *Program Size:* 2
Program ID: 146-55-21-188

Wisconsin

Madison

University of Wisconsin Program
Sponsor: University of Wisconsin Hospital and Clinics
William S Middleton Veterans Hospital
Program Director:
Dennis G Maki, MD
Univ of Wisconsin Hospital and Clinics
600 Highland Ave/Rm H4-574
Madison, WI 53792-0001
Tel: 608 263-1545 *Fax:* 608 263-4464
E-mail: dgmaki@medicine.wisc.edu
Internet: http://www.medicine.wisc.edu/sections/id
Accred Length: 2 Years *Program Size:* 3
Program ID: 146-56-21-120

Milwaukee

Medical College of Wisconsin Program
Sponsor: Medical College of Wisconsin Affiliated Hospitals Inc
Clement J Zablocki Veterans Affairs Medical Center
Froedtert Memorial Lutheran Hospital
Program Director:
David K Wagner, MD
Med Coll of Wisconsin
Dept of Infectious Diseases
5000 W National Ave/CC-111N
Milwaukee, WI 53295
Tel: 414 384-2000, ext 2760 *Fax:* 414 383-8010
Accred Length: 2 Years *Program Size:* 3
Program ID: 146-56-31-039

Internal Medicine

Alabama

Birmingham

Baptist Health System Program

Sponsor: Baptist Health System Inc
Birmingham Baptist Medical Center-Montclair
Birmingham Baptist Medical Center-Princeton
University of Alabama Hospital

Program Director:
Robert A Kreisberg, MD
Birmingham Baptist Med Ctr-Montclair
840 Montclair Rd/Ste 317
Birmingham, AL 35213
Tel: 205 592-5759 *Fax:* 205 592-5694
E-mail: susan.elders@bhsala.com
Internet: http://www.bhsala.com
Accred Length: 3 Years *Program Size:* 36 (*GY1:* 15)
Program ID: 140-01-21-020

Carraway Methodist Medical Center Program

Sponsor: Carraway Methodist Medical Center

Program Director:
Dennis G Delgado, MD
Carraway Methodist Med Ctr
1600 Carraway Blvd
Birmingham, AL 35234
Tel: 205 502-6387 *Fax:* 205 502-5613
E-mail: imres@mail.carraway.com
Internet: http://www.carraway.org
Accred Length: 3 Years *Program Size:* 26 (*GY1:* 10)
Program ID: 140-01-31-021

University of Alabama Medical Center Program

Sponsor: University of Alabama Hospital
Cooper Green Hospital
Veterans Affairs Medical Center (Birmingham)

Program Director:
William E Dismukes, MD
Univ of Alabama
Med House Staff Office
DERB 15
Birmingham, AL 35294-0012
Tel: 205 934-2490 *Fax:* 205 975-6424
E-mail: medres@uab.edu
Internet: http://info.dom.uab.edu/resident.htm
Accred Length: 3 Years *Program Size:* 108 (*GY1:* 41)
Subspecialties: CCM, CD, END, GE, HO, ID, IMG, NEP, PCC, PUD, RHU
Program ID: 140-01-21-022

Mobile

University of South Alabama Program

Sponsor: University of South Alabama Medical Center

Program Director:
John B Bass Jr, MD
Univ of South Alabama Med Ctr
2451 Fillingim St
Mastin 400-L
Mobile, AL 36617
Tel: 334 471-7891 *Fax:* 334 471-1291
E-mail: pgreen@usamail.usouthal.edu
Internet: http://southmed/com/intmed/index.html
Accred Length: 3 Years *Program Size:* 38 (*GY1:* 15)
Subspecialties: CD, GE, HO, ID, PUD
Program ID: 140-01-11-024

Montgomery

University of Alabama Medical Center (Montgomery) Program

Sponsor: University of Alabama Hospital
Baptist Medical Center

Program Director:
J J Kirschenfeld, MD
Univ of Alabama-Montgomery
Dept of Int Med
4371 Narrow Ln Rd/Ste 200
Montgomery, AL 36116-2975
Tel: 334 284-5211, ext 248 *Fax:* 334 284-9020
E-mail: hullhm@uab.edu
Internet: http://www.uabmontgomery.org
Accred Length: 3 Years *Program Size:* 20 (*GY1:* 6)
Program ID: 140-01-21-447

Arizona

Phoenix

Good Samaritan Regional Medical Center Program

Sponsor: Good Samaritan Regional Medical Center
Carl T Hayden Veterans Affairs Medical Center (Phoenix)

Program Director:
Alan I Leibowitz, MD
Good Samaritan Regional Med Ctr
Dept of Med
1111 E McDowell Rd
Phoenix, AZ 85006
Tel: 602 239-2296 *Fax:* 602 239-2084
E-mail: medicine@samaritan.edu
Internet: http://www.samaritan.edu
Accred Length: 3 Years *Program Size:* 59 (*GY1:* 23)
Subspecialties: CD, END, IMG, PUD
Program ID: 140-03-21-025

Maricopa Medical Center Program

Sponsor: Maricopa Medical Center

Program Director:
David B Wisinger, MD
Maricopa Med Ctr
Dept of Int Med
2601 E Roosevelt St
Phoenix, AZ 85008
Tel: 602 267-5768 *Fax:* 602 681-1488
E-mail: erasim@medicine.marocopa.gov
Internet: http://www.azmeded.org
Accred Length: 3 Years *Program Size:* 42 (*GY1:* 14)
Program ID: 140-03-11-026

St Joseph's Hospital and Medical Center Program

Sponsor: St Joseph's Hospital and Medical Center
Carl T Hayden Veterans Affairs Medical Center (Phoenix)

Program Director:
Donald Opila, MD
St Joseph's Hospital and Med Ctr
350 W Thomas Rd
Phoenix, AZ 85013
Tel: 602 406-3375 *Fax:* 602 406-7185
E-mail: intmed@mha.chw.edu
Internet: http://www.chw.edu/mha/mha.html
Accred Length: 3 Years *Program Size:* 36 (*GY1:* 17)
Program ID: 140-03-11-027

Scottsdale

Mayo Graduate School of Medicine (Scottsdale) Program

Sponsor: Mayo Graduate School of Medicine-Mayo Foundation
Mayo Clinic (Scottsdale)
Scottsdale Healthcare-Shea

Program Director:
Philip J Lyng, MD
Mayo Clinic Scottsdale
Dept of Int Med
13400 E Shea Blvd
Scottsdale, AZ 85259
Tel: 602 301-8000, ext 9824 *Fax:* 602 301-4869
E-mail: mgsm.scot.az.internalmed@mayo.edu
Internet: http://www.mayo.edu/
Accred Length: 3 Years *Program Size:* 18 (*GY1:* 6)
Program ID: 140-03-21-512

Tucson

Tucson Hospitals Medical Education Program

Sponsor: Tucson Hospitals Medical Education Program Inc
Kino Community Hospital
Tucson Medical Center

Program Director:
Robert M Aaronson, MD
Tucson Hospitals Med Education Program
Box 42195
5301 E Grant Rd
Tucson, AZ 85733
Tel: 520 324-5095 *Fax:* 520 324-5231
E-mail: eras.thmep@tmcaz.com
Internet: http://www.tmcaz.com/thmep
Accred Length: 3 Years *Program Size:* 19 (*GY1:* 7)
Program ID: 140-03-21-028

University of Arizona Program

Sponsor: University of Arizona College of Medicine
University Medical Center
Veterans Affairs Medical Center (Tucson)

Program Director:
Richard M Mandel, MD
William P Johnson, MD
Univ of Arizona Health Sciences Ctr
Med Education Office
1501 N Campbell Ave/PO Box 245040
Tucson, AZ 85724-5040
Tel: 520 626-7000 *Fax:* 520 626-6020
E-mail: imedprog@u.arizona.edu
Internet:
http://www.medicine.arizona.edu/medicine/residency/
Accred Length: 3 Years *Program Size:* 54 (*GY1:* 19)
Subspecialties: CD, END, GE, HO, ID, IMG, NEP, PCC, RHU
Program ID: 140-03-21-029

Arkansas

Little Rock

University of Arkansas for Medical Sciences Program

Sponsor: University of Arkansas College of Medicine
John L McClellan Memorial Veterans Hospital
University Hospital of Arkansas

Program Director:
Robert W Bradsher Jr, MD
Univ of Arkansas Sch of Med
Med Housestaff Office/Slot 634
4301 W Markham St
Little Rock, AR 72205-7199
Tel: 501 686-5162 *Fax:* 501 686-8188
E-mail: imresident@exchange.uams.edu
Internet: http://www.uams.edu/dim/
Accred Length: 3 Years *Program Size:* 60 (*GY1:* 22)
Subspecialties: CD, END, GE, HEM, ID, IMG, NEP, ON, PCC, RHU
Program ID: 140-04-21-030

California

Bakersfield

Kern Medical Center Program

Sponsor: Kern Medical Center

Program Director:
Jose A Perez Jr, MD MS
Kern Med Ctr
Dept of Med
1830 Flower St
Bakersfield, CA 93305
Tel: 805 326-2202 *Fax:* 805 326-2950
E-mail: greers@kernmedctr.com
Internet:
http://bizweb.lightspeed.net/~kmcmed/kmc.htm
Accred Length: 3 Years *Program Size:* 21 (*GY1:* 7)
Program ID: 140-05-31-031

Fresno

University of California (San Francisco)/Fresno Program

Sponsor: UCSF-Fresno Medical Education Program
University Medical Center
Veterans Affairs Medical Center (Fresno)

Program Director:
Linda Kuribayashi, MD
Univ Med Ctr
445 S Cedar Ave
Fresno, CA 93702
Tel: 209 459-4390 *Fax:* 209 459-6119
Internet: http://www.ucsfresno.edu
Accred Length: 3 Years *Program Size:* 44 (*GY1:* 22)
Program ID: 140-05-31-033

La Jolla

Scripps Clinic/Scripps Green Hospital Program

Sponsor: Scripps Clinic
Scripps Green Hospital

Program Director:
Joel Diamant, MD
Dept of Grad Med Educ/403C
Scripps Clinic-Green Hospital
10666 N Torrey Pines Rd
La Jolla, CA 92037-1093
Tel: 619 455-8090 *Fax:* 619 554-6310
E-mail: bonny@scripps.edu
Internet: http://www.scrippsclinic.com
Accred Length: 3 Years *Program Size:* 19 (*GY1:* 6)
Subspecialties: CD, END, GE, HEM, ON, RHU
Program ID: 140-05-21-490

Loma Linda

Loma Linda University Program

Sponsor: Loma Linda University Medical Center
Jerry L Pettis Memorial Veterans Hospital

Program Director:
Lawrence K Loo, MD
Loma Linda Univ Med Ctr
Dept of Int Med
PO Box 2000
Loma Linda, CA 92354
Tel: 909 824-4636 *Fax:* 909 824-4846
E-mail: twoodruff@ccmail.llu.edu
Internet: http://www.llu.edu/llumc/internal
Accred Length: 3 Years *Program Size:* 94 (*GY1:* 38)
Subspecialties: CCM, CD, GE, PCC, PUD, RHU
Program ID: 140-05-21-038

Long Beach

St Mary Medical Center Program

Sponsor: St Mary Medical Center
Los Angeles County-Harbor-UCLA Medical Center

Program Director:
Peter V Barrett, MD
St Mary Med Ctr
1050 Linden Ave
Long Beach, CA 90801
Tel: 562 491-9350 *Fax:* 562 491-9146
E-mail: stmarylb_meded@chw.edu
Internet:
http://www.geocities.com/collegepark/union/2115/
Accred Length: 3 Years *Program Size:* 30 (*GY1:* 14)
Program ID: 140-05-31-039

Los Angeles

Cedars-Sinai Medical Center Program

Sponsor: Cedars-Sinai Medical Center

Program Director:
Mark S Noah, MD
Cedars-Sinai Med Ctr
Dept of Int Med
8700 Beverly Blvd
Los Angeles, CA 90048
Tel: 310 855-5161 *Fax:* 310 657-6185
Accred Length: 3 Years *Program Size:* 93 (*GY1:* 30)
Subspecialties: CCM, CD, END, HO, ICE, ID, NEP, PCC, RHU
Program ID: 140-05-11-040

Charles R Drew University Program

Sponsor: Charles R Drew University of Medicine and Science
LAC-King/Drew Medical Center

Program Director:
Merlyn Asuncion, MD
Charles R Drew Univ of Med and Science
12021 S Wilmington Ave
Los Angeles, CA 90059
Tel: 310 668-4574 *Fax:* 310 763-8929
Accred Length: 3 Years *Program Size:* 41 (*GY1:* 15)
Subspecialties: END, GE, ID, IMG
Program ID: 140-05-11-045

Southern California Kaiser Permanente Medical Care (Los Angeles) Program

Sponsor: Southern California Kaiser Permanente Medical Group
Kaiser Foundation Hospital (Los Angeles)

Program Director:
Thomas Y Tom, MD
Kaiser Permanente Med Care
393 E Walnut St
Pasadena, CA 91188-8013
Tel: 800 541-7946
Internet: http://www.kpscal.org
Accred Length: 3 Years *Program Size:* 30 (*GY1:* 12)
Subspecialties: CD, GE, ID, NEP
Program ID: 140-05-12-042

UCLA Medical Center Program

Sponsor: UCLA School of Medicine
UCLA Medical Center

Program Director:
Jan H Tillisch, MD
UCLA Med Ctr
Dept of Med
Rm 32-115 CHS
Los Angeles, CA 90095-1736
Tel: 310 825-7375 *Fax:* 310 825-5791
E-mail: troth@medicine.medsch.ucla.edu
Accred Length: 3 Years *Program Size:* 92 (*GY1:* 36)
Subspecialties: CCM, CD, END, GE, HEM, ID, IMG, NEP, ON, PCC, PUD, RHU
Program ID: 140-05-11-046

University of Southern California Program

Sponsor: Los Angeles County-USC Medical Center

Program Director:
Robert A Larsen, MD
Univ of Southern California
2020 Zonal Ave
IRD/Rm 220
Los Angeles, CA 90033
Tel: 213 226-7556 *Fax:* 213 226-2657
E-mail: uscgme@hsc.usc.edu
Accred Length: 3 Years *Program Size:* 160 (*GY1:* 54)
Subspecialties: CD, END, GE, HEM, ICE, ID, IMG, NEP, ON, PCC, RHU
Program ID: 140-05-21-044

VA Greater Los Angeles Healthcare System (Sepulveda) Program

Sponsor: VA Greater Los Angeles Healthcare System
Olive View-UCLA Medical Center

Program Director:
Jill M Klessig, MD
VA Med Ctr
16111 Plummer St/111T
Sepulveda, CA 91343
Tel: 818 895-9397 *Fax:* 818 895-9516
E-mail: jklessig@ucla.edu
Internet: http://www.medsch.ucla.edu/som/ddo/sfvp
Accred Length: 3 Years *Program Size:* 73 (*GY1:* 32)
Subspecialties: END, HO, NEP, PUD, RHU
Program ID: 140-05-21-047

Programs

VA Greater Los Angeles Healthcare System Program

Sponsor: VA Greater Los Angeles Healthcare System

Program Director:
Jane Weinreb, MD
UCLA-VA Med Ctr West Los Angeles
Dept of Med (111A)
11301 Wilshire Blvd
Los Angeles, CA 90073
Tel: 310 268-3034 *Fax:* 310 268-4818
E-mail: dorothy.frazier@med.va.gov
Internet: http://www.va.gov/internalmed/
Accred Length: 3 Years *Program Size:* 61 (*GY1:* 29)
Subspecialties: CD, END, ICE, ID, PUD
Program ID: 140-05-31-048

White Memorial Medical Center Program

Sponsor: White Memorial Medical Center

Program Director:
Michael W Sue, MD
White Memorial Med Ctr
1720 Cesar E Chavez Ave
Los Angeles, CA 90033-2481
Tel: 323 268-5000, ext 1607 *Fax:* 323 881-8702
E-mail: mwsuemd@yahoo.com
Internet: http://www.whitememorial.com
Accred Length: 3 Years *Program Size:* 19 (*GY1:* 9)
Program ID: 140-05-11-049

Oakland

Alameda County Medical Center Program

Sponsor: Alameda County Medical Center
Kaiser Permanente Medical Group (Northern California)

Program Director:
Theodore G Rose Jr, MD
Alameda County Med Ctr-Highland Hospital
1411 E 31st St
Oakland, CA 94602
Tel: 510 437-4268 *Fax:* 510 437-4187
E-mail: trose99@ix.netcom.com
Internet:
http://www.acponline.org/residency/alameda.htm
Accred Length: 3 Years *Program Size:* 50 (*GY1:* 17)
Program ID: 140-05-31-051

Kaiser Permanente Medical Group (Northern California) Program

Sponsor: Kaiser Permanente Medical Group (Northern California)
Kaiser Permanente Medical Center (Oakland)

Program Director:
Stanton T Siu, MD
Kaiser Permanente Med Ctr
Medical Education Office
280 W MacArthur Blvd
Oakland, CA 94611
Tel: 510 596-6126 *Fax:* 510 596-1571
E-mail: medicine.oakmeded@ncal.kaiperm.org
Internet: http://www.kaiserpermanente.org
Accred Length: 3 Years *Program Size:* 33 (*GY1:* 13)
Program ID: 140-05-12-052

Orange

University of California (Irvine) Program

Sponsor: University of California (Irvine) Medical Center
Long Beach Memorial Medical Center

Program Director:
Lloyd Rucker, MD
Univ of California Irvine Med Ctr
101 City Dr S
Rte 1
Orange, CA 92868
Tel: 714 456-5691 *Fax:* 714 456-8874
E-mail: mcrhodes@uci.edu
Internet: http://www.ucihs.uci.edu/intmed
Accred Length: 3 Years *Program Size:* 97 (*GY1:* 38)
Subspecialties: CD, END, GE, HEM, ID, IMG, NEP, ON, PCC, RHU
Program ID: 140-05-21-036

Pasadena

Huntington Memorial Hospital Program

Sponsor: Huntington Memorial Hospital

Program Director:
Myron J Tong, MD
Huntington Memorial Hospital
Med Educ Dept
100 W California Blvd
Pasadena, CA 91109-7013
Tel: 626 397-5166 *Fax:* 626 397-5004
Internet: http://www.huntingtonhospital.com
Accred Length: 3 Years *Program Size:* 21 (*GY1:* 9)
Program ID: 140-05-11-056

Sacramento

University of California (Davis) Program

Sponsor: University of California (Davis) Medical Center
Kaiser Foundation Hospital (Sacramento)

Program Director:
Faith T Fitzgerald, MD
Frederick Meyers, MD
Univ of California Davis Med Ctr
PO Box 179003
4150 V St/Ste 3116
Sacramento, CA 95817-9003
Tel: 916 734-7080 *Fax:* 916 734-1150
E-mail: klthrelkeld@ucdavis.edu
Internet: http://internalmedicine.ucdmc.ucdavis.edu
Accred Length: 3 Years *Program Size:* 91 (*GY1:* 28)
Subspecialties: CD, END, GE, HO, ID, IMG, NEP, PCC
Program ID: 140-05-21-032

San Diego

Naval Medical Center (San Diego) Program

Sponsor: Naval Medical Center (San Diego)

Program Director:
Richard G Osborne, MD
Naval Med Ctr
Int Med Dept/Ste 300
34730 Bob Wilson Drive
San Diego, CA 92134-3300
Tel: 619 532-7504 *Fax:* 619 532-7508
E-mail: rgosborne@nmcsd.med.navy.mil
Accred Length: 3 Years *Program Size:* 43 (*GY1:* 22)
Subspecialties: CD, GE, HO, ID, PCC
Program ID: 140-05-12-012
US Armed Services Program

Scripps Mercy Hospital Program

Sponsor: Scripps Mercy Hospital

Program Director:
Stanley A Amundson, MD
Scripps Mercy Hospital
Dept of Medical Education
4077 Fifth Ave/MER 35
San Diego, CA 92103-2180
Tel: 619 260-7215 *Fax:* 619 260-7305
E-mail: sherylq@mercysd.com
Internet: http://www.mercysdgme.com
Accred Length: 3 Years *Program Size:* 32 (*GY1:* 10)
Program ID: 140-05-11-057

University of California (San Diego) Program

Sponsor: University of California (San Diego) Medical Center
Veterans Affairs Medical Center (San Diego)

Program Director:
Shawn Harrity, MD
UCSD Med Ctr
200 W Arbor Dr/8825
San Diego, CA 92103-8425
Tel: 619 543-6170 *Fax:* 619 543-6529
E-mail: shershman@ucsd.edu
Internet: http://www.medicine.ucsd.edu/medres/
Accred Length: 3 Years *Program Size:* 92 (*GY1:* 33)
Subspecialties: CD, END, GE, HO, ICE, ID, IMG, NEP, PCC, RHU
Program ID: 140-05-21-058

San Francisco

California Pacific Medical Center Program

Sponsor: California Pacific Medical Center
California Pacific Medical Center

Program Director:
Allan Pont, MD
California Pacific Med Ctr
Dept of Med
2351 Clay St/Rm 380
San Francisco, CA 94115
Tel: 415 923-3376 *Fax:* 415 775-7437
Internet: http://www.cpmc.org
Accred Length: 3 Years *Program Size:* 56 (*GY1:* 26)
Subspecialties: CD, GE, PUD
Program ID: 140-05-12-062

Kaiser Permanente Medical Group (Northern California)/San Francisco Program

Sponsor: Kaiser Permanente Medical Group (Northern California)
Kaiser Permanente Medical Center (San Francisco)

Program Director:
Aileen M Dillon, MD
Kaiser Permanente Med Ctr
2425 Geary Blvd/Rm M-160
San Francisco, CA 94115-3395
Tel: 415 202-3034 *Fax:* 415 202-4983
E-mail: sfo.grad.medprg@ncal.kaiperm.org.
Internet: http://ncal.kaiserpermanente.org
Accred Length: 3 Years *Program Size:* 36 (*GY1:* 16)
Program ID: 140-05-12-060

St Mary's Hospital and Medical Center Program
Sponsor: St Mary's Hospital and Medical Center
Program Director:
Mark E Sockell, MD
St Mary's Med Ctr
Med Educ 6-South
450 Stanyan St
San Francisco, CA 94117-1079
Tel: 415 750-5781 *Fax:* 415 750-8149
Accred Length: 3 Years *Program Size:* 36 (*GY1:* 18)
Subspecialties: CD
Program ID: 140-05-22-063

University of California (San Francisco) Program
Sponsor: University of California (San Francisco) School of Medicine
San Francisco General Hospital Medical Center
University of California (San Francisco) Medical Center
Veterans Affairs Medical Center (San Francisco)
Program Director:
Harry Hollander, MD
Dept of Med
505 Parnassus Ave/M-987
Univ of California San Francisco
San Francisco, CA 94143-0119
Tel: 415 476-1528 *Fax:* 415 502-1976
E-mail: jeaniem@medicine.ucsf.edu
Internet: http://www.medicine.ucsf.edu/housestaff/
Accred Length: 3 Years *Program Size:* 141 (*GY1:* 53)
Subspecialties: CCM, CD, END, GE, HEM, HO, ICE, ID, NEP, ON, PCC, RHU
Program ID: 140-05-21-064

University of California (San Francisco)/Mount Zion Program
Sponsor: University of California (San Francisco) School of Medicine
Mount Zion Medical Center of the University of California
Program Director:
Robert B Baron, MD
Univ of California San Francisco-Mount Zion Med Ctr
1600 Divisadero St
San Francisco, CA 94143-1640
Tel: 415 885-7574 *Fax:* 415 885-7724
E-mail: mzmed@itsa.ucsf.edu
Internet:
http://www.medicine.ucsf.edu/housestaff/residency
Accred Length: 3 Years *Program Size:* 30 (*GY1:* 10)
Subspecialties: CD, ID, IMG
Program ID: 140-05-31-061

San Jose

Santa Clara Valley Medical Center Program
Sponsor: Santa Clara Valley Medical Center
Program Director:
Thomas Kelsey, MD
Santa Clara Valley Med Ctr
Dept of Med/4th Fl
751 S Bascom Ave
San Jose, CA 95128
Tel: 408 885-6305 *Fax:* 408 885-6324
Accred Length: 3 Years *Program Size:* 46 (*GY1:* 18)
Program ID: 140-05-31-065

Santa Barbara

Santa Barbara Cottage Hospital Program
Sponsor: Santa Barbara Cottage Hospital
Santa Barbara County Health Care Services
Program Director:
Andrew S Gersoff, MD
Santa Barbara Cottage Hospital
PO Box 689
Santa Barbara, CA 93102
Tel: 805 569-7315 *Fax:* 805 569-8358
E-mail: pkeay@sbch.org
Internet: http://www.sbch.org
Accred Length: 3 Years *Program Size:* 28 (*GY1:* 12)
Program ID: 140-05-22-066

Santa Clara

Kaiser Permanente Medical Group (Northern California)/Santa Clara Program
Sponsor: Kaiser Permanente Medical Group (Northern California)
Kaiser Permanente Medical Center (Santa Clara)
Program Director:
Susan D MacLean, MD
Kaiser Permanente Med Ctr
Grad Med Educ
900 Kiely Blvd/Lower Level
Santa Clara, CA 95051-5386
Tel: 408 236-5720 *Fax:* 408 236-5185
E-mail: scl.gme@ncal.kaiperm.org
Accred Length: 3 Years *Program Size:* 40 (*GY1:* 16)
Program ID: 140-05-21-067

Stanford

Stanford University Program
Sponsor: Stanford University Hospital
Veterans Affairs Palo Alto Health Care System
Program Director:
Kelley M Skeff, MD PhD
Stanford Univ Med Ctr
300 Pasteur Dr
S101 M/C 5109
Stanford, CA 94305
Tel: 650 498-4559 *Fax:* 650 498-6205
E-mail: franb@leland.stanford.edu
Internet:
http://www.med.stanford.edu/school/med/residency
Accred Length: 3 Years *Program Size:* 92 (*GY1:* 36)
Subspecialties: CCM, CD, END, GE, HEM, ICE, ID, IMG, NEP, ON, PCC, RHU
Program ID: 140-05-21-068

Stockton

San Joaquin General Hospital Program
Sponsor: San Joaquin General Hospital
Program Director:
Sheela S Kapre, MD
San Joaquin General Hospital
Int Med Dept
PO Box 1020
Stockton, CA 95201
Tel: 209 468-6624 *Fax:* 209 468-6246
E-mail: sjgh@softcom.net
Internet: http://www.softcom.net/users/sheela
Accred Length: 3 Years *Program Size:* 15 (*GY1:* 5)
Program ID: 140-05-12-069

Torrance

Los Angeles County-Harbor-UCLA Medical Center Program
Sponsor: Los Angeles County-Harbor-UCLA Medical Center
Program Director:
Darryl Y Sue, MD
Harbor-UCLA Med Ctr
1000 W Carson St/Box 400
Torrance, CA 90509
Tel: 310 222-2409 *Fax:* 310 320-9688
Internet:
http://www.medsch.ucla.edu/som/ddo/harbor_med
Accred Length: 3 Years *Program Size:* 51 (*GY1:* 17)
Subspecialties: CCM, CD, END, HO, ICE, ID, NEP, PCC, PUD, RHU
Program ID: 140-05-11-070

Travis AFB

David Grant Medical Center Program
Sponsor: David Grant Medical Center
Program Director:
Kathryn M Amacher, DO
David Grant Med Ctr
60 MDG/SGOM
101 Bodin Cir
Travis AFB, CA 94535-1800
Tel: 707 423-5057 *Fax:* 707 423-5058
E-mail: kathryn.amacher@60mdg.travis.af.mil
Internet:
http://usafsg.satx.disa.mil/~dgmc/sgo/60thmdos.htm
Accred Length: 3 Years *Program Size:* 24 (*GY1:* 8)
Program ID: 140-05-21-465
US Armed Services Program

Colorado

Denver

Exempla St Joseph Hospital Program
Sponsor: Exempla St Joseph Hospital
Program Director:
Robert B Gibbons, MD
Exempla St Joseph Hospital
1835 Franklin St
Denver, CO 80218-1191
Tel: 303 837-7837 *Fax:* 303 866-8044
E-mail: gibbonsr@exempla.org
Accred Length: 3 Years *Program Size:* 34 (*GY1:* 18)
Program ID: 140-07-31-072

University of Colorado Program
Sponsor: University of Colorado Health Sciences Center
Columbia Presbyterian-St Luke's Medical Center
Denver Health and Hospitals
Rose Medical Center
Veterans Affairs Medical Center (Denver)
Program Director:
William Kaehny, MD
Univ of Colorado Med Sch
Box B-177
4200 E Ninth Ave
Denver, CO 80262
Tel: 303 315-7768 *Fax:* 303 315-7653
E-mail: sherry.berka@uchsc.edu
Internet: http://www.uchsc.edu/sm/intmed
Accred Length: 3 Years *Program Size:* 146 (*GY1:* 51)
Subspecialties: CCM, CD, END, GE, HO, ICE, ID, IMG, NEP, PCC, PUD, RHU
Program ID: 140-07-21-073

Connecticut

Bridgeport

St Vincent's Medical Center Program

Sponsor: St Vincent's Medical Center

Program Director:
Brian Kiss, MD
St Vincent's Med Ctr
Dept of Medicine
2800 Main St
Bridgeport, CT 06606
Tel: 203 576-5576 *Fax:* 203 576-5022
Internet: http://www.stvincents.org
Accred Length: 3 Years *Program Size:* 31 (*GY1:* 12)
Program ID: 140-08-11-075

Yale University (Bridgeport) Program

Sponsor: Bridgeport Hospital

Program Director:
David A Baker, MD
Bridgeport Hospital
267 Grant St
Bridgeport, CT 06610-2870
Tel: 203 384-3792 *Fax:* 203 384-4294
Accred Length: 3 Years *Program Size:* 26 (*GY1:* 10)
Subspecialties: CD, GE, PUD
Program ID: 140-08-11-074

Danbury

Danbury Hospital Program

Sponsor: Danbury Hospital

Program Director:
Paul B Iannini, MD
Danbury Hospital
24 Hospital Ave
Danbury, CT 06810
Tel: 203 731-8638 *Fax:* 203 830-2047
E-mail: kerry.cleary@danhosp.org
Internet: http://www.danhosp.org
Accred Length: 3 Years *Program Size:* 36 (*GY1:* 12)
Program ID: 140-08-11-076

Derby

Griffin Hospital Program

Sponsor: Griffin Hospital

Program Director:
Vincent A DeLuca Jr, MD
Griffin Hospital
130 Division St
Derby, CT 06418
Tel: 203 732-7325 *Fax:* 203 732-7185
E-mail: grifdelu@connix.com
Internet: http://www.griffinhealth.org
Accred Length: 3 Years *Program Size:* 21 (*GY1:* 9)
Subspecialties: GE
Program ID: 140-08-31-077

Farmington

University of Connecticut (New Britain) Program

Sponsor: University of Connecticut School of Medicine
Mount Sinai Hospital
New Britain General Hospital
Univ of Connecticut Health Center/John Dempsey Hospital

Program Director:
Michael R Grey, MD MPH
Univ of Connecticut Health Ctr
Primary Care Int Med Res Prog
263 Farmington Ave
Farmington, CT 06030-3935
Tel: 860 679-4017 *Fax:* 860 679-1621
Internet: http://www.uchc.edu
Accred Length: 3 Years *Program Size:* 58 (*GY1:* 18)
Program ID: 140-08-21-499

University of Connecticut Program

Sponsor: University of Connecticut School of Medicine
Hartford Hospital
St Francis Hospital and Medical Center
Univ of Connecticut Health Center/John Dempsey Hospital

Program Director:
Sharon A Diamen, MD
Univ of Connecticut Health Ctr
Dept of Int Med
Rm LG004/MC 3950
Farmington, CT 06030-3950
Tel: 860 679-2562 *Fax:* 860 679-4613
E-mail: diamen@nso.uchc.edu
Internet: http://www.uchc.edu
Accred Length: 3 Years *Program Size:* 109 (*GY1:* 33)
Subspecialties: CD, END, GE, HO, ID, IMG, NEP, PCC, RHU
Program ID: 140-08-31-078

Greenwich

Greenwich Hospital Association Program

Sponsor: Greenwich Hospital

Program Director:
Charles B Seelig, MD MS
Greenwich Hospital
Five Perryridge Rd/Rm 488N
Greenwich, CT 06830
Tel: 203 863-3913 *Fax:* 203 863-3924
E-mail: seelig@idt.net
Internet: http://www.greenhosp.chime.org
Accred Length: 3 Years *Program Size:* 21 (*GY1:* 12)
Program ID: 140-08-21-079

New Haven

Hospital of St Raphael Program

Sponsor: Hospital of St Raphael

Program Director:
Sherri A Clayton, MD
Hospital of St Raphael
Dept of Med
1450 Chapel St
New Haven, CT 06511
Tel: 203 789-3358 *Fax:* 203 789-3222
Internet: http://www.srhs.org
Accred Length: 3 Years *Program Size:* 56 (*GY1:* 26)
Subspecialties: CD, GE, NEP
Program ID: 140-08-31-084

Yale-New Haven Medical Center (Waterbury) Program

Sponsor: Yale-New Haven Hospital
St Mary's Hospital
Waterbury Hospital Health Center

Program Director:
Stephen J Huot, MD PhD
Yale Primary Care Program
Dept of Int Med
PO Box 208033
New Haven, CT 06520-8033
Tel: 203 785-7249 *Fax:* 203 785-7258
E-mail: stephen.huot@yale.edu
Internet: http://cardio.med.yale.edu/pcare/res/home.html
Accred Length: 3 Years *Program Size:* 74 (*GY1:* 30)
Program ID: 140-08-21-496

Yale-New Haven Medical Center Program

Sponsor: Yale-New Haven Hospital
Veterans Affairs Medical Center (West Haven)

Program Director:
Cyrus R Kapadia, MD
Yale-New Haven Hospital
1074 LMP
20 York St
New Haven, CT 06504
Tel: 203 785-7113 *Fax:* 203 785-7030
Internet: http://info.med.yale.edu/intmed/prog
Accred Length: 3 Years *Program Size:* 94 (*GY1:* 37)
Subspecialties: CCM, CD, END, GE, HEM, ID, IMG, NEP, ON, PCC, PUD, RHU
Program ID: 140-08-21-085

Norwalk

Norwalk Hospital Program

Sponsor: Norwalk Hospital

Program Director:
Joseph P Cleary, MD
Dept of Med
Norwalk Hospital
Maple St
Norwalk, CT 06856
Tel: 203 852-2371 *Fax:* 203 855-3589
E-mail: carol.terhune@norwalkhealth.org
Internet: http://www.norwalkhosp.org
Accred Length: 3 Years *Program Size:* 42 (*GY1:* 16)
Subspecialties: CD, GE, PUD
Program ID: 140-08-31-086

Stamford

Stamford Hospital/Columbia University College of Physicians and Surgeons Program

Sponsor: Stamford Hospital

Program Director:
Noel I Robin, MD
Stamford Hospital
Shelburne Rd and W Broad St
Stamford, CT 06904-9317
Tel: 203 325-7485 *Fax:* 203 325-7368
E-mail: drnrobin@stamhosp.chime.org
Accred Length: 3 Years *Program Size:* 19 (*GY1:* 6)
Program ID: 140-08-11-087

Delaware

Wilmington

Christiana Care Health Services Program

Sponsor: Christiana Care Health Services Inc

Program Director:
Virginia U Collier, MD
Christiana Care Health System-Christiana Hospital
4755 Ogletown Stanton Rd
Rm 6339
Newark, DE 19718
Tel: 302 733-6344 *Fax:* 302 733-6386
E-mail: medicine.residency@christianacare.org
Internet: http://www.mcdresidency.org
Accred Length: 3 Years *Program Size:* 39 (*GY1:* 15)
Program ID: 140-09-11-090

District of Columbia

Washington

District of Columbia General Hospital Program

Sponsor: District of Columbia General Hospital
Georgetown University Medical Center

Program Director:
Robin C Newton, MD
DC General Hospital Program-Georgetown Med Service
Rm 6414/Dept of Med
1900 Massachusetts Ave SE
Washington, DC 20003
Tel: 202 675-7172 *Fax:* 202 675-8004
Accred Length: 3 Years *Program Size:* 27 (*GY1:* 11)
Program ID: 140-10-21-460

George Washington University Program

Sponsor: George Washington University School of Medicine
George Washington University Hospital (UHS)
Veterans Affairs Medical Center (Washington, DC)

Program Director:
Jehan ElBayoumi, MD
George Washington Univ
Dept of Med Residency Office
2150 Pennsylvania Ave NW
Washington, DC 20037
Tel: 202 994-3147 *Fax:* 202 994-2938
E-mail: domjeb@gwumc.edu
Internet: http://www.gwu.edu/~gwumc
Accred Length: 3 Years *Program Size:* 75 (*GY1:* 35)
Subspecialties: CCM, CD, END, GE, HO, ICE, ID, IMG, NEP, PCC, RHU
Program ID: 140-10-21-093

Georgetown University Program

Sponsor: Georgetown University Medical Center

Program Director:
Stephen R Mitchell, MD
Georgetown Univ Med Ctr
Dept of Med/PHC-5
3800 Reservoir Rd NW
Washington, DC 20007
Tel: 202 687-5037 *Fax:* 202 687-7797
E-mail: mitchelr@gunet.georgetown.edu
Internet: http://www.dml.georgetown.edu/gumc.html
Accred Length: 3 Years *Program Size:* 105 (*GY1:* 43)
Subspecialties: CD, END, GE, HEM, ICE, ID, NEP, ON, PCC, RHU
Program ID: 140-10-21-091

Howard University Program

Sponsor: Howard University Hospital
District of Columbia General Hospital
Greater Southeast Community Hospital

Program Director:
Adrian O Hosten, MD
Howard Univ Hospital
2041 Georgia Ave NW
Washington, DC 20060
Tel: 202 865-6620
Accred Length: 3 Years *Program Size:* 81 (*GY1:* 33)
Subspecialties: CCM, CD, END, GE, HEM, ID, NEP, ON, PUD
Program ID: 140-10-21-461

Providence Hospital Program

Sponsor: Providence Hospital

Program Director:
Junette C Gibbons, MD
Providence Hospital, Dept of Int Med
1150 Varnum St NE
Washington, DC 20017-2180
Tel: 202 269-7747 *Fax:* 202 269-7892
Accred Length: 3 Years *Program Size:* 21 (*GY1:* 7)
Program ID: 140-10-21-095

Walter Reed Army Medical Center Program

Sponsor: Walter Reed Army Medical Center

Program Director:
Yancy Y Phillips, MD
Dept of Med
Walter Reed Army Med Ctr
6825 16th St NW
Washington, DC 20307-5001
Tel: 202 782-6205 *Fax:* 202 782-6507
E-mail: yancy_y.phillips@wramaa.chcs.amedd.army.mil
Accred Length: 3 Years *Program Size:* 48 (*GY1:* 16)
Subspecialties: CCM, CD, END, GE, HO, ID, NEP, PUD, RHU
Program ID: 140-10-11-006
US Armed Services Program

Washington Hospital Center Program

Sponsor: Washington Hospital Center

Program Director:
Leonard Wartofsky, MD
Dept of Med
Washington Hospital Ctr
110 Irving St NW
Washington, DC 20010-2975
Tel: 202 877-6271 *Fax:* 202 877-6130
Internet: http://www.mhg.edu
Accred Length: 3 Years *Program Size:* 71 (*GY1:* 35)
Subspecialties: CD, GE, HO, ID, NEP, RHU
Program ID: 140-10-11-097

Florida

Fort Lauderdale

Cleveland Clinic Foundation (Florida) Program

Sponsor: Cleveland Clinic Foundation
Cleveland Clinic Florida

Program Director:
Jane D Skelton, MD
Cleveland Clinic Foundation-Florida
3000 W Cypress Creek Rd
Fort Lauderdale, FL 33309
Tel: 954 978-7800 *Fax:* 954 978-7458
E-mail: imprg@cesmtp.ccf.org
Internet: http://www.ccf.org/florida
Accred Length: 3 Years *Program Size:* 21 (*GY1:* 7)
Program ID: 140-11-21-516

Gainesville

University of Florida Program

Sponsor: University of Florida College of Medicine
Shands Hospital at the University of Florida
Veterans Affairs Medical Center (Gainesville)

Program Director:
Craig S Kitchens, MD
Univ of Florida Coll of Med
PO Box 100277
Gainesville, FL 32610-0277
Tel: 352 395-0239 *Fax:* 352 338-9879
E-mail: dealkl@medicine.ufl.edu
Internet: http://www.med.ufl.edu/med/train/
Accred Length: 3 Years *Program Size:* 67 (*GY1:* 27)
Subspecialties: CD, END, GE, HO, ICE, ID, IMG, NEP, ON, PCC, RHU
Program ID: 140-11-21-098

Jacksonville

Mayo Graduate School of Medicine (Jacksonville) Program

Sponsor: Mayo Graduate School of Medicine-Mayo Foundation
Mayo Clinic (Jacksonville)
St Luke's Hospital

Program Director:
Joseph Kaplan, MD
Mayo Clinic Jacksonville
Graduate Resident Education Ctr
4500 San Pablo Rd
Jacksonville, FL 32224
Tel: 904 296-3865 *Fax:* 904 296-3892
E-mail: wilson.barbara@mayo.edu
Internet: http://www.mayo.edu/mgsm/jim.htm
Accred Length: 3 Years *Program Size:* 22 (*GY1:* 8)
Subspecialties: GE, HO
Program ID: 140-11-21-509

University of Florida Health Science Center/Jacksonville Program

Sponsor: University of Florida College of Medicine at Jacksonville
University Medical Center (UFHSC/J)

Program Director:
Linda R Edwards, MD
Univ Med Ctr-UFHSC
653-1 W 8th St
Jacksonville, FL 32209-6511
Tel: 904 549-4985 *Fax:* 904 549-3087
E-mail: llr@umc8.umc.ufl.edu
Internet: http://www.ufhscj.edu
Accred Length: 3 Years *Program Size:* 47 (*GY1:* 21)
Subspecialties: CD, END, GE, ID, ON
Program ID: 140-11-21-099

Miami

University of Miami-Jackson Memorial Medical Center Program

Sponsor: University of Miami-Jackson Memorial Medical Center
Veterans Affairs Medical Center (Miami)

Program Director:
Mark A Gelbard, MD
Univ of Miami-Jackson Memorial Med Ctr
1611 NW 12th Ave
Central Bldg/Rm 600
Miami, FL 33136
Tel: 305 585-5215 *Fax:* 305 326-8302
E-mail: mgelbard@mednet.med.miami.edu
Accred Length: 3 Years *Program Size:* 124 (*GY1:* 48)
Subspecialties: CCM, CD, END, GE, HO, ICE, ID, IMG, NEP, PCC, RHU
Program ID: 140-11-21-100

Miami Beach

Mount Sinai Medical Center of Greater Miami Program
Sponsor: Mount Sinai Medical Center of Greater Miami
Program Director:
Gloria B Weinberg, MD
Mount Sinai Med Ctr
4300 Alton Rd
Miami Beach, FL 33140
Tel: 305 674-2053 *Fax:* 305 674-2057
E-mail: ltrepper@msmc.com
Internet: http://www.mountsinaimiami.org
Accred Length: 3 Years *Program Size:* 34 (*GY1:* 13)
Subspecialties: CD
Program ID: 140-11-12-101

Orlando

Orlando Regional Healthcare System Program
Sponsor: Orlando Regional Medical Center
Program Director:
Jerold J Fadem Jr, MD
Dept of Internal Med
Orlando Regional Healthcare System
86 W Underwood St/Ste 102
Orlando, FL 32806
Tel: 800 895-4613
Internet: http://www.orhs.org/meded/index.html
Accred Length: 3 Years *Program Size:* 24 (*GY1:* 8)
Program ID: 140-11-31-102

Tampa

University of South Florida Program
Sponsor: University of South Florida College of Medicine
James A Haley Veterans Hospital
Tampa General Healthcare
Program Director:
Philip Altus, MD
Univ of South Florida Coll of Med
Harbourside Medical Tower
4 Columbia Dr/Ste 630
Tampa, FL 33606
Tel: 813 251-7419 *Fax:* 813 254-4616
E-mail: paltus@com1.med.usf.edu
Internet:
http://www.med.usf.edu/intmed/resident/index.html
Accred Length: 3 Years *Program Size:* 66 (*GY1:* 22)
Subspecialties: CD, END, GE, HO, ID, IMG, NEP, PCC, RHU
Program ID: 140-11-21-104

Georgia

Atlanta

Emory University Program
Sponsor: Emory University School of Medicine
Crawford Long Hospital of Emory University
Emory University Hospital
Grady Memorial Hospital
Veterans Affairs Medical Center (Atlanta)
Program Director:
Juha P Kokko, MD PhD
Emory Univ Sch of Med
69 Butler St SE
Atlanta, GA 30303-3219
Tel: 404 616-3527 *Fax:* 404 525-2957
Internet: http://www.emory.edu/med/dept
Accred Length: 3 Years *Program Size:* 176 (*GY1:* 62)
Subspecialties: CD, END, GE, HO, ICE, ID, IMG, NEP, PCC, RHU
Program ID: 140-12-21-105

Georgia Baptist Medical Center Program
Sponsor: Georgia Baptist Medical Center
Program Director:
Guillermo E Umpierrez, MD
Georgia Baptist Med Ctr
Dept of Int Med
303 Parkway Dr NE/Box 423
Atlanta, GA 30312-1212
Tel: 404 265-4600 *Fax:* 404 265-4989
Accred Length: 3 Years *Program Size:* 30 (*GY1:* 10)
Program ID: 140-12-12-106

Morehouse School of Medicine Program
Sponsor: Morehouse School of Medicine
Grady Memorial Hospital
Program Director:
Myra E Rose, MD
Morehouse Sch of Med
Internal Medicine Program
720 Westview Dr SW
Atlanta, GA 30310-1495
Tel: 404 756-1325 *Fax:* 404 756-1398
E-mail: medres@msm.edu
Internet: http://www.msm.edu
Accred Length: 3 Years *Program Size:* 38 (*GY1:* 14)
Program ID: 140-12-21-502

Augusta

Medical College of Georgia Program
Sponsor: Medical College of Georgia Hospital and Clinics
Veterans Affairs Medical Center (Augusta)
Program Director:
Peter P Stein, MD
Med Coll of Georgia
Dept of Med/BIW-540
1120 15th St
Augusta, GA 30912
Tel: 706 721-2423 *Fax:* 706 721-6918
Internet:
http://www.mcg.edu/resident/intmed/index.html
Accred Length: 3 Years *Program Size:* 58 (*GY1:* 28)
Subspecialties: CD, END, GE, HO, ID, NEP, PCC, RHU
Program ID: 140-12-21-107

Fort Gordon

Dwight David Eisenhower Army Medical Center Program
Sponsor: Dwight David Eisenhower Army Medical Center
Program Director:
William T Browne, MD
Dwight David Eisenhower Army Med Ctr
Dept of Med
Fort Gordon, GA 30905-5650
Tel: 706 787-6124 *Fax:* 706 787-0005
Accred Length: 3 Years *Program Size:* 15 (*GY1:* 5)
Program ID: 140-12-22-458
US Armed Services Program

Macon

Mercer University School of Medicine Program
Sponsor: Medical Center of Central Georgia
Program Director:
John A Hudson, MD
Med Ctr of Central Georgia
Box 6000/Hospital Box 68
Macon, GA 31208
Tel: 912 633-1822 *Fax:* 912 633-5184
E-mail: mccgintmed@worldnet.att.net
Internet: http://gain.mercer.edu/musm/departments.htm
Accred Length: 3 Years *Program Size:* 25 (*GY1:* 8)
Program ID: 140-12-21-491

Savannah

Memorial Medical Center Program
Sponsor: Memorial Medical Center
Program Director:
Robert J DiBenedetto, MD
Memorial Med Ctr
Internal Med Dept
PO Box 23089
Savannah, GA 31403-3089
Tel: 912 350-7573 *Fax:* 912 350-7270
Internet: http://www.memorialmed.com
Accred Length: 3 Years *Program Size:* 29 (*GY1:* 10)
Program ID: 140-12-12-108

Hawaii

Honolulu

Tripler Army Medical Center Program
Sponsor: Tripler Army Medical Center
Program Director:
Benjamin W Berg, MD
Dept of Med
Tripler Army Med Ctr
Honolulu, HI 96859-5000
Tel: 808 433-5700, ext 5720 *Fax:* 808 433-1555
E-mail:
ltc_benjamin_berg@smtplink.tamc.amedd.army.mil
Internet:
http://www.tamc.army.mil/dpts/medicine/index.html
Accred Length: 3 Years *Program Size:* 24 (*GY1:* 8)
Program ID: 140-14-11-007
US Armed Services Program

University of Hawaii Program
Sponsor: University of Hawaii John A Burns School of Medicine
Kuakini Medical Center
Queen's Medical Center
St Francis Medical Center
Program Director:
Richard I Frankel, MD
Univ of Hawaii
1356 Lusitana St/7th Fl
Honolulu, HI 96813
Tel: 808 558-2910 *Fax:* 808 586-7486
E-mail: uhim@hawaii.edu
Internet: http://uhimrp.hawaii.edu
Accred Length: 3 Years *Program Size:* 61 (*GY1:* 23)
Subspecialties: IMG
Program ID: 140-14-21-109

Illinois

Chicago

Catholic Health Partners Program
Sponsor: Catholic Health Partners
St Joseph Health Centers and Hospital
Program Director:
Joel B Spear, MD
St Joseph Hospital
2900 N Lake Shore Dr
Chicago, IL 60657
Tel: 773 665-3022 *Fax:* 773 665-3384
E-mail: nkeil@cath-health.org
Internet: http://www.cath-health.org
Accred Length: 3 Years *Program Size:* 73 (*GY1:* 28)
Program ID: 140-16-11-122

Cook County Hospital Program
Sponsor: Cook County Hospital
Program Director:
Maurice R Lemon, MD
Cook County Hospital
Dept of Med/Rm 2207
1835 W Harrison St
Chicago, IL 60612-0612
Tel: 312 633-6702 *Fax:* 312 633-5129
E-mail: mlemon@rush.edu
Accred Length: 3 Years *Program Size:* 163 (*GY1:* 52)
Subspecialties: CD, END, GE, HEM, HO, ON, PCC
Program ID: 140-16-12-113

Illinois Masonic Medical Center/Rush Medical College Program
Sponsor: Illinois Masonic Medical Center
Program Director:
Catherine A Kallal, MD
Illinois Masonic Med Ctr
Dept of Int Med
836 W Wellington Ave
Chicago, IL 60657-5193
Tel: 773 296-7046 *Fax:* 773 296-7486
E-mail: eileen.mccormack@immc.org
Internet:
http://www.rush.edu/illinoismasonic/internalmed
Accred Length: 3 Years *Program Size:* 52 (*GY1:* 20)
Subspecialties: CD, ICE
Program ID: 140-16-11-114

McGaw Medical Center of Northwestern University Program
Sponsor: Northwestern University Medical School
Northwestern Memorial Hospital
Veterans Affairs Lakeside Medical Center (Chicago)
Program Director:
Warren H Wallace, MD
250 East Superior/Ste 296
Chicago, IL 60611
Tel: 312 908-8205 *Fax:* 312 503-5230
Internet: http://www.medicine.nwu.edu/
Accred Length: 3 Years *Program Size:* 127 (*GY1:* 47)
Subspecialties: CD, END, GE, HO, ICE, ID, IMG, NEP, PCC, RHU
Program ID: 140-16-21-119

Mercy Hospital and Medical Center Program
Sponsor: Mercy Hospital and Medical Center
Program Director:
Howard E Sweeney, MD
Mercy Hospital and Med Ctr
2525 S Michigan Ave
Chicago, IL 60616-2477
Tel: 312 567-2053 *Fax:* 312 567-2695
Internet: http://members.aol.com/mercyres.html
Accred Length: 3 Years *Program Size:* 48 (*GY1:* 16)
Program ID: 140-16-11-116

Ravenswood Hospital Medical Center Program
Sponsor: Ravenswood Hospital Medical Center
Program Director:
Nikunj N Shah, MD
Ravenswood Hospital Med Ctr
Dept of Med
4550 N Winchester Ave
Chicago, IL 60640
Tel: 773 279-3152 *Fax:* 773 279-3100
E-mail: ravenswoodimr@rhmc.com
Internet:
http://www.advocatehealth.com/residency/index.html
Accred Length: 3 Years *Program Size:* 31 (*GY1:* 12)
Program ID: 140-16-11-120

Rush-Presbyterian-St Luke's Medical Center Program
Sponsor: Rush-Presbyterian-St Luke's Medical Center
Program Director:
Alan A Harris, MD
Rush-Presbyterian-St Luke's Med Ctr
1653 W Congress Pkwy/301 Jones
Chicago, IL 60612
Tel: 312 942-5352 *Fax:* 312 942-5271
E-mail: srosenst@rush.edu
Internet:
http://www.rush.edu/departments/internalmed/residency
Accred Length: 3 Years *Program Size:* 129 (*GY1:* 47)
Subspecialties: CCM, CD, GE, HO, ICE, ID, IMG, NEP, PCC, RHU
Program ID: 140-16-11-121

University of Chicago (Weiss Memorial) Program
Sponsor: Louis A Weiss Memorial Hospital
Program Director:
William D Barnhart, MD MBA
4646 N Marine Dr
Chicago, IL 60640
Tel: 773 564-5225
Accred Length: 3 Years *Program Size:* 32 (*GY1:* 13)
Program ID: 140-16-11-115

University of Chicago Program
Sponsor: University of Chicago Hospitals
Program Director:
Holly J Humphrey, MD
5841 S Maryland Ave/MC 7082
Chicago, IL 60637-1470
Tel: 773 702-1455 *Fax:* 773 834-0464
Internet: http://uhs.bsd.uchicago.edu/program
Accred Length: 3 Years *Program Size:* 77 (*GY1:* 30)
Subspecialties: CCM, CD, END, GE, HO, ICE, IMG, NEP, PCC, RHU
Program ID: 140-16-11-123

University of Illinois College of Medicine at Chicago Program
Sponsor: University of Illinois College of Medicine at Chicago
University of Illinois Hospital and Clinics
Veterans Affairs West Side Medical Center
Program Director:
Linda G Lesky, MD
Univ of Illinois-Chicago
840 S Wood St
1027 CSB M/C 787
Chicago, IL 60612-7323
Tel: 312 996-7408 *Fax:* 312 413-1343
E-mail: resident@uic.edu
Internet:
http://www.uic.edu/depts/mpim/intern/imindex.html
Accred Length: 3 Years *Program Size:* 106 (*GY1:* 40)
Subspecialties: CD, END, GE, HO, ID, IMG, NEP, PCC, RHU
Program ID: 140-16-21-124

University of Illinois College of Medicine at Chicago/Michael Reese Hospital Program
Sponsor: University of Illinois College of Medicine at Chicago
Michael Reese Hospital and Medical Center
Program Director:
John Tulley, MD
Michael Reese Hospital and Med Ctr
Dept of Med
2929 S Ellis Ave
Chicago, IL 60616-3390
Tel: 312 791-4112 *Fax:* 312 791-4178
E-mail: medresidency@michaelreese.com
Internet: http://www.michaelreese.com
Accred Length: 3 Years *Program Size:* 63 (*GY1:* 21)
Subspecialties: CD, END, HO
Program ID: 140-16-11-117

Evanston

McGaw Medical Center of Northwestern University (Evanston) Program
Sponsor: Northwestern University Medical School
Evanston Hospital
Program Director:
E Stephen Kurtides, MD
Evanston Northwestern Healthcare
2650 Ridge Ave
Evanston, IL 60201-1781
Tel: 847 570-2510 *Fax:* 847 570-2905
Internet: http://www.nums.nwu.edu/gme/index.htm
Accred Length: 3 Years *Program Size:* 63 (*GY1:* 29)
Program ID: 140-16-31-125

St Francis Hospital of Evanston Program
Sponsor: St Francis Hospital of Evanston
Program Director:
Fred A Zar, MD
St Francis Hospital of Evanston
355 Ridge Ave
Evanston, IL 60202-3399
Tel: 847 316-6227 *Fax:* 847 316-3307
E-mail: jobradovic@alverno.ssfhs.org
Internet: http://www.reshealth.org
Accred Length: 3 Years *Program Size:* 55 (*GY1:* 22)
Subspecialties: CD, HEM, ON
Program ID: 140-16-11-126

Maywood

Loyola University Program
Sponsor: Loyola University Medical Center
Edward J Hines Jr Veterans Affairs Hospital
MacNeal Memorial Hospital
Program Director:
Kevin P Simpson, MD
Loyola Univ Med Ctr
2160 S First Ave
Bldg 102 Rm 7611A
Maywood, IL 60153
Tel: 708 216-5838 *Fax:* 708 216-9456
E-mail: jpersak@luc.edu
Internet:
http://www.meddean.luc.edu/lumen/deptwebs/medicine/medres/medres.htm
Accred Length: 3 Years *Program Size:* 101 (*GY1:* 33)
Subspecialties: CD, END, GE, HO, ICE, ID, IMG, NEP, PCC, RHU
Program ID: 140-16-21-128

Melrose Park

Resurrection Medical Center Program
Sponsor: Resurrection Medical Center
Westlake Community Hospital
Program Director:
John E Martin, MD
Westlake Community Hospital
1225 Lake St
Melrose Park, IL 60160
Tel: 708 938-7350 *Fax:* 708 938-7098
E-mail: rushwest@worldnet.att.net
Accred Length: 3 Years *Program Size:* 25 (*GY1:* 11)
Program ID: 140-16-11-454

North Chicago

Finch University of Health Sciences/Chicago Medical School Program

Sponsor: Finch University of Health Sciences/Chicago Medical School
Mount Sinai Hospital Medical Center of Chicago
Veterans Affairs Medical Center (North Chicago)

Program Director:
Preston B Cannady Jr, MD
Finch Univ of Health Sciences-Chicago Med Sch
Dept of Med
3333 Green Bay Rd
North Chicago, IL 60064-3095
Tel: 847 578-3227 *Fax:* 847 578-8647
Internet: http://www.finchcms.edu
Accred Length: 3 Years *Program Size:* 65 (*GY1:* 21)
Subspecialties: CCM, CD, END, GE, HO, ID, PUD
Program ID: 140-16-21-111

Oak Lawn

University of Illinois College of Medicine at Chicago/Christ Hospital Program

Sponsor: University of Illinois College of Medicine at Chicago
Christ Hospital and Medical Center

Program Director:
Stanley A Blumenthal, MD
Christ Hospital and Med Ctr
4440 W 95th St
319 South
Oak Lawn, IL 60453-4213
Tel: 708 346-5673 *Fax:* 708 346-2500
Accred Length: 3 Years *Program Size:* 68 (*GY1:* 24)
Program ID: 140-16-21-129

Oak Park

West Suburban Hospital Medical Center Program

Sponsor: West Suburban Hospital Medical Center

Program Director:
Max L Harris, MD
West Suburban Hospital Med Ctr
Ste L-700
Erie at Austin
Oak Park, IL 60302
Tel: 708 763-6908 *Fax:* 708 763-6655
E-mail: gradmeded@yahoo.com
Internet: http://www.wshmc.org
Accred Length: 3 Years *Program Size:* 24 (*GY1:* 8)
Program ID: 140-16-21-467

Park Ridge

Lutheran General Hospital Program

Sponsor: Lutheran General Hospital

Program Director:
Marc S Fine, MD
Lutheran General Hospital
1775 W Dempster St
6 South
Park Ridge, IL 60068-1174
Tel: 847 723-1680 *Fax:* 847 723-5615
Accred Length: 3 Years *Program Size:* 57 (*GY1:* 24)
Subspecialties: CD, GE, IMG
Program ID: 140-16-21-130

Peoria

University of Illinois College of Medicine at Peoria Program

Sponsor: University of Illinois College of Medicine at Peoria
St Francis Medical Center

Program Director:
Sara L Rusch, MD
St Francis Med Ctr
530 NE Glen Oak Ave
Peoria, IL 61637
Tel: 309 655-2730 *Fax:* 309 655-7732
E-mail: pav42991@uic.edu
Internet: http://www.uicomp.uic.edu
Accred Length: 3 Years *Program Size:* 22 (*GY1:* 7)
Program ID: 140-16-31-131

Springfield

Southern Illinois University Program

Sponsor: Southern Illinois University School of Medicine
Memorial Medical Center
St John's Hospital

Program Director:
Andrew J Varney, MD
Southern Illinois Univ Sch of Med
800 N Rutledge
PO Box 19636
Springfield, IL 62794-9636
Tel: 217 782-0193 *Fax:* 217 524-8156
E-mail: cbrower@siumed.edu
Internet: http://www.siumed.edu
Accred Length: 3 Years *Program Size:* 44 (*GY1:* 20)
Subspecialties: END, GE, ID, PUD
Program ID: 140-16-21-132

Urbana

University of Illinois College of Medicine at Urbana Program

Sponsor: University of Illinois College of Medicine at Urbana
Carle Foundation Hospital
Provena Covenant Medical Center
Veterans Affairs Medical Center (Danville)

Program Director:
Robert W Kirby, MD
Univ of Illinois Coll of Med-Urbana
611 W Park St
Urbana, IL 61801
Tel: 217 383-3110 *Fax:* 217 244-0621
E-mail: r-kirby1@uiuc.edu
Internet: http://www.med.uiuc.edu/residency
Accred Length: 3 Years *Program Size:* 46 (*GY1:* 16)
Program ID: 140-16-21-456

Indiana

Indianapolis

Indiana University School of Medicine Program

Sponsor: Indiana University School of Medicine
Clarian IU Hospital
Clarian Methodist Hospital of Indiana
Clarian Riley Hospital for Children
Richard L Roudebush Veterans Affairs Medical Center
William N Wishard Memorial Hospital

Program Director:
Richard B Kohler, MD
Indiana Univ Sch of Med
West Bldg/Rm M200
1001 W 10th St
Indianapolis, IN 46202
Tel: 317 656-4260 *Fax:* 317 630-2667
Internet: http://medicine.iupui.edu/mededuc.html
Accred Length: 3 Years *Program Size:* 105 (*GY1:* 37)
Subspecialties: CD, END, GE, HO, ICE, ID, IMG, NEP, PCC, RHU
Program ID: 140-17-21-133

St Vincent Hospital and Health Care Center Program

Sponsor: St Vincent Hospital and Health Care Center

Program Director:
Robert M Lubitz, MD MPH
St Vincent Hospital and Health Services
2001 W 86th St
Indianapolis, IN 46260
Tel: 317 338-2172 *Fax:* 317 338-6359
E-mail: rmlubitz@stvincent.org
Internet: http://www.stvincent.org
Accred Length: 3 Years *Program Size:* 54 (*GY1:* 24)
Program ID: 140-17-11-135

Muncie

Ball Memorial Hospital Program

Sponsor: Ball Memorial Hospital

Program Director:
William B Fisher, MD
Ball Memorial Hospital
2401 University Ave
Muncie, IN 47303
Tel: 765 747-3367 *Fax:* 765 747-0137
E-mail: jmarsh@hr.cami3.com
Internet: http://www.ballhospital.org/
Accred Length: 3 Years *Program Size:* 19 (*GY1:* 5)
Subspecialties: ISM
Program ID: 140-17-11-136

Iowa

Des Moines

University of Iowa (Des Moines) Program

Sponsor: Iowa Methodist Medical Center
Veterans Affairs Central Iowa Health Care System

Program Director:
Steven R Craig, MD
Iowa Methodist Med Ctr, Dept of Int Med
1200 Pleasant St
Des Moines, IA 50309-1453
Tel: 515 241-6636 *Fax:* 515 241-6576
E-mail: intmedres@ihs.org
Internet: http://www.ihsdesmoines.org
Accred Length: 3 Years *Program Size:* 26 (*GY1:* 10)
Program ID: 140-18-31-137

Iowa City

University of Iowa Hospitals and Clinics Program

Sponsor: University of Iowa Hospitals and Clinics
Veterans Affairs Medical Center (Iowa City)

Program Director:
Janet A Schlechte, MD
Univ of Iowa Hospitals and Clinics
Dept of Int Med
200 Hawkins Dr/E323 GH
Iowa City, IA 52242-1081
Tel: 319 356-2034 *Fax:* 319 384-8955
E-mail: nancy-davin@uiowa.edu
Internet: http://www.int-med.uiowa.edu/trnprgrms.htm
Accred Length: 3 Years *Program Size:* 90 (*GY1:* 29)
Subspecialties: CD, END, GE, HO, ICE, ID, NEP, PCC, RHU
Program ID: 140-18-21-138

Kansas

Kansas City

University of Kansas Medical Center Program

Sponsor: University of Kansas School of Medicine
Bethany Medical Center
Dwight D Eisenhower Veterans Affairs Medical Center
University of Kansas Medical Center
Veterans Affairs Medical Center (Kansas City)

Program Director:
Norton J Greenberger, MD
Univ of Kansas Med Ctr
Dept of Med
3901 Rainbow Blvd
Kansas City, KS 66160-7350
Tel: 913 588-6001 *Fax:* 913 588-3995
E-mail: medresapps@kumc.edu
Internet: http://www.kumc.edu/internal_med/residency/
Accred Length: 3 Years *Program Size:* 64 (*GY1:* 24)
Subspecialties: CD, END, GE, HEM, ID, IMG, NEP, ON, PCC, RHU
Program ID: 140-19-21-139

Wichita

University of Kansas (Wichita) Program

Sponsor: University of Kansas School of Medicine (Wichita)
Columbia Wesley Medical Center
Veterans Affairs Medical Center (Wichita)
Via Christi Regional Medical Center

Program Director:
Garold O Minns, MD
Dept of Int Med
1010 N Kansas
Wichita, KS 67214-3199
Tel: 316 293-2650 *Fax:* 316 293-1878
E-mail: lhudson1@kumc.edu
Internet: http://www.kumc.edu/wichita/dept/intmed
Accred Length: 3 Years *Program Size:* 40 (*GY1:* 18)
Program ID: 140-19-21-140

Kentucky

Lexington

University of Kentucky Medical Center Program

Sponsor: University of Kentucky Hospital
Veterans Affairs Medical Center (Lexington)

Program Director:
Robert W Lightfoot, MD
Univ of Kentucky Coll of Med
Dept of Education
J511 Kentucky Clinic Bldg
Lexington, KY 40536-0284
Tel: 606 323-1003
Internet: http://www.inmed.gws.uky.edu
Accred Length: 3 Years *Program Size:* 60 (*GY1:* 20)
Subspecialties: CD, GE, HO, ID, IMG, NEP, PCC
Program ID: 140-20-21-141

Louisville

University of Louisville Program

Sponsor: University of Louisville School of Medicine
University of Louisville Hospital
Veterans Affairs Medical Center (Louisville)

Program Director:
Lourdes C Corman, MD
Univ of Louisville
Ambulatory Care Bldg/Rm A3K00
530 S Jackson St
Louisville, KY 40292
Tel: 502 852-7041 *Fax:* 502 852-0936
E-mail: rcrade01@med.louisville.edu
Internet:
http://www.louisville.edu/groups/medtrain-www/
Accred Length: 3 Years *Program Size:* 77 (*GY1:* 32)
Subspecialties: CD, END, GE, HO, ICE, ID, NEP, PCC, RHU
Program ID: 140-20-31-142

Louisiana

Baton Rouge

Louisiana State University (Baton Rouge) Program

Sponsor: Earl K Long Medical Center

Program Director:
George H Karam, MD
Earl K Long Med Ctr
Dept of Int Med
5825 Airline Hwy
Baton Rouge, LA 70805-2498
Tel: 504 358-1065
E-mail: gkaram@mail.ekl.lsumc.edu
Accred Length: 3 Years *Program Size:* 28 (*GY1:* 12)
Program ID: 140-21-21-507

Lafayette

Louisiana State University (Lafayette) Program

Sponsor: University Medical Center (Lafayette)

Program Director:
Leela Lakshmi Prasad, MD
Univ Med Ctr
2390 W Congress St
Lafayette, LA 70506
Tel: 318 261-6789 *Fax:* 318 261-6791
E-mail: intmed@umc.lhca.state.la.us
Accred Length: 3 Years *Program Size:* 24 (*GY1:* 10)
Program ID: 140-21-11-144

New Orleans

Alton Ochsner Medical Foundation Program

Sponsor: Alton Ochsner Medical Foundation
Leonard J Chabert Medical Center

Program Director:
Donald T Erwin, MD
Alton Ochsner Med Foundation
Dept of Grad Med Educ
1516 Jefferson Hwy
New Orleans, LA 70121
Tel: 504 842-3260 *Fax:* 504 842-3193
E-mail: derwin@ochsner.org
Internet: http://www.ochsner.org
Accred Length: 3 Years *Program Size:* 48 (*GY1:* 22)
Subspecialties: CD, END, GE, ID, ON, RHU
Program ID: 140-21-22-146

Louisiana State University Program

Sponsor: Louisiana State University School of Medicine
Medical Center of Louisiana at New Orleans

Program Director:
Dayton W Daberkow II, MD
Louisiana State Univ Med Ctr, Dept of Med
1542 Tulane Ave
New Orleans, LA 70112-2822
Tel: 504 568-4600 *Fax:* 504 568-7885
E-mail: ddaberkow@lsumc.edu
Accred Length: 3 Years *Program Size:* 50 (*GY1:* 17)
Subspecialties: CD, END, GE, HEM, ID, NEP, ON, PCC, RHU
Program ID: 140-21-21-143

Tulane University Program

Sponsor: Tulane University School of Medicine
Medical Center of Louisiana at New Orleans
Tulane University Hospital and Clinics
Veterans Affairs Medical Center (New Orleans)
Veterans Affairs Medical Center-LSU Service (New Orleans)

Program Director:
Marc J Kahn, MD
Tulane Univ Med Ctr
Int Med Dept/SL-50
1430 Tulane Ave
New Orleans, LA 70112-2699
Tel: 504 582-7809 *Fax:* 504 586-3971
E-mail: mkahn@tmcpop.tmc.tulane.edu
Internet:
http://www.mcl.tulane.edu/departments/medicine/med_home.htm
Accred Length: 3 Years *Program Size:* 69 (*GY1:* 26)
Subspecialties: CCM, CD, END, GE, HO, ID, IMG, NEP, PUD, TY
Program ID: 140-21-21-147

Shreveport

Louisiana State University (Shreveport) Program

Sponsor: Louisiana State University Hospital-Shreveport
Overton Brooks Veterans Affairs Medical Center

Program Director:
Gerry S San Pedro, MD
Louisiana State Univ Med Ctr
PO Box 33932
1541 Kings Hwy
Shreveport, LA 71130-3932
Tel: 318 675-5857 *Fax:* 318 675-5959
E-mail: gsanpe@lsumc.edu
Internet: http://www.ccm.lsumc.edu/lsumc-im
Accred Length: 3 Years *Program Size:* 58 (*GY1:* 22)
Subspecialties: CCM, CD, END, GE, HO, ID, NEP, PCC, RHU
Program ID: 140-21-21-148

Maine

Portland

Maine Medical Center Program

Sponsor: Maine Medical Center

Program Director:
Robert G Bing-You, MD MEd
Maine Med Ctr
Dept of Med
22 Bramhall St
Portland, ME 04102
Tel: 207 871-2651 *Fax:* 207 871-6788
E-mail: kuchac@mail.mmc.org
Accred Length: 3 Years *Program Size:* 44 (*GYI:* 19)
Subspecialties: CD, END, ID, NEP, PCC
Program ID: 140-22-11-149

Maryland

Baltimore

Franklin Square Hospital Center Program

Sponsor: Franklin Square Hospital Center

Program Director:
Daniel C Hardesty, MD
Franklin Square Hospital Ctr
Dept of Med
9105 Franklin Square Dr/Ste 201
Baltimore, MD 21237-3998
Tel: 410 682-7146 *Fax:* 410 682-8340
E-mail: kendraw@helix.org
Internet: http://www.helixhealth.com
Accred Length: 3 Years *Program Size:* 33 (*GYI:* 13)
Program ID: 140-23-12-151

Good Samaritan Hospital of Maryland Program

Sponsor: Good Samaritan Hospital of Maryland
Johns Hopkins Hospital

Program Director:
Thomas S Wilson, MD PhD
Good Samaritan Hospital
5601 Loch Raven Blvd
Morgan 504
Baltimore, MD 21239-2995
Tel: 410 532-4860 *Fax:* 410 532-3663
Internet: http://www.helixhealth.com
Accred Length: 3 Years *Program Size:* 27 (*GYI:* 10)
Program ID: 140-23-21-489

Greater Baltimore Medical Center Program

Sponsor: Greater Baltimore Medical Center

Program Director:
Thomas F Lansdale III, MD
Greater Baltimore Med Ctr
Internal Med Program
6565 N Charles St/Ste 203
Baltimore, MD 21204
Tel: 410 828-2682 *Fax:* 410 512-8030
E-mail: medres@gbmc.org
Internet: http://www.gbmc.org
Accred Length: 3 Years *Program Size:* 32 (*GYI:* 16)
Program ID: 140-23-31-152

Harbor Hospital Center Program

Sponsor: Harbor Hospital Center

Program Director:
Richard B Williams, MD
Harbor Hospital Ctr
3001 S Hanover St
Baltimore, MD 21225-1290
Tel: 410 350-3565 *Fax:* 410 354-0186
E-mail: terryku@helix.org
Internet:
http://www.helixhealth.com/residency/hh-intmed.htm
Accred Length: 3 Years *Program Size:* 30 (*GYI:* 13)
Program ID: 140-23-31-158

Johns Hopkins University Bayview Medical Center Program

Sponsor: Johns Hopkins University School of Medicine
Johns Hopkins Bayview Medical Center

Program Director:
Roy C Ziegelstein, MD
Johns Hopkins Bayview Med Ctr
Dept of Med
4940 Eastern Ave
Baltimore, MD 21224
Tel: 410 550-0526 *Fax:* 410 550-1094
Internet:
http://www.jhbmc.jhu.edu/medicine/residency.html
Accred Length: 3 Years *Program Size:* 40 (*GYI:* 16)
Subspecialties: GE, NEP
Program ID: 140-23-11-150

Johns Hopkins University Program

Sponsor: Johns Hopkins University School of Medicine
Johns Hopkins Hospital

Program Director:
David B Hellmann, MD
Johns Hopkins Hospital
Dept of Med
1830 E Monument St/9th Fl
Baltimore, MD 21205
Tel: 410 955-7910 *Fax:* 410 955-0430
Internet: http://www.med.jhu.edu/deptmed/housestaff/
Accred Length: 3 Years *Program Size:* 97 (*GYI:* 34)
Subspecialties: CD, END, GE, HEM, ICE, ID, IMG, NEP, ON, PCC, RHU
Program ID: 140-23-11-153

Johns Hopkins University/Sinai Hospital of Baltimore Program

Sponsor: Johns Hopkins University School of Medicine
Sinai Hospital of Baltimore

Program Director:
Steven Gambert, MD
Sinai Health System
Dept of Med
2401 W Belvedere Ave
Baltimore, MD 21215-5271
Tel: 410 601-6256 *Fax:* 410 601-5638
E-mail: dchow@sinai-balt.com
Internet: http://www.sinai-balt.com
Accred Length: 3 Years *Program Size:* 55 (*GYI:* 27)
Program ID: 140-23-12-157

Maryland General Hospital Program

Sponsor: Maryland General Hospital

Program Director:
William C Anthony, MD
Maryland General Hospital
827 Linden Ave
Ste 3B/Armory Bldg
Baltimore, MD 21201
Tel: 410 225-8790 *Fax:* 410 225-8910
Accred Length: 3 Years *Program Size:* 18 (*GYI:* 6)
Program ID: 140-23-11-154

St Agnes HealthCare Program

Sponsor: St Agnes Hospital

Program Director:
Emile R Mohler Jr, MD
St Agnes HealthCare
900 Caton Ave
Baltimore, MD 21229
Tel: 410 368-3120 *Fax:* 410 368-3525
Accred Length: 3 Years *Program Size:* 34 (*GYI:* 12)
Program ID: 140-23-12-156

Union Memorial Hospital Program

Sponsor: Union Memorial Hospital

Program Director:
Robert P Ferguson, MD
Union Memorial Hospital
201 E University Pkwy
Baltimore, MD 21218-2895
Tel: 410 554-2284 *Fax:* 410 554-2184
Internet: http://www.helixhealth.com
Accred Length: 3 Years *Program Size:* 29 (*GYI:* 12)
Subspecialties: IMG
Program ID: 140-23-12-159

University of Maryland Program

Sponsor: University of Maryland Medical System
Mercy Medical Center
Veterans Affairs Medical Center (Baltimore)

Program Director:
Susan D Wolfsthal, MD
Univ of Maryland Hospital
22 S Greene St/Rm N3E09
Baltimore, MD 21201-1595
Tel: 410 328-2388 *Fax:* 410 328-0267
E-mail: umdmed@medicine.ab.umd.edu
Internet: http://www.umm.edu
Accred Length: 3 Years *Program Size:* 83 (*GYI:* 35)
Subspecialties: CD, END, GE, HO, ICE, ID, IMG, NEP, PCC, RHU
Program ID: 140-23-21-160

Bethesda

National Naval Medical Center (Bethesda) Program

Sponsor: National Naval Medical Center (Bethesda)

Program Director:
Angeline A Lazarus, MD
National Naval Med Ctr
Dept of Int Med
8901 Wisconsin Ave
Bethesda, MD 20889-5600
Tel: 301 295-0290 *Fax:* 301 295-5792
E-mail: bth0aal@bth20.med.navy.mil
Accred Length: 3 Years *Program Size:* 36 (*GYI:* 22)
Subspecialties: CD, END, GE, HO, ID, PCC
Program ID: 140-23-11-013
US Armed Services Program

Cheverly

Prince George's Hospital Center Program

Sponsor: Prince George's Hospital Center

Program Director:
Sary O Beidas, MD
Prince George's Hospital Ctr
3001 Hospital Dr
Cheverly, MD 20785
Tel: 301 618-3772
Accred Length: 3 Years *Program Size:* 39 (*GYI:* 15)
Program ID: 140-23-21-161

Massachusetts

Boston

Beth Israel Deaconess Medical Center (East Campus) Program

Sponsor: Beth Israel Deaconess Medical Center

Program Director:
Anthony N Hollenberg, MD
Beth Israel Deaconess Med Ctr
330 Brookline Ave
Boston, MA 02215
Tel: 617 667-4975 *Fax:* 617 667-4921
Internet:
http://www.bidmc.harvard.edu/medicine/training
Accred Length: 3 Years *Program Size:* 164 (*GY1:* 62)
Subspecialties: CD, END, GE, HO, ICE, IMG, NEP
Program ID: 140-24-21-162

Beth Israel Deaconess Medical Center (West Campus) Program

Sponsor: Beth Israel Deaconess Medical Center

Program Director:
Robert C Moellering Jr, MD
Beth Israel Deaconess Med Ctr-West Campus
Dept of Med/LMOB6A
One Deaconess Rd
Boston, MA 02215
Tel: 617 632-0962 *Fax:* 617 632-7442
Accred Length: 3 Years *Program Size:* 23 (*GY1:* 0)
Subspecialties: CD, END, GE, HO, ICE, ID, NEP, PCC, PUD
Program ID: 140-24-21-170

Boston University Medical Center Program

Sponsor: Boston Medical Center
Veterans Affairs Medical Center (Boston)

Program Director:
David L Battinelli, MD
Boston Univ Med Ctr
80 E Concord St/Evans 124
Boston, MA 02118-2393
Tel: 617 638-6500 *Fax:* 617 638-6501
E-mail: internalmed.boston@bmc.org
Accred Length: 3 Years *Program Size:* 151 (*GY1:* 54)
Subspecialties: CD, END, GE, HO, ID, IMG, NEP, PCC, RHU
Program ID: 140-24-31-164

Brigham and Women's Hospital Program

Sponsor: Brigham and Women's Hospital
Brockton-West Roxbury Veterans Affairs Medical Center

Program Director:
Marshall A Wolf, MD
Brigham and Women's Hospital
75 Francis St
Boston, MA 02115
Tel: 617 732-6330 *Fax:* 617 278-6995
Accred Length: 3 Years *Program Size:* 151 (*GY1:* 56)
Subspecialties: CD, END, GE, HO, ICE, ID, NEP, ON, PCC, RHU
Program ID: 140-24-21-172

Carney Hospital Program

Sponsor: Carney Hospital

Program Director:
Michael Barza, MD
Carney Hospital
2100 Dorchester Ave
Boston, MA 02124-5666
Tel: 617 296-4012, ext 2726 *Fax:* 617 298-1547
E-mail: carneymed@aol.com
Accred Length: 3 Years *Program Size:* 43 (*GY1:* 20)
Program ID: 140-24-11-166

Massachusetts General Hospital Program

Sponsor: Massachusetts General Hospital

Program Director:
Hasan Bazari, MD
Massachusetts General Hospital
Fruit St
Boston, MA 02114
Tel: 617 726-2862 *Fax:* 617 724-7441
E-mail: bazari.hasan@mgh.harvard.edu
Internet: http://www.mgh.harvard.edu/depts/medicine
Accred Length: 3 Years *Program Size:* 110 (*GY1:* 46)
Subspecialties: CD, END, GE, HO, ICE, ID, NEP, PCC, RHU
Program ID: 140-24-11-169

New England Medical Center Hospitals Program

Sponsor: New England Medical Center Hospitals
Faulkner Hospital

Program Director:
Richard I Kopelman, MD
New England Med Ctr
750 Washington St/Box 21
Boston, MA 02111
Tel: 617 636-5246 *Fax:* 617 636-7119
E-mail: richard.kopelman@es.nemc.org
Internet: http://www.nemc.org
Accred Length: 3 Years *Program Size:* 63 (*GY1:* 21)
Subspecialties: CD, END, GE, HO, ICE, ID, NEP, PCC, RHU
Program ID: 140-24-21-171

St Elizabeth's Medical Center of Boston Program

Sponsor: St Elizabeth's Medical Center of Boston

Program Director:
Kenneth F MacDonnell, MD
St Elizabeth's Med Ctr
736 Cambridge St
Boston, MA 02135
Tel: 617 789-2548 *Fax:* 617 789-2893
E-mail: med_ed@semc.org
Internet: http://www.semc.org
Accred Length: 3 Years *Program Size:* 54 (*GY1:* 22)
Subspecialties: CD, GE, HEM, HO, ON, PCC
Program ID: 140-24-21-173

Burlington

Lahey Clinic Program

Sponsor: Lahey Clinic

Program Director:
Guy T Napolitana, MD
41 Mall Rd
Burlington, MA 01805
Tel: 781 774-5700
Internet:
http://www.lahey.org/depts/im/resident_im/im.stm
Accred Length: 3 Years *Program Size:* 41 (*GY1:* 18)
Program ID: 140-24-21-511

Cambridge

Cambridge Hospital/Cambridge Health Alliance Program

Sponsor: Cambridge Hospital/Cambridge Health Alliance

Program Director:
Richard J Pels, MD
Cambridge Hospital-Cambridge Health Alliance
Dept of Med
1493 Cambridge St
Cambridge, MA 02139
Tel: 617 498-1021 *Fax:* 617 498-1671
E-mail: imres@challiance.org
Internet: http://www.hmcnet.harvard.edu/cha/med
Accred Length: 3 Years *Program Size:* 24 (*GY1:* 8)
Program ID: 140-24-11-175

Mount Auburn Hospital Program

Sponsor: Mount Auburn Hospital

Program Director:
Eric M Flint, MD
Mount Auburn Hospital
Dept of Med
330 Mount Auburn St
Cambridge, MA 02238
Tel: 617 499-5160 *Fax:* 617 499-5593
Internet: http://www.mtah.org
Accred Length: 3 Years *Program Size:* 44 (*GY1:* 20)
Program ID: 140-24-11-176

Framingham

MetroWest Medical Center Program

Sponsor: MetroWest Medical Center-Framingham Union Hospital

Program Director:
Thomas L Treadwell, MD
MetroWest Med Ctr
115 Lincoln St
Framingham, MA 01702
Tel: 508 383-1572 *Fax:* 508 872-4794
E-mail: thomas_treadwell@mwmc.com
Accred Length: 3 Years *Program Size:* 21 (*GY1:* 8)
Program ID: 140-24-21-177

Newton Lower Falls

Newton-Wellesley Hospital Program

Sponsor: Newton-Wellesley Hospital

Program Director:
Mark S Drapkin, MD
Newton-Wellesley Hospital
2014 Washington St
Newton Lower Falls, MA 02462
Tel: 617 243-6467
E-mail: med.wilm@nwh.org.
Internet: http://www.nwh.org
Accred Length: 3 Years *Program Size:* 27 (*GY1:* 13)
Program ID: 140-24-11-178

Pittsfield

Berkshire Medical Center Program

Sponsor: Berkshire Medical Center

Program Director:
Jack D McCue, MD
Berkshire Med Ctr
725 North St
Pittsfield, MA 01201
Tel: 413 447-2839 *Fax:* 413 447-2088
E-mail: bmcdepmed@bhs1.org
Internet: http://www.bmcdepmed
Accred Length: 3 Years *Program Size:* 34 (*GY1:* 14)
Program ID: 140-24-11-179

Salem

Salem Hospital Program

Sponsor: Salem Hospital

Program Director:
Wayne M Trebbin, MD
Salem Hospital
81 Highland Ave
Salem, MA 01970
Tel: 978 741-1215, ext 4018 *Fax:* 978 740-0418
E-mail: trebbin@nsmc.partners.org
Accred Length: 3 Years *Program Size:* 20 (*GY1:* 9)
Program ID: 140-24-12-180

Springfield

Baystate Medical Center Program

Sponsor: Baystate Medical Center

Program Director:
Robert D Ficalora, MD
Baystate Med Ctr
Dept of Int Med S2570
759 Chestnut St
Springfield, MA 01199
Tel: 413 794-4143 *Fax:* 413 794-8075
E-mail: linda.baillargeon@bhs.org
Internet: http://www.baystatehealth.com
Accred Length: 3 Years *Program Size:* 54 (*GYI:* 18)
Subspecialties: CD, END, HO, ICE, ID
Program ID: 140-24-11-181

Worcester

Memorial Health Care Program

Sponsor: UMass Memorial Health Care (Memorial Campus)

Program Director:
Paula M Cullinane, MD MPH
Memorial Health Care
119 Belmont St
Worcester, MA 01605-2982
Tel: 508 793-6440 *Fax:* 508 792-8271
Accred Length: 3 Years *Program Size:* 57 (*GYI:* 19)
Program ID: 140-24-31-182

St Vincent Hospital Program

Sponsor: St Vincent Hospital

Program Director:
Joel H Popkin, MD
Dept of Med
St Vincent Hospital
25 Winthrop St
Worcester, MA 01604-4593
Tel: 508 798-6208 *Fax:* 508 798-1798
E-mail: jpopkin@massmed.org
Internet: http://www.ultranet.com/~svhimres/
Accred Length: 3 Years *Program Size:* 53 (*GYI:* 25)
Subspecialties: CD
Program ID: 140-24-11-183

University of Massachusetts Program

Sponsor: University of Massachusetts Medical School
UMass Memorial Health Care (University Campus)

Program Director:
Deborah M DeMarco, MD
Univ of Massachusetts Med Sch
Dept of Med
55 Lake Ave N
Worcester, MA 01655
Tel: 508 856-2173 *Fax:* 508 856-6781
Accred Length: 3 Years *Program Size:* 65 (*GYI:* 23)
Subspecialties: CCM, CD, END, GE, HO, ICE, ID, NEP, PUD, RHU
Program ID: 140-24-21-184

Michigan

Ann Arbor

St Joseph Mercy Hospital Program

Sponsor: St Joseph Mercy Health System

Program Director:
Jeffrey A Sanfield, MD
St Joseph Mercy Hospital
5333 McAuley Dr/RHB-3009
PO Box 995
Ann Arbor, MI 48106-9979
Tel: 734 712-3935 *Fax:* 734 712-5583
Internet: http://www.sjmh.com
Accred Length: 3 Years *Program Size:* 53 (*GYI:* 24)
Program ID: 140-25-12-186

University of Michigan Program

Sponsor: University of Michigan Hospitals
Veterans Affairs Medical Center (Ann Arbor)

Program Director:
H David Humes, MD
Univ of Michigan Health System
3110 TC/Box 0368
1500 E Medical Center Dr
Ann Arbor, MI 48109-0368
Tel: 734 936-4385 *Fax:* 734 936-3654
E-mail: sreise@umich.edu
Internet: http://www.med.umich.edu/intmed/resident
Accred Length: 3 Years *Program Size:* 107 (*GYI:* 38)
Subspecialties: CD, END, GE, HO, ICE, ID, IMG, NEP, PCC, RHU
Program ID: 140-25-21-187

Dearborn

Oakwood Hospital Program

Sponsor: Oakwood Hospital

Program Director:
Raphael J Kiel, MD
Oakwood Hospital and Med Ctr
18101 Oakwood Blvd
Dearborn, MI 48124
Tel: 313 593-7796 *Fax:* 313 436-2071
E-mail: mckayv@oakwood.org
Accred Length: 3 Years *Program Size:* 32 (*GYI:* 12)
Program ID: 140-25-31-188

Detroit

Henry Ford Hospital Program

Sponsor: Henry Ford Hospital

Program Director:
Eric Scher, MD
Henry Ford Hospital
2799 W Grand Blvd
Detroit, MI 48202
Tel: 313 876-1888 *Fax:* 313 876-1394
E-mail: ethompsl@hfhs.org
Accred Length: 3 Years *Program Size:* 81 (*GYI:* 26)
Subspecialties: CD, END, GE, HO, ID, NEP, PCC, RHU
Program ID: 140-25-11-189

St John Hospital and Medical Center Program

Sponsor: St John Hospital and Medical Center

Program Director:
Louis D Saravolatz, MD
St John Hospital and Med Ctr
Dept of Med Educ
22101 Moross Rd
Detroit, MI 48236
Tel: 313 343-3875 *Fax:* 313 343-7840
E-mail: sue.moynihan@stjohn.org
Internet: http://www.stjohn.org
Accred Length: 3 Years *Program Size:* 36 (*GYI:* 12)
Subspecialties: CD, ID, NEP
Program ID: 140-25-11-191

Wayne State University/Detroit Medical Center (Grace Hospital) Program

Sponsor: Wayne State University/Detroit Medical Center
Detroit Receiving Hospital and University Health Center
Grace Hospital

Program Director:
Mohamed Siddique, MD
Grace Hospital
6071 W Outer Dr
Detroit, MI 48235
Tel: 313 966-4970 *Fax:* 313 966-1738
Accred Length: 3 Years *Program Size:* 36 (*GYI:* 12)
Program ID: 140-25-21-506

Wayne State University/Detroit Medical Center (Sinai Hospital) Program

Sponsor: Wayne State University/Detroit Medical Center
Sinai Hospital

Program Director:
Mohamed Siddique, MD
Sinai Hospital
Dept of Med
6767 W Outer Dr
Detroit, MI 48235-2899
Tel: 313 493-5780 *Fax:* 313 493-6892
Accred Length: 3 Years *Program Size:* 40 (*GYI:* 12)
Subspecialties: CD, GE, ICE, PUD, RHU
Program ID: 140-25-11-192

Wayne State University/Detroit Medical Center Program

Sponsor: Wayne State University/Detroit Medical Center
Detroit Receiving Hospital and University Health Center
Harper Hospital
Veterans Affairs Medical Center (Detroit)

Program Director:
Ernest Yoder, MD PhD
Detroit Medical Center
4201 St Antoine/ 5-D
Detroit, MI 48201
Tel: 313 745-4896 *Fax:* 313 745-4052
E-mail: intmedresprog@oncgate.wayne.edu
Internet: http://www.intmed.wayne.edu
Accred Length: 3 Years *Program Size:* 98 (*GYI:* 30)
Subspecialties: CCM, CD, END, GE, HEM, ID, IMG, NEP, ON, PCC, PUD, RHU
Program ID: 140-25-21-194

East Lansing

Michigan State University Program

Sponsor: Michigan State University College of Human Medicine
Michigan Capital Medical Center
Michigan State University Clinical Center
Sparrow Hospital

Program Director:
Michael H Zaroukian, MD
B301 Clinical Ctr
Michigan State Univ
East Lansing, MI 48824-1313
Tel: 517 353-5100 *Fax:* 517 432-2759
E-mail: zaroukia@pilot.msu.edu
Internet: http://pilot.msu.edu/user/zaroukia
Accred Length: 3 Years *Program Size:* 27 (*GYI:* 9)
Subspecialties: CD, GE, HEM, HO, ON
Program ID: 140-25-21-195

Flint

Hurley Medical Center/Michigan State University Program

Sponsor: Hurley Medical Center

Program Director:
Barbara A McIntosh, MD
Hurley Med Ctr
Two Hurley Plaza/Ste 212
Flint, MI 48503-5993
Tel: 810 257-9682 *Fax:* 810 762-7245
E-mail: mcintos9@pilot.msu.edu
Internet: http://www.hurleymc.com
Accred Length: 3 Years *Program Size:* 30 (*GYI:* 10)
Program ID: 140-25-31-196

McLaren Regional Medical Center/Michigan State University Program

Sponsor: McLaren Regional Medical Center

Program Director:
Susan J Smith, MD
McLaren Regional Med Ctr-Michigan State Univ
Dept of Int Med
401 S Ballenger Hwy
Flint, MI 48532-3685
Tel: 810 342-2063 *Fax:* 810 342-3659
Accred Length: 3 Years *Program Size:* 36 (*GY1:* 12)
Program ID: 140-25-21-471

Grand Rapids

Spectrum Health-Downtown Campus/Michigan State University Program

Sponsor: Spectrum Health-Downtown Campus

Program Director:
Philip Tate, MD
Spectrum Health-Downtown Campus
21 Michigan Ave
Ste 430
Grand Rapids, MI 49503
Tel: 616 732-3775 *Fax:* 616 732-3130
Internet: http://www.spectrum health.org
Accred Length: 3 Years *Program Size:* 24 (*GY1:* 8)
Program ID: 140-25-31-198

Spectrum Health-East Campus/St Mary's Health Services Program

Sponsor: Spectrum Health-East Campus
St Mary's Health Services

Program Director:
Jeffrey L Wilt, MD
Spectrum Health-East Campus
Med Educ Office
1840 Wealthy St SE
Grand Rapids, MI 49506
Tel: 616 774-7289 *Fax:* 616 774-5290
Accred Length: 3 Years *Program Size:* 25 (*GY1:* 9)
Program ID: 140-25-21-197

Grosse Pointe

Bon Secours Hospital Program

Sponsor: Bon Secours Hospital

Program Director:
Ralph D Cushing, MD
Bon Secours Hospital
468 Cadieux Rd
Grosse Pointe, MI 48230
Tel: 313 343-1490 *Fax:* 313 343-1611
Accred Length: 3 Years *Program Size:* 18 (*GY1:* 6)
Program ID: 140-25-21-469

Kalamazoo

Kalamazoo Center for Medical Studies/Michigan State University Program

Sponsor: Kalamazoo Center for Medical Studies
Borgess Medical Center
Bronson Methodist Hospital

Program Director:
Kenneth A Fisher, MD
Michigan State Univ-Kalamazoo Ctr for Med Studies
Dept of Int Med
1000 Oakland Dr
Kalamazoo, MI 49008-1284
Tel: 616 337-6350 *Fax:* 616 337-4234
E-mail: intmed@kcms.msu.edu
Internet: http://www.kcms.msu.edu
Accred Length: 3 Years *Program Size:* 27 (*GY1:* 9)
Program ID: 140-25-21-199

Pontiac

St Joseph Mercy-Oakland Program

Sponsor: St Joseph Mercy-Oakland

Program Director:
Frank E Check Jr, MD
St Joseph Mercy-Oakland
900 Woodward Ave
Pontiac, MI 48341-2985
Tel: 248 858-6233 *Fax:* 248 858-3244
Accred Length: 3 Years *Program Size:* 34 (*GY1:* 10)
Program ID: 140-25-11-200

Royal Oak

William Beaumont Hospital Program

Sponsor: William Beaumont Hospital

Program Director:
Leslie L Rocher, MD
William Beaumont Hospital
3601 W 13 Mile Rd
Royal Oak, MI 48073-6769
Tel: 248 551-0406 *Fax:* 248 551-5426
Internet: http://www.beaumont.edu/html/gme
Accred Length: 3 Years *Program Size:* 58 (*GY1:* 20)
Subspecialties: CD, GE, ID, IMG, ON
Program ID: 140-25-12-201

Saginaw

Saginaw Cooperative Hospitals Program

Sponsor: Saginaw Cooperative Hospitals Inc
Covenant Medical Center
Saginaw General Hospital
St Mary's Medical Center

Program Director:
Phillip W Lambert, MD
Saginaw Cooperative Hospitals
1000 Houghton Ave
Saginaw, MI 48602
Tel: 517 771-6826
Internet: http://www.chm.msu.edu/saginaw/index.html
Accred Length: 3 Years *Program Size:* 18 (*GY1:* 6)
Program ID: 140-25-31-202

Southfield

Providence Hospital and Medical Centers Program

Sponsor: Providence Hospital and Medical Centers

Program Director:
Neil A Basmaji, MD
Providence Hospital
16001 W Nine Mile Rd
Southfield, MI 48075-4818
Tel: 248 424-3151 *Fax:* 248 424-5324
Accred Length: 3 Years *Program Size:* 30 (*GY1:* 10)
Subspecialties: CD, GE, ON
Program ID: 140-25-11-203

Minnesota

Minneapolis

Abbott-Northwestern Hospital Program

Sponsor: Abbott-Northwestern Hospital

Program Director:
Terry K Rosborough, MD
Abbott-Northwestern Hospital
Grad Med Educ Office (11135)
800 E 28th St
Minneapolis, MN 55407-3799
Tel: 612 863-6766 *Fax:* 612 863-4144
E-mail: aklinkha@allina.com
Internet: http://www.anwim.umn.edu
Accred Length: 3 Years *Program Size:* 30 (*GY1:* 10)
Program ID: 140-26-31-204

Hennepin County Medical Center Program

Sponsor: Hennepin County Medical Center

Program Director:
Morris Davidman, MD
Hennepin County Med Ctr
Internal Med Education #834
701 Park Ave
Minneapolis, MN 55415
Tel: 612 347-2702 *Fax:* 612 904-4577
E-mail: tammy.prose@co.hennepin.mn.us
Internet: http://www.hcmc.org
Accred Length: 3 Years *Program Size:* 55 (*GY1:* 18)
Subspecialties: CCM, RHU
Program ID: 140-26-31-207

University of Minnesota Program

Sponsor: University of Minnesota Medical School
Fairview-University Medical Center
Regions Hospital
Veterans Affairs Medical Center (Minneapolis)

Program Director:
Kathleen V Watson, MD
Univ of Minnesota
Dept of Med/Box 284
420 Delaware St SE
Minneapolis, MN 55455
Tel: 612 624-0691 *Fax:* 612 625-3238
E-mail: ehre0001@tc.umn.edu
Internet: http://www.dept.med.umn.edu/medicine
Accred Length: 3 Years *Program Size:* 75 (*GY1:* 24)
Subspecialties: CCM, CD, END, GE, HO, ICE, ID, IMG, NEP, PCC, PUD, RHU
Program ID: 140-26-21-205

Rochester

Mayo Graduate School of Medicine (Rochester) Program

Sponsor: Mayo Graduate School of Medicine-Mayo Foundation
Mayo Clinic (Rochester)
Rochester Methodist Hospital
St Mary's Hospital of Rochester

Program Director:
Henry J Schultz, MD
Application Processing Ctr
Mayo Graduate Sch of Med
200 First St SW/Siebens 5
Rochester, MN 55905
Tel: 507 284-3126 *Fax:* 507 284-0999
E-mail: res-im@mayo.edu
Internet:
http://www.mayo.edu/int-med/res-program/resid-main.htm
Accred Length: 3 Years *Program Size:* 151 (*GY1:* 55)
Subspecialties: CCM, CD, END, GE, HO, ICE, ID, IMG, NEP, PCC, RHU
Program ID: 140-26-21-208

Mississippi

Jackson

University of Mississippi Medical Center Program

Sponsor: University of Mississippi School of Medicine
University Hospital
Veterans Affairs Medical Center (Jackson)

Program Director:
Shirley Schlessinger, MD
Univ Hospital, Dept of Med
2500 N State St
Jackson, MS 39216-4505
Tel: 601 984-5601 *Fax:* 601 984-5608
E-mail: sschlessinger@medicine.umsmed.edu
Internet: http://www.umc.edu/medicine/housestaff
Accred Length: 3 Years *Program Size:* 62 (*GY1:* 21)
Subspecialties: CD, END, GE, HEM, HO, ID, NEP, ON, PUD
Program ID: 140-27-21-209

Keesler AFB

Keesler Medical Center Program

Sponsor: Keesler Medical Center

Program Director:
Matthew T Carpenter, MD
81 MDOS/SGOM
301 Fisher St/Rm 1A132
Keesler AFB, MS 39534-2519
Tel: 228 377-6075 *Fax:* 228 377-8099
E-mail: carpenter.matthew@keesler.af.mil
Accred Length: 3 Years *Program Size:* 30 (*GY1:* 10)
Program ID: 140-27-12-001
US Armed Services Program

Missouri

Chesterfield

St Luke's Hospital Program

Sponsor: St Luke's Hospital
St Louis ConnectCare

Program Director:
Leon R Robison, MD
222 S Woods Mill Rd/Ste 760N
St Louis, MO 63017
Tel: 314 205-6050 *Fax:* 314 434-5939
E-mail: miklcg@stlo.smhs.com
Accred Length: 3 Years *Program Size:* 38 (*GY1:* 12)
Program ID: 140-28-21-219

Columbia

University of Missouri-Columbia Program

Sponsor: University of Missouri-Columbia School of Medicine
Harry S Truman Memorial Veterans Hospital
University Hospitals and Clinics

Program Director:
John Yanos, MD
Univ of Missouri-Columbia
MA406 Med Science Bldg
One Hospital Dr
Columbia, MO 65212
Tel: 573 882-6198 *Fax:* 573 884-5690
E-mail: im-house@muccmail.missouri.edu
Internet: http://www.imed.missouri.edu
Accred Length: 3 Years *Program Size:* 50 (*GY1:* 20)
Subspecialties: CD, END, GE, HO, ID, NEP, PCC, RHU
Program ID: 140-28-21-210

Kansas City

University of Missouri at Kansas City Program

Sponsor: University of Missouri-Kansas City School of Medicine
Saint Luke's Hospital
Truman Medical Center-West

Program Director:
George R Reisz, MD
Univ of Missouri-Kansas City
2411 Holmes St
Kansas City, MO 64108
Tel: 816 881-6212 *Fax:* 816 881-6209
E-mail: intmed@cctr.umkc.edu
Internet: http://www.research.med.umkc.edu/residency/
Accred Length: 3 Years *Program Size:* 56 (*GY1:* 24)
Subspecialties: CD, END, GE, HO, ICE, ID, NEP, PCC
Program ID: 140-28-31-214

St Louis

Deaconess Hospital Program

Sponsor: Deaconess Hospital

Program Director:
M R Hill, MD
Deaconess Hospital
6150 Oakland Ave
St Louis, MO 63139-3297
Tel: 314 768-3006 *Fax:* 314 768-5632
E-mail: dexascan@geocities.com
Internet:
http://www.geocities.com/hotsprings/2846/homepage.htm
Accred Length: 3 Years *Program Size:* 28 (*GY1:* 12)
Program ID: 140-28-11-216

St John's Mercy Medical Center Program

Sponsor: St John's Mercy Medical Center

Program Director:
Patrick H Henry, MD
Dept of Int Med
615 S New Ballas Rd
St Louis, MO 63141-8277
Tel: 314 569-6959 *Fax:* 314 569-6272
Accred Length: 3 Years *Program Size:* 22 (*GY1:* 7)
Program ID: 140-28-31-217

St Louis University School of Medicine Program

Sponsor: St Louis University School of Medicine
St Louis University School of Medicine
Veterans Affairs Medical Center (St Louis)

Program Director:
Adrian M DiBisceglie, MD
St Louis Univ Sch of Med
Dept of Int Med
1402 S Grand Blvd
St Louis, MO 63104
Tel: 314 577-8762 *Fax:* 314 268-5108
E-mail: stepterc@wpogate.slu.edu
Internet: http://www.slu.edu/departments/medicine/
Accred Length: 3 Years *Program Size:* 74 (*GY1:* 25)
Subspecialties: CCM, CD, END, GE, HO, ID, IMG, NEP, PCC, RHU
Program ID: 140-28-21-218

St Mary's Health Center Program

Sponsor: St Mary's Health Center

Program Director:
Morey Gardner, MD
St Mary's Health Ctr
6420 Clayton Rd
St Louis, MO 63117
Tel: 314 768-8887 *Fax:* 314 768-7101
Accred Length: 3 Years *Program Size:* 28 (*GY1:* 12)
Program ID: 140-28-11-220

Washington University/B-JH/SLCH Consortium (North Campus) Program

Sponsor: Washington University/B-JH/SLCH Consortium
Barnes-Jewish Hospital (North Campus)

Program Director:
Megan Wren, MD
Barnes-Jewish Hospital
Box 8121
660 S Euclid Ave
St Louis, MO 63110
Tel: 314 747-1499 *Fax:* 314 747-4768
E-mail: mwren@imgate.wustl.edu
Accred Length: 3 Years *Program Size:* 46 (*GY1:* 20)
Subspecialties: CD, IMG, NEP
Program ID: 140-28-21-221

Washington University/B-JH/SLCH Consortium (South Campus) Program

Sponsor: Washington University/B-JH/SLCH Consortium
Barnes-Jewish Hospital

Program Director:
Daniel M Goodenberger, MD
Washington Univ Sch of Med
660 S Euclid Ave
Box 8121
St Louis, MO 63110
Tel: 314 362-8064 *Fax:* 314 747-1080
E-mail: tsteinko@im.wustl.edu
Internet:
http://www.internalmed.wustl.edu/divisions/house_staff/menu.html
Accred Length: 3 Years *Program Size:* 102 (*GY1:* 37)
Subspecialties: CD, END, GE, HO, ICE, ID, NEP, PCC, RHU
Program ID: 140-28-21-215

Nebraska

Omaha

Creighton University Program

Sponsor: Creighton University School of Medicine
Tenet St Joseph Hospital at Creighton Univ Medical Center
Veterans Affairs Medical Center (Omaha)

Program Director:
Robert Dunlay, MD
Creighton Univ
601 N 30th St
Omaha, NE 68131
Tel: 402 280-4392 *Fax:* 402 280-4158
E-mail: resapp@creighton.edu
Internet: http://www.medicine.creighton.edu
Accred Length: 3 Years *Program Size:* 53 (*GY1:* 21)
Subspecialties: CD, ID, PUD
Program ID: 140-30-21-222

University of Nebraska Program

Sponsor: University of Nebraska Medical Center
Veterans Affairs Medical Center (Omaha)

Program Director:
James R O'Dell, MD
Univ of Nebraska Hospital and Clinic
Dept of Internal Med Education Office
982055 Nebraska Med Ctr
Omaha, NE 68198-2055
Tel: 402 559-6488 *Fax:* 402 559-6114
E-mail: smaloley@mail.unmc.edu
Internet: http://www.unmc.edu
Accred Length: 3 Years *Program Size:* 42 (*GY1:* 18)
Subspecialties: CD, END, GE, HO, IMG, PCC
Program ID: 140-30-21-224

Nevada

Las Vegas

University of Nevada (Las Vegas) Program

Sponsor: University of Nevada School of Medicine
University Medical Center of Southern Nevada

Program Director:
Lewis B Morrow, MD
Univ of Nevada Sch of Med
Ste 300
2040 W Charleston Blvd
Las Vegas, NV 89102
Tel: 702 671-2345 *Fax:* 702 671-2376
E-mail: lmorrow@med.unr.edu
Accred Length: 3 Years *Program Size:* 45 (*GY1:* 16)
Program ID: 140-31-21-497

Reno

University of Nevada (Reno) Program

Sponsor: University of Nevada School of Medicine
Ioannis A Lougaris Veterans Affairs Medical Center
Washoe Medical Center

Program Director:
Jon P Schrage, MD
Dept of Int Med
VA Med Ctr
1000 Locust St (111)
Reno, NV 89520
Tel: 702 328-1429 *Fax:* 702 328-1769
E-mail: intmed-reno@med.unr.edu
Internet: http://www.unr.edu/med
Accred Length: 3 Years *Program Size:* 35 (*GY1:* 15)
Program ID: 140-31-21-483

New Hampshire

Lebanon

Dartmouth-Hitchcock Medical Center Program

Sponsor: Mary Hitchcock Memorial Hospital
Veterans Affairs Medical Center (White River Junction)

Program Director:
Richard Comi, MD
Dartmouth-Hitchcock Med Ctr
One Medical Center Dr
Lebanon, NH 03756
Tel: 603 650-7684 *Fax:* 603 650-6122
E-mail: richard.comi@dartmouth.edu
Accred Length: 3 Years *Program Size:* 51 (*GY1:* 15)
Subspecialties: CCM, CD, END, GE, HO, ICE, ID, PCC, RHU
Program ID: 140-32-21-225

New Jersey

Atlantic City

Atlantic City Medical Center Program

Sponsor: Atlantic City Medical Center

Program Director:
Paul M Kirschenfeld, MD
Atlantic City Med Ctr
1925 Pacific Ave
Atlantic City, NJ 08401
Tel: 609 441-8074
Accred Length: 3 Years *Program Size:* 28 (*GY1:* 11)
Program ID: 140-33-31-226

Camden

UMDNJ-Robert Wood Johnson Medical School (Camden) Program

Sponsor: Cooper Hospital-University Medical Center

Program Director:
Glenn C Newell, MD
Cooper Hospital-Univ Med Ctr
401 Haddon Ave
E&R Bldg/Rm 242
Camden, NJ 08103
Tel: 609 757-7842 *Fax:* 609 968-9587
E-mail: samahasi@umdnj.edu
Internet: http://www.simon.umdnj.edu/medresidency
Accred Length: 3 Years *Program Size:* 46 (*GY1:* 24)
Subspecialties: CCM, CD, GE, HO, ID, NEP, PCC, RHU
Program ID: 140-33-21-227

Englewood

Mount Sinai School of Medicine (Englewood) Program

Sponsor: Mount Sinai School of Medicine
Englewood Hospital and Medical Center

Program Director:
Robin R Dibner, MD
Englewood Hospital and Med Ctr
PO Box 5479
Englewood, NJ 07631-5479
Tel: 201 894-3664, ext 3664 *Fax:* 201 894-0839
E-mail: margaret.maher@ehmc.com
Internet: http://www.englewoodhospital.com/residency program
Accred Length: 3 Years *Program Size:* 39 (*GY1:* 13)
Program ID: 140-33-21-228

Jersey City

Mount Sinai School of Medicine (Jersey City) Program

Sponsor: Mount Sinai School of Medicine
Jersey City Medical Center

Program Director:
Alan Greenberg, MD
Jersey City Med Ctr
50 Baldwin Ave
Jersey City, NJ 07304
Tel: 201 915-2430 *Fax:* 201 915-2219
Accred Length: 3 Years *Program Size:* 42 (*GY1:* 18)
Subspecialties: CD, GE
Program ID: 140-33-21-232

Livingston

St Barnabas Medical Center Program

Sponsor: St Barnabas Medical Center

Program Director:
Richard S Panush, MD
St Barnabas Med Ctr
Dept of Med
94 Old Short Hills Rd
Livingston, NJ 07039
Tel: 973 322-5645 *Fax:* 973 322-8215
E-mail: ppalma@sbhcs.com
Internet: http://www.saint barnabas medical center.com
Accred Length: 3 Years *Program Size:* 37 (*GY1:* 12)
Program ID: 140-33-12-457

Long Branch

Monmouth Medical Center Program

Sponsor: Monmouth Medical Center

Program Director:
Sara L Wallach, MD
Todd A Gruber, MD MPH
Monmouth Med Ctr
Dept of Med/Rm G-417
300 Second Ave
Long Branch, NJ 07740-9998
Tel: 732 923-6540 *Fax:* 732 923-6536
E-mail: wallach@auhs.edu
Internet: http://www.monmouthmedical.com
Accred Length: 3 Years *Program Size:* 36 (*GY1:* 12)
Program ID: 140-33-11-233

Montclair

Mountainside Hospital Program

Sponsor: Mountainside Hospital

Program Director:
Alan E Matook, MD
Mountainside Hospital
Bay and Highland Aves
Montclair, NJ 07042
Tel: 973 429-6195 *Fax:* 973 680-7970
E-mail: nancy.stio@mtn.ahsys.org
Accred Length: 3 Years *Program Size:* 24 (*GY1:* 8)
Program ID: 140-33-11-234

Morristown

Morristown Memorial Hospital Program

Sponsor: Morristown Memorial Hospital

Program Director:
Albert S Klainer, MD
Morristown Memorial Hospital
100 Madison Ave/PO Box 1956
Morristown, NJ 07962-1956
Tel: 973 971-5136 *Fax:* 973 290-7377
Internet: http://www.atlantichealth.org
Accred Length: 3 Years *Program Size:* 28 (*GY1:* 10)
Program ID: 140-33-11-235

Neptune

Jersey Shore Medical Center Program

Sponsor: Jersey Shore Medical Center

Program Director:
John A Crocco, MD
Jersey Shore Med Ctr, Dept of Med
1945 Rte 33
Neptune, NJ 07754
Tel: 908 776-4420 *Fax:* 908 776-4619
Accred Length: 3 Years *Program Size:* 42 (*GY1:* 16)
Program ID: 140-33-12-236

Newark

Newark Beth Israel Medical Center Program

Sponsor: Newark Beth Israel Medical Center
UMDNJ-University Hospital

Program Director:
Carlo Mainardi, MD
Newark Beth Israel Med Ctr
201 Lyons Ave
Newark, NJ 07112
Tel: 201 926-7333 *Fax:* 201 926-5340
Accred Length: 3 Years *Program Size:* 41 (*GY1:* 15)
Program ID: 140-33-21-518

UMDNJ-New Jersey Medical School Program

Sponsor: UMDNJ-New Jersey Medical School
Hackensack University Medical Center
UMDNJ-University Hospital
Veterans Affairs Medical Center (East Orange)

Program Director:
Marilyn A Miller, MD
UMDNJ-New Jersey Med Sch
150 Bergen St
Level 1/Rm 248
Newark, NJ 07103-2406
Tel: 973 972-6056 *Fax:* 973 972-3129
E-mail: msimmons@umdnj.edu
Internet:
http://www.umdnj.edu/njmsweb/med/medres1.htm
Accred Length: 3 Years *Program Size:* 109 (*GY1:* 39)
Subspecialties: CD, END, GE, ID, IMG, NEP, PCC
Program ID: 140-33-21-237

Paterson

St Joseph's Hospital and Medical Center Program

Sponsor: St Joseph's Hospital and Medical Center

Program Director:
Richard A Gleckman, MD
St Joseph's Hospital and Med Ctr
703 Main St
Paterson, NJ 07503
Tel: 973 754-2476, ext 2431 *Fax:* 973 754-3376
Internet: http://www.sjhmc.org
Accred Length: 3 Years *Program Size:* 41 (*GY1:* 16)
Program ID: 140-33-21-522

Perth Amboy

Raritan Bay Medical Center-Perth Amboy Division Program

Sponsor: Raritan Bay Medical Center-Perth Amboy Division

Program Director:
Purnendu Sen, MD
Raritan Bay Med Ctr-Perth Amboy Div
530 New Brunswick Ave
Perth Amboy, NJ 08861-3685
Tel: 908 324-5080 *Fax:* 908 324-4669
Accred Length: 3 Years *Program Size:* 24 (*GY1:* 7)
Program ID: 140-33-21-466

Piscataway

UMDNJ-Robert Wood Johnson Medical School Program

Sponsor: UMDNJ-Robert Wood Johnson Medical School
Medical Center at Princeton
Robert Wood Johnson University Hospital

Program Director:
Nayan K Kothari, MD
UMDNJ-Robert Wood Johnson Med Sch
One Robert Wood Johnson Pl/PO Box 19
New Brunswick, NJ 08903-0019
Tel: 732 235-7742 *Fax:* 732 235-7427
Accred Length: 3 Years *Program Size:* 112 (*GY1:* 40)
Subspecialties: CD, END, GE, HO, ID, NEP, PCC, RHU
Program ID: 140-33-21-243

Plainfield

Muhlenberg Regional Medical Center Program

Sponsor: Muhlenberg Regional Medical Center

Program Director:
Francis L Griffin, MD
Muhlenberg Regional Med Ctr
Park Ave and Randolph Rd
Plainfield, NJ 07061
Tel: 908 668-2985 *Fax:* 908 668-2814
E-mail: meded@injersey.com
Internet: http://www.muhlenberg.com
Accred Length: 3 Years *Program Size:* 30 (*GY1:* 9)
Program ID: 140-33-11-244

South Orange

Seton Hall University School of Graduate Medical Education Program

Sponsor: Seton Hall University School of Graduate Medical Education
St Elizabeth Hospital
St Joseph's Hospital and Medical Center
St Michael's Medical Center (Cathedral Hlth Srvcs Inc)

Program Director:
Ernest E Federici, MD
Dept of Medicine
400 S Orange Ave
South Orange, NJ 07079
Tel: 908 527-5257 *Fax:* 908 351-7930
Internet: http://www.shu.edu
Accred Length: 3 Years *Program Size:* 78 (*GY1:* 27)
Subspecialties: CCM, CD, END, GE, HEM, ID, ON, PUD, RHU
Program ID: 140-33-21-498

Summit

Overlook Hospital Program

Sponsor: Overlook Hospital

Program Director:
Douglas Ratner, MD
Overlook Hospital
99 Beauvoir Ave
PO Box 220
Summit, NJ 07902-0220
Tel: 908 522-2968 *Fax:* 908 522-0804
E-mail: sharonda.dixon@oh.ahsys.org
Accred Length: 3 Years *Program Size:* 24 (*GY1:* 8)
Program ID: 140-33-11-245

Trenton

Capital Health System-Fuld Campus Program

Sponsor: Capital Health System-Fuld Campus

Program Director:
Martin J Glynn, MD
Capital Health System-Fuld Campus
750 Brunswick Ave
Trenton, NJ 08638
Tel: 609 394-6031 *Fax:* 609 394-6028
Accred Length: 3 Years *Program Size:* 29 (*GY1:* 10)
Program ID: 140-33-21-246

New Mexico

Albuquerque

University of New Mexico Program

Sponsor: University of New Mexico School of Medicine
University Hospital
Veterans Affairs Medical Center (Albuquerque)

Program Director:
Ann Gateley, MD
Univ of New Mexico Sch of Med
Dept of Int Med
2211 Lomas Blvd NE
Albuquerque, NM 87131-5271
Tel: 505 272-6331 *Fax:* 505 272-4628
E-mail: pmcbride@salud.unm.edu
Internet: http://www.unm.edu
Accred Length: 3 Years *Program Size:* 71 (*GY1:* 25)
Subspecialties: CCM, CD, END, GE, HEM, HO, ID, IMG, NEP, ON, PCC, PUD, RHU
Program ID: 140-34-21-247

New York

Albany

Albany Medical Center Program

Sponsor: Albany Medical Center
Veterans Affairs Medical Center (Albany)

Program Director:
Alwin F Steinmann, MD
Albany Med Ctr Hospital
Medicine Education Office/MC-17
47 New Scotland Ave
Albany, NY 12208
Tel: 518 262-5377 *Fax:* 518 262-6873
E-mail: rodi_worgan@ccgateway.amc.edu
Internet: http://www.amc.edu
Accred Length: 3 Years *Program Size:* 61 (*GY1:* 29)
Subspecialties: CD, END, GE, HEM, ID, IMG, NEP, ON, PCC, RHU
Program ID: 140-35-31-248

Binghamton

Wilson Memorial Regional Medical Center (United Health Services) Program

Sponsor: Wilson Memorial Regional Medical Center (United Health Svs)

Program Director:
Roy D Gill, MD
Wilson Hospital
Div of United Health Services
33-57 Harrison St
Johnson City, NY 13790
Tel: 607 763-6391 *Fax:* 607 763-6888
E-mail: linda_kinsey@uhs.org
Accred Length: 3 Years *Program Size:* 28 (*GY1:* 9)
Program ID: 140-35-31-255

Bronx

Albert Einstein College of Medicine (Jacobi) Program

Sponsor: Albert Einstein College of Medicine of Yeshiva University
Jacobi Medical Center
Montefiore Medical Center-Weiler Hospital

Program Director:
Steve C Martin, MD
Dept of Med 3N1
1400 Pelham Pkwy S
Bronx, NY 10461
Tel: 718 918-5640 *Fax:* 718 918-7460
E-mail: smartin@aecom.yu.edu
Internet: http://www.jacobimedicine.com
Accred Length: 3 Years *Program Size:* 100 (*GY1:* 37)
Program ID: 140-35-31-521

Albert Einstein College of Medicine Program

Sponsor: Albert Einstein College of Medicine of Yeshiva University
Montefiore Medical Center-Henry and Lucy Moses Division
Montefiore Medical Center-Weiler Hospital
North Central Bronx Hospital

Program Director:
Joan I Casey, MD
Montefiore Medical Ctr
111 E 210th St
Bronx, NY 10467
Tel: 718 920-6097 *Fax:* 718 515-6103
E-mail: jcasey@aecom.yu.
Internet: http://www.medicine.aecom.yu.edu
Accred Length: 3 Years *Program Size:* 140 (*GY1:* 45)
Subspecialties: CCM, CD, END, GE, HEM, ICE, ID, IMG, NEP, ON, PCC, RHU
Program ID: 140-35-21-287

Bronx-Lebanon Hospital Center Program

Sponsor: Bronx-Lebanon Hospital Center

Program Director:
Jonathan W M Gold, MD
Bronx-Lebanon Hospital Ctr
1650 Grand Concourse/8th Fl
Bronx, NY 10457
Tel: 718 518-5812 *Fax:* 718 518-5001
Accred Length: 3 Years *Program Size:* 84 (*GY1:* 28)
Subspecialties: CD, GE, NEP, PUD
Program ID: 140-35-11-263

Lincoln Medical and Mental Health Center Program

Sponsor: Lincoln Medical and Mental Health Center

Program Director:
Anita Soni, MD
Lincoln Medical and Mental Health Ctr
234 E 149th St
Bronx, NY 10451
Tel: 718 579-5874 *Fax:* 718 579-4836
E-mail: lincoln@lmmhc.org
Internet: http://www.lmmhc.org
Accred Length: 3 Years *Program Size:* 83 (*GY1:* 29)
Subspecialties: CCM, END
Program ID: 140-35-21-470

Mount Sinai School of Medicine (Bronx) Program

Sponsor: Mount Sinai School of Medicine
Veterans Affairs Medical Center (Bronx)

Program Director:
Mark A Korsten, MD
Bronx VA Med Ctr
130 W Kingsbridge Rd
Bronx, NY 10468
Tel: 718 584-9000, ext 6753 *Fax:* 718 579-1635
E-mail: collins.anitra@bronx.va.gov
Accred Length: 3 Years *Program Size:* 24 (*GY1:* 8)
Program ID: 140-35-31-517

New York Medical College (Our Lady of Mercy) Program

Sponsor: New York Medical College
Our Lady of Mercy Medical Center

Program Director:
Barry J Fomberstein, MD
Our Lady of Mercy Med Ctr
Dept of Med
600 E 233rd St
Bronx, NY 10466
Tel: 718 920-9168 *Fax:* 718 920-9036
E-mail: bfomberstein@pol.net
Accred Length: 3 Years *Program Size:* 68 (*GY1:* 28)
Subspecialties: GE, IMG
Program ID: 140-35-21-285

St Barnabas Hospital Program

Sponsor: St Barnabas Hospital

Program Director:
James G Hellerman, MD
St Barnabas Hospital
Third Ave and 183rd St
Bronx, NY 10457
Tel: 718 960-6202 *Fax:* 718 960-3486
Accred Length: 3 Years *Program Size:* 89 (*GY1:* 30)
Program ID: 140-35-21-485

Brooklyn

Brookdale University Hospital Medical Center Program

Sponsor: Brookdale University Hospital Medical Center

Program Director:
Ethan D Fried, MD
Brookdale Univ Hospital and Med Ctr
Dept of Med
One Brookdale Plaza
Brooklyn, NY 11212
Tel: 718 240-6205 *Fax:* 718 240-6505
E-mail: jmcgarit@brookdale.edu
Internet:
http://www.brookdalehospital.com/html/medicine_mission_statement.html
Accred Length: 3 Years *Program Size:* 76 (*GY1:* 28)
Subspecialties: END, HO, NEP, PUD
Program ID: 140-35-11-264

Brooklyn Hospital Center Program

Sponsor: Brooklyn Hospital Center

Program Director:
Eliot J Lazar, MD
Brooklyn Hospital Ctr
121 DeKalb Ave
Brooklyn, NY 11201
Tel: 718 250-6925 *Fax:* 718 250-8120
Internet: http://www.tbh.org
Accred Length: 3 Years *Program Size:* 87 (*GY1:* 35)
Subspecialties: CD, GE, HEM, ON, PUD
Program ID: 140-35-12-265

Coney Island Hospital Program

Sponsor: Coney Island Hospital

Program Director:
Sandor A Friedman, MD
Coney Island Hospital
2601 Ocean Pkwy
Brooklyn, NY 11235
Tel: 718 616-3786 *Fax:* 718 616-3797
Accred Length: 3 Years *Program Size:* 63 (*GY1:* 23)
Subspecialties: CD, END, HEM, PUD
Program ID: 140-35-11-269

Interfaith Medical Center Program

Sponsor: Interfaith Medical Center

Program Director:
Eric A Jaffe, MD
Interfaith Med Ctr
555 Prospect Pl
Brooklyn, NY 11238
Tel: 718 935-7325 *Fax:* 718 935-7323
Accred Length: 3 Years *Program Size:* 83 (*GY1:* 25)
Subspecialties: CD, END, GE, HEM, ON, PUD
Program ID: 140-35-21-276

Kingsbrook Jewish Medical Center Program

Sponsor: Kingsbrook Jewish Medical Center

Program Director:
Mohammad Zahir, MD
Kingsbrook Jewish Med Ctr
David Minkin Plaza
585 Schenectady Ave
Brooklyn, NY 11203-1891
Tel: 718 604-5401 *Fax:* 718 604-5450
E-mail: kjmc.med@mindspring.com
Accred Length: 3 Years *Program Size:* 47 (*GY1:* 13)
Program ID: 140-35-11-277

Long Island College Hospital Program

Sponsor: Long Island College Hospital

Program Director:
Jeffrey S Viera, MD
Long Island College Hospital, Dept of Med
339 Hicks St
Brooklyn, NY 11201
Tel: 718 780-1881 *Fax:* 718 780-1300
Accred Length: 3 Years *Program Size:* 68 (*GY1:* 28)
Subspecialties: CD, GE, HO, ID, NEP, PUD
Program ID: 140-35-11-280

Lutheran Medical Center Program

Sponsor: Lutheran Medical Center

Program Director:
Robert Cucco, MD
Lutheran Med Ctr
Med Educ Office
150 55th St
Brooklyn, NY 11220-2574
Tel: 718 630-7350 *Fax:* 718 630-6322
E-mail: ldamato@lmcmc.com
Internet: http://www.lmcmc.com
Accred Length: 3 Years *Program Size:* 66 (*GY1:* 22)
Program ID: 140-35-11-282

Maimonides Medical Center Program

Sponsor: Maimonides Medical Center

Program Director:
Edgar Lichstein, MD
Maimonides Med Ctr
4802 Tenth Ave
Brooklyn, NY 11219
Tel: 718 283-7074 *Fax:* 718 283-8498
Accred Length: 3 Years *Program Size:* 66 (*GY1:* 22)
Subspecialties: CCM, CD, GE, HO, ID, IMG, NEP, PUD, TY
Program ID: 140-35-11-283

New York Methodist Hospital (Wyckoff Heights) Program

Sponsor: New York Methodist Hospital
Wyckoff Heights Medical Center

Program Director:
Gerald Posner, MD
Dept of Med
374 Stockholm St
Brooklyn, NY 11237
Tel: 718 963-7586 *Fax:* 718 486-4270
Accred Length: 3 Years *Program Size:* 54 (*GY1:* 22)
Program ID: 140-35-21-520

Programs

New York Methodist Hospital Program

Sponsor: New York Methodist Hospital

Program Director:
Harvey Dosik, MD
New York Methodist Hospital
Dept of Med
506 Sixth St
Brooklyn, NY 11215
Tel: 718 780-5246 *Fax:* 718 780-3259
E-mail: hkleinba@nyh.med.cornell.edu
Internet:
http://www.nym.org/education/residencies/residencies.html
Accred Length: 3 Years *Program Size:* 92 (*GY1:* 39)
Subspecialties: HEM, IMG, ON, PUD
Program ID: 140-35-11-284

SUNY Health Science Center at Brooklyn Program

Sponsor: SUNY Health Science Center at Brooklyn
Kings County Hospital Center
University Hospital-SUNY Health Science Center at Brooklyn
Veterans Affairs Medical Center (Brooklyn)

Program Director:
Stephan L Kamholz, MD
SUNY Health Science Ctr-Brooklyn
450 Clarkson Ave
Brooklyn, NY 11203
Tel: 718 270-1574 *Fax:* 718 270-4030
Internet: http://www.hscbklyn.edu/suny
Accred Length: 3 Years *Program Size:* 138 (*GY1:* 52)
Subspecialties: CCM, CD, END, GE, HO, ICE, ID, NEP, PUD, RHU
Program ID: 140-35-21-305

Woodhull Medical and Mental Health Center Program

Sponsor: Woodhull Medical and Mental Health Center

Program Director:
Andres R Hernandez, MD
760 Broadway
Brooklyn, NY 11206
Tel: 718 963-5806 *Fax:* 718 963-8753
Accred Length: 3 Years *Program Size:* 46 (*GY1:* 13)
Program ID: 140-35-21-487

Buffalo

SUNY at Buffalo Graduate Medical-Dental Education Consortium (Mercy Hospital) Program

Sponsor: SUNY at Buffalo Grad Medical-Dental Education Consortium
Mercy Hospital of Buffalo

Program Director:
Thomas A Raab, MD
Mercy Hospital
Dept of Med
565 Abbott Rd
Buffalo, NY 14220
Tel: 716 828-2578 *Fax:* 716 828-2744
E-mail: traab@mercywny.org
Internet: http://wings.buffalo.edu/smbs/med/mhob.htm/
Accred Length: 3 Years *Program Size:* 19 (*GY1:* 7)
Program ID: 140-35-31-249

SUNY at Buffalo Graduate Medical-Dental Education Consortium (Millard Fillmore) Program

Sponsor: SUNY at Buffalo Grad Medical-Dental Education Consortium
CGF Health System (Millard Fillmore Hospitals)

Program Director:
Joseph L Izzo Jr, MD
Millard Fillmore Hospitals
Dept of Int Med
3 Gates Cir
Buffalo, NY 14209
Tel: 716 887-4694 *Fax:* 716 887-4382
Internet: http://www.smbs.buffalo.edu/med/im
Accred Length: 3 Years *Program Size:* 39 (*GY1:* 10)
Program ID: 140-35-31-250

SUNY at Buffalo Graduate Medical-Dental Education Consortium (Sisters of Charity) Program

Sponsor: SUNY at Buffalo Grad Medical-Dental Education Consortium
Sisters of Charity Hospital

Program Director:
Khalid J Qazi, MD
Sisters of Charity Hospital
2157 Main St
Buffalo, NY 14214
Tel: 716 862-2371 *Fax:* 716 862-1420
E-mail: kqazi@acsu.buffalo.edu
Internet: http://www.sisters_buffalo.org
Accred Length: 3 Years *Program Size:* 18 (*GY1:* 7)
Program ID: 140-35-21-251

SUNY at Buffalo Graduate Medical-Dental Education Consortium Program

Sponsor: SUNY at Buffalo Grad Medical-Dental Education Consortium
CGF Health System (Buffalo General Hospital)
Erie County Medical Center
Veterans Affairs Medical Center (Buffalo)

Program Director:
Robert A Klocke, MD
Erie County Med Ctr, Dept of Med
462 Grider St
Buffalo, NY 14215-3098
Tel: 716 898-5210 *Fax:* 716 898-3279
Internet: http://www.smbs.buffalo.edu/med/imrp
Accred Length: 3 Years *Program Size:* 82 (*GY1:* 25)
Subspecialties: CD, END, GE, HEM, ID, IMG, NEP, ON, PCC, RHU
Program ID: 140-35-31-252

Cooperstown

Bassett Healthcare Program

Sponsor: Bassett Healthcare
Mary Imogene Bassett Hospital

Program Director:
Henry F Weil, MD
Office of Med Education
Bassett Healthcare
One Atwell Rd
Cooperstown, NY 13326-1394
Tel: 607 547-3764 *Fax:* 607 547-6612
E-mail: bassedty@telenet.net
Internet: http://www.bassett.edu
Accred Length: 3 Years *Program Size:* 27 (*GY1:* 12)
Program ID: 140-35-11-253

East Meadow

SUNY at Stony Brook (East Meadow) Program

Sponsor: Nassau County Medical Center

Program Director:
Faroque A Khan, MB
Nassau County Med Ctr
2201 Hempstead Trnpk
East Meadow, NY 11554-5400
Tel: 516 572-6501 *Fax:* 516 572-5609
E-mail: mamurphy@ncmc.co.nassau.ny.us
Internet: http://www.ncmc.co.nassau.ny.us
Accred Length: 3 Years *Program Size:* 70 (*GY1:* 25)
Subspecialties: CD, END, GE, HEM, ID, NEP, ON, PUD
Program ID: 140-35-21-254

Elmhurst

Mount Sinai School of Medicine (Elmhurst) Program

Sponsor: Mount Sinai School of Medicine
Elmhurst Hospital Center-Mount Sinai Services
Mount Sinai Medical Center

Program Director:
Rand David, MD
Mount Sinai Sch of Med-Elmhurst
Elmhurst Hospital Ctr
79-01 Broadway/Rm D1-24
Elmhurst, NY 11373
Tel: 718 334-3444 *Fax:* 718 334-5845
Accred Length: 3 Years *Program Size:* 40 (*GY1:* 16)
Subspecialties: CD, GE, PUD
Program ID: 140-35-11-268

Far Rockaway

St John's Episcopal Hospital-South Shore Program

Sponsor: St John's Episcopal Hospital-South Shore
SUNY Health Science Center at Brooklyn

Program Director:
Sheldon Markowitz, MD
Samuel Bavli, MD
St John's Episcopal Hospital-South Shore
Dept of Med
327 Beach 19th St
Far Rockaway, NY 11691
Tel: 718 869-7672 *Fax:* 718 869-8530
E-mail: gmurphy@ehs.org
Internet: http://www.ehs.org/ssmed.htm
Accred Length: 3 Years *Program Size:* 50 (*GY1:* 18)
Program ID: 140-35-21-486

Flushing

New York Flushing Hospital Medical Center Program

Sponsor: New York Flushing Hospital Medical Center

Program Director:
George T Martin, MD
New York Flushing Hospital Med Ctr
Dept of Med
45th Ave at Parsons Blvd
Flushing, NY 11355
Tel: 718 670-5939 *Fax:* 718 670-4510
Accred Length: 3 Years *Program Size:* 52 (*GY1:* 24)
Subspecialties: IMG
Program ID: 140-35-11-272

New York Hospital Medical Center of Queens/Cornell University Medical College Program

Sponsor: New York Hospital Medical Center of Queens

Program Director:
Terence M Brady, MD
New York Hospital Med Ctr of Queens
Dept of Med
56-45 Main St
Flushing, NY 11355-2966
Tel: 718 670-1347 *Fax:* 718 461-2943
Accred Length: 3 Years *Program Size:* 70 (*GY1:* 32)
Subspecialties: GE, ID, NEP, PUD
Program ID: 140-35-11-262

Forest Hills

North Shore University Hospital at Forest Hills Program

Sponsor: North Shore University Hospital at Forest Hills
Syosset Community Hospital

Program Director:
Elizabeth G McDonald, MD
North Shore Univ Hospital at Forest Hills
102-01 66th Rd
Forest Hills, NY 11375
Tel: 718 830-4358 *Fax:* 718 459-9541
Accred Length: 3 Years *Program Size:* 38 (*GY1:* 14)
Program ID: 140-35-21-468

Jamaica

Catholic Medical Center of Brooklyn and Queens Program

Sponsor: Catholic Medical Center of Brooklyn and Queens Inc
Catholic Medical Center (Mary Immaculate Hospital)
Catholic Medical Center (St John's Queens Hospital)

Program Director:
Frantz Duffoo, MD
Catholic Med Ctr of Brooklyn and Queens
88-25 153rd St
Jamaica, NY 11432
Tel: 718 558-7150 *Fax:* 718 558-7156
Accred Length: 3 Years *Program Size:* 69 (*GY1:* 25)
Subspecialties: CD, GE, ID, IMG, PUD
Program ID: 140-35-22-267

Jamaica Hospital Program

Sponsor: Jamaica Hospital

Program Director:
Thomas Santucci Jr, MD
Jamaica Hospital Med Ctr
8900 Van Wyck Expwy
Jamaica, NY 11418-9848
Tel: 718 206-6668 *Fax:* 718 206-6652
E-mail: hrosen1215@aol.com
Internet: http://www.jamaicahospital.org
Accred Length: 3 Years *Program Size:* 42 (*GY1:* 11)
Program ID: 140-35-12-275

Mount Sinai School of Medicine (Jamaica) Program

Sponsor: Mount Sinai School of Medicine
Queens Hospital Center

Program Director:
Fred Rosner, MD
Queens Hospital Ctr
Dept of Med
82-68 164th St
Jamaica, NY 11432
Tel: 718 883-4080 *Fax:* 718 883-6197
Accred Length: 3 Years *Program Size:* 45 (*GY1:* 15)
Subspecialties: HO, ID
Program ID: 140-35-21-510

Manhasset

North Shore University Hospital/NYU School of Medicine Program

Sponsor: North Shore University Hospital

Program Director:
Peter M Reiser, MD
North Shore Univ Hospital
Dept of Med
300 Community Dr
Manhasset, NY 11030
Tel: 516 562-2944 *Fax:* 516 562-3555
E-mail: preiser@nshs.edu
Internet: http://www.nshs.edu
Accred Length: 3 Years *Program Size:* 92 (*GY1:* 34)
Subspecialties: CCM, CD, GE, HEM, HO, ICE, ID, IMG, NEP, ON, PCC, RHU
Program ID: 140-35-21-271

Mineola

Winthrop-University Hospital Program

Sponsor: Winthrop-University Hospital

Program Director:
John F Aloia, MD
Winthrop-Univ Hospital
259 First St
Mineola, NY 11501
Tel: 516 663-2381 *Fax:* 516 663-8796
Internet: http://www.winthrop.org
Accred Length: 3 Years *Program Size:* 81 (*GY1:* 37)
Subspecialties: CD, END, GE, HO, ID, IMG, NEP, PCC, RHU
Program ID: 140-35-11-256

Mount Vernon

Mount Vernon Hospital Program

Sponsor: Mount Vernon Hospital

Program Director:
Zev Carrey, MD
Mount Vernon Hospital
12 N Seventh Ave/Rm 501
Mount Vernon, NY 10550-2098
Tel: 914 664-8000, ext 3276 *Fax:* 914 664-2416
Accred Length: 3 Years *Program Size:* 24 (*GY1:* 8)
Program ID: 140-35-21-482

New Hyde Park

Albert Einstein College of Medicine at Long Island Jewish Medical Center Program

Sponsor: Long Island Jewish Medical Center

Program Director:
Steven J Walerstein, MD
Long Island Jewish Med Ctr
270-05 76th Ave
New Hyde Park, NY 11040
Tel: 718 470-7270 *Fax:* 718 470-0827
E-mail: walerste@lij.edu
Internet: http://www.lij.edu/lij-homepage-ns.html
Accred Length: 3 Years *Program Size:* 62 (*GY1:* 30)
Subspecialties: CD, END, GE, HO, ICE, ID, IMG, NEP, PCC, RHU
Program ID: 140-35-21-281

New Rochelle

New York Medical College (Sound Shore) Program

Sponsor: New York Medical College
Sound Shore Medical Center of Westchester

Program Director:
Jeffrey M Brensilver, MD
Sound Shore Med Ctr of Westchester
Dept of Med
16 Guion Pl
New Rochelle, NY 10802-5500
Tel: 914 637-1681 *Fax:* 914 637-1171
E-mail: ssmcw@cris.com
Internet:
http://www.concentric.net/~ssmcw/residency.shtml
Accred Length: 3 Years *Program Size:* 36 (*GY1:* 16)
Program ID: 140-35-11-258

New York

Albert Einstein College of Medicine at Beth Israel Medical Center Program

Sponsor: Beth Israel Medical Center

Program Director:
Adrienne M Fleckman, MD
Beth Israel Med Ctr
Dept of Med
First Ave at 16th St
New York, NY 10003
Tel: 212 420-4050 *Fax:* 212 420-4615
E-mail: intmed@bethisraelny.org
Internet:
http://www.bethisraelny.org/professionals/residency
Accred Length: 3 Years *Program Size:* 103 (*GY1:* 39)
Subspecialties: CD, END, GE, HO, ID, NEP, PCC
Program ID: 140-35-11-261

Harlem Hospital Center Program

Sponsor: Harlem Hospital Center

Program Director:
Alfred R Ashford, MD
Harlem Hospital Ctr, Dept of Int Med
506 Lenox Ave
New York, NY 10037
Tel: 212 939-1419 *Fax:* 212 939-1053
Accred Length: 3 Years *Program Size:* 74 (*GY1:* 25)
Subspecialties: CD, GE, ID, NEP, PUD
Program ID: 140-35-11-273

Lenox Hill Hospital Program

Sponsor: Lenox Hill Hospital

Program Director:
Michael S Bruno, MD
Lenox Hill Hospital
100 E 77th St
New York, NY 10021-1883
Tel: 212 434-2140 *Fax:* 212 434-2446
E-mail: 105541.1672@compuserve.com
Accred Length: 3 Years *Program Size:* 86 (*GY1:* 38)
Subspecialties: CD, GE, HO, NEP, PUD
Program ID: 140-35-11-278

Mount Sinai School of Medicine (Cabrini) Program

Sponsor: Mount Sinai School of Medicine
Cabrini Medical Center

Program Director:
Wilfredo Talavera, MD
Cabrini Med Ctr
Dept of Med
227 E 19th St/D-301
New York, NY 10003
Tel: 212 995-6629 *Fax:* 212 979-3425
Internet: http://www.cabrininy.org
Accred Length: 3 Years *Program Size:* 66 (*GY1:* 32)
Subspecialties: CD, GE, HO, ID, PUD, RHU
Program ID: 140-35-31-266

Mount Sinai School of Medicine (North General) Program

Sponsor: North General Hospital

Program Director:
Samuel J Daniel, MD
North General Hospital
Dept of Int Med
1879 Madison Ave
New York, NY 10035
Tel: 212 423-4155 *Fax:* 212 423-4399
Accred Length: 3 Years *Program Size:* 31 (*GY1:* 10)
Program ID: 140-35-11-274

Mount Sinai School of Medicine Program

Sponsor: Mount Sinai School of Medicine
Elmhurst Hospital Center-Mount Sinai Services
Mount Sinai Medical Center
Veterans Affairs Medical Center (Bronx)

Program Director:
Lawrence G Smith, MD
Mount Sinai Hospital
One Gustave L Levy Pl
Box 1118
New York, NY 10029-6574
Tel: 212 241-6609 *Fax:* 212 534-3488
E-mail: lsantiago@smtplink.mssm.edu
Internet: http://www.mssm.edu
Accred Length: 3 Years *Program Size:* 124 (*GY1:* 50)
Subspecialties: CCM, CD, END, GE, HO, ICE, ID, IMG, NEP, PCC, RHU
Program ID: 140-35-31-288

New York and Presbyterian Hospital (Columbia Campus) Program

Sponsor: New York and Presbyterian Hospital
New York and Presbyterian Hospital (Columbia Campus)

Program Director:
Peter Gordon, MD
Presbyterian Hospital
622 W 168th St/PH 8/Rm 109
New York, NY 10032
Tel: 212 305-3387 *Fax:* 212 305-8466
Internet: http://cpmcnet.columbia.edu
Accred Length: 3 Years *Program Size:* 129 (*GY1:* 46)
Subspecialties: CCM, CD, END, GE, HO, ICE, ID, NEP, PUD, RHU
Program ID: 140-35-11-297

New York and Presbyterian Hospital (Cornell Campus) Program

Sponsor: New York and Presbyterian Hospital
Memorial Sloan-Kettering Cancer Center
New York and Presbyterian Hospital (Cornell Campus)

Program Director:
Mark S Pecker, MD
New York Presbyterian Hospital (New York-Cornell Campus)
Dept of Med Box 130
525 E 68th St
New York, NY 10021
Tel: 212 746-4749 *Fax:* 212 746-6692
E-mail: jmacalu@mail.med.cornell.edu
Internet: http://www.nycornell.org/medicine
Accred Length: 3 Years *Program Size:* 129 (*GY1:* 43)
Subspecialties: CCM, CD, END, GE, HO, ICE, ID, IMG, NEP, PCC, PUD, RHU
Program ID: 140-35-21-270

New York Medical College (Metropolitan) Program

Sponsor: New York Medical College
Metropolitan Hospital Center

Program Director:
Shobhana A Chaudhari, MD MD
Metropolitan Hospital Ctr
1901 First Ave
New York, NY 10029
Tel: 212 423-6771 *Fax:* 212 423-8099
Accred Length: 3 Years *Program Size:* 56 (*GY1:* 24)
Subspecialties: CD, NEP
Program ID: 140-35-31-290

New York Medical College at St Vincent's Hospital and Medical Center of New York Program

Sponsor: New York Medical College
St Vincent's Hospital and Medical Center of New York

Program Director:
Steven L Sivak, MD
St Vincent's Hospital and Med Ctr
153 W 11th St
New York, NY 10011
Tel: 212 604-7512 *Fax:* 212 604-3286
E-mail: sivak@nymc.edu
Internet: http://svh.nymc.edu
Accred Length: 3 Years *Program Size:* 78 (*GY1:* 34)
Subspecialties: CCM, CD, END, GE, HO, ID, IMG, NEP, PCC
Program ID: 140-35-11-302

New York University Medical Center (Veterans) Program

Sponsor: New York University Medical Center
Veterans Affairs Medical Center (Manhattan)

Program Director:
Robert F Raicht, MD
VA Med Ctr
First Ave at E 24th St
New York, NY 10010
Tel: 212 686-6768, ext 4868 *Fax:* 212 951-5981
Internet: http://www.med.nyu.edu/medicine/page1.html
Accred Length: 3 Years *Program Size:* 40 (*GY1:* 18)
Subspecialties: CD
Program ID: 140-35-21-294

New York University Medical Center Program

Sponsor: New York University Medical Center
Bellevue Hospital Center
Veterans Affairs Medical Center (Manhattan)

Program Director:
Saul J Farber, MD
New York Univ Med Ctr
Dept of Med
550 First Ave
New York, NY 10016
Tel: 212 263-6394 *Fax:* 212 263-7700
Accred Length: 3 Years *Program Size:* 114 (*GY1:* 36)
Subspecialties: CD, END, GE, HEM, ICE, ID, IMG, NEP, ON, PCC, RHU
Program ID: 140-35-21-292

NYU Downtown Hospital Program

Sponsor: NYU Downtown Hospital

Program Director:
Bruce Logan, MD
New York Univ Downtown Hospital
Dept of Med
170 William St
New York, NY 10038
Tel: 212 312-5760
Internet: http://www.nyudh.med.nyu.edu/residency.html
Accred Length: 3 Years *Program Size:* 46 (*GY1:* 18)
Program ID: 140-35-31-289

St Luke's-Roosevelt Hospital Center Program

Sponsor: St Luke's-Roosevelt Hospital Center
St Luke's-Roosevelt Hospital Center-Roosevelt Division
St Luke's-Roosevelt Hospital Center-St Luke's Division

Program Director:
Michael Lesch, MD
St Luke's-Roosevelt Hospital Ctr
1000 Tenth Ave
Rm 3A-02
New York, NY 10019
Tel: 212 523-7333 *Fax:* 212 523-8605
Internet: http://www.docnet.org
Accred Length: 3 Years *Program Size:* 118 (*GY1:* 51)
Subspecialties: CD, END, GE, HEM, ICE, ID, IMG, NEP, ON, PCC, RHU
Program ID: 140-35-21-301

Rochester

Highland Hospital of Rochester Program

Sponsor: Highland Hospital of Rochester

Program Director:
Jamie E Kerr, MD
Highland Hospital of Rochester
1000 South Ave
Rochester, NY 14620
Tel: 716 461-6776 *Fax:* 716 256-3243
E-mail: jkerr@highland.rochester.edu
Accred Length: 3 Years *Program Size:* 6 (*GY1:* 0)
Program ID: 140-35-11-310

St Mary's Hospital Program

Sponsor: St Mary's Hospital (Unity Health System)

Program Director:
Eric A Richard, MD
Unity Health System
Dept of Med
1555 Long Pond Rd
Rochester, NY 14626
Tel: 716 723-7775 *Fax:* 716 723-7834
Accred Length: 3 Years *Program Size:* 37 (*GY1:* 13)
Program ID: 140-35-11-312

University of Rochester (Rochester General) Program

Sponsor: Strong Memorial Hospital of the University of Rochester
Genesee Hospital
Rochester General Hospital

Program Director:
Craig B Kaplan, MD MA
Genesee Hospital
Medical Education
Fifth Fl North Wing
Rochester, NY 14607
Tel: 716 922-7750 *Fax:* 716 922-7710
E-mail: craig.kaplan@viahealth.org
Internet:
http://www.urmc.rochester.edu/smd/medicine/res/residency.htm
Accred Length: 3 Years *Program Size:* 51 (*GY1:* 21)
Program ID: 140-35-31-314

University of Rochester Program

Sponsor: Strong Memorial Hospital of the University of Rochester

Program Director:
Donald R Bordley, MD
Univ of Rochester Med Ctr
601 Elmwood Ave/PO Box MED
Rochester, NY 14642
Tel: 716 275-2873 *Fax:* 716 442-3695
E-mail: donald_bordley@urmc.rochester.edu
Internet:
http://www.urmc.rochester.edu/smd/medicine/res/residency.htm
Accred Length: 3 Years *Program Size:* 69 (*GY1:* 24)
Subspecialties: CCM, CD, END, GE, HO, ICE, ID, IMG, NEP, PCC, RHU
Program ID: 140-35-11-313

Staten Island

New York Medical College (Richmond) Program

Sponsor: New York Medical College
Sisters of Charity Medical Center-St Vincent's Campus

Program Director:
Susan D Grossman, MD
Sisters of Charity Med Ctr-St Vincent's Campus
335 Bard Ave
Staten Island, NY 10310-1699
Tel: 718 876-2416 *Fax:* 718 876-3225
Accred Length: 3 Years *Program Size:* 53 (*GY1:* 27)
Subspecialties: CD
Program ID: 140-35-11-303

Staten Island University Hospital Program

Sponsor: Staten Island University Hospital

Program Director:
Thomas G McGinn, MD
Staten Island Univ Hospital
475 Seaview Ave
Staten Island, NY 10305
Tel: 718 390-9506 *Fax:* 718 226-8966
E-mail: tmcginn@siuh.edu
Internet: http://www.siuh.edu
Accred Length: 3 Years *Program Size:* 78 (*GY1:* 37)
Subspecialties: IMG
Program ID: 140-35-11-304

Stony Brook

SUNY at Stony Brook Program

Sponsor: University Hospital-SUNY at Stony Brook
Veterans Affairs Medical Center (Northport)

Program Director:
Richard Barnett, MD
SUNY-Stony Brook Health Science Ctr
T-16 Rm 020, Dept of Int Med
Stony Brook, NY 11794-8160
Tel: 516 444-9341 *Fax:* 516 444-2493
E-mail: imrp@mail.som.sunysb.edu
Internet:
http://www.informatics.sunysb.edu/internalmed/resident.html
Accred Length: 3 Years *Program Size:* 127 (*GY1:* 53)
Subspecialties: CCM, CD, END, GE, HO, ID, IMG, NEP, PCC, PUD, RHU
Program ID: 140-35-21-315

Syracuse

SUNY Health Science Center at Syracuse Program

Sponsor: University Hospital-SUNY Health Science Center at Syracuse
Crouse Hospital
Veterans Affairs Medical Center (Syracuse)

Program Director:
David G Heisig, MD
SUNY Health Science Ctr-Syracuse
750 E Adams St
Syracuse, NY 13210
Tel: 315 464-4506 *Fax:* 315 464-4484
E-mail: perryk@mailbox.hscsyr.edu
Internet: http://www.hscsyr.edu/%7ewwwhome/uh2/medicine_residency/
Accred Length: 3 Years *Program Size:* 65 (*GY1:* 22)
Subspecialties: CCM, CD, END, GE, HO, ID, IMG, NEP, PCC, RHU
Program ID: 140-35-21-316

Valhalla

New York Medical College at Westchester Medical Center Program

Sponsor: New York Medical College
Westchester Medical Center

Program Director:
Stephen J Peterson, MD
New York Med Coll
Dept of Med
Munger Pavilion Rm 504
Valhalla, NY 10595
Tel: 914 493-8373 *Fax:* 914 594-4434
E-mail: intmed_wmc@nymc.edu
Internet: http://www.nymc.edu
Accred Length: 3 Years *Program Size:* 48 (*GY1:* 24)
Subspecialties: CD, END, GE, HEM, HO, ID, IMG, NEP, ON, PCC, RHU
Program ID: 140-35-11-317

North Carolina

Chapel Hill

University of North Carolina Hospitals Program

Sponsor: University of North Carolina Hospitals

Program Director:
Lee R Berkowitz, MD
Univ of North Carolina Sch of Med
3018 Old Clinic Bldg/CB7005
Chapel Hill, NC 27599-7005
Tel: 919 966-1042 *Fax:* 919 966-5775
E-mail: imresprg@med.unc.edu
Internet:
http://www.med.unc.edu/wrkunits/2depts/medicine/web/hstrain.htm
Accred Length: 3 Years *Program Size:* 74 (*GY1:* 29)
Subspecialties: CD, END, GE, HO, ICE, ID, IMG, NEP, PCC, RHU
Program ID: 140-36-21-318

Charlotte

Carolinas Medical Center Program

Sponsor: Carolinas Medical Center

Program Director:
Raymond F Bianchi, MD
Carolinas Med Ctr
Dept of Int Med
PO Box 32861
Charlotte, NC 28232-2861
Tel: 704 355-3165 *Fax:* 704 355-7626
Internet:
http://www.acponline.org/residency/carolinas.htm
Accred Length: 3 Years *Program Size:* 34 (*GY1:* 13)
Program ID: 140-36-11-319

Durham

Duke University Program

Sponsor: Duke University Medical Center
Veterans Affairs Medical Center (Durham)

Program Director:
Ralph G Corey, MD
Duke Univ Med Ctr
PO Box 3038
Durham, NC 27710
Tel: 919 681-2458 *Fax:* 919 681-6448
E-mail: medresident@medicine.mc.duke.edu
Internet: http://www.medicine.mc.duke.edu/resident
Accred Length: 3 Years *Program Size:* 117 (*GY1:* 41)
Subspecialties: CCM, CD, END, GE, HO, ICE, ID, IMG, NEP, PUD, RHU
Program ID: 140-36-21-320

Greensboro

Moses H Cone Memorial Hospital Program

Sponsor: Moses H Cone Memorial Hospital

Program Director:
Timothy W Lane, MD
Moses H Cone Memorial Hospital
Internal Med Program
1200 N Elm St
Greensboro, NC 27401-1020
Tel: 336 832-7800 *Fax:* 336 832-8026
E-mail: newmanl@med.unc.edu
Internet: http://www.med.unc.edu/gahec/ceimdiv/htm
Accred Length: 3 Years *Program Size:* 20 (*GY1:* 8)
Program ID: 140-36-11-321

Greenville

East Carolina University Program

Sponsor: East Carolina University School of Medicine
Pitt County Memorial Hospital

Program Director:
Peter R Lichstein, MD
East Carolina Univ Sch of Med
Dept of Int Med
Education Office/Rm 340 PCMH-TA
Greenville, NC 27858-4354
Tel: 252 816-4126 *Fax:* 252 816-2280
E-mail: cbyrum@brody.med.ecu.edu
Internet:
http://www.med.ecu.edu/htdocs/int_med/res_pro.htm
Accred Length: 3 Years *Program Size:* 42 (*GY1:* 18)
Subspecialties: CD, END, GE, PUD
Program ID: 140-36-11-323

Wilmington

New Hanover Regional Medical Center Program

Sponsor: New Hanover Regional Medical Center

Program Director:
Jorge J Gonzalez, MD
Peter C Ungaro, MD
New Hanover Regional Med Ctr
Coastal AHEC-Internal Med
2131 S 17th St/PO Box 9025
Wilmington, NC 28402-9025
Tel: 910 343-0161, ext 244 *Fax:* 910 762-6800
Internet: http://www.med.unc.edu/coahec
Accred Length: 3 Years *Program Size:* 20 (*GY1:* 7)
Program ID: 140-36-11-324

Winston-Salem

Wake Forest University School of Medicine Program

Sponsor: Wake Forest University Baptist Medical Center

Program Director:
Mark C Wilson, MD MPH
Wake Forest Univ Baptist Med Ctr
Medical Center Blvd
Winston-Salem, NC 27157-1052
Tel: 336 716-4490 *Fax:* 336 716-4490
E-mail: mwilson@wfubmc.edu
Internet: http://www.wfubmc.edu/intmed/respgm
Accred Length: 3 Years *Program Size:* 85 (*GY1:* 32)
Subspecialties: CCM, CD, END, GE, HO, ICE, ID, IMG, NEP, PCC, RHU
Program ID: 140-36-21-325

North Dakota

Fargo

University of North Dakota Program

Sponsor: Univ of North Dakota School of Medicine & Health Sciences
Veterans Affairs Medical and Regional Office Center (Fargo)
MeritCare Hospital

Program Director:
James Hanley, MD
Univ of North Dakota
Medical Education
720 4th St N
Fargo, ND 58122
Tel: 701 234-5934 *Fax:* 701 234-7230
E-mail: jameshanley@meritcare.com
Internet: http://www.und.nodak.edu
Accred Length: 3 Years *Program Size:* 24 (*GY1:* 8)
Program ID: 140-37-21-326

Ohio

Akron

Akron General Medical Center/NEOUCOM Program

Sponsor: Akron General Medical Center

Program Director:
Irene Chenowith, MD
Akron General Med Ctr
400 Wabash Ave
Akron, OH 44307
Tel: 330 384-6100 *Fax:* 330 384-6820
E-mail: meded@agmc.org
Internet: http://agmc.org
Accred Length: 3 Years *Program Size:* 28 (*GY1:* 12)
Program ID: 140-38-11-328

Summa Health System (Akron City Hospital)/NEOUCOM Program

Sponsor: Summa Health System
Akron City Hospital (Summa Health System)

Program Director:
James S Tan, MD
Summa Health System
Med Educ/Mary Yanik
525 E Market St
Akron, OH 44309
Tel: 800 322-0517
Internet: http://www.summahealth.org/edu/
Accred Length: 3 Years *Program Size:* 48 (*GY1:* 20)
Program ID: 140-38-11-327

Canton

Canton Medical Education Foundation/NEOUCOM Program

Sponsor: Canton Medical Education Foundation
Aultman Hospital
Timken Mercy Medical Center

Program Director:
Frederick C Whittier, MD
Northeastern Ohio Univ Coll of Med Hospitals-Canton
2600 Sixth St SW
Canton, OH 44710
Tel: 330 438-6220 *Fax:* 330 588-2605
E-mail: cantonmedicine@altavista.net
Internet: http://www.acponline.org/residency/
Accred Length: 3 Years *Program Size:* 31 (*GY1:* 10)
Program ID: 140-38-21-330

Cincinnati

Christ Hospital Program

Sponsor: Christ Hospital

Program Director:
Corwin R Dunn, MD
Christ Hospital
2139 Auburn Ave
Cincinnati, OH 45219-8110
Tel: 513 369-2258 *Fax:* 513 369-2673
Internet: http://schneidg@healthall.com
Accred Length: 3 Years *Program Size:* 42 (*GY1:* 21)
Program ID: 140-38-11-331

Good Samaritan Hospital Program

Sponsor: Good Samaritan Hospital

Program Director:
Helen K Koselka, MD
Good Samaritan Hospital
375 Dixmyth Ave
Cincinnati, OH 45220-2489
Tel: 513 872-3229 *Fax:* 513 221-5865
Internet: http://www.trihealth.com
Accred Length: 3 Years *Program Size:* 25 (*GY1:* 12)
Program ID: 140-38-31-332

Jewish Hospital of Cincinnati Program

Sponsor: Jewish Hospital of Cincinnati

Program Director:
Stephen J Goldberg, MD
Jewish Hospital
Dept of Int Med
4777 E Galbraith Rd
Cincinnati, OH 45236
Tel: 513 686-5446 *Fax:* 513 686-5443
E-mail: goldbest@healthall.com
Accred Length: 3 Years *Program Size:* 32 (*GY1:* 12)
Program ID: 140-38-11-333

University Hospital/University of Cincinnati College of Medicine Program

Sponsor: University Hospital Inc
Veterans Affairs Medical Center (Cincinnati)

Program Director:
Gregory W Rouan, MD
Univ of Cincinnati
Dept of Int Med
PO Box 670557
Cincinnati, OH 45267-0557
Tel: 513 558-2590 *Fax:* 513 558-3878
E-mail: ucintmed@uc.edu
Internet: http://www.uc.edu
Accred Length: 3 Years *Program Size:* 69 (*GY1:* 23)
Subspecialties: CD, END, GE, HO, ID, NEP, PCC, RHU
Program ID: 140-38-21-334

Cleveland

Case Western Reserve University (MetroHealth) Program

Sponsor: MetroHealth Medical Center

Program Director:
Michael J McFarlane, MD
MetroHealth Med Ctr
2500 MetroHealth Dr
Cleveland, OH 44109-1998
Tel: 216 778-3886 *Fax:* 216 778-5823
E-mail: medres@metrohealth.org
Internet: http://www.metrohealth.org
Accred Length: 3 Years *Program Size:* 76 (*GY1:* 28)
Subspecialties: CD, GE, IMG, PCC, RHU
Program ID: 140-38-11-336

Case Western Reserve University (Mount Sinai) Program

Sponsor: Mount Sinai Medical Center of Cleveland

Program Director:
D Roy Ferguson, MD
Int Med Dept
Mount Sinai Med Ctr
One Mt Sinai Dr
Cleveland, OH 44106-4198
Tel: 216 421-5768 *Fax:* 216 421-4833
E-mail: egraffein@stratos.net
Internet: http://www.mtsinai.org
Accred Length: 3 Years *Program Size:* 39 (*GY1:* 12)
Program ID: 140-38-21-337

Case Western Reserve University Program

Sponsor: University Hospitals of Cleveland
Veterans Affairs Medical Center (Cleveland)

Program Director:
Keith B Armitage, MD
Thomas R Hornick, MD
Univ Hospitals of Cleveland
11100 Euclid Ave
Cleveland, OH 44106-5029
Tel: 216 844-3833 *Fax:* 216 844-8216
E-mail: kba@po.cwru.edu
Internet: http://www.uhhs.com
Accred Length: 3 Years *Program Size:* 95 (*GY1:* 30)
Subspecialties: CCM, CD, END, GE, HEM, HO, ICE, ID, IMG, NEP, ON, PCC, PUD, RHU
Program ID: 140-38-21-335

Cleveland Clinic Foundation Program
Sponsor: Cleveland Clinic Foundation
Program Director:
Byron J Hoogwerf, MD
Cleveland Clinic Foundation
Dept of Int Med/P39
9500 Euclid Ave
Cleveland, OH 44195
Tel: 216 444-5690 *Fax:* 216 444-1162
E-mail: meded@cesmtp.ccf.org
Internet: http://www.ccf.org/im/res
Accred Length: 3 Years *Program Size:* 110 (*GY1:* 39)
Subspecialties: CD, END, GE, HO, ICE, ID, IMG, NEP, PCC, RHU
Program ID: 140-38-12-339

Fairview Health System Program
Sponsor: Fairview Health System
Fairview Health System (Fairview General Hospital)
Program Director:
Michael Waggoner, MD
Fairview Hospital
18101 Lorain Ave
Cleveland, OH 44111
Tel: 216 476-7369 *Fax:* 216 476-2944
Internet: http://www.webcom.com/fairres
Accred Length: 3 Years *Program Size:* 31 (*GY1:* 10)
Program ID: 140-38-21-340

Meridia Huron Hospital Program
Sponsor: Meridia Huron Hospital
Meridia Hillcrest Hospital
Program Director:
Burton C West, MD
Meridia Huron Hospital
13951 Terrace Rd
Cleveland, OH 44112-4399
Tel: 216 761-2820 *Fax:* 216 761-7579
E-mail: kkorosi@meridia.org
Accred Length: 3 Years *Program Size:* 49 (*GY1:* 16)
Program ID: 140-38-21-476

St Luke's Medical Center Program
Sponsor: St Luke's Medical Center
Program Director:
Richard E Christie, MD
St Luke's Med Ctr
11311 Shaker Blvd
Rm 4135
Cleveland, OH 44104
Tel: 800 368-6886 *Fax:* 216 368-8446
E-mail: slmcim@en.com
Internet: http://en.com/stlukes
Accred Length: 3 Years *Program Size:* 44 (*GY1:* 14)
Program ID: 140-38-11-338

Columbus

Mount Carmel Health Program
Sponsor: Mount Carmel Medical Center
Program Director:
G Patrick Ecklar, MD
Mount Carmel Health System
793 W State St
Columbus, OH 43222
Tel: 614 234-5279 *Fax:* 614 234-2772
E-mail: dsmith@mchs.com
Internet: http://mchsresidency.org
Accred Length: 3 Years *Program Size:* 28 (*GY1:* 12)
Program ID: 140-38-12-341

Ohio State University Program
Sponsor: Ohio State University Medical Center
Program Director:
Evelyn E Pintz, MD
Ohio State Univ Hospital, Dept of Int Med
1654 Upham Dr/209 MEANS
Columbus, OH 43210-1228
Tel: 614 293-3989 *Fax:* 614 293-5118
E-mail: pintz.1@osu.edu
Internet: http://www.med.ohio_state.edu/internal_medicine/intmed.html
Accred Length: 3 Years *Program Size:* 55 (*GY1:* 19)
Subspecialties: CD, END, GE, HO, ICE, ID, NEP, PCC, RHU
Program ID: 140-38-11-342

Riverside Methodist Hospitals (OhioHealth) Program
Sponsor: Riverside Methodist Hospitals (OhioHealth)
Program Director:
Ian M Baird, MD
Riverside Methodist Hospital
Medical Education Dept
3535 Olentangy River Rd
Columbus, OH 43214
Tel: 614 566-5468 *Fax:* 614 566-6852
E-mail: whitfid@ohiohealth.com
Internet: http://www.ohiohealth.com
Accred Length: 3 Years *Program Size:* 52 (*GY1:* 24)
Program ID: 140-38-12-343

Dayton

Wright State University (Miami Valley) Program
Sponsor: Wright State University School of Medicine
Miami Valley Hospital
Veterans Affairs Medical Center (Dayton)
Program Director:
Virginia C Wood, MD
Wright State Univ
Dept of Int Med
One Wyoming St
Dayton, OH 45401-0927
Tel: 937 208-2010 *Fax:* 937 208-2621
E-mail: vwood@discover.wright.edu
Internet: http://users.erinet.com/20475/wsumed/
Accred Length: 3 Years *Program Size:* 42 (*GY1:* 22)
Program ID: 140-38-21-345

Wright State University Program
Sponsor: Wright State University School of Medicine
Good Samaritan Hospital and Health Center
Miami Valley Hospital
Veterans Affairs Medical Center (Dayton)
Program Director:
Timothy B Sorg, MD
Wright State Univ Sch of Med
PO Box 927
Dayton, OH 45401-0927
Tel: 937 208-2010 *Fax:* 937 208-2621
Internet: http://users.erinet.com/20475/wsumed
Accred Length: 3 Years *Program Size:* 36 (*GY1:* 12)
Subspecialties: CD, GE, HO, ID
Program ID: 140-38-21-344

Dayton (Kettering)

Kettering Medical Center Program
Sponsor: Kettering Medical Center
Program Director:
Stephen D McDonald, MD
Kettering Med Ctr
3535 Southern Blvd
Kettering, OH 45429
Tel: 937 296-7293 *Fax:* 937 296-4299
E-mail: delina_unger@ketthealth.com
Internet: http://www.ketthealth.com/meded/edop.htm
Accred Length: 3 Years *Program Size:* 30 (*GY1:* 10)
Program ID: 140-38-21-347

Toledo

Medical College of Ohio Program
Sponsor: Medical College of Ohio
Medical College of Ohio Hospital
St Vincent Mercy Medical Center
Toledo Hospital
Program Director:
Jeffrey Hammersley, MD
Med Coll of Ohio
3000 Arlington Ave
Rm 4143 Hospital
Toledo, OH 43614
Tel: 419 383-3687 *Fax:* 419 383-6180
E-mail: ndrain@.mco.edu
Internet: http://darwin.mco.edu/medicine
Accred Length: 3 Years *Program Size:* 39 (*GY1:* 19)
Subspecialties: CD, END, GE, ICE, ID, NEP, ON, PUD
Program ID: 140-38-21-348

Wright-Patterson AFB

Wright-Patterson Medical Center Program
Sponsor: Wright-Patterson Medical Center
Program Director:
Jose J Gutierrez-Nunez, MD
74th Med Operations Sqd/SGOM
4881 Sugar Maple Dr
Wright-Patterson AFB, OH 45433-5529
Tel: 937 257-9656 *Fax:* 937 257-1529
E-mail: gutierrezj@medcenoa.wpafb.af.mil
Internet: http://www.wpmc1.wpafb.af.mil/
Accred Length: 3 Years *Program Size:* 24 (*GY1:* 8)
Program ID: 140-38-11-002
US Armed Services Program

Youngstown

St Elizabeth Health Center/NEOUCOM Program
Sponsor: St Elizabeth Health Center
Program Director:
Thomas P Marnejon, DO
St Elizabeth Health Ctr
1044 Belmont Ave
PO Box 1790
Youngstown, OH 44501-1790
Tel: 800 837-4783
Accred Length: 3 Years *Program Size:* 24 (*GY1:* 8)
Program ID: 140-38-11-349

Western Reserve Care System/NEOUCOM Program

Sponsor: Western Reserve Care System
Forum Health-Northside Medical Center

Program Director:
L Kevin Nash, MD
Western Reserve Healthcare-Forum Health
500 Gypsy Ln
Youngstown, OH 44501-0990
Tel: 330 740-5813 *Fax:* 330 740-5727
Internet: http://www.wrhc.org
Accred Length: 3 Years *Program Size:* 25 (*GY1:* 8)
Program ID: 140-38-31-350

Oklahoma

Oklahoma City

University of Oklahoma Health Sciences Center Program

Sponsor: University of Oklahoma College of Medicine
University Hospital
Veterans Affairs Medical Center (Oklahoma City)

Program Director:
James H Schmidt, MD
Univ of Oklahoma Coll of Med
PO Box 26901/WP 2040
Oklahoma City, OK 73190
Tel: 405 271-5963 *Fax:* 405 271-3195
E-mail: im-program@ouhsc.edu
Internet: http://dpmed.ouhsc.edu/resinfo/ouimres.htm
Accred Length: 3 Years *Program Size:* 48 (*GY1:* 16)
Subspecialties: CD, END, GE, HO, ICE, ID, IMG, NEP, PCC, RHU
Program ID: 140-39-21-351

Tulsa

University of Oklahoma College of Medicine-Tulsa Program

Sponsor: University of Oklahoma College of Medicine-Tulsa
Hillcrest Medical Center
St Francis Hospital
St John Medical Center
Veterans Affairs Medical Center (Muskogee)

Program Director:
Michael A Weisz, MD
Univ of Oklahoma Coll of Med-Tulsa
Dept of Int Med
2808 S Sheridan Rd
Tulsa, OK 74129
Tel: 918 838-4691 *Fax:* 918 838-4897
Internet: http://www.tulsa.ouhsc.edu
Accred Length: 3 Years *Program Size:* 36 (*GY1:* 12)
Program ID: 140-39-21-352

Oregon

Portland

Legacy Emanuel Hospital and Health Center Program

Sponsor: Legacy Emanuel Hospital and Health Center
Legacy Good Samaritan Hospital and Medical Center

Program Director:
Stephen R Jones, MD
Good Samaritan Hospital and Med Ctr
1015 NW 22nd Ave/R-200
Portland, OR 97210
Tel: 503 413-7036 *Fax:* 503 413-7361
E-mail: imres@lhs.org
Internet: http://legacyhealth.org
Accred Length: 3 Years *Program Size:* 51 (*GY1:* 17)
Program ID: 140-40-11-353

Oregon Health Sciences University Program

Sponsor: Oregon Health Sciences University Hospital
Veterans Affairs Medical Center (Portland)

Program Director:
Thomas G Cooney, MD
Oregon Health Sciences Univ
Dept of Med/L455
3181 SW Sam Jackson Park Rd
Portland, OR 97201-3098
Tel: 503 494-8357 *Fax:* 503 494-5636
E-mail: imresapp@ohsu.edu
Internet: http://www.ohsu.edu/som-medicine
Accred Length: 3 Years *Program Size:* 92 (*GY1:* 29)
Subspecialties: CD, END, GE, HEM, HO, ICE, ID, IMG, NEP, ON, PCC, RHU
Program ID: 140-40-31-357

Providence Medical Center Program

Sponsor: Providence Medical Center

Program Director:
Mark R Rosenberg, MD
Providence Portland Med Ctr
5050 NE Hoyt St/Ste 540
Portland, OR 97213-2967
Tel: 800 642-2131 *Fax:* 503 215-6857
E-mail: imresprog@phsor.org
Internet: http://www.providence.org/portland
Accred Length: 3 Years *Program Size:* 30 (*GY1:* 10)
Program ID: 140-40-31-355

St Vincent Hospital and Medical Center Program

Sponsor: St Vincent Hospital and Medical Center

Program Director:
Kenneth E Melvin, MD
St Vincent Hospital and Med Ctr
9205 SW Barnes/Ste 20
Portland, OR 97225
Tel: 503 216-2401 *Fax:* 503 216-4041
Internet: http://www.phsor.org
Accred Length: 3 Years *Program Size:* 24 (*GY1:* 10)
Program ID: 140-40-31-356

Pennsylvania

Abington

Abington Memorial Hospital Program

Sponsor: Abington Memorial Hospital

Program Director:
David G Smith, MD
Abington Memorial Hospital
1200 Old York Rd/Ste 2B
Abington, PA 19001
Tel: 215 576-2056 *Fax:* 215 576-4361
E-mail: imresidents@amh.org
Internet: http://www.amh.org
Accred Length: 3 Years *Program Size:* 38 (*GY1:* 16)
Program ID: 140-41-12-358

Allentown

Lehigh Valley Hospital/Pennsylvania State University Program

Sponsor: Lehigh Valley Hospital

Program Director:
Richard H Snyder, MD MBA
Lehigh Valley Hospital
Dept of Med
Cedar Crest and I-78/PO Box 689
Allentown, PA 18105-1556
Tel: 610 402-8200 *Fax:* 610 402-1675
E-mail: internalmedres@lvhhn.org
Internet:
http://www.lvhhn.org/academic/residency/medicine/home.html
Accred Length: 3 Years *Program Size:* 45 (*GY1:* 15)
Program ID: 140-41-21-359

Bethlehem

Temple University/St Luke's Hospital Program

Sponsor: St Luke's Hospital

Program Director:
Gloria T Fioravanti, DO
St Luke's Hospital
Dept of Int Med
801 Ostrum St
Bethlehem, PA 18015
Tel: 610 954-4644 *Fax:* 610 954-4979
E-mail: im-residency@slhn.org
Internet: http://slhn-lehighvalley.org
Accred Length: 3 Years *Program Size:* 24 (*GY1:* 8)
Program ID: 140-41-31-360

Danville

Penn State Geisinger Health System/Geisinger Medical Center Program

Sponsor: Penn State Geisinger Health System
Geisinger Medical Center

Program Director:
Robert Palinkas, MD
Geisinger Med Ctr
Dept of Med
100 N Academy Ave
Danville, PA 17822
Tel: 717 271-6787 *Fax:* 717 271-5734
E-mail: ckrebs@psghs.edu
Accred Length: 3 Years *Program Size:* 32 (*GY1:* 10)
Subspecialties: CD, GE, RHU
Program ID: 140-41-11-362

Easton

Easton Hospital Program

Sponsor: Easton Hospital

Program Director:
David G Kemp, MD
Easton Hospital
250 S 21st St
Easton, PA 18042-3892
Tel: 610 250-4013, ext 4517 *Fax:* 610 250-4820
Accred Length: 3 Years *Program Size:* 24 (*GY1:* 8)
Program ID: 140-41-11-363

Harrisburg

PinnacleHealth Hospitals Program
Sponsor: PinnacleHealth System-Polyclinic Hospital
PinnacleHealth System-Harrisburg Hospital
Program Director:
Margaret Kreher, MD
PinnacleHealth-Polyclinic Hospital
2601 N Third St
Harrisburg, PA 17110
Tel: 717 782-5347 *Fax:* 717 782-2186
E-mail: dmauch@pinnaclehealth.org
Internet: http://www.polyclinic.org
Accred Length: 3 Years *Program Size:* 37 (*GY1:* 12)
Program ID: 140-41-11-365

Hershey

Penn State Geisinger Health System/Milton S Hershey Medical Center Program
Sponsor: Penn State Geisinger Health System
Milton S Hershey Medical Center
Program Director:
Richard J Simons, MD
Milton S Hershey Med Ctr
PO Box 850
Hershey, PA 17033
Tel: 717 531-8390 *Fax:* 717 531-5831
E-mail: medres@med.hmc.psghs.edu
Internet: http://www.hmc.psghs.edu/med/residency/
Accred Length: 3 Years *Program Size:* 64 (*GY1:* 28)
Subspecialties: CCM, CD, END, GE, HO, ICE, ID, NEP, PUD
Program ID: 140-41-11-366

Johnstown

Temple University/Conemaugh Valley Memorial Hospital Program
Sponsor: Conemaugh Valley Memorial Hospital
Program Director:
Thomas J McGlynn, MD
Conemaugh Health System-Memorial Med Ctr
1086 Franklin St
Johnstown, PA 15905-4398
Tel: 814 534-9397 *Fax:* 814 534-3290
E-mail: geckenr@conemaugh.org
Accred Length: 3 Years *Program Size:* 22 (*GY1:* 4)
Program ID: 140-41-31-367

McKeesport

McKeesport Hospital/UPMC Program
Sponsor: McKeesport Hospital/UPMC
Program Director:
Usman Ahmad, MD
UPMC McKeesport Hospital
1500 Fifth Ave
McKeesport, PA 15132
Tel: 412 664-2167, ext 2167 *Fax:* 412 664-2164
Accred Length: 3 Years *Program Size:* 27 (*GY1:* 8)
Program ID: 140-41-21-368

Philadelphia

Albert Einstein Medical Center Program
Sponsor: Albert Einstein Medical Center
Program Director:
Lisa Wallenstein, MD
Albert Einstein Med Ctr
Dept of Med
5401 Old York Rd/Ste 363
Philadelphia, PA 19141-3025
Tel: 800 220-2362 *Fax:* 215 455-1933
E-mail: medicine@aehn2.einstein.edu
Internet: http://www.einstein.edu/phl
Accred Length: 3 Years *Program Size:* 60 (*GY1:* 20)
Subspecialties: CD, GE, IMG, NEP, PUD, RHU
Program ID: 140-41-11-369

Episcopal Hospital Program
Sponsor: Episcopal Hospital (TUHS)
Program Director:
David Schlossberg, MD
Episcopal Hospital
100 E Lehigh Ave
MAB Ste107
Philadelphia, PA 19125
Tel: 215 427-7068 *Fax:* 215 427-2927
Accred Length: 3 Years *Program Size:* 31 (*GY1:* 10)
Subspecialties: CD
Program ID: 140-41-11-370

Graduate Hospital Program
Sponsor: Graduate Hospital
Program Director:
Philip O Katz, MD
Ste 504/Pepper Pavilion
MCP Hahnemann Univ Hospital
1800 Lombard St
Philadelphia, PA 19146
Tel: 215 893-2484 *Fax:* 215 893-2472
Internet:
http://www.auhs.edu/resid/gmedres/gmedreshome.html
Accred Length: 3 Years *Program Size:* 47 (*GY1:* 16)
Subspecialties: CD, GE, PUD
Program ID: 140-41-11-371

MCP Hahnemann University Program
Sponsor: MCP Hahnemann University
Hahnemann University Hospital
Medical College of Pennsylvania Hospital
Program Director:
Allan R Tunkel, MD PhD
Dept of Int Med
Med Coll of Pennsylvania Hospital
3300 Henry Ave
Philadelphia, PA 19129
Tel: 215 842-6957 *Fax:* 215 843-6038
E-mail: gallaghera@auhs.edu
Accred Length: 3 Years *Program Size:* 154 (*GY1:* 64)
Subspecialties: CD, END, GE, HEM, HO, ICE, ID, IMG, NEP, ON, PCC, RHU
Program ID: 140-41-21-374

Mercy Catholic Medical Center Program
Sponsor: Mercy Catholic Medical Center Inc
Mercy Hospital of Philadelphia
Mercy Fitzgerald Hospital
Program Director:
M Anthony Albornoz, MD
Mercy Catholic Med Ctr
1500 Lansdowne Ave
Darby, PA 19023
Tel: 610 237-4958 *Fax:* 610 237-5022
Internet: http://www.mercyhealth.org
Accred Length: 3 Years *Program Size:* 62 (*GY1:* 27)
Program ID: 140-41-11-375

Pennsylvania Hospital of the University of Pennsylvania Health System Program
Sponsor: Pennsylvania Hospital (UPHS)
Program Director:
Dennis C Policastro, MD
Pennsylvania Hospital
800 Spruce St
Philadelphia, PA 19107
Tel: 800 832-8364 *Fax:* 215 829-7132
E-mail: depoli@pahosp.com
Internet: http://www.pahosp.com
Accred Length: 3 Years *Program Size:* 46 (*GY1:* 21)
Program ID: 140-41-11-376

Presbyterian Medical Center of the University of Pennsylvania Health System Program
Sponsor: Presbyterian Medical Center (UPHS)
Program Director:
Jack Ende, MD
Univ of Pennsylvania Health System
Presbyterian Med Ctr
39th and Market Sts/Rm W284
Philadelphia, PA 19104-2699
Tel: 215 662-9436 *Fax:* 215 243-3296
Accred Length: 3 Years *Program Size:* 30 (*GY1:* 0)
Subspecialties: CD, GE, ICE, PUD
Program ID: 140-41-11-377

Temple University Program
Sponsor: Temple University Hospital
Fox Chase Cancer Center
Program Director:
Richard S Eisenstaedt, MD
Dept of Int Med
Temple Univ Hospital
3401 N Broad St/8PP
Philadelphia, PA 19140
Tel: 215 707-3397 *Fax:* 215 707-4756
Internet: http://www.blue.vm.temple.edu/˜medres
Accred Length: 3 Years *Program Size:* 72 (*GY1:* 24)
Subspecialties: CD, END, GE, HO, ICE, ID, IMG, NEP, PCC, RHU
Program ID: 140-41-21-378

Thomas Jefferson University Program
Sponsor: Thomas Jefferson University Hospital
Program Director:
Gregory C Kane, MD
Thomas Jefferson Univ Hospital
1025 Walnut St/Rm 801
Philadelphia, PA 19107
Tel: 215 955-8904 *Fax:* 215 955-3890
E-mail: medicine.residency@mail.tju.edu
Accred Length: 3 Years *Program Size:* 120 (*GY1:* 43)
Subspecialties: CD, END, GE, HEM, ID, NEP, ON, PCC, RHU
Program ID: 140-41-21-379

University of Pennsylvania Program
Sponsor: Hospital of the University of Pennsylvania
Veterans Affairs Medical Center (Philadelphia)
Program Director:
Peter G Traber, MD
Hospital of the Univ of Pennsylvania
100 Centrex/Box 708
3400 Spruce St
Philadelphia, PA 19104-4283
Tel: 215 662-3924 *Fax:* 215 662-7919
E-mail: sgmartin@mail.med.upenn.edu
Internet: http://www.med.upenn.edu/medicine
Accred Length: 3 Years *Program Size:* 178 (*GY1:* 72)
Subspecialties: CD, END, GE, HO, ICE, ID, IMG, NEP, PCC, RHU
Program ID: 140-41-21-380

Pittsburgh

Allegheny General Hospital Program

Sponsor: Allegheny General Hospital

Program Director:
Joel T Katz, MD
Allegheny General Hospital
Dept of Internal Med
320 E North Ave
Pittsburgh, PA 15212-9986
Tel: 412 359-4970 *Fax:* 412 359-4983
Accred Length: 3 Years *Program Size:* 67 (*GY1:* 30)
Subspecialties: CD, GE, NEP, ON, PUD
Program ID: 140-41-11-381

Mercy Hospital of Pittsburgh Program

Sponsor: Mercy Hospital of Pittsburgh

Program Director:
Kimball W Mohn, MD
Mercy Hospital of Pittsburgh
Dept of Med
1400 Locust St
Pittsburgh, PA 15219-5166
Tel: 412 232-5533 *Fax:* 412 232-5689
E-mail: internal.medicine.residency@mercy.pmhs.org
Internet: http://www.mercy-meded.com
Accred Length: 3 Years *Program Size:* 52 (*GY1:* 21)
Program ID: 140-41-11-385

St Francis Medical Center Program

Sponsor: St Francis Medical Center

Program Director:
T Michael White, MD
St Francis Med Ctr
400 45th St
Pittsburgh, PA 15201
Tel: 412 622-4388
Internet: http://www.sfhs.edu
Accred Length: 3 Years *Program Size:* 24 (*GY1:* 8)
Program ID: 140-41-11-386

University Health Center of Pittsburgh Program

Sponsor: University Health Center of Pittsburgh
Presbyterian University Hospital/UPMC
Veterans Affairs Medical Center (Pittsburgh)

Program Director:
Frank J Kroboth, MD
Univ Health Ctr of Pittsburgh
3550 Terrace St
1220 Scaife Hall
Pittsburgh, PA 15261
Tel: 412 648-9642 *Fax:* 412 648-2117
Internet: http://www.upmc.edu/medicine
Accred Length: 3 Years *Program Size:* 109 (*GY1:* 39)
Subspecialties: CCM, CD, END, GE, HEM, ICE, ID, IMG, NEP, ON, PCC, RHU
Program ID: 140-41-21-504

Western Pennsylvania Hospital Program

Sponsor: Western Pennsylvania Hospital

Program Director:
Herbert S Diamond, MD
Western Pennsylvania Hospital
Dept of Med
4800 Friendship Ave
Pittsburgh, PA 15224
Tel: 412 578-5750 *Fax:* 412 578-6804
E-mail: intermedwph@yahoo.com
Internet: http://www.westpennhospital.com
Accred Length: 3 Years *Program Size:* 42 (*GY1:* 14)
Subspecialties: CD, GE, HO, PUD
Program ID: 140-41-11-387

Reading

Reading Hospital and Medical Center Program

Sponsor: Reading Hospital and Medical Center

Program Director:
Daniel B Kimball Jr, MD
Reading Hospital and Med Ctr
Sixth Ave and Spruce St
Reading, PA 19611
Tel: 800 592-9943, ext 6133 *Fax:* 610 208-9003
E-mail: kimballd@readinghospital.org
Internet: http://www.readinghospital.org
Accred Length: 3 Years *Program Size:* 20 (*GY1:* 8)
Program ID: 140-41-21-388

Sayre

Guthrie Healthcare System Program

Sponsor: Robert Packer Hospital

Program Director:
Felix J DeSio, MD
Guthrie Healthcare System-Robert Packer Hospital
Medical Education
Guthrie Sq
Sayre, PA 18840
Tel: 717 882-4559 *Fax:* 717 882-5569
E-mail: jwark@inet.guthrie.org
Internet: http://www.guthrie.org/internal.htm
Accred Length: 3 Years *Program Size:* 24 (*GY1:* 8)
Subspecialties: CD, GE, PUD
Program ID: 140-41-12-389

Scranton

Scranton-Temple Residency Program

Sponsor: Scranton-Temple Residency Program Inc
Mercy Hospital
Moses Taylor Hospital

Program Director:
Robert E Wright, MD
Scranton-Temple Residency Program
746 Jefferson Ave
Scranton, PA 18510
Tel: 717 343-2383 *Fax:* 717 963-6133
E-mail: strp@mhs-nepa.com
Internet: http://www.mhs-nepa.com/strp
Accred Length: 3 Years *Program Size:* 20 (*GY1:* 7)
Program ID: 140-41-21-390

Upland

Crozer-Chester Medical Center Program

Sponsor: Crozer-Chester Medical Center

Program Director:
Susan L Williams, MD
Crozer-Chester Med Ctr
One Medical Center Blvd
Third Floor/East Wing
Upland, PA 19013
Tel: 800 225-1171 *Fax:* 610 447-6373
E-mail: ccmcdom@crozer.org
Internet:
http://www.crozer.org/educate/resprog/intmed/intmed.htm
Accred Length: 3 Years *Program Size:* 22 (*GY1:* 7)
Program ID: 140-41-31-514

Wilkes-Barre

Northeastern Pennsylvania Hospitals Program

Sponsor: Veterans Affairs Medical Center (Wilkes-Barre)
Community Medical Center

Program Director:
Ramesh M Shah, MD
VA Med Ctr
1111 E End Blvd
Wilkes-Barre, PA 18711
Tel: 717 821-7291, ext 7601 *Fax:* 717 821-7255
Accred Length: 3 Years *Program Size:* 54 (*GY1:* 14)
Subspecialties: PUD
Program ID: 140-41-31-391

Wynnewood

Lankenau Hospital Program

Sponsor: Lankenau Hospital

Program Director:
Clifford H Pemberton, MD
Lankenau Hospital
100 Lancaster Ave/Ste 114
Wynnewood, PA 19096
Tel: 610 645-2008 *Fax:* 610 649-8201
E-mail: chpemberton @ pol.net
Accred Length: 3 Years *Program Size:* 46 (*GY1:* 22)
Subspecialties: CD, GE, HO, ICE, NEP
Program ID: 140-41-11-373

York

York Hospital Program

Sponsor: York Hospital

Program Director:
J Wolfe Blotzer, MD
York Hospital
1001 S George St
York, PA 17405
Tel: 717 851-2164 *Fax:* 717 851-2843
E-mail: dm_arenninge@yorkhospital.edu
Internet: http://www.yorkhealth.org
Accred Length: 3 Years *Program Size:* 21 (*GY1:* 8)
Program ID: 140-41-11-392

Puerto Rico

Bayamon

Universidad Central del Caribe Program

Sponsor: University Hospital Ramon Ruiz Arnau

Program Director:
Robert F Hunter-Mellado, MD
Univ Hospital Ramon Ruiz Arnau
Dept of Int Med
PO Box 60-327
Bayamon, PR 00960
Tel: 809 740-4295 *Fax:* 809 269-0050
Accred Length: 3 Years *Program Size:* 36 (*GY1:* 12)
Program ID: 140-42-12-452

Caguas

Caguas Regional Hospital Program

Sponsor: Caguas Regional Hospital

Program Director:
Juan R Otero, MD
Caguas Regional Hospital
Dept of Med
PO Box 5729
Caguas, PR 00726
Tel: 787 744-3169, ext 6030
Accred Length: 3 Years *Program Size:* 20 (*GY1:* 8)
Program ID: 140-42-21-393

Mayaguez

Ramon E Betances Hospital-Mayaguez Medical Center Program

Sponsor: Dr Ramon E Betances Hospital-Mayaguez Medical Center

Program Director:
Sifredo Acaron III, MD
Mayaguez Med Ctr
Dept of Int Med
Carr 2 Num 410
Mayaquez, PR 00680-1522
Tel: 787 834-8686
Accred Length: 3 Years *Program Size:* 15 (*GY1:* 5)
Program ID: 140-42-12-394

Ponce

Hospital de Damas Program

Sponsor: Hospital de Damas

Program Director:
Homero Tarrats-Torres, MD
Hospital Damas
2213 Ponce By Pass (Educ Medica)
Ponce, PR 00731-7779
Tel: 787 840-8686, ext 6123 *Fax:* 787 844-0225
Accred Length: 3 Years *Program Size:* 18 (*GY1:* 6)
Subspecialties: CD, GE, PUD
Program ID: 140-42-11-453

Ponce University Hospital Program

Sponsor: Ponce University Hospital

Program Director:
Lawrence Olsen-Maristany, MD
Ponce Univ Hospital
Dept of Int Med
PO Box 185
Ponce, PR 00733
Tel: 787 844-2080, ext 1310 *Fax:* 787 841-3454
Accred Length: 3 Years *Program Size:* 21 (*GY1:* 7)
Program ID: 140-42-11-395

Rio Piedras

San Juan City Hospital Program

Sponsor: San Juan City Hospital

Program Director:
Jose H Martinez, MD
San Juan Municipal Hospital
Apartado BR
Box 21405
Rio Piedras, PR 00928
Tel: 787 765-5147 *Fax:* 787 763-1778
Accred Length: 3 Years *Program Size:* 44 (*GY1:* 16)
Subspecialties: CD, END, HEM, ON, PUD, RHU
Program ID: 140-42-11-396

San German

Hospital de la Concepcion Program

Sponsor: Hospital de la Concepcion

Program Director:
Francisco Jaume, MD
Hospital de la Concepcion
St Luna #41/Box 285
San German, PR 00683
Tel: 787 892-1860 *Fax:* 787 892-2538
Accred Length: 3 Years *Program Size:* 15 (*GY1:* 4)
Program ID: 140-42-21-488

San Juan

University of Puerto Rico Program

Sponsor: University of Puerto Rico School of Medicine
Dr Federico Trilla - Carolina Regional Hospital
University Hospital

Program Director:
Carlos E Girod, MD
Univ Hospital, Dept of Med, Univ of Puerto Rico
Box 365067
San Juan, PR 00936-5067
Tel: 787 751-6034 *Fax:* 787 754-1739
E-mail: gcolonr@coqui.net
Accred Length: 3 Years *Program Size:* 45 (*GY1:* 15)
Subspecialties: CD, END, GE, HO, ID, IMG, NEP, PUD, RHU
Program ID: 140-42-21-397

Veterans Affairs Medical and Regional Office Center Program

Sponsor: Veterans Affairs Medical Center (San Juan)

Program Director:
Carlos H Ramirez-Ronda, MD
VA Med Ctr
One Veterans Plaza
San Juan, PR 00927-5800
Tel: 787 758-6900 *Fax:* 787 771-3602
Accred Length: 3 Years *Program Size:* 54 (*GY1:* 18)
Subspecialties: CD, ID, NEP, PUD
Program ID: 140-42-31-398

Rhode Island

Pawtucket

Brown University (Memorial) Program

Sponsor: Memorial Hospital of Rhode Island

Program Director:
Robert S Crausman, MD
Memorial Hospital of Rhode Island
111 Brewster St
Pawtucket, RI 02860
Tel: 401 729-2522 *Fax:* 401 729-2202
Accred Length: 3 Years *Program Size:* 30 (*GY1:* 10)
Program ID: 140-43-21-473

Providence

Brown University (Miriam) Program

Sponsor: Miriam Hospital

Program Director:
Fred J Schiffman, MD
Miriam Hospital
164 Summit Ave
Providence, RI 02906
Tel: 401 793-4035 *Fax:* 401 793-4049
E-mail: catmed@brown.edu or gimmed@brown.edu
Internet: http://www.brown.edu
Accred Length: 3 Years *Program Size:* 20 (*GY1:* 0)
Subspecialties: CCM, TY
Program ID: 140-43-11-399

Brown University Program

Sponsor: Rhode Island Hospital

Program Director:
Edward Wing, MD
Rhode Island Hospital
Dept of Med
593 Eddy St
Providence, RI 02903-4923
Tel: 401 444-5577 *Fax:* 401 444-4730
Internet: http://www.brown.edu
Accred Length: 3 Years *Program Size:* 128 (*GY1:* 50)
Subspecialties: CCM, CD, END, GE, NEP
Program ID: 140-43-11-400

Roger Williams Medical Center Program

Sponsor: Roger Williams Medical Center

Program Director:
Alan B Weitberg, MD
Boston Univ Program C, Dept of Int Med
Roger Williams Hospital
825 Chalkstone Ave
Providence, RI 02908-4735
Tel: 401 456-2000, ext 2033 *Fax:* 401 456-6719
E-mail: rwmc residency@ids.com
Internet: http://www.rwmc.com
Accred Length: 3 Years *Program Size:* 44 (*GY1:* 21)
Subspecialties: CD, HEM, HO, ID, ON, PUD, RHU
Program ID: 140-43-31-401

South Carolina

Charleston

Medical University of South Carolina Program

Sponsor: Medical University of South Carolina College of Medicine
MUSC Medical Center
Ralph H Johnson Dept of Veterans Affairs Med Center

Program Director:
Donald L Fox, MD
Med Univ of South Carolina
Dept of Int Med
171 Ashley Ave/205 S IOP
Charleston, SC 29425-2220
Tel: 803 792-7281 *Fax:* 803 792-7285
Accred Length: 3 Years *Program Size:* 58 (*GY1:* 21)
Subspecialties: CD, END, GE, HO, ID, NEP, PCC, RHU
Program ID: 140-45-21-403

Columbia

Palmetto Health Alliance/University of South Carolina School of Medicine Program

Sponsor: Palmetto Health Alliance
Palmetto Richland Memorial Hospital
William Jennings Bryan Dorn Veterans Hospital

Program Director:
Michael Stinson, MD
Dept of Med
2 Richland Medical Pk/Ste 502
Columbia, SC 29203
Tel: 803 540-1000 *Fax:* 803 540-1050
E-mail: sstinson@richmed.medpark.sc.edu
Internet: http://www.rmh.edu
Accred Length: 3 Years *Program Size:* 34 (*GY1:* 12)
Subspecialties: CD, END, GE, IMG, ON, PUD
Program ID: 140-45-21-404

Greenville

Greenville Hospital System Program

Sponsor: Greenville Hospital System

Program Director:
Shawn A Chillag, MD
Greenville Hospital System
Dept of Int Med
701 Grove Rd
Greenville, SC 29605
Tel: 864 455-7882 *Fax:* 864 455-8404
E-mail: nhultz@ghsms.ghs.org
Accred Length: 3 Years *Program Size:* 31 (*GY1:* 10)
Program ID: 140-45-11-405

South Dakota

Sioux Falls

University of South Dakota Program
Sponsor: University of South Dakota School of Medicine
Avera McKennan Hospital
Royal C Johnson Veterans Affairs Medical Center
Sioux Valley Hospital
Program Director:
John L Boice, MD
Univ of South Dakota, Dept of Int Med
Health Science Ctr
1400 W 22nd St
Sioux Falls, SD 57105-1570
Tel: 605 357-1558 *Fax:* 605 357-1365
E-mail: dstegeng@usd.edu
Accred Length: 3 Years *Program Size:* 24 (*GY1:* 8)
Program ID: 140-46-21-406

Tennessee

Chattanooga

University of Tennessee College of Medicine at Chattanooga Program
Sponsor: University of Tennessee College of Medicine-Chattanooga Unit
Erlanger Medical Center
Program Director:
Roger C Jones, MD
Univ of Tennessee Coll of Med
Dept of Med
975 E Third St
Chattanooga, TN 37403
Tel: 423 778-2998 *Fax:* 423 756-0361
E-mail: utintmed@erlanger.org
Internet: http://www.erlanger.org/utcom/intermed.html
Accred Length: 3 Years *Program Size:* 30 (*GY1:* 10)
Program ID: 140-47-11-407

Johnson City

East Tennessee State University Program
Sponsor: James H Quillen College of Medicine
Bristol Regional Medical Center
Johnson City Medical Center Hospital
Veterans Affairs Medical Center (Mountain Home)
Wellmont Health System-Holston Valley
Program Director:
Richard Jordan, MD
East Tennessee State Univ
Box 70 622
Johnson City, TN 37614-0622
Tel: 423 439-6282 *Fax:* 423 439-6387
Accred Length: 3 Years *Program Size:* 54 (*GY1:* 25)
Subspecialties: CD, GE, HO, ID, PUD
Program ID: 140-47-21-408

Knoxville

University of Tennessee Medical Center at Knoxville Program
Sponsor: University of Tennessee Graduate School of Medicine
University of Tennessee Memorial Hospital
Program Director:
Warren G Thompson, MD
Univ of Tennessee Grad Sch of Med
1924 Alcoa Hwy
Knoxville, TN 37920-6999
Tel: 423 544-9340
Internet:
http://www.utmck.edu/docs/deptofmed/dom.htm
Accred Length: 3 Years *Program Size:* 25 (*GY1:* 8)
Program ID: 140-47-11-409

Memphis

Methodist Hospitals of Memphis-Central Program
Sponsor: Methodist Hospitals of Memphis-Central
Program Director:
Stephen T Miller, MD
Med Education Dept/1 Tower
Methodist Hospital-Central Unit
1265 Union Ave
Memphis, TN 38104-3499
Tel: 901 726-8255 *Fax:* 901 726-8254
E-mail: millers@methodisthealth.org
Internet: http://www.methodisthealth.org
Accred Length: 3 Years *Program Size:* 28 (*GY1:* 9)
Program ID: 140-47-31-411

University of Tennessee Program
Sponsor: University of Tennessee College of Medicine
Baptist Memorial Hospital
Regional Medical Center at Memphis
University of Tennessee Medical Center (UT Bowld Hospital)
Veterans Affairs Medical Center (Memphis)
Program Director:
Kevin M McKown, MD
Univ of Tennessee
Med Educ Office
956 Court Ave/B318
Memphis, TN 38163
Tel: 901 448-5814 *Fax:* 901 448-7836
E-mail: kconlee@utmem1.utmem.edu
Internet:
http://www.utmem.edu/internal/internalmed.html
Accred Length: 3 Years *Program Size:* 70 (*GY1:* 32)
Subspecialties: CCM, CD, END, GE, HEM, ID, IMG, NEP, ON, PUD, RHU
Program ID: 140-47-21-412

Nashville

Meharry Medical College Program
Sponsor: Meharry Medical College
Alvin C York Veterans Affairs Medical Center
Metropolitan Nashville General Hospital
Program Director:
Robert E Hardy, MD
Meharry Med Coll, Dept of Int Med
1005 D B Todd Jr Blvd
Nashville, TN 37208
Tel: 615 327-6277 *Fax:* 615 327-6417
Internet: http://www.mmc.edu
Accred Length: 3 Years *Program Size:* 30 (*GY1:* 10)
Program ID: 140-47-11-413

University of Tennessee (Nashville) Program
Sponsor: University of Tennessee College of Medicine
Baptist Hospital
Program Director:
Cheryl A Fassler, MD
Dept of Medicine
2000 Church St
Nashville, TN 37236
Tel: 615 329-5663 *Fax:* 615 329-5984
E-mail: intmedicine@email.baptist-hosp.org
Internet: http://www.baptist-hosp.org/residents
Accred Length: 3 Years *Program Size:* 18 (*GY1:* 6)
Program ID: 140-47-21-478

Vanderbilt University Program
Sponsor: Vanderbilt University Medical Center
St Thomas Hospital
Veterans Affairs Medical Center (Nashville)
Program Director:
John M Leonard, MD
D-3100 Vanderbilt Med Ctr North
21st Ave S and Garland Ave
Nashville, TN 37232-2358
Tel: 615 322-3146 *Fax:* 615 343-7550
E-mail: glenna.gant@mcmail.vanderbilt.edu
Internet: http://www.mc.vanderbilt.edu/im/housestaff
Accred Length: 3 Years *Program Size:* 104 (*GY1:* 36)
Subspecialties: CD, END, GE, HO, ICE, ID, IMG, NEP, PCC, RHU
Program ID: 140-47-31-414

Texas

Amarillo

Texas Tech University (Amarillo) Program
Sponsor: Texas Tech University Health Sciences Center at Amarillo
Northwest Texas Health Care System
Veterans Affairs Medical Center (Amarillo)
Program Director:
Dave G Muthali, MD
Texas Tech Univ Health Sciences Ctr
1400 Wallace Blvd
Amarillo, TX 79106
Tel: 806 354-5489 *Fax:* 806 354-5764
E-mail: sherry@cortex.ama.ttuhsc.edu
Internet: http://www.ama.ttuhsc.edu
Accred Length: 3 Years *Program Size:* 25 (*GY1:* 11)
Program ID: 140-48-21-477

Austin

CTMF of Seton Healthcare Network Program
Sponsor: CTMF of Seton Healthcare Network
Brackenridge Hospital
Program Director:
Beth W Miller, MD
Brackenridge Hospital
601 E 15th St
Austin, TX 78701
Tel: 512 324-7868 *Fax:* 512 477-8933
E-mail: jhauschild@seton.org
Internet: http://www.goodhealth.com/CTMF
Accred Length: 3 Years *Program Size:* 24 (*GY1:* 8)
Program ID: 140-48-12-415

Dallas

Baylor University Medical Center Program
Sponsor: Baylor University Medical Center
Program Director:
Michael Emmett, MD
Baylor Univ Med Ctr
Dept of Int Med
3500 Gaston Ave
Dallas, TX 75246
Tel: 214 820-6202 *Fax:* 214 820-6385
E-mail: as.drew@baylordallas.edu
Internet:
http://www.baylordallas.edu/bumc/medicaleducation/imed
Accred Length: 3 Years *Program Size:* 38 (*GY1:* 20)
Subspecialties: CD, GE, ON
Program ID: 140-48-31-416

Methodist Hospitals of Dallas Program
Sponsor: Methodist Hospitals of Dallas
Program Director:
Jack A Barnett, MD
Methodist Hospitals of Dallas
Medical Education Dept
PO Box 655999
Dallas, TX 75265-5999
Tel: 214 947-2306 *Fax:* 214 947-2361
E-mail: dorthy@mhdcme.org
Internet: http://www.mhdcme.org
Accred Length: 3 Years *Program Size:* 18 (*GY1:* 6)
Program ID: 140-48-12-417

Presbyterian Hospital of Dallas Program
Sponsor: Presbyterian Hospital of Dallas
Program Director:
James P Knochel, MD
Presbyterian Hospital of Dallas
Dept of Int Med
8200 Walnut Hill Ln
Dallas, TX 75231-4496
Tel: 214 345-7881 *Fax:* 214 345-5167
E-mail: harrelc@phscare.org
Internet: http://www.phscare.org/gradmed
Accred Length: 3 Years *Program Size:* 24 (*GY1:* 12)
Program ID: 140-48-11-420

St Paul Medical Center Program
Sponsor: St Paul Medical Center
Program Director:
Randall L Rosenblatt, MD
St Paul Med Ctr
Dept of Int Med
5909 Harry Hines Blvd
Dallas, TX 75235
Tel: 214 879-3788 *Fax:* 214 879-3069
E-mail: susanthompson@hmhs.com
Internet: http://www.stpaulmc.org/gradmed/
Accred Length: 3 Years *Program Size:* 18 (*GY1:* 6)
Program ID: 140-48-11-418

University of Texas Southwestern Medical School Program
Sponsor: University of Texas Southwestern Medical School
Dallas County Hospital District-Parkland Memorial Hospital
Veterans Affairs Medical Center (Dallas)
Program Director:
Daniel Foster, MD
Univ of Texas Southwestern Med Sch
PO Box 36423
Dallas, TX 75235
Tel: 214 648-3483 *Fax:* 214 648-9100
E-mail: rtally@mednet.swmed.edu
Internet: http://www.swmed.edu
Accred Length: 3 Years *Program Size:* 133 (*GY1:* 47)
Subspecialties: CD, END, GE, HO, ICE, ID, NEP, PCC, RHU
Program ID: 140-48-21-419

El Paso

Texas Tech University (El Paso) Program
Sponsor: Texas Tech University Health Sciences Center at El Paso
R E Thomason General Hospital
Program Director:
Hoi Ho, MD
Tamis Bright, MD
Texas Tech Univ Health Sciences Ctr
4800 Alberta Ave
El Paso, TX 79905
Tel: 915 545-6630 *Fax:* 915 545-6634
Accred Length: 3 Years *Program Size:* 27 (*GY1:* 10)
Program ID: 140-48-11-424

William Beaumont Army Medical Center Program
Sponsor: William Beaumont Army Medical Center
Program Director:
Col Donald R Skillman, MD
William Beaumont Army Med Ctr
Dept of Med
5005 N Piedras St
El Paso, TX 79920-5001
Tel: 915 569-2504 *Fax:* 915 569-1943
E-mail: dskill@pol.net
Internet: http://www.wbamc.amedd.army.mil/
Accred Length: 3 Years *Program Size:* 22 (*GY1:* 7)
Program ID: 140-48-12-008
US Armed Services Program

Fort Sam Houston

San Antonio Uniformed Services Health Education Consortium (BAMC) Program
Sponsor: San Antonio Uniformed Services Health Education Consortium
Brooke Army Medical Center
Program Director:
Col James E Johnson, MD
Brooke Army Med Ctr
MCHE-MD
3851 Roger Brooke Dr
Fort Sam Houston, TX 78234-6260
Tel: 210 916-3856 *Fax:* 210 916-0700
E-mail:
col_james_e_johnson@bamc.smtplink.amedd.army.mil
Internet: http://www.acponline.org/residency/brooke.htm
Accred Length: 3 Years *Program Size:* 36 (*GY1:* 12)
Subspecialties: CCM, CD, GE, HO, ID, PCC
Program ID: 140-48-12-009
US Armed Services Program

Galveston

University of Texas Medical Branch Hospitals Program
Sponsor: University of Texas Medical Branch Hospitals
Program Director:
Thomas A Blackwell, MD
Univ of Texas Med Branch
Dept of Int Med
301 University Blvd
Galveston, TX 77555-0570
Tel: 409 772-2653 *Fax:* 409 772-5462
Internet: http://www.intmed.utmb.edu
Accred Length: 3 Years *Program Size:* 91 (*GY1:* 37)
Subspecialties: CCM, CD, END, GE, ID, IMG, NEP, ON, PCC, PUD, RHU
Program ID: 140-48-21-421

Houston

Baylor College of Medicine Program
Sponsor: Baylor College of Medicine
Harris County Hospital District-Ben Taub General Hospital
Methodist Hospital
St Luke's Episcopal Hospital
Veterans Affairs Medical Center (Houston)
Program Director:
Edward C Lynch, MD
Baylor Coll of Med
Dept of Med B-501
6565 Fannin St
Houston, TX 77030-2707
Tel: 713 790-3217 *Fax:* 713 793-1522
E-mail: mro@bcm.tmc.edu
Internet: http://www.bcm.tmc.edu/medicine/residency
Accred Length: 3 Years *Program Size:* 155 (*GY1:* 49)
Subspecialties: CCM, CD, END, GE, HEM, ICE, ID, IMG, NEP, ON, PCC, RHU
Program ID: 140-48-21-422

University of Texas at Houston Program
Sponsor: University of Texas Medical School at Houston
Lyndon B Johnson General Hospital
Memorial Hermann Healthcare System
Program Director:
Victor R Lavis, MD
6431 Fannin St/Rm 1.150
Houston, TX 77030
Tel: 713 500-6522 *Fax:* 713 500-6530
Internet:
http://www.uth.tmc.edu/schools/med/imed/index.htm
Accred Length: 3 Years *Program Size:* 97 (*GY1:* 32)
Subspecialties: CD, END, GE, HEM, ICE, ID, NEP, ON, PCC, RHU
Program ID: 140-48-31-423

Lackland AFB

San Antonio Uniformed Services Health Education Consortium (WHMC) Program
Sponsor: San Antonio Uniformed Services Health Education Consortium
Wilford Hall Medical Center (AETC)
Program Director:
Jay B Higgs, MD
Wilford Hall Med Ctr
59th Medical Wing/MMIMR
2200 Bergquist Dr/Ste 1
Lackland, TX 78236-5300
Tel: 210 292-5336 *Fax:* 210 670-7662
E-mail: higgs@whmc-lafb.af.mil
Internet: http://www.whmc.lak.aetc.af.mil
Accred Length: 3 Years *Program Size:* 57 (*GY1:* 23)
Subspecialties: CD, END, GE, HO, ID, NEP, PCC, RHU
Program ID: 140-48-12-003
US Armed Services Program

Lubbock

Texas Tech University (Lubbock) Program
Sponsor: Texas Tech University Health Sciences Center at Lubbock
University Medical Center
Program Director:
Kenneth M Nugent, MD
Texas Tech Univ Health Sciences Ctr
Dept of Med
3601 Fourth St
Lubbock, TX 79430
Tel: 806 743-3155 *Fax:* 806 743-3148
E-mail: medkmn@ttuhsc.edu
Internet: http://ttuhsc.edu/internal medicine
Accred Length: 3 Years *Program Size:* 23 (*GY1:* 9)
Subspecialties: CD, GE, NEP
Program ID: 140-48-21-459

Odessa

Texas Tech University (Odessa) Program
Sponsor: Texas Tech University Health Sciences Center at Odessa
Medical Center Hospital
Memorial Hospital and Medical Center
Program Director:
James Burks, MD
Texas Tech Univ Health Sciences Ctr
800 W Fourth St
Odessa, TX 79763
Tel: 915 335-5250 *Fax:* 915 335-5262
E-mail: medojkb@tthsc8.odessa.ttuhsc.edu
Accred Length: 3 Years *Program Size:* 24 (*GY1:* 8)
Program ID: 140-48-21-519

San Antonio

University of Texas Health Science Center at San Antonio Program

Sponsor: University of Texas Medical School at San Antonio
Audie L Murphy Memorial Veterans Hospital (San Antonio)
University Hospital-South Texas Medical Center

Program Director:
Mark C Henderson, MD
Univ of Texas Health Science Ctr
Office of Educational Programs
7703 Floyd Curl Dr
San Antonio, TX 78284-7871
Tel: 210 567-4820 *Fax:* 210 567-4856
E-mail: henderson@uthscsa.edu
Internet:
http://www.macorb.uthscsa.edu/medres/main.htm
Accred Length: 3 Years *Program Size:* 94 (*GY1:* 39)
Subspecialties: CD, END, GE, HEM, HO, ID, IMG, NEP, ON, PCC, RHU
Program ID: 140-48-21-425

Temple

Texas A&M College of Medicine-Scott and White Program

Sponsor: Scott and White Memorial Hospital
Central Texas Veterans Affairs Healthcare System

Program Director:
Phillip T Cain, MD
Texas A&M-Scott and White
Grad Med Educ
2401 S 31st St
Temple, TX 76508-0001
Tel: 254 724-2364 *Fax:* 254 724-4079
E-mail: intmed@bellnet.tamu.edu
Internet: http://www.sw.org
Accred Length: 3 Years *Program Size:* 38 (*GY1:* 14)
Subspecialties: CD, GE, HEM, ON, PUD
Program ID: 140-48-21-426

Utah

Salt Lake City

LDS Hospital Program

Sponsor: LDS Hospital

Program Director:
G Michael Vincent, MD
LDS Hospital
Eighth Ave and C St
Salt Lake City, UT 84143
Tel: 801 321-1077 *Fax:* 801 321-2361
E-mail: ldmgardn@ihc.com
Internet: http://www.ihc.com/ldsh/residency
Accred Length: 3 Years *Program Size:* 24 (*GY1:* 8)
Program ID: 140-49-11-428

University of Utah Program

Sponsor: University of Utah Medical Center
Veterans Affairs Medical Center (Salt Lake City)

Program Director:
H James Williams, MD
Univ of Utah Med Ctr
50 N Medical Dr/Rm 4C104
Salt Lake City, UT 84132
Tel: 801 581-7899 *Fax:* 801 581-5393
E-mail: improg.dir@hsc.utah.edu
Internet: http://www.int.med.utah.edu
Accred Length: 3 Years *Program Size:* 63 (*GY1:* 28)
Subspecialties: CD, GE, HO, ICE, ID, IMG, NEP, PCC, RHU
Program ID: 140-49-21-427

Vermont

Burlington

University of Vermont Program

Sponsor: Fletcher Allen Health Care

Program Director:
Mark A Levine, MD
Fletcher Allen Health Care
111 Colchester Ave
Dept of Medicine/Brown 330
Burlington, VT 05401
Tel: 802 656-4953 *Fax:* 802 656-5927
E-mail: medicine-resprog@vtmednet.org
Internet:
http://www.vtmednet.org/~p159517/residency.html
Accred Length: 3 Years *Program Size:* 43 (*GY1:* 19)
Subspecialties: CD, END, GE, HO, ID, NEP, PCC, PUD, RHU
Program ID: 140-50-21-429

Virginia

Charlottesville

University of Virginia Program

Sponsor: University of Virginia Medical Center

Program Director:
Cynthia M Yoshida, MD
Univ of Virginia Health Sciences Ctr
PO Box 10013
Charlottesville, VA 22906-0013
Tel: 804 924-5911 *Fax:* 804 924-0401
E-mail: cmy8x@virginia.edu
Internet:
http://www.med.virginia.edu/medicine/clinical/internal/residency/home.html
Accred Length: 3 Years *Program Size:* 78 (*GY1:* 30)
Subspecialties: CCM, CD, END, GE, HO, ICE, ID, IMG, NEP, PCC, RHU
Program ID: 140-51-21-430

Norfolk

Eastern Virginia Medical School Program

Sponsor: Eastern Virginia Medical School
DePaul Medical Center
Sentara Norfolk General Hospital
Veterans Affairs Medical Center (Hampton)

Program Director:
Thomas J Manser, MD
Eastern Virginia Med Sch
Hofheimer Hall
825 Fairfax Ave
Norfolk, VA 23507
Tel: 757 446-8910 *Fax:* 757 446-5242
E-mail: esheridan@intmed1.evms.edu
Internet:
http://www.evms.edu/intmed/residents/index.htm
Accred Length: 3 Years *Program Size:* 30 (*GY1:* 10)
Program ID: 140-51-21-432

Portsmouth

Naval Medical Center (Portsmouth) Program

Sponsor: Naval Medical Center (Portsmouth)

Program Director:
Capt Stephen C Beuttel, MD
Naval Hospital
Dept of Med
620 John Paul Jones Cir
Portsmouth, VA 23708-5100
Tel: 757 953-5067 *Fax:* 757 953-5070
E-mail: pnh0scb@pnh10.med.navy.mil
Internet:
http://www-nmcp.med.navy.mil/intmed/im_index.htm
Accred Length: 3 Years *Program Size:* 40 (*GY1:* 22)
Program ID: 140-51-11-014
US Armed Services Program

Richmond

Medical College of Virginia/Virginia Commonwealth University Program

Sponsor: Medical College of Virginia/Virginia Commonwealth University
Hunter Holmes McGuire VA Medical Center (Richmond)
Medical College of Virginia Hospitals

Program Director:
Michael B Edmond, MD MPH
Med Coll of Virginia
Dept of Int Med
PO Box 980509
Richmond, VA 23298-0509
Tel: 804 828-9726 *Fax:* 804 828-4926
E-mail: medmond@hsc.vcu.edu
Internet:
http://www.views.vcu.edu/internal-medicine/homepage.html
Accred Length: 3 Years *Program Size:* 111 (*GY1:* 50)
Subspecialties: CD, END, GE, HO, ICE, ID, IMG, NEP, PCC, RHU
Program ID: 140-51-21-433

Roanoke

University of Virginia (Roanoke-Salem) Program

Sponsor: Carilion Health System
Carilion Roanoke Community Hospital
Carilion Roanoke Memorial Hospital
Veterans Affairs Medical Center (Salem)

Program Director:
Neil K Dorsey, MD
Univ of Virginia (Roanoke-Salem) Program
Carilion Roanoke Memorial Hospital
PO Box 13367
Roanoke, VA 24033
Tel: 540 981-7120 *Fax:* 540 983-1133
E-mail: njames@carilion.com
Internet: http://www.carilion.com/residency
Accred Length: 3 Years *Program Size:* 38 (*GY1:* 16)
Subspecialties: CD, ID
Program ID: 140-51-31-431

Washington

Seattle

University of Washington Program

Sponsor: University of Washington School of Medicine
Harborview Medical Center
Providence Seattle Medical Center
Swedish Medical Center-Seattle
University of Washington Medical Center
Veterans Affairs Medical Center (Boise)
Veterans Affairs Medical Center (Seattle)

Program Director:
James F Wallace, MD
Univ of Washington
Box 356421
Seattle, WA 98195-6421
Tel: 206 543-3605 *Fax:* 206 685-8652
Internet: http://weber.u.washington.edu/~medweb
Accred Length: 3 Years *Program Size:* 172 (*GY1:* 67)
Subspecialties: CCM, CD, END, GE, HEM, ICE, ID, IMG, NEP, ON, PCC, RHU
Program ID: 140-54-21-434

Virginia Mason Medical Center Program

Sponsor: Virginia Mason Medical Center

Program Director:
Roger W Bush, MD
Virginia Mason Med Ctr
Office of Housestaff Affairs H8-ME
925 Seneca St
Seattle, WA 98111
Tel: 206 583-6079 *Fax:* 206 583-2307
E-mail: gimkmt@vmmc.org
Internet: http://www.vmmc.org/meded/internal.htm
Accred Length: 3 Years *Program Size:* 35 (*GY1:* 14)
Program ID: 140-54-12-435

Spokane

Inland Empire Hospital Services Association Program

Sponsor: Inland Empire Hospital Services Association
Deaconess Medical Center
Sacred Heart Medical Center

Program Director:
George Novan, MD
Internal Medicine Spokane
W 101-8th Ave
Spokane, WA 99204
Tel: 509 455-3022 *Fax:* 509 458-5316
E-mail: intmed@inhs.org
Internet: http://www.internalmedspokane.org
Accred Length: 3 Years *Program Size:* 21 (*GY1:* 7)
Program ID: 140-54-31-436

Tacoma

Madigan Army Medical Center Program

Sponsor: Madigan Army Medical Center

Program Director:
Bernard J Roth, MD
Madigan Army Med Ctr
Dept of Med
Tacoma, WA 98431
Tel: 253 968-0208 *Fax:* 253 968-1168
Internet: http://192.138.33.222
Accred Length: 3 Years *Program Size:* 27 (*GY1:* 9)
Subspecialties: CD, HO, IMG, PUD
Program ID: 140-54-12-010
US Armed Services Program

West Virginia

Charleston

West Virginia University (Charleston Division) Program

Sponsor: Charleston Area Medical Center

Program Director:
Greg Rosencrance, MD
Dept of Int Med
Robert C Byrd Health Sciences Ctr
3110 MacCorkle Ave SE
Charleston, WV 25304
Tel: 304 347-1315 *Fax:* 304 347-1344
Internet: http://www.camcare.com
Accred Length: 3 Years *Program Size:* 29 (*GY1:* 12)
Program ID: 140-55-11-438

Huntington

Marshall University School of Medicine Program

Sponsor: Marshall University School of Medicine
Cabell Huntington Hospital
St Mary's Hospital
Veterans Affairs Medical Center (Huntington)

Program Director:
Kevin W Yingling, MD
Marshall Univ Sch of Med
Dept of Int Med
1600 Medical Center Dr/Ste G-500
Huntington, WV 25701-3655
Tel: 304 691-1086 *Fax:* 304 691-1693
E-mail: yingling@marshall.edu
Accred Length: 3 Years *Program Size:* 32 (*GY1:* 12)
Subspecialties: CD, END, PUD
Program ID: 140-55-21-439

Morgantown

West Virginia University Program

Sponsor: West Virginia University Hospitals

Program Director:
Maria Munoz Kolar, MD
West Virginia Univ Hospital
Dept of Int Med
Rm 4082 Health Sciences Center North
Morgantown, WV 26506-9168
Tel: 304 293-4239 *Fax:* 304 293-3530
E-mail: mkolar@wvu.edu
Internet: http://intramed.hsc.wvu.edu
Accred Length: 3 Years *Program Size:* 39 (*GY1:* 13)
Subspecialties: CD, END, GE, HO, ID, NEP, ON, PCC
Program ID: 140-55-11-440

Wheeling

Ohio Valley Medical Center Program

Sponsor: Ohio Valley Medical Center

Program Director:
Jeffrey S Shultz, MD
Ohio Valley Med Ctr
Dept of Int Med
2000 Eoff St
Wheeling, WV 26003
Tel: 304 234-1835 *Fax:* 304 234-8455
Accred Length: 3 Years *Program Size:* 21 (*GY1:* 6)
Program ID: 140-55-11-441

Wisconsin

La Crosse

Gundersen Lutheran Medical Foundation Program

Sponsor: Gundersen Lutheran Medical Foundation
Gundersen Clinic
Lutheran Hospital-La Crosse

Program Director:
Robert S Witte, MD
Lutheran Hospital-LaCrosse
1836 South Ave
La Crosse, WI 54601-5429
Tel: 608 782-7300, ext 2923 *Fax:* 608 791-4457
E-mail: robert_s_witte@gundluth.org
Internet: http://www.gundluth.org
Accred Length: 3 Years *Program Size:* 22 (*GY1:* 8)
Program ID: 140-56-12-442

Madison

University of Wisconsin Program

Sponsor: University of Wisconsin Hospital and Clinics
William S Middleton Veterans Hospital

Program Director:
Bennett S Vogelman, MD
Univ of Wisconsin Hospital and Clinics
600 Highland Ave
Madison, WI 53792-2454
Tel: 608 263-7350 *Fax:* 608 262-6743
Internet: http://www.medicine.wisc.edu
Accred Length: 3 Years *Program Size:* 75 (*GY1:* 25)
Subspecialties: CD, END, GE, HEM, ID, IMG, NEP, ON, PCC, RHU
Program ID: 140-56-21-443

Marshfield

Marshfield Clinic-St Joseph's Hospital Program

Sponsor: Marshfield Clinic-St Joseph's Hospital

Program Director:
John L Olson, MD
Marshfield Clinic
Dept of Int Med 3K2
1000 N Oak Ave
Marshfield, WI 54449
Tel: 715 387-5511 *Fax:* 715 387-5163
E-mail: millerd@mfldclin.edu
Internet:
http://www.marshmed.org/mfldclin/education/med_ed/residency/resident.htm
Accred Length: 3 Years *Program Size:* 18 (*GY1:* 6)
Program ID: 140-56-31-444

Milwaukee

Aurora Health Care Program

Sponsor: Aurora Health Care
Sinai Samaritan Medical Center

Program Director:
Mark A Gennis, MD
Sinai Samaritan Med Ctr
Attn: Rebecca Young
945 N 12th St/PO Box 342
Milwaukee, WI 53201-0342
Tel: 414 219-7635 *Fax:* 414 219-6078
Internet: http://www.aurorahealthcare.org
Accred Length: 3 Years *Program Size:* 39 (*GY1:* 13)
Subspecialties: CD, GE, ICE, IMG
Program ID: 140-56-21-446

Medical College of Wisconsin Program
Sponsor: Medical College of Wisconsin Affiliated Hospitals Inc
Clement J Zablocki Veterans Affairs Medical Center
Froedtert Memorial Lutheran Hospital
Program Director:
James M Cerletty, MD
Med Coll of Wisconsin
8700 W Wisconsin Ave
Milwaukee, WI 53226
Tel: 414 257-6050 *Fax:* 414 257-6445
E-mail: immcw@mcw.edu
Internet: http://www.mcw.edu
Accred Length: 3 Years *Program Size:* 84 (*GYI:* 28)
Subspecialties: CD, END, GE, HEM, HO, ID, IMG, NEP, ON, PCC, RHU
Program ID: 140-56-31-445

Medical Genetics

Alabama

Birmingham

University of Alabama Medical Center Program
Sponsor: University of Alabama Hospital
Program Director:
Wayne H Finley, MD PhD
Sparks Ctr
1720 Seventh Ave S
Birmingham, AL 35294
Tel: 205 934-4011
E-mail: gene001@uabdpo.dpo.uab.edu
Accred Length: 2 Years *Program Size:* 2
Program ID: 130-01-21-014

California

Los Angeles

Cedars-Sinai Medical Center Program
Sponsor: Cedars-Sinai Medical Center
Los Angeles County-Harbor-UCLA Medical Center
UCLA Medical Center
Program Director:
David L Rimoin, MD PhD
Cedars-Sinai Med Ctr
8700 Beverly Blvd/Ste 4310
Los Angeles, CA 90048
Tel: 310 855-6350 *Fax:* 310 289-8591
E-mail: pkearney@xchg.csmc.edu
Internet: http://www.csmc.edu/genetics
Accred Length: 2 Years *Program Size:* 6
Program ID: 130-05-21-010

Orange

University of California (Irvine) Program
Sponsor: University of California (Irvine) Medical Center
Program Director:
Maureen Bocian, MD
101 The City Dr
Orange, CA 92868
Tel: 714 456-5791 *Fax:* 714 456-5330
E-mail: mebocian@uci.edu
Accred Length: 2 Years *Program Size:* 2 (*GYI:* 1)
Program ID: 130-05-21-042

San Diego

University of California (San Diego) Program
Sponsor: University of California (San Diego) Medical Center
Children's Hospital and Health Center
Program Director:
Marilyn C Jones, MD
3020 Children's Way/MC 5031
San Diego, CA 92123
Tel: 619 576-5840 *Fax:* 619 495-8550
Accred Length: 2 Years *Program Size:* 3 (*GYI:* 1)
Program ID: 130-05-31-019

San Francisco

University of California (San Francisco) Program
Sponsor: University of California (San Francisco) School of Medicine
Stanford University Hospital
University of California (San Francisco) Medical Center
Program Director:
H E Hoyme, MD
Dept of Pediatrics/H-315
Stanford Univ Sch of Med
Stanford, CA 94305-5208
Tel: 650 723-6858 *Fax:* 650 498-4555
Accred Length: 2 Years *Program Size:* 13 (*GYI:* 10)
Program ID: 130-05-31-039

Colorado

Denver

University of Colorado Program
Sponsor: University of Colorado Health Sciences Center
Program Director:
Eva Sujansky, MD
Box B300
1056 E 19th Ave
Denver, CO 80218
Tel: 303 861-6395 *Fax:* 303 861-3921
E-mail: sujansky.eva@tchden.org
Accred Length: 2 Years *Program Size:* 2 (*GYI:* 1)
Program ID: 130-07-21-027

Connecticut

Farmington

University of Connecticut Program
Sponsor: University of Connecticut School of Medicine
Connecticut Children's Medical Center
Univ of Connecticut Health Center/John Dempsey Hospital
Program Director:
Robert M Greenstein, MD
Connecticut Children's Med Ctr
282 Washington St
Hartford, CT 06106
Tel: 860 545-9580 *Fax:* 860 545-9590
E-mail: rgreens@ccmckids.org
Internet: http://www.ccmckids.org
Accred Length: 2 Years *Program Size:* 1 (*GYI:* 1)
Program ID: 130-08-21-041

New Haven

Yale-New Haven Medical Center Program
Sponsor: Yale-New Haven Hospital
Program Director:
Barbara R Pober, MD
Dept of Genetics
PO Box 208005
333 Cedar St
New Haven, CT 06520-8005
Tel: 203 785-5749 *Fax:* 203 785-7227
E-mail: betsy.jasiorkowski@yale.edu
Internet: http://info.med.yale.edu/genetics/clinical
Accred Length: 2 Years *Program Size:* 4
Program ID: 130-08-21-021

Georgia

Atlanta

Emory University Program

Sponsor: Emory University School of Medicine

Program Director:
Louis J Elsas, MD
Emory Univ Sch of Med
Pediatrics/Medical Genetics
2040 Ridgewood Dr
Atlanta, GA 30322
Tel: 404 727-5863 *Fax:* 404 727-5783
E-mail: lje@rw.ped.emory.edu
Internet:
http://www.cc.emory.edu/pediatrics/medgen/medgen.htm
Accred Length: 2 Years *Program Size:* 3 (*GY1:* 1)
Program ID: 130-12-21-048

Illinois

Chicago

University of Illinois College of Medicine at Chicago Program

Sponsor: University of Illinois College of Medicine at Chicago
Michael Reese Hospital and Medical Center
University of Illinois Hospital and Clinics

Program Director:
Barbara K Burton, MD
Div of Genetics M/C 857
Univ of Illinois Coll of Med
840 S Wood St
Chicago, IL 60612
Tel: 312 355-0732 *Fax:* 312 355-0739
E-mail: bkburton@uic.edu
Accred Length: 2 Years *Program Size:* 2
Program ID: 130-16-21-017

Indiana

Indianapolis

Indiana University School of Medicine Program

Sponsor: Indiana University School of Medicine
Clarian IU Hospital
Clarian Riley Hospital for Children

Program Director:
Merrill D Benson, MD MD
Indiana Univ Sch of Med
Dept of Medical/Molecular Genetics
975 W Walnut St/IB 130
Indianapolis, IN 46202-5251
Tel: 317 274-2241 *Fax:* 317 274-2387
E-mail: mbenson@medgen.iupui.edu
Internet: http://medgen.iupui.edu
Accred Length: 2 Years *Program Size:* 2
Program ID: 130-17-21-015

Iowa

Iowa City

University of Iowa Hospitals and Clinics Program

Sponsor: University of Iowa Hospitals and Clinics

Program Director:
William J Rhead, MD
Univ of Iowa Hospitals and Clinics
Dept of Pediatrics
200 Hawkins Dr
Iowa City, IA 52242-1083
Tel: 319 356-2674 *Fax:* 319 356-3347
E-mail: william-rhead@uiowa.edu
Accred Length: 2 Years *Program Size:* 2
Program ID: 130-18-21-004

Louisiana

New Orleans

Tulane University Program

Sponsor: Tulane University School of Medicine
Medical Center of Louisiana at New Orleans

Program Director:
Hans C Andersson, MD
Tulane Univ Sch of Med
Human Genetics Program
1430 Tulane Ave
New Orleans, LA 70112
Tel: 504 588-5229 *Fax:* 504 584-1763
E-mail: handers@tmcpop.tmc.tulane.edu
Internet: http://www.tmc.tulane.edu/departments/human_genetics/main.htm
Accred Length: 2 Years *Program Size:* 2 (*GY1:* 1)
Program ID: 130-21-21-025

Maryland

Baltimore

Johns Hopkins University Program

Sponsor: Johns Hopkins University School of Medicine
Johns Hopkins Hospital

Program Director:
Garry R Cutting, MD
600 N Wolfe St
Baltimore, MD 21287
Tel: 410 955-1773 *Fax:* 410 955-0484
E-mail: gcutting@welchlink.welch.jhu.edu
Accred Length: 2 Years *Program Size:* 16 (*GY1:* 6)
Program ID: 130-23-21-043

Bethesda

National Institutes of Health Clinical Center Program

Sponsor: NIH Warren Grant Magnuson Clinical Center

Program Director:
Maximilian Muenke, MD
National Institutes of Health
NIH Bldg 10/Rm 10C101
Bethesda, MD 20892-1852
Tel: 301 402-8255
E-mail: mmuenke@nhgri.nih.gov
Internet:
http://www.training.nih.gov/postdoctoral/index.html
Accred Length: 2 Years *Program Size:* 8 (*GY1:* 4)
Program ID: 130-23-21-022

Massachusetts

Boston

Boston University Medical Center Program

Sponsor: Boston Medical Center

Program Director:
Aubrey Milunsky, MD
Ctr For Human Genetics
715 Albany St
Ste 408
Boston, MA 02118-2394
Tel: 617 638-7083 *Fax:* 617 638-7092
E-mail: amilunsk@bu.edu
Internet: http://med-info.bu.edu/dna-labs.htm
Accred Length: 2 Years *Program Size:* 1 (*GY1:* 0)
Program ID: 130-24-31-029

Harvard Medical School Program

Sponsor: Children's Hospital
Massachusetts General Hospital

Program Director:
Bruce R Korf, MD
Children's Hospital
300 Longwood Ave
Boston, MA 02115
Tel: 617 355-6091 *Fax:* 617 355-7588
E-mail: korf@hub.tch.harvard.edu
Accred Length: 2 Years *Program Size:* 6 (*GY1:* 3)
Program ID: 130-24-21-024

Michigan

Ann Arbor

University of Michigan Program

Sponsor: University of Michigan Hospitals

Program Director:
Jeffrey W Innis, MD
Univ of Michigan
TC 1924/Box 0318
Ann Arbor, MI 48109-0318
Tel: 734 764-0579 *Fax:* 734 936-6897
E-mail: innis@umich.edu
Accred Length: 2 Years *Program Size:* 4
Program ID: 130-25-21-030

Detroit

Henry Ford Hospital Program

Sponsor: Henry Ford Hospital

Program Director:
Gerald L Feldman, MD PhD
Henry Ford Hospital
Dept of Med Genetics
2799 W Grand Blvd
Detroit, MI 48202
Tel: 313 916-3188 *Fax:* 313 916-2076
E-mail: glfeldman@pol.net
Internet: http://www.henryfordhealth.org
Accred Length: 2 Years *Program Size:* 3
Program ID: 130-25-21-001

Wayne State University/Detroit Medical Center Program

Sponsor: Wayne State University/Detroit Medical Center
Hutzel Hospital

Program Director:
Mark I Evans, MD
4707 St Antoine Blvd
Detroit, MI 48201
Tel: 313 745-7067 *Fax:* 313 993-0153
Accred Length: 2 Years *Program Size:* 1 (*GY1:* 1)
Program ID: 130-25-21-047

Minnesota

Minneapolis

University of Minnesota Program

Sponsor: University of Minnesota Medical School
Fairview-University Medical Center

Program Director:
Susan A Berry, MD
420 Delaware St SE/Box 75
Minneapolis, MN 55455
Tel: 612 624-7144 *Fax:* 612 624-5409
Accred Length: 2 Years *Program Size:* 0
Program ID: 130-26-21-044

Rochester

Mayo Graduate School of Medicine (Rochester) Program

Sponsor: Mayo Graduate School of Medicine-Mayo Foundation
Mayo Clinic (Rochester)
Rochester Methodist Hospital
St Mary's Hospital of Rochester

Program Director:
Virginia V Michels, MD
Mayo Graduate Sch of Med
200 First St SW
Siebens 5
Rochester, MN 55905
Tel: 507 284-3108 *Fax:* 507 284-0999
E-mail: mgsm.medlab.specialties@mayo.edu
Internet: http://www.mayo.edu/
Accred Length: 2 Years *Program Size:* 2
Program ID: 130-26-21-011

New Jersey

Newark

UMDNJ-New Jersey Medical School Program

Sponsor: UMDNJ-New Jersey Medical School
St Peter's University Hospital
UMDNJ-Robert Wood Johnson Medical School

Program Director:
Franklin Desposito, MD
185 S Orange Ave/MSB F-540
Newark, NJ 08903
Tel: 201 982-5276
Accred Length: 2 Years *Program Size:* 0
Program ID: 130-33-21-037

New York

Bronx

Albert Einstein College of Medicine Program

Sponsor: Albert Einstein College of Medicine of Yeshiva University
Montefiore Medical Center-Weiler Hospital

Program Director:
Susan J Gross, MD
Div of Reproductive Genetics
1695 Eastchester Rd/Ste 301
Bronx, NY 10461
Tel: 718 405-8150 *Fax:* 718 405-8154
E-mail: suedoc1@aol.com
Internet:
http://www.aecom.yu.edu/obgyn/divdep/index.html
Accred Length: 2 Years *Program Size:* 4
Program ID: 130-35-31-008

Brooklyn

Maimonides Medical Center Program

Sponsor: Maimonides Medical Center

Program Director:
Gabriel Kupchik, MD
Maimonides Med Ctr
4802 Tenth Ave
Brooklyn, NY 11219
Tel: 718 283-8423, ext 8423 *Fax:* 718 283-6268
E-mail: gabriel@mem.po.com
Accred Length: 2 Years *Program Size:* 2
Program ID: 130-35-21-016

New York

Mount Sinai School of Medicine Program

Sponsor: Mount Sinai School of Medicine
Mount Sinai Medical Center

Program Director:
Robert J Desnick, MD
Mount Sinai Med Ctr
Box 1497
One Gustave L Levy Pl
New York, NY 10029
Tel: 212 241-6944 *Fax:* 212 860-3316
Accred Length: 4 Years *Program Size:* 6 (*GY1:* 1)
Program ID: 130-35-21-006

North Carolina

Chapel Hill

University of North Carolina Hospitals Program

Sponsor: University of North Carolina Hospitals

Program Director:
Arthur S Aylsworth, MD
Univ of North Carolina Hospitals
CB 7487 Med Research Bldg A
Chapel Hill, NC 27599-7487
Tel: 919 966-4202
Accred Length: 2 Years *Program Size:* 1 (*GY1:* 1)
Program ID: 130-36-21-031

Durham

Duke University Program

Sponsor: Duke University Medical Center

Program Director:
Yuan T Chen, MD PhD
Duke Univ
Div of Med Genetics
Box 3528
Durham, NC 27710
Tel: 919 684-2036 *Fax:* 919 684-8944
E-mail: chen0010@mc.duke.edu
Internet: http://www.duke.edu/~ytchen/mghome.html
Accred Length: 2 Years *Program Size:* 2 (*GY1:* 1)
Program ID: 130-36-21-018

Ohio

Cincinnati

Children's Hospital Medical Center/University of Cincinnati College of Medicine Program

Sponsor: Children's Hospital Medical Center

Program Director:
Howard M Saal, MD
Children's Hospital Med Ctr
Div of Human Genetics
3333 Burnet Ave/PAV 3-52
Cincinnati, OH 45229-3039
Tel: 513 636-4760 *Fax:* 513 636-7297
E-mail: saalhm@chmcc.org
Accred Length: 4 Years *Program Size:* 4 (*GY1:* 2)
Program ID: 130-38-21-013

Cleveland

Case Western Reserve University Program

Sponsor: University Hospitals of Cleveland
MetroHealth Medical Center

Program Director:
Suzanne B Cassidy, MD
Ctr for Human Genetics-Univ Hospitals of Cleveland
11100 Euclid Ave/Lakeside 1500
Cleveland, OH 44106-1655
Tel: 216 844-3936 *Fax:* 216 844-7497
E-mail: sbc2@po.cwru.edu
Internet:
http://mediswww.meds.cwru.edu/dept/genetics/ and http://www.uhhs.com
Accred Length: 2 Years *Program Size:* 4
Program ID: 130-38-21-007

Oregon

Portland

Oregon Health Sciences University Program

Sponsor: Oregon Health Sciences University Hospital
Shriners Hospitals for Children (Portland)

Program Director:
Robert S Wildin, MD
Oregon Health Sciences Univ
3181 SW Sam Jackson Park Rd/L103
Portland, OR 97201-3098
Tel: 503 494-4416 *Fax:* 503 494-6886
E-mail: wildinr@ohsu.edu
Internet: http://www.ohsu.edu/som-medgen/genpage.htm
Accred Length: 2 Years *Program Size:* 1
Program ID: 130-40-21-009

Pennsylvania

Philadelphia

Children's Hospital of Philadelphia Program

Sponsor: Children's Hospital of Philadelphia
Hospital of the University of Pennsylvania

Program Director:
Haig H Kazazian Jr, MD
Univ of Pennsylvania Sch of Med
Dept of Genetics
415 Curie Blvd/475 Clinical Research Bldg
Philadelphia, PA 19104-6145
Tel: 215 898-3582 *Fax:* 215 573-7760
E-mail: kazazian@mail.med.upenn.edu
Accred Length: 2 Years *Program Size:* 6
Program ID: 130-41-21-002

Pittsburgh

Allegheny General Hospital Program

Sponsor: Allegheny General Hospital
Hahnemann University Hospital
St Christopher's Hospital for Children

Program Director:
Reed E Pyeritz, MD PhD
Allegheny General Hospital
Dept of Human Genetics
320 E North Ave
Pittsburgh, PA 15212
Tel: 412 359-6388 *Fax:* 412 359-6488
E-mail: pyeritz@pgh.auhs.edu
Internet: http://www.pgh.auhs.edu/res/
Accred Length: 2 Years *Program Size:* 4
Program ID: 130-41-21-020

South Carolina

Greenwood

Greenwood Genetic Center Program

Sponsor: Greenwood Genetic Center
Self Memorial Hospital

Program Director:
Robert A Saul, MD
Greenwood Genetic Ctr
1 Gregor Mendel Cir
Greenwood, SC 29646
Tel: 864 941-8100 *Fax:* 864 941-8114
E-mail: rsaul@ggc.org or ksweet@ggc.org
Internet: http://www.ggc.org/
Accred Length: 2 Years *Program Size:* 1
Program ID: 130-45-21-005

Tennessee

Nashville

Vanderbilt University Program

Sponsor: Vanderbilt University Medical Center

Program Director:
John A Phillips, MD
Vanderbilt Univ
DD-2205 Med Ctr North
Nashville, TN 37232-2578
Tel: 615 322-7601 *Fax:* 615 343-9951
Accred Length: 2 Years *Program Size:* 3 (*GY1:* 1)
Program ID: 130-47-21-033

Texas

Houston

Baylor College of Medicine Program

Sponsor: Baylor College of Medicine
Harris County Hospital District-Ben Taub General Hospital
St Luke's Episcopal Hospital
Texas Children's Hospital

Program Director:
Hagop Youssoufian, MD
Baylor Coll of Med
Dept of Molecular/Human Genetics Rm S842
One Baylor Plaza/Mail Stop BCM225
Houston, TX 77030-3498
Tel: 713 798-8311 *Fax:* 713 798-5386
E-mail: hagopy@bcm.tmc.edu
Internet: http://www.bcm.tmc.edu/molgen/
Accred Length: 4 Years *Program Size:* 8
Program ID: 130-48-21-012

University of Texas at Houston Program

Sponsor: University of Texas Medical School at Houston
Lyndon B Johnson General Hospital
Memorial Hermann Healthcare System

Program Director:
Hope Northrup, MD
6431 Fannin St/MSB 3.144
Houston, TX 77030
Tel: 713 500-5760 *Fax:* 713 500-5689
E-mail: hnorthru@ped1.med.uth.tmc.edu
Accred Length: 4 Years *Program Size:* 4 (*GY1:* 1)
Program ID: 130-48-21-034

Virginia

Richmond

Medical College of Virginia/Virginia Commonwealth University Program

Sponsor: Medical College of Virginia/Virginia Commonwealth University
Medical College of Virginia Hospitals

Program Director:
Walter E Nance, MD PhD
Joann N Bodurtha, MD MPH
Box 980033
1101 E Marshall St
Richmond, VA 23298-0033
Tel: 804 828-9632, ext 112 *Fax:* 804 828-3760
E-mail: bodurtha@hsc.vcu.edu
Accred Length: 2 Years *Program Size:* 1
Program ID: 130-51-21-003

Washington

Seattle

University of Washington Program

Sponsor: University of Washington School of Medicine
Children's Hospital and Medical Center
University of Washington Medical Center

Program Director:
Peter H Byers, MD
Box 357470
Seattle, WA 98195
Tel: 206 543-4206 *Fax:* 206 616-1899
E-mail: pbeyers@u.washington.edu
Internet: http://depts.washington.edu/medgeu
Accred Length: 2 Years *Program Size:* 8 (*GY1:* 4)
Program ID: 130-54-21-040

Wisconsin

Madison

University of Wisconsin Program

Sponsor: University of Wisconsin Hospital and Clinics

Program Director:
Richard M Pauli, MD
Univ of Wisconsin Hospital and Clinics
1500 Highland Ave/#353
Madison, WI 53705
Tel: 608 263-6874 *Fax:* 608 263-3496
E-mail: pauli@waisman.misc.edu
Accred Length: 2 Years *Program Size:* 0
Program ID: 130-56-21-036

Medical Microbiology (Pathology)

Connecticut

Hartford

Hartford Hospital Program
Sponsor: Hartford Hospital
Program Director:
William T Pastuszak, MD
Hartford Hospital
Div of Microbiology
80 Seymour St/PO Box 5037
Hartford, CT 06102-5037
Tel: 860 545-2223 *Fax:* 860 545-2204
Accred Length: 1 Year *Program Size:* 1
Program ID: 314-08-11-003

New Haven

Yale-New Haven Medical Center Program
Sponsor: Yale-New Haven Hospital
Program Director:
Sheldon M Campbell, MD PhD
333 Cedar St
PO Box 3333
New Haven, CT 06511
Tel: 203 932-5711, ext 4122 *Fax:* 203 937-3449
E-mail: sheldon.campbell@yale.edu
Internet:
http://info.med.yale.edu/labmed/microbiology_fellowship.htm
Accred Length: 1 Year *Program Size:* 1
Program ID: 314-08-21-011

Illinois

Chicago

McGaw Medical Center of Northwestern University Program
Sponsor: Northwestern University Medical School
Northwestern Memorial Hospital
Program Director:
Lance R Peterson, MD
Microbiology Sect
Northwestern Memorial Hospital
250 E Superior St/Wesley 565
Chicago, IL 60611
Tel: 312 908-3205 *Fax:* 312 908-4137
E-mail: lancer@nwu.edu
Accred Length: 1 Year *Program Size:* 2
Program ID: 314-16-21-009

Indiana

Indianapolis

Indiana University School of Medicine Program
Sponsor: Indiana University School of Medicine
Clarian IU Hospital
Clarian Riley Hospital for Children
Richard L Roudebush Veterans Affairs Medical Center
William N Wishard Memorial Hospital
Program Director:
Stephen D Allen, MD
Indiana Univ Med Ctr-Univ Hospital
Div of Clin Microbiology Rm 4430
550 N University Blvd
Indianapolis, IN 46202-5283
Tel: 317 274-2557 *Fax:* 317 278-0049
E-mail: sallen@iupui.edu
Internet: http://www.pathology.iupui.edu/fellowship.html
Accred Length: 1 Year *Program Size:* 2
Program ID: 314-17-21-001

Minnesota

Rochester

Mayo Graduate School of Medicine (Rochester) Program
Sponsor: Mayo Graduate School of Medicine-Mayo Foundation
Mayo Clinic (Rochester)
Program Director:
Jon E Rosenblatt, MD
Application Processing Ctr
Mayo Graduate Sch of Med
200 First St SW
Rochester, MN 55905
Tel: 507 284-3108 *Fax:* 507 284-0999
E-mail: mgsm.medlab.specialties@mayo.edu
Internet: http://www.mayo.edu/
Accred Length: 1 Year *Program Size:* 1
Program ID: 314-26-21-006

North Carolina

Chapel Hill

University of North Carolina Hospitals Program
Sponsor: University of North Carolina Hospitals
Program Director:
Peter H Gilligan, PhD
Univ of North Carolina Hospitals
101 Manning Dr
Chapel Hill, NC 27514-7600
Tel: 919 966-2317 *Fax:* 919 966-6407
E-mail: celtsfan@med.unc.edu
Internet: http://www.pathology.med.unc.edu
Accred Length: 1 Year *Program Size:* 1
Program ID: 314-36-31-005

Durham

Duke University Program
Sponsor: Duke University Medical Center
Program Director:
L Barth Reller, MD
Duke Univ Med Ctr
Dept of Pathology
Box 3938
Durham, NC 27710
Tel: 919 684-6474 *Fax:* 919 684-8519
E-mail: relle001@mc.duke.edu
Accred Length: 1 Year *Program Size:* 2
Program ID: 314-36-21-004

Ohio

Cleveland

Cleveland Clinic Foundation Program
Sponsor: Cleveland Clinic Foundation
Program Director:
Gary Procop, MD
Cleveland Clinic Foundation
Section of Microbiology/L40
9500 Euclid Ave
Cleveland, OH 44195-5242
Tel: 216 444-5690 *Fax:* 216 444-1162
E-mail: meded@cestmp.ccf.org
Internet: http://www.ccf.org
Accred Length: 1 Year *Program Size:* 1
Program ID: 314-38-21-008

Texas

Galveston

University of Texas Medical Branch Hospitals Program
Sponsor: University of Texas Medical Branch Hospitals
Program Director:
Gail L Woods, MD
Univ of Texas Med Branch
301 University Blvd
Galveston, TX 77555-0740
Tel: 409 772-4851 *Fax:* 409 772-5683
E-mail: gwoods@beach.utmb.edu
Accred Length: 1 Year *Program Size:* 1
Program ID: 314-48-21-010

Musculoskeletal Oncology (Orthopaedic Surgery)

Florida

Gainesville

University of Florida Program
Sponsor: University of Florida College of Medicine
Shands Hospital at the University of Florida
Program Director:
Mark T Scarborough, MD
Univ of Florida
PO Box 100246/JHMHC
Gainesville, FL 32610
Tel: 352 392-8619 *Fax:* 352 392-8637
E-mail: mark-scarborough@ufl.edu
Internet: http://www.med.ufl.edu/ortho
Accred Length: 1 Year *Program Size:* 2
Program ID: 270-11-21-009

Illinois

Chicago

University of Chicago Program
Sponsor: University of Chicago Hospitals
Program Director:
Michael A Simon, MD
Univ of Chicago Hospitals
5841 S Maryland Ave/MC3079
Chicago, IL 60637-1470
Tel: 773 834-1634 *Fax:* 773 702-4384
E-mail: tsmith@surgery.bsd.uchicago.edu
Accred Length: 1 Year *Program Size:* 1
Program ID: 270-16-21-001

Massachusetts

Boston

Harvard Medical School Program
Sponsor: Massachusetts General Hospital
Children's Hospital
Program Director:
Henry J Mankin, MD
Massachusetts General Hospital
Orthopaedic Surgery
Gray 604
Boston, MA 02114
Tel: 617 724-3700 *Fax:* 617 726-6823
E-mail: mankinh@medex.mgh.harvard.edu
Accred Length: 1 Year *Program Size:* 2
Program ID: 270-24-21-003

Minnesota

Rochester

Mayo Graduate School of Medicine (Rochester) Program
Sponsor: Mayo Graduate School of Medicine-Mayo Foundation
Mayo Clinic (Rochester)
Rochester Methodist Hospital
St Mary's Hospital of Rochester
Program Director:
Michael G Rock, MD
Mayo Graduate Sch of Med
Application Processing Ctr
200 First St SW
Rochester, MN 55905
Tel: 507 284-4331 *Fax:* 507 284-0999
Internet: http://www.mayo.edu/
Accred Length: 1 Year *Program Size:* 1
Program ID: 270-26-21-004

New York

New York

Memorial Sloan-Kettering Cancer Center Program
Sponsor: Memorial Sloan-Kettering Cancer Center
Hospital for Special Surgery
Program Director:
John H Healey, MD
Memorial Sloan Kettering Cancer Ctr
1275 York Ave/A-675
New York, NY 10021
Tel: 212 639-7610 *Fax:* 212 794-4015
Accred Length: 1 Year *Program Size:* 1
Program ID: 270-35-21-005

Ohio

Cleveland

Case Western Reserve University Program
Sponsor: University Hospitals of Cleveland
MetroHealth Medical Center
Veterans Affairs Medical Center (Cleveland)
Program Director:
John T Makley, MD
Univ Hospitals of Cleveland
11100 Euclid Ave
Cleveland, OH 44106
Tel: 216 844-3233 *Fax:* 216 844-5970
Accred Length: 1 Year *Program Size:* 1
Program ID: 270-38-21-006

Texas

Dallas

University of Texas Southwestern Medical School Program
Sponsor: University of Texas Southwestern Medical School
Presbyterian Hospital of Dallas
Program Director:
Gerhard E Maale, MD
8230 Walnut Hill Ln/Ste 514
Dallas, TX 75231
Tel: 214 891-1700 *Fax:* 214 891-0984
Accred Length: 1 Year *Program Size:* 1
Program ID: 270-48-21-008

Musculoskeletal Radiology (Radiology-Diagnostic)

Michigan

Detroit

Henry Ford Hospital Program
Sponsor: Henry Ford Hospital
Program Director:
Marnix T van Holsbeeck, MD
Henry Ford Hospital
2799 W Grand Blvd
Detroit, MI 48202
Tel: 313 556-9848 *Fax:* 313 556-9842
Accred Length: 1 Year *Program Size:* 2
Program ID: 426-25-21-001

New York

Bronx

Albert Einstein College of Medicine Program
Sponsor: Albert Einstein College of Medicine of Yeshiva University
Montefiore Medical Center-Weiler Hospital
Program Director:
Nogah Haramati, MD
111 E 210th St
Bronx, NY 10467
Tel: 718 920-5506 *Fax:* 718 920-4854
Accred Length: 1 Year *Program Size:* 1
Program ID: 426-35-21-002

New York

New York University Medical Center Program
Sponsor: New York University Medical Center
Bellevue Hospital Center
Hospital for Joint Diseases Orthopaedic Institute
Program Director:
Hossein Firooznia, MD
560 First Ave
New York, NY 10016
Tel: 212 263-5217 *Fax:* 212 263-8978
Accred Length: 1 Year *Program Size:* 1
Program ID: 426-35-11-006

Rochester

University of Rochester Program
Sponsor: Strong Memorial Hospital of the University of Rochester
Program Director:
Stuart J Rubin, MD
Box 648
601 Elmwood Ave
Rochester, NY 14642
Tel: 716 275-0872 *Fax:* 716 273-1033
Accred Length: 1 Year *Program Size:* 1
Program ID: 426-35-31-003

Ohio

Cleveland

Cleveland Clinic Foundation Program
Sponsor: Cleveland Clinic Foundation
Program Director:
Bradford J Richmond, MD
9500 Euclid Ave/A21
Cleveland, OH 44195
Tel: 216 444-3931 *Fax:* 216 445-9445
E-mail: richmob@ccisd3.ccf.org
Internet: http://www.ccf.org
Accred Length: 1 Year *Program Size:* 1
Program ID: 426-38-21-007

Pennsylvania

Philadelphia

Temple University Program
Sponsor: Temple University Hospital
Shriners Hospital for Children (Philadelphia)
Program Director:
Akbar Bonakdarpour, MD
Temple Univ
Broad and Ontario Sts
Philadelphia, PA 19140
Tel: 215 707-4220 *Fax:* 215 707-5851
Accred Length: 1 Year *Program Size:* 1
Program ID: 426-41-21-005

Wisconsin

Madison

University of Wisconsin Program
Sponsor: University of Wisconsin Hospital and Clinics
Program Director:
Arthur A De Smet, MD
600 Highland Ave (E3/311 CSC)
Madison, WI 53792-3252
Tel: 608 263-9387 *Fax:* 608 263-0876
E-mail: adesmet@facstaff.wisc.edu
Accred Length: 1 Year *Program Size:* 1
Program ID: 426-56-21-008

Neonatal-Perinatal Medicine (Pediatrics)

Alabama

Birmingham

University of Alabama Medical Center Program
Sponsor: University of Alabama Hospital
Children's Hospital of Alabama
Program Director:
Waldemar A Carlo, MD
Div of Neonatalogy
Univ of Alabama
Univ Hospital/Rm NHB 525
Birmingham, AL 35233-7335
Tel: 205 934-4680 *Fax:* 205 934-3100
E-mail: wcarlo@peds.uab.edu
Accred Length: 3 Years *Program Size:* 6
Program ID: 329-01-21-001

Arkansas

Little Rock

University of Arkansas for Medical Sciences Program
Sponsor: University of Arkansas College of Medicine
Arkansas Children's Hospital
University Hospital of Arkansas
Program Director:
Bonnie J Taylor, MD
Arkansas Children's Hospital
800 Marshall St/Rm S-470
Little Rock, AR 72202-3591
Tel: 501 320-1028 *Fax:* 501 320-4264
E-mail: bjtaylor@achasc.uams.edu
Accred Length: 3 Years *Program Size:* 3
Program ID: 329-04-21-105

California

Loma Linda

Loma Linda University Program
Sponsor: Loma Linda University Medical Center
Program Director:
Douglas D Deming, MD
Loma Linda Univ Med Ctr
Dept of Pediatrics
11234 Anderson St
Loma Linda, CA 92354
Tel: 909 824-0800, ext 42853 *Fax:* 909 478-4298
E-mail: ddeming@ahs.llumc.edu
Accred Length: 3 Years *Program Size:* 3
Program ID: 329-05-21-062

Los Angeles

Cedars-Sinai Medical Center Program

Sponsor: Cedars-Sinai Medical Center

Program Director:
Augusto Sola, MD
Cedars-Sinai Med Ctr
8700 Beverly Blvd
North Tower Rm 4310
Los Angeles, CA 90048
Tel: 310 855-4434 *Fax:* 310 967-0145
E-mail: asola@xchg.peds.csmc.edu
Internet: http://www.csmc.edu/pediatrics
Accred Length: 3 Years *Program Size:* 3
Program ID: 329-05-21-113

UCLA Medical Center Program

Sponsor: UCLA School of Medicine
Olive View-UCLA Medical Center
UCLA Medical Center

Program Director:
Cynthia T Barrett, MD
UCLA Children's Hospital
Ped Neonatology
10833 Le Conte Ave/B2-375 MDCC
Los Angeles, CA 90095-1752
Tel: 310 825-7763 *Fax:* 310 825-6394
E-mail: cbarrett@pediatrics.medsch.ucla.edu
Internet: http://www.peds.medsch.ucla.edu
Accred Length: 3 Years *Program Size:* 3
Program ID: 329-05-21-005

University of Southern California Program

Sponsor: Los Angeles County-USC Medical Center

Program Director:
Manuel Durand, MD
Los Angeles County-USC Med Ctr
Women's and Children's Hospital
1240 N Mission Rd/Rm L-919
Los Angeles, CA 90033
Tel: 323 226-3403 *Fax:* 323 226-3440
Accred Length: 3 Years *Program Size:* 8
Program ID: 329-05-21-004

Orange

University of California (Irvine) Program

Sponsor: University of California (Irvine) Medical Center
Long Beach Memorial Medical Center

Program Director:
Houchang D Modanlou, MD
Univ of California Irvine Med Ctr
101 The City Dr
Bldg 2/Rte 81
Orange, CA 92868
Tel: 714 456-6933 *Fax:* 714 456-8850
E-mail: modanlou@uci.edu
Accred Length: 3 Years *Program Size:* 6
Program ID: 329-05-31-114

Sacramento

University of California (Davis) Program

Sponsor: University of California (Davis) Medical Center

Program Director:
Boyd W Goetzman, MD PhD
Univ of California Davis Sch of Med
Research Lab TB 193
Davis, CA 95616
Tel: 530 752-3441 *Fax:* 530 752-6215
E-mail: bwgoetzman@ucdavis.edu
Accred Length: 3 Years *Program Size:* 9
Program ID: 329-05-21-007

San Diego

University of California (San Diego) Program

Sponsor: University of California (San Diego) Medical Center
Children's Hospital and Health Center

Program Director:
Neil N Finer, MD
Dept of Ped/Neonatology
200 W Arbor Dr/#8774
San Diego, CA 92103-8774
Tel: 619 543-3794 *Fax:* 619 543-3812
E-mail: choliday@ucsd.edu
Accred Length: 3 Years *Program Size:* 6
Program ID: 329-05-31-096

San Francisco

University of California (San Francisco) Program

Sponsor: University of California (San Francisco) School of Medicine
University of California (San Francisco) Medical Center

Program Director:
Joseph A Kitterman, MD
Univ of California San Francisco
503-U/Box 0734
533 Parnassus Ave
San Francisco, CA 94143-0734
Tel: 415 476-1888 *Fax:* 415 476-9976
E-mail: cory@itsa.ucsf.edu
Accred Length: 3 Years *Program Size:* 7
Program ID: 329-05-21-009

Stanford

Stanford University Program

Sponsor: Stanford University Hospital

Program Director:
Louis P Halamek, MD
Stanford Univ Sch of Med
750 Welch Rd/Ste 315
Palo Alto, CA 94304
Tel: 650 723-5711 *Fax:* 650 725-8351
Internet:
http://www-leland.stanford.edu/group/neomed/index.html
Accred Length: 3 Years *Program Size:* 6
Program ID: 329-05-21-010

Torrance

Los Angeles County-Harbor-UCLA Medical Center Program

Sponsor: Los Angeles County-Harbor-UCLA Medical Center
LAC-King/Drew Medical Center

Program Director:
J Usha Raj, MD
Harbor-UCLA Med Ctr
1124 W Carson St/RB-1
Torrance, CA 90502
Tel: 310 222-1969 *Fax:* 310 533-0627
E-mail: raj@afp76.humc.edu
Accred Length: 3 Years *Program Size:* 4
Program ID: 329-05-21-101

Colorado

Denver

University of Colorado Program

Sponsor: University of Colorado Health Sciences Center

Program Director:
William W Hay Jr, MD
Univ of Colorado Health Sciences Ctr
4200 E Ninth Ave
B-195
Denver, CO 80262
Tel: 303 315-5981 *Fax:* 303 315-3851
E-mail: bill.hay@uchsc.edu
Internet: http://www.uchsc.edu
Accred Length: 3 Years *Program Size:* 5
Program ID: 329-07-21-012

Connecticut

Farmington

University of Connecticut Program

Sponsor: University of Connecticut School of Medicine
Connecticut Children's Medical Center
Univ of Connecticut Health Center/John Dempsey Hospital

Program Director:
Isabella Knox, MD EdM
Univ of Connecticut Sch of Med
Div of Neonatology
263 Farmington Ave
Farmington, CT 06030-2948
Tel: 860 679-3105 *Fax:* 860 679-1403
E-mail: jcianciolo@nso1.uchc.edu
Accred Length: 3 Years *Program Size:* 5
Program ID: 329-08-21-013

New Haven

Yale-New Haven Medical Center Program

Sponsor: Yale-New Haven Hospital

Program Director:
Ian Gross, MD
Yale Univ Sch of Med
Dept of Pediatrics
PO Box 208064
New Haven, CT 06520-8064
Tel: 203 688-2320 *Fax:* 203 688-5426
E-mail: ian.gross@yale.edu
Internet:
http://www.info.med.yale.edu/pediat/newborn.html
Accred Length: 3 Years *Program Size:* 6
Program ID: 329-08-21-014

District of Columbia

Washington

George Washington University Program

Sponsor: Children's National Medical Center
George Washington University Hospital (UHS)

Program Director:
Khodayar Rais-Bahrami, MD
Children's Hospital National Med Ctr
Dept of Neonatology
111 Michigan Ave NW
Washington, DC 20010
Tel: 202 884-4764 *Fax:* 202 884-3459
E-mail: kraisbah@cnmc.org
Accred Length: 3 Years *Program Size:* 6
Program ID: 329-10-21-015

Georgetown University Program
Sponsor: Georgetown University Medical Center
Program Director:
Martin Keszler, MD
Georgetown Univ Med Ctr
3800 Reservoir Rd NW/Rm M3400
Washington, DC 20007-2197
Tel: 202 687-8569 *Fax:* 202 784-4747
E-mail: keszlerm@medlib.georgetown.edu
Accred Length: 3 Years *Program Size:* 4
Program ID: 329-10-21-066

Florida

Gainesville

University of Florida Program
Sponsor: University of Florida College of Medicine
Shands Hospital at the University of Florida
Program Director:
Josef Neu, MD
Univ of Florida Coll of Med
Dept of Ped/Neonatology
PO Box 100296
Gainesville, FL 32610-0296
Tel: 352 392-4195 *Fax:* 352 392-4533
E-mail: neuj@peds.ufl.edu
Accred Length: 3 Years *Program Size:* 4
Program ID: 329-11-21-016

Miami

University of Miami-Jackson Memorial Medical Center Program
Sponsor: University of Miami-Jackson Memorial Medical Center
Program Director:
Eduardo Bancalari, MD
Univ of Miami Sch of Med
Dept of Ped/Neonatology (R131)
PO Box 016960
Miami, FL 33101
Tel: 305 585-6408 *Fax:* 305 545-6581
E-mail: ebanca@peds.med.miami.edu
Internet: http://neonatology.med.miami.edu
Accred Length: 3 Years *Program Size:* 6
Program ID: 329-11-21-017

Tampa

University of South Florida Program
Sponsor: University of South Florida College of Medicine
Tampa General Healthcare
Program Director:
Lance E Wyble, MD MS
Univ of South Florida Coll of Med
17 Davis Blvd/2nd Fl
Tampa, FL 33606-3309
Tel: 813 272-3903 *Fax:* 813 272-3832
E-mail: cgroh@com1.med.usf.edu
Internet: http://usfpeds.med.usf.edu
Accred Length: 3 Years *Program Size:* 3
Program ID: 329-11-21-018

Georgia

Atlanta

Emory University Program
Sponsor: Emory University School of Medicine
Grady Memorial Hospital
Program Director:
Lucky Jain, MD
Emory Univ Sch of Med, Dept of Ped/Neonatology
2040 Ridgewood Dr NE
Atlanta, GA 30322-1028
Tel: 404 727-1471 *Fax:* 404 727-1981
E-mail: ljain@emory.edu
Accred Length: 3 Years *Program Size:* 3
Program ID: 329-12-21-085

Augusta

Medical College of Georgia Program
Sponsor: Medical College of Georgia Hospital and Clinics
Program Director:
Jatinder Bhatia, MB BS
Med Coll of Georgia
Dept of Pediatrics
BIW 8078
Augusta, GA 30912-3740
Tel: 706 721-2331 *Fax:* 706 721-7531
E-mail: jatindeb@mail.mcg.edu
Accred Length: 3 Years *Program Size:* 4
Program ID: 329-12-21-067

Hawaii

Honolulu

University of Hawaii Program
Sponsor: University of Hawaii John A Burns School of Medicine
Kapiolani Medical Center for Women and Children
Tripler Army Medical Center
Program Director:
Kenneth T Nakamura, MD
Kapiolani Med Ctr for Women and Children
1319 Punahou St
Honolulu, HI 96826-1032
Tel: 808 983-8020 *Fax:* 808 949-4232
E-mail: kennethn@kapiolani.org
Accred Length: 3 Years *Program Size:* 6
Program ID: 329-14-21-019

Illinois

Chicago

Cook County Hospital Program
Sponsor: Cook County Hospital
Program Director:
Suma P Pyati, MD
Div of Neonatology
Cook County Children's Hospital
700 S Wood St
Chicago, IL 60612-9985
Tel: 312 633-6545 *Fax:* 312 572-3814
Accred Length: 3 Years *Program Size:* 6
Program ID: 329-16-21-020

McGaw Medical Center of Northwestern University Program
Sponsor: Northwestern University Medical School
Children's Memorial Medical Center
Evanston Hospital
Northwestern Memorial Hospital
Program Director:
Daniel H Polk, MD
Children's Memorial Hospital
Div of Neonatology/#45
2300 Children's Plaza
Chicago, IL 60614
Tel: 773 880-4142 *Fax:* 773 880-3061
E-mail: dpolk@nwu.edu
Accred Length: 3 Years *Program Size:* 6
Program ID: 329-16-21-021

University of Chicago Program
Sponsor: University of Chicago Hospitals
University of Chicago Children's Hospital
Program Director:
Kwang-Sun Lee, MD
Univ of Chicago Children's Hospital
5841 S Maryland Ave
MC6060
Chicago, IL 60637-1470
Tel: 773 702-6210 *Fax:* 773 702-0764
Accred Length: 3 Years *Program Size:* 5
Program ID: 329-16-11-098

University of Illinois College of Medicine at Chicago Program
Sponsor: University of Illinois College of Medicine at Chicago
University of Illinois Hospital and Clinics
Program Director:
Vidyasagar Dharmapuri, MD
Univ of Illinois-Chicago Med Ctr
Div of Neonatology
840 S Wood St (M/C 856)
Chicago, IL 60612
Tel: 312 996-4185 *Fax:* 312 413-7901
E-mail: dsagar@uic.edu
Accred Length: 3 Years *Program Size:* 8
Program ID: 329-16-21-022

Maywood

Loyola University Program
Sponsor: Loyola University Medical Center
Program Director:
Jonathan K Muraskas, MD
Foster G McGaw Hospital
2160 S First Ave
Maywood, IL 60153
Tel: 708 216-1067 *Fax:* 708 216-5602
E-mail: tmyers@luc.edu
Internet: http://www.lumc.edu
Accred Length: 3 Years *Program Size:* 6
Program ID: 329-16-21-069

Park Ridge

Lutheran General Hospital Program
Sponsor: Lutheran General Hospital
Program Director:
David Sheftel, MD
Lutheran General Hospital
1775 Dempster St
Park Ridge, IL 60068-1174
Tel: 847 723-5313 *Fax:* 847 723-2338
Accred Length: 3 Years *Program Size:* 6
Program ID: 329-16-21-070

Indiana

Indianapolis

Indiana University School of Medicine Program

Sponsor: Indiana University School of Medicine
Clarian Riley Hospital for Children
William N Wishard Memorial Hospital
Program Director:
Mervin C Yoder, MD
Sect of Neonatal-Perinatal Med
Cancer Research Inst
1044 W Walnut/Rm 419
Indianapolis, IN 46202-5254
Tel: 317 274-4719 *Fax:* 317 274-8679
E-mail: myoder@indyvax.iupui.edu
Accred Length: 3 Years *Program Size:* 3
Program ID: 329-17-21-023

Iowa

Iowa City

University of Iowa Hospitals and Clinics Program

Sponsor: University of Iowa Hospitals and Clinics
Program Director:
Edward F Bell, MD
Univ of Iowa Hospitals and Clinics
200 Hawkins Dr
W215 General Hospital
Iowa City, IA 52242-1009
Tel: 319 356-4006 *Fax:* 319 356-4685
E-mail: edward-bell@uiowa.edu
Internet:
http://www.vh.org/welcome/uihc/uihcmeddepts/peds/neonatology.html
Accred Length: 3 Years *Program Size:* 6
Program ID: 329-18-11-087

Kentucky

Lexington

University of Kentucky Medical Center Program

Sponsor: University of Kentucky Hospital
Program Director:
Alastair A Hutchison, MD MD
Albert B Chandler Med Ctr
Univ of Kentucky
Neonatology MS 472
Lexington, KY 40536-0084
Tel: 606 323-5530 *Fax:* 606 323-8031
E-mail: aahutch@msn.com
Accred Length: 3 Years *Program Size:* 4
Program ID: 329-20-21-024

Louisville

University of Louisville Program

Sponsor: University of Louisville School of Medicine
Kosair Children's Hospital (Alliant Health System)
University of Louisville Hospital
Program Director:
David H Adamkin, MD
Dept of Pediatrics
Univ of Louisville
571 S Floyd St/Ste 300
Louisville, KY 40202-3830
Tel: 502 852-8470 *Fax:* 502 852-8473
E-mail: restoc01@gwise.louisville.edu
Accred Length: 3 Years *Program Size:* 6
Program ID: 329-20-21-025

Louisiana

New Orleans

Louisiana State University/Tulane University Program

Sponsor: Louisiana State University School of Medicine
Childrens Hospital
Medical Center of Louisiana at New Orleans
Tulane University Hospital and Clinics
Program Director:
Duna Penn, MD
Louisiana State Univ Sch of Med
1542 Tulane Ave
New Orleans, LA 70112
Tel: 504 568-4421 *Fax:* 504 568-7532
Accred Length: 3 Years *Program Size:* 3
Program ID: 329-21-21-106

Shreveport

Louisiana State University (Shreveport) Program

Sponsor: Louisiana State University Hospital-Shreveport
Program Director:
Arun K Pramanik, MD
Louisiana State Univ Med Ctr Hospital
Med Educ/Neo-Perinatal
1501 Kings Hwy/PO Box 33932
Shreveport, LA 71130-3932
Tel: 318 675-7276 *Fax:* 318 675-4660
E-mail: aprama@lsumc.edu
Accred Length: 3 Years *Program Size:* 3
Program ID: 329-21-11-088

Maryland

Baltimore

Johns Hopkins University Program

Sponsor: Johns Hopkins University School of Medicine
Johns Hopkins Bayview Medical Center
Johns Hopkins Hospital
Program Director:
Estelle B Gauda, MD
Johns Hopkins Hospital
Eudowood Neonatal Pulmonary Div
600 N Wolfe St/CMSC 210
Baltimore, MD 21287-3200
Tel: 410 955-5259 *Fax:* 410 955-0298
E-mail: egauda@welchlink.welch.jhu.edu
Internet:
http://www.med.jhu.edu/peds/neonatology/neo.html
Accred Length: 3 Years *Program Size:* 4
Program ID: 329-23-21-026

University of Maryland Program

Sponsor: University of Maryland Medical System
Mercy Medical Center
Program Director:
Ira H Gewolb, MD
Dept of Pediatrics/UMMS N5W68
22 S Greene St
Baltimore, MD 21201-1595
Tel: 410 328-6356 *Fax:* 410 328-1076
Internet:
http://www.mdkids.ab.umd.edu/neo/neofel~1.htm
Accred Length: 3 Years *Program Size:* 6
Program ID: 329-23-21-027

Bethesda

National Capital Consortium Program

Sponsor: National Capital Consortium
National Naval Medical Center (Bethesda)
USUHS F Edward Hebert School of Medicine
Walter Reed Army Medical Center
Program Director:
Jerri Curtis, MD
Uniformed Services Univ of Health Sciences
Dept of Pediatrics/Rm C1066
4301 Jones Bridge Rd
Bethesda, MD 20814-4799
Tel: 301 295-3174 *Fax:* 301 319-8214
E-mail: jcurtis@usuhs.mil
Internet: http://www.usuhs.mil/ped/neonatol.html
Accred Length: 3 Years *Program Size:* 6
Program ID: 329-10-11-090
US Armed Services Program

Massachusetts

Boston

Children's Hospital/Boston Medical Center Program

Sponsor: Children's Hospital
Beth Israel Deaconess Medical Center
Brigham and Women's Hospital
Program Director:
Charles F Simmons Jr, MD
Children's Hospital
Newborn Med, Enders 961
300 Longwood Ave
Boston, MA 02115
Tel: 617 355-7667 *Fax:* 617 355-7677
E-mail: simmonsc@a1.tch.harvard.edu
Internet: http://web1.tch.harvard.edu/jpn
Accred Length: 3 Years *Program Size:* 18
Program ID: 329-24-21-028

New England Medical Center Hospitals Program

Sponsor: New England Medical Center Hospitals
Boston Medical Center
Program Director:
Ivan D Frantz III, MD
New England Med Ctr
750 Washington St/Box 44
Boston, MA 02111-9915
Tel: 617 636-5322 *Fax:* 617 636-1456
E-mail: ivan.frantz@es.nemc.org
Accred Length: 3 Years *Program Size:* 9
Program ID: 329-24-21-071

Worcester

University of Massachusetts Program
Sponsor: University of Massachusetts Medical School
UMass Memorial Health Care (Memorial Campus)
UMass Memorial Health Care (University Campus)
Program Director:
Francis J Bednarek, MD
Univ of Massachusetts Memorial Health Care
119 Belmont St
Worcester, MA 01605
Tel: 508 793-6206 *Fax:* 508 793-6083
E-mail: franktia@aol.com
Accred Length: 3 Years *Program Size:* 2
Program ID: 329-24-21-029

Michigan

Ann Arbor

University of Michigan Program
Sponsor: University of Michigan Hospitals
Program Director:
Roger G Faix, MD
F5790 Mott Hospital 0254
200 E Hospital Dr
Ann Arbor, MI 48109-0254
Tel: 313 763-4109 *Fax:* 313 763-7728
E-mail: ped-npm-general@umich.edu
Accred Length: 3 Years *Program Size:* 4
Program ID: 329-25-21-030

Detroit

Wayne State University/Detroit Medical Center Program
Sponsor: Wayne State University/Detroit Medical Center
Children's Hospital of Michigan
Hutzel Hospital
Program Director:
Seetha Shankaran, MD
Children's Hospital
3901 Beaubien Blvd
Detroit, MI 48201
Tel: 313 745-1436 *Fax:* 313 745-5867
E-mail: s_shankaran@wayne.edu
Accred Length: 3 Years *Program Size:* 5
Program ID: 329-25-21-031

East Lansing

Michigan State University Program
Sponsor: Michigan State University College of Human Medicine
Sparrow Hospital
Program Director:
J M Lorenz, MD
Sparrow Hospital
1215 E Michigan Ave
PO Box 30480
Lansing, MI 48909-7980
Tel: 517 483-2670 *Fax:* 517 483-3994
Accred Length: 3 Years *Program Size:* 3
Program ID: 329-25-21-032

Minnesota

Minneapolis

University of Minnesota Program
Sponsor: University of Minnesota Medical School
Children's Health Care (St Paul)
Fairview-University Medical Center
Program Director:
Michael K Georgieff, MD
Box 39
420 Delaware St SE
Minneapolis, MN 55455
Tel: 612 626-0644 *Fax:* 612 624-8176
E-mail: georg001@maroon.tc.umn.edu
Internet:
http://www.peds.umn.edu/divisions/neonatology/default.html
Accred Length: 3 Years *Program Size:* 5
Program ID: 329-26-21-033

Missouri

Columbia

University of Missouri-Columbia Program
Sponsor: University of Missouri-Columbia School of Medicine
University Hospitals and Clinics
Program Director:
Elizabeth P James, MD
Univ of Missouri-Columbia Sch of Med
Child Health Dept of Neonatology
One Hospital Dr
Columbia, MO 65212
Tel: 573 882-2272 *Fax:* 573 884-5226
E-mail: elizabeth_james@muccmail.missouri.edu
Internet: http://www.choir.missouri.edu
Accred Length: 3 Years *Program Size:* 3
Program ID: 329-28-21-035

Kansas City

University of Missouri at Kansas City Program
Sponsor: University of Missouri-Kansas City School of Medicine
Children's Mercy Hospital
Truman Medical Center-West
Program Director:
William E Truog, MD
Children's Mercy Hospital
Dept of Neonatology
Kansas City, MO 64108-9898
Tel: 816 234-3592 *Fax:* 816 234-3590
Internet: http://www.cmh.edu
Accred Length: 3 Years *Program Size:* 3
Program ID: 329-28-11-091

St Louis

St Louis University School of Medicine Program
Sponsor: St Louis University School of Medicine
SSM Cardinal Glennon Children's Hospital
Program Director:
William J Keenan, MD
Akihiko Noguchi, MD
Cardinal Glennon Children's Hospital
1465 S Grand Blvd
St Louis, MO 63104
Tel: 314 577-5642 *Fax:* 314 268-6410
Accred Length: 3 Years *Program Size:* 3
Program ID: 329-28-21-036

Washington University/B-JH/SLCH Consortium Program
Sponsor: Washington University/B-JH/SLCH Consortium
St Louis Children's Hospital
Program Director:
Brian P Hackett, MD PhD
Div of Newborn Med
St Louis Children's Hospital
One Children's Pl
St Louis, MO 63110
Tel: 314 454-4168 *Fax:* 314 454-4633
E-mail: hackett@kids.wustl.edu
Internet: http://www.peds.wustl.edu/newborn/
Accred Length: 3 Years *Program Size:* 9
Program ID: 329-28-21-037

New Hampshire

Lebanon

Dartmouth-Hitchcock Medical Center Program
Sponsor: Mary Hitchcock Memorial Hospital
Program Director:
Robert A Darnall, MD
Dartmouth-Hitchcock Med Ctr
Dept of Pediatrics
HB 7445
Lebanon, NH 03756
Tel: 603 650-6385 *Fax:* 603 650-6130
E-mail: robert.a.darnall@dartmouth.edu
Accred Length: 3 Years *Program Size:* 1
Program ID: 329-32-21-111

New Jersey

New Brunswick

UMDNJ-Robert Wood Johnson Medical School Program
Sponsor: UMDNJ-Robert Wood Johnson Medical School
St Peter's University Hospital
Program Director:
Thomas Hegyi, MD
St Peter's Med Ctr, Div of Neonatology
254 Easton Ave
New Brunswick, NJ 08903
Tel: 732 745-8523 *Fax:* 732 249-6306
E-mail: tomhegyi@aol.com
Accred Length: 3 Years *Program Size:* 8
Program ID: 329-33-21-092

New Mexico

Albuquerque

University of New Mexico Program
Sponsor: University of New Mexico School of Medicine
University Hospital
Program Director:
Lu-Ann Papile, MD
Univ of New Mexico Sch of Med
Dept of Pediatrics
Ambulatory Care Ctr 3 W
Albuquerque, NM 87131-5311
Tel: 505 272-5551 *Fax:* 505 272-6845
E-mail: papile@unm.edu
Accred Length: 3 Years *Program Size:* 3
Program ID: 329-34-21-072

New York

Albany

Albany Medical Center Program

Sponsor: Albany Medical Center

Program Director:
Joaquim M Pinheiro, MD
Albany Med Coll
Div of Neonatology/Mail Code-101
47 New Scotland Ave
Albany, NY 12208-3479
Tel: 518 262-5421 *Fax:* 518 262-5881
E-mail: joaquim_pinheiro@ccgateway.amc.edu
Accred Length: 3 Years *Program Size:* 1
Program ID: 329-35-21-038

Bronx

Albert Einstein College of Medicine Program

Sponsor: Albert Einstein College of Medicine of Yeshiva University
Montefiore Medical Center-Weiler Hospital

Program Director:
Luc P Brion, MD
Jack D Weiler Hospital
1825 Eastchester Rd/Rm 725
Bronx, NY 10461
Tel: 718 904-4105 *Fax:* 718 904-2659
E-mail: brion@aecom.yu.edu
Accred Length: 3 Years *Program Size:* 4
Program ID: 329-35-21-039

Brooklyn

SUNY Health Science Center at Brooklyn Program

Sponsor: SUNY Health Science Center at Brooklyn
Kings County Hospital Center
University Hospital-SUNY Health Science Center at Brooklyn

Program Director:
Nathan Rudolph, MD
SUNY Health Science Ctr
450 Clarkson Ave/Box 49
Brooklyn, NY 11203
Tel: 718 270-1912 *Fax:* 718 270-1985
E-mail: z666666@pol.net
Accred Length: 3 Years *Program Size:* 6
Program ID: 329-35-21-040

Buffalo

SUNY at Buffalo Graduate Medical-Dental Education Consortium Program

Sponsor: SUNY at Buffalo Grad Medical-Dental Education Consortium
CGF Health System (Children's Hospital of Buffalo)

Program Director:
Corinne L Leach, MD PhD
Children's Hospital
219 Bryant St
Buffalo, NY 14222
Tel: 716 878-7673 *Fax:* 716 878-7945
E-mail: clleach@upa.chob.edu
Accred Length: 3 Years *Program Size:* 5
Program ID: 329-35-21-041

Manhasset

North Shore University Hospital/NYU School of Medicine Program

Sponsor: North Shore University Hospital

Program Director:
Rita G Harper, MD
North Shore Univ Hospital-Manhasset
Div of Perinatal Med
300 Community Dr
Manhasset, NY 11030
Tel: 516 562-4665 *Fax:* 516 562-4516
Internet: http://www.home page 11 ww.med help.org/nsuh/peds.htm
Accred Length: 3 Years *Program Size:* 5
Program ID: 329-35-21-073

New Hyde Park

Albert Einstein College of Medicine at Long Island Jewish Medical Center Program

Sponsor: Long Island Jewish Medical Center
Schneider Children's Hosp (Long Island Jewish Med Ctr)

Program Director:
Dennis Davidson, MD
Schneider Children's Hospital
270-05 76th Ave/Rm 344
New Hyde Park, NY 11040
Tel: 718 470-3440 *Fax:* 718 347-3850
Internet: http://www.lij.edu/lij-homepage-ns.html
Accred Length: 3 Years *Program Size:* 6
Program ID: 329-35-21-074

New York

Mount Sinai School of Medicine Program

Sponsor: Mount Sinai School of Medicine
Beth Israel Medical Center
Elmhurst Hospital Center-Mount Sinai Services
Mount Sinai Medical Center

Program Director:
Ian R Holzman, MD
Mount Sinai Med Ctr, Dept of Pediatrics
One Gustave L Levy Pl
New York, NY 10029-6574
Tel: 212 241-6186 *Fax:* 212 534-5207
E-mail: ian_holzman@smtplink.mssm.edu
Internet: http://www.mssm.edu/peds/newborn.html
Accred Length: 3 Years *Program Size:* 4
Program ID: 329-35-21-075

New York and Presbyterian Hospital (Columbia Campus) Program

Sponsor: New York and Presbyterian Hospital
New York and Presbyterian Hospital (Columbia Campus)

Program Director:
S David Rubenstein, MD
Babies Hospital-North
3959 Broadway/Rm 1201
New York, NY 10032
Tel: 212 305-8500, ext 5827 *Fax:* 212 305-8796
Accred Length: 3 Years *Program Size:* 8
Program ID: 329-35-21-076

New York and Presbyterian Hospital (Cornell Campus) Program

Sponsor: New York and Presbyterian Hospital
New York and Presbyterian Hospital (Cornell Campus)

Program Director:
Peter M Auld, MD
New York Hospital-Cornell Med Ctr
Perinatology
525 E 68th St
New York, NY 10021
Tel: 212 746-3530 *Fax:* 212 746-8605
Accred Length: 3 Years *Program Size:* 8
Program ID: 329-35-21-042

New York University Medical Center Program

Sponsor: New York University Medical Center
Bellevue Hospital Center

Program Director:
Karen D Hendricks-Munoz, MD
560 First Ave/TH 553
New York, NY 10016
Tel: 212 263-7477 *Fax:* 212 263-1009
Accred Length: 3 Years *Program Size:* 3
Program ID: 329-35-21-108

Rochester

University of Rochester Program

Sponsor: Strong Memorial Hospital of the University of Rochester

Program Director:
Rita M Ryan, MD
Univ of Rochester Sch of Med and Dentistry
Dept of Pediatrics
601 Elmwood Ave/Box 651
Rochester, NY 14642
Tel: 716 275-5884 *Fax:* 716 461-3614
E-mail: rita_ryan@urmc.rochester.edu
Accred Length: 3 Years *Program Size:* 6
Program ID: 329-35-21-043

Stony Brook

SUNY at Stony Brook Program

Sponsor: University Hospital-SUNY at Stony Brook

Program Director:
Edmund F LaGamma, MD
Dept of Pediatrics
SUNY-Stony Brook
HSC 11T-060
Stony Brook, NY 11794-8111
Tel: 516 444-7653 *Fax:* 516 444-8968
E-mail: elagamma@mail.som.sunysb.edu
Internet: http://www.uhmc.sunysb.edu/pediatrics
Accred Length: 3 Years *Program Size:* 8
Program ID: 329-35-21-093

Valhalla

New York Medical College at Westchester Medical Center Program

Sponsor: New York Medical College
Westchester Medical Center

Program Director:
Edmund F LaGamma, MD
Westchester Med Ctr
Regional Neonatal Intensive Care Unit
Grasslands Rd
Valhalla, NY 10595
Tel: 914 493-8558 *Fax:* 914 493-1488
E-mail: reale @nymc.edu
Accred Length: 3 Years *Program Size:* 5
Program ID: 329-35-21-077

North Carolina

Chapel Hill

University of North Carolina Hospitals Program

Sponsor: University of North Carolina Hospitals

Program Director:
Alan D Stiles, MD
Univ of North Carolina Sch of Med
Dept of Pediatrics/CB#7596
Div of Neonatal-Perinatal Med
Chapel Hill, NC 27599-7596
Tel: 919 966-5570 *Fax:* 919 966-2423
Accred Length: 3 Years *Program Size:* 6
Program ID: 329-36-21-045

Durham

Duke University Program

Sponsor: Duke University Medical Center

Program Director:
Ronald N Goldberg, MD
Maria A Pane, MD
Duke Univ Med Ctr
Box 3179
Attn: Layne Baker
Durham, NC 27710
Tel: 919 681-5218 *Fax:* 919 681-6065
E-mail: baker023@mc.duke.edu
Accred Length: 3 Years *Program Size:* 5
Program ID: 329-36-21-046

Greenville

East Carolina University Program

Sponsor: East Carolina University School of Medicine
Pitt County Memorial Hospital

Program Director:
James J Cummings, MD
East Carolina Univ Sch of Med
Ped/Neonatology
600 Moye Blvd
Greenville, NC 27858-4354
Tel: 252 816-4787 *Fax:* 252 816-3806
E-mail: staton@brody.med.ecu.edu
Accred Length: 3 Years *Program Size:* 1
Program ID: 329-36-21-078

Winston-Salem

Wake Forest University School of Medicine Program

Sponsor: Wake Forest University Baptist Medical Center

Program Director:
Judy L Aschner, MD
Wake Forest Univ Baptist Med Ctr
Medical Center Blvd
Winston-Salem, NC 27157
Tel: 336 716-4663 *Fax:* 336 716-7100
E-mail: jaschner@bgsm.edu
Internet:
http://www.wfubmc.edu/wfubmc/neonatal/nnhome.html
Accred Length: 3 Years *Program Size:* 3
Program ID: 329-36-11-103

Ohio

Cincinnati

Children's Hospital Medical Center/University of Cincinnati College of Medicine Program

Sponsor: Children's Hospital Medical Center
Good Samaritan Hospital
University Hospital Inc

Program Director:
Ward R Rice, MD PhD
Children's Hospital Med Ctr
Neonatology/CHRF-4
3333 Burnet Ave
Cincinnati, OH 45229-3039
Tel: 513 636-7992 *Fax:* 513 636-7868
E-mail: ward.rice@chmcc.org
Internet: http://www.chmcc.org
Accred Length: 3 Years *Program Size:* 10
Program ID: 329-38-21-047

Cleveland

Case Western Reserve University (MetroHealth) Program

Sponsor: MetroHealth Medical Center

Program Director:
John J Moore, MD
MetroHealth Med Ctr
2500 MetroHealth Dr
Cleveland, OH 44109-1998
Tel: 216 778-5909 *Fax:* 216 778-3252
E-mail: jjm6@po.cwru.edu
Accred Length: 3 Years *Program Size:* 5
Program ID: 329-38-21-089

Case Western Reserve University Program

Sponsor: University Hospitals of Cleveland

Program Director:
Avroy A Fanaroff, MD
Rainbow Babies and Childrens Hospital
11100 Euclid Ave/Rm 3100 RBC
Cleveland, OH 44106-6010
Tel: 216 844-3387 *Fax:* 216 844-3380
E-mail: aaf2@po.cwru.ed
Accred Length: 3 Years *Program Size:* 7
Program ID: 329-38-21-048

Columbus

Children's Hospital/Ohio State University Program

Sponsor: Children's Hospital

Program Director:
James Menke, MD
Children's Hospital
700 Children's Dr
Columbus, OH 43205
Tel: 614 722-4530 *Fax:* 614 722-4541
E-mail: jmenke@ch.dsu.edu
Accred Length: 3 Years *Program Size:* 1
Program ID: 329-38-21-049

Oklahoma

Oklahoma City

University of Oklahoma Health Sciences Center Program

Sponsor: University of Oklahoma College of Medicine
Children's Hospital of Oklahoma

Program Director:
Rita P Raman, MD JD
Children's Hospital
Rm 2-B 307
PO Box 26307
Oklahoma City, OK 73126
Tel: 405 271-5215 *Fax:* 405 271-1236
E-mail: rita-raman@ouhsc.edu
Accred Length: 3 Years *Program Size:* 0
Program ID: 329-39-21-079

Oregon

Portland

Oregon Health Sciences University Program

Sponsor: Oregon Health Sciences University Hospital

Program Director:
Linda D Wallen, MD
Oregon Health Sciences Univ
Dept of Pediatrics (NRC5)
3181 SW Sam Jackson Park Rd
Portland, OR 97201-3098
Tel: 503 494-1077 *Fax:* 503 494-0714
E-mail: wallen@ohsu.edu
Accred Length: 3 Years *Program Size:* 3
Program ID: 329-40-21-081

Pennsylvania

Hershey

Penn State Geisinger Health System/Milton S Hershey Medical Center Program

Sponsor: Penn State Geisinger Health System
Milton S Hershey Medical Center

Program Director:
Keith H Marks, MD PhD
Penn State Geisinger Health System-Hershey Med Ctr
PO Box 850/MC H085
Hershey, PA 17033-0850
Tel: 717 531-8412 *Fax:* 717 531-1533
E-mail: nz9@psu.edu
Internet: http://www.hmc.psu.edu/depts/peds/index.htm
Accred Length: 3 Years *Program Size:* 2
Program ID: 329-41-21-050

Philadelphia

Albert Einstein Medical Center Program

Sponsor: Albert Einstein Medical Center

Program Director:
Hallam Hurt, MD
Albert Einstein Med Ctr
Div of Neonatology
5501 Old York Rd
Philadelphia, PA 19141
Tel: 215 456-6695 *Fax:* 215 456-6769
E-mail: melnykj@aehn2.einstein.edu
Accred Length: 3 Years *Program Size:* 4
Program ID: 329-41-11-097

Children's Hospital of Philadelphia Program
Sponsor: Children's Hospital of Philadelphia
Hospital of the University of Pennsylvania
Program Director:
Roberta A Ballard, MD
Children's Hospital
Div of Neonatology
34th St and Civic Center Blvd
Philadelphia, PA 19104-4399
Tel: 215 590-1653 *Fax:* 215 590-3051
E-mail: ballard@email.chop.edu
Internet:
http://www.med.upenn.edu/~neonate/index.html
Accred Length: 3 Years *Program Size:* 8
Program ID: 329-41-21-051

St Christopher's Hospital for Children Program
Sponsor: St Christopher's Hospital for Children
Temple University Hospital
Program Director:
Eileen Tyrala, MD
St Christopher's Hospital for Children
Erie Ave at Front St
Philadelphia, PA 19134-1095
Tel: 215 427-5202 *Fax:* 215 427-8192
E-mail: tyralae@wpo.auhs.edu
Accred Length: 3 Years *Program Size:* 7
Program ID: 329-41-21-082

Thomas Jefferson University/duPont Hospital for Children Program
Sponsor: Thomas Jefferson University Hospital
Christiana Care Health Services Inc
Program Director:
Stephen Pearlman, MD
Christiana Hospital
4755 Ogletown Stanton Rd
PO Box 6001
Newark, DE 19718
Tel: 302 733-2410 *Fax:* 302 733-2602
E-mail: spearlma@christianacare.org.smtp
Accred Length: 3 Years *Program Size:* 9
Program ID: 329-41-21-104

Pittsburgh

University Health Center of Pittsburgh Program
Sponsor: University Health Center of Pittsburgh
Magee-Women's Hospital
Program Director:
Jon F Watchko, MD
Magee-Womens Hospital
Div of Neonatology/Develop Biology
300 Halket St
Pittsburgh, PA 15213-3180
Tel: 412 641-1834 *Fax:* 412 641-5313
E-mail: watchko+@pitt.edu
Internet: http://www.magee.edu/research/research.html
Accred Length: 3 Years *Program Size:* 6
Program ID: 329-41-21-052

Puerto Rico

San Juan

University of Puerto Rico Program
Sponsor: University of Puerto Rico School of Medicine
University Pediatric Hospital
Program Director:
Marta Valcarcel, MD
Univ of Puerto Rico Med Science Campus
GPO Box 365067
San Juan, PR 00936-5067
Tel: 809 754-3535
E-mail: mivalcar@prtc.net
Accred Length: 3 Years *Program Size:* 2
Program ID: 329-42-21-112

Rhode Island

Providence

Brown University Program
Sponsor: Women and Infants Hospital of Rhode Island
Program Director:
Barbara S Stonestreet, MD
Women and Infant's Hospital
101 Dudley St
Providence, RI 02905-2499
Tel: 401 274-1122, ext 1229 *Fax:* 401 453-7571
E-mail: barbara_stonestreet@brown.edu
Accred Length: 3 Years *Program Size:* 7
Program ID: 329-43-21-053

South Carolina

Charleston

Medical University of South Carolina Program
Sponsor: Medical University of South Carolina College of Medicine
MUSC Medical Center
Program Director:
David J Annibale, MD
Med Univ Hospital
672 Children's Hospital
171 Ashley Ave
Charleston, SC 29425
Tel: 843 792-9744 *Fax:* 843 792-8801
E-mail: annibald@musc.edu
Accred Length: 3 Years *Program Size:* 6
Program ID: 329-45-21-100

Tennessee

Memphis

University of Tennessee Program
Sponsor: University of Tennessee College of Medicine
Regional Medical Center at Memphis
Program Director:
Sheldon B Korones, MD
Newborn Ctr
853 Jefferson/2nd Fl
Memphis, TN 38163
Tel: 901 448-5950 *Fax:* 901 448-1691
E-mail: skorones@utmem1.utmem.edu
Internet: http://newborn2.utmem.edu
Accred Length: 3 Years *Program Size:* 6
Program ID: 329-47-21-083

Nashville

Vanderbilt University Program
Sponsor: Vanderbilt University Medical Center
Program Director:
Robert B Cotton, MD
Vanderbilt Univ
Sch of Med/A-0105 MCN
21st Ave S and Garland Ave
Nashville, TN 37232-2370
Tel: 615 322-2823 *Fax:* 615 343-1763
E-mail: robert.cotton@mcmail.vanderbilt.edu
Accred Length: 3 Years *Program Size:* 7
Program ID: 329-47-21-054

Texas

Dallas

University of Texas Southwestern Medical School Program
Sponsor: University of Texas Southwestern Medical School
Dallas County Hospital District-Parkland Memorial Hospital
Program Director:
Charles R Rosenfeld, MD
Univ of Texas Southwestern Med Ctr
5323 Harry Hines Blvd
Dallas, TX 75235-9063
Tel: 214 648-3903 *Fax:* 214 648-2481
E-mail: bbueg@mednet.swmed.edu
Internet:
http://www.swmed.edu/home-pages/peds/clinical.html
Accred Length: 3 Years *Program Size:* 6
Program ID: 329-48-21-055

Galveston

University of Texas Medical Branch Hospitals Program
Sponsor: University of Texas Medical Branch Hospitals
Program Director:
C Joan Richardson, MD
Dept of Pediatrics
301 University Blvd
Galveston, TX 77555-0526
Tel: 409 772-2815 *Fax:* 409 772-0747
E-mail: jrich@utmb.edu
Accred Length: 3 Years *Program Size:* 3
Program ID: 329-48-21-056

Houston

Baylor College of Medicine Program
Sponsor: Baylor College of Medicine
Harris County Hospital District-Ben Taub General Hospital
Texas Children's Hospital
Program Director:
Leonard E Weisman, MD
Baylor Coll of Med
One Baylor Plaza
Houston, TX 77030-3498
Tel: 713 770-1309 *Fax:* 713 770-2799
E-mail: fellowship-program@neo.bcm.tmc.edu
Internet: http://www.neo.tch.tmc.edu/
Accred Length: 3 Years *Program Size:* 15
Program ID: 329-48-21-057

University of Texas at Houston Program
Sponsor: University of Texas Medical School at Houston
Lyndon B Johnson General Hospital
Memorial Hermann Healthcare System
Program Director:
Fernando R Moya, MD
Univ of Texas-Houston Med Sch
PO Box 20708
Houston, TX 77225
Tel: 713 500-5727 *Fax:* 713 500-5794
E-mail: fmoya@ped1.med.uth.tmc.edu
Internet: http://www.ped1.med.uth.tmc.edu
Accred Length: 3 Years *Program Size:* 7
Program ID: 329-48-21-058

Lackland AFB

San Antonio Uniformed Services Health Education Consortium Program
Sponsor: San Antonio Uniformed Services Health Education Consortium
Program Director:
Bradley A Yoder, MD
59th Med Wing
Dept of Pediatrics/PSP
2200 Bergquist Dr/Ste 1
Lackland AFB, TX 78236-5300
Tel: 210 670-6679 *Fax:* 210 670-7933
E-mail: yoder_b@whmc-lafb.af.mil
Accred Length: 3 Years *Program Size:* 5
Program ID: 329-48-21-059
US Armed Services Program

San Antonio

University of Texas Health Science Center at San Antonio Program
Sponsor: University of Texas Medical School at San Antonio
University Hospital-South Texas Medical Center
Program Director:
Marilyn B Escobedo, MD
Univ of Texas Health Science Ctr-San Antonio
7703 Floyd Curl Dr
San Antonio, TX 78284-7812
Tel: 210 567-5225 *Fax:* 210 567-5169
E-mail: gunkel@uthscsa.edu
Accred Length: 3 Years *Program Size:* 1
Program ID: 329-48-21-115

Utah

Salt Lake City

University of Utah Program
Sponsor: University of Utah Medical Center
Primary Children's Medical Center
Program Director:
J Ross Milley, MD PhD
Univ of Utah Sch of Med
Dept of Pediatrics
50 N Medical Dr
Salt Lake City, UT 84132
Tel: 801 581-7052 *Fax:* 801 585-7395
E-mail: jmilley@hsc.utah.edu
Accred Length: 3 Years *Program Size:* 6
Program ID: 329-49-21-094

Vermont

Burlington

University of Vermont Program
Sponsor: Fletcher Allen Health Care
Program Director:
Roger F Soll, MD
Univ of Vermont Coll of Med
Dept of Pediatrics
A-121 Given Bldg
Burlington, VT 05405
Tel: 802 656-2392 *Fax:* 802 656-5225
E-mail: rsoll@salus.med.uvm.edu
Accred Length: 3 Years *Program Size:* 2
Program ID: 329-50-21-060

Virginia

Charlottesville

University of Virginia Program
Sponsor: University of Virginia Medical Center
Program Director:
John Kattwinkel, MD
Univ of Virginia Sch of Med
Dept of Pediatrics
Charlottesville, VA 22908
Tel: 804 924-5428 *Fax:* 804 924-2816
E-mail: jk3f@virginia.edu
Accred Length: 3 Years *Program Size:* 2
Program ID: 329-51-21-084

Richmond

Medical College of Virginia/Virginia Commonwealth University Program
Sponsor: Medical College of Virginia/Virginia Commonwealth University
Medical College of Virginia Hospitals
Program Director:
Henry J Rozycki, MD
Med Coll of Virginia
Children's Med Ctr
PO Box 980276
Richmond, VA 23298-0276
Tel: 804 828-9964 *Fax:* 804 828-6662
E-mail: hrozycki@hsc.vcu.edu
Accred Length: 3 Years *Program Size:* 3
Program ID: 329-51-21-061

Washington

Seattle

University of Washington Program
Sponsor: University of Washington School of Medicine
University of Washington Medical Center
Program Director:
Christine A Gleason, MD
Univ of Washington
Div of Neonatology
Box 356320
Seattle, WA 98195-6320
Tel: 206 543-3200 *Fax:* 206 543-8926
E-mail: cgleason@u.washington.edu
Internet: http://weber.u.washington.edu/~neonatal/
Accred Length: 3 Years *Program Size:* 2
Program ID: 329-54-21-095

Wisconsin

Madison

University of Wisconsin Program
Sponsor: University of Wisconsin Hospital and Clinics
Program Director:
Frank R Greer, MD
Meriter Hospital-Perinatal Ctr
202 S Park St
Madison, WI 53715
Tel: 608 262-6561 *Fax:* 608 267-6377
E-mail: frgreer@facstaff.wisc.edu
Accred Length: 3 Years *Program Size:* 2
Program ID: 329-56-21-099

Milwaukee

Medical College of Wisconsin Program
Sponsor: Medical College of Wisconsin Affiliated Hospitals Inc
Children's Hospital of Wisconsin
Froedtert Memorial Lutheran Hospital
Program Director:
Candice D Fike, MD
MS 213A Dept of Pediatrics
Med Coll of Wisconsin
8701 Watertown Plank Rd
Milwaukee, WI 53226
Tel: 414 266-6719 *Fax:* 414 266-6979
E-mail: cfike@mcw.edu
Internet: http://www.mcw.edu/peds/neonate
Accred Length: 3 Years *Program Size:* 4
Program ID: 329-56-21-110

Nephrology (Internal Medicine)

Alabama

Birmingham

University of Alabama Medical Center Program
Sponsor: University of Alabama Hospital
Program Director:
James L Lewis, MD
Div of Nephrology
THT 647
1900 University Blvd
Birmingham, AL 35294-0007
Tel: 205 934-3217 *Fax:* 205 934-7742
E-mail: jlewis@nrtc.dom.uab.edu
Internet: http://www.nephaux.dom.uab.edu
Accred Length: 2 Years *Program Size:* 13
Program ID: 148-01-21-107

Arizona

Tucson

University of Arizona Program
Sponsor: University of Arizona College of Medicine
University Medical Center
Veterans Affairs Medical Center (Tucson)
Program Director:
Y Howard Lien, MD PhD
Univ of Arizona, Dept of Int Med
1501 N Campbell Ave
Tucson, AZ 85724
Tel: 520 626-6370 *Fax:* 520 626-2024
E-mail: lien.@u.arizona.edu
Internet: http://www.ahsc.arizona.edu/nephrology
Accred Length: 2 Years *Program Size:* 3
Program ID: 148-03-21-091

Arkansas

Little Rock

University of Arkansas for Medical Sciences Program
Sponsor: University of Arkansas College of Medicine
John L McClellan Memorial Veterans Hospital
University Hospital of Arkansas
Program Director:
Sudhir V Shah, MD
Univ of Arkansas for Med Sciences
4301 W Markham St/Slot 501
Little Rock, AR 72205
Tel: 501 671-2517 *Fax:* 501 671-2503
E-mail: shahsudhirv@exchange.uams.edu
Accred Length: 2 Years *Program Size:* 4
Program ID: 148-04-21-092

California

Los Angeles

Cedars-Sinai Medical Center Program
Sponsor: Cedars-Sinai Medical Center
VA Greater Los Angeles Healthcare System
Program Director:
Harvey C Gonick, MD
Cedars-Sinai Med Ctr
8700 Beverly Blvd
Becker Rm 227
Los Angeles, CA 90048-1869
Tel: 310 855-7880 *Fax:* 310 967-0427
E-mail: hgonick@ucla.edu
Internet: http://www.ucla.edu
Accred Length: 2 Years *Program Size:* 2
Program ID: 148-05-11-093

Southern California Kaiser Permanente Medical Care (Los Angeles) Program
Sponsor: Southern California Kaiser Permanente Medical Group
Kaiser Foundation Hospital (Los Angeles)
Program Director:
Scott Rasgon, MD
Kaiser Foundation Hospital
Dept of Nephrology
4700 Sunset Blvd
Los Angeles, CA 90027-6082
Tel: 323 783-4516
Accred Length: 2 Years *Program Size:* 2
Program ID: 148-05-12-029

UCLA Medical Center Program
Sponsor: UCLA School of Medicine
UCLA Medical Center
VA Greater Los Angeles Healthcare System
Program Director:
Ira Kurtz, MD
UCLA Sch of Med
Ctr for Health Sciences
7-155 Factor
Los Angeles, CA 90095-1736
Tel: 310 206-6741 *Fax:* 310 825-6309
E-mail: ikurtz@medl.medsch.ucla.edu
Internet:
http://www.mednet.ucla.edu/som/medicinestarprgm/star_pg1.htp
Accred Length: 2 Years *Program Size:* 5
Program ID: 148-05-11-110

University of Southern California Program
Sponsor: Los Angeles County-USC Medical Center
St Vincent Medical Center
Program Director:
Shaul Massry, MD
Univ of Southern California Med Ctr
1200 N State St
Los Angeles, CA 90033
Tel: 323 226-7337 *Fax:* 323 226-5390
Accred Length: 2 Years *Program Size:* 6
Program ID: 148-05-21-042

VA Greater Los Angeles Healthcare System (Sepulveda) Program
Sponsor: VA Greater Los Angeles Healthcare System
Cedars-Sinai Medical Center
UCLA Medical Center
Program Director:
David B N Lee, MD
VA Med Ctr
16111 Plummer St
Sepulveda, CA 91343-2099
Tel: 818 895-9386 *Fax:* 818 895-9511
E-mail: dbnlee@ucla.edu
Accred Length: 2 Years *Program Size:* 6
Program ID: 148-05-21-111

Orange

University of California (Irvine) Program
Sponsor: University of California (Irvine) Medical Center
Veterans Affairs Medical Center (Long Beach)
Program Director:
N D Vaziri, MD
Univ of California Irvine Med Ctr
101 The City Dr
Bldg 53/Rt 81
Orange, CA 92868
Tel: 714 456-5142 *Fax:* 714 456-6034
E-mail: tabotten@uci.edu
Internet: http://www.ucihs.uci.edu/nephrology
Accred Length: 2 Years *Program Size:* 4
Program ID: 148-05-21-125

Sacramento

University of California (Davis) Program
Sponsor: University of California (Davis) Medical Center
Program Director:
Jane Y Yeun, MD MD
Univ of California Davis Med Ctr
Div of Nephrology, Patient Support Services Building
4150 V St
Sacramento, CA 95817
Tel: 916 734-3774 *Fax:* 916 734-7920
E-mail: jyyeun@ucdavis.edu
Accred Length: 2 Years *Program Size:* 5
Program ID: 148-05-21-082

San Diego

University of California (San Diego) Program
Sponsor: University of California (San Diego) Medical Center
Naval Medical Center (San Diego)
Veterans Affairs Medical Center (San Diego)
Program Director:
Roland C Blantz, MD
VA San Diego Healthcare System
3350 La Jolla Village Dr
San Diego, CA 92161
Tel: 619 552-7528 *Fax:* 619 552-7549
E-mail: rblantz@ucsd.edu
Internet: http://www.medicine.ucsd.edu/nephrology
Accred Length: 2 Years *Program Size:* 8
Program ID: 148-05-21-149

San Francisco

University of California (San Francisco) Program
Sponsor: University of California (San Francisco) School of Medicine
San Francisco General Hospital Medical Center
University of California (San Francisco) Medical Center
Veterans Affairs Medical Center (San Francisco)
Program Director:
Harlan E Ives, MD PhD
Univ of California San Francisco
Dept of Nephrology
Third and Parnassus/Box 0532
San Francisco, CA 94143-0532
Tel: 415 476-2172 *Fax:* 415 476-3381
E-mail: ives@itsa.ucsf.edu
Accred Length: 2 Years *Program Size:* 12
Program ID: 148-05-21-127

Stanford

Stanford University Program

Sponsor: Stanford University Hospital

Program Director:
Rex L Jamison, MD
Stanford Univ Med Ctr
Dept of Med
300 Pasteur Dr
Stanford, CA 94305-5114
Tel: 650 723-6248 *Fax:* 650 723-7917
Accred Length: 2 Years *Program Size:* 13
Program ID: 148-05-21-019

Torrance

Los Angeles County-Harbor-UCLA Medical Center Program

Sponsor: Los Angeles County-Harbor-UCLA Medical Center

Program Director:
Joel D Kopple, MD
Los Angeles County-Harbor-UCLA Med Ctr
Bin 400
1000 W Carson St
Torrance, CA 90509
Tel: 310 222-3891 *Fax:* 310 782-1837
E-mail: kopple@afp76.humc.edu
Accred Length: 2 Years *Program Size:* 4
Program ID: 148-05-11-150

Colorado

Denver

University of Colorado Program

Sponsor: University of Colorado Health Sciences Center
Denver Health and Hospitals
Veterans Affairs Medical Center (Denver)

Program Director:
Stuart L Linas, MD
Univ of Colorado Health Sciences Ctr
4200 E Ninth Ave
C-281
Denver, CO 80262
Tel: 303 315-6734 *Fax:* 303 436-7249
E-mail: stuart.linas@uchsc.edu
Accred Length: 2 Years *Program Size:* 13
Program ID: 148-07-21-051

Connecticut

Farmington

University of Connecticut Program

Sponsor: University of Connecticut School of Medicine
Univ of Connecticut Health Center/John Dempsey Hospital

Program Director:
Nancy D Adams, MD
Joseph Palmisano, MD
Univ of Connecticut Health Ctr
Div of Nephrology/MC-1405
Farmington, CT 06030-1405
Tel: 860 679-2799 *Fax:* 860 679-3968
E-mail: neiman@nso.uchc.edu
Internet: http://www.uchc.edu
Accred Length: 2 Years *Program Size:* 2
Program ID: 148-08-31-001

New Haven

Hospital of St Raphael Program

Sponsor: Hospital of St Raphael

Program Director:
Frederic O Finkelstein, MD
Hospital of St Raphael
Dept of Med
1450 Chapel St
New Haven, CT 06511
Tel: 203 787-0117 *Fax:* 203 777-3559
Internet: http://www.srhs.org
Accred Length: 2 Years *Program Size:* 3
Program ID: 148-08-31-112

Yale-New Haven Medical Center Program

Sponsor: Yale-New Haven Hospital
Veterans Affairs Medical Center (West Haven)

Program Director:
Rex L Mahnensmith, MD
Yale Univ Sch of Med
Dept of Int Med/Nephrology
PO Box 208029
New Haven, CT 06520-8029
Tel: 203 785-4186 *Fax:* 203 785-7068
Internet: http://www.info.med.yale.edu/intmed/nephrol
Accred Length: 2 Years *Program Size:* 11
Program ID: 148-08-21-020

District of Columbia

Washington

George Washington University Program

Sponsor: George Washington University School of Medicine
George Washington University Hospital (UHS)
Veterans Affairs Medical Center (Washington, DC)

Program Director:
Susie Q Lew, MD
George Washington Univ Med Ctr
2150 Pennsylvania Ave NW/Ste 4-425
Washington, DC 20037
Tel: 202 994-4244 *Fax:* 202 994-2972
Accred Length: 2 Years *Program Size:* 4
Program ID: 148-10-21-095

Georgetown University Program

Sponsor: Georgetown University Medical Center
Arlington Hospital
District of Columbia General Hospital

Program Director:
Nicolas J Guzman, MD
Georgetown Univ Med Ctr
Div of Nephrology/Hypertension
3800 Reservoir Rd NW/Ste F6003
Washington, DC 20007
Tel: 202 687-4034 *Fax:* 202 687-7797
E-mail: steelewe@gunet.georgetown.edu
Accred Length: 2 Years *Program Size:* 3
Program ID: 148-10-21-073

Walter Reed Army Medical Center Program

Sponsor: Walter Reed Army Medical Center

Program Director:
Christina M Yuan, MD
Nephrology Service
Walter Reed Army Med Ctr
6825 16th St NW
Washington, DC 20307-5001
Tel: 202 782-6462 *Fax:* 202 782-0185
Internet:
http://www.wramc.amedd.army.mil/departments/medicine/nephro/nephrology/nephrome.htm
Accred Length: 2 Years *Program Size:* 6
Program ID: 148-10-11-113
US Armed Services Program

Washington Hospital Center Program

Sponsor: Washington Hospital Center

Program Director:
Jack Moore Jr, MD
Washington Hospital Ctr
110 Irving St NW/#2A70
Washington, DC 20010
Tel: 202 877-6034 *Fax:* 202 877-8329
Accred Length: 2 Years *Program Size:* 2
Program ID: 148-10-11-114

Florida

Gainesville

University of Florida Program

Sponsor: University of Florida College of Medicine
Shands Hospital at the University of Florida
Veterans Affairs Medical Center (Gainesville)

Program Director:
I David Weiner, MD
Univ of Florida
Div of Nephrology
PO Box 100224
Gainesville, FL 32610
Tel: 352 374-6102 *Fax:* 352 379-4048
E-mail: dweiner@nervm.nerdc.ufl.edu
Internet: http://www.med.ufl.edu/med/neph/neph.htm
Accred Length: 2 Years *Program Size:* 7
Program ID: 148-11-21-031

Miami

University of Miami-Jackson Memorial Medical Center Program

Sponsor: University of Miami-Jackson Memorial Medical Center
Veterans Affairs Medical Center (Miami)

Program Director:
Jacques J Bourgoignie, MD
Univ of Miami Sch of Med
PO Box 016960 (R126)
Miami, FL 33101
Tel: 305 243-6251 *Fax:* 305 243-3506
E-mail: jbourgoi@mednet.med.miami.edu
Accred Length: 2 Years *Program Size:* 8
Program ID: 148-11-21-151

Tampa

University of South Florida Program
Sponsor: University of South Florida College of Medicine
James A Haley Veterans Hospital
Tampa General Healthcare
Veterans Affairs Medical Center (Bay Pines)
Program Director:
German Ramirez, MD
Univ of South Florida Coll of Med
12901 Bruce B Downs Blvd/Box 19
Tampa, FL 33612-4799
Tel: 813 978-5947 *Fax:* 813 978-5850
Accred Length: 2 Years *Program Size:* 4
Program ID: 148-11-21-032

Georgia

Atlanta

Emory University Program
Sponsor: Emory University School of Medicine
Emory University Hospital
Grady Memorial Hospital
Program Director:
Jeff M Sands, MD
Emory Univ
Renal Div
1639 Pierce Dr NE/WMB Rm 338
Atlanta, GA 30322
Tel: 404 727-2525 *Fax:* 404 727-3425
E-mail: nephron @ccms-renal.physio.emory.edu.
Internet: http://www.cc.emory.edu/renal/home.html
Accred Length: 2 Years *Program Size:* 18
Program ID: 148-12-21-115

Augusta

Medical College of Georgia Program
Sponsor: Medical College of Georgia Hospital and Clinics
Veterans Affairs Medical Center (Augusta)
Program Director:
Laura L Mulloy, DO
Med Coll of Georgia
Sect of Nephrology
1120 15th St/BAA909
Augusta, GA 30912-3140
Tel: 706 721-2861 *Fax:* 706 721-7136
Accred Length: 2 Years *Program Size:* 5
Program ID: 148-12-21-002

Illinois

Chicago

McGaw Medical Center of Northwestern University Program
Sponsor: Northwestern University Medical School
Northwestern Memorial Hospital
Veterans Affairs Lakeside Medical Center (Chicago)
Program Director:
Daniel C Batlle, MD
Northwestern Univ Med Sch
320 E Superior
Chicago, IL 60611
Tel: 312 908-8328 *Fax:* 312 503-0622
Accred Length: 2 Years *Program Size:* 4
Program ID: 148-16-21-058

Rush-Presbyterian-St Luke's Medical Center Program
Sponsor: Rush-Presbyterian-St Luke's Medical Center
Program Director:
Susan H Hou, MD
Rush-Presbyterian-St Luke's Med Ctr
1753 W Congress Pkwy
Chicago, IL 60612
Tel: 312 942-6685 *Fax:* 312 942-2881
E-mail: shou@rush.edu
Accred Length: 2 Years *Program Size:* 6
Program ID: 148-16-11-116

University of Chicago Program
Sponsor: University of Chicago Hospitals
Program Director:
Fredric L Coe, MD
Univ of Chicago Hospitals and Clinics
5841 S Maryland Ave/MC5100
Chicago, IL 60637-1470
Tel: 773 702-3630 *Fax:* 773 702-5818
Internet: http://leslie.bsd.uchicago.edu
Accred Length: 2 Years *Program Size:* 8
Program ID: 148-16-11-052

University of Illinois College of Medicine at Chicago Program
Sponsor: University of Illinois College of Medicine at Chicago
Cook County Hospital
University of Illinois Hospital and Clinics
Veterans Affairs West Side Medical Center
Program Director:
Jose A Arruda, MD
Univ of Illinois Hospital
840 S Wood St/MC 793
Chicago, IL 60612
Tel: 312 996-6775 *Fax:* 312 996-7378
E-mail: jaarruda@uic.edu
Accred Length: 2 Years *Program Size:* 6
Program ID: 148-16-21-117

Maywood

Loyola University Program
Sponsor: Loyola University Medical Center
Edward J Hines Jr Veterans Affairs Hospital
Program Director:
Karen A Griffin, MD BS
Loyola Univ Med Ctr, Sect of Nephrology
2160 S First Ave
Maywood, IL 60153
Tel: 708 216-3306 *Fax:* 708 216-4060
E-mail: kgriffi@wpo.it.luc.edu
Accred Length: 2 Years *Program Size:* 5
Program ID: 148-16-21-003

Indiana

Indianapolis

Indiana University School of Medicine Program
Sponsor: Indiana University School of Medicine
Program Director:
Robert L Bacallao, MD
Indiana Univ Sch of Med
Fesler Hall 115
1120 South Dr
Indianapolis, IN 46202-5116
Tel: 317 274-7097 *Fax:* 317 274-8575
E-mail: ccastigl@iupui.edu
Internet: http://www.iupui.edu/~nephrolo/
Accred Length: 2 Years *Program Size:* 8
Program ID: 148-17-21-129

Iowa

Iowa City

University of Iowa Hospitals and Clinics Program
Sponsor: University of Iowa Hospitals and Clinics
Program Director:
John B Stokes, MD
Univ of Iowa Hospitals and Clinics
Dept of Int Med
200 Hawkins Dr/E300 GH
Iowa City, IA 52242-1009
Tel: 319 356-4409 *Fax:* 319 353-6343
E-mail: john-stokes@uiowa.edu
Internet:
http://www.indy.radiology.uiowa.edu/welcome/uihc/uihcmeddepts/intmed/nephrology/nephrology.html
Accred Length: 2 Years *Program Size:* 6
Program ID: 148-18-21-083

Kansas

Kansas City

University of Kansas Medical Center Program
Sponsor: University of Kansas School of Medicine
University of Kansas Medical Center
Program Director:
Arnold M Chonko, MD
Univ of Kansas Med Ctr
3901 Rainbow Blvd
Kansas City, KS 66160-7382
Tel: 913 588-6074 *Fax:* 913 588-3867
E-mail: achonko@kumc.edu
Accred Length: 2 Years *Program Size:* 4
Program ID: 148-19-21-096

Kentucky

Lexington

University of Kentucky Medical Center Program
Sponsor: University of Kentucky Hospital
Veterans Affairs Medical Center (Lexington)
Program Director:
B Peter E Sawaya, MD
Univ of Kentucky Med Ctr
800 Rose St/MN 569
Lexington, KY 40536-0084
Tel: 606 323-5048 *Fax:* 606 323-0232
E-mail: besawa0@pop.uky.edu
Accred Length: 2 Years *Program Size:* 4
Program ID: 148-20-21-152

Louisville

University of Louisville Program

Sponsor: University of Louisville School of Medicine
Jewish Hospital
Kosair Children's Hospital (Alliant Health System)
Norton Hospital (Alliant Health System)
University of Louisville Hospital
Veterans Affairs Medical Center (Louisville)

Program Director:
George R Aronoff, MD
Univ of Louisville Sch of Med
Kidney Disease Program
615 S Preston St
Louisville, KY 40202
Tel: 502 852-5757 *Fax:* 502 852-7643
E-mail: graron01@ulkyvm.louisville.edu
Internet: http://www.kdp-baptist.louisville.edu
Accred Length: 2 Years *Program Size:* 7
Program ID: 148-20-31-075

Louisiana

New Orleans

Louisiana State University Program

Sponsor: Louisiana State University School of Medicine
Alton Ochsner Medical Foundation
Medical Center of Louisiana at New Orleans

Program Director:
John D Wallin, MD
Louisiana State Univ Med Ctr
1542 Tulane Ave/Rm 354
Box T3M-2
New Orleans, LA 70112-2822
Tel: 504 568-8655 *Fax:* 504 568-4749
Accred Length: 2 Years *Program Size:* 5
Program ID: 148-21-21-164

Tulane University Program

Sponsor: Tulane University School of Medicine
Medical Center of Louisiana at New Orleans
Veterans Affairs Medical Center-LSU Service (New Orleans)

Program Director:
L Lee Hamm, MD
Tulane Med Ctr
Sect of Nephrology
1430 Tulane Ave
New Orleans, LA 70112
Tel: 504 588-5346 *Fax:* 504 584-1909
E-mail: lhamm@tmcpop.tmc.tulane.edu
Internet:
http://www.mcl.tulane.edu//departments/nephrology/neph.htm
Accred Length: 2 Years *Program Size:* 5
Program ID: 148-21-21-090

Shreveport

Louisiana State University (Shreveport) Program

Sponsor: Louisiana State University Hospital-Shreveport
Overton Brooks Veterans Affairs Medical Center

Program Director:
Ken Abreo, MD
Louisiana State Univ Med Ctr
Med Educ Dept (Nephrology)
1501 Kings Hwy/PO Box 33932
Shreveport, LA 71130-3932
Tel: 318 674-5910 *Fax:* 318 675-5913
Internet: http://www.med.lsumc.edu/
Accred Length: 2 Years *Program Size:* 4
Program ID: 148-21-21-053

Maine

Portland

Maine Medical Center Program

Sponsor: Maine Medical Center

Program Director:
Jonathan Himmelfarb, MD
Div of Nephrology
Maine Med Ctr
22 Bramhall St
Portland, ME 04102
Tel: 207 871-2417 *Fax:* 207 871-6306
E-mail: himmej@mail.mmc.org
Accred Length: 2 Years *Program Size:* 5
Program ID: 148-22-21-168

Maryland

Baltimore

Johns Hopkins University Bayview Medical Center Program

Sponsor: Johns Hopkins University School of Medicine
Johns Hopkins Bayview Medical Center

Program Director:
David A Spector, MD
Div of Renal Med
Johns Hopkins Bayview Med Ctr
4940 Eastern Ave
Baltimore, MD 21224
Tel: 410 550-0614 *Fax:* 410 550-0979
E-mail: lshir@welchlink.welch.jhu.edu
Accred Length: 2 Years *Program Size:* 4
Program ID: 148-23-11-153

Johns Hopkins University Program

Sponsor: Johns Hopkins University School of Medicine
Johns Hopkins Hospital

Program Director:
Michael J Choi, MD
Johns Hopkins Univ
Dept of Med
1830 E Monument St/Ste 416
Baltimore, MD 21205
Tel: 410 955-5268 *Fax:* 410 955-0485
E-mail: mjchoi@welchlink.welch.jhu.edu
Accred Length: 2 Years *Program Size:* 7
Program ID: 148-23-11-059

University of Maryland Program

Sponsor: University of Maryland Medical System

Program Director:
Matthew R Weir, MD
Univ of Maryland Sch of Med
22 S Greene St
Rm N3W143
Baltimore, MD 21201
Tel: 410 328-5720 *Fax:* 410 328-5685
E-mail: lherbert@umppa1.ab.umd.edu
Accred Length: 2 Years *Program Size:* 4
Program ID: 148-23-21-033

Massachusetts

Boston

Beth Israel Deaconess Medical Center (East Campus) Program

Sponsor: Beth Israel Deaconess Medical Center

Program Director:
Vikas P Sukhatme, MD PhD
Beth Israel Deaconess Med Ctr
330 Brookline Ave/DA 517
Boston, MA 02215
Tel: 617 667-2105 *Fax:* 617 667-7843
E-mail: vsukhatm@bidmc.harvard.edu
Internet: http://www.bidmc.harvard.edu
Accred Length: 2 Years *Program Size:* 11
Program ID: 148-24-21-004

Boston University Medical Center Program

Sponsor: Boston Medical Center
Veterans Affairs Medical Center (Boston)

Program Director:
David J Salant, MD
Boston Med Ctr
Dept of Int Med
88 E Newton St
Boston, MA 02118
Tel: 617 638-7330 *Fax:* 617 638-7326
E-mail: bunephron@med-med1.bu.edu
Accred Length: 2 Years *Program Size:* 11
Program ID: 148-24-21-130

Brigham and Women's Hospital Program

Sponsor: Brigham and Women's Hospital
Massachusetts General Hospital

Program Director:
Barry M Brenner, MD
Hasan Bazari, MD
Brigham and Women's Hospital
Dept of Med
75 Francis St
Boston, MA 02115
Tel: 617 732-5850 *Fax:* 617 732-6392
Accred Length: 2 Years *Program Size:* 21
Program ID: 148-24-21-005

New England Medical Center Hospitals Program

Sponsor: New England Medical Center Hospitals

Program Director:
Nicolaos E Madias, MD
New England Med Ctr
750 Washington St
NEMCH Box 172
Boston, MA 02111
Tel: 617 636-5897 *Fax:* 617 636-1355
E-mail: nicolaos.madias@es.nemc.org
Internet: http://www.nemc.org
Accred Length: 2 Years *Program Size:* 7
Program ID: 148-24-21-006

Worcester

University of Massachusetts Program

Sponsor: University of Massachusetts Medical School
UMass Memorial Health Care (University Campus)

Program Director:
Jeffrey S Stoff, MD
Univ of Massachusetts Med Sch
Div of Renal Medicine
55 Lake Ave N
Worcester, MA 01655
Tel: 508 856-3156 *Fax:* 508 856-3111
E-mail: jeffrey.stoff@banyan.ummed.edu
Accred Length: 2 Years *Program Size:* 3
Program ID: 148-24-21-007

Michigan

Ann Arbor

University of Michigan Program

Sponsor: University of Michigan Hospitals
Veterans Affairs Medical Center (Ann Arbor)

Program Director:
Frank C Brosius, MD
Univ of Michigan Hospitals
1570 MSRB II/Box 0676
1150 W Medical Center Dr
Ann Arbor, MI 48109-0364
Tel: 734 764-3157 *Fax:* 734 936-9621
E-mail: fbrosius@umich.edu
Internet: http://www.med.umich.edu/intmed/nephrology
Accred Length: 2 Years *Program Size:* 10
Program ID: 148-25-21-061

Detroit

Henry Ford Hospital Program

Sponsor: Henry Ford Hospital

Program Director:
Robert G Narins, MD
Henry Ford Hospital
2799 W Grand Blvd/CFP-5
Detroit, MI 48202
Tel: 313 876-9405 *Fax:* 313 876-2554
Accred Length: 2 Years *Program Size:* 7
Program ID: 148-25-11-118

St John Hospital and Medical Center Program

Sponsor: St John Hospital and Medical Center

Program Director:
Robert Provenzano, MD
St John Hospital and Med Ctr
Dept of Med Educ
22101 Moross Rd
Detroit, MI 48236
Tel: 313 343-3875 *Fax:* 313 343-7840
E-mail: sue.moynihan@stjohn.org
Internet: http://www.stjohn.org
Accred Length: 2 Years *Program Size:* 4
Program ID: 148-25-21-174

Wayne State University/Detroit Medical Center Program

Sponsor: Wayne State University/Detroit Medical Center
Detroit Receiving Hospital and University Health Center
Harper Hospital
Veterans Affairs Medical Center (Detroit)

Program Director:
Stephen D Migdal, MD
Harper Hospital
4160 John R St/Ste 908
Detroit, MI 48201
Tel: 313 745-7145 *Fax:* 313 745-8041
E-mail: migdal@oncgate.roc.wayne.edu
Accred Length: 2 Years *Program Size:* 6
Program ID: 148-25-21-040

Minnesota

Minneapolis

University of Minnesota Program

Sponsor: University of Minnesota Medical School
Fairview-University Medical Center
Hennepin County Medical Center
Veterans Affairs Medical Center (Minneapolis)

Program Director:
Mark E Rosenberg, MD
Univ of Minnesota Hospital and Clinics
Box 736
420 Delaware St SE
Minneapolis, MN 55455
Tel: 612 624-9444 *Fax:* 612 626-3840
E-mail: rosen001@maroon.tc.umn.edu
Accred Length: 2 Years *Program Size:* 8
Program ID: 148-26-21-098

Rochester

Mayo Graduate School of Medicine (Rochester) Program

Sponsor: Mayo Graduate School of Medicine-Mayo Foundation
Mayo Clinic (Rochester)
Rochester Methodist Hospital
St Mary's Hospital of Rochester

Program Director:
Thomas R Schwab, MD
Application Processing Ctr
Siebens 5th Fl
Mayo Graduate Sch of Med
Rochester, MN 55905
Tel: 507 284-3126 *Fax:* 507 284-5470
E-mail: mgsm.intmed.specialties@mayo.edu
Internet: http://www.mayo.edu
Accred Length: 2 Years *Program Size:* 6
Program ID: 148-26-21-046

Mississippi

Jackson

University of Mississippi Medical Center Program

Sponsor: University of Mississippi School of Medicine
University Hospital

Program Director:
John D Bower, MD
Univ of Mississippi Med Ctr
2500 N State St
Jackson, MS 39216-4505
Tel: 601 984-5670 *Fax:* 601 984-5765
E-mail: jdbower@teclink.net
Accred Length: 2 Years *Program Size:* 6
Program ID: 148-27-21-062

Missouri

Columbia

University of Missouri-Columbia Program

Sponsor: University of Missouri-Columbia School of Medicine
University Hospitals and Clinics

Program Director:
Karl D Nolph, MD
Univ of Missouri Health Sciences Ctr
MA436 Health Science Ctr
Columbia, MO 65212
Tel: 573 882-7991 *Fax:* 573 884-4820
E-mail: karl_nolph@muccmail.missouri.edu
Internet:
http://www.hsc.missouri.edu/internal_medicine/neph/
Accred Length: 2 Years *Program Size:* 6
Program ID: 148-28-21-063

St Louis

St Louis University School of Medicine Program

Sponsor: St Louis University School of Medicine
St Louis University School of Medicine
Veterans Affairs Medical Center (St Louis)

Program Director:
Kevin J Martin, MB BCh
St Louis Univ Sch of Med
Div of Nephrology (9-FDT)
3635 Vista Ave
St Louis, MO 63110-0250
Tel: 314 577-8765 *Fax:* 314 771-0784
E-mail: martinkj@wpogate.slu.edu
Accred Length: 2 Years *Program Size:* 6
Program ID: 148-28-21-076

Washington University/B-JH/SLCH Consortium (South Campus) Program

Sponsor: Washington University/B-JH/SLCH Consortium
Barnes-Jewish Hospital
Barnes-Jewish Hospital (North Campus)

Program Director:
Marc R Hammerman, MD
Barnes Hospital Group
Dept of Int Med
4989 Barnes Hospital Plaza
St Louis, MO 63110
Tel: 314 362-8231 *Fax:* 314 362-8237
Internet:
http://www.internmed.wustl.edu/division/renal/index.html
Accred Length: 2 Years *Program Size:* 16
Program ID: 148-28-21-131

New Jersey

Camden

UMDNJ-Robert Wood Johnson Medical School (Camden) Program

Sponsor: Cooper Hospital-University Medical Center

Program Director:
Lawrence S Weisberg, MD
UMDNJ-Robert Wood Johnson Med Sch
Educ and Research Bldg
401 Haddon Ave
Camden, NJ 08103
Tel: 609 757-7844 *Fax:* 609 757-7803
E-mail: weisberg@umdnj.edu
Accred Length: 2 Years *Program Size:* 2
Program ID: 148-33-21-160

Programs

Newark

UMDNJ-New Jersey Medical School Program

Sponsor: UMDNJ-New Jersey Medical School
Newark Beth Israel Medical Center
UMDNJ-University Hospital
Veterans Affairs Medical Center (East Orange)

Program Director:
Leonard Meggs, MD MD
UMDNJ-New Jersey Med Sch
185 S Orange Ave
MSB-I524
Newark, NJ 07103
Tel: 973 972-4100 *Fax:* 973 972-3578
Accred Length: 2 Years *Program Size:* 5
Program ID: 148-33-21-159

Piscataway

UMDNJ-Robert Wood Johnson Medical School Program

Sponsor: UMDNJ-Robert Wood Johnson Medical School
Robert Wood Johnson University Hospital
St Peter's University Hospital

Program Director:
John A Walker, MD
UMDNJ-Robert Wood Johnson Med Sch
One Robert Wood Johnson Pl/CN19
New Brunswick, NJ 08903-0019
Tel: 732 235-7778 *Fax:* 732 235-6124
E-mail: mobleycl@umdnj.edu
Accred Length: 2 Years *Program Size:* 4
Program ID: 148-33-21-021

New Mexico

Albuquerque

University of New Mexico Program

Sponsor: University of New Mexico School of Medicine
University Hospital
Veterans Affairs Medical Center (Albuquerque)

Program Director:
Philip G Zager, MD
Univ of New Mexico Sch of Med
Dept of Int Med
2211 Lomas Blvd NE
Albuquerque, NM 87131
Tel: 505 272-4750 *Fax:* 505 272-2349
E-mail: pgzager@medusa.unm.edu
Accred Length: 2 Years *Program Size:* 4
Program ID: 148-34-21-119

New York

Bronx

Albert Einstein College of Medicine Program

Sponsor: Albert Einstein College of Medicine of Yeshiva University
Jacobi Medical Center
Montefiore Medical Center-Henry and Lucy Moses Division
Montefiore Medical Center-Weiler Hospital

Program Director:
Vaughn W Folkert, MD
Albert Einstein Coll of Med
Div of Nephrology
1325 Morris Park Ave
Bronx, NY 10461
Tel: 718 430-3158 *Fax:* 718 430-8963
E-mail: vaughnwf@earthlink.net
Accred Length: 2 Years *Program Size:* 8
Program ID: 148-35-21-086

Bronx-Lebanon Hospital Center Program

Sponsor: Bronx-Lebanon Hospital Center

Program Director:
Mahendraray B Dave, MD
Bronx-Lebanon Hospital Ctr
1650 Grand Concourse
Bronx, NY 10457
Tel: 718 518-5232 *Fax:* 718 518-5244
Accred Length: 2 Years *Program Size:* 3
Program ID: 148-35-11-162

Brooklyn

Brookdale University Hospital Medical Center Program

Sponsor: Brookdale University Hospital Medical Center

Program Director:
Jerome G Porush, MD
Brookdale Univ Hospital and Med Ctr
One Brookdale Plaza
Brooklyn, NY 11212-3198
Tel: 718 240-5615 *Fax:* 718 485-4064
E-mail: jporush@brookdale.edu
Accred Length: 2 Years *Program Size:* 5
Program ID: 148-35-11-134

Long Island College Hospital Program

Sponsor: Long Island College Hospital

Program Director:
Morrell M Avram, MD
Long Island Coll Hospital
Div of Nephrology/Othmer 407
339 Hicks St
Brooklyn, NY 11201
Tel: 718 780-1247 *Fax:* 718 780-1415
Accred Length: 2 Years *Program Size:* 5
Program ID: 148-35-11-023

SUNY Health Science Center at Brooklyn Program

Sponsor: SUNY Health Science Center at Brooklyn
Kings County Hospital Center
University Hospital-SUNY Health Science Center at Brooklyn
Veterans Affairs Medical Center (Brooklyn)

Program Director:
Eli A Friedman, MD
SUNY Health Science Ctr-Brooklyn
450 Clarkson Ave
Box 52
Brooklyn, NY 11203-2098
Tel: 718 270-1584 *Fax:* 718 270-3327
E-mail: elifriedmn@aol.com
Accred Length: 2 Years *Program Size:* 8
Program ID: 148-35-21-008

Buffalo

SUNY at Buffalo Graduate Medical-Dental Education Consortium Program

Sponsor: SUNY at Buffalo Grad Medical-Dental Education Consortium
Erie County Medical Center
Veterans Affairs Medical Center (Buffalo)

Program Director:
James W Lohr, MD
VA Med Ctr
3495 Bailay Ave
Buffalo, NY 14215
Tel: 716 862-3334 *Fax:* 716 862-4794
Accred Length: 2 Years *Program Size:* 4
Program ID: 148-35-31-034

East Meadow

SUNY at Stony Brook (East Meadow) Program

Sponsor: Nassau County Medical Center

Program Director:
Christos P Carvounis, MD
Nassau County Med Ctr
2201 Hempstead Trnpk
East Meadow, NY 11554-5400
Tel: 516 572-8879 *Fax:* 516 572-5609
E-mail: christos@ncmc.co.nassau.ny.us
Accred Length: 2 Years *Program Size:* 3
Program ID: 148-35-21-077

Flushing

New York Hospital Medical Center of Queens/Cornell University Medical College Program

Sponsor: New York Hospital Medical Center of Queens

Program Director:
Marilyn Galler, MD
New York Hospital Med Ctr of Queens
56-45 Main St
Flushing, NY 11355
Tel: 718 670-1151 *Fax:* 718 353-9819
Accred Length: 2 Years *Program Size:* 3
Program ID: 148-35-11-078

Manhasset

North Shore University Hospital/NYU School of Medicine Program

Sponsor: North Shore University Hospital

Program Director:
Alessandro Bellucci, MD
Robert T Mossey, MD
North Shore Univ Hospital
Div of Nephrology/Hypertension
100 Community Dr
Great Neck, NY 11021
Tel: 516 465-8200 *Fax:* 516 465-8203
E-mail: bellucci@nshs.edu
Accred Length: 2 Years *Program Size:* 4
Program ID: 148-35-21-143

Mineola

Winthrop-University Hospital Program

Sponsor: Winthrop-University Hospital

Program Director:
John K Maesaka, MD
Winthrop-Univ Hospital
Dept of Nephrology
259 First St
Mineola, NY 11501
Tel: 516 663-2169 *Fax:* 516 663-2179
Accred Length: 2 Years *Program Size:* 4
Program ID: 148-35-11-064

New Hyde Park

Albert Einstein College of Medicine at Long Island Jewish Medical Center Program

Sponsor: Long Island Jewish Medical Center

Program Director:
Pravin C Singhal, MD
Long Island Jewish Med Ctr
270-05 76th Ave
New Hyde Park, NY 11040
Tel: 718 470-7360 *Fax:* 718 470-6849
E-mail: wagner@lij.edu
Internet: http://www.lij.edu/lij-homepage-ns.html
Accred Length: 2 Years *Program Size:* 3
Program ID: 148-35-21-120

New York

Albert Einstein College of Medicine at Beth Israel Medical Center Program

Sponsor: Beth Israel Medical Center

Program Director:
Allen Kaufman, MD
Beth Israel Med Ctr
350 E 17th St
17th Fl Baird Hall/Rm 50
New York, NY 10003
Tel: 212 420-4070 *Fax:* 212 420-4117
E-mail: syemma@bethisraelny.org
Accred Length: 2 Years *Program Size:* 2
Program ID: 148-35-11-055

Harlem Hospital Center Program

Sponsor: Harlem Hospital Center

Program Director:
Velvie A Pogue, MD
Harlem Hospital Ctr
506 Lenox Ave
Rm 12-101KP
New York, NY 10037
Tel: 212 939-1449 *Fax:* 212 939-1306
E-mail: vap1@columbia.edu
Accred Length: 2 Years *Program Size:* 2
Program ID: 148-35-11-147

Lenox Hill Hospital Program

Sponsor: Lenox Hill Hospital

Program Director:
Michael F Michelis, MD
Lenox Hill Hospital
100 E 77th St
New York, NY 10021-1883
Tel: 212 434-3266 *Fax:* 212 434-4528
E-mail: richard@dr-chan.com
Internet:
http://dr-chan.com/nephrology/nephrohome.html
Accred Length: 2 Years *Program Size:* 4
Program ID: 148-35-11-155

Mount Sinai School of Medicine Program

Sponsor: Mount Sinai School of Medicine
Elmhurst Hospital Center-Mount Sinai Services
Mount Sinai Medical Center
Veterans Affairs Medical Center (Bronx)

Program Director:
Paul E Klotman, MD
Mount Sinai Sch of Med
One Gustave L Levy Pl
Box 1243
New York, NY 10029
Tel: 212 241-8004 *Fax:* 212 987-0389
E-mail: pklotma@smtplink.mssm.edu
Internet:
http://www.mssm.edu/medicine/nephrology/home-page.html
Accred Length: 2 Years *Program Size:* 8
Program ID: 148-35-31-136

New York and Presbyterian Hospital (Columbia Campus) Program

Sponsor: New York and Presbyterian Hospital
New York and Presbyterian Hospital (Columbia Campus)

Program Director:
Qais Al-Awqati, MD
Presbyterian Hospital
622 W 168th St
New York, NY 10032
Tel: 212 305-3512 *Fax:* 212 305-3475
E-mail: qa1@columbia.edu
Accred Length: 2 Years *Program Size:* 4
Program ID: 148-35-11-079

New York and Presbyterian Hospital (Cornell Campus) Program

Sponsor: New York and Presbyterian Hospital
New York and Presbyterian Hospital (Cornell Campus)

Program Director:
Manikkam Suthanthiran, MD
New York Presbyterian Hospital
525 E 68th St
New York, NY 10021
Tel: 212 746-4430 *Fax:* 212 746-8091
E-mail: msuthan@mail.med.cornell.edu
Accred Length: 2 Years *Program Size:* 8
Program ID: 148-35-21-144

New York Medical College (Metropolitan) Program

Sponsor: New York Medical College
Metropolitan Hospital Center
Sisters of Charity Medical Center-St Vincent's Campus

Program Director:
Alf M Tannenberg, MD
Metropolitan Hospital Ctr
1901 First Ave
New York, NY 10029
Tel: 212 423-6401 *Fax:* 212 423-7923
Accred Length: 2 Years *Program Size:* 6
Program ID: 148-35-31-047

New York Medical College at St Vincent's Hospital and Medical Center of New York Program

Sponsor: New York Medical College
St Vincent's Hospital and Medical Center of New York

Program Director:
Godfrey Burns, MD
St Vincent's Hospital and Med Ctr
153 W 11th St
New York, NY 10011
Tel: 212 604-8322 *Fax:* 212 604-3322
Internet: http://svh.nymc.edu
Accred Length: 2 Years *Program Size:* 2
Program ID: 148-35-11-024

New York University Medical Center Program

Sponsor: New York University Medical Center
Bellevue Hospital Center
Veterans Affairs Medical Center (Manhattan)

Program Director:
David S Baldwin, MD
Jerome Lowenstein, MD
New York Univ Med Ctr, Renal Sect
550 First Ave
New York, NY 10016
Tel: 212 263-5635 *Fax:* 212 263-6859
Accred Length: 2 Years *Program Size:* 5
Program ID: 148-35-21-101

St Luke's-Roosevelt Hospital Center Program

Sponsor: St Luke's-Roosevelt Hospital Center
St Luke's-Roosevelt Hospital Center-St Luke's Division

Program Director:
Vinita Sehgal, MD
St Luke's Hospital
1111 Amsterdam Ave
New York, NY 10025
Tel: 212 523-3530 *Fax:* 212 523-3945
Internet:
http://www.users.aol.com/rathid/dialysis/umdc.htm
Accred Length: 2 Years *Program Size:* 2
Program ID: 148-35-21-088

Rochester

University of Rochester Program

Sponsor: Strong Memorial Hospital of the University of Rochester

Program Director:
David A Bushinsky, MD
Strong Memorial Hospital
Nephrology Unit/Box 675
601 Elmwood Ave
Rochester, NY 14642-8675
Tel: 716 275-3660 *Fax:* 716 442-9201
E-mail: david_bushinsky@urmc.rochester.edu
Accred Length: 2 Years *Program Size:* 4
Program ID: 148-35-11-157

Stony Brook

SUNY at Stony Brook Program

Sponsor: University Hospital-SUNY at Stony Brook
Veterans Affairs Medical Center (Northport)

Program Director:
Edward P Nord, MD
Health Science Ctr
Div of Nephrology/HSC T15-020
Stony Brook, NY 11794-8152
Tel: 516 444-2038 *Fax:* 516 444-6174
E-mail: enord@mail.som.sunysb.edu
Accred Length: 2 Years *Program Size:* 5
Program ID: 148-35-21-009

Syracuse

SUNY Health Science Center at Syracuse Program

Sponsor: University Hospital-SUNY Health Science Center at Syracuse
Veterans Affairs Medical Center (Syracuse)

Program Director:
Steven J Scheinman, MD
Dept of Med
SUNY Health Science Ctr
750 E Adams St
Syracuse, NY 13210
Tel: 315 464-5290 *Fax:* 315 464-5295
E-mail: scheinms@vax.cs.hscsyr.edu
Internet: http://www.hscsyr.edu
Accred Length: 2 Years *Program Size:* 4
Program ID: 148-35-21-089

Valhalla

New York Medical College at Westchester Medical Center Program
Sponsor: New York Medical College
Westchester Medical Center
Program Director:
Alvin I Goodman, MD
New York Med Coll
Sect of Nephrology
Valhalla, NY 10595
Tel: 914 493-7701 *Fax:* 914 493-8502
Accred Length: 2 Years *Program Size:* 4
Program ID: 148-35-11-010

North Carolina

Chapel Hill

University of North Carolina Hospitals Program
Sponsor: University of North Carolina Hospitals
Program Director:
Romulo E Colindres, MD MPH
Univ of North Carolina Sch of Med
348 MacNider Bldg
CB 7155
Chapel Hill, NC 27599-7155
Tel: 919 966-2561 *Fax:* 919 966-4251
Accred Length: 2 Years *Program Size:* 4
Program ID: 148-36-21-121

Durham

Duke University Program
Sponsor: Duke University Medical Center
Veterans Affairs Medical Center (Durham)
Program Director:
Thomas M Coffman, MD
Duke Univ Med Ctr
Box 3014
Durham, NC 27710
Tel: 919 660-6850 *Fax:* 919 660-6888
E-mail: coffm002@mc.duke.edu
Internet: http://medicine.mc.dukeedu/nephrol
Accred Length: 2 Years *Program Size:* 6
Program ID: 148-36-21-122

Winston-Salem

Wake Forest University School of Medicine Program
Sponsor: Wake Forest University Baptist Medical Center
Program Director:
Vardaman M Buckalew, MD
Wake Forest Univ Baptist Med Ctr
Medical Center Blvd
Winston-Salem, NC 27157-1053
Tel: 336 716-2062 *Fax:* 336 716-4318
E-mail: buckalew@wfubmc.edu
Accred Length: 2 Years *Program Size:* 5
Program ID: 148-36-21-011

Ohio

Cincinnati

University Hospital/University of Cincinnati College of Medicine Program
Sponsor: University Hospital Inc
Veterans Affairs Medical Center (Cincinnati)
Program Director:
Satwant Singh, MD
Univ of Cincinnati
PO Box 670585
Cincinnati, OH 45267-0585
Tel: 513 558-5471 *Fax:* 513 558-4309
E-mail: cinneph@uc.edu
Accred Length: 2 Years *Program Size:* 4
Program ID: 148-38-21-066

Cleveland

Case Western Reserve University Program
Sponsor: University Hospitals of Cleveland
MetroHealth Medical Center
Veterans Affairs Medical Center (Cleveland)
Program Director:
Donald E Hricik, MD
Univ Hospitals of Cleveland
Lakeside Bldg/Rm 8124-C Bennett
11100 Euclid Ave
Cleveland, OH 44106-5048
Tel: 216 844-8060 *Fax:* 216 844-5204
E-mail: deh5@po.cwru.edu
Accred Length: 2 Years *Program Size:* 6
Program ID: 148-38-21-137

Cleveland Clinic Foundation Program
Sponsor: Cleveland Clinic Foundation
Program Director:
Joseph V Nally, MD
Cleveland Clinic Foundation
Dept of Hypertension/Nephrology/A101
9500 Euclid Ave
Cleveland, OH 44195-5242
Tel: 216 444-5690 *Fax:* 216 444-1162
E-mail: meded@cesmtp.ccf.org
Internet: http://www.ccf.org
Accred Length: 2 Years *Program Size:* 6
Program ID: 148-38-12-139

Columbus

Ohio State University Program
Sponsor: Ohio State University Medical Center
Program Director:
N Stanley Nahman Jr, MD
Ohio State Univ Hospital
1654 Upham Dr/Rm N210
Columbus, OH 43210-1228
Tel: 614 293-4997 *Fax:* 614 293-3073
Accred Length: 2 Years *Program Size:* 6
Program ID: 148-38-11-080

Toledo

Medical College of Ohio Program
Sponsor: Medical College of Ohio
Program Director:
Deepak Malhotra MD, PhD
Med Coll of Ohio, Dept of Med
Rupert Health Ctr
3120 Glendale Ave
Toledo, OH 43614-5809
Tel: 419 383-3724 *Fax:* 419 383-6244
E-mail: dmalhotra@mco.edu
Accred Length: 2 Years *Program Size:* 3
Program ID: 148-38-21-012

Oklahoma

Oklahoma City

University of Oklahoma Health Sciences Center Program
Sponsor: University of Oklahoma College of Medicine
University Hospital
Veterans Affairs Medical Center (Oklahoma City)
Program Director:
Chris Kaufman, MD
Univ of Oklahoma Coll of Med
PO Box 26901/WP 2250
Oklahoma City, OK 73190
Tel: 405 271-6842 *Fax:* 405 271-6496
E-mail: chris_kaufman@uokhsc.edu
Accred Length: 2 Years *Program Size:* 3
Program ID: 148-39-21-067

Oregon

Portland

Oregon Health Sciences University Program
Sponsor: Oregon Health Sciences University Hospital
Veterans Affairs Medical Center (Portland)
Program Director:
David A McCarron, MD
Oregon Health Sciences Univ/PP262
3314 SW US Veterans Hospital Rd
Portland, OR 97201
Tel: 503 494-8490 *Fax:* 503 494-5330
E-mail: vandervs@ohsu.edu
Accred Length: 2 Years *Program Size:* 5
Program ID: 148-40-31-140

Pennsylvania

Hershey

Penn State Geisinger Health System/Milton S Hershey Medical Center Program
Sponsor: Penn State Geisinger Health System
Milton S Hershey Medical Center
Program Director:
Joseph Y Cheung, MD PhD
Milton S Hershey Med Ctr
Sect of Nephrology
PO Box 850
Hershey, PA 17033-0850
Tel: 717 531-8156 *Fax:* 717 531-6776
E-mail: jcheung@med.hmc.psghs.edu
Accred Length: 2 Years *Program Size:* 2
Program ID: 148-41-11-013

Philadelphia

Albert Einstein Medical Center Program
Sponsor: Albert Einstein Medical Center
Program Director:
Rasib M Raja, MD
Albert Einstein Med Ctr
Kraftsow Div of Nephrology
5501 Old York Rd
Philadelphia, PA 19141-3098
Tel: 215 456-6970
Accred Length: 2 Years *Program Size:* 4
Program ID: 148-41-11-056

MCP Hahnemann University Program
Sponsor: MCP Hahnemann University
Medical College of Pennsylvania Hospital
Program Director:
Sandra P Levinson, MD
Med Coll of Pennsylvania Hospital
3300 Henry Ave
Philadelphia, PA 19129
Tel: 215 842-6988 *Fax:* 215 842-9439
E-mail: leej1@auhs.edu
Internet: http://www.auhs.edu
Accred Length: 2 Years *Program Size:* 8
Program ID: 148-41-21-102

Temple University Program
Sponsor: Temple University Hospital
Program Director:
Patricio Silva, MD
Temple Univ Hospital
Dept of Nephrology
3401 N Broad St
Philadelphia, PA 19140
Tel: 215 707-3381 *Fax:* 215 707-4148
Accred Length: 2 Years *Program Size:* 9
Program ID: 148-41-21-026

Thomas Jefferson University Program
Sponsor: Thomas Jefferson University Hospital
Program Director:
James F Burke Jr, MD
Thomas Jefferson Univ
Nephrology/Rm 353 JAH
1020 Locust St
Philadelphia, PA 19107
Tel: 215 503-6950, ext 6950 *Fax:* 215 923-7212
E-mail: dunns@jeflin.tju.edu
Accred Length: 2 Years *Program Size:* 6
Program ID: 148-41-21-027

University of Pennsylvania Program
Sponsor: Hospital of the University of Pennsylvania
Program Director:
Michael P Madaio, MD
Renal Electrolyte/Hypertention Div
Univ of Pennsylvania
415 Curie Blvd/700 Clin Res Bldg
Philadelphia, PA 19104-6144
Tel: 215 662-3612 *Fax:* 215 898-0189
E-mail: madaio@mail.med.upenn.edu
Internet: http://www.rehd.med.upenn.edu
Accred Length: 2 Years *Program Size:* 20
Program ID: 148-41-21-018

Pittsburgh

Allegheny General Hospital Program
Sponsor: Allegheny General Hospital
Program Director:
Douglas M Landwehr, MD
Allegheny General Hospital
Div of Nephrology/Hypertension
320 E North Ave
Pittsburgh, PA 15212-9986
Tel: 412 359-4008 *Fax:* 412 359-4136
Accred Length: 2 Years *Program Size:* 5
Program ID: 148-41-11-036

University Health Center of Pittsburgh Program
Sponsor: University Health Center of Pittsburgh
Presbyterian University Hospital/UPMC
Veterans Affairs Medical Center (Pittsburgh)
Program Director:
Beth Piraino, MD
Hospital of Univ Health Ctr of Pittsburgh
A915 Scaife Hall
3550 Terrace St
Pittsburgh, PA 15261
Tel: 412 647-7157 *Fax:* 412 647-6222
E-mail: cable@med1.dept-me.pitt.edu
Accred Length: 2 Years *Program Size:* 8
Program ID: 148-41-21-037

Wynnewood

Lankenau Hospital Program
Sponsor: Lankenau Hospital
Program Director:
Miles H Sigler, MD
Ste 130/Lankenau Med Bldg W
100 Lancaster Ave
Wynnewood, PA 19096-3426
Tel: 610 649-1175 *Fax:* 610 896-8753
Accred Length: 2 Years *Program Size:* 3
Program ID: 148-41-11-028

Puerto Rico

San Juan

University of Puerto Rico Program
Sponsor: University of Puerto Rico School of Medicine
University Hospital
Program Director:
Rafael Burgos-Calderson, MD
Univ Hospital-Puerto Rico Med Ctr
Box 5067
San Juan, PR 00935
Tel: 787 754-3661
Accred Length: 2 Years *Program Size:* 5
Program ID: 148-42-21-104

Veterans Affairs Medical and Regional Office Center Program
Sponsor: Veterans Affairs Medical Center (San Juan)
Program Director:
Hector R Cordova, MD
VA Med Ctr
One Veterans Plaza (111)
San Juan, PR 00927
Tel: 787 785-7575, ext 3456 *Fax:* 787 766-6021
Accred Length: 2 Years *Program Size:* 3
Program ID: 148-42-31-103

Rhode Island

Providence

Brown University Program
Sponsor: Rhode Island Hospital
Miriam Hospital
Program Director:
J Gary Abuelo, MD
Rhode Island Hospital
593 Eddy St
Providence, RI 02903
Tel: 401 444-5033 *Fax:* 401 444-8453
E-mail: jgabuelo@brown.edu
Internet: http://biomed.brown.edu/medicine_programs nephrologyfellowship/index.htm
Accred Length: 2 Years *Program Size:* 6
Program ID: 148-43-11-105

South Carolina

Charleston

Medical University of South Carolina Program
Sponsor: Medical University of South Carolina College of Medicine
MUSC Medical Center
Ralph H Johnson Dept of Veterans Affairs Med Center
Program Director:
David W Ploth, MD
Med Univ of South Carolina
Div of Nephrology Rm 829 CSB
171 Ashley Ave
Charleston, SC 29425-2225
Tel: 803 792-4123 *Fax:* 803 792-8399
E-mail: plothdw@musc.edu
Accred Length: 2 Years *Program Size:* 8
Program ID: 148-45-21-156

Tennessee

Memphis

University of Tennessee Program
Sponsor: University of Tennessee College of Medicine
Regional Medical Center at Memphis
Veterans Affairs Medical Center (Memphis)
Program Director:
Sergio Acchiardo, MD
Univ of Tennessee
951 Court Ave/Rm D649
Memphis, TN 38163
Tel: 901 448-5764 *Fax:* 901 448-5513
E-mail: sacchiardo@utmem1.utmem.edu
Accred Length: 2 Years *Program Size:* 3
Program ID: 148-47-21-123

Nashville

Vanderbilt University Program
Sponsor: Vanderbilt University Medical Center
Veterans Affairs Medical Center (Nashville)
Program Director:
Steven C Hebert, MD
Vanderbilt Univ
21st Ave S and Garland Ave/S-3223 MCN
Nashville, TN 37232-2372
Tel: 615 343-5028 *Fax:* 615 343-7156
E-mail: susan.britt@mcmail.vanderbilt.edu
Internet: http://www.vanderbilt.edu./nephrol
Accred Length: 2 Years *Program Size:* 11
Program ID: 148-47-31-014

Texas

Dallas

University of Texas Southwestern Medical School Program

Sponsor: University of Texas Southwestern Medical School
Dallas County Hospital District-Parkland Memorial Hospital
Veterans Affairs Medical Center (Dallas)
Program Director:
Biff F Palmer, MD
Univ of Texas Southwestern Med Ctr
5323 Harry Hines Blvd
Dallas, TX 75235-8856
Tel: 214 648-2754 *Fax:* 214 648-2071
E-mail: dedrian.copeland@email.swmed.edu
Accred Length: 2 Years *Program Size:* 13
Program ID: 148-48-21-084

Galveston

University of Texas Medical Branch Hospitals Program

Sponsor: University of Texas Medical Branch Hospitals
Program Director:
Mahendra Govani, MD
Univ of Texas Med Branch
4200 John Sealy Annex
301 University Blvd
Galveston, TX 77555-0562
Tel: 409 772-1811 *Fax:* 409 772-5451
E-mail: mgovani@utmb.edu
Accred Length: 2 Years *Program Size:* 4
Program ID: 148-48-21-049

Houston

Baylor College of Medicine Program

Sponsor: Baylor College of Medicine
Harris County Hospital District-Ben Taub General Hospital
Methodist Hospital
Veterans Affairs Medical Center (Houston)
Program Director:
Wadi N Suki, MD
Baylor Coll of Med-Methodist Hospital
6550 Fannin St/Ste 1275
Houston, TX 77030
Tel: 713 790-3275 *Fax:* 713 790-5053
E-mail: wsuki@bcm.tmc.edu
Accred Length: 2 Years *Program Size:* 6
Program ID: 148-48-21-070

University of Texas at Houston Program

Sponsor: University of Texas Medical School at Houston
Lyndon B Johnson General Hospital
Memorial Hermann Healthcare System
University of Texas M D Anderson Cancer Center
Program Director:
Thomas D DuBose Jr, MD
Univ of Texas Med Sch
6431 Fannin St/MSB 4130
Houston, TX 77030
Tel: 713 500-6868 *Fax:* 713 500-6882
E-mail: galletti@heart.med.uth.tmc.edu
Internet:
http://www.uth.tmc.edu/schools/med/imed/neph/index.htm
Accred Length: 2 Years *Program Size:* 7
Program ID: 148-48-31-015

Lubbock

Texas Tech University (Lubbock) Program

Sponsor: Texas Tech University Health Sciences Center at Lubbock
University Medical Center
Program Director:
Donald E Wesson, MD
Texas Tech Univ Health Sciences Ctr
Dept of Med
3601 Fourth St
Lubbock, TX 79430
Tel: 806 743-3155 *Fax:* 806 743-3148
Accred Length: 2 Years *Program Size:* 2
Program ID: 148-48-21-081

San Antonio

University of Texas Health Science Center at San Antonio Program

Sponsor: University of Texas Medical School at San Antonio
Audie L Murphy Memorial Veterans Hospital (San Antonio)
University Hospital-South Texas Medical Center
Wilford Hall Medical Center (AETC)
Program Director:
Hanna E Abboud, MD
Univ of Texas Health Science Ctr
Div of Nephrology
7703 Floyd Curl Dr
San Antonio, TX 78284-7882
Tel: 210 567-4700 *Fax:* 210 567-4712
E-mail: abboud@uthscsa.edu
Internet:
http://www.homepage-internalmed-fellowshipthrumeded
Accred Length: 2 Years *Program Size:* 10
Program ID: 148-48-21-057

Utah

Salt Lake City

University of Utah Program

Sponsor: University of Utah Medical Center
Veterans Affairs Medical Center (Salt Lake City)
Program Director:
Fuad S Shihab, MD
Univ of Utah Med Ctr
50 N Medical Dr
4R 312 SOM
Salt Lake City, UT 84132
Tel: 801 581-6709 *Fax:* 801 581-4343
E-mail: fuad.shihab@hsc.utah.edu
Accred Length: 2 Years *Program Size:* 3
Program ID: 148-49-21-141

Vermont

Burlington

University of Vermont Program

Sponsor: Fletcher Allen Health Care
Program Director:
F John Gennari, MD
Univ of Vermont Coll of Med
Burgess 318 MCHV Campus
111 Colchester Ave
Burlington, VT 05401
Tel: 802 656-2534 *Fax:* 802 656-8736
E-mail: fgennari@zoo.uvm.edu
Accred Length: 2 Years *Program Size:* 3
Program ID: 148-50-21-142

Virginia

Charlottesville

University of Virginia Program

Sponsor: University of Virginia Medical Center
Program Director:
Mark D Okusa, MD
Div of Nephrology
Univ of Virginia
Box 133
Charlottesville, VA 22908
Tel: 804 924-5124 *Fax:* 804 924-5848
E-mail: mdo7y@virginia.edu
Internet:
http://www.med.virginia.edu/medicine/clinical/internal/nephrology/
Accred Length: 2 Years *Program Size:* 8
Program ID: 148-51-21-016

Richmond

Medical College of Virginia/Virginia Commonwealth University Program

Sponsor: Medical College of Virginia/Virginia Commonwealth University
Medical College of Virginia Hospitals
Program Director:
Anton C Schoolwerth, MD
Med Coll of Virginia
PO Box 980160
Richmond, VA 23298-0160
Tel: 804 828-9682, ext 26 *Fax:* 804 828-7567
E-mail: aschoolwerth@hsc.vcu.edu
Internet: http://www.vcu.edu
Accred Length: 2 Years *Program Size:* 6
Program ID: 148-51-21-017

Washington

Seattle

University of Washington Program

Sponsor: University of Washington School of Medicine
University of Washington Medical Center
Program Director:
William G Couser, MD
Univ of Washington Med Ctr
1959 NE Pacific St/BB 1265 HSB
Box 356521
Seattle, WA 98195
Tel: 206 543-3792 *Fax:* 206 685-8661
E-mail: wgc@u.washington.edu
Internet: http://weber.u.washington.edu/~nephron/
Accred Length: 2 Years *Program Size:* 9
Program ID: 148-54-21-072

West Virginia

Morgantown

West Virginia University Program

Sponsor: West Virginia University Hospitals
Program Director:
Karen MacKay, MD
Dept of Med
Robert C Byrd Health Sciences Ctr
PO Box 9165
Morgantown, WV 26506
Tel: 304 293-2551 *Fax:* 304 293-7373
E-mail: kmackay2@wvu.edu
Internet: http://www.hsc.wvu.edu/medicine/
Accred Length: 2 Years *Program Size:* 2
Program ID: 148-55-11-165

Wisconsin

Madison

University of Wisconsin Program

Sponsor: University of Wisconsin Hospital and Clinics
William S Middleton Veterans Hospital

Program Director:
Richard E Rieselbach, MD
Univ of Wisconsin Hospital and Clinics
600 Highland Ave/Rm H4-510
Madison, WI 53792-0001
Tel: 608 263-3315 *Fax:* 608 263-0568
E-mail: re.rieselbach@hosp.wisc.edu
Internet: http://www.medicine.wisc.edu
Accred Length: 2 Years *Program Size:* 4
Program ID: 148-56-21-106

Milwaukee

Medical College of Wisconsin Program

Sponsor: Medical College of Wisconsin Affiliated Hospitals Inc
Clement J Zablocki Veterans Affairs Medical Center
Froedtert Memorial Lutheran Hospital

Program Director:
Virginia J Savin, MD
Med Coll of Wisconsin
Froedtert Memorial Lutheran Hospital
9200 W Wisconsin Ave
Milwaukee, WI 53226
Tel: 414 259-3070 *Fax:* 414 259-1937
Accred Length: 2 Years *Program Size:* 4
Program ID: 148-56-31-039

Neurological Surgery

Alabama

Birmingham

University of Alabama Medical Center Program

Sponsor: University of Alabama Hospital
Children's Hospital of Alabama
Veterans Affairs Medical Center (Birmingham)

Program Director:
Timothy B Mapstone, MD
Children's Hospital
1600 Seventh Ave S/ACC 400
Birmingham, AL 35233
Tel: 205 939-9653 *Fax:* 205 939-9972
E-mail: timothy.mapstone@ccc.uab.edu
Accred Length: 5 Years *Program Size:* 8
Program ID: 160-01-21-003

Arizona

Phoenix

St Joseph's Hospital and Medical Center Program

Sponsor: St Joseph's Hospital and Medical Center
Maricopa Medical Center

Program Director:
Volker K H Sonntag, MD
St Joseph's Hospital and Med Ctr
PO Box 2071
Phoenix, AZ 85001-2071
Tel: 602 406-3196 *Fax:* 602 406-4104
Internet: http://www.chw.edu/mha/mha.html
Accred Length: 5 Years *Program Size:* 14
Program ID: 160-03-12-004

Arkansas

Little Rock

University of Arkansas for Medical Sciences Program

Sponsor: University of Arkansas College of Medicine
Arkansas Children's Hospital
John L McClellan Memorial Veterans Hospital
University Hospital of Arkansas

Program Director:
Ossama Al-Mefty, MD
Univ of Arkansas for Med Sciences
4301 W Markham St/Slot 507
Little Rock, AR 72205-7199
Tel: 501 686-8757 *Fax:* 501 686-8767
Accred Length: 5 Years *Program Size:* 5
Program ID: 160-04-21-005

California

Loma Linda

Loma Linda University Program

Sponsor: Loma Linda University Medical Center
Jerry L Pettis Memorial Veterans Hospital

Program Director:
Wolff M Kirsch, MD
Loma Linda Univ Sch of Med
Div of Neurosurgery/Rm 2539
Loma Linda, CA 92354
Tel: 909 478-8743 *Fax:* 909 824-4825
Accred Length: 5 Years *Program Size:* 4
Program ID: 160-05-11-008

Los Angeles

UCLA Medical Center Program

Sponsor: UCLA School of Medicine
Los Angeles County-Harbor-UCLA Medical Center
UCLA Medical Center
VA Greater Los Angeles Healthcare System

Program Director:
Donald P Becker, MD
UCLA Sch of Med
Div of Neurological Surgery
18-228NPI
Los Angeles, CA 90095-7039
Tel: 310 206-8093 *Fax:* 310 794-2147
E-mail: macdonal@surgery.medsch.ucla.edu
Internet: http://neurosun.medsch.ucla.edu
Accred Length: 5 Years *Program Size:* 10
Program ID: 160-05-21-010

University of Southern California Program

Sponsor: Los Angeles County-USC Medical Center
Children's Hospital of Los Angeles
USC University Hospital

Program Director:
Martin H Weiss, MD
Los Angeles County-USC Med Ctr
1200 N State St/Ste 5046
Los Angeles, CA 90033
Tel: 213 226-7421 *Fax:* 213 226-7833
Internet: http://www.usc.edu/hsc/neurosurgery
Accred Length: 5 Years *Program Size:* 14
Program ID: 160-05-21-009

Sacramento

University of California (Davis) Program

Sponsor: University of California (Davis) Medical Center
Kaiser Foundation Hospital (Sacramento)

Program Director:
Jan P Muizelaar, MD PhD
Univ of California Sch of Med
4860 Y St
Ste 3740
Sacramento, CA 95817
Tel: 916 734-3658 *Fax:* 916 452-2580
E-mail: clabericci@ucdavis.edu
Accred Length: 5 Years *Program Size:* 7
Program ID: 160-05-11-006

San Diego

University of California (San Diego) Program
Sponsor: University of California (San Diego) Medical Center
Children's Hospital and Health Center
Kaiser Foundation Hospital (San Diego)
Program Director:
Lawrence F Marshall, MD
UCSD Med Ctr
Div of Neurological Surgery
200 W Arbor Dr
San Diego, CA 92103-8893
Tel: 619 543-5540 *Fax:* 619 543-2769
E-mail: mmclaughlin@ucsd.edu
Accred Length: 5 Years *Program Size:* 6
Program ID: 160-05-21-100

San Francisco

University of California (San Francisco) Program
Sponsor: University of California (San Francisco) School of Medicine
Mount Zion Medical Center of the University of California
San Francisco General Hospital Medical Center
University of California (San Francisco) Medical Center
Veterans Affairs Medical Center (San Francisco)
Program Director:
Mitchel S Berger, MD
505 Parnassus Ave/Rm M-779
San Francisco, CA 94143-0112
Tel: 415 476-1087 *Fax:* 415 753-1772
E-mail: stubblebinem@neuro.ucsf.edu
Internet: http://www.som.ucsf.edu/neuros/index.htm
Accred Length: 5 Years *Program Size:* 14 (*GY1:* 2)
Program ID: 160-05-21-011

Stanford

Stanford University Program
Sponsor: Stanford University Hospital
Veterans Affairs Palo Alto Health Care System
Program Director:
Gary K Steinberg, MD
Stanford Univ Med Ctr, Dept of Neurosurgery
300 Pasteur Dr
Edwards Bldg R281
Stanford, CA 94305-5327
Tel: 650 723-5575 *Fax:* 650 723-2815
Internet:
http://www-leland.stanford.edu/dept/neurosurgery/index2.html
Accred Length: 5 Years *Program Size:* 6
Program ID: 160-05-21-012

Colorado

Denver

University of Colorado Program
Sponsor: University of Colorado Health Sciences Center
Children's Hospital
Denver Health and Hospitals
Veterans Affairs Medical Center (Denver)
Program Director:
Glenn Kindt, MD
Univ of Colorado Health Sciences Ctr
Dept of Neurosurgery
4200 E Ninth Ave/Box C307
Denver, CO 80262
Tel: 303 270-7577 *Fax:* 303 270-6197
E-mail: kathy.klutsch@uchsc.edu
Internet:
http://www.uchsc.edu/sm/sm/surgery/neurosur/index.htm
Accred Length: 5 Years *Program Size:* 5 (*GY1:* 1)
Program ID: 160-07-21-102

Connecticut

New Haven

Yale-New Haven Medical Center Program
Sponsor: Yale-New Haven Hospital
Veterans Affairs Medical Center (West Haven)
Program Director:
Charles C Duncan, MD
Yale Univ Sch of Med
333 Cedar St
PO Box 208082
New Haven, CT 06520-8082
Tel: 203 785-2811 *Fax:* 203 785-6916
E-mail: charles.duncan@yale.edu
Internet:
http://info.med.yale.edu/neurosur/neuresi/res-home.htm
Accred Length: 5 Years *Program Size:* 7
Program ID: 160-08-21-015

District of Columbia

Washington

George Washington University Program
Sponsor: George Washington University School of Medicine
Children's National Medical Center
George Washington University Hospital (UHS)
Washington Hospital Center
Program Director:
Laligam N Sekhar, MD
Dept of Neurosurgery
2150 Pennsylvania Ave NW/Rm 7-420
Washington, DC 20037
Tel: 202 994-9147 *Fax:* 202 994-9944
Internet: http://www.ninet.gwumc.edu
Accred Length: 5 Years *Program Size:* 12
Program ID: 160-10-21-017

Georgetown University Program
Sponsor: Georgetown University Medical Center
Children's National Medical Center
Program Director:
Robert L Martuza, MD
Georgetown Univ Med Ctr
Dept of Neurosurgery
3800 Reservoir Rd NW/1-PHC
Washington, DC 20007
Tel: 202 687-4972 *Fax:* 202 687-3744
Accred Length: 5 Years *Program Size:* 6
Program ID: 160-10-21-016

Florida

Gainesville

University of Florida Program
Sponsor: University of Florida College of Medicine
Shands Hospital at the University of Florida
Veterans Affairs Medical Center (Gainesville)
Program Director:
William A Friedman, MD
Univ of Florida, Dept of Neurosurgery
PO Box 100265
Gainesville, FL 32610-0265
Tel: 352 392-4331 *Fax:* 352 392-8156
E-mail: frazier@neocortex.health.ufl.edu
Internet: http://www.neurosurgery.ufl.edu/
Accred Length: 5 Years *Program Size:* 14 (*GY1:* 2)
Program ID: 160-11-21-018

Miami

University of Miami-Jackson Memorial Medical Center Program
Sponsor: University of Miami-Jackson Memorial Medical Center
Veterans Affairs Medical Center (Miami)
Program Director:
Roberto C Heros, MD
Univ of Miami Sch of Med
1501 NW 9th Ave
PO Box 016960 (D4-6)
Miami, FL 33136
Tel: 305 243-6672 *Fax:* 305 243-3180
Internet: http://www.med.miami.edu/neurosurgery/
Accred Length: 5 Years *Program Size:* 10 (*GY1:* 2)
Program ID: 160-11-21-019

Tampa

University of South Florida Program
Sponsor: University of South Florida College of Medicine
All Children's Hospital
H Lee Moffitt Cancer Center
James A Haley Veterans Hospital
Tampa General Healthcare
Program Director:
David W Cahill, MD
Univ of South Florida Coll of Med
Div of Neurological Surgery
4 Columbia Dr/Ste 730
Tampa, FL 33606
Tel: 813 259-0904 *Fax:* 813 259-0858
E-mail: dcahill@com1.med.usf.edu
Internet: http://www.med.usf.edu/surgery/hmpg.html
Accred Length: 5 Years *Program Size:* 6
Program ID: 160-11-21-109

Georgia

Atlanta

Emory University Program
Sponsor: Emory University School of Medicine
Crawford Long Hospital of Emory University
Egleston Children's Hospital at Emory University
Emory University Hospital
Grady Memorial Hospital

Program Director:
Daniel L Barrow, MD
Emory Univ
1365-B Clifton Rd NE
Ste 6400
Atlanta, GA 30322
Tel: 404 778-3895 *Fax:* 404 778-4472
E-mail: dbarr01@emory.edu
Internet: http://www.emory.edu/whsc/neurosurgery
Accred Length: 5 Years *Program Size:* 12
Program ID: 160-12-21-020

Augusta

Medical College of Georgia Program
Sponsor: Medical College of Georgia Hospital and Clinics
Veterans Affairs Medical Center (Augusta)

Program Director:
Dennis E McDonnell, MD
Med Coll of Georgia Hospital and Clinics
1120 15th St
Augusta, GA 30912-4010
Tel: 706 721-3071 *Fax:* 706 721-8084
E-mail: dmcdonel@mail.mcg.edu
Internet:
http://www.mcg.edu/som/surgery/neuros/index.html
Accred Length: 5 Years *Program Size:* 6 (*GYI:* 1)
Program ID: 160-12-21-021

Illinois

Chicago

McGaw Medical Center of Northwestern University Program
Sponsor: Northwestern University Medical School
Children's Memorial Medical Center
Evanston Hospital
Northwestern Memorial Hospital
Veterans Affairs Lakeside Medical Center (Chicago)

Program Director:
Stephen L Ondra, MD
233 E Erie/Ste 614
Chicago, IL 60611
Tel: 312 908-8699 *Fax:* 312 908-0225
E-mail: sondra@nmff.nwu.edu
Accred Length: 5 Years *Program Size:* 14
Program ID: 160-16-21-022

Rush-Presbyterian-St Luke's Medical Center Program
Sponsor: Rush-Presbyterian-St Luke's Medical Center
Cook County Hospital

Program Director:
Walter W Whisler, MD PhD
Rush-Presbyterian-St Luke's Med Ctr
1653 W Congress Pkwy
Rm 1491 Jelke
Chicago, IL 60612
Tel: 312 942-6628 *Fax:* 312 942-2266
E-mail: shadley@rush.edu
Accred Length: 5 Years *Program Size:* 5
Program ID: 160-16-11-023

University of Chicago Program
Sponsor: University of Chicago Hospitals

Program Director:
Bryce Weir, MD
Univ of Chicago Med Ctr
5841 S Maryland Ave/MC3026
Chicago, IL 60637-1470
Tel: 773 702-2123 *Fax:* 773 702-3518
Internet:
http://www.hospitals.uchicago.edu/neurosurgery
Accred Length: 5 Years *Program Size:* 5
Program ID: 160-16-11-024

University of Illinois College of Medicine at Chicago Program
Sponsor: University of Illinois College of Medicine at Chicago
Michael Reese Hospital and Medical Center
University of Illinois Hospital and Clinics

Program Director:
James I Ausman, MD PhD
Univ of Illinois
4th Fl-N NPI M/C 799
912 S Wood St
Chicago, IL 60612
Tel: 312 996-4712 *Fax:* 312 996-9018
E-mail: cgerby@uic.edu
Internet: http://www.uic.edu/depts/mcns
Accred Length: 5 Years *Program Size:* 5
Program ID: 160-16-21-025

Maywood

Loyola University Program
Sponsor: Loyola University Medical Center
Cook County Hospital
West Suburban Hospital Medical Center

Program Director:
T C Origitano, MD PhD
Foster G McGaw Hospital
2160 S First Ave/Bldg 54
Maywood, IL 60153
Tel: 708 216-8235 *Fax:* 708 216-4948
Internet: http://www.bsd.med.dean.luc.ecu/
Accred Length: 5 Years *Program Size:* 10
Program ID: 160-16-21-026

Peoria

University of Illinois College of Medicine at Peoria Program
Sponsor: University of Illinois College of Medicine at Peoria
Methodist Medical Center of Illinois
St Francis Medical Center

Program Director:
Patrick W Elwood, MD
Univ of Illinois Coll of Med
PO Box 1649
Peoria, IL 61656-1649
Tel: 309 655-2642 *Fax:* 309 655-7696
E-mail: jmja@uic.edu
Internet: http://www.uicomp.uic.edu/uicomp.htm
Accred Length: 5 Years *Program Size:* 5
Program ID: 160-16-21-099

Indiana

Indianapolis

Indiana University School of Medicine Program
Sponsor: Indiana University School of Medicine
Clarian IU Hospital
Clarian Methodist Hospital of Indiana
Clarian Riley Hospital for Children
Richard L Roudebush Veterans Affairs Medical Center
William N Wishard Memorial Hospital

Program Director:
Paul B Nelson, MD
Indiana Univ Med Ctr
545 Barnhill Dr/Rm 139
Indianapolis, IN 46202-5124
Tel: 317 274-5723 *Fax:* 317 274-7351
E-mail: mjgallag@iupui.edu
Internet: http://www.iupui.edu/~neurosur/
Accred Length: 5 Years *Program Size:* 9
Program ID: 160-17-11-027

Iowa

Iowa City

University of Iowa Hospitals and Clinics Program
Sponsor: University of Iowa Hospitals and Clinics
Veterans Affairs Medical Center (Iowa City)

Program Director:
John C VanGilder, MD
Univ of Iowa Hospitals and Clinics
Dept of Neurosurgery
200 Hawkins Dr
Iowa City, IA 52242-1009
Tel: 319 356-2772 *Fax:* 319 353-6605
Accred Length: 5 Years *Program Size:* 12 (*GYI:* 2)
Program ID: 160-18-11-028

Kansas

Kansas City

University of Kansas Medical Center Program
Sponsor: University of Kansas School of Medicine
Children's Mercy Hospital
University of Kansas Medical Center
Veterans Affairs Medical Center (Kansas City)

Program Director:
Paul L O'Boynick, MD
Univ of Kansas Med Ctr
3901 Rainbow Blvd.
Kansas City, KS 66160-7383
Tel: 913 588-6119 *Fax:* 913 588-7580
Accred Length: 5 Years *Program Size:* 5
Program ID: 160-19-21-029

Kentucky

Lexington

University of Kentucky Medical Center Program

Sponsor: University of Kentucky Hospital
Veterans Affairs Medical Center (Lexington)

Program Director:
Byron Young, MD
Univ of Kentucky Med Ctr
Div of Neurosurgery MS101
Lexington, KY 40536-0084
Tel: 606 323-5864 *Fax:* 606 257-8011
E-mail: byoun1@pop.uky.edu
Internet: http://www.mc.uky.edu/surgery/
Accred Length: 5 Years *Program Size:* 8 (*GY1:* 1)
Program ID: 160-20-21-030

Louisville

University of Louisville Program

Sponsor: University of Louisville School of Medicine
Kosair Children's Hospital (Alliant Health System)
Norton Hospital (Alliant Health System)
University of Louisville Hospital

Program Director:
Christopher B Shields, MD
Dept of Neurological Surgery
210 E Gray St/Ste 1102
Louisville, KY 40202
Tel: 502 629-5510 *Fax:* 502 629-5512
Internet: http://www.niky.com
Accred Length: 5 Years *Program Size:* 7
Program ID: 160-20-31-031

Louisiana

New Orleans

Louisiana State University Program

Sponsor: Louisiana State University School of Medicine
Alton Ochsner Medical Foundation
Medical Center of Louisiana at New Orleans

Program Director:
David G Kline, MD
Louisiana State Univ Med Ctr
Dept of Neurological Surgery
1542 Tulane Ave
New Orleans, LA 70112-2822
Tel: 504 568-6120 *Fax:* 504 568-6127
E-mail: cdixon@lsumc.edu
Internet:
http://www.lsumc.edu/campus/nsurgery/index.html
Accred Length: 5 Years *Program Size:* 5
Program ID: 160-21-21-032

Tulane University Program

Sponsor: Tulane University School of Medicine
Childrens Hospital
Medical Center of Louisiana at New Orleans
Tulane University Hospital and Clinics
Veterans Affairs Medical Center-LSU Service (New Orleans)

Program Director:
Dzung H Dinh, MD
Tulane Univ Med Ctr
Dept of Neurosurgery-SL47
1430 Tulane Ave
New Orleans, LA 70112-2699
Tel: 504 588-5565 *Fax:* 504 588-5793
E-mail: jcomer@tmcpop.tmc.tulane.edu
Internet: http://www.nsurg.tulane.edu
Accred Length: 5 Years *Program Size:* 5
Program ID: 160-21-21-033

Maryland

Baltimore

Johns Hopkins University Program

Sponsor: Johns Hopkins University School of Medicine
Johns Hopkins Bayview Medical Center
Johns Hopkins Hospital

Program Director:
Donlin M Long, MD PhD
Johns Hopkins Hospital
Meyer 7-109
600 N Wolfe St
Baltimore, MD 21287-7709
Tel: 410 955-2252 *Fax:* 410 955-6407
Internet:
http://hopkins.med.jhu.edu/healthcarepros/neuro/neurosurg.htm
Accred Length: 5 Years *Program Size:* 16
Program ID: 160-23-21-034

University of Maryland Program

Sponsor: University of Maryland Medical System
Veterans Affairs Medical Center (Baltimore)

Program Director:
Howard M Eisenberg, MD
Univ of Maryland Med System
Dept of Neurosurgery
22 S Greene St/Ste S-12-D
Baltimore, MD 21201-1595
Tel: 410 328-8621 *Fax:* 410 328-0756
E-mail: neuralnetwork@surgery1.umaryland.edu
Internet: http://www.neurosurgery-umms.com
Accred Length: 5 Years *Program Size:* 7
Program ID: 160-23-21-035

Bethesda

National Capital Consortium Program

Sponsor: National Capital Consortium
Children's Hospital of Philadelphia
Children's National Medical Center
National Naval Medical Center (Bethesda)
Walter Reed Army Medical Center

Program Director:
James M Ecklund, MD
Walter Reed Army Med Ctr
6825 16th St NW
Washington, DC 20307-5001
Tel: 202 782-9805 *Fax:* 202 782-0713
E-mail: ecklund@vs.wramc.amedd.army.mil/
Internet:
http://www.wrumc.amedd.army.mil/departments/surgery/neuro/index.htm
Accred Length: 5 Years *Program Size:* 6 (*GY1:* 1)
Program ID: 160-10-21-118
US Armed Services Program

Massachusetts

Boston

Children's Hospital/Brigham and Women's Hospital Program

Sponsor: Children's Hospital
Brigham and Women's Hospital

Program Director:
Peter M Black, MD PhD
Children's Hospital
Dept of Neurosurgery
300 Longwood Ave/Bader 3
Boston, MA 02115
Tel: 617 355-6008 *Fax:* 617 730-0419
Internet: http://www.boston-neurosurg.org
Accred Length: 5 Years *Program Size:* 5
Program ID: 160-24-21-036

Massachusetts General Hospital Program

Sponsor: Massachusetts General Hospital

Program Director:
Nicholas T Zervas, MD
Massachusetts General Hospital
55 Fruit St/WH 502
Boston, MA 02114-2696
Tel: 617 726-8581 *Fax:* 617 726-6789
Internet:
http://www.neurosurgery.mgh.harvard.edu./res-hp.htm
Accred Length: 5 Years *Program Size:* 12
Program ID: 160-24-31-037

Tufts University Program

Sponsor: New England Medical Center Hospitals
Beth Israel Deaconess Medical Center

Program Director:
William A Shucart, MD
New England Med Ctr
750 Washington St/Box 178
Boston, MA 02111
Tel: 617 636-5858 *Fax:* 617 636-7587
E-mail: sandra.navarroli@es.nemc.org
Accred Length: 5 Years *Program Size:* 5
Program ID: 160-24-31-038

Michigan

Ann Arbor

University of Michigan Program

Sponsor: University of Michigan Hospitals

Program Director:
Julian T Hoff, MD
Univ of Michigan Hospitals
Sect of Neurosurgery
1500 E Medical Center Dr
Ann Arbor, MI 48109-0338
Tel: 734 936-5015 *Fax:* 734 936-9294
Accred Length: 5 Years *Program Size:* 10 (*GY1:* 2)
Program ID: 160-25-21-039

Detroit

Henry Ford Hospital Program

Sponsor: Henry Ford Hospital

Program Director:
Mark L Rosenblum, MD
Henry Ford Hospital
2799 W Grand Blvd
Detroit, MI 48202
Tel: 313 876-1340 *Fax:* 313 876-7139
E-mail: nsser@neuro.hfh.edu
Accred Length: 5 Years *Program Size:* 12
Program ID: 160-25-11-040

Wayne State University/Detroit Medical Center Program

Sponsor: Wayne State University/Detroit Medical Center
Children's Hospital of Michigan
Detroit Receiving Hospital and University Health Center
Harper Hospital

Program Director:
Fernando Diaz, MD PhD
Univ Health Ctr
4201 St Antoine/6E
Detroit, MI 48201
Tel: 313 745-4661 *Fax:* 313 745-4099
E-mail: diaz@neurosurg.wayne.edu
Internet: http://www.neurosurg.wayne.edu
Accred Length: 5 Years *Program Size:* 5
Program ID: 160-25-21-041

Minnesota

Minneapolis

University of Minnesota Program

Sponsor: University of Minnesota Medical School
Fairview-University Medical Center
Hennepin County Medical Center
Veterans Affairs Medical Center (Minneapolis)

Program Director:
Robert E Maxwell, MD PhD
Univ of Minnesota Med Sch
Dept of Neurosurgery
420 Delaware St SE/Box 96 Mayo
Minneapolis, MN 55455-0392
Tel: 612 624-6666 *Fax:* 612 624-0644
E-mail: balkc002@maroon.tc.umn.edu
Internet: http://www.neuro.umn.edu
Accred Length: 5 Years *Program Size:* 11
Program ID: 160-26-21-042

Rochester

Mayo Graduate School of Medicine (Rochester) Program

Sponsor: Mayo Graduate School of Medicine-Mayo Foundation
Mayo Clinic (Rochester)
St Mary's Hospital of Rochester

Program Director:
David G Piepgras, MD
Application Processing Ctr
Mayo Graduate Sch of Med
200 First St SW/Siebens 5
Rochester, MN 55905
Tel: 507 284-4331 *Fax:* 507 284-0999
E-mail: mgsm.roch.mnneurosurgery@mayo.edu
Internet: http://www.mayo.edu/
Accred Length: 5 Years *Program Size:* 17 (*GY1:* 2)
Program ID: 160-26-21-043

Mississippi

Jackson

University of Mississippi Medical Center Program

Sponsor: University of Mississippi School of Medicine
University Hospital
Veterans Affairs Medical Center (Jackson)

Program Director:
Andrew D Parent, MD
Univ of Mississippi Med Ctr
2500 N State St
Jackson, MS 39206
Tel: 601 984-5705 *Fax:* 601 984-6986
E-mail: rfrench@neurosurgery.umsmed.edu
Internet: http://fiona.umsmed.edu/~ebpneuro
Accred Length: 5 Years *Program Size:* 7
Program ID: 160-27-21-044

Missouri

Columbia

University of Missouri-Columbia Program

Sponsor: University of Missouri-Columbia School of Medicine
Boone Hospital Center
Harry S Truman Memorial Veterans Hospital
University Hospitals and Clinics

Program Director:
David Jimenez, MD
Univ of Missouri Health Sciences Ctr
One Hospital Dr/N521
Columbia, MO 65212
Tel: 573 882-4908 *Fax:* 573 884-5184
E-mail: jimenezd@health.missouri.edu
Internet: http://www.surgery.missouri.edu/ns/education/resident.html
Accred Length: 5 Years *Program Size:* 5
Program ID: 160-28-21-045

St Louis

St Louis University School of Medicine Program

Sponsor: St Louis University School of Medicine
SSM Cardinal Glennon Children's Hospital
St Louis University School of Medicine

Program Director:
Kenneth R Smith Jr, MD
St Louis Univ Sch of Med, Div of Neurosurgery
3635 Vista Ave
PO Box 15250
St Louis, MO 63110-0250
Tel: 314 577-8795, ext 8796 *Fax:* 314 268-5061
E-mail: surgweb@slu.edu
Internet: http://www.slu.edu/colleges/med/departments/surgery
Accred Length: 5 Years *Program Size:* 6
Program ID: 160-28-21-047

Washington University/B-JH/SLCH Consortium Program

Sponsor: Washington University/B-JH/SLCH Consortium
Barnes-Jewish Hospital
St Louis Children's Hospital

Program Director:
Ralph G Dacey Jr, MD
Washington Univ Sch of Med
660 S Euclid Ave
Campus Box 8057
St Louis, MO 63110-1093
Tel: 314 362-3571 *Fax:* 314 362-2107
E-mail: castillo_c@kids.wustl.edu
Internet: http://plexus.wustl.edu
Accred Length: 5 Years *Program Size:* 12
Program ID: 160-28-11-046

Nebraska

Omaha

University of Nebraska Program

Sponsor: University of Nebraska Medical Center
Childrens Memorial Hospital
Methodist Hospital

Program Director:
Lyal G Leibrock, MD
Univ of Nebraska Hospital and Clinic
Sect of Neurosurgery
982035 Nebraska Med Ctr
Omaha, NE 68198-2035
Tel: 402 559-9605 *Fax:* 402 559-7779
E-mail: kbard@mail.unmc.edu
Internet: http://www.unmc.edu/neurosurgery/
Accred Length: 5 Years *Program Size:* 6
Program ID: 160-30-21-111

New Hampshire

Lebanon

Dartmouth-Hitchcock Medical Center Program

Sponsor: Mary Hitchcock Memorial Hospital

Program Director:
David W Roberts, MD
Dartmouth-Hitchcock Med Ctr
Sect of Neurosurgery
One Medical Center Dr
Lebanon, NH 03756-0001
Tel: 603 650-8730 *Fax:* 603 650-4547
E-mail: david.w.roberts@dartmouth.edu
Internet: http://www.hitchcock.org
Accred Length: 5 Years *Program Size:* 5
Program ID: 160-32-21-048

New Jersey

Newark

UMDNJ-New Jersey Medical School Program

Sponsor: UMDNJ-New Jersey Medical School
Hackensack University Medical Center
UMDNJ-University Hospital

Program Director:
Peter W Carmel, MD
UMDNJ-New Jersey Med Sch
90 Bergen St/Ste 7300
Newark, NJ 07103-2499
Tel: 973 972-2323 *Fax:* 973 972-2333
E-mail: caudle@umdnj.edu
Internet: http://www.umdnj.edu/nsurgweb/neurohome.html
Accred Length: 5 Years *Program Size:* 6
Program ID: 160-33-21-106

New Mexico

Albuquerque

University of New Mexico Program

Sponsor: University of New Mexico School of Medicine
Lovelace Medical Center
University Hospital

Program Director:
Edward C Benzel, MD
Univ of New Mexico
Neurosurgery 2ACC
2211 Lomas NE
Albuquerque, NM 87131-5341
Tel: 505 272-3401 *Fax:* 505 272-6091
E-mail: pcleve@salud.unm.edu
Accred Length: 5 Years *Program Size:* 5
Program ID: 160-34-21-115

New York

Albany

Albany Medical Center Program

Sponsor: Albany Medical Center

Program Director:
A John Popp, MD
Albany Med Coll
Div of Neurosurgery/Mail Code 61
47 New Scotland Ave
Albany, NY 12208
Tel: 518 262-5088 *Fax:* 518 262-5692
Accred Length: 5 Years *Program Size:* 5
Program ID: 160-35-21-049

Bronx

Albert Einstein College of Medicine Program

Sponsor: Albert Einstein College of Medicine of Yeshiva University
Jacobi Medical Center
Montefiore Medical Center-Henry and Lucy Moses Division

Program Director:
Patrick A LaSala, MD
Montefiore Med Ctr-Albert Einstein Coll of Med
Dept of Neurological Surgery
111 E 210th St
Bronx, NY 10467-2490
Tel: 718 920-7400 *Fax:* 718 519-6876
Accred Length: 5 Years *Program Size:* 8
Program ID: 160-35-21-051

Brooklyn

SUNY Health Science Center at Brooklyn Program

Sponsor: SUNY Health Science Center at Brooklyn
Kings County Hospital Center
University Hospital-SUNY Health Science Center at Brooklyn

Program Director:
Thomas H Milhorat, MD
SUNY Health Science Ctr-Brooklyn
450 Clarkson Ave/Box 1189
Brooklyn, NY 11203
Tel: 718 270-2111 *Fax:* 718 270-3922
Accred Length: 5 Years *Program Size:* 6
Program ID: 160-35-21-056

Buffalo

SUNY at Buffalo Graduate Medical-Dental Education Consortium Program

Sponsor: SUNY at Buffalo Grad Medical-Dental Education Consortium
CGF Health System (Buffalo General Hospital)
CGF Health System (Children's Hospital of Buffalo)
Erie County Medical Center

Program Director:
Kevin J Gibbons, MD
Millard Fillmore Hospitals
Three Gates Cir
Buffalo, NY 14209-1194
Tel: 716 887-5210 *Fax:* 716 887-4378
E-mail: lawilson1@aol.com
Internet: http://wings.buffalo.edu/smbs/nsur
Accred Length: 5 Years *Program Size:* 7
Program ID: 160-35-21-050

New York

Mount Sinai School of Medicine Program

Sponsor: Mount Sinai School of Medicine
Elmhurst Hospital Center-Mount Sinai Services
Mount Sinai Medical Center

Program Director:
Kalmon D Post, MD
Mount Sinai Hospital
Box 1136
One Gustave L Levy Pl
New York, NY 10029-6574
Tel: 212 241-0933 *Fax:* 212 831-3324
E-mail: neurosurgery@smtplink.mssm.edu
Internet: http://www.mssm.edu
Accred Length: 5 Years *Program Size:* 10
Program ID: 160-35-21-053

New York and Presbyterian Hospital (Columbia Campus) Program

Sponsor: New York and Presbyterian Hospital
New York and Presbyterian Hospital (Columbia Campus)

Program Director:
Donald O Quest, MD
Neurological Inst
710 W 168th St
New York, NY 10032
Tel: 212 305-5543 *Fax:* 212 305-2026
Internet: http://cpmcnet/dept/nsg/
Accred Length: 5 Years *Program Size:* 10
Program ID: 160-35-11-055

New York and Presbyterian Hospital (Cornell Campus) Program

Sponsor: New York and Presbyterian Hospital
Hospital for Special Surgery
Memorial Sloan-Kettering Cancer Center
New York and Presbyterian Hospital (Cornell Campus)

Program Director:
Richard A Fraser, MD
New York Hospital
525 E 68th St
New York, NY 10021
Tel: 212 746-2385 *Fax:* 212 746-8849
E-mail: rfraser@mail.meacornell.edu
Internet: http://surgery.med.cornell.edu/neuro/home.htm
Accred Length: 5 Years *Program Size:* 12
Program ID: 160-35-21-052

New York University Medical Center Program

Sponsor: New York University Medical Center
Bellevue Hospital Center
Veterans Affairs Medical Center (Manhattan)

Program Director:
Patrick J Kelly, MD
New York Univ Med Ctr
Dept of Neurosurgery
550 First Ave
New York, NY 10016
Tel: 212 263-6414 *Fax:* 212 263-8225
E-mail: kelly@mcns04.med.nyu.edu
Internet: http://www.mcns10.med.nyu.edu
Accred Length: 5 Years *Program Size:* 12
Program ID: 160-35-21-054

Rochester

University of Rochester Program

Sponsor: Strong Memorial Hospital of the University of Rochester

Program Director:
Robert Maciunas, MD PhD
Univ of Rochester Med Ctr
601 Elmwood Ave/Box 670
Rochester, NY 14642-8670
Tel: 716 275-5709 *Fax:* 716 275-8545
Internet:
http://www.urmc.rochester.edu/smd/neursurg/residency.htm
Accred Length: 5 Years *Program Size:* 6
Program ID: 160-35-11-057

Syracuse

SUNY Health Science Center at Syracuse Program

Sponsor: University Hospital-SUNY Health Science Center at Syracuse
Crouse Hospital
Veterans Affairs Medical Center (Syracuse)

Program Director:
Charles J Hodge Jr, MD
Dept of Neurosurgery
Health Science Ctr-Syracuse
750 E Adams St
Syracuse, NY 13210
Tel: 315 464-4470 *Fax:* 315 464-5520
E-mail: iwanskik@mailbox.hscsyr.edu
Internet: http://www.neuro.hscsyr.edu
Accred Length: 5 Years *Program Size:* 10
Program ID: 160-35-21-058

Valhalla

New York Medical College at Westchester Medical Center Program

Sponsor: New York Medical College
St Vincent's Hospital and Medical Center of New York
Westchester Medical Center

Program Director:
William T Couldwell, MD PhD
New York Med Coll-Westchester County Med Ctr
Munger Pavilion
Valhalla, NY 10595
Tel: 914 493-8392 *Fax:* 914 594-3641
E-mail: william_couldwell@nymc.edu
Accred Length: 5 Years *Program Size:* 5
Program ID: 160-35-21-108

North Carolina

Chapel Hill

University of North Carolina Hospitals Program

Sponsor: University of North Carolina Hospitals

Program Director:
Estrada J Bernard Jr, MD
Univ of North Carolina Sch of Med
Div of Neurosurgery
148 Burnett-Womack Bldg/CB#7060
Chapel Hill, NC 27599-7060
Tel: 919 966-1374 *Fax:* 919 966-6627
E-mail: bern999@med.unc.edu
Internet: http://www.//sunsite.unc.edu/neuro
Accred Length: 5 Years *Program Size:* 6
Program ID: 160-36-11-059

Durham

Duke University Program

Sponsor: Duke University Medical Center
Durham Regional Hospital
Veterans Affairs Medical Center (Durham)

Program Director:
Allan H Friedman, MD
Duke Univ Med Ctr
Box 3807
Durham, NC 27710
Tel: 919 684-3271 *Fax:* 919 681-7973
Internet:
http://surgery.dev.mc.duke.edu/people/fried010.htm
Accred Length: 5 Years *Program Size:* 11
Program ID: 160-36-21-060

Winston-Salem

Wake Forest University School of Medicine Program

Sponsor: Wake Forest University Baptist Medical Center

Program Director:
David L Kelly Jr, MD
Wake Forest Univ Sch of Med
Dept of Neurosurgery
Medical Center Blvd
Winston-Salem, NC 27157-1029
Tel: 336 716-4038 *Fax:* 336 716-3065
E-mail: fcasstev@wfubmc.edu
Internet:
http://www.wfubmc.edu/bgsm/surg-sci/ns/ns/html
Accred Length: 5 Years *Program Size:* 6
Program ID: 160-36-11-061

Ohio

Cincinnati

University Hospital/University of Cincinnati College of Medicine Program

Sponsor: University Hospital Inc
Christ Hospital
Good Samaritan Hospital

Program Director:
John M Tew Jr, MD
Univ of Cincinnati
PO Box 670515
Cincinnati, OH 45267-0515
Tel: 513 558-5387 *Fax:* 513 558-7702
E-mail: john.tew@uc.edu
Internet: http://www.mayfieldclinic.com
Accred Length: 5 Years *Program Size:* 13 (*GYI:* 2)
Program ID: 160-38-21-064

Cleveland

Case Western Reserve University Program

Sponsor: University Hospitals of Cleveland
MetroHealth Medical Center
Veterans Affairs Medical Center (Cleveland)

Program Director:
Robert A Ratcheson, MD
Case Western Univ
Dept of Neurosurgery
11100 Euclid Ave
Cleveland, OH 44106
Tel: 216 844-5747 *Fax:* 216 844-3014
Accred Length: 5 Years *Program Size:* 13
Program ID: 160-38-21-065

Cleveland Clinic Foundation Program

Sponsor: Cleveland Clinic Foundation

Program Director:
Gene H Barnett, MD
Cleveland Clinic Foundation
Dept of Neurosurgery/S80
9500 Euclid Ave
Cleveland, OH 44195-5014
Tel: 216 444-5690 *Fax:* 216 444-1162
E-mail: meded@cesmtp.ccf.org
Internet: http://www.ccf.org
Accred Length: 5 Years *Program Size:* 9
Program ID: 160-38-22-066

Columbus

Ohio State University Program

Sponsor: Ohio State University Medical Center
Children's Hospital
Riverside Methodist Hospitals (OhioHealth)

Program Director:
Michael E Miner, MD PhD
Ohio State Univ Hospitals
N-1021 Doan Hall
410 W Tenth Ave
Columbus, OH 43210-1228
Tel: 614 293-8714 *Fax:* 614 293-4281
E-mail: mine01@surgdo.surgpo1
Internet: http://www-surgery.med.ohio-state.edu
Accred Length: 5 Years *Program Size:* 10
Program ID: 160-38-21-067

Oklahoma

Oklahoma City

University of Oklahoma Health Sciences Center Program

Sponsor: University of Oklahoma College of Medicine
Children's Hospital of Oklahoma
Columbia Presbyterian Hospital
University Hospital
Veterans Affairs Medical Center (Oklahoma City)

Program Director:
Christopher M Loftus, MD
Univ of Oklahoma Health Sciences Ctr
Dept of Neurosurgery
711 Stanton L Young Blvd/Ste 206
Oklahoma City, OK 73104
Tel: 405 271-4912 *Fax:* 405 271-3091
Internet: http://w3.ouhsc.edu/neurosurgery
Accred Length: 5 Years *Program Size:* 5
Program ID: 160-39-21-068

Oregon

Portland

Oregon Health Sciences University Program

Sponsor: Oregon Health Sciences University Hospital
Veterans Affairs Medical Center (Portland)

Program Director:
Kim J Burchiel, MD
Oregon Health Sciences Univ
Div of Neurosurgery/L-472
3181 SW Sam Jackson Park Rd
Portland, OR 97201-3098
Tel: 503 494-8070 *Fax:* 503 494-7161
E-mail: burchiek@ohsu.edu
Internet: http://www.ohsu.edu/som-surgery/neurosurgery
Accred Length: 5 Years *Program Size:* 6 (*GYI:* 1)
Program ID: 160-40-21-070

Pennsylvania

Hershey

Penn State Geisinger Health System/Milton S Hershey Medical Center Program

Sponsor: Penn State Geisinger Health System
Milton S Hershey Medical Center

Program Director:
Stephen K Powers, MD
500 University Dr/PO Box 850
BMR Bldg/Rm C3830
Hershey, PA 17033
Tel: 717 531-4384 *Fax:* 717 531-3858
Accred Length: 5 Years *Program Size:* 5
Program ID: 160-41-21-110

Philadelphia

MCP Hahnemann University Program

Sponsor: MCP Hahnemann University
Hahnemann University Hospital
Medical College of Pennsylvania Hospital
St Christopher's Hospital for Children

Program Director:
Thomas A Gennarelli, MD
MCP Hahnemann Univ Hospital
Broad and Vine St/MS 455
Philadelphia, PA 19102-1192
Tel: 215 762-3130 *Fax:* 215 762-3132
Internet:
http://www.allegheny.edu/medschool/depts/neurosrg/front.htm
Accred Length: 5 Years *Program Size:* 5
Program ID: 160-41-11-117

Temple University Program

Sponsor: Temple University Hospital
Abington Memorial Hospital
St Christopher's Hospital for Children

Program Director:
Raj K Narayan, MD
Temple Univ Hospital
3401 N Broad St
Parkinson Pavilion/#658
Philadelphia, PA 19140
Tel: 215 707-7200 *Fax:* 215 707-3831
E-mail: neurosrg@blue.temple.edu
Internet: http://www.temple.edu.neurosurgery
Accred Length: 5 Years *Program Size:* 5
Program ID: 160-41-21-073

Thomas Jefferson University Program
Sponsor: Thomas Jefferson University Hospital
Pennsylvania Hospital (UPHS)
Wills Eye Hospital
Program Director:
William A Buchheit, MD
1015 Chestnut St/14th Fl
Philadelphia, PA 19107-4302
Tel: 215 955-6744 *Fax:* 215 923-8071
Internet: http://nsi.tjh.tju.edu
Accred Length: 5 Years *Program Size:* 10
Program ID: 160-41-21-074

University of Pennsylvania Program
Sponsor: Hospital of the University of Pennsylvania
Children's Hospital of Philadelphia
Veterans Affairs Medical Center (Philadelphia)
Program Director:
Eric Zager, MD
Hospital of the Univ of Pennsylvania
3400 Spruce St
5th Fl/Silverstein
Philadelphia, PA 19104-4283
Tel: 215 662-3497 *Fax:* 215 349-5534
E-mail: zager@mail.med.upenn.edu
Internet: http://www.med.upenn.edu/neursurg
Accred Length: 5 Years *Program Size:* 12
Program ID: 160-41-21-075

Pittsburgh

Allegheny General Hospital Program
Sponsor: Allegheny General Hospital
Program Director:
Jack E Wilberger Jr, MD
Allegheny General Hospital
Dept of Neurological Surgery
320 E North Ave
Pittsburgh, PA 15212
Tel: 412 359-6200, ext 8081 *Fax:* 412 359-6615
E-mail: wilberj@wpo.auhs.edu
Accred Length: 5 Years *Program Size:* 5
Program ID: 160-41-31-116

University Health Center of Pittsburgh Program
Sponsor: University Health Center of Pittsburgh
Children's Hospital of Pittsburgh
Presbyterian University Hospital/UPMC
Veterans Affairs Medical Center (Pittsburgh)
Program Director:
L Dade Lunsford, MD
Univ of Pittsburgh
200 Lothrop St/Ste B-400
Pittsburgh, PA 15213-2582
Tel: 412 647-6781 *Fax:* 412 647-0989
Internet: http://www.neuronet.pitt.edu
Accred Length: 5 Years *Program Size:* 17
Program ID: 160-41-31-076

Puerto Rico

San Juan

University of Puerto Rico Program
Sponsor: University of Puerto Rico School of Medicine
San Juan City Hospital
University Hospital
University Pediatric Hospital
Veterans Affairs Medical Center (San Juan)
Program Director:
Nathan Rifkinson, MD
Univ of Puerto Rico Sch of Med
Dept of Neurosurgery
PO Box 365067
San Juan, PR 00936-5067
Tel: 787 765-8276 *Fax:* 787 765-8276
Accred Length: 5 Years *Program Size:* 4
Program ID: 160-42-21-078

Rhode Island

Providence

Brown University Program
Sponsor: Rhode Island Hospital
Program Director:
Mel H Epstein, MD
Brown Univ Program
593 Eddy St
Providence, RI 02903
Tel: 401 444-8701 *Fax:* 401 444-8719
Internet:
http://www.brown.edu/departments/neurosurgery/
Accred Length: 5 Years *Program Size:* 6
Program ID: 160-43-21-103

South Carolina

Charleston

Medical University of South Carolina Program
Sponsor: Medical University of South Carolina College of Medicine
MUSC Medical Center
Program Director:
Stephen J Haines, MD
Med Univ of South Carolina
171 Ashley Ave
Charleston, SC 29425-2272
Tel: 843 792-1471 *Fax:* 843 792-0468
E-mail: terrykl@musc.edu
Internet: http://www.musc.edu/neurosurg
Accred Length: 5 Years *Program Size:* 5 (*GY1:* 0)
Program ID: 160-45-11-079

Tennessee

Memphis

University of Tennessee Program
Sponsor: University of Tennessee College of Medicine
Baptist Memorial Hospital
Methodist Hospitals of Memphis-Central
Regional Medical Center at Memphis
Veterans Affairs Medical Center (Memphis)
Program Director:
Jon H Robertson, MD
Dept of Neurosurgery
847 Monroe Ave/Rm 427
Memphis, TN 38163
Tel: 901 448-6374 *Fax:* 901 448-8468
E-mail: jorobertson@utmem1.utmem.edu
Accred Length: 5 Years *Program Size:* 15
Program ID: 160-47-21-080

Nashville

Vanderbilt University Program
Sponsor: Vanderbilt University Medical Center
St Thomas Hospital
Veterans Affairs Medical Center (Nashville)
Program Director:
George S Allen, MD PhD
Vanderbilt Univ Med Ctr
T-4224 Med Ctr N
Nashville, TN 37232-2380
Tel: 615 322-7423 *Fax:* 615 343-8104
Accred Length: 5 Years *Program Size:* 12
Program ID: 160-47-21-081

Texas

Dallas

University of Texas Southwestern Medical School Program
Sponsor: University of Texas Southwestern Medical School
Children's Medical Center of Dallas
Dallas County Hospital District-Parkland Memorial Hospital
Veterans Affairs Medical Center (Dallas)
Zale-Lipshy University Hospital
Program Director:
Eugene D George, MD
Univ of Texas Southwestern Med Ctr
Dept of Neurological Surgery
5323 Harry Hines Blvd
Dallas, TX 75235-8855
Tel: 214 648-4579 *Fax:* 214 648-2822
E-mail: mcook@mednet.swmed.edu
Internet: http://neuro3.swmed.edu
Accred Length: 5 Years *Program Size:* 10
Program ID: 160-48-21-082

Galveston

University of Texas Medical Branch Hospitals Program
Sponsor: University of Texas Medical Branch Hospitals
Program Director:
Haring J W Nauta, MD PhD
Univ of Texas Med Branch
301 University Blvd
Galveston, TX 77555-0517
Tel: 409 772-1500 *Fax:* 409 772-6352
Internet: http://www.utmb.edu/surgery/
Accred Length: 5 Years *Program Size:* 6
Program ID: 160-48-21-083

Houston

Baylor College of Medicine Program

Sponsor: Baylor College of Medicine
Harris County Hospital District-Ben Taub General Hospital
Methodist Hospital
Veterans Affairs Medical Center (Houston)

Program Director:
Robert G Grossman, MD
Dept of Neurosurgery
Baylor Coll of Med
6560 Fannin/Ste 944
Houston, TX 77030
Tel: 713 798-4696 *Fax:* 713 798-3739
E-mail: grossman@bcm.tmc.edu
Internet: http://www.bcm.tmc.edu/neurosurgery
Accred Length: 5 Years *Program Size:* 15
Program ID: 160-48-21-084

San Antonio

University of Texas Health Science Center at San Antonio Program

Sponsor: University of Texas Medical School at San Antonio
Audie L Murphy Memorial Veterans Hospital (San Antonio)
University Hospital-South Texas Medical Center

Program Director:
Dennis G Vollmer, MD
Univ of Texas Health Science Ctr
7703 Floyd Curl Dr
San Antonio, TX 78284-7843
Tel: 210 567-5625 *Fax:* 210 567-6066
E-mail: mccaffrey@uthscsa.edu
Internet: http://surg62.uthscsa.edu
Accred Length: 5 Years *Program Size:* 6
Program ID: 160-48-21-085

Utah

Salt Lake City

University of Utah Program

Sponsor: University of Utah Medical Center
Primary Children's Medical Center
Veterans Affairs Medical Center (Salt Lake City)

Program Director:
Ronald I Apfelbaum, MD
Univ of Utah Health Sciences Ctr
50 N Medical Dr
Ste 3B-409
Salt Lake City, UT 84132
Tel: 801 581-6908 *Fax:* 801 581-4385
E-mail: julie@suzy.med.utah.edu
Accred Length: 5 Years *Program Size:* 11
Program ID: 160-49-31-086

Vermont

Burlington

University of Vermont Program

Sponsor: Fletcher Allen Health Care

Program Director:
Paul L Penar, MD
Univ of Vermont Coll of Med
Given Bldg D-319
Burlington, VT 05405-0068
Tel: 802 656-8447 *Fax:* 802 656-0680
E-mail: ppenar@uvm.edu
Internet: http://vtmednet.org.:80/surgery/nsinfo.htm
Accred Length: 5 Years *Program Size:* 6 (*GY1:* 1)
Program ID: 160-50-21-101

Virginia

Charlottesville

University of Virginia Program

Sponsor: University of Virginia Medical Center

Program Director:
John A Jane, MD PhD
Univ of Virginia Health Sciences Ctr
Box 212
Charlottesville, VA 22908
Tel: 804 924-2203 *Fax:* 804 924-9656
Accred Length: 5 Years *Program Size:* 12 (*GY1:* 1)
Program ID: 160-51-21-088

Richmond

Medical College of Virginia/Virginia Commonwealth University Program

Sponsor: Medical College of Virginia/Virginia Commonwealth University
Hunter Holmes McGuire VA Medical Center (Richmond)
Medical College of Virginia Hospitals

Program Director:
Harold F Young, MD
Med Coll of Virginia
PO Box 980631
Richmond, VA 23298-0631
Tel: 804 828-9165 *Fax:* 804 828-0374
Internet: http://www.surgery.vcu.edu
Accred Length: 5 Years *Program Size:* 10
Program ID: 160-51-21-089

Washington

Seattle

University of Washington Program

Sponsor: University of Washington School of Medicine
Children's Hospital and Medical Center
Harborview Medical Center
University of Washington Medical Center
Veterans Affairs Medical Center (Seattle)

Program Director:
H Richard Winn, MD
Harborview Med Ctr
Neurological Surgery/Box 359766
325 Ninth Ave
Seattle, WA 98104-2499
Tel: 206 521-1833 *Fax:* 206 521-1881
E-mail: hrwinn@u.washington.edu
Internet: http://www.neurosurgery.washington.edu/
Accred Length: 5 Years *Program Size:* 12 (*GY1:* 2)
Program ID: 160-54-21-090

West Virginia

Morgantown

West Virginia University Program

Sponsor: West Virginia University Hospitals

Program Director:
Howard H Kaufman, MD
Health Science Ctr
Dept of Neurosurgery
PO Box 9183
Morgantown, WV 26506-9183
Tel: 304 293-5042 *Fax:* 304 293-4819
E-mail: lfletcher@hsc.wvu.edu
Accred Length: 5 Years *Program Size:* 5
Program ID: 160-55-11-091

Wisconsin

Madison

University of Wisconsin Program

Sponsor: University of Wisconsin Hospital and Clinics
Meriter Hospital
William S Middleton Veterans Hospital

Program Director:
Robert J Dempsey, MD
Univ of Wisconsin
Clinical Science Ctr H4/342
600 Highland Ave
Madison, WI 53792-3232
Tel: 608 263-1410 *Fax:* 608 263-1728
E-mail: liebman@neurosurg.wisc.edu
Internet: http://www.medsch.wisc.edu/neurosurg
Accred Length: 5 Years *Program Size:* 6 (*GY1:* 1)
Program ID: 160-56-21-092

Milwaukee

Medical College of Wisconsin Program

Sponsor: Medical College of Wisconsin Affiliated Hospitals Inc
Children's Hospital of Wisconsin
Clement J Zablocki Veterans Affairs Medical Center
Froedtert Memorial Lutheran Hospital

Program Director:
Sanford J Larson, MD PhD
Froedtert West Clinic
9200 W Wisconsin Ave
Milwaukee, WI 53226
Tel: 414 454-5407 *Fax:* 414 258-6266
Accred Length: 5 Years *Program Size:* 8 (*GY1:* 1)
Program ID: 160-56-21-093

Neurology

Alabama

Birmingham

University of Alabama Medical Center Program
Sponsor: University of Alabama Hospital
Veterans Affairs Medical Center (Birmingham)
Program Director:
John N Whitaker, MD
Univ of Alabama Med Ctr
625 S 19th St
Birmingham, AL 35294-0007
Tel: 205 934-2402 *Fax:* 205 975-6030
Internet: http://www.neuro.uab.edu
Accred Length: 3 Years *Program Size:* 15
Subspecialties: CHN, CN
Program ID: 180-01-31-004

Mobile

University of South Alabama Program
Sponsor: University of South Alabama Medical Center
Program Director:
William J Hamilton, DO
2451 Fillingim St
MCSB 1215
Mobile, AL 36617
Tel: 334 471-7839 *Fax:* 334 471-7838
E-mail: whamilton@usamail.usouthal.edu
Accred Length: 3 Years *Program Size:* 7
Program ID: 180-01-21-123

Arizona

Phoenix

St Joseph's Hospital and Medical Center Program
Sponsor: St Joseph's Hospital and Medical Center
Program Director:
William R Shapiro, MD
Barrow Neurological Inst
St Joseph's Hospital and Med Ctr
PO Box 2071
Phoenix, AZ 85001-2071
Tel: 602 406-3196 *Fax:* 602 406-4104
E-mail: wshapir@mha.chw.edu
Internet: http://www.chw.edu/mha/mha.html
Accred Length: 3 Years *Program Size:* 9
Subspecialties: CHN
Program ID: 180-03-12-005

Tucson

University of Arizona Program
Sponsor: University of Arizona College of Medicine
University Medical Center
Veterans Affairs Medical Center (Tucson)
Program Director:
David M Labiner, MD
Dept of Neurology
Arizona Health Sciences Ctr
1501 N Campbell Ave
Tucson, AZ 85724
Tel: 520 626-2006 *Fax:* 520 626-2111
E-mail: labinerd@u.arizona.edu
Internet: http://www.ahsc.arizona.edu/neurology/
Accred Length: 3 Years *Program Size:* 9
Program ID: 180-03-21-006

Arkansas

Little Rock

University of Arkansas for Medical Sciences Program
Sponsor: University of Arkansas College of Medicine
John L McClellan Memorial Veterans Hospital
University Hospital of Arkansas
Program Director:
Stacy A Rudnicki, MD
Univ of Arkansas for Med Sciences
4301 W Markham St/Slot 500
Little Rock, AR 72205-7199
Tel: 501 686-5135 *Fax:* 501 686-8689
E-mail: srudnicki@neurology.uams.edu
Internet: http://www.uams.edu/neuro/index.htm
Accred Length: 4 Years *Program Size:* 16
Subspecialties: CHN
Program ID: 180-04-21-007

California

Loma Linda

Loma Linda University Program
Sponsor: Loma Linda University Medical Center
Jerry L Pettis Memorial Veterans Hospital
Kaiser Foundation Hospital (Riverside)
Program Director:
Gordon W Peterson, MD
Loma Linda Univ Med Ctr
Dept of Neurology/Rm 11108 Coleman
PO Box 2000
Loma Linda, CA 92354
Tel: 909 558-4907 *Fax:* 909 558-4207
E-mail: dgiang@ahs.llumc.edu
Internet: http://www.llu.edu
Accred Length: 3 Years *Program Size:* 7
Subspecialties: CHN
Program ID: 180-05-21-124

Los Angeles

Southern California Kaiser Permanente Medical Care (Los Angeles) Program
Sponsor: Southern California Kaiser Permanente Medical Group
Kaiser Foundation Hospital (Los Angeles)
Program Director:
Richard M Green, MD
Kaiser Permanente Med Care
393 E Walnut St
Pasadena, CA 91188-8013
Tel: 800 541-7946
Accred Length: 4 Years *Program Size:* 8 (*GY1:* 2)
Program ID: 180-05-12-010

UCLA Medical Center Program
Sponsor: UCLA School of Medicine
UCLA Medical Center
Program Director:
Andrew Charles, MD
Reed Neurological Research Ctr
710 Westwood Plaza
Los Angeles, CA 90095
Tel: 310 825-6681 *Fax:* 310 206-4733
Accred Length: 3 Years *Program Size:* 19
Subspecialties: CHN, CN
Program ID: 180-05-21-012

University of Southern California Program
Sponsor: Los Angeles County-USC Medical Center
Program Director:
Christi N Heck, MD
Univ of Southern California
Dept of Neurology
1975 Zonal Ave/KAM 410
Los Angeles, CA 90033
Tel: 323 442-3020 *Fax:* 323 442-3015
E-mail: ebueno@hsc.usc.edu
Internet: http://www.usc.edu/hsc/medicine/neurology
Accred Length: 3 Years *Program Size:* 12
Subspecialties: CHN
Program ID: 180-05-21-011

VA Greater Los Angeles Healthcare System Program
Sponsor: VA Greater Los Angeles Healthcare System
Program Director:
Claude G Westerlain, MD
Neurology Service (127A)
VA Med Ctr West Los Angeles
11301 Wilshire Blvd
Los Angeles, CA 90073
Tel: 310 268-3595 *Fax:* 310 268-4611
E-mail: wasterla@ucla.edu
Accred Length: 3 Years *Program Size:* 8
Program ID: 180-05-31-013

Orange

University of California (Irvine) Program
Sponsor: University of California (Irvine) Medical Center
Veterans Affairs Medical Center (Long Beach)
Program Director:
Robert R Young, MD
Univ of California Irvine
Dept of Neurology
105 Irvine Hall
Irvine, CA 92697-4275
Tel: 949 824-3406 *Fax:* 949 824-2076
E-mail: rryoung@uci.edu
Accred Length: 3 Years *Program Size:* 9
Subspecialties: CHN
Program ID: 180-05-21-009

Sacramento

University of California (Davis) Program
Sponsor: University of California (Davis) Medical Center
David Grant Medical Center
Program Director:
David P Richman, MD
Dept of Neurology
4860 Y St/Ste 3700
Sacramento, CA 95817
Tel: 916 734-3514 *Fax:* 916 734-6525
E-mail: dprichman@ucdavis.edu
Internet: http://www.neurology.ucdavis.edu
Accred Length: 4 Years *Program Size:* 15
Subspecialties: CN
Program ID: 180-05-12-008

San Diego

University of California (San Diego) Program
Sponsor: University of California (San Diego) Medical Center
Veterans Affairs Medical Center (San Diego)
Program Director:
Mark Kritchevsky, MD
UCSD Med Ctr
200 W Arbor Dr/8465
San Diego, CA 92103-8465
Tel: 619 543-6266 *Fax:* 619 543-5793
E-mail: jhays@ucsd.edu
Accred Length: 3 Years *Program Size:* 9
Subspecialties: CHN
Program ID: 180-05-21-014

San Francisco

University of California (San Francisco) Program
Sponsor: University of California (San Francisco) School of Medicine
San Francisco General Hospital Medical Center
University of California (San Francisco) Medical Center
Veterans Affairs Medical Center (San Francisco)
Program Director:
John W Engstrom, MD
Univ of California
505 Parnassus Ave
Rm M798
San Francisco, CA 94143-0114
Tel: 415 476-1487 *Fax:* 415 476-3428
Accred Length: 3 Years *Program Size:* 17
Subspecialties: CHN, CN
Program ID: 180-05-21-016

Stanford

Stanford University Program
Sponsor: Stanford University Hospital
Santa Clara Valley Medical Center
Veterans Affairs Palo Alto Health Care System
Program Director:
Jaime R Lopez, MD
Stanford Univ Med Ctr
Dept of Neurology/H3160
300 Pasteur Dr
Stanford, CA 94305-5235
Tel: 650 725-6688 *Fax:* 650 725-7459
E-mail: lopezjr@stanford.edu
Internet: http://www.-leland/group/neurology/res
Accred Length: 3 Years *Program Size:* 15
Subspecialties: CHN, CN
Program ID: 180-05-21-017

Torrance

Los Angeles County-Harbor-UCLA Medical Center Program
Sponsor: Los Angeles County-Harbor-UCLA Medical Center
Program Director:
Mark A Goldberg, MD PhD
Los Angeles County-Harbor-UCLA Med Ctr
1000 W Carson St
Torrance, CA 90509
Tel: 310 222-3897 *Fax:* 310 533-8905
E-mail: m_goldberg@humc.edu
Accred Length: 3 Years *Program Size:* 9
Subspecialties: CHN
Program ID: 180-05-11-018

Colorado

Denver

University of Colorado Program
Sponsor: University of Colorado Health Sciences Center
Denver Health and Hospitals
Veterans Affairs Medical Center (Denver)
Program Director:
John R Corboy, MD
Univ of Colorado Health Sciences Ctr
4200 E Ninth Ave/B-183
Denver, CO 80262
Tel: 303 315-8760 *Fax:* 303 315-5867
E-mail: john.corboy@uchsc.edu
Internet: http://www.uchsc.edu/sm/neuro/index.html
Accred Length: 3 Years *Program Size:* 12
Subspecialties: CHN
Program ID: 180-07-21-019

Connecticut

Farmington

University of Connecticut Program
Sponsor: University of Connecticut School of Medicine
Hartford Hospital
Univ of Connecticut Health Center/John Dempsey Hospital
Program Director:
Leslie I Wolfson, MD
Hartford Hospital
80 Seymour St/Box 5037
Hartford, CT 06102-5037
Tel: 860 545-3621 *Fax:* 860 545-5003
Accred Length: 3 Years *Program Size:* 9
Program ID: 180-08-21-139

New Haven

Yale-New Haven Medical Center Program
Sponsor: Yale-New Haven Hospital
Veterans Affairs Medical Center (West Haven)
Program Director:
George B Richerson, MD PhD
Yale Univ Sch of Med
Dept of Neurology LCI-712
PO Box 208018
New Haven, CT 06520-8018
Tel: 203 785-6054 *Fax:* 203 785-5694
E-mail: clp4@email.med.yale.edu
Internet: http://www.info.med.yale.edu/neurol
Accred Length: 3 Years *Program Size:* 15
Subspecialties: CHN, CN
Program ID: 180-08-21-021

District of Columbia

Washington

George Washington University Program
Sponsor: George Washington University School of Medicine
Children's National Medical Center
George Washington University Hospital (UHS)
Washington Hospital Center
Program Director:
Perry K Richardson, MD
George Washington Univ Med Ctr
2150 Pennsylvania Ave NW/Ste 7-404
Washington, DC 20037
Tel: 202 994-4063 *Fax:* 202 994-3638
E-mail: neupkr@gwumc.edu
Internet: http://www.ninet.gwumc.edu
Accred Length: 3 Years *Program Size:* 7
Subspecialties: CHN
Program ID: 180-10-21-023

Georgetown University Program
Sponsor: Georgetown University Medical Center
Veterans Affairs Medical Center (Washington, DC)
Program Director:
Stanley L Cohan, MD PhD
Georgetown Univ Hospital
Dept of Neurology
3800 Reservoir Rd NW
Washington, DC 20007-2197
Tel: 202 687-8525 *Fax:* 202 784-2261
Accred Length: 3 Years *Program Size:* 18
Program ID: 180-10-21-022

Howard University Program
Sponsor: Howard University Hospital
District of Columbia General Hospital
Program Director:
Annapurni Jayam-Trouth, MD
Howard Univ Hospital
2041 Georgia Ave NW
Washington, DC 20060
Tel: 202 865-1546 *Fax:* 202 865-4395
E-mail: jayamt@aol.com
Accred Length: 3 Years *Program Size:* 8
Program ID: 180-10-21-024

Florida

Fort Lauderdale

Cleveland Clinic Foundation (Florida) Program
Sponsor: Cleveland Clinic Foundation
Cleveland Clinic Florida
Program Director:
Maurice Hanson, MD
3000 W Cypress Creek Rd
Fort Lauderdale, FL 33309
Tel: 945 978-5178 *Fax:* 945 978-7421
Internet: http://www.ccf.org/ed/ccfed.htm
Accred Length: 3 Years *Program Size:* 6
Program ID: 180-11-21-146

Gainesville

University of Florida Program

Sponsor: University of Florida College of Medicine
Shands Hospital at the University of Florida
Veterans Affairs Medical Center (Gainesville)

Program Director:
Edward Valenstein, MD
Univ of Florida Coll of Med
Dept of Neurology
Box 100236/UFHSC
Gainesville, FL 32610-0236
Tel: 352 392-3491 *Fax:* 352 392-6893
E-mail: valene@medicine.ufl.edu
Internet: http://www.med.ufl.edu/med/neuro
Accred Length: 3 Years *Program Size:* 8
Subspecialties: CHN, CN
Program ID: 180-11-21-025

Miami

University of Miami-Jackson Memorial Medical Center Program

Sponsor: University of Miami-Jackson Memorial Medical Center
Veterans Affairs Medical Center (Miami)

Program Director:
Bruce Nolan, MD
Jackson Memorial Hospital
VA Med Ctr/EEG Sleep Lab
1201 NW 16th St/A212
Miami, FL 33125
Tel: 305 324-3371 *Fax:* 305 324-3210
E-mail: bnolan@mednet.med.miami.edu
Internet: http://www.tt.med.miami.edu/organizations/department_of_neurology/residency_program/index.html
Accred Length: 3 Years *Program Size:* 24
Subspecialties: CHN
Program ID: 180-11-21-026

Tampa

University of South Florida Program

Sponsor: University of South Florida College of Medicine
James A Haley Veterans Hospital
Tampa General Healthcare

Program Director:
Shashidhar H Kori, MD
James A Haley Veterans Hospital
Dept of Neurology (127)
13000 Bruce B Downs Blvd
Tampa, FL 33612-4798
Tel: 813 972-7633 *Fax:* 813 978-5995
Internet: http://www.med.usf.edu
Accred Length: 3 Years *Program Size:* 12
Program ID: 180-11-21-027

Georgia

Atlanta

Emory University Program

Sponsor: Emory University School of Medicine
Egleston Children's Hospital at Emory University
Emory University Hospital
Grady Memorial Hospital

Program Director:
Sarah E DeRossett, MD PhD
Emory University
Dept of Neurology/WMRB 6000
1639 Pierce Dr NE
Atlanta, GA 30322
Tel: 404 727-5004 *Fax:* 404 727-3157
E-mail: neuro_res@emory.edu
Internet:
http://www1.cc.emory.edu/neurology/resprog.html
Accred Length: 3 Years *Program Size:* 21
Subspecialties: CHN
Program ID: 180-12-21-028

Augusta

Medical College of Georgia Program

Sponsor: Medical College of Georgia Hospital and Clinics
University Hospital
Veterans Affairs Medical Center (Augusta)

Program Director:
Thomas R Swift, MD
Med Coll of Georgia
Dept of Neurology/BIW 340
1120 15th St
Augusta, GA 30912-3200
Tel: 706 721-1990 *Fax:* 706 721-6757
E-mail: wgarrett@neuro.mcg.edu
Internet: http://www.neuro.mcg.edu
Accred Length: 4 Years *Program Size:* 10
Subspecialties: CHN, CN
Program ID: 180-12-21-029

Illinois

Chicago

McGaw Medical Center of Northwestern University Program

Sponsor: Northwestern University Medical School
Evanston Hospital
Northwestern Memorial Hospital
Veterans Affairs Lakeside Medical Center (Chicago)

Program Director:
James P Kelly, MD
Dept of Neurology
645 N Michigan/Ste 1058
Chicago, IL 60611
Tel: 312 908-7823 *Fax:* 312 908-5073
Accred Length: 3 Years *Program Size:* 15
Subspecialties: CHN, CN, TY
Program ID: 180-16-21-032

Rush-Presbyterian-St Luke's Medical Center Program

Sponsor: Rush-Presbyterian-St Luke's Medical Center
Christ Hospital and Medical Center
Cook County Hospital

Program Director:
Kathleen M Shannon, MD
Russell E Bartt, MD
Rush-Presbyterian-St Luke's Med Ctr
Dept of Neurology
1725 W Harrison St/Ste 1106
Chicago, IL 60612
Tel: 312 942-4500 *Fax:* 312 942-2380
Accred Length: 3 Years *Program Size:* 6
Subspecialties: CN
Program ID: 180-16-11-033

University of Chicago Program

Sponsor: University of Chicago Hospitals

Program Director:
Anthony T Reder, MD
Univ of Chicago Hospitals
5841 S Maryland Ave/MC2030
Chicago, IL 60637-1470
Tel: 773 702-0151 *Fax:* 773 702-9076
E-mail: areder@neurology.bsd.uchicago.edu
Internet: http://neurology.bsd.uchicago.edu/~nuerowww/resident.html
Accred Length: 3 Years *Program Size:* 15
Subspecialties: CHN
Program ID: 180-16-21-034

University of Illinois College of Medicine at Chicago Program

Sponsor: University of Illinois College of Medicine at Chicago
Christ Hospital and Medical Center
University of Illinois Hospital and Clinics

Program Director:
Steven U Brint, MD
Univ of Illinois-Chicago
Dept of Neurology (M/C 796)
912 S Wood St
Chicago, IL 60612-7330
Tel: 312 996-6906 *Fax:* 312 413-1388
E-mail: sbrint@uic.edu
Internet: http://www.uic.edu/depts/mcne
Accred Length: 3 Years *Program Size:* 9
Subspecialties: CN
Program ID: 180-16-21-035

Maywood

Loyola University Program

Sponsor: Loyola University Medical Center
Edward J Hines Jr Veterans Affairs Hospital

Program Director:
Gregory Gruener, MD
Loyola Univ-Stritch Sch of Med
Dept of Neurology
2160 S First Ave
Maywood, IL 60153
Tel: 708 216-5332 *Fax:* 708 216-5617
E-mail: ggruene@luc.edu
Internet: http://www.lumc.edu/neurology
Accred Length: 3 Years *Program Size:* 13
Subspecialties: CHN, CN
Program ID: 180-16-21-036

Peoria

University of Illinois College of Medicine at Peoria Program

Sponsor: University of Illinois College of Medicine at Peoria
Methodist Medical Center of Illinois
St Francis Medical Center

Program Director:
Jorge C Kattah, MD
Univ of Illinois Coll of Med-Peoria
One Illini Dr/Box 1649
Peoria, IL 61656
Tel: 309 655-2702 *Fax:* 309 655-3069
Accred Length: 4 Years *Program Size:* 0
Program ID: 180-16-21-147

Springfield

Southern Illinois University Program

Sponsor: Southern Illinois University School of Medicine
Memorial Medical Center
St John's Hospital

Program Director:
Rodger J Elble, MD PhD
Southern Illinois Univ Sch of Med
Dept of Neurology
PO Box 19637
Springfield, IL 62794-9637
Tel: 217 782-0168 *Fax:* 217 524-4539
Internet: http://www.siumed.edu/neuro
Accred Length: 4 Years *Program Size:* 8 (*GY1:* 2)
Subspecialties: CN
Program ID: 180-16-21-134

Indiana

Indianapolis

Indiana University School of Medicine Program

Sponsor: Indiana University School of Medicine
Clarian Riley Hospital for Children
Richard L Roudebush Veterans Affairs Medical Center
William N Wishard Memorial Hospital

Program Director:
Jose Biller, MD
Dept of Neurology
Indiana Univ Med Ctr
545 Barnhill Dr/EM 125
Indianapolis, IN 46202-5124
Tel: 317 274-4455 *Fax:* 317 274-2384
E-mail: jbiller@indyvax.iupui.edu
Internet: http://www.medlib.iupui.edu/neuro/
Accred Length: 3 Years *Program Size:* 15
Subspecialties: CHN, CN
Program ID: 180-17-21-038

Iowa

Iowa City

University of Iowa Hospitals and Clinics Program

Sponsor: University of Iowa Hospitals and Clinics
Veterans Affairs Medical Center (Iowa City)

Program Director:
Robert L Rodnitzky, MD
Univ of Iowa Hospitals and Clinics
Dept of Neurology
200 Hawkins Dr
Iowa City, IA 52242
Tel: 319 356-3424 *Fax:* 319 356-4505
E-mail: robert-rodnitzky@uiowa.edu
Accred Length: 4 Years *Program Size:* 17 (*GY1:* 2)
Subspecialties: CHN, CN
Program ID: 180-18-21-039

Kansas

Kansas City

University of Kansas Medical Center Program

Sponsor: University of Kansas School of Medicine
University of Kansas Medical Center
Veterans Affairs Medical Center (Kansas City)

Program Director:
Sharon G Lynch, MD
Univ of Kansas Med Ctr
3901 Rainbow Blvd
Kansas City, KS 66160-7314
Tel: 913 588-6970 *Fax:* 913 588-6965
E-mail: slynch@kumc.edu
Internet:
http://www.kumc.edu/instruction/medicine/neurology/index.html
Accred Length: 3 Years *Program Size:* 9
Program ID: 180-19-22-040

Kentucky

Lexington

University of Kentucky Medical Center Program

Sponsor: University of Kentucky Hospital
Veterans Affairs Medical Center (Lexington)

Program Director:
Joseph R Berger, MD MS
Univ of Kentucky Med Ctr
Dept of Neurology
Kentucky Clinic/L-445
Lexington, KY 40536-0284
Tel: 606 323-6702, ext 240 *Fax:* 606 323-5943
E-mail: jrbneuro@pop.uky.edu
Internet: http://www.comed.uky.edu
Accred Length: 4 Years *Program Size:* 12 (*GY1:* 3)
Program ID: 180-20-21-041

Louisville

University of Louisville Program

Sponsor: University of Louisville School of Medicine
Norton Hospital (Alliant Health System)
University of Louisville Hospital
Veterans Affairs Medical Center (Louisville)

Program Director:
Michael R Swenson, MD
Univ of Louisville
Dept of Neurology
Health Sciences Ctr 113A
Louisville, KY 40292-0001
Tel: 502 852-7981 *Fax:* 502 852-6344
E-mail: mrswen01@ulkyvm.louisville.edu
Internet: http://www.louisville.edu/medschool/neuro
Accred Length: 3 Years *Program Size:* 8
Program ID: 180-20-21-042

Louisiana

New Orleans

Louisiana State University Program

Sponsor: Louisiana State University School of Medicine
Medical Center of Louisiana at New Orleans

Program Director:
Amparo Gutierrez, MD
Dept of Neurology
Louisiana State Univ Sch of Med
1542 Tulane Ave
New Orleans, LA 70112-2822
Tel: 504 568-4081 *Fax:* 504 568-7130
Internet:
http://www.lsumc.edu/campus/neur/neurology/lsuneuro.htm
Accred Length: 3 Years *Program Size:* 9
Subspecialties: CHN, CN
Program ID: 180-21-21-043

Tulane University Program

Sponsor: Tulane University School of Medicine
Medical Center of Louisiana at New Orleans
Tulane University Hospital and Clinics
Veterans Affairs Medical Center-LSU Service (New Orleans)

Program Director:
Anne L Foundas, MD
Tulane Univ Sch of Med
Dept of Neurology TB-52
1430 Tulane Ave
New Orleans, LA 70112-2699
Tel: 504 588-2241 *Fax:* 504 584-3695
E-mail: neuro@mailhost.tcs.tulane.edu
Accred Length: 3 Years *Program Size:* 13
Subspecialties: CHN
Program ID: 180-21-21-044

Maryland

Baltimore

Johns Hopkins University Program

Sponsor: Johns Hopkins University School of Medicine
Johns Hopkins Bayview Medical Center
Johns Hopkins Hospital

Program Director:
Justin C McArthur, MB BS
Johns Hopkins Hospital
600 N Wolfe St
Meyer 6-109
Baltimore, MD 21287-7609
Tel: 410 955-3730 *Fax:* 410 955-0672
E-mail: jm@jhmi.edu
Internet:
http://hopkins.med.jhu.edu/healthcarepros/neuro/neurotr.htm
Accred Length: 3 Years *Program Size:* 15
Subspecialties: CHN, CN
Program ID: 180-23-21-045

University of Maryland Program

Sponsor: University of Maryland Medical System
Veterans Affairs Medical Center (Baltimore)

Program Director:
Janine L Good, MD
Univ of Maryland Sch of Med
22 S Greene St/N4W46
Baltimore, MD 21201-1595
Tel: 410 328-6483 *Fax:* 410 328-5589
Accred Length: 3 Years *Program Size:* 13
Subspecialties: CN
Program ID: 180-23-31-046

Bethesda

National Capital Consortium Program

Sponsor: National Capital Consortium
National Naval Medical Center (Bethesda)
Walter Reed Army Medical Center

Program Director:
Capt Andrew J Dutka, MD
Dept of Neurology
8901 Wisconsin Ave
Bethesda, MD 20889-5006
Tel: 301 295-4760 *Fax:* 301 295-0274
Internet: http://131.158.88.90
Accred Length: 4 Years *Program Size:* 17 (*GY1:* 2)
Subspecialties: CHN, CN
Program ID: 180-10-21-144
US Armed Services Program

Massachusetts

Boston

Beth Israel Deaconess Medical Center/Harvard Medical School Program

Sponsor: Beth Israel Deaconess Medical Center
Children's Hospital

Program Director:
Clifford B Saper, MD PhD
Dept of Neurology
Beth Israel Deaconess Med Ctr
330 Brookline Ave
Boston, MA 02215
Tel: 617 667-2268 *Fax:* 617 975-5161
E-mail: csaper@bidmc.harvard.edu
Internet: http://www.bidmc.harvard.edu/neurology
Accred Length: 3 Years *Program Size:* 14
Subspecialties: CHN
Program ID: 180-24-21-049

Boston University Medical Center Program

Sponsor: Boston Medical Center
Veterans Affairs Medical Center (Boston)

Program Director:
Robert G Feldman, MD
Boston Univ Sch of Med
Dept of Neurology
715 Albany St/C-314
Boston, MA 02118-2394
Tel: 617 638-5350 *Fax:* 617 638-5354
Internet: http://med-amsa.bu.edu/neurology/main.html
Accred Length: 3 Years *Program Size:* 18
Program ID: 180-24-21-145

Massachusetts General Hospital Program

Sponsor: Massachusetts General Hospital
Brigham and Women's Hospital

Program Director:
David M Dawson, MD
Massachusetts General Hospital
Kennedy 915
Fruit St
Boston, MA 02114
Tel: 617 726-1067 *Fax:* 617 726-2353
Internet: http://www.mgh.harvard.edu/
Accred Length: 3 Years *Program Size:* 33
Subspecialties: CHN
Program ID: 180-24-31-050

Tufts University Program

Sponsor: New England Medical Center Hospitals
Lahey Clinic
St Elizabeth's Medical Center of Boston

Program Director:
Allan H Ropper, MD
St Elizabeth's Med Ctr
Div of Neurology
736 Cambridge St
Boston, MA 02135
Tel: 617 789-2696 *Fax:* 617 789-5177
E-mail: aropper@aol.com
Internet: http://web.mit.edu/pandre/www/neuro
Accred Length: 3 Years *Program Size:* 15
Subspecialties: CHN, TY
Program ID: 180-24-21-051

Worcester

University of Massachusetts Program

Sponsor: University of Massachusetts Medical School
St Vincent Hospital
UMass Memorial Health Care (University Campus)

Program Director:
David A Drachman, MD
Univ of Massachusetts Med Sch
55 Lake Ave N
Worcester, MA 01655-0318
Tel: 508 856-3081 *Fax:* 508 856-6778
Accred Length: 3 Years *Program Size:* 11
Subspecialties: CHN, CN
Program ID: 180-24-21-121

Michigan

Ann Arbor

University of Michigan Program

Sponsor: University of Michigan Hospitals
Veterans Affairs Medical Center (Ann Arbor)

Program Director:
Sid Gilman, MD
Univ of Michigan Hospitals
1500 E Medical Center Dr
1914 Taubman Ctr/Box 0316
Ann Arbor, MI 48109-0316
Tel: 734 936-9070 *Fax:* 734 936-8763
E-mail: sgilman@umich.edu
Internet: http://www.med.umich.edu/neuro/
Accred Length: 3 Years *Program Size:* 16
Subspecialties: CHN, CN
Program ID: 180-25-31-052

Detroit

Henry Ford Hospital Program

Sponsor: Henry Ford Hospital

Program Director:
Ivo Drury, MD
Henry Ford Hospital
2799 W Grand Blvd/K-11
Detroit, MI 48202
Tel: 313 916-2468 *Fax:* 313 916-3014
Accred Length: 3 Years *Program Size:* 18
Subspecialties: CN
Program ID: 180-25-21-129

Wayne State University/Detroit Medical Center Program

Sponsor: Wayne State University/Detroit Medical Center
Detroit Receiving Hospital and University Health Center
Harper Hospital

Program Director:
Robert P Lisak, MD
4201 St Antoine/UHC-6E
Detroit, MI 48201
Tel: 313 577-1245 *Fax:* 313 745-4216
E-mail: swashing@med.wayne.edu
Internet:
http://www.med.wayne.edu/phymac/departments/neurology
Accred Length: 3 Years *Program Size:* 16
Subspecialties: CHN, CN
Program ID: 180-25-31-054

Minnesota

Minneapolis

University of Minnesota Program

Sponsor: University of Minnesota Medical School
Fairview-University Medical Center
Hennepin County Medical Center
Veterans Affairs Medical Center (Minneapolis)

Program Director:
Praful Kelkar, MD
Univ of Minnesota
Dept of Neurology/Box 284
420 Delaware St SE
Minneapolis, MN 55455-0323
Tel: 612 624-0691 *Fax:* 612 625-3238
E-mail: ehre0001@tc.umn.edu
Internet: http://www.dept.med.umn.edu/neurology
Accred Length: 4 Years *Program Size:* 12
Subspecialties: CHN
Program ID: 180-26-21-055

Rochester

Mayo Graduate School of Medicine (Rochester) Program

Sponsor: Mayo Graduate School of Medicine-Mayo Foundation
Mayo Clinic (Rochester)
St Mary's Hospital of Rochester

Program Director:
Robert Brown Jr, MD
Application Processing Ctr
Mayo Graduate Sch of Med
200 First St SW
Rochester, MN 55905
Tel: 507 284-4205 *Fax:* 507 284-2203
Internet: http://www.mayo.edu/
Accred Length: 3 Years *Program Size:* 37
Subspecialties: CHN, CN
Program ID: 180-26-21-057

Mississippi

Jackson

University of Mississippi Medical Center Program

Sponsor: University of Mississippi School of Medicine
University Hospital
Veterans Affairs Medical Center (Jackson)

Program Director:
James J Corbett, MD
2500 N State St
Jackson, MS 39216-4505
Tel: 601 984-5500 *Fax:* 601 984-5503
Accred Length: 4 Years *Program Size:* 12 (*GY1:* 3)
Subspecialties: CHN, CN
Program ID: 180-27-21-058

Missouri

Columbia

University of Missouri-Columbia Program

Sponsor: University of Missouri-Columbia School of Medicine
Harry S Truman Memorial Veterans Hospital
University Hospitals and Clinics

Program Director:
Steven Horowitz, MD
Univ of Missouri-Columbia
Dept of Psych/Neurology
1 Hospital Dr/DCO67.00
Columbia, MO 65212
Tel: 573 882-8907 *Fax:* 573 884-5936
E-mail: horows@brain.missouri.edu
Internet: http://www.hsc.missouri.edu/~dmhs/psychneur/
Accred Length: 3 Years *Program Size:* 8
Program ID: 180-28-21-059

St Louis

St Louis University School of Medicine Program

Sponsor: St Louis University School of Medicine
St Louis University School of Medicine
Veterans Affairs Medical Center (St Louis)

Program Director:
John B Selhorst, MD
St Louis Univ Sch of Med
Dept of Neurology
3635 Vista Ave
St Louis, MO 63110-0250
Tel: 314 577-8026 *Fax:* 314 268-5101
E-mail: selhorjb@slucare1.sluh.edu
Internet:
http://medschool.slu.edu/departments/neurology
Accred Length: 4 Years *Program Size:* 12
Subspecialties: CHN, CN
Program ID: 180-28-21-060

Washington University/B-JH/SLCH Consortium Program

Sponsor: Washington University/B-JH/SLCH Consortium
Barnes-Jewish Hospital
St Louis ConnectCare

Program Director:
David B Clifford, MD
Washington Univ Sch of Med
Dept of Neurology
660 S Euclid Ave/Box 8111
St Louis, MO 63110-1091
Tel: 314 362-3296 *Fax:* 314 362-2826
E-mail: cliffordd@neuro.wustl.edu
Internet: http://www.neuro.wustl.edu
Accred Length: 3 Years *Program Size:* 24
Subspecialties: CHN, CN
Program ID: 180-28-21-061

Nebraska

Omaha

University of Nebraska/Creighton University Program

Sponsor: University of Nebraska Medical Center
Tenet St Joseph Hospital at Creighton Univ Medical Center

Program Director:
Rifaat M Bashir, MD
Univ of Nebraska Coll of Med
UNMC Neurology
982045 Nebraska Med Ctr
Omaha, NE 68198-2045
Tel: 402 559-4496 *Fax:* 402 559-9213
E-mail: rbashir@unmc.edu
Internet: http://www.unmc.edu/gme/neurohm.htm
Accred Length: 3 Years *Program Size:* 6
Program ID: 180-30-21-062

New Hampshire

Lebanon

Dartmouth-Hitchcock Medical Center Program

Sponsor: Mary Hitchcock Memorial Hospital
Veterans Affairs Medical Center (White River Junction)

Program Director:
Alexander G Reeves, MD
Dartmouth-Hitchcock Med Ctr
Sect of Neurology
One Medical Center Dr
Lebanon, NH 03756-0001
Tel: 603 650-7916 *Fax:* 603 650-0458
E-mail: alexander.g.reeves@hitchcock.org
Accred Length: 3 Years *Program Size:* 6
Program ID: 180-32-21-063

New Jersey

Edison

Seton Hall University School of Graduate Medical Education Program

Sponsor: Seton Hall University School of Graduate Medical Education
JFK Medical Center

Program Director:
Martin Gizzi, MD PhD
65 James St
PO Box 3059
Edison, NJ 08818
Tel: 732 632-1685 *Fax:* 732 632-1584
E-mail: mgizzi@jfk.hbocvan.com
Internet: http://www.jfkhs.org/neuro
Accred Length: 3 Years *Program Size:* 12
Program ID: 180-33-21-142

Newark

UMDNJ-New Jersey Medical School Program

Sponsor: UMDNJ-New Jersey Medical School
Robert Wood Johnson University Hospital
UMDNJ-University Hospital
Veterans Affairs Medical Center (East Orange)

Program Director:
Stuart D Cook, MD
UMDNJ-New Jersey Med Sch
185 S Orange Ave/MSB H-506
Newark, NJ 07103-2714
Tel: 973 972-5208 *Fax:* 973 972-5059
E-mail: cooksd@umdnj.edu
Internet: http://www.umdnj.edu
Accred Length: 4 Years *Program Size:* 22 (*GY1:* 5)
Subspecialties: CHN
Program ID: 180-33-21-064

New Mexico

Albuquerque

University of New Mexico Program

Sponsor: University of New Mexico School of Medicine
University Hospital
Veterans Affairs Medical Center (Albuquerque)

Program Director:
Gary A Rosenberg, MD
Dept of Neurology
2211 Lomas Blvd NE
Ambulatory Care Ctr 2-E
Albuquerque, NM 87106
Tel: 505 272-3342
E-mail: adair, john@albuquerque.va.gov
Internet: http://salud.unm.edu/neuro/
Accred Length: 3 Years *Program Size:* 10
Subspecialties: CHN, CN
Program ID: 180-34-21-065

New York

Albany

Albany Medical Center Program

Sponsor: Albany Medical Center
Veterans Affairs Medical Center (Albany)

Program Director:
Mark P Dentinger, MD
Albany Med Ctr
Dept of Neurology/MC-70
47 New Scotland Ave
Albany, NY 12208
Tel: 518 262-6488 *Fax:* 518 262-5041
Accred Length: 3 Years *Program Size:* 9
Program ID: 180-35-21-066

Bronx

Albert Einstein College of Medicine Program

Sponsor: Albert Einstein College of Medicine of Yeshiva University
Jacobi Medical Center
Montefiore Medical Center-Henry and Lucy Moses Division

Program Director:
Steve Sparr, MD
Albert Einstein Coll of Med
1300 Morris Park Ave
Bronx, NY 10461
Tel: 718 430-3166 *Fax:* 718 430-8784
E-mail: schaumbu@aecom.yu.edu
Accred Length: 3 Years *Program Size:* 23
Subspecialties: CHN, CN
Program ID: 180-35-21-070

Brooklyn

SUNY Health Science Center at Brooklyn Program

Sponsor: SUNY Health Science Center at Brooklyn
Kings County Hospital Center
University Hospital-SUNY Health Science Center at Brooklyn

Program Director:
Lisa R Merlin, MD
SUNY Health Science Ctr-Brooklyn
450 Clarkson Ave
Box 1213
Brooklyn, NY 11203-2098
Tel: 718 270-2945 *Fax:* 718 270-3840
E-mail: lmerlin@netmail.hscbklyn.edu
Internet: http://www.hscbklyn.edu
Accred Length: 3 Years *Program Size:* 14
Subspecialties: CHN, CN
Program ID: 180-35-21-079

Buffalo

SUNY at Buffalo Graduate Medical-Dental Education Consortium Program

Sponsor: SUNY at Buffalo Grad Medical-Dental Education Consortium
CGF Health System (Buffalo General Hospital)
CGF Health System (Millard Fillmore Hospitals)

Program Director:
Patrick M Pullicino, MD PhD
Dept of Neurology
219 Bryant St
Buffalo, NY 14222
Tel: 716 878-7848 *Fax:* 716 878-7326
E-mail: ppullici@ubmedd.buffalo.edu
Accred Length: 4 Years *Program Size:* 10
Subspecialties: CHN, CN
Program ID: 180-35-21-067

East Meadow

Nassau County Medical Center Program

Sponsor: Nassau County Medical Center

Program Director:
Joel S Delfiner, MD
Nassau County Med Ctr
Dept of Neurology
2201 Hempstead Trnpk
East Meadow, NY 11554-5400
Tel: 516 572-3107 *Fax:* 516 572-5715
Accred Length: 3 Years *Program Size:* 8
Subspecialties: CHN
Program ID: 180-35-21-069

Manhasset

North Shore University Hospital/NYU School of Medicine Program

Sponsor: North Shore University Hospital
Memorial Sloan-Kettering Cancer Center

Program Director:
John J Halperin, MD
North Shore Univ Hospital
Dept of Neurology
300 Community Dr
Manhasset, NY 11030
Tel: 516 562-4300 *Fax:* 516 562-2635
E-mail: halperin@nshs.edu
Internet: http://www.nsuh.edu/neurology
Accred Length: 3 Years *Program Size:* 7
Program ID: 180-35-21-073

New Hyde Park

Albert Einstein College of Medicine at Long Island Jewish Medical Center Program

Sponsor: Long Island Jewish Medical Center
Montefiore Medical Center-Henry and Lucy Moses Division

Program Director:
Ronald M Kanner, MD
Long Island Jewish Med Ctr
Dept of Neurology
270-05 76th Ave
New Hyde Park, NY 11040-8110
Tel: 718 470-7311 *Fax:* 718 347-3016
E-mail: ronchefdoc@aol.com
Internet: http://www.lijiedu/lij-homepage-ns.html
Accred Length: 3 Years *Program Size:* 11
Subspecialties: CHN
Program ID: 180-35-21-074

New York

Mount Sinai School of Medicine Program

Sponsor: Mount Sinai School of Medicine
Mount Sinai Medical Center

Program Director:
C Warren Olanow, MD
Mount Sinai Hospital
Dept of Neurology
One Gustave L Levy Pl
New York, NY 10029
Tel: 212 241-7317 *Fax:* 212 987-7635
Accred Length: 4 Years *Program Size:* 19
Subspecialties: CHN
Program ID: 180-35-21-075

New York and Presbyterian Hospital (Columbia Campus) Program

Sponsor: New York and Presbyterian Hospital
New York and Presbyterian Hospital (Columbia Campus)

Program Director:
Timothy A Pedley, MD
Columbia-Presbyterian Med Ctr
Dept of Neurology
710 W 168th St
New York, NY 10032-2603
Tel: 212 305-8550 *Fax:* 212 305-6978
E-mail: tap1@columbia.edu
Internet:
http://www.cpmcnet.columbia.edu/dept/neurology/
Accred Length: 3 Years *Program Size:* 24
Subspecialties: CHN, CN
Program ID: 180-35-31-071

New York and Presbyterian Hospital (Cornell Campus) Program

Sponsor: New York and Presbyterian Hospital
Memorial Sloan-Kettering Cancer Center
New York and Presbyterian Hospital (Cornell Campus)

Program Director:
M Flint Beal, MD
New York Hospital
525 E 68th St/Rm A-569
New York, NY 10021
Tel: 212 746-6575, ext 6141 *Fax:* 212 746-8532
E-mail: moconnor@mail.med.cornell.edu
Accred Length: 3 Years *Program Size:* 18
Subspecialties: CHN, CN
Program ID: 180-35-21-072

New York Medical College at St Vincent's Hospital and Medical Center of New York Program

Sponsor: New York Medical College
St Vincent's Hospital and Medical Center of New York

Program Director:
Joseph C Masdeu, MD PhD
St Vincents Hospital and Med Ctr
153 W 11th St
New York, NY 10011-8397
Tel: 212 604-2400, ext 2400 *Fax:* 212 604-3101
E-mail: masdeu@nymc.edu
Internet: http://svh.nymc.edu/
Accred Length: 3 Years *Program Size:* 9
Program ID: 180-35-11-078

New York University Medical Center Program

Sponsor: New York University Medical Center
Bellevue Hospital Center

Program Director:
Edwin H Kolodny, MD
New York Univ Med Ctr, Dept of Neurology
550 First Ave
New York, NY 10016
Tel: 212 263-8223 *Fax:* 212 263-8228
E-mail: neurology.training@med.nyu.edu
Internet: http://www.med.nyu.edu/neuro
Accred Length: 3 Years *Program Size:* 18
Subspecialties: CHN, CN
Program ID: 180-35-21-077

Rochester

University of Rochester Program

Sponsor: Strong Memorial Hospital of the University of Rochester

Program Director:
Ralph F Jozefowicz, MD
Univ of Rochester Med Ctr
Dept of Neurology
601 Elmwood Ave/PO Box 673
Rochester, NY 14642
Tel: 716 275-2545 *Fax:* 716 244-2529
E-mail: rjozef@mail.neurology.rochester.edu
Internet: http://www.urmc.rochester.edu/smd/neuro
Accred Length: 3 Years *Program Size:* 12
Subspecialties: CHN, CN
Program ID: 180-35-31-082

Stony Brook

SUNY at Stony Brook Program

Sponsor: University Hospital-SUNY at Stony Brook
Veterans Affairs Medical Center (Northport)

Program Director:
James N Davis, MD
Mark A Kaufman, MD
SUNY-Stony Brook
HSC T12/Rm 020
Stony Brook, NY 11794-8121
Tel: 516 444-7878 *Fax:* 516 444-1474
E-mail: jdavis@neuro.som.sunysb.edu
Internet: http://www.uhmc.sunysb.edu/neurology
Accred Length: 3 Years *Program Size:* 12
Subspecialties: CHN, CN
Program ID: 180-35-21-081

Syracuse

SUNY Health Science Center at Syracuse Program

Sponsor: University Hospital-SUNY Health Science Center at Syracuse
Crouse Hospital
Veterans Affairs Medical Center (Syracuse)

Program Director:
Burk Jubelt, MD
SUNY Health Science Ctr-Syracuse
Dept of Neurology
750 E Adams St
Syracuse, NY 13210
Tel: 315 464-4627 *Fax:* 315 464-5006
E-mail: jubeltb@vax.cs.hscsyr.edu
Internet: http://www.hscsyr.edu/neurology/index.html
Accred Length: 3 Years *Program Size:* 12
Program ID: 180-35-21-083

Valhalla

New York Medical College at Westchester Medical Center Program

Sponsor: New York Medical College
Metropolitan Hospital Center
Westchester Medical Center

Program Director:
Moris J Danon, MD
New York Med Coll
Dept of Neurology
Munger Pavilion/4th Fl
Valhalla, NY 10595
Tel: 914 594-4293 *Fax:* 914 594-4295
E-mail: morisjdanon_@nymc.edu
Internet: http://www.nymc.edu/
Accred Length: 3 Years *Program Size:* 10
Program ID: 180-35-21-076

North Carolina

Chapel Hill

University of North Carolina Hospitals Program

Sponsor: University of North Carolina Hospitals

Program Director:
Albert R Hinn, MD
Univ of North Carolina Sch of Med
751 Burnett-Womack Bldg/CB7025
Chapel Hill, NC 27599-7025
Tel: 919 966-5547 *Fax:* 919 966-2922
E-mail: arh@med.unc.edu
Internet: http://www.med.unc.edu/neurolog/
Accred Length: 3 Years *Program Size:* 10
Subspecialties: CHN
Program ID: 180-36-11-084

Durham

Duke University Program

Sponsor: Duke University Medical Center
Veterans Affairs Medical Center (Durham)

Program Director:
Joel C Morgenlander, MD
Duke Univ Med Ctr
Box 3637
122 Baker House
Durham, NC 27710
Tel: 919 684-6666 *Fax:* 919 681-7936
Internet: http://www2.mc.duke.edu/neurology
Accred Length: 3 Years *Program Size:* 12
Subspecialties: CHN
Program ID: 180-36-21-085

Winston-Salem

Wake Forest University School of Medicine Program

Sponsor: Wake Forest University Baptist Medical Center

Program Director:
Peter D Donofrio, MD
Wake Forest Univ Sch of Med
Medical Center Blvd
Winston-Salem, NC 27157-1078
Tel: 336 716-2330 *Fax:* 336 716-9489
E-mail: donofrio@wfubmc.edu
Internet: http://www.wfubmc.edu/neurology
Accred Length: 4 Years *Program Size:* 9
Subspecialties: CHN
Program ID: 180-36-21-086

Ohio

Cincinnati

University Hospital/University of Cincinnati College of Medicine Program

Sponsor: University Hospital Inc
Veterans Affairs Medical Center (Cincinnati)

Program Director:
John G Quinlan, MD
Univ of Cincinnati Med Ctr
231 Bethesda Ave/Rm 4010
PO Box 670525
Cincinnati, OH 45267-0525
Tel: 513 558-2968 *Fax:* 513 558-4305
E-mail: quinlajg@ucmail.uc.edu
Internet:
http://www.med.uc.edu/htdocs/medicine/departme/neuro/neuro3.htm
Accred Length: 3 Years *Program Size:* 11
Subspecialties: CHN
Program ID: 180-38-21-088

Cleveland

Case Western Reserve University Program

Sponsor: University Hospitals of Cleveland
MetroHealth Medical Center
Veterans Affairs Medical Center (Cleveland)

Program Director:
Robert L Ruff, MD PhD
Univ Hospitals of Cleveland
Dept of Neurology
11100 Euclid Ave/HanHse 5040
Cleveland, OH 44106
Tel: 216 844-5550 *Fax:* 216 844-5066
E-mail: jeanette.bartunek@uhhs.com
Internet:
http://mediswww.cwru.edu/dept/neurology/residency.html
Accred Length: 3 Years *Program Size:* 16
Subspecialties: CN
Program ID: 180-38-21-089

Cleveland Clinic Foundation Program

Sponsor: Cleveland Clinic Foundation

Program Director:
Patrick J Sweeney, MD
Cleveland Clinic Foundation
Dept of Neurology/S91
9500 Euclid Ave
Cleveland, OH 44195-5242
Tel: 216 444-2435 *Fax:* 216 444-0230
E-mail: tripepl@cesmtp.ccf.org
Internet: http://www.ccf.org
Accred Length: 3 Years *Program Size:* 24 (*GY1:* 6)
Subspecialties: CHN, CN
Program ID: 180-38-11-090

Programs

Columbus

Ohio State University Program

Sponsor: Ohio State University Medical Center

Program Director:
Andrew L Reeves, MD
Ohio State Univ
411 Means Hall
1654 Upham Dr
Columbus, OH 43210-1250
Tel: 614 293-6127 *Fax:* 614 293-4688
E-mail: reeves-1@medctr.osu.edu
Internet: http://www-neuro.med.ohio-state.edu
Accred Length: 3 Years *Program Size:* 9
Subspecialties: CHN
Program ID: 180-38-21-092

Toledo

Medical College of Ohio Program

Sponsor: Medical College of Ohio
Medical College of Ohio Hospital
Toledo Hospital

Program Director:
Gretchen Tietjen, MD
Div of Neurology
3120 Glendale Ave
Toledo, OH 43614
Tel: 419 383-3544 *Fax:* 419 383-3093
E-mail: gtietjen@mco.edu
Internet: http://www.mco.edu/depts/neurology
Accred Length: 4 Years *Program Size:* 8 (*GY1:* 2)
Program ID: 180-38-21-143

Oklahoma

Oklahoma City

University of Oklahoma Health Sciences Center Program

Sponsor: University of Oklahoma College of Medicine
Columbia Presbyterian Hospital
University Hospital
Veterans Affairs Medical Center (Oklahoma City)

Program Director:
James R Couch Jr, MD PhD
Univ of Oklahoma Coll of Med
711 Stanton L Young Blvd
Ste 215
Oklahoma City, OK 73104-5023
Tel: 405 271-4113 *Fax:* 405 271-5723
E-mail: james-couch@ouhsc.edu
Internet: http://w3.ouhsc.edu/neurology
Accred Length: 4 Years *Program Size:* 9
Subspecialties: CHN
Program ID: 180-39-21-141

Oregon

Portland

Oregon Health Sciences University Program

Sponsor: Oregon Health Sciences University Hospital
Veterans Affairs Medical Center (Portland)

Program Director:
Ruth Whitham, MD
Oregon Health Sciences Univ
Dept of Neurology/L226
3181 SW Sam Jackson Park Rd
Portland, OR 97201-3098
Tel: 503 494-5753 *Fax:* 503 494-7242
E-mail: whitham.ruth_h@portland.va.gov
Internet: http://www.ohsu.edu/som-neuro/residency
Accred Length: 4 Years *Program Size:* 8
Program ID: 180-40-31-095

Pennsylvania

Hershey

Penn State Geisinger Health System/Milton S Hershey Medical Center Program

Sponsor: Penn State Geisinger Health System
Milton S Hershey Medical Center

Program Director:
Richard B Tenser, MD
Pennsylvania State Univ
Coll of Med
Div of Neurology
Hershey, PA 17033
Tel: 717 531-8692 *Fax:* 717 531-4694
Accred Length: 3 Years *Program Size:* 7
Subspecialties: CN
Program ID: 180-41-11-096

Philadelphia

MCP Hahnemann University Program

Sponsor: MCP Hahnemann University
Hahnemann University Hospital
Medical College of Pennsylvania Hospital

Program Director:
Robert J Schwartzman, MD
MCP Hahnemann Univ Hospital
Broad and Vine Sts/MS 423
Philadelphia, PA 19102-1192
Tel: 215 762-7090 *Fax:* 215 762-3161
E-mail: schwartzman@auhs.edu
Internet:
http://www.auhs.edu/medschool/depts/neurology/home.htm
Accred Length: 3 Years *Program Size:* 24
Subspecialties: CN
Program ID: 180-41-21-097

Temple University Program

Sponsor: Temple University Hospital
Albert Einstein Medical Center

Program Director:
Jeffrey I Greenstein, MD
Temple Univ Hospital
Ste 558 Parkinson Palivion
3401 N Broad St
Philadelphia, PA 19140
Tel: 215 707-7847 *Fax:* 215 707-8235
E-mail: greenstn@astro.ocis.temple.edu
Internet: http://www.temple.edu/neuro
Accred Length: 3 Years *Program Size:* 12
Subspecialties: CHN, CN
Program ID: 180-41-21-100

Thomas Jefferson University Program

Sponsor: Thomas Jefferson University Hospital
Christiana Care Health Services Inc
Veterans Affairs Medical Center (Wilmington)

Program Director:
Joyce Liporace, MD
Thomas Jefferson Univ
1025 Walnut St
Ste 310
Philadelphia, PA 19107-5083
Tel: 215 955-9425 *Fax:* 215 923-6792
E-mail: joayn.hill@mail.tju.edu
Accred Length: 3 Years *Program Size:* 17
Subspecialties: CHN
Program ID: 180-41-21-101

University of Pennsylvania Program

Sponsor: Hospital of the University of Pennsylvania
Children's Hospital of Philadelphia
Graduate Hospital

Program Director:
Steven L Galetta, MD
Hospital of Univ of Pennsylvania
Dept of Neurology/3 W Gates
3400 Spruce St
Philadelphia, PA 19104-4283
Tel: 215 662-3370 *Fax:* 215 662-3362
E-mail: lizotte@mail.med.upenn.edu
Internet: http://www.med.upenn.edu/neuro
Accred Length: 4 Years *Program Size:* 26
Subspecialties: CHN
Program ID: 180-41-21-102

Pittsburgh

Allegheny General Hospital Program

Sponsor: Allegheny General Hospital

Program Director:
Thomas Scott, MD
Allegheny General Hospital
Neurology Program
320 E North Ave/7th Fl ST
Pittsburgh, PA 15212-9986
Tel: 412 359-6527 *Fax:* 412 359-8477
Accred Length: 3 Years *Program Size:* 6
Program ID: 180-41-21-140

University Health Center of Pittsburgh Program

Sponsor: University Health Center of Pittsburgh
Veterans Affairs Medical Center (Pittsburgh)

Program Director:
Marina Mata, MD
Univ Health Ctr of Pittsburgh
Dept of Neurology
811 Lilliane Kaufmann Bldg
Pittsburgh, PA 15213
Tel: 412 648-2022 *Fax:* 412 648-1239
E-mail: jgkant+@pitt.edu
Internet: http://www.neurology.pitt.edu
Accred Length: 3 Years *Program Size:* 13
Subspecialties: CHN
Program ID: 180-41-21-103

Puerto Rico

San Juan

University of Puerto Rico Program

Sponsor: University of Puerto Rico School of Medicine
San Juan City Hospital
University Hospital
Veterans Affairs Medical Center (San Juan)
Program Director:
Jesus R Velez-Borras, MD
Univ of Puerto Rico Med Science Campus
GPO Box 5067/Dept of Med
San Juan, PR 00936
Tel: 787 756-3175 *Fax:* 787 751-3911
E-mail: velez_jesus @fstrf.org
Accred Length: 4 Years *Program Size:* 12 (*GY1:* 3)
Program ID: 180-42-21-104

Rhode Island

Providence

Brown University Program

Sponsor: Rhode Island Hospital
Veterans Affairs Medical Center (Providence)
Program Director:
Janet L Wilterdink, MD
Rhode Island Hospital
Physicians Office Bldg/Ste 324
110 Lockwood St
Providence, RI 02903
Tel: 401 444-8795 *Fax:* 401 444-8781
E-mail: neurology_dept@brown.edu
Internet:
http://www.brown.edu/departments/clinical_neurosciences
Accred Length: 3 Years *Program Size:* 9
Subspecialties: CHN, CN
Program ID: 180-43-21-131

South Carolina

Charleston

Medical University of South Carolina Program

Sponsor: Medical University of South Carolina College of Medicine
MUSC Medical Center
Ralph H Johnson Dept of Veterans Affairs Med Center
Program Director:
Timothy D Carter, MD
Med Univ of South Carolina
96 Jonathan Lucas St
Ste 309/PO Box 250606
Charleston, SC 29425-2232
Tel: 843 792-3221 *Fax:* 843 792-8626
E-mail: carterle@musc.edu
Internet: http://www.musc.edu/neurology/
Accred Length: 4 Years *Program Size:* 9
Subspecialties: CN
Program ID: 180-45-21-105

Tennessee

Memphis

University of Tennessee Program

Sponsor: University of Tennessee College of Medicine
Baptist Memorial Hospital
Regional Medical Center at Memphis
University of Tennessee Medical Center (UT Bowld Hospital)
Veterans Affairs Medical Center (Memphis)
Program Director:
Michael Jacewicz, MD
Univ of Tennessee
Dept of Neurology
855 Monroe Ave/Rm 415
Memphis, TN 38163
Tel: 901 448-6661 *Fax:* 901 448-7440
E-mail: hham@utmem1.utmem.edu
Internet: http://www.utmem.edu/neurology
Accred Length: 3 Years *Program Size:* 11
Subspecialties: CHN
Program ID: 180-47-21-106

Nashville

Vanderbilt University Program

Sponsor: Vanderbilt University Medical Center
Veterans Affairs Medical Center (Nashville)
Program Director:
Gerald M Fenichel, MD
Vanderbilt Univ Med Ctr
2100 Pierce Ave
Nashville, TN 37212
Tel: 615 936-0060 *Fax:* 615 936-0223
E-mail: gerald.fenichel@mcmail.vanderbilt.edu
Accred Length: 3 Years *Program Size:* 9
Subspecialties: CHN, CN
Program ID: 180-47-21-107

Texas

Dallas

University of Texas Southwestern Medical School Program

Sponsor: University of Texas Southwestern Medical School
Dallas County Hospital District-Parkland Memorial Hospital
Zale-Lipshy University Hospital
Program Director:
Gil I Wolfe, MD
Dion Graybeal, MD
Univ of Texas Southwestern Med Ctr
Dept of Neurology
5323 Harry Hines Blvd
Dallas, TX 75235-9036
Tel: 214 648-4775 *Fax:* 214 648-5080
E-mail: gwolfe@mednet.swmed.edu
Internet: http://www.nuaserver1.swmed.edu/index.htm
Accred Length: 3 Years *Program Size:* 12
Subspecialties: CHN, CN, TY
Program ID: 180-48-21-108

Galveston

University of Texas Medical Branch Hospitals Program

Sponsor: University of Texas Medical Branch Hospitals
Program Director:
John R Calverley, MD
Univ of Texas Med Branch Hospitals
Dept of Neurology
9128 John Sealy Hospital/E39
Galveston, TX 77555-0539
Tel: 409 772-2746 *Fax:* 409 772-6940
E-mail: jcalverl@utmb.edu
Internet: http://www.neuro.utmb.edu
Accred Length: 3 Years *Program Size:* 8
Program ID: 180-48-11-109

Houston

Baylor College of Medicine Program

Sponsor: Baylor College of Medicine
Harris County Hospital District-Ben Taub General Hospital
Methodist Hospital
Veterans Affairs Medical Center (Houston)
Program Director:
Clifton L Gooch, MD
Dept of Neurology
6501 Fannin
MS-NB302
Houston, TX 77030-3498
Tel: 713 798-8574 *Fax:* 713 798-8530
E-mail: ctorres@bcm.tmc.edu
Internet:
http://www.bcm.tmc.edu/neurol/training/residenc
Accred Length: 3 Years *Program Size:* 18
Subspecialties: CHN, CN
Program ID: 180-48-21-110

University of Texas at Houston Program

Sponsor: University of Texas Medical School at Houston
Lyndon B Johnson General Hospital
Memorial Hermann Healthcare System
University of Texas M D Anderson Cancer Center
Program Director:
Staley A Brod, MD
Univ of Texas-Houston Med Sch
Dept of Neurology
6431 Fannin St/7044/MSB
Houston, TX 77030-1501
Tel: 713 500-7100, ext 7024 *Fax:* 713 500-7019
E-mail: jhaas@neuro.med.uth.tmc.edu
Internet: http://www.neurology.uth.tmc.edu/index.htm
Accred Length: 3 Years *Program Size:* 12
Subspecialties: CHN
Program ID: 180-48-31-111

Lackland AFB

San Antonio Uniformed Services Health Education Consortium Program

Sponsor: San Antonio Uniformed Services Health Education Consortium
Wilford Hall Medical Center (AETC)
Program Director:
Gary S Gronseth, MD
59th Medical Wing/MMCNN
2200 Bergquist Dr/Ste 1
Lackland AFB
San Antonio, TX 78236-5300
Tel: 210 292-3947 *Fax:* 210 292-6953
E-mail: gronseth@whmc-lafb.af.mil
Accred Length: 3 Years *Program Size:* 7
Program ID: 180-48-21-127
US Armed Services Program

San Antonio

University of Texas Health Science Center at San Antonio Program
Sponsor: University of Texas Medical School at San Antonio
Audie L Murphy Memorial Veterans Hospital (San Antonio)
University Hospital-South Texas Medical Center
Program Director:
Merrill K Carolin, MD
Univ of Texas Health Science Ctr
7703 Floyd Curl Dr
San Antonio, TX 78284-7790
Tel: 210 617-5161 *Fax:* 210 567-4659
E-mail: carolin@uthscsa.edu
Accred Length: 3 Years *Program Size:* 10
Program ID: 180-48-21-112

Utah

Salt Lake City

University of Utah Program
Sponsor: University of Utah Medical Center
Veterans Affairs Medical Center (Salt Lake City)
Program Director:
J Richard Baringer, MD
Univ of Utah Sch of Med
Dept of Neurology
50 N Medical Dr
Salt Lake City, UT 84132
Tel: 801 585-5405 *Fax:* 801 581-4192
E-mail: neurology.residency.recruitment@hsc.utah.edu
Internet: http://medstat.med.utah.edu/neuro/
Accred Length: 3 Years *Program Size:* 12
Subspecialties: CHN
Program ID: 180-49-21-113

Vermont

Burlington

University of Vermont Program
Sponsor: Fletcher Allen Health Care
Program Director:
Robert W Hamill, MD
Fletcher Allen Health Care-MCHV Campus
Brown 313
Colchester Ave
Burlington, VT 05401
Tel: 802 656-4588 *Fax:* 802 656-5678
E-mail: robert.hamill@vtmednet.org
Accred Length: 3 Years *Program Size:* 6
Program ID: 180-50-11-114

Virginia

Charlottesville

University of Virginia Program
Sponsor: University of Virginia Medical Center
Program Director:
G Frederick Wooten, MD
Neurology Dept-#394
Univ of Virginia Med Ctr
Charlottesville, VA 22908
Tel: 804 924-5818 *Fax:* 804 982-1726
E-mail: pan@virginia.edu
Internet:
http://www.med.virginia.edu/medicine/clinical/neurology/
Accred Length: 3 Years *Program Size:* 15
Subspecialties: CN
Program ID: 180-51-11-115

Richmond

Medical College of Virginia/Virginia Commonwealth University Program
Sponsor: Medical College of Virginia/Virginia Commonwealth University
Hunter Holmes McGuire VA Medical Center (Richmond)
Medical College of Virginia Hospitals
Program Director:
Robert J DeLorenzo, MD PhD MPH
E C Myer, MD
Med Coll of Virginia Hospital-Virginia Commonwealth Univ
Box 980599
Richmond, VA 23298-0599
Tel: 804 828-9720 *Fax:* 804 828-6373
Accred Length: 4 Years *Program Size:* 16
Subspecialties: CHN, CN
Program ID: 180-51-21-116

Washington

Seattle

University of Washington Program
Sponsor: University of Washington School of Medicine
Children's Hospital and Medical Center
Harborview Medical Center
University of Washington Medical Center
Veterans Affairs Medical Center (Seattle)
Program Director:
Phillip D Swanson, MD PhD
Univ of Washington Sch of Med
Dept of Neurology/Box 356465
1959 NE Pacific St
Seattle, WA 98195
Tel: 206 543-2340 *Fax:* 206 685-8100
E-mail: swansonp@u.washington.edu
Accred Length: 3 Years *Program Size:* 15
Subspecialties: CHN
Program ID: 180-54-21-117

Tacoma

Madigan Army Medical Center Program
Sponsor: Madigan Army Medical Center
Harborview Medical Center
Program Director:
Frederick G Flynn, DO
Madigan Army Med Ctr
Neurology Serv
Attn: MCHJ-MNR
Tacoma, WA 98431-5000
Tel: 253 968-1399 *Fax:* 253 968-2729
E-mail: col_fred_flynn@smtplink.mamc.amedd.army.mil
Internet:
http://www.mamc.amedd.army.mil/gme/gme.htm
Accred Length: 4 Years *Program Size:* 8 (*GY1:* 2)
Program ID: 180-54-21-138
US Armed Services Program

West Virginia

Morgantown

West Virginia University Program
Sponsor: West Virginia University Hospitals
Program Director:
John Brick, MD
West Virginia Univ Health Sciences Ctr
Dept of Neurology
PO Box 9180
Morgantown, WV 26506-9180
Tel: 304 293-2341 *Fax:* 304 293-3352
E-mail: madamsmi@wvu.edu or mgarlick@wvuhsc1.hsc.wvu.edu
Internet: http://www.hsc.wvu.edu
Accred Length: 4 Years *Program Size:* 2
Subspecialties: CHN, CN
Program ID: 180-55-11-118

Wisconsin

Madison

University of Wisconsin Program
Sponsor: University of Wisconsin Hospital and Clinics
William S Middleton Veterans Hospital
Program Director:
Brad R Beinlich, MD
Univ of Wisconsin Hospital and Clinics
H6/568 CSC
600 Highland Ave
Madison, WI 53792-5132
Tel: 608 263-5448 *Fax:* 608 263-0412
Internet: http://www.neurology.wisc.edu
Accred Length: 4 Years *Program Size:* 15 (*GY1:* 3)
Subspecialties: CHN
Program ID: 180-56-21-119

Milwaukee

Medical College of Wisconsin Program
Sponsor: Medical College of Wisconsin Affiliated Hospitals Inc
Clement J Zablocki Veterans Affairs Medical Center
Froedtert Memorial Lutheran Hospital
Program Director:
Wendy L Larson, MD
Froedtert Memorial Lutheran Hospital
9200 W Wisconsin Ave
Milwaukee, WI 53226
Tel: 414 452-5202 *Fax:* 414 259-0469
E-mail: wlarson@mcw.edu
Accred Length: 4 Years *Program Size:* 12 (*GY1:* 3)
Subspecialties: CHN, CN
Program ID: 180-56-21-120

Neuropathology (Pathology)

Alabama

Birmingham

University of Alabama Medical Center Program
Sponsor: University of Alabama Hospital
Veterans Affairs Medical Center (Birmingham)
Program Director:
Cheryl A Palmer, MD
Univ of Alabama Hospitals
Div of Neuropathology
703 S 19th St/UAB Station
Birmingham, AL 35294
Tel: 205 934-2164 *Fax:* 205 975-7548
E-mail: palmer@path.uab.edu
Internet: http://www.path.uab.edu/index.htm
Accred Length: 2 Years *Program Size:* 2
Program ID: 315-01-21-061

California

Los Angeles

UCLA Medical Center Program
Sponsor: UCLA School of Medicine
UCLA Medical Center
Program Director:
Harry V Vinters, MD
UCLA Sch of Med
Div of Neuropathology
Rm 18-170 CHS
Los Angeles, CA 90095-1732
Tel: 310 825-6191 *Fax:* 310 206-8290
E-mail: hvinters@pathology.medsdi.ucla.edu
Accred Length: 2 Years *Program Size:* 1
Program ID: 315-05-21-068

University of Southern California Program
Sponsor: Los Angeles County-USC Medical Center
Program Director:
Carol A Miller, MD
Los Angeles County-USC Med Ctr
1200 N State St/Box 159
Los Angeles, CA 90033
Tel: 323 226-7123 *Fax:* 323 226-2737
E-mail: carolmile@hsc.usc.edu
Accred Length: 2 Years *Program Size:* 2
Program ID: 315-05-11-003

San Diego

University of California (San Diego) Program
Sponsor: University of California (San Diego) Medical Center
Veterans Affairs Medical Center (San Diego)
Program Director:
Henry C Powell, MD DSc
UCSD Med Ctr
Dept of Pathology
PO Box 3385
San Diego, CA 92163-1385
Tel: 619 543-5966 *Fax:* 619 543-3730
E-mail: mfoberg@ucsd.edu
Accred Length: 2 Years *Program Size:* 1
Program ID: 315-05-21-005

San Francisco

University of California (San Francisco) Program
Sponsor: University of California (San Francisco) School of Medicine
San Francisco General Hospital Medical Center
University of California (San Francisco) Medical Center
Veterans Affairs Medical Center (San Francisco)
Program Director:
Stephen J DeArmond, MD PhD
Univ of California San Francisco
HSW 430
Neuropathology Unit
San Francisco, CA 94143-0506
Tel: 415 476-5236 *Fax:* 415 476-7963
E-mail: sdearmo@itsa.ucsf.edu
Accred Length: 2 Years *Program Size:* 1
Program ID: 315-05-21-006

Stanford

Stanford University Program
Sponsor: Stanford University Hospital
Veterans Affairs Palo Alto Health Care System
Program Director:
Dikran S Horoupian, MD
Stanford Univ Med Ctr
Path/Neuropathology
300 Pasteur Dr/Rm R-241
Stanford, CA 94305-5324
Tel: 415 723-6041 *Fax:* 415 725-6902
Accred Length: 2 Years *Program Size:* 2
Program ID: 315-05-21-007

District of Columbia

Washington

Armed Forces Institute of Pathology Program
Sponsor: Armed Forces Institute of Pathology
Program Director:
Hernando Mena, MD
Armed Forces Inst of Pathology
Dept of Neuropathology/G 051
6825 16th St NW
Washington, DC 20306-6000
Tel: 202 782-1620 *Fax:* 202 782-4099
E-mail: mena@email.afip.osd.mil
Internet: http://www.afip.org/neuropath
Accred Length: 2 Years *Program Size:* 4
Program ID: 315-10-12-001
US Armed Services Program

Florida

Gainesville

University of Florida Program
Sponsor: University of Florida College of Medicine
Shands Hospital at the University of Florida
Veterans Affairs Medical Center (Gainesville)
Program Director:
Thomas A Eskin, MD
Univ of Florida
Sect of Neuropathology
PO Box 100275
Gainesville, FL 32610-0275
Tel: 352 395-0238 *Fax:* 352 395-0437
E-mail: eskin.pathology@mail.health.ufl.edu
Internet: http://www.med.ufl.edu/path/homepage
Accred Length: 2 Years *Program Size:* 1
Program ID: 315-11-21-010

Georgia

Atlanta

Emory University Program
Sponsor: Emory University School of Medicine
Emory University Hospital
Grady Memorial Hospital
Veterans Affairs Medical Center (Atlanta)
Program Director:
Stephen B Hunter, MD
H-189 Emory Univ Hospital
Dept of Path Education Office
1364 Clifton Rd NE
Atlanta, GA 30322-8110
Tel: 404 727-4283 *Fax:* 404 727-2519
E-mail: aboyett@emory.edu
Internet: http://www.emory.edu/pathology/residency/
Accred Length: 2 Years *Program Size:* 1
Program ID: 315-12-21-012

Illinois

Chicago

Cook County Hospital Program
Sponsor: Cook County Hospital
Program Director:
Saroja Ilangovan, MD
Cook County Hospital
Div of Pathology
627 S Wood St/Rm 423
Chicago, IL 60612-9985
Tel: 312 633-7166 *Fax:* 312 633-7154
E-mail: mgreyes@uic.edu
Accred Length: 2 Years *Program Size:* 2
Program ID: 315-16-21-074

University of Chicago Program
Sponsor: University of Chicago Hospitals
Program Director:
Robert L Wollmann, MD PhD
Univ of Chicago Hospitals
5841 S Maryland Ave/MC6101
Chicago, IL 60637-1470
Tel: 773 702-6166 *Fax:* 773 702-9903
E-mail: rwollman@mcis.bsd.uchicago.edu
Accred Length: 2 Years *Program Size:* 2
Program ID: 315-16-21-076

Maywood

Loyola University Program
Sponsor: Loyola University Medical Center
Edward J Hines Jr Veterans Affairs Hospital
Program Director:
Chinnamma Thomas, MD
Loyola Univ Med Ctr
Dept of Path/Neuropathology
2160 S First Ave
Maywood, IL 60153
Tel: 708 327-2574 *Fax:* 708 327-2620
Accred Length: 2 Years *Program Size:* 1
Program ID: 315-16-21-014

Programs

Iowa

Iowa City

University of Iowa Hospitals and Clinics Program

Sponsor: University of Iowa Hospitals and Clinics
Veterans Affairs Medical Center (Iowa City)
Program Director:
Gary L Baumbach, MD
Univ of Iowa Hospitals and Clinics
Div of Neuropathology
5232A RCP
Iowa City, IA 52242-1009
Tel: 319 384-9083 *Fax:* 319 356-8470
E-mail: g-baumbach@uiowa.edu
Accred Length: 2 Years *Program Size:* 4
Program ID: 315-18-21-016

Maryland

Baltimore

Johns Hopkins University Program

Sponsor: Johns Hopkins University School of Medicine
Johns Hopkins Hospital
Program Director:
Donald L Price, MD
Johns Hopkins Univ Sch of Med
558 Ross Research Bldg
720 Rutland Ave
Baltimore, MD 21205-2196
Tel: 410 955-5632 *Fax:* 410 955-9777
E-mail: adrc@welchlink.welch.jhu.edu
Accred Length: 2 Years *Program Size:* 1
Program ID: 315-23-11-020

Massachusetts

Boston

Brigham and Women's Hospital Program

Sponsor: Brigham and Women's Hospital
Children's Hospital
Program Director:
Umberto De Girolami, MD
William J Krupsky, MD
Brigham and Women's Hospital
Neuropathology Div
75 Francis St
Boston, MA 02115
Tel: 617 732-7532 *Fax:* 617 975-0944
Accred Length: 2 Years *Program Size:* 2
Program ID: 315-24-12-024

Massachusetts General Hospital Program

Sponsor: Massachusetts General Hospital
Program Director:
E Tessa Hedley-Whyte, MD
Massachusetts General Hospital
Dept of Path/Neuropathology
14 Fruit St
Boston, MA 02114-2696
Tel: 617 726-5154 *Fax:* 617 724-1813
Accred Length: 2 Years *Program Size:* 2
Program ID: 315-24-21-062

Michigan

Ann Arbor

University of Michigan Program

Sponsor: University of Michigan Hospitals
Program Director:
Paul E McKeever, MD
M3218 Med Science I Bldg
1301 Catherine Rd/Box 0602
Ann Arbor, MI 48109-0602
Tel: 734 936-1889 *Fax:* 734 763-6476
E-mail: paulmcke@umich.edu
Accred Length: 2 Years *Program Size:* 0
Program ID: 315-25-21-084

Minnesota

Rochester

Mayo Graduate School of Medicine (Rochester) Program

Sponsor: Mayo Graduate School of Medicine-Mayo Foundation
Mayo Clinic (Rochester)
Program Director:
Joseph E Parisi, MD
Mayo Graduate Sch of Med
200 First St SW
Rochester, MN 55905
Tel: 507 284-3885 *Fax:* 507 284-1599
E-mail: mgsm.medlab.specialties@mayo.edu
Internet: http://www.mayo.edu/
Accred Length: 2 Years *Program Size:* 2
Program ID: 315-26-21-081

Missouri

St Louis

Washington University/B-JH/SLCH Consortium Program

Sponsor: Washington University/B-JH/SLCH Consortium
Barnes-Jewish Hospital
Program Director:
Robert E Schmidt, MD PhD
Barnes-Jewish Hospital
One Barnes-Jewish Hospital Plaza
St Louis, MO 63110
Tel: 314 362-7429 *Fax:* 314 362-4096
E-mail: reschmidt@pathology.wustl.edu
Accred Length: 2 Years *Program Size:* 2
Program ID: 315-28-11-026

New York

Bronx

Albert Einstein College of Medicine Program

Sponsor: Albert Einstein College of Medicine of Yeshiva University
Jacobi Medical Center
Montefiore Medical Center-Henry and Lucy Moses Division
Montefiore Medical Center-Weiler Hospital
Program Director:
Karen M Weidenheim, MD
Asao Hirano, MD
Montefiore Med Ctr
111 E 210th St
Bronx, NY 10467-2400
Tel: 718 920-4446 *Fax:* 718 653-3409
E-mail: weidenhe@aecom.yu.edu
Internet: http://www.aecom.yu.edu
Accred Length: 2 Years *Program Size:* 1
Program ID: 315-35-21-028

Brooklyn

SUNY Health Science Center at Brooklyn Program

Sponsor: SUNY Health Science Center at Brooklyn
Kings County Hospital Center
University Hospital-SUNY Health Science Center at Brooklyn
Program Director:
Chandrakant Rao, MD
450 Clarkson Ave/Box 25
Brooklyn, NY 11203
Tel: 718 270-1410 *Fax:* 718 270-1410
Accred Length: 2 Years *Program Size:* 2
Program ID: 315-35-21-032

Buffalo

SUNY at Buffalo Graduate Medical-Dental Education Consortium Program

Sponsor: SUNY at Buffalo Grad Medical-Dental Education Consortium
CGF Health System (Buffalo General Hospital)
Erie County Medical Center
Program Director:
Reid R Heffner Jr, MD
100 High St
Buffalo, NY 14203
Tel: 716 829-3090 *Fax:* 716 829-2086
Accred Length: 2 Years *Program Size:* 0
Program ID: 315-35-21-085

New York

Mount Sinai School of Medicine Program

Sponsor: Mount Sinai School of Medicine
Mount Sinai Medical Center
Program Director:
Daniel P Perl, MD
Mount Sinai Med Ctr
Neuropathology Div
Annenberg 15-76/Box 1134
New York, NY 10029
Tel: 212 241-7371 *Fax:* 212 996-1343
E-mail: dperl@smtplink.mssm.edu
Accred Length: 2 Years *Program Size:* 2
Program ID: 315-35-31-086

New York and Presbyterian Hospital (Columbia Campus) Program

Sponsor: New York and Presbyterian Hospital
New York and Presbyterian Hospital (Columbia Campus)

Program Director:
James E Goldman, MD
Columbia Presbyterian Med Ctr
630 W 168th St
New York, NY 10032
Tel: 212 305-4531 *Fax:* 212 305-4548
E-mail: jeg5@columbia.edu
Accred Length: 2 Years *Program Size:* 2
Program ID: 315-35-21-029

New York University Medical Center Program

Sponsor: New York University Medical Center
Bellevue Hospital Center

Program Director:
Douglas C Miller, MD
New York Univ Med Ctr
550 First Ave
New York, NY 10016
Tel: 212 263-6449 *Fax:* 212 263-8994
Accred Length: 2 Years *Program Size:* 2
Program ID: 315-35-21-031

Rochester

University of Rochester Program

Sponsor: Strong Memorial Hospital of the University of Rochester

Program Director:
James M Powers, MD
Dept of Pathology/Neurology
Univ of Rochester Med Ctr
601 Elmwood Ave
Rochester, NY 14642
Tel: 716 275-3202 *Fax:* 716 273-1027
E-mail: jpowers@pathology.rochester.edu
Internet:
http://www.urmc.rochester.edu/smd/path/resprog.html
Accred Length: 2 Years *Program Size:* 2
Program ID: 315-35-11-087

Stony Brook

SUNY at Stony Brook Program

Sponsor: University Hospital-SUNY at Stony Brook
Veterans Affairs Medical Center (Northport)

Program Director:
Nancy S Peress, MD
SUNY-Stony Brook Health Science Ctr
Dept of Pathology HSC T2
Univ Hospital
Stony Brook, NY 11794-7025
Tel: 516 444-2227 *Fax:* 516 444-3419
Accred Length: 2 Years *Program Size:* 1
Program ID: 315-35-21-065

Syracuse

SUNY Health Science Center at Syracuse Program

Sponsor: University Hospital-SUNY Health Science Center at Syracuse

Program Director:
Ann Marie Kazee, MD
SUNY Health Science Ctr
750 E Adams St
Syracuse, NY 13210
Tel: 315 464-5170 *Fax:* 315 464-7130
E-mail: kazeea@vax.cs.hscsyr.edu
Accred Length: 2 Years *Program Size:* 1
Program ID: 315-35-11-034

North Carolina

Chapel Hill

University of North Carolina Hospitals Program

Sponsor: University of North Carolina Hospitals

Program Director:
Thomas W Bouldin, MD
Kinuko I Suzuki, MD
Univ of North Carolina Hospitals
Dept of Pathology/Lab Med
CB 7525
Chapel Hill, NC 27599-7525
Tel: 919 966-4584 *Fax:* 919 966-6718
E-mail: tbouldin@med.unc.edu
Internet:
http://www.pathology.med.unc.edu/path/fellowsp/neuropath.htm
Accred Length: 2 Years *Program Size:* 1
Program ID: 315-36-21-060

Durham

Duke University Program

Sponsor: Duke University Medical Center

Program Director:
Roger E McLendon, MD
Duke Univ Med Ctr
Box 3712/M216 Davison Bldg
Durham, NC 27710
Tel: 919 684-6940 *Fax:* 919 681-7634
E-mail: mclen001@mc.duke.edu
Accred Length: 2 Years *Program Size:* 2
Program ID: 315-36-11-035

Ohio

Cincinnati

University Hospital/University of Cincinnati College of Medicine Program

Sponsor: University Hospital Inc

Program Director:
Gabrielle M de Courten-Myers, MD
Univ of Cincinnati Med Ctr
231 Bethesda Ave
PO Box 670529
Cincinnati, OH 45267-0529
Tel: 513 558-7109 *Fax:* 513 558-2289
Internet:
http://www.med.uc/htdocs/medicine/departme/pathdept/web/resident/respage.htm
Accred Length: 2 Years *Program Size:* 1
Program ID: 315-38-21-036

Cleveland

Case Western Reserve University Program

Sponsor: University Hospitals of Cleveland

Program Director:
Mark L Cohen, MD
Univ Hospitals of Cleveland
Div of Neuropathology
11100 Euclid Ave
Cleveland, OH 44106-5077
Tel: 216 844-8928 *Fax:* 216 844-1810
E-mail: mlc11@po.cwrv.edu
Accred Length: 2 Years *Program Size:* 1
Program ID: 315-38-11-037

Columbus

Ohio State University Program

Sponsor: Ohio State University Medical Center

Program Director:
Carl P Boesel, MD
Ohio State Univ Med Ctr
333 W 10th Ave
4169 Graves Hall
Columbus, OH 43210-1239
Tel: 614 292-5884 *Fax:* 614 292-5849
E-mail: boesel-1@medctr.osu.edu
Accred Length: 2 Years *Program Size:* 1
Program ID: 315-38-21-040

Oklahoma

Oklahoma City

University of Oklahoma Health Sciences Center Program

Sponsor: University of Oklahoma College of Medicine
St Anthony Hospital
University Hospital
Veterans Affairs Medical Center (Oklahoma City)

Program Director:
Roger A Brumback, MD
Univ of Oklahoma Health Sciences Ctr
Dept of Pathology/PO Box 26901
BMSB 451
Oklahoma City, OK 73190
Tel: 405 271-2422 *Fax:* 405 271-2568
Accred Length: 2 Years *Program Size:* 0
Program ID: 315-39-21-080

Pennsylvania

Philadelphia

University of Pennsylvania Program

Sponsor: Hospital of the University of Pennsylvania

Program Director:
Nicholas K Gonatas, MD
Univ of Pennsylvania Sch of Med
418 Johnson Pavilion
36th and Hamilton Walk
Philadelphia, PA 19104-6079
Tel: 215 662-6695 *Fax:* 215 573-2059
E-mail: gonatas@pobox.upenn.edu
Accred Length: 2 Years *Program Size:* 4
Program ID: 315-41-21-041

Pittsburgh

University Health Center of Pittsburgh Program

Sponsor: University Health Center of Pittsburgh
Children's Hospital of Pittsburgh
Magee-Women's Hospital
Presbyterian University Hospital/UPMC
Veterans Affairs Medical Center (Pittsburgh)

Program Director:
Clayton A Wiley, MD PhD
Univ of Pittsburgh Med Ctr
Div of Neuropathology
200 Lothrop St/A-506
Pittsburgh, PA 15213-2582
Tel: 412 647-3745 *Fax:* 412 647-5602
E-mail: wiley@np.awing.upmc.edu
Internet: http://www.path.upmc.edu
Accred Length: 2 Years *Program Size:* 2
Program ID: 315-41-21-042

Rhode Island

Providence

Brown University Program
Sponsor: Rhode Island Hospital
Program Director:
Edward G Stopa, MD
Rhode Island Hospital
593 Eddy St
Providence, RI 02903
Tel: 401 444-5155 *Fax:* 401 444-8514
Accred Length: 2 Years *Program Size:* 2
Program ID: 315-43-21-043

Tennessee

Nashville

Vanderbilt University Program
Sponsor: Vanderbilt University Medical Center
Veterans Affairs Medical Center (Nashville)
Program Director:
Thomas J Montine, MD
Vanderbilt Univ Med Ctr
21st Ave S and Garland Ave
Rm T-3218 MCN
Nashville, TN 37232-2561
Tel: 615 322-3998 *Fax:* 615 343-7089
E-mail: tom.montine@mcmail.vanderbilt.edu
Accred Length: 2 Years *Program Size:* 2
Program ID: 315-47-21-073

Texas

Dallas

University of Texas Southwestern Medical School Program
Sponsor: University of Texas Southwestern Medical School
Dallas County Hospital District-Parkland Memorial Hospital
Zale-Lipshy University Hospital
Program Director:
Charles L White III, MD
Univ of Texas Southwestern Med Ctr
5323 Harry Hines Blvd
Dallas, TX 75235-9073
Tel: 214 648-2148 *Fax:* 214 648-6325
E-mail: charles.white@email.swmed.edu
Accred Length: 2 Years *Program Size:* 2
Program ID: 315-48-21-083

Houston

Baylor College of Medicine Program
Sponsor: Baylor College of Medicine
Harris County Hospital District-Ben Taub General Hospital
Methodist Hospital
Texas Children's Hospital
Veterans Affairs Medical Center (Houston)
Program Director:
J Clay Goodman, MD
Baylor Coll of Med
Dept of Pathology
One Baylor Plaza
Houston, TX 77030
Tel: 713 798-4083 *Fax:* 713 798-5838
E-mail: jgoodman@bcm.tmc.edu
Internet: http://www.bcm.tmc.edu/pathology
Accred Length: 2 Years *Program Size:* 2
Program ID: 315-48-21-047

Virginia

Charlottesville

University of Virginia Program
Sponsor: University of Virginia Medical Center
Program Director:
Scott R VandenBerg, MD PhD
Univ of Virginia Health Sciences Ctr
Div of Neuropathology
Box 214
Charlottesville, VA 22908
Tel: 804 924-9175 *Fax:* 804 924-9177
E-mail: srv@virginia.edu
Internet:
http://www.med.virginia.edu/som-cl/pathology/resident/trnneur.htm
Accred Length: 2 Years *Program Size:* 2
Program ID: 315-51-21-063

Richmond

Medical College of Virginia/Virginia Commonwealth University Program
Sponsor: Medical College of Virginia/Virginia Commonwealth University
Medical College of Virginia Hospitals
Program Director:
Nitya R Ghatak, MD
Med Coll of Virginia
Div of Neuropathology
PO Box 980017
Richmond, VA 23298
Tel: 804 828-9735 *Fax:* 804 828-3299
E-mail: nrghatak@hsc.vcu.edu
Accred Length: 2 Years *Program Size:* 1
Program ID: 315-51-11-051

Washington

Seattle

University of Washington Program
Sponsor: University of Washington School of Medicine
University of Washington Medical Center
Program Director:
Ellsworth C Alvord Jr, MD
Univ of Washington Med Ctr
Neuropathology/Box 356480
1959 NE Pacific St
Seattle, WA 98195-6480
Tel: 206 543-1910 *Fax:* 206 685-7271
E-mail: alvord@u.washington.edu
Internet: http://www.larry.pathology.washington.edu/
Accred Length: 2 Years *Program Size:* 2
Program ID: 315-54-11-052

West Virginia

Morgantown

West Virginia University Program
Sponsor: West Virginia University Hospitals
Program Director:
Sydney S Schochet Jr, MD
Robert C Byrd Health Sciences Ctr-North
Dept of Pathology
PO Box 9203
Morgantown, WV 26506
Tel: 304 293-3592 *Fax:* 304 293-6249
Accred Length: 2 Years *Program Size:* 1
Program ID: 315-55-21-082

Neuroradiology (Radiology-Diagnostic)

Alabama

Birmingham

University of Alabama Medical Center Program
Sponsor: University of Alabama Hospital
Children's Hospital of Alabama
Veterans Affairs Medical Center (Birmingham)
Program Director:
Taher El Gammal, MD
Dept of Radiology
Univ of Alabama
619 S 19th St
Birmingham, AL 35233-6830
Tel: 205 934-3144 *Fax:* 205 975-4413
Internet: http://www.rad.uab.edu
Accred Length: 1 Year *Program Size:* 2
Program ID: 423-01-21-001

Arizona

Phoenix

St Joseph's Hospital and Medical Center Program
Sponsor: St Joseph's Hospital and Medical Center
Program Director:
John A Hodak, MD
St Joseph's Hospital and Med Ctr
350 W Thomas Rd
PO Box 2071
Phoenix, AZ 85001-2071
Tel: 602 406-6994 *Fax:* 602 406-7147
E-mail: jhodak@thebni.com
Internet: http://www.chw.edu/mha/mha.html
Accred Length: 1 Year *Program Size:* 7
Program ID: 423-03-21-002

Tucson

University of Arizona Program
Sponsor: University of Arizona College of Medicine
University Medical Center
Veterans Affairs Medical Center (Tucson)
Program Director:
Joachim F Seeger, MD
Sect of Neuroradiology
Arizona Health Sciences Ctr
PO Box 245067
Tucson, AZ 85724-5067
Tel: 520 626-7368 *Fax:* 520 626-1945
E-mail: jsmerz@radiology.arizona.edu
Accred Length: 1 Year *Program Size:* 1
Program ID: 423-03-21-023

Arkansas

Little Rock

University of Arkansas for Medical Sciences Program

Sponsor: University of Arkansas College of Medicine
Arkansas Children's Hospital
John L McClellan Memorial Veterans Hospital
University Hospital of Arkansas

Program Director:
Edgardo J Angtuaco, MD
Univ Hospital for Med Sciences
4301 W Markham St/Slot 596
Little Rock, AR 72205
Tel: 501 686-6932 *Fax:* 501 686-8932
Accred Length: 1 Year *Program Size:* 8
Program ID: 423-04-21-043

California

Loma Linda

Loma Linda University Program

Sponsor: Loma Linda University Medical Center

Program Director:
Joseph R Thompson, MD
Neuroradiology B-621
11234 Anderson St
Loma Linda, CA 92354-2870
Tel: 909 824-4394 *Fax:* 909 824-4149
Accred Length: 1 Year *Program Size:* 1
Program ID: 423-05-21-085

Los Angeles

UCLA Medical Center Program

Sponsor: UCLA School of Medicine
UCLA Medical Center

Program Director:
Gary R Duckwiler, MD
UCLA Sch of Med
Dept of Rad Sciences/BL-133 CHS
10833 Le Conte Ave
Los Angeles, CA 90095-1721
Tel: 310 268-4505 *Fax:* 310 268-3258
E-mail: selsaden@mail.rad.ucla.edu
Internet: http://radsci.ucla.edu
Accred Length: 1 Year *Program Size:* 4
Program ID: 423-05-21-081

University of Southern California Program

Sponsor: Los Angeles County-USC Medical Center
Children's Hospital of Los Angeles

Program Director:
Hervey D Segall, MD
Los Angeles County-USC Med Ctr
1200 N State St/Rm 3750C
Box 762
Los Angeles, CA 90033
Tel: 323 226-7425 *Fax:* 323 226-4059
E-mail: segall@hsc.usc.edu
Accred Length: 1 Year *Program Size:* 5
Program ID: 423-05-21-024

San Diego

University of California (San Diego) Program

Sponsor: University of California (San Diego) Medical Center

Program Director:
John R Hesselink, MD
UCSD Med Ctr
Dept of Radiology 8756
200 W Arbor Dr
San Diego, CA 92103-8756
Tel: 619 543-3856 *Fax:* 619 543-5345
E-mail: jhesselink@ucsd.edu
Accred Length: 1 Year *Program Size:* 0
Program ID: 423-05-21-074

San Francisco

University of California (San Francisco) Program

Sponsor: University of California (San Francisco) School of Medicine
Mount Zion Medical Center of the University of California
University of California (San Francisco) Medical Center
Veterans Affairs Medical Center (San Francisco)

Program Director:
William P Dillon, MD
Univ of California San Francisco
505 Parnassus Ave/L-358
San Francisco, CA 94143-0628
Tel: 415 476-6556 *Fax:* 415 476-4690
E-mail: bill_dillon@radiology.ucsf.edu
Internet: http://www.neurorad.ucsf.edu
Accred Length: 1 Year *Program Size:* 7
Program ID: 423-05-21-044

Stanford

Stanford University Program

Sponsor: Stanford University Hospital

Program Director:
Scott Atlas, MD
Stanford Univ, Dept of Neuroradiology
S-047
300 Pasteur Dr
Stanford, CA 94305-5105
Tel: 650 723-7426 *Fax:* 650 498-5374
E-mail: swatlas@stanford.edu
Internet: http://www-radiology.stanford.edu
Accred Length: 1 Year *Program Size:* 4
Program ID: 423-05-21-075

Torrance

Los Angeles County-Harbor-UCLA Medical Center Program

Sponsor: Los Angeles County-Harbor-UCLA Medical Center

Program Director:
C Mark Mehringer, MD
Los Angeles County-Harbor-UCLA Med Ctr
1000 W Carson St
Box 27
Torrance, CA 90509-2910
Tel: 310 222-2808 *Fax:* 310 618-9500
E-mail: phamm@4link.net
Accred Length: 1 Year *Program Size:* 1
Program ID: 423-05-21-003

Colorado

Denver

University of Colorado Program

Sponsor: University of Colorado Health Sciences Center

Program Director:
Jack H Simon, MD
Univ of Colorado Health Sciences Ctr
Dept of Radiology
4200 E Ninth Ave/Box A 034
Denver, CO 80262-0034
Tel: 303 372-6221 *Fax:* 303 372-6148
Accred Length: 1 Year *Program Size:* 2
Program ID: 423-07-21-084

Connecticut

New Haven

Yale-New Haven Medical Center Program

Sponsor: Yale-New Haven Hospital

Program Director:
Gordon Sze, MD
Yale Univ Sch of Med
333 Cedar St
PO Box 208042
New Haven, CT 06520-8042
Tel: 203 785-5102 *Fax:* 203 737-1241
E-mail: gsze@biomed.med.yale.edu
Accred Length: 1 Year *Program Size:* 5
Program ID: 423-08-21-025

District of Columbia

Washington

George Washington University Program

Sponsor: George Washington University School of Medicine
Children's National Medical Center
George Washington University Hospital (UHS)

Program Director:
William O Bank, MD
George Washington Univ Hospital
Dept of Radiology
901 23rd St NW
Washington, DC 20037
Tel: 202 994-0382 *Fax:* 202 994-0695
E-mail: wobmd@gwis2.circ.gwu.edu
Accred Length: 1 Year *Program Size:* 2
Program ID: 423-10-21-045

Georgetown University Program

Sponsor: Georgetown University Medical Center
Children's National Medical Center
NIH Warren Grant Magnuson Clinical Center

Program Director:
Dieter Schellinger, MD
Georgetown Univ Hospital
3800 Reservoir Rd NW
Washington, DC 20007
Tel: 202 784-3492 *Fax:* 202 687-1804
Accred Length: 1 Year *Program Size:* 4
Program ID: 423-10-21-026

Florida

Gainesville

University of Florida Program
Sponsor: University of Florida College of Medicine
Shands Hospital at the University of Florida
Veterans Affairs Medical Center (Gainesville)
Program Director:
Ronald G Quisling, MD
Univ of Florida
Box J-374
Gainesville, FL 32610
Tel: 352 395-0291 *Fax:* 352 395-0279
Internet: http://www.xray.ufl.edu/index.html
Accred Length: 1 Year *Program Size:* 3
Program ID: 423-11-21-046

Miami

University of Miami-Jackson Memorial Medical Center Program
Sponsor: University of Miami-Jackson Memorial Medical Center
Baptist Hospital of Miami
Program Director:
M Judith D Post, MD
Univ of Miami-Jackson Memorial Med Ctr
1115 NW 14th St
Miami, FL 33136
Tel: 305 243-4702 *Fax:* 305 243-4673
Accred Length: 1 Year *Program Size:* 6
Program ID: 423-11-21-076

Tampa

University of South Florida Program
Sponsor: University of South Florida College of Medicine
James A Haley Veterans Hospital
Tampa General Healthcare
Program Director:
F Reed Murtagh, MD
Univ of South Florida
12901 Bruce B Downs Blvd
Box 17
Tampa, FL 33612-9413
Tel: 813 974-2538 *Fax:* 813 974-3482
E-mail: rtuttle@com1.med.usf.edu
Accred Length: 1 Year *Program Size:* 1
Program ID: 423-11-21-027

Georgia

Atlanta

Emory University Program
Sponsor: Emory University School of Medicine
Grady Memorial Hospital
Program Director:
Patricia Hudgins, MD
Emory Univ Sch of Med, Dept of Radiology
1364 Clifton Rd NE
Atlanta, GA 30322
Tel: 404 712-4583 *Fax:* 404 712-7957
E-mail: patricia_hudgins@emory.org
Internet: http://www.emory.edu/radiology/resident.html
Accred Length: 1 Year *Program Size:* 6
Program ID: 423-12-21-005

Augusta

Medical College of Georgia Program
Sponsor: Medical College of Georgia Hospital and Clinics
Veterans Affairs Medical Center (Augusta)
Program Director:
Ramon E Figueroa, MD
Med Coll of Georgia
1120 15th St
Augusta, GA 30912-3910
Tel: 706 721-2076 *Fax:* 706 721-7319
E-mail: rfiguero@mail.mcg.edu
Internet: http://www.mcg.edu
Accred Length: 1 Year *Program Size:* 1
Program ID: 423-12-21-006

Illinois

Chicago

McGaw Medical Center of Northwestern University Program
Sponsor: Northwestern University Medical School
Children's Memorial Medical Center
Northwestern Memorial Hospital
Program Director:
Eric J Russell, MD
Northwestern Memorial Hospital
Olson Pavilion/Dept of Radiology
710 N Fairbanks Ct/Ste 3425
Chicago, IL 60611
Tel: 312 908-1292 *Fax:* 312 503-1813
E-mail: e-russell@nwu.edu
Accred Length: 1 Year *Program Size:* 3
Program ID: 423-16-21-072

Rush-Presbyterian-St Luke's Medical Center Program
Sponsor: Rush-Presbyterian-St Luke's Medical Center
Program Director:
Michael S Huckman, MD
Rush-Presbyterian-St Luke's Med Ctr
1653 W Congress Pkwy
Chicago, IL 60612
Tel: 312 942-5781 *Fax:* 312 942-2114
E-mail: mhuckman@rush.edu
Internet: http://www.rad.rpslmc.edu
Accred Length: 1 Year *Program Size:* 3
Program ID: 423-16-21-008

University of Chicago Program
Sponsor: University of Chicago Hospitals
Program Director:
Ruth G Ramsey, MD
Univ of Chicago
5841 S Maryland Ave/MC2026
Chicago, IL 60637-1470
Tel: 773 702-3654 *Fax:* 773 702-1161
E-mail: r-ramsey@uchicago.edu
Internet: http://www.radiology.uchicago.edu
Accred Length: 1 Year *Program Size:* 3
Program ID: 423-16-21-009

Maywood

Loyola University Program
Sponsor: Loyola University Medical Center
Program Director:
Behrooz Azar-Kia, MD
Loyola Univ Med Ctr
Dept of Radiology
2160 S First Ave
Maywood, IL 60153
Tel: 708 216-5206 *Fax:* 708 216-8394
Accred Length: 1 Year *Program Size:* 1
Program ID: 423-16-21-010

Peoria

University of Illinois College of Medicine at Peoria Program
Sponsor: University of Illinois College of Medicine at Peoria
St Francis Medical Center
Program Director:
Ken Flaser, MD
OSF St Francis Med Ctr
530 NE Glen Oak Ave
Peoria, IL 61637
Tel: 309 655-7768 *Fax:* 309 655-7365
E-mail: lorid@uic.edu
Accred Length: 1 Year *Program Size:* 2
Program ID: 423-16-21-095

Indiana

Indianapolis

Indiana University School of Medicine Program
Sponsor: Indiana University School of Medicine
Clarian IU Hospital
Clarian Riley Hospital for Children
William N Wishard Memorial Hospital
Program Director:
Vincent P Mathews, MD
Indiana Univ Sch of Med
550 N University Blvd/Rm 0279
Indianapolis, IN 46202-5253
Tel: 317 274-1846 *Fax:* 317 274-1848
E-mail: mathewsv@iupui.edu
Internet: http://www.indyrad.iupui.edu/homepage.htm
Accred Length: 1 Year *Program Size:* 4
Program ID: 423-17-21-028

Iowa

Iowa City

University of Iowa Hospitals and Clinics Program
Sponsor: University of Iowa Hospitals and Clinics
Veterans Affairs Medical Center (Iowa City)
Program Director:
William T Yuh, MD
Univ of Iowa Hospitals and Clinics
3893 JPP
200 Hawkins Dr
Iowa City, IA 52242
Tel: 319 356-3126 *Fax:* 319 353-6275
Internet: http://www.vh.radiology.uiowa.edu
Accred Length: 1 Year *Program Size:* 2
Program ID: 423-18-21-011

Louisiana

New Orleans

Louisiana State University Program

Sponsor: Louisiana State University School of Medicine
Medical Center of Louisiana at New Orleans
Veterans Affairs Medical Center-LSU Service (New Orleans)

Program Director:
Albert E Alexander Jr, MD
Louisiana State Univ Med Ctr
Rm 212 Dept of Radiology
1542 Tulane Ave
New Orleans, LA 70112
Tel: 504 568-4646 *Fax:* 504 568-6536
E-mail: aalexa@lsumc.edu
Accred Length: 1 Year *Program Size:* 2
Program ID: 423-21-21-077

Maryland

Baltimore

Johns Hopkins University Program

Sponsor: Johns Hopkins University School of Medicine
Johns Hopkins Hospital

Program Director:
David M Yousem, MD
Johns Hopkins Hospital
Houck B-112
600 N Wolfe St
Baltimore, MD 21287
Tel: 410 955-2685 *Fax:* 410 955-0962
E-mail: rnbryan@rad.jhu.edu
Accred Length: 1 Year *Program Size:* 6
Program ID: 423-23-21-078

University of Maryland Program

Sponsor: University of Maryland Medical System
Veterans Affairs Medical Center (Baltimore)

Program Director:
Gregg H Zoarski, MD
Univ of Maryland Med Ctr
22 S Greene St
Baltimore, MD 21201-1595
Tel: 410 328-5052 *Fax:* 410 328-3168
E-mail: gzoarski@radiology.ab.umd.edu
Internet: http://www.umm.edu
Accred Length: 1 Year *Program Size:* 4
Program ID: 423-23-21-029

Massachusetts

Boston

Boston University Medical Center Program

Sponsor: Boston Medical Center

Program Director:
Shripad P Tilak, MD
Boston Med Ctr
Dept of Radiology
One Boston Medical Center Pl
Boston, MA 02118
Tel: 617 638-6610 *Fax:* 617 638-6616
Accred Length: 1 Year *Program Size:* 1
Program ID: 423-24-21-091

Brigham and Women's Hospital/Harvard Medical School Program

Sponsor: Brigham and Women's Hospital
Beth Israel Deaconess Medical Center
Children's Hospital

Program Director:
Amir A Zamani, MD
Patrick Barnes, MD
Brigham and Women's Hospital
75 Francis St
Boston, MA 02115
Tel: 617 732-7260 *Fax:* 617 264-5151
E-mail: aazamani@bics.bwh.harvard.edu
Internet: http://www.med.harvard.edu/bwhrad/
Accred Length: 1 Year *Program Size:* 6
Program ID: 423-24-21-065

Massachusetts General Hospital/Harvard Medical School Program

Sponsor: Massachusetts General Hospital

Program Director:
Pamela Schaefer, MD MD
Massachusetts General Hospital
Gray Bldg 2nd Fl Rm B285
Fruit St
Boston, MA 02114
Tel: 617 726-8320 *Fax:* 617 724-3338
E-mail: pschaefer@partners.org
Accred Length: 1 Year *Program Size:* 8
Program ID: 423-24-21-047

Tufts University Program

Sponsor: New England Medical Center Hospitals

Program Director:
Eddie S Kwan, MD
750 Washington St
Box 299
Boston, MA 02111
Tel: 617 636-5000, ext 0040 *Fax:* 617 636-0041
Accred Length: 1 Year *Program Size:* 3
Program ID: 423-24-21-073

Worcester

University of Massachusetts Program

Sponsor: University of Massachusetts Medical School
UMass Memorial Health Care (University Campus)

Program Director:
John Knorr, DO
Univ of Massachusetts Med Sch
55 Lake Ave N
Worcester, MA 01655
Tel: 508 856-2215 *Fax:* 508 856-4669
Internet:
http://www.ummed.edu/dept/radiology/fellow.htm
Accred Length: 1 Year *Program Size:* 1
Program ID: 423-24-21-048

Michigan

Ann Arbor

University of Michigan Program

Sponsor: University of Michigan Hospitals
Veterans Affairs Medical Center (Ann Arbor)

Program Director:
Stephen S Gebarski, MD
Univ of Michigan Hospitals
1500 E Medical Center Dr
UH B2B311
Ann Arbor, MI 48109-0030
Tel: 313 936-4484 *Fax:* 313 764-2412
E-mail: gebarski@umich.edu
Internet:
http://www.rad.med.umich.edu/neurorad/fellowship.html
Accred Length: 1 Year *Program Size:* 4
Program ID: 423-25-21-012

Detroit

Henry Ford Hospital Program

Sponsor: Henry Ford Hospital

Program Director:
Suresh C Patel, MD
Henry Ford Hospital
Dept of Radiology
2799 W Grand Blvd
Detroit, MI 48202
Tel: 313 876-1374 *Fax:* 313 876-1444
E-mail: spatel @ rad.hfh.edu
Accred Length: 1 Year *Program Size:* 4
Program ID: 423-25-21-067

Wayne State University/Detroit Medical Center Program

Sponsor: Wayne State University/Detroit Medical Center
Children's Hospital of Michigan
Harper Hospital

Program Director:
Jeffrey Wilseck, MD
Wayne State Univ-Detroit Med Ctr
Dept of Radiology (c/o Sandy Sees)
4201 St Antoine/DRH 3L-8
Detroit, MI 48201
Tel: 313 745-8411 *Fax:* 313 745-8919
E-mail: ssees@med.wayne.edu
Internet:
http://www.med.wayne.edu/diagradiology/wsuhomepage.html
Accred Length: 1 Year *Program Size:* 2
Program ID: 423-25-21-066

Royal Oak

William Beaumont Hospital Program

Sponsor: William Beaumont Hospital

Program Director:
Ay-Ming Wang, MD
William Beaumont Hospital
3601 W 13 Mile Rd
Royal Oak, MI 48073
Tel: 248 551-1005 *Fax:* 248 551-1154
Internet: http://www.beaumont.edu/html/gme
Accred Length: 1 Year *Program Size:* 2
Program ID: 423-25-21-050

Minnesota

Minneapolis

University of Minnesota Program

Sponsor: University of Minnesota Medical School
Fairview-University Medical Center
Hennepin County Medical Center
Veterans Affairs Medical Center (Minneapolis)

Program Director:
Charles L Truwit, MD
Univ of Minnesota Hospital and Clinics
Dept of Radiology
420 Delaware St SE/Box 292
Minneapolis, MN 55455
Tel: 612 626-4092 *Fax:* 612 624-8495
E-mail: truwit@sparky.drad.umn.edu
Internet: http://www.med.umn.edu/radiology/
Accred Length: 1 Year *Program Size:* 4
Program ID: 423-26-21-090

Programs

Rochester

Mayo Graduate School of Medicine (Rochester) Program
Sponsor: Mayo Graduate School of Medicine-Mayo Foundation
Mayo Clinic (Rochester)
Rochester Methodist Hospital
St Mary's Hospital of Rochester
Program Director:
Patrick H Luetmer, MD
Application Processing Ctr
Mayo Graduate Sch of Med
200 First St SW
Rochester, MN 55905
Tel: 507 284-3108 *Fax:* 507 284-0999
E-mail: mgsm.roch.mn.diagnosticrad@mayo.edu
Internet: http://www.mayo.edu/
Accred Length: 1 Year *Program Size:* 6
Program ID: 423-26-21-013

Missouri

St Louis

St Louis University School of Medicine Program
Sponsor: St Louis University School of Medicine
SSM Cardinal Glennon Children's Hospital
St John's Mercy Medical Center
St Louis University School of Medicine
Program Director:
David S Martin, MD
Dept of Radiology
St Louis Univ Hospital
3635 Vista Ave
St Louis, MO 63110-0250
Tel: 314 268-5781 *Fax:* 314 268-5116
E-mail: diagrad@slu.edu
Internet: http://www.slu.edu
Accred Length: 1 Year *Program Size:* 1
Program ID: 423-28-21-040

Washington University/B-JH/SLCH Consortium Program
Sponsor: Washington University/B-JH/SLCH Consortium
Barnes-Jewish Hospital
Mallinckrodt Institute of Radiology
Program Director:
Mokhtar H Gado, MD
Barnes-Jewish Hospital
Neuroradiology Box 8131
One Barnes-Jewish Hospital Plaza
St Louis, MO 63110
Tel: 314 362-5950 *Fax:* 314 362-4886
Accred Length: 1 Year *Program Size:* 10
Program ID: 423-28-21-079

New Mexico

Albuquerque

University of New Mexico Program
Sponsor: University of New Mexico School of Medicine
University Hospital
Veterans Affairs Medical Center (Albuquerque)
Program Director:
Blaine L Hart, MD
Univ of New Mexico
Dept of Radiology
915 Camino de Salud NE
Albuquerque, NM 87131-5336
Tel: 505 272-0932 *Fax:* 505 277-5821
E-mail: raderas@salud.unm.edu
Accred Length: 1 Year *Program Size:* 1
Program ID: 423-34-21-049

New York

Albany

Albany Medical Center Program
Sponsor: Albany Medical Center
Program Director:
William A Wagle, MD
Albany Med Ctr
Dept of Radiology
43 New Scotland Ave/A-113
Albany, NY 12208
Tel: 518 262-3371 *Fax:* 518 262-8203
Accred Length: 1 Year *Program Size:* 1
Program ID: 423-35-21-014

Bronx

Albert Einstein College of Medicine Program
Sponsor: Albert Einstein College of Medicine of Yeshiva University
Montefiore Medical Center-Henry and Lucy Moses Division
Program Director:
Jacqueline A Bello, MD
Montefiore Med Ctr
Dept of Radiology
111 E 210th St
Bronx, NY 10467
Tel: 718 920-4640 *Fax:* 718 798-7983
Accred Length: 1 Year *Program Size:* 2
Program ID: 423-35-21-051

Manhasset

North Shore University Hospital/NYU School of Medicine Program
Sponsor: North Shore University Hospital
Program Director:
Karen S Black, MD
North Shore Univ Hospital
Dept of Radiology
300 Community Dr
Manhasset, NY 11030
Tel: 516 562-4800 *Fax:* 516 562-4794
Internet: http://www.nshs.edu
Accred Length: 1 Year *Program Size:* 2
Program ID: 423-35-21-015

New Hyde Park

Albert Einstein College of Medicine at Long Island Jewish Medical Center Program
Sponsor: Long Island Jewish Medical Center
Program Director:
Mahendra Patel, MD
Long Island Jewish Med Ctr
Dept of Radiology
New Hyde Park, NY 11040
Tel: 718 470-7175 *Fax:* 718 343-7463
Internet: http://www.lij.edu
Accred Length: 1 Year *Program Size:* 2
Program ID: 423-35-21-033

New York

Albert Einstein College of Medicine at Beth Israel Medical Center Program
Sponsor: Beth Israel Medical Center
Program Director:
Wen C Yang, MD
Beth Israel Med Ctr
16th St at First Ave
New York, NY 10003
Tel: 212 420-2544 *Fax:* 212 420-2510
Accred Length: 1 Year *Program Size:* 2
Program ID: 423-35-21-030

Mount Sinai School of Medicine Program
Sponsor: Mount Sinai School of Medicine
Mount Sinai Medical Center
Program Director:
Michael Sacher, MD
Mount Sinai Med Ctr
Dept of Radiology/Box 1234
One Gustave L Levy Pl
New York, NY 10029-6574
Tel: 212 241-5837 *Fax:* 212 427-8137
E-mail: michael_sacher@smtplink.mssm.edu
Internet: http://www.mssm.edu/radiology/faculty.html
Accred Length: 1 Year *Program Size:* 4
Program ID: 423-35-21-034

New York and Presbyterian Hospital (Columbia Campus) Program
Sponsor: New York and Presbyterian Hospital
New York and Presbyterian Hospital (Columbia Campus)
Program Director:
William S Millar, MD MS
New York Presbyterian Hospital (Columbia-Presbyterian)
Dept of Rad/Neuroradiology
177 Fort Washington Ave/MHB 3-111
New York, NY 10032
Tel: 212 305-9820 *Fax:* 212 305-9785
E-mail: wsm8@columbia.edu
Internet: http://cpmcnet.columbia.edu/dept/radiology/
Accred Length: 1 Year *Program Size:* 4
Program ID: 423-35-21-068

New York and Presbyterian Hospital (Cornell Campus) Program
Sponsor: New York and Presbyterian Hospital
Memorial Sloan-Kettering Cancer Center
New York and Presbyterian Hospital (Cornell Campus)
Program Director:
Michael D Deck, MD
New York Hospital-Cornell Med Ctr
525 E 68th St/Box 141
New York, NY 10021
Tel: 212 746-2575 *Fax:* 212 746-8597
E-mail: mdfdeck@mail.med.cornell.edu
Accred Length: 1 Year *Program Size:* 3
Program ID: 423-35-21-052

New York University Medical Center Program
Sponsor: New York University Medical Center
Bellevue Hospital Center
Veterans Affairs Medical Center (Manhattan)
Program Director:
Irvin I Kricheff, MD
New York Univ Med Ctr
560 First Ave
New York, NY 10016
Tel: 212 263-5219 *Fax:* 212 263-8137
E-mail: kricheff@mri.med.nyu.edu
Accred Length: 1 Year *Program Size:* 6
Program ID: 423-35-21-016

Rochester

University of Rochester Program
Sponsor: Strong Memorial Hospital of the University of Rochester
Program Director:
Henry Z Wang, MD PhD
Strong Memorial Hospital
601 Elmwood Ave
Box 648
Rochester, NY 14642-8648
Tel: 716 275-1839 *Fax:* 716 473-4861
E-mail: henry_wang@urmc.rochester.edu
Accred Length: 1 Year *Program Size:* 3
Program ID: 423-35-21-031

Stony Brook

SUNY at Stony Brook Program
Sponsor: University Hospital-SUNY at Stony Brook
Program Director:
Clemente T Roque, MD
Univ Hospital-SUNY Stony Brook
Level 4/Rm 092
Health Science Ctr
Stony Brook, NY 11794-8460
Tel: 516 444-2484 *Fax:* 516 444-7538
E-mail: croque@radiol.som.sunsb.edu
Internet: http://www.informatics.sunysb.edu/
Accred Length: 1 Year *Program Size:* 2
Program ID: 423-35-21-053

Syracuse

SUNY Health Science Center at Syracuse Program
Sponsor: University Hospital-SUNY Health Science Center at Syracuse
Veterans Affairs Medical Center (Syracuse)
Program Director:
Ja Kwei Chang, MD
SUNY Health Science Ctr-Syracuse
750 E Adams St
Syracuse, NY 13210-2339
Tel: 315 464-7437 *Fax:* 315 464-7398
E-mail: changja@vax.cs.hscsyr.edu
Accred Length: 1 Year *Program Size:* 1
Program ID: 423-35-21-032

Valhalla

New York Medical College at Westchester Medical Center Program
Sponsor: New York Medical College
Westchester Medical Center
Program Director:
Michael S Tenner, MD
Westchester Med Ctr
Dept of Radiology
Valhalla, NY 10595
Tel: 914 493-8549 *Fax:* 914 493-7994
E-mail: tennerm@wcmc.com
Accred Length: 1 Year *Program Size:* 1
Program ID: 423-35-21-035

North Carolina

Chapel Hill

University of North Carolina Hospitals Program
Sponsor: University of North Carolina Hospitals
Program Director:
Mauricio Castillo, MD
Univ of North Carolina
Dept of Radiology
3324 Old Infirmary
Chapel Hill, NC 27599-7510
Tel: 919 966-3085 *Fax:* 919 966-1994
E-mail: castillo@med.unc.edu
Internet: http://www.med.unc.edu/radiology/
Accred Length: 1 Year *Program Size:* 2
Program ID: 423-36-31-088

Durham

Duke University Program
Sponsor: Duke University Medical Center
Program Director:
James M Provenzale, MD
Duke Univ
PO Box 3808
Durham, NC 27710
Tel: 919 681-2711 *Fax:* 919 684-7138
Accred Length: 1 Year *Program Size:* 5
Program ID: 423-36-21-070

Winston-Salem

Wake Forest University School of Medicine Program
Sponsor: Wake Forest University Baptist Medical Center
Program Director:
Allen D Elster, MD
Wake Forest Univ Sch of Med
Dept of Radiology
Medical Center Blvd
Winston-Salem, NC 27157-1088
Tel: 336 716-3294 *Fax:* 336 716-2870
E-mail: ade@rad.wfubmc.edu
Internet: http://www.rad.bgsm.edu
Accred Length: 1 Year *Program Size:* 6
Program ID: 423-36-21-080

Ohio

Cincinnati

University Hospital/University of Cincinnati College of Medicine Program
Sponsor: University Hospital Inc
Program Director:
Thomas A Tomsick, MD
Univ Hospital-Univ of Cincinnati Coll of Med
Sect of Neuroradiology
234 Goodman St/ML 742
Cincinnati, OH 45267-0742
Tel: 513 584-7544 *Fax:* 513 584-9100
E-mail: tomsicta@healthall.com
Internet:
http://www.med.uc.edu/htdocs/medicine/departme/radiol/neurorad/fellow.htm
Accred Length: 1 Year *Program Size:* 2
Program ID: 423-38-21-082

Cleveland

Case Western Reserve University Program
Sponsor: University Hospitals of Cleveland
Veterans Affairs Medical Center (Cleveland)
Program Director:
Charles F Lanzieri, MD
Univ Hospitals of Cleveland
Dept of Radiology
11100 Euclid Ave
Cleveland, OH 44106-5000
Tel: 216 844-3113 *Fax:* 216 844-3905
E-mail: slater@uhrad.com
Internet: http://www.uhrad.com
Accred Length: 1 Year *Program Size:* 17
Program ID: 423-38-21-017

Cleveland Clinic Foundation Program
Sponsor: Cleveland Clinic Foundation
Program Director:
Paul M Ruggieri, MD
Cleveland Clinic Foundation
Dept of Neuroradiology/L10
9500 Euclid Ave
Cleveland, OH 44195-5103
Tel: 216 445-7035 *Fax:* 216 444-3466
E-mail: meded@cesmtp.ccf.org
Internet: http://www.ccf.org
Accred Length: 1 Year *Program Size:* 2
Program ID: 423-38-21-054

Columbus

Ohio State University Program
Sponsor: Ohio State University Medical Center
Program Director:
Donald W Chakeres, MD
Ohio State Univ
Dept of Radiology RH-S-209
450 W Tenth Ave
Columbus, OH 43210
Tel: 614 293-8315 *Fax:* 614 293-6935
E-mail: chakeres-1@medctr.osu.edu
Accred Length: 1 Year *Program Size:* 1
Program ID: 423-38-21-018

Oregon

Portland

Oregon Health Sciences University Program
Sponsor: Oregon Health Sciences University Hospital
Veterans Affairs Medical Center (Portland)
Program Director:
Gary M Nesbit, MD
Oregon Health Sciences Univ
Div of Neuroradiology CR-135
3181 SW Sam Jackson Park Rd
Portland, OR 97201-3098
Tel: 503 494-7576 *Fax:* 503 494-7129
Accred Length: 1 Year *Program Size:* 3
Program ID: 423-40-21-096

Pennsylvania

Hershey

Penn State Geisinger Health System/Milton S Hershey Medical Center Program

Sponsor: Penn State Geisinger Health System
Milton S Hershey Medical Center

Program Director:
Kevin P McNamara, MD
Penn State Ledner Health System
Miron S Hershey Med Ctr
500 University Dr/PO Box 850
Hershey, PA 17033
Tel: 717 531-4087 *Fax:* 717 531-4605
Accred Length: 1 Year *Program Size:* 1
Program ID: 423-41-21-097

Philadelphia

MCP Hahnemann University Program

Sponsor: MCP Hahnemann University
Hahnemann University Hospital

Program Director:
Beverly L Hershey, MD
Hahnemann Univ Hospital
Broad and Vine Sts/MS 206
Philadelphia, PA 19102-1192
Tel: 215 762-8746 *Fax:* 215 762-4092
Accred Length: 1 Year *Program Size:* 1
Program ID: 423-41-21-036

Temple University Program

Sponsor: Temple University Hospital

Program Director:
Orest B Boyko, MD phD
Temple Univ Hospital
3401 N Broad St
Philadelphia, PA 19140
Tel: 215 707-7002 *Fax:* 215 707-2428
Accred Length: 1 Year *Program Size:* 3
Program ID: 423-41-21-056

Thomas Jefferson University Program

Sponsor: Thomas Jefferson University Hospital
Children's Hospital of Philadelphia

Program Director:
David P Friedman, MD
Thomas Jefferson Univ Hospital
132 S Tenth St/Ste 1072
Main Bldg 10th Fl
Philadelphia, PA 19107
Tel: 215 955-5448 *Fax:* 215 955-5329
E-mail: friedm11@jeflin.tju.edu
Internet: http://www.rad.tju.edu
Accred Length: 1 Year *Program Size:* 6
Program ID: 423-41-21-083

University of Pennsylvania Program

Sponsor: Hospital of the University of Pennsylvania
Children's Hospital of Philadelphia
Veterans Affairs Medical Center (Philadelphia)

Program Director:
Robert I Grossman, MD
Hospital of Univ of Pennsylvania
Dept of Radiology
3400 Spruce St
Philadelphia, PA 19104-4283
Tel: 215 662-6865 *Fax:* 215 662-3283
Internet: http://www.rad.upenn.edu/neuro.html
Accred Length: 1 Year *Program Size:* 8
Program ID: 423-41-21-037

Pittsburgh

Allegheny General Hospital Program

Sponsor: Allegheny General Hospital

Program Director:
Ziad L Deeb, MD
Allegheny General Hospital
Dept of Radiology
320 E North Ave
Pittsburgh, PA 15212-4772
Tel: 412 359-4113 *Fax:* 412 359-6912
Accred Length: 1 Year *Program Size:* 1
Program ID: 423-41-21-019

University Health Center of Pittsburgh Program

Sponsor: University Health Center of Pittsburgh
Presbyterian University Hospital/UPMC
Veterans Affairs Medical Center (Pittsburgh)

Program Director:
Melanie B Fukui, MD
Univ of Pittsburgh Med Ctr
Dept of Radiology D-132 PUH
200 Lothrop St
Pittsburgh, PA 15213
Tel: 412 647-3540 *Fax:* 412 647-5359
Accred Length: 1 Year *Program Size:* 4
Program ID: 423-41-21-057

South Carolina

Charleston

Medical University of South Carolina Program

Sponsor: Medical University of South Carolina College of Medicine
MUSC Medical Center

Program Director:
Joseph A Horton, MD
Med Univ of South Carolina Med Ctr
171 Ashley Ave
Charleston, SC 29425-2266
Tel: 843 792-1524 *Fax:* 843 792-5067
E-mail: hortonja@musc.edu
Accred Length: 1 Year *Program Size:* 4
Program ID: 423-45-21-093

Tennessee

Nashville

Vanderbilt University Program

Sponsor: Vanderbilt University Medical Center
Program Director:
Thomas S Dina, MD
Vanderbilt Univ Med Ctr
Dept of Rad/Neuroradiology
1161 21st Ave S/Rm R-1318 MCN
Nashville, TN 37232-2675
Tel: 615 322-3780 *Fax:* 615 322-3764
E-mail: radprogram@mcmail.vanderbilt.edu
Internet: http://www.mc.vanderbilt.edu/radiology/
Accred Length: 1 Year *Program Size:* 2
Program ID: 423-47-21-058

Texas

Dallas

University of Texas Southwestern Medical School Program

Sponsor: University of Texas Southwestern Medical School
Dallas County Hospital District-Parkland Memorial Hospital
Zale-Lipshy University Hospital

Program Director:
Phillip Purdy, MD
Univ of Texas Southwestern Med Ctr
Radiology Dept
5323 Harry Hines Blvd
Dallas, TX 75235-8896
Tel: 214 648-3928 *Fax:* 214 648-3904
E-mail: lmihal@mednet.swmed.edu
Internet: http://www.rad.swmed.edu/resident.html
Accred Length: 1 Year *Program Size:* 4
Program ID: 423-48-21-059

Galveston

University of Texas Medical Branch Hospitals Program

Sponsor: University of Texas Medical Branch Hospitals

Program Director:
Leena Ketonen, MD PhD
Univ of Texas Med Branch
Dept of Radiology/G-09
301 University Blvd
Galveston, TX 77555-0709
Tel: 409 772-7159 *Fax:* 409 772-3229
E-mail: rcoble@utmb.edu
Internet: http://www.utmb.edu/
Accred Length: 1 Year *Program Size:* 2
Program ID: 423-48-21-020

Houston

Baylor College of Medicine Program

Sponsor: Baylor College of Medicine
Methodist Hospital

Program Director:
Michel E Mawad, MD
Baylor Coll of Med-Methodist Hospital
6565 Fannin St/MS 033
Houston, TX 77030
Tel: 713 790-4826 *Fax:* 713 790-4688
E-mail: mmawad@tmh.tmc.edu
Accred Length: 1 Year *Program Size:* 5
Program ID: 423-48-21-060

University of Texas at Houston Program

Sponsor: University of Texas Medical School at Houston
Lyndon B Johnson General Hospital
Memorial Hermann Healthcare System
University of Texas M D Anderson Cancer Center

Program Director:
Joel W Yeakley, MD
Univ of Texas Health Sciences Ctr
6431 Fannin St/2100 MSB
Houston, TX 77030
Tel: 713 500-7640 *Fax:* 713 500-7647
E-mail: tcarter@msrad3.med.uth.tmc.edu
Internet: http://www.msrad3
Accred Length: 1 Year *Program Size:* 1
Program ID: 423-48-21-041

San Antonio

University of Texas Health Science Center at San Antonio Program
Sponsor: University of Texas Medical School at San Antonio
Audie L Murphy Memorial Veterans Hospital (San Antonio)
University Hospital-South Texas Medical Center
Program Director:
J Randy Jinkins, MD
Univ of Texas Health Science Ctr
7703 Floyd Curl Dr
San Antonio, TX 78284-7800
Tel: 210 567-6488 *Fax:* 210 567-5908
Accred Length: 1 Year *Program Size:* 2
Program ID: 423-48-21-061

Utah

Salt Lake City

University of Utah Program
Sponsor: University of Utah Medical Center
Veterans Affairs Medical Center (Salt Lake City)
Program Director:
H Ric Harnsberger, MD
Dept of Radiology/Rm 1A71 SOM
Univ of Utah Health Sciences Ctr
50 N Medical Dr
Salt Lake City, UT 84132
Tel: 801 581-4624 *Fax:* 801 585-7330
E-mail: ric.harnsberger@hsc.utah.edu
Internet: http://www.wwrad.med.utah.edu/
Accred Length: 1 Year *Program Size:* 6
Program ID: 423-49-21-062

Virginia

Charlottesville

University of Virginia Program
Sponsor: University of Virginia Medical Center
Program Director:
Wayne S Cail, MD
Univ of Virginia Hospital
Dept of Radiology/Box 170
Charlottesville, VA 22908
Tel: 804 924-9373 *Fax:* 804 982-1618
E-mail: wsc@virginia.edu
Accred Length: 1 Year *Program Size:* 4
Program ID: 423-51-21-063

Richmond

Medical College of Virginia/Virginia Commonwealth University Program
Sponsor: Medical College of Virginia/Virginia Commonwealth University
Medical College of Virginia Hospitals
Program Director:
Wendy R Smoker, MD MS
Med Coll of Virginia
PO Box 980615
Richmond, VA 23298-0615
Tel: 804 828-3246 *Fax:* 804 828-6066
Accred Length: 1 Year *Program Size:* 2
Program ID: 423-51-21-021

Washington

Seattle

University of Washington Program
Sponsor: University of Washington School of Medicine
Harborview Medical Center
University of Washington Medical Center
Veterans Affairs Medical Center (Seattle)
Program Director:
Jeffrey G Jarvik, MD MPH
Univ of Washington
Dept of Radiology/Box 357115
Seattle, WA 98195-7115
Tel: 206 543-3320 *Fax:* 206 543-6317
Accred Length: 1 Year *Program Size:* 4
Program ID: 423-54-21-038

West Virginia

Morgantown

West Virginia University Program
Sponsor: West Virginia University Hospitals
Program Director:
Judith S Schreiman, MD
Dept of Radiology
West Virginia Univ
PO Box 9235
Morgantown, WV 26506-9235
Tel: 304 293-3091 *Fax:* 304 293-3899
E-mail: jfast@wvu.edu
Accred Length: 1 Year *Program Size:* 1
Program ID: 423-55-21-094

Wisconsin

Madison

University of Wisconsin Program
Sponsor: University of Wisconsin Hospital and Clinics
William S Middleton Veterans Hospital
Program Director:
Virgil B Graves, MD
E3/311 Clinical Science Ctr
600 Highland Ave
Madison, WI 53792-3252
Tel: 608 263-8308 *Fax:* 608 869-0876
E-mail: vbgraves@facstaff.wisc.edu
Accred Length: 1 Year *Program Size:* 4
Program ID: 423-56-21-022

Milwaukee

Medical College of Wisconsin Program
Sponsor: Medical College of Wisconsin Affiliated Hospitals Inc
Froedtert Memorial Lutheran Hospital
Program Director:
David L Daniels, MD
Med Coll of Wisconsin-Froedtert Memorial Luth Hosp
9200 W Wisconsin Ave
Milwaukee, WI 53226
Tel: 414 805-3122 *Fax:* 414 259-9290
Accred Length: 1 Year *Program Size:* 2
Program ID: 423-56-21-039

Nuclear Medicine

Alabama

Birmingham

University of Alabama Medical Center Program
Sponsor: University of Alabama Hospital
Veterans Affairs Medical Center (Birmingham)
Program Director:
Charles Russell, MD
Div of Nuclear Med
619 19th St S
Birmingham, AL 35233
Tel: 205 934-2140 *Fax:* 205 934-5589
Accred Length: 2 Years *Program Size:* 3
Program ID: 200-01-21-007

Arizona

Tucson

University of Arizona Program
Sponsor: University of Arizona College of Medicine
University Medical Center
Veterans Affairs Medical Center (Tucson)
Program Director:
James M Woolfenden, MD
Univ of Arizona
Dept of Nuclear Med
PO Box 245068
Tucson, AZ 85724-5068
Tel: 520 626-7709 *Fax:* 520 694-2412
E-mail: woolfenden@radiology.arizona.edu
Accred Length: 2 Years *Program Size:* 0
Program ID: 200-03-21-008

Arkansas

Little Rock

University of Arkansas for Medical Sciences Program
Sponsor: University of Arkansas College of Medicine
John L McClellan Memorial Veterans Hospital
University Hospital of Arkansas
Program Director:
Gary L Purnell, MD
Univ of Arkansas for Med Sciences
4301 W Markham St/Slot 581
Little Rock, AR 72205-7199
Tel: 501 686-6652 *Fax:* 501 686-6296
Accred Length: 2 Years *Program Size:* 1
Program ID: 200-04-21-009

California

Long Beach

Veterans Affairs Medical Center (Long Beach) Program

Sponsor: Veterans Affairs Medical Center (Long Beach)
University of California (Irvine) Medical Center
Program Director:
Sing Yung Wu, MD PhD
Philip Braunstein, MD
VA Med Ctr
5901 E Seventh St
Long Beach, CA 90822
Tel: 562 494-5565 *Fax:* 562 494-5675
E-mail: sywu@pop.long-beach.va.gov
Accred Length: 2 Years *Program Size:* 1
Program ID: 200-05-31-012

Los Angeles

Cedars-Sinai Medical Center Program

Sponsor: Cedars-Sinai Medical Center
Program Director:
Daniel S Berman, MD
Cedars-Sinai Med Ctr
8700 Beverly Blvd/Rm 5416
Los Angeles, CA 90048
Tel: 310 855-3616 *Fax:* 310 967-0695
E-mail: imaging.housestaff@cshs.org
Internet: http://www.csmc.edu
Accred Length: 2 Years *Program Size:* 2
Program ID: 200-05-21-089

UCLA Medical Center Program

Sponsor: UCLA School of Medicine
UCLA Medical Center
Program Director:
Johannes Czernin, MD
Dept of Molecular/Med Pharmacology
UCLA Sch of Med/Rm AR-128 CHS
10833 Le Conte Ave
Los Angeles, CA 90095-6942
Tel: 310 794-7631 *Fax:* 310 206-4899
E-mail: jczernin@mednet.ucla.edu
Internet: http://www.nuc.ucla.edu
Accred Length: 2 Years *Program Size:* 4
Program ID: 200-05-11-013

VA Greater Los Angeles Healthcare System Program

Sponsor: VA Greater Los Angeles Healthcare System
Program Director:
William H Blahd, MD
VA Greater Los Angeles Healthcare System
Nuclear Med Dept 115
11301 Wilshire Blvd
Los Angeles, CA 90073
Tel: 310 268-3587 *Fax:* 310 268-4916
Accred Length: 2 Years *Program Size:* 3
Program ID: 200-05-31-014

Sacramento

University of California (Davis) Program

Sponsor: University of California (Davis) Medical Center
Program Director:
David K Shelton, MD
Univ of California Davis Med Ctr
4860 Y St
Ste 3100
Sacramento, CA 95817-2282
Tel: 916 734-2754 *Fax:* 916 734-7936
E-mail: david.shelton@ucdmc.ucdavis.edu
Accred Length: 2 Years *Program Size:* 2
Program ID: 200-05-21-010

San Diego

University of California (San Diego) Program

Sponsor: University of California (San Diego) Medical Center
Veterans Affairs Medical Center (San Diego)
Program Director:
David W Yeung, MB BS
UCSD Med Ctr
Nuclear Med Div
200 W Arbor Dr
San Diego, CA 92103-8758
Tel: 619 543-6682 *Fax:* 619 543-1975
Accred Length: 2 Years *Program Size:* 2
Program ID: 200-05-31-015

San Francisco

University of California (San Francisco) Program

Sponsor: University of California (San Francisco) School of Medicine
University of California (San Francisco) Medical Center
Program Director:
Robert J Lull, MD
San Francisco General Hospital
1001 Potrero Ave
Bldg NH/Rm G100
San Francisco, CA 94110-3594
Tel: 415 206-8580 *Fax:* 415 206-6929
E-mail: rlull@sfghsom.ucsf.edu
Accred Length: 2 Years *Program Size:* 5
Program ID: 200-05-21-016

Stanford

Stanford University Program

Sponsor: Stanford University Hospital
Veterans Affairs Palo Alto Health Care System
Program Director:
I Ross McDougall, MD PhD
Stanford Univ Sch of Med
Div of Nuclear Med
H-0101 Rte 8
Stanford, CA 94305-5281
Tel: 650 723-6882 *Fax:* 650 498-5047
Accred Length: 2 Years *Program Size:* 3
Program ID: 200-05-21-018

Colorado

Denver

University of Colorado Program

Sponsor: University of Colorado Health Sciences Center
Veterans Affairs Medical Center (Denver)
Program Director:
Robert A Quaife, MD
4200 E 9th Ave/Box A-034
Denver, CO 80262
Tel: 303 372-6210 *Fax:* 303 372-6271
Accred Length: 2 Years *Program Size:* 1
Program ID: 200-07-21-108

Connecticut

Danbury

University of Connecticut (Danbury) Program

Sponsor: University of Connecticut School of Medicine
Danbury Hospital
Program Director:
Shiv M Gupta, MD
Danbury Hosptial
24 Hospital Ave
Danbury, CT 06810
Tel: 203 797-7222 *Fax:* 203 744-3708
Accred Length: 2 Years *Program Size:* 2
Program ID: 200-08-21-103

Farmington

University of Connecticut Program

Sponsor: University of Connecticut School of Medicine
Hartford Hospital
St Francis Hospital and Medical Center
Univ of Connecticut Health Center/John Dempsey Hospital
Program Director:
Richard P Spencer, MD PhD
Univ of Connecticut Health Ctr
Farmington Ave
Farmington, CT 06030-2804
Tel: 860 679-3120, ext 2768 *Fax:* 860 679-2164
E-mail: rspencer@adp.uchc.edu
Accred Length: 2 Years *Program Size:* 3
Program ID: 200-08-21-020

New Haven

Yale-New Haven Medical Center Program

Sponsor: Yale-New Haven Hospital
Veterans Affairs Medical Center (West Haven)
Program Director:
Holley M Dey, MD
Yale Univ Sch of Med
PO Box 208042
New Haven, CT 06520-8042
Tel: 203 937-3427 *Fax:* 203 937-4509
Accred Length: 2 Years *Program Size:* 1
Program ID: 200-08-11-021

District of Columbia

Washington

Georgetown University Program

Sponsor: Georgetown University Medical Center
Program Director:
Harvey A Ziessman, MD
Georgetown Univ Hospital
Div of Nuclear Med
3800 Reservoir Rd NW/#2005 Gorman
Washington, DC 20007
Tel: 202 784-3360 *Fax:* 202 784-4667
Accred Length: 2 Years *Program Size:* 2
Program ID: 200-10-21-023

Walter Reed Army Medical Center Program

Sponsor: Walter Reed Army Medical Center

Program Director:
Ana A Rodriguez, MD
Walter Reed Army Med Ctr
6825 16th St NW
Washington, DC 20307-5001
Tel: 202 782-0176 *Fax:* 202 782-9061
E-mail: colanarodriguez@wramc13_washdc
Internet: http://www.wramc.amedd.army.mil/departments/nuclear/
Accred Length: 2 Years *Program Size:* 4
Program ID: 200-10-12-002
US Armed Services Program

Florida

Gainesville

University of Florida Program

Sponsor: University of Florida College of Medicine
Shands Hospital at the University of Florida
Veterans Affairs Medical Center (Gainesville)

Program Director:
Suzanne T Mastin, MD
Univ of Florida
Dept of Radiology
Box 100374
Gainesville, FL 32610-0374
Tel: 352 395-0291 *Fax:* 352 395-0279
Accred Length: 2 Years *Program Size:* 2
Program ID: 200-11-21-113

Miami

University of Miami-Jackson Memorial Medical Center Program

Sponsor: University of Miami-Jackson Memorial Medical Center

Program Director:
George N Sfakianakis, MD
Jackson Memorial Hospital, Div of Nuclear Med
1611 NW 12th Ave
Miami, FL 33101
Tel: 305 549-7955 *Fax:* 305 547-2323
Internet: http://www.med.miami.edu/radiology
Accred Length: 2 Years *Program Size:* 11
Program ID: 200-11-21-087

Georgia

Atlanta

Emory University Program

Sponsor: Emory University School of Medicine
Crawford Long Hospital of Emory University
Emory University Hospital
Grady Memorial Hospital

Program Director:
Naomi P Alazraki, MD
Emory Univ Sch of Med
Div of Nuclear Med
1364 Clifton Rd NE
Atlanta, GA 30322
Tel: 404 728-5082 *Fax:* 404 728-5082
E-mail: sfrieso@eagle.cc.emory.edu
Accred Length: 2 Years *Program Size:* 2
Program ID: 200-12-21-083

Illinois

Chicago

McGaw Medical Center of Northwestern University Program

Sponsor: Northwestern University Medical School
Northwestern Memorial Hospital

Program Director:
William G Spies, MD
Northwestern Memorial Hospital
Dept of Nuclear Med
250 E Superior St/W484
Chicago, IL 60611
Tel: 312 908-2514 *Fax:* 312 908-8118
Accred Length: 2 Years *Program Size:* 3
Program ID: 200-16-31-026

Rush-Presbyterian-St Luke's Medical Center Program

Sponsor: Rush-Presbyterian-St Luke's Medical Center

Program Director:
Amjad Ali, MD
Rush-Presbyterian-St Luke's Med Ctr
1653 W Congress Pkwy
Chicago, IL 60612
Tel: 312 942-5757 *Fax:* 312 942-2114
E-mail: aali@rad.rpslmc.edu
Accred Length: 2 Years *Program Size:* 2
Program ID: 200-16-11-027

University of Illinois College of Medicine at Chicago/Michael Reese Hospital Program

Sponsor: University of Illinois College of Medicine at Chicago
Michael Reese Hospital and Medical Center

Program Director:
Carlos Bekerman, MD
Michael Reese Hospital and Med Ctr
Div of Nuclear Med
2929 S Ellis Ave
Chicago, IL 60616
Tel: 312 791-2520 *Fax:* 312 791-8178
Accred Length: 2 Years *Program Size:* 2
Program ID: 200-16-11-025

Maywood

Loyola University Program

Sponsor: Loyola University Medical Center
Edward J Hines Jr Veterans Affairs Hospital

Program Director:
Robert E Henkin, MD
Foster G McGaw Hospital
Loyola Univ Med Ctr
2160 S First Ave
Maywood, IL 60153
Tel: 708 216-3777 *Fax:* 708 216-5813
E-mail: rehenkin@lunis.luc.edu
Accred Length: 2 Years *Program Size:* 5
Program ID: 200-16-21-101

Indiana

Indianapolis

Indiana University School of Medicine Program

Sponsor: Indiana University School of Medicine
Clarian IU Hospital
Clarian Riley Hospital for Children
Richard L Roudebush Veterans Affairs Medical Center
William N Wishard Memorial Hospital

Program Director:
Donald S Schauwecker, MD PhD
Richard L Roudebush VA Med Ctr
Dept of Nuclear Med
1101 W 10th St (115)
Indianapolis, IN 46202
Tel: 317 554-0000, ext 2726
E-mail: dschauwe@iupui.edu
Internet: http://www.indyrad.iupui.edu/homepage.htm
Accred Length: 2 Years *Program Size:* 2
Program ID: 200-17-21-093

Iowa

Iowa City

University of Iowa Hospitals and Clinics Program

Sponsor: University of Iowa Hospitals and Clinics
Veterans Affairs Medical Center (Iowa City)

Program Director:
David Bushnell, MD
Univ of Iowa Hospitals and Clinics
Dept of Radiology
200 Hawkins Dr
Iowa City, IA 52242-1009
Tel: 319 356-4302
E-mail: david-bushnell@uiowa.edu
Accred Length: 2 Years *Program Size:* 2
Program ID: 200-18-21-030

Kansas

Kansas City

University of Kansas Medical Center Program

Sponsor: University of Kansas School of Medicine
University of Kansas Medical Center

Program Director:
Kirkman G Baxter, MD
Univ of Kansas Med Ctr
Div of Nuclear Med
3901 Rainbow Blvd
Kansas City, KS 66160-7234
Tel: 913 588-6810 *Fax:* 913 588-7899
E-mail: kbaxter@kumc.edu
Accred Length: 2 Years *Program Size:* 2
Program ID: 200-19-11-031

Maryland

Baltimore

Johns Hopkins University Program

Sponsor: Johns Hopkins University School of Medicine
Johns Hopkins Hospital

Program Director:
Zsolt Szabo, MD
Johns Hopkins Med Insts
600 N Wolfe St/Nelson B1-126
Baltimore, MD 21287
Tel: 410 955-8448 *Fax:* 410 614-2972
Accred Length: 2 Years *Program Size:* 2
Program ID: 200-23-11-035

Massachusetts

Boston

Harvard Medical School Program

Sponsor: Brigham and Women's Hospital
Beth Israel Deaconess Medical Center
Brockton-West Roxbury Veterans Affairs Medical Center
Children's Hospital
Dana-Farber Cancer Institute

Program Director:
S Ted Treves, MD
Div of Nuclear Medicine
Children's Hospital
300 Longwood Ave
Boston, MA 02115
Tel: 617 355-7935 *Fax:* 617 355-6627
E-mail: treves@al.tch.harvard.edu
Internet: http://www.med.harvard.edu/jpnm/jpnm.html
Accred Length: 2 Years *Program Size:* 6
Program ID: 200-24-21-038

Michigan

Ann Arbor

University of Michigan Program

Sponsor: University of Michigan Hospitals
Veterans Affairs Medical Center (Ann Arbor)

Program Director:
David E Kuhl, MD
Univ of Michigan Hospitals
1500 E Medical Center Dr
B1G 412/Box 0028
Ann Arbor, MI 48109-0028
Tel: 734 936-5387 *Fax:* 734 936-8182
Accred Length: 2 Years *Program Size:* 4
Program ID: 200-25-11-039

Detroit

Henry Ford Hospital Program

Sponsor: Henry Ford Hospital

Program Director:
Kastytis C Karvelis, MD
Henry Ford Hospital
Nuclear Med
2799 W Grand Blvd
Detroit, MI 48202
Tel: 313 876-3436 *Fax:* 313 876-1087
E-mail: karvelis@rad.hfh.edu
Accred Length: 2 Years *Program Size:* 2
Program ID: 200-25-21-106

Royal Oak

William Beaumont Hospital Program

Sponsor: William Beaumont Hospital

Program Director:
Howard J Dworkin, MD
William Beaumont Hospital
Dept of Nuclear Med
3601 W 13 Mile Rd
Royal Oak, MI 48073-6769
Tel: 248 551-4126 *Fax:* 248 551-7344
E-mail: hbalon@beaumont.edu
Internet: http://www.beaumont.edu/html/gme
Accred Length: 2 Years *Program Size:* 2
Program ID: 200-25-11-040

Missouri

Columbia

University of Missouri-Columbia Program

Sponsor: University of Missouri-Columbia School of Medicine
University Hospitals and Clinics

Program Director:
Amolak Singh, MD
Univ Hospital and Clinics
One Hospital Dr
DC06910
Columbia, MO 65212
Tel: 573 882-7955 *Fax:* 573 884-4729
E-mail: singha@health.missouri.edu
Accred Length: 2 Years *Program Size:* 2
Program ID: 200-28-21-094

St Louis

St Louis University School of Medicine Program

Sponsor: St Louis University School of Medicine
St Louis University School of Medicine
Veterans Affairs Medical Center (St Louis)

Program Director:
Henry M Goodgold, MD
VA Med Ctr
3635 Vista St
PO Box 15250
St Louis, MO 63110
Tel: 314 377-8047 *Fax:* 314 268-5144
Internet: http://nucmed.slu.edu
Accred Length: 2 Years *Program Size:* 2
Program ID: 200-28-21-042

Washington University/B-JH/SLCH Consortium Program

Sponsor: Washington University/B-JH/SLCH Consortium
Barnes-Jewish Hospital

Program Director:
Tom R Miller, MD PhD
Div of Nuclear Med
Mallinckrodt Inst of Radiology
510 S Kingshighway
St Louis, MO 63110-1076
Tel: 314 362-2809 *Fax:* 314 362-2806
Accred Length: 2 Years *Program Size:* 5
Program ID: 200-28-11-043

Nebraska

Omaha

University of Nebraska Program

Sponsor: University of Nebraska Medical Center
Veterans Affairs Medical Center (Omaha)

Program Director:
Lisa S Gobar, MD
Sect of Nuclear Med
Univ of Nebraska Med Ctr
600 S 42nd St
Omaha, NE 68198-1045
Tel: 402 559-4341 *Fax:* 402 559-1011
E-mail: lgobar@unmc.edu
Accred Length: 2 Years *Program Size:* 2
Program ID: 200-30-11-044

New York

Bronx

Albert Einstein College of Medicine Program

Sponsor: Albert Einstein College of Medicine of Yeshiva University
Jacobi Medical Center
Montefiore Medical Center-Henry and Lucy Moses Division
Montefiore Medical Center-Weiler Hospital

Program Director:
David M Milstein, MD
Montefiore Med Ctr
1825 Eastchester Rd
Bronx, NY 10461
Tel: 718 904-4058 *Fax:* 718 904-2354
E-mail: huvane@aecom.yu.edu
Accred Length: 2 Years *Program Size:* 5
Program ID: 200-35-21-047

Buffalo

SUNY at Buffalo Graduate Medical-Dental Education Consortium Program

Sponsor: SUNY at Buffalo Grad Medical-Dental Education Consortium
CGF Health System (Buffalo General Hospital)
Mercy Hospital of Buffalo
Roswell Park Cancer Institute
Veterans Affairs Medical Center (Buffalo)

Program Director:
Hani H Abdel Nabi, MD PhD
105 Parker Hall
3435 Main St
Buffalo, NY 14214-3007
Tel: 716 838-5889 *Fax:* 716 838-4918
E-mail: hani@nucmed.buffalo.edu
Internet: http://www.nucmed.buffalo.edu
Accred Length: 2 Years *Program Size:* 3
Program ID: 200-35-21-046

Manhasset

North Shore University Hospital/NYU School of Medicine Program

Sponsor: North Shore University Hospital

Program Director:
Donald Margouleff, MD
North Shore Univ Hospital
300 Community Dr
Manhasset, NY 11030
Tel: 516 562-4400 *Fax:* 516 562-1608
Accred Length: 2 Years *Program Size:* 2
Program ID: 200-35-21-102

New Hyde Park

Albert Einstein College of Medicine at Long Island Jewish Medical Center Program

Sponsor: Long Island Jewish Medical Center

Program Director:
Christopher J Palestro, MD
Long Island Jewish Med Ctr
270-05 76th Ave
New Hyde Park, NY 11042
Tel: 718 470-7081 *Fax:* 718 470-9247
Internet: http://www.lij.edu/lij-homepag
Accred Length: 2 Years *Program Size:* 4
Program ID: 200-35-11-049

New York

Memorial Sloan-Kettering Cancer Center Program

Sponsor: Memorial Sloan-Kettering Cancer Center

Program Director:
Steven M Larson, MD
Memorial Sloan-Kettering Cancer Ctr
Nuclear Med Service
1275 York Ave
New York, NY 10021
Tel: 212 639-7373 *Fax:* 212 717-3263
E-mail: larsons@mskcc.org
Internet: http://www.mskcc.org
Accred Length: 2 Years *Program Size:* 5
Program ID: 200-35-11-050

Mount Sinai School of Medicine Program

Sponsor: Mount Sinai School of Medicine
Mount Sinai Medical Center
Veterans Affairs Medical Center (Bronx)

Program Director:
Josef Machac, MD
Mount Sinai Med Ctr
One Gustave L Levy Pl
Box 1141
New York, NY 10029-6574
Tel: 212 241-7888 *Fax:* 212 831-2851
E-mail: josef_machac@smtplink.mssm.edu
Accred Length: 2 Years *Program Size:* 3
Program ID: 200-35-21-051

New York and Presbyterian Hospital (Columbia Campus) Program

Sponsor: New York and Presbyterian Hospital
New York and Presbyterian Hospital (Columbia Campus)

Program Director:
Ronald L Van Heertum, MD
Presbyterian Hospital
Milstein Hospital Bldg/2-131
177 Fort Washington Ave
New York, NY 10032
Tel: 212 305-7132 *Fax:* 212 305-4244
E-mail: vanheer@cucis.columbia.edu
Accred Length: 2 Years *Program Size:* 1
Program ID: 200-35-21-099

New York and Presbyterian Hospital (Cornell Campus) Program

Sponsor: New York and Presbyterian Hospital
New York and Presbyterian Hospital (Cornell Campus)

Program Director:
Stanley J Goldsmith, MD
Div of Nuclear Med/Rm ST221
New York Hospital
525 E 68th St
New York, NY 10021
Tel: 212 746-4588 *Fax:* 212 746-9010
E-mail: sgoldsmi@nyh.med.cornell.edu
Accred Length: 2 Years *Program Size:* 2
Program ID: 200-35-11-052

New York Medical College at St Vincent's Hospital and Medical Center of New York Program

Sponsor: New York Medical College
St Vincent's Hospital and Medical Center of New York

Program Director:
Hussein M Abdel-Dayem, MD
St Vincent's Hospital and Med Ctr
Dept of Nuclear Med
153 W 11th St
New York, NY 10011-8397
Tel: 212 604-8783 *Fax:* 212 604-3119
Accred Length: 2 Years *Program Size:* 2
Program ID: 200-35-12-054

St Luke's-Roosevelt Hospital Center Program

Sponsor: St Luke's-Roosevelt Hospital Center
St Luke's-Roosevelt Hospital Center-Roosevelt Division
St Luke's-Roosevelt Hospital Center-St Luke's Division

Program Director:
Gordon DePuey, MD
St Luke's-Roosevelt Hospital Ctr
Amsterdam Ave at 114th St
New York, NY 10025
Tel: 212 523-3398 *Fax:* 212 523-3949
Accred Length: 2 Years *Program Size:* 0
Program ID: 200-35-11-084

Northport

Veterans Affairs Medical Center (Northport) Program

Sponsor: Veterans Affairs Medical Center (Northport)
South Nassau Communities Hospital
University Hospital-SUNY at Stony Brook

Program Director:
Mohamed A Antar, MD PhD
VA Med Ctr
79 Middleville Rd (632)
Northport, NY 11768-2290
Tel: 516 261-4400, ext 7819 *Fax:* 516 266-6091
E-mail: antar@northport,va.gov
Accred Length: 2 Years *Program Size:* 4
Program ID: 200-35-21-056

Rochester

University of Rochester Program

Sponsor: Strong Memorial Hospital of the University of Rochester

Program Director:
Robert E O'Mara, MD
Box 620
575 Elmwood Ave
Rochester, NY 14642-8648
Tel: 716 275-4741 *Fax:* 716 273-1022
E-mail: omara@rad.rochester.edu
Accred Length: 2 Years *Program Size:* 2
Program ID: 200-35-11-057

North Carolina

Chapel Hill

University of North Carolina Hospitals Program

Sponsor: University of North Carolina Hospitals

Program Director:
William H McCartney, MD
Univ of North Carolina Hospitals
CB 7510 Old Clinic Bldg
Chapel Hill, NC 27599-7510
Tel: 919 966-4384 *Fax:* 919 966-5934
Accred Length: 2 Years *Program Size:* 1
Program ID: 200-36-21-114

Durham

Duke University Program

Sponsor: Duke University Medical Center
Veterans Affairs Medical Center (Durham)

Program Director:
R Edward Coleman, MD
Duke Univ Med Ctr
Dept of Nuclear Med
Box 3949
Durham, NC 27710
Tel: 919 684-7244 *Fax:* 919 684-7135
E-mail: colem010@mc.duke.edu
Accred Length: 2 Years *Program Size:* 4
Program ID: 200-36-21-060

Winston-Salem

Wake Forest University School of Medicine Program

Sponsor: Wake Forest University Baptist Medical Center

Program Director:
Nat E Watson Jr, MD
WFU-Baptist Med Ctr
Dept of Nuclear Med
Medical Center Blvd
Winston-Salem, NC 27157-1088
Tel: 336 716-4932 *Fax:* 336 716-6108
Accred Length: 2 Years *Program Size:* 1
Program ID: 200-36-11-061

Ohio

Cincinnati

Christ Hospital Program

Sponsor: Christ Hospital

Program Director:
Parshan (Paul) S Ramsingh, MD
Christ Hospital
Dept of Nuclear Med
2139 Auburn Ave
Cincinnati, OH 45219-2989
Tel: 513 369-2938 *Fax:* 513 369-8414
E-mail: kramerb@healthall.com
Internet: http://www.health-alliance.com
Accred Length: 2 Years *Program Size:* 4
Program ID: 200-38-21-112

Oklahoma

Oklahoma City

University of Oklahoma Health Sciences Center Program

Sponsor: University of Oklahoma College of Medicine
Children's Hospital of Oklahoma
University Hospital
Veterans Affairs Medical Center (Oklahoma City)

Program Director:
Joe C Leonard, MD
Univ of Oklahoma Health Sciences Ctr
PO Box 26901
Rm 2NP602
Oklahoma City, OK 73190-3020
Tel: 405 271-5141 *Fax:* 405 271-3533
Accred Length: 2 Years *Program Size:* 2
Program ID: 200-39-21-064

Oregon

Portland

Oregon Health Sciences University Program

Sponsor: Oregon Health Sciences University Hospital
Veterans Affairs Medical Center (Portland)
Program Director:
Jeffrey S Stevens, MD
Oregon Health Sciences Univ
Nuclear Med (OP23)
3181 SW Sam Jackson Park Rd
Portland, OR 97201-3098
Tel: 503 494-8468 *Fax:* 503 271-7883
E-mail: stevensj@ohsu.edu
Accred Length: 2 Years *Program Size:* 4
Program ID: 200-40-21-065

Pennsylvania

Philadelphia

MCP Hahnemann University Program

Sponsor: MCP Hahnemann University
Hahnemann University Hospital
Program Director:
Simin Dadparvar, MD
Hahnemann Univ Hospital
Broad and Vine Sts/MS 309
Philadelphia, PA 19102-1192
Tel: 215 762-7678 *Fax:* 215 246-5926
Accred Length: 2 Years *Program Size:* 2
Program ID: 200-41-11-066

Temple University Program

Sponsor: Temple University Hospital
Program Director:
Alan H Maurer, MD
Temple Univ Hospital
3401 N Broad St
Philadelphia, PA 19140
Tel: 215 707-8269 *Fax:* 215 707-2059
E-mail: amaurer@thunder.temple.edu
Accred Length: 2 Years *Program Size:* 2
Program ID: 200-41-11-088

Thomas Jefferson University Program

Sponsor: Thomas Jefferson University Hospital
Program Director:
Charles M Intenzo, MD
Thomas Jefferson Univ Hospital
132 S Tenth St
861 Main Bldg
Philadelphia, PA 19107
Tel: 215 955-6707 *Fax:* 215 923-0268
Accred Length: 2 Years *Program Size:* 2
Program ID: 200-41-21-100

University of Pennsylvania Program

Sponsor: Hospital of the University of Pennsylvania
Children's Hospital of Philadelphia
Graduate Hospital
Veterans Affairs Medical Center (Philadelphia)
Program Director:
Abass Alavi, MD
Div of Nuclear Med
Hospital of Univ of Pennsylvania
3400 Spruce St
Philadelphia, PA 19104
Tel: 215 662-3069 *Fax:* 215 349-5843
E-mail: alavi@oasis.rad.upenn.edu
Internet: http://www.pet.upenn.edu
Accred Length: 2 Years *Program Size:* 5
Program ID: 200-41-21-067

Puerto Rico

San Juan

University of Puerto Rico Program

Sponsor: University of Puerto Rico School of Medicine
University Hospital
Veterans Affairs Medical Center (San Juan)
Program Director:
Frieda Silva de Roldan, MD
Univ of Puerto Rico Med Science Campus
GPO Box 5067
San Juan, PR 00936
Tel: 787 767-0382 *Fax:* 787 767-0382
Accred Length: 2 Years *Program Size:* 2
Program ID: 200-42-21-069

South Carolina

Charleston

Medical University of South Carolina Program

Sponsor: Medical University of South Carolina College of Medicine
MUSC Medical Center
Ralph H Johnson Dept of Veterans Affairs Med Center
Program Director:
Kenneth M Spicer, MD PhD
Med Univ of South Carolina
171 Ashley Ave
Charleston, SC 29425
Tel: 843 792-1957 *Fax:* 843 792-1746
E-mail: spicerk@musc.edu
Internet: http://www.musc.edu/radiology/nuclear/fellowship.html
Accred Length: 2 Years *Program Size:* 1
Program ID: 200-45-21-070

Tennessee

Knoxville

University of Tennessee Medical Center at Knoxville Program

Sponsor: University of Tennessee Graduate School of Medicine
University of Tennessee Memorial Hospital
Program Director:
Gary T Smith, MD
Univ of Tennessee Grad Sch of Med
1924 Alcoa Hwy
Knoxville, TN 37920-6999
Tel: 423 544-9000 *Fax:* 423 544-8883
Internet: http://www.ipl.utmck.edu/radiology
Accred Length: 2 Years *Program Size:* 2
Program ID: 200-47-21-109

Nashville

Vanderbilt University Program

Sponsor: Vanderbilt University Medical Center
Veterans Affairs Medical Center (Nashville)
Program Director:
Dominique Delbeke, MD PhD
Vanderbilt Univ
Nuclear Med
R-1318 Med Ctr North
Nashville, TN 37232-2675
Tel: 615 322-3780 *Fax:* 615 322-3764
E-mail: radprogram@mcmail.vanderbilt.edu
Internet: http://www.mc.vanderbilt.edu/vumcdept/radio.html
Accred Length: 2 Years *Program Size:* 3
Program ID: 200-47-21-072

Texas

Dallas

University of Texas Southwestern Medical School Program

Sponsor: University of Texas Southwestern Medical School
Dallas County Hospital District-Parkland Memorial Hospital
Veterans Affairs Medical Center (Dallas)
Program Director:
William A Erdman, MD
Univ of Texas Southwestern Med Sch
Dept of Radiology
5323 Harry Hines Blvd
Dallas, TX 75235-8896
Tel: 214 648-8022 *Fax:* 214 648-2678
E-mail: dotter@mednet.swmed.edu
Internet: http://www.rad.swmed.edu/residen.html
Accred Length: 2 Years *Program Size:* 2
Program ID: 200-48-21-073

Houston

Baylor College of Medicine Program

Sponsor: Baylor College of Medicine
Harris County Hospital District-Ben Taub General Hospital
St Luke's Episcopal Hospital
Texas Children's Hospital
Veterans Affairs Medical Center (Houston)
Program Director:
Warren H Moore, MD
Baylor Coll of Med
Grad Med Educ 183A
One Baylor Plaza
Houston, TX 77030
Tel: 713 791-3126 *Fax:* 713 791-3363
Accred Length: 2 Years *Program Size:* 4
Program ID: 200-48-21-075

San Antonio

University of Texas Health Science Center at San Antonio Program
Sponsor: University of Texas Medical School at San Antonio
Brooke Army Medical Center
University Hospital-South Texas Medical Center
Wilford Hall Medical Center (AETC)
Program Director:
Ralph Blumhardt, MD
Kathleen A Hancock, MD
Univ of Texas Health Science Ctr
Dept of Radiology
7703 Floyd Curl Dr
San Antonio, TX 78284-7800
Tel: 210 567-5600 *Fax:* 210 567-6418
Accred Length: 2 Years *Program Size:* 3
Program ID: 200-48-31-085

Utah

Salt Lake City

University of Utah Program
Sponsor: University of Utah Medical Center
Veterans Affairs Medical Center (Salt Lake City)
Program Director:
Sonia Valdivia, MD
Univ of Utah Med Ctr
50 N Medical Dr
Rm 1B622
Salt Lake City, UT 84132
Tel: 801 581-2369 *Fax:* 801 585-2403
Internet: http://www.rad.med.utah.edu
Accred Length: 2 Years *Program Size:* 2
Program ID: 200-49-21-107

Virginia

Richmond

Medical College of Virginia/Virginia Commonwealth University Program
Sponsor: Medical College of Virginia/Virginia Commonwealth University
Hunter Holmes McGuire VA Medical Center (Richmond)
Medical College of Virginia Hospitals
Program Director:
Paul R Jolles, MD
Med Coll of Virginia
PO Box 980615
Richmond, VA 23298-0615
Tel: 804 828-3525 *Fax:* 804 828-6066
E-mail: mdbaker@hsc.vcu.edu
Internet: http://www.vcu.edu/nucmed
Accred Length: 2 Years *Program Size:* 2
Program ID: 200-51-21-077

Washington

Seattle

University of Washington Program
Sponsor: University of Washington School of Medicine
Harborview Medical Center
University of Washington Medical Center
Veterans Affairs Medical Center (Seattle)
Program Director:
Michael M Graham, MD
Univ of Washington
Div of Nuclear Med
Box 356113
Seattle, WA 98195
Tel: 206 548-4240 *Fax:* 206 548-4496
Accred Length: 2 Years *Program Size:* 5
Program ID: 200-54-21-078

Wisconsin

Madison

University of Wisconsin Program
Sponsor: University of Wisconsin Hospital and Clinics
William S Middleton Veterans Hospital
Program Director:
Scott B Perlman, MD
Univ of Wisconsin Hospital and Clinics
Dept of Nuclear Med
600 Highland Ave
Madison, WI 53792-3252
Tel: 608 263-5306 *Fax:* 608 262-0907
E-mail: sperlman@facstaff.wisc.edu
Accred Length: 2 Years *Program Size:* 2
Program ID: 200-56-21-079

Milwaukee

Aurora Health Care Program
Sponsor: Aurora Health Care
St Luke's Medical Center
Program Director:
David L Yuille, MD
St Luke's Med Ctr
2900 W Oklahoma Ave
Milwaukee, WI 53215
Tel: 414 649-6418 *Fax:* 414 649-5993
E-mail: kpslmc@execpc.com
Internet: http://www.aurorahealthcare.org
Accred Length: 2 Years *Program Size:* 4
Program ID: 200-56-12-081

Medical College of Wisconsin Program
Sponsor: Medical College of Wisconsin Affiliated Hospitals Inc
Clement J Zablocki Veterans Affairs Medical Center
Froedtert Memorial Lutheran Hospital
Program Director:
Arthur Z Krasnow, MD
Froedtert Memorial Lutheran Hospital
9200 W Wisconsin Ave
Milwaukee, WI 53226
Tel: 414 805-3774 *Fax:* 414 771-3460
Accred Length: 2 Years *Program Size:* 2
Program ID: 200-56-21-080

Nuclear Radiology (Radiology-Diagnostic)

Connecticut

New Haven

Yale-New Haven Medical Center Program
Sponsor: Yale-New Haven Hospital
Program Director:
Holley M Dey, MD
333 Cedar St
PO Box 208042
New Haven, CT 06520-8042
Tel: 203 937-3427 *Fax:* 203 937-4509
Accred Length: 1 Year *Program Size:* 2
Program ID: 425-08-11-002

Georgia

Atlanta

Emory University Program
Sponsor: Emory University School of Medicine
Emory University Hospital
Grady Memorial Hospital
Program Director:
Naomi P Alazraki, MD
1364 Clifton Rd NE
Atlanta, GA 30322
Tel: 404 728-5082 *Fax:* 404 728-4846
Accred Length: 1 Year *Program Size:* 3
Program ID: 425-12-21-056

Illinois

Chicago

McGaw Medical Center of Northwestern University Program
Sponsor: Northwestern University Medical School
Northwestern Memorial Hospital
Program Director:
William G Spies, MD
Northwestern Memorial Hospital
Dept of Nuclear Med
250 E Superior St/W484
Chicago, IL 60611
Tel: 312 908-2514 *Fax:* 312 908-8118
Accred Length: 1 Year *Program Size:* 3
Program ID: 425-16-21-052

Rush-Presbyterian-St Luke's Medical Center Program
Sponsor: Rush-Presbyterian-St Luke's Medical Center
Program Director:
Amjad Ali, MD
Rush-Presbyterian-St Luke's Med Ctr
1653 W Congress Pkwy
Chicago, IL 60612
Tel: 312 942-5781 *Fax:* 312 942-2114
E-mail: aali@rad.rpslmc.edu
Accred Length: 1 Year *Program Size:* 1
Program ID: 425-16-21-049

Programs

Kansas

Kansas City

University of Kansas Medical Center Program

Sponsor: University of Kansas School of Medicine
University of Kansas Medical Center

Program Director:
Kirkman G Baxter, MD
Univ of Kansas Med Ctr
Div of Nuclear Med
3901 Rainbow Blvd
Kansas City, KS 66160-7234
Tel: 913 588-6810 *Fax:* 913 588-7899
E-mail: kbaxter@kumc.edu
Accred Length: 1 Year *Program Size:* 1
Program ID: 425-19-11-015

Maryland

Baltimore

Johns Hopkins University Program

Sponsor: Johns Hopkins University School of Medicine
Johns Hopkins Hospital

Program Director:
Zsolt Szabo, MD
Johns Hopkins Med Insts
600 N Wolfe St
Nelson B1-126
Baltimore, MD 21287
Tel: 410 955-8448 *Fax:* 410 955-8597
Accred Length: 1 Year *Program Size:* 1
Program ID: 425-23-21-004

University of Maryland Program

Sponsor: University of Maryland Medical System
Veterans Affairs Medical Center (Baltimore)

Program Director:
Lawrence E Holder, MD
22 S Greene St
Baltimore, MD 21201
Tel: 410 328-6890 *Fax:* 410 328-1600
E-mail: lholder@radiology.ab.umd.edu
Internet: http://umm.edu/center/departments/diag_radiology/fel-radioltoc.html
Accred Length: 1 Year *Program Size:* 1
Program ID: 425-23-21-061

Massachusetts

Boston

Beth Israel Deaconess Medical Center (West Campus) Program

Sponsor: Beth Israel Deaconess Medical Center

Program Director:
Thomas C Hill, MD
Beth Israel Deaconess Med Ctr
One Deaconess Rd
Boston, MA 02215
Tel: 617 754-2615 *Fax:* 617 754-2545
Accred Length: 1 Year *Program Size:* 1
Program ID: 425-24-21-045

Brigham and Women's Hospital/Harvard Medical School Program

Sponsor: Brigham and Women's Hospital
Children's Hospital

Program Director:
James S Nagel, MD
Dept of Radiology
Brigham and Women's Hospital
75 Francis St
Boston, MA 02115
Tel: 617 732-6215 *Fax:* 617 732-6099
E-mail: jsnagel@bics.bwh.harvard.edu
Accred Length: 1 Year *Program Size:* 2
Program ID: 425-24-21-036

Michigan

Royal Oak

William Beaumont Hospital Program

Sponsor: William Beaumont Hospital

Program Director:
Howard J Dworkin, MD
Helena R Balon, MD
William Beaumont Hospital
3601 W 13 Mile Rd
Royal Oak, MI 48073-6769
Tel: 248 551-4126 *Fax:* 248 551-7344
E-mail: hbalon@beaumont.edu
Internet: http://www.beaumont.edu/html/gme
Accred Length: 1 Year *Program Size:* 2
Program ID: 425-25-21-018

Minnesota

Rochester

Mayo Graduate School of Medicine (Rochester) Program

Sponsor: Mayo Graduate School of Medicine-Mayo Foundation
Mayo Clinic (Rochester)

Program Director:
Douglas A Collins, MD
Application Processing Ctr
Mayo Graduate Sch of Med
200 First St SW
Rochester, MN 55905
Tel: 507 284-3108 *Fax:* 507 284-0999
E-mail: mgsm.roch.mn.diagnosticrad@mayo.edu
Internet: http://www.mayo.edu/
Accred Length: 1 Year *Program Size:* 1
Program ID: 425-26-21-019

Missouri

St Louis

Washington University/B-JH/SLCH Consortium Program

Sponsor: Washington University/B-JH/SLCH Consortium
Barnes-Jewish Hospital
Mallinckrodt Institute of Radiology

Program Director:
Tom R Miller, MD PhD
Mallinckrodt Inst of Radiology
510 S Kingshighway Blvd
St Louis, MO 63110-1076
Tel: 314 362-2809 *Fax:* 314 362-2806
Accred Length: 1 Year *Program Size:* 5
Program ID: 425-28-11-021

New Jersey

Livingston

St Barnabas Medical Center Program

Sponsor: St Barnabas Medical Center

Program Director:
Letty G Lutzker, MD
St Barnabas Med Ctr, Dept of Radiology
94 Old Short Hills Rd
Livingston, NJ 07039
Tel: 973 322-5957 *Fax:* 973 322-5867
Accred Length: 1 Year *Program Size:* 1
Program ID: 425-33-21-037

New York

Brooklyn

New York Methodist Hospital Program

Sponsor: New York Methodist Hospital

Program Director:
David C Yang, MD
New York Methodist Hospital
506 Sixth St
Brooklyn, NY 11215-3645
Tel: 718 780-5882 *Fax:* 718 780-3245
E-mail: dcyangmd@ix.netcom.com
Accred Length: 1 Year *Program Size:* 2
Program ID: 425-35-21-047

New York

New York and Presbyterian Hospital (Columbia Campus) Program

Sponsor: New York and Presbyterian Hospital
New York and Presbyterian Hospital (Columbia Campus)

Program Director:
Ronald L Van Heertum, MD
Columbia Presbyterian Med Ctr
Milstein Hospital Bldg/2-131
177 Fort Washington Ave
New York, NY 10032
Tel: 212 305-7132 *Fax:* 212 305-4244
E-mail: vanheer@cucis.columbia.edu
Accred Length: 1 Year *Program Size:* 1
Program ID: 425-35-21-042

New York Medical College at St Vincent's Hospital and Medical Center of New York Program

Sponsor: New York Medical College
St Vincent's Hospital and Medical Center of New York

Program Director:
Hussein M Abdel-Dayem, MD
St Vincent's Hospital and Med Ctr
153 W 11th St/Cronin #327
New York, NY 10011-8397
Tel: 212 604-8783 *Fax:* 212 604-3119
Accred Length: 1 Year *Program Size:* 0
Program ID: 425-35-12-023

New York University Medical Center Program

Sponsor: New York University Medical Center

Program Director:
Joseph Sanger, MD
New York Univ Med Ctr
560 First Ave
New York, NY 10016
Tel: 212 263-7410 *Fax:* 212 263-7519
Accred Length: 1 Year *Program Size:* 1
Program ID: 425-35-21-007

St Luke's-Roosevelt Hospital Center Program
Sponsor: St Luke's-Roosevelt Hospital Center
St Luke's-Roosevelt Hospital Center-Roosevelt Division
St Luke's-Roosevelt Hospital Center-St Luke's Division
Program Director:
E Gordon DePuey, MD
St Luke's-Roosevelt Hospital Ctr
Amsterdam Ave at 114th St
New York, NY 10025
Tel: 212 523-3398 *Fax:* 212 523-3949
Accred Length: 1 Year *Program Size:* 0
Program ID: 425-35-21-060

Stony Brook

SUNY at Stony Brook Program
Sponsor: University Hospital-SUNY at Stony Brook
Program Director:
Zvi H Oster, MD
SUNY-Stony Brook
Level 4/Rm 092
Stony Brook, NY 11794-8460
Tel: 516 444-2484 *Fax:* 516 444-7538
E-mail: zvi.oster@sunysb.edu
Internet: http://www.informatics.sunysb.edu/radiology/
Accred Length: 1 Year *Program Size:* 1
Program ID: 425-35-21-044

Syracuse

SUNY Health Science Center at Syracuse Program
Sponsor: University Hospital-SUNY Health Science Center at Syracuse
Program Director:
F Deaver Thomas, MD
SUNY Health Science Ctr-Syracuse
750 E Adams St
Syracuse, NY 13210
Tel: 315 464-7031 *Fax:* 315 464-7068
E-mail: thomasd@vax.cs.hscsyr.edu
Accred Length: 1 Year *Program Size:* 2
Program ID: 425-35-21-008

North Carolina

Durham

Duke University Program
Sponsor: Duke University Medical Center
Program Director:
R Edward Coleman, MD
Duke Univ Med Ctr
Dept of Radiology
Box 3949
Durham, NC 27710
Tel: 919 684-7244 *Fax:* 919 684-7135
E-mail: colem010@mc.duke.edu
Accred Length: 1 Year *Program Size:* 2
Program ID: 425-36-21-024

Winston-Salem

Wake Forest University School of Medicine Program
Sponsor: Wake Forest University Baptist Medical Center
Program Director:
Nat Watson, MD
Bowman Gray Sch of Med
Dept of Rad/Nuclear Med
Medical Center Blvd
Winston-Salem, NC 27157-1088
Tel: 336 716-4932 *Fax:* 336 716-6108
Accred Length: 1 Year *Program Size:* 1
Program ID: 425-36-21-025

Ohio

Cleveland

Cleveland Clinic Foundation Program
Sponsor: Cleveland Clinic Foundation
Program Director:
Donald R Neumann, MD PHD
Cleveland Clinic Foundation
Dept of Nuclear Rad/HB6
9500 Euclid Ave
Cleveland, OH 44195
Tel: 216 444-2193 *Fax:* 216 444-9307
E-mail: meded@cesmtp.ccf.org
Internet: http://www.ccf.org
Accred Length: 1 Year *Program Size:* 2
Program ID: 425-38-21-062

Pennsylvania

Philadelphia

University of Pennsylvania Program
Sponsor: Hospital of the University of Pennsylvania
Program Director:
Abass Alavi, MD
Hospital of Univ of Pennsylvania
Div of Nuclear Med
3400 Spruce St
Philadelphia, PA 19104
Tel: 215 662-3069 *Fax:* 215 349-5843
E-mail: alavi@oasis.rad.upenn.edu
Internet: http://www.pet.upenn.edu
Accred Length: 1 Year *Program Size:* 5
Program ID: 425-41-21-043

Texas

Dallas

University of Texas Southwestern Medical School Program
Sponsor: University of Texas Southwestern Medical School
Dallas County Hospital District-Parkland Memorial Hospital
Veterans Affairs Medical Center (Dallas)
Program Director:
William A Erdman, MD
Univ of Texas Southwestern Med Sch
Dept of Radiology
5323 Harry Hines Blvd
Dallas, TX 75235-8896
Tel: 214 590-6397 *Fax:* 214 590-2720
Internet: http://www.rad.sw.med.edu/residen
Accred Length: 1 Year *Program Size:* 1
Program ID: 425-48-21-027

Utah

Salt Lake City

University of Utah Program
Sponsor: University of Utah Medical Center
Veterans Affairs Medical Center (Salt Lake City)
Program Director:
Sonia Valdivia, MD
Univ of Utah Health Sciences Ctr
1B647 Medical Ctr
50 N Medical Dr
Salt Lake City, UT 84132
Tel: 801 581-2369 *Fax:* 801 585-2403
Internet: http://www.rad.med.utah.edu
Accred Length: 1 Year *Program Size:* 1
Program ID: 425-49-21-059

Virginia

Charlottesville

University of Virginia Program
Sponsor: University of Virginia Medical Center
Program Director:
Charles D Teates, MD
Univ of Virginia Sch of Med
Dept of Radiology/Box 170
Charlottesville, VA 22908
Tel: 804 924-9391 *Fax:* 804 982-1618
E-mail: ssd7n@virginia.edu
Accred Length: 1 Year *Program Size:* 1
Program ID: 425-51-11-028

West Virginia

Morgantown

West Virginia University Program
Sponsor: West Virginia University Hospitals
St Joseph's Hospital
Program Director:
Naresh C Gupta, MD
G-201 Health Sciences South
West Virginia Univ Med Ctr
PO Box 9236
Morgantown, WV 26506
Tel: 304 293-7798 *Fax:* 304 293-7142
E-mail: ngupta@wvu.edu
Accred Length: 1 Year *Program Size:* 1
Program ID: 425-55-21-063

Obstetrics and Gynecology

Alabama

Birmingham

University of Alabama Medical Center Program
Sponsor: University of Alabama Hospital
Cooper Green Hospital
Program Director:
Larry C Kilgore, MD
Univ of Alabama
618 S 20th St/OHB 340
Birmingham, AL 35294-7333
Tel: 205 934-5631 *Fax:* 205 975-6411
E-mail: resident@hsf.uab.edu
Accred Length: 4 Years *Program Size:* 28 (*GY1:* 7)
Program ID: 220-01-11-018

Mobile

University of South Alabama Program
Sponsor: University of South Alabama Medical Center
USA Doctors Hospital
Program Director:
Ian H Thorneycroft, PhD MD
Univ of South Alabama
Dept of Ob/Gyn
2451 Fillingim St
Mobile, AL 36617
Tel: 334 471-7943 *Fax:* 334 471-7740
Internet: http://www.southalabama.edu/residencyprograms/obgyn .html
Accred Length: 4 Years *Program Size:* 16 (*GY1:* 4)
Program ID: 220-01-21-020

Arizona

Phoenix

Good Samaritan Regional Medical Center Program
Sponsor: Good Samaritan Regional Medical Center
Program Director:
John H Mattox, MD
Good Samaritan Regional Med Ctr
Dept of Ob/Gyn
1111 E McDowell Rd
Phoenix, AZ 85006-2666
Tel: 602 239-4344 *Fax:* 602 239-2359
E-mail: jhm@samaritan.edu
Internet: http://www.samaritan.edu
Accred Length: 4 Years *Program Size:* 24 (*GY1:* 6)
Program ID: 220-03-21-024

Phoenix Hospitals Program
Sponsor: Maricopa Medical Center
St Joseph's Hospital and Medical Center
Program Director:
John I Fishburne Jr, MD
Maricopa Med Ctr
Dept of Ob/Gyn
2601 E Roosevelt St
Phoenix, AZ 85008
Tel: 602 267-5119 *Fax:* 602 681-1324
E-mail: jfishbur@medicine.maricopa.gov
Internet: http://www.maricopa.gov/medcenter/mmc/html
Accred Length: 4 Years *Program Size:* 28 (*GY1:* 7)
Program ID: 220-03-21-328

Tucson

University of Arizona Program
Sponsor: University of Arizona College of Medicine
University Medical Center
Program Director:
Kenneth D Hatch, MD
Univ of Arizona Health Sciences Ctr
Dept of Ob/Gyn, PO Box 245078
1501 N Campbell Ave
Tucson, AZ 85724
Tel: 520 626-6636 *Fax:* 520 626-2514
E-mail: varela@u.arizona.edu
Internet: http://www.arizona.edu/acaddepts.html
Accred Length: 4 Years *Program Size:* 17 (*GY1:* 5)
Program ID: 220-03-21-025

Arkansas

Little Rock

University of Arkansas for Medical Sciences Program
Sponsor: University of Arkansas College of Medicine
University Hospital of Arkansas
Program Director:
Tim H Parmley, MD
Univ of Arkansas for Med Sciences
4301 W Markham St/Slot 518
Little Rock, AR 72205
Tel: 501 686-6799 *Fax:* 501 686-8107
E-mail: parmleytimh@exchange.uams.edu
Accred Length: 4 Years *Program Size:* 16 (*GY1:* 4)
Program ID: 220-04-11-026

California

Bakersfield

Kern Medical Center Program
Sponsor: Kern Medical Center
Program Director:
Antonio L Garcia, MD
Kern Med Ctr
Dept of Ob/Gyn 4th Fl
1830 Flower St
Bakersfield, CA 93305-4197
Tel: 805 326-2236 *Fax:* 805 326-2235
E-mail: rugnaoa@kernmedctr.com
Accred Length: 4 Years *Program Size:* 12 (*GY1:* 3)
Program ID: 220-05-31-027

Fresno

University of California (San Francisco)/Fresno Program
Sponsor: UCSF-Fresno Medical Education Program
University Medical Center
Program Director:
J Kenneth Cooke, MD
Univ Med Ctr
Ob/Gyn Program
445 S Cedar Ave
Fresno, CA 93702
Tel: 209 459-5720 *Fax:* 209 459-6815
Accred Length: 4 Years *Program Size:* 12 (*GY1:* 3)
Program ID: 220-05-31-029

Glendale

Glendale Adventist Medical Center Program
Sponsor: Glendale Adventist Medical Center
Loma Linda University Medical Center
Program Director:
Hugo D Riffel, MD
Glendale Adventist Med Ctr
Ob/Gyn Residency
1509 Wilson Terrace
Glendale, CA 91206
Tel: 818 409-8083 *Fax:* 818 546-5606
Accred Length: 4 Years *Program Size:* 8 (*GY1:* 2)
Program ID: 220-05-31-030

Loma Linda

Loma Linda University Program
Sponsor: Loma Linda University Medical Center
Riverside County Regional Medical Center
San Bernardino County Medical Center
Program Director:
Robert J Wagner, MD
Loma Linda Univ Med Ctr
Dept of Ob/Gyn
PO Box 2000
Loma Linda, CA 92354
Tel: 909 824-4763 *Fax:* 909 824-4167
Accred Length: 4 Years *Program Size:* 24 (*GY1:* 6)
Program ID: 220-05-21-329

Los Angeles

Cedars-Sinai Medical Center Program
Sponsor: Cedars-Sinai Medical Center
Program Director:
Lawrence D Platt, MD
8635 W Third St/Ste 160W
Los Angeles, CA 90048
Tel: 310 855-7415 *Fax:* 310 967-0142
E-mail: platt@cshs.org
Internet: http://www.csmc.edu
Accred Length: 4 Years *Program Size:* 20 (*GY1:* 5)
Program ID: 220-05-31-034

Charles R Drew University Program
Sponsor: Charles R Drew University of Medicine and Science
LAC-King/Drew Medical Center
Program Director:
Rosetta Hassan, MD
Martin Luther King Jr-Drew Med Ctr
Dept of Ob/Gyn
12021 S Wilmington Ave
Los Angeles, CA 90059
Tel: 310 668-4634 *Fax:* 310 898-1854
Accred Length: 4 Years *Program Size:* 16 (*GY1:* 4)
Program ID: 220-05-21-037

Southern California Kaiser Permanente Medical Care (Los Angeles) Program
Sponsor: Southern California Kaiser Permanente Medical Group
Kaiser Foundation Hospital (Los Angeles)
Program Director:
Carol Scherfenberg, MD
Kaiser Foundation Hospital
393 E Walnut St
Pasadena, CA 91188-8013
Tel: 800 541-7946
Internet: http://www.kpscal.org
Accred Length: 4 Years *Program Size:* 17 (*GY1:* 4)
Program ID: 220-05-12-035

UCLA Medical Center Program
Sponsor: UCLA School of Medicine
Olive View-UCLA Medical Center
UCLA Medical Center
Program Director:
Jonathan S Berek, MD
10833 Le Conte Ave
27-139 CHS
Los Angeles, CA 90095-1740
Tel: 310 825-9945 *Fax:* 310 206-6531
Accred Length: 4 Years *Program Size:* 29 (*GY1:* 8)
Program ID: 220-05-31-038

University of Southern California Program
Sponsor: Los Angeles County-USC Medical Center
Program Director:
Daniel R Mishell Jr, MD
Women's and Children's Hospital
Rm L1009
1240 N Mission Rd
Los Angeles, CA 90033
Tel: 323 226-3416 *Fax:* 323 226-3509
Accred Length: 4 Years *Program Size:* 51 (*GY1:* 12)
Program ID: 220-05-11-036

White Memorial Medical Center Program
Sponsor: White Memorial Medical Center
Program Director:
Ronald M Nelson, MD
White Memorial Med Ctr
1720 Cesar E Chavez Ave
Los Angeles, CA 90033
Tel: 323 268-5000 *Fax:* 323 264-5592
Internet: http://www.whitememorial.com
Accred Length: 4 Years *Program Size:* 12 (*GY1:* 3)
Program ID: 220-05-21-039

Oakland

Kaiser Permanente Medical Group (Northern California) Program
Sponsor: Kaiser Permanente Medical Group (Northern California)
Kaiser Permanente Medical Center (Oakland)
Program Director:
Lesley R Levine, MD
Dept of Ob/Gyn
Kaiser Permanente Med Ctr
280 W MacArthur Blvd
Oakland, CA 94611-5693
Tel: 510 596-7826 *Fax:* 510 596-1571
E-mail: obgyn.oakmeded@ncal.kaiperm.org
Internet: http://www.kaiserpermanente.org
Accred Length: 4 Years *Program Size:* 12 (*GY1:* 3)
Program ID: 220-05-12-040

Orange

University of California (Irvine) Program
Sponsor: University of California (Irvine) Medical Center
Long Beach Memorial Medical Center
Program Director:
Kirk A Keegan Jr, MD
Univ of California Irvine Med Ctr
Bldg 22A 3rd Fl
101 City Dr S
Orange, CA 92868-3298
Tel: 714 456-6707 *Fax:* 714 456-8360
E-mail: dogarcia@uci.edu
Internet: http://www.med.uci.edu/~ob-gyn/
Accred Length: 4 Years *Program Size:* 24 (*GY1:* 6)
Program ID: 220-05-21-031

Sacramento

University of California (Davis) Program
Sponsor: University of California (Davis) Medical Center
Kaiser Foundation Hospital (Sacramento)
Program Director:
Lloyd H Smith, MD PhD
Dept of Ob/Gyn
4860 Y St/Ste 2500
Sacramento, CA 95817
Tel: 916 734-6930 *Fax:* 916 734-6666
E-mail: obg@ucdavis.edu
Accred Length: 4 Years *Program Size:* 18 (*GY1:* 4)
Program ID: 220-05-21-028

San Diego

Naval Medical Center (San Diego) Program
Sponsor: Naval Medical Center (San Diego)
Program Director:
Manuel E Rivera-Alsina, MD
Naval Med Ctr
Ob/Gyn Service
34730 Bob Wilson Dr/Ste 100
San Diego, CA 92134-3100
Tel: 619 532-7004 *Fax:* 619 532-6587
E-mail: merivera@snd10.med.navy.mil
Accred Length: 4 Years *Program Size:* 21 (*GY1:* 6)
Program ID: 220-05-11-012
US Armed Services Program

University of California (San Diego) Program
Sponsor: University of California (San Diego) Medical Center
Kaiser Foundation Hospital (San Diego)
Program Director:
Charles W Nager, MD
UCSD Med Ctr
200 W Arbor Dr/#8434
San Diego, CA 92103-8434
Tel: 619 543-6922 *Fax:* 619 543-2638
E-mail: ghydoski@ucsd.edu
Internet: http://www.medicine.ucsd.edu/repromed/
Accred Length: 4 Years *Program Size:* 20 (*GY1:* 5)
Program ID: 220-05-21-044

San Francisco

Kaiser Permanente Medical Group (Northern California)/San Francisco Program
Sponsor: Kaiser Permanente Medical Group (Northern California)
Kaiser Permanente Medical Center (San Francisco)
Program Director:
David R Field, MD
Kaiser Permanente Med Ctr
Dept of Ob/Gyn
2200 O'Farrell
San Francisco, CA 94115
Tel: 415 202-4677 *Fax:* 415 202-4983
E-mail: sfo.grad.medprg@ncal.kaiperm.org
Internet: http://ncal.kaiserpermanente.org
Accred Length: 4 Years *Program Size:* 16 (*GY1:* 4)
Program ID: 220-05-12-045

University of California (San Francisco) Program
Sponsor: University of California (San Francisco) School of Medicine
Mount Zion Medical Center of the University of California
San Francisco General Hospital Medical Center
University of California (San Francisco) Medical Center
Program Director:
A Eugene Washington, MD MSc
Dept of Ob/Gyn
505 Parnassus Ave/Box 0132
San Francisco, CA 94143-0132
Tel: 415 476-5192 *Fax:* 415 476-1811
Accred Length: 4 Years *Program Size:* 32 (*GY1:* 8)
Program ID: 220-05-21-047

San Jose

Santa Clara Valley Medical Center Program
Sponsor: Santa Clara Valley Medical Center
Program Director:
Roger A Spencer, MD
Santa Clara Valley Med Ctr
751 S Bascom Ave
San Jose, CA 95128-2699
Tel: 408 885-5550 *Fax:* 408 885-5577
E-mail: obresvmc@wpgate.hhs.co.santa-clara.ca.
Accred Length: 4 Years *Program Size:* 12 (*GY1:* 3)
Program ID: 220-05-21-333

Santa Clara

Kaiser Permanente Medical Group (Northern California)/Santa Clara Program
Sponsor: Kaiser Permanente Medical Group (Northern California)
Kaiser Permanente Medical Center (Santa Clara)
Program Director:
David K Levin, MD
Kaiser Permanente Med Ctr
Office of Grad Med Educ
900 Kiely Blvd/Lower Level
Santa Clara, CA 95051-5386
Tel: 408 236-4921 *Fax:* 408 236-5185
Accred Length: 4 Years *Program Size:* 16 (*GY1:* 4)
Program ID: 220-05-12-311

Stanford

Stanford University Program
Sponsor: Stanford University Hospital
Program Director:
Mary Lake Polan, MD PhD
Stanford Univ Sch of Med
Dept of Ob/Gyn
300 Pasteur Dr/HH333
Stanford, CA 94305-5317
Tel: 650 723-5533 *Fax:* 650 723-7737
Internet: http://obgyn.stanford.edu
Accred Length: 4 Years *Program Size:* 16 (*GY1:* 4)
Program ID: 220-05-21-048

Torrance

Los Angeles County-Harbor-UCLA Medical Center Program
Sponsor: Los Angeles County-Harbor-UCLA Medical Center
Program Director:
David D Deutsch, MD
Los Angeles County-Harbor-UCLA Med Ctr
1000 W Carson St
Harbor Box #3
Torrance, CA 90509-2910
Tel: 310 222-3591 *Fax:* 310 320-6043
Accred Length: 4 Years *Program Size:* 20 (*GY1:* 5)
Program ID: 220-05-21-050

Travis AFB

David Grant Medical Center Program
Sponsor: David Grant Medical Center
Program Director:
Turgut Alagoz, MD
60 MSGS/SGCG
101 Bodin Cir
Travis AFB, CA 94535-1800
Tel: 707 423-5330 *Fax:* 707 423-7356
Accred Length: 4 Years *Program Size:* 12 (*GY1:* 3)
Program ID: 220-05-21-001
US Armed Services Program

Colorado

Denver

Exempla St Joseph Hospital Program
Sponsor: Exempla St Joseph Hospital
Program Director:
Richard Allen, MD
Exempla St Joseph Hospital
Ob/Gyn Med Educ
1835 Franklin St
Denver, CO 80218-1191
Tel: 303 837-7595 *Fax:* 303 837-6677
E-mail: notchj@exempla.org
Internet: http://www.saintjosephdenver.org
Accred Length: 4 Years *Program Size:* 16 (*GY1:* 4)
Program ID: 220-07-21-051

University of Colorado Program
Sponsor: University of Colorado Health Sciences Center
Denver Health and Hospitals
Rose Medical Center
Program Director:
Ronald S Gibbs, MD
Univ of Colorado Health Sciences Ctr
Ob/Gyn Program
4200 E Ninth Ave/Campus Box B-198
Denver, CO 80262
Tel: 303 315-3169 *Fax:* 303 372-6696
E-mail: alicia.gore@uchsc.edu
Accred Length: 4 Years *Program Size:* 36 (*GY1:* 9)
Program ID: 220-07-31-052

Connecticut

Bridgeport

Bridgeport Hospital Program
Sponsor: Bridgeport Hospital
Program Director:
John C Whetham, MD
Dept of Ob/Gyn
PO Box 5000
Bridgeport, CT 06610
Tel: 203 384-3042 *Fax:* 203 384-3264
E-mail: pjwhet@bptiosp.org
Accred Length: 4 Years *Program Size:* 8 (*GY1:* 2)
Program ID: 220-08-11-054

Danbury

Danbury Hospital Program
Sponsor: Danbury Hospital
Program Director:
Lester Silberman, MD
Danbury Hospital
24 Hospital Ave
Danbury, CT 06810
Tel: 203 797-7466 *Fax:* 203 731-8799
E-mail: mcguires@danhosp.chime.org
Accred Length: 4 Years *Program Size:* 8 (*GY1:* 2)
Program ID: 220-08-21-055

Farmington

University of Connecticut Program
Sponsor: University of Connecticut School of Medicine
Hartford Hospital
New Britain General Hospital
Univ of Connecticut Health Center/John Dempsey Hospital
Program Director:
John F Rodis, MD
Univ of Connecticut Health Ctr
Dept of Ob/Gyn
263 Farmington Ave
Farmington, CT 06030-1230
Tel: 860 679-2853 *Fax:* 860 679-1228
E-mail: giove@nso1.uchc.edu
Accred Length: 4 Years *Program Size:* 24 (*GY1:* 8)
Program ID: 220-08-21-355

Hartford

St Francis Hospital and Medical Center Program
Sponsor: St Francis Hospital and Medical Center
Program Director:
Ganson Purcell Jr, MD
St Francis Hospital and Med Ctr
114 Woodland St
Hartford, CT 06105-1299
Tel: 860 714-4457 *Fax:* 860 714-8008
E-mail: obgyn@stfranciscare.org
Internet: http://www.stfranciscare.org/~obgyn
Accred Length: 4 Years *Program Size:* 12 (*GY1:* 3)
Program ID: 220-08-11-059

New Haven

Yale-New Haven Medical Center Program
Sponsor: Yale-New Haven Hospital
Program Director:
Ray Bahado-Singh, MD
Yale Univ Sch of Med
Dept of Ob/Gyn
333 Cedar St/PO Box 208063
New Haven, CT 06520-8063
Tel: 203 785-3091 *Fax:* 203 785-6885
E-mail: ray.bahado-singh@yale.edu
Accred Length: 4 Years *Program Size:* 25 (*GY1:* 7)
Program ID: 220-08-21-060

Stamford

Stamford Hospital/Columbia University College of Physicians and Surgeons Program
Sponsor: Stamford Hospital
Program Director:
Frances W Ginsburg, MD
Stamford Hospital
Shelburne Rd and W Broad St
Stamford, CT 06902
Tel: 203 325-7462 *Fax:* 203 325-7259
Internet: http://www.stamhealth.org
Accred Length: 4 Years *Program Size:* 9 (*GY1:* 3)
Program ID: 220-08-11-061

Delaware

Wilmington

Christiana Care Health Services Program
Sponsor: Christiana Care Health Services Inc
Program Director:
Paul Kaminski, MD
Christiana Hospital
4755 Ogletown Stanton Rd
PO Box 6001
Newark, DE 19718
Tel: 302 733-6565 *Fax:* 302 733-3340
E-mail: pkaminski@christianacare.org
Internet: http://www.mcdresidency.org
Accred Length: 4 Years *Program Size:* 16 (*GY1:* 4)
Program ID: 220-09-11-062

District of Columbia

Washington

George Washington University Program
Sponsor: George Washington University School of Medicine
Fairfax Hospital
George Washington University Hospital (UHS)
Holy Cross Hospital of Silver Spring
Program Director:
John W Larsen Jr, MD
Dept of Ob/Gyn
2150 Pennsylvania Ave NW
Washington, DC 20037
Tel: 202 994-8283 *Fax:* 202 994-0815
E-mail: obgbcb@gwumc.edu
Internet: http://www.gwu.edu/~resobgyn
Accred Length: 4 Years *Program Size:* 36 (*GY1:* 9)
Program ID: 220-10-21-064

Georgetown University Program
Sponsor: Georgetown University Medical Center
Arlington Hospital
Providence Hospital
Program Director:
Anthony R Scialli, MD
Georgetown Univ Med Ctr
Dept of Ob/Gyn
3800 Reservoir Rd NW/3 PHC
Washington, DC 20007-2197
Tel: 202 687-8533 *Fax:* 202 687-4018
E-mail: everettm@gunet.georgetown.edu
Accred Length: 4 Years *Program Size:* 24 (*GY1:* 6)
Program ID: 220-10-21-063

Howard University Program
Sponsor: Howard University Hospital
Prince George's Hospital Center
Program Director:
Deborah M Smith, MD MPH
Howard Univ Hospital
2041 Georgia Ave NW
Washington, DC 20060
Tel: 202 865-4162 *Fax:* 202 865-6922
Accred Length: 4 Years *Program Size:* 16 (*GY1:* 4)
Program ID: 220-10-21-065

Washington Hospital Center Program
Sponsor: Washington Hospital Center
Program Director:
Phillip J Goldstein, MD
Washington Hospital Ctr
110 Irving St NW/Ste 5B-63
Washington, DC 20010-2975
Tel: 202 877-6054 *Fax:* 202 877-5435
E-mail: pjg2@mhg.edu
Internet: http://www.whc.mhg.edu/womens_index.html
Accred Length: 4 Years *Program Size:* 16 (*GY1:* 4)
Program ID: 220-10-31-067

Florida

Gainesville

University of Florida Program
Sponsor: University of Florida College of Medicine
Shands Hospital at the University of Florida
Program Director:
W Patrick Duff, MD
Univ of Florida Coll of Med, Dept of Ob/Gyn
PO Box 100294
1600 SW Archer Rd
Gainesville, FL 32610-0294
Tel: 352 392-9449 *Fax:* 352 392-2808
E-mail: snydermc@obgyn.med.ufl.edu
Internet: http://www.med.ufl.edu/obgyn
Accred Length: 4 Years *Program Size:* 16 (*GY1:* 4)
Program ID: 220-11-11-068

Jacksonville

University of Florida Health Science Center/Jacksonville Program
Sponsor: University of Florida College of Medicine at Jacksonville
University Medical Center (UFHSC/J)
Program Director:
Guy Benrubi, MD
Univ of Florida Health Science Ctr-Jacksonville
653-1 W 8th St
Jacksonville, FL 32209
Tel: 904 549-3112 *Fax:* 904 549-3124
E-mail: glh@umc2.umc.ufl.edu
Internet: http://www.ufhscj.edu/obgyn
Accred Length: 4 Years *Program Size:* 24 (*GY1:* 6)
Program ID: 220-11-21-069

Miami

University of Miami-Jackson Memorial Medical Center Program
Sponsor: University of Miami-Jackson Memorial Medical Center
Program Director:
Allan G W McLeod, MD
Jackson Memorial Med Ctr
1611 NW 12th Ave
East Tower/Rm 3003
Miami, FL 33136
Tel: 305 585-5130 *Fax:* 305 324-8558
E-mail: vlegge@obgyn.med.miami.edu
Accred Length: 4 Years *Program Size:* 36 (*GY1:* 9)
Program ID: 220-11-21-070

Orlando

Orlando Regional Healthcare System Program
Sponsor: Orlando Regional Medical Center
Program Director:
Stephen J Carlan, MD
Orlando Regional Healthcare System
105 W Miller St
Orlando, FL 32806-2093
Tel: 407 841-5297 *Fax:* 407 425-5947
E-mail: scarlan@orhs.org
Internet: http://www.meded-obgyn.orhs.org
Accred Length: 4 Years *Program Size:* 16 (*GY1:* 4)
Program ID: 220-11-12-072

Pensacola

University of Florida College of Medicine (Pensacola) Program
Sponsor: University of Florida College of Medicine
Sacred Heart Hospital of Pensacola
Program Director:
Jorge D Blanco, MD
Univ of Florida Coll of Med-Pensacola
Dept of Ob/Gyn
5045 Carpenter Creek Dr
Pensacola, FL 32503
Tel: 850 416-2418 *Fax:* 850 416-2467
E-mail: jlaurene@sacred-heart.org
Internet: http://www.sacred-heart.org/obgynres.html
Accred Length: 4 Years *Program Size:* 12 (*GY1:* 3)
Program ID: 220-11-21-073

St Petersburg

Bayfront Medical Center Program
Sponsor: Bayfront Medical Center
Program Director:
Karen A Raimer, MD
Bayfront Med Ctr
Ob/Gyn Residency
700 6th St S
St Petersburg, FL 33701
Tel: 813 893-6917 *Fax:* 813 893-6978
E-mail: obres@bayfront.org
Internet: http://www.bayfront.org
Accred Length: 4 Years *Program Size:* 12 (*GY1:* 3)
Program ID: 220-11-11-074

Tampa

University of South Florida Program
Sponsor: University of South Florida College of Medicine
H Lee Moffitt Cancer Center
Tampa General Healthcare
Program Director:
William N Spellacy, MD
Univ of South Florida
Harbourside Medical Tower #500
4 Columbia Dr
Tampa, FL 33606
Tel: 813 254-7774 *Fax:* 813 254-0940
E-mail: mcochran@com1.med.usf.edu
Accred Length: 4 Years *Program Size:* 24 (*GY1:* 6)
Program ID: 220-11-21-075

Georgia

Atlanta

Emory University Program
Sponsor: Emory University School of Medicine
Grady Memorial Hospital
Program Director:
Hugh W Randall, MD
Dept of Ob/Gyn
69 Butler St SE
Atlanta, GA 30303
Tel: 404 616-3540 *Fax:* 404 521-3589
E-mail: gynobresidency@emory.edu
Internet: http://www.emory.edu/whsc/med/gyn-ob
Accred Length: 4 Years *Program Size:* 41 (*GY1:* 10)
Program ID: 220-12-21-076

Georgia Baptist Medical Center Program
Sponsor: Georgia Baptist Medical Center
Program Director:
David C Richardson, MD
Georgia Baptist Med Ctr
Dept of Ob/Gyn
303 Parkway Dr NE/Box 423
Atlanta, GA 30312
Tel: 404 265-4600 *Fax:* 404 265-4989
E-mail: sockness@mindspring.com
Accred Length: 4 Years *Program Size:* 12 (*GY1:* 3)
Program ID: 220-12-22-077

Morehouse School of Medicine Program
Sponsor: Morehouse School of Medicine
Grady Memorial Hospital
Program Director:
Franklyn H Geary Jr, MD
Dept of Ob/Gyn
720 Westview Dr SW
Atlanta, GA 30310-1495
Tel: 404 616-6634 *Fax:* 404 616-6633
E-mail: www.gearyf@msm.edu
Accred Length: 4 Years *Program Size:* 6 (*GY1:* 3)
Program ID: 220-12-21-348

Augusta

Medical College of Georgia Program
Sponsor: Medical College of Georgia Hospital and Clinics
University Hospital
Program Director:
Michael S Macfee, MD
Med Coll of Georgia Hospital and Clinics
Dept of Ob/Gyn
Rm BAA 700
Augusta, GA 30912-3305
Tel: 706 721-3591 *Fax:* 706 721-6211
E-mail: obgyn.mmacfee@mail.mcg.edu
Internet: http://www.mcg.edu/som/obgyn/index.html
Accred Length: 4 Years *Program Size:* 16 (*GY1:* 4)
Program ID: 220-12-21-078

Macon

Mercer University School of Medicine Program
Sponsor: Medical Center of Central Georgia

Program Director:
George D Haber, MD
Med Ctr of Central Georgia
792 Pine St
Macon, GA 31201
Tel: 912 633-1056 *Fax:* 912 749-9171
E-mail: ghaber@mccgobgyn.com
Internet: http://www.mccgobgyn.com
Accred Length: 4 Years *Program Size:* 12 (*GY1:* 3)
Program ID: 220-12-11-079

Savannah

Memorial Medical Center Program
Sponsor: Memorial Medical Center

Program Director:
Donald G Gallup, MD
Memorial Med Ctr
PO Box 23089
Savannah, GA 31403-3089
Tel: 912 350-3595 *Fax:* 912 350-3932
Accred Length: 4 Years *Program Size:* 12 (*GY1:* 3)
Program ID: 220-12-11-080

Hawaii

Honolulu

Tripler Army Medical Center Program
Sponsor: Tripler Army Medical Center

Program Director:
Michael K Yancey, MD
Dept of Ob/Gyn (Attn: MCHK-OB)
Tripler Army Med Ctr
1 Jarrett White Rd
Honolulu, HI 96859-5000
Tel: 808 433-6621 *Fax:* 808 433-1552
E-mail: michael_k.yancey@tamc.chcs.amedd.army.mil
Internet: http://204.208.13.60/obgyn/index.html
Accred Length: 4 Years *Program Size:* 20 (*GY1:* 5)
Program ID: 220-14-12-007
US Armed Services Program

University of Hawaii Program
Sponsor: University of Hawaii John A Burns School of Medicine
Kapiolani Medical Center for Women and Children
Queen's Medical Center

Program Director:
Roy T Nakayama, MD
Univ of Hawaii
Dept of Ob/Gyn
1319 Punahou St/Rm 824
Honolulu, HI 96826
Tel: 808 956-7457
E-mail: kamikawa@jabsom.biomed.hawaii.edu
Internet: http://medworld.biomed.hawaii.edu/hrp/hrp.html
Accred Length: 4 Years *Program Size:* 24 (*GY1:* 6)
Program ID: 220-14-31-081

Illinois

Chicago

Catholic Health Partners Program
Sponsor: Catholic Health Partners

Program Director:
Abdol H Hosseinian, MD
St Joseph Hospital
2900 N Lake Shore Dr
Chicago, IL 60657-6274
Tel: 773 665-3132 *Fax:* 773 665-3718
E-mail: stjobgyn@interaccess.com
Internet: http://www.cath-health.org
Accred Length: 4 Years *Program Size:* 18 (*GY1:* 4)
Program ID: 220-16-11-091

Cook County Hospital Program
Sponsor: Cook County Hospital

Program Director:
Julie B Schmidt, MD
Cook County Hospital
1835 W Harrison St
Chicago, IL 60612-9985
Tel: 312 633-8638 *Fax:* 312 633-5652
Accred Length: 4 Years *Program Size:* 22 (*GY1:* 4)
Program ID: 220-16-31-084

Illinois Masonic Medical Center Program
Sponsor: Illinois Masonic Medical Center

Program Director:
Stephen R Locher, MD
Illinois Masonic Med Ctr
Dept of Ob/Gyn
836 W Wellington Ave
Chicago, IL 60657-5193
Tel: 773 296-5590 *Fax:* 773 296-7207
Internet: http://www.signetusa.net/immcobg
Accred Length: 4 Years *Program Size:* 12 (*GY1:* 3)
Program ID: 220-16-21-085

McGaw Medical Center of Northwestern University Program
Sponsor: Northwestern University Medical School
Evanston Hospital
Northwestern Memorial Hospital

Program Director:
Sharon L Dooley, MD MPH
Northwestern Univ Med Sch
Prentice Women's Hospital
333 E Superior St/#404-F
Chicago, IL 60611
Tel: 312 926-7522 *Fax:* 312 926-1416
E-mail: nu-obgyn@nmh.org
Internet: http://www.nums.nwu.edu/gme/obgyn.htm
Accred Length: 4 Years *Program Size:* 32 (*GY1:* 8)
Program ID: 220-16-21-089

Mercy Hospital and Medical Center Program
Sponsor: Mercy Hospital and Medical Center

Program Director:
Donna S Kirz, MD
Mercy Hospital and Med Ctr
2525 S Michigan Ave
Chicago, IL 60616-2477
Tel: 312 567-2490 *Fax:* 312 567-2628
E-mail: apage@mercy-chicago.org
Accred Length: 4 Years *Program Size:* 12 (*GY1:* 3)
Program ID: 220-16-11-086

Mount Sinai Hospital Medical Center of Chicago Program
Sponsor: Mount Sinai Hospital Medical Center of Chicago

Program Director:
Josef Blankstein, MD
Mount Sinai Hospital Med Ctr
Dept of Ob/Gyn
California Ave at 15th St (F208)
Chicago, IL 60608
Tel: 773 257-6727 *Fax:* 773 257-6359
E-mail: walsh@sinai.org
Internet: http://www./hfnet.sinai.org/
Accred Length: 4 Years *Program Size:* 12 (*GY1:* 3)
Program ID: 220-16-11-088

Rush-Presbyterian-St Luke's Medical Center Program
Sponsor: Rush-Presbyterian-St Luke's Medical Center
Rush North Shore Medical Center

Program Director:
Dee E Fenner, MD
Rush-Presbyterian-St Luke's Med Ctr
1653 W Congress Pkwy
Chicago, IL 60612
Tel: 312 942-6610 *Fax:* 312 942-6606
E-mail: jrodney@rush.edu
Accred Length: 4 Years *Program Size:* 24 (*GY1:* 6)
Program ID: 220-16-21-090

University of Chicago Program
Sponsor: University of Chicago Hospitals
MacNeal Memorial Hospital

Program Director:
Arthur L Herbst, MD
Univ of Chicago Hospitals
5841 S Maryland Ave/MC2050
Chicago, IL 60637-1470
Tel: 773 702-3409 *Fax:* 773 702-0840
Internet: http://bsd.uchicago.edu/~obgyn/
Accred Length: 4 Years *Program Size:* 24 (*GY1:* 6)
Program ID: 220-16-11-092

University of Illinois College of Medicine at Chicago Program
Sponsor: University of Illinois College of Medicine at Chicago
Christ Hospital and Medical Center
Michael Reese Hospital and Medical Center
University of Illinois Hospital and Clinics

Program Director:
Gloria Elam, MD
Univ of Illinois Hospital
Dept of Ob/Gyn (M/C 808)
820 S Wood St
Chicago, IL 60612
Tel: 312 996-7430 *Fax:* 312 996-4238
E-mail: jclark@uic.edu
Internet: http://www.obgyn.uic.edu
Accred Length: 4 Years *Program Size:* 40 (*GY1:* 10)
Program ID: 220-16-11-093

Evanston

St Francis Hospital of Evanston Program
Sponsor: St Francis Hospital of Evanston
Evanston Hospital

Program Director:
John V Knaus, DO
St Francis Hospital of Evanston
Dept of Ob/Gyn
355 Ridge Ave
Evanston, IL 60202
Tel: 847 316-6227 *Fax:* 847 316-3307
E-mail: jobbradovic@alverno.ssfhs.org
Internet: http://www.reshealth.org
Accred Length: 4 Years *Program Size:* 8 (*GY1:* 2)
Program ID: 220-16-21-094

Maywood

Loyola University Program

Sponsor: Loyola University Medical Center
MacNeal Memorial Hospital
West Suburban Hospital Medical Center
Program Director:
John G Gianopoulos, MD
Loyola Univ Med Ctr
Dept of Ob/Gyn
2160 S First Ave
Maywood, IL 60153
Tel: 708 216-5459 *Fax:* 708 216-5669
E-mail: lmerril@wpo.it.edu
Accred Length: 4 Years *Program Size:* 14 (*GY1:* 3)
Program ID: 220-16-21-095

Park Ridge

Lutheran General Hospital Program

Sponsor: Lutheran General Hospital
Program Director:
James D Keller, MD
Lutheran General Hospital
Dept of Ob/Gyn 4-S
1775 W Dempster St
Park Ridge, IL 60068
Tel: 847 723-6994 *Fax:* 847 723-1658
E-mail: obgyn-lghedu@advocatehealth.com
Accred Length: 4 Years *Program Size:* 12 (*GY1:* 3)
Program ID: 220-16-21-325

Peoria

University of Illinois College of Medicine at Peoria Program

Sponsor: University of Illinois College of Medicine at Peoria
St Francis Medical Center
Program Director:
Kenneth A Hodel, MD
St Francis Med Ctr, Dept of Ob/Gyn
530 NE Glen Oak Ave
Peoria, IL 61637
Tel: 309 655-4163 *Fax:* 309 655-3739
Internet: http://www.uicomp.uic.edu/uicomp.htm
Accred Length: 4 Years *Program Size:* 8 (*GY1:* 2)
Program ID: 220-16-11-096

Springfield

Southern Illinois University Program

Sponsor: Southern Illinois University School of Medicine
Memorial Medical Center
St John's Hospital
Program Director:
Robert C Kaufmann, MD
Southern Illinois Univ Sch of Med
Dept of Ob/Gyn
PO Box 19230
Springfield, IL 62794
Tel: 217 524-6498 *Fax:* 217 557-0906
E-mail: phellmers@wpsmtp.siumed.edu
Accred Length: 4 Years *Program Size:* 16 (*GY1:* 4)
Program ID: 220-16-21-097

Indiana

Indianapolis

Indiana University School of Medicine Program

Sponsor: Indiana University School of Medicine
Clarian IU Hospital
Clarian Methodist Hospital of Indiana
Clarian Riley Hospital for Children
William N Wishard Memorial Hospital
Program Director:
Richard S Hansell, MD
Wishard Memorial Hospital
Dept of Ob/Gyn
1001 W 10th St/F-5
Indianapolis, IN 46202-2879
Tel: 317 630-6594 *Fax:* 317 630-6524
E-mail: obrespgm@iupui.edu
Internet: http://www.medlib.iupui.edu/obgyn/reside.html#menu
Accred Length: 4 Years *Program Size:* 40 (*GY1:* 10)
Program ID: 220-17-21-099

St Vincent Hospital and Health Care Center Program

Sponsor: St Vincent Hospital and Health Care Center
Program Director:
Haywood L Brown Sr, MD
Raymond D Rice, MD
Dept of Ob/Gyn
2001 W 86th St
Indianapolis, IN 46260
Tel: 317 338-3745 *Fax:* 317 338-6358
E-mail: hbrown@stvincent.org
Internet: http://www.stvincent.org
Accred Length: 4 Years *Program Size:* 12 (*GY1:* 3)
Program ID: 220-17-11-101

Iowa

Iowa City

University of Iowa Hospitals and Clinics Program

Sponsor: University of Iowa Hospitals and Clinics
Program Director:
Joel I Sorosky, MD
Univ of Iowa Hospitals and Clinics
Dept of Ob/Gyn
200 Hawkins Dr
Iowa City, IA 52242-1009
Tel: 319 356-3617 *Fax:* 319 356-3901
E-mail: joel-sorosky@uiowa.edu
Accred Length: 4 Years *Program Size:* 20 (*GY1:* 5)
Program ID: 220-18-21-102

Kansas

Kansas City

University of Kansas Medical Center Program

Sponsor: University of Kansas School of Medicine
University of Kansas Medical Center
Program Director:
Sterling B Williams, MD
Univ of Kansas Med Ctr
3901 Rainbow Blvd
Dept of Ob/Gyn
Kansas City, KS 66160-7316
Tel: 913 588-6250 *Fax:* 913 588-6271
E-mail: vdodd@kumc.edu
Accred Length: 4 Years *Program Size:* 12 (*GY1:* 3)
Program ID: 220-19-11-103

Wichita

University of Kansas (Wichita) Program

Sponsor: University of Kansas School of Medicine (Wichita)
Columbia Wesley Medical Center
Program Director:
Travis W Stembridge, MD
Wesley Med Ctr
550 N Hillside
Wichita, KS 67214
Tel: 316 688-3182 *Fax:* 316 688-3152
E-mail: dhorbelt@kumc.edu
Internet: http://www.kumc.edu/wichita/dept/obgyn/
Accred Length: 4 Years *Program Size:* 20 (*GY1:* 5)
Program ID: 220-19-11-104

Kentucky

Lexington

University of Kentucky Medical Center Program

Sponsor: University of Kentucky Hospital
Program Director:
Paul DePriest, MD
Univ of Kentucky-Chandler Med Ctr
800 Rose St
Lexington, KY 40536-0084
Tel: 606 323-5389 *Fax:* 606 323-1931
Accred Length: 4 Years *Program Size:* 20 (*GY1:* 5)
Program ID: 220-20-11-105

Louisville

University of Louisville Program

Sponsor: University of Louisville School of Medicine
Kosair Children's Hospital (Alliant Health System)
Norton Hospital (Alliant Health System)
University of Louisville Hospital
Program Director:
Stanley A Gall, MD
Dept of Ob/Gyn
Univ of Louisville
550 S Jackson
Louisville, KY 40292
Tel: 502 852-5811 *Fax:* 502 852-1451
Accred Length: 4 Years *Program Size:* 24 (*GY1:* 6)
Program ID: 220-20-21-106

Louisiana

New Orleans

Alton Ochsner Medical Foundation Program

Sponsor: Alton Ochsner Medical Foundation
Leonard J Chabert Medical Center
Program Director:
Wallace P Begneaud, MD
Alton Ochsner Med Foundation
Dept of Grad Med Educ
1516 Jefferson Hwy
New Orleans, LA 70121
Tel: 504 842-3260 *Fax:* 504 842-3193
E-mail: dlambert@ochsner.org
Internet: http://www.ochsner.org
Accred Length: 4 Years *Program Size:* 16 (*GY1:* 4)
Program ID: 220-21-22-109

Louisiana State University Program
Sponsor: Louisiana State University School of Medicine
Earl K Long Medical Center
Medical Center of Louisiana at New Orleans
University Medical Center (Lafayette)
Program Director:
Ralph Chesson, MD
Louisiana State Univ Med Ctr
Dept of Ob/Gyn
1542 Tulane Ave
New Orleans, LA 70112
Tel: 504 599-1339 *Fax:* 504 599-1340
E-mail: lhull@lsumc.edu
Accred Length: 4 Years *Program Size:* 36 (*GY1:* 9)
Program ID: 220-21-21-107

Tulane University Program
Sponsor: Tulane University School of Medicine
Huey P Long Regional Medical Center
Medical Center of Louisiana at New Orleans
Tulane University Hospital and Clinics
Program Director:
April G O'Quinn, MD
Tulane Univ Sch of Med
1430 Tulane Ave/Box SL-11
New Orleans, LA 70112-2699
Tel: 504 588-5216 *Fax:* 504 584-1846
E-mail: dclaver@tmcpop.tmc.tulane.edu
Internet: http://ww1.omi.tulane.edu/departments/ob-gyn/outline.htm
Accred Length: 4 Years *Program Size:* 36 (*GY1:* 9)
Program ID: 220-21-21-108

Shreveport

Louisiana State University (Shreveport) Program
Sponsor: Louisiana State University Hospital-Shreveport
E A Conway Medical Center
Program Director:
Steve London, MD
Louisiana State Univ Med Ctr Hospital
Medical Education Dept
1501 Kings Hwy/PO Box 33932
Shreveport, LA 71130-3932
Tel: 318 675-5379 *Fax:* 318 675-4671
Internet: http://155.58.115.122/obg/index.html
Accred Length: 4 Years *Program Size:* 24 (*GY1:* 6)
Program ID: 220-21-11-110

Maine

Portland

Maine Medical Center Program
Sponsor: Maine Medical Center
Program Director:
Alan R Alexander, MD
Maine Med Ctr
Dept of Ob/Gyn
22 Bramhall St
Portland, ME 04102
Tel: 207 871-2749 *Fax:* 207 871-6252
E-mail: data.crotec@mail.mmc.org
Internet: http://www.mmc.org
Accred Length: 4 Years *Program Size:* 12 (*GY1:* 3)
Program ID: 220-22-11-111

Maryland

Baltimore

Franklin Square Hospital Center Program
Sponsor: Franklin Square Hospital Center
Program Director:
Gerald A Glowacki, MD MBA
Franklin Square Hospital Ctr
Dept of Ob/Gyn
9000 Franklin Square Dr
Baltimore, MD 21237-3998
Tel: 410 682-7061 *Fax:* 410 682-8180
E-mail: fshobgyn@helix.org
Internet: http://www.helixhealth.com
Accred Length: 4 Years *Program Size:* 12 (*GY1:* 3)
Program ID: 220-23-21-112

Greater Baltimore Medical Center Program
Sponsor: Greater Baltimore Medical Center
University of Maryland School of Medicine
Program Director:
Alfred E Bent, MD
Greater Baltimore Med Ctr
6569 N Charles St/Ste 307
Baltimore, MD 21204
Tel: 410 828-2386 *Fax:* 410 512-8068
Accred Length: 4 Years *Program Size:* 13 (*GY1:* 4)
Program ID: 220-23-31-113

Johns Hopkins University Program
Sponsor: Johns Hopkins University School of Medicine
Johns Hopkins Bayview Medical Center
Johns Hopkins Hospital
Program Director:
Harold E Fox, MD
Johns Hopkins Hospital
Dept of Ob/Gyn
600 N Wolfe St/Harvey 302
Baltimore, MD 21287
Tel: 410 614-0950 *Fax:* 410 955-1003
Internet: http://www.med.jhu.edu/obgyn-residency/
Accred Length: 4 Years *Program Size:* 28 (*GY1:* 7)
Program ID: 220-23-21-114

Maryland General Hospital Program
Sponsor: Maryland General Hospital
Program Director:
Bruce S Gneshin, MD
Maryland General Hospital
827 Linden Ave
Baltimore, MD 21201
Tel: 410 225-8475 *Fax:* 410 225-8754
E-mail: mghlib@earthlink.net
Accred Length: 4 Years *Program Size:* 8 (*GY1:* 2)
Program ID: 220-23-11-115

Sinai Hospital of Baltimore Program
Sponsor: Sinai Hospital of Baltimore
Program Director:
Marc Lowen, MD
Sinai Hospital
Med Staff/Educ Office
2401 W Belvedere Ave
Baltimore, MD 21215-5271
Tel: 410 601-9720 *Fax:* 410 601-6308
Internet: http://www.sinai-balt.com
Accred Length: 4 Years *Program Size:* 16 (*GY1:* 4)
Program ID: 220-23-12-118

Union Memorial Hospital Program
Sponsor: Union Memorial Hospital
Program Director:
Sanford M Markham, MD
Union Memorial Hospital
201 E University Pkwy
Baltimore, MD 21218-2895
Tel: 410 554-2824 *Fax:* 410 554-2255
E-mail: maryken@helix.org
Accred Length: 4 Years *Program Size:* 8 (*GY1:* 2)
Program ID: 220-23-12-120

University of Maryland Program
Sponsor: University of Maryland Medical System
Mercy Medical Center
Program Director:
Harry W Johnson Jr, MD
Univ of Maryland Med System
22 S Greene St
Baltimore, MD 21201
Tel: 410 328-5959 *Fax:* 410 328-8389
Internet: http://www.umm.edu/obgyn/main.html
Accred Length: 4 Years *Program Size:* 24 (*GY1:* 6)
Program ID: 220-23-21-121

Bethesda

National Capital Consortium Program
Sponsor: National Capital Consortium
National Naval Medical Center (Bethesda)
Walter Reed Army Medical Center
Program Director:
Andrew J Satin, MD
Dept of Ob/Gyn
4301 Jones Bridge Rd
Bethesda, MD 20814-4799
Tel: 301 295-4390 *Fax:* 301 295-6240
Accred Length: 4 Years *Program Size:* 27 (*GY1:* 6)
Program ID: 220-10-21-354
US Armed Services Program

Massachusetts

Boston

Beth Israel Deaconess Medical Center (East Campus) Program
Sponsor: Beth Israel Deaconess Medical Center
Program Director:
Henry Klapholz, MD
Beth Israel Deaconess Med Ctr
Harvard Med Sch
330 Brookline Ave
Boston, MA 02215
Tel: 617 667-2285 *Fax:* 617 667-5011
E-mail: hklaphol@bidmc.harvard.edu
Accred Length: 4 Years *Program Size:* 20 (*GY1:* 5)
Program ID: 220-24-11-123

Boston University Medical Center Program
Sponsor: Boston Medical Center
Malden Hospital
Program Director:
Phillip G Stubblefield, MD
Boston Univ Med Ctr
One Boston Medical Center Pl/Mat-3
Boston, MA 02118-2393
Tel: 617 534-5167 *Fax:* 617 534-7300
E-mail: phillip.stubblefield@bmc.org
Accred Length: 4 Years *Program Size:* 17 (*GY1:* 5)
Program ID: 220-24-21-124

Brigham and Women's Hospital Program
Sponsor: Brigham and Women's Hospital
Massachusetts General Hospital
Program Director:
Robert L Barbieri, MD
Brigham and Women's Hospital
Dept of Ob/Gyn
75 Francis St
Boston, MA 02115
Tel: 617 732-7801 *Fax:* 617 730-2833
Accred Length: 4 Years *Program Size:* 36 *(GY1:* 9)
Program ID: 220-24-11-125

Tufts University Program
Sponsor: New England Medical Center Hospitals
St Elizabeth's Medical Center of Boston
Program Director:
Robert D Kennison, MD
New England Med Ctr
750 Washington St
NEMC Box 022
Boston, MA 02111
Tel: 617 636-0265 *Fax:* 617 636-8315
E-mail: starla.pathak@es.nemc.org
Accred Length: 4 Years *Program Size:* 20 *(GY1:* 5)
Program ID: 220-24-21-128

Springfield

Baystate Medical Center Program
Sponsor: Baystate Medical Center
Program Director:
Ronald Burkman, MD
Baystate Med Ctr
Dept of Ob/Gyn
759 Chestnut St
Springfield, MA 01199
Tel: 413 784-5321 *Fax:* 413 784-8166
Accred Length: 4 Years *Program Size:* 20 *(GY1:* 5)
Program ID: 220-24-12-129

Worcester

University of Massachusetts Program
Sponsor: University of Massachusetts Medical School
UMass Memorial Health Care (Memorial Campus)
UMass Memorial Health Care (University Campus)
Program Director:
Jeffrey Riley, MD
Univ of Massachusetts Memorial Health Care
Memorial Campus
119 Belmont St
Worcester, MA 01655
Tel: 508 792-8459 *Fax:* 508 793-6063
Accred Length: 4 Years *Program Size:* 20 *(GY1:* 5)
Program ID: 220-24-21-130

Michigan

Ann Arbor

St Joseph Mercy Hospital Program
Sponsor: St Joseph Mercy Health System
University of Michigan Hospitals
Program Director:
Daniel G McMurtrie, MD
St Joseph Mercy Hospital
5333 McAuley Dr/Ste R-2112
Ypsilanti, MI 48197
Tel: 734 712-3793 *Fax:* 734 712-4151
E-mail: sjmhob@rust.net
Internet: http://www.rust.net/~sjmhob
Accred Length: 4 Years *Program Size:* 12 *(GY1:* 3)
Program ID: 220-25-31-131

University of Michigan Program
Sponsor: University of Michigan Hospitals
Program Director:
John F Randolph Jr, MD
Univ of Michigan Med Sch
L4000 Women's Hospital
1500 E Medical Ctr Dr
Ann Arbor, MI 48109-0276
Tel: 734 936-9434 *Fax:* 734 647-1006
E-mail: mhardy@umich.edu
Internet: http://www.med.umich.edu/obgyn/
Accred Length: 4 Years *Program Size:* 20 *(GY1:* 5)
Program ID: 220-25-31-132

Dearborn

Oakwood Hospital Program
Sponsor: Oakwood Hospital
Program Director:
Sami Guindi, MD
Oakwood Hospital and Med Ctr
18101 Oakwood Blvd
PO Box 2500
Dearborn, MI 48123-2500
Tel: 313 593-7815 *Fax:* 313 436-2783
E-mail: chwalekm@oakwood.org
Internet: http://www.oakwood.org
Accred Length: 4 Years *Program Size:* 16 *(GY1:* 4)
Program ID: 220-25-31-133

Detroit

Henry Ford Hospital Program
Sponsor: Henry Ford Hospital
Program Director:
David A Richardson, MD
Henry Ford Hospital
2799 W Grand Blvd
Detroit, MI 48202
Tel: 313 916-1023 *Fax:* 313 916-2984
E-mail: drichar1@hfhs.org
Internet: http://www.henryfordhealth.org
Accred Length: 4 Years *Program Size:* 12 *(GY1:* 3)
Program ID: 220-25-11-136

St John Hospital and Medical Center Program
Sponsor: St John Hospital and Medical Center
Program Director:
Minuchehr Kashef, MD
St John Hospital and Med Ctr
Dept of Med Educ
22101 Moross Rd
Detroit, MI 48236-2172
Tel: 313 343-3875 *Fax:* 313 343-7840
E-mail: sue.moynihan@stjohn.org
Internet: http://www.stjohn.org
Accred Length: 4 Years *Program Size:* 12 *(GY1:* 3)
Program ID: 220-25-11-137

Wayne State University/Detroit Medical Center (Sinai Hospital) Program
Sponsor: Wayne State University/Detroit Medical Center
Sinai Hospital
Program Director:
David B Schwartz, MD
Sinai Hospital
6767 W Outer Dr
Detroit, MI 48235-2899
Tel: 313 493-5220 *Fax:* 313 493-7503
E-mail: mzakalat@dmc.org
Accred Length: 4 Years *Program Size:* 16 *(GY1:* 4)
Program ID: 220-25-11-138

Wayne State University/Detroit Medical Center Program
Sponsor: Wayne State University/Detroit Medical Center
Grace Hospital
Hutzel Hospital
Program Director:
Carl Christensen, MD
Carole Kowalczyk, MD
Hutzel Hospital
4704 St Antoine Blvd
Detroit, MI 48201
Tel: 313 966-0149 *Fax:* 313 993-7801
E-mail: ccmdphd@aol.com
Internet: http://www.compb10.med.wayne.edu/obgyn/educ.htm/
Accred Length: 4 Years *Program Size:* 47 *(GY1:* 11)
Program ID: 220-25-21-139

Flint

Hurley Medical Center/Michigan State University Program
Sponsor: Hurley Medical Center
Program Director:
John Hebert, MD
Hurley Med Ctr
One Hurley Plaza
Dept of OBG
Flint, MI 48502-5993
Tel: 810 762-6426 *Fax:* 810 235-1210
Accred Length: 4 Years *Program Size:* 12 *(GY1:* 3)
Program ID: 220-25-31-140

Grand Rapids

Spectrum Health-Downtown Campus Program
Sponsor: Spectrum Health-Downtown Campus
Program Director:
Dorsey Ligon, MD
Spectrum Health-Downtown
OB/Gyn Residency/MC 128
100 Michigan NE
Grand Rapids, MI 49503
Tel: 616 391-1929 *Fax:* 616 391-3174
E-mail: lori.marks@spectrum-health.org
Accred Length: 4 Years *Program Size:* 16 *(GY1:* 4)
Program ID: 220-25-11-142

Spectrum Health-East Campus/St Mary's Health Services Program
Sponsor: Spectrum Health-East Campus
St Mary's Health Services
Program Director:
Charles W Newton III, MD
Spectrum Health-East Campus
Medical Education Office
1840 Wealthy St SE
Grand Rapids, MI 49506
Tel: 616 774-7732 *Fax:* 616 774-5290
E-mail: charles_newton@blodgett.com
Accred Length: 4 Years *Program Size:* 16 *(GY1:* 4)
Program ID: 220-25-21-141

Lansing

Sparrow Hospital/Michigan State University Program
Sponsor: Sparrow Hospital
Program Director:
Albert T Shiu, MD
Dept of Ob/Gyn
Sparrow Hospital
1215 E Michigan Ave
Lansing, MI 48909-7980
Tel: 517 483-2577 *Fax:* 517 485-3558
E-mail: albertshiu@prodigy.net
Accred Length: 4 Years *Program Size:* 12 (*GY1:* 3)
Program ID: 220-25-31-143

Pontiac

North Oakland Medical Center Program
Sponsor: North Oakland Medical Center
Program Director:
Leonard Dorey, MD
North Oakland Med Ctrs
461 W Huron
Pontiac, MI 48341
Tel: 248 857-7262 *Fax:* 248 857-6895
E-mail: obgyn@nomc.org
Accred Length: 4 Years *Program Size:* 8 (*GY1:* 2)
Program ID: 220-25-11-144

Royal Oak

William Beaumont Hospital Program
Sponsor: William Beaumont Hospital
Program Director:
John R Musich, MD
William Beaumont Hospital
3601 W 13 Mile Rd
Royal Oak, MI 48073
Tel: 248 551-0427 *Fax:* 248 551-5426
E-mail: jmusich@beaumont.edu
Internet: http://www.beaumont.edu/html/gme
Accred Length: 4 Years *Program Size:* 24 (*GY1:* 6)
Program ID: 220-25-11-146

Saginaw

Saginaw Cooperative Hospitals Program
Sponsor: Saginaw Cooperative Hospitals Inc
Saginaw General Hospital
Program Director:
Joseph F Marshall, MD
Saginaw Cooperative Hospitals
1000 Houghton Ave
Saginaw, MI 48602
Tel: 517 771-6828 *Fax:* 517 771-6941
E-mail: clarkca@pilot.msu.edu
Internet: http://www.chm.msu.edu:80/saginaw/index.html
Accred Length: 4 Years *Program Size:* 12 (*GY1:* 3)
Program ID: 220-25-21-147

Southfield

Providence Hospital and Medical Centers Program
Sponsor: Providence Hospital and Medical Centers
Program Director:
Paul Schnatz, MD
Providence Hospital
Med Educ
16001 W Nine Mile Rd
Southfield, MI 48075-4818
Tel: 248 424-3014 *Fax:* 248 424-5398
E-mail: pschnatz@ic.net
Accred Length: 4 Years *Program Size:* 16 (*GY1:* 4)
Program ID: 220-25-21-148

Minnesota

Minneapolis

University of Minnesota Program
Sponsor: University of Minnesota Medical School
Fairview-University Medical Center
Hennepin County Medical Center
Program Director:
Leo B Twiggs, MD
Univ of Minnesota
420 Delaware St SE
Box 395 UMHC
Minneapolis, MN 55455
Tel: 612 626-3111 *Fax:* 612 626-0665
E-mail: johns586@gold.tc.umn.edu
Internet: http://www.med.umn.edu/obgyn
Accred Length: 4 Years *Program Size:* 24 (*GY1:* 6)
Program ID: 220-26-21-149

Rochester

Mayo Graduate School of Medicine (Rochester) Program
Sponsor: Mayo Graduate School of Medicine-Mayo Foundation
Rochester Methodist Hospital
Program Director:
Timothy O Wilson, MD
Application Processing Ctr
Mayo Graduate Sch of Med
200 First St SW/Siebens 5
Rochester, MN 55905
Tel: 507 284-4331 *Fax:* 507 284-0999
E-mail: mgsm.surgical.specialties@mayo.edu
Internet: http://www.mayo.edu/
Accred Length: 4 Years *Program Size:* 16 (*GY1:* 4)
Program ID: 220-26-21-150

St Paul

HealthPartners Institute for Medical Education Program
Sponsor: HealthPartners Institute for Medical Education
Regions Hospital
United Hospital
Program Director:
John J Yeh, MD
Regions Hospital
Ste 5
640 Jackson St
St Paul, MN 55101-2595
Tel: 612 221-3475 *Fax:* 612 221-8963
E-mail: ob.residency@healthpartners.com
Internet: http://www.healthpartners.com/group/ob/
Accred Length: 4 Years *Program Size:* 12 (*GY1:* 3)
Program ID: 220-26-21-314

Mississippi

Jackson

University of Mississippi Medical Center Program
Sponsor: University of Mississippi School of Medicine
University Hospital
Program Director:
John C Morrison, MD
Univ of Mississippi Med Ctr
Dept of Ob/Gyn
2500 N State St
Jackson, MS 39216
Tel: 601 984-5342 *Fax:* 601 984-5301
E-mail: hmorton@ob-gyn.umsmed.edu
Internet: http://www.obgyn.umsmed.edu
Accred Length: 4 Years *Program Size:* 24 (*GY1:* 6)
Program ID: 220-27-11-151

Keesler AFB

Keesler Medical Center Program
Sponsor: Keesler Medical Center
Program Director:
Lt Col Melissa H Fries, MD
81 MSGS/SGCG
301 Fisher St/Ste 107
Keesler AFB, MS 39534-2576
Tel: 601 377-6396, ext 6730 *Fax:* 601 377-6543
E-mail: fries.melissa@keesler.af.mil
Accred Length: 4 Years *Program Size:* 12 (*GY1:* 3)
Program ID: 220-27-21-002
US Armed Services Program

Missouri

Columbia

University of Missouri-Columbia Program
Sponsor: University of Missouri-Columbia School of Medicine
University Hospitals and Clinics
Program Director:
John W Gay, MD MPH
Univ of Missouri-Columbia
Dept of Ob/Gyn
One Hospital Dr
Columbia, MO 65212
Tel: 573 884-2454 *Fax:* 573 882-9010
E-mail: gayj@health.missouri.edu
Internet: http://www.obgyn.hsc.missouri.edu
Accred Length: 4 Years *Program Size:* 12 (*GY1:* 3)
Program ID: 220-28-11-152

Kansas City

University of Missouri at Kansas City Program
Sponsor: University of Missouri-Kansas City School of Medicine
Saint Luke's Hospital
Truman Medical Center-West
Program Director:
James P Youngblood, MD
Truman Med Ctr
Dept of Ob/Gyn
2301 Holmes St
Kansas City, MO 64108
Tel: 816 556-3454 *Fax:* 816 556-3556
E-mail: jyoungblood@cctr.umkc.edu
Internet: http://www.research.med.umkc.edu/obgyn.ntmc
Accred Length: 4 Years *Program Size:* 32 (*GY1:* 8)
Program ID: 220-28-21-154

St Louis

St John's Mercy Medical Center Program

Sponsor: St John's Mercy Medical Center

Program Director:
Martin L Gimovsky, MD
St John's Mercy Med Ctr
615 S New Ballas Rd
Ste 2009/Tower B
St Louis, MO 63141
Tel: 314 569-6826 *Fax:* 314 995-4376
E-mail: edwakr@stlo.smhs.com
Accred Length: 4 Years *Program Size:* 16 (*GY1:* 4)
Program ID: 220-28-22-157

St Louis University School of Medicine Program

Sponsor: St Louis University School of Medicine
Deaconess Hospital
St Mary's Health Center

Program Director:
Raul Artal, MD
Dept of Ob/Gyn
1031 Bellevue/Ste 290
St Louis, MO 63117
Tel: 314 781-4772, ext 60 *Fax:* 314 781-8582
E-mail: kirchojm@slucare1.sluh.edu.
Internet: http://www.slu.edu/colleges/med/department/obgyn.html
Accred Length: 4 Years *Program Size:* 20 (*GY1:* 5)
Subspecialties: TY
Program ID: 220-28-22-158

Washington University/B-JH/SLCH Consortium Program

Sponsor: Washington University/B-JH/SLCH Consortium
Barnes-Jewish Hospital
Barnes-Jewish Hospital (North Campus)
St Louis ConnectCare

Program Director:
Rebecca P McAlister, MD
Barnes-Jewish Hospital
Box 8064
4911 Barnes-Jewish Hospital Plaza
St Louis, MO 63110
Tel: 314 362-1016 *Fax:* 314 362-0049
E-mail: mcalisterr@msnotes.wustl.edu
Internet: http://www.wumshome.wustl.edu
Accred Length: 4 Years *Program Size:* 33 (*GY1:* 8)
Program ID: 220-28-21-155

Nebraska

Omaha

Creighton University Program

Sponsor: Creighton University School of Medicine
Bergan Mercy Medical Center
Tenet St Joseph Hospital at Creighton Univ Medical Center

Program Director:
Alfred D Fleming, MD
Creighton Univ Med Ctr
601 N 30th St/Ste 4700
Omaha, NE 68131
Tel: 402 280-4438 *Fax:* 402 280-4496
E-mail: kshaul@creightoon.edu
Internet: http://147.134.92.45/obgyn
Accred Length: 4 Years *Program Size:* 12 (*GY1:* 3)
Program ID: 220-30-21-160

University of Nebraska Program

Sponsor: University of Nebraska Medical Center
Methodist Hospital

Program Director:
Carl V Smith, MD
Univ of Nebraska Hospital and Clinic
Dept of Ob/Gyn
983255 Nebraska Med Ctr
Omaha, NE 68198-3255
Tel: 402 559-6150 *Fax:* 402 559-7126
E-mail: cvsmith@mail.unmc.edu
Internet: http://www.unmc.edu
Accred Length: 4 Years *Program Size:* 12 (*GY1:* 3)
Program ID: 220-30-21-161

Nevada

Las Vegas

University of Nevada Program

Sponsor: University of Nevada School of Medicine
University Medical Center of Southern Nevada

Program Director:
Joseph A Rojas, MD
Univ Med Ctr of Southern Nevada
2040 W Charleston Blvd/#200
Las Vegas, NV 89102
Tel: 702 671-2300 *Fax:* 702 671-2333
Internet: http://www.unr.edu/med/residency/southobg.html
Accred Length: 4 Years *Program Size:* 12 (*GY1:* 3)
Program ID: 220-31-21-318

New Hampshire

Lebanon

Dartmouth-Hitchcock Medical Center Program

Sponsor: Mary Hitchcock Memorial Hospital

Program Director:
Emily R Baker, MD
Dartmouth-Hitchcock Med Ctr
Dept of Ob/Gyn
One Medical Center Dr
Lebanon, NH 03756
Tel: 603 650-4658 *Fax:* 603 650-7795
E-mail: meg.m.parker@hitchcock.org
Internet: http://www.hitchcock.org/pages/phys.guide/obstetrics- gynecology.html
Accred Length: 4 Years *Program Size:* 12 (*GY1:* 4)
Program ID: 220-32-12-352

New Jersey

Camden

UMDNJ-Robert Wood Johnson Medical School (Camden) Program

Sponsor: Cooper Hospital-University Medical Center

Program Director:
Ronald M Jaffe, MD
Cooper Hospital-Univ Med Ctr
Dept of Ob/Gyn
3 Cooper Plaza/Ste 211
Camden, NJ 08103
Tel: 609 342-2965 *Fax:* 609 365-1967
Accred Length: 4 Years *Program Size:* 16 (*GY1:* 4)
Program ID: 220-33-11-162

Jersey City

Mount Sinai School of Medicine (Jersey City) Program

Sponsor: Mount Sinai School of Medicine
Jersey City Medical Center

Program Director:
Rhonda R Nichols, MD
Jersey City Med Ctr
Dept of Ob/Gyn
50 Baldwin Ave
Jersey City, NJ 07304
Tel: 201 915-2000, ext 2466 *Fax:* 201 915-2481
Accred Length: 4 Years *Program Size:* 12 (*GY1:* 3)
Program ID: 220-33-21-324

Livingston

St Barnabas Medical Center Program

Sponsor: St Barnabas Medical Center

Program Director:
James L Breen, MD
St Barnabas Med Ctr
94 Old Short Hills Rd
Livingston, NJ 07039
Tel: 973 322-5282 *Fax:* 973 533-4492
E-mail: agundy@spacegate.com
Accred Length: 4 Years *Program Size:* 20 (*GY1:* 5)
Program ID: 220-33-12-163

Long Branch

Monmouth Medical Center Program

Sponsor: Monmouth Medical Center

Program Director:
David M Wallace, MD
Monmouth Med Ctr
Dept of Ob/Gyn Rm 225SW
300 Second Ave
Long Branch, NJ 07740-9998
Tel: 732 923-6795 *Fax:* 732 923-6793
E-mail: wallace@auhs.edu
Accred Length: 4 Years *Program Size:* 8 (*GY1:* 2)
Program ID: 220-33-11-164

Neptune

Jersey Shore Medical Center Program

Sponsor: Jersey Shore Medical Center

Program Director:
Paul G Stumpf, MD
Jersey Shore Med Ctr, Dept of Ob/Gyn
1945 Corlies Ave
Neptune, NJ 07753
Tel: 732 776-4128 *Fax:* 732 776-4525
E-mail: nvalentin@monmouth.com
Internet: http://www.jsmc.com
Accred Length: 4 Years *Program Size:* 8 (*GY1:* 2)
Program ID: 220-33-12-165

Newark

Newark Beth Israel Medical Center Program

Sponsor: Newark Beth Israel Medical Center
St Barnabas Medical Center

Program Director:
Kenneth A Kappy, MD
Newark Beth Israel Med Ctr
201 Lyons Ave
Newark, NJ 07112
Tel: 973 926-4882 *Fax:* 973 705-8650
Internet: http://www.sbhcs.com
Accred Length: 4 Years *Program Size:* 9 (*GY1:* 3)
Program ID: 220-33-21-321

Seton Hall University School of Graduate Medical Education Program
Sponsor: Seton Hall University School of Graduate Medical Education
St Michael's Medical Center (Cathedral Hlth Srvcs Inc)
St Elizabeth Hospital
St James Hospital of Newark
Program Director:
Peter A Beaugard, MD
St Michael's Med Ctr
268 Martin Luther King Blvd/MS 9
Newark, NJ 07102
Tel: 201 877-5350 *Fax:* 201 877-2744
E-mail: janp@tao.agaron.com
Accred Length: 4 Years *Program Size:* 9 (*GY1:* 3)
Program ID: 220-33-21-322

UMDNJ-New Jersey Medical School Program
Sponsor: UMDNJ-New Jersey Medical School
Hackensack University Medical Center
Morristown Memorial Hospital
UMDNJ-University Hospital
Program Director:
Gerson Weiss, MD
UMDNJ-New Jersey Med Sch
185 S Orange Ave/Rm E506
Newark, NJ 07103-2714
Tel: 973 972-5266 *Fax:* 973 972-4574
E-mail: weissge@umdnj.edu
Internet: http://www.umdnj.edu/njmsweb/obgyn
Accred Length: 4 Years *Program Size:* 28 (*GY1:* 7)
Program ID: 220-33-31-166

Paterson

St Joseph's Hospital and Medical Center Program
Sponsor: St Joseph's Hospital and Medical Center
Program Director:
Roger P Kierce, MD
Dept of Ob/Gyn
703 Main St
Paterson, NJ 07503
Tel: 973 754-2700 *Fax:* 973 754-2725
E-mail: kiercer@sjhmc.org
Internet: http://www.sjhmc.org
Accred Length: 4 Years *Program Size:* 8 (*GY1:* 2)
Program ID: 220-33-21-323

Piscataway

UMDNJ-Robert Wood Johnson Medical School (New Brunswick) Program
Sponsor: UMDNJ-Robert Wood Johnson Medical School
Robert Wood Johnson University Hospital
St Peter's University Hospital
Program Director:
Robert A Knuppel, MD MPH
UMDNJ-Robert Wood Johnson Med Sch
125 Paterson St
New Brunswick, NJ 08901-1977
Tel: 732 235-7628 *Fax:* 732 235-7054
E-mail: knuppero@rwja.umdnj.edu
Internet: http://www.rwj-obgyn.umdnj.edu
Accred Length: 4 Years *Program Size:* 24 (*GY1:* 6)
Program ID: 220-33-21-167

New Mexico

Albuquerque

University of New Mexico Program
Sponsor: University of New Mexico School of Medicine
University Hospital
USAF Hospital (Kirtland)
Program Director:
Maxine H Dorin, MD
Univ of New Mexico Sch of Med
Dept of Ob/Gyn ACC-4
2211 Lomas Blvd NE
Albuquerque, NM 87131-5286
Tel: 505 272-6883 *Fax:* 505 272-6385
E-mail: rescoord@somasf.unm.edu
Internet: http://obgyn.unm.edu/obgyn
Accred Length: 4 Years *Program Size:* 24 (*GY1:* 6)
Program ID: 220-34-21-169

New York

Albany

Albany Medical Center Program
Sponsor: Albany Medical Center
St Peter's Hospital
Program Director:
Daniel I Edelstone, MD
Albany Med Ctr
47 New Scotland Ave
Mail Code 74
Albany, NY 12208
Tel: 518 262-5587 *Fax:* 518 262-5292
E-mail: lheckman@ccgateway.amc.edu
Accred Length: 4 Years *Program Size:* 24 (*GY1:* 6)
Program ID: 220-35-21-170

Bronx

Albert Einstein College of Medicine (Jacobi) Program
Sponsor: Albert Einstein College of Medicine of Yeshiva University
Jacobi Medical Center
Montefiore Medical Center-Weiler Hospital
Program Director:
Irwin R Merkatz, MD
Albert Einstein Coll of Med
Belfer/Rm 502
1300 Morris Park Ave
Bronx, NY 10461
Tel: 718 430-4192 *Fax:* 718 931-6670
Internet: http://www.bcohen@aecom.yu.edu
Accred Length: 4 Years *Program Size:* 28 (*GY1:* 7)
Program ID: 220-35-21-178

Albert Einstein College of Medicine Program
Sponsor: Albert Einstein College of Medicine of Yeshiva University
Montefiore Medical Center-Henry and Lucy Moses Division
North Central Bronx Hospital
Program Director:
Richard J Scotti, MD
Albert Einstein Coll of Med-West Campus
111 E 210th St
Rosenthal 4
Bronx, NY 10467
Tel: 718 920-6311 *Fax:* 718 920-6313
E-mail: hlieman@aol.com
Accred Length: 4 Years *Program Size:* 8 (*GY1:* 2)
Program ID: 220-35-21-332

Bronx-Lebanon Hospital Center Program
Sponsor: Bronx-Lebanon Hospital Center
Program Director:
Magdy Mikhail, MD
Bronx Lebanon Hospital Ctr
Dept of Ob/Gyn
1650 Grand Concourse
Bronx, NY 10457
Tel: 718 239-8383 *Fax:* 718 239-8360
E-mail: blhc-ob2@erols.com
Accred Length: 4 Years *Program Size:* 16 (*GY1:* 4)
Program ID: 220-35-11-180

Lincoln Medical and Mental Health Center Program
Sponsor: Lincoln Medical and Mental Health Center
Program Director:
Huseyin Copur, MD
Lincoln Med and Mental Health Ctr
Dept of Ob/Gyn/Rm 518
234 E 149th St
Bronx, NY 10451
Tel: 718 579-5552 *Fax:* 718 579-4699
Accred Length: 4 Years *Program Size:* 12 (*GY1:* 3)
Program ID: 220-35-21-326

New York Medical College (Our Lady of Mercy) Program
Sponsor: New York Medical College
Our Lady of Mercy Medical Center
Program Director:
Kevin D Reilly, MD
Our Lady of Mercy Med Ctr
600 E 233rd St
Bronx, NY 10466
Tel: 718 920-9649
Accred Length: 4 Years *Program Size:* 9 (*GY1:* 3)
Program ID: 220-35-21-330

Brooklyn

Brookdale University Hospital Medical Center Program
Sponsor: Brookdale University Hospital Medical Center
Program Director:
Norma Veridiano, MD
Dept of Ob/Gyn
One Brookdale Plaza
Brooklyn, NY 11212
Tel: 718 240-5978 *Fax:* 718 240-6610
Internet: http://www.brookdalehospital.com
Accred Length: 4 Years *Program Size:* 16 (*GY1:* 4)
Program ID: 220-35-11-181

Brooklyn Hospital Center Program
Sponsor: Brooklyn Hospital Center
Program Director:
George D Kofinas, MD
Brooklyn Hospital Ctr
Dept of Ob/Gyn
121 DeKalb Ave
Brooklyn, NY 11201
Tel: 718 250-6930 *Fax:* 718 250-8881
Accred Length: 4 Years *Program Size:* 17 (*GY1:* 8)
Program ID: 220-35-12-182

Long Island College Hospital Program
Sponsor: Long Island College Hospital
Program Director:
John P Brennan, MD
Long Island College Hospital
339 Hicks St
Brooklyn, NY 11201
Tel: 718 780-1884 *Fax:* 718 780-1392
E-mail: jbrennan@panix.com
Accred Length: 4 Years *Program Size:* 9 (*GY1:* 3)
Program ID: 220-35-12-189

Lutheran Medical Center Program
Sponsor: Lutheran Medical Center

Program Director:
Donald M Zarou, MD
Lutheran Med Ctr
150 55th St
Brooklyn, NY 11220-2574
Tel: 718 630-7350 *Fax:* 718 630-6322
E-mail: ldamato@lmcmc.com
Internet: http://www.lmcmc.com
Accred Length: 4 Years *Program Size:* 12 (*GY1:* 3)
Program ID: 220-35-11-191

Maimonides Medical Center Program
Sponsor: Maimonides Medical Center
Coney Island Hospital

Program Director:
Howard L Minkoff, MD
Maimonides Med Ctr
Dept of Ob/Gyn
4802 Tenth Ave
Brooklyn, NY 11219
Tel: 718 283-7048 *Fax:* 718 283-8468
Accred Length: 4 Years *Program Size:* 20 (*GY1:* 5)
Program ID: 220-35-31-192

New York Methodist Hospital Program
Sponsor: New York Methodist Hospital

Program Director:
Richard H Schwarz, MD
New York Methodist Hospital
506 Sixth St
Brooklyn, NY 11215-9008
Tel: 718 780-3272 *Fax:* 718 780-3079
Accred Length: 4 Years *Program Size:* 13 (*GY1:* 4)
Program ID: 220-35-31-339

SUNY Health Science Center at Brooklyn Program
Sponsor: SUNY Health Science Center at Brooklyn
Kings County Hospital Center
University Hospital-SUNY Health Science Center at Brooklyn

Program Director:
John G Boyce, MD
SUNY Health Science Ctr-Brooklyn
450 Clarkson Ave
Box 24
Brooklyn, NY 11203-2098
Tel: 718 270-3117 *Fax:* 718 270-4223
E-mail: rmatthews@netmail.hscbklyn.edu
Internet: http://www.hscbklyn.edu
Accred Length: 4 Years *Program Size:* 20 (*GY1:* 5)
Program ID: 220-35-21-208

Buffalo

SUNY at Buffalo Graduate Medical-Dental Education Consortium (Sisters of Charity) Program
Sponsor: SUNY at Buffalo Grad Medical-Dental Education Consortium
Sisters of Charity Hospital

Program Director:
Michael Ray, MD
Sisters of Charity Hospital, Dept of Ob/Gyn
2157 Main St
Buffalo, NY 14214
Tel: 716 862-1500 *Fax:* 716 862-1881
Accred Length: 4 Years *Program Size:* 8 (*GY1:* 2)
Program ID: 220-35-21-171

SUNY at Buffalo Graduate Medical-Dental Education Consortium Program
Sponsor: SUNY at Buffalo Grad Medical-Dental Education Consortium
CGF Health System (Buffalo General Hospital)
CGF Health System (Children's Hospital of Buffalo)
CGF Health System (Millard Fillmore Hospitals)

Program Director:
John Choate, MD PHD
Children's Hospital
Dept of Ob/Gyn
219 Bryant St
Buffalo, NY 14222
Tel: 716 878-7138 *Fax:* 716 878-3833
Accred Length: 4 Years *Program Size:* 36 (*GY1:* 8)
Program ID: 220-35-21-172

East Meadow

Nassau County Medical Center Program
Sponsor: Nassau County Medical Center
Mercy Medical Center

Program Director:
Elsie Santana-Fox, MD
Nassau County Med Ctr
2201 Hempstead Turnpike
East Meadow, NY 11554
Tel: 516 572-6255 *Fax:* 516 572-3124
Accred Length: 4 Years *Program Size:* 16 (*GY1:* 4)
Program ID: 220-35-31-174

Flushing

New York Flushing Hospital Medical Center Program
Sponsor: New York Flushing Hospital Medical Center

Program Director:
Joseph A Pennisi, MD
Flushing Hospital Med Ctr
45th Ave at Parsons Blvd
Flushing, NY 11355
Tel: 718 670-5440 *Fax:* 718 670-5780
Accred Length: 4 Years *Program Size:* 13 (*GY1:* 4)
Program ID: 220-35-11-184

Jamaica

Catholic Medical Center of Brooklyn and Queens Program
Sponsor: Catholic Medical Center of Brooklyn and Queens Inc
Catholic Medical Center (Mary Immaculate Hospital)
Catholic Medical Center (St John's Queens Hospital)
Catholic Medical Center (St Mary's Hospital)

Program Director:
Luis A Bracero, MD
Catholic Med Ctr of Brooklyn and Queens
88-25 153rd St
Jamaica, NY 11432
Tel: 718 558-7296 *Fax:* 718 558-5963
E-mail: lbracero@cmcny.com
Accred Length: 4 Years *Program Size:* 18 (*GY1:* 6)
Program ID: 220-35-21-183

Jamaica Hospital Program
Sponsor: Jamaica Hospital

Program Director:
M Maurice Abitbol, MD
Jamaica Hospital Med Ctr
89th Ave and Van Wyck Expwy
Jamaica, NY 11418
Tel: 718 206-6808 *Fax:* 718 206-6829
Accred Length: 4 Years *Program Size:* 8 (*GY1:* 2)
Program ID: 220-35-21-186

Mount Sinai School of Medicine (Jamaica) Program
Sponsor: Mount Sinai School of Medicine
Queens Hospital Center
Mount Sinai Medical Center

Program Director:
Mark Spitzer, MD
Queens Hospital Ctr
82-68 164th St/B 210
Jamaica, NY 11432
Tel: 718 883-4035 *Fax:* 718 883-6129
Accred Length: 4 Years *Program Size:* 12 (*GY1:* 3)
Program ID: 220-35-21-342

Manhasset

North Shore University Hospital/NYU School of Medicine Program
Sponsor: North Shore University Hospital

Program Director:
S Theodore Horwitz, MD
North Shore Univ Hospital
Dept of Ob/Gyn
Manhasset, NY 11030
Tel: 516 562-4435 *Fax:* 516 562-1299
E-mail: cmims@nshs.edu
Internet: http://www.nshs.edu
Accred Length: 4 Years *Program Size:* 17 (*GY1:* 5)
Program ID: 220-35-31-175

Mineola

Winthrop-University Hospital Program
Sponsor: Winthrop-University Hospital

Program Director:
Dev Maulik, MD
Winthrop-Univ Hospital
Dept of Ob/Gyn
259 First St
Mineola, NY 11501
Tel: 516 663-2264 *Fax:* 516 742-7821
Internet: http://www.winthrop.org
Accred Length: 4 Years *Program Size:* 12 (*GY1:* 3)
Program ID: 220-35-12-176

New Hyde Park

Albert Einstein College of Medicine at Long Island Jewish Medical Center Program
Sponsor: Long Island Jewish Medical Center
Syosset Community Hospital

Program Director:
Vicki L Seltzer, MD
Long Island Jewish Med Ctr
270-05 76th Ave
New Hyde Park, NY 11040
Tel: 718 470-7661 *Fax:* 718 962-6739
E-mail: folmer@lij.edu
Internet: http://www.lij.edu/lij-homepage-ns.html
Accred Length: 4 Years *Program Size:* 21 (*GY1:* 6)
Program ID: 220-35-21-190

New York

Albert Einstein College of Medicine at Beth Israel Medical Center Program
Sponsor: Beth Israel Medical Center

Program Director:
David Baram, MD
Beth Israel Med Ctr
First Ave at 16th St
New York, NY 10003
Tel: 212 420-4236 *Fax:* 212 420-2980
E-mail: dbaram@bethisraelny.org
Accred Length: 4 Years *Program Size:* 20 (*GY1:* 5)
Program ID: 220-35-11-179

Harlem Hospital Center Program

Sponsor: Harlem Hospital Center

Program Director:
Barbara Lanzara, MD
Harlem Hospital Ctr
506 Lenox Ave
MLK Pavillion Dept of Ob/Gyn
New York, NY 10037
Tel: 212 939-4336 *Fax:* 212 939-4344
E-mail: obgynharlem@columbia.edu
Accred Length: 4 Years *Program Size:* 6 (*GY1:* 0)
Program ID: 220-35-21-185

Lenox Hill Hospital Program

Sponsor: Lenox Hill Hospital

Program Director:
Michael Y Divon, MD
Dept of Ob/Gyn
Lenox Hill Hospital
100 E 77th St
New York, NY 10021-1883
Tel: 212 434-2160 *Fax:* 212 434-2180
E-mail: lhhobgyn@idt.net
Accred Length: 4 Years *Program Size:* 12 (*GY1:* 3)
Program ID: 220-35-11-188

Mount Sinai School of Medicine Program

Sponsor: Mount Sinai School of Medicine
Elmhurst Hospital Center-Mount Sinai Services
Mount Sinai Medical Center

Program Director:
Michael L Brodman, MD
Mount Sinai Med Ctr
Box 1170
One Gustave L Levy Pl
New York, NY 10029-6574
Tel: 212 241-3144 *Fax:* 212 360-6917
E-mail: mbrodman@smtplink.mssm.edu
Internet: http://www.mssm.edu/obgyn/
Accred Length: 4 Years *Program Size:* 28 (*GY1:* 7)
Program ID: 220-35-21-196

New York and Presbyterian Hospital (Columbia Campus) Program

Sponsor: New York and Presbyterian Hospital
New York and Presbyterian Hospital (Columbia Campus)

Program Director:
Jodi P Lerner, MD
Presbyterian Hospital
Dept of Ob/Gyn
622 W 168th St
New York, NY 10032
Tel: 212 305-2376 *Fax:* 212 305-3869
E-mail: lernerj@columbia3.cis.columbia.edu
Internet: http://cpmcnet.columbia.edu/dept/obgyn/
Accred Length: 4 Years *Program Size:* 20 (*GY1:* 5)
Program ID: 220-35-21-201

New York and Presbyterian Hospital (Cornell Campus) Program

Sponsor: New York and Presbyterian Hospital
New York and Presbyterian Hospital (Cornell Campus)
New York Hospital Medical Center of Queens

Program Director:
William J Ledger, MD
New York Presbyterian Hospital-Cornell Campus
Dept of Ob/Gyn
525 E 68th St/Rm J-130
New York, NY 10021
Tel: 212 746-3058 *Fax:* 212 746-8490
E-mail: cumc-obgyn@mail.med.cornell.edu
Internet: http://www.med.cornell.edu
Accred Length: 4 Years *Program Size:* 25 (*GY1:* 7)
Program ID: 220-35-21-197

New York Medical College at St Vincent's Hospital and Medical Center of New York Program

Sponsor: New York Medical College
St Vincent's Hospital and Medical Center of New York

Program Director:
John Koulos, MD
St Vincent's Hospital and Med Ctr
Dept of Ob/Gyn
153 W 11th St
New York, NY 10011
Tel: 212 604-2070 *Fax:* 212 604-2777
Accred Length: 4 Years *Program Size:* 9 (*GY1:* 3)
Program ID: 220-35-21-205

New York University Medical Center Program

Sponsor: New York University Medical Center
Bellevue Hospital Center

Program Director:
Scott W Smilen, MD
New York Univ Med Ctr
550 First Ave
New York, NY 10016
Tel: 212 562-6594 *Fax:* 212 263-8251
E-mail: scott.smilen@mcobg.med.nyu.edu
Internet: http://www.med.nyu.edu/obgyn/residencytrainprog.html
Accred Length: 4 Years *Program Size:* 25 (*GY1:* 7)
Program ID: 220-35-21-200

NYU Downtown Hospital Program

Sponsor: NYU Downtown Hospital

Program Director:
Iffath A Hoskins, MD PhD
NYU Downtown Hospital
Dept of Ob/Gyn
170 Williams St (8/F)
New York, NY 10038
Tel: 212 312-5880 *Fax:* 212 312-5878
E-mail: nydh-ob@ixnetcom.com
Accred Length: 4 Years *Program Size:* 13 (*GY1:* 4)
Program ID: 220-35-21-198

St Luke's-Roosevelt Hospital Center Program

Sponsor: St Luke's-Roosevelt Hospital Center
St Luke's-Roosevelt Hospital Center-Roosevelt Division
St Luke's-Roosevelt Hospital Center-St Luke's Division

Program Director:
Veronica Gomez-Lobo, MD
Dept of Ob/Gyn
1000 Tenth Ave/Ste 10C01
New York, NY 10019
Tel: 212 523-3348 *Fax:* 212 523-8066
Internet: http://www.wehealny.org
Accred Length: 4 Years *Program Size:* 24 (*GY1:* 6)
Program ID: 220-35-11-204

Rochester

Rochester General Hospital Program

Sponsor: Rochester General Hospital

Program Director:
Fred M Howard, MD MS
Rochester General Hospital
Dept of Ob/Gyn, Box 249
1425 Portland Ave
Rochester, NY 14621-3095
Tel: 716 338-4683 *Fax:* 716 338-3798
E-mail: darbbie.thomas@viahealth.org
Internet: http://www.viahealth.org/rgh/obgyn-residency
Accred Length: 4 Years *Program Size:* 10 (*GY1:* 2)
Program ID: 220-35-31-343

University of Rochester Program

Sponsor: Strong Memorial Hospital of the University of Rochester
Genesee Hospital
Highland Hospital of Rochester

Program Director:
Diane M Hartmann, MD
Strong Memorial Hospital
601 Elmwood Ave
Box 668
Rochester, NY 14642
Tel: 716 275-3733 *Fax:* 716 756-4967
E-mail: jean_boedecker@urmc.rochester.edu
Internet: http://www.rochester.edu/smd/obgyn/obgynhome.html
Accred Length: 4 Years *Program Size:* 38 (*GY1:* 9)
Program ID: 220-35-21-213

Staten Island

New York Medical College (Richmond) Program

Sponsor: New York Medical College
Sisters of Charity Medical Center-St Vincent's Campus

Program Director:
Vincent T Pillari, MD
Sisters of Charity Med Ctr-St Vincent's Campus
355 Bard Ave
Staten Island, NY 10310-1699
Tel: 718 876-4293 *Fax:* 718 876-2865
E-mail: pillari@admin.con2.com
Accred Length: 4 Years *Program Size:* 9 (*GY1:* 3)
Program ID: 220-35-12-206

Staten Island University Hospital Program

Sponsor: Staten Island University Hospital

Program Director:
Mitchell Maiman, MD
Staten Island Univ Hospital
475 Seaview Ave
Staten Island, NY 10305
Tel: 718 226-8074 *Fax:* 718 226-6873
E-mail: smangus@siuh.edu
Internet: http://www.siuh.edu
Accred Length: 4 Years *Program Size:* 9 (*GY1:* 3)
Program ID: 220-35-11-207

Stony Brook

SUNY at Stony Brook Program

Sponsor: University Hospital-SUNY at Stony Brook

Program Director:
Bruce A Meyer, MD
University Hospital
SUNY-Stony Brook
Dept of Ob/Gyn
Stony Brook, NY 11794-8091
Tel: 516 444-2783 *Fax:* 516 444-8954
E-mail: bmeyer@mail.som.sunysb.edu
Internet: http://www.uhmc.sunysb.edu/obgyn/
Accred Length: 4 Years *Program Size:* 16 (*GY1:* 4)
Program ID: 220-35-21-316

Syracuse

SUNY Health Science Center at Syracuse Program
Sponsor: University Hospital-SUNY Health Science Center at Syracuse
Crouse Hospital
Program Director:
Shawky Badawy, MD
SUNY Health Science Ctr-Syracuse
Dept of Ob/Gyn
750 E Adams St
Syracuse, NY 13210
Tel: 315 470-7904 *Fax:* 315 464-4734
Internet: http://www.hscsyr.edu
Accred Length: 4 Years *Program Size:* 20 (*GY1:* 5)
Program ID: 220-35-21-215

Valhalla

New York Medical College at Westchester Medical Center Program
Sponsor: New York Medical College
Metropolitan Hospital Center
Westchester Medical Center
Program Director:
Sari Kaminsky, MD
Metropolitan Hospital Ctr
Dept of Ob/Gyn
1901 First Ave/Rm 3A7
New York, NY 10029
Tel: 212 423-6796 *Fax:* 212 423-8121
Accred Length: 4 Years *Program Size:* 17 (*GY1:* 5)
Program ID: 220-35-21-199

North Carolina

Asheville

Mountain Area Health Education Center Program
Sponsor: Mountain Area Health Education Center
Memorial Mission Hospital
Program Director:
Hal C Lawrence III, MD
MAHEC Dept of Ob/Gyn
60 Livingston St/Ste 100
Asheville, NC 28801
Tel: 828 257-4720 *Fax:* 828 251-0024
E-mail: hall@orca.mtn.ncahec.org
Internet: http://www.mtn.ncahec.org
Accred Length: 4 Years *Program Size:* 16 (*GY1:* 4)
Program ID: 220-36-21-340

Chapel Hill

University of North Carolina Hospitals Program
Sponsor: University of North Carolina Hospitals
Wake Medical Center
Program Director:
Jeffrey A Kuller, MD
CB 7570 MacNider Hall
Univ of North Carolina Sch of Med
Chapel Hill, NC 27599-7570
Tel: 919 966-5096 *Fax:* 919 966-6049
E-mail: kuller@med.unc.edu
Internet: http://www.med.unc.edu/obgyn/resid.htm
Accred Length: 4 Years *Program Size:* 24 (*GY1:* 6)
Program ID: 220-36-21-216

Charlotte

Carolinas Medical Center Program
Sponsor: Carolinas Medical Center
Program Director:
Wallace C Nunley Jr, MD
Dept of Ob/Gyn
PO Box 32861
1000 Blythe Blvd
Charlotte, NC 28232-2861
Tel: 704 355-3153 *Fax:* 704 355-1941
Internet: http://www.carolinas.org
Accred Length: 4 Years *Program Size:* 20 (*GY1:* 5)
Program ID: 220-36-31-217

Durham

Duke University Program
Sponsor: Duke University Medical Center
Program Director:
Charles B Hammond, MD
Duke Univ Med Ctr
Dept of Ob/Gyn
PO Box 3853
Durham, NC 27710-3853
Tel: 919 684-3008 *Fax:* 919 684-6161
E-mail: hammo005@mc.duke.edu
Accred Length: 4 Years *Program Size:* 28 (*GY1:* 7)
Program ID: 220-36-21-219

Greenville

East Carolina University Program
Sponsor: East Carolina University School of Medicine
Pitt County Memorial Hospital
Program Director:
Samuel M Atkinson Jr, MD
Dept of Ob/Gyn
Sch of Med
East Carolina Univ
Greenville, NC 27858-4354
Tel: 252 816-4669 *Fax:* 252 816-5329
E-mail: crichards@brody.med.ecu.edu
Accred Length: 4 Years *Program Size:* 17 (*GY1:* 5)
Program ID: 220-36-21-220

Wilmington

New Hanover Regional Medical Center Program
Sponsor: New Hanover Regional Medical Center
Program Director:
Brent D Wright, MD
New Hanover Regional Med Ctr
Coastal AHEC-Ob/Gyn
PO Box 9025
Wilmington, NC 28402-9025
Tel: 910 343-0161, ext 237 *Fax:* 910 762-2896
Internet: http://www.unc.edu/coahec
Accred Length: 4 Years *Program Size:* 12 (*GY1:* 3)
Program ID: 220-36-11-218

Winston-Salem

Wake Forest University School of Medicine Program
Sponsor: Wake Forest University Baptist Medical Center
Forsyth Memorial Hospital
Program Director:
Joseph M Ernest III, MD
Wake Forest Univ Sch of Med
Dept of Ob/Gyn
Medical Center Blvd
Winston-Salem, NC 27157
Tel: 336 716-4291 *Fax:* 336 716-6937
E-mail: jernest@wfubmc.edu
Internet: http://www.wfubmc.edu
Accred Length: 4 Years *Program Size:* 20 (*GY1:* 5)
Program ID: 220-36-21-221

Ohio

Akron

Akron General Medical Center/NEOUCOM Program
Sponsor: Akron General Medical Center
Program Director:
Michael P Hopkins, MD
Akron General Med Ctr
400 Wabash Ave
Akron, OH 44307
Tel: 330 384-6050 *Fax:* 330 384-1529
E-mail: meded@agmc.org
Internet: http://agmc.org
Accred Length: 4 Years *Program Size:* 12 (*GY1:* 3)
Program ID: 220-38-11-224

Summa Health System (Akron City Hospital)/NEOUCOM Program
Sponsor: Summa Health System
Akron City Hospital (Summa Health System)
Program Director:
Robert F Flora, MD
Summa Health System
Med Educ/Mary Yanik
525 E Market St
Akron, OH 44309
Tel: 800 322-0517
Internet: http://www.summahealth.org/edu/
Accred Length: 4 Years *Program Size:* 16 (*GY1:* 4)
Program ID: 220-38-21-223

Canton

Aultman Hospital/NEOUCOM Program
Sponsor: Aultman Hospital
Program Director:
Alvin Langer, MD
Aultman Hospital
2600 Sixth St SW
Canton, OH 44710-1799
Tel: 330 438-6214 *Fax:* 330 580-5513
E-mail: cdorsey@aultman.com
Internet: http://www.aultmanresidencies.com
Accred Length: 4 Years *Program Size:* 13 (*GY1:* 3)
Program ID: 220-38-21-226

Cincinnati

Bethesda Hospital Program

Sponsor: Bethesda Hospital Inc

Program Director:
Harold E Johnstone, MD
Bethesda Oak Hospital
Dept of Ob/Gyn
619 Oak St/1 West
Cincinnati, OH 45206-1690
Tel: 513 569-6249 *Fax:* 513 569-4072
E-mail: harold_johnstone@trihealth.com
Accred Length: 4 Years *Program Size:* 16 (*GY1:* 4)
Program ID: 220-38-21-227

Good Samaritan Hospital Program

Sponsor: Good Samaritan Hospital

Program Director:
Michael S Baggish, MD
Good Samaritan Hospital
375 Dixmyth Ave
Cincinnati, OH 45220-2489
Tel: 513 872-2750 *Fax:* 513 221-5865
Accred Length: 4 Years *Program Size:* 16 (*GY1:* 4)
Program ID: 220-38-11-228

University Hospital/University of Cincinnati College of Medicine Program

Sponsor: University Hospital Inc
Christ Hospital

Program Director:
Robert W Rebar, MD
Univ of Cincinnati Med Ctr, Dept of Ob/Gyn
PO Box 670526
231 Bethesda Ave
Cincinnati, OH 45267-0526
Tel: 513 558-7653 *Fax:* 513 558-6138
E-mail: lewijj@ucmail.uc.edu
Accred Length: 4 Years *Program Size:* 33 (*GY1:* 9)
Program ID: 220-38-21-229

Cleveland

Case Western Reserve University (MetroHealth) Program

Sponsor: MetroHealth Medical Center
Cleveland Clinic Foundation

Program Director:
Patrick M Catalano, MD
MetroHealth Med Ctr
2500 MetroHealth Dr
Cleveland, OH 44109-1998
Tel: 216 778-4876 *Fax:* 216 778-8847
Accred Length: 4 Years *Program Size:* 20 (*GY1:* 5)
Program ID: 220-38-21-327

Case Western Reserve University Program

Sponsor: University Hospitals of Cleveland

Program Director:
Laszlo Sogor, MD PhD
Univ MacDonald Womens Hospital
11100 Euclid Ave
Cleveland, OH 44106
Tel: 216 844-1692 *Fax:* 216 844-7590
E-mail: lxs12@po.cwru.edu
Accred Length: 4 Years *Program Size:* 16 (*GY1:* 4)
Program ID: 220-38-21-230

Mount Sinai Medical Center of Cleveland Program

Sponsor: Mount Sinai Medical Center of Cleveland

Program Director:
Ori Kushnir, MD
Mt Sinai Med Ctr
Dept of Ob/Gyn
One Mt Sinai Dr
Cleveland, OH 44106-4198
Tel: 216 421-4607 *Fax:* 216 421-3765
Accred Length: 4 Years *Program Size:* 8 (*GY1:* 2)
Program ID: 220-38-11-231

Columbus

Ohio State University Program

Sponsor: Ohio State University Medical Center
Arthur G James Cancer Hospital and Research Institute
Grant Medical Center (OhioHealth)

Program Director:
Philip Samuels, MD
Ohio State Univ Hospital
1654 Upham Dr
507 Means Hall
Columbus, OH 43210
Tel: 614 293-3773 *Fax:* 614 293-5877
E-mail: samuels.8@osu.edu
Accred Length: 4 Years *Program Size:* 36 (*GY1:* 9)
Program ID: 220-38-11-234

Riverside Methodist Hospitals (OhioHealth)/St Ann's Hospital of Columbus Program

Sponsor: Riverside Methodist Hospitals (OhioHealth)
St Ann's Hospital of Columbus

Program Director:
Jeffrey G Bell, MD
Riverside Methodist Hospital
3535 Olentangy River Rd
Columbus, OH 43214
Tel: 614 566-5762 *Fax:* 614 566-5862
E-mail: engelr@ohiohealth.com
Internet: http://www.ohiohealth.com
Accred Length: 4 Years *Program Size:* 16 (*GY1:* 4)
Program ID: 220-38-32-235

Dayton

Wright State University Program

Sponsor: Wright State University School of Medicine
Miami Valley Hospital
Wright-Patterson Medical Center

Program Director:
Stephen H Cruikshank, MD
Wright State Univ, Dept of Ob/Gyn
Miami Valley Hospital
128 E Apple St/Ste 3800 CHE
Dayton, OH 45409-2793
Tel: 937 208-2850 *Fax:* 937 222-7255
E-mail: kluttrell@desire.wright.edu
Accred Length: 4 Years *Program Size:* 24 (*GY1:* 6)
Program ID: 220-38-21-236

Toledo

Medical College of Ohio Program

Sponsor: Medical College of Ohio
St Vincent Mercy Medical Center
Toledo Hospital

Program Director:
Terrence J Horrigan, MD
Med Coll of Ohio, Dept of Ob/Gyn
3120 Glendale Ave
Toledo, OH 43614-5809
Tel: 419 383-4590 *Fax:* 419 383-3090
Accred Length: 4 Years *Program Size:* 19 (*GY1:* 4)
Program ID: 220-38-22-237

Youngstown

St Elizabeth Health Center/NEOUCOM Program

Sponsor: St Elizabeth Health Center

Program Director:
Edmund S Petrilli, MD
St Elizabeth Health Ctr
1044 Belmont Ave
Youngstown, OH 44501-1790
Tel: 330 480-3280 *Fax:* 330 480-2708
Accred Length: 4 Years *Program Size:* 12 (*GY1:* 3)
Program ID: 220-38-11-238

Oklahoma

Oklahoma City

University of Oklahoma Health Sciences Center Program

Sponsor: University of Oklahoma College of Medicine
University Hospital

Program Director:
Robert Mannel, MD
Univ of Oklahoma Health Sciences Ctr
PO Box 26901
Oklahoma City, OK 73190
Tel: 405 271-8787 *Fax:* 405 271-8547
E-mail: faye-smith@ouhsc.edu
Accred Length: 4 Years *Program Size:* 20 (*GY1:* 5)
Program ID: 220-39-11-239

Tulsa

University of Oklahoma College of Medicine-Tulsa Program

Sponsor: University of Oklahoma College of Medicine-Tulsa
Hillcrest Medical Center
St Francis Hospital
St John Medical Center

Program Director:
Howard Shaw, MD PhD
Univ of Oklahoma Coll of Med-Tulsa
Dept of Ob/Gyn
1145 S Utica/Ste 600
Tulsa, OK 74104
Tel: 918 838-4658 *Fax:* 918 831-4464
E-mail: james-beeson@uokhsc.edu
Internet: http://www.online.uokhsc.edu/
Accred Length: 4 Years *Program Size:* 16 (*GY1:* 4)
Program ID: 220-39-21-240

Oregon

Portland

Oregon Health Sciences University Program

Sponsor: Oregon Health Sciences University Hospital
Legacy Emanuel Hospital and Health Center
Legacy Good Samaritan Hospital and Medical Center

Program Director:
E Paul Kirk, MD
Oregon Health Sciences Univ
3181 SW Sam Jackson Park Rd/L466
Portland, OR 97201-3098
Tel: 503 494-3106 *Fax:* 503 494-3111
E-mail: curtinl@ohsu.edu
Internet: http://www.ohsu.edu/som-obgyn/obres.html
Accred Length: 4 Years *Program Size:* 24 (*GY1:* 6)
Program ID: 220-40-21-241

Pennsylvania

Abington

Abington Memorial Hospital Program
Sponsor: Abington Memorial Hospital
Program Director:
Joel I Polin, MD
Dept of Ob/Gyn
Abington Memorial Hospital
1200 Old York Rd
Abington, PA 19001
Tel: 215 572-6222 *Fax:* 215 576-2048
Internet: http://www.amh.com
Accred Length: 4 Years *Program Size:* 12 (*GY1:* 3)
Program ID: 220-41-12-242

Allentown

Lehigh Valley Hospital/Pennsylvania State University Program
Sponsor: Lehigh Valley Hospital
Program Director:
Stephen K Klasko, MD MBA
Lehigh Valley Hospital
17th and Chew Sts
PO Box 7017
Allentown, PA 18105-7017
Tel: 610 402-9520 *Fax:* 610 402-9688
E-mail: obgyn@lvhhn.org
Internet:
http://www.lvhhn.org/academic/residency/ob_gyn/home.html
Accred Length: 4 Years *Program Size:* 16 (*GY1:* 4)
Program ID: 220-41-11-243

Bethlehem

St Luke's Hospital Program
Sponsor: St Luke's Hospital
Program Director:
James N Anasti, MD
St Luke's Hospital
801 Ostrum St
Bethlehem, PA 18015
Tel: 610 954-4670 *Fax:* 610 954-2381
E-mail: obgyn-residency@slhn.org
Internet: http://slhn-lehighvalley.org
Accred Length: 4 Years *Program Size:* 12 (*GY1:* 3)
Subspecialties: TY
Program ID: 220-41-31-244

Danville

Penn State Geisinger Health System/Geisinger Medical Center Program
Sponsor: Penn State Geisinger Health System
Geisinger Medical Center
Program Director:
Tarit K Ghosh, MD
Dept of Ob/Gyn
100 N Academy Ave
Danville, PA 17822-1329
Tel: 717 271-6296 *Fax:* 717 271-5841
E-mail: ckrebs@psghs.edu
Accred Length: 4 Years *Program Size:* 11 (*GY1:* 3)
Program ID: 220-41-12-245

Hershey

Penn State Geisinger Health System/Milton S Hershey Medical Center Program
Sponsor: Penn State Geisinger Health System
Milton S Hershey Medical Center
Program Director:
Matthew Davies, MD
Penn State Geisinger Health System
Milton S Hershey Med Ctr, Dept of Ob/Gyn
500 University Dr
Hershey, PA 17033-0850
Tel: 717 531-8141 *Fax:* 717 531-6752
Internet: http://www.hmc.psu.edu/obgyn/
Accred Length: 4 Years *Program Size:* 16 (*GY1:* 4)
Program ID: 220-41-21-246

Philadelphia

Albert Einstein Medical Center Program
Sponsor: Albert Einstein Medical Center
Chestnut Hill Hospital
Program Director:
Sze-ya Yeh, MD
Albert Einstein Med Ctr
5501 Old York Rd
Philadelphia, PA 19141-3098
Tel: 215 456-8261 *Fax:* 215 456-2386
E-mail: hewlettg@aehn2.einstein.edu
Accred Length: 4 Years *Program Size:* 16 (*GY1:* 4)
Program ID: 220-41-21-247

MCP Hahnemann University Program
Sponsor: MCP Hahnemann University
Crozer-Chester Medical Center
Hahnemann University Hospital
Medical College of Pennsylvania Hospital
Program Director:
David M Goodner, MD
Allegheny Univ Hospitals-City Ave
4150 City Ave
Philadelphia, PA 19131
Tel: 215 871-2041 *Fax:* 215 871-2069
E-mail: goodned@wpo.auhs.edu
Accred Length: 4 Years *Program Size:* 36 (*GY1:* 9)
Subspecialties: TY
Program ID: 220-41-21-250

Pennsylvania Hospital of the University of Pennsylvania Health System Program
Sponsor: Pennsylvania Hospital (UPHS)
Program Director:
Mark B Woodland, MD
Pennsylvania Hospital
800 Spruce St/2 Pine East
Philadelphia, PA 19107
Tel: 215 829-3470 *Fax:* 215 829-7543
Internet: http://www.pahosp.com
Accred Length: 4 Years *Program Size:* 24 (*GY1:* 6)
Program ID: 220-41-11-252

Temple University Program
Sponsor: Temple University Hospital
Frankford Hospital (Torresdale Campus)
Program Director:
Ashwin Chatwani, MD
Temple Univ Hospital
3401 N Broad St
7th Fl-OPB
Philadelphia, PA 19140
Tel: 215 221-3187 *Fax:* 215 707-1516
E-mail: rrobin00@nimbus.ocis.temple.edu
Accred Length: 4 Years *Program Size:* 21 (*GY1:* 6)
Program ID: 220-41-21-254

Thomas Jefferson University Program
Sponsor: Thomas Jefferson University Hospital
Methodist Hospital
West Jersey Health System
Program Director:
Cynthia G Silber, MD
834 Chestnut St/Ste 400
Benjamin Franklin House
Philadelphia, PA 19107
Tel: 215 955-1085 *Fax:* 215 955-5041
Accred Length: 4 Years *Program Size:* 32 (*GY1:* 8)
Program ID: 220-41-21-255

University of Pennsylvania Program
Sponsor: Hospital of the University of Pennsylvania
Program Director:
William W Beck Jr, MD
Hospital of Univ of Pennsylvania
106 Dulles Bldg
3400 Spruce St
Philadelphia, PA 19104-4283
Tel: 215 662-2459 *Fax:* 215 614-0486
E-mail: residency@obgyn.upenn.edu
Internet: http://www.obgyn.upenn.edu
Accred Length: 4 Years *Program Size:* 24 (*GY1:* 6)
Program ID: 220-41-11-256

Pittsburgh

Allegheny General Hospital Program
Sponsor: Allegheny General Hospital
Program Director:
Joseph S Sanfilippo, MD
Allegheny General Hospital
Dept of Ob/Gyn
320 E North Ave
Pittsburgh, PA 15212
Tel: 412 359-6890 *Fax:* 412 359-5133
Accred Length: 4 Years *Program Size:* 8 (*GY1:* 2)
Program ID: 220-41-12-257

University Health Center of Pittsburgh Program
Sponsor: University Health Center of Pittsburgh
Magee-Women's Hospital
Program Director:
William R Crombleholme, MD
Univ Health Ctr of Pittsburgh
Magee-Women's Hospital
300 Halket St
Pittsburgh, PA 15213-3180
Tel: 412 641-1674 *Fax:* 412 641-1133
E-mail: dbrucha@mail.magee.edu
Internet: http://www.pitt.edu/~bruchad
Accred Length: 4 Years *Program Size:* 32 (*GY1:* 8)
Program ID: 220-41-11-258

Western Pennsylvania Hospital Program
Sponsor: Western Pennsylvania Hospital
Program Director:
Gregorio Delgado, MD
Western Pennsylvania Hospital
4800 Friendship Ave
Pittsburgh, PA 15224
Tel: 412 578-5504 *Fax:* 412 578-4477
Accred Length: 4 Years *Program Size:* 12 (*GY1:* 3)
Program ID: 220-41-11-261

Reading

Reading Hospital and Medical Center Program

Sponsor: Reading Hospital and Medical Center

Program Director:
Peter A Schwartz, MD
Reading Hospital and Med Ctr
Dept of Ob/Gyn
Box 16052
West Reading, PA 19612-6052
Tel: 610 378-6827 *Fax:* 610 607-9292
E-mail: schwartzp@readinghospital.org
Accred Length: 4 Years *Program Size:* 12 (*GY1:* 3)
Subspecialties: TY
Program ID: 220-41-12-262

Wynnewood

Lankenau Hospital Program

Sponsor: Lankenau Hospital

Program Director:
Patricia H McConnell, MD
Dept of Ob/Gyn
Lankenau Medical Bldg South
100 Lancaster Ave/Ste 301
Wynnewood, PA 19096
Tel: 610 645-2325 *Fax:* 610 645-2422
E-mail: jcrvisa@mlhs.org
Accred Length: 4 Years *Program Size:* 12 (*GY1:* 3)
Program ID: 220-41-11-249

York

York Hospital Program

Sponsor: York Hospital

Program Director:
Nicolas V Simon, MD
York Hospital
1001 S George St
York, PA 17405
Tel: 717 851-2348 *Fax:* 717 851-2426
E-mail: mf_nsimon@yorkhospital.edu
Internet: http://www.yorkhealth.org
Accred Length: 4 Years *Program Size:* 12 (*GY1:* 3)
Program ID: 220-41-11-263

Puerto Rico

Ponce

Ponce University Hospital Program

Sponsor: Ponce University Hospital

Program Director:
Alberto Aviles-Collado, MD
Ponce Regional Hospital
Dept of Ob/Gyn
State Rd 14
Ponce, PR 00731
Tel: 787 844-2080 *Fax:* 787 841-3454
Accred Length: 4 Years *Program Size:* 16 (*GY1:* 4)
Program ID: 220-42-21-346

Rio Piedras

San Juan City Hospital Program

Sponsor: San Juan City Hospital

Program Director:
Jorge Gandia, MD
San Juan Municipal Hospital
CMM 370
PO Box 70344
San Juan, PR 00936
Tel: 787 767-3733 *Fax:* 787 753-0054
Accred Length: 4 Years *Program Size:* 16 (*GY1:* 4)
Program ID: 220-42-12-267

San Juan

University of Puerto Rico Program

Sponsor: University of Puerto Rico School of Medicine
Caguas Regional Hospital
Dr Federico Trilla - Carolina Regional Hospital
University Hospital

Program Director:
Karlis Adamsons, MD PhD
Univ of Puerto Rico
Med Sciences Campus/Ste 887-A
PO Box 365067
San Juan, PR 00936
Tel: 787 767-8740 *Fax:* 787 764-7881
Internet: http://www.obgyntoday.org
Accred Length: 4 Years *Program Size:* 32 (*GY1:* 8)
Program ID: 220-42-11-268

Rhode Island

Providence

Brown University Program

Sponsor: Women and Infants Hospital of Rhode Island
Rhode Island Hospital

Program Director:
Donald R Coustan, MD
Brown Univ
Women and Infants Hospital, Dept of Ob/Gyn
101 Dudley St
Providence, RI 02905-2401
Tel: 401 274-1122, ext 1575 *Fax:* 401 453-7599
Internet:
http://www.brown.edu/departments/obstetrics_gynecology/
Accred Length: 4 Years *Program Size:* 28 (*GY1:* 7)
Program ID: 220-43-21-269

South Carolina

Charleston

Medical University of South Carolina Program

Sponsor: Medical University of South Carolina College of Medicine
Charleston Memorial Hospital
MUSC Medical Center

Program Director:
J Peter VanDorsten, MD
Med Univ of South Carolina
171 Ashley Ave
Charleston, SC 29425-2233
Tel: 843 792-7108 *Fax:* 843 792-0533
E-mail: dunbarm@musc.edu
Accred Length: 4 Years *Program Size:* 20 (*GY1:* 5)
Program ID: 220-45-21-270

Columbia

Palmetto Health Alliance/University of South Carolina School of Medicine Program

Sponsor: Palmetto Health Alliance
Palmetto Richland Memorial Hospital

Program Director:
S T Smith, MD
Palmetto Richland Memorial Hospital
Dept of Ob/Gyn
2 Medical Pk/Ste 208
Columbia, SC 29203
Tel: 803 779-4928, ext 240 *Fax:* 803 434-4699
Accred Length: 4 Years *Program Size:* 16 (*GY1:* 4)
Program ID: 220-45-11-271

Greenville

Greenville Hospital System Program

Sponsor: Greenville Hospital System

Program Director:
Robert V Cummings, MD
Greenville Hospital System
701 Grove Rd
Greenville, SC 29605
Tel: 864 455-7887, ext 7887 *Fax:* 864 455-5075
Internet: http://www.ghs.org
Accred Length: 4 Years *Program Size:* 16 (*GY1:* 4)
Program ID: 220-45-11-272

Tennessee

Chattanooga

University of Tennessee College of Medicine at Chattanooga Program

Sponsor: University of Tennessee College of Medicine-Chattanooga Unit
Erlanger Medical Center

Program Director:
M Mark Taslimi, MD
Univ of Tennessee Coll of Med
Dept of Ob/Gyn
975 E Third St/Box 221
Chattanooga, TN 37403
Tel: 423 778-7515 *Fax:* 423 267-6244
E-mail: utobgyn@chattanooga.org
Internet: http://www.erlanger.org/utcom/obgyn.html
Accred Length: 4 Years *Program Size:* 13 (*GY1:* 3)
Program ID: 220-47-21-274

Johnson City

East Tennessee State University Program

Sponsor: James H Quillen College of Medicine
Johnson City Medical Center Hospital

Program Director:
Martin E Olsen, MD
East Tennessee State Univ
Dept of Ob/Gyn
PO Box 70 569
Johnson City, TN 37614-0569
Tel: 423 439-6262 *Fax:* 423 439-6766
E-mail: etsustork@washington.xtn.net
Internet: http://www.etsu-tn.edu/ob-gyn/
Accred Length: 4 Years *Program Size:* 12 (*GY1:* 3)
Program ID: 220-47-21-341

Knoxville

University of Tennessee Medical Center at Knoxville Program

Sponsor: University of Tennessee Graduate School of Medicine
University of Tennessee Memorial Hospital

Program Director:
Ran Neiger, MD
Univ of Tennessee Grad Sch of Med
1924 Alcoa Hwy
Knoxville, TN 37920
Tel: 423 544-9306 *Fax:* 423 544-6822
E-mail: utobgyn@mc.utmck.edu
Accred Length: 4 Years *Program Size:* 12 (*GY1:* 3)
Program ID: 220-47-11-275

Memphis

University of Tennessee Program

Sponsor: University of Tennessee College of Medicine
Regional Medical Center at Memphis
University of Tennessee Medical Center (UT Bowld Hospital)

Program Director:
Robert L Summitt Jr, MD
Univ of Tennessee
Dept of Ob/Gyn
853 Jefferson Ave/1st Fl
Memphis, TN 38163
Tel: 901 448-5497 *Fax:* 901 448-4701
E-mail: eperkins@utmem1.utmem.edu
Accred Length: 4 Years *Program Size:* 43 (*GY1:* 10)
Program ID: 220-47-21-276

Nashville

Vanderbilt University Program

Sponsor: Vanderbilt University Medical Center
Baptist Hospital

Program Director:
Stephen Entman, MD
Vanderbilt Univ Hospital, Dept of Ob/Gyn
1161 21st Ave
R1214/MCN
Nashville, TN 37232-2521
Tel: 615 343-8801 *Fax:* 615 343-8806
E-mail: debby.scraggins@mcmail.vanderbilt.edu
Accred Length: 4 Years *Program Size:* 24 (*GY1:* 6)
Program ID: 220-47-21-278

Texas

Amarillo

Texas Tech University (Amarillo) Program

Sponsor: Texas Tech University Health Sciences Center at Amarillo
Northwest Texas Health Care System

Program Director:
Raymond M Hampton II, MD
Texas Tech Univ Health Sciences Ctr
Dept of Ob/Gyn
1400 Wallace Blvd
Amarillo, TX 79106
Tel: 806 354-5502 *Fax:* 806 354-5516
E-mail: judy@cortex.ama.ttuhsc.edu
Internet: http://www.ama.ttuhsc.edu
Accred Length: 4 Years *Program Size:* 14 (*GY1:* 3)
Program ID: 220-48-21-320

Dallas

Baylor University Medical Center Program

Sponsor: Baylor University Medical Center

Program Director:
Carolyn M Matthews, MD
Baylor Univ Med Ctr
Dept of Ob/Gyn
3500 Gaston Ave
Dallas, TX 75246
Tel: 214 820-6226 *Fax:* 214 820-6080
E-mail: mj.beyer@baylordallas.edu
Internet:
http://www.bhcs.com/bumc/medicaleducation/residencies.htm
Accred Length: 4 Years *Program Size:* 16 (*GY1:* 4)
Program ID: 220-48-31-280

Methodist Hospitals of Dallas Program

Sponsor: Methodist Hospitals of Dallas
Dallas County Hospital District-Parkland Memorial Hospital

Program Director:
Clare D Edman, MD
Methodist Med Ctr
1441 N Beckley Ave
PO Box 659999
Dallas, TX 75265-9999
Tel: 214 947-2300 *Fax:* 214 947-2361
E-mail: edman@mhdcme.org
Internet: http://www.mhdcme.org
Accred Length: 4 Years *Program Size:* 9 (*GY1:* 3)
Program ID: 220-48-31-281

St Paul Medical Center Program

Sponsor: St Paul Medical Center
Dallas County Hospital District-Parkland Memorial Hospital

Program Director:
Larry E Word, MD
St Paul Med Ctr
Grad Med Educ Services
5909 Harry Hines Blvd
Dallas, TX 75235
Tel: 214 879-3786 *Fax:* 214 879-3069
Accred Length: 4 Years *Program Size:* 8 (*GY1:* 2)
Program ID: 220-48-31-283

University of Texas Southwestern Medical School Program

Sponsor: University of Texas Southwestern Medical School
Dallas County Hospital District-Parkland Memorial Hospital

Program Director:
George D Wendel Jr, MD
Univ of Texas Southwestern Med Sch
5323 Harry Hines Blvd
Dallas, TX 75235-9032
Tel: 214 648-4866 *Fax:* 214 648-4566
E-mail: gwende@mednet.swmed.edu
Internet:
http://www.swmed.edu/home_pages/obgyn/resident.htm
Accred Length: 4 Years *Program Size:* 56 (*GY1:* 14)
Program ID: 220-48-31-282

El Paso

Texas Tech University (El Paso) Program

Sponsor: Texas Tech University Health Sciences Center at El Paso
R E Thomason General Hospital

Program Director:
Jose L Gonzalez, MD
Texas Tech Univ Health Sciences Ctr-El Paso
Dept of Ob/Gyn
4800 Alberta Ave
El Paso, TX 79905
Tel: 915 545-6708 *Fax:* 915 545-6946
E-mail: obgeib2@ttuhsc.edu
Accred Length: 4 Years *Program Size:* 16 (*GY1:* 4)
Program ID: 220-48-11-315

Fort Worth

Fort Worth Hospitals Program

Sponsor: John Peter Smith Hospital (Tarrant County Hospital District)
Harris Methodist Fort Worth

Program Director:
Ralph J Anderson, MD
John Peter Smith Hospital
1500 S Main St
Fort Worth, TX 76104
Tel: 817 927-1173 *Fax:* 817 927-1668
E-mail: bamckeon@aol.com
Internet: http://jpshealthnet.org
Accred Length: 4 Years *Program Size:* 16 (*GY1:* 4)
Program ID: 220-48-22-284

Galveston

University of Texas Medical Branch Hospitals Program

Sponsor: University of Texas Medical Branch Hospitals

Program Director:
John C Jennings, MD
Univ of Texas Med Branch Hospitals
Dept of Ob/Gyn
301 University Blvd
Galveston, TX 77555-0587
Tel: 409 772-2999 *Fax:* 409 747-0366
E-mail: dfisher@utmb.edu
Internet: http://www.utmb.edu/obgyn
Accred Length: 4 Years *Program Size:* 37 (*GY1:* 9)
Program ID: 220-48-21-285

Houston

Baylor College of Medicine Program

Sponsor: Baylor College of Medicine
Harris County Hospital District-Ben Taub General Hospital

Program Director:
L Russell Malinak, MD
Baylor Coll of Med
Dept of Ob/Gyn
One Baylor Plaza
Houston, TX 77030
Tel: 713 798-7517 *Fax:* 713 798-6044
E-mail: levesque@bcm.tmc.edu
Internet:
http://www.bcm.tmc.edu/obgyn/obgyn-ce/ob-gyn.html
Accred Length: 4 Years *Program Size:* 48 (*GY1:* 12)
Program ID: 220-48-31-286

St Joseph Hospital Program

Sponsor: St Joseph Hospital
Brackenridge Hospital

Program Director:
Benton Baker III, MD
St Joseph Hospital
1819 Crawford/Ste 1708
Houston, TX 77002
Tel: 713 757-7478 *Fax:* 713 657-7191
E-mail: dottie.mersinger@stjoe.sch.org
Accred Length: 4 Years *Program Size:* 16 (*GY1:* 4)
Program ID: 220-48-31-288

University of Texas at Houston Program A

Sponsor: University of Texas Medical School at Houston
Lyndon B Johnson General Hospital
Memorial Hermann Healthcare System

Program Director:
Robert C Maier, MD
Lyndon B Johnson General Hospital
Ob/Gyn Dept/Rm 2LD80001
5656 Kelley St
Houston, TX 77026
Tel: 713 636-5735 *Fax:* 713 636-4521
E-mail: jhayes@obg.med.uth.tmc.edu
Internet: http://www.obg.med.uth.tmc.edu/misc/lbj.htm
Accred Length: 4 Years *Program Size:* 20 (*GYI:* 5)
Program ID: 220-48-21-334

University of Texas at Houston Program B

Sponsor: University of Texas Medical School at Houston
Lyndon B Johnson General Hospital
Memorial Hermann Healthcare System

Program Director:
Allan R Katz, MD
Univ of Texas Med Sch
6431 Fannin St/Ste 3306
Houston, TX 77030
Tel: 713 500-6432 *Fax:* 713 500-7859
E-mail: bdevore@obg.med.uth.tmc.edu
Internet: http://www.obg.med.uth.tmc.edu
Accred Length: 4 Years *Program Size:* 24 (*GYI:* 6)
Program ID: 220-48-21-289

Lackland AFB

San Antonio Uniformed Services Health Education Consortium Program

Sponsor: San Antonio Uniformed Services Health Education Consortium
Brooke Army Medical Center
Darnall Army Community Hospital
Wilford Hall Medical Center (AETC)

Program Director:
Randal D Robinson, MD
859 MDOS/MMNO
2200 Bergquist Dr/Ste 1
Lackland AFB, TX 78236-5300
Tel: 210 292-6136 *Fax:* 210 292-7547
E-mail: robinson_r@whmc-lafb.af.mil
Accred Length: 4 Years *Program Size:* 6 (*GYI:* 6)
Program ID: 220-48-21-356
US Armed Services Program

Lubbock

Texas Tech University (Lubbock) Program

Sponsor: Texas Tech University Health Sciences Center at Lubbock
University Medical Center
US Air Force Hospital (Reese)

Program Director:
Kathy B Porter, MD
Texas Tech Univ Health Sciences Ctr
Dept of Ob/Gyn
3601 Fourth St
Lubbock, TX 79430
Tel: 806 743-3039 *Fax:* 806 743-3200
E-mail: obghrr@ttuhsc.edu
Internet: http://members.tripod.com/~prien
Accred Length: 4 Years *Program Size:* 12 (*GYI:* 3)
Program ID: 220-48-21-290

Odessa

Texas Tech University (Odessa) Program

Sponsor: Texas Tech University Health Sciences Center at Odessa
Medical Center Hospital

Program Director:
Carol A Bergquist, MD
Texas Tech Univ Health Sciences Ctr
Dept of Ob/Gyn
800 W Fourth St
Odessa, TX 79763-4362
Tel: 915 335-5200 *Fax:* 915 335-5240
E-mail: obgonwl@tthsc8.odessa.ttuhsc.edu
Accred Length: 4 Years *Program Size:* 8 (*GYI:* 2)
Program ID: 220-48-21-331

San Antonio

University of Texas Health Science Center at San Antonio Program

Sponsor: University of Texas Medical School at San Antonio
University Hospital-South Texas Medical Center

Program Director:
Elly Xenakis, MD
Univ of Texas Health Science Ctr
Dept of Ob/Gyn
7703 Floyd Curl Dr
San Antonio, TX 78284-7836
Tel: 210 567-4953 *Fax:* 210 567-3406
E-mail: brewerk@uthscsa.edu
Internet: http://macorb.uthscsa.edu/obgyn/obgyn.html
Accred Length: 4 Years *Program Size:* 25 (*GYI:* 6)
Program ID: 220-48-21-292

Temple

Texas A&M College of Medicine-Scott and White Program

Sponsor: Scott and White Memorial Hospital

Program Director:
Steven R Allen, MD
Scott and White Memorial Hospital
2401 S 31st St
Temple, TX 76508-0001
Tel: 254 724-2589 *Fax:* 254 724-7976
E-mail: pmorrise@swmail.sw.org
Internet:
http://www.sw.org/depts/obgyn/gme/obgynres.htm
Accred Length: 4 Years *Program Size:* 16 (*GYI:* 4)
Program ID: 220-48-21-293

Utah

Salt Lake City

University of Utah Program

Sponsor: University of Utah Medical Center
LDS Hospital

Program Director:
Robert M Silver, MD
Univ of Utah Med Ctr
Dept of Ob/Gyn
50 N Medical Dr/Rm 2B200
Salt Lake City, UT 84132
Tel: 801 581-5501 *Fax:* 801 585-5146
E-mail: julie.andrews@hsc.utah.edu
Internet: http://www.med.utah.edu/obgyn/
Accred Length: 4 Years *Program Size:* 16 (*GYI:* 4)
Program ID: 220-49-21-294

Vermont

Burlington

University of Vermont Program

Sponsor: Fletcher Allen Health Care

Program Director:
Marjorie Meyer, MD
Univ of Vermont
Fletcher Allen Health Care/Shep 625
111 Colchester Ave
Burlington, VT 05401
Tel: 802 656-4736 *Fax:* 802 656-5626
Internet: http://salus.uvm.edu:80/obgyn/whcs/whcs.htm
Accred Length: 4 Years *Program Size:* 18 (*GYI:* 5)
Program ID: 220-50-21-295

Virginia

Charlottesville

University of Virginia Program

Sponsor: University of Virginia Medical Center

Program Director:
James D Kitchin III, MD
Univ of Virginia Health Sciences Ctr
PO Box 10016
Charlottesville, VA 22906
Tel: 804 982-3701 *Fax:* 804 982-1840
E-mail: mlp2b@virginia.edu
Accred Length: 4 Years *Program Size:* 20 (*GYI:* 5)
Program ID: 220-51-11-296

Newport News

Riverside Regional Medical Center Program

Sponsor: Riverside Regional Medical Center

Program Director:
William J Mann Jr, MD MBA
Riverside Ob/Gyn and Family Care
316 Main St
2nd Fl
Newport News, VA 23601-3808
Tel: 757 594-4737 *Fax:* 757 594-3835
E-mail: wjmmd@worldnet.att.net
Internet: http://www.riversideobgyn.org
Accred Length: 5 Years *Program Size:* 14 (*GYI:* 4)
Subspecialties: TY
Program ID: 220-51-11-297

Norfolk

Eastern Virginia Medical School Program

Sponsor: Eastern Virginia Medical School
DePaul Medical Center
Portsmouth General Hospital
Sentara Norfolk General Hospital

Program Director:
William E Gibbons, MD
Eastern Virginia Med Sch
601 Colley Ave
Ste 243
Norfolk, VA 23507
Tel: 757 446-8934 *Fax:* 757 446-8998
E-mail: weg@jones1.evms.edu
Internet: http://www.evms.edu./jones/depthome/htm
Accred Length: 4 Years *Program Size:* 17 (*GYI:* 4)
Program ID: 220-51-21-298

Portsmouth

Naval Medical Center (Portsmouth) Program

Sponsor: Naval Medical Center (Portsmouth)

Program Director:
Robert E Ricks Jr, MD
Dept of Ob/Gyn
620 John Paul Jones Cir
Portsmouth, VA 23708-2197
Tel: 757 889-2604 *Fax:* 757 889-2608
E-mail: pnh0rer@pnh10.med.navy.mil
Accred Length: 4 Years *Program Size:* 20 *(GY1:* 5)
Program ID: 220-51-11-014
US Armed Services Program

Richmond

Medical College of Virginia/Virginia Commonwealth University Program

Sponsor: Medical College of Virginia/Virginia Commonwealth University
Medical College of Virginia Hospitals

Program Director:
Stephen Cohen, MD
Med Coll of Virginia Hospitals
PO Box 980034
Richmond, VA 23298-0034
Tel: 804 828-7877 *Fax:* 804 828-5076
E-mail: jwittersheim@hsc.vcu.edu
Internet: http://www.vcu.edu
Accred Length: 4 Years *Program Size:* 26 *(GY1:* 6)
Program ID: 220-51-11-299

Roanoke

Carilion Health System Program

Sponsor: Carilion Health System
Carilion Roanoke Community Hospital
Carilion Roanoke Memorial Hospital

Program Director:
Mark C Arner, MD
Carilion Health System-Carilion Roanoke Community Hospital
102 Highland Ave SE/Ste 435
Roanoke, VA 24013
Tel: 540 985-9977 *Fax:* 540 983-1192
E-mail: marner@carilion.com
Internet: http://www.carilion.com/residency
Accred Length: 4 Years *Program Size:* 12 *(GY1:* 3)
Program ID: 220-51-31-300

Washington

Seattle

University of Washington Program

Sponsor: University of Washington School of Medicine
Swedish Medical Center-Seattle
University of Washington Medical Center

Program Director:
Steven G Gabbe, MD
Louis A Vontver, MD
Univ of Washington
BB617/Health Sciences Bldg
Box 356460
Seattle, WA 98195-6460
Tel: 206 543-9626 *Fax:* 206 543-3915
E-mail: chawes@u.washington.edu
Accred Length: 4 Years *Program Size:* 24 *(GY1:* 6)
Program ID: 220-54-21-301

Tacoma

Madigan Army Medical Center Program

Sponsor: Madigan Army Medical Center

Program Director:
Milo L Hibbert, MD
Madigan Army Med Ctr
Dept of Ob/Gyn
Attn: MCHJ-OG
Tacoma, WA 98431
Tel: 253 968-1315 *Fax:* 253 968-2558
Internet: http://www.mamc.amedd.army.mil
Accred Length: 4 Years *Program Size:* 20 *(GY1:* 5)
Program ID: 220-54-12-010
US Armed Services Program

West Virginia

Charleston

West Virginia University (Charleston Division) Program

Sponsor: Charleston Area Medical Center

Program Director:
E R Heywood, MD
Dept of Ob/Gyn
Robert C Byrd Health Sciences Ctr
830 Pennsylvania Ave/#304
Charleston, WV 25302-3390
Tel: 304 342-0816 *Fax:* 304 342-0828
Accred Length: 4 Years *Program Size:* 12 *(GY1:* 3)
Program ID: 220-55-11-303

Huntington

Marshall University School of Medicine Program

Sponsor: Marshall University School of Medicine
Cabell Huntington Hospital

Program Director:
Robert C Nerhood, MD
Marshall Univ Sch of Med
Dept of Ob/Gyn
1600 Medical Center Dr
Huntington, WV 25701
Tel: 304 691-1400, ext 1454 *Fax:* 304 691-1453
E-mail: kjones@musom02.mu.wvnet.edu
Internet: http://meb.marshall.edu/resident/ob.htm
Accred Length: 4 Years *Program Size:* 12 *(GY1:* 3)
Program ID: 220-55-21-344

Morgantown

West Virginia University Program

Sponsor: West Virginia University Hospitals

Program Director:
Andrew P Soisson, MD
West Virginia Univ Hospitals
4601 Health Services North
PO Box 9186
Morgantown, WV 26506-9186
Tel: 304 293-3141 *Fax:* 304 293-2225
E-mail: tharvey@wvumbrcc1.hsc.wvu.edu
Accred Length: 4 Years *Program Size:* 12 *(GY1:* 3)
Program ID: 220-55-11-304

Wisconsin

Madison

University of Wisconsin Program

Sponsor: University of Wisconsin Hospital and Clinics
Meriter Hospital
St Marys Hospital Medical Center

Program Director:
Sabine Droste, MD
Ob/Gyn Div, Meriter Hospital-Park
202 S Park St
Madison, WI 53715
Tel: 608 263-1228 *Fax:* 608 263-1228
E-mail: wildes@obgyn.wisc.edu
Accred Length: 4 Years *Program Size:* 20 *(GY1:* 5)
Program ID: 220-56-21-306

Milwaukee

Aurora Health Care Program

Sponsor: Aurora Health Care
Sinai Samaritan Medical Center

Program Director:
Betty Amuzu, MD
Milwaukee Clinical Campus
950 N 12th St
PO Box 342
Milwaukee, WI 53201-0342
Tel: 414 219-5725 *Fax:* 414 219-5611
E-mail: jdwatson@facstaff.wisc.edu
Internet: http://www.aurorahealthcare.com
Accred Length: 4 Years *Program Size:* 12 *(GY1:* 3)
Program ID: 220-56-12-308

Medical College of Wisconsin Program

Sponsor: Medical College of Wisconsin Affiliated Hospitals Inc
Froedtert Memorial Lutheran Hospital

Program Director:
Dwight P Cruikshank, MD
Med Coll of Wisconsin
Dept of Ob/Gyn FMLH East
9200 W Wisconsin Ave
Milwaukee, WI 53226
Tel: 414 257-5560 *Fax:* 414 257-5686
E-mail: kuhlmann@mcw.edu
Internet: http://www.mcw.edu/obgyn
Accred Length: 4 Years *Program Size:* 24 *(GY1:* 6)
Subspecialties: TY
Program ID: 220-56-31-307

Oncology (Internal Medicine)

Arkansas

Little Rock

University of Arkansas for Medical Sciences Program
Sponsor: University of Arkansas College of Medicine
John L McClellan Memorial Veterans Hospital
University Hospital of Arkansas
Program Director:
Susan Guba, MD
Clive Zent, MD
Univ of Arkansas for Med Sciences
Mail Slot 508
4301 W Markham St
Little Rock, AR 72205-7199
Tel: 501 686-8511 *Fax:* 501 686-7861
Accred Length: 2 Years *Program Size:* 6
Program ID: 147-04-21-097

California

La Jolla

Scripps Clinic/Scripps Green Hospital Program
Sponsor: Scripps Clinic
Scripps Green Hospital
Program Director:
Michael P Kosty, MD
Dept of Grad Med Educ/403C
Scripps Clinic-Green Hospital
10666 N Torrey Pines Rd
La Jolla, CA 92037-1093
Tel: 619 554-8582 *Fax:* 619 554-6310
E-mail: gme@scripps.edu
Internet: http://scrippsclinic.com
Accred Length: 2 Years *Program Size:* 4
Program ID: 147-05-21-065

Los Angeles

UCLA Medical Center Program
Sponsor: UCLA School of Medicine
UCLA Medical Center
VA Greater Los Angeles Healthcare System
Program Director:
Robert A Figlin, MD
UCLA Med Ctr
Dept of Med/Hem-Onc
10945 Le Conte Ave/Ste 2333
Los Angeles, CA 90095
Tel: 310 825-5788 *Fax:* 310 206-5414
E-mail: rfiglin@med1.medsch.ucla.edu
Accred Length: 2 Years *Program Size:* 17
Program ID: 147-05-11-114

University of Southern California Program
Sponsor: Los Angeles County-USC Medical Center
Program Director:
Christy A Russell, MD
Univ of Southern California Med Ctr
1441 Eastlake Ave/#3448
Los Angeles, CA 90033
Tel: 323 865-3903 *Fax:* 323 865-0061
E-mail: carussel@hsc.usc.edu
Accred Length: 2 Years *Program Size:* 5
Program ID: 147-05-21-045

Orange

University of California (Irvine) Program
Sponsor: University of California (Irvine) Medical Center
Long Beach Memorial Medical Center
Veterans Affairs Medical Center (Long Beach)
Program Director:
Randall F Holcombe, MD
Univ of California Irvine Med Ctr
Div of Hematology/Oncology
101 City Dr S/Bldg 23 Rm 244
Orange, CA 92868-3298
Tel: 714 456-5153 *Fax:* 714 456-7142
E-mail: rholcomb@uci.edu
Accred Length: 2 Years *Program Size:* 0
Program ID: 147-05-21-170

Stanford

Stanford University Program
Sponsor: Stanford University Hospital
Veterans Affairs Palo Alto Health Care System
Program Director:
Sandra J Horning, MD
Stanford Univ
Med/Oncology
1000 Welch Rd/Ste 202
Palo Alto, CA 94304-5756
Tel: 650 725-6456 *Fax:* 650 725-8222
E-mail: hf.drj@forsythe.stanford.edu
Accred Length: 2 Years *Program Size:* 12
Program ID: 147-05-21-020

Connecticut

New Haven

Yale-New Haven Medical Center Program
Sponsor: Yale-New Haven Hospital
Veterans Affairs Medical Center (West Haven)
Program Director:
Jill Lacy, MD
333 Cedar St/PO Box 208032
New Haven, CT 06520-8032
Tel: 203 737-5608 *Fax:* 203 737-5698
Accred Length: 2 Years *Program Size:* 15
Program ID: 147-08-21-021

District of Columbia

Washington

Georgetown University Program
Sponsor: Georgetown University Medical Center
Program Director:
Kevin J Cullen, MD
Georgetown Univ Med Ctr
Div of Hem/Onc LCC Podium Corridor B
3800 Reservoir Rd NW
Washington, DC 20007-2197
Tel: 202 687-1686 *Fax:* 202 687-4429
E-mail: hussc@gunet.georgetown.edu
Accred Length: 2 Years *Program Size:* 12
Program ID: 147-10-21-078

Howard University Program
Sponsor: Howard University Hospital
District of Columbia General Hospital
Program Director:
Elliott Perlin, MD
Howard Univ Hospital
2041 Georgia Ave NW
Washington, DC 20060
Tel: 202 865-1511 *Fax:* 202 865-4607
Accred Length: 2 Years *Program Size:* 2
Program ID: 147-10-21-116

Florida

Jacksonville

University of Florida Health Science Center/Jacksonville Program
Sponsor: University of Florida College of Medicine at Jacksonville
University Medical Center (UFHSC/J)
Baptist Medical Center (UFHSC/J)
Program Director:
Troy H Guthrie Jr, MD
Div of Hematology/Oncology
653-1 W Eighth St
Jacksonville, FL 32209-6511
Tel: 904 549-3072 *Fax:* 904 549-3087
Internet: http://www.ufhscj.edu
Accred Length: 2 Years *Program Size:* 3
Program ID: 147-11-21-022

Kansas

Kansas City

University of Kansas Medical Center Program
Sponsor: University of Kansas School of Medicine
University of Kansas Medical Center
Program Director:
Stephen K Williamson, MD
Univ of Kansas Med Ctr
Clinical Oncology Div
3901 Rainbow Blvd
Kansas City, KS 66160-7353
Tel: 913 588-6029 *Fax:* 913 588-4085
E-mail: swilliam@kumc.edu
Accred Length: 2 Years *Program Size:* 5
Program ID: 147-19-21-102

Louisiana

New Orleans

Alton Ochsner Medical Foundation Program
Sponsor: Alton Ochsner Medical Foundation
Program Director:
John T Cole, MD
Alton Ochsner Med Foundation
Dept of Grad Med Educ
1516 Jefferson Hwy
New Orleans, LA 70121
Tel: 504 842-3260 *Fax:* 504 842-3193
E-mail: dlambert@ochsner.org
Internet: http://www.ochsner.org
Accred Length: 2 Years *Program Size:* 2
Program ID: 147-21-22-131

Louisiana State University Program
Sponsor: Louisiana State University School of Medicine
Medical Center of Louisiana at New Orleans
Program Director:
Richard H Vial, MD
Louisiana State Univ Med Ctr
1542 Tulane Ave
New Orleans, LA 70112
Tel: 504 568-7544 *Fax:* 504 568-7755
E-mail: rvial@lsumc.edu
Accred Length: 2 Years *Program Size:* 5
Program ID: 147-21-21-058

Maryland

Baltimore

Johns Hopkins University Program
Sponsor: Johns Hopkins University School of Medicine
Johns Hopkins Hospital
Program Director:
Ross C Donehower, MD
Johns Hopkins Oncology Ctr
600 N Wolfe St
Rm 124
Baltimore, MD 21287-8936
Tel: 410 614-4459 *Fax:* 410 955-0125
E-mail: blessed@welchlink.welch.jhu.edu
Accred Length: 2 Years *Program Size:* 24
Program ID: 147-23-11-067

Bethesda

National Institutes of Health Clinical Center Program
Sponsor: NIH Warren Grant Magnuson Clinical Center
National Naval Medical Center (Bethesda)
Program Director:
Michael Hamilton, MD
NIH Warren Grant Magnuson Clinical Ctr
Bldg 10/Rm 12N226
9000 Rockville Pike
Bethesda, MD 20892
Tel: 301 496-4916 *Fax:* 301 402-0172
E-mail: mike_hamilton@nih.gov
Accred Length: 2 Years *Program Size:* 29
Program ID: 147-23-21-183

Michigan

Detroit

Wayne State University/Detroit Medical Center Program
Sponsor: Wayne State University/Detroit Medical Center
Detroit Receiving Hospital and University Health Center
Harper Hospital
Veterans Affairs Medical Center (Detroit)
Program Director:
Antoinette J Wozniak, MD
Div of Hematology/Oncology
Wayne State Univ Sch of Med
Box 02143
Detroit, MI 48201-0188
Tel: 313 993-8541 *Fax:* 313 993-0559
E-mail: wozniaka@karmanos.org
Accred Length: 2 Years *Program Size:* 8
Program ID: 147-25-21-042

Royal Oak

William Beaumont Hospital Program
Sponsor: William Beaumont Hospital
Program Director:
David A Decker, MD
William Beaumont Hospital
3601 W 13 Mile Rd
Royal Oak, MI 48073
Tel: 248 288-0800 *Fax:* 248 288-0803
Internet: http://www.beaumont.edu/html/gme
Accred Length: 2 Years *Program Size:* 4
Program ID: 147-25-12-161

Southfield

Providence Hospital and Medical Centers Program
Sponsor: Providence Hospital and Medical Centers
Program Director:
Howard Terebelo, DO
Providence Hospital
Med Education
16001 W Nine Mile Rd
Southfield, MI 48075-4818
Tel: 248 424-3216 *Fax:* 248 424-5324
Accred Length: 2 Years *Program Size:* 4
Program ID: 147-25-21-185

New Jersey

South Orange

Seton Hall University School of Graduate Medical Education Program
Sponsor: Seton Hall University School of Graduate Medical Education
St Joseph's Hospital and Medical Center
St Michael's Medical Center (Cathedral Hlth Srvcs Inc)
Program Director:
Arnold D Rubin, MD
St Joseph's Hospital and Med Ctr
703 Main St
Paterson, NJ 07503
Tel: 973 754-2431 *Fax:* 973 754-2444
Accred Length: 2 Years *Program Size:* 4
Program ID: 147-33-21-043

New York

Albany

Albany Medical Center Program
Sponsor: Albany Medical Center
Veterans Affairs Medical Center (Albany)
Program Director:
David Mastrianni, MD
Albany Med Coll
Div of Med Oncology
47 New Scotland Ave
Albany, NY 12208
Tel: 518 262-5355 *Fax:* 518 262-6770
E-mail: dmastrian@ccgateway.amc.edu
Accred Length: 2 Years *Program Size:* 3
Program ID: 147-35-31-026

Bronx

Albert Einstein College of Medicine Program
Sponsor: Albert Einstein College of Medicine of Yeshiva University
Jacobi Medical Center
Montefiore Medical Center-Henry and Lucy Moses Division
Montefiore Medical Center-Weiler Hospital
North Central Bronx Hospital
Program Director:
Joseph A Sparano, MD
Montefiore Med Ctr-Weiler Div
1825 Eastchester Rd
Bronx, NY 10461
Tel: 718 904-2555 *Fax:* 718 904-2892
E-mail: sparano@jimmy.harvard.edu
Accred Length: 2 Years *Program Size:* 12
Program ID: 147-35-21-091

Brooklyn

Brooklyn Hospital Center Program
Sponsor: Brooklyn Hospital Center
Woodhull Medical and Mental Health Center
Program Director:
Perry C Cook, MD
Brooklyn Hospital Ctr
121 DeKalb Ave
Brooklyn, NY 11201
Tel: 718 250-6960 *Fax:* 718 250-6492
E-mail: percook@earthlink.net
Accred Length: 2 Years *Program Size:* 2
Program ID: 147-35-12-165

New York Methodist Hospital Program
Sponsor: New York Methodist Hospital
Program Director:
Muthuswamy Krishnamurthy, MD
New York Methodist Hospital
506 Sixth St
Brooklyn, NY 11215
Tel: 718 780-5246 *Fax:* 718 780-3259
Accred Length: 2 Years *Program Size:* 4
Program ID: 147-35-11-126

Buffalo

SUNY at Buffalo Graduate Medical-Dental Education Consortium Program
Sponsor: SUNY at Buffalo Grad Medical-Dental Education Consortium
Roswell Park Cancer Institute
Veterans Affairs Medical Center (Buffalo)
Program Director:
Ellis G Levine, MD
Roswell Park Cancer Inst
Dept of Med
Elm and Carlton Sts
Buffalo, NY 14263
Tel: 716 845-8547 *Fax:* 716 845-3423
E-mail: levine@sc3101.med.buffalo.edu
Internet: http://www.smbs.buffalo.edu/med/onc
Accred Length: 2 Years *Program Size:* 6
Program ID: 147-35-31-008

East Meadow

SUNY at Stony Brook (East Meadow) Program

Sponsor: Nassau County Medical Center

Program Director:
Stephen Feffer, MD
Nassau County Med Ctr
2201 Hempstead Trnpk
East Meadow, NY 11554-5400
Tel: 516 572-4713 *Fax:* 516 572-5609
Accred Length: 2 Years *Program Size:* 2
Program ID: 147-35-21-085

New York

New York University Medical Center Program

Sponsor: New York University Medical Center
Bellevue Hospital Center
Veterans Affairs Medical Center (Manhattan)

Program Director:
Franco M Muggia, MD
New York Univ Med Ctr
Div of Oncology
550 First Ave
New York, NY 10016
Tel: 212 263-6485 *Fax:* 212 263-8210
Accred Length: 2 Years *Program Size:* 7
Program ID: 147-35-21-106

St Luke's-Roosevelt Hospital Center Program

Sponsor: St Luke's-Roosevelt Hospital Center
St Luke's-Roosevelt Hospital Center-Roosevelt Division
St Luke's-Roosevelt Hospital Center-St Luke's Division

Program Director:
Arthur Karanas, MD
St Luke's-Roosevelt Hospital Ctr
1000 Tenth Ave
Ste 3B-20
New York, NY 10019
Tel: 212 523-7281 *Fax:* 212 523-6677
Accred Length: 2 Years *Program Size:* 5
Program ID: 147-35-11-092

Pennsylvania

Philadelphia

Thomas Jefferson University Program

Sponsor: Thomas Jefferson University Hospital

Program Director:
Rita Axelrod, MD
Thomas Jefferson Univ
Div of Med Oncology
1015 Walnut S/Rm 705
Philadelphia, PA 19107-5099
Tel: 215 955-7786 *Fax:* 215 955-2366
E-mail: rita.axelrod@mail.tju.edu
Accred Length: 2 Years *Program Size:* 12
Program ID: 147-41-21-029

Pittsburgh

Allegheny General Hospital Program

Sponsor: Allegheny General Hospital

Program Director:
David Friedland, MD PhD
Allegheny General Hospital
Dept of Med Oncology
320 E North Ave
Pittsburgh, PA 15212-9986
Tel: 412 359-8934 *Fax:* 412 359-6654
Internet: http://www.cancerlinks.edu
Accred Length: 2 Years *Program Size:* 4
Program ID: 147-41-11-036

University Health Center of Pittsburgh Program

Sponsor: University Health Center of Pittsburgh
Presbyterian University Hospital/UPMC
Veterans Affairs Medical Center (Pittsburgh)

Program Director:
Robert L Redner, MD
Univ of Pittsburgh Med Ctr
Div of Hematology/Oncology
200 Lothrop St
Pittsburgh, PA 15213-2592
Tel: 412 648-6686 *Fax:* 412 692-2757
E-mail: redner+@pitt.edu
Accred Length: 2 Years *Program Size:* 12
Program ID: 147-41-21-037

Puerto Rico

Rio Piedras

San Juan City Hospital Program

Sponsor: San Juan City Hospital
I Gonzalez Martinez Oncologic Hospital
University Hospital Ramon Ruiz Arnau
Veterans Affairs Medical Center (San Juan)

Program Director:
Luis Baez, MD
Puerto Rico Med Ctr
Rio Piedras, PR 00935
Tel: 787 758-7348 *Fax:* 787 758-7348
Accred Length: 2 Years *Program Size:* 2
Program ID: 147-42-11-088

South Carolina

Columbia

Palmetto Health Alliance/University of South Carolina School of Medicine Program

Sponsor: Palmetto Health Alliance
Palmetto Richland Memorial Hospital
William Jennings Bryan Dorn Veterans Hospital

Program Director:
James A McFarland, MD
Ctr for Cancer Treatment and Research
Seven Richland Medical Park/Ste 202
Columbia, SC 29203
Tel: 803 434-4532 *Fax:* 803 434-4767
E-mail: james.mcfarland@rmh.edu
Accred Length: 2 Years *Program Size:* 0
Program ID: 147-45-21-080

Tennessee

Johnson City

East Tennessee State University Program

Sponsor: James H Quillen College of Medicine
Johnson City Medical Center Hospital
Veterans Affairs Medical Center (Mountain Home)

Program Director:
Anand B Karnad, MD
Div of Medical Oncology/Box 70
622 James H Quillen Coll
Johnson City, TN 37614-0622
Tel: 423 439-6362 *Fax:* 423 439-6387
Accred Length: 2 Years *Program Size:* 2
Program ID: 147-47-21-195

Memphis

University of Tennessee Program

Sponsor: University of Tennessee College of Medicine
Baptist Memorial Hospital
Regional Medical Center at Memphis
Veterans Affairs Medical Center (Memphis)

Program Director:
Harvey B Niell, MD
Univ of Tennessee
3 N Dunlap/Rm 327
Memphis, TN 38163
Tel: 901 448-5798 *Fax:* 901 448-5033
Accred Length: 2 Years *Program Size:* 4
Program ID: 147-47-21-129

Texas

Dallas

Baylor University Medical Center Program

Sponsor: Baylor University Medical Center

Program Director:
Marvin J Stone, MD
Baylor Univ Med Ctr
3500 Gaston Ave
Dallas, TX 75246
Tel: 214 820-3445 *Fax:* 214 820-2780
Internet:
http://www.bhcs.com/bumc/medicaleducation/residencies.htm
Accred Length: 2 Years *Program Size:* 4
Program ID: 147-48-31-076

Galveston

University of Texas Medical Branch Hospitals Program

Sponsor: University of Texas Medical Branch Hospitals

Program Director:
Thomas Blackwell Jr, MD PhD
Univ of Texas Med Branch
4164 John Sealy Hospital/R-0565
Galveston, TX 77555-0565
Tel: 409 772-1164 *Fax:* 409 772-3533
E-mail: jprice@utmb.edu
Accred Length: 2 Years *Program Size:* 6
Program ID: 147-48-21-053

Houston

Baylor College of Medicine Program

Sponsor: Baylor College of Medicine
Harris County Hospital District-Ben Taub General Hospital
Methodist Hospital
Veterans Affairs Medical Center (Houston)

Program Director:
Garrett R Lynch, MD
Baylor Coll of Med
6550 Fannin St/Ste 1053
Houston, TX 77030
Tel: 713 798-8275 *Fax:* 713 798-3342
E-mail: ecamacho@bcm.tmc.edu
Accred Length: 2 Years *Program Size:* 7
Program ID: 147-48-21-077

University of Texas at Houston Program

Sponsor: University of Texas Medical School at Houston
University of Texas M D Anderson Cancer Center

Program Director:
Richard Pazdur, MD
Univ of Texas-MD Anderson Cancer Ctr
1515 Holcombe Blvd/Box 92
Houston, TX 77030
Tel: 713 792-7246 *Fax:* 713 745-1827
E-mail: rpazdur@mdanderson.org
Accred Length: 2 Years *Program Size:* 30
Program ID: 147-48-31-039

Temple

Texas A&M College of Medicine-Scott and White Program

Sponsor: Scott and White Memorial Hospital

Program Director:
Mark Holguin, MD
Scott and White Memorial Hospital
2401 S 31st St
Temple, TX 76508
Tel: 800 299-4463, ext 45817 *Fax:* 254 724-4079
E-mail: bamerman@swmail.sw.org
Internet: http://www.sw.org
Accred Length: 2 Years *Program Size:* 6
Program ID: 147-48-21-186

Washington

Seattle

University of Washington Program

Sponsor: University of Washington School of Medicine
Fred Hutchinson Cancer Research Center
University of Washington Medical Center

Program Director:
Effie W Petersdorf, MD
Fred Hutchinson Cancer Research Ctr
1101 Fairview Avenue N/D5-310
PO Box 19024
Seattle, WA 98109-1024
Tel: 206 667-5244 *Fax:* 206 667-5255
E-mail: epetersd@fhcrc.org
Internet: http://www.fhcrc.org
Accred Length: 2 Years *Program Size:* 18
Program ID: 147-54-21-175

Wisconsin

Madison

University of Wisconsin Program

Sponsor: University of Wisconsin Hospital and Clinics
William S Middleton Veterans Hospital

Program Director:
James A Stewart, MD
Univ of Wisconsin Hospital and Clinics
600 Highland Ave/Rm K6-544
Madison, WI 53792-0001
Tel: 608 263-1399 *Fax:* 608 265-8133
E-mail: stewart@biostat.wisc.edu
Accred Length: 2 Years *Program Size:* 6
Program ID: 147-56-21-111

Ophthalmology

Alabama

Birmingham

University of Alabama Medical Center Program

Sponsor: University of Alabama Hospital
Cooper Green Hospital
Eye Foundation Hospital
Veterans Affairs Medical Center (Birmingham)

Program Director:
Andrew J Mays, MD
Eye Foundation Hospital
700 S 18th St/Ste 300
Birmingham, AL 35233
Tel: 205 325-8507 *Fax:* 205 325-8654
Accred Length: 3 Years *Program Size:* 15
Program ID: 240-01-21-015

Arizona

Tucson

University of Arizona Program

Sponsor: University of Arizona College of Medicine
Kino Community Hospital
University Medical Center
Veterans Affairs Medical Center (Tucson)

Program Director:
Robert J Noecker, MD
Univ of Arizona Coll of Med
Dept of Ophthalmology
1801 N Campbell Ave
Tucson, AZ 85719-3758
Tel: 520 321-3677, ext 204 *Fax:* 520 321-3665
E-mail: rnoecker@eyes.arizona.edu
Internet: http://www.eyes.arizona.edu
Accred Length: 3 Years *Program Size:* 6
Program ID: 240-03-21-171

Arkansas

Little Rock

University of Arkansas for Medical Sciences Program

Sponsor: University of Arkansas College of Medicine
Arkansas Children's Hospital
John L McClellan Memorial Veterans Hospital
University Hospital of Arkansas

Program Director:
Richard A Harper, MD
Univ of Arkansas for Med Sciences
4301 W Markham St/Slot 523
Little Rock, AR 72205-7199
Tel: 501 686-5150 *Fax:* 501 686-7037
E-mail: harperrichardа@exchange.uams.edu
Internet: http://www.uams.edu/jei/home.htm
Accred Length: 3 Years *Program Size:* 9
Program ID: 240-04-21-018

California

Loma Linda

Loma Linda University Program

Sponsor: Loma Linda University Medical Center
Jerry L Pettis Memorial Veterans Hospital
Riverside County Regional Medical Center

Program Director:
Kimber Schneider, MD
Dept of Ophthalmology
11370 Anderson St/#1800
Loma Linda, CA 92354
Tel: 909 799-8414 *Fax:* 909 796-8294
Accred Length: 3 Years *Program Size:* 9
Program ID: 240-05-21-023

Los Angeles

Charles R Drew University Program

Sponsor: Charles R Drew University of Medicine and Science
LAC-King/Drew Medical Center

Program Director:
Glenville A March Jr, MD
Martin Luther King Jr-Drew Med Ctr
12021 S Wilmington Ave
Los Angeles, CA 90059
Tel: 310 668-4531 *Fax:* 310 638-6947
Accred Length: 3 Years *Program Size:* 6
Program ID: 240-05-21-026

UCLA Medical Center Program

Sponsor: UCLA School of Medicine
Los Angeles County-Harbor-UCLA Medical Center
VA Greater Los Angeles Healthcare System

Program Director:
Anthony C Arnold, MD
Jules Stein Eye Inst-UCLA
100 Stein Plaza/Rm 3-223
Los Angeles, CA 90095-7000
Tel: 310 206-6138 *Fax:* 310 206-8015
E-mail: twitchel@ucla.edu
Internet: http://www.medsch.ucla.edu/som/jsei.residpro.html
Accred Length: 3 Years *Program Size:* 21
Program ID: 240-05-21-027

University of Southern California Program

Sponsor: Los Angeles County-USC Medical Center

Program Director:
Alfredo A Sadun, MD PhD
Doheny Eye Inst
1450 San Pablo St
Los Angeles, CA 90033
Tel: 323 442-6417 *Fax:* 323 442-6440
E-mail: asadun@hsc.usc.edu
Internet: http://www.usc.edu/hsc/doheny
Accred Length: 3 Years *Program Size:* 15
Program ID: 240-05-21-025

Orange

University of California (Irvine) Program

Sponsor: University of California (Irvine) Medical Center
Long Beach Memorial Medical Center
Veterans Affairs Medical Center (Long Beach)

Program Director:
Richard A Hill, MD
Univ of California Irvine Coll of Med
Dept of Ophthalmology
118 Med Surge I
Irvine, CA 92697-4375
Tel: 949 824-6109 *Fax:* 949 824-4015
E-mail: alane@uci.edu
Internet: http://uceye.com/
Accred Length: 3 Years *Program Size:* 9
Program ID: 240-05-21-022

Sacramento

University of California (Davis) Program
Sponsor: University of California (Davis) Medical Center

Program Director:
Jeffrey J Caspar, MD
Dept of Ophthalmology
4860 Y St/Ste 2400
Sacramento, CA 95817
Tel: 916 734-6060 *Fax:* 916 734-6992
E-mail: wmreed@ucdavis.edu
Internet: http://www.eyecenter@ucdmc.ucdavis.edu
Accred Length: 3 Years *Program Size:* 9
Program ID: 240-05-21-020

San Diego

Naval Medical Center (San Diego) Program
Sponsor: Naval Medical Center (San Diego)

Program Director:
Neil T Choplin, MD
Naval Med Ctr
Dept of Ophthalmology
34800 Bob Wilson Dr
San Diego, CA 92134-5000
Tel: 619 532-6702 *Fax:* 619 532-7272
E-mail: snd1ntc@snd10.med.navy.mil
Accred Length: 3 Years *Program Size:* 9
Program ID: 240-05-32-008
US Armed Services Program

University of California (San Diego) Program
Sponsor: University of California (San Diego) Medical Center
Veterans Affairs Medical Center (San Diego)

Program Director:
Don O Kikkawa, MD
Shiley Eye Ctr
Dept of Ophthalmology
9500 Gilman Dr (0946)
La Jolla, CA 92093-0946
Tel: 619 534-2238 *Fax:* 619 534-7859
Accred Length: 3 Years *Program Size:* 8
Program ID: 240-05-21-030

San Francisco

California Pacific Medical Center Program
Sponsor: California Pacific Medical Center
Alameda County Medical Center
California Pacific Medical Center

Program Director:
Susan Day, MD
California Pacific Med Ctr
Dept of Med Educ
2351 Clay St/Rm 362
San Francisco, CA 94115
Tel: 800 743-7707 *Fax:* 415 775-7437
Internet: http://www.cpmc.org
Accred Length: 3 Years *Program Size:* 6
Program ID: 240-05-22-031

University of California (San Francisco) Program
Sponsor: University of California (San Francisco) School of Medicine
San Francisco General Hospital Medical Center
University of California (San Francisco) Medical Center
Veterans Affairs Medical Center (San Francisco)

Program Director:
Susan R Carter, MD
Univ of California San Francisco Sch of Med
10 Kirkham St
K-301
San Francisco, CA 94143-0730
Tel: 415 476-1921 *Fax:* 415 476-0336
Internet: http://www.ucsfeye.net
Accred Length: 3 Years *Program Size:* 12
Program ID: 240-05-21-032

Stanford

Stanford University Program
Sponsor: Stanford University Hospital
Santa Clara Valley Medical Center
Veterans Affairs Palo Alto Health Care System

Program Director:
Michael Marmor, MD
Stanford Univ Med Ctr
300 Pasteur Dr/Rm A157
Stanford, CA 94305-5308
Tel: 650 723-5517 *Fax:* 650 723-7918
Accred Length: 3 Years *Program Size:* 9
Program ID: 240-05-21-033

Colorado

Denver

University of Colorado Program
Sponsor: University of Colorado Health Sciences Center
Denver Health and Hospitals
Veterans Affairs Medical Center (Denver)

Program Director:
Caoline J Shea, MD
Dept of Ophthalmology
4200 E Ninth Ave
Box B-204
Denver, CO 80262
Tel: 303 315-8260 *Fax:* 303 315-5644
E-mail: caroline.shea@uchsc.edu
Accred Length: 3 Years *Program Size:* 12
Program ID: 240-07-21-035

Connecticut

New Haven

Yale-New Haven Medical Center Program
Sponsor: Yale-New Haven Hospital
Veterans Affairs Medical Center (West Haven)

Program Director:
Marc Weitzman, MD
Yale Eye Ctr
PO Box 208061
New Haven, CT 06520-8061
Tel: 203 737-1161 *Fax:* 203 785-7694
Internet: http://www.pandora.med.yale.edu/ophtha/
Accred Length: 3 Years *Program Size:* 16
Program ID: 240-08-21-036

District of Columbia

Washington

George Washington University Program
Sponsor: George Washington University School of Medicine
Children's National Medical Center
George Washington University Hospital (UHS)
Veterans Affairs Medical Center (Martinsburg)

Program Director:
John Zacharia, MD
2150 Pennsylvania Ave NW/Fl 2A
Washington, DC 20037
Tel: 202 994-4048 *Fax:* 202 994-6209
Accred Length: 3 Years *Program Size:* 12
Program ID: 240-10-21-039

Georgetown University Program
Sponsor: Georgetown University Medical Center
District of Columbia General Hospital
Veterans Affairs Medical Center (Washington, DC)

Program Director:
Georgia A Chrousos, MD
Ctr for Sight
3800 Reservoir Rd NW
PAC 7th Fl
Washington, DC 20007
Tel: 202 687-4614 *Fax:* 202 687-4978
Accred Length: 3 Years *Program Size:* 12
Program ID: 240-10-21-038

Howard University Program
Sponsor: Howard University Hospital
District of Columbia General Hospital

Program Director:
Brian A Phillpotts, MD
Howard Univ Hospital, Div of Ophthalmology
2041 Georgia Ave NW
Washington, DC 20060
Tel: 202 865-1257 *Fax:* 202 865-4259
Accred Length: 3 Years *Program Size:* 8
Program ID: 240-10-21-040

Walter Reed Army Medical Center Program
Sponsor: Walter Reed Army Medical Center

Program Director:
William P Madigan Jr, MD
Ophthalmology Service
Walter Reed Army Med Ctr
6825 16th St NW
Washington, DC 20307-5001
Tel: 202 782-6960 *Fax:* 202 782-6156
Accred Length: 3 Years *Program Size:* 10
Program ID: 240-10-12-004
US Armed Services Program

Washington Hospital Center Program
Sponsor: Washington Hospital Center

Program Director:
Francis G LaPiana, MD
Washington Hospital Ctr
110 Irving St NW
Ste 1A-19
Washington, DC 20010-2975
Tel: 202 877-6159 *Fax:* 202 877-7743
E-mail: pah6@mhg.edu
Internet: http://www.whc.mhg.edu/wnec
Accred Length: 3 Years *Program Size:* 12
Program ID: 240-10-32-041

Florida

Gainesville

University of Florida Program
Sponsor: University of Florida College of Medicine
Shands Hospital at the University of Florida
University Medical Center (UFHSC/J)
Veterans Affairs Medical Center (Gainesville)

Program Director:
Mary Fran Smith, MD
Univ of Florida
Dept of Ophthalmology
Box 100284 JHMHC
Gainesville, FL 32610-0284
Tel: 352 392-3451 *Fax:* 352 392-7839
E-mail: kjanick@eye1.eye.ufl.edu
Internet: http://www.eye.ufl.edu
Accred Length: 3 Years *Program Size:* 15
Program ID: 240-11-21-042

Miami

University of Miami-Jackson Memorial Medical Center Program
Sponsor: University of Miami-Jackson Memorial Medical Center
Bascom Palmer Eye Institute-Anne Bates Leach Eye Hospital
Veterans Affairs Medical Center (Miami)

Program Director:
Richard K Parrish, MD
Bascom Palmer Eye Inst
PO Box 016880
Miami, FL 33101-6880
Tel: 305 326-6389 *Fax:* 305 326-6306
E-mail: rparrish@bpei.med.miami.edu.
Internet: http://www.bpei.med.miami.edu
Accred Length: 3 Years *Program Size:* 18
Program ID: 240-11-11-043

Tampa

University of South Florida Program
Sponsor: University of South Florida College of Medicine
James A Haley Veterans Hospital
Tampa General Healthcare

Program Director:
Lewis R Groden, MD
Univ of South Florida
Dept of Ophthalmology
12901 Bruce B Downs Blvd/Box 21
Tampa, FL 33612-4799
Tel: 813 974-3820 *Fax:* 813 974-5621
Accred Length: 3 Years *Program Size:* 10
Program ID: 240-11-21-044

Georgia

Atlanta

Emory University Program
Sponsor: Emory University School of Medicine
Emory University Hospital
Grady Memorial Hospital
Veterans Affairs Medical Center (Atlanta)

Program Director:
Geoffrey Broocker, MD
Emory Univ
1365-B Clifton Rd NE
Ste 2400
Atlanta, GA 30322
Tel: 404 778-4530 *Fax:* 404 778-5128
E-mail: sande05@emory.edu
Internet:
http://www.cc.emory.edu/emory_center/index.html
Accred Length: 3 Years *Program Size:* 15
Program ID: 240-12-21-045

Augusta

Medical College of Georgia Program
Sponsor: Medical College of Georgia Hospital and Clinics
Veterans Affairs Medical Center (Augusta)

Program Director:
Malcolm N Luxenberg, MD
Med Coll of Georgia
1120 15th St
Augusta, GA 30912-3400
Tel: 706 721-1148 *Fax:* 706 721-1158
E-mail: mluxenberg@mail.mcg.edu
Internet: http://www.mcg.edu/som/eye/index.html.
Accred Length: 3 Years *Program Size:* 9
Program ID: 240-12-21-046

Illinois

Chicago

Cook County Hospital Program
Sponsor: Cook County Hospital

Program Director:
Alan J Axelrod, MD
Cook County Hospital
1835 W Harrison St
Chicago, IL 60612-9985
Tel: 312 633-6383 *Fax:* 312 572-4962
Accred Length: 3 Years *Program Size:* 9
Program ID: 240-16-22-047

McGaw Medical Center of Northwestern University Program
Sponsor: Northwestern University Medical School
Children's Memorial Medical Center
Evanston Hospital
Northwestern Memorial Hospital
Veterans Affairs Lakeside Medical Center (Chicago)

Program Director:
Michael Rosenberg, MD
Northwestern Univ Med Sch
Dept of Ophthalmology
645 N Michigan Ave/Ste 440
Chicago, IL 60611
Tel: 312 908-8152 *Fax:* 312 503-8152
E-mail: gail-weber@nwu.edu
Accred Length: 3 Years *Program Size:* 12
Program ID: 240-16-21-049

Rush-Presbyterian-St Luke's Medical Center Program
Sponsor: Rush-Presbyterian-St Luke's Medical Center

Program Director:
Jack A Cohen, MD
Rush-Presbyterian-St Luke's Med Ctr
Ste 906/Professional Bldg
1653 W Congress Pkwy
Chicago, IL 60612-3864
Tel: 312 942-5370 *Fax:* 312 942-2140
E-mail: jcohen@rush.edu
Internet:
http://www.rush.edu/departments/ophthalmology/
Accred Length: 3 Years *Program Size:* 6
Program ID: 240-16-11-050

University of Chicago Program
Sponsor: University of Chicago Hospitals
Oak Forest Hospital of Cook County

Program Director:
Samir C Patel, MD
Univ of Chicago-Visual Sciences Ctr
939 E 57th St/MC2114
Chicago, IL 60637-1470
Tel: 773 702-1985 *Fax:* 773 834-0714
E-mail: spatel1@midway.uchicago.edu
Internet: http://bsd.uchicago.edu/oph/
Accred Length: 3 Years *Program Size:* 9
Program ID: 240-16-21-174

University of Illinois College of Medicine at Chicago Program
Sponsor: University of Illinois College of Medicine at Chicago
Michael Reese Hospital and Medical Center
University of Illinois Hospital and Clinics

Program Director:
Mark T Duffy, MD PhD
Univ of Illinois Eye and Ear Infirmary
1855 W Taylor St/1.59
Chicago, IL 60612
Tel: 312 996-8023 *Fax:* 312 996-7770
E-mail: mtd@uic.edu
Internet: http://www.uic.edu/com/eye
Accred Length: 3 Years *Program Size:* 21
Program ID: 240-16-21-052

Maywood

Loyola University Program
Sponsor: Loyola University Medical Center
Edward J Hines Jr Veterans Affairs Hospital

Program Director:
Charles S Bouchard, MD
Loyola Univ-Stritch Sch of Med
Foster G McGaw Hospital
2160 S First Ave
Maywood, IL 60153-5585
Tel: 708 216-3408 *Fax:* 708 216-3557
E-mail: cboucha@luc.edu
Internet:
http://www.meddean.luc.edu/lumen/deptwebs/ophthalmology/general.htm
Accred Length: 3 Years *Program Size:* 9
Program ID: 240-16-21-054

Programs

Indiana

Indianapolis

Indiana University School of Medicine Program

Sponsor: Indiana University School of Medicine
Clarian IU Hospital
Clarian Methodist Hospital of Indiana
Clarian Riley Hospital for Children
Richard L Roudebush Veterans Affairs Medical Center
William N Wishard Memorial Hospital

Program Director:
Louis B Cantor, MD
Indiana Univ Med Ctr
Attn: Peggy Hannah
702 Rotary Circle
Indianapolis, IN 46202-5175
Tel: 317 274-2128 *Fax:* 317 274-2277
E-mail: phannah@.iupui.edu
Internet: http://www.iupui.edu/it/eye/
Accred Length: 3 Years *Program Size:* 18
Program ID: 240-17-21-055

Iowa

Iowa City

University of Iowa Hospitals and Clinics Program

Sponsor: University of Iowa Hospitals and Clinics

Program Director:
Keith D Carter, MD
Univ of Iowa Hospitals and Clinics
Dept of Ophthalmology
200 Hawkins Dr
Iowa City, IA 52242-1091
Tel: 319 356-0453 *Fax:* 319 356-0363
E-mail: e-diane-anderson@uiowa.edu
Internet: http://www.webeye.ophth.uiowa.edu
Accred Length: 3 Years *Program Size:* 17
Program ID: 240-18-11-056

Kansas

Kansas City

University of Kansas Medical Center Program

Sponsor: University of Kansas School of Medicine
University of Kansas Medical Center
Veterans Affairs Medical Center (Kansas City)

Program Director:
Keith A Warren, MD
Univ of Kansas Med Ctr
3901 Rainbow Blvd
Kansas City, KS 66160-7379
Tel: 913 588-6605 *Fax:* 913 588-6615
Internet: http://www.kumc.edu
Accred Length: 3 Years *Program Size:* 6
Program ID: 240-19-21-057

Kentucky

Lexington

University of Kentucky Medical Center Program

Sponsor: University of Kentucky Hospital
Veterans Affairs Medical Center (Lexington)

Program Director:
Julia L Stevens, MD
Univ of Kentucky-Kentucky Clinic
Dept of Ophthalmology
E 306 Kentucky Clinic
Lexington, KY 40536-0284
Tel: 606 323-6438 *Fax:* 606 323-1122
E-mail: jlstev@pop.uky.edu
Internet:
http://www.comed.uky.edu/medicine/departments/ophthalmology/ophthalmology.html
Accred Length: 3 Years *Program Size:* 9
Program ID: 240-20-21-058

Louisville

University of Louisville Program

Sponsor: University of Louisville School of Medicine
Kosair Children's Hospital (Alliant Health System)
University of Louisville Hospital
Veterans Affairs Medical Center (Louisville)

Program Director:
John W Gamel, MD
Univ of Louisville Sch of Med
Dept of Ophthalmology
301 E Muhammad Ali Blvd
Louisville, KY 40202
Tel: 502 852-0710 *Fax:* 502 852-7298
E-mail: jwgame01@homer.louisville.edu
Internet:
http://www.louisville.edu/medschool/ophthalmology/resident.htm
Accred Length: 3 Years *Program Size:* 9
Program ID: 240-20-21-059

Louisiana

New Orleans

Louisiana State University/Alton Ochsner Medical Foundation Program

Sponsor: Louisiana State University School of Medicine
Alton Ochsner Medical Foundation
LSU/Ochsner Opthalmology Center
Medical Center of Louisiana at New Orleans

Program Director:
Donald R Bergsma, MD
Louisiana State Univ Eye Ctr
2020 Gravier St/Ste B
New Orleans, LA 70112
Tel: 504 568-6700, ext 349 *Fax:* 504 568-4210
E-mail: bhill@lsumc.edu
Accred Length: 3 Years *Program Size:* 25
Program ID: 240-21-21-177

Tulane University Program

Sponsor: Tulane University School of Medicine
Medical Center of Louisiana at New Orleans
Tulane University Hospital and Clinics
Veterans Affairs Medical Center-LSU Service (New Orleans)

Program Director:
Zeynel Karcioglu, MD
Tulane Univ Sch of Med
Dept of Ophthalmology
1430 Tulane Ave
New Orleans, LA 70112-2699
Tel: 504 588-5804 *Fax:* 504 584-2684
Internet:
http://www.omi.tulane.edu/department/ophthalmology/fac.html
Accred Length: 3 Years *Program Size:* 27
Program ID: 240-21-21-062

Shreveport

Louisiana State University (Shreveport) Program

Sponsor: Louisiana State University Hospital-Shreveport
Overton Brooks Veterans Affairs Medical Center

Program Director:
Thomas B Redens, MD
Louisiana State Univ Med Ctr, Med Education
1501 Kings Hwy
PO Box 33932
Shreveport, LA 71130-3932
Tel: 318 675-5010 *Fax:* 318 675-6000
E-mail: bplyan@lsumc.edu
Accred Length: 3 Years *Program Size:* 12
Program ID: 240-21-21-063

Maryland

Baltimore

Johns Hopkins University/Sinai Hospital of Baltimore Program

Sponsor: Johns Hopkins University School of Medicine
Greater Baltimore Medical Center
Johns Hopkins Hospital
Sinai Hospital of Baltimore

Program Director:
James P Dunn Jr, MD
Donald A Abrams, MD
Wilmer Eye Inst-Johns Hopkins Hospital
550 N Broadway
Ste 700
Baltimore, MD 21205
Tel: 410 955-1966 *Fax:* 410 955-0629
E-mail: jpdunn@jhmi.edu
Accred Length: 3 Years *Program Size:* 23
Program ID: 240-23-21-065

Maryland General Hospital Program

Sponsor: Maryland General Hospital

Program Director:
Samuel D Friedel, MD
Maryland General Hospital
827 Linden Ave
Baltimore, MD 21201
Tel: 410 225-8077 *Fax:* 410 225-8785
Accred Length: 3 Years *Program Size:* 6
Subspecialties: TY
Program ID: 240-23-12-066

University of Maryland Program
Sponsor: University of Maryland Medical System
Program Director:
Ramzi K Hemady, MD
Univ of Maryland
Dept of Ophthalmology
22 S Greene St
Baltimore, MD 21201-1590
Tel: 410 328-5929 *Fax:* 410 328-6346
Accred Length: 3 Years *Program Size:* 9
Program ID: 240-23-21-068

Massachusetts

Boston

Boston University Medical Center Program
Sponsor: Boston Medical Center
Program Director:
Ippolit C Matjucha, MD
Boston Univ Sch of Med
715 Albany St
L-907
Boston, MA 02118-2398
Tel: 617 638-4550 *Fax:* 617 638-5337
E-mail: ophthalm@bu.edu
Internet: http://www.bumc.bu.edu/ophthalmology
Accred Length: 3 Years *Program Size:* 12
Program ID: 240-24-21-069

Massachusetts Eye and Ear Infirmary Program
Sponsor: Massachusetts Eye and Ear Infirmary
Program Director:
Anthony P Adamis, MD
Massachusetts Eye and Ear Infirmary
243 Charles St
Boston, MA 02114-3096
Tel: 617 573-3529 *Fax:* 617 573-3364
Accred Length: 3 Years *Program Size:* 21
Program ID: 240-24-21-070

Tufts University Program
Sponsor: New England Medical Center Hospitals
UMass Memorial Health Care (University Campus)
Veterans Affairs Medical Center (Boston)
Program Director:
Joel S Schuman, MD
New England Eye Ctr
New England Med Ctr Hospitals
750 Washington St/Box 450
Boston, MA 02111
Tel: 617 636-7950 *Fax:* 617 636-4866
E-mail: joel.schuman@es.nemc.org
Internet: http://www.neec.com
Accred Length: 3 Years *Program Size:* 12
Program ID: 240-24-21-071

Michigan

Ann Arbor

University of Michigan Program
Sponsor: University of Michigan Hospitals
Veterans Affairs Medical Center (Ann Arbor)
Program Director:
Michael Roth, MD
Univ of Michigan Med Sch
W K Kellogg Eye Ctr/Box 0714
1000 Wall St
Ann Arbor, MI 48105
Tel: 313 764-5208 *Fax:* 313 936-2340
E-mail: kwhitney@www.med.umich.edu
Internet: http://www.med.umich.edu/kec/html
Accred Length: 3 Years *Program Size:* 18
Program ID: 240-25-11-072

Detroit

Henry Ford Hospital Program
Sponsor: Henry Ford Hospital
Program Director:
J David Carey, MD
Henry Ford Hospital
2799 W Grand Blvd
Detroit, MI 48202
Tel: 313 876-3239 *Fax:* 313 876-1327
Accred Length: 3 Years *Program Size:* 15
Subspecialties: TY
Program ID: 240-25-12-073

Wayne State University/Detroit Medical Center (Sinai Hospital) Program
Sponsor: Wayne State University/Detroit Medical Center
Sinai Hospital
Program Director:
Hugh Beckman, MD
Sinai Hospital
6767 W Outer Dr
Detroit, MI 48235-2899
Tel: 313 493-5187
Accred Length: 3 Years *Program Size:* 6
Program ID: 240-25-31-074

Wayne State University/Detroit Medical Center Program
Sponsor: Wayne State University/Detroit Medical Center
Children's Hospital of Michigan
Hutzel Hospital
Sinai Hospital
Program Director:
Mark S Juzych, MD
Kresge Eye Inst
4717 St Antoine Blvd
Detroit, MI 48201
Tel: 313 577-7614 *Fax:* 313 577-4991
E-mail: mjuzych@med.wayne.edu
Internet: http://www.med.wayne.edu/kresgeeye
Accred Length: 3 Years *Program Size:* 21
Program ID: 240-25-21-075

Royal Oak

William Beaumont Hospital Program
Sponsor: William Beaumont Hospital
Program Director:
Raymond R Margherio, MD
William Beaumont Hospital
Beaumont Eye Inst
3535 W 13 Mile Rd/#555
Royal Oak, MI 48073
Tel: 248 551-2175 *Fax:* 248 551-4362
E-mail: margheri@oakland.edu
Internet: http://www.beaumont.edu/html/gme
Accred Length: 3 Years *Program Size:* 6
Program ID: 240-25-21-165

Minnesota

Minneapolis

University of Minnesota Program
Sponsor: University of Minnesota Medical School
Fairview-University Medical Center
Hennepin County Medical Center
Regions Hospital
Veterans Affairs Medical Center (Minneapolis)
Program Director:
Martha M Wright, MD
Univ of Minnesota
UMHC Box 493
420 Delaware St SE
Minneapolis, MN 55455-0501
Tel: 612 625-4400 *Fax:* 612 626-3119
E-mail: wrigh004@maroon.tc.umn.edu
Internet: http://www.med.umn.edu/ophthalmology
Accred Length: 3 Years *Program Size:* 14
Program ID: 240-26-21-077

Rochester

Mayo Graduate School of Medicine (Rochester) Program
Sponsor: Mayo Graduate School of Medicine-Mayo Foundation
Mayo Clinic (Rochester)
Rochester Methodist Hospital
St Mary's Hospital of Rochester
Program Director:
John M Pach, MD
Application Processing Ctr
Mayo Graduate Sch of Med
200 First St SW
Rochester, MN 55905
Tel: 507 284-1709 *Fax:* 507 284-0161
E-mail: mgsm.surgical.specialties@mayo.edu
Internet: http://www.mayo.edu/
Accred Length: 3 Years *Program Size:* 12
Program ID: 240-26-21-078

Mississippi

Jackson

University of Mississippi Medical Center Program
Sponsor: University of Mississippi School of Medicine
University Hospital
Veterans Affairs Medical Center (Jackson)
Program Director:
Samuel B Johnson, MD
Univ of Mississippi Med Ctr
2500 N State St
McBryde Bldg
Jackson, MS 39216
Tel: 601 984-5020, ext 5023 *Fax:* 601 984-5031
Accred Length: 3 Years *Program Size:* 9
Program ID: 240-27-21-079

Missouri

Columbia

University of Missouri-Columbia Program

Sponsor: University of Missouri-Columbia School of Medicine
Harry S Truman Memorial Veterans Hospital
University Hospitals and Clinics
Program Director:
John W Cowden, MD
Mason Eye Inst-Univ of Missouri Columbia
One Hospital Dr
Columbia, MO 65212
Tel: 573 882-9678 *Fax:* 573 882-8474
E-mail: jill_hickam@muccmail.missouri.edu
Internet:
http://www.hsc.missouri.edu/~ophthalmology/index.html
Accred Length: 3 Years *Program Size:* 9
Program ID: 240-28-22-080

Kansas City

University of Missouri at Kansas City Program

Sponsor: University of Missouri-Kansas City School of Medicine
Children's Mercy Hospital
Truman Medical Center-West
Program Director:
Nelson R Sabates, MD
Eye Foundation of Kansas City
2300 Holmes St
Kansas City, MO 64108
Tel: 816 881-6150 *Fax:* 816 881-6167
E-mail: nsabates@umkc-efkc.org
Internet: http://www.umkc-efkc.org
Accred Length: 3 Years *Program Size:* 9
Program ID: 240-28-21-081

St Louis

St Louis University School of Medicine Program

Sponsor: St Louis University School of Medicine
Anheuser-Busch Eye Institute
Program Director:
Sophia M Chung, MD
St Louis Univ Sch of Med
1755 S Grand Blvd
St Louis, MO 63104
Tel: 314 577-8260 *Fax:* 314 771-0596
Internet: http://www.slucare.edu/clinical/eye/
Accred Length: 3 Years *Program Size:* 12
Program ID: 240-28-21-083

Washington University/B-JH/SLCH Consortium Program

Sponsor: Washington University/B-JH/SLCH Consortium
Barnes-Jewish Hospital
Veterans Affairs Medical Center (St Louis)
Program Director:
Carla J Siegfried, MD
Washington Univ Sch of Med
660 S Euclid Ave
Campus Box 8096
St Louis, MO 63110
Tel: 314 362-5722 *Fax:* 314 362-3725
E-mail: siegfriedc@am.seer.wustl.edu
Internet: http://www.ophthalmology.wustl.edu
Accred Length: 3 Years *Program Size:* 15
Program ID: 240-28-21-084

Nebraska

Omaha

University of Nebraska Program

Sponsor: University of Nebraska Medical Center
Veterans Affairs Medical Center (Omaha)
Program Director:
Thomas W Hejkal, MD
Univ of Nebraska Med Ctr
985540 Nebraska Med Ctr
Omaha, NE 68198-5540
Tel: 402 559-4276 *Fax:* 402 559-5514
E-mail: twhejkal@unmc.edu
Internet: http://www.unmc.edu/eye
Accred Length: 3 Years *Program Size:* 6
Program ID: 240-30-21-085

New Jersey

Camden

UMDNJ-Robert Wood Johnson Medical School (Camden) Program

Sponsor: Cooper Hospital-University Medical Center
Elkins Park Hospital
Frankford Hospital (Torresdale Campus)
Program Director:
David B Soll, MD
Div of Ophthalmology
3 Cooper Plaza/Ste 510
Camden, NJ 08103
Tel: 609 288-5000 *Fax:* 215 288-5601
Accred Length: 3 Years *Program Size:* 9
Program ID: 240-33-21-172

Newark

UMDNJ-New Jersey Medical School Program

Sponsor: UMDNJ-New Jersey Medical School
Jersey City Medical Center
UMDNJ-University Hospital
Veterans Affairs Medical Center (East Orange)
Program Director:
Paul D Langer, MD
UMDNJ-New Jersey Med Sch
Dept of Ophthalmology/6th Fl DOC
90 Bergen St
Newark, NJ 07103-2499
Tel: 973 982-2036 *Fax:* 973 982-2068
E-mail: planger@umdnj.edu
Internet: http://www.umdnj.edu
Accred Length: 3 Years *Program Size:* 15
Program ID: 240-33-21-086

New York

Albany

Albany Medical Center Program

Sponsor: Albany Medical Center
Veterans Affairs Medical Center (Albany)
Program Director:
Martha G Farber, MD
Lions Eye Inst
35 Hackett Blvd
Albany, NY 12208
Tel: 518 262-2519 *Fax:* 518 262-2516
E-mail: judy_whalen@ccgateway.amc.edu
Accred Length: 3 Years *Program Size:* 9
Program ID: 240-35-21-087

Bronx

Albert Einstein College of Medicine Program

Sponsor: Albert Einstein College of Medicine of Yeshiva University
Jacobi Medical Center
Montefiore Medical Center-Henry and Lucy Moses Division
Montefiore Medical Center-Weiler Hospital
North Central Bronx Hospital
Program Director:
Harry M Engel, MD
Montefiore Med Ctr
Centennial Bldg/Rm 306
111 E 210th St
Bronx, NY 10467
Tel: 718 920-7646 *Fax:* 718 515-3734
E-mail: burde@aecom.yu.edu
Internet: http://www.montefiore.org
Accred Length: 3 Years *Program Size:* 12
Program ID: 240-35-21-093

Bronx-Lebanon Hospital Center Program

Sponsor: Bronx-Lebanon Hospital Center
Program Director:
Martin Mayers, MD
Bronx-Lebanon Hospital Ctr
1650 Selwyn Ave/Apt 10G
Bronx, NY 10457
Tel: 718 960-2041 *Fax:* 718 960-2045
Accred Length: 3 Years *Program Size:* 6
Program ID: 240-35-21-095

Brooklyn

Brookdale University Hospital Medical Center Program

Sponsor: Brookdale University Hospital Medical Center
Program Director:
George F Hyman, MD
Brookdale Univ Hospital and Med Ctr
One Brookdale Plaza
Rm 104
Brooklyn, NY 11212-3198
Tel: 718 240-5827 *Fax:* 718 240-6625
Accred Length: 3 Years *Program Size:* 6
Program ID: 240-35-11-096

Interfaith Medical Center Program

Sponsor: Interfaith Medical Center
Program Director:
Wally Kopelowitz, MD
Interfaith Med Ctr
Dept of Ophthalmology
555 Prospect Pl
Brooklyn, NY 11238
Tel: 718 935-7293 *Fax:* 718 935-7763
Accred Length: 3 Years *Program Size:* 6
Program ID: 240-35-11-100

SUNY Health Science Center at Brooklyn Program

Sponsor: SUNY Health Science Center at Brooklyn
Brooklyn Hospital Center
Coney Island Hospital
Kings County Hospital Center
Long Island College Hospital
Maimonides Medical Center
University Hospital-SUNY Health Science Center at Brooklyn
Veterans Affairs Medical Center (Brooklyn)
Program Director:
Monica Dweck, MD
450 Clarkson Ave
Brooklyn, NY 11203-2098
Tel: 718 270-1961 *Fax:* 718 270-2972
Accred Length: 3 Years *Program Size:* 20
Program ID: 240-35-21-113

Buffalo

SUNY at Buffalo Graduate Medical-Dental Education Consortium Program
Sponsor: SUNY at Buffalo Grad Medical-Dental Education Consortium
CGF Health System (Children's Hospital of Buffalo)
Erie County Medical Center
Veterans Affairs Medical Center (Buffalo)
Program Director:
Scott E Olitsky, MD
Children's Hospital
219 Bryant St
Buffalo, NY 14222
Tel: 716 878-7204 *Fax:* 716 888-3807
E-mail: solitsky@acsu.buffalo.edu
Internet: http://www.smbs.buffalo/ophthalmology
Accred Length: 3 Years *Program Size:* 8
Program ID: 240-35-11-170

East Meadow

Nassau County Medical Center Program
Sponsor: Nassau County Medical Center
Veterans Affairs Medical Center (Northport)
Program Director:
Elsa K Rahn, MD
Nassau County Med Ctr
2201 Hempstead Trnpk
East Meadow, NY 11554-5400
Tel: 516 572-6706 *Fax:* 516 572-5140
Accred Length: 3 Years *Program Size:* 12
Program ID: 240-35-31-091

Jamaica

Catholic Medical Center of Brooklyn and Queens Program
Sponsor: Catholic Medical Center of Brooklyn and Queens Inc
Catholic Medical Center (Mary Immaculate Hospital)
Program Director:
Cono M Grasso, MD
Laurence R Weissman, MD
Catholic Med Ctr of Brooklyn and Queens
88-25 153rd St
Jamaica, NY 11432
Tel: 718 380-8050 *Fax:* 718 558-6276
E-mail: docgrasso@attworldnet.net
Accred Length: 3 Years *Program Size:* 6
Program ID: 240-35-21-098

Manhasset

North Shore University Hospital/NYU School of Medicine Program
Sponsor: North Shore University Hospital
Program Director:
Steven Rubin, MD
North Shore Univ Hospital
#306
600 Northern Blvd
Great Neck, NY 11021
Tel: 516 456-8500 *Fax:* 516 465-8505
E-mail: ardenh@nshs.edu
Accred Length: 3 Years *Program Size:* 6
Program ID: 240-35-11-092

New Hyde Park

Albert Einstein College of Medicine at Long Island Jewish Medical Center Program
Sponsor: Long Island Jewish Medical Center
Queens Hospital Center
Program Director:
Michael L Slavin, MD
Long Island Jewish Med Ctr
Dept of Ophthalmology
600 Northern Blvd/Ste 214
Great Neck, NY 11021
Tel: 516 470-2020 *Fax:* 516 470-2000
Internet:
http://www.lij.edu/lij/ophthalmology/ophthalmology.html
Accred Length: 3 Years *Program Size:* 7
Program ID: 240-35-21-102

New York

Lenox Hill Hospital Program
Sponsor: Lenox Hill Hospital
Program Director:
Stephen A Obstbaum, MD
Dept of Ophthalmology
Lenox Hill Hospital
100 E 77th St
New York, NY 10021
Tel: 212 434-2385 *Fax:* 212 434-3464
Accred Length: 3 Years *Program Size:* 5
Program ID: 240-35-11-101

Manhattan Eye, Ear and Throat Hospital Program
Sponsor: Manhattan Eye, Ear and Throat Hospital
Program Director:
David R Guyer, MD
Manhattan Eye, Ear and Throat Hospital
210 E 64th St
New York, NY 10021
Tel: 212 605-3760 *Fax:* 212 753-7699
Accred Length: 3 Years *Program Size:* 18
Program ID: 240-35-21-168

Mount Sinai School of Medicine Program
Sponsor: Mount Sinai School of Medicine
Elmhurst Hospital Center-Mount Sinai Services
Mount Sinai Medical Center
Veterans Affairs Medical Center (Bronx)
Program Director:
Donna J Galiuso, MD
Mount Sinai Sch of Med
One Gustave L Levy Pl
Box 1183
New York, NY 10029
Tel: 212 241-6752 *Fax:* 212 289-5945
Accred Length: 3 Years *Program Size:* 13
Program ID: 240-35-21-104

New York and Presbyterian Hospital (Columbia Campus) Program
Sponsor: New York and Presbyterian Hospital
New York and Presbyterian Hospital (Columbia Campus)
Program Director:
Stanley Chang, MD
Presbyterian Hospital
635 W 165th St
New York, NY 10032
Tel: 212 305-2725 *Fax:* 212 305-5962
E-mail: sc434@columbia.edu
Internet: http://cpmcnet.cpmc.columbia.edu/dept/eye
Accred Length: 3 Years *Program Size:* 9
Program ID: 240-35-11-109

New York and Presbyterian Hospital (Cornell Campus) Program
Sponsor: New York and Presbyterian Hospital
New York and Presbyterian Hospital (Cornell Campus)
Program Director:
Kip Dolphin, MD
New York Hospital
525 E 68th St
New York, NY 10021
Tel: 212 746-2444 *Fax:* 212 746-8921
E-mail: kdolphin@mail.med.cornell.edu
Accred Length: 3 Years *Program Size:* 9
Program ID: 240-35-21-169

New York Eye and Ear Infirmary Program
Sponsor: New York Eye and Ear Infirmary
Program Director:
Richard B Rosen, MD
New York Eye and Ear Infirmary
310 E 14th St
New York, NY 10003-4201
Tel: 212 979-4495 *Fax:* 212 979-4268
E-mail: rrosen@nyee.edu
Accred Length: 3 Years *Program Size:* 20
Program ID: 240-35-22-105

New York Medical College at St Vincent's Hospital and Medical Center of New York Program
Sponsor: New York Medical College
St Vincent's Hospital and Medical Center of New York
Bayley Seton Hospital
Cabrini Medical Center
Program Director:
Robert A D'Amico, MD
St Vincents Hospital and Med Ctr
Dept of Ophthalmology
153 W 11th St
New York, NY 10011-8305
Tel: 212 604-8041 *Fax:* 212 604-8711
Accred Length: 3 Years *Program Size:* 10
Program ID: 240-35-22-112

New York University Medical Center Program
Sponsor: New York University Medical Center
Bellevue Hospital Center
Veterans Affairs Medical Center (Manhattan)
Program Director:
Kenneth G Noble, MD
New York Univ Med Ctr
550 First Ave
New York, NY 10016
Tel: 212 263-6433 *Fax:* 212 263-8749
Accred Length: 3 Years *Program Size:* 17
Program ID: 240-35-21-108

St Luke's-Roosevelt Hospital Center Program
Sponsor: St Luke's-Roosevelt Hospital Center
St Luke's-Roosevelt Hospital Center-Roosevelt Division
St Luke's-Roosevelt Hospital Center-St Luke's Division
Program Director:
James C Newton, MD
St Luke's-Roosevelt Hospital Ctr
1111 Amsterdam Ave
New York, NY 10025
Tel: 212 523-2562 *Fax:* 212 523-2478
Accred Length: 3 Years *Program Size:* 6
Program ID: 240-35-31-111

Rochester

University of Rochester Program

Sponsor: Strong Memorial Hospital of the University of Rochester
Rochester General Hospital
St Mary's Hospital (Unity Health System)

Program Director:
Donald A Grover, MD
Univ of Rochester Med Ctr
PO Box 659
601 Elmwood Ave
Rochester, NY 14642
Tel: 716 275-3256 *Fax:* 716 273-1043
E-mail: magin@ophth.rochester.edu
Internet: http://www.urmc.rochester.edu/smd/ophthal
Accred Length: 3 Years *Program Size:* 9
Program ID: 240-35-21-115

Syracuse

SUNY Health Science Center at Syracuse Program

Sponsor: University Hospital-SUNY Health Science Center at Syracuse
Crouse Hospital
Veterans Affairs Medical Center (Syracuse)

Program Director:
John A Hoepner, MD
SUNY Health Science Ctr-Syracuse
Dept of Ophthalmology
750 E Adams St
Syracuse, NY 13210
Tel: 315 464-5253 *Fax:* 315 464-6663
E-mail: ophthalm@vax.cs.hscsyr.edu
Internet: http://www.hscsyr.edu/~eye/
Accred Length: 3 Years *Program Size:* 6
Program ID: 240-35-21-116

Valhalla

New York Medical College at Westchester Medical Center Program

Sponsor: New York Medical College
Metropolitan Hospital Center
Our Lady of Mercy Medical Center
Westchester Medical Center

Program Director:
Steven B Zabin, MD
New York Med Coll
Westchester Med Ctr
Valhalla, NY 10595
Tel: 914 493-7671 *Fax:* 914 493-7445
Internet: http://www.nymc.edu
Accred Length: 3 Years *Program Size:* 12
Program ID: 240-35-21-107

North Carolina

Chapel Hill

University of North Carolina Hospitals Program

Sponsor: University of North Carolina Hospitals

Program Director:
David K Wallace, MD
Univ of North Carolina
617 Burnett-Womack Bldg/CB7040
Chapel Hill, NC 27599-7040
Tel: 919 966-5296, ext 241 *Fax:* 919 966-1908
E-mail: dkwallace@med.unc.edu
Internet: http://www.med.unc.edu/ophth/
Accred Length: 3 Years *Program Size:* 9
Program ID: 240-36-31-119

Durham

Duke University Program

Sponsor: Duke University Medical Center
Veterans Affairs Medical Center (Durham)

Program Director:
Terry Kim, MD
Duke Univ Med Ctr
Box 3802
Durham, NC 27710
Tel: 919 681-5995 *Fax:* 919 684-8509
Accred Length: 3 Years *Program Size:* 13
Program ID: 240-36-31-118

Winston-Salem

Wake Forest Universtiy School of Medicine Program

Sponsor: Wake Forest University Baptist Medical Center

Program Director:
Timothy J Martin, MD
Wake Forest Univ Eye Ctr
Medical Center Blvd
Winston-Salem, NC 27157-1033
Tel: 336 716-4091 *Fax:* 336 716-7994
E-mail: eye@wfubmc.edu
Internet: http://www.wfubmc.edu/eye
Accred Length: 3 Years *Program Size:* 6
Program ID: 240-36-11-120

Ohio

Akron

Summa Health System (Akron City Hospital)/NEOUCOM Program

Sponsor: Summa Health System
Akron City Hospital (Summa Health System)
Children's Hospital Medical Center of Akron

Program Director:
James H Bates, MD
Summa Health System
Med Educ/Mary Yanik
525 E Market St
Akron, OH 44309
Tel: 800 322-0517
Internet: http://www.summahealth.org/edu/
Accred Length: 3 Years *Program Size:* 6
Program ID: 240-38-21-121

Cincinnati

University Hospital/University of Cincinnati College of Medicine Program

Sponsor: University Hospital Inc
Veterans Affairs Medical Center (Cincinnati)

Program Director:
Karl Golnik, MD
Dept of Ophthalmology
231 Bethesda Ave (ML 527)
Cincinnati, OH 45267-0527
Tel: 513 558-5151 *Fax:* 513 558-3108
E-mail: mary.choromokos@uc.edu
Accred Length: 3 Years *Program Size:* 9
Program ID: 240-38-21-122

Cleveland

Case Western Reserve University Program

Sponsor: University Hospitals of Cleveland
MetroHealth Medical Center
Mount Sinai Medical Center of Cleveland
Veterans Affairs Medical Center (Cleveland)

Program Director:
Jonathan H Lass, MD
Case Western Reserve Univ
Dept of Ophthalmology
11100 Euclid Ave
Cleveland, OH 44106-5068
Tel: 216 844-8577 *Fax:* 216 844-7117
E-mail: jhl7@po.cwru.edu
Internet: http://mediswww.meds.cwru.edu/dept/eye
Accred Length: 3 Years *Program Size:* 18
Program ID: 240-38-21-123

Cleveland Clinic Foundation Program

Sponsor: Cleveland Clinic Foundation
MetroHealth Medical Center
St Vincent Charity Hospital and Health Center

Program Director:
Roger H S Langston, MD
Cleveland Clinic Foundation
Div of Ophthalmology/A31
9500 Euclid Ave
Cleveland, OH 44195-5242
Tel: 216 444-5690 *Fax:* 216 444-1162
E-mail: meded@cesmtp.ccf.org
Internet: http://www.ccf.org
Accred Length: 3 Years *Program Size:* 12
Program ID: 240-38-22-124

St Luke's Medical Center Program

Sponsor: St Luke's Medical Center

Program Director:
Howard D Kohn, MD
St Luke's Med Ctr
11311 Shaker Blvd
Cleveland, OH 44104
Tel: 216 368-7146
Accred Length: 3 Years *Program Size:* 6
Program ID: 240-38-11-126

Columbus

Ohio State University Program

Sponsor: Ohio State University Medical Center

Program Director:
Robert B Chambers, DO
William H Havener Eye Ctr
456 W 10th Ave
Columbus, OH 43210-1228
Tel: 614 293-8159 *Fax:* 614 293-4579
E-mail: meck.1@osu.edu
Internet: http://www.med.ohio-state/ophtho/cec.htm
Accred Length: 3 Years *Program Size:* 12
Program ID: 240-38-21-127

Oklahoma

Oklahoma City

University of Oklahoma Health Sciences Center Program

Sponsor: University of Oklahoma College of Medicine
Children's Hospital of Oklahoma
McGee Eye Institute
University Hospital
Veterans Affairs Medical Center (Oklahoma City)

Program Director:
Scott C Sigler, MD
Dean A McGee Eye Inst
608 Stanton L Young Blvd
Oklahoma City, OK 73104-9939
Tel: 405 271-1096 *Fax:* 405 271-3680
E-mail: scott-sigler@ouhsc.edu
Accred Length: 3 Years *Program Size:* 9
Program ID: 240-39-21-129

Oregon

Portland

Oregon Health Sciences University Program

Sponsor: Oregon Health Sciences University Hospital
Legacy Good Samaritan Hospital and Medical Center
Veterans Affairs Medical Center (Portland)

Program Director:
David J Wilson, MD
Casey Eye Inst
3375 SW Terwilliger Blvd
Portland, OR 97201-4197
Tel: 503 494-3394 *Fax:* 503 494-7233
E-mail: robinsoa@ohsu.edu
Internet: http://www.ohsu.edu/cei
Accred Length: 3 Years *Program Size:* 12
Program ID: 240-40-21-131

Pennsylvania

Danville

Penn State Geisinger Health System/Geisinger Medical Center Program

Sponsor: Penn State Geisinger Health System
Geisinger Medical Center

Program Director:
Herbert J Ingraham, MD
Geisinger Med Ctr
Dept of Ophthalmology
100 N Academy Ave
Danville, PA 17822-2120
Tel: 717 271-6531 *Fax:* 717 271-5813
E-mail: ckrebs@psghs.edu
Accred Length: 3 Years *Program Size:* 6
Program ID: 240-41-21-132

Hershey

Penn State Geisinger Health System/Milton S Hershey Medical Center Program

Sponsor: Penn State Geisinger Health System
Milton S Hershey Medical Center
Veterans Affairs Medical Center (Lebanon)

Program Director:
David A Quillen, MD
Milton S Hershey Med Ctr
Dept of Ophthalmology
PO Box 850
Hershey, PA 17033
Tel: 717 531-6051 *Fax:* 717 531-5475
E-mail: daq2@psu.edu
Internet: http://www.hmc.psu.edu/ophth/
Accred Length: 3 Years *Program Size:* 6
Program ID: 240-41-11-133

Philadelphia

MCP Hahnemann University Program

Sponsor: MCP Hahnemann University
Hahnemann University Hospital
Veterans Affairs Medical Center (Wilkes-Barre)

Program Director:
Myron Yanoff, MD
Hahnemann Univ Hospital
Broad and Vine Sts/MS 209
Philadelphia, PA 19102-1192
Tel: 215 762-1863 *Fax:* 215 762-4090
Accred Length: 3 Years *Program Size:* 9
Program ID: 240-41-21-134

Temple University Program

Sponsor: Temple University Hospital
Christiana Care Health Services Inc
Lankenau Hospital

Program Director:
Stephen W Wong, MD
Dept of Ophthalmology
Temple Univ Sch of Med
Broad and Tioga Sts/6PP
Philadelphia, PA 19140
Tel: 215 707-4829 *Fax:* 215 707-1684
E-mail: pvd1994@aol.com
Accred Length: 3 Years *Program Size:* 9
Program ID: 240-41-21-164

University of Pennsylvania Program

Sponsor: Hospital of the University of Pennsylvania
Presbyterian Medical Center (UPHS)
Scheie Eye Institute
Veterans Affairs Medical Center (Philadelphia)

Program Director:
Nicholas J Volpe, MD
Scheie Eye Inst
51 N 39th St
Philadelphia, PA 19104
Tel: 215 662-8042 *Fax:* 215 662-0133
E-mail: nickvolp@mail.med.upenn.edu
Internet: http://www.med.upenn.edu/~ophth/scheie
Accred Length: 3 Years *Program Size:* 15
Program ID: 240-41-21-136

Wills Eye Hospital Program

Sponsor: Wills Eye Hospital

Program Director:
John B Jeffers, MD DVM
Wills Eye Hospital
900 Walnut St
Philadelphia, PA 19107-5598
Tel: 215 440-3167 *Fax:* 215 440-3176
E-mail: maus1@att.net
Internet: http://jeffline.tju.edu/wills
Accred Length: 3 Years *Program Size:* 24
Program ID: 240-41-11-137

Pittsburgh

St Francis Medical Center Program

Sponsor: St Francis Medical Center
Allegheny General Hospital

Program Director:
John C Barber, MD
St Francis Med Ctr
Med Education Office
400 45th St
Pittsburgh, PA 15201
Tel: 412 622-4490 *Fax:* 412 622-7092
E-mail: ophres@sfhs.edu
Internet: http://www.sfhs.edu
Accred Length: 3 Years *Program Size:* 6
Program ID: 240-41-21-139

University Health Center of Pittsburgh Program

Sponsor: University Health Center of Pittsburgh
Presbyterian University Hospital/UPMC
Veterans Affairs Medical Center (Pittsburgh)

Program Director:
Randall L Beatty, MD
Dept of Ophthalmology
Eye and Ear Inst Bldg
203 Lothrop St/Rm 817
Pittsburgh, PA 15213
Tel: 412 647-2256 *Fax:* 412 647-5119
Internet: http://visualeyes.upmc.edu
Accred Length: 3 Years *Program Size:* 15
Program ID: 240-41-21-138

Puerto Rico

San Juan

University of Puerto Rico Program

Sponsor: University of Puerto Rico School of Medicine
San Juan City Hospital
University Hospital
Veterans Affairs Medical Center (San Juan)

Program Director:
William Townsend, MD
Univ of Puerto Rico Sch of Med
GPO Box 5067
San Juan, PR 00936
Tel: 787 756-7090 *Fax:* 787 758-3488
Accred Length: 4 Years *Program Size:* 18
Program ID: 240-42-21-141

Rhode Island

Providence

Brown University Program

Sponsor: Rhode Island Hospital
Veterans Affairs Medical Center (Providence)

Program Director:
King W To, MD
Rhode Island Hospital
593 Eddy St/APC-744
Providence, RI 02903
Tel: 401 444-8987 *Fax:* 401 444-6187
Accred Length: 3 Years *Program Size:* 6
Program ID: 240-43-11-142

South Carolina

Charleston

Medical University of South Carolina Program

Sponsor: Medical University of South Carolina College of Medicine
MUSC Medical Center
Ralph H Johnson Dept of Veterans Affairs Med Center
Program Director:
Amy K Hutchinson, MD
Med Univ of South Carolina
Dept of Ophthalmology
171 Ashley Ave
Charleston, SC 29425-2236
Tel: 843 792-8864 *Fax:* 843 792-3903
E-mail: hutchiak@musc.edu
Internet: http://www.stormeye.musc.edu
Accred Length: 3 Years *Program Size:* 12
Program ID: 240-45-21-143

Columbia

Palmetto Health Alliance/University of South Carolina School of Medicine Program

Sponsor: Palmetto Health Alliance
Palmetto Richland Memorial Hospital
William Jennings Bryan Dorn Veterans Hospital
Program Director:
Kakarla V Chalam, MD
South Carolina Eye Inst
Four Richland Medical Park
Ste 300
Columbia, SC 29203
Tel: 803 434-6836, ext 7063 *Fax:* 803 434-2387
E-mail: btandon@richmed.medpark.sc.edu
Internet:
http://www.rmh.edu/res.../newophthalmology.html
Accred Length: 4 Years *Program Size:* 8
Program ID: 240-45-21-163

Tennessee

Chattanooga

University of Tennessee College of Medicine at Chattanooga Program

Sponsor: University of Tennessee College of Medicine-Chattanooga Unit
Erlanger Medical Center
T C Thompson Children's Hospital Medical Center
Willie D Miller Eye Center
Program Director:
Harry M Lawrence, MD
Univ of Tennessee Coll of Med
Dept of Ophthalmology
975 E 3rd St
Chattanooga, TN 37403
Tel: 423 778-6163 *Fax:* 423 778-2260
E-mail: utophth@erlanger.org
Internet: http://www.erlanger.org/utcom/opthal.html
Accred Length: 3 Years *Program Size:* 6
Program ID: 240-47-11-144

Memphis

University of Tennessee Program

Sponsor: University of Tennessee College of Medicine
Methodist Hospitals of Memphis-Central
Regional Medical Center at Memphis
Veterans Affairs Medical Center (Memphis)
Program Director:
R Christopher Walton, MD
Univ of Tennessee Coll of Med
956 Court Ave/Rm D228
Memphis, TN 38163
Tel: 901 448-5884 *Fax:* 901 448-1299
E-mail: cwalton@mail.eye.utmem.edu
Internet: http://www.eye.utmem.edu
Accred Length: 3 Years *Program Size:* 10
Program ID: 240-47-21-145

Nashville

Vanderbilt University Program

Sponsor: Vanderbilt University Medical Center
Veterans Affairs Medical Center (Nashville)
Program Director:
Ming X Wang, MD PhD
Vanderbilt Univ Sch of Med
Dept of Ophthalmology/Vis Sci
8000 Medical Center E
Nashville, TN 37232-8808
Tel: 615 936-1451 *Fax:* 615 936-1544
Internet:
http://www.mc.vanderbilt.edu/vumcdept/ophthal/
Accred Length: 3 Years *Program Size:* 12
Program ID: 240-47-31-147

Texas

Dallas

University of Texas Southwestern Medical School Program

Sponsor: University of Texas Southwestern Medical School
Dallas County Hospital District-Parkland Memorial Hospital
Veterans Affairs Medical Center (Dallas)
Program Director:
David Weakley Jr, MD
5323 Harry Hines Blvd
Dallas, TX 75235-9057
Tel: 214 648-3837
Accred Length: 3 Years *Program Size:* 24
Program ID: 240-48-21-148

Galveston

University of Texas Medical Branch Hospitals Program

Sponsor: University of Texas Medical Branch Hospitals
Program Director:
Stefan D Trocme, MD
Univ of Texas Med Branch
301 University Blvd
Galveston, TX 77555-0787
Tel: 409 772-8104 *Fax:* 409 772-8106
E-mail: strocme@msp01.med.utmb.edu
Internet: http://www.utmb.edu/ovs
Accred Length: 3 Years *Program Size:* 12
Program ID: 240-48-21-149

Houston

Baylor College of Medicine Program

Sponsor: Baylor College of Medicine
Harris County Hospital District-Ben Taub General Hospital
Methodist Hospital
Veterans Affairs Medical Center (Houston)
Program Director:
Andrew G Lee, MD
Baylor Coll of Med
6565 Fannin St/NC 205
Houston, TX 77030
Tel: 713 798-5945 *Fax:* 713 798-8763
E-mail: alee@bcm.tmc.edu
Accred Length: 3 Years *Program Size:* 18
Program ID: 240-48-21-150

University of Texas at Houston Program

Sponsor: University of Texas Medical School at Houston
Memorial Hermann Healthcare System
Program Director:
Richard S Ruiz, MD
Univ of Texas-Houston Med Sch
Dept of Ophthalmology
6431 Fannin St/MSB 7024
Houston, TX 77030
Tel: 713 500-6000 *Fax:* 713 500-0682
E-mail: sabayrac@eye.med.uth.tmc.edu
Internet: http://eye.med.uth.tmc.edu/
Accred Length: 3 Years *Program Size:* 9
Program ID: 240-48-21-151

Lackland AFB

San Antonio Uniformed Services Health Education Consortium Program

Sponsor: San Antonio Uniformed Services Health Education Consortium
Program Director:
Jane B Ward, MD
Wilford Hall Med Ctr
59th MDW/MRPK
2200 Bergquist Dr/Ste 1
Lackland AFB, TX 78236-5300
Tel: 210 292-6573 *Fax:* 210 292-6569
E-mail: ward_ja@whmc.af.mil.
Accred Length: 3 Years *Program Size:* 15
Program ID: 240-48-11-001
US Armed Services Program

Lubbock

Texas Tech University (Lubbock) Program

Sponsor: Texas Tech University Health Sciences Center at Lubbock
University Medical Center
Veterans Affairs Medical Center (Big Spring)
Program Director:
Aziz S Abdul-Rahim, MD
Texas Tech Univ Health Sciences Ctr
10th and Flint
Lubbock, TX 79430
Tel: 806 743-2400, ext 259 *Fax:* 806 743-1782
E-mail: eyesar@ttuhsc.edu
Internet: http://www.eye.ttu.edu
Accred Length: 3 Years *Program Size:* 9
Program ID: 240-48-21-152

San Antonio

University of Texas Health Science Center at San Antonio Program

Sponsor: University of Texas Medical School at San Antonio
Audie L Murphy Memorial Veterans Hospital (San Antonio)
University Health Center-Downtown
University Hospital-South Texas Medical Center

Program Director:
Elmer Y Tu, MD
Univ of Texas Health Science Ctr
Dept of Ophthalmology
7703 Floyd Curl Dr
San Antonio, TX 78284-6230
Tel: 210 567-8406 *Fax:* 210 567-8413
Internet: http://macorb.uthscsa.edu/eye/
Accred Length: 3 Years *Program Size:* 12
Program ID: 240-48-21-153

Temple

Texas A&M College of Medicine-Scott and White Program

Sponsor: Scott and White Memorial Hospital
Central Texas Veterans Affairs Healthcare System

Program Director:
J Paul Dieckert, MD
Texas A&M-Scott and White
Grad Med Educ
2401 S 31st St
Temple, TX 76508-0001
Tel: 254 724-1058 *Fax:* 254 724-9050
E-mail: rcliett@swmail.sw.org
Internet:
http://www.sw.org.tamu.edu/gme/ophth/front.html
Accred Length: 3 Years *Program Size:* 6
Program ID: 240-48-21-154

Utah

Salt Lake City

University of Utah Program

Sponsor: University of Utah Medical Center
Veterans Affairs Medical Center (Salt Lake City)

Program Director:
Randall J Olson, MD
Univ of Utah Health Sciences Ctr
Dept of Ophthalmology/JMEC
75 N Medical Dr
Salt Lake City, UT 84132
Tel: 801 581-6384 *Fax:* 801 581-3357
E-mail: kim.nalewaja@hsc.utah.edu
Internet: http://www.insight.med.utah.edu/
Accred Length: 3 Years *Program Size:* 6
Program ID: 240-49-21-155

Virginia

Charlottesville

University of Virginia Program

Sponsor: University of Virginia Medical Center

Program Director:
Sara A Kaltreider, MD
Univ of Virginia Health System
Dept of Ophthalmology
Box 10009
Charlottesville, VA 22906-0009
Tel: 804 982-1086 *Fax:* 804 924-5180
Internet: http://www.med.virginia.edu/medicine/clinical/ophthalmology/home.html
Accred Length: 3 Years *Program Size:* 9
Program ID: 240-51-21-156

Norfolk

Eastern Virginia Medical School Program

Sponsor: Eastern Virginia Medical School
Sentara Norfolk General Hospital
Veterans Affairs Medical Center (Hampton)

Program Director:
Earl R Crouch, MD
Eastern Virginia Med Sch
880 Kempsville Rd/Ste 2500
Norfolk, VA 23502-3931
Tel: 757 461-0050 *Fax:* 757 461-4538
Internet: http://www.evms.edu
Accred Length: 3 Years *Program Size:* 6
Program ID: 240-51-21-157

Richmond

Medical College of Virginia/Virginia Commonwealth University Program

Sponsor: Medical College of Virginia/Virginia Commonwealth University
Hunter Holmes McGuire VA Medical Center (Richmond)
Medical College of Virginia Hospitals

Program Director:
John D Wright Jr, MD
Med Coll of Virginia-Virginia Commonwealth Univ
PO Box 980012
Richmond, VA 23298-0012
Tel: 804 828-9318 *Fax:* 804 828-3477
E-mail: jdwright@hsc.vcu.edu
Internet: http://views.vcu.edu/eye
Accred Length: 3 Years *Program Size:* 11
Program ID: 240-51-21-158

Washington

Seattle

University of Washington Program

Sponsor: University of Washington School of Medicine
Children's Hospital and Medical Center
Harborview Medical Center
University of Washington Medical Center
Veterans Affairs Medical Center (Seattle)

Program Director:
James L Kinyoun, MD
Ophthalmology
Box 356485
1959 NE Pacific St
Seattle, WA 98195-6485
Tel: 206 685-4749 *Fax:* 206 543-4414
E-mail: lsd1@u.washington.edu
Internet:
http://www.weber.u.washington.edu/~ophthweb/
Accred Length: 3 Years *Program Size:* 12
Program ID: 240-54-21-159

Tacoma

Madigan Army Medical Center Program

Sponsor: Madigan Army Medical Center

Program Director:
Thomas H Mader, MD
Madigan Army Med Ctr
Attn: MCHJ-SOU
Ophthalmology Service
Tacoma, WA 98431
Tel: 253 968-1770 *Fax:* 253 968-1451
Accred Length: 3 Years *Program Size:* 6
Program ID: 240-54-21-175
US Armed Services Program

West Virginia

Morgantown

West Virginia University Program

Sponsor: West Virginia University Hospitals
Louis A Johnson Veterans Affairs Medical Center

Program Director:
Brian Ellis, MD
Dept of Ophthalmology
West Virginia Univ Health Sciences Ctr
PO Box 9193
Morgantown, WV 26506-9193
Tel: 304 293-3757 *Fax:* 304 293-7139
Accred Length: 3 Years *Program Size:* 6
Program ID: 240-55-21-160

Wisconsin

Madison

University of Wisconsin Program

Sponsor: University of Wisconsin Hospital and Clinics
William S Middleton Veterans Hospital

Program Director:
Neal P Barney, MD MD
Univ of Wisconsin Hospital and Clinics
Dept of Ophthalmology
2870 University Ave/Ste 206
Madison, WI 53792-3611
Tel: 608 263-5339 *Fax:* 608 263-7694
E-mail: npbarney@facstaff.wisc.edu
Internet: http://www.medsch.wisc.edu/ophth/
Accred Length: 3 Years *Program Size:* 10
Program ID: 240-56-21-161

Milwaukee

Medical College of Wisconsin Program

Sponsor: Medical College of Wisconsin Affiliated Hospitals Inc
Clement J Zablocki Veterans Affairs Medical Center
Froedtert Memorial Lutheran Hospital

Program Director:
James C Robinson, MD
Dept of Ophthalmology
925 N 87th St
Milwaukee, WI 53226-4812
Tel: 414 456-7876 *Fax:* 414 456-6300
E-mail: kwerner@post.its.mcw.edu
Internet: http://www.mcw.edu/ophthalmology
Accred Length: 3 Years *Program Size:* 12
Program ID: 240-56-21-162

Orthopaedic Sports Medicine (Orthopaedic Surgery)

Alabama

Birmingham

American Sports Medicine Institute Program
Sponsor: American Sports Medicine Institute
Program Director:
James R Andrews, MD
American Sports Med Inst
1313 13th St S
Birmingham, AL 35205
Tel: 205 918-0000 *Fax:* 205 918-0800
E-mail: llevine@asmi.org
Internet: http://asmi.org
Accred Length: 1 Year *Program Size:* 9
Program ID: 268-01-31-026

California

Inglewood

Kerlan-Jobe Orthopaedic Clinic Program
Sponsor: Kerlan-Jobe Orthopaedic Clinic
Centinela Hospital Medical Center
Program Director:
Ronald S Kvitne, MD
Kerlan-Jobe Orthopaedic Clinic
6801 Park Terr
Los Angeles, CA 90045
Tel: 310 665-7200 *Fax:* 310 671-4791
Accred Length: 1 Year *Program Size:* 9
Program ID: 268-05-21-030

Long Beach

Long Beach Memorial Medical Center Program
Sponsor: Long Beach Memorial Medical Center
Southern California Center for Sports Medicine
Program Director:
Douglas W Jackson, MD
Memorial Orthopedic Surgical Group
2760 Atlantic Ave
Long Beach, CA 90806
Tel: 562 424-6666 *Fax:* 562 989-0027
Accred Length: 1 Year *Program Size:* 2
Program ID: 268-05-21-013

San Diego

Alvarado Hospital Medical Center Program
Sponsor: Alvarado Hospital Medical Center
University of California (San Diego) Medical Center
Program Director:
James P Tasto, MD
San Diego Sports Med and Orthopaedic Ctr
6719 Alvarado Rd/Ste 200
San Diego, CA 92120
Tel: 619 229-3932 *Fax:* 619 582-2860
Accred Length: 1 Year *Program Size:* 2
Program ID: 268-05-21-066

Van Nuys

Southern California Orthopaedic Institute Program
Sponsor: Southern California Orthopedic Institute
Program Director:
Richard D Ferkel, MD
Southern California Orthopaedic Inst
6815 Noble St
Van Nuys, CA 91405
Tel: 818 901-6600, ext 1512 *Fax:* 818 901-6660
E-mail: eleanor@scoi.com
Accred Length: 1 Year *Program Size:* 4
Program ID: 268-05-21-043

Colorado

Aspen

Orthopaedic Associates of Aspen and Glenwood Program
Sponsor: University of Colorado Health Sciences Center
Orthopaedic Associates of Aspen and Glenwood
Program Director:
Robert E Hunter, MD
D J King, BS
Aspen Foundation for Sports Med Educ and Research
100 E Main St/#102
Aspen, CO 81611
Tel: 970 925-4141 *Fax:* 970 925-4233
E-mail: afsmer@rof.net
Internet: http://www.aspen.com/orthopaedic
Accred Length: 1 Year *Program Size:* 2
Program ID: 268-07-21-035

Vail

Steadman Hawkins Clinic Program
Sponsor: Steadman Hawkins Clinic
Vail Valley Medical Center
Program Director:
Richard J Hawkins, MD
Steadman Hawkins Clinic
Attn: Greta D Pfendt
181 W Meadow Dr/Ste 1000
Vail, CO 81657
Tel: 970 476-1100, ext 5788 *Fax:* 970 479-9753
E-mail: greta@steadman-hawkins.com
Internet: http://www.steadman-hawkins.com
Accred Length: 1 Year *Program Size:* 6
Program ID: 268-07-21-063

Connecticut

Farmington

University of Connecticut Program
Sponsor: University of Connecticut School of Medicine
Univ of Connecticut Health Center/John Dempsey Hospital
Program Director:
John P Fulkerson, MD
Orthopedic Associates of Hartford
270 Farmington Ave
Ste 364
Farmington, CT 06032
Tel: 860 549-3210 *Fax:* 860 677-9094
E-mail: patelladoc@aol.com
Accred Length: 1 Year *Program Size:* 1
Program ID: 268-08-21-006

New Haven

Yale-New Haven Medical Center Program
Sponsor: Yale-New Haven Hospital
Program Director:
Peter Jokl, MD
Yale Sports Medicine Ctr
1 Long Wharf Dr
6th Fl
New Haven, CT 06511
Tel: 203 764-9771 *Fax:* 203 764-9779
E-mail: marc_galloway@yale.edu
Accred Length: 1 Year *Program Size:* 1
Program ID: 268-08-21-012

Florida

Coral Gables

HealthSouth Doctor's Hospital Program
Sponsor: HealthSouth Doctors' Hospital
Program Director:
Harlan Selesnick, MD
Healthsouth Med Office Bldg
1150 Campo Sano Ave/Ste 301
Coral Cables, FL 33146
Tel: 305 662-2424 *Fax:* 305 666-6185
Accred Length: 1 Year *Program Size:* 1
Program ID: 268-11-21-074

Gainesville

University of Florida Program
Sponsor: University of Florida College of Medicine
Shands Hospital at the University of Florida
Program Director:
Keith Meister, MD
Univ of Florida
Hampton Oaks Sports Med Ctr
Box 100241
Gainesville, FL 32610
Tel: 352 395-0645 *Fax:* 352 395-0657
Accred Length: 1 Year *Program Size:* 1
Program ID: 268-11-21-010

Miami

University of Miami-Jackson Memorial Medical Center Program
Sponsor: University of Miami-Jackson Memorial Medical Center
HealthSouth Doctors' Hospital
Program Director:
John W Uribe, MD
HealthSouth Doctors' Hospital
Div of Sports Med
1150 Campo Sano Ave/Ste 200
Coral Gables, FL 33146
Tel: 305 669-3320 *Fax:* 305 669-3352
Accred Length: 1 Year *Program Size:* 1
Program ID: 268-11-21-015

Georgia

Columbus

Hughston Sports Medicine Foundation Program
Sponsor: Hughston Sports Medicine Foundation
Hughston Sports Medicine Hospital
Program Director:
Glenn C Terry, MD
Hughston Sports Med Foundation
PO Box 9517
Columbus, GA 31908-9517
Tel: 706 576-3365 *Fax:* 706 576-3379
E-mail: gcterry@hughston.com
Internet: http://www.hughston.com
Accred Length: 1 Year *Program Size:* 6
Program ID: 268-12-21-046

Illinois

Chicago

McGaw Medical Center of Northwestern University Program
Sponsor: Northwestern University Medical School
Northwestern Memorial Hospital
Program Director:
Gordon W Nuber, MD
Dept of Orthopaedic Surgery
645 N Michigan Ave
Ste 1058B
Chicago, IL 60611
Tel: 312 908-7937 *Fax:* 312 908-8479
E-mail: orthopaedic@nwu.edu
Internet: http://www.orthopaedics@nwu.edu
Accred Length: 1 Year *Program Size:* 1
Program ID: 268-16-21-072

Rush-Presbyterian-St Luke's Medical Center Program
Sponsor: Rush-Presbyterian-St Luke's Medical Center
Program Director:
Bernard R Bach Jr, MD
Rush-Presbyterian-St Luke's Med Ctr
1725 W Harrison St/Ste 1063
Chicago, IL 60612
Tel: 312 243-4244 *Fax:* 312 942-1517
Accred Length: 1 Year *Program Size:* 2
Program ID: 268-16-31-064

University of Chicago Program
Sponsor: University of Chicago Hospitals
Program Director:
Bruce Reider, MD
Univ of Chicago Hospitals
5841 S Maryland Ave/MC3079
Chicago, IL 60637
Tel: 773 702-6346 *Fax:* 773 702-0076
Accred Length: 1 Year *Program Size:* 1
Program ID: 268-16-21-034

University of Illinois College of Medicine at Chicago Program
Sponsor: University of Illinois College of Medicine at Chicago
Columbus Hospital
St Joseph Health Centers and Hospital
University of Illinois Hospital and Clinics
Program Director:
Preston M Wolin, MD
711 W North Ave/Ste 206
Chicago, IL 60610
Tel: 312 337-0516 *Fax:* 312 787-5073
Accred Length: 1 Year *Program Size:* 1
Program ID: 268-16-31-075

Indiana

Indianapolis

Indiana University School of Medicine Program
Sponsor: Indiana University School of Medicine
Clarian Methodist Hospital of Indiana
Program Director:
K Donald Shelbourne, MD
Clarian Methodist Hospital
Methodist Sports Med Ctr
1815 N Capitol Ave/Ste 530
Indianapolis, IN 46202
Tel: 317 921-3729 *Fax:* 317 921-0230
Accred Length: 1 Year *Program Size:* 2
Program ID: 268-17-21-003

Iowa

Iowa City

University of Iowa Hospitals and Clinics Program
Sponsor: University of Iowa Hospitals and Clinics
Program Director:
John P Albright, MD
David S Tearse, MD
Univ of Iowa Hospitals and Clinics
Dept of Ortho Surgery
200 Hawkins Dr
Iowa City, IA 52242
Tel: 319 356-3471
E-mail: john-albright@uiowa.edu
Accred Length: 1 Year *Program Size:* 1
Program ID: 268-18-21-067

Kentucky

Lexington

Kentucky Sports Medicine Clinic Program
Sponsor: Kentucky Sports Medicine Clinic
Central Baptist Hospital
Program Director:
Mary Lloyd Ireland, MD
Kentucky Sports Medicine Clinic
601 Perimeter Dr
Lexington, KY 40517
Tel: 606 268-0268 *Fax:* 606 268-4519
E-mail: ksportsmed@aol.com
Accred Length: 1 Year *Program Size:* 2
Program ID: 268-20-21-038

University of Kentucky Medical Center Program
Sponsor: University of Kentucky Hospital
Program Director:
Darren Johnson, MD
Univ Hospital-Albert B Chandler Med Ctr
740 S Limestone
Kentucky Clinic/Rm 429
Lexington, KY 40536-0284
Tel: 606 323-5533, ext 250 *Fax:* 606 323-2412
E-mail: dljohns@pop.uky.edu
Accred Length: 1 Year *Program Size:* 1
Program ID: 268-20-21-016

Louisiana

Lake Charles

Louisiana State University Program
Sponsor: Louisiana State University School of Medicine
Lake Charles Memorial Hospital
Louisiana State University Medical College Campus
Program Director:
David Drez Jr, MD
Louisiana State Univ Med Ctr
2025 Gravier St/Ste 400
New Orleans, LA 70112
Tel: 318 494-4902 *Fax:* 318 494-4936
Accred Length: 1 Year *Program Size:* 1
Program ID: 268-21-31-002

New Orleans

Tulane University Program
Sponsor: Tulane University School of Medicine
Tulane University Hospital and Clinics
Program Director:
Michael E Brunet, MD
Tulane Med Ctr
Dept of Orthopaedics/SL32
1430 Tulane Ave
New Orleans, LA 70112-2699
Tel: 504 588-5807, ext 85770 *Fax:* 504 584-3517
E-mail: mbrunet@mailhost.tcs.tulane.edu
Internet:
http://www.mcl.tulane.edu/departments/orthopaedics
Accred Length: 1 Year *Program Size:* 1
Program ID: 268-21-21-020

Maryland

Baltimore

Union Memorial Hospital Program
Sponsor: Union Memorial Hospital
Program Director:
Leslie S Matthews, MD
Union Memorial Hospital
Dept of Ortho Surgery
3333 N Calvert St/Ste 400
Baltimore, MD 21218
Tel: 410 554-6865 *Fax:* 410 554-2853
E-mail: dawng@helix.org
Internet: http://www.helixhealth.com
Accred Length: 1 Year *Program Size:* 2
Program ID: 268-23-21-058

Massachusetts

Boston

Harvard Medical School Program
Sponsor: Massachusetts General Hospital
Program Director:
Bertram Zarins, MD
Massachusetts General Hospital
Sports Med Unit
15 Parkman St/Ste 514
Boston, MA 02114
Tel: 617 726-3421 *Fax:* 617 726-3438
E-mail: zarins.bertram@mgh.harvard.edu
Internet:
http://www.mgh.harvard.edu/depts/sports/default.htm
Accred Length: 1 Year *Program Size:* 2
Program ID: 268-24-31-049

New England Baptist Hospital Program
Sponsor: New England Baptist Hospital

Program Director:
Arnold D Scheller, MD
830 Boylston St
Chestnut Hill, MA 02167
Tel: 617 738-8642 *Fax:* 617 738-5045
Accred Length: 1 Year *Program Size:* 2
Program ID: 268-24-21-044

Tufts University Program
Sponsor: New England Medical Center Hospitals
Veterans Affairs Medical Center (Boston)

Program Director:
John C Richmond, MD
New England Med Ctr Hospital
Dept of Ortho Surgery
750 Washington St/Box 189
Boston, MA 02111
Tel: 617 636-6014 *Fax:* 617 636-5178
E-mail: john.richmond@es.nemc.org
Accred Length: 1 Year *Program Size:* 1
Program ID: 268-24-31-059

Worcester

University of Massachusetts Program
Sponsor: University of Massachusetts Medical School
UMass Memorial Health Care (University Campus)

Program Director:
Arthur M Pappas, MD
Univ of Massachusetts Med Sch
Dept of Ortho Surgery
55 Lake Ave N
Worcester, MA 01165
Tel: 508 856-4262
Accred Length: 1 Year *Program Size:* 1
Program ID: 268-24-31-047

Michigan

Detroit

Wayne State University/Detroit Medical Center Program
Sponsor: Wayne State University/Detroit Medical Center
Hutzel Hospital

Program Director:
Robert A Teitge, MD
Hutzel Health Ctr
Attn: Rose Bachan
4050 E 12 Mile Rd/Ste 110
Warren, MI 48092
Tel: 810 573-3100 *Fax:* 810 573-7924
Accred Length: 1 Year *Program Size:* 1
Program ID: 268-25-21-065

Minnesota

Minneapolis

Minneapolis Sports Medicine Center Program
Sponsor: Minneapolis Sports Medicine Center
Abbott-Northwestern Hospital
Fairview-University Medical Center

Program Director:
David A Fischer, MD
Minneapolis Sports Med Ctr
Ste 400
701 25th Ave S
Minneapolis, MN 55454-1443
Tel: 612 336-9491 *Fax:* 612 339-5391
Accred Length: 1 Year *Program Size:* 3
Program ID: 268-26-21-048

Missouri

Kansas City

University of Missouri at Kansas City Program
Sponsor: University of Missouri-Kansas City School of Medicine
Baptist Medical Center
Saint Luke's Hospital
Truman Medical Center-West

Program Director:
Jon E Browne, MD
Univ of Missouri-Kansas City
6675 Homes St/Ste 400
Kansas City, MO 64131
Tel: 816 444-8300 *Fax:* 816 444-0607
Accred Length: 1 Year *Program Size:* 1
Program ID: 268-28-21-051

St Louis

Washington University/B-JH/SLCH Consortium Program
Sponsor: Washington University/B-JH/SLCH Consortium
Barnes West County Hospital
Barnes-Jewish Hospital
Veterans Affairs Medical Center (St Louis)

Program Director:
Geoge A Paletta, MD
Washington Univ
One Barnes Hospital Plaza/Ste 11300
St Louis, MO 63110
Tel: 314 747-2543 *Fax:* 314 747-2800
E-mail: orthsurg@msnotes.wustl.edu
Accred Length: 1 Year *Program Size:* 1
Program ID: 268-28-21-076

New York

New York

Hospital for Joint Diseases Orthopaedic Institute Program
Sponsor: Hospital for Joint Diseases Orthopaedic Institute

Program Director:
Mark I Pitman, MD
Hospital for Joint Diseases
Sports Med Ctr
301 E 17th St
New York, NY 10003
Tel: 212 598-6497 *Fax:* 212 598-6581
Accred Length: 1 Year *Program Size:* 1
Program ID: 268-35-31-056

Hospital for Special Surgery/Cornell Medical Center Program
Sponsor: Hospital for Special Surgery

Program Director:
Thomas L Wickiewicz, MD
Hospital for Special Surgery
Sports Med/Shoulder Service
535 E 70th St
New York, NY 10021
Tel: 212 606-1466
Internet: http://www.hss.edu
Accred Length: 1 Year *Program Size:* 5
Program ID: 268-35-21-025

Lenox Hill Hospital Program
Sponsor: Lenox Hill Hospital

Program Director:
Barton Nisonson, MD
Lenox Hill Hospital
130 E 77th St
11th Fl
New York, NY 10021
Tel: 212 434-2710 *Fax:* 212 434-2687
E-mail: orthopedics@mindspring.com
Accred Length: 1 Year *Program Size:* 2
Program ID: 268-35-11-004

New York University Medical Center Program
Sponsor: New York University Medical Center
Bellevue Hospital Center
Hospital for Joint Diseases Orthopaedic Institute

Program Director:
Orrin H Sherman, MD
New York Univ Med Ctr-Hospital for Joint Diseases
301 E 17th St
New York, NY 10003
Tel: 212 598-6509 *Fax:* 212 598-6581
Accred Length: 1 Year *Program Size:* 2
Program ID: 268-35-21-005

Rochester

University of Rochester Program
Sponsor: Strong Memorial Hospital of the University of Rochester

Program Director:
Kenneth E DeHaven, MD
Strong Memorial Hospital
Dept of Orthopaedics
601 Elmwood Ave/Box 665
Rochester, NY 14642
Tel: 716 275-2970 *Fax:* 716 242-0763
Accred Length: 1 Year *Program Size:* 1
Program ID: 268-35-21-060

West Point

Keller Army Community Hospital Program
Sponsor: Keller Army Community Hospital

Program Director:
Robert A Arciero, MD
Keller Army Hospital
Orthopaedic Dept
Bldg 900
West Point, NY 10996-1197
Tel: 914 938-4821 *Fax:* 914 938-6806
E-mail: col_robert_arciero@mercy.westpoint.army.mil
Accred Length: 1 Year *Program Size:* 2
Program ID: 268-35-21-055
US Armed Services Program

Ohio

Cincinnati

Christ Hospital/University of Cincinnati School of Medicine Program
Sponsor: Christ Hospital
University of Cincinnati College of Medicine

Program Director:
Robert S Heidt Jr, MD
Christ Hospital
Bone and Joint Inst
2139 Auburn Ave
Cincinnati, OH 45219
Tel: 513 369-2742 *Fax:* 513 629-4892
E-mail: lippsdl@healthall.com
Accred Length: 1 Year *Program Size:* 2
Program ID: 268-38-21-031

Cincinnati Sportsmedicine and Orthopaedic Center Program
Sponsor: Cincinnati Sportsmedicine and Orthopaedic Center
Program Director:
Frank R Noyes, MD
Cincinnati SportsMed and Orthopaedic Ctr
Deaconess Hospital
311 Straight St
Cincinnati, OH 45219
Tel: 513 559-2818 *Fax:* 513 475-5263
E-mail: sankerjuls@aol.com
Accred Length: 1 Year *Program Size:* 4
Program ID: 268-38-21-041

Cleveland

Cleveland Clinic Foundation Program
Sponsor: Cleveland Clinic Foundation
Program Director:
John A Bergfeld, MD
Cleveland Clinic Foundation
Dept of Ortho/Sports Med/A41
9500 Euclid Ave
Cleveland, OH 44195-5242
Tel: 216 444-5690 *Fax:* 216 444-1162
E-mail: baumanc@cesmtp.ccf.org
Internet: http://www.ccf.org
Accred Length: 1 Year *Program Size:* 3
Program ID: 268-38-21-028

Columbus

Ohio State University Program
Sponsor: Ohio State University Medical Center
Program Director:
Christopher C Kaeding, MD
Ohio State Univ Hospital
OSU Sports Med Ctr
2050 Kenny Rd
Columbus, OH 43221
Tel: 614 293-8813 *Fax:* 614 293-4399
Accred Length: 1 Year *Program Size:* 1
Program ID: 268-38-21-008

Oklahoma

Oklahoma City

University of Oklahoma Health Sciences Center Program
Sponsor: University of Oklahoma College of Medicine
Columbia Presbyterian Hospital
Program Director:
William A Grana, MD MPH
Univ of Oklahoma Health Sciences Ctr
1000 N Lincoln Blvd
Ste 200
Oklahoma City, OK 73104
Tel: 405 232-4641 *Fax:* 405 552-0046
Accred Length: 1 Year *Program Size:* 2
Program ID: 268-39-21-007

Pennsylvania

Philadelphia

Graduate Hospital Program
Sponsor: Graduate Hospital
Program Director:
Vincent Di Stefano, MD
Graduate Hospital
Pepper Memorial Pavilion/Ste 802
One Graduate Plaza
Philadelphia, PA 19146
Tel: 215 893-0132 *Fax:* 215 893-0510
Accred Length: 1 Year *Program Size:* 2
Program ID: 268-41-21-014

Temple University Program
Sponsor: Temple University Hospital
Program Director:
Ray A Moyer, MD
Temple Univ Hospital
Dept of Ortho Surgery/Sports Med
3401 N Broad St
Philadelphia, PA 19140
Tel: 215 707-8331 *Fax:* 215 707-2324
E-mail: mkilbrid@vm.temple.edu
Internet:
http://www.temple.edu/orthopaedics/index.html
Accred Length: 1 Year *Program Size:* 2
Program ID: 268-41-21-040

Thomas Jefferson University Program
Sponsor: Thomas Jefferson University Hospital
Christiana Care Health Services Inc
Lankenau Hospital
Pennsylvania Hospital (UPHS)
Program Director:
Phillip J Marone, MD
Thomas Jefferson Univ
925 Chestnut St/Rm 606
Philadelphia, PA 19107
Tel: 215 955-1500 *Fax:* 215 503-0566
E-mail: susan.randolph@mail.tju.edu
Internet: http://www.tjuhortho.org
Accred Length: 1 Year *Program Size:* 2
Program ID: 268-41-21-054

Pittsburgh

University Health Center of Pittsburgh Program
Sponsor: University Health Center of Pittsburgh
Presbyterian University Hospital/UPMC
Program Director:
Christopher D Harner, MD
Ctr for Sports Med and Rehabilitation
4601 Baum Blvd
Pittsburgh, PA 15213-1217
Tel: 412 578-3309 *Fax:* 412 578-3160
Accred Length: 1 Year *Program Size:* 3
Program ID: 268-41-21-018

Tennessee

Knoxville

University of Tennessee College of Medicine at Chattanooga Program
Sponsor: University of Tennessee College of Medicine-Chattanooga Unit
Knoxville Orthopedic Clinic
Erlanger Medical Center
St Mary's Health System
Program Director:
William T Youmans, MD
Knoxville Orthopedic Clinic
1128 Weisgarber Rd
Knoxville, TN 37909
Tel: 423 558-4425 *Fax:* 423 558-4421
Internet: http://www.erlanger.org/utcom
Accred Length: 1 Year *Program Size:* 2
Program ID: 268-47-21-033

Nashville

Southern Sports Medicine and Orthopaedic Center Program
Sponsor: Southern Sports Medicine & Orthopaedic Center
Baptist Hospital
Program Director:
Burton F Elrod, MD
Southern Sports Med and Orthopaedic Ctr
Baptist Medical Plaza II/2nd Fl
2021 Church St
Nashville, TN 37203
Tel: 615 342-0201 *Fax:* 615 284-2003
Accred Length: 1 Year *Program Size:* 1
Program ID: 268-47-21-069

Texas

Houston

Baylor College of Medicine Program
Sponsor: Baylor College of Medicine
Methodist Hospital
Program Director:
James R Bocell, MD
Baylor Coll of Med
Dept of Ortho Surgery
6550 Fannin St/Ste 2625
Houston, TX 77030
Tel: 713 986-7390 *Fax:* 713 986-7391
Accred Length: 1 Year *Program Size:* 3
Program ID: 268-48-31-027

San Antonio

University of Texas Health Science Center at San Antonio (Nix) Program
Sponsor: University of Texas Medical School at San Antonio
Methodist Healthcare
Nix Medical Center
St Luke's Baptist Hospital
Program Director:
Jesse C DeLee, MD
Huebner Med Ctr
9150 Huebner Rd/Ste 250-A
San Antonio, TX 78240
Tel: 210 561-7100 *Fax:* 210 561-7121
Accred Length: 1 Year *Program Size:* 2
Program ID: 268-48-21-042

Utah

Murray

The Orthopedic Specialty Hospital Program

Sponsor: The Orthopedic Specialty Hospital

Program Director:
Lonnie E Paulos, MD
Thomas D Rosenberg, MD
Orthopedic Specialty Hospital
5848 S 300 East
Salt Lake City, UT 84107
Tel: 801 269-4030 *Fax:* 801 269-4015
Accred Length: 1 Year *Program Size:* 3
Program ID: 268-49-31-011

Salt Lake City

University of Utah Program

Sponsor: University of Utah Medical Center

Program Director:
Robert T Burks, MD
Univ of Utah Med Ctr
Dept of Orthopaedics
50 N Medical Dr
Salt Lake City, UT 84132-0001
Tel: 801 581-7601 *Fax:* 801 581-6178
E-mail: robert.burks@hsc.utah.edu
Accred Length: 1 Year *Program Size:* 2
Program ID: 268-49-21-022

Virginia

Arlington

Georgetown University Program

Sponsor: Arlington Hospital
Nirschl Orthopedic Clinic

Program Director:
Robert P Nirschl, MD MS
Nirschl Orthopedic and SportsMed Clinic
1715 N George Mason Dr
Ste 504
Arlington, VA 22205-3609
Tel: 703 525-2200 *Fax:* 703 522-2603
E-mail: nirschl@erols.com
Internet: http://www.nirschl.com
Accred Length: 1 Year *Program Size:* 2
Program ID: 268-51-21-062

Charlottesville

University of Virginia Program

Sponsor: University of Virginia Medical Center

Program Director:
Frank C McCue III, MD
Univ of Virginia Sch of Med
Dept of Orthopaedics
Box 243
Charlottesville, VA 22908
Tel: 804 243-5045 *Fax:* 804 243-5070
Accred Length: 1 Year *Program Size:* 1
Program ID: 268-51-21-057

Richmond

Orthopaedic Research of Virginia Program

Sponsor: Orthopaedic Research of Virginia
Tuckahoe Orthopaedic Associates

Program Director:
John F Meyers, MD
Tuckahoe Orthopaedic Associates
MOB I
7660 E Parham Rd/Ste 207
Richmond, VA 23294
Tel: 804 527-5960 *Fax:* 804 527-5961
E-mail: fellowship@orv.com
Accred Length: 1 Year *Program Size:* 3
Program ID: 268-51-21-039

Wisconsin

Madison

University of Wisconsin Program

Sponsor: University of Wisconsin Hospital and Clinics

Program Director:
John F Orwin, MD
Univ of Wisconsin Clinical Sciences Ctr
600 Highland Ave
G5/314
Madison, WI 53792-3228
Tel: 608 263-5636 *Fax:* 608 265-6450
E-mail: murphy@surgery.wisc.edu
Internet: http://www.biostat.wisc.edu/surgery/sports.html
Accred Length: 1 Year *Program Size:* 1
Program ID: 268-56-21-017

Orthopaedic Surgery

Alabama

Birmingham

University of Alabama Medical Center Program

Sponsor: University of Alabama Hospital
Children's Hospital of Alabama
Cooper Green Hospital
Veterans Affairs Medical Center (Birmingham)

Program Director:
John Cuckler, MD
Univ of Alabama
1813 6th Ave S/MEB 508
Birmingham, AL 35294-3295
Tel: 205 975-9694 *Fax:* 205 975-4701
E-mail: barbara.rivers@ortho.uab.edu
Internet: http://www.ortho.uab.edu
Accred Length: 5 Years *Program Size:* 14
Subspecialties: HSO
Program ID: 260-01-21-044

Mobile

University of South Alabama Program

Sponsor: University of South Alabama Medical Center
USA Doctors Hospital
USA Knollwood Park Hospital

Program Director:
Arthur Manoli II, MD
Univ of South Alabama Med Ctr
2451 Fillingim St
Mastin Bldg/Ste 503
Mobile, AL 36617-2293
Tel: 334 471-7938 *Fax:* 334 471-7477
E-mail: gdriver@usamail.usouthal.edu
Internet: http://www.usouthal.edu/
Accred Length: 5 Years *Program Size:* 10 (*GYI:* 2)
Program ID: 260-01-11-182

Arizona

Phoenix

Maricopa Medical Center Program

Sponsor: Maricopa Medical Center
Carl T Hayden Veterans Affairs Medical Center (Phoenix)
Children's Rehabilitative Services
Harrington Arthritis Research Center

Program Director:
Alex McLaren, MD MD
Ortho Care International
418 N 19th St
Phoenix, AZ 85006
Tel: 602 254-9646, ext 18 *Fax:* 602 254-8835
Internet: http://www.maricopa.gov/medcenter/mmc.html
Accred Length: 5 Years *Program Size:* 16
Subspecialties: HSO
Program ID: 260-03-22-073

Tucson

University of Arizona Program

Sponsor: University of Arizona College of Medicine
Tucson Medical Center
University Medical Center
Veterans Affairs Medical Center (Tucson)

Program Director:
John T Ruth, MD
Arizona Health Sci Ctr (Attn: Sue Ellen Fest)
Sect of Orthopedic Surgery
PO Box 245064
Tucson, AZ 85724-5064
Tel: 520 626-7644 *Fax:* 520 626-2668
E-mail: sfest@u.arizona.edu
Internet: http://www.ahsc.arizona.edu/ortho_residency
Accred Length: 5 Years *Program Size:* 10
Program ID: 260-03-31-054

Arkansas

Little Rock

University of Arkansas for Medical Sciences Program

Sponsor: University of Arkansas College of Medicine
Arkansas Children's Hospital
John L McClellan Memorial Veterans Hospital
University Hospital of Arkansas

Program Director:
Carl L Nelson, MD
Univ of Arkansas for Med Sciences
4301 W Markham St/Slot 531
Little Rock, AR 72205
Tel: 501 686-5251 *Fax:* 501 603-1984
E-mail: orawyvonnes@exchange.uams.edu
Internet: http://www.uams.edu/ortho/ortho.htm
Accred Length: 5 Years *Program Size:* 21 (*GY1:* 4)
Subspecialties: HSO, TY
Program ID: 260-04-21-094

California

Loma Linda

Loma Linda University Program

Sponsor: Loma Linda University Medical Center
Jerry L Pettis Memorial Veterans Hospital
San Bernardino County Medical Center

Program Director:
Christopher M Jobe, MD
Loma Linda Univ Med Ctr
Dept of Ortho Surgery/RmA525
11234 Anderson St
Loma Linda, CA 92354
Tel: 909 824-4413, ext 6074 *Fax:* 909 824-4820
E-mail: dsimmons@som.llu.edu
Internet: http://www.llu.edu/llumc/residency.html
Accred Length: 5 Years *Program Size:* 20 (*GY1:* 4)
Subspecialties: HSO
Program ID: 260-05-21-063

Los Angeles

Charles R Drew University Program

Sponsor: Charles R Drew University of Medicine and Science
LAC-King/Drew Medical Center
LAC-Rancho Los Amigos Medical Center
Orthopaedic Hospital

Program Director:
Clarence Woods, MD
Martin Luther King Jr-Drew Med Ctr
12021 S Wilmington Ave
Los Angeles, CA 90059
Tel: 310 668-4535 *Fax:* 310 223-0733
Accred Length: 5 Years *Program Size:* 10
Program ID: 260-05-22-069

UCLA Medical Center Program

Sponsor: UCLA School of Medicine
Shriners Hospital for Children (Los Angeles)
UCLA Medical Center
VA Greater Los Angeles Healthcare System

Program Director:
Gerald A M Finerman, MD
UCLA Sch of Med
Dept of Ortho Surgery
76-134 CHS
Los Angeles, CA 90095-6902
Tel: 310 825-6986 *Fax:* 310 825-1311
E-mail: jderenne@mednet.ucla.edu
Internet: http://149.142.183.2
Accred Length: 5 Years *Program Size:* 30 (*GY1:* 6)
Subspecialties: HSO
Program ID: 260-05-21-078

University of Southern California Program

Sponsor: Los Angeles County-USC Medical Center
Children's Hospital of Los Angeles
LAC-Rancho Los Amigos Medical Center
Orthopaedic Hospital
USC University Hospital

Program Director:
Michael J Patzakis, MD
Univ of Southern California
2025 Zonal Ave/COH 3900
Los Angeles, CA 90033
Tel: 323 226-7210 *Fax:* 323 226-4051
E-mail: orthopod@hsc.usc.edu
Internet:
http://www.usc.edu/hsc/medicine/orthopaedic_surgery
Accred Length: 5 Years *Program Size:* 52 (*GY1:* 10)
Subspecialties: HSO
Program ID: 260-05-21-193

Orange

University of California (Irvine) Program

Sponsor: University of California (Irvine) Medical Center
Children's Hospital of Orange County
LAC-Rancho Los Amigos Medical Center
Veterans Affairs Medical Center (Long Beach)

Program Director:
Harry B Skinner, MD PhD
Univ of California Irvine Med Ctr
Dept of Ortho Surgery
101 City Dr S/Pavilion III 2nd Fl
Orange, CA 92868
Tel: 714 456-5754 *Fax:* 714 456-7547
Internet: http://www.com.uci.edu/~ortho/
Accred Length: 4 Years *Program Size:* 16
Program ID: 260-05-21-064

Sacramento

University of California (Davis) Program

Sponsor: University of California (Davis) Medical Center
Shriners Hospitals for Children (Sacramento)

Program Director:
Michael W Chapman, MD
Univ of California Davis Med Ctr
Dept of Orthopaedics
4860 Y St/Ste 3800
Sacramento, CA 95817
Tel: 916 734-2709 *Fax:* 916 734-7904
E-mail: wsfeldman@ucdavis.edu
Accred Length: 5 Years *Program Size:* 20 (*GY1:* 4)
Subspecialties: HSO
Program ID: 260-05-21-133

San Diego

Naval Medical Center (San Diego) Program

Sponsor: Naval Medical Center (San Diego)

Program Director:
John S Webster, MD
Naval Med Ctr
34800 Bob Wilson Dr
San Diego, CA 92134-5000
Tel: 619 532-8427 *Fax:* 619 532-8467
E-mail: jswebster@nmcsd.med.navy.mil
Accred Length: 4 Years *Program Size:* 20
Subspecialties: HSO
Program ID: 260-05-31-079
US Armed Services Program

University of California (San Diego) Program

Sponsor: University of California (San Diego) Medical Center
Children's Hospital and Health Center
Veterans Affairs Medical Center (San Diego)

Program Director:
Steven R Garfin, MD
UCSD Med Ctr
Business Office
200 W Arbor Dr/8894
San Diego, CA 92103-8894
Tel: 619 543-5944 *Fax:* 619 543-7510
Internet: http://www.medicine.ucsd.edu/ortho
Accred Length: 4 Years *Program Size:* 13
Subspecialties: HSO, OP, OSM
Program ID: 260-05-21-109

San Francisco

San Francisco Program

Sponsor: St Mary's Hospital and Medical Center
Alameda County Medical Center
Kaiser Permanente Medical Center (San Francisco)

Program Director:
Garnet F Wynne, MD
St Mary's Med Ctr
450 Stanyan St
San Francisco, CA 94117-4160
Tel: 415 750-5782 *Fax:* 415 750-5938
E-mail: sforp@sforp.com
Internet: http://www.sforp.com
Accred Length: 4 Years *Program Size:* 12
Program ID: 260-05-22-108

University of California (San Francisco) Program

Sponsor: University of California (San Francisco) School of Medicine
Alameda County Medical Center
San Francisco General Hospital Medical Center
University of California (San Francisco) Medical Center
Veterans Affairs Medical Center (San Francisco)

Program Director:
David S Bradford, MD
Univ of California San Francisco
Dept of Ortho Surgery
500 Parnassus Ave/Box 0728
San Francisco, CA 94143-0728
Tel: 415 476-1166 *Fax:* 415 476-1304
E-mail: resident1@orthosurg.ucsf.edu
Internet: http://itssrv1.ucsf.edu.orthopedics
Accred Length: 5 Years *Program Size:* 28 (*GY1:* 4)
Subspecialties: HSO
Program ID: 260-05-21-002

Stanford

Stanford University Program

Sponsor: Stanford University Hospital
Lucile Salter Packard Children's Hospital at Stanford
Santa Clara Valley Medical Center
Veterans Affairs Palo Alto Health Care System

Program Director:
Stuart B Goodman, MD
Stanford University
Div of Ortho Surgery
300 Pasteur Dr/Rm R-171
Stanford, CA 94305-5326
Tel: 650 725-5903 *Fax:* 650 723-9805
E-mail: ml.res@forsythe
Internet:
http://www.med.stanford.edu/shc/ortho/residency.html
Accred Length: 5 Years *Program Size:* 21 (*GY1:* 3)
Subspecialties: HSO, OAR
Program ID: 260-05-21-098

Torrance

Los Angeles County-Harbor-UCLA Medical Center Program

Sponsor: Los Angeles County-Harbor-UCLA Medical Center

Program Director:
Daniel M Zinar, MD
Los Angeles County-Harbor-UCLA Med Ctr
1000 W Carson St
Box 422
Torrance, CA 90509
Tel: 310 222-2716 *Fax:* 310 533-8791
Accred Length: 5 Years *Program Size:* 15 (*GY1:* 3)
Program ID: 260-05-31-122

Colorado

Denver

University of Colorado Program

Sponsor: University of Colorado Health Sciences Center
Children's Hospital
Denver Health and Hospitals
Veterans Affairs Medical Center (Denver)

Program Director:
Jerome D Wiedel, MD
Univ of Colorado Health Sciences Ctr
4200 E Ninth Ave
UCHSC Container B202
Denver, CO 80262
Tel: 303 315-6593 *Fax:* 303 315-8600
Accred Length: 4 Years *Program Size:* 16 (*GY1:* 4)
Subspecialties: OSM
Program ID: 260-07-21-004

Connecticut

Farmington

University of Connecticut Program

Sponsor: University of Connecticut School of Medicine
Connecticut Children's Medical Center
Hartford Hospital
St Francis Hospital and Medical Center
Univ of Connecticut Health Center/John Dempsey Hospital

Program Director:
Courtland G Lewis, MD
Univ of Connecticut Health Ctr
Dept of Orthopaedics
PO Box 4037
Farmington, CT 06034-4037
Tel: 860 679-6640 *Fax:* 860 679-6649
E-mail: gcooper@nso.uchc.edu
Accred Length: 5 Years *Program Size:* 19 (*GY1:* 4)
Subspecialties: HSO, OP, OSM
Program ID: 260-08-21-172

New Haven

Yale-New Haven Medical Center Program

Sponsor: Yale-New Haven Hospital
Hospital of St Raphael
Veterans Affairs Medical Center (West Haven)

Program Director:
Gary E Friedlaender, MD
Yale Univ Sch of Med
Dept of Ortho/Rehabilitation
PO Box 208071
New Haven, CT 06520-8071
Tel: 203 785-2579 *Fax:* 203 785-7132
Internet: http://www.info.med.yale.edu/ortho/
Accred Length: 4 Years *Program Size:* 20
Subspecialties: HSO, OSM
Program ID: 260-08-21-005

District of Columbia

Washington

George Washington University Program

Sponsor: George Washington University School of Medicine
Children's National Medical Center
Fairfax Hospital
George Washington University Hospital (UHS)
Washington Hospital Center

Program Director:
Robert J Neviaser, MD
George Washington Univ
2150 Pennsylvania Ave NW
Rm 7-416
Washington, DC 20037
Tel: 202 994-4386 *Fax:* 202 994-1599
E-mail: orthores@gwumc.edu
Accred Length: 4 Years *Program Size:* 16
Subspecialties: OP
Program ID: 260-10-21-083

Georgetown University Program

Sponsor: Georgetown University Medical Center
Arlington Hospital
Sibley Memorial Hospital

Program Director:
Sam W Wiesel, MD
Georgetown Univ Hospital
Office of Education/Dept of Ortho Surgery
3800 Reservoir Rd NW
Washington, DC 20007-2197
Tel: 202 687-1233 *Fax:* 202 687-4287
Accred Length: 5 Years *Program Size:* 15 (*GY1:* 3)
Subspecialties: OSM
Program ID: 260-10-21-014

Howard University Program

Sponsor: Howard University Hospital
Children's National Medical Center
District of Columbia General Hospital
Providence Hospital
Veterans Affairs Medical Center (Washington, DC)

Program Director:
Richard E Grant, MD
Howard Univ Hospital
Div of Ortho Surgery
2041 Georgia Ave NW
Washington, DC 20060
Tel: 202 865-1182 *Fax:* 202 865-4904
Accred Length: 4 Years *Program Size:* 16
Program ID: 260-10-21-115

Walter Reed Army Medical Center Program

Sponsor: Walter Reed Army Medical Center
duPont Hospital for Children

Program Director:
Kathleen A McHale, MD
Walter Reed Army Med Ctr
Orthopaedic Service/Bldg 2
Washington, DC 20307-5001
Tel: 202 782-5848 *Fax:* 202 782-6945
Accred Length: 5 Years *Program Size:* 15
Subspecialties: HSO, OSM
Program ID: 260-10-11-075
US Armed Services Program

Florida

Gainesville

University of Florida Program

Sponsor: University of Florida College of Medicine
Shands Hospital at the University of Florida
Veterans Affairs Medical Center (Gainesville)

Program Director:
B. Hudson Berrey Jr, MD
Univ of Florida Coll of Med
Dept of Ortho/Rehab
PO Box 100246
Gainesville, FL 32610-0246
Tel: 352 392-4251 *Fax:* 352 392-8637
E-mail: hudson-berrey@ufl.edu
Internet: http://www.ufl.edu.ortho
Accred Length: 5 Years *Program Size:* 15 (*GY1:* 3)
Subspecialties: HSO, OAR, OMO, OSM
Program ID: 260-11-21-123

Jacksonville

University of Florida Health Science Center/Jacksonville Program
Sponsor: University of Florida College of Medicine at Jacksonville
University Medical Center (UFHSC/J)
Nemours Children's Clinic (UFHSC/J)
Program Director:
Samuel Agnew, MD
Univ of Florida Health Science Ctr-Jacksonville
653-II W 8th St
Jacksonville, FL 32209-6511
Tel: 904 549-3965 *Fax:* 904 549-3457
Accred Length: 5 Years *Program Size:* 10 (*GYI:* 2)
Program ID: 260-11-21-062

Miami

University of Miami-Jackson Memorial Medical Center Program
Sponsor: University of Miami-Jackson Memorial Medical Center
Cedars Medical Center
HealthSouth Doctors' Hospital
Miami Children's Hospital
Veterans Affairs Medical Center (Miami)
Program Director:
Frank J Eismont, MD
Univ of Miami Sch of Med
Dept of Ortho/Rehab
PO Box 016960/D-27
Miami, FL 33101
Tel: 305 585-1315 *Fax:* 305 324-7658
Accred Length: 5 Years *Program Size:* 30 (*GYI:* 6)
Subspecialties: HSO, OSM, OSS
Program ID: 260-11-21-076

Orlando

Orlando Regional Healthcare System Program
Sponsor: Orlando Regional Medical Center
Florida Elks Children's Hospital
Program Director:
John F Connolly, MD
Orlando Regional Healthcare System
Medical Education Orthopaedics
1414 Kuhl Ave
Orlando, FL 32806
Tel: 407 649-6885 *Fax:* 407 843-7381
E-mail: pdavis@orhs.org
Internet: http://www.orhs.org
Accred Length: 5 Years *Program Size:* 10 (*GYI:* 2)
Subspecialties: OP
Program ID: 260-11-22-184

Georgia

Atlanta

Emory University Program
Sponsor: Emory University School of Medicine
Crawford Long Hospital of Emory University
Egleston Children's Hospital at Emory University
Emory University Hospital
Grady Memorial Hospital
Program Director:
Lamar L Fleming, MD
Emory Univ
Dept of Ortho Surg/402 Glenn Bldg
69 Butler St SE
Atlanta, GA 30303
Tel: 404 616-4475 *Fax:* 404 659-3995
E-mail: lleach@emory.edu
Internet: http://www.emory.edu/whsc/ortho/xxx.html
Accred Length: 5 Years *Program Size:* 26 (*GYI:* 5)
Program ID: 260-12-21-039

Georgia Baptist Medical Center Program
Sponsor: Georgia Baptist Medical Center
Scottish Rite Children's Medical Center
Program Director:
John A Ogden, MD
Dept of Med Educ
303 Parkway Dr NE
PO Box 423
Atlanta, GA 30312
Tel: 404 265-1579 *Fax:* 404 265-4989
Accred Length: 5 Years *Program Size:* 15 (*GYI:* 3)
Program ID: 260-12-22-113

Augusta

Medical College of Georgia Program
Sponsor: Medical College of Georgia Hospital and Clinics
Veterans Affairs Medical Center (Augusta)
Program Director:
Monroe I Levine, MD
Med Coll of Georgia
Dept of Orthopaedic Surgery
1120 15th St
Augusta, GA 30912-4030
Tel: 706 721-4680 *Fax:* 706 721-1794
E-mail: mlevine@mail.mcg.edu
Accred Length: 5 Years *Program Size:* 12 (*GYI:* 3)
Program ID: 260-12-21-114

Fort Gordon

Dwight David Eisenhower Army Medical Center Program
Sponsor: Dwight David Eisenhower Army Medical Center
Scottish Rite Children's Medical Center
Program Director:
Arlon H Jahnke Jr, MD
Dwight David Eisenhower Army Med Ctr
Orthopaedic Surgery Services
Rm 2F31
Fort Gordon, GA 30905-5650
Tel: 706 787-1859 *Fax:* 706 787-8087
Accred Length: 4 Years *Program Size:* 8
Program ID: 260-12-21-192
US Armed Services Program

Hawaii

Honolulu

Tripler Army Medical Center Program
Sponsor: Tripler Army Medical Center
Program Director:
William E Burkhalter Jr, MD
CDR TAMC
1 Jarrett White Rd
Honolulu, HI 96859-5000
Tel: 808 433-6727 *Fax:* 808 433-1554
E-mail: gregg_w.taylor@tamc.chcs.amedd.army.mil
Internet: http://www.tamc.amedd.army.mil
Accred Length: 4 Years *Program Size:* 12
Program ID: 260-14-31-086
US Armed Services Program

University of Hawaii Program
Sponsor: University of Hawaii John A Burns School of Medicine
LAC-Rancho Los Amigos Medical Center
Queen's Medical Center
Shriners Hospitals for Children (Honolulu)
Tripler Army Medical Center
Program Director:
Allen B Richardson, MD
Univ of Hawaii John A Burns Sch of Med
1356 Lusitana St/6th Fl
Honolulu, HI 96813-2478
Tel: 808 586-8233 *Fax:* 808 536-1140
E-mail: fredricksenv@jabsom.biomed.hawaii.edu
Internet:
http://www.medworld.biomed.hawaii.edu/hrp.html
Accred Length: 4 Years *Program Size:* 8
Subspecialties: OP
Program ID: 260-14-21-068

Illinois

Chicago

McGaw Medical Center of Northwestern University Program
Sponsor: Northwestern University Medical School
Children's Memorial Medical Center
Cook County Hospital
Evanston Hospital
Northwestern Memorial Hospital
Veterans Affairs Lakeside Medical Center (Chicago)
Program Director:
Michael F Schafer, MD
Northwestern Univ Med Sch
Dept of Orthopaedics
645 N Michigan Ave/Ste1058B
Chicago, IL 60611
Tel: 312 908-7937 *Fax:* 312 908-8479
E-mail: orthopaedics@nwu.edu
Internet: http://www.orthopaedics.nwu.edu
Accred Length: 5 Years *Program Size:* 45 (*GYI:* 9)
Subspecialties: OP, OSM
Program ID: 260-16-21-007

Programs

Rush-Presbyterian-St Luke's Medical Center Program
Sponsor: Rush-Presbyterian-St Luke's Medical Center
Cook County Hospital
Shriners Hospitals for Children (Chicago)
Program Director:
Joshua Jacobs, MD
Rush-Presbyterian-St Luke's Med Ctr
1653 W Congress Pkwy
Rm 1471 Jelke
Chicago, IL 60612
Tel: 312 942-5850 *Fax:* 312 942-2101
E-mail: jacobs@ortho4.pro.rpslmc.edu
Accred Length: 5 Years *Program Size:* 20 (*GY1:* 4)
Subspecialties: OSM, OSS
Program ID: 260-16-31-174

University of Chicago Program
Sponsor: University of Chicago Hospitals
Louis A Weiss Memorial Hospital
Program Director:
Michael A Simon, MD
5841 S Maryland Ave/MC 3079
Chicago, IL 60637
Tel: 773 834-1634 *Fax:* 773 702-4384
E-mail: msimon@surgery.bsd.uchicago.edu
Accred Length: 5 Years *Program Size:* 18 (*GY1:* 4)
Subspecialties: HSO, OAR, OMO, OSM
Program ID: 260-16-21-136

University of Illinois College of Medicine at Chicago Program
Sponsor: University of Illinois College of Medicine at Chicago
Cook County Hospital
Michael Reese Hospital and Medical Center
Ravenswood Hospital Medical Center
Shriners Hospitals for Children (Chicago)
University of Illinois Hospital and Clinics
Veterans Affairs West Side Medical Center
Program Director:
Edward Abraham, MD
Univ of Illinois Hospital
Dept of Orthopaedics
901 S Wolcott/Rm 209 (M/C 844)
Chicago, IL 60612
Tel: 312 996-7160, ext 7160 *Fax:* 312 996-9025
Internet: http://www.uic.edu/com/ors
Accred Length: 5 Years *Program Size:* 34 (*GY1:* 7)
Subspecialties: OSM, TY
Program ID: 260-16-21-047

Maywood

Loyola University Program
Sponsor: Loyola University Medical Center
Edward J Hines Jr Veterans Affairs Hospital
Shriners Hospitals for Children (Chicago)
Program Director:
Terry R Light, MD
Loyola Univ Med Ctr
2160 S First Ave/Bldg 54
Maywood, IL 60153
Tel: 708 216-6906 *Fax:* 708 216-5858
E-mail: mshanah@luc.edu
Internet: http://www.lumc.edu/orthopaedics
Accred Length: 5 Years *Program Size:* 20 (*GY1:* 4)
Program ID: 260-16-21-050

Springfield

Southern Illinois University Program
Sponsor: Southern Illinois University School of Medicine
Memorial Medical Center
St John's Hospital
Program Director:
D Gordon Allan, MD
Southern Illinois Univ Sch of Med
PO Box 19638
Springfield, IL 62794-9638
Tel: 217 782-8865 *Fax:* 217 524-1793
E-mail: aweinhoeft@siumed.edu
Internet: http://www.siumed.edu/
Accred Length: 5 Years *Program Size:* 15 (*GY1:* 3)
Subspecialties: OSS
Program ID: 260-16-21-110

Indiana

Fort Wayne

Fort Wayne Medical Education Program
Sponsor: Fort Wayne Medical Education Program
Fort Wayne State Development Center
Parkview Memorial Hospital
St Joseph's Medical Center
Program Director:
Daniel Cummiskey, MD
Fort Wayne Med Education Program
2448 Lake Ave
Fort Wayne, IN 46805
Tel: 219 422-6573
E-mail: niccum@fwmep.edu
Internet: http://www.fwmep.edu
Accred Length: 4 Years *Program Size:* 8
Program ID: 260-17-22-138

Indianapolis

Indiana University School of Medicine Program
Sponsor: Indiana University School of Medicine
Clarian IU Hospital
Clarian Methodist Hospital of Indiana
Clarian Riley Hospital for Children
Richard L Roudebush Veterans Affairs Medical Center
William N Wishard Memorial Hospital
Program Director:
Richard E Lindseth, MD
Indiana Univ Med Ctr
541 N Clinical Dr/Rm 600
Indianapolis, IN 46202-5111
Tel: 317 274-8318 *Fax:* 317 274-3702
E-mail: ortho@indyunix.iupui.edu
Internet:
http://www.iupui.edu/it/iuortho/orthohome.html
Accred Length: 5 Years *Program Size:* 25 (*GY1:* 5)
Subspecialties: HSO, OSM
Program ID: 260-17-21-008

Iowa

Iowa City

University of Iowa Hospitals and Clinics Program
Sponsor: University of Iowa Hospitals and Clinics
Veterans Affairs Medical Center (Iowa City)
Program Director:
Reginald R Cooper, MD
Univ of Iowa Hospitals and Clinics
Dept of Ortho Surgery
200 Hawkins Dr
Iowa City, IA 52242-1009
Tel: 319 356-3470 *Fax:* 319 353-6754
E-mail: reginald-cooper@uiowa.edu
Accred Length: 5 Years *Program Size:* 25 (*GY1:* 5)
Subspecialties: HSO, OSM
Program ID: 260-18-21-139

Kansas

Kansas City

University of Kansas Medical Center Program
Sponsor: University of Kansas School of Medicine
University of Kansas Medical Center
Veterans Affairs Medical Center (Kansas City)
Program Director:
Brad Olney, MD
Univ of Kansas Med Ctr
39th and Rainbow Blvd
Kansas City, KS 66160-7387
Tel: 913 588-6138 *Fax:* 913 588-6178
E-mail: llerner@kumc.edu
Accred Length: 5 Years *Program Size:* 12 (*GY1:* 3)
Program ID: 260-19-21-140

Wichita

University of Kansas (Wichita) Program
Sponsor: University of Kansas School of Medicine (Wichita)
Columbia Wesley Medical Center
Shriners Hospitals for Children (St Louis)
Veterans Affairs Medical Center (Wichita)
Via Christi Regional Medical Center
Program Director:
George L Lucas, MD
Univ of Kansas Sch of Med-Wichita
1010 N Kansas
Wichita, KS 67214
Tel: 316 268-5988 *Fax:* 316 291-7799
E-mail: jridgewa@kumc.educ
Internet: http://www.kumc.edu/wichita/dept/ortho
Accred Length: 5 Years *Program Size:* 20 (*GY1:* 4)
Program ID: 260-19-31-106

Kentucky

Lexington

University of Kentucky Medical Center Program

Sponsor: University of Kentucky Hospital
Shriners Hospital for Children (Lexington)
Veterans Affairs Medical Center (Lexington)

Program Director:
Darren L Johnson, MD
Kentucky Clinic
740 S Limestone/K401
Lexington, KY 40536-0284
Tel: 606 323-5533 *Fax:* 606 323-2412
Internet: http://www.uky.edu
Accred Length: 5 Years *Program Size:* 15 (*GY1:* 3)
Subspecialties: OP, OSM
Program ID: 260-20-21-059

Louisville

University of Louisville Program

Sponsor: University of Louisville School of Medicine
Alliant Medical Pavilion
Jewish Hospital
Kosair Children's Hospital (Alliant Health System)
University of Louisville Hospital
Veterans Affairs Medical Center (Louisville)

Program Director:
John R Johnson, MD
Univ of Louisville Sch of Med
ACB/3rd Fl Bridge/HSC
530 S Jackson St
Louisville, KY 40292
Tel: 502 852-5319 *Fax:* 502 852-7227
E-mail: ulortho@ulkyvm.louisville.edu
Internet: http://www.louisville.edu/medschool/orthos
Accred Length: 5 Years *Program Size:* 20
Subspecialties: OSS
Program ID: 260-20-21-009

Louisiana

New Orleans

Alton Ochsner Medical Foundation Program

Sponsor: Alton Ochsner Medical Foundation
Leonard J Chabert Medical Center
Shriners Hospital for Children (Shreveport)

Program Director:
Michael R Wilson, MD
Alton Ochsner Med Foundation
Dept of Grad Med Educ
1516 Jefferson Hwy
New Orleans, LA 70121
Tel: 504 842-3260 *Fax:* 504 842-3193
E-mail: dlambert@ochsner.org
Internet: http://www.ochsner.org
Accred Length: 5 Years *Program Size:* 10 (*GY1:* 2)
Program ID: 260-21-22-056

Louisiana State University Program

Sponsor: Louisiana State University School of Medicine
Childrens Hospital
Earl K Long Medical Center
Medical Center of Louisiana at New Orleans
University Medical Center (Lafayette)

Program Director:
Mitchel B Harris, MD
Dept of Orthopaedic Surgery
2025 Gravier St/Ste 400
New Orleans, LA 70112
Tel: 504 568-4680 *Fax:* 504 568-4466
E-mail: kledet@.lsumc.edu
Internet: http://www.lsumc.edu/campus/orth/surg/
Accred Length: 5 Years *Program Size:* 20 (*GY1:* 4)
Subspecialties: OP, OSM
Program ID: 260-21-21-141

Tulane University Program

Sponsor: Tulane University School of Medicine
Huey P Long Regional Medical Center
Medical Center of Louisiana at New Orleans
Scottish Rite Children's Medical Center
Tulane University Hospital and Clinics
Veterans Affairs Medical Center (Alexandria)
Veterans Affairs Medical Center-LSU Service (New Orleans)

Program Director:
Robert L Barrack, MD
Tulane Univ Sch of Med
1430 Tulane Ave
New Orleans, LA 70112
Tel: 504 588-5192 *Fax:* 504 584-3517
E-mail: limiller@tmcpop.tmc.tulane.edu
Internet: http://www.mcl.tulane.edu/orthopaedics
Accred Length: 4 Years *Program Size:* 24
Subspecialties: OSM, TY
Program ID: 260-21-31-010

Shreveport

Louisiana State University (Shreveport) Program

Sponsor: Louisiana State University Hospital-Shreveport
Overton Brooks Veterans Affairs Medical Center
Shriners Hospital for Children (Shreveport)

Program Director:
James A Albright, MD
Louisiana State Univ Med Ctr Hospital
1501 Kings Hwy
PO Box 33932
Shreveport, LA 71130-3932
Tel: 318 675-6180 *Fax:* 318 675-6186
E-mail: jalbri@lsumc.edu
Internet: http://www.ortho.lsumc.edu/ortho.html
Accred Length: 5 Years *Program Size:* 15 (*GY1:* 3)
Program ID: 260-21-21-043

Maryland

Baltimore

Johns Hopkins University Program

Sponsor: Johns Hopkins University School of Medicine
Children's Hospital and Center for Reconstructive Surgery
Good Samaritan Hospital of Maryland
Johns Hopkins Bayview Medical Center
Johns Hopkins Hospital

Program Director:
Lee Riley III, MD
601 N Caroline St
JHOC/5235
Baltimore, MD 21287-0881
Tel: 410 955-6930 *Fax:* 410 955-1719
Internet: http://www.med.jhu.edu/ortho/
Accred Length: 5 Years *Program Size:* 25 (*GY1:* 5)
Subspecialties: OSM
Program ID: 260-23-21-057

Union Memorial Hospital Program

Sponsor: Union Memorial Hospital
Children's Hospital and Center for Reconstructive Surgery
Johns Hopkins Bayview Medical Center
Johns Hopkins Hospital

Program Director:
Leslie S Matthews, MD
Union Memorial Hospital
Dept of Orthopaedics
3333 N Calvert St/Ste 400
Baltimore, MD 21218
Tel: 410 554-2857 *Fax:* 410 554-2853
Internet: http://www.helixhealth.com
Accred Length: 4 Years *Program Size:* 8
Subspecialties: OSM
Program ID: 260-23-31-087

University of Maryland Program

Sponsor: University of Maryland Medical System
James Lawrence Kernan Hospital
St Agnes Hospital

Program Director:
Andrew Burgess, MD
Univ of Maryland Med System
Div of Ortho Surgery
22 S Greene St
Baltimore, MD 21201
Tel: 410 328-6040 *Fax:* 410 328-0534
Accred Length: 4 Years *Program Size:* 16
Subspecialties: OTR
Program ID: 260-23-31-088

Bethesda

National Naval Medical Center (Bethesda) Program

Sponsor: National Naval Medical Center (Bethesda)

Program Director:
Frederick G Lippert, MD
Frederick B Shannon, MD
National Naval Med Ctr
Dept of Orthopaedics
8901 Wisconsin Ave
Bethesda, MD 20889-5000
Tel: 301 295-4493 *Fax:* 301 295-4141
E-mail: flippert@compuserve.com
Accred Length: 4 Years *Program Size:* 12
Program ID: 260-23-21-183
US Armed Services Program

Programs

Massachusetts

Boston

Boston University Medical Center Program

Sponsor: Boston Medical Center
Lahey Clinic
Shriners Hospitals for Children (Springfield)
Veterans Affairs Medical Center (Boston)

Program Director:
Thomas A Einhorn, MD
Boston Med Ctr
720 Harrison Ave/Ste 808
Boston, MA 02118
Tel: 617 638-8934 *Fax:* 617 638-8493
E-mail: melissa.martin@bmc.org
Accred Length: 5 Years *Program Size:* 20 (*GY1:* 4)
Subspecialties: OP
Program ID: 260-24-31-066

Harvard Medical School Program

Sponsor: Massachusetts General Hospital
Beth Israel Deaconess Medical Center
Brigham and Women's Hospital
Brockton-West Roxbury Veterans Affairs Medical Center
Children's Hospital

Program Director:
James H Herndon, MD
Massachusetts General Hospital
55 Fruit St
GRB 624
Boston, MA 02114
Tel: 617 726-2942 *Fax:* 617 726-6823
E-mail: dsheehan@partners.org
Accred Length: 5 Years *Program Size:* 50 (*GY1:* 10)
Subspecialties: HSO, OMO, OP, OSM
Program ID: 260-24-21-011

Tufts University Program

Sponsor: New England Medical Center Hospitals
New England Baptist Hospital
Newton-Wellesley Hospital
Veterans Affairs Medical Center (Boston)

Program Director:
Michael J Goldberg, MD
New England Med Ctr
Dept of Orthopaedics
750 Washington St/Box 202
Boston, MA 02111
Tel: 617 636-5172 *Fax:* 617 636-5178
E-mail: jane.dolph@es.nemc.org
Accred Length: 5 Years *Program Size:* 16
Subspecialties: HSO, OSM
Program ID: 260-24-21-013

Worcester

University of Massachusetts Program

Sponsor: University of Massachusetts Medical School
UMass Memorial Health Care (Memorial Campus)
UMass Memorial Health Care (University Campus)

Program Director:
Arthur M Pappas, MD
Univ of Massachusetts Med Sch
55 Lake Ave N
Worcester, MA 01655
Tel: 508 856-2171 *Fax:* 508 856-5916
Accred Length: 4 Years *Program Size:* 16
Subspecialties: OSM
Program ID: 260-24-21-170

Michigan

Ann Arbor

University of Michigan Program

Sponsor: University of Michigan Hospitals
St Joseph Mercy Health System
Veterans Affairs Medical Center (Ann Arbor)

Program Director:
Larry S Matthews, MD
Univ of Michigan Hospitals
1500 E Medical Center Dr
2207 Taubman 0342
Ann Arbor, MI 48109-0328
Tel: 734 936-5733 *Fax:* 734 936-5725
Internet: http://www.med.umich.edu/surg/ortho
Accred Length: 5 Years *Program Size:* 30 (*GY1:* 6)
Program ID: 260-25-21-074

Detroit

Grace Hospital Program

Sponsor: Grace Hospital
Providence Hospital and Medical Centers
Sinai Hospital

Program Director:
Ralph B Blasier, MD
Metropolitan NW Detroit Hospitals
Grace Hospital, Orthopedics Dept
6071 W Outer Dr
Detroit, MI 48235
Tel: 313 966-4750 *Fax:* 313 966-4760
Accred Length: 5 Years *Program Size:* 16 (*GY1:* 3)
Program ID: 260-25-21-177

Henry Ford Hospital Program

Sponsor: Henry Ford Hospital

Program Director:
Eric L Radin, MD
Henry Ford Hospital
Orthopedic Surgery/K-12
2799 W Grand Blvd
Detroit, MI 48202
Tel: 313 876-7520 *Fax:* 313 556-8278
E-mail: radin@bjc.hfh.edu
Accred Length: 5 Years *Program Size:* 30 (*GY1:* 6)
Subspecialties: OTR
Program ID: 260-25-11-142

Wayne State University/Detroit Medical Center Program

Sponsor: Wayne State University/Detroit Medical Center
Children's Hospital of Michigan
Detroit Receiving Hospital and University Health Center
Hutzel Hospital
Veterans Affairs Medical Center (Detroit)

Program Director:
Stephen P DeSilva, MD
Hutzel Hospital
4707 St Antoine Blvd
Detroit, MI 48201
Tel: 313 745-8248 *Fax:* 313 993-0857
Accred Length: 4 Years *Program Size:* 25 (*GY1:* 4)
Subspecialties: OAR, OMO, OP
Program ID: 260-25-21-012

Flint

McLaren Regional Medical Center Program

Sponsor: McLaren Regional Medical Center
Hurley Medical Center
Michigan State University Clinical Center

Program Director:
Norman E Walter, MD
McLaren Regional Med Ctr
401 Ballenger Hwy
Flint, MI 48532-3685
Tel: 810 342-2111 *Fax:* 810 342-3659
Accred Length: 4 Years *Program Size:* 10 (*GY1:* 2)
Program ID: 260-25-12-089

Grand Rapids

Spectrum Health-East Campus Program

Sponsor: Spectrum Health-East Campus
Spectrum Health-Downtown Campus
St Mary's Health Services

Program Director:
Alfred B Swanson, MD
Grand Rapids Orthopaedic Program
Med Educ Office
1840 Wealthy St SE/Rm 3E-69
Grand Rapids, MI 49506
Tel: 616 774-7426 *Fax:* 616 774-5337
Accred Length: 5 Years *Program Size:* 20 (*GY1:* 4)
Subspecialties: HSO
Program ID: 260-25-21-195

Kalamazoo

Kalamazoo Center for Medical Studies/Michigan State University Program

Sponsor: Kalamazoo Center for Medical Studies
Borgess Medical Center
Bronson Methodist Hospital

Program Director:
E Dennis Lyne, MD
Michigan State Univ Kalamazoo Ctr for Med Studies
Dept of Ortho Surgery
1000 Oakland Dr
Kalamazoo, MI 49008-1284
Tel: 616 337-6250 *Fax:* 616 337-6441
E-mail: ortho_surg@kcms.msu.edu
Internet: http://www.kcms.msu.edu/orthsurg.html
Accred Length: 5 Years *Program Size:* 10 (*GY1:* 2)
Program ID: 260-25-21-126

Royal Oak

William Beaumont Hospital Program

Sponsor: William Beaumont Hospital

Program Director:
Harry N Herkowitz, MD
William Beaumont Hospital-MOB
3535 W 13 Mile Rd/Ste 604
Royal Oak, MI 48073
Tel: 248 551-0426 *Fax:* 248 551-5404
E-mail: cmusich@beaumont.edu
Internet: http://www.beaumont.edu/html/gme
Accred Length: 5 Years *Program Size:* 10 (*GY1:* 2)
Subspecialties: OSS
Program ID: 260-25-12-173

Minnesota

Minneapolis

University of Minnesota Program

Sponsor: University of Minnesota Medical School
Abbott-Northwestern Hospital
Fairview-University Medical Center
Gillette Children's Speciality Healthcare
Hennepin County Medical Center
Shriners Hospital for Children (Twin Cities Unit)
Veterans Affairs Medical Center (Minneapolis)

Program Director:
Marc F Swiontkowski, MD
Fairview Univ Med Ctr
420 Delaware St SE
PO Box 492
Minneapolis, MN 55455
Tel: 612 625-2157 *Fax:* 612 626-6032
Internet: http://www.med.umn.edu/ortho
Accred Length: 5 Years *Program Size:* 30
Subspecialties: HSO, OSS
Program ID: 260-26-21-080

Rochester

Mayo Graduate School of Medicine (Rochester) Program

Sponsor: Mayo Graduate School of Medicine-Mayo Foundation
Mayo Clinic (Rochester)
Rochester Methodist Hospital
St Mary's Hospital of Rochester

Program Director:
Arlen D Hanssen, MD
Mayo Graduate Sch of Med
Application Processing Ctr
200 First St SW
Rochester, MN 55905
Tel: 507 284-4331 *Fax:* 507 284-0999
E-mail: mgsm.surgical.specialties@mayuo.edu
Internet: http://www.mayo.edu/
Accred Length: 5 Years *Program Size:* 54 (*GY1:* 10)
Subspecialties: HSO, OAR, OMO
Program ID: 260-26-21-121

Mississippi

Jackson

University of Mississippi Medical Center Program

Sponsor: University of Mississippi School of Medicine
University Hospital
Veterans Affairs Medical Center (Jackson)

Program Director:
James L Hughes, MD
Univ of Mississippi Med Ctr
2500 N State St
Jackson, MS 39216-4505
Tel: 601 984-5135 *Fax:* 601 984-5151
E-mail: jmuzzi@orthopedics.umsmed.edu
Accred Length: 5 Years *Program Size:* 15 (*GY1:* 3)
Program ID: 260-27-21-006

Missouri

Columbia

University of Missouri-Columbia Program

Sponsor: University of Missouri-Columbia School of Medicine
Harry S Truman Memorial Veterans Hospital
University Hospitals and Clinics

Program Director:
Walter B Greene, MD
Univ of Missouri-Columbia
One Hospital Dr
Columbia, MO 65212
Tel: 573 882-3104 *Fax:* 573 882-1760
E-mail: hallb@health.missouri.edu
Internet: http://www.hsc.missouri.edu/~/ortho
Accred Length: 4 Years *Program Size:* 12
Program ID: 260-28-21-148

Kansas City

University of Missouri at Kansas City Program

Sponsor: University of Missouri-Kansas City School of Medicine
Children's Mercy Hospital
Saint Luke's Hospital
Truman Medical Center-West

Program Director:
James J Hamilton, MD
Truman Med Ctr
Dept of Ortho Surgery
2301 Holmes St
Kansas City, MO 64108
Tel: 816 556-3561 *Fax:* 816 556-3347
E-mail: hamiltjj@trumed1.trumanmed.org
Accred Length: 4 Years *Program Size:* 12
Subspecialties: OSM
Program ID: 260-28-21-018

St Louis

St Louis University School of Medicine Program

Sponsor: St Louis University School of Medicine
SSM Cardinal Glennon Children's Hospital
St Louis University School of Medicine
St Mary's Health Center

Program Director:
Robert E Burdge, MD
St Louis Univ Sch of Med
3635 Vista Ave
PO Box 15250
St Louis, MO 63110-0250
Tel: 314 577-8850 *Fax:* 314 268-5121
E-mail: ortho@wpogate.slu.edu
Internet: http://medschool.slu.edu/orthosurg
Accred Length: 5 Years *Program Size:* 15 (*GY1:* 3)
Program ID: 260-28-21-046

Washington University/B-JH/SLCH Consortium Program

Sponsor: Washington University/B-JH/SLCH Consortium
Barnes-Jewish Hospital
Shriners Hospitals for Children (St Louis)

Program Director:
Richard H Gelberman, MD
Barnes-Jewish Hospital
One Barnes Hospital Plaza
Ste 11300
St Louis, MO 63110
Tel: 314 747-2543 *Fax:* 314 747-2597
E-mail: orthsurg@msnotes.wustl.edu
Internet: http://www.ortho.wustl.edu
Accred Length: 4 Years *Program Size:* 20
Subspecialties: HSO, OP, OSS
Program ID: 260-28-21-060

Nebraska

Omaha

University of Nebraska/Creighton University Program

Sponsor: University of Nebraska Medical Center
Childrens Memorial Hospital
Tenet St Joseph Hospital at Creighton Univ Medical Center
Veterans Affairs Medical Center (Omaha)

Program Director:
James R Neff, MD
Creighton-Nebraska Health Foundation
Dept of Ortho Surgery
600 S 42nd St/PO Box 981080
Omaha, NE 68198-1080
Tel: 402 559-8000 *Fax:* 402 559-5511
E-mail: jrneff@unmcvm.unmc.edu
Internet: http://www.unmc.edu/orthosurgery/
Accred Length: 5 Years *Program Size:* 21 (*GY1:* 4)
Program ID: 260-30-21-001

New Hampshire

Lebanon

Dartmouth-Hitchcock Medical Center Program

Sponsor: Mary Hitchcock Memorial Hospital
Connecticut Children's Medical Center
Veterans Affairs Medical Center (White River Junction)

Program Director:
Philip M Bernini, MD
Dartmouth-Hitchcock Med Ctr
One Medical Center Dr
Lebanon, NH 03756-0001
Tel: 603 650-5970 *Fax:* 603 650-2097
E-mail: philip.m.bernini@hitchcock.org
Accred Length: 5 Years *Program Size:* 10 (*GY1:* 2)
Program ID: 260-32-21-082

New Jersey

Long Branch

Monmouth Medical Center Program

Sponsor: Monmouth Medical Center
Children's Hospital of Philadelphia

Program Director:
Angelo J Lopano, MD
Monmouth Med Ctr
Dept of Orthopedics/Rm 225SW
300 Second Ave
Long Branch, NJ 07740-9998
Tel: 732 923-6780 *Fax:* 732 923-6788
Accred Length: 5 Years *Program Size:* 5 (*GY1:* 1)
Program ID: 260-33-11-146

Newark

UMDNJ-New Jersey Medical School Program

Sponsor: UMDNJ-New Jersey Medical School
Hospital Center at Orange
Jersey City Medical Center
UMDNJ-University Hospital
Veterans Affairs Medical Center (East Orange)

Program Director:
Fred F Behrens, MD
UMDNJ-New Jersey Med Sch
Dept of Orthopaedics
90 Bergen St/DOC Ste 5200
Newark, NJ 07103
Tel: 973 972-5350 *Fax:* 973 972-9367
E-mail: tabakimd@umdnj.edu
Internet:
http://www.umdnj.edu/~chowchovg/homepage.html
Accred Length: 5 Years *Program Size:* 24
Program ID: 260-33-31-102

Paterson

St Joseph's Hospital and Medical Center Program

Sponsor: St Joseph's Hospital and Medical Center

Program Director:
Vincent K McInerney, MD
St Joseph's Hospital and Med Ctr
703 Main St
Paterson, NJ 07503
Tel: 973 754-2926 *Fax:* 973 754-2934
Accred Length: 5 Years *Program Size:* 4
Program ID: 260-33-12-147

Piscataway

UMDNJ-Robert Wood Johnson Medical School Program

Sponsor: UMDNJ-Robert Wood Johnson Medical School
Children's Hospital of Philadelphia
Robert Wood Johnson University Hospital
St Peter's University Hospital

Program Director:
Joseph P Leddy, MD
UMDNJ-Robert Wood Johnson Med Sch
PO Box 19
New Brunswick, NJ 08903-0019
Tel: 732 235-7869 *Fax:* 732 235-6002
E-mail: rwjortho@umdnj.edu
Internet: http://www2.umdnj.edu/orthoweb/index.htm
Accred Length: 4 Years *Program Size:* 12
Program ID: 260-33-21-149

New Mexico

Albuquerque

University of New Mexico Program

Sponsor: University of New Mexico School of Medicine
Carrie Tingley Hospital
University Hospital
Veterans Affairs Medical Center (Albuquerque)

Program Director:
Moheb S Moneim, MD
Univ of New Mexico Health Sciences Ctr
Dept of Orthopaedic/Rehab
ACC 2 West
Albuquerque, NM 87131-5296
Tel: 505 272-4107 *Fax:* 505 272-3581
E-mail: hpargas@salud.unm.edu
Internet: http://www.unm.edu/~ortho
Accred Length: 5 Years *Program Size:* 20 (*GY1:* 4)
Program ID: 260-34-31-093

New York

Albany

Albany Medical Center Program

Sponsor: Albany Medical Center
Ellis Hospital
St Peter's Hospital
Veterans Affairs Medical Center (Albany)

Program Director:
Richard L Uhl, MD
Albany Med Ctr
Dept of Ortho Surgery/A-61
47 New Scotland Ave/Rm A300A
Albany, NY 12208-3478
Tel: 518 262-5219 *Fax:* 518 262-5400
E-mail: richard_uhl@ccgateway.amc.edu
Accred Length: 5 Years *Program Size:* 19 (*GY1:* 3)
Program ID: 260-35-21-055

Bronx

Albert Einstein College of Medicine Program

Sponsor: Albert Einstein College of Medicine of Yeshiva University
Jacobi Medical Center
Montefiore Medical Center-Henry and Lucy Moses Division
Montefiore Medical Center-Weiler Hospital

Program Director:
Edward T Habermann, MD
Montefiore Med Ctr
111 E 210th St
Bronx, NY 10467
Tel: 718 920-4961 *Fax:* 718 231-2243
Accred Length: 5 Years *Program Size:* 35 (*GY1:* 6)
Program ID: 260-35-21-187

Bronx-Lebanon Hospital Center Program

Sponsor: Bronx-Lebanon Hospital Center

Program Director:
Harvey P Insler, MD
Bronx-Lebanon Hospital Ctr
1650 Selwyn Ave/Ste 5C
Bronx, NY 10457
Tel: 718 960-1300 *Fax:* 718 960-1390
E-mail: emkinsler@erols.com
Accred Length: 4 Years *Program Size:* 8
Program ID: 260-35-11-134

Brooklyn

Kingsbrook Jewish Medical Center Program

Sponsor: Kingsbrook Jewish Medical Center
Beth Israel Medical Center

Program Director:
Eli Bryk, MD
Kingsbrook Jewish Med Ctr
585 Schenectady Ave
Brooklyn, NY 11203
Tel: 718 604-5483 *Fax:* 718 604-5575
Accred Length: 4 Years *Program Size:* 4
Program ID: 260-35-31-185

Maimonides Medical Center Program

Sponsor: Maimonides Medical Center
Coney Island Hospital
Shriners Hospital for Children (Twin Cities Unit)

Program Director:
Allan Strongwater, MD
Maimonides Med Ctr
4802 Tenth Ave
Brooklyn, NY 11219
Tel: 718 283-7400 *Fax:* 718 283-6199
E-mail: astrongwater@maimonidesmed.org
Accred Length: 4 Years *Program Size:* 8
Program ID: 260-35-21-107

SUNY Health Science Center at Brooklyn Program

Sponsor: SUNY Health Science Center at Brooklyn
Brookdale University Hospital Medical Center
Kings County Hospital Center
Long Island College Hospital
University Hospital-SUNY Health Science Center at Brooklyn
Veterans Affairs Medical Center (Brooklyn)

Program Director:
Stanley L Gordon, MD
Dept of Ortho/Rehab Med
450 Clarkson Ave
Box 30
Brooklyn, NY 11203-2098
Tel: 718 270-2179 *Fax:* 718 270-3983
Accred Length: 5 Years *Program Size:* 28 (*GY1:* 5)
Program ID: 260-35-21-144

Buffalo

SUNY at Buffalo Graduate Medical-Dental Education Consortium Program

Sponsor: SUNY at Buffalo Grad Medical-Dental Education Consortium
CGF Health System (Buffalo General Hospital)
CGF Health System (Children's Hospital of Buffalo)
Erie County Medical Center
Veterans Affairs Medical Center (Buffalo)

Program Director:
Robert Gillespie, MD MB ChB
Children's Hospital
Dept of Orthopaedics
82 Hodge St
Buffalo, NY 14222-2098
Tel: 716 878-7722 *Fax:* 716 878-7724
E-mail: orthopaedics@buffalo.edu
Accred Length: 4 Years *Program Size:* 16
Subspecialties: HSO, OP
Program ID: 260-35-21-024

Jamaica

Catholic Medical Center of Brooklyn and Queens Program

Sponsor: Catholic Medical Center of Brooklyn and Queens Inc
Catholic Medical Center (Mary Immaculate Hospital)
Catholic Medical Center (St John's Queens Hospital)
Catholic Medical Center (St Mary's Hospital)

Program Director:
John R Denton, MD
Catholic Med Ctr of Brooklyn and Queens
88-25 153rd St
Jamaica, NY 11432
Tel: 718 558-7241 *Fax:* 718 558-6181
E-mail: jdenton@cmcny.com
Accred Length: 4 Years *Program Size:* 8
Program ID: 260-35-21-124

New Hyde Park

Albert Einstein College of Medicine at Long Island Jewish Medical Center Program

Sponsor: Long Island Jewish Medical Center
Jamaica Hospital
Schneider Children's Hosp (Long Island Jewish Med Ctr)
Program Director:
David M Dines, MD
Long Island Jewish Med Ctr
270-05 76th Ave
New Hyde Park, NY 11040
Tel: 718 470-7020 *Fax:* 718 962-2809
Internet: http://www.lij.edu
Accred Length: 4 Years *Program Size:* 13 (*GY1:* 3)
Program ID: 260-35-21-152

New York

Hospital for Joint Diseases Orthopaedic Institute Program

Sponsor: Hospital for Joint Diseases Orthopaedic Institute
Program Director:
Joseph D Zuckerman, MD
New York Univ Med Ctr-Hospital for Joint Diseases
Orthopaedic Dept
301 E 17th St
New York, NY 10003
Tel: 212 598-6497 *Fax:* 212 598-6581
Accred Length: 4 Years *Program Size:* 46 (*GY1:* 10)
Subspecialties: HSO, OAR, OFA, OP, OSM, OSS
Program ID: 260-35-12-125

Hospital for Special Surgery/Cornell Medical Center Program

Sponsor: Hospital for Special Surgery
New York and Presbyterian Hospital (Cornell Campus)
Program Director:
Russell F Warren, MD
Hospital for Special Surgery
535 E 70th St
New York, NY 10021
Tel: 212 606-1466
Internet: http://www.hss.edu
Accred Length: 4 Years *Program Size:* 35
Subspecialties: HSO, OMO, OP, OSM, OSS
Program ID: 260-35-21-022

Lenox Hill Hospital Program

Sponsor: Lenox Hill Hospital
Children's Hospital
Program Director:
Chitranjan S Ranawat, MD
Lenox Hill Hospital
Dept of Ortho Surgery
100 E 77th St
New York, NY 10021-1883
Tel: 212 434-2710 *Fax:* 212 434-2687
E-mail: orthopedics@mindspring.com
Accred Length: 5 Years *Program Size:* 11 (*GY1:* 2)
Subspecialties: OSM
Program ID: 260-35-11-175

Mount Sinai School of Medicine Program

Sponsor: Mount Sinai School of Medicine
Elmhurst Hospital Center-Mount Sinai Services
Mount Sinai Medical Center
Program Director:
Dempsey S Springfield, MD
Mount Sinai Sch of Med
Dept of Orthopaedics/Box 1188
5 E 98th St
New York, NY 10029-6574
Tel: 212 241-1621 *Fax:* 212 534-6091
E-mail: barbara_walker@smtplink.mssm.edu
Internet: http://www.mssm.edu/orthsurg/home-page.html
Accred Length: 4 Years *Program Size:* 15
Program ID: 260-35-21-065

New York and Presbyterian Hospital (Columbia Campus) Program

Sponsor: New York and Presbyterian Hospital
Harlem Hospital Center
New York and Presbyterian Hospital (Columbia Campus)
Program Director:
Louis U Bigliani, MD
Columbia Univ
622 W 168th St
11-1131
New York, NY 10032-2694
Tel: 212 305-5974 *Fax:* 212 305-6193
E-mail: orthosrg@ortho1.cpmc.columbia.edu
Internet:
http://cpmcnet.columbia.edu/dept/ortho/residency.html
Accred Length: 4 Years *Program Size:* 26
Subspecialties: HSO, OAR
Program ID: 260-35-31-128

New York University Medical Center Program

Sponsor: New York University Medical Center
Bellevue Hospital Center
Veterans Affairs Medical Center (Manhattan)
Program Director:
Joseph B Zuckerman, MD
New York Univ Med Ctr-Hospital for Joint Diseases
Dept of Orthopedic Surgery
301 E 17th St
New York, NY 10016
Tel: 212 598-6497 *Fax:* 212 598-6581
Internet: http://www.med.nyu.edu/ortho/
Accred Length: 5 Years *Program Size:* 58 (*GY1:* 10)
Subspecialties: HSO, OSM
Program ID: 260-35-21-051

St Luke's-Roosevelt Hospital Center Program

Sponsor: St Luke's-Roosevelt Hospital Center
duPont Hospital for Children
St Luke's-Roosevelt Hospital Center-Roosevelt Division
St Luke's-Roosevelt Hospital Center-St Luke's Division
Program Director:
Andrew H Patterson, MD
St Luke's-Roosevelt Hospital Ctr-St Luke's Div
1111 Amsterdam Ave
New York, NY 10025
Tel: 212 523-2650 *Fax:* 212 523-4676
Accred Length: 4 Years *Program Size:* 12 (*GY1:* 3)
Subspecialties: HSO
Program ID: 260-35-11-041

Rochester

University of Rochester Program

Sponsor: Strong Memorial Hospital of the University of Rochester
Highland Hospital of Rochester
Rochester General Hospital
Program Director:
Richard I Burton, MD
Dept of Orthopaedics
601 Elmwood Ave
Box 665
Rochester, NY 14642
Tel: 716 275-5168 *Fax:* 716 756-4721
E-mail: wsaetta@orthomail.ortho.rochester.edu
Internet:
http://www.urmc.rochester.edu/smd/ortho/orthohome.html
Accred Length: 4 Years *Program Size:* 21
Subspecialties: HSO, OSM
Program ID: 260-35-21-031

Stony Brook

SUNY at Stony Brook Program

Sponsor: University Hospital-SUNY at Stony Brook
Nassau County Medical Center
Program Director:
Lawrence C Hurst, MD
Steven Sampson, MD
SUNY-Stony Brook Health Science Ctr
T-18/Rm 020
Stony Brook, NY 11794-8181
Tel: 516 444-1487 *Fax:* 516 444-8894
E-mail: jferguso@surg.som.sunysb.edu
Accred Length: 4 Years *Program Size:* 20
Subspecialties: HSO, OP
Program ID: 260-35-21-181

Syracuse

SUNY Health Science Center at Syracuse Program

Sponsor: University Hospital-SUNY Health Science Center at Syracuse
Crouse Hospital
Veterans Affairs Medical Center (Syracuse)
Program Director:
David G Murray, MD
SUNY Health Science Ctr-Syracuse
Dept of Ortho Surgery
750 E Adams St
Syracuse, NY 13210
Tel: 315 464-5226 *Fax:* 315 464-6470
E-mail: addisonm@vax.cs.hscsyr.edu
Internet: http://www.ec.hscyr.edu:8001/worksin
Accred Length: 4 Years *Program Size:* 16
Subspecialties: HSO, OSS
Program ID: 260-35-21-048

Valhalla

New York Medical College at Westchester Medical Center Program

Sponsor: New York Medical College
Westchester Medical Center
Program Director:
Robert E Zickel, MD
Westchester Med Ctr
Macy Pavilion/Rm S106
Valhalla Campus
Valhalla, NY 10595
Tel: 914 493-8743 *Fax:* 914 493-1230
E-mail: orthsurg@erols
Accred Length: 4 Years *Program Size:* 12
Program ID: 260-35-21-067

North Carolina

Chapel Hill

University of North Carolina Hospitals Program

Sponsor: University of North Carolina Hospitals
Wake Medical Center
Program Director:
Edmund R Campion, MD
Univ of North Carolina Sch of Med
236 Burnett-Womack Bldg 229 H
CB7055
Chapel Hill, NC 27599-7055
Tel: 919 966-9071 *Fax:* 919 966-8731
E-mail: tmh@med.unc.edu
Internet: http://www.med.unc.edu/ortho
Accred Length: 5 Years *Program Size:* 22 (*GY1:* 4)
Program ID: 260-36-21-081

Programs

Charlotte

Carolinas Medical Center Program

Sponsor: Carolinas Medical Center
Shriners Hospital for Children (Greenville)

Program Director:
Edward N Hanley Jr, MD
Carolinas Med Ctr
PO Box 32861
Charlotte, NC 28232-2861
Tel: 704 355-3184 *Fax:* 704 355-6041
E-mail: amyers@mail.carolinas.org
Internet: http://www.carolinas.org
Accred Length: 5 Years *Program Size:* 16 (*GY1:* 3)
Subspecialties: OTR
Program ID: 260-36-22-104

Durham

Duke University Program

Sponsor: Duke University Medical Center
Durham Regional Hospital
Shriners Hospital for Children (Greenville)
Veterans Affairs Medical Center (Asheville)
Veterans Affairs Medical Center (Durham)

Program Director:
James R Urbaniak, MD
Duke Univ Med Ctr
Div of Ortho Surg/Box 2912
Durham, NC 27710
Tel: 919 684-3170 *Fax:* 919 684-8280
Internet:
http://surgery.mc.duke.edu/orthopaedics/residency
Accred Length: 5 Years *Program Size:* 33 (*GY1:* 8)
Subspecialties: HSO, OSM
Program ID: 260-36-31-019

Winston-Salem

Wake Forest University School of Medicine Program

Sponsor: Wake Forest University Baptist Medical Center

Program Director:
Gary G Poehling, MD
Dept of Orthopedic Surgery
Wake Forest Univ Sch of Med
Medical Center Blvd/Box 1070
Winston-Salem, NC 27157-1070
Tel: 336 716-3946 *Fax:* 336 716-6286
E-mail: hermance@wfubmc.edu
Internet: http://www.bgsm.edu/ortho
Accred Length: 5 Years *Program Size:* 15 (*GY1:* 3)
Subspecialties: HSO
Program ID: 260-36-21-077

Ohio

Akron

Akron General Medical Center/NEOUCOM Program

Sponsor: Akron General Medical Center
Children's Hospital Medical Center of Akron

Program Director:
Mark C Leeson, MD FACS
Akron General Med Ctr
400 Wabash Ave
Akron, OH 44307
Tel: 330 384-6055 *Fax:* 330 996-2973
E-mail: meded@agmc.org
Internet: http://agmc.org
Accred Length: 5 Years *Program Size:* 15 (*GY1:* 3)
Program ID: 260-38-21-058

Summa Health System (Akron City Hospital)/NEOUCOM Program

Sponsor: Summa Health System
Akron City Hospital (Summa Health System)
Children's Hospital Medical Center of Akron

Program Director:
J Patrick Flanagan, MD
Summa Health System
Med Educ/Mary Yanik
525 E Market St
Akron, OH 44309
Tel: 800 322-0517
Internet: http://www.summahealth.org/edu/
Accred Length: 5 Years *Program Size:* 15 (*GY1:* 3)
Program ID: 260-38-21-015

Cincinnati

University Hospital/University of Cincinnati College of Medicine Program

Sponsor: University Hospital Inc
Children's Hospital Medical Center
Christ Hospital
Veterans Affairs Medical Center (Cincinnati)

Program Director:
Peter J Stern, MD
Univ of Cincinnati Med Ctr
231 Bethesda Ave
PO Box 670212
Cincinnati, OH 45267-0212
Tel: 513 558-4592 *Fax:* 513 558-2220
E-mail: valeal@ucmail.uc.edu
Internet: http://www.med.uc.edu/departme/ortho/
Accred Length: 5 Years *Program Size:* 17 (*GY1:* 4)
Subspecialties: HSO
Program ID: 260-38-21-017

Cleveland

Case Western Reserve University Program

Sponsor: University Hospitals of Cleveland
MetroHealth Medical Center
Veterans Affairs Medical Center (Cleveland)

Program Director:
Victor M Goldberg, MD
Univ Hospitals of Cleveland
11100 Euclid Ave
Cleveland, OH 44106
Tel: 216 844-5900 *Fax:* 216 844-5970
Accred Length: 4 Years *Program Size:* 30 (*GY1:* 6)
Subspecialties: OMO
Program ID: 260-38-21-027

Cleveland Clinic Foundation Program

Sponsor: Cleveland Clinic Foundation
MetroHealth Medical Center

Program Director:
John J Brems, MD
Cleveland Clinic Foundation
Dept of Ortho Surgery/A41
9500 Euclid Ave
Cleveland, OH 44195
Tel: 216 444-5690 *Fax:* 216 444-1162
E-mail: meded@cesmtp.ccf.org
Internet: http://www.ccf.org
Accred Length: 5 Years *Program Size:* 20 (*GY1:* 4)
Subspecialties: HSO, OSM
Program ID: 260-38-22-042

Mount Sinai Medical Center of Cleveland Program

Sponsor: Mount Sinai Medical Center of Cleveland
University Hospitals of Cleveland

Program Director:
William H Seitz Jr, MD
Mt Sinai Med Ctr
One Mt Sinai Dr
Cleveland, OH 44106-4198
Tel: 216 421-3775 *Fax:* 216 421-3739
E-mail: msmcorth@stratos.net
Accred Length: 5 Years *Program Size:* 10 (*GY1:* 2)
Program ID: 260-38-21-101

St Luke's Medical Center Program

Sponsor: St Luke's Medical Center
Christ Hospital
University Hospitals of Cleveland

Program Director:
Timothy L Stephens Jr, MD
11311 Shaker Blvd/Ste 2204
Cleveland, OH 44104
Tel: 216 368-8466 *Fax:* 216 368-7969
E-mail: orthodaum@bbs2.rmrc.net
Accred Length: 5 Years *Program Size:* 10 (*GY1:* 2)
Program ID: 260-38-11-153

Columbus

Mount Carmel Health Program

Sponsor: Mount Carmel Medical Center
Children's Hospital

Program Director:
Richard A Fankhauser, MD
Mount Carmel Health System
793 W State St
Columbus, OH 43222
Tel: 614 234-5354 *Fax:* 614 234-2772
E-mail: jhill@mchs.com
Internet: http://mchsresidency.org
Accred Length: 5 Years *Program Size:* 10 (*GY1:* 2)
Program ID: 260-38-32-025

Ohio State University Program

Sponsor: Ohio State University Medical Center
Children's Hospital
Riverside Methodist Hospitals (OhioHealth)

Program Director:
Ray C Wasielewski, MD
Ohio State Univ Hospital
N839 Doan Hall
410 W Tenth Ave
Columbus, OH 43210
Tel: 614 293-6194 *Fax:* 614 293-3596
E-mail: surgery-orthores@medctr.osu.edu
Internet: http://www.ortho.ohio-state.edu/
Accred Length: 4 Years *Program Size:* 16
Subspecialties: HSO, OSM
Program ID: 260-38-21-099

Dayton

Wright State University Program

Sponsor: Wright State University School of Medicine
Children's Medical Center
Miami Valley Hospital
Veterans Affairs Medical Center (Dayton)

Program Director:
Hjalmar F Pompe van Meerdervoort, MD MD
Wright State Univ
30 E Apple St/Ste L-200
Dayton, OH 45409
Tel: 937 208-2127 *Fax:* 937 208-2920
Accred Length: 5 Years *Program Size:* 10 (*GY1:* 2)
Program ID: 260-38-21-105

Toledo

Medical College of Ohio Program
Sponsor: Medical College of Ohio
St Vincent Mercy Medical Center
Toledo Hospital
Program Director:
Nabil A Ebraheim, MD
Med Coll of Ohio
3065 Arlington Ave
Rm 2401 Dowling Hall
Toledo, OH 43614-5807
Tel: 419 383-3590 *Fax:* 419 383-3526
Accred Length: 5 Years *Program Size:* 15 (*GY1:* 3)
Subspecialties: OTR
Program ID: 260-38-31-176

Oklahoma

Oklahoma City

University of Oklahoma Health Sciences Center Program
Sponsor: University of Oklahoma College of Medicine
Bone and Joint Hospital
Children's Hospital of Oklahoma
University Hospital
Veterans Affairs Medical Center (Oklahoma City)
Program Director:
J Andy Sullivan, MD
Dept of Orthopedic Surgery
Attn: Virginia Gregory
PO Box 26901/Ste WP-1380
Oklahoma City, OK 73190
Tel: 405 271-4426 *Fax:* 405 271-3461
E-mail: virginia-gregory@ouhsc.edu
Accred Length: 5 Years *Program Size:* 24 (*GY1:* 4)
Subspecialties: OSM
Program ID: 260-39-21-053

Oregon

Portland

Oregon Health Sciences University Program
Sponsor: Oregon Health Sciences University Hospital
Legacy Emanuel Hospital and Health Center
Shriners Hospitals for Children (Portland)
Veterans Affairs Medical Center (Portland)
Program Director:
Charles B Bird, MD
Oregon Health Sciences Univ
3181 SW Sam Jackson Park Rd/L477
Portland, OR 97201-3098
Tel: 503 494-6406 *Fax:* 503 494-5050
Accred Length: 4 Years *Program Size:* 12
Subspecialties: OP
Program ID: 260-40-21-028

Pennsylvania

Danville

Penn State Geisinger Health System/Geisinger Medical Center Program
Sponsor: Penn State Geisinger Health System
Geisinger Medical Center
Program Director:
John Parenti, MD
Geisinger Med Ctr
Dept of Ortho Surgery
100 N Academy Ave
Danville, PA 17821
Tel: 717 271-6541 *Fax:* 717 271-5269
E-mail: ckrebs@psghs.edu
Accred Length: 5 Years *Program Size:* 10 (*GY1:* 2)
Program ID: 260-41-22-155

Erie

Hamot Medical Center Program
Sponsor: Hamot Medical Center
Shriners Hospital for Children (Erie)
Program Director:
John D Lubahn, MD
Hamot Med Ctr
201 State St
Erie, PA 16550-0001
Tel: 814 877-6257 *Fax:* 814 877-4699
E-mail: patricia.rogers@hamot.org
Internet: http://www.hamot.org
Accred Length: 4 Years *Program Size:* 9
Subspecialties: TY
Program ID: 260-41-22-156

Hershey

Penn State Geisinger Health System/Milton S Hershey Medical Center Program
Sponsor: Penn State Geisinger Health System
Milton S Hershey Medical Center
Program Director:
Vincent D Pellegrini Jr, MD
Pennsylvania State Univ Coll of Med
Milton S Hershey Med Ctr
500 University Dr/PO Box 850 MC H089
Hershey, PA 17033-0850
Tel: 717 531-4833 *Fax:* 717 531-7583
E-mail: residency@ortho.hmc.psu.edu
Internet: http://www.ortho.hmc.psu.edu
Accred Length: 5 Years *Program Size:* 17 (*GY1:* 3)
Subspecialties: OSM
Program ID: 260-41-21-151

Philadelphia

Albert Einstein Medical Center Program
Sponsor: Albert Einstein Medical Center
Moss Rehabilitation Hospital
Shriners Hospital for Children (Philadelphia)
Program Director:
John A Handal, MD
Albert Einstein Med Ctr-Northern Div
5501 Old York Rd
Willowcrest 4
Philadelphia, PA 19141-3098
Tel: 215 456-6051 *Fax:* 215 324-2426
E-mail: ortho@aehn2.einstein.edu
Internet: http://www.einstein.edu/phl/1225.html
Accred Length: 4 Years *Program Size:* 8
Program ID: 260-41-11-157

MCP Hahnemann University Program
Sponsor: MCP Hahnemann University
Hahnemann University Hospital
Medical College of Pennsylvania Hospital
Milton S Hershey Medical Center
Shriners Hospital for Children (Philadelphia)
Program Director:
Stephen J Bosacco, MD
Alleghany Univ Hospital
Broad and Vine Sts/MS 420
Philadelphia, PA 19102
Tel: 215 762-8443 *Fax:* 215 762-3442
Accred Length: 4 Years *Program Size:* 16
Program ID: 260-41-21-026

Temple University Program
Sponsor: Temple University Hospital
Abington Memorial Hospital
Shriners Hospital for Children (Philadelphia)
St Christopher's Hospital for Children
Program Director:
Michael Clancy, MD
Temple Univ Hospital
3401 N Broad St
Philadelphia, PA 19140
Tel: 215 707-7208 *Fax:* 215 707-2324
E-mail: sporter@nimbus.temple.edu
Internet:
http://www.temple.edu/orthopaedics/index.html
Accred Length: 4 Years *Program Size:* 16
Subspecialties: OSM
Program ID: 260-41-21-029

Thomas Jefferson University Program
Sponsor: Thomas Jefferson University Hospital
Bryn Mawr Hospital
Cooper Hospital-University Medical Center
duPont Hospital for Children
Methodist Hospital
Pennsylvania Hospital (UPHS)
Program Director:
Michael G Ciccotti, MD
Thomas Jefferson Univ
925 Chestnut St/Rm 606
Philadelphia, PA 19107
Tel: 215 955-1500 *Fax:* 215 503-0566
E-mail: susan.randolph@mail.tju.edu
Internet: http://www.tjuhortho.org
Accred Length: 4 Years *Program Size:* 24
Subspecialties: HSO, OAR, OP, OSM
Program ID: 260-41-21-021

University of Pennsylvania Program
Sponsor: Hospital of the University of Pennsylvania
Children's Hospital of Philadelphia
Veterans Affairs Medical Center (Philadelphia)
Program Director:
Robert H Fitzgerald Jr, MD
Hospital of Univ of Pennsylvania
3400 Spruce St
2 Silverstein
Philadelphia, PA 19104-4283
Tel: 215 662-3350 *Fax:* 215 349-5890
Internet: http://www.med.upenn.edu./ortho/
Accred Length: 5 Years *Program Size:* 40 (*GY1:* 8)
Subspecialties: HSO, OAR
Program ID: 260-41-21-023

Pittsburgh

Allegheny General Hospital Program
Sponsor: Allegheny General Hospital

Program Director:
James H McMaster, MD
Allegheny General Hospital
Dept of Ortho Surgery
320 E North Ave
Pittsburgh, PA 15212-4772
Tel: 412 359-6501 *Fax:* 412 359-6265
E-mail: lhays@aherf.edu
Accred Length: 5 Years *Program Size:* 10 (*GY1:* 2)
Subspecialties: HSO
Program ID: 260-41-21-201

University Health Center of Pittsburgh Program
Sponsor: University Health Center of Pittsburgh
Children's Hospital of Pittsburgh
Presbyterian University Hospital/UPMC
University of Pittsburgh Medical Center (St Margaret)
Veterans Affairs Medical Center (Pittsburgh)

Program Director:
Kenneth M Yaw, MD
Dept of Orthopaedic Surgery
Kaufmann Bldg/Ste 1010
3471 Fifth Ave
Pittsburgh, PA 15213-3221
Tel: 412 605-3267 *Fax:* 412 687-5255
E-mail: pbigenho@uoi.upmc.edu
Internet: http://www.orthonet.upmc.edu
Accred Length: 5 Years *Program Size:* 37 (*GY1:* 8)
Subspecialties: HSO, OSM
Program ID: 260-41-21-030

Puerto Rico

San Juan

University of Puerto Rico Program
Sponsor: University of Puerto Rico School of Medicine
San Juan City Hospital
University Hospital
University Pediatric Hospital
Veterans Affairs Medical Center (San Juan)

Program Director:
Rafael Fernandez-Feliberti, MD
Univ of Puerto Rico Med Sciences Campus
Orthopaedic Surgery Dept
GPO Box 365067
San Juan, PR 00936
Tel: 787 764-5095 *Fax:* 787 759-6681
Accred Length: 4 Years *Program Size:* 16
Program ID: 260-42-21-161

Rhode Island

Providence

Brown University Program
Sponsor: Rhode Island Hospital
Veterans Affairs Medical Center (Providence)

Program Director:
Michael G Ehrlich, MD
Rhode Island Hospital
Dept of Orthopaedics
593 Eddy St
Providence, RI 02903
Tel: 401 444-4030 *Fax:* 401 444-6243
E-mail: michael_ehrlich@brown.edu
Internet: http://www.brown.edu
Accred Length: 4 Years *Program Size:* 18
Program ID: 260-43-11-162

South Carolina

Charleston

Medical University of South Carolina Program
Sponsor: Medical University of South Carolina College of Medicine
Charleston Memorial Hospital
MUSC Medical Center
Naval Hospital (Charleston)
Ralph H Johnson Dept of Veterans Affairs Med Center

Program Director:
Angus M McBryde Jr, MD
Med Univ of South Carolina
Dept of Ortho Surgery
600 MUSC Complex/Ste 708
Charleston, SC 29425
Tel: 843 792-0245 *Fax:* 843 792-7794
Accred Length: 4 Years *Program Size:* 15 (*GY1:* 3)
Program ID: 260-45-21-052

Columbia

Palmetto Health Alliance/University of South Carolina School of Medicine Program
Sponsor: Palmetto Health Alliance
Palmetto Richland Memorial Hospital
Shriners Hospital for Children (Greenville)
William Jennings Bryan Dorn Veterans Hospital

Program Director:
John Eady, MD
Richland Memorial Hospital
2 Richland Medical Pk/Ste 404
Columbia, SC 29203
Tel: 803 434-6812 *Fax:* 803 434-7829
Internet:
http://www.conterra.com/rmh/ridency/orthopaedics.html
Accred Length: 5 Years *Program Size:* 10 (*GY1:* 2)
Program ID: 260-45-31-163

Greenville

Greenville Hospital System Program
Sponsor: Greenville Hospital System
Shriners Hospital for Children (Greenville)

Program Director:
Edward W Bray III, MD
Greenville Hospital System
Ortho Surgery Education
701 Grove Rd
Greenville, SC 29605-5601
Tel: 864 455-7878 *Fax:* 864 455-7082
E-mail: erasort@ghsms.ghs.org
Internet: http://www.ghs.org
Accred Length: 5 Years *Program Size:* 15 (*GY1:* 3)
Program ID: 260-45-21-033

Tennessee

Chattanooga

University of Tennessee College of Medicine at Chattanooga Program
Sponsor: University of Tennessee College of Medicine-Chattanooga Unit
Erlanger Medical Center
T C Thompson Children's Hospital Medical Center

Program Director:
Lynn A Crosby, MD
Univ of Tennessee Coll of Med
Dept of Ortho Surgery
975 E Third St/Hospital Box 260
Chattanooga, TN 37403
Tel: 423 778-9008 *Fax:* 423 778-9009
E-mail: utorthosurg@elranger.org
Internet:
http://www.erlanger.org/utcom/orthopaedic.html
Accred Length: 5 Years *Program Size:* 10
Subspecialties: OSM
Program ID: 260-47-11-164

Memphis

University of Tennessee Program
Sponsor: University of Tennessee College of Medicine
Baptist Memorial Hospital
LeBonheur Children's Medical Center
Regional Medical Center at Memphis
University of Tennessee-Campbell Clinic

Program Director:
James H Beaty, MD
Univ of Tennessee-Campbell Clinic
Dept of Ortho Surgery
910 Madison Ave/Ste 500
Memphis, TN 38113-3403
Tel: 901 759-3274 *Fax:* 901 759-3278
Accred Length: 4 Years *Program Size:* 40
Subspecialties: HSO, OP
Program ID: 260-47-21-061

Nashville

Vanderbilt University Program
Sponsor: Vanderbilt University Medical Center
Veterans Affairs Medical Center (Nashville)

Program Director:
Dan M Spengler, MD
Vanderbilt Univ
Dept of Ortho/Rehab
137A Medical Center S
Nashville, TN 37232-2550
Tel: 615 936-0100 *Fax:* 615 936-0117
E-mail: michelle.lennon@mcmail.vanderbilt.edu
Accred Length: 5 Years *Program Size:* 20
Program ID: 260-47-11-116

Texas

Dallas

University of Texas Southwestern Medical School Program

Sponsor: University of Texas Southwestern Medical School
Baylor University Medical Center
Dallas County Hospital District-Parkland Memorial Hospital
Texas Scottish Rite Hospital for Children
Veterans Affairs Medical Center (Dallas)

Program Director:
Robert W Bucholz, MD
Univ of Texas Southwestern Med Ctr
5323 Harry Hines Blvd
Dallas, TX 75235-8883
Tel: 214 648-4712 *Fax:* 214 648-3008
E-mail: rebecca.gibbs@email.swmed.edu
Internet: http://www.swmed.edu/home_pages/orthosurg/
Accred Length: 4 Years *Program Size:* 20
Subspecialties: OMO, OP
Program ID: 260-48-21-032

El Paso

William Beaumont Army Medical Center/Texas Tech University (El Paso) Program

Sponsor: William Beaumont Army Medical Center
R E Thomason General Hospital
Shriners Hospitals for Children (Spokane)
Texas Tech University Health Sciences Center at El Paso

Program Director:
Paul J Dougherty, MD
William Beaumont Army Med Ctr
5005 N Piedras St
El Paso, TX 79920-5001
Tel: 915 569-2288 *Fax:* 915 569-1931
E-mail: orteedl@ttuhsc.edu
Internet: http://www.erteedl@ttuhsc.edu
Accred Length: 4 Years *Program Size:* 17
Program ID: 260-48-21-198
US Armed Services Program

Fort Sam Houston

San Antonio Uniformed Services Health Education Consortium (BAMC) Program

Sponsor: San Antonio Uniformed Services Health Education Consortium
Brooke Army Medical Center
Children's Hospital
Santa Rosa Health Care Corporation

Program Director:
Lt Col Theodore W Parsons III, MD
Brooke Army Med Ctr
3851 Roger Brooke Dr
Fort Sam Houston, TX 78234-6200
Tel: 210 916-5666 *Fax:* 210 916-0559
Accred Length: 4 Years *Program Size:* 34
Program ID: 260-48-32-117
US Armed Services Program

Fort Worth

Fort Worth Hospitals Program

Sponsor: John Peter Smith Hospital (Tarrant County Hospital District)
Cook-Fort Worth Children's Medical Center
Harris Methodist Fort Worth

Program Director:
David M Lichtman, MD
John Peter Smith Hospital
1500 S Main St
Fort Worth, TX 76104
Tel: 817 927-1173 *Fax:* 817 927-1668
E-mail: bamckeon@aol.com
Internet: http://www.jpshealthnet.org
Accred Length: 5 Years *Program Size:* 15 (*GY1:* 3)
Subspecialties: TY
Program ID: 260-48-22-100

Galveston

University of Texas Medical Branch Hospitals Program

Sponsor: University of Texas Medical Branch Hospitals

Program Director:
Jason H Calhoun, MD
Univ of Texas Med Branch
301 University Blvd
Galveston, TX 77555-0792
Tel: 409 772-2565 *Fax:* 409 772-2266
E-mail: kflesher@utmb.edu
Internet: http://www.utmb.edu/ortho
Accred Length: 5 Years *Program Size:* 20 (*GY1:* 4)
Subspecialties: OSS
Program ID: 260-48-21-165

Houston

Baylor College of Medicine Program

Sponsor: Baylor College of Medicine
Harris County Hospital District-Ben Taub General Hospital
Methodist Hospital
Shriners Hospitals for Children (Houston)
Texas Children's Hospital
Veterans Affairs Medical Center (Houston)

Program Director:
Stephen I Esses, MD
Baylor Coll of Med
Dept of Ortho Surgery
6550 Fannin St/Ste 2625
Houston, TX 77030
Tel: 713 986-7390 *Fax:* 713 986-7391
E-mail: judyo@bcm.tmc.edu
Accred Length: 5 Years *Program Size:* 20
Subspecialties: HSO, OP, OSM, OTR
Program ID: 260-48-31-049

University of Texas at Houston Program

Sponsor: University of Texas Medical School at Houston
Lyndon B Johnson General Hospital
Memorial Hermann Healthcare System
Shriners Hospitals for Children (Houston)

Program Director:
Thomas O Clanton, MD
Dept of Orthopaedic Surgery
Univ of Texas Houston Med Sch
6431 Fannin St/Ste 6142
Houston, TX 77030-1501
Tel: 713 500-7012 *Fax:* 713 500-7012
E-mail: orsurg@ortho1.med.uth.tmc.edu
Internet: http://www.ortho1.med.uth.tmc.edu/newpage
Accred Length: 5 Years *Program Size:* 15 (*GY1:* 3)
Program ID: 260-48-21-166

Lackland AFB

San Antonio Uniformed Services Health Education Consortium (WHMC) Program

Sponsor: San Antonio Uniformed Services Health Education Consortium
Wilford Hall Medical Center (AETC)

Program Director:
Lt Col Theodore W Parsons III, MD BS
59th Med Wing/MMKO
2200 Bergquist Dr/Ste 1
Lackland AFB
San Antonio, TX 78236-5300
Tel: 210 292-5875 *Fax:* 210 292-5844
E-mail: parsons@whmc.af.mil
Internet: http://www.whmc.af.mil
Accred Length: 4 Years *Program Size:* 19
Program ID: 260-48-31-120
US Armed Services Program

Lubbock

Texas Tech University (Lubbock) Program

Sponsor: Texas Tech University Health Sciences Center at Lubbock

Program Director:
Eugene J Dabezies, MD
Texas Tech Univ Health Sciences Ctr
Dept of Ortho Surgery
3601 Fourth St
Lubbock, TX 79430
Tel: 806 743-2465 *Fax:* 806 743-1305
Internet:
http://www.ttuhsc.edu/pages/ortho/welcome.htm
Accred Length: 5 Years *Program Size:* 10 (*GY1:* 2)
Program ID: 260-48-31-160

San Antonio

University of Texas Health Science Center at San Antonio Program

Sponsor: University of Texas Medical School at San Antonio
Audie L Murphy Memorial Veterans Hospital (San Antonio)
Santa Rosa Health Care Corporation
University Hospital-South Texas Medical Center

Program Director:
James D Heckman, MD
Univ of Texas Health Science Ctr
7703 Floyd Curl Dr
San Antonio, TX 78284-7774
Tel: 210 567-5125 *Fax:* 210 567-5167
E-mail: orthopresprg@uthscsa.edu
Internet: http://www.mabrey.uthscsa.edu/ortho2000/
Accred Length: 5 Years *Program Size:* 30 (*GY1:* 6)
Subspecialties: HSO, OAR, OSM
Program ID: 260-48-31-095

Temple

Texas A&M College of Medicine-Scott and White Program

Sponsor: Scott and White Memorial Hospital
Central Texas Veterans Affairs Healthcare System
Shriners Hospitals for Children (Houston)

Program Director:
Hanes H Brindley Jr, MD
Texas A&M-Scott and White
Grad Med Educ
2401 S 31st St
Temple, TX 76508-0001
Tel: 254 724-5455 *Fax:* 254 724-7119
E-mail: ngrisham@swmail.sw.org
Internet: http://www.sw.org
Accred Length: 5 Years *Program Size:* 15 (*GY1:* 3)
Program ID: 260-48-21-171

Utah

Salt Lake City

University of Utah Program

Sponsor: University of Utah Medical Center
LDS Hospital
Primary Children's Medical Center
Salt Lake Regional Medical Center
Shriners Hospital for Children (Intermountain Unit)
Veterans Affairs Medical Center (Salt Lake City)

Program Director:
Harold K Dunn, MD
Univ of Utah Med Ctr
50 N Medical Dr/Rm 3B165
Salt Lake City, UT 84132-0001
Tel: 801 581-7601 *Fax:* 801 581-6178
E-mail: barbara.morzelewski@hsc.utah.edu
Internet: http://www.medstat.med.utah.edu/orthopedics
Accred Length: 4 Years *Program Size:* 15
Subspecialties: HSO, OP, OSM
Program ID: 260-49-31-034

Vermont

Burlington

University of Vermont Program

Sponsor: Fletcher Allen Health Care

Program Director:
James G Howe, MD
Claude E Nichols III, MD
Univ of Vermont Coll of Med
Stafford Hall
Burlington, VT 05405-0084
Tel: 802 656-2250 *Fax:* 802 656-4247
E-mail: ybruley@zoo.uvm.edu
Internet: http://www.vtmednet.org/~g136911
Accred Length: 4 Years *Program Size:* 12
Program ID: 260-50-11-167

Virginia

Charlottesville

University of Virginia Program

Sponsor: University of Virginia Medical Center
Carilion Roanoke Memorial Hospital
Veterans Affairs Medical Center (Salem)

Program Director:
Gwo-Jaw Wang, MD
Univ of Virginia Health Sciences Ctr
Dept of Ortho Surgery
Box 159
Charlottesville, VA 22908
Tel: 804 924-2935 *Fax:* 804 924-5613
E-mail: bjl7e@virginia.edu
Internet:
http://www.med.va.edu/medicine/clinical/orthopaedics
Accred Length: 4 Years *Program Size:* 20
Subspecialties: OAR, OSM
Program ID: 260-51-21-129

Portsmouth

Naval Medical Center (Portsmouth) Program

Sponsor: Naval Medical Center (Portsmouth)

Program Director:
Martin K Deafenbaugh, MD
Naval Medical Center Portsmouth
Orthopaedic Surgery Dept
620 John Paul Jones Cir
Portsmouth, VA 23708-5000
Tel: 804 398-7316 *Fax:* 804 398-6075
E-mail: mdeafenbaugh@med.navy.mil
Internet:
http://www.nmcp.med.navy.mil/ortho/orthohome.htm
Accred Length: 4 Years *Program Size:* 12
Program ID: 260-51-12-130
US Armed Services Program

Richmond

Medical College of Virginia/Virginia Commonwealth University Program

Sponsor: Medical College of Virginia/Virginia Commonwealth University
Children's Hospital
Hunter Holmes McGuire VA Medical Center (Richmond)
Medical College of Virginia Hospitals

Program Director:
John A Cardea, MD
Med Coll of Virgina, Dept of Ortho Surgery
1200 E Broad St/PO Box 980153
9th Fl/East Wing
Richmond, VA 23298
Tel: 804 828-6784 *Fax:* 804 828-4762
E-mail: jcardea@hsc
Accred Length: 5 Years *Program Size:* 20
Program ID: 260-51-21-035

Washington

Seattle

University of Washington Program

Sponsor: University of Washington School of Medicine
Children's Hospital and Medical Center
Harborview Medical Center
University of Washington Medical Center
Veterans Affairs Medical Center (Seattle)

Program Director:
Frederick A Matsen III, MD
Univ Hospital, Dept of Orthopaedics
1959 NE Pacific St
Box 356500
Seattle, WA 98195
Tel: 206 543-3690 *Fax:* 206 685-3139
Internet: http://www.weber.u.washington.edu/~bone.jnt/
Accred Length: 5 Years *Program Size:* 20
Subspecialties: HSO
Program ID: 260-54-21-036

Tacoma

Madigan Army Medical Center Program

Sponsor: Madigan Army Medical Center
Children's Hospital and Medical Center
Shriners Hospitals for Children (Spokane)

Program Director:
Lt Col Frederic L Johnstone II, MD
Madigan Army Med Ctr
Commander
Attn: MCHJ-SOP
Tacoma, WA 98431
Tel: 253 968-3121 *Fax:* 253 968-1586
E-mail: ltc frederic
johnstone@smtplink,mamc.amedd.army.mil
Accred Length: 4 Years *Program Size:* 12
Program ID: 260-54-32-178
US Armed Services Program

West Virginia

Morgantown

West Virginia University Program

Sponsor: West Virginia University Hospitals
Monongalia General Hospital

Program Director:
J David Blaha, MD
West Virginia Univ Sch of Med
Dept of Orthopedics
RC Byrd Hlth Sci Ctr/PO Box 9196
Morgantown, WV 26506-9196
Tel: 304 293-3908 *Fax:* 304 293-7042
E-mail: asummers@wvuortho1.hsc.wvu.edu
Internet: http://www.hsc.wvu.edu./som/orthopedics.html
Accred Length: 5 Years *Program Size:* 15 (*GY1:* 3)
Program ID: 260-55-21-169

Wisconsin

Madison

University of Wisconsin Program

Sponsor: University of Wisconsin Hospital and Clinics
Meriter Hospital
St Marys Hospital Medical Center
William S Middleton Veterans Hospital

Program Director:
Andrew A McBeath, MD
G5-361 Clinical Science Ctr
600 Highland Ave
Madison, WI 53792-3228
Tel: 608 263-1348 *Fax:* 608 263-0454
E-mail: mcbeath@surgery.wisc.edu
Internet: http://www.biostat.wisc.edu/surgery/home.html
Accred Length: 5 Years *Program Size:* 20 (*GY1:* 4)
Subspecialties: OSM
Program ID: 260-56-21-097

Milwaukee

Medical College of Wisconsin Program
Sponsor: Medical College of Wisconsin Affiliated Hospitals Inc
Children's Hospital of Wisconsin
Clement J Zablocki Veterans Affairs Medical Center
Froedtert Memorial Lutheran Hospital
Program Director:
Gregory J Schmeling, MD
Med Coll of Wisconsin
9200 W Wisconsin Ave
PO Box 26099
Milwaukee, WI 53226-0099
Tel: 414 257-7399 *Fax:* 414 257-7861
E-mail: resaps@mcw.edu
Internet: http://www.mcw.edu/ortho
Accred Length: 5 Years *Program Size:* 22 (*GY1:* 4)
Subspecialties: OP, OSS
Program ID: 260-56-21-037

Orthopaedic Surgery of the Spine (Orthopaedic Surgery)

Florida

Gainesville

University of Florida Program
Sponsor: University of Florida College of Medicine
Shands Hospital at the University of Florida
Program Director:
B Hudson Berrey Jr, MD
Richard G Fessler, MD
Univ of Florida
Box 100246/JHMHC
Gainesville, FL 32610-0246
Tel: 352 392-4251 *Fax:* 352 392-8637
Accred Length: 1 Year *Program Size:* 2
Program ID: 267-11-31-005

Miami

University of Miami-Jackson Memorial Medical Center Program
Sponsor: University of Miami-Jackson Memorial Medical Center
Program Director:
Frank J Eismont, MD
Univ of Miami Sch of Med
Dept of Ortho/Rehab
PO Box 016960 (D-27)
Miami, FL 33101
Tel: 305 585-7138 *Fax:* 305 324-7658
Accred Length: 1 Year *Program Size:* 1
Program ID: 267-11-21-004

Illinois

Chicago

Rush-Presbyterian-St Luke's Medical Center Program
Sponsor: Rush-Presbyterian-St Luke's Medical Center
Shriners Hospitals for Children (Chicago)
Program Director:
Ronald L DeWald, MD
Rush-Presbyterian-St Luke's Med Ctr
1725 W Harrison St/Ste 440
Chicago, IL 60612
Tel: 312 738-2903 *Fax:* 312 738-0133
E-mail: cmarth@rush.edu
Internet: http://www.orthopaedics-scoliosis.com
Accred Length: 1 Year *Program Size:* 2
Program ID: 267-16-21-015

Springfield

Southern Illinois University Program
Sponsor: Southern Illinois University School of Medicine
Memorial Medical Center
St John's Hospital
Program Director:
John R Fisk, MD
Southern Illinois Univ Sch of Med
Dept of Ortho Surgery
PO Box 19638
Springfield, IL 62794-9638
Tel: 217 524-6504 *Fax:* 217 524-1793
E-mail: jfisk@siumed.edu
Internet: http://www.siumed.edu/
Accred Length: 1 Year *Program Size:* 2
Program ID: 267-16-21-001

Michigan

Royal Oak

William Beaumont Hospital Program
Sponsor: William Beaumont Hospital
Program Director:
Harry N Herkowitz, MD
William Beaumont Hospital
3535 W 13 Mile Rd/#604
Royal Oak, MI 48073
Tel: 248 551-0426 *Fax:* 248 551-5404
E-mail: cmusich@beaumont.edu
Internet: http://www.beaumont.edu/html/gme
Accred Length: 1 Year *Program Size:* 1
Program ID: 267-25-21-007

Minnesota

Minneapolis

Minnesota Spine Center Program
Sponsor: Minnesota Spine Center
Program Director:
Ensor E Transfeldt, MD
Twin Cities Spine Ctr
913 E 26th St/Ste 600
Minneapolis, MN 55404
Tel: 612 775-6200 *Fax:* 612 775-6222
E-mail: informat@tcspine.com
Internet: http://www.tcspine.com
Accred Length: 1 Year *Program Size:* 3
Program ID: 267-26-21-010

Missouri

St Louis

Washington University/B-JH/SLCH Consortium Program
Sponsor: Washington University/B-JH/SLCH Consortium
Barnes-Jewish Hospital
Shriners Hospitals for Children (St Louis)
St Louis Children's Hospital
Program Director:
Keith H Bridwell, MD
Washington Univ Sch of Med
Ste 11300 West Pavilion
One Barnes-Jewish Hospital Plaza
St Louis, MO 63110
Tel: 314 747-2536 *Fax:* 314 747-2599
E-mail: iffrigt@msnotes.wustl.edu
Internet: http://www.ortho.wustl.edu
Accred Length: 1 Year *Program Size:* 3
Program ID: 267-28-21-016

New York

New York

Hospital for Joint Diseases Orthopaedic Institute Program
Sponsor: Hospital for Joint Diseases Orthopaedic Institute
Program Director:
Thomas Errico, MD
Hospital for Joint Diseases Orthopaedic Inst
Spine Surgery/Ste 1402
301 E 17th St
New York, NY 10003
Tel: 212 263-7182 *Fax:* 212 263-7180
Accred Length: 1 Year *Program Size:* 1
Program ID: 267-35-21-011

Hospital for Special Surgery/Cornell Medical Center Program
Sponsor: Hospital for Special Surgery
Program Director:
Frank P Cammisa Jr, MD
Hospital for Special Surgery
535 E 70th St
New York, NY 10021
Tel: 212 606-1466
Internet: http://www.hss.edu
Accred Length: 1 Year *Program Size:* 3
Program ID: 267-35-21-022

Rochester

University of Rochester Program
Sponsor: Strong Memorial Hospital of the University of Rochester
Program Director:
M Gordon Whitbeck, MD
Dept of Orthopaedics
601 Elmwood Ave/Box 665
Rochester, NY 14642
Tel: 716 275-2446 *Fax:* 716 756-4726
Accred Length: 1 Year *Program Size:* 1
Program ID: 267-35-31-025

Syracuse

SUNY Health Science Center at Syracuse Program
Sponsor: University Hospital-SUNY Health Science Center at Syracuse
Crouse Hospital
Program Director:
Bruce E Fredrickson, MD
Inst for Spine Care
550 Harrison St/Ste 130
Syracuse, NY 13202
Tel: 315 472-2225, ext 322 *Fax:* 315 471-3259
Accred Length: 1 Year *Program Size:* 1
Program ID: 267-35-11-019

Texas

Galveston

University of Texas Medical Branch Hospitals Program
Sponsor: University of Texas Medical Branch Hospitals
Program Director:
Alexander G Hadjipavlou, MD
Univ of Texas Med Branch-Galveston
301 University Blvd
Galveston, TX 77555-0792
Tel: 409 747-0122 *Fax:* 409 772-2266
E-mail: ahadjipa@utmb.edu
Accred Length: 1 Year *Program Size:* 1
Program ID: 267-48-21-023

Virginia

Charlottesville

University of Virginia Program
Sponsor: University of Virginia Medical Center
Program Director:
Donald P Chan, MD
Univ of Virginia
Spine Surgery Div
HSC Box 159
Charlottesville, VA 22908
Tel: 804 982-4242 *Fax:* 804 243-6674
E-mail: slb2b@virginia.edu
Internet:
http://www.med.va.edu/medicine/clinical/orthopaedics
Accred Length: 1 Year *Program Size:* 1
Program ID: 267-51-21-024

Wisconsin

Milwaukee

Medical College of Wisconsin Program
Sponsor: Medical College of Wisconsin Affiliated Hospitals Inc
Froedtert Memorial Lutheran Hospital
Program Director:
Edward P Southern, MD
Med Coll of Wisconsin, Dept of Ortho Surgery
9200 W Wisconsin Ave
PO Box 26099
Milwaukee, WI 53226
Tel: 414 257-6655 *Fax:* 414 257-7861
E-mail: southern@mcw.edu
Internet: http://www.mcw.edu/ortho
Accred Length: 1 Year *Program Size:* 1
Program ID: 267-56-21-018

Orthopaedic Trauma (Orthopaedic Surgery)

Maryland

Baltimore

University of Maryland Program
Sponsor: University of Maryland Medical System
Program Director:
Clifford H Turen, MD
R Adams Cowley Shock Trauma Ctr
22 S Greene St/Rm T3R56
Baltimore, MD 21201-1595
Tel: 410 328-6280 *Fax:* 410 328-2893
E-mail: cturen@surgery1.umaryland.edu
Accred Length: 1 Year *Program Size:* 3
Program ID: 269-23-21-008

North Carolina

Charlotte

Carolinas Medical Center Program
Sponsor: Carolinas Medical Center
Program Director:
James F Kellam, MD
Carolinas Med Ctr
Dept of Ortho Surg/Trauma
PO Box 32861
Charlotte, NC 28232-2861
Tel: 704 355-3184 *Fax:* 704 355-6041
Internet: http://www.carolinas.org
Accred Length: 1 Year *Program Size:* 1
Program ID: 269-36-21-001

Ohio

Toledo

Medical College of Ohio Program
Sponsor: Medical College of Ohio
St Vincent Mercy Medical Center
Program Director:
Nabil A Ebraheim, MD
Med Coll of Ohio
3065 Arlington Ave
Toledo, OH 43699-0000
Tel: 419 381-3590, ext 3590 *Fax:* 419 381-3526
Accred Length: 1 Year *Program Size:* 1
Program ID: 269-38-21-007

Otolaryngology

Alabama

Birmingham

University of Alabama Medical Center Program
Sponsor: University of Alabama Hospital
Children's Hospital of Alabama
Cooper Green Hospital
Veterans Affairs Medical Center (Birmingham)
Program Director:
Glenn E Peters, MD
Univ of Alabama Med Ctr
Div of Oto/Head and Neck Surg
1501 5th Ave S
Birmingham, AL 35233-6889
Tel: 205 934-9765 *Fax:* 205 934-3992
E-mail: rick.carroll@ccc.uab.edu
Accred Length: 4 Years *Program Size:* 12
Program ID: 280-01-21-010

Arkansas

Little Rock

University of Arkansas for Medical Sciences Program
Sponsor: University of Arkansas College of Medicine
Arkansas Children's Hospital
John L McClellan Memorial Veterans Hospital
University Hospital of Arkansas
Program Director:
John L Dornhoffer, MD
Univ of Arkansas for Med Sciences
4301 W Markham St/Slot 543
Little Rock, AR 72205-7199
Tel: 501 686-5140 *Fax:* 501 686-8029
E-mail: dornhofferjohnl@exchange.uams.edu
Internet: http://www.otolaryngology.uams.edu
Accred Length: 4 Years *Program Size:* 10
Program ID: 280-04-21-012

California

Loma Linda

Loma Linda University Program
Sponsor: Loma Linda University Medical Center
Jerry L Pettis Memorial Veterans Hospital
Riverside County Regional Medical Center
Program Director:
George D Chonkich, MD
Loma Linda Univ Med Ctr
11234 Anderson St/Ste 2584
Loma Linda, CA 92354
Tel: 909 558-8558, ext 8558 *Fax:* 909 558-4819
Internet: http://www.llu.edu
Accred Length: 4 Years *Program Size:* 7
Program ID: 280-05-21-117

Los Angeles

Charles R Drew University Program
Sponsor: Charles R Drew University of Medicine and Science
Children's Hospital of Los Angeles
LAC-King/Drew Medical Center
San Bernardino County Medical Center
Program Director:
Jimmy Brown, MD DDS
Martin Luther King Jr-Drew Med Ctr
12021 S Wilmington Ave
RM 5004
Los Angeles, CA 90059
Tel: 310 668-4536 *Fax:* 310 668-4554
E-mail: jibrown@cdrewu.edu
Internet: http://www.cdrewu.edu
Accred Length: 4 Years *Program Size:* 6
Program ID: 280-05-11-016

UCLA Medical Center Program
Sponsor: UCLA School of Medicine
Los Angeles County-Harbor-UCLA Medical Center
Olive View-UCLA Medical Center
UCLA Medical Center
VA Greater Los Angeles Healthcare System
Program Director:
Gerald S Berke, MD
UCLA Med Ctr
Div of Head/Neck Surgery
10833 Le Conte Ave/62-132 CHS
Los Angeles, CA 90095-1624
Tel: 310 825-5179 *Fax:* 310 206-1393
E-mail: rmontoya@surgery.medsch.ucla.edu
Accred Length: 4 Years *Program Size:* 20
Program ID: 280-05-21-017

University of Southern California Program
Sponsor: Los Angeles County-USC Medical Center
USC University Hospital
VA Greater Los Angeles Healthcare System
Program Director:
Dale H Rice, MD
Univ of Southern California Sch of Med
1200 N State St/Box 795
Los Angeles, CA 90033-1029
Tel: 323 226-7315 *Fax:* 323 226-2780
Accred Length: 4 Years *Program Size:* 20
Program ID: 280-05-21-015

Oakland

Kaiser Permanente Medical Group (Northern California) Program
Sponsor: Kaiser Permanente Medical Group (Northern California)
Kaiser Permanente Medical Center (Oakland)
Kaiser Permanente Medical Center (Redwood City)
Kaiser Permanente Medical Center (San Francisco)
Program Director:
Raymond L Hilsinger Jr, MD
Kaiser Permanente Med Ctr
Med Educ Dept
280 W MacArthur Blvd
Oakland, CA 94611-5693
Tel: 510 596-6126 *Fax:* 510 596-1571
Internet: http://www.best.com/~smui/kaiseroakhns.shtml
Accred Length: 4 Years *Program Size:* 8
Program ID: 280-05-22-020

Texas

Houston

Baylor College of Medicine Program
Sponsor: Baylor College of Medicine
Harris County Hospital District-Ben Taub General Hospital
Methodist Hospital
Program Director:
Ronald W Lindsey, MD
Baylor Coll of Med
Dept of Ortho Surgery
6550 Fannin St/Ste 2625
Houston, TX 77030
Tel: 713 986-7390 *Fax:* 713 986-7391
Accred Length: 1 Year *Program Size:* 1
Program ID: 269-48-21-004

Programs

Orange

University of California (Irvine) Program

Sponsor: University of California (Irvine) Medical Center
Veterans Affairs Medical Center (Long Beach)

Program Director:
Jack A Shohet, MD
Univ of California Irvine Med Ctr
Dept of Otolaryngology/5386
101 City Dr S/Rte 81 BL 25
Orange, CA 92868-3298
Tel: 714 456-8450 *Fax:* 714 456-5747
E-mail: jshohet@uci.edu
Internet: http://www.otohns.uci.edu
Accred Length: 4 Years *Program Size:* 10
Program ID: 280-05-21-014

Sacramento

University of California (Davis) Program

Sponsor: University of California (Davis) Medical Center

Program Director:
Craig W Senders, MD MD
Univ of California Davis
Dept of Otolaryngology
2521 Stockton Blvd/Ste 7200
Sacramento, CA 95817
Tel: 916 734-2801 *Fax:* 916 456-7509
Accred Length: 4 Years *Program Size:* 8
Program ID: 280-05-21-013

San Diego

Naval Medical Center (San Diego) Program

Sponsor: Naval Medical Center (San Diego)
Kaiser Foundation Hospital (San Diego)

Program Director:
D Richard Kang, MD
Naval Med Ctr
Dept of Otolaryngology
34520 Bob Wilson Dr/Ste 200
San Diego, CA 92134-2200
Tel: 619 532-9604 *Fax:* 619 532-6088
E-mail: drkang@nmcsd.med.navy.mil
Accred Length: 4 Years *Program Size:* 10
Program ID: 280-05-11-007
US Armed Services Program

University of California (San Diego) Program

Sponsor: University of California (San Diego) Medical Center
Kaiser Foundation Hospital (San Diego)
Veterans Affairs Medical Center (San Diego)

Program Director:
Jeffrey P Harris, MD PhD
UCSD Med Ctr
200 W Arbor Dr/#8895
San Diego, CA 92103-8895
Tel: 619 543-5910 *Fax:* 619 543-5521
E-mail: kcrockett@ucsd.edu
Internet:
http://www.surgery.ucsd.edu/residen/ent/otores.htm
Accred Length: 4 Years *Program Size:* 10
Program ID: 280-05-21-021

San Francisco

University of California (San Francisco) Program

Sponsor: University of California (San Francisco) School of Medicine
San Francisco General Hospital Medical Center
University of California (San Francisco) Medical Center
Veterans Affairs Medical Center (San Francisco)

Program Director:
Andrew H Murr, MD
Univ of California San Francisco
400 Parnassus Ave
Rm A-730
San Francisco, CA 94143-0342
Tel: 415 476-4952 *Fax:* 415 502-6437
E-mail: otweiss@orca.ucsf.edu
Accred Length: 4 Years *Program Size:* 12
Program ID: 280-05-21-022

Stanford

Stanford University Program

Sponsor: Stanford University Hospital
Santa Clara Valley Medical Center
Veterans Affairs Palo Alto Health Care System

Program Director:
Willard E Fee, MD
Stanford Univ Med Ctr
Div of Otolaryngology
300 Pasteur Dr/Edwards R135
Stanford, CA 94305-5328
Tel: 650 725-6500 *Fax:* 650 725-8502
Accred Length: 4 Years *Program Size:* 12
Program ID: 280-05-21-023

Colorado

Denver

University of Colorado Program

Sponsor: University of Colorado Health Sciences Center
Children's Hospital
Denver Health and Hospitals
Veterans Affairs Medical Center (Denver)

Program Director:
Kenny Chan, MD
Glen Y Yoshida, MD
Univ of Colorado Health Sciences Ctr
4200 E Ninth Ave/B-205
Denver, CO 80262
Tel: 303 315-7988 *Fax:* 303 315-8787
Internet: http://www.uchsc.edu/fm/otolaryn/index.html
Accred Length: 4 Years *Program Size:* 10
Program ID: 280-07-21-024

Connecticut

Farmington

University of Connecticut Program

Sponsor: University of Connecticut School of Medicine
Hartford Hospital
New Britain General Hospital
St Francis Hospital and Medical Center
Univ of Connecticut Health Center/John Dempsey Hospital

Program Director:
Gerald Leonard, MD
Univ of Connecticut Sch of Med
263 Farmington Ave
Farmington, CT 06030-3955
Tel: 860 679-3372 *Fax:* 860 679-1276
E-mail: thorp@nso.uchc.edu
Internet: http://www3.uchc.edu/otomain/
Accred Length: 4 Years *Program Size:* 8
Program ID: 280-08-21-025

New Haven

Yale-New Haven Medical Center Program

Sponsor: Yale-New Haven Hospital
Hospital of St Raphael
Veterans Affairs Medical Center (West Haven)

Program Director:
Clarence T Sasaki, MD
Yale Univ Sch of Med, Sect of Otolaryngology
333 Cedar St
PO Box 208041
New Haven, CT 06520-8041
Tel: 203 785-2593 *Fax:* 203 785-3970
E-mail: carmella.smagu6@yale.edu
Internet: http://www.info.med.yale.edu/surgery/otolar
Accred Length: 4 Years *Program Size:* 11
Program ID: 280-08-21-026

District of Columbia

Washington

George Washington University Program

Sponsor: George Washington University School of Medicine
Children's National Medical Center
George Washington University Hospital (UHS)
Howard University Hospital

Program Director:
William R Wilson, MD
Div of Otolaryngology
George Washington Univ
2150 Pennsylvania Ave NW/6B
Washington, DC 20037
Tel: 202 994-5573 *Fax:* 202 994-0567
E-mail: sursab@gwumc.edu
Accred Length: 4 Years *Program Size:* 5
Program ID: 280-10-21-130

Georgetown University Program

Sponsor: Georgetown University Medical Center
Veterans Affairs Medical Center (Washington, DC)
Washington Hospital Center

Program Director:
Kenneth M Grundfast, MD
Georgetown Univ Hospital
Dept of Otolaryngology
3800 Reservoir Rd NW
Washington, DC 20007
Tel: 202 687-8186 *Fax:* 202 687-0162
Accred Length: 4 Years *Program Size:* 12
Program ID: 280-10-32-027

Florida

Gainesville

University of Florida Program

Sponsor: University of Florida College of Medicine
Shands Hospital at the University of Florida
University Medical Center (UFHSC/J)
Veterans Affairs Medical Center (Gainesville)

Program Director:
Scott P Stringer, MD MS
J Hillis Miller Health Ctr
Box 100264
Gainesville, FL 32610-0264
Tel: 352 392-4461 *Fax:* 352 392-6781
E-mail: stringer@ent.health.ufl.edu
Internet: http://www.ent.health.ufl.edu
Accred Length: 4 Years *Program Size:* 10
Program ID: 280-11-21-028

Miami

University of Miami-Jackson Memorial Medical Center Program

Sponsor: University of Miami-Jackson Memorial Medical Center
Veterans Affairs Medical Center (Miami)

Program Director:
Thomas J Balkany, MD
Univ of Miami
Dept of Otolaryngology (D-48)
PO Box 016960
Miami, FL 33101
Tel: 305 585-7127 *Fax:* 305 326-7610
E-mail: vkerwin@mednet.med.miami.edu
Internet:
http://www.med.miami.edu/otolaryngology/otoindex.htm
Accred Length: 4 Years *Program Size:* 17
Program ID: 280-11-21-029

Tampa

University of South Florida Program

Sponsor: University of South Florida College of Medicine
All Children's Hospital
H Lee Moffitt Cancer Center
James A Haley Veterans Hospital
Tampa General Healthcare

Program Director:
Thomas V McCaffrey, MD PhD
Univ of South Florida Coll of Med
12902 Magnolia Dr/Ste 3057
Tampa, FL 33612-9497
Tel: 813 972-8463 *Fax:* 813 979-3830
E-mail: sullivdl@moffitt.usf.edu
Accred Length: 4 Years *Program Size:* 8
Program ID: 280-11-31-030

Georgia

Atlanta

Emory University Program

Sponsor: Emory University School of Medicine
Egleston Children's Hospital at Emory University
Emory University Hospital
Grady Memorial Hospital
Veterans Affairs Medical Center (Atlanta)

Program Director:
Douglas E Mattox, MD
Emory Clinic
Dept of Otolaryngology
1365 Clifton Rd NE
Atlanta, GA 30322-1013
Tel: 404 778-3939 *Fax:* 404 778-4295
E-mail: lesley_graham@emory.org
Internet:
http://www.emory.edu/eushc/med/surgery/resident_book/n_oto.html
Accred Length: 4 Years *Program Size:* 10
Program ID: 280-12-21-031

Augusta

Medical College of Georgia Program

Sponsor: Medical College of Georgia Hospital and Clinics
Veterans Affairs Medical Center (Augusta)

Program Director:
Edward S Porubsky, MD
Med Coll of Georgia Hospital and Clinics
BP 4109
Augusta, GA 30912-4060
Tel: 706 721-2047 *Fax:* 706 721-0112
Accred Length: 4 Years *Program Size:* 8
Program ID: 280-12-21-032

Hawaii

Honolulu

Tripler Army Medical Center Program

Sponsor: Tripler Army Medical Center

Program Director:
Michael R Holtel, MD
Tripler Army Med Ctr
Dept of Surgery
Attn: MCHK-DSH
Tripler AMC, HI 96859-5000
Tel: 808 433-3170 *Fax:* 808 433-9033
E-mail: michael_r.holtel@tamc.chcs.amedd.army.mil
Internet: http://www.tamc.amedd.army.mil
Accred Length: 4 Years *Program Size:* 6
Program ID: 280-14-11-116
US Armed Services Program

Illinois

Chicago

McGaw Medical Center of Northwestern University Program

Sponsor: Northwestern University Medical School
Cook County Hospital
Northwestern Memorial Hospital
Veterans Affairs Lakeside Medical Center (Chicago)

Program Director:
David G Hanson, MD
Northwestern Univ Med Sch
303 E Chicago Ave
Searle Bldg 12-561
Chicago, IL 60611-3008
Tel: 312 503-8920 *Fax:* 312 503-1616
E-mail: oto-hns@nwu.edu
Internet: http://www.oto-hns.nwu.edu
Accred Length: 4 Years *Program Size:* 15
Program ID: 280-16-21-033

Rush-Presbyterian-St Luke's Medical Center Program

Sponsor: Rush-Presbyterian-St Luke's Medical Center

Program Director:
David D Caldarelli, MD
Rush-Presbyterian-St Luke's Med Ctr
1653 W Congress Pkwy
Chicago, IL 60612-3864
Tel: 312 942-6303 *Fax:* 312 243-8280
Internet: http://www.rush.edu/med/ent
Accred Length: 4 Years *Program Size:* 5
Program ID: 280-16-21-034

University of Chicago Program

Sponsor: University of Chicago Hospitals

Program Director:
Robert M Naclerio, MD
Dept of Otolaryngology (MC 1035)
5841 S Maryland Ave/Rm E-102
Chicago, IL 60637
Tel: 773 702-6143 *Fax:* 773 702-6809
Internet:
http://www.surgery.bsd.uchicago.edu/ohns-www/
Accred Length: 4 Years *Program Size:* 6
Program ID: 280-16-21-035

University of Illinois College of Medicine at Chicago Program

Sponsor: University of Illinois College of Medicine at Chicago
Cook County Hospital
Michael Reese Hospital and Medical Center
University of Illinois Hosp-Illinois Eye and Ear Infirmary
Veterans Affairs West Side Medical Center

Program Director:
Edward L Applebaum, MD
Eye and Ear Infirmary
1855 W Taylor St (M/C 648)
Chicago, IL 60612
Tel: 312 996-6582 *Fax:* 312 996-1282
E-mail: sfrazier@uic.edu
Accred Length: 4 Years *Program Size:* 23
Program ID: 280-16-21-036

Maywood

Loyola University Program
Sponsor: Loyola University Medical Center
Edward J Hines Jr Veterans Affairs Hospital
Program Director:
James A Stankiewicz, MD
Loyola Univ Med Ctr
Bldg 105/Rm 1870
2160 S First Ave
Maywood, IL 60153
Tel: 708 216-9183
E-mail: jstank@luc.edu
Internet: http://www.lumc.edu/ent
Accred Length: 4 Years *Program Size:* 15
Program ID: 280-16-31-037

Springfield

Southern Illinois University Program
Sponsor: Southern Illinois University School of Medicine
Memorial Medical Center
St John's Hospital
Program Director:
Horst R Konrad, MD
Southern Illinois Univ Sch of Med
PO Box 19662
Springfield, IL 62794-9662
Tel: 217 785-3833 *Fax:* 217 524-0253
E-mail: hkonrad@siumed.edu
Accred Length: 4 Years *Program Size:* 6
Program ID: 280-16-21-118

Indiana

Indianapolis

Indiana University School of Medicine Program
Sponsor: Indiana University School of Medicine
Clarian IU Hospital
Clarian Riley Hospital for Children
Richard L Roudebush Veterans Affairs Medical Center
William N Wishard Memorial Hospital
Program Director:
Richard T Miyamoto, MD
702 Barnhill Dr/Rm 0860
Indianapolis, IN 46202-5230
Tel: 317 630-8966 *Fax:* 317 630-8958
E-mail: rmiyamot@iupui.edu
Internet: http://www.iupui.edu/it/oto/
Accred Length: 4 Years *Program Size:* 12
Program ID: 280-17-21-038

Iowa

Iowa City

University of Iowa Hospitals and Clinics Program
Sponsor: University of Iowa Hospitals and Clinics
Veterans Affairs Medical Center (Iowa City)
Program Director:
Bruce J Gantz, MD
Univ of Iowa Hospitals and Clinics
Dept of Oto/Head and Neck Surg
200 Hawkins Dr/E230 GH
Iowa City, IA 52242-1009
Tel: 319 356-2173 *Fax:* 319 356-3967
E-mail: bruce-gantz@uiowa.edu
Internet: http://www.medicine.uiowa.edu/otolaryngology
Accred Length: 4 Years *Program Size:* 20
Program ID: 280-18-21-039

Kansas

Kansas City

University of Kansas Medical Center Program
Sponsor: University of Kansas School of Medicine
Children's Mercy Hospital
University of Kansas Medical Center
Veterans Affairs Medical Center (Kansas City)
Program Director:
Terance T Tsue, MD
Univ of Kansas Med Ctr
3901 Rainbow Blvd
Kansas City, KS 66160-7380
Tel: 913 588-6739 *Fax:* 913 588-6708
E-mail: nmccall@kumc.edu
Internet: http://www2.kumc.edu/otolaryngology/
Accred Length: 4 Years *Program Size:* 8
Program ID: 280-19-31-040

Kentucky

Lexington

University of Kentucky Medical Center Program
Sponsor: University of Kentucky Hospital
Veterans Affairs Medical Center (Lexington)
Program Director:
Raleigh O Jones Jr, MD
Univ of Kentucky Med Ctr
800 Rose St/Rm C236
Lexington, KY 40536-0084
Tel: 606 257-5097 *Fax:* 606 257-5096
Accred Length: 4 Years *Program Size:* 6
Program ID: 280-20-21-127

Louisville

University of Louisville Program
Sponsor: University of Louisville School of Medicine
Kosair Children's Hospital (Alliant Health System)
Norton Hospital (Alliant Health System)
University of Louisville Hospital
Veterans Affairs Medical Center (Louisville)
Program Director:
Toni M Ganzel, MD
Univ of Louisville Health Science Ctr
Div of Otolaryngology
Myers Hall
Louisville, KY 40292
Tel: 502 852-6994 *Fax:* 502 852-0865
Internet:
http://www.louisville.edu/medschool/surgery/otolaryngology
Accred Length: 4 Years *Program Size:* 8
Program ID: 280-20-21-041

Louisiana

New Orleans

Louisiana State University Program
Sponsor: Louisiana State University School of Medicine
Medical Center of Louisiana at New Orleans
University Medical Center (Lafayette)
Veterans Affairs Medical Center-LSU Service (New Orleans)
Program Director:
Daniel W Nuss, MD
Louisiana State Univ Sch of Med
Dept of Otolaryngology
2020 Gravier St/Ste A
New Orleans, LA 70112-2234
Tel: 504 568-4785 *Fax:* 504 568-4460
E-mail: ent@lsumc.edu
Internet: http://www.lsumc.edu
Accred Length: 4 Years *Program Size:* 12
Program ID: 280-21-31-042

Tulane University Program
Sponsor: Tulane University School of Medicine
Alton Ochsner Medical Foundation
Medical Center of Louisiana at New Orleans
Tulane University Hospital and Clinics
Veterans Affairs Medical Center (Biloxi)
Program Director:
Ronald G Amedee, MD
Tulane Univ Med Ctr
1430 Tulane Ave/SL59
New Orleans, LA 70112-2699
Tel: 504 588-5454 *Fax:* 504 582-7846
E-mail: ramedee@tmcpop.tmc.tulane.edu
Internet:
http://ww1.omi.tulane.edu/departments/otolaryng
Accred Length: 4 Years *Program Size:* 12
Program ID: 280-21-21-043

Shreveport

Louisiana State University (Shreveport) Program
Sponsor: Louisiana State University Hospital-Shreveport
Overton Brooks Veterans Affairs Medical Center
Program Director:
William E Pate, MD
Louisiana State Univ Med Ctr Hospital
Dept of Otolaryngology
1501 Kings Hwy/PO Box 33932
Shreveport, LA 71130-3932
Tel: 318 675-6262 *Fax:* 318 675-6260
Accred Length: 4 Years *Program Size:* 10
Program ID: 280-21-21-121

Maryland

Baltimore

Johns Hopkins University Program
Sponsor: Johns Hopkins University School of Medicine
Greater Baltimore Medical Center
Johns Hopkins Bayview Medical Center
Johns Hopkins Hospital
Program Director:
Wayne M Koch, MD
Johns Hopkins Hospital
Dept of Otolaryngology
PO Box 41402
Baltimore, MD 21203-6402
Tel: 410 955-4906 *Fax:* 410 614-9825
Internet: http://www.med.jhu.edu/otolar/resident.html
Accred Length: 4 Years *Program Size:* 19
Program ID: 280-23-21-047

University of Maryland Program
Sponsor: University of Maryland Medical System
Maryland General Hospital
Veterans Affairs Medical Center (Baltimore)
Program Director:
Paul F Castellanos, MD
Univ of Maryland Med System
16 S Eutaw St
Ste 500
Baltimore, MD 21201
Tel: 410 328-5828 *Fax:* 410 328-5827
E-mail: jliverman@surgery.umaryland.edu
Internet:
http://www.umm.edu/center/training/residency.html
Accred Length: 4 Years *Program Size:* 10
Program ID: 280-23-21-048

Bethesda

National Capital Consortium Program
Sponsor: National Capital Consortium
National Naval Medical Center (Bethesda)
Walter Reed Army Medical Center
Program Director:
David H Thompson, MD
National Naval Med Ctr
8901 Wisconsin Ave
Bethesda, MD 20889-5600
Tel: 301 295-4670 *Fax:* 301 295-6666
Accred Length: 4 Years *Program Size:* 16
Program ID: 280-10-31-132
US Armed Services Program

Massachusetts

Boston

Boston University Medical Center Program
Sponsor: Boston Medical Center
Lahey Clinic
Veterans Affairs Medical Center (Boston)
Program Director:
Gregory A Grillone, MD
Boston Univ Med Ctr
88 E Newton St
Boston, MA 02118
Tel: 617 638-7933 *Fax:* 617 638-7965
E-mail: gregory.grillone@bmc.org
Internet: http://www.bu.edu/orl/default.html
Accred Length: 4 Years *Program Size:* 8
Program ID: 280-24-31-051

Harvard Medical School Program
Sponsor: Massachusetts Eye and Ear Infirmary
Beth Israel Deaconess Medical Center
Program Director:
Marvin P Fried, MD
Massachusetts Eye and Ear Infirmary
243 Charles St
Boston, MA 02114
Tel: 617 573-3654 *Fax:* 617 573-3939
E-mail: bbbeard@meei.harvard.edu
Internet: http://www.meei-ent.harvard.edu
Accred Length: 4 Years *Program Size:* 17
Program ID: 280-24-21-049

Tufts University Program
Sponsor: New England Medical Center Hospitals
Brockton Hospital
Rhode Island Hospital
Program Director:
Stanley M Shapshay, MD
New England Med Ctr
750 Washington St
Box 850
Boston, MA 02111
Tel: 617 636-8814 *Fax:* 617 636-1479
E-mail: kathleen.winslow@es.nemc.org
Internet: http://www.nemc.org/ent/oto-hns.htm
Accred Length: 4 Years *Program Size:* 8
Program ID: 280-24-31-050

Michigan

Ann Arbor

University of Michigan Program
Sponsor: University of Michigan Hospitals
Veterans Affairs Medical Center (Ann Arbor)
Program Director:
Gregory T Wolf, MD
Univ of Michigan
1904 Taubman Ctr/Box 0312
1500 E Medical Center Dr
Ann Arbor, MI 48109-0312
Tel: 734 936-8029 *Fax:* 734 647-9691
E-mail: gregwolf@umich.edu
Internet:
http://www.umich.edu/oto/residencyprogram.htm
Accred Length: 4 Years *Program Size:* 16
Program ID: 280-25-21-052

Detroit

Henry Ford Hospital Program
Sponsor: Henry Ford Hospital
Program Director:
Elizabeth R Ransom, MD
Henry Ford Hospital
Dept of Otolaryngology
2799 W Grand Blvd
Detroit, MI 48202-2689
Tel: 313 916-2761 *Fax:* 313 916-7263
Accred Length: 4 Years *Program Size:* 11
Program ID: 280-25-12-053

Wayne State University/Detroit Medical Center Program
Sponsor: Wayne State University/Detroit Medical Center
Children's Hospital of Michigan
Detroit Receiving Hospital and University Health Center
Harper Hospital
Veterans Affairs Medical Center (Detroit)
Program Director:
Robert H Mathog, MD
Wayne State Univ Hospitals
Dept of Otolaryngology
4201 St Antoine/5E-UHC
Detroit, MI 48201
Tel: 313 577-0804 *Fax:* 313 577-8555
E-mail: rmathog@med.wayne.edu
Internet:
http://www.med.wayne.edu/otohns/otohnsmain.html
Accred Length: 4 Years *Program Size:* 16
Program ID: 280-25-21-054

Minnesota

Minneapolis

University of Minnesota Program
Sponsor: University of Minnesota Medical School
Fairview-University Medical Center
Hennepin County Medical Center
Regions Hospital
Veterans Affairs Medical Center (Minneapolis)
Program Director:
George L Adams, MD
Dept of Otolaryngology
Box 396 Mayo Bldg
420 Delaware St SE
Minneapolis, MN 55455
Tel: 612 625-3200 *Fax:* 612 625-2101
E-mail: peter096@tc.umn.edu
Internet: http://www.med.umn.edu/otol/
Accred Length: 4 Years *Program Size:* 16
Program ID: 280-26-31-055

Rochester

Mayo Graduate School of Medicine (Rochester) Program
Sponsor: Mayo Graduate School of Medicine-Mayo Foundation
Mayo Clinic (Jacksonville)
Mayo Clinic (Rochester)
Mayo Clinic (Scottsdale)
Rochester Methodist Hospital
St Mary's Hospital of Rochester
Program Director:
Charles W Beatty, MD
Mayo Graduate Sch of Med
Application Processing Ctr
200 First St SW
Rochester, MN 55905
Tel: 507 284-4331 *Fax:* 507 284-0999
E-mail: mgsm.roch.mn.ent@mayo.edu
Internet: http://www.mayo.edu/
Accred Length: 4 Years *Program Size:* 20
Program ID: 280-26-21-056

Mississippi

Jackson

University of Mississippi Medical Center Program
Sponsor: University of Mississippi School of Medicine
University Hospital
Veterans Affairs Medical Center (Jackson)
Program Director:
Vinod Kumar Anand, MD
Univ of Mississippi Med Ctr
2500 N State St
Jackson, MS 39216-4505
Tel: 601 984-5162 *Fax:* 601 984-5085
E-mail: vanand@surgery.umsmed.edu
Internet: http://fiona.umsmed.edu/~alemar/oto.html
Accred Length: 4 Years *Program Size:* 10
Program ID: 280-27-21-122

Programs

Missouri

Columbia

University of Missouri-Columbia Program

Sponsor: University of Missouri-Columbia School of Medicine
Ellis Fischel Cancer Center
Harry S Truman Memorial Veterans Hospital
University Hospitals and Clinics

Program Director:
William E Davis, MD
Univ of Missouri Med Ctr
Otolaryngology/MA314
One Hospital Dr
Columbia, MO 65212
Tel: 573 882-8173 *Fax:* 573 884-4205
E-mail: daviswe@health.missouri.edu
Accred Length: 4 Years *Program Size:* 10
Program ID: 280-28-21-058

St Louis

St Louis University School of Medicine Program

Sponsor: St Louis University School of Medicine
SSM Cardinal Glennon Children's Hospital
St John's Mercy Medical Center
St Louis University School of Medicine

Program Director:
Gregory H Branham, MD
St Louis Univ Med Ctr
Dept of Oto/Head and Neck Surg
3635 Vista Ave
St Louis, MO 63110-0250
Tel: 314 577-8884 *Fax:* 314 268-5111
E-mail: rowejr@slucare1.sluh.edu
Internet: http://medschool.slu.edu/ent/training
Accred Length: 4 Years *Program Size:* 8
Program ID: 280-28-21-059

Washington University/B-JH/SLCH Consortium Program

Sponsor: Washington University/B-JH/SLCH Consortium
Barnes-Jewish Hospital
Barnes-Jewish Hospital (North Campus)
St Louis Children's Hospital
Veterans Affairs Medical Center (St Louis)

Program Director:
Joel A Goebel, MD
Barnes-Jewish Hospital
517 S Euclid
Campus Box 8115
St Louis, MO 63110
Tel: 314 747-0553 *Fax:* 314 362-7522
E-mail: harringm@msnotes.wustl.edu
Internet: http://www.oto.wustl.edu
Accred Length: 4 Years *Program Size:* 24
Program ID: 280-28-21-060

Nebraska

Omaha

University of Nebraska Program

Sponsor: University of Nebraska Medical Center
Boys Town National Research Hospital
Ehrling Bergquist Hospital
Veterans Affairs Medical Center (Omaha)

Program Director:
Anthony J Yonkers, MD
Univ of Nebraska Med Ctr
Dept of Oto-Head and Neck Surg
981225 Nebraska Med Ctr
Omaha, NE 68198-1225
Tel: 402 559-8007 *Fax:* 402 559-8940
E-mail: ayonkers@mail.unmc.com
Internet: http://www.unmc.edu/gme/gme home.htm
Accred Length: 4 Years *Program Size:* 8
Program ID: 280-30-21-061

New Jersey

Newark

UMDNJ-New Jersey Medical School Program

Sponsor: UMDNJ-New Jersey Medical School
Hackensack University Medical Center
Newark Eye and Ear Infirmary (United Hospitals Med Ctr)
St Barnabas Medical Center
UMDNJ-University Hospital
Veterans Affairs Medical Center (East Orange)

Program Director:
Soly Baredes, MD
UMDNJ-New Jersey Med Sch
Sect of Oto/Head and Neck Surg
185 S Orange Ave/Rm H-592
Newark, NJ 07103-2714
Tel: 973 972-4588 *Fax:* 973 972-3767
E-mail: conawajr@umdnj.edu
Internet: http://www.umdnj.edu/snjmsweb/title.htm
Accred Length: 4 Years *Program Size:* 8
Program ID: 280-33-31-062

New Mexico

Albuquerque

University of New Mexico Program

Sponsor: University of New Mexico School of Medicine
Lovelace Medical Center
University Hospital
Veterans Affairs Medical Center (Albuquerque)

Program Director:
Fred S Herzon, MD
Univ of New Mexico Health Sciences Ctr
2211 Lomas Blvd NE/ACC-2
Albuquerque, NM 87131-5341
Tel: 505 272-6452 *Fax:* 505 272-6493
Internet: http://www.unm.edu/~jpatk/unmoto.html
Accred Length: 4 Years *Program Size:* 4
Program ID: 280-34-21-126

New York

Albany

Albany Medical Center Program

Sponsor: Albany Medical Center
Child's Hospital
St Peter's Hospital
Veterans Affairs Medical Center (Albany)

Program Director:
Steven M Parnes, MD
Albany Med Coll
47 New Scotland Ave/MC-41
Albany, NY 12208-3479
Tel: 518 262-5897 *Fax:* 518 262-6670
E-mail: dianna_wilder@ccgateway.amc.edu
Accred Length: 4 Years *Program Size:* 8
Program ID: 280-35-21-063

Bronx

Albert Einstein College of Medicine Program

Sponsor: Albert Einstein College of Medicine of Yeshiva University
Beth Israel Medical Center
Jacobi Medical Center
Long Island Jewish Medical Center
Montefiore Medical Center-Henry and Lucy Moses Division
Montefiore Medical Center-Weiler Hospital
North Central Bronx Hospital

Program Director:
Richard V Smith, MD
Montefiore Med Ctr
Dept of Otolaryngology
111 E 210th St
Bronx, NY 10467-2490
Tel: 718 920-2991 *Fax:* 718 405-9014
Accred Length: 4 Years *Program Size:* 18
Program ID: 280-35-21-133

Brooklyn

SUNY Health Science Center at Brooklyn Program

Sponsor: SUNY Health Science Center at Brooklyn
Kings County Hospital Center
Long Island College Hospital
Veterans Affairs Medical Center (Brooklyn)

Program Director:
Frank E Lucente, MD
Long Island Coll Hospital
Dept of Otolaryngology
339 Hicks St
Brooklyn, NY 11201
Tel: 718 780-1281 *Fax:* 718 780-1488
Accred Length: 4 Years *Program Size:* 15
Program ID: 280-35-21-123

Buffalo

SUNY at Buffalo Graduate Medical-Dental Education Consortium Program

Sponsor: SUNY at Buffalo Grad Medical-Dental Education Consortium
CGF Health System (Children's Hospital of Buffalo)
Dent Neurological Institute (of Millard Fillmore Hospitals)
Erie County Medical Center
Sisters of Charity Hospital
Veterans Affairs Medical Center (Buffalo)

Program Director:
Charles W Pruet, MD
Buffalo General Hospital
100 High St
Buffalo, NY 14203
Tel: 716 859-1218 *Fax:* 716 859-1214
E-mail: waxmk@ascu.buffalo.edu
Accred Length: 4 Years *Program Size:* 10
Program ID: 280-35-21-064

New York

Manhattan Eye, Ear and Throat Hospital Program

Sponsor: Manhattan Eye, Ear and Throat Hospital
Lenox Hill Hospital
Memorial Sloan-Kettering Cancer Center
New York and Presbyterian Hospital (Cornell Campus)

Program Director:
David R Edelstein, MD
Manhattan Eye Ear and Throat Hospital
Dept of Otolaryngology
210 E 64th St
New York, NY 10021
Tel: 212 838-9200, ext 2445 *Fax:* 212 838-6239
Accred Length: 4 Years *Program Size:* 16
Program ID: 280-35-21-068

Mount Sinai School of Medicine Program

Sponsor: Mount Sinai School of Medicine
Elmhurst Hospital Center-Mount Sinai Services
Mount Sinai Medical Center
Veterans Affairs Medical Center (Bronx)

Program Director:
Mark L Urken, MD
Mount Sinai Med Ctr
One Gustave L Levy Pl
Box 1189
New York, NY 10029
Tel: 212 241-5944 *Fax:* 212 369-5701
E-mail: erika_markowitz@smtplink.mssm.edu
Internet: http://www.mssm.edu/ent/
Accred Length: 4 Years *Program Size:* 16
Program ID: 280-35-21-069

New York and Presbyterian Hospital (Columbia Campus) Program

Sponsor: New York and Presbyterian Hospital
New York and Presbyterian Hospital (Columbia Campus)
St Luke's-Roosevelt Hospital Center-Roosevelt Division
St Luke's-Roosevelt Hospital Center-St Luke's Division

Program Director:
Lanny G Close, MD
New York Presbyterian Hospital
630 W 168th St
New York, NY 10032
Tel: 212 305-5820 *Fax:* 212 305-2249
Internet: http://cpmcnet.columbia.edu/dept/ent
Accred Length: 4 Years *Program Size:* 10
Program ID: 280-35-11-074

New York Medical College (New York Eye and Ear Infirmary) Program

Sponsor: New York Medical College
New York Eye and Ear Infirmary
Lincoln Medical and Mental Health Center
St Vincent's Hospital and Medical Center of New York
Westchester Medical Center

Program Director:
Steven D Schaefer, MD
New York Eye and Ear Infirmary
310 E 14th St/6th Fl
New York, NY 10003-4201
Tel: 212 979-4200 *Fax:* 212 979-4315
Internet: http://www.nyee.edu
Accred Length: 4 Years *Program Size:* 15
Program ID: 280-35-21-072

New York University Medical Center Program

Sponsor: New York University Medical Center
Bellevue Hospital Center
Veterans Affairs Medical Center (Manhattan)

Program Director:
Noel L Cohen, MD
New York Univ Med Ctr
550 First Ave
New York, NY 10016
Tel: 212 263-6344 *Fax:* 212 263-8257
E-mail: n.cohen@mcfpo.med.nyu.edu
Internet: http://www.med.nyu.edu/ent/home page.i
Accred Length: 4 Years *Program Size:* 14
Program ID: 280-35-21-073

Rochester

University of Rochester Program

Sponsor: Strong Memorial Hospital of the University of Rochester
Genesee Hospital
Rochester General Hospital

Program Director:
Arthur S Hengerer, MD
Univ of Rochester Med Ctr
601 Elmwood Ave
Box 629
Rochester, NY 14642-8629
Tel: 716 275-2754 *Fax:* 716 271-8552
E-mail: ent@surgery.urmc.rochester.edu
Internet: http://www.urmc.rochester.edu/smd/ent/
Accred Length: 4 Years *Program Size:* 8
Program ID: 280-35-21-078

Stony Brook

SUNY at Stony Brook Program

Sponsor: University Hospital-SUNY at Stony Brook
Veterans Affairs Medical Center (Northport)

Program Director:
Arnold E Katz, MD
SUNY-Stony Brook
HSC, T19-090
Div of Otolaryngology-HNS
Stony Brook, NY 11794-8191
Tel: 516 444-3993 *Fax:* 516 444-7635
E-mail: hogan@surg.som.sunysb.edu
Internet:
http://www.uhmc.sunysb.edu/surgery/edu/otolaryngology/residoto.html
Accred Length: 4 Years *Program Size:* 5
Program ID: 280-35-31-128

Syracuse

SUNY Health Science Center at Syracuse Program

Sponsor: University Hospital-SUNY Health Science Center at Syracuse
Crouse Hospital
Veterans Affairs Medical Center (Syracuse)

Program Director:
Robert M Kellman, MD
SUNY Health Science Ctr-Syracuse
750 E Adams St
Syracuse, NY 13210
Tel: 315 464-7281 *Fax:* 315 464-7298
Accred Length: 4 Years *Program Size:* 12
Program ID: 280-35-21-079

North Carolina

Chapel Hill

University of North Carolina Hospitals Program

Sponsor: University of North Carolina Hospitals
Wake Medical Center

Program Director:
Harold C Pillsbury III, MD
Univ of North Carolina Hospitals
CB 7070/610 Burnett-Womack Bldg
Chapel Hill, NC 27599-7070
Tel: 919 966-8926 *Fax:* 919 966-7656
E-mail: hcp@med.unc.edu
Internet:
http://www.med.unc.edu/wrkunits/2depts/surgery/oto-hns
Accred Length: 4 Years *Program Size:* 15
Program ID: 280-36-21-080

Durham

Duke University Program

Sponsor: Duke University Medical Center
Veterans Affairs Medical Center (Durham)

Program Director:
William J Richtsmeier, MD PhD
Duke Univ Med Ctr
PO Box 3805
Durham, NC 27710
Tel: 919 681-6820 *Fax:* 919 681-6881
E-mail: richt001@mc.duke.edu
Internet: http://thor.oit.duke.edu/dumc-ohns/
Accred Length: 4 Years *Program Size:* 10
Program ID: 280-36-21-081

Winston-Salem

Wake Forest University School of Medicine Program

Sponsor: Wake Forest University Baptist Medical Center

Program Director:
W Fred McGuirt Sr, MD
Wake Forest Univ Sch of Med
Medical Center Blvd
Winston-Salem, NC 27157-1034
Tel: 336 716-3854 *Fax:* 336 716-3857
E-mail: preece@wfubmc.edu
Internet: http://www.wfubmc.edu
Accred Length: 4 Years *Program Size:* 10
Program ID: 280-36-11-082

Ohio

Cincinnati

University Hospital/University of Cincinnati College of Medicine Program

Sponsor: University Hospital Inc
Children's Hospital Medical Center
Veterans Affairs Medical Center (Cincinnati)

Program Director:
Thomas A Tami, MD
Univ of Cincinnati Med Ctr
PO Box 670528
231 Bethesda Ave
Cincinnati, OH 45267-0528
Tel: 513 558-4198 *Fax:* 513 558-5203
E-mail: tamita@uc.edu
Internet: http://www.med.uc.edu/departme/ent/ent.htm/
Accred Length: 4 Years *Program Size:* 14
Program ID: 280-38-21-083

Cleveland

Case Western Reserve University Program

Sponsor: University Hospitals of Cleveland
MetroHealth Medical Center
Veterans Affairs Medical Center (Cleveland)

Program Director:
David W Stepnick, MD
Univ Hospitals of Cleveland
Dept of Oto/Head and Neck Surg
11100 Euclid Ave
Cleveland, OH 44106-5045
Tel: 216 844-5004 *Fax:* 216 844-5727
E-mail: natalie.wheeler@uhhs.com
Internet: http://www.cwru-ent.comm
Accred Length: 4 Years *Program Size:* 12
Program ID: 280-38-21-124

Cleveland Clinic Foundation Program

Sponsor: Cleveland Clinic Foundation

Program Director:
Gordon B Hughes, MD
Cleveland Clinic Foundation
Dept of Otolaryngology/A71
9500 Euclid Ave
Cleveland, OH 44195-5242
Tel: 216 444-5690 *Fax:* 216 444-1162
E-mail: meded@cesmtp.ccf.org
Internet: http://www.ccf.org
Accred Length: 4 Years *Program Size:* 18
Program ID: 280-38-22-085

Columbus

Ohio State University Program

Sponsor: Ohio State University Medical Center
Children's Hospital

Program Director:
David E Schuller, MD
Ohio State Univ Hospital
Rm 4100/Univ Hospital Clinic
456 W Tenth Ave
Columbus, OH 43210-1282
Tel: 614 293-8150 *Fax:* 614 293-3193
Accred Length: 4 Years *Program Size:* 12
Program ID: 280-38-31-087

Oklahoma

Oklahoma City

University of Oklahoma Health Sciences Center Program

Sponsor: University of Oklahoma College of Medicine
Children's Hospital of Oklahoma
Integris Baptist Medical Center
University Hospital
Veterans Affairs Medical Center (Oklahoma City)

Program Director:
Jesus E Medina, MD
Univ of Oklahoma Health Sciences Ctr
PO Box 26901/WP1360
Oklahoma City, OK 73190-3048
Tel: 405 271-5504 *Fax:* 405 271-3248
E-mail: jesus-medina@ouhsc.edu
Internet: http://www.ouhsc.edu/depts/laryn/index.htm
Accred Length: 4 Years *Program Size:* 11
Program ID: 280-39-21-088

Oregon

Portland

Oregon Health Sciences University Program

Sponsor: Oregon Health Sciences University Hospital
Veterans Affairs Medical Center (Portland)

Program Director:
Alexander J Schleuning, MD
Oregon Health Sciences Univ
3181 SW Sam Jackson Park Rd/PV-01
Portland, OR 97201-3098
Tel: 503 494-5674 *Fax:* 503 494-4631
E-mail: schleuni@ohsu.edu
Internet: http://www.sfmatch.org/r-oto/574-13
oregonhsu.htm
Accred Length: 4 Years *Program Size:* 10
Program ID: 280-40-21-089

Pennsylvania

Danville

Penn State Geisinger Health System/Geisinger Medical Center Program

Sponsor: Penn State Geisinger Health System
Geisinger Medical Center

Program Director:
Donald P Vrabec, MD
Geisinger Med Ctr
100 N Academy Ave
Danville, PA 17822
Tel: 717 271-6429 *Fax:* 717 271-6854
E-mail: ckrebs@psghs.edu
Accred Length: 4 Years *Program Size:* 9
Program ID: 280-41-12-090

Hershey

Penn State Geisinger Health System/Milton S Hershey Medical Center Program

Sponsor: Penn State Geisinger Health System
Milton S Hershey Medical Center
Lehigh Valley Hospital

Program Director:
Fred G Fedok, MD
Milton S Hershey Med Ctr
Sect of Oto/Head and Neck Surgery
PO Box 850
Hershey, PA 17033-0850
Tel: 717 531-8946 *Fax:* 717 531-6160
E-mail: ffedok@psghs.edu
Internet: http://webserv.surg.hmc.psu.edu
Accred Length: 4 Years *Program Size:* 5
Program ID: 280-41-11-091

Philadelphia

Temple University Program

Sponsor: Temple University Hospital
Hahnemann University Hospital
St Christopher's Hospital for Children

Program Director:
Glenn C Isaacson, MD
Temple Univ Sch of Med
3400 N Broad St
1st Fl/Kresge West Bldg
Philadelphia, PA 19140-5104
Tel: 215 707-3665 *Fax:* 215 707-7523
E-mail: anita@flower.aud.temple.edu
Accred Length: 4 Years *Program Size:* 8
Program ID: 280-41-21-092

Thomas Jefferson University Program

Sponsor: Thomas Jefferson University Hospital
duPont Hospital for Children
Pennsylvania Hospital (UPHS)
Veterans Affairs Medical Center (Wilmington)

Program Director:
William M Keane, MD
Louis D Lowry, MD
Thomas Jefferson Univ, Dept of Otolaryngology
925 Chestnut St
6th Fl
Philadelphia, PA 19107
Tel: 215 955-6784 *Fax:* 215 923-4532
Accred Length: 4 Years *Program Size:* 16
Program ID: 280-41-21-093

University of Pennsylvania Program

Sponsor: Hospital of the University of Pennsylvania
Children's Hospital of Philadelphia
Pennsylvania Hospital (UPHS)
Veterans Affairs Medical Center (Philadelphia)

Program Director:
David W Kennedy, MD
Univ of Pennsylvania Med Ctr
3400 Spruce St
5 Ravdin
Philadelphia, PA 19104
Tel: 215 349-5382 *Fax:* 215 349-5977
E-mail: mwinberg@mail.med.upenn.edu
Internet:
http://www.med.upenn.edu/~pennorl/welcome.html
Accred Length: 4 Years *Program Size:* 21
Program ID: 280-41-21-095

Pittsburgh

University Health Center of Pittsburgh Program

Sponsor: University Health Center of Pittsburgh
Allegheny General Hospital
Children's Hospital of Pittsburgh
Presbyterian University Hospital/UPMC
Veterans Affairs Medical Center (Pittsburgh)

Program Director:
Jonas T Johnson, MD
Univ of Pittsburgh Sch of Med
Eye and Ear Inst/Ste 500
200 Lothrop St
Pittsburgh, PA 15213
Tel: 412 647-2130 *Fax:* 412 647-2080
E-mail: jtj@med.pitt.edu
Internet:
http://www.wwwdev.upmc.edu/programs/otolaryngology/otoresbrochure
Accred Length: 4 Years *Program Size:* 13
Program ID: 280-41-21-096

Puerto Rico

San Juan

University of Puerto Rico Program

Sponsor: University of Puerto Rico School of Medicine
San Juan City Hospital
University Hospital
Veterans Affairs Medical Center (San Juan)

Program Director:
Juan Trinidad-Pinedo, MD
Univ of Puerto Rico Sch of Med
Dept of Orolaryngology
GPO Box 5867
San Juan, PR 00936
Tel: 787 765-0240 *Fax:* 787 753-3957
Accred Length: 4 Years *Program Size:* 8
Program ID: 280-42-31-098

South Carolina

Charleston

Medical University of South Carolina Program

Sponsor: Medical University of South Carolina College of Medicine
Charleston Memorial Hospital
MUSC Medical Center
Naval Hospital (Charleston)
Ralph H Johnson Dept of Veterans Affairs Med Center

Program Director:
Peter C Weber, MD
Med Univ of South Carolina
Dept of Oto/Communicative Science
171 Ashley Ave
Charleston, SC 29425
Tel: 803 792-7156 *Fax:* 803 792-0546
Accred Length: 4 Years *Program Size:* 8
Program ID: 280-45-21-100

Tennessee

Memphis

University of Tennessee Program

Sponsor: University of Tennessee College of Medicine
Baptist Memorial Hospital
Methodist Hospitals of Memphis-Central
Regional Medical Center at Memphis
University of Tennessee Medical Center (UT Bowld Hospital)
Veterans Affairs Medical Center (Memphis)

Program Director:
K Thomas Robbins, MD
Univ of Tennessee Med Ctr
Dept of Otolaryngology
956 Court Ave/Rm B224 Coleman
Memphis, TN 38163
Tel: 901 448-5886 *Fax:* 901 448-5120
E-mail: krobbins@utmem.edu
Internet: http://www.ent.utmem.edu
Accred Length: 4 Years *Program Size:* 12
Program ID: 280-47-21-101

Nashville

Vanderbilt University Program

Sponsor: Vanderbilt University Medical Center
Veterans Affairs Medical Center (Nashville)

Program Director:
Brian Burkey, MD
Vanderbilt Univ Sch of Med
Dept of Otolaryngology/S2100 MCN
Nashville, TN 37232-2559
Tel: 615 322-7267 *Fax:* 615 343-9556
Internet: http://www.sfmatch.org
Accred Length: 4 Years *Program Size:* 12
Program ID: 280-47-21-125

Texas

Dallas

University of Texas Southwestern Medical School Program

Sponsor: University of Texas Southwestern Medical School
Children's Medical Center of Dallas
Dallas County Hospital District-Parkland Memorial Hospital
Veterans Affairs Medical Center (Dallas)
Zale-Lipshy University Hospital

Program Director:
William L Meyerhoff, MD PhD
Univ of Texas Southwestern Med Ctr
5323 Harry Hines Blvd
Dallas, TX 75235-9035
Tel: 214 648-2432 *Fax:* 214 648-9122
E-mail: wmeyer@mednet.swmed.edu
Internet:
http://www.swmed.edu/home_pages/oto/oto.html
Accred Length: 4 Years *Program Size:* 16
Program ID: 280-48-21-102

Galveston

University of Texas Medical Branch Hospitals Program

Sponsor: University of Texas Medical Branch Hospitals

Program Director:
Byron J Bailey, MD
Univ of Texas Med Branch Hospitals
301 University Blvd/Rt 0521
Galveston, TX 77555-0521
Tel: 409 772-2701 *Fax:* 409 772-1715
E-mail: lrohacek@utmb.edu
Internet: http://www.utmb.edu/oto/
Accred Length: 4 Years *Program Size:* 12
Program ID: 280-48-11-103

Houston

Baylor College of Medicine Program

Sponsor: Baylor College of Medicine
Harris County Hospital District-Ben Taub General Hospital
Methodist Hospital
Veterans Affairs Medical Center (Houston)

Program Director:
Bobby R Alford, MD
Baylor Coll of Med
Dept of Otorhinolaryngology
One Baylor Plaza/NA102
Houston, TX 77030
Tel: 713 798-5906 *Fax:* 713 798-3403
E-mail: balford@bcm.tmc.edu
Internet: http://www.bcm.tmc.edu/oto/
Accred Length: 4 Years *Program Size:* 16
Subspecialties: PDO
Program ID: 280-48-31-104

University of Texas at Houston Program

Sponsor: University of Texas Medical School at Houston
Lyndon B Johnson General Hospital
Memorial Hermann Healthcare System
University of Texas M D Anderson Cancer Center

Program Director:
Charles M Stiernberg, MD
Dept of Oto/Head and Neck Surg
Univ of Texas-Houston Med Sch
6431 Fannin St/MSB 6133
Houston, TX 77030-1501
Tel: 713 500-5410 *Fax:* 713 500-0661
E-mail: sfoster@oto.med.uth.tmc.edu
Internet: http://oto.med.uth.tmc.edu
Accred Length: 4 Years *Program Size:* 11
Program ID: 280-48-21-105

Lackland AFB

San Antonio Uniformed Services Health Education Consortium Program

Sponsor: San Antonio Uniformed Services Health Education Consortium

Program Director:
William D Clark, MD
Wilford Hall Med Ctr
2200 Bergquist Dr/Ste 1
Lackland AFB, TX 78236-5300
Tel: 210 292-5623 *Fax:* 210 292-5621
E-mail: clark_w@whmc-lafb.af.mil
Accred Length: 4 Years *Program Size:* 12
Program ID: 280-48-21-131
US Armed Services Program

San Antonio

University of Texas Health Science Center at San Antonio Program
Sponsor: University of Texas Medical School at San Antonio
Audie L Murphy Memorial Veterans Hospital (San Antonio)
University Hospital-South Texas Medical Center
Program Director:
Robert A Dobie, MD
Univ of Texas Health Science Ctr
Dept of Otolaryngology
7703 Floyd Curl Dr
San Antonio, TX 78284-7777
Tel: 210 567-5655 *Fax:* 210 567-3617
E-mail: dobie@uthscsa.edu
Internet: http://macorb.uthscsa.edu/oto/index.htm
Accred Length: 4 Years *Program Size:* 10
Program ID: 280-48-21-106

Utah

Salt Lake City

University of Utah Program
Sponsor: University of Utah Medical Center
Primary Children's Medical Center
Salt Lake Regional Medical Center
Veterans Affairs Medical Center (Salt Lake City)
Program Director:
R Kim Davis, MD
Univ of Utah Sch of Med
Div of Oto/Head and Neck Surg
50 N Medical Dr/Rm 3C120
Salt Lake City, UT 84132
Tel: 801 581-7514 *Fax:* 801 585-5744
E-mail: illene.rawlings@hsc.utah.edu
Accred Length: 4 Years *Program Size:* 8
Program ID: 280-49-21-107

Vermont

Burlington

University of Vermont Program
Sponsor: Fletcher Allen Health Care
Mary Hitchcock Memorial Hospital
Program Director:
Robert A Sofferman, MD
Fletcher Allen Health Care
1 S Prospect St
Burlington, VT 05401
Tel: 802 656-4535 *Fax:* 802 656-8198
E-mail: robert.sofferman@vtmednet.org
Accred Length: 4 Years *Program Size:* 5
Program ID: 280-50-11-108

Virginia

Charlottesville

University of Virginia Program
Sponsor: University of Virginia Medical Center
Program Director:
Paul A Levine, MD
Univ of Virginia
Attn: Gil Pearman
PO Box 10008
Charlottesville, VA 22906-0008
Tel: 804 924-5594 *Fax:* 804 243-6522
E-mail: jgp8e@virginia.edu
Internet: http://www.med.virginia.edu/medicine/clinic/otolaryngology
Accred Length: 4 Years *Program Size:* 12
Subspecialties: NO
Program ID: 280-51-21-109

Norfolk

Eastern Virginia Medical School Program
Sponsor: Eastern Virginia Medical School
Naval Medical Center (Portsmouth)
Sentara Norfolk General Hospital
Program Director:
David H Darrow, MD DDS
825 Fairfax Ave/Ste 510
Norfolk, VA 23507-1912
Tel: 757 446-5934 *Fax:* 757 446-5968
Internet: http://www.evms.edu
Accred Length: 4 Years *Program Size:* 8
Program ID: 280-51-21-110

Portsmouth

Naval Medical Center (Portsmouth) Program
Sponsor: Naval Medical Center (Portsmouth)
Program Director:
Lorenz F Lassen, MD
Naval Med Ctr
Dept of Oto/HNS (Code 0609)
620 John Paul Jones Cir
Portsmouth, VA 23708-2197
Tel: 757 953-5980 *Fax:* 757 953-7993
E-mail: pnh1lfl@pnh10.med.navy.mil
Internet: http://164.167.49.31/ent/otohns.html
Accred Length: 4 Years *Program Size:* 7
Program ID: 280-51-21-120
US Armed Services Program

Richmond

Medical College of Virginia/Virginia Commonwealth University Program
Sponsor: Medical College of Virginia/Virginia Commonwealth University
Hunter Holmes McGuire VA Medical Center (Richmond)
Medical College of Virginia Hospitals
Program Director:
Aristides Sismanis, MD
Med Coll of Virginia
Box 980146
Richmond, VA 23298-0146
Tel: 804 828-3965 *Fax:* 804 828-5779
Accred Length: 4 Years *Program Size:* 8
Program ID: 280-51-21-111

Washington

Seattle

University of Washington Program
Sponsor: University of Washington School of Medicine
University of Washington Medical Center
Veterans Affairs Medical Center (Seattle)
Program Director:
Ernest A Weymuller Jr, MD
Dept of Oto/Head and Neck Surg
Univ of Washington
Box 356515
Seattle, WA 98195-6515
Tel: 206 543-5230 *Fax:* 206 543-5152
E-mail: peterson@otomail.u.washington.edu
Internet: http://www.weber.u.washington.edu/~otoweb
Accred Length: 4 Years *Program Size:* 15
Program ID: 280-54-21-112

Tacoma

Madigan Army Medical Center Program
Sponsor: Madigan Army Medical Center
Program Director:
Vincent D Eusterman, DDS MD
Madigan Army Med Ctr
Oto/Head and Neck Surgery
Attn: MCHJ-SET
Tacoma, WA 98431-5000
Tel: 253 968-1430 *Fax:* 253 968-3154
E-mail: veusterman@aol.com
Accred Length: 4 Years *Program Size:* 8
Program ID: 280-54-31-005
US Armed Services Program

West Virginia

Morgantown

West Virginia University Program
Sponsor: West Virginia University Hospitals
Louis A Johnson Veterans Affairs Medical Center
Program Director:
Stephen J Wetmore, MD
West Virginia Univ
2222 Health Sciences South
PO Box 9200
Morgantown, WV 26506-9200
Tel: 304 293-3457 *Fax:* 304 293-2902
E-mail: jmorency@mail.hsc.wvu.edu
Internet:
http://www.hsc.wvu.edu/som/otolaryngology/main.htm
Accred Length: 4 Years *Program Size:* 7
Program ID: 280-55-11-113

Otology-Neurotology (Otolaryngology)

Iowa

Iowa City

University of Iowa Hospitals and Clinics Program
Sponsor: University of Iowa Hospitals and Clinics
Program Director:
Bruce J Gantz, MD
Univ of Iowa Hospitals and Clinics
Dept of Otolaryngology
200 Hawkins Dr
Iowa City, IA 52242
Tel: 319 356-2173 *Fax:* 319 356-3967
E-mail: bruce-gantz@uiowa.edu
Internet: http://www.medicine.uiowa.edu/otolaryngology/
Accred Length: 2 Years *Program Size:* 1
Program ID: 286-18-21-003

Michigan

Ann Arbor

University of Michigan Program
Sponsor: University of Michigan Hospitals
Program Director:
Steven A Telian, MD
1500 E Medical Center Dr
Ann Arbor, MI 48109-0312
Tel: 313 936-8006 *Fax:* 313 936-9625
E-mail: telian@umich.edu
Accred Length: 2 Years *Program Size:* 1
Program ID: 286-25-21-001

New York

New York

New York University Medical Center Program
Sponsor: New York University Medical Center
Bellevue Hospital Center
Program Director:
Ronald A Hoffman, MD
New York Univ Med Ctr
Dept of Otolaryngology
550 First Ave
New York, NY 10016
Tel: 212 263-6344 *Fax:* 212 263-8257
Internet: http://www.med.nyu.edu/ent
Accred Length: 2 Years *Program Size:* 2
Program ID: 286-35-21-004

Ohio

Columbus

Ohio State University Program
Sponsor: Ohio State University Medical Center
Program Director:
D Bradley Welling, MD
4100 University Hospitals Clinic
456 W 10th Ave
Columbus, OH 43210
Tel: 614 293-8706 *Fax:* 614 293-3193
E-mail: welling.1@osu.edu
Accred Length: 2 Years *Program Size:* 2
Program ID: 286-38-21-002

Virginia

Charlottesville

University of Virginia Program
Sponsor: University of Virginia Medical Center
Program Director:
Paul R Lambert, MD
Dept of Otolaryngology-HNS
PO Box 10008
Charlottesville, VA 22906-0008
Tel: 804 924-2040 *Fax:* 804 982-4257
E-mail: prl@virginia.edu
Accred Length: 2 Years *Program Size:* 1
Program ID: 286-51-21-005

Wisconsin

Madison

University of Wisconsin Program
Sponsor: University of Wisconsin Hospital and Clinics
Meriter Hospital
William S Middleton Veterans Hospital
Program Director:
Charles N Ford, MD
Univ of Wisconsin Hospital
Oto/Head and Neck Surg H4/310
600 Highland Ave
Madison, WI 53792-3236
Tel: 608 263-7064 *Fax:* 608 263-0454
E-mail: zabel@surgadmin.surgery.wisc.edu
Internet:
http://www.medsch.wisc.edu/otoweb/rbrochur/resident.html
Accred Length: 4 Years *Program Size:* 8
Program ID: 280-56-21-114

Milwaukee

Medical College of Wisconsin Program
Sponsor: Medical College of Wisconsin Affiliated Hospitals Inc
Children's Hospital of Wisconsin
Clement J Zablocki Veterans Affairs Medical Center
Froedtert Memorial Lutheran Hospital
Program Director:
Bruce H Campbell, MD
Med Coll of Wisconsin
Dept of Oto/Communication Sciences
9200 W Wisconsin Ave
Milwaukee, WI 53226
Tel: 414 454-5583 *Fax:* 414 454-5259
E-mail: bcampbel@mcw.edu
Accred Length: 4 Years *Program Size:* 14
Program ID: 280-56-21-115

Programs

Pain Management (Anesthesiology)

Alabama

Birmingham

University of Alabama Medical Center Program
Sponsor: University of Alabama Hospital
Program Director:
Timothy J Ness, MD PhD
845 Jefferson Tower
619 19th St S
Birmingham, AL 35233-6810
Tel: 205 975-9643 *Fax:* 205 934-7437
E-mail: tim.ness@ccc.uab.edu
Accred Length: 1 Year *Program Size:* 2
Program ID: 048-01-21-094

Arizona

Tucson

University of Arizona Program
Sponsor: University of Arizona College of Medicine
Maricopa Medical Center
Mayo Clinic (Scottsdale)
Program Director:
Bennet Davis, MD
Arizona Health Sciences Ctr
1501 N Campbell Ave
PO Box 245114
Tucson, AZ 85724-5114
Tel: 520 626-5119 *Fax:* 520 626-3007
Internet: http://www.ahsc.arizona.edu/anesth
Accred Length: 1 Year *Program Size:* 2
Program ID: 048-03-21-080

California

Loma Linda

Loma Linda University Program
Sponsor: Loma Linda University Medical Center
Program Director:
Daniel J Cole, MD
Loma Linda Univ Med Ctr
Dept of Anesthesiology
PO Box 2000
Loma Linda, CA 92354
Tel: 909 824-4475 *Fax:* 909 824-4143
Accred Length: 1 Year *Program Size:* 2
Program ID: 048-05-21-001

Los Angeles

UCLA Medical Center Program
Sponsor: UCLA School of Medicine
Program Director:
Eric Hsu, MD
Ctr for Health Sciences
10833 Le Conte Ave
Los Angeles, CA 90024
Tel: 310 825-3316 *Fax:* 310 267-1790
Accred Length: 1 Year *Program Size:* 3
Program ID: 048-05-21-076

Orange

University of California (Irvine) Program
Sponsor: University of California (Irvine) Medical Center
Program Director:
Paul T Le, MD
Univ of California Irvine Med Ctr
101 City Dr S/Rte 81A
Orange, CA 92668
Tel: 714 456-5164, ext 7568 *Fax:* 714 456-7702
Accred Length: 1 Year *Program Size:* 0
Program ID: 048-05-31-002

Sacramento

University of California (Davis) Program
Sponsor: University of California (Davis) Medical Center
Program Director:
Peter G Moore, MD PhD
Univ of California Davis Med Ctr
Dept of Anesthesiology
4150 V St/Ste 1200
Sacramento, CA 95817
Tel: 916 734-5169 *Fax:* 916 734-7980
E-mail: blmyers@ucdavis.edu
Internet: http://www.anesthesiology.ucdmc.ucdavis.edu/
Accred Length: 1 Year *Program Size:* 24
Program ID: 048-05-21-064

San Diego

University of California (San Diego) Program
Sponsor: University of California (San Diego) Medical Center
Veterans Affairs Medical Center (San Diego)
Program Director:
Mark S Wallace, MD
Dept of Anesthesiology
200 W Arbor Dr
San Diego, CA 92103-8812
Tel: 619 543-7336 *Fax:* 619 543-6947
E-mail: lsutherland@ucsd.edu
Accred Length: 1 Year *Program Size:* 2
Program ID: 048-05-21-047

San Francisco

University of California (San Francisco) Program
Sponsor: University of California (San Francisco) School of Medicine
Mount Zion Medical Center of the University of California
Program Director:
Robert W Allen, MD
2255 Post St
San Francisco, CA 94143-1654
Tel: 415 885-7246 *Fax:* 415 885-7575
E-mail: randyc@email.his.ucsf.edu
Internet:
http://mzweb.his.ucsf.edu/clin_departments/anesthesia/pain
Accred Length: 1 Year *Program Size:* 2
Program ID: 048-05-31-082

Stanford

Stanford University Program
Sponsor: Stanford University Hospital
Program Director:
Raymond R Gaeta, MD
Dept of Anes/Pain Management
Stanford Univ Sch of Med
300 Pasteur Dr/Boswell A408
Stanford, CA 94305
Tel: 650 725-5852 *Fax:* 650 725-8052
Accred Length: 1 Year *Program Size:* 4
Program ID: 048-05-21-059

Colorado

Denver

University of Colorado Program
Sponsor: University of Colorado Health Sciences Center
Children's Hospital
Veterans Affairs Medical Center (Denver)
Program Director:
Jose M Angel, MD
East Pavillion
4701 E 9th Ave/E113
Denver, CO 80262
Tel: 303 372-1650 *Fax:* 303 372-1732
E-mail: jmangel@ski.uhcolorado.edu
Accred Length: 1 Year *Program Size:* 2
Program ID: 048-07-21-090

Connecticut

New Haven

Yale-New Haven Medical Center Program
Sponsor: Yale-New Haven Hospital
Program Director:
Steven C Levin, MD
333 Cedar St
PO Box 208051
New Haven, CT 06520-6897
Tel: 203 785-2802 *Fax:* 203 785-6897
Accred Length: 1 Year *Program Size:* 1
Program ID: 048-08-21-083

District of Columbia

Washington

Georgetown University Program
Sponsor: Georgetown University Medical Center
Fairfax Hospital
NIH Warren Grant Magnuson Clinical Center
Program Director:
Veronica D Mitchell, MD
Georgetown Univ Med Ctr
3800 Reservoir Rd NW
S Level/CCC
Washington, DC 20007
Tel: 202 784-3348 *Fax:* 202 784-1340
E-mail: mitchellv@medlib.georgetown.edu
Internet:
http://www.dmlgeorgetown.edu/depts/anesthesia/residency
Accred Length: 1 Year *Program Size:* 2
Program ID: 048-10-21-055

Florida

Gainesville

University of Florida Program
Sponsor: University of Florida College of Medicine
Shands Hospital at the University of Florida
Veterans Affairs Medical Center (Gainesville)
Program Director:
Jerry J Berger, MD
Dept of Anesthesia
JHMHSC
PO Box 100254
Gainesville, FL 32610-0254
Tel: 352 395-0077 *Fax:* 352 338-9880
Internet: http://www.anest.ufl.edu
Accred Length: 1 Year *Program Size:* 2
Program ID: 048-11-21-046

Jacksonville

Mayo Graduate School of Medicine (Jacksonville) Program
Sponsor: Mayo Graduate School of Medicine-Mayo Foundation
Mayo Clinic (Jacksonville)
St Luke's Hospital
St Mary's Hospital of Rochester
Program Director:
Kenneth A Marshall, MD
Mayo Clinic Jacksonville
4500 San Pablo Rd
Jacksonville, FL 32224
Tel: 904 296-5287 *Fax:* 904 296-3877
Internet: http://www.mayo.edu/
Accred Length: 1 Year *Program Size:* 2
Program ID: 048-11-31-054

Miami

University of Miami-Jackson Memorial Medical Center Program
Sponsor: University of Miami-Jackson Memorial Medical Center
Program Director:
Vincent Pallares, MD
Univ of Miami Sch of Med
Dept of Anesth (R-370)
PO Box 016370
Miami, FL 33101
Tel: 305 585-6970 *Fax:* 305 545-6753
E-mail: lpatton@umdas.med.miami.edu
Internet: http://umdas.med.miami.edu
Accred Length: 1 Year *Program Size:* 3
Program ID: 048-11-21-003

Tampa

University of South Florida Program
Sponsor: University of South Florida College of Medicine
H Lee Moffitt Cancer Center
James A Haley Veterans Hospital
Program Director:
Rafael V Miguel, MD
Univ of South Florida Coll of Med
12901 Bruce B Downs Blvd/MDC 59
Tampa, FL 33612-4799
Tel: 813 251-7438 *Fax:* 813 251-7418
E-mail: casanova@com1.med.usf.edu
Internet: http://www.med.usf.edu/anesthesiology/index.
Accred Length: 1 Year *Program Size:* 3
Program ID: 048-11-21-050

Georgia

Atlanta

Emory University Program
Sponsor: Emory University School of Medicine
Crawford Long Hospital of Emory University
Emory University Hospital
Program Director:
Allen H Hord, MD
Emory Univ
Dept of Anesthesiology/3 B South
1364 Clifton Rd NE
Atlanta, GA 30322
Tel: 404 778-5582 *Fax:* 404 778-5194
E-mail: ann_murray@emory.org
Internet:
http://www.emory.edu/whsc/med/anesthesiology
Accred Length: 1 Year *Program Size:* 5
Program ID: 048-12-21-004

Augusta

Medical College of Georgia Program
Sponsor: Medical College of Georgia Hospital and Clinics
Program Director:
Dan C Martin, MD
1120 15th St
Augusta, GA 30912
Tel: 706 721-4544 *Fax:* 706 721-7753
Accred Length: 1 Year *Program Size:* 0
Program ID: 048-12-21-105

Illinois

Chicago

Cook County Hospital Program
Sponsor: Cook County Hospital
Program Director:
Silvio Glusman, MD PhD
Cook County Hospital
1835 W Harrison
Chicago, IL 60612
Tel: 312 633-6173 *Fax:* 312 633-5165
Accred Length: 1 Year *Program Size:* 3
Program ID: 048-16-21-077

McGaw Medical Center of Northwestern University Program
Sponsor: Northwestern University Medical School
Northwestern Memorial Hospital
Program Director:
Honorio T Benzon, MD
Northwestern Univ Med Sch
303 E Superior St/Rm 360
Chicago, IL 60611-3053
Tel: 312 908-8254 *Fax:* 312 908-3233
E-mail: hbenzon@nmff.nwu.edu
Accred Length: 1 Year *Program Size:* 4
Program ID: 048-16-21-005

Rush-Presbyterian-St Luke's Medical Center Program
Sponsor: Rush-Presbyterian-St Luke's Medical Center
Rush North Shore Medical Center
Program Director:
Timothy R Lubenow, MD
1653 W Congress Pkwy
Chicago, IL 60612
Tel: 312 942-3134 *Fax:* 312 942-8858
Accred Length: 1 Year *Program Size:* 3
Program ID: 048-16-21-095

University of Chicago Program
Sponsor: University of Chicago Hospitals
Louis A Weiss Memorial Hospital
Program Director:
Friedl Pantle-Fisher, MD
Univ of Chicago Hospitals
5841 S Maryland Ave
Chicago, IL 60637
Tel: 773 702-6842 *Fax:* 773 834-0063
Accred Length: 1 Year *Program Size:* 4
Program ID: 048-16-31-098

University of Illinois College of Medicine at Chicago/Michael Reese Hospital Program
Sponsor: University of Illinois College of Medicine at Chicago
Michael Reese Hospital and Medical Center
Program Director:
Charles E Laurito, MD
Univ of Illinois-Chicago
901 S Wolcott Ave (M/C 845)
Chicago, IL 60612-7319
Tel: 312 996-1128 *Fax:* 312 996-1158
E-mail: sharps@uic.edu
Accred Length: 1 Year *Program Size:* 2
Program ID: 048-16-31-006

Maywood

Loyola University Program
Sponsor: Loyola University Medical Center
Program Director:
Maridas Chinthagada, MD
Dept of Anesthesiology
2160 S First Ave
Maywood, IL 60153
Tel: 708 216-9169 *Fax:* 708 216-1249
Accred Length: 1 Year *Program Size:* 2
Program ID: 048-16-31-078

Indiana

Indianapolis

Indiana University School of Medicine Program
Sponsor: Indiana University School of Medicine
Clarian IU Hospital
Clarian Riley Hospital for Children
Program Director:
John B Ward, MD
Indiana Univ Med Ctr
1120 South Dr
Fesler Hall 204
Indianapolis, IN 46202-5115
Tel: 317 274-0275 *Fax:* 317 274-0256
Internet: http://www.iupui.edu/~anesth/index.html
Accred Length: 1 Year *Program Size:* 1
Program ID: 048-17-21-039

Iowa

Iowa City

University of Iowa Hospitals and Clinics Program
Sponsor: University of Iowa Hospitals and Clinics
Program Director:
Burnett Porter, MD
Univ of Iowa Hospitals and Clinics
Dept of Anesthesia
200 Hawkins Dr
Iowa City, IA 52242-1009
Tel: 319 356-2633 *Fax:* 319 356-2940
Internet:
http://www.anesth.uiowa.edu/anesthesia/painfell.h
Accred Length: 1 Year *Program Size:* 2
Program ID: 048-18-21-007

Kentucky

Lexington

University of Kentucky Medical Center Program

Sponsor: University of Kentucky Hospital

Program Director:
William O Witt, MD
Univ of Kentucky
Albert B Chandler Med Ctr
800 Rose St/Rm N-202
Lexington, KY 40536-0293
Tel: 606 323-5956, ext 123 *Fax:* 606 323-1080
Internet: http://www.anes.uky.edu
Accred Length: 1 Year *Program Size:* 2
Program ID: 048-20-21-035

Louisiana

Shreveport

Louisiana State University (Shreveport) Program

Sponsor: Louisiana State University Hospital-Shreveport
Schumpert Medical Center
Willis-Knighton Medical Center

Program Director:
Randall C Cork, MD PhD
1501 S Kings Hwy
Shreveport, LA 71130
Tel: 318 675-7195 *Fax:* 318 675-6681
E-mail: rcork@lsumc.edu
Internet: http://www.anesthesia.lsumc.edu
Accred Length: 1 Year *Program Size:* 2
Program ID: 048-21-21-099

Maryland

Baltimore

Johns Hopkins University Program

Sponsor: Johns Hopkins University School of Medicine
Johns Hopkins Hospital

Program Director:
Sunil Panchal, MD
Johns Hopkins Univ
550 N Broadway
Ste 301
Baltimore, MD 21205
Tel: 410 955-1818 *Fax:* 410 502-6730
E-mail: slpancha@jhmi.edu
Accred Length: 1 Year *Program Size:* 4
Program ID: 048-23-21-008

University of Maryland Program

Sponsor: University of Maryland Medical System

Program Director:
Joel Kent, MD
Univ of Maryland
419 W Redwood St
Suite 550
Baltimore, MD 21201-1595
Tel: 410 328-8451 *Fax:* 410 328-0230
E-mail: jkent@anesth.ab.umd.edu
Internet: http://anesthesia.ummc.ab.umd.edu
Accred Length: 1 Year *Program Size:* 3
Program ID: 048-23-31-009

Bethesda

National Capital Consortium Program

Sponsor: National Capital Consortium
National Naval Medical Center (Bethesda)
USUHS F Edward Hebert School of Medicine
Walter Reed Army Medical Center

Program Director:
Dominique Schiffer, MD
6900 Georgia Ave NW
Washington, DC 20307-5001
Tel: 202 782-0039 *Fax:* 202 782-9301
Accred Length: 1 Year *Program Size:* 1
Program ID: 048-10-21-101
US Armed Services Program

Massachusetts

Boston

Beth Israel Deaconess Medical Center (East Campus) Program

Sponsor: Beth Israel Deaconess Medical Center
Brigham and Women's Hospital
Children's Hospital

Program Director:
Carol A Warfield, MD
Beth Israel Deaconess Med Ctr
Pain Management Ctr
330 Brookline Ave
Boston, MA 02215
Tel: 617 754-2713 *Fax:* 617 754-2677
Accred Length: 1 Year *Program Size:* 8
Program ID: 048-24-21-010

Brigham and Women's Hospital Program

Sponsor: Brigham and Women's Hospital

Program Director:
Srdjan Nedeljkovic, MD
Pain Management Ctr
Brigham and Women's Hospital
75 Francis St
Boston, MA 02115
Tel: 617 732-5500, ext 2247 *Fax:* 617 731-5453
E-mail: ssnedeljko@bics.bwh.harvard.edu
Internet: http://www.zeus.bwh.harvard.edu
Accred Length: 1 Year *Program Size:* 8
Program ID: 048-24-31-043

Massachusetts General Hospital Program

Sponsor: Massachusetts General Hospital

Program Director:
Shihab U Ahmed, MD
Massachusetts General Hospital
MGH Pain Ctr
15 Parkman St/WAC-324
Boston, MA 02114
Tel: 617 726-8810 *Fax:* 617 724-2719
Accred Length: 1 Year *Program Size:* 4
Program ID: 048-24-21-040

New England Medical Center Hospitals Program

Sponsor: New England Medical Center Hospitals

Program Director:
Andrew W Sukiennik, MD
New England Med Ctr
Dept of Anesthesia/Box 298
750 Washington St
Boston, MA 02111
Tel: 617 636-6044 *Fax:* 617 636-8384
E-mail: andrew.sukiennik@es.nemc.org
Internet: http://www.nemc.org/anes/painmgt.htm
Accred Length: 1 Year *Program Size:* 4
Program ID: 048-24-21-091

Springfield

Baystate Medical Center Program

Sponsor: Baystate Medical Center

Program Director:
Robert B Steinberg, PhD MD
Baystate Med Ctr
Dept of Anesthesiology
759 Chestnut St
Springfield, MA 01199
Tel: 413 794-4326 *Fax:* 413 794-5349
E-mail: kristen.kolb@bhs.org
Internet: http://www.baystatehealth.com
Accred Length: 1 Year *Program Size:* 3
Program ID: 048-24-31-011

Worcester

University of Massachusetts Program

Sponsor: University of Massachusetts Medical School
Health Alliance Hospital-Leominster
UMass Memorial Health Care (University Campus)

Program Director:
Donald S Stevens, MD
Univ of Massachusetts Med Sch
Dept of Anesthesia
55 Lake Ave N
Worcester, MA 01655
Tel: 508 856-2640
E-mail: donald.stevens@banyan.ummed.edu
Accred Length: 1 Year *Program Size:* 2
Program ID: 048-24-21-079

Michigan

Ann Arbor

University of Michigan Program

Sponsor: University of Michigan Hospitals

Program Director:
Vildan Mullin, MD
Univ of Michigan Health System
1500 E Medical Center Dr
C223 Med Inn Bldg
Ann Arbor, MI 48109-0824
Tel: 734 763-5459 *Fax:* 734 936-6585
Accred Length: 1 Year *Program Size:* 5
Program ID: 048-25-31-065

Detroit

Henry Ford Hospital Program

Sponsor: Henry Ford Hospital

Program Director:
Vikas Shah, MD
Henry Ford Hospital
2799 W Grand Blvd
Detroit, MI 48202
Tel: 313 916-8234 *Fax:* 313 876-8023
Accred Length: 1 Year *Program Size:* 3
Program ID: 048-25-21-061

Minnesota

Rochester

Mayo Graduate School of Medicine (Rochester) Program

Sponsor: Mayo Graduate School of Medicine-Mayo Foundation
Mayo Clinic (Rochester)
Rochester Methodist Hospital
St Mary's Hospital of Rochester

Program Director:
Jack L Wilson, MD
Mayo Clinic
St Mary's/Mary Brigh/Rm 2-500
Rochester, MN 55905
Tel: 507 284-4331 *Fax:* 507 284-0999
E-mail: mgsm.roch.mn.anesthesiology@mayo.edu
Internet: http://www.mayo.edu/
Accred Length: 1 Year *Program Size:* 4
Program ID: 048-26-21-012

Mississippi

Jackson

University of Mississippi Medical Center Program

Sponsor: University of Mississippi School of Medicine
University Hospital

Program Director:
Sarah H Hines, MD
2500 N State St
Dept of Anesthesiology
Jackson, MS 39216
Tel: 601 984-5950 *Fax:* 601 984-5939
E-mail: shines@anesthesia.umsmed.edu
Accred Length: 1 Year *Program Size:* 1
Program ID: 048-27-21-104

Missouri

St Louis

Washington University/B-JH/SLCH Consortium Program

Sponsor: Washington University/B-JH/SLCH Consortium
Barnes-Jewish Hospital
St Louis Children's Hospital

Program Director:
Robert A Swarm, MD
Washington Univ Sch of Med
660 S Euclid Ave
Campus Box 8054
St Louis, MO 63110-1093
Tel: 314 747-0202 *Fax:* 314 362-9471
E-mail: swarmr @ msnotes.wustl.edu
Accred Length: 1 Year *Program Size:* 2
Program ID: 048-28-21-013

Nebraska

Omaha

University of Nebraska Program

Sponsor: University of Nebraska Medical Center

Program Director:
Christopher M Criscuolo, MD
984455 Nebraska Med Ctr
Omaha, NE 68198-4455
Tel: 402 559-7405 *Fax:* 402 559-7372
E-mail: ccriscuo@unmc.edu
Accred Length: 1 Year *Program Size:* 2
Program ID: 048-30-21-100

New Hampshire

Lebanon

Dartmouth-Hitchcock Medical Center Program

Sponsor: Mary Hitchcock Memorial Hospital

Program Director:
Gilbert J Fanciullo, MD MS
Dartmouth-Hitchcock Med Ctr
One Medical Center Dr
Lebanon, NH 03756
Tel: 603 650-6040 *Fax:* 603 650-8199
E-mail: gilbert.j.fanciullo@hitchcock.org
Internet:
http://www.hitchcock.org/pages/anes/deptofanes.html
Accred Length: 1 Year *Program Size:* 2
Program ID: 048-32-21-044

New Jersey

Newark

UMDNJ-New Jersey Medical School Program

Sponsor: UMDNJ-New Jersey Medical School
UMDNJ-University Hospital

Program Director:
Wen-hsien Wu, MD MS
UMDNJ-New Jersey Med Sch
Dept of Anesthesiology
185 S Orange Ave/MSB E-538
Newark, NJ 07103-2714
Tel: 973 972-2080 *Fax:* 973 972-4172
E-mail: liuph@umdnj.edu
Accred Length: 1 Year *Program Size:* 2
Program ID: 048-33-21-014

Piscataway

UMDNJ-Robert Wood Johnson Medical School Program

Sponsor: UMDNJ-Robert Wood Johnson Medical School
Robert Wood Johnson University Hospital

Program Director:
Young Choi, MD
Clinical Academic Bldg
125 Paterson St/Ste 6100
New Brunswick, NJ 08901-1977
Tel: 732 235-6444 *Fax:* 732 235-6432
E-mail: choiyo@umdnj.edu
Internet: http://www2.umdnj.edu/pappde/watchfire.htm
Accred Length: 1 Year *Program Size:* 3
Program ID: 048-33-21-063

New Mexico

Albuquerque

University of New Mexico Program

Sponsor: University of New Mexico School of Medicine
University Hospital
Veterans Affairs Medical Center (Albuquerque)

Program Director:
Stephen E Abram, MD
2211 Lomas Blvd NE
Albuquerque, NM 87106
Tel: 505 272-2611 *Fax:* 505 272-1300
Internet:
http://macbeth.unm.edu/som/gme/anesthesiology.html
Accred Length: 1 Year *Program Size:* 2
Program ID: 048-34-21-015

New York

Albany

Albany Medical Center Program

Sponsor: Albany Medical Center

Program Director:
Howard S Smith, MD
Albany Med Coll
Dept of Anesth (PMP)/A-131
47 New Scotland Ave
Albany, NY 12208
Tel: 518 262-4302 *Fax:* 518 262-4736
E-mail: kushniv@mail.amc.edu
Accred Length: 1 Year *Program Size:* 1
Program ID: 048-35-21-016

Bronx

Albert Einstein College of Medicine Program

Sponsor: Albert Einstein College of Medicine of Yeshiva University
Montefiore Medical Center-Henry and Lucy Moses Division
Montefiore Medical Center-Weiler Hospital

Program Director:
Carole W Agin, MD
Montefiore Med Ctr
111 E 210th St
Bronx, NY 10467-0467
Tel: 718 920-5868 *Fax:* 718 547-4641
E-mail: cagin@montefiore.org
Accred Length: 1 Year *Program Size:* 3
Program ID: 048-35-21-062

Brooklyn

Brookdale University Hospital Medical Center Program

Sponsor: Brookdale University Hospital Medical Center

Program Director:
Michael Dibawy, MD
Dept of Anesth/Pain Management
Brookdale Hospital Med Ctr
1 Brookdale Plaza
Brooklyn, NY 11212
Tel: 718 240-5356 *Fax:* 718 240-5367
Accred Length: 1 Year *Program Size:* 1
Program ID: 048-35-21-060

Programs

SUNY Health Science Center at Brooklyn Program
Sponsor: SUNY Health Science Center at Brooklyn
Kings County Hospital Center
Long Island College Hospital
University Hospital-SUNY Health Science Center at Brooklyn
Program Director:
Ravi Venkataraman, MD
SUNY Health Science Ctr
450 Clarkson Ave
Brooklyn, NY 11203
Tel: 718 270-1525 *Fax:* 718 270-3928
Accred Length: 1 Year *Program Size:* 3
Program ID: 048-35-31-056

Buffalo

SUNY at Buffalo Graduate Medical-Dental Education Consortium Program
Sponsor: SUNY at Buffalo Grad Medical-Dental Education Consortium
CGF Health System (Buffalo General Hospital)
Roswell Park Cancer Institute
Program Director:
Mark J Lema, MD PhD
Dept of Anesthesiology
BGH-Hamlin House
100 High St
Buffalo, NY 14203
Tel: 716 859-4525 *Fax:* 716 859-4529
E-mail: brozanski@ubmedd.buffalo.edu
Internet: http://www.wings.buffalo.edu/smbs/anest
Accred Length: 1 Year *Program Size:* 3
Program ID: 048-35-31-017

New York

Mount Sinai School of Medicine Program
Sponsor: Mount Sinai School of Medicine
Mount Sinai Medical Center
Program Director:
Joel M Kreitzer, MD
Mount Sinai Hospital
Box 1192
One Gustave L Levy Pl
New York, NY 10029-6574
Tel: 212 241-6372 *Fax:* 212 348-8695
E-mail: joel_kreitzer@smtplink.mssm.edu
Internet: http://www.mssm.edu/anesthesia
Accred Length: 1 Year *Program Size:* 5
Program ID: 048-35-31-066

New York and Presbyterian Hospital (Columbia Campus) Program
Sponsor: New York and Presbyterian Hospital
New York and Presbyterian Hospital (Columbia Campus)
Program Director:
Richard N Siegfried, MD
622 W 168th St
PH5-500
New York, NY 10032-3784
Tel: 212 305-7114 *Fax:* 212 305-8883
Internet: http://columbia.edu
Accred Length: 1 Year *Program Size:* 1
Program ID: 048-35-31-085

New York and Presbyterian Hospital (Cornell Campus) Program
Sponsor: New York and Presbyterian Hospital
Memorial Sloan-Kettering Cancer Center
New York and Presbyterian Hospital (Cornell Campus)
Program Director:
Subhash Jain, MD
Memorial Sloan-Kettering Cancer Ctr
1275 York Ave
New York, NY 10021
Tel: 212 639-6851 *Fax:* 212 717-3206
E-mail: jains@mskcc.org
Accred Length: 1 Year *Program Size:* 4
Program ID: 048-35-11-073

New York and Presbyterian Hospital (Cornell Campus) Program
Sponsor: New York and Presbyterian Hospital
New York and Presbyterian Hospital (Cornell Campus)
Program Director:
Howard L Rosner, MD
New York Presbyterian Hospital
Dept of Anesthesiology
525 E 68th St/M-0026
New York, NY 10021
Tel: 212 746-2960 *Fax:* 212 746-2023
E-mail: hlrosner@mail.med.cornell.edu
Accred Length: 1 Year *Program Size:* 4
Program ID: 048-35-21-049

New York Medical College at St Vincent's Hospital and Medical Center of New York Program
Sponsor: New York Medical College
St Vincent's Hospital and Medical Center of New York
Program Director:
John M Stamatos, MD
St Vincent's Hospital and Med Ctr
Nurses's Residence/Rm 408
153 W 11th St
New York, NY 10011
Tel: 212 604-7566 *Fax:* 212 604-2637
Internet: http://www.pain-center.com
Accred Length: 1 Year *Program Size:* 2
Program ID: 048-35-21-070

New York University Medical Center Program
Sponsor: New York University Medical Center
Program Director:
Michel Y Dubois, MD
New York Univ Med Ctr
530 1st Ave/Ste 9T
New York, NY 10016
Tel: 212 263-7316 *Fax:* 212 263-7901
E-mail: mdubois@anes.med.nyu.edu
Internet: http://mcrcr4.med.nyu.edu/painmanagement/
Accred Length: 1 Year *Program Size:* 3
Program ID: 048-35-21-084

St Luke's-Roosevelt Hospital Center Program
Sponsor: St Luke's-Roosevelt Hospital Center
Program Director:
Ronny Hertz, MD
St Luke's-Roosevelt Hospital Ctr
Dept of Anesthesiology
1000 Tenth Ave
New York, NY 10019
Tel: 212 523-6357 *Fax:* 212 523-6217
Internet:
http://www.docnet.org/dept/anesthesia/pain.html
Accred Length: 1 Year *Program Size:* 2
Program ID: 048-35-11-018

Rochester

University of Rochester Program
Sponsor: Strong Memorial Hospital of the University of Rochester
Monroe Community Hospital
Program Director:
Frederick M Perkins, MD
Univ of Rochester Med Ctr
Dept of Anesth/Box 604
601 Elmwood Ave
Rochester, NY 14642
Tel: 716 275-2141 *Fax:* 716 244-7271
Accred Length: 1 Year *Program Size:* 3
Program ID: 048-35-21-051

Stony Brook

SUNY at Stony Brook Program
Sponsor: University Hospital-SUNY at Stony Brook
Program Director:
Farrokh R Maneksha, MD
Health Science Ctr
SUNY-Stony Brook/L4-060
Stony Brook, NY 11794-8480
Tel: 516 444-2975 *Fax:* 516 444-2907
Accred Length: 1 Year *Program Size:* 1
Program ID: 048-35-11-067

Syracuse

SUNY Health Science Center at Syracuse Program
Sponsor: University Hospital-SUNY Health Science Center at Syracuse
Veterans Affairs Medical Center (Syracuse)
Program Director:
P Sebastian Thomas, MD
SUNY Health Science Ctr-Syracuse
750 E Adams St
WKH/Rm 1219
Syracuse, NY 13210
Tel: 315 464-4259 *Fax:* 315 464-4905
E-mail: sopchak@vax.cs.hscsyr.edu
Internet: http://www.hscsyr.edu
Accred Length: 1 Year *Program Size:* 3
Program ID: 048-35-21-092

Valhalla

New York Medical College at Westchester Medical Center Program
Sponsor: New York Medical College
Lincoln Medical and Mental Health Center
St Agnes Hospital
Westchester Medical Center
Program Director:
Gregory Kizelshteyn, MD
New York Med Coll
Dept of Anesthesiology/Rm 2395
Grasslands Rd/Macy West Pavilion
Valhalla, NY 10595
Tel: 914 483-7692 *Fax:* 914 493-7927
E-mail: elizabeth frost@nymc.edu
Internet: http://www.nymc.edu
Accred Length: 1 Year *Program Size:* 2
Program ID: 048-35-32-019

North Carolina

Chapel Hill

University of North Carolina Hospitals Program

Sponsor: University of North Carolina Hospitals

Program Director:
William S Blau, MD PhD
Univ of North Carolina Hospitals
223 Burnett-Womack Bldg/CB7010
Chapel Hill, NC 27599-7010
Tel: 919 966-3371, ext 228 *Fax:* 919 966-7006
E-mail: bblau@aims.unc.edu
Internet:
http://www.aims.unc.edu/dept/fellowships/pain/painman.html
Accred Length: 1 Year *Program Size:* 2
Program ID: 048-36-21-088

Durham

Duke University Program

Sponsor: Duke University Medical Center
Veterans Affairs Medical Center (Durham)

Program Director:
Joel Goldberg, MD
Duke Univ Med Ctr
Dept of Anesthesiology
Box 3094
Durham, NC 27710
Tel: 919 684-6542 *Fax:* 919 681-8398
Accred Length: 1 Year *Program Size:* 1
Program ID: 048-36-21-020

Winston-Salem

Wake Forest University School of Medicine Program

Sponsor: Wake Forest University Baptist Medical Center

Program Director:
Richard L Rauck, MD
Pain Control Ctr
Medical Center Blvd
Winston-Salem, NC 27157-1077
Tel: 336 716-5530 *Fax:* 336 716-5537
E-mail: rrack@bgsm.edu
Accred Length: 1 Year *Program Size:* 4
Program ID: 048-36-21-036

Ohio

Cincinnati

University Hospital/University of Cincinnati College of Medicine Program

Sponsor: University Hospital Inc
Children's Hospital Medical Center

Program Director:
Karen Krone, MD
231 Bethesda Ave
PO Box 670531
Cincinnati, OH 45267-0531
Tel: 513 558-4194 *Fax:* 513 558-0995
E-mail: fischecg@email.uc.edu
Internet:
http://www.med.uc.edu/htdocs/medicine/anesthesia/index.htm
Accred Length: 1 Year *Program Size:* 5
Program ID: 048-38-21-021

Cleveland

Case Western Reserve University Program

Sponsor: University Hospitals of Cleveland

Program Director:
Mark V Boswell, MD PhD
Dept of Anesthesiology
Univ Hospitals
11100 Euclid Ave
Cleveland, OH 44106
Tel: 216 844-3771 *Fax:* 216 844-8593
E-mail: mvb2@po.cwru.edu
Internet: http://www.anesth.com
Accred Length: 1 Year *Program Size:* 2
Program ID: 048-38-21-097

Cleveland Clinic Foundation Program

Sponsor: Cleveland Clinic Foundation

Program Director:
Nagy A Mekhail, MD PhD
Cleveland Clinic Foundation
Pain Management Ctr/C25
9500 Euclid Ave
Cleveland, OH 44195
Tel: 216 444-3769 *Fax:* 216 444-9248
E-mail: omabegb@cesmtp.ccf.org
Internet: http://www.anesthesia.ccf.org
Accred Length: 1 Year *Program Size:* 10
Program ID: 048-38-31-022

Columbus

Ohio State University Program

Sponsor: Ohio State University Medical Center

Program Director:
Rao P Lingam, MD
N416 Doan Hall
410 W 10th Ave
Columbus, OH 43210
Tel: 614 293-8487 *Fax:* 614 293-8153
Accred Length: 1 Year *Program Size:* 3
Program ID: 048-38-21-048

Toledo

Medical College of Ohio Program

Sponsor: Medical College of Ohio
Flower Hospital
Medical College of Ohio Hospital

Program Director:
Marc Huntoon, MD
3000 Arlington Ave
Toledo, OH 43614-2598
Tel: 419 383-3556 *Fax:* 419 383-3550
Accred Length: 1 Year *Program Size:* 2
Program ID: 048-38-21-071

Oklahoma

Oklahoma City

University of Oklahoma Health Sciences Center Program

Sponsor: University of Oklahoma College of Medicine
Children's Hospital of Oklahoma
Veterans Affairs Medical Center (Oklahoma City)

Program Director:
Badie S Mansour, MD
Univ of Oklahoma Health Sciences Ctr
PO Box 53188
Oklahoma City, OK 73152-3188
Tel: 405 271-4354 *Fax:* 405 271-1216
Accred Length: 1 Year *Program Size:* 1
Program ID: 048-39-21-087

Oregon

Portland

Oregon Health Sciences University Program

Sponsor: Oregon Health Sciences University Hospital
Veterans Affairs Medical Center (Portland)

Program Director:
Harry G Kingston, MB BCh MBA
Oregon Health Sciences Univ
Dept of Anesth UHS-2
3181 SW Sam Jackson Park Rd
Portland, OR 97201-3098
Tel: 503 494-7641 *Fax:* 503 494-4588
Accred Length: 1 Year *Program Size:* 1
Program ID: 048-40-21-023

Pennsylvania

Hershey

Penn State Geisinger Health System/Milton S Hershey Medical Center Program

Sponsor: Penn State Geisinger Health System
Milton S Hershey Medical Center

Program Director:
Philip D Lumb, MB BS
Penn State Univ-Hershey Med Ctr
Dept of Anesthesia/H187
500 University Dr
Hershey, PA 17033
Tel: 800 206-7718 *Fax:* 717 531-6221
Internet: http://www.anes.hmc.psu.edu
Accred Length: 1 Year *Program Size:* 3
Program ID: 048-41-21-024

Philadelphia

Temple University Program

Sponsor: Temple University Hospital

Program Director:
Timothy O'Grady, MD
3401 N Broad St
Philadelphia, PA 19140
Tel: 215 707-1407 *Fax:* 215 707-8298
Accred Length: 1 Year *Program Size:* 2
Program ID: 048-41-31-025

Thomas Jefferson University Program

Sponsor: Thomas Jefferson University Hospital

Program Director:
Evan D Frank, MD PhD
Thomas Jefferson Univ
Jefferson Pain Ctr
834 Chestnut St/Ste T150
Philadelphia, PA 19107-5127
Tel: 215 955-7246 *Fax:* 215 923-5086
Internet:
http://jeffline.tju.edu/cwis/dept/anesthesiology/pain/painmain.html
Accred Length: 1 Year *Program Size:* 4
Program ID: 048-41-21-041

University of Pennsylvania Program
Sponsor: Hospital of the University of Pennsylvania
Children's Hospital of Philadelphia
Veterans Affairs Medical Center (Philadelphia)
Program Director:
F Michael Ferrante, MD
Univ of Pennsylvania
Dept of Anesthesiology
3400 Spruce St
Philadelphia, PA 19104-4283
Tel: 215 662-3742 *Fax:* 215 349-8133
E-mail: apfeifer@mail.med.upenn.edu
Accred Length: 1 Year *Program Size:* 4
Program ID: 048-41-11-026

Pittsburgh

Allegheny General Hospital Program
Sponsor: Allegheny General Hospital
Program Director:
Lynn R Johnson, MD
Allegheny General Hospital
Dept of Anesthesia
320 E North Ave
Pittsburgh, PA 15212
Tel: 412 359-3155 *Fax:* 412 359-3483
Internet:
http://www.wizard.asri.edu/aghanes/brochure/contac/html
Accred Length: 1 Year *Program Size:* 2
Program ID: 048-41-21-058

University Health Center of Pittsburgh Program
Sponsor: University Health Center of Pittsburgh
Presbyterian University Hospital/UPMC
Program Director:
Doris K Cope, MD MS
UPMC Health System
UPMC Shadyside
5200 Centre Ave/Ste 415
Pittsburgh, PA 15232
Tel: 412 623-1204 *Fax:* 412 623-1262
E-mail: bloomber@smtp.anes.upmc.edu
Internet: http://www.anes.upmc.edu
Accred Length: 1 Year *Program Size:* 6
Program ID: 048-41-32-027

South Carolina

Charleston

Medical University of South Carolina Program
Sponsor: Medical University of South Carolina College of Medicine
MUSC Medical Center
Program Director:
Jeffrey W Folk, MD
Med Univ of South Carolina
525 Children's Hospital
171 Ashley Ave
Charleston, SC 29425-2207
Tel: 843 792-2322 *Fax:* 843 792-2726
Internet: http://www.musc.com/ane/index.htm
Accred Length: 1 Year *Program Size:* 3
Program ID: 048-45-21-074

Tennessee

Nashville

Vanderbilt University Program
Sponsor: Vanderbilt University Medical Center
Program Director:
Benjamin W Johnson Jr, MD MBA
1211 21st Ave S
Medical Arts Bldg/Ste 324
Nashville, TN 37232-4125
Tel: 615 936-1206 *Fax:* 615 936-1198
E-mail: benjamin.johnson@mcmail.vanderbilt.edu
Accred Length: 1 Year *Program Size:* 4
Program ID: 048-47-21-038

Texas

Dallas

University of Texas Southwestern Medical School Program
Sponsor: University of Texas Southwestern Medical School
Dallas County Hospital District-Parkland Memorial Hospital
Texas Scottish Rite Hospital for Children
Zale-Lipshy University Hospital
Program Director:
Dennis F Landers, MD PhD
Univ of Texas Southwestern Med Ctr
5323 Harry Hines Blvd
Dallas, TX 75235-9068
Tel: 214 648-5411 *Fax:* 214 648-5461
Internet: http://www.swmed.edu/home_pages/anesth
Accred Length: 1 Year *Program Size:* 3
Program ID: 048-48-21-052

Galveston

University of Texas Medical Branch Hospitals Program
Sponsor: University of Texas Medical Branch Hospitals
Program Director:
Courtney G Williams, MD
Univ of Texas Med Branch
Dept of Anes/Pain Clinic
301 University Blvd
Galveston, TX 77555-0591
Tel: 409 772-1221 *Fax:* 409 772-1224
E-mail: cbreish@utmb.edu
Internet: http://www.utmb.edu
Accred Length: 1 Year *Program Size:* 1
Program ID: 048-48-21-103

Houston

Baylor College of Medicine Program
Sponsor: Baylor College of Medicine
Methodist Hospital
Program Director:
William F Childres, MD
Baylor Coll of Med
Smith Tower/Ste 1003
6550 Fannin St
Houston, TX 77030
Tel: 713 798-7356 *Fax:* 713 798-7345
E-mail: chilton@bcm.tmc.edu
Internet: http://www.bcm.tmc.edu/anesth/
Accred Length: 1 Year *Program Size:* 2
Program ID: 048-48-21-045

University of Texas at Houston (M D Anderson Cancer Center) Program
Sponsor: University of Texas Medical School at Houston
Memorial Hermann Healthcare System
University of Texas M D Anderson Cancer Center
Program Director:
Suresh K Reddy, MD
Univ of Texas-MD Anderson Ctr
1515 Holcombe Blvd
Box 42
Houston, TX 77030
Tel: 713 792-6911 *Fax:* 713 794-4590
Accred Length: 1 Year *Program Size:* 4
Program ID: 048-48-21-093

University of Texas at Houston Program
Sponsor: University of Texas Medical School at Houston
Memorial Hermann Healthcare System
Program Director:
Michelle Bricker, MD
6410 Fannin St/Ste 470
Houston, TX 77030-3003
Tel: 713 704-7246 *Fax:* 713 704-5711
Internet: http://www.-anes.uth.tmc.edu
Accred Length: 1 Year *Program Size:* 3
Program ID: 048-48-21-029

Lubbock

Texas Tech University (Lubbock) Program
Sponsor: Texas Tech University Health Sciences Center at Lubbock
University Medical Center
Program Director:
Gabor B Racz, MD
Texas Tech Univ Health Sciences Ctr
3601 4th St/Rm 1C282
Lubbock, TX 79430
Tel: 806 743-2981 *Fax:* 806 743-2984
Internet: http://www.ane001.ttuhsc.edu/
Accred Length: 1 Year *Program Size:* 4
Program ID: 048-48-21-030

San Antonio

University of Texas Health Science Center at San Antonio Program
Sponsor: University of Texas Medical School at San Antonio
Audie L Murphy Memorial Veterans Hospital (San Antonio)
University Hospital-South Texas Medical Center
Wilford Hall Medical Center (AETC)
Program Director:
Somayaji Ramamurthy, MD
Univ of Texas Health Science Ctr
Dept of Anes/Pain Management
7703 Floyd Curl Dr
San Antonio, TX 78284-7838
Tel: 210 567-4543 *Fax:* 210 567-4471
E-mail: ramamurthy@uthscsa.edu
Internet: http://www.anesthesia.uthscsa.edu
Accred Length: 1 Year *Program Size:* 2
Program ID: 048-48-31-031

Utah

Salt Lake City

University of Utah Program

Sponsor: University of Utah Medical Center
Primary Children's Medical Center

Program Director:
Michael A Ashburn, MD MPH
Dept of Anesthesiology
546 Chipeta Way/Ste 2000
Salt Lake City, UT 84108
Tel: 801 585-7690 *Fax:* 801 585-7694
E-mail: mashburn01@aol.com
Internet: http://www.med.utah.edu
Accred Length: 1 Year *Program Size:* 1
Program ID: 048-49-21-086

Vermont

Burlington

University of Vermont Program

Sponsor: Fletcher Allen Health Care

Program Director:
James P Rathmell, MD
Univ of Vermont
111 Colchester Ave
Burlington, VT 05401
Tel: 802 656-3737 *Fax:* 802 656-5324
Accred Length: 1 Year *Program Size:* 1
Program ID: 048-50-21-069

Virginia

Charlottesville

University of Virginia Program

Sponsor: University of Virginia Medical Center

Program Director:
John C Rowlingson, MD
Dept of Anesthesiology
Univ of Virginia Health Science Ctr
PO Box 10010
Charlottesville, VA 22906-0010
Tel: 804 982-4307 *Fax:* 804 982-0019
E-mail: cjc7j@virginia.edu
Internet:
http://www.med.virginia.edu/som-cl/anesth/index.html
Accred Length: 1 Year *Program Size:* 3
Program ID: 048-51-21-075

Portsmouth

Naval Medical Center (Portsmouth) Program

Sponsor: Naval Medical Center (Portsmouth)

Program Director:
Robert J Mendez, DO
Dept of Anesthesiology
620 John Paul Jones Cir
Portsmouth, VA 23708-5100
Tel: 757 398-7266
E-mail: pnh0w11@pnh10.med.navy.mil
Accred Length: 1 Year *Program Size:* 1
Program ID: 048-51-21-032
US Armed Services Program

Richmond

Medical College of Virginia/Virginia Commonwealth University Program

Sponsor: Medical College of Virginia/Virginia Commonwealth University
Medical College of Virginia Hospitals

Program Director:
Wayne Marshall, MD
Med Coll of Virginia Campus/VCU
PO Box 980459
Richmond, VA 23298-0459
Tel: 804 828-0733 *Fax:* 804 828-8682
E-mail: jdunaway@hsc.edu.vcu
Internet: http://views.vcu.edu/~aneweb
Accred Length: 1 Year *Program Size:* 3
Program ID: 048-51-31-033

Washington

Seattle

University of Washington Program

Sponsor: University of Washington School of Medicine
University of Washington Medical Center
Veterans Affairs Medical Center (Seattle)

Program Director:
Stephen H Butler, MD
Univ of Washington
Multidisciplinary Pain Ctr
4245 Roosevelt Way NE
Seattle, WA 98105-6920
Tel: 206 548-4429 *Fax:* 206 548-8776
E-mail: stress@u.washington.edu
Accred Length: 1 Year *Program Size:* 4
Program ID: 048-54-21-034

Virginia Mason Medical Center Program

Sponsor: Virginia Mason Medical Center

Program Director:
Hugh W Allen, MD
Virginia Mason Med Ctr
B2-AN
1100 Ninth Ave/PO Box 900
Seattle, WA 98111
Tel: 206 223-6980 *Fax:* 206 223-6982
Internet: http://www.vmmc.org
Accred Length: 1 Year *Program Size:* 2
Program ID: 048-54-21-053

West Virginia

Morgantown

West Virginia University Program

Sponsor: West Virginia University Hospitals

Program Director:
Lynn M Broadman, MD
2 West
Ruby Memorial Hospital
1 Stadium Dr
Morgantown, WV 26506
Tel: 304 598-6244 *Fax:* 304 598-6231
E-mail: kidpain@aol.com
Accred Length: 1 Year *Program Size:* 2
Program ID: 048-55-21-102

Wisconsin

Milwaukee

Medical College of Wisconsin Program

Sponsor: Medical College of Wisconsin Affiliated Hospitals Inc
Froedtert Memorial Lutheran Hospital

Program Director:
Quinn H Hogan, MD
Med Coll of Wisconsin
Dept of Anesthesiology
9200 W Wisconsin Ave
Milwaukee, WI 53226
Tel: 414 257-6259 *Fax:* 414 257-5454
Accred Length: 1 Year *Program Size:* 2
Program ID: 048-56-21-042

Pathology-Anatomic and Clinical

Alabama

Birmingham

Baptist Health System Program
Sponsor: Baptist Health System Inc
Birmingham Baptist Medical Center-Montclair
Birmingham Baptist Medical Center-Princeton
Program Director:
Mary Louise Guerry Force, MD
Birmingham Baptist Med Ctr-Montclair
Dept of Pathology
800 Montclair Rd
Birmingham, AL 35213
Tel: 205 592-5052 *Fax:* 205 592-5646
E-mail: debra.d.smith@bhsala.com
Internet: http://www.bhsala.com
Accred Length: 4 Years *Program Size:* 10 (*GY1:* 2)
Program ID: 300-01-21-017

University of Alabama Medical Center Program
Sponsor: University of Alabama Hospital
Veterans Affairs Medical Center (Birmingham)
Program Director:
C Bruce Alexander, MD
Univ of Alabama
Dept of Pathology/WP P220
Univ Station
Birmingham, AL 35233-7331
Tel: 205 934-4303 *Fax:* 205 934-5499
E-mail: kcoker@wp.path.uab.edu
Internet: http://www.path.uab.edu
Accred Length: 4 Years *Program Size:* 24 (*GY1:* 6)
Subspecialties: BBK, FOP, HMP, NP, PCP
Program ID: 300-01-31-018

Mobile

University of South Alabama Program
Sponsor: University of South Alabama Medical Center
Program Director:
Joseph A Tucker, MD
Univ of South Alabama Med Ctr
Dept of Pathology
2451 Fillingim St
Mobile, AL 36617
Tel: 334 471-7799 *Fax:* 334 471-7884
E-mail: jtucker@usamail.usouthal.edu
Internet: http://www.usouthal.edu
Accred Length: 4 Years *Program Size:* 12 (*GY1:* 2)
Program ID: 300-01-11-019

Arizona

Phoenix

St Joseph's Hospital and Medical Center Program
Sponsor: St Joseph's Hospital and Medical Center
Program Director:
William D Anderson, MD
St Joseph's Hospital and Med Ctr
Dept of Pathology
PO Box 2071
Phoenix, AZ 85001-2071
Tel: 602 406-6994 *Fax:* 602 406-7132
Internet: http://www.chw.edu/mha/mha.html
Accred Length: 4 Years *Program Size:* 8 (*GY1:* 1)
Program ID: 300-03-12-022

Tucson

University of Arizona Program
Sponsor: University of Arizona College of Medicine
University Medical Center
Veterans Affairs Medical Center (Tucson)
Program Director:
Richard E Sobonya, MD
Univ of Arizona Health Sciences Ctr
Dept of Pathology
1501 N Campbell Ave
Tucson, AZ 85724-5108
Tel: 520 626-3100 *Fax:* 520 626-2521
E-mail: rsobonya@umcaz.edu
Internet: http://www.ahsc.arizona.edu/pathology/
Accred Length: 4 Years *Program Size:* 13 (*GY1:* 3)
Program ID: 300-03-21-023

Arkansas

Little Rock

University of Arkansas for Medical Sciences Program
Sponsor: University of Arkansas College of Medicine
Arkansas Children's Hospital
John L McClellan Memorial Veterans Hospital
University Hospital of Arkansas
Program Director:
Aubrey J Hough Jr, MD
Univ of Arkansas for Med Sciences
Dept of Pathology
4301 W Markham St/Slot 517
Little Rock, AR 72205-7199
Tel: 501 686-5170 *Fax:* 501 296-1184
Internet: http://www.rss.uams.edu/path/home.htm
Accred Length: 4 Years *Program Size:* 16 (*GY1:* 3)
Subspecialties: FOP, HMP, PCP
Program ID: 300-04-21-024

California

Loma Linda

Loma Linda University Program
Sponsor: Loma Linda University Medical Center
Jerry L Pettis Memorial Veterans Hospital
Program Director:
Brian S Bull, MD
Loma Linda Univ Med Ctr
Dept of Pathology/Rm 2516
11234 Anderson St
Loma Linda, CA 92350
Tel: 909 824-4094 *Fax:* 909 824-4189
Accred Length: 4 Years *Program Size:* 12 (*GY1:* 3)
Program ID: 300-05-21-028

Los Angeles

Cedars-Sinai Medical Center Program
Sponsor: Cedars-Sinai Medical Center
Program Director:
Ellen B Klapper, MD
Cedars-Sinai Med Ctr
8700 Beverly Blvd
Los Angeles, CA 90048
Tel: 310 855-7469 *Fax:* 310 659-2751
Accred Length: 4 Years *Program Size:* 16 (*GY1:* 4)
Program ID: 300-05-12-030

UCLA Medical Center Program
Sponsor: UCLA School of Medicine
UCLA Medical Center
Program Director:
Scott D Nelson, MD
A2-179 Ctr for the Health Sciences
10833 Le Conte Ave
Los Angeles, CA 90095-1713
Tel: 310 794-1489 *Fax:* 310 206-5178
E-mail: snelson@pathology.medsch.ucla.edu
Internet: http://www.pathnet.medsch.ucla.edu
Accred Length: 4 Years *Program Size:* 19 (*GY1:* 3)
Subspecialties: BBK, HMP, NP, PCP
Program ID: 300-05-11-034

University of Southern California Program
Sponsor: Los Angeles County-USC Medical Center
Program Director:
Clive R Taylor, MD PhD
Los Angeles County-USC Med Ctr
1200 N State St/Rm 2900
Los Angeles, CA 90033
Tel: 323 226-7148 *Fax:* 323 226-5925
E-mail: taylor@pathfinder.hsc.usc.edu
Internet: http://www.usc.edu/hsc/medicine/pathology
Accred Length: 4 Years *Program Size:* 24 (*GY1:* 4)
Subspecialties: NP, PCP
Program ID: 300-05-21-033

VA Greater Los Angeles Healthcare System Program
Sponsor: VA Greater Los Angeles Healthcare System
UCLA Medical Center
Program Director:
Thomas M Stanley, MD
UCLA-VA Med Ctr West Los Angeles
Dept of Path/Lab Med (113)
11301 Wilshire Blvd
Los Angeles, CA 90073-1005
Tel: 310 268-3570 *Fax:* 310 268-4983
E-mail: stanley.thomas_m@west-la.va.gov
Accred Length: 4 Years *Program Size:* 8 (*GY1:* 1)
Program ID: 300-05-31-035

Orange

University of California (Irvine) Program
Sponsor: University of California (Irvine) Medical Center
Long Beach Memorial Medical Center
Veterans Affairs Medical Center (Long Beach)
Program Director:
Fritz Lin, MD
Univ of California Irvine Med Ctr
Bldg 10/Rm 101
101 City Dr S
Orange, CA 92868
Tel: 714 456-6411 *Fax:* 714 456-5873
E-mail: dlspeake@uci.edu
Internet: http://www.med.uci.edu//~path//
Accred Length: 4 Years *Program Size:* 18 (*GY1:* 2)
Subspecialties: NP
Program ID: 300-05-21-407

Sacramento

University of California (Davis) Program
Sponsor: University of California (Davis) Medical Center
David Grant Medical Center
Program Director:
Ralph Green, MD
Univ of California Davis Med Ctr
2315 Stockton Blvd
Sacramento, CA 95817
Tel: 916 734-3330 *Fax:* 916 734-0320
E-mail: ewilliam@clb.ucdmc.ucdavis.edu
Internet: http://www.pathology.ucdmc.ucdavis.edu
Accred Length: 4 Years *Program Size:* 10 (*GY1:* 2)
Program ID: 300-05-11-025

San Diego

Naval Medical Center (San Diego) Program

Sponsor: Naval Medical Center (San Diego)

Program Director:
Frank W Hall, MD
Naval Med Ctr
34800 Bob Wilson Dr
San Diego, CA 92134-5000
Tel: 619 532-9300 *Fax:* 619 532-9403
E-mail: fhall@snd10.med.navy.mil
Accred Length: 4 Years *Program Size:* 12 (*GY1:* 3)
Program ID: 300-05-12-011
US Armed Services Program

University of California (San Diego) Program

Sponsor: University of California (San Diego) Medical Center
Veterans Affairs Medical Center (San Diego)

Program Director:
David N Bailey, MD
UCSD Med Ctr
Dept of Pathology 8320
200 W Arbor Dr
San Diego, CA 92103-8320
Tel: 619 543-5966 *Fax:* 619 543-3730
E-mail: mfoberg@ucsd.edu
Accred Length: 4 Years *Program Size:* 17 (*GY1:* 4)
Program ID: 300-05-21-040

San Francisco

Kaiser Permanente Medical Group (Northern California)/San Francisco Program

Sponsor: Kaiser Permanente Medical Group (Northern California)
Kaiser Permanente Medical Center (San Francisco)
Permanente Medical Group Regional Laboratory

Program Director:
Milton L Bassis, MD
Kaiser Foundation Hospital
Dept of Pathology
350 St Joseph's St
San Francisco, CA 94115-3395
Tel: 415 202-3870 *Fax:* 415 202-3871
Accred Length: 4 Years *Program Size:* 1 (*GY1:* 0)
Program ID: 300-05-12-041

University of California (San Francisco) Program

Sponsor: University of California (San Francisco) School of Medicine
San Francisco General Hospital Medical Center
University of California (San Francisco) Medical Center
Veterans Affairs Medical Center (San Francisco)

Program Director:
Carolyn K Montgomery, MD
C Diana Nicoll, MD PhD
Univ of California San Francisco
Dept of Laboratory Med
505 Parnassus Ave
San Francisco, CA 94143-0134
Tel: 415 502-5324 *Fax:* 415 476-9625
E-mail: ushijima@labmed2.ucsf.edu
Internet: http://www.pangloss.ucsf.edu/
Accred Length: 4 Years *Program Size:* 31 (*GY1:* 7)
Subspecialties: HMP
Program ID: 300-05-21-044

Stanford

Stanford University Program

Sponsor: Stanford University Hospital
Veterans Affairs Palo Alto Health Care System

Program Director:
Klaus G Bensch, MD
Stanford Univ Sch of Med
Dept of Pathology/L-235
300 Pasteur Dr
Stanford, CA 94305-5324
Tel: 415 723-7975 *Fax:* 415 725-6902
Internet: http://pathology.stanford.edu/
Accred Length: 4 Years *Program Size:* 26 (*GY1:* 7)
Program ID: 300-05-21-046

Torrance

Los Angeles County-Harbor-UCLA Medical Center Program

Sponsor: Los Angeles County-Harbor-UCLA Medical Center

Program Director:
Marcia E Cornford, MD
Harbor-UCLA Med Ctr
Dept of Pathology
1000 W Carson St
Torrance, CA 90509-2510
Tel: 310 222-2632 *Fax:* 310 222-5333
Accred Length: 4 Years *Program Size:* 15 (*GY1:* 5)
Subspecialties: BBK
Program ID: 300-05-11-047

Colorado

Colorado Springs

Penrose-St Francis Healthcare System Program

Sponsor: Penrose-St Francis Healthcare System

Program Director:
Tobias Kircher, MD
Penrose Hospital
Dept of Pathology
PO Box 7021
Colorado Springs, CO 80933
Tel: 719 776-5816 *Fax:* 719 776-2108
Accred Length: 4 Years *Program Size:* 6 (*GY1:* 2)
Program ID: 300-07-12-048

Denver

University of Colorado Program

Sponsor: University of Colorado Health Sciences Center
Denver Health and Hospitals
Veterans Affairs Medical Center (Denver)

Program Director:
Hannis W Thompson, MD
Univ of Colorado Health Sciences Ctr
Dept of Pathology Box B216
4200 E Ninth Ave
Denver, CO 80262
Tel: 303 315-7636 *Fax:* 303 315-6795
E-mail: hannis.thompson@uchsc.edu
Internet: http://www.uchsc.edu/sm/patholog/
Accred Length: 4 Years *Program Size:* 21 (*GY1:* 4)
Program ID: 300-07-21-055

Connecticut

Danbury

Danbury Hospital Program

Sponsor: Danbury Hospital

Program Director:
Ramon N Kranwinkel, MD
Danbury Hospital
Dept of Pathology
24 Hospital Ave
Danbury, CT 06810
Tel: 203 797-7338 *Fax:* 203 731-5343
E-mail: kranwinr@danhosp.org
Accred Length: 4 Years *Program Size:* 7 (*GY1:* 2)
Program ID: 300-08-11-057

Hartford

Hartford Hospital Program

Sponsor: Hartford Hospital

Program Director:
William T Pastuszak, MD
Hartford Hospital
80 Seymour St
PO Box 5037
Hartford, CT 06102-5037
Tel: 860 545-2249 *Fax:* 860 545-2204
Accred Length: 4 Years *Program Size:* 12 (*GY1:* 2)
Subspecialties: BBK, HMP, MM, PCP
Program ID: 300-08-11-059

New Haven

Yale-New Haven Medical Center Program

Sponsor: Yale-New Haven Hospital
Veterans Affairs Medical Center (West Haven)

Program Director:
Jose Costa, MD
Yale-New Haven Med Ctr
Dept of Pathology/PO Box 208070
310 Cedar St
New Haven, CT 06520-8070
Tel: 203 785-5803 *Fax:* 203 785-3585
E-mail: jose.costa@yale.edu
Internet: http://www.info.med.yale.edu/pathol/
Accred Length: 4 Years *Program Size:* 26 (*GY1:* 6)
Subspecialties: MM
Program ID: 300-08-21-062

District of Columbia

Washington

George Washington University Program

Sponsor: George Washington University School of Medicine
George Washington University Hospital (UHS)
Veterans Affairs Medical Center (Washington, DC)

Program Director:
Herschel Sidransky, MD
George Washington Univ Med Ctr
2300 Eye St NW
Ross Hall/Rm 502
Washington, DC 20037
Tel: 202 994-3391 *Fax:* 202 944-2618
Internet: http://www.gwumc.edu/dept/path
Accred Length: 4 Years *Program Size:* 14 (*GY1:* 2)
Subspecialties: PCP
Program ID: 300-10-31-069

Programs

Georgetown University Program
Sponsor: Georgetown University Medical Center
Program Director:
Adam Bagg, MD
Alfred B Jenson, MD
Georgetown Univ Med Ctr
Rm 118 Basic Science Bldg
3900 Reservoir Rd NW
Washington, DC 20007-2197
Tel: 202 687-1294 *Fax:* 202 687-7078
E-mail: smithtm@gunet.georgetown.edu
Internet:
http://www.dml.georgetown.edu/depts/pathology/
Accred Length: 4 Years *Program Size:* 12 (*GY1:* 4)
Subspecialties: BBK
Program ID: 300-10-11-068

Howard University Program
Sponsor: Howard University Hospital
Program Director:
Josephine J Marshalleck, MD
Howard Univ Hospital
Dept of Pathology
2041 Georgia Ave NW
Washington, DC 20060
Tel: 202 806-6306 *Fax:* 202 806-7022
Accred Length: 4 Years *Program Size:* 8 (*GY1:* 2)
Program ID: 300-10-21-070

Washington Hospital Center Program
Sponsor: Washington Hospital Center
Program Director:
Mary E Kass, MD
Washington Hospital Center
Dept of Pathology
110 Irving St NW
Washington, DC 20010-2975
Tel: 202 877-6190 *Fax:* 202 877-3820
Accred Length: 4 Years *Program Size:* 9 (*GY1:* 2)
Program ID: 300-10-12-071

Florida

Gainesville

University of Florida Program
Sponsor: University of Florida College of Medicine
Shands Hospital at the University of Florida
Veterans Affairs Medical Center (Gainesville)
Program Director:
William E Winter, MD MD
Univ of Florida Coll of Med
Box 100275
1600 SW Archer Rd
Gainesville, FL 32610-0275
Tel: 352 392-4053 *Fax:* 352 392-6249
E-mail: winter.pathology@mail.health.ufl.edu
Internet: http://www.med.ufl.edu/path/homepage/htw
Accred Length: 4 Years *Program Size:* 11 (*GY1:* 1)
Subspecialties: HMP, PCP
Program ID: 300-11-21-073

Jacksonville

University of Florida Health Science Center/Jacksonville Program
Sponsor: University of Florida College of Medicine at Jacksonville
University Medical Center (UFHSC/J)
Program Director:
Shahla Masood, MD
Ronald M Rhatigan, MD
Univ of Florida Health Science Ctr-Jacksonville
Dept of Pathology
655 W Eighth St
Jacksonville, FL 32209-6511
Tel: 904 549-4387 *Fax:* 904 549-4060
E-mail: sm.umc5@mail.health.ufl.edu
Internet: http://www.ufhscj.edu/path/index.html
Accred Length: 4 Years *Program Size:* 8 (*GY1:* 0)
Subspecialties: PCP
Program ID: 300-11-31-074

Miami

University of Miami-Jackson Memorial Medical Center Program
Sponsor: University of Miami-Jackson Memorial Medical Center
Veterans Affairs Medical Center (Miami)
Program Director:
Gerald E Byrne Jr, MD
Dept of Pathology
Jackson Memorial Hospital
1611 NW 12th Ave/East Tower Rm 2053
Miami, FL 33136
Tel: 305 585-7242 *Fax:* 305 324-9932
E-mail: gbyrne@newssun.med.miami.edu
Internet: http://pat.med.miami.edu
Accred Length: 4 Years *Program Size:* 18 (*GY1:* 3)
Subspecialties: PCP, PIP
Program ID: 300-11-21-075

Miami Beach

Mount Sinai Medical Center of Greater Miami Program
Sponsor: Mount Sinai Medical Center of Greater Miami
Program Director:
Morton J Robinson, MD
Mount Sinai Med Ctr
Dept of Pathology
4300 Alton Rd
Miami Beach, FL 33140
Tel: 305 674-2277 *Fax:* 305 674-2999
Internet: http://www.mountsinaimiami.org
Accred Length: 4 Years *Program Size:* 8 (*GY1:* 2)
Program ID: 300-11-31-076

Orlando

Orlando Regional Healthcare System Program
Sponsor: Orlando Regional Medical Center
Program Director:
Gary S Pearl, MD PhD
Orlando Regional Healthcare System
Dept of Pathology
1414 Kuhl Ave
Orlando, FL 32806
Tel: 407 841-5217 *Fax:* 407 843-2447
Accred Length: 4 Years *Program Size:* 12 (*GY1:* 4)
Program ID: 300-11-12-077

Tampa

University of South Florida Program
Sponsor: University of South Florida College of Medicine
H Lee Moffitt Cancer Center
James A Haley Veterans Hospital
Tampa General Healthcare
Program Director:
Philip R Foulis, MD
Jane L Messina, MD
Univ of South Florida Coll of Med
Dept of Path/Lab Med
12901 Bruce B Downs Blvd/Box 11
Tampa, FL 33612-4799
Tel: 813 972-2000, ext 6468 *Fax:* 813 974-5536
E-mail: pfoulis@coml.med.usf.edu
Accred Length: 4 Years *Program Size:* 18 (*GY1:* 3)
Subspecialties: PCP, PP
Program ID: 300-11-31-078

Georgia

Atlanta

Emory University Program
Sponsor: Emory University School of Medicine
Emory University Hospital
Grady Memorial Hospital
Veterans Affairs Medical Center (Atlanta)
Program Director:
C Whitaker Sewell, MD
Emory Univ Sch of Med
Emory Univ Hospital/Rm H-189
1364 Clifton Rd NE
Atlanta, GA 30322-8110
Tel: 404 727-4283 *Fax:* 404 727-2519
E-mail: aboyett@emory.edu
Internet: http://www.emory.edu/pathology/residency/
Accred Length: 4 Years *Program Size:* 45 (*GY1:* 6)
Subspecialties: BBK, DMP, PCP, PP
Program ID: 300-12-21-080

Augusta

Medical College of Georgia Program
Sponsor: Medical College of Georgia Hospital and Clinics
Veterans Affairs Medical Center (Augusta)
Program Director:
D Greer Falls III, MD
Med Coll of Georgia
1120 15th St (BAE-104)
Augusta, GA 30912
Tel: 706 721-7453 *Fax:* 706 721-2358
E-mail: gfalls@mail.mcg.edu
Accred Length: 4 Years *Program Size:* 12 (*GY1:* 4)
Subspecialties: BBK
Program ID: 300-12-21-082

Hawaii

Honolulu

University of Hawaii Program

Sponsor: University of Hawaii John A Burns School of Medicine
Kaiser Foundation Hospital (Moanalua)
Queen's Medical Center
St Francis Medical Center
Tripler Army Medical Center

Program Director:
John M Hardman, MD
Univ of Hawaii Integrated Pathology Residency
1960 East-West Rd
Biomed Tower 512-B
Honolulu, HI 96822
Tel: 808 956-8970 *Fax:* 808 956-5465
E-mail: bohlem@jabsom.biomed.hawaii.edu
Internet:
http://www.medworld.biomed.hawaii.edu/hrp.html
Accred Length: 4 Years *Program Size:* 11 (*GY1:* 3)
Program ID: 300-14-21-085

Illinois

Chicago

Cook County Hospital Program

Sponsor: Cook County Hospital
Mount Sinai Hospital Medical Center of Chicago

Program Director:
Bourke L Firfer, MD
Cook County Hospital
Hektoen Bldg
627 S Wood St/Hekteon Bldg Rm 411
Chicago, IL 60612
Tel: 312 633-3144 *Fax:* 312 633-7154
E-mail: blfmdms@pol.net
Accred Length: 4 Years *Program Size:* 7 (*GY1:* 0)
Program ID: 300-16-21-088

McGaw Medical Center of Northwestern University Program

Sponsor: Northwestern University Medical School
Children's Memorial Medical Center
Northwestern Memorial Hospital
Veterans Affairs Lakeside Medical Center (Chicago)

Program Director:
G Kenneth Haines III, MD
Northwestern Univ Med Sch
Pathology Dept/Ward 6-204
303 E Chicago Ave
Chicago, IL 60611-3008
Tel: 312 908-7572 *Fax:* 312 908-3127
E-mail: gkhainesiii@nwu.edu
Accred Length: 4 Years *Program Size:* 20 (*GY1:* 4)
Subspecialties: HMP, MM
Program ID: 300-16-21-094

Rush-Presbyterian-St Luke's Medical Center Program

Sponsor: Rush-Presbyterian-St Luke's Medical Center

Program Director:
Melvin M Schwartz, MD
Rush-Presbyterian-St Luke's Med Ctr
1653 W Congress Pkwy
Chicago, IL 60612-3833
Tel: 312 942-5254 *Fax:* 312 942-4228
Accred Length: 4 Years *Program Size:* 16 (*GY1:* 4)
Program ID: 300-16-11-095

University of Chicago Program

Sponsor: University of Chicago Hospitals

Program Director:
Wendy Recant, MD
Univ of Chicago Hospitals
5841 S Maryland Ave/MC6101
Chicago, IL 60637-1470
Tel: 773 702-0967 *Fax:* 773 702-9903
Accred Length: 4 Years *Program Size:* 25 (*GY1:* 5)
Subspecialties: BBK, HMP, NP, PCP
Program ID: 300-16-21-097

University of Illinois College of Medicine at Chicago Metropolitan Group Hospitals Program

Sponsor: University of Illinois College of Medicine at Chicago
Illinois Masonic Medical Center
Lutheran General Hospital
Mercy Hospital and Medical Center

Program Director:
Douglas P Rhone, MD
Metropolitan Group Hospitals
836 W Wellington Ave
Rm 4813
Chicago, IL 60657-5193
Tel: 773 296-7898 *Fax:* 773 296-7444
Accred Length: 4 Years *Program Size:* 16 (*GY1:* 4)
Subspecialties: PCP
Program ID: 300-16-21-409

University of Illinois College of Medicine at Chicago Program

Sponsor: University of Illinois College of Medicine at Chicago
Michael Reese Hospital and Medical Center
University of Illinois Hospital and Clinics
Veterans Affairs West Side Medical Center

Program Director:
Wellington Jao, MD
Univ of Illinois Hospital
Dept of Pathology (M/C 847)
1819 W Polk St
Chicago, IL 60612-7335
Tel: 312 996-7312 *Fax:* 312 996-7586
Accred Length: 4 Years *Program Size:* 24 (*GY1:* 4)
Subspecialties: HMP
Program ID: 300-16-21-098

Evanston

McGaw Medical Center of Northwestern University (Evanston) Program

Sponsor: Northwestern University Medical School
Evanston Hospital

Program Director:
Karen Kaul, MD PhD
Evanston Hospital
Dept of Pathology
2650 Ridge Ave
Evanston, IL 60201-1783
Tel: 847 570-2052 *Fax:* 847 570-1938
E-mail: k-kaul@nwu.edu
Accred Length: 4 Years *Program Size:* 8 (*GY1:* 1)
Program ID: 300-16-21-412

Maywood

Loyola University Program

Sponsor: Loyola University Medical Center
Edward J Hines Jr Veterans Affairs Hospital

Program Director:
Kenneth D McClatchey, DDS MD
Loyola Univ Med Ctr
2160 S First Ave
Maywood, IL 60153
Tel: 708 216-3250 *Fax:* 708 216-8225
E-mail: mpelc@luc.edu
Internet:
http://www.meddean.luc.edu.deptwebs/pathology/pathhome.htm
Accred Length: 4 Years *Program Size:* 14 (*GY1:* 3)
Subspecialties: PCP
Program ID: 300-16-21-394

Indiana

Indianapolis

Indiana University School of Medicine Program

Sponsor: Indiana University School of Medicine
Clarian IU Hospital
Clarian Methodist Hospital of Indiana
Clarian Riley Hospital for Children
Richard L Roudebush Veterans Affairs Medical Center
William N Wishard Memorial Hospital

Program Director:
John N Eble, MD MD
Indiana Univ Sch of Med
Dept of Pathology
635 N Barnhill Dr
Indianapolis, IN 46202-5120
Tel: 317 274-1743 *Fax:* 317 278-2018
E-mail: jeble@iupui.edu
Internet: http://www.pathology.iupui.edu
Accred Length: 4 Years *Program Size:* 20 (*GY1:* 5)
Subspecialties: BBK, HMP, MM, PCP, PP
Program ID: 300-17-21-111

Muncie

Ball Memorial Hospital Program

Sponsor: Ball Memorial Hospital

Program Director:
Douglas A Triplett, MD
Ball Memorial Hospital
2401 W University Ave
Muncie, IN 47303-3499
Tel: 765 747-3246 *Fax:* 765 747-0137
E-mail: dtriplett@cami3.com
Internet: http://www.ballhospital.org
Accred Length: 4 Years *Program Size:* 13 (*GY1:* 3)
Subspecialties: TY
Program ID: 300-17-21-114

Iowa

Iowa City

University of Iowa Hospitals and Clinics Program

Sponsor: University of Iowa Hospitals and Clinics
Veterans Affairs Medical Center (Iowa City)

Program Director:
Fred Dick, MD
Univ of Iowa Hospitals and Clinics
200 Hawkins Dr
Iowa City, IA 52242-1181
Tel: 319 356-2991 *Fax:* 319 356-2243
E-mail: carla-hartl@uiowa.edu
Internet: http://www.medicine.uiowa.edu/pathology
Accred Length: 4 Years *Program Size:* 20 (*GY1:* 4)
Subspecialties: BBK, HMP, PCP, PIP
Program ID: 300-18-21-116

Kansas

Kansas City

University of Kansas Medical Center Program

Sponsor: University of Kansas School of Medicine
University of Kansas Medical Center
Veterans Affairs Medical Center (Kansas City)

Program Director:
James L Fishback, MD
Univ of Kansas Med Ctr
3901 Rainbow Blvd
Kansas City, KS 66160-7410
Tel: 913 588-7070 *Fax:* 913 588-7073
E-mail: jfishbac@kumc.edu
Internet: http://www.kumc.edu/pathology/
Accred Length: 4 Years *Program Size:* 11 (*GY1:* 3)
Program ID: 300-19-21-117

Kentucky

Lexington

University of Kentucky Medical Center Program

Sponsor: University of Kentucky Hospital
Veterans Affairs Medical Center (Lexington)

Program Director:
William O'Connor, MD
Univ of Kentucky
Dept of Pathology
800 Rose St/Ste MS117
Lexington, KY 40536-0084
Tel: 606 323-6183, ext 226 *Fax:* 606 323-2094
E-mail: woconno@pop.uky.edu
Internet:
http://www.uky.edu/medicine/departments/pathology/pathology.html
Accred Length: 4 Years *Program Size:* 13 (*GY1:* 2)
Subspecialties: PCP
Program ID: 300-20-21-120

Louisville

University of Louisville Program

Sponsor: University of Louisville School of Medicine
Kosair Children's Hospital (Alliant Health System)
Norton Hospital (Alliant Health System)
University of Louisville Hospital
Veterans Affairs Medical Center (Louisville)

Program Director:
Ronald J Elin, MD PhD
Dept of Pathology (Attn: Mary Gunter)
Sch of Med
Univ of Louisville
Louisville, KY 40292
Tel: 502 852-8203, ext 8203 *Fax:* 502 852-8299
E-mail: msdixo01@gwise.louisville.edu
Accred Length: 4 Years *Program Size:* 10 (*GY1:* 2)
Subspecialties: HMP, PCP
Program ID: 300-20-21-121

Louisiana

New Orleans

Louisiana State University Program

Sponsor: Louisiana State University School of Medicine
Medical Center of Louisiana at New Orleans
Veterans Affairs Medical Center-LSU Service (New Orleans)

Program Director:
Gary E Lipscomb, MD
Louisiana State Univ Sch of Med
Dept of Pathology Box P5-1
1901 Perdido St
New Orleans, LA 70112-1393
Tel: 504 568-6031 *Fax:* 504 568-6037
E-mail: glipsc@lsumc.edu
Internet: http://www.lsumc.edu/campus/path/
Accred Length: 4 Years *Program Size:* 12 (*GY1:* 3)
Subspecialties: BBK, FOP, PCP, PP
Program ID: 300-21-21-123

Tulane University Program

Sponsor: Tulane University School of Medicine
Medical Center of Louisiana at New Orleans

Program Director:
Krzysztof Moroz, MD
Tulane Univ Med Ctr
Dept of Pathology
1430 Tulane Ave/Rm 6519
New Orleans, LA 70112-2699
Tel: 504 588-5224 *Fax:* 504 587-7389
Accred Length: 4 Years *Program Size:* 14 (*GY1:* 3)
Subspecialties: DMP, HMP, PCP
Program ID: 300-21-21-122

Shreveport

Louisiana State University (Shreveport) Program

Sponsor: Louisiana State University Hospital-Shreveport

Program Director:
Warren D Grafton, MD
Louisiana State Univ Med Ctr Hospital
Med Educ Dept (Pathology)
1501 Kings Hwy/PO Box 33932
Shreveport, LA 71130-3932
Tel: 318 675-5865 *Fax:* 318 675-7662
Internet: http://www.softdisk.com/sites/path
Accred Length: 4 Years *Program Size:* 10 (*GY1:* 2)
Program ID: 300-21-31-126

Maryland

Baltimore

Johns Hopkins University Program

Sponsor: Johns Hopkins University School of Medicine
Johns Hopkins Hospital

Program Director:
Risa B Mann, MD
James R Eshleman, MD PhD
Johns Hopkins Hospital
Dept of Pathology
600 N Wolfe St
Baltimore, MD 21287-6417
Tel: 410 955-3439 *Fax:* 410 614-9011
E-mail: dbooton@pathlan.path.jhu.edu
Internet: http://pathology.jhu.edu
Accred Length: 4 Years *Program Size:* 30 (*GY1:* 8)
Subspecialties: BBK, NP, PCP, PIP
Program ID: 300-23-11-129

University of Maryland Program

Sponsor: University of Maryland Medical System
Veterans Affairs Medical Center (Baltimore)

Program Director:
Steven G Silverberg, MD
Univ of Maryland Med System
Dept of Pathology/Rm NBW43
22 S Greene St
Baltimore, MD 21201
Tel: 410 328-5555 *Fax:* 410 328-5508
Accred Length: 4 Years *Program Size:* 11 (*GY1:* 1)
Subspecialties: HMP
Program ID: 300-23-31-135

Bethesda

National Capital Consortium Program

Sponsor: National Capital Consortium
National Naval Medical Center (Bethesda)
Armed Forces Institute of Pathology
Walter Reed Army Medical Center

Program Director:
Michael R Henry, MD
National Naval Med Ctr
Laboratory Dept/Bldg 9
8901 Wisconsin Ave
Bethesda, MD 20889-5000
Tel: 301 295-5774 *Fax:* 301 295-1397
E-mail: bth0mrh@bth20.med.navy.mil
Accred Length: 4 Years *Program Size:* 24 (*GY1:* 6)
Program ID: 300-10-21-416
US Armed Services Program

National Institutes of Health Clinical Center Program

Sponsor: NIH Warren Grant Magnuson Clinical Center

Program Director:
Lance A Liotta, MD
Elaine S Jaffe, MD
Bldg 10/Rm 2A33
10 Center Dr
Bethesda, MD 20892
Tel: 301 496-3185 *Fax:* 301 402-0043
Accred Length: 3 Years *Program Size:* 9 (*GY1:* 3)
Program ID: 300-23-12-015

Massachusetts

Boston

Beth Israel Deaconess Medical Center/Harvard Medical School Program

Sponsor: Beth Israel Deaconess Medical Center
Lahey Clinic

Program Director:
Donald A Antonioli, MD
Beth Israel Deaconess Med Ctr-East Campus
330 Brookline Ave
Boston, MA 02215-5491
Tel: 617 667-5754 *Fax:* 617 667-7120
E-mail: dantonio@bidmc.harvard.edu
Accred Length: 4 Years *Program Size:* 29 (*GY1:* 7)
Program ID: 300-24-31-419

Boston University Medical Center Program

Sponsor: Boston Medical Center
Veterans Affairs Medical Center (Boston)

Program Director:
Carl O'Hara, MD
Boston Med Ctr-Mallory Inst of Pathology
784 Massachusetts Ave
Boston, MA 02118
Tel: 617 414-5314 *Fax:* 617 414-5315
Accred Length: 4 Years *Program Size:* 15 (*GY1:* 3)
Subspecialties: FOP, HMP, PCP
Program ID: 300-24-21-139

Brigham and Women's Hospital Program

Sponsor: Brigham and Women's Hospital
Brockton-West Roxbury Veterans Affairs Medical Center

Program Director:
Ramzi S Cotran, MD
Brigham and Women's Hospital
Dept of Pathology
75 Francis St
Boston, MA 02115
Tel: 617 732-7514 *Fax:* 617 732-7513
E-mail: rscotran@bics.bwh.harvard.edu
Accred Length: 4 Years *Program Size:* 43 (*GY1:* 8)
Subspecialties: BBK, HMP, NP, PCP
Program ID: 300-24-31-146

Massachusetts General Hospital Program

Sponsor: Massachusetts General Hospital

Program Director:
Nancy Lee Harris, MD
Massachusetts General Hospital
55 Fruit St
WRN Bldg Rm 211
Boston, MA 02114-2696
Tel: 617 726-5155 *Fax:* 617 726-7474
E-mail: harris@helix.mgh.harvard.edu
Internet: http://www.path.mgh.harvard.edu
Accred Length: 4 Years *Program Size:* 30 (*GY1:* 7)
Subspecialties: BBK, NP, PCP, PIP
Program ID: 300-24-31-143

New England Medical Center Hospitals Program

Sponsor: New England Medical Center Hospitals

Program Director:
Angelo A Ucci, MD PhD
Dept of Pathology
800 Washington St
Boston, MA 02111
Tel: 617 636-5828 *Fax:* 617 636-8302
Accred Length: 4 Years *Program Size:* 12 (*GY1:* 2)
Program ID: 300-24-21-145

Pittsfield

Berkshire Medical Center Program

Sponsor: Berkshire Medical Center

Program Director:
Rebecca L Johnson, MD
Berkshire Med Ctr
725 North St
Pittsfield, MA 01201
Tel: 413 447-2565 *Fax:* 413 447-2097
Internet: http://www.bhs1.org
Accred Length: 4 Years *Program Size:* 8 (*GY1:* 2)
Program ID: 300-24-11-153

Springfield

Baystate Medical Center Program

Sponsor: Baystate Medical Center

Program Director:
Shirin V Nash, MD
Baystate Med Ctr
Dept of Pathology
759 Chestnut St
Springfield, MA 01199
Tel: 413 794-5085 *Fax:* 413 794-5893
E-mail: csullivan@bhs.org
Internet: http://www.baystatehealth.com
Accred Length: 4 Years *Program Size:* 10 (*GY1:* 2)
Subspecialties: BBK, PCP
Program ID: 300-24-21-413

Worcester

University of Massachusetts Program

Sponsor: University of Massachusetts Medical School
UMass Memorial Health Care (Memorial Campus)
UMass Memorial Health Care (University Campus)

Program Director:
Armando E Fraire, MD
Univ of Massachusetts Med Sch
55 Lake Ave N
Worcester, MA 01655
Tel: 508 856-6491 *Fax:* 508 856-2968
Accred Length: 4 Years *Program Size:* 12 (*GY1:* 3)
Program ID: 300-24-21-400

Michigan

Ann Arbor

University of Michigan Program

Sponsor: University of Michigan Hospitals
Veterans Affairs Medical Center (Ann Arbor)

Program Director:
Joseph C Fantone III, MD
Univ of Michigan Med Sch
1500 E Medical Center Dr
2G332/Box 0054
Ann Arbor, MI 48109-0054
Tel: 313 936-1888 *Fax:* 313 763-4095
E-mail: jfantone@umich.edu
Internet: http://www.pathology.med.umich.edu
Accred Length: 4 Years *Program Size:* 25 (*GY1:* 5)
Subspecialties: NP, PCH, PCP
Program ID: 300-25-21-158

Detroit

Henry Ford Hospital Program

Sponsor: Henry Ford Hospital

Program Director:
Kenneth A Greenawald, MD
2799 W Grand Blvd
Detroit, MI 48202
Tel: 313 916-3106 *Fax:* 313 916-2385
Accred Length: 4 Years *Program Size:* 15 (*GY1:* 3)
Subspecialties: PCP
Program ID: 300-25-12-160

St John Hospital and Medical Center Program

Sponsor: St John Hospital and Medical Center

Program Director:
Bruce A Jones, MD
St John Hospital and Med Ctr
Dept of Med Educ
22101 Moross Rd
Detroit, MI 48236
Tel: 313 343-3875 *Fax:* 313 343-7840
E-mail: sue.moynihan@stjohn.org
Internet: http://www.stjohn.org
Accred Length: 4 Years *Program Size:* 10 (*GY1:* 2)
Program ID: 300-25-12-162

Wayne State University/Detroit Medical Center Program

Sponsor: Wayne State University/Detroit Medical Center
Children's Hospital of Michigan
Detroit Receiving Hospital and University Health Center
Harper Hospital
Hutzel Hospital

Program Director:
Richard Vander Heide, MD PhD
Wayne State Univ, Dept of Pathology
540 E Canfield
Detroit, MI 48201
Tel: 313 745-8555 *Fax:* 313 577-0057
E-mail: vanderheide@oncvx1.roc.wayne.edu
Internet: http://www.wayne.edu
Accred Length: 4 Years *Program Size:* 12 (*GY1:* 3)
Subspecialties: PCP, PP
Program ID: 300-25-21-165

Royal Oak

William Beaumont Hospital Program

Sponsor: William Beaumont Hospital

Program Director:
Rebecca C Hankin, MD
William Beaumont Hospital
3601 W 13 Mile Rd
Royal Oak, MI 48073
Tel: 248 551-9060 *Fax:* 248 551-9054
E-mail: rhankin@beaumont.edu
Internet: http://www.beaumont.edu/html/gme
Accred Length: 4 Years *Program Size:* 11 (*GY1:* 3)
Subspecialties: HMP, PCP
Program ID: 300-25-21-173

Programs

Minnesota

Minneapolis

Hennepin County Medical Center Program

Sponsor: Hennepin County Medical Center
Abbott-Northwestern Hospital

Program Director:
John T Crosson, MD
Hennepin County Med Ctr
701 Park Ave
Minneapolis, MN 55415-1829
Tel: 612 347-6479 *Fax:* 612 904-4282
E-mail: linda.moyer@co.hennepin.mn.us
Accred Length: 4 Years *Program Size:* 8 (*GY1:* 2)
Program ID: 300-26-21-405

University of Minnesota Program

Sponsor: University of Minnesota Medical School
Fairview-University Medical Center
Veterans Affairs Medical Center (Minneapolis)

Program Director:
Sue A Bartow, MD
Univ of Minnesota
Box 609 Mayo
420 Delaware St SE
Minneapolis, MN 55455-0385
Tel: 612 624-8133 *Fax:* 612 625-0617
E-mail: vjohn@lenti.med.umn.edu
Internet:
http://www.borg.labmed.umn.edu/residency/index.html
Accred Length: 4 Years *Program Size:* 20 (*GY1:* 4)
Subspecialties: NP, SP
Program ID: 300-26-31-178

Rochester

Mayo Graduate School of Medicine (Rochester) Program

Sponsor: Mayo Graduate School of Medicine-Mayo Foundation
Mayo Clinic (Rochester)
Rochester Methodist Hospital
St Mary's Hospital of Rochester

Program Director:
John G Strickler, MD
Application Processing Ctr
Mayo Graduate Sch of Med
200 First St SW
Rochester, MN 55905
Tel: 507 284-3108 *Fax:* 507 284-0999
E-mail: mgsm.medlab.specialties@mayo.edu
Internet: http://www.mayo.edu/
Accred Length: 4 Years *Program Size:* 16 (*GY1:* 4)
Subspecialties: MM, NP
Program ID: 300-26-21-179

St Paul

HealthPartners Institute for Medical Education Program

Sponsor: HealthPartners Institute for Medical Education
Regions Hospital

Program Director:
Erhard Haus, MD PhD
Regions Hospital
640 Jackson St
St Paul, MN 55101
Tel: 651 221-8539 *Fax:* 651 221-2741
E-mail: vicki.x.krstich@healthpartners.com
Internet:
http://www.healthpartners.com/sprmc/pathology/home.htm
Accred Length: 4 Years *Program Size:* 8 (*GY1:* 0)
Program ID: 300-26-21-180

Mississippi

Jackson

University of Mississippi Medical Center Program

Sponsor: University of Mississippi School of Medicine
University Hospital
Veterans Affairs Medical Center (Jackson)

Program Director:
Marian Petrides, MD
Univ of Mississippi Med Ctr
2500 N State St
Jackson, MS 39216-4505
Tel: 601 984-1530 *Fax:* 601 984-1531
E-mail: mpetrides@pathology.umsmed.edu
Accred Length: 4 Years *Program Size:* 12 (*GY1:* 4)
Subspecialties: PCP
Program ID: 300-27-21-182

Missouri

Columbia

University of Missouri-Columbia Program

Sponsor: University of Missouri-Columbia School of Medicine
Harry S Truman Memorial Veterans Hospital
University Hospitals and Clinics

Program Director:
John F Townsend, MD
Univ of Missouri Hospital and Clinics
M263 Med Science Bldg
One Hospital Dr
Columbia, MO 65212
Tel: 573 882-1201 *Fax:* 573 884-4612
Accred Length: 4 Years *Program Size:* 16 (*GY1:* 4)
Program ID: 300-28-21-185

Kansas City

University of Missouri at Kansas City Program

Sponsor: University of Missouri-Kansas City School of Medicine
Children's Mercy Hospital
Saint Luke's Hospital
Truman Medical Center-West

Program Director:
Russell M Fiorella, MD MBA
Truman Med Ctr
Dept of Pathology
2301 Holmes St
Kansas City, MO 64108
Tel: 816 556-3212 *Fax:* 816 556-3942
Accred Length: 4 Years *Program Size:* 10 (*GY1:* 2)
Program ID: 300-28-21-408

St Louis

St Louis University School of Medicine Program

Sponsor: St Louis University School of Medicine
SSM Cardinal Glennon Children's Hospital
St Louis University School of Medicine
St Mary's Health Center
Veterans Affairs Medical Center (St Louis)

Program Director:
Carole Vogler, MD
St Louis Univ Sch of Med
Dept of Pathology
1402 S Grand Blvd
St Louis, MO 63104
Tel: 314 577-8694 *Fax:* 314 268-5645
Internet:
http://www.slu.edu/colleges/med/departments/path/
Accred Length: 4 Years *Program Size:* 13 (*GY1:* 3)
Subspecialties: PCP, PP
Program ID: 300-28-21-192

Washington University/B-JH/SLCH Consortium Program

Sponsor: Washington University/B-JH/SLCH Consortium
Barnes-Jewish Hospital
Barnes-Jewish Hospital (North Campus)

Program Director:
Emil R Unanue, MD
Joseph P Miletich, MD PhD
Dept of Pathology
660 S Euclid Ave
Box 8118
St Louis, MO 63110
Tel: 314 362-7472
E-mail: weber@pathbox.wush.edu
Internet:
http://www.medinfo.wustl.edu/~/abmed/trainprog.html
Accred Length: 4 Years *Program Size:* 50 (*GY1:* 12)
Subspecialties: NP, PCP, PP
Program ID: 300-28-11-193

Nebraska

Omaha

Creighton University Program

Sponsor: Creighton University School of Medicine
Tenet St Joseph Hospital at Creighton Univ Medical Center
Veterans Affairs Medical Center (Omaha)

Program Director:
Kenneth L Sims, MD
St Joseph Hospital
Dept of Pathology
601 N 30th St
Omaha, NE 68131-2197
Tel: 402 449-4963 *Fax:* 402 280-5247
E-mail: ksims@pathology.creighton.edu
Internet:
http://www.medicine.creighton.edu/medschool/path/pathology.html
Accred Length: 4 Years *Program Size:* 8 (*GY1:* 3)
Program ID: 300-30-21-195

University of Nebraska Program

Sponsor: University of Nebraska Medical Center
Veterans Affairs Medical Center (Omaha)

Program Director:
Mary E Fidler, MD
Univ of Nebraska Hospital and Clinic
983135 Nebraska Med Ctr
Omaha, NE 68198-3135
Tel: 402 559-9295 *Fax:* 402 559-6018
E-mail: mefidler@mail.unmc.edu
Internet: http://www.unmc.edu/gme/path.htm
Accred Length: 4 Years *Program Size:* 11 (*GY1:* 3)
Subspecialties: HMP
Program ID: 300-30-21-197

New Hampshire

Lebanon

Dartmouth-Hitchcock Medical Center Program

Sponsor: Mary Hitchcock Memorial Hospital
Veterans Affairs Medical Center (White River Junction)

Program Director:
James P AuBuchon, MD
Dartmouth-Hitchcock Med Ctr
One Medical Center Dr
Lebanon, NH 03756-0001
Tel: 603 650-8623 *Fax:* 603 650-4845
Internet:
http://www.hitchcock.org/pages/path/index.html
Accred Length: 4 Years *Program Size:* 12 (*GY1:* 3)
Program ID: 300-32-21-198

New Jersey

Livingston

St Barnabas Medical Center Program

Sponsor: St Barnabas Medical Center
Newark Beth Israel Medical Center

Program Director:
Jonathan F Lara, MD
94 Old Short Hills Rd
Livingston, NJ 07039
Tel: 973 322-5762 *Fax:* 973 322-5564
Accred Length: 4 Years *Program Size:* 14 (*GY1:* 4)
Program ID: 300-33-21-418

Long Branch

Monmouth Medical Center Program

Sponsor: Monmouth Medical Center

Program Director:
Louis J Zinterhofer, MD
Monmouth Med Ctr
Dept of Pathology
300 Second Ave
Long Branch, NJ 07740-9998
Tel: 732 923-7352 *Fax:* 732 923-7355
E-mail: lzinterhofer@monmouth.com
Accred Length: 4 Years *Program Size:* 8 (*GY1:* 2)
Program ID: 300-33-11-207

Newark

UMDNJ-New Jersey Medical School Program

Sponsor: UMDNJ-New Jersey Medical School
Hackensack University Medical Center
UMDNJ-University Hospital
Veterans Affairs Medical Center (East Orange)

Program Director:
Kenneth M Klein, MD
UMDNJ-New Jersey Med Sch
Dept of Path/Laboratory Med
185 S Orange Ave
Newark, NJ 07103-2714
Tel: 973 972-4716 *Fax:* 973 972-5724
E-mail: kklein@.umdnj.edu
Accred Length: 4 Years *Program Size:* 15 (*GY1:* 2)
Program ID: 300-33-21-381

Piscataway

UMDNJ-Robert Wood Johnson Medical School Program

Sponsor: UMDNJ-Robert Wood Johnson Medical School
Robert Wood Johnson University Hospital
St Peter's University Hospital

Program Director:
Peter S Amenta, MD PhD
UMDNJ-Robert Wood Johnson Med Sch
Dept of Pathology/MEB 212
New Brunswick, NJ 08903-0019
Tel: 732 235-8121 *Fax:* 732 235-8124
Accred Length: 4 Years *Program Size:* 9 (*GY1:* 1)
Subspecialties: HMP
Program ID: 300-33-21-215

New Mexico

Albuquerque

University of New Mexico Program

Sponsor: University of New Mexico School of Medicine
University Hospital
Veterans Affairs Medical Center (Albuquerque)

Program Director:
Therese J Bocklage, MD
Univ of New Mexico Health Sciences Ctr
Dept of Pathology
BMSB 337
Albuquerque, NM 87131-5301
Tel: 505 272-2201 *Fax:* 505 272-2235
E-mail: jlusk@salud.unm.edu
Internet: http://thor.unm.edu/sites/resprog.nsf
Accred Length: 4 Years *Program Size:* 16 (*GY1:* 2)
Subspecialties: HMP
Program ID: 300-34-21-218

New York

Albany

Albany Medical Center Program

Sponsor: Albany Medical Center
Veterans Affairs Medical Center (Albany)

Program Director:
Barbara McKenna, MD
Albany Med Ctr Hospital
47 New Scotland Ave
Mail Code 81
Albany, NY 12208-3479
Tel: 518 262-5436 *Fax:* 518 262-3663
E-mail: dee_burkins@ccgateway.amc.edu
Accred Length: 4 Years *Program Size:* 15 (*GY1:* 3)
Subspecialties: HMP
Program ID: 300-35-21-219

Bronx

Albert Einstein College of Medicine Program

Sponsor: Albert Einstein College of Medicine of Yeshiva University
Jacobi Medical Center
Montefiore Medical Center-Henry and Lucy Moses Division
Montefiore Medical Center-Weiler Hospital
North Central Bronx Hospital

Program Director:
Jacob J Steinberg, MD
Montefiore Med Ctr-Albert Einstein Coll of Med
Dept of Pathology C312
111 E 210th St
Bronx, NY 10467-2490
Tel: 718 920-6573 *Fax:* 718 547-8349
E-mail: steinber@aecom.yu.edu
Internet: http://www.aecom.yu.edu
Accred Length: 4 Years *Program Size:* 25 (*GY1:* 4)
Program ID: 300-35-21-230

Bronx-Lebanon Hospital Center Program

Sponsor: Bronx-Lebanon Hospital Center

Program Director:
Young J Choi, MD
Bronx-Lebanon Hospital Ctr
1650 Grand Concourse
Ground Fl
Bronx, NY 10457
Tel: 718 518-5148 *Fax:* 718 716-8242
Accred Length: 4 Years *Program Size:* 7 (*GY1:* 2)
Subspecialties: PIP
Program ID: 300-35-12-233

Brooklyn

Brooklyn Hospital Center Program

Sponsor: Brooklyn Hospital Center
Lutheran Medical Center
Wyckoff Heights Medical Center

Program Director:
Robert D Kalter, MD
121 DeKalb Ave
Brooklyn, NY 11201
Tel: 718 250-8207 *Fax:* 718 250-8056
Accred Length: 4 Years *Program Size:* 2 (*GY1:* 0)
Program ID: 300-35-11-235

SUNY Health Science Center at Brooklyn Program

Sponsor: SUNY Health Science Center at Brooklyn
Kings County Hospital Center
University Hospital-SUNY Health Science Center at Brooklyn

Program Director:
Peter J Howanitz, MD
SUNY Health Science Ctr-Brooklyn
450 Clarkson Ave/Box 25
Brooklyn, NY 11203-2098
Tel: 718 270-4522 *Fax:* 718 270-4524
Accred Length: 4 Years *Program Size:* 19 (*GY1:* 3)
Subspecialties: PP
Program ID: 300-35-21-260

Programs

Buffalo

SUNY at Buffalo Graduate Medical-Dental Education Consortium Program

Sponsor: SUNY at Buffalo Grad Medical-Dental Education Consortium
CGF Health System (Buffalo General Hospital)
Roswell Park Cancer Institute
Veterans Affairs Medical Center (Buffalo)

Program Director:
Reid R Heffner Jr, MD
Dept of Pathology
SUNY-Buffalo
204 Farber Hall
Buffalo, NY 14214-3000
Tel: 716 829-3090 *Fax:* 716 829-2086
Accred Length: 4 Years *Program Size:* 13 (*GY1:* 3)
Subspecialties: NP
Program ID: 300-35-21-224

East Meadow

Nassau County Medical Center Program

Sponsor: Nassau County Medical Center

Program Director:
Richard J Stenger, MD
Nassau County Med Ctr
Dept of Path/Laboratories
2201 Hempstead Trnpk
East Meadow, NY 11554-5400
Tel: 516 572-3201 *Fax:* 516 572-5614
Accred Length: 4 Years *Program Size:* 9 (*GY1:* 2)
Program ID: 300-35-21-225

Flushing

New York Hospital Medical Center of Queens/Cornell University Medical College Program

Sponsor: New York Hospital Medical Center of Queens
New York and Presbyterian Hospital (Cornell Campus)

Program Director:
Thomas A Godwin, MD
New York Hospital Med Ctr of Queens
Dept of Pathology
56-45 Main St
Flushing, NY 11355-5095
Tel: 718 670-1374, ext 1307 *Fax:* 718 359-7691
E-mail: nyhq_path@yahoo.com
Accred Length: 4 Years *Program Size:* 7 (*GY1:* 0)
Program ID: 300-35-11-232

Manhasset

North Shore University Hospital/NYU School of Medicine Program

Sponsor: North Shore University Hospital

Program Director:
John D Broome, MD
North Shore Univ Hospital
300 Community Dr
Manhasset, NY 11030
Tel: 516 562-1277 *Fax:* 516 562-4591
Internet: http://www.nshs.edu
Accred Length: 4 Years *Program Size:* 12 (*GY1:* 6)
Program ID: 300-35-11-228

Mineola

Winthrop-University Hospital Program

Sponsor: Winthrop-University Hospital

Program Director:
Lucien Nochomovitz, MD
Winthrop-Univ Hospital
259 First St
222 Bldg/Ste 618
Mineola, NY 11501
Tel: 516 663-2450 *Fax:* 516 663-4581
Internet: http://www.winthrop.org
Accred Length: 4 Years *Program Size:* 8 (*GY1:* 2)
Program ID: 300-35-12-229

New Hyde Park

Albert Einstein College of Medicine at Long Island Jewish Medical Center Program

Sponsor: Long Island Jewish Medical Center

Program Director:
Leonard B Kahn, MD
Long Island Jewish Med Ctr
270-05 76th Ave/Rm B67
New Hyde Park, NY 11040-1433
Tel: 718 470-7709 *Fax:* 718 347-9171
Internet: http://www.lij.edu
Accred Length: 4 Years *Program Size:* 9 (*GY1:* 1)
Subspecialties: PCP
Program ID: 300-35-21-245

New York

Harlem Hospital Center Program

Sponsor: Harlem Hospital Center

Program Director:
Carlos Navarro, MD
MLK Pavilion/8th Fl Rm 8115
506 Lenox Ave
New York, NY 10037
Tel: 212 939-3630 *Fax:* 212 939-3629
E-mail: bo9760@mem.po.com
Accred Length: 4 Years *Program Size:* 0
Program ID: 300-35-11-239

Lenox Hill Hospital Program

Sponsor: Lenox Hill Hospital

Program Director:
Harry L Ioachim, MD
Dept of Pathology
Lenox Hill Hospital
100 E 77th St
New York, NY 10021-1883
Tel: 212 434-2330 *Fax:* 212 434-2497
Accred Length: 4 Years *Program Size:* 8 (*GY1:* 2)
Program ID: 300-35-11-243

Mount Sinai School of Medicine Program

Sponsor: Mount Sinai School of Medicine
Mount Sinai Medical Center
Veterans Affairs Medical Center (Bronx)

Program Director:
James A Strauchen, MD
Mount Sinai Med Ctr
One Gustave L Levy Pl
Box 1194
New York, NY 10029-6574
Tel: 212 241-8014 *Fax:* 212 534-7491
Internet:
http://academic.mssm.edu/path/home.page.html
Accred Length: 4 Years *Program Size:* 28 (*GY1:* 5)
Subspecialties: NP, PCP
Program ID: 300-35-21-251

New York and Presbyterian Hospital (Columbia Campus) Program

Sponsor: New York and Presbyterian Hospital
New York and Presbyterian Hospital (Columbia Campus)

Program Director:
Charles C Marboe, MD
New York Presbyterian Hospital
Dept of Pathology
630 W 168th St/PH15 West
New York, NY 10032
Tel: 212 305-5697
E-mail: ccm1@columbia.edu
Internet: http://156.111.205.100/resprog.html
Accred Length: 4 Years *Program Size:* 18 (*GY1:* 4)
Program ID: 300-35-11-237

New York and Presbyterian Hospital (Cornell Campus) Program

Sponsor: New York and Presbyterian Hospital
New York and Presbyterian Hospital (Cornell Campus)

Program Director:
Daniel M Knowles, MD
New York Hospital-Cornell Med Ctr
Dept of Pathology/Rm C-306
525 E 68th St
New York, NY 10021
Tel: 212 746-6464 *Fax:* 212 746-8192
E-mail: glimpera@mail.med.cornell.edu
Internet: http://www.nycornell.org/pathology/
Accred Length: 4 Years *Program Size:* 20 (*GY1:* 4)
Subspecialties: PCP
Program ID: 300-35-11-253

New York Medical College at St Vincent's Hospital and Medical Center Program

Sponsor: New York Medical College
St Vincent's Hospital and Medical Center of New York

Program Director:
John F Gillooley, MD
St Vincents Hospital and Med Ctr
153 W 11th St
New York, NY 10011
Tel: 212 604-8384 *Fax:* 212 604-8426
Accred Length: 4 Years *Program Size:* 7 (*GY1:* 2)
Program ID: 300-35-21-259

New York University Medical Center Program

Sponsor: New York University Medical Center
Bellevue Hospital Center
Veterans Affairs Medical Center (Manhattan)

Program Director:
Douglas C Miller, MD PhD
New York Univ Med Ctr
550 First Ave
New York, NY 10016
Tel: 212 263-5376 *Fax:* 212 263-8211
Accred Length: 4 Years *Program Size:* 21 (*GY1:* 4)
Subspecialties: HMP, NP, PCP, PIP, PP
Program ID: 300-35-21-255

St Luke's-Roosevelt Hospital Center Program

Sponsor: St Luke's-Roosevelt Hospital Center
St Luke's-Roosevelt Hospital Center-Roosevelt Division
St Luke's-Roosevelt Hospital Center-St Luke's Division

Program Director:
Neville Colman, MD PhD
St Luke's-Roosevelt Hospital Ctr
1111 Amsterdam Ave
New York, NY 10025
Tel: 212 523-4330 *Fax:* 212 523-4829
E-mail: ncolman@slrhc.org
Internet:
http://www.wehealnewyork.org/professionals/pathology
Accred Length: 4 Years *Program Size:* 10 (*GY1:* 3)
Program ID: 300-35-21-398

Rochester

University of Rochester Program
Sponsor: Strong Memorial Hospital of the University of Rochester
Program Director:
James M Powers, MD
Strong Memorial Hospital
Dept of Path/Lab Med
601 Elmwood Ave/PO Box 626
Rochester, NY 14642
Tel: 716 275-3202 *Fax:* 716 273-1027
E-mail: jpowers@pathology.rochester.edu
Internet:
http://www.urmc.rochester.edu/smd/path/resprog.html
Accred Length: 4 Years *Program Size:* 12 (*GY1:* 3)
Subspecialties: FOP, NP, PCP
Program ID: 300-35-21-263

Stony Brook

SUNY at Stony Brook Program
Sponsor: University Hospital-SUNY at Stony Brook
Program Director:
Bernard P Lane, MD
SUNY-Stony Brook Health Science Ctr
Dept of Pathology/HSC T2
Univ Hospital
Stony Brook, NY 11794-7025
Tel: 516 444-2224 *Fax:* 516 444-3419
Accred Length: 4 Years *Program Size:* 15 (*GY1:* 3)
Subspecialties: BBK, NP
Program ID: 300-35-21-396

Syracuse

SUNY Health Science Center at Syracuse Program
Sponsor: University Hospital-SUNY Health Science Center at Syracuse
Community-General Hospital of Greater Syracuse
Veterans Affairs Medical Center (Syracuse)
Program Director:
Frederick R Davey, MD
SUNY Health Science Ctr-Syracuse
Dept of Pathology
750 E Adams St
Syracuse, NY 13210
Tel: 315 464-5170 *Fax:* 315 464-7130
E-mail: daveyf@mailbox.hscsyr.edu
Accred Length: 4 Years *Program Size:* 16 (*GY1:* 5)
Subspecialties: BBK, PCP
Program ID: 300-35-21-265

Valhalla

New York Medical College at Westchester Medical Center Program
Sponsor: New York Medical College
Westchester Medical Center
Program Director:
Muhammad B Zaman, MD
New York Med Coll
Dept of Pathology
Basic Sci Bldg/Rm 411
Valhalla, NY 10595
Tel: 914 594-4148 *Fax:* 914 594-4163
Accred Length: 4 Years *Program Size:* 9 (*GY1:* 1)
Subspecialties: PCP
Program ID: 300-35-11-266

North Carolina

Chapel Hill

University of North Carolina Hospitals Program
Sponsor: University of North Carolina Hospitals
Program Director:
Thomas W Bouldin, MD
Univ of North Carolina Sch of Med
303 Brinkhous-Bullitt Bldg/CB7525
Chapel Hill, NC 27599-7525
Tel: 919 966-4676 *Fax:* 919 966-6718
E-mail: tbouldin@med.unc.edu
Internet:
http://www.pathology.med.unc.edu/path/welcome.htm
Accred Length: 4 Years *Program Size:* 11 (*GY1:* 3)
Subspecialties: HMP, MM, PCH, PCP, PIP
Program ID: 300-36-11-267

Durham

Duke University Program
Sponsor: Duke University Medical Center
Veterans Affairs Medical Center (Durham)
Program Director:
William D Bradford, MD
Duke Univ Med Ctr
Dept of Pathology
Box 3712
Durham, NC 27710
Tel: 919 684-5112 *Fax:* 919 681-7377
Accred Length: 4 Years *Program Size:* 17 (*GY1:* 4)
Subspecialties: HMP, MM, NP, PCP
Program ID: 300-36-21-269

Greenville

East Carolina University Program
Sponsor: East Carolina University School of Medicine
Pitt County Memorial Hospital
Program Director:
Gregory A Gagnon, MD
Pitt County Memorial Hospital, Dept of Pathology
PO Box 6028
2100 Stantonsburg Rd
Greenville, NC 27835-6028
Tel: 252 816-5006 *Fax:* 252 816-8200
Internet: http://www.med.ecu.edu
Accred Length: 4 Years *Program Size:* 10 (*GY1:* 2)
Subspecialties: PCP
Program ID: 300-36-21-404

Winston-Salem

Wake Forest University School of Medicine Program
Sponsor: Wake Forest University Baptist Medical Center
Program Director:
Marbry B Hopkins III, MD
Wake Forest Univ Sch of Med
Dept of Pathology
Medical Center Blvd
Winston-Salem, NC 27157-1072
Tel: 336 716-2650 *Fax:* 336 716-7595
Internet: http://pandoras_box.bgsm.edu
Accred Length: 4 Years *Program Size:* 20 (*GY1:* 4)
Program ID: 300-36-11-270

Ohio

Akron

Summa Health System (Akron City Hospital)/NEOUCOM Program
Sponsor: Summa Health System
Akron City Hospital (Summa Health System)
Children's Hospital Medical Center of Akron
Program Director:
Raymond E Clarke, MD
Summa Health System
Dept of Pathology
525 E Market St
Akron, OH 44309
Tel: 800 322-0517 *Fax:* 330 375-4874
Internet: http://www.summahealth.org/edu/
Accred Length: 4 Years *Program Size:* 10 (*GY1:* 2)
Subspecialties: PCP
Program ID: 300-38-11-272

Cincinnati

University Hospital/University of Cincinnati College of Medicine Program
Sponsor: University Hospital Inc
Veterans Affairs Medical Center (Cincinnati)
Program Director:
Amy Noffsinger, MD
Univ of Cincinnati Med Ctr
Dept of Pathology
231 Bethesda Ave/PO Box 670529
Cincinnati, OH 45267-0529
Tel: 513 558-7113 *Fax:* 513 558-2289
E-mail: bishopjc@ucmail.uc.edu
Internet:
http://www.med.uc.edu/departme/pathdept/web/resident/respage.htm
Accred Length: 4 Years *Program Size:* 12 (*GY1:* 4)
Subspecialties: HMP, PCP
Program ID: 300-38-21-276

Cleveland

Case Western Reserve University (MetroHealth) Program
Sponsor: MetroHealth Medical Center
Program Director:
Joseph F Tomashefski Jr, MD
MetroHealth Med Ctr
2500 MetroHealth Dr
Cleveland, OH 44109-1998
Tel: 216 778-5181 *Fax:* 216 778-5701
Internet: http://www.pathology.metrohealth.org
Accred Length: 4 Years *Program Size:* 8 (*GY1:* 2)
Subspecialties: HMP, PCP
Program ID: 300-38-11-279

Case Western Reserve University Program
Sponsor: University Hospitals of Cleveland
Program Director:
Robert D Hoffman, MD PhD
Univ Hospitals of Cleveland
Dept of Pathology
11100 Euclid Ave
Cleveland, OH 44106-5077
Tel: 216 844-3478 *Fax:* 216 844-1810
E-mail: robert.hoffman@uhhs.com
Internet:
http://www.uhhs.com/toteach/pathology/index.html
Accred Length: 4 Years *Program Size:* 23 (*GY1:* 5)
Subspecialties: NP
Program ID: 300-38-21-277

Cleveland Clinic Foundation Program
Sponsor: Cleveland Clinic Foundation

Program Director:
Robert E Petras, MD
Cleveland Clinic Foundation
Dept of Pathology/L25
9500 Euclid Ave
Cleveland, OH 44195-5242
Tel: 216 444-5690 *Fax:* 216 444-1162
E-mail: meded@cesmtp.ccf.org
Internet: http://www.ccf.org
Accred Length: 4 Years *Program Size:* 28 (*GY1:* 6)
Subspecialties: HMP, MM
Program ID: 300-38-12-278

Columbus

Ohio State University Program
Sponsor: Ohio State University Medical Center

Program Director:
William J Becker, DO
Ohio State Univ Med Ctr
E-310 Doan Hall
410 W Tenth Ave
Columbus, OH 43210
Tel: 614 293-2458 *Fax:* 614 293-7273
E-mail: becker-1@medctr.osu.edu
Internet: http://www.medinfo.ohio-state.edu
Accred Length: 4 Years *Program Size:* 12 (*GY1:* 3)
Subspecialties: BBK, HMP
Program ID: 300-38-21-286

Toledo

Medical College of Ohio Program
Sponsor: Medical College of Ohio
Medical College of Ohio Hospital
St Vincent Mercy Medical Center

Program Director:
Aiman Zaher, MD
Med Coll of Ohio
3000 Arlington Ave
Toledo, OH 43614-2598
Tel: 419 383-3478 *Fax:* 419 383-6183
E-mail: ajacobs@mco.edu
Internet: http://www.mco.edu/depts/path
Accred Length: 4 Years *Program Size:* 8 (*GY1:* 2)
Program ID: 300-38-11-290

Youngstown

Western Reserve Care System/NEOUCOM Program
Sponsor: Western Reserve Care System
Forum Health-Northside Medical Center

Program Director:
Shokat Fatteh, MD
Western Reserve Care System
Dept of Laboratories
500 Gypsy Ln
Youngstown, OH 44501
Tel: 330 740-3815 *Fax:* 330 740-3790
Internet: http://www.wrhc.org/pathology.html
Accred Length: 4 Years *Program Size:* 8 (*GY1:* 2)
Program ID: 300-38-11-292

Oklahoma

Oklahoma City

University of Oklahoma Health Sciences Center Program
Sponsor: University of Oklahoma College of Medicine
Children's Hospital of Oklahoma
Integris Baptist Medical Center
University Hospital
Veterans Affairs Medical Center (Oklahoma City)

Program Director:
Anna E Sienko, MD
Univ of Oklahoma Health Sciences Ctr
Dept of Pathology
PO Box 26901 (BMSB 451)
Oklahoma City, OK 73190
Tel: 405 271-2422 *Fax:* 405 271-2568
E-mail: dianne-wright@ouhsc.edu
Internet: http://www.ouhsc.edu/depts/pathology
Accred Length: 4 Years *Program Size:* 18 (*GY1:* 4)
Subspecialties: NP
Program ID: 300-39-21-295

Oregon

Portland

Oregon Health Sciences University Program
Sponsor: Oregon Health Sciences University Hospital
Kaiser Foundation Hospitals-Northwest Region
Veterans Affairs Medical Center (Portland)

Program Director:
Christopher L Corless, MD PhD
Oregon Health Sciences Univ
Pathology/L113
3181 SW Sam Jackson Park Rd
Portland, OR 97201-3098
Tel: 503 494-8276 *Fax:* 503 494-2025
E-mail: pathrap@ohsu.edu
Internet:
http://www.ohsu.edu/som-pathology/pathpage.htm
Accred Length: 4 Years *Program Size:* 12 (*GY1:* 2)
Program ID: 300-40-11-302

St Vincent Hospital and Medical Center Program
Sponsor: St Vincent Hospital and Medical Center

Program Director:
James L Booth, MD
9205 SW Barnes Rd
Portland, OR 97225
Tel: 503 291-2301 *Fax:* 503 216-2305
Accred Length: 4 Years *Program Size:* 3 (*GY1:* 0)
Program ID: 300-40-12-301

Pennsylvania

Danville

Penn State Geisinger Health System/Geisinger Medical Center Program
Sponsor: Penn State Geisinger Health System
Geisinger Medical Center

Program Director:
Steven C Meschter, MD
Geisinger Med Ctr
100 N Academy Ave
Danville, PA 17822
Tel: 717 271-6338 *Fax:* 717 271-6105
E-mail: ckrebs@psghs.edu
Accred Length: 4 Years *Program Size:* 3 (*GY1:* 0)
Subspecialties: PCP
Program ID: 300-41-12-306

Hershey

Penn State Geisinger Health System/Milton S Hershey Medical Center Program
Sponsor: Penn State Geisinger Health System
Milton S Hershey Medical Center

Program Director:
Richard J Zaino, MD
Milton S Hershey Med Ctr
500 University Dr
PO Box 850
Hershey, PA 17033-0850
Tel: 717 531-8351 *Fax:* 717 531-5021
Accred Length: 4 Years *Program Size:* 10 (*GY1:* 2)
Program ID: 300-41-11-308

Johnstown

Conemaugh Valley Memorial Hospital Program
Sponsor: Conemaugh Valley Memorial Hospital
Temple University Hospital

Program Director:
Sidney A Goldblatt, MD
Conemaugh Health System-Memorial Med Ctr
1086 Franklin St
Johnstown, PA 15905-4398
Tel: 814 534-9817 *Fax:* 814 534-9372
Accred Length: 4 Years *Program Size:* 8 (*GY1:* 2)
Subspecialties: TY
Program ID: 300-41-21-397

Philadelphia

MCP Hahnemann University Program
Sponsor: MCP Hahnemann University
Graduate Hospital
Hahnemann University Hospital
Medical College of Pennsylvania Hospital

Program Director:
Kathleen Sazama, MD
Med Coll of Pennsylvania-Hahnemann Univ
Dept of Pathology/6th Fl Rm 207C
3300 Henry Ave
Philadelphia, PA 19129
Tel: 215 762-8521 *Fax:* 215 843-0590
Accred Length: 4 Years *Program Size:* 23 (*GY1:* 5)
Subspecialties: PCP
Program ID: 300-41-21-316

Pennsylvania Hospital of the University of Pennsylvania Health System Program
Sponsor: Pennsylvania Hospital (UPHS)
Program Director:
Helen M Haupt, MD
Pennsylvania Hospital
Ayer Laboratories
8th and Spruce Sts
Philadelphia, PA 19107
Tel: 215 829-3544 *Fax:* 215 829-7564
Accred Length: 4 Years *Program Size:* 10 (*GY1:* 2)
Program ID: 300-41-11-318

Temple University Program
Sponsor: Temple University Hospital
Program Director:
James G Caya, MD
Temple Univ Hospital
Dept of Path/Lab Med
3401 N Broad St
Philadelphia, PA 19140
Tel: 215 707-4994 *Fax:* 215 707-2781
E-mail: rredd@nimbus.ocis.temple.edu
Accred Length: 4 Years *Program Size:* 11 (*GY1:* 4)
Subspecialties: HMP
Program ID: 300-41-11-321

Thomas Jefferson University Program
Sponsor: Thomas Jefferson University Hospital
Program Director:
Peter McCue, MD PhD
132 S 10th St
Ste 285 Main Bldg
Philadelphia, PA 19107
Tel: 215 955-5588 *Fax:* 215 923-1969
E-mail: peter.mccue@mail.tju.edu
Accred Length: 4 Years *Program Size:* 17 (*GY1:* 3)
Subspecialties: PCP, SP
Program ID: 300-41-11-322

University of Pennsylvania Program
Sponsor: Hospital of the University of Pennsylvania
Program Director:
James E Wheeler, MD
Hospital of Univ of Pennsylvania
Dept of Path/Lab Med
3400 Spruce St
Philadelphia, PA 19104-4283
Tel: 215 662-6506 *Fax:* 215 614-1856
Internet: http://www.med.upenn.edu/~path/
Accred Length: 4 Years *Program Size:* 39 (*GY1:* 9)
Subspecialties: PCP
Program ID: 300-41-21-314

Pittsburgh

Allegheny General Hospital Program
Sponsor: Allegheny General Hospital
Program Director:
Jan F Silverman, MD
Allegheny General Hospital
Dept of Laboratory Med
320 E North Ave
Pittsburgh, PA 15212-9986
Tel: 412 359-6886 *Fax:* 412 359-3598
Accred Length: 4 Years *Program Size:* 8 (*GY1:* 2)
Subspecialties: HMP
Program ID: 300-41-12-323

University Health Center of Pittsburgh Program
Sponsor: University Health Center of Pittsburgh
Children's Hospital of Pittsburgh
Magee-Women's Hospital
Presbyterian University Hospital/UPMC
Veterans Affairs Medical Center (Pittsburgh)
Program Director:
Jeffrey Kant, MD PhD
Univ of Pittsburgh
Dept of Pathology
3550 Terrace St/S707 Scaife Hall
Pittsburgh, PA 15213-2582
Tel: 412 648-9699 *Fax:* 412 624-0614
E-mail: tietsworthml@msx.upmc.edu
Internet: http://www.path.upmc.edu/brochure/residency
Accred Length: 4 Years *Program Size:* 32 (*GY1:* 7)
Subspecialties: HMP, PCH, PCP
Program ID: 300-41-21-324

Puerto Rico

San Juan

University of Puerto Rico Program
Sponsor: University of Puerto Rico School of Medicine
San Juan City Hospital
University Hospital
Veterans Affairs Medical Center (San Juan)
Program Director:
Roman Velez Rosario, MD
Univ of Puerto Rico Sch of Med
PO Box 365067
San Juan, PR 00936-5067
Tel: 787 758-2525, ext 1329 *Fax:* 787 754-0710
Accred Length: 4 Years *Program Size:* 9 (*GY1:* 3)
Subspecialties: FOP
Program ID: 300-42-21-385

Rhode Island

Providence

Brown University Program
Sponsor: Rhode Island Hospital
Memorial Hospital of Rhode Island
Miriam Hospital
Roger Williams Medical Center
Women and Infants Hospital of Rhode Island
Program Director:
Thomas C King, MD PhD
Rhode Island Hospital
593 Eddy St
Providence, RI 02903
Tel: 401 444-5151 *Fax:* 401 444-8514
Internet: http://klahanie.com/bpathres.htm
Accred Length: 4 Years *Program Size:* 16 (*GY1:* 4)
Subspecialties: PP
Program ID: 300-43-21-414

South Carolina

Charleston

Medical University of South Carolina Program
Sponsor: Medical University of South Carolina College of Medicine
MUSC Medical Center
Ralph H Johnson Dept of Veterans Affairs Med Center
Program Director:
Clay A Nichols, MD
Med Univ of South Carolina
171 Ashley Ave
Charleston, SC 29425-0701
Tel: 803 792-3121 *Fax:* 803 792-0555
Internet: http://www.musc.edu/path.html
Accred Length: 4 Years *Program Size:* 17 (*GY1:* 3)
Subspecialties: HMP, PCP
Program ID: 300-45-21-332

South Dakota

Sioux Falls

University of South Dakota Program
Sponsor: University of South Dakota School of Medicine
Royal C Johnson Veterans Affairs Medical Center
Sioux Valley Hospital
Program Director:
Karl G Peterson, MD
Univ of South Dakota
PO Box 5134
Sioux Falls, SD 57117-5134
Tel: 605 333-1720 *Fax:* 605 333-1966
Accred Length: 4 Years *Program Size:* 5 (*GY1:* 1)
Program ID: 300-46-21-333

Tennessee

Johnson City

East Tennessee State University Program
Sponsor: James H Quillen College of Medicine
Johnson City Medical Center Hospital
Veterans Affairs Medical Center (Mountain Home)
Program Director:
Philip S Coogan, MD
East Tennessee State Univ Quillen Coll of Med
Dept of Pathology
PO Box 70568
Johnson City, TN 37614-0568
Tel: 423 439-6210 *Fax:* 423 439-4195
E-mail: mcfeatur@etsu.edu
Accred Length: 4 Years *Program Size:* 9 (*GY1:* 4)
Program ID: 300-47-21-399

Knoxville

University of Tennessee Medical Center at Knoxville Program
Sponsor: University of Tennessee Graduate School of Medicine
University of Tennessee Memorial Hospital
Program Director:
Frances K Patterson, MD
Univ of Tennessee Grad Sch of Med
1924 Alcoa Hwy
Knoxville, TN 37920-6999
Tel: 423 544-9080 *Fax:* 423 544-6866
E-mail: fpatters@utk.edu
Internet: http://www.mc.utk.edu
Accred Length: 4 Years *Program Size:* 10 (*GY1:* 2)
Program ID: 300-47-11-335

Memphis

University of Tennessee Program

Sponsor: University of Tennessee College of Medicine
Baptist Memorial Hospital
Regional Medical Center at Memphis
Veterans Affairs Medical Center (Memphis)
Program Director:
John B Schweitzer, MD
899 Madison Ave/Rm 504-M
Memphis, TN 38163
Tel: 901 448-6300 *Fax:* 901 448-6979
Internet:
http://www.pathology.utmem.edu/hospit~1/residenc.htm
Accred Length: 4 Years *Program Size:* 16 (*GY1:* 3)
Program ID: 300-47-12-336

Nashville

Vanderbilt University Program

Sponsor: Vanderbilt University Medical Center
St Thomas Hospital
Veterans Affairs Medical Center (Nashville)
Program Director:
Joyce Johnson, MD
Vanderbilt Univ Med Ctr
Dept of Pathology/C-3321 MCN
1161 21st Ave S
Nashville, TN 37232-2561
Tel: 615 343-4882 *Fax:* 615 343-7023
E-mail: joyce.johnson@mcmail.vanderbilt.edu
Internet: http://www.mc.vanderbilt.edu
Accred Length: 4 Years *Program Size:* 20 (*GY1:* 5)
Subspecialties: NP
Program ID: 300-47-21-341

Texas

Dallas

Baylor University Medical Center Program

Sponsor: Baylor University Medical Center
Program Director:
Glenn W Tillery, MD
Baylor Univ Med Ctr
Dept of Pathology
3500 Gaston Ave
Dallas, TX 75246
Tel: 214 820-3021 *Fax:* 214 820-2535
Internet:
http://www.bhcs.com/bumc/medicaleducation/residencies.htm
Accred Length: 4 Years *Program Size:* 18 (*GY1:* 4)
Program ID: 300-48-12-343

University of Texas Southwestern Medical School Program

Sponsor: University of Texas Southwestern Medical School
Dallas County Hospital District-Parkland Memorial Hospital
Program Director:
Geralyn M Meny, MD
Dept of Pathology
5323 Harry Hines Blvd
Dallas, TX 75235-9072
Tel: 214 648-4141 *Fax:* 214 648-4070
Internet: http://www.swmed.edu/
Accred Length: 4 Years *Program Size:* 41 (*GY1:* 11)
Subspecialties: BBK, HMP, NP, PCP, PIP, PP
Program ID: 300-48-11-345

Galveston

University of Texas Medical Branch Hospitals Program

Sponsor: University of Texas Medical Branch Hospitals
Program Director:
Marjorie R Grafe, MD PhD
Univ of Texas Med Branch
301 University Blvd
Galveston, TX 77555-0609
Tel: 409 772-2870 *Fax:* 409 747-2400
E-mail: mgrafe@utmb.edu
Internet: http://vaxpc.utmb.edu/pathology
Accred Length: 4 Years *Program Size:* 24 (*GY1:* 4)
Subspecialties: DMP, MM
Program ID: 300-48-11-349

Houston

Baylor College of Medicine Program

Sponsor: Baylor College of Medicine
Harris County Hospital District-Ben Taub General Hospital
Methodist Hospital
Texas Children's Hospital
Veterans Affairs Medical Center (Houston)
Program Director:
Mary R Schwartz, MD
Baylor Coll of Med
One Baylor Plaza
Houston, TX 77030
Tel: 713 798-4083 *Fax:* 713 798-5838
E-mail: melindaf@bcm.tmc.edu
Internet: http://www.bcm.tmc.edu/pathology
Accred Length: 4 Years *Program Size:* 27 (*GY1:* 4)
Subspecialties: DMP, HMP, NP, PCP, PP
Program ID: 300-48-31-350

University of Texas at Houston Program

Sponsor: University of Texas Medical School at Houston
Lyndon B Johnson General Hospital
Memorial Hermann Healthcare System
St Luke's Episcopal Hospital
Program Director:
Margaret Uthman, MD
Univ of Texas Med Sch
Dept of Pathology
6431 Fannin St/MSB 2120
Houston, TX 77030
Tel: 713 500-5402 *Fax:* 713 500-0730
Internet: http://dpalm.med.uth.tmc.edu
Accred Length: 4 Years *Program Size:* 26 (*GY1:* 5)
Program ID: 300-48-11-352

Lackland AFB

San Antonio Uniformed Services Health Education Consortium Program

Sponsor: San Antonio Uniformed Services Health Education Consortium
Program Director:
Dennis M Drehner, DO
2200 Bergquist Dr/Ste 1
Lackland AFB, TX 78236-5300
Tel: 210 292-7741 *Fax:* 210 292-7484
E-mail: drehner@whmc-lafb.af.mil
Accred Length: 4 Years *Program Size:* 19 (*GY1:* 1)
Program ID: 300-48-11-417
US Armed Services Program

Lubbock

Texas Tech University (Lubbock) Program

Sponsor: Texas Tech University Health Sciences Center at Lubbock
University Medical Center
Program Director:
David Morgan, MD
Dept of Pathology
Texas Tech Univ Health Science Ctr
3601 Fourth St
Lubbock, TX 79430
Tel: 806 743-2155 *Fax:* 806 743-2117
E-mail: pthcat@ttuhsc.edu
Accred Length: 4 Years *Program Size:* 8 (*GY1:* 2)
Program ID: 300-48-31-415

San Antonio

University of Texas Health Science Center at San Antonio Program

Sponsor: University of Texas Medical School at San Antonio
Audie L Murphy Memorial Veterans Hospital (San Antonio)
Baptist Memorial Healthcare System
University Hospital-South Texas Medical Center
Program Director:
Larry J Fowler, MD
Univ of Texas Health Science Ctr-San Antonio
7703 Floyd Curl Dr
San Antonio, TX 78284-7750
Tel: 210 567-4025 *Fax:* 210 567-2478
E-mail: fowler@uthscsa.edu
Internet: http://pathologyweb.uthscsa.edu/residency.html
Accred Length: 4 Years *Program Size:* 11 (*GY1:* 3)
Subspecialties: HMP, PCP, PP
Program ID: 300-48-21-356

Temple

Texas A&M College of Medicine-Scott and White Program

Sponsor: Scott and White Memorial Hospital
Program Director:
V O Speights, DO DO
Texas A&M-Scott and White
Grad Med Educ
2401 S 31st St
Temple, TX 76508
Tel: 800 299-4463 *Fax:* 817 724-4391
E-mail: dhinson@swmail.sw.org
Internet: http://www.swinfo.tamu.edu
Accred Length: 4 Years *Program Size:* 10 (*GY1:* 2)
Subspecialties: HMP
Program ID: 300-48-12-357

Utah

Salt Lake City

University of Utah Program

Sponsor: University of Utah Medical Center
Veterans Affairs Medical Center (Salt Lake City)
Program Director:
Edward R Ashwood, MD
Univ of Utah Sch of Med
ARUP-500 Chipeta Way
Salt Lake City, UT 84108
Tel: 801 583-2787, ext 2105 *Fax:* 801 584-5207
E-mail: ashwood@med.utah.edu
Internet:
http://www.telpath2.med.utah.edu/study/resident.htm
Accred Length: 4 Years *Program Size:* 20 (*GY1:* 4)
Subspecialties: HMP, PIP
Program ID: 300-49-21-360

Vermont

Burlington

University of Vermont Program

Sponsor: Fletcher Allen Health Care

Program Director:
Sharon L Mount, MD
Univ of Vermont Coll of Med
Soule Med Alumni Bldg
Burlington, VT 05405-0068
Tel: 802 656-0392 *Fax:* 802 656-8892
E-mail: jlarivee@zoo.uvm.edu
Accred Length: 4 Years *Program Size:* 15 (*GY1:* 4)
Subspecialties: PCP
Program ID: 300-50-11-361

Virginia

Charlottesville

University of Virginia Program

Sponsor: University of Virginia Medical Center

Program Director:
Mark A Lovell, MD
Univ of Virginia
Dept of Pathology/Box 214
UVA Health Sciences Ctr
Charlottesville, VA 22908
Tel: 804 924-2291 *Fax:* 804 982-1880
E-mail: mal3u@virginia.edu
Internet:
http://www.med.virginia.edu/medicine/clinical/pathology/home.html
Accred Length: 4 Years *Program Size:* 16 (*GY1:* 4)
Subspecialties: BBK, NP, PCP
Program ID: 300-51-11-362

Norfolk

Eastern Virginia Medical School Program

Sponsor: Eastern Virginia Medical School
Children's Hospital of the King's Daughters
Sentara Norfolk General Hospital
Veterans Affairs Medical Center (Hampton)

Program Director:
Roy C Sutton III, MD
Dept of Pathology/Anatomy
Eastern Virginia Grad Sch of Med
PO Box 1980
Norfolk, VA 23501-1980
Tel: 757 446-7251 *Fax:* 757 446-5719
E-mail: violama@borg.evms.edu
Internet: http://www.evms.edu
Accred Length: 4 Years *Program Size:* 8 (*GY1:* 3)
Program ID: 300-51-21-365

Portsmouth

Naval Medical Center (Portsmouth) Program

Sponsor: Naval Medical Center (Portsmouth)

Program Director:
Dennis A Rowley, MD
Naval Med Ctr
Laboratory Med Dept
620 John Paul Jones Cir
Portsmouth, VA 23708-2197
Tel: 757 953-5594 *Fax:* 757 953-5608
E-mail: pnh@dar@pnh1@.med.navy.mil
Accred Length: 4 Years *Program Size:* 0
Program ID: 300-51-21-013
US Armed Services Program

Richmond

Medical College of Virginia/Virginia Commonwealth University Program

Sponsor: Medical College of Virginia/Virginia Commonwealth University
Medical College of Virginia Hospitals

Program Director:
Margaret M Grimes, MD
Virginia Commonwealth Univ
1101 E Marshall St/Rm 4-009
PO Box 980662
Richmond, VA 23298-0662
Tel: 804 828-9746 *Fax:* 804 828-9749
Internet: http://views.vcu.edu/mded/mdeduc.html
Accred Length: 4 Years *Program Size:* 20 (*GY1:* 4)
Subspecialties: PCH, PCP
Program ID: 300-51-11-366

Washington

Seattle

University of Washington Program

Sponsor: University of Washington School of Medicine
Children's Hospital and Medical Center
Harborview Medical Center
University of Washington Medical Center
Veterans Affairs Medical Center (Seattle)

Program Director:
Lawrence D True, MD
Univ of Washington Sch of Med
Div of Hospital Pathology/Box 356100
1959 NE Pacific St/Rm BB220
Seattle, WA 98195-6100
Tel: 206 548-4933 *Fax:* 206 548-7321
E-mail: msrme@u.washington.edu
Internet: http://www.pathology.washington.edu
Accred Length: 4 Years *Program Size:* 24 (*GY1:* 5)
Program ID: 300-54-21-367

Tacoma

Madigan Army Medical Center Program

Sponsor: Madigan Army Medical Center

Program Director:
Mark D Brissette, MD
Madigan Army Med Ctr
Dept of Pathology
Box 283
Tacoma, WA 98431
Tel: 253 968-1723 *Fax:* 253 968-1084
E-mail:
ltc_mark.brissette@smtplink.mamc.amedd.army.mil
Accred Length: 4 Years *Program Size:* 8 (*GY1:* 2)
Program ID: 300-54-12-009
US Armed Services Program

West Virginia

Huntington

Marshall University School of Medicine Program

Sponsor: Marshall University School of Medicine
Cabell Huntington Hospital
Charleston Area Medical Center
St Mary's Hospital
Veterans Affairs Medical Center (Huntington)

Program Director:
Gerald E Vanston, MD MD MD
Marshall Univ Sch of Med
1542 Spring Valley Dr
Huntington, WV 25704-9388
Tel: 304 696-7346 *Fax:* 304 696-6777
Accred Length: 4 Years *Program Size:* 8 (*GY1:* 2)
Program ID: 300-55-21-372

Morgantown

West Virginia University Program

Sponsor: West Virginia University Hospitals

Program Director:
Jeffrey A Stead, MD
West Virginia Univ
Robert C Byrd Health Sciences Ctr
PO Box 9203
Morgantown, WV 26506-9203
Tel: 304 293-3212 *Fax:* 304 293-1627
E-mail: ltomago@hsc.wvu.edu
Accred Length: 4 Years *Program Size:* 8 (*GY1:* 2)
Subspecialties: NP
Program ID: 300-55-11-373

Wisconsin

Madison

University of Wisconsin Program

Sponsor: University of Wisconsin Hospital and Clinics
Meriter Hospital
William S Middleton Veterans Hospital

Program Director:
Patrick J Buckley, MD PhD
Univ Hospital and Clinics
B4/243 CSC
600 Highland Ave
Madison, WI 53792-2472
Tel: 608 262-7158 *Fax:* 608 263-1568
E-mail: ck.feuling@hosp.wisc.edu
Internet: http://www.biostat.wisc.edu/path
Accred Length: 4 Years *Program Size:* 15 (*GY1:* 3)
Subspecialties: HMP, PCP
Program ID: 300-56-31-376

Milwaukee

Medical College of Wisconsin Program

Sponsor: Medical College of Wisconsin Affiliated Hospitals Inc
Clement J Zablocki Veterans Affairs Medical Center
Froedtert Memorial Lutheran Hospital
St Luke's Medical Center

Program Director:
Richard A Komorowski, MD
Froedtert Memorial Lutheran Hospital
Dept of Pathology
9200 W Wisconsin Ave
MIlwaukee, WI 53226
Tel: 414 257-6201 *Fax:* 414 257-7815
Accred Length: 4 Years *Program Size:* 10 (*GY1:* 2)
Program ID: 300-56-21-377

Pediatric Anesthesiology (Anesthesiology)

Arkansas

Little Rock

University of Arkansas for Medical Sciences Program

Sponsor: University of Arkansas College of Medicine
Arkansas Children's Hospital

Program Director:
Jeffrey L Koh, MD
Dept of Anesthesiology/Slot 203
800 Marshall St
Little Rock, AR 72202
Tel: 501 320-2938 *Fax:* 501 320-2939
Accred Length: 1 Year *Program Size:* 2
Program ID: 042-04-21-023

California

Stanford

Stanford University Program

Sponsor: Stanford University Hospital
Lucile Salter Packard Children's Hospital at Stanford

Program Director:
Elliot J Krane, MD
Dept of Anesthesiology/Rm H3580
300 Pasteur Dr
Stanford, CA 94305-5640
Tel: 650 723-5728 *Fax:* 650 725-8544
E-mail: krane@stanford.edu
Internet: http://pedsanesthesia.stanford.edu/
Accred Length: 1 Year *Program Size:* 2
Program ID: 042-05-31-019

Colorado

Denver

University of Colorado Program

Sponsor: University of Colorado Health Sciences Center
Children's Hospital

Program Director:
Desmond B Henry, MD
1056 E 19th Ave
Denver, CO 80218
Tel: 303 861-6224 *Fax:* 303 837-2899
Accred Length: 1 Year *Program Size:* 2
Program ID: 042-07-21-020

Connecticut

New Haven

Yale-New Haven Medical Center Program

Sponsor: Yale-New Haven Hospital

Program Director:
Zeev Kain, MD
PO Box 208051
New Haven, CT 06520
Tel: 203 785-2802 *Fax:* 203 785-6664
Accred Length: 1 Year *Program Size:* 2
Program ID: 042-08-21-005

District of Columbia

Washington

George Washington University Program

Sponsor: George Washington University School of Medicine
Children's National Medical Center

Program Director:
Raafat S Hannallah, MD
Children's National Med Ctr
111 Michigan Ave NW
Washington, DC 20010
Tel: 202 884-2025 *Fax:* 202 884-5999
Accred Length: 1 Year *Program Size:* 4
Program ID: 042-10-21-006

Florida

Gainesville

University of Florida Program

Sponsor: University of Florida College of Medicine
Nemours Children's Clinic (UFHSC/J)
Shands Hospital at the University of Florida

Program Director:
Shirley A Graves, MD
Box 100254
1600 SW Archer Rd
Gainesville, FL 32610
Tel: 352 395-0462 *Fax:* 352 395-0443
E-mail: graves@anest1.anest.ufl.edu
Accred Length: 1 Year *Program Size:* 1
Program ID: 042-11-21-001

Miami

University of Miami-Jackson Memorial Medical Center Program

Sponsor: University of Miami-Jackson Memorial Medical Center
Miami Children's Hospital

Program Director:
Nancy Setzer-Saade, MD
3100 SW 62nd Ave
Miami, FL 33155
Tel: 305 666-6511 *Fax:* 305 663-8573
Accred Length: 1 Year *Program Size:* 2
Program ID: 042-11-31-007

Maryland

Baltimore

Johns Hopkins University Program

Sponsor: Johns Hopkins University School of Medicine
Johns Hopkins Hospital

Program Director:
Donald H Shaffner Jr, MD
Johns Hopkins Hospital
600 N Wolfe St
Halsted 842E
Baltimore, MD 21287-5842
Tel: 410 955-2393 *Fax:* 410 614-2911
E-mail: dshaffner@welchlink.welch.jhu.edu
Internet:
http://www.med.jhu.edu/anesthesiology/pediatri.htm
Accred Length: 1 Year *Program Size:* 3
Program ID: 042-23-21-028

Massachusetts

Boston

Beth Israel Deaconess Medical Center Program

Sponsor: Beth Israel Deaconess Medical Center
Children's Hospital

Program Director:
Mark A Rockoff, MD
Children's Hospital
300 Longwood Ave
Boston, MA 02115
Tel: 617 355-7051 *Fax:* 617 355-7887
Accred Length: 1 Year *Program Size:* 0
Program ID: 042-24-21-004

New England Medical Center Hospitals Program

Sponsor: New England Medical Center Hospitals

Program Director:
Maureen Strafford, MD
Dept of Anesthesiology/Box 298
750 Washington St
Boston, MA 02111
Tel: 617 636-6044 *Fax:* 617 636-8384
Accred Length: 1 Year *Program Size:* 2
Program ID: 042-24-21-026

Michigan

Ann Arbor

University of Michigan Program

Sponsor: University of Michigan Hospitals

Program Director:
Paul I Reynolds, MD
Dept of Anesthesiology
F3900 Mott/Box 0211
1500 E Medical Dr
Ann Arbor, MI 48109
Tel: 734 936-4280 *Fax:* 734 763-6651
Accred Length: 1 Year *Program Size:* 7
Program ID: 042-25-21-029

New Mexico

Albuquerque

University of New Mexico Program
Sponsor: University of New Mexico School of Medicine
University Hospital
Program Director:
Joyce Phillips, MD
2701 Frontier Blvd NE
Albuquerque, NM 87131
Tel: 505 272-2610 *Fax:* 505 272-1300
E-mail: jphillips@salud.unm.edu
Accred Length: 1 Year *Program Size:* 1
Program ID: 042-34-21-012

Ohio

Cincinnati

University Hospital/University of Cincinnati College of Medicine Program
Sponsor: University Hospital Inc
Children's Hospital Medical Center
Program Director:
Theodore W Striker, MD
3333 Burnet Ave
Cincinnati, OH 45229
Tel: 513 636-4408 *Fax:* 513 636-7337
Accred Length: 1 Year *Program Size:* 3
Program ID: 042-38-21-009

Cleveland

Case Western Reserve University Program
Sponsor: University Hospitals of Cleveland
Program Director:
Paul Tripi, MD
Dept of Anesthesiology
11100 Euclid Ave
Cleveland, OH 44106
Tel: 216 844-7338 *Fax:* 216 844-3781
Internet: http://www.anesth.com
Accred Length: 1 Year *Program Size:* 2
Program ID: 042-38-21-015

Pennsylvania

Pittsburgh

University Health Center of Pittsburgh Program
Sponsor: University Health Center of Pittsburgh
Children's Hospital of Pittsburgh
Program Director:
Peter J Davis, MD
3705 Fifth Ave
Pittsburgh, PA 15213
Tel: 412 692-5260 *Fax:* 412 692-8658
E-mail: davis@smtp.anes.upmc.edu
Accred Length: 1 Year *Program Size:* 12
Program ID: 042-41-21-010

Pediatric Cardiology (Pediatrics)

California

Los Angeles

Children's Hospital of Los Angeles Program
Sponsor: Children's Hospital of Los Angeles
Program Director:
Alan B Lewis, MD
Children's Hospital
PO Box 54700
Los Angeles, CA 90054
Tel: 323 669-2461 *Fax:* 323 669-7317
E-mail: alewis@chla.usc.edu
Accred Length: 3 Years *Program Size:* 3
Program ID: 325-05-11-001

UCLA Medical Center Program
Sponsor: UCLA School of Medicine
UCLA Medical Center
Program Director:
Vivek Allada, MD
UCLA Med Ctr
Div of Ped Cardiology
675 Circle Dr S/3754 MRL
Los Angeles, CA 90095-7045
Tel: 310 794-9738 *Fax:* 310 825-7458
E-mail: valLada@pediatrics.medsch.ucla.edu
Internet: http://www.peds.medsch.ucla.edu
Accred Length: 3 Years *Program Size:* 7
Program ID: 325-05-21-002

San Diego

University of California (San Diego) Program
Sponsor: University of California (San Diego) Medical Center
Program Director:
Abraham Rothman, MD
UCSD Med Ctr
200 W Arbor Dr/8445
San Diego, CA 92103-8445
Tel: 619 543-2927 *Fax:* 619 543-5994
Accred Length: 3 Years *Program Size:* 3
Program ID: 325-05-11-003

San Francisco

University of California (San Francisco) Program
Sponsor: University of California (San Francisco) School of Medicine
University of California (San Francisco) Medical Center
Program Director:
David F Teitel, MD
Univ of California San Francisco
Div of Ped Cardiology
Box 0130/Rm M-1305
San Francisco, CA 94143-0130
Tel: 415 476-8488 *Fax:* 415 502-8710
E-mail: dfteitel@pedcard.ucsf.edu
Internet: http://www.pedcard.ucsf.edu
Accred Length: 3 Years *Program Size:* 7
Program ID: 325-05-21-004

Stanford

Stanford University Program
Sponsor: Stanford University Hospital
Program Director:
Daniel Bernstein, MD
750 Welch Rd/Ste 305
Palo Alto, CA 94304
Tel: 650 723-7913 *Fax:* 650 725-8343
E-mail: dan.bernstein@stanford.edu
Accred Length: 3 Years *Program Size:* 3
Program ID: 325-05-21-062

Colorado

Denver

University of Colorado Program
Sponsor: University of Colorado Health Sciences Center
Children's Hospital
Program Director:
Mark M Boucek, MD
Children's Hospital
1056 E 19th Ave
Box B 100
Denver, CO 80218-1088
Tel: 303 837-2940 *Fax:* 303 837-2595
E-mail: boucek.mark@tchden.org
Accred Length: 3 Years *Program Size:* 3
Program ID: 325-07-21-054

Connecticut

New Haven

Yale-New Haven Medical Center Program
Sponsor: Yale-New Haven Hospital
Program Director:
Charles S Kleinman, MD
Dept of Pediatrics
333 Cedar St
PO Box 208064
New Haven, CT 06520-8064
Tel: 203 785-2022 *Fax:* 203 737-2786
E-mail: charles_kleinman@qm.yale.edu
Internet: http://www.info.med.yale.edu/pediat/
Accred Length: 3 Years *Program Size:* 4
Program ID: 325-08-11-006

District of Columbia

Washington

George Washington University Program
Sponsor: Children's National Medical Center
Program Director:
Gerard R Martin, MD
Children's National Med Ctr
111 Michigan Ave NW
Washington, DC 20010
Tel: 202 884-2020 *Fax:* 202 884-5700
E-mail: gmartin@cnmc.org
Accred Length: 3 Years *Program Size:* 3
Program ID: 325-10-21-007

Florida

Gainesville

University of Florida Program
Sponsor: University of Florida College of Medicine
Shands Hospital at the University of Florida
Program Director:
Barry J Byrne, MD PhD
Univ of Florida
Div of Ped Cardiology
PO Box 100296
Gainesville, FL 32610-0296
Tel: 352 392-6431 *Fax:* 352 392-0547
E-mail: byrne@college.med.ufl.edu
Internet: http://www.shandskids.com
Accred Length: 3 Years *Program Size:* 6
Program ID: 325-11-11-008

Miami

University of Miami-Jackson Memorial Medical Center Program
Sponsor: University of Miami-Jackson Memorial Medical Center
Program Director:
Grace S Wolff, MD
Univ of Miami-Jackson Memorial Med Ctr
PO Box 016960 (R-76)
E Tower Rm 5043
Miami, FL 33101
Tel: 305 585-6683 *Fax:* 305 324-6012
E-mail: gwolff@mednet.med.miami.edu
Internet: http://members.aol.com/sueming/main.html
Accred Length: 3 Years *Program Size:* 6
Program ID: 325-11-21-009

Georgia

Atlanta

Emory University Program
Sponsor: Emory University School of Medicine
Egleston Children's Hospital at Emory University
Grady Memorial Hospital
Program Director:
David W Jones, MD
Children's Heart Ctr
2040 Ridgewood Dr NE
Atlanta, GA 30322
Tel: 404 778-5111 *Fax:* 404 778-5110
Accred Length: 3 Years *Program Size:* 0
Program ID: 325-12-21-010

Augusta

Medical College of Georgia Program
Sponsor: Medical College of Georgia Hospital and Clinics
Program Director:
William B Strong, MD
Med Coll of Georgia Hospital and Clinics
Ped Cardiology
1120 15th St/BAA800W
Augusta, GA 30912-3710
Tel: 706 721-2336 *Fax:* 706 721-3838
E-mail: wstrong@mail.mcg.edu
Accred Length: 3 Years *Program Size:* 3
Program ID: 325-12-11-011

Illinois

Chicago

McGaw Medical Center of Northwestern University Program
Sponsor: Northwestern University Medical School
Children's Memorial Medical Center
Program Director:
Samuel S Gidding, MD
Div of Cardiology #21
Children's Memorial Hospital
2300 Children's Plaza
Chicago, IL 60614
Tel: 773 880-4553 *Fax:* 773 880-8111
E-mail: s.giddding@nwu.edu
Accred Length: 3 Years *Program Size:* 4
Program ID: 325-16-11-013

Oak Lawn

Christ Hospital and Medical Center Program
Sponsor: Christ Hospital and Medical Center
Program Director:
Earl P Ow, MD
4440 W 95th St
Oak Lawn, IL 60453
Tel: 708 346-5580 *Fax:* 708 361-4068
E-mail: phil@thic.com
Accred Length: 3 Years *Program Size:* 12
Program ID: 325-16-21-067

Indiana

Indianapolis

Indiana University School of Medicine Program
Sponsor: Indiana University School of Medicine
Clarian IU Hospital
Clarian Riley Hospital for Children
Program Director:
Roger A Hurwitz, MD
Indiana Univ Med Ctr-Riley Hospital for Children
702 Barnhill Dr
Riley Research/104
Indianapolis, IN 46202-5225
Tel: 317 274-8906 *Fax:* 317 274-4022
Accred Length: 3 Years *Program Size:* 4
Program ID: 325-17-11-017

Iowa

Iowa City

University of Iowa Hospitals and Clinics Program
Sponsor: University of Iowa Hospitals and Clinics
Program Director:
Larry T Mahoney, MD
Univ of Iowa Hospitals and Clinics
Dept of Pediatrics
200 Hawkins Dr
Iowa City, IA 52242-1009
Tel: 319 356-2837 *Fax:* 319 356-4693
E-mail: larry-mahoney@uiowa.edu
Accred Length: 3 Years *Program Size:* 3
Program ID: 325-18-11-018

Louisiana

New Orleans

Tulane University Program
Sponsor: Tulane University School of Medicine
Alton Ochsner Medical Foundation
Tulane Hospital for Children
Program Director:
Arthur S Pickoff, MD
Walter S Culpepper, MD
Dept of Ped Cardiology
1430 Tulane Ave/SL-37
New Orleans, LA 70112-2699
Tel: 504 584-3617 *Fax:* 504 584-2950
E-mail: apickof@tmcpop.tmc.tulane.edu
Accred Length: 3 Years *Program Size:* 6
Program ID: 325-21-21-064

Maryland

Baltimore

Johns Hopkins University Program
Sponsor: Johns Hopkins University School of Medicine
Johns Hopkins Hospital
Program Director:
Jean S Kan, MD
Johns Hopkins Univ
600 N Wolfe St
Brady 516
Baltimore, MD 21287
Tel: 410 955-5987 *Fax:* 410 955-0897
E-mail: pedscard@jhmi.edu
Accred Length: 3 Years *Program Size:* 3
Program ID: 325-23-11-021

Massachusetts

Boston

Children's Hospital/Boston Medical Center Program
Sponsor: Children's Hospital
Program Director:
James E Lock, MD
Children's Hospital
300 Longwood Ave
Boston, MA 02115
Tel: 617 355-7313 *Fax:* 617 355-7513
E-mail: lang@a1.tch.harvard.edu
Accred Length: 3 Years *Program Size:* 18
Program ID: 325-24-11-022

Michigan

Ann Arbor

University of Michigan Program
Sponsor: University of Michigan Hospitals
Program Director:
Macdonald Dick II, MD
C S Mott Children's Hospital
F1310 Mott Box 0204
1500 E Medical Center Dr
Ann Arbor, MI 48109-0204
Tel: 734 936-8993 *Fax:* 734 936-9470
E-mail: mdick@umich.edu
Internet:
http://www.ped.med.umich.edu/divisions/cardio/card,html
Accred Length: 3 Years *Program Size:* 9
Program ID: 325-25-11-023

Detroit

Wayne State University/Detroit Medical Center Program
Sponsor: Wayne State University/Detroit Medical Center
Children's Hospital of Michigan
Program Director:
Michael L Epstein, MD
3901 Beaubien Blvd
Detroit, MI 48201-2196
Tel: 313 745-5956 *Fax:* 313 993-0894
E-mail: mepstein@dmc.org
Accred Length: 3 Years *Program Size:* 4
Program ID: 325-25-21-061

Minnesota

Minneapolis

University of Minnesota Program
Sponsor: University of Minnesota Medical School
Fairview-University Medical Center
Program Director:
John L Bass, MD
420 Delaware St SE
Box 94 UMHC
Minneapolis, MN 55455
Tel: 612 626-2755 *Fax:* 612 626-2467
Accred Length: 3 Years *Program Size:* 6
Program ID: 325-26-21-024

Rochester

Mayo Graduate School of Medicine (Rochester) Program
Sponsor: Mayo Graduate School of Medicine-Mayo Foundation
Mayo Clinic (Rochester)
St Mary's Hospital of Rochester
Program Director:
Coburn J Porter, MD
Application Processing Ctr
Mayo Graduate Sch of Med
200 First St SW
Rochester, MN 55905
Tel: 507 284-3379 *Fax:* 507 284-0999
Internet: http://mgsm.roch.mn.pediatrics@mayo.edu
Accred Length: 3 Years *Program Size:* 3
Program ID: 325-26-21-025

Missouri

St Louis

Washington University/B-JH/SLCH Consortium Program
Sponsor: Washington University/B-JH/SLCH Consortium
St Louis Children's Hospital
Program Director:
Mark C Johnson, MD
Children's Hospital
Div of Cardiology
One Children's Pl
St Louis, MO 63110
Tel: 314 454-6095 *Fax:* 314 454-2561
Internet: http://www.wumshome.wustl.edu/peds.html
Accred Length: 3 Years *Program Size:* 7
Program ID: 325-28-11-027

New York

Brooklyn

SUNY Health Science Center at Brooklyn Program
Sponsor: SUNY Health Science Center at Brooklyn
Kings County Hospital Center
University Hospital-SUNY Health Science Center at Brooklyn
Program Director:
Dov B Nudel, MD
SUNY Health Science Ctr-Brooklyn
450 Clarkson Ave/Box 1200
Brooklyn, NY 11203
Tel: 718 270-2882 *Fax:* 718 270-1985
Accred Length: 3 Years *Program Size:* 3
Program ID: 325-35-21-059

Manhasset

North Shore University Hospital/NYU School of Medicine Program
Sponsor: North Shore University Hospital
Program Director:
Rubin S Cooper, MD
North Shore Univ Hospital
Ped Cardiology
300 Community Dr
Manhasset, NY 11030
Tel: 516 562-3078 *Fax:* 516 562-2922
Internet: http://www.nsuh.edu
Accred Length: 3 Years *Program Size:* 3
Program ID: 325-35-21-069

New Hyde Park

Albert Einstein College of Medicine at Long Island Jewish Medical Center Program
Sponsor: Long Island Jewish Medical Center
Schneider Children's Hosp (Long Island Jewish Med Ctr)
Program Director:
Fredrick Z Bierman, MD
Schneider Children's Hospital
269-01 76th Ave
New Hyde Park, NY 11040
Tel: 718 470-7350 *Fax:* 718 343-9419
E-mail: bierman@lij.edu
Internet: http://www.lij.edu
Accred Length: 3 Years *Program Size:* 3
Program ID: 325-35-21-030

New York

Mount Sinai School of Medicine Program
Sponsor: Mount Sinai School of Medicine
Mount Sinai Medical Center
Program Director:
Ira A Parness, MD
Mount Sinai Med Ctr
One Gustave L Levy Pl/Box 1201
New York, NY 10029-6574
Tel: 212 241-8662 *Fax:* 212 534-2659
E-mail: gelb@msvax.mssm.edu
Internet: http://www.mssm.edu/peds/cardfell.html
Accred Length: 3 Years *Program Size:* 5
Program ID: 325-35-11-060

New York and Presbyterian Hospital (Columbia Campus) Program
Sponsor: New York and Presbyterian Hospital
New York and Presbyterian Hospital (Columbia Campus)
New York and Presbyterian Hospital (Cornell Campus)
Program Director:
Welton M Gersony, MD
Columbia Univ Coll of Physicians and Surgeons
630 W 168th St
New York, NY 10032
Tel: 212 305-8509 *Fax:* 212 305-4429
Accred Length: 3 Years *Program Size:* 14
Program ID: 325-35-11-034

New York University Medical Center Program
Sponsor: New York University Medical Center
Bellevue Hospital Center
Program Director:
Michael Artman, MD
New York Univ Med Ctr
530 First Ave/FPO Ste 9-V
New York, NY 10016
Tel: 212 263-5993 *Fax:* 212 263-5808
E-mail: michael.artman@mcfpo.med.nyu.edu
Internet: http://www.pedcard.med.nyu.edu
Accred Length: 3 Years *Program Size:* 4
Program ID: 325-35-21-033

Rochester

University of Rochester Program
Sponsor: Strong Memorial Hospital of the University of Rochester
Program Director:
Roger P Vermilion, MD
Univ of Rochester Sch of Med and Dentistry
Div of Ped Cardiology
601 Elmwood Ave/Box 631
Rochester, NY 14642
Tel: 716 275-6096 *Fax:* 716 275-7436
E-mail: rvermilion@mail.urmc.rochester.edu
Accred Length: 3 Years *Program Size:* 2
Program ID: 325-35-21-035

Syracuse

SUNY Health Science Center at Syracuse Program
Sponsor: University Hospital-SUNY Health Science Center at Syracuse
Crouse Hospital
Program Director:
Winston E Gaum, MD
725 Irving Ave/Ste 804
Syracuse, NY 13210
Tel: 315 470-7487 *Fax:* 315 464-5761
Accred Length: 3 Years *Program Size:* 3
Program ID: 325-35-21-053

North Carolina

Durham

Duke University Program
Sponsor: Duke University Medical Center
Program Director:
Brenda E Armstrong, MD
Duke Univ Med Ctr
PO Box 3090
Durham, NC 27710
Tel: 919 681-3781 *Fax:* 919 681-8927
E-mail: armst002@onyx.mc.duke.edu
Accred Length: 3 Years *Program Size:* 5
Program ID: 325-36-11-037

Ohio

Cincinnati

Children's Hospital Medical Center/University of Cincinnati College of Medicine Program

Sponsor: Children's Hospital Medical Center
Program Director:
Robert H Beekman, MD
Div of Cardiology
Children's Hospital Med Ctr
3333 Burnet Ave
Cincinnati, OH 45229-3039
Tel: 513 636-7072 *Fax:* 513 636-3952
Internet: http://www.chmcc.org
Accred Length: 3 Years *Program Size:* 9
Program ID: 325-38-11-038

Cleveland

Case Western Reserve University Program

Sponsor: University Hospitals of Cleveland
Program Director:
Kenneth G Zahka, MD
Rainbow Babies and Children's Hospital
Div of Ped Cardiology
11100 Euclid Ave/MS RBC 6011
Cleveland, OH 44106-6011
Tel: 216 844-3275 *Fax:* 216 844-5478
E-mail: kgz@po.cwru.edu
Accred Length: 3 Years *Program Size:* 3
Program ID: 325-38-11-039

Columbus

Children's Hospital/Ohio State University Program

Sponsor: Children's Hospital
Program Director:
Hugh D Allen, MD
Sect of Ped Cardiology
Columbus Children's Hospital
700 Children's Dr
Columbus, OH 43205
Tel: 614 722-2530 *Fax:* 614 722-2549
E-mail: hallen@chi.osu.edu
Internet: http://www.childrenscolumbus.org
Accred Length: 3 Years *Program Size:* 3
Program ID: 325-38-21-070

Oregon

Portland

Oregon Health Sciences University Program

Sponsor: Oregon Health Sciences University Hospital
Program Director:
Mark D Reller, MD
Oregon Health Sciences Univ
Ped Cardiology/UHN-60
3181 SW Sam Jackson Park Rd
Portland, OR 97201
Tel: 503 494-8094 *Fax:* 503 494-2190
E-mail: sahnd@ohsu.edu
Accred Length: 3 Years *Program Size:* 4
Program ID: 325-40-11-040

Pennsylvania

Philadelphia

Children's Hospital of Philadelphia Program

Sponsor: Children's Hospital of Philadelphia
Program Director:
Paul M Weinberg, MD
Children's Hospital of Philadelphia
One Children's Ctr
34th St and Civic Center Blvd
Philadelphia, PA 19104
Tel: 215 590-3274 *Fax:* 215 590-5825
E-mail: weinberg@email.chop.edu
Internet:
http://www.chop.edu/clinical/cardiac/cardfel.htm
Accred Length: 3 Years *Program Size:* 10
Program ID: 325-41-11-041

St Christopher's Hospital for Children Program

Sponsor: St Christopher's Hospital for Children
Program Director:
Bradley W Robinson, MD
Heart Ctr for Children
St Christopher's Hospital for Children
Erie Ave at Front St
Philadelphia, PA 19134-1095
Tel: 215 427-4816 *Fax:* 215 427-4822
E-mail: brobin7001@aol.com
Accred Length: 3 Years *Program Size:* 3
Program ID: 325-41-11-042

Pittsburgh

University Health Center of Pittsburgh Program

Sponsor: University Health Center of Pittsburgh
Children's Hospital of Pittsburgh
Program Director:
Frederick S Sherman, MD
Children's Hospital
Dept of Cardiology
3705 Fifth Ave
Pittsburgh, PA 15213-2583
Tel: 412 692-5540 *Fax:* 412 692-5138
E-mail: shermaf_at_chpcard@chplink.chp.edu
Accred Length: 3 Years *Program Size:* 3
Program ID: 325-41-11-043

South Carolina

Charleston

Medical University of South Carolina Program

Sponsor: Medical University of South Carolina College of Medicine
MUSC Medical Center
Program Director:
J Philip Saul, MD
Med Univ of South Carolina
Div of Ped Cardiology
165 Ashley Ave
Charleston, SC 29403
Tel: 803 792-3287 *Fax:* 803 792-3284
E-mail: saulp@musc.edu
Internet: http://www.pediatrics.musc.edu/pedscard
Accred Length: 3 Years *Program Size:* 8
Program ID: 325-45-11-044

Tennessee

Nashville

Vanderbilt University Program

Sponsor: Vanderbilt University Medical Center
Program Director:
Thomas P Graham Jr, MD
Vanderbilt Univ Med Ctr
Div of Ped Cardiology
D-2220 MCN
Nashville, TN 37232-2572
Tel: 615 322-7447 *Fax:* 615 343-9951
E-mail: tom.graham@mcmail.vanderbilt.edu
Accred Length: 3 Years *Program Size:* 4
Program ID: 325-47-11-045

Texas

Dallas

University of Texas Southwestern Medical School Program

Sponsor: University of Texas Southwestern Medical School
Children's Medical Center of Dallas
Program Director:
Lynn Mahony, MD
Univ of Texas Southwestern Med Ctr
Dept of Pediatrics
5323 Harry Hines Blvd
Dallas, TX 75235-9063
Tel: 214 539-2333 *Fax:* 214 539-6154
E-mail: lmahony@childmed.dallas.tx.us
Internet: http://www.swmed.edu/home_pages/pedicardio
Accred Length: 3 Years *Program Size:* 3
Program ID: 325-48-21-058

Houston

Baylor College of Medicine Program

Sponsor: Baylor College of Medicine
Texas Children's Hospital
Program Director:
Thomas A Vargo, MD
Baylor Coll of Med, Pediatric Cardiology Sect
6621 Fannin St/MC 2-2280
Houston, TX 77030
Tel: 713 770-5642 *Fax:* 713 770-5630
E-mail: mcruz@msmail.card.tch.tmc.edu
Internet: http://www.bcm.tmc.edu/pedi/cardio/
Accred Length: 3 Years *Program Size:* 11
Program ID: 325-48-11-047

Virginia

Charlottesville

University of Virginia Program

Sponsor: University of Virginia Medical Center
Program Director:
Howard P Gutgesell, MD
Dept of Pediatrics/Box 386
Univ of Virginia Health Science Ctr
Charlottesville, VA 22908
Tel: 804 924-2486 *Fax:* 804 924-5656
Accred Length: 3 Years *Program Size:* 2
Program ID: 325-51-21-050

Richmond

Medical College of Virginia/Virginia Commonwealth University Program
Sponsor: Medical College of Virginia/Virginia Commonwealth University
Medical College of Virginia Hospitals
Program Director:
Richard M Schieken, MD MS
Med Coll of Virginia
PO Box 980026
Richmond, VA 23298-0026
Tel: 804 828-1374 *Fax:* 804 828-8517
E-mail: schieken@hsc.vcu.edu
Internet: http://www.littlehearts.com/
Accred Length: 3 Years *Program Size:* 2
Program ID: 325-51-11-051

Pediatric Critical Care Medicine (Pediatrics)

Alabama

Birmingham

University of Alabama Medical Center Program
Sponsor: University of Alabama Hospital
Children's Hospital of Alabama
Program Director:
Scott E Curtis, MD
Children's Hospital
1600 Seventh Ave S
ACC 504
Birmingham, AL 35233
Tel: 205 939-9387 *Fax:* 205 975-6505
Accred Length: 3 Years *Program Size:* 3
Program ID: 323-01-21-040

Arkansas

Little Rock

University of Arkansas for Medical Sciences Program
Sponsor: University of Arkansas College of Medicine
Arkansas Children's Hospital
Program Director:
Kanwaljeet S Anand, MB BS DPh
Arkansas Children's Hospital
800 Marshall St/Slot 512-12
Little Rock, AR 72202-3591
Tel: 501 320-1846 *Fax:* 501 320-3188
E-mail: sms@george.ach.uams.edu
Accred Length: 3 Years *Program Size:* 3
Program ID: 323-04-21-006

California

Loma Linda

Loma Linda University Program
Sponsor: Loma Linda University Medical Center
Program Director:
Ronald M Perkin, MD
Loma Linda Univ Sch of Med
Ped Critical Care Med
11175 Campus St/Coleman Pav
Loma Linda, CA 92354
Tel: 714 824-4250 *Fax:* 714 824-4818
E-mail: picu@ccmail.llumc.edu
Internet: http://www.llu.edu/lluch/picu
Accred Length: 3 Years *Program Size:* 3
Program ID: 323-05-31-057

Los Angeles

Children's Hospital of Los Angeles Program
Sponsor: Children's Hospital of Los Angeles
Program Director:
Randall C Wetzel, MB BS
Childrens Hospital Los Angeles
Div of Critical Care Med
4650 Sunset Blvd MS12
Los Angeles, CA 90027-6062
Tel: 323 669-2557 *Fax:* 323 664-0728
E-mail: rwetzel@chla.usc.edu
Internet: http://www.usc.edu
Accred Length: 3 Years *Program Size:* 7
Program ID: 323-05-31-047

UCLA Medical Center Program
Sponsor: UCLA School of Medicine
Long Beach Memorial Medical Center
UCLA Medical Center
Program Director:
Judith E Brill, MD
UCLA Sch of Med
Ped Critical Care
Box 951752
Los Angeles, CA 90095-1752
Tel: 310 825-6752 *Fax:* 310 794-6623
Accred Length: 3 Years *Program Size:* 7
Program ID: 323-05-21-023

San Diego

Naval Medical Center (San Diego) Program
Sponsor: Naval Medical Center (San Diego)
Children's Hospital and Health Center
Program Director:
Bradley M Peterson, MD
3020 Children's Way/MC 5065
San Diego, CA 92123
Tel: 619 576-5863 *Fax:* 619 279-8415
E-mail: bcfisher@popmail.ucsd.edu
Accred Length: 3 Years *Program Size:* 6
Program ID: 323-05-21-042
US Armed Services Program

San Francisco

University of California (San Francisco) Program
Sponsor: University of California (San Francisco) School of Medicine
Children's Hospital-Oakland
University of California (San Francisco) Medical Center
Program Director:
Maurice S Zwass, MD
Timothy S Yeh, MD
Univ of California San Francisco
505 Parnassus Ave/Moffitt 680
San Francisco, CA 94143-0106
Tel: 415 476-5153 *Fax:* 415 502-4186
E-mail: maurice_zwass@quickmail.ucsf.edu
Accred Length: 3 Years *Program Size:* 9
Program ID: 323-05-21-021

Stanford

Stanford University Program
Sponsor: Stanford University Hospital
Lucile Salter Packard Children's Hospital at Stanford
Program Director:
Lorry R Frankel, MD
Dept of Pediatrics
725 Welch Rd
Palo Alto, CA 94304
Tel: 650 723-5495 *Fax:* 650 725-8343
E-mail: lrf@leland.stanford.edu
Accred Length: 3 Years *Program Size:* 2
Program ID: 323-05-21-056

Torrance

Los Angeles County-Harbor-UCLA Medical Center Program
Sponsor: Los Angeles County-Harbor-UCLA Medical Center
Children's Hospital of Orange County
LAC-King/Drew Medical Center
Program Director:
Richard B Mink, MD
Harbor-UCLA Med Ctr
1000 W Carson St/Box 491
Torrance, CA 90509
Tel: 310 222-4002 *Fax:* 310 320-2271
E-mail: rmink@ucla.edu
Accred Length: 3 Years *Program Size:* 6
Program ID: 323-05-21-033

Colorado

Denver

University of Colorado Program
Sponsor: University of Colorado Health Sciences Center
Children's Hospital
National Jewish Ctr for Immunology and Respiratory Medicine
Program Director:
Anthony G Durmowicz, MD
Kurt R Stenmark, MD
Children's Hospital
Box B530/Critical Care
1056 E 19th Ave
Denver, CO 80218
Tel: 303 861-6211 *Fax:* 303 764-8074
E-mail: tony.durmowicz@uchsc.edu
Accred Length: 3 Years *Program Size:* 5
Program ID: 323-07-21-034

Connecticut

New Haven

Yale-New Haven Medical Center Program
Sponsor: Yale-New Haven Hospital
Program Director:
George Lister, MD
Yale Univ Sch of Med
Dept of Pediatrics
333 Cedar St
New Haven, CT 06520-8064
Tel: 203 785-4651 *Fax:* 203 785-5833
E-mail: george.lister@yale.edu
Accred Length: 3 Years *Program Size:* 6
Program ID: 323-08-21-036

District of Columbia

Washington

George Washington University Program
Sponsor: Children's National Medical Center
Program Director:
Murray M Pollack, MD
Children's National Med Ctr
111 Michigan Ave NW
Washington, DC 20010-2970
Tel: 202 884-2130 *Fax:* 202 884-5724
E-mail: mpollack@cnmc.org
Internet: http://www.cnmc.org
Accred Length: 3 Years *Program Size:* 4
Program ID: 323-10-21-035

Georgetown University Program
Sponsor: Georgetown University Medical Center
Program Director:
Gabriel J Hauser, MD
Georgetown Univ Hospital
3800 Reservoir Rd NW
Ste CCC 5414
Washington, DC 20007
Tel: 202 784-2468 *Fax:* 202 784-2613
E-mail: hauserg@gunet.georgetown.edu
Accred Length: 3 Years *Program Size:* 2
Program ID: 323-10-21-058

Florida

Gainesville

University of Florida Program
Sponsor: University of Florida College of Medicine
Shands Hospital at the University of Florida
Program Director:
Salvatore R Goodwin, MD
Univ of Florida Coll of Med
PO Box 100254 JHMHC
Gainesville, FL 32610-0254
Tel: 352 395-0462 *Fax:* 352 395-0443
E-mail: goodwin@anest1.anest.ufl.edu
Internet: http://www.anest.ufl.edu
Accred Length: 3 Years *Program Size:* 4
Program ID: 323-11-21-020

Jacksonville

University of Florida Health Science Center/Jacksonville Program
Sponsor: University of Florida College of Medicine at Jacksonville
University Medical Center (UFHSC/J)
Baptist Medical Center (UFHSC/J)
Program Director:
Michael O Gayle, MD
Univ of Florida Health Science Ctr-Jacksonville
820 Prudential Dr
Ste 203
Jacksonville, FL 32207
Tel: 904 202-8332 *Fax:* 904 396-1630
E-mail: mogayle@nemours.org
Accred Length: 3 Years *Program Size:* 2
Program ID: 323-11-21-045

Miami

Miami Children's Hospital Program
Sponsor: Miami Children's Hospital
Program Director:
Jack Wolfsdorf, MD
3100 SW 62nd Ave
Miami, FL 33155
Tel: 305 662-2639 *Fax:* 305 663-0530
Accred Length: 3 Years *Program Size:* 6
Program ID: 323-11-21-061

University of Miami-Jackson Memorial Medical Center Program
Sponsor: University of Miami-Jackson Memorial Medical Center
Program Director:
Charles L Schleien, MD
Univ of Miami Sch of Med
Dept of Pediatrics (R-131)
PO Box 016960
Miami, FL 33101
Tel: 305 585-6051 *Fax:* 305 325-0293
E-mail: cschleie@peds.med.miami.edu
Accred Length: 3 Years *Program Size:* 6
Program ID: 323-11-21-012

Georgia

Atlanta

Emory University Program
Sponsor: Emory University School of Medicine
Egleston Children's Hospital at Emory University
Program Director:
James D Fortenberry, MD
Dept of Ped Critical Care
Egleston Children's Hospital
1405 Clifton Rd NE
Atlanta, GA 30322
Tel: 404 315-2212 *Fax:* 404 325-6233
E-mail: jfortenb@mail.egleston.org
Accred Length: 3 Years *Program Size:* 2
Program ID: 323-12-21-030

Augusta

Medical College of Georgia Program
Sponsor: Medical College of Georgia Hospital and Clinics
Program Director:
Lyle E Fisher Jr, MD
Children's Med Ctr-Med Coll of Georgia
1120 15th St
BIW 6033
Augusta, GA 30912-3758
Tel: 706 721-4402 *Fax:* 706 721-7872
E-mail: lfisher@mail.mcg.edu
Accred Length: 3 Years *Program Size:* 3
Program ID: 323-12-21-010

Illinois

Chicago

McGaw Medical Center of Northwestern University Program

Sponsor: Northwestern University Medical School
Children's Memorial Medical Center

Program Director:
Harris P Baden, MD
Children's Memorial Hospital
2300 Children's Plaza/Box 73
Chicago, IL 60614
Tel: 773 880-4780 *Fax:* 773 880-4057
E-mail: hbaden@nwu.edu
Accred Length: 3 Years *Program Size:* 6
Program ID: 323-16-21-032

Rush-Presbyterian-St Luke's Medical Center Program

Sponsor: Rush-Presbyterian-St Luke's Medical Center
Cook County Hospital

Program Director:
Phillip Jacobson, MD
Rush Med Coll
1653 W Congress Pkwy
622 Murdock
Chicago, IL 60612-3864
Tel: 312 942-6194 *Fax:* 312 942-4370
Accred Length: 3 Years *Program Size:* 0
Program ID: 323-16-21-065

University of Chicago Program

Sponsor: University of Chicago Hospitals
University of Chicago Children's Hospital

Program Director:
Brian F Rudinsky, MD
Univ of Chicago-Children's Hospital
5841 S Maryland Ave
MC 4064
Chicago, IL 60637-1470
Tel: 773 702-9659 *Fax:* 773 702-2488
E-mail: brudinsk@midway.uchicago.edu
Internet:
http://peds-www.bsd.uchicago.edu/sections/pulmcrit/index.html
Accred Length: 3 Years *Program Size:* 3
Program ID: 323-16-21-031

Oak Lawn

Christ Hospital and Medical Center Program

Sponsor: Christ Hospital and Medical Center

Program Director:
Gerardo Reyes, MD
Hope Children's Hospital-Christ Hospital
4440 W 95th St
Oak Lawn, IL 60453
Tel: 708 346-5685 *Fax:* 708 346-4712
E-mail: gerardo.reyes-md@advocatehealth.com
Accred Length: 3 Years *Program Size:* 3
Program ID: 323-16-21-073

Park Ridge

Lutheran General Hospital Program

Sponsor: Lutheran General Hospital

Program Director:
Elizabeth Bello, MD
Lutheran General Children's Hospital
Ped ICU
1775 W Dempster St
Park Ridge, IL 60068
Tel: 847 723-7682 *Fax:* 847 723-2325
E-mail: elizabeth.bello-md@advocatehealth.com
Accred Length: 3 Years *Program Size:* 3
Program ID: 323-16-21-046

Kentucky

Louisville

University of Louisville Program

Sponsor: University of Louisville School of Medicine
Kosair Children's Hospital (Alliant Health System)

Program Director:
Mitchell P Ross, MD
Univ of Louisville
Div of Critical Care Med
571 S Floyd St/Ste 332
Louisville, KY 40202
Tel: 502 852-3720 *Fax:* 502 852-3998
Accred Length: 3 Years *Program Size:* 1
Program ID: 323-20-21-071

Maryland

Baltimore

Johns Hopkins University Program

Sponsor: Johns Hopkins University School of Medicine
Johns Hopkins Hospital

Program Director:
Donald H Shaffner Jr, MD
Johns Hopkins Hospital
600 N Wolfe St
Halsted 842
Baltimore, MD 21287-5842
Tel: 410 955-2393 *Fax:* 410 614-2911
E-mail: dshaffne@welchlink.welch.jhu.edu
Internet:
http://www.med.jhu.edu/anesthesiology/pediatri.htm
Accred Length: 3 Years *Program Size:* 8
Program ID: 323-23-21-009

University of Maryland Program

Sponsor: University of Maryland Medical System

Program Director:
Alice D Ackerman, MD
Univ of Maryland Med Ctr
22 S Greene St
Rm S5D18
Baltimore, MD 21201-1595
Tel: 410 328-6957 *Fax:* 410 328-0680
E-mail: aackerma@umms001.ab.umd.edu
Accred Length: 3 Years *Program Size:* 2
Program ID: 323-23-21-070

Massachusetts

Boston

Children's Hospital/Boston Medical Center Program

Sponsor: Children's Hospital

Program Director:
Jeffrey P Burns, MD MPH
Children's Hospital
MICU Office/FA-517
300 Longwood Ave
Boston, MA 02115
Tel: 617 355-7327 *Fax:* 617 734-3863
E-mail: burnsj@a1.tch.harvard.edu
Accred Length: 3 Years *Program Size:* 6
Program ID: 323-24-21-019

Massachusetts General Hospital Program

Sponsor: Massachusetts General Hospital

Program Director:
I David Todres, MD
Massachusetts General Hospital
Ped ICU
Ellison 317
Boston, MA 02114
Tel: 617 724-4380 *Fax:* 617 724-4391
E-mail: todres@etherdome.mgh.harvard.edu
Accred Length: 3 Years *Program Size:* 5
Program ID: 323-24-21-048

Michigan

Ann Arbor

University of Michigan Program

Sponsor: University of Michigan Hospitals

Program Director:
Joseph R Custer, MD
Univ of Michigan Med Ctr
F6884 Mott/0243
1500 E Medical Center Dr
Ann Arbor, MI 48109-0243
Tel: 313 764-5302 *Fax:* 313 763-7359
Accred Length: 3 Years *Program Size:* 4
Program ID: 323-25-21-008

Detroit

Wayne State University/Detroit Medical Center Program

Sponsor: Wayne State University/Detroit Medical Center
Children's Hospital of Michigan

Program Director:
Ashok P Sarnaik, MD
Children's Hospital
3901 Beaubien Blvd
Detroit, MI 48201-2196
Tel: 313 745-5629 *Fax:* 313 966-0105
E-mail: asarnaik@med.wayne.edu
Accred Length: 3 Years *Program Size:* 4
Program ID: 323-25-21-039

Minnesota

Minneapolis

University of Minnesota Program

Sponsor: University of Minnesota Medical School
Fairview-University Medical Center

Program Director:
David N Cornfield, MD
Box 742 UMHC
420 Delaware St SE
Minneapolis, MN 55455
Tel: 612 626-2916 *Fax:* 612 624-0696
E-mail: cornf001@tc.umn.edu
Accred Length: 3 Years *Program Size:* 4
Program ID: 323-26-21-005

Missouri

St Louis

Washington University/B-JH/SLCH Consortium Program

Sponsor: Washington University/B-JH/SLCH Consortium
St Louis Children's Hospital
Program Director:
J Julio Perez Fontan, MD
Washington Univ Sch of Med
Critical Care Med
One Children's Pl/Ste 5S20
St Louis, MO 63110
Tel: 314 454-2527 *Fax:* 314 361-0733
Accred Length: 3 Years *Program Size:* 6
Program ID: 323-28-21-060

New Jersey

Camden

UMDNJ-Robert Wood Johnson Medical School (Camden) Program

Sponsor: Cooper Hospital-University Medical Center
St Christopher's Hospital for Children
Program Director:
Farrukh Mirza, MD
Children's Regional Hospital
Cooper Hospital-UMC
3 Cooper Plaza/Ste 520
Camden, NJ 08103-1489
Tel: 609 342-2530 *Fax:* 609 963-2514
Accred Length: 3 Years *Program Size:* 3
Program ID: 323-33-31-049

Piscataway

UMDNJ-Robert Wood Johnson Medical School Program

Sponsor: UMDNJ-Robert Wood Johnson Medical School
Robert Wood Johnson University Hospital
Program Director:
Frank Castello, MD
UMDNJ-Robert Wood Johnson Med Sch
One Robert Wood Johnson Pl/CN-19
New Brunswick, NJ 08903-0019
Tel: 732 235-7887 *Fax:* 732 235-7345
E-mail: castelfr@umdnj.edu
Accred Length: 3 Years *Program Size:* 3
Program ID: 323-33-21-074

New York

Bronx

Albert Einstein College of Medicine Program

Sponsor: Albert Einstein College of Medicine of Yeshiva University
Montefiore Medical Center-Henry and Lucy Moses Division
Program Director:
Jacqueline S Weingarten-Arams, MD
Montefiore Med Ctr
111 E 210th St
NW 556
Bronx, NY 10467-2490
Tel: 718 920-4999 *Fax:* 718 920-4351
E-mail: jwarams@pol.net
Accred Length: 3 Years *Program Size:* 3
Program ID: 323-35-21-004

Buffalo

SUNY at Buffalo Graduate Medical-Dental Education Consortium Program

Sponsor: SUNY at Buffalo Grad Medical-Dental Education Consortium
CGF Health System (Children's Hospital of Buffalo)
Program Director:
Bradley P Fuhrman, MD
Children's Hospital
Dept of Ped Critical Care Med
219 Bryant St
Buffalo, NY 14222
Tel: 716 878-7442 *Fax:* 716 878-7101
Accred Length: 3 Years *Program Size:* 6
Program ID: 323-35-31-055

New Hyde Park

Albert Einstein College of Medicine at Long Island Jewish Medical Center Program

Sponsor: Long Island Jewish Medical Center
Schneider Children's Hosp (Long Island Jewish Med Ctr)
Program Director:
Mayer Sagy, MD
Schneider Children's Hospital
Long Island Jewish Med Ctr
269-01 76th Ave
New Hyde Park, NY 11040-1432
Tel: 718 470-3330 *Fax:* 718 470-0159
E-mail: sagy@lij.edu
Internet: http://www.lij.edu
Accred Length: 3 Years *Program Size:* 5
Program ID: 323-35-32-059

New York

New York and Presbyterian Hospital (Cornell Campus) Program

Sponsor: New York and Presbyterian Hospital
New York and Presbyterian Hospital (Cornell Campus)
Program Director:
Bruce M Greenwald, MD
New York Hospital-Cornell Med Ctr
Div of Ped Critical Care Med
525 E 68th St/Box 437
New York, NY 10021
Tel: 212 746-3056 *Fax:* 212 746-8332
E-mail: bmgreen@mail.med.cornell.edu
Accred Length: 3 Years *Program Size:* 6
Program ID: 323-35-21-037

Rochester

University of Rochester Program

Sponsor: Strong Memorial Hospital of the University of Rochester
Program Director:
Heidi V Connolly, MD
Univ of Rochester Med Ctr
Ped Intensive Care Unit
601 Elmwood Ave/Box 667
Rochester, NY 14642
Tel: 716 275-8138 *Fax:* 716 275-8706
E-mail: heidi_connolly@urmc.rochester.edu
Accred Length: 3 Years *Program Size:* 3
Program ID: 323-35-21-053

North Carolina

Chapel Hill

University of North Carolina Hospitals Program

Sponsor: University of North Carolina Hospitals
Program Director:
Lewis H Romer, MD
Univ of North Carolina Sch of Med
North Carolina Children's Hospital
7701A 7th Fl CB#7220
Chapel Hill, NC 27599-7220
Tel: 919 966-7495 *Fax:* 919 966-6164
E-mail: lrcc@med.unc.edu
Internet: http://www.bio.med.unc.edu/romer/romer.htm
Accred Length: 3 Years *Program Size:* 3
Program ID: 323-36-21-016

Durham

Duke University Program

Sponsor: Duke University Medical Center
Program Director:
Eva N Grayck, MD
Box 3046
Duke Univ
Durham, NC 27710
Tel: 919 681-3543 *Fax:* 919 681-8357
E-mail: grayc001@mc.duke.edu
Accred Length: 3 Years *Program Size:* 6
Program ID: 323-36-21-038

Winston-Salem

Wake Forest University School of Medicine Program

Sponsor: Wake Forest University Baptist Medical Center
Program Director:
Loren A Bauman, MD
Wake Forest Univ Sch of Med
Dept of Anesthesiology
Medical Center Blvd
Winston-Salem, NC 27157-1009
Tel: 336 716-4684 *Fax:* 336 716-8190
E-mail: lbauman@wfubmc.edu
Accred Length: 3 Years *Program Size:* 3
Program ID: 323-36-21-067

Ohio

Cincinnati

Children's Hospital Medical Center/University of Cincinnati College of Medicine Program

Sponsor: Children's Hospital Medical Center
Program Director:
Hector R Wong, MD
Children's Hospital Med Ctr
3333 Burnet Ave
OSB-5
Cincinnati, OH 45229-2899
Tel: 513 636-4259 *Fax:* 513 636-4267
E-mail: wonghr@chmcc.org
Internet: http://www.chmcc.org
Accred Length: 3 Years *Program Size:* 5
Program ID: 323-38-21-015

Cleveland

Case Western Reserve University Program

Sponsor: University Hospitals of Cleveland
MetroHealth Medical Center

Program Director:
Jeffrey L Blumer, MD
Rainbow Babies and Children's Hospital
11100 Euclid Ave
Cleveland, OH 44106-6010
Tel: 216 844-3310 *Fax:* 216 844-5122
E-mail: mxa35@po.cwru.edu
Accred Length: 3 Years *Program Size:* 6
Program ID: 323-38-21-051

Cleveland Clinic Foundation Program

Sponsor: Cleveland Clinic Foundation

Program Director:
Steven Davis, MD
Cleveland Clinic Foundation
Dept of Ped Critical Care/M43
9500 Euclid Ave
Cleveland, OH 44195-5242
Tel: 216 444-5690 *Fax:* 216 444-1162
E-mail: meded@cestmp.ccf.org
Internet: http://www.ccf.org
Accred Length: 3 Years *Program Size:* 6
Program ID: 323-38-31-052

Columbus

Children's Hospital/Ohio State University Program

Sponsor: Children's Hospital

Program Director:
Diane P Begany, MD
Children's Hospital
Sect of Critical Care Med
700 Children's Dr
Columbus, OH 43205-2696
Tel: 614 722-3435 *Fax:* 614 722-3443
E-mail: dbegany@chi.osu.edu
Accred Length: 3 Years *Program Size:* 0
Program ID: 323-38-31-054

Pennsylvania

Philadelphia

Children's Hospital of Philadelphia Program

Sponsor: Children's Hospital of Philadelphia

Program Director:
Andrew T Costarino, MD
Children's Hospital of Philadelphia
34th St and Civic Center Blvd
Philadelphia, PA 19104-4399
Tel: 215 590-1868 *Fax:* 215 590-4327
E-mail: costarino@email.chop.edu
Accred Length: 3 Years *Program Size:* 9
Program ID: 323-41-21-014

Pittsburgh

University Health Center of Pittsburgh Program

Sponsor: University Health Center of Pittsburgh
Children's Hospital of Pittsburgh

Program Director:
Ann E Thompson, MD
Children's Hospital of Pittsburgh
Ped Critical Care Med
3705 Fifth Ave
Pittsburgh, PA 15213-2583
Tel: 412 692-5164 *Fax:* 412 692-6076
E-mail: thompson@smtp.anes.upmc.edu
Accred Length: 3 Years *Program Size:* 9
Program ID: 323-41-21-028

Puerto Rico

San Juan

University of Puerto Rico Program

Sponsor: University of Puerto Rico School of Medicine
University Pediatric Hospital

Program Director:
Felicita Gotay-Cruz, MD
Univ of Puerto Rico
PO Box 365067
San Juan, PR 00936-5067
Tel: 787 281-2705 *Fax:* 787 751-5306
E-mail: irmamd@tld2.tld.net
Accred Length: 3 Years *Program Size:* 2
Program ID: 323-42-21-069

Tennessee

Memphis

University of Tennessee Program

Sponsor: University of Tennessee College of Medicine
LeBonheur Children's Medical Center

Program Director:
Stephanie A Storgion, MD
Univ of Tennessee, Dept of Pediatrics
50 N Dunlap
Memphis, TN 38103
Tel: 901 572-3132 *Fax:* 901 572-5198
E-mail: sstorgion@utmem1.utmem.edu
Accred Length: 3 Years *Program Size:* 6
Program ID: 323-47-21-027

Nashville

Vanderbilt University Program

Sponsor: Vanderbilt University Medical Center

Program Director:
Kevin B Churchwell, MD
Vanderbilt Children's Hospitlal
Div of Ped Critical Care/Anesthesia
714 Medical Arts Bldg
Nashville, TN 37232-1565
Tel: 615 936-3968 *Fax:* 615 936-3467
E-mail: kevin.churchwell@mcmail.vanderbilt.edu
Accred Length: 3 Years *Program Size:* 5
Program ID: 323-47-21-062

Texas

Dallas

University of Texas Southwestern Medical School Program

Sponsor: University of Texas Southwestern Medical School
Children's Medical Center of Dallas
Dallas County Hospital District-Parkland Memorial Hospital

Program Director:
Brett P Giroir, MD
Univ of Texas Southwestern Med Ctr
5323 Harry Hines Blvd
Dallas, TX 75235-9063
Tel: 214 648-8552 *Fax:* 214 648-8617
E-mail: bgiroi@mednet.swmed.edu
Accred Length: 3 Years *Program Size:* 12
Program ID: 323-48-21-041

Houston

Baylor College of Medicine Program

Sponsor: Baylor College of Medicine
Texas Children's Hospital

Program Director:
Mary M Mariscalco, MD
Baylor Coll of Med
Pediatric Critical Care
One Baylor Plaza
Houston, TX 77030-2399
Tel: 713 770-6230 *Fax:* 713 770-6229
E-mail: marym@bcm.tmc.edu
Internet: http://www.bcm.tmc.edu/pedi/ccare
Accred Length: 3 Years *Program Size:* 7
Program ID: 323-48-31-044

San Antonio

University of Texas Health Science Center at San Antonio Program

Sponsor: University of Texas Medical School at San Antonio
Santa Rosa Health Care Corporation
University Hospital-South Texas Medical Center

Program Director:
Richard P Taylor, MD
Univ of Texas Health Science Ctr
7703 Floyd Curl Dr
San Antonio, TX 78284-7829
Tel: 210 567-5314 *Fax:* 210 567-5311
E-mail: taylorr@uthscsa.edu
Accred Length: 3 Years *Program Size:* 3
Program ID: 323-48-21-072

Utah

Salt Lake City

University of Utah Program

Sponsor: University of Utah Medical Center
Primary Children's Medical Center

Program Director:
Madolin Witte, MD
Univ of Utah
100 N Medical Dr
Salt Lake City, UT 84113-1103
Tel: 801 588-3286 *Fax:* 801 588-3297
E-mail: witte@med.utah.edu
Accred Length: 3 Years *Program Size:* 4
Program ID: 323-49-21-003

Programs

Virginia

Charlottesville

University of Virginia Program
Sponsor: University of Virginia Medical Center
Program Director:
Douglas F Willson, MD
Children's Med Ctr
Box 386
Charlottesville, VA 22908
Tel: 804 982-1707 *Fax:* 804 924-2940
E-mail: dfw4m@virginia.edu
Accred Length: 3 Years *Program Size:* 2
Program ID: 323-51-21-026

Richmond

Medical College of Virginia/Virginia Commonwealth University Program
Sponsor: Medical College of Virginia/Virginia Commonwealth University
Medical College of Virginia Hospitals
Program Director:
Sara L White, MD
Med Coll of Virginia
Box 980530
Richmond, VA 23298-0530
Tel: 804 828-4529 *Fax:* 804 828-4509
Accred Length: 3 Years *Program Size:* 1
Program ID: 323-51-21-025

Washington

Seattle

University of Washington Program
Sponsor: University of Washington School of Medicine
Children's Hospital and Medical Center
Program Director:
Lynn D Martin, MD
Children's Hospital and Regional Med Ctr
Dept of Anesthesia/Critical Care Med
4800 Sand Point Way NE (M/S CH-05)
Seattle, WA 98105
Tel: 206 526-2170 *Fax:* 206 527-3935
E-mail: tmcall@chmc.org
Internet:
http://weber.u.washington.edu/~chmcacc/web/picu.htm
Accred Length: 3 Years *Program Size:* 6
Program ID: 323-54-21-013

Wisconsin

Madison

University of Wisconsin Program
Sponsor: University of Wisconsin Hospital and Clinics
Program Director:
Gregory A Hollman, MD PhD
Univ of Wisconsin
H4/470 Clinical Sci Ctr
600 Highland Ave
Madison, WI 53792-4108
Tel: 608 263-8832 *Fax:* 608 263-0440
E-mail: ghollman@facstaff.wisc.edu
Accred Length: 3 Years *Program Size:* 3
Program ID: 323-56-21-001

Milwaukee

Medical College of Wisconsin Program
Sponsor: Medical College of Wisconsin Affiliated Hospitals Inc
Children's Hospital of Wisconsin
Program Director:
Karen J Wendelberger, MD
PO Box 1997 MS#681
9000 W Wisconsin Ave
Milwaukee, WI 53201
Tel: 414 266-3360 *Fax:* 414 266-3563
E-mail: kwendel@post.its.mcw.edu
Internet: http://www.mcw.edu/peds/cc/
Accred Length: 3 Years *Program Size:* 7
Program ID: 323-56-21-002

Pediatric Endocrinology (Pediatrics)

Arkansas

Little Rock

University of Arkansas for Medical Sciences Program
Sponsor: University of Arkansas College of Medicine
Arkansas Children's Hospital
Program Director:
Stephen F Kemp, MD PhD
Arkansas Children's Hospital
800 Marshall St
Little Rock, AR 72202-3591
Tel: 501 320-1430 *Fax:* 501 320-6299
E-mail: kempstephenf@exchange.uams.edu
Accred Length: 3 Years *Program Size:* 3
Program ID: 326-04-21-040

California

Los Angeles

Children's Hospital of Los Angeles Program
Sponsor: Children's Hospital of Los Angeles
Program Director:
Kaufman R Francine, MD
Children's Hospital
Div of Endocrinology/MS 61
4650 Sunset Blvd
Los Angeles, CA 90027
Tel: 323 669-4606 *Fax:* 323 953-1349
E-mail: ucmg@chlais.usc.edu
Accred Length: 3 Years *Program Size:* 1
Program ID: 326-05-11-001

UCLA Medical Center Program
Sponsor: UCLA School of Medicine
UCLA Medical Center
Program Director:
Mitchell E Geffner, MD
Div of Endocrinology
UCLA Children's Hospital
Los Angeles, CA 90095-1752
Tel: 310 825-6496 *Fax:* 310 206-5843
E-mail: mgeffner@pediatrics.medsch.ucla.edu
Internet: http://www.peds.medsch.ucla.edu
Accred Length: 3 Years *Program Size:* 2
Program ID: 326-05-21-003

San Diego

University of California (San Diego) Program
Sponsor: University of California (San Diego) Medical Center
Children's Hospital and Health Center
Program Director:
Kenneth Lee Jones, MD
UCSD Med Ctr
Div of Endocrinology
9500 Gilman Dr/0831
La Jolla, CA 92093-0831
Tel: 619 543-5238 *Fax:* 619 543-3575
E-mail: kljones@ucsd.edu
Accred Length: 3 Years *Program Size:* 3
Program ID: 326-05-31-004

San Francisco

University of California (San Francisco) Program
Sponsor: University of California (San Francisco) School of Medicine
University of California (San Francisco) Medical Center
Program Director:
Walter L Miller, MD
Univ of California San Francisco
Dept of Pediatrics/Box 0978
San Francisco, CA 94143-0978
Tel: 415 476-2598 *Fax:* 415 476-6286
Internet: http://itsa.ucsf.edu/ pedendo
Accred Length: 3 Years *Program Size:* 5
Program ID: 326-05-21-005

Stanford

Stanford University Program
Sponsor: Stanford University Hospital
Lucile Salter Packard Children's Hospital at Stanford
Program Director:
Raymond L Hintz, MD
Stanford Univ
Dept of Pediatrics
Med Ctr/Rm S-302
Stanford, CA 94305-5208
Tel: 650 723-5791 *Fax:* 650 725-8375
E-mail: hintz@forsythe.stanford.edu
Internet: http://www.med2.stanford.edu/lpch/pedres/
Accred Length: 3 Years *Program Size:* 3
Program ID: 326-05-21-055

Torrance

Los Angeles County-Harbor-UCLA Medical Center Program
Sponsor: Los Angeles County-Harbor-UCLA Medical Center
Program Director:
Jo Anne Brasel, MD
Harbor-UCLA Med Ctr
1000 W Carson St/Box 446
Torrance, CA 90509-2910
Tel: 310 222-1971 *Fax:* 310 533-0627
E-mail: brasel@gcrc.humc.edu
Accred Length: 3 Years *Program Size:* 1
Program ID: 326-05-11-006

Colorado

Denver

University of Colorado Program
Sponsor: University of Colorado Health Sciences Center
Children's Hospital
Program Director:
Michael S Kappy, MD
Children's Hospital
1056 E 19th Ave/Box B-265
Denver, CO 80218-1088
Tel: 303 861-6061 *Fax:* 303 864-5679
E-mail: flores.ampard@tchden.org
Accred Length: 3 Years *Program Size:* 2
Program ID: 326-07-21-007

Connecticut

Farmington

University of Connecticut Program
Sponsor: University of Connecticut School of Medicine
Connecticut Children's Medical Center
Program Director:
Karen R Rubin, MD
Connecticut Children's Med Ctr
Ped Endocrinology
282 Washington St
Hartford, CT 06106
Tel: 860 545-9370 *Fax:* 860 545-9371
E-mail: krubin@ccmckids.org
Accred Length: 3 Years *Program Size:* 2
Program ID: 326-08-21-054

New Haven

Yale-New Haven Medical Center Program
Sponsor: Yale-New Haven Hospital
Program Director:
Thomas O Carpenter, MD
Yale Univ Sch of Med
Ped Endocrinology/3103 LMP
PO Box 208064
New Haven, CT 06520-8064
Tel: 203 785-4648 *Fax:* 203 737-1998
E-mail: kathryn.holthausen@yale.edu
Accred Length: 3 Years *Program Size:* 4
Program ID: 326-08-21-053

Florida

Gainesville

University of Florida Program
Sponsor: University of Florida College of Medicine
Shands Hospital at the University of Florida
Program Director:
Janet H Silverstein, MD
J Hillis Miller Health Ctr
Box 100296
Gainesville, FL 32610-0296
Tel: 352 334-1390 *Fax:* 352 334-1325
E-mail: silvejh@peds.ufl.edu
Accred Length: 3 Years *Program Size:* 3
Program ID: 326-11-31-008

Miami

University of Miami-Jackson Memorial Medical Center Program
Sponsor: University of Miami-Jackson Memorial Medical Center
Program Director:
Gary D Berkovitz, MD
PO Box 016820
1601 NW 12th Ave
Miami, FL 33101
Tel: 305 243-6936 *Fax:* 305 243-6309
E-mail: gberkov@peds.med.miami.edu
Accred Length: 3 Years *Program Size:* 3
Program ID: 326-11-21-067

Tampa

University of South Florida Program
Sponsor: University of South Florida College of Medicine
All Children's Hospital
Program Director:
John I Malone, MD
Allen W Root, MD
All Children's Hospital
801 Sixth St S/6900
St Petersburg, FL 33701
Tel: 727 892-4237 *Fax:* 727 892-4219
E-mail: jmalone@com1.usf.edu
Accred Length: 3 Years *Program Size:* 0
Program ID: 326-11-21-048

Georgia

Atlanta

Emory University Program
Sponsor: Emory University School of Medicine
Egleston Children's Hospital at Emory University
Grady Memorial Hospital
Program Director:
John S Parks, MD PhD
Emory Univ Sch of Med, Dept of Pediatrics
2040 Ridgewood Dr NE
Atlanta, GA 30322
Tel: 404 727-5753 *Fax:* 404 727-3423
E-mail: jparks@emory.edu
Accred Length: 3 Years *Program Size:* 2
Program ID: 326-12-21-042

Illinois

Chicago

McGaw Medical Center of Northwestern University Program
Sponsor: Northwestern University Medical School
Children's Memorial Medical Center
Program Director:
Bernard L Silverman, MD
Children's Memorial Hospital
Div of Endocrinology
2300 Children's Plaza/Box 54
Chicago, IL 60614
Tel: 773 880-4440 *Fax:* 773 880-4063
E-mail: bsilver@nwu.edu
Accred Length: 3 Years *Program Size:* 2
Program ID: 326-16-21-060

University of Chicago Program
Sponsor: University of Chicago Hospitals
University of Chicago Children's Hospital
Program Director:
Robert L Rosenfield, MD
Univ of Chicago-Children's Hospital
5839 S Maryland Ave/MC5053
Chicago, IL 60637-1470
Tel: 773 702-6432 *Fax:* 773 702-0443
E-mail: jmoore@peds.bsd.uchicago.edu
Internet: http://peds-www.bsd.uchicago.edu/
Accred Length: 3 Years *Program Size:* 3
Program ID: 326-16-11-010

Programs

University of Illinois College of Medicine at Chicago Program
Sponsor: University of Illinois College of Medicine at Chicago
Michael Reese Hospital and Medical Center
University of Illinois Hospital and Clinics
Program Director:
Songya Pang, MD
Univ of Illinois-Chicago
Dept of Pediatrics
840 S Wood St (M/C 856)
Chicago, IL 60612
Tel: 312 996-1795 *Fax:* 312 996-8218
E-mail: spang@uic.edu
Accred Length: 3 Years *Program Size:* 1
Program ID: 326-16-31-062

Maywood

Loyola University Program
Sponsor: Loyola University Medical Center
Program Director:
W Patrick Zeller, MD
Loyola Univ-Stritch Sch of Med
Ped Endocrinology
2160 S First Ave
Maywood, IL 60153
Tel: 708 216-5080 *Fax:* 708 216-1114
E-mail: lodenba@wpo.it.luc.edu
Internet: http://www.lumc.edu/childhospital
Accred Length: 3 Years *Program Size:* 0
Program ID: 326-16-21-058

Indiana

Indianapolis

Indiana University School of Medicine Program
Sponsor: Indiana University School of Medicine
Clarian Riley Hospital for Children
Program Director:
Ora Pescovitz, MD
Riley Hospital for Children
702 Barnhill Dr/Rm 5984
Indianapolis, IN 46202-5225
Tel: 317 274-3889 *Fax:* 317 274-3882
Accred Length: 3 Years *Program Size:* 3
Program ID: 326-17-21-052

Iowa

Iowa City

University of Iowa Hospitals and Clinics Program
Sponsor: University of Iowa Hospitals and Clinics
Program Director:
Eva Tsalikian, MD
Univ of Iowa Hospitals and Clinics
Dept of Pediatrics
200 Hawkins Dr
Iowa City, IA 52242-1009
Tel: 319 356-1833 *Fax:* 319 356-8170
E-mail: eva-tsalikian@uiowa.edu
Accred Length: 3 Years *Program Size:* 1
Program ID: 326-18-11-011

Maryland

Baltimore

Johns Hopkins University Program
Sponsor: Johns Hopkins University School of Medicine
Johns Hopkins Hospital
Program Director:
Michael A Levine, MD
Johns Hopkins Hospital
600 N Wolfe St/Park 211
Baltimore, MD 21287-3311
Tel: 410 955-6463 *Fax:* 410 955-9773
E-mail: mlevine@jhu.edu
Accred Length: 3 Years *Program Size:* 10
Program ID: 326-23-21-012

University of Maryland Program
Sponsor: University of Maryland Medical System
Program Director:
Debra Counts, MD
Univ of Maryland Med System
22 S Greene St/Rm N5E13
Baltimore, MD 21201-1595
Tel: 410 328-3410 *Fax:* 410 328-0679
Accred Length: 3 Years *Program Size:* 2
Program ID: 326-23-21-013

Bethesda

National Capital Consortium Program
Sponsor: National Capital Consortium
USUHS F Edward Hebert School of Medicine
Walter Reed Army Medical Center
Program Director:
Gary Francis, MD PhD
Uniformed Services Univ of Health Sciences
4301 Jones Bridge Rd
Bethesda, MD 20814
Tel: 301 295-9716 *Fax:* 301 295-6770
E-mail: gfrancis@usuhs.mil
Accred Length: 3 Years *Program Size:* 6
Program ID: 326-10-11-041
US Armed Services Program

NICHD/Georgetown University Program
Sponsor: NIH Warren Grant Magnuson Clinical Center
Georgetown University Medical Center
Program Director:
George P Chrousos, MD
Bldg 10/Rm 10-N-262
National Institutes of Health
Bethesda, MD 20892-1862
Tel: 301 496-2427 *Fax:* 301 402-0574
E-mail: george.chrousos@nih.gov
Accred Length: 3 Years *Program Size:* 6
Program ID: 326-23-21-056

Massachusetts

Boston

Children's Hospital/Boston Medical Center Program
Sponsor: Children's Hospital
Program Director:
Joseph A Majzoub, MD
Children's Hospital-Harvard Med Sch
300 Longwood Ave
Boston, MA 02115
Tel: 617 355-6421 *Fax:* 617 355-3741
E-mail: majzoub@a1.tch.harvard.edu.
Accred Length: 3 Years *Program Size:* 8
Program ID: 326-24-11-014

Massachusetts General Hospital Program
Sponsor: Massachusetts General Hospital
Program Director:
Lynne L Levitsky, MD
WACC 709
15 Parkman St
Boston, MA 02114
Tel: 617 726-5790 *Fax:* 617 726-3044
E-mail: levitskyl@a1.mgh.harvard.edu
Accred Length: 3 Years *Program Size:* 3
Program ID: 326-24-31-015

Michigan

Ann Arbor

University of Michigan Program
Sponsor: University of Michigan Hospitals
Program Director:
Nancy J Hopwood, MD
Dept of Pediatrics
Univ of Michigan Med Ctr
D3252 MPB/Box 0718
Ann Arbor, MI 48109-0718
Tel: 734 764-5175 *Fax:* 734 436-7035
Accred Length: 3 Years *Program Size:* 2
Program ID: 326-25-21-016

Minnesota

Minneapolis

University of Minnesota Program
Sponsor: University of Minnesota Medical School
Fairview-University Medical Center
Program Director:
David M Brown, MD
Univ of Minnesota Hospital and Clinics
Box 404
420 Delaware St SE
Minneapolis, MN 55455
Tel: 612 624-5409 *Fax:* 612 624-2682
E-mail: dmbrown@maroon.tc.umn.edu
Accred Length: 3 Years *Program Size:* 1
Program ID: 326-26-21-043

Rochester

Mayo Graduate School of Medicine (Rochester) Program
Sponsor: Mayo Graduate School of Medicine-Mayo Foundation
Mayo Clinic (Rochester)
St Mary's Hospital of Rochester
Program Director:
Donald Zimmerman, MD
Application Processing Ctr
Mayo Graduate Sch of Med
200 First St SW
Rochester, MN 55905
Tel: 507 284-3379 *Fax:* 507 284-0727
E-mail: mgsm.roch.mn.pediatrics@mayo.edu
Internet: http://www.mayo.edu/
Accred Length: 3 Years *Program Size:* 2
Program ID: 326-26-21-017

Missouri

Kansas City

University of Missouri at Kansas City Program

Sponsor: University of Missouri-Kansas City School of Medicine
Children's Mercy Hospital

Program Director:
Campbell P Howard, MD
Children's Mercy Hospital
Div of Endocrinology
2401 Gillham Rd
Kansas City, MO 64108-9898
Tel: 816 234-3072 *Fax:* 816 855-1919
Internet: http://www.cmh.edu
Accred Length: 3 Years *Program Size:* 1
Program ID: 326-28-11-018

St Louis

Washington University/B-JH/SLCH Consortium Program

Sponsor: Washington University/B-JH/SLCH Consortium
St Louis Children's Hospital

Program Director:
Neil H White, MD
Washington Univ-St Louis Children's Hospital
One Children's Pl
Campus Box 8116
St Louis, MO 63110
Tel: 314 454-6046 *Fax:* 314 454-4185
E-mail: white_n@kids.wustl.edu
Internet: http://www.wumshome.wustl.edu/peds.
Accred Length: 3 Years *Program Size:* 5
Program ID: 326-28-11-019

New York

Bronx

Albert Einstein College of Medicine Program

Sponsor: Albert Einstein College of Medicine of Yeshiva University
Jacobi Medical Center
Montefiore Medical Center-Henry and Lucy Moses Division
Montefiore Medical Center-Weiler Hospital
North Central Bronx Hospital

Program Director:
Paul Saenger, MD
Montefiore Med Ctr
111 E 210th St
Bronx, NY 10467-2490
Tel: 718 920-4664 *Fax:* 718 405-5609
Accred Length: 3 Years *Program Size:* 3
Program ID: 326-35-21-020

Brooklyn

Maimonides Medical Center Program

Sponsor: Maimonides Medical Center

Program Director:
Henry Anhalt, DO
Maimonides Med Ctr
Dept of Pediatrics
4802 Tenth Ave
Brooklyn, NY 11219
Tel: 718 283-7500, ext 8143 *Fax:* 718 283-6268
E-mail: hanhalt@maimonidesmed.org
Accred Length: 3 Years *Program Size:* 3
Program ID: 326-35-31-064

SUNY Health Science Center at Brooklyn Program

Sponsor: SUNY Health Science Center at Brooklyn
Brookdale University Hospital Medical Center
Kings County Hospital Center
University Hospital-SUNY Health Science Center at Brooklyn

Program Director:
Henry Anhalt, DO
4802 Tenth Ave
Brooklyn, NY 11219
Tel: 718 283-8143 *Fax:* 718 283-6268
Accred Length: 3 Years *Program Size:* 6
Program ID: 326-35-21-022

Buffalo

SUNY at Buffalo Graduate Medical-Dental Education Consortium Program

Sponsor: SUNY at Buffalo Grad Medical-Dental Education Consortium
CGF Health System (Children's Hospital of Buffalo)

Program Director:
Margaret H MacGillivray, MD
Children's Hospital
219 Bryant St
Buffalo, NY 14222
Tel: 716 878-7588 *Fax:* 716 888-3827
Accred Length: 3 Years *Program Size:* 4
Program ID: 326-35-21-021

Manhasset

North Shore University Hospital/NYU School of Medicine Program

Sponsor: North Shore University Hospital

Program Director:
Phyllis W Speiser, MD
North Shore Univ Hospital
300 Community Dr
Manhasset, NY 11030
Tel: 516 562-4635 *Fax:* 516 562-4029
E-mail: speiser@nshs.edu
Internet: http://www.medhelp.org/nsuh/pedsendo.htm
Accred Length: 3 Years *Program Size:* 2
Program ID: 326-35-21-044

Mineola

Winthrop-University Hospital Program

Sponsor: Winthrop-University Hospital

Program Director:
Mariano Castro-Magana, MD
Winthrop-Univ Hospital
120 Mineola Blvd
Mineola, NY 11501
Tel: 516 663-3069 *Fax:* 516 663-3070
E-mail: ggrella@winthrop.org
Internet: http://www.winthrop.org
Accred Length: 3 Years *Program Size:* 3
Program ID: 326-35-31-057

New Hyde Park

Albert Einstein College of Medicine at Long Island Jewish Medical Center Program

Sponsor: Long Island Jewish Medical Center
Schneider Children's Hosp (Long Island Jewish Med Ctr)

Program Director:
Dennis E Carey, MD
Schneider Children's Hospital
Rm CH234
269-01 76th Ave
New Hyde Park, NY 11040
Tel: 718 470-3290 *Fax:* 718 470-9173
E-mail: carey@lij.edu
Internet: http://www.lij.edu/-homepage-ns.html
Accred Length: 3 Years *Program Size:* 2
Program ID: 326-35-21-050

New York

Mount Sinai School of Medicine Program

Sponsor: Mount Sinai School of Medicine
Mount Sinai Medical Center

Program Director:
Robert C McEvoy, MD
Mount Sinai Sch of Med
One Gustave L Levy Pl/Box 1659
New York, NY 10029-6574
Tel: 212 241-6936 *Fax:* 212 831-2501
E-mail: bmcevoy103@aol.com
Internet: http://www.mssm.edu/peds/endo-fel.html
Accred Length: 3 Years *Program Size:* 1
Program ID: 326-35-11-023

New York and Presbyterian Hospital (Columbia Campus) Program

Sponsor: New York and Presbyterian Hospital
New York and Presbyterian Hospital (Columbia Campus)

Program Director:
Sharon E Oberfield, MD
Felicia A Cuomo, MD
630 W 168th St/BHN-Box 50
New York, NY 10032
Tel: 212 305-6559 *Fax:* 212 305-4778
E-mail: seo8@columbia.edu
Accred Length: 3 Years *Program Size:* 2
Program ID: 326-35-21-070

New York and Presbyterian Hospital (Cornell Campus) Program

Sponsor: New York and Presbyterian Hospital (Cornell Campus)

Program Director:
Maria I New, MD
New York Presbyterian Hospital-Cornell Campus
Dept of Pediatrics
525 E 68th St
New York, NY 10021
Tel: 212 746-3450 *Fax:* 212 746-0300
E-mail: minew@mail.med.cornell.edu
Accred Length: 3 Years *Program Size:* 7
Program ID: 326-35-21-049

New York University Medical Center Program

Sponsor: New York University Medical Center
Bellevue Hospital Center

Program Director:
Raphael David, MD
New York Univ Med Ctr
550 First Ave
New York, NY 10016
Tel: 212 263-6462 *Fax:* 212 562-3273
E-mail: raphael.david@mcped.med.nyu.edu
Accred Length: 3 Years *Program Size:* 2
Program ID: 326-35-21-045

Stony Brook

SUNY at Stony Brook Program
Sponsor: University Hospital-SUNY at Stony Brook
Program Director:
Thomas A Wilson, MD
Dept of Pediatrics
SUNY-Stony Brook
Stony Brook, NY 11794-8111
Tel: 516 444-3429 *Fax:* 516 444-6045
E-mail: twilson@mail.som.sunysb.edu
Internet: http://www.uhmc.sunysb.edu/pediatrics/
Accred Length: 3 Years *Program Size:* 3
Program ID: 326-35-21-061

Syracuse

SUNY Health Science Center at Syracuse Program
Sponsor: University Hospital-SUNY Health Science Center at Syracuse
Crouse Hospital
Program Director:
Robert A Richman, MD
SUNY Health Science Ctr
Dept of Pediatrics
750 E Adams St
Syracuse, NY 13210-2339
Tel: 315 464-6064 *Fax:* 315 464-6065
E-mail: richmanr@vax.cs.hscsyr.edu
Accred Length: 3 Years *Program Size:* 1
Program ID: 326-35-21-046

North Carolina

Chapel Hill

University of North Carolina Hospitals Program
Sponsor: University of North Carolina Hospitals
Program Director:
Augustine J D'Ercole, MD
Univ of North Carolina Sch of Med
509 Burnett-Womack Bldg/CB7220
Chapel Hill, NC 27599-7220
Tel: 919 966-4435, ext 221 *Fax:* 919 966-2423
Accred Length: 3 Years *Program Size:* 6
Program ID: 326-36-21-025

Durham

Duke University Program
Sponsor: Duke University Medical Center
Program Director:
Michael S Freemark, MD
Duke Univ Med Ctr
Box 3080
Durham, NC 27710
Tel: 919 684-3772 *Fax:* 919 684-8613
E-mail: freem001@mc.duke.edu
Accred Length: 3 Years *Program Size:* 2
Program ID: 326-36-21-026

Ohio

Cincinnati

Children's Hospital Medical Center/University of Cincinnati College of Medicine Program
Sponsor: Children's Hospital Medical Center
Program Director:
Steven D Chernausek, MD
Children's Hospital Med Ctr
3333 Burnet Ave
Cincinnati, OH 45229-3039
Tel: 513 636-4209 *Fax:* 513 636-7486
E-mail: chernasd@ucbeh.san.uc.edu
Accred Length: 3 Years *Program Size:* 6
Program ID: 326-38-21-027

Cleveland

Case Western Reserve University Program
Sponsor: University Hospitals of Cleveland
Program Director:
William T Dahms, MD
Rainbow Babies and Children's Hospital
11100 Euclid Ave
Cleveland, OH 44106
Tel: 216 844-3661 *Fax:* 216 844-8900
Accred Length: 3 Years *Program Size:* 1
Program ID: 326-38-21-028

Columbus

Children's Hospital/Ohio State University Program
Sponsor: Children's Hospital
Program Director:
William B Zipf, MD
Children's Hospital
Div of Ped Endocrinology
700 Children's Dr
Columbus, OH 43205-2696
Tel: 614 722-4425 *Fax:* 614 722-4565
Accred Length: 3 Years *Program Size:* 0
Program ID: 326-38-21-063

Oregon

Portland

Oregon Health Sciences University Program
Sponsor: Oregon Health Sciences University Hospital
Program Director:
Stephen LaFranchi, MD
Dept of Pediatrics (NRC-5)
3181 SW Sam Jackson Park Rd
Portland, OR 97201-3098
Tel: 503 494-1927 *Fax:* 503 494-1933
Internet:
http://www.ohsu.edu/som-pediatrics/homepge/.htm
Accred Length: 3 Years *Program Size:* 5
Program ID: 326-40-12-031

Pennsylvania

Philadelphia

Children's Hospital of Philadelphia Program
Sponsor: Children's Hospital of Philadelphia
Program Director:
Pinchas Cohen, MD
Childrens Hospital
Rm 410-D/ARC
3400 Civic Center Blvd
Philadelphia, PA 19104
Tel: 215 590-3420 *Fax:* 215 590-1605
E-mail: cohenp@email.chop.edu
Internet: http://www.chop.edu
Accred Length: 3 Years *Program Size:* 3
Program ID: 326-41-21-032

Pittsburgh

University Health Center of Pittsburgh Program
Sponsor: University Health Center of Pittsburgh
Children's Hospital of Pittsburgh
Program Director:
Silva A Arslanian, MD
Children's Hospital of Pittsburgh
3705 Fifth Ave
Pittsburgh, PA 15213
Tel: 412 692-5170 *Fax:* 412 692-5834
E-mail: arslans@chplink.chp.edu
Accred Length: 3 Years *Program Size:* 4
Program ID: 326-41-21-033

Rhode Island

Providence

Brown University Program
Sponsor: Rhode Island Hospital
Program Director:
Philip A Gruppuso, MD
Dept of Pediatrics
Rhode Island Hospital
593 Eddy St
Providence, RI 02903
Tel: 401 444-5504 *Fax:* 401 444-2534
E-mail: philip_gruppuso@brown.edu
Accred Length: 3 Years *Program Size:* 3
Program ID: 326-43-21-034

Tennessee

Memphis

University of Tennessee Program
Sponsor: University of Tennessee College of Medicine
LeBonheur Children's Medical Center
Program Director:
George A Burghen, MD
LeBonheur Children's Med Ctr
Div of Endocrinology/Metabolism
50 N Dunlap
Memphis, TN 38103
Tel: 901 572-3292 *Fax:* 901 572-5198
E-mail: gburghen@utmem1.utmem.edu
Accred Length: 3 Years *Program Size:* 2
Program ID: 326-47-31-035

Nashville

Vanderbilt University Program

Sponsor: Vanderbilt University Medical Center

Program Director:
Rodney A Lorenz, MD
Vanderbilt Univ Sch of Med
T-0107 Medical Ctr N
Nashville, TN 37232-2579
Tel: 615 322-7427 *Fax:* 615 343-5845
E-mail: rod.lorenz@mcmail.vanderbilt.edu
Accred Length: 3 Years *Program Size:* 3
Program ID: 326-47-21-036

Texas

Dallas

University of Texas Southwestern Medical School Program

Sponsor: University of Texas Southwestern Medical School
Dallas County Hospital District-Parkland Memorial Hospital

Program Director:
Perrin C White, MD
Univ of Texas Southwestern Med Sch
5323 Harry Hines Blvd
Dallas, TX 75235-9063
Tel: 214 648-3501 *Fax:* 214 648-9772
E-mail: pwhit2@mednet.swmed.edu
Accred Length: 3 Years *Program Size:* 3
Program ID: 326-48-31-069

Galveston

University of Texas Medical Branch Hospitals Program

Sponsor: University of Texas Medical Branch Hospitals

Program Director:
Bruce S Keenan, MD
Univ of Texas Med Branch
Ped Endocrinology/Diabetes
301 University Blvd
Galveston, TX 77555-0363
Tel: 409 772-3365 *Fax:* 409 747-2213
E-mail: bkeenan@utmb.edu
Internet: http://www.utmb.edu/pedi/
Accred Length: 3 Years *Program Size:* 1
Program ID: 326-48-11-037

Houston

Baylor College of Medicine Program

Sponsor: Baylor College of Medicine
Texas Children's Hospital

Program Director:
John L Kirkland, MD
Baylor Coll of Med
Dept of Pediatrics
One Baylor Plaza
Houston, TX 77030-3498
Tel: 713 798-4793 *Fax:* 713 798-7493
E-mail: kirkland@bcm.tmc.edu
Internet: http://www.bcm.tmc.edu/pedi/
Accred Length: 3 Years *Program Size:* 1
Program ID: 326-48-21-051

University of Texas at Houston Program

Sponsor: University of Texas Medical School at Houston
Lyndon B Johnson General Hospital
Memorial Hermann Healthcare System

Program Director:
Dana S Hardin, MD
Dept of Pediatrics
Univ of Texas Med School
PO Box 20708
Houston, TX 77025
Tel: 713 500-5646 *Fax:* 713 500-5646
E-mail: dhardin@ped1.med.uth.tmc.edu
Accred Length: 3 Years *Program Size:* 2
Program ID: 326-48-21-066

Virginia

Charlottesville

University of Virginia Program

Sponsor: University of Virginia Medical Center

Program Director:
Alan D Rogol, MD PhD
Div of Ped Endo/Metabolism
Univ of Virginia Hospitals
Box 386
Charlottesville, VA 22908-0001
Tel: 804 924-5895 *Fax:* 804 924-2940
E-mail: adr@virginia.edu
Accred Length: 3 Years *Program Size:* 3
Program ID: 326-51-11-039

Wisconsin

Madison

University of Wisconsin Program

Sponsor: University of Wisconsin Hospital and Clinics

Program Director:
Michael J MacDonald, MD
3459 Med Sci Ctr
Univ of Wisconsin Sch of Med
1300 University Ave
Madison, WI 53706
Tel: 608 262-6762 *Fax:* 608 262-9300
Accred Length: 3 Years *Program Size:* 1
Program ID: 326-56-21-059

Pediatric Gastroenterology (Pediatrics)

Alabama

Birmingham

University of Alabama Medical Center Program

Sponsor: University of Alabama Hospital
Children's Hospital of Alabama

Program Director:
Frank A Franklin Jr, MD PhD
Div of Ped Gastro/Nutrition
1600 7th Ave S/Ste 618
Birmingham, AL 35233
Tel: 205 934-6558 *Fax:* 205 939-9919
Accred Length: 3 Years *Program Size:* 0
Program ID: 332-01-21-001

Arkansas

Little Rock

University of Arkansas for Medical Sciences Program

Sponsor: University of Arkansas College of Medicine
Arkansas Children's Hospital

Program Director:
Dennis D Black, MD PhD
Sect of Gastroenterology
800 Marshall St
Little Rock, AR 72202-3591
Tel: 501 320-5985 *Fax:* 501 320-6291
E-mail: ddblack@achasc.hans.edu
Accred Length: 3 Years *Program Size:* 1
Program ID: 332-04-21-002

California

Long Beach

University of California (Irvine) Program

Sponsor: University of California (Irvine) Medical Center
Long Beach Memorial Medical Center

Program Director:
Richard K Mathis, MD
Univ of California Irvine Med Ctr
2801 Atlantic Ave
Long Beach, CA 90801-1428
Tel: 562 933-3009 *Fax:* 562 492-6089
Accred Length: 3 Years *Program Size:* 0
Program ID: 332-05-31-054

Programs

Los Angeles

Children's Hospital of Los Angeles Program
Sponsor: Children's Hospital of Los Angeles
Program Director:
Frank R Sinatra, MD
Women's and Children's Hospital
Los Angeles County-USC Med Ctr
1240 N Mission Rd
Los Angeles, CA 90033
Tel: 213 226-3801 *Fax:* 213 226-4380
E-mail: sinatra@hsc.usc.edu
Accred Length: 3 Years *Program Size:* 3
Program ID: 332-05-21-051

UCLA Medical Center Program
Sponsor: UCLA School of Medicine
UCLA Medical Center
Program Director:
Marvin E Ament, MD
Div of Gastro/Nutrition
10833 Le Conte Ave/MDCC 12-383
Los Angeles, CA 90095-1752
Tel: 310 206-6134 *Fax:* 310 206-0203
Accred Length: 3 Years *Program Size:* 6
Program ID: 332-05-31-004

San Diego

University of California (San Diego) Program
Sponsor: University of California (San Diego) Medical Center
Children's Hospital and Health Center
Program Director:
Joel E Lavine, MD PhD
200 W Arbor Dr/MC8450
San Diego, CA 92103
Tel: 619 543-7544 *Fax:* 619 543-7537
E-mail: jolavine@ucsd.edu
Accred Length: 3 Years *Program Size:* 3
Program ID: 332-05-11-055

San Francisco

University of California (San Francisco) Program
Sponsor: University of California (San Francisco) School of Medicine
University of California (San Francisco) Medical Center
Program Director:
Melvin B Heyman, MD MPH
Univ of California San Francisco
Ped Gastro/Hepatology/Nutrition
500 Parnassus Ave/MU406E Rm 406 Box 0136
San Francisco, CA 94143-0136
Tel: 415 476-5892 *Fax:* 415 476-1343
E-mail: mheyman@peds.ucsf.edu
Accred Length: 3 Years *Program Size:* 5
Program ID: 332-05-21-047

Stanford

Stanford University Program
Sponsor: Stanford University Hospital
Lucile Salter Packard Children's Hospital at Stanford
Program Director:
John Alan Kerner Jr, MD
William Berquist, MD
Stanford Univ Med Ctr
750 Welch Rd/Ste 116
Palo Alto, CA 94304
Tel: 650 723-5070 *Fax:* 650 498-5608
E-mail: md.kerjo@lpch.stanford.edu
Accred Length: 3 Years *Program Size:* 2
Program ID: 332-05-11-005

Colorado

Denver

University of Colorado Program
Sponsor: University of Colorado Health Sciences Center
Children's Hospital
Denver Health and Hospitals
Program Director:
Ronald J Sokol, MD
Sect of Ped Gastro/Nutrition
Children's Hospital/Box B290
1056 E 19th Ave
Denver, CO 80218
Tel: 303 861-6669 *Fax:* 303 764-8025
E-mail: sokol.ronald@tchden.org
Accred Length: 3 Years *Program Size:* 3
Program ID: 332-07-21-006

Connecticut

New Haven

Yale-New Haven Medical Center Program
Sponsor: Yale-New Haven Hospital
Program Director:
M Susan Moyer, MD
Dept of Pediatrics
Yale Univ Sch of Med
333 Cedar St
New Haven, CT 06510-8064
Tel: 203 785-4649 *Fax:* 203 737-1384
E-mail: susan.moyer@qm.yale.edu
Accred Length: 3 Years *Program Size:* 3
Program ID: 332-08-21-007

District of Columbia

Washington

George Washington University Program
Sponsor: Children's National Medical Center
Program Director:
Benny Kerzner, MD
Dept of Gastro/Nutrition
Children's National Med Ctr
111 Michigan Ave NW/Ste 4277
Washington, DC 20010
Tel: 202 884-3031 *Fax:* 202 884-4156
Accred Length: 3 Years *Program Size:* 2
Program ID: 332-10-21-008

Florida

Gainesville

University of Florida Program
Sponsor: University of Florida College of Medicine
Shands Hospital at the University of Florida
Program Director:
Regino P Gonzalez-Peralta, MD
Univ of Florida Coll of Med
Dept of Ped Gastroenterology
PO Box 100296
Gainesville, FL 32610-0296
Tel: 352 392-6410 *Fax:* 352 846-2147
E-mail: regino@peds.ufl.edu
Accred Length: 3 Years *Program Size:* 2
Program ID: 332-11-21-011

Illinois

Chicago

McGaw Medical Center of Northwestern University Program
Sponsor: Northwestern University Medical School
Children's Memorial Medical Center
Program Director:
Peter F Whitington, MD
Children's Memorial Hospital
2300 Children's Plaza/Box 57
Chicago, IL 60614
Tel: 773 880-4643
E-mail: p-whitington@nwu.edu
Accred Length: 3 Years *Program Size:* 3
Program ID: 332-16-21-056

University of Chicago Program
Sponsor: University of Chicago Hospitals
Program Director:
Stefano Guandalini, MD
Univ of Chicago Children's Hospital
Dept of Pediatrics
5841 S Maryland Ave/MC4065
Chicago, IL 60637-1470
Tel: 773 702-6418 *Fax:* 773 702-0668
E-mail: sguandal@peds.bsd.uchicago.edu
Accred Length: 3 Years *Program Size:* 2
Program ID: 332-16-21-012

Indiana

Indianapolis

Indiana University School of Medicine Program
Sponsor: Indiana University School of Medicine
Clarian Riley Hospital for Children
Program Director:
Joseph F Fitzgerald, MD
Riley Hospital for Children
Dept of Pediatrics
702 Barnhill Dr/Rm 2728
Indianapolis, IN 46202-5225
Tel: 317 274-3774 *Fax:* 317 274-8521
Accred Length: 3 Years *Program Size:* 2
Program ID: 332-17-21-013

Iowa

Iowa City

University of Iowa Hospitals and Clinics Program
Sponsor: University of Iowa Hospitals and Clinics
Program Director:
Warren P Bishop, MD
Univ of Iowa Hospitals and Clinics
Dept of Pediatrics
200 Hawkins Dr
Iowa City, IA 52242
Tel: 319 356-2950
E-mail: warren-bishop@uiowa.edu
Accred Length: 3 Years *Program Size:* 0
Program ID: 332-18-21-053

Kentucky

Louisville

University of Louisville Program

Sponsor: University of Louisville School of Medicine
Kosair Children's Hospital (Alliant Health System)

Program Director:
Thomas C Stephen, MD
Dept of Ped Gastroenterology
571 S Floyd/Rm 325
Louisville, KY 40202
Tel: 502 852-3874 *Fax:* 502 852-4093
Accred Length: 3 Years *Program Size:* 1
Program ID: 332-20-21-014

Louisiana

New Orleans

Louisiana State University/Tulane University Program

Sponsor: Louisiana State University School of Medicine
Childrens Hospital
Tulane University Hospital and Clinics

Program Director:
John N Udall Jr, MD PhD
Dept of Ped Gastro/Nutrition
Louisiana State Univ Sch of Med
1542 Tulane Ave
New Orleans, LA 70112-2822
Tel: 504 568-6224 *Fax:* 504 568-6330
E-mail: judall@mail.peds.lsumc.edu
Accred Length: 3 Years *Program Size:* 0
Program ID: 332-21-21-015

Maryland

Baltimore

Johns Hopkins University Program

Sponsor: Johns Hopkins University School of Medicine
Johns Hopkins Hospital

Program Director:
Kathleen B Schwarz, MD
Johns Hopkins Hospital
600 N Wolfe St/Brady 320
Baltimore, MD 21287-2631
Tel: 410 955-8769 *Fax:* 410 955-1464
E-mail: kschwarz@welchlink.welch.jhu.edu
Accred Length: 3 Years *Program Size:* 4
Program ID: 332-23-21-016

Bethesda

National Capital Consortium Program

Sponsor: National Capital Consortium
USUHS F Edward Hebert School of Medicine
Walter Reed Army Medical Center

Program Director:
Victor M Pineiro, MD
Uniformed Services Univ of Health Sciences
Dept of Pediatrics
4301 Jones Bridge Rd
Bethesda, MD 20814-4799
Tel: 301 295-3130 *Fax:* 301 295-3898
E-mail: vpineiro@usuhs.mil
Internet: http://www.usuhs.mil
Accred Length: 3 Years *Program Size:* 4
Program ID: 332-10-21-010
US Armed Services Program

Massachusetts

Boston

Children's Hospital/Boston Medical Center Program

Sponsor: Children's Hospital
Massachusetts General Hospital

Program Director:
W Allan Walker, MD
Dept of Ped Gastroenterology
Massachusetts General Hospital
Bldg 149/13th St/Rm 3401
Charlestown, MA 02129
Tel: 617 726-7988 *Fax:* 617 726-4172
E-mail: walker@helix.mgh.harvard.edu
Accred Length: 3 Years *Program Size:* 12
Program ID: 332-24-31-018

New England Medical Center Hospitals Program

Sponsor: New England Medical Center Hospitals

Program Director:
Richard J Grand, MD
Dept Ped Gastro/Nutrition
New England Med Ctr
750 Washington St/Box 213
Boston, MA 02111-1533
Tel: 617 636-0130 *Fax:* 617 636-8718
Accred Length: 3 Years *Program Size:* 2
Program ID: 332-24-21-017

Michigan

Ann Arbor

University of Michigan Program

Sponsor: University of Michigan Hospitals

Program Director:
Chris J Dickinson, MD MD
Dept of Pediatrics
Univ of Michigan Med Ctr
F6854 Mott/0200
Ann Arbor, MI 48109-0200
Tel: 313 763-9650 *Fax:* 313 763-7359
E-mail: chrisjd@umich.edu
Accred Length: 3 Years *Program Size:* 3
Program ID: 332-25-21-019

Detroit

Wayne State University/Detroit Medical Center Program

Sponsor: Wayne State University/Detroit Medical Center
Children's Hospital of Michigan

Program Director:
Vasundhara Tolia, MD
Wayne State Univ-Children's Hospital
3901 Beaubien Blvd
Detroit, MI 48201
Tel: 313 745-5585 *Fax:* 313 745-5155
E-mail: vtolia@med.wayne.edu
Accred Length: 3 Years *Program Size:* 1
Program ID: 332-25-21-020

Minnesota

Minneapolis

University of Minnesota Program

Sponsor: University of Minnesota Medical School
Fairview-University Medical Center

Program Director:
Harvey L Sharp, MD
Div of Ped Gastro/Nutrition
Box 185 UMHC
420 Delaware St SE
Minneapolis, MN 55455
Tel: 612 624-1133 *Fax:* 612 626-0639
E-mail: sharp001@maroon.tc.umn.edu
Accred Length: 3 Years *Program Size:* 2
Program ID: 332-26-21-048

Rochester

Mayo Graduate School of Medicine (Rochester) Program

Sponsor: Mayo Graduate School of Medicine-Mayo Foundation
Mayo Clinic (Rochester)
St Mary's Hospital of Rochester

Program Director:
Deborah K Freese, MD
Mayo Graduate Sch of Med
200 First St SW
Siebens 5
Rochester, MN 55905
Tel: 507 284-3108 *Fax:* 507 284-0999
E-mail: mgsm.roch.mn.pediatrics@mayo.edu
Internet: http://www.mayo.edu/
Accred Length: 3 Years *Program Size:* 2
Program ID: 332-26-21-021

Missouri

St Louis

Washington University/B-JH/SLCH Consortium Program

Sponsor: Washington University/B-JH/SLCH Consortium
St Louis Children's Hospital

Program Director:
David H Perlmutter, MD
Dept of Pediatrics
Washington Univ Sch of Med
One Children's Pl
St Louis, MO 63110
Tel: 314 454-6033 *Fax:* 314 454-4218
E-mail: perlmutter@kids.wustl.edu
Accred Length: 3 Years *Program Size:* 6
Program ID: 332-28-31-023

Nebraska

Omaha

University of Nebraska/Creighton University Program

Sponsor: University of Nebraska Medical Center
Childrens Memorial Hospital

Program Director:
Jon A Vanderhoof, MD
Joint Sect of Pediatric Gastroenterology
8300 Dodge St/Ste 330
Omaha, NE 68114-4126
Tel: 402 354-3560 *Fax:* 402 354-3574
E-mail: jvanderh@mail.unmc.edu
Accred Length: 3 Years *Program Size:* 2
Program ID: 332-30-21-024

New York

Bronx

Albert Einstein College of Medicine Program
Sponsor: Albert Einstein College of Medicine of Yeshiva University
Montefiore Medical Center-Henry and Lucy Moses Division
North Central Bronx Hospital

Program Director:
William Spivak, MD
111 E 210th St
Bronx, NY 10467
Tel: 718 920-6606 *Fax:* 718 547-2158
Accred Length: 3 Years *Program Size:* 3
Program ID: 332-35-21-050

Brooklyn

SUNY Health Science Center at Brooklyn Program
Sponsor: SUNY Health Science Center at Brooklyn
Kings County Hospital Center
University Hospital-SUNY Health Science Center at Brooklyn

Program Director:
Simon S Rabinowitz, MD PhD
Dept of Ped Gastro/Nutrition
SUNY Health Science Ctr-Brooklyn
450 Clarkson Ave/Box 49
Brooklyn, NY 11203
Tel: 718 270-1625 *Fax:* 718 270-1985
E-mail: rabins08@hscbklyn.edu
Accred Length: 3 Years *Program Size:* 3
Program ID: 332-35-21-026

Manhasset

North Shore University Hospital/NYU School of Medicine Program
Sponsor: North Shore University Hospital

Program Director:
Fredric Daum, MD
Div of Ped Gastroenterology
North Shore Univ Hosp
300 Community Dr
Manhasset, NY 11030
Tel: 516 562-4642 *Fax:* 516 562-2527
Accred Length: 3 Years *Program Size:* 2
Program ID: 332-35-31-027

New York

Mount Sinai School of Medicine Program
Sponsor: Mount Sinai School of Medicine
Mount Sinai Medical Center

Program Director:
Neal S LeLeiko, MD PhD
Mount Sinai Sch of Med
One Gustave L Levy Pl
New York, NY 10029
Tel: 212 241-5415 *Fax:* 212 876-5631
E-mail: neal.leleiko@smtplink.mssm.edu
Accred Length: 3 Years *Program Size:* 3
Program ID: 332-35-11-028

New York and Presbyterian Hospital (Columbia Campus) Program
Sponsor: New York and Presbyterian Hospital
New York and Presbyterian Hospital (Columbia Campus)

Program Director:
Richard J Deckelbaum, MD
Div of Gastro/Nutrition
Columbia Univ, Dept of Pediatrics
3959 Broadway/BHN 7-702
New York, NY 10032
Tel: 212 305-7082 *Fax:* 212 305-8995
Accred Length: 3 Years *Program Size:* 4
Program ID: 332-35-21-030

New York and Presbyterian Hospital (Cornell Campus) Program
Sponsor: New York and Presbyterian Hospital
New York and Presbyterian Hospital (Cornell Campus)

Program Director:
Marta Illueca, MD
Dept of Pediatrics
New York Hospital-Cornell Med Ctr
525 E 68th St/M610
New York, NY 10021
Tel: 212 746-3520 *Fax:* 212 746-8577
E-mail: millueca@mail.med.cornell.edu
Accred Length: 3 Years *Program Size:* 3
Program ID: 332-35-32-029

Valhalla

New York Medical College at Westchester Medical Center Program
Sponsor: New York Medical College
Westchester Medical Center

Program Director:
Stuart H Berezin, MD
Div of Ped Gastro/Nutrition
New York Med Coll
Munger Pavilion/Rm 101
Valhalla, NY 10595
Tel: 914 594-4610 *Fax:* 914 594-4392
E-mail: marvin_medow@nymc.edu
Accred Length: 3 Years *Program Size:* 2
Program ID: 332-35-31-031

North Carolina

Chapel Hill

University of North Carolina Hospitals Program
Sponsor: University of North Carolina Hospitals

Program Director:
Jon M Rhoads, MD
Dept of Ped Gastroenterology
Univ of North Carolina
CB 7220/310 Burnett-Womack Bldg
Chapel Hill, NC 27599-7220
Tel: 919 966-1343 *Fax:* 919 966-8641
E-mail: rhoads.pedslan@mhs.unc.edu
Accred Length: 3 Years *Program Size:* 0
Program ID: 332-36-21-032

Ohio

Cincinnati

Children's Hospital Medical Center/University of Cincinnati College of Medicine Program
Sponsor: Children's Hospital Medical Center

Program Director:
Mitchell B Cohen, MD
Children's Hospital Med Ctr
Div of Ped GI/Nutrition
3333 Burnet Ave
Cincinnati, OH 45229-3039
Tel: 513 636-4415 *Fax:* 513 636-7805
E-mail: mitchell.cohen@chmcc.org
Accred Length: 3 Years *Program Size:* 7
Program ID: 332-38-21-033

Cleveland

Case Western Reserve University Program
Sponsor: University Hospitals of Cleveland

Program Director:
Steven J Czinn, MD
Div of Ped Gastro/Nutrition
Rainbow Babies and Children's Hospital
11100 Euclid Ave/RBC 6004
Cleveland, OH 44106-6004
Tel: 216 844-1765 *Fax:* 216 844-8397
E-mail: sjc3@po.cwru.edu
Accred Length: 3 Years *Program Size:* 1
Program ID: 332-38-11-035

Cleveland Clinic Foundation Program
Sponsor: Cleveland Clinic Foundation

Program Director:
Robert Wyllie, MD
Sect of Ped Gastro/Nutrition
Cleveland Clinic Foundation/A120
9500 Euclid Ave
Cleveland, OH 44195
Tel: 216 444-2237 *Fax:* 216 445-7792
E-mail: wyllier@cesmtp.ccf.org
Internet: http://www.ccf.org
Accred Length: 3 Years *Program Size:* 3
Program ID: 332-38-31-034

Pennsylvania

Philadelphia

Children's Hospital of Philadelphia Program
Sponsor: Children's Hospital of Philadelphia

Program Director:
Andrew E Mulberg, MD
Children's Hospital of Philadelphia
Abramson 416B
34th St and Civic Center Blvd
Philadelphia, PA 19104-4399
Tel: 215 590-3247 *Fax:* 215 590-3680
E-mail: mulberg@email.chop.edu
Accred Length: 3 Years *Program Size:* 6
Program ID: 332-41-21-038

Pittsburgh

University Health Center of Pittsburgh Program
Sponsor: University Health Center of Pittsburgh
Children's Hospital of Pittsburgh
Program Director:
Samuel A Kocoshis, MD
Dept of Ped Gastroenterology
Children's Hospital
3705 Fifth Ave
Pittsburgh, PA 15213-2583
Tel: 412 692-5180 *Fax:* 412 692-7355
E-mail: aldersd@chplink.chp.edu
Accred Length: 3 Years *Program Size:* 3
Program ID: 332-41-21-040

Rhode Island

Providence

Brown University Program
Sponsor: Rhode Island Hospital
Women and Infants Hospital of Rhode Island
Program Director:
Linda B Shalon, MD MS
Rhode Island Hospital
Div of Ped Gastroenterology
593 Eddy St/MPB 126
Providence, RI 02903
Tel: 401 444-8306 *Fax:* 401 444-8845
E-mail: lshalon@lifespan.org
Accred Length: 3 Years *Program Size:* 3
Program ID: 332-43-21-041

South Carolina

Charleston

Medical University of South Carolina Program
Sponsor: Medical University of South Carolina College of Medicine
Program Director:
Robert Baker, MD PhD
158 Rutledge Ave
Charleston, SC 29403
Tel: 843 792-7653 *Fax:* 843 792-6472
E-mail: bakerrd@musc.edu
Accred Length: 3 Years *Program Size:* 2
Program ID: 332-45-21-052

Tennessee

Nashville

Vanderbilt University Program
Sponsor: Vanderbilt University Medical Center
Program Director:
John A Barnard, MD
Dept of Ped Gastro/Nutrition
Vanderbilt Univ Sch of Med
21st Ave S and Garland Ave/4322 Med Ctr N
Nashville, TN 37232-2576
Tel: 615 322-7449 *Fax:* 615 343-8915
E-mail: john.barnard@mcmail.vanderbilt.edu
Internet:
http://www.peds.mc.vanderbilt.edu/vchweb-1/gastroen.html
Accred Length: 3 Years *Program Size:* 4
Program ID: 332-47-21-042

Texas

Dallas

University of Texas Southwestern Medical School Program
Sponsor: University of Texas Southwestern Medical School
Children's Medical Center of Dallas
Program Director:
John M Andersen, MD
Div of Ped Gastro/Nutrition
Children's Med Ctr
1935 Motor St
Dallas, TX 75235
Tel: 214 640-8000 *Fax:* 214 640-8006
E-mail: jandersen@chilmed.dallas.tx.us
Accred Length: 3 Years *Program Size:* 1
Program ID: 332-48-11-045

Houston

Baylor College of Medicine Program
Sponsor: Baylor College of Medicine
Harris County Hospital District-Ben Taub General Hospital
Texas Children's Hospital
Program Director:
William J Klish, MD
Baylor Coll of Med
Texas Children's Hospital
6621 Fannin St/MC 3-3391
Houston, TX 77030-2399
Tel: 713 770-3600 *Fax:* 713 770-3633
E-mail: mgilger@msmail.is5.tch.tcm.edu
Internet: http://www.mgilger@msmail.is5.tch.tmc.
Accred Length: 3 Years *Program Size:* 6
Program ID: 332-48-21-043

Wisconsin

Madison

University of Wisconsin Program
Sponsor: University of Wisconsin Hospital and Clinics
Program Director:
Glenn R Gourley, MD
Univ of Wisconsin
1500 Highland Ave
Waisman Ctr/Rm 609
Madison, WI 53705-2280
Tel: 608 263-9166 *Fax:* 608 265-4103
E-mail: gourley@waisman.wisc.edu
Accred Length: 3 Years *Program Size:* 1
Program ID: 332-56-31-049

Milwaukee

Medical College of Wisconsin Program
Sponsor: Medical College of Wisconsin Affiliated Hospitals Inc
Children's Hospital of Wisconsin
Program Director:
Steven L Werlin, MD
Dept of Pediatrics
Med Coll of Wisconsin
8701 Watertown Plank Rd
Milwaukee, WI 53226
Tel: 414 456-4160 *Fax:* 414 456-6328
E-mail: swerlin@mcw.edu
Accred Length: 3 Years *Program Size:* 2
Program ID: 332-56-21-046

Pediatric Hematology/Oncology (Pediatrics)

Alabama

Birmingham

University of Alabama Medical Center Program
Sponsor: University of Alabama Hospital
Children's Hospital of Alabama
Program Director:
Roger L Berkow, MD
Univ of Alabama Med Ctr
Children's Hospital/651
1600 7th Ave S
Birmingham, AL 35233
Tel: 205 939-9285 *Fax:* 205 975-6377
E-mail: rberkow@peds.uab.edu
Internet: http://www.peds.uab.edu
Accred Length: 3 Years *Program Size:* 3
Program ID: 327-01-21-043

Arizona

Tucson

University of Arizona Program
Sponsor: University of Arizona College of Medicine
University Medical Center
Program Director:
John J Hutter Jr, MD
1501 N Campbell Ave
PO Box 245073
Tucson, AZ 85724-5073
Tel: 520 626-6527 *Fax:* 520 626-4220
Accred Length: 3 Years *Program Size:* 0
Program ID: 327-03-21-073

California

Los Angeles

Children's Hospital of Los Angeles Program
Sponsor: Children's Hospital of Los Angeles
Program Director:
Walter E Laug, MD
Children's Hospital
Div of Hem/Onc
4650 Sunset Blvd
Los Angeles, CA 90027
Tel: 323 669-2163 *Fax:* 323 660-7128
E-mail: jorgtega%smtpgate@chlais.usc.edu
Accred Length: 3 Years *Program Size:* 8
Program ID: 327-05-11-001

UCLA Medical Center Program
Sponsor: UCLA School of Medicine
UCLA Medical Center
Program Director:
Stephen A Feig, MD
UCLA Sch of Med
10833 Le Conte Ave/A2-410 MDCC
Los Angeles, CA 90095-1752
Tel: 310 825-6708 *Fax:* 310 206-8089
Accred Length: 3 Years *Program Size:* 3
Program ID: 327-05-21-003

Oakland

Children's Hospital-Oakland Program
Sponsor: Children's Hospital-Oakland
Program Director:
Caroline A Hastings, MD
Children's Hospital
747 52nd St
Oakland, CA 94609
Tel: 510 428-3631 *Fax:* 510 601-3916
Accred Length: 3 Years *Program Size:* 4
Program ID: 327-05-31-056

Orange

Children's Hospital of Orange County Program
Sponsor: Children's Hospital of Orange County
Program Director:
Diane Nugent, MD
Children's Hospital
455 S Main St
Orange, CA 92868-3874
Tel: 714 532-8541 *Fax:* 714 532-8771
E-mail: djnugent@pacbell.net
Accred Length: 3 Years *Program Size:* 2
Program ID: 327-05-21-057

San Francisco

University of California (San Francisco) Program
Sponsor: University of California (San Francisco) School of Medicine
San Francisco General Hospital Medical Center
University of California (San Francisco) Medical Center
Program Director:
William C Mentzer, MD
San Francisco General Hospital Med Ctr
1001 Potrero Ave/Rm 331
Bldg 100
San Francisco, CA 94110
Tel: 415 206-5169 *Fax:* 415 206-3071
E-mail: wmentzer@sfghpeds.ucsf.edu
Accred Length: 3 Years *Program Size:* 5
Program ID: 327-05-21-006

Stanford

Stanford University Program
Sponsor: Stanford University Hospital
Lucile Salter Packard Children's Hospital at Stanford
Program Director:
Bertil E Glader, MD
Dept of Ped Hem-Onc
300 Pasteur Dr
Stanford, CA 94305-5119
Tel: 415 723-5535 *Fax:* 415 723-5231
Accred Length: 3 Years *Program Size:* 6
Program ID: 327-05-21-004

Colorado

Denver

University of Colorado Program
Sponsor: University of Colorado Health Sciences Center
Children's Hospital
Program Director:
Robert L Garcea, MD
Univ of Colorado Health Sciences Ctr
4200 E Ninth Ave
A036/B-115
Denver, CO 80262
Tel: 303 861-6770 *Fax:* 303 837-2831
E-mail: bob.garcea@uchsc.edu
Accred Length: 3 Years *Program Size:* 6
Program ID: 327-07-21-007

Connecticut

New Haven

Yale-New Haven Medical Center Program
Sponsor: Yale-New Haven Hospital
Program Director:
Diana S Beardsley, MD PhD
Yale Univ Sch of Med
333 Cedar St/LMP 4087
PO Box 208064
New Haven, CT 06520-8064
Tel: 203 785-4640 *Fax:* 203 737-2228
Accred Length: 3 Years *Program Size:* 3
Program ID: 327-08-21-008

District of Columbia

Washington

George Washington University Program
Sponsor: Children's National Medical Center
Program Director:
Nita L Seibel, MD
Children's National Med Ctr
111 Michigan Ave NW
Washington, DC 20010
Tel: 202 884-2147 *Fax:* 202 884-5685
E-mail: nseibel@cnmc.org
Accred Length: 3 Years *Program Size:* 6
Program ID: 327-10-21-009

Florida

Gainesville

University of Florida Program
Sponsor: University of Florida College of Medicine
Shands Hospital at the University of Florida
Program Director:
Paulette S Mehta, MD
Univ of Florida
Box 100296 JHMHC
Gainesville, FL 32610-0296
Tel: 352 392-5633 *Fax:* 352 392-8725
E-mail: mehtaps@peds.ufl.edu
Accred Length: 3 Years *Program Size:* 3
Program ID: 327-11-31-010

Georgia

Atlanta

Emory University Program
Sponsor: Emory University School of Medicine
Egleston Children's Hospital at Emory University
Grady Memorial Hospital
Program Director:
Thomas C Abshire, MD
Emory Univ Sch of Med, Dept of Pediatrics
2040 Ridgewood Dr NE
Ste 100
Atlanta, GA 30322
Tel: 404 727-4451 *Fax:* 404 727-4455
E-mail: thomas_abshire@oz.ped.emory.edu
Internet:
http://www.emory.edu:80/peds/hemonc/hem3.htm
Accred Length: 3 Years *Program Size:* 5
Program ID: 327-12-21-041

Illinois

Chicago

McGaw Medical Center of Northwestern University Program
Sponsor: Northwestern University Medical School
Children's Memorial Medical Center
Program Director:
Sharon B Murphy, MD
Div of Hematology/Oncology
Children's Memorial Hospital
2300 Children's Plaza/Box 30
Chicago, IL 60614
Tel: 312 880-4562, ext 3694 *Fax:* 312 880-3053
E-mail: sbmurphy@nwu.edu
Accred Length: 3 Years *Program Size:* 3
Program ID: 327-16-21-011

University of Chicago Program
Sponsor: University of Chicago Hospitals
University of Chicago Children's Hospital
Program Director:
Charles M Rubin, MD
Univ of Chicago Children's Hospital
MC4060
5841 S Maryland Ave
Chicago, IL 60637-1470
Tel: 773 702-6808 *Fax:* 773 702-9881
E-mail: crubin@peds.bsd.uchicago.edu
Internet: http://wed-www.bsd.uchicago.edu
Accred Length: 3 Years *Program Size:* 3
Program ID: 327-16-11-050

Indiana

Indianapolis

Indiana University School of Medicine Program
Sponsor: Indiana University School of Medicine
Clarian Riley Hospital for Children
Program Director:
Mary C Dinauer, MD PhD
Indiana Univ Med Ctr
Riley Hospital for Children-Cancer Research Inst
1044 W Walnut/#466
Indianapolis, IN 46202-5225
Tel: 317 274-8645 *Fax:* 317 274-8679
E-mail: mdinauer@iupui.edu
Accred Length: 3 Years *Program Size:* 2
Program ID: 327-17-21-012

Iowa

Iowa City

University of Iowa Hospitals and Clinics Program

Sponsor: University of Iowa Hospitals and Clinics

Program Director:
Thomas W Loew, MD
Univ of Iowa Hospitals and Clinics
Dept of Pediatrics 2530 JCP
200 Hawkins Dr
Iowa City, IA 52242-1009
Tel: 319 356-2437 *Fax:* 319 356-7659
E-mail: thomas-loew@uiowa.edu
Accred Length: 3 Years *Program Size:* 0
Program ID: 327-18-11-013

Louisiana

New Orleans

Louisiana State University/Tulane University Program

Sponsor: Louisiana State University School of Medicine
Childrens Hospital
Tulane University Hospital and Clinics

Program Director:
Raj P Warrier, MD
Charles Scher, MD
Louisiana State Univ Med Ctr
Dept of Pediatrics
1542 Tulane Ave
New Orleans, LA 70112
Tel: 504 568-4561 *Fax:* 504 568-3078
E-mail: warrier@mail.peds.lsumc.edu
Accred Length: 3 Years *Program Size:* 2
Program ID: 327-21-21-048

Maryland

Baltimore

Johns Hopkins University Program

Sponsor: Johns Hopkins University School of Medicine
Johns Hopkins Hospital

Program Director:
Curt I Civin, MD
James F Casella, MD
Johns Hopkins Oncology Ctr
Oncology 3-109
600 N Wolfe St
Baltimore, MD 21287-5001
Tel: 410 955-8816 *Fax:* 410 955-8897
E-mail: civinci@aol.com
Internet: http://www.med.jhu.edu.cancerctr/peds
Accred Length: 3 Years *Program Size:* 9
Program ID: 327-23-21-014

Johns Hopkins University Program

Sponsor: Johns Hopkins University School of Medicine
NIH Warren Grant Magnuson Clinical Center

Program Director:
Lee J Helman, MD
Felicia A Cuomo, MD
Pediatric Oncology Branch National Cancer Inst
Bldg 10 Rm 13N240
10 Center Dr/MSC 1928
Bethesda, MD 20892
Tel: 301 496-4257 *Fax:* 301 402-0575
Internet: http://www.training.nih.gov/clinical/clin20.html
Accred Length: 3 Years *Program Size:* 9
Program ID: 327-23-21-074

Bethesda

National Capital Consortium Program

Sponsor: National Capital Consortium
National Naval Medical Center (Bethesda)
Walter Reed Army Medical Center

Program Director:
Capt Bertrand J Duval-Arnould, MD
Dept of Ped Hem-Onc
Walter Reed Army Med Ctr
6825 16th St NW
Washington, DC 20307-5001
Tel: 202 782-0421 *Fax:* 202 782-7020
E-mail: lesduval@pop.erols.com
Internet: http://www.usuhs.mil/ped/hemonc_fellow.html
Accred Length: 3 Years *Program Size:* 6
Program ID: 327-10-21-044
US Armed Services Program

Massachusetts

Boston

Children's Hospital/Boston Medical Center Program

Sponsor: Children's Hospital
Dana-Farber Cancer Institute

Program Director:
Samuel E Lux IV, MD
Children's Hospital
300 Longwood Ave
Enders 7
Boston, MA 02115
Tel: 617 355-7904 *Fax:* 617 355-7262
E-mail: lux@rascal.med.harvard.edu
Accred Length: 3 Years *Program Size:* 14
Program ID: 327-24-11-015

Michigan

Ann Arbor

University of Michigan Program

Sponsor: University of Michigan Hospitals

Program Director:
Laurence A Boxer, MD
Dept of Ped Hem-Onc
Univ of Michigan Hospitals
1500 E Medical Center Dr/L2110
Ann Arbor, MI 48109-0238
Tel: 734 764-7127 *Fax:* 734 615-0464
E-mail: laboxer@umich.edu
Accred Length: 3 Years *Program Size:* 6
Program ID: 327-25-21-016

Detroit

Wayne State University/Detroit Medical Center Program

Sponsor: Wayne State University/Detroit Medical Center
Children's Hospital of Michigan

Program Director:
Yaddanapudi Ravindranath, MD
Attn: Mary F Euth
Grad Med Educ 9C UHC
4201 St Antoine
Detroit, MI 48201
Tel: 313 745-5147
Accred Length: 3 Years *Program Size:* 4
Program ID: 327-25-21-017

Minnesota

Minneapolis

University of Minnesota Program

Sponsor: University of Minnesota Medical School
Fairview-University Medical Center

Program Director:
Jospeh P Neglia, MD MPH
Norma K C Ramsay, MD
Univ of Minnesota Med Sch
Box 484 Mayo Bldg
420 Delaware St SE
Minneapolis, MN 55455
Tel: 612 626-2778 *Fax:* 612 626-2815
Accred Length: 3 Years *Program Size:* 6
Program ID: 327-26-21-018

Rochester

Mayo Graduate School of Medicine (Rochester) Program

Sponsor: Mayo Graduate School of Medicine-Mayo Foundation
Mayo Clinic (Rochester)
St Mary's Hospital of Rochester

Program Director:
Carola A S Arndt, MD
Siebens 5th Fl Registrar
Mayo Graduate Sch of Med
200 First St SW
Rochester, MN 55905
Tel: 507 284-3379 *Fax:* 507 284-0727
Internet: http://www.mayo.edu/
Accred Length: 3 Years *Program Size:* 2
Program ID: 327-26-21-019

Mississippi

Jackson

University of Mississippi Medical Center Program

Sponsor: University of Mississippi School of Medicine
University Hospital

Program Director:
Jeanette Pullen, MD
Univ of Mississippi Med Ctr
2500 N State St
Jackson, MS 39216-4505
Tel: 601 984-5220 *Fax:* 601 984-5279
E-mail: jpullen@ped.umsmed.edu
Accred Length: 3 Years *Program Size:* 2
Program ID: 327-27-12-055

Missouri

Kansas City

University of Missouri at Kansas City Program

Sponsor: University of Missouri-Kansas City School of Medicine
Children's Mercy Hospital

Program Director:
Gerald M Woods, MD
Children's Mercy Hospital
Hematology/Oncology
2401 Gillham Rd
Kansas City, MO 64108-9898
Tel: 816 816-3265 *Fax:* 816 855-1700
E-mail: gwoods@cmh.edu
Internet: http://www.cmh.edu
Accred Length: 3 Years *Program Size:* 1
Program ID: 327-28-21-060

St Louis

Washington University/B-JH/SLCH Consortium Program

Sponsor: Washington University/B-JH/SLCH Consortium
St Louis Children's Hospital

Program Director:
Craig A MacArthur, MD PhD
Washington Univ
Ped Hem/Onc
One Children's Pl/CB 8116
St Louis, MO 63110
Tel: 314 454-2891 *Fax:* 314 454-2685
E-mail: dixon_p@kids.wustl.edu
Internet: http://www.peds.wustl.edu/hemonc
Accred Length: 3 Years *Program Size:* 4
Program ID: 327-28-11-020

New Mexico

Albuquerque

University of New Mexico Program

Sponsor: University of New Mexico School of Medicine
University Hospital

Program Director:
Susan Scott, MD
Univ of New Mexico
Dept of Pediatrics
Albuquerque, NM 87131-5311
Tel: 505 272-4461 *Fax:* 505 272-8699
Accred Length: 3 Years *Program Size:* 0
Program ID: 327-34-21-070

New York

Bronx

Albert Einstein College of Medicine Program

Sponsor: Albert Einstein College of Medicine of Yeshiva University
Jacobi Medical Center
Montefiore Medical Center-Henry and Lucy Moses Division
Montefiore Medical Center-Weiler Hospital
North Central Bronx Hospital

Program Director:
Eva Radel, MD
Dept of Pediatrics
111 E 210th St
Bronx, NY 10467
Tel: 718 920-7844 *Fax:* 718 920-6506
E-mail: radel@aecom.yu.edu
Accred Length: 3 Years *Program Size:* 3
Program ID: 327-35-21-071

Brooklyn

SUNY Health Science Center at Brooklyn Program

Sponsor: SUNY Health Science Center at Brooklyn
Kings County Hospital Center
University Hospital-SUNY Health Science Center at Brooklyn

Program Director:
Sreedhar P Rao, MD
SUNY Health Science Ctr
450 Clarkson Ave/Box 49
Brooklyn, NY 11203
Tel: 718 270-1692 *Fax:* 718 270-1985
E-mail: spulluru@pol.net
Accred Length: 3 Years *Program Size:* 2
Program ID: 327-35-21-022

Buffalo

SUNY at Buffalo Graduate Medical-Dental Education Consortium Program

Sponsor: SUNY at Buffalo Grad Medical-Dental Education Consortium
CGF Health System (Children's Hospital of Buffalo)
Roswell Park Cancer Institute

Program Director:
Sharon Smith, MD
Children's Hospital
Hematology/Oncology
219 Bryant St
Buffalo, NY 14222-2099
Tel: 716 878-7349 *Fax:* 716 888-3801
Accred Length: 3 Years *Program Size:* 2
Program ID: 327-35-21-021

New Hyde Park

Albert Einstein College of Medicine at Long Island Jewish Medical Center Program

Sponsor: Long Island Jewish Medical Center
Schneider Children's Hosp (Long Island Jewish Med Ctr)

Program Director:
Philip Lanzkowsky, MD
Long Island Jewish Med Ctr
270-05 76th Ave
New Hyde Park, NY 11040
Tel: 718 470-3201 *Fax:* 718 343-8542
Internet: http://www.lij.edu/lij-homepage-ns.html
Accred Length: 3 Years *Program Size:* 6
Program ID: 327-35-21-023

New York

Mount Sinai School of Medicine Program

Sponsor: Mount Sinai School of Medicine
Mount Sinai Medical Center

Program Director:
Jeffrey M Lipton, MD PhD
Mount Sinai Sch of Med
Mount Sinai Med Ctr
One Gustave L Levy Pl/Box 1208
New York, NY 10029
Tel: 212 241-6031 *Fax:* 212 360-6921
E-mail: pho@smtplink.mssm.edu
Internet: http://www.mssm.edu/
Accred Length: 3 Years *Program Size:* 3
Program ID: 327-35-11-025

New York and Presbyterian Hospital (Columbia Campus) Program

Sponsor: New York and Presbyterian Hospital
New York and Presbyterian Hospital (Columbia Campus)

Program Director:
Sergio Piomelli, MD
Presbyterian Hospital
622 W 168th St
Rm HP 546
New York, NY 10032
Tel: 212 305-6531 *Fax:* 212 305-8408
E-mail: sp23@columbia.edu
Accred Length: 3 Years *Program Size:* 3
Program ID: 327-35-11-027

New York and Presbyterian Hospital (Cornell Campus) Program

Sponsor: Memorial Sloan-Kettering Cancer Center
New York and Presbyterian Hospital (Cornell Campus)

Program Director:
Paul A Meyers, MD
Patricia Giardina, MD
Memorial Sloan-Kettering Cancer Ctr
1275 York Ave
New York, NY 10021
Tel: 212 639-5966 *Fax:* 212 717-3447
E-mail: wernerw@mskcc.org
Accred Length: 3 Years *Program Size:* 18
Program ID: 327-35-21-024

New York University Medical Center Program

Sponsor: New York University Medical Center
Bellevue Hospital Center

Program Director:
Margaret Karpatkin, MD
New York Univ Med Ctr
Pediatric Hem/Onc
550 First Ave
New York, NY 10016-6402
Tel: 212 263-6428 *Fax:* 212 263-8099
E-mail: ped.hemeonc@ccmail.med.nyu.edu
Internet: http://www.med.nyu.edu/pedho/
Accred Length: 3 Years *Program Size:* 3
Program ID: 327-35-21-026

Rochester

University of Rochester Program

Sponsor: Strong Memorial Hospital of the University of Rochester

Program Director:
George B Segel, MD
Dept of Pediatrics/Box 777
Univ of Rochester Med Ctr
601 Elmwood Ave
Rochester, NY 14642
Tel: 716 275-0515 *Fax:* 716 273-1039
E-mail: george_segel@urmc.rochester.edu
Accred Length: 3 Years *Program Size:* 3
Program ID: 327-35-21-049

Syracuse

SUNY Health Science Center at Syracuse Program
Sponsor: University Hospital-SUNY Health Science Center at Syracuse
Crouse Hospital
Program Director:
Ronald L Dubowy, MD
SUNY Health Science Ctr
750 E Adams St
Syracuse, NY 13210
Tel: 315 464-5294 *Fax:* 315 464-7238
Accred Length: 3 Years *Program Size:* 1
Program ID: 327-35-21-028

North Carolina

Chapel Hill

University of North Carolina Hospitals Program
Sponsor: University of North Carolina Hospitals
Program Director:
Joseph M Wiley, MD
Univ of North Carolina Hospitals
418 Macnider Bldg, Dept of Pediatrics
CB# 7220
Chapel Hill, NC 27599-7220
Tel: 919 966-1103 *Fax:* 919 966-7629
E-mail: jmw@med.unc.edu
Internet: http://www.med.unc.edu/peds/hemonc/
Accred Length: 3 Years *Program Size:* 3
Program ID: 327-36-21-058

Durham

Duke University Program
Sponsor: Duke University Medical Center
Program Director:
Philip M Rosoff, MD
Duke Univ Med Ctr
PO Box 2916
Durham, NC 27710
Tel: 919 684-3401 *Fax:* 919 681-7950
E-mail: rosof001@mc.duke.edu
Internet: http://www.canctr.mc.duke.edu/pho
Accred Length: 3 Years *Program Size:* 9
Program ID: 327-36-21-029

Ohio

Cincinnati

Children's Hospital Medical Center/University of Cincinnati College of Medicine Program
Sponsor: Children's Hospital Medical Center
Program Director:
Cynthia A DeLaat, MD MD
Children's Hospital Med Ctr
3333 Burnet Ave
Cincinnati, OH 45229-3039
Tel: 513 636-7287 *Fax:* 513 636-5845
E-mail: cadelaat@chmcc.org
Internet: http://www.chmcc.org
Accred Length: 3 Years *Program Size:* 9
Program ID: 327-38-21-030

Cleveland

Case Western Reserve University Program
Sponsor: University Hospitals of Cleveland
Program Director:
Susan B Shurin, MD
Rainbow Babies and Children's Hospital
11100 Euclid Ave
Cleveland, OH 44106-3440
Tel: 216 844-3345 *Fax:* 216 844-5431
Accred Length: 3 Years *Program Size:* 6
Program ID: 327-38-21-031

Columbus

Children's Hospital/Ohio State University Program
Sponsor: Children's Hospital
Program Director:
Frederick Ruymann, MD
700 Children's Dr
Columbus, OH 43205-2696
Tel: 614 722-3564 *Fax:* 614 722-3699
E-mail: fruymann@chi.osu.edu
Accred Length: 3 Years *Program Size:* 6
Program ID: 327-38-21-042

Oregon

Portland

Oregon Health Sciences University Program
Sponsor: Oregon Health Sciences University Hospital
Program Director:
Gary R Jones, MD
3181 SW Sam Jackson Park Rd/NRC5
Portland, OR 97201-3098
Tel: 503 494-1543 *Fax:* 503 494-0714
E-mail: jonesga@ohsu.edu
Internet:
http://www.ohsu.edu/som-pediatrics/training/fellow.htm
Accred Length: 3 Years *Program Size:* 3
Program ID: 327-40-21-072

Pennsylvania

Philadelphia

Children's Hospital of Philadelphia Program
Sponsor: Children's Hospital of Philadelphia
Program Director:
Alan R Cohen, MD
34th St and Civic Ctr Blvd
Philadelphia, PA 19104-9786
Tel: 215 590-4993 *Fax:* 215 590-3992
Accred Length: 3 Years *Program Size:* 12
Program ID: 327-41-21-032

St Christopher's Hospital for Children Program
Sponsor: St Christopher's Hospital for Children
Program Director:
Frank E Shafer, MD
St Christopher's Hospital for Children
Sect of Hematology/Oncology
Erie Ave at Front St
Philadelphia, PA 19134-1095
Tel: 215 427-4399 *Fax:* 215 427-6684
E-mail: frank.shafer@tenethealth.com
Accred Length: 3 Years *Program Size:* 2
Program ID: 327-41-12-051

Pittsburgh

University Health Center of Pittsburgh Program
Sponsor: University Health Center of Pittsburgh
Children's Hospital of Pittsburgh
Program Director:
Arthur K Ritchey, MD
Children's Hospital
Div of Hematology/Oncology
3705 Fifth Ave
Pittsburgh, PA 15213-2583
Tel: 412 692-5055 *Fax:* 412 692-7693
Accred Length: 3 Years *Program Size:* 3
Program ID: 327-41-21-066

Puerto Rico

San Juan

University of Puerto Rico Program
Sponsor: University of Puerto Rico School of Medicine
University Pediatric Hospital
Program Director:
Pedro J Santiago-Borrero, MD
Univ of Puerto Rico Sch of Med
PO Box 365067
San Juan, PR 00936-5067
Tel: 787 754-3623 *Fax:* 787 751-5812
Accred Length: 3 Years *Program Size:* 2
Program ID: 327-42-21-065

Rhode Island

Providence

Brown University Program
Sponsor: Rhode Island Hospital
Program Director:
Edwin N Forman, MD
Rhode Island Hospital
593 Eddy St
Providence, RI 02903-4923
Tel: 401 444-5171 *Fax:* 401 444-8845
E-mail: eforman@lifespan.org
Accred Length: 3 Years *Program Size:* 3
Program ID: 327-43-21-033

South Carolina

Charleston

Medical University of South Carolina Program
Sponsor: Medical University of South Carolina College of Medicine
MUSC Medical Center
Program Director:
Joseph H Laver, MD
Med Univ of South Carolina
Children's Hospital
171 Ashley Ave/Rm 510B
Charleston, SC 29425-3311
Tel: 803 792-2957 *Fax:* 803 792-8871
E-mail: laverjh@musc.edu
Accred Length: 3 Years *Program Size:* 3
Program ID: 327-45-21-068

Tennessee

Memphis

University of Tennessee Program

Sponsor: University of Tennessee College of Medicine
LeBonheur Children's Medical Center
St Jude Children's Research Hospital

Program Director:
Jeffrey E Rubnitz, MD
332 N Lauderdale
PO Box 318
Memphis, TN 38101-0318
Tel: 901 495-2388 *Fax:* 901 521-9005
Accred Length: 3 Years *Program Size:* 12
Program ID: 327-47-31-034

Nashville

Vanderbilt University Program

Sponsor: Vanderbilt University Medical Center

Program Director:
John N Lukens, MD
Vanderbilt Univ Sch of Med
Ped Hematology/Oncology 525 MRB II
2220 Pierce Ave
Nashville, TN 37232-6310
Tel: 615 936-1762 *Fax:* 615 936-1767
Accred Length: 3 Years *Program Size:* 3
Program ID: 327-47-21-035

Texas

Dallas

University of Texas Southwestern Medical School Program

Sponsor: University of Texas Southwestern Medical School
Children's Medical Center of Dallas

Program Director:
George R Buchanan, MD
Univ of Texas Southwestern Med Sch
Dept of Pediatrics
5323 Harry Hines Blvd
Dallas, TX 75235-9063
Tel: 214 648-8594 *Fax:* 214 648-3122
E-mail: gbuch2@mednet.swmed.edu
Accred Length: 3 Years *Program Size:* 5
Program ID: 327-48-21-046

Galveston

University of Texas Medical Branch Hospitals Program

Sponsor: University of Texas Medical Branch Hospitals

Program Director:
Blanche P Alter, MD
Univ of Texas Med Branch
301 University Blvd/Rm 3.270
Galveston, TX 77555-0361
Tel: 409 772-2341 *Fax:* 409 747-6618
Internet: http://www.utmb.edu/pedi
Accred Length: 3 Years *Program Size:* 1
Program ID: 327-48-11-036

Houston

Baylor College of Medicine Program

Sponsor: Baylor College of Medicine
Texas Children's Hospital

Program Director:
David G Poplack, MD
Baylor Coll of Med
Dept of Ped Hem/Onc
6621 Fannin St/MC 3-3320
Houston, TX 77030-2399
Tel: 713 770-4200 *Fax:* 713 770-4202
Internet: http://www.tccc.tch.tmc.edu
Accred Length: 3 Years *Program Size:* 15
Program ID: 327-48-21-037

University of Texas at Houston Program

Sponsor: University of Texas Medical School at Houston
Memorial Hermann Healthcare System
University of Texas M D Anderson Cancer Center

Program Director:
William K Hoots, MD
Univ of Texas-MD Anderson Cancer Ctr
Div of Pediatrics/Box 87
1515 Holcombe Blvd
Houston, TX 77030
Tel: 713 792-6613 *Fax:* 713 792-0608
E-mail: khoots@ped1.med.uth.tmc.edu
Accred Length: 3 Years *Program Size:* 1
Program ID: 327-48-21-038

San Antonio

University of Texas Health Science Center at San Antonio Program

Sponsor: University of Texas Medical School at San Antonio
Santa Rosa Health Care Corporation
University Hospital-South Texas Medical Center

Program Director:
Anne-Marie Langevin, MD
Univ of Texas Health Science Ctr
Dept of Ped Hem/Onc
7703 Floyd Curl Dr
San Antonio, TX 78284-7810
Tel: 210 567-5265 *Fax:* 210 567-5339
E-mail: langevin@uthscsa.edu
Accred Length: 3 Years *Program Size:* 1
Program ID: 327-48-21-047

Utah

Salt Lake City

University of Utah Program

Sponsor: University of Utah Medical Center
Primary Children's Medical Center

Program Director:
Richard T O'Brien, MD
Primary Children's Med Ctr
100 N Medical Dr
Salt Lake City, UT 84113
Tel: 801 588-2680 *Fax:* 801 588-2662
Accred Length: 3 Years *Program Size:* 1
Program ID: 327-49-21-039

Virginia

Charlottesville

University of Virginia Program

Sponsor: University of Virginia Medical Center

Program Director:
Pedro A de Alarcon, MD
Dept of Pediatrics/Box 386
Children's Med Ctr
Univ of Virginia Hospital
Charlottesville, VA 22908
Tel: 804 982-1930 *Fax:* 804 982-1927
Accred Length: 3 Years *Program Size:* 2
Program ID: 327-51-21-069

Washington

Seattle

University of Washington Program

Sponsor: University of Washington School of Medicine
Children's Hospital and Medical Center
Fred Hutchinson Cancer Research Center

Program Director:
Irwin D Bernstein, MD
Fred Hutchinson Cancer Research Ctr
1100 Fairview Ave N
PO Box 19024
Seattle, WA 98109-1024
Tel: 206 667-4886 *Fax:* 206 667-6084
E-mail: ibernste@fhcrc.org
Internet: http://www.fhcrc.org
Accred Length: 3 Years *Program Size:* 9
Program ID: 327-54-21-040

Wisconsin

Madison

University of Wisconsin Program

Sponsor: University of Wisconsin Hospital and Clinics

Program Director:
Timothy Cripe, MD PhD
Univ of Wisconsin Hospital and Clinics
K4/530 Clinical Sci Ctr
600 Highland Ave
Madison, WI 53792-4108
Tel: 608 263-6691 *Fax:* 608 265-9721
E-mail: tcripe@facstaff.wisc.edu
Accred Length: 3 Years *Program Size:* 3
Program ID: 327-56-21-059

Milwaukee

Medical College of Wisconsin Program

Sponsor: Medical College of Wisconsin Affiliated Hospitals Inc
Children's Hospital of Wisconsin

Program Director:
J Paul Scott, MD
Sect of Ped Hematology-Oncology
Med Coll of Wisconsin
8701 Watertown Plank Rd
Milwaukee, WI 53226-3548
Tel: 414 937-3896 *Fax:* 414 937-6284
E-mail: paul@smtpgate.bcsew.edu
Accred Length: 3 Years *Program Size:* 3
Program ID: 327-56-21-063

Pediatric Infectious Diseases (Pediatrics)

Alabama

Birmingham

University of Alabama Medical Center Program
Sponsor: University of Alabama Hospital
Children's Hospital of Alabama
Program Director:
Robert F Pass, MD
1600 7th Ave S/Ste 752
Birmingham, AL 35233
Tel: 205 939-9593 *Fax:* 205 975-6549
E-mail: rpass@ped.uab.edu
Accred Length: 3 Years *Program Size:* 3
Program ID: 335-01-21-001

Arkansas

Little Rock

University of Arkansas for Medical Sciences Program
Sponsor: University of Arkansas College of Medicine
Arkansas Children's Hospital
University Hospital of Arkansas
Program Director:
Richard F Jacobs, MD
Arkansas Children's Hospital
800 Marshall St
Little Rock, AR 72202
Tel: 501 320-1416 *Fax:* 501 320-3551
E-mail: jacobsrichard@exchange.uams.edu
Accred Length: 3 Years *Program Size:* 2
Program ID: 335-04-21-002

California

Los Angeles

Children's Hospital of Los Angeles Program
Sponsor: Children's Hospital of Los Angeles
Program Director:
Kwang Sik Kim, MD
4650 Sunset Blvd/MS#51
Los Angeles, CA 90027
Tel: 323 669-2509 *Fax:* 323 660-2661
Accred Length: 3 Years *Program Size:* 3
Program ID: 335-05-31-004

UCLA Medical Center Program
Sponsor: UCLA School of Medicine
UCLA Medical Center
Program Director:
James D Cherry, MD
10833 LeConte Ave
MDCC Rm 22-442
Los Angeles, CA 90095
Tel: 310 825-5226 *Fax:* 310 206-4764
Accred Length: 3 Years *Program Size:* 2
Program ID: 335-05-11-005

Oakland

Children's Hospital-Oakland Program
Sponsor: Children's Hospital-Oakland
Program Director:
Parvin H Azimi, MD
747 52nd St
Oakland, CA 94609
Tel: 510 428-3336 *Fax:* 510 601-3957
Accred Length: 3 Years *Program Size:* 6
Program ID: 335-05-12-006

San Diego

University of California (San Diego) Program
Sponsor: University of California (San Diego) Medical Center
Children's Hospital and Health Center
Program Director:
Stephen A Spector, MD
9500 Gilman Dr
La Jolla, CA 92093
Tel: 619 534-7170 *Fax:* 619 534-7411
Accred Length: 3 Years *Program Size:* 3
Program ID: 335-05-13-007

San Francisco

University of California (San Francisco) Program
Sponsor: University of California (San Francisco) School of Medicine
Mount Zion Medical Center of the University of California
San Francisco General Hospital Medical Center
University of California (San Francisco) Medical Center
Program Director:
Peggy Sue Weintrub, MD
500 Parnassus Ave/MU4 East
San Francisco, CA 94143
Tel: 415 476-8016 *Fax:* 415 476-1343
E-mail: pweintru@peds.ucsf.edu
Accred Length: 3 Years *Program Size:* 3
Program ID: 335-05-22-008

Stanford

Stanford University Program
Sponsor: Stanford University Hospital
Lucile Salter Packard Children's Hospital at Stanford
Program Director:
Yvonne A Maldonado, MD
Dept of Pediatrics
Stanford Univ Hospital
300 Pasteur Dr
Stanford, CA 94305
Tel: 415 723-5682 *Fax:* 415 725-8040
Accred Length: 3 Years *Program Size:* 0
Program ID: 335-05-23-009

Torrance

Los Angeles County-Harbor-UCLA Medical Center Program
Sponsor: Los Angeles County-Harbor-UCLA Medical Center
Program Director:
Joel Ward, MD
1124 W Carson St/E-6
Torrance, CA 90502
Tel: 310 222-2346 *Fax:* 310 782-8776
E-mail: joelward@ucla.edu
Accred Length: 3 Years *Program Size:* 0
Program ID: 335-05-21-010

Colorado

Denver

University of Colorado Program
Sponsor: University of Colorado Health Sciences Center
Children's Hospital
Program Director:
Eric A F Simoes, MD
Children's Hospital
1056 E 19th Ave/B055
Denver, CO 80218
Tel: 303 837-2838 *Fax:* 303 837-2707
E-mail: beam.kristin@tchden.org
Accred Length: 3 Years *Program Size:* 3
Program ID: 335-07-21-011

Connecticut

New Haven

Yale-New Haven Medical Center Program
Sponsor: Yale-New Haven Hospital
Program Director:
George Miller, MD
Yale Univ Sch of Med
Dept of Pediatrics
333 Cedar St/Box 208064
New Haven, CT 06520
Tel: 203 785-4758 *Fax:* 203 785-6961
E-mail: george.miller@yale.edu
Accred Length: 3 Years *Program Size:* 3
Program ID: 335-08-21-012

District of Columbia

Washington

George Washington University Program
Sponsor: Children's National Medical Center
Program Director:
William J Rodriguez, MD
111 Michigan Ave NW
Washington, DC 20010
Tel: 202 884-5051 *Fax:* 202 884-3850
Accred Length: 3 Years *Program Size:* 6
Program ID: 335-10-21-013

Florida

Jacksonville

University of Florida Health Science Center/Jacksonville Program
Sponsor: University of Florida College of Medicine at Jacksonville
Baptist Medical Center (UFHSC/J)
University Medical Center (UFHSC/J)
Program Director:
Mobeen H Rathore, MD
653-1 W 8th St
Jacksonville, FL 32209
Tel: 904 549-3051 *Fax:* 904 549-5341
E-mail: mobeen.rathore@jax.ufl.edu
Accred Length: 3 Years *Program Size:* 3
Program ID: 335-11-21-015

Georgia

Atlanta

Emory University Program
Sponsor: Emory University School of Medicine
Egleston Children's Hospital at Emory University
Grady Memorial Hospital

Program Director:
Andre J Nahmias, MD
69 Butler St SE
Atlanta, GA 30303
Tel: 404 616-4997 *Fax:* 404 659-0129
Accred Length: 3 Years *Program Size:* 0
Program ID: 335-12-21-017

Illinois

Chicago

McGaw Medical Center of Northwestern University Program
Sponsor: Northwestern University Medical School
Children's Memorial Medical Center

Program Director:
Stanford T Shulman, MD
2300 Children's Plaza/Box #90
Chicago, IL 60614
Tel: 773 880-4187 *Fax:* 773 880-8226
E-mail: sshulman@nwu.edu
Accred Length: 3 Years *Program Size:* 3
Program ID: 335-16-21-018

University of Chicago Program
Sponsor: University of Chicago Hospitals
University of Chicago Children's Hospital

Program Director:
Robert S Daum, MD
Univ of Chicago Hospitals
5841 S Maryland Ave (MC 6054)
Chicago, IL 60637
Tel: 773 702-6176 *Fax:* 773 702-1196
Accred Length: 3 Years *Program Size:* 0
Program ID: 335-16-31-019

Kentucky

Louisville

University of Louisville Program
Sponsor: University of Louisville School of Medicine
Kosair Children's Hospital (Alliant Health System)

Program Director:
Gary S Marshall, MD
571 S Floyd St/Ste 300
Louisville, KY 40202
Tel: 502 852-3774 *Fax:* 502 852-3939
Accred Length: 3 Years *Program Size:* 1
Program ID: 335-20-21-021

Louisiana

New Orleans

Tulane University/Louisiana State University Program
Sponsor: Tulane University School of Medicine
Medical Center of Louisiana at New Orleans
Tulane Hospital for Children
Tulane University Hospital and Clinics

Program Director:
James Robinson, MD
Rudolfo Begue, MD
1430 Tulane Ave
SL 64
New Orleans, LA 70112
Tel: 504 588-5422 *Fax:* 504 584-2613
E-mail: jrobins@tmcpop.tmc.tulane.edu
Accred Length: 3 Years *Program Size:* 2
Program ID: 335-21-21-022

Maryland

Baltimore

Johns Hopkins University Program
Sponsor: Johns Hopkins University School of Medicine
Johns Hopkins Hospital

Program Director:
Rodney E Willoughby, MD
600 N Wolfe St/Park 256
Baltimore, MD 21287
Tel: 410 614-3917 *Fax:* 410 614-1491
Accred Length: 3 Years *Program Size:* 3
Program ID: 335-23-21-023

University of Maryland Program
Sponsor: University of Maryland Medical System

Program Director:
Margaret B Rennels, MD
22 S Greene St/Rm N5W70
Baltimore, MD 21201
Tel: 410 328-6919 *Fax:* 410 328-1072
E-mail: mrennels@umaryland.edu
Accred Length: 3 Years *Program Size:* 3
Program ID: 335-23-31-024

Bethesda

National Capital Consortium Program
Sponsor: National Capital Consortium
National Naval Medical Center (Bethesda)
Walter Reed Army Medical Center

Program Director:
Martin Gerard Ottolini, MD
4301 Jones Bridge Rd
Bethesda, MD 20814
Tel: 301 295-9721 *Fax:* 301 295-3898
Accred Length: 3 Years *Program Size:* 0
Program ID: 335-10-31-014
US Armed Services Program

Massachusetts

Boston

Children's Hospital/Boston Medical Center Program 1
Sponsor: Children's Hospital

Program Director:
Kenneth McIntosh, MD
300 Longwood Ave/Rm 609
Enders Bldg
Boston, MA 02115
Tel: 617 355-7621 *Fax:* 617 355-8387
Accred Length: 3 Years *Program Size:* 6
Program ID: 335-24-21-025

Children's Hospital/Boston Medical Center Program 2
Sponsor: Boston Medical Center

Program Director:
Stephen I Pelton, MD
Boston Med Ctr
1 Boston Medical Center Pl
Boston, MA 02118
Tel: 617 414-7408 *Fax:* 617 414-5806
Accred Length: 3 Years *Program Size:* 3
Program ID: 335-24-31-026

Michigan

Ann Arbor

University of Michigan Program
Sponsor: University of Michigan Hospitals

Program Director:
Janet Gilsdorf, MD
1500 E Medical Center Dr
F6854 C S Mott
Ann Arbor, MI 48109
Tel: 734 763-2440 *Fax:* 734 763-7359
Accred Length: 3 Years *Program Size:* 3
Program ID: 335-25-21-027

Detroit

Wayne State University/Detroit Medical Center Program
Sponsor: Wayne State University/Detroit Medical Center
Children's Hospital of Michigan

Program Director:
Basim I Asmar, MD
Children's Hospital of Michigan
Div of Infectious Diseases
3901 Beaubien Blvd
Detroit, MI 48201
Tel: 313 745-5863 *Fax:* 313 993-8846
E-mail: basmar@wayne .edu
Accred Length: 3 Years *Program Size:* 1
Program ID: 335-25-31-028

Minnesota

Minneapolis

University of Minnesota Program
Sponsor: University of Minnesota Medical School
Fairview-University Medical Center
Program Director:
G Scott Giebink, MD
420 Delaware St SE
Box 296 UMHC
Minneapolis, MN 55455
Tel: 612 624-1112 *Fax:* 612 624-8927
E-mail: giebi001@tc.umn.edu
Accred Length: 3 Years *Program Size:* 6
Program ID: 335-26-21-029

Missouri

St Louis

Washington University/B-JH/SLCH Consortium Program
Sponsor: Washington University/B-JH/SLCH Consortium
St Louis Children's Hospital
Program Director:
Joseph W St Geme, MD
One Children's Pl
St Louis, MO 63110
Tel: 314 454-6050 *Fax:* 314 454-2836
E-mail: stgeme@borcim.wustl.edu
Accred Length: 3 Years *Program Size:* 6
Program ID: 335-28-21-030

Nebraska

Omaha

University of Nebraska/Creighton University Program
Sponsor: University of Nebraska Medical Center
Childrens Memorial Hospital
Tenet St Joseph Hospital at Creighton Univ Medical Center
Program Director:
Stephen A Chartrand, MD
2500 California Plaza
Criss II RM 409
Omaha, NE 68178
Tel: 402 280-1231 *Fax:* 402 280-1234
Accred Length: 3 Years *Program Size:* 2
Program ID: 335-30-21-031

New Jersey

Newark

UMDNJ-New Jersey Medical School Program
Sponsor: UMDNJ-New Jersey Medical School
Program Director:
Barry Dashefsky, MD
185 S Orange Ave
Newark, NJ 07103
Tel: 973 972-5066 *Fax:* 973 972-6443
Accred Length: 3 Years *Program Size:* 3
Program ID: 335-33-21-062

New York

Bronx

Albert Einstein College of Medicine Program
Sponsor: Albert Einstein College of Medicine of Yeshiva University
Montefiore Medical Center-Henry and Lucy Moses Division
North Central Bronx Hospital
Program Director:
Nathan Litman, MD
Albert Einstein Coll of Med
111 E 210 St
Bronx, NY 10467
Tel: 718 519-3822 *Fax:* 718 519-4713
Accred Length: 3 Years *Program Size:* 0
Program ID: 335-35-21-034

Brooklyn

SUNY Health Science Center at Brooklyn Program
Sponsor: SUNY Health Science Center at Brooklyn
Kings County Hospital Center
University Hospital-SUNY Health Science Center at Brooklyn
Program Director:
Margaret R Hammerschlag, MD
450 Clarkson Ave/Box 49
Brooklyn, NY 11203
Tel: 718 245-4074 *Fax:* 718 245-2118
E-mail: mhammerschlag@pol.net
Accred Length: 3 Years *Program Size:* 1
Program ID: 335-35-11-036

Manhasset

North Shore University Hospital/NYU School of Medicine Program
Sponsor: North Shore University Hospital
Program Director:
Leonard R Krilov, MD
865 Northern Blvd
Great Neck, NY 11021
Tel: 516 622-5094 *Fax:* 516 622-5074
E-mail: lkrilov@nshs.edu
Accred Length: 3 Years *Program Size:* 1
Program ID: 335-35-21-061

New Hyde Park

Albert Einstein College of Medicine at Long Island Jewish Medical Center Program
Sponsor: Long Island Jewish Medical Center
Schneider Children's Hosp (Long Island Jewish Med Ctr)
Program Director:
Lorry G Rubin, MD
Long Island Jewish Med Ctr
269-01 76th Ave
New Hyde Park, NY 11040
Tel: 718 470-3480 *Fax:* 718 470-8007
Accred Length: 3 Years *Program Size:* 0
Program ID: 335-35-12-037

New York

Mount Sinai School of Medicine Program
Sponsor: Mount Sinai School of Medicine
Mount Sinai Medical Center
Program Director:
Anne Moscona, MD
Mount Sinai Med Ctr
One Gustave L Levy Pl/Box 1657
New York, NY 10029
Tel: 212 241-6930 *Fax:* 212 426-4813
E-mail: a_moscona@smtplink.mssm.edu
Internet: http://www.mssm.edu/peds/idfell.html
Accred Length: 3 Years *Program Size:* 3
Program ID: 335-35-13-038

New York and Presbyterian Hospital (Columbia Campus) Program
Sponsor: New York and Presbyterian Hospital
New York and Presbyterian Hospital (Columbia Campus)
Program Director:
Lisa Saiman, MD
650 W 168th St (BB4-427)
New York, NY 10032
Tel: 212 305-1556 *Fax:* 212 305-2284
E-mail: ls5@columbia.edu
Accred Length: 3 Years *Program Size:* 0
Program ID: 335-35-21-040

New York and Presbyterian Hospital (Cornell Campus) Program
Sponsor: New York and Presbyterian Hospital
New York and Presbyterian Hospital (Cornell Campus)
Program Director:
Gary J Noel, MD
525 E 68th St
Box 596
New York, NY 10021
Tel: 212 746-3326 *Fax:* 212 746-8716
E-mail: gjnoel@mail.med.cornell.edu
Accred Length: 3 Years *Program Size:* 4
Program ID: 335-35-22-039

Rochester

University of Rochester Program
Sponsor: Strong Memorial Hospital of the University of Rochester
Program Director:
Francis Gigliotti, MD
601 Elmwood Ave/Box 690
Rochester, NY 14642
Tel: 716 275-5944 *Fax:* 716 273-1104
E-mail: francis_gigliotti@urmc.rochester.edu
Accred Length: 3 Years *Program Size:* 3
Program ID: 335-35-31-041

Syracuse

SUNY Health Science Center at Syracuse Program
Sponsor: University Hospital-SUNY Health Science Center at Syracuse
Crouse Hospital
St Joseph's Hospital Health Center
Program Director:
Leonard B Weiner, MD
SUNY Health Science Ctr-Syracuse
750 E Adams St
Syracuse, NY 13210
Tel: 315 464-6331 *Fax:* 315 464-7564
E-mail: weinerl@mailbox.hscsyr.edu
Internet: http://www.hscsyr.edu/peds/
Accred Length: 3 Years *Program Size:* 3
Program ID: 335-35-11-042

North Carolina

Durham

Duke University Program

Sponsor: Duke University Medical Center

Program Director:
Ross E McKinney, MD
Box 3461 Rm 1080
Duke South Hospital
Durham, NC 27710
Tel: 919 684-6335 *Fax:* 919 684-8514
E-mail: ross.mckinney@duke.edu
Accred Length: 3 Years *Program Size:* 4
Program ID: 335-36-31-044

Ohio

Cincinnati

Children's Hospital Medical Center/University of Cincinnati College of Medicine Program

Sponsor: Children's Hospital Medical Center

Program Director:
Beverly L Connelly, MD
Children's Hospital Med Ctr
3333 Burnet Ave
Cincinnati, OH 45229
Tel: 513 559-4578 *Fax:* 513 559-7682
Accred Length: 3 Years *Program Size:* 0
Program ID: 335-38-21-045

Cleveland

Case Western Reserve University Program

Sponsor: University Hospitals of Cleveland
Cleveland Clinic Foundation

Program Director:
John R Schreiber, MD
11100 Euclid Ave
Mail Stop 8A
Cleveland, OH 44106
Tel: 216 884-3645 *Fax:* 216 844-8362
Accred Length: 3 Years *Program Size:* 4
Program ID: 335-38-31-046

Pennsylvania

Philadelphia

Children's Hospital of Philadelphia Program

Sponsor: Children's Hospital of Philadelphia

Program Director:
Paul A Offit, MD
34th St and Civic Center Blvd
Rm 1202C Abramson Research Ctr
Philadelphia, PA 19104
Tel: 215 590-2020 *Fax:* 215 590-2025
E-mail: offit@email.chop.edu
Accred Length: 3 Years *Program Size:* 3
Program ID: 335-41-21-047

St Christopher's Hospital for Children Program

Sponsor: St Christopher's Hospital for Children

Program Director:
Sarah S Long, MD
Erie Ave at Front St
Philadelphia, PA 19134
Tel: 215 427-5204 *Fax:* 215 427-8389
Accred Length: 3 Years *Program Size:* 2
Program ID: 335-41-31-048

Pittsburgh

University Health Center of Pittsburgh Program

Sponsor: University Health Center of Pittsburgh
Children's Hospital of Pittsburgh

Program Director:
Marian G Michaels, MD MPH
3705 Fifth Ave
Pittsburgh, PA 15213-2583
Tel: 412 692-5930 *Fax:* 412 692-8499
E-mail: krused@chplink.chp.edu
Internet: http://www.chp.edu
Accred Length: 3 Years *Program Size:* 2
Program ID: 335-41-11-049

Rhode Island

Providence

Brown University Program

Sponsor: Rhode Island Hospital

Program Director:
Georges Peter, MD
Rhode Island Hospital
Div of Ped Infectious Diseases
593 Eddy St
Providence, RI 02903
Tel: 401 444-8360 *Fax:* 401 444-5650
E-mail: georges_peter@brown.edu
Accred Length: 3 Years *Program Size:* 3
Program ID: 335-43-21-050

Tennessee

Memphis

University of Tennessee Program

Sponsor: University of Tennessee College of Medicine
LeBonheur Children's Medical Center
St Jude Children's Research Hospital

Program Director:
Christian C Patrick, MD
332 N Lauderdale St
Memphis, TN 38105
Tel: 901 495-2755
Accred Length: 3 Years *Program Size:* 0
Program ID: 335-47-21-051

Nashville

Vanderbilt University Program

Sponsor: Vanderbilt University Medical Center

Program Director:
Terence S Dermody, MD
Lamb Ctr for Pediatric Research
Vanderbilt Univ Sch of Med
1161 21st Ave S
Nashville, TN 37232-2581
Tel: 615 322-2250 *Fax:* 615 343-9723
E-mail: terry.dermody@mcmail.vanderbilt.edu
Accred Length: 3 Years *Program Size:* 4
Program ID: 335-47-31-052

Texas

Dallas

University of Texas Southwestern Medical School Program

Sponsor: University of Texas Southwestern Medical School
Children's Medical Center of Dallas
Dallas County Hospital District-Parkland Memorial Hospital

Program Director:
George H McCracken Jr, MD
5323 Harry Hines Blvd
Dallas, TX 75235-9063
Tel: 214 648-3439 *Fax:* 214 648-2961
Accred Length: 3 Years *Program Size:* 6
Program ID: 335-48-21-053

Galveston

University of Texas Medical Branch Hospitals Program

Sponsor: University of Texas Medical Branch Hospitals

Program Director:
Tasnee Chonmaitree, MD
301 University Blvd
Galveston, TX 77555
Tel: 409 772-2798 *Fax:* 409 747-1753
E-mail: tchonmai@utmb.edu
Accred Length: 3 Years *Program Size:* 1
Program ID: 335-48-31-054

Houston

Baylor College of Medicine Program

Sponsor: Baylor College of Medicine
Harris County Hospital District-Ben Taub General Hospital
Texas Children's Hospital

Program Director:
Judith R Campbell, MD
One Baylor Plaza/Rm 312E
Houston, TX 77030
Tel: 713 798-4790 *Fax:* 713 798-6407
E-mail: judithc@bcm.tmc.edu
Accred Length: 3 Years *Program Size:* 8
Program ID: 335-48-11-055

University of Texas at Houston Program

Sponsor: University of Texas Medical School at Houston
Lyndon B Johnson General Hospital
Memorial Hermann Healthcare System

Program Director:
Thomas G Cleary, MD
6431 Fannin/JFB 1.739
Houston, TX 77030
Tel: 713 792-5330 *Fax:* 713 792-5199
Accred Length: 3 Years *Program Size:* 0
Program ID: 335-48-12-056

San Antonio

University of Texas Health Science Center at San Antonio Program
Sponsor: University of Texas Medical School at San Antonio
Methodist Healthcare
Santa Rosa Health Care Corporation
University Hospital-South Texas Medical Center
Program Director:
Hal B Jenson, MD
Univ of Texas Health Science Ctr
Dept of Pediatrics
7703 Floyd Curl Dr
San Antonio, TX 78284-7811
Tel: 210 567-5301 *Fax:* 210 567-6305
E-mail: jenson@uthscsa.edu
Accred Length: 3 Years *Program Size:* 1
Program ID: 335-48-13-057

Virginia

Norfolk

Eastern Virginia Medical School Program
Sponsor: Eastern Virginia Medical School
Children's Hospital of the King's Daughters
Sentara Norfolk General Hospital
Program Director:
Larry K Pickering, MD
EVMS
Ctr for Pediatric Research
855 W Brambleton Ave
Norfolk, VA 23510
Tel: 757 668-6400 *Fax:* 757 668-6476
E-mail: lpickeri@chkd.com
Internet: http://www.chkd.org or http://www.pediatricresearch.org
Accred Length: 3 Years *Program Size:* 3
Program ID: 335-51-21-058

Richmond

Medical College of Virginia/Virginia Commonwealth University Program
Sponsor: Medical College of Virginia/Virginia Commonwealth University
Medical College of Virginia Hospitals
Program Director:
Stuart P Adler, MD
Med Coll of Virginia
PO Box 98163 MCV Station
Richmond, VA 23298
Tel: 804 828-1807 *Fax:* 804 828-6455
Accred Length: 3 Years *Program Size:* 0
Program ID: 335-51-31-059

Washington

Seattle

University of Washington Program
Sponsor: University of Washington School of Medicine
Children's Hospital and Medical Center
University of Washington Medical Center
Program Director:
Craig E Rubens, MD
4800 Sand Point Way NE/CH-32
Seattle, WA 98105
Tel: 206 526-2073 *Fax:* 206 527-3890
Accred Length: 3 Years *Program Size:* 2
Program ID: 335-54-21-060

Pediatric Nephrology (Pediatrics)

California

Los Angeles

Cedars-Sinai Medical Center Program
Sponsor: Cedars-Sinai Medical Center
Program Director:
Stanley C Jordan, MD
Cedars-Sinai Med Ctr
Div of Ped Nephrology
8700 Beverly Blvd/NT4310
Los Angeles, CA 90048
Tel: 310 855-4747 *Fax:* 310 967-0145
E-mail: sjordan@xchg.csmc.edu
Accred Length: 3 Years *Program Size:* 1
Program ID: 328-05-21-052

Children's Hospital of Los Angeles Program
Sponsor: Children's Hospital of Los Angeles
Program Director:
Carl M Grushkin, MD
Children's Hospital Los Angeles
Div of Nephrology/Mail Stop #40
4650 Sunset Blvd
Los Angeles, CA 90027
Tel: 323 669-2102 *Fax:* 323 668-1829
Accred Length: 3 Years *Program Size:* 3
Program ID: 328-05-11-001

UCLA Medical Center Program
Sponsor: UCLA School of Medicine
UCLA Medical Center
Program Director:
Robert B Ettenger, MD
UCLA Sch of Med
Rm A2-383 MDCC
10833 Le Conte Ave
Los Angeles, CA 90095-1752
Tel: 310 206-6987 *Fax:* 310 825-0442
E-mail: rettenge@pediatrics.medsch.ucla.edu
Accred Length: 3 Years *Program Size:* 4
Program ID: 328-05-21-002

San Diego

University of California (San Diego) Program
Sponsor: University of California (San Diego) Medical Center
Children's Hospital and Health Center
Program Director:
Jacques M Lemire, MD
UCSD Med Ctr
Div of Nephrology
9500 Gilman Dr/0831
La Jolla, CA 92093-0831
Tel: 619 543-5218 *Fax:* 619 543-3575
E-mail: jalemire@ucsd.edu
Accred Length: 3 Years *Program Size:* 2
Program ID: 328-05-21-047

San Francisco

University of California (San Francisco) Program
Sponsor: University of California (San Francisco) School of Medicine
University of California (San Francisco) Medical Center
Program Director:
Anthony A Portale, MD
Univ of California San Francisco
Children's Renal Ctr
533 Parnassus Ave/Rm U 585
San Francisco, CA 94143-0748
Tel: 415 476-2423 *Fax:* 415 476-9976
E-mail: aportale@peds.ucsf.edu
Accred Length: 3 Years *Program Size:* 3
Program ID: 328-05-11-022

Stanford

Stanford University Program
Sponsor: Stanford University Hospital
Lucile Salter Packard Children's Hospital at Stanford
Program Director:
Steven R Alexander, MD
Dept of Pediatrics/G306
Stanford Univ Med Ctr
300 Pasteur Dr
Stanford, CA 94305
Tel: 650 723-7903 *Fax:* 650 723-2137
Accred Length: 3 Years *Program Size:* 2
Program ID: 328-05-21-029

Colorado

Denver

University of Colorado Program
Sponsor: University of Colorado Health Sciences Center
Children's Hospital
Program Director:
Douglas M Ford, MD
Kidney Ctr B328
1056 E 19th Ave
Denver, CO 80218
Tel: 303 861-6263 *Fax:* 303 837-2541
E-mail: ford.douglas@tchdes.org
Accred Length: 3 Years *Program Size:* 1
Program ID: 328-07-21-003

Connecticut

New Haven

Yale-New Haven Medical Center Program
Sponsor: Yale-New Haven Hospital
Program Director:
Norman J Siegel, MD
Yale Univ Sch of Med
Dept of Pediatrics/PO Box 208064
333 Cedar St
New Haven, CT 06520-8064
Tel: 203 785-4643 *Fax:* 203 785-3462
E-mail: norman.siegel@yale.edu
Accred Length: 3 Years *Program Size:* 3
Program ID: 328-08-21-004

District of Columbia

Washington

George Washington University Program
Sponsor: Children's National Medical Center

Program Director:
Marva M Moxey-Mims, MD
Children's National Med Ctr
Dept of Nephrology
111 Michigan Ave NW
Washington, DC 20010-2970
Tel: 202 884-5058 *Fax:* 202 884-3621
E-mail: mmoxeymi@cnmc.org
Internet: http://www.mmoxeymi@cnmc.org
Accred Length: 3 Years *Program Size:* 0
Program ID: 328-10-21-023

Georgetown University Program
Sponsor: Georgetown University Medical Center

Program Director:
Pedro A Jose, MD PhD
Georgetown Univ Hospital
Dept of Pediatrics
3800 Reservoir Rd NW
Washington, DC 20007-2197
Tel: 202 687-8675 *Fax:* 202 687-7161
E-mail: josep@gunet.georgetown.edu
Accred Length: 3 Years *Program Size:* 0
Program ID: 328-10-21-005

Florida

Gainesville

University of Florida Program
Sponsor: University of Florida College of Medicine
Shands Hospital at the University of Florida

Program Director:
George A Richard, MD
Univ of Florida Coll of Med
Div of Ped Nephrology
PO Box 100296 JHMHC
Gainesville, FL 32610-0296
Tel: 352 392-4434 *Fax:* 352 392-7107
E-mail: richaga@peds.ufl.edu
Accred Length: 3 Years *Program Size:* 3
Program ID: 328-11-31-006

Miami

University of Miami-Jackson Memorial Medical Center Program
Sponsor: University of Miami-Jackson Memorial Medical Center

Program Director:
Gaston E Zilleruelo, MD
Univ of Miami-Jackson Memorial Med Ctr
Div of Ped Nephrology
PO Box 016960 (R-131)
Miami, FL 33101
Tel: 305 585-6726 *Fax:* 305 547-1709
E-mail: pedneph@mednet.med.miami.edu
Accred Length: 3 Years *Program Size:* 3
Program ID: 328-11-21-032

Illinois

Chicago

McGaw Medical Center of Northwestern University Program
Sponsor: Northwestern University Medical School
Children's Memorial Medical Center

Program Director:
H William Schnaper, MD
Children's Memorial Hospital
2300 Children's Plaza
Box 37
Chicago, IL 60614-3318
Tel: 773 880-4326 *Fax:* 773 880-6776
E-mail: dmuse@nwu.edu
Accred Length: 3 Years *Program Size:* 3
Program ID: 328-16-21-030

Indiana

Indianapolis

Indiana University School of Medicine Program
Sponsor: Indiana University School of Medicine
Clarian Riley Hospital for Children

Program Director:
Sharon P Andreoli, MD
Indiana Univ Med Ctr
Riley Hospital for Children
702 Barnhill Dr/Rm 5816
Indianapolis, IN 46202-5225
Tel: 317 274-2563 *Fax:* 317 278-3599
Accred Length: 3 Years *Program Size:* 0
Program ID: 328-17-21-007

Iowa

Iowa City

University of Iowa Hospitals and Clinics Program
Sponsor: University of Iowa Hospitals and Clinics

Program Director:
Craig C Porter, MD
Univ of Iowa Hospitals and Clinics
Dept of Pediatrics
200 Hawkins Dr
Iowa City, IA 52242-1083
Tel: 319 356-3988 *Fax:* 319 384-9616
E-mail: craig-porter@uiowa.edu
Accred Length: 3 Years *Program Size:* 1
Program ID: 328-18-11-008

Louisiana

New Orleans

Tulane University Program
Sponsor: Tulane University School of Medicine
Medical Center of Louisiana at New Orleans
Tulane Hospital for Children

Program Director:
Frank G Boineau, MD
Tulane Univ Med Ctr
Dept of Pediatrics
1430 Tulane Ave/SL-37
New Orleans, LA 70112
Tel: 504 588-5377 *Fax:* 504 584-1852
E-mail: fboinea@tmcpop.tmc.tulane.edu
Accred Length: 3 Years *Program Size:* 3
Program ID: 328-21-21-009

Massachusetts

Boston

Children's Hospital/Boston Medical Center Program
Sponsor: Children's Hospital

Program Director:
William E Harmon, MD
Children's Hospital
300 Longwood Ave
Boston, MA 02115
Tel: 617 355-6129 *Fax:* 617 730-0657
E-mail: harmon@a1.hub.harvard.edu
Accred Length: 3 Years *Program Size:* 6
Program ID: 328-24-11-010

Massachusetts General Hospital Program
Sponsor: Massachusetts General Hospital

Program Director:
Julie R Ingelfinger, MD
WACC 709
15 Parkman St
Boston, MA 02114
Tel: 617 726-2908 *Fax:* 617 726-3044
E-mail: ingelfinger@helix.mgh.harvard.edu
Accred Length: 3 Years *Program Size:* 3
Program ID: 328-24-21-048

Michigan

Ann Arbor

University of Michigan Program
Sponsor: University of Michigan Hospitals

Program Director:
William E Smoyer, MD
1500 E Medical Center Dr
Ann Arbor, MI 48109-0318
Tel: 734 936-4210 *Fax:* 734 763-6997
E-mail: pediatric.nephrology@umich.edu
Internet: http://www.ped.med.umich.edu/pednephz.html
Accred Length: 3 Years *Program Size:* 3
Program ID: 328-25-21-034

Minnesota

Minneapolis

University of Minnesota Program

Sponsor: University of Minnesota Medical School
Fairview-University Medical Center
Program Director:
S Michael Mauer, MD
Youngki Kim, MD
Univ of Minnesota Med Sch
Box 491 UMHC
420 Delaware St SE
Minneapolis, MN 55455-0392
Tel: 612 626-2922 *Fax:* 612 626-2791
E-mail: erick024@maroon.tc.umn.edu
Accred Length: 3 Years *Program Size:* 4
Program ID: 328-26-21-035

Missouri

Kansas City

University of Missouri at Kansas City Program

Sponsor: University of Missouri-Kansas City School of Medicine
Children's Mercy Hospital
Program Director:
Uri S Alon, MD
Children's Mercy Hospital
Dept of Nephrology
2401 Gillham Rd
Kansas City, MO 64108-9898
Tel: 816 234-3010 *Fax:* 816 234-3494
E-mail: ualon@cmh.edu
Internet: http://www.cmh.edu
Accred Length: 3 Years *Program Size:* 3
Program ID: 328-28-11-038

St Louis

Washington University/B-JH/SLCH Consortium Program

Sponsor: Washington University/B-JH/SLCH Consortium
St Louis Children's Hospital
Program Director:
Barbara R Cole, MD
Washington Univ-St Louis Children's Hospital
One Children's Pl
Rm 1060
St Louis, MO 63110
Tel: 314 454-6043 *Fax:* 314 454-4283
E-mail: cole_b@a1.kids.wustl.edu
Internet:
http://www.wumshome.wustl.edu/peds/renal.html
Accred Length: 3 Years *Program Size:* 1
Program ID: 328-28-21-031

New York

Bronx

Albert Einstein College of Medicine Program

Sponsor: Albert Einstein College of Medicine of Yeshiva University
Jacobi Medical Center
Montefiore Medical Center-Weiler Hospital
Program Director:
Frederick J Kaskel, MD
Albert Einstein Coll of Med
1410 Pelham Pkwy S
Rm K721
Bronx, NY 10461
Tel: 718 430-2511 *Fax:* 718 824-2392
Accred Length: 3 Years *Program Size:* 5
Program ID: 328-35-21-011

Brooklyn

SUNY Health Science Center at Brooklyn Program

Sponsor: SUNY Health Science Center at Brooklyn
Kings County Hospital Center
University Hospital-SUNY Health Science Center at Brooklyn
Program Director:
Baqi Noosha, MD
SUNY-Brooklyn
450 Clarkson Ave/Box 49
Brooklyn, NY 11203
Tel: 718 270-1913 *Fax:* 718 270-2826
Accred Length: 3 Years *Program Size:* 6
Program ID: 328-35-21-012

Buffalo

SUNY at Buffalo Graduate Medical-Dental Education Consortium Program

Sponsor: SUNY at Buffalo Grad Medical-Dental Education Consortium
CGF Health System (Children's Hospital of Buffalo)
Program Director:
James E Springate, MD
Children's Hospital
Dept of Ped Nephrology
219 Bryant St
Buffalo, NY 14222
Tel: 716 878-7274 *Fax:* 716 878-1445
Accred Length: 3 Years *Program Size:* 1
Program ID: 328-35-21-024

New York

Mount Sinai School of Medicine Program

Sponsor: Mount Sinai School of Medicine
Mount Sinai Medical Center
Program Director:
Lisa M Satlin, MD
Mount Sinai Sch of Med
One Gustave L Levy Pl
Box 1664
New York, NY 10029-6574
Tel: 212 241-6187 *Fax:* 212 369-7387
E-mail: lisa_satlin@smtplink.mssm.edu
Internet: http://www.mssm.edu/peds/kidney.html
Accred Length: 3 Years *Program Size:* 2
Program ID: 328-35-31-051

New York and Presbyterian Hospital (Cornell Campus) Program

Sponsor: New York and Presbyterian Hospital
New York and Presbyterian Hospital (Cornell Campus)
Program Director:
Valerie L Johnson, MD PhD
525 E 68th St/Rm N-0008
New York, NY 10021
Tel: 212 746-3260 *Fax:* 212 746-8861
E-mail: vljohns@cumc.cornell.edu
Accred Length: 3 Years *Program Size:* 1
Program ID: 328-35-31-049

Rochester

University of Rochester Program

Sponsor: Strong Memorial Hospital of the University of Rochester
Program Director:
George J Schwartz, MD
Univ of Rochester Med Ctr
Div of Ped Nephrology
601 Elmwood Ave/Box 777
Rochester, NY 14642
Tel: 716 275-9784 *Fax:* 716 756-8054
E-mail: gesc@bphvax.biophysics.rochester.edu
Accred Length: 3 Years *Program Size:* 3
Program ID: 328-35-21-050

Stony Brook

SUNY at Stony Brook Program

Sponsor: University Hospital-SUNY at Stony Brook
Program Director:
Richard N Fine, MD
Children's Med Ctr
HSC T-11 Dept of Pediatrics
SUNY-Stony Brook
Stony Brook, NY 11794-8111
Tel: 516 444-7884 *Fax:* 516 444-8968
E-mail: dwhyte@mail.som.sunysb.edu
Accred Length: 3 Years *Program Size:* 2
Program ID: 328-35-21-033

North Carolina

Durham

Duke University Program

Sponsor: Duke University Medical Center
Program Director:
John W Foreman, MD
Duke Univ Med Ctr
Ped Nephrology Dept
Box 3959
Durham, NC 27710
Tel: 919 684-4246 *Fax:* 919 681-6446
E-mail: forem001@mc.duke.edu
Accred Length: 3 Years *Program Size:* 2
Program ID: 328-36-21-044

Ohio

Cincinnati

Children's Hospital Medical Center/University of Cincinnati College of Medicine Program

Sponsor: Children's Hospital Medical Center

Program Director:
Paul T McEnery, MD MBA
Children's Hospital Med Ctr
3333 Burnet Ave
CHRF 5392
Cincinnati, OH 45229-3039
Tel: 513 636-4531 *Fax:* 513 636-7407
E-mail: mcenp0@chmcc.org
Internet: http://www.chmcc.org
Accred Length: 3 Years *Program Size:* 2
Program ID: 328-38-21-015

Cleveland

Case Western Reserve University Program

Sponsor: University Hospitals of Cleveland

Program Director:
Ira D Davis, MD
Univ Hospitals of Cleveland
11100 Euclid Ave
Cleveland, OH 44106
Tel: 216 844-1389 *Fax:* 216 844-8977
Accred Length: 3 Years *Program Size:* 1
Program ID: 328-38-21-054

Cleveland Clinic Foundation Program

Sponsor: Cleveland Clinic Foundation

Program Director:
Robert Cunningham, MD
Cleveland Clinic Foundation
Dept of Pediatrics/A120
9500 Euclid Ave
Cleveland, OH 44195-5242
Tel: 216 444-2200 *Fax:* 216 445-7561
E-mail: meded@cesmtp.ccf.org
Internet: http://www.ccf.org
Accred Length: 3 Years *Program Size:* 0
Program ID: 328-38-31-040

Pennsylvania

Philadelphia

Children's Hospital of Philadelphia Program

Sponsor: Children's Hospital of Philadelphia

Program Director:
Bernard S Kaplan, MD
Children's Hospital
Div of Nephrology
34th St and Civic Center Blvd
Philadelphia, PA 19104
Tel: 215 590-2449 *Fax:* 215 590-3705
E-mail: kaplanb@email.chop.edu
Internet: http://www.chop.edu
Accred Length: 3 Years *Program Size:* 3
Program ID: 328-41-21-025

St Christopher's Hospital for Children Program

Sponsor: St Christopher's Hospital for Children

Program Director:
Susan B Conley, MD
St Christopher's Hospital for Children
Front and Erie Aves
Philadelphia, PA 19134-1092
Tel: 215 427-5190 *Fax:* 215 427-5351
E-mail: sueconley@email.msn.com
Accred Length: 3 Years *Program Size:* 1
Program ID: 328-41-12-017

Pittsburgh

University Health Center of Pittsburgh Program

Sponsor: University Health Center of Pittsburgh
Children's Hospital of Pittsburgh

Program Director:
Demetrius Ellis, MD
Children's Hospital
One Children's Pl
3705 Fifth Ave
Pittsburgh, PA 15213-2583
Tel: 412 692-5182 *Fax:* 412 692-7443
Accred Length: 3 Years *Program Size:* 0
Program ID: 328-41-21-036

Tennessee

Memphis

University of Tennessee Program

Sponsor: University of Tennessee College of Medicine
LeBonheur Children's Medical Center

Program Director:
Deborah P Jones, MD
Univ of Tennessee
50 N Dunlap
CCRF Research Ctr/Rm 301
Memphis, TN 38103
Tel: 901 572-5366 *Fax:* 901 572-5036
Accred Length: 3 Years *Program Size:* 3
Program ID: 328-47-31-018

Nashville

Vanderbilt University Program

Sponsor: Vanderbilt University Medical Center

Program Director:
Iekuni Ichikawa, MD
Vanderbilt Univ
C-4204 Medical Ctr N
1161 21st Ave S
Nashville, TN 37232-2584
Tel: 615 322-7416 *Fax:* 615 322-7929
E-mail: iekuni.ichikawa@mcmail.vanderbilt.edu
Accred Length: 3 Years *Program Size:* 5
Program ID: 328-47-21-046

Texas

Dallas

University of Texas Southwestern Medical School Program

Sponsor: University of Texas Southwestern Medical School
Children's Medical Center of Dallas

Program Director:
Michel G Baum, MD
Univ of Texas Southwestern Med Ctr
Dept of Pediatrics
5323 Harry Hines Blvd
Dallas, TX 75235-9063
Tel: 214 648-3438 *Fax:* 214 648-2034
E-mail: mbaum@mednet.swmed.edu
Accred Length: 3 Years *Program Size:* 6
Program ID: 328-48-21-019

Galveston

University of Texas Medical Branch Hospitals Program

Sponsor: University of Texas Medical Branch Hospitals

Program Director:
Alok Kalia, MD
Children's Hospital
Dept of Pediatrics
301 University Blvd
Galveston, TX 77555-0373
Tel: 409 772-2538 *Fax:* 409 772-5293
E-mail: akalia@utmb.edu
Internet: http://www.utmb.edu/pedi
Accred Length: 3 Years *Program Size:* 4
Program ID: 328-48-11-020

Houston

Baylor College of Medicine Program

Sponsor: Baylor College of Medicine
Texas Children's Hospital

Program Director:
Eileen D Brewer, MD
Baylor Coll of Med
Texas Children's Hospital
6621 Fannin/MC 3-2482
Houston, TX 77030-2399
Tel: 713 770-3800 *Fax:* 713 770-3889
E-mail: ebrewer@bcm.tmc.edu
Accred Length: 3 Years *Program Size:* 3
Program ID: 328-48-21-026

University of Texas at Houston Program

Sponsor: University of Texas Medical School at Houston
Memorial Hermann Healthcare System

Program Director:
Ronald J Portman, MD
Univ of Texas Med Sch
6431 Fannin St
Houston, TX 77030
Tel: 713 500-5670 *Fax:* 713 500-5680
E-mail: rportman@ped1.med.uth.tmc.edu
Accred Length: 3 Years *Program Size:* 5
Program ID: 328-48-21-041

Virginia

Charlottesville

University of Virginia Program
Sponsor: University of Virginia Medical Center
Program Director:
Victoria F Norwood, MD
Univ of Virginia
MR4 Bldg/Rm 2001
Charlottesville, VA 22908
Tel: 804 982-0078 *Fax:* 804 982-4328
E-mail: vfn6t@virginia.edu
Accred Length: 3 Years *Program Size:* 3
Program ID: 328-51-11-027

Richmond

Medical College of Virginia/Virginia Commonwealth University Program
Sponsor: Medical College of Virginia/Virginia Commonwealth University
Medical College of Virginia Hospitals
Program Director:
James C Chan, MD
Med Coll of Virginia
Children's Med Ctr
PO Box 980498
Richmond, VA 23298-0498
Tel: 804 828-9608 *Fax:* 804 828-6455
E-mail: jchan@hsc.vcu.edu
Accred Length: 3 Years *Program Size:* 1
Program ID: 328-51-21-021

Washington

Seattle

University of Washington Program
Sponsor: University of Washington School of Medicine
Children's Hospital and Medical Center
Program Director:
Allison A Eddy, MD
Children's Hospital and Med Ctr
Div of Nephrology CH-46
4800 Sand Point Way NE
Seattle, WA 98105-0371
Tel: 206 526-2524 *Fax:* 206 528-2636
E-mail: aeddy@chmc.org
Accred Length: 3 Years *Program Size:* 5
Program ID: 328-54-21-042

Pediatric Orthopaedics (Orthopaedic Surgery)

California

San Diego

University of California (San Diego) Program
Sponsor: University of California (San Diego) Medical Center
Children's Hospital and Health Center
Program Director:
Dennis R Wenger, MD
Children's Hospital
3030 Children's Way/Ste 410
MC 5062
San Diego, CA 92123-4293
Tel: 619 576-5822 *Fax:* 619 974-6706
Accred Length: 1 Year *Program Size:* 3
Program ID: 265-05-21-009

Connecticut

Farmington

University of Connecticut Program
Sponsor: University of Connecticut School of Medicine
Connecticut Children's Medical Center
Program Director:
John V Banta, MD
Connecticut Children's Med Ctr
282 Washington St
Hartford, CT 06106
Tel: 860 545-8640
Accred Length: 1 Year *Program Size:* 1
Program ID: 265-08-21-020

Delaware

Wilmington

duPont Hospital for Children Program
Sponsor: duPont Hospital for Children
Program Director:
William G Mackenzie, MD
duPont Hospital for Children
PO Box 269
Wilmington, DE 19899
Tel: 302 651-5890 *Fax:* 302 651-5951
E-mail: wmackenz@nemours.org
Internet: http://www.gait.aidi.udel.edu
Accred Length: 1 Year *Program Size:* 10
Program ID: 265-09-31-004

District of Columbia

Washington

George Washington University Program
Sponsor: Children's National Medical Center
Program Director:
William W Robertson Jr, MD
111 Michigan Ave NW
Washington, DC 20010-2970
Tel: 202 884-4152 *Fax:* 202 884-6520
Accred Length: 1 Year *Program Size:* 1
Program ID: 265-10-21-031

Florida

Jacksonville

University of Florida Health Science Center/Jacksonville Program
Sponsor: University of Florida College of Medicine at Jacksonville
Nemours Children's Clinic (UFHSC/J)
Program Director:
R Jay Cummings, MD
807 Nira St
Jacksonville, FL 32207
Tel: 904 390-3548 *Fax:* 904 390-3699
E-mail: jcummings@nemours.org
Accred Length: 1 Year *Program Size:* 1
Program ID: 265-11-31-026

Orlando

Orlando Regional Healthcare System Program
Sponsor: Orlando Regional Medical Center
Florida Elks Children's Hospital
Program Director:
Charles T Price, MD
Nemours Children's Clinic
83 W Columbia St
Orlando, FL 32806
Tel: 407 650-7518 *Fax:* 407 650-7377
E-mail: bmedlin@nemours.org
Accred Length: 1 Year *Program Size:* 1
Program ID: 265-11-11-037

Tampa

Shriners Hospitals for Children (Tampa) Program
Sponsor: Shriners Hospitals for Children (Tampa)
Program Director:
Dennis P Grogan, MD
Shriners Hospital for Children
12502 N Pine Dr
Tampa, FL 33612-9499
Tel: 813 972-2250
Accred Length: 1 Year *Program Size:* 2
Program ID: 265-11-31-035

Georgia

Atlanta

Scottish Rite Children's Medical Center Program

Sponsor: Scottish Rite Children's Medical Center
Program Director:
Raymond T Morrissy, MD
Scottish Rite Children's Med Ctr
5455 Meridian Mark Rd
Ste 440
Atlanta, GA 30342
Tel: 404 250-2022 *Fax:* 404 531-9803
Accred Length: 1 Year *Program Size:* 2
Program ID: 265-12-21-022

Hawaii

Honolulu

Shriners Hospitals for Children (Honolulu) Program

Sponsor: Shriners Hospitals for Children (Honolulu)
Program Director:
Kent A Reinker, MD
Shriners Hospital for Children
1310 Punahou St
Honolulu, HI 96826-1099
Tel: 808 941-4466 *Fax:* 808 942-8573
E-mail: reinkerk@gte.net
Internet: http://davinci.pixi.com/~shriners
Accred Length: 1 Year *Program Size:* 1
Program ID: 265-14-21-029

Illinois

Chicago

McGaw Medical Center of Northwestern University Program

Sponsor: Northwestern University Medical School
Children's Memorial Medical Center
Program Director:
John F Sarwark, MD
Children's Memorial Hospital
2300 Children's Plaza
Box 69
Chicago, IL 60614
Tel: 773 880-4213 *Fax:* 773 880-3064
E-mail: j-sarwark@nwu.edu
Internet: http://www.hsinfo.ghsl.nwu.edu/orthopaedics/
Accred Length: 1 Year *Program Size:* 1
Program ID: 265-16-21-019

Shriners Hospitals for Children (Chicago) Program

Sponsor: Shriners Hospitals for Children (Chicago)
Program Director:
John P Lubicky, MD
Chicago Shriners Hospital for Children
2211 N Oak Park Ave
Chicago, IL 60707-3392
Tel: 773 385-5500 *Fax:* 773 385-5488
Accred Length: 1 Year *Program Size:* 1
Program ID: 265-16-21-027

Louisiana

New Orleans

Louisiana State University Program

Sponsor: Louisiana State University School of Medicine
Childrens Hospital
Program Director:
R B Willis, MD
Children's Hospital
200 Henry Clay Ave
New Orleans, LA 70118
Tel: 504 896-9569 *Fax:* 504 896-9849
Accred Length: 1 Year *Program Size:* 1
Program ID: 265-21-21-016

Massachusetts

Boston

Children's Hospital Program

Sponsor: Children's Hospital
Program Director:
James R Kasser, MD
Children's Hospital
Dept of Ortho Surgery
300 Longwood Ave
Boston, MA 02115
Tel: 617 355-8213 *Fax:* 617 739-3338
E-mail: kasser@a1.tch.harvard.edu
Internet: http://www.11web1.tch.harvard.edu/
Accred Length: 1 Year *Program Size:* 2
Program ID: 265-24-21-008

Springfield

Shriners Hospitals for Children (Springfield) Program

Sponsor: Shriners Hospitals for Children (Springfield)
Program Director:
David M Drvaric, MD
Shriners Hospital for Children
516 Carew St
Springfield, MA 01104
Tel: 413 787-2058 *Fax:* 413 787-2054
E-mail: ddrvaric@shrinerspfld.org
Accred Length: 1 Year *Program Size:* 1
Program ID: 265-24-31-001

Michigan

Detroit

Wayne State University/Detroit Medical Center Program

Sponsor: Wayne State University/Detroit Medical Center
Children's Hospital of Michigan
Hutzel Hospital
Program Director:
Carl L Stanitski, MD
Children's Hospital
3901 Beaubien Blvd
Detroit, MI 49201
Tel: 313 745-5581 *Fax:* 313 745-5742
Accred Length: 1 Year *Program Size:* 1
Program ID: 265-25-21-038

Missouri

St Louis

Shriners Hospitals for Children (St Louis) Program

Sponsor: Shriners Hospitals for Children (St Louis)
St Louis Children's Hospital
Program Director:
Perry L Schoenecker, MD
Shriners Hospital for Children
2001 S Lindbergh Blvd
St Louis, MO 63131-3597
Tel: 314 432-3600 *Fax:* 314 872-7808
Accred Length: 1 Year *Program Size:* 1
Program ID: 265-28-21-006

New York

Buffalo

SUNY at Buffalo Graduate Medical-Dental Education Consortium Program

Sponsor: SUNY at Buffalo Grad Medical-Dental Education Consortium
CGF Health System (Children's Hospital of Buffalo)
Program Director:
Robert Gillespie, MD ChB
Dept of Orthopaedics
SUNY-Buffalo
82 Hodge St
Buffalo, NY 14222-2016
Tel: 716 878-7722 *Fax:* 716 878-7724
E-mail: akoenig@acsu.buffalo.edu
Accred Length: 1 Year *Program Size:* 0
Program ID: 265-35-21-023

New York

Hospital for Joint Diseases Orthopaedic Institute Program

Sponsor: Hospital for Joint Diseases Orthopaedic Institute
Program Director:
Wallace B Lehman, MD
Hospital for Joint Diseases Orthopaedic Inst
Ped Orthopaedic Fellowship
301 E 17th St
New York, NY 10003
Tel: 212 598-6497 *Fax:* 212 598-6581
Internet: http://www.hjd.edu
Accred Length: 1 Year *Program Size:* 1
Program ID: 265-35-12-007

Hospital for Special Surgery/Cornell Medical Center Program

Sponsor: Hospital for Special Surgery
Program Director:
Stephen W Burke, MD
Hospital for Special Surgery
535 E 70th St
New York, NY 10021
Tel: 212 606-1466 *Fax:* 212 472-6023
Internet: http://www.hss.edu
Accred Length: 1 Year *Program Size:* 1
Program ID: 265-35-12-024

Stony Brook

SUNY at Stony Brook Program
Sponsor: University Hospital-SUNY at Stony Brook

Program Director:
Martin A Gruber, MD
SUNY-Stony Brook
Dept of Ortho Surgery
Health Sciences Ctr/T-18 080
Stony Brook, NY 11794-8181
Tel: 516 444-1487 *Fax:* 516 444-8894
Accred Length: 1 Year *Program Size:* 1
Program ID: 265-35-21-033

Ohio

Cincinnati

Children's Hospital Medical Center/University of Cincinnati College of Medicine Program
Sponsor: Children's Hospital Medical Center

Program Director:
Alvin H Crawford, MD
Children's Hospital Med Ctr
Dept of Ped Orthopaedics
3333 Burnet Ave
Cincinnati, OH 45229
Tel: 513 636-4785 *Fax:* 513 636-3928
E-mail: singso@chmcc.org
Internet: http://www.chmcc.org
Accred Length: 1 Year *Program Size:* 2
Program ID: 265-38-21-039

Oregon

Portland

Shriners Hospitals for Children (Portland) Program
Sponsor: Shriners Hospitals for Children (Portland)

Program Director:
Michael D Sussman, MD
Shriners Hospital for Children
3101 SW Sam Jackson Park Rd
Portland, OR 97201
Tel: 503 221-3424 *Fax:* 503 221-3490
E-mail: mds@shcc.org
Accred Length: 1 Year *Program Size:* 1
Program ID: 265-40-21-005

Pennsylvania

Philadelphia

Children's Hospital of Philadelphia Program
Sponsor: Children's Hospital of Philadelphia
Children's Seashore House

Program Director:
John P Dormans, MD
Children's Hospital of Philadelphia
34th and Civic Center Blvd
Wood Bldg 2nd Fl
Philadelphia, PA 19104
Tel: 215 590-1534 *Fax:* 215 590-1501
E-mail: dormans@email.chop.edu
Internet: http://www.chop.edu/clinical/cortho.htm
Accred Length: 1 Year *Program Size:* 1
Program ID: 265-41-21-040

Tennessee

Memphis

University of Tennessee Program
Sponsor: University of Tennessee College of Medicine
LeBonheur Children's Medical Center
University of Tennessee-Campbell Clinic

Program Director:
S Terry Canale, MD
James H Beaty, MD
Univ of Tennessee-Campbell Clinic
Dept of Ped/Ortho Surgery
910 Madison Ave/Ste 500
Memphis, TN 38104-3403
Tel: 901 759-3274 *Fax:* 901 759-3278
Accred Length: 1 Year *Program Size:* 40
Program ID: 265-47-21-034

Texas

Dallas

University of Texas Southwestern Medical School Program
Sponsor: University of Texas Southwestern Medical School
Dallas County Hospital District-Parkland Memorial Hospital
Texas Scottish Rite Hospital for Children

Program Director:
John A Herring, MD
Texas Scottish Rite Hospital for Children
2222 Welborn Ave
Dallas, TX 75219-3993
Tel: 214 559-7604 *Fax:* 214 559-7570
E-mail: tsrorth1@airmail.net
Internet: http://tsrh.org
Accred Length: 1 Year *Program Size:* 4
Program ID: 265-48-21-013

Houston

Baylor College of Medicine Program
Sponsor: Baylor College of Medicine
Harris County Hospital District-Ben Taub General Hospital
Shriners Hospitals for Children (Houston)
Texas Children's Hospital

Program Director:
Wendell D Erwin, MD
Baylor Coll of Med
Dept of Ortho Surgery
6621 Fannin St/MC 3-2295
Houston, TX 77030
Tel: 713 770-3110 *Fax:* 713 770-3127
E-mail: werwin@bcm.tmc.edu
Accred Length: 1 Year *Program Size:* 2
Program ID: 265-48-31-002

Utah

Salt Lake City

University of Utah Program
Sponsor: University of Utah Medical Center
Primary Children's Medical Center
Shriners Hospital for Children (Intermountain Unit)

Program Director:
Peter F Armstrong, MD
Shriners Hospital for Children-Intermountain
Fairfax Rd at Virginia St
Salt Lake City, UT 84103-4399
Tel: 801 536-3600 *Fax:* 801 536-3799
E-mail: peter.armstrong@m.cc.utah.edu
Accred Length: 1 Year *Program Size:* 2
Program ID: 265-49-31-015

Wisconsin

Milwaukee

Medical College of Wisconsin Program
Sponsor: Medical College of Wisconsin Affiliated Hospitals Inc
Children's Hospital of Wisconsin

Program Director:
John Thometz, MD
MACC Fund Research Bldg
8701 Watertown Plank Rd/Ste 3018
Milwaukee, WI 53226
Tel: 414 266-4967 *Fax:* 414 456-6541
E-mail: jthometz@mcw.edu
Internet: http://www.mcw.edu/ortho
Accred Length: 1 Year *Program Size:* 1
Program ID: 265-56-21-036

Pediatric Otolaryngology (Otolaryngology)

Iowa

Iowa City

University of Iowa Hospitals and Clinics Program
Sponsor: University of Iowa Hospitals and Clinics
Program Director:
Richard J H Smith, MD
Nancy M Bauman, MD
Univ of Iowa Hospital and Clinics
Dept of Otolaryngology E230 GH
200 Hawkins Dr
Iowa City, IA 52240
Tel: 319 356-3612 *Fax:* 319 356-4547
Accred Length: 2 Years *Program Size:* 2
Program ID: 288-18-21-003

Ohio

Cincinnati

Children's Hospital Medical Center/University of Cincinnati College of Medicine Program
Sponsor: Children's Hospital Medical Center
Program Director:
Robin T Cotton, MD
Children's Hospital Med Ctr
3333 Burnet Ave
Cincinnati, OH 45229-3039
Tel: 513 636-4355 *Fax:* 513 636-8133
E-mail: chmcent@chmcc.org
Internet: http://www.chmcc.org
Accred Length: 2 Years *Program Size:* 4
Program ID: 288-38-21-004

Pennsylvania

Pittsburgh

University Health Center of Pittsburgh Program
Sponsor: University Health Center of Pittsburgh
Children's Hospital of Pittsburgh
Program Director:
Margaretha L Casselbrant, MD PhD
Children's Hospital of Pittsburgh
3705 Fifth Ave
Pittsburgh, PA 15213
Tel: 412 692-8577 *Fax:* 412 692-6074
E-mail: casselm@chplink.chp.edu
Accred Length: 2 Years *Program Size:* 4
Program ID: 288-41-21-001

Texas

Houston

Baylor College of Medicine Program
Sponsor: Baylor College of Medicine
Texas Children's Hospital
Program Director:
Ellen M Friedman, MD
1102 Bates/Ste 340
Houston, TX 77030
Tel: 713 770-3268 *Fax:* 713 770-3251
Accred Length: 2 Years *Program Size:* 2
Program ID: 288-48-21-005

Pediatric Pathology (Pathology)

Colorado

Denver

Children's Hospital Program
Sponsor: Children's Hospital
Program Director:
Edmund N Orsini Jr, MD
Children's Hospital
Dept of Pathology B120
1056 E 19th Ave
Denver, CO 80218
Tel: 303 861-6712 *Fax:* 303 831-4112
Accred Length: 1 Year *Program Size:* 1
Program ID: 316-07-21-022

Connecticut

Hartford

Hartford Hospital Program
Sponsor: Hartford Hospital
Program Director:
Vijay V Joshi, MD
Hartford Hospital
Dept of Pathology
80 Seymour St/PO Box 5037
Hartford, CT 06102-5037
Tel: 860 545-3530 *Fax:* 860 545-5206
Accred Length: 1 Year *Program Size:* 1
Program ID: 316-08-21-023

Florida

Miami

University of Miami-Jackson Memorial Medical Center Program
Sponsor: University of Miami-Jackson Memorial Medical Center
Program Director:
Maria M Rodriguez, MD
Univ of Miami-Jackson Memorial Med Ctr
1611 NW 12th Ave
East Tower 2142
Miami, FL 33136
Tel: 305 585-6637 *Fax:* 305 545-6735
E-mail: mrodrig3@mednet.med.miami.edu
Accred Length: 1 Year *Program Size:* 1
Program ID: 316-11-21-026

Tampa

University of South Florida Program
Sponsor: University of South Florida College of Medicine
All Children's Hospital
Tampa General Healthcare
Program Director:
Enid Gilbert-Barness, MD
Univ of South Florida
Tampa General Hospital
PO Box 1289
Tampa, FL 33601
Tel: 813 251-7431 *Fax:* 813 253-4073
Accred Length: 1 Year *Program Size:*
Program ID: 316-11-21-015

Illinois

Chicago

McGaw Medical Center of Northwestern University Program

Sponsor: Northwestern University Medical School
Children's Memorial Medical Center
Northwestern Memorial Hospital

Program Director:
Frank Gonzalez-Crussi, MD
McGaw Med Ctr
2300 Children's Plaza/Box 17
Chicago, IL 60614
Tel: 773 880-4439, ext 4276 *Fax:* 773 880-8127
Accred Length: 1 Year *Program Size:* 1
Program ID: 316-16-21-024

Indiana

Indianapolis

Indiana University School of Medicine Program

Sponsor: Indiana University School of Medicine
Clarian Riley Hospital for Children

Program Director:
Mary M Davis, MD
Riley Hospital for Children
Pediatric Pathology
702 Barnhill Dr/Rm 2536
Indianapolis, IN 46202-5200
Tel: 317 274-7001 *Fax:* 317 274-2810
E-mail: mdavis2@iupui.edu
Accred Length: 1 Year *Program Size:* 1
Program ID: 316-17-21-002

Louisiana

New Orleans

Louisiana State University Program

Sponsor: Louisiana State University School of Medicine
Childrens Hospital
Medical Center of Louisiana at New Orleans

Program Director:
Randall D Craver, MD
Louisiana State Univ Med Ctr, Dept of Pathology
1901 Perdido St
New Orleans, LA 70112-1393
Tel: 504 891-7863 *Fax:* 504 896-9704
E-mail: rdcraver@accesscom.net
Accred Length: 1 Year *Program Size:* 1
Program ID: 316-21-21-001

Maryland

Baltimore

Johns Hopkins University Program

Sponsor: Johns Hopkins University School of Medicine
Office of the Chief Medical Examiner

Program Director:
Elizabeth J Perlman, MD
Pathology Bldg/Rm 612
600 N Wolfe St
Baltimore, MD 21287
Tel: 410 955-5327 *Fax:* 410 614-9386
E-mail: eperlman@welchlink.welch.jhu.edu
Accred Length: 1 Year *Program Size:* 1
Program ID: 316-23-21-025

Massachusetts

Boston

Children's Hospital Program

Sponsor: Children's Hospital
Brigham and Women's Hospital

Program Director:
Antonio R Perez-Atayde, MD
Children's Hospital
Dept of Pathology
300 Longwood Ave
Boston, MA 02115
Tel: 617 355-7431 *Fax:* 617 731-0954
E-mail: curtin@a1.tch.harvard.edu
Accred Length: 1 Year *Program Size:* 4
Program ID: 316-24-21-017

Michigan

Detroit

Wayne State University/Detroit Medical Center Program

Sponsor: Wayne State University/Detroit Medical Center
Children's Hospital of Michigan
Hutzel Hospital

Program Director:
Raja Rabah, MD
Children's Hospital
Dept of Ped Pathology
3901 Beaubien Blvd
Detroit, MI 48201-2196
Tel: 313 745-5491 *Fax:* 313 993-8745
Accred Length: 1 Year *Program Size:* 1
Program ID: 316-25-21-004

Missouri

St Louis

St Louis University School of Medicine Program

Sponsor: St Louis University School of Medicine
SSM Cardinal Glennon Children's Hospital

Program Director:
Cirilo Sotelo-Avila, MD
St Louis Univ Sch of Med-Cardinal Glennon Hospital
1465 S Grand Blvd
St Louis, MO 63104-1095
Tel: 314 268-6424 *Fax:* 314 268-6471
Accred Length: 1 Year *Program Size:* 1
Program ID: 316-28-21-008

Washington University/B-JH/SLCH Consortium Program

Sponsor: Washington University/B-JH/SLCH Consortium
Barnes-Jewish Hospital

Program Director:
Louis P Dehner, MD
Barnes-Jewish Hospital
One Barnes Hospital Plaza
St Louis, MO 63110
Tel: 314 362-0101
Accred Length: 1 Year *Program Size:* 1
Program ID: 316-28-21-019

New York

Brooklyn

SUNY Health Science Center at Brooklyn Program

Sponsor: SUNY Health Science Center at Brooklyn
Kings County Hospital Center
Maimonides Medical Center
University Hospital-SUNY Health Science Center at Brooklyn

Program Director:
Virginia M Anderson, MD
SUNY Health Science Ctr-Brooklyn
450 Clarkson Ave/Box 25
Brooklyn, NY 11203
Tel: 718 270-1294 *Fax:* 718 270-3313
E-mail: vanderson@netmail.hscbkyn.edu
Accred Length: 1 Year *Program Size:* 1
Program ID: 316-35-31-018

Buffalo

Children's Hospital of Buffalo Program

Sponsor: CGF Health System (Children's Hospital of Buffalo)

Program Director:
John E Fisher, MD
Children's Hospital of Buffalo
Dept of Pathology
219 Bryant St
Buffalo, NY 14222
Tel: 716 878-7777 *Fax:* 716 888-3802
E-mail: jefisher@buffalo.edu
Accred Length: 1 Year *Program Size:* 1
Program ID: 316-35-21-027

New York

New York University Medical Center Program

Sponsor: New York University Medical Center
North Shore University Hospital

Program Director:
M Alba Greco, MD
560 First Ave
New York, NY 10016
Tel: 212 263-6443 *Fax:* 212 263-8284
E-mail: mag10@is6.nyu.edu
Accred Length: 1 Year *Program Size:* 1
Program ID: 316-35-21-007

Ohio

Akron

Children's Hospital Medical Center of Akron/NEOUCOM Program

Sponsor: Children's Hospital Medical Center of Akron

Program Director:
Dimitris P Agamanolis, MD
Children's Hospital Med Ctr
One Perkins Sq
Akron, OH 44308-1062
Tel: 330 379-8219 *Fax:* 330 258-3226
Accred Length: 1 Year *Program Size:* 1
Program ID: 316-38-31-012

Cincinnati

Children's Hospital Medical Center/University of Cincinnati College of Medicine Program
Sponsor: Children's Hospital Medical Center
Hamilton County Coroner's Office
University of Cincinnati College of Medicine
Program Director:
David P Witte, MD
Children's Hospital Med Ctr
Univ of Cincinnati Coll of Med
3333 Burnet Ave
Cincinnati, OH 45229-3039
Tel: 513 636-4261 *Fax:* 513 636-3924
E-mail: david.witte@uc.edu
Internet: http://www.chmcc.org/departments/43/
Accred Length: 1 Year *Program Size:* 2
Program ID: 316-38-21-021

Columbus

Children's Hospital/Ohio State University Program
Sponsor: Children's Hospital
Program Director:
Sue Hammond, MD
700 Children's Dr
Columbus, OH 43205
Tel: 614 722-5450 *Fax:* 614 722-2899
E-mail: hammonds@chi.osu.edu
Accred Length: 1 Year *Program Size:* 2
Program ID: 316-38-21-010

Pennsylvania

Philadelphia

Children's Hospital of Philadelphia Program
Sponsor: Children's Hospital of Philadelphia
Program Director:
Eduardo D Ruchelli, MD
34th St and Civic Ctr Blvd
Philadelphia, PA 19104
Tel: 215 590-1728 *Fax:* 215 590-1736
E-mail: ruchelli@email.chop.edu
Accred Length: 1 Year *Program Size:* 1
Program ID: 316-41-31-014

St Christopher's Hospital for Children Program
Sponsor: St Christopher's Hospital for Children
Program Director:
Bruce R Pawel, MD
St Christopher's Hospital for Children
Erie Ave at Front St
Philadelphia, PA 19134-1095
Tel: 215 427-5272 *Fax:* 215 427-4284
Accred Length: 1 Year *Program Size:* 1
Program ID: 316-41-21-013

Pittsburgh

University Health Center of Pittsburgh Program
Sponsor: University Health Center of Pittsburgh
Children's Hospital of Pittsburgh
Magee-Women's Hospital
Program Director:
Ronald Jaffe, MD
Children's Hospital of Pittsburgh
3705 Fifth Ave
Pittsburgh, PA 15213-2583
Tel: 412 692-5655 *Fax:* 412 692-6550
Accred Length: 1 Year *Program Size:* 1
Program ID: 316-41-11-016

Rhode Island

Providence

Brown University Program
Sponsor: Women and Infants Hospital of Rhode Island
Rhode Island Hospital
Program Director:
Halit Pinar, MD
101 Dudley St
Providence, RI 02905
Tel: 401 274-1122, ext 1190 *Fax:* 401 453-7681
E-mail: hpinar@wihri.org
Accred Length: 1 Year *Program Size:* 2
Program ID: 316-43-21-005

Texas

Dallas

University of Texas Southwestern Medical School Program
Sponsor: University of Texas Southwestern Medical School
Children's Medical Center of Dallas
Program Director:
Arthur G Weinberg, MD
Children's Med Ctr
1935 Motor St
Dallas, TX 75235
Tel: 214 640-2324 *Fax:* 214 640-6199
Accred Length: 1 Year *Program Size:* 1
Program ID: 316-48-21-003

Houston

Baylor College of Medicine Program
Sponsor: Baylor College of Medicine
Texas Children's Hospital
Program Director:
Milton J Finegold, MD
Texas Children's Hospital
6621 Fannin St/MC 1-2261
Houston, TX 77030
Tel: 713 770-1856 *Fax:* 713 770-1032
E-mail: finegold@bcm.tmc.edu
Internet:
http://www.bcm.edu/pathology/prog/path-res.htm/
Accred Length: 1 Year *Program Size:* 2
Program ID: 316-48-31-009

San Antonio

University of Texas Health Science Center at San Antonio Program
Sponsor: University of Texas Medical School at San Antonio
Santa Rosa Health Care Corporation
Program Director:
Victor A Saldivar, MD
Univ of Texas Health Science Ctr
519 W Houston St
San Antonio, TX 78207-3108
Tel: 210 704-3565 *Fax:* 210 704-3180
E-mail: victor_saldivar@srhc.iwhs.org
Accred Length: 1 Year *Program Size:* 1
Program ID: 316-48-21-020

Pediatric Pulmonology (Pediatrics)

Alabama

Birmingham

University of Alabama Medical Center Program
Sponsor: University of Alabama Hospital
Children's Hospital of Alabama
Program Director:
Raymond K Lyrene, MD
Children's Hospital
1600 Seventh Ave S
Ste 620/Ambulatory Care Ctr
Birmingham, AL 35233-0011
Tel: 205 939-9583 *Fax:* 205 975-5983
E-mail: rlyrene@peds.uab.edu
Accred Length: 3 Years *Program Size:* 1
Program ID: 330-01-21-001

Arizona

Tucson

University of Arizona Program
Sponsor: University of Arizona College of Medicine
University Medical Center
Program Director:
Mark A Brown, MD
Univ of Arizona Health Sciences Ctr
1501 N Campbell Ave
Tucson, AZ 85724-5093
Tel: 520 626-6754 *Fax:* 520 626-6970
E-mail: mabrown@resp-sci.arizona.edu
Internet: http://www.resp-sci.arizona.edu
Accred Length: 3 Years *Program Size:* 2
Program ID: 330-03-21-002

California

Long Beach

University of California (Irvine) Program
Sponsor: University of California (Irvine) Medical Center
Long Beach Memorial Medical Center
Program Director:
Eliezer Nussbaum, MD
Miller Children's Hospital-Long Beach Memorial Med Ctr
Ped Pulmonary 3rd Fl
2801 Atlantic Ave
Long Beach, CA 90801-1428
Tel: 562 933-8740 *Fax:* 562 933-8744
E-mail: enussbaum@memorialcare.org
Accred Length: 3 Years *Program Size:* 2
Program ID: 330-05-21-003

Los Angeles

Children's Hospital of Los Angeles Program
Sponsor: Children's Hospital of Los Angeles
Program Director:
Thomas G Keens, MD
Children's Hospital
4650 Sunset Blvd/MS 83
Los Angeles, CA 90027
Tel: 323 669-2101 *Fax:* 323 664-9758
E-mail: tkeens@chla.usc.edu
Accred Length: 3 Years *Program Size:* 5
Program ID: 330-05-21-004

San Francisco

University of California (San Francisco) Program
Sponsor: University of California (San Francisco) School of Medicine
University of California (San Francisco) Medical Center
Program Director:
Gerd J Cropp, MD
505 Parnassus Ave/Box 0106
650 Moffitt Hospital
San Francisco, CA 94143-0106
Tel: 415 476-2072 *Fax:* 415 476-4009
Accred Length: 3 Years *Program Size:* 2
Program ID: 330-05-21-005

Colorado

Denver

University of Colorado Program
Sponsor: University of Colorado Health Sciences Center
Children's Hospital
National Jewish Ctr for Immunology and Respiratory Medicine
Program Director:
Robin R Deterding, MD
Children's Hospital
Div of Pulmonary Med
1056 E 19th Ave/B395
Denver, CO 80218
Tel: 303 861-6181 *Fax:* 303 837-2924
E-mail: kennedy.juanita@tchden.org
Accred Length: 3 Years *Program Size:* 3
Program ID: 330-07-21-008

Connecticut

Farmington

University of Connecticut Program
Sponsor: University of Connecticut School of Medicine
Connecticut Children's Medical Center
Program Director:
Craig M Schramm, MD
Connecticut Children's Med Ctr
Pediatric Pulmonology / 2B
282 Washington St
Hartford, CT 06106-3322
Tel: 860 545-9440 *Fax:* 860 545-9445
E-mail: cschram@ccmckids.org
Accred Length: 3 Years *Program Size:* 1
Program ID: 330-08-21-007

New Haven

Yale-New Haven Medical Center Program
Sponsor: Yale-New Haven Hospital
Program Director:
Gabriel G Haddad, MD
Yale Univ Sch of Med
Fitkin Bldg/Rm 506
333 Cedar St
New Haven, CT 06520
Tel: 203 785-5444 *Fax:* 203 785-6337
E-mail: gabriel.haddad@yale.edu
Accred Length: 3 Years *Program Size:* 3
Program ID: 330-08-21-014

District of Columbia

Washington

George Washington University Program
Sponsor: Children's National Medical Center
Program Director:
Robert J Fink, MD
Children's National Med Ctr
111 Michigan Ave NW
Washington, DC 20010
Tel: 202 884-2128 *Fax:* 202 884-3461
E-mail: rfink@cnmc.org
Accred Length: 3 Years *Program Size:* 3
Program ID: 330-10-21-049

Florida

Gainesville

University of Florida Program
Sponsor: University of Florida College of Medicine
Shands Hospital at the University of Florida
Program Director:
Sarah E Chesrown, MD PhD
Univ of Florida Coll of Med
Dept of Pediatrics
PO Box 100296
Gainesville, FL 32610-0296
Tel: 352 392-4458 *Fax:* 352 392-4450
E-mail: chesrse@peds.ufl.edu
Accred Length: 3 Years *Program Size:* 4
Program ID: 330-11-21-017

Miami

University of Miami-Jackson Memorial Medical Center Program
Sponsor: University of Miami-Jackson Memorial Medical Center
Program Director:
Giovanni Piedimonte, MD
Katherine A King, MD
Mailman Ctr for Child Development (D-820)
1601 NW 12th Ave/Rm 2008A
Miami, FL 33136
Tel: 305 243-3176 *Fax:* 305 243-6708
E-mail: gpiedimo@peds.med.miami.edu
Accred Length: 3 Years *Program Size:* 3
Program ID: 330-11-21-054

Illinois

Chicago

McGaw Medical Center of Northwestern University Program
Sponsor: Northwestern University Medical School
Children's Memorial Medical Center
Program Director:
Thomas P Green, MD
Div of Pulm/Critical Care #73
2300 Children's Plaza
Chicago, IL 60614
Tel: 773 880-4780 *Fax:* 773 880-4057
Accred Length: 3 Years *Program Size:* 3
Program ID: 330-16-21-052

University of Chicago Program
Sponsor: University of Chicago Hospitals
University of Chicago Children's Hospital
Program Director:
Marc B Hershenson, MD
Univ of Chicago
5841 S Maryland Ave/MC 4064
Chicago, IL 60637-0000
Tel: 773 702-9659 *Fax:* 773 702-4041
E-mail: mhershen@midway.uchicago.edu
Internet:
http://peds-www.bsd.uchicago.edu/sections/pulmcrit/index.html
Accred Length: 3 Years *Program Size:* 1
Program ID: 330-16-21-048

Indiana

Indianapolis

Indiana University School of Medicine Program
Sponsor: Indiana University School of Medicine
Clarian Riley Hospital for Children
Program Director:
Howard Eigen, MD
Riley Hospital for Children
702 Barnhill Dr/Rm 2750
Indianapolis, IN 46202-5225
Tel: 317 274-3434 *Fax:* 317 274-3442
Accred Length: 3 Years *Program Size:* 2
Program ID: 330-17-21-016

Iowa

Iowa City

University of Iowa Hospitals and Clinics Program
Sponsor: University of Iowa Hospitals and Clinics
Program Director:
Miles M Weinberger, MD
Univ of Iowa Hospitals and Clinics
Ped Dept/2449 JCP
200 Hawkins Dr
Iowa City, IA 52242-1009
Tel: 319 356-3485 *Fax:* 319 353-6217
E-mail: miles-weinberger@uiowa.edu
Internet:
http://www.vh.org/welcome/uihc/uihcmeddepts/peds/allergy.html
Accred Length: 3 Years *Program Size:* 3
Program ID: 330-18-21-013

Louisiana

New Orleans

Tulane University Program
Sponsor: Tulane University School of Medicine
Tulane Hospital for Children
Program Director:
David Gozal, MD
Tulane Univ Sch of Med
Dept of Pediatrics/SL-37
1430 Tulane Ave
New Orleans, LA 70112-2699
Tel: 504 588-5601 *Fax:* 504 588-5490
E-mail: dgozal@tmcpop.tmc.tulane.edu
Accred Length: 3 Years *Program Size:* 7
Program ID: 330-21-21-012

Maryland

Baltimore

Johns Hopkins University Program
Sponsor: Johns Hopkins University School of Medicine
Johns Hopkins Hospital
Program Director:
Gerald M Loughlin, MD
Johns Hopkins Hospital
Park 316
600 N Wolfe St
Baltimore, MD 21287-2533
Tel: 410 955-2035 *Fax:* 410 955-1030
E-mail: gloughli@welchlink.welch.jhu.edu
Accred Length: 3 Years *Program Size:* 5
Program ID: 330-23-21-015

Massachusetts

Boston

Children's Hospital/Boston Medical Center Program
Sponsor: Children's Hospital
Program Director:
David A Waltz, MD
Children's Hospital
300 Longwood Ave
Boston, MA 02115
Tel: 617 355-8630 *Fax:* 617 355-6109
Accred Length: 3 Years *Program Size:* 10
Program ID: 330-24-21-009

Massachusetts General Hospital Program
Sponsor: Massachusetts General Hospital
Program Director:
Daniel C Shannon, MD
Massachusetts General Hospital
VBKBA015
Fruit St
Boston, MA 02114
Tel: 617 726-5576 *Fax:* 617 726-1036
E-mail: shannond.daniel@mgh.harvard.edu
Internet: http://www.partners.org
Accred Length: 3 Years *Program Size:* 3
Program ID: 330-24-21-036

Michigan

Ann Arbor

University of Michigan Program
Sponsor: University of Michigan Hospitals
Program Director:
Dietrich W Roloff, MD
Univ of Michigan Med Ctr
D1109 Med Professional Bldg
200 E Medical Center Dr
Ann Arbor, MI 48109-0718
Tel: 313 764-4123 *Fax:* 313 936-7635
E-mail: droloff@umich.edu
Accred Length: 3 Years *Program Size:* 2
Program ID: 330-25-21-010

Minnesota

Minneapolis

University of Minnesota Program
Sponsor: University of Minnesota Medical School
Fairview-University Medical Center
Program Director:
Warren E Regelmann, MD
Univ of Minnesota Med Sch
Box 742
420 Delaware St SE
Minneapolis, MN 55455
Tel: 612 624-0962 *Fax:* 612 624-0696
E-mail: regel001@maroon.tc.umn.edu
Accred Length: 3 Years *Program Size:* 3
Program ID: 330-26-21-018

Missouri

St Louis

Washington University/B-JH/SLCH Consortium Program
Sponsor: Washington University/B-JH/SLCH Consortium
St Louis Children's Hospital
Program Director:
George B Mallory, MD
St Louis Children's Hospital
One Children's Pl
St Louis, MO 63110
Tel: 314 454-2694 *Fax:* 314 464-2515
Accred Length: 3 Years *Program Size:* 2
Program ID: 330-28-21-020

New Mexico

Albuquerque

University of New Mexico Program
Sponsor: University of New Mexico School of Medicine
University Hospital
Program Director:
Robert W Katz Sr, MD
Univ of New Mexico Hospital
Ambulatory Care Ctr/3rd Fl
2211 Lomas Blvd NE
Albuquerque, NM 87131-5311
Tel: 505 272-5551 *Fax:* 505 272-0329
E-mail: rkatz@salud.unm.edu
Internet: http://som.unm.edu/asthma/ppc.htm
Accred Length: 3 Years *Program Size:* 1
Program ID: 330-34-21-039

New York

Brooklyn

SUNY Health Science Center at Brooklyn Program
Sponsor: SUNY Health Science Center at Brooklyn
Kings County Hospital Center
University Hospital-SUNY Health Science Center at Brooklyn
Program Director:
Phillip Steiner, MD
SUNY Health Sciences Ctr-Brooklyn
Ped Dept/Box 49
450 Clarkson Ave
Brooklyn, NY 11203-2098
Tel: 718 279-2908 *Fax:* 718 270-4785
E-mail: steiner@hscbklyn.edu
Accred Length: 3 Years *Program Size:* 2
Program ID: 330-35-21-021

Mineola

Winthrop-University Hospital Program
Sponsor: Winthrop-University Hospital
Program Director:
Haesoon Lee, MD
Winthrop-Univ Hospital
222 Station Plaza N/Ste 603
Mineola, NY 11501
Tel: 516 663-4937 *Fax:* 516 663-3826
E-mail: worosenfeld@winthrop.org
Internet: http://www.winthrop.org
Accred Length: 3 Years *Program Size:* 3
Program ID: 330-35-21-050

New York

Mount Sinai School of Medicine Program
Sponsor: Mount Sinai School of Medicine
Mount Sinai Medical Center
Program Director:
Meyer Kattan, MD
Mount Sinai Sch of Med
One Gustave L Levy Pl
New York, NY 10029-6574
Tel: 212 241-7788 *Fax:* 212 876-3255
E-mail: mk3@doc.mssm.edu
Internet: http://mssm.edu/peds/pulm-ctr.html
Accred Length: 3 Years *Program Size:* 3
Program ID: 330-35-32-042

New York and Presbyterian Hospital (Columbia Campus) Program
Sponsor: New York and Presbyterian Hospital
New York and Presbyterian Hospital (Columbia Campus)
Program Director:
Michael R Bye, MD
Columbia Univ Coll of Physicians and Surgeons
Ped Pulmonary Div BHS 101
630 W 168th St
New York, NY 10032
Tel: 212 305-6551 *Fax:* 212 305-6103
E-mail: mb255@columbia.edu
Accred Length: 3 Years *Program Size:* 3
Program ID: 330-35-21-040

New York and Presbyterian Hospital (Cornell Campus) Program
Sponsor: New York and Presbyterian Hospital
New York and Presbyterian Hospital (Cornell Campus)
Program Director:
David J Valacer, MD
525 E 68th St/Box 586
New York, NY 10021
Tel: 212 746-3313 *Fax:* 212 746-3988
Accred Length: 3 Years *Program Size:* 2
Program ID: 330-35-31-051

Rochester

University of Rochester Program

Sponsor: Strong Memorial Hospital of the University of Rochester

Program Director:
John T McBride, MD
Univ of Rochester Med Ctr
601 Elmwood Ave
Box 667/Rm 4-3226
Rochester, NY 14642-8667
Tel: 716 275-2464 *Fax:* 716 275-8706
E-mail: john_mcbride@urmc.rochester.edu
Accred Length: 3 Years *Program Size:* 3
Program ID: 330-35-21-023

Valhalla

New York Medical College at Westchester Medical Center Program

Sponsor: New York Medical College
Westchester Medical Center

Program Director:
Allen J Dozor, MD
New York Med Coll
Munger Pavilion/Rm 106
Valhalla, NY 10595
Tel: 914 493-7585 *Fax:* 914 594-4336
E-mail: allen_dozor@nymc.edu
Accred Length: 3 Years *Program Size:* 4
Program ID: 330-35-31-041

North Carolina

Chapel Hill

University of North Carolina Hospitals Program

Sponsor: University of North Carolina Hospitals

Program Director:
Margaret W Leigh, MD
Univ of North Carolina
635 Burnett-Womack Bldg/CB7220
Chapel Hill, NC 27599-7220
Tel: 919 966-1055 *Fax:* 919 966-6179
Accred Length: 3 Years *Program Size:* 3
Program ID: 330-36-21-019

Durham

Duke University Program

Sponsor: Duke University Medical Center

Program Director:
Thomas Murphy, MD
Duke Univ Med Ctr
Ped Pulmonary Med
PO Box 2994
Durham, NC 27710
Tel: 919 684-3364 *Fax:* 919 684-2292
Accred Length: 3 Years *Program Size:* 1
Program ID: 330-36-21-044

Ohio

Cincinnati

Children's Hospital Medical Center/University of Cincinnati College of Medicine Program

Sponsor: Children's Hospital Medical Center

Program Director:
Robert W Wilmott, MD PhD
Children's Hospital Med Ctr
Div of Pulmonary Med
3333 Burnet Ave
Cincinnati, OH 45229-3039
Tel: 513 636-6771 *Fax:* 513 636-4615
Accred Length: 3 Years *Program Size:* 6
Program ID: 330-38-21-026

Cleveland

Case Western Reserve University Program

Sponsor: University Hospitals of Cleveland

Program Director:
Pamela B Davis, MD PhD
Dept of Ped Pulmonology
CWRU Sch of Med/BRB 8
10900 Euclid Ave
Cleveland, OH 44106-4948
Tel: 216 368-4370 *Fax:* 216 368-4223
E-mail: pbd@po.cwru.edu
Accred Length: 3 Years *Program Size:* 6
Program ID: 330-38-21-027

Columbus

Children's Hospital/Ohio State University Program

Sponsor: Children's Hospital

Program Director:
Karen S McCoy, MD
Children's Hospital
Sect of Pulmonary Med
700 Children's Dr/ED 442
Columbus, OH 43205-2696
Tel: 614 722-4766 *Fax:* 614 722-4755
E-mail: mccoyk@pediatrics.ohio-state.edu
Accred Length: 3 Years *Program Size:* 4
Program ID: 330-38-21-043

Oregon

Portland

Oregon Health Sciences University Program

Sponsor: Oregon Health Sciences University Hospital

Program Director:
Michael R Powers, MD
Oregon Health Sciences Univ
3181 SW Sam Jackson Park Rd/UHN 56
Portland, OR 97201
Tel: 503 494-8898 *Fax:* 503 494-6670
Accred Length: 3 Years *Program Size:* 1
Program ID: 330-40-21-025

Pennsylvania

Philadelphia

Children's Hospital of Philadelphia Program

Sponsor: Children's Hospital of Philadelphia

Program Director:
Michael M Grunstein, MD PhD
Div of Pulmonary Med
Children's Hospital
34th St and Civic Center Blvd
Philadelphia, PA 19104
Tel: 215 590-3749 *Fax:* 215 590-1605
E-mail: grunstein@email.chop.edu
Accred Length: 3 Years *Program Size:* 3
Program ID: 330-41-21-034

St Christopher's Hospital for Children Program

Sponsor: St Christopher's Hospital for Children

Program Director:
Howard B Panitch, MD
St Christopher's Hospital for Children
Erie Ave at Front St
Philadelphia, PA 19134-1095
Tel: 215 427-5183 *Fax:* 215 427-4621
E-mail: panitch@wpo.auhs.edu
Accred Length: 3 Years *Program Size:* 4
Program ID: 330-41-21-033

Pittsburgh

University Health Center of Pittsburgh Program

Sponsor: University Health Center of Pittsburgh
Children's Hospital of Pittsburgh

Program Director:
Geoffrey Kurland, MD
Children's Hospital of Pittsburgh
3705 Fifth Ave
Pittsburgh, PA 15213-2583
Tel: 412 692-5630 *Fax:* 412 692-6645
Accred Length: 3 Years *Program Size:* 3
Program ID: 330-41-21-035

Puerto Rico

San Juan

University of Puerto Rico Program

Sponsor: University of Puerto Rico School of Medicine
University Pediatric Hospital

Program Director:
Jose R Rodriguez-Santana, MD
Univ Pediatric Hospital
PO Box 365067
San Juan, PR 00936-5067
Tel: 787 754-8500 *Fax:* 787 743-1917
Accred Length: 3 Years *Program Size:* 3
Program ID: 330-42-21-038

Tennessee

Nashville

Vanderbilt University Program
Sponsor: Vanderbilt University Medical Center
Program Director:
Thomas A Hazinski, MD
Div of Ped Pulmonary Med
S-0119 Medical Ctr N
Vanderbilt Univ
Nashville, TN 37232-2586
Tel: 615 343-7617 *Fax:* 615 343-1763
Accred Length: 3 Years *Program Size:* 0
Program ID: 330-47-21-037

Texas

Houston

Baylor College of Medicine Program
Sponsor: Baylor College of Medicine
Texas Children's Hospital
Program Director:
Leland L Fan, MD
Dept of Pediatrics
Baylor Coll of Med
One Baylor Plaza
Houston, TX 77030-2399
Tel: 713 770-3300 *Fax:* 713 770-3308
E-mail: lfan@msmailpo2.is5.tch.tmc.edu
Accred Length: 3 Years *Program Size:* 6
Program ID: 330-48-21-029

Utah

Salt Lake City

University of Utah Program
Sponsor: University of Utah Medical Center
Primary Children's Medical Center
Program Director:
Dennis W Nielson, MD
Univ of Utah Health Sciences Ctr
50 N Medical Dr/2A122SOM
Salt Lake City, UT 84132
Tel: 801 581-2410 *Fax:* 801 581-4920
E-mail: dennis.nielson@hsc.utah.edu
Accred Length: 3 Years *Program Size:* 1
Program ID: 330-49-21-032

Virginia

Charlottesville

University of Virginia Program
Sponsor: University of Virginia Medical Center
Program Director:
Benjamin M Gaston, MD
Felicia A Cuomo, MD
Pediatric Respiratory Med
Box 386
Charlottesville, VA 22908
Tel: 804 924-1820 *Fax:* 804 243-6618
E-mail: bmg@virginia.edu
Accred Length: 3 Years *Program Size:* 8
Program ID: 330-51-21-053

Washington

Seattle

University of Washington Program
Sponsor: University of Washington School of Medicine
Children's Hospital and Medical Center
University of Washington Medical Center
Program Director:
Gregory J Redding, MD
Ronald L Gibson, MD PhD
Div of Ped Pulmonology
Children's Hospital and Regional Med Ctr
4800 Sand Point Way NE/CH-68
Seattle, WA 98195
Tel: 206 526-2174, ext 1 *Fax:* 206 528-2639
E-mail: gredding@u.washington.edu
Internet:
http://weber.u.washington.edu/~ped/divisions/pulmon/pulmon.htm
Accred Length: 3 Years *Program Size:* 3
Program ID: 330-54-21-031

Wisconsin

Madison

University of Wisconsin Program
Sponsor: University of Wisconsin Hospital and Clinics
Program Director:
Michael J Rock, MD
Univ of Wisconsin Hospital and Clinics
Rm H4/436 4108 CSC
600 Highland Ave
Madison, WI 53792-4801
Tel: 608 263-8555 *Fax:* 608 263-0510
E-mail: mjrock@facstaff.wisc.edu
Internet:
http://www2.medsch.wisc.edu/childrenshosp/ppc/ppchome.html
Accred Length: 3 Years *Program Size:* 2
Program ID: 330-56-21-030

Milwaukee

Medical College of Wisconsin Program
Sponsor: Medical College of Wisconsin Affiliated Hospitals Inc
Children's Hospital of Wisconsin
Program Director:
William M Gershan, MD
Dept of Pediatrics
Children's Hospital
9000 W Wisconsin Ave
Milwaukee, WI 53226
Tel: 414 266-6730 *Fax:* 414 266-6742
Accred Length: 3 Years *Program Size:* 1
Program ID: 330-56-21-047

Pediatric Radiology (Radiology-Diagnostic)

Alabama

Birmingham

University of Alabama Medical Center Program
Sponsor: University of Alabama Hospital
Program Director:
Stuart A Royal, MD
Children's Hospital
Dept of Ped Imaging
1600 7th Ave S/Ste 206
Birmingham, AL 35233
Tel: 205 939-9730 *Fax:* 205 939-6998
E-mail: sroyal@uab.edu
Accred Length: 1 Year *Program Size:* 1
Program ID: 424-01-21-004

Arkansas

Little Rock

University of Arkansas for Medical Sciences Program
Sponsor: University of Arkansas College of Medicine
Arkansas Children's Hospital
University Hospital of Arkansas
Program Director:
Theodora Vanderzalm, MD
Arkansas Children's Hospital
Dept of Radiology
800 Marshall St/Slot 105
Little Rock, AR 72202-3591
Tel: 501 320-4911 *Fax:* 501 320-1513
Accred Length: 1 Year *Program Size:* 1
Program ID: 424-04-21-005

California

Loma Linda

Loma Linda University Program
Sponsor: Loma Linda University Medical Center
Program Director:
Lionel W Young, MD
Loma Linda Univ Med Ctr
Dept of Radiology
11234 Anderson St
Loma Linda, CA 92354
Tel: 909 824-4281, ext 45510 *Fax:* 909 478-4266
E-mail: lwyoung@ahs.llumc.edu
Internet: http://www.llu.edu/llumc/radiology/
Accred Length: 1 Year *Program Size:* 1
Program ID: 424-05-31-049

Los Angeles

Children's Hospital of Los Angeles Program
Sponsor: Children's Hospital of Los Angeles
Program Director:
Marvin D Nelson, MD
Childrens Hospital
Dept of Radiology
4650 Sunset Blvd/MS 81
Los Angeles, CA 90027
Tel: 323 669-4572 *Fax:* 323 666-4655
E-mail: mdnelson%smtpgate@chlais.usc.edu
Internet: http://www.chla.org
Accred Length: 1 Year *Program Size:* 3
Program ID: 424-05-21-003

UCLA Medical Center Program
Sponsor: UCLA School of Medicine
Olive View-UCLA Medical Center
UCLA Medical Center
Program Director:
M Ines Boechat, MD
UCLA Med Ctr
Dept of Rad Sciences
10833 Le Conte Ave
Los Angeles, CA 90095-1721
Tel: 310 825-6798 *Fax:* 310 206-5725
E-mail: iboechat@mail.rad.ucla.edu
Internet: http://www.radsci.ucla.edu
Accred Length: 1 Year *Program Size:* 1
Program ID: 424-05-21-022

San Francisco

University of California (San Francisco) Program
Sponsor: University of California (San Francisco) School of Medicine
Children's Hospital-Oakland
University of California (San Francisco) Medical Center
Program Director:
Charles A Gooding, MD
Univ of California
Dept of Radiology
505 Parnassus Ave
San Francisco, CA 94143-0628
Tel: 415 476-1918 *Fax:* 415 476-0616
E-mail: charles.gooding@radiology.ucsf.edu
Accred Length: 1 Year *Program Size:* 1
Program ID: 424-05-21-042

Stanford

Stanford University Program
Sponsor: Stanford University Hospital
Lucile Salter Packard Children's Hospital at Stanford
Program Director:
William H Northway Jr, MD
Lucile S Packard Children's Hospital-Stanford
Dept of Radiology
725 Welch Rd
Palo Alto, CA 94304
Tel: 415 497-8601 *Fax:* 415 497-8745
Accred Length: 1 Year *Program Size:* 1
Program ID: 424-05-21-023

Colorado

Denver

University of Colorado Program
Sponsor: University of Colorado Health Sciences Center
Children's Hospital
Program Director:
John D Strain, MD
Children's Hospital
1056 E 19th Ave
Denver, CO 80218
Tel: 303 861-6541 *Fax:* 303 764-8669
Accred Length: 1 Year *Program Size:* 1
Program ID: 424-07-21-037

Connecticut

New Haven

Yale-New Haven Medical Center Program
Sponsor: Yale-New Haven Hospital
Program Director:
Marc S Keller, MD
Children's Hospital
Dept of Ped Diagnostic Imaging
20 York St
New Haven, CT 06510
Tel: 203 785-2688 *Fax:* 203 785-4328
E-mail: keller@biomed.med.yale.edu
Internet: http://www.into.med.yale.edu/diagrad
Accred Length: 1 Year *Program Size:* 1
Program ID: 424-08-21-040

District of Columbia

Washington

George Washington University Program
Sponsor: Children's National Medical Center
Program Director:
David C Kushner, MD
Children's National Med Ctr
Dept of Diagnostic Imaging/Rad
111 Michigan Ave NW
Washington, DC 20010-2970
Tel: 202 884-5430 *Fax:* 202 884-3644
E-mail: dkushner@cnmc.org
Accred Length: 1 Year *Program Size:* 4
Program ID: 424-10-21-024

Florida

Miami

Miami Children's Hospital Program
Sponsor: Miami Children's Hospital
Program Director:
D H Altman, MD
Miami Children's Hospital
3100 SW 62nd Ave
Miami, FL 33155-3009
Tel: 305 666-6511, ext 4338 *Fax:* 305 667-8689
Accred Length: 1 Year *Program Size:* 2
Program ID: 424-11-21-025

University of Miami-Jackson Memorial Medical Center Program
Sponsor: University of Miami-Jackson Memorial Medical Center
Program Director:
Amal Jabra, MD
Univ of Miami-Jackson Memorial Med Ctr
Dept of Radiology
1611 NW 12th Ave
Miami, FL 33136
Tel: 305 585-6894 *Fax:* 305 325-8591
E-mail: ajabra@mednet.med.miami.edu
Accred Length: 1 Year *Program Size:* 1
Program ID: 424-11-21-006

Georgia

Atlanta

Emory University Program
Sponsor: Emory University School of Medicine
Egleston Children's Hospital at Emory University
Program Director:
Stephen F Simoneaux, MD
Egleston Children's Hospital
1405 Clifton Rd NE
Atlanta, GA 30322-1101
Tel: 404 325-6532 *Fax:* 404 315-2216
E-mail: ssimonea@mail.egleston.org
Accred Length: 1 Year *Program Size:* 1
Program ID: 424-12-21-035

Illinois

Chicago

McGaw Medical Center of Northwestern University Program
Sponsor: Northwestern University Medical School
Children's Memorial Medical Center
Program Director:
Andrew K Poznanski, MD
Children's Memorial Hospital
Dept of Radiology
2300 Children's Plaza/# 9
Chicago, IL 60614-3394
Tel: 312 880-3520 *Fax:* 312 880-3517
E-mail: sgartman@nwu.edu
Accred Length: 1 Year *Program Size:* 3
Program ID: 424-16-21-017

Indiana

Indianapolis

Indiana University School of Medicine Program
Sponsor: Indiana University School of Medicine
Clarian Riley Hospital for Children
Program Director:
John A Smith, MD
Dept of Radiology
702 Barnhill Dr
Indianapolis, IN 46202-5200
Tel: 317 274-2951 *Fax:* 317 274-2920
E-mail: joasmith@iupui.edu
Internet: http://www.indyrad.iupui.edu/homepage.htm
Accred Length: 1 Year *Program Size:* 2
Program ID: 424-17-21-007

Programs

Iowa

Iowa City

University of Iowa Hospitals and Clinics Program

Sponsor: University of Iowa Hospitals and Clinics

Program Director:
Yutaka Sato, MD
Univ of Iowa Hospitals and Clinics
Dept of Radiology
200 Hawkins Dr
Iowa City, IA 52242-1009
Tel: 319 356-3396 *Fax:* 319 356-2220
E-mail: yutaka-sato@uiowa.edu
Accred Length: 1 Year *Program Size:* 1
Program ID: 424-18-21-008

Maryland

Baltimore

Johns Hopkins University Program

Sponsor: Johns Hopkins University School of Medicine
Johns Hopkins Hospital

Program Director:
Jane E Benson, MD
Johns Hopkins Hospital
600 N Wolfe St
Baltimore, MD 21287
Tel: 410 955-6140 *Fax:* 410 614-2972
E-mail: jebenson@rad.jhu.edu
Accred Length: 1 Year *Program Size:* 1
Program ID: 424-23-21-038

Massachusetts

Boston

Children's Hospital Program

Sponsor: Children's Hospital

Program Director:
Carlo Buonomo, MD
Children's Hospital
Dept of Radiology
300 Longwood Ave
Boston, MA 02115
Tel: 617 355-6496 *Fax:* 617 730-0465
E-mail: buonomo@al.tch.harvard.edu
Internet: http://web1.tch.harvard.edu/radiology/
Accred Length: 1 Year *Program Size:* 14
Program ID: 424-24-21-027

Michigan

Ann Arbor

University of Michigan Program

Sponsor: University of Michigan Hospitals

Program Director:
R J Hernandez, MD
CS Mott Children's Hospital Ctr
Univ of Michigan Hospitals
1500 E Medical Center Dr
Ann Arbor, MI 48109-0252
Tel: 734 763-2570 *Fax:* 734 764-9351
E-mail: rjhm@umich.edu
Accred Length: 1 Year *Program Size:* 1
Program ID: 424-25-21-018

Detroit

Wayne State University/Detroit Medical Center Program

Sponsor: Wayne State University/Detroit Medical Center
Children's Hospital of Michigan

Program Director:
Thomas L Slovis, MD
Children's Hospital
Dept of Ped Imaging
3901 Beaubien Blvd
Detroit, MI 48201-2196
Tel: 313 745-0094 *Fax:* 313 993-0393
E-mail: tslovis@med.wayne.edu
Accred Length: 1 Year *Program Size:* 2
Program ID: 424-25-21-019

Minnesota

Minneapolis

University of Minnesota Program

Sponsor: University of Minnesota Medical School
Children's Health Care (Minneapolis)
Fairview-University Medical Center

Program Director:
Stephen H Hite, MD
Univ of Minnesota
Box 292 Mayo Bldg
420 Delaware St SE
Minneapolis, MN 55455
Tel: 612 273-1944 *Fax:* 612 273-8495
Internet:
http://www.umn.edu/nehome/mi22/hitex001/pedsimage/peds.htme
Accred Length: 1 Year *Program Size:* 2
Program ID: 424-26-21-036

Missouri

St Louis

St Louis University School of Medicine Program

Sponsor: St Louis University School of Medicine
SSM Cardinal Glennon Children's Hospital

Program Director:
E R Graviss, MD
Cardinal Glennon Children's Hospital
1465 S Grand Blvd
St Louis, MO 63104
Tel: 314 577-5654 *Fax:* 314 268-6472
E-mail: diagrad@slu.edu
Internet: http://www.slu.edu
Accred Length: 1 Year *Program Size:* 2
Program ID: 424-28-21-041

Washington University/B-JH/SLCH Consortium Program

Sponsor: Washington University/B-JH/SLCH Consortium
Barnes-Jewish Hospital
Mallinckrodt Institute of Radiology

Program Director:
William H McAlister, MD
St Louis Children's Hospital
One Children's Pl
St Louis, MO 63110
Tel: 314 454-6229 *Fax:* 314 454-2868
E-mail: mcalister@mirlink.wustl.edu
Internet:
http://www.mir.wustl.edu/residency/fellowships.html
Accred Length: 1 Year *Program Size:* 1
Program ID: 424-28-21-009

New York

Buffalo

Children's Hospital of Buffalo Program

Sponsor: CGF Health System (Children's Hospital of Buffalo)

Program Director:
Jan S Najdzionek, MD MD
Children's Hospital
219 Bryant St
Buffalo, NY 14222-2099
Tel: 716 878-7525 *Fax:* 716 878-7001
E-mail: najdzion@acsu.buffalo.edu
Accred Length: 1 Year *Program Size:* 2
Program ID: 424-35-21-029

New Hyde Park

Albert Einstein College of Medicine at Long Island Jewish Medical Center Program

Sponsor: Long Island Jewish Medical Center

Program Director:
John C Leonidas, MD
Long Island Jewish Med Ctr
Dept of Radiology
New Hyde Park, NY 11040
Tel: 718 470-3404 *Fax:* 718 343-7463
Internet: http://www.lij.edu/lij-homepage-ns.html
Accred Length: 1 Year *Program Size:* 1
Program ID: 424-35-21-010

New York

Mount Sinai School of Medicine Program

Sponsor: Mount Sinai School of Medicine
Mount Sinai Medical Center

Program Director:
Karen I Norton, MD
Mount Sinai Hospital
One Gustave L Levy Pl
New York, NY 10029-6574
Tel: 212 241-7418 *Fax:* 212 427-8137
E-mail: karen_norton@smtplink.mssm.edu
Internet: http://www.mssm.edu/radiology/faculty.html
Accred Length: 1 Year *Program Size:* 1
Program ID: 424-35-21-051

New York and Presbyterian Hospital (Columbia Campus) Program

Sponsor: New York and Presbyterian Hospital
New York and Presbyterian Hospital (Columbia Campus)

Program Director:
Walter E Berdon, MD
Babies Hospital
3959 Broadway
New York, NY 10032
Tel: 212 305-9864 *Fax:* 212 305-7233
Accred Length: 1 Year *Program Size:* 1
Program ID: 424-35-21-011

New York University Medical Center Program

Sponsor: New York University Medical Center
Bellevue Hospital Center

Program Director:
Nancy Genieser, MD
New York Univ Med Ctr
Dept of Radiology
560 First Ave
New York, NY 10016
Tel: 212 263-5362 *Fax:* 212 263-7348
E-mail: nancy.genieser@med.nyu.edu
Internet:
http://nucmed.med.nyu.edu/radmain/res-desc.html
Accred Length: 1 Year *Program Size:* 1
Program ID: 424-35-21-030

Rochester

University of Rochester Program

Sponsor: Strong Memorial Hospital of the University of Rochester

Program Director:
Nina B Klionsky, MD
Strong Memorial Hospital
Dept of Radiology
601 Elmwood Ave
Rochester, NY 14642-8648
Tel: 716 275-3000 *Fax:* 716 273-1033
E-mail: klionsky@orion.rad.rochester.edu
Accred Length: 1 Year *Program Size:* 1
Program ID: 424-35-21-012

North Carolina

Durham

Duke University Program

Sponsor: Duke University Medical Center

Program Director:
George S Bisset III, MD
Dept of Radiology
Duke Univ Med Ctr
Box 3808
Durham, NC 27710
Tel: 919 684-7289 *Fax:* 919 684-7127
Accred Length: 1 Year *Program Size:* 1
Program ID: 424-36-21-031

Winston-Salem

Wake Forest University School of Medicine Program

Sponsor: Wake Forest University Baptist Medical Center

Program Director:
Thomas E Sumner, MD
Wake Forest Univ Baptist Med Ctr
Medical Center Blvd
Winston-Salem, NC 27157-1088
Tel: 336 716-2463 *Fax:* 336 716-2029
E-mail: carole carr@medcenter.wpmail.wfu.edu
Internet: http://www.rad.bgsm.edu/radmain/htmls/
Accred Length: 1 Year *Program Size:* 1
Program ID: 424-36-21-043

Ohio

Akron

Children's Hospital Medical Center of Akron/NEOUCOM Program

Sponsor: Children's Hospital Medical Center of Akron

Program Director:
Godfrey Gaisie, MD
Children's Hospital Med Ctr
One Perkins Sq
Akron, OH 44308
Tel: 330 379-8778 *Fax:* 330 258-3760
E-mail: ggaisie@chmca.org
Accred Length: 1 Year *Program Size:* 1
Program ID: 424-38-21-020

Cincinnati

Children's Hospital Medical Center/University of Cincinnati College of Medicine Program

Sponsor: Children's Hospital Medical Center

Program Director:
Janet L Strife, MD
Children's Hospital Med Ctr
3333 Burnet Ave
Cincinnati, OH 45229-3039
Tel: 513 636-8703 *Fax:* 513 636-8145
E-mail: strife.jl@chmcc.org
Accred Length: 1 Year *Program Size:* 6
Program ID: 424-38-21-001

Cleveland

Case Western Reserve University Program

Sponsor: University Hospitals of Cleveland

Program Director:
Carlos J Sivit, MD
Rainbow Babies and Children's Hospital
Dept of Radiology
11100 Euclid Ave
Cleveland, OH 44106-5056
Tel: 216 844-1172 *Fax:* 216 844-5474
E-mail: sivit@uhrad.com
Internet: http://www.uhrad.com
Accred Length: 1 Year *Program Size:* 1
Program ID: 424-38-31-052

Cleveland Clinic Foundation Program

Sponsor: Cleveland Clinic Foundation
Children's Hospital Medical Center

Program Director:
Marilyn Goske, MD
Janet Strife, MD
Cleveland Clinic Foundation
Children's Hospital/HB6
9500 Euclid Ave
Cleveland, OH 44195
Tel: 216 445-9597 *Fax:* 216 445-4432
E-mail: goskem@ccisd1.ccf.org
Internet: http://www.ccf.org
Accred Length: 1 Year *Program Size:* 1
Program ID: 424-38-21-050

Pennsylvania

Philadelphia

Children's Hospital of Philadelphia Program

Sponsor: Children's Hospital of Philadelphia

Program Director:
Sandra S Kramer, MD
Dept of Radiology
Children's Hospital
34th St and Civic Center Blvd
Philadelphia, PA 19104-4399
Tel: 215 590-2575 *Fax:* 215 590-4318
Accred Length: 1 Year *Program Size:* 4
Program ID: 424-41-21-032

St Christopher's Hospital for Children Program

Sponsor: St Christopher's Hospital for Children

Program Director:
Eleanor M Smergel, MD
St Christopher's Hospital for Children
Erie Ave at Front St
Philadelphia, PA 19134-1095
Tel: 215 427-5230 *Fax:* 215 427-5407
Accred Length: 1 Year *Program Size:* 2
Program ID: 424-41-21-039

Pittsburgh

University Health Center of Pittsburgh Program

Sponsor: University Health Center of Pittsburgh
Children's Hospital of Pittsburgh

Program Director:
Richard B Towbin, MD
Children's Hospital
3705 Fifth Ave
Pittsburgh, PA 15213-2583
Tel: 412 692-5510 *Fax:* 412 692-6929
E-mail: priatkd@chplink.chp.edu
Accred Length: 1 Year *Program Size:* 3
Program ID: 424-41-21-002

Texas

Dallas

University of Texas Southwestern Medical School Program

Sponsor: University of Texas Southwestern Medical School
Children's Medical Center of Dallas
Dallas County Hospital District-Parkland Memorial Hospital

Program Director:
Nancy Rollins, MD
Children's Med Ctr
Dept of Radiology
1935 Motor St
Dallas, TX 75235
Tel: 214 640-2308 *Fax:* 214 640-6015
Internet: http://www.rad.swmed.edu/residen.html
Accred Length: 1 Year *Program Size:* 2
Program ID: 424-48-21-015

Galveston

University of Texas Medical Branch Hospitals Program

Sponsor: University of Texas Medical Branch Hospitals

Program Director:
Leonard E Swischuck, MD
Univ of Texas Med Branch
Dept of Radiology/G-09
301 University Blvd
Galveston, TX 77555-0709
Tel: 409 747-2849 *Fax:* 409 747-2825
E-mail: rcoble@utmb.edu
Internet: http://www.utmb.edu/
Accred Length: 1 Year *Program Size:* 1
Program ID: 424-48-21-014

Houston

Baylor College of Medicine Program

Sponsor: Baylor College of Medicine
Texas Children's Hospital

Program Director:
Bruce R Parker, MD
Texas Children's Hospital
Diagnostic Imaging
6621 Fannin St/MC 2-2521
Houston, TX 77030-2399
Tel: 713 770-5324 *Fax:* 713 770-5241
E-mail: brucep@bcm.tmc.edu
Accred Length: 1 Year *Program Size:* 3
Program ID: 424-48-21-016

Programs

Washington

Seattle

University of Washington Program
Sponsor: University of Washington School of Medicine
Children's Hospital and Medical Center
Program Director:
C Benjamin Graham, MD
Children's Hospital and Med Ctr
Dept of Radiology CH-69
PO Box 5371
Seattle, WA 98105-0371
Tel: 206 526-2166 *Fax:* 206 528-2730
E-mail: bgraham@u.washington.edu
Accred Length: 1 Year *Program Size:* 3
Program ID: 424-54-21-033

Wisconsin

Milwaukee

Medical College of Wisconsin Program
Sponsor: Medical College of Wisconsin Affiliated Hospitals Inc
Children's Hospital of Wisconsin
Program Director:
David C Gregg, MD
Children's Hospital
Dept of Radiology/MS 721
9000 W Wisconsin Ave
Milwaukee, WI 53226
Tel: 414 266-3110 *Fax:* 414 266-1525
E-mail: jsty@chw.org
Accred Length: 1 Year *Program Size:* 2
Program ID: 424-56-21-034

Pediatric Rheumatology (Pediatrics)

California

Orange

Children's Hospital of Orange County Program
Sponsor: Children's Hospital of Orange County
St Joseph Hospital
University of California (Irvine) Medical Center
Program Director:
Deborah McCurdy, MD
Children's Hospital
455 S Main St
Orange, CA 92668
Tel: 714 532-8617 *Fax:* 714 532-8883
Accred Length: 3 Years *Program Size:* 1
Program ID: 331-05-21-001

San Francisco

University of California (San Francisco) Program
Sponsor: University of California (San Francisco) School of Medicine
Shriners Hospitals for Children (Sacramento)
University of California (San Francisco) Medical Center
Program Director:
Helen Emery, MD
Univ of California San Francisco
Dept of Ped Rheumatology
505 Parnassus Ave
San Francisco, CA 94143-0107
Tel: 415 476-1736 *Fax:* 415 476-3466
E-mail: hemery@peds.ucsf.edu
Accred Length: 3 Years *Program Size:* 2
Program ID: 331-05-31-002

Illinois

Chicago

McGaw Medical Center of Northwestern University Program
Sponsor: Northwestern University Medical School
Children's Memorial Medical Center
Rehabilitation Institute of Chicago
Program Director:
Lauren M Pachman, MD
Northwestern Univ Med Sch-Children's Memorial Hospital
Div of Immunology/Rheumatology
2300 Children's Plaza/Box 50
Chicago, IL 60614
Tel: 773 880-4303 *Fax:* 773 880-6179
E-mail: pachman@nwu.edu
Internet:
http://www.childmmc.edu/cmhweb/cmhdepts/immunology web/immunologyhome.html
Accred Length: 3 Years *Program Size:* 1
Program ID: 331-16-21-004

University of Chicago Program
Sponsor: University of Chicago Hospitals
University of Chicago Children's Hospital
Program Director:
C Egla Rabinovich, MD MPH
Univ of Chicago-La Rabida
E 65th St at Lake Michigan
Chicago, IL 60649
Tel: 773 753-8644 *Fax:* 773 363-0427
E-mail: cderabin@midway.uchicago.edu
Accred Length: 3 Years *Program Size:* 1
Program ID: 331-16-31-005

Kansas

Kansas City

University of Kansas Medical Center Program
Sponsor: University of Kansas School of Medicine
Children's Mercy Hospital
University of Kansas Medical Center
Program Director:
Carol Lindsley, MD
Univ of Kansas Med Ctr
3901 Rainbow Blvd
Kansas City, KS 66160
Tel: 913 588-6325 *Fax:* 913 588-6319
Accred Length: 3 Years *Program Size:* 3
Program ID: 331-19-21-006

Massachusetts

Boston

Children's Hospital/Boston Medical Center Program
Sponsor: Children's Hospital
Brigham and Women's Hospital
Program Director:
Robert Sundel, MD
300 Longwood Ave
Boston, MA 02115
Tel: 617 355-6524 *Fax:* 617 730-0449
E-mail: sundel@a1.tch.harvard.edu
Accred Length: 3 Years *Program Size:* 3
Program ID: 331-24-21-007

New England Medical Center Hospitals Program
Sponsor: New England Medical Center Hospitals
Program Director:
Jane G Schaller, MD
750 Washington St
Box 8683
Boston, MA 02111
Tel: 617 636-7285 *Fax:* 617 636-8388
E-mail: jane.schaller@es.nemc.org
Accred Length: 3 Years *Program Size:* 3
Program ID: 331-24-31-008

Missouri

St Louis

St Louis University School of Medicine Program

Sponsor: St Louis University School of Medicine
SSM Cardinal Glennon Children's Hospital
St Louis University School of Medicine

Program Director:
Terry L Moore, MD
St Louis Univ Sch of Med
1402 S Grand Blvd
R211A Doisy Hall
St Louis, MO 63104
Tel: 314 577-8467 *Fax:* 314 268-5117
E-mail: mooretl@wpogate.slu.edu
Accred Length: 3 Years *Program Size:* 1
Program ID: 331-28-21-009

Washington University/B-JH/SLCH Consortium Program

Sponsor: Washington University/B-JH/SLCH Consortium
Shriners Hospitals for Children (St Louis)
St Louis Children's Hospital

Program Director:
Jonathan D Gitlin, MD
Washington Univ
One Children's Pl
St Louis, MO 63110
Tel: 314 454-6124 *Fax:* 314 454-4861
E-mail: gitlin@kidsa1.wustl.edu
Accred Length: 3 Years *Program Size:* 3
Program ID: 331-28-31-010

New York

New Hyde Park

Albert Einstein College of Medicine at Long Island Jewish Medical Center Program

Sponsor: Long Island Jewish Medical Center
Schneider Children's Hosp (Long Island Jewish Med Ctr)

Program Director:
Norman T Ilowite, MD
Long Island Jewish Med Ctr
269-10 76th Ave
New Hyde Park, NY 11040
Tel: 718 470-3530 *Fax:* 718 831-0182
E-mail: ilowite@lij.edu
Internet: http://www.lij.edu
Accred Length: 3 Years *Program Size:* 1
Program ID: 331-35-21-011

New York

New York and Presbyterian Hospital (Columbia Campus) Program

Sponsor: New York and Presbyterian Hospital
New York and Presbyterian Hospital (Columbia Campus)

Program Director:
J Imundo, MD
630 W 168th St/BHN 106
New York, NY 10032
Tel: 212 305-4932 *Fax:* 212 305-9078
Accred Length: 3 Years *Program Size:* 1
Program ID: 331-35-11-013

New York and Presbyterian Hospital (Cornell Campus) Program

Sponsor: New York and Presbyterian Hospital
Hospital for Special Surgery
New York and Presbyterian Hospital (Cornell Campus)

Program Director:
Thomas J A Lehman, MD
535 E 70th St
New York, NY 10021
Tel: 212 606-1151 *Fax:* 212 606-1938
E-mail: goldscout@aol.com
Internet: http://www.hss.edu
Accred Length: 3 Years *Program Size:* 3
Program ID: 331-35-31-012

North Carolina

Durham

Duke University Program

Sponsor: Duke University Medical Center
University of North Carolina Hospitals

Program Director:
Deborah W Kredich, MD
Duke Univ Med Ctr
Box 3212
Durham, NC 27710
Tel: 919 684-6575 *Fax:* 919 684-6616
E-mail: kredi002@mc.duke.edu
Accred Length: 3 Years *Program Size:* 1
Program ID: 331-36-21-015

Ohio

Cincinnati

Children's Hospital Medical Center/University of Cincinnati College of Medicine Program

Sponsor: Children's Hospital Medical Center

Program Director:
Murray H Passo, MD
Children's Hospital Med Ctr
3333 Burnet Ave
Cincinnati, OH 45229-3039
Tel: 513 636-4676 *Fax:* 513 636-5568
Accred Length: 3 Years *Program Size:* 5
Program ID: 331-38-21-016

Tennessee

Memphis

University of Tennessee Program

Sponsor: University of Tennessee College of Medicine
LeBonheur Children's Medical Center
Regional Medical Center at Memphis

Program Director:
Linda K Myers, MD
50 N Dunlap
Rm 301 W Pt Tower
Memphis, TN 38103
Tel: 901 572-5366 *Fax:* 901 572-5036
Accred Length: 3 Years *Program Size:* 1
Program ID: 331-47-21-017

Texas

Dallas

University of Texas Southwestern Medical School Program

Sponsor: University of Texas Southwestern Medical School
Children's Medical Center of Dallas
Texas Scottish Rite Hospital for Children

Program Director:
Maria Virginia Pascual, MD
Felicia A Cuomo, MD
Dept of Pediatrics
5323 Harry Hines Blvd/MC 9063
Dallas, TX 75235
Tel: 214 648-8996 *Fax:* 214 820-4813
Accred Length: 3 Years *Program Size:* 6
Program ID: 331-48-31-021

Houston

Baylor College of Medicine Program

Sponsor: Baylor College of Medicine
Harris County Hospital District-Ben Taub General Hospital
Texas Children's Hospital

Program Director:
Maria D Perez, MD
6621 Fannin/Mail Code 3-2290
Houston, TX 77030
Tel: 713 770-3830 *Fax:* 713 770-3837
Accred Length: 3 Years *Program Size:* 0
Program ID: 331-48-21-020

Washington

Seattle

University of Washington Program

Sponsor: University of Washington School of Medicine
Children's Hospital and Medical Center
University of Washington Medical Center

Program Director:
David D Sherry, MD
Dept of Ped Rheumatology
1959 NE Pacific St
Seattle, WA 98195
Tel: 206 526-2057 *Fax:* 206 527-3852
E-mail: dsherry@u.washington.edu
Accred Length: 3 Years *Program Size:* 2
Program ID: 331-54-21-019

Pediatric Surgery (General Surgery)

Alabama

Birmingham

University of Alabama Medical Center Program
Sponsor: University of Alabama Hospital
Children's Hospital of Alabama
Program Director:
Keith E Georgeson, MD
Univ of Alabama at Birmingham-Children's Hospital
1600 Seventh Ave S/ACC 300
Birmingham, AL 35233
Tel: 205 939-9688 *Fax:* 205 975-4972
E-mail: helen.cobb@ccc.uab.edu
Internet: http://www.pedsurg.surgery.uab
Accred Length: 2 Years *Program Size:* 2
Program ID: 445-01-21-032

Arkansas

Little Rock

University of Arkansas for Medical Sciences Program
Sponsor: University of Arkansas College of Medicine
Arkansas Children's Hospital
Program Director:
Samuel D Smith, MD
Arkansas Children's Hospital
Dept of Ped Surgery
800 Marshall St
Little Rock, AR 72202-3591
Tel: 501 320-2943 *Fax:* 501 320-1516
E-mail: smithsamueld@exchange.uams.edu
Accred Length: 2 Years *Program Size:* 2
Program ID: 445-04-21-028

California

Los Angeles

Children's Hospital of Los Angeles Program
Sponsor: Children's Hospital of Los Angeles
Program Director:
Kathryn D Anderson, MD
Children's Hospital
4650 Sunset Blvd/Box 72
Los Angeles, CA 90027-6016
Tel: 213 669-2104 *Fax:* 213 666-3466
E-mail: kdanderson@chla.usc.edu
Accred Length: 2 Years *Program Size:* 2
Program ID: 445-05-21-001

Colorado

Denver

University of Colorado Program
Sponsor: University of Colorado Health Sciences Center
Children's Hospital
Program Director:
Frederick M Karrer, MD
Children's Hospital
Dept of Ped Surgery
1950 Ogden St/B-323
Denver, CO 80218
Tel: 303 861-6530 *Fax:* 303 764-8077
E-mail: spaulding.deanna@tchden.org
Accred Length: 2 Years *Program Size:* 1
Program ID: 445-07-21-027

Connecticut

New Haven

Yale-New Haven Medical Center Program
Sponsor: Yale-New Haven Hospital
Program Director:
Robert J Touloukian, MD
Yale Univ Sch of Med, Dept of Surgery
333 Cedar St
PO Box 3333
New Haven, CT 06510
Tel: 203 785-2701 *Fax:* 203 785-3820
Accred Length: 2 Years *Program Size:* 1
Program ID: 445-08-21-030

District of Columbia

Washington

Children's National Medical Center Program
Sponsor: Children's National Medical Center
Program Director:
Gary E Hartman, MD
Children's National Med Ctr
111 Michigan Ave NW
Washington, DC 20010-2970
Tel: 202 884-2151 *Fax:* 202 884-4174
E-mail: ghartman@cnmc.org
Accred Length: 2 Years *Program Size:* 2
Program ID: 445-10-21-015

Georgia

Atlanta

Emory University Program
Sponsor: Emory University School of Medicine
Program Director:
Richard R Ricketts, MD
Emory Children's Ctr
Div of Pediatric Surgery
2040 Ridgewood Dr NE
Atlanta, GA 30322
Tel: 404 727-3779 *Fax:* 404 727-8213
E-mail: richard.ricketts@oz.ped.emory.edu
Accred Length: 2 Years *Program Size:* 1
Program ID: 445-12-21-033

Illinois

Chicago

McGaw Medical Center of Northwestern University Program
Sponsor: Northwestern University Medical School
Children's Memorial Medical Center
Program Director:
Robert M Arensman, MD
2300 Children's Plaza/#115
Chicago, IL 60614
Tel: 312 880-4999 *Fax:* 312 880-4588
E-mail: raresman@nwu.edu
Accred Length: 2 Years *Program Size:* 2
Program ID: 445-16-21-002

University of Chicago Program
Sponsor: University of Chicago Hospitals
Lutheran General Hospital
University of Chicago Children's Hospital
Program Director:
Walter J Chwals, MD
Wyler Children's Hospital
5841 S Maryland Ave
Chicago, IL 60637
Tel: 773 702-6471 *Fax:* 773 702-2140
E-mail: wchwals@surgery.uchicago.edu
Accred Length: 2 Years *Program Size:* 1
Program ID: 445-16-21-026

Indiana

Indianapolis

Indiana University School of Medicine Program
Sponsor: Indiana University School of Medicine
Clarian Riley Hospital for Children
William N Wishard Memorial Hospital
Program Director:
Jay L Grosfeld, MD
Riley Hospital for Children
702 Barnhill Dr/Rm 2500
Indianapolis, IN 46202-5200
Tel: 317 274-4682 *Fax:* 317 274-4491
E-mail: sandyd@iupui.edu
Internet: http://scalpel.med.iupui.edu/peds.info.html
Accred Length: 2 Years *Program Size:* 2
Program ID: 445-17-21-019

Maryland

Baltimore

Johns Hopkins University Program
Sponsor: Johns Hopkins University School of Medicine
Johns Hopkins Hospital
University of Maryland Medical System
Program Director:
Paul M Colombani, MD
Johns Hopkins Hospital
Dept of Ped Surgery
600 N Wolfe St/CMSC 7-113
Baltimore, MD 21287-3716
Tel: 410 955-2717 *Fax:* 410 502-5314
E-mail: pc@jhmi.edu
Internet: http://www.med.jhu/pediatric_surgery
Accred Length: 2 Years *Program Size:* 2
Program ID: 445-23-21-003

Massachusetts

Boston

Children's Hospital Program

Sponsor: Children's Hospital

Program Director:
Moritz M Ziegler, MD
Children's Hospital
300 Longwood Ave
Boston, MA 02115
Tel: 617 355-2469 *Fax:* 617 232-4440
Internet:
http://www.childrenshospital.org/surgery/pedsurg.html
Accred Length: 2 Years *Program Size:* 2
Program ID: 445-24-21-016

New England Medical Center Hospitals Program

Sponsor: New England Medical Center Hospitals

Program Director:
Neil R Feins, MD
New England Med Ctr
750 Washington St/Box 344
Boston, MA 02111
Tel: 617 636-5025 *Fax:* 617 636-8122
E-mail: neil.feins@es.nemc.org
Accred Length: 2 Years *Program Size:* 1
Program ID: 445-24-21-023

Michigan

Ann Arbor

University of Michigan Program

Sponsor: University of Michigan Hospitals

Program Director:
Arnold G Coran, MD
Office of Surgical Education
Univ of Michigan Hospitals
1500 E Medical Center Dr
Ann Arbor, MI 48109-0342
Tel: 734 936-5733 *Fax:* 734 936-5725
E-mail: surgery.ed@umich.edu
Internet: http://www.med.umich.edu/surg/peds/
Accred Length: 2 Years *Program Size:* 2
Program ID: 445-25-21-018

Detroit

Wayne State University/Detroit Medical Center Program

Sponsor: Wayne State University/Detroit Medical Center
Children's Hospital of Michigan

Program Director:
Michael D Klein, MD
Children's Hospital
Dept of Pediatric Surgery
3901 Beaubien Blvd
Detroit, MI 48201-2196
Tel: 313 745-5840 *Fax:* 313 831-3908
E-mail: mklein@dmc.org
Accred Length: 2 Years *Program Size:* 2
Subspecialties: CCS
Program ID: 445-25-11-004

Missouri

Kansas City

University of Missouri at Kansas City Program

Sponsor: University of Missouri-Kansas City School of Medicine
Children's Mercy Hospital

Program Director:
Keith W Ashcraft, MD
Children's Mercy Hospital
Dept of Surgery
2401 Gillham Rd
Kansas City, MO 64108
Tel: 816 234-3579 *Fax:* 816 234-3821
Accred Length: 2 Years *Program Size:* 2
Subspecialties: CCS
Program ID: 445-28-11-005

St Louis

St Louis University School of Medicine Program

Sponsor: St Louis University School of Medicine
SSM Cardinal Glennon Children's Hospital

Program Director:
Thomas R Weber, MD
St Louis Univ Sch of Med
Dept of Ped Surgery
1465 S Grand Blvd
St Louis, MO 63104
Tel: 314 577-5629 *Fax:* 314 268-5466
E-mail: surgweb@slu.edu
Internet:
http://www.slu.edu/colleges/med/departments/surgery
Accred Length: 2 Years *Program Size:* 1
Program ID: 445-28-21-029

Washington University/B-JH/SLCH Consortium Program

Sponsor: Washington University/B-JH/SLCH Consortium
St Louis Children's Hospital

Program Director:
Robert P Foglia, MD
St Louis Children's Hospital
1 Children's Pl
Ste 5S60
St Louis, MO 63110
Tel: 314 454-6022 *Fax:* 314 454-2442
E-mail: fogliar@msnotes.wustl.edu
Accred Length: 2 Years *Program Size:* 1
Program ID: 445-28-21-034

New York

Brooklyn

SUNY Health Science Center at Brooklyn Program

Sponsor: SUNY Health Science Center at Brooklyn
Kings County Hospital Center
University Hospital-SUNY Health Science Center at Brooklyn

Program Director:
Max L Ramenofsky, MD
SUNY Health Science Ctr-Brooklyn
450 Clarkson Ave/Box 40
Brooklyn, NY 11203-2098
Tel: 718 270-1386 *Fax:* 718 270-4197
E-mail: pedtraum@earthlink.net
Accred Length: 2 Years *Program Size:* 1
Program ID: 445-35-11-007

Buffalo

SUNY at Buffalo Graduate Medical-Dental Education Consortium Program

Sponsor: SUNY at Buffalo Grad Medical-Dental Education Consortium
CGF Health System (Children's Hospital of Buffalo)

Program Director:
Richard G Azizkhan, MD
Children's Hospital
219 Bryant St
Buffalo, NY 14222
Tel: 716 878-7790 *Fax:* 716 878-7809
Accred Length: 2 Years *Program Size:* 2
Program ID: 445-35-21-017

New York

New York and Presbyterian Hospital (Columbia Campus) Program

Sponsor: New York and Presbyterian Hospital
New York and Presbyterian Hospital (Columbia Campus)

Program Director:
R Peter Altman, MD
Presbyterian Hospital
3959 Broadway/Rm 204 N
New York, NY 10032-3784
Tel: 212 305-5804 *Fax:* 212 305-9305
E-mail: rpa1@columbia.edu
Internet:
http://www.cpmcnet.columbia.edu/dept/surgery/peds
Accred Length: 2 Years *Program Size:* 2
Program ID: 445-35-11-006

Ohio

Cincinnati

Children's Hospital Medical Center/University of Cincinnati College of Medicine Program

Sponsor: Children's Hospital Medical Center

Program Director:
Richard G Azizkhan, MD
Div of Ped Surgery
Children's Hospital Med Ctr
3333 Burnet Ave
Cincinnati, OH 45229-3039
Tel: 513 636-4371 *Fax:* 513 636-7657
Internet: http://www.chmcc.org
Accred Length: 2 Years *Program Size:* 2
Program ID: 445-38-11-008

Columbus

Children's Hospital/Ohio State University Program

Sponsor: Children's Hospital

Program Director:
Donna A Caniano, MD
Columbus Children's Hospital
700 Children's Dr/ED379
Columbus, OH 43205
Tel: 614 722-3900 *Fax:* 614 722-3903
Accred Length: 2 Years *Program Size:* 3
Program ID: 445-38-21-012

Oklahoma

Oklahoma City

University of Oklahoma Health Sciences Center Program

Sponsor: University of Oklahoma College of Medicine
Children's Hospital of Oklahoma

Program Director:
David W Tuggle, MD
Children's Hospital of Oklahoma
PO Box 26307
Oklahoma City, OK 73126
Tel: 405 271-5922 *Fax:* 405 271-3278
E-mail: david-tuggle@ouhsc.edu
Accred Length: 2 Years *Program Size:* 1
Program ID: 445-39-11-009

Pennsylvania

Philadelphia

Children's Hospital of Philadelphia Program

Sponsor: Children's Hospital of Philadelphia

Program Director:
Alan W Flake, MD
Children's Hospital
One Children's Ctr
34th St and Civic Center Blvd
Philadelphia, PA 19104-4399
Tel: 215 590-2727 *Fax:* 215 590-4875
E-mail: flake@email.chop.edu
Accred Length: 2 Years *Program Size:* 2
Program ID: 445-41-11-014

St Christopher's Hospital for Children Program

Sponsor: St Christopher's Hospital for Children

Program Director:
William H Weintraub, MD
St Christopher's Hospital for Children
Erie Ave at Front St
Philadelphia, PA 19134-1095
Tel: 215 427-5293 *Fax:* 215 427-4616
E-mail: weintrw@wpo.auhs.edu
Accred Length: 2 Years *Program Size:* 2
Program ID: 445-41-21-010

Pittsburgh

University Health Center of Pittsburgh Program

Sponsor: University Health Center of Pittsburgh
Children's Hospital of Pittsburgh

Program Director:
Eugene S Wiener, MD
Univ Health Ctr of Pittsburgh
Dept of Surgery
497 Scaife Hall
Pittsburgh, PA 15261
Tel: 412 692-7288 *Fax:* 412 692-6069
E-mail: eugene_wiener@poplar.chp.edu
Accred Length: 2 Years *Program Size:* 2
Program ID: 445-41-11-013

Rhode Island

Providence

Brown University Program

Sponsor: Rhode Island Hospital

Program Director:
Thomas F Tracy Jr, MD MS
Div of Pediatric Surgery
Hasbro Children's Hospital/Rm 147
593 Eddy St
Providence, RI 02903
Tel: 401 444-7605 *Fax:* 401 444-7629
E-mail: thomas_tracy@brown.edu
Accred Length: 2 Years *Program Size:* 1
Program ID: 445-43-21-031

Tennessee

Memphis

University of Tennessee Program

Sponsor: University of Tennessee College of Medicine
LeBonheur Children's Medical Center
St Jude Children's Research Hospital
University of Tennessee Medical Center (UT Bowld Hospital)

Program Director:
Thom E Lobe, MD
Univ of Tennessee
Sect of Ped Surgery
777 Washington Ave/Ste P220
Memphis, TN 38105
Tel: 901 572-3300 *Fax:* 901 572-5191
E-mail: tlobe@utmem1.utmem.edu
Accred Length: 2 Years *Program Size:* 2
Program ID: 445-47-21-025

Texas

Dallas

University of Texas Southwestern Medical School Program

Sponsor: University of Texas Southwestern Medical School
Children's Medical Center of Dallas

Program Director:
Philip C Guzzetta, MD
1935 Motor St/CMC
3rd Fl W Tower
Dallas, TX 75235
Tel: 214 640-6040 *Fax:* 214 640-6320
Accred Length: 2 Years *Program Size:* 1
Program ID: 445-48-21-022

Houston

Baylor College of Medicine Program

Sponsor: Baylor College of Medicine
Harris County Hospital District-Ben Taub General Hospital
Texas Children's Hospital

Program Director:
David E Wesson, MD
Baylor Coll of Med-Texas Children's Hospital
Clinical Care Ctr #245/MC 3-2325
6621 Fannin St
Houston, TX 77030
Tel: 713 770-3146 *Fax:* 713 770-3141
E-mail: germg@mailpo1.is6.tch.tmc.edu
Internet: http://www.bcm.tmc.edu/surgery
Accred Length: 2 Years *Program Size:* 2
Program ID: 445-48-21-020

Washington

Seattle

Children's Hospital and Medical Center Program

Sponsor: Children's Hospital and Medical Center

Program Director:
David Tapper, MD
Children's Hospital and Regional Med Ctr
4800 Sand Point Way NE
Seattle, WA 98105-0371
Tel: 206 526-2039 *Fax:* 206 526-2257
E-mail: dtappe@chmc.org
Internet: http://www.home.chmc.org
Accred Length: 2 Years *Program Size:* 2
Program ID: 445-54-11-011

Pediatric Urology (Urology)

California

San Diego

Naval Medical Center (San Diego) Program
Sponsor: Naval Medical Center (San Diego)
Children's Hospital and Health Center
Program Director:
George W Kaplan, MD
7930 Frost St
Ste 407
San Diego, CA 92123
Tel: 619 279-8527 *Fax:* 619 279-8876
Accred Length: 1 Year *Program Size:* 1
Program ID: 485-05-21-004
US Armed Services Program

San Francisco

University of California (San Francisco) Program
Sponsor: University of California (San Francisco) School of Medicine
University of California (San Francisco) Medical Center
Program Director:
Laurence Baskin, MD
Rm U-575/Box 0738
533 Parnassus Ave
San Francisco, CA 94143-0738
Tel: 415 476-1611 *Fax:* 415 476-8849
Accred Length: 1 Year *Program Size:* 1
Program ID: 485-05-21-011

Indiana

Indianapolis

Indiana University School of Medicine Program
Sponsor: Indiana University School of Medicine
Clarian Riley Hospital for Children
Program Director:
Michael O Koch, MD
535 N Barnhill Dr/Ste 420
Indianapolis, IN 46202
Tel: 317 274-7338 *Fax:* 317 274-0174
Accred Length: 1 Year *Program Size:* 0
Program ID: 485-17-21-015

Maryland

Baltimore

Johns Hopkins University Program
Sponsor: Johns Hopkins University School of Medicine
Johns Hopkins Hospital
Program Director:
John P Gearhart, MD
Dept of Ped Urology
Johns Hopkins Hospital
600 N Wolfe St/Marburg 149
Baltimore, MD 21287-2101
Tel: 410 955-5358 *Fax:* 410 955-0833
E-mail: jpgearha@jhu.edu
Internet: http://www.med.ju.edu/pediurol/
Accred Length: 1 Year *Program Size:* 1
Program ID: 485-23-21-009

Massachusetts

Boston

Harvard Medical School Program
Sponsor: Children's Hospital
Program Director:
Alan B Retik, MD
Dept. of Urology
Children's Hospital
300 Longwood Ave
Boston, MA 02115
Tel: 617 355-7796 *Fax:* 617 355-8336
E-mail: retik@a!.tch.harvard.edu
Accred Length: 1 Year *Program Size:* 2
Program ID: 485-24-21-006

Michigan

Detroit

Wayne State University/Detroit Medical Center Program
Sponsor: Wayne State University/Detroit Medical Center
Children's Hospital of Michigan
Harper Hospital
Program Director:
Ricardo Gonzalez, MD
Div of Ped Urology
3901 Beaubien Blvd
Detroit, MI 48201
Tel: 313 745-5588 *Fax:* 313 993-8738
E-mail: rgonzale@med.wayne.edu
Accred Length: 1 Year *Program Size:* 2
Program ID: 485-25-21-010

Ohio

Cincinnati

University Hospital/University of Cincinnati College of Medicine Program
Sponsor: Children's Hospital Medical Center
University Hospital Inc
Program Director:
Curtis A Sheldon, MD
Children's Hospital Med Ctr
3333 Burnet Ave/PW-5SE
Cincinnati, OH 45229
Tel: 513 636-7143 *Fax:* 513 636-6753
Internet: http://www.chmcc.org
Accred Length: 1 Year *Program Size:* 1
Program ID: 485-38-21-014

Pennsylvania

Philadelphia

University of Pennsylvania Program
Sponsor: Hospital of the University of Pennsylvania
Children's Hospital of Philadelphia
Program Director:
Douglas A Canning, MD
Children's Hospital
Dept of Ped Urology
34th St and Civic Center Blvd
Philadelphia, PA 19104
Tel: 215 590-2767 *Fax:* 215 590-3985
E-mail: canning@email.chop.edu
Internet: http://www.chop.edu
Accred Length: 1 Year *Program Size:* 2
Program ID: 485-41-21-002

Tennessee

Memphis

University of Tennessee Program
Sponsor: University of Tennessee College of Medicine
LeBonheur Children's Medical Center
Program Director:
H Norman Noe, MD
Univ of Tennessee
Div of Ped Urology
770 Estate Pl
Memphis, TN 38120
Tel: 901 681-4030 *Fax:* 901 681-4094
Accred Length: 1 Year *Program Size:* 1
Program ID: 485-47-21-007

Texas

Houston

Baylor College of Medicine Program
Sponsor: Baylor College of Medicine
Texas Children's Hospital
Program Director:
Edmond T Gonzales Jr, MD
Scott Dept of Urology
6621 Fannin St
Feigin Ctr/Ste 270
Houston, TX 77030
Tel: 713 770-3160 *Fax:* 713 770-3159
E-mail: gonzales@bcm.tmc.edu
Internet: http://www.bcm.tmc.edu/urol
Accred Length: 1 Year *Program Size:* 2
Program ID: 485-48-21-008

Washington

Seattle

University of Washington Program
Sponsor: University of Washington School of Medicine
Children's Hospital and Medical Center
Program Director:
Michael E Mitchell, MD
Children's Hospital and Regional Med Ctr
Div of Ped Urology
PO Box 5371
Seattle, WA 98105
Tel: 206 526-2039 *Fax:* 206 527-3955
E-mail: mmitch@chmc.org
Internet:
http://www.home.chmc.org/department/surgery/urology.htm
Accred Length: 1 Year *Program Size:* 2
Program ID: 485-54-21-012

Pediatrics

Alabama

Birmingham

University of Alabama Medical Center Program
Sponsor: University of Alabama Hospital
Children's Hospital of Alabama
Program Director:
Michele H Nichols, MD
Univ of Alabama
1600 Seventh Ave S/Ste 604-ACC
Birmingham, AL 35233-1711
Tel: 205 939-9589 *Fax:* 205 939-9977
E-mail: uabkids@peds.uab.edu
Internet: http://www.peds.uab.edu
Accred Length: 3 Years *Program Size:* 48 (*GY1:* 16)
Subspecialties: CCP, NPM, PDI, PDP, PG, PHO
Program ID: 320-01-21-017

Mobile

University of South Alabama Program
Sponsor: University of South Alabama Medical Center
Program Director:
Franklin Trimm, MD
Univ of South Alabama
1504 Spring Hill Ave/Rm 5326
Mobile, AL 36604
Tel: 334 434-3961 *Fax:* 334 434-3980
Internet: http://www.usouthal.edu/residencyprograms
Accred Length: 3 Years *Program Size:* 20 (*GY1:* 6)
Program ID: 320-01-21-019

Arizona

Phoenix

Phoenix Hospitals Program
Sponsor: Phoenix Children's Hospital
Maricopa Medical Center
Program Director:
Grace L Caputo, MD MPH
Phoenix Children's Hospital
Medical Education Dept
909 E Brill
Phoenix, AZ 85006
Tel: 602 239-5781 *Fax:* 602 239-4806
E-mail: dlove@phxchildrens.com
Internet: http://www.maricopa.gov/medcenter/mmc/html
Accred Length: 3 Years *Program Size:* 36 (*GY1:* 12)
Program ID: 320-03-32-020

St Joseph's Hospital and Medical Center Program
Sponsor: St Joseph's Hospital and Medical Center
Program Director:
Matilda Garcia, MD
350 W Thomas Rd
Phoenix, AZ 85013
Tel: 602 406-3122 *Fax:* 602 406-4102
E-mail: jgaffne@mha.chw.edu
Internet: http://www.chw.edu/mha/mha.html
Accred Length: 3 Years *Program Size:* 18 (*GY1:* 6)
Program ID: 320-03-21-371

Tucson

University of Arizona Program
Sponsor: University of Arizona College of Medicine
Tucson Medical Center
University Medical Center
Program Director:
Leslie L Barton, MD
Univ of Arizona Health Sciences Ctr
Dept of Pediatrics
1501 N Campbell Ave/PO Box 245073
Tucson, AZ 85724-5073
Tel: 520 626-7944 *Fax:* 520 626-3636
E-mail: cfrost@peds.arizona.edu
Internet: http://www.ahsc.arizona.edu/peds.resid/
Accred Length: 3 Years *Program Size:* 38 (*GY1:* 12)
Subspecialties: CCP, NPM, PDP, PHO
Program ID: 320-03-21-021

Arkansas

Little Rock

University of Arkansas for Medical Sciences Program
Sponsor: University of Arkansas College of Medicine
Arkansas Children's Hospital
University Hospital of Arkansas
Program Director:
Gordon E Schutze, MD
Univ of Arkansas for Med Sciences
Arkansas Children's Hospital
800 Marshall St
Little Rock, AR 72202-3591
Tel: 501 320-1875 *Fax:* 501 320-3196
E-mail: pedshousestaff@exchange.uams.edu
Internet: http://www.ach.uams.edu/
Accred Length: 3 Years *Program Size:* 53 (*GY1:* 18)
Subspecialties: CCP, NPM, PDE, PDI, PG
Program ID: 320-04-21-022

California

Fresno

University of California (San Francisco)/Fresno Program
Sponsor: UCSF-Fresno Medical Education Program
University Medical Center
Valley Children's Hospital
Program Director:
Bjorn W Nilson, MD MPH
Univ Med Ctr
Dept of Pediatrics
445 S Cedar Ave
Fresno, CA 93702
Tel: 209 459-5751 *Fax:* 209 459-3852
Accred Length: 3 Years *Program Size:* 23 (*GY1:* 8)
Subspecialties: TY
Program ID: 320-05-11-024

Loma Linda

Loma Linda University Program
Sponsor: Loma Linda University Medical Center
Riverside County Regional Medical Center
Program Director:
Richard E Chinnock, MD
Loma Linda Univ Med Ctr-Children's Hospital
11175 Campus St/Coleman Rm A1111
Loma Linda, CA 92354
Tel: 909 824-4174 *Fax:* 909 824-4184
E-mail: amelia_maeda@ccmail.llu.edu
Internet: http://www.llu.edu/lluch/pedres/
Accred Length: 3 Years *Program Size:* 60 (*GY1:* 20)
Subspecialties: CCP, NPM
Program ID: 320-05-11-026

Los Angeles

Cedars-Sinai Medical Center Program
Sponsor: Cedars-Sinai Medical Center
Program Director:
Lee Todd Miller, MD
Cedars Sinai Med Ctr
Dept of Pediatrics/Rm 4310
8700 Beverly Blvd
Los Angeles, CA 90048
Tel: 310 855-4780 *Fax:* 310 967-0145
E-mail: lee.miller@cshs.org
Internet: http://www.csmc.edu/pediatrics
Accred Length: 3 Years *Program Size:* 28 (*GY1:* 10)
Subspecialties: NPM, PN
Program ID: 320-05-31-027

Charles R Drew University Program
Sponsor: Charles R Drew University of Medicine and Science
LAC-King/Drew Medical Center
Program Director:
Glenda Lindsey, MD
Martin Luther King Jr-Drew Med Ctr
12021 S Wilmington Ave
Los Angeles, CA 90059
Tel: 310 668-4664 *Fax:* 310 668-3108
E-mail: galindsey@pol.net
Accred Length: 3 Years *Program Size:* 33 (*GY1:* 11)
Program ID: 320-05-11-031

Children's Hospital of Los Angeles Program
Sponsor: Children's Hospital of Los Angeles
Program Director:
Eyal Ben-Isaac, MD
Childrens Hospital Los Angeles
4650 Sunset Blvd/MS 68
Los Angeles, CA 90027
Tel: 323 669-2122 *Fax:* 323 668-7926
Internet: http://www.chla.org
Accred Length: 3 Years *Program Size:* 76 (*GY1:* 26)
Subspecialties: ADL, CCP, PDC, PDE, PDI, PDP, PG, PHO, PN
Program ID: 320-05-11-028

Southern California Kaiser Permanente Medical Care (Los Angeles) Program
Sponsor: Southern California Kaiser Permanente Medical Group
Kaiser Foundation Hospital (Los Angeles)
Program Director:
Steven D Woods, MD
Kaiser Permanente Med Care
393 E Walnut St
Pasadena, CA 91188-8013
Tel: 800 541-7946
Internet: http://www.kpscal.org
Accred Length: 3 Years *Program Size:* 18 (*GY1:* 6)
Program ID: 320-05-12-029

UCLA Medical Center Program
Sponsor: UCLA School of Medicine
Olive View-UCLA Medical Center
UCLA Medical Center
Program Director:
Stuart Slavin, MD
Univ of California Sch of Med
Dept of Pediatrics
10833 Le Conte Ave
Los Angeles, CA 90095-1752
Tel: 310 794-2169 *Fax:* 310 825-6394
E-mail: epotter@pediatrics.medsch.ucla.edu
Internet: http://www.peds.medsch.ucla.edu
Accred Length: 3 Years *Program Size:* 57 (*GY1:* 19)
Subspecialties: CCP, NPM, PDC, PDE, PDI, PG, PHO, PN
Program ID: 320-05-21-032

University of Southern California Program
Sponsor: Los Angeles County-USC Medical Center
Program Director:
Lawrence M Opas, MD
Los Angeles County-USC Med Ctr
1240 N Mission Rd
L-902
Los Angeles, CA 90033-1084
Tel: 213 226-3691, ext 3691 *Fax:* 213 226-4380
Accred Length: 3 Years *Program Size:* 30 (*GY1:* 10)
Subspecialties: NPM, PHO
Program ID: 320-05-11-030

White Memorial Medical Center Program
Sponsor: White Memorial Medical Center
Program Director:
Anthony T Hirsch, MD
White Memorial Med Ctr
1720 Cesar E Chavez Ave
Los Angeles, CA 90033
Tel: 323 268-5000 *Fax:* 323 881-8601
Internet: http://www. whitememorial.com
Accred Length: 3 Years *Program Size:* 13 (*GY1:* 4)
Program ID: 320-05-11-033

Oakland

Children's Hospital-Oakland Program
Sponsor: Children's Hospital-Oakland
Program Director:
Theodore J Chaconas, MD
Children's Hospital
747 52nd St
Oakland, CA 94609
Tel: 510 428-3786 *Fax:* 510 601-3979
Accred Length: 3 Years *Program Size:* 68 (*GY1:* 23)
Subspecialties: PDI, PHO
Program ID: 320-05-31-034

Kaiser Permanente Medical Group (Northern California) Program
Sponsor: Kaiser Permanente Medical Group (Northern California)
Kaiser Permanente Medical Center (Oakland)
Program Director:
Stuart A Zangwill, MD MPH
Kaiser Permanente Med Ctr
Dept of Pediatrics
280 W MacArthur Blvd
Oakland, CA 94611-5693
Tel: 510 596-6126 *Fax:* 510 596-1571
Accred Length: 3 Years *Program Size:* 15 (*GY1:* 5)
Program ID: 320-05-12-035

Orange

Children's Hospital of Orange County Program
Sponsor: Children's Hospital of Orange County
St Joseph Hospital
Program Director:
David J Lang, MD
Children's Hospital
Residency Program
455 S Main St
Orange, CA 92868
Tel: 714 532-8338 *Fax:* 714 289-4010
Accred Length: 3 Years *Program Size:* 36 (*GY1:* 12)
Subspecialties: PHO, PPR
Program ID: 320-05-21-386

University of California (Irvine) Program
Sponsor: University of California (Irvine) Medical Center
Long Beach Memorial Medical Center
Program Director:
Jennifer Johnson, MD
Univ of California Irvine Med Ctr
Ped Residency Office/4482
101 City Dr S/Bldg 2 Rte 81
Orange, CA 92868-3298
Tel: 714 456-5631 *Fax:* 714 456-6660
E-mail: lmphilli@uci.edu
Internet: http://www.ucihs.uci.edu/pediatrics
Accred Length: 3 Years *Program Size:* 48 (*GY1:* 16)
Subspecialties: NPM, PDP, PG
Program ID: 320-05-21-025

Sacramento

University of California (Davis) Program
Sponsor: University of California (Davis) Medical Center
Program Director:
Daniel C West, MD
Univ of California Davis Med Ctr
Dept of Pediatrics
2516 Stockton Blvd
Sacramento, CA 95817
Tel: 916 734-2428 *Fax:* 916 456-2236
E-mail: dcwest@ucdavis.edu
Internet: http://children.ucdmc.ucdavis.edu/
Accred Length: 3 Years *Program Size:* 34 (*GY1:* 11)
Subspecialties: NPM, PHO
Program ID: 320-05-11-023

San Diego

Naval Medical Center (San Diego) Program
Sponsor: Naval Medical Center (San Diego)
Program Director:
Capt Norman J Waecker, MD
Naval Med Ctr
Dept of Pediatrics/Suite 100
34520 Bob Wilson Dr
San Diego, CA 92134-2100
Tel: 619 532-6474 *Fax:* 619 532-9902
E-mail: nwaecker@snd10.med.navy.mil
Accred Length: 3 Years *Program Size:* 20 (*GY1:* 8)
Program ID: 320-05-11-012
US Armed Services Program

University of California (San Diego) Program
Sponsor: University of California (San Diego) Medical Center
Children's Hospital and Health Center
Program Director:
Michael Gottschalk, MD PhD
UCSD Med Ctr
Dept of Pediatrics
PO Box 3729
San Diego, CA 92163-1729
Tel: 619 543-5881 *Fax:* 619 543-6824
E-mail: lkadane@ucsd.edu
Accred Length: 3 Years *Program Size:* 42 (*GY1:* 14)
Subspecialties: CCP, NPM, PDC, PDE, PDI, PG, PN, TY
Program ID: 320-05-31-036

San Francisco

University of California (San Francisco) Program
Sponsor: University of California (San Francisco) School of Medicine
Mount Zion Medical Center of the University of California
San Francisco General Hospital Medical Center
University of California (San Francisco) Medical Center
Program Director:
Robert K Kamei, MD
Dept of Pediatrics
505 Parnassus Ave/Box 0110
San Francisco, CA 94143-0110
Tel: 415 476-5001 *Fax:* 415 476-4009
Internet: http://www.ucsf.edu
Accred Length: 3 Years *Program Size:* 81 (*GY1:* 28)
Subspecialties: CCP, NPM, PDC, PDE, PDI, PDP, PG, PHO, PN, PPR
Program ID: 320-05-21-040

Stanford

Stanford University Program
Sponsor: Stanford University Hospital
Lucile Salter Packard Children's Hospital at Stanford
Santa Clara Valley Medical Center
Program Director:
Theodore C Sectish, MD
Lucile S Packard Children's Health Services
725 Welch Rd
Palo Alto, CA 94304
Tel: 650 497-8979 *Fax:* 650 497-8228
E-mail: peds.res@lpch.stanford.edu
Internet: http://www.-med.stanford.edu/lpch/pedsres/
Accred Length: 3 Years *Program Size:* 59 (*GY1:* 19)
Subspecialties: CCP, NPM, PDC, PDE, PDI, PDP, PG, PHO, PN, TY
Program ID: 320-05-21-041

Torrance

Los Angeles County-Harbor-UCLA Medical Center Program
Sponsor: Los Angeles County-Harbor-UCLA Medical Center
Program Director:
Carol D Berkowitz, MD
Los Angeles County-Harbor-UCLA Med Ctr
1000 W Carson St/Box 437
Torrance, CA 90509-2910
Tel: 310 222-3091 *Fax:* 310 533-8579
Internet: http://www.salu.net/hucla_peds
Accred Length: 3 Years *Program Size:* 30 (*GY1:* 10)
Subspecialties: CCP, NPM, PDE, PDI
Program ID: 320-05-11-042

Travis AFB

David Grant Medical Center Program
Sponsor: David Grant Medical Center
Program Director:
Col Richard L Friederich, MD
Dept of Pediatrics
David Grant Med Ctr/60MDOS/SGOC
101 Bodin Cir
Travis AFB, CA 94535-1800
Tel: 707 423-7176 *Fax:* 707 423-5314
Accred Length: 3 Years *Program Size:* 19 (*GY1:* 6)
Program ID: 320-05-11-001
US Armed Services Program

Colorado

Denver

University of Colorado Program
Sponsor: University of Colorado Health Sciences Center
Children's Hospital
Denver Health and Hospitals
Program Director:
Mary P Glode, MD
Univ of Colorado Health Sciences Ctr-TCH
1056 E 19th Ave/Box 158
Denver, CO 80218
Tel: 303 861-6884 *Fax:* 303 764-8189
E-mail: celio.janet@tchden.org
Internet: http://www.uchsc.edu/sm/gme/peds.html
Accred Length: 3 Years *Program Size:* 63 (*GY1:* 20)
Subspecialties: CCP, NPM, PDC, PDE, PDI, PDP, PG, PHO, PN
Program ID: 320-07-21-043

Connecticut

Bridgeport

Yale University (Bridgeport) Program
Sponsor: Bridgeport Hospital
Program Director:
Thomas L Kennedy, MD
Bridgeport Hospital
267 Grant St
Bridgeport, CT 06610-2870
Tel: 203 384-3712 *Fax:* 203 384-4031
Accred Length: 3 Years *Program Size:* 11 (*GY1:* 3)
Program ID: 320-08-31-044

Farmington

University of Connecticut Program
Sponsor: University of Connecticut School of Medicine
Connecticut Children's Medical Center
St Francis Hospital and Medical Center
Program Director:
Edwin L Zalneraitis, MD
Connecticut Children's Med Ctr
Ctr for Education
282 Washington St
Hartford, CT 06106-3316
Tel: 860 545-9970 *Fax:* 860 545-9975
E-mail: avelez@ccmckids.org
Accred Length: 3 Years *Program Size:* 42 (*GY1:* 13)
Subspecialties: NPM, PDE, PDP
Program ID: 320-08-21-045

New Haven

Yale-New Haven Medical Center Program
Sponsor: Yale-New Haven Hospital
Hospital of St Raphael
Program Director:
Alan H Friedman, MD
Yale-New Haven Med Ctr, Dept of Pediatrics
333 Cedar St
PO Box 208064
New Haven, CT 06520-8064
Tel: 203 785-6662 *Fax:* 203 737-2461
E-mail: alan.friedman@yale.edu
Internet: http://info.med.yale.edu/pediat/residency.html
Accred Length: 3 Years *Program Size:* 51 (*GY1:* 15)
Subspecialties: CCP, NPM, PDC, PDE, PDI, PDP, PG, PHO, PN
Program ID: 320-08-21-046

Delaware

Wilmington

Thomas Jefferson University/duPont Hospital for Children Program
Sponsor: Thomas Jefferson University Hospital
duPont Hospital for Children
Christiana Care Health Services Inc
Program Director:
Steven M Selbst, MD
Alfred I duPont Hospital for Children
PO Box 269
Wilmington, DE 19899
Tel: 302 651-5874 *Fax:* 302 651-5954
E-mail: kwaite@nemours.org
Internet: http://www.kidshealth.org
Accred Length: 3 Years *Program Size:* 56 (*GY1:* 18)
Subspecialties: NPM
Program ID: 320-41-21-210

District of Columbia

Washington

George Washington University Program
Sponsor: Children's National Medical Center
Program Director:
Bernhard L Wiedermann, MD
Children's National Med Ctr
111 Michigan Ave NW
Ste W 3.5-600
Washington, DC 20010-2970
Tel: 202 884-3950 *Fax:* 202 884-4741
Internet: http://www.cnmc.org
Accred Length: 3 Years *Program Size:* 72 (*GY1:* 24)
Subspecialties: CCP, NPM, PDC, PDI, PDP, PG, PHO, PN
Program ID: 320-10-21-051

Georgetown University Program
Sponsor: Georgetown University Medical Center
Program Director:
Dorothy A Richmond, MD
Georgetown Univ Hospital
Dept of Pediatrics
3800 Reservoir Rd NW/2 PHC
Washington, DC 20007-2197
Tel: 202 687-8882 *Fax:* 202 784-1359
Internet: http://gucfm.georgetown.edu/pedres.html
Accred Length: 3 Years *Program Size:* 32 (*GY1:* 10)
Subspecialties: CCP, NPM, PDE, PN, TY
Program ID: 320-10-21-050

Howard University Program
Sponsor: Howard University Hospital
District of Columbia General Hospital
Program Director:
Renee R Jenkins, MD
Howard Univ Hospital
Dept of Pediatrics/Child Health
2041 Georgia Ave NW
Washington, DC 20060
Tel: 202 865-1592 *Fax:* 202 865-4558
Internet: http://138.238.107.150/huhosp/
Accred Length: 3 Years *Program Size:* 44 (*GY1:* 12)
Program ID: 320-10-21-049

Florida

Gainesville

University of Florida Program
Sponsor: University of Florida College of Medicine
Shands Hospital at the University of Florida
Program Director:
James M Sherman, MD
Univ of Florida-Shands Hospital
Ped Education Box 100296
1600 SW Archer Rd
Gainesville, FL 32610-0296
Tel: 352 395-0451 *Fax:* 352 395-0621
E-mail: sherman.peds@mail.health.ufl.edu
Accred Length: 3 Years *Program Size:* 45 (*GY1:* 15)
Subspecialties: CCP, NPM, PDC, PDE, PDP, PG, PHO, PN
Program ID: 320-11-31-053

Jacksonville

University of Florida Health Science Center/Jacksonville Program
Sponsor: University of Florida College of Medicine at Jacksonville
University Medical Center (UFHSC/J)
Baptist Medical Center (UFHSC/J)
Nemours Children's Clinic (UFHSC/J)
Program Director:
James Kirk, DO
Office of Med Education
655 W 8th St
Jacksonville, FL 32209-6511
Tel: 904 549-3049 *Fax:* 904 549-4845
E-mail: job@umc8.umc.ufl.edu
Internet: http://www.ufhscj,edu
Accred Length: 3 Years *Program Size:* 30 (*GY1:* 10)
Subspecialties: CCP, PDI
Program ID: 320-11-21-055

Miami

Miami Children's Hospital Program
Sponsor: Miami Children's Hospital
Program Director:
Fima Lifshitz, MD
Miami Children's Hospital
3100 SW 62nd St
Miami, FL 33155-3009
Tel: 305 666-6511, ext 2565 *Fax:* 305 669-6531
E-mail: cynthia.gibson@mch.com
Accred Length: 3 Years *Program Size:* 60 (*GY1:* 20)
Subspecialties: CCP
Program ID: 320-11-12-057

University of Miami-Jackson Memorial Medical Center Program
Sponsor: University of Miami-Jackson Memorial Medical Center
Program Director:
Charles H Pegelow, MD
Univ of Miami Sch of Med
Dept of Pediatrics
PO Box 016960 (R131)
Miami, FL 33101-6960
Tel: 305 585-6042 *Fax:* 305 545-6018
E-mail: cpegelow@mednet.med.miami.edu
Accred Length: 3 Years *Program Size:* 62 (*GY1:* 20)
Subspecialties: CCP, NPM, PDC, PDE, PDP, PN
Program ID: 320-11-11-056

Orlando

Orlando Regional Healthcare System Program
Sponsor: Orlando Regional Medical Center
Arnold Palmer Hospital for Children and Women
Program Director:
Michael J Muszynski, MD
86 W Underwood St/Ste 202
Orlando, FL 32806
Tel: 407 649-6876 *Fax:* 407 872-0544
E-mail: pedsres@orhs.org
Internet: http://www.orhs.org
Accred Length: 3 Years *Program Size:* 30 (*GY1:* 10)
Program ID: 320-11-31-058

Pensacola

University of Florida College of Medicine (Pensacola) Program
Sponsor: University of Florida College of Medicine
Sacred Heart Hospital of Pensacola
Program Director:
Robert K Wilson Jr, MD
Sacred Heart Children's Hospital
5151 N Ninth Ave
Pensacola, FL 32504
Tel: 850 416-7658 *Fax:* 850 416-6708
Internet: http://www.sacred-heart.org
Accred Length: 3 Years *Program Size:* 15 (*GY1:* 5)
Program ID: 320-11-21-059

Tampa

University of South Florida Program
Sponsor: University of South Florida College of Medicine
All Children's Hospital
Tampa General Healthcare
Program Director:
Lynn Ringenberg, MD
801 Sixth St S
PO Box 31020
St Petersburg, FL 33731-8920
Tel: 727 892-4106 *Fax:* 727 892-8804
E-mail: millerd@allkids.org
Internet: http://www.usfpeds.med.usf.edu
Accred Length: 3 Years *Program Size:* 57 (*GY1:* 18)
Subspecialties: NPM, PDE
Program ID: 320-11-21-060

Georgia

Atlanta

Emory University Program
Sponsor: Emory University School of Medicine
Egleston Children's Hospital at Emory University
Grady Memorial Hospital
Program Director:
Susie Buchter, MD
Emory Univ Sch of Med
Dept of Pediatrics
69 Butler St SE
Atlanta, GA 30303-2607
Tel: 404 616-5133 *Fax:* 404 525-2816
E-mail: mbrad01@emory.edu
Internet: http://www.emory.edu/peds/resid/pag1.htm
Accred Length: 3 Years *Program Size:* 54 (*GY1:* 18)
Subspecialties: CCP, NPM, PDC, PDE, PDI, PHO, TY
Program ID: 320-12-21-061

Augusta

Medical College of Georgia Program
Sponsor: Medical College of Georgia Hospital and Clinics
University Hospital
Program Director:
Valera L Hudson, MD
Med Coll of Georgia
1120 15th St/BG 122
Augusta, GA 30912-3700
Tel: 706 721-9442 *Fax:* 706 721-9463
E-mail: internet:deptped.vhudson@mail.mcg.edu
Internet: http://www.mcg.edu/resident/pedsresidency/
Accred Length: 3 Years *Program Size:* 30 (*GY1:* 10)
Subspecialties: CCP, NPM, PDC
Program ID: 320-12-21-062

Macon

Mercer University School of Medicine Program
Sponsor: Medical Center of Central Georgia
Program Director:
Marcia B Guzzardo, MD
Med Ctr of Central Georgia
777 Hemlock St
Hospital Box 42
Macon, GA 31201
Tel: 912 633-7500 *Fax:* 912 633-5002
E-mail: beard.teresa@mail.mccg.org
Internet:
http://gain.mercer.edu/musm/pediatrics/pediares.htm
Accred Length: 3 Years *Program Size:* 12 (*GY1:* 4)
Program ID: 320-12-21-398

Savannah

Memorial Medical Center Program
Sponsor: Memorial Medical Center
Program Director:
Martin H Greenberg, MD
Memorial Med Ctr
4700 Waters Ave
PO Box 23089
Savannah, GA 31404
Tel: 912 350-8193 *Fax:* 912 350-7221
Accred Length: 3 Years *Program Size:* 12 (*GY1:* 4)
Program ID: 320-12-21-400

Hawaii

Honolulu

Tripler Army Medical Center Program

Sponsor: Tripler Army Medical Center

Program Director:
Lt Col Charles W Callahan, DO
Tripler Army Med Ctr
Dept of Pediatrics
1 Jarrett White Rd
Tripler AMC, HI 96859-5000
Tel: 808 433-6407 *Fax:* 808 433-4837
E-mail: charles_w.callahan@tamc.chcs.amedd.army.mil
Internet:
http://www.tamc.amedd.army.mil/dpts/peds/peds.htm
Accred Length: 3 Years *Program Size:* 18 (*GY1:* 6)
Subspecialties: TY
Program ID: 320-14-21-007
US Armed Services Program

University of Hawaii Program

Sponsor: University of Hawaii John A Burns School of Medicine
Kapiolani Medical Center for Women and Children

Program Director:
Christian Derauf, MD
Kapiolani Med Ctr for Women and Children
1319 Punahou St
Honolulu, HI 96826
Tel: 808 973-8387 *Fax:* 808 949-4232
E-mail: deraufc@jabsom.biomed.hawaii.edu
Internet:
http://www.medworld.biomed.hawaii.edu/hrp.html
Accred Length: 3 Years *Program Size:* 19 (*GY1:* 6)
Subspecialties: NPM
Program ID: 320-14-21-063

Illinois

Chicago

Catholic Health Partners Program

Sponsor: Catholic Health Partners
Columbus Hospital
St Anthony Hospital

Program Director:
Howard Weiss, MD
Dept of Pediatrics
Columbus Hospital
2520 N Lakeview Ave
Chicago, IL 60614
Tel: 773 388-5908 *Fax:* 773 883-8023
Internet: http://www.cath-health.org
Accred Length: 3 Years *Program Size:* 12 (*GY1:* 4)
Program ID: 320-16-31-064

Cook County Hospital Program

Sponsor: Cook County Hospital

Program Director:
Richard C Mervis, MD
Cook County Hospital
Dept of Planning Educ and Research
1900 W Polk St/Rm 408
Chicago, IL 60612
Tel: 312 633-6705
Internet: http://www.countypeds.org
Accred Length: 3 Years *Program Size:* 41 (*GY1:* 13)
Subspecialties: NPM
Program ID: 320-16-11-065

McGaw Medical Center of Northwestern University Program

Sponsor: Northwestern University Medical School
Children's Memorial Medical Center
Evanston Hospital

Program Director:
Sharon M Unti, MD
Children's Memorial Hospital
2300 Children's Plaza/Box 18
Chicago, IL 60614-2620
Tel: 773 880-4302 *Fax:* 773 880-3067
Accred Length: 3 Years *Program Size:* 73 (*GY1:* 24)
Subspecialties: CCP, NPM, PDC, PDE, PDI, PDP, PHO, PN, PPR
Program ID: 320-16-21-070

Mount Sinai Hospital Medical Center of Chicago Program

Sponsor: Mount Sinai Hospital Medical Center of Chicago
Schwab Rehabilitation Hospital and Care Network

Program Director:
Gopal Srinivasan, MD
Mount Sinai Hospital Med Ctr
Dept of Pediatrics/OS451
California Ave at 15th St
Chicago, IL 60608-1797
Tel: 773 257-6474 *Fax:* 773 257-6193
Accred Length: 3 Years *Program Size:* 15 (*GY1:* 5)
Program ID: 320-16-21-408

Rush-Presbyterian-St Luke's Medical Center Program

Sponsor: Rush-Presbyterian-St Luke's Medical Center

Program Director:
Karen R Judy, MD
Rush-Presbyterian-St Luke's Med Ctr
1653 W Congress Pkwy
Jones Bldg/Rm 770
Chicago, IL 60612-3833
Tel: 312 942-8928 *Fax:* 312 942-2243
Internet:
http://www.rush.edu/departments/peditric/residency
Accred Length: 3 Years *Program Size:* 33 (*GY1:* 11)
Subspecialties: CCP
Program ID: 320-16-31-069

University of Chicago Program

Sponsor: University of Chicago Hospitals
University of Chicago Children's Hospital

Program Director:
Patrick T Horn, MD PhD
Univ of Chicago Children's Hospital
5839 S Maryland Ave/MC6380
Chicago, IL 60637-1470
Tel: 773 702-5444 *Fax:* 773 834-0748
E-mail: phorn@babies.bsd.uchicago.edu
Internet:
http://peds-www.bsd.uchicago.edu/residency/index.htm/
Accred Length: 3 Years *Program Size:* 60 (*GY1:* 20)
Subspecialties: CCP, NPM, PDE, PDI, PDP, PG, PHO, PPR
Program ID: 320-16-11-073

University of Illinois College of Medicine at Chicago Program

Sponsor: University of Illinois College of Medicine at Chicago
Michael Reese Hospital and Medical Center
Ravenswood Hospital Medical Center
University of Illinois Hospital and Clinics

Program Director:
Peter Noronha, MD PhD
Univ of Illinois Hospital
840 S Wood St (M/C 856)
Chicago, IL 60612
Tel: 312 996-8297 *Fax:* 312 413-1526
E-mail: pan@uic.edu
Internet: http://www.uic.edu/com/mcpd/
Accred Length: 3 Years *Program Size:* 66 (*GY1:* 22)
Subspecialties: NPM, PDE
Program ID: 320-16-11-074

Maywood

Loyola University Program

Sponsor: Loyola University Medical Center

Program Director:
Simon P Ros, MD
Foster G McGaw Hospital
Dept of Pediatrics
2160 S First Ave
Maywood, IL 60153-6015
Tel: 708 327-9124 *Fax:* 708 327-9132
E-mail: adevitt@lumc.edu
Internet: http://www.luc.edu/childhospital
Accred Length: 3 Years *Program Size:* 27 (*GY1:* 9)
Subspecialties: NPM, PDE
Program ID: 320-16-21-075

Oak Lawn

Christ Hospital and Medical Center Program

Sponsor: Christ Hospital and Medical Center

Program Director:
Larry M Roy, MD
Christ Hospital and Med Ctr
4440 W 95th St/Rm 3175H
Oak Lawn, IL 60453
Tel: 708 346-5825 *Fax:* 708 346-3142
Accred Length: 3 Years *Program Size:* 38 (*GY1:* 12)
Subspecialties: PDC
Program ID: 320-16-21-382

Park Ridge

Lutheran General Hospital Program

Sponsor: Lutheran General Hospital

Program Director:
Jerome R Kraut, MD
Lutheran General Children's Hospital
1775 Dempster St
Park Ridge, IL 60068-1174
Tel: 847 723-5986 *Fax:* 847 723-2325
E-mail: judy.fregetto@advocatehealth.com
Internet:
http://www.advocatehealth.com/residency/residency.html
Accred Length: 3 Years *Program Size:* 33 (*GY1:* 12)
Subspecialties: CCP, NPM
Program ID: 320-16-12-077

Peoria

University of Illinois College of Medicine at Peoria Program

Sponsor: University of Illinois College of Medicine at Peoria
St Francis Medical Center

Program Director:
Jalayne M Lapke, MD
Univ of Illinois Coll of Med-Peoria
Children's Hospital-OSF St Francis Med Ctr
530 NE Glen Oak Ave
Peoria, IL 61637
Tel: 800 599-7337
Internet: http://www.uicomp.uic.edu/uicomp.html
Accred Length: 3 Years *Program Size:* 15 (*GY1:* 5)
Program ID: 320-16-21-078

Springfield

Southern Illinois University Program

Sponsor: Southern Illinois University School of Medicine
St John's Hospital

Program Director:
Scott S MacGilvray, MD
Southern Illinois Univ Sch of Med
PO Box 19230
301 N Eighth St
Springfield, IL 62794-1614
Tel: 217 782-1957 *Fax:* 217 785-4117
E-mail: mcorrigan@pav-nt1.siumed.edu
Internet: http://www.siumed.edu/peds/hompage.htm
Accred Length: 3 Years *Program Size:* 13 (*GY1:* 4)
Program ID: 320-16-21-079

Indiana

Indianapolis

Indiana University School of Medicine Program

Sponsor: Indiana University School of Medicine
Clarian Methodist Hospital of Indiana
Clarian Riley Hospital for Children
William N Wishard Memorial Hospital

Program Director:
Suzanne L Bowyer, MD
Indiana Univ Med Ctr
702 Barnhill Dr/Rm 5867
Indianapolis, IN 46202-5225
Tel: 317 274-4034 *Fax:* 317 274-1476
Internet: http://www.iupui.edu/it/deptpeds/
Accred Length: 3 Years *Program Size:* 70 (*GY1:* 24)
Subspecialties: ADL, NPM, PDC, PDE, PDP, PG, PHO, PN
Program ID: 320-17-21-080

Iowa

Des Moines

Iowa Methodist Medical Center Program

Sponsor: Iowa Methodist Medical Center

Program Director:
William G Bartlett, DO
Raymond Blank Children's Hospital
1200 Pleasant St
Des Moines, IA 50309
Tel: 515 241-4497 *Fax:* 515 241-5127
E-mail: pedresid@ihs.org
Internet: http://www.ihsdesmoines.org
Accred Length: 3 Years *Program Size:* 18 (*GY1:* 6)
Program ID: 320-18-31-082

Iowa City

University of Iowa Hospitals and Clinics Program

Sponsor: University of Iowa Hospitals and Clinics

Program Director:
Gail A McGuinness, MD
Univ of Iowa Hospitals and Clinics
Dept of Pediatrics
200 Hawkins Dr
Iowa City, IA 52242-1009
Tel: 319 356-3568 *Fax:* 319 356-4855
E-mail: twila-hobbs@uiowa.edu
Internet: http://www.vch.vh.org
Accred Length: 3 Years *Program Size:* 36 (*GY1:* 12)
Subspecialties: NPM, PDC, PDE, PDP, PG, PHO, PN
Program ID: 320-18-11-083

Kansas

Kansas City

University of Kansas Medical Center Program

Sponsor: University of Kansas School of Medicine
University of Kansas Medical Center

Program Director:
Pamela K Shaw, MD
Univ of Kansas Med Ctr
Dept of Pediatrics
3901 Rainbow Blvd
Kansas City, KS 66160-7330
Tel: 913 588-6917 *Fax:* 913 588-6319
E-mail: pshaw@kumc.edu
Internet: http://www.kumc.edu/~kumcpeds
Accred Length: 3 Years *Program Size:* 19 (*GY1:* 6)
Subspecialties: PPR
Program ID: 320-19-11-084

Wichita

University of Kansas (Wichita) Program

Sponsor: University of Kansas School of Medicine (Wichita)
Columbia Wesley Medical Center

Program Director:
Katherine J Melhorn, MD
Univ of Kansas Sch of Med-Wichita
Dept of Pediatrics
1010 N Kansas
Wichita, KS 67214-3199
Tel: 316 293-2631 *Fax:* 316 293-2689
E-mail: peds@kumc.edu
Internet:
http://www.kumc.edu/wichita/dept/peds/index.htm
Accred Length: 3 Years *Program Size:* 15 (*GY1:* 5)
Program ID: 320-19-21-086

Kentucky

Lexington

University of Kentucky Medical Center Program

Sponsor: University of Kentucky Hospital

Program Director:
Robert A Broughton, MD
Univ of Kentucky Med Ctr
Pediatrics Program MS 456
Lexington, KY 40536-0298
Tel: 606 323-5157 *Fax:* 606 323-8031
E-mail: lhfogl1@pop.uky.edu
Accred Length: 3 Years *Program Size:* 18 (*GY1:* 6)
Subspecialties: NPM
Program ID: 320-20-21-087

Louisville

University of Louisville Program

Sponsor: University of Louisville School of Medicine
Kosair Children's Hospital (Alliant Health System)

Program Director:
John L Roberts, MD
Univ of Louisville Sch of Med
Dept of Pediatrics
571 S Floyd St/Ste 300
Louisville, KY 40202-3830
Tel: 502 629-8828 *Fax:* 502 629-6783
E-mail: j0ashl01@ulkyvm.louisville.edu
Internet:
http://www.louisville.edu/medschool/pediatrics/residency
Accred Length: 3 Years *Program Size:* 48 (*GY1:* 16)
Subspecialties: CCP, NPM, PDI, PG
Program ID: 320-20-21-088

Louisiana

New Orleans

Louisiana State University Program

Sponsor: Louisiana State University School of Medicine
Childrens Hospital
Medical Center of Louisiana at New Orleans

Program Director:
Alfonso Vargas, MD
Louisiana State Univ Med Ctr
Dept of Pediatrics
1542 Tulane Ave
New Orleans, LA 70112-2822
Tel: 504 568-2569 *Fax:* 504 568-6330
E-mail: swack@lsumc.edu
Internet: http://www.medschool.lsumc.edu/pedresidency
Accred Length: 3 Years *Program Size:* 50 (*GY1:* 16)
Subspecialties: NPM, PG, PHO, TY
Program ID: 320-21-21-090

Tulane University Program

Sponsor: Tulane University School of Medicine
Alton Ochsner Medical Foundation
Medical Center of Louisiana at New Orleans
Tulane Hospital for Children

Program Director:
Hosea J Doucet III, MD
Tulane Univ Sch of Med
Dept of Pediatrics
1430 Tulane Ave/SL-37
New Orleans, LA 70112
Tel: 504 588-5458 *Fax:* 504 988-6808
E-mail: hdoucet@tmcpop.tmc.tulane.edu
Internet:
http://ww1.omi.tulane.edu/departments/pediatrics/resident.htm
Accred Length: 3 Years *Program Size:* 38 (*GY1:* 12)
Subspecialties: PDC, PDI, PDP, PN
Program ID: 320-21-21-092

Shreveport

Louisiana State University (Shreveport) Program

Sponsor: Louisiana State University Hospital-Shreveport

Program Director:
Catrell J McCulloch, MD
Louisiana State Univ Med Ctr Hospital
Med Educ/Pediatrics
1501 Kings Hwy/PO Box 33932
Shreveport, LA 71130-3932
Tel: 318 675-6073
Accred Length: 3 Years *Program Size:* 24 (*GY1:* 8)
Subspecialties: NPM, TY
Program ID: 320-21-11-093

Programs

Maine

Portland

Maine Medical Center Program

Sponsor: Maine Medical Center

Program Director:
Barbara A Chilmonczyk, MD
Maine Med Ctr
Dept of Pediatrics
22 Bramhall St
Portland, ME 04102-3175
Tel: 207 871-2353 *Fax:* 207 871-6272
E-mail: munsor@mail.mmc.org
Accred Length: 3 Years *Program Size:* 19 (*GY1:* 6)
Program ID: 320-22-11-094

Maryland

Baltimore

Johns Hopkins University Program

Sponsor: Johns Hopkins University School of Medicine
Johns Hopkins Hospital

Program Director:
Julia A McMillan, MD
Johns Hopkins Hospital
CMSC 2-124
600 N Wolfe St
Baltimore, MD 21287-3224
Tel: 410 614-4493 *Fax:* 410 955-9850
E-mail: kmm@jhmi.edu
Internet: http://www.med.jhu.edu/peds/pedspage.html
Accred Length: 3 Years *Program Size:* 68 (*GY1:* 23)
Subspecialties: ADL, CCP, NPM, PDC, PDE, PDI, PDP, PG, PHO, PN
Program ID: 320-23-21-096

Sinai Hospital of Baltimore Program

Sponsor: Sinai Hospital of Baltimore

Program Director:
Ina Stephens, MD
Sinai Hospital
Med Staff/Educ Office
2401 W Belvedere Ave
Baltimore, MD 21215
Tel: 410 601-9720 *Fax:* 410 601-6308
Accred Length: 3 Years *Program Size:* 22 (*GY1:* 7)
Program ID: 320-23-11-099

University of Maryland Program

Sponsor: University of Maryland Medical System
Mercy Medical Center

Program Director:
Carol L Carraccio, MD
Univ of Maryland Med System
Dept of Pediatrics
22 S Greene St
Baltimore, MD 21201
Tel: 410 328-6662 *Fax:* 410 328-0646
E-mail: pschmidt@peds.umaryland.edu
Internet: http://www.mdkids.ab.umd.edu
Accred Length: 3 Years *Program Size:* 41 (*GY1:* 13)
Subspecialties: CCP, NPM, PDE, PDI
Program ID: 320-23-21-100

Bethesda

National Capital Consortium Program

Sponsor: National Capital Consortium
National Naval Medical Center (Bethesda)
USUHS F Edward Hebert School of Medicine
Walter Reed Army Medical Center

Program Director:
Capt Richard A Moriarty, MD
Dept of Pediatrics
National Naval Med Ctr
Bethesda, MD 20889-5600
Tel: 301 295-4924 *Fax:* 301 295-6173
Internet: http://www.usuhs.mil/pediatrics/ncures.html
Accred Length: 3 Years *Program Size:* 31 (*GY1:* 11)
Subspecialties: NPM, PDE, PDI, PG, PHO
Program ID: 320-10-21-401
US Armed Services Program

Massachusetts

Boston

Children's Hospital/Boston Medical Center Program

Sponsor: Children's Hospital
Boston Medical Center

Program Director:
Frederick H Lovejoy Jr, MD
Children's Hospital
300 Longwood Ave
Boston, MA 02115
Tel: 617 355-8241 *Fax:* 617 738-7066
E-mail: lovejoy@a1.tch.harvard.edu
Internet: http://www.childrenshospital.org/
Accred Length: 3 Years *Program Size:* 105 (*GY1:* 37)
Subspecialties: ADL, CCP, NPM, PDC, PDE, PDI, PDP, PG, PHO, PN, PPR
Program ID: 320-24-21-403

Massachusetts General Hospital Program

Sponsor: Massachusetts General Hospital

Program Director:
Emmett V Schmidt, MD PhD
15 Parkman St/WAC 731
Boston, MA 02114
Tel: 617 724-7505 *Fax:* 617 726-4466
E-mail: schmidt.emmett@mgh.harvard.edu
Internet:
http://www.partners.org/cgi-view/dbml.exe?template=/p
Accred Length: 3 Years *Program Size:* 42 (*GY1:* 14)
Subspecialties: CCP, PDE, PDP, PN, TY
Program ID: 320-24-31-103

New England Medical Center Hospitals Program

Sponsor: New England Medical Center Hospitals

Program Director:
Lynne Karlson, MD
New England Med Ctr
750 Washington St/Box 286
Boston, MA 02111
Tel: 617 636-5256, ext 5256 *Fax:* 617 636-8388
Accred Length: 3 Years *Program Size:* 37 (*GY1:* 12)
Subspecialties: NPM, PG, PPR
Program ID: 320-24-21-104

Springfield

Baystate Medical Center Program

Sponsor: Baystate Medical Center

Program Director:
Barbara W Stechenberg, MD
Baystate Med Ctr
Dept of Pediatrics
759 Chestnut St
Springfield, MA 01199
Tel: 800 959-4232 *Fax:* 413 784-3623
E-mail: barbara.stechenberg@bhs.org
Internet: http://www.baystatehealth.com
Accred Length: 3 Years *Program Size:* 24 (*GY1:* 8)
Program ID: 320-24-12-106

Worcester

University of Massachusetts Program

Sponsor: University of Massachusetts Medical School
UMass Memorial Health Care (Memorial Campus)
UMass Memorial Health Care (University Campus)

Program Director:
William J Durbin Jr, MD
Univ of Massachusetts Med Sch
55 Lake Ave N
Worcester, MA 01655
Tel: 508 856-3590 *Fax:* 508 856-3779
E-mail: vwhite@banyan.ummed.edu
Internet: http://www.ummed.edu/dept/cmc
Accred Length: 3 Years *Program Size:* 22 (*GY1:* 7)
Subspecialties: NPM
Program ID: 320-24-21-107

Michigan

Ann Arbor

University of Michigan Program

Sponsor: University of Michigan Hospitals

Program Director:
Mary Ellen Bozynski, MD MS
1500 W Medical Center Dr/D3224
Ann Arbor, MI 48109-0718
Tel: 313 764-1258 *Fax:* 313 763-4208
E-mail: umpedsed@umich.edu
Internet: http://www.ped.med.umich.edu
Accred Length: 3 Years *Program Size:* 36 (*GY1:* 12)
Subspecialties: CCP, NPM, PDC, PDE, PDI, PDP, PG, PHO, PN
Program ID: 320-25-21-109

Detroit

Henry Ford Hospital Program

Sponsor: Henry Ford Hospital
St Joseph Mercy-Oakland

Program Director:
Annamaria Church, MD
Henry Ford Hospital
2799 W Grand Blvd/CFP-239
Detroit, MI 48202
Tel: 313 916-3003 *Fax:* 313 916-1771
E-mail: achurch1@hfhs.org
Internet:
http://www.henryfordhealth.org/gme/pediatrics.htm
Accred Length: 3 Years *Program Size:* 52 (*GY1:* 16)
Program ID: 320-25-31-392

St John Hospital and Medical Center Program
Sponsor: St John Hospital and Medical Center
Program Director:
Douglas K Ziegler, MD
St John Hospital and Med Ctr
Dept of Med Educ
22101 Moross Rd
Detroit, MI 48236-2172
Tel: 313 343-3875 *Fax:* 313 343-7840
E-mail: sue.moynihan@stjohn.org
Internet: http://www.stjohn.org
Accred Length: 3 Years *Program Size:* 15 (*GY1:* 5)
Program ID: 320-25-11-113

Wayne State University/Detroit Medical Center Program
Sponsor: Wayne State University/Detroit Medical Center
Children's Hospital of Michigan
Program Director:
Mary W LiehLai, MD
Children's Hospital of Michigan
3901 Beaubien Blvd
Detroit, MI 48201-2196
Tel: 313 745-5533 *Fax:* 313 993-7118
E-mail: mliehlai@med.wayne.edu
Internet: http://www.shiffman.wayne.edu/chm/
Accred Length: 3 Years *Program Size:* 64 (*GY1:* 20)
Subspecialties: CCP, NPM, PDC, PDI, PG, PHO
Program ID: 320-25-21-110

East Lansing

Michigan State University Program
Sponsor: Michigan State University College of Human Medicine
Michigan State University Clinical Center
Sparrow Hospital
Program Director:
Ajovi Scott-Emuakpor, MD PhD
Michigan State Univ
Pediatric Program
1215 E Michigan Ave
Lansing, MI 48912
Tel: 517 483-2856 *Fax:* 517 483-2763
E-mail: pedsres@pilot.msu.edu
Accred Length: 3 Years *Program Size:* 21 (*GY1:* 7)
Subspecialties: NPM, TY
Program ID: 320-25-21-114

Flint

Hurley Medical Center/Michigan State University Program
Sponsor: Hurley Medical Center
Program Director:
Melissa Hamp, MD
Hurley Med Ctr
Dept of Pediatrics
One Hurley Plaza
Flint, MI 48503-5993
Tel: 810 257-9283 *Fax:* 810 257-9736
E-mail: mhamp1@hurleymc.com
Internet: http://www.hurleymc.com
Accred Length: 3 Years *Program Size:* 15 (*GY1:* 5)
Subspecialties: TY
Program ID: 320-25-31-115

Grand Rapids

Spectrum Health-Downtown Campus/Michigan State University Program
Sponsor: Spectrum Health-Downtown Campus
Program Director:
Gary M Kirk, MD
DeVos Children's Hospital
100 Michigan Ave NE/MC11
Grand Rapids, MI 49503
Tel: 616 391-3670 *Fax:* 616 391-3105
E-mail: kimberly.longstreet@spectrum-health.org
Internet: http://www.spectrum-health.org
Accred Length: 3 Years *Program Size:* 24 (*GY1:* 8)
Subspecialties: TY
Program ID: 320-25-21-116

Kalamazoo

Kalamazoo Center for Medical Studies/Michigan State University Program
Sponsor: Kalamazoo Center for Medical Studies
Bronson Methodist Hospital
Program Director:
Donald E Greydanus, MD
Michigan State Univ-Kalamazoo Ctr for Med Studies
Dept of Pediatrics
1000 Oakland Dr
Kalamazoo, MI 49008-1284
Tel: 616 337-6450 *Fax:* 616 337-6474
E-mail: bowman@kcms.msu.edu
Internet: http://www.kcms.msu.edu
Accred Length: 3 Years *Program Size:* 15 (*GY1:* 5)
Program ID: 320-25-21-391

Royal Oak

William Beaumont Hospital Program
Sponsor: William Beaumont Hospital
Program Director:
M Jeffrey Maisels, MD
William Beaumont Hospital
3601 W 13 Mile Rd
Royal Oak, MI 48073-6769
Tel: 248 551-0413 *Fax:* 248 551-5978
E-mail: thill@beaumont.edu
Internet: http://www.beaumont.edu/html/gme
Accred Length: 3 Years *Program Size:* 15 (*GY1:* 5)
Program ID: 320-25-12-119

Minnesota

Minneapolis

University of Minnesota Program
Sponsor: University of Minnesota Medical School
Children's Health Care (Minneapolis)
Children's Health Care (St Paul)
Fairview-University Medical Center
Program Director:
Julie M Hauer, MD
Univ of Minnesota
420 Delaware St SE
Box 391 Mayo
Minneapolis, MN 55455
Tel: 612 626-5655 *Fax:* 612 626-7042
E-mail: peds-res@tc.umn.edu
Internet: http://www.peds.umn.edu/
Accred Length: 3 Years *Program Size:* 67 (*GY1:* 21)
Subspecialties: CCP, NPM, PDC, PDE, PDI, PDP, PG, PHO, PN
Program ID: 320-26-21-120

Rochester

Mayo Graduate School of Medicine (Rochester) Program
Sponsor: Mayo Graduate School of Medicine-Mayo Foundation
Mayo Clinic (Rochester)
Rochester Methodist Hospital
St Mary's Hospital of Rochester
Program Director:
Garth F Asay, MD
Application Processing Ctr
Mayo Graduate Sch of Med
200 First St SW
Rochester, MN 55905
Tel: 507 284-3108 *Fax:* 507 284-0999
E-mail: mgsm.medlab.specialties@mayo.edu
Internet: http://www.mayo.edu/
Accred Length: 3 Years *Program Size:* 24 (*GY1:* 8)
Subspecialties: PDC, PDE, PG, PHO
Program ID: 320-26-21-121

Mississippi

Jackson

University of Mississippi Medical Center Program
Sponsor: University of Mississippi School of Medicine
University Hospital
Program Director:
Gail C Megason, MD
Univ of Mississippi Med Ctr
2500 N State St
Jackson, MS 39216-4505
Tel: 601 984-6562 *Fax:* 601 984-2086
E-mail: nfrohn@ped.umsmed.edu
Accred Length: 3 Years *Program Size:* 30 (*GY1:* 10)
Subspecialties: NPM, PHO
Program ID: 320-27-12-122

Keesler AFB

Keesler Medical Center Program
Sponsor: Keesler Medical Center
Program Director:
Lt Col Gary D Crouch, MD
81st MDOS/SGOC
301 Fisher St/Rm 1A132
Keesler AFB, MS 39534-2519
Tel: 601 377-6621 *Fax:* 601 377-6304
E-mail: crouch.gary@keesler.af.mil
Internet: http://81mdg06.keesler.af.mil/index.cgi
Accred Length: 3 Years *Program Size:* 24 (*GY1:* 8)
Program ID: 320-27-12-002
US Armed Services Program

Missouri

Columbia

University of Missouri-Columbia Program

Sponsor: University of Missouri-Columbia School of Medicine
University Hospitals and Clinics

Program Director:
Sara S Viessman, MD
Child Health Dept
One Hospital Dr
Rm N708
Columbia, MO 65212
Tel: 573 882-4438 *Fax:* 573 884-5226
E-mail: adamskrausp@missouri.edu
Internet: http://www.choir.missouri.edu
Accred Length: 3 Years *Program Size:* 24 (*GY1:* 8)
Subspecialties: NPM
Program ID: 320-28-11-123

Kansas City

University of Missouri at Kansas City Program

Sponsor: University of Missouri-Kansas City School of Medicine
Children's Mercy Hospital

Program Director:
Frederick T Klingbeil, MD
Children's Mercy Hospital
2401 Gillham Rd
Kansas City, MO 64108-9898
Tel: 816 234-3371 *Fax:* 816 346-1328
Internet: http://www.cmh.edu
Accred Length: 3 Years *Program Size:* 49 (*GY1:* 16)
Subspecialties: NPM, PDE, PHO, PN
Program ID: 320-28-11-124

St Louis

St Louis University School of Medicine Program

Sponsor: St Louis University School of Medicine
SSM Cardinal Glennon Children's Hospital

Program Director:
Richard C Barry, MD
Gregory J Mantych, MD
SSM Cardinal Glennon Children's Hospital
1465 S Grand Blvd
St Louis, MO 63104
Tel: 314 577-5634 *Fax:* 314 577-5379
Accred Length: 3 Years *Program Size:* 39 (*GY1:* 13)
Subspecialties: NPM, PDP, PG, PPR
Program ID: 320-28-21-127

Washington University/B-JH/SLCH Consortium Program

Sponsor: Washington University/B-JH/SLCH Consortium
St Louis Children's Hospital

Program Director:
James P Keating, MD
St Louis Children's Hospital
One Children's Place
St Louis, MO 63110
Tel: 314 454-6006 *Fax:* 314 454-4102
E-mail: curtis_p@kids.wustl.edu
Internet: http://www.peds.wustl.edu
Accred Length: 3 Years *Program Size:* 62 (*GY1:* 22)
Subspecialties: CCP, NPM, PDC, PDE, PDI, PDP, PG, PHO, PN, PPR
Program ID: 320-28-11-125

Nebraska

Omaha

University of Nebraska/Creighton University Program

Sponsor: University of Nebraska Medical Center
Childrens Memorial Hospital
Tenet St Joseph Hospital at Creighton Univ Medical Center

Program Director:
John N Walburn, MD MD
Creighton-Nebraska Univ Health Foundation
982185 Nebraska Med Ctr
Omaha, NE 68198-2185
Tel: 402 559-5380 *Fax:* 402 559-9201
E-mail: jwalburn@unmc.edu
Internet: http://www.unmc.edu/pediatrics/residency/
Accred Length: 3 Years *Program Size:* 32 (*GY1:* 10)
Subspecialties: PDI, PG, PHO
Program ID: 320-30-21-383

Nevada

Las Vegas

University of Nevada Program

Sponsor: University of Nevada School of Medicine
University Medical Center of Southern Nevada
Sunrise Hospital and Medical Center

Program Director:
Bernard H Feldman, MD MPH
Univ of Nevada Sch of Med
2040 W Charleston Blvd/#402
Las Vegas, NV 89102-2206
Tel: 702 671-2231 *Fax:* 702 671-2233
E-mail: feldman@med.unr.edu
Internet: http://www.unr.edu/med
Accred Length: 3 Years *Program Size:* 16 (*GY1:* 6)
Program ID: 320-31-21-407

New Hampshire

Lebanon

Dartmouth-Hitchcock Medical Center Program

Sponsor: Mary Hitchcock Memorial Hospital

Program Director:
Carole A Stashwick, MD PhD
Dept of Pediatrics
Dartmouth-Hitchcock Med Ctr
One Medical Center Dr
Lebanon, NH 03756-0001
Tel: 603 650-5475 *Fax:* 603 650-5458
E-mail: carole.a.stashwick@hitchcock.org
Internet: http://www.hitchcock.org
Accred Length: 3 Years *Program Size:* 18 (*GY1:* 6)
Subspecialties: NPM
Program ID: 320-32-22-130

New Jersey

Camden

UMDNJ-Robert Wood Johnson Medical School (Camden) Program

Sponsor: Cooper Hospital-University Medical Center

Program Director:
William G Sharrar, MD
Children's Regional Hospital
Educ and Research Bldg/3rd Fl
401 Haddon Ave
Camden, NJ 08103-1489
Tel: 609 757-7904 *Fax:* 609 757-9647
E-mail: sharrar-william@cooperhealth.org
Accred Length: 3 Years *Program Size:* 30 (*GY1:* 10)
Subspecialties: CCP
Program ID: 320-33-31-251

Florham

Atlantic Health System Program

Sponsor: Atlantic Health System
Atlantic Health System
Morristown Memorial Hospital
Overlook Hospital

Program Director:
Leonard G Feld, MD PhD
Overlook Hospital-Atlantic Health Systems
Dept of Medical Education
99 Beauvoir Ave
Summit, NJ 07902-0220
Tel: 908 522-2187 *Fax:* 908 522-0804
E-mail: marybatjer@oh.ahsys.org
Internet: http://www.atlantichealth.org/pediatrics
Accred Length: 3 Years *Program Size:* 32 (*GY1:* 10)
Program ID: 320-33-21-412

Jersey City

Mount Sinai School of Medicine (Jersey City) Program

Sponsor: Mount Sinai School of Medicine
Jersey City Medical Center

Program Director:
Richard Bonforte, MD
Jersey City Med Ctr
50 Baldwin Ave
Jersey City, NJ 07304
Tel: 201 915-2455 *Fax:* 201 915-2459
Accred Length: 3 Years *Program Size:* 21 (*GY1:* 8)
Program ID: 320-33-21-131

Long Branch

Monmouth Medical Center Program

Sponsor: Monmouth Medical Center

Program Director:
Howard A Fox, MD
Monmouth Med Ctr
Dept of Pediatrics/Rm 209-SW
300 Second Ave
Long Branch, NJ 07740-9998
Tel: 732 923-7250 *Fax:* 732 923-7255
E-mail: foxh@auhs.edu
Accred Length: 3 Years *Program Size:* 18 (*GY1:* 6)
Program ID: 320-33-11-133

Neptune

Jersey Shore Medical Center Program

Sponsor: Jersey Shore Medical Center

Program Director:
Alan Cabasso, MD MD
Jersey Shore Med Ctr
1945 Rte 33
Neptune, NJ 07754
Tel: 908 776-4267 *Fax:* 908 776-4867
E-mail: jsmcped@aol.com
Internet: http://www.jsmc.com
Accred Length: 3 Years *Program Size:* 18 (*GY1:* 6)
Subspecialties: TY
Program ID: 320-33-11-134

Newark

Newark Beth Israel Medical Center Program

Sponsor: Newark Beth Israel Medical Center
Elizabeth General Medical Center

Program Director:
Joshua S Rosenblatt, MD
Children's Hospital
201 Lyons Ave
Newark, NJ 07112
Tel: 973 926-7040 *Fax:* 973 923-2441
E-mail: josh@bethi.com
Accred Length: 3 Years *Program Size:* 45 (*GY1:* 15)
Program ID: 320-33-21-362

UMDNJ-New Jersey Medical School Program

Sponsor: UMDNJ-New Jersey Medical School
UMDNJ-University Hospital

Program Director:
Susan G Mautone, MD
UMDNJ-New Jersey Med Sch
185 S Orange Ave/F509
Newark, NJ 07103
Tel: 973 972-6015 *Fax:* 973 972-0178
E-mail: mautonsu@umdnj.edu
Accred Length: 3 Years *Program Size:* 48 (*GY1:* 16)
Subspecialties: CCP, PDI
Program ID: 320-33-21-135

Paterson

St Joseph's Hospital and Medical Center Program

Sponsor: St Joseph's Hospital and Medical Center

Program Director:
Thomas E Potter, MD
St Joseph's Children's Hospital
703 Main St
Paterson, NJ 07503
Tel: 973 754-2544 *Fax:* 973 754-2546
Internet: http://www.sjhmc.org
Accred Length: 3 Years *Program Size:* 29 (*GY1:* 9)
Program ID: 320-33-21-364

Piscataway

UMDNJ-Robert Wood Johnson Medical School Program

Sponsor: UMDNJ-Robert Wood Johnson Medical School
Robert Wood Johnson University Hospital
St Peter's University Hospital

Program Director:
Dalya L Chefitz, MD
UMDNJ-Robert Wood Johnson Med Sch
Dept of Pediatrics/MEB Rm 308
One Robert Wood Johnson Pl/PO Box 19
New Brunswick, NJ 08903-0019
Tel: 732 235-7883 *Fax:* 732 235-7345
E-mail: mooreke@umdnj.edu
Accred Length: 3 Years *Program Size:* 38 (*GY1:* 12)
Subspecialties: CCP, NPM
Program ID: 320-33-21-136

New Mexico

Albuquerque

University of New Mexico Program

Sponsor: University of New Mexico School of Medicine
University Hospital

Program Director:
Gary D Overturf, MD
Univ of New Mexico Sch of Med
Dept of Pediatrics
Ambulatory Care Ctr/3rd Fl
Albuquerque, NM 87131-5311
Tel: 505 272-3909 *Fax:* 505 272-6845
E-mail: lthompson@salud.unm.edu
Internet:
http://macbeth.unm.edu/som/gme/pedshome.html
Accred Length: 3 Years *Program Size:* 33 (*GY1:* 10)
Subspecialties: NPM, PDP, PHO
Program ID: 320-34-11-138

New York

Albany

Albany Medical Center Program

Sponsor: Albany Medical Center

Program Director:
Elaine Schulte, MD MPH
Albany Med Coll
Dept of Pediatrics/A-88
47 New Scotland Ave
Albany, NY 12208-3479
Tel: 518 262-5626 *Fax:* 518 262-6776
E-mail: pam_demers@ccgateway.amc.edu
Accred Length: 3 Years *Program Size:* 33 (*GY1:* 10)
Subspecialties: NPM
Program ID: 320-35-21-139

Bronx

Albert Einstein College of Medicine (Jacobi) Program

Sponsor: Albert Einstein College of Medicine of Yeshiva University
Jacobi Medical Center

Program Director:
Daniel A Rauch, MD
Dept of Pediatrics
Jacobi Med Ctr
1400 Pelham Pkwy S
Bronx, NY 10461
Tel: 718 918-6986 *Fax:* 718 918-7510
E-mail: rauch@aecom.yu.edu
Accred Length: 3 Years *Program Size:* 39 (*GY1:* 13)
Program ID: 320-35-21-410

Albert Einstein College of Medicine Program

Sponsor: Albert Einstein College of Medicine of Yeshiva University
Jacobi Medical Center
Montefiore Medical Center-Henry and Lucy Moses Division
Montefiore Medical Center-Weiler Hospital

Program Director:
Henry M Adam, MD
Montefiore Med Ctr
111 E 210th St
Bronx, NY 10467
Tel: 718 920-6490 *Fax:* 718 654-6692
E-mail: adam@aecom.yu.edu
Accred Length: 3 Years *Program Size:* 110 (*GY1:* 23)
Subspecialties: ADL, CCP, NPM, PDE, PDI, PG, PHO, PN
Program ID: 320-35-21-363

Bronx-Lebanon Hospital Center Program

Sponsor: Bronx-Lebanon Hospital Center

Program Director:
Thomas J Daley, MD
Bronx-Lebanon Hospital Ctr
1650 Grand Concourse
Bronx, NY 10457
Tel: 718 518-5760 *Fax:* 718 518-5124
E-mail: tomdaley@aol.com
Accred Length: 3 Years *Program Size:* 42 (*GY1:* 13)
Program ID: 320-35-11-146

Lincoln Medical and Mental Health Center Program

Sponsor: Lincoln Medical and Mental Health Center

Program Director:
Ronald Bainbridge, MD
Lincoln Med and Mental Health Ctr
Dept of Pediatrics
234 E 149th St
Bronx, NY 10451
Tel: 718 579-5800 *Fax:* 718 579-4700
Accred Length: 3 Years *Program Size:* 63 (*GY1:* 23)
Program ID: 320-35-31-394

Brooklyn

Brookdale University Hospital Medical Center Program

Sponsor: Brookdale University Hospital Medical Center

Program Director:
Theodore W AvRuskin, MD
Brookdale Univ Hospital and Med Ctr
Linden Blvd at Brookdale Plaza
Brooklyn, NY 11212
Tel: 718 240-5244 *Fax:* 718 240-6515
E-mail: esanchez@brookdale.edu
Accred Length: 3 Years *Program Size:* 41 (*GY1:* 13)
Program ID: 320-35-11-147

Brooklyn Hospital Center Program

Sponsor: Brooklyn Hospital Center

Program Director:
Michael LaCorte, MD
Brooklyn Hospital Ctr
Dept of Pediatrics
121 DeKalb Ave
Brooklyn, NY 11201
Tel: 718 250-6935 *Fax:* 718 250-8735
Accred Length: 3 Years *Program Size:* 38 (*GY1:* 12)
Program ID: 320-35-11-148

Long Island College Hospital Program
Sponsor: Long Island College Hospital
Program Director:
Steven M Schwarz, MD
Long Island College Hospital
339 Hick St/Fuller Bldg Rm 401
Brooklyn, NY 11201
Tel: 718 780-1146 *Fax:* 718 780-2569
Accred Length: 3 Years *Program Size:* 29 (*GY1:* 9)
Program ID: 320-35-11-154

Maimonides Medical Center Program
Sponsor: Maimonides Medical Center
Coney Island Hospital
Program Director:
Henry A Schaeffer, MD
Maimonides Med Ctr
4802 Tenth Ave
Brooklyn, NY 11219
Tel: 718 283-8090, ext 8090 *Fax:* 718 283-6268
E-mail: vpolynice@maimonidesmed.or
Internet: http://www.maimonidesmed.org/peds
Accred Length: 3 Years *Program Size:* 75 (*GY1:* 21)
Subspecialties: PDE
Program ID: 320-35-21-157

New York Methodist Hospital Program
Sponsor: New York Methodist Hospital
New York and Presbyterian Hospital (Cornell Campus)
Program Director:
Leonard Glass, MD
New York Methodist Hospital
506 Sixth St
Brooklyn, NY 11215-9008
Tel: 718 780-5260 *Fax:* 718 780-3266
Accred Length: 3 Years *Program Size:* 27 (*GY1:* 7)
Program ID: 320-35-11-158

SUNY Health Science Center at Brooklyn Program
Sponsor: SUNY Health Science Center at Brooklyn
Kings County Hospital Center
University Hospital-SUNY Health Science Center at Brooklyn
Program Director:
Stephen Wadowski, MD
SUNY Health Science Ctr-Brooklyn
Children's Med Ctr
450 Clarkson Ave/Box 49
Brooklyn, NY 11203-2098
Tel: 718 270-2078 *Fax:* 718 270-1985
Internet: http://www.hscbklyn.edu/peds/
Accred Length: 3 Years *Program Size:* 84 (*GY1:* 30)
Subspecialties: NPM, PDC, PDE, PDI, PDP, PG, PHO, PN
Program ID: 320-35-21-173

Woodhull Medical and Mental Health Center Program
Sponsor: Woodhull Medical and Mental Health Center
Program Director:
John W Moohr, MD
Woodhull Med and Mental Health Ctr
Dept of Pediatrics
760 Broadway
Brooklyn, NY 11206-5317
Tel: 718 963-8652 *Fax:* 718 963-7957
Accred Length: 3 Years *Program Size:* 27 (*GY1:* 9)
Program ID: 320-35-32-387

Buffalo

SUNY at Buffalo Graduate Medical-Dental Education Consortium Program
Sponsor: SUNY at Buffalo Grad Medical-Dental Education Consortium
CGF Health System (Children's Hospital of Buffalo)
Program Director:
Gerald E Daigler, MD
Pediatric Med Education
Children's Hospital
219 Bryant St
Buffalo, NY 14222-2099
Tel: 716 878-7355 *Fax:* 716 878-7185
E-mail: cfarley@upa.chob.edu
Internet: http://www.chob.edu
Accred Length: 3 Years *Program Size:* 50 (*GY1:* 16)
Subspecialties: CCP, NPM, PDE, PHO, PN
Program ID: 320-35-21-140

East Meadow

Nassau County Medical Center Program
Sponsor: Nassau County Medical Center
Program Director:
Stephen P Katz, MD
Nassau County Med Ctr
2201 Hempstead Trnpk
East Meadow, NY 11554-5400
Tel: 516 572-6177 *Fax:* 516 572-5483
Accred Length: 3 Years *Program Size:* 34 (*GY1:* 10)
Program ID: 320-35-21-141

Elmhurst

Mount Sinai School of Medicine (Elmhurst) Program
Sponsor: Mount Sinai School of Medicine
Elmhurst Hospital Center-Mount Sinai Services
Mount Sinai Medical Center
Program Director:
Melvin Gertner, MD
Elmhurst Hospital Ctr-Mount Sinai Services
79-01 Broadway
Elmhurst, NY 11373
Tel: 718 334-3380 *Fax:* 718 334-2862
Accred Length: 3 Years *Program Size:* 39 (*GY1:* 13)
Program ID: 320-35-21-162

Flushing

New York Flushing Hospital Medical Center Program
Sponsor: New York Flushing Hospital Medical Center
Wyckoff Heights Medical Center
Program Director:
Susana Rapaport, MD
4500 Parsons Blvd
Flushing, NY 11355
Tel: 718 670-5535 *Fax:* 718 670-3031
Accred Length: 3 Years *Program Size:* 24 (*GY1:* 5)
Subspecialties: TY
Program ID: 320-35-31-261

Manhasset

North Shore University Hospital/NYU School of Medicine Program
Sponsor: North Shore University Hospital
Program Director:
Harvey Aiges, MD
North Shore Univ Hospital
Dept of Pediatrics
300 Community Dr
Manhasset, NY 11030
Tel: 516 562-4630, ext 4640 *Fax:* 516 562-1518
E-mail: aiges@nshs.edu
Internet: http://www.medhelp.org/nsuh/peds.html
Accred Length: 3 Years *Program Size:* 49 (*GY1:* 16)
Subspecialties: ADL, NPM, PDC, PDE, PDI, PG
Program ID: 320-35-21-150

Mineola

Winthrop-University Hospital Program
Sponsor: Winthrop-University Hospital
Program Director:
Joseph Greensher, MD
Winthrop-Univ Hospital
259 First St
Mineola, NY 11501
Tel: 516 663-2288 *Fax:* 516 663-8955
E-mail: wrosenfeld@winthrop.org
Internet: http://www.winthrop.org
Accred Length: 3 Years *Program Size:* 36 (*GY1:* 12)
Subspecialties: PDE, PDP
Program ID: 320-35-11-143

New Hyde Park

Albert Einstein College of Medicine at Long Island Jewish Medical Center Program
Sponsor: Long Island Jewish Medical Center
Schneider Children's Hosp (Long Island Jewish Med Ctr)
Program Director:
Philip Lanzkowsky, MD
Schneider Children's Hospital
Long Island Jewish Med Ctr
269-01 76th Ave
New Hyde Park, NY 11040
Tel: 718 470-3204 *Fax:* 718 343-8542
E-mail: katz@lij.edu
Internet: http://www.lij.edu
Accred Length: 3 Years *Program Size:* 76 (*GY1:* 25)
Subspecialties: ADL, CCP, NPM, PDC, PDE, PDI, PHO, PPR
Program ID: 320-35-21-155

New York

Albert Einstein College of Medicine at Beth Israel Medical Center Program
Sponsor: Beth Israel Medical Center
Program Director:
Andrew P Mezey, MD
Beth Israel Med Ctr
First Ave at 16th St
New York, NY 10003
Tel: 212 420-4018 *Fax:* 212 420-2560
E-mail: amezey@bethisrael.ny
Accred Length: 3 Years *Program Size:* 24 (*GY1:* 7)
Program ID: 320-35-11-145

Harlem Hospital Center Program
Sponsor: Harlem Hospital Center

Program Director:
Margaret C Heagarty, MD
Harlem Hospital Ctr
506 Lenox Ave
New York, NY 10037
Tel: 212 939-4012, ext 4013 *Fax:* 212 939-4015
E-mail: mxh@wonder.em.cdc.gov
Accred Length: 3 Years *Program Size:* 18 (*GY1:* 6)
Program ID: 320-35-11-151

Mount Sinai School of Medicine Program
Sponsor: Mount Sinai School of Medicine
Mount Sinai Medical Center

Program Director:
Scott H Barnett, MD
Mount Sinai Med Ctr
Dept of Pediatrics
One Gustave L Levy Pl/Box 1512
New York, NY 10029
Tel: 212 241-6934 *Fax:* 212 241-4309
E-mail: s_barnett@smtplink.mssm.edu
Internet: http://www.mssm.edu
Accred Length: 3 Years *Program Size:* 47 (*GY1:* 15)
Subspecialties: NPM, PDC, PDE, PDI, PDP, PG, PHO, PN, TY
Program ID: 320-35-11-161

New York and Presbyterian Hospital (Columbia Campus) Program
Sponsor: New York and Presbyterian Hospital
Metropolitan Hospital Center
New York and Presbyterian Hospital (Columbia Campus)

Program Director:
John M Driscoll Jr, MD
New York Presbyterian Hospital
622 W 168th St
New York, NY 10032-3784
Tel: 212 305-2934 *Fax:* 212 305-3020
Accred Length: 3 Years *Program Size:* 59 (*GY1:* 20)
Subspecialties: NPM, PDC, PDE, PDI, PDP, PG, PHO, PPR
Program ID: 320-35-11-167

New York and Presbyterian Hospital (Cornell Campus) Program
Sponsor: New York and Presbyterian Hospital
New York and Presbyterian Hospital (Cornell Campus)

Program Director:
Patrick A Flynn, MD
New York Presbyterian Hospital (New York-Cornell Campus)
Dept of Pediatrics/F695B
525 E 68th St
New York, NY 10021
Tel: 212 746-3131
E-mail: paflynn@mail.med.cornell.edu
Internet: http://www.nycornell.org/dept/pediatrics
Accred Length: 3 Years *Program Size:* 54 (*GY1:* 19)
Subspecialties: CCP, NPM, PDC, PDE, PDI, PDP, PG, PHO, PN, PPR
Program ID: 320-35-21-149

New York Medical College (Metropolitan) Program
Sponsor: New York Medical College
Metropolitan Hospital Center

Program Director:
Jason Mack, MD
Metropolitan Hospital Ctr
1901 First Ave
New York, NY 10029
Tel: 212 423-6228
Accred Length: 3 Years *Program Size:* 20 (*GY1:* 8)
Program ID: 320-35-21-393

New York Medical College at St Vincent's Hospital and Medical Center of New York Program
Sponsor: New York Medical College
St Vincent's Hospital and Medical Center of New York

Program Director:
Jayne D Rivas, MD
St Vincent's Hospital and Med Ctr
Dept of Pediatrics
153 W 11th St
New York, NY 10011
Tel: 212 604-3750 *Fax:* 212 604-2254
Accred Length: 3 Years *Program Size:* 16 (*GY1:* 5)
Program ID: 320-35-11-170

New York University Medical Center Program
Sponsor: New York University Medical Center
Bellevue Hospital Center

Program Director:
Robert M Lembo, MD
New York Univ Med Ctr
Dept of Pediatrics
550 First Ave
New York, NY 10016
Tel: 212 263-6425 *Fax:* 212 263-8172
Accred Length: 3 Years *Program Size:* 50 (*GY1:* 15)
Subspecialties: NPM, PDC, PDE, PHO
Program ID: 320-35-21-166

St Luke's-Roosevelt Hospital Center Program
Sponsor: St Luke's-Roosevelt Hospital Center
St Luke's-Roosevelt Hospital Center-Roosevelt Division
St Luke's-Roosevelt Hospital Center-St Luke's Division

Program Director:
Andrew P Mezey, MD
St Luke's-Roosevelt Hospital Ctr
1000 Tenth Ave/Rm 11c02
New York, NY 10019
Tel: 212 523-8050
Accred Length: 3 Years *Program Size:* 30 (*GY1:* 12)
Program ID: 320-35-11-168

Rochester

University of Rochester Program
Sponsor: Strong Memorial Hospital of the University of Rochester
Rochester General Hospital

Program Director:
J Peter Harris, MD
Children's Hospital
601 Elmwood Ave/PO Box 777R
Rochester, NY 14642
Tel: 800 871-7337 *Fax:* 716 442-6580
E-mail: chaspedres@urmc.rochester.edu
Internet:
http://www.urmc.rochester.edu/smd/peds/pedshome.htm
Accred Length: 3 Years *Program Size:* 49 (*GY1:* 15)
Subspecialties: ADL, CCP, NPM, PDC, PDE, PDI, PDP, PHO, PN
Program ID: 320-35-21-174

Staten Island

Sisters of Charity Medical Center-St Vincent's Campus/New York University Medical Center Program
Sponsor: Sisters of Charity Medical Center-St Vincent's Campus

Program Director:
Robert J Leggiadro, MD
Sisters of Charity Med Ctr-St Vincent's Campus
355 Bard Ave
Staten Island, NY 10310-1699
Tel: 718 876-4638 *Fax:* 718 876-2739
Accred Length: 3 Years *Program Size:* 18 (*GY1:* 6)
Program ID: 320-35-11-171

Stony Brook

SUNY at Stony Brook Program
Sponsor: University Hospital-SUNY at Stony Brook

Program Director:
Susan Guralnick, MD
SUNY-Stony Brook
Dept of Pediatrics
HSC T11/Rm 040
Stony Brook, NY 11794-8111
Tel: 516 444-2020 *Fax:* 516 444-2894
E-mail: sguralnick@mail.som.sunysb.edu
Internet: http://www.umc.sunysb.edu/pediatrics
Accred Length: 3 Years *Program Size:* 38 (*GY1:* 11)
Subspecialties: NPM, PDE, PN
Program ID: 320-35-21-365

Syracuse

SUNY Health Science Center at Syracuse Program
Sponsor: University Hospital-SUNY Health Science Center at Syracuse
Crouse Hospital

Program Director:
John S Andrake, MD
SUNY Health Science Ctr-Syracuse
750 E Adams St
Syracuse, NY 13210
Tel: 315 464-5800 *Fax:* 315 464-7564
E-mail: mondorep@vax.cs.hscsyr.edu
Internet: http://www.hscsyr.edu/~mondorep/
Accred Length: 3 Years *Program Size:* 36 (*GY1:* 12)
Subspecialties: PDC, PDE, PDI, PHO
Program ID: 320-35-21-175

Valhalla

New York Medical College at Westchester Medical Center Program
Sponsor: New York Medical College
Our Lady of Mercy Medical Center
Westchester Medical Center

Program Director:
Paul K Woolf, MD
New York Med Coll
Dept of Pediatrics
Munger Pavilion/Rm 129
Valhalla, NY 10595
Tel: 914 493-1166 *Fax:* 914 594-3400
E-mail: paul_woolf@nymc.edu
Internet: http://www.nymc.edu
Accred Length: 3 Years *Program Size:* 45 (*GY1:* 15)
Subspecialties: NPM, PDP, PG
Program ID: 320-35-11-176

North Carolina

Chapel Hill

University of North Carolina Hospitals Program
Sponsor: University of North Carolina Hospitals

Program Director:
Harvey J Hamrick, MD
Univ of North Carolina Sch of Med
Old Clinic Bldg/CB#7593
Chapel Hill, NC 27599-7593
Tel: 919 966-3172 *Fax:* 919 966-8419
E-mail: sport@med.unc.edu
Internet: http://www.pediatrics.med.unc.edu
Accred Length: 3 Years *Program Size:* 46 (*GY1:* 16)
Subspecialties: CCP, NPM, PDE, PDP, PG, PHO
Program ID: 320-36-21-178

Programs

Charlotte

Carolinas Medical Center Program

Sponsor: Carolinas Medical Center

Program Director:
Michael E Norman, MD
Carolinas Med Ctr
Dept of Pediatrics/PO Box 32861
Charlotte, NC 28232-2861
Tel: 704 355-3156 *Fax:* 704 355-5429
E-mail: valtoonian@carolinas.org
Internet: http://www.carolinas.org
Accred Length: 3 Years *Program Size:* 21 (*GYI:* 7)
Program ID: 320-36-11-179

Durham

Duke University Program

Sponsor: Duke University Medical Center

Program Director:
Deborah W Kredich, MD
Duke Univ Med Ctr
Dept of Pediatrics
Box 3127
Durham, NC 27710
Tel: 919 684-2356 *Fax:* 919 681-2714
Accred Length: 3 Years *Program Size:* 42 (*GYI:* 14)
Subspecialties: CCP, NPM, PDC, PDE, PDI, PDP, PHO, PN, PPR
Program ID: 320-36-21-180

Greenville

East Carolina University Program

Sponsor: East Carolina University School of Medicine
Pitt County Memorial Hospital

Program Director:
Lorraine Basnight, MD
Univ Health Systems of Eastern Carolina
Dept of Pediatrics
Brody 3E139
Greenville, NC 27858-4354
Tel: 252 816-4169 *Fax:* 252 816-8377
E-mail: basnight@brody.med.ecu.edu
Internet:
http://www.med.ecu.edu/htdocs/peds/residpgm.htm
Accred Length: 3 Years *Program Size:* 26 (*GYI:* 8)
Subspecialties: NPM
Program ID: 320-36-12-182

Winston-Salem

Wake Forest University School of Medicine Program

Sponsor: Wake Forest University Baptist Medical Center

Program Director:
David D Berry, MD
Dept of Pediatrics
Medical Center Blvd
Winston-Salem, NC 27157
Tel: 336 716-4495 *Fax:* 336 716-7100
E-mail: dberry@bgsm.edu
Internet: http://www.bgsm.edu
Accred Length: 3 Years *Program Size:* 36 (*GYI:* 12)
Subspecialties: CCP, NPM
Program ID: 320-36-11-183

Ohio

Akron

Children's Hospital Medical Center of Akron/NEOUCOM Program

Sponsor: Children's Hospital Medical Center of Akron

Program Director:
Ian G Dresner, MD PhD
Children's Hospital Med Ctr of Akron
One Perkins Sq
Akron, OH 44308-1062
Tel: 330 379-8200, ext 8693 *Fax:* 330 379-8157
E-mail: jdouglas@chmca.org
Accred Length: 3 Years *Program Size:* 31 (*GYI:* 11)
Program ID: 320-38-11-184

Cincinnati

Children's Hospital Medical Center/University of Cincinnati College of Medicine Program

Sponsor: Children's Hospital Medical Center

Program Director:
Michael K Farrell, MD
Univ of Cincinnati Hospital
Children's Hospital Med Ctr
3333 Burnet Ave/7th Fl CH
Cincinnati, OH 45229-3039
Tel: 513 636-4315 *Fax:* 513 636-7905
E-mail: michael.farrell@chmcc.org
Internet: http://www.cincinnati.childrens.org
Accred Length: 3 Years *Program Size:* 81 (*GYI:* 26)
Subspecialties: ADL, CCP, NPM, PDC, PDE, PDI, PDP, PG, PHO, PN, PPR
Program ID: 320-38-21-185

Cleveland

Case Western Reserve University (MetroHealth) Program

Sponsor: MetroHealth Medical Center

Program Director:
David G Roberts, MD
MetroHealth Med Ctr
Ped Educ Office-H-457
2500 MetroHealth Dr
Cleveland, OH 44109-1998
Tel: 216 778-5906 *Fax:* 216 778-8520
Accred Length: 3 Years *Program Size:* 24 (*GYI:* 8)
Subspecialties: NPM
Program ID: 320-38-21-369

Case Western Reserve University Program

Sponsor: University Hospitals of Cleveland

Program Director:
Michael L Nieder, MD
Rainbow Babies and Children's Hospital
Dept of Pediatrics
11100 Euclid Ave/Rm 865
Cleveland, OH 44106-6002
Tel: 216 844-3641 *Fax:* 216 844-7166
E-mail: bridget.johnson@uhhs.com
Internet: http://www.uhhs.com/rainbow
Accred Length: 3 Years *Program Size:* 64 (*GYI:* 21)
Subspecialties: CCP, NPM, PDC, PDE, PDI, PDP, PG, PHO, PN
Program ID: 320-38-21-367

Cleveland Clinic Foundation Program

Sponsor: Cleveland Clinic Foundation

Program Director:
Gary D Williams, MD
Cleveland Clinic Foundation
Dept of Pediatrics/M3
9500 Euclid Ave
Cleveland, OH 44195-5242
Tel: 216 444-5690 *Fax:* 216 444-1162
E-mail: meded@cestmp.ccf.org
Internet: http://www.ccf.org
Accred Length: 3 Years *Program Size:* 32 (*GYI:* 11)
Subspecialties: CCP, PG, PN
Program ID: 320-38-31-189

Columbus

Children's Hospital/Ohio State University Program

Sponsor: Children's Hospital

Program Director:
John D Mahan Jr, MD
Children's Hospital
Rm ED615
700 Children's Dr
Columbus, OH 43205-2696
Tel: 614 722-4414 *Fax:* 614 722-6132
E-mail: bozmand@chi.osu.edu
Internet: http://www.childrenscolumbus.org
Accred Length: 3 Years *Program Size:* 60 (*GYI:* 20)
Subspecialties: CCP, NPM, PDC, PDE, PDP, PHO
Program ID: 320-38-21-192

Dayton

Wright State University Program

Sponsor: Wright State University School of Medicine
Children's Medical Center
Wright-Patterson Medical Center

Program Director:
Sherman Alter, MD
Children's Med Ctr
One Children's Plaza
Dayton, OH 45404-1815
Tel: 937 226-8433 *Fax:* 937 463-5408
E-mail: salter@discover.wright.edu
Accred Length: 3 Years *Program Size:* 36 (*GYI:* 12)
Program ID: 320-38-21-193

Toledo

Medical College of Ohio Program

Sponsor: Medical College of Ohio
Toledo Hospital

Program Director:
Donald L Batisky, MD
Med Coll of Ohio
Richard D Ruppert Ctr/Rm 1600
3120 Glendale Ave
Toledo, OH 43614-5809
Tel: 419 383-5264 *Fax:* 419 383-3091
E-mail: dbatisky@mco.edu
Internet: http://www.mco.edu/depts/peds/residency
Accred Length: 3 Years *Program Size:* 19 (*GYI:* 6)
Program ID: 320-38-21-194

Youngstown

Western Reserve Care System/NEOUCOM Program
Sponsor: Western Reserve Care System
Forum Health-Tod Children's Hospital
Program Director:
Eugene M Mowad, MD
Tod Children's Hospital
Western Reserve Care System
500 Gypsy Ln
Youngstown, OH 44501
Tel: 330 740-3832 *Fax:* 330 740-5717
Internet: http://www.wrhc.org
Accred Length: 3 Years *Program Size:* 24 (*GY1:* 8)
Program ID: 320-38-21-195

Oklahoma

Oklahoma City

University of Oklahoma Health Sciences Center Program
Sponsor: University of Oklahoma College of Medicine
Children's Hospital of Oklahoma
Program Director:
Kendall L Stanford, MD
Univ of Oklahoma Health Sciences Ctr
PO Box 26901
Oklahoma City, OK 73190
Tel: 405 271-4417 *Fax:* 405 271-2920
Accred Length: 3 Years *Program Size:* 33 (*GY1:* 11)
Subspecialties: NPM, PDE, PG, PHO
Program ID: 320-39-11-196

Tulsa

University of Oklahoma College of Medicine-Tulsa Program
Sponsor: University of Oklahoma College of Medicine-Tulsa
St Francis Hospital
Program Director:
Robert W Block, MD
Univ of Oklahoma Coll of Med-Tulsa
Dept of Pediatrics
2815 S Sheridan Rd
Tulsa, OK 74129-1077
Tel: 918 838-4838 *Fax:* 918 838-4729
E-mail: connie-johnson@ouhsc.edu
Internet: http://www.tulsa.ouhsc.edu
Accred Length: 3 Years *Program Size:* 16 (*GY1:* 5)
Program ID: 320-39-21-197

Oregon

Portland

Oregon Health Sciences University Program
Sponsor: Oregon Health Sciences University Hospital
Program Director:
Joseph T Gilhooly, MD
Oregon Health Sciences Univ
Dept of Pediatrics
3181 SW Sam Jackson Park Rd/DC10S
Portland, OR 97201
Tel: 503 418-5170 *Fax:* 503 418-5199
E-mail: pedsres@ohsu.edu
Internet: http://www.ohsu.edu/som-pediatrics/training/resident.htm
Accred Length: 3 Years *Program Size:* 36 (*GY1:* 12)
Subspecialties: NPM, PDC, PDE, PDP, PHO
Program ID: 320-40-12-199

Pennsylvania

Danville

Penn State Geisinger Health System/Geisinger Medical Center Program
Sponsor: Penn State Geisinger Health System
Geisinger Medical Center
Program Director:
Janis M Maksimak, MD
Geisinger Med Ctr
Dept of Pediatrics
100 N Academy Ave
Danville, PA 17822-2701
Tel: 717 271-5606 *Fax:* 717 271-5885
E-mail: dfasold@psghs.edu
Accred Length: 3 Years *Program Size:* 22 (*GY1:* 7)
Program ID: 320-41-11-200

Hershey

Penn State Geisinger Health System/Milton S Hershey Medical Center Program
Sponsor: Penn State Geisinger Health System
Milton S Hershey Medical Center
Program Director:
Steven J Wassner, MD
Milton S Hershey Med Ctr
University Dr
PO Box 850
Hershey, PA 17033
Tel: 717 531-8603 *Fax:* 717 531-8985
E-mail: sjw6@psu.edu.
Internet: http://www.hmc.psu.edu/peds/
Accred Length: 3 Years *Program Size:* 32 (*GY1:* 10)
Subspecialties: CCP
Program ID: 320-41-21-372

Philadelphia

Albert Einstein Medical Center Program
Sponsor: Albert Einstein Medical Center
Program Director:
Robert S Wimmer, MD
Albert Einstein Med Ctr
5501 Old York Rd
Philadelphia, PA 19141-3098
Tel: 215 456-7595 *Fax:* 215 456-3436
Accred Length: 3 Years *Program Size:* 23 (*GY1:* 7)
Subspecialties: NPM
Program ID: 320-41-11-204

Children's Hospital of Philadelphia Program
Sponsor: Children's Hospital of Philadelphia
Program Director:
Stephen Ludwig, MD
Children's Hospital of Philadelphia
Dept of Pediatrics
34th St and Civic Center Blvd
Philadelphia, PA 19104
Tel: 215 590-2162 *Fax:* 215 590-2768
E-mail: ludwig@emil.chop.edu.
Internet: http://www.chop.edu/profs-residency
Accred Length: 3 Years *Program Size:* 96 (*GY1:* 30)
Subspecialties: ADL, CCP, NPM, PDC, PDE, PDI, PDP, PG, PHO, PN
Program ID: 320-41-21-205

St Christopher's Hospital for Children Program
Sponsor: St Christopher's Hospital for Children
Program Director:
Robert S McGregor, MD
St Christopher's Hospital for Children
Erie Ave at Front St
Philadelphia, PA 19134-1095
Tel: 215 427-5127 *Fax:* 215 427-4805
E-mail: mcgregor@auhs.edu
Accred Length: 3 Years *Program Size:* 70 (*GY1:* 20)
Subspecialties: NPM, PDC, PDE, PDI, PDP, PG, PHO, PN
Program ID: 320-41-12-209

Pittsburgh

Mercy Hospital of Pittsburgh Program
Sponsor: Mercy Hospital of Pittsburgh
Program Director:
Bradley J Bradford, MD
Mercy Hospital of Pittsburgh
Dept of Pediatrics
1515 Locust St
Pittsburgh, PA 15219-5166
Tel: 412 232-5881 *Fax:* 412 232-7389
E-mail: pediatric.residency@mercy.pmhs.org
Internet: http://www.mercy-meded.com
Accred Length: 3 Years *Program Size:* 19 (*GY1:* 6)
Program ID: 320-41-11-212

University Health Center of Pittsburgh Program
Sponsor: University Health Center of Pittsburgh
Children's Hospital of Pittsburgh
Magee-Women's Hospital
Program Director:
Dena Hofkosh, MD
Children's Hospital
Dept of Pediatrics
3705 Fifth Ave
Pittsburgh, PA 15213-2583
Tel: 412 692-5159 *Fax:* 412 692-7231
E-mail: sandera@chplink.chp.edu
Internet: http://www.chp.edu
Accred Length: 3 Years *Program Size:* 52 (*GY1:* 17)
Subspecialties: CCP, NPM, PDC, PDE, PDI, PDP, PG, PHO, PN
Program ID: 320-41-21-211

Upland

Crozer-Chester Medical Center Program
Sponsor: Crozer-Chester Medical Center
Program Director:
Kathleen A Reeves, MD
Crozer-Chester Med Ctr
One Medical Center Blvd
Ste 402
Upland, PA 19013-3995
Tel: 610 447-6680 *Fax:* 610 447-6677
E-mail: sandfree@hotmail.com
Internet: http://www.crozer.org
Accred Length: 3 Years *Program Size:* 19 (*GY1:* 6)
Subspecialties: TY
Program ID: 320-41-21-206

Puerto Rico

Bayamon

Universidad Central del Caribe Program

Sponsor: University Hospital Ramon Ruiz Arnau

Program Director:
Jose G Rodriguez, MD
Univ Hospital Ramon Ruiz Arnau
Dept of Pediatrics
Ave Laurel/Santa Juanita
Bayamon, PR 00960
Tel: 787 787-4414 *Fax:* 787 787-4414
E-mail: 105531.2675@compuserve.com
Accred Length: 3 Years *Program Size:* 24 (*GY1:* 8)
Subspecialties: TY
Program ID: 320-42-21-255

Caguas

Caguas Regional Hospital Program

Sponsor: Caguas Regional Hospital

Program Director:
Angel L Senquiz, MD
Caguas Regional Hospital
Dept of Pediatrics
PO Box 5729
Caguas, PR 00725
Tel: 787 744-3141 *Fax:* 787 746-3440
Accred Length: 3 Years *Program Size:* 24 (*GY1:* 8)
Subspecialties: TY
Program ID: 320-42-31-213

Mayaguez

Ramon E Betances Hospital-Mayaguez Medical Center Program

Sponsor: Dr Ramon E Betances Hospital-Mayaguez Medical Center

Program Director:
Arturo M Lopez, MD
Mayaguez Med Ctr
410 Hostos Ave
Mayaguez, PR 00680
Tel: 787 834-8689 *Fax:* 787 834-3010
Accred Length: 3 Years *Program Size:* 15 (*GY1:* 5)
Program ID: 320-42-12-214

Ponce

Ponce University Hospital Program

Sponsor: Ponce University Hospital

Program Director:
Ivonne Villafane, MD
Ponce Univ Hospital
Ave Tito Castro 917
Ponce, PR 00731
Tel: 787 844-2080, ext 1650 *Fax:* 787 841-4037
Accred Length: 3 Years *Program Size:* 21 (*GY1:* 7)
Subspecialties: TY
Program ID: 320-42-11-215

Rio Piedras

San Juan City Hospital Program

Sponsor: San Juan City Hospital

Program Director:
Miladi Lugo, MD
San Juan Municipal Hospital
CMMS #79
PO Box 70344
San Juan, PR 00936-8344
Tel: 787 765-7618 *Fax:* 787 751-5149
Accred Length: 3 Years *Program Size:* 27 (*GY1:* 9)
Program ID: 320-42-11-216

San Juan

University of Puerto Rico Program

Sponsor: University of Puerto Rico School of Medicine
University Pediatric Hospital

Program Director:
Yolanda Gomez, MD
Univ of Puerto Rico Med Science Campus
GPO Box 5067
San Juan, PR 00936
Tel: 787 756-3202 *Fax:* 787 756-3394
Accred Length: 3 Years *Program Size:* 42 (*GY1:* 12)
Subspecialties: CCP, NPM, PDP, PHO
Program ID: 320-42-11-217

Rhode Island

Providence

Brown University Program

Sponsor: Rhode Island Hospital
Women and Infants Hospital of Rhode Island

Program Director:
Edwin N Forman, MD
Rhode Island Hospital
593 Eddy St
Providence, RI 02903-4923
Tel: 401 444-5171 *Fax:* 401 444-8845
E-mail: eforman@lifespan.org
Accred Length: 3 Years *Program Size:* 45 (*GY1:* 15)
Subspecialties: NPM, PDE, PDI, PG, PHO
Program ID: 320-43-21-218

South Carolina

Charleston

Medical University of South Carolina Program

Sponsor: Medical University of South Carolina College of Medicine
MUSC Medical Center

Program Director:
George M Johnson, MD
Med Univ of South Carolina
Dept of Pediatrics
171 Ashley Ave
Charleston, SC 29425-2248
Tel: 803 792-8972 *Fax:* 803 792-9223
E-mail: johnsogm@musc.edu
Accred Length: 3 Years *Program Size:* 36 (*GY1:* 12)
Subspecialties: NPM, PDC, PG, PHO
Program ID: 320-45-11-219

Columbia

Palmetto Health Alliance/University of South Carolina School of Medicine Program

Sponsor: Palmetto Health Alliance
Palmetto Richland Memorial Hospital

Program Director:
Roger C Taylor, MD
Univ of South Carolina-Children's Hospital
Dept of Pediatrics
5 Richland Medical Pk/ACC2 Area K
Columbia, SC 29203
Tel: 803 434-7606 *Fax:* 803 434-3855
E-mail: juliegoe@cae1.rmh.edu
Internet:
http://www.rmh.edu/rmh/residency/pediatrics/htm
Accred Length: 3 Years *Program Size:* 24 (*GY1:* 8)
Program ID: 320-45-21-220

Greenville

Greenville Hospital System Program

Sponsor: Greenville Hospital System

Program Director:
John P Matthews Jr, MD
Greenville Hospital System
701 Grove Rd
Balcony Ste 4
Greenville, SC 29605-4295
Tel: 864 455-7879 *Fax:* 864 455-3884
E-mail: shazelwood@ghs.org
Internet: http://www.ghs.org
Accred Length: 3 Years *Program Size:* 24 (*GY1:* 8)
Subspecialties: TY
Program ID: 320-45-12-221

Tennessee

Chattanooga

University of Tennessee College of Medicine at Chattanooga Program

Sponsor: University of Tennessee College of Medicine-Chattanooga Unit
T C Thompson Children's Hospital Medical Center

Program Director:
Billy S Arant Jr, MD
Univ of Tennessee Coll of Med-Chattanooga
T C Thompson Children's Hospital
910 Blackford St
Chattanooga, TN 37403
Tel: 423 778-6217 *Fax:* 423 778-6020
E-mail: utpediat@erlanger.org
Internet: http://www.erlanger.org/utcom/pediatrics.html
Accred Length: 3 Years *Program Size:* 24 (*GY1:* 8)
Program ID: 320-47-11-222

Johnson City

East Tennessee State University Program

Sponsor: James H Quillen College of Medicine
Johnson City Medical Center Hospital

Program Director:
David T Price, MD
James H Quillen Coll of Med
East Tennessee State Univ
PO Box 70578
Johnson City, TN 37614-0578
Tel: 423 439-6763 *Fax:* 423 439-6158
E-mail: priced@etsu.edu
Accred Length: 3 Years *Program Size:* 15 (*GY1:* 4)
Program ID: 320-47-21-381

Knoxville

University of Tennessee Medical Center at Knoxville Program

Sponsor: University of Tennessee Graduate School of Medicine
University of Tennessee Memorial Hospital

Program Director:
Patricia A Mohr, MD
Univ of Tennessee Graduate Sch of Med
Dept of Pediatrics
1924 Alcoa Hwy
Knoxville, TN 37920
Tel: 423 544-9330 *Fax:* 423 544-8879
E-mail: pchadwic@mc.utmck.edu
Accred Length: 3 Years *Program Size:* 18 (*GY1:* 6)
Program ID: 320-47-21-396

Memphis

University of Tennessee Program

Sponsor: University of Tennessee College of Medicine
LeBonheur Children's Medical Center
Regional Medical Center at Memphis

Program Director:
Russell W Chesney, MD
LeBonheur Children's Med Ctr
50 N Dunlap
Memphis, TN 38103-2893
Tel: 901 572-3106 *Fax:* 901 572-5036
E-mail: rchesney@utmem1.utmem.edu
Internet:
http://www.utmem.edu/pediatricsrcoord@utmem1.utmem.edu
Accred Length: 3 Years *Program Size:* 42 (*GY1:* 14)
Subspecialties: CCP, NPM, PDE, PDI, PHO, PN, PPR
Program ID: 320-47-31-225

Nashville

Vanderbilt University Program

Sponsor: Vanderbilt University Medical Center
Metropolitan Nashville General Hospital

Program Director:
James C Gay, MD
Vanderbilt Univ Hospital
Dept of Pediatrics
AA-0216 MCN
Nashville, TN 37232-2574
Tel: 615 322-3377 *Fax:* 615 343-6249
Internet: http://www.peds.mc.vanderbilt.edu/vchweb-1/
Accred Length: 3 Years *Program Size:* 68 (*GY1:* 18)
Subspecialties: CCP, NPM, PDC, PDE, PDI, PDP, PG, PHO, PN
Program ID: 320-47-21-227

Texas

Amarillo

Texas Tech University (Amarillo) Program

Sponsor: Texas Tech University Health Sciences Center at Amarillo
Northwest Texas Health Care System

Program Director:
Tribhawan S Vats, MD
Texas Tech Univ Health Sciences Ctr
Dept of Pediatrics
1400 Wallace Blvd
Amarillo, TX 79106
Tel: 806 354-5432 *Fax:* 806 354-5536
E-mail: trib@cortex.ama.ttuhsc.edu
Internet: http://www.ama.ttuhsc.edu
Accred Length: 3 Years *Program Size:* 12 (*GY1:* 4)
Program ID: 320-48-21-370

Austin

CTMF of Seton Healthcare Network Program

Sponsor: CTMF of Seton Healthcare Network
Brackenridge Hospital

Program Director:
George A Edwards, MD
Children's Hospital of Austin
Austin Pediatric Education Program
601 E 15th St
Austin, TX 78701
Tel: 512 324-8565 *Fax:* 512 324-8634
E-mail: apepfac@tcms.com
Accred Length: 3 Years *Program Size:* 25 (*GY1:* 8)
Subspecialties: TY
Program ID: 320-48-31-228

Corpus Christi

Driscoll Children's Hospital Program

Sponsor: Driscoll Children's Hospital

Program Director:
William J Riley, MD
Driscoll Children's Hospital
3533 S Alameda
PO Drawer 6530
Corpus Christi, TX 78466-6530
Tel: 512 694-5465 *Fax:* 512 694-5466
E-mail: rileyw@driscollchildrens.org
Internet: http://www.driscollchildrens.org
Accred Length: 3 Years *Program Size:* 42 (*GY1:* 14)
Program ID: 320-48-11-229

Dallas

University of Texas Southwestern Medical School Program

Sponsor: University of Texas Southwestern Medical School
Children's Medical Center of Dallas

Program Director:
Charles M Ginsburg, MD
Univ of Texas Southwestern Med Sch
5323 Harry Hines Blvd
Dallas, TX 75235-9063
Tel: 214 648-3563 *Fax:* 214 648-8617
Internet: http://www.peds.swmed.edu
Accred Length: 3 Years *Program Size:* 78 (*GY1:* 26)
Subspecialties: CCP, NPM, PDC, PDE, PDI, PG, PHO, PN, PPR
Program ID: 320-48-21-230

El Paso

Texas Tech University (El Paso) Program

Sponsor: Texas Tech University Health Sciences Center at El Paso
R E Thomason General Hospital

Program Director:
Gilbert A Handal, MD
Texas Tech Univ Health Sciences Ctr
Dept of Pediatrics
4800 Alberta Ave
El Paso, TX 79905
Tel: 915 545-6785 *Fax:* 915 545-6976
E-mail: pedelf@ttuhsc.edu
Internet: http://www.ttuhsc.edu/pages/el paso ped/default.htm
Accred Length: 3 Years *Program Size:* 26 (*GY1:* 8)
Program ID: 320-48-11-234

Galveston

University of Texas Medical Branch Hospitals Program

Sponsor: University of Texas Medical Branch Hospitals

Program Director:
Susan E Keeney, MD
Univ of Texas Med Branch
301 University Blvd
Galveston, TX 77555-0354
Tel: 409 772-1398 *Fax:* 409 772-4599
E-mail: skeeney@utmb.edu
Internet: http://www.utmb.edu/pedi
Accred Length: 3 Years *Program Size:* 36 (*GY1:* 12)
Subspecialties: NPM, PDE, PDI, PHO, PN
Program ID: 320-48-11-231

Houston

Baylor College of Medicine Program

Sponsor: Baylor College of Medicine
Harris County Hospital District-Ben Taub General Hospital
Texas Children's Hospital

Program Director:
Ralph D Feigin, MD
Baylor Coll of Med
Dept of Pediatrics
One Baylor Plaza
Houston, TX 77030-3498
Tel: 713 770-1170 *Fax:* 713 770-1187
E-mail: parker@bcm.tmc.edu
Internet: http://www.bcm.tmc.edu/pedi/res
Accred Length: 3 Years *Program Size:* 108 (*GY1:* 36)
Subspecialties: CCP, NPM, PDC, PDE, PDI, PDP, PG, PHO, PN, PPR
Program ID: 320-48-21-232

University of Texas at Houston Program

Sponsor: University of Texas Medical School at Houston
Lyndon B Johnson General Hospital
Memorial Hermann Healthcare System

Program Director:
Sharon S Crandell, MD
Univ of Texas Health Science Ctr
6431 Fannin St/MSB 3244
Houston, TX 77030
Tel: 713 500-5800 *Fax:* 713 500-5805
E-mail: sknight@ped1.med.uth.tmc.edu
Internet:
http://ped1.med.uth.tmc.edu/resident/resident.html
Accred Length: 3 Years *Program Size:* 42 (*GY1:* 14)
Subspecialties: NPM, PDE, PDI, PHO, PN
Program ID: 320-48-21-233

Lackland AFB

San Antonio Uniformed Services Health Education Consortium Program

Sponsor: San Antonio Uniformed Services Health Education Consortium

Program Director:
Col John D Roscelli, MD
59th Med Wing/MNP
2200 Bergquist Dr/Ste 1
Lackland AFB, TX 78236-5300
Tel: 210 292-5097 *Fax:* 210 292-5238
E-mail: john_d.roscelli@sa chcs.mednet.af.mil
Accred Length: 3 Years *Program Size:* 41 (*GY1:* 14)
Subspecialties: NPM
Program ID: 320-48-21-406
US Armed Services Program

Lubbock

Texas Tech University (Lubbock) Program

Sponsor: Texas Tech University Health Sciences Center at Lubbock
University Medical Center

Program Director:
Surendra K Varma, MD
Texas Tech Univ Health Sciences Ctr
Dept of Pediatrics
3601 Fourth St
Lubbock, TX 79430
Tel: 806 743-2244, ext 291 *Fax:* 806 743-2314
E-mail: pedskv@ttuhsc.edu
Accred Length: 3 Years *Program Size:* 18 (*GY1:* 6)
Program ID: 320-48-21-260

San Antonio

University of Texas Health Science Center at San Antonio Program

Sponsor: University of Texas Medical School at San Antonio
Santa Rosa Health Care Corporation
University Hospital-South Texas Medical Center

Program Director:
Robert J Nolan Jr, MD
Univ of Texas Health Science Ctr
7703 Floyd Curl Dr
San Antonio, TX 78284-7816
Tel: 210 567-5187 *Fax:* 210 567-6921
E-mail: nolanr@uthscsa.edu
Internet: http://www./macorb.uthscsa.edu/pedi/
Accred Length: 3 Years *Program Size:* 48 (*GY1:* 16)
Subspecialties: CCP, NPM, PDE, PDI, PHO
Program ID: 320-48-21-235

Temple

Texas A&M College of Medicine-Scott and White Program

Sponsor: Scott and White Memorial Hospital

Program Director:
Denise FitzSimon-Williams, MD
Texas A&M-Scott and White
Grad Med Educ
2401 S 31st St
Temple, TX 76508-0001
Tel: 800 299-4463, ext 5092 *Fax:* 817 724-0274
E-mail: saddington@swmail.sw.org
Internet: http://www.swinfo.tamu.edu
Accred Length: 3 Years *Program Size:* 18 (*GY1:* 6)
Program ID: 320-48-21-236

Utah

Salt Lake City

University of Utah Program

Sponsor: University of Utah Medical Center
Primary Children's Medical Center

Program Director:
Ronald S Bloom, MD
Univ of Utah Health Sciences Ctr
Dept of Pediatrics
50 N Medical Dr/Rm 2A152
Salt Lake City, UT 84132
Tel: 801 581-7572 *Fax:* 801 581-4920
E-mail: peds.res@hsc.utah.edu
Internet: http://www.ped.med.utah.edu
Accred Length: 3 Years *Program Size:* 42 (*GY1:* 14)
Subspecialties: CCP, NPM, PDP, PHO
Program ID: 320-49-21-237

Vermont

Burlington

University of Vermont Program

Sponsor: Fletcher Allen Health Care

Program Director:
Ann P Guillot, MD
Univ of Vermont Coll of Med
Dept of Pediatrics
Given Medical Bldg/A-121
Burlington, VT 05405-0068
Tel: 802 656-3544 *Fax:* 802 656-5557
E-mail: ann.guillot@vtmednet.org
Internet:
http://www.vtmednet.org/children/uvmresid.htm
Accred Length: 3 Years *Program Size:* 18 (*GY1:* 6)
Subspecialties: NPM
Program ID: 320-50-11-238

Virginia

Charlottesville

University of Virginia Program

Sponsor: University of Virginia Medical Center

Program Director:
Richard W Kesler, MD
Univ of Virginia Hospitals
Box 386
Charlottesville, VA 22908
Tel: 804 924-2357 *Fax:* 804 924-5244
E-mail: rwk@virginia.edu
Internet: http://ww.hsc.virginia.edu/cmc/residency/
Accred Length: 3 Years *Program Size:* 34 (*GY1:* 11)
Subspecialties: CCP, NPM, PDC, PDE, PDP, PHO, PN
Program ID: 320-51-11-239

Falls Church

Fairfax Hospital Program

Sponsor: Fairfax Hospital

Program Director:
Michael F Altieri, MD
Fairfax Hospital
3300 Gallows Rd
Falls Church, VA 22042
Tel: 703 204-6652 *Fax:* 703 204-6078
Accred Length: 3 Years *Program Size:* 28 (*GY1:* 10)
Program ID: 320-51-21-399

Norfolk

Eastern Virginia Medical School Program

Sponsor: Eastern Virginia Medical School
Children's Hospital of the King's Daughters

Program Director:
Clarence W Gowen Jr, MD
Children's Hospital of the King's Daughters
601 Children's Ln
Norfolk, VA 23507
Tel: 757 668-7272 *Fax:* 757 668-9766
E-mail: cgowen@chkd.com
Internet: http://www.chkd.org
Accred Length: 3 Years *Program Size:* 45 (*GY1:* 15)
Subspecialties: PDI
Program ID: 320-51-21-240

Portsmouth

Naval Medical Center (Portsmouth) Program

Sponsor: Naval Medical Center (Portsmouth)

Program Director:
Lt Col Robert Ellis, MD
Naval Med Ctr
Dept of Pediatrics
620 John Paul Jones Cir
Portsmouth, VA 23708-2197
Tel: 757 953-7358 *Fax:* 757 953-5964
E-mail: pnh0rwe@pnh10.med.navy.mil
Internet: http://www.nmcp.med.navy.mil/peds/peds.htm
Accred Length: 3 Years *Program Size:* 20 (*GY1:* 8)
Program ID: 320-51-21-014
US Armed Services Program

Richmond

Medical College of Virginia/Virginia Commonwealth University Program

Sponsor: Medical College of Virginia/Virginia Commonwealth University
Medical College of Virginia Hospitals

Program Director:
Richard R Brookman, MD
Med Coll of Virginia-Children's Med Ctr
PO Box 980264
Richmond, VA 23298-0264
Tel: 804 828-3282 *Fax:* 804 828-2435
E-mail: sbjones@hsc.vcu.edu
Internet: http://822p://views.vcu./pediatrics/.
Accred Length: 3 Years *Program Size:* 50 (*GY1:* 16)
Subspecialties: CCP, NPM, PDC, PDI, PN
Program ID: 320-51-21-241

Washington

Seattle

University of Washington Program

Sponsor: University of Washington School of Medicine
Children's Hospital and Medical Center
University of Washington Medical Center

Program Director:
Richard P Shugerman, MD
Children's Hospital and Regional Med Ctr
4800 Sand Point Way NE
PO Box C-5371/CH-30
Seattle, WA 98105-0371
Tel: 206 526-2525 *Fax:* 206 527-3843
Internet: http://www.washington.edu
Accred Length: 3 Years *Program Size:* 66 (*GY1:* 24)
Subspecialties: CCP, NPM, PDI, PDP, PHO, PN, PPR
Program ID: 320-54-21-358

Tacoma

Madigan Army Medical Center Program

Sponsor: Madigan Army Medical Center

Program Director:
William O Walker Jr, MD
Attn: MCHJ-P Dept of Pediatrics
Madigan Army Med Ctr
Tacoma, WA 98431
Tel: 253 968-0220 *Fax:* 253 968-0384
E-mail: wotisw@u.washington.edu
Accred Length: 3 Years *Program Size:* 16 (*GY1:* 6)
Program ID: 320-54-11-010
US Armed Services Program

West Virginia

Charleston

West Virginia University (Charleston Division) Program
Sponsor: Charleston Area Medical Center
Program Director:
Raheel R Khan, MD
Dept of Pediatrics
Robert C Byrd Health Sciences Ctr
830 Pennsylvania Ave/#104
Charleston, WV 25302
Tel: 304 342-8272 *Fax:* 304 342-8288
Accred Length: 3 Years *Program Size:* 12 (*GY1:* 4)
Program ID: 320-55-21-243

Huntington

Marshall University School of Medicine Program
Sponsor: Marshall University School of Medicine
Cabell Huntington Hospital
Program Director:
James M Waldeck, MD
Dept of Pediatrics
1600 Medical Center Dr/Ste 3500
Huntington, WV 25701-3655
Tel: 304 691-1371 *Fax:* 304 691-1375
E-mail: dchapman@marshall.edu
Internet:
http://www.musom.marshall.edu/peds/general.htm
Accred Length: 3 Years *Program Size:* 12 (*GY1:* 4)
Program ID: 320-55-21-380

Morgantown

West Virginia University Program
Sponsor: West Virginia University Hospitals
Program Director:
Martin E Weisse, MD
West Virginia Univ Sch of Med
Robert C Byrd Health Sciences Ctr
PO Box 9214
Morgantown, WV 26506-9214
Tel: 304 293-1198 *Fax:* 304 293-1216
E-mail: nkimble@hsc.wvu.edu
Internet: http://www.hsc.wvu.edu/som/pediatrics/peds
Accred Length: 3 Years *Program Size:* 12 (*GY1:* 4)
Subspecialties: CCP, NPM, PDC
Program ID: 320-55-11-245

Wisconsin

Madison

University of Wisconsin Program
Sponsor: University of Wisconsin Hospital and Clinics
Meriter Hospital
Program Director:
David B Allen, MD
Univ of Wisconsin Hospital and Clinics
Dept of Pediatrics/H4/447 CSC
600 Highland Ave
Madison, WI 53792-4108
Tel: 608 263-8557 *Fax:* 608 263-0440
E-mail: bschwarz@facstaff.wisc.edu
Accred Length: 3 Years *Program Size:* 39 (*GY1:* 13)
Subspecialties: CCP, NPM, PDE, PDP, PG, PHO
Program ID: 320-56-21-247

Marshfield

Marshfield Clinic-St Joseph's Hospital Program
Sponsor: Marshfield Clinic-St Joseph's Hospital
Program Director:
Edna O DeVries, MD
Marshfield Clinic
Dept of Pediatrics 1A4
1000 N Oak Ave
Marshfield, WI 54449-5777
Tel: 715 387-5267 *Fax:* 715 387-5240
E-mail: schaefec@mfldclin.edu
Internet:
http://www.marshmed.org/mfldclin/education/med_ed/residency/resident.htm
Accred Length: 3 Years *Program Size:* 12 (*GY1:* 4)
Program ID: 320-56-31-248

Milwaukee

Medical College of Wisconsin Program
Sponsor: Medical College of Wisconsin Affiliated Hospitals Inc
Children's Hospital of Wisconsin
Program Director:
David A Lewis, MD
Children's Hospital
Med Educ Ste 214
9000 W Wisconsin Ave/PO Box 1997
Milwaukee, WI 53226-1997
Tel: 414 266-6800 *Fax:* 414 266-6749
E-mail: dlewis@post.its.mcw.edu
Internet: http://www.mcw.edu/peds/residency
Accred Length: 3 Years *Program Size:* 48 (*GY1:* 16)
Subspecialties: CCP, NPM, PDP, PG, PHO
Program ID: 320-56-21-249

Physical Medicine and Rehabilitation

Alabama

Birmingham

University of Alabama Medical Center Program
Sponsor: University of Alabama Hospital
Program Director:
Laura B Kezar, MD
Univ of Alabama
Spain Rehabilitation Ctr
1717 Sixth Ave S
Birmingham, AL 35233-7330
Tel: 205 934-3450 *Fax:* 205 975-9754
E-mail: spains@sun.rehabm.uab.edu
Accred Length: 3 Years *Program Size:* 9
Program ID: 340-01-21-002

Arkansas

Little Rock

University of Arkansas for Medical Sciences Program
Sponsor: University of Arkansas College of Medicine
Arkansas Children's Hospital
Baptist Rehabilitation Institute
John L McClellan Memorial Veterans Hospital
University Hospital of Arkansas
Program Director:
Kevin M Means, MD
Univ of Arkansas for Med Sciences
Dept of Phys Med/Rehab
4301 W Markham St/Slot 602B
Little Rock, AR 72205
Tel: 501 661-1202, ext 2373 *Fax:* 501 671-2585
Internet: http://www.uams.edu/pmr
Accred Length: 4 Years *Program Size:* 16
Program ID: 340-04-21-083

California

Loma Linda

Loma Linda University Program
Sponsor: Loma Linda University Medical Center
Jerry L Pettis Memorial Veterans Hospital
Program Director:
Murray E Brandstater, MD PhD
Loma Linda Univ Med Ctr
Dept of Physical Med
11234 Anderson St/PO Box 2000
Loma Linda, CA 92354
Tel: 909 824-4009 *Fax:* 909 824-4133
Internet: http://www.llu.edu/llumc/rehabilitation
Accred Length: 4 Years *Program Size:* 18 (*GY1:* 4)
Program ID: 340-05-21-077

Los Angeles

VA Greater Los Angeles Healthcare System Program

Sponsor: VA Greater Los Angeles Healthcare System
Cedars-Sinai Medical Center

Program Director:
A M Erika Scremin, MD
UCLA-VA Multicampus Program
VA Greater Los Angeles Healthcare System
11301 Wilshire Blvd
Los Angeles, CA 90073
Tel: 310 268-3342 *Fax:* 310 268-4935
Accred Length: 3 Years *Program Size:* 25
Program ID: 340-05-21-007

Orange

University of California (Irvine) Program

Sponsor: University of California (Irvine) Medical Center
Long Beach Memorial Medical Center
Veterans Affairs Medical Center (Long Beach)

Program Director:
Phyllis E Page, MD
Univ of California Irvine Med Ctr
Dept of Phys Med/Rehab
101 The City Dr S/Rte 81 Bldg #53 Rm B-17
Orange, CA 92868
Tel: 714 456-6444 *Fax:* 714 456-6557
E-mail: amlievan@uci.edu
Accred Length: 3 Years *Program Size:* 15
Program ID: 340-05-21-005

Sacramento

University of California (Davis) Program

Sponsor: University of California (Davis) Medical Center

Program Director:
David D Kilmer, MD
Univ of California Davis Med Ctr
Ellison Ambulatory Care Ctr
4860 Y St/Ste 3850
Sacramento, CA 95817-2282
Tel: 916 734-8723 *Fax:* 916 734-7838
E-mail: dmwilliams@ucdavis.edu
Accred Length: 4 Years *Program Size:* 10 (*GY1:* 1)
Program ID: 340-05-21-004

Stanford

Stanford University Program

Sponsor: Stanford University Hospital
Santa Clara Valley Medical Center
Veterans Affairs Palo Alto Health Care System

Program Director:
Elaine S Date, MD
Stanford Univ-Palo Alto VA Med Ctr
Phys Med/Rehab (117)
3801 Miranda Ave
Palo Alto, CA 94304
Tel: 650 493-5000, ext 65469 *Fax:* 650 852-3470
Accred Length: 3 Years *Program Size:* 20
Subspecialties: SCI
Program ID: 340-05-21-008

Colorado

Denver

University of Colorado Program

Sponsor: University of Colorado Health Sciences Center
Veterans Affairs Medical Center (Denver)

Program Director:
Donna Jo Blake, MD
Dan Scott, MD
Univ of Colorado Health Sciences Ctr
4200 E Ninth Ave
Campus Box C279
Denver, CO 80262
Tel: 303 372-5610 *Fax:* 303 372-5605
E-mail: lxweil@ski.uhcolorado.edu
Internet: http://www.uchsc.edu./sm/gme/index.html
Accred Length: 3 Years *Program Size:* 12
Program ID: 340-07-21-009

District of Columbia

Washington

National Rehabilitation Hospital Program

Sponsor: National Rehabilitation Hospital
Washington Hospital Center

Program Director:
Susan M Miller, MD
National Rehabilitation Hospital
102 Irving St NW/#2159
Washington, DC 20010-2949
Tel: 202 877-1627 *Fax:* 202 877-1166
Accred Length: 3 Years *Program Size:* 14
Program ID: 340-10-21-087

Georgia

Atlanta

Emory University Program

Sponsor: Emory University School of Medicine
Emory University Hospital
Grady Memorial Hospital
Veterans Affairs Medical Center (Atlanta)

Program Director:
Dale C Strasser, MD
Dept of Phys Med/Rehab
1441 Clifton Rd NE/Rm 118
Atlanta, GA 30322
Tel: 404 712-5507 *Fax:* 404 712-5895
Accred Length: 3 Years *Program Size:* 13
Program ID: 340-12-21-011

Illinois

Chicago

McGaw Medical Center of Northwestern University Program

Sponsor: Northwestern University Medical School
Northwestern Memorial Hospital
Rehabilitation Institute of Chicago

Program Director:
James A Sliwa, DO
Office of Grad Med Educ
Northwestern Univ Med Sch
303 E Chicago Ave/#932
Chicago, IL 60611
Tel: 312 503-4748 *Fax:* 312 503-5230
E-mail: r-bailey@nwu.edu
Internet: http://www.nwu.edu/pmr
Accred Length: 4 Years *Program Size:* 40 (*GY1:* 4)
Program ID: 340-16-21-014

Rush-Presbyterian-St Luke's Medical Center Program

Sponsor: Rush-Presbyterian-St Luke's Medical Center
Marianjoy Rehabilitation Hospital and Clinics
Oak Forest Hospital of Cook County

Program Director:
R Samuel Mayer, MD
Rush-Presbyterian-St Luke's Med Ctr
1725 W Harrison St
Ste 1018
Chicago, IL 60612
Tel: 312 942-3675 *Fax:* 312 942-4234
E-mail: bcook@rush.edu.
Accred Length: 4 Years *Program Size:* 17
Program ID: 340-16-21-082

Schwab Rehabilitation Hospital and Care Network/University of Chicago Program

Sponsor: Schwab Rehabilitation Hospital and Care Network
Mount Sinai Hospital Medical Center of Chicago

Program Director:
Michelle S Gittler, MD
Schwab Rehabilitation Hospital and Care Network
1401 S California Blvd
Chicago, IL 60608-1612
Tel: 773 522-5856, ext 5238 *Fax:* 773 522-5886
Accred Length: 3 Years *Program Size:* 18
Program ID: 340-16-22-012

University of Illinois College of Medicine at Chicago Program

Sponsor: University of Illinois College of Medicine at Chicago
Michael Reese Hospital and Medical Center
University of Illinois Hospital and Clinics
Veterans Affairs West Side Medical Center

Program Director:
Jessica Tinianow, MD MD
Univ of Illinois Hospital
Dept of Rehab Med/Restorative Sciences
840 S Wood St (M/C 888)
Chicago, IL 60612
Tel: 312 996-7211 *Fax:* 312 996-4829
E-mail: rehab@uic.edu
Accred Length: 3 Years *Program Size:* 12
Program ID: 340-16-21-015

Maywood

Loyola University Program
Sponsor: Loyola University Medical Center
Edward J Hines Jr Veterans Affairs Hospital
Marianjoy Rehabilitation Hospital and Clinics
Program Director:
Jay Subbarao, MD
Loyola Univ Med Ctr
Div of Phys Med/Rehab
2160 S First Ave
Maywood, IL 60153
Tel: 708 216-4994 *Fax:* 708 216-9348
Accred Length: 4 Years *Program Size:* 12 (*GYI:* 3)
Program ID: 340-16-31-016

Wheaton

Rehabilitation Foundation Program
Sponsor: Rehabilitation Foundation Inc
Marianjoy Rehabilitation Hospital and Clinics
Program Director:
Dennis J Keane, MD
Rehabilitation Foundation
PO Box 675
26 W 171 Roosevelt Rd
Wheaton, IL 60189
Tel: 800 462-5655 *Fax:* 630 462-4547
E-mail: resident@rfi.org
Internet: http://www.rfi.org
Accred Length: 3 Years *Program Size:* 9
Program ID: 340-16-21-097

Indiana

Indianapolis

Indiana University School of Medicine Program
Sponsor: Indiana University School of Medicine
Clarian IU Hospital
Clarian Riley Hospital for Children
Community Hospitals of Indianapolis
Richard L Roudebush Veterans Affairs Medical Center
Program Director:
Ralph M Buschbacher, MD
Dept of Phys Med/Rehab
541 N Clinical Dr/Rm 368
Indianapolis, IN 46202-5111
Tel: 317 278-0200 *Fax:* 317 278-0206
Internet: http://www.iupui.edu/it/deptpmr/index.htm
Accred Length: 3 Years *Program Size:* 6
Program ID: 340-17-21-098

Kansas

Kansas City

University of Kansas Medical Center Program
Sponsor: University of Kansas School of Medicine
Bethany Medical Center
Dwight D Eisenhower Veterans Affairs Medical Center
University of Kansas Medical Center
Veterans Affairs Medical Center (Kansas City)
Program Director:
Lisa A McPeak, MD
Rehabilitation Med Dept
Univ of Kansas Med Ctr
3901 Rainbow Blvd
Kansas City, KS 66160-7306
Tel: 913 588-6777 *Fax:* 913 588-6765
E-mail: ttipton@kumc.edu
Accred Length: 3 Years *Program Size:* 12
Program ID: 340-19-21-018

Kentucky

Lexington

University of Kentucky Medical Center Program
Sponsor: University of Kentucky Hospital
Cardinal Hill Hospital
Veterans Affairs Medical Center (Lexington)
Program Director:
Susan McDowell, MD
Robert Nickerson, MD
Univ of Kentucky Med Ctr
Dept of Phys Med/Rehab
Kentucky Clinic/Wing B
Lexington, KY 40536-0284
Tel: 606 257-4890 *Fax:* 606 323-1123
Internet: http://www.mcpmr.uky.edu
Accred Length: 4 Years *Program Size:* 12 (*GYI:* 3)
Program ID: 340-20-21-079

Louisville

University of Louisville Program
Sponsor: University of Louisville School of Medicine
Amelia Brown Frazier Rehabilitation Center
Program Director:
Karen K Bloom, MD
Frazier Rehabilitation Ctr
220 Abraham Flexner Way
Louisville, KY 40202
Tel: 502 582-7465 *Fax:* 502 582-7477
Accred Length: 3 Years *Program Size:* 7
Program ID: 340-20-11-019

Louisiana

New Orleans

Louisiana State University Program
Sponsor: Louisiana State University School of Medicine
Louisiana Rehabilitation Institute
Medical Center of Louisiana at New Orleans
Touro Infirmary
Program Director:
Robert C Mipro Jr, MD
Louisiana State Univ Med Ctr
Sect of Phys Med/Rehab
1542 Tulane Ave/Box T6M-2
New Orleans, LA 70112-2822
Tel: 504 568-2688 *Fax:* 504 568-7839
E-mail: pmr@lsumc.edu
Accred Length: 4 Years *Program Size:* 20 (*GYI:* 4)
Program ID: 340-21-21-020

Maryland

Baltimore

Sinai Hospital of Baltimore/Johns Hopkins University Program
Sponsor: Sinai Hospital of Baltimore
Good Samaritan Hospital of Maryland
Johns Hopkins Hospital
Program Director:
Gerald Felsenthal, MD
Sinai Hospital
Dept of Rehab Med
2401 W Belvedere Ave
Baltimore, MD 21215-5271
Tel: 410 601-5584 *Fax:* 410 601-9939
E-mail: gfelsent@sinai-balt.com
Internet: http://www.sinai-balt.com
Accred Length: 3 Years *Program Size:* 13
Program ID: 340-23-22-021

Bethesda

National Capital Consortium Program
Sponsor: National Capital Consortium
Walter Reed Army Medical Center
Program Director:
Steven E Braverman, MD
Phys Med/Rehabilitation Service
Walter Reed Army Med Ctr
6825 16th St NW
Washington, DC 20307-5001
Tel: 202 782-2747 *Fax:* 202 782-0970
E-mail:
maj_steven_braverman@wramc1-amedd.army.mil
Internet:
http://www.wramc.amedd.army.mil/departments/physmed/resprgrm.htm
Accred Length: 3 Years *Program Size:* 11
Program ID: 340-10-21-074
US Armed Services Program

Massachusetts

Boston

Boston University Medical Center Program
Sponsor: Boston Medical Center
Braintree Hospital
Program Director:
Susan Biener-Bergman, MD
Boston Med Ctr
One Boston Medical Center Pl
Rm 511
Boston, MA 02118-2398
Tel: 617 638-7310 *Fax:* 617 638-7313
Internet:
http://www.bumc.bu.edu/departments/homemain.asp?departmentid=91
Accred Length: 3 Years *Program Size:* 13
Program ID: 340-24-11-024

Harvard Medical School Program
Sponsor: Spaulding Rehabilitation Hospital
Program Director:
David T Burke, MD
Spaulding Rehabilitation Hospital
125 Nashua St
Boston, MA 02114
Tel: 617 573-2759 *Fax:* 617 573-2769
Accred Length: 3 Years *Program Size:* 19
Program ID: 340-24-21-094

Tufts University Program
Sponsor: New England Medical Center Hospitals
New England Sinai Hospital and Rehabilitation Center
Veterans Affairs Medical Center (Boston)

Program Director:
Parminder S Phull, MD
Dept of Phys Med/Rehab
New England Med Ctr
750 Washington St/Box 387
Boston, MA 02111
Tel: 617 636-5634 *Fax:* 617 636-5056
E-mail: parminder.phull@es.nemc.org
Internet: http://www.nemc.org/rehab/resprog.htm
Accred Length: 3 Years *Program Size:* 14
Program ID: 340-24-21-023

Michigan

Ann Arbor

University of Michigan Program
Sponsor: University of Michigan Hospitals

Program Director:
M Catherine Spires, MD
Univ of Michigan Health System
1500 E Medical Center Dr/Box 0042
Ann Arbor, MI 48109-0042
Tel: 734 936-7201 *Fax:* 734 936-6121
E-mail: alchees@umich.edu
Internet: http://med.umich.edu/pmr/
Accred Length: 3 Years *Program Size:* 18
Program ID: 340-25-21-025

Detroit

Wayne State University/Detroit Medical Center (Sinai Hospital) Program
Sponsor: Wayne State University/Detroit Medical Center
Sinai Hospital

Program Director:
Maury R Ellenberg, MD
Sinai Hospital
6767 W Outer Dr
Detroit, MI 48235-2899
Tel: 313 493-6554 *Fax:* 313 493-3871
Accred Length: 4 Years *Program Size:* 9
Program ID: 340-25-31-026

Wayne State University/Detroit Medical Center Program
Sponsor: Wayne State University/Detroit Medical Center
Rehabilitation Institute

Program Director:
Bruce E Becker, MD
Rehabilitation Inst of Michigan
261 Mack Blvd
Detroit, MI 48201-9903
Tel: 313 745-1095 *Fax:* 313 745-1063
E-mail: 75143,1020@compuserve.com
Accred Length: 3 Years *Program Size:* 18
Program ID: 340-25-21-027

East Lansing

Michigan State University Program
Sponsor: Michigan State University College of Osteopathic Medicine
Ingham Regional Medical Center

Program Director:
Michael T Andary, MD
B401 W Fee Hall, Dept of Phys Med/Rehab
Michigan State Univ
Coll of Osteopathic Med
East Lansing, MI 48824
Tel: 517 353-0713 *Fax:* 517 432-1339
E-mail: andary@com.msu.edu
Accred Length: 3 Years *Program Size:* 8
Program ID: 340-25-21-100

Royal Oak

William Beaumont Hospital Program
Sponsor: William Beaumont Hospital
William Beaumont Hospital-Troy

Program Director:
Myron M LaBan, MD
William Beaumont Hospital
3601 W 13 Mile Rd
Royal Oak, MI 48073-6769
Tel: 248 551-0161 *Fax:* 248 551-3631
E-mail: thaggerty@beaumont.edu
Internet: http://www.beaumont.edu/html/gme
Accred Length: 4 Years *Program Size:* 12 (*GYI:* 3)
Program ID: 340-25-21-076

Minnesota

Minneapolis

University of Minnesota Program
Sponsor: University of Minnesota Medical School
Fairview-University Medical Center
Veterans Affairs Medical Center (Minneapolis)

Program Director:
Dennis D Dykstra, MD
Univ of Minnesota
Box 297 UMHC 500
420 Delaware St SE
Minneapolis, MN 55455
Tel: 612 626-4913 *Fax:* 612 624-6686
E-mail: olsen014@maroon.tc.umn.edu
Accred Length: 3 Years *Program Size:* 12
Program ID: 340-26-21-028

Rochester

Mayo Graduate School of Medicine (Rochester) Program
Sponsor: Mayo Graduate School of Medicine-Mayo Foundation
Mayo Clinic (Rochester)
Rochester Methodist Hospital
St Mary's Hospital of Rochester

Program Director:
Stephen F Noll, MD
Application Processing Ctr
Mayo Graduate Sch of Med
200 First St SW
Rochester, MN 55905
Tel: 507 284-3108 *Fax:* 507 284-0999
E-mail: mgsm.medlab.specialties@mayo.edu
Internet: http://www.mayo.edu/
Accred Length: 3 Years *Program Size:* 26
Program ID: 340-26-21-030

Missouri

Columbia

University of Missouri-Columbia Program
Sponsor: University of Missouri-Columbia School of Medicine
Harry S Truman Memorial Veterans Hospital
University Hospitals and Clinics

Program Director:
Robert Conway, MD
Rusk Rehabilitation Ctr
1 Hospital Dr/DCO 4600
Columbia, MO 65212
Tel: 573 882-3101 *Fax:* 573 884-4540
E-mail: conway@health.missouri.edu
Internet: http://www.hsc.missouri.edu/som/pmr
Accred Length: 3 Years *Program Size:* 11
Program ID: 340-28-21-031

St Louis

Washington University/B-JH/SLCH Consortium Program
Sponsor: Washington University/B-JH/SLCH Consortium
Barnes-Jewish Hospital (North Campus)

Program Director:
Oksana Volshteyn, MD
Barnes-Jewish Hospital
216 S Kingshighway
St Louis, MO 63110
Tel: 314 454-7755 *Fax:* 314 454-5277
E-mail: oav1549@bjcmail.carenet.org
Accred Length: 4 Years *Program Size:* 15 (*GYI:* 3)
Program ID: 340-28-11-032

New Jersey

Edison

JFK Medical Center Program
Sponsor: JFK Medical Center
JFK Johnson Rehabilitation Institute

Program Director:
Thomas E Strax, MD
JFK Johnson Rehabilitation Inst
65 James St
Edison, NJ 08818-3059
Tel: 732 321-7000, ext 2133 *Fax:* 732 906-4910
Accred Length: 3 Years *Program Size:* 12
Program ID: 340-33-21-033

Newark

UMDNJ-New Jersey Medical School Program
Sponsor: UMDNJ-New Jersey Medical School
Kessler Institute for Rehabilitation
UMDNJ-University Hospital
Veterans Affairs Medical Center (East Orange)

Program Director:
Steven Kirshblum, MD
UMDNJ-New Jersey Med Sch
150 Bergen St/UH B261
Newark, NJ 07103
Tel: 973 972-3606 *Fax:* 973 972-5148
E-mail: leckyal@umdnj.edu
Internet: http://njmsa.umdnj.edu
Accred Length: 3 Years *Program Size:* 28
Program ID: 340-33-32-034

New York

Albany

Albany Medical Center Program

Sponsor: Albany Medical Center
St Peter's Hospital
Sunnyview Hospital and Rehabilitation Center
Veterans Affairs Medical Center (Albany)

Program Director:
George F Gombas, MD
Albany Med Ctr
Dept of Phys Med/Rehab
43 New Scotland Ave
Albany, NY 12208-3479
Tel: 518 262-3291 *Fax:* 518 262-4492
Accred Length: 4 Years *Program Size:* 8 (*GY1:* 2)
Program ID: 340-35-21-035

Bronx

Albert Einstein College of Medicine Program

Sponsor: Albert Einstein College of Medicine of Yeshiva University
Jacobi Medical Center
Montefiore Medical Center-Henry and Lucy Moses Division
Montefiore Medical Center-Weiler Hospital
North Central Bronx Hospital

Program Director:
Mark A Thomas, MD
Montefiore Med Ctr
Rehabilitation Med Admin
111 E 210th St
Bronx, NY 10467-2490
Tel: 718 920-2753 *Fax:* 718 920-5048
Accred Length: 3 Years *Program Size:* 22
Program ID: 340-35-21-043

Brooklyn

Kingsbrook Jewish Medical Center Program

Sponsor: Kingsbrook Jewish Medical Center
Staten Island University Hospital

Program Director:
Zoraida Navarro, MD
Kingsbrook Jewish Med Ctr
Dept of Phys Med/Rehab
585 Schenectady Ave
Brooklyn, NY 11203-1891
Tel: 718 604-5341 *Fax:* 718 604-5272
Accred Length: 3 Years *Program Size:* 17
Program ID: 340-35-22-041

SUNY Health Science Center at Brooklyn Program

Sponsor: SUNY Health Science Center at Brooklyn
Kings County Hospital Center

Program Director:
Tsai C Chao, MD
SUNY Health Science Ctr
450 Clarkson Ave/Box 30
Brooklyn, NY 11203
Tel: 718 245-5165 *Fax:* 718 245-5164
E-mail: hrmb4@ingress.com
Accred Length: 3 Years *Program Size:* 9
Program ID: 340-35-21-048

Buffalo

SUNY at Buffalo Graduate Medical-Dental Education Consortium Program

Sponsor: SUNY at Buffalo Grad Medical-Dental Education Consortium
CGF Health System (Buffalo General Hospital)
Erie County Medical Center
Veterans Affairs Medical Center (Buffalo)

Program Director:
Gary S Clark, MD
Erie County Med Ctr
462 Grider St
Buffalo, NY 14215
Tel: 716 898-3218 *Fax:* 716 898-3652
Internet: http://www.udsmr.org
Accred Length: 4 Years *Program Size:* 10 (*GY1:* 3)
Program ID: 340-35-21-036

East Meadow

Nassau County Medical Center Program

Sponsor: Nassau County Medical Center

Program Director:
Lyn Weiss, MD
Nassau County Med Ctr
Dept of Phys Med/Rehab
2201 Hempstead Trnpk
East Meadow, NY 11554-5400
Tel: 516 572-6525 *Fax:* 516 572-3170
Accred Length: 3 Years *Program Size:* 13
Program ID: 340-35-11-037

New Hyde Park

Albert Einstein College of Medicine at Long Island Jewish Medical Center Program

Sponsor: Long Island Jewish Medical Center
Jamaica Hospital
Southside Hospital

Program Director:
Daniel Fechtner, MD
Long Island Jewish Med Ctr
270-05 76th Ave/CH005
New Hyde Park, NY 11040
Tel: 718 470-3020 *Fax:* 718 962-6233
E-mail: fechtner@lij.edu
Internet: http://www.lij.edu
Accred Length: 3 Years *Program Size:* 11
Program ID: 340-35-21-042

New York

Mount Sinai School of Medicine Program

Sponsor: Mount Sinai School of Medicine
Beth Israel Medical Center
Elmhurst Hospital Center-Mount Sinai Services
Mount Sinai Medical Center
Veterans Affairs Medical Center (Bronx)

Program Director:
Kristjan T Ragnarsson, MD
Mount Sinai Hospital
One Gustave L Levy Pl/Box 1240
New York, NY 10029-6574
Tel: 212 241-9654 *Fax:* 212 348-5901
Accred Length: 3 Years *Program Size:* 18
Program ID: 340-35-21-044

New York and Presbyterian Hospital (Columbia Campus) Program

Sponsor: New York and Presbyterian Hospital
New York and Presbyterian Hospital (Columbia Campus)

Program Director:
Nancy E Strauss, MD
New York Presbyterian Hospital
630 W 168th St
Unit 38
New York, NY 10032
Tel: 212 305-8592 *Fax:* 212 305-3916
Accred Length: 3 Years *Program Size:* 15
Program ID: 340-35-21-039

New York and Presbyterian Hospital (Cornell Campus) Program

Sponsor: New York and Presbyterian Hospital
Memorial Sloan-Kettering Cancer Center
New York and Presbyterian Hospital (Cornell Campus)

Program Director:
Willibald Nagler, MD
New York Hospital-Cornell Med Ctr
525 E 68th St/Box 142
New York, NY 10021-8110
Tel: 212 746-1500 *Fax:* 212 746-8900
Accred Length: 3 Years *Program Size:* 15
Program ID: 340-35-21-040

New York Medical College (Metropolitan) Program

Sponsor: New York Medical College
Metropolitan Hospital Center
Our Lady of Mercy Medical Center

Program Director:
Maria P de Araujo, MD
New York Med Coll
Dept of Rehab Med
Rm 557 Munger Pavilion
Valhalla, NY 10595
Tel: 914 594-4275 *Fax:* 914 594-4276
Accred Length: 4 Years *Program Size:* 11 (*GY1:* 2)
Program ID: 340-35-21-045

New York Medical College at St Vincent's Hospital and Medical Center Program

Sponsor: New York Medical College
St Vincent's Hospital and Medical Center of New York

Program Director:
Lakshmi Murali, MD
St Vincent's Hospital and Med Ctr
153 W 11th St
New York, NY 10011
Tel: 212 604-8682 *Fax:* 212 604-3272
E-mail: lmurali106aol.com
Accred Length: 3 Years *Program Size:* 11
Program ID: 340-35-11-047

New York University Medical Center Program

Sponsor: New York University Medical Center
Bellevue Hospital Center
Goldwater Memorial Hospital
Rusk Institute of Rehabilitation Medicine
Veterans Affairs Medical Center (Manhattan)

Program Director:
Howard G Thistle, MD
New York Univ Med Ctr
Dept of Rehab Med
400 E 34th St/Ste 600
New York, NY 10016-4998
Tel: 212 263-6110 *Fax:* 212 263-8815
Accred Length: 4 Years *Program Size:* 41 (*GY1:* 1)
Program ID: 340-35-21-046

Rochester

University of Rochester Program

Sponsor: Strong Memorial Hospital of the University of Rochester
St Mary's Hospital (Unity Health System)

Program Director:
Kanakadurga Rao Poduri, MD
Univ of Rochester Med Ctr
601 Elmwood Ave/Box 664
Rochester, NY 14642
Tel: 716 275-3271 *Fax:* 716 442-2949
E-mail: cpappert@cc.urmc.rochester.edu
Internet: http://www.urmc.rochester.edu
Accred Length: 4 Years *Program Size:* 11
Program ID: 340-35-21-051

Stony Brook

SUNY at Stony Brook Program

Sponsor: University Hospital-SUNY at Stony Brook
Veterans Affairs Medical Center (Northport)

Program Director:
Craig H Rosenberg, MD
St Charles Hospital
200 Belle Terre Rd
Port Jefferson, NY 11777
Tel: 516 474-6146 *Fax:* 516 474-6413
E-mail: stace868@aol.com
Internet: http://www.stcharles.org
Accred Length: 4 Years *Program Size:* 12 (*GY1:* 3)
Program ID: 340-35-21-103

Syracuse

SUNY Health Science Center at Syracuse Program

Sponsor: University Hospital-SUNY Health Science Center at Syracuse
St Camillus Health and Rehabilitation Center
Veterans Affairs Medical Center (Syracuse)

Program Director:
Robert J Weber, MD
SUNY Health Science Ctr-Syracuse
750 E Adams St
Syracuse, NY 13210-2375
Tel: 315 464-5820 *Fax:* 315 464-8699
E-mail: weberr@mailbox.hscsyr.edu
Accred Length: 3 Years *Program Size:* 10
Program ID: 340-35-21-093

North Carolina

Chapel Hill

University of North Carolina Hospitals Program

Sponsor: University of North Carolina Hospitals

Program Director:
Michael Y Lee, MD
Univ of North Carolina at Chapel Hill
Dept of Physical Med/Rehabilitation
CB#7200 1148 UNC-H
Chapel Hill, NC 27599-7200
Tel: 919 966-5164 *Fax:* 919 966-0083
E-mail: mylee@med.unc.edu
Internet: http://www.med.unc.edu/wrkunits/z depts/phyrehab/
Accred Length: 4 Years *Program Size:* 6 (*GY1:* 3)
Program ID: 340-36-21-104

Charlotte

Carolinas Medical Center Program

Sponsor: Carolinas Medical Center
Charlotte Institute of Rehabilitation

Program Director:
William L Bockenek, MD
Charlotte Inst of Rehabilitation
Dept of Phys Med/Rehab
1100 Blythe Blvd
Charlotte, NC 28203
Tel: 704 355-4406 *Fax:* 704 355-0709
E-mail: wbockenek@carolinas.org
Internet: http://www.charweb.org/health/rehab
Accred Length: 4 Years *Program Size:* 11 (*GY1:* 3)
Program ID: 340-36-21-095

Greenville

East Carolina University Program

Sponsor: East Carolina University School of Medicine
Pitt County Memorial Hospital

Program Director:
Joseph B Webster, MD MD
East Carolina Univ Sch of Med
Dept of Phys Med/Rehab
Moye Blvd
Greenville, NC 27858-4354
Tel: 919 816-7907 *Fax:* 919 816-8108
E-mail: dgrady@brody.med.ecu.edu or dbgrady.general.services.pcmh
Internet: http://www.med.ecu.edu/htdocs/rehab/index.htm
Accred Length: 4 Years *Program Size:* 15 (*GY1:* 3)
Program ID: 340-36-21-091

Ohio

Cincinnati

University Hospital/University of Cincinnati College of Medicine Program

Sponsor: University Hospital Inc

Program Director:
Mary E Dillon, MD
Univ Hospital-Univ of Cincinnati Coll of Med
Dept of Phys Med/Rehab
PO Box 670530
Cincinnati, OH 45267-0530
Tel: 513 558-7635 *Fax:* 513 558-4458
E-mail: williapa@email.uc.edu
Internet: http://www.med.uc.edu/htdocs/medicine/departme/pmr/pmrres.htm
Accred Length: 4 Years *Program Size:* 9 (*GY1:* 2)
Program ID: 340-38-21-086

Cleveland

Case Western Reserve University Program

Sponsor: MetroHealth Medical Center

Program Director:
Shu Q Huang, MD
MetroHealth Med Ctr
2500 MetroHealth Dr
Cleveland, OH 44109-1998
Tel: 216 778-3219 *Fax:* 216 778-3262
Accred Length: 4 Years *Program Size:* 15 (*GY1:* 2)
Program ID: 340-38-31-053

Columbus

Ohio State University Program

Sponsor: Ohio State University Medical Center
Grant Medical Center (OhioHealth)
Mount Carmel Medical Center
Riverside Methodist Hospitals (OhioHealth)

Program Director:
William S Pease, MD
Dodd Hall
480 W Ninth Ave
Columbus, OH 43210-1245
Tel: 614 293-3433 *Fax:* 614 293-3809
E-mail: pease.2@osu.edu
Internet: http://axon.med.ohio-state.edu/physmed
Accred Length: 4 Years *Program Size:* 20 (*GY1:* 6)
Program ID: 340-38-21-054

Toledo

Medical College of Ohio Program

Sponsor: Medical College of Ohio
Flower Hospital
St Vincent Mercy Medical Center
Toledo Hospital

Program Director:
Greg Nemunaitis, MD
Med Coll of Ohio
3065 Arlington Ave
Toledo, OH 43614
Tel: 419 383-5090 *Fax:* 419 383-3106
E-mail: csmith@gemini.mco.edu
Accred Length: 4 Years *Program Size:* 8 (*GY1:* 2)
Program ID: 340-38-21-080

Pennsylvania

Philadelphia

Graduate Hospital Program

Sponsor: Graduate Hospital

Program Director:
Francis J Bonner Jr, MD
Pepper Pavilion, Suite 1000B
1800 Lombard St
Philadelphia, PA 19146
Tel: 215 893-7559 *Fax:* 215 893-2503
Accred Length: 3 Years *Program Size:* 15
Program ID: 340-41-21-088

Temple University Program

Sponsor: Temple University Hospital
Albert Einstein Medical Center
Moss Rehabilitation Hospital

Program Director:
James Demopoulos, MD
Dept of Phys Med/Rehab
Temple Univ Hospital
3401 N Broad St
Philadelphia, PA 19140
Tel: 215 707-7022 *Fax:* 215 707-7661
Accred Length: 3 Years *Program Size:* 27
Program ID: 340-41-21-056

Thomas Jefferson University Program
Sponsor: Thomas Jefferson University Hospital
Magee Rehabilitation Hospital

Program Director:
Christopher S Formal, MD
Thomas Jefferson Univ Hospital
Dept of Rehab Med
925 S 9th St
Philadelphia, PA 19107
Tel: 215 955-6585 *Fax:* 215 923-3729
E-mail: tabitha.mays@mail.tju.edu
Internet:
http://oac1.oac.tju.edu/cwis/dept/rehab/res/index.htm
Accred Length: 3 Years *Program Size:* 12
Program ID: 340-41-21-057

University of Pennsylvania Program
Sponsor: Hospital of the University of Pennsylvania
Children's Seashore House
Our Lady of Lourdes Medical Center
Veterans Affairs Medical Center (Philadelphia)

Program Director:
Keith M Robinson, MD
Hospital of Univ of Pennsylvania
5th Fl W Gates Bldg
3400 Spruce St
Philadelphia, PA 19104-4283
Tel: 215 349-5574 *Fax:* 215 349-8944
Accred Length: 3 Years *Program Size:* 12
Program ID: 340-41-21-058

Pittsburgh

St Francis Medical Center Program
Sponsor: St Francis Medical Center
Mercy Hospital of Pittsburgh
University of Pittsburgh Medical Center (St Margaret)

Program Director:
Joseph K Eshleman, DO
St Francis Med Ctr
Med Education Office
400 45th St
Pittsburgh, PA 15201
Tel: 412 622-7187
Accred Length: 4 Years *Program Size:* 13 (*GY1:* 3)
Program ID: 340-41-22-059

University Health Center of Pittsburgh Program
Sponsor: University Health Center of Pittsburgh
Harmarville Rehabilitation Center
Presbyterian University Hospital/UPMC

Program Director:
Louis E Penrod, MD
Hospital of Univ Health Ctr of Pittsburgh
PMR Residency
1405 Shady Ave
Pittsburgh, PA 15217
Tel: 412 420-2171 *Fax:* 412 420-2269
E-mail: walkerjl@msx.upmc.edu
Internet: http://www.dev.upmc.edu/rehabmed
Accred Length: 4 Years *Program Size:* 16 (*GY1:* 4)
Program ID: 340-41-21-075

Puerto Rico

San Juan

University of Puerto Rico Program
Sponsor: University of Puerto Rico School of Medicine
University Hospital
University Pediatric Hospital
Vocational Rehabilitation Center

Program Director:
William F Micheo, MD
Univ of Puerto Rico Sch of Med
Caparra Heights Station
PO Box 365067
Rio Piedras, PR 00936-5067
Tel: 787 751-9625 *Fax:* 787 751-9625
Accred Length: 4 Years *Program Size:* 12 (*GY1:* 3)
Program ID: 340-42-31-062

Veterans Affairs Medical and Regional Office Center Program
Sponsor: Veterans Affairs Medical Center (San Juan)

Program Director:
William Acevedo, MD
VA Med Ctr
Phys Med/Rehab Service (117)
One Veterans Plaza
San Juan, PR 00927-5800
Tel: 787 758-7575, ext 3317 *Fax:* 787 766-6100
E-mail: acevedo,william@san-juan.va.gov
Accred Length: 4 Years *Program Size:* 12 (*GY1:* 3)
Program ID: 340-42-31-063

South Carolina

Charleston

Medical University of South Carolina Program
Sponsor: Medical University of South Carolina College of Medicine
MUSC Medical Center

Program Director:
James E Warmoth, MD
Med Univ of South Carolina
St Francis Annex/4th Fl
150 Ashley Ave/PO Box 250583
Charleston, SC 29425
Tel: 803 792-2792 *Fax:* 803 792-5549
E-mail: danielr@musc.edu
Accred Length: 3 Years *Program Size:* 6
Program ID: 340-45-21-092

Tennessee

Chattanooga

University of Tennessee College of Medicine at Chattanooga Program
Sponsor: University of Tennessee College of Medicine-Chattanooga Unit
Erlanger Medical Center

Program Director:
James P Little, MD
Univ of Tennessee Coll of Med
Siskin Hospital for Physical Rehab
One Siskin Plaza
Chattanooga, TN 37403
Tel: 423 634-1554 *Fax:* 423 634-1508
E-mail: aharper@siskinrehab.org
Internet: http://www.erlanger.org/utcom/rehab.html
Accred Length: 3 Years *Program Size:* 12
Program ID: 340-47-21-099

Texas

Dallas

Baylor University Medical Center Program
Sponsor: Baylor University Medical Center
Baylor Institute for Rehabilitation

Program Director:
Barry S Smith, MD
Baylor Univ Med Ctr
Dept of Phys Med/Rehab
3500 Gaston Ave
Dallas, TX 75246-2088
Tel: 214 820-7192 *Fax:* 214 820-8892
E-mail: drbssmith@aol.com
Accred Length: 3 Years *Program Size:* 9
Program ID: 340-48-31-064

University of Texas Southwestern Medical School Program
Sponsor: University of Texas Southwestern Medical School
Dallas County Hospital District-Parkland Memorial Hospital
Healthsouth Dallas Rehabilitation Institute
Veterans Affairs Medical Center (Dallas)

Program Director:
Geetha Pandian, MD
Univ of Texas Southwestern Med Ctr
Dept of Phys Med/Rehab
5323 Harry Hines Blvd
Dallas, TX 75235-9055
Tel: 214 648-8826 *Fax:* 214 648-8828
E-mail: ccowar@mednet.swmed.edu
Internet: http://www.swmed.edu:80/index.html
Accred Length: 3 Years *Program Size:* 19
Program ID: 340-48-21-065

Houston

Baylor College of Medicine Program
Sponsor: Baylor College of Medicine
Methodist Hospital
St Luke's Episcopal Hospital
The Institute for Rehabilitation and Research (TIRR)
Veterans Affairs Medical Center (Houston)

Program Director:
Carol Bodenheimer, MD
Dept of Phys Med/Rehab
Education/Rm B-107 TIRR
1333 Moursund
Houston, TX 77030-3405
Tel: 713 799-5034 *Fax:* 713 797-5982
E-mail: mckenzie@bcm.tmc.edu
Internet: http://www.bcm.tmc/pm&r/
Accred Length: 3 Years *Program Size:* 29
Program ID: 340-48-21-066

University of Texas at Houston Program
Sponsor: University of Texas Medical School at Houston
Lyndon B Johnson General Hospital
Memorial Hermann Healthcare System
The Institute for Rehabilitation and Research (TIRR)

Program Director:
Kenneth C Parsons, MD
Dept. of Phys Med/Rehab
Education/RM B-107 TIRR
1333 Moursund
Houston, TX 77030-3405
Tel: 713 799-5034 *Fax:* 713 797-5982
E-mail: mckenzie@bcm.tmc.edu
Internet: http://www.bcm.tmc/pm&r/
Accred Length: 3 Years *Program Size:* 9
Program ID: 340-48-21-101

San Antonio

University of Texas Health Science Center at San Antonio Program

Sponsor: University of Texas Medical School at San Antonio
Audie L Murphy Memorial Veterans Hospital (San Antonio)
San Antonio Warm Springs Rehabilitation Hospital
University Hospital-South Texas Medical Center

Program Director:
Daniel Dumitru, MD
Univ of Texas Health Science Ctr
Dept of Rehab Med
7703 Floyd Curl Dr
San Antonio, TX 78284-7798
Tel: 210 567-5300 *Fax:* 210 567-5354
E-mail: dumitru@uthscsa.edu
Internet: http://daffodil.uthscsa.edu/
Accred Length: 4 Years *Program Size:* 24 (*GYI:* 6)
Program ID: 340-48-21-067

Utah

Salt Lake City

University of Utah Program

Sponsor: University of Utah Medical Center
Primary Children's Medical Center
Veterans Affairs Medical Center (Salt Lake City)

Program Director:
James R Swenson, MD
Univ of Utah Med Ctr, Div of Phys Med/Rehab
50 N Medical Dr
Salt Lake City, UT 84132
Tel: 801 581-7985 *Fax:* 801 585-5757
E-mail: james.swenson@hsc.utah.edu
Internet: http://www.hsc.med.utah.edu
Accred Length: 3 Years *Program Size:* 8
Program ID: 340-49-21-068

Virginia

Charlottesville

University of Virginia Program

Sponsor: University of Virginia Medical Center
Mount Vernon Hospital

Program Director:
Paul T Diamond, MD
Univ of Virginia Health Sciences Ctr
Dept of Phys Med/Rehabilitation
545 Ray C Hunt Dr/Ste 240
Charlottesville, VA 22903-2981
Tel: 804 243-5627 *Fax:* 804 243-5639
E-mail: pmrmd@virginia.edu
Internet:
http://www.med.virginia.edu/medicine/clinical/phys-med-rehab
Accred Length: 4 Years *Program Size:* 14 (*GYI:* 2)
Program ID: 340-51-21-089

Norfolk

Eastern Virginia Medical School Program

Sponsor: Eastern Virginia Medical School
Sentara Norfolk General Hospital
Veterans Affairs Medical Center (Hampton)

Program Director:
Cynthia L Flick, MD
Eastern Virginia Med Sch
Dept of Phys Med/Rehab
825 Fairfax Ave
Norfolk, VA 23507-1912
Tel: 757 446-5915 *Fax:* 757 446-5089
E-mail: braceyml@mccoy.evms.edu
Internet: http://www.evms.edu
Accred Length: 3 Years *Program Size:* 9
Program ID: 340-51-21-081

Richmond

Medical College of Virginia/Virginia Commonwealth University Program

Sponsor: Medical College of Virginia/Virginia Commonwealth University
Hunter Holmes McGuire VA Medical Center (Richmond)
Medical College of Virginia Hospitals

Program Director:
William O McKinley, MD
Med Coll of Virginia
PO Box 980661
Richmond, VA 23298-0677
Tel: 804 828-4233 *Fax:* 804 828-5074
Internet:
http://www.griffin.vcu.edu/html/pmr/residents/pmrres.html
Accred Length: 4 Years *Program Size:* 10
Program ID: 340-51-21-069

Washington

Seattle

University of Washington Program

Sponsor: University of Washington School of Medicine
Children's Hospital and Medical Center
Harborview Medical Center
University of Washington Medical Center
Veterans Affairs Medical Center (Seattle)

Program Director:
Teresa L Massagli, MD
Univ of Washington
Dept of Rehab Med
Box 356490
Seattle, WA 98195
Tel: 206 685-0936 *Fax:* 206 685-3244
E-mail: massagli@u.washington.edu
Internet: http://www.weber.u.washington.edu/~rehab/
Accred Length: 4 Years *Program Size:* 32 (*GYI:* 3)
Program ID: 340-54-21-070

Wisconsin

Madison

University of Wisconsin Program

Sponsor: University of Wisconsin Hospital and Clinics

Program Director:
Keith B Sperling, MD
Univ of Wisconsin Hospital and Clinics
600 Highland Ave/Rm E3-348
Madison, WI 53792-0001
Tel: 608 263-8640 *Fax:* 608 263-9271
E-mail: cj.kaltenberg@hosp.wisc.edu
Internet: http://www.biostat.wisc.edu/rehab
Accred Length: 4 Years *Program Size:* 13 (*GYI:* 3)
Program ID: 340-56-21-072

Milwaukee

Medical College of Wisconsin Program

Sponsor: Medical College of Wisconsin Affiliated Hospitals Inc
Clement J Zablocki Veterans Affairs Medical Center
Froedtert Memorial Lutheran Hospital
St Luke's Medical Center

Program Director:
Gerda E Klingbeil, MD
Med Coll of Wisconsin
Froedtert Memorial Lutheran Hospital
9200 W Wisconsin Ave
Milwaukee, WI 53226
Tel: 414 257-5439 *Fax:* 414 454-4043
E-mail: jpierson@post.its.mcw.edu
Accred Length: 4 Years *Program Size:* 11 (*GYI:* 1)
Program ID: 340-56-21-071

Plastic Surgery

Alabama

Birmingham

University of Alabama Medical Center Program

Sponsor: University of Alabama Hospital
Children's Hospital of Alabama
Veterans Affairs Medical Center (Birmingham)

Program Director:
Luis Vasconez, MD
Univ of Alabama, Div of Plastic Surgery
Med Educ Bldg 524
1813 6th Ave S
Birmingham, AL 35294-3295
Tel: 205 934-3245 *Fax:* 205 975-6155
Accred Length: 2 Years *Program Size:* 4
Program ID: 360-01-21-121

California

Loma Linda

Loma Linda University Program

Sponsor: Loma Linda University Medical Center
Jerry L Pettis Memorial Veterans Hospital
Kaiser Foundation Hospital (Fontana)
Riverside County Regional Medical Center

Program Director:
Robert A Hardesty, MD
Loma Linda Univ Med Ctr
11175 Coleman Pav #21126
Loma Linda, CA 92354
Tel: 909 824-4176 *Fax:* 909 824-4175
Internet: http://www.llu.edu/llu/medicine/plastic
Accred Length: 6 Years *Program Size:* 8 (*GY1:* 2)
Program ID: 360-05-21-133
Integrated model

Los Angeles

UCLA Medical Center Program

Sponsor: UCLA School of Medicine
Los Angeles County-Harbor-UCLA Medical Center
Olive View-UCLA Medical Center
UCLA Medical Center
VA Greater Los Angeles Healthcare System

Program Director:
William W Shaw, MD
UCLA Med Ctr
10833 Le Conte Ave
64-140 CHS
Los Angeles, CA 90095-1665
Tel: 310 206-3656 *Fax:* 310 825-2785
E-mail: dlondon@surgery.medsch.ucla.edu
Accred Length: 2 Years *Program Size:* 6
Program ID: 360-05-21-009

University of Southern California Program

Sponsor: Los Angeles County-USC Medical Center
Children's Hospital of Los Angeles
City of Hope National Medical Center
Kaiser Foundation Hospital (West Los Angeles)
LAC-Rancho Los Amigos Medical Center
USC University Hospital

Program Director:
Randolph Sherman, MD
Univ of Southern California
Div of Plastic Surgery
1450 San Pablo St/Ste 2000
Los Angeles, CA 90033-4680
Tel: 323 442-6482 *Fax:* 323 442-6481
E-mail: randys@hsc.usc.edu
Accred Length: 3 Years *Program Size:* 9
Subspecialties: HSP
Program ID: 360-05-21-118

Orange

University of California (Irvine) Program

Sponsor: University of California (Irvine) Medical Center
Veterans Affairs Medical Center (Long Beach)

Program Director:
David W Furnas, MD
Univ of California Irvine Med Ctr
101 The City Dr
Orange, CA 92868
Tel: 714 456-5755 *Fax:* 714 456-7718
Accred Length: 2 Years *Program Size:* 2
Program ID: 360-05-21-008

Sacramento

University of California (Davis) Program

Sponsor: University of California (Davis) Medical Center

Program Director:
Thomas R Stevenson, MD
Univ of California Davis Med Ctr
Residency Office
2315 Stockton Blvd/Rm 6309
Sacramento, CA 95817
Tel: 916 734-2724 *Fax:* 916 734-5633
E-mail: kathleen.kelly@ucdmc.ucdavis.edu
Internet: http://web.ucdmc.ucdavis.edu/surgery
Accred Length: 2 Years *Program Size:* 4
Program ID: 360-05-21-113

San Diego

University of California (San Diego) Program

Sponsor: University of California (San Diego) Medical Center
Children's Hospital and Health Center
Veterans Affairs Medical Center (San Diego)

Program Director:
Jack C Fisher, MD
Div of Plastic Surgery
UCSD Med Ctr
200 W Arbor Dr
San Diego, CA 92103-8890
Tel: 619 543-6084 *Fax:* 619 543-3645
E-mail: rholmes@ucsd.edu
Internet: http://www.ucsd.edu
Accred Length: 2 Years *Program Size:* 2
Program ID: 360-05-21-010

San Francisco

University of California (San Francisco) Program

Sponsor: University of California (San Francisco) School of Medicine
Davies Medical Center
San Francisco General Hospital Medical Center
University of California (San Francisco) Medical Center
Veterans Affairs Medical Center (San Francisco)

Program Director:
Stephen J Mathes, MD
Univ of California San Francisco
Div of Plastic Surgery
350 Parnassus/#509
San Francisco, CA 94117
Tel: 415 476-3061 *Fax:* 415 476-9241
Accred Length: 2 Years *Program Size:* 6
Subspecialties: HSP
Program ID: 360-05-22-012

Stanford

Stanford University Program

Sponsor: Stanford University Hospital
Kaiser Permanente Medical Center (Santa Clara)
Veterans Affairs Palo Alto Health Care System

Program Director:
Barry Press, MD
Stanford Health Services
Div of Plastic Surgery
Rm NC-104/Hoover Pavilion
Stanford, CA 94305-5715
Tel: 650 723-5824 *Fax:* 650 725-6605
Accred Length: 2 Years *Program Size:* 6
Program ID: 360-05-31-013

Colorado

Denver

University of Colorado Program

Sponsor: University of Colorado Health Sciences Center
Children's Hospital
Denver Health and Hospitals
Veterans Affairs Medical Center (Denver)

Program Director:
Lawrence L Ketch, MD
Univ of Colorado Health Sciences Ctr
4200 E Ninth Ave/C-309
Denver, CO 80262
Tel: 303 315-6668 *Fax:* 303 315-4502
E-mail: lawrence.ketch@uchsc.edu
Accred Length: 2 Years *Program Size:* 2
Program ID: 360-07-21-122

Connecticut

New Haven

Yale-New Haven Medical Center Program

Sponsor: Yale-New Haven Hospital
Hospital of St Raphael
Veterans Affairs Medical Center (West Haven)
Program Director:
John A Persing, MD
Yale Univ Sch of Med
Dept of Surg/Plastics
333 Cedar St/YPB-2
New Haven, CT 06520-8041
Tel: 203 785-2570 *Fax:* 203 785-5714
E-mail: john.persing@yale.edu
Internet:
http://yalesurgery.med.yale.edu/surgery/sections.htm
Accred Length: 3 Years *Program Size:* 7
Subspecialties: HSP
Program ID: 360-08-21-015

District of Columbia

Washington

George Washington University Program

Sponsor: George Washington University School of Medicine
Children's National Medical Center
George Washington University Hospital (UHS)
Program Director:
Mary H McGrath, MD MPH
George Washington Univ Med Ctr
2150 Pennsylvania Ave NW
ACC 6B-422
Washington, DC 20037
Tel: 202 994-5573 *Fax:* 202 994-0567
E-mail: sursab@gwumc.edu
Accred Length: 2 Years *Program Size:* 2
Program ID: 360-10-21-018

Georgetown University Program

Sponsor: Georgetown University Medical Center
Fairfax Hospital
Suburban Hospital
Union Memorial Hospital
Veterans Affairs Medical Center (Washington, DC)
Washington Hospital Center
Program Director:
Scott L Spear, MD
Office of Surgical Education
Georgetown Univ Med Ctr
3800 Reservoir Rd NW/4th Fl PHC Bldg
Washington, DC 20007
Tel: 202 687-1233 *Fax:* 202 687-4287
Accred Length: 6 Years *Program Size:* 4 (*GY1:* 2)
Program ID: 360-10-21-017
Integrated model

Florida

Gainesville

University of Florida Program

Sponsor: University of Florida College of Medicine
Shands Hospital at the University of Florida
Veterans Affairs Medical Center (Gainesville)
Program Director:
H Hollis Caffee, MD
Univ of Florida
Div of Plastic Surgery
Box 100286 JHMHC
Gainesville, FL 32610-0286
Tel: 352 846-0372 *Fax:* 352 846-0387
Accred Length: 3 Years *Program Size:* 2
Program ID: 360-11-21-019

Miami

University of Miami-Jackson Memorial Medical Center Program

Sponsor: University of Miami-Jackson Memorial Medical Center
Program Director:
Seth R Thaller, MD DMD
Univ of Miami Sch of Med
Div of Plastic Surgery (R-88)
PO Box 016960
Miami, FL 33101
Tel: 305 585-5285 *Fax:* 305 324-7384
E-mail: sthaller@mednet.med.miami.edu
Accred Length: 2 Years *Program Size:* 6
Program ID: 360-11-21-022

Tampa

University of South Florida Program

Sponsor: University of South Florida College of Medicine
All Children's Hospital
Florida Hospital
H Lee Moffitt Cancer Center
James A Haley Veterans Hospital
Tampa General Healthcare
Veterans Affairs Medical Center (Bay Pines)
Program Director:
Wyatt G Payne, MD
Bay Pines VA Medical Center
10,000 Bay Pines Blvd., Box 5005
Bay Pines, FL 33744
Tel: 813 259-0986 *Fax:* 813 259-0985
Accred Length: 3 Years *Program Size:* 9
Subspecialties: HSP
Program ID: 360-11-21-128

Georgia

Atlanta

Emory University Program

Sponsor: Emory University School of Medicine
Crawford Long Hospital of Emory University
Emory University Hospital
Grady Memorial Hospital
Scottish Rite Children's Medical Center
Veterans Affairs Medical Center (Atlanta)
Program Director:
John Bostwick III, MD
Div of Plastic Surgery
1365 Clifton Rd NE/Ste B-2100
Atlanta, GA 30322
Tel: 404 778-3832 *Fax:* 404 778-5018
Accred Length: 2 Years *Program Size:* 4
Program ID: 360-12-21-024

Augusta

Medical College of Georgia Program

Sponsor: Medical College of Georgia Hospital and Clinics
Veterans Affairs Medical Center (Augusta)
Program Director:
Kenna S Given, MD
Med Coll of Georgia
Div of Plastic Surgery
1115 15th St
Augusta, GA 30912
Tel: 706 721-4620 *Fax:* 706 721-6931
E-mail: deptsurg.kgiven@mail.mcg.edu
Accred Length: 2 Years *Program Size:* 4
Program ID: 360-12-21-111

Illinois

Chicago

McGaw Medical Center of Northwestern University Program

Sponsor: Northwestern University Medical School
Children's Memorial Medical Center
Evanston Hospital
Northwestern Memorial Hospital
Shriners Hospitals for Children (Chicago)
Program Director:
Thomas A Mustoe, MD
Northwestern Univ Med Ctr
707 N Fairbanks Ct
Ste 811
Chicago, IL 60611
Tel: 312 908-6022 *Fax:* 312 908-5022
Internet: http://www.hsinfo.ghsl.nwu.edu/plast_surg/
Accred Length: 6 Years *Program Size:* 12 (*GY1:* 2)
Program ID: 360-16-21-025
Integrated model

Rush-Presbyterian-St Luke's Medical Center Program

Sponsor: Rush-Presbyterian-St Luke's Medical Center
Program Director:
Randall I McNally, MD
Rush-Presbyterian-St Luke's Med Ctr
Dept of Plastic/Reconstr Surg
1725 W Harrison St/Ste 106
Chicago, IL 60612
Tel: 312 942-6542 *Fax:* 312 666-6328
Accred Length: 2 Years *Program Size:* 2
Subspecialties: HSP
Program ID: 360-16-11-026

University of Chicago Program

Sponsor: University of Chicago Hospitals
Lutheran General Hospital
Program Director:
Robert L Walton, MD
Univ of Chicago Med Ctr
5841 S Maryland Ave/MC6035
Chicago, IL 60637
Tel: 773 702-6302 *Fax:* 773 702-1634
E-mail: jtomczak@surgery.bsd.uchicago.edu
Internet: http://www.surgery.bsd.uchicago.edu
Accred Length: 2 Years *Program Size:* 4
Program ID: 360-16-11-027

University of Illinois College of Medicine at Chicago Program
Sponsor: University of Illinois College of Medicine at Chicago
Cook County Hospital
Michael Reese Hospital and Medical Center
University of Illinois Hospital and Clinics
Program Director:
Mimis N Cohen, MD
Univ of Illinois-Chicago
Div of Plastic Surgery (M/C 958)
820 S Wood St/Ste 515 CSN
Chicago, IL 60612-7316
Tel: 312 996-9313 *Fax:* 312 413-0495
E-mail: mncohen@uic.edu
Internet: http://www.uic.edu/com/surgery/_private
Accred Length: 3 Years *Program Size:* 6
Program ID: 360-16-21-028

Maywood

Loyola University Program
Sponsor: Loyola University Medical Center
Children's Memorial Medical Center
Cook County Hospital
Edward J Hines Jr Veterans Affairs Hospital
Program Director:
Raymond L Warpeha, MD DDS PhD
Foster G McGaw Hospital
2160 S First Ave
Bldg 110/Rm 3255
Maywood, IL 60153
Tel: 708 327-2654 *Fax:* 708 327-2698
Accred Length: 3 Years *Program Size:* 3
Program ID: 360-16-21-029

Springfield

Southern Illinois University Program
Sponsor: Southern Illinois University School of Medicine
Memorial Medical Center
St John's Hospital
Program Director:
Michael W Neumeister, MD
Southern Illinois Univ Sch of Med
747 N Rutledge St
PO Box 19653
Springfield, IL 62794-9653
Tel: 217 524-6314, ext 4009 *Fax:* 217 524-2588
E-mail: mkoster@wpsmtp.siumed.med
Accred Length: 6 Years *Program Size:* 4 (*GY1:* 2)
Program ID: 360-16-21-030
Integrated model

Indiana

Indianapolis

Indiana University School of Medicine Program
Sponsor: Indiana University School of Medicine
Clarian IU Hospital
Clarian Riley Hospital for Children
Richard L Roudebush Veterans Affairs Medical Center
William N Wishard Memorial Hospital
Program Director:
John J Coleman III, MD
Indiana Univ Sch of Med
Emerson Hall/Rm 235
545 Barnhill Dr
Indianapolis, IN 46202-5124
Tel: 317 274-8106 *Fax:* 317 274-2227
Internet: http://www.iupui.edu/~mney/plassur.html
Accred Length: 2 Years *Program Size:* 6
Program ID: 360-17-11-031

Kansas

Kansas City

University of Kansas Medical Center Program
Sponsor: University of Kansas School of Medicine
University of Kansas Medical Center
Veterans Affairs Medical Center (Kansas City)
Program Director:
Ned W Garrigues, MD
Kansas Univ Med Ctr
3901 Rainbow Blvd
Kansas City, KS 66160-7389
Tel: 913 588-2071 *Fax:* 913 588-2061
E-mail: ngarrigu@kumc.edu
Accred Length: 2 Years *Program Size:* 4
Program ID: 360-19-11-032

Kentucky

Lexington

University of Kentucky Medical Center Program
Sponsor: University of Kentucky Hospital
Veterans Affairs Medical Center (Lexington)
Program Director:
Henry C Vasconez, MD
Univ of Kentucky
Kentucky Clinic/Ste K454
Lexington, KY 40536-0284
Tel: 606 323-5887 *Fax:* 606 323-3823
Internet: http://www.uky.edu/medicalcenter/plasurgy
Accred Length: 2 Years *Program Size:* 2
Program ID: 360-20-21-033

Louisville

University of Louisville Program
Sponsor: University of Louisville School of Medicine
Jewish Hospital
Kosair Children's Hospital (Alliant Health System)
Norton Hospital (Alliant Health System)
University of Louisville Hospital
Veterans Affairs Medical Center (Louisville)
Program Director:
Gordon R Tobin, MD
Div of Plastic/Recon Surgery
Univ of Louisville
Louisville, KY 40292
Tel: 502 852-6880 *Fax:* 502 852-8915
E-mail: grtobi01@ulkyvm.louisville.edu
Internet: http://www.plastics.louisville.edu/plastics/
Accred Length: 2 Years *Program Size:* 4
Program ID: 360-20-21-034

Louisiana

New Orleans

Louisiana State University Program
Sponsor: Louisiana State University School of Medicine
Medical Center of Louisiana at New Orleans
Veterans Affairs Medical Center-LSU Service (New Orleans)
Program Director:
Charles L Dupin, MD
Louisiana State Univ Sch of Med
1542 Tulane Ave/Rm 719
New Orleans, LA 70112
Tel: 504 568-7638 *Fax:* 504 568-4633
Accred Length: 2 Years *Program Size:* 4
Program ID: 360-21-11-035

Maryland

Baltimore

Johns Hopkins University/University of Maryland Program
Sponsor: Johns Hopkins University School of Medicine
Children's Hospital and Center for Reconstructive Surgery
Johns Hopkins Bayview Medical Center
Johns Hopkins Hospital
Union Memorial Hospital
University of Maryland Medical System
Program Director:
Paul N Manson, MD
Nelson H Goldberg, MD
Johns Hopkins Hospital
Div of Plastic Surgery
601 N Caroline St
Baltimore, MD 21287-0980
Tel: 410 955-6897 *Fax:* 410 614-1296
Internet: http://www.med.jhu.edu/plasticsurg
Accred Length: 2 Years *Program Size:* 6
Program ID: 360-23-21-037

Massachusetts

Boston

Beth Israel Deaconess Medical Center (West Campus) Program
Sponsor: Beth Israel Deaconess Medical Center
Cambridge Hospital/Cambridge Health Alliance
Program Director:
Francis G Wolfort, MD
Beth Israel Deaconess Med Ctr
Lowry Medical Office Bldg Ste 9E
110 Francis St
Boston, MA 02215
Tel: 617 632-8039 *Fax:* 617 632-0793
E-mail: btierney@bidmc.harvard.edu
Internet: http://www.bidmc.harvard.edu
Accred Length: 2 Years *Program Size:* 2
Subspecialties: HSP
Program ID: 360-24-21-124

Brigham and Women's Hospital/Children's Hospital Program
Sponsor: Brigham and Women's Hospital
Brockton-West Roxbury Veterans Affairs Medical Center
Children's Hospital
Program Director:
Julian Pribaz, MD
Brigham and Women's Hospital
Surgery Education Office
75 Francis St
Boston, MA 02115
Tel: 617 732-6861 *Fax:* 617 264-6850
E-mail: surgery@bics.bwh.harvard.edu
Internet: http://www.bwh.partners.org/surged
Accred Length: 2 Years *Program Size:* 4
Subspecialties: HSP
Program ID: 360-24-21-040

Programs

Harvard Medical School Program
Sponsor: Brigham & Women's Hospital
Beth Israel Deaconess Medical Center
Children's Hospital
Massachusetts General Hospital
Shriners Hospital for Children-Boston
Program Director:
Julian Pribaz, MD
Dept of Plastic Surgery
Brigham & Women's Hospital
75 Francis St
Boston, MA 02115
Tel: 617 732-6390
Accred Length: 6 Years *Program Size:* 24 *(GY1:* 3)
Program ID: 360-24-21-135
Integrated model

Massachusetts General Hospital Program
Sponsor: Massachusetts General Hospital
New England Medical Center Hospitals
Program Director:
James W May Jr, MD
Massachusetts General Hospital-Harvard Med Sch
Div of Plastic Surgery
15 Parkman St/Ste 453
Boston, MA 02114
Tel: 617 726-8220 *Fax:* 617 726-5365
Accred Length: 2 Years *Program Size:* 4
Subspecialties: HSP
Program ID: 360-24-21-039

Burlington

Lahey Clinic Program
Sponsor: Lahey Clinic
Brigham and Women's Hospital
Children's Hospital
Maine Medical Center
Program Director:
Brooke R Seckel, MD
Lahey Clinic
Dept of Plastic/Reconstructive Surgery
41 Mall Rd
Burlington, MA 01805
Tel: 781 744-8940 *Fax:* 781 744-1052
E-mail: christine.l.holman@lahey.hitchcock.org
Internet: http://www.lahey.hitchcock.org
Accred Length: 2 Years *Program Size:* 4
Program ID: 360-24-21-125

Worcester

University of Massachusetts Program
Sponsor: University of Massachusetts Medical School
Lenox Hill Hospital
UMass Memorial Health Care (University Campus)
Program Director:
W Thomas Lawrence, MD MPH
Univ of Massachusetts Med Sch
Dept of Plastic Surgery
55 Lake Ave N
Worcester, MA 01655-0328
Tel: 508 856-6644 *Fax:* 508 856-5250
Accred Length: 2 Years *Program Size:* 4
Program ID: 360-24-21-117

Michigan

Ann Arbor

University of Michigan Program
Sponsor: University of Michigan Hospitals
St Joseph Mercy Health System
Veterans Affairs Medical Center (Ann Arbor)
Program Director:
David J Smith Jr, MD
Univ of Michigan Hospitals
2207 TC/O342
1500 E Medical Center Dr
Ann Arbor, MI 48109-0342
Tel: 734 936-5733 *Fax:* 734 936-5725
E-mail: surged@umich.edu
Internet:
http://www.surg.med.umich.edu/plastic/plastic.home.html
Accred Length: 6 Years *Program Size:* 14 *(GY1:* 2)
Program ID: 360-25-21-042
Integrated model

Detroit

Wayne State University/Detroit Medical Center Program
Sponsor: Wayne State University/Detroit Medical Center
Children's Hospital of Michigan
Detroit Receiving Hospital and University Health Center
Grace Hospital
Harper Hospital
Veterans Affairs Medical Center (Detroit)
Program Director:
Eti Gursel, MD
Wayne State Univ Sch of Med
Div of Plastic Surg, Harper Hospital
3990 John R St
Detroit, MI 48201
Tel: 313 745-8773 *Fax:* 313 745-1873
Accred Length: 2 Years *Program Size:* 8
Subspecialties: HSP
Program ID: 360-25-21-043

Grand Rapids

Grand Rapids Area Medical Education Consortium Program
Sponsor: Grand Rapids Area Medical Education Consortium
Spectrum Health-Downtown Campus
Spectrum Health-East Campus
St Mary's Health Services
Program Director:
Steven L Ringler, MD
Grand Rapids Area Med Educ Consortium
240 Cherry St SE
Grand Rapids, MI 49503
Tel: 616 732-6246 *Fax:* 616 732-6255
E-mail: dubois@gramec.msu.edu
Accred Length: 2 Years *Program Size:* 4
Program ID: 360-25-22-044

Southfield

Providence Hospital and Medical Centers Program
Sponsor: Providence Hospital and Medical Centers
Grace Hospital
Program Director:
Ian T Jackson, MD
Providence Hospital
16001 W Nine Mile Rd
Southfield, MI 48075-4818
Tel: 248 424-3403 *Fax:* 248 424-5881
Accred Length: 2 Years *Program Size:* 4
Program ID: 360-25-31-046

Minnesota

Minneapolis

University of Minnesota Program
Sponsor: University of Minnesota Medical School
Fairview-University Medical Center
North Memorial Health Care
Regions Hospital
Veterans Affairs Medical Center (Minneapolis)
Program Director:
Bruce L Cunningham, MD MS
Univ of Minnesota Hospital
420 Delaware St SE/Box 122
Rm 11-248 Moos Tower
Minneapolis, MN 55455
Tel: 612 625-1188 *Fax:* 612 624-4441
E-mail: cunni001@tc.umn.edu
Internet: http://www.med.umn.edu/surg/
Accred Length: 3 Years *Program Size:* 3
Program ID: 360-26-21-131

Rochester

Mayo Graduate School of Medicine (Rochester) Program
Sponsor: Mayo Graduate School of Medicine-Mayo Foundation
Mayo Clinic (Rochester)
Rochester Methodist Hospital
St Mary's Hospital of Rochester
Program Director:
Uldis Bite, MD
Mayo Graduate Sch of Med
Application Processing Ctr
200 First St SW
Rochester, MN 55905
Tel: 507 284-4331 *Fax:* 507 284-0999
E-mail: mgsm.roch.mnsurgery@mayo.edu
Internet: http://www.mayo.edu/
Accred Length: 2 Years *Program Size:* 8
Program ID: 360-26-21-047

Mississippi

Jackson

University of Mississippi Medical Center Program
Sponsor: University of Mississippi School of Medicine
Mississippi Baptist Medical Center
St Dominic-Jackson Memorial Hospital
University Hospital
Veterans Affairs Medical Center (Jackson)
Program Director:
Michael F Angel, MD
Univ of Mississippi Med Ctr
2500 N State St
Jackson, MS 39216-4505
Tel: 601 984-5180 *Fax:* 601 984-5183
Accred Length: 2 Years *Program Size:* 2
Program ID: 360-27-21-126

Missouri

Columbia

University of Missouri-Columbia Program

Sponsor: University of Missouri-Columbia School of Medicine
Harry S Truman Memorial Veterans Hospital
University Hospitals and Clinics

Program Director:
Charles L Puckett, MD
Univ of Missouri-Columbia
One Hospital Dr
Columbia, MO 65212
Tel: 573 882-2275 *Fax:* 573 884-4788
E-mail: puckettc@health.missouri.edu
Internet:
http://www.surgery.missouri.edu/departments/resident/resbps.htm
Accred Length: 6 Years *Program Size:* 7 (*GY1:* 1)
Program ID: 360-28-21-049
Integrated model

St Louis

St Louis University School of Medicine Program

Sponsor: St Louis University School of Medicine
SSM Cardinal Glennon Children's Hospital
St Louis University School of Medicine
St Mary's Health Center
Veterans Affairs Medical Center (St Louis)

Program Director:
Christian E Paletta, MD
St Louis Univ Sch of Med
3635 Vista Ave
PO Box 15250
St Louis, MO 63110-0250
Tel: 314 511-8317 *Fax:* 314 268-5466
E-mail: surgweb@slu.edu
Internet:
http://www.slu.edu/colleges/med/departments/surgery
Accred Length: 2 Years *Program Size:* 4
Program ID: 360-28-21-051

Washington University/B-JH/SLCH Consortium Program

Sponsor: Washington University/B-JH/SLCH Consortium
Barnes West County Hospital
Barnes-Jewish Hospital
St Louis Children's Hospital
St Louis ConnectCare

Program Director:
Susan E Mackinnon, MD
Barnes-Jewish Hospital
One Barnes-Jewish Hospital Plaza
Box 8238
St Louis, MO 63110
Tel: 314 362-7388 *Fax:* 314 362-7491
E-mail: woltmanr@msnotes.wustl.edu
Internet: http://www.surgery.wustl.edu/residenc
Accred Length: 2 Years *Program Size:* 6
Subspecialties: HSP
Program ID: 360-28-21-052

New Hampshire

Lebanon

Dartmouth-Hitchcock Medical Center Program

Sponsor: Mary Hitchcock Memorial Hospital
Shriners Hospitals for Children (Boston)
Shriners Hospitals for Children (Springfield)
Veterans Affairs Medical Center (White River Junction)

Program Director:
Carolyn L Kerrigan, MD
Dartmouth-Hitchcock Med Ctr
One Medical Center Dr
Lebanon, NH 03756-0001
Tel: 603 650-8068 *Fax:* 603 650-5809
E-mail: carolyn.kerrigan@hitchcock.org/pages/physician
Internet: http://www.hitchcock.org/pages/physician guide/surgery/plastic/dept-plastic.html
Accred Length: 2 Years *Program Size:* 2
Program ID: 360-32-21-129

New Jersey

Camden

UMDNJ-Robert Wood Johnson Medical School (Camden) Program

Sponsor: Cooper Hospital-University Medical Center
Children's Hospital of Philadelphia
St Agnes Medical Center

Program Director:
Martha S Matthews, MD
Cooper Hospital-Univ Med Ctr
Div of Plastic/Recon Surgery
3 Cooper Plaza/Ste 411
Camden, NJ 08103
Tel: 609 342-3114 *Fax:* 609 365-7582
E-mail: kochey-carol@cooperhealth.edu
Accred Length: 2 Years *Program Size:* 2
Program ID: 360-33-21-132

Newark

UMDNJ-New Jersey Medical School Program

Sponsor: UMDNJ-New Jersey Medical School
Hackensack University Medical Center
UMDNJ-University Hospital

Program Director:
Marek K Dobke, MD
Doctors Office Ctr
90 Bergen St/Ste 7200
Newark, NJ 07103-2499
Tel: 973 972-2541 *Fax:* 973 972-2407
Accred Length: 2 Years *Program Size:* 4
Program ID: 360-33-21-119

New Mexico

Albuquerque

University of New Mexico Program

Sponsor: University of New Mexico School of Medicine
Lovelace Medical Center
University Hospital
Veterans Affairs Medical Center (Albuquerque)

Program Director:
Bret R Baack, MD
Univ of New Mexico Sch of Med
Div of Plastic Surgery
2211 Lomas Blvd NE
Albuquerque, NM 87131-5341
Tel: 505 272-4264 *Fax:* 505 272-6493
Internet:
http://medlab1.unm.edu/index.html/gme/gmetraining.html
Accred Length: 2 Years *Program Size:* 1
Program ID: 360-34-21-054

New York

Albany

Albany Medical Center Program

Sponsor: Albany Medical Center
Child's Hospital
St Peter's Hospital
Veterans Affairs Medical Center (Albany)

Program Director:
James G Hoehn, MD
Albany Med Coll
Div of Plastic Surgery/Mail Code 61-PL
47 New Scotland Ave
Albany, NY 12208-3479
Tel: 518 262-5752 *Fax:* 518 262-5692
Accred Length: 6 Years *Program Size:* 12 (*GY1:* 2)
Program ID: 360-35-21-055
Integrated model

Bronx

Albert Einstein College of Medicine Program

Sponsor: Albert Einstein College of Medicine of Yeshiva University
Fishkill Correctional Facility-NY State Dept of Correction
Jacobi Medical Center
Montefiore Medical Center-Henry and Lucy Moses Division
Montefiore Medical Center-Weiler Hospital
North Central Bronx Hospital

Program Director:
Berish Strauch, MD
Montefiore Med Ctr
Dept of Plastic Surgery
3331 Bainbridge Ave
Bronx, NY 10467
Tel: 718 920-5551 *Fax:* 718 798-0909
E-mail: bstrauch351@pol.net
Accred Length: 2 Years *Program Size:* 8
Program ID: 360-35-21-064

Programs

Brooklyn

SUNY Health Science Center at Brooklyn Program

Sponsor: SUNY Health Science Center at Brooklyn
Kings County Hospital Center
Maimonides Medical Center
New York Methodist Hospital
University Hospital-SUNY Health Science Center at Brooklyn
Veterans Affairs Medical Center (Brooklyn)

Program Director:
David L Abramson, MD
SUNY Health Science Ctr-Brooklyn
450 Clarkson Ave
Box 40
Brooklyn, NY 11203
Tel: 718 270-1965 *Fax:* 718 270-2826
Accred Length: 2 Years *Program Size:* 6
Program ID: 360-35-21-069

East Meadow

Nassau County Medical Center Program

Sponsor: Nassau County Medical Center
North Shore University Hospital
Winthrop-University Hospital

Program Director:
Roger L Simpson, MD
Nassau County Med Ctr
2201 Hempstead Trnpk
8th Fl DCB
East Meadow, NY 11554
Tel: 516 572-6703 *Fax:* 516 572-5140
Accred Length: 2 Years *Program Size:* 5
Program ID: 360-35-21-058

New York

Harlem Hospital Center Program

Sponsor: Harlem Hospital Center

Program Director:
Ferdinand A Ofodile, MD
Harlem Hospital Ctr
506 Lenox Ave
New York, NY 10037
Tel: 212 939-3537 *Fax:* 212 939-3536
Accred Length: 2 Years *Program Size:* 2
Program ID: 360-35-21-120

Mount Sinai School of Medicine Program

Sponsor: Mount Sinai School of Medicine
Elmhurst Hospital Center-Mount Sinai Services
Mount Sinai Medical Center
Veterans Affairs Medical Center (Bronx)
Westchester Medical Center

Program Director:
Lester Silver, MD
Mount Sinai Med Ctr
One Gustave L Levy Pl
Box 1259
New York, NY 10029-6574
Tel: 212 241-5873 *Fax:* 212 534-2654
Internet: http://mssm.edu
Accred Length: 3 Years *Program Size:* 5
Program ID: 360-35-21-065

New York and Presbyterian Hospital (Cornell Campus) Program

Sponsor: New York and Presbyterian Hospital
Memorial Sloan-Kettering Cancer Center
New York and Presbyterian Hospital (Cornell Campus)

Program Director:
Lloyd A Hoffman, MD
New York Hospital
525 E 68th St
Box 115
New York, NY 10021
Tel: 212 746-5511 *Fax:* 212 746-8666
E-mail: lcamacho@surgery.med.cornell.edu
Internet: http://surgery.med.cornell.edu
Accred Length: 2 Years *Program Size:* 5
Program ID: 360-35-21-060

New York University Medical Center Program

Sponsor: New York University Medical Center
Bellevue Hospital Center

Program Director:
Joseph G McCarthy, MD
New York Univ Med Ctr
Inst of Reconst Plastic Surgery
550 First Ave
New York, NY 10016
Tel: 212 263-5207 *Fax:* 212 263-5400
Accred Length: 3 Years *Program Size:* 8
Subspecialties: HSP
Program ID: 360-35-21-066

St Luke's-Roosevelt Hospital Center Program

Sponsor: St Luke's-Roosevelt Hospital Center
St Luke's-Roosevelt Hospital Center-Roosevelt Division
St Luke's-Roosevelt Hospital Center-St Luke's Division

Program Director:
Peter B Cinelli, MD
St Luke's-Roosevelt Hospital Ctr
1111 Amsterdam Ave
Clark Bldg/Rm 51002 10th Fl
New York, NY 10025
Tel: 212 523-7783 *Fax:* 212 523-1844
Accred Length: 2 Years *Program Size:* 0
Program ID: 360-35-21-068

Rochester

University of Rochester Program

Sponsor: Strong Memorial Hospital of the University of Rochester
Genesee Hospital
Rochester General Hospital

Program Director:
Joseph M Serletti Jr, MD
Univ of Rochester Med Ctr
601 Elmwood Ave/Box 661
Rochester, NY 14642-8661
Tel: 716 275-5818 *Fax:* 716 273-1064
Accred Length: 2 Years *Program Size:* 4
Program ID: 360-35-12-070

North Carolina

Chapel Hill

University of North Carolina Hospitals Program

Sponsor: University of North Carolina Hospitals
Carolinas Medical Center

Program Director:
Gerald M Sloan, MD
Univ of North Carolina-Chapel Hill
181 Medical School Wing D
CB 7195
Chapel Hill, NC 27599-7195
Tel: 919 966-4446 *Fax:* 919 966-3814
E-mail: gsloan@med.unc.edu
Internet: http://www.med.unc.edu/surgery/res-pgms.htm
Accred Length: 2 Years *Program Size:* 4
Program ID: 360-36-11-072

Durham

Duke University Program

Sponsor: Duke University Medical Center
Durham Regional Hospital
Kleinert, Kutz, and Associates
Veterans Affairs Medical Center (Durham)

Program Director:
Lawrence S Levin, MD
Div of Plastic Surgery
Duke Univ Med Ctr
Box 3945
Durham, NC 27710
Tel: 919 681-5079 *Fax:* 919 681-7340
E-mail: levin001@mc.duke.edu
Internet: http://www.duke.edu/~klitz
Accred Length: 6 Years *Program Size:* 9
Program ID: 360-36-21-073
Integrated model

Winston-Salem

Wake Forest University School of Medicine Program

Sponsor: Wake Forest University Baptist Medical Center

Program Director:
Louis C Argenta, MD
Wake Forest Univ Baptist Med Ctr
Medical Center Blvd
Winston-Salem, NC 27157-1075
Tel: 910 716-4416 *Fax:* 910 716-6646
Accred Length: 2 Years *Program Size:* 4
Program ID: 360-36-11-074

Ohio

Akron

Summa Health System (Akron City Hospital)/NEOUCOM Program

Sponsor: Summa Health System
Akron City Hospital (Summa Health System)
Akron General Medical Center
Children's Hospital Medical Center of Akron

Program Director:
James M Lewis, MD
Summa Health System
Med Educ/Mary Yanik
525 E Market St
Akron, OH 44309
Tel: 800 322-0517
Internet: http://www.summahealth.org/edu/
Accred Length: 4 Years *Program Size:* 4
Program ID: 360-38-21-075

Cincinnati

University Hospital/University of Cincinnati College of Medicine Program

Sponsor: University Hospital Inc

Program Director:
Henry W Neale, MD
Univ of Cincinnati Med Ctr
Mail Location 558
Cincinnati, OH 45267-0558
Tel: 513 558-0984 *Fax:* 513 558-0570
Accred Length: 6 Years *Program Size:* 2 (*GY1:* 1)
Program ID: 360-38-21-112
Integrated model

Cleveland

Case Western Reserve University Program

Sponsor: University Hospitals of Cleveland
MetroHealth Medical Center
Mount Sinai Medical Center of Cleveland
Veterans Affairs Medical Center (Cleveland)

Program Director:
Edward A Luce, MD
Univ Hospitals of Cleveland
Plastic/Reconstructive Surgery
11100 Euclid Ave
Cleveland, OH 44106-5044
Tel: 216 844-4780 *Fax:* 216 844-8667
Internet: http://www.cwru.edu/som/dept.html
Accred Length: 2 Years *Program Size:* 4
Program ID: 360-38-21-078

Cleveland Clinic Foundation Program

Sponsor: Cleveland Clinic Foundation
St Vincent Charity Hospital and Health Center

Program Director:
Randall J Yetman, MD
Cleveland Clinic Foundation
Dept of Plastic Surgery/A60
9500 Euclid Ave
Cleveland, OH 44195-5242
Tel: 216 444-5960 *Fax:* 216 444-1162
E-mail: meded@cesmtp.ccf.org
Internet: http://www.ccf.org
Accred Length: 2 Years *Program Size:* 4
Program ID: 360-38-21-079

Columbus

Ohio State University Program

Sponsor: Ohio State University Medical Center
Children's Hospital
Mount Carmel Medical Center
Riverside Methodist Hospitals (OhioHealth)

Program Director:
Robert L Ruberg, MD
Ohio State Univ
Rm N-809/Doan Hall
410 W Tenth Ave
Columbus, OH 43210-1228
Tel: 614 293-8566 *Fax:* 614 293-3381
E-mail: glowry@medctr.osu.edu
Accred Length: 2 Years *Program Size:* 5
Program ID: 360-38-21-081

Toledo

Medical College of Ohio Program

Sponsor: Medical College of Ohio
St Vincent Mercy Medical Center

Program Director:
John H Robinson, MD
St Vincent Mercy Med Ctr
Sect of Plastic Surgery
2213 Cherry St
Toledo, OH 43608
Tel: 419 251-4613 *Fax:* 419 251-3856
E-mail: karen_bash@svmc.org
Accred Length: 2 Years *Program Size:* 4
Subspecialties: HSP
Program ID: 360-38-21-084

Oklahoma

Oklahoma City

University of Oklahoma Health Sciences Center Program

Sponsor: University of Oklahoma College of Medicine
Children's Hospital of Oklahoma
University Hospital
Veterans Affairs Medical Center (Oklahoma City)

Program Director:
Norman S Levine, MD
Univ of Oklahoma Health Sciences Ctr
WP2220/PO Box 26901
Oklahoma City, OK 73190
Tel: 405 271-4864 *Fax:* 405 271-2737
Accred Length: 2 Years *Program Size:* 4
Program ID: 360-39-21-085

Oregon

Portland

Oregon Health Sciences University Program

Sponsor: Oregon Health Sciences University Hospital
Veterans Affairs Medical Center (Portland)

Program Director:
Alan E Seyfer, MD
Oregon Health Sciences Univ
3181 SW Sam Jackson Park Rd/L352A
Portland, OR 97201-3098
Tel: 503 494-7824 *Fax:* 503 494-0441
E-mail: seyfera@ohsu.edu
Internet: http://www.ohsu.edu/som-plasticsurg
Accred Length: 2 Years *Program Size:* 4
Subspecialties: HSP
Program ID: 360-40-21-116

Pennsylvania

Allentown

Lehigh Valley Hospital/Pennsylvania State University Program

Sponsor: Lehigh Valley Hospital

Program Director:
Walter J Okunski, MD
Lehigh Valley Hospital
Cedar Crest and I78/PO Box 689
Allentown, PA 18105-1556
Tel: 610 402-8966 *Fax:* 610 402-1667
E-mail: plasticres@lvhhn.org
Internet: http://www.lvhhn.org/academic/residency/plastic/home.html
Accred Length: 3 Years *Program Size:* 3
Program ID: 360-41-22-086

Hershey

Penn State Geisinger Health System/Milton S Hershey Medical Center Program

Sponsor: Penn State Geisinger Health System
Milton S Hershey Medical Center
PinnacleHealth System-Harrisburg Hospital
PinnacleHealth System-Polyclinic Hospital
York Hospital

Program Director:
William P Graham III, MD
Penn State Geisinger Health System-Hershey Med Ctr
500 University Dr
PO Box 850/MC-H071
Hershey, PA 17033-0850
Tel: 717 531-8372 *Fax:* 717 531-4339
E-mail: mkatrak@psghs.edu
Internet: http://www.prs.hmc.psghs.edu
Accred Length: 2 Years *Program Size:* 4
Program ID: 360-41-21-087

Philadelphia

Temple University Program

Sponsor: Temple University Hospital
Abington Memorial Hospital
St Christopher's Hospital for Children

Program Director:
Amitabha Mitra, MD MS
Temple Univ Hospital
Dept of Plastic Surgery
3322 N Broad St/3rd Fl
Philadelphia, PA 19140
Tel: 215 707-3933 *Fax:* 215 707-2531
Accred Length: 2 Years *Program Size:* 4
Program ID: 360-41-21-088

University of Pennsylvania Program

Sponsor: Hospital of the University of Pennsylvania
Bryn Mawr Hospital
Children's Hospital of Philadelphia

Program Director:
Linton A Whitaker, MD
Univ of Pennsylvania Med Ctr
Div of Plastic Surgery
3400 Spruce St/10 Penn Tower
Philadelphia, PA 19104-4385
Tel: 215 662-7075 *Fax:* 215 662-2172
E-mail: lwhitake@mail.med.upenn.edu
Accred Length: 3 Years *Program Size:* 6
Program ID: 360-41-21-089

Pittsburgh

University Health Center of Pittsburgh Program

Sponsor: University Health Center of Pittsburgh
Allegheny General Hospital
Children's Hospital of Pittsburgh
Presbyterian University Hospital/UPMC
Western Pennsylvania Hospital

Program Director:
Michael Bentz, MD
Univ of Pittsburgh
3705 Fifth Ave
Pittsburgh, PA 15261
Tel: 412 648-9673 *Fax:* 412 648-1987
E-mail: bentzm@chplink.chp.edu
Accred Length: 2 Years *Program Size:* 8
Subspecialties: HSP
Program ID: 360-41-21-090

Rhode Island

Providence

Brown University Program

Sponsor: Rhode Island Hospital
Roger Williams Medical Center
Veterans Affairs Medical Center (Providence)

Program Director:
Lee E Edstrom, MD
Rhode Island Hospital
2 Dudley St/MOC Ste 450
Providence, RI 02905
Tel: 401 444-4188 *Fax:* 401 444-4863
Internet: http://www.brown.edu/department/plastic
Accred Length: 2 Years *Program Size:* 4
Program ID: 360-43-21-092

South Carolina

Charleston

Medical University of South Carolina Program

Sponsor: Medical University of South Carolina College of Medicine
Charleston Memorial Hospital
MUSC Medical Center
Ralph H Johnson Dept of Veterans Affairs Med Center

Program Director:
David J Barillo, MD
Med Univ of South Carolina
600 MUSC Complex
Ste 426
Charleston, SC 29425-2271
Tel: 843 792-4274 *Fax:* 843 792-3080
E-mail: rollinrp@musc.edu
Accred Length: 2 Years *Program Size:* 4
Program ID: 360-45-22-093

Tennessee

Chattanooga

University of Tennessee College of Medicine at Chattanooga Program

Sponsor: University of Tennessee College of Medicine-Chattanooga Unit
Erlanger Medical Center

Program Director:
Larry A Sargent, MD
Univ of Tennessee Coll of Med
Dept of Plastic Surgery
979 E 3rd St/Ste 900
Chattanooga, TN 37403
Tel: 423 778-9047 *Fax:* 423 778-9984
E-mail: utplastics@erlanger.org
Internet: http://www.erlanger.org/utcom/plastics.html
Accred Length: 2 Years *Program Size:* 4
Program ID: 360-47-11-094

Memphis

University of Tennessee Program

Sponsor: University of Tennessee College of Medicine
Baptist Memorial Hospital
Regional Medical Center at Memphis
University of Tennessee Medical Center (UT Bowld Hospital)
Veterans Affairs Medical Center (Memphis)

Program Director:
Robert D Wallace, MD
Univ of Tennessee
956 Court Ave/Rm G230
Memphis, TN 38163
Tel: 901 448-4541 *Fax:* 901 448-7306
Accred Length: 2 Years *Program Size:* 4
Program ID: 360-47-31-095

Nashville

Vanderbilt University Program

Sponsor: Vanderbilt University Medical Center
Baptist Hospital
Metropolitan Nashville General Hospital
Veterans Affairs Medical Center (Nashville)

Program Director:
R Bruce Shack, MD
Vanderbilt Univ Hospital
2100 Pierce Ave
230 MCS
Nashville, TN 37232-3631
Tel: 615 936-0160 *Fax:* 615 936-0167
E-mail: jammie.baber@surgery.mc.vanderbilt.edu
Internet:
http://www.mc.vanderbilt.edu/surgery/plastic/index.html
Accred Length: 2 Years *Program Size:* 6
Program ID: 360-47-21-096

Texas

Dallas

University of Texas Southwestern Medical School Program

Sponsor: University of Texas Southwestern Medical School
Baylor University Medical Center
Children's Medical Center of Dallas
Dallas County Hospital District-Parkland Memorial Hospital
Veterans Affairs Medical Center (Dallas)
Zale-Lipshy University Hospital

Program Director:
Rod J Rohrich, MD
Univ of Texas Southwestern Med Ctr
Dept of Plastic Surgery
5323 Harry Hines Blvd
Dallas, TX 75235-9132
Tel: 214 648-3571 *Fax:* 214 648-6776
E-mail: rrohrich@mednet.swmed.edu
Internet: http://www.swmed.edu/home_pages/plastsurg
Accred Length: 2 Years *Program Size:* 8
Subspecialties: HSP
Program ID: 360-48-21-097

Galveston

University of Texas Medical Branch Hospitals Program

Sponsor: University of Texas Medical Branch Hospitals
Shriners Hospitals for Children (Galveston Burns Institute)
University of Texas M D Anderson Cancer Center

Program Director:
Linda G Phillips, MD
Div of Plastic Surgery
Univ of Texas Med Branch
301 University Blvd
Galveston, TX 77555-0724
Tel: 409 772-1255 *Fax:* 409 772-1872
Accred Length: 5 Years *Program Size:* 9
Program ID: 360-48-11-098
Integrated model

Houston

Baylor College of Medicine Program

Sponsor: Baylor College of Medicine
Harris County Hospital District-Ben Taub General Hospital
Methodist Hospital
St Luke's Episcopal Hospital
Veterans Affairs Medical Center (Houston)

Program Director:
Saleh M Shenaq, MD
Baylor Coll of Med
Div of Plastic Surgery
6560 Fannin/Ste 800
Houston, TX 77030
Tel: 713 798-8555 *Fax:* 713 798-3806
E-mail: sshenaq@bcm.tmc.edu
Internet: http://www.bcm.tmc.edu/plastic.surgery
Accred Length: 6 Years *Program Size:* 18 (*GY1:* 3)
Subspecialties: HSP
Program ID: 360-48-31-099
Integrated model

St Joseph Hospital Program
Sponsor: St Joseph Hospital
Program Director:
Benjamin E Cohen, MD
St Joseph Hospital
1315 Calhoun/Ste 920
Houston, TX 77002
Tel: 713 951-0400 *Fax:* 713 951-0314
Accred Length: 2 Years *Program Size:* 4
Program ID: 360-48-12-100

University of Texas at Houston Program
Sponsor: University of Texas Medical School at Houston
Lyndon B Johnson General Hospital
Memorial Hermann Healthcare System
Program Director:
Donald H Parks, MD
Univ of Texas Med Sch
6431 Fannin St/Ste 4152
Houston, TX 77030-1503
Tel: 713 792-5414 *Fax:* 713 500-0716
Accred Length: 2 Years *Program Size:* 4
Program ID: 360-48-31-101

Temple

Texas A&M College of Medicine-Scott and White Program
Sponsor: Scott and White Memorial Hospital
Central Texas Veterans Affairs Healthcare System
Program Director:
Peter C Grothaus, MD
Texas A&M-Scott and White
Grad Med Educ
2401 S 31st St
Temple, TX 76508-0001
Tel: 817 724-1695 *Fax:* 817 724-5245
E-mail: plassurgresi@bellnet.tamu.edu
Internet: http://www.swinfo.tamu.edu
Accred Length: 3 Years *Program Size:* 2
Program ID: 360-48-21-130

Utah

Salt Lake City

University of Utah Program
Sponsor: University of Utah Medical Center
Primary Children's Medical Center
Salt Lake Regional Medical Center
Veterans Affairs Medical Center (Salt Lake City)
Program Director:
W Bradford Rockwell, MD
Div of Plastic/Recon Surgery
50 N Medical Dr/Rm 3C127
Salt Lake City, UT 84132
Tel: 801 581-7719 *Fax:* 801 581-5794
E-mail: brad.rockwell@hsc.utah.edu
Internet:
http://www.medlib.med.utah.edu/plastic_surgery
Accred Length: 2 Years *Program Size:* 4
Program ID: 360-49-21-103

Virginia

Charlottesville

University of Virginia Program
Sponsor: University of Virginia Medical Center
Program Director:
Raymond F Morgan, MD
Univ of Virginia Health Sciences Ctr
Box 376
Charlottesville, VA 22908
Tel: 804 924-1234 *Fax:* 804 924-1333
Internet: http://www.med.virginia.edu/medicine/clinical/plasticsurgery/
Accred Length: 6 Years *Program Size:* 4
Subspecialties: HSP
Program ID: 360-51-11-104
Integrated model

Richmond

Medical College of Virginia/Virginia Commonwealth University Program
Sponsor: Medical College of Virginia/Virginia Commonwealth University
Hunter Holmes McGuire VA Medical Center (Richmond)
Medical College of Virginia Hospitals
St Mary's Hospital
Program Director:
Austin I Mehrhof Jr, DDS MD
Med Coll of Virginia-Virginia Commonwealth Univ
Div of Plastic Surgery
401 N 11th St/Ste 520
Richmond, VA 23298
Tel: 804 828-3030 *Fax:* 804 828-3045
E-mail: aimehrho@hsc.vcu.edu
Accred Length: 2 Years *Program Size:* 3
Program ID: 360-51-21-108

Washington

Seattle

University of Washington Program
Sponsor: University of Washington School of Medicine
Children's Hospital and Medical Center
Harborview Medical Center
University of Washington Medical Center
Valley Medical Center
Veterans Affairs Medical Center (Seattle)
Program Director:
Loren H Engrav, MD
Univ of Washington
Sch of Med
Box 359796
Seattle, WA 98104
Tel: 206 731-3209 *Fax:* 206 731-3656
Internet: http://www.weber.u.washington.edu/nengrev
Accred Length: 3 Years *Program Size:* 3
Program ID: 360-54-21-123

Wisconsin

Madison

University of Wisconsin Program
Sponsor: University of Wisconsin Hospital and Clinics
Meriter Hospital
St Marys Hospital Medical Center
Program Director:
David G Dibbell Sr, MD
Univ of Wisconsin Hospital and Clinics
600 Highland Ave/Rm G5-355
Madison, WI 53792
Tel: 608 263-1367 *Fax:* 608 265-9695
E-mail: kopelber@surgery.wisc.edu
Internet: http://www.biostat.wisc.edu/surgery/home.html
Accred Length: 2 Years *Program Size:* 4
Program ID: 360-56-21-109
Integrated model

Milwaukee

Medical College of Wisconsin Program
Sponsor: Medical College of Wisconsin Affiliated Hospitals Inc
Children's Hospital of Wisconsin
Clement J Zablocki Veterans Affairs Medical Center
Froedtert Memorial Lutheran Hospital
Program Director:
David L Larson, MD
Med Coll of Wisconsin Clinics-Froedtert East
Dept of Plastic Surgery
9200 W Wisconsin Ave
Milwaukee, WI 53226-3596
Tel: 414 454-5447 *Fax:* 414 259-0901
E-mail: cromellp@mcw.edu
Accred Length: 5 Years *Program Size:* 4
Subspecialties: HSP
Program ID: 360-56-21-110

Preventive Medicine (Gen Prev Med, Occupational Med, Aerospace Med, & Pub Hlth)

Alabama

Birmingham

University of Alabama Medical Center Program

Sponsor: University of Alabama Hospital
University of Alabama at Birmingham School of Public Health
University of Alabama School of Medicine

Program Director:
Timothy J Key, MD MPH
Univ of Alabama
Rm 119
930 20th St S
Birmingham, AL 35205
Tel: 205 934-7303 *Fax:* 205 975-4377
E-mail: tjk@fms.uab.edu
Accred Length: 2 Years *Program Size:* 6
Program ID: 380-01-77-054
Occupational medicine program

Arizona

Tucson

University of Arizona Program

Sponsor: University of Arizona College of Medicine
University Medical Center

Program Director:
Wayne F Peate, MD MS
General Preventive Med Program
4001 N 3rd St
Ste 415
Phoenix, AZ 85012
Tel: 602 631-6550 *Fax:* 602 631-6560
E-mail: gpmres@u.arizona.edu
Internet: http://www.ahsc.arizona.edu/apc/
Accred Length: 2 Years *Program Size:* 4
Program ID: 380-03-21-007
General preventive medicine program

California

Berkeley

University of California School of Public Health Program

Sponsor: University of California School of Public Health

Program Director:
George W Rutherford, MD
Univ of California Berkeley
Sch of Public Health
140 Warren Hall
Berkeley, CA 94720-7360
Tel: 510 643-2700 *Fax:* 510 643-8753
E-mail: gruther@socrates.berkeley.edu
Internet: http://www.garnet.berkeley.edu/sph
Accred Length: 2 Years *Program Size:* 8
Program ID: 380-05-32-008
General preventive medicine program

Davis

University of California (Davis) Program

Sponsor: University of California (Davis) School of Medicine
University of California (Davis) Medical Center
University of California School of Public Health

Program Director:
Stephen A McCurdy, MD
Univ of California Davis Med Ctr
Epidemiology/Prev Med
Sch of Med/TB 168
Davis, CA 95616-8638
Tel: 916 752-8051 *Fax:* 916 752-3239
E-mail: samccurdy@ucdavis.edu
Accred Length: 2 Years *Program Size:* 0
Program ID: 380-05-77-056
Occupational medicine program

Loma Linda

Loma Linda University Program

Sponsor: Loma Linda University Medical Center

Program Director:
Linda H Ferry, MD MPH
Loma Linda Univ Med Ctr
Nichol Hall/Rm 1516
Loma Linda, CA 92350
Tel: 909 558-4918 *Fax:* 909 558-4087
E-mail: lferry@sph.llu.edu
Internet: http://www.llu.edu
Accred Length: 3 Years *Program Size:* 14 (*GY1:* 2)
Program ID: 380-05-21-033
General preventive medicine program

Los Angeles

UCLA Medical Center Program

Sponsor: UCLA School of Medicine
UCLA School of Public Health

Program Director:
Charles E Lewis, MD ScD
UCLA Schs of Med and Public Health
Box 951772
Los Angeles, CA 90095-1772
Tel: 310 825-5081 *Fax:* 310 206-5717
E-mail: lewis@admin.ph.ucla.edu
Internet: http://www.ph.ucla.edu/pmr/
Accred Length: 2 Years *Program Size:* 4
Program ID: 380-05-21-010
General preventive medicine program

University of Southern California Program

Sponsor: University of Southern California School of Medicine
UCLA School of Public Health

Program Director:
John M Peters, MD
Div of Occup/Environmental Med
Univ of Southern California Sch of Med
1540 Alcazar St/Ste 236
Los Angeles, CA 90033
Tel: 323 442-1096 *Fax:* 323 442-3272
E-mail: jpeters@hsc.usc.edu
Accred Length: 2 Years *Program Size:* 6
Program ID: 380-05-77-057
Occupational medicine program

Orange

University of California (Irvine) Program

Sponsor: University of California (Irvine) Medical Center
University of California (Irvine) College of Medicine

Program Director:
Dean B Baker, MD
19722 MacArthur Blvd
Irvine, CA 92612
Tel: 949 824-8641 *Fax:* 949 824-2345
E-mail: dbaker@edu.uci
Accred Length: 2 Years *Program Size:* 5
Program ID: 380-05-77-058
Occupational medicine program

Sacramento

California Department of Health Services Program

Sponsor: California Department of Health Services
UCLA School of Public Health
University of California School of Public Health

Program Director:
Kathleen H Acree, MD MPH JD
Nathalie Bera, MD MPH
Chronic Disease Control Branch/MS-725
California Dept of Health Services
PO Box 942732
Sacramento, CA 94234-7320
Tel: 916 327-6985 *Fax:* 916 324-7764
E-mail: kacree@pacbell.net
Accred Length: 2 Years *Program Size:* 6
Program ID: 380-05-88-097
Public health program

San Diego

University of California (San Diego)/San Diego State University Program

Sponsor: University of California (San Diego) Medical Center
Graduate School of Public Health

Program Director:
Linda Hill, MD MPH
San Diego State Univ
5500 Campanile Dr
San Diego, CA 92182-4701
Tel: 619 594-5332 *Fax:* 619 594-5613
E-mail: pmr@mail.sdsu.edu
Internet: http://www.shs.sdsu.edu/pmr
Accred Length: 2 Years *Program Size:* 12
Program ID: 380-05-21-038
General preventive medicine program

San Francisco

University of California (San Francisco) Program
Sponsor: University of California (San Francisco) School of Medicine
San Francisco General Hospital Medical Center
University of California School of Public Health
Program Director:
John R Balmes, MD
Univ of California San Francisco
Campus Box 0843
San Francisco, CA 94143-0843
Tel: 415 206-8950 *Fax:* 415 206-8949
E-mail: dsilva@sfghoem.ucsf.edu
Internet: http://ehs.sph.berkeley.edu/coeh/ucsfoem
Accred Length: 2 Years *Program Size:* 4
Program ID: 380-05-77-059
Occupational medicine program

Colorado

Denver

University of Colorado Program A
Sponsor: University of Colorado Health Sciences Center
National Jewish Ctr for Immunology and Respiratory Medicine
Program Director:
A James Ruttenber, MD PhD
Univ of Colorado Health Sciences Ctr
Campus Box C-245
4200 E Ninth Ave
Denver, CO 80262
Tel: 303 315-5627 *Fax:* 303 315-3183
E-mail: jim.ruttenber@uchsc.edu
Internet:
http://www.uchsc.edu/sm/pmb/pmb/envh/page1.htm
Accred Length: 2 Years *Program Size:* 4
Program ID: 380-07-77-060
Occupational medicine program

University of Colorado Program
Sponsor: University of Colorado Health Sciences Center
Program Director:
William M Marine, MD MPH
Univ of Colorado Health Sciences Ctr
Box C-245
4200 E Ninth Ave
Denver, CO 80262
Tel: 303 315-6850 *Fax:* 303 315-3183
E-mail: william.marine@uchsc.edu
Internet:
http://www.uchsc.edu/sm/pmb/pmb/edpgms/pmres.htm
Accred Length: 2 Years *Program Size:* 7
Program ID: 380-07-21-041
General preventive medicine program

Connecticut

Derby

Griffin Hospital Program
Sponsor: Griffin Hospital
Yale University School of Public Health
Program Director:
James F Jekel, MD MPH
130 Division St
Derby, CT 06418
Tel: 203 732-7325, ext 7220 *Fax:* 203 732-7185
Accred Length: 2 Years *Program Size:* 4 *(GYI: 2)*
Program ID: 380-08-88-119
Public health program

Farmington

University of Connecticut Program
Sponsor: University of Connecticut School of Medicine
Univ of Connecticut Health Center/John Dempsey Hospital
Program Director:
Michael Grey, MD MPH
Univ of Connecticut Health Ctr
Div of Occup/Environ Med
263 Farmington Ave
Farmington, CT 06030-6210
Tel: 860 679-2445 *Fax:* 860 679-1349
E-mail: rieder@nso.uchc.edu
Internet:
http://www.resprog.uchc.edu/md/envir/home.html
Accred Length: 2 Years *Program Size:* 4
Program ID: 380-08-77-061
Occupational medicine program

New Haven

Yale-New Haven Medical Center Program
Sponsor: Yale-New Haven Hospital
Program Director:
Mark R Cullen, MD
Occupational/Environmental Med Program
Yale Univ Sch of Med
135 College St/Rm 366
New Haven, CT 06510-2483
Tel: 203 785-5885 *Fax:* 203 785-7391
E-mail: linda.oliva@yale.edu
Internet: http://info.med.yale.edu/intmed/yoemp
Accred Length: 2 Years *Program Size:* 6
Program ID: 380-08-77-062
Occupational medicine program

District of Columbia

Washington

George Washington University Program
Sponsor: George Washington University School of Medicine
George Washington University Hospital (UHS)
Program Director:
John M Balbus, MD MPH
George Washington Univ
Warwick Bldg
2300 K St NW/Rm 201
Washington, DC 20037
Tel: 202 994-1734 *Fax:* 202 994-0011
E-mail: eohjmb@gwumc.edu
Internet: http://www.gwumc.edu/occenv
Accred Length: 2 Years *Program Size:* 2
Program ID: 380-10-77-063
Occupational medicine program

Walter Reed Army Institute of Research Program
Sponsor: Walter Reed Army Institute of Research
Program Director:
Ralph L Erickson, MD MPH MD
Walter Reed Army Inst of Research
Div of Preventive Med
Attn: MCMR-UWK
Washington, DC 20307-5100
Tel: 202 782-1300 *Fax:* 202 782-0613
E-mail: ltc_loren_erickson@wrsmtp-ccmail.army.mil
Internet: http://wrair-www.army.mil
Accred Length: 2 Years *Program Size:* 7
Program ID: 380-10-21-002
US Armed Services Program
General preventive medicine program

Florida

Pensacola

Naval Aerospace and Operational Medical Institute Program
Sponsor: Naval Aerospace and Operational Medical Institute
Program Director:
Michael R Valdez, MD MPH
Naval Operational Medicine Inst
Aerospace Med Residency/Code 32
220 Hovey Rd/Ste A
Pensacola, FL 32508-1047
Tel: 850 452-8212 *Fax:* 850 452-5194
E-mail: code030@nomi.med.navy.mil
Internet: http://www.nomi.navy.mil
Accred Length: 1 Year *Program Size:* 19
Program ID: 380-11-66-051
US Armed Services Program
Aerospace medicine program

Tampa

University of South Florida Program
Sponsor: University of South Florida College of Medicine
Tampa General Healthcare
University of South Florida College of Public Health
Program Director:
Stuart M Brooks, MD
Dept of Environment/Occup Health
Univ of South Florida Coll of Pub Hlth
13201 Bruce B Downs Blvd/MDC56
Tampa, FL 33612-3805
Tel: 813 974-6626 *Fax:* 813 974-4986
E-mail: sbrooks@com1.med.usf.edu
Internet: http://www.hsc.usf.edu/erc/omr.html
Accred Length: 2 Years *Program Size:* 8
Program ID: 380-11-77-064
Occupational medicine program

West Palm Beach

Palm Beach County Public Health Unit Program
Sponsor: Palm Beach County Public Health Unit
Program Director:
Jean Marie Malecki, MD MPH
Palm Beach County Health Dept
PO Box 29
West Palm Beach, FL 33402
Tel: 561 355-3120 *Fax:* 561 355-3165
Accred Length: 2 Years *Program Size:* 2
Program ID: 380-11-88-098
Public health program

Georgia

Atlanta

Centers for Disease Control and Prevention Program
Sponsor: Centers for Disease Control and Prevention
Program Director:
Andrew L Dannenberg, MD MPH
Ctrs for Disease Control and Prevention
1600 Clifton Rd/MS D-18
Atlanta, GA 30333
Tel: 404 639-3187 *Fax:* 404 639-2222
E-mail: acd7@cdc.gov
Internet: http://inside.cdc.gov/intranet/epo/pmr.htm
Accred Length: 1 Year *Program Size:* 15
Program ID: 380-12-88-109
Public health program

Emory University Program A
Sponsor: Emory University School of Medicine
Georgia Dept of Human Resources-Division of Public Health
Grady Memorial Hospital
Rollins School of Public Health of Emory University
Program Director:
Erica Frank, MD MPH
Emory Univ Sch of Med
69 Butler St SE
Atlanta, GA 30303
Tel: 404 616-5603 *Fax:* 404 616-6847
E-mail: efrank@fpm.eushc.org
Accred Length: 2 Years *Program Size:* 4
Program ID: 380-12-88-110
Public health program

Emory University Program
Sponsor: Rollins School of Public Health of Emory University
Program Director:
Fredric Gerr, MD
Rollins Sch of Public Health-Emory Univ
1518 Clifton Rd
Atlanta, GA 30322
Tel: 404 727-3697 *Fax:* 404 727-8744
E-mail: fgerr@sph.emory.edu
Internet: http://www.sph.emory.edu/eoh/residence.html
Accred Length: 2 Years *Program Size:* 4
Program ID: 380-12-77-065
Occupational medicine program

Morehouse School of Medicine Program
Sponsor: Morehouse School of Medicine
Georgia Dept of Human Resources-Division of Public Health
Program Director:
Beverly D Taylor, MD
Dept of Com Health/Prev Med
720 Westview Dr SW
Atlanta, GA 30310-1495
Tel: 404 752-1852 *Fax:* 404 752-1160
E-mail: durhamc@link.msm.edu
Accred Length: 2 Years *Program Size:* 6
Program ID: 380-12-88-108
Public health program

Illinois

Chicago

Cook County Board of Commissioners Program
Sponsor: Cook County Hospital
University of Illinois School of Public Health
Program Director:
Rachel Rubin, MD MPH
Cook County Hospital
1900 W Polk St/Ste 500
Chicago, IL 60612
Tel: 312 633-5310 *Fax:* 312 633-6442
E-mail: rrubin@uic.edu
Accred Length: 2 Years *Program Size:* 7 (*GY1:* 1)
Program ID: 380-16-77-067
Occupational medicine program

Cook County Hospital Program
Sponsor: Cook County Hospital
University of Illinois School of Public Health
Program Director:
Arthur Hoffman, MD MPH
1835 W Harrison
Chicago, IL 60612
Tel: 312 633-5627 *Fax:* 312 572-4964
E-mail: arthurhoffman@pol.net
Accred Length: 2 Years *Program Size:* 4
Program ID: 380-16-21-050
General preventive medicine program

University of Illinois College of Medicine at Chicago Program
Sponsor: University of Illinois College of Medicine at Chicago
University of Illinois Hospital and Clinics
University of Illinois School of Public Health
Program Director:
Linda S Forst, MD MPH MS
Univ of Illinois-Chicago Sch of Public Health
Great Lakes Ctr for Occupational Safety and Health
2121 W Taylor (M/C 922)
Chicago, IL 60612-7321
Tel: 312 996-1283 *Fax:* 312 413-8485
E-mail: forst-l@uic.edu
Accred Length: 2 Years *Program Size:* 4
Program ID: 380-16-77-066
Occupational medicine program

Springfield

Illinois Department of Public Health Program
Sponsor: Illinois Department of Public Health
University of Illinois School of Public Health
Program Director:
Byron J Francis, MD MPH
Illinois Dept of Public Health
525 W Jefferson St
1st Fl
Springfield, IL 62761
Tel: 217 557-4049 *Fax:* 217 524-6090
E-mail: bfrancis@idph.state.il.us
Accred Length: 2 Years *Program Size:* 0
Program ID: 380-16-88-099
Public health program

Iowa

Iowa City

University of Iowa Hospitals and Clinics Program
Sponsor: University of Iowa Hospitals and Clinics
Program Director:
Nancy L Sprince, MD MPH
Univ of Iowa Hospitals and Clinics
Occupational Med Program
100 Oakdale Campus/124 IREH
Iowa City, IA 52242-5000
Tel: 319 335-4422 *Fax:* 319 335-4225
E-mail: nancy-sprince@uiowa.edu
Internet:
http://www.info.pmeh.uiowa.edu/gradprog/gradpro1.htm
Accred Length: 2 Years *Program Size:* 2
Program ID: 380-18-77-069
Occupational medicine program

Kentucky

Lexington

University of Kentucky Medical Center Program A
Sponsor: University of Kentucky Hospital
University of Kentucky College of Medicine
Program Director:
Timothy S Prince, MD
Univ of Kentucky Coll of Med
1141 Red Mile Rd/Ste 201
Lexington, KY 40504
Tel: 606 257-5150 *Fax:* 606 257-8982
E-mail: tprince@pop.uky.edu
Accred Length: 2 Years *Program Size:* 2
Program ID: 380-20-77-070
Occupational medicine program

University of Kentucky Medical Center Program
Sponsor: University of Kentucky Hospital
University of Kentucky College of Medicine
Program Director:
Terence R Collins, MD MPH
Univ of Kentucky Coll of Med
Dept of Preventive Med
1141 Red Mile Rd/Ste 201
Lexington, KY 40504
Tel: 606 323-5166 *Fax:* 606 323-1038
E-mail: trcoll01@pop.uky.edu
Accred Length: 2 Years *Program Size:* 2
Program ID: 380-20-21-039
General preventive medicine program

Louisiana

New Orleans

Tulane University School of Public Health and Tropical Medicine Program
Sponsor: Tulane Univ School of Public Health and Tropical Medicine
Program Director:
Marie A Krousel-Wood, MD MPH
Dept of Family/Community Med
1430 Tulane Ave/TB3
New Orleans, LA 70112-2699
Tel: 504 584-2556 *Fax:* 504 586-3801
E-mail: jmitche3@mailhost.tcs.tulane.edu
Internet:
http://www.tmc.tulane.edu/departments/fammed/
Accred Length: 2 Years *Program Size:* 6
Program ID: 380-21-21-014
General preventive medicine program

Maryland

Baltimore

Johns Hopkins University School of Hygiene and Public Health Program A
Sponsor: Johns Hopkins University School of Hygiene/Public Health
Program Director:
Clifford S Mitchell, MS MD MPH
Sch of Hygiene and Public Health
615 N Wolfe St/Rm 7041
Baltimore, MD 21205
Tel: 410 955-4157 *Fax:* 410 955-1811
E-mail: cmitchel@jhsph.edu
Accred Length: 2 Years *Program Size:* 12
Program ID: 380-23-77-072
Occupational medicine program

Johns Hopkins University School of Hygiene and Public Health Program
Sponsor: Johns Hopkins University School of Hygiene/Public Health
Program Director:
Miriam H Alexander, MD MPH
Johns Hopkins Univ Sch of Hygiene and Public Health
624 N Broadway/Rm 527
Baltimore, MD 21205
Tel: 410 955-3630 *Fax:* 410 614-1582
E-mail: mhalexan@jhsph.edu
Internet: http://www.med.jhu.edu/prevention
Accred Length: 2 Years *Program Size:* 20
Program ID: 380-23-11-015
General preventive medicine program

Maryland State Department of Health and Mental Hygiene Program

Sponsor: Maryland State Department of Health and Mental Hygiene
George Washington University School of Medicine
Johns Hopkins University School of Hygiene/Public Health
Program Director:
Diane L Matuszak, MD MPH
Maryland Dept of Health and Mental Hygiene
201 W Preston St
Baltimore, MD 21201
Tel: 410 767-5300 *Fax:* 410 333-7106
E-mail: matuszd@dhmh.state.md.us
Accred Length: 2 Years *Program Size:* 2
Program ID: 380-23-88-100
Public health program

University of Maryland Program

Sponsor: University of Maryland School of Medicine
Program Director:
Judith D Rubin, MD MPH
Dept of Epidemiology/Prev Med
Univ of Maryland Sch of Med
660 W Redwood St/Rm 102H
Baltimore, MD 21201-1596
Tel: 410 706-2864 *Fax:* 410 706-8013
E-mail: jrubin@epi.umaryland.edu
Internet:
http://soml.ab.umd.edu/epidemiology/depm.html
Accred Length: 2 Years *Program Size:* 8
Program ID: 380-23-11-016
General preventive medicine program

Bethesda

Uniformed Services University of the Health Sciences Program A

Sponsor: USUHS F Edward Hebert School of Medicine
Program Director:
Gail M Gullickson, MD MPH
Uniformed Services Univ of Hlth Sciences
4301 Jones Bridge Rd/Rm A1040A
Bethesda, MD 20814-4799
Tel: 301 295-3717 *Fax:* 301 295-0335
E-mail: ggullickson@usuhs.mil
Internet: http://www.usuhs.mil/prevmed.html
Accred Length: 2 Years *Program Size:* 16
Program ID: 380-23-77-073
US Armed Services Program
Occupational medicine program

Uniformed Services University of the Health Sciences Program

Sponsor: USUHS F Edward Hebert School of Medicine
Program Director:
R Kevin Hanson, MD MPH
Uniformed Services Univ of Health Sciences
Rm A1040-A/PMB
4301 Jones Bridge Rd
Bethesda, MD 20814-4799
Tel: 301 295-3717 *Fax:* 301 295-0335
E-mail: khanson@usuhs.mil
Internet: http://www.usuhs.mil/prevmed/prevmed.html
Accred Length: 2 Years *Program Size:* 16
Program ID: 380-23-21-044
US Armed Services Program
General preventive medicine program

Massachusetts

Boston

Boston University Medical Center Program

Sponsor: Boston Medical Center
Boston University School of Public Health
Public Health Commission
Program Director:
Jane M Liebschutz, MD MPH
715 Albany St
Boston, MA 02118-2526
Tel: 617 638-8080 *Fax:* 617 638-8076
E-mail: jliebs@bu.edu
Accred Length: 2 Years *Program Size:* 6
Program ID: 380-24-21-037
General preventive medicine program

Carney Hospital Program

Sponsor: Carney Hospital
Boston University School of Public Health
Program Director:
Anthony L Schlaff, MD MPH
Carney Hospital-Tufts Univ Preventive Med Residency
Carney Hospital
2100 Dorchester Ave
Boston, MA 02124-5666
Tel: 617 296-4220 *Fax:* 617 296-4222
E-mail: aschlaff@massmed.org
Accred Length: 2 Years *Program Size:* 13
Program ID: 380-24-21-043
General preventive medicine program

Center for Community Responsive Care Program

Sponsor: Center for Community Responsive Care Inc
UMass Memorial Health Care (University Campus)
Program Director:
Hugh S Fulmer, MD MPH
Ctr for Community Responsive Care
90 Cushing Ave
Boston, MA 02125
Tel: 617 265-4400 *Fax:* 617 265-7060
E-mail: copc1@aol.com
Accred Length: 2 Years *Program Size:* 12
Program ID: 380-24-88-101
Public health program

Harvard School of Public Health Program

Sponsor: Harvard School of Public Health
Program Director:
Howard Hu, MD MPH ScD
Harvard Univ Sch of Public Health
665 Huntington Ave
Boston, MA 02115-9957
Tel: 617 432-3327 *Fax:* 617 432-0219
E-mail: hhu@hohp.harvard.edu
Internet: http://www.hsph.harvard.edu/erc
Accred Length: 2 Years *Program Size:* 10
Program ID: 380-24-77-074
Occupational medicine program

Worcester

University of Massachusetts Program A

Sponsor: University of Massachusetts Medical School
UMass Memorial Health Care (University Campus)
University of Massachusetts School of Public Health
Program Director:
Thomas K Hicks, MD MPH
Univ of Massachusetts Med Sch
Dept of Family Med/Community Health
55 Lake Ave N
Worcester, MA 01655
Tel: 508 856-4159 *Fax:* 508 856-1680
E-mail: tom.hicks@banyan.ummed.edu
Internet:
http://www.ummed.edu:8000/dept/f+cmmm/index.htmll
Accred Length: 2 Years *Program Size:* 3
Program ID: 380-24-77-076
Occupational medicine program

University of Massachusetts Program

Sponsor: University of Massachusetts Medical School
UMass Memorial Health Care (University Campus)
Program Director:
Jacalyn Coghlin-Strom, MD MPH
Dept of Family/Com Med
Univ of Massachusetts Med Sch
55 Lake Ave N
Worcester, MA 01655-0309
Tel: 508 856-6163 *Fax:* 508 856-1212
E-mail: jackie.coghlinstrom@banyan.ummed.edu
Accred Length: 2 Years *Program Size:* 4
Program ID: 380-24-21-018
General preventive medicine program

Michigan

Ann Arbor

University of Michigan School of Public Health Program

Sponsor: University of Michigan School of Public Health
Program Director:
Alfred Franzblau, MD
Univ of Mich Sch of Pub Hlth
M6206 SPH II
1420 Washington Heights
Ann Arbor, MI 48109-2029
Tel: 734 936-0749 *Fax:* 734 763-8095
E-mail: mbartolo@umich.edu
Internet: http://www.sph.umich.edu/eih
Accred Length: 2 Years *Program Size:* 8
Program ID: 380-25-77-077
Occupational medicine program

Detroit

Wayne State University/Detroit Medical Center Program

Sponsor: Wayne State University/Detroit Medical Center
Detroit Receiving Hospital and University Health Center
Program Director:
Mark J Upfal, MD MPH
Occupational/Environmental Med
4201 St Antoine/UHC 4J
Detroit, MI 48201
Tel: 313 577-6852 *Fax:* 313 577-3070
E-mail: marufa@med.wayne.edu
Accred Length: 2 Years *Program Size:* 4
Program ID: 380-25-77-078
Occupational medicine program

Minnesota

Rochester

Mayo Graduate School of Medicine (Rochester) Program

Sponsor: Mayo Graduate School of Medicine-Mayo Foundation
Mayo Clinic (Rochester)
University of Minnesota School of Public Health
Program Director:
Philip Hagen, MD
Application Processing Ctr
Mayo Graduate Sch of Med
200 First St SW
Rochester, MN 55905
Tel: 507 284-3195 *Fax:* 507 284-5470
E-mail: mgsm.intmed.specialties@mayo.edu
Internet: http://www.mayo.edu/
Accred Length: 2 Years *Program Size:* 3
Program ID: 380-26-21-020
General preventive medicine program

St Paul

HealthPartners Institute for Medical Education Program

Sponsor: HealthPartners Institute for Medical Education
Regions Hospital
University of Minnesota School of Public Health
Program Director:
William H Lohman, MD
Regions Hospital
640 Jackson St
St Paul, MN 55101
Tel: 612 221-3771 *Fax:* 612 221-8848
E-mail: william.h.lohman@healthpartners.com
Accred Length: 2 Years *Program Size:* 6
Program ID: 380-26-77-079
Occupational medicine program

Missouri

St Louis

St Louis University School of Medicine Program

Sponsor: St Louis University School of Medicine
Missouri Department of Health
St Louis City Department of Health and Hospitals
St Louis University School of Public Health
Program Director:
A Lesley McLaren, MD MPH
St Louis Univ Sch of Med
Dept of Community/Family Med
1402 S Grand Blvd
St Louis, MO 63104
Tel: 314 577-8527, ext 8527 *Fax:* 314 268-5168
Internet: http://www.slu.edu
Accred Length: 2 Years *Program Size:* 2
Program ID: 380-28-88-102
Public health program

St Louis University School of Medicine Program

Sponsor: St Louis University School of Medicine
Program Director:
Rebecca L Tominack, MD MPH
St Louis Univ Sch of Med
1402 S Grand Blvd
St Louis, MO 63104
Tel: 314 577-8527, ext 8527 *Fax:* 314 268-5168
E-mail: engelhk@slu.edu
Internet: http://www.slu.edu
Accred Length: 2 Years *Program Size:* 4
Program ID: 380-28-77-080
Occupational medicine program

New Jersey

Morristown

Columbia University School of Public Health Program

Sponsor: Columbia University School of Public Health
Morristown Memorial Hospital
Program Director:
Jan Schwarz-Miller, MD MPH
Columbia Univ Sch of Public Health
60 H Ave/B-1
New York, NY 10032
Tel: 973 971-5441 *Fax:* 973 290-7078
Accred Length: 2 Years *Program Size:* 3 (*GY1:* 1)
Program ID: 380-35-77-083
Occupational medicine program

Piscataway

UMDNJ-Robert Wood Johnson Medical School Program

Sponsor: UMDNJ-Robert Wood Johnson Medical School
Program Director:
Michael Gochfeld, MD PhD
UMDNJ-Robert Wood Johnson Med Sch
Environ/Com Med EOHSI Bldg
170 Frelinghuysen Rd
Piscataway, NJ 08854
Tel: 732 445-0123, ext 627 *Fax:* 732 445-0130
E-mail: gochfeld@eohsi.rutgers.edu
Internet: http://www.eohsi.rutgers.edu
Accred Length: 2 Years *Program Size:* 5
Program ID: 380-33-77-081
Occupational medicine program

Trenton

New Jersey Department of Health and Senior Services Program

Sponsor: State of New Jersey Department of Health and Senior Services
Johns Hopkins University School of Hygiene/Public Health
Program Director:
Sindy M Paul, MD MPH
New Jersey Dept of Health
Div of AIDS Prevention/Control
50 E State St/4th Fl
Trenton, NJ 08625-0363
Tel: 609 984-2455 *Fax:* 609 292-4244
Accred Length: 2 Years *Program Size:* 3
Program ID: 380-33-88-103
Public health program

New York

Albany

SUNY at Albany School of Public Health Program

Sponsor: New York State Department of Health
SUNY at Albany School of Public Health
Program Director:
Mary S Applegate, MD MPH
New York State Dept of Health
Empire State Plaza
1882 Corning Tower
Albany, NY 12237
Tel: 518 474-1911 *Fax:* 518 474-3180
E-mail: qej03@health.state.ny.us
Internet: http://www.albany.edu/sph/pmrhome.html
Accred Length: 2 Years *Program Size:* 4
Program ID: 380-35-88-111
Public health program

Buffalo

SUNY at Buffalo Graduate Medical-Dental Education Consortium Program

Sponsor: SUNY at Buffalo Grad Medical-Dental Education Consortium
CGF Health System (Buffalo General Hospital)
Program Director:
Michael F Noe, MD MPH
SUNY-Buffalo
Dept of Social/Prev Med
3435 Main St/270 Farber Hall
Buffalo, NY 14214
Tel: 716 829-2975 *Fax:* 716 831-2979
Accred Length: 2 Years *Program Size:* 4
Program ID: 380-35-21-045
General preventive medicine program

New York

Mount Sinai School of Medicine Program A

Sponsor: Mount Sinai School of Medicine
Mount Sinai Medical Center
Program Director:
Jacqueline M Moline, MD MS
Mount Sinai Sch of Med
One Gustave L Levy Pl/Box 1057
New York, NY 10029
Tel: 212 241-4792 *Fax:* 212 996-0407
E-mail: jacqueline.moline@mssm.edu
Internet:
http://www.mssm.edu/commed/home-page.htmc
Accred Length: 2 Years *Program Size:* 5
Program ID: 380-35-77-082
Occupational medicine program

Mount Sinai School of Medicine Program

Sponsor: Mount Sinai School of Medicine
Mount Sinai Medical Center
Program Director:
Elizabeth J Garland, MD
Mount Sinai Sch of Med
One Gustave L Levy Pl/Box 1043
New York, NY 10029
Tel: 212 241-6442 *Fax:* 212 360-6965
E-mail: elizabeth.garland@mountsinai.org
Internet:
http://www.mssm.edu/commed/home.page.htmc
Accred Length: 2 Years *Program Size:* 3
Program ID: 380-35-21-024
General preventive medicine program

New York and Presbyterian Hospital (Cornell Campus) Program
Sponsor: New York and Presbyterian Hospital
Cornell University Medical College
New York and Presbyterian Hospital (Cornell Campus)
Program Director:
Lewis M Drusin, MD MPH
New York Presbyterian Hospital New York-Cornell Campus
525 E 68th St
New York, NY 10021
Tel: 212 746-1264 *Fax:* 212 746-8544
E-mail: mmontalv@mail.med.cornell.edu
Accred Length: 2 Years *Program Size:* 2
Program ID: 380-35-21-023
General preventive medicine program

New York City Department of Health Program
Sponsor: New York City Department of Health
Columbia University School of Public Health
Program Director:
Katherine Kaye, MD MPH
New York City Dept of Health
346 Broadway
CN-12 Rm 707B
New York, NY 10013
Tel: 212 442-3524 *Fax:* 212 442-3535
E-mail: kkaye@dohlan.nycnet.ci.nyc.ny.us
Internet: http://www.ci.nyc.ny.us/health
Accred Length: 2 Years *Program Size:* 5
Program ID: 380-35-88-104
Public health program

Stony Brook

SUNY at Stony Brook Program
Sponsor: University Hospital-SUNY at Stony Brook
Columbia University School of Public Health
Nassau County Department of Health
Suffolk County Department of Health Services
Program Director:
Dorothy S Lane, MD MPH
SUNY-Stony Brook
Sch of Med
Stony Brook, NY 11794-8036
Tel: 516 444-3902 *Fax:* 516 444-7525
E-mail: dlane@uhmc.sunysb.edu
Internet:
http://www.uhmc.sunysb.edu/prevmed/residency/
Accred Length: 2 Years *Program Size:* 8
Program ID: 380-35-88-112
Public health program

Valhalla

New York Medical College Program
Sponsor: New York Medical College
Hudson Valley Healthcare System
Mount Vernon Hospital
Our Lady of Mercy Medical Center
Westchester County Department of Health
Program Director:
Joseph A Cimino, MD
Dept of Com/Prev Med
New York Med Coll
Munger Pavilion
Valhalla, NY 10595
Tel: 914 594-4253 *Fax:* 914 594-4576
E-mail: joseph_cimino@nymc.edu
Accred Length: 1 Year *Program Size:* 4
Program ID: 380-35-31-047
General preventive medicine program

North Carolina

Chapel Hill

University of North Carolina Hospitals Program
Sponsor: University of North Carolina Hospitals
University of North Carolina School at Chapel Hill
University of North Carolina School of Medicine
Program Director:
Linda S Kinsinger, MD MPH
Preventive Med Residency Program
Wing D/CB#7240
Univ of North Carolina
Chapel Hill, NC 27599-7240
Tel: 919 962-1136 *Fax:* 919 966-7499
E-mail: jmtj@med.unc.edu
Internet:
http://www.med.unc.edu/wrkunits/2depts/soclmed/prevmedresidency.html
Accred Length: 2 Years *Program Size:* 8
Program ID: 380-36-21-026
General preventive medicine program

Durham

Duke University Program
Sponsor: Duke University Medical Center
University of North Carolina School at Chapel Hill
Program Director:
Dennis Darcey, MD
Duke Univ Med Ctr
PO Box 3834
Durham, NC 27710
Tel: 919 286-1722 *Fax:* 919 286-1021
E-mail: darce001@mc.duke.edu
Internet: http://occ-env-med.mc.duke.edu/oem
Accred Length: 2 Years *Program Size:* 2
Program ID: 380-36-77-084
Occupational medicine program

Ohio

Cincinnati

University Hospital/University of Cincinnati College of Medicine Program
Sponsor: University Hospital Inc
Program Director:
James R Donovan Jr, MD MS
Occupational/Environmental Med
Univ of Cincinnati Coll of Med
PO Box 670056
Cincinnati, OH 45267-0056
Tel: 513 558-0030 *Fax:* 513 558-6272
E-mail: millerdb@ucmail.uc.edu
Accred Length: 2 Years *Program Size:* 9
Program ID: 380-38-77-085
Occupational medicine program

Columbus

Ohio State University Program
Sponsor: Ohio State University Medical Center
Ohio State University College of Medicine
Program Director:
Benita M Jackson, MD MPH
Ohio State Univ
Sch of Public Health
B-115 Starling Loving Hall
Columbus, OH 43210-1240
Tel: 614 293-3913 *Fax:* 614 293-3937
E-mail: jackson-3@medctr.osu.edu
Internet:
http://www.med.ohio-state.edu/progs/pmr/pmrpage.html
Accred Length: 2 Years *Program Size:* 4
Program ID: 380-38-88-114
Public health program

Dayton

Wright State University Program
Sponsor: Wright State University School of Medicine
Program Director:
Stanley R Mohler, MD
Wright State Univ Sch of Med
Aerospace Med
PO Box 927
Dayton, OH 45401-0927
Tel: 937 276-8338 *Fax:* 937 275-5420
Internet:
http://www.med.wright.edu/som/resident/asm/asmhome.html
Accred Length: 2 Years *Program Size:* 6
Program ID: 380-38-66-052
Aerospace medicine program

Oklahoma

Oklahoma City

University of Oklahoma Health Sciences Center Program
Sponsor: University of Oklahoma College of Medicine
University Hospital
WorkMed Occupational Health Network (Tulsa)
Program Director:
Roy L DeHart, MD MPH
Univ of Oklahoma Health Sciences Ctr
900 NE 10th St/Rm 2400
Oklahoma City, OK 73104
Tel: 405 271-6177 *Fax:* 405 271-4125
E-mail: belinda-pfeiffer@ouhsc.edu
Internet:
http://www.fammed.uokhsc.edu/occmed/occmed.htm
Accred Length: 2 Years *Program Size:* 6
Program ID: 380-39-77-086
Occupational medicine program

Oregon

Portland

Oregon Health Sciences University Program

Sponsor: Oregon Health Sciences University Hospital

Program Director:
Jay D Kravitz, MD MPH
Oregon Health Sciences Univ
Dept of Public Health/Prev Med
3181 SW Sam Jackson Park Rd/CB 669
Portland, OR 97201-3098
Tel: 503 494-8257 *Fax:* 503 494-4981
E-mail: kravitzj@ohsu.edu
Internet:
http://www.ohsu.edu/som-pubhealth/residency.html
Accred Length: 2 Years *Program Size:* 4
Program ID: 380-40-88-115
Public health program

Pennsylvania

Philadelphia

Thomas Jefferson University Program

Sponsor: Thomas Jefferson University Hospital

Program Director:
Edward A Emmett, MD
Jefferson Med Coll
Rm 381 Jefferson Alumni Hall
1020 Locust St
Philadelphia, PA 19107-6799
Tel: 215 955-0577 *Fax:* 215 955-0575
Accred Length: 1 Year *Program Size:* 8
Program ID: 380-41-77-120
Occupational medicine program

Pittsburgh

University of Pittsburgh Graduate School of Public Health Program

Sponsor: University of Pittsburgh Graduate School of Public Health

Program Director:
Joseph J Schwerha, MD MPH
Univ of Pittsburgh Graduate Sch of Public Health
A718
130 Desoto St
Pittsburgh, PA 15261
Tel: 412 624-3155 *Fax:* 412 624-3040
Accred Length: 2 Years *Program Size:* 6
Program ID: 380-41-77-087
Occupational medicine program

South Carolina

Columbia

University of South Carolina School of Medicine Program

Sponsor: University of South Carolina School of Medicine

Program Director:
Gary B Ewing, MD MPH
Univ of South Carolina Sch of Med
Dept of Family/Prev Med
6 Richland Medical Pk
Columbia, SC 29203
Tel: 803 434-2447 *Fax:* 803 434-7776
E-mail: gewing@fpgw.rmh.edu
Internet: http://www.prevmend.scarolina.edu/
Accred Length: 2 Years *Program Size:* 6
Program ID: 380-45-88-116
Public health program

Tennessee

Nashville

Meharry Medical College Program

Sponsor: Meharry Medical College

Program Director:
Robert Levine, MD
George W Hubbard Hospital
1005 D B Todd Jr Blvd
Nashville, TN 37208
Tel: 615 327-6737 *Fax:* 615 327-5834
Accred Length: 3 Years *Program Size:* 8 (*GYI:* 2)
Program ID: 380-47-21-028
General preventive medicine program

Meharry Medical College Program A

Sponsor: Meharry Medical College

Program Director:
Otis Cosby, MD
Meharry Med Coll
Dept of Occup/Prev Med
1005 Dr D B Todd Jr Blvd
Nashville, TN 37208
Tel: 615 327-6736, ext 6831 *Fax:* 615 327-6717
Accred Length: 3 Years *Program Size:* 6 (*GYI:* 2)
Program ID: 380-47-77-088
Occupational medicine program

Texas

Austin

Texas Department of Health Program

Sponsor: Texas Department of Health
University of Texas School of Public Health

Program Director:
William S Riggins Jr, MD MPH
Texas Dept of Health
7430 Louis Pasteur
San Antonio, TX 78229
Tel: 210 949-2003 *Fax:* 210 949-2015
Internet: http://www.tdh.state.tx.us
Accred Length: 1 Year *Program Size:* 4
Program ID: 380-48-88-105
Public health program

Brooks AFB

USAF School of Aerospace Medicine Program

Sponsor: USAF School of Aerospace Medicine

Program Director:
Michael R Mork, MD MPH
USAF Sch of Aerospace Med
USAFSAM/AF
2602 Westgate Rd
Brooks AFB, TX 78235-5252
Tel: 210 536-3314 *Fax:* 210 536-2017
E-mail: mike.mork@mirage.brooks.af.mil
Internet: http://www.sam.brooks.af.mil/ram
Accred Length: 1 Year *Program Size:* 61
Program ID: 380-48-66-053
US Armed Services Program
Aerospace medicine program

USAF School of Aerospace Medicine Program A

Sponsor: USAF School of Aerospace Medicine

Program Director:
Richard H Stoller, MD MPH
USAF Sch of Aerospace Med/AF
2602 W Gate Rd
Brooks AFB, TX 78235
Tel: 210 536-1554 *Fax:* 210 536-2017
E-mail: richard.stoller@mirage.brooks.af.mil
Accred Length: 1 Year *Program Size:* 18
Program ID: 380-48-77-089
US Armed Services Program
Occupational medicine program

Galveston

University of Texas Medical Branch at Galveston Program

Sponsor: University of Texas Medical Branch Hospitals
University of Texas Medical School at Galveston

Program Director:
A Nelson Avery, MD
Univ of Texas Med Branch
Office of Preventive Med Residencies
301 University Blvd
Galveston, TX 77555-1150
Tel: 409 747-5351 *Fax:* 409 747-6129
E-mail: anwhorto@utmb.edu
Internet:
http://snapper.utmb.edu/pmch/areas/residencies
Accred Length: 2 Years *Program Size:* 2
Program ID: 380-48-77-121
Occupational medicine program

University of Texas Medical Branch Hospitals (NASA) Program

Sponsor: University of Texas Medical Branch Hospitals
NASA Johnson Space Center
University of Texas Medical School at Galveston

Program Director:
Jeffrey R Davis, MD MS
Univ of Texas Med Branch
Office of Preventive Med Residencies
301 University Blvd
Galveston, TX 77555-1150
Tel: 409 747-5351 *Fax:* 409 747-6129
E-mail: anwhorto@utmb.edu
Internet: http://www.utmb.edu/asm
Accred Length: 2 Years *Program Size:* 5
Program ID: 380-48-66-118
Aerospace medicine program

University of Texas Medical Branch Hospitals Program

Sponsor: University of Texas Medical Branch Hospitals

Program Director:
Tufail Q Shaikh, MD MPH
Univ of Texas Med Branch
Office of Preventive Med Residencies
301 University Blvd
Galveston, TX 77555-1150
Tel: 409 747-5351 *Fax:* 409 747-6129
Internet:
http://snapper.utmb.edu/pmch/areas/residencies
Accred Length: 2 Years *Program Size:* 2
Program ID: 380-48-21-049
General preventive medicine program

Houston

University of Texas School of Public Health Program

Sponsor: University of Texas School of Public Health

Program Director:
Arch I Carson, MD PhD
Univ of Texas Sch of Public Health
PO Box 20186
Houston, TX 77225-0186
Tel: 713 500-9440 *Fax:* 713 500-9442
E-mail: ccarson@utsph.sph.uth.tmc.edu
Internet:
http://www.sph.uth.tmc.edu/www/ctr/swcoeh/delweb.htm
Accred Length: 2 Years *Program Size:* 5
Program ID: 380-48-77-090
Occupational medicine program

Tyler

University of Texas Health Center at Tyler Program

Sponsor: University of Texas Health Center at Tyler
Stephen F Austin State University
University of Texas School of Public Health

Program Director:
Jeffrey L Levin, MD MPH
Univ of Texas Health Ctr-Tyler
11937 Hwy 271
Tyler, TX 75708-3154
Tel: 903 877-5900 *Fax:* 903 877-7060
E-mail: levin@uthct.edu
Internet: http://www.uthct.edu
Accred Length: 2 Years *Program Size:* 3
Program ID: 380-48-77-091
Occupational medicine program

Utah

Salt Lake City

University of Utah Program

Sponsor: University of Utah Medical Center
University of Utah School of Medicine

Program Director:
Anthony J Suruda, MD MPH
Univ of Utah
Occupational Med/RMCOEH/DFPM
75 S 2000 East
Salt Lake City, UT 84112-5120
Tel: 801 581-3841 *Fax:* 801 585-3759
E-mail: kbradakis@rmcoeh.utah.edu
Internet: http://www.rmcoeh.utah.edu
Accred Length: 2 Years *Program Size:* 6
Program ID: 380-49-77-092
Occupational medicine program

Virginia

Richmond

Medical College of Virginia/Virginia Commonwealth University Program

Sponsor: Medical College of Virginia/Virginia Commonwealth University
Commonwealth of Virginia Department of Health
Medical College of Virginia Hospitals

Program Director:
Christopher M Buttery, MD MPH
PO Box 980212
1008 E Clay St
Richmond, VA 23298-0212
Tel: 804 758-0707 *Fax:* 804 758-0507
E-mail: kimro@crosslink.net
Internet: http://views.vcu.edu/views/prevmed/
Accred Length: 2 Years *Program Size:* 4
Program ID: 380-51-88-106
Public health program

Washington

Seattle

University of Washington School of Public Health and Community Medicine Program A

Sponsor: University of Washington School of Public Health

Program Director:
Gary M Goldbaum, MD MPH
Sch of Public Health
Box 357230
Seattle, WA 98195-7230
Tel: 206 543-1144 *Fax:* 206 543-3813
E-mail: gary.goldbaum@matrokc.gov
Internet:
http://weber.u.washington.edu/~sphcm/academic/prevmed.html
Accred Length: 2 Years *Program Size:* 6
Program ID: 380-54-88-117
Public health program

University of Washington School of Public Health and Community Medicine Program

Sponsor: University of Washington School of Public Health

Program Director:
Scott Barnhart, MD MPH
Harborview Med Ctr
325 Ninth Ave/Box 359739
415 Harborview Hall
Seattle, WA 98104-2499
Tel: 206 731-3388 *Fax:* 206 731-8247
E-mail: oemp@u.washington.edu
Internet:
http://www.sphcm.washington.edu/dehweb/om.html
Accred Length: 2 Years *Program Size:* 6
Program ID: 380-54-77-093
Occupational medicine program

Tacoma

Madigan Army Medical Center Program

Sponsor: Madigan Army Medical Center
University of Washington School of Public Health

Program Director:
Jeffrey D Gunzenhauser, MD MPH
Madigan Army Med Ctr
Preventive Med Service
Tacoma, WA 98431
Tel: 253 968-4479 *Fax:* 253 968-4483
Accred Length: 2 Years *Program Size:* 8
Program ID: 380-54-88-107
US Armed Services Program
Public health program

West Virginia

Morgantown

West Virginia University Program

Sponsor: West Virginia University School of Medicine

Program Director:
John D Meyer, MD MPH
Inst of Occup/Environmental Med
West Virginia Univ Sch of Med
PO Box 9190
Morgantown, WV 26506-9190
Tel: 304 293-3693 *Fax:* 304 293-2629
Internet: http://www.hsc.wvu.edu/ioeh
Accred Length: 2 Years *Program Size:* 6
Program ID: 380-55-77-094
Occupational medicine program

Wisconsin

Milwaukee

Medical College of Wisconsin Program

Sponsor: Medical College of Wisconsin Affiliated Hospitals Inc
Medical College of Wisconsin

Program Director:
Dale A Tavris, MD MPH
Dept of Preventive Med
8701 Watertown Plank Rd
Milwaukee, WI 53226
Tel: 414 456-4500 *Fax:* 414 456-6547
E-mail: drtavris@post.its.mcw.edu
Internet: http://www.mcw.edu/prevmed/index.htm
Accred Length: 2 Years *Program Size:* 2
Program ID: 380-56-21-031
General preventive medicine program

Medical College of Wisconsin Program

Sponsor: Medical College of Wisconsin Affiliated Hospitals Inc
Medical College of Wisconsin

Program Director:
Ross L Clay, MD MPH
Med Coll of Wisconsin
8701 Watertown Plank Rd
Milwaukee, WI 53226
Tel: 414 456-4500 *Fax:* 414 456-6547
E-mail: rclay@post.its.mcw.edu
Internet: http://www.mcw.edu/orevmed/wdex.ht
Accred Length: 2 Years *Program Size:* 2
Program ID: 380-56-77-095
Occupational medicine program

Psychiatry

Alabama

Birmingham

University of Alabama Medical Center Program

Sponsor: University of Alabama Hospital
Veterans Affairs Medical Center (Birmingham)

Program Director:
Margaret M Scalise, MD
Univ of Alabama Sch of Med
121 Smolian Psychiatric Clinic
1700 Seventh Ave S/UAB Station
Birmingham, AL 35294-0018
Tel: 205 934-3041 *Fax:* 205 934-4659
E-mail: mscalise@psych.uabmc.edu
Internet: http://www.uaab.edu/psychiatry/resident.htm
Accred Length: 4 Years *Program Size:* 24 (*GY1:* 6)
Subspecialties: PYG
Program ID: 400-01-11-009

Mobile

University of South Alabama Program

Sponsor: University of South Alabama Medical Center
Searcy State Hospital
USA Doctors Hospital
USA Knollwood Park Hospital

Program Director:
Dirk M Dhossche, MD
Univ of South Alabama
3421 Medical Park Dr W
Ste 2
Mobile, AL 36693
Tel: 334 660-5157 *Fax:* 334 660-5198
E-mail: ddhossch@jaguar1.usouthal.edu
Internet: http://www.southalabama.edu/psychiatry
Accred Length: 4 Years *Program Size:* 12 (*GY1:* 3)
Program ID: 400-01-22-232

Arizona

Phoenix

Good Samaritan Regional Medical Center Program

Sponsor: Good Samaritan Regional Medical Center

Program Director:
James B McLoone, MD
Good Samaritan Regional Med Ctr
Samaritan Behavioral Health Ctr
925 E McDowell Rd/4th Fl
Phoenix, AZ 85006
Tel: 602 239-6880 *Fax:* 602 239-6988
E-mail: andreaw@samaritan.edu
Internet: http://www.samaritan.edu
Accred Length: 4 Years *Program Size:* 16 (*GY1:* 4)
Program ID: 400-03-12-010

Maricopa Medical Center Program

Sponsor: Maricopa Medical Center

Program Director:
Glenn Lippman, MD
Maricopa Med Ctr
Psychiatric Ctr
2601 E Roosevelt St
Phoenix, AZ 85008
Tel: 602 267-5751 *Fax:* 602 267-5891
Internet: http://www.maricopa.gov/medcenter/mmc.html
Accred Length: 4 Years *Program Size:* 16 (*GY1:* 4)
Program ID: 400-03-22-011

Tucson

University of Arizona Program

Sponsor: University of Arizona College of Medicine
Kino Community Hospital
University Medical Center
Veterans Affairs Medical Center (Tucson)

Program Director:
Rebecca L Potter, MD
Univ of Arizona Coll of Med
1501 N Campbell Ave
PO Box 245002
Tucson, AZ 85724-5002
Tel: 520 626-6795 *Fax:* 520 626-2004
E-mail: potter@u.arizona.edu
Accred Length: 4 Years *Program Size:* 24 (*GY1:* 6)
Program ID: 400-03-21-012

Arkansas

Little Rock

University of Arkansas for Medical Sciences Program

Sponsor: University of Arkansas College of Medicine
Arkansas Children's Hospital
Arkansas State Hospital-Little Rock Hospital
John L McClellan Memorial Veterans Hospital
University Hospital of Arkansas

Program Director:
Frederick G Guggenheim, MD
Univ of Arkansas Med Sch
4301 W Markham St/Slot 589
Little Rock, AR 72205
Tel: 501 686-6196 *Fax:* 501 686-7424
E-mail: guggenheimfrederick@exchange.uams.edu
Accred Length: 4 Years *Program Size:* 24 (*GY1:* 6)
Program ID: 400-04-22-014

California

Fresno

University of California (San Francisco)/Fresno Program

Sponsor: UCSF-Fresno Medical Education Program
University Medical Center
Veterans Affairs Medical Center (Fresno)

Program Director:
Hoyle Leigh, MD
Univ of California San Francisco-Fresno
Dept of Psychiatry/116A
2615 E Clinton Ave
Fresno, CA 93703-2223
Tel: 209 228-6931 *Fax:* 209 228-6979
E-mail: leigh@ucsfresno.edu
Internet: http://www.ucsfresno.edu/psychiatry
Accred Length: 4 Years *Program Size:* 16 (*GY1:* 4)
Program ID: 400-05-21-018

Loma Linda

Loma Linda University Program

Sponsor: Loma Linda University Medical Center
Jerry L Pettis Memorial Veterans Hospital

Program Director:
David Schultz, MD
Dept of Psychiatry
Loma Linda Univ
PO Box 1007
Loma Linda, CA 92354
Tel: 909 799-6094 *Fax:* 909 799-6093
Accred Length: 4 Years *Program Size:* 24 (*GY1:* 6)
Program ID: 400-05-21-021

Los Angeles

Cedars-Sinai Medical Center Program

Sponsor: Cedars-Sinai Medical Center

Program Director:
Lawrence S Gross, MD
Thalians Mental Health Ctr
8730 Alden Dr/Ste W-101
Los Angeles, CA 90048-0750
Tel: 310 855-3461 *Fax:* 310 967-0114
E-mail: grossl@csme.edu
Accred Length: 4 Years *Program Size:* 20 (*GY1:* 4)
Program ID: 400-05-11-022

Charles R Drew University Program

Sponsor: Charles R Drew University of Medicine and Science
LAC-King/Drew Medical Center

Program Director:
Gregory Gray, MD
King-Drew Med Ctr, Dept of Psychiatry
1720 E 120th St
Los Angeles, CA 90059
Tel: 310 668-3588 *Fax:* 310 668-4805
Accred Length: 4 Years *Program Size:* 28 (*GY1:* 7)
Program ID: 400-05-32-024

UCLA Medical Center Program

Sponsor: UCLA School of Medicine
UCLA Neuropsychiatric Hospital

Program Director:
James E Spar, MD
UCLA Neuropsychiatric Inst
Attn: Sandra Lipschultz, Admin
760 Westwood Plaza/Rm C8-852
Los Angeles, CA 90024-1759
Tel: 310 825-0548 *Fax:* 310 825-0340
E-mail: sandrajl@npih.medsch.ucla.edu
Internet: http://www.mental health.ucla.edu/trainees
Accred Length: 4 Years *Program Size:* 56 (*GY1:* 14)
Subspecialties: PYG
Program ID: 400-05-21-025

University of Southern California Program

Sponsor: Los Angeles County-USC Medical Center

Program Director:
Charles W Patterson, MD
Dept of Psychiatry
Los Angeles County-USC Med Ctr
1937 Hospital Pl
Los Angeles, CA 90033
Tel: 323 226-4945 *Fax:* 323 226-4948
Accred Length: 4 Years *Program Size:* 42 (*GY1:* 10)
Program ID: 400-05-11-023

VA Greater Los Angeles Healthcare System Program

Sponsor: VA Greater Los Angeles Healthcare System
Olive View-UCLA Medical Center

Program Director:
Murray Brown, MD
Education Office (116A3) Psychiatry Dept
Sepulveda VA Med Ctr
16111 Plummer St
Sepulveda, CA 91343
Tel: 818 895-9349 *Fax:* 818 895-9437
E-mail: pshah@ucla.edu
Internet: http://www.mentalhealth.ucla.edu
Accred Length: 4 Years *Program Size:* 31 (*GY1:* 8)
Program ID: 400-05-31-032

Orange

University of California (Irvine) Program

Sponsor: University of California (Irvine) Medical Center
Veterans Affairs Medical Center (Long Beach)

Program Director:
Rhoda K Hahn, MD
Univ of California Irvine Med Ctr
Dept of Psychiatry
101 City Dr S
Orange, CA 92697
Tel: 714 456-5770 *Fax:* 714 456-7615
Internet: http://www.med.uci.edu/psych/
Accred Length: 4 Years *Program Size:* 30 (*GY1:* 8)
Program ID: 400-05-21-020

Sacramento

University of California (Davis) Program

Sponsor: University of California (Davis) Medical Center

Program Director:
Mark E Servis, MD
Univ of California Davis Med Ctr
2315 Stockton Blvd
Sacramento, CA 95817
Tel: 916 734-2614 *Fax:* 916 451-9946
E-mail: psychiatry.training@ucdmc.ucdavis.edu
Internet:
http://www.neuroscience.ucdavis.edu/psychiatry
Accred Length: 4 Years *Program Size:* 20 (*GY1:* 4)
Program ID: 400-05-31-017

San Diego

Naval Medical Center (San Diego) Program

Sponsor: Naval Medical Center (San Diego)

Program Director:
Jennifer S Berg, MD MD
Naval Med Ctr
Mental Health Services
34800 Bob Wilson Dr/Ste 108
San Diego, CA 92134-1108
Tel: 619 532-8552 *Fax:* 619 532-8353
E-mail: jsberg@snd10.med.navy.mil
Accred Length: 4 Years *Program Size:* 16 (*GY1:* 4)
Program ID: 400-05-21-253
US Armed Services Program

University of California (San Diego) Program

Sponsor: University of California (San Diego) Medical Center
Veterans Affairs Medical Center (San Diego)

Program Director:
Sidney Zisook, MD
UCSD Med Ctr
Dept of Psychiatry (0603-R)
9500 Gilman Dr
La Jolla, CA 92093-0603
Tel: 619 534-4040 *Fax:* 619 822-0231
E-mail: szisook@ucsd.edu
Internet: http://eugene.ucsd.edu/~psych/index.htm
Accred Length: 4 Years *Program Size:* 38 (*GY1:* 8)
Subspecialties: PYG
Program ID: 400-05-21-026

San Francisco

California Pacific Medical Center Program

Sponsor: California Pacific Medical Center
California Pacific Medical Center

Program Director:
Charles P Fisher, MD
California Pacific Med Ctr-Pacific Campus
2340 Clay St/7th Fl
PO Box 7999
San Francisco, CA 94115
Tel: 415 923-3510 *Fax:* 415 923-3525
E-mail: conleyk@sutterhealth.org
Internet: http://www.cpmc.org
Accred Length: 4 Years *Program Size:* 14 (*GY1:* 14)
Program ID: 400-05-22-028

University of California (San Francisco) Program

Sponsor: University of California (San Francisco) School of Medicine
Langley Porter Psychiatric Hospitals and Clinics
San Francisco General Hospital Medical Center
University of California (San Francisco) Medical Center
Veterans Affairs Medical Center (San Francisco)

Program Director:
Marc Jacobs, MD
Univ of California San Francisico
Langley Porter Psychiatric Inst
401 Parnassus Ave/RTP
San Francisco, CA 94143-0984
Tel: 415 476-7577 *Fax:* 415 476-7722
Internet: http://itsa.ucsf.edu/~lppi/
Accred Length: 4 Years *Program Size:* 63 (*GY1:* 14)
Program ID: 400-05-21-030

San Mateo

San Mateo Community Mental Health Services Program

Sponsor: San Mateo County General Hospital

Program Director:
Deborah J Hales, MD
Psychiatry Training Program
San Mateo County General Hospital
222 W 39th Ave
San Mateo, CA 94403
Tel: 415 573-2530 *Fax:* 415 573-2527
E-mail: hsa*licursi@smtpgate.co.sanmateo.ca.us
Accred Length: 4 Years *Program Size:* 16 (*GY1:* 4)
Program ID: 400-05-22-031

Stanford

Stanford University Program

Sponsor: Stanford University Hospital
Kaiser Permanente Medical Center (Santa Clara)
Veterans Affairs Palo Alto Health Care System

Program Director:
C Barr Taylor, MD
UCSF Stanford Health Care
Dept of Psych/Behav Science
401 Quarry Rd/Rm 2109
Stanford, CA 94305-5723
Tel: 650 725-5591 *Fax:* 650 725-5594
E-mail: faesloss@leland.stanford.edu
Internet: http://www.stanford.edu/dept/pbs/
Accred Length: 4 Years *Program Size:* 45 (*GY1:* 9)
Subspecialties: PYG
Program ID: 400-05-31-033

Torrance

Los Angeles County-Harbor-UCLA Medical Center Program

Sponsor: Los Angeles County-Harbor-UCLA Medical Center

Program Director:
Ira M Lesser, MD
Harbor-UCLA Med Ctr
Dept of Psychiatry/Box 498
1000 W Carson St
Torrance, CA 90509
Tel: 310 222-3137 *Fax:* 310 328-5546
E-mail: lesser@humc.edu
Internet: http://www.humc.edu
Accred Length: 4 Years *Program Size:* 27 (*GY1:* 8)
Program ID: 400-05-11-035

Colorado

Denver

University of Colorado Program

Sponsor: University of Colorado Health Sciences Center
Denver Health and Hospitals
Veterans Affairs Medical Center (Denver)

Program Director:
Robert House, MD
Univ of Colorado Sch of Med
4200 E Ninth Ave/Box C-249
Denver, CO 80262
Tel: 303 315-7255 *Fax:* 303 315-5641
E-mail: robert.house@uchsc.edu
Accred Length: 4 Years *Program Size:* 42 (*GY1:* 9)
Subspecialties: ADP, PFP
Program ID: 400-07-21-038

Connecticut

Farmington

Institute of Living/University of Connecticut Program

Sponsor: University of Connecticut School of Medicine
Hartford Hospital
Institute of Living
Univ of Connecticut Health Center/John Dempsey Hospital

Program Director:
David A Goldberg, MD
Univ of Connecticut Health Ctr
Dept of Psychiatry
10 Talcott Notch Rd E/MC 6410
Farmington, CT 06030-1806
Tel: 860 679-6729 *Fax:* 860 679-6675
E-mail: residency@psychiatry.uchc.edu
Accred Length: 4 Years *Program Size:* 32 (*GY1:* 8)
Program ID: 400-08-21-266

New Haven

Yale-New Haven Medical Center Program
Sponsor: Yale-New Haven Hospital
Connecticut Mental Health Center
Greenwich Hospital
Hospital of St Raphael
Norwalk Hospital
Veterans Affairs Medical Center (West Haven)
Yale Psychiatric Institute
Yale University Health Service
Program Director:
Richard Belitsky, MD
Yale Univ Sch of Med
25 Park St/6th Fl GEB
New Haven, CT 06519
Tel: 203 785-2095 *Fax:* 203 785-7357
E-mail: richard.belitsky@yale.edu
Internet: http://www.med.yale.edu/psych
Accred Length: 4 Years *Program Size:* 58 (*GY1:* 10)
Subspecialties: PYG
Program ID: 400-08-21-042

Delaware

New Castle

Delaware State Hospital Program
Sponsor: Delaware State Hospital
Christiana Care Health Services Inc
Program Director:
David T Springer, MD
Delaware Psychiatric Ctr
1901 N DuPont Hwy/Springer #2
New Castle, DE 19720
Tel: 302 577-4316 *Fax:* 302 577-4359
E-mail: dspringer@state.de.us
Accred Length: 4 Years *Program Size:* 12 (*GY1:* 3)
Program ID: 400-09-31-046

District of Columbia

Washington

George Washington University Program
Sponsor: George Washington University School of Medicine
George Washington University Hospital (UHS)
Program Director:
James L Griffith, MD
George Washington Univ Hospital
8-420 Burns Building
2150 Pennsylvania Ave NW
Washington, DC 20037-2396
Tel: 202 994-2956 *Fax:* 202 994-6377
Internet: http://www.gwumc.edu
Accred Length: 4 Years *Program Size:* 16 (*GY1:* 4)
Program ID: 400-10-21-048

Georgetown University Program
Sponsor: Georgetown University Medical Center
Fairfax Hospital
Veterans Affairs Medical Center (Washington, DC)
Program Director:
Thomas S Zaubler, MD MPH
Georgetown Univ Sch of Med
Dept of Psychiatry
3800 Reservoir Rd NW
Washington, DC 20007-2197
Tel: 202 687-8537 *Fax:* 202 687-6658
E-mail: zaublert@gunet.georgetown.edu
Accred Length: 4 Years *Program Size:* 24 (*GY1:* 6)
Program ID: 400-10-21-047

Howard University Program
Sponsor: Howard University Hospital
Veterans Affairs Medical Center (Washington, DC)
Program Director:
William J Klein, MD
Howard Univ Hospital
Dept of Psychiatry
2041 Georgia Ave NW
Washington, DC 20060
Tel: 202 865-6611 *Fax:* 202 865-6212
Accred Length: 4 Years *Program Size:* 15 (*GY1:* 3)
Program ID: 400-10-21-049

St Elizabeth's Hospital Program
Sponsor: DC Commission on Mental Health Services-St Elizabeth Campus
George Washington University Hospital (UHS)
Washington School of Psychiatry
Program Director:
David I Joseph, MD
Barton Hall/Rm 201-A
2700 Martin Luther King Jr SE
Washington, DC 20032
Tel: 202 373-7583 *Fax:* 202 373-6433
Accred Length: 4 Years *Program Size:* 35 (*GY1:* 9)
Program ID: 400-10-21-239

Florida

Gainesville

University of Florida Program
Sponsor: University of Florida College of Medicine
Shands Hospital at the University of Florida
Veterans Affairs Medical Center (Gainesville)
Program Director:
Ross A McElroy Jr, MD
Univ of Florida Health Science Ctr
Dept of Psychiatry
Box 100256
Gainesville, FL 32610-0256
Tel: 352 395-0680, ext 55220 *Fax:* 352 395-6987
E-mail: mcelroy@college.med.ufl.edu
Accred Length: 4 Years *Program Size:* 27 (*GY1:* 7)
Subspecialties: PYG
Program ID: 400-11-21-050

Miami

University of Miami-Jackson Memorial Medical Center Program
Sponsor: University of Miami-Jackson Memorial Medical Center
Veterans Affairs Medical Center (Miami)
Program Director:
Richard M Steinbook, MD
Univ of Miami Sch of Med
D29 Dept of Psychiatry
PO Box 016960
Miami, FL 33101-8110
Tel: 305 585-6335 *Fax:* 305 324-8601
E-mail: cremy@mednet.med.miami.edu
Internet: http://www.med.miami.edu
Accred Length: 4 Years *Program Size:* 46 (*GY1:* 8)
Subspecialties: ADP, PYG
Program ID: 400-11-21-051

Tampa

University of South Florida Program
Sponsor: University of South Florida College of Medicine
James A Haley Veterans Hospital
Tampa General Healthcare
TGH University Psychiatry Center
Program Director:
Kailie R Shaw, MD
Univ of South Florida Psychiatry Ctr
3515 E Fletcher Ave
Tampa, FL 33613
Tel: 813 974-2388 *Fax:* 813 974-3223
E-mail: kshaw@com1.med.usf.edu
Internet: http://www.med.usf.edu/psych/psychome.html
Accred Length: 4 Years *Program Size:* 23 (*GY1:* 5)
Subspecialties: ADP, PYG
Program ID: 400-11-21-052

Georgia

Atlanta

Emory University Program
Sponsor: Emory University School of Medicine
Emory University Hospital
Grady Memorial Hospital
Veterans Affairs Medical Center (Atlanta)
Program Director:
Miles K Crowder, MD
Emory Univ
Dept of Psych/Behav Sciences
1701 Uppergate Dr/Rm 133
Atlanta, GA 30322
Tel: 404 727-5157 *Fax:* 404 727-4746
Internet:
http://www.emory.edu/whsc/med/psychiatry/home.htm
Accred Length: 4 Years *Program Size:* 50 (*GY1:* 12)
Subspecialties: PYG
Program ID: 400-12-21-053

Morehouse School of Medicine Program
Sponsor: Morehouse School of Medicine
Brawner Psychiatric Institute
Central Alabama Veterans Healthcare System
Fulton County Health Department
Georgia Regional Hospital at Atlanta
Grady Memorial Hospital
The Ridgeview Institute
West Paces Ferry Medical Center
Program Director:
John O Gaston Sr, MD
Morehouse Sch of Med
Dept of Psych/Behavioral Sciences
720 Westview Dr/SW
Atlanta, GA 30310-1495
Tel: 404 756-1440
Internet: http://www.msm.edu
Accred Length: 4 Years *Program Size:* 16 (*GY1:* 4)
Program ID: 400-12-21-262

Augusta

Medical College of Georgia Program
Sponsor: Medical College of Georgia Hospital and Clinics
Veterans Affairs Medical Center (Augusta)
Program Director:
Donald A Misch, MD
Med Coll of Georgia
Dept of Psych/Health Behavior
1515 Pope Ave
Augusta, GA 30912-3800
Tel: 706 721-6715 *Fax:* 706 721-1793
E-mail: hosp2.dnewman@mail.mcg.edu
Accred Length: 4 Years *Program Size:* 20 (*GY1:* 5)
Program ID: 400-12-21-054

Fort Gordon

Dwight David Eisenhower Army Medical Center Program

Sponsor: Dwight David Eisenhower Army Medical Center

Program Director:
Douglas A Waldrep, MD
Dwight David Eisenhower Army Med Ctr
Dept of Psych/Neurology
Fort Gordon, GA 30905-5650
Tel: 706 787-2550 *Fax:* 706 787-6004
E-mail:
douglas_a.waldrep@ddeamc-a.chcs.amedd.army.mil
Internet: http://www.ddeamc.amedd.army.mil/
Accred Length: 4 Years *Program Size:* 12 (*GY1:* 0)
Program ID: 400-12-12-004
US Armed Services Program

Hawaii

Honolulu

Tripler Army Medical Center Program

Sponsor: Tripler Army Medical Center

Program Director:
Maj Richard L Jaconette, MD
Dept of Psychiatry
Tripler Army Med Ctr
1 Jarrett White Rd
Honolulu, HI 96859-5000
Tel: 808 433-5780 *Fax:* 808 433-4591
E-mail: richard_l.jaconette@tamc.chcs.amedd.army.mil
Internet:
http://webserver.tamc.amedd.army.mil/psychiatry/index.html
Accred Length: 4 Years *Program Size:* 24 (*GY1:* 6)
Program ID: 400-14-11-233
US Armed Services Program

University of Hawaii Program

Sponsor: University of Hawaii John A Burns School of Medicine
Hawaii State Hospital
Queen's Medical Center

Program Director:
Iqbal Ahmed, MD
Univ of Hawaii
Dept of Psychiatry
1356 Lusitana St/4th Fl
Honolulu, HI 96813
Tel: 808 586-2900 *Fax:* 808 586-2940
Internet:
http://medworld.biomed.hawaii.edu/hrp/hrp.html
Accred Length: 4 Years *Program Size:* 24 (*GY1:* 5)
Subspecialties: ADP, PYG
Program ID: 400-14-31-055

Illinois

Chicago

McGaw Medical Center of Northwestern University Program

Sponsor: Northwestern University Medical School
Evanston Hospital
Northwestern Memorial Hospital
Veterans Affairs Lakeside Medical Center (Chicago)

Program Director:
Ronald F Krasner, MD
McGaw Med Ctr-Northwestern Univ Med Sch
Dept of Psychiatry
303 E Superior St/Rm 594
Chicago, IL 60611-3053
Tel: 312 908-8058 *Fax:* 312 908-4840
E-mail: r-krasner@nwu.edu
Accred Length: 4 Years *Program Size:* 30 (*GY1:* 8)
Subspecialties: ADP, PYG
Program ID: 400-16-21-060

Rush-Presbyterian-St Luke's Medical Center Program

Sponsor: Rush-Presbyterian-St Luke's Medical Center

Program Director:
Daniel Levin, MD
Rush-Presbyterian-St Luke's Med Ctr
1720 W Polk St
Chicago, IL 60612
Tel: 312 942-2099 *Fax:* 312 942-3186
Internet: http://www.rush.edu
Accred Length: 4 Years *Program Size:* 23 (*GY1:* 5)
Program ID: 400-16-11-061

University of Chicago Program

Sponsor: University of Chicago Hospitals

Program Director:
Kathleen M Kelley, MD
Univ of Chicago Hospitals
Dept of Psychiatry
5841 S Maryland Ave/MC3077
Chicago, IL 60637-1470
Tel: 773 702-0529 *Fax:* 773 702-4297
E-mail: education@yoda.bsd.uchicago.edu
Accred Length: 4 Years *Program Size:* 26 (*GY1:* 7)
Program ID: 400-16-31-062

University of Illinois College of Medicine at Chicago Program

Sponsor: University of Illinois College of Medicine at Chicago
University of Illinois Hospital and Clinics
Veterans Affairs West Side Medical Center

Program Director:
Henry W Dove, MD
Univ of Illinois-Chicago
Dept of Psychiatry (M/C 913)
912 S Wood St
Chicago, IL 60612-7327
Tel: 312 996-7380 *Fax:* 312 996-3514
E-mail: recruit@psych.uic.edu.
Internet: http://www.psych.uic.edu
Accred Length: 4 Years *Program Size:* 55 (*GY1:* 12)
Program ID: 400-16-21-063

Evanston

McGaw Medical Center of Northwestern University (Evanston) Program

Sponsor: Northwestern University Medical School
Evanston Hospital

Program Director:
Rachel Yudkowsky, MD
Evanston Hospital
2650 Ridge Ave
Evanston, IL 60201
Tel: 847 570-2683 *Fax:* 847 570-1405
E-mail: r-yudkowsky@nwu.edu
Accred Length: 4 Years *Program Size:* 2 (*GY1:* 0)
Program ID: 400-16-21-280

Maywood

Loyola University Program

Sponsor: Loyola University Medical Center
Edward J Hines Jr Veterans Affairs Hospital

Program Director:
Francisco Fernandez, MD
Loyola Univ Med Ctr
Dept of Psychiatry
2160 S First Ave/Bldg 54
Maywood, IL 60153
Tel: 708 216-3273 *Fax:* 708 216-5885
E-mail: fferna@luc.edu
Internet:
http://www.meddean.luc.edu/lumen/deptwebs/psychiat/psychiat.htm
Accred Length: 4 Years *Program Size:* 29 (*GY1:* 6)
Program ID: 400-16-21-064

North Chicago

Finch University of Health Sciences/Chicago Medical School Program

Sponsor: Finch University of Health Sciences/Chicago Medical School
Mount Sinai Hospital Medical Center of Chicago
Ravenswood Hospital Medical Center
Veterans Affairs Medical Center (North Chicago)

Program Director:
David A Garfield, MD
Finch Univ of Health Sciences-Chicago Med Sch
3333 Green Bay Rd
North Chicago, IL 60064
Tel: 847 578-8705 *Fax:* 847 578-3328
Accred Length: 4 Years *Program Size:* 38 (*GY1:* 9)
Program ID: 400-16-31-056

Park Ridge

Lutheran General Hospital Program

Sponsor: Lutheran General Hospital

Program Director:
Gustavo Hernandez, MD
Lutheran General Hospital
Dept of Psychiatry/8 South
1775 W Dempster St
Park Ridge, IL 60068-1174
Tel: 847 723-5887 *Fax:* 847 723-7312
Accred Length: 4 Years *Program Size:* 12 (*GY1:* 3)
Program ID: 400-16-21-257

Springfield

Southern Illinois University Program
Sponsor: Southern Illinois University School of Medicine
Memorial Medical Center
St John's Hospital
Program Director:
Karen E Broquet, MD
Southern Illinois Univ Sch of Med
PO Box 19642
Springfield, IL 62794-9642
Tel: 217 785-3935, ext 3106 *Fax:* 217 524-4736
E-mail: rstark@wpsmtp.siumed.edu
Internet: http://www.siumed.edu/psych/res
Accred Length: 4 Years *Program Size:* 14 (*GY1:* 3)
Program ID: 400-16-21-065

Indiana

Indianapolis

Indiana University School of Medicine Program
Sponsor: Indiana University School of Medicine
Clarian IU Hospital
Clarian Riley Hospital for Children
Larue D Carter Memorial Hospital
Richard L Roudebush Veterans Affairs Medical Center
William N Wishard Memorial Hospital
Program Director:
Alan D Schmetzer, MD
Indiana Univ Med Ctr
Clinical Bldg/278
541 Clinical Dr
Indianapolis, IN 46202-5111
Tel: 317 274-1224 *Fax:* 317 274-1248
Internet: http://www.iupui.edu/~psych
Accred Length: 4 Years *Program Size:* 28 (*GY1:* 7)
Subspecialties: ADP, PYG
Program ID: 400-17-21-066

Iowa

Iowa City

University of Iowa Hospitals and Clinics Program
Sponsor: University of Iowa Hospitals and Clinics
Veterans Affairs Medical Center (Iowa City)
Program Director:
Catherine Woodman, MD
Univ of Iowa Hospitals and Clinics
Dept of Psychiatry/2887 JPP
200 Hawkins Dr
Iowa City, IA 52242
Tel: 319 339-7146, ext 6415 *Fax:* 319 339-7171
E-mail: catherine-woodman@uiowa.edu
Internet: http://www.uihc.uiowa.edu/pubinfo/psychl.ntm
Accred Length: 4 Years *Program Size:* 24 (*GY1:* 6)
Program ID: 400-18-21-069

Kansas

Kansas City

University of Kansas Medical Center Program
Sponsor: University of Kansas School of Medicine
University of Kansas Medical Center
Veterans Affairs Medical Center (Kansas City)
Program Director:
Jane S Lauchland, MD
Univ of Kansas Med Ctr
3901 Rainbow Blvd
1009 Olathe Pavilion
Kansas City, KS 66160-7341
Tel: 913 588-6412 *Fax:* 913 588-6414
Accred Length: 4 Years *Program Size:* 24 (*GY1:* 6)
Program ID: 400-19-21-070

Topeka

Menninger School of Psychiatry Program
Sponsor: Menninger Clinic
Colmery-O'Neil Veterans Affairs Medical Center
St Joseph's Hospital and Medical Center
Topeka State Hospital
Program Director:
Marceil D Bauman-Bork, MD
Karl Menninger Sch of Psychiatry
Menninger Clinic
Box 829
Topeka, KS 66601-0829
Tel: 785 350-5815 *Fax:* 785 350-5392
E-mail: reppat@menninger.edu
Internet: http://www.menninger.edu
Accred Length: 4 Years *Program Size:* 29 (*GY1:* 7)
Program ID: 400-19-22-071

Wichita

University of Kansas (Wichita) Program
Sponsor: University of Kansas School of Medicine (Wichita)
Charter Hospital of Wichita
Veterans Affairs Medical Center (Wichita)
Via Christi Regional Medical Center
Via Christi Regional Medical Center-St Joseph
Program Director:
John F Bober, MD
Univ of Kansas Sch of Med, Dept of Psychiatry
1010 N Kansas
Wichita, KS 67214-3199
Tel: 316 293-2645 *Fax:* 316 293-1874
E-mail: dappelma@kumc.edu
Internet:
http://www.kumc.edu/wichita/dept/psych/psych.html
Accred Length: 4 Years *Program Size:* 20 (*GY1:* 5)
Subspecialties: PYG
Program ID: 400-19-21-254

Kentucky

Lexington

University of Kentucky Medical Center Program
Sponsor: University of Kentucky Hospital
Veterans Affairs Medical Center (Lexington)
Program Director:
Debra A Katz, MD
Univ Hospital-Albert B Chandler Med Ctr
Dept of Psychiatry
Kentucky Clinic/Wing B
Lexington, KY 40536-0284
Tel: 606 323-6021, ext 272 *Fax:* 606 323-1194
Accred Length: 4 Years *Program Size:* 17 (*GY1:* 4)
Subspecialties: ADP
Program ID: 400-20-21-074

Louisville

University of Louisville Program
Sponsor: University of Louisville School of Medicine
Child Psychiatric Services (Bingham Child Guidance Clinic)
Norton Hospital (Alliant Health System)
University of Louisville Hospital
Veterans Affairs Medical Center (Louisville)
Program Director:
Gordon D Strauss, MD
Univ of Louisville Sch of Med
Dept of Psychiatry
Louisville, KY 40292-0001
Tel: 502 852-5395 *Fax:* 502 852-1115
E-mail: gdstra01@ulkyvm.louisville.edu
Internet: http://www.louisville.edu./medschool/psychiatry
Accred Length: 4 Years *Program Size:* 36 (*GY1:* 8)
Program ID: 400-20-21-075

Louisiana

New Orleans

Alton Ochsner Medical Foundation Program
Sponsor: Alton Ochsner Medical Foundation
Program Director:
Dean A Hickman, MD
Alton Ochsner Med Foundation
Dept of Grad Med Educ
1516 Jefferson Hwy
New Orleans, LA 70121
Tel: 504 842-3260 *Fax:* 504 842-3193
E-mail: dlambert@ochsner.org
Internet: http://www.ochsner.org
Accred Length: 4 Years *Program Size:* 12 (*GY1:* 4)
Program ID: 400-21-12-077

Louisiana State University Program
Sponsor: Louisiana State University School of Medicine
Medical Center of Louisiana at New Orleans
Touro Infirmary
Program Director:
Michael J Prejean, MD
Louisiana State Univ Med Ctr
Dept of Psychiatry
1542 Tulane Ave
New Orleans, LA 70112-2822
Tel: 504 568-6001 *Fax:* 504 568-8647
Internet: http://www.lsumc.edu
Accred Length: 4 Years *Program Size:* 32 (*GY1:* 8)
Subspecialties: PFP, PYG
Program ID: 400-21-21-076

Tulane University Program

Sponsor: Tulane University School of Medicine
Medical Center of Louisiana at New Orleans
Tulane University Hospital and Clinics
Veterans Affairs Medical Center-LSU Service (New Orleans)

Program Director:
Patrick T O'Neill, MD
Tulane Univ Sch of Med
Dept of Psychiatry TB53
1440 Canal St
New Orleans, LA 70112-2715
Tel: 504 894-7269 *Fax:* 504 894-7290
E-mail: poneill@mailhost.tcs.tulane.edu.
Internet: http://www.tulane.edu/
Accred Length: 4 Years *Program Size:* 24 (*GY1:* 5)
Program ID: 400-21-21-078

Shreveport

Louisiana State University (Shreveport) Program

Sponsor: Louisiana State University Hospital-Shreveport
Charter Forest Behavioral Health System
Overton Brooks Veterans Affairs Medical Center

Program Director:
Mary Jo Fitz-Gerald, MD
Louisiana State Univ Med Ctr Hospital
Med Educ/Psychiatry
1501 Kings Hwy/PO Box 33932
Shreveport, LA 71130-3932
Tel: 318 675-6041 *Fax:* 318 675-6148
Accred Length: 4 Years *Program Size:* 14 (*GY1:* 3)
Program ID: 400-21-21-274

Maine

Portland

Maine Medical Center Program

Sponsor: Maine Medical Center

Program Director:
George N McNeil, MD
Maine Med Ctr
22 Bramhall St
Portland, ME 04102
Tel: 207 871-2598 *Fax:* 207 871-6783
E-mail: romanm@mail.mmc.org
Internet: http://www.mmc.org/psych
Accred Length: 4 Years *Program Size:* 12 (*GY1:* 3)
Program ID: 400-22-11-080

Maryland

Baltimore

Johns Hopkins University Program

Sponsor: Johns Hopkins University School of Medicine
Johns Hopkins Bayview Medical Center
Johns Hopkins Hospital

Program Director:
Glenn J Treisman, MD PhD
Johns Hopkins Hospital
600 N Wolfe St
Meyer 4-119
Baltimore, MD 21287-7419
Tel: 410 955-6328 *Fax:* 410 955-0946
E-mail: glenn@welchlink.welch.jhu.edu
Internet:
http://www.med.jhu.edu/jhhpsychiatry/masterl.htm
Accred Length: 4 Years *Program Size:* 44 (*GY1:* 6)
Subspecialties: PYG
Program ID: 400-23-21-081

Sheppard and Enoch Pratt Hospital Program

Sponsor: Sheppard and Enoch Pratt Hospital
Franklin Square Hospital Center

Program Director:
Donald R Ross, MD
Sheppard Pratt Health System
Div of Educ/Residency Training
6501 N Charles St/PO Box 6815
Baltimore, MD 21285-6815
Tel: 410 938-4800 *Fax:* 410 938-4806
E-mail: sduckowitz@sheppardpratt.org
Accred Length: 4 Years *Program Size:* 6 (*GY1:* 0)
Program ID: 400-23-22-085

University of Maryland Program

Sponsor: University of Maryland Medical System
Spring Grove Hospital Center
Veterans Affairs Medical Center (Baltimore)
Walter P Carter Mental Health Center

Program Director:
Lisa Dixon, MD MPH
Univ of Maryland, Dept of Psychiatry
701 W Pratt St/4th Fl
Baltimore, MD 21201
Tel: 410 328-6325 *Fax:* 410 328-1212
Accred Length: 4 Years *Program Size:* 47 (*GY1:* 0)
Subspecialties: ADP
Program ID: 400-23-31-082

University of Maryland/Sheppard and Enoch Pratt Hospital Program

Sponsor: University of Maryland Medical System
Sheppard and Enoch Pratt Hospital
Spring Grove Hospital Center
Veterans Affairs Medical Center (Baltimore)
Walter P Carter Mental Health Center

Program Director:
Lisa Dixon, MD MPH
Sheppard and Enoch Pratt Hospital
Dept of Residency Training
701 W Pratt St/4th Fl
Baltimore, MD 21201
Tel: 410 328-6325 *Fax:* 410 328-1212
E-mail: spearson@umpsy.ab.umd.edu
Internet:
http://www.umm.edu.center/training/psych.contents.html
Accred Length: 4 Years *Program Size:* 54 (*GY1:* 14)
Subspecialties: PYG
Program ID: 400-23-21-289

Bethesda

National Capital Consortium Program

Sponsor: National Capital Consortium
Malcolm Grow Medical Center (SGE)
National Naval Medical Center (Bethesda)
Walter Reed Army Medical Center

Program Director:
Thomas A Grieger, MD
Uniformed Services Univ of Health Sciences
Dept of Psychiatry
4301 Jones-Bridge Rd
Bethesda, MD 20814-4799
Tel: 202 782-5990 *Fax:* 202 782-6480
E-mail: tagrieger@pol.net
Internet: http://www.usuhs.mil
Accred Length: 4 Years *Program Size:* 56 (*GY1:* 14)
Program ID: 400-10-21-287
US Armed Services Program

National Institutes of Health Clinical Center Program

Sponsor: NIH Warren Grant Magnuson Clinical Center

Program Director:
Donald L Rosenstein, MD PhD
NIH Clinical Ctr
Clinical Ctr/10-3N238
Bethesda, MD 20892
Tel: 301 496-9675 *Fax:* 301 402-2588
E-mail: rosend@codon.nih.gov
Accred Length: 1 Year *Program Size:* 4 (*GY1:* 0)
Program ID: 400-23-12-245

Massachusetts

Boston

Boston University Medical Center Program

Sponsor: Boston Medical Center
Edith Nourse Rogers Memorial Veterans Hospital
Solomon Carter Fuller Mental Health Center
Veterans Affairs Medical Center (Boston)

Program Director:
Janet E Osterman, MD MS BS
Boston Univ Med Ctr
Dept of Psychiatry
One Boston Medical Center Pl
Boston, MA 02118-2394
Tel: 617 638-8540 *Fax:* 617 638-8542
E-mail: maria@bu.edu
Internet: http://www.bumc.bu.edu
Accred Length: 4 Years *Program Size:* 32 (*GY1:* 8)
Program ID: 400-24-21-089

Harvard Medical School Program

Sponsor: Brigham and Women's Hospital
Beth Israel Deaconess Medical Center
Carney Hospital
Children's Hospital
Harvard Community Health Plan
Massachusetts Mental Health Center
MetroWest Medical Center-Framingham Union Hospital

Program Director:
William Greenberg, MD
Harvard Longwood Psychiatry Program
330 Brookline Ave
Boston, MA 02215
Tel: 617 667-4630 *Fax:* 617 667-5575
E-mail: wgreenbe@bidmc.harvard.edu
Accred Length: 4 Years *Program Size:* 60 (*GY1:* 15)
Program ID: 400-24-31-277

Massachusetts General Hospital/McLean Hospital Program

Sponsor: Massachusetts General Hospital
Erich Lindemann Mental Health Center
McLean Hospital

Program Director:
John B Herman, MD
Bulfinch 355/Dept of Psychiatry
Massachusetts General Hospital
55 Fruit St
Boston, MA 02114
Tel: 617 726-2972 *Fax:* 617 724-0308
E-mail: jherman@partners.org
Internet: http://www.psych.mgh.harvard.edu/
Accred Length: 4 Years *Program Size:* 64 (*GY1:* 16)
Program ID: 400-24-21-288

St Elizabeth's Medical Center of Boston Program

Sponsor: St Elizabeth's Medical Center of Boston

Program Director:
Gregory F Oxenkrug, MD PhD
Dept of Psychiatry
St Elizabeth's Med Ctr
736 Cambridge St
Boston, MA 02135
Tel: 617 789-3070 *Fax:* 617 789-2168
E-mail: rshostak@semc.org
Accred Length: 4 Years *Program Size:* 17 (*GY1:* 5)
Program ID: 400-24-21-092

Tufts University Program

Sponsor: New England Medical Center Hospitals
Lemuel Shattuck Hospital

Program Director:
Deborah Spitz, MD
New England Med Ctr
Dept of Psychiatry Box 1007
750 Washington St
Boston, MA 02111
Tel: 617 636-1632 *Fax:* 617 636-8442
E-mail: dspitz@opal.tufts.edu
Internet: http://www.nemc.org/psych/training.htlm
Accred Length: 4 Years *Program Size:* 19 (*GY1:* 4)
Program ID: 400-24-21-093

Brockton

Harvard Medical School (South Shore) Program

Sponsor: Brockton-West Roxbury Veterans Affairs Medical Center

Program Director:
Grace J Mushrush, MD
Dept of Psychiatry
VA Med Ctr-Brockton/West Roxbury
940 Belmont St/116A7
Brockton, MA 02401
Tel: 508 583-4500, ext 2458 *Fax:* 508 586-0894
Accred Length: 4 Years *Program Size:* 24 (*GY1:* 6)
Program ID: 400-24-21-279

Cambridge

Cambridge Hospital/Cambridge Health Alliance Program

Sponsor: Cambridge Hospital/Cambridge Health Alliance

Program Director:
Pamela Reeves, MD
Bliss I Rand, MD
Cambridge Hospital
Dept of Psychiatry
1493 Cambridge St
Cambridge, MA 02139
Tel: 617 498-1187 *Fax:* 617 498-1204
Internet: http://adpsychres.cambhosp@cha.org
Accred Length: 4 Years *Program Size:* 22 (*GY1:* 8)
Subspecialties: TY
Program ID: 400-24-11-094

Stockbridge

Austen Riggs Center Program

Sponsor: Austen Riggs Center

Program Director:
James L Sacksteder, MD
Austen Riggs Ctr
Dept of Psychiatry
25 Main St
Stockbridge, MA 01262-0962
Tel: 413 298-5511, ext 212 *Fax:* 413 298-4020
Internet: http://www.austenriggs.org
Accred Length: 1 Year *Program Size:* 1 (*GY1:* 1)
Program ID: 400-24-11-249

Worcester

University of Massachusetts Program

Sponsor: University of Massachusetts Medical School
UMass Memorial Health Care (University Campus)

Program Director:
Sheldon Benjamin, MD
Univ of Massachusetts Med Sch
Dept of Psychiatry
55 Lake Ave N
Worcester, MA 01655
Tel: 508 856-4087 *Fax:* 508 856-6426
E-mail: sheldon.benjamin@banyan.ummed.edu
Internet: http://www.ummed.edu/dept/psychiatry
Accred Length: 4 Years *Program Size:* 24 (*GY1:* 4)
Program ID: 400-24-21-234

Michigan

Ann Arbor

University of Michigan Program

Sponsor: University of Michigan Hospitals
Veterans Affairs Medical Center (Ann Arbor)

Program Director:
Michael Jibson, MD PhD
Univ of Michigan Hospitals
1500 E Medical Center Dr/0118
Ann Arbor, MI 48109-0118
Tel: 734 764-6875 *Fax:* 734 647-8514
Internet: http://www.med.umich.edu/psych/
Accred Length: 4 Years *Program Size:* 46 (*GY1:* 10)
Subspecialties: PYG
Program ID: 400-25-21-097

Detroit

Henry Ford Hospital Program

Sponsor: Henry Ford Hospital
Henry Ford Cottage Hospital
Kingswood Hospital

Program Director:
Cathy Frank, MD
Henry Ford Hospital
Dept of Psychiatry
One Ford Pl/1C
Detroit, MI 48202
Tel: 313 874-6611 *Fax:* 313 874-6655
Accred Length: 4 Years *Program Size:* 24 (*GY1:* 6)
Program ID: 400-25-21-235

Wayne State University/Detroit Medical Center Program

Sponsor: Wayne State University/Detroit Medical Center
Harper Hospital

Program Director:
Elliot Luby, MD
Univ Psychiatric Ctr-Central Campus
101 E Alexandrine
Detroit, MI 48201
Tel: 313 577-5267 *Fax:* 313 577-2233
Internet: http://psychiatry1.med.wayne.edu
Accred Length: 4 Years *Program Size:* 45 (*GY1:* 8)
Subspecialties: PYG
Program ID: 400-25-21-283

East Lansing

Michigan State University Program

Sponsor: Michigan State University College of Human Medicine
Ingham Regional Medical Center
Lansing General Hospital
Michigan State University Clinical Center
Pine Rest Christian Hospital
St Lawrence Hospital and HealthCare Services
St Mary's Health Services

Program Director:
Jed G Magen, DO
Michigan State Univ
Dept of Psychiatry
B-109 W Fee
East Lansing, MI 48824-1316
Tel: 517 353-4362 *Fax:* 517 432-3603
Internet: http://www.chm.msu.edu/psychiatry
Accred Length: 4 Years *Program Size:* 18 (*GY1:* 5)
Program ID: 400-25-21-101

Kalamazoo

Kalamazoo Center for Medical Studies/Michigan State University Program

Sponsor: Kalamazoo Center for Medical Studies
Borgess Medical Center

Program Director:
Steven J Young, MD
Michigan State Univ-Kalamazoo Ctr for Med Studies
Dept of Psychiatry
1000 Oakland Dr
Kalamazoo, MI 49008-1284
Tel: 800 275-5267, ext 6375
E-mail: programs@kcms.msu.edu
Internet: http://www.kcms.msu.edu
Accred Length: 4 Years *Program Size:* 16 (*GY1:* 4)
Program ID: 400-25-31-284

Minnesota

Minneapolis

Hennepin County Medical Center/Regions Hospital Program

Sponsor: Hennepin County Medical Center
Regions Hospital

Program Director:
Elizabeth Reeve, MD
Hennepin County Med Ctr
701 Park Ave S
Mail Code 865C
Minneapolis, MN 55415-1829
Tel: 612 347-2617 *Fax:* 612 904-4350
E-mail: steve.glick@co.hennepin.mn.us
Internet: http://www.hcmc.org
Accred Length: 4 Years *Program Size:* 16 (*GY1:* 4)
Program ID: 400-26-21-285

University of Minnesota Program
Sponsor: University of Minnesota Medical School
Fairview-University Medical Center
Hennepin County Medical Center
Regions Hospital
Veterans Affairs Medical Center (Minneapolis)
Program Director:
William L Clapp, MD
William H Meller, MD
Univ of Minnesota
Box 393 Mayo Bldg
420 Delaware St SE
Minneapolis, MN 55455
Tel: 612 626-5185 *Fax:* 612 626-5591
Internet: http://www.med.umn.edu
Accred Length: 4 Years *Program Size:* 32 (*GY1:* 8)
Subspecialties: ADP, PYG
Program ID: 400-26-21-106

Rochester

Mayo Graduate School of Medicine (Rochester) Program
Sponsor: Mayo Graduate School of Medicine-Mayo Foundation
Mayo Clinic (Rochester)
St Mary's Hospital of Rochester
Program Director:
Joyce A Tinsley, MD
Mayo Graduate Sch of Med
Application Processing Ctr
200 First St SW
Rochester, MN 55905
Tel: 507 284-3792 *Fax:* 507 284-0999
E-mail: mgsm.medlab.specialties@mayo.edu
Internet: http://www.mayo.edu/
Accred Length: 4 Years *Program Size:* 31 (*GY1:* 6)
Subspecialties: ADP
Program ID: 400-26-21-107

Mississippi

Jackson

University of Mississippi Medical Center Program
Sponsor: University of Mississippi School of Medicine
University Hospital
Veterans Affairs Medical Center (Jackson)
Program Director:
Robert W Baker, MD
Univ of Mississippi Med Ctr
Psychiatry Box 139
2500 N State St
Jackson, MS 39216-4505
Tel: 601 984-6925, ext 5826 *Fax:* 601 984-5885
Accred Length: 4 Years *Program Size:* 22 (*GY1:* 5)
Program ID: 400-27-11-108

Missouri

Columbia

University of Missouri-Columbia Program
Sponsor: University of Missouri-Columbia School of Medicine
Harry S Truman Memorial Veterans Hospital
Mid-Missouri Mental Health Center
University Hospitals and Clinics
Program Director:
Cheryl A Hemme, MD
Univ of Missouri-Columbia
1 Hospital Dr/DCO67.00
Columbia, MO 65212
Tel: 573 882-8907 *Fax:* 573 884-5396
E-mail: hemmec@brain.missouri.edu
Internet: http://www.hsc.missouri.edu/~dmhs/psychneur/
Accred Length: 4 Years *Program Size:* 24 (*GY1:* 6)
Program ID: 400-28-21-109

Kansas City

University of Missouri at Kansas City Program
Sponsor: University of Missouri-Kansas City School of Medicine
Western Missouri Mental Health Center
Program Director:
Stephen P Jarvis, MD
Univ of Missouri Sch of Med, Dept of Psychiatry
600 E 22nd St
Kansas City, MO 64108-2620
Tel: 816 512-4177 *Fax:* 816 512-4183
E-mail: spjarvis@cctr.umkc.edu
Internet:
http://www.cctr.umkc.edu/user/sajaffri/psy/hpage.htm
Accred Length: 4 Years *Program Size:* 27 (*GY1:* 6)
Program ID: 400-28-21-110

St Louis

St Louis University School of Medicine Program
Sponsor: St Louis University School of Medicine
St Louis University School of Medicine
Veterans Affairs Medical Center (St Louis)
Program Director:
Michal Artal, MD
St Louis Univ Group of Hospitals
David P Wohl Sr Memorial Inst, Dept of Psychiatry
1221 S Grand Blvd
St Louis, MO 63104-1094
Tel: 314 577-8728 *Fax:* 314 664-7248
Internet:
http://slu.edu/colleges/med/departments/psychiatry.html
Accred Length: 4 Years *Program Size:* 16 (*GY1:* 4)
Subspecialties: PYG
Program ID: 400-28-21-113

Washington University/B-JH/SLCH Consortium Program
Sponsor: Washington University/B-JH/SLCH Consortium
Barnes-Jewish Hospital
Barnes-Jewish Hospital (North Campus)
Malcolm Bliss Mental Health Center
Program Director:
Eugene H Rubin, MD PhD
Box 8134
Washington Univ
4940 Children's Pl
St Louis, MO 63110
Tel: 314 362-2462 *Fax:* 314 362-0193
E-mail: residency@psychiatry.wustl.edu
Internet:
http://www.internalmed.wustl.edu/divisions/psychiatry/psych.htm
Accred Length: 4 Years *Program Size:* 40 (*GY1:* 10)
Program ID: 400-28-21-114

Nebraska

Omaha

Creighton University/University of Nebraska Program
Sponsor: Creighton University School of Medicine
St Joseph Center for Mental Health
University of Nebraska Medical Center
Veterans Affairs Medical Center (Omaha)
Program Director:
Carl B Greiner, MD
Creighton-Nebraska Dept of Psychiatry
985582 Nebraska Med Ctr
Omaha, NE 68198-5582
Tel: 402 559-5018 *Fax:* 402 559-6791
E-mail: vthomsen@mail.unmc.edu
Internet: http://www.unmc.edu/gme/gmehome.htm
Accred Length: 4 Years *Program Size:* 24 (*GY1:* 6)
Subspecialties: PYG
Program ID: 400-30-21-116

Nevada

Reno

University of Nevada Program
Sponsor: University of Nevada School of Medicine
BHC Health Services of Nevada
Ioannis A Lougaris Veterans Affairs Medical Center
Nevada Mental Health Institute
Washoe Medical Center
Program Director:
Grant D Miller, MD
Univ of Nevada Sch of Med
Dept of Psych/Behav Science 354
Reno, NV 89557-0046
Tel: 702 784-4919 *Fax:* 702 784-1428
E-mail: gdmiller@unr.edu
Internet: http://www.unr.edu/med
Accred Length: 4 Years *Program Size:* 16 (*GY1:* 4)
Program ID: 400-31-21-263

New Hampshire

Lebanon

Dartmouth-Hitchcock Medical Center Program

Sponsor: Mary Hitchcock Memorial Hospital
New Hampshire Hospital
Veterans Affairs Medical Center (White River Junction)

Program Director:
Ronald L Green, MD
Dartmouth-Hitchcock Med Ctr
One Medical Center Dr
Lebanon, NH 03756
Tel: 603 650-5820 *Fax:* 603 650-5842
E-mail: ronaldlgreen@dartmouth.edu
Internet: http://www.dartmouth.edu/dms/psychtry/stage
Accred Length: 4 Years *Program Size:* 17 (*GY1:* 4)
Subspecialties: PYG
Program ID: 400-32-21-117

New Jersey

Camden

UMDNJ-Robert Wood Johnson Medical School (Camden) Program

Sponsor: Cooper Hospital-University Medical Center
Atlantic City Medical Center

Program Director:
Thomas Newmark, MD
UMDNJ-Robert Wood Johnson Med Sch
Dept of Psychiatry
401 Haddon Ave/3rd Fl
Camden, NJ 08103
Tel: 609 757-7799 *Fax:* 609 757-9651
Accred Length: 4 Years *Program Size:* 12 (*GY1:* 3)
Program ID: 400-33-21-255

Newark

UMDNJ-New Jersey Medical School Program

Sponsor: UMDNJ-New Jersey Medical School
Hackensack University Medical Center
UMDNJ-University Hospital
Veterans Affairs Medical Center (East Orange)

Program Director:
Beverly R Delaney, MD
UMDNJ-New Jersey Med Sch
Univ Hts/1501 Admin Complex
30 Bergen St
Newark, NJ 07107-3000
Tel: 973 972-4670
E-mail: delanebr@umdnj.edu
Internet: http://www.umdnj.edu/njmsweb/psychiatry/
Accred Length: 4 Years *Program Size:* 29 (*GY1:* 6)
Program ID: 400-33-21-119

Paramus

Bergen Regional Medical Center Program

Sponsor: Bergen Regional Medical Center

Program Director:
William Greenberg, MD
Bergen Regional Med Ctr
Psychiatric Education
230 E Ridgewood Ave/Bldg 14
Paramus, NJ 07652
Tel: 201 967-4009
Accred Length: 4 Years *Program Size:* 24 (*GY1:* 7)
Program ID: 400-33-12-120

Piscataway

UMDNJ-Robert Wood Johnson Medical School Program

Sponsor: UMDNJ-Robert Wood Johnson Medical School
Robert Wood Johnson University Hospital

Program Director:
Barbara Palmeri, MD
UMDNJ-Robert Wood Johnson Med Sch
Dept of Psychiatry
671 Hoes Ln/UBHC C-205
Piscataway, NJ 08854-5633
Tel: 732 235-4433 *Fax:* 732 235-4649
E-mail: palmerib@umdnj.edu
Accred Length: 4 Years *Program Size:* 24 (*GY1:* 6)
Subspecialties: PYG
Program ID: 400-33-21-121

New Mexico

Albuquerque

University of New Mexico Program

Sponsor: University of New Mexico School of Medicine
University Hospital
Veterans Affairs Medical Center (Albuquerque)

Program Director:
Nancy K Morrison, MD
Univ of New Mexico Sch of Med, Dept of Psych
Family Practice Bldg/4th Fl
2400 Tucker Ave NE
Albuquerque, NM 87131-5326
Tel: 505 272-5417 *Fax:* 505 272-4639
E-mail: nmorriso@salud.unm.edu
Internet: http://hsc.unm.edu/som/psychiatry/index.htm
Accred Length: 4 Years *Program Size:* 38 (*GY1:* 8)
Program ID: 400-34-21-123

New York

Albany

Albany Medical Center Program

Sponsor: Albany Medical Center
Capital District Psychiatric Center
Veterans Affairs Medical Center (Albany)

Program Director:
Victoria Balkoski, MD
Albany Med Ctr
47 New Scotland Ave/A-164
Albany, NY 12208
Tel: 518 262-5511 *Fax:* 518 262-6111
E-mail: vbalkoski@ccgateway.amc.edu
Accred Length: 4 Years *Program Size:* 22 (*GY1:* 5)
Program ID: 400-35-22-124

Bronx

Albert Einstein College of Medicine at Bronx-Lebanon Hospital Center Program

Sponsor: Bronx-Lebanon Hospital Center

Program Director:
Nalini V Juthani, MD
Bronx-Lebanon Hospital Ctr
1276 Fulton Ave/4S
Bronx, NY 10456
Tel: 718 901-8652 *Fax:* 718 901-8656
E-mail: juthani@aecom.yu.edu
Accred Length: 4 Years *Program Size:* 19 (*GY1:* 6)
Subspecialties: CHP
Program ID: 400-35-21-135

Albert Einstein College of Medicine Program

Sponsor: Albert Einstein College of Medicine of Yeshiva University
Bronx Psychiatric Center
Jacobi Medical Center
Montefiore Medical Center-Henry and Lucy Moses Division

Program Director:
Peter J Buckley, MD
Marny R Cherkasky, MD
Montefiore Med Ctr
Dept of Psychiatry
3317 Rochambeau Ave
Bronx, NY 10467
Tel: 718 920-7967 *Fax:* 718 798-3810
E-mail: nruiz@montefiore.org
Accred Length: 4 Years *Program Size:* 40 (*GY1:* 6)
Subspecialties: PYG
Program ID: 400-35-11-131

Lincoln Medical and Mental Health Center Program

Sponsor: Lincoln Medical and Mental Health Center

Program Director:
Vyas Persaud, MD
Lincoln Med and Mental Health Ctr
234 E 149th St
Bronx, NY 10451
Tel: 718 579-5124 *Fax:* 718 579-4860
Accred Length: 4 Years *Program Size:* 14 (*GY1:* 3)
Program ID: 400-35-11-133

Brooklyn

Brookdale University Hospital Medical Center Program

Sponsor: Brookdale University Hospital Medical Center

Program Director:
Nyapati Rao, MD
Brookdale Univ Hospital and Med Ctr
Dept of Psychiatry
One Brookdale Plaza
Brooklyn, NY 11212-3198
Tel: 718 240-5667 *Fax:* 718 240-5451
E-mail: nrraomd@pol.net
Internet: http://www.brookdalehospital.com
Accred Length: 4 Years *Program Size:* 20 (*GY1:* 6)
Program ID: 400-35-11-136

Maimonides Medical Center Program

Sponsor: Maimonides Medical Center

Program Director:
Jeffrey Goldberg, DO
Maimonides Med Ctr
Dept of Psychiatry
4802 Tenth Ave
Brooklyn, NY 11219
Tel: 718 283-8184, ext 8184 *Fax:* 718 283-6540
Internet: http://www.maimonidesmed.org
Accred Length: 4 Years *Program Size:* 26 (*GY1:* 5)
Program ID: 400-35-21-143

SUNY Health Science Center at Brooklyn Program

Sponsor: SUNY Health Science Center at Brooklyn
Kings County Hospital Center
University Hospital-SUNY Health Science Center at Brooklyn

Program Director:
Eric Weitzner, MD
SUNY Health Science Ctr-Brooklyn
450 Clarkson Ave/Box 1203
Brooklyn, NY 11203
Tel: 718 270-2902 *Fax:* 718 245-2321
Accred Length: 4 Years *Program Size:* 31 (*GY1:* 8)
Subspecialties: PYG
Program ID: 400-35-21-154

Buffalo

SUNY at Buffalo Graduate Medical-Dental Education Consortium Program

Sponsor: SUNY at Buffalo Grad Medical-Dental Education Consortium
Erie County Medical Center
Veterans Affairs Medical Center (Buffalo)

Program Director:
Michele T Pato, MD
462 Grider St
Buffalo, NY 14215
Tel: 716 898-4221 *Fax:* 716 898-5332
E-mail: sunypsyres@aol.com
Accred Length: 4 Years *Program Size:* 23 (*GYI:* 7)
Program ID: 400-35-21-126

East Meadow

Nassau County Medical Center Program

Sponsor: Nassau County Medical Center

Program Director:
Jacob Ninan, MD
Nassau County Med Ctr
2201 Hempstead Trnpk
East Meadow, NY 11554-5400
Tel: 516 572-6511 *Fax:* 516 572-3210
Accred Length: 4 Years *Program Size:* 24 (*GYI:* 6)
Program ID: 400-35-11-128

Elmhurst

Mount Sinai School of Medicine (Elmhurst) Program

Sponsor: Mount Sinai School of Medicine
Elmhurst Hospital Center-Mount Sinai Services

Program Director:
Amy S Hoffman, MD
Mount Sinai Sch of Med
Elmhurst Hospital Ctr
79-01 Broadway/Rm A6-2
Elmhurst, NY 11373
Tel: 718 334-3542 *Fax:* 718 334-3557
Accred Length: 4 Years *Program Size:* 25 (*GYI:* 6)
Program ID: 400-35-11-242

Manhasset

North Shore University Hospital/NYU School of Medicine Program

Sponsor: North Shore University Hospital

Program Director:
Victor M Fornari, MD
North Shore Univ Hospital
Dept of Psychiatry
400 Community Dr
Manhasset, NY 11030
Tel: 516 562-3051 *Fax:* 516 562-3997
E-mail: vfornari@nshs.edu
Internet: http://www.nshs.edu
Accred Length: 4 Years *Program Size:* 20 (*GYI:* 4)
Subspecialties: ADP
Program ID: 400-35-11-129

New Hyde Park

Albert Einstein College of Medicine at Long Island Jewish Medical Center Program

Sponsor: Long Island Jewish Medical Center
Hillside Hospital (Long Island Jewish Medical Center)

Program Director:
Bruce R Levy, MD
Hillside Hospital
New Hyde Park, NY 11042
Tel: 718 470-8005 *Fax:* 718 343-7739
E-mail: levy@lij.edu
Internet: http://www.lij.edu
Accred Length: 4 Years *Program Size:* 38 (*GYI:* 9)
Subspecialties: PYG
Program ID: 400-35-21-142

New York

Albert Einstein College of Medicine at Beth Israel Medical Center Program

Sponsor: Beth Israel Medical Center

Program Director:
Harold Been, MD
Beth Israel Med Ctr
Dept of Psychiatry
First Ave at 16th St
New York, NY 10003
Tel: 212 420-2376 *Fax:* 212 420-3442
E-mail: hbeen@bethisrealny.org
Accred Length: 4 Years *Program Size:* 33 (*GYI:* 7)
Subspecialties: ADP, PYG
Program ID: 400-35-11-134

Harlem Hospital Center Program

Sponsor: Harlem Hospital Center

Program Director:
Henry L McCurtis, MD
Womens Pavilion 542
506 Lenox Ave
New York, NY 10037
Tel: 212 939-3060 *Fax:* 212 939-3064
Accred Length: 4 Years *Program Size:* 20 (*GYI:* 5)
Program ID: 400-35-11-140

Mount Sinai School of Medicine (Cabrini) Program

Sponsor: Mount Sinai School of Medicine
Cabrini Medical Center

Program Director:
Giovanni Caracci, MD
Cabrini Med Ctr
227 E 19th St
New York, NY 10003-2600
Tel: 212 995-6000, ext 6762 *Fax:* 212 995-7031
E-mail: gcaracci@cabrininy.org
Accred Length: 4 Years *Program Size:* 16 (*GYI:* 4)
Program ID: 400-35-31-137

Mount Sinai School of Medicine (North General) Program

Sponsor: North General Hospital

Program Director:
Gregory A Miller, MD
1879 Madison Ave
New York, NY 10035
Tel: 212 423-4474 *Fax:* 212 423-4095
E-mail: a201@hotmail.com
Accred Length: 4 Years *Program Size:* 16 (*GYI:* 4)
Program ID: 400-35-31-278

Mount Sinai School of Medicine Program

Sponsor: Mount Sinai School of Medicine
Mount Sinai Medical Center
Veterans Affairs Medical Center (Bronx)

Program Director:
Michael J Serby, MD
Mount Sinai Hospital
One Gustave L Levy Pl
Box 1230
New York, NY 10029-6574
Tel: 212 824-7026 *Fax:* 212 849-2509
E-mail: mserby@smtplink.mssm.edu
Internet: http://intranet1.online.mssm.edu/
Accred Length: 4 Years *Program Size:* 47 (*GYI:* 6)
Subspecialties: PYG
Program ID: 400-35-11-146

New York and Presbyterian Hospital (Columbia Campus) Program

Sponsor: New York and Presbyterian Hospital
New York and Presbyterian Hospital (Columbia Campus)
New York State Psychiatric Institute

Program Director:
Ronald O Rieder, MD
New York State Psychiatric Inst
1051 Riverside Dr.
New York, NY 10032
Tel: 212 543-5553 *Fax:* 212 543-5356
E-mail: rorl@columbia.edu
Internet:
http://nypisys.cpmc.columbia.edu/development/web/res/train.htm
Accred Length: 4 Years *Program Size:* 46 (*GYI:* 11)
Subspecialties: ADP, PYG
Program ID: 400-35-21-138

New York and Presbyterian Hospital (Cornell Campus) Program

Sponsor: New York and Presbyterian Hospital
New York and Presbyterian Hospital (Cornell Campus)
New York and Presbyterian Hospital-Payne Whitney Clinic

Program Director:
Elizabeth L Auchincloss, MD
New York Presbyterian Hospital-Cornell Campus
525 E 68th St
Box 140
New York, NY 10021
Tel: 212 746-3720 *Fax:* 212 746-8886
E-mail: psych-res@mail.med.cornell.edu
Accred Length: 4 Years *Program Size:* 38 (*GYI:* 10)
Program ID: 400-35-11-147

New York Medical College (Metropolitan) Program

Sponsor: New York Medical College
Metropolitan Hospital Center

Program Director:
Richard A Winters, MD
Metropolitan Hospital Ctr
1901 First Ave
Rm 4M-14-A
New York, NY 10029
Tel: 212 423-7061 *Fax:* 212 423-7434
Accred Length: 4 Years *Program Size:* 24 (*GYI:* 6)
Program ID: 400-35-11-148

New York Medical College at St Vincent's Hospital and Medical Center of New York Program

Sponsor: New York Medical College
St Vincent's Hospital and Medical Center of New York

Program Director:
Brian J Ladds, MD
St Vincent's Hospital and Med Ctr
Training Office-Reiss 175
144 W 12th St
New York, NY 10011
Tel: 212 604-8795 *Fax:* 212 604-8197
Accred Length: 4 Years *Program Size:* 46 (*GY1:* 9)
Subspecialties: PYG
Program ID: 400-35-12-152

New York University Medical Center Program

Sponsor: New York University Medical Center
Bellevue Hospital Center
Manhattan Psychiatric Center
Veterans Affairs Medical Center (Manhattan)

Program Director:
Carol A Bernstein, MD
New York Univ Med Ctr
550 First Ave
NB 20N11
New York, NY 10016
Tel: 212 263-6238 *Fax:* 212 263-6497
E-mail: carol.bernstein@nyu.edu
Accred Length: 4 Years *Program Size:* 65 (*GY1:* 16)
Subspecialties: ADP, PYG
Program ID: 400-35-21-149

St Luke's-Roosevelt Hospital Center Program

Sponsor: St Luke's-Roosevelt Hospital Center
St Luke's-Roosevelt Hospital Center-Roosevelt Division
St Luke's-Roosevelt Hospital Center-St Luke's Division

Program Director:
Steven Wager, MD
St Luke's-Roosevelt Hospital Ctr
Dept of Psychiatry
1111 Amsterdam Ave
New York, NY 10025
Tel: 212 523-5089 *Fax:* 212 523-1685
Internet: http://www.docnet.org/dept/psych
Accred Length: 4 Years *Program Size:* 24 (*GY1:* 6)
Program ID: 400-35-21-270

Queens Village

Creedmoor Psychiatric Center Program

Sponsor: Creedmoor Psychiatric Center
Catholic Medical Center (St John's Queens Hospital)
Wyckoff Heights Medical Center

Program Director:
Mark F Sorensen, MD
Creedmoor Psychiatric Ctr
80-45 Winchester Blvd/Bldg 40 2-a
Queens Village, NY 11427-2199
Tel: 718 264-5030 *Fax:* 718 264-5027
E-mail: crmdmfs%alb4381@omh.mailnet.state.ny.us
Accred Length: 4 Years *Program Size:* 16 (*GY1:* 4)
Program ID: 400-35-12-139

Rochester

University of Rochester Program

Sponsor: Strong Memorial Hospital of the University of Rochester

Program Director:
Rory P Houghtalen, MD
Univ of Rochester Med Ctr
300 Crittenden Blvd
Rochester, NY 14642-8409
Tel: 716 275-4985 *Fax:* 716 273-1066
E-mail: trudy_haseley@urmc.rochester.edu
Internet: http://www.urmc.rochester.edu/smd/psych
Accred Length: 4 Years *Program Size:* 18 (*GY1:* 4)
Subspecialties: PYG
Program ID: 400-35-11-158

Staten Island

New York Medical College (Richmond) Program

Sponsor: New York Medical College
Sisters of Charity Medical Center-St Vincent's Campus
Bayley Seton Hospital

Program Director:
Richard L Pearlman, MD
Sisters of Charity Med Ctr
Dept of Psychiatry
355 Bard Ave
Staten Island, NY 10310
Tel: 718 876-4131 *Fax:* 718 720-6027
E-mail: blackman@admin.con2.com
Internet: http://www.schcs.com
Accred Length: 4 Years *Program Size:* 19 (*GY1:* 4)
Program ID: 400-35-12-153

Stony Brook

SUNY at Stony Brook Program

Sponsor: University Hospital-SUNY at Stony Brook
Veterans Affairs Medical Center (Northport)

Program Director:
Michael Schwartz, MD
SUNY-Stony Brook
Dept of Psychiatry
Health Science Ctr/T-10 020
Stony Brook, NY 11794-8101
Tel: 516 444-3005 *Fax:* 516 444-7534
Accred Length: 4 Years *Program Size:* 25 (*GY1:* 6)
Program ID: 400-35-21-159

Syracuse

SUNY Health Science Center at Syracuse Program

Sponsor: University Hospital-SUNY Health Science Center at Syracuse
Richard H Hutchings Psychiatric Center
Veterans Affairs Medical Center (Syracuse)

Program Director:
Mantosh Dewan, MD
SUNY Health Science Ctr-Syracuse
750 E Adams St
Syracuse, NY 13210
Tel: 315 464-3106 *Fax:* 315 464-3163
E-mail: dewanm@vax.cs.hscsyr.edu.
Internet: http://www.hscsyr.edu
Accred Length: 4 Years *Program Size:* 26 (*GY1:* 6)
Program ID: 400-35-21-160

Valhalla

New York Medical College at Westchester Medical Center Program

Sponsor: New York Medical College
Danbury Hospital
St Vincent's Hospital of New York-Westchester Branch
Stamford Hospital
Westchester Medical Center

Program Director:
Robert E Feinstein, MD
Westchester Med Ctr
Behavioral Health Ctr
3rd Fl/Rm N307
Valhalla, NY 10595
Tel: 914 285-1903 *Fax:* 914 285-1015
Accred Length: 4 Years *Program Size:* 27 (*GY1:* 8)
Program ID: 400-35-21-162

White Plains

New York and Presbyterian Hospital (Cornell Campus)/Westchester Program

Sponsor: New York and Presbyterian Hospital
New York and Presbyterian Hospital-Westchester Division

Program Director:
Kenneth G Terkelsen, MD
New York Presbyterian Hospital-Westchester Div
21 Bloomingdale Rd
White Plains, NY 10605
Tel: 914 997-5710 *Fax:* 914 682-6963
E-mail: kterkels%westnyh@nyh.med.cornell.edu
Accred Length: 4 Years *Program Size:* 13 (*GY1:* 0)
Subspecialties: CHP, PYG
Program ID: 400-35-21-164

North Carolina

Chapel Hill

University of North Carolina Hospitals Program

Sponsor: University of North Carolina Hospitals
Dorothea Dix Hospital

Program Director:
Allan A Maltbie, MD
Univ of North Carolina Sch of Med
CB7160 Dept of Psychiatry
Rm 10602/Neurosciences Hospital
Chapel Hill, NC 27599-7160
Tel: 919 966-2127 *Fax:* 919 966-2220
E-mail: amaltbie@css.unc.edu
Internet: http://www.psychiatry.unc.edu
Accred Length: 4 Years *Program Size:* 56 (*GY1:* 14)
Program ID: 400-36-21-166

Durham

Duke University Program

Sponsor: Duke University Medical Center
Veterans Affairs Medical Center (Durham)

Program Director:
Grace Thrall, MD
Duke Univ Med Ctr
Dept of Psychiatry
PO Box 3837
Durham, NC 27710
Tel: 919 684-2258 *Fax:* 919 684-2290
E-mail: psychres@mc.duke.edu
Internet: http://niles.mc.duke.edu
Accred Length: 4 Years *Program Size:* 43 (*GY1:* 8)
Program ID: 400-36-21-167

Greenville

East Carolina University Program

Sponsor: East Carolina University School of Medicine
Pitt County Memorial Hospital
Pitt County Mental Health Center

Program Director:
Vivian J Weathers, MD
East Carolina Univ Sch of Med
Dept of Psychiatric Med
Six Doctors Pk
Greenville, NC 27858-4354
Tel: 919 816-2663 *Fax:* 919 816-2419
E-mail: vweathers@brody.med.ecu.edu
Accred Length: 4 Years *Program Size:* 24 (*GY1:* 6)
Program ID: 400-36-21-169

Winston-Salem

Wake Forest University School of Medicine Program

Sponsor: Wake Forest University Baptist Medical Center

Program Director:
Stephen I Kramer, MD
Dept of Psychiatry
Wake Forest Univ Sch of Med
Baptist Med Ctr
Winston-Salem, NC 27157-1087
Tel: 336 716-3920 *Fax:* 336 716-6830
E-mail: skramer@wfubmc.edu
Internet: http://www.wfubmc.edu/psychiatry
Accred Length: 4 Years *Program Size:* 23 (*GY1:* 5)
Program ID: 400-36-21-171

North Dakota

Fargo

University of North Dakota Program

Sponsor: Univ of North Dakota School of Medicine & Health Sciences
Veterans Affairs Medical and Regional Office Center (Fargo)
Lakeland Mental Health Center
MeritCare Hospital
Southeast Human Service Center

Program Director:
David W Abbott, MD
Univ of North Dakota Sch of Med and Health Sciences
Dept of Neuroscience
1919 N Elm St
Fargo, ND 58102
Tel: 701 293-4113 *Fax:* 701 293-4109
E-mail: psychres@medicine.nodak.edu
Internet:
http://www.med.und.nodak.edu/depts/neuro/home.htm
Accred Length: 4 Years *Program Size:* 12 (*GY1:* 3)
Subspecialties: TY
Program ID: 400-37-21-251

Ohio

Cincinnati

University Hospital/University of Cincinnati College of Medicine Program

Sponsor: University Hospital Inc
Veterans Affairs Medical Center (Cincinnati)

Program Director:
Warren M Liang, MD
Univ Hospital-Univ of Cincinnati Med Ctr
Dept of Psychiatry
PO Box 670559
Cincinnati, OH 45267-0559
Tel: 513 558-5190 *Fax:* 513 558-3477
E-mail: warren.liang@uc.edu
Internet: http://www.uc.edu/~liang
Accred Length: 4 Years *Program Size:* 19 (*GY1:* 5)
Subspecialties: ADP, PYG
Program ID: 400-38-21-173

Cleveland

Case Western Reserve University (MetroHealth) Program

Sponsor: MetroHealth Medical Center
Cleveland Psychiatric Institute
Cleveland Psychoanalytic Institute

Program Director:
Jonathan E Dunn, MD PhD
MetroHealth Med Ctr
2500 MetroHealth Dr
Cleveland, OH 44109-1998
Tel: 216 778-4823 *Fax:* 216 778-8412
Accred Length: 4 Years *Program Size:* 17 (*GY1:* 5)
Program ID: 400-38-21-240

Case Western Reserve University Program

Sponsor: University Hospitals of Cleveland
Veterans Affairs Medical Center (Cleveland)

Program Director:
Robert J Ronis, MD MPH
Univ Hospitals of Cleveland
11100 Euclid Ave
Cleveland, OH 44106-5080
Tel: 216 844-3450 *Fax:* 216 844-1703
E-mail: cac29@po.cwru.edu
Accred Length: 4 Years *Program Size:* 29 (*GY1:* 5)
Subspecialties: PYG
Program ID: 400-38-21-174

Cleveland Clinic Foundation Program

Sponsor: Cleveland Clinic Foundation

Program Director:
Kathleen N Franco, MD
Cleveland Clinic Foundation
Dept of Psychiatry/P68
9500 Euclid Ave
Cleveland, OH 44195-5242
Tel: 216 445-2997 *Fax:* 216 445-7032
E-mail: meded@cesmtp.ccf.org
Internet: http://www.ccf.org
Accred Length: 4 Years *Program Size:* 24 (*GY1:* 6)
Program ID: 400-38-22-175

Columbus

Ohio State University Program

Sponsor: Ohio State University Medical Center
Harding Hospital
Mount Carmel Medical Center

Program Director:
Radu Saveanu, MD
Dept of Psychiatry
473 West 12th Ave
Columbus, OH 43210-1228
Tel: 614 293-8282 *Fax:* 614 293-4200
Accred Length: 4 Years *Program Size:* 19 (*GY1:* 4)
Program ID: 400-38-21-281

Dayton

Wright State University Program

Sponsor: Wright State University School of Medicine
Good Samaritan Hospital and Health Center
Kettering Medical Center
Veterans Affairs Medical Center (Dayton)
Wright-Patterson Medical Center

Program Director:
David G Bienenfeld, MD
Wright State Univ Sch of Med
Dept of Psychiatry
PO Box 927
Dayton, OH 45401-0927
Tel: 937 276-8329 *Fax:* 937 275-2817
E-mail: dbienenf@alpha.wright.edu
Internet:
http://www.med.wright.edu/som/resident/psych/psychres.htm
Accred Length: 4 Years *Program Size:* 40 (*GY1:* 10)
Program ID: 400-38-21-178

Rootstown

Northeastern Ohio Universities College of Medicine Program

Sponsor: Northeastern Ohio Universities College of Medicine
Akron General Medical Center
Children's Hospital Medical Center of Akron
St Thomas Hospital (Summa Health System)

Program Director:
Joseph D Varley, MD
400 Wabash Ave
Akron, OH 44307-2463
Tel: 330 384-6440 *Fax:* 330 996-2943
E-mail: sland@neoucom.edu
Internet: http://agmc.org
Accred Length: 4 Years *Program Size:* 17 (*GY1:* 4)
Program ID: 400-38-21-180

Toledo

Medical College of Ohio Program

Sponsor: Medical College of Ohio
Northwest Psychiatric Hospital
St Vincent Mercy Medical Center

Program Director:
Ronald A McGinnis, MD
Med Coll of Ohio, Dept of Psychiatry
Ruppert Health Ctr
3120 Glendale Ave
Toledo, OH 43614-5809
Tel: 419 383-5695 *Fax:* 419 383-3031
E-mail: jplummer@gemini.mco.edu
Internet: http://www.mco.edu/depts/psych
Accred Length: 4 Years *Program Size:* 15 (*GY1:* 3)
Program ID: 400-38-21-181

Programs

Oklahoma

Norman

Griffin Memorial Hospital Program
Sponsor: Griffin Memorial Hospital
Children's Hospital of Oklahoma

Program Director:
Ernest G Shadid, MD
Griffin Memorial Hospital
900 E Main
PO Box 151
Norman, OK 73070
Tel: 405 573-6602 *Fax:* 405 573-6684
Accred Length: 4 Years *Program Size:* 20 (*GY1:* 5)
Program ID: 400-39-21-183

Oklahoma City

University of Oklahoma Health Sciences Center Program
Sponsor: University of Oklahoma College of Medicine
Children's Hospital of Oklahoma
University Hospital
Veterans Affairs Medical Center (Oklahoma City)

Program Director:
Jay Lensgraf, MD
Dept of Psychiatry/Behav Sci
Univ of Oklahoma Health Sciences Ctr
PO Box 26901 (WP3440)
Oklahoma City, OK 73190-3048
Tel: 405 271-5251, ext 47683 *Fax:* 405 271-8802
Accred Length: 4 Years *Program Size:* 16 (*GY1:* 4)
Program ID: 400-39-21-184

Tulsa

University of Oklahoma College of Medicine-Tulsa Program
Sponsor: University of Oklahoma College of Medicine-Tulsa
Children's Medical Center
Laureate Psychiatric Clinic and Hospital
Parkside Inc

Program Director:
William R Yates, MD
Univ of Oklahoma Coll of Med-Tulsa
Psychiatry
2808 S Sheridan Rd
Tulsa, OK 74129-1077
Tel: 918 838-4645 *Fax:* 918 838-4653
E-mail: william-yates@ouhsc.edu
Internet: http://www.tulsa.uokhsc.edu
Accred Length: 4 Years *Program Size:* 16 (*GY1:* 4)
Program ID: 400-39-21-246

Oregon

Portland

Oregon Health Sciences University Program
Sponsor: Oregon Health Sciences University Hospital
Veterans Affairs Medical Center (Portland)

Program Director:
George A Keepers, MD
Residency Training Program
3181 SW Sam Jackson Park Rd/UHN 80
Portland, OR 97201-3098
Tel: 503 494-6149 *Fax:* 503 494-6152
E-mail: psychres@ohsu.edu
Accred Length: 4 Years *Program Size:* 34 (*GY1:* 8)
Subspecialties: PYG
Program ID: 400-40-21-185

Pennsylvania

Hershey

Penn State Geisinger Health System/Milton S Hershey Medical Center Program
Sponsor: Penn State Geisinger Health System
Milton S Hershey Medical Center

Program Director:
Enos D Martin, MD
Pennsylvania State Univ, Psychiatry Dept
Milton S Hershey Med Ctr
500 University Dr/PO Box 850
Hershey, PA 17033
Tel: 717 531-8338 *Fax:* 717 531-6491
E-mail: exm6@psw.edu
Accred Length: 4 Years *Program Size:* 20 (*GY1:* 5)
Subspecialties: PYG
Program ID: 400-41-11-187

Philadelphia

Albert Einstein Medical Center Program
Sponsor: Albert Einstein Medical Center
Belmont Center for Comprehensive Treatment

Program Director:
Frederick C Miller, MD
Albert Einstein Med Ctr
5501 Old York Rd
Philadelphia, PA 19141-3098
Tel: 215 456-7045 *Fax:* 215 254-2781
Internet: http://www.einstein.edu/phl/1207a.html
Accred Length: 4 Years *Program Size:* 34 (*GY1:* 8)
Subspecialties: PYG
Program ID: 400-41-31-189

MCP Hahnemann University Program
Sponsor: MCP Hahnemann University
Hahnemann University Hospital
Medical College of Pennsylvania Hospital

Program Director:
Donna M Sudak, MD
Med Coll of Pennsylvania
Dept of Psychiatry
3300 Henry Ave
Philadelphia, PA 19129
Tel: 215 842-4148 *Fax:* 215 991-1795
Accred Length: 4 Years *Program Size:* 54 (*GY1:* 13)
Program ID: 400-41-21-192

Pennsylvania Hospital of the University of Pennsylvania Health System Program
Sponsor: Pennsylvania Hospital (UPHS)

Program Director:
Richard F Summers, MD
Pennsylvania Hospital
800 Spruce St
Philadelphia, PA 19107
Tel: 215 829-7336 *Fax:* 215 829-7315
E-mail: antren@pahosp.com
Internet: http://www.med.upenn.edu/psychres/
Accred Length: 4 Years *Program Size:* 9 (*GY1:* 0)
Program ID: 400-41-11-193

Temple University Program
Sponsor: Temple University Hospital

Program Director:
Ellen H Sholevar, MD
Temple Univ Hospital
Dept of Psychiatry
3401 N Broad St
Philadelphia, PA 19140
Tel: 215 707-3360 *Fax:* 215 707-1557
Accred Length: 4 Years *Program Size:* 19 (*GY1:* 6)
Program ID: 400-41-21-195

Thomas Jefferson University Program
Sponsor: Thomas Jefferson University Hospital
Friends Hospital

Program Director:
Edward K Silberman, MD
Thomas Jefferson Univ Hospital
1020 Sanson St
Rm 1652-G Thompson Bldg
Philadelphia, PA 19107-5004
Tel: 215 955-6104 *Fax:* 215 955-8473
E-mail: edward.k.silberman@mail.tju.edu
Accred Length: 4 Years *Program Size:* 26 (*GY1:* 7)
Program ID: 400-41-21-196

University of Pennsylvania Program
Sponsor: Hospital of the University of Pennsylvania
Philadelphia Child Guidance Center
Veterans Affairs Medical Center (Philadelphia)

Program Director:
Anthony Rostain, MD
Univ of Pennsylvania
8th Fl Dept of Psychiatry
3600 Market St
Philadelphia, PA 19104
Tel: 215 662-3513 *Fax:* 215 662-3512
E-mail: evibber@.mail.med.upenn.edu
Internet: http://www.med.upenn.edu/psych
Accred Length: 4 Years *Program Size:* 35 (*GY1:* 10)
Subspecialties: ADP, PYG
Program ID: 400-41-21-197

Pittsburgh

Allegheny General Hospital Program
Sponsor: Allegheny General Hospital

Program Director:
Gary N Swanson, MD
Allegheny General Hospital
Dept of Psychiatry
4 Allegheny Ctr/8th Fl
Pittsburgh, PA 15212-4772
Tel: 412 330-4242 *Fax:* 412 330-4010
E-mail: gswanson@aherf.edu
Accred Length: 4 Years *Program Size:* 16 (*GY1:* 4)
Program ID: 400-41-21-272

St Francis Medical Center Program
Sponsor: St Francis Medical Center

Program Director:
David J Lynn, MD
Dept of Psychiatry
St Francis Med Ctr
400 45th St
Pittsburgh, PA 15201
Tel: 412 622-4796
E-mail: psyres@sfhs.edu
Internet: http://www.sfhs.edu/meded/psych/index.htm
Accred Length: 4 Years *Program Size:* 16 (*GY1:* 4)
Subspecialties: TY
Program ID: 400-41-21-243

University Health Center of Pittsburgh Program
Sponsor: University Health Center of Pittsburgh
Presbyterian University Hospital/UPMC
Veterans Affairs Medical Center (Pittsburgh)
Western Psychiatric Institute and Clinic/UPMC

Program Director:
Ravinder D Reddy, MD
Western Psychiatric Inst and Clinic
3811 O'Hara St
Pittsburgh, PA 15213-2593
Tel: 412 624-2876 *Fax:* 412 624-0319
E-mail: reddyr@msx.upmc.edu
Internet: http://www.wpic.pitt.edu
Accred Length: 4 Years *Program Size:* 40 (*GY1:* 10)
Subspecialties: PYG
Program ID: 400-41-31-198

Puerto Rico

San Juan

Puerto Rico Institute of Psychiatry Program

Sponsor: Puerto Rico Institute of Psychiatry
State Psychiatric Hospital

Program Director:
Myrna Zegarra Paz, MD
Puerto Rico Inst of Psychiatry
GPO Box 363741
San Juan, PR 00936-3741
Tel: 787 754-5040 *Fax:* 787 754-5041
Accred Length: 3 Years *Program Size:* 30 (*GY1:* 10)
Program ID: 400-42-22-200

University of Puerto Rico Program

Sponsor: University of Puerto Rico School of Medicine
University Hospital
Veterans Affairs Medical Center (San Juan)

Program Director:
Luz Colon, MD
Univ of Puerto Rico
Dept of Psychiatry
GPO Box 5067
San Juan, PR 00936
Tel: 809 766-0940
Accred Length: 4 Years *Program Size:* 14 (*GY1:* 3)
Program ID: 400-42-31-201

Rhode Island

Providence

Brown University Program

Sponsor: Butler Hospital
Miriam Hospital
Rhode Island Hospital
Roger Williams Medical Center
Veterans Affairs Medical Center (Providence)

Program Director:
Timothy I Mueller, MD
345 Blackstone Blvd
Providence, RI 02906
Tel: 401 455-6375 *Fax:* 401 455-6497
E-mail: timothy_mueller@brown.edu
Internet: http://www.brown.edu/departments/psychiatry
Accred Length: 4 Years *Program Size:* 40 (*GY1:* 10)
Subspecialties: PYG
Program ID: 400-43-21-203

South Carolina

Charleston

Medical University of South Carolina Program

Sponsor: Medical University of South Carolina College of Medicine
Charleston Memorial Hospital
MUSC Medical Center
Ralph H Johnson Dept of Veterans Affairs Med Center

Program Director:
Alberto B Santos, MD
Med Univ of South Carolina
Dept of Psych/Behavioral Science
67 President St/PO Box 250861
Charleston, SC 29425
Tel: 843 792-0192 *Fax:* 843 792-0048
E-mail: putneyms@musc.edu
Internet: http://www.musc.edu/psychiatry
Accred Length: 4 Years *Program Size:* 40 (*GY1:* 10)
Subspecialties: ADP, PYG
Program ID: 400-45-21-204

Columbia

Palmetto Health Alliance/University of South Carolina School of Medicine Program

Sponsor: Palmetto Health Alliance
Palmetto Richland Memorial Hospital
William Jennings Bryan Dorn Veterans Hospital
William S Hall Psychiatric Institute

Program Director:
Ronald E Prier, MD MPH
William S Hall Psychiatric Inst
1800 Colonial Dr
PO Box 202
Columbia, SC 29202
Tel: 803 734-7044 *Fax:* 803 734-4413
E-mail: dks05@wshpi.dmh.state.sc.us
Internet: http://www.ceb.sc.edu
Accred Length: 4 Years *Program Size:* 26 (*GY1:* 6)
Program ID: 400-45-31-205

South Dakota

Sioux Falls

University of South Dakota Program

Sponsor: University of South Dakota School of Medicine
Avera McKennan Hospital
Royal C Johnson Veterans Affairs Medical Center
Southeastern Mental Health Center

Program Director:
K-Lynn Paul, MD
Univ of South Dakota
Dept of Psychiatry
800 E 21st St
Sioux Falls, SD 57101
Tel: 605 367-5950 *Fax:* 605 367-5598
Accred Length: 4 Years *Program Size:* 16 (*GY1:* 4)
Program ID: 400-46-21-260

Tennessee

Johnson City

East Tennessee State University Program

Sponsor: James H Quillen College of Medicine
Johnson City Medical Center Hospital
Veterans Affairs Medical Center (Mountain Home)
Woodridge Hospital

Program Director:
Brent R Coyle, MD
East Tennessee State Univ James H Quillen Coll of Med
Dept of Psychiatry
Box 70567
Johnson City, TN 37614-0567
Tel: 423 439-6305, ext 7362 *Fax:* 423 439-7033
Internet: http://www.etsu-tn.edu/psych/
Accred Length: 4 Years *Program Size:* 18 (*GY1:* 5)
Subspecialties: PYG
Program ID: 400-47-21-258

Memphis

University of Tennessee Program

Sponsor: University of Tennessee College of Medicine
Regional Medical Center at Memphis

Program Director:
David M Allen, MD
135 N Pauline/6th Fl
Memphis, TN 38105
Tel: 901 448-4567 *Fax:* 901 448-4276
E-mail: dmallen@utmem1.utmem.edu
Accred Length: 4 Years *Program Size:* 20 (*GY1:* 5)
Program ID: 400-47-21-206

Nashville

Meharry Medical College Program

Sponsor: Meharry Medical College
Alvin C York Veterans Affairs Medical Center
Centennial Medical Center
Middle Tennessee Mental Health Institute

Program Director:
Zia U Wahid, MD
Meharry Med Coll, Dept of Psychiatry
1005 D B Todd Jr Blvd
Nashville, TN 37208
Tel: 615 327-6491 *Fax:* 615 327-6841
Internet: http://www.meharry.edu
Accred Length: 4 Years *Program Size:* 16 (*GY1:* 4)
Program ID: 400-47-21-207

Vanderbilt University Program

Sponsor: Vanderbilt University Medical Center

Program Director:
James L Nash, MD
Vanderbilt Univ Sch of Med
Dept of Psychiatry
Village at Vanderbilt/Ste 2200
Nashville, TN 37212-7646
Tel: 615 343-3840 *Fax:* 615 343-9038
E-mail: james.nash@mcmail.vanderbilt.edu
Accred Length: 4 Years *Program Size:* 24 (*GY1:* 5)
Program ID: 400-47-11-208

Texas

Austin

Austin State Hospital Program

Sponsor: Austin State Hospital
Austin-Travis County Mental Health and Retardation Center
CTMF of Seton Healthcare Network

Program Director:
Beverly J Sutton, MD
Austin Psychiatric Residency Program
Austin State Hospital
4110 Guadalupe
Austin, TX 78751-4296
Tel: 512 419-2116 *Fax:* 512 419-2432
E-mail: beverly.sutton@mhmr.state.tx.us
Accred Length: 4 Years *Program Size:* 16 (*GY1:* 4)
Program ID: 400-48-12-209

Dallas

University of Texas Southwestern Medical School Program

Sponsor: University of Texas Southwestern Medical School
Dallas County Hospital District-Parkland Memorial Hospital
Presbyterian Hospital of Dallas
Terrell State Hospital
Veterans Affairs Medical Center (Dallas)
Zale-Lipshy University Hospital

Program Director:
Paul C Mohl, MD
Univ of Texas Southwestern Med Sch
5323 Harry Hines Blvd
Dallas, TX 75235-9070
Tel: 214 648-2216 *Fax:* 214 648-4883
E-mail: bmanni@mednet.swmed.edu
Internet:
http://www.swmed.edu/home_pages/psych/resmainpage.html
Accred Length: 4 Years *Program Size:* 59 (*GY1:* 11)
Subspecialties: PYG
Program ID: 400-48-21-211

Programs

El Paso

Texas Tech University (El Paso) Program
Sponsor: Texas Tech University Health Sciences Center at El Paso
R E Thomason General Hospital
Program Director:
David F Briones, MD
Texas Tech Univ Health Sciences Ctr
4800 Alberta Ave
El Paso, TX 79905-1298
Tel: 915 545-6838 *Fax:* 915 545-6442
E-mail: psyega@ttuhsc.com
Internet: http://www.ttuhsc.edu
Accred Length: 4 Years *Program Size:* 14 (*GY1:* 3)
Program ID: 400-48-11-217

Fort Worth

John Peter Smith Hospital (Tarrant County Hospital District) Program
Sponsor: John Peter Smith Hospital (Tarrant County Hospital District)
Program Director:
James K Witschy, MD
Dept of Psychiatry
1500 S Main St
Fort Worth, TX 76104
Tel: 817 921-3431, ext 3050 *Fax:* 817 923-8769
E-mail: jwitschy@airmail.net
Internet: http://jpshealthnet.org
Accred Length: 4 Years *Program Size:* 16 (*GY1:* 4)
Program ID: 400-48-21-282

Galveston

University of Texas Medical Branch Hospitals Program
Sponsor: University of Texas Medical Branch Hospitals
Program Director:
Elinore McCance-Katz, MD MD
Univ of Texas Med Branch
Dept of Psychiatry
Graves Bldg/Rte D-30
Galveston, TX 77555-0430
Tel: 409 772-4833 *Fax:* 409 772-6793
Internet: http://www.psy.utmb.edu
Accred Length: 4 Years *Program Size:* 26 (*GY1:* 6)
Program ID: 400-48-11-212

Houston

Baylor College of Medicine Program
Sponsor: Baylor College of Medicine
Harris County Hospital District-Ben Taub General Hospital
Methodist Hospital
Veterans Affairs Medical Center (Houston)
Program Director:
Linda B Andrews, MD
Baylor Coll of Med
One Baylor Plaza/Ste 622D
Houston, TX 77030
Tel: 713 798-4872 *Fax:* 713 798-1479
E-mail: landrews@bcm.tmc.edu
Accred Length: 4 Years *Program Size:* 46 (*GY1:* 10)
Program ID: 400-48-21-213

University of Texas at Houston Program
Sponsor: University of Texas Medical School at Houston
Harris County Psychiatric Center
Memorial Hermann Healthcare System
University of Texas M D Anderson Cancer Center
Program Director:
Edward Reilly, MD
1300 Moursund/Ste 267
Houston, TX 77030
Tel: 713 794-1463 *Fax:* 713 500-2530
E-mail: ereilly@msi.uth.tmc.edu
Internet: http://oac.hsc.uth.tmc.edu/schools/med/ms
Accred Length: 4 Years *Program Size:* 32 (*GY1:* 8)
Program ID: 400-48-31-215

Lubbock

Texas Tech University (Lubbock) Program
Sponsor: Texas Tech University Health Sciences Center at Lubbock
St Mary of the Plains Hospital
University Medical Center
Program Director:
Elizabeth B Stuyt, MD
Texas Tech Univ Health Sciences Ctr
3601 4th St
Lubbock, TX 79430-0001
Tel: 806 743-2800 *Fax:* 806 743-2784
E-mail: psyebs@ttuhsc.edu
Internet: http://www.pegasus.acs.ttu.edu/~unjas
Accred Length: 4 Years *Program Size:* 16 (*GY1:* 4)
Program ID: 400-48-21-256

San Antonio

University of Texas Health Science Center at San Antonio Program
Sponsor: University of Texas Medical School at San Antonio
Audie L Murphy Memorial Veterans Hospital (San Antonio)
University Hospital-South Texas Medical Center
Program Director:
Kenneth L Matthews, MD
Univ of Texas Health Science Ctr
7703 Floyd Curl Dr
San Antonio, TX 78284-7792
Tel: 210 567-5430 *Fax:* 210 567-6941
E-mail: matthewsk@uthscsa.edu
Internet: http://psych68.uthscsa.edu
Accred Length: 4 Years *Program Size:* 34 (*GY1:* 7)
Subspecialties: ADP
Program ID: 400-48-31-218

Temple

Texas A&M College of Medicine-Scott and White Program
Sponsor: Scott and White Memorial Hospital
Program Director:
Paul B Hicks, MD PhD
Scott and White Memorial Hospital
2401 S 31st St
Temple, TX 76508
Tel: 254 724-1768 *Fax:* 254 724-1747
E-mail: psych@bellnet.tamu.edu
Internet: http://www.sw.org
Accred Length: 4 Years *Program Size:* 16 (*GY1:* 4)
Program ID: 400-48-21-276

Utah

Salt Lake City

University of Utah Program
Sponsor: University of Utah Medical Center
University Counseling Center
University of Utah Neuropsychiatric Institute
Valley Mental Health
Veterans Affairs Medical Center (Salt Lake City)
Program Director:
Craig B Hummel, MD
Univ of Utah Health Sciences Ctr
Dept of Psychiatry
50 N Medical Dr
Salt Lake City, UT 84132
Tel: 801 581-4096 *Fax:* 801 581-5604
E-mail: sue.howard@hsc.utah.edu
Internet:
http://medstat.med.utah.edu/som/education/gme
Accred Length: 4 Years *Program Size:* 19 (*GY1:* 4)
Program ID: 400-49-21-219

Vermont

Burlington

University of Vermont Program
Sponsor: Fletcher Allen Health Care
Program Director:
Richard A Bernstein, MD
Fletcher Allen Health Care
Dept of Psychiatry
1 S Prospect St
Burlington, VT 05401-3456
Tel: 802 656-2259 *Fax:* 802 656-8747
E-mail: carol.allen@vtmednet.org
Internet:
http://www.vtmednet.org./psychiatry/residenc.htm
Accred Length: 4 Years *Program Size:* 20 (*GY1:* 5)
Program ID: 400-50-11-241

Virginia

Charlottesville

University of Virginia Program
Sponsor: University of Virginia Medical Center
Veterans Affairs Medical Center (Salem)
Program Director:
Zachariah C Dameron, MD
Univ of Virginia Sch of Med
Dept of Psychiatric Med
Box 623 HSC
Charlottesville, VA 22908
Tel: 804 924-5408 *Fax:* 804 924-5149
E-mail: psychresidency@virginia.edu
Internet: http://www.hsc.virginia.edu/psychresidency/
Accred Length: 4 Years *Program Size:* 23 (*GY1:* 6)
Subspecialties: PYG
Program ID: 400-51-21-220

Norfolk

Eastern Virginia Medical School Program
Sponsor: Eastern Virginia Medical School
Sentara Norfolk General Hospital
Veterans Affairs Medical Center (Hampton)
Program Director:
Maria R Urbano, MD
Eastern Virginia Med Sch
Dept of Psychiatry
PO Box 1980
Norfolk, VA 23501-1980
Tel: 757 446-5884 *Fax:* 757 446-5918
E-mail: brezinhr@mccoy.evms.edu
Internet: http://www.evms.edu
Accred Length: 4 Years *Program Size:* 16 (*GY1:* 4)
Program ID: 400-51-21-221

Portsmouth

Naval Medical Center (Portsmouth) Program
Sponsor: Naval Medical Center (Portsmouth)
Program Director:
William A McDonald, MD
Naval Med Ctr
Dept of Psychiatry
620 John Paul Jones Cir
Portsmouth, VA 23708-2197
Tel: 757 953-5257 *Fax:* 757 953-7416
E-mail: pnh0wxm@pnh10.med.navy.mil
Internet: http://164.167.49.31/psych/nmcptrn.htm
Accred Length: 4 Years *Program Size:* 16 (*GY1:* 4)
Program ID: 400-51-12-007
US Armed Services Program

Richmond

Medical College of Virginia/Virginia Commonwealth University Program
Sponsor: Medical College of Virginia/Virginia Commonwealth University
Hunter Holmes McGuire VA Medical Center (Richmond)
MCV-Virginia Treatment Center for Children
Medical College of Virginia Hospitals
Program Director:
John R Urbach, MD
Med Coll of Virginia
PO Box 980710
Richmond, VA 23298-0710
Tel: 804 828-9158 *Fax:* 804 828-1472
E-mail: dyeatts@hsc.vcu.edu
Accred Length: 4 Years *Program Size:* 36 (*GY1:* 9)
Program ID: 400-51-21-223

Roanoke

University of Virginia (Roanoke-Salem) Program
Sponsor: Carilion Health System
Carilion Roanoke Memorial Hospital
Veterans Affairs Medical Center (Salem)
Program Director:
J Joe Yazel, MD
VA Med Ctr
Dept of Psychiatry/Bldg 116A7
Salem, VA 24153
Tel: 540 982-2463, ext 1652 *Fax:* 540 983-1086
Internet: http://www.carilion.com/residency
Accred Length: 4 Years *Program Size:* 30 (*GY1:* 6)
Program ID: 400-51-21-267

Washington

Seattle

University of Washington Program
Sponsor: University of Washington School of Medicine
Harborview Medical Center
Sacred Heart Medical Center
University of Washington Medical Center
Veterans Affairs Medical Center (Seattle)
Program Director:
Deborah S Cowley, MD
Dept of Psychiatry/Behav Sci
Univ of Washington/Box 356560
Seattle, WA 98195-6560
Tel: 206 543-6577 *Fax:* 206 685-8952
E-mail: psychres@u.washington.edu
Internet:
http://weber.u.washington.edu/~psychweb/pbsw.html
Accred Length: 4 Years *Program Size:* 56 (*GY1:* 10)
Subspecialties: ADP, PYG
Program ID: 400-54-21-225

West Virginia

Charleston

West Virginia University (Charleston Division) Program
Sponsor: Charleston Area Medical Center
Program Director:
Thomas O Dickey III, MD
501 Morris St/PO Box 1547
Charleston, WV 25326
Tel: 304 341-1500 *Fax:* 304 341-1554
Internet: http://www.camcare.com
Accred Length: 4 Years *Program Size:* 12 (*GY1:* 3)
Program ID: 400-55-21-264

Morgantown

West Virginia University Program
Sponsor: West Virginia University Hospitals
Charleston Area Medical Center
Program Director:
Calvin R Sumner, MD
West Virginia Univ Sch of Med
Dept of Behavioral Med/Psych
930 Chestnut Ridge Rd
Morgantown, WV 26505-2854
Tel: 304 293-2411 *Fax:* 304 293-8724
E-mail: king@wvnvm.wvnet.edu
Internet: http://www.hsc.wvu.edu/som/psychiatry
Accred Length: 4 Years *Program Size:* 12 (*GY1:* 3)
Program ID: 400-55-21-226

Wisconsin

Madison

University of Wisconsin Program
Sponsor: University of Wisconsin Hospital and Clinics
Meriter Hospital
William S Middleton Veterans Hospital
Program Director:
Stephen J Weiler, MD
Univ of Wisconsin-Psychiatric Inst and Clinics
6001 Research Park Blvd
Madison, WI 53719-1179
Tel: 608 263-6092 *Fax:* 608 263-0265
E-mail: sjweiler@facstaff.wisc.edu
Internet: http://www.psychiatry.wisc.edu
Accred Length: 4 Years *Program Size:* 30 (*GY1:* 8)
Subspecialties: PYG
Program ID: 400-56-21-228

Milwaukee

Aurora Health Care Program
Sponsor: Aurora Health Care
Sinai Samaritan Medical Center
University of Wisconsin Hospital and Clinics
Program Director:
Gregory L Schmidt, PhD MD
Sinai Samaritan Med Ctr
PO Box 342
Milwaukee, WI 53201-0342
Tel: 414 219-5479 *Fax:* 414 219-5238
Accred Length: 4 Years *Program Size:* 4 (*GY1:* 0)
Program ID: 400-56-21-259

Medical College of Wisconsin Program
Sponsor: Medical College of Wisconsin Affiliated Hospitals Inc
Clement J Zablocki Veterans Affairs Medical Center
Columbia Hospital
Froedtert Memorial Lutheran Hospital
Milwaukee County Mental Health Complex
Program Director:
Carlyle H Chan, MD
8701 Watertown Plank Rd
Milwaukee, WI 53226
Tel: 414 257-5995 *Fax:* 414 257-7228
E-mail: cchan@post.its.mcw.edu
Internet: http://www.mcw.edu/psych
Accred Length: 4 Years *Program Size:* 32 (*GY1:* 8)
Program ID: 400-56-21-229

Pulmonary Disease (Internal Medicine)

Alabama

Mobile

University of South Alabama Program
Sponsor: University of South Alabama Medical Center
Program Director:
John B Bass Jr, MD
Univ of South Alabama Med Ctr
2451 Fillingim St
10th Fl/Ste H
Mobile, AL 36617
Tel: 334 471-7888 *Fax:* 334 471-7889
E-mail: jbass@usamail.usouthal.edu
Accred Length: 2 Years *Program Size:* 2
Program ID: 149-01-11-048

Arizona

Phoenix

Good Samaritan Regional Medical Center Program
Sponsor: Good Samaritan Regional Medical Center
Carl T Hayden Veterans Affairs Medical Center (Phoenix)
Program Director:
Bernard E Levine, MD
Jay J Rohwedder, MD
Pulmonary Disease Sect (111P)
VA Med Ctr
750 E Indian School Rd
Phoenix, AZ 85012
Tel: 602 277-5551, ext 7388 *Fax:* 602 222-2746
Accred Length: 2 Years *Program Size:* 4
Program ID: 149-03-21-033

California

San Francisco

California Pacific Medical Center Program
Sponsor: California Pacific Medical Center
California Pacific Medical Center
Program Director:
Ronald Elkin, MD
California Pacific Med Ctr
Medical Education
2351 Clay St/#362
San Francisco, CA 94115
Tel: 800 743-7707 *Fax:* 415 775-7437
Internet: http://www.cpmc.org
Accred Length: 2 Years *Program Size:* 2
Program ID: 149-05-12-147

Connecticut

Bridgeport

Yale University (Bridgeport) Program
Sponsor: Bridgeport Hospital
Yale-New Haven Hospital
Program Director:
Raymond G Haddad, MD
Bridgeport Hospital
267 Grant St
Bridgeport, CT 06610
Tel: 203 384-3794 *Fax:* 203 384-4663
Accred Length: 2 Years *Program Size:* 2
Program ID: 149-08-21-199

Norwalk

Norwalk Hospital Program
Sponsor: Norwalk Hospital
Program Director:
Jonathan Fine, MD
Norwalk Hospital
Sect of Pulmonary Med
Maple St
Norwalk, CT 06856
Tel: 203 855-3543 *Fax:* 203 852-2738
E-mail: jonathan.fine@norwalkhealth.org
Internet: http://www.norwalkhosp.org
Accred Length: 2 Years *Program Size:* 4
Program ID: 149-08-31-003

District of Columbia

Washington

Howard University Program
Sponsor: Howard University Hospital
District of Columbia General Hospital
Program Director:
Alvin V Thomas Jr, MD
Howard Univ Hospital
Div of Pulmonary Dis/Ste 5026 Tower
2041 Georgia Ave NW
Washington, DC 20060
Tel: 202 865-6798 *Fax:* 202 865-4669
Internet: http://138.238.107.150/huhosp
Accred Length: 2 Years *Program Size:* 4
Program ID: 149-10-21-086

Illinois

North Chicago

Finch University of Health Sciences/Chicago Medical School Program
Sponsor: Finch University of Health Sciences/Chicago Medical School
Mount Sinai Hospital Medical Center of Chicago
Veterans Affairs Medical Center (North Chicago)
Program Director:
Eric Gluck, MD
Finch Univ of Health Sciences-Chicago Med Sch
Dept of Med
333 Green Bay Rd
North Chicago, IL 60064-3095
Tel: 847 688-1900, ext 6001 *Fax:* 847 578-3848
Accred Length: 2 Years *Program Size:* 4
Program ID: 149-16-21-051

Springfield

Southern Illinois University Program
Sponsor: Southern Illinois University School of Medicine
Memorial Medical Center
St John's Hospital
Program Director:
Lanie E Eagleton, MD
Southern Illinois Univ Sch of Med
701 N. First Street
PO Box 19636
Springfield, IL 62794-9636
Tel: 217 782-0187 *Fax:* 217 788-5543
Accred Length: 2 Years *Program Size:* 2
Program ID: 149-16-21-194

Louisiana

New Orleans

Tulane University Program
Sponsor: Tulane University School of Medicine
Medical Center of Louisiana at New Orleans
Tulane University Hospital and Clinics
Veterans Affairs Medical Center-LSU Service (New Orleans)
Program Director:
Mitchell Friedman, MD
Tulane Med Ctr
1430 Tulane Ave
Box SL9
New Orleans, LA 70112-2699
Tel: 504 588-2250 *Fax:* 504 587-2144
E-mail: ijeffer@tmcpop.tmc.tulane.edu
Accred Length: 2 Years *Program Size:* 9
Program ID: 149-21-21-106

Massachusetts

Boston

Beth Israel Deaconess Medical Center Program
Sponsor: Beth Israel Deaconess Medical Center
Lahey Clinic
Program Director:
Erik Garpestad, MD
Deaconess Hospital
Pulmonary Sect
One Deaconess Rd
Boston, MA 02215
Tel: 617 667-3244
Accred Length: 2 Years *Program Size:* 0
Program ID: 149-24-21-175

Worcester

University of Massachusetts Program
Sponsor: University of Massachusetts Medical School
UMass Memorial Health Care (University Campus)
Program Director:
Oren Schaefer, MD
Univ of Massachusetts Med Ctr
55 Lake Ave N
Worcester, MA 01655
Tel: 508 856-3121 *Fax:* 508 856-3999
E-mail: oren.schaefer@banyan.ummed.edu
Accred Length: 2 Years *Program Size:* 5
Program ID: 149-24-21-008

Mississippi

Jackson

University of Mississippi Medical Center Program

Sponsor: University of Mississippi School of Medicine
University Hospital
Veterans Affairs Medical Center (Jackson)

Program Director:
Deborah Shure, MD
Univ of Mississippi Med Ctr
2500 N State St
Jackson, MS 39216-4505
Tel: 601 984-5650 *Fax:* 601 984-5658
E-mail: dshure@medicine.umsmed.edu
Accred Length: 2 Years *Program Size:* 4
Program ID: 149-27-21-074

Nebraska

Omaha

Creighton University Program

Sponsor: Creighton University School of Medicine
Tenet St Joseph Hospital at Creighton Univ Medical Center
Veterans Affairs Medical Center (Omaha)

Program Director:
Joseph C Campbell Jr, MD
Pulmonary Med/Ste 3820
601 N 30th St
Omaha, NE 68131-2100
Tel: 402 449-4486 *Fax:* 402 280-5256
E-mail: mcoburn@creighton.edu
Accred Length: 2 Years *Program Size:* 3
Program ID: 149-30-21-154

New Jersey

South Orange

Seton Hall University School of Graduate Medical Education Program

Sponsor: Seton Hall University School of Graduate Medical Education
St Joseph's Hospital and Medical Center
St Michael's Medical Center (Cathedral Hlth Srvcs Inc)

Program Director:
M Anees Khan, MD
St Joseph's Hospital and Med Ctr
703 Main St
Paterson, NJ 07503
Tel: 201 754-2450 *Fax:* 201 754-2469
Accred Length: 2 Years *Program Size:* 6
Program ID: 149-33-11-156

New York

Bronx

Bronx-Lebanon Hospital Center Program

Sponsor: Bronx-Lebanon Hospital Center

Program Director:
Jerome Ernst, MD
Bronx-Lebanon Hospital Ctr
1650 Grand Concourse
Bronx, NY 10457
Tel: 718 960-2003 *Fax:* 718 960-1333
E-mail: jerry@aol.com
Accred Length: 2 Years *Program Size:* 5
Program ID: 149-35-11-102

Brooklyn

Brookdale University Hospital Medical Center Program

Sponsor: Brookdale University Hospital Medical Center

Program Director:
Elliott Bondi, MD
Brookdale Univ Hospital and Med Ctr
Linden Blvd at Brookdale Plaza
Brooklyn, NY 11212-3198
Tel: 718 240-5236 *Fax:* 718 240-6592
Accred Length: 2 Years *Program Size:* 6
Program ID: 149-35-11-157

Brooklyn Hospital Center Program

Sponsor: Brooklyn Hospital Center

Program Director:
Marshal S Reminick, MD
Brooklyn Hospital Ctr
121 DeKalb Ave
Brooklyn, NY 11201
Tel: 718 250-6950 *Fax:* 718 250-6110
Internet: http://www.tbh.org//
Accred Length: 2 Years *Program Size:* 3
Program ID: 149-35-12-185

Coney Island Hospital Program

Sponsor: Coney Island Hospital

Program Director:
Santi R Dhar, MD
Coney Island Hospital
2601 Ocean Pkwy
Brooklyn, NY 11235
Tel: 718 616-3171 *Fax:* 718 616-4071
Accred Length: 2 Years *Program Size:* 4
Program ID: 149-35-11-178

Interfaith Medical Center Program

Sponsor: Interfaith Medical Center

Program Director:
Gerald M Greenberg, MD
Interfaith Med Ctr
555 Prospect Pl
Brooklyn, NY 11238
Tel: 718 935-7503 *Fax:* 718 935-7237
Accred Length: 2 Years *Program Size:* 3
Program ID: 149-35-21-179

Long Island College Hospital Program

Sponsor: Long Island College Hospital
Woodhull Medical and Mental Health Center

Program Director:
Ute W Rosa, MD
Long Island College Hospital
339 Hicks St
Brooklyn, NY 11201
Tel: 718 780-1664 *Fax:* 718 780-1256
Accred Length: 2 Years *Program Size:* 4
Program ID: 149-35-11-064

Maimonides Medical Center Program

Sponsor: Maimonides Medical Center

Program Director:
Sidney Tessler, MD
Maimonides Med Ctr
Div of Pulmonary Diseases
4802 Tenth Ave
Brooklyn, NY 11219
Tel: 718 283-8380 *Fax:* 718 283-7884
E-mail: stessler@maimonidesmed.org
Accred Length: 2 Years *Program Size:* 4
Program ID: 149-35-11-158

New York Methodist Hospital Program

Sponsor: New York Methodist Hospital

Program Director:
Nanarao Anandarao, MD MB BS
New York Methodist Hospital
506 Sixth St
Brooklyn, NY 11215
Tel: 718 780-5246 *Fax:* 718 780-3259
Accred Length: 2 Years *Program Size:* 4
Program ID: 149-35-11-091

SUNY Health Science Center at Brooklyn Program

Sponsor: SUNY Health Science Center at Brooklyn
Kings County Hospital Center
St John's Episcopal Hospital-South Shore
University Hospital-SUNY Health Science Center at Brooklyn
Veterans Affairs Medical Center (Brooklyn)

Program Director:
Linda S Efferen, MD
SUNY Health Science Ctr-Brooklyn
450 Clarkson Ave/Box 19
Brooklyn, NY 11203-2098
Tel: 718 270-1770 *Fax:* 718 270-1733
Accred Length: 2 Years *Program Size:* 8
Program ID: 149-35-21-054

East Meadow

SUNY at Stony Brook (East Meadow) Program

Sponsor: Nassau County Medical Center

Program Director:
Suhail Raoof, MD
Nassau County Med Ctr
2201 Hempstead Trnpk
East Meadow, NY 11554-5400
Tel: 516 572-8714 *Fax:* 516 572-5609
E-mail: sraoof@ncmc.co.nassau.ny.us
Internet: http://www.ncmc.co.nassau.ny.us
Accred Length: 2 Years *Program Size:* 2
Program ID: 149-35-21-089

Elmhurst

Mount Sinai School of Medicine (Elmhurst) Program

Sponsor: Mount Sinai School of Medicine
Elmhurst Hospital Center-Mount Sinai Services
Mount Sinai Medical Center

Program Director:
Harvey M Shanies, MD PhD
Elmhurst Hospital Ctr
79-01 Broadway
Elmhurst, NY 11373
Tel: 718 334-3122 *Fax:* 718 334-2879
Accred Length: 2 Years *Program Size:* 2
Program ID: 149-35-11-116

Flushing

New York Hospital Medical Center of Queens/Cornell University Medical College Program

Sponsor: New York Hospital Medical Center of Queens

Program Director:
Stephen Karbowitz, MD
New York Hospital Med Ctr of Queens
56-45 Main St
Flushing, NY 11355-5095
Tel: 718 670-1405 *Fax:* 718 461-2943
E-mail: gtmartin%queens@nyh.med.cornell.edu
Accred Length: 2 Years *Program Size:* 3
Program ID: 149-35-11-090

Jamaica

Catholic Medical Center of Brooklyn and Queens Program

Sponsor: Catholic Medical Center of Brooklyn and Queens Inc
Catholic Medical Center (Mary Immaculate Hospital)
Catholic Medical Center (St John's Queens Hospital)
Program Director:
Luis A Bracero, MD
Catholic Med Ctr of Brooklyn and Queens
88-25 153rd St/Ste 3J
Jamaica, NY 11432
Tel: 718 558-7227 *Fax:* 718 558-6165
Accred Length: 2 Years *Program Size:* 4
Program ID: 149-35-22-047

New York

Harlem Hospital Center Program

Sponsor: Harlem Hospital Center
Program Director:
Jean Ford, MD
Harlem Hospital Ctr
Dept of Med/Rm 12-106
506 Lenox Ave
New York, NY 10037
Tel: 212 939-1459 *Fax:* 212 939-1456
E-mail: jf24@columbia.edu
Accred Length: 2 Years *Program Size:* 4
Program ID: 149-35-11-168

Lenox Hill Hospital Program

Sponsor: Lenox Hill Hospital
Program Director:
Murray R Rogers, MD
Lenox Hill Hospital
Pulmonary Section/6 Black Hall
100 E 77th St
New York, NY 10021-1883
Tel: 212 434-2140 *Fax:* 212 434-2446
Accred Length: 2 Years *Program Size:* 2
Program ID: 149-35-11-181

Mount Sinai School of Medicine (Cabrini) Program

Sponsor: Mount Sinai School of Medicine
Cabrini Medical Center
Program Director:
Ari Klapholz, MD
Cabrini Med Ctr
227 E 19th St
New York, NY 10003
Tel: 212 995-6658 *Fax:* 212 979-3513
Accred Length: 2 Years *Program Size:* 4
Program ID: 149-35-31-096

New York and Presbyterian Hospital (Columbia Campus) Program

Sponsor: New York and Presbyterian Hospital
New York and Presbyterian Hospital (Columbia Campus)
Program Director:
Randolph P Cole, MD
Presbyterian Hospital in the City of New York
630 W 168th St
PH 8 Center
New York, NY 10032-8110
Tel: 212 305-9817 *Fax:* 212 305-8464
Internet:
http://cpmcnet.columbia.edu/dept/pulmonary/fellowship.html
Accred Length: 2 Years *Program Size:* 4
Program ID: 149-35-11-142

New York and Presbyterian Hospital (Cornell Campus) Program

Sponsor: Memorial Sloan-Kettering Cancer Center
Program Director:
Jean T Santamauro, MD
Diane E Stover, MD
Memorial Sloan-Kettering Cancer Ctr
Pulmonary Service
1275 York Ave/Rm C-678
New York, NY 10021
Tel: 212 639-8002 *Fax:* 212 717-3116
Accred Length: 2 Years *Program Size:* 4
Program ID: 149-35-21-173

North Carolina

Greenville

East Carolina University Program

Sponsor: East Carolina University School of Medicine
Pitt County Memorial Hospital
Program Director:
Ralph E Whatley, MD
East Carolina Univ Sch of Med
Brody Bldg 3E111
Greenville, NC 27858
Tel: 919 816-4653 *Fax:* 919 816-4887
Accred Length: 2 Years *Program Size:* 0
Program ID: 149-36-21-203

Ohio

Toledo

Medical College of Ohio Program

Sponsor: Medical College of Ohio
Program Director:
Dan E Olson, MD
Med Coll of Ohio
3000 Arlington Ave
Toledo, OH 43699-0008
Tel: 419 381-3543
Accred Length: 2 Years *Program Size:* 3
Program ID: 149-38-21-202

Pennsylvania

Hershey

Penn State Geisinger Health System/Milton S Hershey Medical Center Program

Sponsor: Penn State Geisinger Health System
Milton S Hershey Medical Center
Program Director:
Rebecca Bascom, MD MPH
Penn State Geisinger Health Systesm
MC HO41
PO Box 850
Hershey, PA 17033-0850
Tel: 717 531-6525 *Fax:* 717 531-5785
E-mail: rbascom@med.hmc.psghs.edu
Accred Length: 2 Years *Program Size:* 6
Program ID: 149-41-11-016

Philadelphia

Albert Einstein Medical Center Program

Sponsor: Albert Einstein Medical Center
Program Director:
Michael Lippman, MD
5401 Old York Rd
Klein Bldg, Ste 363
Philadelphia, PA 19141
Tel: 215 456-6950 *Fax:* 215 455-1933
Accred Length: 2 Years *Program Size:* 3
Program ID: 149-41-21-204

Graduate Hospital Program

Sponsor: Graduate Hospital
Program Director:
Morris A Swartz, MD
Graduate Hospital
Pepper Pavilion/Ste 607
One Graduate Plaza
Philadelphia, PA 19146
Tel: 215 893-2424 *Fax:* 215 893-7220
Accred Length: 2 Years *Program Size:* 4
Program ID: 149-41-11-139

Pittsburgh

Allegheny General Hospital Program

Sponsor: Allegheny General Hospital
Program Director:
Peter Kaplan, MD
Allegheny General Hospital
Dept of Pulmonary Disease
320 E North Ave
Pittsburgh, PA 15212-9986
Tel: 412 359-3038 *Fax:* 412 359-6609
Accred Length: 2 Years *Program Size:* 6
Program ID: 149-41-11-040

Western Pennsylvania Hospital Program

Sponsor: Western Pennsylvania Hospital
Program Director:
Paul C Fiehler, MD
Western Pennsylvania Hospital
Dept of Med
4800 Friendship Ave
Pittsburgh, PA 15224
Tel: 412 578-5750 *Fax:* 412 578-6804
Accred Length: 2 Years *Program Size:* 3
Program ID: 149-41-11-042

Puerto Rico

Ponce

Hospital de Damas Program

Sponsor: Hospital de Damas
Ponce University Hospital
Program Director:
Homero Tarrats, MD
Hospital de Damas
Edif Parra 2225 Ste 407
Ponce Bypass
Ponce, PR 00731
Tel: 787 840-8686, ext 6123
Accred Length: 2 Years *Program Size:* 1
Program ID: 149-42-11-190

Rio Piedras

San Juan City Hospital Program
Sponsor: San Juan City Hospital
University Hospital Ramon Ruiz Arnau
Program Director:
Samuel A Amill, MD
Dept of Medicine
Puerto Rico Med Ctr
Rio Piedras, PR 00935
Tel: 787 765-5147 *Fax:* 787 761-0459
Accred Length: 2 Years *Program Size:* 2
Program ID: 149-42-11-097

San Juan

University of Puerto Rico Program
Sponsor: University of Puerto Rico School of Medicine
University Hospital
Veterans Affairs Medical Center (San Juan)
Program Director:
Yohana De Jesús, MD
Univ of Puerto Rico
Medical Sciences Campus
PO Box 365067
San Juan, PR 00936-5067
Tel: 787 754-3750
E-mail: pcarriat@compuserve.com
Accred Length: 2 Years *Program Size:* 2
Program ID: 149-42-21-121

Veterans Affairs Medical and Regional Office Center Program
Sponsor: Veterans Affairs Medical Center (San Juan)
Program Director:
William Rodriguez, MD
VA Med Ctr
One Veterans Plaza
San Juan, PR 00927-5800
Tel: 787 758-7575, ext 5656 *Fax:* 787 766-6021
E-mail: rodriguez,william@san-juan.va.gov
Internet: http://www.va.gov
Accred Length: 2 Years *Program Size:* 2
Program ID: 149-42-31-120

Rhode Island

Providence

Roger Williams Medical Center Program
Sponsor: Roger Williams Medical Center
Program Director:
Sidney S Braman, MD
Rhode Island Hospital, Div of Pulm/Critical Care
593 Eddy St
Providence, RI 02903
Tel: 401 444-8410 *Fax:* 401 444-5914
E-mail: sidney_braman@brown.edu
Accred Length: 2 Years *Program Size:* 7
Program ID: 149-43-31-043

Tennessee

Johnson City

East Tennessee State University Program
Sponsor: James H Quillen College of Medicine
Bristol Regional Medical Center
Johnson City Medical Center Hospital
Veterans Affairs Medical Center (Mountain Home)
Program Director:
Thomas Roy, MD
Mountain Home VA Med Ctr (111-B)
Mountain Home, TN 37684
Tel: 423 926-1171, ext 2447 *Fax:* 423 461-7939
Accred Length: 2 Years *Program Size:* 4
Program ID: 149-47-21-187

Memphis

University of Tennessee Program
Sponsor: University of Tennessee College of Medicine
Regional Medical Center at Memphis
Veterans Affairs Medical Center (Memphis)
Program Director:
John P Griffin, MD
Univ of Tennessee
956 Court Ave/Rm H314
Memphis, TN 38163
Tel: 901 448-5757 *Fax:* 901 448-7726
Accred Length: 2 Years *Program Size:* 7
Program ID: 149-47-21-140

Texas

Temple

Texas A&M College of Medicine-Scott and White Program
Sponsor: Scott and White Memorial Hospital
Central Texas Veterans Affairs Healthcare System
Program Director:
Richard E Winn, MD
Texas A&M-Scott and White
Grad Med Educ
2401 S 31st St
Temple, TX 76508-0001
Tel: 254 724-7633, ext 5817 *Fax:* 254 724-9280
E-mail: blculp@swmail.sw.org
Internet: http://www.sw.org
Accred Length: 2 Years *Program Size:* 4
Program ID: 149-48-21-019

West Virginia

Huntington

Marshall University School of Medicine Program
Sponsor: Marshall University School of Medicine
Cabell Huntington Hospital
St Mary's Hospital
Veterans Affairs Medical Center (Huntington)
Program Director:
Nancy J Munn, MD
Marshall Univ Sch of Med
Dept of Int Med
1600 Medical Center Dr/Ste G500
Huntington, WV 25701-3655
Tel: 304 691-1084 *Fax:* 304 691-1693
Accred Length: 2 Years *Program Size:* 3
Program ID: 149-55-21-183

Pulmonary Disease and Critical Care Medicine (Internal Medicine)

Alabama

Birmingham

University of Alabama Medical Center Program
Sponsor: University of Alabama Hospital
Veterans Affairs Medical Center (Birmingham)
Program Director:
J Allen D Cooper Jr, MD
Univ of Alabama
215 Tinsley Harrison Tower
1900 University Blvd
Birmingham, AL 35294-0006
Tel: 205 934-5400 *Fax:* 205 934-7315
E-mail: allenc409@aol.com
Internet: http://info.dom.uab.edu/pulm/index.htm
Accred Length: 3 Years *Program Size:* 9
Program ID: 156-01-21-105

Arizona

Tucson

University of Arizona Program
Sponsor: University of Arizona College of Medicine
University Medical Center
Veterans Affairs Medical Center (Tucson)
Program Director:
Stuart F Quan, MD
Univ of Arizona Coll of Med
Respiratory Sciences Ctr
1501 N Campbell Ave/PO Box 245030
Tucson, AZ 85724
Tel: 520 626-6114 *Fax:* 520 626-6970
E-mail: annr@resp-sci.arizona.edu
Internet: http://www.ahsc.arizona.edu
Accred Length: 3 Years *Program Size:* 4
Program ID: 156-03-21-001

Arkansas

Little Rock

University of Arkansas for Medical Sciences Program
Sponsor: University of Arkansas College of Medicine
John L McClellan Memorial Veterans Hospital
University Hospital of Arkansas
Program Director:
Paula J Anderson, MD
4301 W Markham/Slot 555
Little Rock, AR 72205
Tel: 501 686-5525 *Fax:* 501 686-7893
E-mail: paulaanderson@exchange.uams.edu
Accred Length: 3 Years *Program Size:* 6
Program ID: 156-04-21-002

California

Loma Linda

Loma Linda University Program

Sponsor: Loma Linda University Medical Center
Jerry L Pettis Memorial Veterans Hospital

Program Director:
Philip M Gold, MD
Loma Linda Univ Med Ctr
11234 Anderson St/Rm 1521
Loma Linda, CA 92354
Tel: 909 824-4489
Accred Length: 3 Years *Program Size:* 3
Program ID: 156-05-21-113

Los Angeles

Cedars-Sinai Medical Center Program

Sponsor: Cedars-Sinai Medical Center
VA Greater Los Angeles Healthcare System

Program Director:
Zab Mohsenifar, MD
Michael I Lewis, MD
Cedars-Sinai Med Ctr
8700 Beverly Blvd
Rm 6732
Los Angeles, CA 90048
Tel: 310 967-1835 *Fax:* 310 967-0129
E-mail: mohsenifarz@cshs.org
Accred Length: 3 Years *Program Size:* 6
Program ID: 156-05-21-003

UCLA Medical Center Program

Sponsor: UCLA School of Medicine
Olive View-UCLA Medical Center
UCLA Medical Center
VA Greater Los Angeles Healthcare System

Program Director:
Paul E Bellamy, MD
UCLA Sch of Med
Ctr for the Health Sciences
Los Angeles, CA 90024-1736
Tel: 310 825-5988 *Fax:* 310 206-8622
Accred Length: 3 Years *Program Size:* 2
Program ID: 156-05-31-114

University of Southern California Program

Sponsor: Los Angeles County-USC Medical Center
Barlow Respiratory Hospital

Program Director:
Edward D Crandall, PhD MD
Div of Pulm/Critical Care Med
2025 Zonal Ave/GNH 11900
Los Angeles, CA 90033
Tel: 213 226-7924 *Fax:* 213 226-2738
E-mail: ecrandal@hsc.usc.edu
Accred Length: 3 Years *Program Size:* 14
Program ID: 156-05-31-004

Orange

University of California (Irvine) Program

Sponsor: University of California (Irvine) Medical Center
Veterans Affairs Medical Center (Long Beach)

Program Director:
Archie F Wilson, MD PhD
Pulmonary/Critical Care Div
Univ of California Irvine Med Ctr
101 City Dr S
Orange, CA 92868-3298
Tel: 714 456-5150 *Fax:* 714 456-8349
E-mail: pulmdocs@ccmail.hsis.uci.edu
Accred Length: 3 Years *Program Size:* 8
Program ID: 156-05-11-005

Sacramento

University of California (Davis) Program

Sponsor: University of California (Davis) Medical Center

Program Director:
Susan Murin, MD
Univ of California Davis Med Ctr
Div of Pulmonary/Critical Care Med
4150 V St/Ste 3400
Sacramento, CA 95817
Tel: 916 734-3564 *Fax:* 916 734-7924
Internet:
http://internalmedicine.ucdmc.ucdavis.edu/pulmhome.htm
Accred Length: 3 Years *Program Size:* 7
Program ID: 156-05-12-006

San Diego

Naval Medical Center (San Diego) Program

Sponsor: Naval Medical Center (San Diego)

Program Director:
Kevin M Murray, MD
Pulmonary Div
Naval Med Ctr
34730 Bob Wilson Dr/Ste 301
San Diego, CA 92134-3301
Tel: 619 532-9067 *Fax:* 619 532-7606
E-mail: snd1kmm@snd10.med.navy.mil
Accred Length: 3 Years *Program Size:* 6
Program ID: 156-05-13-007
US Armed Services Program

University of California (San Diego) Program

Sponsor: University of California (San Diego) Medical Center
Veterans Affairs Medical Center (San Diego)

Program Director:
Andrew Ries, MD MPH
UCSD Med Ctr
200 W Arbor Dr
San Diego, CA 92103-8372
Tel: 619 543-5970 *Fax:* 619 543-2751
E-mail: aries@ucsd.edu
Accred Length: 3 Years *Program Size:* 16
Program ID: 156-05-22-008

San Francisco

University of California (San Francisco) Program

Sponsor: University of California (San Francisco) School of Medicine
San Francisco General Hospital Medical Center
University of California (San Francisco) Medical Center
Veterans Affairs Medical Center (San Francisco)

Program Director:
H Benfer Kaltrerder, MD
John M Luce, MD
Univ of California San Francisco
Dept of Med
Box 0120
San Francisco, CA 94143
Tel: 415 750-2007 *Fax:* 415 387-3568
Accred Length: 3 Years *Program Size:* 18
Program ID: 156-05-23-009

Stanford

Stanford University Program

Sponsor: Stanford University Hospital

Program Director:
Thomas A Raffin, MD
Stanford Univ Med Ctr
Div of Pulmonary/CCM Med
300 Pasteur Dr/Rm H3151
Stanford, CA 94305-5236
Tel: 650 723-6381 *Fax:* 650 725-5489
Internet: http://www-leland.stanford.edu/dept/pulmonary
Accred Length: 3 Years *Program Size:* 12
Program ID: 156-05-21-010

Torrance

Los Angeles County-Harbor-UCLA Medical Center Program

Sponsor: Los Angeles County-Harbor-UCLA Medical Center

Program Director:
Darryl Y Sue, MD
Los Angeles County-Harbor-UCLA Med Ctr
Respiratory Med/RB-2
1000 W Carson St/Box 405
Torrance, CA 90509-2910
Tel: 310 222-3801
Internet:
http://www.medsch.ucla.edu/som/ddo/harbo_med
Accred Length: 3 Years *Program Size:* 5
Program ID: 156-05-11-115

Colorado

Denver

University of Colorado Program

Sponsor: University of Colorado Health Sciences Center
Denver Health and Hospitals
Rose Medical Center
Veterans Affairs Medical Center (Denver)

Program Director:
Marvin I Schwarz, MD
Univ of Colorado Health Sciences Ctr
Box C272/Rm 5525
4200 E Ninth Ave
Denver, CO 80262
Tel: 303 315-7047 *Fax:* 303 315-5632
E-mail: marvin.schwarz@uchsc.edu
Accred Length: 3 Years *Program Size:* 18
Program ID: 156-07-21-097

Connecticut

Farmington

University of Connecticut Program

Sponsor: University of Connecticut School of Medicine
Mount Sinai Hospital
New Britain General Hospital
St Francis Hospital and Medical Center
Univ of Connecticut Health Center/John Dempsey Hospital

Program Director:
Mark L Metersky, MD
Univ of Connecticut Health Ctr
Div of Pulmonary/Critical Care
263 Farmington Ave
Farmington, CT 06030-1225
Tel: 860 679-3585 *Fax:* 860 679-1103
E-mail: metersky@nso.uchc.edu
Internet: http://www.resprog.uchc.edu/md/
Accred Length: 3 Years *Program Size:* 6
Program ID: 156-08-21-011

New Haven

Yale-New Haven Medical Center Program
Sponsor: Yale-New Haven Hospital
Veterans Affairs Medical Center (West Haven)
Program Director:
RIchard A Matthay, MD
333 Cedar St
New Haven, CT 06520-8057
Tel: 203 785-4196 *Fax:* 203 785-3634
E-mail: matthay@biomed.med.yale.edu
Internet: http://info.med.yale.edu
Accred Length: 3 Years *Program Size:* 17
Program ID: 156-08-21-104

District of Columbia

Washington

George Washington University Program
Sponsor: George Washington University School of Medicine
George Washington University Hospital (UHS)
Veterans Affairs Medical Center (Washington, DC)
Program Director:
Prashant K Rohatgi, MD
2150 Pennsylvania Ave NW/Rm 5-411
Washington, DC 20037
Tel: 202 994-0324 *Fax:* 202 994-3949
Accred Length: 3 Years *Program Size:* 5
Program ID: 156-10-21-080

Georgetown University Program
Sponsor: Georgetown University Medical Center
Fairfax Hospital
Program Director:
Charles A Read, MD
Georgetown Univ Med Ctr
Pulm/Critical Care Med
3800 Reservoir Rd NW
Washington, DC 20007-2197
Tel: 202 687-8830 *Fax:* 202 687-7336
E-mail: steelewe@gunet.georgetown.edu
Accred Length: 3 Years *Program Size:* 4
Program ID: 156-10-21-013

Walter Reed Army Medical Center Program
Sponsor: Walter Reed Army Medical Center
National Naval Medical Center (Bethesda)
Program Director:
Kevin O'Neil, MD
Walter Reed Army Med Ctr
Ward 77
6825 16th St NW
Washington, DC 20307-5001
Tel: 202 782-5731 *Fax:* 202 782-9032
E-mail: cdr_kevin_oneil@wramc1.amedd.army.mil
Internet:
http://www.wramc.amedd.army.mil/departments/medicine/pulm/ftpccc.htm
Accred Length: 3 Years *Program Size:* 15
Program ID: 156-10-21-082
US Armed Services Program

Florida

Gainesville

University of Florida Program
Sponsor: University of Florida College of Medicine
Shands Hospital at the University of Florida
Veterans Affairs Medical Center (Gainesville)
Program Director:
Michael J Cicale, MD
Univ of Florida
PO Box 100225
Gainesville, FL 32610-0225
Tel: 352 846-0754 *Fax:* 352 392-0821
E-mail: cicalmj@medicine.ufl.edu
Internet: http://www.med.ufl.edu/med/train/pulm.htm
Accred Length: 3 Years *Program Size:* 5
Program ID: 156-11-21-014

Miami

University of Miami-Jackson Memorial Medical Center Program
Sponsor: University of Miami-Jackson Memorial Medical Center
Mount Sinai Medical Center of Greater Miami
Veterans Affairs Medical Center (Miami)
Program Director:
Horst J Baier, MD JD
Univ of Miami Sch of Med
PO Box 016960 (R-47)
Miami, FL 33101
Tel: 305 585-7340 *Fax:* 305 324-0869
E-mail: hbaier@mednet.med.miami.edu
Accred Length: 3 Years *Program Size:* 13
Program ID: 156-11-31-015

Tampa

University of South Florida Program
Sponsor: University of South Florida College of Medicine
James A Haley Veterans Hospital
Tampa General Healthcare
Program Director:
David A Solomon, MD
Univ of South Florida
Div of Pulmonary/Critical Care
13000 Bruce B Downs Blvd (111C)
Tampa, FL 33612-4798
Tel: 813 972-7543 *Fax:* 813 979-3606
Accred Length: 3 Years *Program Size:* 6
Program ID: 156-11-21-102

Georgia

Atlanta

Emory University Program
Sponsor: Emory University School of Medicine
Emory University Hospital
Grady Memorial Hospital
Veterans Affairs Medical Center (Atlanta)
Program Director:
Gerald W Staton Jr, MD
Crawford Long Hospital
550 Peachtree St NE
Atlanta, GA 30365-2225
Tel: 404 686-2505 *Fax:* 404 686-4840
E-mail: gerald_staton@emory.org
Internet: http://www.emory.edu/whsc/med/plum
Accred Length: 3 Years *Program Size:* 11
Program ID: 156-12-21-016

Augusta

Medical College of Georgia Program
Sponsor: Medical College of Georgia Hospital and Clinics
Veterans Affairs Medical Center (Augusta)
Program Director:
W Bruce Davis, MD
Med Coll of Georgia
Sect of Pulmonary Dis/BBR5513
1120 15th St
Augusta, GA 30912-3135
Tel: 706 721-2566 *Fax:* 706 721-3069
Accred Length: 3 Years *Program Size:* 6
Program ID: 156-12-31-017

Illinois

Chicago

Cook County Hospital Program
Sponsor: Cook County Hospital
Program Director:
Petham P Muthuswamy, MD
Div of Pulm/Critical Care
Cook County Hospital
1900 W Polk
Chicago, IL 60612
Tel: 312 633-8966 *Fax:* 312 622-3107
E-mail: mswamy@pol.net
Accred Length: 3 Years *Program Size:* 6
Program ID: 156-16-21-018

McGaw Medical Center of Northwestern University Program
Sponsor: Northwestern University Medical School
Northwestern Memorial Hospital
Veterans Affairs Lakeside Medical Center (Chicago)
Program Director:
Peter H Sporn, MD
Northwestern Univ Med Sch
Pulm/Critical Care Div, Passavant 777
303 E Superior St
Chicago, IL 60611-3053
Tel: 312 908-8163 *Fax:* 312 908-4650
E-mail: p-sporn@nwu.edu
Internet: http://www.medicine.nwu.edu
Accred Length: 3 Years *Program Size:* 8
Program ID: 156-16-21-081

Rush-Presbyterian-St Luke's Medical Center Program
Sponsor: Rush-Presbyterian-St Luke's Medical Center
Program Director:
Robert A Balk, MD
Rush-Presbyterian-St Luke's Med Ctr
1653 W Congress Pkwy
Chicago, IL 60612
Tel: 312 942-5092 *Fax:* 312 563-2157
E-mail: rbalk@rush.edu
Accred Length: 3 Years *Program Size:* 6
Program ID: 156-16-31-019

University of Chicago Program
Sponsor: University of Chicago Hospitals
Program Director:
Steven White, MD
Univ of Chicago Hospitals and Clinics
5841 S Maryland Ave
MC6026
Chicago, IL 60637
Tel: 773 702-1454 *Fax:* 773 702-6500
E-mail: swhite@medicine.bsd.uchicago.edu
Accred Length: 3 Years *Program Size:* 9
Program ID: 156-16-21-091

University of Illinois College of Medicine at Chicago Program
Sponsor: University of Illinois College of Medicine at Chicago
Michael Reese Hospital and Medical Center
University of Illinois Hospital and Clinics
Veterans Affairs West Side Medical Center
Program Director:
Ergun Onal, MD
Univ of Illinois
Dept of Med (M/C 787)
840 S Wood St
Chicago, IL 60612-7323
Tel: 312 996-8039 *Fax:* 312 996-4665
E-mail: rccm@uic.edu
Internet: http://www.uic.edu/com/rccm
Accred Length: 3 Years *Program Size:* 9
Program ID: 156-16-21-020

Maywood

Loyola University Program
Sponsor: Loyola University Medical Center
Edward J Hines Jr Veterans Affairs Hospital
Program Director:
Martin J Tobin, MD
Loyola Univ-Stritch Sch of Med
2160 S First Ave
Fahey Ctr/A-351500-1
Maywood, IL 60153
Tel: 708 216-5402 *Fax:* 708 216-6839
Internet:
http://www.meddean.luc.edu/deptwebs/medicine/index.htm
Accred Length: 3 Years *Program Size:* 9
Program ID: 156-16-31-021

Indiana

Indianapolis

Indiana University School of Medicine Program
Sponsor: Indiana University School of Medicine
Clarian IU Hospital
Clarian Methodist Hospital of Indiana
William N Wishard Memorial Hospital
Program Director:
Scott T Pottratz, MD
Indiana Univ Sch of Med
1001 W 10th St/OPW 529
Indianapolis, IN 46202-2879
Tel: 317 630-6445 *Fax:* 317 630-7487
E-mail: spottrat@iupui.edu
Internet: http://medicine.iupui.edu/pulmonar.html
Accred Length: 3 Years *Program Size:* 10
Program ID: 156-17-21-022

Iowa

Iowa City

University of Iowa Hospitals and Clinics Program
Sponsor: University of Iowa Hospitals and Clinics
Program Director:
Michael W Peterson, MD
Univ of Iowa Hospitals and Clinics
Dept of Int Med/Pulmonary
200 Hawkins Dr
Iowa City, IA 52242
Tel: 319 356-1012 *Fax:* 319 353-6406
E-mail: michael-peterson@uiowa.edu
Internet: http://www.int-med.uiowa.edu
Accred Length: 3 Years *Program Size:* 9
Program ID: 156-18-21-023

Kansas

Kansas City

University of Kansas Medical Center Program
Sponsor: University of Kansas School of Medicine
University of Kansas Medical Center
Program Director:
Susan K Pingleton, MD
Univ of Kansas Med Ctr
3901 Rainbow Blvd
Kansas City, KS 66160-7381
Tel: 913 588-6045 *Fax:* 913 588-4098
E-mail: spinglet@kumc.edu
Accred Length: 3 Years *Program Size:* 6
Program ID: 156-19-21-024

Kentucky

Lexington

University of Kentucky Medical Center Program
Sponsor: University of Kentucky Hospital
Veterans Affairs Medical Center (Lexington)
Program Director:
Rolando Berger, MD
Univ of Kentucky Chandler Med Ctr
800 Rose St/MN-614
Lexington, KY 40536-0298
Tel: 606 323-5045 *Fax:* 606 257-2418
Accred Length: 3 Years *Program Size:* 6
Program ID: 156-20-21-101

Louisville

University of Louisville Program
Sponsor: University of Louisville School of Medicine
University of Louisville Hospital
Veterans Affairs Medical Center (Louisville)
Program Director:
Eugene C Fletcher, MD
Univ of Louisville
Ambulatory Care Bldg/Rm A3L01
530 S Jackson St
Louisville, KY 40292
Tel: 502 852-5841 *Fax:* 502 852-1359
E-mail: ecflet01@ulkyvm.louisville.edu
Accred Length: 3 Years *Program Size:* 6
Program ID: 156-20-21-077

Louisiana

New Orleans

Louisiana State University Program
Sponsor: Louisiana State University School of Medicine
Alton Ochsner Medical Foundation
Medical Center of Louisiana at New Orleans
Memorial Medical Center
Program Director:
Karan Omidvari, MD
Louisiana State Univ Med Ctr
Pulm/Critical Care Med
1901 Perdido St/Ste 3205
New Orleans, LA 70112-1393
Tel: 504 568-4634 *Fax:* 504 568-4295
E-mail: komid@lsumc.edu
Accred Length: 3 Years *Program Size:* 8
Program ID: 156-21-21-025

Shreveport

Louisiana State University (Shreveport) Program
Sponsor: Louisiana State University Hospital-Shreveport
Overton Brooks Veterans Affairs Medical Center
Program Director:
Boaz Markewitz, MD
G Douglas Campbell, MD
Louisiana State Univ Med Ctr
Sect of Pulm/Critical Care Med
1501 Kings Hwy
Shreveport, LA 71130-3932
Tel: 318 675-5920 *Fax:* 318 675-5959
E-mail: markewitz.boza@shreveport.va.gov
Accred Length: 3 Years *Program Size:* 6
Program ID: 156-21-31-026

Maine

Portland

Maine Medical Center Program
Sponsor: Maine Medical Center
Program Director:
Stephen A Mette, MD
Maine Med Ctr
22 Bramhall St
Portland, ME 04102-3175
Tel: 207 871-2770 *Fax:* 207 871-4691
Accred Length: 3 Years *Program Size:* 5
Program ID: 156-22-21-027

Maryland

Baltimore

Johns Hopkins University Program
Sponsor: Johns Hopkins University School of Medicine
Johns Hopkins Bayview Medical Center
Johns Hopkins Hospital
Program Director:
Robert Wise, MD
Roy G Brower, MD
Johns Hopkins Univ Sch of Med
Asthma and Allergy Ctr
5501 Hopkins Bayview Cir
Baltimore, MD 21224
Tel: 410 550-0545 *Fax:* 410 550-2612
Accred Length: 3 Years *Program Size:* 22
Program ID: 156-23-21-028

University of Maryland Program
Sponsor: University of Maryland Medical System
Veterans Affairs Medical Center (Baltimore)
Program Director:
Lewis J Rubin, MD
Univ of Maryland
10 S Pine St/Ste 800
Baltimore, MD 21201-1192
Tel: 410 706-3344 *Fax:* 410 706-8162
E-mail: lrubin@umaryland.edu
Accred Length: 3 Years *Program Size:* 8
Program ID: 156-23-21-107

Massachusetts

Boston

Beth Israel Deaconess Medical Center (West Campus) Program

Sponsor: Beth Israel Deaconess Medical Center
Lahey Clinic

Program Director:
Andrew G Villanueva, MD
Lahey Hitchcock Med Ctr
411 Mall Rd
Burlington, MA 01805
Tel: 617 744-8480 *Fax:* 617 744-3443
E-mail: andrew.g.villanueva@lahey.hitchcock.org
Accred Length: 3 Years *Program Size:* 4
Program ID: 156-24-21-029

Boston University Medical Center Program

Sponsor: Boston Medical Center
Veterans Affairs Medical Center (Boston)

Program Director:
Jeffrey S Berman, MD
Pulmonary Ctr/Rm R-304
80 E Concord St
Boston, MA 02118
Tel: 617 638-4860 *Fax:* 617 536-8093
E-mail: jberman@bupula.bu.edu
Accred Length: 3 Years *Program Size:* 19
Program ID: 156-24-21-090

Massachusetts General Hospital Program

Sponsor: Massachusetts General Hospital
Beth Israel Deaconess Medical Center
Brigham and Women's Hospital
Brockton-West Roxbury Veterans Affairs Medical Center

Program Director:
David M Systrom, MD
Massachusetts General Hospital
Pulmonary/Critical Care
55 Fruit St
Boston, MA 02114-2689
Tel: 617 726-3734 *Fax:* 617 724-6954
E-mail: systrom@helix.mgh.harvard.edu
Internet: http://www.mgh.harvard.edu
Accred Length: 3 Years *Program Size:* 12
Program ID: 156-24-21-079

New England Medical Center Hospitals Program

Sponsor: New England Medical Center Hospitals

Program Director:
Leonard Sicilian, MD
New England Med Ctr
Pulm/Critical Care Div #369
750 Washington St
Boston, MA 02111
Tel: 617 636-6382 *Fax:* 617 636-6361
E-mail: leonard.sicilian@es.nemc.org
Accred Length: 3 Years *Program Size:* 10
Program ID: 156-24-21-030

St Elizabeth's Medical Center of Boston Program

Sponsor: St Elizabeth's Medical Center of Boston

Program Director:
Bartolome R Celli, MD
St Elizabeth's Med Ctr
736 Cambridge St
STN 3 P
Boston, MA 02135-2997
Tel: 617 789-2554 *Fax:* 617 562-7756
E-mail: mfarrell@semc.org
Accred Length: 3 Years *Program Size:* 6
Program ID: 156-24-31-031

Michigan

Ann Arbor

University of Michigan Program

Sponsor: University of Michigan Hospitals
Veterans Affairs Medical Center (Ann Arbor)

Program Director:
Marc Peters-Golden, MD
Univ of Michigan
6301 MSRB III
1150 W Medical Center Dr
Ann Arbor, MI 48109-0642
Tel: 734 763-9077 *Fax:* 734 764-4556
E-mail: petersm@umich.edu
Accred Length: 3 Years *Program Size:* 9
Program ID: 156-25-21-032

Detroit

Henry Ford Hospital Program

Sponsor: Henry Ford Hospital

Program Director:
John Popovich Jr, MD
Henry Ford Hospital
2799 W Grand Blvd
Detroit, MI 48202
Tel: 313 876-2428 *Fax:* 313 876-9102
Accred Length: 3 Years *Program Size:* 12
Program ID: 156-25-31-033

Wayne State University/Detroit Medical Center Program

Sponsor: Wayne State University/Detroit Medical Center
Detroit Receiving Hospital and University Health Center
Harper Hospital
Veterans Affairs Medical Center (Detroit)

Program Director:
Basim Dubaybo, MD
Harper Hospital
3 Hudson
3990 John R
Detroit, MI 48201
Tel: 313 745-8471 *Fax:* 313 993-0562
Accred Length: 3 Years *Program Size:* 9
Program ID: 156-25-21-116

Minnesota

Minneapolis

University of Minnesota Program

Sponsor: University of Minnesota Medical School
Fairview-University Medical Center
Hennepin County Medical Center
Regions Hospital
Veterans Affairs Medical Center (Minneapolis)

Program Director:
Peter B Bitterman, MD
Univ of Minnesota
Box 276 F-UMC
420 Delaware Street SE
Minneapolis, MN 55455
Tel: 612 624-0999 *Fax:* 612 625-2174
Internet:
http://www.med.umn.edu/medicine/fel/pulmonary/index.htm
Accred Length: 3 Years *Program Size:* 9
Program ID: 156-26-21-109

Rochester

Mayo Graduate School of Medicine (Rochester) Program

Sponsor: Mayo Graduate School of Medicine-Mayo Foundation
Mayo Clinic (Rochester)
Rochester Methodist Hospital
St Mary's Hospital of Rochester

Program Director:
Andrew H Limper, MD
Application Processing Ctr
Mayo Graduate Sch of Med
200 First St SW/Siebens 5
Rochester, MN 55905
Tel: 507 284-3126 *Fax:* 507 284-0999
E-mail: mgsm.intmed.specialties@mayo.edu
Internet: http://www.mayo.edu/
Accred Length: 3 Years *Program Size:* 12
Program ID: 156-26-21-034

Missouri

Columbia

University of Missouri-Columbia Program

Sponsor: University of Missouri-Columbia School of Medicine
University Hospitals and Clinics

Program Director:
Robert W Lukeman Sr, MD
Univ of Missouri-Columbia
Health Sciences Ctr/MA 417
One Hospital Dr
Columbia, MO 65212
Tel: 573 882-2991 *Fax:* 573 884-4892
E-mail: julie_a._mitchell@muccmail.missouri.edu
Internet:
http://www.hsc.missouri.edu/~internal_medicine/pulm/
Accred Length: 3 Years *Program Size:* 6
Program ID: 156-28-21-035

Kansas City

University of Missouri at Kansas City Program

Sponsor: University of Missouri-Kansas City School of Medicine
Saint Luke's Hospital
Truman Medical Center-West

Program Director:
Gary Salzman, MD
Univ of Missouri-Kansas City Sch of Med
2411 Holmes St
Kansas City, MO 64108
Tel: 816 235-1970 *Fax:* 816 235-5514
E-mail: gsalzman@cctr.umkc.edu
Accred Length: 3 Years *Program Size:* 6
Program ID: 156-28-31-036

St Louis

St Louis University School of Medicine Program
Sponsor: St Louis University School of Medicine
St John's Mercy Medical Center
St Louis University School of Medicine
Program Director:
George M Matuschak, MD
St Louis Univ Sch of Med
3635 Vista Ave/PO Box 15250
Pulmonology/7th Fl
St Louis, MO 63110-0250
Tel: 314 577-8856 *Fax:* 314 577-8859
E-mail: matuscgm@wpogate.slu.edu
Internet: http://www.slu.edu
Accred Length: 3 Years *Program Size:* 6
Program ID: 156-28-12-038

Washington University/B-JH/SLCH Consortium (South Campus) Program
Sponsor: Washington University/B-JH/SLCH Consortium
Barnes-Jewish Hospital
Barnes-Jewish Hospital (North Campus)
Program Director:
Michael J Holtzman, MD
Washington Univ Sch of Med
Box 8052
660 S Euclid Ave
St Louis, MO 63110-1093
Tel: 314 362-0207 *Fax:* 314 362-1334
E-mail: dschuller@pulmonary.wustl.edu
Internet: http://www.pulmonary.wustl.edu
Accred Length: 3 Years *Program Size:* 14
Program ID: 156-28-11-037

Nebraska

Omaha

University of Nebraska Program
Sponsor: University of Nebraska Medical Center
Program Director:
Craig A Piquette, MD MPH
Univ of Nebraska Med Ctr
Pulm/Critical Care Med
985300 Nebraska Med Ctr
Omaha, NE 68198-5300
Tel: 402 346-8800, ext 3817 *Fax:* 402 977-5697
Internet:
http://www.unmc.edu/gme/pumonary-intmed.htm
Accred Length: 3 Years *Program Size:* 4
Program ID: 156-30-21-093

New Hampshire

Lebanon

Dartmouth-Hitchcock Medical Center Program
Sponsor: Mary Hitchcock Memorial Hospital
Veterans Affairs Medical Center (White River Junction)
Program Director:
Donald A Mahler, MD
Dartmouth-Hitchcock Med Ctr
One Medical Center Dr
Lebanon, NH 03756-0001
Tel: 603 650-5533 *Fax:* 603 650-4437
Accred Length: 3 Years *Program Size:* 3
Program ID: 156-32-21-039

New Jersey

Camden

UMDNJ-Robert Wood Johnson Medical School (Camden) Program
Sponsor: Cooper Hospital-University Medical Center
Program Director:
Thaddeus Bartter, MD
UMDNJ-Robert Wood Johnson Med Sch
Three Cooper Plaza/Ste 312
Camden, NJ 08103
Tel: 609 342-2478 *Fax:* 609 541-3968
Accred Length: 3 Years *Program Size:* 3
Program ID: 156-33-21-040

Newark

UMDNJ-New Jersey Medical School Program
Sponsor: UMDNJ-New Jersey Medical School
Hackensack University Medical Center
UMDNJ-University Hospital
Program Director:
Matthew G Marin, MD
UMDNJ-Univ Hospital
150 Bergen St/I-354
Newark, NJ 07103
Tel: 973 972-6111 *Fax:* 973 972-6228
E-mail: marinma@umdnj.edu
Accred Length: 3 Years *Program Size:* 10
Program ID: 156-33-31-041

Piscataway

UMDNJ-Robert Wood Johnson Medical School Program
Sponsor: UMDNJ-Robert Wood Johnson Medical School
Deborah Heart and Lung Center
Robert Wood Johnson University Hospital
St Peter's University Hospital
Veterans Affairs Medical Center (Lyons)
Program Director:
Richard J Strobel, MD
UMDNJ-Robert Wood Johnson Med Sch
MEB 568/PO Box 19
One Robert Wood Johnson Pl
New Brunswick, NJ 08903-0019
Tel: 732 235-7840 *Fax:* 732 235-7048
E-mail: strobel@umdnj.edu
Accred Length: 3 Years *Program Size:* 6
Program ID: 156-33-11-042

New Mexico

Albuquerque

University of New Mexico Program
Sponsor: University of New Mexico School of Medicine
University Hospital
Veterans Affairs Medical Center (Albuquerque)
Program Director:
Helen K Busby, MD MD
Univ of New Mexico, Dept of Int Med
5th Fl Ambulatory Care Ctr
2211 Lomas Blvd NE
Albuquerque, NM 87131-5271
Tel: 505 272-4751 *Fax:* 505 272-8700
E-mail: hbusby@salud.unm.edu
Internet: http://macbeth.unm.edu/som/gme
Accred Length: 3 Years *Program Size:* 3
Program ID: 156-34-21-108

New York

Albany

Albany Medical Center Program
Sponsor: Albany Medical Center
Veterans Affairs Medical Center (Albany)
Program Director:
Anthony L Malanga, MD
Div of Pulm/Critical Care Med
Albany Med Ctr
A-91
Albany, NY 12208
Tel: 518 262-5196 *Fax:* 518 262-6472
Accred Length: 3 Years *Program Size:* 4
Program ID: 156-35-21-043

Bronx

Albert Einstein College of Medicine Program
Sponsor: Albert Einstein College of Medicine of Yeshiva University
Jacobi Medical Center
Montefiore Medical Center-Henry and Lucy Moses Division
Program Director:
Thomas K Aldrich, MD
Montefiore Med Ctr, Pulmonary Div
111 E 210th St
Bronx, NY 10467
Tel: 718 920-6087 *Fax:* 718 652-8384
Accred Length: 3 Years *Program Size:* 10
Program ID: 156-35-21-092

Buffalo

SUNY at Buffalo Graduate Medical-Dental Education Consortium Program
Sponsor: SUNY at Buffalo Grad Medical-Dental Education Consortium
CGF Health System (Buffalo General Hospital)
Erie County Medical Center
Veterans Affairs Medical Center (Buffalo)
Program Director:
Alan T Aquilina, MD
462 Grider St
Buffalo, NY 14215-3021
Tel: 716 898-3199 *Fax:* 716 898-3376
E-mail: aquilina@acsu.buffalo.edu
Internet: http://128.205.200.103/pccm
Accred Length: 3 Years *Program Size:* 6
Program ID: 156-35-31-044

Manhasset

North Shore University Hospital/NYU School of Medicine Program
Sponsor: North Shore University Hospital
Program Director:
Steven Feinsilver, MD
North Shore Univ Hospital
300 Community Dr
Manhasset, NY 11030
Tel: 516 562-4217 *Fax:* 516 562-4908
E-mail: stevenf@nshs.edu
Internet: http://www.nshs.edu
Accred Length: 3 Years *Program Size:* 6
Program ID: 156-35-11-045

Mineola

Winthrop-University Hospital Program

Sponsor: Winthrop-University Hospital

Program Director:
Jonathan S Ilowite, MD
Winthrop-Univ Hospital
222 Station Plaza N
Ste 400
Mineola, NY 11501
Tel: 516 663-2004 *Fax:* 516 663-4888
Accred Length: 3 Years *Program Size:* 7
Program ID: 156-35-12-046

New Hyde Park

Albert Einstein College of Medicine at Long Island Jewish Medical Center Program

Sponsor: Long Island Jewish Medical Center

Program Director:
Harry N Steinberg, MD
Long Island Jewish Med Ctr
270-05 76th Ave
New Hyde Park, NY 11040
Tel: 718 470-7231 *Fax:* 718 470-1035
Internet: http://www.lij.edu.lij-homepage-ns.html
Accred Length: 3 Years *Program Size:* 6
Program ID: 156-35-13-047

New York

Albert Einstein College of Medicine at Beth Israel Medical Center Program

Sponsor: Beth Israel Medical Center

Program Director:
Roslyn F Schneider, MD
Beth Israel Med Ctr
Pulm/Critical Care
First Ave at 16th St
New York, NY 10003
Tel: 212 420-2697 *Fax:* 212 420-4684
E-mail: rscheider@bethisraelny.org
Accred Length: 3 Years *Program Size:* 7
Program ID: 156-35-22-048

Mount Sinai School of Medicine Program

Sponsor: Mount Sinai School of Medicine
Mount Sinai Medical Center
Queens Hospital Center
Veterans Affairs Medical Center (Bronx)

Program Director:
Alvin S Teirstein, MD
Mount Sinai Med Ctr
One Gustave L Levy Pl
Box 1232
New York, NY 10029
Tel: 212 241-5900 *Fax:* 212 987-5584
Accred Length: 3 Years *Program Size:* 13
Program ID: 156-35-23-049

New York and Presbyterian Hospital (Cornell Campus) Program

Sponsor: New York and Presbyterian Hospital
New York and Presbyterian Hospital (Cornell Campus)

Program Director:
Ronald G Crystal, MD
New York Hospital-Cornell Med Ctr
Div of Pulmonary/Critical Care Med
525 E 68th St/Box 96 Starr 505
New York, NY 10021
Tel: 212 746-2250 *Fax:* 212 746-8808
Accred Length: 3 Years *Program Size:* 9
Program ID: 156-35-21-083

New York Medical College at St Vincent's Hospital and Medical Center of New York Program

Sponsor: New York Medical College
St Vincent's Hospital and Medical Center of New York

Program Director:
Patricia A Tietjen, MD
St Vincent's Hospital and Med Ctr
153 W 11th St
New York, NY 10011
Tel: 212 604-2757 *Fax:* 212 604-3667
Internet: http://svh.nymc.edu
Accred Length: 3 Years *Program Size:* 4
Program ID: 156-35-11-052

New York University Medical Center Program

Sponsor: New York University Medical Center
Bellevue Hospital Center
Veterans Affairs Medical Center (Manhattan)

Program Director:
William N Rom, MD
New York Univ Med Ctr
550 First Ave/7N24
New York, NY 10016
Tel: 212 263-6479 *Fax:* 212 263-8442
E-mail: romwo1@gcrc.med.nyu.edu
Accred Length: 3 Years *Program Size:* 15
Program ID: 156-35-21-050

St Luke's-Roosevelt Hospital Center Program

Sponsor: St Luke's-Roosevelt Hospital Center
St Luke's-Roosevelt Hospital Center-St Luke's Division

Program Director:
C Redington Barrett Jr, MD
St Luke's-Roosevelt Hospital Ctr
1111 Amsterdam Ave
New York, NY 10025
Tel: 212 523-3610 *Fax:* 212 523-3609
Accred Length: 3 Years *Program Size:* 6
Program ID: 156-35-31-051

Rochester

University of Rochester Program

Sponsor: Strong Memorial Hospital of the University of Rochester

Program Director:
Mark W Frampton, MD
Univ of Rochester Med Ctr
Pulmonary/Critical Care Unit
601 Elmwood Ave/Box 692
Rochester, NY 14642-8692
Tel: 716 275-4861 *Fax:* 716 273-1058
E-mail: mark_frampton@urmc.rochester.edu
Internet: http://www.urmc.rochester.edu/smd/pulmcc/
Accred Length: 3 Years *Program Size:* 6
Program ID: 156-35-31-099

Stony Brook

SUNY at Stony Brook Program

Sponsor: University Hospital-SUNY at Stony Brook
Veterans Affairs Medical Center (Northport)

Program Director:
Hussein D Foda, MD
SUNY-Stony Brook Health Science Ctr
HSC 17-040
Stony Brook, NY 11794-8172
Tel: 516 444-1776 *Fax:* 516 444-7502
E-mail: hfoda@mail.som.sunysb.edu
Accred Length: 3 Years *Program Size:* 6
Program ID: 156-35-21-106

Syracuse

SUNY Health Science Center at Syracuse Program

Sponsor: University Hospital-SUNY Health Science Center at Syracuse
Veterans Affairs Medical Center (Syracuse)

Program Director:
Edward Sivak, MD
SUNY Health Science Ctr
750 E Adams St
Syracuse, NY 13210
Tel: 315 464-4184 *Fax:* 315 464-5400
Accred Length: 3 Years *Program Size:* 4
Program ID: 156-35-12-053

Valhalla

New York Medical College at Westchester Medical Center Program

Sponsor: New York Medical College
Metropolitan Hospital Center
Westchester Medical Center

Program Director:
George P Maguire, MD
New York Med Coll
Westchester Med Ctr
Pulmonary Lab/Macy Pavilion
Valhalla, NY 10595
Tel: 914 493-7518 *Fax:* 914 493-8130
Accred Length: 3 Years *Program Size:* 7
Program ID: 156-35-13-054

North Carolina

Chapel Hill

University of North Carolina Hospitals Program

Sponsor: University of North Carolina Hospitals

Program Director:
James R Yankaskas, MD
7011 Thurston-Bowles Bldg/CB7248
Univ of North Carolina Sch of Med
Chapel Hill, NC 27599-7248
Tel: 919 966-1077 *Fax:* 919 966-7524
E-mail: pwsjry@med.unc.edu
Accred Length: 3 Years *Program Size:* 9
Program ID: 156-36-21-055

Durham

Duke University Program

Sponsor: Duke University Medical Center
Veterans Affairs Medical Center (Durham)

Program Director:
William Fulkerson, MD
Box 3121
Durham, NC 27710
Tel: 919 681-5850 *Fax:* 919 681-8951
E-mail: fulker003@mc.duke.edu
Internet: http://rheal.mc.duke.edu/
Accred Length: 3 Years *Program Size:* 13
Program ID: 156-36-21-117

Winston-Salem

Wake Forest University School of Medicine Program

Sponsor: Wake Forest University Baptist Medical Center

Program Director:
Edward Haponik, MD
Medical Center Blvd
Winston-Salem, NC 27157-1054
Tel: 336 716-4409 *Fax:* 336 716-7277
Accred Length: 3 Years *Program Size:* 3
Program ID: 156-36-21-094

Ohio

Cincinnati

University Hospital/University of Cincinnati College of Medicine Program

Sponsor: University Hospital Inc
Veterans Affairs Medical Center (Cincinnati)

Program Director:
Stephen B Liggett, MD
Univ of Cincinnati Med Ctr
PO Box 670564
Cincinnati, OH 45267-0564
Tel: 513 558-0477 *Fax:* 513 558-4858
E-mail: mary.rosensweet@uc.edu
Internet: http://www.pulmonary.med.uc.edu
Accred Length: 3 Years *Program Size:* 6
Program ID: 156-38-21-056

Cleveland

Case Western Reserve University (MetroHealth) Program

Sponsor: MetroHealth Medical Center

Program Director:
Gerald Supinski, MD
MetroHealth Med Ctr
2500 MetroHealth Dr
Cleveland, OH 44109
Tel: 216 778-2362 *Fax:* 216 778-8215
Accred Length: 3 Years *Program Size:* 3
Program ID: 156-38-31-057

Case Western Reserve University Program

Sponsor: University Hospitals of Cleveland
MetroHealth Medical Center
Veterans Affairs Medical Center (Cleveland)

Program Director:
E Regis McFadden Jr, MD
Div of Pulm/Critical Care Med
Univ Hospitals of Cleveland
11100 Euclid Ave
Cleveland, OH 44106-5067
Tel: 216 844-8668 *Fax:* 216 844-3226
E-mail: clt4@po.cwru.edu
Accred Length: 3 Years *Program Size:* 8
Program ID: 156-38-21-110

Cleveland Clinic Foundation Program

Sponsor: Cleveland Clinic Foundation

Program Director:
Alejandro C Arroliga, MD
Cleveland Clinic Foundation
Dept of Pulmonary/Critical Care G62
9500 Euclid Ave
Cleveland, OH 44195-5242
Tel: 216 444-5690 *Fax:* 216 444-1162
E-mail: meded@cesmtp.ccf.org
Internet: http://www.ccf.org
Accred Length: 3 Years *Program Size:* 10
Program ID: 156-38-11-058

Columbus

Ohio State University Program

Sponsor: Ohio State University Medical Center

Program Director:
Eric R Pacht, MD
N325 Means Hall
1654 Upham Dr
Columbus, OH 43210-1228
Tel: 614 293-4925 *Fax:* 614 293-4799
Accred Length: 3 Years *Program Size:* 6
Program ID: 156-38-12-059

Oklahoma

Oklahoma City

University of Oklahoma Health Sciences Center Program

Sponsor: University of Oklahoma College of Medicine
University Hospital
Veterans Affairs Medical Center (Oklahoma City)

Program Director:
Jerry D Leu, MD
Univ of Oklahoma Health Sciences Ctr
PO Box 26901
WP 1310
Oklahoma City, OK 73190
Tel: 405 271-6173 *Fax:* 405 297-5974
E-mail: jerry-leu@ouhsc.edu
Accred Length: 3 Years *Program Size:* 6
Program ID: 156-39-21-060

Oregon

Portland

Oregon Health Sciences University Program

Sponsor: Oregon Health Sciences University Hospital
Veterans Affairs Medical Center (Portland)

Program Director:
Mark E Deffebach, MD
3181 SW Sam Jackson Park Rd
Portland, OR 97201-3098
Tel: 503 494-7680 *Fax:* 503 494-6670
Accred Length: 3 Years *Program Size:* 3
Program ID: 156-40-21-061

Pennsylvania

Philadelphia

MCP Hahnemann University Program

Sponsor: MCP Hahnemann University
Hahnemann University Hospital
Medical College of Pennsylvania Hospital

Program Director:
Michael S Sherman, MD
Hahnemann Univ Hospital
Broad and Vine Sts/MS 107
Philadelphia, PA 19102-1192
Tel: 215 762-7013 *Fax:* 215 762-8728
Accred Length: 3 Years *Program Size:* 13
Program ID: 156-41-21-062

Temple University Program

Sponsor: Temple University Hospital
Albert Einstein Medical Center

Program Director:
Gilbert E D'Alonzo, DO
Temple Univ Hospital
3401 N Broad St
9th Fl Parkinson Pavilion
Philadelphia, PA 19140
Tel: 215 707-3332 *Fax:* 215 707-6867
E-mail: gdalonzo@nimbus.ocis.temple.edu
Internet: http://www.temple.edu/pulmonary/
Accred Length: 3 Years *Program Size:* 7
Program ID: 156-41-11-064

Thomas Jefferson University Program

Sponsor: Thomas Jefferson University Hospital
Temple University Hospital

Program Director:
James G Zangrilli, MD
James E Fish, MD
Thomas Jefferson Univ
Rm 805 College
1025 Walnut St
Philadelphia, PA 19107-5083
Tel: 215 955-6591 *Fax:* 215 955-0830
E-mail: james.zangrilli@mail.tju.edu
Accred Length: 3 Years *Program Size:* 8
Program ID: 156-41-12-065

University of Pennsylvania Program

Sponsor: Hospital of the University of Pennsylvania

Program Director:
Robert M Kotloff, MD
Hospital of Univ of Pennsylvania
838 W Gates
3400 Spruce St
Philadelphia, PA 19104-4283
Tel: 215 349-5488 *Fax:* 215 349-5172
E-mail: kotloff@mail.med.upenn.edu
Internet:
http://www.med.upenn.edu/lungctr/academic_programs/pulmonary/
Accred Length: 3 Years *Program Size:* 18
Program ID: 156-41-21-088

Pittsburgh

University Health Center of Pittsburgh Program

Sponsor: University Health Center of Pittsburgh
Presbyterian University Hospital/UPMC
Veterans Affairs Medical Center (Pittsburgh)

Program Director:
Michael P Donahoe, MD
440 Scaife Hall
3550 Terrace St
Pittsburgh, PA 15261
Tel: 412 648-9350 *Fax:* 412 648-9203
E-mail: donahoem@msx.upmc.edu
Accred Length: 3 Years *Program Size:* 9
Program ID: 156-41-13-066

South Carolina

Charleston

Medical University of South Carolina Program

Sponsor: Medical University of South Carolina College of Medicine
Charleston Memorial Hospital
MUSC Medical Center
Ralph H Johnson Dept of Veterans Affairs Med Center
Program Director:
Steven A Sahn, MD
Med Univ of South Carolina
600 MUSC Complex/Ste 812
Charleston, SC 29425
Tel: 803 792-0492 *Fax:* 803 792-0732
Accred Length: 3 Years *Program Size:* 8
Program ID: 156-45-21-067

Tennessee

Nashville

Vanderbilt University Program

Sponsor: Vanderbilt University Medical Center
Veterans Affairs Medical Center (Nashville)
Program Director:
Arthur P Wheeler, MD
Ctr for Lung Research
T-1217 Med Ctr N
Nashville, TN 37232-2650
Tel: 615 322-3412 *Fax:* 615 343-7448
Accred Length: 3 Years *Program Size:* 11
Program ID: 156-47-21-068

Texas

Dallas

University of Texas Southwestern Medical School Program

Sponsor: University of Texas Southwestern Medical School
Dallas County Hospital District-Parkland Memorial Hospital
Veterans Affairs Medical Center (Dallas)
Program Director:
W D Pitcher, MD
Pulmonary/Critical Care Div
5323 Harry Hines Blvd
Dallas, TX 75235-9034
Tel: 214 648-3429 *Fax:* 214 648-2283
E-mail: ncampb@mednet.swmed.edu
Accred Length: 3 Years *Program Size:* 7
Program ID: 156-48-21-069

Fort Sam Houston

San Antonio Uniformed Services Health Education Consortium (BAMC) Program

Sponsor: San Antonio Uniformed Services Health Education Consortium
Brooke Army Medical Center
Program Director:
Daniel R Ouellette, MD
Pulmonary Disease Service
Brooke Army Med Ctr
3851 Roger Brooke Dr
Fort Sam Houston, TX 78234-6200
Tel: 210 916-1136 *Fax:* 210 916-0709
E-mail: ouellette@iname.com
Accred Length: 3 Years *Program Size:* 6
Program ID: 156-48-21-070
US Armed Services Program

Galveston

University of Texas Medical Branch Hospitals Program

Sponsor: University of Texas Medical Branch Hospitals
Program Director:
Victor J Cardenas Jr, MD
Univ of Texas Med Branch
Div of Pulmonary/Critical Care Med
301 University Blvd
Galveston, TX 77555-0561
Tel: 409 772-2436 *Fax:* 409 772-9539
E-mail: vcardena@utmb.edu
Internet: http://www.utmb.edu
Accred Length: 3 Years *Program Size:* 6
Program ID: 156-48-21-112

Houston

Baylor College of Medicine Program

Sponsor: Baylor College of Medicine
Harris County Hospital District-Ben Taub General Hospital
Methodist Hospital
Veterans Affairs Medical Center (Houston)
Program Director:
Joseph R Rodarte, MD
6550 Fannin St/SM 1225
Houston, TX 77030
Tel: 713 790-6218 *Fax:* 713 790-3648
E-mail: rodarte@bcm.tmc.edu
Internet: http://www.bcm.tmc.edu/medicine/pulmonary
Accred Length: 3 Years *Program Size:* 20
Program ID: 156-48-21-084

University of Texas at Houston Program

Sponsor: University of Texas Medical School at Houston
Memorial Hermann Healthcare System
University of Texas M D Anderson Cancer Center
Program Director:
David E Taylor, MD
Univ of Texas-Houston Med Sch
6431 Fannin St/Ste 1274
Houston, TX 77030
Tel: 713 500-6828 *Fax:* 713 500-6829
E-mail: dtaylor@heart.med.uth.tmc.edu
Internet:
http://www.uth.tmc.edu/schools/med/imed/pulmo/fellow.htm
Accred Length: 3 Years *Program Size:* 7
Program ID: 156-48-31-071

Lackland AFB

San Antonio Uniformed Services Health Education Consortium (WHMC) Program

Sponsor: San Antonio Uniformed Services Health Education Consortium
Wilford Hall Medical Center (AETC)
Program Director:
Stephen Derdak, DO
2200 Bergquist Dr
Ste1-PSMP
Lackland AFB, TX 78236-5300
Tel: 210 292-5235 *Fax:* 210 292-6180
E-mail: derdak_s@whmc-lafb.af.mil
Accred Length: 3 Years *Program Size:* 6
Program ID: 156-48-21-095
US Armed Services Program

San Antonio

University of Texas Health Science Center at San Antonio Program

Sponsor: University of Texas Medical School at San Antonio
Audie L Murphy Memorial Veterans Hospital (San Antonio)
University Hospital-South Texas Medical Center
Program Director:
Jay Peters, MD
Univ of Texas Health Science Ctr
Pulm/Critical Care
7703 Floyd Curl Dr
San Antonio, TX 78284-7885
Tel: 210 617-5256 *Fax:* 210 567-6677
E-mail: peters@uthscsa.edu
Accred Length: 3 Years *Program Size:* 6
Program ID: 156-48-11-072

Utah

Salt Lake City

University of Utah Program

Sponsor: University of Utah Medical Center
Program Director:
John R Hoidal, MD
Univ of Utah Health Sciences Ctr
50 N Medical Dr
701 MWB
Salt Lake City, UT 84132-0001
Tel: 801 581-7806 *Fax:* 801 585-3355
E-mail: jhoidal@med.utah.edu
Internet: http://www.med.utah.edu/pulm/pulm.html
Accred Length: 3 Years *Program Size:* 12
Program ID: 156-49-21-089

Vermont

Burlington

University of Vermont Program

Sponsor: Fletcher Allen Health Care
Program Director:
Thomas Bouder, MD
Univ of Vermont Coll of Med
Pulmonary Dis/Critical Care Med
C317 Given Bldg
Burlington, VT 05405-0068
Tel: 802 656-2182 *Fax:* 802 656-3854
E-mail: pulmonary@vtmednet.org
Internet: http://www.vtmednet.org/~p159517/units.html
Accred Length: 3 Years *Program Size:* 6
Program ID: 156-50-21-111

Programs

Virginia

Charlottesville

University of Virginia Program
Sponsor: University of Virginia Medical Center
Program Director:
Sharon A Esau, MD
Univ of Virginia Health Systems
Box 546
Charlottesville, VA 22908-0001
Tel: 804 924-5210 *Fax:* 804 924-9682
E-mail: ilg@virginia.edu
Accred Length: 3 Years *Program Size:* 2
Program ID: 156-51-21-085

Richmond

Medical College of Virginia/Virginia Commonwealth University Program
Sponsor: Medical College of Virginia/Virginia Commonwealth University
Hunter Holmes McGuire VA Medical Center (Richmond)
Medical College of Virginia Hospitals
Program Director:
Kevin R Cooper, MD
Med Coll of Virginia, Div of Pulm/Critical Care Med
1200 E Broad St
PO Box 980050
Richmond, VA 23298-0050
Tel: 804 828-9071 *Fax:* 804 828-2578
E-mail: csmith@hsc.vcu.edu
Accred Length: 3 Years *Program Size:* 5
Program ID: 156-51-21-073

Washington

Seattle

University of Washington Program
Sponsor: University of Washington School of Medicine
University of Washington Medical Center
Program Director:
Leonard D Hudson, MD
Harborview Med Ctr
325 Ninth Ave/Box 359762
Seattle, WA 98104
Tel: 206 731-8483 *Fax:* 206 731-8584
E-mail: kathleen@colossus.pulmcc.washington.edu
Internet: http://www.u.washington.edu/~pulmcc
Accred Length: 3 Years *Program Size:* 17
Program ID: 156-54-21-074

West Virginia

Morgantown

West Virginia University Program
Sponsor: West Virginia University Hospitals
Program Director:
Daniel E Banks, MD
PO Box 9166
West Virginia Univ Sch of Med
Morgantown, WV 26506-9166
Tel: 304 293-4661 *Fax:* 304 293-3724
E-mail: dbanks@wvu.edu
Accred Length: 3 Years *Program Size:* 4
Program ID: 156-55-21-075

Wisconsin

Madison

University of Wisconsin Program
Sponsor: University of Wisconsin Hospital and Clinics
William S Middleton Veterans Hospital
Program Director:
Kenneth E Wood, DO
Univ of Wisconsin Hospital and Clinics
600 Highland Ave
H6-380
Madison, WI 53792-3240
Tel: 608 263-3035 *Fax:* 608 263-3104
E-mail: kew@medicine.wisc.edu
Internet: http://www.medicine.wisc.edu/sections/pulm/
Accred Length: 3 Years *Program Size:* 6
Program ID: 156-56-21-076

Milwaukee

Medical College of Wisconsin Program
Sponsor: Medical College of Wisconsin Affiliated Hospitals Inc
Clement J Zablocki Veterans Affairs Medical Center
Froedtert Memorial Lutheran Hospital
Program Director:
Richard M Effros, MD
Med Coll of Wisconsin
Pulm/Critical Care Med
9200 W Wisconsin Ave
Milwaukee, WI 53226
Tel: 414 454-5260 *Fax:* 414 259-1499
E-mail: effros@mcw.edu
Accred Length: 3 Years *Program Size:* 7
Program ID: 156-56-21-100

Radiation Oncology

Alabama

Birmingham

University of Alabama Medical Center Program
Sponsor: University of Alabama Hospital
Veterans Affairs Medical Center (Birmingham)
Program Director:
James Bonner, MD
Univ of Alabama
619 S 19th St
Birmingham, AL 35233-6832
Tel: 205 934-2760 *Fax:* 205 975-6161
Accred Length: 4 Years *Program Size:* 4
Program ID: 430-01-21-002

Arizona

Tucson

University of Arizona Program
Sponsor: University of Arizona College of Medicine
University Medical Center
Program Director:
John M Anderson, MD PHD
Univ of Arizona Coll of Med
Rad Oncology Dept
PO Box 245081
Tucson, AZ 85724-5081
Tel: 520 626-6724 *Fax:* 520 626-3141
E-mail: janderson@azcc.arizona.edu
Accred Length: 4 Years *Program Size:* 4
Program ID: 430-03-11-003

California

Loma Linda

Loma Linda University Program
Sponsor: Loma Linda University Medical Center
Program Director:
Leslie T Yonemoto, MD
Loma Linda Univ Med Ctr
11234 Anderson St/Rm B121
Loma Linda, CA 92354
Tel: 909 824-4257 *Fax:* 909 824-4083
Accred Length: 4 Years *Program Size:* 5
Program ID: 430-05-21-006

Los Angeles

Southern California Kaiser Permanente Medical Care (Los Angeles) Program
Sponsor: Southern California Kaiser Permanente Medical Group
Kaiser Foundation Hospital (Los Angeles)
Program Director:
Aroor R Rao, MD
Kaiser Permanente Med Care
393 E Walnut St
Pasadena, CA 91188-8013
Tel: 800 541-7946 *Fax:* 213 783-5927
Accred Length: 4 Years *Program Size:* 5
Program ID: 430-05-21-115

UCLA Medical Center Program
Sponsor: UCLA School of Medicine
UCLA Medical Center
VA Greater Los Angeles Healthcare System
Program Director:
Michael T Selch, MD
Dept of Rad Oncology
200 UCLA Med Plaza/Ste B265
Box 956951
Los Angeles, CA 90095-6951
Tel: 310 825-4966 *Fax:* 310 794-9795
E-mail: selch@radonc.ucla.edu
Internet:
http://www.radonc.ucla.edu/rowww/rohome.html
Accred Length: 4 Years *Program Size:* 5
Program ID: 430-05-21-008

University of Southern California Program
Sponsor: Los Angeles County-USC Medical Center
Kenneth Norris Jr Cancer Hospital and Research Institute
Program Director:
Vaclav Klement, MD PhD
Univ of Southern California Sch of Med
Dept of Rad Oncology
1441 Eastlake Ave/NOR G355
Los Angeles, CA 90033-0804
Tel: 323 865-3092 *Fax:* 323 865-3037
E-mail: thsu@hsc.usc.edu
Internet: http://norm28.hsc.usc.edu/uscradonc.html
Accred Length: 4 Years *Program Size:* 5
Program ID: 430-05-11-007

Orange

University of California (Irvine) Program
Sponsor: University of California (Irvine) Medical Center
City of Hope National Medical Center
Long Beach Memorial Medical Center
Veterans Affairs Medical Center (Long Beach)
Program Director:
Nilam S Ramsinghani, MD
Univ of California Irvine Med Ctr
Dept of Rad Onc/Bldg 23 Rte 26
101 The City Dr S
Orange, CA 92868
Tel: 714 456-5508 *Fax:* 714 456-7170
E-mail: nsramsin@uci.edu
Accred Length: 4 Years *Program Size:* 5
Program ID: 430-05-21-005

San Francisco

St Mary's Hospital and Medical Center Program
Sponsor: St Mary's Hospital and Medical Center
Seton Medical Center
Program Director:
John L Meyer, MD
St Mary's Hospital and Med Ctr
Dept of Rad Oncology
450 Stanyan St
San Francisco, CA 94117
Tel: 415 775-4321 *Fax:* 415 750-4831
Accred Length: 4 Years *Program Size:* 3
Program ID: 430-05-22-012

University of California (San Francisco) Program
Sponsor: University of California (San Francisco) School of Medicine
Mount Zion Medical Center of the University of California
University of California (Davis) Medical Center
University of California (San Francisco) Medical Center
Program Director:
David A Larson, MD PHD
Long Hospital
Dept of Rad Oncology/Rm L75
San Francisco, CA 94143-0226
Tel: 415 476-4815 *Fax:* 415 476-9069
Internet: http://itsa.ucsf.edu/~radonc/index.html
Accred Length: 4 Years *Program Size:* 8
Program ID: 430-05-21-013

Stanford

Stanford University Program
Sponsor: Stanford University Hospital
Program Director:
Joseph C Poen, MD
Stanford Univ Med Ctr, Dept of Radiation
300 Pasteur Dr
Stanford, CA 94305
Tel: 650 723-2107 *Fax:* 650 725-8231
E-mail: poen@reyes.stanford.edu
Internet: http://www.-radonc.stanford.edu
Accred Length: 4 Years *Program Size:* 11
Program ID: 430-05-11-014

Connecticut

New Haven

Yale-New Haven Medical Center Program
Sponsor: Yale-New Haven Hospital
Uncas on Thames Hospital
Program Director:
Bruce G Haffty, MD
Yale-New Haven Hospital
20 York St
New Haven, CT 06504
Tel: 203 785-2959 *Fax:* 203 785-4622
E-mail: bruce.haffty@yale.edu
Internet:
http://info.med.yale.edu/therarad/train_prog.html#resident
Accred Length: 4 Years *Program Size:* 6
Program ID: 430-08-11-017

District of Columbia

Washington

Georgetown University Program
Sponsor: Georgetown University Medical Center
Program Director:
K William Harter, MD
Georgetown Univ Med Ctr
Dept of Radiation Med
3800 Reservoir Rd NW
Washington, DC 20007-2197
Tel: 202 784-3320 *Fax:* 202 784-3323
Accred Length: 4 Years *Program Size:* 4
Program ID: 430-10-21-112

Howard University Program
Sponsor: Howard University Hospital
Program Director:
Olubunmi K Abayomi, MD
Howard Univ Hospital, Dept of Rad Oncology
2041 Georgia Ave NW
Washington, DC 20060
Tel: 202 865-1421 *Fax:* 202 865-1723
Accred Length: 4 Years *Program Size:* 5
Program ID: 430-10-11-021

Florida

Gainesville

University of Florida Program
Sponsor: University of Florida College of Medicine
Shands Hospital at the University of Florida
Program Director:
Robert B Marcus Jr, MD
Dept of Rad Oncology
Shands Cancer Ctr
PO Box 100385
Gainesville, FL 32610-0385
Tel: 904 395-0287 *Fax:* 904 395-0546
Accred Length: 4 Years *Program Size:* 8
Program ID: 430-11-12-022

Miami

University of Miami-Jackson Memorial Medical Center Program
Sponsor: University of Miami-Jackson Memorial Medical Center
Program Director:
Aaron H Wolfson, MD
Dept of Rad Oncology
Sylvester Comprehensive Cancer Ctr
PO Box 016960 (D-31)
Miami, FL 33101
Tel: 305 243-4210 *Fax:* 305 243-4363
Internet: http://www.radonc.miami.med.edu
Accred Length: 4 Years *Program Size:* 5
Program ID: 430-11-21-023

Georgia

Atlanta

Emory University Program
Sponsor: Emory University School of Medicine
Crawford Long Hospital of Emory University
Grady Memorial Hospital
Veterans Affairs Medical Center (Atlanta)
Program Director:
Karen D Godette, MD
Emory Univ Sch of Med
Dept of Rad Oncology
1365 Clifton Rd NE
Atlanta, GA 30322
Tel: 404 778-4763 *Fax:* 404 778-5152
Accred Length: 4 Years *Program Size:* 8
Program ID: 430-12-21-125

Programs

Illinois

Chicago

McGaw Medical Center of Northwestern University Program

Sponsor: Northwestern University Medical School
Evanston Hospital
Northwestern Memorial Hospital

Program Director:
Maryanne H Marymont, MD
Dept of Rad Oncology
Rm 44/Wesley Pavilion
250 E Superior St
Chicago, IL 60611
Tel: 312 908-2520 *Fax:* 312 908-6374
E-mail: mmarymon@nmh.org
Accred Length: 4 Years *Program Size:* 4
Program ID: 430-16-21-027

Rush-Presbyterian-St Luke's Medical Center Program

Sponsor: Rush-Presbyterian-St Luke's Medical Center

Program Director:
Shalina Gupta-Burt, MD
Rush-Presbyterian-St Luke's Med Ctr
1653 W Congress Pkwy
Atrium Bldg
Chicago, IL 60612
Tel: 312 942-5751, ext 29226 *Fax:* 312 942-2339
E-mail: sburt@therad.rpslmc.edu
Internet:
http://www.eve.therad.rpslmc.edu/gmep/gmep.html
Accred Length: 4 Years *Program Size:* 7
Program ID: 430-16-11-028

University of Chicago/Michael Reese Program

Sponsor: University of Chicago Hospitals
Michael Reese Hospital and Medical Center

Program Director:
Srinivasan Vijayakumar, MD
Univ of Chicago
5758 S Maryland Ave/MC9006
Chicago, IL 60637-1470
Tel: 773 702-6819 *Fax:* 773 702-0610
Internet: http://www.radonc.uchicago.edu/resporg/
Accred Length: 4 Years *Program Size:* 12
Program ID: 430-16-11-116

Maywood

Loyola University Program

Sponsor: Loyola University Medical Center
Edward J Hines Jr Veterans Affairs Hospital

Program Director:
Bahman Emami, MD
Loyola Univ Med Ctr Dept of Radiorapy
2160 S First Ave
Hines 114B
Maywood, IL 60153
Tel: 708 216-2649 *Fax:* 708 216-2647
Internet:
http://www.lumc.edu/lumc/patcar/clinserv/csradioth.htm
Accred Length: 4 Years *Program Size:* 5
Program ID: 430-16-22-031

Indiana

Indianapolis

Indiana University School of Medicine Program

Sponsor: Indiana University School of Medicine
Clarian IU Hospital
Clarian Riley Hospital for Children
Richard L Roudebush Veterans Affairs Medical Center
William N Wishard Memorial Hospital

Program Director:
Mark P Langer, MD
Indiana Univ Sch of Med
Dept of Rad Oncology
535 Barnhill Dr/RT 041
Indianapolis, IN 46202-5289
Tel: 317 274-1315 *Fax:* 317 274-2486
E-mail: cspring@radonc.uh.iupui.edu
Internet: http://www.radonc.iupui.edu
Accred Length: 4 Years *Program Size:* 5
Program ID: 430-17-11-032

Iowa

Iowa City

University of Iowa Hospitals and Clinics Program

Sponsor: University of Iowa Hospitals and Clinics

Program Director:
David H Hussey, MD
Univ of Iowa Hospitals and Clinics
Dept of Radiology
200 Hawkins Dr
Iowa City, IA 52242-1009
Tel: 319 356-2699 *Fax:* 319 356-1530
E-mail: david-hussey@uiowa.edu
Accred Length: 4 Years *Program Size:* 4
Program ID: 430-18-11-033

Kansas

Kansas City

University of Kansas Medical Center Program

Sponsor: University of Kansas School of Medicine
University of Kansas Medical Center

Program Director:
Leela Krishnan, MD
Univ of Kansas Med Ctr
3901 Rainbow Blvd
Kansas City, KS 66160-7321
Tel: 913 588-3609 *Fax:* 913 588-3663
E-mail: lkrishna@kumc.edu
Accred Length: 4 Years *Program Size:* 4
Program ID: 430-19-21-034

Kentucky

Lexington

University of Kentucky Medical Center Program

Sponsor: University of Kentucky Hospital

Program Director:
Pushpa Patel, MD
Univ of Kentucky
Dept of Radiation Med
800 Rose St
Lexington, KY 40536-0084
Tel: 606 323-6880 *Fax:* 606 257-4931
E-mail: ppate@pop.uky.edu
Accred Length: 4 Years *Program Size:* 5
Program ID: 430-20-11-035

Louisville

University of Louisville Program

Sponsor: University of Louisville School of Medicine
University of Louisville Hospital

Program Director:
Kristie J Paris, MD
Brown Cancer Ctr
529 S Jackson St
Louisville, KY 40292
Tel: 502 852-7171 *Fax:* 502 852-7760
E-mail: kjp@bcc.louisville.edu
Internet: http://bcc.louisville.edu
Accred Length: 4 Years *Program Size:* 5
Program ID: 430-20-11-036

Maryland

Baltimore

Johns Hopkins University Program

Sponsor: Johns Hopkins University School of Medicine
Johns Hopkins Hospital

Program Director:
Ding-Jen Lee, MD PhD
Johns Hopkins Hospital
600 N Wolfe St
Baltimore, MD 21287-8922
Tel: 410 955-8062 *Fax:* 410 955-3691
E-mail: leedj@welchlink.welch.jhu.edu
Accred Length: 4 Years *Program Size:* 7
Program ID: 430-23-11-039

University of Maryland Program

Sponsor: University of Maryland Medical System

Program Director:
Andrew Kennedy, MD
Univ of Maryland Med System
Dept of Rad Oncology
22 S Greene St
Baltimore, MD 21201-1595
Tel: 410 328-2328 *Fax:* 410 328-5279
Accred Length: 4 Years *Program Size:* 6
Program ID: 430-23-21-040

Bethesda

National Capital Consortium Program
Sponsor: National Capital Consortium
National Cancer Institute
National Naval Medical Center (Bethesda)
Walter Reed Army Medical Center

Program Director:
Rosemary M Altemus, MD
National Cancer Institute/NIH
9000 Rockville Pike
Bldg 10 Rm B3B69
Bethesda, MD 20892
Tel: 301 496-5457 *Fax:* 301 480-5439
Accred Length: 4 Years *Program Size:* 6
Program ID: 430-10-21-113
US Armed Services Program

Massachusetts

Boston

Joint Center for Radiation Therapy Program
Sponsor: Joint Center for Radiation Therapy
Beth Israel Deaconess Medical Center
Brigham and Women's Hospital
Children's Hospital
Dana-Farber Cancer Institute

Program Director:
Jay R Harris, MD
Joint Ctr for Radiation Therapy
330 Brookline Ave
Boston, MA 02215
Tel: 617 667-9550 *Fax:* 617 667-9551
E-mail: rmurphy@jcrt.harvard.edu
Internet: http://www.jcrt.harvard.edu/jcrt/
Accred Length: 4 Years *Program Size:* 13
Program ID: 430-24-21-042

Massachusetts General Hospital Program
Sponsor: Massachusetts General Hospital

Program Director:
Anthony L Zietman, MD
Massachusetts General Hospital
100 Blossom St
Cox 3
Boston, MA 02114
Tel: 617 724-1158 *Fax:* 617 726-3603
Internet: http://www.mgh.harvard.edu
Accred Length: 4 Years *Program Size:* 11
Program ID: 430-24-31-043

Tufts University Program
Sponsor: New England Medical Center Hospitals
Veterans Affairs Medical Center (Boston)

Program Director:
David E Wazer, MD
New England Med Ctr
750 Washington St
Boston, MA 02111
Tel: 617 636-7673 *Fax:* 617 636-4513
E-mail: david.wazer@es.nemc.org
Accred Length: 4 Years *Program Size:* 8
Program ID: 430-24-21-044

Michigan

Ann Arbor

University of Michigan Program
Sponsor: University of Michigan Hospitals
Providence Hospital and Medical Centers

Program Director:
Avraham Eisbruch, MD
Univ of Michigan Med Sch
UH B2C490/Box 0010
1500 E Medical Center Dr
Ann Arbor, MI 48109-0010
Tel: 734 936-7810 *Fax:* 734 763-7370
E-mail: eisbruch@umich.edu
Accred Length: 4 Years *Program Size:* 10
Program ID: 430-25-11-045

Detroit

Henry Ford Hospital Program
Sponsor: Henry Ford Hospital

Program Director:
Vinay Sharma, MD
Henry Ford Hospital
2799 W Grand Blvd
Detroit, MI 48202
Tel: 313 876-1015 *Fax:* 313 876-3235
Accred Length: 4 Years *Program Size:* 6
Program ID: 430-25-12-046

Wayne State University/Detroit Medical Center Program
Sponsor: Wayne State University/Detroit Medical Center
Grace Hospital
Harper Hospital

Program Director:
Amr Aref, MD
Wayne State Univ Hospitals
Dept of Rad Oncology
4201 St Antoine
Detroit, MI 48201
Tel: 313 745-1985 *Fax:* 313 745-2314
Accred Length: 4 Years *Program Size:* 6
Program ID: 430-25-21-048

Royal Oak

William Beaumont Hospital Program
Sponsor: William Beaumont Hospital
William Beaumont Hospital-Troy

Program Director:
Frank A Vicini, MD
William Beaumont Hospital
Dept of Rad Oncology
3601 W 13 Mile Rd
Royal Oak, MI 48073
Tel: 248 551-1219 *Fax:* 248 551-0089
Internet: http://www.beaumont.edu/html/gme
Accred Length: 4 Years *Program Size:* 8
Program ID: 430-25-12-049

Minnesota

Minneapolis

University of Minnesota Program
Sponsor: University of Minnesota Medical School
Fairview-University Medical Center

Program Director:
Kwan H Cho, MD
UMHC Box 494
420 Delaware St SE
Minneapolis, MN 55455
Tel: 612 626-2631 *Fax:* 612 624-8994
E-mail: thomp182@tc.umn.edu
Accred Length: 4 Years *Program Size:* 6
Program ID: 430-26-21-050

Rochester

Mayo Graduate School of Medicine (Rochester) Program
Sponsor: Mayo Graduate School of Medicine-Mayo Foundation
Mayo Clinic (Rochester)

Program Director:
Ivy A Petersen, MD
Application Processing Ctr
Mayo Graduate Sch of Med
200 First St SW
Rochester, MN 55905
Tel: 507 284-3108 *Fax:* 507 284-0999
E-mail: mgsm.medlab.specialties@mayo.edu
Internet: http://www.mayo.edu/
Accred Length: 4 Years *Program Size:* 9
Program ID: 430-26-21-051

Missouri

St Louis

Washington University/B-JH/SLCH Consortium Program
Sponsor: Washington University/B-JH/SLCH Consortium
Barnes-Jewish Hospital
Barnes-Jewish Hospital (North Campus)
Mallinckrodt Institute of Radiology
St Louis Children's Hospital
Washington University School of Medicine

Program Director:
Carlos A Perez, MD
Rad Oncology Ctr
Washington Univ-Barnes Hospital
4939 Children's Pl/Ste 5500
St Louis, MO 63110
Tel: 314 362-8503 *Fax:* 314 362-8521
Accred Length: 4 Years *Program Size:* 12
Program ID: 430-28-11-054

New Jersey

Camden

UMDNJ-Robert Wood Johnson Medical School (Camden) Program
Sponsor: Cooper Hospital-University Medical Center

Program Director:
Jeffrey S Wenger, MD
Cooper Hospital-Univ Med Ctr
Dept of Rad Oncology
One Cooper Plaza
Camden, NJ 08103-1489
Tel: 609 342-2300, ext 2581 *Fax:* 609 365-8504
Accred Length: 4 Years *Program Size:* 6
Program ID: 430-33-21-114

Livingston

St Barnabas Medical Center Program
Sponsor: St Barnabas Medical Center
Program Director:
Andrew I Zablow, MD
St Barnabas Med Ctr
94 Old Short Hills Rd
Livingston, NJ 07039
Tel: 973 533-5637 *Fax:* 973 533-5648
Accred Length: 4 Years *Program Size:* 4
Program ID: 430-33-31-057

New York

Bronx

Albert Einstein College of Medicine Program
Sponsor: Albert Einstein College of Medicine of Yeshiva University
Montefiore Medical Center-Henry and Lucy Moses Division
Montefiore Medical Center-Weiler Hospital
Program Director:
James S Butler, MD
Montefiore Med Ctr-Albert Einstein Cancer Ctr
1825 E Chester Rd
Bronx, NY 10467-2490
Tel: 718 904-2921 *Fax:* 718 904-2911
E-mail: jbutler.montefiore.org
Accred Length: 4 Years *Program Size:* 3
Program ID: 430-35-21-061

Brooklyn

New York Methodist Hospital Program
Sponsor: New York Methodist Hospital
Lutheran Medical Center
Program Director:
Hosny Selim, MD
New York Methodist Hospital
506 Sixth St
Box 159-008
Brooklyn, NY 11215-9008
Tel: 718 780-3677 *Fax:* 718 780-3637
Accred Length: 4 Years *Program Size:* 4
Program ID: 430-35-22-064

SUNY Health Science Center at Brooklyn Program
Sponsor: SUNY Health Science Center at Brooklyn
Kings County Hospital Center
Long Island College Hospital
University Hospital-SUNY Health Science Center at Brooklyn
Program Director:
Marvin Rotman, MD
SUNY Health Science Ctr-Brooklyn
450 Clarkson Ave/Box 1211
Brooklyn, NY 11203-2098
Tel: 718 270-2181 *Fax:* 718 270-1535
E-mail: mrotman@netmail.hscbklyn.edu
Accred Length: 4 Years *Program Size:* 5
Program ID: 430-35-21-070

Buffalo

SUNY at Buffalo Graduate Medical-Dental Education Consortium Program
Sponsor: SUNY at Buffalo Grad Medical-Dental Education Consortium
CGF Health System (Buffalo General Hospital)
Roswell Park Cancer Institute
Veterans Affairs Medical Center (Buffalo)
Program Director:
R Jeffrey Lee, MD
Dept of Rad Oncology
Roswell Park Cancer Inst
Elm and Carlton Sts
Buffalo, NY 14263
Tel: 716 845-3172 *Fax:* 716 845-7616
Accred Length: 4 Years *Program Size:* 4
Program ID: 430-35-21-122

Flushing

New York Hospital Medical Center of Queens/Cornell University Medical College Program
Sponsor: New York Hospital Medical Center of Queens
New York and Presbyterian Hospital (Cornell Campus)
Program Director:
Mary Katherine Hayes, MD
New York Presbyterian Hospital-New York Cornell Campus
525 E 68th St
New York, NY 10021
Tel: 212 746-3610 *Fax:* 212 746-8749
Accred Length: 4 Years *Program Size:* 6
Program ID: 430-35-22-126

New York

Memorial Sloan-Kettering Cancer Center Program
Sponsor: Memorial Sloan-Kettering Cancer Center
Program Director:
Michael J Zelefsky, MD
Memorial Sloan-Kettering Cancer Ctr
1275 York Ave
Mailbox 22
New York, NY 10021
Tel: 212 639-5834, ext 5834 *Fax:* 212 639-2417
E-mail: larssonm@mskcc.org
Accred Length: 4 Years *Program Size:* 13
Program ID: 430-35-21-063

Mount Sinai School of Medicine Program
Sponsor: Mount Sinai School of Medicine
Mount Sinai Medical Center
Program Director:
Richard G Stock, MD
Box 1236
One Gustave L Levy Pl
New York, NY 10029-6574
Tel: 212 241-7818 *Fax:* 212 410-7194
Accred Length: 4 Years *Program Size:* 6
Program ID: 430-35-21-119

New York and Presbyterian Hospital (Columbia Campus) Program
Sponsor: New York and Presbyterian Hospital
New York and Presbyterian Hospital (Columbia Campus)
St Luke's-Roosevelt Hospital Center
Program Director:
Peter B Schiff, MD PhD
Dept of Radiation Oncology
622 W 168th St
New York, NY 10032-3784
Tel: 212 305-8096 *Fax:* 212 305-5935
E-mail: pbs1@columbia.edu
Internet:
http://cait.cpmc.columbia.edu/dept/radoncology/
Accred Length: 4 Years *Program Size:* 6
Program ID: 430-35-11-068

New York University Medical Center Program
Sponsor: New York University Medical Center
Bellevue Hospital Center
Program Director:
Jay S Cooper, MD
New York Univ Med Ctr
Div of Rad Oncology
566 First Ave
New York, NY 10016
Tel: 212 263-5055 *Fax:* 212 263-6274
E-mail: jay.cooper@med.nyu.edu
Internet: http://www.med.nyu.edu/radonc/nyurad.html.
Accred Length: 4 Years *Program Size:* 5
Program ID: 430-35-21-067

Rochester

University of Rochester Program
Sponsor: Strong Memorial Hospital of the University of Rochester
Program Director:
Ralph A Brasacchio, MD
Louis S Constine, MD
Strong Memorial Hospital
601 Elmwood Ave
Box 647
Rochester, NY 14642-8647
Tel: 716 275-5575 *Fax:* 716 275-1531
E-mail: rasb@radonc.medinfo.rochester.edu
Accred Length: 4 Years *Program Size:* 6
Program ID: 430-35-11-071

Syracuse

SUNY Health Science Center at Syracuse Program
Sponsor: University Hospital-SUNY Health Science Center at Syracuse
Program Director:
Jeffrey A Bogart, MD
SUNY Health Science Ctr-Syracuse
750 E Adams St
Syracuse, NY 13210
Tel: 315 464-5276 *Fax:* 315 464-5943
E-mail: bogartj@vax.cs.hscsyr.edu
Internet: http://www.ec.hscsyr.edu/~bogartj/
Accred Length: 4 Years *Program Size:* 5
Program ID: 430-35-11-072

Valhalla

New York Medical College at Westchester Medical Center Program
Sponsor: New York Medical College
Westchester Medical Center
Program Director:
Chitti R Moorthy, MD
Dept of Radiation Medicine
New York Med Coll-Westchester Med Ctr
Macy Pavilion
Valhalla, NY 10595
Tel: 914 493-8561 *Fax:* 914 493-8352
E-mail: moorthyc@wcmc.com
Accred Length: 4 Years *Program Size:* 4
Program ID: 430-35-21-117

North Carolina

Chapel Hill

University of North Carolina Hospitals Program
Sponsor: University of North Carolina Hospitals
Program Director:
Mahesh A Varia, MD
Univ of North Carolina Hospitals
Dept of Rad Oncology/CB#7512
Chapel Hill, NC 27599-7512
Tel: 919 966-7700, ext 263 *Fax:* 919 966-7681
E-mail: grundman@radonc.unc.edu
Internet: http://www.med.unc.edu/wrkunits/2depts
Accred Length: 4 Years *Program Size:* 4
Program ID: 430-36-11-073

Durham

Duke University Program
Sponsor: Duke University Medical Center
Veterans Affairs Medical Center (Durham)
Program Director:
Lawrence B Marks, MD
Duke Univ Med Ctr
Dept of Rad Oncology
Box 3085
Durham, NC 27710
Tel: 919 660-2110 *Fax:* 919 684-3953
Internet: http://www.radonc.duke.edu
Accred Length: 4 Years *Program Size:* 8
Program ID: 430-36-21-074

Winston-Salem

Wake Forest University School of Medicine Program
Sponsor: Wake Forest University Baptist Medical Center
Program Director:
W Robert Lee, MD
Wake Forest Univ Sch of Med
Medical Center Blvd
Winston-Salem, NC 27157-1030
Tel: 336 716-4981 *Fax:* 336 716-5972
E-mail: wrlee@wfubmc.edu
Accred Length: 4 Years *Program Size:* 4
Program ID: 430-36-11-075

Ohio

Cincinnati

University Hospital/University of Cincinnati College of Medicine Program
Sponsor: University Hospital Inc
Veterans Affairs Medical Center (Cincinnati)
Program Director:
Kevin P Redmond, MD
Univ of Cincinnati
Rad Oncology/ML 0757
234 Goodman St
Cincinnati, OH 45267-0757
Tel: 513 558-5668 *Fax:* 513 558-4007
E-mail: redmondkp@healthall.com
Internet: http://www.ucradonc.org
Accred Length: 4 Years *Program Size:* 4
Program ID: 430-38-21-076

Cleveland

Case Western Reserve University Program
Sponsor: University Hospitals of Cleveland
Program Director:
Michael A Samuels, MD
Univ Hospitals of Cleveland
11100 Euclid Ave
Cleveland, OH 44106-5056
Tel: 216 844-3103 *Fax:* 216 844-1038
Accred Length: 4 Years *Program Size:* 1
Program ID: 430-38-11-077

Cleveland Clinic Foundation Program
Sponsor: Cleveland Clinic Foundation
Program Director:
John Suh, MD
Cleveland Clinic Foundation
Dept of Radiation Oncology/T28
9500 Euclid Ave
Cleveland, OH 44195-5242
Tel: 216 444-5690 *Fax:* 216 444-1162
E-mail: meded@cesmtp.ccf.org
Internet: http://www.ccf.org
Accred Length: 4 Years *Program Size:* 10
Program ID: 430-38-12-078

Columbus

Ohio State University Program
Sponsor: Ohio State University Medical Center
Program Director:
Reinhard Gahbauer, MD
Arthur G James Cancer Hospital and Research Inst
Ohio State Univ
300 W Tenth Ave
Columbus, OH 43210
Tel: 614 293-8415 *Fax:* 614 293-4044
E-mail: gahbauer.1@osu.edu
Internet: http://www-radonc.med.ohio-state.edu
Accred Length: 4 Years *Program Size:* 4
Program ID: 430-38-11-079

Oregon

Portland

Oregon Health Sciences University Program
Sponsor: Oregon Health Sciences University Hospital
Program Director:
Kenneth R Stevens Jr, MD
Oregon Health Sciences Univ
Dept of Rad Oncology/L337
3181 SW Sam Jackson Park Rd
Portland, OR 97201-3098
Tel: 503 494-8758 *Fax:* 503 494-6967
E-mail: stevenk@ohsu.edu
Accred Length: 4 Years *Program Size:* 4
Program ID: 430-40-21-081

Pennsylvania

Philadelphia

Fox Chase Cancer Center Program
Sponsor: Fox Chase Cancer Center
Program Director:
Wayne Pinover, DO
7701 Burholme Ave
Philadelphia, PA 19111
Tel: 215 728-3692 *Fax:* 215 214-4038
E-mail: d_elder@fccc.edu
Internet: http://www.fccc.edu
Accred Length: 4 Years *Program Size:* 7
Program ID: 430-41-21-123

MCP Hahnemann University Program
Sponsor: MCP Hahnemann University
Hahnemann University Hospital
Program Director:
Bizhan Micaily, MD
Hahnemann Univ Hospital
Dept of Rad Oncology
Broad and Vine Sts/MS 200
Philadelphia, PA 19102-1192
Tel: 215 762-3089 *Fax:* 215 762-8523
Accred Length: 4 Years *Program Size:* 5
Program ID: 430-41-11-084

Thomas Jefferson University Program
Sponsor: Thomas Jefferson University Hospital
Program Director:
Lydia Komarnicky, MD
Bodine Ctr for Cancer Treatment
111 S 11th St
Philadelphia, PA 19107
Tel: 215 955-6644 *Fax:* 215 955-0412
Accred Length: 4 Years *Program Size:* 7
Program ID: 430-41-11-086

University of Pennsylvania Program
Sponsor: Hospital of the University of Pennsylvania
Veterans Affairs Medical Center (Philadelphia)
Program Director:
Joel W Goldwein, MD
Dept of Rad Oncology
3400 Spruce St
Donner 2
Philadelphia, PA 19104
Tel: 215 662-2428 *Fax:* 215 349-5445
Internet: http://www.xrt.upenn.edu/
Accred Length: 4 Years *Program Size:* 16
Program ID: 430-41-21-087

Pittsburgh

Allegheny General Hospital Program
Sponsor: Allegheny General Hospital
Program Director:
Shalom Kalnicki, MD
Allegheny General Hospital
Dept of Radiation Oncology
320 E North Ave
Pittsburgh, PA 15212-9986
Tel: 412 359-3400 *Fax:* 412 359-3981
E-mail: skalnick@pgh.auhs.edu
Accred Length: 4 Years *Program Size:* 4
Program ID: 430-41-31-127

South Carolina

Charleston

Medical University of South Carolina Program
Sponsor: Medical University of South Carolina College of Medicine
MUSC Medical Center
Program Director:
Stephen J Milito, MD
Med Univ of South Carolina
Dept of Rad Oncology
171 Ashley Ave
Charleston, SC 29425
Tel: 803 792-3271 *Fax:* 803 792-5498
E-mail: milito@radonc.musc.edu
Internet: http://www.radonc.musc.edu/
Accred Length: 4 Years *Program Size:* 4
Program ID: 430-45-21-092

Texas

Galveston

University of Texas Medical Branch Hospitals Program
Sponsor: University of Texas Medical Branch Hospitals
Program Director:
Martin Colman, MD
Univ of Texas Med Branch
301 University Blvd
3354 Gail Borden Bldg/Rte 0656
Galveston, TX 77555-0656
Tel: 409 772-6723 *Fax:* 409 747-0064
E-mail: mcolman@utmb.edu
Accred Length: 4 Years *Program Size:* 4
Program ID: 430-48-11-097

Houston

Baylor College of Medicine Program
Sponsor: Baylor College of Medicine
Harris County Hospital District-Ben Taub General Hospital
Methodist Hospital
Veterans Affairs Medical Center (Houston)
Program Director:
Shiao Y Woo, MD
Baylor Coll of Med
One Baylor Plaza/165B
Houston, TX 77030-3498
Tel: 713 790-2091 *Fax:* 713 793-1301
E-mail: sclark@bcm.tmc.edu
Accred Length: 4 Years *Program Size:* 6
Program ID: 430-48-21-098

University of Texas M D Anderson Cancer Center Program
Sponsor: University of Texas M D Anderson Cancer Center
Program Director:
Alan Pollack, MD PhD
Univ of Texas-MD Anderson Cancer Ctr
1515 Holcombe Blvd
Box 97
Houston, TX 77030
Tel: 713 792-2534 *Fax:* 713 792-3642
E-mail: temshoff@notes.mdacc.tmc.edu
Accred Length: 4 Years *Program Size:* 17
Program ID: 430-48-22-099

San Antonio

University of Texas Health Science Center at San Antonio Program
Sponsor: University of Texas Medical School at San Antonio
University Hospital-South Texas Medical Center
Program Director:
Terence S Herman, MD
Univ of Texas Health Science Ctr
Rad Oncology
7703 Floyd Curl Dr
San Antonio, TX 78284-7800
Tel: 210 616-5648 *Fax:* 210 949-5085
Accred Length: 4 Years *Program Size:* 5
Program ID: 430-48-21-100

Utah

Salt Lake City

University of Utah Program
Sponsor: University of Utah Medical Center
LDS Hospital
Program Director:
Lynn M Smith, MD
Univ of Utah Med Ctr
Dept of Rad Oncology
50 N Medical Dr
Salt Lake City, UT 84132
Tel: 801 581-8793 *Fax:* 801 585-3502
E-mail: lynn.m.smith.@hsc.utah.edu
Internet: http://www.med.utah.edu/radoncol/
Accred Length: 4 Years *Program Size:* 4
Program ID: 430-49-12-102

Virginia

Charlottesville

University of Virginia Program
Sponsor: University of Virginia Medical Center
Program Director:
Tyvin A Rich, MD
Dept of Rad Oncology/Box 383
Univ of Virginia
Jefferson Park Ave
Charlottesville, VA 22908
Tel: 804 924-9412 *Fax:* 804 982-3262
E-mail: tar4d@virginia.edu
Accred Length: 4 Years *Program Size:* 5
Program ID: 430-51-11-104

Norfolk

Eastern Virginia Medical School Program
Sponsor: Eastern Virginia Medical School
Maryview Hospital
Sentara Norfolk General Hospital
Virginia Beach General Hospital
Program Director:
Jock R Wheeler, MD
Deborah A Kuban, MD
Eastern Virginia Med Sch
Dept of Rad Oncology
600 Gresham Dr
Norfolk, VA 23507-1999
Tel: 757 668-2075 *Fax:* 757 627-0334
Accred Length: 4 Years *Program Size:* 0
Program ID: 430-51-11-105

Richmond

Medical College of Virginia/Virginia Commonwealth University Program
Sponsor: Medical College of Virginia/Virginia Commonwealth University
Hunter Holmes McGuire VA Medical Center (Richmond)
Medical College of Virginia Hospitals
Program Director:
Douglas W Arthur, MD
Med Coll of Virginia
PO Box 980058
Richmond, VA 23298-0058
Tel: 804 828-7232 *Fax:* 804 828-6042
E-mail: dwarthur@hsc.vcu.edu
Internet: http://views.vcu.edu/mcvro/
Accred Length: 4 Years *Program Size:* 7
Program ID: 430-51-11-106

Washington

Seattle

University of Washington Program
Sponsor: University of Washington School of Medicine
University of Washington Medical Center
Program Director:
Karen L Lindsley, MD
Univ of Washington
Dept of Rad Oncology/BX356043
1959 NE Pacific St
Seattle, WA 98195-6043
Tel: 206 548-4115 *Fax:* 206 548-6218
E-mail: shawna@radonc.washington.edu
Internet: http://www.radonc.washington.edu
Accred Length: 4 Years *Program Size:* 8
Program ID: 430-54-21-107

Wisconsin

Madison

University of Wisconsin Program
Sponsor: University of Wisconsin Hospital and Clinics
Program Director:
Paul M Harari, MD
Univ of Wisconsin Hospital and Clinics
600 Highland Ave/Rm K4-B100
Madison, WI 53792-8310
Tel: 608 263-8500 *Fax:* 608 263-9167
E-mail: harari@humonc.wisc.edu
Internet: http://www.humonc.wisc.edu
Accred Length: 4 Years *Program Size:* 7
Program ID: 430-56-21-108

Milwaukee

Medical College of Wisconsin Program
Sponsor: Medical College of Wisconsin Affiliated Hospitals Inc
Clement J Zablocki Veterans Affairs Medical Center
Community Memorial Hospital
Froedtert Memorial Lutheran Hospital
Program Director:
Colleen A Lawton, MD
Med Coll of Wisconsin
Dept of Rad Oncology
8701 Watertown Plank Rd
Milwaukee, WI 53226
Tel: 414 805-4470 *Fax:* 414 805-4369
E-mail: colleen@mcw.edu
Internet: http://www.mcw.edu
Accred Length: 4 Years *Program Size:* 6
Program ID: 430-56-21-109

Radiology-Diagnostic

Alabama

Birmingham

Baptist Health System Program
Sponsor: Baptist Health System Inc
Birmingham Baptist Medical Center-Montclair
Birmingham Baptist Medical Center-Princeton
Program Director:
Bibb Allen Jr, MD
Birmingham Baptist Med Ctr-Montclair
800 Montclair Rd
Birmingham, AL 35213
Tel: 205 592-1257
E-mail: programdir@bbmcradiology.org
Internet: http://www.bbmcradiology.org
Accred Length: 4 Years *Program Size:* 13
Program ID: 420-01-21-006

University of Alabama Medical Center Program
Sponsor: University of Alabama Hospital
Veterans Affairs Medical Center (Birmingham)
Program Director:
Robert E Koehler, MD
Univ of Alabama Med Ctr
Dept of Radiology
619 S 19th St
Birmingham, AL 35233-6830
Tel: 205 934-3240 *Fax:* 205 975-4413
E-mail: rkoehler@uabmc.edu
Internet: http://www.rad.uab.edu
Accred Length: 4 Years *Program Size:* 25
Subspecialties: PDR, RNR, VIR
Program ID: 420-01-11-007

Mobile

University of South Alabama Program
Sponsor: University of South Alabama Medical Center
Program Director:
Jeffrey C Brandon, MD
Univ of South Alabama Med Ctr
Mastin Bldg Rm 315
2451 Fillingim St
Mobile, AL 36617-2293
Tel: 334 471-7866 *Fax:* 334 471-7882
E-mail: jnorthcutt@usamail.usouthal.edu
Internet: http://www.usouthal.edu
Accred Length: 4 Years *Program Size:* 21
Program ID: 420-01-11-008

Arizona

Phoenix

St Joseph's Hospital and Medical Center Program
Sponsor: St Joseph's Hospital and Medical Center
Program Director:
Barry Green, MD
St Joseph's Hospital and Med Ctr
Rad/Diagnostic Imaging
PO Box 2071
Phoenix, AZ 85001-2071
Tel: 602 406-6994 *Fax:* 602 406-7147
Internet: http://www.chw.edu/mha/mha.html
Accred Length: 4 Years *Program Size:* 12
Subspecialties: RNR
Program ID: 420-03-12-010

Tucson

University of Arizona Program
Sponsor: University of Arizona College of Medicine
University Medical Center
Veterans Affairs Medical Center (Tucson)
Program Director:
K Rebecca Hunt, MD
Univ of Arizona Coll of Med
Dept of Radiology
PO Box 245067
Tucson, AZ 85724-5067
Tel: 520 626-7368 *Fax:* 520 626-1945
E-mail: jsmerz@radiology.arizona.edu
Internet: http://zeki.radiology.arizona.edu/
Accred Length: 4 Years *Program Size:* 19
Subspecialties: NR, RNR
Program ID: 420-03-21-011

Arkansas

Little Rock

University of Arkansas for Medical Sciences Program
Sponsor: University of Arkansas College of Medicine
John L McClellan Memorial Veterans Hospital
University Hospital of Arkansas
Program Director:
Sarah G Klein, MD
Univ of Arkansas for Med Sciences
Dept of Radiology
800 Marshall St
Little Rock, AR 72202
Tel: 501 320-4865 *Fax:* 501 320-1513
E-mail: snr@exhange.ach.uams.edu
Internet: http://www.uams.edu/radiology
Accred Length: 4 Years *Program Size:* 21
Subspecialties: PDR, RNR, VIR
Program ID: 420-04-21-012

California

Fresno

University of California (San Francisco)/Fresno Program
Sponsor: UCSF-Fresno Medical Education Program
University Medical Center
Veterans Affairs Medical Center (Fresno)
Program Director:
William J Vlymen, MD PhD
VA Med Ctr
2615 E Clinton Ave
Fresno, CA 93703
Tel: 209 228-5317 *Fax:* 209 228-6911
Accred Length: 4 Years *Program Size:* 5
Program ID: 420-05-21-219

Loma Linda

Loma Linda University Program
Sponsor: Loma Linda University Medical Center
Jerry L Pettis Memorial Veterans Hospital
Program Director:
Douglas C Smith, MD
Loma Linda Univ Med Ctr
11234 Anderson St
2605 Schuman Pavilion
Loma Linda, CA 92354
Tel: 909 824-4370 *Fax:* 909 478-4202
E-mail: rosalyn_hamilton@ccmail.llumc.edu
Internet: http://www.llu.edu/llumc/radiology/
Accred Length: 4 Years *Program Size:* 26
Subspecialties: PDR, RNR, VIR
Program ID: 420-05-21-015

Los Angeles

Cedars-Sinai Medical Center Program
Sponsor: Cedars-Sinai Medical Center
Program Director:
Mitchell S Komaiko, MD
Cedars-Sinai Med Ctr
8700 Beverly Blvd
Rm 5416
Los Angeles, CA 90048-0750
Tel: 310 855-3616 *Fax:* 310 967-8335
E-mail: imaging.housestaff@cshs.org
Internet: http://www.csmc.edu
Accred Length: 4 Years *Program Size:* 12
Program ID: 420-05-21-018

Charles R Drew University Program
Sponsor: Charles R Drew University of Medicine and Science
LAC-King/Drew Medical Center
Program Director:
Janis F Owens, MD
Martin Luther King Jr-Drew Med Ctr
Dept of Radiology
12021 S Wilmington Ave
Los Angeles, CA 90059
Tel: 310 668-4702 *Fax:* 310 632-8068
E-mail: jaowens@cdrewu.edu
Accred Length: 4 Years *Program Size:* 16
Program ID: 420-05-12-022

Southern California Kaiser Permanente Medical Care (Los Angeles) Program
Sponsor: Southern California Kaiser Permanente Medical Group
Kaiser Foundation Hospital (Los Angeles)
Program Director:
Anne Kosco, MD
Kaiser Foundation Hospital
Diagnostic Radiology Dept
1505 N Edgemont/Basement
Los Angeles, CA 90027-5299
Tel: 363 783-5791 *Fax:* 363 783-6908
Accred Length: 4 Years *Program Size:* 10 (*GY1:* 2)
Program ID: 420-05-12-020

UCLA Medical Center Program
Sponsor: UCLA School of Medicine
Olive View-UCLA Medical Center
UCLA Medical Center
VA Greater Los Angeles Healthcare System
Program Director:
Richard H Gold, MD
UCLA Hospital and Clinics
Dept of Rad Sciences
10833 Le Conte Ave
Los Angeles, CA 90095-1721
Tel: 310 825-7532 *Fax:* 310 794-5734
E-mail: rgold@mail.rad.ucla.edu
Internet: http://www.radsci.ucla.edu
Accred Length: 4 Years *Program Size:* 40
Subspecialties: PDR, RNR, VIR
Program ID: 420-05-11-023

University of Southern California Program
Sponsor: Los Angeles County-USC Medical Center
Program Director:
Deborah M Forrester, MD
Los Angeles County-USC Med Ctr
1200 N State St
Box 481/Rm 3550
Los Angeles, CA 90033
Tel: 323 226-7242 *Fax:* 323 226-2280
E-mail: radiol@hsc.usc.edu
Internet: http://www.usc.edu/hsc/medicine/radiology/
Accred Length: 4 Years *Program Size:* 40
Subspecialties: RNR, VIR
Program ID: 420-05-11-021

Orange

University of California (Irvine) Program
Sponsor: University of California (Irvine) Medical Center
Long Beach Memorial Medical Center
Veterans Affairs Medical Center (Long Beach)
Program Director:
Norah Milne, MD
Univ of California Irvine Med Ctr
Dept of Radiology
101 City Dr S
Orange, CA 92868-3298
Tel: 714 456-6167 *Fax:* 714 456-8908
Internet: http://www.med.uci.edu/~radiosci
Accred Length: 4 Years *Program Size:* 22
Program ID: 420-05-21-014

Sacramento

University of California (Davis) Program
Sponsor: University of California (Davis) Medical Center
Program Director:
John P McGahan, MD
Univ of California Davis Med Ctr
Dept of Radiology
4860 Y St/Ste 3100
Sacramento, CA 95817
Tel: 916 734-5195 *Fax:* 916 734-6548
E-mail: barbara.dyer@ucdmc.ucdavis.edu
Internet: http://www.radiology.ucdmc.ucdavis.edu
Accred Length: 4 Years *Program Size:* 17
Program ID: 420-05-11-013

San Diego

University of California (San Diego) Program
Sponsor: University of California (San Diego) Medical Center
Veterans Affairs Medical Center (San Diego)
Program Director:
Giovanna Casola, MD
UCSD Med Ctr
200 W Arbor Dr
San Diego, CA 92103-8756
Tel: 619 543-3534 *Fax:* 619 543-3746
E-mail: svanburen@ucsd.edu
Internet: http://www.radiology.ucsd.edu
Accred Length: 4 Years *Program Size:* 23
Subspecialties: RNR, VIR
Program ID: 420-05-21-027

US Navy Coordinated Program-Naval Medical Center (San Diego) Program
Sponsor: Naval Medical Center (San Diego)
Program Director:
Timothy L Workman, MD
Naval Med Ctr
Dept of Radiology
Bob Wilson Dr
San Diego, CA 92134-5000
Tel: 619 532-8670 *Fax:* 619 532-8714
Accred Length: 4 Years *Program Size:* 26
Program ID: 420-05-21-914
US Armed Services Program

San Francisco

University of California (San Francisco) Program
Sponsor: University of California (San Francisco) School of Medicine
San Francisco General Hospital Medical Center
University of California (San Francisco) Medical Center
Veterans Affairs Medical Center (San Francisco)
Program Director:
Ruth B Goldstein, MD
Univ of California San Francisco
505 Parnassus Ave/Ste M-391
San Francisco, CA 94143-0628
Tel: 415 476-8358 *Fax:* 415 476-0616
E-mail: elaine.shanahan@radiology.ucsf.edu
Internet: http://www.radiology.ucsf.edu
Accred Length: 4 Years *Program Size:* 35
Subspecialties: PDR, RNR, VIR
Program ID: 420-05-21-031

San Jose

Santa Clara Valley Medical Center Program
Sponsor: Santa Clara Valley Medical Center
Program Director:
Andrew H Koo, MD
Santa Clara Valley Med Ctr
751 S Bascom Ave
San Jose, CA 95128
Tel: 408 885-6370 *Fax:* 408 885-6360
Accred Length: 4 Years *Program Size:* 12
Program ID: 420-05-31-032

Santa Barbara

Santa Barbara Cottage Hospital Program
Sponsor: Santa Barbara Cottage Hospital
Program Director:
Arthur A Lee, MD
Santa Barbara Cottage Hospital
Dept of Radiology
PO Box 689
Santa Barbara, CA 93102-0689
Tel: 805 569-7279 *Fax:* 805 569-8279
E-mail: tpetter@cottagehealthsystem.org
Internet: http://cottagehealthsystem.org
Accred Length: 4 Years *Program Size:* 9
Program ID: 420-05-22-033

Stanford

Stanford University Program
Sponsor: Stanford University Hospital
Veterans Affairs Palo Alto Health Care System
Program Director:
Robert Mindelzun, MD
Stanford Univ Med Ctr
300 Pasteur Dr/Rm H-1307
Stanford, CA 94305-5105
Tel: 650 723-5407 *Fax:* 650 723-1909
E-mail: hidalgo@stanford.edu
Internet:
http://www-radiology.stanford.edu/education/residency.html
Accred Length: 4 Years *Program Size:* 28
Subspecialties: PDR
Program ID: 420-05-21-034

Torrance

Los Angeles County-Harbor-UCLA Medical Center Program
Sponsor: Los Angeles County-Harbor-UCLA Medical Center
Program Director:
Richard Renslo, MD
Los Angeles County-Harbor-UCLA Med Ctr
Dept of Radiology/Box 27
1000 W Carson St
Torrance, CA 90509-2910
Tel: 310 222-2847 *Fax:* 310 618-9500
E-mail: phamm@4link.net
Accred Length: 4 Years *Program Size:* 20
Subspecialties: RNR
Program ID: 420-05-11-035

Travis AFB

David Grant Medical Center Program
Sponsor: David Grant Medical Center
Program Director:
Raymond S Dougherty, MD
60th Med Group
Dept of Radiology (60 MDTS/SGQX)
101 Bodin Cir
Travis AFB, CA 94535-1800
Tel: 707 423-7182 *Fax:* 707 423-7207
E-mail: conte@sparc1.castles.com
Accred Length: 4 Years *Program Size:* 14
Program ID: 420-05-21-001
US Armed Services Program

Colorado

Denver

University of Colorado Program
Sponsor: University of Colorado Health Sciences Center
Denver Health and Hospitals
Veterans Affairs Medical Center (Denver)
Program Director:
Ronald Townsend, MD
Univ of Colorado Health Sciences Ctr
4200 E Ninth Ave
Box C-276
Denver, CO 80262-0030
Tel: 303 372-6137 *Fax:* 303 372-6626
E-mail: ron.townsend@uchsc.edu
Accred Length: 4 Years *Program Size:* 26
Subspecialties: PDR, RNR, VIR
Program ID: 420-07-21-038

Connecticut

Bridgeport

Bridgeport Hospital Program
Sponsor: Bridgeport Hospital
Program Director:
Octavio G Choy, MD
Bridgeport Hospital
267 Grant St
Bridgeport, CT 06610
Tel: 203 384-3834 *Fax:* 203 384-3030
E-mail: raderas@bpthosp.org
Accred Length: 4 Years *Program Size:* 9
Program ID: 420-08-12-039

St Vincent's Medical Center Program
Sponsor: St Vincent's Medical Center
Program Director:
Robert D Russo, MD
St Vincent's Med Ctr
Radiology Dept
2800 Main St
Bridgeport, CT 06606
Tel: 203 576-5062 *Fax:* 203 576-5733
Internet: http://www.stvincents.org
Accred Length: 4 Years *Program Size:* 8
Subspecialties: TY
Program ID: 420-08-11-040

Farmington

University of Connecticut Program
Sponsor: University of Connecticut School of Medicine
St Francis Hospital and Medical Center
Univ of Connecticut Health Center/John Dempsey Hospital
Program Director:
Mary B Friar, MD
Univ of Connecticut Health Ctr
Dept of Radiology
263 Farmington Ave
Farmington, CT 06030-2905
Tel: 860 679-2784 *Fax:* 860 679-3145
Internet:
http://www.resprog.uchc.edu/md/radiology/home.html
Accred Length: 4 Years *Program Size:* 8
Program ID: 420-08-21-225

Hartford

Hartford Hospital Program
Sponsor: Hartford Hospital
Program Director:
Frederick U Conard III, MD
Hartford Hospital
80 Seymour St
PO Box 5037
Hartford, CT 06102-5037
Tel: 860 545-2864 *Fax:* 860 545-1957
E-mail: fconard@harthosp.org
Accred Length: 4 Years *Program Size:* 16
Program ID: 420-08-22-041

New Haven

Hospital of St Raphael Program
Sponsor: Hospital of St Raphael
Program Director:
Lee H Greenwood, MD
Hospital of St Raphael
Dept of Diagnostic Rad
1450 Chapel St
New Haven, CT 06511
Tel: 203 789-3118 *Fax:* 203 789-5161
Internet: http://www:srhs.org
Accred Length: 4 Years *Program Size:* 12
Program ID: 420-08-22-042

Yale-New Haven Medical Center Program
Sponsor: Yale-New Haven Hospital
Veterans Affairs Medical Center (West Haven)
Program Director:
Coralie Shaw, MD
Yale Univ Sch of Med
Dept of Diagnostic Rad
333 Cedar St
New Haven, CT 06520
Tel: 203 785-4746 *Fax:* 203 737-1688
E-mail: shaw@biomed.med.yale.edu
Accred Length: 4 Years *Program Size:* 24
Subspecialties: NR, PDR, RNR, VIR
Program ID: 420-08-21-043

Norwalk

Norwalk Hospital Program
Sponsor: Norwalk Hospital
Program Director:
Edward B Strauss, MD
Dept of Radiology
Norwalk Hospital
Maple St
Norwalk, CT 06856
Tel: 203 852-2715 *Fax:* 203 855-3967
Accred Length: 4 Years *Program Size:* 8
Program ID: 420-08-21-216

Delaware

Wilmington

Christiana Care Health Services Program
Sponsor: Christiana Care Health Services Inc
Program Director:
Sharon W Gould, MD
Christiana Care Health System
Christiana Hospital
PO Box 6001/Rm 1763
Newark, DE 19718
Tel: 302 733-5582 *Fax:* 302 733-5589
E-mail: rad.residency@christianacare.org
Internet: http://www.mcdresidency.org
Accred Length: 4 Years *Program Size:* 20 (*GYI:* 4)
Program ID: 420-09-11-044

District of Columbia

Washington

George Washington University Program
Sponsor: George Washington University School of Medicine
George Washington University Hospital (UHS)
Program Director:
Barry M Potter, MD
George Washington Univ Hospital
901 23rd St NW
Washington, DC 20037
Tel: 202 994-8384 *Fax:* 202 994-8285
E-mail: raderas@gwis2.circ.gwu.edu
Internet: http://www.gwumc.edu/edu/radiology
Accred Length: 4 Years *Program Size:* 15
Subspecialties: PDR, RNR, VIR
Program ID: 420-10-21-046

Georgetown University Program
Sponsor: Georgetown University Medical Center
Program Director:
Rebecca A Zuurbier, MD
Dept of Radiology
3800 Reservoir Rd NW
Washington, DC 20007-2197
Tel: 202 784-3314 *Fax:* 202 687-3081
E-mail: villaros@gunet.georgetown.edu
Accred Length: 4 Years *Program Size:* 16
Subspecialties: RNR, VIR
Program ID: 420-10-11-045

Howard University Program
Sponsor: Howard University Hospital
Program Director:
James S Teal, MD
Howard Univ Hospital
Dept of Radiology
2041 Georgia Ave NW
Washington, DC 20060
Tel: 202 865-1571 *Fax:* 202 865-3285
E-mail: mshelgreen@hotmail.com
Accred Length: 4 Years *Program Size:* 15
Program ID: 420-10-11-047

Florida

Gainesville

University of Florida Program
Sponsor: University of Florida College of Medicine
Shands Hospital at the University of Florida
Veterans Affairs Medical Center (Gainesville)
Program Director:
Jonathan L Williams, MD MBA
Univ of Florida
Dept of Radiology
PO Box 100374
Gainesville, FL 32610-0374
Tel: 352 395-0291 *Fax:* 352 395-0279
E-mail: farmerm@xray.ufl.edu
Internet: http://www.xray.ufl.edu
Accred Length: 4 Years *Program Size:* 24
Subspecialties: NM, NR, PDR, RNR, VIR
Program ID: 420-11-21-048

Jacksonville

University of Florida Health Science Center/Jacksonville Program
Sponsor: University of Florida College of Medicine at Jacksonville
University Medical Center (UFHSC/J)
Program Director:
Frederick S Vines, MD
Dept of Radiology, UFHSC/J
Univ Med Ctr
655 W Eighth St
Jacksonville, FL 32209
Tel: 904 549-4225 *Fax:* 904 549-3186
E-mail: fsv@umc5.umc.ufl.edu
Internet: http://www.ufhscj.edu/radiology/radiology.html
Accred Length: 4 Years *Program Size:* 16
Subspecialties: RNR
Program ID: 420-11-21-223

Miami

University of Miami-Jackson Memorial Medical Center Program
Sponsor: University of Miami-Jackson Memorial Medical Center
Program Director:
Luis A Rivas, MD
Jackson Memorial Hospital
Dept of Radiology
1611 NW 12th Ave/WW 279
Miami, FL 33136
Tel: 305 585-6894 *Fax:* 305 325-8591
E-mail: resident@mednet.med.miami.edu
Internet: http://www.med.miami.edu/radiology
Accred Length: 4 Years *Program Size:* 38
Subspecialties: PDR, RNR, VIR
Program ID: 420-11-21-049

Miami Beach

Mount Sinai Medical Center of Greater Miami Program
Sponsor: Mount Sinai Medical Center of Greater Miami
Program Director:
Manuel Viamonte Jr, MD
Mount Sinai Med Ctr of Greater Miami
Dept of Radiology
4300 Alton Rd
Miami Beach, FL 33140
Tel: 305 674-2950 *Fax:* 305 674-2694
E-mail: mviamonte@msmc.com
Internet: http://www.mountsinaimiami.org
Accred Length: 4 Years *Program Size:* 20
Program ID: 420-11-21-050

Tampa

University of South Florida Program
Sponsor: University of South Florida College of Medicine
H Lee Moffitt Cancer Center
James A Haley Veterans Hospital
Tampa General Healthcare
Program Director:
Robert A Clark, MD
Dept of Radiology
12901 Bruce B Downs Blvd/Box 17
Tampa, FL 33612-4799
Tel: 813 974-6311 *Fax:* 813 979-7231
E-mail: rtuttle@com1.med.usf.edu
Accred Length: 4 Years *Program Size:* 20
Subspecialties: RNR, VIR
Program ID: 420-11-21-051

Georgia

Atlanta

Emory University Program
Sponsor: Emory University School of Medicine
Emory University Hospital
Grady Memorial Hospital
Program Director:
Bruce R Baumgartner, MD
Emory Univ Hospital
Dept of Radiology
1364 Clifton Rd NE
Atlanta, GA 30322-2000
Tel: 404 712-4686 *Fax:* 404 712-7908
E-mail: maryellen_johnson@emory.org
Internet: http://www.emory.edu/radiology.resident.html
Accred Length: 4 Years *Program Size:* 41
Subspecialties: NR, PDR, RNR, VIR
Program ID: 420-12-21-052

Augusta

Medical College of Georgia Program
Sponsor: Medical College of Georgia Hospital and Clinics
Veterans Affairs Medical Center (Augusta)
Program Director:
Edward M Burton, MD
Med Coll of Georgia
1120 15th St
BAN 153
Augusta, GA 30912-3900
Tel: 706 721-3214 *Fax:* 706 721-7319
E-mail: eburton@mail.mcg.edu
Internet:
http://www.mcg.edu/hospital&clinics/residencyprograms
Accred Length: 4 Years *Program Size:* 13
Subspecialties: RNR
Program ID: 420-12-21-053

Savannah

Memorial Medical Center Program
Sponsor: Memorial Medical Center
Program Director:
Terry Reynolds, MD
Memorial Med Ctr
PO Box 23089
Savannah, GA 31403-3089
Tel: 912 350-7394 *Fax:* 912 350-3790
E-mail: mmcrad@g-net.net
Accred Length: 4 Years *Program Size:* 8
Program ID: 420-12-12-054

Hawaii

Honolulu

Tripler Army Medical Center Program
Sponsor: Tripler Army Medical Center
Program Director:
Lt Col Terry D Yeager, MD MS
Dept of Radiology
MCHK: DR CDR TAMC
1 Jarrett White Rd
Tripler AMC, HI 96859-5000
Tel: 808 433-6070 *Fax:* 808 433-4688
E-mail: yeagert@popmail.tamc.amedd.army.mil
Internet: http://www.tamc/radology/rad.html
Accred Length: 4 Years *Program Size:* 15
Program ID: 420-14-21-933
US Armed Services Program

Illinois

Chicago

Cook County Hospital Program

Sponsor: Cook County Hospital

Program Director:
Bradley G Langer, MD
Cook County Hospital
Dept of Radiology
1835 W Harrison St
Chicago, IL 60612-9985
Tel: 312 633-5319 *Fax:* 312 633-8791
Accred Length: 4 Years *Program Size:* 16
Program ID: 420-16-21-055

Illinois Masonic Medical Center Program

Sponsor: Illinois Masonic Medical Center

Program Director:
Kevin J Kirshenbaum, MD
Illinois Masonic Med Ctr
Dept of Radiology
836 W Wellington Ave
Chicago, IL 60657-5193
Tel: 773 296-7820 *Fax:* 773 296-7821
Internet: http://www.immc.org
Accred Length: 4 Years *Program Size:* 10
Program ID: 420-16-21-217

McGaw Medical Center of Northwestern University Program

Sponsor: Northwestern University Medical School
Evanston Hospital
Northwestern Memorial Hospital
Veterans Affairs Lakeside Medical Center (Chicago)

Program Director:
Barry M Rabin, MD
Office of Grad Med Educ
Northwestern Univ Med Sch
303 E Chicago Ave/Ward Bldg 9-332
Chicago, IL 60611-3008
Tel: 312 503-4748 *Fax:* 312 503-5230
E-mail: kku935@nwu.edu
Internet:
http://pubweb.acns.nwu.edu/~dbk675/nwu_radiology.html
Accred Length: 4 Years *Program Size:* 26
Subspecialties: NR, PDR, RNR, VIR
Program ID: 420-16-21-059

Rush-Presbyterian-St Luke's Medical Center Program

Sponsor: Rush-Presbyterian-St Luke's Medical Center

Program Director:
Carolyn Donaldson, MD
Rush-Presbyterian-St Luke's Med Ctr
Diagnostic Radiology Dept
1653 W Congress Pkwy
Chicago, IL 60612
Tel: 312 942-5781 *Fax:* 312 942-2114
E-mail: dwesson@rad.rpslmc.edu
Internet: http://www.rad.rush.edu
Accred Length: 4 Years *Program Size:* 17
Subspecialties: NR, RNR, VIR
Program ID: 420-16-11-060

University of Chicago Program

Sponsor: University of Chicago Hospitals

Program Director:
Tamar Ben-Ami, MD
Univ of Chicago Med Ctr
5841 S Maryland Ave/MC2026
Chicago, IL 60637-1470
Tel: 773 702-3550 *Fax:* 773 702-1161
E-mail: radiology@uchicago.edu
Internet: http://www-radiology.uchicago.edu
Accred Length: 4 Years *Program Size:* 23
Subspecialties: RNR, VIR
Program ID: 420-16-11-061

University of Illinois College of Medicine at Chicago Program

Sponsor: University of Illinois College of Medicine at Chicago
University of Illinois Hospital and Clinics
Veterans Affairs West Side Medical Center

Program Director:
Andrew C Wilbur, MD
Univ of Illinois Hospital
1740 W Taylor
Ste 2483/MC 931
Chicago, IL 60612-7233
Tel: 312 996-0234 *Fax:* 312 996-8097
Internet: http://www.uic.edu/com/uhrd
Accred Length: 4 Years *Program Size:* 16
Program ID: 420-16-21-062

University of Illinois College of Medicine at Chicago/Michael Reese Hospital Program

Sponsor: University of Illinois College of Medicine at Chicago
Mercy Hospital and Medical Center
Michael Reese Hospital and Medical Center

Program Director:
Nancy L Brown, MD
Michael Reese Hospital
Diagnostic Radiology Dept
2929 S Ellis Ave
Chicago, IL 60616
Tel: 312 791-4567 *Fax:* 312 791-3945
Accred Length: 4 Years *Program Size:* 20
Subspecialties: NR, RNR
Program ID: 420-16-12-057

Evanston

St Francis Hospital of Evanston Program

Sponsor: St Francis Hospital of Evanston

Program Director:
Carlos H Escamilla, MD
St Francis Hospital
Dept of Radiology
355 Ridge Ave
Evanston, IL 60202
Tel: 847 316-6101 *Fax:* 847 316-2241
Internet: http://www.reshealth.org
Accred Length: 4 Years *Program Size:* 8
Subspecialties: TY
Program ID: 420-16-12-063

Maywood

Loyola University Program

Sponsor: Loyola University Medical Center

Program Director:
Michael E Flisak, MD
Loyola Univ Med Ctr
Dept of Radiology
2160 S First Ave
Maywood, IL 60153
Tel: 708 216-1084 *Fax:* 708 216-8394
Accred Length: 4 Years *Program Size:* 20
Subspecialties: RNR
Program ID: 420-16-11-064

Peoria

University of Illinois College of Medicine at Peoria Program

Sponsor: University of Illinois College of Medicine at Peoria
St Francis Medical Center

Program Director:
Terry M Brady, MD
St Francis Med Ctr
Radiology Dept
530 NE Glen Oak Ave
Peoria, IL 61637
Tel: 309 655-7768 *Fax:* 309 655-7365
E-mail: lorid@uic.edu
Accred Length: 4 Years *Program Size:* 8
Subspecialties: RNR
Program ID: 420-16-21-243

Springfield

Southern Illinois University Program

Sponsor: Southern Illinois University School of Medicine
Memorial Medical Center
St John's Hospital

Program Director:
Kevin J Coakley, MD
Southern Illinois Univ, Dept of Radiology
Attn: Shelley Brumme
PO Box 19663
Springfield, IL 62794-9663
Tel: 217 785-2434 *Fax:* 217 525-5671
E-mail: sbrumme@siumed.edu
Accred Length: 4 Years *Program Size:* 9
Program ID: 420-16-21-065

Indiana

Indianapolis

Indiana University School of Medicine (Methodist) Program

Sponsor: Indiana University School of Medicine
Clarian Methodist Hospital of Indiana

Program Director:
Gonzalo T Chua, MD
Methodist Hospital of Indiana
I-65 at 21st St
PO Box 1367
Indianapolis, IN 46206-1367
Tel: 317 929-8250 *Fax:* 317 929-6312
E-mail: wgiles@clarian.com
Accred Length: 4 Years *Program Size:* 20
Subspecialties: VIR
Program ID: 420-17-12-067

Indiana University School of Medicine Program

Sponsor: Indiana University School of Medicine
Clarian IU Hospital
Clarian Riley Hospital for Children
Richard L Roudebush Veterans Affairs Medical Center
William N Wishard Memorial Hospital

Program Director:
Valerie P Jackson, MD
Wishard Memorial Hospital
Radiology Admin Rm 1154
1001 W 10th St
Indianapolis, IN 46202-2879
Tel: 317 630-6468 *Fax:* 317 630-7053
E-mail: vjackso@iupui.edu
Internet: http://www.indyrad.iupui.edu/homepage.htm
Accred Length: 4 Years *Program Size:* 43
Subspecialties: PDR, RNR, VIR
Program ID: 420-17-21-066

Programs

Iowa

Iowa City

University of Iowa Hospitals and Clinics Program

Sponsor: University of Iowa Hospitals and Clinics
Veterans Affairs Medical Center (Iowa City)
Program Director:
Brad H Thompson, MD
Univ of Iowa Hospitals and Clinics
Dept of Radiology
200 Hawkins Dr
Iowa City, IA 52242-1009
Tel: 319 356-3396 *Fax:* 319 356-2220
Internet:
http://www.vh.org/welcome/uihc/uihcmeddepts/diagnostic radiology/radatiowa/iowaradhome.html
Accred Length: 4 Years *Program Size:* 25 (*GY1:* 7)
Subspecialties: NR, PDR, RNR, VIR
Program ID: 420-18-21-068

Kansas

Kansas City

University of Kansas Medical Center Program

Sponsor: University of Kansas School of Medicine
University of Kansas Medical Center
Program Director:
Louis H Wetzel, MD
Univ of Kansas Med Ctr
Dept of Radiology
3901 Rainbow Blvd
Kansas City, KS 66160-7234
Tel: 913 588-6805 *Fax:* 913 588-7899
E-mail: mmonroe@kumc.edu
Accred Length: 4 Years *Program Size:* 18
Subspecialties: NR
Program ID: 420-19-11-069

Wichita

University of Kansas (Wichita) Program

Sponsor: University of Kansas School of Medicine (Wichita)
Columbia Wesley Medical Center
Program Director:
Charles W McGuire, MD
Univ of Kansas Sch of Med-Wichita
Wesley Med Ctr
550 N Hillside
Wichita, KS 67214-4976
Tel: 316 688-2211 *Fax:* 316 688-3396
E-mail: ehauserm@kumc.edu
Internet:
http://www.kumc.edu/wichita/dept/rad/radiology.htm
Accred Length: 4 Years *Program Size:* 8
Program ID: 420-19-12-070

Kentucky

Lexington

University of Kentucky Medical Center Program

Sponsor: University of Kentucky Hospital
Program Director:
Andrew M Fried, MD
Univ of Kentucky Med Ctr
Dept of Diagnostic Rad
800 Rose St/HX311
Lexington, KY 40536-0084
Tel: 606 323-5236 *Fax:* 606 323-2510
E-mail: afried@pop.uky.edu
Accred Length: 4 Years *Program Size:* 19 (*GY1:* 4)
Subspecialties: RNR
Program ID: 420-20-21-071

Louisville

University of Louisville Program

Sponsor: University of Louisville School of Medicine
University of Louisville Hospital
Veterans Affairs Medical Center (Louisville)
Program Director:
Gregory C Postel, MD
Univ of Louisville Sch of Med
Dept of Diagnostic Rad/CCB-C07
530 S Jackson St
Louisville, KY 40202-0000
Tel: 502 852-5875 *Fax:* 502 852-1754
E-mail: diagrad@ulkyvm.louisville.edu
Accred Length: 4 Years *Program Size:* 16
Program ID: 420-20-21-230

Louisiana

New Orleans

Alton Ochsner Medical Foundation Program

Sponsor: Alton Ochsner Medical Foundation
Program Director:
Michael A Sullivan, MD
Alton Ochsner Med Foundation
Dept of Grad Med Educ
1516 Jefferson Hwy
New Orleans, LA 70121
Tel: 504 842-3260 *Fax:* 504 842-3193
E-mail: dlambert@ochsner.org
Internet: http://www.ochsner.org
Accred Length: 4 Years *Program Size:* 20 (*GY1:* 4)
Program ID: 420-21-12-074

Louisiana State University Program

Sponsor: Louisiana State University School of Medicine
Childrens Hospital
Medical Center of Louisiana at New Orleans
Veterans Affairs Medical Center-LSU Service (New Orleans)
Program Director:
John N Joslyn, MD
Scott Beech, MD
Louisiana State Univ Med Ctr
Dept of Radiology
1542 Tulane Ave
New Orleans, LA 70112-2822
Tel: 504 568-4968 *Fax:* 504 568-8955
E-mail: kcampb@lsumc.edu
Accred Length: 4 Years *Program Size:* 24
Subspecialties: RNR
Program ID: 420-21-21-234

Tulane University Program

Sponsor: Tulane University School of Medicine
Tulane University Hospital and Clinics
Program Director:
Edward H De Mouy, MD
Tulane Univ Med Ctr
Dept of Radiology
1430 Tulane Ave/Box SL54
New Orleans, LA 70112-2699
Tel: 504 587-7567 *Fax:* 504 587-7616
E-mail: ewalker@tmc.tulane.edu
Internet:
http://www.omi.tulane.edu/departments/radiology/rad_home.htm
Accred Length: 4 Years *Program Size:* 16
Program ID: 420-21-21-235

Shreveport

Louisiana State University (Shreveport) Program

Sponsor: Louisiana State University Hospital-Shreveport
Program Director:
Mardjohan Hardjasudarma, MD
Louisiana State Univ Med Ctr Hospital
Dept of Radiology
1501 Kings Hwy/PO Box 33932
Shreveport, LA 71130-3932
Tel: 318 675-6240 *Fax:* 318 675-6351
E-mail: jhardj.@lsumc.edu
Accred Length: 4 Years *Program Size:* 12
Program ID: 420-21-11-075

Maine

Portland

Maine Medical Center Program

Sponsor: Maine Medical Center
Program Director:
Barbara P Biber, MD
Maine Med Ctr
Dept of Diagnostic Rad
22 Bramhall St
Portland, ME 04102
Tel: 207 871-4279 *Fax:* 207 871-6259
Internet:
http://www.mnetwork.com/mainemedical/lib.html
Accred Length: 4 Years *Program Size:* 14 (*GY1:* 3)
Program ID: 420-22-11-076

Maryland

Baltimore

Johns Hopkins University Program

Sponsor: Johns Hopkins University School of Medicine
Johns Hopkins Hospital
Program Director:
Stanley S Siegelman, MD
Johns Hopkins Hospital
Dept of Radiology
600 N Wolfe St
Baltimore, MD 21287
Tel: 410 955-5525 *Fax:* 410 614-2972
Accred Length: 4 Years *Program Size:* 24
Subspecialties: NR, PDR, RNR, VIR
Program ID: 420-23-11-077

University of Maryland Program
Sponsor: University of Maryland Medical System
Program Director:
Charles S Resnik, MD
Univ of Maryland Med System
22 S Greene St
Baltimore, MD 21201-1595
Tel: 410 328-3477 *Fax:* 410 328-0641
E-mail: resprog@radiology.ab.umd.edu
Internet:
http://umm.edu/center/specialties/departments/diag_radiology/res.toc.html
Accred Length: 4 Years *Program Size:* 24 *(GY1:* 6)
Subspecialties: RNR, VIR
Program ID: 420-23-11-079

Bethesda

National Capital Consortium Program
Sponsor: National Capital Consortium
National Naval Medical Center (Bethesda)
Walter Reed Army Medical Center
Program Director:
Douglas W Fellows, MD
Walter Reed Army Med Ctr
6825 16th St NW
Washington, DC 20307
Tel: 202 782-1699 *Fax:* 202 782-3393
E-mail: fellows@tatrc.org
Accred Length: 4 Years *Program Size:* 26 *(GY1:* 8)
Program ID: 420-10-21-247
US Armed Services Program

Massachusetts

Boston

Beth Israel Deaconess Medical Center Program
Sponsor: Beth Israel Deaconess Medical Center
Program Director:
Ferris M Hall, MD
Beth Israel Deaconess Med Ctr
Dept of Radiology
330 Brookline Ave
Boston, MA 02215
Tel: 617 667-3532 *Fax:* 617 667-8212
E-mail: radresidency@bidmc.harvard.edu
Internet: http://www.bidmc.harvard.edu/radiology
Accred Length: 4 Years *Program Size:* 32
Subspecialties: VIR
Program ID: 420-24-21-080

Boston University Medical Center Program
Sponsor: Boston Medical Center
Program Director:
William R Cranley, MD
Boston Med Ctr
Dept of Radiology
One Boston Medical Center Pl
Boston, MA 02118
Tel: 617 638-6610 *Fax:* 617 638-6616
Internet: http://med-amsa.bu.edu/radiology/main.html
Accred Length: 4 Years *Program Size:* 28
Subspecialties: RNR, TY, VIR
Program ID: 420-24-21-081

Brigham and Women's Hospital/Harvard Medical School Program
Sponsor: Brigham and Women's Hospital
Children's Hospital
Program Director:
Faye C Laing, MD
Brigham and Women's Hospital
Dept of Radiology
75 Francis St
Boston, MA 02115-6195
Tel: 617 278-0702 *Fax:* 617 278-6976
E-mail: laing@ulna.bwh.harvard.edu
Internet: http://www.med.harvard.edu/bwhrad/
Accred Length: 4 Years *Program Size:* 21
Subspecialties: NR, RNR, VIR
Program ID: 420-24-21-085

Massachusetts General Hospital/Harvard Medical School Program
Sponsor: Massachusetts General Hospital
Program Director:
Theresa C McLoud, MD
Massachusetts General Hospital
55 Fruit St
PO Box 9657/MZFND216
Boston, MA 02114-2696
Tel: 617 724-4255 *Fax:* 617 726-3077
E-mail: tmcloud@partners.org
Internet: http://132.183.8.152/mghradiology/
Accred Length: 4 Years *Program Size:* 29
Subspecialties: RNR, VIR
Program ID: 420-24-31-083

Tufts University Program
Sponsor: New England Medical Center Hospitals
Veterans Affairs Medical Center (Boston)
Program Director:
Elizabeth Oates, MD
New England Med Ctr
Dept of Radiology
750 Washington St/#228
Boston, MA 02111
Tel: 617 636-0067 *Fax:* 617 636-0041
E-mail: residency.program@es.nemc.org
Internet: http://www.nemcrad.com
Accred Length: 4 Years *Program Size:* 20
Subspecialties: RNR
Program ID: 420-24-21-086

Burlington

Lahey Clinic Program
Sponsor: Lahey Clinic
Program Director:
Carl R Larsen, MD
Lahey Clinic Med Ctr
Dept of Diagnostic Radiology
41 Mall Rd
Burlington, MA 01805
Tel: 781 744-8170 *Fax:* 781 744-5232
E-mail: carl.r.larsen@lahey.org
Internet: http://www.lahey.org
Accred Length: 4 Years *Program Size:* 12
Subspecialties: RNR
Program ID: 420-24-22-082

Cambridge

Mount Auburn Hospital Program
Sponsor: Mount Auburn Hospital
Program Director:
Michael J Shortsleeve, MD
Mount Auburn Hospital
Dept of Radiology
330 Mount Auburn St
Cambridge, MA 02238
Tel: 617 499-5070 *Fax:* 617 499-5138
E-mail: mta.rad.pmc@mahhosp.org
Internet: http://www.mtah.org
Accred Length: 4 Years *Program Size:* 8
Program ID: 420-24-11-087

Springfield

Baystate Medical Center Program
Sponsor: Baystate Medical Center
Program Director:
Thomas H Parker, MD
Baystate Med Ctr
Dept of Radiology
759 Chestnut St
Springfield, MA 01199
Tel: 413 794-3521 *Fax:* 413 794-5988
E-mail: linda.fratini@bhs.org
Internet: http://www.baystatehealth.com
Accred Length: 4 Years *Program Size:* 12
Program ID: 420-24-12-088

Worcester

St Vincent Hospital Program
Sponsor: St Vincent Hospital
Program Director:
Murray L Janower, MD
St Vincent Hospital
25 Winthrop St
Worcester, MA 01604
Tel: 508 798-6060 *Fax:* 508 798-1236
Accred Length: 4 Years *Program Size:* 8
Program ID: 420-24-12-089

University of Massachusetts Program
Sponsor: University of Massachusetts Medical School
UMass Memorial Health Care (University Campus)
Program Director:
Cynthia B Umali-Torres, MD
Univ of Massachusetts Med Sch
55 Lake Ave N
Worcester, MA 01655
Tel: 508 856-2160 *Fax:* 508 856-4669
E-mail: rad.residency@banyan.ummed.edu
Accred Length: 4 Years *Program Size:* 17
Subspecialties: RNR, VIR
Program ID: 420-24-21-090

Michigan

Ann Arbor

University of Michigan Program
Sponsor: University of Michigan Hospitals
Veterans Affairs Medical Center (Ann Arbor)
Program Director:
Richard H Cohan, MD
Univ of Michigan Health Systems
Dept of Radiology
1500 E Medical Center Dr
Ann Arbor, MI 48109-0030
Tel: 734 936-4474 *Fax:* 734 936-7948
E-mail: rochan@umich.edu
Internet: http://www.rad.med.umich.edu/residency.html
Accred Length: 4 Years *Program Size:* 36
Subspecialties: PDR, RNR, VIR
Program ID: 420-25-21-091

Dearborn

Oakwood Hospital Program
Sponsor: Oakwood Hospital
Program Director:
Sharon R Helmer, MD
Oakwood Healthcare System
18101 Oakwood Blvd
PO Box 2500
Dearborn, MI 48123-2500
Tel: 313 593-7302 *Fax:* 313 436-2071
E-mail: krayewsp@oakwood.org
Internet: http://www.oakwood.org
Accred Length: 4 Years *Program Size:* 20 (*GY1:* 5)
Program ID: 420-25-12-092

Detroit

Henry Ford Hospital Program
Sponsor: Henry Ford Hospital
Program Director:
Robert D Halpert, MD
Henry Ford Hospital
Dept of Radiology
2799 W Grand Blvd
Detroit, MI 48202
Tel: 313 876-9154 *Fax:* 313 556-8857
E-mail: halpert@rad.hfh.edu
Accred Length: 4 Years *Program Size:* 28
Subspecialties: MSR, RNR, VIR
Program ID: 420-25-11-093

Wayne State University/Detroit Medical Center Program
Sponsor: Wayne State University/Detroit Medical Center
Detroit Receiving Hospital and University Health Center
Grace Hospital
Harper Hospital
Program Director:
Lawrence P Davis, MD
Wayne State Univ-Detroit Med Ctr
Dept of Radiology DRH 3 L-8
4201 St Antoine
Detroit, MI 48201
Tel: 313 745-3430 *Fax:* 313 577-8600
E-mail: x-ray@med.wayne.edu
Internet:
http://www.med.wayne.edu/diagradiology/wsuhomepage.html
Accred Length: 4 Years *Program Size:* 32
Subspecialties: NR, RNR
Program ID: 420-25-21-096

Flint

Michigan State University (Flint) Program
Sponsor: Michigan State Univ College of Human Medicine-Flint Campus
Genesys Regional Medical Center-St Joseph Campus
Hurley Medical Center
McLaren Regional Medical Center
Program Director:
Alexander Gottschalk, MD
Michigan State Univ-Flint Campus
One Hurley Plaza
Flint, MI 48503-5902
Tel: 810 232-7000 *Fax:* 810 232-7020
Internet: http://msufame.msu.edu
Accred Length: 4 Years *Program Size:* 12
Program ID: 420-25-31-100

Grand Rapids

Grand Rapids Area Medical Education Consortium/Michigan State University Program
Sponsor: Grand Rapids Area Medical Education Consortium
Michigan State University College of Human Medicine
Spectrum Health-Downtown Campus
Spectrum Health-East Campus
St Mary's Health Services
Program Director:
Alexander Gottschalk, MD
Grand Rapids Area Med Educ Consortium
240 Cherry St SE
Grand Rapids, MI 49503
Tel: 616 732-6232 *Fax:* 616 732-6255
E-mail: kelderdk@gramec.msu.edu
Internet: http://www.radiology.msu.edu
Accred Length: 4 Years *Program Size:* 15 (*GY1:* 3)
Program ID: 420-25-21-099

Pontiac

St Joseph Mercy-Oakland Program
Sponsor: St Joseph Mercy-Oakland
Program Director:
Hugh H Kerr, MD
St Joseph Mercy Oakland
Dept of Radiology
900 Woodward Ave
Pontiac, MI 48341-2985
Tel: 248 858-3040 *Fax:* 248 858-3017
E-mail: creasonl@mercyhealth.com
Accred Length: 4 Years *Program Size:* 16
Program ID: 420-25-32-101

Royal Oak

William Beaumont Hospital Program
Sponsor: William Beaumont Hospital
Program Director:
Duane Mezwa, MD
Donald Gibson, MD
William Beaumont Hospital
Dept of Diagnostic Rad
3601 W 13 Mile Rd
Royal Oak, MI 48073
Tel: 248 551-6051 *Fax:* 248 551-5520
E-mail: diag_rad@beaumont.edu
Internet: http://www.beaumont.edu/html/gme
Accred Length: 4 Years *Program Size:* 28
Subspecialties: NR, RNR
Program ID: 420-25-12-102

Southfield

Providence Hospital and Medical Centers Program
Sponsor: Providence Hospital and Medical Centers
Program Director:
David L Osher, MD
Providence Hospital
Med Educ
16001 W Nine Mile Rd
Southfield, MI 48075-4818
Tel: 248 424-3051 *Fax:* 248 424-5395
Accred Length: 4 Years *Program Size:* 15
Program ID: 420-25-21-103

Minnesota

Minneapolis

University of Minnesota Program
Sponsor: University of Minnesota Medical School
Fairview-University Medical Center
Hennepin County Medical Center
Veterans Affairs Medical Center (Minneapolis)
Program Director:
Charles A Dietz Jr, MD
William M Thompson, MD
Box 292 UMHC
420 Delaware St SE
Minneapolis, MN 55455-0374
Tel: 612 626-3456 *Fax:* 612 624-1470
Accred Length: 4 Years *Program Size:* 40
Subspecialties: PDR, RNR, VIR
Program ID: 420-26-21-104

Rochester

Mayo Graduate School of Medicine (Rochester) Program
Sponsor: Mayo Graduate School of Medicine-Mayo Foundation
Mayo Clinic (Rochester)
Program Director:
Bradley D Lewis, MD
Application Processing Ctr
Mayo Graduate Sch of Med
200 First St SW
Rochester, MN 55905
Tel: 507 284-3108 *Fax:* 507 284-0999
E-mail: mgsm.roch.mn.diagnosticrad@mayo.edu
Internet: http://www.mayo.edu/
Accred Length: 4 Years *Program Size:* 40 (*GY1:* 10)
Subspecialties: NR, RNR, VIR
Program ID: 420-26-21-105

Mississippi

Jackson

University of Mississippi Medical Center Program
Sponsor: University of Mississippi School of Medicine
University Hospital
Program Director:
Lawrence W Dautenhahn, MD
Univ of Mississippi Med Ctr
Attn: Beth Morris, Res Coordinator
2500 N State St
Jackson, MS 39216-4505
Tel: 601 984-2695 *Fax:* 601 984-2683
E-mail: bmorris@radiology.umsmed.edu
Internet:
http://www.fiona.umsmed.edu/~rwiggins/rad.html
Accred Length: 4 Years *Program Size:* 18
Program ID: 420-27-11-107

Missouri

Columbia

University of Missouri-Columbia Program

Sponsor: University of Missouri-Columbia School of Medicine
Harry S Truman Memorial Veterans Hospital
University Hospitals and Clinics

Program Director:
Harry J Griffiths, MD
Univ of Missouri Hospital and Clinics
Radiology Dept/DC069.10
One Hospital Dr
Columbia, MO 65212
Tel: 573 882-7901 *Fax:* 573 884-4729
E-mail: crookj@fsrad1.hsc.missouri.edu
Internet: http://www.miams.missouri.edu/demoproj.html
Accred Length: 4 Years *Program Size:* 16
Subspecialties: NR
Program ID: 420-28-11-108

Kansas City

University of Missouri at Kansas City Program

Sponsor: University of Missouri-Kansas City School of Medicine
Saint Luke's Hospital
Truman Medical Center-West

Program Director:
Martin L Goldman, MD
Truman Med Ctr-West
Dept of Radiology
2301 Holmes St
Kansas City, MO 64108-8110
Tel: 816 556-3926 *Fax:* 816 556-3846
Accred Length: 4 Years *Program Size:* 19
Program ID: 420-28-21-231

St Louis

St Louis University School of Medicine Program

Sponsor: St Louis University School of Medicine
SSM Cardinal Glennon Children's Hospital
St Louis University School of Medicine
Veterans Affairs Medical Center (St Louis)

Program Director:
Murali Sundaram, MD
St Louis Univ Sch of Med, Dept of Radiology
3635 Vista Ave
PO Box 15250
St Louis, MO 63110-0250
Tel: 314 268-5781 *Fax:* 314 268-5116
E-mail: diagrad@slu.edu
Internet: http://www.slu.edu
Accred Length: 4 Years *Program Size:* 23
Subspecialties: PDR, RNR, VIR
Program ID: 420-28-21-110

Washington University/B-JH/SLCH Consortium Program

Sponsor: Washington University/B-JH/SLCH Consortium
Barnes-Jewish Hospital
Barnes-Jewish Hospital (North Campus)
Mallinckrodt Institute of Radiology
St Louis Children's Hospital
Washington University School of Medicine

Program Director:
Dennis M Balfe, MD
Mallinckrodt Inst of Radiology
510 S Kingshighway Blvd
St Louis, MO 63110
Tel: 314 362-2928 *Fax:* 314 362-2976
E-mail: balfe@mirlink.wustl.edu
Accred Length: 4 Years *Program Size:* 64
Subspecialties: NR, PDR, RNR, VIR
Program ID: 420-28-11-111

Nebraska

Omaha

Creighton University Program

Sponsor: Creighton University School of Medicine
Tenet St Joseph Hospital at Creighton Univ Medical Center

Program Director:
Charles Lerner, MD
Creighton Univ Sch of Med
Dept of Radiology
601 N 30th St
Omaha, NE 68131
Tel: 402 449-4753 *Fax:* 402 449-4271
E-mail: hanneman@creighton.edu
Internet: http://www.radiology.creighton.edu
Accred Length: 4 Years *Program Size:* 8
Program ID: 420-30-21-220

University of Nebraska Program

Sponsor: University of Nebraska Medical Center
Veterans Affairs Medical Center (Omaha)

Program Director:
Craig W Walker, MD
Univ of Nebraska Med Ctr
Dept of Radiology
600 S 42nd St
Omaha, NE 68198-1045
Tel: 402 559-6955 *Fax:* 402 559-1011
E-mail: cwwalker@unmc.edu
Internet: http://www.unmc.edu
Accred Length: 4 Years *Program Size:* 16
Subspecialties: VIR
Program ID: 420-30-21-112

New Hampshire

Lebanon

Dartmouth-Hitchcock Medical Center Program

Sponsor: Mary Hitchcock Memorial Hospital

Program Director:
Jocelyn D Chertoff, MD
Dartmouth-Hitchcock Med Ctr
Dept of Radiology
One Medical Center Dr
Lebanon, NH 03756
Tel: 603 650-4477 *Fax:* 603 650-5455
E-mail: jocelyn.d.chertoff@hitchcock.org
Internet:
http://www.hitchcock.org/pages/radiology/radiology.html
Accred Length: 4 Years *Program Size:* 12
Subspecialties: VIR
Program ID: 420-32-11-113

New Jersey

Camden

UMDNJ-Robert Wood Johnson Medical School (Camden) Program

Sponsor: Cooper Hospital-University Medical Center
Children's Hospital of Philadelphia

Program Director:
James H Jacoby, MD
Cooper Hospital-Univ Med Ctr
Diagnostic Radiology Dept
One Cooper Plaza
Camden, NJ 08103
Tel: 609 342-2382 *Fax:* 609 365-0472
E-mail: jacoby-james@cooperhealth.edu
Accred Length: 4 Years *Program Size:* 12
Program ID: 420-33-21-244

Hackensack

Hackensack Medical Center Program

Sponsor: Hackensack University Medical Center

Program Director:
Patrick J Toth, MD
Hackensack Med Ctr
30 Prospect Ave
Hackensack, NJ 07601
Tel: 201 996-2182 *Fax:* 201 996-3976
Accred Length: 4 Years *Program Size:* 8
Program ID: 420-33-12-114

Livingston

St Barnabas Medical Center Program

Sponsor: St Barnabas Medical Center

Program Director:
Lester Kalisher, MD
St Barnabas Med Ctr
94 Old Short Hills Rd
Livingston, NJ 07039
Tel: 973 322-5822 *Fax:* 973 322-5536
Accred Length: 4 Years *Program Size:* 12
Subspecialties: NR
Program ID: 420-33-21-215

Long Branch

Monmouth Medical Center Program

Sponsor: Monmouth Medical Center

Program Director:
Richard B Ruchman, MD
Monmouth Med Ctr
Dept of Radiology
300 Second Ave
Long Branch, NJ 07740-9998
Tel: 732 923-6806 *Fax:* 732 229-7359
E-mail: ruchman@auhs.edu
Accred Length: 4 Years *Program Size:* 8
Program ID: 420-33-31-115

Morristown

Morristown Memorial Hospital Program

Sponsor: Morristown Memorial Hospital

Program Director:
Jeanne R Schwartz, MD
Morristown Memorial Hospital, Dept of Radiology
100 Madison Ave
PO Box 1956
Morristown, NJ 07962-1956
Tel: 973 971-5372 *Fax:* 973 290-7294
Internet: http://www.atlantichealth.org
Accred Length: 4 Years *Program Size:* 8
Program ID: 420-33-11-116

Newark

Newark Beth Israel Medical Center Program

Sponsor: Newark Beth Israel Medical Center

Program Director:
Eva M Horn, MD
Newark Beth Israel Med Ctr
201 Lyons Ave
Newark, NJ 07112
Tel: 973 926-7035 *Fax:* 973 926-1395
Accred Length: 4 Years *Program Size:* 8
Program ID: 420-33-31-118

UMDNJ-New Jersey Medical School Program

Sponsor: UMDNJ-New Jersey Medical School
UMDNJ-University Hospital

Program Director:
Stephen R Baker, MD
UMDNJ-New Jersey Med Sch
Dept of Radiology/C-320
150 Bergen St
Newark, NJ 07103-2406
Tel: 973 972-6025 *Fax:* 973 972-7429
E-mail: williapm@umdnj.edu
Accred Length: 4 Years *Program Size:* 17
Program ID: 420-33-21-226

Piscataway

UMDNJ-Robert Wood Johnson Medical School Program

Sponsor: UMDNJ-Robert Wood Johnson Medical School
Robert Wood Johnson University Hospital
St Peter's University Hospital

Program Director:
Judith K Amorosa, MD
UMDNJ-Robert Wood Johnson Med Sch
Dept of Radiology
One Robert Wood Johnson Pl
New Brunswick, NJ 08903-0019
Tel: 732 235-7721 *Fax:* 732 235-6889
E-mail: tothmc@umdnj.edu
Internet: http://www.rwj-rad.rwjuh.edu
Accred Length: 4 Years *Program Size:* 12
Program ID: 420-33-21-228

Summit

Overlook Hospital Program

Sponsor: Overlook Hospital

Program Director:
William J Esposito, MD
Overlook Hospital
99 Beauvoir Ave
PO Box 220
Summit, NJ 07902-0220
Tel: 908 522-2065 *Fax:* 908 522-0804
Accred Length: 4 Years *Program Size:* 6
Program ID: 420-33-11-119

New Mexico

Albuquerque

University of New Mexico Program

Sponsor: University of New Mexico School of Medicine
University Hospital
Veterans Affairs Medical Center (Albuquerque)

Program Director:
Fred A Mettler Jr, MD
Univ of New Mexico Sch of Med
Dept of Radiology
915 Camino de Salud NE
Albuquerque, NM 87131-5336
Tel: 505 272-0932 *Fax:* 505 272-5821
E-mail: raderas@salud.unm.edu
Internet:
http://medlab1.unm.edu/index.html/gmetraining.html
Accred Length: 4 Years *Program Size:* 21 (*GY1:* 6)
Subspecialties: RNR
Program ID: 420-34-21-120

New York

Albany

Albany Medical Center Program

Sponsor: Albany Medical Center
Veterans Affairs Medical Center (Albany)

Program Director:
Matthew D Rifkin, MD
Albany Med Ctr
Dept of Radiology/MC-113
43 New Scotland Ave
Albany, NY 12208-3478
Tel: 518 445-3371 *Fax:* 518 262-4827
E-mail: kathie_breheny@ccgateway.amc.edu.
Accred Length: 4 Years *Program Size:* 17
Subspecialties: RNR
Program ID: 420-35-11-121

Bronx

Albert Einstein College of Medicine Program

Sponsor: Albert Einstein College of Medicine of Yeshiva University
Jacobi Medical Center
Montefiore Medical Center-Weiler Hospital

Program Director:
Mordecai Koenigsberg, MD
1300 Morris Park Ave
Bronx, NY 10461
Tel: 718 918-4520 *Fax:* 718 920-4854
E-mail: dchinea@worldnet.att.net
Accred Length: 4 Years *Program Size:* 33
Subspecialties: RNR, VIR
Program ID: 420-35-21-126

Bronx-Lebanon Hospital Center Program

Sponsor: Bronx-Lebanon Hospital Center

Program Director:
Harry L Miller, MD
1650 Grand Concourse Ave
Bronx, NY 10457
Tel: 718 518-5053 *Fax:* 718 901-3201
Accred Length: 4 Years *Program Size:* 12
Program ID: 420-35-12-128

Brooklyn

Long Island College Hospital Program

Sponsor: Long Island College Hospital

Program Director:
Deborah L Reede, MD
Neil E Adler, MD
Long Island Coll Hospital
339 Hicks St
Brooklyn, NY 11201
Tel: 718 780-1793 *Fax:* 718 780-1611
Accred Length: 4 Years *Program Size:* 12
Program ID: 420-35-11-131

Maimonides Medical Center Program

Sponsor: Maimonides Medical Center

Program Director:
Steven Shankman, MD
Maimonides Med Ctr
Dept of Radiology
4802 Tenth Ave
Brooklyn, NY 11219
Tel: 718 283-7117 *Fax:* 718 283-8874
Internet: http://www.maimonidesmed.org
Accred Length: 4 Years *Program Size:* 8
Program ID: 420-35-21-221

New York Methodist Hospital Program

Sponsor: New York Methodist Hospital

Program Director:
Helen T Winer Muram, MD
New York Methodist Hospital
506 Sixth St
Brooklyn, NY 11215-9008
Tel: 718 780-5870 *Fax:* 718 780-3494
Accred Length: 4 Years *Program Size:* 9
Subspecialties: NR
Program ID: 420-35-12-133

SUNY Health Science Center at Brooklyn Program

Sponsor: SUNY Health Science Center at Brooklyn
Kings County Hospital Center
University Hospital-SUNY Health Science Center at Brooklyn

Program Director:
David H Gordon, MD
SUNY Health Science Ctr-Brooklyn
Dept of Radiology
450 Clarkson Ave/Box 1198
Brooklyn, NY 11203-2098
Tel: 718 270-1603 *Fax:* 718 270-2667
Internet: http://www.hscbkyln.edu
Accred Length: 4 Years *Program Size:* 27
Program ID: 420-35-21-143

Buffalo

SUNY at Buffalo Graduate Medical-Dental Education Consortium Program

Sponsor: SUNY at Buffalo Grad Medical-Dental Education Consortium
CGF Health System (Buffalo General Hospital)
Erie County Medical Center

Program Director:
Angelo DelBalso, MD DDS
Erie County Med Ctr
Dept of Radiology
462 Grider St
Buffalo, NY 14215
Tel: 716 898-3424 *Fax:* 716 898-5217
Accred Length: 4 Years *Program Size:* 14
Program ID: 420-35-21-122

East Meadow

Nassau County Medical Center Program

Sponsor: Nassau County Medical Center

Program Director:
Dvorah Balsam, MD
Nassau County Med Ctr, Dept of Radiology
2201 Hempstead Trnpk
East Meadow, NY 11554-5400
Tel: 516 572-6633 *Fax:* 516 572-6787
Accred Length: 4 Years *Program Size:* 16
Program ID: 420-35-11-123

Manhasset

North Shore University Hospital/NYU School of Medicine Program

Sponsor: North Shore University Hospital

Program Director:
Mitchell A Goldman, MD
North Shore Univ Hospital
Dept of Radiology
300 Community Dr
Manhasset, NY 11030
Tel: 516 562-4800 *Fax:* 516 562-4794
Internet: http://www.nshs.edu
Accred Length: 4 Years *Program Size:* 20
Subspecialties: RNR
Program ID: 420-35-31-124

Mineola

Winthrop-University Hospital Program

Sponsor: Winthrop-University Hospital

Program Director:
Arthur Fruauff, MD
Winthrop-Univ Hospital
Dept of Radiology
259 First St
Mineola, NY 11501
Tel: 516 663-3800 *Fax:* 516 663-8172
E-mail: radiology@winthrop.org
Internet: http://www.winthrop.org
Accred Length: 4 Years *Program Size:* 12
Program ID: 420-35-21-240

New Hyde Park

Albert Einstein College of Medicine at Long Island Jewish Medical Center Program

Sponsor: Long Island Jewish Medical Center

Program Director:
Peter G Herman, MD
Long Island Jewish Med Ctr
Dept of Radiology
270-05 76th Ave
New Hyde Park, NY 11040
Tel: 718 470-7179 *Fax:* 718 343-7463
Internet: http://www.lij.edu/lij-homepage-ns.html
Accred Length: 4 Years *Program Size:* 17
Subspecialties: NR, PDR, RNR, VIR
Program ID: 420-35-21-132

New York

Albert Einstein College of Medicine at Beth Israel Medical Center Program

Sponsor: Beth Israel Medical Center

Program Director:
Arnold C Friedman, MD
Beth Israel Med Ctr
First Ave at 16th St
New York, NY 10003
Tel: 212 420-4585 *Fax:* 212 420-2510
Accred Length: 4 Years *Program Size:* 20
Subspecialties: RNR
Program ID: 420-35-21-127

Harlem Hospital Center Program

Sponsor: Harlem Hospital Center
New York and Presbyterian Hospital (Columbia Campus)

Program Director:
Roberta C Locko, MD
Harlem Hospital Ctr
506 Lenox Ave
New York, NY 10037
Tel: 212 939-4901 *Fax:* 212 939-4836
Accred Length: 4 Years *Program Size:* 2
Program ID: 420-35-21-214

Lenox Hill Hospital Program

Sponsor: Lenox Hill Hospital

Program Director:
Lewis M Rothman, MD
Lenox Hill Hospital
Dept of Radiology
100 E 77th St
New York, NY 10021-1883
Tel: 212 434-2929 *Fax:* 212 434-2945
Accred Length: 4 Years *Program Size:* 10
Program ID: 420-35-21-218

Mount Sinai School of Medicine Program

Sponsor: Mount Sinai School of Medicine
Elmhurst Hospital Center-Mount Sinai Services
Mount Sinai Medical Center

Program Director:
Kathleen P Halton, MD
Mount Sinai Med Ctr
One Gustave L Levy Pl
New York, NY 10029-6574
Tel: 212 241-4013 *Fax:* 212 427-8137
E-mail: kathleen_halton@smtplink.mssm.edu
Internet: http://www.mssm.edu/radiology/faculty.html
Accred Length: 4 Years *Program Size:* 24
Subspecialties: PDR, RNR, VIR
Program ID: 420-35-21-135

New York and Presbyterian Hospital (Columbia Campus) Program

Sponsor: New York and Presbyterian Hospital
New York and Presbyterian Hospital (Columbia Campus)

Program Director:
Carrie Ruzal Shapiro, MD
Presbyterian Hospital
622 W 168th St
New York, NY 10032
Tel: 212 305-8994 *Fax:* 212 305-4835
Internet: http://cpmcnet.columbia.edu/dept/radiology/
Accred Length: 4 Years *Program Size:* 24
Subspecialties: NR, PDR, RNR, VIR
Program ID: 420-35-11-138

New York and Presbyterian Hospital (Cornell Campus) Program

Sponsor: New York and Presbyterian Hospital
Hospital for Special Surgery
Memorial Sloan-Kettering Cancer Center
New York and Presbyterian Hospital (Cornell Campus)

Program Director:
Nicholas Papanicolau, MD
New York Hospital-Cornell Med Ctr
525 E 68th St
New York, NY 10021
Tel: 212 746-2562 *Fax:* 212 746-8596
Accred Length: 4 Years *Program Size:* 32
Subspecialties: RNR, VIR
Program ID: 420-35-21-129

New York Medical College at St Vincent's Hospital and Medical Center of New York Program

Sponsor: New York Medical College
St Vincent's Hospital and Medical Center of New York

Program Director:
Jeremy J Kaye, MD
St Vincent's Hospital and Med Ctr
153 W 11th St
New York, NY 10011
Tel: 212 604-2416 *Fax:* 212 604-2929
Accred Length: 4 Years *Program Size:* 13
Subspecialties: NR, TY
Program ID: 420-35-12-141

New York University Medical Center Program

Sponsor: New York University Medical Center
Bellevue Hospital Center
Veterans Affairs Medical Center (Manhattan)

Program Director:
Albert F Keegan, MD
New York Univ Med Ctr
550 First Ave
New York, NY 10016
Tel: 212 263-6373 *Fax:* 212 263-7666
Internet:
http://nucmed.med.nyu.edu/ambrosino/ambrosino/index.htm
Accred Length: 4 Years *Program Size:* 32
Subspecialties: MSR, NR, PDR, RNR
Program ID: 420-35-21-137

St Luke's-Roosevelt Hospital Center Program

Sponsor: St Luke's-Roosevelt Hospital Center
St Luke's-Roosevelt Hospital Center-Roosevelt Division
St Luke's-Roosevelt Hospital Center-St Luke's Division

Program Director:
Jeanne W Baer, MD
St Luke's-Roosevelt Hospital Ctr
Dept of Radiology
1111 Amsterdam Ave
New York, NY 10025
Tel: 212 523-4259 *Fax:* 212 523-2433
Accred Length: 4 Years *Program Size:* 20
Subspecialties: NR, VIR
Program ID: 420-35-21-224

Rochester

Rochester General Hospital Program

Sponsor: Rochester General Hospital

Program Director:
Daniel Jacobson, MD
Rochester General Hospital
1425 Portland Ave
Rochester, NY 14621
Tel: 800 393-4874 *Fax:* 716 336-9695
E-mail: daniel.jacobson@viahealth.org
Internet: http://www.viahealth.org/radres
Accred Length: 4 Years *Program Size:* 10
Program ID: 420-35-12-145

University of Rochester Program

Sponsor: Strong Memorial Hospital of the University of Rochester

Program Director:
Jovitas Skucas, MD
Univ of Rochester Med Ctr
601 Elmwood Ave/Box 648
Rochester, NY 14642-8648
Tel: 716 275-2622 *Fax:* 716 273-1033
E-mail: skucas@rad.rochester.edu
Accred Length: 4 Years *Program Size:* 16 (*GYI:* 3)
Subspecialties: PDR, RNR, VIR
Program ID: 420-35-11-146

Staten Island

New York Medical College (Richmond) Program

Sponsor: New York Medical College
Sisters of Charity Medical Center-St Vincent's Campus
Westchester Medical Center

Program Director:
Ruwini D de Silva, MD
St Vincent's Med Ctr of Richmond
355 Bard Ave
Staten Island, NY 10310-1699
Tel: 718 876-3153 *Fax:* 718 876-1869
E-mail: megan@admin.con2.com
Accred Length: 4 Years *Program Size:* 9
Program ID: 420-35-21-229

Stony Brook

SUNY at Stony Brook Program

Sponsor: University Hospital-SUNY at Stony Brook
Veterans Affairs Medical Center (Northport)

Program Director:
Kathleen C Finzel, MD
Univ Hospital
Level 4 Rm 092
Health Science Ctr
Stony Brook, NY 11794-8460
Tel: 516 444-2484 *Fax:* 516 444-7538
Internet: http://www.informatics.sunysb.edu/radiology
Accred Length: 4 Years *Program Size:* 17
Subspecialties: NR, RNR
Program ID: 420-35-21-222

Syracuse

SUNY Health Science Center at Syracuse Program

Sponsor: University Hospital-SUNY Health Science Center at Syracuse
Veterans Affairs Medical Center (Syracuse)

Program Director:
Stuart A Groskin, MD
Kimball G Clark, MD
SUNY Health Science Ctr
Dept of Radiology
750 E Adams St
Syracuse, NY 13210
Tel: 315 464-7434 *Fax:* 315 464-7458
Internet: http://www.hscsyr.edu/-xray/
Accred Length: 4 Years *Program Size:* 20
Subspecialties: NR, RNR
Program ID: 420-35-21-147

Valhalla

New York Medical College at Westchester Medical Center Program

Sponsor: New York Medical College
Westchester Medical Center

Program Director:
Susan A Klein, MD
New York Med Coll
Macy Pavilion
Dept of Radiology
Valhalla, NY 10595
Tel: 914 493-8550 *Fax:* 914 493-7407
Accred Length: 4 Years *Program Size:* 12
Subspecialties: RNR, VIR
Program ID: 420-35-21-136

North Carolina

Chapel Hill

University of North Carolina Hospitals Program

Sponsor: University of North Carolina Hospitals

Program Director:
Paul L Molina, MD
Univ of North Carolina Sch of Med
520 Old Infirmary/CB7510
Chapel Hill, NC 27599-7510
Tel: 919 966-6952 *Fax:* 919 966-0817
E-mail: plmolina@med.unc.edu
Internet: http://www.med.unc.edu/radiology/
Accred Length: 4 Years *Program Size:* 20 (*GY1:* 5)
Subspecialties: PDR, RNR, VIR
Program ID: 420-36-11-148

Durham

Duke University Program

Sponsor: Duke University Medical Center
Veterans Affairs Medical Center (Durham)

Program Director:
Linda Gray Leithe, MD
Duke Univ Med Ctr
Dept of Radiology
Box 3808
Durham, NC 27710
Tel: 919 684-7456 *Fax:* 919 684-7123
Internet:
http://www.radweb.mc.duke.edu/resident/residency.html
Accred Length: 4 Years *Program Size:* 40
Subspecialties: NR, PDR, RNR
Program ID: 420-36-31-149

Winston-Salem

Wake Forest University School of Medicine Program

Sponsor: Wake Forest University Baptist Medical Center

Program Director:
Ronald J Zagoria, MD
Wake Forest Univ Sch of Med
Medical Center Blvd
Winston-Salem, NC 27157-1088
Tel: 336 716-4260 *Fax:* 336 716-0555
E-mail: zagoriar@rad.wfubmc.edu
Internet:
http://www.rad.bgsm.edu/radmain/htmls/resprgm/respgm.html
Accred Length: 4 Years *Program Size:* 30 (*GY1:* 8)
Subspecialties: NR, PDR, RNR, VIR
Program ID: 420-36-11-150

Ohio

Canton

Aultman Hospital/NEOUCOM Program

Sponsor: Aultman Hospital
Timken Mercy Medical Center

Program Director:
Barry S Rose, MD
Canton Affiliated Hospitals-NEOUCOM Radiology Residency Prog
2600 Sixth St SW
Canton, OH 44710
Tel: 330 438-6200 *Fax:* 330 588-2601
Accred Length: 4 Years *Program Size:* 16
Subspecialties: TY
Program ID: 420-38-21-232

Cincinnati

University Hospital/University of Cincinnati College of Medicine Program

Sponsor: University Hospital Inc
Christ Hospital
Veterans Affairs Medical Center (Cincinnati)

Program Director:
Kyuran A Choe, MD
University Hospital
Dept of Radiology
234 Goodman St/ML 0742
Cincinnati, OH 45219-0742
Tel: 513 584-6016 *Fax:* 513 584-0431
E-mail: choeka@healthall.com
Internet:
http://www.med.uc.edu/htdocs/medicine/departme/radiol/radhomep2.htm
Accred Length: 4 Years *Program Size:* 25
Subspecialties: PDR, RNR
Program ID: 420-38-21-152

Cleveland

Case Western Reserve University (MetroHealth) Program

Sponsor: MetroHealth Medical Center

Program Director:
Errol M Bellon, MD
MetroHealth Med Ctr
Dept of Radiology
2500 MetroHealth Dr
Cleveland, OH 44109-1998
Tel: 216 778-4016 *Fax:* 216 778-4072
E-mail: nerwin@metrohealth.org
Internet: http://www.metrohealth.org/clinical/radiology
Accred Length: 4 Years *Program Size:* 16
Program ID: 420-38-21-242

Case Western Reserve University Program

Sponsor: University Hospitals of Cleveland

Program Director:
Charles Lanzieri, MD
Peter B Sachs, MD
Univ Hospitals of Cleveland
Attn: Mattie L Slater
11100 Euclid Ave
Cleveland, OH 44106-5000
Tel: 216 844-3113 *Fax:* 216 844-3905
E-mail: slater@uhrad.com
Internet: http://www.uhrad.com
Accred Length: 4 Years *Program Size:* 24 (*GY1:* 5)
Subspecialties: RNR, VIR
Program ID: 420-38-21-153

Cleveland Clinic Foundation Program

Sponsor: Cleveland Clinic Foundation

Program Director:
David M Einstein, MD
Cleveland Clinic Foundation
Dept of Diagnostic Rad/HB6
9500 Euclid Ave
Cleveland, OH 44195-5242
Tel: 216 444-5690 *Fax:* 216 444-1162
E-mail: meded@cesmtp.ccf.org
Internet: http://www.ccf.org
Accred Length: 4 Years *Program Size:* 24 (*GY1:* 6)
Subspecialties: PDR, RNR, VIR
Program ID: 420-38-12-154

Mount Sinai Medical Center of Cleveland Program

Sponsor: Mount Sinai Medical Center of Cleveland

Program Director:
Avram E Pearlstein, MD
Mt Sinai Med Ctr
One Mt Sinai Dr
Cleveland, OH 44106-4198
Tel: 216 421-5903 *Fax:* 216 421-5343
Accred Length: 4 Years *Program Size:* 11
Subspecialties: TY
Program ID: 420-38-11-155

Columbus

Ohio State University Program

Sponsor: Ohio State University Medical Center

Program Director:
Charles F Mueller, MD
Ohio State Univ
Dept of Radiology/RH S-209
410 W Tenth Ave
Columbus, OH 43210
Tel: 614 293-8369 *Fax:* 614 293-6935
Accred Length: 4 Years *Program Size:* 20
Subspecialties: RNR
Program ID: 420-38-21-156

Toledo

Medical College of Ohio Program

Sponsor: Medical College of Ohio
St Vincent Mercy Medical Center

Program Director:
Lee S Woldenberg, MD
Med Coll of Ohio
Dept of Radiology
3000 Arlington Ave/Rm 1217
Toledo, OH 43614-2598
Tel: 419 383-3428 *Fax:* 419 383-6422
E-mail: cfrench@opus.mco.edu
Accred Length: 4 Years *Program Size:* 11
Program ID: 420-38-21-157

Youngstown

St Elizabeth Health Center/NEOUCOM Program

Sponsor: St Elizabeth Health Center
Forum Health-Northside Medical Center

Program Director:
Steven Aubel, MD
St Elizabeth Health Ctr
1044 Belmont Ave
PO Box 1790
Youngstown, OH 44501
Tel: 330 480-3631 *Fax:* 330 480-2912
E-mail: rosey_hilland@hmis.org
Accred Length: 4 Years *Program Size:* 6
Program ID: 420-38-21-233

Oklahoma

Oklahoma City

Integris Baptist Medical Center Program

Sponsor: Integris Baptist Medical Center

Program Director:
Jay A Harolds, MD
Baptist Med Ctr of Oklahoma
Dept of Radiology
3300 NW Expressway
Oklahoma City, OK 73112
Tel: 405 951-2272 *Fax:* 405 949-3939
E-mail: fayssj@integris-health.com
Internet: http://www.integris-health.com
Accred Length: 4 Years *Program Size:* 16
Program ID: 420-39-12-158

University of Oklahoma Health Sciences Center Program

Sponsor: University of Oklahoma College of Medicine
Children's Hospital of Oklahoma
University Hospital
Veterans Affairs Medical Center (Oklahoma City)

Program Director:
Bob G Eaton, MD
Univ of Oklahoma Health Sciences Ctr
Dept of Radiological Sciences
PO Box 26901
Oklahoma City, OK 73190-3020
Tel: 405 271-5125 *Fax:* 405 271-3462
Accred Length: 4 Years *Program Size:* 24
Subspecialties: VIR
Program ID: 420-39-21-159

Oregon

Portland

Oregon Health Sciences University Program

Sponsor: Oregon Health Sciences University Hospital
Veterans Affairs Medical Center (Portland)

Program Director:
Paul C Lakin, MD
Oregon Health Sciences Univ
Dept of Diagnostic Rad/L340
3181 SW Sam Jackson Park Rd
Portland, OR 97201-3098
Tel: 503 494-5266 *Fax:* 503 494-4982
E-mail: lakinp@ohsu.edu
Internet: http://www.ohsu.edu/ps-diagradiol/radres.htm
Accred Length: 4 Years *Program Size:* 16
Program ID: 420-40-31-160

Pennsylvania

Bryn Mawr

Bryn Mawr Hospital Program

Sponsor: Bryn Mawr Hospital

Program Director:
Vikram S Dravid, MD
Bryn Mawr Hospital
Dept of Radiology
130 S Bryn Mawr Ave
Bryn Mawr, PA 19010-3160
Tel: 610 526-3436 *Fax:* 610 526-4590
E-mail: thompsonl2@mlhs.org
Accred Length: 4 Years *Program Size:* 8
Program ID: 420-41-21-162

Danville

Penn State Geisinger Health System/Geisinger Medical Center Program

Sponsor: Penn State Geisinger Health System
Geisinger Medical Center

Program Director:
Anne P Dunne, MD
Geisinger Med Ctr
100 N Academy Ave
Danville, PA 17822
Tel: 717 271-5976
E-mail: adunne@psghs.edu
Accred Length: 4 Years *Program Size:* 12
Program ID: 420-41-21-163

Hershey

Penn State Geisinger Health System/Milton S Hershey Medical Center Program

Sponsor: Penn State Geisinger Health System
Milton S Hershey Medical Center

Program Director:
Rickhesvar P Mahraj, MD
Coll of Med-Univ Hospital
Milton S Hershey Med Ctr
PO Box 850
Hershey, PA 17033
Tel: 717 531-6896 *Fax:* 717 531-4605
Internet: http://www.xray.hmc.psu.edu
Accred Length: 4 Years *Program Size:* 22
Subspecialties: VIR
Program ID: 420-41-21-164

Philadelphia

Albert Einstein Medical Center Program

Sponsor: Albert Einstein Medical Center

Program Director:
William Herring, MD
Albert Einstein Med Ctr
5501 Old York Rd
Philadelphia, PA 19141-3098
Tel: 215 456-6200 *Fax:* 215 456-6227
E-mail: radiology@aehn2.einstein.edu
Internet: http://www.einstein.edu
Accred Length: 4 Years *Program Size:* 16
Program ID: 420-41-21-165

MCP Hahnemann University Program

Sponsor: MCP Hahnemann University
Hahnemann University Hospital
Medical College of Pennsylvania Hospital

Program Director:
Beverly L Hershey, MD
Hahnemann Univ Hospital
Dept of Rad Sciences
Broad and Vine Sts
Philadelphia, PA 19102
Tel: 215 762-8746 *Fax:* 215 762-4092
Accred Length: 4 Years *Program Size:* 30
Program ID: 420-41-21-169

Mercy Catholic Medical Center Program

Sponsor: Mercy Catholic Medical Center Inc
Mercy Hospital of Philadelphia
Mercy Fitzgerald Hospital

Program Director:
Michael L Brooks, MD
1500 Lansdowne Ave
Darby, PA 19023
Tel: 610 237-4355 *Fax:* 610 237-2599
Internet: http://www.mercyhealth.org as well as vs012057@mindspring.com
Accred Length: 4 Years *Program Size:* 9
Subspecialties: TY
Program ID: 420-41-21-170

Pennsylvania Hospital of the University of Pennsylvania Health System Program
Sponsor: Pennsylvania Hospital (UPHS)
Program Director:
Geoffrey A Agrons, MD
Christine Emery, MD
Pennsylvania Hospital
800 Spruce St
Philadelphia, PA 19107-6192
Tel: 215 829-3201 *Fax:* 215 829-7482
Accred Length: 4 Years *Program Size:* 16
Program ID: 420-41-31-171

Temple University Program
Sponsor: Temple University Hospital
Program Director:
Michael B Love, MD
Dept of Diagnostic Imaging
Temple Univ Hospital
Broad and Ontario Sts
Philadelphia, PA 19140
Tel: 215 707-2586 *Fax:* 215 707-5851
E-mail: radiores@blue.temple.edu
Internet: http://www.temple.edu/radiology
Accred Length: 4 Years *Program Size:* 24
Subspecialties: NR, RNR
Program ID: 420-41-11-173

Thomas Jefferson University Program
Sponsor: Thomas Jefferson University Hospital
Program Director:
Vijay M Rao, MD
Thomas Jefferson Univ
132 S Tenth St
Rm 1092 Main Bldg
Philadelphia, PA 19107-8110
Tel: 215 955-4804 *Fax:* 215 955-5329
Internet: http://www.rad.tju.edu
Accred Length: 4 Years *Program Size:* 24
Subspecialties: RNR, VIR
Program ID: 420-41-11-174

University of Pennsylvania Program
Sponsor: Hospital of the University of Pennsylvania
Program Director:
Igor Laufer, MD
Hospital of Univ of Pennsylvania
Dept of Radiology
3400 Spruce St
Philadelphia, PA 19104
Tel: 215 662-3263 *Fax:* 215 349-5925
E-mail: laufer@oasis.rad.upenn.edu
Internet: http://www.rad.upenn.edu/rrphome.html
Accred Length: 4 Years *Program Size:* 32
Subspecialties: NR, PDR, RNR, VIR
Program ID: 420-41-21-175

Pittsburgh

Allegheny General Hospital Program
Sponsor: Allegheny General Hospital
Program Director:
Andrew L Goldberg, MD
Allegheny General Hospital
Dept of Radiology
320 E North Ave
Pittsburgh, PA 15212-9986
Tel: 412 359-4113 *Fax:* 412 359-6912
Accred Length: 4 Years *Program Size:* 16
Subspecialties: RNR
Program ID: 420-41-21-176

Mercy Hospital of Pittsburgh Program
Sponsor: Mercy Hospital of Pittsburgh
Program Director:
William R Poller, MD
Mercy Hospital of Pittsburgh
Dept of Radiology
1400 Locust St
Pittsburgh, PA 15219-5166
Tel: 412 232-7909 *Fax:* 412 232-7914
E-mail: diagnostic.radiology.residency@mercy.pmhs.org
Internet: http://www.mercy-meded.com
Accred Length: 4 Years *Program Size:* 12
Program ID: 420-41-11-178

St Francis Medical Center Program
Sponsor: St Francis Medical Center
Allegheny University Hospitals-Forbes Regional
Program Director:
Gerald J Ross, MD
St Francis Med Ctr
Med Educ Office
400 45th St
Pittsburgh, PA 15201
Tel: 412 622-6748
E-mail: radres@sfhs.edu
Internet: http://www.sfhs.edu
Accred Length: 4 Years *Program Size:* 15 (*GY1:* 3)
Program ID: 420-41-21-179

University Health Center of Pittsburgh Program
Sponsor: University Health Center of Pittsburgh
Presbyterian University Hospital/UPMC
Program Director:
James H Oliver III, MD
Univ of Pittsburgh Med Ctr
Dept of Radiology
200 Lothrop St
Pittsburgh, PA 15213-2582
Tel: 412 647-7338 *Fax:* 412 647-1137
E-mail: oliverjh@radserv.arad.upmc.edu
Internet: http://radserv.arad.upmc.edu/residency/
Accred Length: 4 Years *Program Size:* 28
Subspecialties: PDR, RNR, VIR
Program ID: 420-41-21-177

Western Pennsylvania Hospital Program
Sponsor: Western Pennsylvania Hospital
Program Director:
Ellen B Mendelson, MD
Western Pennsylvania Hospital
4800 Friendship Ave
Pittsburgh, PA 15224
Tel: 412 578-4810 *Fax:* 412 578-1693
E-mail: wphradrs@usaor.net
Internet: http://www.westpennhospital.com
Accred Length: 4 Years *Program Size:* 12
Subspecialties: VIR
Program ID: 420-41-21-241

Reading

Reading Hospital and Medical Center Program
Sponsor: Reading Hospital and Medical Center
Program Director:
Thomas G Helinek, MD PhD
Reading Hospital and Med Ctr
PO Box 16052
Sixth Ave and Spruce St
Reading, PA 19612-6052
Tel: 610 378-6108 *Fax:* 610 378-6400
E-mail: helinekt@readinghospital.org
Accred Length: 4 Years *Program Size:* 6 (*GY1:* 1)
Program ID: 420-41-22-181

Puerto Rico

San Juan

University of Puerto Rico Program
Sponsor: University of Puerto Rico School of Medicine
San Juan City Hospital
University Hospital
Veterans Affairs Medical Center (San Juan)
Program Director:
Edgar Colon Negron, MD
PO Box 365067
Medical Sciences Campus
San Juan, PR 00936-5067
Tel: 787 754-3576 *Fax:* 787 754-4093
Accred Length: 4 Years *Program Size:* 16 (*GY1:* 5)
Program ID: 420-42-21-182

Rhode Island

Providence

Brown University Program
Sponsor: Rhode Island Hospital
Program Director:
John J Cronan, MD
Dept of Diagnostic Imaging
Rhode Island Hospital
593 Eddy St
Providence, RI 02903
Tel: 401 444-5184 *Fax:* 401 444-5017
E-mail: gpascetta@lifespan.org
Internet: http://www.brown.edu/departments/diagnostic imaging/
Accred Length: 4 Years *Program Size:* 19
Subspecialties: VIR
Program ID: 420-43-21-183

South Carolina

Charleston

Medical University of South Carolina Program
Sponsor: Medical University of South Carolina College of Medicine
Charleston Memorial Hospital
MUSC Medical Center
Ralph H Johnson Dept of Veterans Affairs Med Center
Program Director:
Jeanne G Hill, MD
Med Univ of South Carolina
Dept of Radiology
171 Ashley Ave
Charleston, SC 29425-0720
Tel: 843 792-7179 *Fax:* 843 792-6414
E-mail: radresid@musc.edu
Internet: http://www.musc.edu/radiology/residency
Accred Length: 4 Years *Program Size:* 21
Subspecialties: PDR, RNR, VIR
Program ID: 420-45-21-184

Tennessee

Knoxville

University of Tennessee Medical Center at Knoxville Program

Sponsor: University of Tennessee Graduate School of Medicine
University of Tennessee Memorial Hospital

Program Director:
Anton Allen, MD
Kathleen B Hudson, MD
Univ of Tennessee Grad Sch of Med
1924 Alcoa Hwy
Knoxville, TN 37920-6999
Tel: 423 544-9062 *Fax:* 423 544-9025
Internet: http://scanner.hosp.utk.edu/radiology/
Accred Length: 4 Years *Program Size:* 16
Program ID: 420-47-21-236

Memphis

Baptist Memorial Hospital Program

Sponsor: Baptist Memorial Hospital

Program Director:
Allen K Tonkin, MD
Baptist Memorial Hospital
Dept of Radiology
899 Madison Ave
Memphis, TN 38146
Tel: 901 227-3000 *Fax:* 901 227-3009
E-mail: imaging@magibox.net
Internet: http://www.msit.com
Accred Length: 4 Years *Program Size:* 20
Program ID: 420-47-12-186

Methodist Hospitals of Memphis-Central Program

Sponsor: Methodist Hospitals of Memphis-Central

Program Director:
Robert E Laster Jr, MD MD
Methodist Healthcare-Central Unit
Dept of Radiology
1265 Union Ave
Memphis, TN 38104
Tel: 901 726-8529 *Fax:* 901 726-7490
E-mail: barnsl@mhsgate.meth-mem.org
Internet: http://www.meth-mem.org
Accred Length: 4 Years *Program Size:* 12
Program ID: 420-47-21-187

University of Tennessee Program

Sponsor: University of Tennessee College of Medicine
LeBonheur Children's Medical Center
Regional Medical Center at Memphis
University of Tennessee Medical Center (UT Bowld Hospital)
Veterans Affairs Medical Center (Memphis)

Program Director:
John D King, MD
Univ of Tennessee
Dept of Radiology
800 Madison Ave/150 Chandler
Memphis, TN 38163
Tel: 901 448-8248 *Fax:* 901 448-5352
E-mail: pfelix@utmem.edu
Internet:
http://www2.utmem.edu/radiology/utradhome.htm
Accred Length: 4 Years *Program Size:* 17
Subspecialties: PDR, VIR
Program ID: 420-47-21-188

Nashville

Vanderbilt University Program

Sponsor: Vanderbilt University Medical Center
Veterans Affairs Medical Center (Nashville)

Program Director:
Thomas S Dina, MD
Vanderbilt Univ Sch of Med
Dept of Radiology/R-1318 MCN
21st Ave S and Garland Ave
Nashville, TN 37232-2675
Tel: 615 322-3780 *Fax:* 615 322-3764
E-mail: radprogram@mcmail.vanderbilt.edu
Internet: http://www.mc.vanderbilt.edu/radiology/
Accred Length: 4 Years *Program Size:* 26
Subspecialties: PDR, RNR, VIR
Program ID: 420-47-21-189

Texas

Dallas

Baylor University Medical Center Program

Sponsor: Baylor University Medical Center

Program Director:
Mark Zibilich, MD
Baylor Univ Med Ctr
Dept of Radiology
3500 Gaston Ave
Dallas, TX 75246
Tel: 214 820-3219 *Fax:* 214 820-7437
Internet:
http://www.bhcs.com/bumc/medicaleducation/residencies.htm
Accred Length: 4 Years *Program Size:* 18
Subspecialties: VIR
Program ID: 420-48-22-190

University of Texas Southwestern Medical School Program

Sponsor: University of Texas Southwestern Medical School
Dallas County Hospital District-Parkland Memorial Hospital
Veterans Affairs Medical Center (Dallas)

Program Director:
George C Curry, MD
Univ of Texas Southwestern Med Ctr
Dept of Radiology
5323 Harry Hines Blvd
Dallas, TX 75235-8896
Tel: 214 648-8022 *Fax:* 214 648-2678
E-mail: dotter@mednet.swmed.edu
Internet: http://www.rad.swmed.edu/residen.html
Accred Length: 4 Years *Program Size:* 50 (*GYI:* 12)
Subspecialties: NR, PDR, RNR, VIR
Program ID: 420-48-21-192

Fort Sam Houston

San Antonio Uniformed Services Health Education Consortium Program

Sponsor: San Antonio Uniformed Services Health Education Consortium
Brooke Army Medical Center
Wilford Hall Medical Center (AETC)

Program Director:
Michael A Cawthon, DO
Dept of Radiology (MCHE-DR)
Brooke Army Med Ctr
3851 Roger Brooke Dr
Fort Sam Houston, TX 78234-6200
Tel: 210 916-3290 *Fax:* 210 916-5193
E-mail: cawthon@tatrc.org
Accred Length: 4 Years *Program Size:* 38
Program ID: 420-48-21-248
US Armed Services Program

Galveston

University of Texas Medical Branch Hospitals Program

Sponsor: University of Texas Medical Branch Hospitals

Program Director:
Brian W Goodacre, MD
Univ of Texas Med Branch Hospitals
Dept of Radiology G-09
Galveston, TX 77555-0709
Tel: 409 747-2849 *Fax:* 409 747-2825
E-mail: rcoble@utmb.edu
Internet: http://utmb.edu/
Accred Length: 4 Years *Program Size:* 22
Subspecialties: PDR, RNR
Program ID: 420-48-11-194

Houston

Baylor College of Medicine Program

Sponsor: Baylor College of Medicine
Harris County Hospital District-Ben Taub General Hospital
Methodist Hospital
St Luke's Episcopal Hospital
Texas Children's Hospital
Veterans Affairs Medical Center (Houston)

Program Director:
Neela Lamki, MD
Baylor Coll of Med
Dept of Radiology
One Baylor Plaza
Houston, TX 77030-3498
Tel: 713 798-6362 *Fax:* 713 798-8359
E-mail: nlamki@bcm.tmc.edu
Internet: http://www.bcm.tmc.edu/radiology/
Accred Length: 4 Years *Program Size:* 26
Subspecialties: PDR, RNR, TY
Program ID: 420-48-21-195

University of Texas at Houston Program

Sponsor: University of Texas Medical School at Houston
Lyndon B Johnson General Hospital
Memorial Hermann Healthcare System
St Joseph Hospital
University of Texas M D Anderson Cancer Center

Program Director:
Sandra A Oldham, MD
Univ of Texas Med Sch
Dept of Radiology
6431 Fannin/Ste 2.026
Houston, TX 77030
Tel: 713 500-7640 *Fax:* 713 500-7647
E-mail: tcarter@msrad3.med.uth.tmc.edu
Internet: http://www.msrad3
Accred Length: 4 Years *Program Size:* 39
Subspecialties: RNR
Program ID: 420-48-21-196

San Antonio

University of Texas Health Science Center at San Antonio Program
Sponsor: University of Texas Medical School at San Antonio
Audie L Murphy Memorial Veterans Hospital (San Antonio)
University Hospital-South Texas Medical Center
Program Director:
Ewell A Clarke, MD
Univ of Texas Health Science Ctr
7703 Floyd Curl Dr
San Antonio, TX 78284-7800
Tel: 210 567-6482 *Fax:* 210 567-6469
E-mail: freabe@uthscsa.edu
Internet: http://www.uthscsa.edu
Accred Length: 4 Years *Program Size:* 25 (*GY1:* 5)
Subspecialties: RNR, VIR
Program ID: 420-48-21-197

Temple

Texas A&M College of Medicine-Scott and White Program
Sponsor: Scott and White Memorial Hospital
Program Director:
Bryan Maupin, MD
Scott and White Memorial Hospital
2401 S 31st St
Temple, TX 76508-0001
Tel: 254 724-4507 *Fax:* 254 724-5385
E-mail: p.marek@swmail.sw.org
Internet: http://www.sw.org
Accred Length: 4 Years *Program Size:* 20 (*GY1:* 4)
Program ID: 420-48-11-198

Utah

Salt Lake City

University of Utah Program
Sponsor: University of Utah Medical Center
Veterans Affairs Medical Center (Salt Lake City)
Program Director:
Paula J Woodward, MD
Univ of Utah Sch of Med
Dept of Radiology
50 N Medical Dr
Salt Lake City, UT 84132
Tel: 801 581-7553 *Fax:* 801 581-2414
E-mail: renate.hulen@hsc.utah.edu
Internet: http://www.rad.med.utah.edu/
Accred Length: 4 Years *Program Size:* 16
Subspecialties: NR, RNR, VIR
Program ID: 420-49-21-199

Vermont

Burlington

University of Vermont Program
Sponsor: Fletcher Allen Health Care
Program Director:
Charles N Pappas, MD
Univ of Vermont Coll of Med, Dept of Radiology
FAHC/MCHV Campus/Patrick 1
111 Colchester Ave
Burlington, VT 05401
Tel: 802 656-3593 *Fax:* 802 656-4822
E-mail: cpappas@vtmednet.org
Accred Length: 4 Years *Program Size:* 12
Subspecialties: VIR
Program ID: 420-50-31-200

Virginia

Charlottesville

University of Virginia Program
Sponsor: University of Virginia Medical Center
Program Director:
Spencer B Gay, MD
Univ of Virginia Health System
Dept of Radiology/Box 170
Lee St
Charlottesville, VA 22908
Tel: 804 924-9372 *Fax:* 804 982-1618
E-mail: smy@virginia.edu
Internet:
http://www.virginia.edu/medicine/clinical/radiology/uvaprogram
Accred Length: 4 Years *Program Size:* 28 (*GY1:* 7)
Subspecialties: NR, RNR, VIR
Program ID: 420-51-11-201

Norfolk

Eastern Virginia Medical School Program
Sponsor: Eastern Virginia Medical School
DePaul Medical Center
Sentara Norfolk General Hospital
Veterans Affairs Medical Center (Hampton)
Program Director:
Michael E Katz, MD
Hofheimer Hall/Ste 541
825 Fairfax Ave
Norfolk, VA 23507-1912
Tel: 757 446-8990 *Fax:* 757 446-8441
E-mail: radpro@mccoy.evms.edu
Internet: http://www.evms.edu
Accred Length: 4 Years *Program Size:* 12 (*GY1:* 2)
Program ID: 420-51-21-202

Richmond

Medical College of Virginia/Virginia Commonwealth University Program
Sponsor: Medical College of Virginia/Virginia Commonwealth University
Hunter Holmes McGuire VA Medical Center (Richmond)
Medical College of Virginia Hospitals
Program Director:
Fred J Laine, MD
Med Coll of Virginia
Box 980615
Richmond, VA 23298-0615
Tel: 804 828-3525 *Fax:* 804 828-6066
E-mail: mdbaker@hsc.vcu.edu
Internet: http://views.vcu.edu/~mcvrad/residency.htm
Accred Length: 4 Years *Program Size:* 29
Subspecialties: RNR
Program ID: 420-51-21-203

Washington

Seattle

University of Washington Program
Sponsor: University of Washington School of Medicine
Children's Hospital and Medical Center
Harborview Medical Center
University of Washington Medical Center
Veterans Affairs Medical Center (Seattle)
Program Director:
Charles A Rohrmann Jr, MD
Lee B Talner, MD
Univ Hospital
Dept of Radiology/Box 357115
1959 NE Pacific St
Seattle, WA 98195
Tel: 206 543-3320 *Fax:* 206 543-6317
E-mail: bstumpf@u.washington.edu
Internet: http://www.rad.washington.edu
Accred Length: 4 Years *Program Size:* 38
Subspecialties: PDR, RNR, VIR
Program ID: 420-54-21-205

Virginia Mason Medical Center Program
Sponsor: Virginia Mason Medical Center
Program Director:
Ingrid M Peterson, MD
Virginia Mason Med Ctr
Grad Med Educ/H8-GME
925 Seneca St
Seattle, WA 98111
Tel: 206 583-6079 *Fax:* 206 583-2307
Internet: http://www.vmmc.org
Accred Length: 4 Years *Program Size:* 10 (*GY1:* 2)
Program ID: 420-54-12-206

Spokane

Inland Empire Hospital Services Association Program
Sponsor: Inland Empire Hospital Services Association
Sacred Heart Medical Center
Program Director:
Royce L Zobell, MD
Sacred Heart Med Ctr
101 W Eighth Ave
PO Box 2555
Spokane, WA 99220-2555
Tel: 509 455-3330 *Fax:* 509 458-5316
E-mail: shmcradr@inhs.org
Internet: http://www.spokanehealth.org
Accred Length: 4 Years *Program Size:* 8 (*GY1:* 2)
Subspecialties: TY
Program ID: 420-54-21-207

Tacoma

Madigan Army Medical Center Program
Sponsor: Madigan Army Medical Center
Program Director:
Lt Col Miguel J Rovira, MD
Madigan Army Med Ctr
Attn Commander: MCHJ-R (Radiology)
Tacoma, WA 98431
Tel: 253 968-2130 *Fax:* 253 968-3140
E-mail: miguel_rovira@smtplink.mamc.amedd.army.mil
Internet:
http://www.mamc.amedd.army.mil/williams/index1.htm
Accred Length: 4 Years *Program Size:* 14
Program ID: 420-54-21-239
US Armed Services Program

West Virginia

Morgantown

West Virginia University Program

Sponsor: West Virginia University Hospitals

Program Director:
Judith S Schreiman, MD
Robert C Byrd Health Sciences Ctr
PO Box 9235
Morgantown, WV 26506-9235
Tel: 304 293-3092 *Fax:* 304 293-3899
E-mail: jfast@wvu.edu
Internet: http://www.hsc.wvu.edu/som/radio
Accred Length: 4 Years *Program Size:* 10
Subspecialties: RNR
Program ID: 420-55-21-208

Wisconsin

Madison

University of Wisconsin Program

Sponsor: University of Wisconsin Hospital and Clinics
William S Middleton Veterans Hospital

Program Director:
Jannette Collins, MD EdD
Michael J Tuite, MD
Univ Hospital and Clinics
E3-311 Clin Sci Ctr
600 Highland Ave
Madison, WI 53792-3252
Tel: 608 263-8310 *Fax:* 608 262-0907
E-mail: rad-app@facstaff.wisc.edu
Internet: http://www.radres.radiology.wisc.edu
Accred Length: 4 Years *Program Size:* 32
Subspecialties: MSR, RNR, VIR
Program ID: 420-56-21-210

Milwaukee

Aurora Health Care Program

Sponsor: Aurora Health Care
St Luke's Medical Center

Program Director:
David L Olson, MD
St Luke's Med Ctr
2900 W Oklahoma Ave
Milwaukee, WI 53215
Tel: 414 649-6298 *Fax:* 414 649-7981
Internet: http://www.aurorahealthcare.org
Accred Length: 4 Years *Program Size:* 16
Subspecialties: TY
Program ID: 420-56-12-213

Medical College of Wisconsin Program

Sponsor: Medical College of Wisconsin Affiliated Hospitals Inc
Children's Hospital of Wisconsin
Clement J Zablocki Veterans Affairs Medical Center
Froedtert Memorial Lutheran Hospital

Program Director:
Guillermo F Carrera, MD
Med Coll of Wisconsin-Froedtert Memorial Lutheran Hospital
9200 W Wisconsin Ave
Milwaukee, WI 53226
Tel: 414 805-3750 *Fax:* 414 259-9290
E-mail: jyouker@mcw.edu
Accred Length: 4 Years *Program Size:* 20
Subspecialties: PDR, RNR, VIR
Program ID: 420-56-21-211

St Joseph's Hospital Program

Sponsor: St Joseph's Hospital

Program Director:
Steven M Gryniewicz, MD
St Joseph's Hospital
5000 W Chambers St
Milwaukee, WI 53210
Tel: 414 447-2195 *Fax:* 414 874-4348
Accred Length: 4 Years *Program Size:* 8
Program ID: 420-56-22-212

Rheumatology (Internal Medicine)

Alabama

Birmingham

University of Alabama Medical Center Program

Sponsor: University of Alabama Hospital

Program Director:
Dennis W Boulware, MD
Univ of Alabama
Div of Rheumatology
Univ Station/VH L205
Birmingham, AL 35294-0019
Tel: 205 934-9498 *Fax:* 205 934-3278
E-mail: boulware@uab.edu
Internet: http://info.dom.uab.edu/rheum/index.htm
Accred Length: 2 Years *Program Size:* 6
Program ID: 150-01-21-088

Arizona

Tucson

University of Arizona Program

Sponsor: University of Arizona College of Medicine
University Medical Center
Veterans Affairs Medical Center (Tucson)

Program Director:
Michael J Maricic, MD
Univ of Arizona
Rheum/Allergy/Immunology Sect
1501 N Campbell Ave
Tucson, AZ 85724
Tel: 520 626-7527 *Fax:* 520 626-7114
Accred Length: 2 Years *Program Size:* 2
Program ID: 150-03-21-076

Arkansas

Little Rock

University of Arkansas for Medical Sciences Program

Sponsor: University of Arkansas College of Medicine
John L McClellan Memorial Veterans Hospital
University Hospital of Arkansas

Program Director:
Hugo E Jasin, MD
Univ of Arkansas for Med Sciences
Div of Rheumatology/509
4301 W Markham St
Little Rock, AR 72205-7199
Tel: 501 686-6770 *Fax:* 501 603-1380
E-mail: jasin hugo e@exchange.uams.edu
Internet: http://www.uams.edu/dim/rheum.htm
Accred Length: 2 Years *Program Size:* 3
Program ID: 150-04-21-145

California

La Jolla

Scripps Clinic/Scripps Green Hospital Program
Sponsor: Scripps Clinic
Scripps Green Hospital
Program Director:
Ken D Pischel, MD PhD
Dept of Grad Med Educ/403C
Scripps Clinic and Research Foundation
10666 N Torrey Pines Rd
La Jolla, CA 92037-1093
Tel: 619 554-8819 *Fax:* 619 554-6390
E-mail: gme@scripps.edu
Internet: http://www.scrippsclinic.com
Accred Length: 2 Years *Program Size:* 4
Program ID: 150-05-21-042

Loma Linda

Loma Linda University Program
Sponsor: Loma Linda University Medical Center
Jerry L Pettis Memorial Veterans Hospital
Program Director:
Edwin H Krick, MD MPH
Loma Linda Univ
Dept of Int Med
PO Box 2000
Loma Linda, CA 92354
Tel: 909 824-4909 *Fax:* 909 478-4219
Accred Length: 2 Years *Program Size:* 2
Program ID: 150-05-21-090

Los Angeles

Cedars-Sinai Medical Center Program
Sponsor: Cedars-Sinai Medical Center
Program Director:
James R Klinenberg, MD
Cedars-Sinai Med Ctr
Dept of Int Med/Rheumatology
8700 Beverly Blvd
Los Angeles, CA 90048-0750
Tel: 310 855-5141 *Fax:* 310 358-0480
Accred Length: 2 Years *Program Size:* 2
Program ID: 150-05-11-078

UCLA Medical Center Program
Sponsor: UCLA School of Medicine
UCLA Medical Center
VA Greater Los Angeles Healthcare System
Program Director:
Bevra H Hahn, MD
UCLA Med Ctr
Dept of Med/Rheumatology
Los Angeles, CA 90095-1736
Tel: 310 825-7375
Accred Length: 2 Years *Program Size:* 6
Program ID: 150-05-11-091

University of Southern California Program
Sponsor: Los Angeles County-USC Medical Center
LAC-Rancho Los Amigos Medical Center
Program Director:
David A Horwitz, MD
Univ of Southern California Med Ctr
2011 Zonal Ave/HMR 711
Los Angeles, CA 90033
Tel: 323 442-1946 *Fax:* 323 442-2874
E-mail: dhorwitz@hsc.usc.edu
Accred Length: 2 Years *Program Size:* 4
Program ID: 150-05-21-031

VA Greater Los Angeles Healthcare System (Sepulveda) Program
Sponsor: VA Greater Los Angeles Healthcare System
Olive View-UCLA Medical Center
Program Director:
Richard Weisbart, MD
VA Med Ctr
16111 Plummer St
Sepulveda, CA 91343
Tel: 818 895-9384 *Fax:* 818 895-9423
E-mail: weisbart.richard@sepulveda.va.gov
Accred Length: 2 Years *Program Size:* 2
Program ID: 150-05-21-092

Orange

University of California (Irvine) Program
Sponsor: University of California (Irvine) Medical Center
Veterans Affairs Medical Center (Long Beach)
Program Director:
Brian S Andrews, MB BS MD
Univ of California Irvine Med Ctr
101 City Dr S
Bldg 53/RT81
Orange, CA 92868
Tel: 949 824-5907 *Fax:* 949 824-5639
E-mail: bsandrew@uci.edu
Accred Length: 2 Years *Program Size:* 2
Program ID: 150-05-21-108

San Diego

University of California (San Diego) Program
Sponsor: University of California (San Diego) Medical Center
Veterans Affairs Medical Center (San Diego)
Program Director:
Robert Terkeltaub, MD
UCSD Med Ctr
Div of Rheumatic Dis
9500 Gilman Dr
La Jolla, CA 92093-0656
Tel: 619 543-2359 *Fax:* 619 534-2606
Accred Length: 2 Years *Program Size:* 3
Program ID: 150-05-21-123

San Francisco

University of California (San Francisco) Program
Sponsor: University of California (San Francisco) School of Medicine
San Francisco General Hospital Medical Center
University of California (San Francisco) Medical Center
Veterans Affairs Medical Center (San Francisco)
Program Director:
David Wofsy, MD
Univ of California San Francisco
4150 Clement St (111R)
San Francisco, CA 94121
Tel: 415 750-2104 *Fax:* 415 750-6920
E-mail: dwofsy@itsa.ucsf.edu
Accred Length: 2 Years *Program Size:* 9
Program ID: 150-05-21-109

Stanford

Stanford University Program
Sponsor: Stanford University Hospital
Veterans Affairs Palo Alto Health Care System
Program Director:
Ronald F van Vollenhoven, MD PhD
Stanford Univ Med Ctr
300 Pasteur Dr
Grant Bldg Rm S021
Stanford, CA 94305-5111
Tel: 650 725-5957 *Fax:* 650 725-4114
E-mail: ml.rfv@forsythe.stanford.edu
Accred Length: 2 Years *Program Size:* 4
Program ID: 150-05-21-016

Colorado

Denver

University of Colorado Program
Sponsor: University of Colorado Health Sciences Center
Denver Health and Hospitals
Veterans Affairs Medical Center (Denver)
Program Director:
Sterling G West, MD
Univ of Colorado Health Sciences Ctr
4200 E Ninth Ave/B-115
Denver, CO 80262
Tel: 303 315-6665 *Fax:* 303 315-5540
E-mail: helen.martinez@uchsc.edu
Accred Length: 2 Years *Program Size:* 3
Program ID: 150-07-21-036

Connecticut

Farmington

University of Connecticut Program
Sponsor: University of Connecticut School of Medicine
Univ of Connecticut Health Center/John Dempsey Hospital
Program Director:
Naomi F Rothfield, MD
Univ of Connecticut Health Ctr
Dept of Med
263 Farmington Ave
Farmington, CT 06030-1310
Tel: 860 679-3605 *Fax:* 860 679-1287
E-mail: rothfield@nso.uchc.edu
Internet: http://www2.uchc.edu/~rheum
Accred Length: 2 Years *Program Size:* 2
Program ID: 150-08-31-001

New Haven

Yale-New Haven Medical Center Program
Sponsor: Yale-New Haven Hospital
Veterans Affairs Medical Center (West Haven)
Waterbury Hospital Health Center
Program Director:
Linda K Bockenstedt, MD
Yale Univ Sch of Med
333 Cedar St
PO Box 208031
New Haven, CT 06520-8031
Tel: 203 785-2454 *Fax:* 203 785-7053
Internet: http://www.info.med.yale.edu/intmed/rheumat/
Accred Length: 2 Years *Program Size:* 5
Program ID: 150-08-21-017

District of Columbia

Washington

George Washington University Program

Sponsor: George Washington University School of Medicine
Children's National Medical Center
George Washington University Hospital (UHS)
Program Director:
Arthur Weinstein, MD
George Washington Univ Med Ctr
2150 Pennsylvania Ave NW/Ste 5-405
Washington, DC 20037
Tel: 202 994-4624 *Fax:* 202 994-9953
E-mail: domaxw@gwumc.edu
Accred Length: 2 Years *Program Size:* 1
Program ID: 150-10-21-079

Georgetown University Program

Sponsor: Georgetown University Medical Center
Veterans Affairs Medical Center (Washington, DC)
Program Director:
Daniel J Clauw, MD
Georgetown Univ Hospital
Dept of Med/Rheumatology
3800 Reservoir Rd NW
Washington, DC 20007-2197
Tel: 202 687-4034 *Fax:* 202 687-7797
E-mail: steelewe@gunet.georgetown.edu
Accred Length: 2 Years *Program Size:* 4
Program ID: 150-10-21-060

Walter Reed Army Medical Center Program

Sponsor: Walter Reed Army Medical Center
Program Director:
Gregory J Dennis, MD
Rheumatology Service
Walter Reed Hospital and Med Ctr
6825 16th St NW
Washington, DC 20307-5001
Tel: 202 782-5690 *Fax:* 202 782-0594
E-mail: gdennis@ibm.net
Internet: http://www.wramc.amedd.army.mil
Accred Length: 2 Years *Program Size:* 4
Program ID: 150-10-11-093
US Armed Services Program

Washington Hospital Center Program

Sponsor: Washington Hospital Center
Program Director:
Werner F Barth, MD
Washington Hospital Ctr
110 Irving St NW
Washington, DC 20010
Tel: 202 877-6274
E-mail: wfb2@mhg.edu
Internet: http://www.mhg.edu/gme/
Accred Length: 2 Years *Program Size:* 2
Program ID: 150-10-11-094

Florida

Gainesville

University of Florida Program

Sponsor: University of Florida College of Medicine
Shands Hospital at the University of Florida
Veterans Affairs Medical Center (Gainesville)
Program Director:
N Lawrence Edwards Sr, MD
Univ of Florida, Dept of Med
Box 100277
J Hillis Miller Health Ctr
Gainesville, FL 32610
Tel: 904 392-8600
E-mail: lee.med@shands.ufl.edu
Internet: http://www.med.ufl.edu/med/rheum/
Accred Length: 2 Years *Program Size:* 3
Program ID: 150-11-21-025

Miami

University of Miami-Jackson Memorial Medical Center Program

Sponsor: University of Miami-Jackson Memorial Medical Center
Veterans Affairs Medical Center (Miami)
Program Director:
Carlos J Lozada, MD
Univ of Miami
1150 NW 14th St/Ste 310
Miami, FL 33136
Tel: 305 243-7547 *Fax:* 305 243-7546
Accred Length: 2 Years *Program Size:* 3
Program ID: 150-11-21-125

Tampa

University of South Florida Program

Sponsor: University of South Florida College of Medicine
James A Haley Veterans Hospital
Tampa General Healthcare
Program Director:
Frank B Vasey, MD
Univ of South Florida Coll of Med
12901 Bruce B Downs Blvd/Box 19
Tampa, FL 33612-4799
Tel: 813 974-2681 *Fax:* 813 974-5229
Accred Length: 2 Years *Program Size:* 1
Program ID: 150-11-21-026

Georgia

Atlanta

Emory University Program

Sponsor: Emory University School of Medicine
Emory University Hospital
Grady Memorial Hospital
Veterans Affairs Medical Center (Atlanta)
Program Director:
Carlos A Agudelo, MD
Rheumatology Div
VA Med Ctr
1670 Clairmont Rd
Atlanta, GA 30030
Tel: 404 321-6121, ext 2074 *Fax:* 404 235-3011
Accred Length: 2 Years *Program Size:* 4
Program ID: 150-12-21-095

Augusta

Medical College of Georgia Program

Sponsor: Medical College of Georgia Hospital and Clinics
Program Director:
Joseph P Bailey Jr, MD
Med Coll of Georgia
Dept of Med
1120 15th St/BIW 558
Augusta, GA 30912-3146
Tel: 706 721-2981 *Fax:* 706 721-6314
E-mail: jbailey@mail.mcg.edu
Accred Length: 2 Years *Program Size:* 3
Program ID: 150-12-21-002

Illinois

Chicago

McGaw Medical Center of Northwestern University Program

Sponsor: Northwestern University Medical School
Northwestern Memorial Hospital
Veterans Affairs Lakeside Medical Center (Chicago)
Program Director:
Alisa E Koch, MD
Northwestern Univ Med Sch
303 E Chicago Ave
Ward 3-315
Chicago, IL 60611
Tel: 312 503-8197 *Fax:* 312 503-0994
E-mail: ae-koch@nwu.edu
Internet: http://www.medicine.nwu.edu/rheumatology/
Accred Length: 2 Years *Program Size:* 3
Program ID: 150-16-21-051

Rush-Presbyterian-St Luke's Medical Center Program

Sponsor: Rush-Presbyterian-St Luke's Medical Center
Program Director:
Calvin R Brown Jr, MD
Rush-Presbyterian-St Luke's Med Ctr
1725 W Harrison St/Ste 1017
Chicago, IL 60612-3864
Tel: 312 942-8268 *Fax:* 312 563-2075
E-mail: cbrown@rush.edu
Internet: http://www.rush.edu
Accred Length: 2 Years *Program Size:* 4
Program ID: 150-16-11-096

University of Chicago Program

Sponsor: University of Chicago Hospitals
Program Director:
Michael A Becker, MD
Univ of Chicago
5841 S Maryland Ave/MC4055
NO29
Chicago, IL 60637-1470
Tel: 773 702-5390 *Fax:* 773 702-8702
Accred Length: 2 Years *Program Size:* 2
Program ID: 150-16-21-138

Programs

University of Illinois College of Medicine at Chicago Program
Sponsor: University of Illinois College of Medicine at Chicago
Mercy Hospital and Medical Center
Michael Reese Hospital and Medical Center
University of Illinois Hospital and Clinics
Veterans Affairs West Side Medical Center
Program Director:
John Varga, MD
Univ of Illinois-Chicago
Med/Rheumatology
900 S Ashland Ave/MBRB 1158 M/C 733
Chicago, IL 60607-7171
Tel: 312 413-9310 *Fax:* 312 413-9271
E-mail: jvarga@uic.edu
Accred Length: 2 Years *Program Size:* 3
Program ID: 150-16-21-097

Maywood

Loyola University Program
Sponsor: Loyola University Medical Center
Edward J Hines Jr Veterans Affairs Hospital
Program Director:
Elaine M Adams, MD
Loyola Univ Med Ctr
2160 S First Ave
Bldg 54 Rm 121
Maywood, IL 60153
Tel: 708 216-3313 *Fax:* 708 216-1085
E-mail: eadams2@luc.edu
Accred Length: 2 Years *Program Size:* 2
Program ID: 150-16-21-003

Indiana

Indianapolis

Indiana University School of Medicine Program
Sponsor: Indiana University School of Medicine
Clarian IU Hospital
Clarian Riley Hospital for Children
Richard L Roudebush Veterans Affairs Medical Center
William N Wishard Memorial Hospital
Program Director:
Kenneth D Brandt, MD
Indiana Univ Sch of Med
541 N Clinical Dr/Rm 492
Indianapolis, IN 46202-5103
Tel: 317 274-4225 *Fax:* 317 274-7792
E-mail: kbrandt@iupui.edu
Internet:
http://medicine.iupui.edu/fellow.html#rheumatology
Accred Length: 2 Years *Program Size:* 4
Program ID: 150-17-21-110

Iowa

Iowa City

University of Iowa Hospitals and Clinics Program
Sponsor: University of Iowa Hospitals and Clinics
Program Director:
Robert F Ashman, MD
Univ of Iowa Hospitals and Clinics
Dept of Int Med
200 Hawkins Dr
Iowa City, IA 52242-1009
Tel: 319 356-2287 *Fax:* 319 353-6290
Accred Length: 2 Years *Program Size:* 3
Program ID: 150-18-21-067

Kansas

Kansas City

University of Kansas Medical Center Program
Sponsor: University of Kansas School of Medicine
University of Kansas Medical Center
Program Director:
Daniel J Stechschulte, MD
Univ of Kansas Med Ctr
3901 Rainbow Blvd
Rm 4035 Wescoe
Kansas City, KS 66160-7317
Tel: 913 588-6008 *Fax:* 913 588-3987
E-mail: dstechsc@kumc.edu
Accred Length: 2 Years *Program Size:* 2
Program ID: 150-19-21-080

Kentucky

Louisville

University of Louisville Program
Sponsor: University of Louisville School of Medicine
University of Louisville Hospital
Veterans Affairs Medical Center (Louisville)
Program Director:
Steven H Stern, MD
Univ of Louisville, Div of Rheumatology
Ambulatory Care Bldg/3rd Fl
530 S Jackson St
Louisville, KY 40292
Tel: 502 852-5233 *Fax:* 502 852-1638
Accred Length: 2 Years *Program Size:* 2
Program ID: 150-20-31-062

Louisiana

New Orleans

Alton Ochsner Medical Foundation Program
Sponsor: Alton Ochsner Medical Foundation
Program Director:
Robert J Quinet, MD
Alton Ochsner Med Foundation
Dept of Grad Med Educ
1516 Jefferson Hwy
New Orleans, LA 70121
Tel: 504 842-3260 *Fax:* 504 842-3193
E-mail: rquinet@ochsner.org
Internet: http://www.ochsner.org
Accred Length: 2 Years *Program Size:* 2
Program ID: 150-21-22-106

Louisiana State University Program
Sponsor: Louisiana State University School of Medicine
Medical Center of Louisiana at New Orleans
Program Director:
Luis R Espinoza, MD
Louisiana State Univ Med Ctr
1542 Tulane Ave/Box T4M-4
New Orleans, LA 70112-2822
Tel: 504 568-4630 *Fax:* 504 568-4642
Accred Length: 2 Years *Program Size:* 2
Program ID: 150-21-21-037

Shreveport

Louisiana State University (Shreveport) Program
Sponsor: Louisiana State University Hospital-Shreveport
Overton Brooks Veterans Affairs Medical Center
Program Director:
Robert E Wolf, MD
Louisiana State Univ Med Ctr Hospital
Med Educ (Rheumatology)
PO Box 33932
Shreveport, LA 71130-3932
Tel: 318 675-5930 *Fax:* 318 675-6980
Accred Length: 2 Years *Program Size:* 2
Program ID: 150-21-21-063

Maryland

Baltimore

Johns Hopkins University Program
Sponsor: Johns Hopkins University School of Medicine
Johns Hopkins Hospital
Program Director:
Fredrick M Wigley, MD
Johns Hopkins Univ
Div of Rheumatology
1830 E Monument St/Ste 7300
Baltimore, MD 21205
Tel: 410 955-3375 *Fax:* 410 614-7285
E-mail: fwig@welchlink.welch.jhu.edu
Accred Length: 2 Years *Program Size:* 3
Program ID: 150-23-11-052

University of Maryland Program
Sponsor: University of Maryland Medical System
Veterans Affairs Medical Center (Baltimore)
Program Director:
Raymond H Flores, MD
Univ of Maryland
10S Pine St
MSTF 8-34
Baltimore, MD 21201-1734
Tel: 410 706-6474 *Fax:* 410 706-0231
Accred Length: 2 Years *Program Size:* 4
Program ID: 150-23-21-131

Bethesda

National Institutes of Health Clinical Center Program
Sponsor: NIH Warren Grant Magnuson Clinical Center
Program Director:
John H Klippel, MD
NIH Warren Grant Magnuson Clinical Ctr
Bldg 10/Rm 9-S-205
Bethesda, MD 20892
Tel: 301 496-3374 *Fax:* 301 402-0765
E-mail: klippelj@arb.niams.nih.gov
Internet: http://www.nih.gov/niams/about/irp/clinfel.htm
Accred Length: 2 Years *Program Size:* 12
Program ID: 150-23-21-141

Massachusetts

Boston

Boston University Medical Center Program

Sponsor: Boston Medical Center
Veterans Affairs Medical Center (Boston)
Program Director:
Joseph H Korn, MD
Arthritis Ctr
Conte Bldg
715 Albany St
Boston, MA 02118-2394
Tel: 617 638-4310 *Fax:* 617 638-5226
Accred Length: 2 Years *Program Size:* 3
Program ID: 150-24-21-111

Brigham and Women's Hospital Program

Sponsor: Brigham and Women's Hospital
Beth Israel Deaconess Medical Center
Program Director:
Ronald J Anderson, MD
Brigham and Women's Hospital
Dept of Rheumatology
75 Francis St
Boston, MA 02115
Tel: 617 732-5345 *Fax:* 617 732-5505
E-mail: rjanderson@bics.bwh.harvard.edu
Accred Length: 2 Years *Program Size:* 7
Program ID: 150-24-21-004

Massachusetts General Hospital Program

Sponsor: Massachusetts General Hospital
Program Director:
Dwight R Robinson, MD
Bulfinch 165
Massachusetts General Hospital
Fruit St
Boston, MA 02114
Tel: 617 726-2870 *Fax:* 617 726-2872
Accred Length: 2 Years *Program Size:* 6
Program ID: 150-24-11-038

New England Medical Center Hospitals Program

Sponsor: New England Medical Center Hospitals
Program Director:
Allen C Steere, MD
New England Med Ctr
750 Washington St/Box 406
Boston, MA 02111
Tel: 617 636-5789 *Fax:* 617 636-4252
E-mail: elena.massarotti@es.nemc.org
Internet:
http://www.nemc.org/home/departments/aduls/rheumato.htm
Accred Length: 2 Years *Program Size:* 2
Program ID: 150-24-21-005

Worcester

University of Massachusetts Program

Sponsor: University of Massachusetts Medical School
UMass Memorial Health Care (University Campus)
Program Director:
Robert B Zurier, MD
Univ of Massachusetts Med Sch
Div of Rheumatology
55 Lake Ave N
Worcester, MA 01655-0317
Tel: 508 856-6246 *Fax:* 508 856-1983
E-mail: robert.zurier@banyan.ummed.edu
Accred Length: 2 Years *Program Size:* 2
Program ID: 150-24-21-006

Michigan

Ann Arbor

University of Michigan Program

Sponsor: University of Michigan Hospitals
Veterans Affairs Medical Center (Ann Arbor)
Program Director:
David A Fox, MD
Univ of Michigan Hospitals
TC 3918/Box 0358
1500 E Medical Center Dr
Ann Arbor, MI 48109-0358
Tel: 734 936-5566 *Fax:* 734 763-1253
E-mail: dfox@umich.edu
Internet: http://www.med.umich.edu/rheum/
Accred Length: 2 Years *Program Size:* 6
Program ID: 150-25-21-053

Detroit

Henry Ford Hospital Program

Sponsor: Henry Ford Hospital
Program Director:
James Leisen, MD
Henry Ford Hospital
2799 W Grand Blvd
Detroit, MI 48202
Tel: 313 876-2646 *Fax:* 313 876-6065
Accred Length: 2 Years *Program Size:* 0
Program ID: 150-25-11-099

Wayne State University/Detroit Medical Center Program

Sponsor: Wayne State University/Detroit Medical Center
Detroit Receiving Hospital and University Health Center
Harper Hospital
Hutzel Hospital
Veterans Affairs Medical Center (Detroit)
Program Director:
Jose L Granda, MD PhD
Hutzel Hospital
4707 St Antoine Blvd
Detroit, MI 48201
Tel: 313 577-1134 *Fax:* 313 577-1938
Accred Length: 2 Years *Program Size:* 6
Program ID: 150-25-21-030

Minnesota

Minneapolis

University of Minnesota Program

Sponsor: University of Minnesota Medical School
Fairview-University Medical Center
Regions Hospital
Veterans Affairs Medical Center (Minneapolis)
Program Director:
Maren L Mahowald, MD
VA Med Ctr
Sect of Rheumatology-111R
1 Veterans Dr
Minneapolis, MN 55417
Tel: 612 725-2000, ext 4190 *Fax:* 612 725-2267
E-mail: maho001@maroon.tc.umn.edu
Accred Length: 2 Years *Program Size:* 3
Program ID: 150-26-21-082

Rochester

Mayo Graduate School of Medicine (Rochester) Program

Sponsor: Mayo Graduate School of Medicine-Mayo Foundation
Mayo Clinic (Rochester)
Rochester Methodist Hospital
St Mary's Hospital of Rochester
Program Director:
Thomas G Mason III, MD
Application Processing Ctr
Siebens 5th Fl
Mayo Graduate Sch of Med
Rochester, MN 55905
Tel: 507 284-3126 *Fax:* 507 284-0999
E-mail: mgsm.intmed.specialties@mayo.edu
Internet: http://www.mayo.edu/
Accred Length: 2 Years *Program Size:* 4
Program ID: 150-26-21-032

Missouri

Columbia

University of Missouri-Columbia Program

Sponsor: University of Missouri-Columbia School of Medicine
Harry S Truman Memorial Veterans Hospital
University Hospitals and Clinics
Program Director:
Sara E Walker, MD
Univ of Missouri-Columbia
Dept of Int Med
One Hospital Dr/MA427 HSC
Columbia, MO 65212
Tel: 573 884-8792 *Fax:* 573 884-0304
E-mail: peggy_young@muccmail.missouri.edu
Internet:
http://www.hfc.missouri.edu/internal_medicine/rheum/
Accred Length: 2 Years *Program Size:* 4
Program ID: 150-28-21-054

St Louis

St Louis University School of Medicine Program

Sponsor: St Louis University School of Medicine
SSM Cardinal Glennon Children's Hospital
St Louis University School of Medicine
Program Director:
Terry L Moore, MD
St Louis Univ Sch of Med
1402 S Grand Blvd
R211A Doisy Hall
St Louis, MO 63104-1028
Tel: 314 577-8467 *Fax:* 314 268-5117
E-mail: mooretl@sluwpogate.slu.edu
Accred Length: 2 Years *Program Size:* 3
Program ID: 150-28-21-064

Programs

Washington University/B-JH/SLCH Consortium (South Campus) Program
Sponsor: Washington University/B-JH/SLCH Consortium
Barnes-Jewish Hospital
Program Director:
Richard D Brasington Jr, MD
Washington Univ Sch of Med
Rheumatology/Box 8045
660 S Euclid Ave
St Louis, MO 63110
Tel: 314 454-7279 *Fax:* 314 454-1091
E-mail: rbrasing@imgate.wustl.edu
Internet:
http://www.internalmed.wustl.edu/divisions/rheum/brochure.htm
Accred Length: 2 Years *Program Size:* 9
Program ID: 150-28-21-112

New Hampshire

Lebanon

Dartmouth-Hitchcock Medical Center Program
Sponsor: Mary Hitchcock Memorial Hospital
Veterans Affairs Medical Center (White River Junction)
Program Director:
Lin A Brown, MD
Dartmouth-Hitchcock Med Ctr
Connective Tissue Disease Sect
One Medical Center Dr
Lebanon, NH 03756-0001
Tel: 603 650-7700 *Fax:* 603 650-6223
Accred Length: 2 Years *Program Size:* 2
Program ID: 150-32-21-107

New Jersey

Camden

UMDNJ-Robert Wood Johnson Medical School (Camden) Program
Sponsor: Cooper Hospital-University Medical Center
Program Director:
Antonio J Reginato, MD
Carolyn R O'Connor, MD
Cooper Hospital-Univ Med Ctr
Educ and Research Bldg
401 Haddon Ave
Camden, NJ 08103
Tel: 609 757-4818 *Fax:* 609 757-7803
Accred Length: 2 Years *Program Size:* 2
Program ID: 150-33-21-132

Piscataway

UMDNJ-Robert Wood Johnson Medical School Program
Sponsor: UMDNJ-Robert Wood Johnson Medical School
Robert Wood Johnson University Hospital
Program Director:
Leonard H Sigal, MD
UMDNJ-Robert Wood Johnson Med Sch
Div of Rheumatology
One Robert Wood Johnson Pl/PO Box 19
New Brunswick, NJ 08903-0019
Tel: 732 235-7702 *Fax:* 732 235-7238
Accred Length: 2 Years *Program Size:* 4
Program ID: 150-33-21-019

New Mexico

Albuquerque

University of New Mexico Program
Sponsor: University of New Mexico School of Medicine
University Hospital
Veterans Affairs Medical Center (Albuquerque)
Program Director:
Arthur D Bankhurst, MD
Univ of New Mexico Sch of Med
Div of Rheumatology/5th Fl ACC
2211 Lomas Blvd NE
Albuquerque, NM 87131
Tel: 505 272-4761 *Fax:* 505 271-4628
Accred Length: 2 Years *Program Size:* 2
Program ID: 150-34-21-100

New York

Albany

Albany Medical Center Program
Sponsor: Albany Medical Center
Veterans Affairs Medical Center (Albany)
Program Director:
Joel M Kremer, MD
Albany Med Coll
Div of Rheumatology/Mail Code 100
47 New Scotland Ave
Albany, NY 12208-3479
Tel: 518 445-5342 *Fax:* 518 262-6473
Accred Length: 2 Years *Program Size:* 2
Program ID: 150-35-31-020

Bronx

Albert Einstein College of Medicine Program
Sponsor: Albert Einstein College of Medicine of Yeshiva University
Jacobi Medical Center
Montefiore Medical Center-Henry and Lucy Moses Division
Montefiore Medical Center-Weiler Hospital
North Central Bronx Hospital
Program Director:
Anne Davidson, MD
Albert Einstein Coll of Med
Div of Rheumatology
1300 Morris Park Ave/Ull 505
Bronx, NY 10461
Tel: 718 430-4107 *Fax:* 718 430-8789
E-mail: davidson@aecom.yu.edu
Accred Length: 2 Years *Program Size:* 4
Program ID: 150-35-21-072

Brooklyn

SUNY Health Science Center at Brooklyn Program
Sponsor: SUNY Health Science Center at Brooklyn
Kings County Hospital Center
University Hospital-SUNY Health Science Center at Brooklyn
Veterans Affairs Medical Center (Brooklyn)
Program Director:
Ellen M Ginzler, MD MPH
SUNY Health Science Ctr-Brooklyn
450 Clarkson Ave/Box 42
Brooklyn, NY 11203
Tel: 718 270-1662 *Fax:* 718 270-1562
Accred Length: 2 Years *Program Size:* 4
Program ID: 150-35-21-009

Buffalo

SUNY at Buffalo Graduate Medical-Dental Education Consortium Program
Sponsor: SUNY at Buffalo Grad Medical-Dental Education Consortium
Erie County Medical Center
Veterans Affairs Medical Center (Buffalo)
Program Director:
Alan N Baer, MD
Erie County Med Ctr
462 Grider St
Buffalo, NY 14215
Tel: 716 898-4694 *Fax:* 716 898-3074
E-mail: alanbaer@acsu.buffalo.edu
Accred Length: 2 Years *Program Size:* 2
Program ID: 150-35-31-007

Manhasset

North Shore University Hospital/NYU School of Medicine Program
Sponsor: North Shore University Hospital
Program Director:
Richard A Furie, MD
Nicholas Chiorazzi, MD
North Shore Univ Hospital
Dept of Med
300 Community Dr
Manhasset, NY 11030
Tel: 516 562-4392 *Fax:* 516 562-2807
E-mail: furie@nshs.edu
Internet: http://www.nshs.edu
Accred Length: 2 Years *Program Size:* 2
Program ID: 150-35-21-121

Mineola

Winthrop-University Hospital Program
Sponsor: Winthrop-University Hospital
Nassau County Medical Center
Program Director:
Steven E Carsons, MD
Winthrop-Univ Hospital
Rm 430
222 Station Plaza N
Mineola, NY 11501
Tel: 516 663-2098 *Fax:* 516 663-2946
E-mail: scarsons@winthrop.org
Internet: http://www.winthrop.org
Accred Length: 2 Years *Program Size:* 3
Program ID: 150-35-21-142

New York

Mount Sinai School of Medicine (Cabrini) Program
Sponsor: Mount Sinai School of Medicine
Cabrini Medical Center
Program Director:
Girolamo G Cuppari, MD
Cabrini Med Ctr
227 E 19th St
New York, NY 10003
Tel: 212 995-6686 *Fax:* 212 979-3540
Accred Length: 2 Years *Program Size:* 2
Program ID: 150-35-31-068

Mount Sinai School of Medicine Program
Sponsor: Mount Sinai School of Medicine
Elmhurst Hospital Center-Mount Sinai Services
Mount Sinai Medical Center
Queens Hospital Center
Veterans Affairs Medical Center (Bronx)
Program Director:
Peter Gorevic, MD
Mount Sinai Med Ctr
Annenberg 5 Rm 207-P
One Gustave L Levy Pl/Box 1244
New York, NY 10029-6574
Tel: 212 241-6792 *Fax:* 212 987-5584
E-mail: dcalto@smtplink.mssm.edu
Internet: http://www.mssm.edu
Accred Length: 2 Years *Program Size:* 2
Program ID: 150-35-31-114

New York and Presbyterian Hospital (Columbia Campus) Program
Sponsor: New York and Presbyterian Hospital
New York and Presbyterian Hospital (Columbia Campus)
Program Director:
Leonard Chess, MD
Presbyterian Hospital
622 W 168th St
PH8-E Ste 101
New York, NY 10032
Tel: 212 305-9986 *Fax:* 212 305-4943
E-mail: lc19@columbia.edu
Accred Length: 2 Years *Program Size:* 2
Program ID: 150-35-11-039

New York and Presbyterian Hospital (Cornell Campus) Program
Sponsor: New York and Presbyterian Hospital
New York and Presbyterian Hospital (Cornell Campus)
Program Director:
Stephen A Paget, MD
New York Hospital
525 E 68th St
New York, NY 10021
Tel: 212 606-1845 *Fax:* 212 606-1170
E-mail: pagets@hss.edu
Internet: http://www.hss.edu
Accred Length: 2 Years *Program Size:* 6
Program ID: 150-35-21-122

New York University Medical Center Program
Sponsor: New York University Medical Center
Bellevue Hospital Center
Hospital for Joint Diseases Orthopaedic Institute
Veterans Affairs Medical Center (Manhattan)
Program Director:
Gerald Weissmann, MD
Steven B Abramson, MD
New York Univ Med Ctr
550 First Ave
New York, NY 10016
Tel: 212 263-6403 *Fax:* 212 598-6582
E-mail: steven.abramson@ccmail.med.nyu.edu
Internet: http://www.hjd.edu
Accred Length: 2 Years *Program Size:* 7
Program ID: 150-35-21-083

Rochester

University of Rochester Program
Sponsor: Strong Memorial Hospital of the University of Rochester
Program Director:
Christopher T Ritchlin, MD
Clinical Immunology/Rheumatology Unit
Univ of Rochester Med Ctr
601 Elmwood Ave/Box 695
Rochester, NY 14642-8695
Tel: 716 275-1649 *Fax:* 716 442-3214
Internet: http://www.urmc.rochester.edu/smd/air
Accred Length: 2 Years *Program Size:* 3
Program ID: 150-35-11-127

Stony Brook

SUNY at Stony Brook Program
Sponsor: University Hospital-SUNY at Stony Brook
Veterans Affairs Medical Center (Northport)
Program Director:
Barry L Gruber, MD
Div of Rheumatology
SUNY Health Sciences Ctr
T16-040
Stony Brook, NY 11794-8161
Tel: 516 444-8366 *Fax:* 516 444-3475
E-mail: bgruber@mail.som.sunysb.edu
Accred Length: 2 Years *Program Size:* 2
Program ID: 150-35-21-010

Syracuse

SUNY Health Science Center at Syracuse Program
Sponsor: University Hospital-SUNY Health Science Center at Syracuse
Veterans Affairs Medical Center (Syracuse)
Program Director:
Paul E Phillips, MD
SUNY Health Science Ctr
Dept of Med
750 E Adams St
Syracuse, NY 13210
Tel: 315 464-4194 *Fax:* 315 464-4176
Accred Length: 2 Years *Program Size:* 2
Program ID: 150-35-21-074

Valhalla

New York Medical College at Westchester Medical Center Program
Sponsor: New York Medical College
Westchester Medical Center
Program Director:
L Frank Cavaliere, MD
New York Med Coll
Div of Rheumatic Diseases
Munger Pavilion G73
Valhalla, NY 10595
Tel: 914 594-4444 *Fax:* 914 594-4277
E-mail: frank_cavaliere@nymc.edu
Accred Length: 2 Years *Program Size:* 2
Program ID: 150-35-11-040

North Carolina

Chapel Hill

University of North Carolina Hospitals Program
Sponsor: University of North Carolina Hospitals
Program Director:
John B Winfield, MD
Univ of North Carolina Sch of Med
Div of Rheumatology/Immunology
3330 Thurston Bldg/CB#7280
Chapel Hill, NC 27599-7280
Tel: 919 966-0568 *Fax:* 919 966-0572
Internet: http://www.med.unc.edu
Accred Length: 2 Years *Program Size:* 3
Program ID: 150-36-21-102

Durham

Duke University Program
Sponsor: Duke University Medical Center
Veterans Affairs Medical Center (Durham)
Program Director:
David S Pisetsky, MD PhD
Duke Univ Med Ctr
Box 3544
Durham, NC 27710
Tel: 919 684-5546 *Fax:* 919 684-6891
Accred Length: 2 Years *Program Size:* 6
Program ID: 150-36-21-103

Winston-Salem

Wake Forest University School of Medicine Program
Sponsor: Wake Forest University Baptist Medical Center
Program Director:
Kenneth S O'Rourke, MD
Wake Forest Univ Sch of Med
Sect on Rheumatology
Medical Center Blvd
Winston-Salem, NC 27157-1058
Tel: 336 716-4209 *Fax:* 336 716-9821
E-mail: korourke@wfubmc.edu
Accred Length: 2 Years *Program Size:* 2
Program ID: 150-36-21-011

Ohio

Cleveland

Case Western Reserve University Program
Sponsor: University Hospitals of Cleveland
Veterans Affairs Medical Center (Cleveland)
Program Director:
Roland W Moskowitz, MD
Univ Hospitals of Cleveland
Dept of Med/Rheumatology
11100 Euclid Ave
Cleveland, OH 44106-5000
Tel: 216 844-3168 *Fax:* 216 844-5172
E-mail: rwm3@po.cwru.edu
Internet:
http://www.cwru.edu/cwru/med/medicine/divrheu.htm
Accred Length: 2 Years *Program Size:* 2
Program ID: 150-38-21-115

Cleveland Clinic Foundation Program
Sponsor: Cleveland Clinic Foundation
Program Director:
Brian F Mandell, MD PhD
Cleveland Clinic Foundation
Dept of Rheumatology/A50
9500 Euclid Ave
Cleveland, OH 44195-5242
Tel: 216 444-5690 *Fax:* 216 444-1162
E-mail: mandelb@cesmtp.ccf.org
Internet: http://www.ccf.org
Accred Length: 2 Years *Program Size:* 4
Program ID: 150-38-12-117

Columbus

Ohio State University Program
Sponsor: Ohio State University Medical Center
Program Director:
Ronald L Whisler, MD
Ohio State Univ
Davis Med Research Ctr
480 W Ninth Ave
Columbus, OH 43210
Tel: 614 293-8093 *Fax:* 614 293-5631
Accred Length: 2 Years *Program Size:* 2
Program ID: 150-38-21-144

Oklahoma

Oklahoma City

University of Oklahoma Health Sciences Center Program
Sponsor: University of Oklahoma College of Medicine
University Hospital
Veterans Affairs Medical Center (Oklahoma City)
Program Director:
Morris Reichlin, MD
Univ of Oklahoma Health Sciences Ctr
PO Box 26901
OMRF Mail Stop 24/C-308
Oklahoma City, OK 73190
Tel: 405 271-7766 *Fax:* 405 271-4110
E-mail: donna_whitbeck@omrf.uokhsc.edu
Accred Length: 2 Years *Program Size:* 2
Program ID: 150-39-21-056

Oregon

Portland

Oregon Health Sciences University Program
Sponsor: Oregon Health Sciences University Hospital
Veterans Affairs Medical Center (Portland)
Program Director:
Robert M Bennett, MD
Oregon Health Sciences Univ
Dept of Med/L329A
Portland, OR 97201
Tel: 503 494-8963 *Fax:* 503 494-1022
Accred Length: 2 Years *Program Size:* 2
Program ID: 150-40-31-118

Pennsylvania

Danville

Penn State Geisinger Health System/Geisinger Medical Center Program
Sponsor: Penn State Geisinger Health System
Geisinger Medical Center
Program Director:
Thomas M Harrington, MD
Geisinger Med Ctr
100 N Academy Ave
Danville, PA 17822
Tel: 717 271-6416 *Fax:* 717 271-5940
E-mail: ckrebs@psghs.edu
Accred Length: 2 Years *Program Size:* 2
Program ID: 150-41-11-104

Philadelphia

Albert Einstein Medical Center Program
Sponsor: Albert Einstein Medical Center
Moss Rehabilitation Hospital
Program Director:
Lawrence H Brent, MD
Albert Einstein Med Ctr
Einstein Arthritis Ctr
5501 Old York Rd/Korman 103
Philadelphia, PA 19141-3098
Tel: 215 456-7380 *Fax:* 215 456-3898
Accred Length: 2 Years *Program Size:* 2
Program ID: 150-41-11-033

MCP Hahnemann University Program
Sponsor: MCP Hahnemann University
Hahnemann University Hospital
Medical College of Pennsylvania Hospital
Veterans Affairs Medical Center (Philadelphia)
Program Director:
Bruce I Hoffman, MD
MCP Hahnemann Univ Hospital
3300 Henry Ave
Philadelphia, PA 19129
Tel: 215 842-6449 *Fax:* 215 843-6924
Accred Length: 2 Years *Program Size:* 4
Program ID: 150-41-21-084

Temple University Program
Sponsor: Temple University Hospital
Program Director:
Steven Berney, MD
Temple Univ Hospital, Sect of Rheumatology
1316 W Ontario St
8th Fl Rheumatology
Philadelphia, PA 19140
Tel: 215 707-3635 *Fax:* 215 707-1694
Accred Length: 2 Years *Program Size:* 1
Program ID: 150-41-21-023

Thomas Jefferson University Program
Sponsor: Thomas Jefferson University Hospital
Program Director:
Raphael J DeHoratius, MD
Div of Rheumatology
613 Curtis Bldg
1015 Walnut St
Philadelphia, PA 19107
Tel: 215 955-1410 *Fax:* 215 923-7885
E-mail: raphael.dehoratius@mail.tju.edu
Internet:
http://www.jeffline.tju.edu/cwis/dept/rheumatology
Accred Length: 2 Years *Program Size:* 2
Program ID: 150-41-21-024

University of Pennsylvania Program
Sponsor: Hospital of the University of Pennsylvania
Program Director:
Joan M Von Feldt, MD
Univ of Pennsylvania Sch of Med
5 Maloney/Ste 504
3600 Spruce St
Philadelphia, PA 19104-4283
Tel: 215 662-2789 *Fax:* 215 662-4500
E-mail: rheum@mail.med.upenn.edu
Internet: http://www.med.upenn.edu/rheum/
Accred Length: 2 Years *Program Size:* 9
Program ID: 150-41-21-015

Pittsburgh

University Health Center of Pittsburgh Program
Sponsor: University Health Center of Pittsburgh
Presbyterian University Hospital/UPMC
Veterans Affairs Medical Center (Pittsburgh)
Program Director:
Timothy M Wright, MD
Hospital of Univ Health Ctr of Pittsburgh
3471 Fifth Ave
Kaufmann Bldg/Ste 502
Pittsburgh, PA 15213
Tel: 412 692-4343 *Fax:* 412 692-4350
E-mail: twrightt@pitt.edu
Accred Length: 2 Years *Program Size:* 5
Program ID: 150-41-21-027

Puerto Rico

Rio Piedras

San Juan City Hospital Program
Sponsor: San Juan City Hospital
University Hospital
Veterans Affairs Medical Center (San Juan)
Program Director:
Rodolfo Concepcion, MD
San Juan Municipal Hospital, Dept of Med
Box 21405
Puerto Rico Med Ctr
Rio Piedras, PR 00928
Tel: 787 766-2222, ext 3110 *Fax:* 787 763-1778
Accred Length: 2 Years *Program Size:* 2
Program ID: 150-42-11-069

San Juan

University of Puerto Rico Program
Sponsor: University of Puerto Rico School of Medicine
University Hospital
Program Director:
Esther N Gonzalez-Pares, MD
Univ Hospital, Dept of Med
Box 5067
San Juan, PR 00936
Tel: 809 758-2525
E-mail: e_gonzalez@rcmaca.upr.clu.edu
Accred Length: 2 Years *Program Size:* 1
Program ID: 150-42-21-085

Rhode Island

Providence

Roger Williams Medical Center Program

Sponsor: Roger Williams Medical Center
Rhode Island Hospital
Veterans Affairs Medical Center (Providence)

Program Director:
Edward V Lally, MD
Roger Williams Med Ctr
Div of Rheumatology
825 Chalkstone Ave
Providence, RI 02908-4735
Tel: 401 456-2069 *Fax:* 401 456-2016
Accred Length: 2 Years *Program Size:* 3
Program ID: 150-43-31-028

South Carolina

Charleston

Medical University of South Carolina Program

Sponsor: Medical University of South Carolina College of Medicine
MUSC Medical Center
Ralph H Johnson Dept of Veterans Affairs Med Center

Program Director:
Richard M Silver, MD
Med Univ of South Carolina
Div of Rheumatology/Immunology
600 MUSC Complex/Ste 912
Charleston, SC 29425-2229
Tel: 843 792-1991 *Fax:* 843 792-7121
E-mail: kivettv@musc.edu
Internet: http://www.musc.edu/rheumatology
Accred Length: 2 Years *Program Size:* 4
Program ID: 150-45-21-075

Tennessee

Memphis

University of Tennessee Program

Sponsor: University of Tennessee College of Medicine
Baptist Memorial Hospital
Regional Medical Center at Memphis
Veterans Affairs Medical Center (Memphis)

Program Director:
Kristine M Lohr, MD
Univ of Tennessee
Dept of Med
956 Court Ave/Rm E320
Memphis, TN 38163
Tel: 901 448-5780 *Fax:* 901 448-7265
E-mail: klohr@utmem1.utmem.edu
Accred Length: 2 Years *Program Size:* 2
Program ID: 150-47-21-105

Nashville

Vanderbilt University Program

Sponsor: Vanderbilt University Medical Center
St Thomas Hospital
Veterans Affairs Medical Center (Nashville)

Program Director:
Howard A Fuchs, MD
Vanderbilt University Med Ctr
T3219 MCN
Nashville, TN 37232-2681
Tel: 615 322-4746 *Fax:* 615 322-6248
E-mail: fuchsha@ctrvax.vanderbilt.edu
Accred Length: 2 Years *Program Size:* 2
Program ID: 150-47-31-012

Texas

Dallas

University of Texas Southwestern Medical School Program

Sponsor: University of Texas Southwestern Medical School
Dallas County Hospital District-Parkland Memorial Hospital
Veterans Affairs Medical Center (Dallas)

Program Director:
Peter E Lipsky, MD
Univ of Texas Southwestern Med Ctr
5323 Harry Hines Blvd
Dallas, TX 75235-8884
Tel: 214 648-9110 *Fax:* 214 648-7995
E-mail: peter.lipsky@email.swmed.edu
Accred Length: 2 Years *Program Size:* 15
Program ID: 150-48-21-070

Galveston

University of Texas Medical Branch Hospitals Program

Sponsor: University of Texas Medical Branch Hospitals

Program Director:
Bruce Baethge, MD
Univ of Texas Med Branch
301 University Blvd
Galveston, TX 77555-0759
Tel: 409 772-2865 *Fax:* 409 772-7355
E-mail: bbaethge@utmb.edu
Accred Length: 2 Years *Program Size:* 2
Program ID: 150-48-21-147

Houston

Baylor College of Medicine Program

Sponsor: Baylor College of Medicine
Harris County Hospital District-Ben Taub General Hospital

Program Director:
Donald M Marcus, MD
Baylor Coll of Med-Texas Med Ctr
One Baylor Plaza
FBRN B567
Houston, TX 77030
Tel: 713 790-5310 *Fax:* 713 793-1445
E-mail: dhouston@bcm.tmc.edu
Internet:
http://www.bcm.tmc.edu/medicine/residency/subspecialty
Accred Length: 2 Years *Program Size:* 3
Program ID: 150-48-21-058

University of Texas at Houston Program

Sponsor: University of Texas Medical School at Houston
Lyndon B Johnson General Hospital
Memorial Hermann Healthcare System

Program Director:
Frank C Arnett Jr, MD
Univ of Texas-Houston Med Sch
PO Box 20708
Houston, TX 77025
Tel: 713 500-6900 *Fax:* 713 500-0580
E-mail: arnett@heart.med.uth.tmc.edu
Internet:
http://www.uth.tmc.edu/schools/med/imed/rheuma/index.htm
Accred Length: 2 Years *Program Size:* 3
Program ID: 150-48-31-130

Lackland AFB

San Antonio Uniformed Services Health Education Consortium (WHMC) Program

Sponsor: San Antonio Uniformed Services Health Education Consortium
Wilford Hall Medical Center (AETC)

Program Director:
Ramon A Arroyo, MD
759 MDOS/MMIR
2200 Bergquist Dr/Ste 1
Lackland AFB, TX 78236-5300
Tel: 210 292-7307 *Fax:* 210 292-7662
E-mail: arroyo@whmc-lafb.af.mil
Accred Length: 2 Years *Program Size:* 2
Program ID: 150-48-12-065
US Armed Services Program

San Antonio

University of Texas Health Science Center at San Antonio Program

Sponsor: University of Texas Medical School at San Antonio
Audie L Murphy Memorial Veterans Hospital (San Antonio)
University Hospital-South Texas Medical Center

Program Director:
Michael Fischbach, MD
Univ of Texas Health Science Ctr
Dept of Med/Rheumatology
7703 Floyd Curl Dr
San Antonio, TX 78284-7874
Tel: 210 567-4658 *Fax:* 210 567-4721
E-mail: boyle@uthscsa
Accred Length: 2 Years *Program Size:* 2
Program ID: 150-48-21-041

Utah

Salt Lake City

University of Utah Program

Sponsor: University of Utah Medical Center
Veterans Affairs Medical Center (Salt Lake City)

Program Director:
H James Williams, MD
Univ of Utah Med Ctr
50 N Medical Dr/4B218
Salt Lake City, UT 84132
Tel: 801 581-4333 *Fax:* 801 581-6069
E-mail: james.williams@hsc.utah.edu
Accred Length: 2 Years *Program Size:* 4
Program ID: 150-49-21-148

Vermont

Burlington

University of Vermont Program
Sponsor: Fletcher Allen Health Care
Program Director:
Sheldon M Cooper, MD
Univ of Vermont Coll of Med
Dept of Med
Given Bldg D-301
Burlington, VT 05405-0068
Tel: 802 656-2144 *Fax:* 802 656-3854
E-mail: scooper@zoo.uvm.edu
Accred Length: 2 Years *Program Size:* 2
Program ID: 150-50-21-120

Virginia

Charlottesville

University of Virginia Program
Sponsor: University of Virginia Medical Center
Program Director:
Martha L Barnett, MD
Univ of Virginia Health Sciences Ctr
Div of Rheumatology/Box 412
Charlottesville, VA 22908
Tel: 804 924-5214 *Fax:* 804 924-2327
E-mail: mbarnett@virginia.edu
Accred Length: 2 Years *Program Size:* 2
Program ID: 150-51-21-013

Richmond

Medical College of Virginia/Virginia Commonwealth University Program
Sponsor: Medical College of Virginia/Virginia Commonwealth University
Medical College of Virginia Hospitals
Program Director:
W. Neal Roberts, MD
Med Coll of Virginia, Dept of Med
Box 980263/MCV Station
Richmond, VA 23298-0263
Tel: 804 828-9685 *Fax:* 804 828-0283
E-mail: prob@aol.com
Internet: http://www.views.vcu.edu/internal-medicine
Accred Length: 2 Years *Program Size:* 2
Program ID: 150-51-21-014

Washington

Seattle

University of Washington Program
Sponsor: University of Washington School of Medicine
University of Washington Medical Center
Veterans Affairs Medical Center (Seattle)
Program Director:
Mart Mannik, MD
Div of Rheumatology
Dept of Med Box 356428
Univ of Washington
Seattle, WA 98195-6428
Tel: 206 543-3414 *Fax:* 206 685-9397
E-mail: mannik@u.washington.edu
Internet: http://weber.washington.edu/~medweb
Accred Length: 2 Years *Program Size:* 4
Program ID: 150-54-21-059

Wisconsin

Madison

University of Wisconsin Program
Sponsor: University of Wisconsin Hospital and Clinics
William S Middleton Veterans Hospital
Program Director:
Frank M Graziano, MD PhD
Univ of Wisconsin Hospital
600 Highland Ave/Rm H6-367
Madison, WI 53792-3244
Tel: 608 263-3457 *Fax:* 608 263-3104
E-mail: jae@parc.medicine.wisc.edu
Internet: http://www.medicine.wisc.edu/sections/rheum
Accred Length: 2 Years *Program Size:* 2
Program ID: 150-56-21-087

Milwaukee

Medical College of Wisconsin Program
Sponsor: Medical College of Wisconsin Affiliated Hospitals Inc
Clement J Zablocki Veterans Affairs Medical Center
Froedtert Memorial Lutheran Hospital
Program Director:
Lawrence M Ryan, MD
Med Coll of Wisconsin
9200 W Wisconsin Ave/MOB 4760
Milwaukee, WI 53226
Tel: 414 456-7010 *Fax:* 414 456-6205
E-mail: lryan@mcw.edu
Accred Length: 2 Years *Program Size:* 2
Program ID: 150-56-31-029

Selective Pathology (Pathology)

California

Los Angeles

Children's Hospital of Los Angeles Program
Sponsor: Children's Hospital of Los Angeles
Program Director:
Jon M Rowland, MD PhD
Dept of Pathology/Box 103
4650 Sunset Blvd
Los Angeles, CA 90027
Tel: 323 669-4623 *Fax:* 323 667-1123
Internet:
http://www.usc.edu/hsc/chla/path/demo/chlapages/
Accred Length: 1 Year *Program Size:* 2
Program ID: 301-05-21-001

Massachusetts

Boston

Brigham and Women's Hospital Program
Sponsor: Brigham and Women's Hospital
Program Director:
Christopher Crum, MD
Brigham and Women's Hospital
75 Francis St
Boston, MA 02115
Tel: 617 732-7530 *Fax:* 617 975-0864
E-mail: cpcrum@bics.bwh.harvard.edu
Accred Length: 1 Year *Program Size:* 2
Program ID: 301-24-11-003

Minnesota

Minneapolis

University of Minnesota Program
Sponsor: University of Minnesota Medical School
Fairview-University Medical Center
Program Director:
Phuong Nguyen, MD
Univ of Minnesota
420 Delaware St SE
Box 609 Mayo
Minneapolis, MN 55455-0392
Tel: 612 626-5704 *Fax:* 612 625-0617
E-mail: vjohn@lenti.med.umn.edu
Accred Length: 1 Year *Program Size:* 2
Program ID: 301-26-21-020

New York

Buffalo

Roswell Park Cancer Institute Program
Sponsor: Roswell Park Cancer Institute
Program Director:
Janet S Winston, MD
Roswell Park Cancer Inst
666 Elm and Carlton St
Buffalo, NY 14263-0000
Tel: 716 845-7700 *Fax:* 716 845-3427
E-mail: winston@sc3102.med.buffalo.edu
Accred Length: 1 Year *Program Size:* 4
Program ID: 301-35-31-016

New York

Hospital for Joint Diseases Orthopaedic Institute Program
Sponsor: Hospital for Joint Diseases Orthopaedic Institute
Program Director:
German C Steiner, MD
Hospital for Joint Diseases Orthopaedic Inst
Dept of Path/Lab Med
301 E 17th St/Bernard Aronson Pl
New York, NY 10003
Tel: 212 598-6231 *Fax:* 212 598-6057
Accred Length: 1 Year *Program Size:* 1
Program ID: 301-35-21-005

Memorial Sloan-Kettering Cancer Center Program
Sponsor: Memorial Sloan-Kettering Cancer Center
Program Director:
David Klimstra, MD
Memorial Sloan-Kettering Cancer Ctr
1275 York Ave
New York, NY 10021
Tel: 212 639-8410 *Fax:* 212 772-8521
E-mail: klimstrd@mskcc.org
Internet: http://www.mskcc.org/mp.htm
Accred Length: 1 Year *Program Size:* 15
Program ID: 301-35-21-011

New York Medical College (Manhattan) Program
Sponsor: New York Medical College
New York Eye and Ear Infirmary
Program Director:
Steven A McCormick, MD
New York Med Coll
Second Ave at 14th St
New York, NY 10003
Tel: 212 979-4156 *Fax:* 212 677-1284
E-mail: smccormick@nyee.edu
Accred Length: 1 Year *Program Size:* 1
Program ID: 301-35-11-017

North Carolina

Charlotte

Carolinas Medical Center Program
Sponsor: Carolinas Medical Center
Program Director:
Peter M Banks, MD
Carolinas Med Ctr
1000 Blythe Blvd
Charlotte, NC 28203
Tel: 704 355-2251 *Fax:* 704 355-2156
Accred Length: 1 Year *Program Size:* 2
Program ID: 301-36-21-019

Pennsylvania

Philadelphia

Thomas Jefferson University Program
Sponsor: Thomas Jefferson University Hospital
Fox Chase Cancer Center
Program Director:
Peter McCue, MD
132 S 10th St/Ste 285
Philadelphia, PA 19107
Tel: 215 955-9544 *Fax:* 215 923-6039
Accred Length: 1 Year *Program Size:* 2
Program ID: 301-41-21-018

Texas

Houston

University of Texas M D Anderson Cancer Center Program
Sponsor: University of Texas M D Anderson Cancer Center
Program Director:
Aysegul Sahin, MD
Univ of Texas-MD Anderson Cancer Ctr
Dept of Pathology/Box 85
1515 Holcombe Blvd
Houston, TX 77030-4095
Tel: 713 792-3108 *Fax:* 713 745-0789
E-mail: jknight@notes.mdacc.tmc.edu
Accred Length: 1 Year *Program Size:* 13
Subspecialties: PCP
Program ID: 301-48-21-010

Spinal Cord Injury Medicine (Physical Medicine and Rehabilitation)

Alabama

Birmingham

University of Alabama Medical Center Program
Sponsor: University of Alabama Hospital
Children's Hospital of Alabama
Program Director:
Amie B Jackson, MD
Univ of Alabama
1717 6th Ave S
Birmingham, AL 35233-7330
Tel: 205 934-3450 *Fax:* 205 975-9754
E-mail: jackson@sun.rehabm.uab.edu
Accred Length: 1 Year *Program Size:* 1
Program ID: 345-01-21-001

California

Stanford

Stanford University Program
Sponsor: Stanford University Hospital
Veterans Affairs Palo Alto Health Care System
Program Director:
Inder Perkash, MD
3801 Maranda Ave
SCIM Service (128)
Palo Alto, CA 94304
Tel: 650 493-5000 *Fax:* 650 852-3455
E-mail: perkash@pobox4.stanford.edu
Accred Length: 1 Year *Program Size:* 2
Program ID: 345-05-21-007

Massachusetts

Boston

Harvard Medical School Program
Sponsor: Spaulding Rehabilitation Hospital
Brigham and Women's Hospital
Brockton-West Roxbury Veterans Affairs Medical Center
Program Director:
Dominic K Foo, MD
Spinal Cord Injury Service
Brockton-West Roxbury VA Med Ctr
1400 VFW Pkwy
West Roxbury, MA 02132
Tel: 617 323-7700, ext 5128 *Fax:* 617 363-5552
E-mail: foo_md.dominic@brockton.va.gov
Accred Length: 1 Year *Program Size:* 1
Program ID: 345-24-21-002

New Jersey

Newark

UMDNJ-New Jersey Medical School Program
Sponsor: UMDNJ-New Jersey Medical School
Kessler Institute for Rehabilitation
Program Director:
Steven Kirshblum, MD
150 Bergen St/Rm B-261
Newark, NJ 07103
Tel: 973 972-3606 *Fax:* 973 972-5148
E-mail: leckyal@umdnj.edu
Accred Length: 1 Year *Program Size:* 2
Program ID: 345-33-21-003

Pennsylvania

Philadelphia

Thomas Jefferson University Program
Sponsor: Thomas Jefferson University Hospital
Magee Rehabilitation Hospital
Program Director:
William E Stass Jr, MD
6 Franklin Plaza
Philadelphia, PA 19102
Tel: 215 587-3099 *Fax:* 215 587-9154
E-mail: magee@mageerehab.org
Accred Length: 1 Year *Program Size:* 0
Program ID: 345-41-21-005

Virginia

Richmond

Medical College of Virginia/Virginia Commonwealth University Program
Sponsor: Medical College of Virginia/Virginia Commonwealth University
Hunter Holmes McGuire VA Medical Center (Richmond)
Medical College of Virginia Hospitals
Program Director:
Meena Midha, MD
Hunter Holmes McGuire VA Med Ctr
1201 Broad Rock Blvd
Richmond, VA 23249
Tel: 804 675-5128, ext 3380 *Fax:* 804 675-5223
E-mail: midha.meena nmn@richmond.va.gov
Accred Length: 1 Year *Program Size:* 3
Program ID: 345-51-21-004

Sports Medicine (Emergency Medicine)

Pennsylvania

Pittsburgh

Allegheny General Hospital Program
Sponsor: Allegheny General Hospital
Program Director:
Edward D Snell, MD
Allegheny General Hospital
390 E North Ave
Ste 500
Pittsburgh, PA 15212
Tel: 412 359-6501 *Fax:* 412 359-6265
Accred Length: 1 Year *Program Size:* 1
Program ID: 116-41-21-001

Sports Medicine (Family Practice)

Alabama

Huntsville

University of Alabama Medical Center (Huntsville) Program
Sponsor: University of Alabama Hospital
Huntsville Hospital
Program Director:
Michael M Linder, MD
Huntsville Hospital
201 Governors Dr
Huntsville, AL 35801-9990
Tel: 256 551-4632 *Fax:* 256 551-4633
E-mail: edwardsh@email.uah.edu
Accred Length: 1 Year *Program Size:* 1
Program ID: 127-01-21-002

California

Fontana

Southern California Kaiser Permanente Medical Care (Fontana) Program
Sponsor: Southern California Kaiser Permanente Medical Group
Kaiser Foundation Hospital (Fontana)
Program Director:
Aaron Rubin, MD
9985 Sierra Ave
Fontana, CA 92335
Tel: 909 427-5083 *Fax:* 909 427-5619
E-mail: aaron.l.rubin@kp.org
Accred Length: 1 Year *Program Size:* 2
Program ID: 127-05-21-003

La Mesa

Sharp HealthCare (La Mesa) Program
Sponsor: Sharp HealthCare
Grossmont Hospital
Alvarado Hospital Medical Center
Naval Hospital (Camp Pendleton)
Program Director:
E Lee Rice, DO
6719 Alvarado Rd/Ste 200
San Diego, CA 92120-5289
Tel: 619 229-3909 *Fax:* 619 582-1497
E-mail: erice6719@aol.com
Accred Length: 1 Year *Program Size:* 1
Program ID: 127-05-21-034

Los Angeles

UCLA Medical Center Program
Sponsor: UCLA School of Medicine
UCLA Medical Center
Program Director:
James C Puffer, MD
10833 Le Conte Ave
Los Angeles, CA 90095-1683
Tel: 310 825-8848 *Fax:* 310 206-5351
E-mail: jpuffer@mednet.ucla.edu
Internet: http://www.ucla.edu
Accred Length: 1 Year *Program Size:* 4
Program ID: 127-05-21-018

San Diego

University of California (San Diego) Program
Sponsor: University of California (San Diego) Medical Center
Program Director:
Mark D Bracker, MD
UCSD Med Ctr, Dept of Family/Prev Med
9500 Gilman M/C 0807
La Jolla, CA 92093-0622
Tel: 619 543-5476 *Fax:* 619 543-5996
E-mail: lmoore@ucsd.edu
Internet: http://www.orpheus.ucsd.edu/famed/resident
Accred Length: 1 Year *Program Size:* 2
Program ID: 127-05-31-004

San Jose

San Jose Medical Center Program
Sponsor: San Jose Medical Center
Program Director:
Michael J Henehan, DO
25 N 14th St/Ste 1060
San Jose, CA 95112
Tel: 408 977-4507 *Fax:* 408 977-4456
Internet: http://www_leland.stanford.edu/group/fpecs/sjfamilypracticeresidency.html
Accred Length: 1 Year *Program Size:* 2
Program ID: 127-05-31-019

Delaware

Wilmington

Christiana Care Health Services Program
Sponsor: Christiana Care Health Services Inc
Program Director:
Lisa C Barkley, MD
4755 Ogletown-Stanton Rd
PO Box 6001/Rm 4100-4C
Newark, DE 19718
Tel: 302 733-4109 *Fax:* 302 733-4174
Accred Length: 1 Year *Program Size:* 2
Program ID: 127-09-21-038

Florida

Daytona Beach

Halifax Medical Center Program
Sponsor: Halifax Medical Center
Program Director:
John Shelton, MD
Halifax Med Ctr
303 N Clyde Morris Blvd
Daytona Beach, FL 32114-2732
Tel: 904 254-4047 *Fax:* 904 258-4867
Internet: http://www.halifax.org
Accred Length: 1 Year *Program Size:* 1
Program ID: 127-11-21-036

St Petersburg

Bayfront Medical Center Program
Sponsor: Bayfront Medical Center
Program Director:
Russell D White, MD
Bayfront Med Ctr
700 Sixth St S
St Petersburg, FL 33701
Tel: 813 893-6156 *Fax:* 813 553-7340
E-mail: whiter@bayfront.org
Internet: http://www.bayfront.org
Accred Length: 1 Year *Program Size:* 2
Program ID: 127-11-21-041

Illinois

Berwyn

MacNeal Memorial Hospital Program
Sponsor: MacNeal Memorial Hospital
Rush-Presbyterian-St Luke's Medical Center
Program Director:
Thomas Wang, MD
3231 S Euclid Ave
Berwyn, IL 60402
Tel: 708 783-3425 *Fax:* 708 783-3656
Accred Length: 1 Year *Program Size:* 1
Program ID: 127-16-21-040

Park Ridge

Lutheran General Hospital Program
Sponsor: Lutheran General Hospital
Program Director:
William W Briner Jr, MD
Lutheran General Hospital
1775 Dempster St/6 South
Park Ridge, IL 60068-1100
Tel: 847 723-7969 *Fax:* 847 723-5615
E-mail: marie.markovich@advocatehealth.com
Internet: http://www.lghfpres.com
Accred Length: 1 Year *Program Size:* 1
Program ID: 127-16-21-006

Indiana

Indianapolis

Indiana University School of Medicine Program
Sponsor: Indiana University School of Medicine
Clarian Methodist Hospital of Indiana
Program Director:
Douglas W Robertson, MD
Gregory A Rowdon, MD
Indiana Univ Sch of Med
1815 N Capitol Ave/Ste 401
Indianapolis, IN 46202
Tel: 317 921-3729 *Fax:* 317 921-0230
Accred Length: 1 Year *Program Size:* 2
Program ID: 127-17-21-021

South Bend

Memorial Hospital of South Bend Program
Sponsor: Memorial Hospital of South Bend
St Joseph's Regional Medical Center of South Bend
Program Director:
Mark E Lavallee, MD
Memorial Hospital
714 N Michigan St
South Bend, IN 46601
Tel: 219 284-7913 *Fax:* 219 284-6819
E-mail: mlavamd@aol.com
Internet: http://www.qualityoflife.org/fpc.htm
Accred Length: 1 Year *Program Size:* 1
Program ID: 127-17-21-042

St Joseph's Medical Center of South Bend Program
Sponsor: St Joseph's Regional Medical Center of South Bend
Memorial Hospital of South Bend
Program Director:
Stephen M Simons, MD
837 E Cedar
Ste 125
South Bend, IN 46617
Tel: 219 237-7749 *Fax:* 219 239-6088
E-mail: simonss@sjcg.org
Accred Length: 1 Year *Program Size:* 2
Program ID: 127-17-31-043

Maine

Portland

Maine Medical Center Program
Sponsor: Maine Medical Center
Program Director:
William W Dexter, MD
Maine Med Ctr
103 India St
Portland, ME 04101
Tel: 207 871-6839 *Fax:* 207 874-1918
E-mail: dexterw@mail.mmc.org
Accred Length: 1 Year *Program Size:* 2
Program ID: 127-22-21-035

Maryland

Baltimore

University of Maryland Program
Sponsor: University of Maryland Medical System
James Lawrence Kernan Hospital
Program Director:
Andrew M Tucker, MD
2200 Kernan Dr/2nd Fl
Baltimore, MD 21207
Tel: 410 448-6296 *Fax:* 410 448-6789
Accred Length: 1 Year *Program Size:* 1
Program ID: 127-23-21-051

Michigan

Ann Arbor

University of Michigan Program
Sponsor: University of Michigan Hospitals
Program Director:
Robert B Kiningham, MD MA
Univ of Michigan
1018 Fuller St
Box 0708
Ann Arbor, MI 48109
Tel: 313 998-7128 *Fax:* 313 998-7335
Internet: http://www.med.umich.edu/fp/
Accred Length: 1 Year *Program Size:* 1
Program ID: 127-25-21-007

Kalamazoo

Kalamazoo Center for Medical Studies/Michigan State University Program
Sponsor: Kalamazoo Center for Medical Studies
Borgess Medical Center
Bronson Methodist Hospital
Program Director:
Dilip Patel, MD
MSU/KCMS
1000 Oakland Dr
Kalamazoo, MI 49008
Tel: 616 337-6550 *Fax:* 616 337-6565
E-mail: dickson@kcms.msu.edu
Internet: http://www.kcms.msu.edu
Accred Length: 1 Year *Program Size:* 1
Program ID: 127-25-21-050

Lansing

Sparrow Hospital Program
Sponsor: Sparrow Hospital
St Lawrence Hospital and HealthCare Services
Program Director:
Jeffrey R Kovan, DO
Michigan State Univ
2900 Hannah Blvd/Ste 104
East Lansing, MI 48823
Tel: 517 336-4520 *Fax:* 517 332-4576
Accred Length: 1 Year *Program Size:* 3
Program ID: 127-25-21-001

Southfield

Providence Hospital and Medical Centers Program
Sponsor: Providence Hospital and Medical Centers
Program Director:
Scott Eathorne, MD
Providence Hospital
16001 W Nine Mile Rd
Southfield, MI 48075
Tel: 248 424-3216 *Fax:* 248 424-5324
Accred Length: 1 Year *Program Size:* 1
Program ID: 127-25-21-022

Minnesota

Minneapolis

Hennepin County Medical Center Program
Sponsor: Hennepin County Medical Center
Program Director:
Robert J Johnson, MD
Family Med Ctr
5 W Lake St
Minneapolis, MN 55408
Tel: 612 827-9777 *Fax:* 612 827-9734
Accred Length: 1 Year *Program Size:* 3
Program ID: 127-26-21-008

New Jersey

Piscataway

UMDNJ-Robert Wood Johnson Medical School Program
Sponsor: UMDNJ-Robert Wood Johnson Medical School
Hospital for Special Surgery
St Peter's University Hospital
Program Director:
Brian Halpern, MD
UMDNJ-Robert Wood Johnson Med Sch
Dept of Family Medicine
One Robert Wood Johnson Pl
New Brunswick, NJ 08903-0019
Tel: 732 235-7669 *Fax:* 732 246-8084
Internet: http://www2.umdnj.edu/fmedweb/smfell.htm
Accred Length: 1 Year *Program Size:* 1
Program ID: 127-33-21-030

North Carolina

Greensboro

Moses H Cone Memorial Hospital Program
Sponsor: Moses H Cone Memorial Hospital
Program Director:
Karl B Fields, MD
1125 N Church St
Greensboro, NC 27401
Tel: 910 574-8133 *Fax:* 910 574-7078
Accred Length: 1 Year *Program Size:* 1
Program ID: 127-36-21-023

Winston-Salem

Wake Forest University School of Medicine Program
Sponsor: Wake Forest University Baptist Medical Center
Program Director:
Douglas G Browning, MD
Wake Forest Univ Baptist Med Ctr
Medical Center Blvd
Winston-Salem, NC 27157
Tel: 336 716-2794 *Fax:* 336 716-9126
Accred Length: 1 Year *Program Size:* 0
Program ID: 127-36-21-048

Ohio

Cleveland

Fairview Health System Program
Sponsor: Fairview Health System
Cleveland Clinic Foundation
Program Director:
Robert J Dimeff, MD
Cleveland Clinic Foundation
9500 Euclid Ave/A41
Cleveland, OH 44195-5027
Tel: 216 444-2185 *Fax:* 216 445-7460
E-mail: dimeffr@cesmtp.ccf.org or baumanc@cesmtp.ccf.org
Internet: http://www.ccf.org
Accred Length: 1 Year *Program Size:* 2
Program ID: 127-38-21-047

Columbus

Ohio State University Program
Sponsor: Ohio State University Medical Center
Program Director:
John A Lombardo, MD
2050 Kenny Rd
Columbus, OH 43221
Tel: 614 293-5260 *Fax:* 614 293-4399
Accred Length: 1 Year *Program Size:* 4
Program ID: 127-38-21-031

Dayton

Franciscan Medical Center (Dayton) Program
Sponsor: Franciscan Medical Center-Dayton Campus
Program Director:
James Tytko, MD
Franciscan Med Ctr
One Franciscan Way
Dayton, OH 45408
Tel: 937 229-6670 *Fax:* 937 229-7425
Accred Length: 1 Year *Program Size:* 1
Program ID: 127-38-21-010

Toledo

Toledo Hospital Program
Sponsor: Toledo Hospital
Program Director:
Roger J Kruse, MD
2051 W Central Ave
Toldeo, OH 43606
Tel: 419 471-5905 *Fax:* 419 479-6055
E-mail: roger.kruse.md@promedica.org
Accred Length: 1 Year *Program Size:* 3
Program ID: 127-38-31-011

Oklahoma

Oklahoma City

University of Oklahoma Health Sciences Center Program

Sponsor: University of Oklahoma College of Medicine
Columbia Presbyterian Hospital
University Hospital
Program Director:
James R Barrett, MD
Univ of Oklahoma Health Sciences Ctr
Dept of Family/Prev Med
900 NE 10th St
Oklahoma City, OK 73104
Tel: 405 271-8818 *Fax:* 405 271-4366
E-mail: sports-medicine@ouhsc.edu
Accred Length: 1 Year *Program Size:* 3
Program ID: 127-39-21-012

Tulsa

University of Oklahoma College of Medicine-Tulsa Program

Sponsor: University of Oklahoma College of Medicine-Tulsa
St Francis Hospital
Program Director:
T Jeffrey Emel, MD
6585 S Yale/Ste 500
Tulsa, OK 74136
Tel: 918 494-9300 *Fax:* 918 494-9359
E-mail: eooc@ionet.net
Accred Length: 1 Year *Program Size:* 3
Program ID: 127-39-31-013

Pennsylvania

Philadelphia

Thomas Jefferson University Program

Sponsor: Thomas Jefferson University Hospital
Pennsylvania Hospital (UPHS)
Program Director:
John McShane, MD
Thomas Jefferson Univ Hospital
1015 Walnut St/Ste 401
Philadelphia, PA 19107
Tel: 215 955-0641 *Fax:* 215 923-6256
Accred Length: 1 Year *Program Size:* 2
Program ID: 127-41-21-024

Pittsburgh

Shadyside Hospital/UPMC Program

Sponsor: Shadyside Hospital/UPMC
Program Director:
Douglas B McKeag, MD MS
UPMC Shadyside
Dept of Family Practice
5230 Centre Ave
Pittsburgh, PA 15232
Tel: 412 623-2028 *Fax:* 412 623-6253
E-mail: mckeagdb@msx.upmc.edu
Internet: http://www.sportsmed.upmc.edu/pcsm
Accred Length: 1 Year *Program Size:* 1
Program ID: 127-41-21-014

University of Pittsburgh Medical Center (St Margaret) Program

Sponsor: University of Pittsburgh Medical Center (St Margaret)
Program Director:
Douglas B McKeag, MD
Rm 215 Son-Shady Hospital
5230 Centre Ave
Pittsburgh, PA 15232
Tel: 412 623-2028 *Fax:* 412 623-6253
Accred Length: 1 Year *Program Size:* 1
Program ID: 127-41-31-025

Upland

Crozer-Keystone Health System Program

Sponsor: Crozer-Chester Medical Center
Crozer-Keystone Health System
Program Director:
Brian J Shiple, DO
1260 E Woodland Ave/Ste 200
Springfield, PA 19064
Tel: 610 690-4480 *Fax:* 610 328-9391
E-mail: bshiple@crozer.org
Internet: http://www.hslc.org/ccm/ccm.html
Accred Length: 1 Year *Program Size:* 1
Program ID: 127-41-21-033

South Carolina

Columbia

Palmetto Health Alliance/University of South Carolina School of Medicine Program

Sponsor: Palmetto Health Alliance
Palmetto Richland Memorial Hospital
Program Director:
Mark J Leski, MD
6 Richland Medical Pk
Columbia, SC 29203
Tel: 803 434-6116 *Fax:* 803 434-7529
Internet: http://www.rmh.edu
Accred Length: 1 Year *Program Size:* 2
Program ID: 127-45-21-015

Tennessee

Knoxville

University of Tennessee Medical Center at Knoxville Program

Sponsor: University of Tennessee Graduate School of Medicine
University of Tennessee Memorial Hospital
Program Director:
Kenneth M Bielak, MD
Univ of Tennessee Graduate Sch of Med
Sports Med Family Practice/U-67
Knoxville, TN 37920
Tel: 423 544-9352 *Fax:* 423 544-6532
E-mail: utfprp@mc.utmck.edu
Internet: http://www.mc.utk.edu
Accred Length: 1 Year *Program Size:* 1
Program ID: 127-47-21-044

Texas

Dallas

University of Texas Southwestern Medical Center (Methodist) Program

Sponsor: Methodist Hospitals of Dallas
Charlton Methodist Hospital
Program Director:
David S Ross, MD
3400 W Wheatland Rd
Dallas, TX 75237
Tel: 214 947-5420 *Fax:* 214 947-5425
E-mail: helenmalone@mhdcme.org
Internet: http://www.mhdcme.org
Accred Length: 1 Year *Program Size:* 2
Program ID: 127-48-21-016

San Antonio

University of Texas Health Science Center at San Antonio Program

Sponsor: University of Texas Medical School at San Antonio
Methodist Healthcare
San Antonio Community Hospital
St Luke's Baptist Hospital
Program Director:
Walter L Calmbach, MD
Univ of Texas Health Science Ctr
Dept of Family Practice
7703 Floyd Curl Dr
San Antonio, TX 78284-7795
Tel: 210 567-4550 *Fax:* 210 567-4579
E-mail: calmbach@uthscsa.edu
Accred Length: 1 Year *Program Size:* 1
Program ID: 127-48-21-027

Virginia

Fort Belvoir

DeWitt Army Community Hospital Program

Sponsor: DeWitt Army Community Hospital
Arlington Hospital
Malcolm Grow Medical Center (SGE)
Program Director:
Francis G O'Connor, MD
Uniformed Services Univ of Health Sciences
4301 Jones Bridge Rd
Bethesda, MD 20814
Tel: 301 295-3632 *Fax:* 301 295-3100
E-mail: foconnor@.usuhs.mil
Internet: http://www.usuhs.mil
Accred Length: 1 Year *Program Size:* 3
Program ID: 127-51-21-037
US Armed Services Program

Programs

Washington

Seattle

University of Washington Program
Sponsor: University of Washington School of Medicine
University of Washington Medical Center
Program Director:
Michael K Eshleman, MD
Hall Health Primary Care Ctr
Box 354410
Univ of Washington
Seattle, WA 98195-4410
Tel: 206 685-1044 *Fax:* 206 616-4683
E-mail: eshleman@u.washington.edu
Accred Length: 1 Year *Program Size:* 1
Program ID: 127-54-21-039

Wisconsin

Janesville

Mercy Health System Program
Sponsor: Mercy Health System
Program Director:
David A Braunreiter, MD
Mercy Sports Medicine Ctr
557 N Washington St
Janesville, WI 53545-2907
Tel: 608 754-6000 *Fax:* 608 755-7892
E-mail: dbraunreiter@mhsjvl.org
Internet: http://www.mercyhealthsystem.org
Accred Length: 1 Year *Program Size:* 2
Program ID: 127-56-21-046

Milwaukee

Medical College of Wisconsin (St Mary's) Program
Sponsor: Medical College of Wisconsin Affiliated Hospitals Inc
Froedtert Memorial Lutheran Hospital
Program Director:
Craig C Young, MD
Sports Med Clinic
9200 W Wisconsin Ave
Milwaukee, WI 53226
Tel: 414 257-5115 *Fax:* 414 257-7861
Internet: http://www.mcw.edu/ortho
Accred Length: 1 Year *Program Size:* 1
Program ID: 127-56-21-029

Sports Medicine (Internal Medicine)

Indiana

Muncie

Ball Memorial Hospital Program
Sponsor: Ball Memorial Hospital
Program Director:
Thomas L Sevier, MD
Ball Memorial Hospital
Central Indiana Sports Med
3600 W Bethel Ave
Muncie, IN 47304-5407
Tel: 765 213-3770 *Fax:* 765 284-4266
E-mail: tomsevier@iquest.net
Internet: http://www.ballhospital.org
Accred Length: 1 Year *Program Size:* 2
Program ID: 157-17-21-002

Surgery-General

Alabama

Birmingham

Baptist Health System Program
Sponsor: Baptist Health System Inc
Birmingham Baptist Medical Center-Montclair
Birmingham Baptist Medical Center-Princeton
Program Director:
Roy Gandy, MD
Birmingham Baptist Med Ctr-Princeton
817 Princeton Ave SW
POB 2/Ste 105
Birmingham, AL 35211
Tel: 205 783-3191 *Fax:* 205 783-7399
E-mail: renay.reeves@bhsala.com
Internet: http://www.bhsala.com
Accred Length: 5 Years *Program Size:* 15 (*GY1:* 6)
Subspecialties: TY
Program ID: 440-01-21-020

Carraway Methodist Medical Center Program
Sponsor: Carraway Methodist Medical Center
Program Director:
Henry L Laws, MD
Carraway Methodist Med Ctr
Office of Surgical Education
1600 Carraway Blvd
Birmingham, AL 35234
Tel: 205 502-6230 *Fax:* 205 502-6389
E-mail: gsres@mail.carraway.com
Internet: http://www.carraway.org
Accred Length: 5 Years *Program Size:* 17 (*GY1:* 5)
Subspecialties: TY
Program ID: 440-01-12-021

University of Alabama Medical Center Program
Sponsor: University of Alabama Hospital
Cooper Green Hospital
Lloyd Noland Hospital and Health Centers
Veterans Affairs Medical Center (Birmingham)
Program Director:
Marshall M Urist, MD
Univ of Alabama Med Ctr
Div of General Surgery
1922 S 7th Ave/301 Kracke Bldg
Birmingham, AL 35294-0016
Tel: 205 934-9600 *Fax:* 205 975-5867
E-mail: lajean.bartlett@ccc.uab.edu
Internet: http://www.surgery.uab.edu
Accred Length: 5 Years *Program Size:* 44 (*GY1:* 14)
Subspecialties: PDS
Program ID: 440-01-21-022

Mobile

University of South Alabama Program
Sponsor: University of South Alabama Medical Center
St Joseph's Hospital and Medical Center
Program Director:
Arnold Luterman, MD
Univ of South Alabama Med Ctr
2451 Fillingim St
Mastin 709
Mobile, AL 36617
Tel: 334 471-7990 *Fax:* 334 471-7022
E-mail: cdavis@usamail.usouthal.edu
Internet: http://www.usouth.edu/residency programs/surgery.html
Accred Length: 5 Years *Program Size:* 24 (*GY1:* 8)
Program ID: 440-01-11-024

Arizona

Phoenix

Good Samaritan Regional Medical Center Program

Sponsor: Good Samaritan Regional Medical Center
Carl T Hayden Veterans Affairs Medical Center (Phoenix)
Mayo Clinic (Scottsdale)

Program Director:
H Harlan Stone, MD
Phoenix Integrated Surgical Residency
1300 N 12th St
Ste 619
Phoenix, AZ 85006-2849
Tel: 602 239-2282 *Fax:* 602 495-9112
E-mail: isr@goodnet.com
Accred Length: 5 Years *Program Size:* 30 (*GY1:* 9)
Subspecialties: TY
Program ID: 440-03-22-026

Maricopa Medical Center Program

Sponsor: Maricopa Medical Center
Mayo Clinic (Scottsdale)

Program Director:
Marco V Canulla, MD
Maricopa Med Ctr
Dept of Surgery
2601 E Roosevelt St
Phoenix, AZ 85008
Tel: 602 267-5600 *Fax:* 602 392-0942
Internet:
http://www.maricopa.gov/medcenter/surgery/surg.html
Accred Length: 5 Years *Program Size:* 26 (*GY1:* 10)
Subspecialties: TY
Program ID: 440-03-22-025

Scottsdale

Mayo Graduate School of Medicine (Scottsdale) Program

Sponsor: Mayo Graduate School of Medicine-Mayo Foundation
Mayo Clinic (Scottsdale)
Scottsdale Healthcare-Shea

Program Director:
Keith A Kelly, MD
Dept of Surgery
Mayo Clinic Scottsdale
13400 E Shea Blvd
Scottsdale, AZ 85259
Tel: 602 301-8254 *Fax:* 602 301-8414
E-mail: mgsm.scot.az.surgery@mayo.edu
Internet: http://www.mayo.edu/
Accred Length: 5 Years *Program Size:* 16 (*GY1:* 4)
Subspecialties: TY
Program ID: 440-03-21-402

Tucson

University of Arizona Program

Sponsor: University of Arizona College of Medicine
Tucson Medical Center
University Medical Center
Veterans Affairs Medical Center (Tucson)

Program Director:
John B Fortune, MD
Univ of Arizona-AHSC
Dept of Surgery Residency
1501 N Campbell Ave/Rm 5335 PO Box 245058
Tucson, AZ 85724-5058
Tel: 520 626-7747 *Fax:* 520 626-2247
E-mail: kristyh@u.arizona.edu
Internet: http://www.surgery.arizona.edu/gsresident/
Accred Length: 5 Years *Program Size:* 34 (*GY1:* 8)
Subspecialties: TY, VS
Program ID: 440-03-21-027

Arkansas

Little Rock

University of Arkansas for Medical Sciences Program

Sponsor: University of Arkansas College of Medicine
Arkansas Children's Hospital
John L McClellan Memorial Veterans Hospital
University Hospital of Arkansas

Program Director:
Robert W Barnes, MD
Univ of Arkansas for Med Sciences
4301 W Markham St/Slot 520
Little Rock, AR 72205
Tel: 501 686-5610 *Fax:* 501 686-5696
Accred Length: 5 Years *Program Size:* 30 (*GY1:* 12)
Subspecialties: PDS, VS
Program ID: 440-04-21-029

California

Bakersfield

Kern Medical Center Program

Sponsor: Kern Medical Center

Program Director:
Jack H Bloch, MD
1830 Flower St
Bakersfield, CA 93305-4197
Tel: 805 326-2274 *Fax:* 805 326-2282
E-mail: alefor@ucsd.edu
Internet: http://bizweb.lightspeed.net/~kmcsurgery
Accred Length: 5 Years *Program Size:* 12 (*GY1:* 4)
Subspecialties: TY
Program ID: 440-05-31-030

Fresno

University of California (San Francisco)/Fresno Program

Sponsor: UCSF-Fresno Medical Education Program
University Medical Center
Valley Children's Hospital
Veterans Affairs Medical Center (Fresno)

Program Director:
Steven N Parks, MD
University Med Ctr
Department of Surgery
445 S Cedar Ave
Fresno, CA 93702-2998
Tel: 209 459-4490, ext 5196 *Fax:* 209 459-3719
E-mail: bgardner@chsnet.com
Internet: http://www.ucsfresno.edu
Accred Length: 5 Years *Program Size:* 15 (*GY1:* 3)
Program ID: 440-05-21-032

Loma Linda

Loma Linda University Program

Sponsor: Loma Linda University Medical Center
Jerry L Pettis Memorial Veterans Hospital
Kaiser Foundation Hospital (Fontana)
Riverside County Regional Medical Center
San Bernardino County Medical Center

Program Director:
Bryan Fandrich, MD
Loma Linda Univ Med Ctr
Dept of Surgery/Rm 21108 CP
11175 Campus
Loma Linda, CA 92354
Tel: 909 824-4289 *Fax:* 909 824-4872
Internet: http://www.llu.edu
Accred Length: 5 Years *Program Size:* 45 (*GY1:* 18)
Subspecialties: TY, VS
Program ID: 440-05-21-034

Los Angeles

Cedars-Sinai Medical Center Program

Sponsor: Cedars-Sinai Medical Center

Program Director:
Alan T Lefor, MD PhD
Cedars-Sinai Med Ctr
8700 Beverly Blvd/Ste 8215
Los Angeles, CA 90048
Tel: 310 855-5874 *Fax:* 310 967-0139
Internet: http://www.csmc.edu
Accred Length: 5 Years *Program Size:* 20 (*GY1:* 6)
Subspecialties: CCS
Program ID: 440-05-11-037

Charles R Drew University Program

Sponsor: Charles R Drew University of Medicine and Science
California Hospital Medical Center
LAC-King/Drew Medical Center
Long Beach Memorial Medical Center

Program Director:
Arthur W Fleming, MD
Martin Luther King Jr-Drew Med Ctr
12021 S Wilmington Ave
Ste 3015
Los Angeles, CA 90059
Tel: 310 668-4520 *Fax:* 310 635-2079
E-mail: afleming@dhs.co.la.ca.us
Accred Length: 5 Years *Program Size:* 38 (*GY1:* 12)
Program ID: 440-05-11-040

Southern California Kaiser Permanente Medical Care (Los Angeles) Program

Sponsor: Southern California Kaiser Permanente Medical Group
Kaiser Foundation Hospital (Los Angeles)
Los Angeles County-USC Medical Center

Program Director:
Theodore X O'Connell, MD
Kaiser Permanente Med Ctr
4747 Sunset Blvd/3rd Fl
Los Angeles, CA 90027
Tel: 323 783-4924 *Fax:* 323 783-8747
Accred Length: 5 Years *Program Size:* 21 (*GY1:* 6)
Program ID: 440-05-12-038

UCLA Medical Center Program

Sponsor: UCLA School of Medicine
Olive View-UCLA Medical Center
UCLA Medical Center
VA Greater Los Angeles Healthcare System

Program Director:
Darryl T Hiyama, MD MD
Dept of Surgery
UCLA Sch of Med
PO Box 951749
Los Angeles, CA 90095-1749
Tel: 310 825-6557 *Fax:* 310 206-7024
E-mail: gensurg@surgery.medsch.ucla.edu
Internet: http://www.surgery.medsch.ucla.edu
Accred Length: 5 Years *Program Size:* 48 (*GY1:* 12)
Subspecialties: VS
Program ID: 440-05-21-042

University of Southern California Program

Sponsor: Los Angeles County-USC Medical Center
USC University Hospital

Program Director:
Fred A Weaver, MD
1510 San Pablo St/Ste 514
Los Angeles, CA 90033-4612
Tel: 213 342-5925 *Fax:* 213 342-5872
E-mail: jbash@surgery.hsc.usc.edu
Internet: http://www.usc.edu/divisions/residency
Accred Length: 5 Years *Program Size:* 55 (*GY1:* 24)
Subspecialties: CCS
Program ID: 440-05-11-039

Oakland

University of California (Davis) East Bay Program

Sponsor: University of California (Davis) School of Medicine
Kaiser Permanente Medical Center (Oakland)
Alameda County Medical Center
Naval Hospital (Oakland)
Program Director:
Claude H Organ Jr, MD
Univ of California Davis-East Bay
1411 E 31st St
Oakland, CA 94602
Tel: 510 437-4089 *Fax:* 510 437-5017
Internet: http://www.ucdebsurgery.com
Accred Length: 5 Years *Program Size:* 43 (*GY1:* 12)
Program ID: 440-05-21-389

Orange

University of California (Irvine) Program

Sponsor: University of California (Irvine) Medical Center
Veterans Affairs Medical Center (Long Beach)
Program Director:
Russell A Williams, MD
Univ of California Irvine Med Ctr
Dept of Surgery
101 The City Dr
Orange, CA 92868
Tel: 714 456-7252 *Fax:* 714 456-8205
E-mail: rawillia@uci.edu
Internet: http://www.meded.uci.edu/~surgery/
Accred Length: 5 Years *Program Size:* 38 (*GY1:* 13)
Subspecialties: CCS
Program ID: 440-05-21-033

Pasadena

Huntington Memorial Hospital Program

Sponsor: Huntington Memorial Hospital
Cedars-Sinai Medical Center
Children's Hospital of Los Angeles
City of Hope National Medical Center
Program Director:
Steven C Stain, MD
Huntington Memorial Hospital
Med Educ Dept
100 W California Blvd
Pasadena, CA 91105
Tel: 626 397-5166 *Fax:* 626 397-5004
E-mail: mededu.hmh@schs.com
Internet: http://www.huntingtonhospital.com
Accred Length: 5 Years *Program Size:* 12 (*GY1:* 5)
Program ID: 440-05-11-047

Sacramento

University of California (Davis) Program

Sponsor: University of California (Davis) Medical Center
Kaiser Foundation Hospital (Sacramento)
Kaiser Foundation Hospital (South Sacramento)
Program Director:
Felix D Battistella, MD
Univ of California Davis Med Ctr
Surgery Housestaff Office
2315 Stockton Blvd/Rm 6309
Sacramento, CA 95817
Tel: 916 734-2724 *Fax:* 916 734-5633
E-mail: gensurg.residency@ucdmc.ucdavis.edu
Internet: http://web.ucdmc.ucdavis.edu/surgery/
Accred Length: 5 Years *Program Size:* 56 (*GY1:* 20)
Subspecialties: CCS
Program ID: 440-05-21-031

San Diego

Naval Medical Center (San Diego) Program

Sponsor: Naval Medical Center (San Diego)
Program Director:
Capt James H Carlisle, MD
Naval Med Ctr
Dept of Surgery
34800 Bob Wilson Dr
San Diego, CA 92134-5000
Tel: 619 532-7579 *Fax:* 619 532-7673
E-mail: jhcarlisle@nmcsd.med.navy.mil
Accred Length: 5 Years *Program Size:* 38 (*GY1:* 22)
Subspecialties: TY
Program ID: 440-05-12-013
US Armed Services Program

University of California (San Diego) Program

Sponsor: University of California (San Diego) Medical Center
Veterans Affairs Medical Center (San Diego)
Program Director:
David W Easter, MD
UCSD Med Ctr, Dept of Surgery
Box 34396 No 8402
San Diego, CA 92163-4396
Tel: 619 543-6890 *Fax:* 619 543-3763
E-mail: crunge@ucsd.edu
Internet: http://www.surgery.ucsd.edu
Accred Length: 5 Years *Program Size:* 39 (*GY1:* 13)
Subspecialties: CCS
Program ID: 440-05-21-048

San Francisco

University of California (San Francisco) Program

Sponsor: University of California (San Francisco) School of Medicine
Kaiser Permanente Medical Center (San Francisco)
Mount Zion Medical Center of the University of California
San Francisco General Hospital Medical Center
University of California (San Francisco) Medical Center
Veterans Affairs Medical Center (San Francisco)
Program Director:
Linda Reilly, MD
Univ of California San Francisco
Dept of Surgery 343-S
San Francisco, CA 94143-0470
Tel: 415 476-1239 *Fax:* 415 476-1734
E-mail: ahirano@surgery.ucsf.edu
Accred Length: 5 Years *Program Size:* 77 (*GY1:* 34)
Subspecialties: VS
Program ID: 440-05-21-052

Santa Barbara

Santa Barbara Cottage Hospital Program

Sponsor: Santa Barbara Cottage Hospital
Program Director:
Kenneth Waxman, MD
Santa Barbara Cottage Hospital
PO Box 689
Santa Barbara, CA 93102
Tel: 805 569-7316 *Fax:* 805 569-7317
E-mail: kwaxman@sbch.org
Internet: http://www.sbch.org
Accred Length: 5 Years *Program Size:* 14 (*GY1:* 6)
Program ID: 440-05-12-053

Stanford

Stanford University Program

Sponsor: Stanford University Hospital
Kaiser Permanente Medical Center (Santa Clara)
Santa Clara Valley Medical Center
Veterans Affairs Palo Alto Health Care System
Program Director:
J Augusto Bastidas, MD
Stanford Univ Med Ctr
Dept of Surgery
300 Pasteur Dr/Ste H3680
Stanford, CA 94305
Tel: 650 725-2181 *Fax:* 650 725-0791
Internet: http://www.med.stanford.edu/school/surgery
Accred Length: 5 Years *Program Size:* 53 (*GY1:* 23)
Subspecialties: VS
Program ID: 440-05-21-054

Stockton

San Joaquin General Hospital Program

Sponsor: San Joaquin General Hospital
St Joseph Hospital
Program Director:
Nathaniel M Matolo, MD
San Joaquin General Hospital
Dept of Surgery
PO Box 1020
Stockton, CA 95201-1020
Tel: 209 468-6600 *Fax:* 209 468-6136
E-mail: sjgh@softcom.net
Accred Length: 5 Years *Program Size:* 10 (*GY1:* 2)
Subspecialties: TY
Program ID: 440-05-12-055

Torrance

Los Angeles County-Harbor-UCLA Medical Center Program

Sponsor: Los Angeles County-Harbor-UCLA Medical Center
St Mary Medical Center
Program Director:
Rodney A White, MD
Harbor-UCLA Med Ctr
1000 W Carson St/Box 461
Torrance, CA 90509
Tel: 310 222-2700 *Fax:* 310 533-1841
Internet: http://hucla-surgery.org
Accred Length: 5 Years *Program Size:* 39 (*GY1:* 11)
Subspecialties: VS
Program ID: 440-05-21-056

Travis AFB

David Grant Medical Center Program

Sponsor: David Grant Medical Center
Program Director:
Lt Col David R Arbutina, MD
David Grant Med Ctr-60th MSGS/SGCQR
101 Bodin Cir
Travis AFB, CA 94535-1800
Tel: 707 423-5180 *Fax:* 707 423-7479
E-mail: david.arbutin@60mdg.travis.af.mil
Accred Length: 5 Years *Program Size:* 15 (*GY1:* 6)
Subspecialties: TY
Program ID: 440-05-31-001
US Armed Services Program

Colorado

Denver

Exempla St Joseph Hospital Program
Sponsor: Exempla St Joseph Hospital
Program Director:
Jeffrey R Clark, MD
Exempla St Joseph Hospital
Surgery Education
1835 Franklin St
Denver, CO 80218-1191
Tel: 303 837-7295 *Fax:* 303 866-8044
Accred Length: 5 Years *Program Size:* 29 (*GY1:* 12)
Program ID: 440-07-22-057

University of Colorado Program
Sponsor: University of Colorado Health Sciences Center
Denver Health and Hospitals
Veterans Affairs Medical Center (Denver)
Program Director:
C Edward Hartford, MD
Univ of Colorado Health Sciences Ctr
4200 E Ninth Ave
Campus Box C-302
Denver, CO 80262
Tel: 303 315-7448 *Fax:* 303 315-8098
E-mail: martha.george@uchsc.edu
Internet: http://uchsc.edu
Accred Length: 5 Years *Program Size:* 64 (*GY1:* 20)
Subspecialties: PDS
Program ID: 440-07-21-058

Connecticut

Farmington

University of Connecticut Program
Sponsor: University of Connecticut School of Medicine
Hartford Hospital
New Britain General Hospital
St Francis Hospital and Medical Center
Univ of Connecticut Health Center/John Dempsey Hospital
Program Director:
Joseph M Civetta, MD
Univ of Connecticut Sch of Med
Dept of Surgery
Farmington, CT 06030-3955
Tel: 860 679-3467 *Fax:* 860 679-1276
E-mail: reilly@nso.uchc.edu
Internet: http://www.resprog.uchc.edu/md
Accred Length: 5 Years *Program Size:* 47 (*GY1:* 21)
Subspecialties: CCS, VS
Program ID: 440-08-21-390

New Haven

Hospital of St Raphael Program
Sponsor: Hospital of St Raphael
Program Director:
Randolph B Reinhold, MD
Hospital of St Raphael, Dept of Surgery
Attn: Dana West, Residency Prog Coord
1450 Chapel St
New Haven, CT 06511
Tel: 203 789-3443 *Fax:* 203 867-5248
E-mail: danawest@aol.com
Internet: http://www.srhs.org
Accred Length: 5 Years *Program Size:* 24 (*GY1:* 8)
Subspecialties: TY
Program ID: 440-08-21-063

Yale-New Haven Medical Center Program
Sponsor: Yale-New Haven Hospital
Bridgeport Hospital
Veterans Affairs Medical Center (West Haven)
Program Director:
Ronald C Merrell, MD
Yale Univ Sch of Med
330 Cedar St
102 Farnam Memorial Bldg
New Haven, CT 06520-8062
Tel: 203 785-5479 *Fax:* 203 737-5209
E-mail: ronald.merrell@yale.edu
Internet: http://www.130.132.88.92/
Accred Length: 5 Years *Program Size:* 54 (*GY1:* 22)
Subspecialties: CCS, VS
Program ID: 440-08-21-064

Stamford

Stamford Hospital/Columbia University College of Physicians and Surgeons Program
Sponsor: Stamford Hospital
Program Director:
James E Barone, MD
Stamford Hospital
PO Box 9317
Stamford, CT 06904-9317
Tel: 203 325-7470 *Fax:* 203 325-7089
E-mail: drjbarone@stamhosp.chime.org
Internet: http://www.stamhealth.org/surgery/
Accred Length: 5 Years *Program Size:* 12 (*GY1:* 4)
Program ID: 440-08-21-364

Waterbury

St Mary's Hospital Program
Sponsor: St Mary's Hospital
Program Director:
Stanley J Dudrick, MD
St Mary's Hospital
56 Franklin St
Waterbury, CT 06706
Tel: 203 574-6314 *Fax:* 203 574-6089
E-mail: drdudric@smhosp.chime.org
Internet: http://www.smhosp.chime.org
Accred Length: 5 Years *Program Size:* 14 (*GY1:* 3)
Program ID: 440-08-31-065

Waterbury Hospital Health Center Program
Sponsor: Waterbury Hospital Health Center
Yale-New Haven Hospital
Program Director:
Edward M Kwasnik, MD
Waterbury Hospital Health Ctr
64 Robbins St
Waterbury, CT 06721
Tel: 203 573-7257 *Fax:* 203 573-6073
E-mail: ekwasnik@wtbyhosp.chime.org
Internet: http://katnet.com/whhc
Accred Length: 5 Years *Program Size:* 12 (*GY1:* 4)
Program ID: 440-08-11-066

Delaware

Wilmington

Christiana Care Health Services Program
Sponsor: Christiana Care Health Services Inc
Program Director:
Dennis J Hoelzer, MD
Christiana Care Health System
Dept of Surgery/Ste 129
4745 Ogletown-Stanton Rd
Newark, DE 19713
Tel: 302 733-4500 *Fax:* 302 733-4505
E-mail: hoelzer.d@christianacare.org
Internet: http://www.mcd.gen.de.us/residency/surgery
Accred Length: 5 Years *Program Size:* 23 (*GY1:* 7)
Program ID: 440-09-11-067

District of Columbia

Washington

George Washington University Program
Sponsor: George Washington University School of Medicine
George Washington University Hospital (UHS)
Program Director:
Paul P Lin, MD
Dept of Surgery
2150 Pennsylvania Ave NW
Washington, DC 20037
Tel: 202 994-5573 *Fax:* 202 994-0567
E-mail: sursab@gwumc.edu
Accred Length: 5 Years *Program Size:* 36 (*GY1:* 13)
Program ID: 440-10-21-069

Georgetown University Program
Sponsor: Georgetown University Medical Center
Arlington Hospital
District of Columbia General Hospital
Fairfax Hospital
Veterans Affairs Medical Center (Washington, DC)
Program Director:
James V Sitzmann, MD
Georgetown Univ Hospital
Office of Education 4PHC
3800 Reservoir Rd NW
Washington, DC 20007
Tel: 202 687-1233 *Fax:* 202 687-4287
Accred Length: 5 Years *Program Size:* 44 (*GY1:* 15)
Program ID: 440-10-21-068

Howard University Program
Sponsor: Howard University Hospital
District of Columbia General Hospital
Greater Southeast Community Hospital
Providence Hospital
Program Director:
Haile M Mezghebe, MD
Dept of Surgery 4B02
Howard Univ Hospital
2041 Georgia Ave NW
Washington, DC 20060
Tel: 202 865-1446 *Fax:* 202 865-5396
Accred Length: 5 Years *Program Size:* 36 (*GY1:* 9)
Subspecialties: TY
Program ID: 440-10-21-070

Walter Reed Army Medical Center Program

Sponsor: Walter Reed Army Medical Center

Program Director:
Lt Col Craig D Shriver, MD
Rm 5C27A Heaton Pavilion
Dept of the Army
Washington, DC 20307-5001
Tel: 202 782-9697 *Fax:* 202 782-0759
E-mail: shriver@home.com
Accred Length: 5 Years *Program Size:* 21 (*GY1:* 5)
Subspecialties: TY, VS
Program ID: 440-10-11-007
US Armed Services Program

Washington Hospital Center Program

Sponsor: Washington Hospital Center

Program Director:
John R Kirkpatrick, MD
Washington Hospital Ctr
110 Irving St NW
Ste NAG-253
Washington, DC 20010-2975
Tel: 202 877-3536 *Fax:* 202 877-3699
Accred Length: 5 Years *Program Size:* 41 (*GY1:* 16)
Subspecialties: CCS
Program ID: 440-10-31-071

Florida

Gainesville

University of Florida Program

Sponsor: University of Florida College of Medicine
Shands Hospital at the University of Florida
Veterans Affairs Medical Center (Gainesville)
Veterans Affairs Medical Center (Lake City)

Program Director:
Timothy C Flynn, MD
Univ of Florida
Dept of Surgery
Box 100287
Gainesville, FL 32610-0287
Tel: 352 395-7973, ext 53634 *Fax:* 352 338-9809
E-mail: dot@surgery.ufl.edu
Internet: http://www.surgery.ufl.edu
Accred Length: 5 Years *Program Size:* 39 (*GY1:* 18)
Subspecialties: VS
Program ID: 440-11-21-072

Jacksonville

Mayo Graduate School of Medicine (Jacksonville) Program

Sponsor: Mayo Graduate School of Medicine-Mayo Foundation
Mayo Clinic (Jacksonville)
Orlando Regional Medical Center
St Luke's Hospital

Program Director:
Ronald A Hinder, MD
4500 San Pablo Rd
Jacksonville, FL 32224
Tel: 904 953-2000 *Fax:* 904 953-2432
Accred Length: 5 Years *Program Size:* 11 (*GY1:* 3)
Program ID: 440-11-21-405

University of Florida Health Science Center/Jacksonville Program

Sponsor: University of Florida College of Medicine at Jacksonville
University Medical Center (UFHSC/J)

Program Director:
Joseph J Tepas III, MD
Univ of Florida Health Science Ctr-Jacksonville
655 W 8th St
Jacksonville, FL 32209
Tel: 904 549-3903 *Fax:* 904 549-3870
Internet: http://www.ufhscj.edu
Accred Length: 5 Years *Program Size:* 26 (*GY1:* 7)
Program ID: 440-11-21-073

Miami

University of Miami-Jackson Memorial Medical Center Program

Sponsor: University of Miami-Jackson Memorial Medical Center
Veterans Affairs Medical Center (Miami)

Program Director:
Duane G Hutson, MD
Univ of Miami-Jackson Memorial Med Ctr
Dept of Surgery (Attn: Maria Elias)
PO Box 016310
Miami, FL 33101
Tel: 305 585-1280 *Fax:* 305 324-9779
Accred Length: 5 Years *Program Size:* 53 (*GY1:* 24)
Subspecialties: CCS
Program ID: 440-11-21-074

Miami Beach

Mount Sinai Medical Center of Greater Miami Program

Sponsor: Mount Sinai Medical Center of Greater Miami
Memorial Regional Hospital
University of Miami-Jackson Memorial Medical Center

Program Director:
Manuel Sivina, MD
Mount Sinai Med Ctr of Greater Miami
Dept of General Surgery
4300 Alton Rd/Ste #212-A
Miami Beach, FL 33140
Tel: 305 674-2760 *Fax:* 305 674-2769
Internet: http://www.mountsinaimiami.org
Accred Length: 5 Years *Program Size:* 17 (*GY1:* 6)
Program ID: 440-11-22-075

Orlando

Orlando Regional Healthcare System Program

Sponsor: Orlando Regional Medical Center

Program Director:
Mark L Friedell, MD
Orlando Regional Med Ctr
86 W Underwood St/Ste 201
Orlando, FL 32806
Tel: 407 841-5142 *Fax:* 407 648-3686
E-mail: markf@orhs.org
Internet: http://www.orhs-surged.org
Accred Length: 5 Years *Program Size:* 13 (*GY1:* 5)
Program ID: 440-11-11-076

Tampa

University of South Florida Program

Sponsor: University of South Florida College of Medicine
H Lee Moffitt Cancer Center
James A Haley Veterans Hospital
Tampa General Healthcare
Veterans Affairs Medical Center (Bay Pines)

Program Director:
Larry C Carey, MD
Dept of Surgery
Univ of South Florida
12901 Bruce B Downs Blvd/Box 16
Tampa, FL 33612-4799
Tel: 813 974-6159 *Fax:* 813 974-8106
Accred Length: 5 Years *Program Size:* 29 (*GY1:* 6)
Subspecialties: VS
Program ID: 440-11-31-078

Georgia

Atlanta

Emory University Program

Sponsor: Emory University School of Medicine
Crawford Long Hospital of Emory University
Emory University Hospital
Grady Memorial Hospital
Piedmont Hospital
Veterans Affairs Medical Center (Atlanta)

Program Director:
Thomas F Dodson, MD
Emory Univ
H120 Emory Univ Hospital
1364 Clifton Rd NE
Atlanta, GA 30322
Tel: 404 727-0093 *Fax:* 404 727-3316
E-mail: lynda_watts@emory.org
Accred Length: 5 Years *Program Size:* 48 (*GY1:* 12)
Subspecialties: VS
Program ID: 440-12-21-079

Georgia Baptist Medical Center Program

Sponsor: Georgia Baptist Medical Center

Program Director:
John T Promes, MD
Georgia Baptist Med Ctr, Dept of Med Educ
303 Parkway Dr NE
Box 423
Atlanta, GA 30312
Tel: 404 265-4411 *Fax:* 404 265-4989
Accred Length: 5 Years *Program Size:* 17 (*GY1:* 6)
Subspecialties: TY, VS
Program ID: 440-12-22-080

Morehouse School of Medicine Program

Sponsor: Morehouse School of Medicine
Grady Memorial Hospital

Program Director:
William L Weaver, MD
Morehouse Sch of Med
720 Westview Dr SW
Atlanta, GA 30310-1495
Tel: 404 616-3562 *Fax:* 404 616-3091
Accred Length: 5 Years *Program Size:* 22 (*GY1:* 8)
Program ID: 440-12-21-397

Augusta

Medical College of Georgia Program

Sponsor: Medical College of Georgia Hospital and Clinics
University Hospital
Veterans Affairs Medical Center (Augusta)

Program Director:
Thomas R Gadacz, MD
Med Coll of Georgia
Dept of Surgery/BIW 446
1120 15th St
Augusta, GA 30912-4000
Tel: 706 721-2503 *Fax:* 706 721-6828
Accred Length: 5 Years *Program Size:* 25 (*GY1:* 5)
Program ID: 440-12-31-082

Fort Gordon

Dwight David Eisenhower Army Medical Center Program

Sponsor: Dwight David Eisenhower Army Medical Center

Program Director:
Lt Col James H North Jr, MD
Eisenhower Army Med Ctr
General Surgery Service
Bldg 300
Fort Gordon, GA 30905-5650
Tel: 706 787-2567 *Fax:* 706 787-2347
E-mail: jnorthjr@pol.net
Internet:
http://www.ddeamc.amedd.army.mil/gmep/general.htm
Accred Length: 5 Years *Program Size:* 18 (*GY1:* 6)
Subspecialties: TY
Program ID: 440-12-21-365
US Armed Services Program

Macon

Mercer University School of Medicine Program

Sponsor: Medical Center of Central Georgia

Program Director:
Martin L Dalton, MD
Med Ctr of Central Georgia
777 Hemlock St
PO Box 6000
Macon, GA 31208
Tel: 912 633-1367 *Fax:* 912 633-5153
E-mail: bedgood.sheryl@mccg.org
Internet: http://gain.mercer.edu/musm
Accred Length: 5 Years *Program Size:* 12 (*GY1:* 4)
Subspecialties: TY
Program ID: 440-12-21-083

Savannah

Memorial Medical Center Program

Sponsor: Memorial Medical Center

Program Director:
Carl R Boyd, MD
Memorial Med Ctr
Surgical Education
PO Box 22084
Savannah, GA 31403-2084
Tel: 912 350-8598 *Fax:* 912 350-5984
Accred Length: 5 Years *Program Size:* 13 (*GY1:* 5)
Program ID: 440-12-31-084

Hawaii

Honolulu

Tripler Army Medical Center Program

Sponsor: Tripler Army Medical Center

Program Director:
Paul R Cordts, MD
Tripler Army Med Ctr
CDR TAMC, MCHK-DSG
1 Jarrett White Rd
Honolulu, HI 96859-5000
Tel: 808 433-3435 *Fax:* 808 433-6539
E-mail: cordtsp@chcs.tamc.amedd.army.mil
Internet: http://www.tamc.amedd.army.mil
Accred Length: 5 Years *Program Size:* 19 (*GY1:* 8)
Program ID: 440-14-12-008
US Armed Services Program

University of Hawaii Program

Sponsor: University of Hawaii John A Burns School of Medicine
Kaiser Foundation Hospital (Moanalua)
Kuakini Medical Center
Queen's Medical Center
St Francis Medical Center
Straub Clinic and Hospital

Program Director:
George O McPheeters, MD
Univ of Hawaii
Surgical Program
1356 Lusitana St/6th Fl
Honolulu, HI 96813
Tel: 808 586-2920 *Fax:* 808 536-1140
E-mail: owenss@jabsom.biomed.hawaii.edu
Internet: http://www.careermd.com/profiles/suhi001.htm
Accred Length: 5 Years *Program Size:* 28 (*GY1:* 12)
Subspecialties: CCS, TY
Program ID: 440-14-21-085

Illinois

Chicago

Catholic Health Partners Program

Sponsor: Catholic Health Partners

Program Director:
Mark M Connolly, MD
Columbus Hospital-St Joseph Hospital
Dept of Surgery
2900 N Lake Shore Dr
Chicago, IL 60657
Tel: 773 665-6237 *Fax:* 773 665-6232
Internet: http://www.cath-health.org
Accred Length: 5 Years *Program Size:* 8 (*GY1:* 4)
Subspecialties: TY
Program ID: 440-16-31-086

McGaw Medical Center of Northwestern University Program

Sponsor: Northwestern University Medical School
Evanston Hospital
Northwestern Memorial Hospital
Veterans Affairs Lakeside Medical Center (Chicago)

Program Director:
Raymond J Joehl, MD
Northwestern Univ Med Sch
250 E Superior
Wesley 201
Chicago, IL 60611-2950
Tel: 312 908-2016 *Fax:* 312 908-7404
Internet: http://www.numf.nwu.edu/gme/index.htm
Accred Length: 5 Years *Program Size:* 57 (*GY1:* 30)
Subspecialties: VS
Program ID: 440-16-21-091

Rush-Presbyterian-St Luke's Medical Center Program

Sponsor: Rush-Presbyterian-St Luke's Medical Center
Cook County Hospital

Program Director:
Richard A Prinz, MD
Rush-Presbyterian-St Luke's Med Ctr
1653 W Congress Pkwy
Chicago, IL 60612
Tel: 312 942-6379 *Fax:* 312 942-2867
Internet: http://www.rush.edu
Accred Length: 5 Years *Program Size:* 55 (*GY1:* 21)
Subspecialties: TY, VS
Program ID: 440-16-21-092

University of Chicago Program

Sponsor: University of Chicago Hospitals
Cook County Hospital
Louis A Weiss Memorial Hospital

Program Director:
Fabrizio Michelassi, MD
Univ of Chicago Hospitals
5841 S Maryland Ave/MC 5093
Chicago, IL 60637-1470
Tel: 773 202-6337 *Fax:* 773 702-5909
E-mail: clubert@surgery.bsd.uchicago.edu
Internet: http://www.surgery.bsd.uchicago.edu
Accred Length: 5 Years *Program Size:* 29 (*GY1:* 6)
Subspecialties: TY, VS
Program ID: 440-16-11-094

University of Illinois College of Medicine at Chicago Metropolitan Group Hospitals Program

Sponsor: University of Illinois College of Medicine at Chicago
Illinois Masonic Medical Center
Lutheran General Hospital
Mercy Hospital and Medical Center
St Francis Hospital of Evanston

Program Director:
Joseph F Giannola, MD
Metropolitan Group Hospitals
836 W Wellington Ave/Rm 4813
Chicago, IL 60657-5193
Tel: 773 296-7093 *Fax:* 773 296-5570
Accred Length: 5 Years *Program Size:* 40 (*GY1:* 11)
Subspecialties: CCS, TY
Program ID: 440-16-31-096

University of Illinois College of Medicine at Chicago Program

Sponsor: University of Illinois College of Medicine at Chicago
Christ Hospital and Medical Center
Michael Reese Hospital and Medical Center
University of Illinois Hospital and Clinics
Veterans Affairs West Side Medical Center

Program Director:
Charles L Rice, MD
Univ of Illinois-Chicago
Dept of Surgery (M/C 958)
840 S Wood St/Ste 518-E CSB
Chicago, IL 60612-7322
Tel: 312 996-6765 *Fax:* 312 996-1214
Internet: http://www.uic.edu/com/surgery/_private/
Accred Length: 5 Years *Program Size:* 35 (*GY1:* 7)
Program ID: 440-16-21-395

Maywood

Loyola University Program
Sponsor: Loyola University Medical Center
Edward J Hines Jr Veterans Affairs Hospital
Resurrection Medical Center
Program Director:
Richard L Gamelli, MD
Loyola Univ Med Ctr
Dept of Surgery
2160 S First Ave
Maywood, IL 60153
Tel: 708 327-2690 *Fax:* 708 327-2698
E-mail: surg-res@lumc.edu
Internet: http://www.lumc.edu
Accred Length: 5 Years *Program Size:* 53 (*GY1:* 22)
Subspecialties: TY, VS
Program ID: 440-16-21-099

North Chicago

Finch University of Health Sciences/Chicago Medical School Program
Sponsor: Finch University of Health Sciences/Chicago Medical School
Mount Sinai Hospital Medical Center of Chicago
Swedish Covenant Hospital
Program Director:
Michael J Zdon, MD
Finch Univ of Health Sciences-Chicago Med Sch
Dept of Surgery
California Ave at 15th St
Chicago, IL 60608
Tel: 773 257-4752 *Fax:* 773 257-6548
Internet: http://www.finchcms.edu/
Accred Length: 5 Years *Program Size:* 24 (*GY1:* 6)
Subspecialties: TY
Program ID: 440-16-21-385

Peoria

University of Illinois College of Medicine at Peoria Program
Sponsor: University of Illinois College of Medicine at Peoria
St Francis Medical Center
Program Director:
Norman C Estes, MD
Univ of Illinois Coll of Med
Dept of Surgery
420 NE Glen Oak Ave/Ste 302
Peoria, IL 61603
Tel: 309 655-3971 *Fax:* 309 655-3630
Internet: http://www.uicomp.uic.edu
Accred Length: 5 Years *Program Size:* 16 (*GY1:* 4)
Program ID: 440-16-21-101

Springfield

Southern Illinois University Program
Sponsor: Southern Illinois University School of Medicine
Memorial Medical Center
St John's Hospital
Program Director:
Gary L Dunnington, MD
Southern Illinois Univ Sch of Med
800 N Rutledge/PO Box 19230
Springfield, IL 62794-1312
Tel: 217 524-4401 *Fax:* 217 524-8827
E-mail: bcarter@siumed.edu
Accred Length: 5 Years *Program Size:* 10 (*GY1:* 2)
Subspecialties: VS
Program ID: 440-16-21-102

Indiana

Indianapolis

Indiana University School of Medicine (Methodist) Program
Sponsor: Indiana University School of Medicine
Clarian Methodist Hospital of Indiana
Program Director:
Jay L Grosfeld Sr, MD
Indiana Univ Sch of Med, Surgery Program
545 Barnhill Dr
Emerson Hall/Rm 202
Indianapolis, IN 46202-5125
Tel: 317 274-7262
Accred Length: 5 Years *Program Size:* 29 (*GY1:* 23)
Subspecialties: TY
Program ID: 440-17-11-104

Indiana University School of Medicine Program
Sponsor: Indiana University School of Medicine
Clarian IU Hospital
Clarian Riley Hospital for Children
Richard L Roudebush Veterans Affairs Medical Center
William N Wishard Memorial Hospital
Program Director:
Jay L Grosfeld, MD
Indiana Univ Med Ctr
545 Barnhill Dr
Emerson Hall/Rm 202
Indianapolis, IN 46202-5125
Tel: 317 274-7262 *Fax:* 317 274-8769
E-mail: sdrye@iupui.edu
Internet: http://scalpel.med.iupui.edu
Accred Length: 5 Years *Program Size:* 69 (*GY1:* 23)
Program ID: 440-17-21-103

Iowa

Des Moines

Iowa Methodist Medical Center Program
Sponsor: Iowa Methodist Medical Center
Broadlawns Medical Center
Veterans Affairs Central Iowa Health Care System
Program Director:
Donald W Moorman, MD
Iowa Methodist Med Ctr
Dept of Surgery Educ
1221 Pleasant St/Ste 550
Des Moines, IA 50309-1453
Tel: 515 241-4076 *Fax:* 515 241-4080
E-mail: langstmr@ihs.org
Internet: http://www.ihsdesmoines.org
Accred Length: 5 Years *Program Size:* 19 (*GY1:* 7)
Subspecialties: TY
Program ID: 440-18-22-105

Iowa City

University of Iowa Hospitals and Clinics Program
Sponsor: University of Iowa Hospitals and Clinics
Veterans Affairs Medical Center (Iowa City)
Program Director:
Siroos S Shirazi, MD
Univ of Iowa Hospitals and Clinics
Dept of Surgery
200 Hawkins Dr/#1516 JCP
Iowa City, IA 52242-1086
Tel: 319 353-6425 *Fax:* 319 356-3762
E-mail: sshirazi@surgery.uiowa.edu
Internet: http://www.surgery.uiowa.edu
Accred Length: 5 Years *Program Size:* 34 (*GY1:* 10)
Subspecialties: VS
Program ID: 440-18-21-107

Kansas

Kansas City

University of Kansas Medical Center Program
Sponsor: University of Kansas School of Medicine
Dwight D Eisenhower Veterans Affairs Medical Center
University of Kansas Medical Center
Veterans Affairs Medical Center (Kansas City)
Program Director:
Romano Delcore, MD
Univ of Kansas Med Ctr
3901 Rainbow Blvd
Rm 4945 Murphy Bldg
Kansas City, KS 66160-7309
Tel: 913 588-6124 *Fax:* 913 588-7540
E-mail: gensurgresidency@kumc.edu
Internet: http://www2.edu/surgery/
Accred Length: 5 Years *Program Size:* 34 (*GY1:* 12)
Subspecialties: VS
Program ID: 440-19-21-108

Wichita

University of Kansas (Wichita) Program
Sponsor: University of Kansas School of Medicine (Wichita)
Columbia Wesley Medical Center
Via Christi Regional Medical Center
Program Director:
R Larry Beamer, MD
Dept of Surgery
929 N St Francis
Rm 3082
Wichita, KS 67214-3882
Tel: 316 268-5990 *Fax:* 316 291-7662
E-mail: brunyan@kumc.edu
Internet: http://www.kumc.edu/wichita/dept/surgery
Accred Length: 5 Years *Program Size:* 30 (*GY1:* 6)
Program ID: 440-19-21-387

Kentucky

Lexington

University of Kentucky Medical Center Program

Sponsor: University of Kentucky Hospital
Veterans Affairs Medical Center (Lexington)

Program Director:
Eric D Endean, MD
Rm C 224/Dept of General Surgery
800 Rose St
Lexington, KY 40536-0084
Tel: 606 323-6346 *Fax:* 606 323-6840
E-mail: edende0@pop.uky.edu
Accred Length: 5 Years *Program Size:* 41 (*GY1:* 18)
Subspecialties: VS
Program ID: 440-20-21-112

Louisville

University of Louisville Program

Sponsor: University of Louisville School of Medicine
Kosair Children's Hospital (Alliant Health System)
Norton Hospital (Alliant Health System)
University of Louisville Hospital
Veterans Affairs Medical Center (Louisville)

Program Director:
Hiram C Polk Jr, MD
Univ of Louisville Sch of Med
Dept of Surgery
Louisville, KY 40292
Tel: 502 852-6191 *Fax:* 502 852-8915
E-mail: anjone01@ulkyvm.louisville.edu
Internet: http://www.louisvillesurgery.com
Accred Length: 5 Years *Program Size:* 49 (*GY1:* 16)
Subspecialties: CCS, HSS
Program ID: 440-20-21-113

Louisiana

New Orleans

Alton Ochsner Medical Foundation Program

Sponsor: Alton Ochsner Medical Foundation
Leonard J Chabert Medical Center

Program Director:
George M Fuhrman, MD
Alton Ochsner Med Foundation
Dept of General Surgery
1516 Jefferson Hwy
New Orleans, LA 70121
Tel: 504 842-4620 *Fax:* 504 842-3100
E-mail: agoldman@ochsner.org
Internet: http://www.ochsner.org
Accred Length: 5 Years *Program Size:* 28 (*GY1:* 9)
Subspecialties: VS
Program ID: 440-21-22-115

Louisiana State University Program

Sponsor: Louisiana State University School of Medicine
Earl K Long Medical Center
Medical Center of Louisiana at New Orleans
University Medical Center (Lafayette)
Veterans Affairs Medical Center-LSU Service (New Orleans)

Program Director:
J Patrick O'Leary, MD
Louisiana State Univ Med Ctr, Dept of Surgery
1542 Tulane Ave
New Orleans, LA 70112-2822
Tel: 504 568-4750 *Fax:* 504 568-4633
E-mail: lcapot@lsumc.edu
Internet: http://www.lsumc.edu
Accred Length: 5 Years *Program Size:* 63 (*GY1:* 21)
Subspecialties: VS
Program ID: 440-21-21-114

Tulane University Program

Sponsor: Tulane University School of Medicine
Huey P Long Regional Medical Center
Medical Center of Louisiana at New Orleans
Touro Infirmary
Tulane University Hospital and Clinics

Program Director:
Lewis M Flint, MD
Tulane Univ Sch of Med
Dept of Surgery
1430 Tulane Ave
New Orleans, LA 70112-2699
Tel: 504 584-1982 *Fax:* 504 584-1838
E-mail: lflint@tmcpop.tmc.tulane.edu
Internet:
http://www.mcl.tulane.edu/departments/surgery dept:surg..htm
Accred Length: 5 Years *Program Size:* 52 (*GY1:* 21)
Subspecialties: CCS
Program ID: 440-21-21-116

Shreveport

Louisiana State University (Shreveport) Program

Sponsor: Louisiana State University Hospital-Shreveport
E A Conway Medical Center
Overton Brooks Veterans Affairs Medical Center

Program Director:
John C McDonald, MD
Louisiana State Univ Med Ctr Hospital
Med Educ/Surgery
1501 Kings Hwy/PO Box 33932
Shreveport, LA 71130-3932
Tel: 318 675-6100 *Fax:* 318 675-6141
E-mail: jmcdon@lsumc.edu
Internet: http://www.surgery.lsumc.edu
Accred Length: 5 Years *Program Size:* 31 (*GY1:* 5)
Program ID: 440-21-21-117

Maine

Portland

Maine Medical Center Program

Sponsor: Maine Medical Center

Program Director:
Albert W Dibbins, MD
Maine Med Ctr
22 Bramhall St
Portland, ME 04102-3175
Tel: 207 871-2515 *Fax:* 207 871-6389
E-mail: trembjm@mail.mmc.org
Internet: http://www.mmc.org/surgical/residency
Accred Length: 5 Years *Program Size:* 17 (*GY1:* 4)
Program ID: 440-22-21-119

Maryland

Baltimore

Johns Hopkins University Program

Sponsor: Johns Hopkins University School of Medicine
Johns Hopkins Bayview Medical Center
Johns Hopkins Hospital
Sinai Hospital of Baltimore

Program Director:
John L Cameron, MD
Johns Hopkins Univ Sch of Med
720 Rutland Ave
759 Ross Bldg
Baltimore, MD 21205
Tel: 410 955-5166 *Fax:* 410 955-0834
Accred Length: 5 Years *Program Size:* 77 (*GY1:* 27)
Subspecialties: CCS
Program ID: 440-23-21-392

St Agnes HealthCare Program

Sponsor: St Agnes Hospital

Program Director:
Michael A Zatina, MD
St Agnes HealthCare
Dept of Surgery
900 Caton Ave
Baltimore, MD 21229-5299
Tel: 410 368-2718 *Fax:* 410 368-3569
Internet: http://www.stagnes.org
Accred Length: 5 Years *Program Size:* 19 (*GY1:* 6)
Program ID: 440-23-22-123

Union Memorial Hospital Program

Sponsor: Union Memorial Hospital
Franklin Square Hospital Center

Program Director:
James C A Fuchs, MD
Union Memorial Hospital
201 E University Pkwy
Baltimore, MD 21218-2895
Tel: 410 554-2290 *Fax:* 410 554-2378
Accred Length: 5 Years *Program Size:* 20 (*GY1:* 8)
Subspecialties: HSS, TY
Program ID: 440-23-21-127

University of Maryland Program

Sponsor: University of Maryland Medical System
Mercy Medical Center

Program Director:
Barbara L Bass, MD
Univ of Maryland Med System
Dept of Surgery
22 S Greene St
Baltimore, MD 21201
Tel: 410 328-6442 *Fax:* 410 328-4084
E-mail: jhall@surgery1.ab.umd.edu
Internet: http://som1.ab.umd.edu/surgery/surgery.html
Accred Length: 5 Years *Program Size:* 45 (*GY1:* 18)
Subspecialties: CCS, VS
Program ID: 440-23-21-128

Bethesda

National Naval Medical Center (Bethesda) Program

Sponsor: National Naval Medical Center (Bethesda)

Program Director:
John W DeNobile, MD
Dept of General Surgery
8901 Wisconsin Ave
Bethesda, MD 20889-5600
Tel: 301 295-4435 *Fax:* 301 295-0959
Accred Length: 5 Years *Program Size:* 28 (*GY1:* 16)
Subspecialties: TY
Program ID: 440-23-21-014
US Armed Services Program

Massachusetts

Boston

Beth Israel Deaconess Medical Center (East Campus) Program

Sponsor: Beth Israel Deaconess Medical Center
MetroWest Medical Center-Framingham Union Hospital

Program Director:
Michael D Stone, MD
Beth Israel Deaconess Med Ctr
Surgical Education/Ste 2A
110 Francis St
Boston, MA 02215
Tel: 617 632-9236 *Fax:* 617 632-0064
E-mail: surgedu@west.bidmc.harvard.edu
Internet: http://www.bidmc.harvard.edu
Accred Length: 5 Years *Program Size:* 71 (*GY1:* 22)
Program ID: 440-24-11-130

Beth Israel Deaconess Medical Center (West Campus) Program

Sponsor: Beth Israel Deaconess Medical Center
Cambridge Hospital/Cambridge Health Alliance
Mount Auburn Hospital

Program Director:
Michael D Stone, MD
Beth Israel Deaconess Med Ctr.
Surgical Education Office
110 Francis St/Ste 2A
Boston, MA 02215
Tel: 617 632-9236 *Fax:* 617 632-0064
E-mail: surgedu@west.bidmc.harvard.edu
Internet: http://www.bidmc.harvard.edu
Accred Length: 5 Years *Program Size:* 71 (*GY1:* 22)
Subspecialties: CCS, VS
Program ID: 440-24-21-133

Boston University Medical Center Program

Sponsor: Boston Medical Center
Veterans Affairs Medical Center (Boston)

Program Director:
James M Becker, MD
Boston Univ Surgical Program
Boston Med Ctr
E Newton Campus/Rm C515
Boston, MA 02118-2393
Tel: 617 638-8442 *Fax:* 617 638-8409
E-mail: jennifer.konda@bmc.org
Internet: http://med-www.bu.edu/gensurgery/
Accred Length: 5 Years *Program Size:* 43 (*GY1:* 21)
Subspecialties: CCS, VS
Program ID: 440-24-21-131

Brigham and Women's Hospital Program

Sponsor: Brigham and Women's Hospital
Brockton-West Roxbury Veterans Affairs Medical Center

Program Director:
Michael Belkin, MD
Brigham and Women's Hospital
Carrie Hall Ste CA254
75 Francis St
Boston, MA 02115
Tel: 617 732-6861 *Fax:* 617 264-6850
E-mail: surgery@bics.bwh.harvard.edu
Internet: http://www.bwh.partners.org/surged
Accred Length: 5 Years *Program Size:* 38 (*GY1:* 12)
Subspecialties: TY, VS
Program ID: 440-24-21-135

Massachusetts General Hospital Program

Sponsor: Massachusetts General Hospital

Program Director:
Charles M Ferguson, MD
Massachusetts General Hospital
Surgical Program/GRB 418
Fruit St
Boston, MA 02114
Tel: 617 726-2800 *Fax:* 617 724-3499
Accred Length: 5 Years *Program Size:* 56 (*GY1:* 18)
Subspecialties: CCS, VS
Program ID: 440-24-31-132

New England Medical Center Hospitals Program

Sponsor: New England Medical Center Hospitals
Faulkner Hospital
Newton-Wellesley Hospital

Program Director:
William C Mackey, MD
New England Med Ctr
750 Washington St/Box 437
Boston, MA 02111
Tel: 617 636-5891 *Fax:* 617 636-5498
E-mail: eileen.donovan@es.nemc.org
Accred Length: 5 Years *Program Size:* 24 (*GY1:* 11)
Subspecialties: VS
Program ID: 440-24-21-134

St Elizabeth's Medical Center of Boston Program

Sponsor: St Elizabeth's Medical Center of Boston
Cardinal Cushing General Hospital

Program Director:
James G Petros, MD
St Elizabeth's Med Ctr
736 Cambridge St
Boston, MA 02135-2997
Tel: 617 789-2990 *Fax:* 617 789-3419
E-mail: colon@shore.net
Internet: http://www.semc.org.
Accred Length: 5 Years *Program Size:* 20 (*GY1:* 8)
Program ID: 440-24-21-136

Burlington

Lahey Clinic Program

Sponsor: Lahey Clinic

Program Director:
Desmond H Birkett, MD
Lahey Clinic Med Ctr
Dept of General Surgery
41 Mall Rd
Burlington, MA 01805
Tel: 781 744-8585 *Fax:* 781 744-5636
E-mail: jenni.r.johnston@lahey.org
Accred Length: 5 Years *Program Size:* 15 (*GY1:* 4)
Program ID: 440-24-21-401

Pittsfield

Berkshire Medical Center Program

Sponsor: Berkshire Medical Center

Program Director:
Parvis J Sadighi, MD
Dept of Surgery
Berkshire Med Ctr
725 North St
Pittsfield, MA 01201
Tel: 413 447-2741 *Fax:* 413 447-2766
Accred Length: 5 Years *Program Size:* 13 (*GY1:* 5)
Program ID: 440-24-31-137

Springfield

Baystate Medical Center Program

Sponsor: Baystate Medical Center

Program Director:
Richard B Wait, MD PhD
Baystate Med Ctr
Dept of Surgery
759 Chestnut St
Springfield, MA 01199
Tel: 413 784-5161 *Fax:* 413 784-5940
Accred Length: 5 Years *Program Size:* 28 (*GY1:* 9)
Program ID: 440-24-11-138

Worcester

University of Massachusetts Program

Sponsor: University of Massachusetts Medical School
St Vincent Hospital
UMass Memorial Health Care (Memorial Campus)
UMass Memorial Health Care (University Campus)

Program Director:
Wayne E Silva, MD
Univ of Massachusetts Med Sch
Dept of Surgery
55 Lake Ave N
Worcester, MA 01655-0117
Tel: 508 856-3744 *Fax:* 508 856-5662
Accred Length: 5 Years *Program Size:* 46 (*GY1:* 16)
Subspecialties: CCS, VS
Program ID: 440-24-21-139

Michigan

Ann Arbor

St Joseph Mercy Hospital Program

Sponsor: St Joseph Mercy Health System

Program Director:
Verne L Hoshal Jr, MD
St Joseph Mercy Hospital
PO Box 995-RHB 2115
Ann Arbor, MI 48106-0995
Tel: 734 712-7352 *Fax:* 734 712-2809
Accred Length: 5 Years *Program Size:* 17 (*GY1:* 5)
Subspecialties: TY
Program ID: 440-25-11-140

University of Michigan Program

Sponsor: University of Michigan Hospitals
Veterans Affairs Medical Center (Ann Arbor)

Program Director:
Michael W Mulholland, MD PhD
Univ of Michigan Hospitals
TC2207/Box 0342
1500 E Medical Center Dr
Ann Arbor, MI 48109-0342
Tel: 734 936-5733 *Fax:* 734 936-5725
E-mail: surgery.ed@umich.edu
Internet: http://www.med.umich.edu./surg
Accred Length: 5 Years *Program Size:* 44 (*GY1:* 21)
Subspecialties: CCS, VS
Program ID: 440-25-21-141

Detroit

Henry Ford Hospital Program
Sponsor: Henry Ford Hospital
Program Director:
Frank R Lewis, MD
Henry Ford Hospital
2799 W Grand Blvd
Detroit, MI 48202-2689
Tel: 313 916-3480 *Fax:* 313 916-7354
E-mail: jcesari1@hfhs.org
Internet: http://www.henryfordhealth.org
Accred Length: 5 Years *Program Size:* 33 (*GY1:* 7)
Subspecialties: CCS, VS
Program ID: 440-25-12-143

St John Hospital and Medical Center Program
Sponsor: St John Hospital and Medical Center
Program Director:
Larry R Lloyd, MD
St John Hospital and Med Ctr
Dept of Med Educ
22101 Moross Rd
Detroit, MI 48236
Tel: 313 343-3875 *Fax:* 313 343-7840
E-mail: sue.moynihan@stjohn.org
Internet: http://www.stjohn.org
Accred Length: 5 Years *Program Size:* 24 (*GY1:* 6)
Subspecialties: TY
Program ID: 440-25-11-145

Wayne State University/Detroit Medical Center (Sinai Hospital) Program
Sponsor: Wayne State University/Detroit Medical Center
Sinai Hospital
Program Director:
Andrew Saxe, MD
Sinai Hospital
6767 W Outer Dr
Detroit, MI 48235
Tel: 313 493-5770 *Fax:* 313 493-7526
Accred Length: 5 Years *Program Size:* 7 (*GY1:* 0)
Program ID: 440-25-11-146

Wayne State University/Detroit Medical Center Program
Sponsor: Wayne State University/Detroit Medical Center
Detroit Receiving Hospital and University Health Center
Grace Hospital
Harper Hospital
Veterans Affairs Medical Center (Detroit)
Program Director:
James G Tyburski, MD
Wayne State Univ-Detroit Med Ctr
Dept of Surgery
4201 St Antoine/6C-UHC
Detroit, MI 48201-1928
Tel: 313 745-3486 *Fax:* 313 577-5310
Accred Length: 5 Years *Program Size:* 52 (*GY1:* 17)
Subspecialties: TY, VS
Program ID: 440-25-21-148

East Lansing

Michigan State University Program
Sponsor: Michigan State University College of Human Medicine
McLaren Regional Medical Center
Michigan Capital Medical Center
Sparrow Hospital
St Lawrence Hospital and HealthCare Services
Program Director:
Richard E Dean, MD
Michigan State Univ, Dept of Surgery
B-424 Clinical Ctr
East Lansing, MI 48824-1315
Tel: 517 353-8730 *Fax:* 517 353-6392
Accred Length: 5 Years *Program Size:* 18 (*GY1:* 5)
Program ID: 440-25-21-386

Grand Rapids

Spectrum Health-Downtown Campus Program
Sponsor: Spectrum Health-Downtown Campus
Program Director:
Bruce W Bonnell, MD
Dept of Surgical Education
221 Michigan NE/Ste 200
Grand Rapids, MI 49503
Tel: 616 391-8772 *Fax:* 616 391-8611
E-mail: info@spectrum-health.org
Internet:
http://www.spectrum-health.org/educ/surgedresid/ersrgres.htm
Accred Length: 5 Years *Program Size:* 23 (*GY1:* 8)
Subspecialties: CCS
Program ID: 440-25-31-153

Spectrum Health-East Campus/St Mary's Health Services Program
Sponsor: Spectrum Health-East Campus
St Mary's Health Services
Program Director:
William J Passinault, MD
St Mary's Health Services
Surgery Education Office
200 Jefferson
Grand Rapids, MI 49503
Tel: 616 752-6742
Accred Length: 5 Years *Program Size:* 20 (*GY1:* 5)
Subspecialties: TY
Program ID: 440-25-11-152

Kalamazoo

Kalamazoo Center for Medical Studies/Michigan State University Program
Sponsor: Kalamazoo Center for Medical Studies
Borgess Medical Center
Bronson Methodist Hospital
Program Director:
Duane T Freier, MD
Michigan State Univ Kalamazoo Ctr for Med Studies
Dept of General Surgery
1000 Oakland Dr
Kalamazoo, MI 49008-1284
Tel: 616 337-6260 *Fax:* 616 337-6441
E-mail: gen_surg@kcms.msu.edu
Internet: http://www.kcms.msu.edu/gensurg.html
Accred Length: 5 Years *Program Size:* 12 (*GY1:* 4)
Program ID: 440-25-21-400

Pontiac

North Oakland Medical Center Program
Sponsor: North Oakland Medical Center
Program Director:
Yvan J Silva, MD
North Oakland Med Ctrs
461 W Huron
Pontiac, MI 48341
Tel: 248 857-7314 *Fax:* 248 857-6793
Accred Length: 5 Years *Program Size:* 12 (*GY1:* 4)
Program ID: 440-25-11-156

St Joseph Mercy-Oakland Program
Sponsor: St Joseph Mercy-Oakland
Program Director:
Allen Silbergleit, MD PhD
St Joseph Mercy-Oakland
900 Woodward Ave
Pontiac, MI 48341-2985
Tel: 248 858-3234 *Fax:* 248 858-3244
Accred Length: 5 Years *Program Size:* 14 (*GY1:* 4)
Subspecialties: TY
Program ID: 440-25-11-157

Royal Oak

William Beaumont Hospital Program
Sponsor: William Beaumont Hospital
Program Director:
John L Glover, MD
William Beaumont Hospital
3601 W 13 Mile Rd
Royal Oak, MI 48073-6769
Tel: 248 551-0422 *Fax:* 248 551-5426
Internet: http://www.beaumont.edu/html/gme
Accred Length: 5 Years *Program Size:* 39 (*GY1:* 9)
Program ID: 440-25-12-158

Saginaw

Saginaw Cooperative Hospitals Program
Sponsor: Saginaw Cooperative Hospitals Inc
Covenant Medical Center
Saginaw General Hospital
St Mary's Medical Center
Program Director:
James C Gruenberg, MD
Saginaw Cooperative Hospitals
1000 Houghton Ave/Rm 2061
Saginaw, MI 48602
Tel: 517 771-6827 *Fax:* 517 771-6898
E-mail: jeromel@pilot.msu.edu
Internet: http://www.chm.msu.cdu:80/saginaw/index.html
Accred Length: 5 Years *Program Size:* 10 (*GY1:* 2)
Program ID: 440-25-21-159

Southfield

Providence Hospital and Medical Centers Program
Sponsor: Providence Hospital and Medical Centers
Samaritan Health Center-Mercy Hospital
Program Director:
Shun C Young, MD
Providence Hospital
Med Educ
16001 W Nine Mile Rd
Southfield, MI 48075-4818
Tel: 248 424-3073 *Fax:* 248 424-5380
Accred Length: 5 Years *Program Size:* 24 (*GY1:* 8)
Subspecialties: TY
Program ID: 440-25-21-160

Minnesota

Minneapolis

Hennepin County Medical Center Program
Sponsor: Hennepin County Medical Center
Program Director:
Donald M Jacobs, MD
Hennepin County Med Ctr
701 Park Ave S
Minneapolis, MN 55415
Tel: 612 347-2810, ext 2849 *Fax:* 612 904-4297
Accred Length: 5 Years *Program Size:* 25 (*GY1:* 7)
Subspecialties: TY
Program ID: 440-26-11-161

University of Minnesota Program
Sponsor: University of Minnesota Medical School
Fairview-University Medical Center
North Memorial Health Care
Regions Hospital
Veterans Affairs Medical Center (Minneapolis)
Program Director:
David Dunn, MD PhD
Univ of Minnesota
516 Delaware St SE
11-132 Phillips-Wangensteen Bldg/Box 195
Minneapolis, MN 55455-0321
Tel: 612 626-2590 *Fax:* 612 625-8496
Internet: http://www.surg.umn.edu
Accred Length: 5 Years *Program Size:* 50 (*GY1:* 22)
Subspecialties: CCS
Program ID: 440-26-31-162

Rochester

Mayo Graduate School of Medicine (Rochester) Program
Sponsor: Mayo Graduate School of Medicine-Mayo Foundation
Mayo Clinic (Rochester)
Rochester Methodist Hospital
St Mary's Hospital of Rochester
Program Director:
David R Farley, MD
Application Processing Ctr
Mayo Graduate Sch of Med
200 First St SW
Rochester, MN 55905
Tel: 507 284-4331 *Fax:* 507 284-0999
E-mail: mgsm.roch.mn.surgery@mayo.edu
Internet: http://www.mayo.edu/
Accred Length: 5 Years *Program Size:* 54 (*GY1:* 20)
Subspecialties: CCS, TY, VS
Program ID: 440-26-21-163

Mississippi

Jackson

University of Mississippi Medical Center Program
Sponsor: University of Mississippi School of Medicine
University Hospital
Veterans Affairs Medical Center (Jackson)
Program Director:
Ralph H Didlake, MD
Univ of Mississippi Med Ctr
2500 N State St
Jackson, MS 39216-4505
Tel: 601 984-5102 *Fax:* 601 984-5107
E-mail: rdidlake@surgery.umsmed.edu
Accred Length: 5 Years *Program Size:* 25 (*GY1:* 5)
Program ID: 440-27-21-165

Keesler AFB

Keesler Medical Center Program
Sponsor: Keesler Medical Center
Veterans Affairs Medical Center (Biloxi)
Program Director:
A Letch Kline, MD
81 MSGS/SGCQ
301 Fisher St/Rm 1A132
Keesler AFB, MS 39534-2519
Tel: 228 377-6558 *Fax:* 228 377-7434
E-mail: kline.albert@keesler.af.mil
Internet: http://1mdg06.keesler.af.mil/training/residency/gensurg/index.html
Accred Length: 5 Years *Program Size:* 25 (*GY1:* 8)
Program ID: 440-27-31-002
US Armed Services Program

Missouri

Columbia

University of Missouri-Columbia Program
Sponsor: University of Missouri-Columbia School of Medicine
Harry S Truman Memorial Veterans Hospital
Saint Luke's Hospital
University Hospitals and Clinics
Program Director:
Debra Koivunen, MD
Univ of Missouri Hospitals and Clinics
Div of General Surgery/N323
One Hospital Dr
Columbia, MO 65212
Tel: 573 882-2245 *Fax:* 573 884-4611
Internet: http://www.surgery.missouri.edu
Accred Length: 5 Years *Program Size:* 25 (*GY1:* 13)
Subspecialties: CCS, VS
Program ID: 440-28-21-166

Kansas City

University of Missouri at Kansas City Program
Sponsor: University of Missouri-Kansas City School of Medicine
Saint Luke's Hospital
Truman Medical Center-West
Program Director:
L Beaty Pemberton, MD
Univ of Missouri-Kansas City, Dept of Surgery
2301 Holmes St
Kansas City, MO 64108-2792
Tel: 816 556-3505 *Fax:* 816 556-3347
E-mail: kbailey@cctr.umkc.edu
Internet: http://www.umkc.edu/surgery
Accred Length: 5 Years *Program Size:* 31 (*GY1:* 10)
Program ID: 440-28-21-168

St Louis

St Louis University School of Medicine Program
Sponsor: St Louis University School of Medicine
SSM Cardinal Glennon Children's Hospital
St John's Mercy Medical Center
St Louis University School of Medicine
St Mary's Health Center
Veterans Affairs Medical Center (St Louis)
Program Director:
Rodney M Durham, MD
St Louis Univ Sch of Med
3635 Vista Ave
PO Box 15250
St Louis, MO 63110-0250
Tel: 314 577-8317 *Fax:* 314 268-5466
E-mail: surgweb@slu.edu
Internet:
http://www.slu.edu/colleges/med/departments/surgery
Accred Length: 5 Years *Program Size:* 32 (*GY1:* 10)
Subspecialties: CCS, VS
Program ID: 440-28-21-171

Washington University/B-JH/SLCH Consortium Program
Sponsor: Washington University/B-JH/SLCH Consortium
Barnes-Jewish Hospital
Barnes-Jewish Hospital (North Campus)
St Louis ConnectCare
Veterans Affairs Medical Center (St Louis)
Program Director:
Timothy J Eberlein, MD
Washington Univ Sch of Med
1701 West Bldg
660 S Euclid Ave
St Louis, MO 63110
Tel: 314 362-8028 *Fax:* 314 747-1288
E-mail: resapp@msnotes.wustl.edu
Internet: http://www.surgery.wustl.edu
Accred Length: 5 Years *Program Size:* 73 (*GY1:* 27)
Subspecialties: CCS, PDS, VS
Program ID: 440-28-21-388

Nebraska

Omaha

Creighton University Program
Sponsor: Creighton University School of Medicine
Tenet St Joseph Hospital at Creighton Univ Medical Center
VA Greater Nebraska Health Care System (Lincoln Division)
Veterans Affairs Medical Center (Omaha)
Program Director:
Robert J Fitzgibbons Jr, MD
Creighton Univ, Dept of Surgery
601 N 30th St/Ste 3740
Omaha, NE 68131
Tel: 402 280-4231 *Fax:* 402 280-4593
E-mail: dfrost@creighton.edu
Internet: http://www.creighton.edu/surgery/surgres.html
Accred Length: 5 Years *Program Size:* 23 (*GY1:* 8)
Program ID: 440-30-31-175

University of Nebraska Program
Sponsor: University of Nebraska Medical Center
Childrens Memorial Hospital
Methodist Hospital
Veterans Affairs Medical Center (Omaha)
Program Director:
James A Edney, MD
Univ of Nebraska Med Ctr
Dept of Surgery
600 S 42nd St
Omaha, NE 68198-3280
Tel: 402 559-7272 *Fax:* 402 559-6749
E-mail: nlonerga@unmc.mail.edu
Internet: http://www.unmc.edu/gme/surgery.htm
Accred Length: 5 Years *Program Size:* 31 (*GY1:* 10)
Program ID: 440-30-21-176

Nevada

Las Vegas

University of Nevada Program
Sponsor: University of Nevada School of Medicine
University Medical Center of Southern Nevada
Ioannis A Lougaris Veterans Affairs Medical Center
Program Director:
Alex G Little, MD
Univ of Nevada
2040 W Charleston Blvd/Ste 601
Las Vegas, NV 89102-2214
Tel: 702 671-2339 *Fax:* 702 384-7506
Internet: http://www.unr.edu/med
Accred Length: 5 Years *Program Size:* 19 (*GY1:* 4)
Program ID: 440-31-21-378

New Hampshire

Lebanon

Dartmouth-Hitchcock Medical Center Program

Sponsor: Mary Hitchcock Memorial Hospital
Veterans Affairs Medical Center (White River Junction)

Program Director:
Richard W Dow, MD
Dartmouth-Hitchcock Med Ctr
Dept of Surgery
One Medical Center Dr
Lebanon, NH 03756
Tel: 603 650-7400 *Fax:* 603 650-6061
Accred Length: 5 Years *Program Size:* 33 (*GY1:* 12)
Subspecialties: VS
Program ID: 440-32-21-177

New Jersey

Camden

UMDNJ-Robert Wood Johnson Medical School (Camden) Program

Sponsor: Cooper Hospital-University Medical Center

Program Director:
Thomas V Whalen, MD
Cooper Hospital-Univ Med Ctr
Three Cooper Plaza/Ste 411
Camden, NJ 08103-1489
Tel: 609 342-3012 *Fax:* 609 342-7606
E-mail: whalen@umdnj.edu
Accred Length: 5 Years *Program Size:* 19 (*GY1:* 4)
Subspecialties: CCS
Program ID: 440-33-21-179

Livingston

St Barnabas Medical Center Program

Sponsor: St Barnabas Medical Center
Jersey City Medical Center

Program Director:
Michael A Marano, MD
St Barnabas Med Ctr
Dept of Surgery
94 Old Short Hills Rd
Livingston, NJ 07039
Tel: 973 322-8945 *Fax:* 973 322-2471
Accred Length: 5 Years *Program Size:* 26 (*GY1:* 9)
Subspecialties: TY
Program ID: 440-33-22-181

Long Branch

Monmouth Medical Center Program

Sponsor: Monmouth Medical Center
Newark Beth Israel Medical Center

Program Director:
Charles Sills, MD
Monmouth Med Ctr
Dept of Surgery/Rm 251-SW
300 Second Ave
Long Branch, NJ 07740-9998
Tel: 732 923-6769 *Fax:* 732 923-6768
E-mail: sills@auhs.edu
Accred Length: 5 Years *Program Size:* 20 (*GY1:* 7)
Program ID: 440-33-21-182

Morristown

Morristown Memorial Hospital Program

Sponsor: Morristown Memorial Hospital

Program Director:
Thomas J Smith, MD
Morristown Memorial Hospital
100 Madison Ave
PO Box 1956
Morristown, NJ 07962-1956
Tel: 973 971-5678 *Fax:* 973 290-7066
Internet: http://www. atlantichealth.org
Accred Length: 5 Years *Program Size:* 24 (*GY1:* 6)
Program ID: 440-33-11-183

Newark

UMDNJ-New Jersey Medical School Program

Sponsor: UMDNJ-New Jersey Medical School
Hackensack University Medical Center
UMDNJ-University Hospital
Veterans Affairs Medical Center (East Orange)

Program Director:
Suresh Raina, MD
UMDNJ-New Jersey Med Sch
150 Bergen St/E350
Newark, NJ 07103-2714
Tel: 973 972-6601 *Fax:* 973 972-6591
E-mail: raina@umdnj.edu
Internet: http://www.umdnj.edu/njmsweb/surg/
Accred Length: 5 Years *Program Size:* 45 (*GY1:* 8)
Subspecialties: CCS, TY, VS
Program ID: 440-33-21-184

Piscataway

UMDNJ-Robert Wood Johnson Medical School Program

Sponsor: UMDNJ-Robert Wood Johnson Medical School
Jersey Shore Medical Center
Medical Center at Princeton
Robert Wood Johnson University Hospital
St Peter's University Hospital

Program Director:
Ralph S Greco, MD
UMDNJ-Robert Wood Johnson Med Sch
Dept of Surgery/Rm 594 MEB
One Robert Wood Johnson Pl/PO Box 19
New Brunswick, NJ 08903-0019
Tel: 908 235-7674 *Fax:* 908 235-8372
E-mail: fitzgeck@umdnj.edu
Internet: http://www.rwjsurgery.umdnj.edu
Accred Length: 5 Years *Program Size:* 42 (*GY1:* 13)
Subspecialties: VS
Program ID: 440-33-21-187

Trenton

St Francis Medical Center Program

Sponsor: St Francis Medical Center

Program Director:
Francis John Cottone, MD
St Francis Med Ctr
Dept of Surgery/Rm B154
601 Hamilton Ave
Trenton, NJ 08629
Tel: 609 599-5062 *Fax:* 609 599-6232
Accred Length: 5 Years *Program Size:* 12 (*GY1:* 4)
Program ID: 440-33-31-189

New Mexico

Albuquerque

University of New Mexico Program

Sponsor: University of New Mexico School of Medicine
Lovelace Medical Center
University Hospital
Veterans Affairs Medical Center (Albuquerque)

Program Director:
Mark Langsfeld, MD
Univ of New Mexico Health Sciences Ctr
Dept of Surgery/ACC 2nd Fl
Albuquerque, NM 87131-5341
Tel: 505 272-4161 *Fax:* 505 272-4159
E-mail: pgonzalez@saulud.unm.edu
Accred Length: 5 Years *Program Size:* 28 (*GY1:* 9)
Program ID: 440-34-21-190

New York

Albany

Albany Medical Center Program

Sponsor: Albany Medical Center
St Peter's Hospital
Veterans Affairs Medical Center (Albany)

Program Director:
Dhiraj M Shah, MD
Albany Med Coll
Dept of Surgery/A-61
47 New Scotland Ave
Albany, NY 12208-3479
Tel: 518 262-5905 *Fax:* 518 262-5692
Accred Length: 5 Years *Program Size:* 25 (*GY1:* 9)
Subspecialties: VS
Program ID: 440-35-21-191

Bronx

Albert Einstein College of Medicine Program

Sponsor: Albert Einstein College of Medicine of Yeshiva University
Jacobi Medical Center
Montefiore Medical Center-Henry and Lucy Moses Division
Montefiore Medical Center-Weiler Hospital
North Central Bronx Hospital

Program Director:
Michael Zenilman, MD
Montefiore Med Ctr
111 E 210th St
Bronx, NY 10467
Tel: 718 920-6286 *Fax:* 718 798-1883
Accred Length: 5 Years *Program Size:* 52 (*GY1:* 25)
Subspecialties: VS
Program ID: 440-35-21-202

Bronx-Lebanon Hospital Center Program

Sponsor: Bronx-Lebanon Hospital Center

Program Director:
Paul H Gerst, MD
Bronx-Lebanon Hospital Ctr
1650 Grand Concourse
Bronx, NY 10457
Tel: 718 960-1216 *Fax:* 718 960-1230
E-mail: saunking@aol.com
Accred Length: 5 Years *Program Size:* 26 (*GY1:* 10)
Program ID: 440-35-11-206

Programs

Lincoln Medical and Mental Health Center Program

Sponsor: Lincoln Medical and Mental Health Center
St Joseph's Medical Center

Program Director:
Dennis L Bordan, MD
Lincoln Med and Mental Health Ctr
Dept of Surgery
234 E 149th St/Rm 6-20
Bronx, NY 10451
Tel: 718 579-5890 *Fax:* 718 579-4620
Accred Length: 5 Years *Program Size:* 14 (*GY1:* 6)
Program ID: 440-35-31-407

New York Medical College (Our Lady of Mercy) Program

Sponsor: New York Medical College
Our Lady of Mercy Medical Center
St Agnes Hospital

Program Director:
C Gene Cayten, MD
Our Lady of Mercy Med Ctr
600 E 233rd St
Bronx, NY 10466
Tel: 718 920-9522 *Fax:* 718 920-9837
E-mail: gene-cayten@nymc.edu
Internet: http://www.ourladyofmercy.com
Accred Length: 5 Years *Program Size:* 14 (*GY1:* 5)
Program ID: 440-35-11-408

Brooklyn

Brookdale University Hospital Medical Center Program

Sponsor: Brookdale University Hospital Medical Center

Program Director:
Richard J Fogler, MD
Brookdale Univ Hospital and Med Ctr
Dept of Surgical Services
1 Brookdale Plaza
Brooklyn, NY 11212-3198
Tel: 718 240-6386 *Fax:* 718 240-6389
E-mail: czelazny@brookdale.edu
Accred Length: 5 Years *Program Size:* 28 (*GY1:* 12)
Program ID: 440-35-21-207

Brooklyn Hospital Center Program

Sponsor: Brooklyn Hospital Center

Program Director:
Albert O Duncan, MD
Brooklyn Hospital Ctr
Dept of Surgery
121 DeKalb Ave
Brooklyn, NY 11201
Tel: 718 250-6920 *Fax:* 718 250-6080
Accred Length: 5 Years *Program Size:* 30 (*GY1:* 10)
Program ID: 440-35-31-208

Maimonides Medical Center Program

Sponsor: Maimonides Medical Center
Coney Island Hospital
Lutheran Medical Center

Program Director:
Joseph N Cunningham Jr, MD
Maimonides Med Ctr
4802 Tenth Ave
Brooklyn, NY 11219
Tel: 718 283-7692 *Fax:* 718 283-8909
Accred Length: 5 Years *Program Size:* 41 (*GY1:* 13)
Subspecialties: VS
Program ID: 440-35-21-221

New York Methodist Hospital Program

Sponsor: New York Methodist Hospital

Program Director:
Leslie Wise, MD
New York Methodist Hospital
506 Sixth St
Buckley 6
Brooklyn, NY 11215-9008
Tel: 718 780-3288 *Fax:* 718 780-3154
Accred Length: 5 Years *Program Size:* 17 (*GY1:* 4)
Program ID: 440-35-21-222

SUNY Health Science Center at Brooklyn Program

Sponsor: SUNY Health Science Center at Brooklyn
Kings County Hospital Center
Long Island College Hospital
Sisters of Charity Medical Center-St Vincent's Campus
University Hospital-SUNY Health Science Center at Brooklyn
Veterans Affairs Medical Center (Brooklyn)

Program Director:
Bruce G Sommer, MD MD
SUNY Health Science Ctr-Brooklyn
Dept of Surgery
450 Clarkson Ave/Box 40
Brooklyn, NY 11203
Tel: 718 270-1973, ext 1421 *Fax:* 718 270-2826
Accred Length: 5 Years *Program Size:* 66 (*GY1:* 22)
Subspecialties: VS
Program ID: 440-35-21-237

Buffalo

SUNY at Buffalo Graduate Medical-Dental Education Consortium Program

Sponsor: SUNY at Buffalo Grad Medical-Dental Education Consortium
CGF Health System (Buffalo General Hospital)
CGF Health System (Millard Fillmore Hospitals)
Erie County Medical Center
Veterans Affairs Medical Center (Buffalo)

Program Director:
Eddie L Hoover, MD
Erie County Med Ctr
Dept of Surgery
462 Grider St
Buffalo, NY 14215-3098
Tel: 716 898-3808 *Fax:* 716 898-5029
E-mail: rhn@ubunix.acsu.buffalo.edu
Accred Length: 5 Years *Program Size:* 55 (*GY1:* 19)
Subspecialties: VS
Program ID: 440-35-21-393

Cooperstown

Bassett Healthcare Program

Sponsor: Bassett Healthcare
Mary Imogene Bassett Hospital

Program Director:
Patrick A Dietz, MD
Bassett Healthcare
Med Educ
1 Atwell Rd
Cooperstown, NY 13326-1394
Tel: 607 547-3764 *Fax:* 607 547-6612
E-mail: bassed@telenet.net
Internet: http://www.bassett.edu
Accred Length: 5 Years *Program Size:* 13 (*GY1:* 4)
Subspecialties: TY
Program ID: 440-35-31-197

East Meadow

Nassau County Medical Center Program

Sponsor: Nassau County Medical Center

Program Director:
Gerald W Shaftan, MD
Nassau County Med Ctr
2201 Hempstead Trnpk
East Meadow, NY 11554
Tel: 516 572-6703 *Fax:* 516 572-5140
E-mail: gshaftan@ncmc.co.nassau.ny.us
Accred Length: 5 Years *Program Size:* 26 (*GY1:* 14)
Program ID: 440-35-12-198

Flushing

New York Hospital Medical Center of Queens/Cornell University Medical College Program

Sponsor: New York Hospital Medical Center of Queens
New York Flushing Hospital Medical Center

Program Director:
James W Turner, MD
56-45 Main St
Flushing, NY 11355
Tel: 718 670-1572 *Fax:* 718 670-1864
E-mail: dmdechir%queens@nyh.med.cornell.edu
Internet: http://www.surgeryatnyhq.org
Accred Length: 5 Years *Program Size:* 28 (*GY1:* 12)
Subspecialties: TY
Program ID: 440-35-11-205

Jamaica

Catholic Medical Center of Brooklyn and Queens Program

Sponsor: Catholic Medical Center of Brooklyn and Queens Inc
Catholic Medical Center (Mary Immaculate Hospital)
Catholic Medical Center (St Mary's Hospital)

Program Director:
Walter F Pizzi, MD
Catholic Med Ctr of Brooklyn and Queens
88-25 153rd St
Parsons Manor/Ste 2P
Jamaica, NY 11432
Tel: 718 558-7216 *Fax:* 718 558-7090
E-mail: wpizzi@cmcny.com
Internet: http://www.mcny.com
Accred Length: 5 Years *Program Size:* 13 (*GY1:* 5)
Program ID: 440-35-21-210

Manhasset

North Shore University Hospital/NYU School of Medicine Program

Sponsor: North Shore University Hospital

Program Director:
Naji N Abumrad, MD
North Shore Univ Hospital
Dept of Surgery
300 Community Dr
Manhasset, NY 11030
Tel: 516 562-4863 *Fax:* 516 562-1521
E-mail: drisucci@nshs.edu
Internet: http://www.nshs.edu
Accred Length: 5 Years *Program Size:* 33 (*GY1:* 15)
Subspecialties: CCS, VS
Program ID: 440-35-11-212

New Hyde Park

Albert Einstein College of Medicine at Long Island Jewish Medical Center Program

Sponsor: Long Island Jewish Medical Center
North Shore University Hospital at Forest Hills

Program Director:
Jon R Cohen, MD
Long Island Jewish Med Ctr
270-05 76th Ave
New Hyde Park, NY 11040
Tel: 718 470-7210 *Fax:* 718 343-3429
Internet: http://www.lij.edu
Accred Length: 5 Years *Program Size:* 36 (*GY1:* 18)
Program ID: 440-35-21-219

New Rochelle

New York Medical College (Sound Shore) Program

Sponsor: New York Medical College
Sound Shore Medical Center of Westchester

Program Director:
Burton L Herz, MD
Sound Shore Med Ctr of Westchester
16 Guion Pl
3 Joyce
New Rochelle, NY 10802-1729
Tel: 914 632-5000, ext 3998 *Fax:* 914 637-1639
Accred Length: 5 Years *Program Size:* 15 (*GY1:* 5)
Subspecialties: TY
Program ID: 440-35-21-201

New York

Albert Einstein College of Medicine at Beth Israel Medical Center Program

Sponsor: Beth Israel Medical Center

Program Director:
Moses Nussbaum, MD
Beth Israel Med Ctr
First Ave at 16th St
New York, NY 10003
Tel: 212 420-4044
Internet: http://www.wehealny.org
Accred Length: 5 Years *Program Size:* 25 (*GY1:* 12)
Program ID: 440-35-11-204

Harlem Hospital Center Program

Sponsor: Harlem Hospital Center

Program Director:
Harold P Freeman, MD
Harlem Hospital Ctr
506 Lenox Ave
New York, NY 10037
Tel: 212 939-3533 *Fax:* 212 939-3536
Accred Length: 5 Years *Program Size:* 20 (*GY1:* 5)
Program ID: 440-35-11-214

Lenox Hill Hospital Program

Sponsor: Lenox Hill Hospital

Program Director:
Valavanur A Subramanian, MD
Lenox Hill Hospital
100 E 77th St
New York, NY 10021-1883
Tel: 212 434-2150 *Fax:* 212 434-4559
Accred Length: 5 Years *Program Size:* 20 (*GY1:* 11)
Program ID: 440-35-11-217

Mount Sinai School of Medicine (Cabrini) Program

Sponsor: Mount Sinai School of Medicine
Cabrini Medical Center

Program Director:
Raymond D LaRaja, MD
Cabrini Med Ctr
Dept of Surgery
227 E 19th St/D-309
New York, NY 10003
Tel: 212 995-6727 *Fax:* 212 979-3464
Internet: http://www.cabrininy.org
Accred Length: 5 Years *Program Size:* 13 (*GY1:* 4)
Program ID: 440-35-21-209

Mount Sinai School of Medicine Program

Sponsor: Mount Sinai School of Medicine
Elmhurst Hospital Center-Mount Sinai Services
Mount Sinai Medical Center

Program Director:
Larry H Hollier, MD
Mount Sinai Med Ctr
Dept of Surgery
One Gustave L Levy Pl/Box 1259
New York, NY 10029-6574
Tel: 212 241-5871 *Fax:* 212 987-9310
Accred Length: 5 Years *Program Size:* 63 (*GY1:* 24)
Subspecialties: VS
Program ID: 440-35-21-225

New York and Presbyterian Hospital (Columbia Campus) Program

Sponsor: New York and Presbyterian Hospital
New York and Presbyterian Hospital (Columbia Campus)
Overlook Hospital

Program Director:
Mark Hardy, MD MD
Presbyterian Hospital
177 Fort Washington Ave
Milstein 7GS-313
New York, NY 10032-3784
Tel: 212 305-3038 *Fax:* 212 305-8321
Accred Length: 5 Years *Program Size:* 51 (*GY1:* 21)
Subspecialties: TY
Program ID: 440-35-21-229

New York and Presbyterian Hospital (Cornell Campus) Program

Sponsor: New York and Presbyterian Hospital
Jamaica Hospital
Memorial Sloan-Kettering Cancer Center
New York and Presbyterian Hospital (Cornell Campus)

Program Director:
John M Daly, MD
New York Presbyterian Hospital-Cornell Campus
Dept of Surgery
525 E 68th St/F-739
New York, NY 10021
Tel: 212 746-5144 *Fax:* 212 746-8753
Internet: http://surgery.med.cornell.edu
Accred Length: 5 Years *Program Size:* 59 (*GY1:* 23)
Program ID: 440-35-21-211

New York Medical College at St Vincent's Hospital and Medical Center of New York Program

Sponsor: New York Medical College
St Vincent's Hospital and Medical Center of New York
Huntington Hospital
Metropolitan Hospital Center
St Joseph's Hospital and Medical Center

Program Director:
Marc K Wallack, MD
St Vincent's Hospital and Med Ctr
Dept of Surgery/Cronin 802
153 W 11th St
New York, NY 10011
Tel: 212 604-8344 *Fax:* 212 604-8355
Accred Length: 5 Years *Program Size:* 50 (*GY1:* 20)
Program ID: 440-35-21-234

New York University Medical Center Program

Sponsor: New York University Medical Center
Bellevue Hospital Center
Veterans Affairs Medical Center (Manhattan)

Program Director:
Thomas H Gouge, MD
New York Univ Med Ctr
550 First Ave
New York, NY 10016
Tel: 212 263-7301 *Fax:* 212 253-8216
Accred Length: 5 Years *Program Size:* 65 (*GY1:* 20)
Subspecialties: VS
Program ID: 440-35-21-394

St Luke's-Roosevelt Hospital Center Program

Sponsor: St Luke's-Roosevelt Hospital Center
St Luke's-Roosevelt Hospital Center-Roosevelt Division
St Luke's-Roosevelt Hospital Center-St Luke's Division

Program Director:
David Tilson, MD
St Luke's-Roosevelt Hospital Ctr
1000 Tenth Ave/Ste 2B
New York, NY 10019
Tel: 212 523-7780 *Fax:* 212 523-6495
Accred Length: 5 Years *Program Size:* 37 (*GY1:* 14)
Program ID: 440-35-21-383

Rochester

University of Rochester Program

Sponsor: Strong Memorial Hospital of the University of Rochester
Genesee Hospital
Rochester General Hospital

Program Director:
Oscar Bronsther, MD
Dept of Surgery
Univ of Rochester Med Ctr
601 Elmwood Ave
Rochester, NY 14642-8410
Tel: 716 275-2723 *Fax:* 716 275-8513
E-mail: dplassch@surgery.urmc.rochester.edu
Internet: http://www.urmc.rochester.edu
Accred Length: 5 Years *Program Size:* 34 (*GY1:* 7)
Subspecialties: CCS, VS
Program ID: 440-35-21-240

Staten Island

Staten Island University Hospital Program

Sponsor: Staten Island University Hospital

Program Director:
Gene F Coppa, MD
Staten Island Univ Hospital
475 Seaview Ave
Staten Island, NY 10305-3498
Tel: 718 226-9508 *Fax:* 718 226-8365
Internet: http://www.interstat.net/siuh2/surgery res.html
Accred Length: 5 Years *Program Size:* 21 (*GY1:* 7)
Program ID: 440-35-11-236

Stony Brook

SUNY at Stony Brook Program
Sponsor: University Hospital-SUNY at Stony Brook
Veterans Affairs Medical Center (Northport)
Winthrop-University Hospital
Program Director:
John J Ricotta, MD
SUNY-Stony Brook
Dept of Surgery
HSC T-19/Rm 020
Stony Brook, NY 11794-8191
Tel: 516 444-1791 *Fax:* 516 444-7635
E-mail: brochhau@sunysb.edu/surgery
Internet: http://www.uhmc.sunysb.edu/surgery
Accred Length: 5 Years *Program Size:* 40 (*GY1:* 15)
Subspecialties: VS
Program ID: 440-35-21-242

Syracuse

SUNY Health Science Center at Syracuse Program
Sponsor: University Hospital-SUNY Health Science Center at Syracuse
Community-General Hospital of Greater Syracuse
Crouse Hospital
Veterans Affairs Medical Center (Syracuse)
Program Director:
John C Aust, MD
SUNY Health Science Ctr-Syracuse
Dept of Surgery
750 E Adams St
Syracuse, NY 13210
Tel: 315 464-6289 *Fax:* 315 464-6233
E-mail: smithm@vax.cs.hscsyr.edu
Accred Length: 5 Years *Program Size:* 42 (*GY1:* 17)
Program ID: 440-35-21-244

Valhalla

New York Medical College at Westchester Medical Center Program
Sponsor: New York Medical College
St Vincent's Medical Center
Westchester Medical Center
Program Director:
John A Savino, MD
New York Med Coll
Dept of Surgery
Munger Pavilion
Valhalla, NY 10595
Tel: 914 594-4352
Internet:
http://www.nymc.edu/depthome/academic/surgery/surgery.htm
Accred Length: 5 Years *Program Size:* 28 (*GY1:* 9)
Subspecialties: CCS
Program ID: 440-35-21-227

North Carolina

Chapel Hill

University of North Carolina Hospitals Program
Sponsor: University of North Carolina Hospitals
Wake Medical Center
Program Director:
Anthony A Meyer, MD PhD
Univ of North Carolina Sch of Med
166 Burnett-Womack Bldg/CB#7050
Chapel Hill, NC 27599-7050
Tel: 919 966-4321 *Fax:* 919 966-7841
E-mail: jnorwood@med.unc.edu
Internet: http://www.med.unc.edu/surgery/
Accred Length: 5 Years *Program Size:* 33 (*GY1:* 10)
Subspecialties: CCS, VS
Program ID: 440-36-21-245

Charlotte

Carolinas Medical Center Program
Sponsor: Carolinas Medical Center
Program Director:
Frederick L Greene, MD
Carolinas Med Ctr
Dept of General Surgery
PO Box 32861
Charlotte, NC 28232
Tel: 704 355-3176 *Fax:* 704 355-7833
Accred Length: 5 Years *Program Size:* 16 (*GY1:* 4)
Subspecialties: VS
Program ID: 440-36-12-246

Durham

Duke University Program
Sponsor: Duke University Medical Center
Durham Regional Hospital
Veterans Affairs Medical Center (Asheville)
Veterans Affairs Medical Center (Durham)
Program Director:
Theodore N Pappas, MD
Duke Univ Med Ctr
Dept of Surgery
PO Box 3479
Durham, NC 27710
Tel: 919 681-3816 *Fax:* 919 681-7934
Accred Length: 5 Years *Program Size:* 55 (*GY1:* 28)
Subspecialties: CCS
Program ID: 440-36-21-247

Greenville

East Carolina University Program
Sponsor: East Carolina University School of Medicine
Pitt County Memorial Hospital
Program Director:
W Randolph Chitwood Jr, MD
East Carolina Univ Sch of Med
Dept of Surgery
Greenville, NC 27858-4354
Tel: 252 816-5262 *Fax:* 252 816-3156
E-mail: scox@brody.med.ecu.edu
Internet:
http://www.med.ecu.edu/htdocs/surgery/index.htm
Accred Length: 5 Years *Program Size:* 28 (*GY1:* 6)
Program ID: 440-36-11-248

Wilmington

New Hanover Regional Medical Center Program
Sponsor: New Hanover Regional Medical Center
Program Director:
J Gary Maxwell, MD
New Hanover Regional Med Ctr
Coastal AHEC-Surgery
2131 S 17th St/PO Box 9025
Wilmington, NC 28402-9025
Tel: 910 343-0161, ext 232 *Fax:* 910 763-4630
E-mail: blumax@med.unc.edu
Internet: http://www.med.unc.edu/coahec
Accred Length: 5 Years *Program Size:* 10 (*GY1:* 2)
Program ID: 440-36-31-249

Winston-Salem

Wake Forest University School of Medicine Program
Sponsor: Wake Forest University Baptist Medical Center
Forsyth Memorial Hospital
Program Director:
J Wayne Meredith, MD
Wake Forest Univ Baptist Med Ctr
Dept of General Surgery
Medical Center Blvd
Winston-Salem, NC 27157-1095
Tel: 336 716-7579 *Fax:* 336 716-5414
E-mail: merediw@wfubmc.edu
Accred Length: 5 Years *Program Size:* 34 (*GY1:* 15)
Subspecialties: VS
Program ID: 440-36-31-250

North Dakota

Grand Forks

University of North Dakota Program
Sponsor: Univ of North Dakota School of Medicine & Health Sciences
Altru Health System Hospital
Veterans Affairs Medical and Regional Office Center (Fargo)
Program Director:
William K Becker, MD PhD
Univ of North Dakota
Dept of Surgery
PO Box 9037
Grand Forks, ND 58202-9037
Tel: 701 777-3067 *Fax:* 701 777-2609
E-mail: landersn@mail.med.und.nodak.und
Accred Length: 5 Years *Program Size:* 12 (*GY1:* 4)
Program ID: 440-37-21-379

Ohio

Akron

Akron General Medical Center/NEOUCOM Program
Sponsor: Akron General Medical Center
Program Director:
Daniel P Guyton, MD
Akron General Med Ctr
400 Wabash Ave
Akron, OH 44307
Tel: 330 384-6050 *Fax:* 330 384-1529
E-mail: meded@agmc.org
Internet: http://agmc.org
Accred Length: 5 Years *Program Size:* 14 (*GY1:* 3)
Subspecialties: TY
Program ID: 440-38-11-252

Summa Health System (Akron City Hospital)/NEOUCOM Program

Sponsor: Summa Health System
Akron City Hospital (Summa Health System)

Program Director:
Duane L Donovan, MD
Summa Health System
Med Educ/Mary Yanik
525 E Market St
Akron, OH 44309
Tel: 800 322-0517
Internet: http://www.summahealth.org/edu/
Accred Length: 5 Years *Program Size:* 15 (*GY1:* 3)
Program ID: 440-38-21-251

Cincinnati

Good Samaritan Hospital Program

Sponsor: Good Samaritan Hospital
Franciscan Hospital-Mount Airy Campus

Program Director:
Richard E Welling, MD
Good Samaritan Hospital
375 Dixmyth Ave
Cincinnati, OH 45220-2489
Tel: 513 872-3562 *Fax:* 513 221-5865
E-mail: rebecca_stratmann@trihealth.com
Internet: http://www.trihealth.com
Accred Length: 5 Years *Program Size:* 22 (*GY1:* 6)
Subspecialties: VS
Program ID: 440-38-31-253

Jewish Hospital of Cincinnati Program

Sponsor: Jewish Hospital of Cincinnati

Program Director:
Creighton B Wright, MD
Jewish Hospital
Dept of Surgery
4777 E Galbraith Rd
Cincinnati, OH 45236
Tel: 513 686-5474 *Fax:* 513 686-5469
E-mail: wrightcr@healthall.com
Accred Length: 5 Years *Program Size:* 12 (*GY1:* 4)
Program ID: 440-38-31-254

University Hospital/University of Cincinnati College of Medicine Program

Sponsor: University Hospital Inc
Veterans Affairs Medical Center (Cincinnati)

Program Director:
Josef E Fischer, MD
Univ of Cincinnati Med Ctr
Dept of Surgery
231 Bethesda Ave/ML 0558
Cincinnati, OH 45267-0558
Tel: 513 558-5861 *Fax:* 513 558-3474
Internet: http://www.uc.edu/www/surgery
Accred Length: 5 Years *Program Size:* 30 (*GY1:* 8)
Subspecialties: CCS, VS
Program ID: 440-38-21-255

Cleveland

Case Western Reserve University Program

Sponsor: University Hospitals of Cleveland
MetroHealth Medical Center
Mount Sinai Medical Center of Cleveland
Veterans Affairs Medical Center (Cleveland)

Program Director:
Jerry M Shuck, MD DSc
Univ Hospitals of Cleveland
Dept of Surgery
11100 Euclid Ave
Cleveland, OH 44106-5047
Tel: 216 844-3027 *Fax:* 216 844-8201
Accred Length: 5 Years *Program Size:* 37 (*GY1:* 6)
Subspecialties: CCS
Program ID: 440-38-21-399

Cleveland Clinic Foundation Program

Sponsor: Cleveland Clinic Foundation

Program Director:
J Michael Henderson, MD
Cleveland Clinic Foundation
Dept of Surgery/A80
9500 Euclid Ave
Cleveland, OH 44195-5242
Tel: 216 444-5690 *Fax:* 216 444-1162
E-mail: meded@cesmtp.ccf.org
Internet: http://www.ccf.org
Accred Length: 5 Years *Program Size:* 24 (*GY1:* 8)
Subspecialties: VS
Program ID: 440-38-22-257

Fairview Health System Program

Sponsor: Fairview Health System
Fairview Health System (Fairview General Hospital)

Program Director:
Stephen G ReMine, MD
Fairview Hospital
Dept of Surgery
18101 Lorain Ave
Cleveland, OH 44111-5656
Tel: 216 476-7155 *Fax:* 216 476-7883
E-mail: fhsurgmp@ix.netcom.com
Internet:
http://www.webcom.com/fairres/surgery/default.html
Accred Length: 5 Years *Program Size:* 18 (*GY1:* 6)
Program ID: 440-38-22-258

Meridia Huron Hospital Program

Sponsor: Meridia Huron Hospital
Cleveland Clinic Foundation
Meridia Hillcrest Hospital

Program Director:
Raphael S Chung, MD
Meridia Huron Hospital
13951 Terrace Rd
Cleveland, OH 44112
Tel: 216 761-4223 *Fax:* 216 761-3499
Accred Length: 5 Years *Program Size:* 10 (*GY1:* 2)
Program ID: 440-38-22-259

Columbus

Mount Carmel Health Program

Sponsor: Mount Carmel Medical Center
Mount Carmel East Hospital

Program Director:
Thomas H Hartranft, MD
Mount Carmel Health System
793 W State St
Columbus, OH 43222
Tel: 614 234-5983 *Fax:* 614 234-2772
E-mail: lbadurina@mchs.com
Internet: http://mchsresidency.org
Accred Length: 5 Years *Program Size:* 14 (*GY1:* 6)
Subspecialties: TY
Program ID: 440-38-32-263

Ohio State University Program

Sponsor: Ohio State University Medical Center
Arthur G James Cancer Hospital and Research Institute

Program Director:
E Christopher Ellison, MD
Ohio State Univ
321 Means Hall
1654 Upham Dr
Columbus, OH 43210-1250
Tel: 614 293-8704 *Fax:* 614 293-4063
E-mail: hanson-1@medctr.ohio-state.edu
Internet: http://www.-surgery.med.ohio-state.edu
Accred Length: 5 Years *Program Size:* 41 (*GY1:* 14)
Subspecialties: CCS, VS
Program ID: 440-38-21-264

Riverside Methodist Hospitals (OhioHealth) Program

Sponsor: Riverside Methodist Hospitals (OhioHealth)

Program Director:
James M Blackford, MD
Riverside Methodist Hospital
Medical Education Dept
3535 Olentangy River Rd
Columbus, OH 43214
Tel: 614 566-5762 *Fax:* 614 566-6852
E-mail: engelr@ohiohealth.com
Internet: http://www.ohiohealth.com
Accred Length: 5 Years *Program Size:* 14 (*GY1:* 6)
Subspecialties: TY
Program ID: 440-38-12-265

Dayton

Wright State University Program

Sponsor: Wright State University School of Medicine
Children's Medical Center
Franciscan Medical Center-Dayton Campus
Good Samaritan Hospital and Health Center
Kettering Medical Center
Miami Valley Hospital
Veterans Affairs Medical Center (Dayton)
Wright-Patterson Medical Center

Program Director:
James B Peoples, MD
Wright State Univ
One Wyoming St
CHE Bldg/Ste 7000
Dayton, OH 45409-2793
Tel: 937 208-2177 *Fax:* 937 208-2105
Internet:
http://www.med.wright.edu/som/academic/surg.html
Accred Length: 5 Years *Program Size:* 44 (*GY1:* 16)
Subspecialties: TY
Program ID: 440-38-21-266

Toledo

Medical College of Ohio Program

Sponsor: Medical College of Ohio
St Vincent Mercy Medical Center
Toledo Hospital

Program Director:
Edgar Staren, MD PhD
Dept of Surgery
Dowling Hall
3065 Arlington Ave
Toledo, OH 43614-5807
Tel: 419 383-6298 *Fax:* 419 383-3057
Accred Length: 5 Years *Program Size:* 24 (*GY1:* 5)
Subspecialties: TY
Program ID: 440-38-21-269

Youngstown

St Elizabeth Health Center/NEOUCOM Program

Sponsor: St Elizabeth Health Center

Program Director:
Rashid A Abdu, MD
St Elizabeth Health Center
1044 Belmont Ave
PO Box 1790
Youngstown, OH 44501-1790
Tel: 330 480-3124 *Fax:* 330 480-3640
Accred Length: 5 Years *Program Size:* 15 (*GY1:* 3)
Program ID: 440-38-11-270

Western Reserve Care System/NEOUCOM Program
Sponsor: Western Reserve Care System
Forum Health-Northside Medical Center
Forum Health-Tod Children's Hospital
Program Director:
Jeffrey R Rubin, MD
Western Reserve Care System
Northside Med Ctr
500 Gypsy Ln
Youngstown, OH 44501-0990
Tel: 330 740-3472 *Fax:* 330 740-5690
E-mail: jrr@neoucom.edu
Internet: http://www.wrhc.org
Accred Length: 5 Years *Program Size:* 13 (*GY1:* 4)
Program ID: 440-38-21-271

Oklahoma

Oklahoma City

University of Oklahoma Health Sciences Center Program
Sponsor: University of Oklahoma College of Medicine
Children's Hospital of Oklahoma
University Hospital
Veterans Affairs Medical Center (Oklahoma City)
Program Director:
M Alex Jacocks, MD
Univ of Oklahoma Health Sciences Ctr
PO Box 26901
Oklahoma City, OK 73190
Tel: 405 271-8096 *Fax:* 405 271-3919
E-mail: alex-jacocks@ouhsc.edu
Accred Length: 5 Years *Program Size:* 17 (*GY1:* 3)
Program ID: 440-39-21-273

Tulsa

University of Oklahoma College of Medicine-Tulsa Program
Sponsor: University of Oklahoma College of Medicine-Tulsa
Hillcrest Medical Center
St Francis Hospital
Veterans Affairs Medical Center (Muskogee)
Program Director:
J Michael McGee, MD
Univ of Oklahoma Health Sciences Ctr-Tulsa Campus
Dept of Surgery
2808 S Sheridan Rd
Tulsa, OK 74129-1077
Tel: 918 744-3584 *Fax:* 918 744-3651
E-mail: michael-mcgee@ouhsc.edu
Internet: http://www.tulsa.ouhsc.edu
Accred Length: 5 Years *Program Size:* 13 (*GY1:* 5)
Program ID: 440-39-21-274

Oregon

Portland

Oregon Health Sciences University Program
Sponsor: Oregon Health Sciences University Hospital
Kaiser Foundation Hospitals-Northwest Region
Legacy Good Samaritan Hospital and Medical Center
St Vincent Hospital and Medical Center
Veterans Affairs Medical Center (Portland)
Program Director:
Karen Deveney, MD
Oregon Health Sciences University
Dept of Surgery L223
3181 SW Sam Jackson Park Rd
Portland, OR 97201-3098
Tel: 503 494-7758 *Fax:* 503 494-5615
E-mail: lynchp@ohsu.edu
Internet: http://www.ohsu.edu/
Accred Length: 5 Years *Program Size:* 65 (*GY1:* 18)
Subspecialties: CCS, TY, VS
Program ID: 440-40-21-278

Pennsylvania

Abington

Abington Memorial Hospital Program
Sponsor: Abington Memorial Hospital
Program Director:
Thomas L Dent, MD
Abington Memorial Hospital
Dept of Surgery
1200 Old York Rd
Abington, PA 19001
Tel: 215 576-7464 *Fax:* 215 576-2159
Accred Length: 5 Years *Program Size:* 19 (*GY1:* 7)
Program ID: 440-41-12-279

Allentown

Lehigh Valley Hospital/Pennsylvania State University Program
Sponsor: Lehigh Valley Hospital
Program Director:
Gary G Nicholas, MD
Lehigh Valley Hospital
Cedar Crest and I-78
PO Box 689
Allentown, PA 18105-1556
Tel: 610 402-8966 *Fax:* 610 402-1667
E-mail: surgeryres@lvhhn.org
Internet: http://www.lvhhn.org/academic/residency/general/home.html
Accred Length: 5 Years *Program Size:* 20 (*GY1:* 5)
Subspecialties: CCS, TY
Program ID: 440-41-21-280

Bethlehem

St Luke's Hospital Program
Sponsor: St Luke's Hospital
Program Director:
Joel C Rosenfeld, MD
St Luke's Hospital
801 Ostrum St
Bethlehem, PA 18015
Tel: 610 954-2255 *Fax:* 610 954-6450
E-mail: surgery-residency@slhn.org
Internet: http://slhn-lehighvalley.org
Accred Length: 5 Years *Program Size:* 10 (*GY1:* 2)
Program ID: 440-41-21-398

Danville

Penn State Geisinger Health System/Geisinger Medical Center Program
Sponsor: Penn State Geisinger Health System
Geisinger Medical Center
Program Director:
John E Deitrick, MD
Geisinger Med Ctr
Dept of Surgery
100 N Academy Ave
Danville, PA 17822
Tel: 717 271-6365 *Fax:* 717 271-5785
E-mail: ckrebs@psghs.edu
Accred Length: 5 Years *Program Size:* 10 (*GY1:* 2)
Subspecialties: VS
Program ID: 440-41-21-283

Easton

Easton Hospital Program
Sponsor: Easton Hospital
Program Director:
Manuel H Espinosa, MD
Easton Hospital
250 S 21st St
Easton, PA 18042
Tel: 610 250-4375 *Fax:* 610 250-4851
Internet: http://www.eastonhospital.org/surg_res.htm
Accred Length: 5 Years *Program Size:* 14 (*GY1:* 4)
Subspecialties: TY
Program ID: 440-41-31-284

Harrisburg

PinnacleHealth Hospitals Program
Sponsor: PinnacleHealth System-Polyclinic Hospital
Program Director:
Stephen M Weiss, MD
PinnacleHealth Hospitals Program
Dept of Surgery, Polyclinic Hospital
2601 N Third St
Harrisburg, PA 17110
Tel: 717 782-2828 *Fax:* 717 782-2692
Accred Length: 5 Years *Program Size:* 12 (*GY1:* 4)
Program ID: 440-41-21-384

Hershey

Penn State Geisinger Health System/Milton S Hershey Medical Center Program
Sponsor: Penn State Geisinger Health System
Milton S Hershey Medical Center
Program Director:
Gordon L Kauffman Jr, MD
Milton S Hershey Med Ctr
Dept of Surgery H149
500 University Dr
Hershey, PA 17033-0850
Tel: 717 531-8815 *Fax:* 717 531-4151
E-mail: gkauffman@psghs.edu
Internet: http://www.webserv.surg.hmc.psu.edu
Accred Length: 5 Years *Program Size:* 33 (*GY1:* 14)
Subspecialties: CCS, VS
Program ID: 440-41-21-287

Johnstown

Temple University/Conemaugh Valley Memorial Hospital Program
Sponsor: Conemaugh Valley Memorial Hospital
Program Director:
Richard A Moore, PhD MD
Conemaugh Health System-Memorial Med Ctr
1086 Franklin St
Johnstown, PA 15905-4398
Tel: 814 534-9099 *Fax:* 814 534-3279
Accred Length: 5 Years *Program Size:* 12 (*GY1:* 4)
Program ID: 440-41-11-288

Philadelphia

Albert Einstein Medical Center Program
Sponsor: Albert Einstein Medical Center
Program Director:
Robert G Somers, MD
Albert Einstein Med Ctr
5501 Old York Rd
Klein Bldg/Ste 510
Philadelphia, PA 19141
Tel: 215 456-6930 *Fax:* 215 456-3529
E-mail: joness@aehn2.einstein.edu
Accred Length: 5 Years *Program Size:* 25 (*GY1:* 9)
Subspecialties: TY
Program ID: 440-41-11-291

Episcopal Hospital Program
Sponsor: Episcopal Hospital (TUHS)
St Agnes Medical Center
Program Director:
David H Levien, MD
Episcopal Hospital
100 E Lehigh Ave
Philadelphia, PA 19125-1098
Tel: 215 427-7042 *Fax:* 215 427-9976
E-mail: dlevien@ix.netcom.com
Accred Length: 5 Years *Program Size:* 14 (*GY1:* 6)
Program ID: 440-41-11-292

Graduate Hospital Program
Sponsor: Graduate Hospital
Underwood-Memorial Hospital
Program Director:
Jerome J Vernick, MD
Graduate Hospital
One Graduate Plaza/Ste 1101
1800 Lombard St
Philadelphia, PA 19146
Tel: 215 893-7677 *Fax:* 215 893-2329
Accred Length: 5 Years *Program Size:* 30 (*GY1:* 10)
Program ID: 440-41-21-293

MCP Hahnemann University Program
Sponsor: MCP Hahnemann University
Hahnemann University Hospital
Medical College of Pennsylvania Hospital
Program Director:
Joel J Roslyn, MD
MCP Hahnemann Univ-MCP Div
Dept of General Surgery
3300 Henry Ave/8th Fl
Philadelphia, PA 19129-1191
Tel: 215 842-6640 *Fax:* 215 843-1095
Accred Length: 5 Years *Program Size:* 43 (*GY1:* 16)
Program ID: 440-41-21-295

Mercy Catholic Medical Center Program
Sponsor: Mercy Catholic Medical Center Inc
Mercy Hospital of Philadelphia
Mercy Fitzgerald Hospital
Program Director:
Chris D Tzarnas, MD
Mercy Catholic Med Ctr
1500 Lansdowne Ave
Darby, PA 19023
Tel: 610 237-4950 *Fax:* 610 237-4329
Internet: http://www.mercyhealth.org
Accred Length: 5 Years *Program Size:* 12 (*GY1:* 4)
Program ID: 440-41-31-297

Pennsylvania Hospital of the University of Pennsylvania Health System Program
Sponsor: Pennsylvania Hospital (UPHS)
Program Director:
Alan L Schuricht, MD
Pennsylvania Hospital
Dept of Surgery
301 S 8th St/4th Fl
Philadelphia, PA 19106
Tel: 215 829-6880
Accred Length: 5 Years *Program Size:* 16 (*GY1:* 6)
Subspecialties: VS
Program ID: 440-41-11-298

Temple University Program
Sponsor: Temple University Hospital
Fox Chase Cancer Center
Reading Hospital and Medical Center
Program Director:
Stuart I Myers, MD
Temple Univ Hospital
3401 N Broad St
Philadelphia, PA 19140
Tel: 215 707-5080 *Fax:* 215 707-1915
Accred Length: 5 Years *Program Size:* 38 (*GY1:* 15)
Subspecialties: VS
Program ID: 440-41-21-300

Thomas Jefferson University Program
Sponsor: Thomas Jefferson University Hospital
Bryn Mawr Hospital
Program Director:
John C Kairys Sr, MD
Thomas Jefferson Univ
Dept of Surgery
1025 Walnut St/Ste 605
Philadelphia, PA 19107
Tel: 215 955-6864 *Fax:* 215 923-1420
Internet: http://jeffline.tju.edu/cwis/dept/surgery/
Accred Length: 5 Years *Program Size:* 45 (*GY1:* 16)
Subspecialties: TY
Program ID: 440-41-21-301

University of Pennsylvania Program
Sponsor: Hospital of the University of Pennsylvania
Veterans Affairs Medical Center (Philadelphia)
Program Director:
Clyde F Barker, MD
Hospital of Univ of Pennsylvania
3400 Spruce St
4 Silverstein
Philadelphia, PA 19104
Tel: 215 662-6156 *Fax:* 215 662-7983
Internet: http://www.med.upenn.edu/surgery
Accred Length: 5 Years *Program Size:* 38 (*GY1:* 10)
Subspecialties: CCS, VS
Program ID: 440-41-21-302

Pittsburgh

Allegheny General Hospital Program
Sponsor: Allegheny General Hospital
Program Director:
Charles F Cobb, MD
Allegheny General Hospital
Div of General Surgery
320 E North Ave
Pittsburgh, PA 15212-9986
Tel: 412 359-6907 *Fax:* 412 359-6732
Accred Length: 5 Years *Program Size:* 29 (*GY1:* 8)
Program ID: 440-41-12-303

Mercy Hospital of Pittsburgh Program
Sponsor: Mercy Hospital of Pittsburgh
Program Director:
Charles E Copeland, MD
Mercy Hospital of Pittsburgh
Dept of Surgery
1400 Locust St
Pittsburgh, PA 15219
Tel: 412 232-5528 *Fax:* 412 232-8096
E-mail: general.surgery.residency@mercy.pmhs.org
Internet: http://www.mercy-meded.com
Accred Length: 5 Years *Program Size:* 20 (*GY1:* 8)
Subspecialties: TY
Program ID: 440-41-12-305

University Health Center of Pittsburgh Program
Sponsor: University Health Center of Pittsburgh
Children's Hospital of Pittsburgh
Presbyterian University Hospital/UPMC
Veterans Affairs Medical Center (Pittsburgh)
Program Director:
Marshall W Webster, MD
Attn: Beth A Fischer, Res Coordinator
677 Scaife Hall
3550 Terrace St
Pittsburgh, PA 15261
Tel: 412 648-9900 *Fax:* 412 383-9746
E-mail: fischer@pittsurg.nb.upmc.edu
Internet: http://www.pitt.edu/~surg2/
Accred Length: 5 Years *Program Size:* 48 (*GY1:* 15)
Subspecialties: CCS, TY
Program ID: 440-41-21-304

Western Pennsylvania Hospital Program
Sponsor: Western Pennsylvania Hospital
Program Director:
Joseph F Homann, MD
Western Pennsylvania Hospital
4800 Friendship Ave/Ste 2820
Pittsburgh, PA 15224
Tel: 412 578-6880 *Fax:* 412 578-7212
Accred Length: 5 Years *Program Size:* 25 (*GY1:* 8)
Subspecialties: TY
Program ID: 440-41-12-308

Sayre

Guthrie Healthcare System Program
Sponsor: Robert Packer Hospital
Program Director:
Sushil K Gupta, MD
Guthrie Healthcare System-Robert Packer Hospital
Guthrie Sq
Sayre, PA 18840-1698
Tel: 570 882-5720 *Fax:* 570 882-5695
E-mail: bhornung@inet.guthrie.org
Internet: http://www.guthrie.org/surgery.htm
Accred Length: 5 Years *Program Size:* 19 (*GY1:* 7)
Program ID: 440-41-12-309

Wynnewood

Lankenau Hospital Program
Sponsor: Lankenau Hospital
Bryn Mawr Hospital
Hospital of the University of Pennsylvania
St Christopher's Hospital for Children
Program Director:
Robert D Smink, MD
Lankenau Hospital, Dept of Surgery
100 Lancaster Ave
Wynnewood, PA 19096
Tel: 610 645-2169 *Fax:* 610 642-3304
Accred Length: 5 Years *Program Size:* 12 (*GY1:* 4)
Program ID: 440-41-11-296

York

York Hospital Program
Sponsor: York Hospital
Program Director:
Jonathan E Rhoads Jr, MD
York Hospital
1001 S George St
York, PA 17405
Tel: 717 851-4362 *Fax:* 717 851-4466
E-mail: mf_jrhoads@yorkhospital.edu
Internet: http://www.yorkhealth.org
Accred Length: 5 Years *Program Size:* 16 (*GY1:* 4)
Program ID: 440-41-12-310

Puerto Rico

Mayaguez

Ramon E Betances Hospital-Mayaguez Medical Center Program
Sponsor: Dr Ramon E Betances Hospital-Mayaguez Medical Center
Hospital Pavia
Program Director:
Victor M Carlo, MD
Mayaguez Med Ctr
Dept of Surgery
PO Box 2636
Mayaguez, PR 00681
Tel: 787 833-7013 *Fax:* 787 265-8207
Accred Length: 5 Years *Program Size:* 14 (*GY1:* 4)
Subspecialties: TY
Program ID: 440-42-21-380

San Juan

University of Puerto Rico Program
Sponsor: University of Puerto Rico School of Medicine
University Hospital
Veterans Affairs Medical Center (San Juan)
Program Director:
Juan J Lojo, MD
Univ of Puerto Rico
Med Sci Campus
GPO Box 365067
San Juan, PR 00936-5067
Tel: 809 763-2440 *Fax:* 809 758-1649
E-mail: ju_lojo@rcmaxp.upr.clu.edu
Accred Length: 5 Years *Program Size:* 43 (*GY1:* 16)
Subspecialties: TY
Program ID: 440-42-21-313

Rhode Island

Providence

Brown University Program
Sponsor: Rhode Island Hospital
Miriam Hospital
Veterans Affairs Medical Center (Providence)
Program Director:
Kirby I Bland, MD
Rhode Island Hospital
APC 110
593 Eddy St
Providence, RI 02903
Tel: 401 444-8393 *Fax:* 401 444-6681
Accred Length: 5 Years *Program Size:* 47 (*GY1:* 20)
Subspecialties: CCS, PDS
Program ID: 440-43-21-314

South Carolina

Charleston

Medical University of South Carolina Program
Sponsor: Medical University of South Carolina College of Medicine
Charleston Memorial Hospital
MUSC Medical Center
Naval Hospital (Charleston)
Ralph H Johnson Dept of Veterans Affairs Med Center
Program Director:
David B Adams, MD
Med Univ of South Carolina Med Ctr
600 MUSC Complex
Ste 420
Charleston, SC 29425-2270
Tel: 843 792-3072 *Fax:* 843 792-8286
E-mail: wethersf@musc.edu
Internet: http://www.musc.edu/surgery
Accred Length: 5 Years *Program Size:* 33 (*GY1:* 17)
Program ID: 440-45-21-315

Columbia

Palmetto Health Alliance/University of South Carolina School of Medicine Program
Sponsor: Palmetto Health Alliance
Palmetto Richland Memorial Hospital
William Jennings Bryan Dorn Veterans Hospital
Program Director:
Richard M Bell, MD
Univ of South Carolina-Palmetto Richland Memorial Hosp
Dept of Surgery
2 Richland Medical Pk/Ste 300
Columbia, SC 29203
Tel: 803 256-2657, ext 362 *Fax:* 803 434-7349
E-mail: horne@surgery.rmp2.sc.edu
Internet:
http://www.rmh.edu/rmh/residency/surgical.html
Accred Length: 5 Years *Program Size:* 17 (*GY1:* 4)
Program ID: 440-45-21-316

Greenville

Greenville Hospital System Program
Sponsor: Greenville Hospital System
Program Director:
Spence M Taylor Sr, MD
Greenville Hospital System
Dept of Surgical Educ
701 Grove Rd
Greenville, SC 29605-5601
Tel: 864 455-7886 *Fax:* 864 455-7082
E-mail: sburns@ghs.org
Internet: http://www.ghs.org
Accred Length: 5 Years *Program Size:* 19 (*GY1:* 7)
Program ID: 440-45-11-317

Spartanburg

Spartanburg Regional Medical Center Program
Sponsor: Spartanburg Regional Healthcare System
Program Director:
Sidney R Steinberg, MD
Spartanburg Regional Healthcare System
101 E Wood St
Spartanburg, SC 29303
Tel: 864 560-6285 *Fax:* 864 560-6063
E-mail: slully@srhs.com
Internet: http://www.srhs.com
Accred Length: 5 Years *Program Size:* 13 (*GY1:* 5)
Subspecialties: TY
Program ID: 440-45-31-318

Tennessee

Chattanooga

University of Tennessee College of Medicine at Chattanooga Program
Sponsor: University of Tennessee College of Medicine-Chattanooga Unit
Erlanger Medical Center
Program Director:
Joseph B Cofer, MD
Univ of Tennessee Coll of Med
Dept of Surgery
979 E Third St/Ste 401
Chattanooga, TN 37403
Tel: 423 778-7695 *Fax:* 423 778-2950
E-mail: utsurg@erlanger.org
Internet: http://www.erlanger.org/utcom/surgery.html
Accred Length: 5 Years *Program Size:* 28 (*GY1:* 8)
Subspecialties: TY
Program ID: 440-47-11-320

Johnson City

East Tennessee State University Program
Sponsor: James H Quillen College of Medicine
Johnson City Medical Center Hospital
Veterans Affairs Medical Center (Mountain Home)
Wellmont Health System-Holston Valley
Program Director:
William Browder, MD
East Tennessee State Univ
Dept of Surgery
Box 70575
Johnson City, TN 37614-0575
Tel: 423 439-6267 *Fax:* 423 439-6259
E-mail: wells@etsu.edu
Internet: http://www.etsu.edu/surgery
Accred Length: 5 Years *Program Size:* 26 (*GY1:* 8)
Program ID: 440-47-21-377

Knoxville

University of Tennessee Medical Center at Knoxville Program
Sponsor: University of Tennessee Graduate School of Medicine
University of Tennessee Memorial Hospital
Program Director:
Mitchell H Goldman, MD
Univ of Tennessee Grad Sch of Med
1924 Alcoa Hwy
Knoxville, TN 37920-6999
Tel: 423 544-9230 *Fax:* 423 544-8894
E-mail: hamilto1@utk.edu
Internet: http://www.mc.utk.edu/docs/surgery
Accred Length: 5 Years *Program Size:* 22 (*GY1:* 5)
Subspecialties: CCS, TY, VS
Program ID: 440-47-11-321

Memphis

University of Tennessee Program
Sponsor: University of Tennessee College of Medicine
Baptist Memorial Hospital
Methodist Hospitals of Memphis-Central
Regional Medical Center at Memphis
University of Tennessee Medical Center (UT Bowld Hospital)
Veterans Affairs Medical Center (Memphis)
Program Director:
Eugene Mangiante, MD
956 Court Ave
Memphis, TN 38163
Tel: 901 448-4541 *Fax:* 901 448-7306
Accred Length: 5 Years *Program Size:* 63 (*GY1:* 23)
Subspecialties: CCS, TY, VS
Program ID: 440-47-21-324

Nashville

Vanderbilt University Program
Sponsor: Vanderbilt University Medical Center
St Thomas Hospital
Veterans Affairs Medical Center (Nashville)
Program Director:
James A O'Neill Jr, MD
Vanderbilt Univ Med Ctr
Dept of Surgery/D-4314 MCN
1161 21st Ave S
Nashville, TN 37232-2730
Tel: 615 343-6642 *Fax:* 615 343-0017
E-mail: doris.risley@mcmail.vanderbilt.edu
Internet:
http://www.mc.vanderbilt.edu/surgery/training-program-1.html
Accred Length: 5 Years *Program Size:* 65 (*GY1:* 27)
Subspecialties: CCS, VS
Program ID: 440-47-21-327

Texas

Dallas

Baylor University Medical Center Program
Sponsor: Baylor University Medical Center
John Peter Smith Hospital (Tarrant County Hospital District)
Program Director:
Ronald C Jones, MD
Baylor Univ Med Ctr
Dept of Surgery
3500 Gaston Ave
Dallas, TX 75246-9989
Tel: 214 820-2468 *Fax:* 214 820-4538
E-mail: rh.kenitzer@baylordallas.edu
Internet: http://www.bhcs.com/bumc/medicaleducation/residencies.htm
Accred Length: 5 Years *Program Size:* 40 (*GY1:* 11)
Subspecialties: VS
Program ID: 440-48-21-328

Methodist Hospitals of Dallas Program
Sponsor: Methodist Hospitals of Dallas
Program Director:
Ernest L Dunn, MD
Methodist Hospitals of Dallas, Med Education
PO Box 655999
Dallas, TX 75265-5999
Tel: 214 947-2303 *Fax:* 214 947-2361
E-mail: berta@mhdcme.org
Internet: http://www.mhdcme.org
Accred Length: 5 Years *Program Size:* 12 (*GY1:* 5)
Program ID: 440-48-12-329

University of Texas Southwestern Medical School Program
Sponsor: University of Texas Southwestern Medical School
Dallas County Hospital District-Parkland Memorial Hospital
Veterans Affairs Medical Center (Dallas)
Program Director:
R James Valentine, MD
Univ of Texas Southwestern Med Ctr
Dept of Surgery
5323 Harry Hines Blvd
Dallas, TX 75235-9159
Tel: 214 648-3515 *Fax:* 214 648-7969
E-mail: jcraig@mednet.swmed.edu
Internet: http://www.swmed.edu
Accred Length: 5 Years *Program Size:* 99 (*GY1:* 33)
Subspecialties: CCS, PDS, VS
Program ID: 440-48-21-331

El Paso

Texas Tech University (El Paso) Program
Sponsor: Texas Tech University Health Sciences Center at El Paso
R E Thomason General Hospital
Program Director:
Edward C Saltzstein, MD
Texas Tech Univ Health Sciences Ctr
Dept of Surgery
4800 Alberta Ave
El Paso, TX 79905-1298
Tel: 915 545-6855, ext 6872 *Fax:* 915 545-6864
Accred Length: 5 Years *Program Size:* 12 (*GY1:* 4)
Subspecialties: TY
Program ID: 440-48-11-332

William Beaumont Army Medical Center Program
Sponsor: William Beaumont Army Medical Center
Program Director:
Lt Col Stephen P Hetz, MD
William Beaumont Army Med Ctr
General Surgery Service
5005 N Piedras St
El Paso, TX 79920-5001
Tel: 915 569-2698 *Fax:* 915 569-2602
Internet: http://www.wbamc.amedd.army.mil
Accred Length: 5 Years *Program Size:* 16 (*GY1:* 4)
Subspecialties: TY
Program ID: 440-48-12-009
US Armed Services Program

Fort Sam Houston

San Antonio Uniformed Services Health Education Consortium (BAMC) Program
Sponsor: San Antonio Uniformed Services Health Education Consortium
Brooke Army Medical Center
Program Director:
R Russell Martin, MD
General Surgery Program
Brooke Army Med Ctr
3851 Roger Brooke Dr
Fort Sam Houston, TX 78234-6200
Tel: 210 916-0439 *Fax:* 210 916-2202
Accred Length: 5 Years *Program Size:* 25 (*GY1:* 12)
Subspecialties: CCS, TY
Program ID: 440-48-22-010
US Armed Services Program

Galveston

University of Texas Medical Branch Hospitals Program
Sponsor: University of Texas Medical Branch Hospitals
Program Director:
Courtney M Townsend Jr, MD
Univ of Texas Med Branch Hospitals
Dept of Surgery
301 University Blvd
Galveston, TX 77555-0527
Tel: 409 772-1875 *Fax:* 409 772-6368
Internet: http://www.utmb.edu/surgery
Accred Length: 5 Years *Program Size:* 34 (*GY1:* 15)
Program ID: 440-48-11-333

Houston

Baylor College of Medicine Program
Sponsor: Baylor College of Medicine
Harris County Hospital District-Ben Taub General Hospital
Methodist Hospital
Veterans Affairs Medical Center (Houston)
Program Director:
Charles H McCollum, MD
Baylor Coll of Med
Surgery Education Office
One Baylor Plaza/Rm 404D
Houston, TX 77030
Tel: 713 798-6078 *Fax:* 713 798-8941
E-mail: hchurch@bcm.tmc.edu
Internet:
http://www.bcm.tmc.edu/surgery/edu-residency.html#general
Accred Length: 5 Years *Program Size:* 68 (*GY1:* 25)
Subspecialties: VS
Program ID: 440-48-21-334

St Joseph Hospital Program

Sponsor: St Joseph Hospital
Brackenridge Hospital
University of Texas M D Anderson Cancer Center

Program Director:
Joseph C Gathe, MD
St Joseph Hospital
1919 LaBranch
Houston, TX 77002
Tel: 713 756-5684 *Fax:* 713 657-7136
Accred Length: 5 Years *Program Size:* 18 (*GY1:* 6)
Subspecialties: TY
Program ID: 440-48-22-335

University of Texas at Houston Program

Sponsor: University of Texas Medical School at Houston
Lyndon B Johnson General Hospital
Memorial Hermann Healthcare System
University of Texas M D Anderson Cancer Center

Program Director:
John R Potts III, MD
Univ of Texas-Houston Med Sch
Dept of Surgery
6431 Fannin St/MSB 4268
Houston, TX 77030
Tel: 713 500-7219 *Fax:* 713 500-7239
E-mail: jpotts@utsurg.med.uth.tmc.edu
Internet: http://www.utsurg.edu
Accred Length: 5 Years *Program Size:* 46 (*GY1:* 19)
Subspecialties: CCS, TY
Program ID: 440-48-21-337

Lackland AFB

San Antonio Uniformed Services Health Education Consortium (WHMC) Program

Sponsor: San Antonio Uniformed Services Health Education Consortium
Wilford Hall Medical Center (AETC)

Program Director:
David L Smith, MD
959 MDOS/MMKG
2200 Bergquist Dr/Ste 1
Lackland AFB
San Antonio, TX 78236-5300
Tel: 210 292-5906 *Fax:* 210 292-3893
E-mail: smith_da@whmc-lafb.af.mil
Accred Length: 5 Years *Program Size:* 34 (*GY1:* 16)
Subspecialties: TY
Program ID: 440-48-21-004
US Armed Services Program

Lubbock

Texas Tech University (Lubbock) Program

Sponsor: Texas Tech University Health Sciences Center at Lubbock
University Medical Center

Program Director:
Stuart R Lacey, MD
Texas Tech Univ Health Sciences Ctr
3601 4th St
Lubbock, TX 79430
Tel: 806 743-2370 *Fax:* 806 743-2113
Accred Length: 5 Years *Program Size:* 18 (*GY1:* 5)
Program ID: 440-48-21-363

San Antonio

University of Texas Health Science Center at San Antonio Program

Sponsor: University of Texas Medical School at San Antonio
Audie L Murphy Memorial Veterans Hospital (San Antonio)
University Hospital-South Texas Medical Center

Program Director:
Kenneth R Sirinek, MD PhD
Univ of Texas Health Science Ctr
Dept of Surgery
7703 Floyd Curl Dr
San Antonio, TX 78284-7842
Tel: 210 567-5711 *Fax:* 210 567-6609
E-mail: dahlm@uthscsa.edu
Accred Length: 5 Years *Program Size:* 43 (*GY1:* 21)
Program ID: 440-48-21-338

Temple

Texas A&M College of Medicine-Scott and White Program

Sponsor: Scott and White Memorial Hospital
Central Texas Veterans Affairs Healthcare System

Program Director:
Randall W Smith, MD
Texas A&M-Scott and White
Grad Med Educ
2401 S 31st St
Temple, TX 76508-0001
Tel: 817 724-2366 *Fax:* 817 724-5473
E-mail: lmikeska@swmail.sw.org
Internet: http://www.sw.org
Accred Length: 5 Years *Program Size:* 15 (*GY1:* 3)
Program ID: 440-48-21-339

Utah

Salt Lake City

University of Utah Program

Sponsor: University of Utah Medical Center
LDS Hospital
Salt Lake Regional Medical Center
Veterans Affairs Medical Center (Salt Lake City)

Program Director:
James M McGreevy, MD
Univ of Utah Health Sciences Ctr
50 N Medical Dr
3B324 SOM
Salt Lake City, UT 84132
Tel: 801 581-4488 *Fax:* 801 581-6612
E-mail: mcgreevy@msscc.med.utah.edu
Internet: http://www.utah.med.edu
Accred Length: 5 Years *Program Size:* 40 (*GY1:* 15)
Subspecialties: TY
Program ID: 440-49-21-340

Vermont

Burlington

University of Vermont Program

Sponsor: Fletcher Allen Health Care

Program Director:
James C Hebert, MD
Univ of Vermont-Fletcher Allen Health Care
Surgery Education Office
Fletcher 309/MCHV Campus
Burlington, VT 05401
Tel: 802 656-2566 *Fax:* 802 656-5552
E-mail: judith.mcgivney@vtmednet.org
Internet: http://salus.med.uvm.edu/~cyberdoc/surgery
Accred Length: 5 Years *Program Size:* 26 (*GY1:* 10)
Program ID: 440-50-21-341

Virginia

Charlottesville

University of Virginia Program

Sponsor: University of Virginia Medical Center
Veterans Affairs Medical Center (Salem)

Program Director:
John Minasi, MD
Univ of Virginia Hospitals
Dept of Surgery
PO Box 10005
Charlottesville, VA 22906-0005
Tel: 804 924-2180 *Fax:* 804 924-1238
Internet:
http://www.med.virginia.edu/medicine/clinical/surgery
Accred Length: 5 Years *Program Size:* 46 (*GY1:* 23)
Subspecialties: VS
Program ID: 440-51-21-342

Norfolk

Eastern Virginia Medical School Program

Sponsor: Eastern Virginia Medical School
DePaul Medical Center
Sentara Leigh Hospital
Sentara Norfolk General Hospital
Veterans Affairs Medical Center (Hampton)

Program Director:
L D Britt, MD MPH
Eastern Virginia Med Sch
Dept of Surgery
825 Fairfax Ave
Norfolk, VA 23507-1912
Tel: 757 446-8950 *Fax:* 757 446-5197
E-mail: mem@mccoy.evms.edu
Internet: http://www.evms.edu
Accred Length: 5 Years *Program Size:* 26 (*GY1:* 8)
Subspecialties: VS
Program ID: 440-51-21-343

Portsmouth

Naval Medical Center (Portsmouth) Program

Sponsor: Naval Medical Center (Portsmouth)
Sentara Norfolk General Hospital

Program Director:
William A Liston, MD
Dept of General Surgery
620 John Paul Jones Cir
Portsmouth, VA 23708-2197
Tel: 757 953-5460 *Fax:* 757 953-5463
E-mail: waliston@pnh10.med.navy.mil
Internet: http://www.nmcp.med.navy.mil
Accred Length: 5 Years *Program Size:* 23 (*GY1:* 14)
Subspecialties: TY
Program ID: 440-51-32-015
US Armed Services Program

Richmond

Medical College of Virginia/Virginia Commonwealth University Program

Sponsor: Medical College of Virginia/Virginia Commonwealth University
Hunter Holmes McGuire VA Medical Center (Richmond)
Medical College of Virginia Hospitals

Program Director:
Jeannie F Savas, MD
Box 980135/MCV Station
1200 E Broad St
Richmond, VA 23298-0135
Tel: 804 828-7880 *Fax:* 804 828-2760
E-mail: surgery@gems.vcu.edu
Internet: http://www.surgery.vcu.edu
Accred Length: 5 Years *Program Size:* 55 (*GY1:* 22)
Subspecialties: VS
Program ID: 440-51-21-344

Roanoke

Carilion Health System Program

Sponsor: Carilion Health System
Carilion Roanoke Community Hospital
Carilion Roanoke Memorial Hospital

Program Director:
Ross S Davies, MD
Carilion Roanoke Memorial Hospital
Belleview Ave at Jefferson St
PO Box 13367
Roanoke, VA 24033
Tel: 540 981-8280 *Fax:* 540 981-8681
E-mail: lfeathers@carilion.com
Internet: http://www.carilion.com/residency
Accred Length: 5 Years *Program Size:* 20 (*GY1:* 6)
Subspecialties: TY
Program ID: 440-51-31-345

Washington

Seattle

Swedish Medical Center-Seattle Program

Sponsor: Swedish Medical Center-Seattle
Harborview Medical Center

Program Director:
Michael Hart, MD
Swedish Med Ctr-Seattle
747 Broadway/A Fl W
Seattle, WA 98122-4307
Tel: 206 386-2123 *Fax:* 206 386-3180
E-mail: pbrooks@swedish.org
Accred Length: 5 Years *Program Size:* 13 (*GY1:* 4)
Program ID: 440-54-32-347

University of Washington Program

Sponsor: University of Washington School of Medicine
Harborview Medical Center
Providence Seattle Medical Center
University of Washington Medical Center
Veterans Affairs Medical Center (Seattle)

Program Director:
Hugh M Foy, MD
Univ of Washington
Dept of Surgery/Box 356410
1959 NE Pacific St
Seattle, WA 98195-6410
Tel: 206 543-3687 *Fax:* 206 543-8136
E-mail: hughfoy@u.washington.edu
Internet: http://www.weber.u.washington.edu/~surgweb/
Accred Length: 5 Years *Program Size:* 55 (*GY1:* 24)
Subspecialties: CCS, VS
Program ID: 440-54-21-348

Virginia Mason Medical Center Program

Sponsor: Virginia Mason Medical Center
Harborview Medical Center

Program Director:
Richard C Thirlby, MD
Virginia Mason Med Ctr
Grad Med Educ/H8-GME
925 Seneca St
Seattle, WA 98111
Tel: 206 583-6079 *Fax:* 206 583-2307
Internet: http://www.vmmc.org
Accred Length: 5 Years *Program Size:* 28 (*GY1:* 8)
Subspecialties: TY
Program ID: 440-54-12-349

Tacoma

Madigan Army Medical Center Program

Sponsor: Madigan Army Medical Center

Program Director:
William C Williard III, MD
Madigan Army Med Ctr
Dept of Surgery
Tacoma, WA 98431
Tel: 253 968-2200 *Fax:* 253 968-0232
Internet: http://www.mamc.amedd.army.mil
Accred Length: 5 Years *Program Size:* 21 (*GY1:* 9)
Program ID: 440-54-12-011
US Armed Services Program

West Virginia

Charleston

West Virginia University (Charleston Division) Program

Sponsor: Charleston Area Medical Center

Program Director:
James P Boland, MD
Dept of Surgery
Robert C Byrd Health Sciences Ctr
3110 MacCorkle Ave SE
Charleston, WV 25304
Tel: 304 347-1333 *Fax:* 304 347-1343
E-mail: jwiseman@camcare.com
Accred Length: 5 Years *Program Size:* 17 (*GY1:* 5)
Program ID: 440-55-11-351

Huntington

Marshall University School of Medicine Program

Sponsor: Marshall University School of Medicine
Cabell Huntington Hospital
St Mary's Hospital
Veterans Affairs Medical Center (Huntington)

Program Director:
John T Walker, MD
Marshall Univ Sch of Med
Dept of Surgery
1600 Medical Center Dr/Ste 2500
Huntington, WV 25701-3655
Tel: 304 691-1280 *Fax:* 304 691-1287
E-mail: campbel5@marshall.edu
Internet: http://www.musom.marshall.edu
Accred Length: 5 Years *Program Size:* 18 (*GY1:* 6)
Subspecialties: TY
Program ID: 440-55-21-366

Morgantown

West Virginia University Program

Sponsor: West Virginia University Hospitals
Louis A Johnson Veterans Affairs Medical Center

Program Director:
Ronald C Hill, MD
West Virginia Univ
Dept of Surgery/Rm 4075
PO Box 9238/Hlth Sci Ctr N
Morgantown, WV 26506-9238
Tel: 304 293-3311, ext 1254 *Fax:* 304 293-4711
Accred Length: 5 Years *Program Size:* 22 (*GY1:* 8)
Program ID: 440-55-21-352

Wisconsin

La Crosse

Gundersen Lutheran Medical Foundation Program

Sponsor: Gundersen Lutheran Medical Foundation
Gundersen Clinic
Lutheran Hospital-La Crosse

Program Director:
Thomas H Cogbill, MD
Gundersen Med Foundation
Lutheran Hospital-La Crosse
1836 South Ave
La Crosse, WI 54601-5429
Tel: 608 782-7300, ext 2431 *Fax:* 608 791-4460
E-mail: coheron@gc.gundluth.org
Internet: http://www.gundluth.org
Accred Length: 5 Years *Program Size:* 10 (*GY1:* 2)
Subspecialties: TY
Program ID: 440-56-12-354

Madison

University of Wisconsin Program

Sponsor: University of Wisconsin Hospital and Clinics
William S Middleton Veterans Hospital

Program Director:
James R Starling, MD
Univ of Wisconsin Hospital and Clinics
600 Highland Ave
H4/710 Clinical Science Ctr
Madison, WI 53792-7375
Tel: 608 263-9792 *Fax:* 608 265-5963
Internet:
http://www.medsch.wisc.edu/surgery/home.html
Accred Length: 5 Years *Program Size:* 29 (*GY1:* 5)
Program ID: 440-56-21-355

Marshfield

Marshfield Clinic-St Joseph's Hospital Program

Sponsor: Marshfield Clinic-St Joseph's Hospital

Program Director:
Anselmo Nunez, MD
Marshfield Clinic
Dept of General Surgery 3F1
1000 N Oak Ave
Marshfield, WI 54449
Tel: 715 387-9222 *Fax:* 715 387-5240
E-mail: fuchsk@mfldclin.edu
Internet:
http://www.marshmed.org/mfldclin/education/med_ed/residency/resident.htm
Accred Length: 5 Years *Program Size:* 10 (*GY1:* 2)
Subspecialties: TY
Program ID: 440-56-31-356

Milwaukee

Medical College of Wisconsin Program

Sponsor: Medical College of Wisconsin Affiliated Hospitals Inc
Clement J Zablocki Veterans Affairs Medical Center
Froedtert Memorial Lutheran Hospital

Program Director:
Henry A Pitt, MD
Med Coll of Wisconsin
Dept of Surgery
9200 W Wisconsin Ave
Milwaukee, WI 53226
Tel: 414 454-5751 *Fax:* 414 454-0152
E-mail: mprosper@mcw.edu
Internet: http://www.mcw.edu/tsur
Accred Length: 5 Years *Program Size:* 35 (*GY1:* 8)
Subspecialties: CCS, VS
Program ID: 440-56-21-357

Surgical Critical Care (General Surgery)

California

Fresno

University of California (San Francisco)/Fresno Program

Sponsor: UCSF-Fresno Medical Education Program
University Medical Center

Program Director:
Krista L Kaups, MD
Univ Med Ctr
445 S Cedar Ave
Dept of Surgery
Fresno, CA 93702-2998
Tel: 209 459-3770 *Fax:* 209 459-3719
E-mail: kaups@ucsfresno.edu
Accred Length: 1 Year *Program Size:* 1
Program ID: 442-05-21-067

Los Angeles

Cedars-Sinai Medical Center Program

Sponsor: Cedars-Sinai Medical Center

Program Director:
M Michael Shabot, MD
Cedars-Sinai Med Ctr
Dept of Surgery/Rm 8215
8700 Beverly Blvd
Los Angeles, CA 90048
Tel: 310 855-5873 *Fax:* 310 967-0139
E-mail: shabot@csmc.edu
Internet: http://www.csmc.edu/sicu
Accred Length: 1 Year *Program Size:* 2
Program ID: 442-05-21-046

University of Southern California Program

Sponsor: Los Angeles County-USC Medical Center

Program Director:
Thomas V Berne, MD
Los Angeles County-USC Med Ctr
Dept of Surgery
1200 N State St/Rm 9900
Los Angeles, CA 90033-4525
Tel: 323 226-7720 *Fax:* 323 226-5996
E-mail: berne@usc.edu
Internet:
http://www.usc.edu/hsc/medicine/surgery/trauma.
Accred Length: 1 Year *Program Size:* 2
Program ID: 442-05-31-058

Orange

University of California (Irvine) Program

Sponsor: University of California (Irvine) Medical Center

Program Director:
Marianne Cinat, MD
Univ of California Irvine Med Ctr
101 City Dr S
Route 81/Bldg 53 Rm 211
Orange, CA 92868
Tel: 714 456-7252 *Fax:* 714 456-8205
Internet: http://www.meded.uci.edu/~surgery/
Accred Length: 1 Year *Program Size:* 1
Program ID: 442-05-21-003

Sacramento

University of California (Davis) Program

Sponsor: University of California (Davis) Medical Center

Program Director:
David H Wisner, MD
Univ of California Davis Med Ctr
Dept of Surgery
4301 X St/Rm 2230
Sacramento, CA 95817
Tel: 916 734-8298 *Fax:* 916 734-3951
E-mail: dhwisner@ucdavis.edu
Internet: http://web.ucdmc.ucdavis.edu/surgery
Accred Length: 1 Year *Program Size:* 2
Program ID: 442-05-21-017

San Diego

University of California (San Diego) Program

Sponsor: University of California (San Diego) Medical Center

Program Director:
David B Hoyt, MD
UCSD Med Ctr
200 W Arbor Dr
San Diego, CA 92103-8896
Tel: 619 294-6400 *Fax:* 619 293-0920
E-mail: dhoyt@ucsd.edu
Accred Length: 1 Year *Program Size:* 2
Program ID: 442-05-21-052

Connecticut

Farmington

University of Connecticut Program

Sponsor: University of Connecticut School of Medicine
Hartford Hospital

Program Director:
Kevin P Keating, MD
Hartford Hospital
80 Seymour St
PO Box 5037
Hartford, CT 06102-5037
Tel: 860 545-5201 *Fax:* 860 545-3266
E-mail: kkeatin@harthosp.org
Accred Length: 1 Year *Program Size:* 4
Program ID: 442-08-21-020

New Haven

Yale-New Haven Medical Center Program

Sponsor: Yale-New Haven Hospital
Bridgeport Hospital

Program Director:
Peter B Angood, MD
Yale Univ Sch of Med
Dept of Surgery
333 Cedar St/LH118
New Haven, CT 06520
Tel: 203 785-2572 *Fax:* 203 785-3950
E-mail: peter.angood@yale.edu
Accred Length: 1 Year *Program Size:* 2
Program ID: 442-08-21-045

District of Columbia

Washington

Washington Hospital Center Program

Sponsor: Washington Hospital Center

Program Director:
John R Kirkpatrick, MD
Washington Hospital Ctr
Dept of Surgery
110 Irving St NW/Rm G253
Washington, DC 20010
Tel: 202 877-3536 *Fax:* 202 877-3699
Accred Length: 1 Year *Program Size:* 3
Program ID: 442-10-21-048

Florida

Miami

University of Miami-Jackson Memorial Medical Center Program

Sponsor: University of Miami-Jackson Memorial Medical Center

Program Director:
Mark McKenney, MD
Univ of Miami Sch of Med
PO Box 016960 D-40
Miami, FL 33101
Tel: 305 585-1292 *Fax:* 305 326-7065
E-mail: mark@miami.edu
Internet: http://trauma.med.miami.edu/rtc.htm
Accred Length: 1 Year *Program Size:* 5
Program ID: 442-11-21-004

Orlando

Orlando Regional Healthcare System Program

Sponsor: Orlando Regional Medical Center

Program Director:
Loren D Nelson, MD
Orlando Regional Healthcare System
86 W Underwood St/Ste 201
Orlando, FL 32806
Tel: 407 841-5296 *Fax:* 407 648-3686
E-mail: lorenn@orhs.org
Internet: http://www.orhs-surged.org
Accred Length: 1 Year *Program Size:* 2
Program ID: 442-11-21-068

Georgia

Atlanta

Emory University Program

Sponsor: Emory University School of Medicine
Emory University Hospital
Grady Memorial Hospital

Program Director:
Grace S Rozycki, MD
69 Butler St SE
Room 302
Atlanta, GA 30303
Tel: 404 616-3553 *Fax:* 404 616-7333
E-mail: grozyck@emory.edu
Accred Length: 1 Year *Program Size:* 1
Program ID: 442-12-21-069

Hawaii

Honolulu

University of Hawaii Program

Sponsor: University of Hawaii John A Burns School of Medicine
Queen's Medical Center

Program Director:
Mihae Yu, MD
Univ of Hawaii
John A Burns Sch of Med
1356 Lusitana St/6th Fl
Honolulu, HI 96813
Tel: 808 537-7297 *Fax:* 808 537-7825
E-mail: yum@jabsom.biomed.hawaii.edu
Accred Length: 1 Year *Program Size:* 1
Program ID: 442-14-21-036

Illinois

Chicago

University of Illinois College of Medicine at Chicago Metropolitan Group Hospitals Program

Sponsor: University of Illinois College of Medicine at Chicago
Illinois Masonic Medical Center

Program Director:
Richard J Fantus, MD
Illinois Masonic Med Ctr
836 W Wellington Ave
Chicago, IL 60657
Tel: 773 296-7033 *Fax:* 773 296-7199
E-mail: rfantus@immc.org
Accred Length: 1 Year *Program Size:* 1
Program ID: 442-16-21-060

Kentucky

Louisville

University of Louisville Program

Sponsor: University of Louisville School of Medicine
University of Louisville Hospital

Program Director:
David A Spain, MD
Univ of Louisville Sch of Med
Dept of Surgery
Louisville, KY 40292
Tel: 502 852-5676 *Fax:* 502 852-8915
E-mail: daspai01@ulkyvm.louisville.edu
Internet: http://www.louisvillesurgery.com
Accred Length: 1 Year *Program Size:* 2
Program ID: 442-20-21-059

Louisiana

New Orleans

Tulane University Program

Sponsor: Tulane University School of Medicine
Medical Center of Louisiana at New Orleans
Veterans Affairs Medical Center-LSU Service (New Orleans)

Program Director:
Mary Jo Wright, MD
Tulane Univ Sch of Med
1430 Tulane Ave/Box SL-27
New Orleans, LA 70112
Tel: 504 588-5336 *Fax:* 504 584-1874
Internet: http://www.mcl.tulane.edu/departments/dept surg.htm
Accred Length: 1 Year *Program Size:* 1
Program ID: 442-21-21-057

Maryland

Baltimore

Johns Hopkins University Program

Sponsor: Johns Hopkins University School of Medicine
Johns Hopkins Hospital

Program Director:
Pamela A Lipsett, MD
Johns Hopkins Univ Sch of Med
Blalock 605
600 N Wolfe St
Baltimore, MD 21287-4605
Tel: 410 955-3739 *Fax:* 410 614-9083
E-mail: plipsett@welchlink.welch.edu
Accred Length: 1 Year *Program Size:* 3
Program ID: 442-23-31-009

University of Maryland Program

Sponsor: University of Maryland Medical System

Program Director:
Lena M Napolitano, MD
Univ of Maryland Sch of Med
Dept of Surgery
22 S Greene St
Baltimore, MD 21201
Tel: 410 328-5830 *Fax:* 410 328-0687
E-mail: lnapolitano@surgery1.umaryland.edu
Internet: http://www.umaryland.edu
Accred Length: 1 Year *Program Size:* 8
Program ID: 442-23-21-032

Massachusetts

Boston

Beth Israel Deaconess Medical Center (West Campus) Program

Sponsor: Beth Israel Deaconess Medical Center
Brigham and Women's Hospital

Program Director:
R Armour Forse, MD PhD
Beth Israel Deaconess Med Ctr
110 Francis St/Ste 3A
Boston, MA 02215-2215
Tel: 617 632-9864 *Fax:* 617 632-7424
E-mail: aforse@bidmc.harvard.edu
Accred Length: 1 Year *Program Size:* 1
Program ID: 442-24-21-042

Boston University Medical Center Program
Sponsor: Boston Medical Center
Program Director:
Richard C Dennis, MD
Boston Med Ctr
Critical Care Med A2707
One Boston Medical Center Pl
Boston, MA 02118-2393
Tel: 617 638-6406 *Fax:* 617 638-6452
E-mail: sarah.mccoy@bmc.edu
Internet: http://www.bumc.edu/
Accred Length: 1 Year *Program Size:* 4
Program ID: 442-24-21-011

Massachusetts General Hospital Program
Sponsor: Massachusetts General Hospital
Program Director:
Ralph L Warren, MD
Massachusetts General Hospital, Dept of Surgery
GRB 1302
55 Fruit St
Boston, MA 02114-0000
Tel: 617 726-3712 *Fax:* 617 726-4127
E-mail: rwarren@partners.org
Accred Length: 1 Year *Program Size:* 2
Program ID: 442-24-21-054

Worcester

University of Massachusetts Program
Sponsor: University of Massachusetts Medical School
UMass Memorial Health Care (University Campus)
Program Director:
Paul Bankey, MD
Univ of Massachusetts Med Sch
55 Lake Ave N
Worcester, MA 01655-0000
Tel: 508 856-3682 *Fax:* 508 856-4224
Accred Length: 1 Year *Program Size:* 2
Program ID: 442-24-21-012

Michigan

Ann Arbor

University of Michigan Program
Sponsor: University of Michigan Hospitals
Program Director:
Robert H Bartlett, MD
1500 E Medical Center Dr
TC-2920 Taubman Health Care Ctr
Ann Arbor, MI 48109-0331
Tel: 734 936-5822 *Fax:* 734 936-5830
Accred Length: 1 Year *Program Size:* 6
Program ID: 442-25-21-013

Detroit

Henry Ford Hospital Program
Sponsor: Henry Ford Hospital
Program Director:
H Mathilda Horst, MD
Henry Ford Hospital
2799 W Grand Blvd
Detroit, MI 48202
Tel: 313 916-1052 *Fax:* 313 916-8007
Accred Length: 1 Year *Program Size:* 2
Program ID: 442-25-21-026

Wayne State University/Detroit Medical Center Program
Sponsor: Wayne State University/Detroit Medical Center
Program Director:
Michael D Klein, MD
Children's Hospital
Dept of Ped Surgery
3901 Beaubien Blvd
Detroit, MI 48201
Tel: 313 745-5840 *Fax:* 313 831-3908
Accred Length: 1 Year *Program Size:* 1
Program ID: 442-25-31-027

Grand Rapids

Spectrum Health-Downtown Campus/Michigan State University Program
Sponsor: Spectrum Health-Downtown Campus
Program Director:
Bruce W Bonnell, MD
221 Michigan St NE
Ste 200A
Grand Rapids, MI 49503
Tel: 616 391-3745 *Fax:* 616 391-8611
E-mail: bruce.bonnell@spectrum-health.org
Internet: http://www.spectrum-health.org
Accred Length: 1 Year *Program Size:* 2
Program ID: 442-25-21-014

Minnesota

Minneapolis

University of Minnesota Program
Sponsor: University of Minnesota Medical School
Fairview-University Medical Center
Regions Hospital
Veterans Affairs Medical Center (Minneapolis)
Program Director:
Gregory J Beilman, MD
Univ of Minnesota Hospital and Clinics
420 Delaware St SE
Box 11 UMHC
Minneapolis, MN 55455
Tel: 612 625-7911 *Fax:* 612 626-0439
E-mail: beilm001@maroon.tc.umn.edu
Internet:
http://www.tc.umn.edu/nlhome/g048/buged001/ccm.um/homepage.html
Accred Length: 1 Year *Program Size:* 6
Program ID: 442-26-21-022

Rochester

Mayo Graduate School of Medicine (Rochester) Program
Sponsor: Mayo Graduate School of Medicine-Mayo Foundation
St Mary's Hospital of Rochester
Program Director:
Michael P Bannon, MD
Mayo Graduate Sch of Med
Mayo Clinic
200 First St SW
Rochester, MN 55905
Tel: 507 255-6365 *Fax:* 507 255-9872
E-mail: mgsm.roch.mn.surgery@mayo.edu
Internet: http://www.mayo.edu/
Accred Length: 1 Year *Program Size:* 2
Program ID: 442-26-21-034

Missouri

Columbia

University of Missouri-Columbia Program
Sponsor: University of Missouri-Columbia School of Medicine
University Hospitals and Clinics
Program Director:
Michael H Metzler, MD
Univ of Missouri-Columbia Hospitals and Clinics
Div of General Surgery Rm N323
One Hospital Dr
Columbia, MO 65212
Tel: 573 882-2245 *Fax:* 573 884-4611
E-mail: metzlerm@health.missouri.edu
Internet: http://www.surgery.missouri.edu/
Accred Length: 1 Year *Program Size:* 1
Program ID: 442-28-21-016

Kansas City

University of Missouri at Kansas City Program
Sponsor: University of Missouri-Kansas City School of Medicine
Children's Mercy Hospital
Program Director:
Ronald J Sharp, MD
2401 Gillham Rd
Kansas City, MO 64108
Tel: 816 234-3574 *Fax:* 816 234-3821
Accred Length: 1 Year *Program Size:* 1
Program ID: 442-28-21-071

St Louis

St Louis University School of Medicine Program
Sponsor: St Louis University School of Medicine
St John's Mercy Medical Center
St Louis University School of Medicine
Program Director:
Rodney M Durham, MD
St Louis Univ Sch of Med
3635 Vista Ave
PO Box 15250
St Louis, MO 63110-0250
Tel: 314 577-8317 *Fax:* 314 268-5466
E-mail: surgweb@slu.edu
Internet:
http://www.slu.edu/colleges/med/departments/surgery/
Accred Length: 1 Year *Program Size:* 1
Program ID: 442-28-21-023

Washington University/B-JH/SLCH Consortium Program
Sponsor: Washington University/B-JH/SLCH Consortium
Barnes-Jewish Hospital
Program Director:
Timothy G Buchman, MD PhD
Washington Univ Sch of Med
660 S Euclid Ave/Campus Box 8109
St Louis, MO 63110-1093
Tel: 314 362-9347 *Fax:* 314 362-1185
E-mail: buchman@msnotes.wustl.edu
Internet: http://www.surgery.wustl.edu/criticalcare/
Accred Length: 1 Year *Program Size:* 2
Program ID: 442-28-21-051

New Jersey

Camden

UMDNJ-Robert Wood Johnson Medical School (Camden) Program

Sponsor: Cooper Hospital-University Medical Center

Program Director:
Gus J Slotman, MD
Cooper Hospital-Univ Med Ctr
Div of Surg Crit Care
3 Cooper Plaza/Ste 411
Camden, NJ 08103
Tel: 609 963-3673 *Fax:* 609 541-5379
E-mail: slotman@rwjcam.umdnj.edu
Internet: http://www.umdnj.edu
Accred Length: 1 Year *Program Size:* 3
Program ID: 442-33-21-031

Newark

UMDNJ-New Jersey Medical School Program

Sponsor: UMDNJ-New Jersey Medical School
UMDNJ-University Hospital

Program Director:
David H Livingston, MD
UMDNJ-New Jersey Trauma Ctr
Univ Hospital E-245
150 Bergen St
Newark, NJ 07103-2406
Tel: 973 972-4900 *Fax:* 973 972-7411
E-mail: livingst@umdnj.edu
Internet: http://www.umdnj.edu/snjmsweb/title.htm
Accred Length: 1 Year *Program Size:* 1
Program ID: 442-33-21-049

New Mexico

Albuquerque

University of New Mexico Program

Sponsor: University of New Mexico School of Medicine
University Hospital

Program Director:
Roxie M Albrecht, MD
Univ of New Mexico Health Sciences Ctr
Dept of Surgery ACC 2nd Fl
Albuquerque, NM 87131
Tel: 505 272-4161 *Fax:* 505 272-4159
E-mail: ralbrecht@salud.unm.edu
Accred Length: 1 Year *Program Size:* 1
Program ID: 442-34-21-073

New York

Bronx

Lincoln Medical and Mental Health Center Program

Sponsor: Lincoln Medical and Mental Health Center

Program Director:
Joseph S Edwards, MD
234 E 149th St
Bronx, NY 10451
Tel: 718 579-5890 *Fax:* 718 579-4620
Accred Length: 1 Year *Program Size:* 3
Program ID: 442-35-31-033

Manhasset

North Shore University Hospital/NYU School of Medicine Program

Sponsor: North Shore University Hospital

Program Director:
Akram Talhouk, MD
North Shore Univ Hospital
300 Community Dr
Manhasset, NY 11030
Tel: 516 562-4862 *Fax:* 516 562-1610
E-mail: atalhouk@nshs.edu
Internet: http://www.nshs.edu
Accred Length: 1 Year *Program Size:* 2
Program ID: 442-35-21-015

Rochester

University of Rochester Program

Sponsor: Strong Memorial Hospital of the University of Rochester
Genesee Hospital
Rochester General Hospital

Program Director:
Palmer Q Bessey, MD
Univ of Rochester Med Ctr
Dept of Surgery
601 Elmwood Ave
Rochester, NY 14642-8410
Tel: 716 275-3376 *Fax:* 716 275-8513
E-mail: palmer_bessey@urmc.rochester.edu
Internet:
http://www.urmc.rochester.edu/smd/surg/resprog.html
Accred Length: 1 Year *Program Size:* 1
Program ID: 442-35-21-025

Valhalla

New York Medical College at Westchester Medical Center Program

Sponsor: New York Medical College
Westchester Medical Center

Program Director:
John A Savino, MD
Westchester County Med Ctr
Dept of Surgery
Munger Pavillion
Valhalla, NY 10595
Tel: 914 594-4352
Internet:
http://www.nymc.edu/depthome/academic/surgery/surgery.htm
Accred Length: 1 Year *Program Size:* 2
Program ID: 442-35-11-035

North Carolina

Chapel Hill

University of North Carolina Hospitals Program

Sponsor: University of North Carolina Hospitals

Program Director:
Edmund J Rutherford, MD
Univ of North Carolina Hospitals and Clinics
214 Burnett Womack Bldg/CB #7210
Chapel Hill, NC 27599-7210
Tel: 919 962-7555 *Fax:* 919 966-0369
E-mail: ejruther@med.unc.edu
Internet: http://www.med.unc.edu
Accred Length: 1 Year *Program Size:* 2
Program ID: 442-36-21-028

Durham

Duke University Program

Sponsor: Duke University Medical Center
Veterans Affairs Medical Center (Durham)

Program Director:
Mark W Sebastian, MD
Dept of Surgery
Duke Univ Med Ctr
PO Box 31117
Durham, NC 27710
Tel: 919 681-6096 *Fax:* 919 684-4392
E-mail: sebas002@acpub.duke.edu
Accred Length: 1 Year *Program Size:* 2
Program ID: 442-36-21-037

Ohio

Cincinnati

University Hospital/University of Cincinnati College of Medicine Program

Sponsor: University Hospital Inc

Program Director:
Scott B Frame, MD
Univ of Cincinnati Med Ctr
231 Bethesda Ave
Cincinnati, OH 45267-0558
Tel: 513 558-5661 *Fax:* 513 558-3136
Accred Length: 1 Year *Program Size:* 1
Program ID: 442-38-21-063

Cleveland

Case Western Reserve University Program

Sponsor: University Hospitals of Cleveland
MetroHealth Medical Center

Program Director:
Charles J Yowler, MD
MetroHealth Med Ctr
2500 MetroHealth Dr
Cleveland, OH 44109-1998
Tel: 216 778-5627 *Fax:* 216 778-1099
Accred Length: 1 Year *Program Size:* 1
Program ID: 442-38-21-070

Columbus

Ohio State University Program

Sponsor: Ohio State University Medical Center

Program Director:
Larry C Martin, MD
Ohio State Univ Hospital
410 W Tenth Ave
N-748 Doan Hall
Columbus, OH 43210
Tel: 614 293-3451 *Fax:* 614 293-3425
E-mail: hanson-1@medctr.osu.edu
Accred Length: 1 Year *Program Size:* 4
Program ID: 442-38-21-021

Oregon

Portland

Oregon Health Sciences University Program

Sponsor: Oregon Health Sciences University Hospital
Veterans Affairs Medical Center (Portland)

Program Director:
Richard J Mullins, MD
Oregon Health Sciences Univ
3181 SW Sam Jackson Park Rd/L223A
Portland, OR 97201-3098
Tel: 503 494-5300 *Fax:* 503 494-8884
E-mail: mullinsr@ohsu.edu
Internet: http://www.ohsu.edu
Accred Length: 1 Year *Program Size:* 2
Program ID: 442-40-21-064

Pennsylvania

Allentown

Lehigh Valley Hospital/Pennsylvania State University Program

Sponsor: Lehigh Valley Hospital

Program Director:
Michael D Pasquale, MD
Lehigh Valley Hospital
Cedar Crest and I-78
PO Box 689
Allentown, PA 18105-1556
Tel: 610 402-8966 *Fax:* 610 402-1667
E-mail: traumares@lvhhn.org
Internet:
http://www.lvhhn.org/academic/residency/trauma/home.html
Accred Length: 1 Year *Program Size:* 1
Program ID: 442-41-31-047

Hershey

Penn State Geisinger Health System/Milton S Hershey Medical Center Program

Sponsor: Penn State Geisinger Health System
Milton S Hershey Medical Center

Program Director:
Robert N Cooney, MD
Milton S Hershey Med Ctr
PO Box 850
Hershey, PA 17033
Tel: 717 531-6241 *Fax:* 717 531-3649
Accred Length: 1 Year *Program Size:* 1
Program ID: 442-41-21-041

Philadelphia

MCP Hahnemann University Program

Sponsor: MCP Hahnemann University
Hahnemann University Hospital
Medical College of Pennsylvania Hospital

Program Director:
Thomas A Santora, MD
3300 Henry Ave
Philadelphia, PA 19129
Tel: 215 842-6567 *Fax:* 215 843-1095
E-mail: santora@anhs.edu
Accred Length: 1 Year *Program Size:* 5
Program ID: 442-41-21-065

Thomas Jefferson University Program

Sponsor: Thomas Jefferson University Hospital

Program Director:
Murray J Cohen, MD
Pauline K Park, MD
Div of Trauma/Surgical Critical Care
Thomas Jefferson Univ Hospital
118 S 11th St/1st Fl
Philadelphia, PA 19107
Tel: 215 955-2600 *Fax:* 215 955-5570
E-mail: pauline.k.park@mail.tju.edu
Accred Length: 1 Year *Program Size:* 2
Program ID: 442-41-31-066

University of Pennsylvania Program

Sponsor: Hospital of the University of Pennsylvania

Program Director:
Patrick M Reilly, MD
Univ of Pennsylvania Med Ctr
3440 Market St/First Fl
Philadelphia, PA 19104-4283
Tel: 215 662-7320 *Fax:* 215 349-5917
E-mail: reillyp@mail.med.upenn.edu
Internet:
http://www.med.upenn.edu/~traumacc/fell-tcc.html
Accred Length: 1 Year *Program Size:* 8
Program ID: 442-41-21-056

Pittsburgh

University Health Center of Pittsburgh Program

Sponsor: University Health Center of Pittsburgh
Presbyterian University Hospital/UPMC

Program Director:
Samuel Tisherman, MD
Univ Health Ctr of Pittsburgh
Surgical Critical Care Fellowship
612 Scaife Hall
Pittsburgh, PA 15261
Tel: 412 647-3135 *Fax:* 412 647-8060
E-mail: mcctp@smtp.anes.upmc.edu
Internet: http://www.anes.upmc.edu/mcctp
Accred Length: 1 Year *Program Size:* 4
Program ID: 442-41-21-005

Rhode Island

Providence

Brown University Program

Sponsor: Rhode Island Hospital
Miriam Hospital

Program Director:
H Hank Simms, MD
Div of Surg Critical Care/Trauma
Rhode Island Hospital
593 Eddy St/APC 110
Providence, RI 02903
Tel: 401 444-8393 *Fax:* 401 444-6681
Accred Length: 1 Year *Program Size:* 1
Program ID: 442-43-21-044

Tennessee

Knoxville

University of Tennessee Medical Center at Knoxville Program

Sponsor: University of Tennessee Graduate School of Medicine
University of Tennessee Memorial Hospital

Program Director:
Blaine L Enderson, MD
Div of Trauma/Critical Care
Univ of Tennessee Med Ctr-Knoxville
1924 Alcoa Hwy/U-11
Knoxville, TN 37920
Tel: 423 544-9296 *Fax:* 423 544-8894
E-mail: hamilto1@utk.edu
Internet: http://www.mc.utk.edu/docs/surgery
Accred Length: 1 Year *Program Size:* 1
Program ID: 442-47-21-043

Memphis

University of Tennessee Program

Sponsor: University of Tennessee College of Medicine
Regional Medical Center at Memphis

Program Director:
Timothy C Fabian, MD
Univ of Tennessee
Dept of Surgery
956 Court Ave
Memphis, TN 38163
Tel: 901 448-5914 *Fax:* 901 448-7306
Accred Length: 1 Year *Program Size:* 2
Program ID: 442-47-21-024

Nashville

Vanderbilt University Program

Sponsor: Vanderbilt University Medical Center

Program Director:
Virginia A Eddy, MD
Div of Trauma
Vanderbilt Univ Sch of Med
2100 Pierce Ave/243 MCS
Nashville, TN 37212
Tel: 615 936-0175 *Fax:* 615 936-0185
E-mail: virginia.eddy@surgery.mc.vanderbilt.edu
Internet:
http://www.mc.vanderbilt.edu/surgery/trauma/fellow.html
Accred Length: 1 Year *Program Size:* 2
Program ID: 442-47-21-007

Texas

Dallas

University of Texas Southwestern Medical School Program

Sponsor: University of Texas Southwestern Medical School
Dallas County Hospital District-Parkland Memorial Hospital

Program Director:
Joseph P Minei, MD
Univ of Texas Southwestern Med Ctr
Dept of Surgery
5323 Harry Hines Blvd
Dallas, TX 75235-9158
Tel: 214 648-7295 *Fax:* 214 648-5477
E-mail: joseph.minei@email.swmed.edu
Accred Length: 1 Year *Program Size:* 2
Program ID: 442-48-21-001

Fort Sam Houston

San Antonio Uniformed Services Health Education Consortium (BAMC) Program

Sponsor: San Antonio Uniformed Services Health Education Consortium
Brooke Army Medical Center

Program Director:
Maj Stephen F Flaherty, MD
Critical Care/Surgery Program
Brooke Army Med Ctr
3851 Roger Brooke Dr
Fort Sam Houston, TX 78234-6200
Tel: 210 916-4326 *Fax:* 210 916-1602
Accred Length: 1 Year *Program Size:* 1
Program ID: 442-48-22-008
US Armed Services Program

Houston

University of Texas at Houston Program

Sponsor: University of Texas Medical School at Houston
Lyndon B Johnson General Hospital
Memorial Hermann Healthcare System

Program Director:
Christine S Cocanour, MD
6431 Fannin St/MSB 4284
Houston, TX 77030
Tel: 713 500-7244 *Fax:* 713 500-7268
E-mail: cocanour@utsurg.med.uth.tmc.edu
Internet: http://www.utsurg.med.uth.tmc.edu
Accred Length: 1 Year *Program Size:* 2
Program ID: 442-48-21-038

Washington

Seattle

University of Washington Program

Sponsor: University of Washington School of Medicine
Harborview Medical Center

Program Director:
Ronald V Maier, MD
Dept of Surgery/Box 359796
325 Ninth Ave
Seattle, WA 98104-2499
Tel: 206 731-3299 *Fax:* 206 731-8582
E-mail: ronmaier@u.washington.edu
Internet: http://www.weber.u.washington.edu/~surgweb
Accred Length: 1 Year *Program Size:* 3
Program ID: 442-54-21-050

Wisconsin

Milwaukee

Medical College of Wisconsin Program

Sponsor: Medical College of Wisconsin Affiliated Hospitals Inc
Froedtert Memorial Lutheran Hospital

Program Director:
Edward Quebbeman, MD PhD
9200 W Wisconsin Ave
Milwaukee, WI 53226
Tel: 414 454-5835 *Fax:* 414 454-0152
Accred Length: 1 Year *Program Size:* 0
Program ID: 442-56-21-010

Thoracic Surgery

Alabama

Birmingham

University of Alabama Medical Center Program

Sponsor: University of Alabama Hospital
Veterans Affairs Medical Center (Birmingham)

Program Director:
A D Pacifico, MD
Univ of Alabama Med Ctr
Div of Cardiothoracic Surgery
1900 University Blvd/THT Rm 760
Birmingham, AL 35294-0016
Tel: 205 934-6209
E-mail: thoracic.residency@ccc.uab.edu
Accred Length: 2 Years *Program Size:* 4
Program ID: 460-01-21-007

Arizona

Tucson

University of Arizona Program

Sponsor: University of Arizona College of Medicine
University Medical Center
Veterans Affairs Medical Center (Tucson)

Program Director:
Jack G Copeland III, MD
Univ of Arizona Health Sciences Ctr
Cardiothoracic Surgery
PO Box 245071
Tucson, AZ 85724-5071
Tel: 520 626-4341 *Fax:* 520 626-4042
E-mail: dongm@u.arizona.edu
Accred Length: 2 Years *Program Size:* 2
Program ID: 460-03-21-106

Arkansas

Little Rock

University of Arkansas for Medical Sciences Program

Sponsor: University of Arkansas College of Medicine
Arkansas Children's Hospital
John L McClellan Memorial Veterans Hospital
University Hospital of Arkansas

Program Director:
Tamim Antakli Sr, MD
Univ of Arkansas for Med Sciences
4301 W Markham St
Slot 713
Little Rock, AR 72205
Tel: 501 686-7884 *Fax:* 501 686-8503
E-mail: antaklitamim@exchange.uams.edu
Accred Length: 2 Years *Program Size:* 2
Program ID: 460-04-21-008

California

Loma Linda

Loma Linda University Program

Sponsor: Loma Linda University Medical Center
Jerry L Pettis Memorial Veterans Hospital

Program Director:
Steven R Gundry, MD
Loma Linda Univ Med Ctr
Div of Cardiothoracic Surgery
11234 Anderson St/Rm 21121CP
Loma Linda, CA 92354
Tel: 909 824-4354 *Fax:* 909 558-0348
E-mail: sgundry@som.llu.edu
Accred Length: 3 Years *Program Size:* 3
Program ID: 460-05-21-102

Los Angeles

UCLA Medical Center Program

Sponsor: UCLA School of Medicine
Southern California Kaiser Permanente Medical Group
UCLA Medical Center

Program Director:
Hillel Laks, MD
Cardiothoracic Surgery
10833 Le Conte Ave
Los Angeles, CA 90095-1741
Tel: 310 206-8232 *Fax:* 310 825-7473
E-mail: hlaks@surgery.medsch.ucla.edu
Internet: http://149.142.102.4/ct/ct.htm
Accred Length: 2 Years *Program Size:* 4
Program ID: 460-05-21-013

University of Southern California Program

Sponsor: Los Angeles County-USC Medical Center
Children's Hospital of Los Angeles

Program Director:
Vaughn A Starnes, MD
USA Cardiothoracic Surgery Program
LAC+USC Med Ctr-CHLA-Univ Hospital
1510 San Pablo St/Ste 415
Los Angeles, CA 90033-4612
Tel: 323 442-5850 *Fax:* 323 442-5956
Internet: http://www.cts.usc.edu
Accred Length: 2 Years *Program Size:* 5
Program ID: 460-05-22-011

Sacramento

University of California (Davis) Program

Sponsor: University of California (Davis) Medical Center

Program Director:
David M Follette, MD
Univ of California Davis Med Ctr
Div of Cardiothoracic Surgery
4301 X St/Ste 2250
Sacramento, CA 95817
Tel: 916 734-3635 *Fax:* 916 734-5633
E-mail: david.follette@ucdmc.ucdavis.edu
Internet: http://web.ucdmc.ucdavis.edu/surgery
Accred Length: 2 Years *Program Size:* 2
Program ID: 460-05-21-112

Programs

San Diego

University of California (San Diego) Program
Sponsor: University of California (San Diego) Medical Center
Veterans Affairs Medical Center (San Diego)
Program Director:
Stuart W Jamieson, MD
200 W Arbor Dr
San Diego, CA 92103-8892
Tel: 619 543-7777 *Fax:* 619 543-2652
E-mail: sjamieson@ucsd.edu
Accred Length: 2 Years *Program Size:* 2
Program ID: 460-05-21-109

San Francisco

University of California (San Francisco) Program
Sponsor: University of California (San Francisco) School of Medicine
Mount Zion Medical Center of the University of California
University of California (San Francisco) Medical Center
Veterans Affairs Medical Center (San Francisco)
Program Director:
Frank L Hanley, MD
Timothy S Hall, MD
Univ of California San Francisco (Residency Coordinator)
505 Parnassus/M-593
San Francisco, CA 94143-0118
Tel: 415 476-3501 *Fax:* 415 476-9678
E-mail: vcrase@itsa.ucsf.edu
Accred Length: 2 Years *Program Size:* 2
Program ID: 460-05-21-015

Stanford

Stanford University Program
Sponsor: Stanford University Hospital
Veterans Affairs Palo Alto Health Care System
Program Director:
Bruce A Reitz, MD
Stanford Univ Sch of Med
Dept of Cardiothoracic Surg
300 Pasteur Dr
Stanford, CA 94305-5407
Tel: 415 725-3816 *Fax:* 415 725-3846
E-mail: adena.goodart@forsythe.stanford.edu
Accred Length: 3 Years *Program Size:* 6
Program ID: 460-05-21-016

Colorado

Denver

University of Colorado Program
Sponsor: University of Colorado Health Sciences Center
Children's Hospital
Veterans Affairs Medical Center (Denver)
Program Director:
Frederick L Grover, MD
Univ of Colorado Health Sciences Ctr
4200 E Ninth Ave/Box C-310
Denver, CO 80262
Tel: 303 315-8527 *Fax:* 303 315-3065
Internet: http://www.uchsc.edu/sm/surgery
Accred Length: 3 Years *Program Size:* 9
Program ID: 460-07-21-017

Connecticut

New Haven

Yale-New Haven Medical Center Program
Sponsor: Yale-New Haven Hospital
Program Director:
John A Elefteriades, MD
Yale Univ Sch of Med
333 Cedar St
PO Box 208039
New Haven, CT 06520-8039
Tel: 203 785-2704 *Fax:* 203 785-3346
E-mail: john.elefteriades@yale.edu
Internet: http://yalesurgery.med.yale.edu
Accred Length: 2 Years *Program Size:* 4
Program ID: 460-08-21-018

District of Columbia

Washington

George Washington University Program
Sponsor: George Washington University School of Medicine
Children's National Medical Center
George Washington University Hospital (UHS)
Veterans Affairs Medical Center (Washington, DC)
Washington Hospital Center
Program Director:
E Pendleton Alexander, MD
George Washington Univ Med Ctr
2150 Pennsylvania Ave NW
Washington, DC 20037
Tel: 202 994-5573 *Fax:* 202 994-0567
E-mail: sursab@gwumc.edu
Accred Length: 2 Years *Program Size:* 4
Program ID: 460-10-21-019

Walter Reed Army Medical Center Program
Sponsor: Walter Reed Army Medical Center
Program Director:
Dennis Moritz, MD
Thoracic Surgery Service
Walter Reed Army Med Ctr
6825 16th St NW
Washington, DC 20307-5001
Tel: 202 782-6433 *Fax:* 202 782-8253
E-mail: dmoritz@vs.wramc.amedd.army.mil
Internet: http://www.wramc.amedd.army.mil/departments/surgery/thoracic/
Accred Length: 2 Years *Program Size:* 2
Program ID: 460-10-11-003
US Armed Services Program

Florida

Gainesville

University of Florida Program
Sponsor: University of Florida College of Medicine
Shands Hospital at the University of Florida
Veterans Affairs Medical Center (Gainesville)
Program Director:
James A Alexander, MD
PO Box 100286
Health Science Ctr-Univ of Florida
Gainesville, FL 32610-0286
Tel: 352 846-0364 *Fax:* 352 846-0356
E-mail: sandyw@surgery.ufl.edu
Accred Length: 2 Years *Program Size:* 3
Program ID: 460-11-21-020

Miami

University of Miami-Jackson Memorial Medical Center Program
Sponsor: University of Miami-Jackson Memorial Medical Center
Mount Sinai Medical Center of Greater Miami
Veterans Affairs Medical Center (Miami)
Program Director:
A J Furst, MD
Univ of Miami Sch of Med
PO Box 016960 (R114)
1611 NW 12th Ave/East Tower 3072
Miami, FL 33136-1094
Tel: 305 585-5271 *Fax:* 305 547-2185
Accred Length: 2 Years *Program Size:* 4
Program ID: 460-11-21-021

Georgia

Atlanta

Emory University Program
Sponsor: Emory University School of Medicine
Crawford Long Hospital of Emory University
Egleston Children's Hospital at Emory University
Emory University Hospital
Grady Memorial Hospital
Veterans Affairs Medical Center (Atlanta)
Program Director:
Robert A Guyton, MD
Emory Clinic, Cardiothoracic Surgery
Bldg A Rm 2223
1365 Clifton Rd NE
Atlanta, GA 30322
Tel: 404 778-3836 *Fax:* 404 778-5039
E-mail: whw@williswilliams.net
Internet:
http://www.emory.edu/whsc/med/surgery/cardio_surgery/index.html
Accred Length: 2 Years *Program Size:* 9
Program ID: 460-12-21-022

Augusta

Medical College of Georgia Program
Sponsor: Medical College of Georgia Hospital and Clinics
Veterans Affairs Medical Center (Augusta)
Program Director:
Ganesh Pai, MD
BAA-4300
1120 15th St
Augusta, GA 30912-4040
Tel: 706 721-3226 *Fax:* 706 721-7508
E-mail: cbozeman@mail.mcg.edu
Accred Length: 2 Years *Program Size:* 3
Program ID: 460-12-21-023

Illinois

Chicago

McGaw Medical Center of Northwestern University Program
Sponsor: Northwestern University Medical School
Children's Memorial Medical Center
Evanston Hospital
Northwestern Memorial Hospital
Veterans Affairs Lakeside Medical Center (Chicago)
Program Director:
David A Fullerton, MD
Northwestern Univ Med Sch
251 E Chicago Ave
Wesley Tower/Ste 1030
Chicago, IL 60611
Tel: 312 908-3121 *Fax:* 312 908-1903
E-mail: smontgom@nmh.org
Accred Length: 3 Years *Program Size:* 3
Program ID: 460-16-21-025

Rush-Presbyterian-St Luke's Medical Center Program
Sponsor: Rush-Presbyterian-St Luke's Medical Center
Children's Memorial Medical Center
Program Director:
Verdi J DiSesa, MD
Rush-Presbyterian-St Luke's Med Ctr
1653 W Congress Pkwy
Rm 714 Jelke
Chicago, IL 60612-3833
Tel: 312 942-6373 *Fax:* 312 666-0242
E-mail: cadams@rush.edu
Internet: http://www.rush.edu
Accred Length: 2 Years *Program Size:* 4
Program ID: 460-16-21-027

University of Illinois College of Medicine at Chicago Program
Sponsor: University of Illinois College of Medicine at Chicago
Christ Hospital and Medical Center
Cook County Hospital
University of Illinois Hospital and Clinics
Veterans Affairs West Side Medical Center
Program Director:
Michel Ilbawi, MD MD
Univ of Illinois Hospital
M/C 958 Rm 417 CBS
840 S Wood St
Chicago, IL 60612
Tel: 312 996-4942 *Fax:* 312 996-2013
E-mail: elliesw@uic.edu
Internet: http://www.uic.edu
Accred Length: 2 Years *Program Size:* 2
Program ID: 460-16-21-029

Maywood

Loyola University Program
Sponsor: Loyola University Medical Center
Edward J Hines Jr Veterans Affairs Hospital
Program Director:
Bradford Blakeman, MD MD
Loyola Univ Med Ctr-Foster G McGaw Hospital
2160 S First Ave
Bldg 110 Rm 6246
Maywood, IL 60153
Tel: 708 327-2521 *Fax:* 708 327-2504
E-mail: bblakem@luc.edu
Accred Length: 2 Years *Program Size:* 4
Program ID: 460-16-31-030

Indiana

Indianapolis

Indiana University School of Medicine Program
Sponsor: Indiana University School of Medicine
Clarian IU Hospital
Clarian Riley Hospital for Children
Richard L Roudebush Veterans Affairs Medical Center
Program Director:
John W Brown, MD
Indiana Univ Med Ctr
Emerson Hall 215
545 Barnhill Dr
Indianapolis, IN 46202-5125
Tel: 317 274-7150 *Fax:* 317 274-2940
Accred Length: 2 Years *Program Size:* 4
Program ID: 460-17-21-031

Iowa

Iowa City

University of Iowa Hospitals and Clinics Program
Sponsor: University of Iowa Hospitals and Clinics
Program Director:
Douglas M Behrendt, MD
Univ of Iowa Hospitals and Clinics
Dept of Surgery
200 Hawkins Dr
Iowa City, IA 52242-1009
Tel: 319 356-2761 *Fax:* 319 356-3891
E-mail: dbehrend@surgery.uiowa.edu
Internet: http://www.surgery/ct/index/html
Accred Length: 2 Years *Program Size:* 4
Program ID: 460-18-21-032

Kentucky

Louisville

University of Louisville Program
Sponsor: University of Louisville School of Medicine
Jewish Hospital
Kosair Children's Hospital (Alliant Health System)
University of Louisville Hospital
Veterans Affairs Medical Center (Louisville)
Program Director:
Laman A Gray Jr, MD
Sch of Med, Dept of Surgery
Univ of Louisville
Louisville, KY 40292
Tel: 502 561-2180 *Fax:* 502 561-2190
Accred Length: 2 Years *Program Size:* 4
Program ID: 460-20-21-105

Louisiana

New Orleans

Alton Ochsner Medical Foundation Program
Sponsor: Alton Ochsner Medical Foundation
Program Director:
Clifford Van Meter Jr, MD
Alton Ochsner Med Foundation
Dept of Grad Med Educ
1516 Jefferson Hwy
New Orleans, LA 70121
Tel: 504 842-3260 *Fax:* 504 842-3193
E-mail: dlambert@ochsner.org
Internet: http://www.ochsner.org
Accred Length: 2 Years *Program Size:* 2
Program ID: 460-21-21-036

Maryland

Baltimore

Johns Hopkins University Program
Sponsor: Johns Hopkins University School of Medicine
Johns Hopkins Hospital
Program Director:
William A Baumgartner, MD
Johns Hopkins Hospital
Blalock 618
600 N Wolfe St
Baltimore, MD 21287-4618
Tel: 410 955-5248 *Fax:* 410 955-3809
E-mail: wbaumgar@csurg.jhmi.jhu.edu
Internet: http://www.jhu.edu
Accred Length: 3 Years *Program Size:* 6
Program ID: 460-23-11-037

University of Maryland Program
Sponsor: University of Maryland Medical System
Program Director:
Glenn J Whitman, MD
Univ of Maryland Hospital
22 S Greene St
Baltimore, MD 21201
Tel: 410 328-5842 *Fax:* 410 328-2750
Internet: http://som1.ab.umd.edu/surgery/surgery.html
Accred Length: 2 Years *Program Size:* 2
Program ID: 460-23-11-038

Massachusetts

Boston

Beth Israel Deaconess Medical Center (West Campus) Program
Sponsor: Beth Israel Deaconess Medical Center
Children's Hospital
Program Director:
Robert G Johnson, MD
Beth Israel Deaconess Med Ctr
110 Francis St/Ste 2C
Boston, MA 02215
Tel: 617 632-8385 *Fax:* 617 632-8387
E-mail: rjohnson@bidmc.harvard.edu
Accred Length: 2 Years *Program Size:* 2
Program ID: 460-24-21-041

Boston University Medical Center Program
Sponsor: Boston Medical Center
Children's Hospital
Lahey Clinic
Program Director:
Richard J Shemin, MD
Boston Med Ctr
Cardiothoracic Surgery Dept
88 E Newton St
Boston, MA 02118-2393
Tel: 617 638-7350 *Fax:* 617 638-7228
E-mail: richard.shemin@bmc.org
Internet: http://www.bmc.org/ct
Accred Length: 3 Years *Program Size:* 2
Program ID: 460-24-21-039

Brigham and Women's Hospital/Children's Hospital Program
Sponsor: Brigham and Women's Hospital
Children's Hospital
Program Director:
Lawrence H Cohn, MD
Brigham and Women's Hospital
Surgery Education Office
75 Francis St
Boston, MA 02115
Tel: 617 732-6861 *Fax:* 617 264-6850
E-mail: surgery@bics.bwh.harvard.edu
Internet: http://www.bwh.partners.org/surged
Accred Length: 2 Years *Program Size:* 6
Program ID: 460-24-22-043

Massachusetts General Hospital Program
Sponsor: Massachusetts General Hospital
Children's Hospital
Mount Auburn Hospital
Program Director:
Douglas Mathisen, MD
Massachusetts General Hospital
32 Fruit St
Blake 1570
Boston, MA 02114
Tel: 617 726-2806 *Fax:* 617 726-7667
E-mail: mathisen.douglas@mgh.harvard.edu
Internet: http://www.partners.org/mgh/thoracic
Accred Length: 2 Years *Program Size:* 9
Program ID: 460-24-11-040

New England Medical Center Hospitals Program
Sponsor: New England Medical Center Hospitals
St Elizabeth's Medical Center of Boston
Program Director:
Douglas D Payne, MD
750 Washington St
Boston, MA 02111
Tel: 617 636-5593 *Fax:* 617 636-7616
Accred Length: 2 Years *Program Size:* 2
Program ID: 460-24-21-042

Worcester

University of Massachusetts Program
Sponsor: University of Massachusetts Medical School
Children's Hospital
St Vincent Hospital
UMass Memorial Health Care (University Campus)
Program Director:
Thomas J Vander Salm, MD
Univ of Massachusetts Med Sch
55 Lake Ave N
Worcester, MA 01655
Tel: 508 856-2216 *Fax:* 508 856-3740
Accred Length: 3 Years *Program Size:* 3
Program ID: 460-24-21-111

Michigan

Ann Arbor

University of Michigan Program
Sponsor: University of Michigan Hospitals
Veterans Affairs Medical Center (Ann Arbor)
Program Director:
Mark B Orringer, MD
Univ of Michigan Med Ctr
2110 K-A Alfred Taubman Hlth Care
1500 E Medical Center Dr
Ann Arbor, MI 48109-0344
Tel: 734 936-4975 *Fax:* 734 764-2255
E-mail: morrin@umich.edu
Internet:
http://www.surg.med.umich.edu//thoracic.home.html
Accred Length: 2 Years *Program Size:* 6
Program ID: 460-25-21-044

Detroit

Wayne State University/Detroit Medical Center Program
Sponsor: Wayne State University/Detroit Medical Center
Children's Hospital of Michigan
Detroit Receiving Hospital and University Health Center
Harper Hospital
Program Director:
Larry W Stephenson, MD
3990 John R St/Ste 2102
Detroit, MI 48201
Tel: 313 993-0584 *Fax:* 313 993-0572
E-mail: hammond@cardiology.harper.wayne.edu
Accred Length: 2 Years *Program Size:* 6
Program ID: 460-25-21-045

Minnesota

Minneapolis

University of Minnesota Program
Sponsor: University of Minnesota Medical School
Fairview-University Medical Center
Regions Hospital
Veterans Affairs Medical Center (Minneapolis)
Program Director:
R Morton Bolman III, MD
Univ of Minnesota
Box 207
420 Delaware St SE
Minneapolis, MN 55455
Tel: 612 625-3902 *Fax:* 612 625-1683
E-mail: bolma001@tc.umn.edu
Internet: http://www.umn.edu.med/surg
Accred Length: 3 Years *Program Size:* 6
Program ID: 460-26-21-046

Rochester

Mayo Graduate School of Medicine (Rochester) Program
Sponsor: Mayo Graduate School of Medicine-Mayo Foundation
Mayo Clinic (Rochester)
Rochester Methodist Hospital
St Mary's Hospital of Rochester
Program Director:
Hartzell V Schaff, MD
Application Processing Ctr
Mayo Graduate Sch of Med
200 First St SW/Siebens 5
Rochester, MN 55905
Tel: 507 284-4331 *Fax:* 507 284-0999
E-mail: mgsm.roch.mn.surgery@mayo.edu
Internet: http://www.mayo.edu/
Accred Length: 3 Years *Program Size:* 6
Program ID: 460-26-21-047

Mississippi

Jackson

University of Mississippi Medical Center Program
Sponsor: University of Mississippi School of Medicine
University Hospital
Veterans Affairs Medical Center (Jackson)
Program Director:
Bobby J Heath, MD
Univ of Mississippi Med Ctr
2500 N State St
Jackson, MS 39216-4525
Tel: 601 984-5170 *Fax:* 601 984-5198
Accred Length: 2 Years *Program Size:* 2
Program ID: 460-27-11-048

Missouri

Columbia

University of Missouri-Columbia Program
Sponsor: University of Missouri-Columbia School of Medicine
Harry S Truman Memorial Veterans Hospital
University Hospitals and Clinics
Program Director:
Jack J Curtis, MD
Univ of Missouri Hospitals and Clinics
Dept of Cardiothoracic Surg/MA312
One Hospital Dr
Columbia, MO 65212
Tel: 573 882-6954 *Fax:* 573 884-0437
E-mail: curtisj@health.missouri.edu
Accred Length: 2 Years *Program Size:* 2
Program ID: 460-28-21-049

Kansas City

St Luke's Hospital Program
Sponsor: Saint Luke's Hospital
Program Director:
Jeffrey M Piehler, MD
Medical Plaza II/Ste 50
4320 Wornall Rd
Kansas City, MO 64111
Tel: 816 931-7743 *Fax:* 816 931-0461
Accred Length: 2 Years *Program Size:* 2
Program ID: 460-28-12-050

St Louis

St Louis University School of Medicine Program

Sponsor: St Louis University School of Medicine
SSM Cardinal Glennon Children's Hospital
St Louis University School of Medicine
Veterans Affairs Medical Center (St Louis)

Program Director:
Keith S Naunheim, MD
St Louis Univ Sch of Med
3635 Vista Ave
PO Box 15250
St Louis, MO 63110-0250
Tel: 314 577-8360 *Fax:* 314 268-5466
E-mail: surgweb@slu.edu
Internet:
http://www.slu.edu/colleges/med/departments/surgery
Accred Length: 2 Years *Program Size:* 2
Program ID: 460-28-21-052

Washington University/B-JH/SLCH Consortium Program

Sponsor: Washington University/B-JH/SLCH Consortium
Barnes-Jewish Hospital
Barnes-Jewish Hospital (North Campus)
St Louis Children's Hospital

Program Director:
Joel D Cooper, MD
Barnes-Jewish Hospital
One Barnes Hospital Plaza
Box 8234
St Louis, MO 63110
Tel: 314 362-1935
Accred Length: 2 Years *Program Size:* 6
Program ID: 460-28-21-051

New Jersey

Newark

Newark Beth Israel Medical Center Program

Sponsor: Newark Beth Israel Medical Center

Program Director:
Laszlo Fuzesi, MD
Newark Beth Israel Med Ctr
201 Lyons Ave
Newark, NJ 07112
Tel: 973 926-7325 *Fax:* 973 926-2243
E-mail: lfuzesi@ibm.net
Accred Length: 2 Years *Program Size:* 2
Program ID: 460-33-11-054

UMDNJ-New Jersey Medical School Program

Sponsor: UMDNJ-New Jersey Medical School
Children's Hospital of Philadelphia
Hackensack University Medical Center
St Michael's Medical Center (Cathedral Hlth Srvcs Inc)
UMDNJ-University Hospital
Veterans Affairs Medical Center (East Orange)

Program Director:
John R McCormick, MD
UMDNJ-New Jersey Med Sch
185 S Orange Ave/G-595 MSB
Newark, NJ 07103
Tel: 973 972-5678 *Fax:* 973 972-2925
E-mail: mccormjr@umdnj.edu
Accred Length: 2 Years *Program Size:* 2
Program ID: 460-33-21-053

Piscataway

UMDNJ-Robert Wood Johnson Medical School Program

Sponsor: UMDNJ-Robert Wood Johnson Medical School
Deborah Heart and Lung Center
Robert Wood Johnson University Hospital
St Peter's University Hospital

Program Director:
James W Mackenzie, MD
UMDNJ-Robert Wood Johnson Med Sch
One Robert Wood Johnson Pl/PO Box 19
MEB 508
New Brunswick, NJ 08903-0019
Tel: 732 235-7806 *Fax:* 732 235-7013
E-mail: mackenjw@umdjn.edu
Internet: http://www.rwjsurgery.umdnj.edu/ctweb
Accred Length: 3 Years *Program Size:* 3
Program ID: 460-33-21-110

New Mexico

Albuquerque

University of New Mexico Program

Sponsor: University of New Mexico School of Medicine
University Hospital
Veterans Affairs Medical Center (Albuquerque)

Program Director:
Jorge A Wernly, MD
Univ of New Mexico Med Ctr
Dept of Cardiothoracic Surg/2-ACC
2211 Lomas Blvd NE
Albuquerque, NM 87131-5341
Tel: 505 272-6901 *Fax:* 505 272-6909
E-mail: jwernly@salud.unm.edu
Internet:
http://salud.unm.edu/surgery/thoracic/cardiothoracic
Accred Length: 2 Years *Program Size:* 2
Program ID: 460-34-21-055

New York

Albany

Albany Medical Center Program

Sponsor: Albany Medical Center

Program Director:
Charles C Canver, MD
Albany Med Coll
47 New Scotland Ave
Mail Code 61
Albany, NY 12208-3479
Tel: 518 262-5114 *Fax:* 518 262-5999
E-mail: charles_canver@ccgateway.amc.edu
Accred Length: 2 Years *Program Size:* 2
Program ID: 460-35-11-056

Bronx

Albert Einstein College of Medicine Program

Sponsor: Albert Einstein College of Medicine of Yeshiva University
Jacobi Medical Center
Montefiore Medical Center-Henry and Lucy Moses Division
Montefiore Medical Center-Weiler Hospital

Program Director:
Jeffrey P Gold, MD
Montefiore Med Ctr
111 E 210th St
Bronx, NY 10467-2490
Tel: 718 920-7000 *Fax:* 718 231-7113
E-mail: jpgold@montefiore.org
Accred Length: 2 Years *Program Size:* 4
Program ID: 460-35-21-058

Brooklyn

SUNY Health Science Center at Brooklyn Program

Sponsor: SUNY Health Science Center at Brooklyn
Kings County Hospital Center
Lutheran Medical Center
Maimonides Medical Center
University Hospital-SUNY Health Science Center at Brooklyn

Program Director:
Joseph N Cunningham Jr, MD
SUNY Health Science Ctr-Brooklyn
Div of Cardiothoracic Surgery
450 Clarkson Ave
Brooklyn, NY 11203
Tel: 718 270-1981 *Fax:* 718 270-3843
Accred Length: 2 Years *Program Size:* 4
Program ID: 460-35-11-066

Buffalo

SUNY at Buffalo Graduate Medical-Dental Education Consortium Program

Sponsor: SUNY at Buffalo Grad Medical-Dental Education Consortium
CGF Health System (Buffalo General Hospital)
CGF Health System (Children's Hospital of Buffalo)
CGF Health System (Millard Fillmore Hospitals)
Veterans Affairs Medical Center (Buffalo)

Program Director:
Tomas A Salerno, MD
CGF Health System
100 High St
Buffalo, NY 14203
Tel: 716 859-1080 *Fax:* 716 859-4697
E-mail: sur237@po1.bgh.edu
Accred Length: 2 Years *Program Size:* 4
Program ID: 460-35-21-057

New Hyde Park

Albert Einstein College of Medicine at Long Island Jewish Medical Center Program

Sponsor: Long Island Jewish Medical Center

Program Director:
L Michael Graver, MD
Long Island Jewish Med Ctr
Heart Inst/Rm 2123
270-05 76th Ave
New Hyde Park, NY 11040
Tel: 718 470-7460 *Fax:* 718 831-0260
E-mail: graver@lij.edu
Internet: http://www.lij.edu
Accred Length: 2 Years *Program Size:* 2
Program ID: 460-35-21-062

New York

Mount Sinai School of Medicine Program
Sponsor: Mount Sinai School of Medicine
Mount Sinai Medical Center
Program Director:
Randall B Griepp, MD
M Arisan Ergin, MD
Mount Sinai Med Ctr
One Gustave L Levy Pl
Box 1028
New York, NY 10029-6574
Tel: 212 241-8181 *Fax:* 212 534-3357
Accred Length: 3 Years *Program Size:* 3
Program ID: 460-35-11-064

New York and Presbyterian Hospital (Columbia Campus) Program
Sponsor: New York and Presbyterian Hospital
New York and Presbyterian Hospital (Columbia Campus)
Program Director:
Craig R Smith, MD
Presbyterian Hospital
177 Fort Washington Ave
New York, NY 10032
Tel: 212 305-2633 *Fax:* 212 305-2439
Accred Length: 2 Years *Program Size:* 4
Program ID: 460-35-21-059

New York and Presbyterian Hospital (Cornell Campus) Program
Sponsor: New York and Presbyterian Hospital
Memorial Sloan-Kettering Cancer Center
New York and Presbyterian Hospital (Cornell Campus)
Program Director:
O Wayne Isom, MD
Robert J Ginsberg, MD
New York Presbyterian Hospital-Cornell Campus
525 E 68th St
New York, NY 10021
Tel: 212 746-5151 *Fax:* 212 746-8828
E-mail: owisom@mail.med.cornell.edu
Accred Length: 2 Years *Program Size:* 6
Program ID: 460-35-11-060

New York University Medical Center Program
Sponsor: New York University Medical Center
Bellevue Hospital Center
Veterans Affairs Medical Center (Manhattan)
Program Director:
Stephen B Colvin, MD
New York Univ Med Ctr
530 First Ave/SK-9-V
New York, NY 10016
Tel: 212 263-6384 *Fax:* 212 263-6546
E-mail: colvin@cv.med.nyu.edu
Accred Length: 2 Years *Program Size:* 6
Program ID: 460-35-21-065

Rochester

University of Rochester Program
Sponsor: Strong Memorial Hospital of the University of Rochester
Rochester General Hospital
Program Director:
George L Hicks Jr, MD
Strong Memorial Hospital
Box Surgery
601 Elmwood Ave
Rochester, NY 14642
Tel: 716 275-5384 *Fax:* 716 244-7171
E-mail: joan@ctsurg.urmc.rochester.edu
Accred Length: 2 Years *Program Size:* 4
Program ID: 460-35-21-067

Syracuse

SUNY Health Science Center at Syracuse Program
Sponsor: University Hospital-SUNY Health Science Center at Syracuse
Crouse Hospital
Program Director:
Berkeley Brandt III, MD
SUNY Health Science Ctr
Div of Cardiopulmonary Surgery
750 E Adams St
Syracuse, NY 13210
Tel: 315 464-5812 *Fax:* 315 464-6251
E-mail: brandtb@mailbox.hscsyr.edu
Internet: http://www.hscsyr.edu1/^surgery/maindept md/home.htm
Accred Length: 2 Years *Program Size:* 3
Program ID: 460-35-21-068

North Carolina

Chapel Hill

University of North Carolina Hospitals Program
Sponsor: University of North Carolina Hospitals
Program Director:
Michael R Mill, MD
Univ of North Carolina Sch of Med
108 Burnett-Womack Bldg/CB#7065
Chapel Hill, NC 27599-7065
Tel: 919 966-3381 *Fax:* 919 966-3475
E-mail: mrm@med.unc.edu
Internet:
http://www.med.unc.edu/wrkunits/2depts/surgery/cardioth/welcome.htm
Accred Length: 2 Years *Program Size:* 3
Program ID: 460-36-11-069

Charlotte

Carolinas Medical Center Program
Sponsor: Carolinas Medical Center
Program Director:
Francis Robicsek, MD PhD
Dept of Thoracic/Cardiovascular Surg
Carolinas Med Ctr
PO Box 32861
Charlotte, NC 28232-2861
Tel: 704 355-4005 *Fax:* 704 355-6227
E-mail: spinder@carolinas.org
Accred Length: 2 Years *Program Size:* 4
Program ID: 460-36-12-070

Durham

Duke University Program
Sponsor: Duke University Medical Center
Veterans Affairs Medical Center (Asheville)
Veterans Affairs Medical Center (Durham)
Program Director:
Walter G Wolfe, MD
Peter K Smith, MD
Duke Univ Med Ctr
Dept of Surgery
PO Box 3507
Durham, NC 27710
Tel: 919 684-4117 *Fax:* 919 681-8912
E-mail: wolfe001@mc.duke.edu
Accred Length: 2 Years *Program Size:* 6
Program ID: 460-36-21-071

Winston-Salem

Wake Forest University School of Medicine Program
Sponsor: Wake Forest University Baptist Medical Center
Program Director:
D'Glenn Pennington, MD
Wake Forest University Sch of Med
Medical Center Blvd
Winston-Salem, NC 27157-1096
Tel: 336 716-2124 *Fax:* 336 716-3348
Accred Length: 2 Years *Program Size:* 2
Program ID: 460-36-11-072

Ohio

Cleveland

Case Western Reserve University Program
Sponsor: University Hospitals of Cleveland
MetroHealth Medical Center
Veterans Affairs Medical Center (Cleveland)
Program Director:
Robert W Stewart, MD
Univ Hospitals of Cleveland
11100 Euclid Ave
Cleveland, OH 44106-5011
Tel: 216 844-7268 *Fax:* 216 844-8479
Internet: http://www.uhhs.com
Accred Length: 2 Years *Program Size:* 4
Program ID: 460-38-21-074

Cleveland Clinic Foundation Program
Sponsor: Cleveland Clinic Foundation
Program Director:
Delos M Cosgrove III, MD
Cleveland Clinic Foundation
Dept of Thoracic Surgery/F25
9500 Euclid Ave
Cleveland, OH 44195
Tel: 216 444-6733 *Fax:* 216 444-0777
E-mail: meded@cesmtp.ccf.org
Internet: http://www.ccf.org
Accred Length: 3 Years *Program Size:* 6
Program ID: 460-38-12-075

Columbus

Ohio State University Program
Sponsor: Ohio State University Medical Center
Children's Hospital
Program Director:
Robert Michler, MD
Ohio State Univ Hospital
N-825 Doan Hall
410 W Tenth Ave
Columbus, OH 43210
Tel: 614 293-7277 *Fax:* 614 293-4726
Internet: http://www.surgery.medctr.osu.edu
Accred Length: 2 Years *Program Size:* 3
Program ID: 460-38-21-077

Oklahoma

Oklahoma City

University of Oklahoma Health Sciences Center Program

Sponsor: University of Oklahoma College of Medicine
Children's Hospital of Oklahoma
University Hospital
Veterans Affairs Medical Center (Oklahoma City)

Program Director:
Ronald C Elkins, MD
Univ of Oklahoma Coll of Med
Sect of Thoracic Surg/WP2230
PO Box 26901
Oklahoma City, OK 73190
Tel: 405 271-5789 *Fax:* 405 271-3288
E-mail: ronald-elkins@uokhsc.edu
Accred Length: 2 Years *Program Size:* 2
Program ID: 460-39-21-078

Oregon

Portland

Oregon Health Sciences University Program

Sponsor: Oregon Health Sciences University Hospital
Veterans Affairs Medical Center (Portland)

Program Director:
Adnan Cobanoglu, MD
Oregon Health Sciences Univ/L353
3181 SW Sam Jackson Park Rd
Portland, OR 97201-3098
Tel: 503 494-7820 *Fax:* 503 494-7829
Accred Length: 2 Years *Program Size:* 2
Program ID: 460-40-21-079

Pennsylvania

Hershey

Penn State Geisinger Health System/Milton S Hershey Medical Center Program

Sponsor: Penn State Geisinger Health System
Milton S Hershey Medical Center

Program Director:
Ralph J Damiano, MD
Pennsylvania State Univ-Penn State Geisinger Health System
Milton S Hershey Med Ctr
500 University Dr/ MC H165
Hershey, PA 17033
Tel: 717 531-8330 *Fax:* 717 531-3664
E-mail: rdamiano@psghs.edu
Internet: http://webserv.surg.hmc.psu.edu
Accred Length: 2 Years *Program Size:* 2
Program ID: 460-41-11-080

Philadelphia

MCP Hahnemann University Program

Sponsor: MCP Hahnemann University
Fox Chase Cancer Center
Hahnemann University Hospital
St Christopher's Hospital for Children

Program Director:
Andrew S Wechsler, MD
Hahnemann Univ Hospital
Broad and Vine/MS 111
Philadelphia, PA 19102-1192
Tel: 215 762-4955 *Fax:* 215 762-1858
E-mail: wechsla@wpo.auhs.edu
Accred Length: 3 Years *Program Size:* 3
Program ID: 460-41-21-104

Thomas Jefferson University Program

Sponsor: Thomas Jefferson University Hospital
Children's Hospital of Philadelphia
Christiana Care Health Services Inc

Program Director:
Richard N Edie, MD
Thomas Jefferson Univ
1025 Walnut St/Ste 607
Philadelphia, PA 19107
Tel: 215 955-5654 *Fax:* 215 955-6010
Accred Length: 3 Years *Program Size:* 3
Program ID: 460-41-21-081

University of Pennsylvania Program

Sponsor: Hospital of the University of Pennsylvania
Children's Hospital of Philadelphia

Program Director:
Timothy J Gardner, MD
Univ of Pennsylvania Med Ctr
3400 Spruce St
Four Silverstein Pavilion
Philadelphia, PA 19104
Tel: 215 662-2022 *Fax:* 215 349-5798
E-mail: gardnert@mail.med.upenn.edu
Accred Length: 2 Years *Program Size:* 4
Program ID: 460-41-21-082

Pittsburgh

Allegheny General Hospital Program

Sponsor: Allegheny General Hospital
West Virginia University Hospitals

Program Director:
George J Magovern Jr, MD
Allegheny General Hospital
Dept of Cardiothoracic Surgery
320 E North Ave
Pittsburgh, PA 15212-9986
Tel: 412 359-3711 *Fax:* 412 359-3878
Accred Length: 2 Years *Program Size:* 4
Program ID: 460-41-31-084

University Health Center of Pittsburgh Program

Sponsor: University Health Center of Pittsburgh
Children's Hospital of Pittsburgh
Presbyterian University Hospital/UPMC
Veterans Affairs Medical Center (Pittsburgh)

Program Director:
Bartley P Griffith, MD
Univ Health Ctr of Pittsburgh
Cardiothoracic Surgery
200 Lothrop St/C700 PUH
Pittsburgh, PA 15213
Tel: 412 648-9890 *Fax:* 412 648-4141
E-mail: griffithbp@msx.upmc.edu
Accred Length: 2 Years *Program Size:* 6
Program ID: 460-41-21-085

South Carolina

Charleston

Medical University of South Carolina Program

Sponsor: Medical University of South Carolina College of Medicine
Charleston Memorial Hospital
MUSC Medical Center
Ralph H Johnson Dept of Veterans Affairs Med Center

Program Director:
Fred A Crawford Jr, MD
Med Univ of South Carolina
171 Ashley Ave
Charleston, SC 29425
Tel: 843 792-5897 *Fax:* 843 792-8286
Accred Length: 3 Years *Program Size:* 3
Program ID: 460-45-21-087

Tennessee

Memphis

University of Tennessee Program

Sponsor: University of Tennessee College of Medicine
Baptist Memorial Hospital
LeBonheur Children's Medical Center
Regional Medical Center at Memphis
University of Tennessee Medical Center (UT Bowld Hospital)
Veterans Affairs Medical Center (Memphis)

Program Director:
Donald C Watson, MD
Univ of Tennessee
Div of Thoracic Surgery
956 Court Ave/G230
Memphis, TN 38163
Tel: 901 448-4541 *Fax:* 901 448-7306
Accred Length: 2 Years *Program Size:* 4
Program ID: 460-47-21-088

Nashville

Vanderbilt University Program

Sponsor: Vanderbilt University Medical Center
St Thomas Hospital
Veterans Affairs Medical Center (Nashville)

Program Director:
Davis C Drinkwater Jr, MD
Vanderbilt Univ Med Ctr
2986 TVC
1301 22nd Ave S
Nashville, TN 37232-5734
Tel: 615 322-0064 *Fax:* 615 343-9194
E-mail: davis.drinkwater@mcmail.vanderbilt.edu
Accred Length: 3 Years *Program Size:* 2
Program ID: 460-47-31-089

Texas

Dallas

University of Texas Southwestern Medical School Program

Sponsor: University of Texas Southwestern Medical School
Children's Medical Center of Dallas
Dallas County Hospital District-Parkland Memorial Hospital
St Paul Medical Center
Veterans Affairs Medical Center (Dallas)

Program Director:
Michael E Jessen, MD
Univ of Texas Southwestern Med Sch
Div of Thoracic/Cardiovascular Surgery
5323 Harry Hines Blvd
Dallas, TX 75235-8879
Tel: 214 648-3568 *Fax:* 214 648-2465
E-mail: peggy.thomas@email.swmed.edu
Internet: http://www.swmed.edu
Accred Length: 2 Years *Program Size:* 4
Program ID: 460-48-21-090

Fort Sam Houston

San Antonio Uniformed Services Health Education Consortium Program

Sponsor: San Antonio Uniformed Services Health Education Consortium
Brooke Army Medical Center
Wilford Hall Medical Center (AETC)

Program Director:
David J Cohen, MD
Cardiothoracic Surgery Service
Brooke Army Med Ctr
3851 Roger Brooke Dr
Fort Sam Houston, TX 78234-6200
Tel: 210 916-2412 *Fax:* 210 916-5348
E-mail:
col_david_cohen@smtplink.bamc.amedd.army.mil
Accred Length: 2 Years *Program Size:* 2
Program ID: 460-48-12-004
US Armed Services Program

Galveston

University of Texas Medical Branch Hospitals Program

Sponsor: University of Texas Medical Branch Hospitals

Program Director:
Vincent R Conti, MD
Univ of Texas Med Branch Hospitals
Div of Cardiothoracic Surgery
6120 John Sealy Annex
Galveston, TX 77555-0528
Tel: 409 772-1203 *Fax:* 409 772-1421
E-mail: vconti@utmb.edu
Internet: http://www.utmb.edu
Accred Length: 2 Years *Program Size:* 1
Program ID: 460-48-21-091

Houston

Baylor College of Medicine Program

Sponsor: Baylor College of Medicine
Harris County Hospital District-Ben Taub General Hospital
Methodist Hospital
Texas Children's Hospital
Veterans Affairs Medical Center (Houston)

Program Director:
Michael J Reardon Jr, MD
Baylor Coll of Med
Surgery Education Office
One Baylor Plaza/Rm 404D
Houston, TX 77030
Tel: 713 798-6078 *Fax:* 713 798-8941
E-mail: jcorke@bcm.tmc.edu
Accred Length: 2 Years *Program Size:* 6
Program ID: 460-48-21-092

Texas Heart Institute Program

Sponsor: Texas Heart Institute
Memorial Hermann Healthcare System
St Luke's Episcopal Hospital
Texas Children's Hospital
University of Texas M D Anderson Cancer Center

Program Director:
Denton A Cooley, MD
Texas Heart Inst
PO Box 20345
Houston, TX 77225-0345
Tel: 713 791-4900 *Fax:* 713 791-3770
Internet: http://www.tmc.edu/thi/
Accred Length: 2 Years *Program Size:* 7
Program ID: 460-48-21-093

San Antonio

University of Texas Health Science Center at San Antonio Program

Sponsor: University of Texas Medical School at San Antonio
Audie L Murphy Memorial Veterans Hospital (San Antonio)
University Hospital-South Texas Medical Center

Program Director:
John H Calhoon, MD
Univ of Texas Health Science Ctr
Div of Cardiothoracic Surgery
7703 Floyd Curl Dr
San Antonio, TX 78284-7841
Tel: 210 567-6863 *Fax:* 210 567-2877
E-mail: calhoon@uthscsa.edu
Accred Length: 2 Years *Program Size:* 3
Program ID: 460-48-21-094

Utah

Salt Lake City

University of Utah Program

Sponsor: University of Utah Medical Center
LDS Hospital
Primary Children's Medical Center
Veterans Affairs Medical Center (Salt Lake City)

Program Director:
S V Karwande, MD
Univ of Utah Med Ctr
50 N Medical Dr
Salt Lake City, UT 84132
Tel: 801 581-5311 *Fax:* 801 585-3936
E-mail: martha.noll@hsc.utah.edu
Accred Length: 2 Years *Program Size:* 4
Program ID: 460-49-21-095

Virginia

Charlottesville

University of Virginia Program

Sponsor: University of Virginia Medical Center

Program Director:
Irving L Kron, MD
Univ of Virginia Health Sciences Ctr
Div of Thoracic Cardio Surg
Box 310
Charlottesville, VA 22908
Tel: 804 924-2158 *Fax:* 804 982-3885
Internet:
http://www.med.virginia.edu/docs/heart/docs/profs/tcvresidency
Accred Length: 2 Years *Program Size:* 4
Program ID: 460-51-11-096

Richmond

Medical College of Virginia/Virginia Commonwealth University Program

Sponsor: Medical College of Virginia/Virginia Commonwealth University
Hunter Holmes McGuire VA Medical Center (Richmond)
Medical College of Virginia Hospitals

Program Director:
David Salter, MD
1200 E Broad St
South Wing, 7th Fl. PO Box 980068
Richmond, VA 23298-0068
Tel: 804 828-2768 *Fax:* 804 828-2760
Accred Length: 2 Years *Program Size:* 4
Program ID: 460-51-11-097

Washington

Seattle

University of Washington Program

Sponsor: University of Washington School of Medicine
Children's Hospital and Medical Center
University of Washington Medical Center
Veterans Affairs Medical Center (Seattle)

Program Director:
Edward D Verrier, MD
Div of Cardiothoracic Surgery/Box 356310
Univ of Washington
1959 NE Pacific St/Rm AA115
Seattle, WA 98195
Tel: 206 685-3370 *Fax:* 206 616-9063
E-mail: edver@u.washington.edu
Accred Length: 2 Years *Program Size:* 4
Program ID: 460-54-21-098

West Virginia

Morgantown

West Virginia University Program

Sponsor: West Virginia University Hospitals
Monongalia General Hospital

Program Director:
Gordon F Murray, MD
Dept of Surgery
PO Box 9238 HSCN
West Virginia Univ
Morgantown, WV 26506
Tel: 304 293-4869 *Fax:* 304 293-4711
E-mail: gmurray @wvu.edu
Internet: http://www.hsc.wvu.edu
Accred Length: 2 Years *Program Size:* 2
Program ID: 460-55-11-099

Wisconsin

Madison

University of Wisconsin Program
Sponsor: University of Wisconsin Hospital and Clinics
St Marys Hospital Medical Center
Program Director:
Richard P Cochran, MD
Univ of Wisconsin Hospital and Clinics
Div of Cardiothoracic Surgery
600 Highland Ave/CSC H4/358
Madison, WI 53792-3236
Tel: 608 263-0439 *Fax:* 608 263-0547
E-mail: cochran@surgery.wisc.edu
Internet:
http://www.medsch.wisc.edu/surgery/home.html
Accred Length: 2 Years *Program Size:* 4
Program ID: 460-56-21-100

Milwaukee

Medical College of Wisconsin Program
Sponsor: Medical College of Wisconsin Affiliated Hospitals Inc
Children's Hospital of Wisconsin
Clement J Zablocki Veterans Affairs Medical Center
Froedtert Memorial Lutheran Hospital
Program Director:
Gordon N Olinger, MD
Med Coll of Wisconsin-Milwaukee Regional Med Ctr
9200 W Wisconsin Ave
Milwaukee, WI 53226
Tel: 414 456-6900 *Fax:* 414 456-6217
Accred Length: 2 Years *Program Size:* 3
Program ID: 460-56-21-101

Transitional Year

Alabama

Birmingham

Baptist Health System Program
Sponsor: Baptist Health System Inc
Birmingham Baptist Medical Center-Montclair
Birmingham Baptist Medical Center-Princeton
Program Director:
Elizabeth D Ennis, MD
Birmingham Baptist Med Ctr-Montclair
840 Montclair Rd/Ste 317
Birmingham, AL 35213
Tel: 205 592-5759 *Fax:* 205 592-5694
E-mail: susan@wwisp.com
Internet: http://www.bhsala.com
Accred Length: 1 Year *Program Size:* 16 (*GY1:* 16)
Sponsoring Spec: DR, GS, IM
Program ID: 999-01-00-001

Carraway Methodist Medical Center Program
Sponsor: Carraway Methodist Medical Center
Program Director:
Edward D Haigler Jr, MD
Carraway Methodist Med Ctr
1600 Carraway Blvd
Birmingham, AL 35234
Tel: 205 502-6358 *Fax:* 205 502-5613
E-mail: transres@mail.carraway.com
Internet: http://www.carraway.org
Accred Length: 1 Year *Program Size:* 8 (*GY1:* 8)
Sponsoring Spec: FP, GS, IM, OBG
Program ID: 999-01-00-002

Arizona

Phoenix

Maricopa Medical Center Program
Sponsor: Maricopa Medical Center
Program Director:
Paul A Blackburn, DO
Maricopa Med Ctr
2601 E Roosevelt
Phoenix, AZ 85008
Tel: 602 267-5808 *Fax:* 602 267-5907
E-mail: mmced@mmclib.maricopa.gov
Internet:
http://www.maricopa.gov/medcenter/ed/edhome/html
Accred Length: 1 Year *Program Size:* 0 (*GY1:* 0)
Sponsoring Spec: EM, GS, IM, OBG, PD
Program ID: 999-03-00-005

Phoenix Area Medical Education Consortium Program
Sponsor: Phoenix Area Medical Education Consortium
Good Samaritan Regional Medical Center
Program Director:
Robert A Raschke, MD
Good Samaritan Regional Med Ctr
Dept of Med/Transitional
1111 E McDowell Rd
Phoenix, AZ 85006
Tel: 602 239-2296 *Fax:* 602 239-2084
E-mail: medicine@samaritan.edu
Internet: http://www.samaritan.edu
Accred Length: 1 Year *Program Size:* 5 (*GY1:* 5)
Sponsoring Spec: GS, IM, OBG
Program ID: 999-03-00-004

Scottsdale

Mayo Graduate School of Medicine (Scottsdale) Program
Sponsor: Mayo Graduate School of Medicine-Mayo Foundation
Mayo Clinic (Scottsdale)
Mayo Clinic Hospital
Scottsdale Healthcare-Shea
Program Director:
Donald E Novicki, MD
Mayo Clinic Scottsdale
13400 E Shea Blvd
Scottsdale, AZ 85259
Tel: 602 342-2091 *Fax:* 602 342-2027
E-mail: mgsm.scot.aztransyear@mayo.edu
Internet: http://www.mayo.edu/
Accred Length: 1 Year *Program Size:* 6 (*GY1:* 6)
Sponsoring Spec: D, DR, GS, IM
Program ID: 999-03-00-226

Tucson

Tucson Hospitals Medical Education Program
Sponsor: Tucson Hospitals Medical Education Program Inc
Kino Community Hospital
Tucson Medical Center
Program Director:
Eric G Ramsay, MD
Tucson Hospitals Med Education Program
PO Box 42195
5301 E Grant Rd
Tucson, AZ 85733
Tel: 520 324-5095, ext
E-mail: eras.thmep@tmcaz.com
Internet: http://www.tmcaz.com/thmep
Accred Length: 1 Year *Program Size:* 12 (*GY1:* 12)
Sponsoring Spec: GS, IM
Program ID: 999-03-00-006

Arkansas

Little Rock

University of Arkansas for Medical Sciences Program
Sponsor: University of Arkansas College of Medicine
Arkansas Children's Hospital
Baptist Medical Center
John L McClellan Memorial Veterans Hospital
St Vincent Infirmary Medical Center
Program Director:
Sarah G Klein, MD
Univ of Arkansas Coll of Med
4301 W Markham St/Slot 592
Little Rock, AR 72205-7199
Tel: 501 686-5738 *Fax:* 501 686-8160
E-mail: brazilchristy@exchange.uams.edu
Accred Length: 1 Year *Program Size:* 21 (*GY1:* 21)
Sponsoring Spec: AN, IM, ORS
Program ID: 999-04-00-007

Programs

California

Bakersfield

Kern Medical Center Program

Sponsor: Kern Medical Center

Program Director:
Jennifer J Abraham, MD
Kern Med Ctr
1830 Flower St
Bakersfield, CA 93305
Tel: 805 326-2201 *Fax:* 805 326-2950
E-mail: abrahamj@kernmedctr.com
Internet: http://bizweb.lightspeed.net/~kmcemed
Accred Length: 1 Year *Program Size:* 6 (*GY1:* 6)
Sponsoring Spec: EM, GS, IM, OBG
Program ID: 999-05-00-222

Fresno

University of California (San Francisco)/Fresno Program

Sponsor: UCSF-Fresno Medical Education Program
University Medical Center

Program Director:
James A Comes, MD
Univ Med Ctr
Office of Med Educ
445 S Cedar Ave
Fresno, CA 93702
Tel: 209 459-5005 *Fax:* 209 459-4338
E-mail: transitional@ucsfresno.edu
Internet: http://www.ucsfresno.edu
Accred Length: 1 Year *Program Size:* 9 (*GY1:* 9)
Sponsoring Spec: EM, IM, OBG, PD
Program ID: 999-05-00-149

Oakland

Alameda County Medical Center Program

Sponsor: Alameda County Medical Center

Program Director:
Steven Sackrin, MD
Highland General Hospital-Alameda County Med Ctr
Dept of Med
1411 E 31st St
Oakland, CA 94602
Tel: 510 437-4268 *Fax:* 510 437-4187
Accred Length: 1 Year *Program Size:* 11 (*GY1:* 11)
Sponsoring Spec: EM, IM
Program ID: 999-05-00-185

San Bernardino

San Bernardino County Medical Center Program

Sponsor: San Bernardino County Medical Center

Program Director:
Elizabeth M Richards, MD
San Bernardino County Med Ctr
Dept of Family Med
780 E Gilbert St
San Bernardino, CA 92415-0935
Tel: 909 387-7882 *Fax:* 909 387-0407
E-mail: fammed@co.san-bernardino.ca.us
Internet: http://www.co.san-bernardino.ca.us/cmc/fammed/residency.htm
Accred Length: 1 Year *Program Size:* 12 (*GY1:* 12)
Sponsoring Spec: FP, GS
Program ID: 999-05-00-009

San Diego

Naval Medical Center (San Diego) Program

Sponsor: Naval Medical Center (San Diego)

Program Director:
Cmdr W Bradley Poss, MD
34800 Bob Wilson Dr
San Diego, CA 92134-5000
Tel: 619 532-7936 *Fax:* 619 532-5507
E-mail: wposs@snd10.med.navy.mil
Accred Length: 1 Year *Program Size:* 22 (*GY1:* 22)
Sponsoring Spec: GS, IM
Program ID: 999-05-00-151
US Armed Services Program

Scripps Mercy Hospital Program

Sponsor: Scripps Mercy Hospital

Program Director:
Edwin J Heffernan, MD
Scripps Mercy Hospital
Dept of Med Education
4077 Fifth Ave/MER 35
San Diego, CA 92103-2180
Tel: 619 260-7220 *Fax:* 619 260-7305
E-mail: tedh@mercysd.com
Internet: http://www.mercysdgme.com
Accred Length: 1 Year *Program Size:* 18 (*GY1:* 18)
Sponsoring Spec: IM, PD
Program ID: 999-05-00-010

San Jose

Santa Clara Valley Medical Center Program

Sponsor: Santa Clara Valley Medical Center

Program Director:
Steven S Guest, MD
Santa Clara Valley Med Ctr
Dept of Med
751 S Bascom Ave
San Jose, CA 95128
Tel: 408 885-6305 *Fax:* 408 885-6324
Accred Length: 1 Year *Program Size:* 16 (*GY1:* 16)
Sponsoring Spec: IM, PD
Program ID: 999-05-00-013

Travis AFB

David Grant Medical Center Program

Sponsor: David Grant Medical Center

Program Director:
Lt Col Douglas C Warren, MD
60th Med Group/SGT
101 Bodin Cir
Travis AFB, CA 94535-1800
Tel: 707 423-7947 *Fax:* 707 423-7952
Accred Length: 1 Year *Program Size:* 4 (*GY1:* 4)
Sponsoring Spec: GS, IM, OBG, PD
Program ID: 999-05-00-008
US Armed Services Program

Colorado

Denver

Columbia Presbyterian-St Luke's Medical Center Program

Sponsor: Columbia Presbyterian-St Luke's Medical Center

Program Director:
Gregory J Gahm, MD
1719 E 19th Ave/5C-East
Denver, CO 80218
Tel: 303 839-6741, ext
Accred Length: 1 Year *Program Size:* 13 (*GY1:* 13)
Sponsoring Spec: DR, EM, IM
Program ID: 999-07-00-017

Connecticut

Bridgeport

St Vincent's Medical Center Program

Sponsor: St Vincent's Medical Center

Program Director:
Marvin Garrell, MD
St Vincent's Med Ctr
2800 Main St
Bridgeport, CT 06606
Tel: 203 576-5576 *Fax:* 203 576-5022
Internet: http://www.stvincents.org
Accred Length: 1 Year *Program Size:* 4 (*GY1:* 4)
Sponsoring Spec: DR, IM
Program ID: 999-08-00-018

New Haven

Hospital of St Raphael Program

Sponsor: Hospital of St Raphael

Program Director:
Ernest D Moritz, MD
Hospital of St Raphael
1450 Chapel St
New Haven, CT 06511-4440
Tel: 203 789-3989 *Fax:* 203 789-3222
E-mail: spane@srhs.org
Internet: http://www.srhs.org
Accred Length: 1 Year *Program Size:* 14 (*GY1:* 14)
Sponsoring Spec: GS, IM
Program ID: 999-08-00-020

Delaware

Wilmington

Christiana Care Health Services Program

Sponsor: Christiana Care Health Services Inc

Program Director:
Virginia U Collier, MD
Christiana Care Health System-Christiana Hospital
4755 Ogletown-Stanton Rd
Newark, DE 19718-6001
Tel: 302 733-6339 *Fax:* 302 733-6386
E-mail: transition.residency@christianacare.org
Internet: http://www.mcdresidency.org
Accred Length: 1 Year *Program Size:* 4 (*GY1:* 4)
Sponsoring Spec: FP, IM
Program ID: 999-09-00-021

District of Columbia

Washington

Howard University Program

Sponsor: Howard University Hospital

Program Director:
Adrian O Hosten, MD
Howard Univ Hospital
2041 Georgia Ave NW
Washington, DC 20060
Tel: 202 865-6620 *Fax:* 202 865-4607
Accred Length: 1 Year *Program Size:* 19 (*GY1:* 19)
Sponsoring Spec: GS, IM
Program ID: 999-10-00-022

Walter Reed Army Medical Center Program

Sponsor: Walter Reed Army Medical Center

Program Director:
Mary C Nace, MD
Walter Reed Army Med Ctr
Dept of Ob/Gyn
6825 16th St
Washington, DC 20307-5001
Tel: 202 782-1384 *Fax:* 202 782-8133
Accred Length: 1 Year *Program Size:* 0
Sponsoring Spec: GS, IM, OBG
Program ID: 999-10-00-024
US Armed Services Program

Florida

Jacksonville

Mayo Graduate School of Medicine (Jacksonville) Program

Sponsor: Mayo Graduate School of Medicine-Mayo Foundation
Mayo Clinic (Jacksonville)
St Luke's Hospital

Program Director:
Gary M Lee, MD
Mayo Clinic Jacksonville
Graduate Educ Ctr/Roger Main 250
4500 San Pablo Rd
Jacksonville, FL 32224
Tel: 904 296-3863 *Fax:* 904 296-3892
E-mail: mgsm.jack.fl.transyear@mayo.edu
Internet: http://www.mayo.edu/
Accred Length: 1 Year *Program Size:* 6 (*GY1:* 6)
Sponsoring Spec: AN, GS, IM
Program ID: 999-11-00-228

Georgia

Atlanta

Emory University Program

Sponsor: Emory University School of Medicine
Egleston Children's Hospital at Emory University
Emory University Hospital
Grady Memorial Hospital

Program Director:
H Kenneth Walker, MD
Emory Univ
Transitional Program
69 Butler St SE
Atlanta, GA 30303
Tel: 404 616-3527 *Fax:* 404 525-2957
Internet: http://www.emory.edu/med/dept
Accred Length: 1 Year *Program Size:* 18 (*GY1:* 18)
Sponsoring Spec: IM, PD
Program ID: 999-12-00-026

Georgia Baptist Medical Center Program

Sponsor: Georgia Baptist Medical Center

Program Director:
David L Anders, MD
303 Parkway Dr NE
Med Educ Box 423
Atlanta, GA 30312
Tel: 404 265-4627 *Fax:* 404 265-4989
E-mail: gbmctrans@mindspring.com
Accred Length: 1 Year *Program Size:* 9 (*GY1:* 9)
Sponsoring Spec: GS, IM, OBG
Program ID: 999-12-00-027

Columbus

The Medical Center Program

Sponsor: The Medical Center Inc

Program Director:
John R Bucholtz, DO
Med Ctr Inc
710 Ctr St/Box 100
Columbus, GA 31902-2299
Tel: 706 571-1430 *Fax:* 706 571-1604
Accred Length: 1 Year *Program Size:* 4 (*GY1:* 4)
Sponsoring Spec: FP, ORS
Program ID: 999-12-00-229

Fort Gordon

Dwight David Eisenhower Army Medical Center Program

Sponsor: Dwight David Eisenhower Army Medical Center

Program Director:
Matthew S Bachinski, MD
Dwight David Eisenhower Army Med Ctr
Transitional Year Program
Office of Grad Med Education
Fort Gordon, GA 30905-5650
Tel: 706 787-4657 *Fax:* 706 787-1745
Accred Length: 1 Year *Program Size:* 12 (*GY1:* 12)
Sponsoring Spec: GS, IM, ORS
Program ID: 999-12-00-029
US Armed Services Program

Macon

Mercer University School of Medicine Program

Sponsor: Medical Center of Central Georgia

Program Director:
T W Treadwell Jr, MD
Med Ctr of Central Georgia
3780 Eisenhower Pkwy
Macon, GA 31206-3608
Tel: 912 784-3589 *Fax:* 912 784-3550
E-mail: transyear.residency@mail.mccg.org
Accred Length: 1 Year *Program Size:* 4 (*GY1:* 4)
Sponsoring Spec: FP, GS, IM, OBG
Program ID: 999-12-00-233

Hawaii

Honolulu

Tripler Army Medical Center Program

Sponsor: Tripler Army Medical Center

Program Director:
James M Olsen, MD
Tripler Army Med Ctr
MCHK-ME
1 Jarrett White Rd
Honolulu, HI 96859-5000
Tel: 808 433-2474 *Fax:* 808 433-1559
Accred Length: 1 Year *Program Size:* 15 (*GY1:* 15)
Sponsoring Spec: GS, IM, OBG, PD
Program ID: 999-14-00-030
US Armed Services Program

University of Hawaii Program

Sponsor: University of Hawaii John A Burns School of Medicine
Kaiser Foundation Hospital (Moanalua)
Kapiolani Medical Center for Women and Children
Kuakini Medical Center
Queen's Medical Center
St Francis Medical Center
Straub Clinic and Hospital

Program Director:
James E Hastings, MD
Univ of Hawaii Transitional Residency
University Tower/7th Fl
1356 Lusitana St
Honolulu, HI 96813-2427
Tel: 808 586-2910 *Fax:* 808 586-7486
E-mail: uhtrans@hawaii.edu
Internet:
http://unimrp.hawaii.edu/transitional/trweb98/trwe
Accred Length: 1 Year *Program Size:* 12 (*GY1:* 12)
Sponsoring Spec: GS, IM, OBG, PD
Program ID: 999-14-00-031

Illinois

Berwyn

MacNeal Memorial Hospital Program

Sponsor: MacNeal Memorial Hospital

Program Director:
Katherine Tynus, MD
MacNeal Memorial Hospital
3249 S Oak Park Ave
Berwyn, IL 60402
Tel: 708 795-3400, ext 3403 *Fax:* 708 783-3341
E-mail: ktynus@macneal.com
Internet: http://www.macneal.com
Accred Length: 1 Year *Program Size:* 13 (*GY1:* 13)
Sponsoring Spec: FP, GS, IM, OBG
Program ID: 999-16-00-032

Chicago

Catholic Health Partners Program

Sponsor: Catholic Health Partners
Columbus Hospital

Program Director:
Stephen Grohmann, MD
St Joseph Hospital
2900 N Lake Shore Dr
Chicago, IL 60657
Tel: 773 665-3263 *Fax:* 773 665-3384
Internet: http://www.cath-health.org
Accred Length: 1 Year *Program Size:* 6 (*GY1:* 6)
Sponsoring Spec: GS, IM
Program ID: 999-16-00-033

Illinois Masonic Medical Center Program

Sponsor: Illinois Masonic Medical Center

Program Director:
Frank J Konicek, MD
Illinois Masonic Med Ctr
Transitional Year Program
836 W Wellington Ave
Chicago, IL 60657-5193
Tel: 773 296-5399 *Fax:* 773 296-5051
Internet: http://www.immc.org
Accred Length: 1 Year *Program Size:* 10 (*GY1:* 10)
Sponsoring Spec: AN, DR, EM, FP, GS, IM, OBG, PD, PTH
Program ID: 999-16-00-034

Louis A Weiss Memorial Hospital Program
Sponsor: Louis A Weiss Memorial Hospital
Program Director:
William D Barnhart, MD MBA
Louis A Weiss Memorial Hospital
4646 N Marine Dr
Chicago, IL 60640-9966
Tel: 773 564-5225, ext
E-mail: bfuqua@mcis.bsd.uchicago.edu
Accred Length: 1 Year *Program Size:* 8 *(GY1:* 8)
Sponsoring Spec: GS, IM
Program ID: 999-16-00-035

Ravenswood Hospital Medical Center Program
Sponsor: Ravenswood Hospital Medical Center
Program Director:
Norbert Nadler, MD
Ravenswood Hospital Med Ctr
4550 N Winchester Ave
Chicago, IL 60640-5205
Tel: 773 878-4300, ext 4416 *Fax:* 773 279-4195
E-mail: ravenswoodtyr@rhmc.com
Internet:
http://www.advocatehealth.com/residency/index.html
Accred Length: 1 Year *Program Size:* 9 *(GY1:* 9)
Sponsoring Spec: FP, IM, ORS
Program ID: 999-16-00-153

Resurrection Medical Center Program
Sponsor: Resurrection Medical Center
Loyola University of Chicago Stritch School of Medicine
Program Director:
Joseph L Daddino, MD
Resurrection Med Ctr
Med Educ Office
7435 W Talcott Ave
Chicago, IL 60631
Tel: 773 792-5144 *Fax:* 773 792-9935
E-mail: jdaddino@reshealthcare.org
Accred Length: 1 Year *Program Size:* 6 *(GY1:* 6)
Sponsoring Spec: FP, GS
Program ID: 999-16-00-207

Swedish Covenant Hospital Program
Sponsor: Swedish Covenant Hospital
Program Director:
Michael J Plunkett, MD
Swedish Covenant Hospital
5145 N California Ave
Chicago, IL 60625
Tel: 773 989-3808, ext
E-mail: slasater@schosp.org or rarregui@schosp.org
Accred Length: 1 Year *Program Size:* 6 *(GY1:* 6)
Sponsoring Spec: FP, GS
Program ID: 999-16-00-231

Evanston

McGaw Medical Center of Northwestern University (Evanston) Program
Sponsor: Northwestern University Medical School
Evanston Hospital
Program Director:
James S Grober, MD
Evanston Northwestern Healthcare
2650 Ridge Ave
Evanston, IL 60201-1781
Tel: 847 570-2510 *Fax:* 847 570-2905
Internet: http://www.nums.nwu.edu/gme/index.htm
Accred Length: 1 Year *Program Size:* 10 *(GY1:* 10)
Sponsoring Spec: AN, IM, N
Program ID: 999-16-00-037

St Francis Hospital of Evanston Program
Sponsor: St Francis Hospital of Evanston
Program Director:
Marko Jachtorowycz, MD
St Francis Hospital of Evanston
355 Ridge Ave
Evanston, IL 60602-3399
Tel: 847 316-6227 *Fax:* 847 316-3307
E-mail: jobradovic@alverno.ssfhs.org
Internet: http://www.reshealth.org
Accred Length: 1 Year *Program Size:* 8 *(GY1:* 8)
Sponsoring Spec: DR, IM
Program ID: 999-16-00-038

Oak Park

West Suburban Hospital Medical Center Program
Sponsor: West Suburban Hospital Medical Center
Program Director:
Malcolm A Deam, MD
West Suburban Hospital Med Ctr
Ste L-700
Erie at Austin
Oak Park, IL 60302
Tel: 708 763-6908 *Fax:* 708 383-7655
Accred Length: 1 Year *Program Size:* 8 *(GY1:* 8)
Sponsoring Spec: FP, IM
Program ID: 999-16-00-154

Indiana

Indianapolis

Indiana University School of Medicine (Methodist) Program
Sponsor: Indiana University School of Medicine
Clarian Methodist Hospital of Indiana
Program Director:
Jack K Keene, MD
Clarian Methodist Hospital
I-65 at 21st St
PO Box 1367
Indianapolis, IN 46206-1367
Tel: 317 929-8881 *Fax:* 317 929-2150
E-mail: jkeene@clarian.com
Internet: http://www.iupui.edu/it/medschl/hsprogs.html
Accred Length: 1 Year *Program Size:* 12 *(GY1:* 12)
Sponsoring Spec: EM, FP, GS, IM, OBG, PD
Program ID: 999-17-00-040

St Vincent Hospital and Health Care Center Program
Sponsor: St Vincent Hospital and Health Care Center
Program Director:
Robert H Love, MD
St Vincent Hospital and Health Services
2001 W 86th St
Indianapolis, IN 46260
Tel: 317 338-2172 *Fax:* 317 338-6359
E-mail: rhlove@stvincent.org
Internet: http://www.stvincent.org
Accred Length: 1 Year *Program Size:* 12 *(GY1:* 12)
Sponsoring Spec: FP, IM
Program ID: 999-17-00-041

Muncie

Ball Memorial Hospital Program
Sponsor: Ball Memorial Hospital
Program Director:
Gerard T Costello, MD
Ball Memorial Hospital
2401 University Ave
Muncie, IN 47303
Tel: 765 741-1095 *Fax:* 765 747-0137
E-mail: bmh@iquest.net
Internet: http://www.ballhospital.org/
Accred Length: 1 Year *Program Size:* 8 *(GY1:* 8)
Sponsoring Spec: IM, PTH
Program ID: 999-17-00-157

Iowa

Des Moines

Broadlawns Medical Center Program
Sponsor: Broadlawns Medical Center
Iowa Methodist Medical Center
Program Director:
Nicholas J Galioto, MD
Broadlawns Med Ctr
1801 Hickman Rd
Des Moines, IA 50314
Tel: 515 282-2293 *Fax:* 515 282-2332
E-mail: jriegel@broadlawns.org
Internet: http://broadlawns.org
Accred Length: 1 Year *Program Size:* 2 *(GY1:* 2)
Sponsoring Spec: FP, GS, IM, OBG, PD
Program ID: 999-18-00-042

Iowa Methodist Medical Center Program
Sponsor: Iowa Methodist Medical Center
Veterans Affairs Central Iowa Health Care System
Program Director:
Douglas B Dorner, MD
Iowa Methodist Med Ctr
Med Educ Services Office
1415 Woodland Ave/Ste 140
Des Moines, IA 50309-9976
Tel: 515 241-6266 *Fax:* 515 241-5532
E-mail: qtturner@mail.ihs.org
Internet: http://www.ihsdesmoines.org
Accred Length: 1 Year *Program Size:* 4 *(GY1:* 4)
Sponsoring Spec: GS, IM, PD
Program ID: 999-18-00-220

Louisiana

New Orleans

Tulane University Program
Sponsor: Tulane University School of Medicine
Childrens Hospital
Medical Center of Louisiana at New Orleans
Tulane University Hospital and Clinics
Veterans Affairs Medical Center-LSU Service (New Orleans)
Program Director:
M A Krousel Wood, MD MPH
Transitional Program (TB-3)
Tulane Med Sch
1430 Tulane Ave
New Orleans, LA 70112-2699
Tel: 504 584-2841 *Fax:* 504 586-3801
E-mail: amiester@tmcpop.tmc.tulane.edu
Internet:
http://www.tmc.tulane.edu/departments/fammed/trans
Accred Length: 1 Year *Program Size:* 14 *(GY1:* 14)
Sponsoring Spec: IM, PD
Program ID: 999-21-00-047

Shreveport

Louisiana State University (Shreveport) Program

Sponsor: Louisiana State University Hospital-Shreveport
E A Conway Medical Center
Overton Brooks Veterans Affairs Medical Center

Program Director:
Kevin M Sittig, MD
Louisiana State Univ Med Ctr
1501 Kings Hwy
PO Box 33932
Shreveport, LA 71130-3932
Tel: 318 675-5069 *Fax:* 318 675-5666
E-mail: jevans@lsumc.edu
Accred Length: 1 Year *Program Size:* 8 (*GY1:* 8)
Sponsoring Spec: GS, IM, OBG, PD
Program ID: 999-21-00-048

Maryland

Andrews AFB

National Capital Consortium Program

Sponsor: National Capital Consortium
Malcolm Grow Medical Center (SGE)
National Naval Medical Center (Bethesda)

Program Director:
Kimberly P May, MD
89th Med Group/SGAT
Transitional Year Program
1050 W Perimeter Rd
Andrews AFB, MD 20762-6600
Tel: 301 981-8812 *Fax:* 301 981-4093
E-mail: maykim@mgmc.af.mil
Accred Length: 1 Year *Program Size:* 10 (*GY1:* 10)
Sponsoring Spec: FP, OBG
Program ID: 999-23-00-023
US Armed Services Program

Baltimore

Harbor Hospital Center Program

Sponsor: Harbor Hospital Center
Union Memorial Hospital

Program Director:
Richard B Williams, MD
Harbor Hospital Ctr
3001 S Hanover St
Baltimore, MD 21225-1290
Tel: 410 347-3565 *Fax:* 410 354-0186
E-mail: terryku@helix.org
Internet:
http://www.helixhealth.com/residency/hh-tranyear.h
Accred Length: 1 Year *Program Size:* 3 (*GY1:* 3)
Sponsoring Spec: GS, IM
Program ID: 999-23-00-050

Maryland General Hospital Program

Sponsor: Maryland General Hospital

Program Director:
William C Anthony, MD
Maryland General Hospital
827 Linden Ave/Ste 3B
Baltimore, MD 21201
Tel: 410 225-8790 *Fax:* 410 225-8910
Accred Length: 1 Year *Program Size:* 11 (*GY1:* 11)
Sponsoring Spec: IM, OPH
Program ID: 999-23-00-049

Bethesda

National Naval Medical Center (Bethesda) Program

Sponsor: National Naval Medical Center (Bethesda)

Program Director:
Cdr John M Avallone, MD
National Naval Med Ctr
Dept of Ophthalmology
Bldg 8
Bethesda, MD 20889-5011
Tel: 301 295-0280 *Fax:* 301 295-1481
E-mail: jmava@aol.com
Accred Length: 1 Year *Program Size:* 12 (*GY1:* 12)
Sponsoring Spec: GS, IM, OBG, PD
Program ID: 999-23-00-051
US Armed Services Program

Massachusetts

Boston

Carney Hospital Program

Sponsor: Carney Hospital

Program Director:
Michael Barza, MD
Carney Hospital
2100 Dorchester Ave
Boston, MA 02124-5666
Tel: 617 296-4012, ext 2726 *Fax:* 617 298-1547
E-mail: carneymed@aol.com
Accred Length: 1 Year *Program Size:* 7 (*GY1:* 7)
Sponsoring Spec: GS, IM
Program ID: 999-24-00-159

Tufts University Program

Sponsor: Lemuel Shattuck Hospital

Program Director:
James R Quirk, MD
Lemuel Shattuck Hospital
170 Morton St
Jamaica Plain, MA 02130-3782
Tel: 617 522-8110, ext 338 *Fax:* 617 983-2243
Accred Length: 1 Year *Program Size:* 6 (*GY1:* 6)
Sponsoring Spec: IM, N
Program ID: 999-24-00-199

Brockton

Boston University Medical Center/Brockton Hospital Program

Sponsor: Boston Medical Center
Brockton Hospital

Program Director:
Burton J Polansky, MD
Brockton Hospital
680 Centre St
Brockton, MA 02402
Tel: 508 941-7221 *Fax:* 508 941-6336
E-mail: pgy1broc@erols.com
Internet: http://www.brocktonhospital.com
Accred Length: 1 Year *Program Size:* 7 (*GY1:* 7)
Sponsoring Spec: DR, IM
Program ID: 999-24-00-158

Cambridge

Cambridge Hospital/Cambridge Health Alliance Program

Sponsor: Cambridge Hospital/Cambridge Health Alliance

Program Director:
Ira L Mintzer, MD
Cambridge Hospital
1493 Cambridge St
Cambridge, MA 02139
Tel: 617 498-1021 *Fax:* 617 498-1671
E-mail: transint@challiance.org
Accred Length: 1 Year *Program Size:* 3 (*GY1:* 3)
Sponsoring Spec: IM, P, PD
Program ID: 999-24-00-054

Framingham

MetroWest Medical Center/Harvard Medical School Program

Sponsor: MetroWest Medical Center-Framingham Union Hospital

Program Director:
Joel L Bass, MD
MetroWest Med Ctr-Framingham Union Hospital
Dept of Med Educ
115 Lincoln St
Framingham, MA 01702
Tel: 508 383-1555 *Fax:* 508 383-1548
Accred Length: 1 Year *Program Size:* 12 (*GY1:* 12)
Sponsoring Spec: IM, PD
Program ID: 999-24-00-160

Malden

Malden Hospital/Boston University Medical Center Program

Sponsor: Malden Hospital
Boston Medical Center

Program Director:
Ellen Malsky, MD
Malden Hospital
100 Hospital Rd
Malden, MA 02148
Tel: 617 397-6559 *Fax:* 617 397-6087
Accred Length: 1 Year *Program Size:* 7 (*GY1:* 7)
Sponsoring Spec: FP, IM
Program ID: 999-24-00-161

Michigan

Ann Arbor

St Joseph Mercy Hospital Program

Sponsor: St Joseph Mercy Health System

Program Director:
Jack H Carman, MD
St Joseph Mercy Hospital
RHB-1115
PO Box 995
Ann Arbor, MI 48106
Tel: 734 712-5015 *Fax:* 734 712-8777
E-mail: carman@mercyhealth.com
Accred Length: 1 Year *Program Size:* 12 (*GY1:* 12)
Sponsoring Spec: GS, IM
Program ID: 999-25-00-056

Dearborn

Oakwood Hospital Program
Sponsor: Oakwood Hospital
Program Director:
Lyle D Victor, MD
Oakwood Healthcare System
18101 Oakwood Blvd
PO Box 2500
Dearborn, MI 48123-2500
Tel: 313 593-8435 *Fax:* 313 436-2071
Accred Length: 1 Year *Program Size:* 15 (*GY1:* 15)
Sponsoring Spec: FP, IM
Program ID: 999-25-00-057

Detroit

Henry Ford Hospital Program
Sponsor: Henry Ford Hospital
Program Director:
Bruce M Thompson, MD
Henry Ford Hospital
2799 W Grand Blvd
Detroit, MI 48202
Tel: 313 876-7143 *Fax:* 313 556-8843
Accred Length: 1 Year *Program Size:* 20 (*GY1:* 20)
Sponsoring Spec: AN, EM, IM, OPH
Program ID: 999-25-00-058

St John Hospital and Medical Center Program
Sponsor: St John Hospital and Medical Center
Program Director:
John H Burrows, MD
St John Hospital and Med Ctr
Dept of Med Educ
22101 Moross Rd
Detroit, MI 48236
Tel: 313 343-3875 *Fax:* 313 343-7840
E-mail: sue.moynihan@stjohn.org
Internet: http://www.stjohn.org
Accred Length: 1 Year *Program Size:* 8 (*GY1:* 8)
Sponsoring Spec: GS, IM
Program ID: 999-25-00-059

Wayne State University/Detroit Medical Center Program
Sponsor: Wayne State University/Detroit Medical Center
Children's Hospital of Michigan
Detroit Receiving Hospital and University Health Center
Grace Hospital
Harper Hospital
Hutzel Hospital
Program Director:
Kenneth L Bergsman, MD
Grace Hospital
6071 W Outer Dr
Detroit, MI 48235
Tel: 313 966-4064 *Fax:* 313 966-1738
Internet: http://www.intmed.wayne.edu
Accred Length: 1 Year *Program Size:* 12 (*GY1:* 12)
Sponsoring Spec: EM, GS, IM, OBG
Program ID: 999-25-00-060

Flint

Hurley Medical Center/Michigan State University Program
Sponsor: Hurley Medical Center
Program Director:
Ghassan I Bachuwa, MD
Hurley Med Ctr
Two Hurley Plaza
Flint, MI 48503-5993
Tel: 810 257-9319 *Fax:* 810 762-7245
E-mail: gbachu1@hurleymc.com
Internet: http://www.hurleymc.com
Accred Length: 1 Year *Program Size:* 8 (*GY1:* 8)
Sponsoring Spec: IM, PD
Program ID: 999-25-00-062

Grand Rapids

Spectrum Health-Downtown Campus Program
Sponsor: Spectrum Health-Downtown Campus
Program Director:
Sohail Qadir, MD
Spectrum Health-Downtown Campus
100 Michigan Ave NE/MC41
Grand Rapids, MI 49503
Tel: 616 391-1835 *Fax:* 616 391-2911
Internet: http://www.spectrum-health.org
Accred Length: 1 Year *Program Size:* 5 (*GY1:* 5)
Sponsoring Spec: EM, IM, OBG, PD
Program ID: 999-25-00-190

Spectrum Health-East Campus Program
Sponsor: Spectrum Health-East Campus
Program Director:
Robert L Tupper, MD
Spectrum Health-East Campus
1840 Wealthy St SE
Grand Rapids, MI 49506
Tel: 616 774-7733 *Fax:* 616 774-5290
E-mail: robert_tupper@blodgett.com
Accred Length: 1 Year *Program Size:* 8 (*GY1:* 8)
Sponsoring Spec: GS, IM
Program ID: 999-25-00-063

St Mary's Health Services Program
Sponsor: St Mary's Health Services
Program Director:
Enrico C Sobong, MD
St Mary's Health Services
200 Jefferson Ave SE
Grand Rapids, MI 49503
Tel: 616 752-6420 *Fax:* 616 732-3033
Accred Length: 1 Year *Program Size:* 6 (*GY1:* 6)
Sponsoring Spec: GS, IM
Program ID: 999-25-00-064

Kalamazoo

Kalamazoo Center for Medical Studies/Michigan State University Program
Sponsor: Kalamazoo Center for Medical Studies
Borgess Medical Center
Bronson Methodist Hospital
Program Director:
Marilyn R Terranella, MD
Michigan State Univ-Kalamazoo Ctr for Med Studies
Dept of Transitional Year
1000 Oakland Dr
Kalamazoo, MI 49008-1284
Tel: 616 337-6350 *Fax:* 616 337-4234
E-mail: trans@kcms.msu.edu
Internet: http://www.kcms.msu.edu
Accred Length: 1 Year *Program Size:* 5 (*GY1:* 5)
Sponsoring Spec: FP, IM
Program ID: 999-25-00-065

Lansing

Sparrow Hospital/Michigan State University Program
Sponsor: Sparrow Hospital
Program Director:
Cynthia S Boynton, MD
Sparrow Hospital
Attn: Transitional Year Residency
1215 E Michigan Ave
Lansing, MI 48912-1896
Tel: 517 483-2150 *Fax:* 517 483-2763
E-mail: transres@pilot.msu.edu
Accred Length: 1 Year *Program Size:* 6 (*GY1:* 6)
Sponsoring Spec: EM, FP, IM, OBG, PD
Program ID: 999-25-00-066

Pontiac

St Joseph Mercy-Oakland Program
Sponsor: St Joseph Mercy-Oakland
Program Director:
Bernard A Bercu, MD
St Joseph Mercy Oakland
900 Woodward Ave
Pontiac, MI 48341-2985
Tel: 248 858-3234, ext
Accred Length: 1 Year *Program Size:* 5 (*GY1:* 5)
Sponsoring Spec: GS, IM
Program ID: 999-25-00-067

Royal Oak

William Beaumont Hospital Program
Sponsor: William Beaumont Hospital
William Beaumont Hospital-Troy
Program Director:
Steven C Winokur, MD
William Beaumont Hospital
3601 W 13 Mile Rd
Royal Oak, MI 48073
Tel: 248 551-0431 *Fax:* 248 551-5426
E-mail: sfiore@beaumont.edu
Internet: http://www.beaumont.edu/html/gme
Accred Length: 1 Year *Program Size:* 16 (*GY1:* 16)
Sponsoring Spec: EM, IM
Program ID: 999-25-00-178

Southfield

Providence Hospital and Medical Centers Program
Sponsor: Providence Hospital and Medical Centers
Program Director:
Bruce L Kaplan, DO
Providence Hospital
16001 W Nine Mile Rd
Southfield, MI 48075-4818
Tel: 248 424-3151 *Fax:* 248 424-5324
Accred Length: 1 Year *Program Size:* 10 (*GY1:* 10)
Sponsoring Spec: DR, GS, IM, OBG, P
Program ID: 999-25-00-068

Minnesota

Minneapolis

Hennepin County Medical Center Program

Sponsor: Hennepin County Medical Center

Program Director:
Michael B Belzer, MD
Hennepin County Med Ctr
Med Admin #867A
701 Park Ave S
Minneapolis, MN 55415-1623
Tel: 612 347-2357 *Fax:* 612 904-4401
Internet: http://www.hcmc.org
Accred Length: 1 Year *Program Size:* 21 (*GY1:* 21)
Sponsoring Spec: EM, GS, IM, N, OBG, P, PD
Program ID: 999-26-00-069

Missouri

St Louis

Deaconess Hospital Program

Sponsor: Deaconess Hospital

Program Director:
M R Hill, MD
Deaconess Hospital
6150 Oakland Ave
St Louis, MO 63139-3297
Tel: 314 768-3006 *Fax:* 314 768-5632
E-mail: dexascan@geocities.com
Internet:
http://www.geocities.com/hotsprings/2846/homepage.
Accred Length: 1 Year *Program Size:* 9 (*GY1:* 9)
Sponsoring Spec: FP, IM, OBG
Program ID: 999-28-00-179

St John's Mercy Medical Center Program

Sponsor: St John's Mercy Medical Center

Program Director:
Christopher Veremakis, MD
St John's Mercy Med Ctr
Grad Med Educ
615 S New Ballas Rd
St Louis, MO 63141-8277
Tel: 314 569-6930 *Fax:* 314 995-4288
Accred Length: 1 Year *Program Size:* 10 (*GY1:* 10)
Sponsoring Spec: IM, OBG, PTH
Program ID: 999-28-00-071

New Jersey

Livingston

St Barnabas Medical Center Program

Sponsor: St Barnabas Medical Center

Program Director:
Arthur Maron, MD
St Barnabas Med Ctr
94 Old Short Hills Rd
Livingston, NJ 07039
Tel: 973 322-5777 *Fax:* 973 322-8720
Accred Length: 1 Year *Program Size:* 12 (*GY1:* 12)
Sponsoring Spec: GS, IM
Program ID: 999-33-00-073

Neptune

Jersey Shore Medical Center Program

Sponsor: Jersey Shore Medical Center

Program Director:
Margaret M Quinn, MD
Jersey Shore Med Ctr
Attn: J McCorkel, Acad Affairs
1945 Rte 33
Neptune, NJ 07754
Tel: 908 776-4943 *Fax:* 908 776-4683
E-mail: mquinn@monmouth.com
Internet: http://www.medicalexchange.com/hospital/jsmc
Accred Length: 1 Year *Program Size:* 6 (*GY1:* 6)
Sponsoring Spec: IM, PD
Program ID: 999-33-00-074

New York

Binghamton

Wilson Memorial Regional Medical Center (United Health Services) Program

Sponsor: Wilson Memorial Regional Medical Center (United Health Svs)

Program Director:
David W Towle, DO MS MPH
United Health Services Hospitals
Med Educ Dept
33-57 Harrison St
Johnson City, NY 13790
Tel: 800 338-8471 *Fax:* 607 763-6888
E-mail: linda_kinsey@uhs.org
Accred Length: 1 Year *Program Size:* 7 (*GY1:* 7)
Sponsoring Spec: FP, IM
Program ID: 999-35-00-081

Brooklyn

Maimonides Medical Center Program

Sponsor: Maimonides Medical Center

Program Director:
Joseph N Cunningham Jr, MD
Maimonides Med Ctr
4802 Tenth Ave
Brooklyn, NY 11219
Tel: 718 283-7687 *Fax:* 718 283-8909
Accred Length: 1 Year *Program Size:* 5 (*GY1:* 5)
Sponsoring Spec: AN, GS, IM
Program ID: 999-35-00-204

Cooperstown

Bassett Healthcare Program

Sponsor: Bassett Healthcare
Mary Imogene Bassett Hospital

Program Director:
Eric J DelGiacco, MD
Bassett Healthcare
Medical Education
One Atwell Rd
Cooperstown, NY 13326-1394
Tel: 607 547-3764 *Fax:* 607 547-6612
E-mail: bassedty@telenet.net
Internet: http://www.bassett.edu
Accred Length: 1 Year *Program Size:* 5 (*GY1:* 5)
Sponsoring Spec: GS, IM
Program ID: 999-35-00-080

Flushing

New York Flushing Hospital Medical Center Program

Sponsor: New York Flushing Hospital Medical Center

Program Director:
Robert Golub, MD
Flushing Hospital and Med Ctr
4500 Parsons Blvd
Flushing, NY 11355
Tel: 718 670-5000 *Fax:* 718 670-4449
Accred Length: 1 Year *Program Size:* 10 (*GY1:* 10)
Sponsoring Spec: GS, IM, OBG, PD
Program ID: 999-35-00-196

New York Hospital Medical Center of Queens/Cornell University Medical College Program

Sponsor: New York Hospital Medical Center of Queens

Program Director:
Anthony Somogyi, MD
New York Hospital Med Ctr of Queens
56-45 Main St
Flushing, NY 11355
Tel: 718 670-1477 *Fax:* 718 321-8857
E-mail: mfmarrer%queens@nyh.med.cornell.edu
Accred Length: 1 Year *Program Size:* 12 (*GY1:* 12)
Sponsoring Spec: GS, IM
Program ID: 999-35-00-225

New Rochelle

New York Medical College (Sound Shore) Program

Sponsor: New York Medical College
Sound Shore Medical Center of Westchester

Program Director:
Jeffrey M Brensilver, MD
Sound Shore Med Ctr of Westchester
Dept of Med
16 Guion Pl
New Rochelle, NY 10802-5500
Tel: 914 637-1681 *Fax:* 914 637-1171
E-mail: ssmcw@cris.com
Internet:
http://www.concentric.net/~ssmcw/residency.shtml
Accred Length: 1 Year *Program Size:* 3 (*GY1:* 3)
Sponsoring Spec: GS, IM
Program ID: 999-35-00-216

New York

New York Medical College at St Vincent's Hospital and Medical Center of New York Program

Sponsor: New York Medical College
St Vincent's Hospital and Medical Center of New York

Program Director:
Eric C Rackow, MD
St Vincent's Hospital and Med Ctr
153 W 11th St
New York, NY 10011
Tel: 212 604-7512 *Fax:* 212 604-3286
Internet: http://svh.nymc.edu
Accred Length: 1 Year *Program Size:* 15 (*GY1:* 15)
Sponsoring Spec: AN, CHP, DR, IM, N, NM, OBG, OPH, P, PD, PM, PTH
Program ID: 999-35-00-083

Syracuse

St Joseph's Hospital Health Center Program

Sponsor: St Joseph's Hospital Health Center

Program Director:
Robert T Friedman, MD
St Joseph's Hospital Health Ctr
301 Prospect Ave
Syracuse, NY 13203
Tel: 315 448-5547 *Fax:* 315 448-6313
E-mail: schloc54@sjhsyr.org
Accred Length: 1 Year *Program Size:* 4 (*GY1:* 4)
Sponsoring Spec: EM, FP
Program ID: 999-35-00-084

North Dakota

Fargo

University of North Dakota Program

Sponsor: Univ of North Dakota School of Medicine & Health Sciences
MeritCare Hospital
Veterans Affairs Medical and Regional Office Center (Fargo)

Program Director:
Mark J Tieszen, MD
Merit Care Med Ctr
720 Fourth St N
Fargo, ND 58122
Tel: 701 234-5933 *Fax:* 701 234-7230
E-mail: undtyprog@meritcare.com
Accred Length: 1 Year *Program Size:* 6 (*GY1:* 6)
Sponsoring Spec: FP, IM, P
Program ID: 999-37-00-086

Ohio

Akron

Akron General Medical Center/NEOUCOM Program

Sponsor: Akron General Medical Center

Program Director:
Joseph Finocchio, MD
Akron General Med Ctr
400 Wabash Ave
Akron, OH 44307
Tel: 330 384-6050 *Fax:* 330 384-1529
E-mail: meded@agmc.org
Internet: http://agmc.org
Accred Length: 1 Year *Program Size:* 4 (*GY1:* 4)
Sponsoring Spec: FP, GS, IM
Program ID: 999-38-00-088

Summa Health System (Akron City Hospital)/NEOUCOM Program

Sponsor: Summa Health System
Akron City Hospital (Summa Health System)
St Thomas Hospital (Summa Health System)

Program Director:
Melinda S Phinney, MD
Summa Health System
Med Educ/Mary Yanik
525 E Market St
Akron, OH 44309
Tel: 800 322-0517, ext
Internet: http://www.summahealth.org/edu/
Accred Length: 1 Year *Program Size:* 5 (*GY1:* 5)
Sponsoring Spec: EM, IM
Program ID: 999-38-00-087

Canton

Aultman Hospital/NEOUCOM Program

Sponsor: Aultman Hospital

Program Director:
Ronald D Crock, MD
Aultman Hospital
2600 Sixth St SW
Canton, OH 44710
Tel: 330 438-7434 *Fax:* 330 580-5513
Internet: http://www.aultmanresidencies.com
Accred Length: 1 Year *Program Size:* 4 (*GY1:* 4)
Sponsoring Spec: DR, FP, IM, OBG
Program ID: 999-38-00-191

Cleveland

Mount Sinai Medical Center of Cleveland Program

Sponsor: Mount Sinai Medical Center of Cleveland

Program Director:
D Roy Ferguson, MD
Mt Sinai Med Ctr
One Mt Sinai Dr/ED3
Cleveland, OH 44106-4198
Tel: 216 421-4000 *Fax:* 216 421-4833
E-mail: egraffein@stratos.net
Internet: http://www.mtsinai.org
Accred Length: 1 Year *Program Size:* 5 (*GY1:* 5)
Sponsoring Spec: DR, EM, IM, OBG, OPH, PTH
Program ID: 999-38-00-091

Columbus

Mount Carmel Health Program

Sponsor: Mount Carmel Medical Center

Program Director:
James N Parsons, MD
Mount Carmel Health System
793 W State St
Columbus, OH 43222
Tel: 614 234-5279 *Fax:* 614 234-2772
Internet: http://mchsresidency.org
Accred Length: 1 Year *Program Size:* 5 (*GY1:* 5)
Sponsoring Spec: GS, IM
Program ID: 999-38-00-093

Riverside Methodist Hospitals (OhioHealth) Program

Sponsor: Riverside Methodist Hospitals (OhioHealth)

Program Director:
Thomas J Boes, MD
Riverside Methodist Hospital
Dept of Medical Education
3535 Olentangy River Rd
Columbus, OH 43214
Tel: 614 566-4462 *Fax:* 614 566-6852
Internet: http://www.ohiohealth.com
Accred Length: 1 Year *Program Size:* 12 (*GY1:* 12)
Sponsoring Spec: GS, IM
Program ID: 999-38-00-095

Dayton (Kettering)

Kettering Medical Center Program

Sponsor: Kettering Medical Center
Children's Medical Center
Miami Valley Hospital

Program Director:
John A Shrader, MD
Kettering Med Ctr
3535 Southern Blvd
Kettering, OH 45429-1298
Tel: 800 203-8925 *Fax:* 937 296-4299
E-mail: delina_unger@ketthealth.com/meded/edop.htm
Internet: http://www.ketthealth.com/med/edop.htm
Accred Length: 1 Year *Program Size:* 8 (*GY1:* 8)
Sponsoring Spec: EM, FP, GS, IM, OBG, PD
Program ID: 999-38-00-096

Toledo

Mercy Health Partners Program

Sponsor: St Vincent Mercy Medical Center

Program Director:
Walter R Woodhouse, MD MSA
Mercy Healthcare Ctr
2200 Jefferson Ave
Toledo, OH 43624
Tel: 419 251-1395 *Fax:* 419 251-1351
E-mail: mhptyr @ primenet.com
Internet: http://www.mercyfp@primenet.com
Accred Length: 1 Year *Program Size:* 7 (*GY1:* 7)
Sponsoring Spec: FP, GS
Program ID: 999-38-00-165

Oregon

Portland

Legacy Emanuel Hospital and Health Center Program

Sponsor: Legacy Emanuel Hospital and Health Center
Legacy Good Samaritan Hospital and Medical Center

Program Director:
Geoffrey S Sewell, MD
2801 N Gantenbein Ave
Portland, OR 97227
Tel: 503 413-4692 *Fax:* 503 413-2144
E-mail: tyres@email.lhs.org
Internet: http://www.legacyhealth.org
Accred Length: 1 Year *Program Size:* 7 (*GY1:* 7)
Sponsoring Spec: GS, IM
Program ID: 999-40-00-101

Pennsylvania

Allentown

Lehigh Valley Hospital/Pennsylvania State University Program

Sponsor: Lehigh Valley Hospital

Program Director:
Richard H Snyder, MD MBA
Lehigh Valley Hospital
Dept of Med
Cedar Crest and I-78/PO Box 689
Allentown, PA 18105-1556
Tel: 610 402-8200 *Fax:* 610 402-1675
E-mail: medicaled@lvhhn.org
Internet:
http://www.lvhhn.org/academic/residency/transition
Accred Length: 1 Year *Program Size:* 8 (*GY1:* 8)
Sponsoring Spec: GS, IM, OBG
Program ID: 999-41-00-103

Bethlehem

St Luke's Hospital Program

Sponsor: St Luke's Hospital

Program Director:
Gloria T Fioravanti, DO
St Luke's Hospital
801 Ostrum St
Bethlehem, PA 18015
Tel: 610 954-4644 *Fax:* 610 954-4979
E-mail: im-residency@slhn.org
Internet: http://slhn-lehighvalley.org
Accred Length: 1 Year *Program Size:* 4 (*GY1:* 4)
Sponsoring Spec: IM, OBG
Program ID: 999-41-00-104

Darby

Mercy Catholic Medical Center Program
Sponsor: Mercy Catholic Medical Center Inc
Mercy Fitzgerald Hospital
Program Director:
J. Harris Joseph, DO
Mercy Catholic Med Ctr
1500 Lansdowne Ave
Darby, PA 19023
Tel: 610 237-5090 *Fax:* 610 237-5093
Internet: http://www.mercyhealth.org
Accred Length: 1 Year *Program Size:* 10 (*GY1:* 10)
Sponsoring Spec: DR, IM
Program ID: 999-41-00-106

Easton

Easton Hospital Program
Sponsor: Easton Hospital
Program Director:
Raymond S Buch, MD
Easton Hospital
250 S 21st St
Easton, PA 18042-3892
Tel: 610 250-4517 *Fax:* 610 250-4820
E-mail: jane_grube@valleyhealth.org
Accred Length: 1 Year *Program Size:* 0 (*GY1:* 0)
Sponsoring Spec: GS, IM
Program ID: 999-41-00-218

Erie

Hamot Medical Center Program
Sponsor: Hamot Medical Center
Program Director:
Steven A Levy, MD
Hamot Med Ctr
201 State St
Erie, PA 16550
Tel: 814 877-6055 *Fax:* 814 877-4699
E-mail: kathy.hull@hamot.org
Internet: http://www.hamot.org
Accred Length: 1 Year *Program Size:* 3 (*GY1:* 3)
Sponsoring Spec: FP, ORS
Program ID: 999-41-00-232

Johnstown

Conemaugh Valley Memorial Hospital Program
Sponsor: Conemaugh Valley Memorial Hospital
Program Director:
Joseph T Sobieski, MD MD
Memorial Med Ctr
1086 Franklin St
Johnstown, PA 15905-4398
Tel: 814 534-9408 *Fax:* 814 534-3290
Accred Length: 1 Year *Program Size:* 8 (*GY1:* 8)
Sponsoring Spec: FP, IM, PTH
Program ID: 999-41-00-108

Philadelphia

Albert Einstein Medical Center Program
Sponsor: Albert Einstein Medical Center
Program Director:
Lisa B Wallenstein, MD
Transitional Year Program
Albert Einstein Med Ctr
5401 Old York Rd/Ste 363
Philadelphia, PA 19141-3025
Tel: 800 220-2362 *Fax:* 215 455-1933
E-mail: medicine@aehn2.einstein.edu
Internet: http://www.einstein.edu/phl
Accred Length: 1 Year *Program Size:* 14 (*GY1:* 14)
Sponsoring Spec: GS, IM, PD
Program ID: 999-41-00-224

Chestnut Hill Hospital Program
Sponsor: Chestnut Hill Hospital
Program Director:
Simeon L Bardin, MD
Chestnut Hill Hospital
8835 Germantown Ave
Philadelphia, PA 19118-2767
Tel: 215 248-8265 *Fax:* 215 248-8859
E-mail: pollock@chh.org
Internet: http://www.chh.org
Accred Length: 1 Year *Program Size:* 8 (*GY1:* 8)
Sponsoring Spec: FP, GS
Program ID: 999-41-00-111

Presbyterian Medical Center of the University of Pennsylvania Health System Program
Sponsor: Presbyterian Medical Center (UPHS)
Program Director:
John J Millili, MD
Presbyterian Med Ctr-Univ of Pennsylvania
51 N 39th St
Wright-Saunders Bldg 128
Philadelphia, PA 19104
Tel: 215 662-9784 *Fax:* 215 662-0472
Accred Length: 1 Year *Program Size:* 14 (*GY1:* 14)
Sponsoring Spec: DR, IM
Program ID: 999-41-00-113

Temple University Program
Sponsor: Temple University Hospital
Frankford Hospital (Frankford Campus)
Frankford Hospital (Torresdale Campus)
Program Director:
Ralph R Vassallo Jr, MD
Frankford Hospital
Dept of Med Educ
Red Lion and Knights Rds
Philadelphia, PA 19114-1486
Tel: 215 612-4846 *Fax:* 215 612-4946
E-mail: frnkfrdtyr@aol.com
Accred Length: 1 Year *Program Size:* 29 (*GY1:* 29)
Sponsoring Spec: GS, OBG
Program ID: 999-41-00-112

Pittsburgh

Mercy Hospital of Pittsburgh Program
Sponsor: Mercy Hospital of Pittsburgh
Program Director:
Kimball W Mohn, MD
Mercy Hospital of Pittsburgh
Dept of Med
1400 Locust St
Pittsburgh, PA 15219-5166
Tel: 412 232-5533 *Fax:* 412 232-5689
E-mail: transitional.year@mercy.pmhs.org
Internet: http://www.mercy-meded.com
Accred Length: 1 Year *Program Size:* 10 (*GY1:* 10)
Sponsoring Spec: AN, DR, GS, IM
Program ID: 999-41-00-114

Shadyside Hospital/UPMC Program
Sponsor: Shadyside Hospital/UPMC
Program Director:
Gary H Tabas, MD
UPMC Shadyside
5230 Centre Ave
Pittsburgh, PA 15232
Tel: 412 623-6685 *Fax:* 412 623-2555
Internet: http://ssh.edu
Accred Length: 1 Year *Program Size:* 6 (*GY1:* 6)
Sponsoring Spec: FP, IM
Program ID: 999-41-00-117

St Francis Medical Center Program
Sponsor: St Francis Medical Center
Program Director:
Louis E Leff, MD
St Francis Med Ctr
Med Educ Office
400 45th St
Pittsburgh, PA 15201
Tel: 412 622-4388, ext
E-mail: leff@sfhs.edu
Internet: http://www.sfhs.edu
Accred Length: 1 Year *Program Size:* 10 (*GY1:* 10)
Sponsoring Spec: IM, P
Program ID: 999-41-00-116

University Health Center of Pittsburgh Program
Sponsor: University Health Center of Pittsburgh
Children's Hospital of Pittsburgh
Magee-Women's Hospital
Presbyterian University Hospital/UPMC
Veterans Affairs Medical Center (Pittsburgh)
Western Psychiatric Institute and Clinic/UPMC
Program Director:
Frank J Bruns, MD
Univ Health Ctr of Pittsburgh
3550 Terrace St
1220 Scaife Hall
Pittsburgh, PA 15261
Tel: 412 648-9642 *Fax:* 412 648-2117
Internet: http://www.upmc.edu/medicine
Accred Length: 1 Year *Program Size:* 8 (*GY1:* 8)
Sponsoring Spec: AN, D, DR, GS, IM, N, OBG, OPH, ORS, P, PD, PTH
Program ID: 999-41-00-115

Western Pennsylvania Hospital Program
Sponsor: Western Pennsylvania Hospital
Program Director:
Elliot Goldberg, MD
Western Pennsylvania Hospital
4800 Friendship Ave
Pittsburgh, PA 15224-1793
Tel: 412 578-5750 *Fax:* 412 578-6804
E-mail: intermedwph@yahoo.com
Internet: http://www.westpennhospital.com
Accred Length: 1 Year *Program Size:* 8 (*GY1:* 8)
Sponsoring Spec: AN, DR, EM, FP, GS, IM, OBG
Program ID: 999-41-00-234

Reading

Reading Hospital and Medical Center Program
Sponsor: Reading Hospital and Medical Center
Program Director:
David L George, MD
Reading Hospital and Med Ctr
Sixth Ave and Spruce St
West Reading, PA 19612-6052
Tel: 610 378-6470 *Fax:* 610 208-9003
E-mail: georged@readinghospital.org
Internet: http://www.readinghospital.org
Accred Length: 1 Year *Program Size:* 5 (*GY1:* 5)
Sponsoring Spec: FP, IM, OBG
Program ID: 999-41-00-119

Upland

Crozer-Chester Medical Center Program

Sponsor: Crozer-Chester Medical Center
Program Director:
Susan L Williams, MD
Crozer-Chester Med Ctr
Residency Office 3rd Fl East Wing
One Medical Center Blvd
Upland, PA 19013-8110
Tel: 800 225-1171 *Fax:* 610 447-6373
Internet:
http://www.crozer.org/educate/resprog/tranyear/tra
Accred Length: 1 Year *Program Size:* 12 (*GY1:* 12)
Sponsoring Spec: IM, PD
Program ID: 999-41-00-212

York

York Hospital Program

Sponsor: York Hospital
Program Director:
Peter M Hartmann, MD
York Hospital
1001 S George St
York, PA 17405
Tel: 717 851-2753 *Fax:* 717 851-2968
E-mail: mf_jbergeron@yorkhospital.edu
Internet: http://www.yorkhealth.org
Accred Length: 1 Year *Program Size:* 4 (*GY1:* 4)
Sponsoring Spec: FP, IM
Program ID: 999-41-00-120

Puerto Rico

Bayamon

Universidad Central del Caribe Program

Sponsor: University Hospital Ramon Ruiz Arnau
Program Director:
Ramon A Suarez, MD
Dr Ramon Ruiz Arnau Univ Hospital
Call Box 60-327
Bayamon, PR 00960-6032
Tel: 787 798-3001, ext 268 *Fax:* 787 740-4343
Accred Length: 1 Year *Program Size:* 10 (*GY1:* 10)
Sponsoring Spec: FP, IM, PD
Program ID: 999-42-00-121

Caguas

Caguas Regional Hospital Program

Sponsor: Caguas Regional Hospital
University Hospital
Program Director:
Luis A Medina, MD
Caguas Regional Hospital
PO Box 5729
Caguas, PR 00726
Tel: 787 744-3141, ext 2059 *Fax:* 787 746-3440
Accred Length: 1 Year *Program Size:* 8 (*GY1:* 8)
Sponsoring Spec: FP, IM, PD
Program ID: 999-42-00-122

Mayaguez

Ramon E Betances Hospital-Mayaguez Medical Center Program

Sponsor: Dr Ramon E Betances Hospital-Mayaguez Medical Center
Program Director:
Elba I Morales de Roman, MD
Ramon E Betances Hospital
Mayaguez Med Ctr
410 Hostos Ave
Mayaguez, PR 00680
Tel: 787 834-8686, ext 2950 *Fax:* 787 832-7110
Accred Length: 1 Year *Program Size:* 9 (*GY1:* 9)
Sponsoring Spec: GS, IM, PD
Program ID: 999-42-00-123

Ponce

Hospital de Damas Program

Sponsor: Hospital de Damas
Ponce University Hospital
Program Director:
Hector R Silva, MD
Edificio Parra
2225 Ponce By-Pass
Ste 407
Ponce, PR 00731-7779
Tel: 787 840-8686, ext 6123
Accred Length: 1 Year *Program Size:* 12 (*GY1:* 12)
Sponsoring Spec: IM, PD
Program ID: 999-42-00-236

Ponce University Hospital Program

Sponsor: Ponce University Hospital
Program Director:
Olga Rodriguez, MD
Ponce Univ Hospital
Ave Tito Castro #917
Ponce, PR 00731
Tel: 809 843-3031 *Fax:* 787 841-7165
E-mail: olgita@caribe.net
Accred Length: 1 Year *Program Size:* 12 (*GY1:* 12)
Sponsoring Spec: IM, PD
Program ID: 999-42-00-125

Rio Piedras

San Juan City Hospital Program

Sponsor: San Juan City Hospital
University Hospital
Program Director:
Hilda Rivera-Tubens, MD
San Juan Municipal Hospital
CMMS #79 PO Box 70344
San Juan, PR 00936-8344
Tel: 787 766-0205 *Fax:* 787 764-3643
Accred Length: 1 Year *Program Size:* 10 (*GY1:* 10)
Sponsoring Spec: D, DR, EM, GS, IM, N, OBG, OPH, OTO, PD
Program ID: 999-42-00-213

Rhode Island

Providence

Brown University Program

Sponsor: Miriam Hospital
Program Director:
A Gerson Greenburg, MD PhD
Miriam Hospital
164 Summit Ave
Providence, RI 02906
Tel: 401 793-4510 *Fax:* 401 274-8789
E-mail: tgauvin@lifespan.org
Accred Length: 1 Year *Program Size:* 3 (*GY1:* 3)
Sponsoring Spec: GS, IM
Program ID: 999-43-00-166

South Carolina

Greenville

Greenville Hospital System Program

Sponsor: Greenville Hospital System
Program Director:
J William Kelly, MD
Greenville Hospital System
701 Grove Rd
Greenville, SC 29605-5601
Tel: 864 455-7773 *Fax:* 864 455-5008
Accred Length: 1 Year *Program Size:* 6 (*GY1:* 6)
Sponsoring Spec: IM, PD
Program ID: 999-45-00-126

Spartanburg

Spartanburg Regional Medical Center Program

Sponsor: Spartanburg Regional Healthcare System
Program Director:
Joseph Walton, MD
Spartanburg Regional Healthcare System
101 E Wood St
Spartanburg, SC 29303
Tel: 864 560-6902 *Fax:* 864 560-7015
E-mail: bwest@teleplex.net
Internet: http://www.srhs.com
Accred Length: 1 Year *Program Size:* 6 (*GY1:* 6)
Sponsoring Spec: FP, GS
Program ID: 999-45-00-182

South Dakota

Sioux Falls

University of South Dakota Program

Sponsor: University of South Dakota School of Medicine
Avera McKennan Hospital
Royal C Johnson Veterans Affairs Medical Center
Sioux Valley Hospital
Program Director:
Rodney R Parry, MD
Univ of South Dakota Sch of Med
Office of the Dean
1400 W 22nd St
Sioux Falls, SD 57105-1570
Tel: 605 357-1300 *Fax:* 605 357-1311
E-mail: rparry@sundance.usd.edu
Accred Length: 1 Year *Program Size:* 6 (*GY1:* 6)
Sponsoring Spec: FP, IM
Program ID: 999-46-00-230

Tennessee

Chattanooga

University of Tennessee College of Medicine at Chattanooga Program

Sponsor: University of Tennessee College of Medicine-Chattanooga Unit
Erlanger Medical Center

Program Director:
Mukta Panda, MD
Erlanger Health System
Medicine Clinic
975 E Third St
Chattanooga, TN 37403
Tel: 423 778-6670 *Fax:* 423 778-2586
E-mail: uttrans@erlanger.org
Internet:
http://www.erlanger.org/utcom/transitional.html
Accred Length: 1 Year *Program Size:* 4 (*GY1:* 4)
Sponsoring Spec: GS, IM, OBG, OPH, PD
Program ID: 999-47-00-129

Knoxville

University of Tennessee Medical Center at Knoxville Program

Sponsor: University of Tennessee Graduate School of Medicine
University of Tennessee Memorial Hospital

Program Director:
Lisa L Kirkland, MD
Univ of Tennessee
Graduate Sch of Med
1924 Alcoa Hwy
Knoxville, TN 37920
Tel: 423 544-9340 *Fax:* 423 544-6849
Accred Length: 1 Year *Program Size:* 7 (*GY1:* 7)
Sponsoring Spec: FP, GS, IM, OBG
Program ID: 999-47-00-130

Memphis

Methodist Hospitals of Memphis-Central Program

Sponsor: Methodist Hospitals of Memphis-Central

Program Director:
Stephen T Miller, MD
Methodist Healthcare-Memphis
Med Education/1 Tower
1265 Union Ave
Memphis, TN 38104-3499
Tel: 901 726-8255 *Fax:* 901 726-8254
E-mail: millers@methodisthealth.org
Internet: http://www.methodisthealth.org
Accred Length: 1 Year *Program Size:* 10 (*GY1:* 10)
Sponsoring Spec: DR, GS, IM
Program ID: 999-47-00-131

University of Tennessee Program

Sponsor: University of Tennessee College of Medicine
Baptist Memorial Hospital

Program Director:
Laura R Sprabery, MD
Baptist Memorial Hospital
899 Madison Ave
Memphis, TN 38146
Tel: 901 227-5138 *Fax:* 901 227-4346
E-mail: sandra.stpierre@bmhcc.org
Accred Length: 1 Year *Program Size:* 7 (*GY1:* 7)
Sponsoring Spec: GS, IM
Program ID: 999-47-00-132

Texas

Austin

CTMF of Seton Healthcare Network Program

Sponsor: CTMF of Seton Healthcare Network

Program Director:
Thomas B Coopwood Jr, MD
Central Texas Med Foundation
601 E 15th St
Austin, TX 78701
Tel: 512 324-7870 *Fax:* 512 477-8933
Internet: http://www.ctmf.edu
Accred Length: 1 Year *Program Size:* 6 (*GY1:* 6)
Sponsoring Spec: FP, IM, PD
Program ID: 999-48-00-133

El Paso

Texas Tech University (El Paso) Program

Sponsor: Texas Tech University Health Sciences Center at El Paso
R E Thomason General Hospital

Program Director:
Manuel Schydlower, MD
Texas Tech Univ Health Sciences Ctr
4800 Alberta Ave
El Paso, TX 79905-1298
Tel: 915 545-6520 *Fax:* 915 532-5468
Accred Length: 1 Year *Program Size:* 4 (*GY1:* 4)
Sponsoring Spec: EM, GS, IM, OBG
Program ID: 999-48-00-221

William Beaumont Army Medical Center Program

Sponsor: William Beaumont Army Medical Center

Program Director:
Kevin M Kumke, MD
William Beaumont Army Med Ctr
Office of Grad Med Educ
5005 N Piedras St
El Paso, TX 79920-5001
Tel: 915 569-2521 *Fax:* 915 569-2653
Accred Length: 1 Year *Program Size:* 11 (*GY1:* 11)
Sponsoring Spec: GS, IM, OBG, ORS, PD
Program ID: 999-48-00-137
US Armed Services Program

Fort Sam Houston

San Antonio Uniformed Services Health Education Consortium (BAMC) Program

Sponsor: San Antonio Uniformed Services Health Education Consortium
Brooke Army Medical Center

Program Director:
Maureen K Koops, MD
Transitional Year Program
Brooke Army Med Ctr
3851 Roger Brooke Dr
Fort Sam Houston, TX 78234-6200
Tel: 210 916-5920 *Fax:* 210 916-5187
Accred Length: 1 Year *Program Size:* 25 (*GY1:* 25)
Sponsoring Spec: GS, IM
Program ID: 999-48-00-138
US Armed Services Program

Fort Worth

John Peter Smith Hospital (Tarrant County Hospital District) Program

Sponsor: John Peter Smith Hospital (Tarrant County Hospital District)

Program Director:
Donald K Nelms, MD
John Peter Smith Hospital
1500 S Main St
Fort Worth, TX 76104
Tel: 817 927-1173 *Fax:* 817 927-1668
E-mail: bamckeon@aol.com
Internet: http://www.jpshealthnet.org
Accred Length: 1 Year *Program Size:* 8 (*GY1:* 8)
Sponsoring Spec: FP, OBG, ORS
Program ID: 999-48-00-168

Houston

Baylor College of Medicine Program

Sponsor: Baylor College of Medicine
Harris County Hospital District-Ben Taub General Hospital
Methodist Hospital
St Luke's Episcopal Hospital
Veterans Affairs Medical Center (Houston)

Program Director:
Moise L Levy, MD
Office of Grad Med Educ
1 Baylor Plaza/S-102
Houston, TX 77030-3498
Tel: 713 798-4606 *Fax:* 713 798-4334
Internet: http://www.bcm.tmc.edu/gme/transitional.html
Accred Length: 1 Year *Program Size:* 19 (*GY1:* 19)
Sponsoring Spec: D, DR, IM, OPH, OTO, PD, PTH
Program ID: 999-48-00-139

St Joseph Hospital Program

Sponsor: St Joseph Hospital

Program Director:
Ethan A Natelson, MD
St Joseph Hospital
Medical Education
1919 LaBranch/GWS # 9
Houston, TX 77002
Tel: 713 757-7529 *Fax:* 713 657-7136
Accred Length: 1 Year *Program Size:* 12 (*GY1:* 12)
Sponsoring Spec: FP, GS
Program ID: 999-48-00-140

University of Texas at Houston Program

Sponsor: University of Texas Medical School at Houston
Lyndon B Johnson General Hospital
Memorial Hermann Healthcare System
University of Texas M D Anderson Cancer Center

Program Director:
James D Hefner, MD
Univ of Texas-Houston Med Sch
Lyndon B Johnson General Hospital
5656 Kelley St
Houston, TX 77026
Tel: 713 636-4658 *Fax:* 713 636-4655
E-mail: kleather@utlbj1.lbj.uth.tmc.edu
Internet: http://www.lbj.uth.tmc.edu
Accred Length: 1 Year *Program Size:* 13 (*GY1:* 13)
Sponsoring Spec: GS, IM, OBG, PD
Program ID: 999-48-00-219

Lackland AFB

San Antonio Uniformed Services Health Education Consortium (WHMC) Program

Sponsor: San Antonio Uniformed Services Health Education Consortium
Wilford Hall Medical Center (AETC)

Program Director:
Col Charles T Morton, MD
Wilford Hall USAF Med Ctr
859 MDOS/MMNP
2200 Bergquist Dr/Ste 1
Lackland AFB, TX 78236-5300
Tel: 210 292-7347 *Fax:* 210 292-5238
Accred Length: 1 Year *Program Size:* 8 (*GY1:* 8)
Sponsoring Spec: EM, GS, IM, PD
Program ID: 999-48-00-192
US Armed Services Program

Utah

Salt Lake City

LDS Hospital Program

Sponsor: LDS Hospital
Primary Children's Medical Center

Program Director:
James F Orme, MD
LDS Hospital
8th Ave and C St
Salt Lake City, UT 84143
Tel: 801 321-1077 *Fax:* 801 321-2361
E-mail: ldmgardn@ihc.com
Internet: http://www.ihc.com/losh/residency
Accred Length: 1 Year *Program Size:* 10 (*GY1:* 10)
Sponsoring Spec: GS, IM, PD
Program ID: 999-49-00-142

Virginia

Falls Church

Georgetown University Program

Sponsor: Georgetown University Medical Center
Fairfax Hospital

Program Director:
James N Cooper, MD
Dept of Med
Fairfax Hospital
3300 Gallows Rd
Falls Church, VA 22042-3300
Tel: 703 698-2896 *Fax:* 703 698-3020
E-mail: transitional.residency@inova.com
Internet:
http://www.dml.georgetown.edu/guhifh/transres.html
Accred Length: 1 Year *Program Size:* 10 (*GY1:* 10)
Sponsoring Spec: IM, PD
Program ID: 999-51-00-205

Newport News

Riverside Regional Medical Center Program

Sponsor: Riverside Regional Medical Center

Program Director:
T Eugene Temple Jr, MD
Riverside Regional Med Ctr
500 J Clyde Morris Blvd
Newport News, VA 23601-1976
Tel: 804 594-2041 *Fax:* 804 594-3245
Accred Length: 1 Year *Program Size:* 12 (*GY1:* 12)
Sponsoring Spec: FP, OBG
Program ID: 999-51-00-170

Portsmouth

Naval Medical Center (Portsmouth) Program

Sponsor: Naval Medical Center (Portsmouth)

Program Director:
Thomas K Tandy III, MD
Naval Med Ctr
John Paul Jones Cir
Portsmouth, VA 23708-5000
Tel: 757 953-7218 *Fax:* 757 953-7471
E-mail: pnh0rkc@pnh10.med.navy.mil
Accred Length: 1 Year *Program Size:* 15 (*GY1:* 15)
Sponsoring Spec: EM, GS, IM, OBG, P, PD
Program ID: 999-51-00-193
US Armed Services Program

Roanoke

Carilion Health System Program

Sponsor: Carilion Health System
Carilion Roanoke Community Hospital
Carilion Roanoke Memorial Hospital

Program Director:
William S Erwin Jr, MD
Carilion Health System-Roanoke Memorial Hospital
Med Educ Dept
PO Box 13367
Roanoke, VA 24033-3367
Tel: 800 568-7130 *Fax:* 540 981-8681
E-mail: werwin@carilion.com
Internet: http://www.carilion.com/residency
Accred Length: 1 Year *Program Size:* 10 (*GY1:* 10)
Sponsoring Spec: GS, IM
Program ID: 999-51-00-143

Washington

Seattle

Virginia Mason Medical Center Program

Sponsor: Virginia Mason Medical Center

Program Director:
James W Benson Jr, MD
Virginia Mason Med Ctr
Grad Med Educ/H8-GME
925 Seneca St
Seattle, WA 98101
Tel: 206 583-6079 *Fax:* 206 583-2307
Accred Length: 1 Year *Program Size:* 6 (*GY1:* 6)
Sponsoring Spec: GS, IM, PD
Program ID: 999-54-00-144

Spokane

Deaconess Medical Center Program

Sponsor: Deaconess Medical Center

Program Director:
Judy Benson, MD
Deaconess Med Ctr-Spokane
800 W Fifth Ave
PO Box 248
Spokane, WA 99210-0248
Tel: 509 458-7159 *Fax:* 509 458-7797
E-mail: bensonj@empirehealth.org
Internet: http://www.spokanehealth.org/spokanemed/
Accred Length: 1 Year *Program Size:* 8 (*GY1:* 8)
Sponsoring Spec: FP, IM
Program ID: 999-54-00-169

Inland Empire Hospital Services Association Program

Sponsor: Inland Empire Hospital Services Association
Sacred Heart Medical Center

Program Director:
Lawrence G Schrock, MD
101 W 8th Ave
PO Box 2555
Spokane, WA 99220-2555
Tel: 509 455-3020 *Fax:* 509 458-5316
E-mail: shmctyp@inhs.org
Internet: http://www.spokanehealth.org
Accred Length: 1 Year *Program Size:* 10 (*GY1:* 10)
Sponsoring Spec: DR, FP, IM
Program ID: 999-54-00-145

Tacoma

Madigan Army Medical Center Program

Sponsor: Madigan Army Medical Center

Program Director:
Robert J Newman, MD
Madigan Army Med Ctr
Attn: MCHJ-EDME
Tacoma, WA 98431
Tel: 253 968-1511 *Fax:* 253 968-0365
E-mail:
colleen_johnston@mamc.smtplink.amedd.army.mil
Internet: http://www.mamc.amedd.army.mil
Accred Length: 1 Year *Program Size:* 17 (*GY1:* 17)
Sponsoring Spec: EM, GS, IM, OBG, ORS, OTO, PD, U
Program ID: 999-54-00-146
US Armed Services Program

West Virginia

Huntington

Marshall University School of Medicine Program

Sponsor: Marshall University School of Medicine
Cabell Huntington Hospital
St Mary's Hospital
Veterans Affairs Medical Center (Huntington)

Program Director:
Martin L Evers, MD
Marshall Univ Sch of Med
1600 Medical Center Dr
Ste G-500
Huntington, WV 25701-3655
Tel: 304 691-1084 *Fax:* 304 691-1693
E-mail: martinle@aol.com
Accred Length: 1 Year *Program Size:* 4 (*GY1:* 4)
Sponsoring Spec: GS, IM, PD
Program ID: 999-55-00-194

Wisconsin

La Crosse

Gundersen Lutheran Medical Foundation Program
Sponsor: Gundersen Lutheran Medical Foundation
Gundersen Clinic
Lutheran Hospital-La Crosse
Program Director:
Thomas P Lathrop, MD
Gundersen Med Foundation
Lutheran Hospital-La Crosse
1836 South Ave
La Crosse, WI 54601-5429
Tel: 608 782-7300, ext 2281 *Fax:* 608 791-4457
E-mail: thomas_p_lathrop@gundluth.org
Internet: http://www.gundluth.org
Accred Length: 1 Year *Program Size:* 10 (*GY1:* 10)
Sponsoring Spec: GS, IM
Program ID: 999-56-00-147

Marshfield

Marshfield Clinic-St Joseph's Hospital Program
Sponsor: Marshfield Clinic-St Joseph's Hospital
Program Director:
John L Olson, MD
Marshfield Clinic
Dept of Int Med 3K2
1000 N Oak Ave
Marshfield, WI 54449
Tel: 715 387-5260 *Fax:* 715 387-5163
E-mail: millerd@mfldclin.edu
Internet:
http://www.marshmed.org/mfldclin/education/med_ed/
Accred Length: 1 Year *Program Size:* 4 (*GY1:* 4)
Sponsoring Spec: GS, IM, PD
Program ID: 999-56-00-183

Milwaukee

Aurora Health Care Program
Sponsor: Aurora Health Care
St Luke's Medical Center
Program Director:
Richard J Battiola, MD
St Luke's Med Ctr
2900 W Oklahoma Ave
PO Box 2901
Milwaukee, WI 53201-2901
Tel: 414 649-3323 *Fax:* 414 649-5158
E-mail: rjbatslm@execpc.com
Internet: http://www.aurorahealthcare.org
Accred Length: 1 Year *Program Size:* 13 (*GY1:* 13)
Sponsoring Spec: DR, FP, IM
Program ID: 999-56-00-148

St Joseph's Hospital/Medical College of Wisconsin Program
Sponsor: St Joseph's Hospital
Program Director:
Kesavan Kutty, MD
St Joseph's Hospital
5000 W Chambers St
Milwaukee, WI 53210
Tel: 414 447-2195 *Fax:* 414 874-4352
Accred Length: 1 Year *Program Size:* 12 (*GY1:* 12)
Sponsoring Spec: IM, OBG
Program ID: 999-56-00-184

Urology

Alabama

Birmingham

University of Alabama Medical Center Program
Sponsor: University of Alabama Hospital
Children's Hospital of Alabama
St Vincent's Hospital
Veterans Affairs Medical Center (Birmingham)
Program Director:
L Keith Lloyd, MD
Univ of Alabama
1813 6th Ave S
606 Med Educ Bldg
Birmingham, AL 35294-3296
Tel: 205 934-1459 *Fax:* 205 934-4933
E-mail: klloyd@urology.uab.edu
Internet: http://www.urology.uab.edu
Accred Length: 4 Years *Program Size:* 8
Program ID: 480-01-11-014

Arizona

Tucson

University of Arizona Program
Sponsor: University of Arizona College of Medicine
Tucson Medical Center
University Medical Center
Veterans Affairs Medical Center (Tucson)
Program Director:
Bruce L Dalkin, MD
1501 N Campbell Ave
PO Box 245077
Tucson, AZ 85724-5077
Tel: 520 626-6236, ext 2 *Fax:* 520 626-4933
E-mail: rebalder@u.arizona.edu
Accred Length: 4 Years *Program Size:* 6
Program ID: 480-03-21-015

Arkansas

Little Rock

University of Arkansas for Medical Sciences Program
Sponsor: University of Arkansas College of Medicine
Arkansas Children's Hospital
John L McClellan Memorial Veterans Hospital
University Hospital of Arkansas
Program Director:
Alex E Finbeiner, MD
Univ of Arkansas for Med Sciences
4301 W Markham St/Slot 540
Little Rock, AR 72205-7199
Tel: 501 686-5242 *Fax:* 501 686-5277
E-mail: montgomerymargaretd@exchange.uams.edu
Accred Length: 3 Years *Program Size:* 6
Program ID: 480-04-21-016

California

Loma Linda

Loma Linda University Program
Sponsor: Loma Linda University Medical Center
Jerry L Pettis Memorial Veterans Hospital
San Bernardino County Medical Center
Program Director:
H Roger Hadley, MD
Loma Linda Univ Med Ctr
Div of Urology
11234 Anderson St/Rm A562
Loma Linda, CA 92354
Tel: 909 824-4196 *Fax:* 909 824-4806
Accred Length: 4 Years *Program Size:* 8
Program ID: 480-05-21-019

Los Angeles

Southern California Kaiser Permanente Medical Care (Los Angeles) Program
Sponsor: Southern California Kaiser Permanente Medical Group
Kaiser Foundation Hospital (Los Angeles)
Kaiser Foundation Hospital (Bellflower)
Program Director:
Gary C Bellman, MD
Kaiser Permanente Med Ctr
Dept of Academic Affairs
4733 Sunset Blvd/W Mezzanine
Los Angeles, CA 90027
Tel: 323 783-4516 *Fax:* 323 783-4771
Accred Length: 4 Years *Program Size:* 12
Program ID: 480-05-12-020

UCLA Medical Center Program
Sponsor: UCLA School of Medicine
Los Angeles County-Harbor-UCLA Medical Center
Olive View-UCLA Medical Center
UCLA Medical Center
VA Greater Los Angeles Healthcare System
Program Director:
Robert B Smith, MD
UCLA Med Ctr
Box 951738
CHS 66-124
Los Angeles, CA 90095-1738
Tel: 310 206-8177 *Fax:* 310 206-5343
Accred Length: 4 Years *Program Size:* 18
Program ID: 480-05-21-022

University of Southern California Program
Sponsor: Los Angeles County-USC Medical Center
Kenneth Norris Jr Cancer Hospital and Research Institute
Program Director:
Donald G Skinner, MD
Univ of Southern California-Norris Cancer Ctr
1441 Eastlake Ave/Ste 7414
Los Angeles, CA 90033
Tel: 323 865-3700 *Fax:* 323 865-0120
Accred Length: 4 Years *Program Size:* 18
Program ID: 480-05-21-021

Programs

Orange

University of California (Irvine) Program
Sponsor: University of California (Irvine) Medical Center
Kaiser Foundation Hospitals (Anaheim)
Veterans Affairs Medical Center (Long Beach)
Program Director:
Thomas E Ahlering, MD
Univ of California Irvine Med Ctr
Dept of Surg/Urology
101 City Dr S/Rte 81
Orange, CA 92868-3298
Tel: 714 456-6068 *Fax:* 714 456-7189
Internet: http://www.ucihs.uci.edu/surgery
Accred Length: 4 Years *Program Size:* 7
Program ID: 480-05-21-018

Sacramento

University of California (Davis) Program
Sponsor: University of California (Davis) Medical Center
Kaiser Foundation Hospital (Sacramento)
Kaiser Foundation Hospital (South Sacramento)
Program Director:
Ralph W deVere White, MD
Univ of California Davis
4301 Y St/Ste 3500
Sacramento, CA 95817-2281
Tel: 916 734-2823 *Fax:* 916 734-8094
E-mail: gwendolyn.dennis@ucdmc.ucdavis.edu
Internet: http://web.ucdmc.ucdavis.edu/urology/
Accred Length: 4 Years *Program Size:* 8
Program ID: 480-05-21-017

San Diego

Naval Medical Center (San Diego) Program
Sponsor: Naval Medical Center (San Diego)
Program Director:
Christopher J Kane, MD
Naval Med Ctr San Diego
Urology St 200
34730 Bob Wilson Dr
San Diego, CA 92134-3200
Tel: 619 532-7202 *Fax:* 619 532-7234
Accred Length: 4 Years *Program Size:* 5
Subspecialties: UP
Program ID: 480-05-11-009
US Armed Services Program

University of California (San Diego) Program
Sponsor: University of California (San Diego) Medical Center
Children's Hospital and Health Center
Veterans Affairs Medical Center (San Diego)
Program Director:
Joseph D Schmidt, MD
UCSD Med Ctr
Div of Urology (8897)
200 W Arbor Dr
San Diego, CA 92103-8897
Tel: 619 543-5904 *Fax:* 619 543-6573
Internet: http://www.surgery.ucsd.edu/urology.htm
Accred Length: 4 Years *Program Size:* 6
Program ID: 480-05-21-024

San Francisco

University of California (San Francisco) Program
Sponsor: University of California (San Francisco) School of Medicine
San Francisco General Hospital Medical Center
University of California (San Francisco) Medical Center
Veterans Affairs Medical Center (San Francisco)
Program Director:
Peter R Carroll, MD
Univ of California San Francisco
Dept of Urology
533 Parnassus Ave/U-575 Box 0738
San Francisco, CA 94143-0738
Tel: 415 476-1611 *Fax:* 415 476-8849
Accred Length: 4 Years *Program Size:* 12
Subspecialties: UP
Program ID: 480-05-21-025

Stanford

Stanford University Program
Sponsor: Stanford University Hospital
Lucile Salter Packard Children's Hospital at Stanford
Santa Clara Valley Medical Center
Veterans Affairs Palo Alto Health Care System
Program Director:
Linda M D Shortliffe, MD
Dept of Urology (S287) MC5118
Stanford Univ Sch of Med
300 Pasteur Dr
Stanford, CA 94305-5118
Tel: 650 498-5042 *Fax:* 650 723-4055
E-mail: lindas@leland.stanford.edu
Internet:
http://www.med.stanford.edu:80/medschool/urology
Accred Length: 4 Years *Program Size:* 8
Program ID: 480-05-31-026

Colorado

Denver

University of Colorado Program
Sponsor: University of Colorado Health Sciences Center
Children's Hospital
Denver Health and Hospitals
Exempla St Joseph Hospital
Veterans Affairs Medical Center (Denver)
Program Director:
Paramjit S Chandhoke, MD PhD
Univ of Colorado Health Sciences Ctr
4200 E Ninth Ave
Mail Container C-319
Denver, CO 80262-0319
Tel: 303 315-6321 *Fax:* 303 315-7611
Accred Length: 4 Years *Program Size:* 8
Program ID: 480-07-21-027

Connecticut

Farmington

University of Connecticut Program
Sponsor: University of Connecticut School of Medicine
Connecticut Children's Medical Center
Hartford Hospital
St Francis Hospital and Medical Center
Univ of Connecticut Health Center/John Dempsey Hospital
Program Director:
Peter Albertsen, MD
Univ of Connecticut Health Ctr
263 Farmington Ave/MC 3955
Farmington, CT 06030-3955
Tel: 860 679-3676 *Fax:* 860 679-1318
E-mail: albertsen@nso.uchc.edu
Internet: http://www.resprog.uchc.edu/md
Accred Length: 4 Years *Program Size:* 8
Program ID: 480-08-21-028

New Haven

Yale-New Haven Medical Center Program
Sponsor: Yale-New Haven Hospital
Veterans Affairs Medical Center (West Haven)
Waterbury Hospital Health Center
Program Director:
Robert M Weiss, MD
Yale Univ Sch of Med
PO Box 208041/YPB-#321
New Haven, CT 06520-8041
Tel: 203 785-2815 *Fax:* 203 785-4043
E-mail: robert.weiss@yale.edu
Internet: http://yalesurgery.med.yale.edu
Accred Length: 3 Years *Program Size:* 6
Program ID: 480-08-11-029

District of Columbia

Washington

George Washington University Program
Sponsor: George Washington University School of Medicine
Children's National Medical Center
Fairfax Hospital
George Washington University Hospital (UHS)
Program Director:
Michael J Manyak, MD
George Washington Univ
2150 Pennsylvania Ave NW
Washington, DC 20037
Tel: 202 994-4001 *Fax:* 202 994-3671
Accred Length: 4 Years *Program Size:* 8
Program ID: 480-10-21-031

Georgetown University Program
Sponsor: Georgetown University Medical Center
Sibley Memorial Hospital
Veterans Affairs Medical Center (Washington, DC)
Program Director:
John H Lynch, MD
Georgetown Univ Med Ctr
Office of Education/Dept of Surgery
3800 Reservoir Rd NW/4PHC
Washington, DC 20007-2197
Tel: 202 687-1233 *Fax:* 202 687-4287
Accred Length: 4 Years *Program Size:* 8
Program ID: 480-10-21-030

Howard University Program
Sponsor: Howard University Hospital
District of Columbia General Hospital
Program Director:
Aaron G Jackson, MD
Howard Univ Hospital
2041 Georgia Ave NW
Washington, DC 20060
Tel: 202 865-1314 *Fax:* 202 865-1647
Accred Length: 4 Years *Program Size:* 4
Program ID: 480-10-21-032

Walter Reed Army Medical Center Program
Sponsor: Walter Reed Army Medical Center
Program Director:
Col David G McLeod, MD JD
Urology Service
Walter Reed Army Med Ctr
6825 Georgia Ave NW
Washington, DC 20307-5001
Tel: 202 782-6408 *Fax:* 202 782-4118
E-mail: col_david_mcleod@wramc1-amedd.army.mil
Internet:
http://www.wramc.amedd.army.mil/departments/surgery/urology
Accred Length: 4 Years *Program Size:* 8
Program ID: 480-10-21-004
US Armed Services Program

Washington Hospital Center Program
Sponsor: Washington Hospital Center
Program Director:
Arnold M Kwart, MD
Washington Hospital Ctr
110 Irving St NW
Rm 3B-19
Washington, DC 20010
Tel: 202 877-7011 *Fax:* 202 877-7012
E-mail: amk3@mhg.edu
Internet: http://www.whc.mhg.edu/gme/
Accred Length: 4 Years *Program Size:* 4
Program ID: 480-10-12-033

Florida

Gainesville

University of Florida Program
Sponsor: University of Florida College of Medicine
Shands Hospital at the University of Florida
Veterans Affairs Medical Center (Gainesville)
Program Director:
Zev Wajsman, MD
1600 SW Archer Road, Rm M-351
Gainesville, FL 32610—024
Tel: 352 846-1550 *Fax:* 352 395-0627
E-mail: munoz@surgery.ufl.edu
Accred Length: 3 Years *Program Size:* 6
Program ID: 480-11-21-034

Miami

University of Miami-Jackson Memorial Medical Center Program
Sponsor: University of Miami-Jackson Memorial Medical Center
Cedars Medical Center
Veterans Affairs Medical Center (Miami)
Program Director:
Mark S Soloway, MD
Jackson Memorial Hospital
PO Box 016960 (M814)
Miami, FL 33101
Tel: 305 243-6596 *Fax:* 305 243-4653
E-mail: msoloway@mednet.med.miami.edu
Accred Length: 4 Years *Program Size:* 11
Program ID: 480-11-21-036

Tampa

University of South Florida Program
Sponsor: University of South Florida College of Medicine
H Lee Moffitt Cancer Center
James A Haley Veterans Hospital
Tampa General Healthcare
Veterans Affairs Medical Center (Bay Pines)
Program Director:
Jorge L Lockhart, MD
Univ of South Florida
4 Columbia Dr
Ste 730
Tampa, FL 33606
Tel: 813 259-0862 *Fax:* 813 259-0968
Internet: http://www.med.usf.edu/surgery/hmpg.html
Accred Length: 4 Years *Program Size:* 8
Program ID: 480-11-21-169

Georgia

Atlanta

Emory University Program
Sponsor: Emory University School of Medicine
Emory University Hospital
Grady Memorial Hospital
Veterans Affairs Medical Center (Atlanta)
Program Director:
Harry Clarke, MD
Emory Clinic, Dept of Urology
1365 Clifton Rd NE
Bldg A Rm 3225
Atlanta, GA 30322
Tel: 404 778-5951 *Fax:* 404 778-4336
Accred Length: 4 Years *Program Size:* 12
Program ID: 480-12-21-039

Augusta

Medical College of Georgia Program
Sponsor: Medical College of Georgia Hospital and Clinics
University Hospital
Veterans Affairs Medical Center (Augusta)
Program Director:
Ronald W Lewis, MD
Med Coll of Georgia
Rm BA-8412
1120 15th St
Augusta, GA 30912-4050
Tel: 706 721-0981 *Fax:* 706 721-2548
E-mail: deptsurg.dclark@mail.mcg.edu
Accred Length: 4 Years *Program Size:* 5
Program ID: 480-12-21-040

Hawaii

Honolulu

Tripler Army Medical Center Program
Sponsor: Tripler Army Medical Center
Program Director:
George E Deshon Jr, MD
Tripler Army Med Ctr
MCHK-DSU
1 Jarrett White Rd
Tripler AMC, HI 96859-5000
Tel: 808 433-2972 *Fax:* 808 433-7194
Internet: http://tamc.dsweb/urology/home.html
Accred Length: 3 Years *Program Size:* 3
Program ID: 480-14-32-005
US Armed Services Program

Illinois

Chicago

McGaw Medical Center of Northwestern University Program
Sponsor: Northwestern University Medical School
Children's Memorial Medical Center
Northwestern Memorial Hospital
Veterans Affairs Lakeside Medical Center (Chicago)
Program Director:
Anthony J Schaeffer, MD
Northwestern Univ Med Sch
Dept of Urology
303 E Chicago Ave/Tarry 11-715
Chicago, IL 60611
Tel: 312 908-1998 *Fax:* 312 908-7275
E-mail: p-merced@nwu.edu
Internet: http://www.nums.nwu.edu/~urology/index.html
Accred Length: 4 Years *Program Size:* 12
Program ID: 480-16-21-045

Rush-Presbyterian-St Luke's Medical Center Program
Sponsor: Rush-Presbyterian-St Luke's Medical Center
Program Director:
Charles F McKiel Jr, MD
Rush-Presbyterian-St Luke's Med Ctr
1653 W Congress Pkwy
Chicago, IL 60612-3864
Tel: 312 942-6447 *Fax:* 312 563-0426
Accred Length: 4 Years *Program Size:* 5
Program ID: 480-16-31-046

University of Chicago Program
Sponsor: University of Chicago Hospitals
Louis A Weiss Memorial Hospital
Program Director:
Charles B Brendler, MD
Univ of Chicago Med Ctr
5841 S Maryland Ave/MC6038
Chicago, IL 60637-1470
Tel: 773 702-6105 *Fax:* 773 702-1001
Accred Length: 4 Years *Program Size:* 8
Program ID: 480-16-21-047

University of Illinois College of Medicine at Chicago Program
Sponsor: University of Illinois College of Medicine at Chicago
Christ Hospital and Medical Center
Michael Reese Hospital and Medical Center
University of Illinois Hospital and Clinics
Veterans Affairs West Side Medical Center
Program Director:
Lawrence S Ross, MD
Univ of Illinois Coll of Med
820 S Wood St (M/C955)
Chicago, IL 60612-7316
Tel: 312 996-9330 *Fax:* 312 996-1291
E-mail: cseydel@uic.edu
Accred Length: 4 Years *Program Size:* 13
Program ID: 480-16-21-174

Maywood

Loyola University Program
Sponsor: Loyola University Medical Center
Edward J Hines Jr Veterans Affairs Hospital
Lutheran General Hospital
Program Director:
Robert C Flanigan, MD
Foster G McGaw Hospital
2160 S First Ave
Bldg 54/Rm 237A
Maywood, IL 60153-5585
Tel: 708 216-4076 *Fax:* 708 216-6585
E-mail: rflanig@wpo.it.luc.edu
Internet:
http://www.meddean.luc.edu/lumen/deptwebs/urology/urolfac.htm
Accred Length: 4 Years *Program Size:* 12
Program ID: 480-16-21-166

Springfield

Southern Illinois University Program
Sponsor: Southern Illinois University School of Medicine
Memorial Medical Center
St John's Hospital
Program Director:
Durwood E Neal Jr, MD
Southern Illinois Univ Sch of Med
Div of Urology
PO Box 19230
Springfield, IL 62794-1312
Tel: 217 782-8860 *Fax:* 217 524-1793
E-mail: sgodbey@siumed.edu
Accred Length: 3 Years *Program Size:* 3
Program ID: 480-16-21-050

Indiana

Indianapolis

Indiana University School of Medicine Program
Sponsor: Indiana University School of Medicine
Clarian IU Hospital
Clarian Methodist Hospital of Indiana
Clarian Riley Hospital for Children
Richard L Roudebush Veterans Affairs Medical Center
William N Wishard Memorial Hospital
Program Director:
Michael O Koch, MD
535 N Barnhill Dr/#420
Indianapolis, IN 46202-5289
Tel: 317 274-7338 *Fax:* 317 274-0174
E-mail: miokoch@iupui.edu
Accred Length: 4 Years *Program Size:* 12
Program ID: 480-17-21-051

Iowa

Iowa City

University of Iowa Hospitals and Clinics Program
Sponsor: University of Iowa Hospitals and Clinics
Veterans Affairs Medical Center (Iowa City)
Program Director:
Bernard Fallon, MD
Univ of Iowa Hospitals and Clinics
Dept of Urology
200 Hawkins Dr
Iowa City, IA 52242-1009
Tel: 319 356-2905 *Fax:* 319 353-8564
E-mail: bernard-fallon@uiowa.edu
Accred Length: 4 Years *Program Size:* 15
Program ID: 480-18-21-052

Kansas

Kansas City

University of Kansas Medical Center Program
Sponsor: University of Kansas School of Medicine
University of Kansas Medical Center
Veterans Affairs Medical Center (Kansas City)
Program Director:
J Brantley Thrasher, MD
Univ of Kansas Med Ctr
3901 Rainbow Blvd
Kansas City, KS 66160-7390
Tel: 913 588-6152 *Fax:* 913 588-7625
E-mail: bthrasher@kumc.edu
Internet: http://www.kumc.edu/usurg/
Accred Length: 3 Years *Program Size:* 9
Program ID: 480-19-21-053

Kentucky

Lexington

University of Kentucky Medical Center Program
Sponsor: University of Kentucky Hospital
Central Baptist Hospital
St Joseph Hospital
Veterans Affairs Medical Center (Lexington)
Program Director:
Randall G Rowland, MD PhD
Univ of Kentucky Chandler Med Ctr
800 Rose St/MS283
Lexington, KY 40536-0293
Tel: 606 323-6677 *Fax:* 606 323-1944
E-mail: rrowlan@pop.uky.edu
Internet: http://www.mc.uky.edu/surgery/
Accred Length: 3 Years *Program Size:* 8
Program ID: 480-20-21-054

Louisville

University of Louisville Program
Sponsor: University of Louisville School of Medicine
Jewish Hospital
Kosair Children's Hospital (Alliant Health System)
Norton Hospital (Alliant Health System)
University of Louisville Hospital
Veterans Affairs Medical Center (Louisville)
Program Director:
James I Harty, MD
Div of Urology
Univ of Louisville
Louisville, KY 40292
Tel: 502 852-5447 *Fax:* 502 852-8915
Accred Length: 3 Years *Program Size:* 6
Program ID: 480-20-21-055

Louisiana

New Orleans

Louisiana State University/Alton Ochsner Medical Foundation Program
Sponsor: Alton Ochsner Medical Foundation
Childrens Hospital
Meadowcrest Hospital
Medical Center of Louisiana at New Orleans
Program Director:
Harold A Fuselier Jr, MD
Alton Ochsner Med Foundation
Dept of Grad Med Educ
1516 Jefferson Hwy
New Orleans, LA 70121
Tel: 504 842-3260 *Fax:* 504 842-3193
E-mail: dlambert@ochsner.org
Internet: http://www.ochsner.org
Accred Length: 4 Years *Program Size:* 8
Program ID: 480-21-21-176

Tulane University Program
Sponsor: Tulane University School of Medicine
Medical Center of Louisiana at New Orleans
Tulane University Hospital and Clinics
Veterans Affairs Medical Center-LSU Service (New Orleans)
Program Director:
Raju Thomas, MD MBA
Tulane Univ Sch of Med
Dept of Urology
1430 Tulane Ave/Box SL-42
New Orleans, LA 70112
Tel: 504 584-2794 *Fax:* 504 588-5059
E-mail: mfanning@tmcpop.tmc.tulane.edu
Internet: http://www.tmc.tulane.edu/urology/
Accred Length: 4 Years *Program Size:* 10
Program ID: 480-21-21-058

Shreveport

Louisiana State University (Shreveport) Program
Sponsor: Louisiana State University Hospital-Shreveport
Overton Brooks Veterans Affairs Medical Center
Schumpert Medical Center
Program Director:
Dennis D Venable, MD
Louisiana State Univ Med Ctr Hospital
Med Educ/Urology
1501 Kings Hwy/PO Box 33932
Shreveport, LA 71130-3932
Tel: 318 675-5600 *Fax:* 318 675-5665
Internet: http://sh_aux.lsumc.edu/urology
Accred Length: 3 Years *Program Size:* 10
Program ID: 480-21-21-059

Maryland

Baltimore

Johns Hopkins University Program

Sponsor: Johns Hopkins University School of Medicine
Johns Hopkins Bayview Medical Center
Johns Hopkins Hospital
Program Director:
Patrick C Walsh, MD
Dept of Urology
Johns Hopkins Hospital
600 N Wolfe St
Baltimore, MD 21287-2101
Tel: 410 614-3377 *Fax:* 410 955-0833
E-mail: pwalsh@gwgate1.jhmi.jhu.edu
Internet: http://www.128.220.136.100
Accred Length: 4 Years *Program Size:* 8
Subspecialties: UP
Program ID: 480-23-21-060

University of Maryland Program

Sponsor: University of Maryland Medical System
Johns Hopkins Hospital
Sinai Hospital of Baltimore
Veterans Affairs Medical Center (Baltimore)
Program Director:
Stephen C Jacobs, MD
Division of Urology
22 S Greene St/Rm S8D18
Baltimore, MD 21201-1595
Tel: 410 328-5544 *Fax:* 410 328-0595
E-mail: sjacobs@surgery1.umaryland.edu
Internet:
http://www.umm.edu/center/specialties/departments/clinical-depts-83.html
Accred Length: 4 Years *Program Size:* 8
Program ID: 480-23-21-062

Bethesda

National Naval Medical Center (Bethesda) Program

Sponsor: National Naval Medical Center (Bethesda)
Program Director:
Harold A Frazier, MD
National Naval Med Ctr
Dept of Urology
8901 Wisconsin Ave
Bethesda, MD 20889-5600
Tel: 301 295-6558 *Fax:* 301 295-4280
E-mail: bthohaf@bth20.med.navy.mil
Accred Length: 3 Years *Program Size:* 3
Program ID: 480-23-21-010
US Armed Services Program

Massachusetts

Boston

Boston University Medical Center Program

Sponsor: Boston Medical Center
Children's Hospital
Veterans Affairs Medical Center (Boston)
Program Director:
Robert J Krane, MD
Boston Univ Med Ctr
720 Harrison Ave/Ste 606
Boston, MA 02118-2393
Tel: 617 638-8485 *Fax:* 617 638-8487
Accred Length: 4 Years *Program Size:* 8
Program ID: 480-24-21-063

Harvard Medical School Program

Sponsor: Brigham and Women's Hospital
Beth Israel Deaconess Medical Center
Brockton-West Roxbury Veterans Affairs Medical Center
Children's Hospital
Program Director:
Jerome P Richie, MD
Brigham and Women's Hospital
Surgery Education Office
75 Francis St
Boston, MA 02115
Tel: 617 732-6861 *Fax:* 617 264-6850
E-mail: surgery@bics.bwh.harvard.edu
Internet: http://www.bwh.partners.org/surged
Accred Length: 4 Years *Program Size:* 12
Subspecialties: UP
Program ID: 480-24-21-064

Massachusetts General Hospital/Harvard Medical School Program

Sponsor: Massachusetts General Hospital
Children's Hospital
Program Director:
W Scott McDougal, MD
Massachusetts General Hospital
Dept of Urology/GRB1102
55 Fruit St
Boston, MA 02114
Tel: 617 726-3010 *Fax:* 617 726-6131
E-mail: mcdougalw@al.mgh.harvard.edu
Accred Length: 4 Years *Program Size:* 8
Program ID: 480-24-11-161

Tufts University Program

Sponsor: New England Medical Center Hospitals
St Elizabeth's Medical Center of Boston
Program Director:
Grannum R Sant, MD
New England Med Ctr Hospital
750 Washington St/Box 142
Boston, MA 02111
Tel: 617 636-7956 *Fax:* 617 636-5349
E-mail: grannum.sant@es.nemc.org
Accred Length: 4 Years *Program Size:* 4
Program ID: 480-24-21-162

Burlington

Lahey Clinic Program

Sponsor: Lahey Clinic
Beth Israel Deaconess Medical Center
Program Director:
William Bihrle III, MD
Lahey Clinic Foundation
Dept of Urology
41 Mall Rd
Burlington, MA 01805
Tel: 781 744-8420 *Fax:* 781 744-5429
Internet:
http://www.lahey.org/depts/urology/index_uro.stm
Accred Length: 4 Years *Program Size:* 12
Program ID: 480-24-22-065

Worcester

University of Massachusetts Program

Sponsor: University of Massachusetts Medical School
St Vincent Hospital
UMass Memorial Health Care (Memorial Campus)
UMass Memorial Health Care (University Campus)
Veterans Affairs Medical Center (Togus)
Program Director:
Robert D Blute Jr, MD
Philip Ayvazian, MD
Univ of Massachusetts Med Sch
55 Lake Ave N
Worcester, MA 01655
Tel: 508 856-5295 *Fax:* 508 856-3137
Accred Length: 3 Years *Program Size:* 8
Program ID: 480-24-21-167

Michigan

Ann Arbor

University of Michigan Program

Sponsor: University of Michigan Hospitals
Veterans Affairs Medical Center (Ann Arbor)
Program Director:
James E Montie, MD
Univ of Michigan
TC 2916/0330
1500 E Medical Center Dr
Ann Arbor, MI 48109-0330
Tel: 734 615-0563 *Fax:* 734 936-9127
Internet: http://www.urology.med.umich.edu
Accred Length: 4 Years *Program Size:* 12
Subspecialties: UP
Program ID: 480-25-21-066

Detroit

Henry Ford Hospital Program

Sponsor: Henry Ford Hospital
Program Director:
James O Peabody, MD
Henry Ford Hospital
2799 W Grand Blvd
Detroit, MI 48202
Tel: 313 874-4811 *Fax:* 313 874-4729
Accred Length: 3 Years *Program Size:* 8
Program ID: 480-25-11-067

Wayne State University/Detroit Medical Center Program

Sponsor: Wayne State University/Detroit Medical Center
Children's Hospital of Michigan
Harper Hospital
Veterans Affairs Medical Center (Detroit)
Program Director:
Marko R Gudziak, MD
Wayne State Univ-Detroit Med Ctr
4160 John R St/#1017
Detroit, MI 48201
Tel: 313 745-7381 *Fax:* 313 745-0464
E-mail: mgudziak@med.wayne.edu
Internet: http://www.med.wayne.edu/urology
Accred Length: 4 Years *Program Size:* 12
Subspecialties: UP
Program ID: 480-25-31-069

Programs

Royal Oak

William Beaumont Hospital Program
Sponsor: William Beaumont Hospital
Program Director:
Ananias C Diokno, MD
William Beaumont Hospital
3601 W 13 Mile Rd
Royal Oak, MI 48073-6769
Tel: 248 551-5012 *Fax:* 248 551-8107
Internet: http://www.beaumont.edu/html/gme
Accred Length: 4 Years *Program Size:* 8
Program ID: 480-25-12-071

Minnesota

Minneapolis

University of Minnesota Program
Sponsor: University of Minnesota Medical School
Fairview-University Medical Center
Regions Hospital
Veterans Affairs Medical Center (Minneapolis)
Program Director:
Cesar J Ercole, MD
Paul Gleich, MD
Univ of Minnesota Hospital and Clinics
420 Delaware St SE
Box 394 Mayo Memorial Bldg
Minneapolis, MN 55455
Tel: 612 625-2486 *Fax:* 612 626-0428
E-mail: schmi083@tc.umn.edu
Accred Length: 4 Years *Program Size:* 8
Program ID: 480-26-21-072

Rochester

Mayo Graduate School of Medicine (Rochester) Program
Sponsor: Mayo Graduate School of Medicine-Mayo Foundation
Rochester Methodist Hospital
St Mary's Hospital of Rochester
Program Director:
David M Barrett, MD
Application Processing Ctr
Mayo Graduate Sch of Med
200 First St SW
Rochester, MN 55905
Tel: 507 284-4331 *Fax:* 507 284-0999
E-mail: mgsm.surgical.specialties@mayo.edu
Internet: http://www.mayo.edu/
Accred Length: 4 Years *Program Size:* 30
Subspecialties: UP
Program ID: 480-26-21-073

Mississippi

Jackson

University of Mississippi Medical Center Program
Sponsor: University of Mississippi School of Medicine
University Hospital
Veterans Affairs Medical Center (Jackson)
Program Director:
Jackson E Fowler Jr, MD
Univ of Mississippi Med Ctr
Dept of Urology
2500 N State St
Jackson, MS 39216-4505
Tel: 601 984-5185 *Fax:* 601 984-5190
Accred Length: 4 Years *Program Size:* 11
Program ID: 480-27-21-075

Missouri

Columbia

University of Missouri-Columbia Program
Sponsor: University of Missouri-Columbia School of Medicine
Harry S Truman Memorial Veterans Hospital
University Hospitals and Clinics
Program Director:
Stephen H Weinstein, MD
Univ Hospital and Clinics
Div of Urology
One Hospital Dr/M562 Medical Sciences Bldg
Columbia, MO 65212
Tel: 573 882-1151 *Fax:* 573 884-7453
E-mail: tammy_ellebracht@surgery.missouri.edu
Accred Length: 4 Years *Program Size:* 6
Program ID: 480-28-21-076

St Louis

St Louis University School of Medicine Program
Sponsor: St Louis University School of Medicine
SSM Cardinal Glennon Children's Hospital
St John's Mercy Medical Center
St Louis ConnectCare
St Louis University School of Medicine
Veterans Affairs Medical Center (St Louis)
Program Director:
Raul Parra, MD
St Louis Univ Sch of Med
3635 Vista Ave
PO Box 15250
St Louis, MO 63110-0250
Tel: 314 577-8317 *Fax:* 314 268-5466
E-mail: surgweb@slu.edu
Internet:
http://www.slu.edu/colleges/med/departments/surgery/
Accred Length: 4 Years *Program Size:* 10
Program ID: 480-28-21-078

Washington University/B-JH/SLCH Consortium Program
Sponsor: Washington University/B-JH/SLCH Consortium
Barnes-Jewish Hospital
Veterans Affairs Medical Center (St Louis)
Program Director:
Gerald L Andriole Jr, MD
1 Barnes Hospital Plaza
Ste 5101
St Louis, MO 63110
Tel: 314 362-8212 *Fax:* 314 361-2203
Internet: http://www.surgery.wustl.edu
Accred Length: 4 Years *Program Size:* 12
Program ID: 480-28-21-079

Nebraska

Omaha

University of Nebraska Program
Sponsor: University of Nebraska Medical Center
Methodist Hospital
Veterans Affairs Medical Center (Omaha)
Program Director:
Rodney J Taylor, MD
Univ of Nebraska Med Ctr
Sect of Urologic Surgery
600 S 42nd St
Omaha, NE 68198-2360
Tel: 402 559-4292 *Fax:* 402 559-6529
E-mail: rjtaylor@unmc.edu
Accred Length: 4 Years *Program Size:* 8
Program ID: 480-30-21-081

New Hampshire

Lebanon

Dartmouth-Hitchcock Medical Center Program
Sponsor: Mary Hitchcock Memorial Hospital
Veterans Affairs Medical Center (White River Junction)
Program Director:
John A Heaney, MD
Dartmouth-Hitchcock Med Ctr
One Medical Center Dr
Lebanon, NH 03756
Tel: 603 650-6033 *Fax:* 603 650-4961
Accred Length: 4 Years *Program Size:* 4
Program ID: 480-32-21-082

New Jersey

Newark

UMDNJ-New Jersey Medical School Program
Sponsor: UMDNJ-New Jersey Medical School
Hackensack University Medical Center
UMDNJ-University Hospital
Veterans Affairs Medical Center (East Orange)
Program Director:
Robert J Irwin, MD
UMDNJ-New Jersey Med Sch, Sect of Urology (G-536)
185 S Orange Ave
Newark, NJ 07103-2757
Tel: 973 972-4488 *Fax:* 973 972-3892
E-mail: irwinrj@umdnj.edu
Accred Length: 4 Years *Program Size:* 8
Program ID: 480-33-21-083

Piscataway

UMDNJ-Robert Wood Johnson Medical School Program
Sponsor: UMDNJ-Robert Wood Johnson Medical School
Cooper Hospital-University Medical Center
Medical Center at Princeton
Robert Wood Johnson University Hospital
Program Director:
Kenneth B Cummings, MD
UMDNJ-Robert Wood Johnson Med Sch
One Robert Wood Johnson Pl
Div of Urology/MEB 588
New Brunswick, NJ 08903-0019
Tel: 732 235-7775 *Fax:* 732 235-6042
Accred Length: 4 Years *Program Size:* 8
Program ID: 480-33-21-173

New Mexico

Albuquerque

University of New Mexico Program
Sponsor: University of New Mexico School of Medicine
Lovelace Medical Center
University Hospital
Veterans Affairs Medical Center (Albuquerque)
Program Director:
Thomas A Borden, MD
Univ of New Mexico Sch of Med
Div of Urology
2211 Lomas Blvd NE
Albuquerque, NM 87131-5341
Tel: 505 272-5505 *Fax:* 505 272-6493
Accred Length: 3 Years *Program Size:* 6
Program ID: 480-34-21-084

New York

Albany

Albany Medical Center Program

Sponsor: Albany Medical Center
Veterans Affairs Medical Center (Albany)

Program Director:
Barry A Kogan, MD
Albany Med Coll
47 New Scotland Ave/A-108
Albany, NY 12208-3479
Tel: 518 262-3341 *Fax:* 518 262-6660
E-mail: barry_kogan@ccgateway.amc.edu
Accred Length: 4 Years *Program Size:* 10
Program ID: 480-35-21-085

Bronx

Albert Einstein College of Medicine Program

Sponsor: Albert Einstein College of Medicine of Yeshiva University
Jacobi Medical Center
Montefiore Medical Center-Henry and Lucy Moses Division
Montefiore Medical Center-Weiler Hospital
North Central Bronx Hospital

Program Director:
Arnold Melman, MD
Montefiore Med Ctr
Greene Medical Arts Pavilion
3400 Bainbridge Ave/5th Fl
Bronx, NY 10467
Tel: 718 920-4531 *Fax:* 718 547-2902
Internet: http://www.montefiore.org
Accred Length: 4 Years *Program Size:* 14
Program ID: 480-35-21-089

Brooklyn

Brookdale University Hospital Medical Center Program

Sponsor: Brookdale University Hospital Medical Center

Program Director:
Hong Kim, MD
Brookdale Univ Hospital and Med Ctr
Dept of Urology
Linden Blvd at Brookdale Plaza
Brooklyn, NY 11212
Tel: 718 240-5323 *Fax:* 718 240-6605
Accred Length: 4 Years *Program Size:* 4
Program ID: 480-35-31-091

Maimonides Medical Center Program

Sponsor: Maimonides Medical Center
Coney Island Hospital

Program Director:
Gilbert J Wise, MD
Maimonides Med Ctr
4802 Tenth Ave
Brooklyn, NY 11219
Tel: 718 438-3475 *Fax:* 718 438-0514
E-mail: gjw@mail.idt.net
Accred Length: 4 Years *Program Size:* 8
Program ID: 480-35-21-099

SUNY Health Science Center at Brooklyn Program

Sponsor: SUNY Health Science Center at Brooklyn
Kings County Hospital Center
Long Island College Hospital
University Hospital-SUNY Health Science Center at Brooklyn
Veterans Affairs Medical Center (Brooklyn)

Program Director:
Richard J Macchia, MD
445 Lenox Rd/Box 79
Brooklyn, NY 11203-2098
Tel: 718 270-2554 *Fax:* 718 270-3848
Accred Length: 4 Years *Program Size:* 12
Program ID: 480-35-21-107

Buffalo

SUNY at Buffalo Graduate Medical-Dental Education Consortium Program

Sponsor: SUNY at Buffalo Grad Medical-Dental Education Consortium
CGF Health System (Buffalo General Hospital)
CGF Health System (Children's Hospital of Buffalo)
CGF Health System (Millard Fillmore Hospitals)
Veterans Affairs Medical Center (Buffalo)

Program Director:
Gerald Sufrin, MD
Erie County Med Ctr
462 Grider St
Buffalo, NY 14215
Tel: 716 859-2212 *Fax:* 716 898-5172
Accred Length: 4 Years *Program Size:* 12
Program ID: 480-35-21-087

New Hyde Park

Albert Einstein College of Medicine at Long Island Jewish Medical Center Program

Sponsor: Long Island Jewish Medical Center
Winthrop-University Hospital

Program Director:
Arthur D Smith, MD
Long Island Jewish Med Ctr
Dept of Urology
270-05 76th Ave
New Hyde Park, NY 11040-1496
Tel: 718 470-7220 *Fax:* 718 343-6254
Internet: http://www.lij.edu
Accred Length: 4 Years *Program Size:* 5
Program ID: 480-35-21-098

New York

Albert Einstein College of Medicine at Beth Israel Medical Center Program

Sponsor: Beth Israel Medical Center

Program Director:
Harris M Nagler, MD
Dept of Urology
Beth Israel Med Ctr
10 Union Sq E/Ste 3A
New York, NY 10003
Tel: 212 844-8920 *Fax:* 212 844-8921
E-mail: hnagler@bethisraelny.org
Accred Length: 3 Years *Program Size:* 5
Program ID: 480-35-11-090

Lenox Hill Hospital Program

Sponsor: Lenox Hill Hospital

Program Director:
John A Fracchia, MD
Lenox Hill Hospital
Sect of Urology
100 E 77th St
New York, NY 10021-1883
Tel: 212 434-2190 *Fax:* 212 434-3495
Accred Length: 4 Years *Program Size:* 4
Program ID: 480-35-11-096

Mount Sinai School of Medicine Program

Sponsor: Mount Sinai School of Medicine
Elmhurst Hospital Center-Mount Sinai Services
Mount Sinai Medical Center
Veterans Affairs Medical Center (Bronx)

Program Director:
Michael J Droller, MD
Mount Sinai Med Ctr, Dept of Urology
One Gustave L Levy Pl
Box 1272
New York, NY 10029-6574
Tel: 212 241-8711 *Fax:* 212 876-3246
E-mail: emmacharles@smtplink.mssm.edu
Accred Length: 4 Years *Program Size:* 8
Program ID: 480-35-21-102

New York and Presbyterian Hospital (Columbia Campus) Program

Sponsor: New York and Presbyterian Hospital
St Luke's-Roosevelt Hospital Center

Program Director:
Carl A Olsson, MD
Columbia-Presbyterian Med Ctr
Atchley Pavilion/11th Fl
161 Fort Washington Ave
New York, NY 10032
Tel: 212 305-0100 *Fax:* 212 305-0106
Internet: http://cpmcnet.columbia.edu/dept/urology
Accred Length: 4 Years *Program Size:* 18
Program ID: 480-35-21-092

New York and Presbyterian Hospital (Cornell Campus) Program

Sponsor: New York and Presbyterian Hospital
New York and Presbyterian Hospital (Cornell Campus)

Program Director:
E Darracott Vaughan Jr, MD
New York Presbyterian Hospital-Cornell Campus
525 E 68th St/Box 94
New York, NY 10021
Tel: 212 746-5480 *Fax:* 212 746-8153
E-mail: jbbrady@mail.med.cornell.edu
Accred Length: 4 Years *Program Size:* 12
Program ID: 480-35-21-093

New York University Medical Center Program

Sponsor: New York University Medical Center
Bellevue Hospital Center
Cabrini Medical Center
Veterans Affairs Medical Center (Manhattan)

Program Director:
Herbert Lepor, MD
540 First Ave/Ste 10U
New York, NY 10016
Tel: 212 263-6301 *Fax:* 212 263-6303
Internet:
http://www.mcrcr4.med.nyu.edu/facprac/urolassoc.htm
Accred Length: 4 Years *Program Size:* 12
Program ID: 480-35-21-104

Programs

Rochester

University of Rochester Program
Sponsor: Strong Memorial Hospital of the University of Rochester
Genesee Hospital
Rochester General Hospital
Program Director:
William C Hulbert, MD
Strong Memorial Hospital
601 Elmwood Ave/Box 656
Rochester, NY 14642
Tel: 716 275-7993 *Fax:* 716 273-1068
E-mail: ingrid_mikk@urmc.rochester.edu
Internet:
http://www.urmc.rochester.edu/smd/urol/urolhome.html
Accred Length: 4 Years *Program Size:* 8
Program ID: 480-35-21-108

Stony Brook

SUNY at Stony Brook Program
Sponsor: University Hospital-SUNY at Stony Brook
Veterans Affairs Medical Center (Northport)
Program Director:
Wayne C Waltzer, MD
Dept of Urology
SUNY-Stony Brook Sch of Med
HSC T9-040
Stony Brook, NY 11794-8093
Tel: 516 444-1205 *Fax:* 516 444-7620
Internet: http://www.uhms.sunysb.edu/urology/
Accred Length: 4 Years *Program Size:* 4
Program ID: 480-35-21-175

Syracuse

SUNY Health Science Center at Syracuse Program
Sponsor: University Hospital-SUNY Health Science Center at Syracuse
Veterans Affairs Medical Center (Syracuse)
Program Director:
Gabriel P Haas, MD
SUNY Health Science Ctr-Syracuse
Dept of Urology
750 E Adams St
Syracuse, NY 13210
Tel: 315 464-4473, ext 6106 *Fax:* 315 464-6117
Accred Length: 4 Years *Program Size:* 4
Program ID: 480-35-21-109

Valhalla

New York Medical College at Westchester Medical Center Program
Sponsor: New York Medical College
Lincoln Medical and Mental Health Center
Metropolitan Hospital Center
Westchester Medical Center
Program Director:
Camille Mallouh, MD
New York Med Coll
Dept of Urology
Munger Pavilion/Rm 460
Valhalla, NY 10595
Tel: 914 594-4300 *Fax:* 914 594-4394
E-mail: camille_mallouh@nymc.edu
Accred Length: 4 Years *Program Size:* 12
Program ID: 480-35-21-103

North Carolina

Chapel Hill

University of North Carolina Hospitals Program
Sponsor: University of North Carolina Hospitals
Carolinas Medical Center
Wake Medical Center
Program Director:
Culley C Carson III, MD
Univ of North Carolina, Div of Urology
427 Burnett Womack
Chapel Hill, NC 27599-7235
Tel: 919 966-2571 *Fax:* 919 966-0098
E-mail: carson@med.unc.edu.
Internet: http://www.med.unc.edu/surgery/urology
Accred Length: 4 Years *Program Size:* 8
Program ID: 480-36-21-110

Durham

Duke University Program
Sponsor: Duke University Medical Center
Veterans Affairs Medical Center (Asheville)
Veterans Affairs Medical Center (Durham)
Program Director:
Glenn M Preminger, MD
Duke Univ Med Ctr
PO Box 2922
Durham, NC 27710
Tel: 919 684-5693 *Fax:* 919 681-7423
E-mail: walke043@mc.duke.edu
Accred Length: 4 Years *Program Size:* 16
Program ID: 480-36-21-112

Winston-Salem

Wake Forest University School of Medicine Program
Sponsor: Wake Forest University Baptist Medical Center
Program Director:
R L Kroovand, MD
Wake Forest Univ Sch of Med
Medical Center Blvd
Winston-Salem, NC 27157-1094
Tel: 336 716-4131 *Fax:* 336 716-5711
Internet: http://www.wfubmc.edu/education/admissio
Accred Length: 4 Years *Program Size:* 7
Program ID: 480-36-21-113

Ohio

Akron

Akron General Medical Center/NEOUCOM Program
Sponsor: Akron General Medical Center
Akron City Hospital (Summa Health System)
Children's Hospital Medical Center of Akron
Program Director:
Jack L Summers, MD PhD
Summa Health System-Akron City Hosp
75 Arch St/Ste 101
Akron, OH 44307
Tel: 330 384-6050 *Fax:* 330 384-1529
E-mail: meded@agmc.org
Internet: http://agmc.org
Accred Length: 3 Years *Program Size:* 10
Program ID: 480-38-21-164

Cincinnati

University Hospital/University of Cincinnati College of Medicine Program
Sponsor: University Hospital Inc
Children's Hospital Medical Center
Christ Hospital
Veterans Affairs Medical Center (Cincinnati)
Program Director:
Thomas E Bell, MD
Univ of Cincinnati Med Ctr
Div of Urology
231 Bethesda Ave/ML 589
Cincinnati, OH 45267-0589
Tel: 513 558-0983 *Fax:* 513 558-3575
E-mail: thomas.bell@med.va.gov
Accred Length: 4 Years *Program Size:* 11
Program ID: 480-38-21-117

Cleveland

Case Western Reserve University Program
Sponsor: University Hospitals of Cleveland
MetroHealth Medical Center
Mount Sinai Medical Center of Cleveland
Veterans Affairs Medical Center (Cleveland)
Program Director:
Martin I Resnick, MD
Case Western Reserve Univ
11100 Euclid Ave/LKSD 7112
Cleveland, OH 44106-5046
Tel: 216 844-3011 *Fax:* 216 844-1900
E-mail: mir@po.cwru.edu
Accred Length: 4 Years *Program Size:* 12
Program ID: 480-38-21-118

Cleveland Clinic Foundation Program
Sponsor: Cleveland Clinic Foundation
Program Director:
Drogo K Montague, MD
Cleveland Clinic Foundation
Dept of Urology/A100
9500 Euclid Ave
Cleveland, OH 44195-5242
Tel: 216 444-5690 *Fax:* 216 444-1162
E-mail: meded@cestmp.ccf.org
Internet: http://www.ccf.org
Accred Length: 4 Years *Program Size:* 18
Program ID: 480-38-22-119

Columbus

Ohio State University Program
Sponsor: Ohio State University Medical Center
Children's Hospital
Riverside Methodist Hospitals (OhioHealth)
Program Director:
Robert R Bahnson, MD
4960 UHC
456 W 10th Ave
Columbus, OH 43210-1228
Tel: 614 293-8155 *Fax:* 614 293-5363
E-mail: shull.20@osu.edu
Internet: http://www.surgery.med.ohio-state.edu
Accred Length: 3 Years *Program Size:* 6
Program ID: 480-38-21-120

Toledo

Medical College of Ohio Program

Sponsor: Medical College of Ohio
St Vincent Mercy Medical Center
Toledo Hospital
Program Director:
Kenneth A Kropp, MD
Med Coll of Ohio, Dept of Urology
3065 Arlington Ave
Toledo, OH 43614
Tel: 419 383-5416 *Fax:* 419 383-3785
E-mail: vfine@mco.edu
Accred Length: 4 Years *Program Size:* 12
Program ID: 480-38-21-122

Oklahoma

Oklahoma City

University of Oklahoma Health Sciences Center Program

Sponsor: University of Oklahoma College of Medicine
Children's Hospital of Oklahoma
University Hospital
Veterans Affairs Medical Center (Oklahoma City)
Program Director:
Daniel J Culkin, MD
Univ of Oklahoma Health Sciences Ctr
Dept of Urology
920 Stanton L Young Blvd/WP3150
Oklahoma City, OK 73104
Tel: 405 271-6900 *Fax:* 405 271-3118
E-mail: daniel-culkin@ouhsc.edu
Internet: http://www.urology-okc
Accred Length: 4 Years *Program Size:* 9
Program ID: 480-39-21-123

Oregon

Portland

Oregon Health Sciences University Program

Sponsor: Oregon Health Sciences University Hospital
Kaiser Foundation Hospitals-Northwest Region
Veterans Affairs Medical Center (Portland)
Program Director:
John M Barry, MD
Oregon Health Sciences Univ
3181 SW Sam Jackson Park Rd
Portland, OR 97201-3098
Tel: 503 494-8470 *Fax:* 503 494-8671
E-mail: taylorme@ohsu.edu
Accred Length: 4 Years *Program Size:* 8
Program ID: 480-40-21-124

Pennsylvania

Danville

Penn State Geisinger Health System/Geisinger Medical Center Program

Sponsor: Penn State Geisinger Health System
Geisinger Medical Center
Program Director:
Joseph J Mowad, MD
Geisinger Med Ctr
Dept of Urology
100 N Academy Ave
Danville, PA 17822
Tel: 717 271-6376 *Fax:* 717 271-6955
E-mail: meded@psghs.edu
Accred Length: 4 Years *Program Size:* 6
Program ID: 480-41-11-125

Hershey

Penn State Geisinger Health System/Milton S Hershey Medical Center Program

Sponsor: Penn State Geisinger Health System
Milton S Hershey Medical Center
Lancaster General Hospital
Lehigh Valley Hospital
Program Director:
Ross M Decter Sr, MD
Div of Urology
Univ Hospital
PO Box 850
Hershey, PA 17033
Tel: 717 531-8849 *Fax:* 717 531-4475
E-mail: rdecter@psghs.edu
Accred Length: 4 Years *Program Size:* 8
Subspecialties: TY
Program ID: 480-41-21-127

Philadelphia

Temple University Program

Sponsor: Temple University Hospital
Abington Memorial Hospital
St Christopher's Hospital for Children
Program Director:
Michel A Pontari, MD
Temple Univ Hospital
3401 N Broad St
Ste 350 Parkinson Pavillion
Philadelphia, PA 19140
Tel: 215 707-4445 *Fax:* 215 707-4758
E-mail: mpontari@aol.com
Accred Length: 4 Years *Program Size:* 8
Program ID: 480-41-21-132

Thomas Jefferson University Program

Sponsor: Thomas Jefferson University Hospital
Bryn Mawr Hospital
duPont Hospital for Children
Veterans Affairs Medical Center (Wilmington)
Program Director:
S Grant Mulholland, MD
Thomas Jefferson Univ Hospital, Dept of Urology
1025 Walnut St/1112 Coll Bldg
Philadelphia, PA 19107
Tel: 215 955-6961 *Fax:* 215 923-1884
Accred Length: 4 Years *Program Size:* 8
Program ID: 480-41-21-133

University of Pennsylvania Program

Sponsor: Hospital of the University of Pennsylvania
Children's Hospital of Philadelphia
Pennsylvania Hospital (UPHS)
Veterans Affairs Medical Center (Philadelphia)
Program Director:
Alan J Wein, MD
Hospital of Univ of Pennsylvania
Div of Urology
3400 Spruce St/One Rhoads Pavilion
Philadelphia, PA 19104
Tel: 215 349-5042 *Fax:* 215 662-3955
Accred Length: 4 Years *Program Size:* 12
Subspecialties: UP
Program ID: 480-41-21-134

Pittsburgh

University Health Center of Pittsburgh Program

Sponsor: University Health Center of Pittsburgh
Children's Hospital of Pittsburgh
Presbyterian University Hospital/UPMC
Veterans Affairs Medical Center (Pittsburgh)
Program Director:
Thomas R Hakala, MD
Univ of Pittsburgh
3471 Fifth Ave/Ste 700
Pittsburgh, PA 15213
Tel: 412 692-4092 *Fax:* 412 692-4081
Accred Length: 4 Years *Program Size:* 8
Program ID: 480-41-21-135

Puerto Rico

San Juan

University of Puerto Rico Program

Sponsor: University of Puerto Rico School of Medicine
Hospital Pavia
University Hospital
University Pediatric Hospital
Veterans Affairs Medical Center (San Juan)
Program Director:
Antonio Puras-Baez, MD
Univ of Puerto Rico
Recinto de Ciencias Medicas
Apartado 5067
San Juan, PR 00936
Tel: 787 758-2525
Accred Length: 4 Years *Program Size:* 3
Program ID: 480-42-31-138

Rhode Island

Providence

Brown University Program

Sponsor: Rhode Island Hospital
Roger Williams Medical Center
Veterans Affairs Medical Center (Providence)
Program Director:
Anthony A Caldamone, MD
Rhode Island Hospital
Dept of Urology
2 Dudley St/Ste 174
Providence, RI 02905
Tel: 401 444-5795 *Fax:* 401 444-6947
Accred Length: 4 Years *Program Size:* 8
Program ID: 480-43-31-139

South Carolina

Charleston

Medical University of South Carolina Program

Sponsor: Medical University of South Carolina College of Medicine
MUSC Medical Center
Ralph H Johnson Dept of Veterans Affairs Med Center

Program Director:
William R Turner Jr, MD
Med Univ of South Carolina
171 Ashley Ave
Ste 644 Clinical Sciences Bldg
Charleston, SC 29425-2280
Tel: 803 792-4531 *Fax:* 803 792-8523
E-mail: turnerw@musc.edu
Accred Length: 3 Years *Program Size:* 8
Program ID: 480-45-21-140

Tennessee

Memphis

University of Tennessee Program

Sponsor: University of Tennessee College of Medicine
LeBonheur Children's Medical Center
Regional Medical Center at Memphis
University of Tennessee Medical Center (UT Bowld Hospital)
Veterans Affairs Medical Center (Memphis)

Program Director:
Clair E Cox, MD
Univ of Tennessee Med Ctr
Dept of Urology
956 Court Ave/Rm H216
Memphis, TN 38163
Tel: 901 448-5868 *Fax:* 901 448-8758
Accred Length: 4 Years *Program Size:* 12
Subspecialties: UP
Program ID: 480-47-21-141

Nashville

Vanderbilt University Program

Sponsor: Vanderbilt University Medical Center
Baptist Hospital
Veterans Affairs Medical Center (Nashville)

Program Director:
Joseph A Smith Jr, MD
A-1302 Med Ctr North
21st Ave S and Garland Ave
Nashville, TN 37232-2765
Tel: 615 322-2142 *Fax:* 615 322-8990
E-mail: derenda.gold@mcmail.vanderbilt.edu
Internet:
http://www.mc.vanderbilt.edu/surgery/urol/index.htm
Accred Length: 4 Years *Program Size:* 8
Program ID: 480-47-21-142

Texas

Dallas

University of Texas Southwestern Medical School Program

Sponsor: University of Texas Southwestern Medical School
Baylor University Medical Center
Children's Medical Center of Dallas
Dallas County Hospital District-Parkland Memorial Hospital
Veterans Affairs Medical Center (Dallas)
Zale-Lipshy University Hospital

Program Director:
John D McConnell, MD
Univ of Texas Southwestern Med Sch
5323 Harry Hines Blvd
Dallas, TX 75235-9110
Tel: 214 648-4765 *Fax:* 214 648-3398
Accred Length: 4 Years *Program Size:* 16
Program ID: 480-48-21-143

Galveston

University of Texas Medical Branch Hospitals Program

Sponsor: University of Texas Medical Branch Hospitals

Program Director:
Michael M Warren, MD
Div of Urology/Rte 0540
Univ of Texas Med Branch
301 University Blvd
Galveston, TX 77555-0540
Tel: 409 772-2091 *Fax:* 409 772-5144
E-mail: mwarren@utmb.edu
Internet: http://www.utmb.edu/surgery/
Accred Length: 4 Years *Program Size:* 6
Program ID: 480-48-11-144

Houston

Baylor College of Medicine Program

Sponsor: Baylor College of Medicine
Harris County Hospital District-Ben Taub General Hospital
Methodist Hospital
St Luke's Episcopal Hospital
Texas Children's Hospital
Veterans Affairs Medical Center (Houston)

Program Director:
Brian J Miles, MD
Baylor Coll of Med
Dept of Urology
6560 Fannin St/Ste 2100
Houston, TX 77030
Tel: 713 798-8144 *Fax:* 713 798-5553
E-mail: hartman@bcm.tmc.edu
Internet: http://www.bcm.tmc.edu/urol/
Accred Length: 4 Years *Program Size:* 16
Subspecialties: UP
Program ID: 480-48-21-145

University of Texas at Houston Program

Sponsor: University of Texas Medical School at Houston
Lyndon B Johnson General Hospital
Memorial Hermann Healthcare System
St Joseph Hospital
University of Texas M D Anderson Cancer Center

Program Director:
Edward J McGuire, MD
Univ of Texas Med Sch
6431 Fannin St/MSB 6018
Houston, TX 77030
Tel: 713 500-7333 *Fax:* 713 500-0751
E-mail: lchelett@utsurg.med.uth.tmc.edu
Accred Length: 4 Years *Program Size:* 15
Program ID: 480-48-21-146

Lackland AFB

San Antonio Uniformed Services Health Education Consortium Program

Sponsor: San Antonio Uniformed Services Health Education Consortium

Program Director:
Lt Col Steven C Lynch, MD
Wilford Hall Med Ctr/MMKU
59th Medical Wing
2200 Bergquist Dr/Ste 1
Lackland AFB, TX 78236-5300
Tel: 210 292-7558 *Fax:* 210 292-7199
E-mail: lynch@whmc.af.mil
Accred Length: 4 Years *Program Size:* 12
Program ID: 480-48-21-170
US Armed Services Program

San Antonio

University of Texas Health Science Center at San Antonio Program

Sponsor: University of Texas Medical School at San Antonio
Audie L Murphy Memorial Veterans Hospital (San Antonio)
Methodist Healthcare
San Antonio Community Hospital
Santa Rosa Health Care Corporation
University Hospital-South Texas Medical Center

Program Director:
Thomas P Ball Jr, MD
Univ of Texas Health Science Ctr
Div of Urology
7703 Floyd Curl Dr
San Antonio, TX 78284-7845
Tel: 210 567-5640 *Fax:* 210 567-6868
E-mail: torrey@uthscsa.edu
Accred Length: 4 Years *Program Size:* 8
Program ID: 480-48-21-147

Temple

Texas A&M College of Medicine-Scott and White Program

Sponsor: Scott and White Memorial Hospital
Central Texas Veterans Affairs Healthcare System

Program Director:
Richard C Klugo, MD
Texas A&M-Scott and White
Grad Med Educ
2401 S 31st St
Temple, TX 76508-0001
Tel: 254 724-1695 *Fax:* 254 724-5245
E-mail: urolresi@bellnet.tamu.edu
Internet: http://www.swinfo.tamu.edu
Accred Length: 4 Years *Program Size:* 6
Program ID: 480-48-21-148

Utah

Salt Lake City

University of Utah Program

Sponsor: University of Utah Medical Center
LDS Hospital
Primary Children's Medical Center
Veterans Affairs Medical Center (Salt Lake City)

Program Director:
Richard G Middleton, MD
Univ of Utah Med Ctr
Attn: Anita Gallacher
50 N Medical Dr
Salt Lake City, UT 84132
Tel: 801 581-4703 *Fax:* 801 581-6127
Accred Length: 3 Years *Program Size:* 6
Program ID: 480-49-21-149

Virginia

Charlottesville

University of Virginia Program

Sponsor: University of Virginia Medical Center
Veterans Affairs Medical Center (Salem)

Program Director:
William D Steers, MD
Univ of Virginia Sch of Med
Dept of Urology/Box 422
Charlottesville, VA 22908
Tel: 804 924-2224 *Fax:* 804 982-3652
Internet: http://www.med.virginia.edu:80/som-cl
Accred Length: 4 Years *Program Size:* 8
Program ID: 480-51-21-151

Norfolk

Eastern Virginia Medical School Program

Sponsor: Eastern Virginia Medical School
Children's Hospital of the King's Daughters
Sentara Leigh Hospital
Sentara Norfolk General Hospital

Program Director:
Paul F Schellhammer, MD
Eastern Virginia Graduate Sch of Med
Dept of Urology
600 Gresham Dr/Ste 203
Norfolk, VA 23507
Tel: 757 668-3571 *Fax:* 757 627-3211
Accred Length: 3 Years *Program Size:* 3
Program ID: 480-51-21-153

Portsmouth

Naval Medical Center (Portsmouth) Program

Sponsor: Naval Medical Center (Portsmouth)
Sentara Norfolk General Hospital
Veterans Affairs Medical Center (Hampton)

Program Director:
Capt Leo Kusuda, MD
Naval Med Ctr
620 John Paul Jones Circle
Portsmouth, VA 23708
Tel: 757 953-5234 *Fax:* 757 953-6072
E-mail: lkusuda@pnh10.med.navy.mil
Accred Length: 3 Years *Program Size:* 5
Program ID: 480-51-31-011
US Armed Services Program

Richmond

Medical College of Virginia/Virginia Commonwealth University Program

Sponsor: Medical College of Virginia/Virginia Commonwealth University
Hunter Holmes McGuire VA Medical Center (Richmond)
Medical College of Virginia Hospitals

Program Director:
P Gary Katz, MD
Med Coll of Virginia
PO Box 980118
Richmond, VA 23298-0118
Tel: 804 828-5318 *Fax:* 804 828-2157
Accred Length: 3 Years *Program Size:* 6
Program ID: 480-51-21-154

Washington

Seattle

University of Washington Program

Sponsor: University of Washington School of Medicine
Children's Hospital and Medical Center
Harborview Medical Center
University of Washington Medical Center
Veterans Affairs Medical Center (Seattle)
Virginia Mason Medical Center

Program Director:
Michael E Mayo, MD
Univ of Washington
Dept of Urology/Box 356510
1959 NE Pacific St
Seattle, WA 98195
Tel: 206 685-3245 *Fax:* 206 543-3272
E-mail: hhovey@u.washington.edu
Internet: http://weber.u.washington.edu/~uroweb
Accred Length: 4 Years *Program Size:* 12
Subspecialties: UP
Program ID: 480-54-21-155

Tacoma

Madigan Army Medical Center Program

Sponsor: Madigan Army Medical Center

Program Director:
Robert C Allen Jr, MD
Attn: MCHJ-SU
Madigan Army Med Ctr
Tacoma, WA 98431
Tel: 253 968-4141 *Fax:* 253 968-2444
Internet: http://www.mamc.amedd.army.mil
Accred Length: 3 Years *Program Size:* 4
Subspecialties: TY
Program ID: 480-54-11-007
US Armed Services Program

West Virginia

Morgantown

West Virginia University Program

Sponsor: West Virginia University Hospitals
Louis A Johnson Veterans Affairs Medical Center

Program Director:
Stanley J Kandzari, MD
Robert C Byrd Health Sciences Ctr
Dept of Urology
PO Box 9251
Morgantown, WV 26506-9251
Tel: 304 293-2706 *Fax:* 304 293-2807
Accred Length: 4 Years *Program Size:* 8
Program ID: 480-55-21-157

Wisconsin

Madison

University of Wisconsin Program

Sponsor: University of Wisconsin Hospital and Clinics
Meriter Hospital
St Marys Hospital Medical Center
William S Middleton Veterans Hospital

Program Director:
Reginald C Bruskewitz, MD
Univ of Wisconsin Hospital and Clinics
600 Highland Ave/Rm G5-339 CSC
Madison, WI 53792-3236
Tel: 608 263-9534 *Fax:* 608 263-0454
Accred Length: 3 Years *Program Size:* 10
Program ID: 480-56-21-158

Milwaukee

Medical College of Wisconsin Program

Sponsor: Medical College of Wisconsin Affiliated Hospitals Inc
Children's Hospital of Wisconsin
Clement J Zablocki Veterans Affairs Medical Center
Froedtert Memorial Lutheran Hospital

Program Director:
Frank P Begun, MD
Froedtert Memorial Lutheran Hospital
Div of Urology
9200 W Wisconsin Ave
Milwaukee, WI 53226
Tel: 414 456-6950 *Fax:* 414 456-6217
E-mail: orth@urology.fmlh.edu
Accred Length: 3 Years *Program Size:* 10
Program ID: 480-56-21-159

Vascular and Interventional Radiology (Radiology-Diagnostic)

Alabama

Birmingham

University of Alabama Medical Center Program
Sponsor: University of Alabama Hospital
Veterans Affairs Medical Center (Birmingham)
Program Director:
Souheil Saddekni, MD
Univ of Alabama Med Ctr
619 S 19th St/JT-Rm N312
Birmingham, AL 35233
Tel: 205 975-4850 *Fax:* 205 975-5257
E-mail: ssaddekn@uabmc.edu
Internet: http://www.rad.uab.edu
Accred Length: 1 Year *Program Size:* 3
Program ID: 427-01-21-054

Arizona

Tucson

University of Arizona Program
Sponsor: University of Arizona College of Medicine
Kino Community Hospital
Veterans Affairs Medical Center (Tucson)
Program Director:
Stephen H Smyth, MD
Arizona Health Sciences Ctr, Dept of Radiology
1501 N Campbell Ave
PO Box 245067
Tucson, AZ 85724-5067
Tel: 520 626-6794 *Fax:* 520 626-1945
E-mail: ltaylor@radiology.arizona.edu
Accred Length: 1 Year *Program Size:* 2
Program ID: 427-03-21-074

Arkansas

Little Rock

University of Arkansas for Medical Sciences Program
Sponsor: University of Arkansas College of Medicine
John L McClellan Memorial Veterans Hospital
University Hospital of Arkansas
Program Director:
David R McFarland, MD
Dept of Radiology/Slot 556
5301 W Markham St
Little Rock, AR 72205
Tel: 501 686-6901 *Fax:* 501 320-5000
E-mail: dmcfarland@radlan.uams.edu
Accred Length: 1 Year *Program Size:* 1
Program ID: 427-04-21-007

California

Loma Linda

Loma Linda University Program
Sponsor: Loma Linda University Medical Center
Program Director:
Douglas C Smith, MD
Loma Linda Univ Med Ctr
Dept of Radiology Rm 2605
11234 Anderson St
Loma Linda, CA 92354
Tel: 909 824-4370 *Fax:* 909 478-9202
E-mail: rosalyn_hamilton@ccmail.llumc.edu
Accred Length: 1 Year *Program Size:* 2
Program ID: 427-05-21-026

Los Angeles

UCLA Medical Center Program
Sponsor: UCLA School of Medicine
UCLA Medical Center
Program Director:
Paul Dong, MD
UCLA Hospital and Clinics
Dept of Rad Sciences
10833 Le Conte Ave
Los Angeles, CA 90095-1721
Tel: 310 794-7923 *Fax:* 310 206-2701
E-mail: pdong@mailrad.ucla.edu
Internet: http://www.radsci.ucla.edu
Accred Length: 1 Year *Program Size:* 4
Program ID: 427-05-21-063

University of Southern California Program
Sponsor: Los Angeles County-USC Medical Center
Kenneth Norris Jr Cancer Hospital and Research Institute
USC University Hospital
Program Director:
Michael D Katz, MD
Univ of Southern California Hospital
1500 San Pablo St
Los Angeles, CA 90033
Tel: 323 226-4218 *Fax:* 323 442-8552
Internet: http://www.usc.edu/hsc/medicine/radiology/
Accred Length: 1 Year *Program Size:* 3
Program ID: 427-05-21-013

Orange

University of California (Irvine) Program
Sponsor: University of California (Irvine) Medical Center
Program Director:
Larry Stuart Deutsch, MD
Univ of California Irvine
Dept of Radiological Sciences
101 The City Dr S/Rt 140
Orange, CA 92868-3298
Tel: 714 456-5033 *Fax:* 714 456-7864
Accred Length: 1 Year *Program Size:* 1
Program ID: 427-05-11-089

Sacramento

University of California (Davis) Program
Sponsor: University of California (Davis) Medical Center
Kaiser Foundation Hospital (Sacramento)
Program Director:
Daniel P Link, MD
Univ of California Davis
4860 Y St
Ste 3100
Sacramento, CA 95817
Tel: 916 734-3766 *Fax:* 916 734-8490
E-mail: daniel.link@ucdmc.ucdavis.edu
Internet: http://www-iris.ucdmc.ucdavis.edu
Accred Length: 1 Year *Program Size:* 2
Program ID: 427-05-31-082

San Diego

University of California (San Diego) Program
Sponsor: University of California (San Diego) Medical Center
Veterans Affairs Medical Center (San Diego)
Program Director:
Anne C Roberts, MD
200 W Arbor Dr
San Diego, CA 92103-8756
Tel: 619 543-6607 *Fax:* 619 543-3781
E-mail: pamelarosario@radiology.ucsd.edu
Accred Length: 1 Year *Program Size:* 2
Program ID: 427-05-21-058

San Francisco

University of California (San Francisco) Program
Sponsor: University of California (San Francisco) School of Medicine
University of California (San Francisco) Medical Center
Program Director:
Roy L Gordon, MD
Rm M-361/Box 0628
505 Parnassus Ave
San Francisco, CA 94143-0628
Tel: 415 476-3131 *Fax:* 415 476-1086
E-mail: roy.gordon@radiology.ucsf.edu
Accred Length: 1 Year *Program Size:* 3
Program ID: 427-05-21-009

Stanford

Stanford University Program
Sponsor: Stanford University Hospital
Program Director:
Mahmood Razavi, MD
H3630 Route 2
300 Pasteur Dr
Stanford, CA 94305-5105
Tel: 650 725-5202 *Fax:* 650 725-0533
E-mail: charles.semba@forsythe.stanford.edu
Accred Length: 1 Year *Program Size:* 3
Program ID: 427-05-21-081

Colorado

Denver

University of Colorado Program

Sponsor: University of Colorado Health Sciences Center

Program Director:
David A Kumpe, MD
Dept of Radiology/A030
4200 E Ninth Ave
Denver, CO 80262-0030
Tel: 303 372-6130 *Fax:* 303 372-6275
E-mail: david.kumpe@uchsc.edu
Accred Length: 1 Year *Program Size:* 3
Program ID: 427-07-21-049

Connecticut

New Haven

Yale-New Haven Medical Center Program

Sponsor: Yale-New Haven Hospital
Veterans Affairs Medical Center (West Haven)

Program Director:
Jeffrey S Pollak, MD
Yale-New Haven Hospital
20 York St/SP2-323
New Haven, CT 06504
Tel: 203 785-7026 *Fax:* 203 737-1077
E-mail: melendez@biomed.med.yale.edu
Accred Length: 1 Year *Program Size:* 3
Program ID: 427-08-21-032

District of Columbia

Washington

George Washington University Program

Sponsor: George Washington University School of Medicine

Program Director:
Edward M Druy, MD
901 23rd St NW
Washington, DC 20037
Tel: 202 994-0382 *Fax:* 202 994-0695
E-mail: emdru@gwis2.circ.gwu.edu
Internet: http://www.gwumc.edu/edu/radiology
Accred Length: 1 Year *Program Size:* 1
Program ID: 427-10-21-070

Georgetown University Program

Sponsor: Georgetown University Medical Center

Program Director:
Klemens H Barth, MD
Georgetown Univ Hospital
Dept of Radiology
3800 Reservoir Rd NW
Washington, DC 20007-2197
Tel: 202 784-3420 *Fax:* 202 784-4896
Accred Length: 1 Year *Program Size:* 3
Program ID: 427-10-31-069

Howard University Program

Sponsor: Howard University Hospital
Washington Hospital Center

Program Director:
Richard J Gray, MD
110 Irving St NW
Washington, DC 20060
Tel: 202 877-6495 *Fax:* 202 877-8153
Accred Length: 1 Year *Program Size:* 2
Program ID: 427-10-21-068

Florida

Gainesville

University of Florida Program

Sponsor: University of Florida College of Medicine
Shands Hospital at the University of Florida
Veterans Affairs Medical Center (Gainesville)

Program Director:
James G Caridi, MD
Univ of Florida
Dept of Radiology
Box 100374 JHMHC
Gainesville, FL 32610-0374
Tel: 352 395-0291, ext 52288 *Fax:* 352 395-0279
E-mail: caridij@xray.ufl.edu
Internet: http://www.xray.ufl.edu/index.html
Accred Length: 1 Year *Program Size:* 3
Program ID: 427-11-21-033

Jacksonville

University of Florida Health Science Center/Jacksonville Program

Sponsor: University of Florida College of Medicine at Jacksonville
University Medical Center (UFHSC/J)

Program Director:
Harry M Northup, MD
655 W Eighth St
Jacksonville, FL 32209
Tel: 904 549-4225 *Fax:* 904 549-3186
E-mail: jac@umc5.umc.ufl.edu
Internet: http://www.ufhscj.edu/radiology/radiology.html
Accred Length: 1 Year *Program Size:* 1
Program ID: 427-11-21-086

Miami

University of Miami-Jackson Memorial Medical Center (Baptist) Program

Sponsor: University of Miami-Jackson Memorial Medical Center
Baptist Hospital of Miami

Program Director:
Gary J Becker, MD
Miami Cardiac and Vascular Inst
Baptist Hospital of Miami
8900 N Kendall Dr
Miami, FL 33176
Tel: 305 598-5990 *Fax:* 305 270-3600
E-mail: garyb@bhssf.org
Internet: http://mcvi.baptisthealth.net
Accred Length: 1 Year *Program Size:* 3
Program ID: 427-11-21-025

University of Miami-Jackson Memorial Medical Center Program

Sponsor: University of Miami-Jackson Memorial Medical Center
Cedars Medical Center

Program Director:
Jose M Yrizarry, MD
Univ of Miami-Jackson Memorial Med Ctr
Dept of Radiology (R109)
PO Box 016960
Miami, FL 33101
Tel: 305 585-5507 *Fax:* 305 585-2689
E-mail: hceballo@mednet.med.miami.edu
Accred Length: 1 Year *Program Size:* 4
Program ID: 427-11-31-028

Tampa

University of South Florida Program

Sponsor: University of South Florida College of Medicine
Tampa General Healthcare

Program Director:
Thomas J Black, MD
Radiology Associates of Tampa
511 W Bay St/Ste 301
Tampa, FL 33601
Tel: 813 251-7444 *Fax:* 813 253-4032
Accred Length: 1 Year *Program Size:* 1
Program ID: 427-11-21-092

Georgia

Atlanta

Emory University Program

Sponsor: Emory University School of Medicine
Emory University Hospital
Grady Memorial Hospital

Program Director:
Robert H Smith, MD
Emory Univ Hospital
Dept of Vascular/Interventional Rad
1364 Clifton Rd NE
Atlanta, GA 30322
Tel: 404 712-7033 *Fax:* 404 712-7970
E-mail: robert_h_smith@emory.org
Accred Length: 1 Year *Program Size:* 5
Program ID: 427-12-21-022

Illinois

Chicago

McGaw Medical Center of Northwestern University Program

Sponsor: Northwestern University Medical School
Northwestern Memorial Hospital

Program Director:
Howard B Chrisman, MD
Northwestern Memorial Hospital
Radiology/Olson Pavilion
710 N Fairbanks Ct
Chicago, IL 60611
Tel: 312 908-5659 *Fax:* 312 908-9029
E-mail: h-chrisman@nwu.edu
Accred Length: 1 Year *Program Size:* 4
Program ID: 427-16-21-034

Rush-Presbyterian-St Luke's Medical Center Program

Sponsor: Rush-Presbyterian-St Luke's Medical Center

Program Director:
Virginia McDonald, MD
Rush-Presbyterian-St Luke's Med Ctr
1653 W Congress Pkwy
Chicago, IL 60612-3864
Tel: 312 942-5781, ext 27578 *Fax:* 312 942-2114
E-mail: vmcdonal@rad.rpslmc.edu
Accred Length: 1 Year *Program Size:* 4
Program ID: 427-16-21-023

University of Chicago Program
Sponsor: University of Chicago Hospitals

Program Director:
Jeffrey A Leef, MD
Univ of Chicago Hospitals
MC 2026
5841 S Maryland Ave
Chicago, IL 60637
Tel: 773 702-3550 *Fax:* 773 702-1161
Internet: http://www-radiology.uchicago.edu
Accred Length: 1 Year *Program Size:* 2
Program ID: 427-16-21-059

Indiana

Indianapolis

Indiana University School of Medicine (Methodist) Program
Sponsor: Indiana University School of Medicine
Clarian Methodist Hospital of Indiana

Program Director:
Karen Ehrman, MD
Clarian Methodist Hospital
Dept of Radiology
I-65 at 21st St/PO Box 1367
Indianapolis, IN 46206-1367
Tel: 317 929-8250 *Fax:* 317 929-6312
Accred Length: 1 Year *Program Size:* 1
Program ID: 427-17-21-037

Indiana University School of Medicine Program
Sponsor: Indiana University School of Medicine
Clarian IU Hospital
Clarian Riley Hospital for Children

Program Director:
Matthew S Johnson, MD
Dept of Radiology/UH 0279
550 N University Blvd
Indianapolis, IN 46202-5253
Tel: 317 274-1840 *Fax:* 317 274-1848
E-mail: mjohnson@xray.indyrad.iupui.edu
Internet: http://www.indyrad.iupui.edu/homepage.htm
Accred Length: 1 Year *Program Size:* 4
Program ID: 427-17-21-010

Iowa

Iowa City

University of Iowa Hospitals and Clinics Program
Sponsor: University of Iowa Hospitals and Clinics
Veterans Affairs Medical Center (Iowa City)

Program Director:
Melhem J Sharafuddin, MD
Univ of Iowa Hospitals and Clinics
Dept of Radiology
200 Hawkins Dr
Iowa City, IA 52242
Tel: 319 356-4329
E-mail: mel-sharafuddin@uiowa.edu
Internet: http://www.indy.radiology.uiowa.edu/
Accred Length: 1 Year *Program Size:* 2
Program ID: 427-18-21-065

Louisiana

New Orleans

Louisiana State University Program
Sponsor: Louisiana State University School of Medicine
Medical Center of Louisiana at New Orleans
Veterans Affairs Medical Center-LSU Service (New Orleans)

Program Director:
Wilfrido R Castaneda, MD
Louisiana State Univ Med Ctr
1542 Tulane Ave
Rm 311
New Orleans, LA 70112
Tel: 504 568-4966 *Fax:* 504 568-8955
E-mail: hferra@lsumc.edu
Accred Length: 1 Year *Program Size:* 3
Program ID: 427-21-21-079

Maryland

Baltimore

Johns Hopkins University Program
Sponsor: Johns Hopkins University School of Medicine
Johns Hopkins Hospital

Program Director:
Anthony C Venbrux, MD
Johns Hopkins Hospital
600 N Wolfe St
Blalock 544
Baltimore, MD 21287-2191
Tel: 410 614-2237 *Fax:* 410 955-0233
E-mail: avenbrux@rad.jhu.edu
Internet: http://www.cvdl.rad.jhu.edu
Accred Length: 1 Year *Program Size:* 10
Program ID: 427-23-21-011

University of Maryland Program
Sponsor: University of Maryland Medical System
Mercy Medical Center
Veterans Affairs Medical Center (Baltimore)

Program Director:
Geoffrey S Hastings, MD
Univ of Maryland Med System
22 S Greene St
Baltimore, MD 21201
Tel: 410 328-7490 *Fax:* 410 328-3168
E-mail: ghastings@radiology.umaryland.edu
Internet:
http://umm.edu/center/specialties/departments/diag_radiology/fel-radioltoc.html
Accred Length: 1 Year *Program Size:* 3
Program ID: 427-23-21-053

Massachusetts

Boston

Beth Israel Deaconess Medical Center (West Campus) Program
Sponsor: Beth Israel Deaconess Medical Center

Program Director:
Max P Rosen, MD
Beth Israel Deaconess Med Ctr
Radiology Fellowship Program
330 Brookline Ave
Boston, MA 02215
Tel: 617 754-2523 *Fax:* 617 754-2545
E-mail: mrosen2@bidmc.harvard.edu
Internet: http://www.bidmc.harvard.edu/radiology
Accred Length: 1 Year *Program Size:* 3
Program ID: 427-24-31-042

Boston University Medical Center Program
Sponsor: Boston Medical Center

Program Director:
Heriberto Pagan-Marin, MD
Boston Med Ctr
One Boston Medical Center Pl
Boston, MA 02118
Tel: 617 638-6610 *Fax:* 617 638-6616
E-mail: hpagan@bu.edu
Accred Length: 1 Year *Program Size:* 2
Program ID: 427-24-21-050

Brigham and Women's Hospital/Harvard Medical School Program
Sponsor: Brigham and Women's Hospital

Program Director:
Michael F Meyerovitz, MD
Dept of Radiology
Brigham and Women's Hospital
75 Francis St
Boston, MA 02115
Tel: 617 732-7257 *Fax:* 617 277-8331
E-mail: mfmeyerovi@bics.bwh.harvard.edu
Accred Length: 1 Year *Program Size:* 3
Program ID: 427-24-21-005

Massachusetts General Hospital/Harvard Medical School Program
Sponsor: Massachusetts General Hospital

Program Director:
John A Kaufman, MD
Massachusetts General Hospital
32 Fruit St
Boston, MA 02114
Tel: 617 726-8315 *Fax:* 617 726-8476
E-mail: mrmiller@partners.org
Accred Length: 1 Year *Program Size:* 7
Program ID: 427-24-21-041

Worcester

University of Massachusetts Program
Sponsor: University of Massachusetts Medical School
UMass Memorial Health Care (University Campus)

Program Director:
David A Phillips, MD
Univ of Massachusetts Med Sch
55 Lake Ave N
Worcester, MA 01655
Tel: 508 856-1512 *Fax:* 508 856-4669
Accred Length: 1 Year *Program Size:* 1
Program ID: 427-24-31-052

Michigan

Ann Arbor

University of Michigan Program
Sponsor: University of Michigan Hospitals
Veterans Affairs Medical Center (Ann Arbor)

Program Director:
Kyung J Cho, MD
Univ of Michigan Hospitals
Dept of Radiology/B1-D530
Ann Arbor, MI 48109-0030
Tel: 734 936-4481 *Fax:* 734 936-7948
E-mail: kyungcho@umich.edu
Accred Length: 1 Year *Program Size:* 4
Program ID: 427-25-21-035

Detroit

Henry Ford Hospital Program
Sponsor: Henry Ford Hospital
Program Director:
P C Shetty, MD
Henry Ford Hospital
2799 W Grand Blvd
Detroit, MI 48202
Tel: 313 916-2814
E-mail: shetty@rad.hfhedu
Accred Length: 1 Year *Program Size:* 2
Program ID: 427-25-21-055

Wayne State University/Detroit Medical Center Program
Sponsor: Wayne State University/Detroit Medical Center
Harper Hospital
Program Director:
Monte Harvill, MD
Harper Hospital
Dept of Radiology
3990 John R St
Detroit, MI 48201
Tel: 313 745-8411 *Fax:* 313 745-8919
Accred Length: 1 Year *Program Size:* 1
Program ID: 427-25-31-083

Royal Oak

William Beaumont Hospital Program
Sponsor: William Beaumont Hospital
Program Director:
Matthias J Kirsch, MD
3601 W 13 Mile Rd
Royal Oak, MI 48073
Tel: 248 551-6047 *Fax:* 248 551-2418
E-mail: mkirsch@beaumont.edu
Internet: http://www.beaumont.edu/html/gme
Accred Length: 1 Year *Program Size:* 2
Program ID: 427-25-21-080

Minnesota

Minneapolis

University of Minnesota Program
Sponsor: University of Minnesota Medical School
Fairview-University Medical Center
Hennepin County Medical Center
Veterans Affairs Medical Center (Minneapolis)
Program Director:
David W Hunter, MD
Dept of Radiology
Fairview Univ Med Ctr
420 Delaware St SE/Box 292
Minneapolis, MN 55455-0392
Tel: 612 273-7195 *Fax:* 612 273-4446
E-mail: huntd@rad-gate.drad.umn.edu
Internet: http://www.tc.umn.edu
Accred Length: 1 Year *Program Size:* 4
Program ID: 427-26-21-008

Rochester

Mayo Graduate School of Medicine (Rochester) Program
Sponsor: Mayo Graduate School of Medicine-Mayo Foundation
Mayo Clinic (Rochester)
Rochester Methodist Hospital
St Mary's Hospital of Rochester
Program Director:
Jerome F Breen, MD
Mayo Graduate Sch of Med
Application Processing Center
200 First St SW
Rochester, MN 55905
Tel: 507 255-5659 *Fax:* 507 255-7872
Internet: http://www.mayo.edu/
Accred Length: 1 Year *Program Size:* 2
Program ID: 427-26-21-064

Mississippi

Jackson

University of Mississippi Medical Center Program
Sponsor: University of Mississippi School of Medicine
St Dominic-Jackson Memorial Hospital
University Hospital
Program Director:
James U Morano, MD
Univ of Mississippi Med Ctr
Dept of Radiology
2500 N State St
Jackson, MS 39216
Tel: 601 984-2833 *Fax:* 601 984-2542
E-mail: jum@bellsouth.net
Accred Length: 1 Year *Program Size:* 2
Program ID: 427-27-21-077

Missouri

St Louis

St Louis University School of Medicine Program
Sponsor: St Louis University School of Medicine
St Louis University School of Medicine
Program Director:
Thomas P Bocchini, MD
St Louis Univ Sch of Med
3635 Vista Ave
St Louis, MO 63110-0250
Tel: 314 268-5781 *Fax:* 314 268-5116
E-mail: diagrad@slu.edu
Internet: http://www.slu.edu
Accred Length: 1 Year *Program Size:* 1
Program ID: 427-28-21-071

Washington University/B-JH/SLCH Consortium Program
Sponsor: Washington University/B-JH/SLCH Consortium
Barnes-Jewish Hospital
Mallinckrodt Institute of Radiology
St Louis Children's Hospital
Washington University School of Medicine
Program Director:
Michael D Darcy, MD
Mallinckrodt Inst of Radiology
510 S Kingshighway Blvd
St Louis, MO 63110
Tel: 314 362-2900 *Fax:* 314 362-2276
E-mail: darcy@mirlink.wustl.edu
Accred Length: 1 Year *Program Size:* 6
Program ID: 427-28-21-001

Nebraska

Omaha

University of Nebraska Program
Sponsor: University of Nebraska Medical Center
Program Director:
Timothy C McCowan, MD
Univ of Nebraska Med Ctr
Dept of Radiology
600 S 42nd St
Omaha, NE 68198-1045
Tel: 402 559-6990 *Fax:* 402 559-1011
E-mail: tmccowan@unmc.edu
Accred Length: 1 Year *Program Size:* 1
Program ID: 427-30-21-014

New Hampshire

Lebanon

Dartmouth-Hitchcock Medical Center Program
Sponsor: Mary Hitchcock Memorial Hospital
Program Director:
Michael A Bettmann, MD
Dartmouth-Hitchcock Med Ctr
One Medical Center Dr
Lebanon, NH 03756
Tel: 603 650-4477 *Fax:* 603 650-5455
Accred Length: 1 Year *Program Size:* 2
Program ID: 427-32-21-067

New Jersey

Piscataway

UMDNJ-Robert Wood Johnson Medical School Program
Sponsor: UMDNJ-Robert Wood Johnson Medical School
Robert Wood Johnson University Hospital
St Peter's University Hospital
Program Director:
John L Nosher, MD
UMDNJ-Robert Wood Johnson Med Sch
One Robert Wood Johnson Pl/PO Box 19
New Brunswick, NJ 08903-0019
Tel: 732 235-7721 *Fax:* 732 235-6889
E-mail: lakatofs@umdnj.edu
Internet: http://www.rwj-rad.rwjuh.edu
Accred Length: 1 Year *Program Size:* 1
Program ID: 427-33-21-087

New Mexico

Albuquerque

University of New Mexico Program
Sponsor: University of New Mexico School of Medicine
University Hospital
Veterans Affairs Medical Center (Albuquerque)
Program Director:
Anna M Champlin, MD
Univ of New Mexico Sch of Med
Dept of Radiology
915 Camino de Salud NE
Albuquerque, NM 87131-5336
Tel: 505 272-0931 *Fax:* 505 272-5821
E-mail: raderas@salud.unm.edu
Accred Length: 1 Year *Program Size:* 1
Program ID: 427-34-21-091

New York

Albany

Albany Medical Center Program

Sponsor: Albany Medical Center
Veterans Affairs Medical Center (Albany)

Program Director:
Gary P Siskin, MD
Albany Med Ctr
Dept of Radiology/A-113
47 New Scotland Ave
Albany, NY 12208-3479
Tel: 518 262-3393 *Fax:* 518 262-6773
E-mail: gsiskin@global2000.net
Accred Length: 1 Year *Program Size:* 2
Program ID: 427-35-31-073

Bronx

Albert Einstein College of Medicine Program

Sponsor: Albert Einstein College of Medicine of Yeshiva University
Montefiore Medical Center-Henry and Lucy Moses Division

Program Director:
Jacob Cynamon, MD
Montefiore Med Ctr
Dept of Radiology
111 E 210th St
Bronx, NY 10467
Tel: 718 920-5506 *Fax:* 718 920-4854
E-mail: dchinea@worldnet.att.net
Accred Length: 1 Year *Program Size:* 2
Program ID: 427-35-32-027

New Hyde Park

Albert Einstein College of Medicine at Long Island Jewish Medical Center Program

Sponsor: Long Island Jewish Medical Center

Program Director:
David N Siegel, MD
George Pillari, MD
Long Island Jewish Med Ctr
Dept of Radiology
270-05 76th Ave
New Hyde Park, NY 11040
Tel: 718 470-7134 *Fax:* 718 343-7463
Internet: http://www.lij.edu
Accred Length: 1 Year *Program Size:* 1
Program ID: 427-35-31-024

New York

Mount Sinai School of Medicine Program

Sponsor: Mount Sinai School of Medicine

Program Director:
Harold A Mitty, MD
Mount Sinai Hospital
One Gustave L Levy Pl
New York, NY 10029-6574
Tel: 212 241-7417 *Fax:* 212 427-8137
E-mail: harold_mitty@smtplink.mssm.edu
Internet: http://www.mssm.edu/radiology/faculty.html
Accred Length: 1 Year *Program Size:* 2
Program ID: 427-35-21-048

New York and Presbyterian Hospital (Columbia Campus) Program

Sponsor: New York and Presbyterian Hospital
New York and Presbyterian Hospital (Columbia Campus)

Program Director:
Eric C Martin, MD
Columbia-Presbyterian Med Ctr
Vascular/Interventional Rad/PH3W
177 Fort Washington Ave
New York, NY 10032
Tel: 212 305-5123 *Fax:* 212 305-6184
Accred Length: 1 Year *Program Size:* 2
Program ID: 427-35-21-021

New York and Presbyterian Hospital (Cornell Campus) Program

Sponsor: New York and Presbyterian Hospital
Memorial Sloan-Kettering Cancer Center
New York and Presbyterian Hospital (Cornell Campus)

Program Director:
Neil M Khilnani, MD
New York Hospital-Cornell Med Ctr
525 E 68th St/Rm L-515
New York, NY 10021
Tel: 212 746-2602 *Fax:* 212 746-8463
Accred Length: 1 Year *Program Size:* 4
Program ID: 427-35-21-039

New York University Medical Center Program

Sponsor: New York University Medical Center
Bellevue Hospital Center
Veterans Affairs Medical Center (Manhattan)

Program Director:
Robert J Rosen, MD
560 First Ave
New York, NY 10016
Tel: 212 263-5898 *Fax:* 212 263-7914
Accred Length: 1 Year *Program Size:* 2
Program ID: 427-35-21-090

St Luke's-Roosevelt Hospital Center Program

Sponsor: St Luke's-Roosevelt Hospital Center
St Luke's-Roosevelt Hospital Center-Roosevelt Division
St Luke's-Roosevelt Hospital Center-St Luke's Division

Program Director:
Stanley G Cooper, MD
St Luke's-Roosevelt Hospital Ctr
1000 Tenth Ave
New York, NY 10019
Tel: 212 523-7806 *Fax:* 212 523-8145
E-mail: scooper@slrhc.org
Internet: http://www.wehealny.org
Accred Length: 1 Year *Program Size:* 2
Program ID: 427-35-21-072

Rochester

University of Rochester Program

Sponsor: Strong Memorial Hospital of the University of Rochester

Program Director:
David L Waldman, MD PhD
Univ of Rochester Med Ctr, Dept of Radiology
601 Elmwood Ave
Rochester, NY 14642-8648
Tel: 716 275-4002 *Fax:* 716 273-1033
E-mail: poles@rad.rochester.edu
Accred Length: 1 Year *Program Size:* 2
Program ID: 427-35-21-051

Stony Brook

SUNY at Stony Brook Program

Sponsor: University Hospital-SUNY at Stony Brook

Program Director:
John A Ferretti, MD
SUNY-Stony Brook
HSC Level 4/Rm 092
Stony Brook, NY 11794-8460
Tel: 516 444-2484 *Fax:* 516 444-7538
E-mail: jferretti@radiol.sunysb.edu
Internet: http://www.informatics.sunysb.edu/radiology/
Accred Length: 1 Year *Program Size:* 1
Program ID: 427-35-21-084

Syracuse

SUNY Health Science Center at Syracuse Program

Sponsor: University Hospital-SUNY Health Science Center at Syracuse
Veterans Affairs Medical Center (Syracuse)

Program Director:
Paramjit S Chopra, MD
750 E Adams St
Syracuse, NY 13210
Tel: 315 464-7417 *Fax:* 315 464-7458
Accred Length: 1 Year *Program Size:* 1
Program ID: 427-35-31-085

Valhalla

New York Medical College at Westchester Medical Center Program

Sponsor: New York Medical College
Westchester Medical Center

Program Director:
Grigory Rozenblit, MD
Dept of Radiology
New York Med Coll
Valhalla, NY 10595
Tel: 914 285-1119 *Fax:* 914 285-7561
Accred Length: 1 Year *Program Size:* 1
Program ID: 427-35-31-075

North Carolina

Chapel Hill

University of North Carolina Hospitals Program

Sponsor: University of North Carolina Hospitals

Program Director:
Paul F Jaques, MD
Vascular/Interventional Rad Sect
Radiology #CB 7510
Univ of North Carolina Sch of Med
Chapel Hill, NC 27599-7510
Tel: 919 966-4397 *Fax:* 919 966-5934
E-mail: pfjaques@med.unc.edu
Accred Length: 1 Year *Program Size:* 2
Program ID: 427-36-21-030

Durham

Duke University Program
Sponsor: Duke University Medical Center
Veterans Affairs Medical Center (Durham)
Program Director:
Paul V Suhocki, MD
Duke Univ Med Ctr
Dept of Radiology
Box 3808
Durham, NC 27710
Tel: 919 684-7359 *Fax:* 919 684-7141
Accred Length: 1 Year *Program Size:* 3
Program ID: 427-36-21-088

Winston-Salem

Wake Forest University School of Medicine Program
Sponsor: Wake Forest University Baptist Medical Center
Program Director:
William Douglas Routh, MD
Wake Forest Univ Sch of Med
Medical Center Blvd
Winston-Salem, NC 27157-1088
Tel: 336 716-4435 *Fax:* 336 716-2029
E-mail: wrouth@radmin.rad.wfubmc.edu
Internet: http://www.rad.wfubmc.edu
Accred Length: 1 Year *Program Size:* 2
Program ID: 427-36-21-015

Ohio

Cleveland

Case Western Reserve University Program
Sponsor: University Hospitals of Cleveland
Program Director:
Joseph P LiPuma, MD
Dept of Radiology
Univ Hospitals of Cleveland
11100 Euclid Ave
Cleveland, OH 44106-5000
Tel: 216 844-3113 *Fax:* 216 844-3905
E-mail: slater@uhrad.com
Accred Length: 1 Year *Program Size:* 1
Program ID: 427-38-21-012

Cleveland Clinic Foundation Program
Sponsor: Cleveland Clinic Foundation
Program Director:
Michael A Geisinger, MD
Cleveland Clinic Foundation
Dept of Radiology/Hb6
9500 Euclid Ave
Cleveland, OH 44195
Tel: 216 444-6654 *Fax:* 216 444-9307
E-mail: geisinm@ccisd3.ccf.org
Internet: http://www.ccf.org
Accred Length: 1 Year *Program Size:* 2
Program ID: 427-38-21-002

Oklahoma

Oklahoma City

University of Oklahoma Health Sciences Center Program
Sponsor: University of Oklahoma College of Medicine
Children's Hospital of Oklahoma
University Hospital
Veterans Affairs Medical Center (Oklahoma City)
Program Director:
Tim Tytle, MD
Dept of Rad Sciences
Univ of Oklahoma Health Sciences Ctr
PO Box 26901
Oklahoma City, OK 73190-3020
Tel: 405 271-5136 *Fax:* 405 271-3462
Accred Length: 1 Year *Program Size:* 2
Program ID: 427-39-21-036

Pennsylvania

Hershey

Penn State Geisinger Health System/Milton S Hershey Medical Center Program
Sponsor: Penn State Geisinger Health System
Milton S Hershey Medical Center
Program Director:
John F Cardella, MD
Penn State Geisinger Health System
Dept of Radiology/H066 Rm HG315D
500 University Dr/PO Box 850
Hershey, PA 17033
Tel: 717 531-5415 *Fax:* 717 531-5596
E-mail: jfc8@psu.edu
Accred Length: 1 Year *Program Size:* 1
Program ID: 427-41-21-004

Philadelphia

Temple University Program
Sponsor: Temple University Hospital
Program Director:
David S Ball, DO
3401 N Broad St
Philadelphia, PA 19140
Tel: 215 707-4218 *Fax:* 215 707-2428
Accred Length: 1 Year *Program Size:* 2
Program ID: 427-41-21-076

Thomas Jefferson University Program
Sponsor: Thomas Jefferson University Hospital
Program Director:
Joseph Bonn Sr, MD
Thomas Jefferson Univ Hospital
111 S 11th St
Ste 4200 Gibbon
Philadelphia, PA 19107
Tel: 215 955-6609 *Fax:* 215 923-6754
E-mail: joseph.bonn@mail.tju.edu
Accred Length: 1 Year *Program Size:* 4
Program ID: 427-41-21-040

University of Pennsylvania Program
Sponsor: Hospital of the University of Pennsylvania
Veterans Affairs Medical Center (Philadelphia)
Program Director:
David B Freiman, MD
Univ of Pennsylvania Med Ctr
Dept of Radiology
3400 Spruce St
Philadelphia, PA 19104
Tel: 215 662-4034 *Fax:* 215 662-7110
E-mail: intrad@oasis.rad.upenn.edu
Internet: http://www.rad.upenn.edu
Accred Length: 1 Year *Program Size:* 6
Program ID: 427-41-21-016

Pittsburgh

University Health Center of Pittsburgh Program
Sponsor: University Health Center of Pittsburgh
Presbyterian University Hospital/UPMC
Program Director:
Albert B Zajko, MD
200 Lothrop St
Pittsburgh, PA 15213
Tel: 412 647-3545 *Fax:* 412 647-0878
E-mail: zajko@radserv.arad.upmc.edu
Accred Length: 1 Year *Program Size:* 2
Program ID: 427-41-21-061

Western Pennsylvania Hospital Program
Sponsor: Western Pennsylvania Hospital
Program Director:
Gordon K McLean, MD
Western Pennsylvania Hospital
Dept of Radiology
4800 Friendship Ave
Pittsburgh, PA 15224
Tel: 412 578-1787 *Fax:* 412 578-4064
Internet: http://www.westpennhospital.com
Accred Length: 1 Year *Program Size:* 2
Program ID: 427-41-31-044

Rhode Island

Providence

Brown University Program
Sponsor: Rhode Island Hospital
Program Director:
Timothy P Murphy, MD
Rhode Island Hospital
593 Eddy St
Providence, RI 02903
Tel: 401 444-5194 *Fax:* 401 444-8756
E-mail: tpm@brown.edu
Internet: http://www.brown.edu/departments/diagnostic-imaging/fellows/offered.html
Accred Length: 1 Year *Program Size:* 2
Program ID: 427-43-21-066

South Carolina

Charleston

Medical University of South Carolina Program

Sponsor: Medical University of South Carolina College of Medicine
MUSC Medical Center
Program Director:
Renan Uflacker, MD
Med Univ of South Carolina
171 Ashley Ave
Charleston, SC 29425
Tel: 803 792-5387 *Fax:* 803 792-9503
E-mail: uflackrp@musc.edu
Internet: http://www.musc.edu/intervrad/
Accred Length: 1 Year *Program Size:* 2
Program ID: 427-45-21-056

Tennessee

Memphis

University of Tennessee Program

Sponsor: University of Tennessee College of Medicine
Regional Medical Center at Memphis
University of Tennessee Medical Center (UT Bowld Hospital)
Program Director:
Robert E Gold, MD
Univ of Tennessee
Dept of Radiology
800 Madison Ave/Rm F150C Chandler
Memphis, TN 38163
Tel: 901 448-8248 *Fax:* 901 448-5352
E-mail: rgold@utmem.edu
Accred Length: 1 Year *Program Size:* 3
Program ID: 427-47-21-019

Nashville

Vanderbilt University Program

Sponsor: Vanderbilt University Medical Center
Program Director:
Murray J Mazer, MD
Vanderbilt Univ Hospital
21st Ave S and Garland Ave
R-1318 Med Ctr North
Nashville, TN 37232-2675
Tel: 615 322-3780
E-mail: radprogram@mcmail.vanderbilt.edu
Internet: http://www.mc.vanderbilt.edu/radiology
Accred Length: 1 Year *Program Size:* 2
Program ID: 427-47-21-060

Texas

Dallas

Baylor University Medical Center Program

Sponsor: Baylor University Medical Center
Program Director:
Chet R Rees, MD
Dept of Vascular/Interventional Rad
Baylor Hospital
3500 Gaston Ave
Dallas, TX 75246
Tel: 214 820-3206 *Fax:* 214 820-4626
E-mail: kd.myrick@baylordallas.edu
Accred Length: 1 Year *Program Size:* 2
Program ID: 427-48-21-043

University of Texas Southwestern Medical School Program

Sponsor: University of Texas Southwestern Medical School
Dallas County Hospital District-Parkland Memorial Hospital
Zale-Lipshy University Hospital
Program Director:
George L Miller III, MD
Univ of Texas Southwestern Med Sch
Dept of Radiology
5323 Harry Hines Blvd
Dallas, TX 75235-8896
Tel: 214 648-8022 *Fax:* 214 648-2678
E-mail: gmille@mednet.swmed.edu
Internet: http://www.rad.swmed.edu/residen.html
Accred Length: 1 Year *Program Size:* 1
Program ID: 427-48-21-003

Houston

University of Texas at Houston Program

Sponsor: University of Texas Medical School at Houston
Memorial Hermann Healthcare System
St Luke's Episcopal Hospital
University of Texas M D Anderson Cancer Center
Program Director:
Marshall E Hicks, MD
1515 Holcombe Blvd
Box 57
Houston, TX 77030
Tel: 713 792-8295 *Fax:* 713 745-1151
E-mail: mhicks@di.mdall.tmc.edu
Accred Length: 1 Year *Program Size:* 3
Program ID: 427-48-21-078

Lackland AFB

San Antonio Uniformed Services Health Education Consortium (WHMC) Program

Sponsor: San Antonio Uniformed Services Health Education Consortium
Wilford Hall Medical Center (AETC)
Program Director:
Daniel C Diffin, MD
Dept of Air Force
2200 Bergquist Dr/Ste 1
Lackland AFB, TX 78236-5300
Tel: 210 292-5265 *Fax:* 210 292-3946
E-mail: dandiffin@hotmail.com
Accred Length: 1 Year *Program Size:* 1
Program ID: 427-48-31-006
US Armed Services Program

San Antonio

University of Texas Health Science Center at San Antonio Program

Sponsor: University of Texas Medical School at San Antonio
Audie L Murphy Memorial Veterans Hospital (San Antonio)
University Hospital-South Texas Medical Center
Program Director:
Julio C Palmaz, MD
Univ of Texas Health Science Ctr
Vascular/Interventional Rad
7703 Floyd Curl Dr
San Antonio, TX 78284-7800
Tel: 210 567-5564 *Fax:* 210 567-5541
Accred Length: 1 Year *Program Size:* 3
Program ID: 427-48-21-031

Utah

Salt Lake City

University of Utah Program

Sponsor: University of Utah Medical Center
Veterans Affairs Medical Center (Salt Lake City)
Program Director:
Franklin J Miller Jr, MD
50 N Medical Dr
Salt Lake City, UT 84132
Tel: 801 581-7553
E-mail: frank.miller@hsc.utah.edu
Internet: http://wwrad.med.utah.edu
Accred Length: 1 Year *Program Size:* 1
Program ID: 427-49-21-045

Vermont

Burlington

University of Vermont Program

Sponsor: Fletcher Allen Health Care
Program Director:
Kenneth E Najarian, MD
Fletcher Allen Health Care
111 Colchester Ave
Burlington, VT 05401
Tel: 802 656-3592 *Fax:* 802 656-4822
Accred Length: 1 Year *Program Size:* 2
Program ID: 427-50-21-062

Virginia

Alexandria

George Washington University Program

Sponsor: George Washington University School of Medicine
Alexandria Hospital
Program Director:
Keith M Sterling, MD
INOVA Alexandria Hospital
Dept of Cardiovascular/Interventional Rad
4320 Seminary Rd
Alexandria, VA 22304-1500
Tel: 703 504-7950 *Fax:* 703 504-3287
Accred Length: 1 Year *Program Size:* 2
Program ID: 427-51-21-020

Charlottesville

University of Virginia Program

Sponsor: University of Virginia Medical Center
Program Director:
Alan H Matsumoto, MD
John F Angle, MD
Univ of Virginia Health System
Dept of Radiology/Box 170
Charlottesville, VA 22908
Tel: 804 924-9279 *Fax:* 804 243-2786
E-mail: tla3e@avery.med.virginia.edu
Accred Length: 1 Year *Program Size:* 4
Program ID: 427-51-21-057

Vascular Surgery (General Surgery)

Arizona

Tucson

University of Arizona Program
Sponsor: University of Arizona College of Medicine
University Medical Center
Program Director:
Joseph L Mills, MD
Univ of Arizona Health Sciences Ctr
Sect of Vascular Surgery
1501 N Campbell Ave/PO Box 245072
Tucson, AZ 85724-5072
Tel: 520 626-6670 *Fax:* 520 626-4008
E-mail: jmills@u.arizona.edu
Accred Length: 1 Year *Program Size:* 2
Program ID: 450-03-21-032

Arkansas

Little Rock

University of Arkansas for Medical Sciences Program
Sponsor: University of Arkansas College of Medicine
John L McClellan Memorial Veterans Hospital
University Hospital of Arkansas
Program Director:
John F Eidt, MD
Univ of Arkansas for Med Sciences
4301 W Markham St/Slot 520-2
Little Rock, AR 72205
Tel: 501 686-6176 *Fax:* 501 686-5328
E-mail: eidtjohnf@exchange.uams.edu
Accred Length: 1 Year *Program Size:* 2
Program ID: 450-04-21-055

California

Loma Linda

Loma Linda University Program
Sponsor: Loma Linda University Medical Center
Program Director:
Jeffrey L Ballard, MD
Loma Linda Univ Med Ctr
Div of Vascular Surgery
11234 Anderson St/Rm 21123 CP
Loma Linda, CA 92354
Tel: 909 558-8665 *Fax:* 909 558-0337
E-mail: jballard@ccmail.llu.edu
Internet: http://www.llu.edu
Accred Length: 1 Year *Program Size:* 1
Program ID: 450-05-21-010

Los Angeles

UCLA Medical Center Program
Sponsor: UCLA School of Medicine
UCLA Medical Center
Program Director:
Julie A Freischlag, MD
UCLA Ctr for Health Sciences
200 Medical Plaza/Ste 510-5
PO Box 956908
Los Angeles, CA 90095-6908
Tel: 310 267-0182 *Fax:* 310 267-0189
E-mail: jfreisch@surgery.medsch.ucla.edu
Internet: http://www.surgery.medsch.ucla.edu
Accred Length: 1 Year *Program Size:* 1
Program ID: 450-05-21-011

San Francisco

University of California (San Francisco) Program
Sponsor: University of California (San Francisco) School of Medicine
University of California (San Francisco) Medical Center
Program Director:
Louis M Messina, MD
Univ of California San Francisco
505 Parnassus Ave
Box 0222/Rm M-488
San Francisco, CA 94143-0222
Tel: 415 476-2381 *Fax:* 415 476-4950
E-mail: messina@itsa.ucsf.edu
Accred Length: 1 Year *Program Size:* 1
Program ID: 450-05-21-033

Stanford

Stanford University Program
Sponsor: Stanford University Hospital
Program Director:
Christopher K Zarins, MD
Stanford Univ Med Ctr
Div of Vascular Surgery
300 Pasteur Dr/Ste H3600
Stanford, CA 94305-5642
Tel: 650 723-2185 *Fax:* 650 498-6044
E-mail: hf.sbs@forsythe.stanford.edu
Accred Length: 1 Year *Program Size:* 2
Program ID: 450-05-21-021

Torrance

Los Angeles County-Harbor-UCLA Medical Center Program
Sponsor: Los Angeles County-Harbor-UCLA Medical Center
St Mary Medical Center
Program Director:
Rodney A White, MD
Harbor-UCLA Med Ctr
1000 W Carson St/Box 11
Torrance, CA 90509
Tel: 310 222-2704 *Fax:* 310 787-1889
Accred Length: 1 Year *Program Size:* 2
Program ID: 450-05-21-067

Connecticut

Farmington

University of Connecticut Program

Sponsor: University of Connecticut School of Medicine
Hartford Hospital
Univ of Connecticut Health Center/John Dempsey Hospital

Program Director:
A David Drezner, MD
Hartford Hospital, Dept of Surgery
80 Seymour St/B501
Hartford, CT 06102
Tel: 860 545-2840 *Fax:* 860 545-1568
E-mail: strevis@harthosp.org
Internet: http://www.resprog.uchc.edu/md/
Accred Length: 1 Year *Program Size:* 2
Program ID: 450-08-21-070

New Haven

Yale-New Haven Medical Center Program

Sponsor: Yale-New Haven Hospital

Program Director:
Bauer E Sumpio, MD PhD
Yale Univ Sch of Med, Dept of Surgery
333 Cedar St
FMB 137
New Haven, CT 06510
Tel: 203 785-2561 *Fax:* 203 785-7556
Internet: http://info.med.yale.edu/surgery/vascular
Accred Length: 1 Year *Program Size:* 1
Program ID: 450-08-21-084

District of Columbia

Washington

Walter Reed Army Medical Center Program

Sponsor: Walter Reed Army Medical Center

Program Director:
Lt Col Sean D O'Donnell, MD
Walter Reed Army Med Ctr
Dept of Surg/Peripheral Vascular Surg
6825 16th St NW
Washington, DC 20307-5001
Tel: 202 782-6537 *Fax:* 202 782-3198
E-mail: odonnell@vs.wramc.amedd.army.mil
Internet: http://www.wramc.amedd.army.mil/departments/surgery/vascular
Accred Length: 1 Year *Program Size:* 2
Program ID: 450-10-11-022
US Armed Services Program

Florida

Gainesville

University of Florida Program

Sponsor: University of Florida College of Medicine
Shands Hospital at the University of Florida
Veterans Affairs Medical Center (Gainesville)

Program Director:
James M Seeger, MD
Univ of Florida
Dept of Surgery
Box 100286
Gainesville, FL 32610-0286
Tel: 352 395-0605 *Fax:* 352 338-9818
E-mail: seeger@surgery.ufl.edu
Accred Length: 1 Year *Program Size:* 2
Program ID: 450-11-21-044

Tampa

University of South Florida Program

Sponsor: University of South Florida College of Medicine
Tampa General Healthcare

Program Director:
Dennis Bandyk, MD
Univ of South Florida Coll of Med
Harbourside Medical Tower #730
4 Columbia Dr
Tampa, FL 33606
Tel: 813 259-0921 *Fax:* 813 259-0606
E-mail: dbandyk@com1.med.usf.edu
Accred Length: 1 Year *Program Size:* 2
Program ID: 450-11-21-031

Georgia

Atlanta

Emory University Program

Sponsor: Emory University School of Medicine
Emory University Hospital

Program Director:
Alan B Lumsden, MB ChB MD
Emory Univ Hospital
5105 WMB
1639 Pierce Dr
Atlanta, GA 30322
Tel: 404 727-7246 *Fax:* 404 727-3660
E-mail: alumsden@surgery.eushc.org
Accred Length: 1 Year *Program Size:* 2
Program ID: 450-12-21-012

Georgia Baptist Medical Center Program

Sponsor: Georgia Baptist Medical Center
West Paces Ferry Medical Center

Program Director:
David Rosenthal, MD
Georgia Baptist Med Ctr
315 Boulevard NE/Ste 412
Atlanta, GA 30312
Tel: 404 524-0095 *Fax:* 404 658-9558
E-mail: docro@mindspring.com
Accred Length: 1 Year *Program Size:* 2
Program ID: 450-12-21-079

Illinois

Chicago

McGaw Medical Center of Northwestern University Program

Sponsor: Northwestern University Medical School
Northwestern Memorial Hospital
Veterans Affairs Lakeside Medical Center (Chicago)

Program Director:
William H Pearce, MD
Northwestern Univ Med Sch
251 E Chicago Ave/Ste 628
Chicago, IL 60611
Tel: 312 503-2437 *Fax:* 312 908-9072
Internet: http://www.nums.nwu.edu/gme/index.htm
Accred Length: 1 Year *Program Size:* 2
Program ID: 450-16-21-001

Rush-Presbyterian-St Luke's Medical Center Program

Sponsor: Rush-Presbyterian-St Luke's Medical Center

Program Director:
Walter J McCarthy, MD
Rush-Presbyterian-St Luke's Med Ctr
1653 W Congress Pkwy
Rm 714 Jelke
Chicago, IL 60612-3833
Tel: 312 942-6373 *Fax:* 312 666-0242
E-mail: cadams@rush.edu
Internet: http://www.rush.edu
Accred Length: 1 Year *Program Size:* 1
Program ID: 450-16-21-057

University of Chicago Program

Sponsor: University of Chicago Hospitals

Program Director:
Bruce L Gewertz, MD
Univ of Chicago Med Ctr
5841 S Maryland Ave/MC5028
Chicago, IL 60637-1470
Tel: 773 834-0999 *Fax:* 773 702-0863
E-mail: gewertz@surgery.bsd.uchicago.edu
Internet:
http://www.surgery.bsd.uchicago.edu/sections/vascular
Accred Length: 1 Year *Program Size:* 1
Program ID: 450-16-11-023

Maywood

Loyola University Program

Sponsor: Loyola University Medical Center
Edward J Hines Jr Veterans Affairs Hospital

Program Director:
Fred Littooy, MD
Foster G McGaw Hospital
2160 S First Ave
Maywood, IL 60153
Tel: 708 327-2686 *Fax:* 708 327-2810
Accred Length: 1 Year *Program Size:* 1
Program ID: 450-16-21-002

Springfield

Southern Illinois University Program

Sponsor: Southern Illinois University School of Medicine
Memorial Medical Center
St John's Hospital

Program Director:
Kim J Hodgson, MD
Southern Illinois Univ Sch of Med
Memorial Med Ctr
800 N Rutledge St/Ste D-346
Springfield, IL 62781
Tel: 217 782-8856 *Fax:* 217 524-1793
E-mail: cbuettner@siumed.edu
Accred Length: 1 Year *Program Size:* 2
Program ID: 450-16-21-034

Iowa

Iowa City

University of Iowa Hospitals and Clinics Program

Sponsor: University of Iowa Hospitals and Clinics

Program Director:
John D Corson, MB ChB
Univ of Iowa Hospitals and Clinics
Dept of Surgery/1537 JCP
200 Hawkins Dr
Iowa City, IA 52242-1086
Tel: 319 356-1639 *Fax:* 319 356-8378
E-mail: john-corson@uiowa.edu
Accred Length: 1 Year *Program Size:* 2
Program ID: 450-18-21-048

Kansas

Kansas City

University of Kansas Medical Center Program

Sponsor: University of Kansas School of Medicine
University of Kansas Medical Center

Program Director:
James H Thomas, MD
Univ of Kansas Med Ctr
3901 Rainbow Blvd
4002 Murphy Bldg
Kansas City, KS 66160-7308
Tel: 913 588-6115 *Fax:* 913 588-7540
E-mail: ldoolitt@kumc.edu
Internet: http://www.kumc.edu/vsurg/
Accred Length: 1 Year *Program Size:* 1
Program ID: 450-19-21-060

Kentucky

Lexington

University of Kentucky Medical Center Program

Sponsor: University of Kentucky Hospital
Veterans Affairs Medical Center (Lexington)

Program Director:
Eric D Endean, MD
Univ of Kentucky Med Ctr
Div of General Surgery/Rm C226
Lexington, KY 40536-0084
Tel: 606 323-6346 *Fax:* 606 323-6840
E-mail: edende0@pop.uky.edu
Accred Length: 1 Year *Program Size:* 2
Program ID: 450-20-21-062

Louisiana

New Orleans

Alton Ochsner Medical Foundation Program

Sponsor: Alton Ochsner Medical Foundation

Program Director:
Samuel R Money, MD
Alton Ochsner Med Foundation
Dept of Grad Med Educ
1516 Jefferson Hwy
New Orleans, LA 70121
Tel: 504 842-3260 *Fax:* 504 842-3193
E-mail: dlambert@ochsner.org
Internet: http://www.ochsner.org
Accred Length: 1 Year *Program Size:* 2
Program ID: 450-21-22-024

Louisiana State University Program

Sponsor: Louisiana State University School of Medicine
Medical Center of Louisiana at New Orleans
Veterans Affairs Medical Center-LSU Service (New Orleans)

Program Director:
Robert C Batson, MD
Louisiana State Univ Med Ctr
Div of Vascular Surgery
1542 Tulane Ave
New Orleans, LA 70112-2822
Tel: 504 568-4750 *Fax:* 504 568-4633
E-mail: lcapot@novms.lsumc.edu
Accred Length: 1 Year *Program Size:* 1
Program ID: 450-21-21-058

Maryland

Baltimore

Johns Hopkins University Program

Sponsor: Johns Hopkins University School of Medicine
Johns Hopkins Hospital

Program Director:
Bruce A Perler, MD
600 N Wolfe St/Blalock 685
Johns Hopkins Hospital
Baltimore, MD 21287-4685
Tel: 410 955-2618 *Fax:* 410 614-3537
E-mail: bperler@jhmi.edu
Accred Length: 1 Year *Program Size:* 1
Program ID: 450-23-31-086

University of Maryland Program

Sponsor: University of Maryland Medical System
Mercy Medical Center
Veterans Affairs Medical Center (Baltimore)

Program Director:
William R Flinn, MD
Univ of Maryland Med System
Div of Vascular Surgery
22 S Greene St/Ste N4W66
Baltimore, MD 21201
Tel: 410 328-5840 *Fax:* 410 328-0717
E-mail: wrflinn@surgery1.umd.edu
Accred Length: 1 Year *Program Size:* 2
Program ID: 450-23-21-080

Massachusetts

Boston

Beth Israel Deaconess Medical Center (West Campus) Program

Sponsor: Beth Israel Deaconess Medical Center
Mount Auburn Hospital

Program Director:
Frank W LoGerfo, MD
Beth Israel Deaconess Med Ctr
110 Francis St
Boston, MA 02215
Tel: 617 632-9955 *Fax:* 617 632-7356
E-mail: flogerfo@bidmc.harvard.edu
Accred Length: 1 Year *Program Size:* 2
Program ID: 450-24-21-040

Boston University Medical Center Program

Sponsor: Boston Medical Center

Program Director:
James O Menzoian, MD
Boston Med Ctr
One Boston Medical Center Pl
E Newton St/Campus D506
Boston, MA 02118
Tel: 617 638-8488 *Fax:* 617 638-8469
E-mail: marianne.kitchenka@bmc.org
Accred Length: 1 Year *Program Size:* 2
Program ID: 450-24-21-026

Brigham and Women's Hospital Program

Sponsor: Brigham and Women's Hospital

Program Director:
Anthony D Whittemore, MD
Brigham and Women's Hospital
75 Francis St
Boston, MA 02115
Tel: 617 732-6861 *Fax:* 617 264-6850
E-mail: surgery@bics.bwh.harvard.edu
Internet: http://www.bwh.partners.org/surged
Accred Length: 1 Year *Program Size:* 1
Program ID: 450-24-21-003

Massachusetts General Hospital Program

Sponsor: Massachusetts General Hospital

Program Director:
William M Abbott, MD
Massachusetts General Hospital
15 Parkman St/WAC 458
Boston, MA 02114
Tel: 617 726-8250 *Fax:* 617 726-8700
E-mail: abbott.william@mgh.harvard.edu
Internet: http://www.partners.org
Accred Length: 1 Year *Program Size:* 3
Program ID: 450-24-21-004

New England Medical Center Hospitals Program

Sponsor: New England Medical Center Hospitals

Program Director:
William C Mackey, MD
New England Med Ctr
750 Washington St/Box 437
Boston, MA 02111
Tel: 617 636-5891 *Fax:* 617 636-5498
E-mail: eileen.donovan@es.nemc.org
Accred Length: 1 Year *Program Size:* 2
Program ID: 450-24-21-005

Worcester

University of Massachusetts Program
Sponsor: University of Massachusetts Medical School
UMass Memorial Health Care (University Campus)
Program Director:
Bruce S Cutler, MD
Univ of Massachusetts Med Sch
55 Lake Ave N
Worcester, MA 01655
Tel: 508 856-2219 *Fax:* 508 856-8329
E-mail: bruce.cutler@banyan.ummed.edu
Accred Length: 1 Year *Program Size:* 2
Program ID: 450-24-21-013

Michigan

Ann Arbor

University of Michigan Program
Sponsor: University of Michigan Hospitals
Veterans Affairs Medical Center (Ann Arbor)
Program Director:
James C Stanley, MD
Univ of Michigan Med Ctr
1500 E Medical Center Dr
2210TC/Box 0329
Ann Arbor, MI 48109-0329
Tel: 734 936-5786 *Fax:* 734 647-9867
E-mail: jstanley@umich.edu
Accred Length: 1 Year *Program Size:* 2
Program ID: 450-25-21-035

Detroit

Henry Ford Hospital Program
Sponsor: Henry Ford Hospital
Program Director:
Daniel J Reddy, MD
Dept of Vascular Surg
Henry Ford Hospital
2799 W Grand Blvd
Detroit, MI 48202-2689
Tel: 313 916-3156 *Fax:* 313 916-3023
Internet: http://www.henryfordhealth.org
Accred Length: 1 Year *Program Size:* 2
Program ID: 450-25-12-014

Wayne State University/Detroit Medical Center Program
Sponsor: Wayne State University/Detroit Medical Center
Harper Hospital
Program Director:
Ramon Berguer, MD PhD
Wayne State Univ, Div of Vascular Surgery
Harper Hospital
3990 John R
Detroit, MI 48201
Tel: 313 745-8637 *Fax:* 313 993-0244
E-mail: rberguer@med.wayne.edu
Accred Length: 1 Year *Program Size:* 1
Program ID: 450-25-21-066

Minnesota

Rochester

Mayo Graduate School of Medicine (Rochester) Program
Sponsor: Mayo Graduate School of Medicine-Mayo Foundation
Mayo Clinic (Rochester)
Rochester Methodist Hospital
St Mary's Hospital of Rochester
Program Director:
Thomas C Bower, MD
Application Processing Ctr
Mayo Graduate Sch of Med
200 First St SW
Rochester, MN 55905
Tel: 507 284-8462
E-mail: mgsm.roch.mn.surgery@mayo.edu
Internet: http://www.mayo.edu/
Accred Length: 1 Year *Program Size:* 2
Program ID: 450-26-21-042

Missouri

Columbia

University of Missouri-Columbia Program
Sponsor: University of Missouri-Columbia School of Medicine
University Hospitals and Clinics
Program Director:
Donald Silver, MD
Dept of Surgery N150
Univ of Missouri Health Sci Ctr
1 Hospital Dr
Columbia, MO 65212
Tel: 573 884-1348 *Fax:* 573 884-4585
Internet: http://www.surgery.missouri.edu/vs/home.htm
Accred Length: 1 Year *Program Size:* 2
Program ID: 450-28-21-049

St Louis

St Louis University School of Medicine Program
Sponsor: St Louis University School of Medicine
St John's Mercy Medical Center
St Louis University School of Medicine
Program Director:
Gary J Peterson, MD
St Louis Univ Sch of Med
3635 Vista Ave
PO Box 15250
St Louis, MO 63110-0250
Tel: 314 577-8317 *Fax:* 314 268-5466
E-mail: surgweb@slu.edu
Internet:
http://www.slu.edu/colleges/med/departments/surgery
Accred Length: 1 Year *Program Size:* 1
Program ID: 450-28-21-027

Washington University/B-JH/SLCH Consortium Program
Sponsor: Washington University/B-JH/SLCH Consortium
Barnes-Jewish Hospital
Program Director:
Gregorio A Sicard, MD
Barnes-Jewish Hospital
One Barnes Hospital Plaza
Ste 5103
St Louis, MO 63110
Tel: 314 362-7841 *Fax:* 314 454-3923
E-mail: swapd@msnotes.wustl.edu
Internet: http://www.surgery.wustl.edu
Accred Length: 1 Year *Program Size:* 2
Program ID: 450-28-21-050

New Hampshire

Lebanon

Dartmouth-Hitchcock Medical Center Program
Sponsor: Mary Hitchcock Memorial Hospital
Program Director:
Jack L Cronenwett, MD
Dartmouth-Hitchcock Med Ctr
One Medical Center Dr
Lebanon, NH 03756-0001
Tel: 603 650-8670 *Fax:* 603 650-4973
E-mail: j.cronenwett@hitchcock.org
Accred Length: 1 Year *Program Size:* 2
Program ID: 450-32-21-059

New Jersey

Newark

Newark Beth Israel Medical Center Program
Sponsor: Newark Beth Israel Medical Center
Program Director:
Bruce J Brener, MD
Newark Beth Israel Med Ctr
Dept of Surgery L3
201 Lyons Ave
Newark, NJ 07112
Tel: 973 926-7330 *Fax:* 973 923-8757
Accred Length: 1 Year *Program Size:* 1
Program ID: 450-33-21-087

UMDNJ-New Jersey Medical School Program
Sponsor: UMDNJ-New Jersey Medical School
St Michael's Medical Center (Cathedral Hlth Srvcs Inc)
UMDNJ-University Hospital
Veterans Affairs Medical Center (East Orange)
Program Director:
Robert W Hobson II, MD
UMDNJ-New Jersey Med Sch
185 S Orange Ave/MSB G-532
Newark, NJ 07103-2714
Tel: 973 972-6633 *Fax:* 973 972-5924
E-mail: hobsonrw@umdnj.edu
Internet: http://www.umdnj.edu/njmsweb/vascdoc
Accred Length: 1 Year *Program Size:* 2
Program ID: 450-33-21-036

Piscataway

UMDNJ-Robert Wood Johnson Medical School Program

Sponsor: UMDNJ-Robert Wood Johnson Medical School
Robert Wood Johnson University Hospital

Program Director:
Alan M Graham, MD
UMDNJ-Robert Wood Johnson Med Sch
One Robert Wood Johnson Pl/CN-19
New Brunswick, NJ 08903-0019
Tel: 732 235-7816 *Fax:* 732 235-8538
E-mail: grahamal@umdnj.edu
Internet: http://www.umdnj.edu
Accred Length: 1 Year *Program Size:* 2
Program ID: 450-33-21-037

New York

Albany

Albany Medical Center Program

Sponsor: Albany Medical Center

Program Director:
Dhiraj M Shah, MD
Albany Med Ctr Hospital
Dept of Surgery/Vascular/A-61
43 New Scotland Ave
Albany, NY 12208-3578
Tel: 518 262-5905 *Fax:* 518 262-5692
Accred Length: 1 Year *Program Size:* 2
Program ID: 450-35-21-061

Bronx

Albert Einstein College of Medicine Program

Sponsor: Albert Einstein College of Medicine of Yeshiva University
Montefiore Medical Center-Henry and Lucy Moses Division

Program Director:
Frank J Veith, MD
Montefiore Med Ctr
111 E 210th St
Bronx, NY 10467
Tel: 718 920-4108 *Fax:* 718 231-9811
Accred Length: 1 Year *Program Size:* 2
Program ID: 450-35-21-015

Brooklyn

Maimonides Medical Center Program

Sponsor: Maimonides Medical Center

Program Director:
Enrico Ascher, MD
Maimonides Med Ctr
Div of Vascular Surgery
4802 Tenth Ave
Brooklyn, NY 11219
Tel: 718 283-7957 *Fax:* 718 635-7050
Accred Length: 1 Year *Program Size:* 2
Program ID: 450-35-21-076

SUNY Health Science Center at Brooklyn Program

Sponsor: SUNY Health Science Center at Brooklyn
University Hospital-SUNY Health Science Center at Brooklyn
Veterans Affairs Medical Center (Brooklyn)

Program Director:
Thomas F Panetta, MD
SUNY Health Science Ctr-Brooklyn
Box 40
450 Clarkson Ave
Brooklyn, NY 11203-2098
Tel: 718 270-1035 *Fax:* 718 270-2762
Accred Length: 1 Year *Program Size:* 2
Program ID: 450-35-21-081

Buffalo

SUNY at Buffalo Graduate Medical-Dental Education Consortium Program

Sponsor: SUNY at Buffalo Grad Medical-Dental Education Consortium
CGF Health System (Buffalo General Hospital)
CGF Health System (Millard Fillmore Hospitals)
Veterans Affairs Medical Center (Buffalo)

Program Director:
E L Hoover, MD
Dept of Surgery
Millard Fillmore Hospital
3 Gates Cir
Buffalo, NY 14209
Tel: 716 887-5110 *Fax:* 716 887-4220
E-mail: mshriver@mfhs.edu
Accred Length: 1 Year *Program Size:* 2
Program ID: 450-35-21-069

Manhasset

North Shore University Hospital/NYU School of Medicine Program

Sponsor: North Shore University Hospital

Program Director:
Steven G Friedman, MD
North Shore Univ Hospital
300 Community Dr
Manhasset, NY 11030
Tel: 516 562-2185 *Fax:* 516 562-3787
Internet: http://www.nshs.edu
Accred Length: 1 Year *Program Size:* 2
Program ID: 450-35-31-082

New Hyde Park

Albert Einstein College of Medicine at Long Island Jewish/Beth Israel Medical Center Program

Sponsor: Long Island Jewish Medical Center

Program Director:
Jon R Cohen, MD
Long Island Jewish Med Ctr
270-05 76th Ave
New Hyde Park, NY 11040
Tel: 718 470-8787 *Fax:* 718 343-3429
Internet: http://www.lij.edu
Accred Length: 1 Year *Program Size:* 1
Program ID: 450-35-21-064

New York

Mount Sinai School of Medicine Program

Sponsor: Mount Sinai School of Medicine
Mount Sinai Medical Center

Program Director:
Larry H Hollier, MD
Mount Sinai Sch of Med
One Gustave L Levy Pl
Box 1259
New York, NY 10029
Tel: 212 241-5871 *Fax:* 212 987-9310
Accred Length: 1 Year *Program Size:* 2
Program ID: 450-35-21-038

New York University Medical Center Program

Sponsor: New York University Medical Center
Bellevue Hospital Center

Program Director:
Patrick J Lamparello, MD
New York Univ Med Ctr
530 First Ave/Ste 6F
New York, NY 10016
Tel: 212 263-7312 *Fax:* 212 263-7722
Accred Length: 1 Year *Program Size:* 2
Program ID: 450-35-21-045

Rochester

University of Rochester Program

Sponsor: Strong Memorial Hospital of the University of Rochester
Rochester General Hospital

Program Director:
Richard M Green, MD
Univ of Rochester Med Ctr
Sect of Vascular Surgery
601 Elmwood Ave
Rochester, NY 14642-8410
Tel: 716 275-6772 *Fax:* 716 273-1077
E-mail: barb_love@urmc.rochester.edu
Accred Length: 1 Year *Program Size:* 2
Program ID: 450-35-21-006

Stony Brook

SUNY at Stony Brook Program

Sponsor: University Hospital-SUNY at Stony Brook
Veterans Affairs Medical Center (Northport)

Program Director:
John J Ricotta, MD
SUNY-Stony Brook, Div of Vascular Surg
Health Science Ctr T19/Rm 020
Stony Brook, NY 11794-8191
Tel: 516 444-8477 *Fax:* 516 444-8947
E-mail: ricotta@surg.som.sunysb.edu
Internet: http://www.uhmc.sunysb.edu
Accred Length: 1 Year *Program Size:* 2
Program ID: 450-35-21-051

North Carolina

Chapel Hill

University of North Carolina Hospitals Program

Sponsor: University of North Carolina Hospitals

Program Director:
Blair A Keagy, MD
Univ of North Carolina Hospitals
Campus Box 7212
Burnett-Womack Clinical Sciences
Chapel Hill, NC 27599-7212
Tel: 919 966-3391 *Fax:* 919 966-2898
Accred Length: 1 Year *Program Size:* 2
Program ID: 450-36-21-007

Charlotte

Carolinas Medical Center Program
Sponsor: Carolinas Medical Center
Program Director:
Francis Robicsek, MD PhD
Dept of Thoracic/Cardiovascular Surg
Carolinas Med Ctr
PO Box 32861
Charlotte, NC 28232-2861
Tel: 704 355-4005 *Fax:* 704 355-6227
E-mail: spinder@carolinas.org
Accred Length: 1 Year *Program Size:* 2
Program ID: 450-36-21-008

Winston-Salem

Wake Forest University School of Medicine Program
Sponsor: Wake Forest University Baptist Medical Center
Program Director:
Kimberley J Hansen, MD
Wake Forest Univ Sch of Med
Dept of General Surgery
Medical Center Blvd
Winston-Salem, NC 27157-1095
Tel: 336 716-4151 *Fax:* 336 716-9758
E-mail: kjhansen@wfubmc.edu
Internet: http://www.bgsm.edu/surg-sci/gs/vs11.html
Accred Length: 1 Year *Program Size:* 2
Program ID: 450-36-21-073

Ohio

Cincinnati

Good Samaritan Hospital Program
Sponsor: Good Samaritan Hospital
Program Director:
Richard E Welling, MD
Good Samaritan Hospital
375 Dixmyth Ave
Cincinnati, OH 45220-2489
Tel: 513 872-3562 *Fax:* 513 221-5865
E-mail: rebecca_stratmann@trihealth.com
Accred Length: 1 Year *Program Size:* 2
Program ID: 450-38-31-043

University Hospital/University of Cincinnati College of Medicine Program
Sponsor: University Hospital Inc
Christ Hospital
Program Director:
John D Edwards, MD
Univ of Cincinnati Hospital
Div of Vascular Surgery
PO Box 670558
Cincinnati, OH 45267-0558
Tel: 513 558-5367 *Fax:* 513 558-2967
E-mail: hennesva@ucmail.uc.edu
Accred Length: 1 Year *Program Size:* 1
Program ID: 450-38-31-078

Cleveland

Case Western Reserve University Program
Sponsor: University Hospitals of Cleveland
MetroHealth Medical Center
Program Director:
Henry R Baele, MD
Univ Hospitals of Cleveland
11100 Euclid Ave
Cleveland, OH 44106-5000
Tel: 216 844-3030 *Fax:* 216 844-7716
Accred Length: 1 Year *Program Size:* 2
Program ID: 450-38-21-071

Cleveland Clinic Foundation Program
Sponsor: Cleveland Clinic Foundation
Program Director:
Leonard P Krajewski, MD
Cleveland Clinic Foundation
Dept of Vascular Surgery/S61
9500 Euclid Ave
Cleveland, OH 44195-5242
Tel: 216 444-5690 *Fax:* 216 444-1162
E-mail: meded@cestmp.ccf.org
Internet: http://www.ccf.org
Accred Length: 1 Year *Program Size:* 6
Program ID: 450-38-22-046

Columbus

Ohio State University Program
Sponsor: Ohio State University Medical Center
Program Director:
William L Smead, MD
Ohio State Univ
N708 Doan Hall
410 W Tenth Ave
Columbus, OH 43210-1228
Tel: 614 293-8536 *Fax:* 614 293-8616
Accred Length: 1 Year *Program Size:* 1
Program ID: 450-38-21-056

Oregon

Portland

Oregon Health Sciences University Program
Sponsor: Oregon Health Sciences University Hospital
Program Director:
John M Porter, MD
Oregon Health Sciences Univ
3181 SW Sam Jackson Park Rd/OP-11
Portland, OR 97201-3098
Tel: 503 494-7593 *Fax:* 503 494-4324
E-mail: mcnameeb@ohsu.edu
Internet: http://www.ohsu.edu/
Accred Length: 1 Year *Program Size:* 2
Program ID: 450-40-21-009

Pennsylvania

Danville

Penn State Geisinger Health System/Geisinger Medical Center Program
Sponsor: Penn State Geisinger Health System
Geisinger Medical Center
Program Director:
David P Franklin, MD
Geisinger Med Ctr
100 N Academy Ave
Danville, PA 17822
Tel: 717 271-6367 *Fax:* 717 271-5840
E-mail: ckrebs@psghs.edu
Accred Length: 1 Year *Program Size:* 2
Program ID: 450-41-21-072

Hershey

Penn State Geisinger Health System/Milton S Hershey Medical Center Program
Sponsor: Penn State Geisinger Health System
Milton S Hershey Medical Center
Program Director:
Robert G Atnip, MD
Dept of Surgery
Milton S Hershey Med Ctr
PO Box 850
Hershey, PA 17033-0850
Tel: 717 531-8888 *Fax:* 717 531-4151
E-mail: ratnip@psghs.edu
Accred Length: 1 Year *Program Size:* 2
Program ID: 450-41-21-065

Philadelphia

MCP Hahnemann University Program
Sponsor: MCP Hahnemann University
Crozer-Chester Medical Center
Hahnemann University Hospital
Program Director:
Calvin B Ernst, MD
Hahnemann Univ Hospital
Broad and Vine Sts/MS 468
Philadelphia, PA 19102-1192
Tel: 215 762-8181 *Fax:* 215 762-8682
Accred Length: 1 Year *Program Size:* 2
Program ID: 450-41-21-063

Pennsylvania Hospital of the University of Pennsylvania Health System Program
Sponsor: Pennsylvania Hospital (UPHS)
Program Director:
Keith D Calligaro, MD
Pennsylvania Hospital
Sect of Vascular Surgery
700 Spruce St/Ste 101
Philadelphia, PA 19106-4014
Tel: 215 829-5000 *Fax:* 215 627-3199
Accred Length: 1 Year *Program Size:* 1
Program ID: 450-41-31-074

Temple University Program
Sponsor: Temple University Hospital
Program Director:
Anthony J Comerota, MD
Temple Univ Hospital
3401 N Broad St
Philadelphia, PA 19140
Tel: 215 707-3622 *Fax:* 215 707-4357
Accred Length: 1 Year *Program Size:* 1
Program ID: 450-41-21-054

University of Pennsylvania Program
Sponsor: Hospital of the University of Pennsylvania
Program Director:
Michael A Golden, MD
Hospital of Univ of Pennsylvania
4 Silverstein
3400 Spruce St
Philadelphia, PA 19104-4283
Tel: 215 662-7836 *Fax:* 215 662-7476
Accred Length: 1 Year *Program Size:* 1
Program ID: 450-41-21-052

Pittsburgh

University Health Center of Pittsburgh Program

Sponsor: University Health Center of Pittsburgh
Veterans Affairs Medical Center (Pittsburgh)

Program Director:
Michel S Makaroun, MD
A1011 PUH
200 Lathrop St
Pittsburgh, PA 15213
Tel: 412 648-2060 *Fax:* 412 647-0289
Accred Length: 1 Year *Program Size:* 1
Program ID: 450-41-21-088

Tennessee

Knoxville

University of Tennessee Medical Center at Knoxville Program

Sponsor: University of Tennessee Graduate School of Medicine

Program Director:
Mitchell H Goldman, MD
Univ of Tennessee Med Ctr
Dept of Surgery
1924 Alcoa Hwy
Knoxville, TN 37920
Tel: 423 544-9230 *Fax:* 423 544-8894
E-mail: hamilto1@utk.edu
Internet: http://www.mc.utk.edu/docs/surgery
Accred Length: 1 Year *Program Size:* 2
Program ID: 450-47-21-075

Memphis

University of Tennessee Program

Sponsor: University of Tennessee College of Medicine
Baptist Memorial Hospital
Veterans Affairs Medical Center (Memphis)

Program Director:
H Edward Garrett Jr, MD
Univ of Tennessee
Div of Vascular Surgery
956 Court Ave/G230 Coleman Bldg
Memphis, TN 38163
Tel: 901 448-4541 *Fax:* 901 448-7306
Accred Length: 1 Year *Program Size:* 2
Program ID: 450-47-21-041

Nashville

Vanderbilt University Program

Sponsor: Vanderbilt University Medical Center
St Thomas Hospital

Program Director:
Thomas C Naslund, MD
Vanderbilt Univ
1161 22nd Ave S
D-5237 MCN
Nashville, TN 37232-2735
Tel: 615 322-2343 *Fax:* 615 343-4251
E-mail: thomas.naslund@surgery.mc.vanderbilt.edu
Internet:
http://www.mc.vanderbilt.edu/surgery/training-program-1.html
Accred Length: 1 Year *Program Size:* 1
Program ID: 450-47-21-047

Texas

Dallas

Baylor University Medical Center Program

Sponsor: Baylor University Medical Center

Program Director:
Gregory J Pearl, MD
Baylor Univ Med Ctr
712 N Washington/Ste 509
Dallas, TX 75246-1635
Tel: 214 824-7280
Accred Length: 1 Year *Program Size:* 2
Program ID: 450-48-21-028

University of Texas Southwestern Medical School Program

Sponsor: University of Texas Southwestern Medical School
Dallas County Hospital District-Parkland Memorial Hospital
Veterans Affairs Medical Center (Dallas)
Zale-Lipshy University Hospital

Program Director:
G Patrick Clagett, MD
Univ of Texas Southwestern Med Sch
5323 Harry Hines Blvd
Dallas, TX 75235-9157
Tel: 214 648-3516 *Fax:* 214 648-2790
Accred Length: 1 Year *Program Size:* 1
Program ID: 450-48-21-029

Houston

Baylor College of Medicine Program

Sponsor: Baylor College of Medicine
Methodist Hospital

Program Director:
Hazim J Safi, MD
Baylor Coll of Med
One Baylor Plaza
404D
Houston, TX 77030
Tel: 713 798-6078 *Fax:* 713 798-8941
E-mail: jcorke@bcm.tmc.edu
Accred Length: 1 Year *Program Size:* 6
Program ID: 450-48-21-016

Utah

Salt Lake City

University of Utah Program

Sponsor: University of Utah Medical Center

Program Director:
Spencer W Galt, MD
Univ of Utah Health Sciences Ctr
50 N Medical Dr
Salt Lake City, UT 84132
Tel: 801 581-8301 *Fax:* 801 581-3433
E-mail: spencer.galt@gatormail.cvrti.utah.edu
Accred Length: 1 Year *Program Size:* 1
Program ID: 450-49-21-085

Virginia

Charlottesville

University of Virginia Program

Sponsor: University of Virginia Medical Center

Program Director:
Irving L Kron, MD
Univ of Virginia Health Sciences Ctr
Sect of Vascular Surgery
Box 310
Charlottesville, VA 22908
Tel: 804 924-2158 *Fax:* 804 982-3885
Internet: http://www.med.virginia.edu/heart/docs/profs/vascularresidency.html
Accred Length: 1 Year *Program Size:* 1
Program ID: 450-51-21-083

Norfolk

Eastern Virginia Medical School Program

Sponsor: Eastern Virginia Medical School
Sentara Norfolk General Hospital

Program Director:
Roger T Gregory, MD
Eastern Virginia Med Sch
250 W Brambleton Ave
Norfolk, VA 23510
Tel: 757 622-2649 *Fax:* 757 625-0433
E-mail: vascnsg@aol.com
Accred Length: 1 Year *Program Size:* 2
Program ID: 450-51-21-018

Richmond

Medical College of Virginia/Virginia Commonwealth University Program

Sponsor: Medical College of Virginia/Virginia Commonwealth University
Hunter Holmes McGuire VA Medical Center (Richmond)
Medical College of Virginia Hospitals

Program Director:
Raymond G Makhoul, MD
Med Coll of Virginia
PO Box 980108
Richmond, VA 23298-0108
Tel: 804 828-7749 *Fax:* 804 828-2744
Internet: http://surg.vcu.edu
Accred Length: 1 Year *Program Size:* 2
Program ID: 450-51-21-039

Washington

Seattle

University of Washington Program

Sponsor: University of Washington School of Medicine
University of Washington Medical Center
Veterans Affairs Medical Center (Seattle)

Program Director:
Alexander W Clowes, MD
Univ of Washington Sch of Med
Div of Vascular Surgery
BB442 HSB/Box 356410
Seattle, WA 98195-6410
Tel: 206 543-9890 *Fax:* 206 616-7495
E-mail: kjp@u.washington.edu
Internet:
http://washington.edu./medical/som/som_departments/surgery/index.html
Accred Length: 1 Year *Program Size:* 2
Program ID: 450-54-21-019

Wisconsin

Milwaukee

Medical College of Wisconsin Program

Sponsor: Medical College of Wisconsin Affiliated Hospitals Inc
Froedtert Memorial Lutheran Hospital

Program Director:
Jonathan B Towne, MD
Med Coll of Wisconsin
9200 W Wisconsin Ave
Milwaukee, WI 53226
Tel: 414 257-5518 *Fax:* 414 257-5953
E-mail: jtowne@post.its.mcw.edu
Accred Length: 1 Year *Program Size:* 2
Program ID: 450-56-21-020

Section IV

New and Withdrawn Programs

New Programs

The following programs were accredited by the Accreditation Council for Graduate Medical Education since the publication of the 1998-1999 *Directory*. Additional information on these programs is included in Section III under the applicable specialty listing.

Addiction Psychiatry (Psychiatry)

Albert Einstein College of Medicine Program
Bronx, New York
Program ID: 401-35-21-023

Duke University Program
Durham, North Carolina
Program ID: 401-36-21-035

Indiana University School of Medicine Program
Indianapolis, Indiana
Program ID: 401-17-21-030

Mayo Graduate School of Medicine (Rochester) Program
Rochester, Minnesota
Program ID: 401-26-21-031

New York and Presbyterian Hospital (Columbia Campus) Program
New York, New York
Program ID: 401-35-21-032

New York and Presbyterian Hospital (Cornell Campus) Program
New York, New York
Program ID: 401-35-11-018

University of Hawaii Program
Honolulu, Hawaii
Program ID: 401-14-21-033

University of Miami-Jackson Memorial Medical Center Program
Miami, Florida
Program ID: 401-11-21-029

University of South Florida Program
Tampa, Florida
Program ID: 401-11-21-034

University of Texas Southwestern Medical School Program
Dallas, Texas
Program ID: 401-48-21-028

Adolescent Medicine (Pediatrics)

Albert Einstein College of Medicine at Long Island Jewish Medical Center Program
New Hyde Park, New York
Program ID: 321-35-31-011

Albert Einstein College of Medicine Program
Bronx, New York
Program ID: 321-35-21-008

Children's Hospital Medical Center/University of Cincinnati College of Medicine Program
Cincinnati, Ohio
Program ID: 321-38-21-014

Children's Hospital of Los Angeles Program
Los Angeles, California
Program ID: 321-05-21-018

Children's Hospital of Philadelphia Program
Philadelphia, Pennsylvania
Program ID: 321-41-21-015

Children's Hospital/Boston Medical Center Program
Boston, Massachusetts
Program ID: 321-24-21-002

Indiana University School of Medicine Program
Indianapolis, Indiana
Program ID: 321-17-21-006

Johns Hopkins University Program
Baltimore, Maryland
Program ID: 321-23-21-007

North Shore University Hospital/NYU School of Medicine Program
Manhasset, New York
Program ID: 321-35-21-010

University of Rochester Program
Rochester, New York
Program ID: 321-35-12-013

Allergy and Immunology

Mayo Graduate School of Medicine (Rochester) Program
Rochester, Minnesota
Program ID: 020-26-21-115

University of California (San Francisco)/Stanford University Program
San Francisco, California
Program ID: 020-05-21-116

University of Kansas Medical Center Program
Kansas City, Kansas
Program ID: 020-19-21-117

Anesthesiology

National Capital Consortium Program
Bethesda, Maryland
Program ID: 040-10-21-190

San Antonio Uniformed Services Health Education Consortium Program
Lackland AFB, Texas
Program ID: 040-48-21-091

Cardiovascular Disease (Internal Medicine)

Brown University Program 2
Providence, Rhode Island
Program ID: 141-43-21-260

Child and Adolescent Psychiatry (Psychiatry)

Albert Einstein College of Medicine at Bronx-Lebanon Hospital Center Program
Bronx, New York
Program ID: 405-35-21-177

University of Mississippi Medical Center Program
Jackson, Mississippi
Program ID: 405-27-21-176

Clinical Cardiac Electrophysiology (Internal Medicine)

Penn State Geisinger Health System/Milton S Hershey Medical Center Program
Hershey, Pennsylvania
Program ID: 154-41-21-084

University of Utah Program
Salt Lake City, Utah
Program ID: 154-49-21-075

Clinical Neurophysiology (Neurology)

Beth Israel Deaconess Medical Center/Harvard Medical School Program
Boston, Massachusetts
Program ID: 187-24-21-071

Los Angeles County-Harbor-UCLA Medical Center Program
Torrance, California
Program ID: 187-05-21-068

MCP Hahnemann University (Graduate) Program
Philadelphia, Pennsylvania
Program ID: 187-41-31-089

St Joseph Hospital and Medical Center Program
Phoenix, Arizona
Program ID: 187-03-21-094

Temple University Program
Philadelphia, Pennsylvania
Program ID: 187-41-31-049

Colon and Rectal Surgery

Mount Sinai School of Medicine Program
New York, New York
Program ID: 060-35-21-046

University of Texas Health Sciences Center at San Antonio Program
San Antonio, Texas
Program ID: 060-48-21-044

Washington Hospital Center Program
Washington, District of Columbia
Program ID: 060-10-21-045

Cytopathology (Pathology)

Tulane University Program
New Orleans, Louisiana
Program ID: 307-21-21-080

Dermatology

St Luke's - Roosevelt Hospital Center Program
New York, New York
Program ID: 080-35-21-124

University of Southern California Program
Los Angeles, California
Program ID: 080-05-11-015

Emergency Medicine

Newark Beth Israel Medical Center Program
Newark, New Jersey
Program ID: 110-33-21-158

Saginaw Cooperative Hospitals/Michigan State University Program
Saginaw, Michigan
Program ID: 110-25-11-138

Endocrinology, Diabetes, and Metabolism (Internal Medicine)

Charles R Drew University Program
Los Angeles, California
Program ID: 143-05-21-173

Family Practice

Boston University Medical Center Program
Boston, Massachusetts
Program ID: 120-24-21-644

Kalamazoo Center for Medical Studies/Michigan State University Rural Program
South Haven, Michigan
Program ID: 120-25-21-638

Louisiana State University (Kenner) Program
Kenner, Louisiana
Program ID: 120-21-21-641

Meadville Medical Center Program
Meadville, Pennsylvania
Program ID: 120-41-21-645

Medical College of Georgia (Okefenokee Satilla) Program
Waycross, Georgia
Program ID: 120-12-21-637

Medical College of Wisconsin (Froedtert Memorial) Program
Milwaukee, Wisconsin
Program ID: 120-56-31-639

Northeast Alabama Regional Medical Center Program
Anniston, Alabama
Program ID: 120-01-21-636

Ohio State University Rural Program
Bellefontaine, Ohio
Program ID: 120-38-21-640

Provena St Joseph Medical Center Program
Joliet, Illinois
Program ID: 120-16-21-647

Scripps Memorial Hospital (Chula Vista) Program
Chula Vista, California
Program ID: 120-05-21-632

St Joseph Mercy Hospital Program
Ann Arbor, Michigan
Program ID: 120-25-21-642

University of Minnesota/Fairview-University Medical Center Program
Minneapolis, Minnesota
Program ID: 120-26-21-650

University of Minnesota/HealthEast St Joseph's Hospital Program
St Paul, Minnesota
Program ID: 120-26-12-653

University of Minnesota/North Memorial Health Care Program @LIST TEXT = Robbinsdale, Minnesota
Program ID: 120-26-31-651

University of Minnesota/St John's Hospital Program
Maplewood, Minnesota
Program ID: 120-26-11-652

University of Wisconsin Rural Program
Antigo, Wisconsin
Program ID: 120-56-21-635

Forensic Pathology (Pathology)

Harris County Medical Examiner Department Program
Houston, Texas
Program ID: 310-48-21-080

Forensic Psychiatry (Psychiatry)

Louisiana State University Program
New Orleans, Louisiana
Program ID: 406-21-21-024

University of Colorado Program
Denver, Colorado
Program ID: 406-07-21-004

Geriatric Medicine (Family Practice)

Riverside Regional Medical Center Program
Newport News, Virginia
Program ID: 125-51-21-037

University of Iowa Hospitals and Clinics Program
Iowa City, Iowa
Program ID: 125-18-21-034

University of Louisville Program
Louisville, Kentucky
Program ID: 125-20-21-035

Geriatric Medicine (Internal Medicine)

Catholic Medical Center of Brooklyn and Queens Program
Jamaica, New York
Program ID: 151-35-31-124

Maimonides Medical Center Program
Brooklyn, New York
Program ID: 151-35-11-126

New York and Presbyterian Hospital (Cornell Campus) Program
New York, New York
Program ID: 151-35-12-127

Vanderbilt University Program
Nashville, Tennessee
Program ID: 151-47-21-125

Geriatric Psychiatry (Psychiatry)

East Tennessee State University Program
Johnson City, Tennessee
Program ID: 407-47-21-050

Yale-New Haven Medical Center Program
New Haven, Connecticut
Program ID: 407-08-21-052

Hand Surgery (Plastic Surgery)

Yale-New Haven Medical Center Program
New Haven, Connecticut
Program ID: 363-08-21-024

Hematology (Pathology)

Boston University Medical Center Program
Boston, Massachusetts
Program ID: 311-24-21-077

Tulane University Program
New Orleans, Louisiana
Program ID: 311-21-31-076

Hematology and Oncology (Internal Medicine)

Medical College of Wisconsin Program
Milwaukee, Wisconsin
Program ID: 155-56-21-119

Oregon Health Sciences University Program
Portland, Oregon
Program ID: 155-40-21-118

St Elizabeth's Medical Center of Boston Program
Boston, Massachusetts
Program ID: 155-24-21-124

Infectious Disease (Internal Medicine)

Charles R Drew University Program
Los Angeles, California
Program ID: 146-05-11-123

University of Kentucky Medical Center Program
Lexington, Kentucky
Program ID: 146-20-21-196

Internal Medicine

Albert Einstein College of Medicine (Jacobi) Program
Bronx, New York
Program ID: 140-35-31-521

St Joseph's Hospital and Medical Center Program
Paterson, New Jersey
Program ID: 140-33-21-522

Musculoskeletal Radiology (Radiology-Diagnostic)

Cleveland Clinic Foundation Program
Cleveland, Ohio
Program ID: 426-38-21-007

New York University Medical Center Program
New York, New York
Program ID: 426-35-11-006

University of Rochester Program
Rochester, New York
Program ID: 426-35-31-003

University of Wisconsin Program
Madison, Wisconsin
Program ID: 426-56-21-008

Neonatal-Perinatal Medicine (Pediatrics)

University of Texas Health Science Center at San Antonio Program
San Antonio, Texas
Program ID: 329-48-21-115

Neurological Surgery

National Capital Consortium Program
Bethesda, Maryland
Program ID: 160-10-21-118

Neurology

Cleveland Clinic Foundation (Florida) Program
Fort Lauderdale, Florida
Program ID: 180-11-21-146

University of Illinois College of Medicine at Peoria Program
Peoria, Illinois
Program ID: 180-16-21-147

Obstetrics and Gynecology

University of Connecticut Program
Farmington, Connecticut
Program ID: 220-08-21-355

Orthopaedic Surgery of the Spine (Orthopaedic Surgery)

University of Virginia Program
Charlottesville, Virginia
Program ID: 267-51-21-024

Otology-Neurotology (Otolaryngology)

New York University Medical Center Program
New York, New York
Program ID: 286-35-21-004

Ohio State University Program
Columbus, Ohio
Program ID: 286-38-21-002

University of Virginia Program
Charlottesville, Virginia
Program ID: 286-51-21-005

Pain Management (Anesthesiology)

Medical College of Georgia Program
Augusta, Georgia
Program ID: 048-12-21-105

Ohio State University Program
Columbus, Ohio
Program ID: 048-38-21-048

University of Mississippi Medical Center Program
Jackson, Mississippi
Program ID: 048-27-21-104

Pediatric Anesthesiology (Anesthesiology)

Beth Israel Deaconess Medical Center Program
Boston, Massachusetts
Program ID: 042-24-21-004

Case Western Reserve University Program
Cleveland, Ohio
Program ID: 042-38-21-015

George Washington University Program
Washington, District of Columbia
Program ID: 042-10-21-006

Johns Hopkins University Program
Baltimore, Maryland
Program ID: 042-23-21-028

New England Medical Center Hospitals Program
Boston, Massachusetts
Program ID: 042-24-21-026

Stanford University Program
Stanford, California
Program ID: 042-05-31-019

University Health Center of Pittsburgh Program
Pittsburgh, Pennsylvania
Program ID: 042-41-21-010

University Hospital/University of Cincinnati College of Medicine Program
Cincinnati, Ohio
Program ID: 042-38-21-009

University of Arkansas for Medical Sciences Program
Little Rock, Arkansas
Program ID: 042-04-21-023

University of Colorado Program
Denver, Colorado
Program ID: 042-07-21-020

University of Florida Program
Gainesville, Florida
Program ID: 042-11-21-001

University of Miami-Jackson Memorial Medical Center Program
Miami, Florida
Program ID: 042-11-31-007

University of Michigan Program
Ann Arbor, Michigan
Program ID: 042-25-21-029

University of New Mexico Program
Albuquerque, New Mexico
Program ID: 042-34-21-012

Yale-New Haven Medical Center Program
New Haven, Connecticut
Program ID: 042-08-21-005

Pediatric Endocrinology (Pediatrics)

New York and Presbyterian Hospital (Columbia Campus) Program
New York, New York
Program ID: 326-35-21-070

Pediatric Gastroenterology (Pediatrics)

University of California (San Diego) Program
San Diego, California
Program ID: 332-05-11-055

Pediatric Hematology/Oncology (Pediatrics)

Johns Hopkins University Program
Baltimore, Maryland
Program ID: 327-23-21-074

Pediatric Infectious Diseases (Pediatrics)

Albert Einstein College of Medicine at Long Island Jewish Medical Center Program
New Hyde Park, New York
Program ID: 335-35-12-037

Albert Einstein College of Medicine Program
Bronx, New York
Program ID: 335-35-21-034

Baylor College of Medicine Program
Houston, Texas
Program ID: 335-48-11-055

Brown University Program
Providence, Rhode Island
Program ID: 335-43-21-050

Case Western Reserve University Program
Cleveland, Ohio
Program ID: 335-38-31-046

Children's Hospital Medical Center/University of Cincinnati College of Medicine Program
Cincinnati, Ohio
Program ID: 335-38-21-045

Children's Hospital of Los Angeles Program
Los Angeles, California
Program ID: 335-05-31-004

Children's Hospital of Philadelphia Program
Philadelphia, Pennsylvania
Program ID: 335-41-21-047

Children's Hospital-Oakland Program
Oakland, California
Program ID: 335-05-12-006

Children's Hospital/Boston Medical Center Program 1
Boston, Massachusetts
Program ID: 335-24-21-025

Children's Hospital/Boston Medical Center Program 2
Boston, Massachusetts
Program ID: 335-24-31-026

Duke University Program
Durham, North Carolina
Program ID: 335-36-31-044

Eastern Virginia Medical School Program
Norfolk, Virginia
Program ID: 335-51-21-058

Emory University Program
Atlanta, Georgia
Program ID: 335-12-21-017

George Washington University Program
Washington, District of Columbia
Program ID: 335-10-21-013

Johns Hopkins University Program
Baltimore, Maryland
Program ID: 335-23-21-023

Los Angeles County-Harbor-UCLA Medical Center Program
Torrance, California
Program ID: 335-05-21-010

McGaw Medical Center of Northwestern University Program
Chicago, Illinois
Program ID: 335-16-21-018

Medical College of Virginia/Virginia Commonwealth University Program
Richmond, Virginia
Program ID: 335-51-31-059

Mount Sinai School of Medicine Program
New York, New York
Program ID: 335-35-13-038

National Capital Consortium Program
Bethesda, Maryland
Program ID: 335-10-31-014

New York and Presbyterian Hospital (Columbia Campus) Program
New York, New York
Program ID: 335-35-21-040

New York and Presbyterian Hospital (Cornell Campus) Program
New York, New York
Program ID: 335-35-22-039

North Shore University Hospital/NYU School of Medicine Program
Manhasset, New York
Program ID: 335-35-21-061

St Christopher's Hospital for Children Program
Philadelphia, Pennsylvania
Program ID: 335-41-31-048

Stanford University Program
Stanford, California
Program ID: 335-05-23-009

SUNY Health Science Center at Brooklyn Program
Brooklyn, New York
Program ID: 335-35-11-036

SUNY Health Science Center at Syracuse Program
Syracuse, New York
Program ID: 335-35-11-042

Tulane University/Louisiana State University Program
New Orleans, Louisiana
Program ID: 335-21-21-022

UCLA Medical Center Program
Los Angeles, California
Program ID: 335-05-11-005

UMDNJ-New Jersey Medical School Program
Newark, New Jersey
Program ID: 335-33-21-062

University Health Center of Pittsburgh Program
Pittsburgh, Pennsylvania
Program ID: 335-41-11-049

University of Alabama Medical Center Program
Birmingham, Alabama
Program ID: 335-01-21-001

University of Arkansas for Medical Sciences Program
Little Rock, Arkansas
Program ID: 335-04-21-002

University of California (San Diego) Program
San Diego, California
Program ID: 335-05-13-007

University of California (San Francisco) Program
San Francisco, California
Program ID: 335-05-22-008

University of Chicago Program
Chicago, Illinois
Program ID: 335-16-31-019

University of Colorado Program
Denver, Colorado
Program ID: 335-07-21-011

University of Florida Health Science Center/Jacksonville Program
Jacksonville, Florida
Program ID: 335-11-21-015

University of Louisville Program
Louisville, Kentucky
Program ID: 335-20-21-021

University of Maryland Program
Baltimore, Maryland
Program ID: 335-23-31-024

University of Michigan Program
Ann Arbor, Michigan
Program ID: 335-25-21-027

University of Minnesota Program
Minneapolis, Minnesota
Program ID: 335-26-21-029

University of Nebraska/Creighton University Program
Omaha, Nebraska
Program ID: 335-30-21-031

University of Rochester Program
Rochester, New York
Program ID: 335-35-31-041

University of Tennessee Program
Memphis, Tennessee
Program ID: 335-47-21-051

University of Texas at Houston Program
Houston, Texas
Program ID: 335-48-12-056

University of Texas Health Science Center at San Antonio Program
San Antonio, Texas
Program ID: 335-48-13-057

University of Texas Medical Branch Hospitals Program
Galveston, Texas
Program ID: 335-48-31-054

University of Texas Southwestern Medical School Program
Dallas, Texas
Program ID: 335-48-21-053

University of Washington Program
Seattle, Washington
Program ID: 335-54-21-060

Vanderbilt University Program
Nashville, Tennessee
Program ID: 335-47-31-052

Washington University/B-JH/SLCH Consortium Program
St Louis, Missouri
Program ID: 335-28-21-030

Wayne State University/Detroit Medical Center Program
Detroit, Michigan
Program ID: 335-25-31-028

Yale-New Haven Medical Center Program
New Haven, Connecticut
Program ID: 335-08-21-012

Pediatric Otolaryngology (Otolaryngology)

Baylor College of Medicine Program
Houston, Texas
Program ID: 288-48-21-005

Children's Hospital Medical Center/University of Cincinnati College of Medicine Program
Cincinnati, Ohio
Program ID: 288-38-21-004

University Health Center of Pittsburgh Program
Pittsburgh, Pennsylvania
Program ID: 288-41-21-001

University of Iowa Hospitals and Clinics Program
Iowa City, Iowa
Program ID: 288-18-21-003

Pediatric Pathology (Pathology)

Children's Hospital of Buffalo Program
Buffalo, New York
Program ID: 316-35-21-027

Pediatric Pulmonology (Pediatrics)

University of Miami-Jackson Memorial Medical Center Program
Miami, Florida
Program ID: 330-11-21-054

University of Virginia Program
Charlottesville, Virginia
Program ID: 330-51-21-053

Pediatric Rheumatology (Pediatrics)

Baylor College of Medicine Program
Houston, Texas
Program ID: 331-48-21-020

University of Texas Southwestern Medical School Program
Dallas, Texas
Program ID: 331-48-31-021

Pediatric Urology (Urology)

Indiana University School of Medicine Program
Indianapolis, Indiana
Program ID: 485-17-21-015

Pediatrics

Albert Einstein College of Medicine (Jacobi) Program
Bronx, New York
Program ID: 320-35-21-410

Atlantic Health System Program
Florham, New Jersey
Program ID: 320-33-21-412

Physical Medicine and Rehabilitation

University of North Carolina Hospitals Program
Chapel Hill, North Carolina
Program ID: 340-36-21-104

Preventive Medicine (Gen Prev Med, Occupational Med, Aerospace Med, & Pub Hlth)

Thomas Jefferson University Program
Philadelphia, Pennsylvania
Program ID: 380-41-77-120

University of Texas Medical Branch at Galveston Program
Galveston, Texas
Program ID: 380-48-77-121

Psychiatry

California Pacific Medical Center Program
San Francisco, California
Program ID: 400-05-22-028

Pulmonary Disease (Internal Medicine)

Albert Einstein Medical Center Program
Philadelphia, Pennsylvania
Program ID: 149-41-21-204

East Carolina University Program
Greenville, North Carolina
Program ID: 149-36-21-203

Pulmonary Disease and Critical Care Medicine (Internal Medicine)

Los Angeles County-Harbor-UCLA Medical Center Program
Torrance, California
Program ID: 156-05-11-115

UCLA Medical Center Program
Los Angeles, California
Program ID: 156-05-31-114

Wayne State University/Detroit Medical Center Program
Detroit, Michigan
Program ID: 156-25-21-116

Radiology-Diagnostic

San Antonio Uniformed Services Health Education Consortium Program
Fort Sam Houston, Texas
Program ID: 420-48-21-248

Rheumatology (Internal Medicine)

University of Utah Program
Salt Lake City, Utah
Program ID: 150-49-21-148

Spinal Cord Injury Medicine (Physical Medicine and Rehabilitation)

Stanford University Program
Stanford, California
Program ID: 345-05-21-007

Sports Medicine (Family Practice)

Bayfront Medical Center Program
St Petersburg, Florida
Program ID: 127-11-21-041

Christiana Care Health Services Program
Wilmington, Delaware
Program ID: 127-09-21-038

Fairview Health System Program
Cleveland, Ohio
Program ID: 127-38-21-047

Kalamazoo Center for Medical Studies/Michigan State University Program
Kalamazoo, Michigan
Program ID: 127-25-21-050

MacNeal Memorial Hospital Program
Berwyn, Illinois
Program ID: 127-16-21-040

Memorial Hospital of South Bend Program
South Bend, Indiana
Program ID: 127-17-21-042

Mercy Health System Program
Janesville, Wisconsin
Program ID: 127-56-21-046

St Joseph's Medical Center of South Bend Program
South Bend, Indiana
Program ID: 127-17-31-043

University of Maryland Program
Baltimore, Maryland
Program ID: 127-23-21-051

University of Tennessee Medical Center at Knoxville Program
Knoxville, Tennessee
Program ID: 127-47-21-044

University of Washington Program
Seattle, Washington
Program ID: 127-54-21-039

Wake Forest University School of Medicine Program
Winston-Salem, North Carolina
Program ID: 127-36-21-048

Surgical Critical Care (General Surgery)

Case Western Reserve University Program
Cleveland, Ohio
Program ID: 442-38-21-070

University of New Mexico Program
Albuquerque, New Mexico
Program ID: 442-34-21-073

Transitional Year

Hospital de Damas Program
Ponce, Puerto Rico
Program ID: 999-42-00-236

Vascular and Interventional Radiology (Radiology-Diagnostic)

Duke University Program
Durham, North Carolina
Program ID: 427-36-21-088

New York University Medical Center Program
New York, New York
Program ID: 427-35-21-090

University of Arizona Program
Tucson, Arizona
Program ID: 427-03-21-074

University of California (Irvine) Program
Orange, California
Program ID: 427-05-11-089

University of Florida Health Science Center/Jacksonville Program
Jacksonville, Florida
Program ID: 427-11-21-086

University of New Mexico Program
Albuquerque, New Mexico
Program ID: 427-34-21-091

University of South Florida Program
Tampa, Florida
Program ID: 427-11-21-092

Vascular Surgery (General Surgery)

University Health Center of Pittsburgh Program
Pittsburgh, Pennsylvania
Program ID: 450-41-21-088

Withdrawn Programs

The accreditation of the following programs was withdrawn or voluntarily withdrawn since the publication of the 1998-1999 *Directory.* These programs are not listed in this year's edition.

Allergy and Immunology

Stanford University Program
Stanford, California
Program ID: 020-05-21-006

University of California (San Francisco) Program
San Francisco, California
Program ID: 020-05-21-059

University of Kansas Medical Center/Children's Mercy Hospital Program
Kansas City, Kansas
Program ID: 020-19-21-030

Anesthesiology

Hackensack Medical Center Program
Hackensack, New Jersey
Program ID: 040-33-11-084

Louisiana State University Program
New Orleans, Louisiana
Program ID: 040-21-21-054

National Naval Medical Center (Bethesda) Program
Bethesda, Maryland
Program ID: 040-23-21-007

San Antonio Uniformed Services Health Education Consortium (BAMC) Program
Fort Sam Houston, Texas
Program ID: 040-48-12-004

San Antonio Uniformed Services Health Education Consortium (WHMC) Program
Lackland AFB, Texas
Program ID: 040-48-21-001

Walter Reed Army Medical Center Program
Washington, District of Columbia
Program ID: 040-10-31-003

Blood Banking/Transfusion Medicine (Pathology)

Vanderbilt University Program
Nashville, Tennessee
Program ID: 305-47-31-008

Cardiovascular Disease (Internal Medicine)

Beth Israel Deaconess Medical Center (West Campus) Program
Burlington, Massachusetts
Program ID: 141-24-21-221

Guthrie Healthcare System Program
Sayre, Pennsylvania
Program ID: 141-41-21-249

Hospital of St Raphael Program
New Haven, Connecticut
Program ID: 141-08-31-002

Indiana University School of Medicine (Methodist) Program
Indianapolis, Indiana
Program ID: 141-17-11-135

Norwalk Hospital Program
Norwalk, Connecticut
Program ID: 141-08-31-003

Presbyterian Medical Center of the University of Pennsylvania Health System Program
Philadelphia, Pennsylvania
Program ID: 141-41-11-146

University of Virginia (Roanoke-Salem) Program
Salem, Virginia
Program ID: 141-51-31-085

Wayne State University/Detroit Medical Center (Sinai Hospital) Program
Detroit, Michigan
Program ID: 141-25-11-064

Chemical Pathology (Pathology)

University of Minnesota Program
Minneapolis, Minnesota
Program ID: 306-26-21-001

Clinical and Laboratory Immunology (Allergy and Immunology)

Medical College of Georgia Program
Augusta, Georgia
Program ID: 025-12-21-013

Clinical Cardiac Electrophysiology (Internal Medicine)

Ohio State University Program
Columbus, Ohio
Program ID: 154-38-31-057

Critical Care Medicine (Anesthesiology)

Henry Ford Hospital Program
Detroit, Michigan
Program ID: 045-25-21-055

Mercy Hospital of Pittsburgh Program
Pittsburgh, Pennsylvania
Program ID: 045-41-21-036

Critical Care Medicine (Internal Medicine)

Los Angeles County-Harbor-UCLA Medical Center Program
Torrance, California
Program ID: 142-05-11-014

North Shore University Hospital/NYU School of Medicine Program
Manhasset, New York
Program ID: 142-35-21-062

Cytopathology (Pathology)

Baptist Memorial Hospital Program
Memphis, Tennessee
Program ID: 307-47-21-064

Dermatopathology (Dermatology and Pathology)

University Hospital/University of Cincinnati College of Medicine Program
Cincinnati, Ohio
Program ID: 100-38-11-008

University of Colorado Program
Denver, Colorado
Program ID: 100-07-21-022

Endocrinology, Diabetes, and Metabolism (Internal Medicine)

Coney Island Hospital Program
Brooklyn, New York
Program ID: 143-35-11-138

Shadyside Hospital/UPMC Program
Pittsburgh, Pennsylvania
Program ID: 143-41-22-046

University of Missouri at Kansas City Program
Kansas City, Missouri
Program ID: 143-28-21-168

VA Greater Los Angeles Healthcare System (Sepulveda) Program
Los Angeles (Sepulveda), California
Program ID: 143-05-21-106

West Virginia University Program
Morgantown, West Virginia
Program ID: 143-55-21-158

Family Practice

Polyclinic Medical Center Program
Harrisburg, Pennsylvania
Program ID: 120-41-12-266

St Lawrence Hospital and HealthCare Services/Michigan State University Program
Lansing, Michigan
Program ID: 120-25-31-165

University of Kansas (Wichita) Program
Wichita, Kansas
Program ID: 120-19-11-141

University of Kansas (Wichita)/St Francis Program
Wichita, Kansas
Program ID: 120-19-11-140

University of Minnesota Program
Minneapolis, Minnesota
Program ID: 120-26-21-491

Wayne State University/Detroit Medical Center (Sinai Hospital) Program
Detroit, Michigan
Program ID: 120-25-21-561

Forensic Pathology (Pathology)

Rhode Island Office of State Medical Examiners Program
Providence, Rhode Island
Program ID: 310-43-21-071

Gastroenterology (Internal Medicine)

Griffin Hospital Program
Derby, Connecticut
Program ID: 144-08-31-132

Guthrie Healthcare System Program
Sayre, Pennsylvania
Program ID: 144-41-12-198

Hospital of St Raphael Program
New Haven, Connecticut
Program ID: 144-08-21-209

Wayne State University/Detroit Medical Center (Sinai Hospital) Program
Detroit, Michigan
Program ID: 144-25-11-207

Geriatric Medicine (Internal Medicine)

St Luke's-Roosevelt Hospital Center Program
New York, New York
Program ID: 151-35-21-094

University of Tennessee Program
Memphis, Tennessee
Program ID: 151-47-21-051

Geriatric Psychiatry (Psychiatry)

Mount Sinai School of Medicine Program
New York, New York
Program ID: 407-35-13-026

Hand Surgery (Orthopaedic Surgery)

Naval Medical Center (San Diego) Program
San Diego, California
Program ID: 263-05-21-050

Hand Surgery (Plastic Surgery)

Rush-Presbyterian-St Luke's Medical Center Program
Chicago, Illinois
Program ID: 363-16-21-003

Hematology (Internal Medicine)

Interfaith Medical Center Program
Brooklyn, New York
Program ID: 145-35-21-128

Medical College of Wisconsin Program
Milwaukee, Wisconsin
Program ID: 145-56-31-042

Michigan State University Program
East Lansing, Michigan
Program ID: 145-25-21-068

St Elizabeth's Medical Center of Boston Program
Boston, Massachusetts
Program ID: 145-24-21-048

Hematology (Pathology)

Case Western Reserve University (MetroHealth) Program
Cleveland, Ohio
Program ID: 311-38-11-022

National Naval Medical Center (Bethesda) Program
Bethesda, Maryland
Program ID: 311-23-21-008

Scripps Clinic/Scripps Green Hospital Program
La Jolla, California
Program ID: 311-05-31-054

University of Louisville Program
Louisville, Kentucky
Program ID: 311-20-21-043

Hematology and Oncology (Internal Medicine)

Finch University of Health Sciences/Chicago Medical School Program
North Chicago, Illinois
Program ID: 155-16-12-019

Madigan Army Medical Center Program
Tacoma, Washington
Program ID: 155-54-21-071

Naval Medical Center (San Diego) Program
San Diego, California
Program ID: 155-05-11-006

Immunopathology (Pathology)

New York University Medical Center Program
New York, New York
Program ID: 313-35-21-010

University of Utah Program
Salt Lake City, Utah
Program ID: 313-49-21-016

Infectious Disease (Internal Medicine)

University of Arizona Program
Tucson, Arizona
Program ID: 146-03-21-106

University of Virginia (Roanoke-Salem) Program
Salem, Virginia
Program ID: 146-51-31-030

Internal Medicine

Catholic Health Partners (Columbus) Program
Chicago, Illinois
Program ID: 140-16-21-501

Indiana University School of Medicine (Methodist) Program
Indianapolis, Indiana
Program ID: 140-17-11-134

Shadyside Hospital/UPMC Program
Pittsburgh, Pennsylvania
Program ID: 140-41-22-451

St Francis Medical Center Program
Trenton, New Jersey
Program ID: 140-33-21-508

St Luke's-Roosevelt Hospital Center (Roosevelt) Program
New York, New York
Program ID: 140-35-11-298

Veterans Affairs Medical Center (Washington) Program
Washington, District of Columbia
Program ID: 140-10-21-096

Medical Genetics

University of Arizona Program
Tucson, Arizona
Program ID: 130-03-21-035

Neonatal-Perinatal Medicine (Pediatrics)

University of Mississippi Medical Center Program
Jackson, Mississippi
Program ID: 329-27-21-034

West Virginia University Program
Morgantown, West Virginia
Program ID: 329-55-11-086

Nephrology (Internal Medicine)

Albany Medical Center Program
Albany, New York
Program ID: 148-35-31-022

Beth Israel Deaconess Medical Center (West Campus) Program
Boston, Massachusetts
Program ID: 148-24-21-176

Indiana University School of Medicine (Methodist) Program
Indianapolis, Indiana
Program ID: 148-17-11-094

Maimonides Medical Center Program
Brooklyn, New York
Program ID: 148-35-11-135

University of Missouri at Kansas City Program
Kansas City, Missouri
Program ID: 148-28-21-170

Neurological Surgery

National Naval Medical Center (Bethesda) Program
Bethesda, Maryland
Program ID: 160-23-21-002

University of California (Irvine) Program
Orange, California
Program ID: 160-05-21-007

University of Connecticut Program
Farmington, Connecticut
Program ID: 160-08-21-014

University of Massachusetts Program
Worcester, Massachusetts
Program ID: 160-24-21-105

Walter Reed Army Medical Center Program
Washington, District of Columbia
Program ID: 160-10-11-001

Neuropathology (Pathology)

University of California (Irvine) Program
Orange, California
Program ID: 315-05-21-089

Yale-New Haven Medical Center Program
New Haven, Connecticut
Program ID: 315-08-21-078

Neuroradiology (Radiology-Diagnostic)

University of Florida Health Science Center/Jacksonville Program
Jacksonville, Florida
Program ID: 423-11-21-092

University of Kentucky Medical Center Program
Lexington, Kentucky
Program ID: 423-20-21-089

Nuclear Medicine

Massachusetts General Hospital Program
Boston, Massachusetts
Program ID: 200-24-21-091

National Naval Medical Center (Bethesda) Program
Bethesda, Maryland
Program ID: 200-23-21-004

University of Southern California Program
Los Angeles, California
Program ID: 200-05-21-105

Nuclear Radiology (Radiology-Diagnostic)

Albert Einstein College of Medicine at Long Island Jewish Medical Center Program
New Hyde Park, New York
Program ID: 425-35-21-055

Temple University Program
Philadelphia, Pennsylvania
Program ID: 425-41-21-054

University of Florida Program
Gainesville, Florida
Program ID: 425-11-21-058

University of Illinois College of Medicine at Chicago/Michael Reese Hospital Program
Chicago, Illinois
Program ID: 425-16-12-003

University of Missouri-Columbia Program
Columbia, Missouri
Program ID: 425-28-21-020

Wayne State University/Detroit Medical Center Program
Detroit, Michigan
Program ID: 425-25-21-041

Obstetrics and Gynecology

Catholic Health Partners (Columbus) Program
Chicago, Illinois
Program ID: 220-16-21-083

Oncology (Internal Medicine)

Interfaith Medical Center Program
Brooklyn, New York
Program ID: 147-35-21-124

Medical College of Wisconsin Program
Milwaukee, Wisconsin
Program ID: 147-56-31-040

Michigan State University Program
East Lansing, Michigan
Program ID: 147-25-21-084

St Elizabeth's Medical Center of Boston Program
Boston, Massachusetts
Program ID: 147-24-21-049

Ophthalmology

Greater Baltimore Medical Center Program
Baltimore, Maryland
Program ID: 240-23-12-064

Sinai Hospital of Baltimore Program
Baltimore, Maryland
Program ID: 240-23-21-067

Southern Illinois University Program
Springfield, Illinois
Program ID: 240-16-31-176

Orthopaedic Sports Medicine (Orthopaedic Surgery)

Penn State Geisinger Health System/Milton S Hershey Medical Center Program
Hershey, Pennsylvania
Program ID: 268-41-21-070

Orthopaedic Trauma (Orthopaedic Surgery)

Henry Ford Hospital Program
Detroit, Michigan
Program ID: 269-25-21-005

Pathology-Anatomic and Clinical

Albert Einstein College of Medicine at Beth Israel Medical Center Program
New York, New York
Program ID: 300-35-11-231

Fairfax Hospital Program
Falls Church, Virginia
Program ID: 300-51-12-364

Lankenau Hospital Program
Wynnewood, Pennsylvania
Program ID: 300-41-12-315

Lutheran General Hospital Program
Park Ridge, Illinois
Program ID: 300-16-21-388

Maimonides Medical Center Program
Brooklyn, New York
Program ID: 300-35-11-246

Shadyside Hospital/UPMC Program
Pittsburgh, Pennsylvania
Program ID: 300-41-11-326

St John's Mercy Medical Center Program
St Louis, Missouri
Program ID: 300-28-12-190

William Beaumont Army Medical Center Program
El Paso, Texas
Program ID: 300-48-12-007

Pediatric Cardiology (Pediatrics)

New York and Presbyterian Hospital (Cornell Campus) Program
New York, New York
Program ID: 325-35-11-032

West Virginia University Program
Morgantown, West Virginia
Program ID: 325-55-21-068

Pediatric Critical Care Medicine (Pediatrics)

Penn State Geisinger Health System/Milton S Hershey Medical Center Program
Hershey, Pennsylvania
Program ID: 323-41-21-066

West Virginia University Program
Morgantown, West Virginia
Program ID: 323-55-21-068

Pediatric Endocrinology (Pediatrics)

St Christopher's Hospital for Children Program
Philadelphia, Pennsylvania
Program ID: 326-41-12-047

University of Rochester Program
Rochester, New York
Program ID: 326-35-21-024

University of Texas Health Science Center at San Antonio Program
San Antonio, Texas
Program ID: 326-48-21-038

Pediatric Hematology/Oncology (Pediatrics)

National Capital Consortium Program
Bethesda, Maryland
Program ID: 327-10-21-067

University of Nebraska/Creighton University Program
Omaha, Nebraska
Program ID: 327-30-21-062

Pediatric Pathology (Pathology)

Emory University Program
Atlanta, Georgia
Program ID: 316-12-21-006

Pediatric Radiology (Radiology-Diagnostic)

Medical University of South Carolina Program
Charleston, South Carolina
Program ID: 424-45-21-046

University of Missouri at Kansas City Program
Kansas City, Missouri
Program ID: 424-28-21-028

University of North Carolina Hospitals Program
Chapel Hill, North Carolina
Program ID: 424-36-31-048

University of Tennessee Program
Memphis, Tennessee
Program ID: 424-47-21-013

Vanderbilt University Program
Nashville, Tennessee
Program ID: 424-47-21-021

Pediatrics

Morristown Memorial Hospital Program
Morristown, New Jersey
Program ID: 320-33-21-368

Overlook Hospital Program
Summit, New Jersey
Program ID: 320-33-11-137

Plastic Surgery

San Antonio Uniformed Services Health Education Consortium Program
Lackland AFB, Texas
Program ID: 360-48-12-001

University of Missouri at Kansas City Program
Kansas City, Missouri
Program ID: 360-28-21-050

Wright State University Program
Dayton (Kettering), Ohio
Program ID: 360-38-21-083

Preventive Medicine (Gen Prev Med, Occupational Med, Aerospace Med, & Pub Hlth)

University of Hawaii School of Public Health Program
Honolulu, Hawaii
Program ID: 380-14-12-012

Psychiatry

Mercer University School of Medicine Program
Macon, Georgia
Program ID: 400-12-21-261

Napa State Hospital Program
Napa, California
Program ID: 400-05-22-019

San Antonio Uniformed Services Health Education Consortium Program
Lackland AFB, Texas
Program ID: 400-48-21-001

Trenton Psychiatric Hospital Program
West Trenton, New Jersey
Program ID: 400-33-21-122

Wayne State University/Detroit Medical Center (Sinai Hospital) Program
Detroit, Michigan
Program ID: 400-25-21-100

Pulmonary Disease (Internal Medicine)

Los Angeles County-Harbor-UCLA Medical Center Program
Torrance, California
Program ID: 149-05-11-170

Madigan Army Medical Center Program
Tacoma, Washington
Program ID: 149-54-12-068

Northeastern Pennsylvania Hospitals Program
Wilkes-Barre, Pennsylvania
Program ID: 149-41-31-191

Palmetto Health Alliance/University of South Carolina School of Medicine Program
Columbia, South Carolina
Program ID: 149-45-21-093

Presbyterian Medical Center of the University of Pennsylvania Health System Program
Philadelphia, Pennsylvania
Program ID: 149-41-11-119

UCLA Medical Center Program
Los Angeles, California
Program ID: 149-05-11-127

VA Greater Los Angeles Healthcare System (Sepulveda) Program
Los Angeles (Sepulveda), California
Program ID: 149-05-21-174

VA Greater Los Angeles Healthcare System Program
Los Angeles, California
Program ID: 149-05-31-050

Wayne State University/Detroit Medical Center (Sinai Hospital) Program
Detroit, Michigan
Program ID: 149-25-11-192

Wayne State University/Detroit Medical Center Program
Detroit, Michigan
Program ID: 149-25-21-045

Pulmonary Disease and Critical Care Medicine (Internal Medicine)

Massachusetts General Hospital Program
Boston, Massachusetts
Program ID: 156-24-21-096

Radiation Oncology

Albert Einstein Medical Center Program
Philadelphia, Pennsylvania
Program ID: 430-41-12-082

University of Oklahoma Health Sciences Center Program
Oklahoma City, Oklahoma
Program ID: 430-39-21-080

Radiology-Diagnostic

Beth Israel Deaconess Medical Center (West Campus) Program
Boston, Massachusetts
Program ID: 420-24-21-084

Columbia Presbyterian-St Luke's Medical Center Program
Denver, Colorado
Program ID: 420-07-22-036

San Antonio Uniformed Services Health Education Consortium (BAMC) Program
Fort Sam Houston, Texas
Program ID: 420-48-11-943

San Antonio Uniformed Services Health Education Consortium (WHMC) Program
Lackland AFB, Texas
Program ID: 420-48-12-002

Rheumatology (Internal Medicine)

Wayne State University/Detroit Medical Center (Sinai Hospital) Program
Detroit, Michigan
Program ID: 150-25-11-135

Sports Medicine (Family Practice)

Grant Medical Center (OhioHealth) Program
Columbus, Ohio
Program ID: 127-38-21-009

Surgery-General

Albert Einstein College of Medicine at Long Island Jewish/Beth Israel Medical Center Program
New Hyde Park, New York
Program ID: 440-35-21-406

MCP Hahnemann University (Hahnemann) Program
Philadelphia, Pennsylvania
Program ID: 440-41-21-294

Mount Sinai School of Medicine (North General) Program
New York, New York
Program ID: 440-35-31-215

Thoracic Surgery

Tulane University Program
New Orleans, Louisiana
Program ID: 460-21-21-103

Transitional Year

Lancaster General Hospital Program
Lancaster, Pennsylvania
Program ID: 999-41-00-109

Mount Sinai School of Medicine (Elmhurst) Program
Elmhurst, New York
Program ID: 999-35-00-223

Vascular and Interventional Radiology (Radiology-Diagnostic)

Beth Israel Deaconess Medical Center (East Campus) Program
Boston, Massachusetts
Program ID: 427-24-11-046

Section V

Graduate Medical Education Teaching Institutions

Section V lists hospitals and organizations that sponsor graduate medical education (GME) programs or participate in GME. *Sponsoring institutions* assume final responsibility for a GME program. Most GME programs are sponsored by specific clinical departments within a hospital, another health care institution such as a medical school, or an educational consortium. *Major participating institutions* include hospitals or other sites recognized by at least one residency review committee as providing a major portion of required GME. Hospitals and other institutions that provide rotations of less than one-sixth of the program length or less than a total of 6 months are not listed in the *Directory*.

All institutions that sponsor GME programs or participate in GME are listed in alphabetical order by state and city. Each listing includes the institution name, address, and identification code. Also provided are codes of medical schools affiliated with each institution (where applicable) and abbreviations for the specialty and subspecialty programs affiliated with each institution. (A key for specialty and subspecialty abbreviation codes is provided inside the front cover of this *Directory*).

Candidates seeking a residency should refer to the list of programs in Section III. Applications for a residency position should be addressed to the program director rather than to an institution.

Relationships Between Hospitals and Medical Schools (Medical School Affiliation)

Hospitals that sponsor an accredited program are not required to have a formal relationship with a medical school. Where such a relationship exists, the affiliation is identified by the dean of the medical school as M (major), G (graduate only), or L (limited). The medical school associated with the code number in this listing is identified in Appendix D.

Major affiliation (M) signifies that an institution is an important part of the teaching program of the medical school and is a major unit in the clinical clerkship program. Major teaching institutions provide clerkship experience in two or more of the major specialties: internal medicine, surgery, pediatrics, and obstetrics-gynecology. An institution responsible for most of the teaching in a single specialty, such as psychiatry or pediatrics, may also be considered a major affiliation. In a major teaching institution, medical students serve clinical clerkships regularly on inpatient services, under the direct supervision of medical school faculty. A major teaching institution may or may not be used for medical school residencies.

Graduate affiliation (G) indicates that the institution is affiliated with the medical school only for its graduate programs and that one or more of the following arrangements is in effect:

1. House staff of the GME programs are selected by officials of a medical school department or by a joint committee of the institution teaching staff and medical school faculty.
2. Medical school faculty (other than the institution's attending staff) are regularly scheduled to participate in the teaching programs of the institution. No graduate affiliation is indicated if medical school faculty participation at the institution is limited to an occasional lecture or consultation visit, or if the institution's residents attend medical school teaching conferences only as visitors.
3. A contractual arrangement (with or without financial commitment) specifies the medical school participation in the organization and supervision of the GME program in the institution.
4. There is some degree of exchange of residents between this institution and the principal teaching institution of the medical school.

Limited affiliation (L) signifies that the institution is affiliated with the medical school's teaching program only for brief and/or unique rotations of students or residents.

Teaching Institutions

Alabama

Anniston

Northeast Alabama Regional Medical Center
400 E Tenth St
PO Box 2208
Anniston, AL 36202
Programs sponsored in: FP
Institution ID: 01-0517

Birmingham

American Red Cross Blood Services-Alabama Region
2225 Third Ave N
Birmingham, AL 35203
Major participating institution for programs in: BBK
Institution ID: 01-8004

American Sports Medicine Institute
1313 13th St S
Birmingham, AL 35205
Programs sponsored in: OSM
Institution ID: 01-8009

Baptist Health System Inc
3500 Blue Lake Dr
PO Box 830605
Birmingham, AL 35283
Programs sponsored in: DR, GS, IM, PTH, TY
Institution ID: 01-0519

Birmingham Baptist Medical Center-Montclair
800 Montclair Rd
Birmingham, AL 35213
Med Sch Affil: M-00102
Major participating institution for programs in: DMP, DR, GS, IM, PTH, TY
Institution ID: 01-0307

Birmingham Baptist Medical Center-Princeton
701 Princeton Ave SW
Birmingham, AL 35211
Med Sch Affil: M-00102
Major participating institution for programs in: DR, GS, IM, PTH, TY
Institution ID: 01-0187

Carraway Methodist Medical Center
Academic Affairs
1600 Carraway Blvd
Birmingham, AL 35234
Med Sch Affil: M-00102
Programs sponsored in: FP, GS, IM, TY
Major participating institution for programs in: AN
Institution ID: 01-0132

Children's Hospital of Alabama
1600 7th Ave S
Birmingham, AL 35233
Med Sch Affil: M-00102
Major participating institution for programs in: AN, CCP, CHN, CHP, NPM, NS, ORS, OTO, PD, PDI, PDP, PDS, PG, PHO, PS, RNR, SCI, U
Institution ID: 01-0497

Cooper Green Hospital
1515 6th Ave S
Birmingham, AL 35233-1601
Med Sch Affil: M-00102
Major participating institution for programs in: AN, GS, IM, OBG, OPH, ORS, OTO
Institution ID: 01-0511

Eye Foundation Hospital
1720 University Blvd
Birmingham, AL 35233
Med Sch Affil: M-00102
Major participating institution for programs in: OPH
Institution ID: 01-0502

Jefferson County Coroner/Medical Examiner's Office
1515 6th Ave S
Birmingham, AL 35233
Major participating institution for programs in: FOP
Institution ID: 01-0531

Medical Center East
50 Medical Park East Dr
Birmingham, AL 35235-3499
Med Sch Affil: L-00102
Programs sponsored in: FP
Institution ID: 01-0515

St Vincent's Hospital
2701 9th Ct S
PO Box 12407
Birmingham, AL 35202-2407
Med Sch Affil: G-00102
Major participating institution for programs in: U
Institution ID: 01-0196

University of Alabama at Birmingham School of Public Health
308 Tidwell Hall
720 S 20th St
Birmingham, AL 35294
Major participating institution for programs in: GPM
Institution ID: 01-8008

University of Alabama Hospital
619 19th St S
Birmingham, AL 35233-6805
Med Sch Affil: M-00102
Programs sponsored in: AI, AN, APM, BBK, CCP, CD, CHN, CHP, CN, D, DMP, DR, END, FOP, FP, FSM, GE, GPM, GS, HMP, HO, HSO, ID, IM, IMG, MG, MPD, N, NEP, NM, NP, NPM, NS, OBG, OPH, ORS, OTO, P, PCC, PCP, PD, PDI, PDP, PDR, PDS, PG, PHO, PM, PS, PTH, PYG, RHU, RNR, RO, SCI, TS, U, VIR
Major participating institution for programs in: IM
Institution ID: 01-0498

University of Alabama School of Medicine
306 Medical Education Bldg
1813 Sixth Ave S
Birmingham, AL 35294-3293
Med Sch Affil: M-00102
Programs sponsored in: FP
Major participating institution for programs in: GPM
Institution ID: 01-0527

Veterans Affairs Medical Center (Birmingham)
700 S 19th St
Birmingham, AL 35233
Med Sch Affil: M-00102
Major participating institution for programs in: AN, CN, D, DMP, DR, GS, IM, IMG, N, NM, NP, NS, OPH, ORS, OTO, P, PCC, PCP, PS, PTH, PYG, RNR, RO, TS, U, VIR
Institution ID: 01-0500

Fairfield (Birmingham)

Lloyd Noland Hospital and Health Centers
701 Lloyd Noland Pkwy
Fairfield (Birmingham), AL 35064
Med Sch Affil: L-00102
Major participating institution for programs in: GS
Institution ID: 01-0488

Huntsville

Huntsville Hospital
101 Sivley Rd
Huntsville, AL 35801-9990
Med Sch Affil: M-00102
Major participating institution for programs in: FP, FSM
Institution ID: 01-0507

Mobile

University of South Alabama Medical Center
2451 Fillingim St
Mobile, AL 36617-2293
Med Sch Affil: M-00106
Programs sponsored in: CD, DR, FP, GE, GS, HO, ID, IM, MN, MPD, N, OBG, ORS, P, PD, PTH, PUD
Institution ID: 01-0406

USA Doctors Hospital
1700 Center St
Mobile, AL 36604-3391
Med Sch Affil: M-00106
Major participating institution for programs in: OBG, ORS, P
Institution ID: 01-8011

USA Knollwood Park Hospital
5600 Girby Rd
PO Box 9753
Mobile, AL 36691
Med Sch Affil: M-00106
Major participating institution for programs in: GE, ORS, P
Institution ID: 01-8010

Montgomery

Baptist Medical Center
PO Box 11010
2105 E South Blvd
Montgomery, AL 36111-1010
Med Sch Affil: G-00102
Major participating institution for programs in: FP, IM
Institution ID: 01-0309

Baptist Outreach Services
2055 E South Blvd
PO Box 11010
Montgomery, AL 36111-0010
Programs sponsored in: FP
Institution ID: 01-8012

Central Alabama Veterans Healthcare System
215 Perry Hill Rd
Montgomery, AL 36193
Med Sch Affil: M-01221
Major participating institution for programs in: P
Institution ID: 01-0306

Mount Vernon

Searcy State Hospital
PO Box 1001
Mount Vernon, AL 36560
Med Sch Affil: L-00106
Major participating institution for programs in: P
Institution ID: 01-0530

Selma

Four Rivers Medical Center
1015 Medical Center Pkwy
Selma, AL 36701
Med Sch Affil: G-00102
Programs sponsored in: FP
Institution ID: 01-0514

Vaughan Regional Medical Center
1050 W Dallas Ave
Selma, AL 36701
Med Sch Affil: G-00102
Major participating institution for programs in: FP
Institution ID: 01-0512

Tuscaloosa

DCH Regional Medical Center
809 University Blvd E
Tuscaloosa, AL 35401
Med Sch Affil: M-00102
Major participating institution for programs in: FP
Institution ID: 01-0510

University of Alabama College of Community Health Sciences
PO Box 870326
Tuscaloosa, AL 35487-0326
Med Sch Affil: M-00102
Programs sponsored in: FP
Institution ID: 01-0523

Alaska

Anchorage

Providence Hospital
3200 Provence Dr
PO Box 196604
Anchorage, AK 99519
Programs sponsored in: FP
Institution ID: 02-8001

Arizona

Phoenix

Carl T Hayden Veterans Affairs Medical Center (Phoenix)
650 E Indian School Rd
Phoenix, AZ 85012-1894
Med Sch Affil: L-00301
Major participating institution for programs in: CD, END, GE, GS, IM, IMG, ORS, PUD
Institution ID: 03-0504

Children's Rehabilitative Services
124 W Thomas Rd
Phoenix, AZ 85013-1134
Med Sch Affil: L-00301
Major participating institution for programs in: ORS
Institution ID: 03-0495

Good Samaritan Regional Medical Center
1111 E McDowell Rd
PO Box 52174
Phoenix, AZ 85062-2174
Med Sch Affil: M-00301
Programs sponsored in: CD, END, FP, GS, IM, IMG, MP, MPD, OBG, P, PUD
Major participating institution for programs in: GE, TY
Institution ID: 03-0345

Hand Surgery Associates
2610 N 3rd St
Phoenix, AZ 85004-1198
Major participating institution for programs in: HSO
Institution ID: 03-8023

Harrington Arthritis Research Center
300 N 18th St
Phoenix, AZ 85006
Major participating institution for programs in: ORS
Institution ID: 03-8021

Maricopa Medical Center
2601 E Roosevelt
Phoenix, AZ 85008
Med Sch Affil: M-00301
Programs sponsored in: EM, FP, GS, HSO, IM, MPD, OBG, ORS, P, TY
Major participating institution for programs in: AN, APM, CCA, END, FP, MPD, NS, PD
Institution ID: 03-0253

Mayo Clinic Hospital
5777 E Mayo Blvd
Phoenix, AZ 85054
Major participating institution for programs in: TY
Institution ID: 03-8029

Phoenix Area Medical Education Consortium
4001 N Third St/Ste 405
Phoenix, AZ 85012-2065
Programs sponsored in: TY
Institution ID: 03-8028

Phoenix Baptist Hospital and Medical Center
Family Medicine Ctr
PO Box 11469
Phoenix, AZ 85061
Med Sch Affil: L-00301
Programs sponsored in: FP
Institution ID: 03-0517

Phoenix Children's Hospital
1300 N 12th St/Ste 404
Phoenix, AZ 85006
Programs sponsored in: PD
Major participating institution for programs in: MPD
Institution ID: 03-8015

Phoenix Regional Medical Center
1947 E Thomas Rd
Phoenix, AZ 85016-7795
Institution ID: 03-8030

St Joseph's Hospital and Medical Center
350 W Thomas Rd
PO Box 2071
Phoenix, AZ 85001-2071
Med Sch Affil: M-00301, G-04815
Programs sponsored in: CHN, CN, DR, FP, FPG, IM, N, NS, PD, PTH, RNR
Major participating institution for programs in: GS, OBG, P
Institution ID: 03-0136

Scottsdale

Mayo Clinic (Scottsdale)
13400 E Shea Blvd
Scottsdale, AZ 85259
Med Sch Affil: M-02608
Major participating institution for programs in: AN, APM, GS, IM, OTO, TY
Institution ID: 03-8019

Scottsdale Healthcare Hospitals
7400 E Osborn Rd
Scottsdale, AZ 85251-5672
Med Sch Affil: M-02608
Programs sponsored in: FP
Institution ID: 03-0512

Scottsdale Healthcare-Shea
10450 N 92nd St
PO Box 4500
Scottsdale, AZ 85261
Major participating institution for programs in: AN, FP, GS, IM, TY
Institution ID: 03-8024

Tucson

Kino Community Hospital
2800 E Ajo Way
Tucson, AZ 85713-6289
Med Sch Affil: M-00301
Major participating institution for programs in: IM, OPH, P, TY, VIR
Institution ID: 03-0246

Tucson Hospitals Medical Education Program Inc
5301 E Grant Rd
Box 42195
Tucson, AZ 85733
Programs sponsored in: IM, TY
Institution ID: 03-0497

Tucson Medical Center
5301 E Grant Rd
PO Box 42195
Tucson, AZ 85733-2195
Med Sch Affil: M-00301
Major participating institution for programs in: GS, IM, ORS, PD, TY, U
Institution ID: 03-0235

University Medical Center
1501 N Campbell Ave
PO Box 245128
Tucson, AZ 85724
Med Sch Affil: M-00301
Major participating institution for programs in: AN, CCA, CD, CHP, D, DR, EM, END, FP, GE, GPM, GS, HO, ID, IM, IMG, MN, N, NEP, NM, OBG, OPH, ORS, P, PCC, PD, PDP, PHO, PTH, PYN, RHU, RNR, RO, TS, U, VS
Institution ID: 03-0506

University of Arizona College of Medicine
1501 N Campbell Ave
Tucson, AZ 85724-1111
Programs sponsored in: AN, APM, CCA, CD, CHP, D, DR, EM, END, FP, GE, GPM, GS, HO, ID, IM, IMG, MN, N, NEP, NM, OBG, OPH, ORS, P, PCC, PD, PDP, PHO, PTH, PYN, RHU, RNR, RO, TS, U, VIR, VS
Institution ID: 03-0509

Veterans Affairs Medical Center (Tucson)
3601 S 6th Ave
Tucson, AZ 85723
Med Sch Affil: M-00301
Major participating institution for programs in: AN, CD, D, DR, END, GE, GS, HO, ID, IM, IMG, MN, N, NEP, NM, OPH, ORS, P, PCC, PTH, PYN, RHU, RNR, TS, U, VIR
Institution ID: 03-0501

Teaching Institutions

Arkansas

El Dorado

Area Health Education Center (South Arkansas)
490 W Faulkner
El Dorado, AR 71730
Major participating institution for programs in: FP
Institution ID: 04-0481

Medical Center of South Arkansas
PO Box 1998
El Dorado, AR 71731-1998
Major participating institution for programs in: FP
Institution ID: 04-0476

Medical Center of South Arkansas
PO Box 1998
El Dorado, AR 71731-1998
Major participating institution for programs in: FP
Institution ID: 04-0477

Fayetteville

Area Health Education Center (Northwest)
241 West Spring St
Fayetteville, AR 72701
Major participating institution for programs in: FP
Institution ID: 04-0470

Washington Regional Medical Center
1125 N College
Fayetteville, AR 72703
Major participating institution for programs in: FP
Institution ID: 04-0473

Fort Smith

Sparks Regional Medical Center
PO Box 17006
Fort Smith, AR 72917-7006
Major participating institution for programs in: FP
Institution ID: 04-0467

Jonesboro

St Bernards Regional Medical Center
PO Box 9320
Jonesboro, AR 72403-9320
Major participating institution for programs in: FP
Institution ID: 04-0478

Little Rock

Arkansas Children's Hospital
800 Marshall St
Little Rock, AR 72202-3591
Med Sch Affil: M-00401
Major participating institution for programs in: AN, CCP, CHN, CHP, GS, HSO, MPD, NPM, NS, OPH, ORS, OTO, P, PAN, PD, PDE, PDI, PDR, PDS, PG, PM, PTH, RNR, TS, TY, U
Institution ID: 04-0284

Arkansas State Crime Laboratory
3 Natural Resources Dr
PO Box 5274
Little Rock, AR 72215
Med Sch Affil: G-00401
Major participating institution for programs in: FOP
Institution ID: 04-8021

Arkansas State Hospital-Little Rock Hospital
4313 W Markham St
Little Rock, AR 72205-4096
Med Sch Affil: G-00401
Major participating institution for programs in: CHP, P
Institution ID: 04-0307

Baptist Medical Center
9601 I-630 Exit #7
Little Rock, AR 72205-7299
Med Sch Affil: L-00401
Major participating institution for programs in: TY
Institution ID: 04-0350

Baptist Rehabilitation Institute
9601 I-630 Exit #7
Little Rock, AR 72205-7249
Med Sch Affil: L-00401
Major participating institution for programs in: PM
Institution ID: 04-8015

John L McClellan Memorial Veterans Hospital
4300 W 7th St
Little Rock, AR 72205-5484
Med Sch Affil: M-00401
Major participating institution for programs in: AN, CD, CHN, D, DMP, DR, END, FP, GE, GS, HEM, HMP, HSO, ID, IM, IMG, MPD, N, NEP, NM, NS, ON, OPH, ORS, OTO, P, PCC, PCP, PM, PTH, RHU, RNR, TS, TY, U, VIR, VS
Institution ID: 04-0349

St Vincent Infirmary Medical Center
2 St Vincent Cir
Little Rock, AR 72205-5499
Med Sch Affil: L-00401
Major participating institution for programs in: TY
Institution ID: 04-0463

UAMS-Area Health Education Centers
4301 W Markham St
Slot 599
Little Rock, AR 72205
Med Sch Affil: M-00401
Programs sponsored in: FP
Institution ID: 04-8018

University Hospital of Arkansas
4301 W Markham St
Slot 719
Little Rock, AR 72205
Med Sch Affil: M-00401
Programs sponsored in: MPD
Major participating institution for programs in: AN, CD, CHP, D, DMP, DR, EM, END, FP, GE, GS, HEM, HMP, ID, IM, IMG, N, NEP, NM, NPM, NS, OBG, ON, OPH, ORS, OTO, P, PCC, PD, PDI, PDR, PM, PTH, RHU, RNR, TS, U, VIR, VS
Institution ID: 04-0261

University of Arkansas College of Medicine
4301 W Markham St
Little Rock, AR 72205-7199
Med Sch Affil: M-00401
Programs sponsored in: AN, CCP, CD, CHN, CHP, D, DMP, DR, EM, END, FOP, FP, GE, GS, HEM, HMP, HSO, ID, IM, IMG, N, NEP, NM, NPM, NS, OBG, ON, OPH, ORS, OTO, P, PAN, PCC, PCP, PD, PDE, PDI, PDR, PDS, PG, PM, PTH, RHU, RNR, TS, TY, U, VIR, VS
Institution ID: 04-9501

Pine Bluff

Jefferson Regional Medical Center
1515 W 42nd Ave
Pine Bluff, AR 71603
Major participating institution for programs in: FP
Institution ID: 04-0465

Texarkana

Health Care Center
2600 St Michael Dr
PO Box 1140
Texarkana, TX 75504
Major participating institution for programs in: FP
Institution ID: 04-7012

California

Anaheim

Kaiser Foundation Hospitals (Anaheim)
Anaheim Med Ctr
441 Lakeview Ave
Anaheim, CA 92807
Major participating institution for programs in: FP, IMG, U
Institution ID: 05-8043

Atascadero

Atascadero State Hospital
10333 El Camino Real
PO Box 7001
Atascadero, CA 93423-7001
Major participating institution for programs in: PFP
Institution ID: 05-8097

Bakersfield

Kern Medical Center
1830 Flower St
Bakersfield, CA 93305-4197
Med Sch Affil: G-00518, G-00514
Programs sponsored in: EM, FP, GS, IM, OBG, TY
Institution ID: 05-0120

Bellflower

Kaiser Foundation Hospital (Bellflower)
9400 Rosecrans Ave
Bellflower, CA 90706-2246
Major participating institution for programs in: U
Institution ID: 05-8046

Berkeley

Permanente Medical Group Regional Laboratory
1725 Eastshore Hwy
Berkeley, CA 94710
Major participating institution for programs in: PTH
Institution ID: 05-8036

University of California School of Public Health
140 Earl Warren Hall
Berkeley, CA 94720-7360
Med Sch Affil: L-00502
Programs sponsored in: GPM
Major participating institution for programs in: GPM
Institution ID: 05-0376

Camp Pendleton

Naval Hospital (Camp Pendleton)

Attn: Dir of Med Service
Box 555191
Camp Pendleton, CA 92055-5191
Med Sch Affil: L-00518, G-02312
Programs sponsored in: FP
Major participating institution for programs in: FSM
Institution ID: 05-0320

Cerritos

College Hospital

10802 College Pl
Cerritos, CA 90701
Major participating institution for programs in: CHP
Institution ID: 05-8091

Chula Vista

Scripps Memorial Hospital-Chula Vista

435 H St
Chula Vista, CA 91910-1537
Programs sponsored in: FP
Institution ID: 05-8098

Sharp Chula Vista Medical Center

751 Medical Center Ct
PO Box 1297
Chula Vista, CA 91912
Major participating institution for programs in: FP
Institution ID: 05-8081

Daly City

Seton Medical Center

1900 Sullivan Ave
Daly City, CA 94015
Med Sch Affil: L-00502
Major participating institution for programs in: RO
Institution ID: 05-0494

Davis

Sutter Davis Hospital

Rd 99 at Covell Blvd
PO Box 1617
Davis, CA 95617
Major participating institution for programs in: FP
Institution ID: 05-0728

University of California (Davis) School of Medicine

Health Sciences Dr
Davis, CA 95616
Med Sch Affil: M-00519
Programs sponsored in: GPM, GS
Institution ID: 05-9502

Downey

LAC-Rancho Los Amigos Medical Center

7601 E Imperial Hwy/117HB
Downey, CA 90242
Med Sch Affil: M-00506, G-00515, G-01401
Major participating institution for programs in: END, ID, ORS, PS, RHU
Institution ID: 05-0504

Duarte

City of Hope National Medical Center

1500 E Duarte Rd
Duarte, CA 91010-0269
Med Sch Affil: L-00506, G-00518, G-00515
Programs sponsored in: HMP
Major participating institution for programs in: GS, HO, PS, RO
Institution ID: 05-0233

Fairfield

Solano County Mental Health Clinic

1735-3 Enterprise Dr
Fairfield, CA 94533
Major participating institution for programs in: P
Institution ID: 05-8008

Fontana

Kaiser Foundation Hospital (Fontana)

9961 Sierra Ave
Fontana, CA 92335
Med Sch Affil: L-00512, G-00518
Major participating institution for programs in: FP, FSM, GS, PS
Institution ID: 05-0576

Fresno

UCSF-Fresno Medical Education Program

2615 E Clinton Ave
Fresno, CA 93703
Programs sponsored in: CCS, DR, EM, FP, GS, IM, OBG, P, PD, TY
Institution ID: 05-9501

University Medical Center

445 S Cedar Ave
Fresno, CA 93702-2907
Med Sch Affil: M-00502
Major participating institution for programs in: CCS, DR, EM, FP, GS, IM, OBG, P, PD, TY
Institution ID: 05-0485

Valley Children's Hospital

3151 N Millbrook Ave
Fresno, CA 93703-1497
Med Sch Affil: M-00502
Major participating institution for programs in: GS, PD
Institution ID: 05-7058

Veterans Affairs Medical Center (Fresno)

2615 E Clinton Ave
Fresno, CA 93703
Med Sch Affil: M-00502
Major participating institution for programs in: DR, GS, IM, P
Institution ID: 05-0581

Glendale

Glendale Adventist Medical Center

1509 Wilson Terr
Glendale, CA 91206
Med Sch Affil: L-00512
Programs sponsored in: FP, OBG
Institution ID: 05-0116

Inglewood

Centinela Hospital Medical Center

555 E Hardy St
Inglewood, CA 90307
Major participating institution for programs in: OSM
Institution ID: 05-0792

Kerlan-Jobe Orthopaedic Clinic

501 E Hardy St/Ste 420
Inglewood, CA 90301
Programs sponsored in: OSM
Institution ID: 05-8067

Irvine

University of California (Irvine) College of Medicine

Irvine Hall Bldg
Irvine, CA 92717-4089
Major participating institution for programs in: ALI, GPM
Institution ID: 05-0741

La Jolla

Scripps Clinic

10666 N Torrey Pines Rd/403C
La Jolla, CA 92037-1093
Med Sch Affil: L-00518
Programs sponsored in: AI, CD, END, GE, HEM, IM, ON, RHU
Institution ID: 05-0225

Scripps Green Hospital

10666 N Torrey Pines Rd
La Jolla, CA 92037
Major participating institution for programs in: AI, CD, END, GE, HEM, IM, ON, RHU
Institution ID: 05-8106

La Mesa

Grossmont Hospital

5555 Grossmont Ctr Rd
PO Box 158
La Mesa, CA 91944-0158
Major participating institution for programs in: FP, FSM
Institution ID: 05-0566

Loma Linda

Jerry L Pettis Memorial Veterans Hospital

11201 Benton St
Loma Linda, CA 92357-1111
Med Sch Affil: M-00512
Major participating institution for programs in: CD, D, DR, GE, GS, IM, MPD, N, NS, OPH, ORS, OTO, P, PCC, PM, PS, PTH, RHU, TS, U
Institution ID: 05-0748

Loma Linda University Community Hospital

25333 Barton Rd
Loma Linda, CA 92354
Med Sch Affil: M-00512
Programs sponsored in: FP
Major participating institution for programs in: MPD
Institution ID: 05-8044

Loma Linda University Medical Center

11234 Anderson St
Loma Linda, CA 92354
Med Sch Affil: M-00512, L-02312, G-00515
Programs sponsored in: AN, APM, CCP, CD, CHN, D, DR, EM, GE, GPM, GS, HSO, IM, MPD, N, NPM, NS, OBG, OPH, ORS, OTO, P, PCC, PD, PDR, PM, PS, PTH, RHU, RNR, RO, TS, U, VIR, VS
Major participating institution for programs in: OBG
Institution ID: 05-0238

Long Beach

Long Beach Memorial Medical Center
2801 Atlantic Ave
PO Box 1428
Long Beach, CA 90801-1428
Med Sch Affil: M-00515, L-00514
Programs sponsored in: BBK, FP, OSM
Major participating institution for programs in: CCP, CD, DR, EM, GE, GS, HEM, IM, IMG, MPD, NPM, OBG, ON, OPH, PD, PDP, PG, PM, PTH, RO
Institution ID: 05-0195

Southern California Center for Sports Medicine
2760 Atlantic Ave
Long Beach, CA 90806
Major participating institution for programs in: OSM
Institution ID: 05-8062

St Mary Medical Center
1050 Linden Ave
PO Box 887
Long Beach, CA 90801
Med Sch Affil: L-00514
Programs sponsored in: IM
Major participating institution for programs in: GS, VS
Institution ID: 05-0267

Veterans Affairs Medical Center (Long Beach)
5901 E 7th St
Long Beach, CA 90822-5201
Med Sch Affil: M-00515
Programs sponsored in: NM
Major participating institution for programs in: AI, AN, CCA, CD, D, DMP, DR, END, GE, GS, HEM, ID, N, NEP, ON, OPH, ORS, OTO, P, PCC, PM, PS, PTH, RHU, RO, U
Institution ID: 05-0186

Los Angeles

American Red Cross Blood Services-South Calif Region
1130 S Vermont Ave
Los Angeles, CA 90006-0908
Major participating institution for programs in: BBK
Institution ID: 05-0764

Barlow Respiratory Hospital
2000 Stadium Way
Los Angeles, CA 90026-2696
Med Sch Affil: L-00506
Major participating institution for programs in: PCC
Institution ID: 05-7025

California Hospital Medical Center
1401 S Grand Ave
Los Angeles, CA 90015
Med Sch Affil: G-00506
Programs sponsored in: FP
Major participating institution for programs in: GS
Institution ID: 05-0231

Cedars-Sinai Medical Center
8700 Beverly Blvd
Los Angeles, CA 90048-1869
Med Sch Affil: M-00514, G-04815
Programs sponsored in: BBK, CCM, CCS, CD, CHP, DR, END, GS, HMP, HO, ICE, IM, MG, MPD, NEP, NM, NPM, OBG, P, PCC, PD, PN, PTH, RHU
Major participating institution for programs in: AN, GE, GS, HO, ID, NEP, PM
Institution ID: 05-0545

Central Juvenile Hall
1605 Eastlake Ave
Los Angeles, CA 90033
Institution ID: 05-8101

Charles R Drew University of Medicine and Science
1621 E 120th St
Los Angeles, CA 90059
Med Sch Affil: M-00502
Programs sponsored in: AN, D, DR, EM, END, FP, GE, GS, ID, IM, IMG, OBG, OPH, ORS, OTO, P, PD
Institution ID: 05-0590

Children's Hospital of Los Angeles
4650 Sunset Blvd
Los Angeles, CA 90027
Med Sch Affil: M-00506, G-00515
Programs sponsored in: ADL, CCP, PD, PDC, PDE, PDI, PDP, PDR, PDS, PG, PHO, PN, SP
Major participating institution for programs in: AI, CHN, GS, NS, ORS, OTO, PS, RNR, TS
Institution ID: 05-0344

County of Los Angeles-Department of Coroner
1104 N Mission Rd
Los Angeles, CA 90033
Programs sponsored in: FOP
Institution ID: 05-0553

Joseph H Boyes Foundation
1510 San Pablo/Ste 300
Los Angeles, CA 90033
Major participating institution for programs in: HSO
Institution ID: 05-8075

Kaiser Foundation Hospital (Los Angeles)
4867 Sunset Blvd
Los Angeles, CA 90027
Med Sch Affil: M-00514
Major participating institution for programs in: AI, CD, DR, FP, FPG, GE, GS, ID, IM, N, NEP, OBG, PD, RO, U
Institution ID: 05-0285

Kaiser Foundation Hospital (West Los Angeles)
6041 Cadillac Ave
Los Angeles, CA 90034
Med Sch Affil: G-00514
Major participating institution for programs in: PS
Institution ID: 05-0742

Kenneth Norris Jr Cancer Hospital and Research Institute
1441 Eastlake Ave
Los Angeles, CA 90033
Med Sch Affil: M-00506
Major participating institution for programs in: CRS, RO, U, VIR
Institution ID: 05-0793

LAC-King/Drew Medical Center
12021 S Wilmington Ave
Los Angeles, CA 90059-3019
Med Sch Affil: M-00514, L-00506
Major participating institution for programs in: AN, CCP, D, DR, EM, END, FP, GE, GS, ID, IM, IMG, NPM, OBG, OPH, ORS, OTO, P, PD
Institution ID: 05-0577

Los Angeles County-USC Medical Center
1200 N State St/Rm 1112
Los Angeles, CA 90033
Med Sch Affil: M-00506, G-01401
Programs sponsored in: AI, AN, BBK, CCS, CD, CHN, CHP, CRS, D, DR, EM, END, GE, GS, HEM, HMP, HSO, HSP, ICE, ID, IM, IMG, MN, MPD, N, NEP, NP, NPM, NS, OBG, ON, OPH, ORS, OTO, P, PCC, PCP, PD, PFP, PS, PTH, RHU, RNR, RO, TS, U, VIR
Major participating institution for programs in: FP, GS, P
Institution ID: 05-0557

Orthopaedic Hospital
2400 S Flower St
Los Angeles, CA 90007
Med Sch Affil: M-00506
Major participating institution for programs in: ORS
Institution ID: 05-0347

Shriners Hospital for Children (Los Angeles)
3160 Geneva St
Los Angeles, CA 90020-1199
Med Sch Affil: L-00514
Major participating institution for programs in: ORS
Institution ID: 05-0367

St Vincent Medical Center
2131 W Third St
Los Angeles, CA 90057
Med Sch Affil: L-00506, G-00515
Major participating institution for programs in: CD, NEP
Institution ID: 05-0382

UCLA Medical Center
10833 Le Conte Ave
Los Angeles, CA 90024-1705
Med Sch Affil: M-00514
Major participating institution for programs in: AI, AN, BBK, CCM, CCP, CD, CHN, CN, D, DR, EM, EMP, END, FP, FSM, GE, GS, HEM, HMP, HSO, ID, IM, IMG, MG, N, NEP, NM, NP, NPM, NS, OBG, ON, ORS, OTO, PCC, PCP, PD, PDC, PDE, PDI, PDR, PG, PHO, PN, PS, PTH, RHU, RNR, RO, TS, U, VIR, VS
Institution ID: 05-0555

UCLA Neuropsychiatric Hospital
760 Westwood Plaza/Rm C8-852
Los Angeles, CA 90024-1759
Med Sch Affil: M-00514
Major participating institution for programs in: CHP, P, PYG
Institution ID: 05-0722

UCLA School of Medicine
10833 Le Conte Ave
Los Angeles, CA 90024
Med Sch Affil: L-02312
Programs sponsored in: AI, AN, APM, BBK, CCM, CCP, CD, CHN, CHP, CN, D, DR, EM, EMP, END, FP, FSM, GE, GPM, GS, HEM, HMP, HSO, ID, IM, IMG, N, NEP, NM, NP, NPM, NS, OBG, ON, OPH, ORS, OTO, P, PCC, PCP, PD, PDC, PDE, PDI, PDR, PG, PHO, PN, PS, PTH, PYG, RHU, RNR, RO, TS, U, VIR, VS
Institution ID: 05-9503

UCLA School of Public Health
Dean's Office
16-035 CHS
10833 Le Conte Ave
Los Angeles, CA 90095-1772
Major participating institution for programs in: GPM
Institution ID: 05-0514

University of Southern California School of Medicine
1975 Zonal Ave/KAM 500
Los Angeles, CA 90033
Med Sch Affil: M-00506
Programs sponsored in: FP, GPM
Institution ID: 05-0753

USC University Hospital
1500 San Pablo St
Los Angeles, CA 90033
Med Sch Affil: M-00506
Major participating institution for programs in: END, FP, GS, ICE, NS, ORS, OTO, PS, VIR
Institution ID: 05-8065

VA Greater Los Angeles Healthcare System
11301 Wilshire Blvd
Los Angeles, CA 90073
Programs sponsored in: AI, CD, END, HO, ICE, ID, IM, N, NEP, NM, P, PM, PTH, RHU
Major participating institution for programs in: AN, D, DR, END, GE, GS, HEM, HSO, IMG, NEP, NS, ON, OPH, ORS, OTO, PCC, PS, PYG, RHU, RO, U
Institution ID: 05-8105

White Memorial Medical Center
1720 Brooklyn Ave
Los Angeles, CA 90033-2481
Med Sch Affil: L-00512
Programs sponsored in: FP, IM, OBG, PD
Major participating institution for programs in: FP
Institution ID: 05-0353

Martinez

Contra Costa Regional Medical Center
2500 Alhambra Ave
Martinez, CA 94553-3191
Med Sch Affil: G-00519
Programs sponsored in: FP
Institution ID: 05-0271

Marysville

Rideout Memorial Hospital
726 Fourth St
Box 2128
Marysville, CA 95901-2128
Institution ID: 05-8104

Merced

Sutter Merced Medical Center
301 E 13th St
PO Box 231
Merced, CA 95340
Med Sch Affil: G-00519
Programs sponsored in: FP
Institution ID: 05-0715

Modesto

Doctors Medical Center
1441 Florida Ave
PO Box 4138
Modesto, CA 95352-4138
Major participating institution for programs in: FP
Institution ID: 05-8099

Stanislaus County Health Services
830 Scenic Dr
Modesto, CA 95350
Programs sponsored in: FP
Institution ID: 05-8102

Moreno Valley

Riverside County Regional Medical Center
26520 Cactus Ave
Moreno Valley, CA 92555
Med Sch Affil: M-00512, L-00514
Programs sponsored in: FP
Major participating institution for programs in: EM, GS, MPD, OBG, OPH, OTO, PD, PS
Institution ID: 05-0260

North Hollywood

Medical Center of North Hollywood
1629 Riverside Dr
North Hollywood, CA 91607-3495
Major participating institution for programs in: FP
Institution ID: 05-8095

Northridge

Northridge Hospital Medical Center
18300 Roscoe Blvd
Northridge, CA 91328
Med Sch Affil: L-00514
Programs sponsored in: FP
Institution ID: 05-0726

Oakland

Alameda County Medical Center
1411 E 31st St
Oakland, CA 94602-1093
Med Sch Affil: L-00502, G-00519
Programs sponsored in: EM, IM, TY
Major participating institution for programs in: GS, OPH, ORS
Institution ID: 05-0413

Children's Hospital-Oakland
747 52nd St
Oakland, CA 94609
Med Sch Affil: M-00502
Programs sponsored in: PD, PDI, PHO
Major participating institution for programs in: CCP, PDR
Institution ID: 05-0110

Kaiser Permanente Medical Center (Oakland)
280 W MacArthur Blvd
Oakland, CA 94611-5693
Med Sch Affil: L-00502, G-00519
Major participating institution for programs in: GS, IM, OBG, OTO, PD
Institution ID: 05-0296

Kaiser Permanente Medical Group (Northern California)
1800 Harrison St/21st Fl
Oakland, CA 94612
Programs sponsored in: IM, OBG, OTO, PD, PTH
Major participating institution for programs in: IM
Institution ID: 05-8090

Naval Hospital (Oakland)
8750 Mountain Blvd
Oakland, CA 94627-5000
Med Sch Affil: M-02312
Major participating institution for programs in: GS
Institution ID: 05-0194

Orange

Children's Hospital of Orange County
455 S Main St
Orange, CA 92868
Med Sch Affil: G-00515
Programs sponsored in: PD, PHO, PPR
Major participating institution for programs in: CCP, MPD, ORS
Institution ID: 05-0547

St Joseph Hospital
1100 W Stewart Dr
Orange, CA 92668-5600
Med Sch Affil: L-00515
Major participating institution for programs in: GS, PD, PPR
Institution ID: 05-0749

University of California (Irvine) Medical Center
101 The City Dr
Rte 62
Orange, CA 92868
Med Sch Affil: M-00515
Programs sponsored in: AI, ALI, AN, APM, CCA, CCS, CD, CHN, CHP, D, DMP, DR, EM, END, FP, GE, GPM, GS, HEM, ID, IM, IMG, MG, N, NEP, NPM, OBG, ON, OPH, ORS, OTO, P, PCC, PD, PDP, PG, PM, PS, PTH, RHU, RO, U, VIR
Major participating institution for programs in: NM, PPR
Institution ID: 05-0564

Palo Alto

Lucile Salter Packard Children's Hospital at Stanford
725 Welch Rd
Palo Alto, CA 94304
Med Sch Affil: M-00511
Major participating institution for programs in: AI, CCP, CN, HSO, ORS, PAN, PD, PDE, PDI, PDR, PG, PHO, PN, U
Institution ID: 05-0572

Veterans Affairs Palo Alto Health Care System
3801 Miranda Ave
Palo Alto, CA 94304-1207
Med Sch Affil: M-00511
Major participating institution for programs in: CD, CHN, D, DR, END, GE, GS, HEM, HSO, ICE, ID, IM, IMG, N, NM, NP, NS, ON, OPH, ORS, OTO, P, PM, PS, PTH, RHU, SCI, TS, U
Institution ID: 05-0273

Pasadena

Huntington Memorial Hospital
100 W California Blvd
PO Box 7013
Pasadena, CA 91109-7013
Med Sch Affil: M-00506
Programs sponsored in: GS, IM
Institution ID: 05-0474

Southern California Kaiser Permanente Medical Group
393 E Walnut St/7th Fl
Pasadena, CA 90027
Programs sponsored in: AI, CD, DR, FP, FPG, FSM, GE, GS, ID, IM, N, NEP, OBG, PD, RO, U
Major participating institution for programs in: TS
Institution ID: 05-8072

Patton

Patton State Hospital
3102 E Highland Ave
Patton, CA 92369
Institution ID: 05-0149

Pomona

Pomona Valley Hospital Medical Center
1798 N Garey Ave
Pomona, CA 91767
Programs sponsored in: FP
Institution ID: 05-8094

Redding

Mercy Medical Center
Clairmont Heights
PO Box 496009
Redding, CA 96049-6009
Med Sch Affil: G-00519
Programs sponsored in: FP
Institution ID: 05-0745

Redwood City

Kaiser Permanente Medical Center (Redwood City)
1150 Veterans Blvd
Redwood City, CA 94063
Med Sch Affil: L-00511
Major participating institution for programs in: OTO
Institution ID: 05-8029

Riverside

Kaiser Foundation Hospital (Riverside)
10800 Magnolia Ave
Riverside, CA 92505-3000
Major participating institution for programs in: FP, N
Institution ID: 05-8066

Sacramento

California Department of Health Services
714 P St/Rm 1253
PO Box 942732
Sacramento, CA 94234-7320
Programs sponsored in: GPM
Institution ID: 05-0202

Kaiser Foundation Hospital (Sacramento)
2025 Morse Ave
Sacramento, CA 95825
Med Sch Affil: M-00519
Major participating institution for programs in: GE, GS, HO, IM, MPD, NS, OBG, U, VIR
Institution ID: 05-0578

Kaiser Foundation Hospital (South Sacramento)
6600 Bruceville Rd
Sacramento, CA 95823-4691
Major participating institution for programs in: EM, GS, U
Institution ID: 05-8048

Methodist Hospital of Sacramento
7500 Hospital Dr
Sacramento, CA 95823
Programs sponsored in: FP
Institution ID: 05-8089

North California Forensic Pathology
4400 V St
Sacramento, CA 95817
Programs sponsored in: FOP
Institution ID: 05-0724

Shriners Hospitals for Children (Sacramento)
2425 Stockton Blvd
Sacramento, CA 95817
Med Sch Affil: L-00502
Major participating institution for programs in: ORS, PPR
Institution ID: 05-0239

Sutter General Hospital
2801 L St
Sacramento, CA 95816
Med Sch Affil: M-00519
Major participating institution for programs in: FP
Institution ID: 05-0241

Sutter Health
PO Box 160727
Sacramento, CA 95816
Programs sponsored in: FP
Institution ID: 05-8085

Sutter Memorial Hospital
5151 F Street
Sacramento, CA 95819
Major participating institution for programs in: FP
Institution ID: 05-8084

University of California (Davis) Medical Center
2315 Stockton Blvd
Sacramento, CA 95817
Med Sch Affil: M-00519, L-02312
Programs sponsored in: AI, AN, APM, CCS, CD, CHP, CN, D, DR, EM, END, FP, FPP, GE, GS, HMP, HO, HSO, ID, IM, IMG, MPD, N, NEP, NM, NPM, NS, OBG, OPH, ORS, OTO, P, PCC, PD, PM, PS, PTH, TS, U, VIR
Major participating institution for programs in: FOP, FP, GPM, RO
Institution ID: 05-0436

Salinas

Natividad Medical Center
1330 Natividad Rd
PO Box 81611
Salinas, CA 93912-1611
Med Sch Affil: M-00502
Programs sponsored in: FP
Institution ID: 05-0160

San Bernardino

San Bernardino County Coroner's Office
175 S Lena Rd
San Bernardino, CA 92415-0037
Programs sponsored in: FOP
Institution ID: 05-8073

San Bernardino County Medical Center
780 E Gilbert St
San Bernardino, CA 92415-0935
Med Sch Affil: L-00512, G-00515
Programs sponsored in: FP, FPG, TY
Major participating institution for programs in: AN, GS, HSO, OBG, ORS, OTO, U
Institution ID: 05-0207

San Diego

Alvarado Hospital Medical Center
6655 Alvarado Rd
San Diego, CA 92120
Programs sponsored in: OSM
Major participating institution for programs in: FSM
Institution ID: 05-8086

Children's Hospital and Health Center
3020 Children's Way/Rm 5064
San Diego, CA 92123-4282
Med Sch Affil: M-00518
Major participating institution for programs in: AN, CCP, CHN, CHP, MG, NPM, NS, OP, ORS, PD, PDE, PDI, PG, PN, PS, U, UP
Institution ID: 05-0533

Graduate School of Public Health
5500 Campanile Dr
San Diego, CA 92182
Med Sch Affil: L-00518
Major participating institution for programs in: GPM
Institution ID: 05-8030

Kaiser Foundation Hospital (San Diego)
4647 Zion Ave
San Diego, CA 92120
Med Sch Affil: G-00518
Major participating institution for programs in: NS, OBG, OTO
Institution ID: 05-0760

Naval Medical Center (San Diego)
34800 Bob Wilson Dr
San Diego, CA 92134-5000
Med Sch Affil: M-00518, M-02312, L-02012
Programs sponsored in: AN, CCP, CD, D, DR, EM, GE, GS, ID, IM, OBG, OPH, ORS, OTO, P, PCC, PD, PTH, TY, U, UP
Major participating institution for programs in: NEP
Institution ID: 05-0386

San Diego County Medical Examiner
5555 Overland Ave/Bldg #14
San Diego, CA 92123
Programs sponsored in: FOP
Institution ID: 05-8061

Scripps Mercy Hospital
4077 5th Ave
San Diego, CA 92103-2180
Med Sch Affil: M-00518
Programs sponsored in: IM, TY
Major participating institution for programs in: CD
Institution ID: 05-0397

Sharp HealthCare
3131 Berger Ave
San Diego, CA 92123
Programs sponsored in: FP, FSM
Institution ID: 05-8076

University of California (San Diego) Medical Center
200 W Arbor Dr
San Diego, CA 92103-8970
Med Sch Affil: M-00518
Programs sponsored in: AI, AN, APM, CCS, CD, CHN, CHP, D, DR, EM, END, FP, FPP, FSM, GE, GPM, GS, HO, HSO, ICE, ID, IM, IMG, MG, MPD, N, NEP, NM, NP, NPM, NS, OBG, OP, OPH, ORS, OTO, P, PCC, PD, PDC, PDE, PDI, PG, PN, PS, PTH, PYG, RHU, RNR, TS, U, VIR
Major participating institution for programs in: OSM
Institution ID: 05-0434

Veterans Affairs Medical Center (San Diego)

3350 La Jolla Village Dr
San Diego, CA 92161-4223
Med Sch Affil: M-00518
Major participating institution for programs in: AN, APM, CD, CHN, D, DR, END, GE, GS, HO, HSO, ID, IM, IMG, N, NEP, NM, NP, OPH, ORS, OTO, P, PCC, PS, PTH, PYG, RHU, TS, U, VIR
Institution ID: 05-0589

San Francisco

Blood Centers of the Pacific

270 Masonic Ave
San Francisco, CA 94118-4496
Programs sponsored in: BBK
Institution ID: 05-0767

California Pacific Medical Center

2351 Clay
PO Box 7999
San Francisco, CA 94120
Programs sponsored in: CD, GE, HSO, IM, OPH, P, PUD
Institution ID: 05-8082

California Pacific Medical Center

PO Box 7999
2351 Clay
San Francisco, CA 94120
Med Sch Affil: L-00502
Major participating institution for programs in: CD, GE, HSO, IM, OPH, P, PUD
Institution ID: 05-0432

California Pacific Medical Center (California Campus)

PO Box 7999
2351 Clay
San Francisco, CA 94120
Med Sch Affil: M-00502
Major participating institution for programs in: CN
Institution ID: 05-0190

Davies Medical Center

Castro and Duboce Sts
San Francisco, CA 94114
Med Sch Affil: G-00502
Major participating institution for programs in: HSP, PS
Institution ID: 05-0469

Kaiser Permanente Medical Center (San Francisco)

2425 Geary Blvd
San Francisco, CA 94115-3395
Med Sch Affil: L-00502
Major participating institution for programs in: GS, IM, OBG, ORS, OTO, PTH
Institution ID: 05-0204

Langley Porter Psychiatric Hospitals and Clinics

401 Parnassus Ave/Box ADM-0984
San Francisco, CA 94143-0984
Med Sch Affil: M-00502
Major participating institution for programs in: P
Institution ID: 05-0122

Mount Zion Medical Center of the University of California

PO Box 7921
San Francisco, CA 94120-7921
Med Sch Affil: M-00502
Major participating institution for programs in: AN, APM, GS, ID, IM, IMG, NS, OBG, P, PD, PDI, RNR, RO, TS
Institution ID: 05-0289

San Francisco General Hospital Medical Center

1001 Potrero Avenue
Suite 2A5
San Francisco, CA 94110
Med Sch Affil: M-00502
Major participating institution for programs in: AN, CCA, CD, CHN, CN, D, DR, END, FP, GE, GPM, GS, HO, HSO, ID, IM, MN, N, NEP, NP, NS, OBG, OPH, ORS, OTO, P, PCC, PCP, PD, PDI, PHO, PS, PTH, RHU, U
Institution ID: 05-0334

San Francisco SurgiCentre

1635 Divisadero St
San Francisco, CA 94115
Major participating institution for programs in: HSO
Institution ID: 05-8074

St Mary's Hospital and Medical Center

450 Stanyan St
San Francisco, CA 94117-1079
Med Sch Affil: L-00502
Programs sponsored in: CD, IM, ORS, RO
Institution ID: 05-0163

University of California (San Francisco) Medical Center

500 Parnassus Ave
5th Fl MU East
San Francisco, CA 94143-0296
Med Sch Affil: M-00502
Programs sponsored in: AI
Major participating institution for programs in: AN, BBK, CCA, CCM, CCP, CD, CHN, CHP, CN, D, DR, END, GE, GS, HMP, HO, HSP, ICE, ID, IM, MG, N, NEP, NM, NP, NPM, NS, OBG, OPH, ORS, OTO, P, PCC, PD, PDC, PDE, PDI, PDP, PDR, PG, PHO, PN, PPR, PS, PTH, RHU, RNR, RO, TS, U, UP, VIR, VS
Institution ID: 05-0554

University of California (San Francisco) School of Medicine

513 Parnassus Ave
San Francisco, CA 94143-0410
Med Sch Affil: M-00502
Programs sponsored in: AN, APM, CCA, CCM, CCP, CD, CHN, CHP, CN, D, DMP, DR, END, FP, GE, GPM, GS, HMP, HO, HSO, HSP, ICE, ID, IM, IMG, MG, MN, N, NEP, NM, NP, NPM, NS, OBG, OPH, ORS, OTO, P, PCC, PCP, PD, PDC, PDE, PDI, PDP, PDR, PG, PHO, PN, PPR, PS, PTH, RHU, RNR, RO, TS, U, UP, VIR, VS
Institution ID: 05-0737

Veterans Affairs Medical Center (San Francisco)

4150 Clement St
San Francisco, CA 94121-1598
Med Sch Affil: M-00502
Major participating institution for programs in: CD, CHN, D, DR, END, GE, GS, HO, ID, IM, MN, N, NEP, NP, NS, OPH, ORS, OTO, P, PCC, PS, PTH, RHU, RNR, TS, U
Institution ID: 05-0113

San Jose

San Jose Medical Center

675 E Santa Clara St
San Jose, CA 95112
Med Sch Affil: L-00511
Programs sponsored in: FP, FSM
Institution ID: 05-0723

Santa Clara Valley Medical Center

2220 Moorpark Ave
San Jose, CA 95128-2699
Med Sch Affil: M-00511
Programs sponsored in: DR, IM, OBG, TY
Major participating institution for programs in: AN, CHN, D, END, GE, GS, ID, N, OPH, ORS, OTO, PD, PM, U
Institution ID: 05-0438

Santa Teresa Community Hospital

250 Hospital Pkwy
San Jose, CA 95119
Major participating institution for programs in: ICE
Institution ID: 05-8092

San Mateo

San Mateo County General Hospital

222 W 39th Ave
San Mateo, CA 94403-0222
Programs sponsored in: P
Institution ID: 05-0585

San Rafael

Marin County Mental Health Services

20 N San Pedro Rd/Ste 2028
San Rafael, CA 94903
Major participating institution for programs in: P
Institution ID: 05-8041

Santa Ana

Western Medical Center

1001 N Tustin Ave
Santa Ana, CA 92705
Med Sch Affil: G-00515
Major participating institution for programs in: FP
Institution ID: 05-0747

Santa Barbara

Santa Barbara Cottage Hospital

PO Box 689
Santa Barbara, CA 93102
Med Sch Affil: L-00514, L-00506
Programs sponsored in: DR, GS, IM
Institution ID: 05-0381

Santa Barbara County Health Care Services

300 N San Antonio Rd
Santa Barbara, CA 93110
Major participating institution for programs in: IM
Institution ID: 05-0588

Santa Clara

Kaiser Permanente Medical Center (Santa Clara)

900 Kiely Blvd
Santa Clara, CA 95051-5386
Med Sch Affil: M-00511
Major participating institution for programs in: EM, GS, IM, OBG, P, PS
Institution ID: 05-0571

Santa Monica

Santa Monica-UCLA Medical Center

1250 16th St
Santa Monica, CA 90404
Med Sch Affil: G-00514
Programs sponsored in: FP
Institution ID: 05-0439

Santa Rosa

Sutter Medical Center of Santa Rosa

3325 Chanate Rd
Santa Rosa, CA 95404-1797
Med Sch Affil: M-00502
Programs sponsored in: FP
Institution ID: 05-0152

Stanford

Stanford University Hospital

300 Pasteur Dr
Stanford, CA 94305
Med Sch Affil: M-00511
Programs sponsored in: APM, CCA, CCM, CCP, CD, CHN, CHP, CN, D, DMP, DR, EM, END, GE, GS, HEM, HMP, HSO, ICE, ID, IM, IMG, N, NEP, NM, NP, NPM, NS, OAR, OBG, ON, OPH, ORS, OTO, P, PAN, PCC, PD, PDC, PDE, PDI, PDR, PG, PHO, PM, PN, PS, PTH, PYG, RHU, RNR, RO, SCI, TS, U, VIR, VS
Major participating institution for programs in: AI, MG
Institution ID: 05-0129

Stockton

San Joaquin General Hospital

PO Box 1020
500 W Hospital Rd
Stockton, CA 95201
Med Sch Affil: G-00519
Programs sponsored in: FP, GS, IM
Institution ID: 05-0281

Sylmar

Olive View-UCLA Medical Center

14445 Olive View Dr
Sylmar, CA 91342-1496
Programs sponsored in: MEM, PFP
Major participating institution for programs in: CD, CN, DR, EM, EMP, END, FP, GE, GS, HO, ID, IM, NPM, OBG, OTO, P, PCC, PD, PDR, PS, RHU, U
Institution ID: 05-0216

Torrance

Los Angeles County-Harbor-UCLA Medical Center

1000 W Carson St
Torrance, CA 90509-2910
Med Sch Affil: M-00514
Programs sponsored in: AI, AN, BBK, CCP, CD, CHN, CHP, CN, DR, EM, END, FP, GS, HO, ICE, ID, IM, N, NEP, NPM, OBG, ORS, P, PCC, PD, PDE, PDI, PTH, RNR, VS
Major participating institution for programs in: GE, IM, MG, NS, OPH, OTO, PS, U
Institution ID: 05-0385

Travis AFB

David Grant Medical Center

101 Bodin Cir
Travis AFB, CA 94535-1800
Med Sch Affil: M-02312, M-00519, G-02312
Programs sponsored in: DR, FP, GS, IM, OBG, PD, TY
Major participating institution for programs in: CN, ID, N, PTH
Institution ID: 05-0499

Van Nuys

Southern California Orthopedic Institute

6815 Noble Ave
Van Nuys, CA 91405-3730
Programs sponsored in: OSM
Major participating institution for programs in: HSP
Institution ID: 05-8070

Ventura

Ventura County Medical Center

3291 Loma Vista Rd
Ventura, CA 93003
Programs sponsored in: FP
Institution ID: 05-0324

Whittier

Presbyterian Intercommunity Hospital

12401 E Washington Blvd
Whittier, CA 90602-1099
Med Sch Affil: G-00506
Programs sponsored in: FP
Institution ID: 05-0762

Woodland Hills

Kaiser Foundation Hospital (Woodland Hills)

5601 DeSoto Ave
Woodland Hills, CA 91365-4084
Med Sch Affil: G-00514
Major participating institution for programs in: FP
Institution ID: 05-8068

Yuba City

Fremont Medical Center

970 Plumas St
Yuba City, CA 95991
Institution ID: 05-8103

Colorado

Aspen

Orthopaedic Associates of Aspen and Glenwood

100 E Main St/Ste 101
Aspen, CO 81611
Major participating institution for programs in: OSM
Institution ID: 07-8013

Colorado Springs

Penrose-St Francis Healthcare System

2215 N Cascade Ave
PO Box 7021
Colorado Springs, CO 80933-9939
Med Sch Affil: L-00702
Programs sponsored in: PTH
Institution ID: 07-0327

Denver

Children's Hospital

1056 E 19th Ave
Medical Education Box 158
Denver, CO 80218-1088
Med Sch Affil: M-00702
Programs sponsored in: PP
Major participating institution for programs in: APM, CCP, CHN, NS, ORS, OTO, PAN, PD, PDC, PDE, PDI, PDP, PDR, PDS, PG, PHO, PN, PS, TS, U
Institution ID: 07-0378

Columbia Presbyterian-St Luke's Medical Center

1719 E 19th Ave
Denver, CO 80218-1281
Programs sponsored in: DR, IM, TY
Major participating institution for programs in: IM
Institution ID: 07-0277

Denver Health and Hospitals

777 Bannock St
Denver, CO 80204-4507
Med Sch Affil: M-00702, L-02312
Programs sponsored in: EM
Major participating institution for programs in: AN, CD, CHN, D, DR, END, FP, GE, GS, HO, ID, IM, N, NEP, NS, OBG, OPH, ORS, OTO, P, PCC, PD, PG, PS, PTH, RHU, U
Institution ID: 07-0280

Exempla St Joseph Hospital

1835 Franklin St
Denver, CO 80218-9968
Programs sponsored in: FP, GS, IM, OBG
Major participating institution for programs in: U
Institution ID: 07-0451

Immunological Associates of Denver

101 University Blvd
PO Box 61159
Denver, CO 80206-4632
Major participating institution for programs in: ALI
Institution ID: 07-8014

National Jewish Ctr for Immunology and Respiratory Medicine

1400 Jackson St
Denver, CO 80206-1997
Med Sch Affil: M-00702
Major participating institution for programs in: AI, ALI, CCP, GPM, PDP
Institution ID: 07-0287

Rose Medical Center

4567 E 9th Ave
Denver, CO 80220-3941
Med Sch Affil: G-00702
Major participating institution for programs in: FP, HO, IM, OBG, PCC
Institution ID: 07-0269

St Anthony Hospital Central

4231 W 16th Ave
Denver, CO 80204
Programs sponsored in: FP
Institution ID: 07-0351

University Hospital

4200 E 9th Ave
Denver, CO 80262
Major participating institution for programs in: FP
Institution ID: 07-8022

University of Colorado Health Sciences Center

4200 E 9th Ave
PO Box C-293
Denver, CO 80262
Med Sch Affil: M-00702, L-02312
Programs sponsored in: ADP, AI, ALI, AN, APM, CCP, CD, CHN, CHP, D, DR, END, FP, GE, GPM, GS, HO, ICE, ID, IM, IMG, IPM, MG, N, NEP, NM, NPM, NS, OBG, OPH, ORS, OSM, OTO, P, PAN, PCC, PD, PDC, PDE, PDI, PDP, PDR, PDS, PFP, PG, PHO, PM, PMP, PN, PS, PTH, RHU, RNR, TS, U, VIR
Institution ID: 07-0313

Veterans Affairs Medical Center (Denver)

1055 Clermont St
Denver, CO 80220
Med Sch Affil: M-00702
Major participating institution for programs in: ADP, AN, APM, CD, D, DR, END, FP, GE, GS, HO, ID, IM, IMG, N, NEP, NM, NS, OPH, ORS, OTO, P, PCC, PM, PS, PTH, RHU, TS, U
Institution ID: 07-0157

Englewood

Swedish Medical Center

501 E Hampden Ave
PO Box 2901
Englewood, CO 80150
Med Sch Affil: G-00702
Major participating institution for programs in: FP
Institution ID: 07-8020

Fort Collins

Poudre Valley Hospital

1024 Lemay Ave
Fort Collins, CO 80524-3998
Programs sponsored in: FP
Institution ID: 07-0705

Grand Junction

St Mary's Hospital and Medical Center

PO Box 1628
Grand Junction, CO 81502
Programs sponsored in: FP
Institution ID: 07-0713

Greeley

North Colorado Medical Center

1801 16th St
Greeley, CO 80631-5199
Programs sponsored in: FP
Institution ID: 07-0348

Louisville

Avista Hospital

100 Health Park Dr
Louisville, CO 80027
Major participating institution for programs in: FP
Institution ID: 07-8019

Pueblo

Centura Health St Mary-Corwin Medical Center

1008 Minnequa Ave
Pueblo, CO 81004-3798
Programs sponsored in: FP
Institution ID: 07-0360

Colorado Mental Health Institute at Pueblo

1600 W 24th St
Pueblo, CO 81003-1499
Major participating institution for programs in: PFP
Institution ID: 07-8024

Vail

Steadman Hawkins Clinic

181 W Meadow Dr/Ste 400
Vail, CO 81657
Programs sponsored in: OSM
Institution ID: 07-8018

Vail Valley Medical Center

181 W Meadow Dr
Vail, CO 81657
Major participating institution for programs in: OSM
Institution ID: 07-8017

Westminster

St Anthony Hospital North

2551 W 84th Ave
Westminster, CO 80030
Major participating institution for programs in: FP
Institution ID: 07-8023

Wray

Wray Community District Hospital

340 Birch St
PO Box 65
Wray, CO 80758
Major participating institution for programs in: FP
Institution ID: 07-8016

Connecticut

Bridgeport

Bridgeport Hospital

267 Grant St
Bridgeport, CT 06610-2870
Med Sch Affil: M-00801
Programs sponsored in: CD, DR, GE, IM, MPD, OBG, PD, PUD
Major participating institution for programs in: CCS, EM, GS
Institution ID: 08-0359

St Vincent's Medical Center

2800 Main St
Bridgeport, CT 06606
Med Sch Affil: M-00801, G-03509
Programs sponsored in: DR, IM, TY
Major participating institution for programs in: GS
Institution ID: 08-0341

Danbury

Danbury Hospital

24 Hospital Ave
Danbury, CT 06810-6099
Med Sch Affil: M-00801, G-03509, G-00802
Programs sponsored in: IM, OBG, PTH
Major participating institution for programs in: NM, P
Institution ID: 08-0363

Derby

Griffin Hospital

130 Division St
Derby, CT 06418
Med Sch Affil: M-00801
Programs sponsored in: GPM, IM
Institution ID: 08-0172

Farmington

Connecticut Red Cross Blood Services

209 Farmington Ave
Farmington, CT 06032
Med Sch Affil: G-00802
Major participating institution for programs in: BBK
Institution ID: 08-0723

Univ of Connecticut Health Center/John Dempsey Hospital

263 Farmington Ave
Farmington, CT 06030-1915
Med Sch Affil: M-00802
Programs sponsored in: MPD
Major participating institution for programs in: AN, BBK, CCA, CD, CHP, DR, END, GE, GPM, GS, HO, HSO, ID, IM, IMG, MG, MP, N, NEP, NM, NPM, NS, OBG, ORS, OSM, OTO, P, PCC, RHU, U, VS
Institution ID: 08-0501

University of Connecticut School of Medicine

263 Farmington Ave
Farmington, CT 06030-1915
Programs sponsored in: ADP, AN, BBK, CCA, CCS, CD, CHP, DR, EM, END, FP, GE, GPM, GS, HO, HSO, ID, IM, IMG, MG, MP, N, NEP, NM, NPM, NS, OBG, OP, ORS, OSM, OTO, P, PCC, PD, PDE, PDP, RHU, U, VS
Institution ID: 08-0445

Greenwich

Greenwich Hospital

Dept of Medical Education/Rm 487N
Perryridge Rd
Greenwich, CT 06830
Med Sch Affil: M-00801
Programs sponsored in: IM
Major participating institution for programs in: P
Institution ID: 08-0257

Hartford

Connecticut Children's Medical Center

282 Washington St
Hartford, CT 06106
Med Sch Affil: M-00802, G-03201
Major participating institution for programs in: AN, CHP, MG, NPM, NS, OP, ORS, PD, PDE, PDP, U
Institution ID: 08-0407

Hartford Hospital

80 Seymour St
Hartford, CT 06115-0729
Med Sch Affil: M-00802, L-03201
Programs sponsored in: BBK, DR, HMP, MM, PCP, PP, PTH
Major participating institution for programs in: ADP, AN, BBK, CCA, CCS, CD, EM, END, GE, GS, HO, HSO, ID, IM, MP, N, NM, NS, OBG, ORS, OTO, P, U, VS
Institution ID: 08-0275

Institute of Living

400 Washington St
Hartford, CT 06106-3392
Med Sch Affil: M-00802
Major participating institution for programs in: CHP, P
Institution ID: 08-0400

Mount Sinai Hospital

500 Blue Hills Ave
Hartford, CT 06112-1596
Med Sch Affil: M-00802
Major participating institution for programs in: CD, CHP, ID, IM, PCC
Institution ID: 08-0316

St Francis Hospital and Medical Center

114 Woodland St
Hartford, CT 06105-1299
Med Sch Affil: M-00802
Programs sponsored in: CRS, OBG
Major participating institution for programs in: AN, BBK, CD, DR, EM, END, FP, GE, GS, HO, IM, NM, ORS, OTO, PCC, PD, U
Institution ID: 08-0490

Middletown

Middlesex Hospital
28 Crescent St
Middletown, CT 06457-0650
Med Sch Affil: L-00802
Programs sponsored in: FP
Institution ID: 08-0135

Riverview Hospital for Children
River Rd
Box 621
Middletown, CT 06457
Major participating institution for programs in: CHP
Institution ID: 08-8015

New Britain

New Britain General Hospital
100 Grand St
New Britain, CT 06050-0100
Med Sch Affil: M-00802
Major participating institution for programs in: GE, GS, IM, OBG, OTO, PCC
Institution ID: 08-0372

New Haven

Connecticut Mental Health Center
34 Park St
New Haven, CT 06519
Med Sch Affil: M-00801
Major participating institution for programs in: ADP, P, PFP
Institution ID: 08-0715

Hospital of St Raphael
1450 Chapel St
New Haven, CT 06511-4440
Med Sch Affil: M-00801
Programs sponsored in: CD, DR, GE, GS, IM, NEP, TY
Major participating institution for programs in: HSP, ORS, OTO, P, PD, PS
Institution ID: 08-0244

Yale Psychiatric Institute
184 Liberty St
PO Box 208038
New Haven, CT 06520-8038
Med Sch Affil: M-00801
Major participating institution for programs in: P
Institution ID: 08-0711

Yale University Health Service
17 Hillhouse Ave
New Haven, CT 06520
Med Sch Affil: G-00801
Major participating institution for programs in: P
Institution ID: 08-0716

Yale University School of Public Health
60 College St
PO Box 208034
New Haven, CT 06520-8034
Major participating institution for programs in: GPM
Institution ID: 08-0505

Yale-New Haven Hospital
1063 Clinic Bldg
20 York St
New Haven, CT 06504-1111
Med Sch Affil: M-00801
Programs sponsored in: ADP, AI, AN, APM, BBK, CCA, CCP, CCS, CD, CHN, CHP, CN, D, DMP, DR, EM, END, GE, GPM, GS, HEM, HSO, HSP, ID, IM, IMG, MG, MM, MPD, N, NEP, NM, NPM, NR, NS, OBG, ON, OPH, ORS, OSM, OTO, P, PAN, PCC, PCP, PD, PDC, PDE, PDI, PDP, PDR, PDS, PFP, PG, PHO, PN, PS, PTH, PYG, RHU, RNR, RO, TS, U, VIR, VS
Major participating institution for programs in: GS, PUD
Institution ID: 08-0433

Yale-New Haven Hospital
333 Cedar St
PO Box 3333
New Haven, CT 06510
Med Sch Affil: M-00801
Major participating institution for programs in: MPD
Institution ID: 08-0504

Norwalk

Norwalk Hospital
Maple St
Norwalk, CT 06856-5050
Med Sch Affil: M-00801, L-01642
Programs sponsored in: CD, DR, GE, IM, PUD
Major participating institution for programs in: P
Institution ID: 08-0206

Norwich

Uncas on Thames Hospital
PO Box 711
Norwich, CT 06360
Med Sch Affil: L-00802
Major participating institution for programs in: RO
Institution ID: 08-7003

Stamford

Stamford Hospital
Shelburne Rd and W Broad St
PO Box 9317
Stamford, CT 06904-9317
Med Sch Affil: M-03509
Programs sponsored in: FP, GS, IM, OBG
Major participating institution for programs in: P
Institution ID: 08-0456

Waterbury

St Mary's Hospital
56 Franklin St
Waterbury, CT 06706
Med Sch Affil: M-00802, M-00801
Programs sponsored in: GS
Major participating institution for programs in: IM
Institution ID: 08-0458

Waterbury Hospital Health Center
64 Robbins St
Waterbury, CT 06721
Med Sch Affil: M-00801
Programs sponsored in: GS
Major participating institution for programs in: GE, IM, RHU, U
Institution ID: 08-0131

West Haven

Veterans Affairs Medical Center (West Haven)
950 Campbell Ave
West Haven, CT 06516-2700
Med Sch Affil: M-00801
Major participating institution for programs in: ADP, AN, CD, CHN, CN, D, DR, END, GE, GS, HSP, ID, IM, IMG, N, NEP, NM, NS, ON, OPH, ORS, OTO, P, PCC, PS, PTH, PYG, RHU, U, VIR
Institution ID: 08-0199

Delaware

New Castle

Delaware State Hospital
1901 N DuPont Hwy
New Castle, DE 19720
Programs sponsored in: P
Institution ID: 09-0297

Wilmington

Christiana Care Health Services Inc
501 W 14th St
PO Box 1668
Wilmington, DE 19899
Med Sch Affil: M-04102, G-04113
Programs sponsored in: DR, EM, FP, FSM, GS, IM, MEM, MPD, OBG, TY
Major participating institution for programs in: N, NPM, OPH, OSM, P, PD, TS
Institution ID: 09-0247

duPont Hospital for Children
1600 Rockland Rd
PO Box 269
Wilmington, DE 19899-0269
Med Sch Affil: M-04102, G-04113
Programs sponsored in: OP
Major participating institution for programs in: MPD, ORS, OTO, PD, PMP, U
Institution ID: 09-0340

St Francis Hospital
7th and Clayton Sts
MSB Level 2
Wilmington, DE 19805-0500
Med Sch Affil: M-04113
Programs sponsored in: FP
Institution ID: 09-0709

Veterans Affairs Medical Center (Wilmington)
1601 Kirkwood Hwy
Wilmington, DE 19805-9997
Med Sch Affil: M-04102, G-02301
Major participating institution for programs in: N, OTO, U
Institution ID: 09-0462

District of Columbia

Washington

Armed Forces Institute of Pathology
6825 16th St NW
Washington, DC 20306-6000
Med Sch Affil: L-01001, L-01643, L-02307, G-02012, G-03201
Programs sponsored in: DMP, FOP, NP
Major participating institution for programs in: PCP, PTH
Institution ID: 10-0392

Children's National Medical Center
111 Michigan Ave NW
Washington, DC 20010
Med Sch Affil: M-01001, L-01002
Programs sponsored in: AI, CCP, CHN, CHP, NPM, OP, PD, PDC, PDI, PDP, PDR, PDS, PG, PHO, PN
Major participating institution for programs in: CN, D, N, NS, OPH, ORS, OTO, PAN, PS, RHU, RNR, TS, U
Institution ID: 10-0441

DC Commission on Mental Health Services-St Elizabeth Campus
A Bldg Rm 105
2700 Martin Luther King Ave SE
Washington, DC 20032
Med Sch Affil: L-01001
Programs sponsored in: P
Institution ID: 10-0471

District of Columbia General Hospital
19th St and Massachusetts Ave SE
Washington, DC 20003
Med Sch Affil: L-01002
Programs sponsored in: IM
Major participating institution for programs in: CD, EM, END, GE, GS, HEM, IM, N, NEP, ON, OPH, ORS, PD, PUD, U
Institution ID: 10-0183

George Washington University Hospital (UHS)
901 23rd St NW
Washington, DC 20037
Med Sch Affil: M-01001, G-01002
Major participating institution for programs in: AN, CCA, CCM, CD, CHN, D, DR, EM, END, GE, GPM, GS, HO, ICE, ID, IM, IMG, N, NEP, NPM, NS, OBG, OPH, ORS, OTO, P, PCC, PCP, PS, PTH, RHU, RNR, TS, U
Institution ID: 10-0249

George Washington University School of Medicine
2300 Eye St NW
Washington, DC 20037
Programs sponsored in: AN, CCA, CCM, CD, D, DR, EM, END, FP, GE, GPM, GS, HO, ICE, ID, IM, IMG, N, NEP, NS, OBG, OPH, ORS, OTO, P, PAN, PCC, PCP, PS, PTH, RHU, RNR, TS, U, VIR
Major participating institution for programs in: GPM
Institution ID: 10-9501

Georgetown University Medical Center
1st Fl Main
3800 Reservoir Rd NW
Washington, DC 20007-2194
Med Sch Affil: M-01002, L-02312, G-01001, G-02301
Programs sponsored in: AN, APM, BBK, CCP, CD, DR, END, FPG, GE, GS, HEM, ICE, ID, IM, MPD, N, NEP, NM, NPM, NS, OBG, ON, OPH, ORS, OTO, P, PCC, PCP, PD, PN, PS, PTH, RHU, RNR, RO, TY, U, VIR
Major participating institution for programs in: HSO, IM, PDE
Institution ID: 10-0470

Greater Southeast Community Hospital
1310 Southern Ave SE
Washington, DC 20032
Major participating institution for programs in: GS, IM
Institution ID: 10-0704

Howard University Hospital
2041 Georgia Ave NW
Washington, DC 20060
Med Sch Affil: G-01002
Programs sponsored in: AN, CD, D, DR, EM, END, FP, GE, GS, HEM, ID, IM, N, OBG, ON, OPH, ORS, P, PD, PTH, PUD, RO, TY, U, VIR
Major participating institution for programs in: OTO
Institution ID: 10-0475

National Rehabilitation Hospital
102 Irving St NW
Washington, DC 20010
Med Sch Affil: G-02312
Programs sponsored in: PM
Institution ID: 10-0720

Providence Hospital
1150 Varnum St NE
Washington, DC 20017
Med Sch Affil: L-01001, L-02312, G-01002
Programs sponsored in: FP, IM
Major participating institution for programs in: FPG, GS, OBG, ORS
Institution ID: 10-0412

Sibley Memorial Hospital
5255 Loughboro Rd NW
Washington, DC 20016-2698
Med Sch Affil: L-01002
Major participating institution for programs in: ORS, U
Institution ID: 10-0479

Veterans Affairs Medical Center (Washington, DC)
50 Irving St NW
Washington, DC 20422-0001
Med Sch Affil: M-01001, M-01002
Programs sponsored in: IM
Major participating institution for programs in: CD, D, END, GE, GS, HO, ICE, ID, IM, N, NEP, OPH, ORS, OTO, P, PCC, PS, PTH, RHU, TS, U
Institution ID: 10-0291

Walter Reed Army Institute of Research
Medical Research Fellowship
Walter Reed Army Inst
Washington, DC 20307-5100
Med Sch Affil: G-02312
Programs sponsored in: GPM, MP
Institution ID: 10-0485

Walter Reed Army Medical Center
Bldg 2/Rm 2J35
6825 16th St NW
Washington, DC 20307-5001
Med Sch Affil: M-01002, M-02312, L-01001
Programs sponsored in: AI, ALI, CCM, CD, GS, HSO, ID, IM, NEP, NM, OPH, ORS, PCC, RHU, TS, TY, U, VS
Major participating institution for programs in: ALI, AN, APM, CCA, CHN, CHP, CN, D, DMP, DR, END, HO, N, NPM, NS, OBG, OTO, P, PD, PDE, PDI, PG, PHO, PM, PTH, RO
Institution ID: 10-0242

Washington Hospital Center
110 Irving St NW
Washington, DC 20010-2975
Med Sch Affil: M-02312, L-01001, G-01002
Programs sponsored in: CCS, CD, CRS, D, GE, GS, HO, ID, IM, NEP, OBG, OPH, PTH, RHU, U
Major participating institution for programs in: CCM, N, NS, ORS, OTO, PM, PS, TS, VIR
Institution ID: 10-0377

Washington School of Psychiatry
2025 I St NW/Ste 815
Washington, DC 20006
Major participating institution for programs in: P
Institution ID: 10-0715

Florida

Bay Pines

Veterans Affairs Medical Center (Bay Pines)
Med Ctr (516/11B)
10000 Bay Pines Blvd
Bay Pines, FL 33504
Med Sch Affil: M-01104
Major participating institution for programs in: CCA, D, GS, NEP, PS, U
Institution ID: 11-0302

Clearwater

Morton Plant Hospital
323 Jeffords St
PO Box 219
Clearwater, FL 33065
Major participating institution for programs in: FP
Institution ID: 11-8101

Coral Gables

HealthSouth Doctors' Hospital
5000 University Dr
Coral Gables, FL 33146
Programs sponsored in: OSM
Major participating institution for programs in: ORS, OSM
Institution ID: 11-7024

Coral Springs

Coral Springs Medical Center
3000 Coral Hills Dr
Coral Springs, FL 33065
Med Sch Affil: G-01103
Major participating institution for programs in: FP
Institution ID: 11-8100

Daytona Beach

Halifax Medical Center
303 N Clyde Morris Blvd
PO Box 2830
Daytona Beach, FL 32115-2830
Med Sch Affil: L-01104
Programs sponsored in: FP, FSM
Institution ID: 11-0165

Eglin AFB

Headquarters Air Force Development Test Center (AFMC)
307 Boatner Rd/Ste 114
Eglin AFB, FL 32542-1282
Med Sch Affil: L-02312
Programs sponsored in: FP
Institution ID: 11-0722

Fort Lauderdale

Broward County Medical Examiner's Office

5301 SW 31st Ave
Fort Lauderdale, FL 33312
Programs sponsored in: FOP
Institution ID: 11-0524

Broward General Medical Center

1600 S Andrews Ave
Fort Lauderdale, FL 33316-2510
Major participating institution for programs in: FP
Institution ID: 11-0114

Cleveland Clinic Florida

3000 W Cypress Creek Rd
Fort Lauderdale, FL 33309-1743
Major participating institution for programs in: CRS, IM, N
Institution ID: 11-8092

Cleveland Clinic Hospital

2835 N Ocean Blvd
Fort Lauderdale, FL 33308
Major participating institution for programs in: CRS
Institution ID: 11-8091

Gainesville

Alachua General Hospital

801 SW Second Ave
Gainesville, FL 32601-2666
Med Sch Affil: M-01103
Major participating institution for programs in: FP
Institution ID: 11-0523

Shands Hospital at the University of Florida

PO Box 100326
1600 SW Archer Rd
Gainesville, FL 32610-0326
Med Sch Affil: M-01103
Major participating institution for programs in: AN, APM, CCA, CCP, CD, CHN, CHP, CN, D, DR, END, FP, GE, GS, HMP, HO, HSO, ICE, ID, IM, IMG, MPD, N, NEP, NM, NP, NPM, NS, OAR, OBG, OMO, OPH, ORS, OSM, OSS, OTO, P, PAN, PCC, PCP, PD, PDC, PDE, PDP, PG, PHO, PN, PS, PTH, PYG, RHU, RNR, RO, TS, U, VIR, VS
Institution ID: 11-0461

University of Florida College of Medicine

PO Box 100215
1600 SW Archer Rd
Gainesville, FL 32610-0215
Med Sch Affil: M-01103, L-01104
Programs sponsored in: AN, APM, CCA, CCP, CD, CHN, CHP, CN, D, DR, END, FP, GE, GS, HMP, HO, HSO, ICE, ID, IM, IMG, MPD, N, NEP, NM, NP, NPM, NS, OAR, OBG, OMO, OPH, ORS, OSM, OSS, OTO, P, PAN, PCC, PCP, PD, PDC, PDE, PDP, PFP, PG, PHO, PN, PS, PTH, PYG, RHU, RNR, RO, TS, U, VIR, VS
Institution ID: 11-9501

Veterans Affairs Medical Center (Gainesville)

1601 SW Archer Rd
Gainesville, FL 32608-1197
Med Sch Affil: M-01103
Major participating institution for programs in: AN, APM, CCA, CD, CN, D, DR, END, GE, GS, HO, ICE, ID, IM, IMG, N, NEP, NM, NP, NS, OPH, ORS, OTO, P, PCC, PCP, PS, PTH, PYG, RHU, RNR, TS, U, VIR, VS
Institution ID: 11-0525

Hollywood

Memorial Regional Hospital

3501 Johnson St
Hollywood, FL 33021
Major participating institution for programs in: GS
Institution ID: 11-0276

Jacksonville

Baptist Medical Center (UFHSC/J)

800 Prudential Dr
Jacksonville, FL 32207-8203
Med Sch Affil: G-01103
Major participating institution for programs in: CCP, ID, ON, PD, PDI
Institution ID: 11-0119

Mayo Clinic (Jacksonville)

4500 San Pablo Rd
Jacksonville, FL 32224
Med Sch Affil: M-02608, G-01103
Major participating institution for programs in: AN, APM, FP, GE, GS, HO, IM, OTO, TY
Institution ID: 11-8093

Naval Hospital (Jacksonville)

2080 Child St
Jacksonville, FL 32214-5227
Med Sch Affil: L-01103
Programs sponsored in: FP
Institution ID: 11-0256

Nemours Children's Clinic (UFHSC/J)

807 Nira St
PO Box 5720
Jacksonville, FL 32207-8426
Med Sch Affil: L-01103
Major participating institution for programs in: OP, ORS, PAN, PD
Institution ID: 11-0478

St Luke's Hospital

4201 Belfort Rd
Jacksonville, FL 32216
Med Sch Affil: M-02608
Major participating institution for programs in: AN, APM, FP, GE, GS, HO, IM, TY
Institution ID: 11-0215

St Vincent's Medical Center

PO Box 2982
Jacksonville, FL 32203
Med Sch Affil: L-01104, G-01103
Programs sponsored in: FP
Institution ID: 11-0148

University Medical Center (UFHSC/J)

655 W 8th St
Jacksonville, FL 32209-6597
Med Sch Affil: M-01103
Major participating institution for programs in: CCP, CD, CHP, DR, EM, END, FP, GE, GS, ID, IM, OBG, ON, OPH, ORS, OTO, PCP, PD, PDI, PTH, VIR
Institution ID: 11-0486

University of Florida College of Medicine at Jacksonville

655 W 8th St
Jacksonville, FL 32209
Med Sch Affil: L-02312
Programs sponsored in: CCP, CD, DR, EM, END, FP, GE, GS, ID, IM, OBG, ON, OP, ORS, PCP, PD, PDI, PTH, VIR
Institution ID: 11-9502

Lake City

Veterans Affairs Medical Center (Lake City)

801 S Marion St
Lake City, FL 32025-5898
Major participating institution for programs in: GS
Institution ID: 11-0507

Miami

Baptist Hospital of Miami

8900 N Kendall Dr
Miami, FL 33176
Major participating institution for programs in: RNR, VIR
Institution ID: 11-0511

Bascom Palmer Eye Institute-Anne Bates Leach Eye Hospital

PO Box 016880
Miami, FL 33101-6880
Med Sch Affil: M-01102
Major participating institution for programs in: OPH
Institution ID: 11-0701

Cedars Medical Center

1400 NW 12th Ave
Miami, FL 33136
Med Sch Affil: L-01102
Major participating institution for programs in: ORS, U, VIR
Institution ID: 11-0707

Metropolitan Dade County Office of Medical Examiner

Number One on Bob Hope Rd
Miami, FL 33136-1133
Programs sponsored in: FOP
Institution ID: 11-0496

Miami Children's Hospital

6125 S W 31st St
Miami, FL 33155
Med Sch Affil: L-01102
Programs sponsored in: CCP, PD, PDR
Major participating institution for programs in: AN, ORS, PAN
Institution ID: 11-0311

Miami Jewish Home and Hospital for the Aged

5200 NE 2nd Ave
Miami, FL 33137
Major participating institution for programs in: IMG, PYG
Institution ID: 11-8096

University of Miami Hospital and Clinics

1475 NW 12th Ave
Miami, FL 33136-1002
Med Sch Affil: M-01102
Major participating institution for programs in: CHP
Institution ID: 11-0721

University of Miami-Jackson Memorial Medical Center

1611 NW 12th Ave
Miami, FL 33136
Med Sch Affil: M-01102, L-02312
Programs sponsored in: ADP, AN, APM, CCA, CCM, CCP, CCS, CD, CHN, CHP, D, DMP, DR, END, FP, GE, GS, HO, HSO, ICE, ID, IM, IMG, MPD, N, NEP, NM, NPM, NS, OBG, OPH, ORS, OSM, OSS, OTO, P, PAN, PCC, PCP, PD, PDC, PDE, PDP, PDR, PIP, PN, PP, PS, PTH, PYG, PYN, RHU, RNR, RO, TS, U, VIR
Major participating institution for programs in: GS
Institution ID: 11-0314

Veterans Affairs Medical Center (Miami)
1201 NW 16th St
Miami, FL 33125-1693
Med Sch Affil: M-01102
Major participating institution for programs in: AN, CCM, CD, D, END, GE, GS, HO, HSO, ID, IM, IMG, MPD, N, NEP, NS, OPH, ORS, OTO, P, PCC, PTH, PYG, PYN, RHU, TS, U
Institution ID: 11-0515

Miami Beach
Mount Sinai Medical Center of Greater Miami
4300 Alton Rd
Miami Beach, FL 33140
Med Sch Affil: L-01104, L-01102
Programs sponsored in: CD, DR, GS, IM, PTH
Major participating institution for programs in: ADP, AN, CCM, D, GE, ID, IMG, PCC, PYG, TS
Institution ID: 11-0101

Orlando
Arnold Palmer Hospital for Children and Women
Med Ed Admin MP #7
92 W Miller St
Orlando, FL 32806
Major participating institution for programs in: PD
Institution ID: 11-8095

Florida Hospital
601 E Rollins St
Orlando, FL 32803-1273
Med Sch Affil: L-00512, L-01104
Programs sponsored in: FP, FPG
Major participating institution for programs in: CRS, PS
Institution ID: 11-0513

Office of the Medical Examiner, District Nine
1401 Lucerne Terr
Orlando, FL 32806
Programs sponsored in: FOP
Institution ID: 11-8018

Orlando Regional Medical Center
Med Educ Admin/MP 7
1414 Kuhl Ave
Orlando, FL 32806-2093
Med Sch Affil: L-01103
Programs sponsored in: CCS, CRS, EM, GS, IM, MPD, OBG, OP, ORS, PD, PTH
Major participating institution for programs in: GS
Institution ID: 11-0258

Pensacola
Naval Aerospace and Operational Medical Institute
220 Hovey Rd
Pensacola, FL 32508-1047
Programs sponsored in: GPM
Institution ID: 11-0108

Naval Hospital (Pensacola)
6000 W Hwy 98
Pensacola, FL 32512-0003
Med Sch Affil: G-02312
Programs sponsored in: FP
Institution ID: 11-0159

Sacred Heart Hospital of Pensacola
5151 N 9th Ave
Pensacola, FL 32504
Med Sch Affil: G-01103
Major participating institution for programs in: OBG, PD
Institution ID: 11-0396

St Petersburg
All Children's Hospital
801 6th St S
PO Box 31020
St Petersburg, FL 33731-8920
Med Sch Affil: M-01104
Major participating institution for programs in: AI, ALI, NS, OTO, PD, PDE, PP, PS
Institution ID: 11-0182

Bayfront Medical Center
701 6th St S
St Petersburg, FL 33701-4891
Med Sch Affil: L-01104
Programs sponsored in: FP, FSM, OBG
Institution ID: 11-0440

Tallahassee
Tallahassee Memorial Regional Medical Center
1300 Miccosukee Rd
Tallahassee, FL 32308
Med Sch Affil: L-01104
Programs sponsored in: FP
Institution ID: 11-0522

Tampa
Florida Blood Services
3602 Spectrum Blvd
PO Box 2125
Tampa, FL 33601-2125
Med Sch Affil: L-01104
Programs sponsored in: BBK
Institution ID: 11-8001

H Lee Moffitt Cancer Center
12902 Magnolia Dr
Tampa, FL 33612-9497
Med Sch Affil: M-01104
Major participating institution for programs in: AN, APM, D, DR, GS, HO, ID, NS, OBG, OTO, PCP, PS, PTH, U
Institution ID: 11-8003

Hillsborough County Medical Examiner Department
401 S Morgan St
Tampa, FL 33602
Major participating institution for programs in: FOP
Institution ID: 11-8094

James A Haley Veterans Hospital
13000 Bruce B Downs Blvd
Tampa, FL 33612-4798
Med Sch Affil: M-01104
Major participating institution for programs in: ADP, AI, ALI, APM, CD, D, DR, END, GE, GS, HO, HSP, ID, IM, IMG, N, NEP, NS, OPH, OTO, P, PCC, PS, PTH, PYG, RHU, RNR, U
Institution ID: 11-0521

Shriners Hospitals for Children (Tampa)
12502 N Pine Dr
Tampa, FL 33612-9499
Med Sch Affil: L-01104, G-03519
Programs sponsored in: OP
Major participating institution for programs in: HSP
Institution ID: 11-8002

Tampa General Healthcare
PO Box 1289
Davis Islands
Tampa, FL 33601-1289
Med Sch Affil: L-01104
Major participating institution for programs in: ALI, AN, CCA, CD, CHP, D, DR, END, GE, GPM, GS, HO, HSP, ID, IM, IMG, MPD, N, NEP, NPM, NS, OBG, OPH, OTO, P, PCC, PD, PP, PS, PTH, RHU, RNR, U, VIR, VS
Institution ID: 11-0726

TGH University Psychiatry Center
3515 E Fletcher Ave
Tampa, FL 33613
Major participating institution for programs in: CHP, P, PYG
Institution ID: 11-8016

University of South Florida College of Medicine
12901 Bruce B Downs Blvd
PO Box 2
Tampa, FL 33612-4799
Med Sch Affil: M-01104
Programs sponsored in: ADP, AI, ALI, AN, APM, CCA, CD, CHP, D, DR, END, FOP, FP, GE, GPM, GS, HO, HSP, ID, IM, IMG, MPD, N, NEP, NPM, NS, OBG, OPH, OTO, P, PCC, PCP, PD, PDE, PP, PS, PTH, PYG, RHU, RNR, U, VIR, VS
Institution ID: 11-0184

University of South Florida College of Public Health
13201 Bruce B Downs Blvd
Tampa, FL 33612
Major participating institution for programs in: GPM
Institution ID: 11-8097

Umatilla
Florida Elks Children's Hospital
633 Umatilla Blvd
PO Box 49
Umatilla, FL 32784
Major participating institution for programs in: OP, ORS
Institution ID: 11-8011

West Palm Beach
Palm Beach County Public Health Unit
PO Box 29
826 Evernia St
West Palm Beach, FL 33402
Programs sponsored in: GPM
Institution ID: 11-0729

Georgia
Albany
Phoebe Putney Memorial Hospital
417 Third Ave
PO Box 1828
Albany, GA 31702-1828
Med Sch Affil: L-01222
Programs sponsored in: FP
Institution ID: 12-0315

Atlanta

Centers for Disease Control and Prevention
1600 Clifton Rd/Mail Stop C-08
Atlanta, GA 30333-4016
Med Sch Affil: L-01221, G-02312
Programs sponsored in: GPM
Institution ID: 12-0491

Crawford Long Hospital of Emory University
550 Peachtree St NE
Atlanta, GA 30365-2225
Med Sch Affil: M-01205
Major participating institution for programs in: APM, CCA, CD, EM, FP, GS, ICE, IM, NM, NS, ORS, PS, RO, TS
Institution ID: 12-0173

Egleston Children's Hospital at Emory University
1405 Clifton Rd NE
Atlanta, GA 30322-1101
Med Sch Affil: M-01205
Major participating institution for programs in: AI, AN, CCP, CHN, CHP, N, NS, ORS, OTO, PCP, PD, PDC, PDE, PDI, PDR, PHO, TS, TY
Institution ID: 12-0481

Emory University Hospital
1364 Clifton Rd NE
Atlanta, GA 30322
Med Sch Affil: M-01205
Major participating institution for programs in: AI, AN, APM, CCS, CD, D, DMP, DR, END, GE, GS, HMP, HO, ID, IM, N, NEP, NM, NP, NR, NRN, NS, OPH, ORS, OTO, P, PCC, PCP, PM, PS, PTH, PYG, RHU, TS, TY, U, VIR, VS
Institution ID: 12-0139

Emory University School of Medicine
319 WHSCAB
1440 Clifton Rd NE
Atlanta, GA 30322
Med Sch Affil: M-01205
Programs sponsored in: AI, AN, APM, BBK, CCA, CCP, CCS, CD, CHN, CHP, D, DMP, DR, EM, END, FOP, FP, GE, GPM, GS, HMP, HO, ICE, ID, IM, IMG, MG, N, NEP, NM, NP, NPM, NR, NRN, NS, OBG, OPH, ORS, OTO, P, PCC, PCP, PD, PDC, PDE, PDI, PDR, PDS, PFP, PHO, PM, PS, PTH, PYG, RHU, RNR, RO, TS, TY, U, VIR, VS
Institution ID: 12-0490

Fulton County Health Department
990 Butler St SE
Atlanta, GA 30335
Major participating institution for programs in: P
Institution ID: 12-8021

Fulton County Medical Examiner's Office
50 Coca Cola Pl SE
Atlanta, GA 30303
Med Sch Affil: L-01205
Major participating institution for programs in: FOP
Institution ID: 12-0496

Georgia Baptist Medical Center
303 Parkway Dr NE
Atlanta, GA 30312
Med Sch Affil: M-01201, L-01222
Programs sponsored in: FP, GS, IM, OBG, ORS, TY, VS
Institution ID: 12-0198

Georgia Mental Health Institute
1256 Briarcliff Rd NE
Atlanta, GA 30306-2694
Med Sch Affil: L-01205
Major participating institution for programs in: CHP
Institution ID: 12-0488

Grady Memorial Hospital
80 Butler St SE
PO Box 26189
Atlanta, GA 30335
Med Sch Affil: M-01205, M-01221
Major participating institution for programs in: AI, AN, CCA, CCS, CD, CHN, CHP, D, DMP, DR, EM, END, FOP, FP, GE, GPM, GS, HO, ID, IM, N, NEP, NM, NP, NPM, NR, NRN, NS, OBG, OPH, ORS, OTO, P, PCC, PCP, PD, PDC, PDE, PDI, PFP, PHO, PM, PS, PTH, RHU, RNR, RO, TS, TY, U, VIR
Institution ID: 12-0483

Morehouse School of Medicine
720 Westview Dr SW
Atlanta, GA 30310-1495
Med Sch Affil: M-01221
Programs sponsored in: FP, GPM, GS, IM, OBG, P
Institution ID: 12-0499

Piedmont Hospital
1968 Peachtree Rd NW
Atlanta, GA 30309
Med Sch Affil: G-01205
Major participating institution for programs in: GS
Institution ID: 12-0317

Rollins School of Public Health of Emory University
1518 Clifton Rd NE
Atlanta, GA 30322
Programs sponsored in: GPM
Major participating institution for programs in: GPM
Institution ID: 12-9501

Scottish Rite Children's Medical Center
1001 Johnson Ferry Rd NE
Atlanta, GA 30342-1600
Med Sch Affil: L-02101, G-01205
Programs sponsored in: OP
Major participating institution for programs in: ORS, PS
Institution ID: 12-0111

Southwest Community Hospital and Medical Center
501 Fairburn Rd SW
Atlanta, GA 30331-2099
Med Sch Affil: M-01221
Major participating institution for programs in: FP
Institution ID: 12-0500

Wesley Woods Geriatric Hospital
1821 Clifton Rd NE
Atlanta, GA 30329
Med Sch Affil: G-01205
Major participating institution for programs in: IMG, PYG
Institution ID: 12-7032

West Paces Ferry Medical Center
3200 Howell Mill Rd
Atlanta, GA 30327
Major participating institution for programs in: P, VS
Institution ID: 12-8020

Augusta

Georgia Regional Hospital at Augusta
3405 Old Savannah Rd
Augusta, GA 30906
Major participating institution for programs in: CHP
Institution ID: 12-8013

Medical College of Georgia Hospital and Clinics
1120 15th St
Augusta, GA 30912-5000
Med Sch Affil: M-01201
Programs sponsored in: AI, AN, APM, BBK, CCP, CD, CHN, CHP, CN, D, DR, EM, END, FP, GE, GS, HO, ID, IM, N, NEP, NPM, NS, OBG, OPH, ORS, OTO, P, PCC, PD, PDC, PS, PTH, RHU, RNR, TS, U
Institution ID: 12-0391

University Hospital
1350 Walton Way
Augusta, GA 30901-2629
Med Sch Affil: M-01201
Major participating institution for programs in: CHN, EM, GS, N, OBG, PD, U
Institution ID: 12-0428

Veterans Affairs Medical Center (Augusta)
1 Freedom Way
Augusta, GA 30904-6285
Med Sch Affil: M-01201
Major participating institution for programs in: AN, CD, CHN, D, DR, END, GE, GS, HO, ID, IM, N, NEP, NS, OPH, ORS, OTO, P, PCC, PS, PTH, RNR, TS, U
Institution ID: 12-0272

Columbus

Hughston Sports Medicine Foundation
PO Box 9517
6262 Hamilton Rd
Columbus, GA 31908-9517
Programs sponsored in: OSM
Institution ID: 12-8023

Hughston Sports Medicine Hospital
100 First Ct
PO Box 2319
Columbus, GA 31908-2319
Med Sch Affil: G-02312
Major participating institution for programs in: OSM
Institution ID: 12-0501

The Medical Center Inc
710 Center St
Columbus, GA 31902
Med Sch Affil: L-01222, L-01201, G-01221
Programs sponsored in: FP, TY
Institution ID: 12-0209

Decatur

Georgia Regional Hospital at Atlanta
3073 Panthersville Rd
Decatur, GA 30037-0407
Med Sch Affil: G-01221
Major participating institution for programs in: P
Institution ID: 12-8017

Veterans Affairs Medical Center (Atlanta)
1670 Clairmont Rd
Decatur, GA 30033
Med Sch Affil: M-01205
Major participating institution for programs in: CD, D, DMP, END, GE, GS, IM, IMG, NP, OPH, OTO, P, PCC, PM, PS, PTH, RHU, RO, TS, U
Institution ID: 12-0293

Fort Benning

Martin Army Community Hospital
US Army Med Dept Activity
Bldg 9200
Marne Rd
Fort Benning, GA 31905-6100
Med Sch Affil: G-02312
Programs sponsored in: FP
Institution ID: 12-0357

Fort Gordon

Dwight David Eisenhower Army Medical Center
Graduate Medical Education
Fort Gordon, GA 30905-5650
Med Sch Affil: L-01201, L-02312
Programs sponsored in: FP, FPP, GS, IM, ORS, P, TY
Major participating institution for programs in: CHP
Institution ID: 12-0492

Macon

Medical Center of Central Georgia
777 Hemlock St
PO Box 6000
Macon, GA 31208-6000
Med Sch Affil: M-01222
Programs sponsored in: FP, GS, IM, OBG, PD, TY
Major participating institution for programs in: P
Institution ID: 12-0266

River Edge Behavioral Health Center
175 Emery Hwy
Macon, GA 31201
Major participating institution for programs in: P
Institution ID: 12-8026

Marietta

Georgia Dept of Human Resources-Division of Public Health
1650 County Farm Rd
Marietta, GA 30060-4009
Major participating institution for programs in: GPM
Institution ID: 12-8015

Milledgeville

Central State Hospital
Central State Hospital
Milledgeville, GA 31062
Major participating institution for programs in: P
Institution ID: 12-0346

Rome

Floyd Medical Center
304 Turner McCall Blvd
PO Box 233
Rome, GA 30162-0233
Med Sch Affil: L-01222
Programs sponsored in: FP
Institution ID: 12-0402

Savannah

Memorial Medical Center
PO Box 23089
Savannah, GA 31403-3089
Med Sch Affil: M-01222, L-01201
Programs sponsored in: DR, FP, GS, IM, OBG, PD
Institution ID: 12-0362

Smyrna

Brawner Psychiatric Institute
3180 Atlanta St SE
Smyrna, GA 30080
Major participating institution for programs in: P
Institution ID: 12-8019

The Ridgeview Institute
3995 S Cobb Dr
Smyrna, GA 30080
Med Sch Affil: M-01221, L-01205
Major participating institution for programs in: P
Institution ID: 12-8018

Waycross

Satilla Regional Medical Center
410 Darling Ave
PO Box 139
Waycross, GA 31502-0139
Major participating institution for programs in: FP
Institution ID: 12-8027

Hawaii

Ewa Beach

Kahi Mohala Hospital
91-2301 Ft Weaver Rd
Ewa Beach, HI 96706
Major participating institution for programs in: CHP
Institution ID: 14-8012

Honolulu

Kaiser Foundation Hospital (Moanalua)
3288 Moanalua Rd
Honolulu, HI 96819-1499
Med Sch Affil: M-01401, G-00502
Major participating institution for programs in: GS, IMG, PTH, TY
Institution ID: 14-0431

Kapiolani Medical Center for Women and Children
1319 Punahou St
Honolulu, HI 96826-1032
Med Sch Affil: M-01401
Major participating institution for programs in: CHP, CPP, MPD, NPM, OBG, PD, TY
Institution ID: 14-0371

Kuakini Medical Center
347 N Kuakini St
Honolulu, HI 96817-9980
Med Sch Affil: M-01401
Major participating institution for programs in: GS, IM, IMG, MPD, TY
Institution ID: 14-0425

Leahi Hospital
3675 Kilauea Ave
Honolulu, HI 96816
Med Sch Affil: L-01401
Major participating institution for programs in: CPP
Institution ID: 14-0430

Queen's Medical Center
1301 Punchbowl St
Honolulu, HI 96813-1234
Med Sch Affil: M-01401
Major participating institution for programs in: ADP, CCS, GS, IM, MPD, OBG, ORS, P, PTH, TY
Institution ID: 14-0429

Shriners Hospitals for Children (Honolulu)
1310 Punahou St
Honolulu, HI 96826-1099
Med Sch Affil: L-01401
Programs sponsored in: OP
Major participating institution for programs in: ORS
Institution ID: 14-0300

St Francis Medical Center
2230 Liliha St
Honolulu, HI 96817
Med Sch Affil: M-01401
Major participating institution for programs in: GS, IM, MPD, PTH, TY
Institution ID: 14-0210

Straub Clinic and Hospital
888 S King St
Honolulu, HI 96813
Med Sch Affil: L-01401
Major participating institution for programs in: GS, TY
Institution ID: 14-0440

Tripler Army Medical Center
1 Jarrett White Rd
Honolulu, HI 96859-5000
Med Sch Affil: M-01401, G-02312
Programs sponsored in: CHP, DR, FP, FPP, GS, IM, MP, OBG, ORS, OTO, P, PD, TY, U
Major participating institution for programs in: NPM, ORS, PTH
Institution ID: 14-0426

University of Hawaii John A Burns School of Medicine
1960 East-West Rd
Bio-Med T-101
Honolulu, HI 96822
Med Sch Affil: M-01401
Programs sponsored in: ADP, CCS, CHP, CPP, FP, GS, IM, IMG, MPD, NPM, OBG, ORS, P, PD, PTH, PYG, TY
Institution ID: 14-0439

VA Regional Office-Outpatient Clinic (Honolulu)
PO Box 50188
Honolulu, HI 96850-0002
Med Sch Affil: L-01401
Major participating institution for programs in: PYG
Institution ID: 14-0444

Kaneohe

Hawaii State Hospital
45-710 Keaahala Rd
Kaneohe, HI 96744
Med Sch Affil: M-01401
Major participating institution for programs in: ADP, P, PYG
Institution ID: 14-0268

Wahiawa

Wahiawa General Hospital

128 Lehua St/PO Box 508
Wahiawa, HI 96786
Med Sch Affil: M-01401
Major participating institution for programs in: FP
Institution ID: 14-8014

Idaho

Boise

Family Practice Residency of Idaho

777 N Raymond
Boise, ID 83704
Programs sponsored in: FP
Institution ID: 15-0714

St Alphonsus Regional Medical Center

1055 N Curtis Rd
Boise, ID 83706
Med Sch Affil: L-05404
Major participating institution for programs in: FP
Institution ID: 15-0713

St Luke's Regional Medical Center

190 E Bannock St
Boise, ID 83712
Med Sch Affil: L-05404
Major participating institution for programs in: FP
Institution ID: 15-0711

Veterans Affairs Medical Center (Boise)

500 W Fort St
Boise, ID 83702-4598
Med Sch Affil: M-05404
Major participating institution for programs in: IM
Institution ID: 15-0712

Pocatello

Bannock Regional Medical Center

651 Memorial Dr
Pocatello, ID 83201
Major participating institution for programs in: FP
Institution ID: 15-8002

Idaho State University

Campus Box 8357
Pocatello, ID 83209-8357
Programs sponsored in: FP
Institution ID: 15-8001

Pocatello Regional Medical Center

777 Hospital Way
Pocatello, ID 83201
Major participating institution for programs in: FP
Institution ID: 15-8003

Illinois

Aurora

Copley Memorial Hospital

2000 Ogden Ave
Aurora, IL 60504-4206
Major participating institution for programs in: FP
Institution ID: 16-7005

Belleville

St Elizabeth's Hospital

211 S Third St
Belleville, IL 62222
Major participating institution for programs in: FP
Institution ID: 16-0787

Berwyn

MacNeal Memorial Hospital

3249 S Oak Park Ave
Berwyn, IL 60402
Med Sch Affil: L-01602, L-01643, L-01601, G-01642
Programs sponsored in: FP, FSM, TY
Major participating institution for programs in: CD, HO, IM, OBG
Institution ID: 16-0453

Carbondale

Memorial Hospital of Carbondale

405 W Jackson St
PO Box 10000
Carbondale, IL 62902-9000
Med Sch Affil: M-01645
Major participating institution for programs in: FP
Institution ID: 16-0508

Chicago

Catholic Health Partners

2913 N Commonwealth Ave
Chicago, IL 60657-6274
Programs sponsored in: FP, GS, IM, OBG, PD, TY
Institution ID: 16-8035

Children's Memorial Medical Center

2300 Children's Plaza
Chicago, IL 60614
Med Sch Affil: M-01606, G-01643
Major participating institution for programs in: AI, AN, CCP, CHN, CHP, CN, D, NPM, NS, OP, OPH, ORS, PD, PDC, PDE, PDI, PDP, PDR, PDS, PG, PHO, PN, PP, PPR, PS, PTH, RNR, TS, U
Institution ID: 16-0264

Columbus Hospital

2520 N Lakeview Ave
Chicago, IL 60614-1895
Med Sch Affil: L-01643, G-01606, G-01611
Major participating institution for programs in: OSM, PD, TY
Institution ID: 16-0334

Cook County Hospital

1835 W Harrison St
Chicago, IL 60612-9985
Med Sch Affil: M-01601, M-01642, M-01611, L-01602, G-01606, G-01643
Programs sponsored in: AN, APM, CD, CRS, D, DR, EM, END, FP, GE, GPM, HO, IM, IPM, MPD, NP, NPM, OBG, OPH, PCC, PD, PTH
Major participating institution for programs in: AI, CCM, CCP, GS, ID, N, NEP, NS, ORS, OTO, PS, TS
Institution ID: 16-0164

HCA Chicago Lakeshore Hospital

4840 N Marine Dr
Chicago, IL 60640
Med Sch Affil: L-01602
Major participating institution for programs in: CHP
Institution ID: 16-8028

Illinois Masonic Medical Center

836 W Wellington Ave
Chicago, IL 60657-5193
Med Sch Affil: M-01611, M-01601, L-01642, G-01643
Programs sponsored in: AN, CD, DR, ICE, IM, OBG, TY
Major participating institution for programs in: CCS, EM, FP, GS, PTH
Institution ID: 16-0411

Jackson Park Hospital

7531 S Stony Island Ave
Chicago, IL 60649-3913
Programs sponsored in: FP
Institution ID: 16-0354

Louis A Weiss Memorial Hospital

4646 N Marine Dr
Chicago, IL 60640
Med Sch Affil: M-01602
Programs sponsored in: IM, OAR, TY
Major participating institution for programs in: APM, GS, ORS, U
Institution ID: 16-0123

Mercy Hospital and Medical Center

2525 S Michigan Ave
Chicago, IL 60616-2477
Med Sch Affil: M-01611, M-01643, L-01602, G-01606
Programs sponsored in: IM, OBG
Major participating institution for programs in: DR, EM, GS, MPD, PTH, RHU
Institution ID: 16-0329

Michael Reese Hospital and Medical Center

2929 S Ellis Ave
Chicago, IL 60616-3390
Med Sch Affil: M-01611, G-01602
Major participating institution for programs in: AN, APM, CD, DMP, DR, EM, END, GE, GS, HO, ID, IM, MG, MPD, NM, NS, OBG, OPH, ORS, OTO, PCC, PD, PDE, PM, PS, PTH, RHU, RO, U
Institution ID: 16-0112

Mount Sinai Hospital Medical Center of Chicago

California Ave at 15th St
Chicago, IL 60608-1797
Med Sch Affil: M-01642, G-01602
Programs sponsored in: FP, OBG, PD
Major participating institution for programs in: CCM, CD, END, GE, GS, HO, ID, IM, P, PM, PTH, PUD
Institution ID: 16-0339

Northwestern Memorial Hospital

Wesley Pavilion/Rm 290
250 E Superior St
Chicago, IL 60611
Med Sch Affil: M-01606
Major participating institution for programs in: AN, APM, CCA, CD, CHN, CHP, CN, D, DR, EM, END, GE, GS, HMP, HO, ICE, ID, IM, IMG, MM, N, NEP, NM, NPM, NR, NS, OBG, OPH, ORS, OSM, OTO, P, PCC, PCP, PM, PP, PS, PTH, PYG, RHU, RNR, RO, TS, U, VIR, VS
Institution ID: 16-0286

Northwestern University Medical School

303 E Chicago Ave
Chicago, IL 60611-3008
Med Sch Affil: M-01606
Programs sponsored in: AI, AN, APM, CCA, CCP, CD, CHN, CHP, CN, D, DR, EM, END, GE, GS, HMP, HO, ICE, ID, IM, IMG, MM, N, NEP, NM, NPM, NR, NS, OBG, OP, OPH, ORS, OSM, OTO, P, PCC, PCP, PD, PDC, PDE, PDI, PDP, PDR, PDS, PG, PHO, PM, PN, PP, PPR, PS, PTH, PYG, RHU, RNR, RO, TS, TY, U, VIR, VS
Institution ID: 16-9502

Office of the Medical Examiner of Cook County
2121 W Harrison St
Chicago, IL 60612-3705
Med Sch Affil: G-01643
Programs sponsored in: FOP
Institution ID: 16-0502

Provident Hospital of Cook Country
500 E 51st St
Chicago, IL 60615
Major participating institution for programs in: FP
Institution ID: 16-0201

Ravenswood Hospital Medical Center
4550 N Winchester Ave
Chicago, IL 60640-5205
Med Sch Affil: M-01611, G-01642
Programs sponsored in: IM, TY
Major participating institution for programs in: FP, ORS, P, PD
Institution ID: 16-0115

Rehabilitation Institute of Chicago
345 E Superior St
Chicago, IL 60611
Med Sch Affil: M-01606
Major participating institution for programs in: PM, PPR
Institution ID: 16-0491

Resurrection Medical Center
7435 W Talcott Ave
Chicago, IL 60631
Med Sch Affil: M-01643, G-01642
Programs sponsored in: EM, FP, IM, TY
Major participating institution for programs in: GS
Institution ID: 16-0121

Rush-Presbyterian-St Luke's Medical Center
1653 W Congress Pkwy
Chicago, IL 60612-3833
Med Sch Affil: M-01601
Programs sponsored in: AI, AN, APM, CCM, CCP, CD, CHP, CN, D, DR, FP, GE, GS, HO, HSP, ICE, ID, IM, IMG, MP, MPD, N, NEP, NM, NR, NS, OBG, OPH, ORS, OSM, OSS, OTO, P, PCC, PD, PFP, PM, PS, PTH, RHU, RNR, RO, TS, U, VIR, VS
Major participating institution for programs in: FSM
Institution ID: 16-0278

Schwab Rehabilitation Hospital and Care Network
1401 S California Blvd
Chicago, IL 60608-1612
Programs sponsored in: PM
Major participating institution for programs in: PD
Institution ID: 16-0480

Shriners Hospitals for Children (Chicago)
2211 N Oak Park Ave
Chicago, IL 60635-3392
Med Sch Affil: L-01606, G-01643, G-01611, G-01601
Programs sponsored in: OP
Major participating institution for programs in: ORS, OSS, PS
Institution ID: 16-0312

St Anthony Hospital
2875 W 19th St
Chicago, IL 60623
Major participating institution for programs in: PD
Institution ID: 16-0370

St Elizabeth's Hospital
1431 N Claremont Ave
Chicago, IL 60622
Programs sponsored in: FP
Institution ID: 16-0143

St Joseph Health Centers and Hospital
2900 N Lake Shore Dr
Chicago, IL 60657
Med Sch Affil: M-01606, L-01602, G-01611, G-01643
Major participating institution for programs in: FP, IM, OSM
Institution ID: 16-0310

St Mary of Nazareth Hospital Center
Medical Affairs Office
2233 W Division St
Chicago, IL 60622-3086
Programs sponsored in: FP
Institution ID: 16-0133

Swedish Covenant Hospital
5145 N California Ave
Chicago, IL 60625
Med Sch Affil: L-01642
Programs sponsored in: FP, TY
Major participating institution for programs in: GS
Institution ID: 16-0342

University of Chicago Children's Hospital
5841 S Maryland Ave
Chicago, IL 60637
Med Sch Affil: M-01602
Major participating institution for programs in: CCP, MPD, NPM, PD, PDE, PDI, PDP, PDS, PHO, PPR
Institution ID: 16-0763

University of Chicago Hospitals
5841 S Maryland Ave
Chicago, IL 60637-1470
Med Sch Affil: M-01602, G-01611
Programs sponsored in: APM, BBK, CCM, CCP, CD, CHN, CHP, CN, D, DMP, DR, EM, END, GE, GS, HMP, HO, HSO, ICE, IM, IMG, MPD, N, NEP, NP, NPM, NS, OBG, OMO, OPH, ORS, OSM, OTO, P, PCC, PCP, PD, PDE, PDI, PDP, PDS, PG, PHO, PPR, PS, PTH, RHU, RNR, RO, TS, U, VIR, VS
Major participating institution for programs in: ID
Institution ID: 16-0465

University of Illinois College of Medicine at Chicago
1853 W Polk St/MC 784
Chicago, IL 60612
Med Sch Affil: M-01611
Programs sponsored in: ADP, AN, APM, CCS, CD, CHP, CN, D, DR, EM, END, FP, GE, GPM, GS, HMP, HO, ID, IM, IMG, MEM, MG, MPD, MPM, N, NEP, NM, NPM, NPR, NS, OBG, OPH, ORS, OSM, OTO, P, PCC, PCP, PD, PDE, PM, PS, PTH, PYN, RHU, TS, U
Institution ID: 16-0762

University of Illinois Hosp-Illinois Eye and Ear Infirmary
1855 W Taylor St
Chicago, IL 60612
Med Sch Affil: M-01611, L-01643
Major participating institution for programs in: OTO
Institution ID: 16-0337

University of Illinois Hospital and Clinics
1740 W Taylor St/MC 693
Chicago, IL 60612
Med Sch Affil: M-01611, L-01602
Major participating institution for programs in: ADP, AN, CD, D, DR, EM, END, FP, GE, GPM, GS, HO, ID, IM, IMG, MEM, MG, MPD, MPM, N, NEP, NPM, NPR, NS, OBG, OPH, ORS, OSM, P, PCC, PCP, PD, PDE, PM, PS, PTH, RHU, TS, U
Institution ID: 16-0447

University of Illinois School of Public Health
2121 W Taylor St
Chicago, IL 60612-7260
Major participating institution for programs in: GPM
Institution ID: 16-0769

Veterans Affairs Lakeside Medical Center (Chicago)
333 E Huron St
Chicago, IL 60611
Med Sch Affil: M-01606
Major participating institution for programs in: ADP, AN, CCA, CD, D, DR, END, GE, GS, HO, ID, IM, IMG, N, NEP, NS, OPH, ORS, OTO, P, PCC, PCP, PTH, RHU, TS, U, VS
Institution ID: 16-0243

Veterans Affairs West Side Medical Center
820 S Damen Ave
PO Box 8195
Chicago, IL 60680
Med Sch Affil: M-01611
Major participating institution for programs in: CD, D, DR, END, GE, GS, HO, ID, IM, IMG, MPD, MPM, NEP, ORS, OTO, P, PCC, PM, PTH, RHU, TS, U
Institution ID: 16-0220

Danville

Veterans Affairs Medical Center (Danville)
1900 E Main St
Danville, IL 61832
Med Sch Affil: M-01611, L-01645
Major participating institution for programs in: IM
Institution ID: 16-0766

Decatur

Decatur Memorial Hospital
2300 N Edward St
Decatur, IL 62526
Med Sch Affil: G-01645
Major participating institution for programs in: FP
Institution ID: 16-0158

St Mary's Hospital
1800 E Lake Shore Dr
Decatur, IL 62521
Med Sch Affil: G-01645
Major participating institution for programs in: FP
Institution ID: 16-0767

Evanston

Evanston Hospital
2650 Ridge Ave
Evanston, IL 60201-1781
Med Sch Affil: M-01606, G-01642
Major participating institution for programs in: AN, DR, EM, GS, IM, N, NPM, NS, OBG, OPH, ORS, P, PD, PS, PTH, RO, TS, TY
Institution ID: 16-0145

St Francis Hospital of Evanston
355 Ridge Ave
Evanston, IL 60202-3399
Med Sch Affil: M-01611, L-01602, G-01643
Programs sponsored in: DR, FP, IM, OBG, TY
Major participating institution for programs in: GE, GS
Institution ID: 16-0168

Hines

Edward J Hines Jr Veterans Affairs Hospital
5th Ave and Roosevelt Rd
PO Box 5000
Hines, IL 60141
Med Sch Affil: M-01643, L-01642
Major participating institution for programs in: AN, CD, CHN, CN, D, END, GE, GS, HMP, HO, ID, IM, IMG, N, NEP, NM, NP, OPH, ORS, OTO, P, PCC, PCP, PM, PS, PTH, RHU, RO, TS, U, VS
Institution ID: 16-0259

Hinsdale

Hinsdale Hospital
120 N Oak St
Hinsdale, IL 60521-3829
Med Sch Affil: L-00512, L-01601, L-01642
Programs sponsored in: FP
Institution ID: 16-0369

Joliet

Provena St Joseph Medical Center
333 N Madison St
Joliet, IL 60435-6595
Programs sponsored in: FP
Institution ID: 16-0325

Kewanee

Kewanee Hospital
719 Elliott St
PO Box 747
Kewanee, IL 61443-0747
Major participating institution for programs in: FP
Institution ID: 16-8034

LaGrange

La Grange Memorial Hospital
5101 S Willow Springs Rd
LaGrange, IL 60525-9998
Med Sch Affil: L-01602, L-01601
Programs sponsored in: FP
Major participating institution for programs in: IMG, TS
Institution ID: 16-0175

Maywood

Loyola University Medical Center
2160 S First Ave
Maywood, IL 60153-5585
Med Sch Affil: M-01643
Programs sponsored in: AN, APM, BBK, CD, CHN, CN, DR, END, FP, GE, GS, HMP, HO, ICE, ID, IM, IMG, MPD, N, NEP, NM, NP, NPM, NS, OBG, OPH, ORS, OTO, P, PCC, PCP, PD, PDE, PM, PS, PTH, RHU, RNR, RO, TS, TY, U, VS
Institution ID: 16-0498

Melrose Park

Westlake Community Hospital
1225 Lake St
Melrose Park, IL 60160
Med Sch Affil: L-01601
Major participating institution for programs in: IM
Institution ID: 16-7049

North Chicago

Finch University of Health Sciences/Chicago Medical School
3333 Green Bay Rd
North Chicago, IL 60064
Med Sch Affil: M-01642
Programs sponsored in: CCM, CD, END, GS, HO, ID, IM, P, PUD
Institution ID: 16-0748

Veterans Affairs Medical Center (North Chicago)
3001 Green Bay Rd
North Chicago, IL 60064
Med Sch Affil: M-01642
Major participating institution for programs in: CCM, CD, END, HO, ID, IM, P, PUD
Institution ID: 16-0460

Oak Forest

Oak Forest Hospital of Cook County
15900 S Cicero Ave
Oak Forest, IL 60452
Med Sch Affil: G-01602, G-01601
Major participating institution for programs in: OPH, PM
Institution ID: 16-0732

Oak Lawn

Christ Hospital and Medical Center
4440 W 95th St
Oak Lawn, IL 60453-4213
Med Sch Affil: M-01611, L-01642, L-01601
Programs sponsored in: CCP, EM, PD, PDC
Major participating institution for programs in: CD, END, FP, GS, IM, N, OBG, TS, U
Institution ID: 16-0303

Oak Park

West Suburban Hospital Medical Center
Erie at Austin
Oak Park, IL 60302
Med Sch Affil: L-01601
Programs sponsored in: FP, IM, TY
Major participating institution for programs in: NS, OBG
Institution ID: 16-0454

Park Ridge

Lutheran General Hospital
1775 Dempster St
Park Ridge, IL 60068-1174
Med Sch Affil: M-01642, G-01611, G-01643, G-01606
Programs sponsored in: CCP, CD, FP, FSM, GE, IM, IMG, NPM, OBG, P, PD
Major participating institution for programs in: GS, PDS, PS, PTH, U
Institution ID: 16-0484

Peoria

Methodist Medical Center of Illinois
221 NE Glen Oak Ave
Peoria, IL 61636
Med Sch Affil: M-01611
Major participating institution for programs in: FP, N, NS
Institution ID: 16-0390

St Francis Medical Center
530 NE Glen Oak Ave
Peoria, IL 61637
Med Sch Affil: M-01611
Programs sponsored in: MPD
Major participating institution for programs in: DR, EM, GS, IM, N, NS, OBG, PD, RNR
Institution ID: 16-0398

University of Illinois College of Medicine at Peoria
One Illini Dr
Peoria, IL 61605
Programs sponsored in: DR, EM, FP, GS, IM, N, NS, OBG, PD, RNR
Institution ID: 16-0751

Quincy

Blessing Hospital
Broadway at 11th St
PO Box 7005
Quincy, IL 62305-7005
Med Sch Affil: G-01645
Major participating institution for programs in: FP
Institution ID: 16-7127

Rockford

Swedish American Health System
1400 Charles St
Rockford, IL 61104-2298
Med Sch Affil: M-01611
Major participating institution for programs in: FP
Institution ID: 16-0446

University of Illinois College of Medicine at Rockford
1601 Parkview Ave
Rockford, IL 61107-1897
Programs sponsored in: FP
Institution ID: 16-0504

Scott AFB

375th Medical Group
Scott AFB, IL 62225-5252
Med Sch Affil: G-02312
Major participating institution for programs in: FP
Institution ID: 16-0476

Skokie

Rush North Shore Medical Center
9600 Gross Point Rd
Skokie, IL 60076
Med Sch Affil: M-01601
Major participating institution for programs in: APM, OBG
Institution ID: 16-0753

Springfield

Illinois Department of Public Health
535 W Jefferson St
Springfield, IL 62761
Med Sch Affil: G-01645
Programs sponsored in: GPM
Institution ID: 16-0167

Memorial Medical Center
701 N 1st St
Springfield, IL 62781-0001
Med Sch Affil: M-01645
Major participating institution for programs in: D, DR, END, FP, GE, GS, HSP, ID, IM, MP, MPD, N, OBG, ORS, OSS, OTO, P, PS, PUD, U, VS
Institution ID: 16-0509

Southern Illinois University School of Medicine
800 N Rutledge St/D234
PO Box 19230
Springfield, IL 62794-9230
Med Sch Affil: M-01645
Programs sponsored in: D, DR, END, FP, GE, GS, HSP, ID, IM, MP, MPD, N, OBG, ORS, OSS, OTO, P, PD, PS, PUD, U, VS
Institution ID: 16-0512

St John's Hospital
800 E Carpenter St
Springfield, IL 62769
Med Sch Affil: M-01645
Major participating institution for programs in: D, DR, END, FP, GE, GS, HSP, ID, IM, MP, MPD, N, OBG, ORS, OSS, OTO, P, PD, PS, PUD, U, VS
Institution ID: 16-0503

Urbana

Carle Foundation Hospital
611 W Park St
Urbana, IL 61801-2595
Med Sch Affil: M-01611
Programs sponsored in: CRS, FP
Major participating institution for programs in: IM
Institution ID: 16-0146

Provena Covenant Medical Center
1400 W Park St
Urbana, IL 61801
Med Sch Affil: M-01611
Major participating institution for programs in: IM
Institution ID: 16-0768

University of Illinois College of Medicine at Urbana
190 Medical Sciences Bldg
506 S Mathews St
Urbana, IL 61801
Med Sch Affil: M-01611
Programs sponsored in: IM
Institution ID: 16-0752

Wheaton

Marianjoy Rehabilitation Hospital and Clinics
26 W 171 Roosevelt Rd
PO Box 795
Wheaton, IL 60189-0795
Med Sch Affil: G-01601, G-01643
Major participating institution for programs in: PM
Institution ID: 16-8025

Rehabilitation Foundation Inc
26 W 171 Roosevelt Rd
PO Box 675
Wheaton, IL 60189
Programs sponsored in: PM
Institution ID: 16-8033

Indiana

Beech Grove

St Francis Hospital and Health Centers
1600 Albany St
Beech Grove, IN 46107-1593
Med Sch Affil: L-01720
Programs sponsored in: FP
Institution ID: 17-0125

Evansville

Deaconess Hospital
415 W Columbia St
Evansville, IN 47710
Med Sch Affil: L-01720
Programs sponsored in: FP
Institution ID: 17-0708

St Mary's Medical Center
3700 Washington Ave
Evansville, IN 47750
Med Sch Affil: L-01720
Programs sponsored in: FP
Institution ID: 17-0424

Fort Wayne

Fort Wayne Medical Education Program
2448 Lake Ave
Fort Wayne, IN 46805
Programs sponsored in: FP, ORS
Institution ID: 17-0446

Fort Wayne State Development Center
4900 St Joe Rd
Fort Wayne, IN 46835
Major participating institution for programs in: ORS
Institution ID: 17-8003

Lutheran Hospital of Indiana
7950 W Jefferson Blvd
Fort Wayne, IN 46804
Med Sch Affil: L-01720
Major participating institution for programs in: FP
Institution ID: 17-0228

Parkview Memorial Hospital
2200 Randallia Dr
Fort Wayne, IN 46805
Med Sch Affil: L-01720
Major participating institution for programs in: FP, ORS
Institution ID: 17-0447

St Joseph's Medical Center
700 Broadway
Fort Wayne, IN 46802
Med Sch Affil: L-01720
Major participating institution for programs in: FP, ORS
Institution ID: 17-0422

Gary

Methodist Hospitals
600 Grant St
Gary, IN 46402-1523
Med Sch Affil: L-01720
Programs sponsored in: FP
Institution ID: 17-0236

Indianapolis

Central Indiana Regional Blood Center
3450 N Meridian St
Indianapolis, IN 46208
Major participating institution for programs in: BBK
Institution ID: 17-8008

Clarian IU Hospital
550 N University Blvd
Indianapolis, IN 46202-5250
Med Sch Affil: M-01720
Programs sponsored in: PYN
Major participating institution for programs in: AN, APM, BBK, CD, CN, CPP, D, DMP, DR, END, GE, GS, HMP, HO, HSO, IM, MG, MM, MN, MPD, NM, NS, OBG, OPH, ORS, OTO, P, PCC, PCP, PDC, PM, PS, PTH, PYG, RHU, RNR, RO, TS, U, VIR
Institution ID: 17-0444

Clarian Methodist Hospital of Indiana
I-65 at 21st St
PO Box 1367
Indianapolis, IN 46206-1367
Med Sch Affil: M-01720
Major participating institution for programs in: ADL, DR, EM, EMP, FP, FSM, GS, IM, NS, OBG, OPH, ORS, OSM, PCC, PD, PTH, PYG, TY, U, VIR
Institution ID: 17-0217

Clarian Riley Hospital for Children
702 N Barnhill Dr
Indianapolis, IN 46202-5200
Major participating institution for programs in: ADL, AN, APM, CHN, CHP, CN, CPP, D, DMP, DR, GS, HMP, IM, MG, MM, N, NM, NPM, NS, OBG, OPH, ORS, OTO, P, PCP, PD, PDC, PDE, PDP, PDR, PDS, PG, PHO, PM, PN, PP, PS, PTH, RHU, RNR, RO, TS, U, UP, VIR
Institution ID: 17-8005

Community Hospitals of Indianapolis
1500 N Ritter Ave
Indianapolis, IN 46219-0805
Med Sch Affil: M-01720
Programs sponsored in: FP
Major participating institution for programs in: PM
Institution ID: 17-0710

Indiana Hand Center
8501 Hardcourt Rd
Indianapolis, IN 46260
Major participating institution for programs in: HSO
Institution ID: 17-8007

Indiana University School of Medicine
1120 South Dr
302 Fesler Hall
Indianapolis, IN 46202-5114
Programs sponsored in: ADL, ADP, AN, APM, BBK, CD, CHN, CHP, CN, CPP, D, DMP, DR, EM, EMP, END, FOP, FP, FSM, GE, GS, HMP, HO, HSO, ICE, ID, IM, IMG, MG, MM, MN, MPD, N, NEP, NM, NPM, NS, OBG, OPH, ORS, OSM, OTO, P, PCC, PCP, PD, PDC, PDE, PDP, PDR, PDS, PG, PHO, PM, PN, PP, PS, PTH, PYG, RHU, RNR, RO, TS, TY, U, UP, VIR
Institution ID: 17-9501

Larue D Carter Memorial Hospital
2601 Cold Spring Rd
Indianapolis, IN 46222
Med Sch Affil: M-01720
Major participating institution for programs in: CHP, P
Institution ID: 17-0189

Richard L Roudebush Veterans Affairs Medical Center
1481 W 10th St
Indianapolis, IN 46202-2884
Med Sch Affil: M-01720
Major participating institution for programs in: ADP, AN, D, DMP, DR, END, GE, GS, ICE, IM, IMG, MM, MN, MPD, N, NM, NS, OPH, ORS, OTO, P, PCP, PM, PS, PTH, PYN, RHU, RO, TS, U
Institution ID: 17-0414

St Vincent Hospital and Health Care Center
2001 W 86th St
PO Box 40970
Indianapolis, IN 46240
Med Sch Affil: M-01720
Programs sponsored in: FP, IM, OBG, TY
Major participating institution for programs in: HSO
Institution ID: 17-0421

William N Wishard Memorial Hospital
1001 W 10th St
Indianapolis, IN 46202-2879
Med Sch Affil: M-01720
Major participating institution for programs in: ADL, ADP, AN, CHP, D, DMP, DR, END, GE, GS, IM, IMG, MM, MN, MPD, N, NM, NPM, NS, OBG, OPH, ORS, OTO, P, PCC, PCP, PD, PDS, PS, PTH, PYG, PYN, RHU, RNR, RO, U
Institution ID: 17-0141

Muncie

Ball Memorial Hospital
2401 University Ave
Muncie, IN 47303-3499
Med Sch Affil: L-01720
Programs sponsored in: FP, FPG, IM, ISM, PTH, TY
Institution ID: 17-0150

South Bend

Memorial Hospital of South Bend
714 N Michigan St
South Bend, IN 46601-9986
Med Sch Affil: L-01720
Programs sponsored in: FP, FSM
Major participating institution for programs in: FSM
Institution ID: 17-0335

St Joseph's Regional Medical Center of South Bend
801 E LaSalle St
PO Box 1935
South Bend, IN 46634-1935
Med Sch Affil: L-01720
Programs sponsored in: FP, FSM
Major participating institution for programs in: FSM
Institution ID: 17-0419

Terre Haute

Union Hospital
1606 N 7th St
Terre Haute, IN 47804-2780
Med Sch Affil: L-01720
Programs sponsored in: FP
Institution ID: 17-0709

Iowa

Cedar Rapids

Cedar Rapids Medical Education Foundation
1026 A Ave NE
Cedar Rapids, IA 52402
Programs sponsored in: FP
Institution ID: 18-8002

Mercy Medical Center
701 10th St SE
Cedar Rapids, IA 52403-0003
Major participating institution for programs in: FP
Institution ID: 18-0452

St Luke's Methodist Hospital
1026 A Ave NE
PO Box 3026
Cedar Rapids, IA 52406-3026
Major participating institution for programs in: FP
Institution ID: 18-0417

Davenport

Genesis Medical Center
1227 E Rusholme St
Davenport, IA 52803
Med Sch Affil: L-01803
Major participating institution for programs in: FP
Institution ID: 18-8001

Genesis Medical Education Foundation
1345 W Central Park
Davenport, IA 52804
Programs sponsored in: FP
Institution ID: 18-9501

Des Moines

Broadlawns Medical Center
1801 Hickman Rd
Des Moines, IA 50314-1597
Med Sch Affil: L-01803
Programs sponsored in: FP, TY
Major participating institution for programs in: GS
Institution ID: 18-0240

Iowa Lutheran Hospital
700 E University Ave
Des Moines, IA 50316-2396
Med Sch Affil: L-01803
Programs sponsored in: FP
Institution ID: 18-0496

Iowa Methodist Medical Center
1200 Pleasant St
Des Moines, IA 50309-1453
Med Sch Affil: M-01803
Programs sponsored in: GS, IM, PD, TY
Major participating institution for programs in: TY
Institution ID: 18-0130

Mercy Hospital Medical Center
400 University Ave
Des Moines, IA 50314-3190
Major participating institution for programs in: FP
Institution ID: 18-0356

Veterans Affairs Central Iowa Health Care System
3600 30th St
Des Moines, IA 50310-5774
Med Sch Affil: L-01803
Major participating institution for programs in: GS, IM, TY
Institution ID: 18-0226

Iowa City

Mercy Hospital
500 E Market St
Iowa City, IA 52245
Med Sch Affil: G-01803
Major participating institution for programs in: FP
Institution ID: 18-0416

University of Iowa Hospitals and Clinics
200 Hawkins Dr
Iowa City, IA 52242-1009
Med Sch Affil: M-01803
Programs sponsored in: AI, AN, APM, BBK, CCA, CD, CHP, CN, D, DR, END, FP, FPG, FPP, GE, GPM, GS, HMP, HO, HSO, ICE, ID, IM, MG, MP, N, NEP, NM, NO, NP, NPM, NS, OBG, OPH, ORS, OSM, OTO, P, PCC, PCP, PD, PDC, PDE, PDO, PDP, PDR, PG, PHO, PIP, PN, PTH, RHU, RNR, RO, TS, U, VIR, VS
Institution ID: 18-0415

Veterans Affairs Medical Center (Iowa City)
Highway #6 West
Iowa City, IA 52246
Med Sch Affil: M-01803
Major participating institution for programs in: AN, DR, GS, ICE, IM, MP, N, NM, NP, NS, ORS, OTO, P, PCP, PTH, RNR, U, VIR
Institution ID: 18-0319

Mason City

North Iowa Mercy Health Center
1000 Fourth St SW
Mason City, IA 50401
Med Sch Affil: L-01803
Programs sponsored in: FP
Institution ID: 18-0705

Sioux City

Marian Health Center
801 5th St
PO Box 3168
Sioux City, IA 51101
Med Sch Affil: L-01803
Major participating institution for programs in: FP
Institution ID: 18-0709

St Luke's Regional Medical Center
2720 Stone Park Blvd
Sioux City, IA 51104-9989
Med Sch Affil: L-01803
Programs sponsored in: FP
Institution ID: 18-0710

Waterloo

Allen Memorial Hospital
1825 Logan Ave
Waterloo, IA 50703-1999
Med Sch Affil: L-01803
Major participating institution for programs in: FP
Institution ID: 18-0713

Covenant Medical Center
3421 W 9th St
Waterloo, IA 50702-5499
Med Sch Affil: L-01803
Major participating institution for programs in: FP
Institution ID: 18-0714

Northeast Iowa Medical Education Foundation
441 E San Marman Dr
Waterloo, IA 50702
Programs sponsored in: FP
Institution ID: 18-0712

Kansas

Hays

Hays Medical Center
2220 Canterbury Dr
PO Box 660
Hays, KS 67601
Med Sch Affil: G-01902
Major participating institution for programs in: FP
Institution ID: 19-8004

Junction City

Geary Community Hospital
1102 St Mary's Rd
Box 490
Junction City, KS 66441
Major participating institution for programs in: FP
Institution ID: 19-8003

Kansas City

Bethany Medical Center
51 N 12th St
Kansas City, KS 66102
Med Sch Affil: L-01902
Major participating institution for programs in: IM, PM
Institution ID: 19-0418

University of Kansas Medical Center
3901 Rainbow Blvd
Kansas City, KS 66160-7100
Med Sch Affil: M-01902
Major participating institution for programs in: AI, AN, CD, CHP, D, DR, FP, GE, GS, HEM, ID, IM, IMG, MP, MPD, N, NEP, NM, NR, NS, OBG, ON, OPH, ORS, OTO, P, PCC, PCP, PD, PM, PPR, PS, PTH, RHU, RO, U, VS
Institution ID: 19-0488

University of Kansas School of Medicine
3901 Rainbow Blvd
Kansas City, KS 66160-7100
Med Sch Affil: M-01902
Programs sponsored in: AI, AN, CD, CHP, D, DR, FP, GE, GS, HEM, ID, IM, IMG, MP, MPD, N, NEP, NM, NR, NS, OBG, ON, OPH, ORS, OTO, P, PCC, PCP, PD, PM, PPR, PS, PTH, RHU, RO, U, VS
Institution ID: 19-9501

Leavenworth

Dwight D Eisenhower Veterans Affairs Medical Center
4101 S 4th St Trafficway
Leavenworth, KS 66048-5055
Med Sch Affil: M-01902
Major participating institution for programs in: GS, IM, PM
Institution ID: 19-0406

Salina

Salina Regional Health Center
400 S Santa Fe Ave
PO Box 5080
Salina, KS 67402-5080
Major participating institution for programs in: FP
Institution ID: 19-0518

Topeka

C F Menninger Memorial Hospital
5800 SW 6th Ave
PO Box 829
Topeka, KS 66601-0829
Major participating institution for programs in: CHP
Institution ID: 19-0504

Colmery-O'Neil Veterans Affairs Medical Center
2200 Gage Blvd
Topeka, KS 66622
Major participating institution for programs in: P
Institution ID: 19-0498

Kansas Medical Education Foundation
1505 SW 8th St
Topeka, KS 66606-1630
Programs sponsored in: FP
Institution ID: 19-8002

Menninger Clinic
PO Box 829
Topeka, KS 66601-0829
Programs sponsored in: CHP, P
Institution ID: 19-8005

St Francis Hospital and Medical Center
1700 W 7th St
Topeka, KS 66606-1690
Med Sch Affil: G-01902
Major participating institution for programs in: FP
Institution ID: 19-0513

Stormont-Vail Regional Health Center
1500 SW 10th
Topeka, KS 66604-1353
Med Sch Affil: G-01902
Major participating institution for programs in: FP
Institution ID: 19-0510

Topeka State Hospital
Center Bldg
2700 W 6th St
Topeka, KS 66606-1898
Major participating institution for programs in: P
Institution ID: 19-0138

Wichita

Charter Hospital of Wichita
8901 E Orme
Wichita, KS 67207
Major participating institution for programs in: P
Institution ID: 19-8001

Columbia Wesley Medical Center
550 N Hillside
Wichita, KS 67214-4976
Med Sch Affil: M-01902
Major participating institution for programs in: AN, DR, FP, GS, IM, MPD, OBG, ORS, PD
Institution ID: 19-0500

University of Kansas School of Medicine (Wichita)
1010 N Kansas
Wichita, KS 67214-3199
Med Sch Affil: M-01902
Programs sponsored in: AN, DR, FP, GS, IM, MPD, OBG, ORS, P, PD, PYG
Institution ID: 19-0511

Veterans Affairs Medical Center (Wichita)
5500 E Kellogg
Wichita, KS 67218
Med Sch Affil: L-01902
Major participating institution for programs in: IM, ORS, P
Institution ID: 19-0196

Via Christi Regional Medical Center
929 N St Francis Ave
Wichita, KS 67214-3882
Med Sch Affil: M-01902
Major participating institution for programs in: AN, FP, GS, IM, ORS, P, PYG
Institution ID: 19-0132

Via Christi Regional Medical Center-St Joseph
3600 E Harry St
Wichita, KS 67218-3713
Med Sch Affil: M-01902
Major participating institution for programs in: AN, FP, P, PYG
Institution ID: 19-0306

Kentucky

Edgewood

St Elizabeth Medical Center
One Medical Village Dr
Edgewood, KY 41017-3422
Med Sch Affil: L-03841, G-02012
Programs sponsored in: FP
Institution ID: 20-0463

Glasgow

T J Samspon Community Hospital
1301 N Race St
Glasgow, KY 42141
Major participating institution for programs in: FP
Institution ID: 20-7044

Hazard

ARH Regional Medical Center
100 Medical Center Dr
Hazard, KY 41701
Med Sch Affil: G-02012
Major participating institution for programs in: FP
Institution ID: 20-7045

Lexington

Cardinal Hill Hospital
2050 Versailles Rd
Lexington, KY 40504
Med Sch Affil: G-02012
Major participating institution for programs in: PM
Institution ID: 20-0525

Central Baptist Hospital
1740 Nicholasville Rd
Lexington, KY 40503
Major participating institution for programs in: OSM, U
Institution ID: 20-0248

Charter Ridge Hospital
3050 Rio Dosa Dr
Lexington, KY 40509
Med Sch Affil: G-02012
Major participating institution for programs in: ADP, CHP, CPP
Institution ID: 20-8006

Kentucky Sports Medicine Clinic
601 Perimeter Dr
Lexington, KY 40517
Programs sponsored in: OSM
Institution ID: 20-8010

Shriners Hospital for Children (Lexington)
1900 Richmond Rd
Lexington, KY 40502-1298
Med Sch Affil: G-02012
Major participating institution for programs in: ORS
Institution ID: 20-0284

St Joseph Hospital
1 St Joseph Dr
Lexington, KY 40504-3754
Med Sch Affil: L-02012
Major participating institution for programs in: U
Institution ID: 20-0261

University of Kentucky College of Medicine
800 Rose St/N-106
Lexington, KY 40536-0084
Med Sch Affil: M-02012
Programs sponsored in: FP
Major participating institution for programs in: GPM
Institution ID: 20-0513

University of Kentucky Hospital
800 Rose St/N-106
Lexington, KY 40536-0084
Med Sch Affil: M-02012
Programs sponsored in: ADP, AN, APM, CD, CHP, CPP, DR, EM, FP, GE, GPM, GS, HO, ID, IM, IMG, MPD, N, NEP, NPM, NS, OBG, OPH, ORS, OSM, OTO, P, PCC, PCP, PD, PM, PS, PTH, RO, U, VS
Major participating institution for programs in: FP
Institution ID: 20-0505

Veterans Affairs Medical Center (Lexington)
2250 Leestown Rd
Lexington, KY 40511-1093
Med Sch Affil: M-02012
Major participating institution for programs in: ADP, CD, GE, GS, HO, ID, IM, MPD, N, NEP, NS, OPH, ORS, OTO, P, PCC, PCP, PM, PS, PTH, U, VS
Institution ID: 20-0352

Louisville

Alliant Medical Pavilion
315 E Broadway
PO Box 35070
Louisville, KY 40232
Med Sch Affil: L-02012
Major participating institution for programs in: ORS
Institution ID: 20-8007

Amelia Brown Frazier Rehabilitation Center
220 Abraham Flexner Way
Louisville, KY 40202
Med Sch Affil: G-02002
Major participating institution for programs in: PM
Institution ID: 20-0515

American Red Cross Blood Services (Louisville Region)
520 E Chestnut St
PO Box 3168
Louisville, KY 40201-3168
Programs sponsored in: BBK
Institution ID: 20-8020

Child Psychiatric Services (Bingham Child Guidance Clinic)
200 E Chestnut St
Louisville, KY 40202-1822
Med Sch Affil: L-02002
Major participating institution for programs in: CHP, P
Institution ID: 20-0500

James Graham Brown Medical Center
529 S Jackson St
Louisville, KY 40202
Major participating institution for programs in: HO
Institution ID: 20-8005

Jewish Hospital
217 E Chestnut St
Louisville, KY 40202
Med Sch Affil: G-02002
Major participating institution for programs in: END, FP, GE, HSS, ICE, NEP, ORS, PS, TS, U
Institution ID: 20-0136

Kleinert, Kutz, and Associates
1 Medical Plaza/Ste 850
Louisville, KY 40202
Med Sch Affil: L-03607
Major participating institution for programs in: PS
Institution ID: 20-8003

Kosair Children's Hospital (Alliant Health System)
Medical Towers South/Ste 225
PO Box 35070
Louisville, KY 40232-5070
Med Sch Affil: M-02002
Major participating institution for programs in: AN, BBK, CCP, CHP, EM, GS, MPD, NEP, NPM, NS, OBG, OPH, ORS, OTO, PD, PDI, PG, PS, PTH, TS, U
Institution ID: 20-0345

Norton Hospital (Alliant Health System)
PO Box 35070
200 E Chestnut St
Louisville, KY 40232-5070
Med Sch Affil: M-02002
Major participating institution for programs in: BBK, EM, END, GE, GS, N, NEP, NS, OBG, OTO, P, PS, PTH, U
Institution ID: 20-0235

Office of Chief Medical Examiner
810 Barret Ave
Louisville, KY 40204
Major participating institution for programs in: FOP
Institution ID: 20-8008

University of Louisville Hospital
530 S Jackson St
Louisville, KY 40202-3611
Med Sch Affil: M-02002
Major participating institution for programs in: AN, BBK, CCS, CD, D, DR, EM, END, FOP, FP, FPG, GE, GS, HO, ICE, ID, IM, MPD, N, NEP, NPM, NS, OBG, OPH, ORS, OTO, P, PCC, PS, PTH, RHU, RO, TS, U
Institution ID: 20-0283

University of Louisville School of Medicine
Health Sciences Ctr
Louisville, KY 40292
Med Sch Affil: M-02002
Programs sponsored in: AN, CCP, CCS, CD, CHP, D, DR, EM, END, FOP, FP, FPG, GE, GS, HO, HSS, ICE, ID, IM, MPD, N, NEP, NPM, NS, OBG, OPH, ORS, OTO, P, PCC, PCP, PD, PDI, PG, PM, PS, PTH, RHU, RO, TS, U
Institution ID: 20-0507

Veterans Affairs Medical Center (Louisville)
800 Zorn Ave
Louisville, KY 40206-1499
Med Sch Affil: M-02002
Major participating institution for programs in: AN, CD, D, DR, END, GE, GS, HO, ICE, ID, IM, MPD, N, NEP, OPH, ORS, OTO, P, PCC, PS, PTH, RHU, TS, U
Institution ID: 20-0179

Madisonville

Regional Medical Center of Hopkins County
900 Hospital Dr
Madisonville, KY 42431-1694
Med Sch Affil: L-02002, L-02012
Major participating institution for programs in: FP
Institution ID: 20-0520

Trover Clinic Foundation
900 Hospital Dr
Madisonville, KY 42431-1768
Programs sponsored in: FP
Institution ID: 20-8021

Louisiana

Alexandria

Rapides Regional Medical Center
211 Fourth St
Box 30101
Alexandria, LA 71306
Med Sch Affil: L-02106
Major participating institution for programs in: FP
Institution ID: 21-8028

Veterans Affairs Medical Center (Alexandria)
Shreveport Hwy
Alexandria, LA 71301
Med Sch Affil: G-02101
Major participating institution for programs in: ORS
Institution ID: 21-0100

Baton Rouge

Baton Rouge General Medical Center
3600 Florida Blvd
PO Box 2511
Baton Rouge, LA 70821-2511
Med Sch Affil: M-02105
Programs sponsored in: FP
Major participating institution for programs in: EM
Institution ID: 21-7005

Earl K Long Medical Center
5825 Airline Hwy
Baton Rouge, LA 70805-2498
Med Sch Affil: M-02105
Programs sponsored in: EM, FP, IM, MPD
Major participating institution for programs in: GS, OBG, ORS
Institution ID: 21-0491

Gretna

Meadowcrest Hospital
2500 Belle Chase Hwy
Gretna, LA 70056
Major participating institution for programs in: U
Institution ID: 21-8023

Homer

Homer Memorial Hospital
E College St
Box 809
Homer, LA 71040
Med Sch Affil: L-02106
Major participating institution for programs in: FP
Institution ID: 21-8029

Houma

Leonard J Chabert Medical Center
1978 Industrial Blvd
Houma, LA 70363
Major participating institution for programs in: FP, GS, IFP, IM, OBG, ORS
Institution ID: 21-0735

Kenner

Kenner Regional Medical Center
180 W Esplanade
Kenner, LA 70065
Major participating institution for programs in: FP
Institution ID: 21-8030

Lafayette

University Medical Center (Lafayette)
2390 W Congress
PO Box 4016-C
Lafayette, LA 70502-4016
Med Sch Affil: M-02105
Programs sponsored in: FP, IM
Major participating institution for programs in: GS, OBG, ORS, OTO
Institution ID: 21-0380

Lake Charles

Lake Charles Memorial Hospital
1701 Oak Park Blvd
Drawer M
Lake Charles, LA 70601
Med Sch Affil: L-02105, L-02106
Major participating institution for programs in: FP, OSM
Institution ID: 21-8019

Metairie

East Jefferson General Hospital
4200 Houma Blvd
Metairie, LA 70011
Programs sponsored in: FP
Institution ID: 21-8021

Monroe

E A Conway Medical Center
PO Box 1881
4864 Jackson St
Monroe, LA 71210-1881
Med Sch Affil: G-02106
Programs sponsored in: FP
Major participating institution for programs in: GS, OBG, TY
Institution ID: 21-0344

New Orleans

Alton Ochsner Medical Foundation
1516 Jefferson Hwy
New Orleans, LA 70121
Med Sch Affil: M-02105, L-00106, G-02101
Programs sponsored in: AN, CD, CRS, DR, END, FP, GE, GS, ID, IFP, IM, OBG, ON, ORS, P, PTH, RHU, TS, U, VS
Major participating institution for programs in: HMP, NEP, NS, OPH, OTO, PCC, PD, PDC
Institution ID: 21-0381

Children's Hospital
200 Henry Clay Ave
New Orleans, LA 70118
Med Sch Affil: M-02105, L-00106, G-02101
Major participating institution for programs in: AI, CHN, CN, DR, MPD, NPM, NS, OP, ORS, PD, PG, PHO, PP, TY, U
Institution ID: 21-0731

DePaul/Tulane Behavioral Health Center
1040 Calhoun St
New Orleans, LA 70118
Major participating institution for programs in: ADP
Institution ID: 21-8031

Louisiana Rehabilitation Institute
L M Building
1532 Tulane Ave
New Orleans, LA 70140
Major participating institution for programs in: PM
Institution ID: 21-0734

Louisiana State University Medical College Campus
2021 Perdido St
New Orleans, LA 70112
Major participating institution for programs in: MEM, MPD, MPM, OSM
Institution ID: 21-0231

Louisiana State University Medical College Campus
2021 Perdido St
New Orleans, LA 70112
Med Sch Affil: M-02101
Major participating institution for programs in: AI, MN, MP, PYN
Institution ID: 21-0726

Louisiana State University School of Medicine
1542 Tulane Ave/SL 76
New Orleans, LA 70112-2822
Med Sch Affil: M-02105
Programs sponsored in: AI, AN, BBK, CD, CHN, CHP, CN, D, DR, EM, END, FOP, FP, GE, GS, HEM, ID, IM, MEM, MPD, MPM, N, NEP, NPM, NS, OBG, ON, OP, OPH, ORS, OSM, OTO, P, PCC, PCP, PD, PFP, PG, PHO, PM, PP, PS, PTH, PYG, RHU, RNR, VIR, VS
Major participating institution for programs in: TS
Institution ID: 21-9502

LSU/Ochsner Opthalmology Center
2020 Gravier St/Ste B
New Orleans, LA 70112
Med Sch Affil: M-02105
Major participating institution for programs in: OPH
Institution ID: 21-8015

Medical Center of Louisiana at New Orleans
20021 Perdido St
New Orleans, LA 70112-1396
Med Sch Affil: M-02105
Major participating institution for programs in: AI, AN, BBK, CCS, CD, CHN, CHP, CN, D, DMP, DR, EM, END, FP, GE, GS, HEM, HO, ID, IM, MG, MPD, N, NEP, NPM, NS, OBG, ON, OPH, ORS, OTO, P, PCC, PCP, PD, PDI, PFP, PM, PN, PP, PS, PTH, PUD, RHU, RNR, TS, TY, U, VIR, VS
Institution ID: 21-0727

Medical Center of Louisiana-University Hospital Campus
2021 Perdido St
PO Box 61262
New Orleans, LA 70161-1262
Med Sch Affil: M-02105
Major participating institution for programs in: MEM
Institution ID: 21-0223

Memorial Medical Center
2700 Napoleon Ave
New Orleans, LA 70115
Med Sch Affil: M-02105
Major participating institution for programs in: GE, PCC
Institution ID: 21-0409

New Orleans Adolescent Hospital
210 State St
New Orleans, LA 70118
Institution ID: 21-8017

Parish of Orleans Coroner's Office
Criminal Court Bldg
2700 Tulane Ave
New Orleans, LA 70119
Major participating institution for programs in: FOP
Institution ID: 21-8032

The Blood Center
312 S Galvez St
New Orleans, LA 70119
Major participating institution for programs in: BBK
Institution ID: 21-8026

Touro Infirmary
1401 Foucher St
New Orleans, LA 70115-3593
Med Sch Affil: M-02101, G-02105
Major participating institution for programs in: GS, P, PM, PYG
Institution ID: 21-0193

Tulane Hospital for Children
1415 Tulane Ave
New Orleans, LA 70112
Major participating institution for programs in: PD, PDC, PDI, PDP, PN
Institution ID: 21-8027

Tulane Univ School of Public Health and Tropical Medicine
1430 Tulane Ave
New Orleans, LA 70112
Programs sponsored in: GPM
Major participating institution for programs in: IPM
Institution ID: 21-0493

Tulane University Hospital and Clinics
1415 Tulane Ave/Ste 2700
New Orleans, LA 70112-2632
Med Sch Affil: M-02101
Major participating institution for programs in: AI, AN, CCM, CD, CHN, CHP, D, DR, END, GE, GS, HO, IM, MN, MP, N, NPM, NS, OBG, OPH, ORS, OSM, OTO, P, PDI, PFP, PG, PHO, PUD, PYN, TS, TY, U
Institution ID: 21-0485

Tulane University School of Medicine
1430 Tulane Ave
PO Box SL77
New Orleans, LA 70112-2699
Med Sch Affil: M-02101, L-02312
Programs sponsored in: ADP, AI, AN, CCM, CCS, CD, CHN, CHP, D, DMP, DR, END, GE, GS, HMP, HO, ID, IM, IMG, IPM, MG, MN, MP, MPD, N, NEP, NS, OBG, OPH, ORS, OSM, OTO, P, PCP, PD, PDC, PDI, PDP, PFP, PN, PTH, PUD, PYN, TS, TY, U
Institution ID: 21-9501

Veterans Affairs Medical Center (New Orleans)
1601 Perdido St
New Orleans, LA 70146
Med Sch Affil: M-02101
Major participating institution for programs in: AI, CD, IM, MN, MP, MPD, PYN
Institution ID: 21-0733

Veterans Affairs Medical Center-LSU Service (New Orleans)
1601 Perdido St
New Orleans, LA 70112-1262
Med Sch Affil: M-02105
Major participating institution for programs in: ADP, AI, AN, CCM, CCS, CD, DR, GE, GS, HO, ID, IM, IMG, N, NEP, NS, OPH, ORS, OTO, P, PS, PTH, PUD, RNR, TS, TY, U, VIR, VS
Institution ID: 21-0234

Pineville

Huey P Long Regional Medical Center
PO Box 5352
Pineville, LA 71361-5352
Med Sch Affil: M-02101, L-02105
Major participating institution for programs in: GS, OBG, ORS
Institution ID: 21-0430

Shreveport

Charter Forest Behavioral Health System
9320 Linwood Ave
PO Box 18130
Shreveport, LA 71138-1130
Major participating institution for programs in: P
Institution ID: 21-8024

Louisiana State University Hospital-Shreveport
1501 Kings Hwy
PO Box 33932
Shreveport, LA 71130-3932
Med Sch Affil: M-02106
Programs sponsored in: AI, AN, APM, CCM, CD, CRS, DR, END, FP, GE, GS, HO, ID, IM, MPD, NEP, NPM, OBG, OPH, ORS, OTO, P, PCC, PCP, PD, PTH, RHU, TY, U
Institution ID: 21-0722

Overton Brooks Veterans Affairs Medical Center
510 E Stoner Ave
Shreveport, LA 71101-4295
Med Sch Affil: M-02106
Major participating institution for programs in: CCM, CD, D, GE, GS, ID, IM, NEP, OPH, ORS, OTO, P, PCC, RHU, TY, U
Institution ID: 21-0497

Schumpert Medical Center
1 St Mary Pl
PO Box 21976
Shreveport, LA 71120-1976
Med Sch Affil: L-02106
Major participating institution for programs in: APM, CRS, FP, U
Institution ID: 21-0460

Shriners Hospital for Children (Shreveport)
3100 Samford Ave
Shreveport, LA 71103-4289
Med Sch Affil: L-02106
Major participating institution for programs in: ORS
Institution ID: 21-0410

Willis-Knighton Medical Center
PO Box 32600
Shreveport, LA 71130-2600
Major participating institution for programs in: APM
Institution ID: 21-0459

Maine

Augusta

MaineGeneral Medical Center
6 E Chestnut St
Augusta, ME 04330
Programs sponsored in: FP
Institution ID: 22-0100

Bangor

Eastern Maine Medical Center
489 State St
Bangor, ME 04401
Med Sch Affil: L-02407
Programs sponsored in: FP
Institution ID: 22-0191

Lewiston

Central Maine Medical Center
300 Main St
Lewiston, ME 04240-0001
Med Sch Affil: L-02405
Programs sponsored in: FP
Institution ID: 22-0116

Portland

Maine Medical Center
22 Bramhall St
Portland, ME 04102-3175
Med Sch Affil: M-05002
Programs sponsored in: AN, CD, CHP, DR, EM, END, FP, FSM, GS, ID, IM, NEP, OBG, P, PCC, PD
Major participating institution for programs in: PS
Institution ID: 22-0384

South Portland

Jackson Brook Institute
175 Running Hill Rd
South Portland, ME 04106
Major participating institution for programs in: CHP
Institution ID: 22-8001

Togus

Veterans Affairs Medical Center (Togus)
One VA Center
Togus, ME 04330
Med Sch Affil: G-02416
Major participating institution for programs in: U
Institution ID: 22-0200

Waterville

Maine General Medical Center
149 North St
Waterville, ME 04901
Med Sch Affil: G-03201
Major participating institution for programs in: FP
Institution ID: 22-0260

Maryland

Andrews AFB

Malcolm Grow Medical Center (SGE)
89th Medical Group/SGAT
1050 W Perimeter Rd
Andrews AFB, MD 20762-6600
Med Sch Affil: M-02312
Major participating institution for programs in: FP, FPP, FSM, P, TY
Institution ID: 23-0216

Baltimore

American Red Cross Blood Services
4700 Mount Hope Dr
Baltimore, MD 21215-3200
Med Sch Affil: L-02307
Major participating institution for programs in: BBK
Institution ID: 23-8014

Children's Hospital and Center for Reconstructive Surgery
3825 Greenspring Ave
Baltimore, MD 21211
Med Sch Affil: G-02301
Major participating institution for programs in: ORS, PS
Institution ID: 23-0285

Franklin Square Hospital Center
9000 Franklin Square Dr
Baltimore, MD 21237-3998
Med Sch Affil: L-02307, L-02301
Programs sponsored in: FP, IM, OBG
Major participating institution for programs in: GS, P
Institution ID: 23-0122

Good Samaritan Hospital of Maryland
5601 Loch Raven Blvd
Baltimore, MD 21239-2995
Med Sch Affil: G-02307
Programs sponsored in: IM
Major participating institution for programs in: ORS, PM
Institution ID: 23-0522

Greater Baltimore Medical Center
6701 N Charles St
Baltimore, MD 21204-6808
Med Sch Affil: L-02301, G-02307
Programs sponsored in: CRS, IM, OBG, OPH
Major participating institution for programs in: OPH, OTO
Institution ID: 23-0507

Harbor Hospital Center
3001 S Hanover St
Baltimore, MD 21230
Med Sch Affil: L-02301, L-02307
Programs sponsored in: IM, TY
Institution ID: 23-0459

James Lawrence Kernan Hospital
2200 Kernan Dr
Baltimore, MD 21207-6697
Major participating institution for programs in: FSM, ORS
Institution ID: 23-0238

Johns Hopkins Bayview Medical Center
4940 Eastern Ave
Baltimore, MD 21224
Med Sch Affil: M-02307, L-02301
Major participating institution for programs in: AI, AN, D, DMP, EM, GE, GS, IM, IMG, N, NEP, NPM, NS, OBG, ORS, OTO, P, PCC, PS, U
Institution ID: 23-0118

Johns Hopkins Hospital
600 N Wolfe St/Billings 29
Baltimore, MD 21287-1629
Med Sch Affil: M-02307, G-02301
Major participating institution for programs in: ADL, AI, AN, APM, BBK, CCA, CCP, CCS, CD, CHN, CHP, D, DMP, DR, EM, END, GE, GS, HEM, HMP, ICE, ID, IM, IMG, MG, N, NEP, NM, NP, NPM, NR, NS, OBG, ON, OPH, ORS, OTO, P, PAN, PCC, PCP, PD, PDC, PDE, PDI, PDP, PDR, PDS, PG, PHO, PIP, PM, PS, PTH, PYG, RHU, RNR, RO, TS, U, UP, VIR, VS
Institution ID: 23-0191

Johns Hopkins University School of Hygiene/Public Health
615 N Wolfe St
Baltimore, MD 21205-2179
Med Sch Affil: L-02307
Programs sponsored in: GPM
Major participating institution for programs in: GPM
Institution ID: 23-0503

Johns Hopkins University School of Medicine
720 Rutland Ave
Baltimore, MD 21205-2195
Med Sch Affil: M-02307
Programs sponsored in: ADL, AI, AN, APM, BBK, CCA, CCP, CCS, CD, CHN, CHP, CN, D, DMP, DR, EM, END, GE, GS, HEM, HMP, ICE, ID, IM, IMG, MG, N, NEP, NM, NP, NPM, NR, NS, OBG, ON, OPH, ORS, OTO, P, PAN, PCC, PCP, PD, PDC, PDE, PDI, PDP, PDR, PDS, PG, PHO, PIP, PP, PS, PTH, PYG, RHU, RNR, RO, TS, U, UP, VIR, VS
Institution ID: 23-0703

Maryland General Hospital
827 Linden Ave
Baltimore, MD 21201-4681
Med Sch Affil: L-02312, L-02301
Programs sponsored in: IM, OBG, OPH, TY
Major participating institution for programs in: OTO
Institution ID: 23-0147

Maryland State Department of Health and Mental Hygiene
201 W Preston St
Baltimore, MD 21201-2399
Med Sch Affil: G-02312
Programs sponsored in: GPM
Institution ID: 23-0494

Mercy Medical Center
301 St Paul Pl
Baltimore, MD 21201-2165
Med Sch Affil: M-02301
Major participating institution for programs in: EM, EMP, GS, IM, MEM, NPM, OBG, PD, VIR, VS
Institution ID: 23-0195

Office of the Chief Medical Examiner
111 Penn St
Baltimore, MD 21201
Med Sch Affil: L-02307
Programs sponsored in: FOP
Major participating institution for programs in: PP
Institution ID: 23-0499

Sheppard and Enoch Pratt Hospital
6501 N Charles St
PO Box 6815
Baltimore, MD 21285-6815
Med Sch Affil: G-02301
Programs sponsored in: P
Major participating institution for programs in: CHP, P
Institution ID: 23-0397

Sinai Hospital of Baltimore
2401 W Belvedere Ave
Baltimore, MD 21215-5271
Med Sch Affil: M-02307, L-02301
Programs sponsored in: MPM, OBG, OPH, PD, PM
Major participating institution for programs in: GS, IM, OPH, U
Institution ID: 23-0160

St Agnes Hospital
900 S Caton Ave
Baltimore, MD 21229-5299
Med Sch Affil: L-02301, G-02307
Programs sponsored in: GS, IM
Major participating institution for programs in: ORS
Institution ID: 23-0320

Union Memorial Hospital
201 E University Pkwy
Baltimore, MD 21218-2895
Med Sch Affil: L-02312, L-02307, L-02301
Programs sponsored in: GS, HSS, IM, IMG, OBG, ORS, OSM
Major participating institution for programs in: FP, HSO, PS, TY
Institution ID: 23-0287

University of Maryland Medical System
22 S Greene St
Baltimore, MD 21201-1559
Med Sch Affil: M-02301, G-02307
Programs sponsored in: ADP, AN, APM, CCA, CCP, CCS, CD, CHP, CN, D, DR, EM, EMP, END, FP, FSM, GE, GS, HMP, HO, ICE, ID, IM, IMG, MEM, MN, MPD, N, NEP, NPM, NR, NS, OBG, OPH, ORS, OTO, OTR, P, PCC, PD, PDE, PDI, PTH, PYG, RHU, RNR, RO, TS, U, VIR, VS
Major participating institution for programs in: PDS, PS
Institution ID: 23-0247

University of Maryland School of Medicine
655 W Baltimore St/Rm 14-015
Baltimore, MD 21201-1559
Med Sch Affil: M-02301, L-02312, G-04101
Programs sponsored in: GPM, PFP
Major participating institution for programs in: OBG
Institution ID: 23-0513

Veterans Affairs Medical Center (Baltimore)
10 N Greene St
Baltimore, MD 21201-1524
Med Sch Affil: M-02301, G-02307
Major participating institution for programs in: ADP, CD, D, END, ICE, ID, IM, IMG, MN, N, NR, NS, OTO, P, PCC, PTH, PYG, RHU, RNR, U, VIR, VS
Institution ID: 23-0265

Walter P Carter Mental Health Center
630 W Fayette St
Baltimore, MD 21201-1585
Med Sch Affil: M-02301
Major participating institution for programs in: ADP, P
Institution ID: 23-0713

Bethesda

National Cancer Institute
Bldg 10/Rm 12N-214
9000 Rockville Pike
Bethesda, MD 20892
Major participating institution for programs in: HMP, PCP, RO
Institution ID: 23-8012

National Capital Consortium
4301 Jones Bridge Rd
Bethesda, MD 20814-4799
Programs sponsored in: AN, APM, CCA, CHN, CHP, CN, D, DR, FP, FPP, N, NPM, NS, OBG, OTO, P, PCP, PD, PDE, PDI, PG, PHO, PM, PTH, RO, TY
Major participating institution for programs in: MP
Institution ID: 10-8020

National Naval Medical Center (Bethesda)
8901 Wisconsin Ave
Bethesda, MD 20814-5011
Med Sch Affil: M-01002, M-02312, L-01001
Programs sponsored in: END, GE, GS, HO, IM, OPH, ORS, TY, U
Major participating institution for programs in: AN, APM, CD, CN, D, DR, ID, N, NPM, NS, OBG, ON, OTO, P, PCC, PCP, PD, PDI, PHO, PTH, RO, TY
Institution ID: 23-0275

NIH Warren Grant Magnuson Clinical Center
Bldg 10/Rm 1C129 NIH
10 Center Dr/MSC 1158
Bethesda, MD 20892-1158
Med Sch Affil: L-01001, L-02312, G-01002
Programs sponsored in: AI, ALI, BBK, CCM, D, END, HEM, ID, MG, ON, P, PCP, PDE, PTH, RHU
Major participating institution for programs in: ALI, APM, CN, GE, PHO, RNR
Institution ID: 23-0204

Suburban Hospital
8600 Old Georgetown Rd
Bethesda, MD 20814-1497
Med Sch Affil: G-01002, G-02312
Major participating institution for programs in: PS
Institution ID: 23-0386

USUHS F Edward Hebert School of Medicine
4301 Jones Bridge Rd
Bethesda, MD 20814-4799
Programs sponsored in: GPM
Major participating institution for programs in: APM, NPM, PD, PDE, PG
Institution ID: 23-0714

Catonsville
Spring Grove Hospital Center
Wade Ave
Catonsville, MD 21228
Med Sch Affil: L-02301
Major participating institution for programs in: P
Institution ID: 23-0289

Cheverly
Prince George's Hospital Center
3001 Hospital Dr
Cheverly, MD 20785
Med Sch Affil: L-01001, L-02312
Programs sponsored in: FP, IM
Major participating institution for programs in: EM, OBG
Institution ID: 23-0142

Jessup
Clifton T Perkins Hospital Center
8450 Dorsey Run Rd
PO Box 1000
Jessup, MD 20794-1000
Major participating institution for programs in: PFP
Institution ID: 23-8015

Silver Spring
Holy Cross Hospital of Silver Spring
1500 Forest Glen Rd
Silver Spring, MD 20910-1484
Med Sch Affil: M-01001
Major participating institution for programs in: FP, OBG
Institution ID: 23-0710

Westminster
Carroll County General Hospital
200 Memorial Ave
Westminster, MD 21157-5799
Institution ID: 23-8016

Massachusetts

Amherst
University of Massachusetts School of Public Health
102 Arnold House
Amherst, MA 01003-0430
Major participating institution for programs in: GPM
Institution ID: 24-8067

Bedford
Edith Nourse Rogers Memorial Veterans Hospital
200 Springs Rd
Bedford, MA 01730
Med Sch Affil: L-02405
Major participating institution for programs in: IMG, P
Institution ID: 24-0443

Belmont
McLean Hospital
115 Mill St
Belmont, MA 02178
Med Sch Affil: M-02401
Programs sponsored in: PYG
Major participating institution for programs in: CHP, P
Institution ID: 24-0230

Beverly
Beverly Hospital
85 Herrick St
Beverly, MA 01915
Programs sponsored in: FP
Institution ID: 24-0232

Boston
Beth Israel Deaconess Medical Center
330 Brookline Ave
Boston, MA 02215
Programs sponsored in: AN, APM, BBK, CCA, CCS, CD, DR, END, GE, GS, HMP, HO, HSP, ICE, ID, IM, IMG, N, NEP, NR, OBG, PAN, PCC, PCP, PS, PTH, PUD, TS, VIR, VS
Major participating institution for programs in: CHN, D, DMP, GE, HSO, NM, NPM, NS, ORS, OTO, P, PCC, RHU, RNR, RO, U
Institution ID: 24-8076

Boston Medical Center
One Boston Medical Center Pl
Boston, MA 02118-2393
Programs sponsored in: ADP, AI, AN, CCS, CD, CHP, D, DMP, DR, EM, END, FOP, FP, GE, GPM, GS, HMP, HO, ID, IM, IMG, MG, MN, N, NEP, OBG, OPH, ORS, OTO, P, PCC, PCP, PDI, PM, PTH, RHU, RNR, TS, TY, U, VIR, VS
Major participating institution for programs in: NPM, PD, TY
Institution ID: 24-8077

Boston University School of Public Health
80 E Concord St
Boston, MA 02118
Major participating institution for programs in: GPM
Institution ID: 24-0449

Brigham and Women's Hospital
75 Francis St
Boston, MA 02115
Med Sch Affil: M-02401, M-02401
Programs sponsored in: AI, AN, APM, BBK, CD, DR, EM, END, GE, GS, HMP, HO, HSO, ICE, IM, MPD, NEP, NM, NP, NR, OBG, P, PCP, PS, PTH, RHU, RNR, SP, TS, U, VIR, VS
Major participating institution for programs in: APM, CCS, CHN, D, DMP, ID, N, NPM, NS, ORS, PCC, PIP, PP, PPR, PS, RO, SCI
Institution ID: 24-0438

Carney Hospital
2100 Dorchester Ave
Boston, MA 02124-5666
Med Sch Affil: L-02405, L-02407
Programs sponsored in: GPM, IM, TY
Major participating institution for programs in: P
Institution ID: 24-0239

Center for Community Responsive Care Inc
90 Cushing Ave
Boston, MA 02125
Programs sponsored in: GPM
Institution ID: 24-8075

Children's Hospital
300 Longwood Ave
Boston, MA 02115
Med Sch Affil: M-02401, M-02401, L-03515, G-03201, G-02405, G-02416
Programs sponsored in: ADL, AI, CCP, CHN, CHP, CN, MG, NPM, NS, OP, PD, PDC, PDE, PDI, PDP, PDR, PDS, PG, PHO, PN, PP, PPR, UP
Major participating institution for programs in: APM, BBK, CCA, D, DR, HSO, MPD, N, NM, NP, NR, NS, OMO, ORS, P, PAN, PS, RNR, RO, TS, U
Institution ID: 24-0152

Dana-Farber Cancer Institute
44 Binney St
Boston, MA 02115
Major participating institution for programs in: NM, PHO, RO
Institution ID: 24-0726

Erich Lindemann Mental Health Center
25 Staniford St
Government Ctr
Boston, MA 02114
Major participating institution for programs in: P
Institution ID: 24-0757

Faulkner Hospital
1153 Centre St
Boston, MA 02130
Med Sch Affil: M-02407, L-02401, G-02401
Major participating institution for programs in: GE, GS, IM
Institution ID: 24-0472

Harvard Community Health Plan
Teaching Ctr
2 Fenway Plaza
Boston, MA 02215
Med Sch Affil: M-02401
Major participating institution for programs in: P
Institution ID: 24-0510

Harvard School of Public Health
677 Huntington Ave
Boston, MA 02115
Programs sponsored in: GPM
Institution ID: 24-0124

Jewish Memorial Hospital
59 Townsend St
Boston, MA 02119
Med Sch Affil: G-02405
Major participating institution for programs in: IMG
Institution ID: 24-0753

Joint Center for Radiation Therapy
50 Binney St
Boston, MA 02115
Programs sponsored in: RO
Institution ID: 24-0523

Joslin Diabetes Center
One Joslin Pl
Boston, MA 02215
Major participating institution for programs in: END
Institution ID: 24-8034

Judge Baker Guidance Center
295 Longwood Ave
Boston, MA 02115
Med Sch Affil: M-02401
Major participating institution for programs in: CHP
Institution ID: 24-0212

Lemuel Shattuck Hospital
Medical Services
170 Morton St
Boston, MA 02130
Med Sch Affil: L-02407
Programs sponsored in: TY
Major participating institution for programs in: GE, P
Institution ID: 24-0401

Mallory Institute of Pathology
784 Massachusetts Ave
Boston, MA 02118
Major participating institution for programs in: DMP
Institution ID: 24-8030

Massachusetts Eye and Ear Infirmary
243 Charles St
Boston, MA 02114
Med Sch Affil: M-02401
Programs sponsored in: OPH, OTO
Institution ID: 24-0155

Massachusetts General Hospital
55 Fruit St
Boston, MA 02114
Med Sch Affil: M-02401
Programs sponsored in: AI, AN, APM, BBK, CCA, CCP, CCS, CD, CHN, CHP, D, DMP, DR, END, GE, GS, HSO, HSP, ICE, ID, IM, N, NP, NS, OMO, ORS, OSM, P, PCC, PCP, PD, PDE, PDP, PFP, PIP, PN, PS, PTH, RHU, RNR, RO, TS, U, VIR, VS
Major participating institution for programs in: BBK, EM, HO, MG, MPD, NEP, OBG, PG
Institution ID: 24-0394

Massachusetts Mental Health Center
74 Fenwood Rd
Boston, MA 02115
Med Sch Affil: M-02401
Major participating institution for programs in: CHP, P
Institution ID: 24-0255

New England Baptist Hospital
125 Parker Hill Ave
Boston, MA 02120-2850
Med Sch Affil: L-02407
Programs sponsored in: OSM
Major participating institution for programs in: HSO, ORS
Institution ID: 24-0522

New England Medical Center Hospitals
750 Washington St
Boston, MA 02111-9915
Med Sch Affil: M-02407
Programs sponsored in: AN, APM, CD, CHN, CHP, CPP, DR, END, GE, GS, HO, HSO, ICE, ID, IM, N, NEP, NPM, NS, OBG, OPH, ORS, OSM, OTO, P, PAN, PCC, PD, PDS, PG, PM, PPR, PTH, RHU, RNR, RO, TS, U, VS
Major participating institution for programs in: D, DMP, MPM, PS
Institution ID: 24-0378

Office of the Chief Medical Examiner
720 Albany St
Boston, MA 02118
Major participating institution for programs in: FOP
Institution ID: 24-8006

Public Health Commission
1010 Massachusetts Ave
Boston, MA 02118
Major participating institution for programs in: GPM
Institution ID: 24-8071

Shriners Hospitals for Children (Boston)
51 Blossom St
Boston, MA 02114-2699
Major participating institution for programs in: PS
Institution ID: 24-8073

Solomon Carter Fuller Mental Health Center
85 E Newton St
Boston, MA 02118
Med Sch Affil: G-02405
Major participating institution for programs in: P
Institution ID: 24-0755

Spaulding Rehabilitation Hospital
125 Nashua St
Boston, MA 02114
Programs sponsored in: PM, SCI
Institution ID: 24-8036

St Elizabeth's Medical Center of Boston
736 Cambridge St
Boston, MA 02135-1111
Med Sch Affil: M-02407
Programs sponsored in: AN, CD, GE, GS, HO, IM, P, PCC
Major participating institution for programs in: N, OBG, TS, U
Institution ID: 24-0211

Veterans Affairs Medical Center (Boston)
150 S Huntington Ave
Boston, MA 02130-4893
Med Sch Affil: M-02405, L-02407
Major participating institution for programs in: ADP, AI, CD, D, DR, GE, GS, HO, ID, IM, N, NEP, OPH, ORS, OSM, OTO, P, PCC, PM, PTH, RHU, RO, U
Institution ID: 24-0257

Braintree

Braintree Hospital
250 Pond St
Braintree, MA 02184
Major participating institution for programs in: PM
Institution ID: 24-8070

Brockton

Brockton Hospital
680 Centre St
Brockton, MA 02402-3395
Med Sch Affil: M-02405
Major participating institution for programs in: OTO, TY
Institution ID: 24-0225

Brockton-West Roxbury Veterans Affairs Medical Center
940 Belmont St
Brockton, MA 02401-5596
Med Sch Affil: M-02401, M-02401
Programs sponsored in: P
Major participating institution for programs in: END, GE, GS, HSO, ICE, IM, IMG, NM, ORS, PCC, PS, PTH, SCI, U
Institution ID: 24-0172

Cardinal Cushing General Hospital
235 N Pearl St
Brockton, MA 02401
Med Sch Affil: L-02407
Major participating institution for programs in: GS
Institution ID: 24-8014

Burlington

Lahey Clinic
41 Mall Rd
Burlington, MA 01805
Med Sch Affil: M-02407, L-02401, G-02405, G-02416
Programs sponsored in: CD, CRS, DR, END, GE, GS, ICE, IM, PS, U
Major participating institution for programs in: D, N, ORS, OTO, PCC, PTH, PUD, TS
Institution ID: 24-0163

Cambridge

Cambridge Hospital/Cambridge Health Alliance
1493 Cambridge St
Cambridge, MA 02139
Med Sch Affil: M-02401, M-02401, L-02407
Programs sponsored in: CHP, IM, P, TY
Major participating institution for programs in: D, GS, HSP, PS
Institution ID: 24-0367

Mount Auburn Hospital
330 Mount Auburn St
Cambridge, MA 02238
Med Sch Affil: M-02401
Programs sponsored in: DR, IM
Major participating institution for programs in: GS, TS, VS
Institution ID: 24-0375

Fitchburg

Health Alliance Hospital-Leominster
275 Nichols Rd
Fitchburg, MA 01420-8209
Major participating institution for programs in: APM, FP
Institution ID: 24-0366

Framingham

MetroWest Medical Center-Framingham Union Hospital
115 Lincoln St
Framingham, MA 01701
Med Sch Affil: L-02416, L-02405, G-02401
Programs sponsored in: IM, TY
Major participating institution for programs in: GS, P
Institution ID: 24-0162

Lawrence

Greater Lawrence Family Health Center Inc
150 Park St
Lawrence, MA 01841
Programs sponsored in: FP
Institution ID: 24-8072

Lawrence General Hospital
One General St
Lawrence, MA 01842
Major participating institution for programs in: FP
Institution ID: 24-0330

Malden

Malden Hospital
100 Hospital Rd
Malden, MA 02148-3591
Med Sch Affil: M-02405
Programs sponsored in: FP, TY
Major participating institution for programs in: OBG
Institution ID: 24-0188

Newton Lower Falls

Newton-Wellesley Hospital
2014 Washington St
Newton Lower Falls, MA 02162
Med Sch Affil: M-02407
Programs sponsored in: IM, MPM
Major participating institution for programs in: GS, HSO, ORS
Institution ID: 24-0448

Pittsfield

Berkshire Medical Center
725 North St
Pittsfield, MA 01201
Med Sch Affil: M-02416
Programs sponsored in: GS, IM, PTH
Institution ID: 24-0180

Salem

Salem Hospital
81 Highland Ave
Salem, MA 01970-2768
Med Sch Affil: L-02407
Programs sponsored in: IM
Institution ID: 24-0287

Somerville

Somerville Hospital
230 Highland Ave
Somerville, MA 02143
Major participating institution for programs in: CHP
Institution ID: 24-8074

Springfield

Baystate Medical Center
759 Chestnut St
Springfield, MA 01199-9999
Med Sch Affil: M-02407, L-02416, G-02405
Programs sponsored in: AN, APM, BBK, CCA, CD, DR, EM, END, GS, HO, ICE, ID, IM, MPD, OBG, PCP, PD, PTH
Institution ID: 24-0309

Shriners Hospitals for Children (Springfield)
516 Carew St
Springfield, MA 01104
Med Sch Affil: L-03503, G-02405
Programs sponsored in: OP
Major participating institution for programs in: ORS, PS
Institution ID: 24-0388

Stockbridge

Austen Riggs Center
25 Main St
Stockbridge, MA 01262-0962
Programs sponsored in: P
Institution ID: 24-0435

Stoneham

New England Memorial Hospital
5 Woodland Rd
PO Box 9102
Stoneham, MA 02180-9102
Major participating institution for programs in: CHP
Institution ID: 24-0740

Stoughton

New England Sinai Hospital and Rehabilitation Center
150 York St
Stoughton, MA 02072
Major participating institution for programs in: PM
Institution ID: 24-8035

Worcester

St Vincent Hospital
25 Winthrop St
Worcester, MA 01604-4593
Med Sch Affil: M-02416
Programs sponsored in: CD, DR, IM
Major participating institution for programs in: EM, FP, GE, GS, N, NS, TS, U
Institution ID: 24-0361

UMass Memorial Health Care (Memorial Campus)
119 Belmont St
Worcester, MA 01605-2982
Med Sch Affil: M-02416
Programs sponsored in: IM
Major participating institution for programs in: EM, FP, GS, NPM, OBG, ORS, PD, PTH, U
Institution ID: 24-0113

UMass Memorial Health Care (University Campus)
55 Lake Ave N
Worcester, MA 01655
Med Sch Affil: M-02416, G-02312
Major participating institution for programs in: AN, APM, CCA, CCM, CCS, CD, CHN, CHP, CN, D, DR, EM, END, FP, GE, GPM, GS, HO, ICE, ID, IM, N, NEP, NPM, NS, OBG, OPH, ORS, OSM, P, PD, PFP, PS, PTH, PUD, RHU, RNR, TS, U, VIR, VS
Institution ID: 24-0724

University of Massachusetts Medical School
55 Lake Ave N
Worcester, MA 01655
Programs sponsored in: AN, APM, CCA, CCM, CCS, CD, CHN, CHP, CN, D, DR, EM, END, FP, GE, GPM, GS, HO, ICE, ID, IM, MPD, N, NEP, NPM, NS, OBG, ORS, OSM, P, PD, PFP, PS, PTH, PUD, RHU, RNR, TS, U, VIR, VS
Institution ID: 24-9501

Worcester City Hospital
26 Queen St
Worcester, MA 01610
Major participating institution for programs in: CCA
Institution ID: 24-0140

Michigan

Allen Park

Veterans Affairs Medical Center (Detroit)
Southfield and Outer Dr
Allen Park, MI 48101-3199
Med Sch Affil: M-02507
Major participating institution for programs in: AI, CD, D, END, GE, GS, ID, IM, IMG, MPD, NEP, ON, ORS, OTO, PCC, PS, RHU, U
Institution ID: 25-0108

Ann Arbor

Center for Forensic Psychiatry
3501 Willis Rd
PO Box 2060
Ann Arbor, MI 48106
Programs sponsored in: PFP
Institution ID: 25-8006

St Joseph Mercy Health System
5301 E Huron River Dr
PO Box 995
Ann Arbor, MI 48106
Med Sch Affil: M-02501
Programs sponsored in: FP, GS, IM, OBG, TY
Major participating institution for programs in: MPD, ORS, PS
Institution ID: 25-0487

University of Michigan Hospitals
1500 W Medical Center Dr
M4101 Med Sci Bldg I/0603
Ann Arbor, MI 48109-0603
Med Sch Affil: M-02501
Programs sponsored in: AI, AN, APM, CCA, CCP, CCS, CD, CHN, CHP, CN, D, DR, EM, END, FP, FSM, GE, GS, HMP, HO, ICE, ID, IM, IMG, MG, MPD, N, NEP, NM, NO, NP, NPM, NS, OBG, OPH, ORS, OTO, P, PAN, PCC, PCH, PCP, PD, PDC, PDE, PDI, PDP, PDR, PDS, PG, PHO, PM, PN, PS, PTH, PYG, RHU, RNR, RO, TS, U, VIR, VS
Major participating institution for programs in: OBG, PFP
Institution ID: 25-0256

University of Michigan School of Public Health
109 S Observatory
Ann Arbor, MI 48109-2029
Programs sponsored in: GPM
Institution ID: 25-0526

Veterans Affairs Medical Center (Ann Arbor)
2215 Fuller Rd
Ann Arbor, MI 48105
Med Sch Affil: M-02501
Major participating institution for programs in: CD, D, DR, END, GE, GS, HO, ID, IM, IMG, MPD, N, NEP, NM, OPH, ORS, OTO, P, PCC, PS, PTH, PYG, RHU, RNR, TS, U, VIR, VS
Institution ID: 25-0498

Chelsea

Chelsea Community Hospital
775 S Main St
Chelsea, MI 48118
Med Sch Affil: L-02501
Major participating institution for programs in: FP
Institution ID: 25-0555

Commerce

Huron Valley-Sinai Hospital
1 William Carls Dr
Commerce, MI 48382-1271
Med Sch Affil: G-02507
Major participating institution for programs in: FP
Institution ID: 25-8003

Dearborn

Oakwood Hospital

18101 Oakwood Blvd
PO Box 2500
Dearborn, MI 48123-2500
Med Sch Affil: M-02501, M-02507
Programs sponsored in: DR, FP, IM, OBG, TY
Major participating institution for programs in: ICE
Institution ID: 25-0366

Detroit

American Red Cross Blood Serv-Southeastern Michigan Region

100 Mack Ave
PO Box 33351
Detroit, MI 48232-5351
Major participating institution for programs in: BBK
Institution ID: 25-0550

Children's Hospital of Michigan

3901 Beaubien Blvd
Detroit, MI 48201-2196
Med Sch Affil: M-02507
Programs sponsored in: EMP, MPD, PMP
Major participating institution for programs in: AI, CCP, CHN, CN, D, EM, NPM, NS, OP, OPH, ORS, OTO, PD, PDC, PDI, PDR, PDS, PG, PHO, PP, PS, PTH, RNR, TS, TY, U, UP
Institution ID: 25-0456

Detroit Receiving Hospital and University Health Center

4201 St Antoine Blvd
Detroit, MI 48201
Med Sch Affil: M-02507
Major participating institution for programs in: AI, CCM, CD, CN, D, DR, EM, EMP, END, GE, GPM, GS, ID, IM, MEM, MPD, MPM, N, NEP, NS, OAR, ON, ORS, OTO, PCC, PS, PTH, RHU, TS, TY
Institution ID: 25-0131

Grace Hospital

6071 W Outer Dr
Detroit, MI 48235
Med Sch Affil: M-02507
Programs sponsored in: ORS
Major participating institution for programs in: DR, EM, FP, GS, IM, MPD, OBG, PS, RO, TY
Institution ID: 25-0291

Harper Hospital

3990 John R St
Detroit, MI 48201
Med Sch Affil: M-02507
Major participating institution for programs in: CCM, CD, CHN, D, DR, END, GE, GS, HEM, HSP, ID, IM, MEM, N, NEP, NS, ON, OTO, P, PCC, PCP, PS, PTH, RHU, RNR, RO, TS, TY, U, UP, VIR, VS
Institution ID: 25-0151

Henry Ford Hospital

2799 W Grand Blvd
Detroit, MI 48202-2689
Med Sch Affil: M-03806, L-02501
Programs sponsored in: AI, AN, APM, CCS, CD, CN, CRS, D, DR, EM, END, FP, GE, GS, HO, ID, IM, MEM, MG, MSR, N, NEP, NM, NS, OBG, OPH, ORS, OTO, P, PCC, PCP, PD, PTH, RHU, RNR, RO, TY, U, VIR, VS
Institution ID: 25-0331

Hutzel Hospital

4707 St Antoine Blvd
Detroit, MI 48034
Med Sch Affil: M-02507
Major participating institution for programs in: MG, MPD, NPM, OAR, OBG, OP, OPH, ORS, OSM, PCP, PP, PTH, RHU, TY
Institution ID: 25-0105

Rehabilitation Institute

261 Mack Blvd
Detroit, MI 48201
Med Sch Affil: M-02507
Major participating institution for programs in: MPM, PM, PMP
Institution ID: 25-0210

Samaritan Health Center-Mercy Hospital

5555 Conner Ave
Detroit, MI 48213
Major participating institution for programs in: FP, GS
Institution ID: 25-0165

Sinai Hospital

6767 W Outer Dr
Detroit, MI 48235-2899
Med Sch Affil: M-02507
Major participating institution for programs in: GS, ICE, IM, OBG, OPH, ORS, P, PM
Institution ID: 25-0114

St John Hospital and Medical Center

22101 Morross Rd
Detroit, MI 48236-2172
Med Sch Affil: M-02507
Programs sponsored in: CD, EM, FP, GS, ID, IM, MPD, NEP, OBG, PD, PTH, TY
Major participating institution for programs in: ICE
Institution ID: 25-0486

Wayne County Medical Examiner's Office

600 Randolph Ave
Detroit, MI 48226
Programs sponsored in: FOP
Institution ID: 25-0520

Wayne State University/Detroit Medical Center

Orchestra Pl/Ste 200
3663 Woodward Ave
Detroit, MI 48201-2403
Med Sch Affil: M-02507
Programs sponsored in: AI, AN, CCA, CCM, CCP, CCS, CD, CHN, CHP, CN, D, DR, EM, END, FP, GE, GPM, GS, HEM, HSP, ICE, ID, IM, IMG, MEM, MG, MPM, N, NEP, NPM, NS, OAR, OBG, ON, OP, OPH, ORS, OSM, OTO, P, PCC, PCP, PD, PDC, PDI, PDR, PDS, PG, PHO, PM, PP, PS, PTH, PYG, RHU, RNR, RO, TS, TY, U, UP, VIR, VS
Major participating institution for programs in: EMP
Institution ID: 25-9501

East Lansing

Michigan State University Clinical Center

Human Health Programs
D132 Fee Hall
East Lansing, MI 48824-1316
Med Sch Affil: M-02512
Major participating institution for programs in: IM, MP, MPD, ORS, P, PD
Institution ID: 25-0532

Michigan State University College of Human Medicine

Dean's Office
A-110 E Fee Hall MSU
East Lansing, MI 48824-1316
Med Sch Affil: M-02512
Programs sponsored in: CD, FPP, GE, GS, HO, IM, MP, MPD, NPM, P, PD
Major participating institution for programs in: DR
Institution ID: 25-9502

Michigan State University College of Osteopathic Medicine

A308 E Fee Hall
East Lansing, MI 48824-1316
Programs sponsored in: PM
Institution ID: 25-9503

Ferndale

Kingswood Hospital

10300 W Eight Mile Rd
Ferndale, MI 48220
Major participating institution for programs in: P
Institution ID: 25-8398

Flint

Genesys Regional Medical Center-St Joseph Campus

302 Kensington Ave
Flint, MI 48503-2000
Med Sch Affil: M-02512
Major participating institution for programs in: DR
Institution ID: 25-0480

Hurley Medical Center

One Hurley Plaza
Flint, MI 48503-5993
Med Sch Affil: M-02512, G-02501
Programs sponsored in: IM, MPD, OBG, PD, TY
Major participating institution for programs in: DR, ORS
Institution ID: 25-0304

McLaren Regional Medical Center

401 S Ballenger Hwy
Flint, MI 48532-3685
Med Sch Affil: M-02512
Programs sponsored in: FP, IM, ORS
Major participating institution for programs in: DR, GS
Institution ID: 25-0412

Michigan State Univ College of Human Medicine-Flint Campus

One Hurley Plaza
Flint, MI 48503-5902
Med Sch Affil: M-02512
Programs sponsored in: DR
Institution ID: 25-0562

Grand Blanc

Genesys Regional Medical Center

One Genesys Pkwy
Grand Blanc, MI 48439-1477
Programs sponsored in: FP
Institution ID: 25-8007

Grand Rapids

Grand Rapids Area Medical Education Consortium

240 Cherry St SE
Grand Rapids, MI 49503
Programs sponsored in: PS
Institution ID: 25-0460

Pine Rest Christian Hospital
300 68th St SE
Grand Rapids, MI 49501-0165
Major participating institution for programs in: P
Institution ID: 25-0544

Spectrum Health-Downtown Campus
100 Michigan Ave NE
Grand Rapids, MI 49503
Med Sch Affil: M-02512
Programs sponsored in: CCS, EM, GS, IM, MPD, OBG, PD, TY
Major participating institution for programs in: FP, ORS, PS
Institution ID: 25-0341

Spectrum Health-East Campus
1840 Wealthy St SE
Grand Rapids, MI 49506-2968
Med Sch Affil: M-02512
Programs sponsored in: CRS, GS, HSO, IM, OBG, ORS, TY
Major participating institution for programs in: PS
Institution ID: 25-0395

St Mary's Health Services
200 Jefferson SE
Grand Rapids, MI 49503
Med Sch Affil: M-02512
Programs sponsored in: FP, TY
Major participating institution for programs in: GS, IM, OBG, ORS, P, PS
Institution ID: 25-0473

Grosse Pointe

Bon Secours Hospital
468 Cadieux Rd
Grosse Pointe, MI 48230-1592
Med Sch Affil: M-02507
Programs sponsored in: FP, IM
Institution ID: 25-0103

Grosse Pointe Farms

Henry Ford Cottage Hospital
159 Kercheval Ave
Grosse Pointe Farms, MI 48236-3692
Major participating institution for programs in: FP, P
Institution ID: 25-0493

Kalamazoo

Borgess Medical Center
1521 Gull Rd
Kalamazoo, MI 49001-1640
Med Sch Affil: M-02512, L-02501
Major participating institution for programs in: EM, FP, FSM, GS, IM, ORS, P, TY
Institution ID: 25-0490

Bronson Methodist Hospital
One Healthcare Plaza
Kalamazoo, MI 49007
Med Sch Affil: M-02512
Major participating institution for programs in: EM, FP, FSM, GS, IM, MPD, ORS, PD, TY
Institution ID: 25-0458

Kalamazoo Center for Medical Studies
1000 Oakland Dr
Kalamazoo, MI 49008
Med Sch Affil: M-02512
Programs sponsored in: EM, FP, FSM, GS, IM, MPD, ORS, P, PD, TY
Institution ID: 25-0538

Lansing

Ingham Regional Medical Center
401 W Greenlawn Ave
Lansing, MI 48910
Major participating institution for programs in: P, PM
Institution ID: 25-8004

Lansing General Hospital
2727 S Pennsylvania Ave
Lansing, MI 48910
Major participating institution for programs in: P
Institution ID: 25-9012

Michigan Capital Medical Center
401 W Greenlawn
Lansing, MI 48910-2819
Med Sch Affil: M-02512
Major participating institution for programs in: EM, GS, HO, IM
Institution ID: 25-0183

Sparrow Hospital
PO Box 30480
Lansing, MI 48909-7980
Med Sch Affil: M-02512
Programs sponsored in: EM, FP, FPG, FSM, OBG, TY
Major participating institution for programs in: CD, GS, HO, IM, MPD, NPM, PD
Institution ID: 25-0290

St Lawrence Hospital and HealthCare Services
1210 W Saginaw St
Lansing, MI 48915-1999
Med Sch Affil: M-02512
Major participating institution for programs in: FPG, FPP, FSM, GS, HO, MP, MPD, P
Institution ID: 25-0182

Marquette

Marquette General Hospital
420 W Magnetic St
Marquette, MI 49855-2794
Med Sch Affil: M-02512
Programs sponsored in: FP
Institution ID: 25-0549

Midland

MidMichigan Regional Medical Center
4005 Orchard Dr
Midland, MI 48670
Med Sch Affil: L-02512
Programs sponsored in: FP
Institution ID: 25-0322

Northville

Hawthorn Center Hospital
18471 Haggerty Rd
Northville, MI 48167
Med Sch Affil: G-02507
Major participating institution for programs in: CHP, P
Institution ID: 25-0247

Pontiac

North Oakland Medical Center
461 W Huron
Pontiac, MI 48341-1651
Med Sch Affil: L-02507
Programs sponsored in: FP, GS, OBG
Institution ID: 25-0222

St Joseph Mercy-Oakland
900 Woodward Ave
Pontiac, MI 48341-2985
Med Sch Affil: M-02507
Programs sponsored in: DR, GS, IM, MPD, TY
Major participating institution for programs in: PD
Institution ID: 25-0478

Royal Oak

William Beaumont Hospital
3601 W 13 Mile Rd
Royal Oak, MI 48073-6769
Med Sch Affil: M-02501, M-02507
Programs sponsored in: BBK, CD, CRS, DR, EM, FP, GE, GS, HMP, ID, IM, IMG, MPD, NM, NR, OBG, ON, OPH, ORS, OSS, PCH, PCP, PD, PM, PTH, RNR, RO, TY, U, VIR
Institution ID: 25-0396

Saginaw

Covenant Medical Center
1447 North Harrison
Saginaw, MI 48602
Med Sch Affil: M-02512
Major participating institution for programs in: EM, FP, GS, IM
Institution ID: 25-0314

Saginaw Cooperative Hospitals Inc
1000 Houghton Ave
Saginaw, MI 48602
Programs sponsored in: EM, FP, GS, IM, OBG
Institution ID: 25-0525

Saginaw General Hospital
1447 N Harrison St
Saginaw, MI 48602
Med Sch Affil: M-02512
Major participating institution for programs in: EM, FP, GS, IM, OBG
Institution ID: 25-0200

St Mary's Medical Center
830 S Jefferson St
Saginaw, MI 48601
Med Sch Affil: M-02512
Major participating institution for programs in: EM, GS, IM
Institution ID: 25-0276

South Haven

South Haven Community Hospital
955 S Bailey Ave
South Haven, MI 49090
Major participating institution for programs in: FP
Institution ID: 25-8008

Southfield

Providence Hospital and Medical Centers
16001 W Nine Mile Rd
PO Box 2043
Southfield, MI 48075
Med Sch Affil: M-02507, G-02501
Programs sponsored in: CD, DR, FP, FSM, GE, GS, IM, OBG, ON, PS, TY
Major participating institution for programs in: ORS, RO
Institution ID: 25-0197

Traverse City

Munson Medical Center
1105 6th St
Traverse City, MI 49684
Programs sponsored in: FP
Institution ID: 25-0251

Troy

William Beaumont Hospital-Troy
44201 Dequindre Rd
Troy, MI 48098
Major participating institution for programs in: EM, FP, PM, RO, TY
Institution ID: 25-0551

Westland

Walter P Reuther Psychiatric Hospital
30901 Palmer Rd
Westland, MI 48185
Major participating institution for programs in: PYG
Institution ID: 25-8005

Minnesota

Duluth

St Luke's Hospital
915 E First St
Duluth, MN 55805-2193
Med Sch Affil: M-02607
Programs sponsored in: FP
Institution ID: 26-0209

St Mary's Medical Center
407 E Third St
Duluth, MN 55805
Med Sch Affil: M-02607
Major participating institution for programs in: FP
Institution ID: 26-0346

Fergus Falls

Lakeland Mental Health Center
126 E Alcott Ave
Fergus Falls, MN 56537
Med Sch Affil: G-03701
Major participating institution for programs in: P
Institution ID: 26-8023

Mankato

Immanuel-St Joseph's Hospital
1025 Marsh St
PO Box 8673
Mankato, MN 56002
Med Sch Affil: L-02604
Major participating institution for programs in: FP
Institution ID: 26-8030

Maplewood

St John's Hospital
1575 Beam Ave
Maplewood, MN 55109
Med Sch Affil: G-02604
Major participating institution for programs in: FP
Institution ID: 26-0130

Minneapolis

Abbott-Northwestern Hospital
800 E 28th St
Minneapolis, MN 55407-3799
Med Sch Affil: L-02604, G-01643
Programs sponsored in: IM
Major participating institution for programs in: CRS, ORS, OSM, PTH
Institution ID: 26-0343

Allina Health System
5601 Smetana Dr
Minneapolis, MN 55440-9310
Programs sponsored in: FP
Institution ID: 26-8031

Children's Health Care (Minneapolis)
2525 Chicago Ave S
Minneapolis, MN 55404-9976
Med Sch Affil: L-02604
Major participating institution for programs in: MPD, PD, PDR
Institution ID: 26-0740

Fairview-University Medical Center
420 Delaware St SE
Box 502
Minneapolis, MN 55455-0392
Med Sch Affil: M-02604
Programs sponsored in: MPD
Major participating institution for programs in: ADP, AI, AN, BBK, CCA, CCP, CCS, CD, CHN, CHP, CN, CRS, D, DR, END, FP, FPG, GE, GS, HO, HSO, ICE, ID, IM, MG, N, NEP, NPM, NS, OBG, OPH, ORS, OSM, OTO, P, PD, PDC, PDE, PDI, PDP, PDR, PG, PHO, PM, PN, PS, PTH, RHU, RNR, RO, SP, TS, U, VIR
Institution ID: 26-8033

Hennepin County Medical Center
701 Park Ave S
Minneapolis, MN 55415-1623
Med Sch Affil: M-02604
Programs sponsored in: CCM, EM, EMP, FP, FSM, GS, IM, P, PTH, TY
Major participating institution for programs in: AN, CHN, CN, D, DR, ID, MPD, N, NEP, NS, OBG, OPH, ORS, OTO, P, RNR, VIR
Institution ID: 26-0402

Hennepin County Medical Examiner
730 S 7th St
Minneapolis, MN 55415-1798
Programs sponsored in: FOP
Institution ID: 26-0733

Memorial Blood Centers of Minnesota
2304 Park Ave S
Minneapolis, MN 55404
Med Sch Affil: G-02604
Major participating institution for programs in: BBK
Institution ID: 26-0735

Methodist Hospital
6500 Excelsior Blvd
PO Box 650
Minneapolis, MN 55440-0650
Med Sch Affil: G-02604
Major participating institution for programs in: CCM, FP, HSO
Institution ID: 26-0135

Minneapolis Sports Medicine Center
701 25th Ave S
Minneapolis, MN 55454
Programs sponsored in: OSM
Institution ID: 26-8024

Minnesota Spine Center
913 E 26th St/#600
Minneapolis, MN 55404-4515
Programs sponsored in: OSS
Institution ID: 26-8032

Shriners Hospital for Children (Twin Cities Unit)
2025 E River Pkwy
Minneapolis, MN 55414-3696
Med Sch Affil: G-02604
Major participating institution for programs in: ORS
Institution ID: 26-0481

University of Minnesota Medical School
UMHC Box 293
420 Delaware St SE
Minneapolis, MN 55455
Med Sch Affil: M-02604
Programs sponsored in: ADP, AI, AN, BBK, CCA, CCP, CCS, CD, CHN, CHP, CN, CRS, D, DR, END, FP, FPG, FPP, GE, GS, HO, HSO, ICE, ID, IM, MG, N, NEP, NPM, NS, OBG, OPH, ORS, OTO, P, PCC, PD, PDC, PDE, PDI, PDP, PDR, PG, PHO, PM, PN, PS, PTH, PYG, RHU, RNR, RO, SP, TS, U, VIR
Institution ID: 26-9501

University of Minnesota School of Public Health
Box 197 Mayo Bldg/Rm A-304
420 Delaware St SE
Minneapolis, MN 55455-0381
Major participating institution for programs in: GPM
Institution ID: 26-0495

Veterans Affairs Medical Center (Minneapolis)
One Veterans Dr
Minneapolis, MN 55417
Med Sch Affil: M-02604
Major participating institution for programs in: ADP, BBK, CCA, CCS, CD, CN, CRS, D, DR, END, FPG, GE, GS, ID, IM, MPD, N, NEP, NS, OPH, ORS, OTO, P, PM, PS, PTH, PYG, RHU, RNR, TS, U, VIR
Institution ID: 26-0119

Robbinsdale

North Memorial Health Care
3300 Oakdale Ave N
Robbinsdale, MN 55422-2900
Med Sch Affil: G-02604
Major participating institution for programs in: FP, GS, PS
Institution ID: 26-0498

Rochester

Mayo Clinic (Rochester)
200 First St SW
Rochester, MN 55905
Major participating institution for programs in: AI, AN, APM, BBK, CCA, CCM, CD, CHN, CHP, CN, CRS, D, DMP, DR, END, FP, GE, GPM, GS, HMP, HO, HSO, ID, IM, IMG, MG, MM, N, NEP, NP, NR, NS, OAR, OMO, OPH, ORS, OTO, P, PCC, PD, PDC, PDE, PG, PHO, PM, PS, PTH, RHU, RNR, RO, TS, VIR, VS
Institution ID: 26-0737

Mayo Graduate School of Medicine-Mayo Foundation
Siebens 5th Fl
200 First St SW
Rochester, MN 55905
Med Sch Affil: M-02608, L-02012
Programs sponsored in: ADP, AI, AN, APM, BBK, CCA, CCM, CCS, CD, CHN, CHP, CN, CRS, D, DMP, DR, END, FP, GE, GPM, GS, HMP, HO, HSO, ICE, ID, IM, IMG, MG, MM, N, NEP, NP, NR, NS, OAR, OBG, OMO, OPH, ORS, OTO, P, PCC, PD, PDC, PDE, PG, PHO, PM, PS, PTH, RHU, RNR, RO, TS, TY, U, VIR, VS
Institution ID: 26-0173

Rochester Methodist Hospital
201 W Center St
Rochester, MN 55902
Med Sch Affil: M-02608
Major participating institution for programs in: AI, AN, APM, CCM, CD, CHN, CHP, CN, CRS, D, DMP, END, FP, GE, GS, HO, HSO, ID, IM, IMG, MG, NEP, OAR, OBG, OMO, OPH, ORS, OTO, PCC, PD, PM, PS, PTH, RHU, RNR, TS, U, VIR, VS
Institution ID: 26-0483

St Mary's Hospital of Rochester
1216 Second St SW
Rochester, MN 55902-1970
Med Sch Affil: M-02608
Major participating institution for programs in: ADP, AI, AN, APM, CCM, CCS, CD, CHN, CHP, CN, CRS, D, DMP, END, FP, GE, GS, HO, HSO, ICE, ID, IM, IMG, MG, N, NEP, NS, OMO, OPH, ORS, OTO, P, PCC, PD, PDC, PDE, PG, PHO, PM, PS, PTH, RHU, RNR, TS, U, VIR, VS
Institution ID: 26-0317

St Cloud

St Cloud Hospital
1406 Sixth Ave N
St Cloud, MN 56303
Major participating institution for programs in: FP
Institution ID: 26-7010

St Paul

American Red Cross Blood Services-St Paul Region
100 S Robert St
St Paul, MN 55107-1489
Med Sch Affil: G-02604
Major participating institution for programs in: BBK
Institution ID: 26-0736

Children's Health Care (St Paul)
345 N Smith Ave/Rm 1129
St Paul, MN 55102-9974
Med Sch Affil: L-02604
Major participating institution for programs in: FP, MPD, NPM, PD
Institution ID: 26-0497

Gillette Children's Speciality Healthcare
200 E University Ave
St Paul, MN 55101
Med Sch Affil: G-02604
Major participating institution for programs in: HSO, ORS
Institution ID: 26-0492

Healtheast St Joseph's Hospital
69 W Exchange St
St Paul, MN 55102-9902
Med Sch Affil: G-02604
Major participating institution for programs in: FP
Institution ID: 26-0357

HealthPartners Institute for Medical Education
640 Jackson St
St Paul, MN 55101
Programs sponsored in: EM, FP, GPM, OBG, PTH
Institution ID: 26-8034

Regions Hospital
640 Jackson St
St Paul, MN 55101
Med Sch Affil: M-02604
Major participating institution for programs in: CCA, CCS, CD, CHN, D, EM, FP, FPG, GPM, GS, IM, MPD, OBG, OPH, OTO, P, PS, PTH, RHU, TS, U
Institution ID: 26-0184

United Hospital
333 N Smith Ave
St Paul, MN 55102
Med Sch Affil: L-02604
Major participating institution for programs in: CRS, FP, OBG
Institution ID: 26-0311

Mississippi

Biloxi

Veterans Affairs Medical Center (Biloxi)
400 Veterans Ave
Biloxi, MS 39531-2410
Med Sch Affil: L-00106, G-02101
Major participating institution for programs in: GS, OTO
Institution ID: 27-0425

Jackson

Mississippi Baptist Medical Center
1225 N State St
Jackson, MS 39201-2002
Med Sch Affil: G-02701
Major participating institution for programs in: PS
Institution ID: 27-0374

St Dominic-Jackson Memorial Hospital
969 Lakeland Dr
Jackson, MS 39216
Med Sch Affil: G-02701
Major participating institution for programs in: PS, VIR
Institution ID: 27-0433

University Hospital
2500 N State St
Jackson, MS 39216-4505
Med Sch Affil: M-02701
Programs sponsored in: MPD
Major participating institution for programs in: AN, APM, CD, CHN, CHP, DR, EM, END, FP, GE, GS, HO, HSO, ID, IM, N, NEP, NS, OBG, OPH, ORS, OTO, P, PD, PHO, PS, PTH, PUD, TS, U, VIR
Institution ID: 27-0427

University of Mississippi School of Medicine
2500 N State St
Jackson, MS 39216
Programs sponsored in: AN, APM, CD, CHN, CHP, CN, DR, EM, END, FP, GE, GS, HO, HSO, ID, IM, N, NEP, NS, OBG, OPH, ORS, OTO, P, PCP, PD, PHO, PS, PTH, PUD, TS, U, VIR
Major participating institution for programs in: FP
Institution ID: 27-9501

Veterans Affairs Medical Center (Jackson)
1500 E Woodrow Wilson Dr
Jackson, MS 39216-5199
Med Sch Affil: M-02701
Major participating institution for programs in: CD, END, GE, GS, HO, HSO, ID, IM, N, NS, OPH, ORS, OTO, P, PCP, PS, PTH, PUD, TS, U
Institution ID: 27-0430

Keesler AFB

Keesler Medical Center
81st Medical Group/SGOK
301 Fisher St/Ste 1A132
Keesler AFB, MS 39534-2519
Med Sch Affil: L-00106
Programs sponsored in: GS, IM, OBG, PD
Institution ID: 27-0371

Tupelo

North Mississippi Medical Center
830 S Gloster St
Tupelo, MS 38801
Med Sch Affil: G-02701
Programs sponsored in: FP
Institution ID: 27-7005

Missouri

Berkeley

St Louis County Medical Examiner's Office
6039 Helen Ave
Berkeley, MO 63134
Major participating institution for programs in: FOP
Institution ID: 28-8174

Chesterfield

St Luke's Hospital
232 S Woods Mill Rd
Chesterfield, MO 63017-3480
Med Sch Affil: M-02803
Programs sponsored in: IM
Institution ID: 28-0203

Columbia

Boone Hospital Center
1600 E Broadway
Columbia, MO 65201
Med Sch Affil: L-02803
Major participating institution for programs in: NS
Institution ID: 28-7035

Charter Hospital of Columbia
200 Portland St
Columbia, MO 65201
Major participating institution for programs in: CHP
Institution ID: 28-8017

Ellis Fischel Cancer Center
115 Business Loop 70 West
Columbia, MO 65203-3299
Major participating institution for programs in: HO, OTO
Institution ID: 28-0169

Harry S Truman Memorial Veterans Hospital
800 Hospital Dr
Columbia, MO 65201-5297
Med Sch Affil: M-02803
Major participating institution for programs in: CD, D, DR, END, FPG, GE, GS, HO, ID, IM, N, NS, OPH, ORS, OTO, P, PM, PS, PTH, RHU, TS, U
Institution ID: 28-0178

Mid-Missouri Mental Health Center
3 Hospital Dr
Columbia, MO 65201
Med Sch Affil: M-02803
Major participating institution for programs in: CHP, P
Institution ID: 28-8013

University Hospitals and Clinics
One Hospital Dr, DC031
Columbia, MO 65212
Med Sch Affil: M-02803
Major participating institution for programs in: AN, CCS, CD, CHP, D, DR, END, FP, FPG, GE, GS, HO, ID, IM, MPD, N, NEP, NM, NPM, NS, OBG, OPH, ORS, OTO, P, PCC, PD, PM, PS, PTH, RHU, TS, U, VS
Institution ID: 28-0176

University of Missouri-Columbia School of Medicine
MA202 Med Sciences Bldg
One Hospital Dr
Columbia, MO 65212
Programs sponsored in: AN, CCS, CD, CHP, D, DR, END, FP, FPG, GE, GS, HO, ID, IM, MPD, N, NEP, NM, NPM, NS, OBG, OPH, ORS, OTO, P, PCC, PD, PM, PS, PTH, RHU, TS, U, VS
Institution ID: 28-0709

Jefferson City

Missouri Department of Health
PO Box 570
920 Wildwood Dr
Jefferson City, MO 65102-0570
Major participating institution for programs in: GPM
Institution ID: 28-8016

Kansas City

Baptist Medical Center
6601 Rockhill Rd
Kansas City, MO 64131-1197
Med Sch Affil: M-02846, L-01902
Programs sponsored in: FP
Major participating institution for programs in: OSM
Institution ID: 28-0451

Children's Mercy Hospital
2401 Gillham Rd
Kansas City, MO 64108-9898
Med Sch Affil: M-02846, L-01902, G-03006
Programs sponsored in: MPD
Major participating institution for programs in: AI, CCS, NPM, NS, OPH, ORS, OTO, PD, PDE, PDS, PHO, PN, PPR, PS, PTH
Institution ID: 28-0426

Research Medical Center
2316 E Meyer Blvd
Kansas City, MO 64132-1199
Med Sch Affil: M-02846, L-01902
Major participating institution for programs in: PS
Institution ID: 28-0175

Saint Luke's Hospital
Wornall Rd and 44th
Kansas City, MO 64111
Med Sch Affil: M-02846, L-01902
Programs sponsored in: TS
Major participating institution for programs in: AN, CD, DR, GS, ICE, ID, IM, MPD, NEP, OBG, ORS, OSM, PCC, PS, PTH
Institution ID: 28-0337

Trinity Lutheran Hospital
3030 Baltimore
Kansas City, MO 64108
Med Sch Affil: M-02846, L-01902
Programs sponsored in: FP
Institution ID: 28-0180

Truman Medical Center-East
7900 Lee's Summit Rd
Kansas City, MO 64139
Med Sch Affil: M-02846, L-01902
Major participating institution for programs in: FP, FPG, MPD
Institution ID: 28-8012

Truman Medical Center-West
2301 Holmes St
Kansas City, MO 64108-2640
Med Sch Affil: M-02846
Major participating institution for programs in: AI, AN, CD, DR, EM, FP, GE, GS, HO, ID, IM, NEP, NPM, OBG, OPH, ORS, OSM, PCC, PS, PTH
Institution ID: 28-0263

University of Missouri-Kansas City School of Medicine
2411 Holmes St
Kansas City, MO 64108-2792
Programs sponsored in: AI, AN, CCS, CD, DR, EM, FP, FPG, GE, GS, HO, ICE, ID, IM, NEP, NPM, OBG, OPH, ORS, OSM, P, PCC, PD, PDE, PDS, PHO, PN, PS, PTH
Institution ID: 28-0453

Veterans Affairs Medical Center (Kansas City)
4801 Linwood Blvd
Kansas City, MO 64128-2295
Med Sch Affil: M-01902
Major participating institution for programs in: GS, IM, MP, N, NS, OPH, ORS, OTO, P, PM, PS, PTH, U
Institution ID: 28-0218

Western Missouri Mental Health Center
600 E 22nd St
Kansas City, MO 64108-2620
Med Sch Affil: M-02846
Major participating institution for programs in: P
Institution ID: 28-0433

Springfield

Cox Medical Center North
1423 N Jefferson Ave
Springfield, MO 65802-1988
Programs sponsored in: FP
Institution ID: 28-8168

Cox Medical Center South
3801 S National
Springfield, MO 65807-3801
Major participating institution for programs in: FP
Institution ID: 28-8169

St Louis

Anheuser-Busch Eye Institute
1755 S Grand Blvd
St Louis, MO 63104
Med Sch Affil: M-02834
Major participating institution for programs in: OPH
Institution ID: 28-7025

Barnes West County Hospital
12634 Olive St Rd
St Louis, MO 63146-354
Major participating institution for programs in: OSM, PS
Institution ID: 28-8173

Barnes-Jewish Hospital
One Barnes-Jewish Hospital Plaza
St Louis, MO 63110
Med Sch Affil: M-02802
Major participating institution for programs in: AI, AN, APM, BBK, CCA, CCS, CD, CHN, CHP, CN, D, DMP, DR, EM, END, GE, GS, HMP, HO, HSP, ICE, ID, IM, IMG, N, NEP, NM, NP, NR, NS, OBG, OPH, ORS, OSM, OSS, OTO, P, PCC, PCP, PDR, PP, PS, PTH, RHU, RNR, RO, TS, U, VIR, VS
Institution ID: 28-0210

Barnes-Jewish Hospital (North Campus)
216 S Kingshighway
St Louis, MO 63110
Med Sch Affil: M-02802
Major participating institution for programs in: BBK, CD, CHP, CRS, DR, EM, END, GS, ICE, IM, IMG, NEP, OBG, OTO, P, PCC, PCP, PM, PTH, RO, TS
Institution ID: 28-0146

Deaconess Hospital
6150 Oakland Ave
St Louis, MO 63139-3297
Med Sch Affil: M-02834
Programs sponsored in: FP, IM, TY
Major participating institution for programs in: OBG
Institution ID: 28-0245

Malcolm Bliss Mental Health Center
5400 Arsenal St
St Louis, MO 63139
Med Sch Affil: M-02802
Major participating institution for programs in: P
Institution ID: 28-0214

Mallinckrodt Institute of Radiology
510 S Kingshighway
St Louis, MO 63110
Med Sch Affil: G-02802
Major participating institution for programs in: DR, NR, PDR, RNR, RO, VIR
Institution ID: 28-0211

Shriners Hospitals for Children (St Louis)
2001 S Lindbergh Blvd
St Louis, MO 63131-3597
Med Sch Affil: L-01902
Programs sponsored in: OP
Major participating institution for programs in: ORS, OSS, PPR
Institution ID: 28-0164

SSM Cardinal Glennon Children's Hospital
1465 S Grand Blvd
St Louis, MO 63104-1095
Med Sch Affil: M-02834
Major participating institution for programs in: AI, AN, CHN, CHP, CN, DR, GS, MPD, NPM, NS, ORS, OTO, PD, PDR, PDS, PP, PPR, PS, PTH, RHU, RNR, TS, U
Institution ID: 28-0444

St John's Mercy Medical Center
615 S New Ballas Rd
St Louis, MO 63141-8221
Med Sch Affil: M-02834, G-02803
Programs sponsored in: IM, OBG, PTH, TY
Major participating institution for programs in: CCM, CCS, CRS, GS, OTO, PCC, RNR, U, VS
Institution ID: 28-0231

St Louis Children's Hospital
One Children's Pl
St Louis, MO 63110-1077
Med Sch Affil: M-02802
Major participating institution for programs in: APM, CCP, CHN, CHP, CN, DR, EM, NPM, NS, OP, OSS, OTO, PCP, PD, PDC, PDE, PDI, PDP, PDS, PG, PHO, PN, PPR, PS, RO, TS, VIR
Institution ID: 28-0145

St Louis City Department of Health and Hospitals
PO Box 14702
St Louis, MO 63178
Major participating institution for programs in: GPM
Institution ID: 28-8176

St Louis ConnectCare
5535 Delmar Blvd
St Louis, MO 63112-3095
Med Sch Affil: M-02802, L-02834, L-02803
Major participating institution for programs in: IM, N, OBG, PS, U
Institution ID: 28-0250

St Louis University School of Medicine
1402 S Grand Blvd
St Louis, MO 63104
Med Sch Affil: M-02834
Programs sponsored in: AI, AN, CCM, CCS, CD, CHN, CHP, CN, CRS, D, DR, END, FOP, FP, GE, GPM, GS, HMP, HO, ID, IM, IMG, MPD, N, NEP, NM, NPM, NS, OBG, OPH, ORS, OTO, P, PCC, PCP, PD, PDR, PDS, PP, PPR, PS, PTH, PYG, RHU, RNR, TS, U, VIR, VS
Major participating institution for programs in: FOP
Institution ID: 28-9501

St Louis University School of Medicine
1402 South Grand Blvd
St Louis, MO 63104
Med Sch Affil: M-02834
Major participating institution for programs in: AI, AN, CCM, CCS, CD, CHN, CN, CRS, D, DR, END, GE, GS, HMP, HO, ID, IM, IMG, MPD, N, NEP, NM, NS, ORS, OTO, P, PCC, PCP, PPR, PS, PTH, PYG, RHU, RNR, TS, U, VIR, VS
Institution ID: 28-0167

St Louis University School of Public Health
3663 Lindell Blvd
St Louis, MO 63108-3342
Major participating institution for programs in: GPM
Institution ID: 28-8175

St Mary's Health Center
6420 Clayton Rd
St Louis, MO 63117
Med Sch Affil: M-02834
Programs sponsored in: IM
Major participating institution for programs in: GE, GS, MPD, OBG, ORS, PS, PTH
Institution ID: 28-0442

Veterans Affairs Medical Center (St Louis)
1 Jefferson Barracks Dr
St Louis, MO 63125-4199
Med Sch Affil: M-02834, M-02802
Major participating institution for programs in: CD, CN, DR, GE, GS, ID, IM, IMG, MPD, N, NEP, NM, OPH, OSM, OTO, P, PCP, PS, PTH, TS, U
Institution ID: 28-0354

Washington University School of Medicine
660 S Euclid Ave
St Louis, MO 63110-1093
Med Sch Affil: M-02802
Major participating institution for programs in: DR, RO, VIR
Institution ID: 28-0440

Washington University/B-JH/SLCH Consortium
Campus Box 8064
660 S Euclid Ave
St Louis, MO 63110-1093
Programs sponsored in: AI, AN, APM, BBK, CCA, CCP, CCS, CD, CHN, CHP, CN, CRS, D, DMP, DR, EM, END, GE, GS, HMP, HO, HSO, HSP, ICE, ID, IM, IMG, N, NEP, NM, NP, NPM, NR, NS, OBG, OPH, ORS, OSM, OSS, OTO, P, PCC, PCP, PD, PDC, PDE, PDI, PDP, PDR, PDS, PG, PHO, PM, PN, PP, PPR, PS, PTH, RHU, RNR, RO, TS, U, VIR, VS
Institution ID: 28-9502

Windsor

Royal Oaks Hospital
307 N Main
Windsor, MO 65360
Major participating institution for programs in: CHP
Institution ID: 28-8177

Montana

Billings

Deaconess Medical Center
2800 Tenth Ave N
PO Box 37000
Billings, MT 59107
Med Sch Affil: L-05404
Major participating institution for programs in: FP
Institution ID: 29-8002

Montana Family Practice Residency
PO Box 35500-554
Billings, MT 59107
Programs sponsored in: FP
Institution ID: 29-8001

Glasgow

Frances Mahon Deaconess Hospital
621 Third St S
Glasgow, MT 59230
Major participating institution for programs in: FP
Institution ID: 29-7007

Nebraska

Grand Island

St Francis Medical Center (Grand Island)
2620 W Faidley Ave
Box 9804
Grand Island, NE 68802-9804
Med Sch Affil: G-03005
Major participating institution for programs in: FP
Institution ID: 30-7009

Kearney

Good Samaritan Hospital (Kearney)
31st St and Central Ave
PO Box 1990
Kearney, NE 68848
Med Sch Affil: G-03005
Major participating institution for programs in: FP
Institution ID: 30-7004

Lincoln

BryanLGH Medical Center East
1600 S 48th St
Lincoln, NE 68506
Med Sch Affil: L-03005
Major participating institution for programs in: FP
Institution ID: 30-0329

BryanLGH Medical Center West
2300 S 16th St
Lincoln, NE 68502
Med Sch Affil: L-03005
Major participating institution for programs in: FP
Institution ID: 30-0332

Lincoln Medical Education Foundation
4600 Valley Rd
Lincoln, NE 68510
Programs sponsored in: FP
Institution ID: 30-0706

St Elizabeth Community Health Center
555 S 70th St
Lincoln, NE 68510
Med Sch Affil: L-03005
Major participating institution for programs in: FP
Institution ID: 30-0278

VA Greater Nebraska Health Care System (Lincoln Division)
600 S 70th St
Lincoln, NE 68510-2010
Med Sch Affil: G-03006
Major participating institution for programs in: GS
Institution ID: 30-0115

North Platte

Great Plains Regional Medical Center
601 W Leota St
Box 1167
North Platte, NE 69103
Major participating institution for programs in: FP
Institution ID: 30-8004

Offutt AFB

Ehrling Bergquist Hospital
2501 Capehart Rd
Offutt AFB, NE 68113
Med Sch Affil: M-03005, G-03006
Major participating institution for programs in: AI, FP, OTO
Institution ID: 30-0708

Omaha

Bergan Mercy Medical Center
7500 Mercy Rd
Omaha, NE 68124
Med Sch Affil: M-03006
Major participating institution for programs in: OBG
Institution ID: 30-0452

Boys Town National Research Hospital
555 N 30th St
Omaha, NE 68131
Major participating institution for programs in: MPD, OTO
Institution ID: 30-8003

Children's Memorial Hospital
8301 Dodge St
Omaha, NE 68114-4199
Med Sch Affil: M-03006, M-03005
Major participating institution for programs in: GS, MPD, NS, ORS, PD, PDI, PG
Institution ID: 30-0390

Clarkson Regional Health Service
44th St at Dewey Ave
Omaha, NE 68105-1018
Med Sch Affil: L-03005
Programs sponsored in: FP
Institution ID: 30-0453

Creighton University School of Medicine
California at 24th St
Omaha, NE 68178
Programs sponsored in: ADP, AI, CD, CHP, CRS, DR, FP, GS, ID, IM, OBG, P, PTH, PUD, PYG
Major participating institution for programs in: END
Institution ID: 30-9502

Methodist Hospital
8303 Dodge St
Omaha, NE 68114
Med Sch Affil: M-03005
Major participating institution for programs in: FP, GS, NS, OBG, U
Institution ID: 30-0294

St Joseph Center for Mental Health
819 Dorcas St
Omaha, NE 68108-1137
Med Sch Affil: M-03006
Major participating institution for programs in: ADP, CHP, P
Institution ID: 30-0712

Tenet St Joseph Hospital at Creighton Univ Medical Center
601 N 30th St
Omaha, NE 68131
Med Sch Affil: M-03006, M-03005
Programs sponsored in: MPD
Major participating institution for programs in: AI, CD, CRS, DR, FP, GS, ID, IM, N, OBG, ORS, PD, PDI, PTH, PUD
Institution ID: 30-0709

University of Nebraska Medical Center
600 S 42nd St
Omaha, NE 68198-4285
Med Sch Affil: M-03005, G-03006
Programs sponsored in: AN, APM, CD, DR, END, FP, GE, GS, HMP, HO, IM, IMG, N, NM, NS, OBG, OPH, ORS, OTO, PCC, PD, PDI, PG, PTH, U, VIR
Major participating institution for programs in: ID, P, PYG
Institution ID: 30-0710

Veterans Affairs Medical Center (Omaha)
4101 Woolworth Ave
Omaha, NE 68105-3012
Med Sch Affil: M-03006, M-03005
Major participating institution for programs in: ADP, CD, DR, GE, GS, HO, ID, IM, MPD, NM, OPH, ORS, OTO, P, PTH, PUD, U
Institution ID: 30-0447

Scottsbluff

Regional West Medical Center
4021 Ave B
Scottsbluff, NE 69361-4695
Med Sch Affil: M-03005
Major participating institution for programs in: FP
Institution ID: 30-8005

Nevada

Las Vegas

Sunrise Hospital and Medical Center
3186 Maryland Pkwy
PO Box 98530
Las Vegas, NV 89193-8530
Major participating institution for programs in: PD
Institution ID: 31-8014

University Medical Center of Southern Nevada
1800 W Charleston Blvd
Las Vegas, NV 89102-2386
Med Sch Affil: M-03101
Major participating institution for programs in: FP, GS, IM, OBG, PD
Institution ID: 31-0100

Reno

BHC Health Services of Nevada
West Hills Hospital
1240 E Ninth St
Reno, NV 89512
Med Sch Affil: G-03101
Major participating institution for programs in: P
Institution ID: 31-8013

Ioannis A Lougaris Veterans Affairs Medical Center
1000 Locust St
Reno, NV 89520
Med Sch Affil: M-03101
Major participating institution for programs in: FP, GS, IM, P
Institution ID: 31-0110

University of Nevada School of Medicine
Savitt Med Sci Bldg (332)
Univ of Nevada
Reno, NV 89557-0046
Programs sponsored in: FP, GS, IM, OBG, P, PD
Institution ID: 31-0111

Washoe Medical Center
77 Pringle Way/Rm H166
Reno, NV 89520-0109
Med Sch Affil: M-03101
Major participating institution for programs in: FP, IM, P
Institution ID: 31-7004

Sparks

Nevada Mental Health Institute
480 Galletti Way
Sparks, NV 89431
Med Sch Affil: G-03101
Major participating institution for programs in: P
Institution ID: 31-7002

New Hampshire

Concord

Concord Hospital
250 Pleasant St
Concord, NH 03301
Med Sch Affil: M-03201
Programs sponsored in: FP
Major participating institution for programs in: FP
Institution ID: 32-8002

New Hampshire Hospital
105 Pleasant St
Concord, NH 03301
Med Sch Affil: G-03201
Major participating institution for programs in: P, PYG
Institution ID: 32-0338

Lebanon

Mary Hitchcock Memorial Hospital
One Medical Center Dr
Lebanon, NH 03756
Programs sponsored in: ADP, AN, APM, CCA, CCM, CD, CHP, D, DR, FP, GE, GS, HO, ICE, ID, IM, MP, N, NPM, NS, OBG, ORS, P, PCC, PD, PS, PTH, PYG, RHU, U, VIR, VS
Major participating institution for programs in: OTO
Institution ID: 32-8001

New Jersey

Atlantic City

Atlantic City Medical Center
1925 Pacific Ave
Atlantic City, NJ 08401
Programs sponsored in: IM
Major participating institution for programs in: P
Institution ID: 33-0168

Browns Mills

Deborah Heart and Lung Center
200 Trenton Rd
Browns Mills, NJ 08015-1799
Med Sch Affil: G-03305, G-03306, G-04101
Major participating institution for programs in: CD, PCC, TS
Institution ID: 33-0513

Camden

Atlantic Health System
One Cooper Plaza
Camden, NJ 08103
Major participating institution for programs in: PD
Institution ID: 33-8019

Cooper Hospital-University Medical Center
One Cooper Plaza
Camden, NJ 08103-1489
Med Sch Affil: M-03306, G-04101
Programs sponsored in: CCA, CCM, CCP, CCS, CD, D, DR, EM, GE, GS, HO, ID, IM, MEM, MPD, NEP, OBG, OPH, P, PCC, PD, PS, RHU, RO
Major participating institution for programs in: ORS, U
Institution ID: 33-0465

Our Lady of Lourdes Medical Center
1600 Haddon Ave
Camden, NJ 08103-1111
Med Sch Affil: G-04101
Major participating institution for programs in: PM
Institution ID: 33-0166

West Jersey Health System
1000 Atlantic Ave
Camden, NJ 08104
Med Sch Affil: G-04102
Major participating institution for programs in: OBG
Institution ID: 33-0719

East Orange

Veterans Affairs Medical Center (East Orange)
385 Tremont Ave
East Orange, NJ 07018-1095
Med Sch Affil: M-03305
Major participating institution for programs in: AI, CD, CHN, D, END, GE, GS, ID, IM, MPD, MPM, N, NEP, OPH, ORS, OTO, P, PM, PTH, TS, U, VS
Institution ID: 33-0187

Edison

JFK Johnson Rehabilitation Institute
65 James St
Edison, NJ 08818
Major participating institution for programs in: PM
Institution ID: 33-8017

JFK Medical Center
65 James St
Edison, NJ 08818-3059
Med Sch Affil: G-03306
Programs sponsored in: FP, PM
Major participating institution for programs in: CCM, CRS, N
Institution ID: 33-0714

Elizabeth

Elizabeth General Medical Center
925 E Jersey St
Elizabeth, NJ 07201
Med Sch Affil: G-03305
Major participating institution for programs in: MPD, PD
Institution ID: 33-0454

St Elizabeth Hospital
225 Williamson St
Elizabeth, NJ 07207-0696
Major participating institution for programs in: AN, IM, OBG
Institution ID: 33-0417

Englewood

Englewood Hospital and Medical Center
350 Engle St
Englewood, NJ 07631
Med Sch Affil: M-03547
Major participating institution for programs in: CCM, IM, MPD
Institution ID: 33-0259

Flemington

Hunterdon Medical Center
2100 Wescott Dr
Flemington, NJ 08822-4604
Med Sch Affil: L-03306
Programs sponsored in: FP
Institution ID: 33-0444

Florham

Atlantic Health System
325 Columbia Trnpk
Florham, NJ 07932-0959
Programs sponsored in: PD
Institution ID: 33-8020

Hackensack

Hackensack University Medical Center
30 Prospect Ave
Hackensack, NJ 07601
Med Sch Affil: M-03305
Programs sponsored in: AN, DR
Major participating institution for programs in: CD, GS, ID, IM, IMG, NS, OBG, OTO, P, PCC, PS, PTH, TS, U
Institution ID: 33-0219

Hoboken

St Mary Hospital
308 Willow Ave
Hoboken, NJ 07030-3889
Programs sponsored in: FP
Institution ID: 33-0226

Jersey City

Jersey City Medical Center
50 Baldwin Ave
Jersey City, NJ 07304-3199
Med Sch Affil: L-03547, G-03305
Major participating institution for programs in: CD, GS, IM, OBG, OPH, ORS, PD
Institution ID: 33-0189

Livingston

St Barnabas Medical Center
94 Old Short Hills Rd
Livingston, NJ 07039-5672
Med Sch Affil: M-03547, L-03305
Programs sponsored in: AN, DR, GS, IM, NR, OBG, PTH, RO, TY
Major participating institution for programs in: EM, OBG, OTO, P
Institution ID: 33-0416

Long Branch

Monmouth Medical Center
300 Second Ave
Long Branch, NJ 07740
Med Sch Affil: M-04115
Programs sponsored in: DR, GS, IM, OBG, ORS, PD, PTH
Institution ID: 33-0335

Lyons

Veterans Affairs Medical Center (Lyons)
151 Knollcroft Rd
Lyons, NJ 07939-9988
Med Sch Affil: M-03306, G-03305
Major participating institution for programs in: GE, P, PCC
Institution ID: 33-0132

Montclair

Mountainside Hospital
1 Bay Ave
Montclair, NJ 07042-4898
Med Sch Affil: L-03306, G-03305
Programs sponsored in: FP, IM
Institution ID: 33-0217

Morristown

Morristown Memorial Hospital
100 Madison Ave
PO Box 1956
Morristown, NJ 07962-1956
Med Sch Affil: M-03305, L-03306
Programs sponsored in: DR, EM, GS, IM, MPD
Major participating institution for programs in: GPM, OBG, PD
Institution ID: 33-0236

Mount Holly

Memorial Hospital of Burlington County
175 Madison Ave
Mount Holly, NJ 08060-2099
Med Sch Affil: L-03306
Programs sponsored in: FP
Institution ID: 33-0171

Neptune

Jersey Shore Medical Center
1945 Corlies Ave/Hwy 33
Neptune, NJ 07754-0397
Med Sch Affil: M-03306
Programs sponsored in: IM, OBG, PD, TY
Major participating institution for programs in: GS, ID
Institution ID: 33-0220

New Brunswick

Robert Wood Johnson University Hospital
One Robert Wood Johnson Pl
PO Box 2601
New Brunswick, NJ 08903-2601
Med Sch Affil: M-03306, G-03305
Major participating institution for programs in: AN, APM, CCP, CD, CHP, DR, END, GE, GS, HMP, HO, ID, IM, MP, N, NEP, OBG, ORS, P, PCC, PD, PTH, PYG, RHU, TS, U, VIR, VS
Institution ID: 33-0141

St Peter's University Hospital
254 Easton Ave
New Brunswick, NJ 08901-0591
Med Sch Affil: M-03306
Major participating institution for programs in: DR, END, FP, FPG, FSM, GS, HO, MG, NEP, NPM, OBG, ORS, PCC, PD, PTH, TS, VIR
Institution ID: 33-0107

Newark

Newark Beth Israel Medical Center

201 Lyons Ave
Newark, NJ 07112
Med Sch Affil: M-03547, L-03305
Programs sponsored in: DR, EM, IM, MPD, OBG, PD, TS, VS
Major participating institution for programs in: GS, IMG, MPD, NEP, PTH
Institution ID: 33-0424

Newark Eye and Ear Infirmary (United Hospitals Med Ctr)

15 S 9th St
Newark, NJ 07107
Major participating institution for programs in: OTO
Institution ID: 33-0421

St James Hospital of Newark

155 Jefferson St
Newark, NJ 07105
Major participating institution for programs in: OBG
Institution ID: 33-7053

St Michael's Medical Center (Cathedral Hlth Srvcs Inc)

University Heights
268 King Blvd
Newark, NJ 07102
Med Sch Affil: L-04202, G-03305
Major participating institution for programs in: CCM, CD, HEM, ID, IM, MPD, OBG, ON, PUD, TS, VS
Institution ID: 33-0418

UMDNJ-Community Mental Health Center at Newark

100 Bergen St
Newark, NJ 07103-2770
Med Sch Affil: M-03305, M-03305
Major participating institution for programs in: CHP
Institution ID: 33-8015

UMDNJ-New Jersey Medical School

185 S Orange Ave/Rm C-595
Newark, NJ 07103-2714
Med Sch Affil: M-03305
Programs sponsored in: AI, AN, APM, CCS, CD, CHN, CHP, D, DMP, DR, END, GE, GS, ID, IM, IMG, MG, MPD, MPM, N, NEP, NS, OBG, OPH, ORS, OTO, P, PCC, PD, PDI, PM, PMP, PS, PTH, SCI, TS, U, VS
Institution ID: 33-9502

UMDNJ-University Hospital

65 Bergen St
Newark, NJ 07103-2714
Med Sch Affil: M-03305
Major participating institution for programs in: AI, AN, APM, CCS, CD, CHN, CHP, D, DMP, DR, END, GE, GS, ID, IM, IMG, MPD, MPM, N, NEP, NS, OBG, OPH, ORS, OTO, P, PCC, PD, PM, PS, PTH, TS, U, VS
Institution ID: 33-0274

Orange

Hospital Center at Orange

188 S Essex Ave
Orange, NJ 07051-0001
Med Sch Affil: G-03305
Major participating institution for programs in: ORS
Institution ID: 33-0128

Paramus

Bergen Regional Medical Center

230 E Ridgewood Ave
Paramus, NJ 07652-4131
Med Sch Affil: G-03305
Programs sponsored in: P
Major participating institution for programs in: IMG
Institution ID: 33-0109

Paterson

St Joseph's Hospital and Medical Center

703 Main St
Paterson, NJ 07503-2691
Med Sch Affil: L-03306, L-03547, G-03305
Programs sponsored in: AN, FP, IM, MPD, OBG, ORS, PD
Major participating institution for programs in: CD, GE, GS, HEM, ID, IM, ON, PUD
Institution ID: 33-0319

Perth Amboy

Raritan Bay Medical Center-Perth Amboy Division

530 New Brunswick Ave
Perth Amboy, NJ 08861-3685
Med Sch Affil: L-03306
Programs sponsored in: IM
Institution ID: 33-0144

Phillipsburg

Warren Hospital

185 Roseberry St
Phillipsburg, NJ 08865-1684
Med Sch Affil: L-03306
Programs sponsored in: FP
Institution ID: 33-0138

Piscataway

UMDNJ-Community Behavioral HealthCare at Piscataway

671 Hoes Ln
Piscataway, NJ 08854
Med Sch Affil: M-03306
Major participating institution for programs in: CHP, P
Institution ID: 33-0717

UMDNJ-Robert Wood Johnson Medical School

675 Hoes Ln
Piscataway, NJ 08854-5635
Med Sch Affil: M-03306
Programs sponsored in: AN, APM, CCP, CD, CHP, CRS, DR, END, FP, FPG, FSM, GE, GPM, GS, HMP, HO, ID, IM, MP, NEP, NPM, OBG, ORS, P, PCC, PD, PTH, PYG, RHU, TS, U, VIR, VS
Major participating institution for programs in: MG
Institution ID: 33-0522

Plainfield

Muhlenberg Regional Medical Center

Park Ave and Randolph Rd
Plainfield, NJ 07061-3399
Med Sch Affil: M-03306
Programs sponsored in: IM
Major participating institution for programs in: CRS
Institution ID: 33-0137

Princeton

Medical Center at Princeton

253 Witherspoon St
Princeton, NJ 08540-3213
Med Sch Affil: M-03306
Major participating institution for programs in: GS, HO, IM, PYG, U
Institution ID: 33-0452

Somerville

Somerset Medical Center

110 Rehill Ave
Somerville, NJ 08876
Med Sch Affil: L-03306
Programs sponsored in: FP
Institution ID: 33-0356

South Orange

Seton Hall University School of Graduate Medical Education

400 S Orange Ave
South Orange, NJ 07079-2698
Programs sponsored in: CCM, CD, GE, HEM, ID, IM, N, OBG, ON, PUD
Institution ID: 33-9501

Summit

Overlook Hospital

99 Beauvoir Ave
PO Box 220
Summit, NJ 07902-0220
Med Sch Affil: G-03305
Programs sponsored in: DR, FP, IM, MPD
Major participating institution for programs in: GS, PD
Institution ID: 33-0240

Trenton

Capital Health System-Fuld Campus

750 Brunswick Ave
Trenton, NJ 08638
Med Sch Affil: L-03306
Programs sponsored in: FP, IM
Major participating institution for programs in: P
Institution ID: 33-0150

St Francis Medical Center

601 Hamilton Ave
Trenton, NJ 08629-1986
Med Sch Affil: L-03306
Programs sponsored in: GS, IM
Institution ID: 33-0415

State of New Jersey Department of Health and Senior Services

John Fitch Plaza/CN 360
Trenton, NJ 08625-0360
Programs sponsored in: GPM
Institution ID: 33-0520

Voorhees

West Jersey Hospital-Voorhees

101 Carnie Blvd
Voorhees, NJ 08043
Programs sponsored in: FP
Institution ID: 33-8018

West Orange

Kessler Institute for Rehabilitation

1199 Pleasant Valley Way
West Orange, NJ 07052-1419
Med Sch Affil: M-03305
Major participating institution for programs in: PM, SCI
Institution ID: 33-0726

Woodbury

Underwood-Memorial Hospital

509 N Broad St
Woodbury, NJ 08096
Programs sponsored in: FP
Major participating institution for programs in: GS
Institution ID: 33-7079

New Mexico

Albuquerque

Carrie Tingley Hospital

1127 University Blvd NE
Albuquerque, NM 87102-1715
Med Sch Affil: G-03401
Major participating institution for programs in: ORS
Institution ID: 34-0500

Lovelace Medical Center

5400 Gibson Blvd SE
Albuquerque, NM 87108
Med Sch Affil: L-03401
Major participating institution for programs in: CD, GE, GS, NS, OTO, PS, U
Institution ID: 34-0196

Office of the Medical Investigator

700 Camino de Salud NE
Albuquerque, NM 87131-5091
Med Sch Affil: G-03401
Major participating institution for programs in: FOP
Institution ID: 34-0508

Presbyterian Healthcare Services

5901 Harper Dr NE
PO Box 26666
Albuquerque, NM 87125-6666
Med Sch Affil: L-03401
Major participating institution for programs in: EM
Institution ID: 34-0507

University Hospital

2211 Lomas Blvd NE
Albuquerque, NM 87106-2745
Med Sch Affil: M-03401
Major participating institution for programs in: APM, CCM, CCS, CD, CHN, CHP, D, DR, EM, END, FP, GE, GS, HMP, HO, HSO, ID, IM, IMG, MN, N, NEP, NPM, NS, OBG, ORS, OTO, P, PAN, PCC, PD, PDP, PHO, PS, PTH, RHU, RNR, TS, U, VIR
Institution ID: 34-0498

University of New Mexico School of Medicine

Campus Box 535
Albuquerque, NM 87131
Med Sch Affil: M-03401, G-04815
Programs sponsored in: AN, APM, CCM, CCS, CD, CHN, CHP, CN, D, DR, EM, END, FOP, FP, GE, GS, HMP, HO, HSO, ID, IM, IMG, MN, N, NEP, NPM, NS, OBG, ORS, OTO, P, PAN, PCC, PD, PDP, PHO, PS, PTH, RHU, RNR, TS, U, VIR
Institution ID: 34-0510

Veterans Affairs Medical Center (Albuquerque)

2100 Ridgecrest Dr SE
Albuquerque, NM 87108
Med Sch Affil: M-03401
Major participating institution for programs in: AN, APM, CCM, CD, CN, D, DR, END, GE, GS, ID, IM, IMG, MN, N, NEP, ORS, OTO, P, PCC, PS, PTH, RHU, RNR, TS, U, VIR
Institution ID: 34-0499

Kirtland AFB

USAF Hospital (Kirtland)

1951 Second St SE
Kirtland AFB, NM 87117-5559
Med Sch Affil: L-02312, G-03401
Major participating institution for programs in: OBG
Institution ID: 34-0511

Las Cruces

Memorial Medical Center, Inc

2450 S Telshor Blvd
Las Cruces, NM 88001-5076
Programs sponsored in: FP
Institution ID: 34-8014

Roswell

Eastern New Mexico Medical Center

405 W Country Club Rd
Roswell, NM 88201
Major participating institution for programs in: FP
Institution ID: 34-8016

New York

Albany

Albany Medical Center

43 New Scotland Ave
Albany, NY 12208-3478
Med Sch Affil: M-03503
Programs sponsored in: AN, APM, CCA, CD, D, DMP, DR, EM, END, FP, GE, GS, HEM, HMP, ID, IM, IMG, MPD, N, NPM, NS, OBG, ON, OPH, ORS, OTO, P, PCC, PD, PM, PS, PTH, RHU, RNR, TS, U, VIR, VS
Institution ID: 35-0345

Capital District Psychiatric Center

75 New Scotland Ave
Albany, NY 12208-3474
Med Sch Affil: M-03503
Major participating institution for programs in: P
Institution ID: 35-0815

Child's Hospital

25 Hackett Blvd
Albany, NY 12208-5499
Med Sch Affil: G-03503
Major participating institution for programs in: OTO, PS
Institution ID: 35-0515

New York State Department of Health

651 Corning Tower
Empire State Plaza
Albany, NY 12237
Programs sponsored in: GPM
Institution ID: 35-0456

St Peter's Hospital

315 S Manning Blvd
Albany, NY 12208
Med Sch Affil: M-03503
Major participating institution for programs in: FP, GS, MPD, OBG, ORS, OTO, PM, PS
Institution ID: 35-0103

SUNY at Albany School of Public Health

Executive Park S
Albany, NY 12203-3727
Major participating institution for programs in: GPM
Institution ID: 35-8036

Veterans Affairs Medical Center (Albany)

113 Holland Ave
Albany, NY 12208
Med Sch Affil: M-03503
Major participating institution for programs in: CD, DR, GS, HMP, ID, IM, MPD, N, ON, OPH, ORS, OTO, P, PCC, PM, PS, PTH, RHU, U, VIR
Institution ID: 35-0151

Bay Shore

Southside Hospital

Montauk Hwy
Bay Shore, NY 11706
Med Sch Affil: L-03548
Programs sponsored in: FP
Major participating institution for programs in: PM
Institution ID: 35-0556

Beacon

Fishkill Correctional Facility-NY State Dept of Correction

PO Box 307
Beacon, NY 12508
Major participating institution for programs in: PS
Institution ID: 35-0824

Binghamton

Binghamton Psychiatric Center

425 Robinson St
Binghamton, NY 13901
Major participating institution for programs in: PYG
Institution ID: 35-0261

Wilson Memorial Regional Medical Center (United Health Svs)

20-42 Mitchell Ave
Binghamton, NY 13903
Med Sch Affil: M-03515
Programs sponsored in: FP, IM, TY
Institution ID: 35-0110

Bronx

Albert Einstein College of Medicine of Yeshiva University
1300 Morris Park Ave
Bronx, NY 10461
Med Sch Affil: M-03546
Programs sponsored in: ADL, ADP, AI, AN, APM, CCA, CCM, CCP, CD, CHN, CHP, CN, CPP, D, DR, EM, END, FP, GE, GS, HEM, HMP, ICE, ID, IM, IMG, MG, MP, MSR, N, NEP, NM, NP, NPM, NS, OBG, ON, OPH, ORS, OTO, P, PCC, PCP, PD, PDE, PDI, PFP, PG, PHO, PM, PN, PS, PTH, PYG, RHU, RNR, RO, TS, U, VIR, VS
Institution ID: 35-0745

Bronx Children's Psychiatric Center
1000 Waters Pl
Bronx, NY 10461
Major participating institution for programs in: CHP
Institution ID: 35-8039

Bronx Psychiatric Center
1500 Waters Pl
Bronx, NY 10461
Med Sch Affil: M-03546
Major participating institution for programs in: P, PFP, PYG
Institution ID: 35-0542

Bronx-Lebanon Hospital Center
1276 Fulton Ave
Bronx, NY 10456-3499
Med Sch Affil: M-03546
Programs sponsored in: ADP, CD, CHP, DR, FP, GE, GS, IM, MP, NEP, OBG, OPH, ORS, P, PD, PIP, PTH, PUD
Institution ID: 35-0352

Jacobi Medical Center
Pelham Pkwy S and Eastchester Rd
Bronx, NY 10461
Med Sch Affil: M-03546
Major participating institution for programs in: ADP, AI, AN, CCM, CHN, CHP, CPP, D, DR, EM, END, GE, GS, HEM, ID, IM, MP, N, NEP, NM, NP, NS, OBG, ON, OPH, ORS, OTO, P, PCC, PD, PDE, PHO, PM, PN, PS, PTH, RHU, TS, U
Institution ID: 35-0179

Lincoln Medical and Mental Health Center
234 E 149th St
Bronx, NY 10451
Med Sch Affil: L-03520
Programs sponsored in: CCS, EM, GS, IM, MPD, OBG, P, PD
Major participating institution for programs in: APM, D, GE, OTO, U
Institution ID: 35-0437

Montefiore Medical Center-Henry and Lucy Moses Division
111 E 210th St
Bronx, NY 10467-0001
Med Sch Affil: M-03546
Major participating institution for programs in: ADL, AN, APM, CCA, CCM, CCP, CD, CHN, CHP, CN, D, END, FP, GE, GS, HEM, ICE, ID, IM, IMG, N, NEP, NM, NP, NS, OBG, ON, OPH, ORS, OTO, P, PCC, PCP, PD, PDE, PDI, PG, PHO, PM, PS, PTH, PYG, RHU, RNR, RO, TS, U, VIR, VS
Institution ID: 35-0526

Montefiore Medical Center-Weiler Hospital
1825 Eastchester Rd
Bronx, NY 10461-2373
Med Sch Affil: M-03546
Major participating institution for programs in: AI, AN, APM, CD, CHN, D, DR, END, GS, HMP, IM, MG, MSR, NEP, NM, NP, NPM, OBG, ON, OPH, ORS, OTO, PD, PDE, PHO, PM, PN, PS, PTH, RHU, RO, TS, U
Institution ID: 35-0543

North Central Bronx Hospital
3424 Kossuth Ave
Bronx, NY 10467
Med Sch Affil: M-0346
Major participating institution for programs in: ADP, END, GE, GS, HEM, IM, OBG, ON, OPH, OTO, PDE, PDI, PG, PHO, PM, PS, PTH, RHU, U
Institution ID: 35-0784

Our Lady of Mercy Medical Center
600 E 233rd St
Bronx, NY 10466-2697
Med Sch Affil: M-03509
Major participating institution for programs in: D, EM, GE, GPM, GS, IM, IMG, OBG, OPH, PD, PM
Institution ID: 35-0401

St Barnabas Hospital
4422 Third Ave
Bronx, NY 10457
Med Sch Affil: L-03520
Programs sponsored in: IM
Institution ID: 35-0348

Veterans Affairs Medical Center (Bronx)
130 W Kingsbridge Rd
Bronx, NY 10468
Med Sch Affil: M-03547
Major participating institution for programs in: CCM, CD, D, END, GE, HO, IM, NEP, NM, OPH, OTO, P, PCC, PM, PS, PTH, PYG, RHU, U
Institution ID: 35-0247

Brooklyn

Brookdale University Hospital Medical Center
1 Brookdale Plaza
Brooklyn, NY 11212-3198
Med Sch Affil: M-03508
Programs sponsored in: AN, APM, CHP, GS, HO, IM, MPD, NEP, OBG, OPH, P, PD, PUD, U
Major participating institution for programs in: CD, GE, ORS, PDE
Institution ID: 35-0307

Brooklyn Hospital Center
121 Dekalb Ave
Brooklyn, NY 11201
Med Sch Affil: M-03519, L-03508
Programs sponsored in: CD, EM, FP, GE, GS, HEM, IM, OBG, ON, PD, PTH, PUD
Major participating institution for programs in: OPH
Institution ID: 35-0202

Catholic Medical Center (St Mary's Hospital)
170 Buffalo Ave
Brooklyn, NY 11213-2421
Major participating institution for programs in: GS, OBG, ORS
Institution ID: 35-0395

Children's Medical Center of Brooklyn
340 Clarkson Ave
PO Box 49
Brooklyn, NY 11203
Major participating institution for programs in: MPD
Institution ID: 35-8038

Coney Island Hospital
2601 Ocean Pkwy
Brooklyn, NY 11235
Med Sch Affil: L-03508
Programs sponsored in: CD, END, HEM, IM, PUD
Major participating institution for programs in: AN, END, GS, OBG, OPH, ORS, PD, U
Institution ID: 35-0469

Interfaith Medical Center
555 Prospect Pl
Brooklyn, NY 11238
Med Sch Affil: L-03508
Programs sponsored in: CD, END, GE, IM, OPH, PUD
Institution ID: 35-0347

Kings County Hospital Center
451 Clarkson Ave
Brooklyn, NY 11203-2097
Med Sch Affil: M-03508
Major participating institution for programs in: AI, ALI, AN, APM, CCA, CCM, CD, CHN, CHP, CN, D, DR, EM, END, FP, GE, GS, HO, ID, IM, MP, MPD, N, NEP, NP, NPM, NS, OBG, OPH, ORS, OTO, P, PD, PDC, PDE, PDI, PDP, PDS, PG, PHO, PM, PN, PP, PS, PTH, PUD, RHU, RO, TS, U
Institution ID: 35-0109

Kingsboro Psychiatric Center
681 Clarkson Ave
Brooklyn, NY 11203
Major participating institution for programs in: PYG
Institution ID: 35-0231

Kingsbrook Jewish Medical Center
585 Schenectady Ave
Brooklyn, NY 11203-1891
Med Sch Affil: G-03508
Programs sponsored in: IM, ORS, PM
Institution ID: 35-0387

Long Island College Hospital
339 Hicks St
Brooklyn, NY 11201
Med Sch Affil: M-03508
Programs sponsored in: AI, CD, DR, GE, HO, IM, MPD, NEP, OBG, PD, PUD
Major participating institution for programs in: AN, APM, CCA, CN, GS, OPH, ORS, OTO, RO, U
Institution ID: 35-0439

Lutheran Medical Center
150 55th St
Brooklyn, NY 11220-2574
Med Sch Affil: M-03508
Programs sponsored in: FP, IM, OBG
Major participating institution for programs in: GS, PTH, RO, TS
Institution ID: 35-0449

Maimonides Medical Center
4802 Tenth Ave
Brooklyn, NY 11219-9988
Med Sch Affil: M-03508
Programs sponsored in: AN, CCM, CD, DR, GE, GS, HO, ID, IM, IMG, MG, MPD, NEP, OBG, ORS, P, PD, PDE, PTH, PUD, TY, U, VS
Major participating institution for programs in: CD, OPH, PP, PS, TS
Institution ID: 35-0366

Teaching Institutions

New York Methodist Hospital
506 Sixth St
Box 159008
Brooklyn, NY 11215-9008
Med Sch Affil: L-03508, L-03520
Programs sponsored in: AN, DR, EM, GS, HEM, IM, IMG, MPD, NR, OBG, ON, PD, PUD, RO
Major participating institution for programs in: GE, PS
Institution ID: 35-0267

SUNY Health Science Center at Brooklyn
450 Clarkson Ave/Box 1
Brooklyn, NY 11203
Programs sponsored in: AI, ALI, AN, APM, CCA, CCM, CD, CHN, CHP, CN, D, DR, EM, END, FP, GE, GS, HO, ICE, ID, IM, MP, MPD, N, NEP, NP, NPM, NS, OBG, OPH, ORS, OTO, P, PD, PDC, PDE, PDI, PDP, PDS, PG, PHO, PM, PN, PP, PS, PTH, PUD, PYG, RHU, RO, TS, U, VS
Major participating institution for programs in: IM
Institution ID: 35-9502

University Hospital-SUNY Health Science Center at Brooklyn
445 Lenox Rd
PO Box 23
Brooklyn, NY 11203-2098
Med Sch Affil: M-03508
Major participating institution for programs in: AI, ALI, AN, APM, CCA, CCM, CD, CHN, CHP, CN, D, DR, EM, END, FP, GE, GS, HO, ID, IM, MP, MPD, N, NEP, NP, NPM, NS, OBG, OPH, ORS, P, PD, PDC, PDE, PDI, PDP, PDS, PG, PHO, PN, PP, PS, PTH, PUD, PYG, RHU, RO, TS, U, VS
Institution ID: 35-0541

Veterans Affairs Medical Center (Brooklyn)
Office of Education (141)
800 Poly Pl
Brooklyn, NY 11209
Med Sch Affil: M-03508
Major participating institution for programs in: CCM, CD, D, END, GE, GS, HO, ID, IM, MPD, NEP, OPH, ORS, OTO, PS, PUD, RHU, U, VS
Institution ID: 35-0331

Woodhull Medical and Mental Health Center
760 Broadway/Rm 3BC 360
Brooklyn, NY 11206-5383
Med Sch Affil: L-03508
Programs sponsored in: IM, PD
Major participating institution for programs in: CD, GE, HEM, HO, ON, PUD
Institution ID: 35-0825

Wyckoff Heights Medical Center
374 Stockholm St
Brooklyn, NY 11237
Med Sch Affil: L-03520
Programs sponsored in: FP
Major participating institution for programs in: IM, P, PD, PTH
Institution ID: 35-0412

Buffalo

CGF Health System (Buffalo General Hospital)
100 High St
Buffalo, NY 14203
Med Sch Affil: M-03506
Major participating institution for programs in: AI, AN, APM, CCA, CD, CN, CRS, D, DR, EM, FP, GE, GPM, GS, HEM, IM, IPM, MN, MPD, MPM, N, NM, NP, NPR, NS, OBG, ORS, PCC, PM, PTH, RO, TS, U, VS
Institution ID: 35-0482

CGF Health System (Children's Hospital of Buffalo)
219 Bryant St
Buffalo, NY 14222
Med Sch Affil: M-03506
Programs sponsored in: MPD, PDR, PP
Major participating institution for programs in: AI, AN, CCA, CCP, CHN, CHP, CN, D, NPM, NS, OBG, OP, OPH, ORS, OTO, PD, PDE, PDS, PHO, PN, TS, U
Institution ID: 35-0223

CGF Health System (Millard Fillmore Hospitals)
3 Gates Circle
Buffalo, NY 14209-9986
Med Sch Affil: M-03506
Major participating institution for programs in: AN, CD, CN, EM, FP, GS, HSO, IM, N, OBG, TS, U, VS
Institution ID: 35-0330

Dent Neurological Institute (of Millard Fillmore Hospitals)
3 Gates Cir
Buffalo, NY 14209
Major participating institution for programs in: OTO
Institution ID: 35-8032

Erie County Medical Center
462 Grider St
Buffalo, NY 14215
Med Sch Affil: M-03506
Major participating institution for programs in: AN, CCA, CD, CHN, CN, D, DR, EM, END, FP, GE, GS, HEM, HSO, ID, IM, MN, MPD, MPM, NEP, NP, NPR, NS, OPH, ORS, OTO, P, PCC, PM, RHU
Institution ID: 35-0413

Mercy Hospital of Buffalo
565 Abbott Rd
Buffalo, NY 14220-1234
Med Sch Affil: L-03506
Major participating institution for programs in: IM, NM
Institution ID: 35-0126

Roswell Park Cancer Institute
Elm and Carlton Sts
Buffalo, NY 14263-0001
Med Sch Affil: M-03506
Programs sponsored in: SP
Major participating institution for programs in: AN, APM, CCA, D, GE, NM, ON, PHO, PTH, RO
Institution ID: 35-0451

Sisters of Charity Hospital
2157 Main St
Buffalo, NY 14214-9984
Med Sch Affil: L-03506
Major participating institution for programs in: IM, OBG, OTO
Institution ID: 35-0157

SUNY at Buffalo Grad Medical-Dental Education Consortium
3435 Main St/113 Cary Hall
Buffalo, NY 14214
Med Sch Affil: M-03506
Programs sponsored in: AI, AN, APM, CCA, CCP, CD, CHN, CHP, CN, CRS, D, DR, EM, END, FP, GE, GPM, GS, HEM, HSO, ID, IM, IMG, IPM, MN, MPM, N, NEP, NM, NP, NPM, NPR, NS, OBG, ON, OP, OPH, ORS, OTO, P, PCC, PD, PDE, PDS, PHO, PM, PN, PTH, RHU, RO, TS, U, VS
Institution ID: 35-9501

SUNY at Buffalo School of Medicine
3435 Main St
Buffalo, NY 14214
Med Sch Affil: M-03506
Major participating institution for programs in: CHP
Institution ID: 35-8028

Veterans Affairs Medical Center (Buffalo)
3495 Bailey Ave
Buffalo, NY 14215
Med Sch Affil: M-03506
Major participating institution for programs in: AN, CCA, CD, CHN, CN, D, END, GE, GS, HEM, ID, IM, IMG, MPD, MPM, NEP, NM, NPR, ON, OPH, ORS, OTO, P, PCC, PM, PTH, RHU, RO, TS, U, VS
Institution ID: 35-0466

Canandaigua

Frederick Ferris Thompson Systems
350 Parrish St
Canandaigua, NY 14424
Major participating institution for programs in: FP
Institution ID: 35-7042

Cooperstown

Bassett Healthcare
1 Atwell Rd
Cooperstown, NY 13326-1394
Programs sponsored in: FP, GS, IM, TY
Institution ID: 35-8049

Mary Imogene Bassett Hospital
1 Atwell Rd
Cooperstown, NY 13326-1394
Med Sch Affil: M-03501
Major participating institution for programs in: GS, IM, TY
Institution ID: 35-0134

East Meadow

Nassau County Medical Center
2201 Hempstead Trnpk
East Meadow, NY 11554-5400
Med Sch Affil: M-03548
Programs sponsored in: AI, ALI, AN, CD, CHN, DR, END, GE, GS, HEM, ID, IM, N, NEP, OBG, ON, OPH, P, PD, PM, PS, PTH, PUD
Major participating institution for programs in: ORS, RHU
Institution ID: 35-0162

Nassau County Medical Examiner's Office
Hempstead Trnpk and Franklin Ave
East Meadow, NY 11554
Programs sponsored in: FOP
Institution ID: 35-0577

Elmhurst

Catholic Medical Center (St John's Queens Hospital)
90-02 Queens Blvd
Elmhurst, NY 11373-4941
Major participating institution for programs in: CD, ID, IM, IMG, OBG, ORS, P, PUD
Institution ID: 35-0172

Elmhurst Hospital Center-Mount Sinai Services
79-01 Broadway
Elmhurst, NY 11373
Med Sch Affil: M-03547
Major participating institution for programs in: AN, CCA, CD, CHP, D, DR, EM, GE, GS, HO, ID, IM, MPD, NEP, NPM, NS, OBG, OPH, ORS, OTO, P, PD, PM, PS, PUD, PYG, RHU, TY, U
Institution ID: 35-0271

Far Rockaway

St John's Episcopal Hospital-South Shore
327 Beach 19th St
Far Rockaway, NY 11691
Med Sch Affil: M-03508
Programs sponsored in: IM
Major participating institution for programs in: ADP, CCM, GE, PUD, PYG
Institution ID: 35-0244

Flushing

New York Flushing Hospital Medical Center
45th Ave at Parsons Blvd
Flushing, NY 11355
Med Sch Affil: L-03520
Programs sponsored in: IM, IMG, OBG, PD, TY
Major participating institution for programs in: GS
Institution ID: 35-0364

New York Hospital Medical Center of Queens
56-45 Main St
Flushing, NY 11355-5095
Med Sch Affil: M-03520, G-03519
Programs sponsored in: GE, GS, ID, IM, NEP, PTH, PUD, RO, TY
Major participating institution for programs in: IMG, OBG
Institution ID: 35-0349

Forest Hills

North Shore University Hospital at Forest Hills
102-01 66th Rd
Forest Hills, NY 11375-2029
Programs sponsored in: IM
Major participating institution for programs in: GS
Institution ID: 35-0568

Geneva

Geneva General Hospital
196 North St
Geneva, NY 14456-1694
Major participating institution for programs in: FP
Institution ID: 35-7171

Glen Cove

North Shore University Hospital at Glen Cove
101 St Andrews Ln
Glen Cove, NY 11542-2263
Med Sch Affil: L-03548
Programs sponsored in: FP
Institution ID: 35-0409

Glen Oaks

Hillside Hospital (Long Island Jewish Medical Center)
75-59 263rd St
Glen Oaks, NY 11004
Major participating institution for programs in: P, PYG, PYN
Institution ID: 35-0299

Harrison

St Vincent's Hospital of New York-Westchester Branch
275 North St
Harrison, NY 10528
Med Sch Affil: L-03509
Major participating institution for programs in: P
Institution ID: 35-0490

Hauppauge

Suffolk County Department of Health Services
225 Rabro Dr E
Hauppauge, NY 11788
Med Sch Affil: G-03548
Major participating institution for programs in: GPM
Institution ID: 35-8021

Hawthorne

Westchester County Department of Health
19 Bradhurst Ave
Hawthorne, NY 10532
Major participating institution for programs in: GPM
Institution ID: 35-8044

Huntington

Huntington Hospital
270 Park Ave
Huntington, NY 11743-2799
Major participating institution for programs in: GS
Institution ID: 35-0532

Jamaica

Catholic Medical Center (Mary Immaculate Hospital)
152-11 89th Ave
Jamaica, NY 11432-9998
Major participating institution for programs in: CD, FP, GS, ID, IM, IMG, OBG, OPH, ORS, PUD
Institution ID: 35-0472

Catholic Medical Center of Brooklyn and Queens Inc
88-25 153rd St/Ste 1C
Jamaica, NY 11432-9998
Med Sch Affil: M-03546, L-03508
Programs sponsored in: CD, FP, GS, ID, IM, IMG, OBG, OPH, ORS, PUD
Institution ID: 35-0558

Jamaica Hospital
8900 Van Wyck Expwy
Jamaica, NY 11418-2897
Med Sch Affil: L-03520, L-03508
Programs sponsored in: FP, IM, OBG
Major participating institution for programs in: GS, ORS, PM
Institution ID: 35-0216

Queens Hospital Center
82-68 164th St
Jamaica, NY 11432
Med Sch Affil: M-03547
Major participating institution for programs in: END, GE, IM, OBG, OPH, PCC, PCP, RHU
Institution ID: 35-0220

Kingston

Benedictine Hospital
105 Mary's Ave
Kingston, NY 12401-5894
Med Sch Affil: L-03509
Major participating institution for programs in: FP
Institution ID: 35-0350

Kingston Hospital
396 Broadway
Kingston, NY 12401
Med Sch Affil: L-03509
Major participating institution for programs in: FP
Institution ID: 35-0435

Mid-Hudson Family Health Institute
One Family Practice Dr
Kingston, NY 12401
Programs sponsored in: FP
Institution ID: 35-0432

Manhasset

North Shore University Hospital
300 Community Dr
Manhasset, NY 11030-3876
Med Sch Affil: M-03519
Programs sponsored in: ADL, ADP, CCS, CD, CHP, DR, EM, GE, GS, HO, ICE, ID, IM, IMG, MPD, N, NEP, NM, NPM, OBG, OPH, P, PCC, PD, PDC, PDE, PDI, PG, PTH, RHU, RNR, VS
Major participating institution for programs in: AI, ALI, PP, PS
Institution ID: 35-0467

Mineola

Nassau County Department of Health
240 Old Country Rd
Mineola, NY 11501-4250
Major participating institution for programs in: GPM
Institution ID: 35-8022

Winthrop-University Hospital
259 First St
Mineola, NY 11501-3957
Med Sch Affil: M-03548
Programs sponsored in: CD, DR, END, GE, HO, ID, IM, IMG, NEP, OBG, PCC, PD, PDE, PDP, PTH, RHU
Major participating institution for programs in: CD, GS, PS, U
Institution ID: 35-0375

Montrose

Hudson Valley Healthcare System
PO Box 100
Montrose, NY 10548
Med Sch Affil: L-03509
Major participating institution for programs in: GPM
Institution ID: 35-0251

Mount Vernon

Mount Vernon Hospital
12 N 7th Ave
Mount Vernon, NY 10550-2098
Med Sch Affil: L-03509
Programs sponsored in: IM
Major participating institution for programs in: GPM
Institution ID: 35-0255

New Hyde Park

Long Island Jewish Medical Center
270-05 76th Ave
New Hyde Park, NY 11040
Med Sch Affil: M-03546, L-03508
Programs sponsored in: ADL, AI, CCP, CD, CHN, CHP, DR, EM, END, GE, GS, HO, ICE, ID, IM, IMG, MEM, N, NEP, NM, NPM, OBG, OPH, ORS, P, PCC, PCP, PD, PDC, PDE, PDI, PDR, PHO, PM, PPR, PTH, PYG, PYN, RNR, TS, U, VIR, VS
Major participating institution for programs in: CD, OTO
Institution ID: 35-0232

Schneider Children's Hosp (Long Island Jewish Med Ctr)
270-05 76th Ave
New Hyde Park, NY 11040
Med Sch Affil: M-03546
Major participating institution for programs in: ADL, AI, CCP, CHN, CHP, NPM, ORS, PD, PDC, PDE, PDI, PHO, PPR
Institution ID: 35-8024

New Rochelle

Sound Shore Medical Center of Westchester
16 Guion Pl
New Rochelle, NY 10802-5500
Med Sch Affil: M-03509
Major participating institution for programs in: AN, END, GS, IM, TY
Institution ID: 35-0104

New York

Bellevue Hospital Center
27th St and 1st Ave
New York, NY 10016
Med Sch Affil: M-03519
Major participating institution for programs in: ADP, AN, CCA, CD, CHN, CHP, D, DMP, DR, EM, END, GE, GS, HEM, HMP, HSO, HSP, ICE, ID, IM, IMG, MSR, N, NEP, NO, NP, NPM, NRN, NS, OBG, ON, OPH, ORS, OSM, OTO, P, PCC, PCP, PD, PDC, PDE, PDR, PFP, PHO, PM, PS, PTH, PYG, PYN, RHU, RNR, RO, TS, U, VIR, VS
Institution ID: 35-0235

Beth Israel Medical Center
First Ave at 16th St
New York, NY 10003
Med Sch Affil: M-03546
Programs sponsored in: ADP, AN, CD, DR, EM, END, FP, GE, GS, HMP, HO, ID, IM, MEM, NEP, OAR, OBG, P, PCC, PD, PYG, RNR, U
Major participating institution for programs in: D, NPM, ORS, OTO, PM
Institution ID: 35-0284

Cabrini Medical Center
227 E 19th St
New York, NY 10003
Med Sch Affil: M-03547, G-03519
Major participating institution for programs in: CD, END, GE, GS, HO, ID, IM, OPH, P, PUD, RHU, U
Institution ID: 35-0410

Columbia University School of Public Health
600 W 168th St
New York, NY 10032
Med Sch Affil: L-03501
Programs sponsored in: GPM
Major participating institution for programs in: GPM
Institution ID: 35-0766

Cornell University Medical College
1300 York Ave
New York, NY 10021
Med Sch Affil: M-03520
Major participating institution for programs in: GPM
Institution ID: 35-0791

Goldwater Memorial Hospital
F D Roosevelt Island
New York, NY 10044
Med Sch Affil: G-03519
Major participating institution for programs in: PM, PYG
Institution ID: 35-0122

Harlem Hospital Center
506 Lenox Ave
New York, NY 10037-1003
Med Sch Affil: M-03501
Programs sponsored in: CD, CHP, DR, GE, GS, ID, IM, NEP, OBG, P, PD, PS, PTH, PUD
Major participating institution for programs in: HO, ORS
Institution ID: 35-0195

Hospital for Joint Diseases Orthopaedic Institute
Bernard Aronson Plaza
301 E 17th St
New York, NY 10003
Med Sch Affil: M-03519
Programs sponsored in: HSO, OFA, OP, ORS, OSM, OSS, SP
Major participating institution for programs in: IMG, MSR, OSM, RHU
Institution ID: 35-0289

Hospital for Special Surgery
535 E 70th St
New York, NY 10021-1000
Med Sch Affil: M-03520
Programs sponsored in: HSO, OP, ORS, OSM, OSS
Major participating institution for programs in: CN, DR, FSM, NS, OMO, PPR
Institution ID: 35-0459

Lenox Hill Hospital
100 E 77th St
New York, NY 10021-1883
Med Sch Affil: M-03519, G-02416
Programs sponsored in: CD, DR, GE, GS, HO, IM, NEP, OBG, OPH, ORS, OSM, PTH, PUD, U
Major participating institution for programs in: OTO, PS
Institution ID: 35-0334

Manhattan Eye, Ear and Throat Hospital
210 E 64th St
New York, NY 10021
Med Sch Affil: L-03501, G-03519
Programs sponsored in: OPH, OTO
Institution ID: 35-0367

Manhattan Psychiatric Center
600 E 125th St
Ward's Island
New York, NY 10035
Med Sch Affil: L-03519
Major participating institution for programs in: P, PYG
Institution ID: 35-0239

Memorial Sloan-Kettering Cancer Center
1275 York Ave
New York, NY 10021
Med Sch Affil: M-03520, L-03508, G-03519
Programs sponsored in: CCA, CCM, GE, HO, ID, NM, OMO, PCP, PHO, PUD, RO, SP
Major participating institution for programs in: AN, APM, BBK, DMP, DR, GE, GS, IM, N, NS, OTO, PM, PS, RNR, TS, VIR
Institution ID: 35-0125

Metropolitan Hospital Center
1901 First Ave
New York, NY 10029
Med Sch Affil: M-03509
Programs sponsored in: MPD
Major participating institution for programs in: AN, CHP, D, EM, GE, GS, ID, IM, N, NEP, OBG, OPH, P, PCC, PD, PM, U
Institution ID: 35-0163

Mount Sinai Medical Center
One Gustave L Levy Pl
New York, NY 10029
Med Sch Affil: M-03547, G-03519
Programs sponsored in: CPP
Major participating institution for programs in: AI, AN, APM, BBK, CCA, CCM, CD, CHN, CHP, CRS, D, DMP, DR, EM, END, GE, GPM, GS, HO, HSP, ICE, ID, IM, IMG, MEM, MG, MPD, N, NEP, NM, NP, NPM, NS, OBG, OPH, ORS, OTO, P, PCC, PCP, PD, PDC, PDE, PDI, PDP, PDR, PG, PHO, PM, PMG, PN, PS, PTH, PUD, RHU, RNR, RO, TS, U, VS
Institution ID: 35-0376

Mount Sinai School of Medicine
One Gustave L Levy Pl
New York, NY 10029-6574
Med Sch Affil: M-03547
Programs sponsored in: AI, AN, APM, CCA, CCM, CD, CHN, CHP, CRS, D, DMP, DR, EM, END, FP, GE, GPM, GS, HO, ICE, ID, IM, IMG, MG, MPD, N, NEP, NM, NP, NPM, NS, OBG, OPH, ORS, OTO, P, PCC, PCP, PD, PDC, PDE, PDI, PDP, PDR, PG, PHO, PM, PMG, PN, PS, PTH, PUD, PYG, RHU, RNR, RO, TS, TY, U, VIR, VS
Institution ID: 35-9503

New York and Presbyterian Hospital
525 E 68th St
New York, NY 10021
Programs sponsored in: ADP, AI, AN, APM, CCA, CCM, CCP, CD, CHN, CHP, CN, D, DMP, DR, END, FP, GE, GPM, GS, HO, HSO, ICE, ID, IM, IMG, N, NEP, NM, NP, NPM, NR, NS, OAR, OBG, OPH, ORS, OTO, P, PCC, PCP, PD, PDC, PDE, PDI, PDP, PDR, PDS, PG, PHO, PM, PN, PPR, PS, PTH, PUD, PYG, RHU, RNR, RO, TS, U, VIR
Institution ID: 35-8051

New York and Presbyterian Hospital (Columbia Campus)
622 W 168th St
New York, NY 10032-3784
Med Sch Affil: M-03501
Programs sponsored in: MPM
Major participating institution for programs in: ADP, AI, AN, APM, CCA, CCM, CD, CHN, CHP, CN, D, DR, END, FP, GE, GS, HO, HSO, ICE, ID, IM, N, NEP, NM, NP, NPM, NR, NS, OAR, OBG, OPH, ORS, OTO, P, PD, PDC, PDE, PDI, PDP, PDR, PDS, PG, PHO, PM, PPR, PTH, PUD, PYG, RHU, RNR, RO, TS, VIR
Institution ID: 35-0269

New York and Presbyterian Hospital (Cornell Campus)
525 E 68th St/F-164
New York, NY 10021-1234
Med Sch Affil: M-03520
Programs sponsored in: PDE
Major participating institution for programs in: ADP, AI, AN, APM, CCA, CCP, CD, CHN, CHP, CN, D, DMP, DR, END, GE, GPM, GS, HO, HSO, ICE, ID, IM, IMG, N, NEP, NM, NPM, NS, OBG, OPH, ORS, OTO, P, PCC, PCP, PD, PDC, PDI, PDP, PG, PHO, PM, PN, PPR, PS, PTH, RHU, RNR, RO, TS, U, VIR
Institution ID: 35-0262

New York and Presbyterian Hospital-Payne Whitney Clinic
Box 140
525 E 68th St
New York, NY 10021
Med Sch Affil: M-03520
Major participating institution for programs in: ADP, CHP, P
Institution ID: 35-0823

New York Blood Center
310 E 67th St
New York, NY 10021
Programs sponsored in: BBK
Major participating institution for programs in: BBK
Institution ID: 35-0807

New York City Department of Health
Rm 331/Box 28
125 Worth St
New York, NY 10013
Programs sponsored in: GPM
Institution ID: 35-0394

New York Eye and Ear Infirmary
310 E 14th St
New York, NY 10003-4200
Med Sch Affil: G-03509
Programs sponsored in: OPH
Major participating institution for programs in: OTO, SP
Institution ID: 35-0230

New York State Psychiatric Institute
722 W 168th St
New York, NY 10032
Med Sch Affil: M-03501
Major participating institution for programs in: ADP, CHP, P
Institution ID: 35-0353

New York University Medical Center
550 First Ave
New York, NY 10016-1111
Med Sch Affil: M-03519
Programs sponsored in: ADP, AN, APM, CCA, CD, CHN, CHP, CN, D, DMP, DR, EM, END, GE, GS, HEM, HMP, HSO, HSP, ICE, ID, IM, IMG, MSR, N, NEP, NO, NP, NPM, NR, NRN, NS, OBG, ON, OPH, ORS, OSM, OTO, P, PCC, PCP, PD, PDC, PDE, PDR, PFP, PHO, PIP, PM, PP, PS, PTH, PYG, PYN, RHU, RNR, RO, TS, U, VIR, VS
Major participating institution for programs in: BBK
Institution ID: 35-0450

North General Hospital
1879 Madison Ave
New York, NY 10035
Med Sch Affil: L-03547
Programs sponsored in: IM, P
Institution ID: 35-0808

NYU Downtown Hospital
170 William St
New York, NY 10038-2649
Med Sch Affil: G-03519
Programs sponsored in: IM, OBG
Institution ID: 35-0270

Office of Chief Medical Examiner-City of New York
520 First Ave
New York, NY 10016
Programs sponsored in: FOP
Institution ID: 35-0528

Rockefeller University Hospital
1230 York Ave
New York, NY 10021
Major participating institution for programs in: DMP
Institution ID: 35-0725

Rusk Institute of Rehabilitation Medicine
400 E 34th St/R R615
New York, NY 10016-1111
Med Sch Affil: M-03519
Major participating institution for programs in: PM
Institution ID: 35-0145

St Luke's-Roosevelt Hospital Center
1111 Amsterdam Ave
New York, NY 10025
Med Sch Affil: M-03501
Programs sponsored in: AN, APM, CD, CHP, CRS, D, DR, EM, END, GE, GS, HEM, HSO, ICE, ID, IM, NEP, NM, NR, OBG, ON, OPH, ORS, P, PCC, PD, PS, PTH, VIR
Major participating institution for programs in: CD, HSO, RO, U
Institution ID: 35-8013

St Luke's-Roosevelt Hospital Center-Roosevelt Division
428 W 59th St
New York, NY 10019
Med Sch Affil: M-03501
Major participating institution for programs in: CHP, CRS, D, DR, EM, GE, GS, HEM, HSO, IM, NM, NR, OBG, ON, OPH, ORS, OTO, P, PD, PS, PTH, VIR
Institution ID: 35-0211

St Luke's-Roosevelt Hospital Center-St Luke's Division
1111 Amsterdam Ave
New York, NY 10025
Med Sch Affil: M-03501
Major participating institution for programs in: AN, CD, CHP, D, DR, EM, END, GE, GS, HEM, ICE, ID, IM, NEP, NM, NR, OBG, ON, OPH, ORS, OTO, P, PCC, PD, PS, PTH, VIR
Institution ID: 35-0135

St Vincent's Hospital and Medical Center of New York
153 W 11th St
New York, NY 10011-8397
Med Sch Affil: M-03509, L-03508
Programs sponsored in: MPD
Major participating institution for programs in: AN, APM, CCM, CD, CHP, DR, EM, END, GE, GS, HO, ID, IM, IMG, N, NEP, NM, NR, NS, OBG, OPH, OTO, P, PCC, PD, PM, PTH, PYG, TY
Institution ID: 35-0241

The Institute for Urban Family Health
16 E 16th St
New York, NY 10003
Major participating institution for programs in: FP
Institution ID: 35-8045

The Rogosin Institute
505 E 70th St
New York, NY 10021
Major participating institution for programs in: END
Institution ID: 35-8043

Veterans Affairs Medical Center (Manhattan)
423 E 23rd St
New York, NY 10010
Med Sch Affil: M-03519
Major participating institution for programs in: AN, CD, D, DMP, DR, END, GS, HEM, HSO, ID, IM, MPD, NEP, NRN, NS, ON, OPH, ORS, OTO, P, PCC, PM, PTH, PYN, RHU, RNR, TS, U, VIR
Institution ID: 35-0392

Niagara Falls

Niagara Falls Memorial Medical Center
621 10th St
Niagara Falls, NY 14302-0708
Med Sch Affil: L-03506
Major participating institution for programs in: FP
Institution ID: 35-0448

Northport

Veterans Affairs Medical Center (Northport)
79 Middleville Rd
Northport, NY 11768
Med Sch Affil: M-03548
Programs sponsored in: NM
Major participating institution for programs in: CD, CN, D, DR, END, GE, GS, HO, ID, IM, IMG, MN, N, NEP, NP, OPH, OTO, P, PCC, PM, RHU, U, VS
Institution ID: 35-0441

Oceanside

South Nassau Communities Hospital
2445 Oceanside Rd
Oceanside, NY 11572
Med Sch Affil: L-03548
Programs sponsored in: FP
Major participating institution for programs in: NM
Institution ID: 35-0277

Olean

Olean General Hospital
515 Main St
Olean, NY 14760
Major participating institution for programs in: FP
Institution ID: 35-7243

Orangeburg

Rockland Children's Psychiatric Center
Convent Rd
Orangeburg, NY 10962
Major participating institution for programs in: CHP
Institution ID: 35-8042

Penn Yan

Soldiers and Sailors Memorial Hospital of Yates County
418 N Main St
Penn Yan, NY 14527-1085
Major participating institution for programs in: FP
Institution ID: 35-8050

Poughkeepsie

St Francis Hospital
35 North Rd
Poughkeepsie, NY 12601
Major participating institution for programs in: FP
Institution ID: 35-0443

Vassar Brothers Hospital
Reade Pl
Poughkeepsie, NY 12601
Major participating institution for programs in: FP
Institution ID: 35-0340

Queens Village

Creedmoor Psychiatric Center
80-45 Winchester Blvd
Queens Village, NY 11427-2199
Programs sponsored in: P
Institution ID: 35-0193

Rochester

Genesee Hospital
224 Alexander St
Rochester, NY 14607-4055
Med Sch Affil: M-03545
Major participating institution for programs in: CCA, CCM, CCS, END, GE, GS, IM, MPD, OBG, OTO, PS, U
Institution ID: 35-0120

Highland Hospital of Rochester
1000 South Ave
Rochester, NY 14620-9986
Med Sch Affil: M-03545
Programs sponsored in: FP, IM
Major participating institution for programs in: OBG, ORS
Institution ID: 35-0397

Monroe Community Hospital
435 E Henrietta Rd
Rochester, NY 14620
Med Sch Affil: M-03545
Major participating institution for programs in: APM, IMG
Institution ID: 35-0562

Monroe County Medical Examiners Office
740 E Henrietta Rd
Rochester, NY 14623
Programs sponsored in: FOP
Institution ID: 35-0554

Rochester General Hospital
1425 Portland Ave
Rochester, NY 14621-3095
Med Sch Affil: M-03545
Programs sponsored in: DR, OBG
Major participating institution for programs in: ADL, CCA, CCS, CD, END, FP, GS, IM, MPD, OPH, ORS, OTO, PD, PS, TS, U, VS
Institution ID: 35-0388

Rochester Psychiatric Center
1111 Elmwood Ave
Rochester, NY 14620-3005
Med Sch Affil: L-03545
Major participating institution for programs in: CHP, PFP
Institution ID: 35-0309

St Mary's Hospital (Unity Health System)
89 Genesee St
Rochester, NY 14611-3285
Med Sch Affil: M-03545
Programs sponsored in: IM
Major participating institution for programs in: END, GE, OPH, PFP, PM
Institution ID: 35-0372

Strong Memorial Hospital of the University of Rochester
601 Elmwood Ave
Rochester, NY 14642
Med Sch Affil: M-03545
Programs sponsored in: ADL, AI, AN, APM, CCA, CCM, CCP, CCS, CD, CHN, CHP, CN, D, DR, EM, END, GE, GS, HO, HSO, ICE, ID, IM, IMG, MP, MPD, MSR, N, NEP, NM, NP, NPM, NS, OBG, OPH, ORS, OSM, OSS, OTO, P, PCC, PCP, PD, PDC, PDI, PDP, PDR, PFP, PHO, PM, PN, PS, PTH, PYG, RHU, RNR, RO, TS, U, VIR, VS
Major participating institution for programs in: FP
Institution ID: 35-0493

Rockville Centre

Mercy Medical Center
1000 N Village Ave
Rockville Centre, NY 11570
Major participating institution for programs in: OBG
Institution ID: 35-0212

Schenectady

Ellis Hospital
1101 Nott St
Schenectady, NY 12308
Med Sch Affil: G-03503
Major participating institution for programs in: MPD, ORS
Institution ID: 35-0474

St Clare's Hospital of Schenectady
600 McClellan St
Schenectady, NY 12304
Med Sch Affil: G-03503
Programs sponsored in: FP
Institution ID: 35-0214

Sunnyview Hospital and Rehabilitation Center
1270 Belmont Ave
Schenectady, NY 12308-2198
Med Sch Affil: G-03503
Major participating institution for programs in: PM
Institution ID: 35-0523

Staten Island

Bayley Seton Hospital
75 Vanderbilt Ave
Staten Island, NY 10304-3850
Med Sch Affil: M-03509
Major participating institution for programs in: D, OPH, P
Institution ID: 35-0813

Sisters of Charity Medical Center-St Vincent's Campus
355 Bard Ave
Staten Island, NY 10310
Med Sch Affil: M-03508, M-03509
Programs sponsored in: PD
Major participating institution for programs in: CD, DR, GS, IM, NEP, OBG, P
Institution ID: 35-0458

Staten Island University Hospital
475 Seaview Ave
Staten Island, NY 10305
Med Sch Affil: M-03508
Programs sponsored in: GS, IM, IMG, MPD, OBG
Major participating institution for programs in: GE, PM
Institution ID: 35-0156

Stony Brook

University Hospital-SUNY at Stony Brook
Health Sciences Ctr
Stony Brook, NY 11794-8410
Med Sch Affil: M-03548
Programs sponsored in: AI, AN, APM, BBK, CD, CHN, CHP, CN, D, DR, EM, END, FP, GE, GPM, GS, HO, HSO, ID, IM, IMG, MN, MPD, N, NEP, NP, NPM, NR, OBG, OP, ORS, OTO, P, PCC, PD, PDE, PM, PN, PTH, RHU, RNR, U, VIR, VS
Major participating institution for programs in: NM
Institution ID: 35-0560

Syosset

Syosset Community Hospital
221 Jericho Trnpk
Syosset, NY 11791
Major participating institution for programs in: IM, OBG
Institution ID: 35-8046

Syracuse

American Red Cross Blood Services-Syracuse Region
636 S Warren St
Syracuse, NY 13202-3368
Med Sch Affil: L-03515
Major participating institution for programs in: BBK
Institution ID: 35-8025

Community-General Hospital of Greater Syracuse
Broad Rd
Syracuse, NY 13215
Med Sch Affil: M-03515
Major participating institution for programs in: GS, PTH
Institution ID: 35-0567

Crouse Hospital
736 Irving Ave
Syracuse, NY 13210
Med Sch Affil: M-03515
Programs sponsored in: FP
Major participating institution for programs in: AN, BBK, GS, HSO, ID, IM, N, NS, OBG, OPH, ORS, OSS, OTO, PD, PDC, PDE, PDI, PHO, TS
Institution ID: 35-0566

Richard H Hutchings Psychiatric Center
620 Madison St
Syracuse, NY 13210
Med Sch Affil: M-03515
Major participating institution for programs in: P
Institution ID: 35-0780

St Camillus Health and Rehabilitation Center
813 Fay Rd
Syracuse, NY 13219-3098
Major participating institution for programs in: PM
Institution ID: 35-8037

St Joseph's Hospital Health Center

301 Prospect Ave
Syracuse, NY 13203-1807
Med Sch Affil: M-03515
Programs sponsored in: FP, TY
Major participating institution for programs in: EM, PDI
Institution ID: 35-0445

University Hospital-SUNY Health Science Center at Syracuse

750 E Adams St
Syracuse, NY 13210
Med Sch Affil: M-03515
Programs sponsored in: AN, APM, BBK, CCA, CD, CN, DR, EM, END, GE, GS, HMP, HO, HSO, ID, IM, IMG, N, NEP, NP, NR, NS, OBG, OPH, ORS, OSS, OTO, P, PCC, PCP, PD, PDC, PDE, PDI, PHO, PM, PTH, RHU, RNR, RO, TS, U, VIR
Institution ID: 35-0174

Veterans Affairs Medical Center (Syracuse)

800 Irving Ave
Syracuse, NY 13210
Med Sch Affil: M-03515
Major participating institution for programs in: AN, APM, CD, CN, DR, END, GE, GS, HO, ID, IM, N, NEP, NS, OPH, ORS, OTO, P, PCC, PM, PTH, RHU, RNR, U, VIR
Institution ID: 35-0183

Utica

St Elizabeth Medical Center

2209 Genesee St
Utica, NY 13501-5930
Major participating institution for programs in: FP
Institution ID: 35-0759

Valhalla

New York Medical College

Administration Bldg
Valhalla, NY 10595
Med Sch Affil: M-03509
Programs sponsored in: AN, APM, CCM, CCS, CD, CHP, D, DR, EM, END, FP, GE, GPM, GS, HO, ID, IM, IMG, N, NEP, NM, NPM, NR, NS, OBG, OPH, ORS, OTO, P, PCC, PCP, PD, PDP, PG, PM, PTH, PYG, RHU, RNR, RO, SP, TY, U, VIR
Institution ID: 35-0782

Westchester Medical Center

Valhalla Campus
Valhalla, NY 10595-1689
Med Sch Affil: M-03509
Major participating institution for programs in: AN, APM, BBK, CCS, CD, CHP, D, DR, END, GE, GS, HO, ID, IM, IMG, N, NEP, NPM, NS, OBG, OPH, ORS, OTO, P, PCC, PCP, PD, PDP, PG, PS, PTH, RHU, RNR, RO, U, VIR
Institution ID: 35-0301

West Brentwood

Central Islip Psychiatric Center

998 Crooked Hill Rd
West Brentwood, NY 11717
Major participating institution for programs in: PYG
Institution ID: 35-0233

West Point

Keller Army Community Hospital

US Army Med Dept Activity
West Point, NY 10996-1197
Programs sponsored in: OSM
Institution ID: 35-7271

West Seneca

Western New York Children's Psychiatric Center

1010 East and West Rd
West Seneca, NY 14224
Major participating institution for programs in: CHP
Institution ID: 35-8035

White Plains

New York and Presbyterian Hospital-Westchester Division

21 Bloomingdale Rd
White Plains, NY 10605-1504
Med Sch Affil: M-03520
Major participating institution for programs in: CHP, P, PYG
Institution ID: 35-0378

St Agnes Hospital

305 North St
White Plains, NY 10605
Major participating institution for programs in: APM, GS
Institution ID: 35-7123

Yonkers

St Joseph's Medical Center

127 S Broadway
Yonkers, NY 10701-4080
Med Sch Affil: L-03509
Major participating institution for programs in: FP, GS
Institution ID: 35-0442

North Carolina

Ahoskie

Roanoke-Chowan Hospital

500 S Academy St
PO Box 1385
Ahoskie, NC 27910
Major participating institution for programs in: FP
Institution ID: 36-8013

Asheville

Memorial Mission Hospital

509 Biltmore Ave
Asheville, NC 28801-4690
Med Sch Affil: L-03601
Major participating institution for programs in: FP, OBG
Institution ID: 36-0114

Mountain Area Health Education Center

501 Biltmore Ave
Asheville, NC 28801-4686
Programs sponsored in: FP, OBG
Institution ID: 36-0732

Veterans Affairs Medical Center (Asheville)

1100 Tunnel Rd
Asheville, NC 28805
Med Sch Affil: L-03607
Major participating institution for programs in: GS, ORS, TS, U
Institution ID: 36-0740

Butner

Federal Correctional Institution-Butner

PO Box 1000
Butner, NC 27509-1000
Med Sch Affil: G-03607
Major participating institution for programs in: PFP
Institution ID: 36-8018

John Umstead Hospital

1003 12th St
Butner, NC 27509-1626
Med Sch Affil: G-03607
Major participating institution for programs in: ADP, CHP, PYG
Institution ID: 36-0507

Chapel Hill

Office of the Chief Medical Examiner

Campus Box 7580
Chapel Hill, NC 27599-7580
Major participating institution for programs in: FOP
Institution ID: 36-0514

University of North Carolina Hospitals

101 Manning Dr
Chapel Hill, NC 27514
Med Sch Affil: M-03601, L-03607
Programs sponsored in: AN, APM, BBK, CCA, CCP, CCS, CD, CHN, CHP, D, DR, EM, END, FOP, FP, GE, GPM, GS, HMP, HO, ICE, ID, IM, IMG, MG, MM, MPD, N, NEP, NM, NP, NPM, NS, OBG, OPH, ORS, OTO, P, PCC, PCP, PD, PDE, PDP, PG, PHO, PIP, PM, PS, PTH, RHU, RNR, RO, TS, U, VIR, VS
Major participating institution for programs in: PPR
Institution ID: 36-0478

University of North Carolina School at Chapel Hill

CB No 7400
168 Rosenau Hall
Chapel Hill, NC 27599-7400
Med Sch Affil: L-03607
Major participating institution for programs in: GPM
Institution ID: 36-9502

University of North Carolina School of Medicine

CB 7400 Rosenau Hall
Chapel Hill, NC 27599
Med Sch Affil: M-03601
Major participating institution for programs in: GPM
Institution ID: 36-0511

Charlotte

Carolinas Medical Center

1000 Blythe Blvd
Charlotte, NC 28203
Med Sch Affil: M-03601
Programs sponsored in: EM, FP, GS, HMP, IM, OBG, ORS, OTR, PD, PM, SP, TS, VS
Major participating institution for programs in: PS, U
Institution ID: 36-0291

Charlotte Institute of Rehabilitation

1100 Blythe Blvd
Charlotte, NC 28203
Major participating institution for programs in: PM
Institution ID: 36-8012

Clinton

Sampson County Memorial Hospital

607 Beaman St/Drawer 258
Clinton, NC 28328
Major participating institution for programs in: FP
Institution ID: 36-8017

Concord

Northeast Medical Center

920 Church St N
Concord, NC 28025
Programs sponsored in: FP
Institution ID: 36-8016

Durham

Duke University Medical Center

Box 3708
Durham, NC 27710
Med Sch Affil: L-03608
Programs sponsored in: ADP, AI, AN, APM, CCA, CCP, CCS, CD, CHN, CHP, CN, D, DMP, DR, END, FP, GE, GPM, GS, HMP, HO, HSO, ICE, ID, IM, IMG, MG, MM, MN, MP, MPD, N, NEP, NM, NP, NPM, NR, NS, OBG, OPH, ORS, OTO, P, PCC, PCP, PD, PDC, PDE, PDI, PDP, PDR, PFP, PHO, PN, PPR, PS, PTH, PYG, RHU, RNR, RO, TS, U, VIR
Institution ID: 36-0222

Durham Regional Hospital

3643 N Roxboro St
Durham, NC 27704-2763
Med Sch Affil: M-03607, L-03601
Major participating institution for programs in: FP, GS, NS, ORS, PS
Institution ID: 36-0440

Veterans Affairs Medical Center (Durham)

508 Fulton St
Durham, NC 27705
Med Sch Affil: M-03607
Major participating institution for programs in: ADP, APM, CCA, CCS, CD, CN, D, DMP, DR, END, GE, GS, HMP, ID, IM, IMG, MN, MP, MPD, N, NEP, NM, NS, OPH, ORS, OTO, P, PCC, PS, PTH, PYG, RHU, RO, TS, U, VIR
Institution ID: 36-0473

Fayetteville

Cape Fear Valley Medical Center

PO Box 2000
Fayetteville, NC 28302-2000
Major participating institution for programs in: FP
Institution ID: 36-0731

Southern Regional Health Education Center

1601 Owen Dr
Fayetteville, NC 28304-3482
Programs sponsored in: FP
Institution ID: 36-8020

Fort Bragg

Womack Army Medical Center

Graduate Med Ctr
Womack Army Med Ctr
Fort Bragg, NC 28307-5000
Med Sch Affil: G-02312
Programs sponsored in: FP
Institution ID: 36-0101

Goldsboro

Cherry Hospital

201 Stevens Mill Rd
Goldsboro, NC 27530-1057
Med Sch Affil: L-03608
Major participating institution for programs in: CHP
Institution ID: 36-8001

Greensboro

Moses H Cone Memorial Hospital

1200 N Elm St
Greensboro, NC 27401-1020
Med Sch Affil: M-03601
Programs sponsored in: FP, FSM, IM
Institution ID: 36-0486

Greenville

East Carolina University School of Medicine

Brody Med Sci Bldg/AD48
Greenville, NC 27858-4354
Med Sch Affil: M-03608
Programs sponsored in: AI, CD, CHP, EM, FP, FPG, GE, GS, IM, MP, NPM, OBG, P, PCP, PD, PM, PTH, PUD
Institution ID: 36-9501

Pitt County Memorial Hospital

PO Box 6028
2100 Stantonsburg Rd
Greenville, NC 27835-6028
Med Sch Affil: M-03608
Programs sponsored in: MPD
Major participating institution for programs in: AI, CD, CHP, EM, FP, FPG, GE, GS, IM, MP, NPM, OBG, P, PCP, PD, PM, PTH, PUD
Institution ID: 36-0738

Pitt County Mental Health Center

203 Government Cir
Greenville, NC 27834-7706
Med Sch Affil: L-03608
Major participating institution for programs in: CHP, P
Institution ID: 36-0741

Hendersonville

Margaret R Pardee Memorial Hospital

715 Fleming St
Hendersonville, NC 28739
Major participating institution for programs in: FP
Institution ID: 36-8015

Monroe

Union Regional Medical Center

600 Hospital Dr
Monroe, NC 28111
Major participating institution for programs in: FP
Institution ID: 36-8019

Raleigh

Dorothea Dix Hospital

820 S Boylan Ave
Raleigh, NC 27603-2176
Med Sch Affil: M-03601
Major participating institution for programs in: CHP, P
Institution ID: 36-0377

Wake Medical Center

3000 New Bern Ave
Raleigh, NC 27610
Med Sch Affil: M-03601, L-02312
Major participating institution for programs in: EM, FP, GS, OBG, ORS, OTO, U
Institution ID: 36-0498

Williamston

Martin General Hospital

310 S McCaskey Rd
PO Box 1128
Williamston, NC 27892
Major participating institution for programs in: FP
Institution ID: 36-8014

Wilmington

New Hanover Regional Medical Center

2131 S 17th St
PO Box 9025
Wilmington, NC 28402-9025
Med Sch Affil: M-03601
Programs sponsored in: FP, GS, IM, OBG
Institution ID: 36-0288

Winston-Salem

Forsyth Memorial Hospital

3333 Silas Creek Pkwy
Winston-Salem, NC 27103
Med Sch Affil: M-03605
Major participating institution for programs in: FP, GS, OBG
Institution ID: 36-0242

Wake Forest University Baptist Medical Center

300 S Hawthorne Rd
Winston-Salem, NC 27157-1088
Med Sch Affil: M-03605
Programs sponsored in: AI, AN, APM, CCA, CCM, CCP, CD, CHN, CHP, D, DMP, DR, EM, END, FP, FSM, GE, GS, HO, HSO, ICE, ID, IM, IMG, N, NEP, NM, NPM, NR, NS, OBG, OPH, ORS, OTO, P, PCC, PD, PDR, PS, PTH, RHU, RNR, RO, TS, U, VIR, VS
Institution ID: 36-0480

North Dakota

Bismarck

Medcenter One Inc

300 N 7th St
Bismarck, ND 58501
Med Sch Affil: M-03701
Major participating institution for programs in: FP
Institution ID: 37-0159

St Alexius Medical Center

900 E Broadway
Box 5510
Bismarck, ND 58501-0001
Med Sch Affil: M-03701
Major participating institution for programs in: FP
Institution ID: 37-0108

Fargo

Dakota Hospital
1720 S University Dr
PO Box 6014
Fargo, ND 58108-6014
Med Sch Affil: M-03701
Major participating institution for programs in: FP
Institution ID: 37-0390

MeritCare Hospital
720 N Fourth St
Fargo, ND 58122
Med Sch Affil: M-03701
Major participating institution for programs in: FP, IM, P, TY
Institution ID: 37-0396

Southeast Human Service Center
2624 9th Ave SW
Fargo, ND 58103-2350
Med Sch Affil: G-03701
Major participating institution for programs in: P
Institution ID: 37-8011

Veterans Affairs Medical and Regional Office Center (Fargo)
2101 N Elm St
Fargo, ND 58102
Med Sch Affil: M-03701
Major participating institution for programs in: GS, IM, P, TY
Institution ID: 37-0395

Grand Forks

Altru Health System Hospital
1200 S Columbia Rd
PO Box 6002
Grand Forks, ND 58206-6002
Med Sch Affil: M-03701
Major participating institution for programs in: FP, GS
Institution ID: 37-0403

Univ of North Dakota School of Medicine & Health Sciences
501 N Columbia Rd
Box 9037
Grand Forks, ND 58202-9037
Med Sch Affil: M-03701, L-02312
Programs sponsored in: FP, GS, IM, P, TY
Institution ID: 37-0400

Minot

Trinity Medical Center
PO Box 5020
Minot, ND 58702-5020
Med Sch Affil: M-03701
Major participating institution for programs in: FP
Institution ID: 37-0409

UniMed Medical Center
3rd St SE and Burdick Expwy
Minot, ND 58701
Med Sch Affil: L-03701
Major participating institution for programs in: FP
Institution ID: 37-0408

Ohio

Akron

Akron City Hospital (Summa Health System)
525 E Market St
Akron, OH 44309-2090
Med Sch Affil: M-03844, L-03840
Major participating institution for programs in: EM, FP, GS, IM, OBG, OPH, ORS, PCP, PS, PTH, TY, U
Institution ID: 38-0215

Akron General Medical Center
400 Wabash Ave
Akron, OH 44307
Med Sch Affil: M-03844, L-03840
Programs sponsored in: EM, FP, GS, IM, MPD, OBG, ORS, TY, U
Major participating institution for programs in: P, PS
Institution ID: 38-0124

Children's Hospital Medical Center of Akron
One Perkins Sq
Akron, OH 44308-1062
Med Sch Affil: M-03844
Programs sponsored in: PD, PDR, PP
Major participating institution for programs in: MPD, OPH, ORS, P, PCP, PS, PTH, U
Institution ID: 38-0371

St Thomas Hospital (Summa Health System)
444 N Main St
Akron, OH 44310
Med Sch Affil: M-03844
Major participating institution for programs in: P, TY
Institution ID: 38-0167

Summa Health System
525 E Market St
PO Box 2090
Akron, OH 44309-2090
Programs sponsored in: EM, FP, GS, IM, MPD, OBG, OPH, ORS, PCP, PS, PTH, TY
Institution ID: 38-8066

Barberton

Barberton Citizens Hospital
155 Fifth St NE
Barberton, OH 44203
Med Sch Affil: M-03844
Programs sponsored in: FP
Institution ID: 38-0184

Bellefontaine

Mary Rutan Hospital
205 Palmer Ave
Bellefontaine, OH 43311
Major participating institution for programs in: FP
Institution ID: 38-8069

Canton

Aultman Hospital
2600 6th St SW
Canton, OH 44710
Med Sch Affil: M-03844
Programs sponsored in: DR, FP, OBG, TY
Major participating institution for programs in: IM
Institution ID: 38-0148

Canton Medical Education Foundation
2600 Sixth St SW
Canton, OH 44710
Programs sponsored in: IM
Institution ID: 38-8059

Timken Mercy Medical Center
1320 Mercy Dr NW
Canton, OH 44708-2641
Med Sch Affil: M-03844
Major participating institution for programs in: DR, IM
Institution ID: 38-0426

Cincinnati

Bethesda Hospital Inc
619 Oak St
Cincinnati, OH 45206-1690
Med Sch Affil: L-03841
Programs sponsored in: FP, OBG
Major participating institution for programs in: HSO
Institution ID: 38-0464

Children's Hospital Medical Center
3333 Burnet Ave
Cincinnati, OH 45229-3039
Med Sch Affil: M-03841
Programs sponsored in: ADL, CCP, CHN, MG, NPM, OP, PD, PDC, PDE, PDI, PDO, PDP, PDR, PDS, PG, PHO, PN, PP, PPR, UP
Major participating institution for programs in: AI, AN, APM, CHP, CN, ORS, OTO, PAN, PDR, U
Institution ID: 38-0302

Christ Hospital
2139 Auburn Ave
Cincinnati, OH 45219-2906
Med Sch Affil: M-03841
Programs sponsored in: IM, NM, OSM
Major participating institution for programs in: DR, FPG, NS, OBG, ORS, U, VS
Institution ID: 38-0492

Cincinnati Sportsmedicine and Orthopaedic Center
311 Straight St
Cincinnati, OH 45219
Programs sponsored in: OSM
Institution ID: 38-8058

Drake Center
151 W Galbraith Rd
Cincinnati, OH 45216
Med Sch Affil: L-03841
Major participating institution for programs in: FPG
Institution ID: 38-0368

Franciscan Hospital-Mount Airy Campus
2446 Kipling Ave
Cincinnati, OH 45239-6650
Med Sch Affil: G-03841
Major participating institution for programs in: FP, FPG, GS
Institution ID: 38-0525

Good Samaritan Hospital
375 Dixmyth Ave
Cincinnati, OH 45220-2489
Med Sch Affil: M-03841
Programs sponsored in: GS, IM, OBG, VS
Major participating institution for programs in: NPM, NS
Institution ID: 38-0346

Hamilton County Coroner's Office
3159 Eden Ave
Cincinnati, OH 45219
Programs sponsored in: FOP
Major participating institution for programs in: PP
Institution ID: 38-0541

Hoxworth Blood Center
3130 Highland Ave
PO Box 670055
Cincinnati, OH 45267-0055
Programs sponsored in: BBK
Institution ID: 38-0763

Jewish Hospital of Cincinnati
4777 E Galbraith Rd
Cincinnati, OH 45236
Med Sch Affil: L-03841
Programs sponsored in: GS, IM
Institution ID: 38-0428

University Hospital Inc
234 Goodman St
Cincinnati, OH 45267-0700
Med Sch Affil: M-03841, L-02012
Programs sponsored in: ADP, AI, AN, APM, CCS, CD, CHP, CN, CPP, D, DR, EM, END, FP, FPG, FPP, GE, GPM, GS, HMP, HO, HSO, ID, IM, MPD, MPM, N, NEP, NP, NS, OBG, OPH, ORS, OTO, P, PAN, PCC, PCP, PM, PMP, PS, PTH, PYG, RNR, RO, U, VS
Major participating institution for programs in: CHN, NPM, UP
Institution ID: 38-0405

University of Cincinnati College of Medicine
231 Bethesda Ave
Mail Location 182
Cincinnati, OH 45267-0553
Med Sch Affil: M-03841
Major participating institution for programs in: OSM, PP
Institution ID: 38-0521

Veterans Affairs Medical Center (Cincinnati)
3200 Vine St
Cincinnati, OH 45220-2213
Med Sch Affil: M-03841
Major participating institution for programs in: ADP, AI, CD, CN, DR, END, GE, GS, HO, ID, IM, N, NEP, OPH, ORS, OTO, P, PCC, PTH, RO, U
Institution ID: 38-0329

Cleveland

American Red Cross Northern Ohio Region
3747 Euclid Ave
Cleveland, OH 44115-2501
Programs sponsored in: BBK
Institution ID: 38-8064

Cleveland Clinic Foundation
9500 Euclid Ave/TT32
Cleveland, OH 44195-5242
Med Sch Affil: M-04114, M-03840, L-02312, L-03806
Programs sponsored in: AI, AN, APM, CCA, CCP, CD, CHN, CHP, CN, CRS, D, DMP, DR, END, GE, GS, HMP, HO, HSO, ICE, ID, IM, IMG, MM, MPD, MSR, N, NEP, NR, NRN, NS, OPH, ORS, OSM, OTO, P, PCC, PD, PDR, PG, PN, PS, PTH, RHU, RNR, RO, TS, U, VIR, VS
Major participating institution for programs in: BBK, EM, FSM, GS, OBG, PDI
Institution ID: 38-0393

Cleveland Psychiatric Institute
1708 Aiken Ave
Cleveland, OH 44109
Major participating institution for programs in: P
Institution ID: 38-0391

Cleveland Psychoanalytic Institute
11328 Euclid Ave
Cleveland, OH 44106
Major participating institution for programs in: P
Institution ID: 38-8057

Cuyahoga County Coroner's Office
2121 Adelbert Rd
Cleveland, OH 44106-2624
Programs sponsored in: FOP
Institution ID: 38-0198

Fairview Health System
18101 Lorain Ave
Cleveland, OH 44111-5656
Programs sponsored in: FP, FSM, GS, IM
Institution ID: 38-8021

Fairview Health System (Fairview General Hospital)
18101 Lorain Ave
Cleveland, OH 44111-5656
Med Sch Affil: L-03806
Major participating institution for programs in: FP, GS, IM
Institution ID: 38-0209

Meridia Huron Hospital
13951 Terrace Rd
Cleveland, OH 44112-4399
Med Sch Affil: L-03806
Programs sponsored in: AN, GS, IM
Institution ID: 38-0170

MetroHealth Medical Center
2500 MetroHealth Dr
Cleveland, OH 44109-1998
Med Sch Affil: M-03806
Programs sponsored in: AN, CD, DR, EM, FP, FPG, GE, IFP, IM, MPD, MPM, NPM, OBG, P, PCC, PCP, PD, PM, PMP, PTH
Major participating institution for programs in: CCP, CCS, D, GS, HSO, ID, MG, N, NEP, NS, OMO, OPH, ORS, OTO, PCC, PS, TS, U, VS
Institution ID: 38-0173

Mount Sinai Medical Center of Cleveland
Office of Medical Affairs
One Mt Sinai Dr
Cleveland, OH 44106-4198
Med Sch Affil: M-03806
Programs sponsored in: DR, EM, IM, OBG, ORS, TY
Major participating institution for programs in: CD, FP, GS, OPH, PS, U
Institution ID: 38-0169

St Luke's Medical Center
11311 Shaker Blvd
Cleveland, OH 44104-9989
Med Sch Affil: M-03806
Programs sponsored in: IM, OPH, ORS
Institution ID: 38-0370

St Vincent Charity Hospital and Health Center
2351 E 22nd St
Cleveland, OH 44115
Med Sch Affil: L-03806
Major participating institution for programs in: OPH, PS
Institution ID: 38-0411

University Hospitals of Cleveland
11100 Euclid Ave
Cleveland, OH 44106-2602
Med Sch Affil: M-03806
Programs sponsored in: AN, APM, CCA, CCP, CCS, CD, CHP, CN, D, DR, END, FP, FPP, GE, GS, HMP, HO, ICE, ID, IM, IMG, MG, MPD, N, NEP, NP, NPM, NS, OBG, OMO, OPH, ORS, OTO, P, PAN, PCC, PCP, PD, PDC, PDE, PDI, PDP, PDR, PFP, PG, PHO, PMG, PN, PS, PTH, PYG, RHU, RNR, RO, TS, U, VIR, VS
Major participating institution for programs in: BBK, HSO, ORS
Institution ID: 38-0373

Veterans Affairs Medical Center (Cleveland)
10701 East Blvd
Cleveland, OH 44106
Med Sch Affil: M-03806
Major participating institution for programs in: AN, CD, CN, D, END, GE, GS, HO, ICE, ID, IM, IMG, N, NEP, NS, OMO, OPH, ORS, OTO, P, PCC, PS, RHU, RNR, TS, U
Institution ID: 38-0390

Columbus

American Red Cross Central Ohio Region
995 E Broad St
Columbus, OH 43205
Major participating institution for programs in: BBK
Institution ID: 38-8063

Arthur G James Cancer Hospital and Research Institute
300 W 10th Ave
Columbus, OH 43210
Med Sch Affil: M-03840
Major participating institution for programs in: CCA, GS, HO, OBG
Institution ID: 38-8020

Children's Hospital
700 Children's Dr
Columbus, OH 43205-2596
Med Sch Affil: M-03840
Programs sponsored in: CCP, NPM, PD, PDC, PDE, PDP, PDS, PHO, PMP, PP
Major participating institution for programs in: HSO, MPD, NS, ORS, OTO, PS, TS, U
Institution ID: 38-0491

Grant Medical Center (OhioHealth)
111 S Grant Ave
Columbus, OH 43215
Med Sch Affil: M-03840
Programs sponsored in: CRS, FP
Major participating institution for programs in: OBG, PM
Institution ID: 38-0317

Mount Carmel East Hospital
6001 Broad St
Columbus, OH 43213
Major participating institution for programs in: GS
Institution ID: 38-0761

Mount Carmel Medical Center
793 W State St
Columbus, OH 43222-1560
Med Sch Affil: M-03840
Programs sponsored in: FP, GS, IM, ORS, TY
Major participating institution for programs in: PM, PS
Institution ID: 38-0245

Ohio State University College of Medicine
370 W 9th Ave
Columbus, OH 43210-1228
Med Sch Affil: M-03840
Major participating institution for programs in: GPM
Institution ID: 38-0176

Ohio State University Medical Center
410 W 10th Ave
Columbus, OH 43210
Med Sch Affil: M-03840
Programs sponsored in: APM, BBK, CCA, CCS, CD, CHP, D, DMP, DR, EM, END, FP, FSM, GE, GPM, GS, HMP, HO, HSO, ID, IM, MPD, N, NEP, NO, NP, NS, OBG, OPH, ORS, OSM, OTO, P, PCC, PCP, PM, PS, PTH, RHU, RNR, RO, TS, U, VS
Institution ID: 38-0123

Park Medical Center
1492 E Broad St
Columbus, OH 43205
Major participating institution for programs in: FP
Institution ID: 38-0584

Riverside Methodist Hospitals (OhioHealth)
Medical Education Dept
3535 Olentangy River Rd
Columbus, OH 43214
Med Sch Affil: M-03840
Programs sponsored in: FP, GS, IM, OBG, TY
Major participating institution for programs in: HSO, NS, ORS, PM, PS, U
Institution ID: 38-0383

Dayton

Children's Medical Center
One Children's Plaza
Dayton, OH 45404-1815
Med Sch Affil: M-03845
Programs sponsored in: MPD
Major participating institution for programs in: CHP, D, GS, ORS, PD, TY
Institution ID: 38-0536

Franciscan Medical Center-Dayton Campus
One Franciscan Way
Dayton, OH 45408
Med Sch Affil: M-03845
Programs sponsored in: FP, FSM
Major participating institution for programs in: CHP, D, GS, PS
Institution ID: 38-0303

Good Samaritan Hospital and Health Center
2222 Philadelphia Dr
Dayton, OH 45406-1891
Med Sch Affil: M-03845, L-03840
Programs sponsored in: FP
Major participating institution for programs in: CD, CHP, EM, GS, HO, ID, IM, MPD, P
Institution ID: 38-0315

Miami Valley Hospital
1 Wyoming St
Dayton, OH 45409-2793
Med Sch Affil: M-03845
Programs sponsored in: FP
Major participating institution for programs in: GS, ID, IM, MPD, OBG, ORS, TY
Institution ID: 38-0431

Office of the Montgomery County Coroner
361 W Third St
Dayton, OH 45402
Programs sponsored in: FOP
Institution ID: 38-8060

Veterans Affairs Medical Center (Dayton)
4100 W 3rd St
Dayton, OH 45428
Med Sch Affil: M-03845, L-03840
Major participating institution for programs in: CD, D, GE, GS, HO, ID, IM, MPD, ORS, P
Institution ID: 38-0453

Wright State University School of Medicine
PO Box 927
Dayton, OH 45401-0927
Med Sch Affil: M-03845
Programs sponsored in: CD, CHP, D, EM, GE, GPM, GS, HO, ID, IM, OBG, ORS, P, PD
Institution ID: 38-0756

Dayton (Kettering)

Kettering Medical Center
3535 Southern Blvd
Dayton (Kettering), OH 45429-1298
Med Sch Affil: M-03845
Programs sponsored in: IM, PS, TY
Major participating institution for programs in: EM, GS, P
Institution ID: 38-0515

Mayfield Heights

Meridia Hillcrest Hospital
6780 Mayfield Rd
Mayfield Heights, OH 44124-2202
Major participating institution for programs in: GS, IM
Institution ID: 38-0483

Middletown

Middletown Regional Hospital
105 McKnight Dr
Middletown, OH 45044-4
Major participating institution for programs in: PS
Institution ID: 38-8068

Rootstown

Northeastern Ohio Universities College of Medicine
PO Box 95
Rootstown, OH 44272-0095
Med Sch Affil: M-03844
Programs sponsored in: P
Institution ID: 38-0755

Sylvania

Flower Hospital
5200 Harroun Rd
Sylvania, OH 43560
Med Sch Affil: L-03843
Programs sponsored in: FP
Major participating institution for programs in: AN, APM, PM
Institution ID: 38-0362

Toledo

Medical College of Ohio
3065 Arlington Ave
Toledo, OH 43614-5807
Programs sponsored in: AN, APM, CD, CHP, DR, FP, GS, ID, IM, N, NEP, OBG, ORS, OTR, P, PD, PM, PS, PTH, PUD, U
Institution ID: 38-9501

Medical College of Ohio Hospital
PO Box 10008
Toledo, OH 43699-0008
Med Sch Affil: M-03843
Programs sponsored in: MPD, PMP
Major participating institution for programs in: AN, APM, CD, FP, IM, N, PTH
Institution ID: 38-0533

Northwest Psychiatric Hospital
930 S Detroit Ave
Toledo, OH 43614-2701
Med Sch Affil: M-03843
Major participating institution for programs in: P
Institution ID: 38-0531

St Vincent Mercy Medical Center
2213 Cherry St
Toledo, OH 43608-2691
Med Sch Affil: M-03843
Programs sponsored in: EM, FP, TY
Major participating institution for programs in: DR, FP, GS, IM, MPD, OBG, ORS, OTR, P, PM, PMP, PS, PTH, U
Institution ID: 38-0180

Toledo Hospital
2121 Hughes Dr
Toledo, OH 43606
Med Sch Affil: M-03843
Programs sponsored in: FP, FSM
Major participating institution for programs in: AN, EM, FP, GS, IM, MPD, N, OBG, ORS, PD, PM, PMP, U
Institution ID: 38-0218

Westerville

St Ann's Hospital of Columbus
500 S Cleveland Ave
Westerville, OH 43081-8998
Med Sch Affil: L-03840
Major participating institution for programs in: OBG
Institution ID: 38-0321

Wilmington

Clinton Memorial Hospital
610 W Main St
Wilmington, OH 45177-2194
Programs sponsored in: FP
Institution ID: 38-8067

Worthington

Harding Hospital
445 E Granville Rd
Worthington, OH 43085-3195
Med Sch Affil: M-03840
Major participating institution for programs in: P
Institution ID: 38-0111

Wright-Patterson AFB

Wright-Patterson Medical Center

4881 Sugar Maple Dr
Wright-Patterson AFB, OH 45433-5529
Med Sch Affil: M-02312, M-03845
Programs sponsored in: IM
Major participating institution for programs in: D, EM, GE, GS, MPD, OBG, P, PD
Institution ID: 38-0336

Youngstown

Forum Health-Northside Medical Center

500 Gypsy Ln
Youngstown, OH 44501
Med Sch Affil: M-03844
Major participating institution for programs in: DR, FP, GS, IM, MPD, PTH
Institution ID: 38-8056

Forum Health-Tod Children's Hospital

500 Gypsy Ln
Youngstown, OH 44501
Med Sch Affil: M-03844
Major participating institution for programs in: GS, MPD, PD
Institution ID: 38-0754

Southside Medical Center

345 Oak Hill Ave
PO Box 990
Youngstown, OH 44501-0990
Major participating institution for programs in: FP, MPD
Institution ID: 38-0339

St Elizabeth Health Center

1044 Belmont Ave
PO Box 1790
Youngstown, OH 44501-1790
Med Sch Affil: M-03844
Programs sponsored in: DR, FP, GS, IM, OBG
Institution ID: 38-0145

Western Reserve Care System

345 Oak Hill Ave
Youngstown, OH 44501
Programs sponsored in: FP, GS, IM, MPD, PD, PTH
Institution ID: 38-8061

Oklahoma

Enid

Bass Memorial Baptist Hospital

600 S Monroe
PO Box 3168
Enid, OK 73702-3168
Med Sch Affil: G-03901
Programs sponsored in: FP
Institution ID: 39-0488

St Mary's Mercy Hospital

305 S Fifth St
PO Box 232
Enid, OK 73702
Med Sch Affil: G-03901
Major participating institution for programs in: FP
Institution ID: 39-0489

Muskogee

Veterans Affairs Medical Center (Muskogee)

1011 Honor Heights Dr
Muskogee, OK 74401
Med Sch Affil: L-03901
Major participating institution for programs in: GS, IM, MPD
Institution ID: 39-7021

Norman

Griffin Memorial Hospital

900 E Main St
PO Box 151
Norman, OK 73070-0151
Med Sch Affil: G-03901
Programs sponsored in: P
Institution ID: 39-0286

Oklahoma City

Bone and Joint Hospital

1111 N Dewey Ave
Oklahoma City, OK 73103-2615
Med Sch Affil: G-03901
Major participating institution for programs in: ORS
Institution ID: 39-0294

Children's Hospital of Oklahoma

PO Box 26307
940 NE 13th St
Oklahoma City, OK 73126
Med Sch Affil: M-03901
Major participating institution for programs in: AN, APM, BBK, CHN, CHP, D, DMP, DR, EM, GS, MPD, NM, NPM, NS, OPH, ORS, OTO, P, PD, PDS, PS, PTH, TS, U, VIR
Institution ID: 39-0130

Columbia Presbyterian Hospital

700 NE 13th St
Oklahoma City, OK 73104-5070
Med Sch Affil: G-03901
Major participating institution for programs in: EM, FSM, HSO, N, NS, OSM
Institution ID: 39-0312

Great Plains Medical Foundation

3300 NW 56th St
Oklahoma City, OK 73112
Programs sponsored in: FP
Institution ID: 39-8020

Integris Baptist Medical Center

3300 Northwest Expwy
Oklahoma City, OK 73112
Med Sch Affil: G-03901
Programs sponsored in: DR, HSO
Major participating institution for programs in: EM, FP, OTO, PTH
Institution ID: 39-0475

McGee Eye Institute

608 Stanton L Young Blvd
Oklahoma City, OK 73104
Major participating institution for programs in: OPH
Institution ID: 39-8019

Office of the Chief Medical Examiner-State of Oklahoma

901 N Stonewall
Oklahoma City, OK 73117-1111
Programs sponsored in: FOP
Institution ID: 39-0485

St Anthony Hospital

1000 N Lee
PO Box 205
Oklahoma City, OK 73101-0205
Med Sch Affil: G-03901
Programs sponsored in: FP
Major participating institution for programs in: EM, NP
Institution ID: 39-0115

University Hospital

PO Box 26307
940 NE 13th St
Oklahoma City, OK 73126
Med Sch Affil: M-03901
Programs sponsored in: MPD
Major participating institution for programs in: AN, BBK, CD, CHN, D, DMP, DR, EM, END, FP, FSM, GE, GPM, GS, HO, ICE, ID, IM, IMG, N, NEP, NM, NP, NS, OBG, OPH, ORS, OTO, P, PCC, PS, PTH, RHU, TS, U, VIR
Institution ID: 39-0121

University of Oklahoma College of Medicine

BMSB Rm 357
PO Box 26901
Oklahoma City, OK 73190
Med Sch Affil: M-03901
Programs sponsored in: AN, APM, BBK, CD, CHN, CHP, D, DMP, DR, EM, END, FP, FSM, GE, GPM, GS, HO, ICE, ID, IM, IMG, N, NEP, NM, NP, NPM, NS, OBG, OPH, ORS, OSM, OTO, P, PCC, PD, PDS, PS, PTH, RHU, TS, U, VIR
Institution ID: 39-0477

Veterans Affairs Medical Center (Oklahoma City)

921 NE 13th St
Oklahoma City, OK 73104
Med Sch Affil: M-03901
Major participating institution for programs in: AN, APM, BBK, CD, CHN, D, DMP, DR, END, GE, GS, HO, ICE, ID, IM, IMG, N, NEP, NM, NP, NS, OPH, ORS, OTO, P, PCC, PS, PTH, RHU, TS, U, VIR
Institution ID: 39-0471

Tulsa

Children's Medical Center

5300 E Skelly Dr
PO Box 35648
Tulsa, OK 74145
Med Sch Affil: G-03901
Major participating institution for programs in: P
Institution ID: 39-0181

Hillcrest Medical Center

1120 S Utica Ave
Tulsa, OK 74104
Med Sch Affil: M-03901
Major participating institution for programs in: FP, GS, IM, MPD, OBG
Institution ID: 39-0117

In His Image Inc

7306 S Lewis Ave/Ste 100
Tulsa, OK 74136
Programs sponsored in: FP
Institution ID: 39-8016

Laureate Psychiatric Clinic and Hospital

6655 S Yale
Tulsa, OK 74136
Med Sch Affil: G-03901
Major participating institution for programs in: P
Institution ID: 39-8015

Parkside Inc

1620 E 12th St
Tulsa, OK 74120
Med Sch Affil: G-03901
Major participating institution for programs in: P
Institution ID: 39-0499

St Francis Hospital

6161 S Yale Ave
Tulsa, OK 74136-1992
Med Sch Affil: M-03901
Major participating institution for programs in: FP, FSM, GS, IM, MPD, OBG, PD
Institution ID: 39-0479

St John Medical Center

1923 S Utica Ave
Tulsa, OK 74104
Med Sch Affil: M-03901
Major participating institution for programs in: FP, IM, MPD, OBG
Institution ID: 39-0447

University of Oklahoma College of Medicine-Tulsa

2808 S Sheridan Rd
Tulsa, OK 74129-1077
Med Sch Affil: M-03901
Programs sponsored in: FP, FPP, FSM, GS, IM, MPD, OBG, P, PD
Institution ID: 39-9501

WorkMed Occupational Health Network (Tulsa)

PO Box 14210
Tulsa, OK 74159-1210
Major participating institution for programs in: GPM
Institution ID: 39-8018

Oregon

Bend

St Charles Medical Center

2500 NE Neff Rd
Bend, OR 97701
Major participating institution for programs in: FP
Institution ID: 40-8005

Klamath Falls

Merle West Medical Center

2865 Daggett Ave
Klamath Falls, OR 97601
Major participating institution for programs in: FP
Institution ID: 40-8004

Portland

Kaiser Foundation Hospitals-Northwest Region

500 NE Multnomah St
Portland, OR 97232-2099
Med Sch Affil: G-04002
Major participating institution for programs in: GS, PTH, U
Institution ID: 40-0707

Legacy Emanuel Hospital and Health Center

2801 N Gantenbein Ave
Portland, OR 97227
Med Sch Affil: M-04002
Programs sponsored in: IM, TY
Major participating institution for programs in: OBG, ORS
Institution ID: 40-0229

Legacy Good Samaritan Hospital and Medical Center

1015 NW 22nd Ave
Portland, OR 97210-3090
Med Sch Affil: M-04002
Major participating institution for programs in: GS, IM, OBG, OPH, TY
Institution ID: 40-0102

Oregon Health Sciences University Hospital

3181 SW Sam Jackson Park Rd/L579
Portland, OR 97201-3098
Med Sch Affil: M-04002
Programs sponsored in: AN, APM, CCS, CD, CHP, D, DR, EM, END, FP, GE, GPM, GS, HO, HSP, ICE, IM, IMG, MG, N, NEP, NM, NPM, NS, OBG, OPH, ORS, OTO, P, PCC, PD, PDC, PDE, PDP, PHO, PS, PTH, PYG, RHU, RNR, RO, TS, U, VS
Institution ID: 40-0109

Providence Medical Center

4805 NE Glisan St
Portland, OR 97213-2967
Med Sch Affil: G-04002
Programs sponsored in: IM
Institution ID: 40-0398

Shriners Hospitals for Children (Portland)

3101 SW Sam Jackson Park Rd
Portland, OR 97201-4698
Med Sch Affil: L-04002
Programs sponsored in: OP
Major participating institution for programs in: HSP, MG, ORS
Institution ID: 40-0325

St Vincent Hospital and Medical Center

9205 SW Barnes Rd
Portland, OR 97225-6661
Med Sch Affil: M-04002
Programs sponsored in: IM, PTH
Major participating institution for programs in: GS
Institution ID: 40-0133

Veterans Affairs Medical Center (Portland)

3710 SW US Veterans Hospital Rd
PO Box 1034
Portland, OR 97207
Med Sch Affil: M-04002
Major participating institution for programs in: APM, CCS, CD, D, DR, END, GE, GS, HO, HSP, ICE, IM, IMG, N, NEP, NM, NS, OPH, ORS, OTO, P, PCC, PS, PTH, PYG, RHU, RNR, TS, U
Institution ID: 40-0171

Salem

Oregon State Hospital

2600 Center St NE
Salem, OR 97310
Med Sch Affil: L-04002
Major participating institution for programs in: PYG
Institution ID: 40-0143

Pennsylvania

Abington

Abington Memorial Hospital

1200 Old York Rd
Abington, PA 19001-3788
Med Sch Affil: M-04113, G-04101
Programs sponsored in: FP, GS, IM, OBG
Major participating institution for programs in: NS, ORS, PS, U
Institution ID: 41-0455

Allentown

Lehigh Valley Hospital

Cedar Crest and I-78
PO Box 689
Allentown, PA 18105-1556
Med Sch Affil: M-04114, L-04113, L-04115
Programs sponsored in: CCS, CRS, FP, GS, IM, OBG, PS, TY
Major participating institution for programs in: OTO, U
Institution ID: 41-0724

Sacred Heart Hospital

421 W Chew St
Allentown, PA 18102-3490
Med Sch Affil: M-04113
Programs sponsored in: FP
Institution ID: 41-0179

Altoona

Altoona Hospital

620 Howard Ave
Altoona, PA 16601-4899
Programs sponsored in: FP
Institution ID: 41-0220

Bala Cynwyd

Mercy Catholic Medical Center Inc

One Bala Plaza/Ste 402
Bala Cynwyd, PA 19004-1401
Programs sponsored in: DR, GS, IM, TY
Institution ID: 41-8029

Beaver

The Medical Center (Beaver PA)

1000 Dutch Ridge Rd
Beaver, PA 15009
Med Sch Affil: L-04114
Programs sponsored in: FP
Institution ID: 41-0747

Bethlehem

St Luke's Hospital

801 Ostrum St
Bethlehem, PA 18015-9982
Med Sch Affil: M-04113
Programs sponsored in: EM, FP, GS, IM, OBG, TY
Institution ID: 41-0234

Bryn Mawr

Bryn Mawr Hospital

130 S Bryn Mawr Ave
Bryn Mawr, PA 19010-3160
Med Sch Affil: M-04102, G-04101
Programs sponsored in: DR, FP
Major participating institution for programs in: GS, ORS, PS, U
Institution ID: 41-0274

Danville

Geisinger Medical Center

100 N Academy Ave
Danville, PA 17822-2201
Med Sch Affil: M-04114, M-04102, L-04115
Major participating institution for programs in: CD, D, DR, EM, FP, GE, GS, IM, OBG, OPH, ORS, OTO, PCP, PD, PTH, RHU, U, VS
Institution ID: 41-0240

Penn State Geisinger Health System

100 N Academy Ave
Danville, PA 17822-2201
Programs sponsored in: AN, APM, CCA, CCM, CCS, CD, CHP, CN, D, DR, EM, END, FP, GE, GS, HO, ICE, ID, IM, MPD, N, NEP, NPM, NS, OBG, OPH, ORS, OSM, OTO, P, PCP, PD, PS, PTH, PUD, PYG, RHU, RNR, TS, U, VIR, VS
Institution ID: 41-8036

Darby

Mercy Fitzgerald Hospital

1500 S Lansdowne Ave
Darby, PA 19023
Med Sch Affil: G-04101
Major participating institution for programs in: DR, GS, HSO, IM, TY
Institution ID: 41-0414

Easton

Easton Hospital

250 S 21st St
Easton, PA 18042-3892
Med Sch Affil: M-04115, G-04101
Programs sponsored in: GS, IM, TY
Institution ID: 41-0420

Elkins Park

Elkins Park Hospital

60 E Township Line Rd
Elkins Park, PA 19027-2249
Med Sch Affil: M-04115
Major participating institution for programs in: OPH
Institution ID: 41-0726

Erie

Hamot Medical Center

201 State St
Erie, PA 16550-0001
Med Sch Affil: M-04115
Programs sponsored in: FP, ORS, TY
Institution ID: 41-0452

Shriners Hospital for Children (Erie)

1645 W 8th St
Erie, PA 16505
Major participating institution for programs in: ORS
Institution ID: 41-0526

St Vincent Health Center

232 W 25th St
Erie, PA 16544
Med Sch Affil: L-04114
Programs sponsored in: CRS, FP
Institution ID: 41-0191

Harrisburg

PinnacleHealth System-Harrisburg Hospital

111 S Front St
Harrisburg, PA 17101-2099
Med Sch Affil: M-04115
Programs sponsored in: FP
Major participating institution for programs in: IM, PS
Institution ID: 41-0356

PinnacleHealth System-Polyclinic Hospital

2601 N Third St
Harrisburg, PA 17110
Med Sch Affil: M-04115
Programs sponsored in: FP, GS, IM
Major participating institution for programs in: PS
Institution ID: 41-0463

Hershey

Milton S Hershey Medical Center

500 University Dr/Rm C-1708
PO Box 850
Hershey, PA 17033
Med Sch Affil: M-04114
Major participating institution for programs in: AN, APM, CCA, CCM, CCS, CD, CHP, CN, D, DR, END, FP, GE, GS, HO, ICE, ID, IM, N, NEP, NPM, NS, OBG, OPH, ORS, OSM, OTO, P, PD, PS, PTH, PUD, PYG, RNR, TS, U, VIR, VS
Institution ID: 41-0528

Johnstown

Conemaugh Valley Memorial Hospital

1086 Franklin St
Johnstown, PA 15905-4398
Med Sch Affil: M-04113
Programs sponsored in: FP, GS, IM, PTH, TY
Institution ID: 41-0236

Kingston

WVHCS-Hospital

562 Wyoming Ave
Kingston, PA 18704
Med Sch Affil: L-04115
Major participating institution for programs in: FP
Institution ID: 41-0301

Lancaster

Lancaster General Hospital

555 N Duke St
PO Box 3555
Lancaster, PA 17603
Med Sch Affil: M-04113, L-04114
Programs sponsored in: FP
Major participating institution for programs in: U
Institution ID: 41-0107

Latrobe

Latrobe Area Hospital

121 W Second Ave
Latrobe, PA 15650-1096
Med Sch Affil: M-04102
Programs sponsored in: FP
Institution ID: 41-0715

Lebanon

Good Samaritan Hospital

4th and Walnut Sts
PO Box 1281
Lebanon, PA 17042-1281
Med Sch Affil: G-04114
Major participating institution for programs in: FP
Institution ID: 41-0130

Veterans Affairs Medical Center (Lebanon)

1700 S Lincoln Ave
Lebanon, PA 17042-7597
Med Sch Affil: M-04114
Major participating institution for programs in: GE, OPH
Institution ID: 41-7070

McKeesport

McKeesport Hospital/UPMC

1500 Fifth Ave
McKeesport, PA 15132-2483
Med Sch Affil: M-04113
Programs sponsored in: FP, IM
Institution ID: 41-0497

Meadville

Meadville Medical Center

751 Liberty Ave
Meadville, PA 16335
Programs sponsored in: FP
Institution ID: 41-8037

Monroeville (Pittsburgh)

Allegheny University Hospitals-Forbes Regional

2570 Haymaker Rd
Monroeville (Pittsburgh), PA 15146
Med Sch Affil: L-04115
Programs sponsored in: FP
Major participating institution for programs in: DR
Institution ID: 41-0524

Norristown

Montgomery Hospital

1301 Powell St
Norristown, PA 19401-0992
Med Sch Affil: M-04113
Programs sponsored in: FP
Institution ID: 41-0495

Philadelphia

Albert Einstein Medical Center

5501 Old York Rd
Philadelphia, PA 19141-3098
Med Sch Affil: M-04113
Programs sponsored in: CD, DR, EM, GE, GS, IM, IMG, MP, MPD, MPM, NEP, NPM, OBG, ORS, P, PD, PUD, PYG, RHU, TY
Major participating institution for programs in: MPM, N, P, PCC, PM
Institution ID: 41-0450

American Red Cross Blood Services-Penn-Jersey Region

700 Spring Garden St
Philadelphia, PA 19123-3594
Major participating institution for programs in: BBK
Institution ID: 41-8003

Belmont Center for Comprehensive Treatment
4200 Monument Ave
Philadelphia, PA 19131
Med Sch Affil: L-04113
Major participating institution for programs in: P, PYG
Institution ID: 41-0283

Chestnut Hill Hospital
8835 Germantown Ave
Philadelphia, PA 19118-2767
Med Sch Affil: M-04101
Programs sponsored in: FP, TY
Major participating institution for programs in: OBG
Institution ID: 41-0358

Children's Hospital of Philadelphia
One Children's Ctr
34th St and Civic Center Blvd
Philadelphia, PA 19104
Med Sch Affil: M-04101, L-04115, G-04102
Programs sponsored in: ADL, AI, CCP, CHN, MG, NPM, OP, PD, PDC, PDE, PDI, PDP, PDR, PDS, PG, PHO, PN, PP
Major participating institution for programs in: AN, APM, CCA, CN, D, DR, HSO, N, NM, NS, ORS, OTO, PS, RNR, TS, U, UP
Institution ID: 41-0189

Children's Seashore House
3405 Civic Center Blvd
Philadelphia, PA 19104
Med Sch Affil: G-04101
Major participating institution for programs in: OP, PM
Institution ID: 41-8025

Episcopal Hospital (TUHS)
100 E Lehigh Ave
Philadelphia, PA 19125-1098
Med Sch Affil: M-04102
Programs sponsored in: CD, GS, IM
Major participating institution for programs in: GE
Institution ID: 41-0424

Fox Chase Cancer Center
7701 Burholme Ave
Philadelphia, PA 19111-2497
Med Sch Affil: M-04113, L-04115
Programs sponsored in: RO
Major participating institution for programs in: CCA, GS, HO, IM, SP, TS
Institution ID: 41-0529

Frankford Hospital (Frankford Campus)
Red Lion and Knights Rds
Philadelphia, PA 19114
Med Sch Affil: G-04113
Major participating institution for programs in: TY
Institution ID: 41-8004

Frankford Hospital (Torresdale Campus)
Red Lion and Knights Rds
Philadelphia, PA 19114
Med Sch Affil: G-04101
Major participating institution for programs in: OBG, OPH, TY
Institution ID: 41-0166

Friends Hospital
4641 Roosevelt Blvd
Philadelphia, PA 19124-2399
Major participating institution for programs in: P, PYG
Institution ID: 41-7107

Graduate Hospital
One Graduate Plaza
1800 Lombard St
Philadelphia, PA 19146-1497
Med Sch Affil: M-04113, M-04101, M-04115
Programs sponsored in: CD, GE, GS, IM, OSM, PM, PUD
Major participating institution for programs in: CN, D, N, NM, PTH
Institution ID: 41-0144

Hahnemann University Hospital
3300 Henry Ave
Philadelphia, PA 19129
Med Sch Affil: M-04115, G-04113
Programs sponsored in: MPM
Major participating institution for programs in: AN, CCS, CD, CHP, CN, D, DMP, DR, EM, FOP, GS, HO, ICE, ID, IM, MG, MPD, N, NM, NS, OBG, OPH, ORS, OTO, P, PCC, PCP, PTH, RHU, RNR, RO, TS, VS
Institution ID: 41-0484

Hospital of the University of Pennsylvania
3400 Spruce St
Philadelphia, PA 19104-4283
Med Sch Affil: M-04101
Programs sponsored in: ADP, AI, AN, APM, BBK, CCA, CCS, CD, CN, D, DMP, DR, EM, END, FP, GE, GS, HMP, HO, HSO, ICE, ID, IM, IMG, N, NEP, NM, NP, NPR, NR, NS, OAR, OBG, OPH, ORS, OTO, P, PCC, PCP, PM, PS, PTH, PYG, RHU, RNR, RO, TS, U, UP, VIR, VS
Major participating institution for programs in: ADL, AI, CHN, GS, MG, NPM
Institution ID: 41-0106

Magee Rehabilitation Hospital
6 Franklin Plaza
Philadelphia, PA 19102
Major participating institution for programs in: PM, SCI
Institution ID: 41-0508

MCP Hahnemann University
2900 Queen Ln
Philadelphia, PA 19129
Programs sponsored in: AN, CCS, CD, CHP, CN, D, DMP, DR, EM, END, FOP, FP, GE, GS, HO, ICE, ID, IM, IMG, N, NEP, NM, NS, OBG, OPH, ORS, P, PCC, PCP, PTH, RHU, RNR, RO, TS, VS
Institution ID: 41-9503

Medical College of Pennsylvania Hospital
3300 Henry Ave
Philadelphia, PA 19129
Med Sch Affil: M-04115
Major participating institution for programs in: CCS, CD, CHP, CN, DR, EM, END, FOP, FP, GE, GS, HO, ICE, ID, IM, IMG, MPD, N, NEP, NS, OBG, ORS, P, PCC, PCP, PTH, RHU
Institution ID: 41-0736

Mercy Hospital of Philadelphia
5301 Cedar Ave
Philadelphia, PA 19143
Med Sch Affil: G-04115
Major participating institution for programs in: DR, EM, GS, IM
Institution ID: 41-0499

Methodist Hospital
2301 S Broad St
Philadelphia, PA 19148
Med Sch Affil: M-04102
Major participating institution for programs in: EM, OBG, ORS
Institution ID: 41-0306

Moss Rehabilitation Hospital
1200 W Tabor Rd
Philadelphia, PA 19141
Med Sch Affil: G-04113
Major participating institution for programs in: ORS, PM, RHU
Institution ID: 41-0515

Office of the Medical Examiner
321 University Ave
Philadelphia, PA 19104
Med Sch Affil: G-04115
Major participating institution for programs in: FOP
Institution ID: 41-0136

Pennsylvania Hospital (UPHS)
800 Spruce St
Philadelphia, PA 19107
Med Sch Affil: M-04101
Programs sponsored in: DR, GS, IM, OBG, P, PTH, VS
Major participating institution for programs in: D, FSM, ID, NS, OAR, ORS, OSM, OTO, U
Institution ID: 41-0235

Philadelphia Child Guidance Center
34th St and Civic Center Blvd
Philadelphia, PA 19104-4322
Med Sch Affil: G-04101
Programs sponsored in: CHP
Major participating institution for programs in: P
Institution ID: 41-0127

Presbyterian Medical Center (UPHS)
51 N 39th St
Philadelphia, PA 19104
Med Sch Affil: M-04101
Programs sponsored in: IM, TY
Major participating institution for programs in: FP, GE, OPH
Institution ID: 41-0323

Scheie Eye Institute
51 N 39th St
Philadelphia, PA 19104
Med Sch Affil: M-04101
Major participating institution for programs in: OPH
Institution ID: 41-0532

Shriners Hospital for Children (Philadelphia)
8400 Roosevelt Blvd
Philadelphia, PA 19152-9999
Med Sch Affil: G-04115, G-04113
Major participating institution for programs in: MSR, ORS
Institution ID: 41-0110

St Agnes Medical Center
1900 S Broad St
Philadelphia, PA 19145-3089
Med Sch Affil: L-04115, G-04101
Major participating institution for programs in: GS, PS
Institution ID: 41-0223

St Christopher's Hospital for Children
Erie Ave at Front St
Philadelphia, PA 19134-1095
Med Sch Affil: M-04115, M-04113, G-04102
Programs sponsored in: CHN, MPD, NPM, PD, PDC, PDI, PDP, PDR, PDS, PHO, PN, PP
Major participating institution for programs in: CCA, CCP, CN, GS, HMP, MG, NS, ORS, OTO, PMP, PS, TS, U
Institution ID: 41-0380

Temple University Hospital
Broad and Ontario Sts
Philadelphia, PA 19140-3615
Med Sch Affil: M-04113
Programs sponsored in: AN, APM, CCA, CD, CN, DR, EM, GE, GS, HMP, HO, ICE, ID, IM, IMG, MPM, MSR, N, NEP, NM, NS, OBG, OPH, ORS, OSM, OTO, P, PCC, PM, PMP, PS, PTH, RHU, RNR, TY, U, VIR, VS
Major participating institution for programs in: MPM, NPM, PCC, PTH
Institution ID: 41-0413

Thomas Jefferson University Hospital
111 S 11th St
Philadelphia, PA 19107-5096
Med Sch Affil: M-04102, G-04115
Programs sponsored in: AI, AN, APM, BBK, CCS, CD, CHP, CN, CRS, D, DMP, DR, EM, END, FP, FPG, FSM, GE, GPM, GS, HEM, HSO, ID, IM, N, NEP, NM, NPM, NS, OAR, OBG, ON, ORS, OSM, OTO, P, PCC, PCP, PD, PM, PMP, PTH, RHU, RNR, RO, SCI, SP, TS, U, VIR
Institution ID: 41-0224

Veterans Affairs Medical Center (Philadelphia)
University and Woodland Aves
Philadelphia, PA 19104
Med Sch Affil: M-04115, M-04101
Major participating institution for programs in: ADP, AN, APM, D, END, GS, ICE, ID, IM, IMG, NM, NS, OPH, ORS, OSM, OTO, P, PM, RHU, RNR, RO, U, VIR
Institution ID: 41-0285

Wills Eye Hospital
900 Walnut St
Philadelphia, PA 19107-5598
Med Sch Affil: M-04102
Programs sponsored in: OPH
Major participating institution for programs in: NS
Institution ID: 41-0494

Pittsburgh

Allegheny County Coroner's Office
542 Fourth Ave
Pittsburgh, PA 15219-2186
Programs sponsored in: FOP
Institution ID: 41-0531

Allegheny General Hospital
320 E North Ave
Pittsburgh, PA 15212-4772
Med Sch Affil: M-04115
Programs sponsored in: AN, APM, CD, CHP, DR, EM, ESM, GE, GS, HMP, HSO, IM, MEM, MG, N, NEP, NS, OBG, ON, ORS, P, PCP, PTH, PUD, RNR, RO, TS
Major participating institution for programs in: BBK, OPH, OTO, PS
Institution ID: 41-0465

Central Blood Bank
3636 Blvd of the Allies
Pittsburgh, PA 15213
Programs sponsored in: BBK
Institution ID: 41-8030

Children's Hospital of Pittsburgh
One Children's Pl
3705 Fifth Ave
Pittsburgh, PA 15213-2583
Med Sch Affil: M-04112
Major participating institution for programs in: AI, BBK, CCP, CHN, CN, D, GS, HMP, HSO, MPD, NP, NS, ORS, OTO, PAN, PD, PDC, PDE, PDI, PDO, PDP, PDR, PDS, PG, PHO, PN, PP, PS, PTH, TS, TY, U
Institution ID: 41-0161

Harmarville Rehabilitation Center
PO Box 11460
Guys Run Rd
Pittsburgh, PA 15238-0460
Major participating institution for programs in: PM
Institution ID: 41-0740

Magee-Women's Hospital
300 Halket St
Pittsburgh, PA 15213-3180
Med Sch Affil: M-04112
Major participating institution for programs in: NP, NPM, OBG, PCP, PD, PP, PTH, TY
Institution ID: 41-0208

Mercy Hospital of Pittsburgh
1400 Locust St
Pittsburgh, PA 15219-5166
Med Sch Affil: M-04112
Programs sponsored in: AN, DR, FP, GS, IM, PD, TY
Major participating institution for programs in: EM, PM
Institution ID: 41-0196

Presbyterian University Hospital/UPMC
Desoto at O'Hara Sts
Pittsburgh, PA 15213
Med Sch Affil: M-04112
Major participating institution for programs in: AN, APM, BBK, CCA, CCM, CCS, CD, CHN, CHP, D, DMP, DR, EM, END, GE, GS, HEM, HMP, HSP, ID, IM, IMG, NEP, NP, NS, ON, OPH, ORS, OSM, OTO, P, PCC, PCP, PM, PS, PTH, RHU, RNR, TS, TY, U, VIR
Institution ID: 41-0349

Shadyside Hospital/UPMC
5230 Centre Ave
Pittsburgh, PA 15232
Med Sch Affil: M-04112
Programs sponsored in: CD, END, FP, FSM, GE, IMG, TY
Major participating institution for programs in: MPD
Institution ID: 41-0482

St Francis Medical Center
400 45th St
Pittsburgh, PA 15201
Med Sch Affil: M-04112
Programs sponsored in: ADP, DR, IM, MP, MPM, OPH, P, PM, TY
Institution ID: 41-0271

University Health Center of Pittsburgh
121 Meyran Ave
Pittsburgh, PA 15260
Med Sch Affil: M-04112
Programs sponsored in: AI, AN, APM, CCA, CCM, CCP, CCS, CD, CHN, CHP, CN, D, DMP, DR, EM, END, GE, GS, HEM, HMP, HSO, HSP, ICE, ID, IM, IMG, MPD, N, NEP, NP, NPM, NS, OBG, ON, OPH, ORS, OSM, OTO, P, PAN, PCC, PCP, PD, PDC, PDE, PDI, PDO, PDP, PDR, PDS, PG, PHO, PM, PN, PP, PS, PTH, PYG, RHU, RNR, TS, TY, U, VIR, VS
Institution ID: 41-8024

University of Pittsburgh Graduate School of Public Health
130 De Soto St/111 Parran Hall
Pittsburgh, PA 15261
Programs sponsored in: GPM
Institution ID: 41-0118

University of Pittsburgh Medical Center (St Margaret)
815 Freeport Rd
Pittsburgh, PA 15215-3399
Med Sch Affil: M-04112
Programs sponsored in: FP, FPG, FSM
Major participating institution for programs in: ORS, PM
Institution ID: 41-0324

Veterans Affairs Medical Center (Pittsburgh)
University Dr C
Pittsburgh, PA 15240-1001
Med Sch Affil: M-04112
Major participating institution for programs in: CCM, CD, D, END, GE, GS, HEM, HSO, ID, IM, IMG, N, NEP, NP, NS, ON, OPH, ORS, OTO, P, PCC, PTH, RHU, RNR, TS, TY, U, VS
Institution ID: 41-0296

Western Pennsylvania Hospital
4800 Friendship Ave
Pittsburgh, PA 15224-1793
Med Sch Affil: M-04112
Programs sponsored in: AN, CD, DR, FP, GE, GS, IM, OBG, PUD, TY, VIR
Major participating institution for programs in: EM, PS
Institution ID: 41-0122

Western Psychiatric Institute and Clinic/UPMC
3811 O'Hara St
Pittsburgh, PA 15213-2593
Med Sch Affil: M-04112
Major participating institution for programs in: CHP, CN, P, PYG, TY
Institution ID: 41-0462

Reading

Reading Hospital and Medical Center
PO Box 16052
Reading, PA 19612-6052
Med Sch Affil: M-04114, M-04113, G-04101
Programs sponsored in: DR, FP, IM, OBG, TY
Major participating institution for programs in: GS
Institution ID: 41-0305

St Joseph Medical Center
PO Box 316
12th and Walnut Sts
Reading, PA 19603-0316
Programs sponsored in: FP
Institution ID: 41-0485

Sayre

Guthrie Healthcare System
Guthrie Sq
Sayre, PA 18840
Programs sponsored in: FP
Institution ID: 41-8021

Robert Packer Hospital
Guthrie Sq
Sayre, PA 18840-9984
Med Sch Affil: M-03515, L-04115
Programs sponsored in: CD, GE, GS, IM
Major participating institution for programs in: FP
Institution ID: 41-0352

Scranton

Community Medical Center
1822 Mulberry St
Scranton, PA 18510-2398
Major participating institution for programs in: IM, PUD
Institution ID: 41-0716

Mercy Hospital
Administrative Ste
746 Jefferson Ave
Scranton, PA 18510
Med Sch Affil: M-04113
Major participating institution for programs in: IM
Institution ID: 41-0717

Moses Taylor Hospital
700 Quincy Ave
Scranton, PA 18510-1970
Med Sch Affil: M-04113
Major participating institution for programs in: IM
Institution ID: 41-0718

Scranton-Temple Residency Program Inc
746 Jefferson Ave
Scranton, PA 18510
Programs sponsored in: IM
Institution ID: 41-0719

Upland

Crozer-Chester Medical Center
One Medical Center Blvd
Upland, PA 19013
Med Sch Affil: M-04115, G-04101, G-04102
Programs sponsored in: FP, FSM, IM, PD, TY
Major participating institution for programs in: GS, OBG, VS
Institution ID: 41-0511

Crozer-Keystone Health System
One Medical Center Blvd
Upland, PA 19013-3995
Med Sch Affil: L-04115, G-04113
Major participating institution for programs in: FP, FSM, OAR
Institution ID: 41-0505

Warminster

Warminster Hospital
225 Newtown Rd
Warminster, PA 18974
Major participating institution for programs in: FP
Institution ID: 41-8031

Washington

Washington Hospital
155 Wilson Ave
Washington, PA 15301
Programs sponsored in: FP
Institution ID: 41-0385

Wilkes-Barre

Veterans Affairs Medical Center (Wilkes-Barre)
1111 E End Blvd
Wilkes-Barre, PA 18711-0026
Med Sch Affil: G-04115
Programs sponsored in: IM, PUD
Major participating institution for programs in: OPH
Institution ID: 41-0517

Wyoming Valley Health Care System
North River and Auburn St
Wilkes-Barre, PA 18764
Programs sponsored in: FP
Institution ID: 41-8035

Williamsport

Williamsport Hospital and Medical Center
777 Rural Ave
Williamsport, PA 17701-3198
Programs sponsored in: FP
Institution ID: 41-0147

Wynnewood

Lankenau Hospital
100 Lancaster Ave
Wynnewood, PA 19096-3498
Med Sch Affil: M-04102, G-04113
Programs sponsored in: CD, GE, GS, HO, ICE, IM, NEP, OBG, PCP
Major participating institution for programs in: OPH, OSM
Institution ID: 41-0403

York

York Hospital
1001 S George St
York, PA 17405
Med Sch Affil: M-04114, M-04101, L-02301
Programs sponsored in: EM, FP, GS, IM, OBG, TY
Major participating institution for programs in: PS
Institution ID: 41-0142

Puerto Rico

Bayamon

Hospital San Pablo
Calle Santa Cruz #70
Urb Santa Cruz
Bayamon, PR 00960
Med Sch Affil: L-04203
Programs sponsored in: FP
Institution ID: 42-0473

University Hospital Ramon Ruiz Arnau
Avenidas Laurel y Santa Juanita
Bayamon, PR 00956-6032
Med Sch Affil: M-04203
Programs sponsored in: FP, IM, PD, TY
Major participating institution for programs in: HEM, ON, PUD
Institution ID: 42-7019

Caguas

Caguas Regional Hospital
PO Box 5729
Caguas, PR 00726
Med Sch Affil: M-04201
Programs sponsored in: IM, PD, TY
Major participating institution for programs in: FP, FPG, OBG
Institution ID: 42-0470

Carolina

Dr Federico Trilla - Carolina Regional Hospital
Ave 65th de Infanteria/KM 8 3
PO Box 3869
Carolina, PR 00984-3869
Major participating institution for programs in: EM, IM, IMG, OBG
Institution ID: 42-8015

Manati

Hospital Dr Alejandro Otero Lopez
PO Box 1142
Manati, PR 00674
Med Sch Affil: L-04203
Programs sponsored in: FP
Institution ID: 42-8016

Mayaguez

Bella Vista Hospital
State Rd 349
PO Box 1750
Mayaguez, PR 00681
Programs sponsored in: FP
Institution ID: 42-8022

Dr Ramon E Betances Hospital-Mayaguez Medical Center
410 Carretera #2
Mayaguez, PR 00680-1522
Med Sch Affil: L-04202
Programs sponsored in: GS, IM, PD, TY
Institution ID: 42-0467

Ponce

Dr Pila Hospital
PO Box 1910
Ponce, PR 00733-1910
Med Sch Affil: L-04202
Programs sponsored in: FP
Institution ID: 42-7016

Hospital de Damas
Ponce Bypass
Ponce, PR 00731
Med Sch Affil: M-04202
Programs sponsored in: CD, GE, IM, PUD, TY
Institution ID: 42-0289

Hospital San Lucas
Box 2027
Ponce, PR 00733-2027
Med Sch Affil: L-04202
Major participating institution for programs in: CD
Institution ID: 42-7018

Ponce University Hospital
Bo Machuelo
Carretera 14
Ponce, PR 00731
Med Sch Affil: M-04202
Programs sponsored in: IM, OBG, PD, TY
Major participating institution for programs in: FP, GE, PUD, TY
Institution ID: 42-0194

Rio Piedras

San Juan City Hospital
Hicaco 53
Milaville
Rio Piedras, PR 00926
Med Sch Affil: M-04201, M-04203
Programs sponsored in: CD, END, HEM, IM, OBG, ON, PD, PUD, RHU, TY
Major participating institution for programs in: AN, D, DR, N, NS, OPH, ORS, OTO, PTH
Institution ID: 42-0320

San German

Hospital de la Concepcion
Box 285
San German, PR 00683
Med Sch Affil: L-04202
Programs sponsored in: IM
Institution ID: 42-0478

San Juan

Hospital Pavia
1462 Asia St
Aptdo 11137 Santurce
San Juan, PR 00910
Major participating institution for programs in: GS, U
Institution ID: 42-7006

I Gonzalez Martinez Oncologic Hospital
Puerto Rico Med Ctr
PO Box 191811
San Juan, PR 00919
Med Sch Affil: M-04201
Major participating institution for programs in: ON
Institution ID: 42-0205

Institute of Forensic Sciences of Puerto Rico
Box 11878
Caparra Heights Station
San Juan, PR 00922-1878
Programs sponsored in: FOP
Institution ID: 42-0461

Puerto Rico Institute of Psychiatry
GPO Box 363741
San Juan, PR 00936-3741
Programs sponsored in: P
Institution ID: 42-0387

State Psychiatric Hospital
Call Box 2100
Caparra Heights Station
San Juan, PR 00922-2100
Major participating institution for programs in: P
Institution ID: 42-8019

University Hospital
Puerto Rico Med Ctr
Rio Piedras Station
San Juan, PR 00935
Med Sch Affil: M-04201
Major participating institution for programs in: AN, CD, CHP, D, DR, END, GE, GS, HO, ID, IM, IMG, N, NEP, NM, NS, OBG, OPH, ORS, OTO, P, PM, PTH, PUD, RHU, TY, U
Institution ID: 42-0178

University of Puerto Rico School of Medicine
GPO Box 365067
San Juan, PR 00936-5067
Med Sch Affil: M-04201
Programs sponsored in: AN, CCP, CD, CHP, D, DR, EM, END, FP, FPG, GE, GS, HO, ID, IM, IMG, N, NEP, NM, NPM, NS, OBG, OPH, ORS, OTO, P, PD, PDP, PHO, PM, PTH, PUD, RHU, U
Major participating institution for programs in: CD
Institution ID: 42-0464

University Pediatric Hospital
PO Box 191079
San Juan, PR 00919-1079
Med Sch Affil: M-04201
Major participating institution for programs in: CCP, NPM, NS, ORS, PD, PDP, PHO, PM, U
Institution ID: 42-0477

Veterans Affairs Medical Center (San Juan)
One Veterans Plaza
San Juan, PR 00927-5800
Med Sch Affil: M-04201, L-04203
Programs sponsored in: CD, ID, IM, NEP, PM, PUD
Major participating institution for programs in: AN, DR, GE, GS, HEM, ID, IMG, N, NM, NS, ON, OPH, ORS, OTO, P, PTH, PUD, RHU, U
Institution ID: 42-0265

Vocational Rehabilitation Center
PO Box 191681
San Juan, PR 00919
Major participating institution for programs in: PM
Institution ID: 42-0469

Rhode Island

Cranston

Eleanor Slater Hospital
PO Box 8269
Cranston, RI 02920
Major participating institution for programs in: PYG
Institution ID: 43-8012

East Providence

Emma Pendleton Bradley Hospital
1011 Veterans Memorial Pkwy
East Providence, RI 02915-5099
Med Sch Affil: M-04301
Programs sponsored in: CPP
Major participating institution for programs in: CHP, HO
Institution ID: 43-0432

Pawtucket

Memorial Hospital of Rhode Island
111 Brewster St
Pawtucket, RI 02860
Programs sponsored in: FP, IM
Major participating institution for programs in: CD, D, HO, ID, PTH
Institution ID: 43-0436

Providence

Butler Hospital
345 Blackstone Blvd
Providence, RI 02906
Med Sch Affil: M-04301
Programs sponsored in: P, PYG, PYN
Institution ID: 43-0483

Miriam Hospital
164 Summit Ave
Providence, RI 02906
Med Sch Affil: M-04301
Programs sponsored in: CCM, IM, TY
Major participating institution for programs in: CCS, CD, GS, ID, NEP, P, PTH, PYG
Institution ID: 43-0232

Rhode Island Hospital
593 Eddy St
Providence, RI 02903-4970
Med Sch Affil: M-04301, G-02416
Programs sponsored in: CCS, CD, CHN, CHP, CN, D, DR, EM, END, GE, GS, IM, MPD, N, NEP, NP, NS, OPH, ORS, PD, PDE, PDI, PDS, PG, PHO, PS, PTH, U, VIR
Major participating institution for programs in: CCM, ID, OBG, OTO, P, PP, PYN, RHU
Institution ID: 43-0281

Roger Williams Medical Center
825 Chalkstone Ave
Providence, RI 02908-4735
Med Sch Affil: M-04301, L-04301
Programs sponsored in: D, DMP, HO, ID, IM, PUD, RHU
Major participating institution for programs in: END, GE, P, PS, PTH, U
Institution ID: 43-0438

Veterans Affairs Medical Center (Providence)
830 Chalkstone Ave
Providence, RI 02908-4799
Med Sch Affil: M-04301
Major participating institution for programs in: CD, D, END, GE, GS, HO, ID, N, OPH, ORS, P, PS, RHU, U
Institution ID: 43-0439

Women and Infants Hospital of Rhode Island
101 Dudley St
Providence, RI 02905-2401
Med Sch Affil: M-04301
Programs sponsored in: NPM, OBG, PP
Major participating institution for programs in: PD, PG, PTH
Institution ID: 43-0334

South Carolina

Anderson

Anderson Area Medical Center
800 N Fant St
Anderson, SC 29621
Med Sch Affil: L-04504, L-04501
Programs sponsored in: FP
Institution ID: 45-0732

Charleston

Charleston Memorial Hospital
326 Calhoun St
Charleston, SC 29401
Med Sch Affil: M-04501
Major participating institution for programs in: DR, GS, OBG, ORS, OTO, P, PCC, PS, TS
Institution ID: 45-0483

Medical University of South Carolina College of Medicine
171 Ashley Ave
Charleston, SC 29425-2201
Med Sch Affil: M-04501
Programs sponsored in: ADP, AN, APM, CD, CHP, CN, D, DMP, DR, END, FOP, FP, GE, GS, HMP, HO, ID, IM, MP, N, NEP, NM, NPM, NS, OBG, OPH, ORS, OTO, P, PCC, PCP, PD, PDC, PG, PHO, PM, PS, PTH, PYG, RHU, RNR, RO, TS, U, VIR
Institution ID: 45-9501

MUSC Medical Center
171 Ashley Ave
Charleston, SC 29425-0950
Med Sch Affil: M-04501, L-04504
Major participating institution for programs in: ADP, AN, APM, CD, CHP, CN, D, DMP, DR, END, FOP, GE, GS, HMP, HO, ID, IM, MP, N, NEP, NM, NPM, NS, OBG, OPH, ORS, OTO, P, PCC, PD, PDC, PHO, PM, PS, PTH, RHU, RNR, RO, TS, U, VIR
Institution ID: 45-0152

Naval Hospital (Charleston)
3600 Rivers Ave
Charleston, SC 29405-7744
Med Sch Affil: L-04501
Major participating institution for programs in: GS, ORS, OTO
Institution ID: 45-0134

Ralph H Johnson Dept of Veterans Affairs Med Center
109 Bee St
Charleston, SC 29401-5799
Med Sch Affil: M-04501
Major participating institution for programs in: AN, D, DR, END, GE, GS, HO, ID, IM, MP, N, NEP, NM, OPH, ORS, OTO, P, PCC, PS, PTH, PYG, RHU, TS, U
Institution ID: 45-0485

Columbia

Palmetto Health Alliance
5 Richland Medical Pk
Columbia, SC 29203
Programs sponsored in: CD, CHP, EM, END, FP, FSM, GE, GS, IM, IMG, OBG, ON, OPH, ORS, P, PD, PFP, PUD
Institution ID: 45-8005

Palmetto Richland Memorial Hospital
5 Richland Medical Pk
Columbia, SC 29203
Med Sch Affil: M-04504, L-04501
Major participating institution for programs in: CD, EM, END, FP, FSM, GE, GS, IM, IMG, OBG, ON, OPH, ORS, P, PD, PUD
Institution ID: 45-0366

University of South Carolina School of Medicine
6439 Garners Ferry Rd
Columbia, SC 29209
Med Sch Affil: M-04504
Programs sponsored in: GPM
Institution ID: 45-8001

William Jennings Bryan Dorn Veterans Hospital
6439 Garners Ferry Rd
Columbia, SC 29209
Med Sch Affil: M-04504
Major participating institution for programs in: CD, END, GE, GS, IM, ON, OPH, ORS, P, PUD
Institution ID: 45-0735

William S Hall Psychiatric Institute
1800 Colonial Dr
PO Box 202
Columbia, SC 29202
Med Sch Affil: M-04504, L-04501
Major participating institution for programs in: CHP, P, PFP
Institution ID: 45-0484

Florence

McLeod Regional Medical Center
555 E Cheves St
Florence, SC 29506-2617
Med Sch Affil: L-04504, L-04501
Programs sponsored in: FP
Institution ID: 45-0239

Greenville

Greenville Hospital System
701 Grove Rd
Greenville, SC 29605
Med Sch Affil: M-04504, L-04501
Programs sponsored in: FP, GS, IM, OBG, ORS, PD, TY
Institution ID: 45-0367

Shriners Hospital for Children (Greenville)
950 W Faris Rd
Greenville, SC 29605-4277
Med Sch Affil: L-03607
Major participating institution for programs in: ORS
Institution ID: 45-0174

Greenwood

Greenwood Genetic Center
1 Gregor Mendel Cir
Greenwood, SC 29646
Programs sponsored in: MG
Institution ID: 45-8004

Self Memorial Hospital
1325 Spring St
Greenwood, SC 29646-3875
Med Sch Affil: L-04501, L-04504
Programs sponsored in: FP
Major participating institution for programs in: MG
Institution ID: 45-7024

Spartanburg

Spartanburg Regional Healthcare System
101 E Wood St
Spartanburg, SC 29303-3072
Med Sch Affil: L-04504, L-04501
Programs sponsored in: FP, GS, TY
Institution ID: 45-0162

South Dakota

Rapid City

Rapid City Regional Hospital
353 Fairmont Blvd
PO Box 6000
Rapid City, SD 57709
Med Sch Affil: M-04601
Programs sponsored in: FP
Institution ID: 46-8005

Sioux Falls

Avera McKennan Hospital
PO Box 5045
800 E 21st St
Sioux Falls, SD 57117-5045
Med Sch Affil: M-04601
Major participating institution for programs in: FP, IM, P, TY
Institution ID: 46-0125

Royal C Johnson Veterans Affairs Medical Center
PO Box 5046
2501 W 22nd St
Sioux Falls, SD 57117-5046
Med Sch Affil: M-04601
Major participating institution for programs in: IM, P, PTH, TY
Institution ID: 46-0218

Sioux Valley Hospital
1100 S Euclid Ave
PO Box 5039
Sioux Falls, SD 57117-5039
Med Sch Affil: M-04601
Major participating institution for programs in: CHP, FP, IM, PTH, TY
Institution ID: 46-0212

Southeastern Mental Health Center
2000 S Summit Ave
Sioux Falls, SD 57105
Med Sch Affil: G-04601
Major participating institution for programs in: P
Institution ID: 46-8001

University of South Dakota School of Medicine
1400 W 22nd St
Sioux Falls, SD 57105-1570
Programs sponsored in: CHP, FP, IM, P, PTH, TY
Institution ID: 46-9501

Tennessee

Bristol

Bristol Regional Medical Center
1 Medical Park Blvd
Bristol, TN 37620
Med Sch Affil: M-04720
Major participating institution for programs in: FP, IM, PUD, PYG
Institution ID: 47-0491

Chattanooga

Erlanger Medical Center
975 E Third St
Chattanooga, TN 37403
Med Sch Affil: M-04706
Major participating institution for programs in: FP, GS, IM, OBG, OPH, ORS, OSM, PM, PS, TY
Institution ID: 47-0330

Memorial Hospital
2525 de Sales Ave
Chattanooga, TN 37404
Med Sch Affil: M-04720
Major participating institution for programs in: FP
Institution ID: 47-7001

T C Thompson Children's Hospital Medical Center
910 Blackford St
Chattanooga, TN 37403
Med Sch Affil: M-04706
Major participating institution for programs in: OPH, ORS, PD
Institution ID: 47-0313

University of Tennessee College of Medicine-Chattanooga Unit
975 E Third St
Hospital Box 255
Chattanooga, TN 37403
Med Sch Affil: M-04706
Programs sponsored in: FP, GS, IM, OBG, OPH, ORS, OSM, PD, PM, PS, TY
Institution ID: 47-0490

Willie D Miller Eye Center
975 E Third St
Chattanooga, TN 37403
Major participating institution for programs in: OPH
Institution ID: 47-8016

Jackson

Jackson-Madison County General Hospital
294 Summar Dr
Jackson, TN 38301-3983
Med Sch Affil: G-04706
Major participating institution for programs in: FP
Institution ID: 47-0480

Johnson City

James H Quillen College of Medicine
Box 70571
Johnson City, TN 37614-0571
Med Sch Affil: M-04720
Programs sponsored in: CD, FP, GE, GS, ID, IM, MN, MPD, OBG, ON, P, PD, PTH, PUD, PYG
Institution ID: 47-0492

Johnson City Medical Center Hospital
400 N State
Johnson City, TN 37604-6094
Med Sch Affil: M-04720
Major participating institution for programs in: CD, FP, GE, GS, ID, IM, MN, OBG, ON, P, PD, PTH, PUD
Institution ID: 47-0499

Woodridge Hospital
403 State
Johnson City, TN 37604
Med Sch Affil: M-04720
Major participating institution for programs in: P
Institution ID: 47-0493

Kingsport

Wellmont Health System-Holston Valley
130 W Ravine Rd
PO Box 238
Kingsport, TN 37662-0224
Med Sch Affil: M-04720
Major participating institution for programs in: FP, GS, IM
Institution ID: 47-0379

Knoxville

Knoxville Orthopedic Clinic
PO Box 51090
Knoxville, TN 37950-1090
Major participating institution for programs in: OSM
Institution ID: 47-8022

St Mary's Health System
900 E Oak Hill Ave
Knoxville, TN 37917
Major participating institution for programs in: OSM
Institution ID: 47-0104

University of Tennessee Graduate School of Medicine
1924 Alcoa Hwy/Box 94
Knoxville, TN 37920-6999
Med Sch Affil: M-04706
Programs sponsored in: AN, CCA, CCS, DR, FP, FSM, GS, IM, NM, CCG, PD, PTH, TY, VS
Institution ID: 47-0448

University of Tennessee Memorial Hospital
1924 Alcoa Hwy
Knoxville, TN 37920-6999
Major participating institution for programs in: AN, CCA, CCS, DR, FP, FSM, GS, IM, NM, OBG, PD, PTH, TY
Institution ID: 47-8023

Memphis

Baptist Memorial Hospital
899 Madison Ave
Memphis, TN 38146
Med Sch Affil: M-04706
Programs sponsored in: DR
Major participating institution for programs in: AI, CHN, D, DMP, END, FP, GS, HEM, IM, MN, N, NS, ON, ORS, OTO, PS, PTH, RHU, TS, TY, VS
Institution ID: 47-0382

LeBonheur Children's Medical Center
50 N Dunlap Ave
Memphis, TN 38103-2893
Med Sch Affil: M-04706
Major participating institution for programs in: AI, CCP, CHN, CHP, CN, DR, MPD, OP, ORS, PD, PDE, PDI, PDS, PHO, PN, PPR, TS, U, UP
Institution ID: 47-0186

Methodist Hospitals of Memphis-Central
1265 Union Ave
Memphis, TN 38104-3415
Med Sch Affil: M-04706
Programs sponsored in: DR, IM, TY
Major participating institution for programs in: CN, GS, NS, OPH, OTO
Institution ID: 47-0113

Regional Medical Center at Memphis
877 Jefferson Ave
Memphis, TN 38103-9999
Med Sch Affil: M-04706
Major participating institution for programs in: AN, CCM, CCS, CD, CHN, D, DR, END, GE, GS, HEM, ID, IM, MN, MPD, N, NEP, NPM, NS, OBG, ON, OPH, ORS, OTO, P, PD, PPR, PS, PTH, PUD, RHU, TS, U, VIR
Institution ID: 47-0241

St Francis Hospital
5959 Park Ave
PO Box 171808
Memphis, TN 38187
Med Sch Affil: G-04706
Major participating institution for programs in: FP
Institution ID: 47-0478

St Joseph Hospital
220 Overton Ave
Memphis, TN 38101
Major participating institution for programs in: CHP
Institution ID: 47-0375

St Jude Children's Research Hospital
332 N Lauderdale St
Memphis, TN 38105-0318
Med Sch Affil: M-04706
Major participating institution for programs in: AI, MPD, PDI, PDS, PHO
Institution ID: 47-0482

University of Tennessee College of Medicine
956 Court Ave
PO Box 19A
Memphis, TN 38163-9999
Med Sch Affil: M-04706
Programs sponsored in: AI, AN, CCM, CCP, CCS, CD, CHN, CHP, CN, D, DMP, DR, END, FOP, FP, GE, GS, HEM, HSO, ID, IM, MN, MPD, N, NEP, NPM, NS, OBG, ON, OP, OPH, ORS, OTO, P, PD, PDE, PDI, PDS, PHO, PN, PPR, PS, PTH, PUD, RHU, TS, TY, U, UP, VIR, VS
Institution ID: 47-0474

University of Tennessee Medical Center (UT Bowld Hospital)
951 Court Ave
Memphis, TN 38103
Med Sch Affil: M-04706
Major participating institution for programs in: AI, AN, CHP, D, DR, FP, GS, IM, MN, MPD, N, OBG, OTO, PDS, PS, TS, U, VIR
Institution ID: 47-0269

University of Tennessee-Campbell Clinic
Dept of Orthopedic Surgery
910 Madison Ave/#500
Memphis, TN 38103-3403
Med Sch Affil: M-04706
Major participating institution for programs in: HSO, OP, ORS
Institution ID: 47-0401

Veterans Affairs Medical Center (Memphis)
1030 Jefferson Ave
Memphis, TN 38104
Med Sch Affil: M-04706
Major participating institution for programs in: AI, CCM, CD, CHN, D, DMP, DR, END, GE, GS, HEM, ID, IM, MN, MPD, N, NEP, NS, ON, OPH, OTO, PS, PTH, PUD, RHU, TS, U, VS
Institution ID: 47-0280

Mountain Home

Veterans Affairs Medical Center (Mountain Home)
VA Med Ctr (11C)
Mountain Home, TN 37684-5001
Med Sch Affil: M-04720
Major participating institution for programs in: CD, FP, GE, GS, ID, IM, MN, ON, P, PTH, PUD, PYG
Institution ID: 47-0498

Murfreesboro

Alvin C York Veterans Affairs Medical Center
3400 Lebanon Rd
Murfreesboro, TN 37129
Med Sch Affil: M-04707
Major participating institution for programs in: FP, IM, P
Institution ID: 47-0501

Nashville

Baptist Hospital

2000 Church St
Nashville, TN 37236-0001
Med Sch Affil: M-04706, L-04705
Major participating institution for programs in: IM, OBG, OSM, PS, U
Institution ID: 47-0163

Centennial Medical Center

2300 Patterson St
Nashville, TN 37203
Major participating institution for programs in: P
Institution ID: 47-8028

Meharry Medical College

1005 Dr D B Todd Jr Blvd
Nashville, TN 37208
Programs sponsored in: FP, GPM, IM, P
Institution ID: 47-9501

Metropolitan Nashville General Hospital

72 Hermitage Ave
Nashville, TN 37210-2110
Med Sch Affil: M-04707
Major participating institution for programs in: D, FP, ICE, IM, MPD, PD, PS
Institution ID: 47-0408

Middle Tennessee Mental Health Institute

1501 Murfreesboro Rd
Nashville, TN 37214-3325
Major participating institution for programs in: P
Institution ID: 47-0502

Psychiatric Hospital at Vanderbilt

1601 23rd Ave S
Nashville, TN 37212
Major participating institution for programs in: ADP, CHP
Institution ID: 47-8021

Southern Sports Medicine & Orthopaedic Center

Baptist Medical Plaza II/2nd Fl
2021 Church St
Nashville, TN 37203
Programs sponsored in: OSM
Institution ID: 47-8027

St Thomas Hospital

4220 Harding Rd
PO Box 380
Nashville, TN 37202
Med Sch Affil: M-04705
Major participating institution for programs in: D, GE, GS, HO, ID, IM, NS, PTH, RHU, TS, VS
Institution ID: 47-0262

Vanderbilt University Medical Center

1161 21st Ave S
Nashville, TN 37232
Med Sch Affil: M-04705, L-02012
Programs sponsored in: ADP, AI, AN, APM, CCA, CCP, CCS, CD, CHN, CHP, CN, D, DR, EM, END, GE, GS, HMP, HO, ICE, ID, IM, IMG, MG, MPD, N, NEP, NM, NP, NPM, NS, OBG, OPH, ORS, OTO, P, PCC, PD, PDC, PDE, PDI, PDP, PG, PHO, PN, PS, PTH, PYG, RHU, RNR, TS, U, VIR, VS
Institution ID: 47-0467

Veterans Affairs Medical Center (Nashville)

1310 24th Ave S
Nashville, TN 37212-2637
Med Sch Affil: M-04705
Major participating institution for programs in: D, DR, GE, GS, HMP, HO, ICE, ID, IM, MPD, N, NEP, NM, NP, NS, OPH, ORS, OTO, PCC, PS, PTH, RHU, TS, U
Institution ID: 47-0461

Texas

Amarillo

Northwest Texas Health Care System

PO Box 1110
1501 S Coulter
Amarillo, TX 79175
Med Sch Affil: M-04815
Major participating institution for programs in: FP, IM, OBG, PD
Institution ID: 48-0566

St Anthony's Hospital

PO Box 950
Amarillo, TX 79176
Major participating institution for programs in: FP
Institution ID: 48-7005

Texas Tech University Health Sciences Center at Amarillo

1400 Wallace Blvd
Amarillo, TX 79106
Med Sch Affil: M-04815
Programs sponsored in: FP, IM, OBG, PD
Institution ID: 48-0520

Veterans Affairs Medical Center (Amarillo)

6010 Amarillo Blvd W
Amarillo, TX 79106
Med Sch Affil: M-04815
Major participating institution for programs in: IM
Institution ID: 48-0584

Austin

Austin State Hospital

4110 Guadalupe
Austin, TX 78751-4296
Programs sponsored in: CHP, P
Institution ID: 48-0388

Austin-Travis County Mental Health and Retardation Center

1430 Collier St
Austin, TX 78704
Major participating institution for programs in: P
Institution ID: 48-0586

Brackenridge Hospital

601 E 15th St
Austin, TX 78701
Major participating institution for programs in: CHP, FP, GS, IM, OBG, PD
Institution ID: 48-0563

CTMF of Seton Healthcare Network

601 E 15th St
Austin, TX 78701
Programs sponsored in: FP, IM, PD, TY
Major participating institution for programs in: P
Institution ID: 48-0451

Texas Department of Health

1100 W 49th St
Austin, TX 78756
Programs sponsored in: GPM
Institution ID: 48-0458

Baytown

San Jacinto Methodist Hospital

4401 Garth Rd
Baytown, TX 77521
Med Sch Affil: M-04814
Programs sponsored in: FP
Institution ID: 48-0579

Belton

Cedar Crest Residential Treatment Center

I-35 South
Belton, TX 76513
Major participating institution for programs in: CHP
Institution ID: 48-8065

Big Spring

Veterans Affairs Medical Center (Big Spring)

2400 Gregg St
Big Spring, TX 79720
Med Sch Affil: G-04815
Major participating institution for programs in: OPH
Institution ID: 48-0557

Brooks AFB

USAF School of Aerospace Medicine

USAFSAM/AF
2513 Kennedy Cir
Brooks AFB, TX 78235-5301
Programs sponsored in: GPM
Institution ID: 48-0493

Bryan

St Joseph Regional Health Center

2801 Franciscan Dr
Bryan, TX 77802-2544
Med Sch Affil: G-04816
Major participating institution for programs in: FP
Institution ID: 48-8063

College Station

Family Practice Foundation of the Brazos Valley

147 Joe H Reynolds Medical Bldg
College Station, TX 77843-1114
Programs sponsored in: FP
Institution ID: 48-8062

Conroe

Conroe Regional Medical Center

504 Medical Center Blvd
Conroe, TX 77304
Major participating institution for programs in: FP
Institution ID: 48-0574

Corpus Christi

Driscoll Children's Hospital
3533 S Alameda Ave
PO Box 6530
Corpus Christi, TX 78466-6530
Med Sch Affil: M-04816, L-04802
Programs sponsored in: PD
Institution ID: 48-0157

Spohn Memorial Hospital
2606 Hospital Blvd
Corpus Christi, TX 78405-1818
Med Sch Affil: G-04813
Programs sponsored in: FP
Institution ID: 48-0257

Dallas

Baylor Institute for Rehabilitation
3505 Gaston Ave
Dallas, TX 75246-2018
Major participating institution for programs in: PM
Institution ID: 48-8030

Baylor University Medical Center
3500 Gaston Ave
Dallas, TX 75246-2088
Med Sch Affil: L-04812
Programs sponsored in: CD, CRS, DR, GE, GS, IM, OBG, ON, PM, PTH, VIR, VS
Major participating institution for programs in: PS, U
Institution ID: 48-0351

Charlton Methodist Hospital
3500 W Wheatland Rd
Dallas, TX 75237
Major participating institution for programs in: FP, FSM
Institution ID: 48-0575

Children's Medical Center of Dallas
1935 Motor St
Dallas, TX 75235
Med Sch Affil: M-04812
Major participating institution for programs in: CCP, CHN, CHP, D, END, HMP, NS, OTO, PD, PDC, PDI, PDR, PDS, PG, PHO, PN, PP, PPR, PS, TS, U
Institution ID: 48-0360

Dallas County Hospital District-Parkland Memorial Hospital
5201 Harry Hines Blvd
Dallas, TX 75235
Med Sch Affil: M-04812
Major participating institution for programs in: AN, APM, CCP, CCS, CD, CHN, CHP, CN, CRS, D, DMP, DR, EM, END, FP, GE, GS, HMP, HO, HSP, ICE, ID, IM, N, NEP, NM, NP, NPM, NR, NS, OBG, OP, OPH, ORS, OTO, P, PCC, PCP, PDE, PDI, PDR, PIP, PM, PS, PTH, PYG, RHU, RNR, TS, U, VIR, VS
Institution ID: 48-0400

Dallas County Mental Health and Mental Retardation Center
1341 Mockingbird Ln/Ste 1000-E
Dallas, TX 75247
Major participating institution for programs in: PYG
Institution ID: 48-8052

Healthsouth Dallas Rehabilitation Institute
2124 Research Row
Dallas, TX 75235-2597
Major participating institution for programs in: PM
Institution ID: 48-0545

Methodist Hospitals of Dallas
PO Box 655999
Dallas, TX 75265-5999
Med Sch Affil: L-04812
Programs sponsored in: FP, FSM, GS, IM, OBG
Institution ID: 48-0407

Presbyterian Hospital of Dallas
8200 Walnut Hill Ln
Dallas, TX 75231-4496
Med Sch Affil: L-04812
Programs sponsored in: CRS, IM
Major participating institution for programs in: OMO, P, PYG
Institution ID: 48-0519

Southwestern Institute of Forensic Sciences
5230 Medical Center Dr
PO Box 35728
Dallas, TX 75235-0728
Programs sponsored in: FOP
Institution ID: 48-0536

St Paul Medical Center
5909 Harry Hines Blvd
Dallas, TX 75235-0001
Med Sch Affil: L-04812
Programs sponsored in: FP, IM, OBG
Major participating institution for programs in: TS
Institution ID: 48-0103

Texas Scottish Rite Hospital for Children
2222 Welborn St
Dallas, TX 75219-3993
Med Sch Affil: L-04815, G-04812
Major participating institution for programs in: APM, CHN, HSP, OP, ORS, PPR
Institution ID: 48-0341

University of Texas Southwestern Medical School
5323 Harry Hines Blvd
Dallas, TX 75235-9002
Med Sch Affil: M-04812
Programs sponsored in: AI, AN, APM, BBK, CCP, CCS, CD, CHN, CHP, CN, D, DMP, DR, EM, END, FP, GE, GS, HMP, HO, HSP, ICE, ID, IM, N, NEP, NM, NP, NPM, NR, NS, OBG, OMO, OP, OPH, ORS, OTO, P, PCC, PCP, PD, PDC, PDE, PDI, PDR, PDS, PG, PHO, PIP, PM, PN, PP, PPR, PS, PTH, PYG, RHU, RNR, TS, U, VIR, VS
Institution ID: 48-0316

Veterans Affairs Medical Center (Dallas)
4500 S Lancaster Rd
Dallas, TX 75216
Med Sch Affil: M-04812
Major participating institution for programs in: CD, CN, D, DR, END, GE, GS, HO, ICE, ID, IM, NEP, NM, NR, NS, OPH, ORS, OTO, P, PCC, PM, PS, RHU, TS, U, VS
Institution ID: 48-0290

Zale-Lipshy University Hospital
5151 Harry Hines Blvd
Dallas, TX 75235-7786
Med Sch Affil: M-04812
Major participating institution for programs in: APM, D, N, NP, NS, OTO, P, PS, RNR, U, VIR, VS
Institution ID: 48-8034

El Paso

R E Thomason General Hospital
4815 Alameda Ave
El Paso, TX 79905
Med Sch Affil: M-04815
Major participating institution for programs in: AN, EM, FP, GS, IM, OBG, ORS, P, PD, TY
Institution ID: 48-0442

Texas Tech University Health Sciences Center at El Paso
4800 Alberta Ave
El Paso, TX 79905-2709
Med Sch Affil: M-04815, L-04802
Programs sponsored in: AN, EM, FP, GS, IM, OBG, P, PD, TY
Major participating institution for programs in: ORS
Institution ID: 48-0550

William Beaumont Army Medical Center
5005 N Piedras St
El Paso, TX 79920-5001
Med Sch Affil: M-02312, M-04815
Programs sponsored in: GS, IM, ORS, TY
Institution ID: 48-0318

Fort Hood

Darnall Army Community Hospital
36000 Darnell Loop
Fort Hood, TX 76544-4752
Med Sch Affil: M-04816, G-02312
Programs sponsored in: EM
Major participating institution for programs in: CHP, OBG
Institution ID: 48-0199

Fort Sam Houston

Brooke Army Medical Center
2410 Stanley Rd/Bldg 1029
Fort Sam Houston, TX 78234-6200
Med Sch Affil: M-02312, L-04813
Major participating institution for programs in: AN, CCA, CCM, CCS, CD, DR, GE, GS, HO, ID, IM, NM, OBG, ORS, PCC, PS, TS, TY
Institution ID: 48-0277

Fort Worth

Cook-Fort Worth Children's Medical Center
1400 Cooper St
Fort Worth, TX 76104
Major participating institution for programs in: ORS
Institution ID: 48-0503

Harris Methodist Fort Worth
1301 Pennsylvania Ave
Fort Worth, TX 76104
Major participating institution for programs in: OBG, ORS
Institution ID: 48-0361

John Peter Smith Hospital (Tarrant County Hospital District)
1500 S Main St
Fort Worth, TX 76104-4917
Med Sch Affil: G-04812
Programs sponsored in: FP, OBG, ORS, P, TY
Major participating institution for programs in: GS
Institution ID: 48-0214

Galveston

Shriners Hospitals for Children (Galveston Burns Institute)
815 Market St
Galveston, TX 77550-2725
Med Sch Affil: G-04802
Major participating institution for programs in: PS
Institution ID: 48-8001

University of Texas Medical Branch Hospitals
301 University Blvd/Rte 0138
Galveston, TX 77555-0138
Med Sch Affil: M-04802, L-04815
Programs sponsored in: AI, AN, APM, CCA, CD, CHP, D, DMP, DR, END, FP, GE, GPM, GS, ID, IM, IMG, MM, MN, MPD, N, NEP, NPM, NS, OBG, ON, OPH, ORS, OSS, OTO, P, PCC, PD, PDE, PDI, PDR, PHO, PN, PS, PTH, RHU, RNR, RO, TS, U
Institution ID: 48-0131

University of Texas Medical School at Galveston
604 Administration Bldg
301 University Blvd
Galveston, TX 77555-0129
Major participating institution for programs in: GPM
Institution ID: 48-9502

Garland

Baylor Medical Center at Garland
2300 Marie Curie Blvd
Garland, TX 75042
Programs sponsored in: FP
Institution ID: 48-8058

Family Healthcare Medical Education Center at Garland
2300 Marie Curie Blvd
Garland, TX 75042
Major participating institution for programs in: FP
Institution ID: 48-8057

Harlingen

Valley Baptist Medical Center
2101 Pease St
PO Box 2588
Harlingen, TX 78551
Med Sch Affil: L-04802, G-04813
Programs sponsored in: FP
Institution ID: 48-8060

Houston

AMI Park Plaza Hospital
1313 Hermann Dr
Houston, TX 77004
Med Sch Affil: L-04804
Major participating institution for programs in: FP
Institution ID: 48-8059

Baylor College of Medicine
One Baylor Plaza
Houston, TX 77030-3498
Med Sch Affil: L-02012, G-04815
Programs sponsored in: AI, ALI, AN, APM, CCM, CCP, CD, CHN, CHP, CN, D, DMP, DR, END, FP, GE, GS, HEM, HMP, HSO, HSP, ICE, ID, IM, IMG, IPM, MG, MPD, MPM, N, NEP, NM, NP, NPM, NS, OBG, ON, OP, OPH, ORS, OSM, OTO, OTR, P, PCC, PCP, PD, PDC, PDE, PDI, PDO, PDP, PDR, PDS, PG, PHO, PM, PMP, PN, PP, PPR, PS, PTH, RHU, RNR, RO, TS, TY, U, UP, VS
Institution ID: 48-0211

Harris County Hospital District-Ben Taub General Hospital
1504 Taub Loop
Houston, TX 77030
Med Sch Affil: M-04804, L-02312
Major participating institution for programs in: AN, BBK, CD, D, DMP, DR, END, FP, GE, GS, HEM, HMP, HSO, HSP, ICE, ID, IM, IPM, MG, MPD, N, NEP, NM, NP, NPM, NS, OBG, ON, OP, OPH, ORS, OTO, OTR, P, PCC, PCP, PD, PDI, PDS, PG, PPR, PS, PTH, RHU, RO, TS, TY, U
Institution ID: 48-0363

Harris County Medical Examiner Department
1885 Old Spanish Trail
Houston, TX 77054
Programs sponsored in: FOP
Institution ID: 48-8070

Harris County Psychiatric Center
2800 S MacGregor Dr
PO Box 20249
Houston, TX 77225-0249
Med Sch Affil: M-04814
Major participating institution for programs in: P
Institution ID: 48-8044

Lyndon B Johnson General Hospital
5656 Kelly St
Houston, TX 77026
Med Sch Affil: M-04814
Major participating institution for programs in: CCS, CD, D, DR, EM, END, FP, GE, GS, HEM, ID, IM, MG, N, NEP, NPM, OBG, ORS, OTO, PD, PDE, PDI, PM, PS, PTH, RHU, RNR, TY, U
Institution ID: 48-8045

Memorial Herman Hospital System
7737 SW Freeway/Ste 200
Houston, TX 77074
Med Sch Affil: M-04814
Programs sponsored in: FP
Institution ID: 48-0443

Memorial Hermann Healthcare System
7737 Southwest Freeway/Ste 200
Houston, TX 77074
Med Sch Affil: M-04814
Major participating institution for programs in: AN, APM, CCA, CCS, CD, CHN, CN, CRS, D, DR, EM, END, FP, GE, GS, HEM, ICE, ID, IM, MG, MPD, N, NEP, NPM, OBG, OPH, ORS, OTO, P, PCC, PD, PDE, PDI, PHO, PM, PN, PS, PTH, RHU, RNR, TS, TY, U, VIR
Institution ID: 48-0359

Methodist Hospital
6565 Fannin St
Houston, TX 77030-9979
Med Sch Affil: M-04804
Major participating institution for programs in: AI, ALI, AN, APM, CCM, CD, CN, D, DMP, DR, END, GE, GS, HEM, HMP, HSO, ICE, ID, IM, IPM, MPD, N, NEP, NP, NS, ON, OPH, ORS, OSM, OTO, OTR, P, PCC, PCP, PM, PS, PTH, RNR, RO, TS, TY, U, VS
Institution ID: 48-0172

NASA Johnson Space Center
Johnson Space Ctr
Houston, TX 77058
Major participating institution for programs in: GPM
Institution ID: 48-8067

Shriners Hospitals for Children (Houston)
6977 Main St
Houston, TX 77030-1695
Med Sch Affil: G-04814
Major participating institution for programs in: CHN, OP, ORS
Institution ID: 48-0528

St Joseph Hospital
1919 LaBranch St
Houston, TX 77002
Med Sch Affil: M-04814, L-04802
Programs sponsored in: FP, GS, OBG, PS, TY
Major participating institution for programs in: DR, MPD, U
Institution ID: 48-0206

St Luke's Episcopal Hospital
PO Box 20269
Houston, TX 77225-0269
Med Sch Affil: M-04804, L-01602, L-04815, L-04814
Major participating institution for programs in: CD, DR, FP, HSP, ICE, ID, IM, IPM, MG, MPD, NM, PM, PS, PTH, TS, TY, U, VIR
Institution ID: 48-0395

Texas Children's Hospital
6621 Fannin St
Houston, TX 77030-2399
Med Sch Affil: M-04804, L-04814
Major participating institution for programs in: AI, ALI, CCP, CHN, CHP, CN, DR, HMP, HSP, MG, MPD, NM, NP, NPM, OP, ORS, PD, PDC, PDE, PDI, PDO, PDP, PDR, PDS, PG, PHO, PN, PP, PPR, PTH, TS, U, UP
Institution ID: 48-0456

Texas Heart Institute
PO Box 20345/MC 3-116
Houston, TX 77225-0345
Med Sch Affil: L-01602, L-04814, L-02101, L-04815, L-04802
Programs sponsored in: TS
Major participating institution for programs in: MPD
Institution ID: 48-0529

The Institute for Rehabilitation and Research (TIRR)
1333 Moursund
Houston, TX 77030
Med Sch Affil: M-04804
Major participating institution for programs in: PM
Institution ID: 48-0511

University of Texas M D Anderson Cancer Center
1515 Holcombe Blvd
Houston, TX 77030
Med Sch Affil: M-04814, L-04804, L-02012, L-04802
Programs sponsored in: BBK, HMP, PCH, PCP, RO, SP
Major participating institution for programs in: APM, CHN, D, DR, END, GE, GS, HEM, ID, MPD, N, NEP, ON, OTO, P, PCC, PHO, PS, RNR, TS, TY, U, VIR
Institution ID: 48-0404

University of Texas Medical School at Houston
Ste G.103 MSB
6431 Fannin St
PO Box 20708
Houston, TX 77025
Med Sch Affil: M-04814
Programs sponsored in: AN, APM, CCA, CCS, CD, CHN, CHP, CN, CRS, D, DR, EM, END, FP, GE, GS, HEM, ICE, ID, IM, MG, MPD, N, NEP, NPM, OBG, ON, OPH, ORS, OTO, P, PCC, PD, PDE, PDI, PHO, PM, PN, PS, PTH, RHU, RNR, TY, U, VIR
Institution ID: 48-0547

University of Texas Mental Sciences Institute
1300 Moursund
Houston, TX 77030
Med Sch Affil: M-04814
Major participating institution for programs in: CHP
Institution ID: 48-0525

University of Texas School of Public Health
PO Box 20186
Houston, TX 77225-0186
Med Sch Affil: L-04814
Programs sponsored in: GPM
Major participating institution for programs in: GPM
Institution ID: 48-0560

Veterans Affairs Medical Center (Houston)

2002 Holcombe Blvd
Houston, TX 77030-4298
Med Sch Affil: M-04804
Major participating institution for programs in: AN, CD, D, DR, END, GE, GS, HEM, HSO, HSP, ICE, ID, IM, IMG, IPM, MPD, N, NEP, NM, NP, NS, ON, OPH, ORS, OTO, P, PCC, PCP, PM, PS, PTH, RO, TS, TY, U
Institution ID: 48-0326

Lackland AFB

San Antonio Uniformed Services Health Education Consortium

2200 Bergquist Dr/Ste 1
Lackland AFB, TX 78236-5300
Programs sponsored in: AI, ALI, AN, CCA, CCM, CCS, CD, D, DR, EM, END, GE, GS, HO, ID, IM, N, NPM, OBG, OPH, ORS, OTO, P, PCC, PCP, PD, PS, PTH, RHU, TS, TY, U, VIR
Institution ID: 48-8068

Wilford Hall Medical Center (AETC)

2200 Bergquist Dr/Ste 1
Lackland AFB, TX 78236-5300
Med Sch Affil: M-02312, L-04813
Major participating institution for programs in: AI, ALI, AN, APM, CCA, CN, DR, END, GE, GS, ID, IM, N, NEP, NM, OBG, ORS, P, PCC, PS, RHU, TS, TY, VIR
Institution ID: 48-0287

Lubbock

St Mary of the Plains Hospital

4000 24th St
Lubbock, TX 79410-1208
Med Sch Affil: G-04815
Major participating institution for programs in: FP, P
Institution ID: 48-0561

Texas Tech University Health Sciences Center at Lubbock

3601 4th St
Lubbock, TX 79430
Med Sch Affil: M-04815
Programs sponsored in: AN, APM, CD, D, FP, GE, GS, IM, NEP, OBG, OPH, ORS, P, PD, PTH
Institution ID: 48-0534

University Medical Center

602 Indiana Ave
PO Box 5980
Lubbock, TX 79417-5980
Med Sch Affil: M-04815
Major participating institution for programs in: AN, APM, CD, D, FP, GE, GS, IM, NEP, OBG, OPH, P, PD, PTH
Institution ID: 48-0562

McAllen

McAllen Medical Center

301 W Expressway 83
McAllen, TX 78503
Med Sch Affil: G-04813
Major participating institution for programs in: FP
Institution ID: 48-0548

Midland

Memorial Hospital and Medical Center

2200 W Illinois Ave
Midland, TX 79701-9980
Major participating institution for programs in: IM
Institution ID: 48-8032

Nacogdoches

Stephen F Austin State University

1936 North St
Nacogdoches, TX 75962
Major participating institution for programs in: GPM
Institution ID: 48-8069

Odessa

Medical Center Hospital

PO Drawer 7239
500 W 4th
Odessa, TX 79761
Med Sch Affil: M-04815
Major participating institution for programs in: FP, IM, OBG
Institution ID: 48-0588

Texas Tech University Health Sciences Center at Odessa

800 W Fourth St
Odessa, TX 79763-4362
Med Sch Affil: M-04815
Programs sponsored in: FP, IM, MPD, OBG
Institution ID: 48-0589

Port Arthur

St Mary Hospital

3535 Gates Blvd/Ste 100
Port Arthur, TX 77642-1111
Major participating institution for programs in: FP
Institution ID: 48-7021

Reese AFB

US Air Force Hospital (Reese)

250 13th St
Reese AFB, TX 79489
Major participating institution for programs in: OBG
Institution ID: 48-0578

San Antonio

Audie L Murphy Memorial Veterans Hospital (San Antonio)

7400 Merton Minter Blvd
San Antonio, TX 78284-5799
Med Sch Affil: M-04813
Major participating institution for programs in: ADP, AN, APM, CD, CN, D, DR, END, FP, GE, GS, HMP, HO, ID, IM, IMG, MP, N, NEP, NS, OAR, OPH, ORS, OTO, P, PCC, PCP, PM, PTH, RHU, RNR, TS, U, VIR
Institution ID: 48-0530

Baptist Memorial Healthcare System

111 Dallas St
San Antonio, TX 78205-1230
Med Sch Affil: L-04813
Major participating institution for programs in: PTH
Institution ID: 48-0309

Bexar County Forensic Science Center

7337 Louis Pasteur
San Antonio, TX 78229-4565
Programs sponsored in: FOP
Institution ID: 48-8027

Child Guidance Center of San Antonio

2135 Babcock Rd
San Antonio, TX 78229
Med Sch Affil: L-04813
Major participating institution for programs in: CHP
Institution ID: 48-0531

Methodist Healthcare

7700 Floyd Curl Dr
San Antonio, TX 78229
Med Sch Affil: L-04813
Major participating institution for programs in: FSM, OSM, PDI, U
Institution ID: 48-8051

Nix Medical Center

414 Navarro St
San Antonio, TX 78205
Major participating institution for programs in: OSM
Institution ID: 48-7086

Northeastern Baptist Hospital

6811 Village Dr
San Antonio, TX 78217
Major participating institution for programs in: FP
Institution ID: 48-8064

San Antonio Community Hospital

8026 Floyd Curl Dr
San Antonio, TX 78229
Med Sch Affil: L-04813
Major participating institution for programs in: FSM, U
Institution ID: 48-8031

San Antonio Warm Springs Rehabilitation Hospital

5101 Medical Dr
San Antonio, TX 78229
Major participating institution for programs in: PM
Institution ID: 48-8056

Santa Rosa Health Care Corporation

519 W Houston St
PO Box 7330/Station A
San Antonio, TX 78207-3108
Med Sch Affil: M-04813
Programs sponsored in: FP
Major participating institution for programs in: CCP, ORS, PD, PDI, PHO, PP, U
Institution ID: 48-0468

Southwest Neuropsychiatric Institute

8535 Tom Slick Dr
San Antonio, TX 78229
Major participating institution for programs in: CHP
Institution ID: 48-8028

St Luke's Baptist Hospital

7930 Floyd Curl Dr
Box 29100
San Antonio, TX 78229
Med Sch Affil: L-04813
Major participating institution for programs in: FSM, HO, HSO, OSM
Institution ID: 48-8050

University Health Center-Downtown

District DBA
San Antonio, TX 78229-4493
Med Sch Affil: M-04813
Major participating institution for programs in: FP, OPH
Institution ID: 48-0445

University Hospital-South Texas Medical Center

4502 Medical Dr
San Antonio, TX 78284
Med Sch Affil: M-04813
Major participating institution for programs in: AN, APM, BBK, CCP, CD, CN, CPP, CRS, D, DR, END, FP, GE, GS, HMP, HO, HSO, ID, IM, IMG, MP, N, NEP, NM, NPM, NS, OAR, OBG, OPH, ORS, OTO, P, PCC, PCP, PD, PDI, PHO, PM, PTH, RHU, RNR, RO, TS, U, VIR
Institution ID: 48-0522

University of Texas Medical School at San Antonio

Office of Medical Dean
7703 Floyd Curl Dr
San Antonio, TX 78284-7790
Med Sch Affil: M-04813
Programs sponsored in: ADP, AN, APM, BBK, CCP, CD, CHP, CN, CPP, CRS, D, DR, END, FP, FSM, GE, GS, HMP, HO, HSO, ID, IM, IMG, MP, N, NEP, NM, NPM, NS, OAR, OBG, OPH, ORS, OSM, OTO, P, PCC, PCP, PD, PDI, PHO, PM, PP, PTH, RHU, RNR, RO, TS, U, VIR
Institution ID: 48-9501

Temple

Central Texas Veterans Affairs Healthcare System

1901 S First St
Temple, TX 76504
Med Sch Affil: M-04816
Major participating institution for programs in: AN, GS, HMP, IM, OPH, ORS, PS, PUD, U
Institution ID: 48-0505

Scott and White Memorial Hospital

2401 S 31st St
Temple, TX 76508-0001
Med Sch Affil: M-04816
Programs sponsored in: AN, CD, CHP, DR, EM, FP, GE, GS, HMP, IM, MPD, OBG, ON, OPH, ORS, P, PD, PS, PTH, PUD, U
Institution ID: 48-0140

Terrell

Terrell State Hospital

1200 E Brin St
PO Box 70
Terrell, TX 75160-0070
Med Sch Affil: G-04812
Major participating institution for programs in: P
Institution ID: 48-0515

Texarkana

Wadley Regional Medical Center (Texarkana TX)

1000 Pine St/Box 1878
Texarkana, TX 75504
Major participating institution for programs in: FP
Institution ID: 48-8055

Tyler

Mother Frances Hospital Regional Health Care Center

800 E Dawson
Tyler, TX 75701
Major participating institution for programs in: FP
Institution ID: 48-8037

University of Texas Health Center at Tyler

11937 US Highway 271
Tyler, TX 75708
Programs sponsored in: FP, GPM
Institution ID: 48-0587

Waco

Hillcrest Baptist Medical Center

3000 Herring
PO Box 5100
Waco, TX 76708
Med Sch Affil: G-04812
Major participating institution for programs in: FP
Institution ID: 48-0539

McLennan County Medical Education and Research Foundation

1600 Providence Dr
PO Box 3276
Waco, TX 76707
Programs sponsored in: FP
Institution ID: 48-0533

Providence Health Center

6901 Medical Pkwy
PO Box 2589
Waco, TX 76712
Med Sch Affil: G-04812
Major participating institution for programs in: FP
Institution ID: 48-0540

Wichita Falls

Bethania Regional Health Care Center

1600 11th St
Wichita Falls, TX 76301-4388
Med Sch Affil: G-04812
Major participating institution for programs in: FP
Institution ID: 48-0553

North Central Texas Medical Foundation

1301 3rd St
Wichita Falls, TX 76301
Programs sponsored in: FP
Institution ID: 48-0555

United Regional Health Care System

1600 Tenth Street
Wichita Falls, TX 76301-4307
Med Sch Affil: G-04812
Major participating institution for programs in: FP
Institution ID: 48-0554

Utah

Murray

The Orthopedic Specialty Hospital

5848 S 300 East
Murray, UT 84107
Programs sponsored in: OSM
Institution ID: 49-8013

Ogden

McKay-Dee Hospital Center

3939 Harrison Blvd
Ogden, UT 84409-0370
Programs sponsored in: FP
Institution ID: 49-0304

Provo

Utah Valley Regional Medical Center

1034 N 500 West
Provo, UT 84605
Programs sponsored in: FP
Institution ID: 49-8019

Salt Lake City

Children's Center

1855 Medical Cir
Salt Lake City, UT 84112
Major participating institution for programs in: CHP
Institution ID: 49-0448

LDS Hospital

Eighth Ave and C St
Salt Lake City, UT 84143-1001
Med Sch Affil: M-04901
Programs sponsored in: IM, TY
Major participating institution for programs in: GS, OBG, ORS, RO, TS, U
Institution ID: 49-0340

Primary Children's Medical Center

100 N Medical Dr
Salt Lake City, UT 84113-1100
Med Sch Affil: M-04901
Major participating institution for programs in: APM, CCP, CHN, CHP, CN, D, MPD, NPM, NS, OP, ORS, OTO, PD, PDP, PHO, PM, PS, TS, TY, U
Institution ID: 49-0151

Salt Lake Regional Medical Center

1050 E South Temple
Salt Lake City, UT 84102-1599
Med Sch Affil: L-04901
Major participating institution for programs in: FP, GS, ORS, OTO, PS
Institution ID: 49-0297

Shriners Hospital for Children (Intermountain Unit)

Fairfax Ave and Virginia St
Salt Lake City, UT 84103-4399
Med Sch Affil: G-04901
Major participating institution for programs in: OP, ORS
Institution ID: 49-0331

St Mark's Health Care Foundation

2490 S State St
Salt Lake City, UT 84115
Programs sponsored in: FP
Institution ID: 49-8021

St Mark's Hospital

1200 E 3900 S
Salt Lake City, UT 84124
Major participating institution for programs in: FP
Institution ID: 49-0441

State of Utah Department of Health

288 N 1460 West
Salt Lake City, UT 84116
Programs sponsored in: FOP
Institution ID: 49-0445

University Counseling Center

426 Student Services Bldg
Salt Lake City, UT 84112
Major participating institution for programs in: P
Institution ID: 49-8015

University of Utah Medical Center

50 N Medical Dr
Salt Lake City, UT 84132
Med Sch Affil: M-04901
Programs sponsored in: AN, APM, CCP, CD, CHN, CHP, CN, CPP, D, DR, FP, GE, GPM, GS, HMP, HO, HSO, ICE, ID, IM, IMG, MPD, N, NEP, NM, NPM, NR, NS, OBG, OP, OPH, ORS, OSM, OTO, P, PCC, PD, PDP, PHO, PM, PS, PTH, RHU, RNR, RO, TS, U, VIR, VS
Institution ID: 49-0247

University of Utah Neuropsychiatric Institute

501 Chipeta Way
Salt Lake City, UT 84108
Med Sch Affil: L-04901
Major participating institution for programs in: P
Institution ID: 49-8014

University of Utah School of Medicine
50 N Medical Dr
Salt Lake City, UT 84132
Med Sch Affil: M-04901
Major participating institution for programs in: GPM
Institution ID: 49-9501

Valley Mental Health
2001 S State
Ste S2600
Salt Lake City, UT 84190-2450
Major participating institution for programs in: CHP, P
Institution ID: 49-0140

Veterans Affairs Medical Center (Salt Lake City)
500 Foothill Dr
Salt Lake City, UT 84148-0001
Med Sch Affil: M-04901
Major participating institution for programs in: CD, D, DR, GE, GS, ICE, ID, IM, IMG, MPD, N, NEP, NM, NR, NS, OPH, ORS, OTO, P, PM, PS, PTH, RHU, RNR, TS, U, VIR
Institution ID: 49-0251

Vermont

Brattleboro

Brattleboro Retreat
75 Linden St
Brattleboro, VT 05301
Med Sch Affil: G-03201
Major participating institution for programs in: CHP
Institution ID: 50-7002

Burlington

Fletcher Allen Health Care
111 Colchester Ave
Burlington, VT 05401-1429
Med Sch Affil: M-05002, G-03201
Programs sponsored in: AN, APM, CD, CN, DR, END, FP, GE, GS, HO, ID, IM, N, NEP, NPM, NS, OBG, ORS, OTO, P, PCC, PCP, PD, PTH, RHU, VIR
Institution ID: 50-0480

White River Junction

Veterans Affairs Medical Center (White River Junction)
N Hartland Rd
White River Junction, VT 05009
Med Sch Affil: M-03201
Major participating institution for programs in: ADP, D, GE, GS, HO, ID, IM, MP, N, ORS, P, PCC, PS, PTH, RHU, U
Institution ID: 50-0249

Virginia

Alexandria

Alexandria Hospital
4320 Seminary Rd
Alexandria, VA 22304
Med Sch Affil: L-02312, G-01001
Major participating institution for programs in: EM, VIR
Institution ID: 51-0412

Mount Vernon Hospital
2501 Parker's Ln
Alexandria, VA 22306
Major participating institution for programs in: PM
Institution ID: 51-8015

Arlington

Arlington Hospital
1701 N George Mason Dr
Arlington, VA 22205-3698
Med Sch Affil: M-01002, L-02312, L-02012
Programs sponsored in: OSM
Major participating institution for programs in: FSM, GS, NEP, OBG, ORS
Institution ID: 51-0501

Nirschl Orthopedic Clinic
1715 N George Mason Dr/Ste 504
Arlington, VA 22205
Med Sch Affil: G-02312
Major participating institution for programs in: OSM
Institution ID: 51-8023

Blackstone

Blackstone Family Practice Center
920 S Main St
Blackstone, VA 23824
Major participating institution for programs in: FP
Institution ID: 51-8001

Burkeville

Piedmont Geriatric Hospital
Highway 460/360
Burkeville, VA 23922-9999
Institution ID: 51-7005

Chantilly

American Medical Laboratories
14225 Newbrook Dr
Chantilly, VA 22021-0841
Major participating institution for programs in: PTH
Institution ID: 51-8022

Charlottesville

University of Virginia Medical Center
McKim Hall/Rm 1044
Jefferson Park Ave
Charlottesville, VA 22908
Med Sch Affil: M-05101
Programs sponsored in: AI, AN, APM, BBK, CCA, CCM, CCP, CD, CHP, CN, D, DMP, DR, EM, END, FP, GE, GS, HO, HSP, ICE, ID, IM, IMG, MP, N, NEP, NO, NP, NPM, NR, NS, OAR, OBG, OPH, ORS, OSM, OSS, OTO, P, PCC, PCP, PD, PDC, PDE, PDP, PHO, PM, PN, PS, PTH, PYG, RHU, RNR, RO, TS, U, VIR, VS
Major participating institution for programs in: ID
Institution ID: 51-0124

Falls Church

Fairfax Hospital
3300 Gallows Rd
Falls Church, VA 22046
Med Sch Affil: M-01002, M-01001, L-02312, G-05104
Programs sponsored in: PD, PTH
Major participating institution for programs in: APM, EM, FP, GS, OBG, ORS, P, PCC, PS, TY, U
Institution ID: 51-0492

Fort Belvoir

DeWitt Army Community Hospital
US Army Med Dept Activity
Attn: HSXA-DCCS
Fort Belvoir, VA 22060-5901
Med Sch Affil: G-02312
Programs sponsored in: FP, FSM
Institution ID: 51-0377

Hampton

Veterans Affairs Medical Center (Hampton)
100 Emancipation Dr
Hampton, VA 23667
Med Sch Affil: M-05107
Major participating institution for programs in: DR, GS, IM, OPH, P, PM, PTH, U
Institution ID: 51-0508

Lynchburg

Centra Health Inc
3300 Rivermont Ave
Lynchburg, VA 24503
Med Sch Affil: G-05101
Programs sponsored in: FP
Institution ID: 51-0716

Newport News

Riverside Regional Medical Center
500 J Clyde Morris Blvd
Newport News, VA 23601-1976
Med Sch Affil: L-05107, G-05104
Programs sponsored in: FP, FPG, OBG, TY
Institution ID: 51-0108

Norfolk

Children's Hospital of the King's Daughters
601 Children's Ln
Norfolk, VA 23507-1971
Med Sch Affil: M-05107
Major participating institution for programs in: PD, PDI, PTH, U
Institution ID: 51-0490

DePaul Medical Center
150 Kingsley Ln
Norfolk, VA 23505-4602
Med Sch Affil: M-05107
Major participating institution for programs in: DR, EM, GS, IM, OBG
Institution ID: 51-0242

Eastern Virginia Medical School
PO Box 1980
721 Fairfax Ave
Norfolk, VA 23501
Med Sch Affil: M-05107
Programs sponsored in: DR, EM, FP, GS, IFP, IM, OBG, OPH, OTO, P, PD, PDI, PM, PTH, RO, U, VS
Institution ID: 51-0714

Sentara Leigh Hospital
830 Kempsville Rd
Norfolk, VA 23502
Major participating institution for programs in: GS, U
Institution ID: 51-0713

Sentara Norfolk General Hospital
600 Gresham Dr
Norfolk, VA 23507
Med Sch Affil: M-05107
Major participating institution for programs in: DR, EM, FP, GS, IFP, IM, OBG, OPH, OTO, P, PDI, PM, PTH, RO, U, VS
Institution ID: 51-0276

Portsmouth

Maryview Hospital
3636 High St
Portsmouth, VA 23707
Med Sch Affil: L-05107
Major participating institution for programs in: FP, RO
Institution ID: 51-0480

Naval Medical Center (Portsmouth)
620 John Paul Jones Cir
Portsmouth, VA 23708-2197
Med Sch Affil: M-02312, M-05107
Programs sponsored in: AN, APM, EM, GS, IM, OBG, ORS, OTO, P, PD, PTH, TY, U
Major participating institution for programs in: OTO, PS
Institution ID: 51-0314

Portsmouth General Hospital
850 Crawford Pkwy
Portsmouth, VA 23704-2385
Med Sch Affil: M-05107
Major participating institution for programs in: FP, OBG
Institution ID: 51-0256

Richmond

Children's Hospital
2924 Brook Rd
Richmond, VA 23220-1298
Med Sch Affil: G-05104
Major participating institution for programs in: ORS
Institution ID: 51-0291

Columbia-HCA Chippenham Medical Center
7101 Jahnke Rd
Richmond, VA 23225
Med Sch Affil: G-05104
Major participating institution for programs in: FP
Institution ID: 51-0721

Columbia-HCA Johnston-Willis Hospital
2908 Kensington Ave
Richmond, VA 23221
Major participating institution for programs in: FP
Institution ID: 51-0119

Commonwealth of Virginia Department of Health
Main St Station/Ste 214
PO Box 2448
Richmond, VA 23218
Major participating institution for programs in: GPM
Institution ID: 51-0184

Hunter Holmes McGuire VA Medical Center (Richmond)
1201 Broad Rock Rd
Richmond, VA 23249
Med Sch Affil: M-05104
Major participating institution for programs in: AN, CN, D, DR, END, GS, HO, ICE, ID, IM, IMG, N, NM, NS, OPH, ORS, OTO, P, PCC, PM, PS, RO, SCI, TS, U, VS
Institution ID: 51-0148

MCV-Virginia Treatment Center for Children
Box 980489 MCV
Richmond, VA 23298-0489
Med Sch Affil: G-05104
Major participating institution for programs in: CHP, P
Institution ID: 51-0494

Medical College of Virginia Hospitals
West Hospital/6th Fl/S Wing
PO Box 980257
1200 E Broad St
Richmond, VA 23298-0257
Med Sch Affil: M-05104
Programs sponsored in: MPD
Major participating institution for programs in: AI, ALI, AN, APM, CCP, CD, CHN, CHP, CN, D, DR, END, FOP, FP, GE, GPM, GS, HO, ICE, ID, IM, IMG, MG, N, NEP, NM, NP, NPM, NS, OBG, OPH, ORS, OTO, P, PCC, PCH, PCP, PD, PDC, PDI, PM, PN, PS, PTH, RHU, RNR, RO, SCI, TS, U, VS
Institution ID: 51-0487

Medical College of Virginia/Virginia Commonwealth University
1200 E Broad St
PO Box 9805257
Richmond, VA 23298-0257
Med Sch Affil: M-05104
Programs sponsored in: AI, ALI, AN, APM, CCP, CD, CHN, CHP, CN, D, DR, END, FOP, FP, GE, GPM, GS, HO, ICE, ID, IM, IMG, MG, N, NEP, NM, NP, NPM, NS, OBG, OPH, ORS, OTO, P, PCC, PCH, PCP, PD, PDC, PDI, PM, PN, PS, PTH, RHU, RNR, RO, SCI, TS, U, VS
Institution ID: 51-9501

Orthopaedic Research of Virginia
7660 E Parham Rd
Ste 207
Richmond, VA 23294
Programs sponsored in: OSM
Institution ID: 51-8026

St Mary's Hospital
5801 Bremo Rd
Richmond, VA 23226-1999
Med Sch Affil: G-05104
Major participating institution for programs in: PS
Institution ID: 51-8017

Tuckahoe Orthopaedic Associates
8919 Three Chopt Rd
Richmond, VA 23229
Major participating institution for programs in: OSM
Institution ID: 51-8021

Roanoke

Carilion Health System
PO Box 13367
Roanoke, VA 24033-3367
Programs sponsored in: FP, GS, ID, IM, MP, OBG, P, TY
Institution ID: 51-8024

Carilion Roanoke Community Hospital
101 Elm Ave SE
PO Box 12946
Roanoke, VA 24029
Med Sch Affil: M-05101
Major participating institution for programs in: FP, GS, ID, IM, OBG, TY
Institution ID: 51-0197

Carilion Roanoke Memorial Hospital
Belleview at Jefferson St
PO Box 13367
Roanoke, VA 24033-3367
Med Sch Affil: M-05101
Major participating institution for programs in: FP, GS, ID, IM, MP, OBG, ORS, P, TY
Institution ID: 51-0258

Salem

Veterans Affairs Medical Center (Salem)
1970 Blvd
Salem, VA 24153-6483
Med Sch Affil: M-05101
Major participating institution for programs in: GE, GS, ID, IM, MP, ORS, P, U
Institution ID: 51-0513

Staunton

De Jarnette Center
PO Box 2309
Staunton, VA 24402-2309
Major participating institution for programs in: CHP
Institution ID: 51-8002

Virginia Beach

Virginia Beach General Hospital
1060 First Colonial Rd
Virginia Beach, VA 23454-3002
Med Sch Affil: L-05107
Major participating institution for programs in: RO
Institution ID: 51-0514

Winchester

Valley Health System
1830 Amherst St
PO Box 1334
Winchester, VA 22604
Programs sponsored in: FP
Institution ID: 51-8027

Washington

Bremerton

Naval Hospital (Bremerton)
Boone Rd
Bremerton, WA 98312-1898
Med Sch Affil: L-05404, G-02312
Programs sponsored in: FP
Institution ID: 54-7003

Colville

Mount Carmel Hospital
982 E Columbia St
Box 351
Colville, WA 99114
Major participating institution for programs in: FP
Institution ID: 54-8008

Goldendale

Klickitat Valley Hospital
310 Roosevelt St
PO Box 5
Goldendale, WA 98620
Major participating institution for programs in: FP
Institution ID: 54-8010

Olympia

St Peter Hospital

525 Lilly Rd NE
Olympia, WA 98506
Med Sch Affil: L-05404
Programs sponsored in: FP
Institution ID: 54-8004

Omak

Mid-Valley Hospital

810 Valley Way
Box 793
Omak, WA 98841
Major participating institution for programs in: FP
Institution ID: 54-8011

Renton

Valley Medical Center

400 S 43rd St
Renton, WA 98055
Med Sch Affil: L-05404
Programs sponsored in: FP
Major participating institution for programs in: PS
Institution ID: 54-0519

Seattle

Children's Hospital and Medical Center

4800 Sand Point Way NE
PO Box C-5371
Seattle, WA 98105
Med Sch Affil: M-05404
Programs sponsored in: PDS
Major participating institution for programs in: AI, CCP, CHN, CHP, DR, HMP, MG, N, NS, OPH, ORS, PD, PDI, PDP, PDR, PHO, PM, PN, PPR, PS, PTH, TS, U, UP
Institution ID: 54-0311

Fred Hutchinson Cancer Research Center

1100 Fairview Ave N
PO Box 19024
Seattle, WA 98109-1024
Med Sch Affil: L-05404
Major participating institution for programs in: ON, PHO
Institution ID: 54-8001

Group Health Cooperative of Puget Sound

521 Wall St
Seattle, WA 98121-1536
Med Sch Affil: M-05404
Programs sponsored in: FP
Institution ID: 54-0498

Harborview Medical Center

325 Ninth Ave
Seattle, WA 98104-2499
Med Sch Affil: M-05404
Major participating institution for programs in: AN, CCS, CHN, DR, END, GS, HSO, IM, IMG, N, NM, NS, OPH, ORS, P, PM, PS, PTH, PYG, RNR, U, VIR
Institution ID: 54-0405

King County Medical Examiner's Office

325 Ninth Ave
PO Box 359792
Seattle, WA 98104-2499
Med Sch Affil: L-05404
Programs sponsored in: FOP
Institution ID: 54-0515

Northwest Colon and Rectal Clinic, PS

600 Broadway/Ste 400
Seattle, WA 98122
Programs sponsored in: CRS
Institution ID: 54-8005

Northwest Hospital

1550 N 115th St
Seattle, WA 98133
Major participating institution for programs in: CRS
Institution ID: 54-8006

Providence Seattle Medical Center

500 17th Ave
PO Box 34008
Seattle, WA 98124-1008
Med Sch Affil: M-05404
Programs sponsored in: FP
Major participating institution for programs in: GS, IM
Institution ID: 54-0139

Puget Sound Blood Center

921 Terry Ave
Seattle, WA 98104-1256
Programs sponsored in: BBK
Institution ID: 54-8012

Swedish Medical Center-Seattle

747 Broadway
PO Box 14999
Seattle, WA 98114-0999
Med Sch Affil: M-05404
Programs sponsored in: FP, GS
Major participating institution for programs in: CRS, IM, OBG
Institution ID: 54-0481

University of Washington Medical Center

1959 NE Pacific St
Seattle, WA 98195
Med Sch Affil: M-05404
Major participating institution for programs in: AI, AN, APM, CCM, CD, CHN, CHP, D, DR, END, FP, FSM, GE, GS, HEM, HSO, ICE, ID, IM, MG, N, NEP, NM, NP, NPM, NS, OBG, ON, OPH, ORS, OTO, P, PCC, PD, PDI, PDP, PM, PPR, PS, PTH, PYG, RHU, RNR, RO, TS, U, VIR, VS
Institution ID: 54-0209

University of Washington School of Medicine

Box 356340
1959 NE Pacific St/Rm A300
Seattle, WA 98195
Med Sch Affil: M-05404
Programs sponsored in: ADP, AI, AN, APM, CCM, CCP, CCS, CD, CHN, CHP, D, DR, END, FP, FSM, GE, GS, HEM, HMP, HSO, ICE, ID, IM, IMG, MG, N, NEP, NM, NP, NPM, NS, OBG, ON, OPH, ORS, OTO, P, PCC, PD, PDI, PDP, PDR, PFP, PHO, PM, PN, PPR, PS, PTH, PYG, RHU, RNR, RO, TS, U, UP, VIR, VS
Institution ID: 54-0502

University of Washington School of Public Health

HSC F350/SC-30
Seattle, WA 98195-7230
Med Sch Affil: L-05404
Programs sponsored in: GPM
Major participating institution for programs in: GPM
Institution ID: 54-0505

Veterans Affairs Medical Center (Seattle)

1660 S Columbian Way
Seattle, WA 98108
Med Sch Affil: M-05404
Major participating institution for programs in: ADP, APM, CD, DR, END, GS, IM, IMG, N, NM, NS, OPH, ORS, OTO, P, PM, PS, PTH, RHU, RNR, TS, U, VIR, VS
Institution ID: 54-0362

Virginia Mason Medical Center

925 Seneca St/H7-ME
Seattle, WA 98101
Med Sch Affil: L-05404
Programs sponsored in: AN, APM, DR, GS, IM, TY
Major participating institution for programs in: FP, U
Institution ID: 54-0346

Spokane

Deaconess Medical Center

800 W Fifth Ave
PO Box 248
Spokane, WA 99210-0248
Med Sch Affil: L-05404
Programs sponsored in: TY
Major participating institution for programs in: FP, IM
Institution ID: 54-0302

Inland Empire Hospital Services Association

101 W 8th Ave/TAF C9
Spokane, WA 99200
Programs sponsored in: DR, FP, IM, TY
Institution ID: 54-0516

Sacred Heart Medical Center

101 W 8th Ave
PO Box 2555
Spokane, WA 99220-2555
Med Sch Affil: M-05404
Major participating institution for programs in: CHP, DR, FP, IM, P, TY
Institution ID: 54-0402

Shriners Hospitals for Children (Spokane)

PO Box 2472
Spokane, WA 99210-2472
Major participating institution for programs in: ORS
Institution ID: 54-0198

Tacoma

Madigan Army Medical Center

Attn: MCHJ-CG
Tacoma, WA 98431-5000
Med Sch Affil: M-02312, M-05404
Programs sponsored in: CD, DR, EM, FP, GPM, GS, IM, IMG, N, OBG, OPH, ORS, OTO, PD, PTH, PUD, TY, U
Institution ID: 54-0393

Mary Bridge Children's Hospital and Health Center

315 S L St
PO Box 5299
Tacoma, WA 98405
Med Sch Affil: L-05404
Major participating institution for programs in: FP
Institution ID: 54-0513

MultiCare Medical Center

PO Box 5299
Tacoma, WA 98415
Programs sponsored in: FP
Institution ID: 54-8013

Tacoma General Hospital

315 S K St
PO Box 5277
Tacoma, WA 98405
Med Sch Affil: L-05404
Major participating institution for programs in: FP
Institution ID: 54-0266

VA Puget Sound Health Care System-American Lake Div
American Lake VAMC
Tacoma, WA 98493
Major participating institution for programs in: IMG
Institution ID: 54-8003

Western State Hospital
9601 Steilacoom Blvd SW
Tacoma, WA 98498-7213
Major participating institution for programs in: PFP
Institution ID: 54-8014

Vancouver

Southwest Washington Medical Center
PO Box 1600
Vancouver, WA 98668
Programs sponsored in: FP
Institution ID: 54-8007

Yakima

Providence Yakima Medical Center
110 S Ninth Ave
Yakima, WA 98902-3397
Major participating institution for programs in: FP
Institution ID: 54-0509

Yakima Valley Memorial Hospital
2811 Tieton Dr
Yakima, WA 98902
Programs sponsored in: FP
Institution ID: 54-0510

West Virginia

Buckhannon

St Joseph's Hospital
Amalia Dr
Buckhannon, WV 26201-2222
Major participating institution for programs in: NR
Institution ID: 55-8017

Charleston

Charleston Area Medical Center
501 Morris St
PO Box 1547
Charleston, WV 25326-1547
Med Sch Affil: G-05502
Programs sponsored in: CHP, FP, GS, IM, MP, MPD, OBG, P, PD
Major participating institution for programs in: P, PTH, PYN
Institution ID: 55-0350

Clarksburg

Louis A Johnson Veterans Affairs Medical Center
One Medical Center Dr
Clarksburg, WV 26301-4199
Major participating institution for programs in: GS, OPH, OTO, U
Institution ID: 55-0740

United Hospital Center
3 Hospital Plaza
Box 1680
Clarksburg, WV 26302-1680
Programs sponsored in: FP
Institution ID: 55-0738

Huntington

Cabell Huntington Hospital
1340 Hal Greer Blvd
Huntington, WV 25701-0195
Med Sch Affil: M-05502
Major participating institution for programs in: CD, END, FP, GS, IM, OBG, PD, PTH, PUD, TY
Institution ID: 55-0170

Marshall University School of Medicine
1600 Medical Center Dr
Ste 3400
Huntington, WV 25701-3655
Med Sch Affil: M-05502
Programs sponsored in: CD, END, FP, GS, IM, MPD, OBG, PD, PTH, PUD, TY
Institution ID: 55-9501

St Mary's Hospital
2900 First Ave
Huntington, WV 25702-1271
Med Sch Affil: M-05502
Major participating institution for programs in: CD, END, GS, IM, MPD, PTH, PUD, TY
Institution ID: 55-0300

Veterans Affairs Medical Center (Huntington)
1540 Spring Valley Dr
Huntington, WV 25704-9300
Med Sch Affil: M-05502
Major participating institution for programs in: CD, END, GS, IM, MPD, PTH, PUD, TY
Institution ID: 55-0742

Martinsburg

City Hospital
Dry Run Rd
PO Box 1418
Martinsburg, WV 25401
Major participating institution for programs in: FP
Institution ID: 55-7031

Veterans Affairs Medical Center (Martinsburg)
Charles Town Rd
Martinsburg, WV 25401-0205
Med Sch Affil: G-01001
Major participating institution for programs in: OPH
Institution ID: 55-0210

Morgantown

HealthSouth Mountain Regional Rehabilitation Hospital
1160 Van Voorhis
Morgantown, WV 26505
Institution ID: 55-8018

Monongalia General Hospital
1000 JD Anderson Dr
Morgantown, WV 26505
Major participating institution for programs in: ORS, TS
Institution ID: 55-0745

West Virginia University Hospitals
PO Box 8058
Morgantown, WV 26506-8058
Programs sponsored in: AN, APM, CD, CHN, CN, D, DMP, DR, EM, FP, FPP, GS, HO, ID, IM, MN, MP, MPD, N, NEP, NP, NR, NS, OBG, OPH, ORS, OTO, P, PCC, PD, PTH, PYN, RNR, TS, U
Major participating institution for programs in: TS
Institution ID: 55-0426

West Virginia University School of Medicine
PO Box 9000
Morgantown, WV 26506-9000
Programs sponsored in: GPM
Institution ID: 55-9502

South Charleston

Thomas Memorial Hospital
4605 MacCorkle Ave SE
South Charleston, WV 25309
Major participating institution for programs in: FP
Institution ID: 55-0433

Wheeling

Ohio Valley Medical Center
2000 Eoff St
Wheeling, WV 26003
Programs sponsored in: IM
Institution ID: 55-0425

Wheeling Hospital
40 Medical Pk
Wheeling, WV 26003-8110
Programs sponsored in: FP
Institution ID: 55-0431

Wisconsin

Antigo

Langlade Memorial Hospital
112 E Fifth Ave
Antigo, WI 54409-2796
Major participating institution for programs in: FP
Institution ID: 56-8026

Appleton

Appleton Medical Center
1818 N Meade St
Appleton, WI 54911
Med Sch Affil: G-05605
Major participating institution for programs in: FP
Institution ID: 56-0724

St Elizabeth Hospital
1506 S Oneida St
Appleton, WI 54915-1397
Med Sch Affil: G-05605
Major participating institution for programs in: FP
Institution ID: 56-7001

Baraboo

St Clare Hospital and Health Services
707 14th St
Baraboo, WI 53913-1597
Major participating institution for programs in: FP
Institution ID: 56-8021

Eau Claire

Luther Hospital
1221 Whipple St/Call Box 5
Eau Claire, WI 54702-4105
Med Sch Affil: G-05605
Major participating institution for programs in: FP
Institution ID: 56-0399

Sacred Heart Hospital
900 W Clairemont Ave
Eau Claire, WI 54701
Med Sch Affil: G-05605
Major participating institution for programs in: FP
Institution ID: 56-0716

Janesville

Mercy Health System
1000 Mineral Point Ave
PO Box 5003
Janesville, WI 53547-5003
Programs sponsored in: FP, FSM
Institution ID: 56-0333

Kenosha

Medical College of Wisconsin
900 Wood Rd
Kenosha, WI 53141
Major participating institution for programs in: GPM
Institution ID: 56-0451

St Catherine's Hospital
3556 Seventh Ave
Kenosha, WI 53140
Major participating institution for programs in: FP
Institution ID: 56-0732

La Crosse

Franciscan Skemp Healthcare-La Crosse Campus
700 West Ave S
La Crosse, WI 54601-4783
Programs sponsored in: FP
Institution ID: 56-0718

Gundersen Clinic
1910 South Ave
La Crosse, WI 54601-9980
Major participating institution for programs in: GS, IM, TY
Institution ID: 56-8031

Gundersen Lutheran Medical Foundation
1836 South Ave
La Crosse, WI 54601
Programs sponsored in: GS, IM, TY
Institution ID: 56-8030

Lutheran Hospital-La Crosse
1910 South Ave
La Crosse, WI 54601-9980
Med Sch Affil: M-05605
Major participating institution for programs in: FP, GS, IM, TY
Institution ID: 56-0355

Madison

American Red Cross Blood Services-Badger Region
Sheboygan Ave
PO Box 5905
Madison, WI 53705
Major participating institution for programs in: BBK
Institution ID: 56-8017

HCA Parkway Hospital
6001 Research Park Blvd
Madison, WI 53719
Major participating institution for programs in: CHP
Institution ID: 56-8019

Mendota Mental Health Institute
301 Troy Dr
Madison, WI 53704-1599
Med Sch Affil: L-05605
Major participating institution for programs in: CHP, PFP, PYG
Institution ID: 56-0437

Meriter Hospital
202 S Park St
Madison, WI 53715-1599
Med Sch Affil: M-05605
Major participating institution for programs in: NS, OBG, ORS, OTO, P, PD, PS, PTH, U
Institution ID: 56-8018

St Marys Hospital Medical Center
707 S Mills St
Madison, WI 53715-0450
Med Sch Affil: G-05605
Major participating institution for programs in: FP, OBG, ORS, PS, TS, U
Institution ID: 56-0450

University of Wisconsin Hospital and Clinics
600 Highland Ave/H4/823
Madison, WI 53792-8310
Med Sch Affil: M-05605
Programs sponsored in: AI, AN, BBK, CCA, CCP, CD, CHP, D, DR, END, GE, GS, HEM, HMP, ID, IM, IMG, MG, MSR, N, NEP, NM, NPM, NRN, NS, OBG, ON, OPH, ORS, OSM, OTO, P, PCC, PCP, PD, PDE, PDP, PG, PHO, PM, PS, PTH, PYG, RHU, RNR, RO, TS, U, VIR
Major participating institution for programs in: FP, P
Institution ID: 56-0176

University of Wisconsin Medical School
1300 University Ave
Madison, WI 53706
Programs sponsored in: FP
Institution ID: 56-9501

William S Middleton Veterans Hospital
Attn: Chief of Staff
2500 Overlook Terr
Madison, WI 53705
Med Sch Affil: M-05605
Major participating institution for programs in: AI, AN, CCA, CD, D, DR, END, GE, GS, HEM, ID, IM, IMG, N, NEP, NM, NRN, NS, ON, OPH, ORS, OTO, P, PCC, PTH, PYG, RHU, RNR, U, VIR
Institution ID: 56-0218

Marshfield

Marshfield Clinic-St Joseph's Hospital
1000 N Oak Ave
Marshfield, WI 54449-5777
Med Sch Affil: M-05605
Programs sponsored in: GS, IM, MPD, PD, TY
Major participating institution for programs in: D
Institution ID: 56-0264

Mauston

Mile Bluff Medical Center (Mauston)
1050 Division St
Mauston, WI 53948
Major participating institution for programs in: FP
Institution ID: 56-8024

Menomonee Falls

Community Memorial Hospital
W180 N8085 Town Hall Rd
PO Box 408
Menomonee Falls, WI 53052-0408
Major participating institution for programs in: RO
Institution ID: 56-8029

Menomonie

Myrtle Werth Medical Center
2321 Stout Rd
Menomonie, WI 54751
Major participating institution for programs in: FP
Institution ID: 56-8022

Milwaukee

Aurora Health Care
Outpatient Health Ctr
945 N 12th St
Milwaukee, WI 53201
Programs sponsored in: CD, DR, FP, GE, ICE, IM, IMG, NM, OBG, P, TY
Institution ID: 56-8020

Blood Center of Southeastern Wisconsin
1701 W Wisconsin Ave
Milwaukee, WI 53233-2194
Med Sch Affil: G-05606
Major participating institution for programs in: BBK
Institution ID: 56-0737

Children's Hospital of Wisconsin
9000 W Wisconsin Ave
PO Box 1997
Milwaukee, WI 53201
Med Sch Affil: M-05606, L-05605
Major participating institution for programs in: AI, CCP, CHN, CHP, CN, DR, HSP, NPM, NS, OP, ORS, OTO, PD, PDP, PDR, PG, PHO, PS, TS, U
Institution ID: 56-0237

Clement J Zablocki Veterans Affairs Medical Center
5000 W National Ave
Milwaukee, WI 53295-1000
Med Sch Affil: M-05606
Major participating institution for programs in: AI, AN, CD, CHN, CN, D, DR, END, GE, GS, HO, ID, IM, IMG, MN, N, NEP, NM, NS, OPH, ORS, OTO, P, PCC, PM, PS, PTH, RHU, RO, TS, U, VIR
Institution ID: 56-0354

Columbia Hospital
2025 E Newport Ave
Milwaukee, WI 53211
Med Sch Affil: M-05606
Major participating institution for programs in: FP, P
Institution ID: 56-0433

Froedtert Memorial Lutheran Hospital
9200 W Wisconsin Ave
PO Box 26099
Milwaukee, WI 53226-3522
Med Sch Affil: M-05606
Major participating institution for programs in: AI, AN, APM, BBK, CCA, CCS, CD, CHN, CN, D, DR, EM, END, FP, FSM, GE, GS, HMP, HO, HSP, ID, IM, MN, N, NEP, NM, NPM, NS, OBG, OPH, ORS, OSS, OTO, P, PCC, PM, PS, PTH, RHU, RNR, RO, TS, U, VIR, VS
Institution ID: 56-0739

Medical College of Wisconsin Affiliated Hospitals Inc
8701 Watertown Plank Rd
Milwaukee, WI 53226
Programs sponsored in: AI, AN, APM, BBK, CCA, CCP, CCS, CD, CHN, CHP, CN, D, DR, EM, END, FP, FPP, FSM, GE, GPM, GS, HMP, HO, HSP, ID, IM, IMG, MN, MPD, N, NEP, NM, NPM, NS, OBG, OP, OPH, ORS, OSS, OTO, P, PCC, PD, PDP, PDR, PFP, PG, PHO, PM, PMP, PS, PTH, RHU, RNR, RO, TS, U, VIR, VS
Institution ID: 56-0441

Milwaukee County Medical Examiner's Office
933 W Highland Ave
Milwaukee, WI 53233-1445
Programs sponsored in: FOP
Institution ID: 56-8016

Milwaukee County Mental Health Complex
9455 Watertown Plank Rd
Milwaukee, WI 53226-3559
Med Sch Affil: M-05606
Major participating institution for programs in: P, PFP
Institution ID: 56-0146

Sinai Samaritan Medical Center
945 N 12th St
PO Box 342
Milwaukee, WI 53201-0342
Med Sch Affil: M-05605, G-05606
Major participating institution for programs in: CD, GE, ICE, IM, IMG, OBG, P
Institution ID: 56-0303

St Joseph's Hospital
5000 W Chambers St
Milwaukee, WI 53210
Med Sch Affil: M-05606
Programs sponsored in: DR, TY
Major participating institution for programs in: GE
Institution ID: 56-0370

St Luke's Medical Center
PO Box 2901
Milwaukee, WI 53201-2901
Med Sch Affil: M-05605, G-05606
Major participating institution for programs in: DR, FP, ICE, NM, PM, PTH, TY
Institution ID: 56-0337

St Mary's Hospital of Milwaukee
2323 N Lake Dr
Milwaukee, WI 53211
Med Sch Affil: M-05606
Major participating institution for programs in: FP
Institution ID: 56-0167

St Michael Hospital
2400 W Villard Ave
Milwaukee, WI 53209
Med Sch Affil: G-05606
Major participating institution for programs in: FP
Institution ID: 56-0180

Racine

All Saints Healthcare System, Inc
1320 Wisconsin Ave
Racine, WI 53403-1987
Major participating institution for programs in: FP
Institution ID: 56-8028

St Mary's Medical Center
3801 Spring St
Racine, WI 53405
Major participating institution for programs in: FP
Institution ID: 56-8027

Waukesha

Waukesha Memorial Hospital
725 American Ave
Waukesha, WI 53188-5099
Med Sch Affil: G-05606
Major participating institution for programs in: FP
Institution ID: 56-0722

Wausau

Wausau Hospital
333 Pine Ridge Blvd
Wausau, WI 54401-4187
Med Sch Affil: G-05605
Major participating institution for programs in: FP
Institution ID: 56-0411

Wauwatosa

Milwaukee Psychiatric Hospital-Dewey Center
1220 Dewey Ave
Wauwatosa, WI 53213-2504
Med Sch Affil: G-05606
Major participating institution for programs in: CHP
Institution ID: 56-0400

Wyoming

Casper

Wyoming Medical Center
1233 E 2nd St
Casper, WY 82601
Major participating institution for programs in: FP
Institution ID: 57-0100

Cheyenne

United Medical Center
300 E 23rd St
Cheyenne, WY 82001-3790
Major participating institution for programs in: FP
Institution ID: 57-0106

Veterans Affairs Center
2360 E Pershing Blvd
Cheyenne, WY 82001-5392
Major participating institution for programs in: FP
Institution ID: 57-8001

Laramie

University of Wyoming College of Health Sciences
Box 3432
Laramie, WY 82071
Programs sponsored in: FP
Institution ID: 57-9501

Appendix A Combined Specialty Programs

Combined specialty programs have been approved by each respective specialty board; resident physicians completing these programs are eligible for board certification. Neither the Accreditation Council for Graduate Medical Education (ACGME) nor the Residency Review Committees accredit combined programs; they accredit each specialty program separately. Requests for information about the guidelines for these programs should be directed to the specialty boards at the addresses listed in Appendix B. Applicants to combined specialty programs are encouraged to review requirements for admission to the certification process of each board in Appendix B of this *Directory*.

Internal Medicine/Emergency Medicine

The American Board of Internal Medicine and the American Board of Emergency Medicine offer dual certification for candidates who have completed at least 2 1/2 years of suitable accredited training in each specialty. A combined residency consists of 5 years of balanced education in the two disciplines. It is strongly recommended that the participating residencies be in the same academic health center.

To be eligible for dual certification, the resident must satisfactorily complete 60 months of combined education, which must be verified by the directors of both programs. The certifying examinations cannot be taken until all 5 years are completed.

Internal Medicine/Family Practice

The American Board of Internal Medicine and the American Board of Family Practice offer dual certification for candidates who have satisfactorily completed 4 years of combined training in programs approved by both boards.

To be eligible for dual certification, combined residency training in internal medicine and family practice must include at least 48 months of balanced education in the two disciplines and be verified by the training director(s) of the program. The written certifying examinations cannot be taken until all required years in both specialties are completed.

Internal Medicine/Neurology

The American Board of Internal Medicine and the American Board of Psychiatry and Neurology offer dual certification for candidates who have completed 5 years of combined training suitable to both boards. A combined residency in internal medicine and neurology must include at least 5 years of coherent education integral to residencies in the two disciplines. It is strongly recommended that the participating residencies be in the same institution.

To meet eligibility for dual certification, the resident must satisfactorily complete 60 months of training, which must be verified by the directors of both programs. The written certifying examinations cannot be taken until all required years in both specialties are satisfactorily completed.

Internal Medicine/Pediatrics

The American Board of Internal Medicine and the American Board of Pediatrics offer dual certification in internal medicine and pediatrics. A combined residency must include at least 2 years in each specialty, for a total of 4 years of coherent training integral to residencies in the two disciplines. The participating residencies should be in the same academic health center. Continuity clinics in each specialty should be provided throughout the 4 years.

To meet eligibility requirements for dual certification, the resident must satisfactorily complete 48 months of combined education, and clinical competence in both specialties must be verified by the directors of both programs. The certifying examinations can-

Combined Specialty Programs

not be taken until all required years in both specialties are satisfactorily completed.

Internal Medicine/Physical Medicine and Rehabilitation

The American Board of Internal Medicine and the American Board of Physical Medicine and Rehabilitation offer dual certification for candidates who have completed at least 2 and a half years of suitable accredited training in each specialty. A combined residency must include at least 5 years of coherent training integral to residencies in the two disciplines. It is strongly recommended that the participating residencies be in the same institution.

To meet eligibility requirements for dual certification, the resident must satisfactorily complete 60 months of combined education, which must be verified by the directors of both programs. The written certifying examinations cannot be taken until required training in a specialty has been satisfactorily completed. The certifying examination in internal medicine cannot be taken prior to the fall of the fifth year in the combined program.

Internal Medicine/Preventive Medicine

The American Board of Internal Medicine (ABIM) and the American Board of Preventive Medicine (ABPM) offer dual certification for candidates who have completed a minimum of 4 years of accredited training in combined internal medicine/preventive medicine programs that meet the *Guidelines for Combined Internal Medicine - Preventive Medicine Residency Training Programs* approved by ABPM and ABIM. In addition to satisfactory completion of the combined training programs, applicants for the ABPM certifying examination must have completed the required year of preventive medicine practice to qualify.

Internal Medicine/Psychiatry

The American Board of Internal Medicine and the American Board of Psychiatry and Neurology offer dual certification in internal medicine and psychiatry. A combined residency must include at least 5 years of coherent education integral to residencies in the two disciplines. Participating residencies must be in the same institution.

To meet eligibility requirements for dual certification, the resident must satisfactorily complete 60 months of combined education, which must be verified by the directors of both programs. The written certifying examinations cannot be taken until all required years in both specialties are satisfactorily completed.

Neurology/Physical Medicine and Rehabilitation

The American Board of Psychiatry and Neurology and the American Board of Physical Medicine and Rehabilitation offer dual certification in neurology and physical medicine and rehabilitation. A combined residency must include 5 years of combined education. This combined training must follow a year in a residency program that meets the requirements for neurology and should be completed in the same institution. All required years in both specialties must be satisfactorily completed prior to admission to the certifying examinations of each board.

Neurology/Diagnostic Radiology/Neuroradiology

The American Board of Psychiatry and Neurology and the American Board of Radiology offer certification in neurology, diagnostic radiology, and neuroradiology. The combined residency must include at least 7 years of coherent training integral to all three residencies. It is recommended that the participating residencies be in the same academic health center.

To meet eligibility requirements for triple certification, the resident must satisfactorily complete 84 months of combined training, which must be verified by the directors of each program. Lacking verification of acceptable clinical competence in the combined program, the resident must satisfactorily complete the standard length of residency training and all other requirements before each certifying examination may be taken. Applicants may not take the certifying examination until all required years of training have been completed. In order to be eligible for the neuroradiology exam, a resident must have completed certification in both diagnostic radiology and neurology.

Pediatrics/Emergency Medicine

The American Board of Pediatrics and the American Board of Emergency Medicine offer dual certification for candidates who fulfill the requirements of both boards by completing joint training in 5 years. All 5 years should be completed in the same combined program; exceptions must be approved in advance by both boards. Applicants may not take the certifying examinations until all required years in both specialties have been completed.

Pediatrics/Medical Genetics

The American Board of Pediatrics and the American Board of Medical Genetics offer dual certification for candidates who fulfill the requirements of both boards by completing joint training in 5 years. All 5 years should be completed in the same combined program; exceptions must be approved in advance by both boards. Applicants may not take the certifying examinations until all required years in both specialties have been completed.

Pediatrics/Physical Medicine and Rehabilitation

The American Board of Pediatrics and the American Board of Physical Medicine and Rehabilitation permit applicants interested in pediatric rehabilitation to qualify for admission to the certifying examinations of both boards by completing a 5-year combined program. All 5 years should be completed at one academic institution; exceptions must be approved in advance by both boards.

Applicants may not take the certifying examinations until all required years in both specialties have been completed.

Pediatrics/Psychiatry/Child and Adolescent Psychiatry

The American Board of Pediatrics, the American Board of Psychiatry and Neurology, and the Committee on Certification in Child and Adolescent Psychiatry have developed a committee that is overseeing training via a different format. This is a 5-year curriculum with 24 months of pediatrics, 18 months of adult psychiatry, and 18 months of child and adolescent psychiatry. Completion of the program will satisfy the training requirement for certification in all three areas. Applicants pursuing training in these programs may not take the certifying examinations until all training has been completed. Credit for training via this route may be obtained only by training in one of these programs.

Psychiatry/Family Practice

The American Board of Family Practice and the American Board of Psychiatry and Neurology offer dual certification in family practice and psychiatry. A combined residency in family practice and psychiatry must include at least 5 years of coherent training integral to residencies in the two disciplines. It is required that the combined training be under the aegis of the same academic institution.

To meet eligibility for dual certification, the resident must satisfactorily complete 60 months of combined training, which must be verified by the directors of both programs. The certifying examinations may not be taken until all required years of training in both specialties are satisfactorily completed.

Psychiatry/Neurology

The American Board of Psychiatry and Neurology has established guidelines for combined training in psychiatry and neurology. A combined residency must include one postgraduate year (PGY1) of training that is acceptable to neurology plus a minimum of 5 years of combined residency training. The 5 years of residency training are usually taken at one approved institution but may be taken at no more than two approved institutions.

Combined Specialty Programs

		Accred Length(s)	GY1*	# of Programs	
800	MPD	4	Y	108	Internal Medicine/Pediatrics
805	MEM	5	Y	10	Internal Medicine/Emergency Medicine
810	MPM	5	Y	15	Internal Medicine/Physical Medicine and Rehabilitation
815	MP	5	Y	27	Internal Medicine/Psychiatry
820	FPP	5	Y	13	Psychiatry/Family Practice
825	EMP	5	Y	5	Pediatrics/Emergency Medicine
830	CPP	5	Y	10	Pediatrics/Psychiatry/Child and Adolescent Psychiatry
835	PMP	5	Y	6	Pediatrics/Physical Medicine and Rehabilitation
840	IFP	4	Y	3	Internal Medicine/Family Practice
845	MN	5	Y	15	Internal Medicine/Neurology
850	NPR	5	Y	2	Neurology/Physical Medicine and Rehabilitation
851	IPM	4	Y	5	Internal Medicine/Preventive Medicine
855	PYN	5	Y	9	Psychiatry/Neurology
860	NRN	7	Y	4	Neurology/Diagnostic Radiology/Neuroradiology
865	PMG	5	Y	2	Pediatrics/Medical Genetics
Total				**234**	

Y = Graduate year 1 positions available

Combined Specialty Programs

Internal Medicine/ Emergency Medicine

California

Sylmar

UCLA Medical Center Program
Sponsor: Olive View-UCLA Medical Center
Program Director:
Jill Klessig, MD
14445 Olive View Dr
Sylmar, CA 91342
Tel: 818 895-9397 *Fax:* 818 895-9516
E-mail: jklessig@ucla.edu
Internet: http://www:medsch.ucla.edu/residencies
Accred Length: 5 Years *Program Size:* 6 (*GY1:* 2)
Program ID: 805-05-44-016

Delaware

Wilmington

Christiana Care Health Services Program
Sponsor: Christiana Care Health Services Inc
Program Director:
Charles L Reese IV, MD
Christiana Care Health Services
Emergency Med/Int Med Program
PO Box 6001
Newark, DE 19718-6001
Tel: 302 733-1840 *Fax:* 302 733-1633
E-mail: creese@christianacare.org
Internet: http://www.christianacare.org/residency/emim
Accred Length: 5 Years *Program Size:* 13 (*GY1:* 3)
Program ID: 805-09-44-010

Illinois

Chicago

University of Illinois College of Medicine at Chicago Program
Sponsor: University of Illinois College of Medicine at Chicago
University of Illinois Hospital and Clinics
Program Director:
Craig A Rosenberg, MD
Univ of Illinois Hospital
M/C 722
1740 W Taylor St
Chicago, IL 60612-0612
Tel: 312 996-4160 *Fax:* 312 996-2727
E-mail: car@uic.edu
Internet:
http://www.uic.edu/depts/mpim/imem/ieindex.html
Accred Length: 5 Years *Program Size:* 10 (*GY1:* 2)
Program ID: 805-16-44-012

Louisiana

New Orleans

Louisiana State University Program
Sponsor: Louisiana State University School of Medicine
Louisiana State University Medical College Campus
Medical Center of Louisiana-University Hospital Campus
Program Director:
Dayton W Daberkow II, MD
Jorge Martinez, MD
Louisiana State Univ Med Ctr
1542 Tulane Ave
New Orleans, LA 70112-2822
Tel: 504 568-4600 *Fax:* 504 568-7885
E-mail: ddaberkow@lsumc.edu
Accred Length: 5 Years *Program Size:* 8 (*GY1:* 2)
Program ID: 805-21-44-015

Maryland

Baltimore

University of Maryland Program
Sponsor: University of Maryland Medical System
Mercy Medical Center
Program Director:
Amal Mattu, MD
Univ of Maryland Med Ctr
Div of Emerg Med/Int Med
419 W Redwood St/Ste 280
Baltimore, MD 21201
Tel: 410 328-8025 *Fax:* 410 328-8028
E-mail: emera@surgery1.ab.umd.edu
Internet:
http://www.umm.edu/center/training/residency.html
Accred Length: 5 Years *Program Size:* 7 (*GY1:* 2)
Program ID: 805-23-44-014

Michigan

Detroit

Henry Ford Hospital Program
Sponsor: Henry Ford Hospital
Program Director:
David Portelli, MD
Emergency Med/Int Med Program
Henry Ford Hospital
2799 W Grand Blvd/ECFP-1
Detroit, MI 48202
Tel: 313 916-1553 *Fax:* 313 916-7437
Internet: http://www.henryfordhealth.org
Accred Length: 5 Years *Program Size:* 10 (*GY1:* 2)
Program ID: 805-25-44-003

Wayne State University Program
Sponsor: Wayne State University/Detroit Medical Center
Detroit Receiving Hospital and University Health Center
Harper Hospital
Program Director:
Brooks F Bock, MD
Detroit Receiving Hospital
8D-University Health Ctr
4201 St Antoine
Detroit, MI 48201-2194
Tel: 313 993-2530 *Fax:* 313 993-7703
E-mail: rwahl@med.wayne.edu
Internet: http://www.med.wayne.edu/er/
Accred Length: 5 Years *Program Size:* 5 (*GY1:* 0)
Program ID: 805-25-44-004

New York

New Hyde Park

Albert Einstein College of Medicine at Long Island Jewish Medical Center Program
Sponsor: Long Island Jewish Medical Center
Program Director:
Kumar Alagappan, MD
Long Island Jewish Med Ctr
270-05 76th Ave
New Hyde Park, NY 11040
Tel: 718 470-7873 *Fax:* 718 470-9113
E-mail: alagappa@lij.edu
Internet: http://www.lij.edu/lij-homepage-ns.html
Accred Length: 5 Years *Program Size:* 10 (*GY1:* 2)
Program ID: 805-35-44-011

New York

Beth Israel Medical Center Program
Sponsor: Beth Israel Medical Center
Mount Sinai Medical Center
Program Director:
Marcelo Sandoval, MD
Adrienne M Fleckman, MD
Beth Israel Med Ctr
Dept of Emergency Med
First Ave at 16th St
New York, NY 10003
Tel: 212 420-3948 *Fax:* 212 420-2863
E-mail: emergmedres@bethisraelny.org
Accred Length: 5 Years *Program Size:* 3 (*GY1:* 0)
Program ID: 805-35-44-005

Pennsylvania

Pittsburgh

Allegheny General Hospital Program
Sponsor: Allegheny General Hospital
Program Director:
Dennis P Hanlon, MD
Allegheny General Hospital
Dept of Emergency Med
320 E North Ave
Pittsburgh, PA 15212-9986
Tel: 412 359-4905 *Fax:* 412 359-4963
Accred Length: 5 Years *Program Size:* 10 (*GY1:* 2)
Program ID: 805-41-44-006

Internal Medicine/ Family Practice

Louisiana

New Orleans

Alton Oschner Medical Foundation Program

Sponsor: Alton Ochsner Medical Foundation
Leonard J Chabert Medical Center

Program Director:
Donald T Erwin, MD
William R Brandon, MD MPH
Alton Ochsner Med Foundation
Dept of Grad Med Educ
1516 Jefferson Hwy
New Orleans, LA 70121
Tel: 504 842-3260 *Fax:* 504 842-3193
E-mail: derwin@ochsner.org
Internet: http://www.ochsner.org
Accred Length: 4 Years *Program Size:* 6 (*GY1:* 2)
Program ID: 840-21-44-002

Ohio

Cleveland

Case Western Reserve University (MetroHealth) Program

Sponsor: MetroHealth Medical Center

Program Director:
Michael J McFarlane, MD
Mary Corrigan, MD
MetroHealth Med Ctr
Dept of Med
2500 MetroHealth Dr/G533
Cleveland, OH 44109-1998
Tel: 216 778-3886 *Fax:* 216 778-5823
E-mail: medres@metrohealth.org
Internet: http://www.metrohealth.org
Accred Length: 4 Years *Program Size:* 8 (*GY1:* 2)
Program ID: 840-38-44-004

Virginia

Norfolk

Eastern Virginia Medical School Program

Sponsor: Eastern Virginia Medical School
Sentara Norfolk General Hospital

Program Director:
James G Dixon, MD
Eastern Virginia Med Sch
Dept of Internal Med
825 Fairfax Ave
Norfolk, VA 23507-1912
Tel: 757 446-8910 *Fax:* 757 446-5242
E-mail: lbrennan@intmed1.evms.edu.
Internet:
http://www.evms.edu/intmed/residents/index.htm
Accred Length: 4 Years *Program Size:* 16 (*GY1:* 4)
Program ID: 840-51-44-001

Internal Medicine/ Neurology

Alabama

Mobile

University of South Alabama Program

Sponsor: University of South Alabama Medical Center

Program Director:
Ronald Allison, MD
William Hamilton, DO
Univ of South Alabama
2451 Fillingim St
MCSB 1215
Mobile, AL 36617
Tel: 334 471-7891 *Fax:* 334 471-1291
E-mail: pgreen@usamail.southal.edu
Internet: http://southmed/com/intmed/index.html
Accred Length: 5 Years *Program Size:* 1 (*GY1:* 1)
Program ID: 845-01-44-015

Arizona

Tucson

University of Arizona Program

Sponsor: University of Arizona College of Medicine
University Medical Center
Veterans Affairs Medical Center (Tucson)

Program Director:
David M Labiner, MD
Richard Mandel, MD
Univ of Arizona Health Sciences Ctr
1501 N Campbell Ave
PO Box 245040
Tucson, AZ 85724-5040
Tel: 520 626-2006 *Fax:* 520 626-2111
E-mail: labinerd@u.arizona.edu
Internet: http://www.ahsc.arizona.edu/neurology/
Accred Length: 5 Years *Program Size:* 3 (*GY1:* 1)
Program ID: 845-03-44-010

California

Los Angeles

University of Southern California Program

Sponsor: Los Angeles County-USC Medical Center

Program Director:
Christi Heck, MD
Univ of Southern California Sch of Med
Dept of Neurology
1510 San Pablo St/Ste 646
Los Angeles, CA 90033
Tel: 213 342-5793 *Fax:* 213 342-5794
Accred Length: 5 Years *Program Size:* 3 (*GY1:* 1)
Program ID: 845-05-44-006

San Francisco

University of California (San Francisco) Program

Sponsor: University of California (San Francisco) School of Medicine
San Francisco General Hospital Medical Center
Veterans Affairs Medical Center (San Francisco)

Program Director:
John W Engstrom, MD
Harry Hollander, MD
Univ of California San Francisco
505 Parnassus Ave
Box 0114/Rm M798
San Francisco, CA 94143
Tel: 415 476-1489 *Fax:* 415 502-3428
Accred Length: 5 Years *Program Size:* 3 (*GY1:* 3)
Program ID: 845-05-44-012

Indiana

Indianapolis

Indiana University School of Medicine Program

Sponsor: Indiana University School of Medicine
Clarian IU Hospital
Richard L Roudebush Veterans Affairs Medical Center
William N Wishard Memorial Hospital

Program Director:
Jose Biller, MD
Indiana Univ Sch of Med
Dept of Neurology
545 Barnhill Dr/EM125
Indianapolis, IN 46202-5124
Tel: 317 274-4455 *Fax:* 317 274-2384
E-mail: jbiller@indvax.iupui.edu
Internet: http://www.medlib.iupui.edu/neuro/
Accred Length: 5 Years *Program Size:* 2 (*GY1:* 1)
Program ID: 845-17-44-009

Louisiana

New Orleans

Tulane University Program

Sponsor: Tulane University School of Medicine
Louisiana State University Medical College Campus
Tulane University Hospital and Clinics
Veterans Affairs Medical Center (New Orleans)

Program Director:
Anne L Foundas, MD
Marc J Kahn, MD
Tulane Univ Sch of Med
Dept of Neurology TB-52
1430 Tulane Ave
New Orleans, LA 70112-2699
Tel: 504 588-2241 *Fax:* 504 584-3695
E-mail: neuro@mailhost.tcs.tulane.edu
Accred Length: 5 Years *Program Size:* 3 (*GY1:* 1)
Program ID: 845-21-44-005

Combined Specialty Programs

Maryland

Baltimore

University of Maryland Program
Sponsor: University of Maryland Medical System
Veterans Affairs Medical Center (Baltimore)
Program Director:
Susan D Wolfsthal, MD
Janine L Good, MD
Univ of Maryland
22 S Greene St/Rm N3E09
Baltimore, MD 21201-1595
Tel: 410 328-2388 *Fax:* 410 328-0267
E-mail: umdmed@medicine.ab.umd.edu
Internet: http://www.umm.edu
Accred Length: 5 Years *Program Size:* 2 (*GY1:* 2)
Program ID: 845-23-44-013

Massachusetts

Boston

Boston University Medical Center Program
Sponsor: Boston Medical Center
Program Director:
David Battinelli, MD
Carlos S Kase, MD
Boston Univ Med Ctr
80 E Concord St
Evans 124
Boston, MA 02118
Tel: 617 638-6500 *Fax:* 617 638-6501
Accred Length: 5 Years *Program Size:* 0 (*GY1:* 0)
Program ID: 845-24-44-017

New York

Buffalo

SUNY at Buffalo Graduate Medical-Dental Education Consortium Program
Sponsor: SUNY at Buffalo Grad Medical-Dental Education Consortium
CGF Health System (Buffalo General Hospital)
Erie County Medical Center
Program Director:
Patrick M Pullicino, MD PhD
James P Nolan, MD
SUNY-Buffalo
Sch of Med
219 Bryant St
Buffalo, NY 14222
Tel: 716 878-7848 *Fax:* 716 878-7326
E-mail: ppullici@ubmedd.buffalo.edu
Accred Length: 5 Years *Program Size:* 3 (*GY1:* 0)
Program ID: 845-35-44-001

Stony Brook

SUNY at Stony Brook Program
Sponsor: University Hospital-SUNY at Stony Brook
Veterans Affairs Medical Center (Northport)
Program Director:
James N Davis, MD
Medical House Staff Services
Univ Hospital T14
SUNY-Stony Brook
Stony Brook, NY 11794-7718
Tel: 516 444-1450 *Fax:* 516 444-1474
Internet: http://www.uhmc.sunysb.edu/neurology
Accred Length: 5 Years *Program Size:* 2 (*GY1:* 2)
Program ID: 845-35-44-004

North Carolina

Durham

Duke University Program
Sponsor: Duke University Medical Center
Veterans Affairs Medical Center (Durham)
Program Director:
Joel C Morgenlander, MD
Ralph Corey, MD
Duke Univ Med Ctr
Dept of Neurology
PO Box 3637
Durham, NC 27710
Tel: 919 684-6666 *Fax:* 919 681-7936
Internet: http://www2.mc.duke.edu/neurology
Accred Length: 5 Years *Program Size:* 2 (*GY1:* 0)
Program ID: 845-36-44-003

Tennessee

Memphis

University of Tennessee Program
Sponsor: University of Tennessee College of Medicine
Baptist Memorial Hospital
Regional Medical Center at Memphis
University of Tennessee Medical Center (UT Bowld Hospital)
Veterans Affairs Medical Center (Memphis)
Program Director:
Michael Jacswicz, MD
Kevin McKown, MD
Univ of Tennessee
Dept of Neurology
855 Monroe Ave/Rm 415
Memphis, TN 38163
Tel: 901 448-5814 *Fax:* 901 448-7836
E-mail: mjacewicz@utmem1.utmem.edu
Internet: http://www.utmem.edu/neurology
Accred Length: 5 Years *Program Size:* 9 (*GY1:* 3)
Program ID: 845-47-44-014

Texas

Galveston

University of Texas Medical Branch Hospitals Program
Sponsor: University of Texas Medical Branch Hospitals
Program Director:
John R Calverley, MD
Thomas A Blackwell, MD
Univ of Texas Med Branch
Dept of Neurology/Int Med
301 University Blvd
Galveston, TX 77555-0539
Tel: 409 772-2646, ext 2646 *Fax:* 409 772-6940
E-mail: jcalverl@utmb.edu
Internet: http://www.neuro.utmb.edu
Accred Length: 5 Years *Program Size:* 5 (*GY1:* 1)
Program ID: 845-48-44-007

West Virginia

Morgantown

West Virginia University School of Medicine Program
Sponsor: West Virginia University Hospitals
Program Director:
Maria M Kolar, MD
John F Brick, MD
Robert C Byrd Health Sciences Ctr
Dept of Med
PO Box 9168
Morgantown, WV 26506-9168
Tel: 304 293-4239 *Fax:* 304 293-3530
E-mail: mkolar@wvu.edu
Internet: http://www.hsc.wvu.edu/medicine
Accred Length: 5 Years *Program Size:* 4 (*GY1:* 1)
Program ID: 845-55-44-002

Wisconsin

Milwaukee

Medical College of Wisconsin Program
Sponsor: Medical College of Wisconsin Affiliated Hospitals Inc
Clement J Zablocki Veterans Affairs Medical Center
Froedtert Memorial Lutheran Hospital
Program Director:
Charlotte Heidenreich, MD
Wendy Larson, MD
Educational Affairs/FEH
9200 W Wisconsin Ave
Milwaukee, WI 53226
Tel: 414 257-7287 *Fax:* 414 257-6445
E-mail: cheiden@mcw.edu
Accred Length: 5 Years *Program Size:* 2 (*GY1:* 2)
Program ID: 845-56-44-016

Internal Medicine/ Pediatrics

Alabama

Birmingham

University of Alabama Medical Center Program
Sponsor: University of Alabama Hospital
Program Director:
Raymond G Watts, MD
John I Kennedy Jr, MD
Univ of Alabama, Dept of Pediatrics
1600 7th Ave S
604 ACC
Birmingham, AL 35233-0011
Tel: 205 934-5004 *Fax:* 205 939-9977
E-mail: uabkids@peds.uab.edu
Internet: http://www.peds.uab.edu
Accred Length: 4 Years *Program Size:* 16 *(GY1:* 4)
Program ID: 800-01-44-115

Mobile

University of South Alabama Program
Sponsor: University of South Alabama Medical Center
Program Director:
Franklin Trimm, MD
Ronald C Allison, MD
Univ of South Alabama
Dept of Med/Peds
1504 Springhill Ave/Rm 5326
Mobile, AL 36604
Tel: 334 434-3961 *Fax:* 334 434-3980
Internet: http://www.usouthal.edu/residencyprograms
Accred Length: 4 Years *Program Size:* 13 *(GY1:* 4)
Program ID: 800-01-44-085

Arizona

Phoenix

Maricopa Medical Center Program
Sponsor: Maricopa Medical Center
Phoenix Children's Hospital
Program Director:
Mary E Rimsza, MD
Maricopa Med Ctr, Dept of Pediatrics
2601 E Roosevelt
Phoenix, AZ 85008
Tel: 602 267-5404 *Fax:* 602 267-5859
E-mail: gfeilbac@medcenter.maricopa.gov
Internet: http://www.maricopa.gov/medcenter/mmc.html
Accred Length: 4 Years *Program Size:* 15 *(GY1:* 4)
Program ID: 800-03-44-094

Phoenix Hospitals Program
Sponsor: Good Samaritan Regional Medical Center
Maricopa Medical Center
Phoenix Children's Hospital
Program Director:
Donna L Holland, MD
Good Samaritan Regional Med Ctr
Dept of Med
1111 E McDowell Rd
Phoenix, AZ 85006
Tel: 602 239-2296 *Fax:* 602 239-2084
E-mail: medicine@samaritan.edu
Internet: http://www.samaritan.edu
Accred Length: 4 Years *Program Size:* 24 *(GY1:* 6)
Program ID: 800-03-44-001

Arkansas

Little Rock

University of Arkansas for Medical Sciences Program
Sponsor: University Hospital of Arkansas
Arkansas Children's Hospital
John L McClellan Memorial Veterans Hospital
Program Director:
Robert W Bradsher Jr, MD
Gordon E Schutze, MD
Univ of Arkansas for Med Sciences
4301 W Markham St
H/S Office Slot 634
Little Rock, AR 72205-7199
Tel: 501 686-5162 *Fax:* 501 686-8188
E-mail: imresident@exchange.uams.edu
Internet: http://www.uams.edu./dim/
Accred Length: 4 Years *Program Size:* 19 *(GY1:* 5)
Program ID: 800-04-44-002

California

Loma Linda

Loma Linda University Program
Sponsor: Loma Linda University Medical Center
Jerry L Pettis Memorial Veterans Hospital
Loma Linda University Community Hospital
Riverside County Regional Medical Center
Program Director:
Tamara M Shankel, MD
Richard Chinnock, MD
Loma Linda Univ Med Ctr
Int Med/Peds Combined Program
PO Box 2000
Loma Linda, CA 92354
Tel: 909 824-4174 *Fax:* 909 824-4846
Accred Length: 4 Years *Program Size:* 16 *(GY1:* 4)
Program ID: 800-05-44-003

Los Angeles

Cedars-Sinai Medical Center Program
Sponsor: Cedars-Sinai Medical Center
Program Director:
Brian D Kan, MD
Cedars-Sinai Med Ctr
Med/Ped Combined Prgm
8700 Beverly Blvd/Rm 4310
Los Angeles, CA 90048
Tel: 310 855-4780 *Fax:* 310 967-0145
E-mail: kan@csmc.edu
Internet: http://www.csmc.edu/gme/med-peds
Accred Length: 4 Years *Program Size:* 16 *(GY1:* 4)
Program ID: 800-05-44-004

University of Southern California Program
Sponsor: Los Angeles County-USC Medical Center
Program Director:
Lawrence M Opas, MD
Ron Ben-Ari, MD
Los Angeles County-USC Med Ctr
Women's and Children's Hospital
1240 N Mission Rd/Rm L-902
Los Angeles, CA 90033-1084
Tel: 323 226-3691 *Fax:* 323 226-4380
Accred Length: 4 Years *Program Size:* 32 *(GY1:* 8)
Program ID: 800-05-44-005

Sacramento

University of California (Davis) Program
Sponsor: University of California (Davis) Medical Center
Program Director:
Faith T Fitzgerald, MD
Daniel West, MD
Univ of California Davis Med Ctr
4150 V St/#3116
Sacramento, CA 95817
Tel: 916 734-7080 *Fax:* 916 736-1150
E-mail: imres@ucdavis.edu
Accred Length: 4 Years *Program Size:* 1 *(GY1:* 1)
Program ID: 800-05-44-123

San Diego

University of California (San Diego) Program
Sponsor: University of California (San Diego) Medical Center
Program Director:
Shawn Harrity, MD
UCSD Med Ctr
Combined Med/Peds
200 W Arbor Dr
San Diego, CA 92103-8811
Tel: 619 543-6272 *Fax:* 619 543-6529
Internet: http://www.medicine.ucsd.edu/medres/
Accred Length: 4 Years *Program Size:* 16 *(GY1:* 4)
Program ID: 800-05-44-099

Connecticut

Bridgeport

Yale University (Bridgeport) Program
Sponsor: Bridgeport Hospital
Yale-New Haven Hospital
Program Director:
Michael J Smith, MD
Bridgeport Hospital
267 Grant St
Bridgeport, CT 06610
Tel: 203 384-3495 *Fax:* 203 384-3910
E-mail: pmsmit@bpthosp.org
Accred Length: 4 Years *Program Size:* 14 *(GY1:* 4)
Program ID: 800-08-44-008

Farmington

University of Connecticut Health Center/John Dempsey Hospital Program
Sponsor: Univ of Connecticut Health Center/John Dempsey Hospital
Program Director:
Jacqueline Nissen, MD
John Dempsey Hospital
263 Farmington Ave
Farmington, CT 06030-3950
Tel: 860 679-2437
E-mail: jnissen@nso.uchc.edu
Internet: http://www.uchc.com
Accred Length: 4 Years *Program Size:* 6 *(GY1:* 2)
Program ID: 800-08-44-114

New Haven

Yale-New Haven Medical Center Program

Sponsor: Yale-New Haven Hospital

Program Director:
Stephen Huot, MD PhD
M Susan Moyer, MD
Yale Univ Sch of Med
PO Box 208086
New Haven, CT 06520-8086
Tel: 203 785-7249 *Fax:* 203 785-7258
E-mail: stephen-huot@yale.edu
Accred Length: 4 Years *Program Size:* 4 (*GY1:* 4)
Program ID: 800-08-44-127

Delaware

Wilmington

Christiana Care Health Services Program

Sponsor: Christiana Care Health Services Inc
duPont Hospital for Children

Program Director:
Louis E Bartoshesky, MD MPH
Virginia U Collier, MD
Christiana Care Health Systems
Med/Peds Residency Office
PO Box 6001
Newark, DE 19718
Tel: 302 733-2313 *Fax:* 302 733-4339
E-mail: jbucci@mcd.gen.de.us
Internet: http://www.mcdresidency.org
Accred Length: 4 Years *Program Size:* 16 (*GY1:* 4)
Program ID: 800-09-44-009

District of Columbia

Washington

Georgetown University Medical Center Program

Sponsor: Georgetown University Medical Center

Program Director:
Joseph T Wayne, MD MPH
Georgetown Univ Med Ctr
3800 Reservoir Rd NW/5PHC
Washington, DC 20007-2197
Tel: 202 687-5037 *Fax:* 202 687-7797
Internet: http://www.dml.georgetown.edu/depts/medicine/medpeds
Accred Length: 4 Years *Program Size:* 12 (*GY1:* 4)
Program ID: 800-10-44-129

Florida

Gainesville

University of Florida Program

Sponsor: University of Florida College of Medicine
Shands Hospital at the University of Florida

Program Director:
Craig S Kitchens, MD
Joel M Andres, MD
Univ of Florida Health Science Ctr
Dept of Med
PO Box 100277
Gainesville, FL 32610-0277
Tel: 352 395-0239 *Fax:* 352 338-9884
Accred Length: 4 Years *Program Size:* 4 (*GY1:* 0)
Program ID: 800-11-44-107

Miami

University of Miami-Jackson Memorial Medical Center Program

Sponsor: University of Miami-Jackson Memorial Medical Center
Veterans Affairs Medical Center (Miami)

Program Director:
Mark A Gelbard, MD
Charles H Pegalow, MD
Jackson Memorial Hospital
1611 NW 12th Ave
Miami, FL 33136
Tel: 305 585-5215 *Fax:* 305 326-8302
Accred Length: 4 Years *Program Size:* 16 (*GY1:* 4)
Program ID: 800-11-44-086

Orlando

Orlando Regional Healthcare System Program

Sponsor: Orlando Regional Medical Center

Program Director:
George Everett, MD
Michael Muszynski, MD
Orlando Regional Med Ctr
Dept of Int Med
86 W Underwood St/Ste 102
Orlando, FL 32806-2134
Tel: 800 895-4613
Internet: http://www.orhs.org/meded/index.html
Accred Length: 4 Years *Program Size:* 12 (*GY1:* 4)
Program ID: 800-11-44-112

Tampa

University of South Florida Program

Sponsor: University of South Florida College of Medicine
Tampa General Healthcare

Program Director:
Lynn Ringenberg, MD
Philip Altus, MD
Univ of South Florida Coll of Med
17 Davis Blvd/Ste 200
Tampa, FL 33606
Tel: 813 272-2272 *Fax:* 813 272-2962
E-mail: slamar@com1.med.usf.edu
Internet: http://www.usfpeds.med.usf.edu
Accred Length: 4 Years *Program Size:* 8 (*GY1:* 4)
Program ID: 800-11-44-125

Hawaii

Honolulu

University of Hawaii Program

Sponsor: University of Hawaii John A Burns School of Medicine
Kapiolani Medical Center for Women and Children
Kuakini Medical Center
Queen's Medical Center
St Francis Medical Center

Program Director:
John S Melish, MD
M Stanton Michels, MD
Univ of Hawaii
Dept of Med
1356 Lusitana St/7th Fl
Honolulu, HI 96813
Tel: 808 586-2910 *Fax:* 808 586-7486
E-mail: adzuara@hawaii.edu
Internet: http://uhimrp.hawaii.edu
Accred Length: 4 Years *Program Size:* 11 (*GY1:* 4)
Program ID: 800-14-44-110

Illinois

Chicago

Cook County Hospital Program

Sponsor: Cook County Hospital

Program Director:
Darryl A Woods, MD
Cook County Hospital
1900 W Polk St/Ste 940
Chicago, IL 60612
Tel: 312 633-7946 *Fax:* 312 633-8333
Accred Length: 4 Years *Program Size:* 8 (*GY1:* 2)
Program ID: 800-16-44-011

Rush-Presbyterian-St Luke's Medical Center Program

Sponsor: Rush-Presbyterian-St Luke's Medical Center

Program Director:
Keith M Boyd, MD
Rita Rossi-Foulkes, MD
Rush Combined Int Med/Peds Program
Rush-Presbyterian-St Luke's Med Ctr
1700 W Van Buren St/TOB Ste 457
Chicago, IL 60612-3833
Tel: 312 942-3254 *Fax:* 312 942-3551
E-mail: wshulman@rush.edu
Accred Length: 4 Years *Program Size:* 16 (*GY1:* 4)
Program ID: 800-16-44-103

University of Chicago Program

Sponsor: University of Chicago Hospitals
Mercy Hospital and Medical Center
University of Chicago Children's Hospital

Program Director:
Deborah Burnet, MD
Univ of Chicago Hospitals and Clinics
5841 S Maryland Ave/MC7082
Chicago, IL 60637-1470
Tel: 773 702-0309 *Fax:* 773 702-2230
E-mail: dburnet@uhs.bsd.uchicago.edu
Internet: http://uhs.bsd.uchicago.edu/program
Accred Length: 4 Years *Program Size:* 15 (*GY1:* 4)
Program ID: 800-16-44-012

University of Illinois College of Medicine at Chicago Program

Sponsor: University of Illinois College of Medicine at Chicago
Michael Reese Hospital and Medical Center
University of Illinois Hospital and Clinics
Veterans Affairs West Side Medical Center

Program Director:
Saul J Weiner, MD
Univ of Illinois Med Ctr
840 S Wood St (M/C 787)
Chicago, IL 60612
Tel: 312 413-5454 *Fax:* 312 413-8283
E-mail: sweiner@uic.edu
Internet: http://www.uic.edu/com/dom/res/impeds/
Accred Length: 4 Years *Program Size:* 15 (*GY1:* 4)
Program ID: 800-16-44-013

Maywood

Loyola University Program

Sponsor: Loyola University Medical Center

Program Director:
William Cannon, MD
Kevin P Simpson, MD
Loyola Univ Med Ctr
2160 S First Ave
Bldg 102/Rm 7611A
Maywood, IL 60153
Tel: 708 216-5838 *Fax:* 708 216-9456
Internet: http://www.meddean.luc.edu/lumen/deptwebs/medicine/medres/medres.htm
Accred Length: 4 Years *Program Size:* 16 (*GY1:* 4)
Program ID: 800-16-44-014

Peoria

University of Illinois College of Medicine at Peoria Program
Sponsor: St Francis Medical Center
Program Director:
Richard L Horndasch, MD
Univ of Illinois Coll of Med-Peoria
OSF St Francis Med Ctr
530 NE Glen Oak Ave
Peoria, IL 61637
Tel: 800 301-7531
Internet: http://www.uicomp.uic.edu/uicomp.html
Accred Length: 4 Years *Program Size:* 32 (*GY1:* 8)
Program ID: 800-16-44-015

Springfield

Southern Illinois University Program
Sponsor: Southern Illinois University School of Medicine
Memorial Medical Center
St John's Hospital
Program Director:
Andrew J Varney, MD
Steven R Bowers, MD
Southern Illinois Univ Sch of Med
800 N Rutledge St
PO Box 19636
Springfield, IL 62794-9636
Tel: 217 782-0193 *Fax:* 217 524-8156
E-mail: cbrower@siumed.edu
Internet: http://www.siumed.edu
Accred Length: 4 Years *Program Size:* 16 (*GY1:* 4)
Program ID: 800-16-44-016

Indiana

Indianapolis

Indiana University School of Medicine Program
Sponsor: Indiana University School of Medicine
Clarian IU Hospital
Richard L Roudebush Veterans Affairs Medical Center
William N Wishard Memorial Hospital
Program Director:
Mary R Ciccarelli, MD
Riley Hospital for Children
702 Barnhill Dr/Rm 5900
West Bldg M200
Indianapolis, IN 46202-5225
Tel: 317 274-4034 *Fax:* 317 274-1476
Internet: http://www.iupui.edu/it/deptpeds/home.html
Accred Length: 4 Years *Program Size:* 56 (*GY1:* 16)
Program ID: 800-17-44-018

Kansas

Kansas City

University of Kansas Medical Center Program
Sponsor: University of Kansas School of Medicine
University of Kansas Medical Center
Program Director:
Andreas Deymann, MD
Pamela K Shaw, MD
Univ of Kansas Med Ctr
Dept of Med/Pediatrics
3901 Rainbow Blvd
Kansas City, KS 66160-7350
Tel: 913 588-7309 *Fax:* 913 588-3995
E-mail: sscott5@kumc.edu
Internet: http://www.kumc.edu/internal_med/medpeds/index.html
Accred Length: 4 Years *Program Size:* 20 (*GY1:* 4)
Program ID: 800-19-44-087

Wichita

University of Kansas (Wichita) Program
Sponsor: University of Kansas School of Medicine (Wichita)
Columbia Wesley Medical Center
Program Director:
Garold O Minns, MD
Katherine Melhorn, MD
Univ of Kansas Med Ctr
1010 N Kansas
Wichita, KS 67214-3199
Tel: 316 293-2650 *Fax:* 316 293-1878
E-mail: lhudson1@kumc.edu
Internet: http://www.kumc.edu/dept/intmed
Accred Length: 4 Years *Program Size:* 8 (*GY1:* 2)
Program ID: 800-19-44-124

Kentucky

Lexington

University of Kentucky Medical Center Program
Sponsor: University of Kentucky Hospital
Veterans Affairs Medical Center (Lexington)
Program Director:
Mary M Burke, MD
Jackson Smith Jr, MD
Univ of Kentucky Med Ctr
Kentucky Clinic, Med/Peds Program
RM K512
Lexington, KY 40536-0284
Tel: 606 323-1723 *Fax:* 606 323-1197
Accred Length: 4 Years *Program Size:* 24 (*GY1:* 6)
Program ID: 800-20-44-019

Louisville

University of Louisville Program
Sponsor: University of Louisville School of Medicine
Kosair Children's Hospital (Alliant Health System)
University of Louisville Hospital
Veterans Affairs Medical Center (Louisville)
Program Director:
Charlene K Mitchell, MD
Univ of Louisville Sch of Med
Dept of Med
Rm A3K00 Ambulatory Care Bldg
Louisville, KY 40292
Tel: 502 852-7041 *Fax:* 502 852-8980
E-mail: ckmitc01@ulkyvm.louisville.edu
Internet: http://www.louisville.edu/groups/medschool/gme/med-ped/
Accred Length: 4 Years *Program Size:* 20 (*GY1:* 5)
Program ID: 800-20-44-020

Louisiana

New Orleans

Louisiana State University Program
Sponsor: Louisiana State University School of Medicine
Childrens Hospital
Louisiana State University Medical College Campus
Program Director:
Dayton W Daberkow II, MD
Louisiana State Univ Sch of Med
1542 Tulane Ave
New Orleans, LA 70112
Tel: 504 568-4600 *Fax:* 504 568-7885
E-mail: ddaberkow@lsumc.edu
Internet: http://www.medschool.lsumc.edu/medpeds/
Accred Length: 4 Years *Program Size:* 31 (*GY1:* 8)
Program ID: 800-21-44-022

Tulane University Program
Sponsor: Tulane University School of Medicine
Medical Center of Louisiana at New Orleans
Veterans Affairs Medical Center (New Orleans)
Program Director:
Terry L Cummings, MD
Tulane Univ Sch of Med
1430 Tulane Ave/Box SL37
New Orleans, LA 70112-2699
Tel: 504 988-6689 *Fax:* 504 988-6808
E-mail: tcummin@tmcpop.tmc.tulane.edu
Accred Length: 4 Years *Program Size:* 24 (*GY1:* 6)
Program ID: 800-21-44-023

Shreveport

Louisiana State University (Shreveport) Program
Sponsor: Louisiana State University Hospital-Shreveport
Program Director:
Jacob T Cross Jr, MD MPH
Louisiana State Univ Med Ctr Hospital
Med Educ-Med/Peds
1501 Kings Hwy/PO Box 33932
Shreveport, LA 71130-3932
Tel: 318 675-6073 *Fax:* 318 675-5907
E-mail: tcross@lsumc.edu
Accred Length: 4 Years *Program Size:* 16 (*GY1:* 4)
Program ID: 800-21-44-101

Maryland

Baltimore

University of Maryland Program

Sponsor: University of Maryland Medical System

Program Director:
Susan D Wolfsthal, MD
Carol Carraccio, MD
Univ of Maryland
22 S Greene St/Rm N3E09
Baltimore, MD 21201-1595
Tel: 410 328-2388 *Fax:* 410 328-0267
E-mail: umdmed@medicine.ab.umd.edu
Internet: http://www.umm.edu
Accred Length: 4 Years *Program Size:* 16 (*GY1:* 4)
Program ID: 800-23-44-095

Massachusetts

Boston

Harvard Combined Program

Sponsor: Brigham and Women's Hospital
Children's Hospital
Massachusetts General Hospital

Program Director:
Laurence J Ronan, MD
Massachusetts General Hospital
Ellison 1934 D
Fruit St
Boston, MA 02114
Tel: 617 726-7782 *Fax:* 617 724-9068
E-mail: ronan.laurence@mgh.harvard.edu
Internet: http://www.hmcnet.harvard.edu/medpeds/
Accred Length: 4 Years *Program Size:* 32 (*GY1:* 8)
Program ID: 800-24-44-084

Springfield

Baystate Medical Center Program

Sponsor: Baystate Medical Center

Program Director:
Samuel H Borden, MD
Baystate Med Ctr
759 Chestnut St
Springfield, MA 01199
Tel: 413 794-3998 *Fax:* 413 794-4588
E-mail: samuel.borden@bhs.org
Internet: http://www.baystatehealth.com
Accred Length: 4 Years *Program Size:* 32 (*GY1:* 8)
Program ID: 800-24-44-024

Worcester

University of Massachusetts Program

Sponsor: University of Massachusetts Medical School

Program Director:
Lynn Manfred, MD
John Solomonides, MD
Univ of Massachusetts Med Sch
Dept of Pediatrics
55 Lake Ave N
Worcester, MA 01655
Tel: 508 856-3590 *Fax:* 508 856-1031
E-mail: vickie.white@banyan.ummed.edu
Accred Length: 4 Years *Program Size:* 6 (*GY1:* 2)
Program ID: 800-24-44-111

Michigan

Ann Arbor

University of Michigan Program 1

Sponsor: University of Michigan Hospitals
Veterans Affairs Medical Center (Ann Arbor)

Program Director:
John G Frohna, MD MPH
Univ of Michigan
3110G Taubman Ctr/Box 0368
1500 E Medical Center Dr
Ann Arbor, MI 48109-0368
Tel: 734 936-4385 *Fax:* 734 936-7024
E-mail: medpeds@umich.edu
Internet: http://www.med.umich.edu/intmed/med-peds
Accred Length: 4 Years *Program Size:* 20 (*GY1:* 6)
Program ID: 800-25-44-025

University of Michigan Program 2

Sponsor: University of Michigan Hospitals
St Joseph Mercy Health System

Program Director:
Donald K Martin, MD
St Joseph Mercy Hospital
PO Box 995
5333 McAuley Dr/RHB 3009
Ann Arbor, MI 48106
Tel: 313 712-3935
E-mail: martindk@mercyhealth.com
Internet: http://www.ped.med.umich.edu
Accred Length: 4 Years *Program Size:* 8 (*GY1:* 2)
Program ID: 800-25-44-026

Detroit

St John Hospital and Medical Center Program

Sponsor: St John Hospital and Medical Center

Program Director:
Thomas S Piazza, MD
St John Hospital and Med Ctr
Dept of Med Educ
22101 Moross Rd
Detroit, MI 48236
Tel: 313 343-3875 *Fax:* 313 343-7840
E-mail: sue.moynihan@stjohn.org
Internet: http://www.stjohn.org
Accred Length: 4 Years *Program Size:* 8 (*GY1:* 2)
Program ID: 800-25-44-028

Wayne State University Program

Sponsor: Children's Hospital of Michigan
Detroit Receiving Hospital and University Health Center
Grace Hospital
Hutzel Hospital
Veterans Affairs Medical Center (Detroit)

Program Director:
Howard Schubiner, MD
Wayne State Univ Hospitals
4201 St Antoine/UHC 5C
Detroit, MI 48201-2196
Tel: 313 577-5030 *Fax:* 313 745-4710
E-mail: schubiner@oncgate.roc.wayne.edu
Internet: http://www.intmed.wayne.edu
Accred Length: 4 Years *Program Size:* 28 (*GY1:* 7)
Program ID: 800-25-44-029

East Lansing

Michigan State University Program

Sponsor: Michigan State University College of Human Medicine
Michigan State University Clinical Center
Sparrow Hospital
St Lawrence Hospital and HealthCare Services

Program Director:
Michael H Zaroukian, MD PhD
B301 Clinical Ctr
Michigan State Univ
East Lansing, MI 48824-1313
Tel: 517 353-5100 *Fax:* 517 432-2759
E-mail: zaroukia@pilot.msu.edu
Internet: http://pilot.msu.edu/user/zaroukia/
Accred Length: 4 Years *Program Size:* 8 (*GY1:* 2)
Program ID: 800-25-44-088

Flint

Hurley Medical Center/Michigan State University Program

Sponsor: Hurley Medical Center

Program Director:
Laura A Carravallah, MD
Hurley Med Ctr
3A-W Combined Med/Peds Educ
One Hurley Plaza
Flint, MI 48503-5993
Tel: 810 257-9283 *Fax:* 810 257-9736
E-mail: lcarrav1@hurleymc.com
Internet: http://www.hurleymc.com
Accred Length: 4 Years *Program Size:* 16 (*GY1:* 4)
Program ID: 800-25-44-030

Grand Rapids

Spectrum Health-Downtown Campus Program

Sponsor: Spectrum Health-Downtown Campus

Program Director:
Richard A Switzer, MD
Spectrum Health
21 Michigan St NE/Ste 525
Grand Rapids, MI 49503
Tel: 616 391-3775 *Fax:* 616 391-3130
Internet: http://www.spectrum-health.org
Accred Length: 4 Years *Program Size:* 16 (*GY1:* 4)
Program ID: 800-25-44-098

Kalamazoo

Kalamazoo Center for Medical Studies/Michigan State University Program

Sponsor: Kalamazoo Center for Medical Studies
Bronson Methodist Hospital

Program Director:
Thomas Melgar, MD
Michigan State Univ-Kalamazoo Ctr for Med Studies
Dept of Med/Peds
1000 Oakland Dr
Kalamazoo, MI 49008-1284
Tel: 616 337-6350 *Fax:* 616 337-4234
E-mail: medpeds@kcms.msu.edu
Internet: http://www.kcms.msu.edu
Accred Length: 4 Years *Program Size:* 20 (*GY1:* 5)
Program ID: 800-25-44-089

Pontiac

St Joseph Mercy-Oakland Program
Sponsor: St Joseph Mercy-Oakland
Program Director:
Bernard A Bercu, MD
Annamaria Church, MD
St Joseph Mercy-Oakland
900 Woodward Ave
Pontiac, MI 48341-2985
Tel: 248 858-6233 *Fax:* 248 858-3244
Accred Length: 4 Years *Program Size:* 19 (*GY1:* 5)
Program ID: 800-25-44-032

Royal Oak

William Beaumont Hospital Program
Sponsor: William Beaumont Hospital
Program Director:
Jeffrey D Haller, MD
William Beaumont Hospital
3601 W 13 Mile Rd
Royal Oak, MI 48073-6769
Tel: 248 551-4469 *Fax:* 248 551-8880
E-mail: dvowler@beaumont.edu
Internet: http://www.beaumont.edu/html/gme
Accred Length: 4 Years *Program Size:* 20 (*GY1:* 5)
Program ID: 800-25-44-033

Minnesota

Minneapolis

University of Minnesota Program
Sponsor: Fairview-University Medical Center
Children's Health Care (Minneapolis)
Children's Health Care (St Paul)
Hennepin County Medical Center
Regions Hospital
Veterans Affairs Medical Center (Minneapolis)
Program Director:
Deepak Kamat, MD PhD MD
Med/Peds Residency Program
420 Delaware St SE/Box 391
Minneapolis, MN 55455
Tel: 612 624-0990 *Fax:* 612 626-7042
E-mail: peds-res@tc.umn.edu
Internet: http://www.peds.umn.edu/
Accred Length: 4 Years *Program Size:* 49 (*GY1:* 12)
Program ID: 800-26-44-034

Mississippi

Jackson

University of Mississippi Program
Sponsor: University Hospital
Program Director:
Stephanie L Elkins, MD
Univ of Mississippi Med Ctr
2500 N State St
Jackson, MS 39216-4505
Tel: 601 984-5615 *Fax:* 601 984-5689
E-mail: selkins@medicine.umsmed.edu
Internet: http://www.umsmed.edu
Accred Length: 4 Years *Program Size:* 10 (*GY1:* 4)
Program ID: 800-27-44-035

Missouri

Columbia

University of Missouri-Columbia Program
Sponsor: University of Missouri-Columbia School of Medicine
University Hospitals and Clinics
Program Director:
Sara S Viessman, MD
John Yanos, MD
Univ of Missouri-Columbia
Dept of Child Health
One Hospital Dr/Rm N708
Columbia, MO 65212
Tel: 573 882-4438 *Fax:* 573 884-5666
E-mail: adamskrausp@health.missouri.edu
Accred Length: 4 Years *Program Size:* 16 (*GY1:* 4)
Program ID: 800-28-44-126

Kansas City

University of Missouri at Kansas City Program
Sponsor: Children's Mercy Hospital
Saint Luke's Hospital
Truman Medical Center-East
Program Director:
Frederick Klingbeil, MD
George R Reisz, MD
Univ of Missouri-Kansas City Sch of Med
Combined Int Med/Peds
2411 Holmes St
Kansas City, MO 64108
Tel: 816 881-6212 *Fax:* 816 881-6209
E-mail: intmed@cctr.umkc.edu
Internet: http://www.research.med.umkc.edu/resid
Accred Length: 4 Years *Program Size:* 16 (*GY1:* 4)
Program ID: 800-28-44-036

St Louis

St Louis University School of Medicine Program
Sponsor: St Louis University School of Medicine
SSM Cardinal Glennon Children's Hospital
St Louis University School of Medicine
St Mary's Health Center
Veterans Affairs Medical Center (St Louis)
Program Director:
Adrian M Di Bisceglie, MD
St Louis Univ Sch of Med
Dept of Int Med
1402 S Grand Blvd
St Louis, MO 63104
Tel: 314 577-8762 *Fax:* 314 268-5108
E-mail: stepterc@wpogate.slu.edu
Internet: http://www.slu.edu/departments/medicine
Accred Length: 4 Years *Program Size:* 16 (*GY1:* 4)
Program ID: 800-28-44-037

Nebraska

Omaha

Creighton University Program
Sponsor: Tenet St Joseph Hospital at Creighton Univ Medical Center
Boys Town National Research Hospital
Childrens Memorial Hospital
Veterans Affairs Medical Center (Omaha)
Program Director:
Daniel J Boken, MD
Creighton Univ
601 N 30th St
Ste 5850
Omaha, NE 68131-2197
Tel: 402 280-4392 *Fax:* 402 280-4158
E-mail: resapp@creighton.edu
Internet: http://www.medicine.creighton.edu
Accred Length: 4 Years *Program Size:* 14 (*GY1:* 4)
Program ID: 800-30-44-038

New Jersey

Camden

UMDNJ-Cooper Hospital Program
Sponsor: Cooper Hospital-University Medical Center
Program Director:
Glenn C Newell, MD
Cooper Hospital-Univ Med Ctr
401 Haddon Ave
Camden, NJ 08103
Tel: 609 757-7842 *Fax:* 609 968-9587
E-mail: samahasi@rwjcam.umdj.edu
Internet: http://www.simon.umdnj.edu/medresidency
Accred Length: 4 Years *Program Size:* 14 (*GY1:* 4)
Program ID: 800-33-44-102

Morristown

Morristown Memorial Hospital Program
Sponsor: Morristown Memorial Hospital
Program Director:
Sudhir E Finch, MD
Morristown Memorial Hospital
100 Madison Ave
PO Box 1956
Morristown, NJ 07962-1956
Tel: 973 971-7550 *Fax:* 973 290-7364
Internet: http://www.atlantichealth.org
Accred Length: 4 Years *Program Size:* 10 (*GY1:* 3)
Program ID: 800-33-44-039

Newark

Newark Beth Israel Medical Center Program
Sponsor: Newark Beth Israel Medical Center
Elizabeth General Medical Center
St Michael's Medical Center (Cathedral Hlth Srvcs Inc)
Program Director:
Jules A Titelbaum, MD
Carlo Mainardi, MD
Newark Beth Israel Med Ctr
201 Lyons Ave
Newark, NJ 07112
Tel: 973 926-7333 *Fax:* 973 923-5340
Accred Length: 4 Years *Program Size:* 16 (*GY1:* 4)
Program ID: 800-33-44-041

UMDNJ-New Jersey Medical School Program

Sponsor: UMDNJ-New Jersey Medical School
Newark Beth Israel Medical Center
UMDNJ-University Hospital
Veterans Affairs Medical Center (East Orange)

Program Director:
Marilyn A Miller, MD
Susan Mautone, MD
UMDNJ-Univ Hospital
150 Bergen St
Newark, NJ 07103
Tel: 973 972-6056 *Fax:* 973 972-7160
Accred Length: 4 Years *Program Size:* 16 (*GY1:* 4)
Program ID: 800-33-44-040

Paterson

St Joseph's Hospital and Medical Center Program

Sponsor: St Joseph's Hospital and Medical Center

Program Director:
Naipaul Rambaran, MD
St Joseph's Hospital and Med Ctr
Med/Peds Program
703 Main St/Rm J249
Paterson, NJ 07503
Tel: 973 754-2569 *Fax:* 973 754-2096
Internet: http://www.sjhmc.org
Accred Length: 4 Years *Program Size:* 8 (*GY1:* 2)
Program ID: 800-33-44-042

Summit

Overlook Hospital Program

Sponsor: Overlook Hospital

Program Director:
Rafael E Pajaro, MD MD
99 Beauvoir Ave
PO Box 220
Summit, NJ 07902-0220
Tel: 908 522-2934 *Fax:* 908 522-0804
Accred Length: 4 Years *Program Size:* 8 (*GY1:* 2)
Program ID: 800-33-44-119

New York

Albany

Albany Medical Center Program

Sponsor: Albany Medical Center
Ellis Hospital
St Peter's Hospital
Veterans Affairs Medical Center (Albany)

Program Director:
Elizabeth A Higgins, MD
Paul C Sorum, MD
Albany Med Ctr
Dept of Med/Peds A-130
724 Watervliet-Shaker Rd
Latham, NY 12110
Tel: 518 783-0312 *Fax:* 518 782-7485
E-mail: eahiggins@pol.net
Internet: http://www.amc.edu
Accred Length: 4 Years *Program Size:* 16 (*GY1:* 4)
Program ID: 800-35-44-044

Brooklyn

Brookdale University Hospital Medical Center Program

Sponsor: Brookdale University Hospital Medical Center

Program Director:
Ethan D Fried, MD
T W Avruskin, MD
Brookdale Univ Hospital and Med Ctr
One Brookdale Plaza
Brooklyn, NY 11212
Tel: 718 240-6202, ext 6205 *Fax:* 718 240-6505
Accred Length: 4 Years *Program Size:* 8 (*GY1:* 2)
Program ID: 800-35-44-045

Maimonides Medical Center Program

Sponsor: Maimonides Medical Center

Program Director:
Edgar Lichstein, MD
Henry A Schaeffer, MD
Maimonides Med Ctr
4802 Tenth Ave
Brooklyn, NY 11219
Tel: 718 283-8918 *Fax:* 718 283-6268
E-mail: vpolynice@maimonidesmed.org
Internet: http://www.maimonidesmed.org/peds
Accred Length: 4 Years *Program Size:* 10 (*GY1:* 4)
Program ID: 800-35-44-122

New York Methodist Hospital Program

Sponsor: New York Methodist Hospital

Program Director:
Harvey Dosik, MD
L Glass, MD
New York Methodist Hospital
506 Sixth St
Brooklyn, NY 11215-9008
Tel: 718 780-5246 *Fax:* 718 780-3259
Accred Length: 4 Years *Program Size:* 2 (*GY1:* 2)
Program ID: 800-35-44-130

SUNY Health Science Center at Brooklyn Program

Sponsor: SUNY Health Science Center at Brooklyn
Children's Medical Center of Brooklyn
Kings County Hospital Center
University Hospital-SUNY Health Science Center at Brooklyn
Veterans Affairs Medical Center (Brooklyn)

Program Director:
Stephen Kamholz, MD
Leonard Glass, MD
SUNY Health Science Ctr-Brooklyn
Children's Med Ctr
450 Clarkson Ave/Box 49
Brooklyn, NY 11203
Tel: 718 270-1625 *Fax:* 718 270-1985
Internet: http://www.hscbklyn.edu
Accred Length: 4 Years *Program Size:* 9 (*GY1:* 3)
Program ID: 800-35-44-048

Buffalo

SUNY at Buffalo Graduate Medical-Dental Education Consortium Program

Sponsor: CGF Health System (Children's Hospital of Buffalo)
CGF Health System (Buffalo General Hospital)
Erie County Medical Center
Veterans Affairs Medical Center (Buffalo)

Program Director:
Margaret McAloon, MD
Children's Hospital of Buffalo
140 Hodge
Buffalo, NY 14222
Tel: 716 878-7853 *Fax:* 716 888-3899
Accred Length: 4 Years *Program Size:* 16 (*GY1:* 4)
Program ID: 800-35-44-049

New York

Mount Sinai School of Medicine Program

Sponsor: Mount Sinai School of Medicine
Elmhurst Hospital Center-Mount Sinai Services
Englewood Hospital and Medical Center
Mount Sinai Medical Center
Veterans Affairs Medical Center (Manhattan)

Program Director:
Scott H Barnett, MD
Mount Sinai Med Ctr
One Gustave L Levy Pl
Box 1110
New York, NY 10029
Tel: 212 241-3145 *Fax:* 212 426-7585
Accred Length: 4 Years *Program Size:* 16 (*GY1:* 4)
Program ID: 800-35-44-105

New York Medical College Program

Sponsor: Metropolitan Hospital Center

Program Director:
Peter Reynaud, MD
Shobhana Chaudhari, MD
New York Med Coll-Metropolitan Hospital Ctr
1901 First Ave
New York, NY 10029
Tel: 212 423-6228
Accred Length: 4 Years *Program Size:* 11 (*GY1:* 2)
Program ID: 800-35-44-051

St Vincent's Hospital and Medical Center of New York Program

Sponsor: St Vincent's Hospital and Medical Center of New York

Program Director:
Steven L Sivak, MD
Jayne Rivas, MD
St Vincent's Hospital and Med Ctr
153 W 11th St
New York, NY 10011
Tel: 212 604-7512 *Fax:* 212 604-3286
Internet: http://svh.nymc.edu
Accred Length: 4 Years *Program Size:* 16 (*GY1:* 4)
Program ID: 800-35-44-082

Rochester

University of Rochester Combined Internal Medicine/Pediatrics Program

Sponsor: Strong Memorial Hospital of the University of Rochester
Genesee Hospital
Rochester General Hospital

Program Director:
Lynn C Garfunkel, MD
Brett Robbins, MD
Strong Memorial Hospital
601 Elmwood Ave/Box 702
Rochester, NY 14642-8702
Tel: 716 338-4369 *Fax:* 716 338-2347
E-mail: medped@urmc.rochester.edu
Internet: http://www.urmc.rochester.edu/smd/medicine/res/medped.htm
Accred Length: 4 Years *Program Size:* 30 (*GY1:* 7)
Program ID: 800-35-44-054

Staten Island

Staten Island University Hospital Program

Sponsor: Staten Island University Hospital

Program Director:
Thomas G McGinn, MD
Staten Island Univ Hospital
475 Seaview Ave
Staten Island, NY 10305
Tel: 718 226-9506 *Fax:* 718 226-8966
E-mail: tmcginn@siuh.edu
Internet: http://www.siuh.edu
Accred Length: 4 Years *Program Size:* 16 (*GY1:* 4)
Program ID: 800-35-44-053

Stony Brook

SUNY at Stony Brook Program

Sponsor: University Hospital-SUNY at Stony Brook

Program Director:
Richard Barnett, MD
Susan Guralnick, MD
SUNY-Stony Brook
Sch of Med
HSC T-16/Rm 020
Stony Brook, NY 11794-8160
Tel: 516 444-2065 *Fax:* 516 444-2493
E-mail: dbrand@epo.som.sunysb.edu
Accred Length: 4 Years *Program Size:* 8 (*GY1:* 2)
Program ID: 800-35-44-093

North Carolina

Chapel Hill

University of North Carolina Hospitals Program

Sponsor: University of North Carolina Hospitals

Program Director:
Jim Visser, MD MPH
Univ of North Carolina Sch of Med
Old Clinic Bldg/CB#7593
Chapel Hill, NC 27599-7593
Tel: 919 966-6770 *Fax:* 919 966-8419
E-mail: uncmp@med.unc.edu
Internet: http://www.pediatrics.med.unc.edu
Accred Length: 4 Years *Program Size:* 24 (*GY1:* 6)
Program ID: 800-36-44-055

Durham

Duke University Program

Sponsor: Duke University Medical Center
Veterans Affairs Medical Center (Durham)

Program Director:
Deborah Kredich, MD
Ralph Corey, MD
Duke Univ Med Ctr
Dept of Med/Pediatrics
Box 3127
Durham, NC 27710
Tel: 919 684-2356 *Fax:* 919 681-2714
Accred Length: 4 Years *Program Size:* 23 (*GY1:* 6)
Program ID: 800-36-44-056

Greenville

East Carolina University Program

Sponsor: Pitt County Memorial Hospital

Program Director:
Dale A Newton, MD
East Carolina Univ Sch of Med
Dept of Pediatrics
3E-139 Brody Med Sciences Bldg
Greenville, NC 27858-4354
Tel: 252 816-3041 *Fax:* 252 816-2398
E-mail: newton@brody.med.ecu.edu
Internet: http://www.med.ecu.edu/med_peds/index.htm
Accred Length: 4 Years *Program Size:* 23 (*GY1:* 6)
Program ID: 800-36-44-057

Ohio

Akron

Akron General Medical Center/Children's Hospital Medical Center Program

Sponsor: Akron General Medical Center
Children's Hospital Medical Center of Akron

Program Director:
Irene H Chenowith, MD
Ian Dresner, MD
Akron General Med Ctr
400 Wabash Ave
Akron, OH 44307
Tel: 330 384-6050 *Fax:* 330 384-1529
E-mail: meded@agmc.org
Internet: http://agmc.org
Accred Length: 4 Years *Program Size:* 7 (*GY1:* 2)
Program ID: 800-38-44-058

Summa Health System (Children's Hospital Medical Center) Program

Sponsor: Summa Health System
Children's Hospital Medical Center of Akron

Program Director:
Joseph P Myers, MD
Ian G Dresner, MD
Summa Health System
Med Educ/Mary Yanik
525 E Market St
Akron, OH 44309
Tel: 800 322-0517
Internet: http://www.summahealth.org/edu/
Accred Length: 4 Years *Program Size:* 8 (*GY1:* 2)
Program ID: 800-38-44-059

Cincinnati

University of Cincinnati Hospital Group Program

Sponsor: University Hospital Inc

Program Director:
Caroline V Mueller, MD
Frank M Biro, MD
Univ of Cincinnati
Dept of Int Med
PO Box 670557
Cincinnati, OH 45267-0557
Tel: 513 558-2590 *Fax:* 513 558-3878
E-mail: ucintmed@uc.edu
Internet: http://www.med.uc.edu/peds/medpeds.htm
Accred Length: 4 Years *Program Size:* 28 (*GY1:* 7)
Program ID: 800-38-44-082

Cleveland

Case Western Reserve University (MetroHealth) Program

Sponsor: MetroHealth Medical Center

Program Director:
Holly B Perzy, MD
MetroHealth Med Ctr
Dept of Med/Peds
2500 MetroHealth Dr/H522
Cleveland, OH 44109-1998
Tel: 216 778-2882 *Fax:* 216 778-1384
E-mail: ndacko@metrohealth.org
Internet: http://www.metrohealth.org
Accred Length: 4 Years *Program Size:* 23 (*GY1:* 6)
Program ID: 800-38-44-061

Case Western Reserve University Program

Sponsor: University Hospitals of Cleveland

Program Director:
Pamela B David, MD PhD
Keith Armitage, MD
Dept of Med
11100 Euclid Ave
Cleveland, OH 44106
Tel: 216 844-3833 *Fax:* 216 844-8216
Accred Length: 4 Years *Program Size:* 8 (*GY1:* 4)
Program ID: 800-38-44-121

Cleveland Clinic Foundation Program

Sponsor: Cleveland Clinic Foundation

Program Director:
Gary D Williams, MD
Byron J Hoogwerf, MD
Cleveland Clinic Foundation
Dept of Int Med/Pediatrics/P39
9500 Euclid Ave
Cleveland, OH 44195-5242
Tel: 216 444-5690 *Fax:* 216 444-1162
E-mail: meded@cesmtp.ccf.org
Internet: http://www.ccf.org/im/res
Accred Length: 4 Years *Program Size:* 18 (*GY1:* 4)
Program ID: 800-38-44-060

Columbus

Ohio State University Program

Sponsor: Ohio State University Medical Center
Children's Hospital

Program Director:
Dwight A Powell, MD
Robert Murden, MD
Children's Hospital
OSU IM/Peds Program
700 Children's Dr/ED-577
Columbus, OH 43205
Tel: 614 722-4459 *Fax:* 614 722-4458
E-mail: davisp@pediatrics.ohio-state.edu
Accred Length: 4 Years *Program Size:* 28 (*GY1:* 8)
Program ID: 800-38-44-063

Dayton

Wright State University Program

Sponsor: Children's Medical Center
Good Samaritan Hospital and Health Center
Miami Valley Hospital
Veterans Affairs Medical Center (Dayton)
Wright-Patterson Medical Center

Program Director:
Gary M Onady, MD PhD
Wright State Univ
Med/Peds Program
Ste 126 Frederick A White Health Ctr
Dayton, OH 45401-0927
Tel: 937 775-3875 *Fax:* 937 775-2261
E-mail: medpeds@wright.edu
Internet: http://www.med.wright.edu/som/resident/medped/medped.html
Accred Length: 4 Years *Program Size:* 16 (*GY1:* 4)
Program ID: 800-38-44-064

Toledo

Medical College of Ohio at Toledo Program

Sponsor: Medical College of Ohio Hospital
St Vincent Mercy Medical Center
Toledo Hospital

Program Director:
Judith A Schoonmaker, MD
Med Coll of Ohio
3000 Arlington Ave
Rm 4143 Hospital
Toledo, OH 43614
Tel: 419 383-3687 *Fax:* 419 383-6180
E-mail: ndrain@.mco.edu
Internet: http://darwin.mco.edu/medicine
Accred Length: 4 Years *Program Size:* 16 (*GY1:* 3)
Program ID: 800-38-44-065

Youngstown

Western Reserve Care System/NEOUCOM Program

Sponsor: Western Reserve Care System
Forum Health-Northside Medical Center
Forum Health-Tod Children's Hospital
Southside Medical Center

Program Director:
Mary B Toth, MD
Eugene Mowad, MD
Western Reserve Healthcare-Forum Health
500 Gypsy Ln
Box 240
Youngstown, OH 44501-0240
Tel: 330 740-5813 *Fax:* 330 740-5727
Accred Length: 4 Years *Program Size:* 10 (*GY1:* 4)
Program ID: 800-38-44-066

Oklahoma

Oklahoma City

University of Oklahoma Health Sciences Center Program

Sponsor: University Hospital
Children's Hospital of Oklahoma

Program Director:
Todd A Krehbiel, MD
Univ of Oklahoma Coll of Med
Children's Hospital
PO Box 26901/Rm 2426-B
Oklahoma City, OK 73190
Tel: 405 271-4417 *Fax:* 405 271-2920
Accred Length: 4 Years *Program Size:* 13 (*GY1:* 3)
Program ID: 800-39-44-090

Tulsa

University of Oklahoma College of Medicine-Tulsa Program

Sponsor: University of Oklahoma College of Medicine-Tulsa
Hillcrest Medical Center
St Francis Hospital
St John Medical Center
Veterans Affairs Medical Center (Muskogee)

Program Director:
Michael A Weisz, MD
Gwen Gibson, MD
Univ of Oklahoma Coll of Med-Tulsa
Dept of Int Med
2808 S Sheridan Rd
Tulsa, OK 74129-1077
Tel: 918 838-4691 *Fax:* 918 838-4897
Internet: http://www.tulsa.ouhsc.edu/
Accred Length: 4 Years *Program Size:* 8 (*GY1:* 2)
Program ID: 800-39-44-067

Pennsylvania

Danville

Penn State Geisinger Health System/Geisinger Medical Center Program

Sponsor: Penn State Geisinger Health System

Program Director:
Mark Speake, MD
Geisinger Med Ctr
100 N Academy Ave
Danville, PA 17822
Tel: 717 271-6787 *Fax:* 717 271-5734
E-mail: dkeszkowski@psghs.edu
Accred Length: 4 Years *Program Size:* 16 (*GY1:* 4)
Program ID: 800-41-44-068

Penn State Geisinger Health System/Milton S Hershey Medical Center Program

Sponsor: Penn State Geisinger Health System

Program Director:
Barbara E Ostrov, MD
Milton S Hershey Med Ctr
PO Box 850
500 University Dr
Hershey, PA 17033-0850
Tel: 717 531-8882 *Fax:* 717 531-4096
E-mail: beo3@psu.edu
Accred Length: 4 Years *Program Size:* 16 (*GY1:* 4)
Program ID: 800-41-44-081

Philadelphia

Albert Einstein Medical Center Program

Sponsor: Albert Einstein Medical Center

Program Director:
Uzi M Selcer, MD
Int Med/Pediatrics Program
Albert Einstein Med Ctr
5401 Old York Rd/Ste 363
Philadelphia, PA 19141-3025
Tel: 800 220-2362 *Fax:* 215 455-1933
E-mail: medpeds@aehn2.einstein.edu
Internet: http://www.einstein.edu/phl
Accred Length: 4 Years *Program Size:* 16 (*GY1:* 4)
Program ID: 800-41-44-069

Allegheny University Hospitals/St Christopher's Hospital for Children Program

Sponsor: St Christopher's Hospital for Children
Hahnemann University Hospital
Medical College of Pennsylvania Hospital

Program Director:
Allan R Tunkel, MD PhD
Robert McGregor, MD
Med Coll of Pennsylvania Hospital
3300 Henry Ave
Philadelphia, PA 19129
Tel: 215 842-6957 *Fax:* 215 843-6038
E-mail: gallaghera@auhs.edu
Accred Length: 4 Years *Program Size:* 2 (*GY1:* 0)
Program ID: 800-41-44-117

Pittsburgh

UPMC Health System Program

Sponsor: University Health Center of Pittsburgh
Children's Hospital of Pittsburgh
Shadyside Hospital/UPMC

Program Director:
Gary Tabas, MD
J Carlton Gartner Jr, MD
UPMC Shadyside
5230 Centre Ave
Pittsburgh, PA 15232
Tel: 412 623-6685 *Fax:* 412 623-2555
Internet: http://www.upmc.edu/medicine/pediatrics
Accred Length: 4 Years *Program Size:* 4 (*GY1:* 4)
Program ID: 800-41-44-128

Rhode Island

Providence

Rhode Island Hospital Program

Sponsor: Rhode Island Hospital

Program Director:
Dominick Tammaro, MD
Patricia Flanagan, MD
Rhode Island Hospital
Dept of Med
593 Eddy St
Providence, RI 02903
Tel: 401 444-4083 *Fax:* 401 444-4730
E-mail: dominick_tammaro@brown.edu
Internet: http://www.brown.edu
Accred Length: 4 Years *Program Size:* 14 (*GY1:* 4)
Program ID: 800-43-44-108

Tennessee

Johnson City

East Tennessee State University Program

Sponsor: James H Quillen College of Medicine

Program Director:
Richard M Jordan, MD
David Price, MD
Dept of Int Med
East Tennessee State Univ
Box 70622
Johnson City, TN 37614-0622
Tel: 423 439-6283 *Fax:* 423 439-6387
Accred Length: 4 Years *Program Size:* 3 (*GY1:* 2)
Program ID: 800-47-44-092

Memphis

University of Tennessee Program

Sponsor: University of Tennessee College of Medicine
LeBonheur Children's Medical Center
Regional Medical Center at Memphis
St Jude Children's Research Hospital
University of Tennessee Medical Center (UT Bowld Hospital)
Veterans Affairs Medical Center (Memphis)

Program Director:
Kevin M McKown, MD
Univ of Tennessee
956 Court Ave/Rm B318
Memphis, TN 38163
Tel: 901 448-5814 *Fax:* 901 448-7836
E-mail: kconlee@utmem1.utmem.edu
Internet: http://www.utmem.edu/internal/internalmed.html
Accred Length: 4 Years *Program Size:* 44 (*GY1:* 12)
Program ID: 800-47-44-071

Nashville

Vanderbilt University Program

Sponsor: Vanderbilt University Medical Center
Metropolitan Nashville General Hospital
Veterans Affairs Medical Center (Nashville)

Program Director:
Sandra Moutsios, MD
Ian M Burr, MD
Vanderbilt Univ Med Ctr
AA-0216 MCN
Nashville, TN 37232-2358
Tel: 615 322-3377 *Fax:* 615 343-7550
E-mail: pridgen.dodie@mcmail.vanderbilt.edu
Internet: http://www.mc.vanderbilt.edu
Accred Length: 4 Years *Program Size:* 16 (*GY1:* 4)
Program ID: 800-47-44-070

Texas

Galveston

University of Texas Medical Branch Hospitals Program

Sponsor: University of Texas Medical Branch Hospitals

Program Director:
Susan E Keeney, MD
Univ of Texas Med Branch
Dept of Pediatrics
301 University Blvd
Galveston, TX 77555-0354
Tel: 409 772-1398 *Fax:* 409 772-4599
E-mail: skeeney@utmb.edu
Internet: http://www.utmb.edu/pedi
Accred Length: 4 Years *Program Size:* 15 (*GY1:* 6)
Program ID: 800-48-44-113

Houston

Baylor College of Medicine Program

Sponsor: Baylor College of Medicine
Harris County Hospital District-Ben Taub General Hospital
Methodist Hospital
St Luke's Episcopal Hospital
Texas Children's Hospital
Veterans Affairs Medical Center (Houston)

Program Director:
Charles H Miranda, MD
Edward C Lynch, MD
Baylor Coll of Med
6565 Fannin St/MS B-501
Fondren-Brown Bldg
Houston, TX 77030-2707
Tel: 713 790-3217 *Fax:* 713 793-1522
E-mail: mro@bcm.tmc.edu
Internet: http://www.bcm.tmc.edu/medicine/residency
Accred Length: 4 Years *Program Size:* 31 (*GY1:* 8)
Program ID: 800-48-44-074

University of Texas at Houston Program

Sponsor: University of Texas Medical School at Houston
Memorial Hermann Healthcare System
St Joseph Hospital
St Luke's Episcopal Hospital
Texas Heart Institute
University of Texas M D Anderson Cancer Center

Program Director:
Mark A Farnie, MD
Univ of Texas Med Sch
Dept of Int Med
6431 Fannin St/Ste 1.150
Houston, TX 77030
Tel: 713 500-6522 *Fax:* 713 500-6530
E-mail: imres@heart.med.uth.tmc.edu
Internet: http://www.med.uth.tmc.edu/
Accred Length: 4 Years *Program Size:* 53 (*GY1:* 14)
Program ID: 800-48-44-075

Temple

Texas A&M College of Medicine-Scott and White Program

Sponsor: Scott and White Memorial Hospital

Program Director:
James A Barker, MD
John Blevins, MD
Texas A&M-Scott and White
Grad Med Educ
2401 S 31st St
Temple, TX 76508-0001
Tel: 254 724-7633 *Fax:* 254 724-9280
E-mail: blculp@swmail.sw.org
Internet: http://www.swinfo.tamu.edu/gme
Accred Length: 4 Years *Program Size:* 12 (*GY1:* 3)
Program ID: 800-48-44-083

Utah

Salt Lake City

University of Utah Program

Sponsor: University of Utah Medical Center
Primary Children's Medical Center
Veterans Affairs Medical Center (Salt Lake City)

Program Director:
H James Williams, MD
Ronald S Bloom, MD
Univ of Utah Med Ctr
50 N Medical Dr
Salt Lake City, UT 84132
Tel: 801 581-7899 *Fax:* 801 581-5393
E-mail: improg.dir@hsc.utah.edu or peds.res@hsc.utah.edu
Internet: http://www.int.med.utah.edu and http://www.ped.med.utah.edu
Accred Length: 4 Years *Program Size:* 8 (*GY1:* 2)
Program ID: 800-49-44-091

Virginia

Richmond

Medical College of Virginia Program

Sponsor: Medical College of Virginia Hospitals

Program Director:
Suzanne R Lavoie, MD
Med Coll of Virginia
1101 E Marshall St
Box 980049
Richmond, VA 23298-0049
Tel: 804 828-9711 *Fax:* 804 828-3097
E-mail: slavoie@hsc.vcu.edu
Internet: http://www.views.vcu.edu/internal-medicine/homepage.htm/
Accred Length: 4 Years *Program Size:* 24 (*GY1:* 6)
Program ID: 800-51-44-077

West Virginia

Charleston

West Virginia University (Charleston Division) Program

Sponsor: Charleston Area Medical Center

Program Director:
Gregory D Clarke, MD
James G Rosencrance, MD
West Virginia Univ Health Sciences Ctr
Dept of Int Med
3110 MacCorkle Ave SE
Charleston, WV 25304
Tel: 304 347-1341 *Fax:* 304 347-1344
E-mail: xkff52a@prodigy.com
Internet: http://www.camcare.com/resident.html/#medpeds
Accred Length: 4 Years *Program Size:* 15 (*GY1:* 4)
Program ID: 800-55-44-078

Huntington

Marshall University School of Medicine Program
Sponsor: Marshall University School of Medicine
St Mary's Hospital
Veterans Affairs Medical Center (Huntington)

Program Director:
Kevin W Yingling, MD
Marshall Univ Sch of Med
1600 Medical Center Dr/Ste G-500
Huntington, WV 25701-3655
Tel: 304 691-1084 *Fax:* 304 691-1693
E-mail: yingling@marshall.edu
Accred Length: 4 Years *Program Size:* 7 (*GY1:* 2)
Program ID: 800-55-44-079

Morgantown

West Virginia University Hospitals Program
Sponsor: West Virginia University Hospitals

Program Director:
Christine R Kincaid, MD
West Virginia Univ Hospital
Dept of Med/Peds
PO Box 9214/HSCN
Morgantown, WV 26506-9214
Tel: 304 293-1198 *Fax:* 304 293-1216
E-mail: nkimble@hsc.wvu.edu
Internet: http://www.hsc.wvu.edu/som/pediatrics/peds
Accred Length: 4 Years *Program Size:* 15 (*GY1:* 5)
Program ID: 800-55-44-080

Wisconsin

Marshfield

Marshfield Clinic-St Joseph's Hospital Program
Sponsor: Marshfield Clinic-St Joseph's Hospital

Program Director:
Joseph J Mazza, MD
Marshfield Clinic
Dept of Pediatrics 1A4
1000 N Oak Ave
Marshfield, WI 54449-5777
Tel: 715 387-5267 *Fax:* 715 387-5240
E-mail: schaefec@mfldclin.edu
Internet: http://www.marshmed.org/mfldclin/education/med_ed/residency/resident.htm
Accred Length: 4 Years *Program Size:* 8 (*GY1:* 2)
Program ID: 800-56-44-109

Milwaukee

Medical College of Wisconsin Program
Sponsor: Medical College of Wisconsin Affiliated Hospitals Inc

Program Director:
Charlotte Heidenreich, MD
David Lewis, MD
Dept of Medicine
Div of Educational Affairs
9200 W Wisconsin Ave/FMLH-MOB
Milwaukee, WI 53226
Tel: 414 456-6794 *Fax:* 414 456-6213
Internet: http://www.mcw.edu
Accred Length: 4 Years *Program Size:* 16 (*GY1:* 4)
Program ID: 800-56-44-096

Internal Medicine/ Physical Medicine and Rehabilitation

Illinois

Chicago

University of Illinois College of Medicine at Chicago Program
Sponsor: University of Illinois College of Medicine at Chicago
University of Illinois Hospital and Clinics
Veterans Affairs West Side Medical Center

Program Director:
Jessica F Tinianow, MD
Linda G Lesky, MD
Univ of Illinois Hospital
Dept of Phys Med/Rehab
840 S Wood St (M/C 899)
Chicago, IL 60612
Tel: 312 996-7211 *Fax:* 312 996-4829
E-mail: rehab@uic.edu
Accred Length: 5 Years *Program Size:* 1 (*GY1:* 0)
Program ID: 810-16-44-014

Louisiana

New Orleans

Louisiana State University Program
Sponsor: Louisiana State University School of Medicine
Louisiana State University Medical College Campus

Program Director:
Robert C Mipro Jr, MD
Dayton Daberkow, MD
Louisiana State Univ Med Ctr
Sect of Phys Med/Rehab
1542 Tulane Ave/Box T6M-2
New Orleans, LA 70112-2822
Tel: 504 568-2688 *Fax:* 504 568-7839
E-mail: pmr@lsumc.edu
Accred Length: 5 Years *Program Size:* 8 (*GY1:* 2)
Program ID: 810-21-44-002

Maryland

Baltimore

Sinai Hospital of Baltimore Program
Sponsor: Sinai Hospital of Baltimore

Program Director:
Steven Gambert, MD
Gerald Felsenthal, MD
Sinai Health System
Dept of Med
2435 W Belvedere Ave
Baltimore, MD 21215-5271
Tel: 410 601-6256 *Fax:* 410 601-5638
E-mail: dchow@sinai-balt.com
Internet: http://www.sinai-balt.com
Accred Length: 5 Years *Program Size:* 6 (*GY1:* 0)
Program ID: 810-23-44-011

Massachusetts

Newton Lower Falls

Tufts University Program
Sponsor: Newton-Wellesley Hospital
New England Medical Center Hospitals

Program Director:
Mark S Drapkin, MD
Marvin M Brooke, MD
Tufts Comb Int Med/Phys Med and Rehab
Newton-Wellesley Hospital
2014 Washington St
Newton, MA 02162
Tel: 617 243-6467 *Fax:* 617 243-6701
Internet: http://www.nwh.org
Accred Length: 5 Years *Program Size:* 3 (*GY1:* 0)
Program ID: 810-24-44-012

Michigan

Detroit

Wayne State University Program
Sponsor: Wayne State University/Detroit Medical Center
Detroit Receiving Hospital and University Health Center
Rehabilitation Institute

Program Director:
Bruce E Becker, MD
Rehabilitation Inst of Michigan
261 Mack Ave
Detroit, MI 48201
Tel: 313 745-9852 *Fax:* 313 745-1197
Internet: http://www.med.wayne.edu
Accred Length: 5 Years *Program Size:* 8 (*GY1:* 1)
Program ID: 810-25-44-015

New Jersey

Newark

UMDNJ-New Jersey Medical School Program
Sponsor: UMDNJ-New Jersey Medical School
UMDNJ-University Hospital
Veterans Affairs Medical Center (East Orange)

Program Director:
Steven Kirshblum, MD
Marilyn Miller, MD MD
UMDNJ-New Jersey Med Sch
Univ Hospital
150 Bergen St/B261
Newark, NJ 07103
Tel: 973 972-3606
E-mail: leckyal@umdnj.edu
Accred Length: 5 Years *Program Size:* 10 (*GY1:* 2)
Program ID: 810-33-44-022

New York

Buffalo

SUNY at Buffalo Graduate Medical-Dental Education Consortium Program
Sponsor: SUNY at Buffalo Grad Medical-Dental Education Consortium
CGF Health System (Buffalo General Hospital)
Erie County Medical Center
Veterans Affairs Medical Center (Buffalo)
Program Director:
Gary S Clark, MD MD MD
SUNY-Buffalo
Erie County Med Ctr Rm G223
462 Grider St
Buffalo, NY 14215
Tel: 716 898-3218 *Fax:* 716 898-3652
Accred Length: 5 Years *Program Size:* 5 *(GY1:* 1)
Program ID: 810-35-44-020

New York

Columbia-Presbyterian Medical Center Program
Sponsor: New York and Presbyterian Hospital (Columbia Campus)
Program Director:
Peter Gordon, MD
Nancy E Strauss, MD
Presbyterian Hospital
622 W 168th St/PH8 W
New York, NY 10032
Tel: 212 305-9396 *Fax:* 212 305-9349
E-mail: pgg2@columbia.edu
Accred Length: 5 Years *Program Size:* 1 *(GY1:* 0)
Program ID: 810-35-44-022

Ohio

Cincinnati

University of Cincinnati Medical Center Program
Sponsor: University Hospital Inc
Program Director:
Mary E Dillon, MD
Univ Hospital-Univ of Cincinnati Coll of Med
Dept of Phys Med/Rehab
PO Box 670530
Cincinnati, OH 45267-0530
Tel: 513 558-7635 *Fax:* 513 558-4458
E-mail: williapa@email.uc.edu
Internet: http://www.med.uc.edu/htdocs/medicine/departme/pmr/pmrres.htm
Accred Length: 5 Years *Program Size:* 4 *(GY1:* 1)
Program ID: 810-38-44-019

Cleveland

Case Western Reserve University Program
Sponsor: MetroHealth Medical Center
Program Director:
Michael J McFarlane, MD
Shu Huang, MD
MetroHealth Med Ctr
2500 MetroHealth Dr
Cleveland, OH 44109-1998
Tel: 216 778-3886 *Fax:* 216 778-5823
E-mail: medres@metrohealth.org
Internet: http://www.metrohealth.org
Accred Length: 5 Years *Program Size:* 4 *(GY1:* 0)
Program ID: 810-38-44-016

Pennsylvania

Philadelphia

Albert Einstein Medical Center Program
Sponsor: Albert Einstein Medical Center
Temple University Hospital
Program Director:
Lisa B Wallenstein, MD
James T Demopoulos, MD
Int Med/Phys Med and Rehab Program
Albert Einstein Med Ctr
5401 Old York Rd/Ste 363
Philadelphia, PA 19141-3025
Tel: 800 220-2362 *Fax:* 215 455-1933
E-mail: medicine@aehn2.einstein.edu
Internet: http://www.einstein.edu/phl
Accred Length: 5 Years *Program Size:* 10 *(GY1:* 2)
Program ID: 810-41-44-013

Temple University Program
Sponsor: Temple University Hospital
Program Director:
Richard S Eisenstaedt, MD
James T Demopoulos, MD
Temple Univ Hospital
3401 N Broad St
Parkinson Pavilion/8th Fl
Philadelphia, PA 19140
Tel: 215 707-7021 *Fax:* 215 707-7661
Accred Length: 5 Years *Program Size:* 10 *(GY1:* 2)
Program ID: 810-41-44-006

The Graduate Hospital Program
Sponsor: Hahnemann University Hospital
Program Director:
Eliot H Nierman, MD
Francis J Bonner Jr, MD
Graduate Hospital
1800 Lombard St
Philadelphia, PA 19146-1497
Tel: 215 893-4150 *Fax:* 215 893-6623
Accred Length: 5 Years *Program Size:* 0
Program ID: 810-41-44-021

Pittsburgh

St Francis Medical Center Program
Sponsor: St Francis Medical Center
Program Director:
T Michael White, MD
Joseph Eshleman, DO
St Francis Med Ctr
Med Educ Office
400 45th St
Pittsburgh, PA 15201
Tel: 412 622-4388
Internet: http://www.sfhs.edu
Accred Length: 5 Years *Program Size:* 5 *(GY1:* 1)
Program ID: 810-41-44-008

Texas

Houston

Baylor College of Medicine Program
Sponsor: Baylor College of Medicine
Program Director:
Edward C Lynch, MD
Martin Grabois, MD
Combined Int Med/Phys Med and Rehab
6565 Fannin St/MS B-501
Fondren Brown Bldg
Houston, TX 77030-2707
Tel: 713 790-3217 *Fax:* 713 793-1522
Accred Length: 5 Years *Program Size:* 1 *(GY1:* 0)
Program ID: 810-48-44-009

Internal Medicine/ Preventive Medicine

Colorado

Denver

University of Colorado Program
Sponsor: University of Colorado Health Sciences Center
Program Director:
William D Kaehny, MD
William M Marine, MD
Univ of Colorado Sch of Med
4200 E Ninth Ave/B-177
Denver, CO 80262
Tel: 303 315-7768 *Fax:* 303 315-7653
E-mail: sherry.berka@uchsc.edu
Internet: http://www.uchsc.edu/sm/pmb/pmb/edpgms.htm
Accred Length: 4 Years *Program Size:* 2 *(GY1:* 0)
Program ID: 851-07-44-002

Illinois

Chicago

Cook County Hospital Program
Sponsor: Cook County Hospital
Program Director:
Maurice Lemon, MD
Rachel Rubin, MD
Dept of Medicine
Cook County Hospital
1835 W Harrison
Chicago, IL 60612
Tel: 312 633-5310 *Fax:* 312 633-6442
E-mail: rrubin@uic.edu
Accred Length: 4 Years *Program Size:* 7 *(GY1:* 2)
Program ID: 851-16-44-005

Louisiana

New Orleans

Tulane University Program
Sponsor: Tulane University School of Medicine
Tulane Univ School of Public Health and Tropical Medicine
Program Director:
Mark J Kahn, MD
M Krousel-Wood, MD
Tulane Univ Med Ctr
Dept of Med/SL50
1430 Tulane Ave
New Orleans, LA 70112-2699
Tel: 504 582-7821 *Fax:* 504 586-3971
E-mail: mkahn@tmcpop.tmc.tulane.edu
Accred Length: 4 Years *Program Size:* 4 *(GY1:* 1)
Program ID: 851-21-44-003

New York

Buffalo

SUNY at Buffalo Graduate Medical-Dental Education Consortium Program
Sponsor: SUNY at Buffalo Grad Medical-Dental Education Consortium
CGF Health System (Buffalo General Hospital)
Program Director:
Robert A Klocke, MD
Michael F Noe, MD
Erie County Med Ctr
Dept of Medicine
462 Grider St
Buffalo, NY 14215
Tel: 716 898-5210 *Fax:* 716 898-3279
Accred Length: 4 Years *Program Size:* 1 (*GYI:* 1)
Program ID: 851-35-44-004

Texas

Houston

Baylor College of Medicine Program
Sponsor: Baylor College of Medicine
Harris County Hospital District-Ben Taub General Hospital
Methodist Hospital
St Luke's Episcopal Hospital
Veterans Affairs Medical Center (Houston)
Program Director:
Edward Lynch, MD
George L Delclos, MD
Baylor Coll of Med
6565 Fannin St/MS B-501
Fondren-Brown Bldg
Houston, TX 77030-2707
Tel: 713 790-3217 *Fax:* 713 793-1522
E-mail: mro@bcm.tmc.edu
Internet: http://www.bcm.tmc.edu/medicine/residency
Accred Length: 4 Years *Program Size:* 1 (*GYI:* 1)
Program ID: 851-48-44-001

Internal Medicine/ Psychiatry

Arizona

Phoenix

Good Samaritan Regional Medical Center Program
Sponsor: Good Samaritan Regional Medical Center
Program Director:
James B McLoone, MD
Alan I Leibowitz, MD
Good Samaritan Regional Med Ctr
925 E McDowell Rd/4th Fl
Phoenix, AZ 85006
Tel: 602 239-6880 *Fax:* 602 239-6988
E-mail: andreaw@samaritan.edu
Internet: http://www.samaritan.edu
Accred Length: 5 Years *Program Size:* 6 (*GYI:* 2)
Program ID: 815-03-44-017

Connecticut

Farmington

University of Connecticut Program
Sponsor: University of Connecticut School of Medicine
Hartford Hospital
Univ of Connecticut Health Center/John Dempsey Hospital
Program Director:
Sharon Diamen, MD
10 Talcott Notch Rd
East Wing
Farmington, CT 06030-6410
Tel: 860 679-6729
Accred Length: 5 Years *Program Size:* 10 (*GYI:* 0)
Program ID: 815-08-44-029

District of Columbia

Washington

National Capital Consortium Program
Sponsor: Walter Reed Army Institute of Research
National Capital Consortium
Program Director:
Scott Joslin, MD
James Rundell, MD
Dept of Psychiatry
Walter Reed Army Med Ctr
Washington, DC 20307-5001
Tel: 202 782-6545 *Fax:* 202 782-8396
E-mail: scott25@erols.com
Accred Length: 5 Years *Program Size:* 7 (*GYI:* 1)
Program ID: 815-23-44-021
US Armed Services Program

Hawaii

Honolulu

Tripler Army Medical Center Program
Sponsor: Tripler Army Medical Center
Program Director:
Maj Richard L Jaconette, MD
Lt Col Benjamin W Berg, MD
Tripler Army Med Ctr
1 Jarrett White Rd
Tripler AMC, HI 96589-5000
Tel: 808 433-4049
E-mail: benjamin_w.berg@tamc.chcs.amedd.army.mil
Accred Length: 5 Years *Program Size:* 3 (*GYI:* 3)
Program ID: 815-14-44-019
US Armed Services Program

Illinois

Chicago

Rush-Presbyterian-St Luke's Medical Center Program
Sponsor: Rush-Presbyterian-St Luke's Medical Center
Program Director:
Stephanie V Cavanaugh, MD
Richard Abrams, MD
Rush-Presbyterian-St Luke's Med Ctr
1720 W Polk St
Chicago, IL 60612-3833
Tel: 312 942-5015 *Fax:* 312 942-3113
Accred Length: 5 Years *Program Size:* 10 (*GYI:* 4)
Program ID: 815-16-44-018

Springfield

Southern Illinois University Program
Sponsor: Southern Illinois University School of Medicine
Memorial Medical Center
St John's Hospital
Program Director:
Andrew J Varney, MD
Southern Illinois Univ Sch of Med
800 N Rutledge
PO Box 19636
Springfield, IL 62794-9636
Tel: 217 782-0193 *Fax:* 217 524-8156
E-mail: avarney@siumed.edu
Internet: http://www.siumed.edu
Accred Length: 5 Years *Program Size:* 9 (*GYI:* 2)
Program ID: 815-16-44-009

Iowa

Iowa City

University of Iowa Hospitals and Clinics Program
Sponsor: University of Iowa Hospitals and Clinics
Veterans Affairs Medical Center (Iowa City)
Program Director:
Caroline C Doebbeling, MD
Univ of Iowa Hospitals and Clinics
Dept of Int Med/GH
200 Hawkins Dr
Iowa City, IA 52242-1081
Tel: 319 356-2034 *Fax:* 319 356-7893
E-mail: caroline-carney@uiowa.edu
Accred Length: 5 Years *Program Size:* 10 (*GYI:* 2)
Program ID: 815-18-44-003

Kansas

Kansas City

University of Kansas Medical Center Program

Sponsor: University of Kansas School of Medicine
University of Kansas Medical Center
Veterans Affairs Medical Center (Kansas City)

Program Director:
Teresa D Long, MD
Jane Lauchland, MD
Univ of Kansas Med Ctr
Dept of Psychiatry
3901 Rainbow Blvd
Kansas City, KS 66160-7341
Tel: 913 588-6464 *Fax:* 913 588-6414
Accred Length: 5 Years *Program Size:* 5 (*GY1:* 2)
Program ID: 815-19-44-008

Louisiana

New Orleans

Tulane University Program

Sponsor: Tulane University School of Medicine
Louisiana State University Medical College Campus
Tulane University Hospital and Clinics
Veterans Affairs Medical Center (New Orleans)

Program Director:
Patrick T O'Neill, MD
Marc J Kahn, MD
Tulane Univ Sch of Med
Dept of Psychiatry TB53
1440 Canal St
New Orleans, LA 70112-2715
Tel: 504 894-7269 *Fax:* 504 894-7290
E-mail: poneill@mailhost.tcs.tulane.edu.
Internet: http://www.tulane.edu/
Accred Length: 5 Years *Program Size:* 5 (*GY1:* 2)
Program ID: 815-21-44-010

Michigan

East Lansing

Michigan State University Program

Sponsor: Michigan State University College of Human Medicine
Michigan State University Clinical Center
St Lawrence Hospital and HealthCare Services

Program Director:
Jed Magen, DO
Michael Zaroukian, MD
Michigan State Univ
Dept of Psychiatry
B-109 W Fee
East Lansing, MI 48824-1316
Tel: 517 353-4362
Accred Length: 5 Years *Program Size:* 2 (*GY1:* 0)
Program ID: 815-25-44-011

New Hampshire

Lebanon

Dartmouth-Hitchcock Medical Center Program

Sponsor: Mary Hitchcock Memorial Hospital
Veterans Affairs Medical Center (White River Junction)

Program Director:
Richard Comi, MD
Ronald Green, MD
Dartmouth-Hitchcock Med Ctr
One Medical Center Dr
Lebanon, NH 03756
Tel: 603 650-7688 *Fax:* 603 650-6122
Accred Length: 5 Years *Program Size:* 5 (*GY1:* 2)
Program ID: 815-32-44-016

New Jersey

Piscataway

UMDNJ-Robert Wood Johnson Medical Center Program

Sponsor: UMDNJ-Robert Wood Johnson Medical School
Robert Wood Johnson University Hospital

Program Director:
Barbara Palmeri, MD
UMDNJ-Robert Wood Johnson Med Sch
Dept of Psychiatry
671 Hoes Ln
New Brunswick, NJ 08854-5633
Tel: 732 235-4433 *Fax:* 732 235-4649
Accred Length: 5 Years *Program Size:* 2 (*GY1:* 2)
Program ID: 815-33-44-023

New York

Bronx

Albert Einstein College of Medicine Program

Sponsor: Albert Einstein College of Medicine of Yeshiva University
Jacobi Medical Center

Program Director:
Steven R Hahn, MD
Scott Rogge, MD
Jacobi Med Ctr
Jacobi 3 West-10
Pelham Pkwy S and Eastchester
Bronx, NY 10461
Tel: 718 918-4996 *Fax:* 718 918-7701
Accred Length: 5 Years *Program Size:* 1 (*GY1:* 0)
Program ID: 815-35-44-019

Bronx-Lebanon Hospital Center Program

Sponsor: Bronx-Lebanon Hospital Center

Program Director:
Nalini V Juthani, MD
Sridhar Chilimuri, MD
Bronx-Lebanon Hospital Ctr
Dept of Psychiatry
1276 Fulton Ave
Bronx, NY 10456
Tel: 718 901-8653 *Fax:* 718 901-8656
E-mail: juthani@aecom.yu.edu
Accred Length: 5 Years *Program Size:* 0 (*GY1:* 0)
Program ID: 815-35-44-016

Brooklyn

SUNY Health Science Center at Brooklyn Program

Sponsor: SUNY Health Science Center at Brooklyn
Kings County Hospital Center
University Hospital-SUNY Health Science Center at Brooklyn

Program Director:
Eric Weitzner, MD
Jeanne Macrae, MD
SUNY Health Science Ctr-Brooklyn
450 Clarkson Ave/Box 1203
Brooklyn, NY 11203-2098
Tel: 718 245-2321 *Fax:* 718 778-5397
Accred Length: 5 Years *Program Size:* 4 (*GY1:* 1)
Program ID: 815-35-44-004

Rochester

University of Rochester Program

Sponsor: Strong Memorial Hospital of the University of Rochester

Program Director:
Rory P Houghtalen, MD
Craig B Kaplan, MD
Univ of Rochester Med Ctr
300 Crittenden Blvd
Rochester, NY 14642-8409
Tel: 716 275-4985 *Fax:* 716 273-1066
E-mail: trudy_haseley@urmc.rochester.edu
Internet: http://www.urmc.rochester.edu/smd/psych
Accred Length: 5 Years *Program Size:* 10 (*GY1:* 2)
Program ID: 815-35-44-007

North Carolina

Durham

Duke University Program

Sponsor: Duke University Medical Center
Veterans Affairs Medical Center (Durham)

Program Director:
Grace Thrall, MD
Ralph Corey, MD
Duke Univ Med Ctr
PO Box 3837
Durham, NC 27710
Tel: 919 684-2258 *Fax:* 919 684-2290
E-mail: psychres@mc.duke.edu
Internet: http://niles.mc.duke.edu
Accred Length: 5 Years *Program Size:* 14 (*GY1:* 4)
Program ID: 815-36-44-012

Greenville

East Carolina University Program

Sponsor: East Carolina University School of Medicine
Pitt County Memorial Hospital

Program Director:
James G Peden Jr, MD
East Carolina Univ Sch of Med
Dept of Med
389 PCMH-TA
Greenville, NC 27858
Tel: 919 816-4663
Accred Length: 5 Years *Program Size:* 10 (*GY1:* 2)
Program ID: 815-36-44-005

Pennsylvania

Philadelphia

Albert Einstein Medical Center Program

Sponsor: Albert Einstein Medical Center

Program Director:
Lisa B Wallenstein, MD
Frederick C Miller, MD
Albert Einstein Med Ctr
Dept of Med
5401 Old York Rd/Ste 363
Philadelphia, PA 19141-3025
Tel: 800 220-2362 *Fax:* 215 455-1933
E-mail: medicine@aehn2.einstein.edu
Internet: http://www.einstein.edu/phl
Accred Length: 5 Years *Program Size:* 10 (*GY1:* 2)
Program ID: 815-41-44-001

Pittsburgh

St Francis Health System Program

Sponsor: St Francis Medical Center

Program Director:
David J Lynn, MD
T Michael White, MD
St Francis Med Ctr
Med Educ Office
400 45th St
Pittsburgh, PA 15201-1198
Tel: 412 622-4796
E-mail: psyres@sfhs.edu
Internet: http://www.sfhs.edu/meded/psych/index.htm
Accred Length: 5 Years *Program Size:* 4 (*GY1:* 2)
Program ID: 815-41-44-015

South Carolina

Charleston

Medical University of South Carolina Program

Sponsor: Medical University of South Carolina College of Medicine
MUSC Medical Center
Ralph H Johnson Dept of Veterans Affairs Med Center

Program Director:
Alan Robbins, MD
Alberto Santos, MD
Med Univ of South Carolina
171 Ashley Ave
Charleston, SC 29425-2201
Tel: 843 577-5011, ext 7202 *Fax:* 843 792-2967
Accred Length: 5 Years *Program Size:* 10 (*GY1:* 2)
Program ID: 815-45-44-025

Tennessee

Johnson City

East Tennessee State University Program

Sponsor: James H Quillen College of Medicine
Johnson City Medical Center Hospital
Veterans Affairs Medical Center (Mountain Home)

Program Director:
Richard M Jordan, MD
Brent R Coyle, MD
Dept of Internal Medicine
Box 70622
Johnson City, TN 37614-0622
Tel: 423 439-6282
Accred Length: 5 Years *Program Size:* 10 (*GY1:* 0)
Program ID: 815-47-44-028

Texas

San Antonio

University of Texas Health Science Center at San Antonio Program

Sponsor: University of Texas Medical School at San Antonio
Audie L Murphy Memorial Veterans Hospital (San Antonio)
University Hospital-South Texas Medical Center

Program Director:
Kenneth L Matthews, MD
Univ of Texas Health Science Ctr
Dept of Psychiatry
7703 Floyd Curl Dr
San Antonio, TX 78284-7792
Tel: 210 567-5430 *Fax:* 210 567-6941
E-mail: matthewsk@uthscsa.edu
Internet: http://www.psych68.uthscsa.edu
Accred Length: 5 Years *Program Size:* 4 (*GY1:* 4)
Program ID: 815-48-44-024

Virginia

Charlottesville

University of Virginia Program

Sponsor: University of Virginia Medical Center

Program Director:
Zachariah C Dameron, MD
Univ of Virginia Sch of Med
Dept of Psychiatric Med
Box 623 HSC
Charlottesville, VA 22908
Tel: 804 924-5408 *Fax:* 804 924-5149
E-mail: psychresidency@virginia.edu
Internet: http://www.hsc.virginia.edu/psychresidency/
Accred Length: 5 Years *Program Size:* 17 (*GY1:* 4)
Program ID: 815-51-44-002

Roanoke

University of Virginia-Roanoke/Salem Program

Sponsor: Carilion Health System
Carilion Roanoke Memorial Hospital
Veterans Affairs Medical Center (Salem)

Program Director:
J Joe Yazel, MD
VA Med Ctr
1970 Roanoke Blvd
Salem, VA 24153
Tel: 540 982-2463, ext 1650 *Fax:* 540 983-1086
E-mail: yazel.john_j@salem.va.gov
Internet: http://www.carilion.com/residency
Accred Length: 5 Years *Program Size:* 10 (*GY1:* 2)
Program ID: 815-51-44-027

West Virginia

Charleston

West Virginia University (Charleston Division) Program

Sponsor: Charleston Area Medical Center

Program Director:
T O Dickey III, MD
Shawn Chillag, MD
Med/Psychiatry Program
Robert C Byrd Health Sciences Ctr
501 Morris St/PO Box 1547
Charleston, WV 25326-1547
Tel: 304 341-1500 *Fax:* 304 341-1508
Accred Length: 5 Years *Program Size:* 10 (*GY1:* 2)
Program ID: 815-51-44-014

Morgantown

West Virginia University Program

Sponsor: West Virginia University Hospitals

Program Director:
Calvin R Sumner, MD
Maria Kolar, MD
Dept of Behav Med/Psychiatry
Chestnut Ridge Hospital
930 Chestnut Ridge Rd
Morgantown, WV 26506
Tel: 304 293-2411 *Fax:* 304 293-8724
E-mail: king@wvnvm.wvnet.edu
Internet: http://www.hsc.wvu.edu/som/psychiatry
Accred Length: 5 Years *Program Size:* 10 (*GY1:* 2)
Program ID: 815-55-44-006

Neurology/Diagnostic Radiology/ Neuroradiology

Georgia

Atlanta

Emory University Program
Sponsor: Emory University School of Medicine
Emory University Hospital
Grady Memorial Hospital
Program Director:
Bruce R Baumgartner, MD
Dept of Radiology
Emory Univ Hospital
1364 Clifton Rd NE
Atlanta, GA 30322
Tel: 404 712-4686 *Fax:* 404 712-7908
E-mail: maryellen_johnson@emory.org
Accred Length: 7 Years *Program Size:* 2 (*GY1:* 1)
Program ID: 860-12-44-001

New York

New York

New York University Medical Center Program
Sponsor: New York University Medical Center
Bellevue Hospital Center
Veterans Affairs Medical Center (Manhattan)
Program Director:
Peter K Nelson, MD
New York Univ Med Ctr
Dept of Rad/Neurointerventional Service
560 First Ave
New York, NY 10016
Tel: 212 263-8223 *Fax:* 212 263-8228
E-mail: patricia.szymanski@med.nyu.edu
Accred Length: 7 Years *Program Size:* 2 (*GY1:* 2)
Program ID: 860-35-44-002

Ohio

Cleveland

Cleveland Clinic Foundation Program
Sponsor: Cleveland Clinic Foundation
Program Director:
Paul M Ruggieri, MD
Patrick J Sweeney, MD
Cleveland Clinic Foundation
Dept of Neuroradiology/L10
9500 Euclid Ave
Cleveland, OH 44195
Tel: 216 444-7035 *Fax:* 216 444-5466
E-mail: ruggiep@cesmtp.ccf.org
Internet: http://www.ccf.org
Accred Length: 7 Years *Program Size:* 0 (*GY1:* 0)
Program ID: 860-38-44-003

Wisconsin

Madison

University of Wisconsin Program
Sponsor: University of Wisconsin Hospital and Clinics
William S Middleton Veterans Hospital
Program Director:
Virgil Graves, MD
Lindell Gentry, MD
Univ of Wisconsin
E3-311 CSC
600 Highland Ave
Madison, WI 53792
Tel: 608 263-6457 *Fax:* 608 263-0412
E-mail: vbgraves@facstaff.wisc.edu
Internet: http://www.radres.radiology.wisc.edu
Accred Length: 7 Years *Program Size:* 1 (*GY1:* 1)
Program ID: 860-56-44-004

Neurology/Physical Medicine and Rehabilitation

Illinois

Chicago

University of Illinois College of Medicine at Chicago Program
Sponsor: University of Illinois College of Medicine at Chicago
University of Illinois Hospital and Clinics
Program Director:
Steven Brint, MD
Jessica F Tinianow, MD
Univ of Illinois
Dept of Neurology
912 S Wood St/Rm 855N
Chicago, IL 60612-7330
Tel: 312 996-6906 *Fax:* 312 413-1388
E-mail: neuro@uic.edu
Internet: http://www.uic.edu/depts/mcne
Accred Length: 5 Years *Program Size:* 1 (*GY1:* 1)
Program ID: 850-16-44-003

Pennsylvania

Philadelphia

University of Pennsylvania Program
Sponsor: Hospital of the University of Pennsylvania
Program Director:
Charles R Cantor, MD
Keith M Robinson, MD
Pennsylvania Hospital
Dept of Neurology
8th and Spruce Sts
Philadelphia, PA 19107
Tel: 215 829-7550 *Fax:* 215 625-9187
Accred Length: 5 Years *Program Size:* 3 (*GY1:* 2)
Program ID: 850-41-44-002

Pediatrics/Emergency Medicine

California

Los Angeles

UCLA-Olive View Program
Sponsor: UCLA School of Medicine
Olive View-UCLA Medical Center
UCLA Medical Center
Program Director:
James Korb, MD
Pamela L Dyne, MD
Dept of Pediatrics
10833 Le Conte Ave
Los Angeles, CA 90095-1752
Tel: 310 794-2169 *Fax:* 310 825-6394
Accred Length: 5 Years *Program Size:* 10 (*GY1:* 2)
Program ID: 825-05-44-008

Indiana

Indianapolis

Indiana University School of Medicine (Methodist) Program
Sponsor: Indiana University School of Medicine
Clarian Methodist Hospital of Indiana
Program Director:
Carey D Chisholm, MD
Charlene E Graves, MD
Clarian Methodist Hospital
Emergency Med/Trauma Ctr
1701 N Senate Blvd
Indianapolis, IN 46202
Tel: 317 929-5975 *Fax:* 317 929-2306
E-mail: cchisholm@clarian.com
Accred Length: 5 Years *Program Size:* 11 (*GY1:* 2)
Program ID: 825-17-44-005

Maryland

Baltimore

University of Maryland Program
Sponsor: University of Maryland Medical System
Mercy Medical Center
Program Director:
Carol L Carraccio, MD
Univ of Maryland Med Ctr
Dept of Pediatrics
22 S Greene St
Baltimore, MD 21201
Tel: 410 328-6662 *Fax:* 410 328-0646
E-mail: pschmidt@peds.umaryland.edu
Internet: http://www.mdkids.ab.umd.edu
Accred Length: 5 Years *Program Size:* 10 (*GY1:* 2)
Program ID: 825-23-44-006

Michigan

Detroit

Wayne State University Program
Sponsor: Children's Hospital of Michigan
Detroit Receiving Hospital and University Health Center
Wayne State University/Detroit Medical Center
Program Director:
Brooks F Bock, MD
Alan B Gruskin, MD
Detroit Receiving Hospital
8D-University Health Ctr
4201 St Antoine
Detroit, MI 48201-2194
Tel: 313 993-2530 *Fax:* 313 993-7703
E-mail: rwahl@med.wayne.edu
Internet: http://www.med.wayne.edu/er/
Accred Length: 5 Years *Program Size:* 4 (*GY1:* 0)
Program ID: 825-25-44-001

Minnesota

Minneapolis

Hennepin County Medical Center Program
Sponsor: Hennepin County Medical Center
Program Director:
Douglas D Brunette, MD
Hennepin County Med Ctr
701 Park Ave S
Minneapolis, MN 55415
Tel: 612 347-5683 *Fax:* 612 904-4241
Accred Length: 5 Years *Program Size:* 0 (*GY1:* 0)
Program ID: 825-26-44-007

Pediatrics/Medical Genetics

New York

New York

Mount Sinai Medical Center Program
Sponsor: Mount Sinai School of Medicine
Mount Sinai Medical Center
Program Director:
Margaret Mary McGovern, MD PhD
One Gustave L Levy Pl
Box 1497
New York, NY 10029-6574
Tel: 212 241-6947 *Fax:* 212 860-3316
E-mail: mmcgovern@esmtplink.mssm.edu
Accred Length: 5 Years *Program Size:* 1 (*GY1:* 1)
Program ID: 865-35-44-001

Ohio

Cleveland

Case Western Reserve University Program
Sponsor: University Hospitals of Cleveland
Program Director:
Suzanne B Cassidy, MD
Michael L Nieder, MD
11100 Euclid Ave
Cleveland, OH 44106
Tel: 216 844-3936 *Fax:* 216 844-7497
Accred Length: 5 Years *Program Size:* 2 (*GY1:* 2)
Program ID: 865-38-44-002

Pediatrics/Physical Medicine and Rehabilitation

Colorado

Denver

University of Colorado Program
Sponsor: University of Colorado Health Sciences Center
Program Director:
Mary P Glode, MD
Donna J Blake, MD
Univ of Colorado Health Sciences Ctr
Dept of Pediatrics
1056 E 19th Ave/B158
Denver, CO 80218
Tel: 303 861-6738 *Fax:* 303 764-8189
E-mail: glode.mary@tchden.org
Internet: http://www.uchsc.edu./sm/gme/index.htm
Accred Length: 5 Years *Program Size:* 2 (*GY1:* 1)
Program ID: 835-07-44-001

Michigan

Detroit

Wayne State University Program
Sponsor: Children's Hospital of Michigan
Rehabilitation Institute
Program Director:
Mary W Lieh Lai, MD
Bruce E Becker, MD
Children's Hospital of Michigan
3901 Beaubien Blvd
Detroit, MI 48201-2196
Tel: 313 745-5533 *Fax:* 313 993-7118
E-mail: mliehlai@med.wayne.edu
Internet: http://www.shiffman.wayne.edu/chm/
Accred Length: 5 Years *Program Size:* 5 (*GY1:* 1)
Program ID: 835-25-44-002

Ohio

Cincinnati

University of Cincinnati Hospital Group Program
Sponsor: University Hospital Inc
Program Director:
Mary E Dillon, MD
Univ Hospital-Univ of Cincinnati Coll of Med
Dept of Phys Med/Rehab
PO Box 670530
Cincinnati, OH 45267-0530
Tel: 513 558-7635 *Fax:* 513 558-4458
E-mail: williapa@email.uc.edu
Internet: http://www.med.uc.edu/htdocs/medicine//departme/pmr/pmrres.htm
Accred Length: 5 Years *Program Size:* 5 (*GY1:* 1)
Program ID: 835-38-44-012

Columbus

Children's Hospital/Ohio State University Program
Sponsor: Children's Hospital
Program Director:
John Mahan, MD
William Pease, MD
Columbus Children's Hospital
700 Children's Dr
Columbus, OH 43205
Tel: 614 293-4869 *Fax:* 614 722-6132
Accred Length: 5 Years *Program Size:* 1 (*GY1:* 0)
Program ID: 835-38-44-010

Pennsylvania

Philadelphia

Temple University Program
Sponsor: Temple University Hospital
St Christopher's Hospital for Children
Program Director:
James T Demopoulos, MD
Robert S Wimmer, MD
Temple Univ Hospital
3401 N Broad St
Philadelphia, PA 19140
Tel: 215 707-7021 *Fax:* 215 707-7661
Accred Length: 5 Years *Program Size:* 2 (*GY1:* 1)
Program ID: 835-41-44-021

Thomas Jefferson University/duPont Hospital for Children Program
Sponsor: Thomas Jefferson University Hospital
duPont Hospital for Children
Program Director:
Steven M Selbst, MD
Christopher Formal II, MD
duPont Hospital for Children
PO Box 269
Wilmington, DE 19899
Tel: 302 651-5874 *Fax:* 302 651-5954
E-mail: kwaite@aidi.nemours.org
Accred Length: 5 Years *Program Size:* 1 (*GY1:* 0)
Program ID: 835-41-44-020

Pediatrics/Psychiatry/Child and Adolescent Psychiatry

Hawaii

Honolulu

University of Hawaii Program
Sponsor: University of Hawaii John A Burns School of Medicine
Kapiolani Medical Center for Women and Children
Leahi Hospital
Program Director:
Alayne Yates, MD
Robert J Bidwell Sr, MD
Univ of Hawaii
1319 Punahou St/Rm 635
Honolulu, HI 96826
Tel: 808 983-8375 *Fax:* 808 942-5725
E-mail: yatesa@jabsom.biomed.hawaii.edu
Accred Length: 5 Years *Program Size:* 8 (*GY1:* 2)
Program ID: 830-14-44-007

Indiana

Indianapolis

Indiana University School of Medicine Program
Sponsor: Indiana University School of Medicine
Clarian Riley Hospital for Children
Clarian IU Hospital
Program Director:
David W Dunn, MD
Susan Bowyer, MD
Indiana Univ Sch of Med
Riley Hospital for Children 3701
702 Barnhill Dr
Indianapolis, IN 46202-5200
Tel: 317 274-8162 *Fax:* 317 278-0609
E-mail: jraetz@iupui.edu
Accred Length: 5 Years *Program Size:* 6 (*GY1:* 2)
Program ID: 830-17-44-009

Kentucky

Lexington

University of Kentucky Medical Center Program
Sponsor: University of Kentucky Hospital
Charter Ridge Hospital
Program Director:
H Otto Kaak, MD
Univ of Kentucky Med Ctr
213E Annex 4
Lexington, KY 40536-0226
Tel: 606 323-6021, ext 257 *Fax:* 606 323-1670
E-mail: hokaak@pop.uky.edu
Accred Length: 5 Years *Program Size:* 10 (*GY1:* 2)
Program ID: 830-20-44-001

Massachusetts

Boston

Tufts University Program
Sponsor: New England Medical Center Hospitals
Program Director:
Joseph J Jankowski, MD
New England Med Ctr Hospital
PO Box 1007
750 Washington St
Boston, MA 02111
Tel: 617 636-1635 *Fax:* 617 636-4852
Internet: http://www.nemc.org/psych/training.htm
Accred Length: 5 Years *Program Size:* 10 (*GY1:* 2)
Program ID: 830-24-44-002

New York

Bronx

Albert Einstein College of Medicine Program
Sponsor: Albert Einstein College of Medicine of Yeshiva University
Jacobi Medical Center
Program Director:
Audrey Walker, MD
Montefiore Med Ctr
Office of Residency Training
3317 Rochambeau Ave
Bronx, NY 10467
Tel: 718 920-7970 *Fax:* 718 920-3810
Accred Length: 5 Years *Program Size:* 8 (*GY1:* 2)
Program ID: 830-35-44-003

New York

Mount Sinai School of Medicine Program
Sponsor: Mount Sinai Medical Center
Program Director:
Susan Lurie, MD
Mount Sinai Hospital
Dept of Psychiatry/Box 1230
One Gustave L Levy Pl
New York, NY 10029
Tel: 212 824-7037 *Fax:* 212 348-8436
E-mail: susan_lurie@smtplink.mssm.edu
Internet: http://www.mssm.edu/peds/residenc.html
Accred Length: 5 Years *Program Size:* 10 (*GY1:* 2)
Program ID: 830-35-44-004

Ohio

Cincinnati

University Hospital/University of Cincinnati College of Medicine Program
Sponsor: University Hospital Inc
Program Director:
Warren M Liang, MD
Michael Farrell, MD
Univ Hospital-Univ of Cincinnati
Dept of Psychiatry
231 Bethesda Ave
Cincinnati, OH 45267-0559
Tel: 513 558-5190 *Fax:* 513 558-3477
E-mail: warren.liang@uc.edu
Internet: http://www.uc.edu/~liang/
Accred Length: 5 Years *Program Size:* 6 (*GY1:* 2)
Program ID: 830-38-44-008

Rhode Island

East Providence

Brown University Program
Sponsor: Emma Pendleton Bradley Hospital
Program Director:
Henrietta L Leonard, MD
Rhode Island Hospital
593 Eddy St
Providence, RI 02903
Tel: 401 444-3762 *Fax:* 401 444-8879
Accred Length: 5 Years *Program Size:* 15 (*GY1:* 3)
Program ID: 830-43-44-005

Texas

San Antonio

University of Texas Health Science Center at San Antonio Program
Sponsor: University of Texas Medical School at San Antonio
University Hospital-South Texas Medical Center
Program Director:
Robert J Nolan Jr, MD
Kenneth L Matthews Sr, MD
Univ of Texas Health Science Ctr
7703 Floyd Curl Dr
San Antonio, TX 78284-7816
Tel: 210 567-5185 *Fax:* 210 567-6921
E-mail: nolanr@uthscsa.edu
Internet: http://psych68.uthscsa.edu
Accred Length: 5 Years *Program Size:* 8 (*GY1:* 2)
Program ID: 830-48-44-010

Utah

Salt Lake City

University of Utah Program
Sponsor: University of Utah Medical Center
Program Director:
Bonnie J Flick, MD
Dept of Psychiatry
Univ of Utah Sch of Med
50 N Medical Dr
Salt Lake City, UT 84132
Tel: 801 581-3936 *Fax:* 801 581-5604
E-mail: laura.hart@hsc.utah.edu
Internet: http://www.med.utah.edu/psychiatry
Accred Length: 5 Years *Program Size:* 10 (*GY1:* 2)
Program ID: 830-49-44-006

Psychiatry/Family Practice

California

Sacramento

University of California (Davis) Program
Sponsor: University of California (Davis) Medical Center
Program Director:
Mark Servis, MD
James Nuovo, MD
Univ of California Davis Med Ctr
Dept of Psychiatry
2315 Stockton Blvd
Sacramento, CA 95817
Tel: 916 734-2614 *Fax:* 916 734-3384
E-mail: psychiatry.training@ucdmc.ucdavis.edu
Internet:
http://www.neuroscience.ucdavis.edu/psychiatry
Accred Length: 5 Years *Program Size:* 8 (*GY1:* 2)
Program ID: 820-05-44-004

San Diego

University of California (San Diego) Program
Sponsor: University of California (San Diego) Medical Center
Program Director:
Margaret E McCahill, MD
Stephen Shucter, MD
UCSD Med Ctr
Dept of Family Med
200 W Arbor Dr/Mail Code 8809
San Diego, CA 92103
Tel: 619 543-5487 *Fax:* 619 543-5996
E-mail: mmccahill@ucsd.edu
Internet: http://www.ucsd.edu/famres
Accred Length: 5 Years *Program Size:* 6 (*GY1:* 2)
Program ID: 820-05-44-005

Georgia

Fort Gordon

Dwight David Eisenhower Army Medical Center Program
Sponsor: Dwight David Eisenhower Army Medical Center
Program Director:
Douglas A Waldrep, MD
Brian K Unwin, MD
Dwight David Eisenhower Army Med Ctr
Dept of Psychiatry
Fort Gordon, GA 30905-5650
Tel: 706 787-2550 *Fax:* 706 787-6004
E-mail:
douglas_a.waldrep@ddeamc-a.chcs.amedd.army.mil
Internet: http://www.ddeamc.amedd.army.mil
Accred Length: 5 Years *Program Size:* 0
Program ID: 820-12-44-002
US Armed Services Program

Hawaii

Honolulu

Tripler Army Medical Center Program

Sponsor: Tripler Army Medical Center

Program Director:
Maj Richard L Jaconette, MD
Lt Col Mary J Wyman, MD
Tripler Army Med Ctr
Dept of Psychiatry
1 Jarrett White Rd
Tripler AMC, HI 96859-5000
Tel: 808 433-6413 *Fax:* 808 433-4591
E-mail: mary_j.wyman @tamc.chcs.amedd.army.mil
Internet: http://www.webserver.tamc.amedd.army.mil
Accred Length: 5 Years *Program Size:* 2 (*GY1:* 2)
Program ID: 820-14-44-008
US Armed Services Program

Iowa

Iowa City

University of Iowa Hospitals and Clinics Program

Sponsor: University of Iowa Hospitals and Clinics

Program Director:
George R Bergus, MD
Catherine L Woodman, MD
Univ of Iowa Hospitals and Clinics
Dept of Family Medicine
200 Hawkins Dr/01110-D PFP
Iowa City, IA 52242
Tel: 319 384-7507 *Fax:* 319 384-7822
E-mail: george-bergus@uiowa.edu
Accred Length: 5 Years *Program Size:* 2 (*GY1:* 1)
Program ID: 820-18-44-009

Maryland

Bethesda

National Capital Consortium Program

Sponsor: National Capital Consortium
Malcolm Grow Medical Center (SGE)

Program Director:
William Sykora, MD
James Rundell, MD
1075 W Perimeter Rd
Ste A-01
Andrews AFB, MD 20762
Tel: 240 857-3956 *Fax:* 240 857-3011
Accred Length: 5 Years *Program Size:* 10 (*GY1:* 2)
Program ID: 820-23-44-012
US Armed Services Program

Michigan

East Lansing

Michigan State University Program

Sponsor: Michigan State University College of Human Medicine
St Lawrence Hospital and HealthCare Services

Program Director:
Jed Magen, DO
Randolph Pearson, MD
Michigan State Univ
Dept of Psychiatry
West Fee Hall
East Lansing, MI 48824-1316
Tel: 517 353-4362 *Fax:* 517 432-3603
Accred Length: 5 Years *Program Size:* 2 (*GY1:* 2)
Program ID: 820-25-44-003

Minnesota

Minneapolis

University of Minnesota Program

Sponsor: University of Minnesota Medical School

Program Director:
Sheila Specker, MD
Manuel Idrogo, MD
Univ of Minnesota
Dept of Psychiatry
420 Delaware St SE/Box 393
Minneapolis, MN 55455
Tel: 612 626-3698 *Fax:* 612 626-5591
E-mail: speck001@maroon.tc.umm.edu
Accred Length: 5 Years *Program Size:* 6 (*GY1:* 3)
Program ID: 820-26-44-007

Ohio

Cincinnati

University of Cincinnati Hospital Group Program

Sponsor: University Hospital Inc

Program Director:
Lawson R Wulsin, MD
Jeffrey Heck, MD
Univ of Cincinnati Med Ctr
231 Bethesda Ave
Mail Location 559
Cincinnati, OH 45267-0559
Tel: 513 558-5190 *Fax:* 513 558-3477
E-mail: lawson.wulsin@uc.edu
Internet: http://www.uc.edu/~liang
Accred Length: 5 Years *Program Size:* 9 (*GY1:* 2)
Program ID: 820-38-44-006

Cleveland

Case Western Reserve University/University Hospitals of Cleveland Program

Sponsor: University Hospitals of Cleveland

Program Director:
Michael Rowane, MD
Robert Ronis, MD
Case Western Reserve Univ-Univ Hosp of Cleveland
Dept of Psychiatry
1100 Euclid Ave
Cleveland, OH 44106-5000
Tel: 216 844-1705 *Fax:* 216 844-1703
E-mail: rjr4@po.cwru.edu
Accred Length: 5 Years *Program Size:* 2 (*GY1:* 2)
Program ID: 820-38-44-013

Oklahoma

Tulsa

University of Oklahoma College of Medicine-Tulsa Program

Sponsor: University of Oklahoma College of Medicine-Tulsa

Program Director:
William R Yates, MD
Univ of Oklahoma Health Science Ctr-Tulsa
2808 S Sheridan Rd
Tulsa, OK 74129-1077
Tel: 918 838-4738 *Fax:* 918 838-4653
E-mail: william-yates@ouhsc.edu
Internet: http://www.tuslsa.ouhsc.edu
Accred Length: 5 Years *Program Size:* 10 (*GY1:* 2)
Program ID: 820-39-44-001

West Virginia

Morgantown

West Virginia University Program

Sponsor: West Virginia University Hospitals

Program Director:
Calvin R Sumner, MD
James G Arbogast, MD
WVU School of Med
Behavioral Med/Psych
930 Chestnut Ridge Rd
Morgantown, WV 26506
Tel: 304 293-2411 *Fax:* 304 293-8724
Internet: http://www.hsc.wvu.edu/som/psychiatry
Accred Length: 5 Years *Program Size:* 2 (*GY1:* 1)
Program ID: 820-55-44-010

Wisconsin

Milwaukee

Medical College of Wisconsin Program

Sponsor: Medical College of Wisconsin Affiliated Hospitals Inc

Program Director:
Loren Leshan, MD
Carrlyle Chan, MD
Dept of Psychiatry
8701 Watertown Plank Rd
Milwaukee, WI 53226
Tel: 414 257-5995 *Fax:* 414 257-7228
E-mail: cchan@mcw.edu
Internet: http://www.mcw.edu/psych
Accred Length: 5 Years *Program Size:* 2 (*GY1:* 2)
Program ID: 820-56-44-011

Psychiatry/Neurology

Arizona

Tucson

University of Arizona Program
Sponsor: University of Arizona College of Medicine
University Medical Center
Veterans Affairs Medical Center (Tucson)
Program Director:
David Labiner, MD
Rebecca L Potter, MD
Dept of Neurology
1501 N Campbell Ave
Box 245023
Tucson, AZ 85724-5023
Tel: 520 626-2006 *Fax:* 520 626-2111
Accred Length: 5 Years *Program Size:* 2 (*GY1:* 2)
Program ID: 855-03-44-007

Florida

Miami

University of Miami-Jackson Memorial Medical Center Program
Sponsor: University of Miami-Jackson Memorial Medical Center
Veterans Affairs Medical Center (Miami)
Program Director:
Bruce Nolan, MD
Richard Steinbook, MD
Univ of Miami Sch of Med-Jackson Memorial Hospital
Dept of Psych/Neurology
PO Box 016960/Mental Health Bldg
Miami, FL 33210
Tel: 305 324-3371 *Fax:* 305 324-3210
E-mail: cremy@mednet.mednet.edu
Accred Length: 5 Years *Program Size:* 6 (*GY1:* 1)
Program ID: 855-11-44-009

Illinois

Chicago

University of Illinois College of Medicine at Chicago Program
Sponsor: University of Illinois College of Medicine at Chicago
Program Director:
Steven U Brint, MD
Henry W Dove, MD
Univ of Illinois-Chicago
Dept of Psychiatry (M/C 913)
912 S Wood St
Chicago, IL 60612-7330
Tel: 312 996-6906 *Fax:* 312 996-4169
E-mail: recruit@psych.uic.edu
Internet: http://www.psych.uic.edu
Accred Length: 5 Years *Program Size:* 1 (*GY1:* 1)
Program ID: 855-16-44-006

Indiana

Indianapolis

Indiana University School of Medicine Program
Sponsor: Clarian IU Hospital
Richard L Roudebush Veterans Affairs Medical Center
William N Wishard Memorial Hospital
Program Director:
Alan Schmetzer, MD
Jose Biller, MD
Indiana Univ Sch of Med
541 N Clinical Dr/Rm 278
Indianapolis, IN 46202-5111
Tel: 317 278-3938 *Fax:* 317 274-1248
Internet: http://www.iupui.edu/psych
Accred Length: 5 Years *Program Size:* 2 (*GY1:* 1)
Program ID: 855-17-44-003

Louisiana

New Orleans

Tulane University Program
Sponsor: Tulane University School of Medicine
Louisiana State University Medical College Campus
Tulane University Hospital and Clinics
Veterans Affairs Medical Center (New Orleans)
Program Director:
Patrick T O'Neill, MD
Anne Foundas, MD
Tulane Univ Sch of Med
Dept of Psych/Neuro TB53
1440 Canal St
New Orleans, LA 70112-2715
Tel: 504 894-7269 *Fax:* 504 894-7290
E-mail: poneill@mailhost.tcs.tulane.edu.
Internet: http://www.tulane.edu
Accred Length: 5 Years *Program Size:* 4 (*GY1:* 1)
Program ID: 855-21-44-002

New York

Glen Oaks

Long Island Jewish Medical Center Program
Sponsor: Long Island Jewish Medical Center
Hillside Hospital (Long Island Jewish Medical Center)
Program Director:
Bruce R Levy, MD
Ronald Kanner, MD
Dept of Psychiatry
Hillside Hospital
75-59 263rd St
Glen Oaks, NY 11004
Tel: 718 470-8005 *Fax:* 718 343-7739
E-mail: levy@lij.edu
Internet: http://www.lij.edu
Accred Length: 5 Years *Program Size:* 2 (*GY1:* 2)
Program ID: 855-35-44-004

New York

New York University Medical Center Program
Sponsor: New York University Medical Center
Bellevue Hospital Center
Veterans Affairs Medical Center (Manhattan)
Program Director:
Carol Bernstein, MD
Herman Weinreb, MD
New York Univ Med Ctr
550 First Ave
NB 20N11
New York, NY 10016
Tel: 212 263-6238 *Fax:* 212 263-6497
E-mail: carol.bernstnc@nyu.edu
Accred Length: 5 Years *Program Size:* 2 (*GY1:* 2)
Program ID: 855-35-44-008

Rhode Island

Providence

Brown University Program
Sponsor: Butler Hospital
Rhode Island Hospital
Program Director:
Stephen Salloway, MD
Butler Hospital
Dept of Neurology
345 Blackstone Blvd
Providence, RI 02906
Tel: 401 444-8771 *Fax:* 401 444-8781
E-mail: neurology_dept@brown.edu
Accred Length: 5 Years *Program Size:* 5 (*GY1:* 1)
Program ID: 855-43-44-005

West Virginia

Morgantown

West Virginia University Program
Sponsor: West Virginia University Hospitals
Charleston Area Medical Center
Program Director:
Calvin R Sumner, MD
Ludwig G Gutmann, MD
West Virginia Sch of Med
Behavioral Med/Psychiatry
930 Chestnut Ridge Rd
Morgantown, WV 26505
Tel: 304 293-2411 *Fax:* 304 293-8724
E-mail: king@wvnvm.wvnet.edu
Internet: http://www.hsc.wvu.edu/som/psychiatry
Accred Length: 5 Years *Program Size:* 3 (*GY1:* 1)
Program ID: 855-55-44-001

Appendix B

Medical Specialty Board Certification Requirements

Twenty-four medical specialty boards have been approved by the American Board of Medical Specialties (ABMS) and the American Medical Association (AMA) Council on Medical Education through the Liaison Committee for Specialty Boards (LCSB). Applications for recognition as a specialty board are submitted to the LCSB and reviewed for compliance with the requirements and criteria published in the *Essentials for Approval of New Examining Boards in Medical Specialties* approved by both the ABMS and the AMA. If an applicant is approved for recognition as a medical specialty board by the LCSB, the application must then be approved by the membership of the ABMS and the AMA Council on Medical Education. The *Essentials* may be obtained from the office of the Executive Vice President of the ABMS, 1007 Church St/Ste 404, Evanston, IL 60201-5913, or from the Council on Medical Education, AMA, 515 N State St, Chicago, IL 60610.

The primary objective of medical specialty boards is the improvement of the quality of medical education and medical care. The primary functions of each of the medical specialty boards are to evaluate candidates in a medical specialty field who voluntarily appear for examination and to certify as diplomates those candidates who are qualified. To accomplish these functions, medical specialty boards determine whether candidates have received adequate preparation in accordance with established educational standards; provide comprehensive examinations designed to assess knowledge, skills, and experience required to provide quality patient care in that specialty; and certify those candidates who have satisfied the requirements.

In collaboration with the other organizations and agencies concerned, the approved medical specialty boards assist in improving the quality of medical education by elevating the standards of graduate medical education and approving facilities for specialty training.

The actual accreditation review for the approval of residency programs in each specialty is conducted by a Residency Review Committee on which the respective specialty board has equal representation with the AMA Council on Medical Education and, in some cases, with a related specialty society.

Medical specialty board certification is an additional process to receiving a medical degree, completing residency training, and receiving a license to practice medicine.

Certification requirements of each member board of ABMS are included on subsequent pages. Inquiries regarding specialty board certification requirements should be directed to the specialty board executive offices listed in Table 1. The member boards of ABMS publish materials containing statements on the requirements for certification, which are also reprinted in each edition of the *Official American Board of Medical Specialties Directory of Board Certified Medical Specialists*. This publication contains certification and biographical information on each specialist who has been certified by a member board of ABMS. The *Directory* is available from Marquis Who's Who, 121 Chanlon Rd, New Providence, NJ 07974.

ABMS Information

American Board of Medical Specialties
1007 Church St/Ste 404
Evanston, IL 60201-5913
847 491-9091
847 328-3596 Fax

Table 1. Member Boards of the American Board of Medical Specialties

American Board of Allergy and Immunology
(a Conjoint Board of the American Board of Internal Medicine and the American Board of Pediatrics)
John W Yunginger, MD
Executive Secretary
510 Walnut St/Ste 1701
Philadelphia, PA 19106-3699
215 592-9466
215 592-9411 Fax
E-mail: abai@abai.org
Internet: http://www.abai.org

American Board of Anesthesiology
Francis M James, III, MD
Secretary-Treasurer
4101 Lake Boone Trail
Raleigh, NC 27607-7506
919 881-2570
919 881-2575 Fax

American Board of Colon and Rectal Surgery
Herand Abcarian, MD
Executive Director
20600 Eureka Rd/Ste 713
Taylor, MI 48180
313 282-9400

American Board of Dermatology
Harry J Hurley, MD
Executive Director
Henry Ford Hospital, One Ford Place
Detroit, MI 48202
313 874-1088
313 872-3221 Fax

American Board of Emergency Medicine
Benson S Munger, PhD
Executive Director
3000 Coolidge Rd
East Lansing, MI 48823-6319
517 332-4800
517 332-2234 Fax
Internet: http://www.abem.org

American Board of Family Practice
Paul R Young, MD
Executive Director
2228 Young Dr
Lexington, KY 40505
606 269-5626
Internet: http://www.abfp.org

American Board of Internal Medicine
Harry R Kimball, MD
President
510 Walnut St/Ste 1700
Philadelphia, PA 19106-3699
800 441-2246
215 446-3590 Fax
E-mail: requests@abim.org
Internet: http://www.abim.org

American Board of Medical Genetics
Sharon B Robinson, MS
Administrator
9650 Rockville Pike
Bethesda, MD 20814-3998
301 571-1825
Internet: http://www.faseb.org/genetics

American Board of Neurological Surgery
Donald O Quest, MD
Secretary-Treasurer
6550 Fannin St/Ste 2139
Houston, TX 77030-2701
713 790-6015
Internet: http://www.abns.org

American Board of Nuclear Medicine
William H Blahd, MD
President
900 Veteran Ave
Los Angeles, CA 90024-1786
310 825-7887
310 825-9433 Fax

American Board of Obstetrics and Gynecology
Norman F Gant, MD
Executive Director
2915 Vine St/Ste 300
Dallas, TX 75204-1069
214 871-1619
214 871-1943 Fax

American Board of Ophthalmology
Denis M O'Day, MD
Executive Director
111 Presidential Blvd/Ste 241
Bala Cynwyd, PA 19004
610 664-1175
610 664-6503 Fax
Internet: http://www.abop.org

American Board of Orthopaedic Surgery
G Paul DeRosa, MD
Executive Director
400 Silver Cedar Ct
Chapel Hill, NC 27514
919 929-7103
919 942-8988 Fax

American Board of Otolaryngology
Robert W Cantrell, MD
Executive Vice President
2211 Norfolk/Ste 800
Houston, TX 77098-4044
713 528-6200
713 528-1171 Fax
Internet: http://www.aboto.org

American Board of Pathology
William H Hartmann, MD
Executive Vice President
PO Box 25915
Tampa, FL 33622-5915
813 286-2444
813 289-5279 Fax
Internet: http://www.abpath.org

American Board of Pediatrics
James A Stockman III, MD
President
111 Silver Cedar Ct
Chapel Hill, NC 27514-1651
919 929-0461
919 929-9255 Fax
Internet: http://www.abp.org

American Board of Physical Medicine and Rehabilitation
Mark R Raymond, PhD
Executive Director
Norwest Ctr/Ste 674
21 First St SW
Rochester, MN 55902-3009
507 282-1776
507 282-9242 Fax

American Board of Plastic Surgery
R Barrett Noone, MD
Executive Director
Seven Penn Ctr/Ste 400
1635 Market St
Philadelphia, PA 19103-2204
215 587-9322
215 587-9622 Fax
E-mail: abpsphl@p3.net
Internet: www.abplsurg.org

American Board of Preventive Medicine
Alice R Ring, MD, MPH
Executive Director
9950 W Lawrence Ave/Ste 106
Schiller Park, IL 60176
847 671-1750
847 671-1751 Fax
E-mail: 72370.664@compuserve.com
Internet: http://www.abprevmed.org

American Board of Psychiatry and Neurology
Stephen C Scheiber, MD
Executive Vice President
500 Lake Cook Rd/Ste 335
Deerfield, IL 60015
847 945-7900
847 945-1146 Fax
Internet: http://www.abpn.org

American Board of Radiology
M Paul Capp, MD
Executive Director
5255 E Williams Circle/Ste 6800
Tucson, AZ 85711
520 790-2900
520 790-3200 Fax
Internet: http://www.theabr.org

American Board of Surgery
Wallace P Ritchie, Jr, MD, PhD
Executive Director
1617 John F Kennedy Blvd/Ste 860
Philadelphia, PA 19103-1847
215 568-4000
215 563-5718 Fax
Internet: http://www.absurgery.org

American Board of Thoracic Surgery
Richard J Cleveland, MD
Secretary-Treasurer
One Rotary Ctr/Ste 803
Evanston, IL 60201
847 475-1520
847 475-6240 Fax
E-mail: abts@juno.com

American Board of Urology
Stuart S Howards, MD
Executive Secretary
2216 Ivy Rd/Ste 210
Charlottesville, VA 22903
804 979-0059
804 979-0266 Fax

American Board of Allergy and Immunology

(A Conjoint Board of the American Board of Internal Medicine and the American Board of Pediatrics)
510 Walnut St/Ste 1701
Philadelphia, PA 19106-3699
215 592-9466
215 592-9411 Fax
E-mail: abai@abai.org
Internet: http://www.abai.org

(The Board reserves the right to make changes in its policies and procedures at any time and cannot assume responsibility for giving advance notice thereof. All applicants are advised to contact the American Board of Allergy and Immunology [ABAI] to determine whether the following information remains current.)

Organization and Purpose

The ABAI was established in 1971 as a nonprofit organization and is one of 24 member boards of the American Board of Medical Specialties (ABMS). The ABAI is a Conjoint Board of the ABIM and the ABP and is sponsored jointly by the American Academy of Allergy, Asthma and Immunology (AAAAI), the American Academy of Pediatrics (AAP) - Section on Allergy and Immunology, the American College of Allergy, Asthma and Immunology (ACAAI), the American Medical Association (AMA) - Section Council of Allergy and Immunology, and the Clinical Immunology Society (CIS).

ABAI's major purposes are to

a. establish qualifications and examine physician candidates for certification as specialists in allergy/immunology,
b. serve the public and the health care community by providing the names of physicians certified as allergists/immunologists,
c. improve the quality of health,
d. establish and improve standards for the teaching and practice of allergy/immunology, and
e. establish standards for training programs in allergy/immunology working with the Residency Review Committee for Allergy and Immunology of the Accreditation Council for Graduate Medical Education (ACGME).

Significance of Certification

A certified specialist in allergy and immunology is a physician who previously has passed the certification examination of the ABIM and/or the ABP with additional certification by the ABAI, a Conjoint Board of the ABIM and the ABP. Diplomates of the ABAI have detailed knowledge of the underlying pathophysiology and the diagnosis, treatment, and prevention of allergic diseases such as allergic rhinitis, allergic asthma, urticaria, anaphylaxis, hypersensitivity pneumonitis, atopic and contact dermatitis, and allergic gastrointestinal disorders, as well as comparable clinical problems without an apparent allergic etiology or component such as vasomotor rhinitis, nonallergic asthma, and idiopathic and/or hereditary forms of urticaria and/or angioedema. Diplomates also have expertise in the management of pulmonary complications of certain of these diseases.

Diplomates of the ABAI also possess advanced understanding of immunochemistry, immunobiology, and pharmacology and experience in the application of this knowledge to the diagnosis, management, and therapy of immunologic diseases. This includes inborn or acquired defects of host resistance, autoimmune diseases, bone marrow and solid organ transplantation, gene replacement therapy, adverse drug reactions, and related conditions. Diplomates have demonstrated to the satisfaction of their peers that they possess the general qualifications specified and are ethical and humanistic practitioners of medicine.

Certification

The ABAI serves candidates who have embarked on a graduate program of study with the express purpose of excelling in the practice of the subspecialty of allergy/immunology. The ABAI is responsible for the establishment and maintenance of the standards of knowledge required for certification. The ABAI anticipates that during a post-medical school training program, the candidates will acquire adequate knowledge in basic science, as applied to this discipline. In outlining its requirements, the ABAI assists the candidate to select superior educational programs that will develop his/her competency in allergy/immunology. The ABAI believes that all allergists/immunologists should have a fundamental knowledge of the biological science basic to this discipline. The responsibility of acquiring the knowledge rests with the candidate. Such knowledge is essential to the continued professional progress of any qualified allergist/immunologist.

The candidate must demonstrate competency to the ABAI in order to justify certification in this discipline. Each candidate for certification must satisfy the general and professional qualifications listed below.

Content for Certification

The examination covers all content areas listed in the current Program Requirements for Residency Education in Allergy and Immunology and the Content Outline determined by the Board of Directors, which is distributed with the application, and the following:

Candidates for certification must be familiar with the fundamental elements of the immune system, such as the types of immune cells and the anatomical organs that constitute the immune system, the circulation patterns of immune cells, the biologic roles of products of the immune system, and the abnormal conditions of the immune system that constitute immunopathology. Moreover, the candidate will be expected to be proficient in understanding the molecular basis of allergic and other immune reactions, including interaction between immune cells, cell membrane signal transduction pathways, gene expression, cytokine release, receptor targeting, cellular differentiation, and death. Proficiency must be demonstrated in the diagnosis and treatment of allergic and other immunologic diseases.

Because the ABAI is a conjoint board representing pediatric and adult medicine, the candidate must master the spectrum of allergic and immunologic diseases as it presents in children and adults. In addition to a familiarity with allergic diseases, including allergic rhinitis, asthma, atopic dermatitis, and urticaria, the candidate must be knowledgeable in autoimmune conditions. Equally important as competence in diseases of immune dysfunction is the knowledge of human pathology that results from an absence of immunity, either whole or partial, congenital or acquired. Thus, an understanding of the primary immunodeficiency states is required, including congenital disorders, absence of specific complement components, lack of specific neutrophil function, absence of specific adhesive cellular glycoproteins, and dysfunctional states of the immune system produced by external agents.

It is important for the candidate to demonstrate proficiency in the proper selection of appropriate clinical and laboratory tests, which aid the formulation of a clinical diagnosis based upon first obtaining a detailed medical history and performing a complete physical examination. The candidate must understand the scientific basis of the following list (noninclusive) of tests:

- serum immunoglobulin determination;
- functional antibody measurement;
- complement component and functional assays;
- lymphocyte subset analysis using monoclonal antibodies and flow cytometry;
- lymphocyte proliferation assays with mitogen and antigens; and
- neutrophil and monocyte chemotaxis, phagocytosis, and killing assessment.

In addition, competence must be demonstrated with the use of molecular diagnostic techniques involving the binding of ligands to nucleic acid or polypeptide sequences. The importance of DNA replication technology must be understood. The molecular basis for immediate hypersensitivity skin testing must be understood in the context of the detailed molecular events occurring in the tissue mast cell and blood basophil, particularly the release of preformed mediators, and in the generation of newly formed mediators. Similarly, skin testing for T cell competence with recall antigens must be understood in relation to antigen presentation, cytokine secretion and interaction, and lymphocyte subset activation and function. Candidates must also have familiarity with the misuse of standard tests and with controversial tests in allergy and immunology. The candidate must understand the principles and analytic methods employed in experimental clinical studies for determining the diagnostic utility of specific tests and in evaluating the safety, toxicity, efficacy, and outcomes of treatments and drugs for allergic and immunologic disease. Candidates must be familiar with the principles and methods employed in epidemiologic studies.

A corollary of the competence of the candidate in understanding the pathophysiology, clinical presentation, and immunologic testing of allergic and other immunologic diseases is the knowledge of appropriate treatment options. For example, the common aspect of all types of asthma is the presence of airway inflammation. Definitive treatment of asthma demands that therapies be utilized that include interruption of the inflammatory response. Thus, candidates for certification must understand use of drugs that decrease airway inflammation in asthma. Based upon the molecular knowledge of the allergic response, the candidate must appreciate the importance of allergen avoidance and medical treatment of allergic rhinitis before initiation of the more intense treatment of immunotherapy. In the latter therapy, the candidates must demonstrate competence in allergen selection and administration in successful treatment regimens. Therapy for immunologic diseases must be understood, such as (noninclusive): intravenous immune globulin for antibody deficiency, treatment of immunodeficiency with biologic response modifiers, HLA-identical and HLA-haploidentical (T cell-depleted) bone marrow transplants for cellular immunodeficiencies, and gene replacement therapy currently used for the immunodeficiency associated with adenosine deaminase deficiency as well as theoretical principles/potential approaches in other congenital immune disorders.

Requirements for Certification

The candidate qualifies for examination by:

1. *holding current certification* by the ABIM and/or ABP;
2. presenting evidence acceptable to the Board of Directors of at least 2 years of full-time residency/fellowship in *allergy/immunology programs accredited by the ACGME* or other acceptable training in allergy/immunology programs. These programs are listed in the *Graduate Medical Education Directory*, published by the American Medical Association;
3. documentation and evaluations from the training program director substantiating clinical competence and 2 full-time years of allergy/immunology training. Areas to be reviewed include clinical judgment; medical knowledge; clinical skills of history taking, physical examination, and procedural skills; humanistic qualities, attitudes, and professional behavior; medical care (utilizing laboratory tests and diagnostic procedures); commitment to scholarship; and work habits. Procedural skills to be assessed include immediate hypersensitivity skin testing, delayed hypersensitivity skin testing, specific allergen immunotherapy, drug desensitization, pulmonary function testing, and intravenous immunoglobulin therapy. Rhinoscopy, nasal smears, patch testing, oral food challenge, and immunomodulatory therapy may be assessed in the future;

   The training program director must also provide written evidence of the candidate's clinical experience and readiness to sit for the examination. In compliance with the ACGME Program Requirements for Residency Education in Allergy and Immunology, a semiannual record must be maintained with copies to the ABAI for tracking purposes. The Evaluation Form together with the Explanation of Ratings Scale may be obtained from the ABAI. If a trainee has received two consecutive evaluations with overall unsatisfactory ratings, the training program director must provide the trainee and the ABAI with a written plan for remediation of the trainee's deficiencies. After 6 months, the training program director must provide the ABAI and the trainee with a report of the success or failure of the remediation program, as well as any additional plans for corrective action;
4. documentation from the chief of medicine or pediatrics, ABAI diplomates in the geographical area, chiefs of community hospitals, or officers of state or regional societies to verify the medical, ethical, and moral standing and clinical competence of the candidate as a specialist in allergy/immunology; *and*
5. evidence of a valid (current), unrestricted license to practice medicine in a state, territory, possession, or province of the United States or Canada or providing a written explanation of extenuating circumstances. Candidates with a restricted, suspended, or revoked license at the time of application or examination will not be admitted to the examination or certified.

Conjoint Committees—The nature of a Conjoint Board requires involvement of the sponsoring primary boards in critical areas of decision making. The ABAI has formed two advisory committees with representation from the ABAI, ABIM, and ABP. The Conjoint Credentials Committee reviews the credentials of candidates for the certification examination to the Board for its determination. The Conjoint Standards Committee recommends the passing grade for the certification examination to the Board for its determination.

Pathways for Dual Certification

Formal special pathways exist for individuals wishing to qualify for dual certification in either allergy/immunology and *pediatric pulmonology* or *adult rheumatology*. Additional information regarding special pathways is available upon request to the ABAI.

Recertification

Since 1977, the ABAI has offered its diplomates a recertification process every other year so that the effectiveness of each diplomate's own efforts in continuing education would be evaluated.

Beginning with 1989, new ABAI diplomates receive certificates valid for 10 years. Time-unlimited certificates were issued prior to October 1, 1989. However, all diplomates, especially those involved in training programs, are strongly encouraged to recertify as often as possible, but at a minimum of every 10 years. Maintaining a current certificate is an expression of professional accountability. Presently 1,250 ABAI diplomates hold time-limited certificates; renewal may be achieved in the interim. ABAI recommends recertification for diplomates holding time-unlimited certificates.

The 1998-1999 recertification process is composed of the home study examination (available August 1 with completion by November 30, 1998) and the proctored modular examination (administered August 9, 1999). Recertification candidates will be required to attain an 80% correct score on the home study examination to gain entry to the proctored modular examination. If such an absolute score is not attained, the diplomate will be required to pass a subsequent remedial examination and attain an 80% correct score. Should performance not meet this standard, the candidates will not be permitted entry to the proctored modular examination, and a partial refund will be provided to the recertification candidate.

Upon gaining entry to the proctored modular examination, the recertification candidate will be required to complete a 50-item recent advances module (emphasizing new knowledge in the specialty) and complete one of two 150-item modules (preference as declared upon registration) in either allergy or immunology. The modular format has been designed to ensure that the recertification process is relevant to the diplomate's professional activities—either in the clinical and/or in a laboratory or research setting. The ABAI anticipates that most diplomates seeking recertification will be successful. Recertification candidates will be required to attain an absolute minimum score to ultimately gain recertification in allergy and immunology. Standards are established to justify public confidence.

Content for Recertification

The content of the home study examination covers the broad area of allergy and immunology listed previously under "Content for Certification" and will provide diplomates a learning experience in the following areas of clinical science: immediate hypersensitivity, immunological disorders, pharmacology and therapeutics, specific diagnostic modalities, and allergens and antigens. Attention will also be given to the following areas of basic science: immune mechanisms, cells involved in immune responses, specific immune mechanisms, and laboratory tests.

The proctored examination reflects the current ABAI Content Outline, which is distributed upon successful performance on the Home Study Examination. The recent advances module contains items covering the broad field of allergy and immunology. The allergy module contains basic and clinical items covering immediate hypersensitivity disorders. The immunology module contains items covering both basic and clinical immunology.

Requirements for Recertification

The diplomate qualifies for examination:

1. by having previously been certified by the ABAI (recertification in internal medicine or pediatrics is encouraged of ABAI diplomates); *and*
2. by presenting documentation from physicians in the ABAI diplomate's community that he/she currently practices the specialty of allergy and immunology; *and*
3. by presenting evidence of a valid (current), unrestricted license to practice medicine in a state, territory, possession, or province of the United States or Canada or by providing a written explanation of extenuating circumstances. Diplomates with a restricted, suspended, or revoked license at the time of application or examination will not be admitted to the examination or recertified.

Clinical and Laboratory Immunology (CLI)

In 1983 the ABMS approved Certification of Special Qualification in Diagnostic Laboratory Immunology (DLI) for Diplomates of the ABAI, ABIM, and ABP. Such recognition was awarded in 1986, 1988, and 1990 following successful examination performance to specialists with significant experience (at least 4 years) in comprehensive DLI or at least 1 year's training in DLI who were involved in the teaching, research, or practice settings in which the diagnostic immunology laboratory is of central importance, and were recognized by their peers as competent by way of their significant contributions to DLI.

In 1991 ABMS approved the change to a Certificate of Added Qualification in Clinical and Laboratory Immunology (CLI) for those specialists with 1 year of formal training following subspecialty certification in an immunologically based subspecialty in order to recognize the clinical interpretative skills inherent with such training. The first CLI examination was administered in 1994.

Content for Clinical and Laboratory Immunology (CLI)

With the goal of certifying candidates in the broader sense of clinical skills and laboratory expertise in clinical immunology, the ABAI recommends that CLI candidates be prepared to demonstrate competency by examination in the theory and practice of the following (noninclusive) clinical areas:

1. allergic diseases;
2. primary and secondary immunodeficiency diseases;
3. autoimmune diseases;
4. immunologic aspects of bone marrow and organ transplantation;
5. immune aspects of gene replacement therapy;
6. immunologic aspects of organ-specific inflammatory conditions; and
7. immune aspects of malignancy and cancer.

Although these clinical areas of competence are expected of the traditional candidate in allergy/immunology, the candidate for CLI will be expected to master these concepts to a far greater degree. Moreover, because upon certification the CLI candidate should be competent to supervise an immunology laboratory, evidence of competence will be required in the following (noninclusive) areas:

1. quantitation of immunoglobulins;
2. measurement of specific antibodies;
3. functional and quantitative complement tests;
4. assays of lymphocyte, monocyte, neutrophil, and basophil function and quantitation;
5. autoantibody measurement;
6. rapid tests for infectious diseases;
7. DNA amplification and binding tests;
8. genetic testing;
9. histocompatibility testing;
10. prenatal diagnosis;
11. quality control testing;

Certification Requirements

12. data management and statistical analysis; and
13. regulatory agency interactions.

The examination reflects the current ACGME Program Requirements for Residency Education in CLI and the Content Outline determined by the Joint Testing Committee of the ABAI, ABIM, and ABP, which is distributed with the application.

Requirements for Clinical and Laboratory Immunology (CLI)

The 1999 examination will be administered to those ABAI, ABIM, and ABP diplomates following a 2-year allergy/immunology training program or immunologically related subspecialty training, eg, rheumatology, infectious diseases, etc, with subspecialty certification, and a third year of CLI training. Competence must be verified by the program director responsible for the third year of training. Candidates whose applications were previously accepted and whose training meets the Program Requirements for Residency Education in CLI may also file an application.

Physicians qualified for examination are expected to be involved with applying laboratory methods to problems in human diseases involving changes in immune responses and will be able to perform, develop, interpret, and evaluate the clinical relevance of special laboratory procedures related to immunologically based diseases.

Examination Methodology

Announcements

The proctored certification and recertification examination is administered simultaneously in several US locations in alternate years. The times and places are determined by the ABAI and announced in the appropriate specialty journals.

Applications

The act of filing an application is the candidate's responsibility. Application forms are available from the ABAI. They must be accompanied by two recently signed photographs and the necessary fees. Completed applications must be received on or before the close of registration (postmark applicable).

Board Review Courses

The ABAI does not sponsor or maintain any records on any courses that claim to be review courses in preparation for its examinations nor does it offer or endorse any specific publications or courses to prepare for its examinations.

Cancellations

Candidates who are accepted for examination, but fail to appear or who withdraw after the deadline for cancellation, will have their examination fee placed into an escrow account for the next examination. For each subsequent examination, candidates will be required to pay the current registration and examination fees.

Certificates

Candidates/diplomates who pass the examinations will be certified or recertified in the specialty of allergy/immunology or CLI as of the date of the examination and receive a 10-year time limited certificate, subject to revocation by the ABAI for cause. This information becomes public information and will be listed in the *Official ABMS Directory of Board Certified Specialists*.

Description

The written examinations vary in length, certification being two 4-hour sessions, recertification being one 4-hour session, and CLI being two 3-hour sessions. The multiple-choice questions are objective and designed to test the individual's knowledge through recall, interpretation, and problem solving. Each examination may contain previously used questions, new questions, or questions undergoing field-testing. The individual's performance on field test questions will not be counted in determining results.

Candidates with Disabilities

Individuals who may need accommodation during the examination must provide written details to the ABAI at the time of application for examination in order to receive information about ABAI's disability policy and approval.

Fees

The fees are set forth in the instruction sheet included with the application. Candidates whose applications are rejected will receive a refund of the examination fee; however, the ABAI will retain the registration fee to cover the processing and evaluation costs. A nonrefundable late fee will apply to those applications received after the close of registration and prior to the cancellation deadline.

Irregular Behavior

All Board examinations are supervised by proctors, who are required to report any irregular behavior, which includes, but is not limited to, giving or obtaining unauthorized information or aid before, during, or after the examination as evidenced by observation or subsequent statistical analysis of answer sheets. Offering financial or other benefit to a proctor, employee, or agent of the ABAI is forbidden.

Rescores

On written request and payment of a nominal fee, candidates may obtain rescoring within 3 months of receiving results. Answer sheets will be destroyed 12 months after administration of the examination.

Results

Individuals will be informed of the results of the examinations within 3 months of administration. The validity of the individual's performance on the examination is secured by every means available.

Special Policies

Verification of Board Status

Based on ABMS-recommended policy, the ABAI does not issue statements of or implying "Board Eligibility" for any reason. Medical specialty certification is a process of advancement through several individual steps including examination. Having completed one step, such as the minimal educational requirements, should not imply that a candidate is now possessed of some special qualification that is more or less equivalent to certification. For written verification of the status of an allergist/immunologist, ABAI charges a nominal fee per name.

Revocation of Certificate

Certificates issued by the ABAI shall be subject to revocation under specific circumstances, including but not limited to a state medical license revocation or revocation of certification by either the ABIM or ABP.

Absences During Residency

Absences in excess of a total of 2 months over the 2-year allergy/immunology training program, whether for vacation, sick leave, maternity leave, etc, should be made up. If the training program director believes that an absence of more than 2 months is justified, a letter of explanation should be sent by the director for review by the Conjoint Credentials Committee.

Changes in Policies and Procedures

The ABAI reserves the right to make changes in its Policies and Procedures and fees at any time, and cannot assume responsibility for giving advance notice thereof. The provisions of this publication are not to be construed as a contract between any candidate and the ABAI.

Examination Schedule

Certification
Date: August 9, 1999
Registration period: November 1, 1998 - January 31, 1999
Fee: US $1,500
Cancellation Date: July 15, 1999

Recertification
Home Study Examination: available August 1, 2000
Proctored Modular Examination: August 2001 (to be determined)
Registration period: January 1 - June 30, 2000
Fee: (to be determined)
Cancellation date: July 15, 2001

Clinical and Laboratory Immunology
Date: August 9, 1999
Registration Period: November 1, 1998 - January 31, 1999
Fee: US $1,500
Cancellation Date: July 15, 1999

American Board of Anesthesiology

4101 Lake Boone Trail/Suite 510
Raleigh, NC 27607-7506
919 881-2570
919 881-2575 Fax
Internet: http://www.abanes.org

(These criteria and conditions are subject to change without notice. All applicants are advised to contact the American Board of Anesthesiology [ABA] to ascertain whether the information below is current.)

Introduction

The chair of the anesthesiology department is the director of the residency program. Although the department chair may delegate responsibility for administering the program, the ABA corresponds officially about training matters only with the department chair.

The department chair must ensure that each resident's training fulfills all criteria for entering the ABA examination system. However, it is crucial that the resident know the requirements described in the Booklet of Information since *the resident ultimately bears responsibility for compliance with the requirements and bears the consequences if one or more aspects of training prove unacceptable.* This is especially important when requests are made for special training sequences or sites or for exemptions. *If, after speaking with the department chair, there is any question about the acceptability of any portion of training, the resident should write the Secretary of the ABA directly at the ABA office.*

Applicants and candidates for ABA examinations have the ultimate responsibility to know and comply with the Board's policies, procedures, requirements, and deadlines regarding admission to and opportunities for examination.

Primary Certification in Anesthesiology Certification Requirements

At the time of certification by the ABA, the candidate shall be capable of performing independently the entire scope of anesthesiology practice and must:

A. Hold a permanent, unconditional, unrestricted and unexpired license to practice medicine or osteopathy in one state or jurisdiction of the United States or province of Canada.
B. Have fulfilled all the requirements of the Continuum of Education in Anesthesiology.
C. Have on file with the ABA a Certificate of Clinical Competence with an overall satisfactory rating covering the final 6-month period of clinical anesthesia training in each anesthesiology residency program.

D. Have satisfied all examination requirements of the Board.
E. Have a moral, ethical, and professional standing satisfactory to the ABA.

A person certified by the ABA is designated a diplomate in publications of the American Board of Medical Specialties and the American Society of Anesthesiologists.

Continuum of Education in Anesthesiology

The continuum of education in anesthesiology consists of 4 years of training subsequent to the date that the medical or osteopathic degree has been conferred. The continuum consists of a clinical base year (CBY) and 36 months approved training in anesthesia (CA-1, CA-2, and CA-3 years).

A. The **clinical base year** must be devoted to clinical training of which at most 1 month may involve the administration of anesthesia. Acceptable training for the 12 months of Clinical Base includes training in a transitional year, internal or emergency medicine, pediatrics, surgery or any of the surgical specialties, obstetrics and gynecology, neurology, family practice, or any combination of these as approved for the individual resident by the director of his or her training program in anesthesiology.

The clinical base year must be spent in residency programs in the United States or its territories accredited by the Accreditation Council for Graduate Medical Education (ACGME) or approved by the American Osteopathic Association, or outside the United States and its territories in institutions affiliated with medical schools approved by the Liaison Committee on Medical Education (LCME).

Clinical base training must be completed before clinical rotations in fulfillment of the CA-3 year are begun.

B. The 3-year **clinical anesthesia** curriculum (CA 1-3) consists of experience in basic anesthesia training, subspecialty anesthesia training, and advanced anesthesia training. It is a graded curriculum of increasing difficulty and learning that is progressively more challenging of the resident's intellect and technical skills.

1. Experience in **basic anesthesia training** is intended to emphasize basic and fundamental aspects of the management of anesthesia. It is recommended that at least 12 months of the CA-1 and CA-2 years be spent in basic anesthesia training with a majority of this time occurring during the CA-1 year.
2. **Subspecialty anesthesia training** is required to emphasize the theoretical background, subject material, and practice of subdisciplines of anesthesiology. These subdisciplines include obstetric anesthesia, pediatric anesthesia, cardiothoracic anesthesia, neuroanesthesia, anesthesia for outpatient surgery, recovery room care, regional anesthesia, and pain management. It is recommended that these experiences be subspecialty rotations and occupy 7 to 12 months of the CA-1 and CA-2 years. The sequencing of these rotations in the CA-1 and CA-2 years is left to the discretion of the program director.

   In addition to the above requirements for subspecialty experiences, 2 months of training in *critical care medicine* are required during clinical anesthesia years. An acceptable critical care rotation should include active participation in patient care, active involvement by anesthesia faculty experienced in the practice and teaching of critical care, and an appropriate population of critically ill patients. Experience in short-term overnight postanesthesia units, intermediate step-down units, or emergency rooms does *not* fulfill this requirement.
3. Experience in **advanced anesthesia training** constitutes the CA-3 year. *Clinical rotations in fulfillment of the CA-3 year requirement must follow completion of the Clinical Base and CA-1 and CA-2 years*. The program director, in collaboration with the resident, will select one of three tracks designated as the advanced clinical track, subspecialty clinical track, or clinical scientist track. Regardless of the track selected, resident assignments in the CA-3 year should include the more difficult or complex anesthetic procedures and care of the most seriously ill patients.

   Residents in the **advanced clinical track** are required to complete a minimum of 6 months of experience in advanced and complex clinical anesthesia assignments. The remaining 6 months may be spent in one to three selected subspecialty rotations. Alternatively, additional complex clinical anesthesia assignments may be selected.

   Residents in the **subspecialty clinical track** should complete 9 to 12 months of experience in one subspecialty rotation or 6 months of experience in each of two subspecialty rotations. Such rotations may include time assigned to medical or surgical activities directly related to the anesthesia subspecialty.

   The **clinical scientist track** consists of clinical training in combination with research experience occurring at any time during the period the physician is enrolled and training as a resident in an ACGME-accredited anesthesiology program. There are two options for fulfilling the requirements of this track.

   Option A of the clinical scientist track may be fulfilled by completing 6 months of clinical or laboratory research experience during 48 months of training, which must include 12 months of clinical base and a minimum of 30 months of clinical anesthesia.

   Option B of the clinical scientist track, intended for residents who plan careers as academic investigators, may be fulfilled by completing 18 months of clinical or laboratory research at any time during 60 months of training, which must include 12 months of clinical base and a minimum of 30 months of clinical anesthesia. They are eligible for entrance into the ABA examination system after they have completed their clinical base requirement, 30 months of clinical anesthesia satisfactorily, and a minimum of 6 months of research experience.

   The anesthesiology program director may request 6 months of credit toward the research component of Option B for a resident with a PhD degree in a discipline relevant to anesthesiology. Documents supporting this request should include documentation of the PhD degree, a description of the current research, and a copy of the resident's curriculum vitae. Approval is at the discretion of the Credentials Committee and must be obtained prior to the start of the last 12 months of residency training. Credit will be granted only upon *completion* of all other requirements of Option B of the clinical scientist track.

   Regardless of which clinical scientist option is chosen, a resident who elects this track must not have an unsatisfactory Clinical Competence Committee report for the 6 months of clinical anesthesia training immediately preceding any research period.

C. Credit toward the CA 1-3 year requirements is granted by the ABA for clinical anesthesia training that satisfies *all* of the following conditions:

1. The CA 1-3 years of training are spent as a resident enrolled with the ABA by no more than two ACGME-accredited residency programs in the United States or its territories.
2. The period of clinical anesthesia training as an enrolled resident of any single program is at least 6 months of uninterrupted training.

3. The final 6 months of clinical anesthesia training in each program ends with receipt of a satisfactory Certificate of Clinical Competence. When the final period of training in any program is not satisfactory, the ABA grants credit for clinical anesthesia training in that program only to the date of the most recent satisfactory certificate received for the resident from that program.

   To receive credit from the ABA for a period of clinical anesthesia that is not satisfactory, the resident must immediately complete an additional 6 months of uninterrupted clinical anesthesia training in the same program with receipt of a satisfactory Certificate of Clinical Competence.
4. No more than 6 months during the first two clinical anesthesia years, and a maximum of 12 months during the 3 years of clinical anesthesia training, are spent training outside the parent programs in affiliated or nonaffiliated institutions. *The Credentials Committee of the ABA must prospectively approve clinical anesthesia training in nonaffiliated programs.* The prospective request for approval must include a chronological description of the rotations, information about the supervision of the resident, and assurances that the resident will be in compliance with the limits on training outside the parent program. Further, the resident must remain enrolled in the parent program while training at an affiliated or nonaffiliated institution, and the parent program must report the training on the Clinical Competence Committee report filed for the period involved.

D. Prospective approval is required for exceptions to policies regarding the training planned for residents. The Credentials Committee of the ABA considers requests for prospective approval on an individual basis. The ABA office must receive the request from the department chair on behalf of a resident at least 2 months before the resident begins the training in question. It is the responsibility of the department chair and the resident to assure that the request is received in a timely manner.

Principal Objectives

The examination system for the ABA's primary certificate has two distinct parts, the written examination and the oral examination. Each is designed to assess different qualities of a Board-certified anesthesiologist.

A Board-certified anesthesiologist is a physician who provides medical management and consultation during the perioperative period, in pain management, and in critical care medicine. A diplomate of the Board must possess knowledge, judgment, adaptability, clinical skills, technical facility, and personal characteristics sufficient to carry out the entire scope of anesthesiology practice. An ABA diplomate must logically organize and effectively present rational diagnoses and appropriate treatment protocols to peers, patients, their families, and others involved in the medical community. A diplomate of the Board can serve as an expert in matters related to anesthesiology, deliberate with others, and provide advice and defend opinions in all aspects of the specialty of anesthesiology. A Board-certified anesthesiologist is able to function as the leader of the anesthesiology care team.

Because of the nature of anesthesiology, the ABA diplomate must be able to manage emergent life-threatening situations in an independent and timely fashion. The ability to independently acquire and process information in a timely manner is central to assure individual responsibility for all aspects of anesthesiology care. Adequate physical and sensory faculties, such as eyesight, hearing, speech, and coordinated function of the extremities, are essential to the independent performance of the Board-certified anesthesiologist. Freedom from the influence of or dependency on chemical substances that impair cognitive, physical, sensory, or motor function also is an essential characteristic of the Board-certified anesthesiologist.

The written examination is designed to assess the candidate's knowledge of basic and clinical sciences as applied to anesthesiology.

It is necessary for candidates to pass the written examination to qualify for the oral examination. Candidates must wait at least 6 months after passing the written examination to be eligible to appear for the oral examination.

The oral examination is designed to assess the candidate's ability to manage patients presented in clinical scenarios, with particular emphasis on the scientific and clinical rationale that supports the management.

Irregular Behavior

The Board acts to maintain the integrity of its examination and certification process and to ensure the equitable and objective administration of its examinations to all candidates. Information about behavior the Board considers a violation of the integrity of its examination and certification process is sent to all candidates scheduled for examination. Statistical analyses may be conducted to verify observations and reports of suspected irregularities in the conduct of an examination. The examination of a candidate whose conduct, in the Board's judgment, violates or attempts to violate the integrity of its examination and certification process will be invalidated and no results will be reported. Furthermore, the candidate will be subject to punitive action as determined by the Board. In that event the candidate would be informed of the reasons for the Board's actions and could request an opportunity to present information deemed relevant to the issue and to petition the Board to reconsider its decision.

Nonstandard Examination Administration

The ABA supports the intent of the Americans with Disabilities Act (ADA) and has a process for considering requests that its assessment programs be modified to accommodate an individual with a disability. Anyone having questions about the process should write or call the executive vice president of the Board at the ABA office.

Unforeseeable Events

In the event a natural disaster, war, government regulations, strikes, civil disorders, curtailment of transportation facilities, or other unforeseeable events make it inadvisable, illegal, or impossible for the ABA to administer an examination to a candidate at the appointed date, time, and location, or to conclude a candidate's examination, the ABA is not responsible for any personal expense the candidate may have incurred to be present for the examination nor for any such expense the candidate may incur for any substitute examination.

Application Form

Application for admission to the examination system of the ABA must be made to the secretary on a form prescribed by the Board. *Photocopies or facsimiles of the application form are not acceptable.*

The proper application form and other information may be obtained by writing to the Secretary, American Board of Anesthesiology, 4101 Lake Boone Trail, Suite 510, Raleigh, NC 27607-7506. An applicant must request an application form by writing to the Board. *Telephone requests are not acceptable.*

Filing and Documentation Deadlines

The ABA must receive the completed application and the appropriate fee on or before January 10 of the year in which the written examination is to be administered. *The January 10 deadline for receipt of completed applications is absolute, and no application will be accepted after that date for any reason.*

The ABA must receive all documentation it requires to make a determination about an applicant's qualifications for admission to examination no later than March 10 of the year in which the written examination is to be administered. This includes but is not limited to references and evidence of medical licensure or of having qualified for such licensure. An application will not be accepted if the required documentation is not received by that date. *It ultimately is the responsibility of every applicant to ensure that the ABA receives all required documentation in a timely manner.*

Applicant Declaration and Consent

The application form includes the following declaration, which the applicant shall be required to sign:

I hereby make application to The American Board of Anesthesiology, Inc., for the issuance to me of a Certificate, and for examination relative thereto, all in accordance with and subject to its rules and regulations, and the fee requested. I agree to disqualification from examination or from the issuance of a Certificate or to forfeiture and redelivery of such Certification in the event that any of the statements heretofore made by me are false or in the event that any of the rules governing such examinations are violated by me or in the event that I did not comply with or shall violate any of the provisions of the Certificate of Incorporation or By-Laws of The American Board of Anesthesiology, Inc., or both, as then constituted. I understand that the American Board of Anesthesiology, Inc., may report my status in the examination system, including the result of any written or oral examination, to the Director of the program in which I completed my training in clinical anesthesiology either routinely or upon the request of such program director, use any score in psychometric analyses to confirm observations and reports of suspected irregularities in the conduct of an examination, and respond to any inquiry about my status in its examination system in accordance with its policy as then constituted. I authorize any and all repositories to grant access to or to produce copies for The American Board of Anesthesiology, Inc., of all documents and records containing information and data pertaining to my practice of the medical specialty of anesthesiology and its subdisciplines. I understand that such information and data will be used exclusively for current and longitudinal studies to assess the certification processes of The American Board of Anesthesiology, Inc. More particularly, such information as it pertains to me shall be held in confidence and shall be reported or released only as a part of the aggregate of such information gathered and studied without specific reference to myself or any other individuals. Such information and data will not bear in any way whatsoever upon the decision of The American Board of Anesthesiology, Inc., whether or not to grant me a certificate. I agree to hold The American Board of Anesthesiology, Inc., its members, examiners, officers, and agents free from any damage or complaint by reason of any action they, or any of them, take in connection with this application, such examinations, the grade or grades given with respect to any examination, the failure of said Board or Corporation to issue to me such certification, the gathering and collecting of information and data about my practice of anesthesiology, or the use of such information or data in studies of the certification processes of The American Board of Anesthesiology, Inc., as described above.

The application form also includes the following consent, which the applicant shall be required to sign:

I, the undersigned, in connection with my application for certification by The American Board of Anesthesiology, Inc., hereby authorize The American Board of Anesthesiology, Inc., now and in the future, to request, procure and review any information regarding my medical practice, professional standing and character, including any information related to any disciplinary action related to the practice of medicine by any state licensing agency or any institution in which I have practiced medicine and any information related to any history of alcoholism or illegal use of drugs and any treatment or rehabilitation related thereto.

I hereby authorize The American Board of Anesthesiology, Inc., now and in the future, to request and procure such information from any individual or institution, each of which shall be absolutely immune from civil liability arising from any act, communication, report, recommendation or disclosure of any such information even where the information involved would otherwise be deemed privileged so long as any such act, communication, report, recommendation or disclosure is performed or made in good faith and without malice.

I hereby authorize The American Board of Anesthesiology, Inc., to supply a copy of this consent, which has been executed by me, to any individual or institution from which it requests information relating to me.

Entrance Requirements

At the time of application to enter the examination system of the ABA, the applicant shall be capable of performing independently the entire scope of anesthesiology practice and must:

A. Have graduated from a medical school in a state or jurisdiction of the United States or in Canada that was accredited at the date of graduation by the LCME, the Committee on Accreditation of Canadian Medical Schools, or the American Osteopathic Association. Graduates of medical schools outside the jurisdiction of the United States and Canada must have one of the following: a permanent (valid indefinitely) certificate from the Educational Commission for Foreign Medical Graduates, comparable credentials from the Medical Council of Canada, or documentation of training for those who entered postdoctoral medical training in the United States via the Fifth Pathway as proposed by the American Medical Association.

B. Provide evidence satisfactory to the Board of having been awarded a medical or osteopathic degree acceptable to the Board.

C. Provide evidence acceptable to the Board of having satisfied the licensure requirement for certification. The applicant must inform the ABA of any conditions or restrictions in force on any active medical license he or she holds. When there is a restriction or condition in force on any of the applicant's medical licenses, the Credentials Committee of the ABA will determine whether the applicant shall be admitted to the ABA examination system.

   Residents in training may submit evidence with their application of having qualified on examinations that provide eligibility for medical licensure (eg, USMLE Steps 1, 2, and 3). Residents who do so must have evidence of permanent, unconditional, unrestricted, and currently unexpired medical licensure on file in the ABA office by November 30 of the year in which the written examination for which they applied is administered.

D. Have on file in the Board office evidence of having satisfactorily fulfilled all requirements of the Continuum of Education in Anesthesiology before the date of examination and after receiving a medical or osteopathic degree acceptable to the ABA. Such evidence must include a satisfactory Certificate of Clinical Competence covering the final 6 months of clinical anesthesia training in each residency program. A grace period will be permitted so that applicants completing this requirement by August 31 may apply for the immediately preceding July written examination.

E. Have on file with the Board evaluations of various aspects of his or her current practice of anesthesiology as solicited by the Board in determining the applicant's qualifications for admission to the examination system. The ABA may request such evaluations from the residency program director or others familiar with the applicant's current practice of anesthesiology. The Clinical Competence Committee Report from the department and the evaluation of the program director and others will be used as the basis for assessing admission qualifications.

F. If residency training was completed more than 12 years before the date of application or if a second or subsequent application has been declared void, the applicant must submit proof of having reestablished his or her qualifications for admission to the examination system. Acceptable proof consists of documentation of having qualified on an entry examination designated by the Board. The Board has designated the examination administered annually by the Joint Council on In-Training Examinations as the entry examination. Information about the entry examination and a registration form may be obtained by writing the Joint Council c/o the American Society of Anesthesiologists.

Alternatively, the applicant may complete 12 consecutive months of additional clinical training in anesthesia as a CA-3 year resident in one ACGME-accredited program with receipt of a satisfactory Certificate of Clinical Competence covering the final 6 months. The applicant must qualify on the entry examination or satisfactorily complete the year of additional training after the date the ABA declared her or his most recent application void and within the 3 years immediately preceding the next application.

The ABA will *not* validate or report the results to applicants who sit for the written examination and do not fulfill those conditions by the deadlines.

The Board shall determine that entry into the examination system is merited when a judgment of adequate levels of scholarship and clinical competence can be made from the information submitted. After approval of all of their credentials, the ABA will notify applicants that they are accepted as candidates for certification.

The Board, acting as a committee of the whole, reserves the right not to accept an application for any reason deemed appropriate.

The Board reserves the right to correct clerical errors affecting its decisions.

Certificate of Clinical Competence

The Board requires every residency training program to file, on forms provided by the Board, an Evaluation of Clinical Competence in January and July on behalf of each resident who has spent any portion of the prior 6 months in clinical anesthesia training in or under the sponsorship of the residency program and its affiliates. The program director (department chair) must not chair the Clinical Competence Committee.

Entry into the examination system is contingent upon the applicant having a Certificate of Clinical Competence on file with the Board attesting to satisfactory clinical competence during the final period of clinical anesthesia training in or under the sponsorship of each program. The Board, therefore, will deny entry into the examination system until this requirement is fulfilled.

Absence From Training

The total of any and all absences during clinical anesthesia training may not exceed the equivalent of 20 working days per year. Attendance at scientific meetings, not to exceed 5 working days per year, shall be considered a part of the training program. Duration of absence during the clinical base year may conform to the policy of the institution and department in which that portion of the training is served. Absences in excess of those specified will require lengthening of the total training time to the extent of the additional absence.

A lengthy interruption in training may have a deleterious effect upon the resident's knowledge or clinical competence. Therefore, when there is an absence for a period in excess of 6 months, the Credentials Committee of the ABA shall determine the number of months of training the resident will have to complete subsequent to resumption of the residency program to satisfy the training required for admission to the ABA examination system.

Entrance Into the System

The examination system for the ABA's primary certificate has two distinct parts, the written examination and the oral examination. Each is designed to assess different qualities of a Board-certified anesthesiologist.

The written examination is designed to assess the candidate's knowledge of basic and clinical sciences as applied to anesthesiology. Written examinations are held annually in locations throughout the United States and Canada on a Saturday in July. A passing grade, as determined by the Board, is required.

It is necessary for candidates to pass the written examination to qualify for the oral examination. Candidates must wait at least 6 months after passing the written examination to be eligible to appear for the oral examination.

The oral examination is designed to assess the candidate's ability to manage patients presented in clinical scenarios with particular emphasis on the scientific and clinical rationale that supports the management. The ABA conducts oral examinations in the spring and fall of each year at a single location in the United States. Examiners consist of directors of the Board and other ABA diplomates who assist as associate examiners. A passing grade, as determined by the Board, is required.

The ABA will *not* schedule candidates to appear at consecutive oral examinations. Candidates who do not take or do not pass an oral examination for which they are scheduled, for whatever reason, are not eligible to appear at the next regularly scheduled oral examination.

A. The duration of candidate status is limited. Candidates are given one opportunity a calendar year, for 3 years, to successfully complete each examination requirement. They must satisfactorily complete the written examination within 4 years of the date of the first examination that follows acceptance of the application, and they must satisfactorily complete the oral examination within 7 years of that date. The ABA will declare the candidate's application void if the candidate does not satisfy an examination requirement within the prescribed number of opportunities or time, whichever comes first.

B. The ABA sends notification of an examination and a reply form to every candidate eligible to appear for the examination at least 4 months prior to the examination date. The notification is sent to candidates at their address of record on file in the Board office.

Candidates are *required* to respond to every written and oral examination notice by the response date established by the ABA, whether or not they accept the examination opportunity. The ABA will acknowledge every reply to an examination notice within 2 weeks of the response deadline.

Candidates scheduled to appear for examination are notified of the exact date, time, and location of their examination and the rules for its conduct at least 2 months before the date of examination.

The Board office is not responsible for an interruption in communication with a candidate that is due to circumstances beyond its control. Candidates must send the Board written notice of an address change immediately. Candidates must call the Board office if they do not receive an examination notice they are expecting within the time frame described above. The candidate's Social Security number is used by the Board for identification purposes and should be included on all correspondence with the Board.

C. The ABA requires each candidate to accept each opportunity offered by the Board to appear for examination. The ABA must receive the candidate's written response to the notice of opportunity for examination by the deadline specified in the notification. The candidate forfeits the examination opportunity if the ABA does *not* receive acceptance of the examination opportunity or a request to be excused from the examination by the response deadline. A candidate who accepts the opportunity and fails to appear for the examination forfeits the opportunity and the examination fee.

Under certain circumstances the ABA, at its discretion, may grant a candidate's request for an excused absence from any scheduled examination without forfeiture of the opportunity or fee. Such a request must be filed in writing, include the candidate's reason, and arrive in the ABA office by the response deadline specified in the examination notice or, for scheduled candidates, by the examination date. A candidate may be excused from examination if it is determined the reason warrants such a decision and there is sufficient time remaining in the application period to provide the number of examination opportunities the candidate is permitted. Candidates excused from an examination are required to appear at the next examination for which they are eligible.

The Board reserves the right to limit the number of candidates to be admitted to any examination. Places in the oral examination schedule are assigned randomly when more candidates request the examination than can be accommodated. Candidates who are not given an examination appointment, whether or not they accepted the examination opportunity, are required to appear at the next examination for which they are eligible.

Fees

The application fee for primary certification in anesthesiology is $1,700. It must accompany the application.

For completed applications received between January 11 and November 20 of the previous year, the application fee is $1,600—a reduction of $100 for early filing.

The application fee includes a nonrefundable fee for administrative services. It is $200 for applications for primary certification that arrive after November 20 and $100 for those received on or before that date. In the event an application is not accepted, or the application is accepted and subsequently withdrawn by the candidate, the fee for administrative services will be retained and the balance of the application fee will be refunded. No fee will be remitted if the candidate's notice of withdrawal from the examination system is received in the Board office after the deadline by which candidates must notify the Board of their choice of test center for the first written examination for which they are eligible.

The **reexamination fee** is $400 for the anesthesiology written examination and $1,100 for the oral examination. The reexamination fee will be charged to candidates whether they have failed a previous examination, canceled a scheduled appointment for examination, or failed to appear for any examination for which they were properly scheduled.

A charge of $50 will be made whenever a check is returned for nonpayment.

The ABA is a nonprofit organization. The fees for application and examination are computed on a basis of cost of maintaining the functions of the Board. The Board reserves the right to change the fees when necessary.

Reapplication

The ABA declares void the application of a candidate who does not satisfy the examination requirements in the prescribed number of opportunities or time for whatever reason. The physician may reapply by submitting a new application. Such application shall be subject to the fees, rules, privileges, and requirements that apply at the time of reapplication. The applicant who meets existing requirements will be readmitted into the examination system.

The reapplicant for primary certification who has had a second or subsequent application declared void for any cause, or has completed anesthesia residency training more than 12 years before the date of reapplication, must reestablish his or her qualifications for admission to the examination system before filing another application. In all instances, the candidate must pass both the written and oral examinations under the new application.

Status of Individuals

The ABA reserves to itself exclusively the right to define and confer "Board eligible" status whenever such status refers to an individual's relationship to the ABA examination and certification system. The ABA shall confer Board eligible status only on physicians who have a current accepted application in its examination system. *Thus, physicians are Board eligible only when they are eligible to appear for an ABA examination.* Board eligible status is not conferred indefinitely.

Inquiries about the current status of individuals should be addressed to the ABA office, which will respond with one of the following statements:

- The physician is certified by the American Board of Anesthesiology.
- The physician is Board eligible in anesthesiology.
- The physician is neither certified by the American Board of Anesthesiology nor Board eligible.

The fee for written confirmation of an individual's status is $10.

Alcoholism and Substance Abuse

The Americans with Disabilities Act (ADA) protects individuals with a history of alcoholism or substance abuse who are not currently abusing alcohol or using drugs illegally. The ABA supports the intent of the ADA.

The ABA will admit qualified applicants and candidates with a history of alcoholism to its examination system and to examination if, in response to its inquiries, the ABA receives acceptable documentation that they do not currently pose a direct threat to the health and safety of others.

The ABA will admit qualified applicants and candidates with a history of illegal use of drugs to its examination system and to examination if, in response to its inquiries, the ABA receives acceptable documentation that they are not currently engaged in the illegal use of drugs.

After a candidate with a history of alcoholism or illegal use of drugs satisfies the examination requirements for certification, the ABA will determine whether it should defer awarding its certification to the candidate for a period of time to avoid certifying a candidate who poses a direct threat to the health and safety of others. If the ABA determines that deferral of the candidate's certification is appropriate because the candidate does currently pose a threat to the health and safety of others, the ABA will assess the specific circumstances of the candidate's history of alcoholism or illegal use of drugs to determine when the candidate should write the Board to request issuance of its certification.

Revocation of Certificate

A certificate is issued by the Board with the understanding that it remains the property of the Board during the life of the diplomate. Any certificate issued by the Board shall be subject to revocation in the event that:

A. The issuance of such certificate or its receipt by the person so certified shall have been contrary to, or in violation of, any provision of the Certificate of Incorporation of this Board or its By-Laws; or

B. The person certified shall not have been eligible to receive such certificate whether or not the facts making him or her ineligible were known to, or could have been ascertained by, the Board or any of the directors at the time of issuance of such certificate; or

C. The person certified shall have made any misstatement of fact in his or her application for such certificate or in any other statement or representation to the Board or its representatives; or

D. The person certified shall fail to maintain moral, ethical, or professional behavior satisfactory to the Board.

The Board shall be the sole judge of whether the evidence or information before it is sufficient to require or permit revocation of any certificate issued by the Board, and the decision of the Board shall be final.

Certification by Other Organizations

The ABA will make no statement about the comparability of the ABA certificate and another organization's certificate. The ABA will not accept certification by another entity as meeting the requirements for entrance into the ABA examination system for specialty or subspecialty certification or recertification.

Records Retention

The ABA retains documents pertaining to an individual's residency training, application for certification, examination opportunities, and examination results for the sole purpose of determining that its requirements for admission to examination and for certification are fulfilled.

In the absence of an application for certification, documents pertaining to the ABA entrance requirements are retained for 7 years from the date of the most recent correspondence to or from the ABA regarding the requirements. Documents pertaining to an unsuccessful application are retained until the individual submits another application to the ABA or the aforementioned 7-year period expires, whichever occurs first. Documentation corroborating the results of a candidate's examination is retained until 1 year after the date of the most recent correspondence to or from the ABA regarding the results. Documentation corroborating the candidate's fulfillment of the ABA certification requirements is retained until 1 year after the date of the most recent correspondence to or from the ABA regarding the candidate's certification by the ABA. The ABA sees to the secure destruction of the documents in its file for an individual when the period specified for retention of the documents has expired.

The ABA retains indefinitely an electronic record for residents who trained in an ACGME-accredited anesthesiology program. This record includes entries that identify the training program, the dates of training, and the overall evaluation of the resident.

The ABA retains indefinitely microfiche and electronic records for candidates issued its certification. These records include documents and entries attesting that each certification requirement was met.

Appeals

An individual has the right to appeal an interpretation of ABA policy. The individual must write the ABA secretary stating the basis for appeal within 30 days of receiving the decision under appeal.

Subspecialty Certification in Critical Care Medicine

A. Definition of Critical Care Medicine

The discipline of critical care medicine has evolved over the last few decades in parallel with the development of techniques and technology for acute and long-term life support of patients with multiple organ system derangement. Because the problems encountered in the critically ill patient encompass aspects of many different specialties, critical care medicine is a multidisciplinary endeavor that crosses traditional department and specialty lines.

The critical care medicine physician is a specialist whose knowledge is of necessity broad, involving all aspects of management of the critically ill patient, and whose primary base of operation is the intensive care unit (ICU). This physician has completed training in a primary specialty and has received additional training in critical care medicine aspects of many disciplines. This background enables the physician to work in concert with the various specialists on the patient care team in the ICU; to utilize recognized techniques for vital support; to teach other physicians, nurses, and health professionals the practice of intensive care; and to foster research.

B. Certification Requirements

At the time of subspecialty certification in critical care medicine by the ABA, each candidate shall be capable of performing independently the entire scope of anesthesiology critical care medicine practice and must:

- Be a diplomate of the ABA.
- Fulfill the licensure requirement for certification.
- Have fulfilled the requirement of the continuum of education in critical care medicine as defined by the ABA.
- Have satisfied the critical care medicine examination requirement of the ABA.

C. Continuum of Education in Critical Care Medicine

The continuum of education in critical care medicine consists of 12 months of full-time training in critical care medicine. The training must be in an anesthesiology critical care medicine program in the United States or its territories accredited by the ACGME. The training must follow completion of the continuum of education in anesthesiology (ie, clinical base and CA 1-3 years) unless the Credentials Committee of the ABA prospectively approves a different training sequence for the resident.

Training in critical care medicine must *not* be interrupted by frequent or prolonged periods of absence. When there is an absence for a period in excess of 2 months, the Credentials Committee of the ABA shall determine the number of months of training the resident will have to complete subsequent to resumption of the residency program to satisfy the training required for admission to the ABA subspecialty examination system.

D. Entrance Requirements

At the time of application to enter the critical care medicine examination system of the ABA, the applicant shall be capable of performing independently the entire scope of anesthesiology critical care medicine practice and must:

- Be certified by the ABA.
- Submit proof of having fulfilled the licensure requirement for certification. The applicant must inform the ABA of any conditions or restrictions in force on any active medical license he or she holds. When there is a restriction or condition in force on any of the applicant's medical licenses, the Credentials Committee of the ABA will determine whether the applicant shall be admitted to the ABA examination system.
- Have on file in the ABA office documentation of having fulfilled the requirement of the continuum of education in critical care medicine.

The ABA will solicit evaluations of various aspects of the applicant's current practice of anesthesiology critical care medicine as part of its assessment of the applicant's qualifications for admission to its critical care medicine examination system. The Board shall determine that entry into its critical care medicine examination system is merited when a judgment of clinical competence can be made from the information submitted.

The ABA will notify an applicant who is accepted as a candidate for its critical care medicine examination after approval of all credentials. The Board, acting as a committee of the whole, reserves the right not to accept an application for any reason deemed appropriate. The Board reserves the right to correct clerical errors affecting its decisions.

E. Application Procedure

1. The proper application form and other information may be obtained by writing to the Secretary of the ABA at 4101 Lake Boone Trail, Suite 510, Raleigh, NC 27607-7506. An applicant must request an application form by writing to the Board. *Telephone requests are not acceptable.*

Application for admission to the examination system of the ABA must be made to the secretary upon a form prescribed by the Board. *Photocopies or facsimiles of the application form are not acceptable.*

2. The application form includes the identical statements of declaration and consent included in the application for primary certification. The applicant for examination in critical care medicine shall be required to sign each statement.

F. Filing and Documentation Deadlines

The ABA must receive the completed application and the appropriate fee for the 1999 critical care medicine examination on or before March 1, 1999. *Applications received after the deadline will not be accepted.*

The ABA must receive all documentation it requires to make a determination about an applicant's qualifications for admission to the examination no later than May 1, 1999. This includes but is not limited to references, evidence of medical licensure, and verification that the training requirement is met. An application will not be accepted if the required documentation is not received by that date. *It ultimately is the responsibility of every applicant to assure that the ABA receives all required documentation in a timely manner.*

G. Fees

The application fee for admission to the critical care medicine examination system is $1,000. It must accompany the application.

The application fee includes a nonrefundable fee for administrative services of $250. The reexamination fee for the critical care medicine examination is $750.

A charge of $50 will be made whenever a check is returned for nonpayment.

H. Examination System

The written examination in critical care medicine is designed to test for the presence of knowledge that is considered essential for the ABA diplomate to function as a practitioner of critical care medicine. The examination analyzes the cognitive and deductive skills as well as the clinical judgment of the candidates.

The critical care medicine examination is administered once every 2 years. The ABA will mail notice to all eligible candidates announcing the location(s) and date of the critical care medicine examination approximately 4 months prior to the date of its scheduled administration.

Every candidate is given three opportunities to satisfy the critical care medicine examination requirement. The ABA will declare the candidate's application void if the candidate does not satisfy the examination requirement within the three opportunities or the prescribed time, whichever comes first.

The prescribed period of time for the successful completion of the examination for subspecialty certification in critical care medicine is the time between the date of the examination for which the candidate applied and the next three consecutive administrations of the critical care medicine examination. Thus, the ABA, at its discretion, may excuse a candidate from at most one critical care medicine examination without forfeiture of an opportunity.

I. Status of Individual

Inquiries about the current status of physicians relative to the ABA critical care medicine certification system should be addressed to the ABA office. The ABA will affirm the status of physicians who are certified in critical care medicine by the ABA. For others, the response to the inquiry will be in keeping with the ABA policy.

J. Reapplication

The ABA declares void the application of a candidate who has failed to satisfy the examination requirement in the prescribed number of opportunities or time for any reason. The physician may reapply by submitting a new application. Such application shall be subject to the fees, rules, privileges, and requirements that apply at the time of reapplication. The applicant who is judged to meet existing requirements will be readmitted into the examination system.

Every reapplicant who qualified previously by temporary criteria is required to have completed satisfactorily the 1-year continuum of education in critical care medicine before reapplying for the subspecialty certificate.

Subspecialty Certification in Pain Management

A. Definition of Pain Management

Pain management is the medical discipline concerned with the diagnosis and treatment of the entire range of painful disorders. Because of the vast scope of the field, pain management is a multidisciplinary subspecialty. The expertise of several disciplines is brought together in an effort to provide the maximum benefit to each patient. Although the care of patients is heavily influenced by the primary specialty of physicians who subspecialize in pain management, each member of the pain treatment team understands the anatomical and physiological basis of pain perception, the psychological factors that modify the pain experience, and the basic principles of pain management.

B. Certification Requirements

At the time of subspecialty certification in pain management by the ABA, each candidate shall be capable of performing independently the entire scope of anesthesiology pain management practice and must:

- Be a diplomate of the ABA.
- Fulfill the licensure requirement for certification.
- Have fulfilled the requirement of the continuum of education in pain management as defined by the ABA.

- Have satisfied the pain management examination requirement of the ABA.

The ABA subspecialty certificate in pain management is valid for a period of 10 years after the year the candidate passes the examination for certification. It is left to the holder of the subspecialty certificate when to reapply to the ABA for examination and renewal of the pain management certification.

C. Continuum of Education in Pain Management

The continuum of education in pain management consists of 12 months of full-time training in acute, chronic, and oncology pain management. The training must be in an anesthesiology pain management program in the United States or its territories accredited by the ACGME. The training must follow completion of the continuum of education in anesthesiology (ie, clinical base and CA 1-3 years), unless the Credentials Committee of the ABA prospectively approves a different training sequence for the resident.

Training in pain management must *not* be interrupted by frequent or prolonged periods of absence. When there is an absence for a period in excess of 2 months, the Credentials Committee of the ABA shall determine the number of months of training the resident will have to complete subsequent to resumption of the residency program to satisfy the training required for admission to the ABA subspecialty examination system.

D. Entrance Requirements

At the time of application to enter the pain management examination system of the ABA, the applicant shall be capable of performing independently the entire scope of anesthesiology pain management practice and must:

- Be certified by the ABA.
- Submit proof of having fulfilled the licensure requirement for certification. The applicant must inform the ABA of any conditions or restrictions in force on any active medical license he or she holds. When there is a restriction or condition in force on any of the applicant's medical licenses, the Credentials Committee of the ABA will determine whether the applicant shall be admitted to the ABA examination system.
- Have on file in the Board office documentation of having fulfilled the requirement of the continuum of education in pain management.

The ABA will solicit evaluations of various aspects of the applicant's current practice of anesthesiology pain management as part of its assessment of the applicant's qualifications for admission to its pain management examination system. The Board shall determine that entry into its pain management examination system is merited when a judgment of clinical competence can be made from the information submitted.

The ABA will notify an applicant who is accepted as a candidate for its pain management examination after approval of all credentials. The Board, acting as a committee of the whole, reserves the right not to accept an application for any reason deemed appropriate. The Board reserves the right to correct clerical errors affecting its decisions.

E. Application Procedure

1. The proper application form and other information may be obtained by writing to the secretary of the ABA at 4101 Lake Boone Trail, Suite 510, Raleigh, NC 27607-7506. An applicant must request an application form by writing to the Board. *Telephone requests are not acceptable.*

   Application for admission to the examination system of the ABA must be made to the secretary upon a form prescribed by the Board. *Photocopies or facsimiles of the application form are not acceptable.*
2. The application form includes the identical statements of declaration and consent included in the application for primary certification. The applicant for examination in pain management shall be required to sign each statement.

F. Filing and Documentation Deadlines

The completed application and the appropriate fee for the year 2000 pain management examination must be received by the ABA on or before March 1, 2000. *Applications received after the deadline will not be accepted.*

The ABA must receive all documentation it requires to make a determination about an applicant's qualifications for admission to the examination no later than May 1, 2000. This includes but is not limited to references, evidence of medical licensure, and verification that the training requirement is met. An application will not be accepted if the required documentation is not received by that date. *It ultimately is the responsibility of every applicant to ensure that the ABA receives all required documentation in a timely manner.*

G. Fees

The application fee for admission to the pain management examination system is $1,000. The fee must accompany the application.

The application fee includes a nonrefundable fee for administrative services of $250. The reexamination fee for the pain management examination is $750.

A charge of $50 will be made whenever a check is returned for nonpayment.

H. Examination System

The written examination in pain management is designed to test for the presence of knowledge that is considered essential for the ABA diplomate to function as a practitioner of pain management. The examination analyzes the cognitive and deductive skills as well as the clinical judgment of the candidates.

The ABA will administer the pain management examination annually, beginning with the examination in the year 2000. The ABA will mail notice to all eligible candidates announcing the location(s) and date of the pain management examination approximately 4 months prior to the date of its scheduled administration.

Every candidate is given three opportunities to satisfy the pain management examination requirement. The ABA will declare the candidate's application void if the candidate does not satisfy the examination requirement within the three opportunities or the prescribed time, whichever comes first.

The prescribed period of time for the successful completion of the examination for subspecialty certification in pain management is the time between the date of the examination for which the candidate applied and the next three consecutive administrations of the pain management examination. Thus, the ABA, at its discretion, may excuse a candidate from at most one pain management examination without forfeiture of an opportunity.

I. Status of Individuals

Inquiries about the current status of physicians relative to the ABA pain management certification system should be addressed to the ABA office. The ABA will affirm the status of physicians who are certified in pain management by the ABA. For others, the response to the inquiry will be in keeping with ABA policy.

J. Reapplication

The ABA declares void the application of a candidate who has failed to satisfy the examination requirement in the prescribed number of opportunities or time for whatever reason. The physician may reapply by submitting a new application. Such application shall be subject to the fees, rules, privileges, and requirements that apply at the time of reapplication. The applicant who is judged to meet existing requirements will be readmitted into the examination system.

Every reapplicant who qualified previously by temporary criteria is required to have completed satisfactorily the 1-year continuum of education in pain management before reapplying for the subspecialty certificate.

Program for Recertification

A. Background

Initiatives at federal, state, and local levels convinced the ABA that some of its diplomates would need or desire a mechanism to demonstrate their continuing qualifications. In May 1989, the ABA announced its intent to develop a program for continued demonstration of qualifications (CDQ), which would afford its diplomates the opportunity to *voluntarily* demonstrate current knowledge and quality of practice.

The ABA approved a policy of time-limited certification in 1994-1995. All certificates issued by the ABA on or after January 1, 2000, will expire 10 years after the year the candidate passed the certification examination. The ABA took this step to reassure the public that the diplomate continues to demonstrate the attributes of a Board-certified anesthesiologist.

The ABMS approved the ABA recertification proposal in March 1996. Subsequently, the ABA changed the name of the CDQ program to recertification.

The ABA recertification program includes a commitment to continued education in anesthesiology, assessment of the quality of practice in the local environment, and evaluation of knowledge. *Diplomates who hold a certificate that is not time-limited may voluntarily elect to apply to the ABA for recertification. The ABA will not alter the status of their certification if they do not recertify.*

B. Requirements

The recertification program includes two major components: an evaluation of the quality of current practice conducted at the local level and a secure written examination.

To be admissible to the recertification examination of the ABA, the applicant shall be capable of performing independently the entire scope of anesthesiology practice and must:

- Be a physician to whom the ABA previously awarded certification.
- Submit evidence that he or she holds a permanent, unconditional, unrestricted, and unexpired license to practice medicine in the state or jurisdiction of the United States or the province of Canada where the principal hospital or facility in which he or she practices anesthesiology is located. The applicant must inform the ABA of any conditions or restrictions in force on any active medical license he or she holds. When there is a restriction or condition in force on any of the applicant's medical licenses, the Credentials Committee of the ABA will determine whether the applicant shall be admitted to the recertification examination.
- Have on file in the ABA office documentation solicited by the ABA from the hospital/facility chief of staff or others attesting to the applicant's current hospital/facility credentials and privileges, where applicable.

The ABA shall issue a recertification certificate to the applicant who is accepted for and satisfies the recertification examination requirement established by the ABA.

C. The Application Procedure

Physicians previously certified by the ABA may apply for admission to the recertification program at whatever interval they prefer following certification by the ABA.

The proper application form and other information may be obtained by writing to the secretary of the ABA at 4101 Lake Boone Trail, Suite 510, Raleigh, NC 27607-7506. An applicant must request an application form by writing to the Board. *Telephone requests are not acceptable.*

Application for admission to the ABA recertification program must be made to the secretary upon a form prescribed by the Board. *Photocopies or facsimiles of the application form are not acceptable.*

The application form includes the identical statements of declaration and consent included in the application for primary certification. The recertification applicant shall be required to sign each statement.

D. Filing and Documentation Deadlines

The ABA must receive the completed application and the appropriate fee for the May 2000 recertification examination on or before November 15, 1999. *Applications received after the deadline will not be accepted.*

The ABA must receive all the documentation it requires to make a determination about an applicant's qualifications for admission to the examination no later than January 15, 2000. This includes but is not limited to evidence of medical licensure and verification of current credentialing/hospital privileges. An application will not be accepted if the required documentation is not received by that date. *It ultimately is the responsibility of every applicant to ensure that the ABA receives all required documentation in a timely manner.*

E. Fees

The application fee for admission to the recertification program is $700. The fee must accompany the application.

The application fee includes a nonrefundable fee for administrative services of $200.

A charge of $50 will be made whenever a check is returned for nonpayment.

F. The Examination System

The ABA shall determine that admission to the recertification examination is warranted when a judgment of clinical competence can be made from the information submitted by and on behalf of the applicant.

The ABA will notify an applicant who is accepted as a candidate for its recertification examination after approval of all credentials. The Board, acting as a committee of the whole, reserves the right not to accept an application for any reason deemed appropriate. If the applicant wishes to exercise the right to appeal this decision, the applicant must inform the Board of this intention within 30 days of the date of receipt of written notification of the decision not to accept the application. The Board reserves the right to correct clerical errors affecting its decisions.

The recertification examination is designed to assess current knowledge of the breadth of anesthesia practice. The examination presents clinically relevant items that apply to all types of anesthesia practice.

The recertification examination is administered once each year. The ABA will mail notice to all eligible candidates announcing the location(s) and date of the recertification examination approximately 4 months prior to the date of its scheduled administration.

It is intended that the recertification program be a contemporaneous evaluation of the quality of practice and assessment of knowledge. Therefore, every candidate is given one opportunity per application to satisfy the examination requirement.

Every candidate must satisfy the recertification examination requirement within 1 year of the date of the examination for which he/she applied. At its discretion the ABA may excuse a candidate from at most one recertification examination.

G. Status of Individuals

Inquiries about the current status of physicians relative to the ABA voluntary program for recertification should be addressed to the ABA office. For physicians certified by the ABA who subsequently complete the recertification program, the ABA will affirm their diplomate status and the year of their recertification. For others, the response to the inquiry will be in keeping with ABA policy.

H. Reapplication

Physicians who previously completed the ABA recertification program, and those who did not, may apply for recertification at whatever interval they prefer. To reapply, the physician must submit a new application. Such application shall be subject to the fees, rules, privileges, and requirements that apply at the time of reapplication. The applicant who is judged to meet existing requirements will be accepted into the program for recertification.

Test Dates and Deadlines

Written Examinations

November 20, 1999—Early filing deadline for application with reduced fee
January 10, 2000—Application deadline
March 10, 2000—Documents deadline
May 1, 1999—Deadline for reply to examination notice
July 8, 2000—Examination date

Recertification Examinations

November 15, 1999—Application deadline
January 15, 2000—Documents deadline
March 1, 1999—Deadline for reply to examination notice
May 6-20, 2000—Examination dates

Oral Examinations

April 19-23, 1999—Examination dates
September 27-October 1, 1999—Examination dates
April 10-14, 2000—Examination dates
September 11-15, 2000—Examination dates

Critical Care Medicine Examination

March 1, 1999—Application deadline
May 1, 1999—Documents deadline
July 1, 1999—Deadline for reply to examination notice
September 18, 1999—Examination date

Pain Management Examination

March 1, 2000—Application deadline
May 1, 2000—Documents deadline
July 1, 2000—Deadline for reply to examination notice
September 9, 2000—Examination date

American Board of Colon and Rectal Surgery

20600 Eureka Rd/Ste 713
Taylor, MI 48180
734 282-9400

Marvin L Corman, MD, President, Los Angeles, California
Robert W Beart, Jr, MD, Vice President, Los Angeles, California
Herand Abcarian, MD, Secretary-Treasurer/Executive Director, Taylor, Michigan
Yanek S Y Chiu, MD, San Francisco, California
James W Fleshman, MD, St Louis, Missouri
Robert D Fry, MD, Philadelphia, Pennsylvania
Philip H Gordon, MD, Montreal, Quebec
Donald L Kaminski, MD, St Louis, Missouri
Ian C Lavery, MD, Cleveland, Ohio
Richard L Nelson, MD, Chicago, Illinois
David A Rothenberger, MD, St Paul, Minnesota
Alan G Thorson, MD, Omaha, Nebraska

(These criteria and conditions are subject to change without notice. All applicants are advised to contact the American Board of Colon and Rectal Surgery [ABCRS] to ascertain whether the information below is current.)

Qualifications of Candidates

All candidates shall comply with the following regulations:

General Requirements

1. A candidate shall appear personally before the Board and shall submit to the required examinations.
2. A candidate shall limit the majority of his/her practice to colon and rectal surgery.
3. A candidate may be required to deliver to the Board sufficient case reports to demonstrate proficiency in colon and rectal surgery.
4. A bibliography of papers and books published by the candidate shall be submitted to the Board upon its request.
5. The moral and ethical fitness of a candidate must be satisfactory to the Board and in conformity with the *Statements on Principles* of the American College of Surgeons and the *Principles of Medical Ethics* of the American Medical Association. Practices not conforming therewith may result in rejection of an application or in deferral of examination until such matters have been resolved satisfactorily.

Professional Qualifications

1. A candidate must have completed an accredited residency program in colon and rectal surgery.
2. All candidates must have a currently *valid* registered, full, and unrestricted license to practice medicine in a state, territory, or possession of the United States or in a Canadian province and must continue to be licensed throughout the certification process.
3. A candidate must successfully complete the Qualifying Examination of the American Board of Surgery before being admitted to the ABCRS Written Examination (Part I).
4. A candidate must achieve certification by the American Board of Surgery before being admitted to the ABCRS Oral Examination (Part II).

Application for Examination

Each candidate for examination must complete and submit an Application for Examination, which may be obtained from the secretary of the Board. Applications must be submitted before July 15 of each year.

The application must be accompanied by two unmounted, recent photographs of the applicant and the required application fee.

Within 2 weeks after conclusion of the training program, the applicant must submit to the secretary of the Board a prescribed form, listing all operative procedures performed during the training period. This form is available from the secretary of the Board and must be countersigned by the program director.

The acceptability of a candidate for examination depends not only upon completion of the requirements listed under "Qualifications for Candidates" but also upon information available to the Board regarding the candidate's professional maturity, surgical judgment, and technical competence.

Examinations

To achieve certification by the ABCRS, a candidate must pass a Written Examination (Part I) and an Oral Examination (Part II). The Written Examination is offered in the spring of the year, and a candidate is required to pass this examination before being permitted to take the Oral Examination, which is given in the fall of the year.

Examinations are conducted at times and places determined by the Board, and this information may be obtained from the Board office. It is also published in *Diseases of the Colon and Rectum* and in the *Journal of the American Medical Association.* Examinations will be held in one designated city in the United States.

Part I—Written Examination

The Written Examination is an assessment of a candidate's knowledge of the theory and practice of colon and rectal surgery, with separate examinations in pathology and radiology. The written portion of the examination is a 4-hour test of multiple-choice questions covering the spectrum of colon and rectal surgery and the body of basic science pertinent to it. The pathology and radiology portions of the examination are each 1 hour in length and consist of questions and slide presentations.

Part II—Oral Examination

The Oral Examination is conducted by members of the Board or its designated examiners. Its objective is to evaluate the candidate's clinical experience, problem-solving ability, and surgical judgment and to ascertain the candidate's knowledge of current literature on colon and rectal diseases and surgery. Each candidate will undergo at least three 30-minute oral examinations by three 2-member examining teams.

Examination Results

The Board makes every effort to be as prompt as possible in notifying candidates of their examination results, and letters of notification may be expected within 4 to 6 weeks following the examination.

Reexaminations

A candidate who has failed either the written or oral part of the examination may be reexamined after 1 year has elapsed.

A candidate who fails to pass either the written or oral portion of the examination may repeat that part of the examination twice, thus offering the candidate three opportunities to pass each part of the examination.

A candidate who fails to pass either the written or oral portion of the examination three times may not repeat the examination without satisfactory completion of an approved colon and rectal surgery residency program and submission of a new application for examination.

Status of Applicant

The Board does not use or sanction the terms "Board eligible" or "Board qualified." The status of an applicant with the Board is determined by and varies with the current status of his/her credentials.

A candidate must apply to the Board's certification process within 5 years after completion of approved colon and rectal surgery training.

The entire certification process with the Board must be successfully completed within 7 years following approval of the formal application. In addition, a candidate whose application for examination has been approved but who does not take the examination within 3 years must submit a new application.

In exceptional or unusual circumstances, the Board may, at its discretion, waive one or more of the limitations specified under "Status of Applicant."

Fees

Application fee: A nonrefundable fee of $300 shall accompany the application.

Written Examination fee (Part I): A fee of $400 is due and payable when the candidate is notified of approval to take the Written Examination.

Oral Examination fee (Part II): A fee of $500 is due and payable when the candidate is notified of approval to take the Oral Examination.

Reexamination fee: Fees for reexamination are the same as shown above for each examination.

Withdrawal from examination: A candidate who withdraws must notify the Board office at least 10 business days before a scheduled examination. A candidate who fails to appear for examination or who withdraws without giving at least 10 days' notice as defined above will forfeit $100 of the designated examination fee and will have to resubmit the forfeited amount before being admitted to the next scheduled examination.

Late applications: Recognizing that a situation may arise that prevents an applicant from meeting the July 15 deadline, the Board has a provision for late applications. Late applications are those that are postmarked from July 16 through August 15 each year. There is a nonrefundable late application fee of $100, bringing the total processing fee for a late application to $400. No applications postmarked after August 15 will be accepted.

Fees are subject to change as directed by the Board.

Reconsideration and Appeals

The Board has adopted a policy with regard to reconsideration and appeals of decisions adverse to applicants. A request for reconsideration, which is the first step, must be made in writing and received by the Board office within 60 days of the date of notice from the Board of the action in question. A copy of the Reconsideration and Appeals Policy may be obtained from the Board office upon request.

Certification

A candidate who has met all the requirements and successfully completed the examinations of the ABCRS will be issued a certificate attesting to his/her qualifications in colon and rectal surgery. The certificate shall be signed by the president or vice president and the secretary and shall bear the corporate seal of the Board.

The certificate granted by the Board does not confer privilege or license to practice colon and rectal surgery but is evidence that a physician's qualifications for specialty practice are recognized by his/her peers. It is not intended to define the requirements for membership on hospital staffs, to gain special recognition or privileges for its diplomates, to define the scope of specialty practice, or to state who may or may not engage in the practice of the specialty.

Unless the candidate specifies otherwise, the Board forwards the names of candidates who have achieved certification to the American Board of Medical Specialties (ABMS) for publication in the *Official ABMS Directory of Board Certified Medical Specialists,* published jointly by the ABMS and Marquis Who's Who.

Time-Limited Certification

Beginning with those candidates who passed the certifying examination in 1990 and thereafter, the ABCRS will issue time-limited certificates. Certificates will be valid for 8 years from the date of certification, after which the certificates will no longer be valid. (*Note*: Time-limited certification will not affect diplomates holding certificates issued prior to 1990.)

Recertification

The ABCRS offers recertification in the specialty. Certificates can be renewed prior to expiration by fulfilling the requirements for recertification specified by the Board. The recertification examination is offered annually, on a voluntary basis, to all certified colon and rectal surgeons who apply and meet the Board's requirements. A recertification information booklet, which outlines the requirements and procedures, is available by writing to the Board office.

Revocation of Certificates

The filing of an application for examination, participating in examination, and accepting a certificate are voluntary acts. Therefore, the Board assumes no responsibility for any effect that certification or failure to obtain certification may have on the private or professional activities of candidates.

When an application is submitted, candidates are required to sign an agreement, a portion of which reads as follows: "I agree to disqualification from examination or from the issuance of a certificate, and I agree to the forfeiture and redelivery of such certificate in the event that any of the statements herein made by me at this time or at any time in the past or future in regard to my application for a certificate are false or in the event that any of the rules and regulations of the Board governing such examinations and certificate are violated by me."

Certificates that have been issued are subject to the provisions of the Articles of Incorporation and the Constitution and Bylaws of the American Board of Colon and Rectal Surgery, Inc, and may be revoked for violation of any of these provisions.

Examination of Candidates With Disabilities

The ABCRS supports the intent of the Americans with Disabilities Act. The Board will make a reasonable effort to provide Board applicants who have documented disabilities with modifications in its examination process that are appropriate for such disabilities but that do not alter the measurement of the skills or knowledge that the examination process is intended to test.

American Board of Dermatology

Henry Ford Hospital
1 Ford Place
Detroit, MI 48202-3450
313 874-1088
313 872-3221 Fax

(These criteria and conditions are subject to change without notice. All applicants are advised to contact the American Board of Dermatology [ABD] to ascertain whether the information below is current.)

Requirements for Eligibility to Take the Examination

Each applicant must satisfy the following requirements before he/she is eligible to take the certifying examination of the Board.

General Qualifications

1. The candidate must have graduated from a medical school in the United States accredited by the Liaison Committee for Medical Education (LCME), an accredited medical school in Canada, or an accredited osteopathic school in the United States; if a graduate of a foreign medical school, the candidate must possess the standard certificate of the Educational Commission for Foreign Medical Graduates (ECFMG). If, however, the foreign medical school graduate is in training in an accredited program in Canada, the Board will recognize the certificate of the Medical Council of Canada.
2. The candidate must hold a currently valid, full, and unrestricted license to practice medicine or osteopathy in either the United States or Canada.

Residency Training Requirements

1. Candidates for certification by the ABD are required to have a total of 4 years of postgraduate training, as described below in Sections (a) and (b).
   a. The first year must consist of clinical training in one of the following types of broad-based programs in the United States accredited by the Accreditation Council for Graduate Medical Education (ACGME) or a similar program in Canada accredited by the Royal College of Physicians and Surgeons of Canada (RCPSC): transitional year (formerly called flexible first postgraduate year) or a first-year residency in internal medicine, general surgery, family practice, obstetrics and gynecology, pediatrics, or emergency medicine.

b. Three years of full-time training as a resident in a dermatology residency training program in the United States accredited by the ACGME or 3 years of full-time training as a resident in a dermatology residency training program in Canada accredited by the RCPSC. Accreditation of dermatology training programs in the United States is the responsibility of the Residency Review Committee (RRC) for Dermatology acting with authority delegated to it by the ACGME (accredited dermatology residency training programs and clinical programs for first post-graduate year credit are listed in this directory.

At least 75% of the resident's time throughout each year of dermatology residency training must be related to the direct care of dermatologic outpatients and inpatients; this includes clinical conferences directly related to patient care, consultations, and inpatient rounds.

Dermatopathology, microbiology, and other basic science lectures, seminars, and conferences are essential components of the resident's training (see the Program Requirements for Residency Education in Dermatology).

The Board also emphasizes the importance of basic and clinical investigation in the educational experience of trainees. Accordingly, all residents should participate in basic and/or clinical research during their training.

For those candidates whose career plans involve a primary commitment to investigative or academic dermatology, a special training track, which must assure adequate clinical education and experience in accordance with the general requirements described above, may also be acceptable. The first year (PGY2) of this track must be at least 75% clinical in character. Investigative or academic experience can be integrated with the required additional clinical training during the second (PGY3) and/or third (PGY4) year(s). Requests for approval of this special track must be submitted *prospectively*, at least 4 months prior to the beginning of such training. This will be on or before March 1 of the PGY2 year for a special track beginning on July 1 of the PGY3 year, or later if special track training is to begin later. Requests earlier than February 1 of the PGY2 year will not be considered because the program director must have had an opportunity to judge the clinical potential of the trainee. The request for consideration of this investigative/academic track must include details of the scheduled program and time commitments during the entire training period of these candidates. It is incumbent upon program directors to select candidates for this special training track whose skills and learning capabilities permit the acquisition of clinical competence as well as the execution of their investigative or academic responsibilities. Moreover, the program director must monitor the training of these residents throughout their residency and must validate their clinical experience at the completion of their residencies.

2. A preliminary registration form must be filed by the candidate and signed by his/her training director shortly after the resident begins residency training in dermatology (ie, by August 1 or within 30 days of the start of training).
3. It is mandatory that the training director submit a yearly report form for each resident to the Board office by August 1 after completion of the first and second year of training and by May 15 for residents who will complete their third year of training on June 30. In order for a candidate to take the certifying examination, the training director must certify that each year of training was completed in a satisfactory manner.
4. Training must be completed within 5 years after the beginning of dermatology residency, except when military service or other compelling circumstances intervene.
5. It is the responsibility of the residency program director to determine if a resident has satisfactorily completed the required 3 years of dermatology training and is therefore eligible to sit for the certifying examination of the ABD.

Guidelines for Determining Adequacy of Clinical Training

The following guidelines are designed to assist program directors in their determination of the adequacy of the clinical training of residents and to assure satisfaction of the eligibility requirements for certification by the ABD. Of special concern are those residents on the special investigative/academic track or those residents whose training experience differs from the standard 36 months of full-time clinical training, as approved for each program by the RRC of the ACGME:

a. In general, high priority should be given to completing 36 continuous months of full-time dermatology training. For most residents, this will consist of full-time clinical training; for residents with a primary commitment to investigative or academic dermatology, this may be a special training track, as defined previously.
b. Any departure from (a), as required, for example, for a medical leave of absence, should be documented and fully justified in the resident evaluation forms filed annually with the Board by the training program director.
c. An absence exceeding 6 weeks in any 1 academic year or a total of 14 weeks over 3 years, including vacation, should be approved only under truly exceptional circumstances. In addition, any resident approved to sit for the certifying examination despite such an absence should have completed each year of training in an above-average or excellent manner, as recorded on the residency evaluation forms.
d. Any resident who will have been absent more than 6 weeks in 1 year or 14 weeks over 3 years and whose performance has not been uniformly above average or excellent throughout residency training should be required to complete an additional period of training at least equal in length to the total period of absence in excess of routinely provided total vacation time. If the program director anticipates that this additional training will be completed in a satisfactory manner before September 1, the director may approve the resident to sit for the certifying examination in that year, just as if training had been completed by July 1.

Registration for the Examination of the Board

Candidates who have completed the training requirements as outlined above are eligible to apply for examination by the Board. Candidates should request an Application for Certification Form from the office of the executive director of the Board. However, for those candidates who are completing their residency training, application forms will be sent to the program directors for distribution to each candidate. The completed application must be filed with the Board office before May 1 of the year in which the candidate plans to take the examination. Physicians who complete their residency training in dermatology by July 1 of a given year are eligible to apply to take the examination in the fall of that year. Under the special conditions described previously ("Guidelines for Determining Adequacy of Training"), candidates completing additional (make-up) training before September 1 may also be eligible to take the fall certifying examination. It is emphasized that it is the candidate's responsibility to send a completed application form to the Board if he/she plans to take the certifying examination of the Board.

A candidate is not considered an "active" candidate until his/her application has been received and approved by the Board. This approval includes a review of the application and annual evaluation reports from the candidate's training director. After the application is approved, the candidate is required to take the examination within 3 years. Candidates who do not exercise the examination privilege within 3 years of the date they are declared eligible will be required to file a new application and have their eligibility for examination reviewed by the Requirements Committee. If the reapplication is approved by the Board, the candidate is again eligible to take the examination within another 3-year period.

The Board does not use the term "Board eligible" in corresponding with directors of hospitals or others who send inquiries to the Board office. On written request by a candidate, the Board will send the candidate a letter stating his/her status with the Board at any given time.

Board Examination

The certifying examination in dermatology, which is administered over a period of 2 days, includes the following:

1. Comprehensive Multiple-Choice Examination in Dermatology: This is a 3-hour comprehensive examination, and was formerly referred to as the Written or Part I examination. It tests the candidate's knowledge of the basic science and clinical aspects of dermatology, including all the related disciplines. Among the topics included in this part of the examination are clinical dermatology, pediatric dermatology, preventive dermatology, entomology, epidemiology, dermatopathology, cutaneous allergy and immunology, dermatologic surgery, cutaneous oncology, sexually transmitted diseases, internal medicine as it pertains to dermatology, medical ethics, photobiology, and cutaneous microbiology, as well as anatomy, physiology, biochemistry, molecular biology, radiation physics, radiation therapy, physical therapy, pharmacology, genetics, and electron microscopy as related to dermatology. Considerable emphasis is placed on comprehensive knowledge of the literature.
2. Examination in Clinical and Laboratory Dermatology: Projected Kodachrome slides are utilized in this part of the examination. Candidates must answer multiple-choice-type questions about the projected pictorial material, which is drawn from all areas of clinical and laboratory dermatology. Examples of the types of slides used include photographs of patients; diagrams and illustrative drawings and pictures of dermatologic surgical procedures, histopathologic sections, fungal cultures, culture mounts, bacterial cultures, Tzanck preparations, skin scrapings and smears, roentgenograms, histochemical and fluorescent photomicrographs, electron micrographs, darkfield micrographs; and drawings or photographs of organisms, including viruses, rickettsiae, bacteria, and parasites that affect the skin.
3. Examination in Dermatopathology: In this section, candidates are questioned on histopathologic slides that they examine microscopically, utilizing personal or rented microscopes. This section of the examination encompasses the entire spectrum of dermatopathology.

For the purposes of scoring, the Examination in Clinical and Laboratory Dermatology is combined with the Examination in Dermatopathology, and candidates must pass this combined examination (formerly designated the Part II examination) as well as the Comprehensive Multiple Choice Examination in Dermatology (formerly designated the Part I examination) in order to be certified. If a candidate fails either the combined Examination in Clinical and Laboratory Dermatology/Examination in Dermatopathology or the Comprehensive Multiple Choice Examination in Dermatology, only the failed component must be repeated.

The examination is given annually in the fall over a 2-day period and lasts a total of approximately 10 hours. In 1998, it will be held on October 18 and 19 at the Holiday Inn O'Hare in Rosemont, Illinois, which is in the O'Hare International Airport area of Chicago.

Reexamination

With their initial examination application, candidates have a 3-year period during which they may take the examination or any necessary reexamination on either a failed part (see above) or both parts of the examination. For a reexamination, they must notify the Board office by May 1 of the year they plan to retake the examination. A candidate who has not passed or does not take the examination during this 3-year period must reapply and complete the necessary forms, after which he/she will have another 3-year period of eligibility during which to take the examination or reexamination. For further information concerning this as well as the appropriate fees required, the Board office should be contacted.

Candidates With Disabilities

The ABD supports the intent of the Americans with Disabilities Act (ADA) and, therefore, will provide or allow the use of necessary auxiliary aids, services, or testing conditions that do not fundamentally alter the measurement of the skills or knowledge the Board assessment program is intended to test. In order to implement this policy, notification of the need for special testing circumstances must be given to the ABD by a candidate for certification at the time that he/she submits the application for any of the Board's certifying examinations. This deadline is necessary in order to allow the Board to request the necessary documentation, to review the records, and to verify the disability, if necessary. In addition, since this policy also applies to the In-Training Examination, which is under the jurisdiction of the ABD, appropriate advance notification of the need for special testing circumstances must be provided when the application for the In-Training Examination is submitted by the department.

Upon receipt of such request, the ABD will initiate the appropriate procedural steps, but it should be understood that all special arrangements must be made and agreed upon in advance; special arrangements cannot be made at the time the examination is given. Therefore, early notification of the need for special testing circumstances is encouraged.

Chemical Dependency or Substance Abuse

A candidate with a chemical dependency or substance abuse problem will not be permitted to take the examination unless he/she can submit evidence, which must be verifiable, that the disorder is being treated and is under control. Individuals with such problems or a history thereof must provide the necessary documentation at the time of application to take the examination. A confirmatory letter from a licensed physician within 1 month of the examination stating that the disorder no longer exists or is currently controlled is also necessary.

Certification

After meeting the above requirements and passing the examination, the candidate will be awarded a certificate that acknowledges that he/she has completed the required course of graduate study and clinical training, has met other specific standards and qualifications, and has passed the examination conducted by the Board. The candidate is then referred to as a diplomate of the American Board of Dermatology, Inc. The names of diplomates of the Board appear in *The Official ABMS Directory of Board Certified Medical Specialists,* published by Marquis Who's Who in cooperation with the American Board of Medical Specialties (ABMS).

Each certificate is subject to revocation in the event that (a) the physician so certified shall not have been eligible to receive such certificate, whether or not the facts concerning his/her ineligibility were known or could have been ascertained by the directors of the Board at the time of the issuance of the certificate; (b) the physician so certified shall have made any material misrepresentation or omission in the application for such certificate or in any other statement to the Board or its representatives; (c) the physician so certified shall have been convicted by a court of competent jurisdiction, or pleads nolo contendere to said crime, which in the judgment of the Board is related to or arises out of the practice of medicine.

Appeals Procedure

The ABD recognizes a candidate's right of appeal following an adverse action at any stage of the certification process. Within the residency program, trainees must be accorded due process in compliance with provisions established by the parent institution and as stipulated in the Essentials of Accredited Residencies in Graduate Medical Education (July 1, 1982) of the ACGME.

Candidates whom the Board has declared ineligible to sit for the certifying examination on the basis of qualifications may appeal such decisions by written request within 90 days of the date of notification of the Board's ruling.

A candidate failing a certifying examination may request in writing that his/her examination be rescored by hand to verify the accuracy of the results as reported. Such requests must be received in the Board office within 30 days of the date of mailing of the examination results to the candidates. A check in the amount of $35 payable to the American Board of Dermatology must accompany this written request. There shall be no further appeal from failure of an examination.

Recertification

The Board began issuing time-limited certificates, valid for 10 years, in 1991, and its process of voluntary recertification was approved by the ABMS in 1994. The first recertification examination, which will be a clinically focused, take-home, open-book examination tailored to the candidate's practice profile, will be administered in 1999 and biennially thereafter. There is no limit on the number of times diplomates may undertake the recertification process. If the candidate does not successfully complete the recertification process prior to expiration of his/her time-limited certificate, he/she will remain eligible to participate in the recertification process but will cease to be Board certified until the process is successfully completed and a new time-limited certificate is issued. If the candidate successfully completes the recertification process before expiration of his/her certificate, eg, in year 8 or 9 of the 10 years, the new certificate will be issued for 10 years commencing on the expiration date of the prior certificate.

Diplomates with lifetime certification may elect to pursue voluntary recertification in any given year after the process has been implemented. Any questions or correspondence relating to the recertification process should be directed to the executive director of the ABD.

It is to be noted that at this time a recertification process has not been approved for Special Qualifications in Dermatopathology or Clinical and Laboratory Dermatological Immunology.

Fees for Examination and Reexamination

The directors of the Board serve without compensation. Fees are based on the actual expenses incurred in administration of the Board office and related activities and on the costs of development and administration of the Board examinations.

All fees are payable when the application for an examination is submitted and are applied to the first examination of that type given after approval of the application. Except as indicated below, or because of verifiable extenuating circumstances, there will be no refunds of any of these fees. Contact the Board office for the current fee schedule.

All checks are to be made payable to The American Board of Dermatology, Inc.

When a candidate's application for the Certifying Examination in Dermatology or a Special Qualification Examination is disapproved, the Board retains an administrative fee of $100 and will refund the balance to the candidate.

Candidates who fail the certifying examination in Dermatology retain the right to *apply* to retake the examination in subsequent years. For further information concerning Board policy in effect and for the applicable examination fee, candidates are advised to write or call the Board office (313 874-1088). Candidates who *do not take* the certifying examination at the first opportunity after completion of their training are also advised to contact the Board office for clarification of Board policy and the examination fee if they intend to apply to take the certifying examination in any given year.

Publication

The ABD publishes a booklet of information, which may be obtained from the Board office.

All correspondence should be sent to

Harry J Hurley, MD
Executive Director
The American Board of Dermatology, Inc
Henry Ford Hospital
1 Ford Place
Detroit, MI 48202-3450

Certification for Special Qualification in Dermatopathology

Special Qualification certification in Dermatopathology is a joint and equal function of the ABD and the American Board of Pathology (ABP). Such function will relate to qualifications of candidates, standards of examination, and the form of the certificate.

All candidates applying to sit for this certifying examination must hold a currently valid, full, and unrestricted license to practice medicine or osteopathy in either the United States or Canada.

All candidates for this certification must satisfy the following requirements:

Prerequisites

1. Primary certification by both the ABD and the ABP (anatomic pathology or anatomic and clinical pathology).
2. Primary certification by either the ABD or the ABP (anatomic pathology or anatomic and clinical pathology) and the satisfactory completion of 1 year of training in dermatopathology in a program accredited for such training (see below) by the ACGME. This additional training must be taken after the candidate has met the full training requirements for certification in dermatology or pathology. The dermatologist applicant must spend one-half of the required training time in pathology. The pathologist applicant must spend one-half of the required training time in clinical dermatology.

Training

Accredited institutional training programs in dermatopathology are an equal and joint function of the departments of dermatology and pathology of that institution. Training programs in dermatopathology are reviewed and accredited by the Residency Review Subcommittee for Dermatopathology, which includes three members from the RRC for Dermatology and three members from the RRC for Pathology. Upon recommendation by this subcommittee, training programs in dermatopathology are accredited by conjoint action of the RRCs for Dermatology and Pathology acting with authority delegated by the ACGME. Information concerning accredited dermatopathology training programs may be found in this directory.

Examination: Deadline for Application and Date of Examination

Candidates who have satisfied the above requirements are eligible to apply to the Board to take the examination for Special Qualification in Dermatopathology, which is a comprehensive assessment of the candidates' knowledge of dermatopathology, including the related basic sciences, and laboratory and clinical areas pertaining to this discipline.

Candidates planning to take the Special Qualification examination should request an application from the office of the executive director of the ABD. The deadline for receipt of applications is July 1 of the year in which the candidate plans to take the examination. The date of the next examination has not been determined at this time.

Certification for Special Qualification in Clinical and Laboratory Dermatological Immunology (CLDI)

Prerequisites

The requirements for Special Qualification certification in CLDI are as follows:

1. A currently valid, full, and unrestricted license to practice medicine or osteopathy in either the United States or Canada.
2. Primary certification by the ABD and the satisfactory completion of at least 1 year of training in an accredited fellowship in CLDI. This additional training must be taken after the candidate has met the full training requirements for certification in dermatology.

Training

Information concerning accredited training programs in CLDI is available from the office of the ABD. As stated above, a minimum of 1 year of full-time training in a CLDI training program is required of all candidates.

Examination: Deadline for Application and Date of Examination

Candidates who have satisfied the above requirements are eligible to apply to the Board to take the Special Qualification Examination in CLDI. The deadline for receipt of applications to take the examination for Special Qualification in CLDI is April 1 of the year in which the examination is given. The date of the next examination has not been determined at this time.

American Board of Emergency Medicine

3000 Coolidge Rd
East Lansing, MI 48823-6319
517 332-4800
517 332-2234 Fax
Internet: http://www.abem.org

(These criteria and conditions are subject to change without notice. All applicants are advised to contact the American Board of Emergency Medicine [ABEM] to ascertain whether the information below is current.)

Requirements for Certification in Emergency Medicine

An applicant must satisfy all credential requirements at the time the application is submitted. Requirements fulfilled after the date of application will not be considered.

The applicant must have graduated from medical school.

1. Graduates of approved schools of osteopathic medicine in the United States are considered when they have satisfactorily met the credential requirements as outlined.
2. An applicant graduating from a medical school other than one in the United States, its territories, or Canada must provide the Board with a verified and translated diploma.

Throughout the certification process, applicants and candidates practicing medicine in the United States, its territories, or Canada must hold a current, valid, unrestricted, and unqualified license to practice medicine in the jurisdiction(s) in which they practice. A physician who is not currently practicing medicine or is practicing medicine outside the United States, its territories, or Canada must hold a current, valid, unrestricted, and unqualified license to practice medicine in at least one jurisdiction in the United States, its territories, or Canada.

The applicant must have successfully completed a total of 36 months of postmedical school training, under the control of an accredited emergency medicine residency program. Emergency medicine programs must be accredited by the Accreditation Council for Graduate Medical Education (ACGME) or the Royal College of Physicians and Surgeons of Canada for Canadian programs.

If the emergency medicine residency training program is structured so that it exceeds the length of training specified above, the resident must successfully complete the requirements of his/her residency program to apply under the emergency medicine residency category of application.

(*Note*: For residents who began their emergency medicine training prior to July 1, 1987, the candidate must have successfully completed a total of 36 months of postmedical school training, at least 24 months of which were under the control of an accredited emergency medicine residency program at the PGY2 level and above.)

The applicant must submit evidence of 50 hours of continuing medical education in emergency medicine annually, acceptable to the Board, starting 1 year from the date of graduation from the emergency medicine residency program and continuing until the date of application. If a resident applies to the Board within 1 year of graduation, no continuing medical education is required.

Combined Training Programs

A special agreement exists between the ABEM and the American Board of Pediatrics whereby an applicant may fulfill the training requirements of both Boards by completing joint training in 5 years. Training programs must be approved prospectively by both Boards. Guidelines for combined training have been approved by both Boards and are available by writing either Board office. Applicants may not appear for the certifying examination until all training has been satisfactorily completed.

A special agreement exists between the ABEM and the American Board of Internal Medicine whereby an applicant may fulfill the training requirements of both Boards by completing joint training in 5 years. Training programs must be approved prospectively by both Boards. Guidelines for combined training have been approved by both Boards and are available by writing to either Board office. Applicants may not appear for the certifying examination until all training has been satisfactorily completed.

Applications

Applications are distributed in the spring of each year (mid April) and are available from the Board office. Applications are accepted from April 15 through July 31 of each year. A mailing list is maintained throughout the year for requests received during times when applications are not available.

A nonrefundable processing fee must accompany the application at the time it is submitted.

Applicants wishing to be considered for examination must submit a fully completed application form to the Board. The Board will not be responsible for any opinion expressed concerning the individual's credentials for the examination unless it is in writing and over the signature of the president or secretary of the Board.

Examination Information

The certification examination in emergency medicine is composed of two parts, a written examination and an oral examination.

The written certification examination is a 6.5-hour comprehensive examination that is administered once a year. It includes approximately 335 single-best-answer, multiple-choice test items. Approximately 10% to 15% of the items have a pictorial stimulus.

The oral certification examination is administered twice a year. It includes five simulated patient encounters, each involving one patient, and two simulated situation encounters, each involving more than one patient.

A candidate must successfully complete the fall written examination to be scheduled for either the spring or fall oral examination the following year.

Examination fees are due upon assignment to an examination administration.

Certification

All candidates who successfully complete both the written and the oral certification examinations shall be known as diplomates of the ABEM. Diplomates receive an appropriate certificate, which shall remain the property of ABEM. Certification is for a period of 10 years.

Any certificate issued by the Board shall be subject to revocation at any time, should the Board determine, in its sole judgment, that a candidate who has received a certificate was in some respect not properly qualified to receive or retain it.

Recertification

To achieve recertification, successful completion of one of the following three examinations is required: the written or oral certification examination or the written recertification examination. In order to maintain diplomate status without lapse, diplomates must successfully complete an examination prior to the expiration of their certificate. If a diplomate does not take a recertification examination within 3 years of the expiration of the certificate, the certification examination (both the written and the oral portions) must be successfully completed to regain diplomate status. Recertification is for a period of 10 years.

American Board of Family Practice

2228 Young Dr
Lexington, KY 40505-4294
606 269-5626
888 995-5700 (toll-free)
E-mail: general@abfp.org
Internet: http://www.abfp.org

(These criteria and conditions are subject to change without notice. All applicants are advised to contact the American Board of Family Practice [ABFP] to ascertain whether the information below is current.)

ABFP Official Definition of Family Practice

"Family practice is the medical specialty which is concerned with the total health care of the individual and the family. It is the specialty in breadth which integrates the biological, clinical, and behavioral sciences. The scope of family practice is not limited by age, sex, organ system, or disease entity."

Board Eligibility

The ABFP does not recognize or use the term "Board eligible" and does not issue statements concerning "Board eligibility." The Board informs an applicant of admissibility to an examination to be given on a specified date after a formal application has been reviewed and approved.

Certification Process

The ABFP administers the certification and recertification examinations in various centers throughout the United States annually, on the second Friday in July.

The ABFP certification and recertification examinations are written tests of cognitive knowledge and problem-solving abilities relevant to family practice. Appropriate subject areas of the following disciplines are included: internal medicine, pediatrics, surgery, obstetrics, gynecology, psychiatry and behavioral sciences, community medicine, and geriatrics. Elements of the examination include but are not limited to diagnosis, management, and prevention of disease.

General Requirements for Certification

All candidates for the ABFP certification examination must have satisfactorily completed 3 years of training (a full 36 calendar months with 12 months in each of the GY1, GY2, and GY3 years) in a family practice residency program accredited by the Accreditation Council for Graduate Medical Education (ACGME) subsequent to receipt of the MD or DO degree from an accredited institution and, when applicable, a Fifth Pathway year, or receipt of a standard certificate from the Educational Commission for Foreign Medical Graduates, or compliance with other ACGME requirements for entry into graduate medical training in the United States. If a physician does not meet the eligibility requirements of the ACGME for entry into resident training, his/her training will not be recognized by the Board.

Candidates who obtained their MD degree from medical schools in the United States or Canada must have attended a school accredited by the Liaison Committee on Medical Education or the Committee for Accreditation of Canadian Medical Schools. Candidates who obtained a DO degree must have graduated from a college of osteopathic medicine accredited by the American Osteopathic Association (AOA).

The Board prefers all 3 years of postgraduate training to be in the same ACGME-accredited family practice program; however, other training may be considered as equivalent (eg, flexible/transitional year, AOA osteopathic internship). In these cases, and for physicians who have had international training, each individual's training will be evaluated by the Board. Internationally trained physicians must provide all of the required documentation of education and training to receive any credit toward certification for prior training. The ABFP requires residency programs to submit prospective requests for advanced placement of residents. Program directors are responsible for notifying the Board prior to the entry of the transferring resident. If a program director fails to comply, the Board will determine the amount of transfer credit at the time of its discovery of the transfer. Consequently, the resident may receive less credit toward certification than anticipated and may be required to extend the duration of training.

The last 2 years of family practice residency training must be completed in the same accredited program. Transfers after the beginning of the GY2 year are approved only in extraordinary circumstances.

Verification of satisfactory completion of residency training must be stated in writing by the program director. All applicants for the certification examination are subject to the approval of the Board, and the final decision regarding any application rests solely with the ABFP.

All candidates' education and training experiences are subject to review and approval by the ABFP. Any variance from the above must have prior written approval of the Board. No credit may be given for any previous training as equivalent to family practice training without the written approval of the Board.

Candidates must complete all requirements of the Board no later than June 30 of the year of the examination. Complete documentation from the program director that the resident has or is expected to have satisfactorily completed the residency must be received by the Board by June 30. Applications, supplied to the residents directly through the program director, are made available only to residents expected to complete the required training by June 30 of the current year. Residents who complete their training at an interim date must write to the Board for an application.

All candidates must hold a currently valid, full, and unrestricted license to practice medicine in the United States or Canada. Furthermore, every license to practice medicine held by the candidate in any state or territory of the United States or province of Canada must be currently valid, full, and unrestricted, whether or not the candidate in effect practices in such state, territory, or province. Candidates shall be required to maintain a full and unrestricted medical license in the United States or Canada even if they are out of the country for extended periods of time.

Any candidate whose license to practice medicine has been revoked, suspended, or restricted in any state or territory of the United States or province of Canada shall be ineligible for certification until such time as the encumbered license is reinstated in full. Should a license be revoked, suspended, or restricted following the submission of an application for certification but prior to the notification of examination results, the application and certification will be simultaneously invalidated.

It is the responsibility of the candidate to inform the Board immediately upon a change in licensure status. If the candidate fails to notify the Board of any suspension, revocation, restriction, or probation within 60 days after the effective date, the candidate shall be ineligible to seek certification for up to 1 year following the reinstatement of full and unrestricted licensure. A restricted medical license is any adverse action by a state licensing agency that encumbers the ability of a physician to diagnose, manage, and/or treat patients. An action by a state licensing agency that is taken against a canceled or inactive license is *not* considered a violation of ABFP policy. An action by a state licensing agency that limits the practice of medicine to the specialty of family medicine may not necessarily be considered a violation of ABFP policy. However, any action by a state licensing agency that restricts a physician from prescribing medications to the physician's immediate family *is* considered a violation of ABFP policy and will be enforced accordingly. In cases where a physician has changed the physician's residence deliberately to avoid prosecution, loss of license, or disciplinary action by a state licensing agency, the Board reserves the right to revoke or suspend diplomate status, and/or prohibit application for certification.

An opportunity for certification will be denied to any physician otherwise eligible who has been involved in the fraudulent misrepresentation of certification by the ABFP. Eligibility to make application for certification will be denied to the offending party for a period not to exceed 6 years from the date of discovery of the offense. In the event the individual appeals or otherwise challenges the declaration of ineligibility, the 6-year period shall be tolled until the action of the Board is determined to be final and enforceable. Questions about licensure should be presented to the Board in writing.

No candidate will be allowed to take the examination until all fees are paid and all of the above requirements have been satisfactorily met.

Candidates who apply for the Certification Examination within 3 years of completion of an ACGME-accredited family practice residency are not required to document any continuing medical education (CME). Candidates who apply after the 3-year period must provide documentation of 50 hours of CME for each subsequent year. Residents completing training on or before June 30 receive an application through their residency program. Physicians completing training after June 30 must request an application directly from the Board.

Osteopathic Physicians

Physicians who have graduated from an AOA-approved school of osteopathic medicine in the United States may qualify for certification if they meet all the same requirements as specified for allopathic medical school graduates. They may apply to ACGME-accredited family practice programs for entry into the first year (GY1). Osteopathic physicians who have documented satisfactory completion of an AOA-approved internship (GY1) year may receive credit for the portion of the GY1 year that meets the ABFP guidelines for advanced-level entry or interprogram transfers.

All candidates (MD or DO) must satisfactorily complete at least 36 calendar months of accredited graduate medical education. Only the GY1 year may be fulfilled by an AOA-approved internship year. Training beyond the GY1 year must be in continuity in an ACGME-accredited family practice residency program.

Reciprocity Agreements

The ABFP has developed reciprocity agreements with the College of Family Physicians of Canada (CFPC), the Royal College of General Practitioners of Great Britain, the Royal New Zealand College of General Practitioners, and the Royal Australian College of General Practitioners. Diplomates of the ABFP may be eligible to seek certification by these colleges, and members in good standing of these colleges who meet all of the other requirements of the ABFP and reside in the United States may be eligible to take the certification examination. Eligibility to sit for the ABFP certification examination through reciprocity will be available only to physicians who have satisfactorily completed formal training in family practice accredited by a nationally recognized accrediting organization within the country in which they are certified.

Canadian Applicants

1. Physicians who have satisfactorily completed 2 years of training in a program accredited by the CFPC must have a third year of accredited family practice residency. The third year of training must be satisfactorily completed in an ACGME-accredited family practice program or, if taken in Canada, must be approved by the CFPC and must have prior approval of the ABFP. The third year must bring the total experience into compliance with the ACGME's Program Requirements for Residency Education in Family Practice. The request must be accompanied by documentation of satisfactory performance of the first 2 years of training (including a description of the curriculum) signed by the program director.
2. Physicians who have passed the CFPC Certification Examination in Family Medicine and who (a) are members in good standing of the CFPC, (b) have completed family practice training accredited by the CFPC, (c) have been residents of the United States for at least 6 months, (d) hold a valid and unrestricted license to practice medicine in the United States, and, (e) are actively involved in family practice in the United States may apply to sit for the ABFP certification examination.

Registrants of the Royal College of General Practitioners of Great Britain

Physicians who have been certified by the Royal College of General Practitioners by examination may be permitted to apply for certification by the ABFP if they (1) are members in good standing of the Royal College of General Practitioners, (2) possess a certificate of prescribed/equivalent experience issued by the Joint Committee on Postgraduate Training for General Practice, (3) reside in the United States, (4) hold a valid and unrestricted license to practice medicine in the United States, and (5) are actively involved in family practice in the United States.

Members of the Royal New Zealand College of General Practitioners

Physicians who are members of the Royal New Zealand College of General Practitioners may be permitted to apply for examination for certification by the ABFP if they (1) are members in good standing of the Royal New Zealand College of General Practitioners, (2) have completed the General Practice Training Programme (GPTP), (3) reside in the United States, (4) hold a valid and unrestricted license to practice medicine in the United States, and (5) are actively involved in family practice in the United States.

Fellows of the Royal Australian College of General Practitioners

Physicians who are fellows of the Royal Australian College of General Practitioners may be permitted to apply for examination for certification by the ABFP if they (1) are members in good standing of the Royal Australian College of General Practitioners, (2) have completed the GPTP, (3) reside in the United States, (4) hold a valid and unrestricted license to practice medicine in the United States, and (5) are actively involved in family practice in the United States.

Recertification Process

The ABFP confers diplomate status for the specified period of time noted on the certificate, which is dated for a 7-year period. In order to maintain diplomate status, the diplomate must be recertified before the certificate expires. Although the certificate is dated for 7 years, the Board routinely administers the recertification process on a 6-year cycle. This allows a "reserve" year for those diplomates who for some reason are unable to participate in the sixth year or in cases where the diplomate fails to receive a satisfactory score in the sixth year.

Should a diplomate not be recertified by the end of the seventh year, the certificate will expire and the physician will lose diplomate status. However, the physician may reapply for the recertification process, but he/she must meet all criteria in effect at that time.

For diplomates who participate in the recertification process during the sixth year and pass, the new certificate of 7 years' duration is dated from the time of that examination.

Requirements for Recertification

A. Submission of a formal application.
B. Documentation of 300 hours of approvable continuing medical education.
C. Submission of statement of acknowledgment and compliance with Board policy regarding medical licensure.
D. Satisfactory completion of the office record review portion of the recertification process.
E. Satisfactory performance on the written test of cognitive knowledge.

Diplomates will be given advance notice of any changes in the recertification requirements.

Reexamination

Candidates who fail the examination may apply for admission to the next annual examination. There is no limit to the number of times a qualified candidate may take the examination when it is offered, provided the qualifications are met with each reapplication. In addition to valid and unrestricted licensure status, 50 hours per year of CME since the last application are required for reexamination. Full fees are charged for each examination.

Certificates of Added Qualifications

Geriatric Medicine

The ABFP and the American Board of Internal Medicine in a joint venture offer a Certificate of Added Qualifications (CAQ) in Geriatric Medicine. The "added certificate" is designed to recognize excellence among those diplomates who provide care to the elderly. The Geriatric Medicine Examinations will be given annually beginning November 1998. Announcements will be made in the *Journal of the American Board of Family Practice* concerning exact dates and the application process.

Certification Requirements

1. Family physicians must be certified by the ABFP and must be diplomates in good standing at the time of the examination.
2. The diplomate must hold a currently valid, full, and unrestricted license to practice medicine in the United States or Canada.
3. Diplomates may qualify by satisfactory completion of an ACGME-accredited fellowship training program in geriatric medicine.
4. Diplomates must achieve a satisfactory score on a 1-day written examination.

Recertification Requirements

The recertification process for the geriatric medicine certificate is completed over a 2-year period and may begin in the eighth year of the 10-year certificate and includes the following requirements.

1. Current primary certification in family practice at the time of the examination.
2. Completion of a geriatric medicine recertification preapplication form and submission of a self-evaluation fee.
3. Successful completion of three Self-Evaluation Process (SEP) modules (*see explanation below*).
4. Completion of a formal geriatric medicine examination application form and submission of an examination fee.
5. Verification that all licenses held in the United States and Canada are currently valid, full, and unrestricted.
6. Successful completion of a half-day written examination.

The SEP modules are at-home, open book examinations of 60 questions each. All candidates must successfully complete three modules to be eligible to sit for the examination. The SEP modules will be scored and incorrect answers will be identified. No references to the literature will be given with the score report. Should a candidate be unsuccessful on any of the SEP modules, the candidate will be required to repeat the particular module until successful.

Sports Medicine

The ABFP offers certification in sports medicine. The CAQ in Sports Medicine is offered biennially in odd-numbered years in conjunction with the American Board of Emergency Medicine, the American Board of Internal Medicine, and the American Board of Pediatrics.

Certification Requirements

1. Family physicians must be certified by the ABFP and must be diplomates in good standing at the time of the examination.
2. The diplomate must hold a currently valid, full, and unrestricted license to practice medicine in the United States or Canada.
3. Family physicians must qualify through one of the following:
   a. Fellowship Pathway*: A candidate must have satisfactorily completed, or will have completed by June 30 of the examination year, a minimum of 1 year in a sports medicine fellowship program associated with an ACGME-accredited residency in emergency medicine, family practice, internal medicine, or pediatrics. (If the sports medicine program is not currently accredited by the ACGME, or has not previously provided candidates for examination, the program director should seek prior ABFP approval of the curriculum to be completed.)

   ** Effective July 1, 1998, family practice sports medicine fellowship training must be accredited by the ACGME to be used toward training requirements for admission to the examination.*

   b. Practice Pathway**: A candidate must have 5 years of practice experience (exclusive of residency or fellowship training) consisting of at least 20% professional time devoted to sports medicine defined as one or more of the following: (1) field supervision of athletes; (2) emergency assessment and care of acutely injured athletes; (3) diagnosis, treatment, management, and disposition of common sports injuries and illness; (4) management of medical problems in the athlete; (5) rehabilitation of ill and injured athletes; and (6) exercise as treatment. In addition, a candidate must show evidence of participation in 30 hours of sports medicine-related American Medical Association Category 1 (or its equivalent) CME during the past 5 years.

*** Plan II will be available through the 1999 examination. After 1999, diplomates may qualify only via the Fellowship Pathway.*

4. Diplomates must achieve a satisfactory score on a half-day written examination.

Recognition of Successful Candidates

Successful CAQ candidates will be awarded the ABFP Certificate of Added Qualifications. The certificate will be valid for 10 years at which time recertification is required for renewal of the certificate.

If for any reason *primary* certification in family practice is lost (eg, expired, revoked, etc) the CAQ will be simultaneously withdrawn. With restoration of the primary certificate, the CAQ will be reinstated for the remaining period of time, if any, on the CAQ certificate.

Questions or comments about the CAQ in geriatrics or sports medicine may be addressed to ABFP staff at 888 995-5700, extension 264.

Revocation

General

Each certificate issued by the Board of Directors of the ABFP shall be subject to revocation in any of the following circumstances:

1. The issuance of such certificate or its receipt by the person so certified shall have been contrary to, or in violation of, any provision of the Articles of Incorporation of the ABFP, Inc, or of the Bylaws of the ABFP.
2. The person so certified shall not have been eligible to receive such certificate, irrespective of whether the facts constituting such ineligibility were known to, or could have been ascertained by, the directors of the corporation or its representatives.
3. The person so certified shall have made a misstatement of fact in the application for such certificate or in any other statement or representation to the corporation or its representatives.
4. The person so certified shall at any time have neglected to maintain the degree of competency in the field of family practice as established by the Board.
5. The person so certified has fraudulently altered, copied, or changed a certificate of the ABFP, or has fraudulently presented, or allowed to be presented on behalf of the individual, an altered, copied, or changed certificate of the Board. In such cases, the Board reserves the right to revoke, suspend, and/or prohibit subsequent certification of the offending party for a period not to exceed 6 years from the date of discovery of the offense. In the event the individual appeals or otherwise challenges the suspension, the 6-year period shall be tolled until the action of the Board is determined to be final and enforceable.

Licensure Status

A diplomate of the ABFP shall be required to hold a currently valid, full, and unrestricted license to practice medicine in the United States or Canada. Furthermore, every license to practice medicine held by a diplomate in any state or territory of the United States or province of Canada must be currently valid, full, and unrestricted, whether or not the diplomate in effect practices in such state, territory, or province. Diplomates shall be required to retain a full and unrestricted medical license in the United States or Canada even if they are out of the country for extended periods of time. Failure to retain a license will result in loss of diplomate status and will result in loss of the ability to make application for certification, recertification, or other examinations offered by the Board.

In the event a diplomate's license to practice in *any* state or territory of the United States or province of Canada is revoked, restricted, or suspended, the diplomate's certificate is simultaneously rescinded at the time of the licensure revocation, restriction, or suspension. The physician must advise the ABFP within 60 days and cease immediately identifying himself/herself in any way directly or indirectly as a diplomate of the ABFP. If the physician fails to notify the ABFP of any revocation, restriction, or suspension within 60 days after the effective date, he/she shall be ineligible to seek reinstatement of diplomate status for up to 1 year following the reinstatement of full and unrestricted licensure.

A restricted medical license is any adverse action by a state licensing agency that encumbers the ability of a physician to diagnose, manage, and/or treat patients. An action by a state licensing agency that is taken against a canceled or inactive license is *not* considered a violation of ABFP policy. An action by a state licensing agency that limits the practice of medicine to the specialty of family medicine may not necessarily be considered a violation of ABFP policy. However, any action by a state licensing agency that restricts a physician from prescribing medications to the physician's immediate family *is* considered a violation of ABFP policy and will be enforced accordingly. In cases where a physician has changed the physician's residence deliberately to avoid prosecution, loss of license, or disciplinary action by a state licensing agency, the Board reserves the right to revoke or suspend diplomate status and/or prohibit application for certification. Questions about licensure should be presented to the Board in writing.

If and when the physician's revoked, restricted, or suspended license is reinstated in full (with no restrictions) and official written documentation of reinstatement is provided, the ABFP will honor the remainder of the current certificate and the diplomate will not be required to be reexamined. If the current certificate has expired prior to the reinstatement of the license, the physician may make application for the next annual examination. Successful compliance with all application requirements in effect at that time will be expected.

Authority

The Board of Directors of the ABFP shall have sole power and authority to determine whether or not the evidence or information before it is sufficient to constitute grounds for revocation of any certificate issued by this Corporation. The Board of Directors may, however, at its discretion, require any person so certified to appear before the Board of Directors, upon not less than 30 days' written notice by registered mail, and to show cause, at the time and place specified in such notice, why the certificate should not be revoked. The failure of any person so notified to appear as required in such notice shall, at the discretion of the Board of Directors, constitute cause for revocation of the certificate. The decision of the Board of Directors in all such matters shall be final.

Applications and Additional Information

Applications and additional information may be obtained by writing to

Robert F Avant, MD, Executive Director
American Board of Family Practice
2228 Young Dr
Lexington, KY 40505-4294

American Board of Internal Medicine

510 Walnut St/Ste 1700
Philadelphia, PA 19106-3699
800 441-ABIM (2246)
215 446-3500
215 446-3470 Fax
E-mail: request@abim.org
Internet: http://www.abim.org

(These criteria and conditions are subject to change without notice. All applicants are advised to contact the American Board of Internal Medicine [ABIM] to ascertain whether the information below is current.)

Preface

The Board's decision about a candidate's eligibility for certification is determined by the policies and procedures described in this document. This edition of policies and procedures supersedes all previous publications.

The Board reserves the right to make changes in its fees, examinations, policies, and procedures at any time without advance notice. The Board also reserves the right, under extraordinary circumstances, to waive certain of its requirements. Admission to the Board's examinations will be determined under policies in force at the time of application.

Introduction

The ABIM was established in 1936 and is a private, nonprofit corporation that is not a part of or affiliated with any other organization. Its members are elected by the Board of Directors and serve 2-year terms. The Board receives no public funds and has no licensing authority or function.

The mission of the ABIM is to enhance the quality of health care available to the American public by continuously improving the process and maintaining high standards for certifying internists and subspecialists who possess the knowledge, skills, and attitudes essential for the provision of excellent care.

The Board's core values are: assuring the public of the highest quality patient care; professionalism and excellence in the practice of medicine; science-based medicine and intellectual rigor; leadership in evaluation and standard setting; and maintaining autonomy to preserve these values.

Certification by the ABIM recognizes excellence in the discipline of internal medicine, its subspecialties, and areas of added qualifications. Certification by the Board is not a requirement to practice internal medicine, nor does the Board confer privilege to practice. The Board does not intend either to interfere with or to restrict the professional activities of a licensed physician because the physician is not certified.

The ABIM administers the certification and recertification processes by (1) establishing training requirements, (2) assessing the credentials of candidates, (3) obtaining substantiation by appropriate authorities of the clinical competence and professional standing of candidates, and (4) developing and conducting examinations for certification and recertification.

The duration of the validity of all certificates issued by the Board in 1990 (1987 for critical care medicine and 1988 for geriatric medicine) and thereafter is 10 years, and the dates of validity are noted on the certificates. Certificates issued before these dates will continue to be valid indefinitely. Diplomates with certificates that are valid indefinitely will be offered the same opportunity to recertify as those who hold time-limited certificates.

Information about the Board's recertification program is available on request.

Training Requirements for Certification

Internal Medicine

Physicians who are awarded a certificate in internal medicine must have completed the required predoctoral medical education, met the postdoctoral training requirements, demonstrated clinical competence in the care of patients, and passed the certification examination in internal medicine.

Predoctoral Medical Education

Candidates from medical schools in the United States or Canada must have attended a school accredited at the date of graduation by the Liaison Committee on Medical Education (LCME), the Committee for Accreditation of Canadian Medical Schools, or the American Osteopathic Association.

Graduates of international medical schools are required to submit one of the following:

1. A permanent (valid indefinitely) certificate from the Educational Commission for Foreign Medical Graduates; or
2. Comparable credentials from the Medical Council of Canada; or
3. Documentation of training for candidates who entered postdoctoral medical training in the United States via the Fifth Pathway, as defined by the American Medical Association.

For those entering training prior to June 1999, the following training requirements apply:

Postdoctoral Training Requirements

To be admitted to an examination, physicians must have completed 3 years of accredited training before July 1 of the year of examination. Residency training or research experience occurring before the completion of the requirements for the MD or DO degree cannot be credited toward the Board's training requirements.

The 3 years of required training must satisfy *all* the following conditions:

1. The director of the accredited internal medicine training program must have had responsibility for the educational process during the entire 36 months of training. The program director may assign up to 6 months to training in specialties other than internal medicine.
2. The 36 months of training must have included a minimum of 24 months of meaningful patient responsibility. Of these 24 months, at least 20 must occur in the following settings: (a) inpatient services in which disorders of general internal medicine or its subspecialties are managed; (b) emergency medicine, general medical, or subspecialty ambulatory settings; and (c) dermatology or neurology services. Four months of meaningful patient responsibility may be taken outside the above areas with the approval of the internal medicine program director.
3. The training must be completed in an internal medicine program accredited by the Accreditation Council for Graduate Medical Education (ACGME), the Royal College of Physicians and Surgeons of Canada (RCPSC), or the Professional Corporation of Physicians of Quebec.
4. The level of responsibility for patient care must increase in each year of training.

Training Taken in Accredited Programs Other Than Categorical Internal Medicine

For residents transferring to the first- or second-year level of internal medicine training from other ACGME-accredited residencies, the internal medicine program director may recommend to the Board that credit be granted toward the internal medicine requirements according to the following guidelines:

- For ACGME-accredited programs sponsored by internal medicine, month-for-month up to 12 months for the internal medicine rotations and up to 2 months for other specialties to a maximum of 6 months.
- For ACGME-accredited programs sponsored by specialties other than internal medicine, month-for-month up to 2 months per specialty to a maximum of 6 months.
- No credit is granted for training in non-ACGME-accredited programs.

For those entering training June 1999 and after, the following training requirements printed in italics will apply:

Standard Postdoctoral Training Requirements

To be admitted to a certification examination in internal medicine physicians must have completed, by August 31 of the year of examination, 36 months of graduate medical education accredited by the ACGME, the RCPSC, or the Professional Corporation of Physicians of Quebec. Residency training or research experience occurring before the completion of the requirements for the MD or DO degree cannot be credited toward the Board's training requirements.

The 36 months of required training must include (1) a maximum of 12 months of internal medicine rotations at the R-1 level, and (2) a minimum of 24 months of training in an accredited internal medicine program, 12 months at the R-2 level and 12 months at the R-3 level.

Minimum Content of Training

The 36 months of full-time medical residency education must include the following:

- *Thirty months of internal medicine rotations in general internal medicine, subspecialty internal medicine, critical care medicine, geriatric medicine, and emergency medicine, which may include a maximum of 4 months of non-internal medicine primary care skill areas (eg, neurology, dermatology, office gynecology, or pediatrics); up to 3 months of other electives approved by the internal medicine program director; and up to 3 months of leave for vacation time or illnesses (including pregnancy-related disabilities). Vacation and other leave cannot be forfeited to reduce training requirements.*
- *Twenty-four months of direct patient responsibility: 20 of the 24 months of direct patient responsibility must occur in general internal medicine, subspecialty internal medicine, emergency medicine, critical care medicine, and geriatric medicine; the remaining 4 months may occur on non-internal medicine rotations. Direct patient responsibility may occur in either inpatient or ambulatory settings.*
- *A minimum of 6 months of the direct patient responsibility on internal medicine rotations* ***must*** *occur during the R-1 year.*

Credit for Training Taken Prior to Entering Internal Medicine Residency

Upon the receipt of a proposal from the director of an accredited internal medicine residency program, the Board may grant credit for some or all of the R-1 training requirement for training taken prior to entering R-2 internal medicine training as described below.

Month-for-month credit for R-1 training may be granted for satisfactory completion of internal medicine rotations taken during an accredited non-internal medicine residency program:

- *if the internal medicine training occurred under the direction of a program director of an accredited internal medicine program, and*
- *if the training occurred in an institution accredited for training internal medicine residents, and*
- *if the rotations were identical to the rotations of the residents enrolled in the accredited internal medicine residency program.*

In addition to month-for-month credit for internal medicine rotations:

- *up to 6 months credit may be granted for satisfactory completion of 12 months of an accredited family practice or pediatrics program; or*
- *up to 3 months credit for satisfactory completion of 12 months in an accredited residency program other than family practice or pediatrics.*

Up to 12 months credit may be granted for 3 or more years of US- or Canadian-accredited training in another clinical specialty and certification by an ABMS member Board in that specialty.

Twelve months credit may be granted for 3 or more years of verified internal medicine training abroad.

No credit may be granted to substitute for 24 months of R-2 and R-3 internal medicine training.

Requirements for Full-time Faculty Trained Abroad

Full time internal medicine faculty members in an LCME-accredited medical school or an accredited Canadian medical school may qualify for admission to the certification examination in internal medicine if they:

- *Are proposed by the chair of the department of internal medicine in an accredited medical school or the program director of an accredited internal medicine residency;*
- *Have completed 3 or more years of verified internal medicine training abroad;*
- *Hold an appointment at the level of Associate Professor or higher at the time of proposal; and*

- *Have completed 8 years of post-formal training experience as a clinician-educator or a clinical investigator in internal medicine with a full-time appointment on a medical school faculty.*

Credit for Training in Combined Programs

Training guidelines and requirements for credit toward the ABIM certification examination in internal medicine are available on request in the following combined programs:

- Emergency medicine/internal medicine
- Family practice/internal medicine
- Internal medicine/neurology
- Internal medicine/pediatrics
- Internal medicine/physical medicine and rehabilitation
- Internal medicine/preventive medicine
- Internal medicine/psychiatry

Subspecialties and Added Qualifications

In addition to the primary certificate in internal medicine, the Board offers subspecialty certificates and certificates of added qualifications. Subspecialty certificates are offered in cardiovascular disease; endocrinology, diabetes, and metabolism; gastroenterology; hematology; infectious disease; medical oncology; nephrology; pulmonary disease; and rheumatology.

The certificates of added qualifications recognize special expertise in areas that have a fundamental practice-oriented relationship to an underlying discipline, and are offered currently in adolescent medicine, clinical cardiac electrophysiology, critical care medicine, clinical and laboratory immunology, geriatric medicine, and sports medicine. A new certificate of added qualifications in interventional cardiology will be offered in 1999.

Physicians who are awarded a certificate in a subspecialty or an area of added qualifications must have been previously certified in internal medicine by the ABIM, completed the requisite training, demonstrated clinical competence in the care of patients, and passed the subspecialty or added qualifications examination.

Information regarding each of the added qualifications examinations is available from the Board upon request.

For information and application forms for the clinical and laboratory immunology examination, please contact the American Board of Allergy and Immunology, 510 Walnut St, Ste 1701, Philadelphia, PA 19106-3699.

Subspecialty training initiated July 1, 1989, and after must be accredited by the ACGME, the RCPSC, or the Professional Corporation of Physicians of Quebec. Subspecialty training completed prior to July 1, 1989, must have been completed in a program associated with an accredited residency in internal medicine in the United States or Canada.

Candidates for certification in the subspecialties must meet the Board's requirements for the total duration of training as well as minimum clinical training. Clinical training requirements may be met by aggregating clinical training that occurs throughout the entire fellowship training period; clinical training need not be completed in successive months.

Fellowship training taken before the date of completion of the requirements for the MD or DO degree and training as a chief medical resident do not count toward the requirements for subspecialty certification. In addition, practice experience and attendance at postgraduate courses cannot be credited.

Educational experience in a subspecialty during a full-time junior faculty appointment in an accredited medical school in the United States or Canada may be applicable toward the training requirements. Such clinical experience must be approved by the appropriate program director and be reviewed prospectively by the Board.

To be admitted to an examination, candidates must have completed the required subspecialty training by July 1 of the year of examination.

Training Requirements for Each Subspecialty

Cardiovascular disease requires 3 years of accredited training, of which a minimum of 24 months is clinical training, in the diagnosis and management of a broad spectrum of cardiovascular diseases.

(Two years of accredited cardiology training completed before July 1990 may be acceptable through the year 2000. Contact the Board for details.)

Gastroenterology requires 3 years of accredited training, of which a minimum of 18 months is clinical training, in the diagnosis and management of a broad spectrum of gastroenterological diseases.

(Two years of accredited gastroenterology training is required for candidates who initiated fellowship training prior to June 1996.)

Endocrinology, diabetes, and metabolism; hematology; infectious disease; medical oncology; nephrology; pulmonary disease; and rheumatology require 2 years of accredited training, of which a minimum of 12 months is clinical training, in the diagnosis and management of a broad spectrum of medical diseases. Additionally, hematology and medical oncology each require experience in an ambulatory care setting and a minimum of 1 half day per week spent in a continuity outpatient clinic during the entire 2-year training period.

Dual Certification Requirements

Hematology and Medical Oncology

Dual certification in hematology and medical oncology requires 3 years of full-time combined fellowship training, which must include: (a) a minimum of 18 months of prospectively designed full-time clinical training with patient care responsibility, (b) a minimum of 12 months in the diagnosis and management of a broad spectrum of neoplastic diseases, including hematological malignancies, and (c) a minimum of 6 months of training in the diagnosis and management of a broad spectrum of non-neoplastic hematological disorders.

Full-time clinical training is defined as at least 80% of the trainee's professional time during a working week dedicated to clinical (patient care or educational) activities. During the entire 3 years the candidate must attend at least one outpatient clinic for a minimum of 1 half day per week and have the responsibility for providing continuous care to a defined cohort of patients being managed for neoplastic and hematological disorders.

The ABIM recommends that the 3 years of combined training be taken in programs in the same institution that is accredited both in hematology and medical oncology by the ACGME, the RCPSC, or the Professional Corporation of Physicians of Quebec. If circumstances dictate that this training be taken in two different programs, 24 continuous months must be in one institution, and both institutions must be accredited in hematology and medical oncology.

Candidates must complete all 3 years of required combined training before being admitted to an examination in either subspecialty. Those who elect to undertake an examination in one subspecialty following only 2 years of fellowship training will be required to complete 4 years of accredited training for dual certification. Candidates who have completed all 3 years of required combined training may take the hematology and medical oncology examinations in the same year or in different years.

Rheumatology and Allergy and Immunology

Dual certification in rheumatology and allergy and immunology requires a minimum of 3 years of full-time training which must include (a) at least 12 months full-time clinical rheumatology supervised by the director of an accredited rheumatology training program, (b) weekly attendance for 18 consecutive months in an ambulatory care program supervised by rheumatology faculty, which must include continuity of patient care within ambulatory clinics, and (c) at least 18 months of full-time allergy and immunology training supervised by the training program director of an accredited program in allergy and immunology.

Plans for combined training should be approved in writing by both the rheumatology and the allergy and immunology training program directors and by the ABIM Subspecialty Board on Rheumatology and the American Board of Allergy and Immunology before training begins. Admission to either examination requires (1) certification in internal medicine, (2) satisfactory clinical competence, and (3) completion of the entire 3-year combined program.

Candidates seeking dual certification for other subspecialty combinations should write to the Board for information.

Research Pathway

In recognition of the importance of training general and subspecialist internists as research scientists, the Board established a new research pathway to certification that became effective July 1997.

The new research pathway is intended for trainees who seek academic careers as investigators in basic science or clinical research. The research pathway integrates training in clinical medicine with 3 years in basic or clinical research. Although prospective planning of this pathway by trainees and program directors is necessary, prospective approval by the Board is no longer a requirement. Program directors will document the training experience of these individuals through the Board's tracking program.

Training for the research pathway is longer in duration than standard clinical training (ie, a total of 5 years for general internal medicine and 6 or 7 years for the subspecialties and/or added qualifications depending on the discipline), and the curriculum is not optimal preparation for clinical practice. Candidates who change their career path from investigator to clinician must meet all the requirements for the standard clinical pathway.

Requirements for the research pathway are summarized below.

General Internal Medicine Requirements

Candidates must complete the following:

- Two-years of full-time clinical training in an accredited internal medicine program, which includes at least 20 months of direct patient responsibility in an appropriately balanced curriculum.
- Three years of research training at a minimum of 80% full-time commitment. During research training, at least 20% of each year must be spent in clinical experiences, including at least 1 half day per week in a continuity clinic.

Trainees in the general internal medicine research pathway may be admitted to the certification examination in internal medicine in the fall of graduate year 5 as long as the candidate can provide documentation of commitment to 80% research time in either a trainee or full-time faculty position for the duration of the fifth year.

Subspecialty Internal Medicine Requirements

Candidates must complete the following:

- Two years of full-time clinical training in an accredited internal medicine program, which includes at least 20 months of direct patient responsibility in an appropriately balanced curriculum.
- One year of accredited clinical fellowship training in allergy and immunology; critical care medicine; endocrinology, diabetes, and metabolism; geriatric medicine; hematology; infectious disease, medical oncology; nephrology; pulmonary disease; and rheumatology; or

  Two years of accredited fellowship training in gastroenterology; hematology/oncology; pulmonary/critical care medicine; and rheumatology/allergy and immunology, 18 months of which must be clinical training; or

  Two years of accredited clinical fellowship training in cardiovascular disease.
- At least 3 years of subspecialty-related research training at a minimum of 80% full-time commitment. During research training responsibility for ambulatory clinic must be maintained at the level of at least 1 half day per week.

Trainees in the subspecialty internal medicine research pathway may be admitted to the certification examination in internal medicine in the fall of graduate year 4 as long as the 2 required years in internal medicine have been successfully completed. After certification in internal medicine, the subspecialty examination may be taken in the fall of their last year of training (GY6 or GY7, depending on the subspecialty), as long as the candidate can provide documentation of commitment to 80% research time in either a trainee or a full-time faculty position for the duration of the sixth or seventh year.

More information about the research pathway is available on request.

Candidates for Special Consideration

The Board will only review proposals on behalf of candidates with nonstandard training who meet the following criteria:

1. At least 2 years of full-time formal training in internal medicine in accredited programs in the United States or Canada that have occurred after (a) 3 or more years of verified foreign training in internal medicine or (b) 3 or more years of US- or Canadian-accredited training in another specialty, and certification by an ABMS member Board in that specialty. Or
2. Full-time internal medicine faculty members in an LCME-accredited US medical school or an accredited Canadian medical school who (a) have completed 3 or more years of training in internal medicine abroad, (b) hold an appointment at the level of associate professor or higher, and (c) have completed 8 years of experience after formal training as a full-time clinician-educator or a clinical investigator in internal medicine with an appointment on a medical school faculty.

No other exceptions to the Board's standard training requirements will be considered.

Candidates must be proposed by the chair of a department of internal medicine in an accredited medical school or the program director of an accredited internal medicine residency. Guidelines for proposing candidates for special consideration for certification in internal medicine should be obtained prior to submitting a proposal.

Guidelines for proposing candidates for special consideration for the subspecialties and added qualifications are also available upon request.

Substantiation of Clinical Competence

Components of Clinical Competence

The Board requires substantiation that candidates for certification are competent in the following:

Internal medicine: clinical judgment, medical knowledge, clinical skills (medical interviewing, physical examination, and procedural skills), humanistic qualities, professionalism, and provision of medical care.

Subspecialties: clinical judgment, medical knowledge, clinical skills (medical interviewing, physical examination, and procedural skills), humanistic qualities, professionalism, provision of medical care, and continuing scholarship.

All trainees must receive a satisfactory rating of overall clinical competence, humanistic qualities, and moral and ethical behavior in each of the required years of training. In addition, during the final year of required training they must receive satisfactory ratings in each of the components of competence.

Procedural Skills Required for Certification

Internal Medicine: The diagnostic and therapeutic procedures listed below are required for certification. Although the Board does not prescribe an absolute number of times a procedure must be done to ensure competence, it has developed the following guidelines (indicated in parentheses) for the minimum number of directly supervised, successfully performed procedures, below which the confirmation of proficiency is not credible: abdominal paracentesis (3), arterial puncture for blood gas analysis (5), arthrocentesis of the knee joint (3), central venous line placement (5), lumbar puncture (5), nasogastric intubation (3), thoracentesis (5), and critical life-saving procedures (this requirement can be met by documentation of successful training in advanced cardiac life support). Additional procedures required for those entering residency training in June 1997 and after are breast examinations (5), rectal examinations (5), pelvic examinations and pap smear including wet mount (5).

Subspecialties and Added Qualifications: The diagnostic and therapeutic procedures required for certification in the subspecialties and added qualifications follow.

Cardiovascular Disease: advanced cardiac life support (ACLS), including cardioversion; electrocardiography, including ambulatory monitoring and exercise testing; echocardiography; arterial catheter insertion; and right-heart catheterization, including insertion and management of temporary pacemakers.

Clinical Cardiac Electrophysiology: electrophysiologic studies, including mapping, both with a catheter and intraoperatively; surgical and other ablation procedures; and implantation of pacemakers, cardioverters, and defibrillators (a minimum of 100 intracardiac procedures in at least 50 patients, of whom at least 25% had supraventricular tachycardia).

Critical Care Medicine: maintenance of open airway; oral/nasal intubation; ventilator management, including experience with various modes; insertion and management of chest tubes; ACLS; placement of arterial, central venous, and pulmonary artery balloon flotation catheters; and calibration and operation of hemodynamic recording systems.

Endocrinology, Diabetes, and Metabolism: thyroid aspiration biopsy.

Gastroenterology: proctoscopy and/or flexible sigmoidoscopy; diagnostic upper gastrointestinal endoscopy; colonoscopy, including biopsy and polypectomy; esophageal dilation; therapeutic upper and lower gastrointestinal endoscopy; and liver biopsy.

Hematology: bone marrow aspiration and biopsy, including preparation, staining, examination, and interpretation of blood smears, bone marrow aspirates, and touch preparations of bone marrow biopsies; measurement of complete blood count, including platelets and white cell differential, using automated or manual techniques with appropriate quality control; administration of chemotherapeutic agents and biological products through all therapeutic routes; and management and care of indwelling venous access catheters.

Infectious Disease: microscopic evaluation of diagnostic specimens, including preparation, staining, and interpretation; management, maintenance, and removal of indwelling venous access catheters; and administration of antimicrobial and biologic products via all routes.

Interventional Cardiology: a minimum of 250 cardiac interventional procedures during 12 months of acceptable interventional cardiology fellowship training.

Medical Oncology: bone marrow aspiration and biopsy; administration of chemotherapeutic agents and biological products through all therapeutic routes; and management and care of indwelling venous access catheters.

Nephrology: placement of temporary vascular access for hemodialysis and related procedures; acute and chronic hemodialysis; peritoneal dialysis (excluding placement of temporary peritoneal catheters); continuous renal replacement therapy (CRRT); and percutaneous biopsy of both autologous and transplanted kidneys.

Pulmonary Disease: oral/nasal intubation; fiberoptic bronchoscopy and accompanying procedures; ventilator management; thoracentesis and percutaneous pleural biopsy; arterial puncture; placement of arterial and pulmonary artery balloon flotation catheters; calibration and operation of hemodynamic recording systems; supervision of the technical aspects of pulmonary function testing; progressive exercise testing; and insertion and management of chest tubes.

Rheumatology: diagnostic aspiration of and analysis by light and polarized light microscopy of synovial fluid from diarthrodial joints, bursae, and tenosynovial structures; and therapeutic injection of diarthrodial joints, bursae, tenosynovial structures, and entheses.

Annual Evaluation of Trainees

Through its tracking process, the Board requires program directors to complete evaluation forms annually attesting to the clinical competence of internal medicine and subspecialty trainees.

For subspecialty trainees, verification of their clinical competence is sought from both the director of the subspecialty training program and the chair of the department of medicine.

For trainees planning to change programs, the Board expects the trainee to request that a written evaluation of past performance be sent from the previous training program to the new training program. Upon the request of the new program director, the Board will provide (when available) a summary of the previous performance ratings and the total credits accumulated toward the Board's training requirements. In addition, at the trainee's request, the Board will provide the new program director with comments or other information obtained from previous training programs.

Marginal Ratings: Internal medicine trainees rated as marginal in either their GY1 or GY2 will receive credit for that year of training. However, if they receive marginal ratings in *both* GY1 and GY2, an additional year of accredited internal medicine training will be required. Marginal ratings do not apply to subspecialty trainees.

Additional Training and Deficiencies: The Board requires trainees with documented deficiencies in clinical competence to obtain additional accredited training. One additional year of accredited training (including satisfactory completion and performance) is required for each unsatisfactory year. It is the trainee's responsibility to arrange for this training.

Trainees demonstrating deficiencies solely in the areas of humanistic qualities or moral and ethical behavior may, at the discretion of the Board, be required to complete additional training and/or a specified period of close observation.

Due Process: The responsibility for the evaluation of a trainee rests with the training program, not with the Board. The Board is not in a position to reexamine the facts and circumstances of an individual's training and evaluation. As required by the ACGME in its *Essentials of Accredited Residencies in Graduate Medical Education*, trainees must be provided due process at the educational institution. In the event that a trainee disagrees with a rating, the appropriate course of redress is the due process procedure at that institution.

Professional Standing of Practitioners

Every 4 years following formal training, the Board requires verification that candidates applying for certification are recognized as specialists or subspecialists in good standing. Verification is sought from the chief of medical service at the institution where the candidate's principal staff appointment is held. Any challenge to good standing must be resolved locally to the Board's satisfaction before admission to the examination. For example, substance abuse, convictions for felonies related to medical practice, or substantial disciplinary action by the institution may lead to deferred admission or rejection.

Licensure

A valid, unrestricted, and unchallenged license to practice medicine in a state, territory, commonwealth, possession, or province of the United States or Canada is required of all candidates. Candidates with a restricted, suspended, or revoked license in any jurisdiction will not be admitted to the examination or certified. Restrictions include but are not limited to conditions, contingencies, probation, and stipulated agreements.

Special Policies

Board Eligibility

The Board does not use, define, or recognize the term "Board eligible." Admissibility to certifying examinations is not affected by prior examination attempts, nor will it be time-limited. Candidates will be admissible to certifying examinations provided they meet all the requirements of the Board as set forth in its *Policies and Procedures* brochure and on ABIM's home page (http://www.abim.org).

The Board will routinely report by mail, fax, or internet (http://www.abim.org) whether candidates are certified (including dates) or not certified. If a diplomate was previously certified, this fact and dates of former certification will be noted. If certification is suspended or revoked, this also will be reported.

On a candidate's written request to the Board, the following information will also be reported: (1) that an application is currently in process and/or (2) the year the candidate was last admitted to examination.

Disclosure of Information

The Board provides information to program directors each year regarding both the certification status of individuals who trained in their programs and took the examination and the program's overall performance. This information is helpful to the program in evaluating its educational effectiveness. The Board also provides internal medicine program pass rate information to the Residency Review Committee for Internal Medicine, Association of American Medical Colleges, and American Medical Association and via the internet (http://www.abim.org). In addition, at its discretion, the Board may release examination results, examination scores, and other pertinent candidate information to those whom it deems have a legitimate need for such information.

Disabled Candidates

The Board recognizes that some candidates may be unable to fulfill the requirement for proficiency in performing procedures because of disability. For such individuals, the procedural skills requirement may be waived. Program directors should write to the Board for approval before the individual enters training.

The Board is committed to offering suitable accommodations for all candidates, including individuals with disabilities. When necessary, alternative arrangements under comparable conditions to those provided for nondisabled individuals are offered to disabled individuals. Candidates who need accommodation during the examination for a disability must provide a written request to the Board at the time of application for examination. Documentation must be received no later than 4 months prior to the date of examination.

Substance Abuse

If a history of substance abuse exists, candidates must provide documentation that they can safely and effectively perform the duties and responsibilities of an ABIM diplomate. Evidence of successful completion of a treatment program and/or a documented period of abstinence, usually 1 year, is required. The Board treats such information as confidential.

Leave of Absence

Up to 1 month of credit may be granted in any 1 year for vacation time or illnesses (including pregnancy-related disabilities). Vacation time cannot be forfeited to reduce training requirements. Up to 6 weeks' credit may also be granted for leave relating to care for a newborn or newly adopted child.

Reduced-Schedule Training

Part-time training, even though continuous, is not acceptable. Interrupted full-time training, however, is acceptable, provided that no period of full-time training is shorter than 1 month. In any 12-month period, at least 6 months must be spent in training. Patient care responsibilities should be maintained in a continuity clinic during the nontraining component of the year. Board approval must be obtained before initiating an interrupted training program.

Revocation of Certificates

The Board may at its discretion revoke certification if the diplomate was not qualified to receive the certificate at the time it was issued, even if the certificate was issued as a result of a mistake on the part of the Board. It may revoke or suspend the certificate if (1) the diplomate made any material misstatement of fact or omission of fact to the Board in connection with application or otherwise, or to any third party concerning the diplomate's certification status; or (2) the diplomate's license to practice medicine has been revoked in any jurisdiction.

Reexamination

Candidates who are unsuccessful on any certification examination may apply for reexamination. There is no restriction on the number of opportunities for reexamination. Once admitted to an examination, candidates will be considered to have fulfilled the training requirements for future examinations in that discipline. All candidates for examination and reexamination must meet the requirements for licensure status and professional standing.

Late Applications

Awareness of and meeting registration deadlines are the candidate's responsibility. There is a nonrefundable penalty fee of $300 for any application postmarked between November 2, 1998, and December 1, 1998, for the April sports medicine examination; December 2, 1998, and February 1, 1999, for the August internal medicine examination; and April 2, 1998, and July 1, 1998, for the November certification examinations.

Additional Information and Inquiries

Please address all inquiries concerning examination applications to

American Board of Internal Medicine
510 Walnut St, Ste 1700
Philadelphia, PA 19106-3699
215 446-3500 or 800 441-2246
215 446-3470 or 215 446-3590 Fax
E-mail: request@abim.org

The following Board publications are available upon request. These are not designed to aid in preparation for examinations.

ABIM Policies and Procedures for Certification
ABIM Recertification Program
Guidelines and Criteria for the ABIM General and Subspecialty Internal Medicine Research Pathway
Guide to Evaluation of Residents in Internal Medicine
Residents: Evaluating Your Clinical Competence
Attending Physicians: Your Role in Evaluating Residents
Resource Document for Subspecialty Program Directors: Clinical Competence Guidelines and Other Information
Care Competencies in Women's Health: What Internists Need to Know
Project Professionalism
Caring for the Dying: Identification and Promotion of Physician Competency—Educational Resources and Personal Narratives
Promoting Medical Interviewing Skills in Internal Medicine
Guide to Awareness and Evaluation of Humanistic Qualities
Certification in Added Qualifications of:

- Adolescent Medicine
- *Clinical Cardiac Electrophysiology*
- *Critical Care Medicine*
- *Geriatric Medicine*
- *Interventional Cardiology*
- *Sports Medicine*

Examination Schedule

Certification examination in

Internal Medicine

August 24-25, 1999
Registration period: September 1 to December 1, 1998
Fee (US): $855
Cancellation deadline: July 1, 1999
August 22-23, 2000
Registration period: September 1 to December 1, 1999
Fee (US): Not determined
Cancellation deadline: July 1, 2000

Adolescent Medicine

November 15, 1999
Registration period: January 1 to April 1, 1999
Fee (US): $1,080
Cancellation deadline: October 1, 1999

Cardiovascular Disease

November 3-4, 1999
Registration period: January 1 to April 1, 1999
Fee (US): $1,080
Cancellation deadline: September 15, 1999

Clinical Cardiac Electrophysiology

November 3, 1999
Registration period: January 1 to April 1, 1999
Fee (US): $1,080
Cancellation deadline: September 15, 1999

Critical Care Medicine

November 3, 1999
Registration period: January 1 to April 1, 1999
Fee (US): $1,080
Cancellation deadline: September 15, 1999

Endocrinology, Diabetes, and Metabolism

November 3, 1999
Registration period: January 1 to April 1, 1999
Fee (US): $1,080
Cancellation deadline: September 15, 1999

Gastroenterology

November 3, 1999
Registration period: January 1 to April 1, 1999
Fee (US): $1,080
Cancellation deadline: September 15, 1999

Geriatric Medicine

November 3, 1999
Registration period: January 1 to April 1, 1999
Fee (US): $1,080
Cancellation deadline: September 15, 1999

Hematology

November 3, 1999
Registration period: January 1 to April 1, 1999
Fee (US): $1,080
Cancellation deadline: September 15, 1999

Infectious Disease

November 3, 1999
Registration period: January 1 to April 1, 1999
Fee (US): $1,080
Cancellation deadline: September 15, 1999

Interventional Cardiology

November 3, 1999
Registration period: January 1 to April 1, 1999
Fee (US): $1,080
Cancellation deadline: September 15, 1999

Medical Oncology

November 3, 1999
Registration period: January 1 to April 1, 1999
Fee (US): $1,080
Cancellation deadline: September 15, 1999

Nephrology

November 3, 1999
Registration period: January 1 to April 1, 1999
Fee (US): $1,080
Cancellation deadline: September 15, 1999

Pulmonary Disease

November 3, 1999
Registration period: January 1 to April 1, 1999
Fee (US): $1,080
Cancellation deadline: September 15, 1999

Rheumatology

November 3, 1999
Registration period: January 1 to April 1, 1999
Fee (US): $1,080
Cancellation deadline: September 15, 1999

Sports Medicine

April 16, 1999
Registration period: July 1 to November 1, 1998
Fee (US): $1,080
Cancellation deadline: March 1, 1999
Please see previous section for penalty fee for late applications.

American Board of Medical Genetics

Sharon B Robinson, MS, Administrator
9650 Rockville Pike
Bethesda, MD 20814-3998
301 571-1825
301 571-1895 Fax
Internet: http://www.faseb.org/genetics/abmg/abmgmenu.htm

(These criteria and conditions apply to the 1999 examination cycle and are subject to change without notice. The American Board of Medical Genetics [ABMG] offers exams every 3 years; the next examination cycle will be June 1999. All applicants are advised to contact the Board to ascertain whether the information below is current.)

General Information

The American Board of Medical Genetics, Inc, incorporated in 1980 under the sponsorship of the American Society of Human Genetics, Inc, prepares and administers examinations to certify individuals who provide services in medical genetics and provides accreditation of medical genetics training programs. The certification program consists of a general (core) examination, taken by all examinees, and specialty examinations in the following areas: (1) clinical genetics, (2) PhD medical genetics, (3) clinical biochemical genetics, (4) clinical cytogenetics, and (5) clinical molecular genetics.

General Candidacy Requirements

"Active Candidate Status"

Once the application has been approved, the applicant is considered an active candidate for ABMG certification. The term "Board eligible" is not used to describe this status. If a candidate fails to achieve certification for any reason (including withdrawing from the examination process), the individual loses his/her active candidate status. Such individuals may reapply for active candidate status, as described below.

First-time Applicants

Candidacy for the 1999 examination requires successful completion of an Accreditation Council for Graduate Medical Education (ACGME)-accredited or ABMG-accredited medical genetics training program by June 30, 1999. All graduates of an accredited training program are considered for active candidate status for the certification examinations provided they submit acceptable supporting credentials. It is strongly recommended that the application be submitted to ABMG within 5 years of completion of the training program. Changes in the field are incorporated into the examinations and applicants may be held responsible for revisions in certification requirements.

The ABMG limits active candidacy to individuals who demonstrate to its satisfaction that specific criteria for certification have been met. Those practitioners working in genetics who, despite academic or clinical backgrounds, do not meet specific criteria described herein will not be permitted to sit for any examination.

If an applicant's background is found to be deficient, the ABMG may require additional training and/or clinical experience before allowing the applicant to sit for the examination. The ABMG also reserves the right to declare a candidate ineligible if training, background, or references are deemed inadequate or otherwise unacceptable.

Individuals who have received equivalent training in other countries and who complete their logbooks under the auspices of ABMG-accredited training programs may also be granted candidacy to sit for the examinations. Individuals are strongly encouraged to seek evaluation of the equivalency of their foreign training prior to starting their training in the United States. Such candidates must submit an Information Supplement form with their formal application. The ABMG reserves the right to grant or deny such candidacy.

Applicants for Reexamination

Reexaminees are those individuals who failed the examination for the first time in 1996. Reexaminees must retake all examinations for specialties in which they desire certification, as well as the general examination. They cannot carry over a passed examination to the next cycle. Refer to the "Requirements for Reexaminees Within One Cycle" for specific application requirements.

Applicants Who Fail to Achieve Certification Within 6 Years of Application

Applicants are required to pass the certification examination within two successive examination cycles or within 6 years of application, whichever comes first. Failure to achieve certification in two cycles, including, but not limited to, failing both cycles of the examination or withdrawing from one cycle and failing the other, require the applicant to begin again as a "New Applicant."

Failure to achieve certification during this period is taken as evidence of inadequate knowledge or training in medical genetics and an indication of the need for additional training. To qualify for candidacy to resit the Board examinations, the applicant must complete the equivalent of 1 year of additional training in an ABMG- or ACGME-accredited medical genetics program, and generate a logbook of 150 new cases seen under the auspices of that program. The additional training must be approved by the director of the training program and documented to the ABMG at the onset of training. The applicant should contact the ABMG Administrative Office to clarify additional training requirements.

Applicants for Certification in an Additional Specialty

Doctoral diplomates previously certified in one (or more) ABMG specialty who desire to take another specialty examination must submit new credentials, including evidence of 1 additional year of *full-time training* in the additional specialty at an ABMG-accredited training program, and include a new logbook of recent cases completed at the ABMG-accredited training program during that period of training. Applicants must pass both the general examination and the additional specialty examination to be certified in the additional area.

General Instructions

Deadline for Applications

Complete applications must be **postmarked no later than December 31, 1998**. Applications postmarked between January 1 and January 31, 1999, must be accompanied by a $250 late fee. Applications postmarked February 1, 1999, or later will be returned to the applicant without review. Incomplete applications will not be reviewed. *All information, including logbooks and letters of endorsement, must be submitted before the deadline.*

Applicants who have completed training must submit a completed logbook by December 31, 1998. Applicants whose training ends between January 1, 1999, and June 30, 1999, are permitted to submit logbooks with at least 100 cases per specialty by December 31, 1998, and must submit the remainder of their cases by March 15, 1999. No late fee will be assessed if the remaining cases are submitted by stated deadlines.

It is recommended that candidates send their applications via US Postal Service certified mail, with a return receipt of delivery. It is the applicant's responsibility to assure delivery of the application on time.

Receipt of Application

Upon receipt of completed application and appropriate application review fees, credentials are evaluated by the ABMG and, at its discretion, are approved or disapproved. Once an application is approved, the applicant achieves "Active Candidate" status. The term "Board eligible" is not to be used to describe this status. At this point, the individual is advised of the deadline to remit examination fees.

When all fees have been received from the active candidate, he or she is assigned to an examination center and notified of the site. An admission card is mailed to the candidate approximately 3 weeks before the examination. *No candidate will be admitted to any examination without an admission card.* It is the candidate's responsibility to notify ABMG of any change of address or if an admission card is not received.

Fees

All applicants must register for the general examination and at least one specialty examination. Fees must be paid in US currency by check or money order. The candidate's canceled check is considered the receipt.

Application Review Fee

One specialty	$450
Two specialties	$500
Three specialties	$550
Four specialties	$600

This fee is nonrefundable and must accompany the application.

Examination Fees

General Examination	$400
Specialties	
Clinical genetics	$500
PhD medical genetics	$500
Clinical cytogenetics	$500
Clinical biochemical genetics	$500
Clinical molecular genetics	$500

Late Fees

A late fee of $250 must accompany any application postmarked between January 1, 1999, and January 31, 1999. Applications postmarked after January 31, 1999, will be returned without review.

Fee Payment Schedule

First Time Applicants: Submit application review fee with your application; examination fees will be requested once your application has been approved.

Reexaminees: Submit examination fees with your application. The application fee is not required.

Request to Withdraw

If an approved applicant withdraws from the examination, examination fees may be refunded at the applicant's request. It is the applicant's responsibility to notify the ABMG Administrative Office in writing no less than 3 weeks prior to the examination date. A fee of $100 is retained to cover administrative costs. Fees are not refunded to examinees who withdraw within 3 weeks of the examination date. A candidate who fails to appear for an examination will forfeit all examination fees.

Active candidate status is not maintained after examination results are released. Such applicants may reapply for "active candidate status." Applicants are required to achieve certification within two successive examination cycles or within 6 years of achieving active candidate status, whichever comes first. Credentials carry an applicant for two cycles. Withdrawing from an examination cycle is counted as failure to achieve certification during that cycle.

Applicants With Special Disabilities

The ABMG supports the intent of the Americans with Disabilities Act (ADA) and will attempt to make reasonable accommodation for applicants with disabilities. The ABMG offers examinations in a place and manner accessible to persons with disabilities or offers alternative accessible arrangements for such individuals. Auxiliary aids and services will be offered only if they do not fundamentally alter the measurement of skills or knowledge the examination is intended to test.

Applicants with a physical or mental disability who need special accommodation during the examinations are requested to check the appropriate box on the application form and to request an "Application for Special Accommodation" from the ABMG Administrative Office. This form should be completed and submitted with the application.

If circumstances arise that cause the applicant to request accommodation after completion of the application, the applicant should notify the ABMG Administrative Office immediately.

Certificates

Candidates who pass the general examination and at least one specialty examination will become diplomates of the ABMG. This information becomes public information and is listed in the official *ABMS Directory of Board Certified Medical Specialists*. Any certificate issued by the ABMG shall be subject to revocation at any time should the ABMG determine, in its sole judgment, that a candidate who has received a certificate was in some respect not properly qualified to receive or retain it.

Time-limited Certification

As of the 1993 certification examination, all certificates are time-limited for a period of 10 years from the date of the examination.

Final Decisions by the American Board of Medical Genetics

Final decisions regarding candidacy (active candidate status) for certifying examinations and certification of applicants will be made by the Board of Directors of the ABMG. Appeals of ABMG decisions may be made in writing to the ABMG Review Committee at the ABMG Administrative Office address. *Failure to pass a certifying examination is not appealable.* Write to the Administrative Office to obtain a copy of the "Appeal Process for Adverse Decisions Affecting Certification."

Canadian College of Medical Genetics (CCMG) and ABMG Reciprocity

Beginning with the 1996 cycle of certifying examinations, trainees completing CCMG-accredited postdoctoral training programs are eligible to apply for admission to ABMG examinations, and trainees completing ABMG-accredited postdoctoral training programs are eligible to apply for admission to CCMG examinations; the ABMG and CCMG now recognize each other's training as provided by accredited programs. Candidates from such accredited training programs may seek admission to the certifying examinations of either country or of both countries. Candidates from accredited programs in the United States and Canada who seek certification in the country other than that of their training are required to meet all of the credentialing requirements and pay all of the applicable fees to the certifying body.

Canadian-trained candidates for the ABMG certifying examinations must submit logbooks, laboratory method competency lists, and other required documents signed by their program directors. Letters of recommendation may be submitted by CCMG- or ABMG-certified colleagues, one of whom must be the program director of their training. In addition, Canadian-trained candidates must submit an "Information Supplement Form" for special consideration.

Individuals who hold certificates from the ABMG or CCMG in one of the recognized specialties may apply to the certifying body of the other country for admission to the certifying examination for that specialty. A valid certificate, however, serves only as evidence of appropriate prior training. Candidates must meet all of the credentialing requirements of the certifying body to which they apply. ABMG applicants must pass both the general examination and at least one specialty examination in order to be certified.

Requirements

A. Requirements for First-time Applicants, Those Requesting an Additional Specialty, and Those Who Have Failed to Achieve Certification Within 6 Years of Application

1. Applicants must submit a notarized application indicating intent to sit the certification examination.
2. Applicants for the Clinical Genetics specialty must have a US- or Canadian-earned, or the equivalent of an earned, MD or DO degree. Applicants for the PhD medical genetics specialty must have a US- or Canadian-earned, or the equivalent of an earned, PhD in genetics, human genetics, or a related field. Applicants for the laboratory specialty examinations must have a US- or Canadian-earned, or the equivalent of an earned, MD, DO, or PhD. All applicants are required to submit an official transcript of the MD, DO, or PhD program, indicating date of graduation.
3. Applicants must submit a current curriculum vitae and bibliography.
4. Applicants for PhD medical genetics or laboratory specialties are required to complete at least 2 years in an ABMG-accredited training program. Clinical genetics applicants are required to complete 2 years in an ACGME-accredited clinical genetics residency and submit verification of satisfactory completion of at least 2 years in an ACGME-accredited residency training program in any clinical specialty. The program director must certify that the candidate has had ongoing assessment during training, has satisfactorily completed the requirements of the program, has the clinical skills necessary for the specialty (or specialties) of interest, and that for each laboratory specialty the applicant has had at least 1 full year of *clinical* laboratory bench experience as a fellow or resident in the training program. The program director may also write one of the letters of endorsement.

   Applicants completing their training between January 1, 1999, and June 30, 1999, may apply for the 1999 examinations and supply current training information. The ABMG will contact the program director at the conclusion of the training period for verification of successful completion of training.

   Some applicants will not complete their fellowship before sitting for the examination (eg, they will have finished only 2 or 3 years of a longer fellowship). If this is the case, a letter from the program director must clarify how the fellow has met *all* of the requirements for candidacy in the specialties for which he/she is applying.
5. Applicants are required to submit at least three letters of endorsement from ABMG-certified diplomates who are familiar with the applicant's medical genetics experience. Diplomates, in the letters, must attest to the applicant's character, honesty, and integrity and support the application for candidacy. One or more letters must be from ABMG-certified program faculty who were directly responsible for training in each specialty (or specialties) for which the applicant is seeking candidacy.

   The letters of endorsement, and any letter from the program director, must be sealed and signed by the author over the seal and submitted with the application.
6. All applicants are required to submit a logbook of 150 clinical cases per specialty. See the "Instructions for Completion of Logbook of Medical Genetics Experience" for further instructions.
7. Laboratory specialty applicants are required to submit a competency list for each laboratory specialty in which certification is requested. This list is to be signed by the program director and by the ABMG laboratory specialist in charge of that part of the training program (ie, the person specified in the program's application for accreditation).
8. Clinical genetics specialty applicants are required to submit verification of satisfactory completion of at least 2 years in an ACGME-accredited clinical residency program in another medical specialty or 4 years in an ACGME-accredited clinical genetics residency program.
9. Clinical genetics specialty applicants must be able to practice medicine at the time they will sit the examination. Clinical genetics applicants are required to submit a copy of their current unrestricted and valid medical license.
10. Applicants are required to submit an acknowledgment card along with the application. If applying for more than one specialty, only one card is necessary.
11. First-time applicants must submit an application fee along with their application.

B. Requirements for Reexaminees Within One Cycle

1. Applicants must submit a notarized application indicating intent to sit the certification examination.
2. Applicants must submit an official transcript of a US- or Canadian-earned, or the equivalent of an earned MD, DO, or PhD training program, indicating date of graduation.
3. Applicants must submit a current curriculum vitae and bibliography.
4. Laboratory specialty applicants are required to submit a competency list for each laboratory specialty in which certification is requested. This list is to be signed by the program director and by the ABMG laboratory specialist in charge of that part of the training program (ie, the person specified in the program's application for accreditation).
5. Applicants are required to submit an acknowledgment card along with the application. If applying for more than one specialty, only one card is necessary.
6. Reexaminees are required to submit the appropriate examination fee with the application.

Description of Specialties in Medical Genetics

To be an active candidate for certification by the ABMG, an individual must meet the criteria in the area of desired certification and provide the required supporting documentation. Certification is offered in clinical genetics, PhD medical genetics, clinical cytogenetics, clinical biochemical genetics, and clinical molecular genetics.

Clinical Geneticist

A clinical geneticist is an individual who holds a US- or Canadian-earned, or the equivalent of an earned, MD or DO degree, has had 2 years in an ACGME-accredited clinical residency program in another medical specialty, 2 years in an ACGME-accredited residency in clinical genetics (or 4 years in an accredited clinical genetics residency program), a valid medical license, and demonstrates competence to provide comprehensive genetic diagnostic, management, therapeutic, and counseling services.

These requirements imply that the individual possesses

- broad knowledge in human and medical genetics, including an understanding of heterogeneity, variability, and natural history of genetic disorders;
- diagnostic and therapeutic skills in a wide range of genetic disorders;
- the ability to elicit and interpret individual and family histories;
- the ability to integrate clinical and genetic information and understand the uses, limitations, interpretation, and significance of specialized laboratory and clinical procedures;
- expertise in genetic and mathematical principles to perform risk assessment;
- skills in interviewing and counseling techniques required to (1) elicit from the patient or family the information necessary to reach an appropriate conclusion; (2) anticipate areas of difficulty and conflict; (3) help families and individuals recognize and cope with their emotional and psychological needs; (4) recognize situations requiring psychiatric referral; and (5) transmit pertinent information in a way that is comprehensible to the individual or family; and
- knowledge of available health care resources (community, regional, and national) required for appropriate referral or support.

PhD Medical Geneticist

A PhD medical geneticist is an individual with a US- or Canadian-earned, or the equivalent of an earned, PhD degree in genetics, human genetics, or a related field, who demonstrates competence to provide comprehensive genetic diagnostic, management, and counseling services, as well as expertise in complex risk assessments and in the integration of clinical and genetic information.

These requirements imply that the individual possesses

- broad knowledge in human and medical genetics, including an understanding of heterogeneity, variability, and natural history of genetic disorders;
- the ability to elicit and interpret individual and family histories;
- the ability to integrate clinical and genetic information and understand the uses, limitations, interpretation, and significance of specialized laboratory and clinical procedures;
- expertise in genetic and mathematical principles to perform complex risk assessments, paternity and forensic computations, interpret pedigree analysis (both segregation and linkage), and understand the principles of medical genetics;
- skills in interviewing and counseling techniques required to (1) elicit from the patient or family the information necessary to reach an appropriate conclusion, (2) anticipate areas of difficulty and conflict, (3) help families and individuals recognize and cope with their emotional and psychological needs, (4) recognize situations requiring psychiatric referral, and (5) transmit pertinent information in a comprehensible way to the individual or family; and
- knowledge of available health care resources (community, regional, and national) required for appropriate referral or support.

Clinical Biochemical Geneticist

A clinical biochemical geneticist is an individual with a US- or Canadian-earned, or the equivalent of an earned, doctoral degree (MD, DO, PhD) who can correctly perform and interpret biochemical analyses relevant to the diagnosis and management of human genetic diseases and who acts as a consultant regarding laboratory diagnosis of a broad range of biochemical genetic disorders.

These requirements imply that the individual possesses

- the ability to supervise and direct the operations of a clinical biochemical genetics diagnostic laboratory, including technical expertise and knowledge in quality control and quality assessment procedures;
- broad knowledge of (1) basic biochemistry and genetics, (2) the application of biochemical techniques to the diagnosis and management of genetic diseases, and (3) the etiology, pathogenesis, clinical manifestations, and management of human inherited biochemical disorders;
- an understanding of the heterogeneity, variability, and natural history of biochemical genetic disorders;
- diagnostic and interpretive skills in a wide range of biochemical genetic problems; and
- the ability to communicate biochemical laboratory results in the capacity of consultant to medical genetics professionals and other clinicians, and directly to patients in concert with other professional staff.

Clinical Cytogeneticist

A clinical cytogeneticist is an individual with a US- or Canadian-earned, or the equivalent of an earned, doctoral degree (MD, DO, PhD) who can correctly perform and interpret cytogenetic analyses relevant to the diagnosis and management of human genetic diseases, and who acts as a consultant regarding laboratory diagnosis for a broad range of cytogenetic disorders, including inherited and acquired conditions.

These requirements imply that the individual possesses

- the ability to supervise and direct the operations of a clinical cytogenetic diagnostic laboratory and has technical expertise and knowledge in quality control and quality assessment procedures;
- broad knowledge in human cytogenetics, including prenatal and postnatal cytogenetic diagnosis, infertility and pregnancy loss, cancer, and leukemia;
- an understanding of the heterogeneity, variability, and natural history of cytogenetic disorders;
- diagnostic and interpretive skills in a wide range of cytogenetic problems; and
- the ability to communicate cytogenetic laboratory results in the capacity of consultant to medical genetics professionals and other clinicians and directly to patients in concert with other professional staff.

Clinical Molecular Geneticist

A clinical molecular geneticist is an individual with a US- or Canadian-earned, or the equivalent of an earned, doctoral degree (MD, DO, PhD) who can correctly perform and interpret molecular analyses relevant to the diagnosis and management of human genetic diseases and who can act as a consultant regarding laboratory diagnosis of a broad range of molecular genetic disorders.

These requirements imply that the individual possesses

- the ability to supervise and direct the operations of a clinical molecular genetics diagnostic laboratory and has technical experience and knowledge in quality control and quality assessment procedures;
- the ability to perform a variety of molecular diagnostic assays;
- an understanding of the heterogeneity, variability, and natural history of molecular genetic disorders;
- a broad knowledge of (1) basic molecular biology and genetics; (2) the application of recombinant DNA techniques and linkage analysis to the diagnosis of genetic diseases; and (3) the etiology,

pathogenesis, clinical manifestations, and management of human genetic disorders;
- diagnostic and interpretive skills in a wide range of clinical molecular genetics problems; and
- the ability to communicate molecular diagnostic laboratory results in the capacity of a consultant to medical genetics professionals and other clinicians and directly to patients in concert with other professional staff.

American Board of Neurological Surgery

6550 Fannin St/Ste 2139
Houston, TX 77030-2701
713 790-6015
713 794-0207 Fax
E-mail: abns@tmh.tmc.edu
Internet: http://www.abns.org

(These criteria and conditions are subject to change without notice. All applicants are advised to contact the American Board of Neurological Surgery to ascertain whether the information below is current.)

Diplomates

A list of diplomates and the bylaws of the American Board of Neurological Surgery (ABNS) appear in the *Official American Board of Medical Specialties Directory of Board Certified Medical Specialists,* which can be obtained from Marquis Who's Who, Inc (121 Chanlon Rd, New Providence, NJ 07974). In addition, a list of new diplomates is published in the *Journal of Neurosurgery* shortly after each examination.

Information regarding training programs acceptable for certification can be found in the *Graduate Medical Education Directory*. This directory can be purchased from the American Medical Association (515 N State St, Chicago, IL 60610).

Qualifications

The ABNS evaluates all qualified applicants for their proficiency in neurosurgery.

The minimum educational requirements of the Board should not be interpreted as restricting programs to these standards. If necessary, neurosurgical program directors may retain residents in their programs beyond the required 5 years of residency training in order to ensure satisfactory competence in neurosurgery.

It is the responsibility of the candidate to seek information concerning current requirements for certification by the ABNS. Even though directors of approved neurosurgical residency programs are well informed regarding requirements for certification, placement in an approved program does not guarantee adequate training for certification. The candidate must make sure he/she receives such training.

Training Prior to Neurosurgery Residency

1. Graduation from a medical school that is acceptable to the Board.
2. Currently valid license to practice medicine in the state, province, or country of residence.

3. Twelve months devoted to acquiring adequate knowledge of fundamental clinical skills. This is known as postgraduate year one (PGY1), general surgery year one, or internship; it is recommended for completion prior to beginning neurosurgical training but must be completed prior to beginning the third year of that training. This may be achieved by 1 year of training in an Accreditation Council for Graduate Medical Education (ACGME)-accredited general surgery program in the United States or, for applicants entering training programs prior to July 16, 1997, a Canadian equivalent. It may also be acquired during the course of training in an ACGME-accredited neurosurgical residency program in the US or, for applicants entering training programs prior to July 16, 1997, a Canadian equivalent. Such training must include not less than 6 months in surgical disciplines other than neurosurgery; the remaining 6 months should include fundamental clinical skills considered appropriate by the program director, but this portion may not include more than 6 weeks of neurosurgery; it may include up to 3 months of neurology.

Neurological Surgery Training Requirements

For residents beginning the neurosurgery portion of their training on or after July 1, 1979:

1. Completion of 5 years of training following PGY1. Neurosurgery training must occur in residency programs accredited by the Residency Review Committee for Neurosurgery or, for applicants entering training prior to July 16, 1997, its Canadian equivalent.
2. The 60 months of training must include at least 36 months of clinical neurosurgery in accredited programs; 12 months of this period must be served as a senior resident.
3. The training in clinical neurosurgery must be progressive and not obtained during repeated short intervals in a number of institutions. At least 24 months of training in clinical neurosurgery must be obtained in one institution.
4. At least 3 months must be devoted to training in clinical neurology. Six months is recommended. This training may be undertaken during PGY1.
5. The unobligated 21 months may be devoted to neuropathology, neuroradiology, basic neurosciences, research, or other disciplines related to neurological surgery.
6. Rotations by residents outside of their neurosurgical residency program may be arranged by the respective training program directors with the consent of the Board. In such instances, the secretary of the Board must be notified of the rotation prospectively. Such training may in no way compromise the 36 months of core neurosurgery. Training in any institution other than in the parent institution and its affiliated hospitals will not be considered as counting toward the requirements unless specified in advance by the program director and approved in writing by the Board.
7. The program director must notify the Board of the appointment of each new neurosurgical resident and whether he/she is entering the program with intent to obtain certification and, if so, whether the director has informed the trainee of the requirements necessary to obtain such certification.
8. Residents in training after June 30, 1983, are required to record, in a fashion determined by the Board, their operative procedures.
9. Prior to acceptance for the certification process, the Board requires a statement from the candidate's program director to the effect that the candidate has met the minimum time requirements, has performed in training in a satisfactory manner, and, in the judgment of the program director, is well prepared to enter into the independent practice of neurosurgery.

Exceptional Modifying Circumstances

Upon recommendation of the program director and ratification by the Board, credit may be given for previous training if a candidate

1. before entering an approved neurosurgical training program, has had substantially more than the prerequisite training in general surgery, medical neurology, or the basic neurological sciences (such credit must be approved by the Board);
2. transfers from one approved neurosurgical training program to another approved program
   a. with the consent of the directors of both programs, or
   b. without the consent of one of the program directors, but with the approval of the Board.

In both cases, the director of the program from which the candidate transfers must indicate in writing to the new program director the credit for training, in time and category, that he/she is prepared to certify that the candidate has successfully completed. A copy of such statement must be submitted to the secretary of the Board. The new program director may or may not honor such credit, depending upon appraisal of the resident's professional and educational progress in the new program; a statement of how much training credit will be accepted must also be submitted to the secretary of the Board.

Requests for training away from a parent institution or for transfer from one program to another should be submitted in writing to the Board prospectively, not retroactively.

Training by preceptorship is not considered as fulfilling certification requirements. No credit is given for time spent in such training.

Credit for elective training in foreign or other nonapproved centers may be granted by the Board on an individual basis when this training is carried out as an integral part of the training program and with the advice and approval of the candidate's program director. The Board must be informed of such a rotation prior to its occurrence (see 6 under "Neurological Surgery Training Requirements").

The above provisions in no way alter the basic minimum requirement of 60 months of residency training in neurosurgery, including a minimum of 3 months of training in clinical neurology and 36 months of clinical neurosurgery in accredited institutions, 12 months of which must be as senior resident and 24 months in one institution.

Primary Examination

Each applicant for the Board's oral examination must first pass for credit the primary examination, which is a written examination prepared by the Board with the assistance of a professional testing organization. The examination includes information on neuroanatomy, neurobiology, neurochemistry, neurology, neuropathology, neuropharmacology, neurophysiology, neuroradiology, neurosurgery, fundamental clinical skills, critical care, and material from other relevant disciplines deemed suitable and important by the Board.

The primary examination is given in March each year at training programs throughout the United States and Canada. Residents in accredited training programs may take it for self-assessment or credit toward certification at the discretion of their program directors. It is also open for all neurosurgeons who have successfully completed training at accredited programs; they may take it as often as desired for self-assessment or credit. An application must be filed to take the primary examination. The deadline for receipt of this application by the Board is the first of January. The form must be accompanied by the fee set by the Board. This fee will be refunded only if the candidate informs the secretary's office prior to the deadline date for receipt of applications that he/she is not going to sit for the examination. Examinees are required to sign a pledge that states that they agree to be bound by the Board's ruling regarding credentials, irrespective of scores on the examination. By signing the pledge, candidates also grant permission to the ABNS and its testing organization to release the results, either for credit or self-assessment, to the examinee's program director, and they pledge not to reproduce or copy the examination in any form in part or in whole.

Practice Requirements

After beginning practice, the candidate shall furnish to the Board the names of three physicians in the community (two neurosurgeons, including one ABNS diplomate) who are knowledgeable about the quality of the candidate's practice. The Board will request reference letters from these physicians and other physicians in the candidate's community. It is the prerogative of the Board to send representatives to review the candidate's practice.

In addition, the candidate shall submit the names and addresses of each hospital where the candidate has or has had privileges. Letters will be requested to advise the Board of the candidate's status regarding admitting and operating privileges in each hospital where he/she practices. At the time of credentialing, each candidate must be in possession of hospital staff privileges in all hospitals in which he/she cares for patients. Such privileges must be unrestricted in respect to the hospital's requirements for a neurosurgeon.

The candidate must also forward to the Board a typewritten, chronological list of all inpatients for whom he/she has been the responsible physician or surgeon for a current, 12-consecutive-month period. The total experience must be tabulated by the candidate in a format defined by the Board. The case material must be accompanied by a form signed by the chief of staff, chief of service, president of the medical staff, or hospital administrator of each hospital where the candidate practices in verification of the essential accuracy of the data. These data must be approved by the Board prior to scheduling for oral examination. Candidates are responsible for retaining duplicate copies of these records.

Candidates must be scheduled for oral examination by the Board within 5 years of completing an accredited training program. Compliance with this regulation requires early submission of applications for oral examination and certification after training. If a candidate cannot be scheduled within the 5-year limit due to late submission of an application, he/she must once again pass the primary examination for credit before being scheduled for oral examination within the succeeding 3-year period. Candidates should also keep in mind that usually 12 months are required between submission of a complete application and oral examination.

Certification of Those Training in Canadian Programs

Those who began neurological residency training in approved Canadian programs before July 16, 1997, and who satisfactorily completed such training, and who hold a fellowship in neurosurgery from the Royal College of Physicians and Surgeons (Canada) are eligible for certification through the same route as candidates training in the United States, as outlined above.

Applications

Applications for oral examination and certification are automatically sent to residents in July after their last year of training. Additional applications and practice data information are available from the Board's office. The entire application and data should be filled out and returned to the Board as soon as possible after beginning practice.

A pledge is part of the application for oral examination. By signing the application, the applicant agrees to abide by all Bylaws and Rules and Regulations of the Board.

Upon receipt of an application, the Board takes such steps as deemed appropriate to verify the statements of facts made in the application. Inquiries are made from references and others familiar with the candidate to obtain information relevant to the requirements for examination. The Board makes the final decision regarding a candidate's eligibility for oral examination and potential certification after considering all available information pertaining to the entire process of certification.

Application fees, once received, will not be refunded.

Oral Examination

The oral examination, a clinical problem-solving and patient-management examination, is given twice a year. Candidates are given case histories and, where appropriate, x-rays, scans, and other visual aids to augment the presentation and development of cases. The candidate must be able to explain verbally how he/she would proceed in evaluating and managing a case, and in planning and performing any proposed operation or operations, if indicated. One hour is devoted to neurological surgery-intracranial diseases; 1 hour to neurological surgery-spinal and peripheral nerve diseases; and 1 hour to a mixture. Neurosurgical neurology is included in all sections. Each of the 3 hours is conducted in an interview setting with two examiners.

A candidate who passes the oral examination and is thereby certified will be forwarded the Board's certificate, once it has been suitably engrossed and signed by the officers of the Board.

Reexamination Rules

A candidate failing the oral examination once may request reexamination within 3 years. A minimum of 1 year must elapse before taking the examination for the second time. The examination fee must be paid.

A candidate who has failed the oral examination on two or more occasions must pass the primary examination for credit again before becoming eligible to retake the oral examination. Two letters of reference from neurosurgeons certifying the nature and quality of the candidate's practice must be submitted to the Board, as well as hospital privilege letters and a year of current practice data. In addition, the candidate must pay the oral examination fee. Under these circumstances, candidates must take the oral exam within 3 years of repassing the primary examination. Should the candidate not apply for or fail to appear for oral examination within the 3-year period, the candidate must repass the primary examination before being eligible for the oral examination once again.

Payment of Fees

Fees for filing an application and for oral examination will be determined by the Board. They reflect costs that the Board incurs through obligations associated with the certification process. The application fee will not be returned even when the application for examination is denied.

Revocation of Certification

Pursuant to the rules and regulations established by the ABNS, the Board has the authority to revoke any certificate issued by it for various reasons, including: the person to whom the certificate was issued is convicted of a felony, or his/her license to practice medicine has been lost or encumbered, or false information was given on the application for oral examination and certification. Should revocation be disputed, there is a hearing mechanism for such an action.

American Board of Nuclear Medicine

900 Veteran Ave
Los Angeles, CA 90024-1786
310 825-6787
310 825-9433 Fax

(These criteria and conditions are subject to change without notice. All applicants are advised to contact the American Board of Nuclear Medicine [ABNM] to ascertain whether the information below is current.)

General Requirements for Each Candidate

Assurance that the applicant represents himself/herself to be a specialist in nuclear medicine.

General Professional Education

Graduation from a medical school approved by the Liaison Committee on Medical Education or from a school of osteopathy. If the applicant is a graduate of a medical school outside the United States or Canada, he/she must hold a currently valid ECFMG certificate issued by the Educational Commission for Foreign Medical Graduates, 3624 Market St, Philadelphia, PA 19104-2685; 215 386-5900.

Preparatory Postdoctoral Training

Training required for admission to the certifying examination in nuclear medicine shall comprise 1 or more years of preparatory postdoctoral training and 2 or more years of residency training in nuclear medicine.

Preparatory postdoctoral training shall consist of 1 or more years of residency training in programs satisfactory to the ABNM. Such programs shall provide broad experience in clinical medicine in which the primary emphasis is on the patient and his/her clinical problems. Preparatory training may be in any specialty in a residency program in the United States approved by the Accreditation Council for Graduate Medical Education (ACGME) or in programs in Canada approved by the Royal College of Physicians and Surgeons of Canada (RCPSC) or the Professional Corporation of Physicians of Quebec (PCPQ). One year of preparatory postdoctoral training must precede training in nuclear medicine.

Each nuclear medicine residency training program director must ensure that for each resident entering his or her program the preparatory postdoctoral training has been in a United States program approved by the ACGME or in a Canadian program approved by the RCPSC or the PCPQ.

Special Postdoctoral Training in Nuclear Medicine

1. After completion of the preparatory postdoctoral training programs, there shall be satisfactory completion of a 2-year formal residency training program in nuclear medicine in a nuclear medicine residency training program recognized and approved by the Residency Review Committee (RRC) for Nuclear Medicine of the ACGME or in a Canadian program approved by the RCPSC or the PCPQ as competent to provide a satisfactory training in nuclear medicine.
2. The 2-year formal residency training program in nuclear medicine must include the following:
   a. Training in clinical nuclear medicine that will include, but not be limited to, performance and interpretation of in vivo imaging studies of body organs and systems using radiopharmaceuticals; training and experience in the application of nonimaging procedures, including radioimmunoassay and receptor assay technology; radiopharmaceutical absorption, dilution, excretion, and organ function studies; and therapeutic uses of unsealed radiopharmaceuticals, including patient selection, dosimetry, and dose administration in the treatment of cancer, hematologic and metabolic disorders. In vivo studies will include use of external detectors and scintillation cameras, including single-photon tomography and positron emission tomography; cardiovascular nuclear medicine procedures, including exercise and pharmacologic stress testing, as well as management of cardiac emergencies related to such testing; and correlation of nuclear medicine procedures with other imaging modalities such as computed tomography, ultrasonography, nuclear magnetic resonance imaging, and angiography.
   b. Training in basic and allied sciences that will include medical nuclear physics; instrumentation; radiopharmaceutical chemistry, including reactor, cyclotron, and generator production of radionuclides; computer sciences; statistics; radiation biology; and radiation safety, including safe management and disposal of radioactive substances. Training in allied sciences may include pathology, physiology, and other basic sciences associated with nuclear medicine. The time spent in training in allied sciences may be spaced throughout the period of training in nuclear medicine and in a manner that does not exceed 6 months of training.
   c. For applicants who have completed residency training programs in clinical disciplines closely related to nuclear medicine in residency programs approved by the ACGME, the RCPSC, or the PCPQ, credit may be given for some of that training. Applicants desiring credit toward the nuclear medicine requirement should write to the Board requesting such credit.
   d. Applicants who have completed an accredited program in diagnostic radiology, which includes 6 months of nuclear medicine training, 3 months of correlative imaging, and 3 months of basic science, may apply to take the examination upon completion of a further 12 months of nuclear medicine training in an accredited nuclear medicine program. All training must be accredited by the ACGME, RCPSC, or PCPQ.

      Applicants who have completed an accredited program in internal medicine/cardiology, which includes 3 months in the clinical subspecialties of internal medicine, 3 months of invasive cardiology, and 6 months of noninvasive cardiology (with an emphasis on nuclear cardiology), may apply to take the examination upon completion of a further 12 months of nuclear medicine training (with an emphasis on noncardiac aspects of nuclear medicine) in an accredited nuclear medicine program. All training must be in programs accredited by the ACGME, RCPSC, or PCPQ.

      Credit for training taken in diagnostic radiology and cardiology must be reviewed and approved by the Board. Applicants requesting credit for such training must provide details of the training to the Board.

3. Evaluation of clinical training in nuclear medicine: The Board considers demonstration of clinical competence in the management of the nuclear medicine patient of paramount importance in its qualification of the applicant to take the certifying examination. The Board designates the directors of nuclear medicine residency programs and their supporting evaluation committees as the authorities who most appropriately can provide to the Board the necessary documentation of competence in clinical nuclear medicine and also requires that all program directors certify to the Board that each applicant from their programs is competent in clinical nuclear medicine. These reports will be reviewed by the Board before accepting an applicant to take the certifying examination.

If a residency program director's evaluation indicates that an applicant's competence in clinical nuclear medicine is unsatisfactory, the applicant will not be admitted to the examination unless the Board finds that the applicant's overall performance meets its standards. An applicant not admitted to an examination on the basis of these findings may appeal in writing to the Board for a special evaluation of competence in clinical nuclear medicine within 45 days of receipt of notification. The appeal should state that a request is made for review of the decision not to admit to the examination and why the applicant considers the decision to be in error. Applicants whose clinical competence is judged satisfactory in this evaluation will be admitted to the next examination for which they apply. Applicants judged not satisfactory in this evaluation are advised to spend an additional year training before applying again for special evaluation of competence.

Applicants submitting false credentials are subject to disqualification from examination or revocation of certification.

Patient Care Responsibility

Applicants for certification in nuclear medicine will have 1 or more years of training in which the primary emphasis is on the patient and his/her clinical problems.

Canadian Training

Physicians who satisfactorily complete training in Canadian nuclear medicine programs approved by the RCPSC or the PCPQ are eligible for admission to the ABNM certifying examinations.

Completion of Training

All preliminary and nuclear medicine residency training must be completed prior to September 1 of the year the candidate takes the certifying examination.

Licensure Requirement

A valid, unrestricted license to practice medicine in a state, territory, possession, or province of the United States or Canada will be required of all applicants for the certifying or recertifying examinations. If a candidate is licensed in more than one such jurisdiction, each license must be valid and unrestricted. A photocopy of every license held by the candidate must be submitted to the Board.

Approved Residency Training Programs

Residency training programs in nuclear medicine accredited by the ACGME may be found in the *Graduate Medical Education Directory*, published annually by the American Medical Association, or may be obtained by contacting the Secretary, Residency Review Committee for Nuclear Medicine, ACGME, 515 N State St/Ste 2000, Chicago, IL 60610.

Admissibility to Examination

An applicant is admissible to the examination only when all of the preliminary and graduate educational requirements of the Board currently in force at the time of receipt of the formal application have been satisfactorily fulfilled and deemed acceptable.

Examination

An objective type examination is administered in a morning and an afternoon session. The examination evaluates the applicant's knowledge of and competence in the management of patients in the area of clinical nuclear medicine, including, but not limited to, radioassay/radiobioassay, in vitro and in vivo measurements, nuclear imaging, the principles of nuclear magnetic resonance imaging, therapy with unsealed radionuclides, the medical effects of exposure to ionizing radiation, the medical management of persons exposed to ionizing radiation, radiation safety, and the safe management and disposal of radioactive substances. Also included is an evaluation of the candidate's knowledge in the related sciences of medical nuclear physics, radiation biology, radiation protection, instrumentation, radiopharmaceutical chemistry, computer sciences, and statistics; the examination may also include pathology, physiology, and other basic sciences associated with nuclear medicine.

Applications

Applicants who wish to be examined by the Board must complete, sign, and file with the Board office an application on the official form together with the supporting data required by the application. It is the responsibility of the applicant to make certain that the required evaluation forms have been completed by his/her program director and sent to and received by the ABNM.

As soon as determination is made concerning admission or nonadmission to the examination, the applicant will be notified by mail, and, if admitted, assignment of the candidate number and notification of the examination site will be given. Applications must be complete with *all* required documentation by August 1.

Before the final action on applications, officers, members, and employees of the Board are not authorized to estimate the eligibility of applicants. Applicants are requested not to discuss or write for opinions regarding the status of their applications. The Board decides on eligibility to take the examination only by approving or disapproving individual applications and accordingly has no "Board-eligible" category.

Inquiries concerning the applicability of previous training and experience should be sent with complete documentation of all education and training to the Board office. A copy of the Board's response to these inquiries should be forwarded with any subsequent examination application.

Release of Information

Candidates will receive the results of their examinations (pass/fail letter) approximately 4 months after the examination.

A list of diplomates of the ABNM will be found in the *Official American Board of Medical Specialties Directory of Board Certified Medical Specialists*, published by the American Board of Medical Specialties and Marquis Who's Who.

Upon request, and with the approval of the Board chairman, the Board releases information on diplomates to federal and state licensing bodies and to educational and professional organizations for specific, limited, and appropriate professional use. An authorization for release of this information is a part of the examination application form.

Policy on Reexamination

Candidates who fail the examination are eligible for reexamination. An examination fee must accompany each completed application for reexamination. If a candidate is disqualified from the examination by reason of dishonesty in the application or in taking the examination and his/her examination is invalidated by the Board, reexamination shall be at the Board's discretion.

Recertification

The ABNM offers its diplomates voluntary recertification based upon fulfillment of certain requirements, including passing an objective cognitive examination. The ABNM will not rescind initial certification granted prior to 1992. Beginning in 1992 certification will be valid for a period of 10 years and may be revalidated by recertification.

Journals Publishing Information on Application and Examination Schedules

Annals of Internal Medicine (Medical News Section)
Journal of the American Medical Association (Examinations and Licensure Monthly Section)
Journal of Nuclear Medicine
Radiology
Journal of Clinical Pathology

Changes in Policies and Procedures

The Board reserves the right to make changes in its fees, policies, and procedures at any time and cannot assume responsibility for giving advance notice thereof. The provisions of this publication are not to be construed as a contract between any candidate and the ABNM.

Fees

The examination fee must accompany the application. If the applicant is rejected by the Board or withdraws prior to August 1, the application processing fee will be retained by the Board. If the applicant withdraws after August 1, the entire examination fee will be retained by the Board.

American Board of Obstetrics and Gynecology

2915 Vine St/Ste 300
Dallas, TX 75204
214 871-1619
214 871-1943 Fax

Gerson Weiss, MD, President, Newark, New Jersey
Philip J DiSaia, MD, Vice President, Orange, California
William Droegemueller, MD, Director of Evaluation, Chapel Hill, North Carolina
Ronald S Gibbs, MD, Treasurer, Denver, Colorado
Robert C Cefalo, MD, PhD, Chairman of the Board, Chapel Hill, North Carolina
Haywood L Brown, MD, Indianapolis, Indiana
Alan H DeCherney, MD, Los Angeles, California
Sharon L Dooley, MD, MPH, Chicago, Illinois
Sherman Elias, MD, Chicago, Illinois
Wesley C Fowler, Jr, MD, Chapel Hill, North Carolina
Larry C Gilstrap III, MD, Houston, Texas
Arthur F Haney, MD, Durham, North Carolina
Michael T Mennuti, MD, Philadelphia, Pennsylvania
Kenneth L Noller, MD, Worcester, Massachusetts
Valerie M Parisi, MD, MPH, Chapel Hill, North Carolina
Donald K Rahhal, MD, Oklahoma City, Oklahoma
Morton A Stenchever, MD, , Seattle, Washington
Norman F Gant, MD, Executive Director, Dallas, Texas
Alvin L Brekken, MD, Assistant to the Executive Director, Dallas, Texas
Laurie Daniels, Assistant Executive Director, Dallas, Texas
Deborah L Burkett, EdD, Educational Associate, Troup, Texas
Barry Hornburg, Systems Analyst

Division of Gynecologic Oncology
Philip J DiSaia, MD, Director and Representative
Patricia Braly, MD
Larry J Copeland, MD
William J Hoskins, MD
Stephen C Rubin, MD, PhD

Division of Maternal and Fetal Medicine
Valerie M Parisi, MD, Director and Representative
Eleanor L Capeless, MD
Thomas J Garite, MD
Ronald S Gibbs, MD
Michael L Socol, MD

Division of Reproductive Endocrinology
Arthur F Haney, MD, Director and Representative
Rogerio A Lobo, MD
James R Schreiber, MD
Daniel H Riddick, MD
Nanette Santoro, MD

Urogynecology/Reconstructive Pelvic Surgery Committee
Morton A Stenchever, MD, Director and Representative
Richard C Bump, MD
Wesley C Fowler, Jr, MD
Nicolette S Horbach, MD
Raymond A Lee, MD

(These criteria and conditions are subject to change without notice. All applicants are advised to contact the American Board of Obstetrics and Gynecology to ascertain whether the information below is current.)

Types of Board Status

Residency Graduate

An individual is registered with the Board when, upon application, the Board rules that he/she has fulfilled the requirements to take the written examination (see "Requirements" for the written examination).

Active Candidate

1. An individual achieves active candidate status by passing the written examination.
2. To maintain active candidate status, the candidate must fulfill all requirements for admission to the oral examination and must not have exceeded the *limitations* to admissibility for the oral examination (see "Limitations").
3. Active candidate status that has expired may be regained by repeating and passing the Board's written examination.

Diplomate

1. An individual becomes a diplomate of the Board when the written and the oral examinations have been satisfactorily completed and the Board's certifying diploma has been awarded.
2. Certificates have limited duration of validity. Certificates will bear a limiting date of 10 years, after which they are no longer valid. Each diplomate must be evaluated again to receive a new certificate.

Expired Certificate

1. An individual has failed to complete successfully a certificate renewal examination prior to the expiration date printed on their time-limited certifying diploma.
2. Individuals in this category are *not* diplomates of the American Board of Obstetrics and Gynecology.

Certification Process

Certification as a specialist in obstetrics and gynecology is the end of a process lasting many years. The required minimum duration of graduate education is 4 years.

Written Examination

During the final year of graduate training, it is necessary to initiate certain measures. Candidates due to complete their graduate training program prior to September 30 should, between September 1 and November 30 of the final year of residency, request and complete the application for the written examination. If ruled admissible to take the examination, the candidate will do so in June of the final year of residency.

For candidates who will complete their residency training after September 30, application for the written examination must be delayed until the following year. If ruled admissible to take the examination, the candidate will do so in June of the following year.

Oral Examination

To be ruled admissible to take the oral examination, candidates are required to provide a list of patients under their care for a 12-month period beginning on July 1 of the second year of practice after the written examination is passed. After November 1 of this second year of practice and before the following February 28, candidates should request and complete the application (November 1-February 28).

The candidate's list of patients must be mailed to the Board office between July 1 and August 1, following the completion of the 12-month period of patient care. The case lists should not be mailed until the candidate is notified of approval to submit their case list. If ruled admissible, the candidate thus takes the subspecialty oral examination in November.

Important Dates in the Certification Process

A. Final Year of Residency

July 1—Commence
September 1 to November 30—Apply for written examination
June—Take written examination

B. Practice

1. First year of practice
   No Board activities necessary
2. Second year of practice
   July 1 to June 30—Patient list
   November 1 to February 28—Apply for oral examination
3. Third year of practice
   August 15—Deadline for submission of patient list
   November—Take oral examination

C. Fellowship in Subspecialty

1. First year (fellowship)
   No Board activities
2. Second year (fellowship)
   No basic Board activities
   September 1 to November 30—Apply for subspecialty written examination
3. Third year—First year of practice
   January 1 to February 28—Apply for the oral examination
   January 1 to December 31—Patient list
4. Fourth year—Second year of practice
   January 1—Deadline for submission of thesis
   February 1—Deadline for submission of patient list
   March or April—Take oral examination

Responsibility of a Candidate

It is the responsibility of the candidate to seek information concerning the current requirements for certification as an obstetrician and gynecologist. The Board does not assume responsibility for notifying a candidate of changing requirements or the impending loss of a candidate's admissibility to an examination.

Duration of Certificate Validity

Certificates have a limited valid duration of 10 years, after which they are no longer valid. Each diplomate must undergo a Board-approved method of certificate renewal in order to receive a new certificate.

Certificate Renewal

A certificate renewal and a voluntary recertification evaluation process are available for diplomates certified by this Board. Participation for some may be voluntary, but beginning in 1986, 10-year time-limited certificates were issued by the Board. Thus, for continued certification, diplomates certified in or after 1986 must renew their certification at least every 10 years.

Certificate renewal or voluntary recertification may be achieved in one of three different ways. These methods are

1. a cognitive written examination; or
2. a 1 ½-hour oral examination; or
3. Annual Board Certification (ABC), a continuous certificate renewal, achieved by reviews of assigned scientific and/or clinical publications.

More specific information can be obtained about these methods of certificate renewal/voluntary recertification by *writing* the executive director at the Board address.

Fees

The application fee for the written or the oral examination is due with the application. This fee is $560. Additionally, an examination fee of $400 is due prior to either the written or the oral examination. The fees for the Annual Board Certification (ABC), a form of continuous certification, will be $150 per year for general obstetrics and gynecology and $200 per year for subspecialists (includes general and subspecialty items).

An application form and application fee are required for each cycle of the written or the oral examination and are not refundable.

Written Examination

The written examination is a 3-hour 20-minute examination consisting of questions of the objective (multiple-choice) type. Questions will be chosen from each of the following areas of knowledge:

1. Basic science
2. Endocrinology, fertility
3. Primary/preventive medicine
4. Clinical gynecology
5. Clinical obstetrics
6. Medical, surgical, and psychiatric diseases in the nonpregnant woman and medical, surgical, and psychiatric diseases in pregnancy and complications of pregnancy
7. Oncology and pathology

The candidate will be expected to demonstrate skills necessary to apply basic knowledge to the management of clinical problems.

These skills include:

1. Obtaining needed information
2. Interpretation and use of data obtained
3. Selecting, instituting, and implementing care
4. Management of complications
5. Following and continuing care

The areas of information and skills examined are further outlined in *Educational Objectives for Resident Education in Obstetrics and Gynecology*, published by the Council on Resident Education in Obstetrics and Gynecology.

Requirements

1. Degree of doctor of medicine, or an equivalent degree, and unrestricted license (an educational or institutional license will suffice) to practice medicine in all states or territories of the United States or a province of Canada in which the candidate holds a license.

   The requirement of unrestricted license must have been met prior to the time that the application is submitted. An educational or institutional license is satisfactory.

   Candidates with a DO degree must have graduated from a school of osteopathy accredited by the American Osteopathic Association.
2. The candidate will be required to have completed or be near completion (see "Application for Examination in 1999") of no less than 4 years in clinical programs accredited by the Accreditation Council for Graduate Medical Education (ACGME) or no less than 5 years in clinical obstetrical or gynecological programs accredited by the Council of the Royal College of Physicians and Surgeons of Canada. This must include at least 36 months of obstetrics and gynecology, including the usual time as chief (senior) resident in the program. Completion of a year of GY1 plus a 3-year residency program or a 4-year residency program will fulfill this requirement, but if the program consists of more than 4 years, the entire program must be completed.

   Time spent in an osteopathic hospital or in any program not accredited by the ACGME will not fulfill this requirement.
3. A statement signed by the program director certifying that the candidate has
   A. followed satisfactorily the course of instruction designed for this program;
   B. taken leaves of absence and vacation not exceeding 8 weeks in any of the first 3 years, 6 weeks in the final year, or 20 weeks total for the overall 4-year period;
   C. completed and submitted to the program director a satisfactory resident experience log;
   D. achieved the appropriate knowledge, ability, and judgment in order to provide competent clinical care in obstetrics and gynecology, as documented by ongoing evaluation during the entire resident program; and
   E. demonstrated the necessary technical skills to competently perform
      1. major abdominal and vaginal surgical procedures on the female pelvis and related structures;
      2. spontaneous and operative obstetric deliveries;
      3. surgical exploration of the abdomen;
      4. endoscopic procedures of proven value in the pelvis;
      5. diagnostic evaluation, including electronic monitoring, ultrasound, colposcopy, and amniocentesis;
      6. diagnosis and treatment of complications of the above; and
      7. demonstrated good moral and ethical character.

Application for Examination in 1999

A candidate who has completed an accredited residency program and a candidate scheduled to complete an accredited residency program on or before September 30, 1999, may apply on or before November 30, 1998, to write the examination on June 28, 1999.

The requirement of an unrestricted license must have been met prior to the time that the application is submitted. An educational or institutional license is satisfactory.

The form on which to apply to write the examination on June 28, 1999, may be obtained by writing to the Board office after September 1, 1998. Each applicant must meet the requirements effective in the year of requested admission to the examination. As a part of the application form, endorsement and verification of the resident's experience, competence, satisfactory performance, and confirmation of the scheduled date for completion of the candidate's residency are required to be affirmed by the current director of the obstetric and gynecologic residency program.

The Board will make the final decision concerning the applicant's admission to the examination after considering all circumstances affecting the application.

A candidate's application to write the examination on June 28, 1999, completed in all details, together with payment of the application fee, must be received in the Board office before November 30, 1998. Application fees must accompany the application. Application fees sent prior to the mailing of an application are subject to late charges. A copy of the candidate's current license registration also is required.

Late fees will be applied to applicants who have not submitted all required materials by November 30, 1998.

The candidate ruled admissible to the examination will be notified by April 15

1. that the examination is scheduled to be written in June;
2. that the examination fee is payable and the date the fee must be paid; and
3. that two 2x2-inch photographs should accompany the examination fee.

If a candidate has not been contacted by the board by May 3, 1999, concerning admissibility for the June 28, 1999, written examination, it is *the candidate's* responsibility to contact the Board office in writing or by fax no later than May 10, 1999, in order to ascertain why they have not received notification. It also is the candidate's responsibility to inform the Board of a change of address in writing in order to receive notifications in a timely manner.

If a candidate is found to be involved in litigation or investigation regarding ethical or moral issues, the application will be reviewed. Typically, the Credentials Committee will defer a decision for entry to the examination to gain further information.

Falsification of data (including case lists) or evidence of other egregious ethical, moral, or professional misbehavior may result in a deferral of a candidate's application for at least 3 years. The candidate must meet all eligibility requirements in effect at the end of the deferred period.

When the Credentials Committee rules an applicant not admissible to the written examination, a new application and fee must be submitted for the next examination. The candidate must fulfill the requirements in effect the year of the new application.

Admission to the Written Examination

The candidate ruled admissible to the examination will be sent an "Authorization for Admission" form, which must be presented to the proctor at the time and place of examination. When a candidate is scheduled to complete residency, after submission of the application (but before October of that year), verification that the candidate is completing residency in a satisfactory manner must be reaffirmed by the signature of the director of the residency program on the Authorization for Admission form, dated within the month the candidate is scheduled to write the examination.

Results of the Examination

The results of the written examination will be reported confidentially to each candidate within 9 weeks from the date of the examination.

A passing grade on the written examination does not ensure a candidate's admissibility to the oral examination for certification, nor does it allow the use of the term "Board eligible." The term "Board eligible" is *not* approved by the Board for any individual seeking Board certification or for those who have only completed residency training. An individual who has completed residency training, but not yet passed the written examination, should be referred to as a "residency graduate." An individual who has passed the written examination should be referred to as an "active candidate."

Requests for Reexamination

A candidate previously scheduled to write the examination who does not do so, as well as the candidate who writes but does not pass the examination, must write the Board office after September 1 to request reapplication materials for the next examination. It is necessary for each applicant to meet the requirements in effect the year of the requested admission to the examination. The reapplicant must have submitted completed reapplication materials, a copy of current license registration, and the reapplication fee prior to the November 30 deadline. There is no limit to the number of times a candidate may take a written examination.

The application and examination fees (see "Fees") must be paid each year a candidate is to be scheduled to write an examination.

Written Examination Fees

Fees have been computed to cover the costs of examination and administrative expenses. They will not, therefore, be refunded or credited. All fees must be paid in United States currency. The candidate's canceled check is to be considered the receipt.

The application fee must be enclosed with each application or reapplication to write the examination. The candidate will be notified by April 15 of the approval of the application or reapplication, at which time the examination fee will be due. If payment of the examination fee has not been *received* in the Board office on or before May 14, the candidate will not be scheduled to write the examination in June.

No application fees will be credited against a future application or refunded.

Examination fees may be refunded, provided candidates inform the Board office *in writing* of their inability to write the examination prior to May 14.

Dates, Deadlines, Fees, and Late Fees for Written Examination

September 1—November 30, 1998
Candidate must request in writing an application form

November 30, 1998
Application and application fee of $320 must be received in the Board office

December 1, 1998—January 29, 1999
Application, application fee ($320), and late fee ($215) must be received in the Board office

January 30, 1999—March 30, 1999
Application, application fee ($320), and late fee ($530) must be received in the Board office

April 1, 1999
No applications accepted after this date

April 15, 1999—May 15, 1999
Candidates notified to submit two 2x2 photographs and examination fee ($430)

May 14, 1999
No examination fees accepted after this date

June 28, 1999
Written examination at various sites

Oral Examination

All correspondence, applications, and information directed to the Board must be in English.

All fees must be paid in United States currency.

The oral examination is designed to evaluate the candidate's knowledge and ability to solve clinical problems in obstetrics and gynecology. It is emphasized that candidates will be examined in all areas of obstetrics and gynecology, to evaluate actual behavior in independent practice. More than half the examination will consist of questions concerning patient management problems. The candidate's list of patients will be used by the examiners for this purpose. In addition, other clinical problems will be included in the examination. The remainder of the examination will include basic knowledge in obstetrics and gynecology and interpretation of sonograms and Kodachromes of various conditions.

Slide projectors will be used. The knowledge required for passing the oral examination is the same as those categories listed in regard to the written examination.

Recording devices will not be permitted during the oral examination.

Candidates will be expected to demonstrate that they have acquired the capability to perform, independently, major gynecologic operations and spontaneous and operative obstetric deliveries, to manage the complications thereof, and to perform the essential diagnostic procedures required of a consultant in obstetrics and gynecology.

Candidates will be expected to demonstrate a level of competence that allows them to serve as consultants to physicians who are non-obstetrician-gynecologists in their community.

The report of the examining team will be reviewed by the Board of Directors, and each candidate is passed or failed by vote of the Board.

The examination will be completed within one-half day.

At the completion of the oral examination, if a candidate believes the examination has not been conducted in a fair and unprejudiced manner, a second examination may be requested. The request must be made within 1 hour. To do so, a candidate may go to a hotel phone and request to be connected to the offices of the Board within the hotel. If the request is granted

a. a second examination will be provided at the next regularly scheduled annual oral examination at no additional charge;

b. the repeat examination will be conducted by an entirely different team of examiners, no one of whom shall have previously participated in an examination of the candidate or know that this examination is being conducted as an appeal examination;

c. neither the questions nor the candidate's answers on the first examination will be known to or taken into account by the second group of examiners; and

d. the decision of the examiners conducting the second examination will determine the results of the candidate's oral examination.

Requirements

1. Passing grade on the written examination prior to making application for the oral examination.
2. Good moral and ethical character.
3. Unrestricted license to practice medicine in each state or territory (United States or a province of Canada) in which the candidate has held a medical license since at least February 28, 1998. An educational or institutional license does *not* meet this requirement.
4. A written explanation must be provided with the application of the circumstances involved if a candidate has ever had his/her medical license restricted or revoked in any territory, province, or state in the United States or Canada. A written explanation also must be provided with the application of the circumstances involved if a candidate has ever had his/her hospital practice terminated or restricted because of personal physical or mental impairments, excessive operative complications, or disciplinary reasons.
5. Actively engaged in unsupervised practice, defined as:
   a. Independent, continuous, unsupervised patient care in obstetrics and gynecology
      1. for at least the time from February 28, 1998, through June 30, 1999 (time spent in a critical care fellowship does not meet this requirement); or
      2. for at least the time from July 1, 1998, through June 30, 1999, for candidates who have successfully completed a Board-approved fellowship (this includes critical care fellowship *only* if taken in continuity with a Board-approved subspecialty fellowship).

   b. Unrestricted hospital privileges to practice as an obstetrician-gynecologist since at least February 28, 1998. Such privileges must be granted in each of the hospitals in which the candidate has been responsible for patient care during this time. If the candidate is under investigation or on probation, the examination will be deferred until the investigation is completed, the probation is lifted, and full and unrestricted privileges are granted.
6. Submission of typewritten lists (three copies) and summary sheets (seven copies), on or before August 1 preceding an examination, of all patients dismissed from care in all hospitals during the 12 months ending June 30 prior to the scheduled examination, and a list of 40 patients from office practice, unless a 24-month patient list is submitted.

   The candidate is personally responsible for the proper preparation, accuracy, and completeness of the case lists, which will reflect the unsupervised practice (private or nonprivate) activity following residency and fellowship.
7. On the day of the examination, the candidate will be expected to sign the following statement: "There have been no restrictions in my hospital privileges or restrictions placed on any license I have to practice medicine in any state or country since the date of my application." Candidates who are unable to sign this statement will not be admitted to the examination until and unless they present evidence that full and unrestricted privileges have been restored.
8. Practice that consists of ambulatory care exclusively will not be considered adequate to fulfill these requirements.
9. Candidates practicing in a country other than the United States or Canada must submit, with the application, a letter(s) from a senior responsible officer in the hospital(s) where the candidate practices, verifying the candidate's responsibility for independent, unsupervised care of obstetric and gynecologic patients.

Limitations

Duration of active candidate status is limited. Candidates must pass the oral examination within 6 years of passing the written examination and may take the oral examination only three times. Time spent in Board-approved fellowship training is excluded from this 6-year limitation. If a candidate fails the oral examination three times, or fails to pass the oral examination within 6 years, the candidate becomes ineligible to repeat the examination at that time. The candidate must repeat and pass the written examination to become admissible to the oral examination again. There is no limit to the number of times the written examination and the 6-year cycle to pass the oral examination can be repeated.

Determination of Qualifications

The Board will require, by confidential inquiry, documented evidence concerning a candidate's professional reputation, moral and ethical character, and in-hospital practice privileges from administrative officers of organizations and institutions to whom the candidate and his/her conduct of practice is known.

Time spent as a resident in excess of that necessary to fulfill the requirements to take the written examination is not acceptable. Time spent in a teaching or research appointment that does not involve appointment to the staff of an approved hospital with unrestricted privileges to practice as an obstetrician and gynecologist will not be sufficient evidence of responsibility for patient care, that is, acceptable to fulfill the requirement of "independent practice."

Each candidate will be required to furnish the Board with certain prescribed information concerning performance in practice (maternal mortality rate, perinatal mortality rate, cesarean delivery rate, etc).

If a candidate is involved in litigation or investigation regarding ethical or moral issues, the individual will not be scheduled for examination and the application will be reexamined. The Credentials Committee usually will defer such a decision for 1 year to gain further information.

Falsification of data (including case lists) or evidence of other egregious ethical, moral, or professional misbehavior may result in deferral of a candidate's application for at least 3 years. The candidate must meet all requirements in effect at the end of the deferred period.

Patient lists (a) not providing the information required; (b) not prepared in accordance with the format requested; (c) not having sufficient numbers of patients; or (d) not including sufficient breadth and depth of clinical problems may disqualify the candidate for admission to the oral examination.

Application for Examination in 1999

Application to take the oral examination on November 8-12, 1999, must be obtained by writing to the Board office after November 1, 1998. The application, complete in all details, with payment of the application fee of $450, a copy of a current medical license, and two 2x2-inch passport-sized photographs, with the candidate's signature across the front, must be received in the Board office on or before February 26, 1999.

The application fee must accompany the oral examination application. Application fees sent prior to the mailing of an application are subject to a late charge. The deadline for receipt of applications in the board office is February 26, 1999.

Late fees will apply for late or incomplete applications.

Admission to the Oral Examination

The Board will make the final decision concerning the applicant's admission to the oral examination after considering all circumstances affecting the individual situation.

A candidate ruled admissible to the oral examination in November 1999, will be so notified in July 1999. On or before August 2, 1999, the candidate must submit

(a) triplicate, typewritten, and verified lists of all patients dismissed from the candidate's care in all hospitals during the 12 months preceding June 30, 1999, and a list of 40 patients from the candidate's office practice. Seven copies of the summary sheet also must be submitted. The candidate's lists of patients will be used as a basis for questions during the oral examination and will not be returned to the candidate.

(If, but only if, the list of all patients dismissed from the candidate's care during this 12-month period does not achieve the minimum 50 hospitalized and/or short-stay patients as defined in this document, an additional list of all patients dismissed from the candidate's care during the year immediately prior to the 12-month period preceding June 30, 1999, may also be submitted. This will require the preparation and submission of two separate 1-year patient case lists in triplicate, each with a separate summary sheet, *plus seven copies of a combined summary sheet* that includes the cases from both yearly case lists. The minimum requirement of 50 patients as defined elsewhere in this document will still apply.)

(b) payment of the examination fee and late fee, if applicable, by personal check or money order in US funds.

Patient Lists for the Oral Examination

Each candidate for the oral examination must prepare the following patient lists for review by the examiners at the time of examination. The candidate's list of patients will be freely used as a basis for questions that will be patient-management oriented. Questions will be developed that test the ability of the candidate to

1. develop a diagnosis, including the necessary clinical, laboratory, and diagnostic procedures;
2. select and apply proper treatment under elective and emergency conditions;
3. prevent, recognize, and manage complications; and
4. plan and direct follow-up and continuing care.

Carelessly prepared or incomplete case lists may contribute to failure to pass the oral examination.

The candidate should bring a copy of his/her patient list to the oral examination for personal reference. Information should not be included on this duplicate list that did not appear on the case lists sent to the Board office.

All candidates must have an office and a hospital practice. Thus, case lists must consist of office practice plus hospitalized and day (short-stay) surgery patients in obstetrics and gynecology, or obstetrics alone, or gynecology alone. If a candidate practices both obstetrics and gynecology, case lists must be submitted in (1) office practice, (2) obstetrics, and (3) gynecology. Case lists limited to office practice and obstetrics or gynecology can be submitted only by those individuals who limit their practice to either gynecology or obstetrics. It is to the candidate's advantage to submit case lists containing obstetrical, gynecological, and office practice patients. If a candidate submits only a case list limited to office practice and obstetrics or gynecology, the examiners will necessarily have to present hypothetical cases to the candidate in the area without cases. The candidate will be examined in all three areas. The case lists must have sufficient numbers and sufficient breadth and depth of clinical experience. All day surgery and hospitalized patients must be reported. The case list must include 40 office practice patients and a minimum of 50 hospitalized and/or ambulatory, gynecological, or obstetrical patients with significant problems. If, but only if, a minimum of 50 such patients can not be obtained during the 12-month period from July 1, 1998, through June 30, 1999, the candidate may submit a complete 24-month case list dating from July 1, 1997, through June 30, 1999. This will require the preparation and submission of two separate 1-year patient case lists, in triplicate, each with a separate summary sheet, plus seven copies of a combined summary sheet that includes the cases from both yearly case lists. The minimum requirement of 50 patients will still apply. The clinical problems will vary according to the nature of the candidates' practices. The problems must be of sufficient variety and severity, however, to permit the evaluation of a candidate's ability to function as a consultant.

For candidates who have successfully completed a Board-approved fellowship and who are active candidates for certification in one of these subspecialties, case lists may be submitted in a single subspecialty within obstetrics and gynecology. If a qualified candidate chooses to submit a case list limited (ie, a "limited case list") to a single subspecialty, the limited case list must include a minimum of 50 cases of hospitalized or ambulatory surgical patients in that subspecialty, but *all day surgery and hospitalized patients must be reported*. Moreover, the 50 cases must represent the breadth and depth of that subspecialty. For a limited case list, a mixture of subspecialty and normal gynecological or obstetrical cases will not meet this 50-case requirement. A list of office patients should be submitted (see below). The candidate will be examined in all three areas. For example, if the candidate has only a gynecologic oncology case list, the candidate will be presented hypothetical cases in obstetrics, office practice, and general gynecology, as well as selected cases from their own case list.

The patients listed must be only those for whom the candidate has had personal responsibility for professional management and care. Recording such professional responsibility implies that the candidate has personally controlled the medical and/or surgical management of each patient listed. In the case of a partnership or group practice, the patients listed should be only those managed by the candidate.

The case list must be received in the Board office on or before August 2 preceding the November examinations, but only after receipt of approval.

Procedure

A patient list should be accurately typed across unbound sheets of white paper 8 1/2 by 11 inches. Type size must be at least 12 point. The headings must conform in all details and provide the information indicated by the format of the forms enclosed with the oral application. Three copies of the complete list must be submitted, as well as seven copies of the summary sheet.

Standard nomenclature should be used. Only approved abbreviations supplied with the instructions for completion of the patient forms are acceptable. Only English language will be acceptable.

The triplicate lists of patients will not be returned to the candidate after the examination. The candidate should bring a copy of the case list supplied to the Board to the examination.

1. Office Practice Patients

A list of 40 patients from the candidate's office practice should be prepared using the format accompanying the application. List separately patients who have presented with any of the following prob-

lems. List no more than four patients from any one category. Do not include any patients who appear on the hospital lists.
Preventive care and health maintenance

Obesity
Sexual dysfunction
Contraceptive complications
Psychosomatic problems
Genetic problems
Primary or secondary amenorrhea
Infertility
Endometriosis
Menopausal problems
Office surgery
Abnormal uterine bleeding
Abnormal cervical cytology
Pelvic pain
Vaginal discharge
Vulvar skin disease
Breast diseases
Urinary incontinence/pelvic relaxation
Urinary tract infections
Sexually transmitted diseases
Medical complications of pregnancy
Preconceptional counseling
Immunizations
Pediatric gynecology
Rape
Spousal abuse
Dysmenorrhea
Premenstrual syndrome
Benign pelvic masses
Abnormal vaginal ultrasonography
Abnormal fetal growth
Substance abuse

List separately each patient and include the problem (one of the listed categories), diagnostic procedures, treatment, results, and number of office visits during the 12-month period. Group patients together under each separate category.

2. Gynecology

A list of all gynecologic patients should be prepared in the format accompanying the application and listed in order as follows:

I. Hospitalized patients
  a. Major operative procedures
  b. Minor operative procedures
  c. Nonsurgical admissions
  d. Total number of ultrasound and Doppler examinations performed upon hospitalized gynecological patients

II. Ambulatory or short-stay surgery

The preoperative diagnosis should appear for all major and minor surgical procedures. The size of ovarian cysts and neoplasms must be recorded. For nonsurgical conditions, the admission diagnosis should be recorded. The treatment recorded should include all surgical procedures, as well as primary nonsurgical therapy. Surgical diagnosis refers to the pathology diagnosis. For hysterectomy specimens, the uterine weight in grams must be recorded. In cases without tissue for histologic diagnosis, the final clinical diagnosis should be listed.

Days in hospital on this listing of patients, as well as on all other lists, is the arithmetic difference between date of discharge and date of admission.

3. Obstetrics

A list of obstetric patients should be prepared in the format accompanying the application. List separately each patient with a complication or abnormality, as well as medical and surgical intervention during pregnancy, labor, delivery, and the puerperium. In addition, a total of the number of normal, uncomplicated obstetric patients, managed during the same 12-month period (or 24-month period, if a 2-year case list is submitted), should appear at the end of the obstetric list.

Interpretation of "normal obstetric patients" for this listing implies that

a. pregnancy, labor, delivery, and the puerperium were uncomplicated and labor began spontaneously between the 37th and 42nd weeks of gestation;
b. membranes ruptured or were ruptured after labor began;
c. presentation was vertex, position was occiput anterior or transverse, and labor was less than 24 hours in duration;
d. delivery was spontaneous or by outlet forceps, with or without episiotomy, from an anterior position;
e. infant had a 5-minute Apgar score of 7 or more, weighed between 2,500 and 4,500 gm, and was healthy; and
f. placental delivery was uncomplicated and blood loss was less than 500 mL.

Deliveries not fulfilling these criteria must be listed individually. Include gestational age at admission.

4. Cover Sheets

Each list of patients, (a) gynecological (hospitalized and ambulatory) and (b) obstetrical, from each hospital, should be verified on the form accompanying the application. On this form, the record librarian or other similar hospital official must submit a statement attesting that (1) the patients listed were cared for by the candidate and (2) that all of the hospitalized patients dismissed from the candidate's care have been separately listed or reported in the totals reported for the period indicated. If the candidate is submitting a 2-year case list, separate attestations must be obtained for each year.

5. Summary Sheet

Using the form provided for this purpose, prepare a summary of all cases for all hospitals combined. If a 2-year case list is submitted, this will require the preparation and submission of a summary sheet for each year, as well as seven copies of a combined summary sheet for both years.

Admission to the Oral Examination

If the examination fee has been paid and the three copies of lists of patients have been submitted by August 15, 1997, and are approved by the Board, the candidate will receive an authorization for admission form and a reservation card for the hotel at least 1 month prior to the examination, indicating the day, time, and place to report for the examination. Please keep the Board informed of current mailing address.

Ruling Not Admissible

A candidate not admitted to an oral examination may reapply by submitting a new application, paying the application fee, and meeting the requirements applicable at the time of the reapplication.

If the candidate was disqualified because the case lists were judged insufficient for a comprehensive examination, the new case lists should be added to those previously submitted. Thus, the requirement of sufficient numbers, breadth, and depth in the case lists makes time in practice the variable and experience the constant.

Reexaminations

A candidate who is disqualified or fails to pass the oral examination must reapply by submitting a new application, paying the reapplication fee, and meeting the requirements applicable at the time of reapplication.

A candidate reapplying for examination will be asked to provide verification of responsibilities for patient care and will be notified in July of admissibility to the next examination.

A candidate accepted for reexamination must submit, by the August 1 prior to the examination, a new case list for the 12 months (or 24-month period, if a 2-year case list is submitted) preceding the June 30 before the oral examination.

The examination fee is due each time a candidate receives notification of admissibility to take the oral examination. Each reexamination will be conducted by examiners who have no knowledge of the fact or circumstances of a candidate's previous failure.

Postponement of Oral Examination

A candidate failing to take a scheduled oral examination must submit a new application during January or February of the following year. Admissibility to the next examination will be determined on the basis of the candidate's professional activities as reported during the current year. Payment of the reapplication fee must accompany each reapplication.

If notified of admissibility to the next oral examination, the candidate must again submit, before August 11, a listing of all patients dismissed from the candidate's care in all hospitals during the 12 months (or 24-month period, if a 2-year case list is submitted) ending June 30 prior to the oral examination and a list of 40 patients from office practice.

Oral Examination Fees

Fees have been computed to cover the costs of examination and administrative expenses. They will not be refunded or credited. All fees must be paid in United States currency. The candidate's canceled check is to be considered the receipt.

The application fee must be enclosed with each application to take the oral examination. A candidate notified in July of admissibility to the oral examination in November is required to pay the examination fee before being scheduled to take the oral examination. If the examination fee and case list have not been received in the Board office on or before August 2, or if these items, including the late fee, have not been received in the Board office on or before August 31, the candidate will not be scheduled to take the examination in November.

No application fees will be credited against a future application or refunded.

Examination fees may be refunded, provided candidates inform the Board office in writing prior to September 24 of their inability to write the examination.

Oral Examination Dates

November 1, 1998
- Request application
- Deadline for receipt—February 15, 1999

November 1, 1998-February 26, 1999
- Application, current medical license, two 2x2 photographs, plus application fee
- Deadline for receipt—February 26, 1999
- Fee—$480

February 27-April 30, 1999
- Application, current medical license, two 2x2 photographs, application fee plus late fee ($215)
- Deadline for receipt—April 30, 1999
- Fee—$695 ($480 plus $215)

May 1-June 15, 1999
- Application, current medical license, two 2x2 photographs, application fee plus late fee ($530)
- Deadline for receipt—June 15, 1999
- Fee— $1,010 ($480 plus $530)

June 15
- No applications accepted after this date

July 1999
- Candidates notified to submit properly formatted case lists and examination fee
- Deadline for receipt—August 2, 1999
- Fee—$530

August 3-31, 1999
- Candidates notified by the Board in July to submit their properly formatted case lists and examination fee must include a late fee ($215)
- Deadline for receipt—August 31, 1999
- Fee—$745 ($530 plus $215)

August 31, 1999
- No case lists or examination fees accepted after this date

November 8-12, 1999
- Oral Examination, Chicago, Illinois

Listings of Certified Diplomates

Each year the Board office notifies the American College of Obstetricians and Gynecologists of the names and addresses of the diplomates certified in that year. A list of the names of the most recently certified diplomates is also sent to the American Medical Association and to the American Board of Medical Specialties with the request that they be included in the next issues of (1) the *Directory of Physicians in the United States* and (2) the *Official ABMS Directory of Board Certified Obstetrician-Gynecologists*.

After this effort to ensure initial listings of the newly certified diplomates, the Board assumes no responsibility for a diplomate's listing in subsequent issues of any directory.

Revocation of Diploma or Certificate

Each candidate, when making application, signs an agreement regarding disqualification or revocation of the candidate's diploma, certificate, or other evidence of qualification for cause. Revocation may occur whenever

a. The physician shall not in fact have been eligible to receive the diploma or certificate, irrespective of whether or not the facts constituting such ineligibility were known to or could have been ascertained by this Board, its members, directors, examiners, officers, or agents at or before the time of issuance of such diploma or certificate.
b. Any rule governing examination for a diploma or certificate shall have been violated by the physician but the fact of such violation shall not have been ascertained until after the issuance of his/her diploma or certificate.
c. The physician shall have violated the moral or ethical standards of the practice of medicine then accepted by organized medicine in the locality where the diplomate is practicing and, without limitation of the foregoing, the forfeiture, revocation, or suspension of the diplomate's license to practice medicine, or the expulsion from, or suspension from, the rights and privileges of membership in a local, regional, or national organization of professional peers shall be evidence of a violation of such standards of the ethical practice of medicine.
d. The physician shall fail to comply with the rules and regulations of this Board.
e. The issuance or receipt of such diploma, certificate, or other evidence of qualification shall have been contrary to or in violation of the Certificate of Incorporation or the Bylaws of this Board.

f. The physician shall have violated any of *The Ethical Considerations in the Practice of Obstetrics and Gynecology* currently published by the American College of Obstetricians and Gynecologists and adhered to by the Board.

Upon revocation of any diploma or certificate by this Board as aforesaid, the holder shall return the diploma or certificate and other evidence of qualification to the executive director of the Board, and the holder's name shall be removed from the list of certified specialists.

American Board of Ophthalmology

111 Presidential Blvd/Ste 241
Bala Cynwyd, PA 19004
610 664-1175
610 664-6503 Fax
E-mail: mrladden@abop.org
Internet: http://www.abop.org

Governing Rules and Regulations

The Rules and Regulations of the American Board of Ophthalmology (ABO), which are subject to change from time to time without notice, contain specific provisions concerning eligibility for the examinations administered by the Board; an admission appeals process, which is available under certain circumstances; the application process; the examination processes (initial and renewal); a description of the circumstances under which candidates will be required to reactivate an existing application, submit a new application, or repeat an examination; a list of occurrences that could lead the Board to revoke a certificate previously issued by it to a diplomate or to place the diplomate on probation; and other matters relating to the Board's examination and certification/recertification processes. Many, but not all, of those provisions are summarized or described in this publication. In the event of any inconsistency between the Board's Rules and Regulations and this publication, or any omission from this publication of any provision of the Rules and Regulations, the Rules and Regulations shall govern. Copies of the Rules and Regulations are available upon request from the Board's executive office.

Certification Requirements

Many physicians write to the Board outlining their training and asking for an estimate of their qualifications and whether further training is required. The Board's requirements, as published herewith, provide this information, and any potential candidate should be able to determine his/her status after studying these requirements. Individual officers or directors of the Board cannot and will not make such determinations. All evaluations of an applicant's status will be made by the Committee on Admissions in accordance with the rules and regulations of the Board, after submission of an application for examination and payment of the registration fee, which must accompany the application. Personal interviews with officers and directors of the Board should not be requested at any time.

It is the responsibility of the candidate to seek information concerning the current requirements for certification as an ophthalmologist. The Board does not assume responsibility for notifying a candidate of changing requirements or the impending loss of his/her eligibility to take an examination.

Educational

All applicants must have graduated from a medical school or from a school of osteopathy.

All applicants entering ophthalmology training programs must have completed a graduate clinical year (GY1) in a program in the United States accredited by the Accreditation Council for Graduate Medical Education (ACGME) or a program in Canada approved by the appropriate accrediting body in Canada. The GY1 year must be composed of training in which the resident has primary responsibility for patient care in fields such as internal medicine, neurology, pediatrics, surgery, family practice, or emergency medicine. As a minimum, 6 months of this year must consist of broad experience in direct patient care. It is a requirement of the Board that the program chairman ascertain that an individual has completed an accredited GY1 year in the United States or in Canada prior to the start of the ophthalmology residency.

In addition to a GY1 year, all applicants must have satisfactorily completed an entire formal graduated residency training program in ophthalmology of at least 36 months duration (GY4 or better) in either the United States accredited by the Accreditation Council for Graduate Medical Education, or in Canada accredited by the Royal College of Physicians and Surgeons of Canada (RCPSC). No other training, *including any form of fellowship*, is acceptable.

The applicant's chairman is required to verify satisfactory completion of an entire formal graduated ophthalmology residency training program of at least 36 months' duration. When a resident's graduate education and clinical experience have been gained in more than one residency program, each chairman will be required to complete a satisfactory completion form. Less than 6 months' service in an accredited program is not acceptable as a part of the required training in ophthalmology. The chairman's verification form(s) cannot be submitted to the Board until the applicant has completed the entire residency training program.

If a program is disapproved or withdrawn during the course of a resident's training, he/she must complete the remaining required number of months of training in another accredited program.

Only those applicants who have completed their GY1 and entire ophthalmology training program, GY4 or beyond, by August 1 are eligible to apply for the Written Qualifying Examination given in April of the following year.

Licensure

Graduates of United States and Canadian Medical Schools

A person shall be eligible to apply for and to take any examination administered by the Board only if, as of the date of application and at all times thereafter through and including the date of administration of each examination of the Board taken by the person, the person has a valid and unrestricted license to practice medicine in the place or places in which the person's practice of medicine is regularly conducted in the United States, any of its territories, or Canada and in each other place in which the person practices or has practiced medicine and has an unexpired license. Individuals in the military will meet the valid and unrestricted licensing condition if they are on full-time active duty as a physician at a military installation in any branch of the US Armed Services and submit a valid and unrestricted military medical license. Accompanying this military license must be a signed document from the individual's commanding officer stating that he/she solely provides medical care and treatment on the military installation to members of the US Services and their dependents. Information concerning the Board's Rules and Regulations with respect to definitions of an invalid or restricted license is available upon request from the Board's executive office.

Other Medical Graduates

An applicant may have graduated from a medical school of a country other than the United States or Canada. Graduates of foreign medical schools must have a valid and unrestricted license to practice medicine (as defined above and in the Rules and Regulations of the Board); they are also required to have a certificate from the Educational Commission for Foreign Medical Graduates (ECFMG).

Applicant Disclosure Obligations

At the time a person submits an application to the Board and at all times thereafter, the person shall have a continuing obligation to disclose promptly to the Board the existence or occurrence of any circumstances causing the person to fail to satisfy the foregoing condition of eligibility to apply for and take any examination administered by the Board. A person submitting an application to the Board shall inform the Board on, or in a written submission accompanying, the person's application or in a written submission to the Board before taking any examination administered by the Board, as the case may be, if the person's license to practice medicine in the United States, any of its territories, or Canada has previously been surrendered or not renewed upon its expiration or if the person's practice of medicine or license to practice medicine in the United States, any of its territories, or Canada has previously been revoked, restricted, conditioned, suspended, limited, qualified, or subject to the terms of probation.

Applications

An applicant who wishes to be examined by the Board shall complete, sign and file with the executive director an application on the official form then in use by the Board. The application shall be considered complete only when all supporting data required by the application, including the chairman's verification form, are also filed with the executive director. Applications can be obtained from the chairmen of accredited residency programs or from the office of the Board.

Written Examination Deadline

If an applicant wishes to be considered for a Written Qualifying Examination to be conducted in a particular year, his/her application and all supporting data, including supporting data furnished directly by others with respect to the applicant, must be postmarked between March 1 and August 1 except for the chairman's verification form, which must be postmarked on or before October 1 of the calendar year immediately preceding the calendar year in which the Written Qualifying Examination is to be conducted. By paying a late fee (see "Fees for Examinations") the deadline for postmarking the completed application may be extended from August 1 to September 1. No other exceptions to, or extensions of, these requirements will be made for any reason. The dates of future examinations can be found on the internet at http://www.abop.org and will be announced in the *Journal of the American Medical Association.*

An applicant who does not receive notification from the Board office by January 15 of the acceptance or rejection of his/her application must contact the Board office in writing to inquire about the status of the application. Failure to contact the Board office in writing by February 15 will result in such applicant's removal from the examination roster.

If a completed application and all required supporting data are not timely postmarked, the application will not be valid and the application fee shall be returned. It is best not to mail application materials just before the postmark deadline because packets are sometimes postmarked a day or two after mailing. Caution: If there is a discrepancy between a metered postmark and an official US Postal Service postmark, the latter will be considered official.

The application shall be accompanied by a check payable to the Board for the application fee. No application will be considered to be complete until the fee and all required supporting data, including a copy of your current registration to practice medicine and two recent photographs for identification at the Written Qualifying Examination and the Oral Examination, have been received by the executive director.

The application form contains a pledge that explains the prohibitions regarding improper conduct before, during, and after examinations. Candidates must certify that the information they provide in their applications is true and accurate. If (1) any misrepresentation is discovered in the application, in any other information submitted to the Board, or in the identity of a person applying to take or taking the examinations, (2) any financial or other benefit is offered by a candidate to any director, officer, employee, proctor, or other agent or representative of the Board in order to obtain a right, privilege, or benefit not usually granted by the Board to similarly situated candidates, or (3) any irregular behavior during the examination, such as copying answers, sharing information, using notes, or otherwise giving or receiving aid is discovered by observation, statistical analysis of answer sheets, or otherwise, the candidate in question shall be given written notice of the charges and an opportunity to respond in accordance with the procedures set forth in the rules and regulations of the Board. If the Board determines that a violation has occurred, the Board may permanently bar the person(s) involved in the violation from all future examinations, invalidate the results of prior examinations taken by the person(s), withhold or revoke the certificate of the person(s), or take other appropriate action. If sanctions are imposed pursuant to the rules and regulations of the Board, the Board may notify legitimately interested third parties of its action.

When the Board determines that irregular behavior has occurred during an examination, the Board will make every effort to withhold the scores of only those candidates directly implicated in the irregularity. Nevertheless, in some instances the evidence of irregularity, though sufficiently strong to cast doubt on the validity of scores, may not enable the Board to identify the specific candidates involved in the irregularity. In such circumstances, the Board may withhold the scores of candidates not directly implicated in the irregularity and, if necessary, may require those candidates to take an additional examination at a later date to ensure the validity of all scores.

The examination booklets used in the Written Qualifying Examination and the illustrative materials and questions asked in the Oral Examination are copyrighted as the sole property of the Board and must not be removed by the candidate from the test area or reproduced in any way. Any reproduction, in whole or in part, of the written test booklet or Oral Examination materials and questions is a federal offense and also may subject the candidate to the sanctions listed above. No notes, textbooks, other reference materials, scratch paper or recording devices may be taken into either the Written or the Oral Examinations.

Disabilities

The ABO supports the intent of the Americans with Disabilities Act (ADA) to mitigate the effects of the disability on the testing activity. To accommodate individuals with disabilities the Board will make reasonable modifications to its examinations that do not fundamentally alter the requirements of the examination or the measurement of the skills or knowledge the Board examinations are intended to test.

A candidate for Board certification who believes that he or she is disabled within the meaning of the ADA, and who requests an examination under nonstandard conditions, shall specify on (or in a supplement submitted with) the application form the existence, specific nature, and extent of their disability and the specific modification requested. The candidate shall also submit either with the timely filed application, or no later than 30 days after the deadline for applying for a particular examination, all independent documentary evidence substantiating the individual's disabilities.

Documentation includes, but is not limited to

1. Name, address, telephone number, and qualifications of each expert who provides a report documenting the individual's disabilities.
2. Dates and locations of all assessments performed and included in the documentation.
3. Copies of evaluation reports with scores or ratings for each standard instrument or assessment method used. The Board requires that this documentation be no more than 3 years old.
4. A full description of any nonstandard instruments and assessment methods used to determine the disabilities and diagnoses.
5. Any diagnoses of the individual's disabilities using standard nomenclature, ie, International Classification of Diseases (ICD); American Psychiatric Association, Diagnostic and Statistical Manual (DSM).
6. A description of the individual's functional limitations owing to any disabilities.
7. Reports of any past accommodations on examinations the individuals received because of the disabilities.

The ABO will verify the documentation of the disability and reserves the right to have the individual independently evaluated at its own expense.

Fees for Examinations

Written Qualifying Examination

- Review of application and registration, $985, payable with application
- Review of late application and registration (after August 1 to September 1 postmark), $1,255
- Repeat registration fee, $715
- Late repeat registration fee, (after August 1 to September 1 postmark), $870

Oral Examination

Due to time constraints, there is no late filing period for oral candidates

- Registration fee, $985, payable on successful completion of the Written Qualifying Examination
- Repeat entire examination, $985
- Repeat one subject, $355
- Repeat two subjects, $540

Cancellations

To cover administrative expenses an additional charge equal to 50% of the original application and registration fee (or repeat registration fee) for that particular Written Qualifying Examination or Oral Examination will be imposed on any candidate who cancels or fails to keep an examination assignment, regardless of the reason. This fee is due at the time of cancellation.

Fees for accepted candidates for the Written Qualifying Examination and the Oral Examination are not refundable.

The fees for examinations shall be established annually by the Board of Directors on the basis of the actual and anticipated costs of the Board in the examination of candidates and the administration of its business. The directors of the Board serve without compensation except for reimbursement of expenses.

Time Limit

On January 23, 1993, the American Board of Ophthalmology instituted a 6-year time limit in which to complete the certification process. This affects the following four groups of individuals:

1. New Applicants

New applicants are those individuals who completed their residency programs after this rule was instituted; that is, those graduating in the year 1993 or thereafter. They must successfully complete the Written Qualifying Examination and the entire Oral Examination by December 31 of the sixth year following completion of accredited training in ophthalmology.

2. Active Candidates

Active candidates are those individuals who had an approved active application on file with the Board when this 6-year rule was instituted on January 23, 1993. They must successfully complete the Written Qualifying Examination and the entire Oral Examination within 6 years or by December 31, 1999.

3. Inactive Candidates

Inactive candidates are those individuals who had an approved inactive application on file with the Board when this 6-year rule was instituted on January 23, 1993. They must successfully complete the Written Qualifying Examination and the entire Oral Examination within 6 years or by December 31, 1999.

4. Individuals Who Have Never Applied

All individuals who completed their residency prior to 1993 but have never applied to the Board have until August 1, 1998, to submit a completed application and until December 31, 1999, to successfully complete the Written Qualifying Examination and the entire Oral Examination.

Reentry Process

Candidates failing to achieve certification within the initial 6-year period may reenter the process for one additional 6-year period by completing a reentry process. During the period when an individual is in the reentry process, he/she is not considered to be scheduled for a certification examination. If a candidate completes the reentry process but does not attain certification within the second 6-year period, the individual will not be given another opportunity to reenter the process until he/she has satisfactorily completed an additional accredited residency program.

Those individuals who have completed their residency prior to 1993 and have not applied to the Board by August 1, 1998 (see above paragraph, "Individuals Who Have Never Applied") will be able to enter the system for one 6-year period if they complete the reentry process.

The requirements for reentry into the examination process are as follows:

1. A waiting period of 1 year is required before an individual can apply to take their first reentry examination.
2. All reentry applicants must file a timely application with the Board. The filing period is the same as the initial application process (March 1 to August 1) of the year preceding the reentry examination.
3. An individual must provide a copy of a valid and unrestricted license to practice medicine as described under "Licensure."
4. An individual must attain 100 category 1 CME credits, accredited by the Accreditation Council for Continuing Medical Education (ACCME) during the 1-year waiting period.
5. An individual must pass the Written Reentry Examination given in the spring of each year.

Successful completion of the reentry process including the Written Reentry Examination will qualify the individual to make an application to take the Oral Examination.

Written Qualifying Examination

In order to qualify for an Oral Examination, each candidate must pass a Written Qualifying Examination. The Written Qualifying Examination consists of 250 multiple-choice questions. The purpose of the Written Qualifying Examination is to evaluate the breadth and depth of the basic science and clinical knowledge of candidates who have satisfactorily completed an accredited program of education in ophthalmology. Candidates who successfully complete the Written Qualifying Examination will be further evaluated in an Oral Examination.

Aspects of the candidate's ability that are tested include:

1. recall of information;
2. understanding and application of basic knowledge;
3. relation of pathogenesis to disease process;
4. evaluation of clinical data;
5. utilization of diagnostic and therapeutic procedures;
6. anticipation and recognition of complications;
7. ethics of ophthalmic practice.

Topics covered include:

1. optics, visual physiology, and correction of refractive errors;
2. retina, vitreous, and uvea;
3. neuro-ophthalmology;
4. pediatric ophthalmology;
5. external disease and cornea;
6. glaucoma, cataract, and anterior segment;
7. plastic surgery and orbital diseases;
8. ophthalmic pathology.

The Written Qualifying Examination is given simultaneously in designated cities in the United States in March or April of each year.

Oral Examination

Upon successful completion of the Written Qualifying Examination candidates will be sent specific instructions for registration for the Oral Examination. A check payable to the Board for the amount then in effect for the Oral Examination must accompany the completed registration form and be forwarded to the Board office within the appropriate time frame.

Oral Examination Schedule

It has been the custom of the Board to hold two oral examinations a year with candidates who have passed the March or April Written Qualifying Examination assigned either to a group taking the Oral Examinations in the fall of that year or to a group taking the Oral Examinations in the spring of the following year. Candidates who pass the April 1999 Written will be assigned to either the Fall 1999 Oral or the Spring 2000 Oral. The Board reserves the right to limit the number of candidates admitted to any scheduled examination and to designate the candidates to be examined.

Oral Examination Subjects

The Oral Examination will be divided into the subjects listed and described in the following paragraphs. All subjects are given by appointment within a half-day period utilizing a panel system. Information about the examination procedures and scheduling is sent to all candidates after they have been registered for the Oral Examinations.

1. optics, visual physiology and correction of refractive errors
2. pediatric ophthalmology and strabismus
3. neuro-ophthalmology and orbit
4. external eye and adnexa
5. anterior segment of the eye
6. posterior segment of the eye

In each of the oral examinations emphasis will be placed upon the following:

I. Data Acquisition
Recognition by the candidate of depicted abnormalities and diseases that affect the eye, ocular adnexa, and the visual pathways. Candidates will be asked for historical information and examination data that might be obtained on a patient with a particular condition depicted or described.

II. Diagnosis
The ability of candidates to synthesize historical and physical evaluation information, along with the appropriate laboratory data, to arrive at correct diagnoses and differential diagnoses.

III. Treatment
Candidates will be expected to provide a reasonable and appropriate plan for medical and/or surgical management of patients with the conditions depicted or described and be able to discuss the prognosis and/or therapeutic complications for the particular condition.

These examinations will include developmental, dystrophic, degenerative, inflammatory, infectious, toxic, traumatic, neoplastic, and vascular diseases affecting the eye and its surrounding structures.

1. Optics, Visual Physiology, and Correction of Refractive Errors
Candidates should be familiar with the basic principles of physical and geometrical optics and the operation of standard optical instruments. They should understand the essentials of visual physiology, including visual acuity, light and dark adaptation, accommodation, and color vision. They should know the various forms of ametropia, principles and techniques of refraction, principles of lens design, and methods of correction of ametropia, including spectacles, contact lenses, intraocular lenses, and keratorefractive surgery. Candidates should be familiar with the methods for prescribing protective lenses, absorptive lenses, and aids for low vision.

2. Pediatric Ophthalmology and Strabismus
Candidates should be familiar with diseases affecting the eyes of infants and children and associated systemic abnormalities. Candidates should understand the anatomy, pathology, and physiology of the neuromuscular mechanisms subserving ocular motility and binocular vision. Candidates should be familiar with the methods of examination for detection and assessment of sensory and ocular motor disorders. They should also know the clinical features, differential diagnosis, and natural course and management of the various types of comitant and noncomitant deviations. They should be familiar with the principles and complications of surgery upon the extraocular muscles.

3. Neuro-Ophthalmology and Orbit
Candidates should know the anatomy of the orbit and the neuroanatomy of the afferent and efferent visual systems. They should understand the principles and techniques of various diagnostic procedures and be able to interpret visual field testing, visually evoked responses, ultrasonography, conventional X-ray imaging, CT scanning, and magnetic resonance imaging. Candidates should be familiar with the clinical features, pathology, differential diagnosis, and management of disorders of the orbit, visual pathways, oculomotor system, and pupillomotor pathways, including the indications for, principles of, and complications of orbital surgery.

4. External Eye and Adnexa
Candidates should understand the anatomy, embryology, physiology, and pathology of the structures composing the lacrimal system, lids, cornea, conjunctiva, and sclera. They will be expected to discuss conditions affecting these structures and provide an appropriate differential diagnosis. Candidates should also be able to describe and discuss medical and surgical treatment for diseases and abnormalities involving these tissues, including indications for and complications of surgery.

5. Anterior Segment of the Eye
This examination concerns the anatomy, embryology, physiology, and pathology of abnormalities and diseases of the cornea, anterior chamber angle, iris, ciliary body, and lens.

Candidates will be expected to discuss conditions affecting these structures and those to be considered in their differential diagnosis. They should also be able to describe and provide indications for medical and surgical therapy directed toward alleviating or curing these conditions.

6. Posterior Segment of the Eye
This examination concerns the anatomy, embryology, physiology, and pathology of abnormalities and diseases of the vitreous, retina, choroid, and posterior sclera.

Candidates will be expected to discuss conditions affecting these structures and those to be considered in their differential diagnosis. They should also be able to describe and provide indications for medical and surgical therapy directed toward alleviating or curing these conditions.

Reactivation

Written Qualifying Examination

An applicant shall be required to reactivate his/her application for approval and submit an additional application fee under the following circumstances, which relate to the Written Qualifying Examination:

1. If a candidate fails to take the Written Qualifying Examination within 24 months after notice has been sent to him/her that his/her application has been accepted
2. If a candidate does not repeat the Written Qualifying Examination within 24 months after failing
3. If a candidate receives two consecutive failures on a Written Qualifying Examination on the same application.

Oral Examination

Beginning with the administration of the November 1997 oral examination the grading process was changed to an overall pass/fail grade. The Board continues to require that each candidate is examined in six separate subsections of the oral examination. A percent correct is calculated for each subject and these six scores are averaged to arrive at a total score. Failure to achieve the necessary overall passing score requires that an individual repeat the entire six subjects of the oral examination. Additional information on grading is specified in the "Rules for Grading," which are sent to all candidates at the time of their Oral Examination registration.

An applicant shall be required to reactivate his/her application for approval, submit an additional application fee, and pass another Written Qualifying Examination before being admitted to the Oral Examination under the following circumstances:

1. If a candidate does not take the Oral Examination within 24 months after notice has been sent to the candidate that he/she has passed the Written Qualifying Examination
2. If a candidate who is eligible to do so fails to repeat the Oral Examination within 24 months after failing such examination
3. If the candidate does not pass the entire examination in three attempts.

Reactivation Procedure

In order to reactivate an application the following actions must be completed by the postmarked August 1 registration deadline:

1. File a new application
2. Remit the current fee

3. Submit a copy of a current valid and unrestricted license to practice medicine in the United States, its territories, or in a province of Canada (see "Licensure")
4. Provide letters of endorsement from two ABO-certified ophthalmologists in the community in which the applicant practices

Inactive Applications

When an application has not been reactivated it is considered by the Board to have lapsed. Inquiries to the Board by outside agencies about the certification status of a physician with an inactive application will be answered by stating that said physician is not certified and is not scheduled for an examination.

Cancellation of Examination

If the ABO is unable to administer or complete the administration of a Written or Oral Examination at the scheduled date, time, and location due to circumstances beyond the Board's control, the examination may be cancelled at the sole discretion of the Board, and if the examination is cancelled, the Board is not responsible for any expense an affected candidate may have incurred in connection with the cancelled examination or for any expense the candidate may incur in connection with any substitute examination.

Results of Examinations

Within a reasonable time after completion of the Written and/or Oral Examinations, the candidate shall be notified by the executive director as to the results thereof. The decision of the Board as to these results shall be final and conclusive. Grades are not subject to appeal. Because such is the case, individual directors of the Board or associate examiners should not be contacted about specific examination results. To preserve confidentiality, results of an examination will not be given over the telephone or by facsimile.

Certification

A candidate who successfully passes both the Written Qualifying and Oral Examinations within the required time limitations hereinabove set forth, as determined by the Board in its sole discretion, shall be entitled to receive a certificate without further consideration of his/her qualifications by the Board. Physicians who have received the certificate are diplomates of the Board.

Duration of Certification

Certificates issued by the Board after July 1, 1992, are valid for a period of 10 years. Thereafter, a diplomate will be required to satisfactorily complete a designated renewal program every 10 years in order to extend the validity of his/her certificate. Certificates issued prior to July 1, 1992, are valid during the diplomate's lifetime.

Disciplinary Sanctions

The Board shall have the authority to impose disciplinary sanctions upon a candidate or a diplomate for any of the following reasons:

1. Violation of rules and regulations of the Board relating to the Written Qualifying, Oral, and Certificate Renewal Examinations and applications to take the examinations
2. Substantial misstatement or omission of a material fact to the Board in an application or in any other information submitted to the Board
3. Presenting or distributing, or aiding or assisting another person(s) to present or distribute, a forged document or other written instrument purporting to have been issued by or under the authority of the Board to evidence that a candidate, diplomate, or any other person(s) is currently or was previously certified by the Board, when that is not the case, or claiming orally or in writing, or assisting another person(s) to claim, that a candidate, diplomate, or any other person(s) is currently or was previously certified by the Board, when that is not the case
4. Revocation of license(s) to practice of a person to whom a certificate was issued
5. Issuance of a certificate contrary to or in violation of the rules and regulations of the Board
6. Ineligibility of the person to whom the certificate was issued to receive the certificate

Statements of Eligibility

The Board does not issue statements of eligibility for its examinations. The only information the Board will divulge is whether a physician is or is not certified or has an active application on file.

The ABO charges a $25 fee for each formal verification of a physician's certification.

American Board of Medical Specialties

The American Board of Medical Specialties (ABMS) was established in 1933 to serve in an advisory capacity to the American specialty boards and to cooperate with organizations that seek its advice concerning the certification of medical specialists. The ABO is officially recognized by the ABMS and contributes an annual fee of $2,000 in addition to a per capita fee for each new diplomate certified, as do all other medical specialty boards, to the ABMS in support of the activities of the ABMS.

The ABO provides an annual listing of new diplomates for inclusion in the *Official ABMS Directory of Board Certified Medical Specialists* and in the *Official ABMS Directory of Board Certified Ophthalmologists*. Both are published by Marquis Who's Who. Each diplomate will be contacted directly for biographical information and to update information every year.

Certificate Renewal—Background

Periodic certificate renewal is meant to assure that members of the profession continue their education, keep current in information and skills, and practice in a contemporary manner. Thus the process expects continued update of relevant knowledge and requires participation in educational experience. It expects that the educational experience has been assimilated and documents the assimilation by testing. It expects the updated knowledge to be applied in practice. As is feasible, it may also assess whether the practice reflects a caring attitude toward patients and ethical behavior appropriate to a profession, or at least ascertain a commitment to these goals.

Guiding Principles

1. *Primary purpose.* The primary purpose of the certificate renewal process is to promote optimum delivery of competent care by certified members of the ophthalmic profession. The intent of the process is to set a goal that will guide all members of the profession as they strive to keep up-to-date in knowledge and skills and to practice competently. Another function is to identify any who are severely wanting in professional capabilities or behavior and to provide incentive and opportunity to improve. The Board is not to be viewed as responsible for discovering, correcting, and disciplining all who are unacceptable practitioners. Licensing boards, professional societies, quality assurance committees of medical care facilities, and the legal system share in this responsibility.

   The process is primarily to act as an incentive to all in the profession. The goal is that all who are willing and able will achieve renewal. The exceptions are those who have become infirm and are therefore unable to maintain certain required qualities and those who are unwilling to participate in the process of continued growth in the professional capabilities that they once demonstrated. Opportunity for remediation rather than exclusion from renewal certification is the mechanism for elevating those who have slipped below the standard of their peers. Nonrenewal is the action designed to remove the individual who is uncorrectably wanting.

2. *Flexibility by practice.* The process is intended to take into account that individual practitioners may have developed differently in the types of patients they serve, diagnostic problems that present to them, and the therapeutic methods required by the population they serve. The process therefore contains flexible requirements that to some degree can be modified to suit the nature of individual practices.
3. *Flexibility by individual preference.* Alternate pathways or components are provided to permit some selection according to individual preference. For example, individual practitioners may have different means for maintaining their knowledge or may have preference with regard to how they might like to have their continued abilities evaluated.
4. *Sequential process.* It is desirable that the process of maintaining intellectual and professional qualities be a continual process. The educational and the assessment requirements of the plan can be satisfied over a period of time with completed items accumulated until the requirement is satisfied, with opportunity to repeat and strive for improvement in any element that is not accomplished satisfactorily at first.
5. *Time for remediation.* Standards need to be sufficiently high that they are meaningful and thus sometimes might not be met on first attempt. For elements that are judged unsatisfactory, timely opportunities need to be provided for satisfactory performance. The result should be a higher level for the profession as a whole than might have occurred without time-limited certificates and the renewal process. This is in fact the primary purpose of the certificate renewal process.

Requirements

Certificates issued by the ABO in 1992 and thereafter are time-limited, expiring in 10 years, and are subject to renewal. All evaluations of a candidate's status will be made by the Committee on Admissions in accordance with the rules and regulations of the Board, after submission of an application for examination and payment of the renewal fee, which must accompany the application. Personal interviews with officers and directors of the Board should not be requested at any time.

Additionally, it is the responsibility of the candidate to seek information concerning the current requirements for certificate renewal. The Board does not assume responsibility for notifying a candidate of changing requirements or the impending loss of his/her eligibility to take an examination.

The first certificate renewal will be required in 2002, therefore, the following ABO renewal process will be available beginning in 1999:

Eligibility

1. The individual must hold a time-limited certificate issued by the ABO in 1992 or thereafter. Requirements for certificate renewal can be achieved before or after the expiration date of the time-limited certificate. Renewal is for 10 years from the date of completion of the requirements or 10 years from the expiration of the previous certificate, whichever is later.

   Requests for recertification from ophthalmologists who hold lifetime certificates issued before 1992 are considered on a case-by-case basis. The duration of recertification and the examination process is identical to that offered to holders of time-limited certificates. Lifetime certificate holders who fail to pass the recertification process do not place their initial certificate in jeopardy. They merely are not listed in the Board directory as being recertified.
2. The applicant must hold a valid, unrestricted license to practice medicine in the United States or Canada in every jurisdiction in which the applicant practices medicine, in keeping with the ABO requirements for certification. This valid, unrestricted licensure requirement applies to the time at which knowledge assessment and review of practice requirements are conducted and also to the date on which certificate renewal is issued. Loss of valid, unrestricted licensure after certification or certificate renewal may result in loss of certification. Individuals in the military will meet the valid and unrestricted licensing condition if they are on full-time active duty as a physician at a military installation in any branch of the US Armed Services and submit a valid and unrestricted military medical license. Accompanying this military license must be a signed document from the individual's commanding officer stating that he/she solely provides medical care and treatment on the military installation to members of the US Services and their dependents. A copy of a current valid and unrestricted registration to practice medicine in the United States, its territories, or Canada in which he/she primarily practices must accompany the application.
3. During the renewal process, the candidate must sign a statement affirming commitment to practice in an ethical manner. This can be found on the application's "Agreement for Recertification."

Applications

The application filing period runs from January through June 1 each year. Since the knowledge and practice assessment components for certificate renewal can be accomplished within 2 years (this includes time for remediation, if necessary), all eligible certificate renewal holders will be notified 3 years prior to expiration of their certificate that they may make application. Ultimately, it is the diplomate's responsibility to obtain an application. If a completed application and all required supporting data are not timely postmarked the application will not be valid, and the application fee shall be returned. It is best not to mail application materials just before the postmark deadline because packets are sometimes postmarked a day or two after mailing. Caution: If there is a discrepancy between a metered postmark and an official US Postal Service postmark, the latter will be considered official.

Educational Requirements

Although exposure to an educational experience does not assure assimilation or utilization of knowledge, a high standard of ophthalmic care can better be rendered with an ongoing educational experience that is relevant to the individual's practice. Therefore it is required that the candidate have an average of 50 hours per year of CME credits granted by an ACCME-accredited institution since the date of time-limited certification. At least 60% of the hours must be met from among category I CME activity, and the remaining 40% may be met by programs composed of category II or category I credits. (These requirements are subject to change based on revisions of ACCME classifications.) The educational experience should be of a type and content appropriate for the practice of ophthalmology. It should include educational programs in general ophthalmology, any subspecialty interest of the applicant, in general medicine, and ethics and humanitarianism. At least 80% of category I and 80% of category II hours are to be ophthalmology related. At least 250 hours of the required CME must be obtained in the 5 years prior to the date of issue of the renewed certificate. A listing of the approved educational experience is required.

Knowledge Assessment

As an encouragement to utilize continuing education resources of quality, as an encouragement for self study, and as a verification of the effectiveness of these educational endeavors, an evaluation of knowledge is required. This requirement can be satisfied by any *one* of three methods:

1. *Certificate Renewal Written Examination*: The examination concentrates on, but is not limited to, clinically relevant new information disseminated in clinical journals and educational media during the preceding decade. The examination consists of several parts: a general examination required of all candidates choosing this pathway and a spectrum of modules dealing with different categories of disease from which the candidate selects the most relevant to his or her practice. This annually administered general and modular test is an open-book, multiple-choice question test mailed to candidates to be taken during a 2-month time period of February and March. The candidate must take and pass an examination that includes both general and modular components in order to achieve certificate renewal. The general and modular test may be taken annually as often as needed, until passed. If a candidate wishes to be considered for the Certificate Renewal Examination, Written (CREW) to be conducted in a particular year, his/her application and all supporting data must be approved and his/her registration form for this pathway must be postmarked on or before October 1 to be eligible for the following year's CREW examination. Or,
2. The *Oral Examination* currently used for candidates undergoing initial certification. This examination is offered annually in the spring with a registration deadline of December 1 of the year immediately preceding the Spring Oral Examination. Or,
3. *Certificate Renewal Oral Examination:* This pathway consists of patient management problems (PMPs) dealing with common general ophthalmological topics. Candidates are allowed some latitude in the selection of subjects to emphasize their areas of interest. This examination is offered annually in the spring with a registration deadline of December 1 of the year immediately preceding the spring Certificate Renewal Oral Examination.

To satisfy this knowledge assessment requirement, the candidate must satisfactorily pass any one of these three examination methods before achieving certificate renewal. If a candidate fails in any one of the three examinations, the examination may be repeated as often as required, or a different option may be selected.

Review of Practice

All candidates are asked to complete scan sheets from representative office patient records so that the Board can determine the practice pattern of each candidate. The ABO reserves the right to make site visits to the office of candidates to verify the validity of the scan sheet method of reviewing office practice.

The application form surveys the categories of patients that are seen in the applicant's practice commonly, occasionally, or rarely (if ever). This information helps in the selection of patient types for office record review. In registering for office record scan review, each candidate selects three diagnoses-related categories from an available list of categories. Representative patient records from each category (with patient identification masked for confidentiality) are to be selected, copied, and submitted to the Board office. Corresponding office record scan forms are then sent to the candidate in order to assess the patient's proper history, treatment, management, and diagnosis. The candidate will have 1 month to complete and return all office record scan review forms. Beginning in 1999 the office record scan review process will be offered twice yearly during the months of January and July.

If a candidate wishes to be considered for the January office record scan review, a registration form with all supporting data must be received in the Board office postmarked on or before November 1 of the calendar year immediately preceding the January review. Likewise, if a candidate wishes to be considered for the July office record scan review, a registration form with all supporting data must be received in the Board office postmarked on or before May 1 immediately preceding the July review.

The renewal certificate for all successful candidates is identical, and the characterization of practice in the application is only for the purpose of guiding the mechanism for certificate renewal.

Synopsis of Certificate Renewal

Along with eligibility requirements, completion of requirements in each of four areas:

1. *Licensure:* A candidate must possess and maintain a valid and unrestricted license to participate in the renewal process. During periods of discontinuity of unrestricted licensure, no participation in knowledge assessment or practice review is permitted or credited.
2. *Continuing Medical Education (CME):* An average of 50 ACCME-approved credit hours per year is required: Minimum of 60% in category I. Minimum of 50% of the 500 hours achieved in the 5 years prior to the renewal date. Eighty percent of category I and 80% of category II hours must be relevant to the practice of ophthalmology.
3. *Knowledge Assessment:* Any one of the following three methods satisfies this requirement: Certificate renewal written examination (take home); certificate renewal oral examination (patient management problem format emphasizing the areas of interest applicable to the candidate's practice); certification oral examination.
4. *Practice Assessment:* An office record scan review is required.

Associates

All associates, whether examiners or members of special committees, are informed by the Board that they shall not promote, or permit others to promote, his/her participation in commercial or educational activities under circumstances that exploit, or might be perceived to exploit, his/her familiarity with examinations administered by the ABO or otherwise compromise the integrity of those examinations.

American Board of Orthopaedic Surgery

400 Silver Cedar Ct
Chapel Hill, NC 27514
919 929-7103
919 942-8988 Fax
Internet: http://www.abos.org

Andrew J Weiland, MD, President, New York, New York
Robert H Cofield, MD, President-Elect, Rochester, Minnesota
James H Beaty, MD, Secretary, Memphis, Tennessee
Richard E Grant, Treasurer, Washington, District of Columbia
Directors
Gordon M Aamoth, MD, Minneapolis, Minnesota
Robert W Bucholz, MD, Dallas, Texas
Frank J Eismont, MD, Miami, Florida
William E Garrett, Jr, MD, PhD, Chapel Hill, North Carolina
Mark C Gebhardt, MD, Boston, Massachusetts
Richard H Gelberman, MD, St. Louis, Missouri
Robert Poss, MD, Boston, Massachusetts
Stuart L Weinstein, MD, Iowa City, Iowa
Senior Directors
Joseph A Buckwalter, MD, Iowa City, Iowa
Harold M Dick, MD, New York, New York
Donald C Ferlic, MD, Denver, Colorado
Michael A Simon, MD, Chicago, Illinois
James H Van Olst, MD, Corvallis, Oregon
Executive Director
G Paul DeRosa, MD, Chapel Hill, North Carolina

(These criteria and conditions are subject to change without notice. All applicants are advised to contact the American Board of Orthopaedic Surgery [ABOS] to ascertain whether the information below is current.)

I. Introduction

A. Definition

Orthopaedic surgery is the medical specialty that includes the preservation, investigation, and restoration of the form and function of the extremities, spine, and associated structures by medical, surgical, and physical methods.

B. Purpose

The ABOS was founded in 1934 as a private, voluntary, nonprofit, autonomous organization. It exists to serve the best interest of the public and of the medical profession by establishing educational standards for orthopaedic residents and by evaluating the initial and continuing qualifications and competence of orthopaedic surgeons. For this purpose, the Board reviews the credentials and practices of voluntary candidates and issues certificates as appropriate. It defines minimum educational requirements in the specialty, stimulates graduate medical education and continuing medical education, and aids in the evaluation of educational facilities and programs.

The Board does not confer any rights on its diplomates, nor does it purport to direct licensed physicians in any way in the conduct of their professional duties or lives. It is neither the intent nor the purpose of the Board to define requirements for membership in any organization or for staff privileges at any hospital.

C. Directors

The directors of the ABOS are elected from diplomates of the Board who are nominated by the American Orthopaedic Association, the American Medical Association, and the American Academy of Orthopaedic Surgeons. They serve without salary.

D. Organization

Directors of the Board elect a president, president-elect, secretary, and treasurer annually. An executive director, who is a diplomate, serves as an ex officio director of the Board. The president appoints directors to serve on standing committees on credentials, examinations, finance, graduate education, and research. Other committees may be formed as deemed necessary. The Board holds regularly scheduled meetings yearly.

E. Directory

A current directory of certified orthopaedic surgeons is maintained and published by the Board. The names of diplomates also appear in the *Official ABMS Directory of Board Certified Medical Specialists*.

II. General Statement of Educational Goal for Orthopaedic Surgery

The goal of orthopaedic education is to prepare orthopaedic residents to be competent and ethical practitioners of orthopaedic surgery. In fulfillment of this goal, applicants for certification must have received through orthopaedic residency

A. education in the entire field of orthopaedic surgery, including inpatient and outpatient diagnosis and care as well as operative and nonoperative management and rehabilitation;
B. the opportunity to develop, through experience, the necessary cognitive, technical, interpersonal, teaching, and research skills;
C. the opportunity to create new knowledge and to become skilled in the critical evaluation of information;
D. education in the recognition and management of basic medical and surgical problems;
E. an evaluation of ethical performance.

III. Minimum Educational Requirements for Board Certification

The Board has established the following minimum educational requirements for certification. These requirements should not be interpreted as restricting programs to minimum standards.

Throughout these rules, the term "accredited" denotes approval by the Accreditation Council for Graduate Medical Education (ACGME).

A. Time Requirements

1. Five years (60 months) of accredited postdoctoral residency are required.
2. Prior to July 1, 2000, 4 of these years (48 months) must be served in a program whose curriculum is determined by the director of an accredited orthopaedic surgery residency.
   a. Three of these years (36 months) must be served in an accredited orthopaedic surgery residency program.
   b. One year (12 months) may be served in an accredited graduate medical program whose educational content is determined by the director of an accredited orthopaedic surgery residency program.

   Beginning on July 1, 2000, 1 year (12 months) must be served in an accredited graduate medical education program whose curriculum fulfills the content requirements for the graduate year 1 (GY1) (see B.1, below) and is determined or approved by the director of an accredited orthopaedic surgery residency program. An additional 4 years (48 months) must be served in an accredited orthopaedic surgery residency program. An additional 4 years (48 months) must be served in an accredited orthopaedic

Certification Requirements

surgery residency program whose curriculum is determined by the director of the accredited orthopaedic surgery residency.

3. Each program may provide individual sick and vacation times for the resident in accordance with overall institutional policy. However, 1 year of credit must include at least 46 weeks of full-time orthopaedic education. Vacation or leave time may not be accumulated to reduce the 5-year requirement.
4. Program directors may retain a resident for as long as needed beyond the minimum required time to ensure the necessary degree of competence in orthopaedic surgery. According to the current Program Requirements for Residency Education in Orthopaedic Surgery, the committee must be notified of such retention. This information must also be provided to the Board on the Record of Residency Assignment form.

B. Content Requirements

1. Requirements for GY1
   Prior to July 1, 2000, a minimum of 9 months during the GY1 must be based in clinical services other than orthopaedics. This requirement may be fulfilled by a year of accredited residency in any broad-based program involving patient care.
   Beginning on July 1, 2000, the residency program director should be responsible for the design, implementation, and oversight of the GY1. The GY1 must include
   a. a minimum of 6 months of structured education in surgery to include multisystem trauma, plastic surgery/burn care, intensive care, and vascular surgery;
   b. a minimum of 1 month of structured education in at least three of the following—emergency medicine, medical/cardiac intensive care, internal medicine, neurology, neurological surgery, rheumatology, anesthesiology, musculoskeletal imaging, and rehabilitation;
   c. a maximum of 3 months of orthopaedic surgery.
2. Orthopaedic requirements beyond the GY1
   a. Minimum distribution. Orthopaedic education must be broadly representative of the entire field of orthopaedic surgery. The minimum distribution of educational experience must include
      1. 12 months of adult orthopaedics;
      2. 12 months of fractures/trauma;
      3. 6 months of children's orthopaedics;
      4. 6 months of basic science and/or clinical specialties.
      Experience may be received in two or more subject areas concurrently. Concurrent or integrated programs must allocate time by proportion of experience.
   b. Scope. Orthopaedic education must provide experience with all of the following:
      1. Children's orthopaedics. The educational experience in children's orthopaedics must be obtained either in an accredited position in the specific residency program in which the resident is enrolled or in a children's hospital in an assigned accredited residency position.
      2. Anatomic areas. All aspects of diagnosis and care of disorders affecting the bones, joints, and soft tissues of the upper and lower extremities, including the hand and foot; the entire spine, including intervertebral discs; and the bony pelvis.
      3. Acute and chronic care. Diagnosis and care, both operative and nonoperative, of acute trauma (including athletic injuries), infectious disease, neurovascular impairment, and chronic orthopaedic problems including reconstructive surgery, neuromuscular disease, metabolic bone disease, benign and malignant tumors, and rehabilitation.
      4. Related clinical subjects. Musculoskeletal imaging procedures, use and interpretation of clinical laboratory tests, prosthetics, orthotics, physical modalities and exercises, and neurological and rheumatological disorders.
      5. Research. Exposure to clinical and/or laboratory research.
      6. Basic science. Instruction in anatomy, biochemistry, biomaterials, biomechanics, microbiology, pathology, pharmacology, physiology, and other basic sciences related to orthopaedic surgery. The resident must have the opportunity to apply these basic sciences to all phases of orthopaedic surgery.
   c. Options. Twelve months of the 4 required years under the direction of the orthopaedic surgery residency program director may be spent on services consisting partially or entirely of:
      1. additional experience in general adult or children's orthopaedics or fractures/trauma;
      2. an orthopaedic clinical specialty;
      3. orthopaedics-related research;
      4. experience in an accredited graduate medical education program whose educational content is preapproved by the director of the orthopaedic surgery residency program.

C. Accreditation Requirements

1. The educational experience in orthopaedic surgery obtained in the United States must be in an approved position in programs accredited by the RRC for Orthopaedic Surgery and by the ACGME.
   All other clinical education obtained in the United States must be in programs accredited by the ACGME and the appropriate RRC. The *Graduate Medical Education Directory*, published annually by the American Medical Association, 515 N State St, Chicago, IL 60610, lists accredited rotations of 6 months or longer.
2. During the 5 years of accredited residency, a total period of no more than 6 months may be served in unaccredited institutions.
3. Credit for time spent in residency education will be granted only for the period during which the residency program is accredited, and only for time served in an approved position within an accredited program.
4. If an orthopaedic residency program has its accreditation withdrawn by the RRC for Orthopaedic Surgery and the ACGME, no educational credit will be granted past the effective date of withdrawal of accreditation.
5. Educational credit may be granted for clinical experience in the US military and/or public health services if the experience is accepted by the director of the orthopaedic surgery residency program that the applicant enters. Up to 1 month of credit may be granted for every 2 months of clinical experience, not to exceed 12 months of credit. Credit earned in this manner is subject to approval by the Board's Credentials Committee. This approval should be sought prior to entry into the program.
6. Educational experience obtained in Canada must be on services approved by the Royal College of Physicians and Surgeons of Canada (RCPSC) and must extend over a minimum of 5 years. The content requirements outlined in III.B must be met.
7. The Board does not grant credit for foreign educational experience, other than as permitted in 2 and 6, above.
8. The term "fellow" is not synonymous with the term "resident" for the purpose of obtaining Board credit for educational experience. A resident is an individual enrolled in an approved position in an accredited educational program.

D. Achievement Requirements

1. The director of the program providing general graduate medical education must certify the satisfactory completion of that segment of education.

2. In orthopaedic surgery residency programs, the program director must certify the satisfactory completion of each rotation for which credit is awarded. (See III.F, below.)
3. The program director responsible for the final year of the resident's education must certify that the resident has achieved a satisfactory level of competence and is qualified for the certifying process.
4. The certification referred to in 2 and 3, above, must be made on the appropriate Record of Residency Assignment form.
5. Medical practice activity outside of residency duties must not be allowed to interfere with the educational experience. Residents may not engage in such activities without the specific prior approval of the program director. Approval must be based on the judgment that rotations are being completed without compromise and that the circumstances of the resident warrant such activity.

E. Continuity Requirements

The resident should have progressively increasing patient care responsibility. A part-time or piecemeal approach to residency requirements is discouraged. The final 24 months of orthopaedic residency education must be obtained in a single orthopaedic residency program unless prior approval of the Credentials Committee is obtained.

F. Documentation Requirements

1. For orthopaedic education obtained in the United States, the program director must provide the Board with yearly documentation during the residency. Each May, directors will receive Record of Residency Assignment forms on which the required information will be recorded. The appropriate forms are to be signed by the program director and the resident. The original, signed forms are to be returned to the Board office within 30 days of the end of the academic year (August 1).
2. The Record of Residency Assignment forms are to be completed for each resident as follows:
   a. Form 1 will be submitted the year the resident enters the program.
   b. Form 1-A must be provided for residents receiving educational credit in a nonorthopaedic ACGME-accredited program and for nonorthopaedic education received within the ACGME-accredited orthopaedic residency.
   c. Form 2-A must be completed yearly for each resident in the orthopaedic program. It must indicate the content and time spent on rotations, information on any unaccredited rotations, and whether or not credit was granted for a full year.
   d. Form 3 is the final evaluation form.
3. The original, signed forms are due in the Board office within 30 days of completion of the academic year. Part I examination results for candidates who take the examination in the same year they complete their residencies will not be mailed either to the candidates or to the program directors until the forms have been received in the Board office.
4. When a resident leaves a program prematurely, the program director must notify the Board office in writing within 30 days. The letter must record the reasons for leaving and confirm credit granted for rotations during the academic year in which the resident left. At the end of the academic year, Form 2-A and Form 3 must be completed.
5. Before a resident enters a new program, the new program director must obtain copies of the resident's Record of Residency Assignment forms from the Board office and review them thoroughly in order to develop an appropriate individual program that will meet the minimum educational requirements and include progressively increasing responsibility.

IV. Requirements for Taking the Certifying Examinations

The certifying examination is divided into two parts. Part I is a written examination, which may be taken at any time after the completion of the educational requirements. Part II is an oral examination, which may be taken after passing Part I, completion of the 22-month practice requirement, evaluation of the applicant's practice, and admission to the examination. A candidate must pass both parts of the certifying examination to be certified.

After taking and passing the written examination, candidates have 5 years to take or retake the oral examination. Candidates who do not pass the oral examination within those 5 years must retake and repass the written examination before applying to take the oral examination. Time spent in fellowship education after passing Part I will not count as a part of the 5-year time limit.

An applicant seeking certification by the ABOS must satisfy the educational requirements that were in effect when he/she first enrolled in an accredited orthopaedic residency. For all other requirements, an applicant must meet the specifications in effect at the time of application.

A. Educational Requirements

1. An applicant must satisfactorily complete and document the minimum educational requirements in effect when he/she first enrolled in an accredited orthopaedic residency.
2. Upon successful completion of 54 of the 60 months of required education and on the recommendation of the program director, a candidate may apply to take Part I of the examination.
3. In order to be admitted to the examination, the candidate must complete the full 60 months of required education.
4. An applicant who has received orthopaedic surgery residency education in Canada must have fulfilled the requirements of the ABOS and must have passed the qualifying examination in orthopaedic surgery of the RCPSC before applying for either part of the Board's certifying examination.

B. License Requirement

Applicants who are in practice at the time they apply for Part I and all applicants for Part II must either possess a full and unrestricted license to practice medicine in the United States or Canada or be engaged in full-time practice in the US federal government, for which licensure is not required. An applicant will be rendered ineligible for any part of the certifying examination by limitation, suspension, or termination of any right associated with the practice of medicine in any state, province, or country due to a violation of a medical practice act or other statute or governmental regulation; to disciplinary action by any medical licensing authority; by entry into a consent order; or by voluntary surrender while under investigation, or suspension of license.

C. Board Eligible Status

Effective July 1, 1996, the Board will recognize those candidates who have successfully completed Part I and are awaiting to take Part II as being "Board eligible." The limit of Board eligibility is the 5 years candidates have to take or retake the oral examination (Part II) after passing Part I. Candidates who do not pass the oral examination (Part II) within those 5 years will lose their Board-eligible status. (See "IV. Requirements for Taking the Certifying Examinations," above.)

D. Practice Requirements

1. The applicant must be continuously and actively engaged in the practice of operative orthopaedic surgery other than as a resident or fellow (or equivalent) for at least 22 full months immediately prior to the Part II examination. An applicant must have started practice on or before September 1, 1997, in order to qual-

ify for the 1999 Part II Examination. An applicant who interrupts the 22 months of practice with a fellowship can count the months of practice that preceded the fellowship as part of the 22-month requirement.

2. The applicant must be in one practice location for a minimum of 12 consecutive months during the required 22-month period. A change in location, type of hospital practice, or practice association may result in deferral. The practice must be located in the United States or its territories, Canada, or a US service installation.
3. The practice must include hospital admitting and surgical privileges (temporary privileges acceptable) in effect at the time of application and at the time of examination. The practice must allow independent decision making in matters of patient care.
4. The applicant must demonstrate professional competence and adherence to acceptable ethical and professional standards. It is the responsibility of the applicant to provide documentation that he/she is an ethical and competent practitioner.
5. A reduction, restriction, suspension, termination, or resignation at the request of a hospital of all or any portion of an applicant's surgical staff privileges, or pending action to do so, will normally result in a deferral until such action is finally resolved and the applicant's practice has stabilized sufficiently for it to be evaluated.
6. An applicant in the US uniformed services may satisfy the practice requirement if assigned as an orthopaedic surgeon for at least 22 full months prior to the date of the Part II examination. The applicant must submit a letter from his/her immediate supervisor evaluating his/her capability in the practice of orthopaedic surgery, as well as any other documentation the Credentials Committee may require to demonstrate professional competence and adherence to acceptable ethical and professional standards.

E. Evaluation of Applicant

1. Individuals who do not engage in active orthopaedic surgery cannot be adequately evaluated for the Part II examination and will not be certified.
2. Qualifications for taking the Part II examination will be determined by the Credentials Committee after review of the application, letters of recommendation, and other relevant information.
3. It is the responsibility of the applicant to provide the information on which the Credentials Committee bases its evaluation of the qualifications of the applicant. This responsibility extends to information that the Credentials Committee requests from other persons. If the Credentials Committee does not receive requested information from the applicant, a program director, a reference, a hospital representative, or another source, the Board will notify the applicant and defer the decision on admission to the examination until the information has been received. The applicant may be required to authorize release of peer review information to the Board.
4. Representatives of the Board may visit the site of an applicant's practice if the Credentials Committee believes that this is necessary for adequate evaluation of the applicant's work.

V. Impaired Physicians

A. Chemical Dependency

Applicants for either part of the certifying examination who, within 3 years of their application, have been diagnosed as chemically dependent and/or have been treated for drug or other substance abuse will be required, as part of their demonstration that they meet the practice requirements in IV.D., to present evidence from the appropriate agencies, hospitals, and physicians demonstrating to the satisfaction of the Board that they have both (1) satisfactorily completed the program of treatment prescribed for their condition, and (2) been free of chemical dependency for a period sufficient to establish that they are not currently using illegal drugs and/or that the use of illegal drugs or other substance abuse is not an ongoing problem. This documentation must accompany the completed application form. The maintenance of any such applicant's certification may be conditional upon periodic drug testing.

B. Mental and Physical Condition

Applicants for either part of the certifying examination who have a mental or physical condition that could affect their ability to practice orthopaedic surgery will be required, as part of their demonstration that they meet the practice requirements in IV.D., to present medical evidence from the appropriate physicians, treatment centers, and hospitals demonstrating to the Board that the impairment does not compromise their ability to render safe and effective care to their patients. This documentation must accompany the completed application form.

VI. Procedure for Application for Part I and Part II of the Certifying Examinations

A. Application Dates and Requests

1. The dates, locations, and application deadlines for Part I and Part II of the certifying examination are announced in the Journal of Bone and Joint Surgery. They are also listed on the Board's website: www.abos.org. Examination dates may be changed at the discretion of the Board. Confirmation of published examination dates can be obtained from the Board's office.
2. All applications must be requested in writing.

B. Application Deadlines

1. Part I. A completed application on an original form provided by the Board for Part I must be postmarked by registered mail on or before March 1 of the year of the examination. The application must be accompanied by a nonrefundable examination fee of $770.
2. Part II. A completed application on an original form provided by the Board for Part II must be postmarked by registered mail on or before October 31 of the year preceding the examination. The application must be accompanied by a nonrefundable application and credentialing fee of $700.
3. Late or incomplete applications. Applications postmarked after the deadlines for Part I or Part II of the certifying examination and applications received incomplete will be returned to the applicant together with the fee check.
   a. If a Part I applicant wishes to resubmit the Part I application by registered mail postmarked on or before March 31, the nonrefundable examination fee of $770 and a nonrefundable late fee of $250 must be enclosed.
   b. If a Part II applicant wishes to resubmit the Part II application by registered mail postmarked on or before November 30, the nonrefundable application and credentialing fee of $700 and a nonrefundable late fee of $250 must be enclosed.
   c. No applications will be accepted after the late deadlines.

C. Notifying the Board of Application Changes

1. It is the responsibility of all applicants to notify the Board office of any change of address, practice association, or hospital affiliation.
2. If a Part II applicant changes practice location or practice association or acquires new hospital staff affiliations, new references will be solicited by the Board.
3. An applicant is also required to notify the Board of the denial of any request for hospital privileges; of any action to restrict, suspend, or terminate all or any portion of surgical staff privileges; of any request by a hospital to resign all or any portion of surgical

staff privileges; and of any action by a governmental agency that would result in the restriction, suspension, or probation of the applicant's license or any right associated with the practice of medicine.

D. Notifying the Applicant of Examination Admission

1. For Part I, the applicant will receive examination information, an assigned examination number, and an admission card not later than 30 days prior to the examination date.
2. For Part II, the decision of the Credentials Committee is mailed to the applicant not later than 60 days prior to the examination date.

E. Fees

1. For Part I, the nonrefundable examination fee of $770 must be submitted with the application form.
2. For Part II:
   a. The nonrefundable application and credentialing fee of $700 must be submitted with the application form.
   b. The candidate must also submit an examination fee of $770 on or before the date specified in the letter of notification of admission to the examination. This fee will be forfeited if the candidate fails to appear for the examination or cancels after being scheduled.
3. There will be a $50 charge levied for any application or examination fee check that is returned not paid by the Board's bank.
4. The fees paid to the ABOS are not tax deductible as a charitable contribution, but may be deductible under some other provision of the Internal Revenue Service code.

Fees

Part I examination fee	$770
Part II application and credentialing fee	$700
Part II examination fee	$770
Late fee	$250
Returned check service charge	$50

F. Practice-Based Oral Examination

The Part II examination is practice based. The purpose of the practice-based examination is to evaluate a candidate's own practice as broadly as possible. This exercise will be conducted much as rounds or conferences are during residency, with the candidate presenting his/her cases and responding to the examiner's questions and comments. Applicants are urged to attend to details and follow procedures carefully and exactly to ensure admission to the examination.

1. Case collection: Each applicant will receive case collection software diskettes with their application. This is the program that the applicant must use to enter his/her 6-month case list information. The applicant is to collect all operative cases, including same-day surgery, for which he/she was the responsible operating surgeon for 6 consecutive months beginning July 1 of the year before the Part II examination. If time is taken off during those 6 months, the starting point for the collection period must be backed up by the amount of time missed. For example, case collection for an applicant who took a 2-week vacation in August would begin in mid June.

   All cases must be collected from each hospital or surgery center at which the applicant has operated during the 6-month period. If the applicant did no cases during the case collection period, this fact must be verified by a letter from the hospital and/or surgery center. The letter(s) must be sent to the Board office along with the case lists.

   Case lists: Once all cases have been entered into the case collection program, the applicant will print out his/her complete case list(s) by hospital. No changes can be made to the case list(s) after this is done. Each complete hospital list must then be certified by the director of medical records. The director of medical records signature must then be notarized. When the applicant has each hospital list certified and notarized, he/she must then save the complete case list to a 3.5-inch diskette.
2. Case submission: By January 31 of the year of the Part II examination, the applicant must submit to the Board:
   a. The complete printed case list(s) for the required 6-month period. Each hospital list must be stapled separately and have the required signatures and notarization. Before mailing, the applicant should make a copy of the complete case list(s), as the copies the applicant must bring to the examination must be of these printed and certified lists.
   b. A 3.5-inch diskette containing his/her complete case list. The case information on the printed lists and on the diskette must be identical.
   c. For each hospital or surgery center where no cases were performed, a letter stating that no cases were performed there during the 6-month period.

   This information must be sent to the Board office by registered mail or courier of your choice (ie, Federal Express, Express Mail, certified mail, etc) to ABOS, Part II Exam, 400 Silver Cedar Ct, Chapel Hill, NC 27514. Case lists must be postmarked by January 31 of the year of the examination. The Board office will not verify receipt of case lists.
3. Case Selection: The Board will select 12 cases from the applicant's 6-month case list(s). The list of 12 cases selected by the Board will be sent to the candidate in mid May. From the list of 12, the applicant will then select ten cases to bring to the examination for detailed presentation.
4. Examination Materials/Preparation: Once the candidate has received the list of the 12 cases selected by the Board, he/she must gather all of the following to bring to the examination:
   a. Three copies of the list of 12 selected cases.
   b. Three copies of the applicant's complete case list that was submitted to the Board in January.
   c. Images (including x-rays) for the 10 cases selected by the candidate—the pertinent pre-, intra-, or immediate post-operative and most recent follow-up x-rays for each case selected by the candidate for presentation. Before the examination begins, x-rays should be arranged in order of presentation and clearly marked in terms of date, pre- and postoperative. Pertinent images in CT and MRI panels must also be marked.
   d. Two copies of notes for the 10 cases selected by the applicant—this includes admission and discharge notes, operative notes, office notes, and any other patient chart material that will aid in case presentation.
   e. Video prints or photographic prints for arthroscopy cases selected that show the initial lesion(s) and the lesion(s) after treatment.
   f. For cases with complications, images (including x-rays) pertinent to the complication and its treatment and two copies of any consultation report(s).

   Please note: Because the examination is to be anonymous, the candidate should obliterate his/her name wherever it appears on any material brought to the examination, including the 6-month case list(s) and the Board's list of 12 selected cases.

   Although the examiners will concentrate on cases brought for presentation, they may also ask questions pertaining to a candidate's case lists or practice. The candidate should not be concerned if all material brought to the examination is not covered. Discussion may focus on one area, or candidate and examiners may become involved in a few cases in such detail that time will not allow presentation of all patients. The candidate will not be penalized for this during the grading.

Applicants who have questions about materials and procedures for the practice-based oral Part II examination should call or write the Board office well before the examination. Failure to comply with the steps outlined may invalidate an examination.

VII. Falsified Information and Irregular Behavior

A. If it is determined that an applicant has falsified information on the application form or failed to provide material information, the applicant will not be considered for either part of the examination not already passed and must wait 3 years before being allowed to file a new application.

B. Examination applicants should understand that the following may be sufficient cause to bar them from future examinations, terminate participation in the examination, invalidate the results of an examination, withhold or revoke scores or certificates, or take other appropriate action:

1. The giving or receiving of aid in the examination, as evidenced either by observation or by statistical analysis of answers of one or more participants in the examination
2. The unauthorized possession, reproduction, or disclosure of any materials, including, but not limited to, examination questions or answers, before, during, or after the examination
3. The offering of any benefit to any agent of the Board in return for any right, privilege, or benefit that is not usually granted by the Board to other similarly situated candidates or persons.
4. The engaging in irregular behavior in connection with the administration of the examination

C. The following are examples of behavior considered to be irregular and that may be cause for invalidation of the examination or imposition of a penalty:

1. Referring to books, notes, or other devices at any time during the examination. This prohibited material includes written information or information transferred by electronic, acoustical, or other means.
2. Any transfer of information or signals between candidates during the test. This prohibition includes any transfer of information between the candidate and any other person at any time during the testing period, including bathroom breaks.
3. Any appearance of looking at the answer sheet or the examination booklet of another candidate during the examination.
4. Allowing another candidate to view one's answer sheet or examination booklet or otherwise assisting another candidate in the examination.
5. Taking any examination material outside the examination room. All examination materials are the property of the Board and must be left in the room at the end of the examination.

D. Applicants should also understand that the Board may or may not require a candidate to retake one or more portions of the examination if presented with sufficient evidence that the security of the examination has been compromised, notwithstanding the absence of any evidence of a candidate's personal involvement in such activities.

VIII. Credentials Decisions

A. Determining Admission to Examinations

1. The Credentials Committee meets at least once each year to consider applications for the examinations. At this meeting, a decision about each applicant will be made either to approve admission to the next examination, to deny admission, or to defer decision pending further evaluation.
2. A decision approving admission to an examination applies only until the next available examination and does not carry over from one examination until the next. A new application is required for each examination.

B. Deferral of Admission Decision

A decision on an applicant's admission to either Part I or Part II of the examination may be deferred if information received by the Credentials Committee is insufficient for the Committee to make a judgment and/or warrants further investigation. Typically, the committee will defer such a decision for 1 year to gain further information. If information is still insufficient, the decision will be deferred for a second year to enable representatives of the Board to conduct a site visit as described in IV.E.4. A deferral of not more than 2 consecutive years is not viewed by the Board as an adverse action; thus, no appeal of a decision of the Credentials Committee is permitted unless an applicant has been denied admission or has been deferred for more than 2 consecutive years.

C. Appeal of Admission Decision

An applicant denied admission to the examination or deferred for more than 2 years will be informed of the basis for such action and may request a hearing by an appeals committee of the ABOS. (See XII, below.)

IX. Certificates and Certificate Renewal

A. Awarding Certificates

The ABOS awards a certificate to a candidate who specializes in orthopaedic surgery, has met the educational requirements of the Board, has demonstrated competence in orthopaedic surgery and adherence to ethical and professional standards, and has passed both parts of the certifying examination. Certificates awarded after 1985 are valid for 10 years. This portion of the Board's responsibility is discharged by issuance of a certificate to an individual found qualified as of the date of certification.

B. Certificate Revocation

At its discretion, the Board may revoke a certificate for due causes, including, but not limited to the following:

1. The diplomate did not possess the required qualifications and requirements for examination, whether or not such deficiency was known to the Board or any committee thereof prior to examination or at the time of issuance of the certificate, as the case may be.
2. The diplomate made an intentional and material misrepresentation or withheld information in the application to either part of the examination or in any other representation to the Board or any committee thereof.
3. The diplomate made a misrepresentation to the Board or any third party as to his/her status as a diplomate of the Board or his/her receipt of or eligibility for certification by the Board.
4. The diplomate engaged in irregular behavior in connection with an examination of the Board (as described in VII.C), whether or not such practice had an effect on the performance of the candidate on an examination.
5. The diplomate was convicted by a court of competent jurisdiction of a felony or misdemeanor involving moral turpitude and, in the opinion of the Board, having a material relationship to the practice of medicine.
6. There has been a limitation, suspension, or termination of any right of the diplomate associated with the practice of medicine in any state, province, or country, including the imposition of any requirement of surveillance, supervision, or review due to a violation of a medical practice act, or other statute or governmental regulation, disciplinary action by any medical licensing authority, entry into a consent order, or voluntary surrender of license.

A diplomate may appeal the revocation of his/her certificates pursuant to the procedures set forth in Section XII.

C. Certificate Reinstatement

Should the circumstances that justified revocation or surrender of the diplomate's certificate be corrected, the Board may reinstate the certificate after appropriate review of the individual's qualifications and performance, using the same standard applied to other applicants for certification.

D. Certificate Renewal

Diplomates are encouraged to renew their credentials periodically through the Board's recertification process. Information about recertification options can be obtained from the Board office.

X. Unsuccessful Candidates

Unsuccessful Part I candidates may repeat the examination by submitting a new application form for the examination and again being found admissible. (See VI.B.1.)

Unsuccessful Part II candidates may repeat the examination by submitting a new application form for the examination and again being found admissible. (See VI.B.2 and VIII.) Candidates who do not pass Part II within 5 years (as measured in Section IV) of passing Part I must retake and repass Part I before applying to take Part II.

XI. Program Accreditation

Institutions offering orthopaedic education must meet the Institutional and Program Requirements of the ACGME and the RRC for Orthopaedic Surgery as stated in the *Graduate Medical Education Directory*. (See III.C.)

A. RRC for Orthopaedic Surgery

Program accreditation is issued by the RRC for Orthopaedic Surgery, an autonomous committee composed of three representatives from each of the three sponsoring organizations: the ABOS, the Council on Medical Education of the American Medical Association, and the American Academy of Orthopaedic Surgeons. In evaluating orthopaedic residency programs, the RRC considers the number of residents, training period, program organization, educational experience, and institutional responsibility. The committee meets twice yearly.

B. Changes in Accreditation

Programs seeking changes in accredited positions or institutional affiliations can obtain information and application forms from the secretary of the RRC for Orthopaedic Surgery at the ACGME, 515 N State St, Chicago, IL 60610. Completed forms are to be returned to the secretary at the above address.

C. Program Surveys

Programs applying for accreditation or changes in accreditation will be surveyed at the earliest feasible date by a specialist site visitor or by a field representative for the ACGME. A report of the survey is submitted to the RRC for Orthopaedic Surgery for evaluation and official action. The RRC makes a determination regarding the accreditation of the program under authority delegated by the ACGME, and it notifies the program director and the sponsoring institutions.

D. Number of Residents

The total number of residents assigned to any orthopaedic residency program and the number at each level of education must have prior approval by the RRC for Orthopaedic Surgery.

XII. Appeals Procedure

A. An individual who has received an unfavorable ruling from a committee of the Board may appeal such determination by mailing a notice of appeal to the office of the ABOS within 60 days of the date such ruling was mailed to him or her. Exception: The decisions by the Examinations Committee that a candidate has failed either part of the certifying examination may be appealed only in the manner and to the extent provided in G and H, below.

B. Upon receipt of a notice of appeal, the concerned Board committee shall consider any information submitted therewith by the individual in support of his/her appeal and make such further investigation as it deems appropriate. If the committee then decides in a manner favorable to the individual, it shall so notify the individual. If the committee does not so determine, it shall notify the individual and the president of the ABOS.

C. The individual shall then have the right to an appeals hearing to decide whether the determination of the concerned Board committee shall be confirmed, modified, or overruled in accordance with the hearing process described in this appeals procedure.

1. The president of the ABOS shall appoint an ad hoc appeals committee consisting of three directors of the Board who did not participate in making the determination being appealed, one of whom shall be designated by the president as chairman of the appeals committee.
2. In the event that the subject matter of the appeal involves complex issues of fact or issues not solely dependent upon medical, surgical, or professional standards, the president of the ABOS, at his/her sole discretion, may appoint a hearing officer to conduct the appeals hearing and to submit a full written report and a recommended decision to the ad hoc appeals committee. The hearing officer appointed at the discretion of the president shall be an impartial physician, lawyer, or other professional.
3. The chairman of the appeals committee shall convene a hearing before the appeals committee or the hearing officer, if one is appointed, within a reasonable time after their respective appointments, but not less than 60 days after the appointment of the appeals committee and the hearing officer, whichever is later.

D. Prior to the hearing

1. The concerned Board committee shall provide the executive director with such written information concerning its decision as it deems appropriate; a list of witnesses, if any, whom it expects to call to testify; copies of any written material that it considered in making the determination appealed (but only if it intends to present such material at the hearing); and a list of information and documents the individual is required to produce at the hearing. This material, together with written notice stating the time and place of the hearing, shall be sent to the individual by the executive director not less than 30 days prior to the hearing. Not less than 7 days prior to the hearing, the concerned Board committee shall provide the executive director and the individual with copies of any written reports, affidavits, or statements of experts that the concerned Board committee intends to present at the hearing.
2. Not less than 7 days prior to the hearing, the individual shall provide the executive director and the concerned Board committee with such written information concerning his/her position as he/she deems appropriate; a list of witnesses, if any, whom he/she expects to call to testify; and copies of any written reports, affidavits, or statements of experts that he/she intends to present at the hearing.
3. The executive director shall submit the written material referred to in this section D to the members of the appeals committee or to the hearing officer, if one has been appointed, prior to the hearing. Copies of this material must also be submitted to the individual and to the concerned Board committee no later than the time when submitted to the appeals committee or the hearing officer.

E. The hearing, whether conducted before the appeals committee or a hearing officer, shall be a hearing de novo. The concerned Board committee and the individual shall have the right to present all relevant information and evidence in support of their respective positions, and neither the concerned Board committee nor the individual shall be limited to the information and evidence considered by the concerned Board committee in making its original determination or its reconsideration of the original decision.

1. The concerned Board committee shall have the burden of proving at the hearing that the determination being appealed should be confirmed. The standard of proof to be applied by the appeals committee and the hearing officer in deciding whether the information and evidence presented at the hearing is sufficient to warrant confirmation of the determination being appealed is by the preponderance or greater weight of the evidence.
2. At the hearing, the concerned Board committee and its legal or other representatives shall present such relevant information and evidence as it deems appropriate to support its previously made determination. However, the committee shall not have the right to present any information or evidence not previously provided as required in D.1. The committee may call, examine, and cross-examine witnesses.
3. The individual shall have the right to be represented at the hearing by legal counsel or any person of his/her choice. He/she may present such relevant information and evidence as he/she deems appropriate in support of his/her position. However, the individual shall not have the right to present any information or evidence if not previously provided as required in D.2. The failure of the individual to produce information or documents requested by the concerned Board committee as required in D.2 shall be grounds for upholding and confirming the determinations of the concerned Board committee. The individual may call, examine, and cross-examine witnesses.
4. The individual and the concerned Board committee may submit written statements at the close of the hearing. A written record of the hearing shall be made available to the individual at one half the cost of its preparation.

F. After the conclusion of the hearing

1. If the hearing has been conducted before a hearing officer, the hearing officer shall prepare a written report based on the information and evidence presented, including the findings of fact determined by the hearing officer and a recommended decision as to whether the determination being appealed should be confirmed, modified, or overruled. The hearing officer shall submit the written report to the appeals committee and send copies to the individual and the concerned Board committee. The individual and/or the concerned Board committee may file objections to the report and recommendations of the hearing officer with the appeals committee within 10 days after receipt of the report. The opposing party shall then have 10 days to file its response to such objections with the appeals committee.
2. The appeals committee shall make its decisions following the hearing. If the hearing has been conducted before a hearing officer, the appeals committee will first receive the written report and recommendations of the hearing officer and the objections and responses filed thereto by the parties. If a majority of the members of the appeals committee determine, on the basis of the information and evidence presented, including, when applicable, the report and recommendations of the hearing officer, that the determination of the concerned Board committee should be confirmed or modified, the appeals committee shall so declare. If a majority determines that the concerned Board committee's determination should be overruled, the appeals committee shall so declare. The appeals committee shall inform the individual and the concerned Board committee of its decision in writing within a reasonable time following the hearing, explaining the basis for its judgment. The decision of the appeals committee shall be final and binding.

G. A candidate who believes that the Part II examination was administered in an unfair or inaccurate manner or that one or more of his/her oral examiners was acquainted with him or her or was not impartial may immediately, upon completion of the examination, request that he/she be reexamined. The request shall be made to the chairman of the Oral Examinations Committee and reviewed by the president and the secretary. If, after discussing the matter with the candidate and making such other investigation as they may deem appropriate, a majority of the president, the secretary, and the chairman of the Oral Examinations Committee determine that reasonable grounds exist for the candidate's request, he/she shall be immediately reexamined by another panel of oral examiners. In such event, the first oral examination will be disregarded and only the candidate's performance on the reexamination shall be considered in determining his/her score on the examination.

H. A candidate who fails the Part I examination may request in writing that his/her examination be rescored by hand to verify the accuracy of the results as reported to him or her. Such a request is to be made within 60 days of his/her being notified of the results of the examination. The request must be accompanied by a check for $100 payable to the ABOS to cover the cost of hand scoring. There shall be no further appeal of a failure on the Part I examination.

American Board of Otolaryngology

2211 Norfolk/Ste 800
Houston, TX 77098-4044
713 528-6200
713 528-1171 Fax
Internet: http://www.aboto.org

(These criteria and conditions are subject to change without notice. All applicants are advised to contact the American Board of Otolaryngology [ABOto] to ascertain whether the information below is correct.)

Important Dates

April 10, 1998	Applications for 1998 Written Examination become available
July 10, 1998	Applications due. To avoid late fees, the envelope must be postmarked July 10 or before, and all required items must be enclosed with the application, including the $1,800 fee
July 10, 1998	Operative Experience Report diskettes & printouts due from all residents and new applicants
July 10, 1998	Resident Registry forms due from program directors
July 11-20 1998	Applications postmarked between these dates (inclusive) accepted with $200 late fee
July 20, 1998	Applications postmarked after this date not accepted
August 5, 1998	Applicants notified of acceptance for examination
September 1, 1998	Operative Experience Report diskettes issued to new residents or returned to returning residents
September 19, 1998	Written Examination
March 27, 1999	Otolaryngology Training Examination
April 17-18, 1999	Oral Exam for qualifying candidates from 1998 Written Exam

Board Eligibility and Status Inquiries

The ABOto does not recognize or use the term "Board eligible." The Board states whether an individual is certified, is not certified, or is in the process of being examined (ie, between written and oral examinations).

Examination

The ABOto certification process consists of two phases: a written qualifying examination and an oral certifying examination.

All candidates must take a written examination, which is offered in the fall of each year. Candidates who do not achieve the qualifying score fail the exam and are not eligible to take the oral examination. They may retake the written exam in a subsequent year.

Candidates who meet or exceed the qualifying score must then successfully complete an oral examination, which is offered in the spring of each year, in order to become certified. Qualified candidates are given three consecutive opportunities to take the oral exam. If a passing score is not achieved after three exam cycles, the candidate must reapply to take the written exam and must again achieve a qualifying score in order to be permitted to retake the oral exam.

Written and oral examination scores are *not* combined. An individual must successfully complete both the written and the oral exam in order to be certified. A certificate is granted by the ABOto to a candidate who has met all the requirements and has satisfactorily passed its exams.

Prerequisite Requirements

1. Resident Registry

All residents must be registered with the ABOto during the first year of otolaryngology training in order to subsequently apply to take the certification examination.

A New Resident Form must be filed for each new resident by the program director by July 10 of the first year of otolaryngology-head and neck surgery training. The form must be signed by both the program director and the resident.

The program director subsequently submits a Resident Evaluation Form for each returning resident by July 10 of each year. It must be noted whether the previous year was successfully completed, and the form must be signed by both the program director and the resident.

Resident Evaluation Forms become part of the individual's ABOto file and are a prerequisite for application for the certification examination.

Credit may not be granted by the ABOto for any year of training for which an Evaluation Form is not received.

2. Operative Experience Report (OER)

All residents maintain a log of their surgical procedures on a computer diskette during otolaryngology-head and neck surgery training.

A disk is prepared at the ABOto office for each new resident and disks are sent to the resident's program director for distribution in early September.

Throughout the year, each resident maintains a record of his or her surgical procedures on the computer disk.

All residents return their disks to the ABOto by July 10 of each year. A printout, signed by the resident and the program director, is also submitted by July 10.

Residents who complete a full year of research between years of otolaryngology training and who perform no surgical cases during that year need not submit a disk for that year. However, a letter must be submitted by July 10 explaining this.

Data from the disk is transferred to a master database for review by the Credentials Committee. Disks are then returned to residents in early September.

A fee of $25 is charged for lost disks. A fee of $200 is charged for disks and/or printouts not received by the July 10 deadline.

Completion and return of OER data annually is a prerequisite for application for the certification examination.

Credit may not be granted by the ABOto for any year of training for which OER data is not recorded.

3. Transfers

A resident wishing to transfer from one residency program to another must notify the ABOto in writing and explain the circumstances of the proposed transfer.

Letters from the current and prospective directors of training must also be submitted:

- The letter from the current program director must verify the exact amount of training successfully completed in the program.
- The letter from the prospective program director must verify that sufficient residency positions, accredited by the Residency Review Committee for Otolaryngology of the Accreditation Council for Graduate Medical Education (ACGME), exist in the program to provide the transferring resident with the training necessary to meet the requirements of the ABOto for certification.

Leaves of Absence

Leave of absence and vacation may be granted to residents at the discretion of the program director in accordance with local rules. The total of such leaves and vacation may not exceed 6 weeks in any one year. If a longer leave of absence is granted in any year, the required period of graduate medical education may be extended accordingly.

Training Requirements

All training specified below must be successfully completed in ACGME-accredited programs.

Training programs in otolaryngology-head and neck surgery in the United States are evaluated by the Residency Review Committee for Otolaryngology, which consists of representatives from the American Medical Association, the American College of Surgeons, and the ABOto and are accredited by the ACGME. Information concerning approved educational programs is contained in the *Graduate Medical Education Directory*, published by the American Medical Association.

The applicant whose residency training began July 1, 1997, or thereafter must have satisfactorily completed a minimum of 5 years of residency training as follows:

1. At least *1 year* of general surgical training. It is preferred that the general surgical residency be taken prior to otolaryngologic training, but it may not be taken after otolaryngologic training.
2. At least 4 years of residency training in otolaryngology-head and neck surgery. This training must involve increasing responsibility each year and must include a final year of senior experience. This final year must be spent within the accredited program in which the previous year of training was spent, unless prior approval is obtained from the ABOto.

All residency training must be completed in a manner acceptable to the head of that residency program.

Foreign Training

An applicant who completed otolaryngologic training in the United Kingdom or the Republic of Ireland prior to January 1, 1997, in a program accredited by the Specialist Advisory Committee and who has received a certificate of accreditation in otolaryngology from the Joint Committee on Higher Surgical Training in the United Kingdom and the Republic of Ireland may be considered for examination.

An applicant who completed otolaryngologic training under the New Zealand program after January 1, 1984, but before July 1, 1998, and who has passed the examination leading to Fellowship in the Royal Australasian College of Surgeons may be considered for examination.

An applicant who completed training under the Australian program after January 1, 1986, but before July 1, 1998, and who has passed the examination leading to fellowship in the Royal Australasian College of Surgeons may be considered for examination.

Application for Examination

There is no required time interval between completion of the residency program and application for examination. However, all residency training must be successfully completed before the date of the examination in any given year.

Application materials for the written examination in any given year become available April 10 and must be completed and returned (postmarked) by July 10 of that year. The application consists of the following:

1. Application form, signed by the program director and another ABOto diplomate
2. Verification of medical degree (official transcript or letter from Dean) from an approved school of medicine or osteopathy
3. Verification of Otolaryngology Residency Form, signed by the program director, attesting to satisfactory completion of the training program
4. Verification of Surgery Residency Form, signed by the chief of surgery, attesting to satisfactory completion of the training program
5. Verification of Additional Residency Form, signed by the appropriate program director, attesting to satisfactory completion of the training program or internship
6. Verification of all licenses to practice medicine, showing nonrestricted status and date of expiration

   Individuals who have completed residency training but who will enter a fellowship program utilizing an institutional license must submit a statement from the program director as evidence of this fact.

   Individuals who have completed residency training but who will go on to practice medicine in a foreign country not requiring licensure must make a written request to be accepted for the examination without medical license. Such requests must be submitted with the application.
7. Operative Experience Report (diskette and printout), which lists procedures assisted in and performed by the applicant during otolaryngology residency
8. The applicant must possess high moral, ethical and professional qualifications as determined by, and the sole discretion of the Board. Additional information may be requested by the Board from the following: local medical society, Board-certified otolaryngologists from the geographical area in which the applicant practices, the director of the applicant's training program, hospital chiefs of staff, and/or other individuals and entities who may have knowledge of the applicant's moral and ethical standing, qualifications, or abilities.

Applications are approved by the Credentials Committee in August, and applicants are then notified if they have been approved for examination. The Board reserves the right to reject any application.

Applications are valid for one written exam and three oral exams. At the conclusion of this period, or upon failure of the written exam, the application expires, and individuals are required to submit new forms.

Applicants With Special Disabilities

The ABOto fully supports the intent of the Americans with Disabilities Act (ADA). Upon request, it will make reasonable accommodations in its examination procedures for candidates with documented disabilities. A candidate for certification who believes that he/she is disabled within the meaning of the ADA law should request detailed information concerning ABOto's policy regarding accommodation so that his/her special needs can be met in a timely manner. Documentation of the disability must accompany the application.

Fees

1. General Information

a. Fees are *not refundable*, nor can they be "held over" to a subsequent exam.
b. All fees must be paid in US funds. Applicants residing outside the United States must submit payment by International Money Order.
c. Fees must be paid in full by the stated deadlines. Applications without payment will not be processed.
d. A fee of $200 will be charged for any application or portion thereof postmarked between July 11 and July 20 (inclusive). *Applications postmarked after July 20 are not accepted.*
e. A fee of $25 will be charged for any check returned by the bank for insufficient funds.
f. Fees are subject to change at the discretion of the Board.

2. New Applicants

a. The examination fee of $1,800 is due with the application by July 10.
b. Individuals who become candidates for the oral examination (by achieving the qualifying score on the written exam) take their first oral examination at no additional cost.
c. Candidates are given three consecutive opportunities to take the oral examination. A fee of $1,000 will be charged for the second and/or third oral exam.

3. Reapplicants

a. If an individual fails the written examination, or if a passing score is not achieved after three oral exams, the individual must reapply to take the written exam, and $1,800 must accompany the reapplication form.
b. Individuals who again become oral candidates follow the same procedure and pay the same fees as outlined in paragraph 2b and c of the "New Applicants" section above.

Purpose of Examination

The purpose of the examination is to determine the candidate's knowledge, skill, and understanding in the following categories:

1. Morphology, physiology, pharmacology, pathology, microbiology, biochemistry, genetics, and immunology relevant to the head and neck; the respiratory and upper alimentary systems; the communication sciences, including knowledge of audiology and speech-language pathology; the chemical senses and allergy, endocrinology, and neurology as they relate to the head and neck
2. Diagnosis and diagnostic methods including audiologic and vestibular assessments, electrophysiologic techniques, and other related laboratory procedures for diseases and disorders of the ears, the respiratory and upper alimentary systems, and the head and neck
3. Therapeutic and diagnostic radiology, including the interpretation of medical imaging techniques relevant to the head, neck, and thorax, including the temporal bone, skull, nose, paranasal sinuses, salivary and thyroid glands, larynx, neck, lungs, and esophagus
4. Diagnostic evaluation and management of congenital anomalies, allergy, trauma, and other diseases in the regions and systems mentioned above
5. The cognitive management, including operative intervention with its preoperative and postoperative care, of congenital, inflammatory, endocrine, neoplastic, degenerative, and traumatic states, including:
   a. temporal bone surgery;
   b. paranasal sinus and nasal surgery;
   c. skull-base surgery;
   d. maxillofacial surgery including the orbits, jaws, and facial skeleton;
   e. aesthetic, plastic, and reconstructive surgery of the face, head, and neck;
   f. surgery of the thyroid, parathyroid, pituitary, and salivary glands;
   g. head and neck reconstructive surgery relating to the restoration of form and function in congenital anomalies and head and neck trauma, and associated with ablative operations
   h. endoscopy, both diagnostic and therapeutic;
   i. surgery of the lymphatic tissues of the head and neck
6. The habilitation and rehabilitation techniques and procedures pertaining to respiration, deglutition, chemoreception, balance, speech, and hearing
7. The current literature, especially pertaining to the areas listed above
8. Research methodology

In order to assist otolaryngology program directors in evaluating their programs, the Board reports each applicant's examination results to the director of the program in which the applicant completed his/her senior resident year.

Examination Procedure

The Board vigorously enforces the highest standards of honesty and integrity in its examination process. Accordingly, the following are considered a breach of ABOto policy and are forbidden and may be sufficient cause for the ABOto to terminate an applicant's participation in the examination, to invalidate the results of the examination, to withhold an applicant's score or certificate, to bar an applicant permanently from all future examinations, to revoke a certificate, or to take other appropriate action:

1. Falsification of the application or the submission of any falsified documents to the ABOto
2. The giving or receiving of aid in the examination, including but not limited to copying answers from another candidate or permitting one's answers to be copied, as evidenced by observation at the time of the examination or by statistical analysis afterward
3. The offer of any financial or other benefit to any director, officer, employee, proctor, or other agent or representative of the ABOto in return for any right, privilege, or benefit that is not usually granted by the ABOto to other similarly situated candidates or persons
4. The unauthorized possession, reproduction, recording, discussion, or disclosure of any material, including but not limited to written or oral examination questions or answers before, during, or after the examination

Proctors are required to report any suspected irregularity during an examination. A candidate may be moved to a more isolated area, or his/her participation in the examination may be terminated. Additionally, the ABOto's educational consultants may undertake statistical studies of a candidate's answers compared with the answers of other participants in the examination to provide evidence that would support or fail to support a suspected irregularity. If, in the opinion of the ABOto, there exists a probability that an irregularity occurred, the ABOto will afford the suspected individual(s) procedural due process in order to assure fairness in the determination as to whether an irregularity occurred.

The ABOto will not report scores or grant certification on the basis of scores that it determines to be invalid, and reserves the right to take whatever legal action is indicated with regard to violation of ABOto copyright or examination violations.

Certification, Rejection, and Revocation from The Bylaws, Article VI)

The Board shall issue an appropriate certificate of qualification in otolaryngology (or in a subdivision thereof) to those who show themselves worthy of such certification according to the requirements of training, experience, and demonstrated competence as stated in the current ABOto *Booklet of Information*.

No certificate shall be issued, and any certificate issued by the Board shall be subject to revocation at any time by the Board, if it shall determine that the person involved:

1. did not possess the required qualifications and requirements for examination, whether or not such deficiency was known to the Board or any director thereof, or could have been ascertained by the Board prior to examination or at the time of the issuance of a certificate as the case may be;
2. made a material misstatement or withheld information in his/her application or any other representation to the Board or any Committee thereof, whether intentional or unintentional;
3. has been convicted by a court of competent jurisdiction of any felony or misdemeanor involving moral turpitude and, in the opinion of the Board, having a material relationship to the practice of medicine; or
4. had a license to practice medicine revoked or shall have been disciplined or censured by any court or other body having proper jurisdiction and authority because of any act or omission arising from the practice of medicine.

If the Board determines to withhold or revoke any certificate for any reason, the person affected thereby shall be given written notice of the reasons therefor. Such actions by the Board shall be regarded as final unless such person requests a review of such action within 30 days after notice thereof has been mailed by the Board.

American Board of Pathology

PO Box 25915
Tampa, FL 33622-5915
813 286-2444
813 286-5279 Fax
Internet: http://www.abpath.org

(These criteria and conditions are subject to change without notice. Please contact the American Board of Pathology [ABP] for current requirements.)

Qualification Requirements for Examination

All applications for certification are evaluated by the Credentials Committee of the ABP. The evaluation process includes the consideration of the following four requirements:

I. Professional Education
II. Medical Licensure
III. Pathology Training Requirements
IV. The Credentialing Year

I. Professional Education

A candidate must have graduated from a medical school in the United States or Canada accredited by the Liaison Committee on Medical Education, graduated from an osteopathic college of medicine accredited by the Bureau of Professional Education of the American Osteopathic Association, or graduated from a medical school outside the United States or Canada acceptable to the ABP.

A graduate of a medical school outside the United States or Canada must submit with the application a notarized copy of the medical school diploma, along with an English translation, showing the medical degree and the date that it was awarded. A certificate showing that the applicant has passed a final examination is not acceptable.

II. Medical Licensure

The candidate must hold a currently valid, full, and unrestricted license to practice medicine or osteopathy issued by one of the licensing agencies of the United States or Canada.

III. Pathology Training Requirements

To acknowledge the diverse activities in the practice of pathology and to accommodate the interests of individuals wanting to enter the field, the ABP offers primary certification through one of the following three routes: combined anatomic pathology and clinical pathology, anatomic pathology only, and clinical pathology only. A variety of specialty certificates is offered. Under certain circumstances, primary certification in anatomic pathology or clinical pathology can be combined with one of the subspecialty certificates.

Only pathology training taken in the United States or, in certain circumstances, in Canada is acceptable toward meeting the ABP requirements. The training must be in programs that have been inspected and accredited by the Accreditation Council for Graduate Medical Education (ACGME) or the Royal College of Physicians and Surgeons of Canada (RCPSC) or specifically approved by the ABP.

A. Primary Certification

In addition to accredited pathology training, all applicants for primary certification must meet the 1-full-year credentialing requirement as defined under Section IV, "The Credentialing Year."

1. *Training.* The candidate must satisfactorily complete pathology training in a program accredited by the ACGME or the RCPSC as follows:
   a. Combined Anatomic Pathology and Clinical Pathology (AP/CP) Certification
   Four full years of full-time, approved training in an accredited APCP-4 program that includes at least 18 months of structured training in anatomic pathology and 18 months of structured training in clinical pathology, and either an additional 12 months of full-time, continued structured training in anatomic pathology and/or clinical pathology or 12 months of full-time, approved flexible training in a specific area of pathology as part of the defined 4-year accredited AP/CP training program.
   b. Anatomic Pathology (AP) Certification
      1. Three full years of full-time, approved training in anatomic pathology in an accredited APCP-4 or AP-3 program that includes at least 24 months of structured training in anatomic pathology, and either an additional 12 months of full-time, continued structured training in anatomic pathology *or* 12 months of full-time, approved flexible training in a specific area of pathology as part of the defined accredited training program.
      2. Primary certification in clinical pathology and 2 full years of full-time, approved training in anatomic pathology in an accredited APCP-4 or AP-3 program, with at least 18 months of structured training in anatomic pathology. Six months may be full-time, approved training in a specific area of pathology as part of the defined accredited training program.
   c. Clinical Pathology (CP) Certification
      1. Three full years of full-time, approved training in clinical pathology in an accredited APCP-4 program that includes at least 24 months of structured training in clinical pathology, and either an additional 12 months of full-time, continued structured training in clinical pathology or 12 months of full-time, approved flexible training in a specific area of pathology as part of the defined accredited training program.
      2. Primary certification in anatomic pathology and 2 full years of full-time, approved training in clinical pathology in an accredited APCP-4 program, with at least 18 months of structured training in clinical pathology. Six months may be full-time, approved training in a specific area of pathology as part of the defined accredited training program.
2. *Advanced Pathology Training Credit Mechanisms.* Under special circumstances, advanced credit will be given by the mechanisms described hereafter. Advanced credit is any medically relevant, postbaccalaureate, 12-month experience that is not approved by the ACGME for training in pathology and is relevant to the education of pathologists as determined by the ABP and can be applied to satisfy the flexible year in pathology. The acceptance of advanced credits as substitutes for accredited pathology training toward primary certification is not automatic and is evaluated on an individual basis. Advanced credit is given only for activities that have occurred in either the United States or Canada. The total combined period of advanced pathology training credit allowed for in paragraphs a and b in this section will not exceed 12 months and can be applied only to the flexible year of required pathology training necessary for certification in AP/CP, AP, or CP.
   To avoid any misunderstanding, potential applicants should communicate with the ABP early in the training period to ascertain whether credit may be acceptable. The pathology training program director will be asked to assess the proposal and to provide a recommendation as to the amount of credit that the director believes the candidate should receive. The recommendation should be made only after the pathology training program director has observed the performance of the applicant.
   The ABP will notify the director of the pathology training program of such potential credit. Prior to the candidate's admission to the certifying examination, the director of the final year of training must certify that the candidate is fully qualified to sit for the examination.
   a. Candidates holding a PhD degree in a special discipline of pathology or a basic science related to pathology may, under certain circumstances, obtain pathology training credit. The evaluation and granting of the amount of training credit will depend on an assessment by the ABP regarding relevance of the field of study to anatomic pathology or clinical pathology.
   b. Research with a direct application to the practice of anatomic pathology or clinical pathology and not leading to an advanced degree may be considered for credit not to exceed 12 months in combination with other advanced credits. The research must be full time, and the applicant must be able to demonstrate active participation in the generation of the hypothesis and development of the protocol. No credit is given for research employment as a technician or technologist. The ABP encourages research and believes that candidates should carry on investigation, teaching, and the publication of scientific papers during primary training.
3. *Postpathology-course Fellowship and Student Fellowship Training During Medical School—Criteria for Acceptance.* Under certain circumstances, candidates may receive advanced pathology training credit toward the primary certification requirements for postpathology-course fellowship training or research in pathology. Such credit is *not* given toward the requirements for subspecialty certification. The credit is assessed on an individual basis. Granted credit will be assigned only to the flexible year of required primary training. Credit will not be given toward the required 18 months of structured anatomic pathology training or the required 18 months of structured clinical pathology training necessary to qualify for combined anatomic pathology and clinical pathology certification.
   Advanced credit toward single certification in anatomic pathology or single certification in clinical pathology will be given toward only the flexible year of required pathology training and not toward the 24 months of required structured training.
   The guidelines for acceptable postpathology-course fellowship training for credit are:
   a. The fellow must have fully and satisfactorily completed the medical school year in which the pathology course is given.
   b. The fellow must not receive credit for fellowship activities toward the requirements for graduation from medical school.
   c. Training must be full-time in a department of pathology that has a fully accredited pathology training program.
   d. Training must be validated by the director of the student fellowship program and be approved as an acceptable experience by the director of the accredited pathology training program in which the candidate is registered.

e. No credit is given for electives or for courses that are part of the medical school curriculum.
f. Training must be under the direction of the director of the pathology training program or the chair of the department of pathology.
g. A description of proposed activities, responsibilities, and assignments for anatomic pathology, clinical pathology, and research must be available and on file prior to the beginning of the fellowship. If a formal institutional program exists, a copy should be filed with the ABP.
h. A validation and evaluation report must be submitted on completion of the fellowship by the pathology training program director or chair of the department of pathology if the fellow is seeking credit toward certification requirements.

4. *Interval of Training.* A candidate for primary certification who completed the required pathology training 5 years or more prior to the date of submission of an application for certification must have 1 year of additional training in pathology in a program accredited for such training by the ACGME or the RCPSC. This additional requirement must be met during the 5-year period immediately preceding the date of submission of an application.

B. Subspecialty (Formerly Special or Added Qualification) Certification

All candidates applying for subspecialty certification must hold a primary certificate from the ABP or, where indicated, from another member medical specialty board of the American Board of Medical Specialties (ABMS).

Credit is not given for pathology training taken outside of the United States, nor is credit given for training in a subspecialty area that was part of the training program for the primary examination in AP and/or CP.

No advanced credit will be given toward the requirements for subspecialty certification by the mechanisms described in Section III.A.2, "Advanced Pathology Training Credit Mechanisms."

1. *Blood Banking/Transfusion Medicine (BB/TM)*
   a. For applicants who hold a certificate in anatomic pathology and clinical pathology, clinical pathology only, or a primary certificate plus a subspecialty certificate in hematology from another member medical specialty board of the ABMS:
      1. One full year of additional training in blood banking/transfusion medicine in a program accredited for such training by the ACGME or
      2. Two additional years of full-time experience or its equivalent in blood banking/transfusion medicine under circumstances acceptable to the ABP. This by-experience route to blood banking/transfusion medicine certification will not be available for applications received after the deadline for the 1999 blood banking/transfusion medicine examination.
   b. For diplomates of the American Board of Anesthesiology: 1 full year of additional training in blood banking/transfusion medicine in a program accredited for such training by the ACGME.
   c. For applicants, other than those described in 1.a or 1.b, who hold a primary certificate from a member medical specialty board of the ABMS: 2 full years of full-time training in blood banking/transfusion medicine in a program accredited for such training by the ACGME.
   d. For applicants seeking combined certification in clinical pathology and blood banking/transfusion medicine, see Section III.C, "Combined Primary and Subspecialty Certification."
2. *Chemical Pathology (Chem P)*
   a. For applicants who hold a certificate in anatomic pathology and clinical pathology or clinical pathology only:
      1. One full year of additional training in chemical pathology in a program accredited for such training by the ACGME or
      2. Two additional years of full-time experience or its equivalent in chemical pathology under circumstances acceptable to the ABP. This by-experience route to chemical pathology certification will not be available for applications received after the deadline for the 1999 chemical pathology examination.
   b. For applicants, other than those described in 2.a, who hold a primary certificate from a member medical specialty board of the ABMS: 2 full years of full-time training in chemical pathology in a program accredited for such training by the ACGME.
   c. For applicants seeking combined certification in clinical pathology and chemical pathology, see Section III.C, "Combined Primary and Subspecialty Certification."
3. *Dermatopathology (DP)*

   Certification in dermatopathology is a joint and equal function of the ABP and the American Board of Dermatology (ABD). Such function relates to qualifications of candidates, standards of examinations, and the form of the certificate.

   All candidates applying for examination must hold a currently valid, full, and unrestricted license to practice medicine or osteopathy in the United States or Canada.
   a. Prerequisites

      The ABP and the ABD will admit candidates to examination for subspecialty certificates in dermatopathology who are otherwise qualified and who
      1. are diplomates of the ABP and the ABD;
      2. hold a primary certificate from the ABP (anatomic pathology or combined anatomic pathology and clinical pathology) or the ABD and have completed at least 1 year of training in dermatopathology in a program accredited for such training by the ACGME. This additional training must be taken after the candidate has met the full training requirements for certification in pathology or dermatology.
   b. Training

      Training programs in dermatopathology are a joint and equal function of the departments of pathology and dermatology. The pathologist applicant must spend half of the required training time in clinical dermatology.

   Committee for Dermatopathology
   Juan Rosai, MD, Chair (ABP)
   John C Maize, MD, Vice Chair (ABD)
   Ronald J Barr, MD (ABD)
   Ronald P Rapini, MD (ABD)
   David B Troxel, MD (ABP)
   Kay Herrin Woodruff, MD (ABP)
   Candidates may obtain an application as follows:

   Pathologists
   William H Hartmann, MD
   Executive Vice President
   American Board of Pathology
   PO Box 25915
   Tampa, FL 33622-5915

   Dermatologists
   Harry J Hurley, MD
   Executive Director
   American Board of Dermatology
   Henry Ford Hospital
   1 Ford Place
   Detroit, MI 48202-3450
4. *Forensic Pathology (FP)*
   a. For applicants who hold a certificate in anatomic pathology and clinical pathology or anatomic pathology only:

1. One full year of additional supervised training in forensic pathology in a program accredited for such training by the ACGME, or
2. Two additional years of full-time experience in forensic pathology or its equivalent in a situation comparable to that of a program accredited for such training by the ACGME. This by-experience route to forensic pathology certification will not be available for applications received after the deadline for the 1999 forensic pathology examination.

b. For applicants seeking combined certification in anatomic pathology and forensic pathology, see Section III.C, "Combined Primary and Subspecialty Certification."

5. Hematology (HEM)

a. For applicants who hold a certificate in anatomic pathology and clinical pathology, anatomic pathology only, clinical pathology only, or a primary certificate plus a subspecialty certificate in hematology from another member medical specialty board of the ABMS:
1. One full year of additional supervised training in hematology (pathology) in a program accredited for such training by the ACGME, or
2. Two additional years of full-time experience or its equivalent in clinical laboratory hematology under circumstances acceptable to the ABP. This by-experience route to hematology certification will not be available for applications received after the deadline for the 1999 hematology examination.

b. For applicants, other than those described in 5.a, who hold a primary certificate from a member medical specialty board of the ABMS: 2 full years of full-time training in hematology (pathology) in a program accredited for such training by the ACGME.

c. For applicants seeking combined certification in clinical pathology or anatomic pathology and hematology, see Section III.C, "Combined Primary and Subspecialty Certification."

6. Immunopathology (IP)

(Note: The last anticipated immunopathology certification examination will be held in 1999. Please check with the ABP for more information.)

a. For applicants who hold a certificate in anatomic pathology and clinical pathology:
1. One full year of additional supervised training in immunopathology in a program accredited for such training by the ACGME, or
2. Two additional years of full-time experience in immunopathology or its equivalent under circumstances acceptable to the ABP. This by-experience route to immunopathology certification will not be available for applications received after the deadline for the 1999 immunopathology examination.

b. For applicants who hold a certificate in anatomic pathology only or clinical pathology only:
1. Two full years of additional supervised training in immunopathology in a program accredited for such training by the ACGME, or
2. Four additional years of full-time experience in immunopathology or its equivalent under circumstances acceptable to the ABP. This by-experience route to immunopathology certification will not be available for applications received after the deadline for the 1999 immunopathology examination.

c. For applicants who hold a certificate in anatomic pathology only or clinical pathology only plus a subspecialty certificate in blood banking/transfusion medicine, hematology, medical microbiology, or chemical pathology:
1. One full year of additional supervised training in immunopathology in a program accredited for such training by the ACGME, or
2. Two additional years of full-time experience in immunopathology or its equivalent under circumstances acceptable to the ABP. This by-experience route to immunopathology certification will not be available for applications received after the deadline for the 1999 immunopathology examination.

d. For applicants seeking combined certification in anatomic pathology or clinical pathology and immunopathology, see Section III.C, "Combined Primary and Subspecialty Certification."

7. Medical Microbiology (MMB)

a. For applicants who hold a certificate in anatomic pathology and clinical pathology, anatomic pathology only, clinical pathology only, or a primary certificate plus a subspecialty certificate in infectious disease from another member medical specialty board of the ABMS:
1. One full year of additional training in medical microbiology in a program accredited for such training by the ACGME, or
2. Two additional years of full-time experience or its equivalent in clinical laboratory medical microbiology under circumstances acceptable to the ABP. This by-experience route to medical microbiology certification will not be available for applications received after the deadline for the 1999 medical microbiology examination.

b. For applicants, other than those described in 7.a, who hold a primary certificate from a member medical specialty board of the ABMS: 2 full years of full-time training in medical microbiology in a program accredited for such training by the ACGME.

c. For applicants seeking combined certification in clinical pathology and medical microbiology, see Section III.C, "Combined Primary and Subspecialty Certification."

8. Neuropathology (NP)

a. For applicants who hold a certificate in anatomic pathology and clinical pathology or anatomic pathology only: 2 full years of additional supervised training in neuropathology in a program accredited for such training by the ACGME.

b. For applicants who hold a certificate in clinical pathology or a primary certificate from another member medical specialty board of the ABMS:
1. One full year of approved training in anatomic pathology in a program accredited for such training by the ACGME and
2. Two full years of additional supervised training in neuropathology in a program accredited for such training by the ACGME.

c. For applicants seeking combined certification in anatomic pathology and neuropathology, see Section III.C, "Combined Primary and Subspecialty Certification."

9. Pediatric Pathology (PP)

a. For applicants who hold a certificate in anatomic pathology and clinical pathology or anatomic pathology only from the ABP or anatomic pathology or general pathology from the RCPSC:
1. One full year of additional supervised training in pediatric pathology in a program accredited for such training by the ACGME, or
2. Two additional years of full-time practice experience in pediatric pathology or its equivalent in a situation offering experience opportunities comparable to those of an accredited or approved training program in pediatric pathology and acceptable to the ABP. This by-experience route to pediatric pathology certification will not be available for applications received after the deadline for the 1999 pediatric pathology examination.

b. The pediatric pathology training or experience should occur after the completion of the full training requirements necessary to qualify for certification in AP/CP or AP.

10. Cytopathology (CYP)

a. For applicants who hold a certificate in anatomic pathology or combined anatomic and clinical pathology:
   1. One full year of full-time supervised training in cytopathology in a program accredited for such training by the ACGME.

b. For applicants seeking combined certification in anatomic pathology and cytopathology, see Section III.C, "Combined Primary and Subspecialty Certification."

C. Combined Primary and Subspecialty Certification

Under certain circumstances, subspecialty training may be arranged in conjunction with the primary training requirements, permitting a candidate to qualify for a combined certificate. All applicants for combined certification must also meet the additional credentialing year requirement. (See Section IV, "The Credentialing Year.")

Advanced credit will *not* be given toward the requirements for combined certification (involving primary training and subspecialty training) by the mechanisms described in Section III.A.2, "Advanced Pathology Training Credit Mechanisms."

The acceptable combinations of certification and required training are:

1. Anatomic Pathology and Cytopathology—3 full years of approved training in anatomic pathology in a program accredited for such training by the ACGME and 1 full year of approved training in cytopathology in a program accredited for such training by the ACGME
2. Anatomic Pathology and Forensic Pathology—2 full years of approved training in anatomic pathology in a program accredited for such training by the ACGME, 1 full year of approved training in forensic pathology in a program accredited for such training by the ACGME, and 1 additional year of approved training in anatomic pathology or in a specific area of pathology such as neuropathology, toxicology, or chemical pathology
3. Anatomic Pathology and Neuropathology—2 full years of approved training in anatomic pathology and 2 full years of approved training in neuropathology in a program accredited for such training by the ACGME with adequate experience in diagnostic neuropathology
4. Anatomic Pathology and Hematology—2 full years of approved training in anatomic pathology in a program accredited for such training by the ACGME and 2 full years of approved training in hematology in a program accredited for such training by the ACGME
5. Anatomic Pathology and Immunopathology—2 full years of approved training in anatomic pathology in a program accredited for such training by the ACGME and 2 full years of approved training in immunopathology in a program accredited for such training by the ACGME (Note: The last anticipated immunopathology certification examination will be held in 1999. Please check with the ABP for more information.)
6. Anatomic Pathology and Medical Microbiology—2 full years of approved training in anatomic pathology in a progam accredited for such training by the ACGME and 2 full years of approved training in medical microbiology in a program accredited for such training by the ACGME
7. Clinical Pathology and Subspecialty Certification—3 full years of approved training in clinical pathology in a program accredited for such training by the ACGME and 1 full year of approved subspecialty training in blood banking/transfusion medicine, chemical pathology, hematology, or medical microbiology in a program accredited for such training by the ACGME, as defined in Section III.B, "Subspecialty Certification," or 2 full years of approved training in clinical pathology and 2 full years of approved subspecialty training in blood banking/transfusion medicine, chemical pathology, hematology, immunopathology, or medical microbiology in a program accredited for such training by the ACGME, as defined in Section III.B, "Subspecialty Certification"

IV. The Credentialing Year

The 12-month credentialing year requirement is in addition to the required pathology training and can be satisfied only after the candidate has obtained the medical degree.

The ABP considers the most appropriate and, for applicants, the most beneficial approach to meeting this requirement to be 1 full year of full-time, approved clinical training in the United States or Canada (Pathway A). The ABP recognizes that such is not always possible and therefore offers alternative pathways to meeting the requirement.

The requirement can be met by

A. One full year of full-time, approved graduate medical education in a transitional year training program or in a clinical area of medicine such as internal medicine, surgery, obstetrics and gynecology, pediatrics, emergency medicine, or family practice, or

B. One full year of full-time research in pathology or in another clinical discipline, provided that the research was done in the United States or Canada and has clearly defined clinical implications.

   The guidelines for acceptance of research activity are:
   1. The research activity must have taken place after the candidate has obtained a recognized medical degree.
   2. The candidate must have had a clearly defined investigator role in the research program.
   3. The research must have directly involved patients, or materials obtained from patients, or techniques that can be applied directly to the diagnosis of human disease or to the understanding of the basic mechanisms of disease.
   4. Prior approval of a research program for credentialing credit must have been given in writing by the director of the pathology training program.
   5. Credit for research activity completed prior to entering a pathology training program must be approved by the director of the pathology training program and the ABP. Such research must have occurred in an institution in the United States or Canada; or

C. One year of training in one of the recognized subspecialty fields of pathology that includes clinical correlation and patient contact. (This year cannot be used to meet the requirements for both the credentialing year and subspecialty certification.) Or

D. The satisfactory completion of 1 full year of a combination of clinical training, clinical research, or subspecialty pathology training in addition to the required pathology training necessary to qualify for certification in anatomic pathology and clinical pathology, anatomic pathology, or clinical pathology. The pathology training program director is responsible for defining and justifying this year to the ABP. The ABP recommends that for applicants meeting the credentialing year requirement by combinations of pathways A, B, and C (shown above), the periods of activity be at least 4 months in duration wherever possible.

Under certain circumstances, credit toward the credentialing year may be given for pathology experience if the applicant holds a primary certificate in pathology issued by the independent national certifying body in a country other than the United States or Canada, provided that the certification was by national examination following 4 full years of approved training in pathology.

E. Under certain circumstances, clinical training taken outside the United States and Canada may be acceptable toward meeting the ABP credentialing year requirement of clinical training, provided that the following criteria are fully met and validated:
1. Clinical training taken after the candidate obtained a medical degree acceptable to the ABP
2. Satisfactory completion of 1 full year of full-time training in clinical medicine in a multidisciplinary training program (internship) or in a training program in internal medicine, pediatric medicine, general surgery, or obstetrics and gynecology
3. Documentation from the training institution that the program in question has been inspected and approved for graduate medical education
4. Indication from the director of the clinical training program that the candidate was registered in the program, completed the training satisfactorily, and was the physician of record in the diagnosis and treatment of patients throughout the full 12 months
5. Recommendation from the pathology training program director in regard to the person's request

The acceptability of clinical training toward meeting the ABP requirements is assessed on an individual basis, and it is imperative that an opinion be obtained from the ABP well in advance of the submission of an application for certification. The amount of advanced credit for clinical training outside the United States and Canada toward the ABP requirements for certification cannot exceed a total of 12 months.

It is the responsibility of the person seeking credit to ensure that all validating items for these criteria are submitted to the ABP for consideration. No assessment of possible credit will be given until all validating and reference information has been received.

Application for Examination

Requests for application forms must be made in writing to the ABP. Completed original application forms should be returned with the required credentials and the application-examination fee. An application cannot be given consideration unless it is accompanied by the application-examination fee.

Reporting of Results

Coinciding with the accreditation visit from the ACGME, each pathology training program director and the RRC will receive a report of the cumulative examination performance of graduates of that training program.

Fees

The application-examination fee schedule for 1999 is as follows:

Anatomic pathology only	$1,000
Clinical pathology only	$1,000
Anatomic pathology portion of combined AP/CP	$1,000
Clinical pathology portion of combined AP/CP	$1,000
Combined anatomic pathology and clinical pathology	$1,200
Subspecialty	$1,200
Anatomic pathology or clinical pathology combined with subspecialty	$1,400

(For this fee to apply, the primary and the subspecialty examinations should be taken in sequence as offered, AP or CP examination first and the subspecialty examination the next time offered and only if the application is for the combined examination.)

The application-examination fee includes a nonrefundable processing fee of $100. If the different divisions of the AP/CP and the combined primary and subspecialty examinations are taken at separate sittings, there is a separate examination fee for each sitting. If the candidate fails in the examination, admission to a repeat examination is permitted, but any reexamination must occur within the 3-year period of qualification described under "Qualification Period for Examination." The applicant must pay the examination fee according to the current fee schedule before another examination can be taken. If, after having applied for a specific examination, the candidate requests, in writing, a transfer to a future examination prior to the final filing date, there is a transfer fee of $100.

In the event of the candidate's illness at the time of the examination, validated by the candidate's attending physician, a major portion of the application-examination fee will be either transferred to the next examination or refunded.

Vacation, Maternity, and Other Leave

Each institution sponsoring a pathology training program should develop individual sick, vacation, and other leave policies for the resident. However, 1 year of approved training credit toward ABP certification requirements must be 52 weeks in duration and must include at least 48 weeks of full-time pathology training. Furthermore, unused vacation and other leave time may not be accumulated to reduce the overall duration of training.

Irregular Behavior

In the interest of protecting the integrity of the ABP and its certification examinations, the following irregular behaviors may be sufficient to bar a person from future examinations, terminate participation in an examination, invalidate the results of a candidate's examination, cause the withholding or revocation of scores or certificates, or merit other appropriate action by the ABP:
1. The giving or receiving of aid in the examination as evidenced either by observation or by statistical analysis of candidates' answers
2. The unauthorized possession, reproduction, or disclosure of any ABP examination-related materials, including, but not limited to, examination questions or answers, before, during, or after the examination
3. The offering of any benefit to any agent of the ABP in return for any right, privilege, or benefit that is not usually granted by the ABP to other similarly situated candidates or persons
4. Possession of notes, books, or any other examination aid in the vicinity of the examination room

In addition, the ABP may withhold a candidate's scores and require that the candidate retake one or more portions of the examination if presented with sufficient evidence that the security of the examination has been compromised, notwithstanding the absence of any evidence of the candidate's personal involvement in such activities.

Chemical Dependency

Applications for certification from individuals with a history of chemical dependency as reported to the ABP will not be accepted unless the applicant submits documentation acceptable to the ABP that the applicant
1. has satisfactorily completed the program of treatment prescribed for the applicant's condition and
2. has been drug-free for a period sufficient to indicate recovery, which, in most cases, would be at least 3 years.

Candidates who have been declared qualified to sit for a certifying examination and who have a current problem of chemical dependency as reported to the ABP will not be admitted to the examination. Denial of admission to examination may result in the loss of opportunities for examination and, ultimately, in the decision to declare the candidate's application void for failure to complete the requirements for certification within the qualification time period allotted to every candidate.

Qualification Period for Examination

The ABP does not recognize or use the term "board eligible" and does not issue statements concerning "board eligibility." An applicant is declared qualified for examination only after an application has been received and approved by the Credentials Committee.

The ABP will permit a candidate who has qualified for examination on the basis of approved training and/or experience to sit for the examination during a period not to exceed 3 years after being declared qualified to take the examination. For candidates who have been unsuccessful in the subspecialty examinations given biennially, the period of qualification will be extended to include three administrations of the subspecialty examination. When this period has expired and the candidate has been unsuccessful, additional periods of qualification for examination will be permitted on submission of documentation that the candidate has obtained further training or experience subsequent to the beginning of the period of qualification.

At any time after declaring a candidate qualified for examination, the Credentials Committee, at its discretion, may withdraw such qualification or, as a condition, may require satisfaction by the candidate of specified conditions. In the exercise of its discretion under this regulation, the Credentials Committee shall be entitled to act without reason assigned.

If it is determined that an applicant has falsified information in the application form, the applicant will not be approved for the certifying examination and must wait a period of 3 years before being permitted to file a new application. The applicant will not be considered qualified to sit for the certifying examination during the 3-year interim.

Unsuccessful Candidates

Once the initial period of qualification has terminated, candidates who have been unsuccessful in any of the certification examinations may apply for one additional period of qualification based on satisfactory experience in the field of pathology in question. A one-time extension of 3 years will be granted on the submission of appropriate and acceptable documentation of 2 years of full-time experience in the discipline of requested certification, *or* candidates may apply for one additional period of qualification based on satisfactory completion of 1 additional year of training in an ACGME-accredited training program in the discipline of the application.

Candidates who continue to be unsuccessful in the certification examination may apply for an additional period of qualification, which may be granted only to those who submit evidence of satisfactory completion of 1 additional year of training in an ACGME-accredited training program in the discipline of the application.

Examination Dates and Sites

Examinations are held at the discretion of the ABP. The tentative schedules for forthcoming examinations are:

Anatomic Pathology and Clinical Pathology Examinations

All primary certification examinations are administered via the computer system in the ABP Examination Center in Tampa, Florida.

The spring 1999 examinations will be begin on Monday, June 7, 1999, and the fall examinations will begin on Monday, October 4, 1999. Both examinations will continue on a Monday, Tuesday, Wednesday weekly cycle until all qualified candidates have been examined.

Subspecialty Examinations

All subspecialty examinations are computer-based and administered at the ABP Examination Center in Tampa, Florida. The cytopathology examination will be computer-based beginning in 2000.

The subspecialty examinations in chemical pathology, immunopathology, medical microbiology, neuropathology, and pediatric pathology are given every 2 years.

IP—July 8, 1999
CYP—July 12, 1999
BB/TM—July 29, 1999
HEM—August 12, 1999
PP—August 19, 1999
Chem P—August 26, 1999
FP—September 9, 1999
MMB—September 16, 1999
NP—September 23, 1999

Final Filing and Cutoff Dates

The final filing dates for receipt of applications or registrations are as follows:

- February 1 for spring primary examinations for all candidates
- April 1 for subspecialty examinations
- July 1 for dermatopathology examinations
- August for fall primary examinations for initial applicants, September 1 for all others

If the candidate cancels an appearance for the examination after these dates or does not appear for the examination, the entire application-examination fee is forfeited.

Issuance of Certificate

On satisfactorily passing the appropriate examination(s), a candidate will be issued a certificate by the ABP in those fields of pathology for which the ABP accepted the credentials. Thus, a candidate who is qualified for the combined examination in anatomic pathology and clinical pathology, having fulfilled the minimum pathology requirement of 48 months and the credentialing year requirement of 12 months, will receive a certificate only after both parts (anatomic pathology and clinical pathology) of the examination have been passed.

Candidates qualified for examination in anatomic pathology or clinical pathology and a subspecialty area of pathology on the basis of the required training in each area will receive a certificate only after each of the examinations has been passed.

A candidate who has fulfilled all the prerequisites, including the minimum requirement of 36 months of approved training in anatomic pathology only or clinical pathology only, and the credentialing year activity will receive a certificate after passing the examination in anatomic pathology or clinical pathology.

Candidates qualified for combined AP/CP who pass only the AP portion or the CP portion of the examination may request an application for consideration of awarding a single certificate. Consideration will be given only to candidates who meet the requirements for the single certificate. For additional information on the awarding of single certificates, please contact the ABP.

If a candidate's certificate is lost or destroyed, the ABP will issue a duplicate certificate on written request and justification, together with an engraving and handling charge of $50.

Revocation of Certificate

At its discretion, the ABP may revoke a certificate for due cause, including, but not limited to:

a. The diplomate did not possess the required qualifications and requirements for examination, whether or not such deficiency was known to the ABP or any committee thereof prior to examination or at the time of the issuance of the certificate, as the case may be.

b. The diplomate made a material misstatement or withheld information in the application or in any other representation to the ABP or any committee thereof, whether intentional or unintentional.

c. The diplomate engaged in irregular behavior in connection with an examination of the ABP (as described under "Irregular Behavior"), whether or not such practice had an effect on the performance of the candidate on an examination.

d. The diplomate was convicted by a court of competent jurisdiction of a felony or misdemeanor involving moral turpitude and, in the opinion of the ABP, having a material relationship to the practice of medicine.

e. There has been a limitation or termination of any right of the diplomate associated with the practice of medicine in any state, province, or country, including the imposition of any requirement of surveillance, supervision, or review by reason of violation of a medical practice act or other statute or governmental regulation, disciplinary action by any medical licensing authority, entry into a consent order, or voluntary surrender of license.

Revocation of certificates will be governed by procedures set forth in the ABP bylaws as amended from time to time.

Update of the ABP Certificate

The ABP will permit its diplomates to retake the examination in the area of pathology in which they are already certified for the purpose of updating their certificate(s). The application-examination fee and the passing requirements are the same as for initial candidates. Successful candidates will be issued new, currently dated certificates.

Recertification

To enable diplomates to demonstrate continued competence in the practice of pathology, the ABP offers a voluntary process of recertification. For additional information on the recertification process, please request the ABP booklet on recertification.

Limitation of Subspecialty (SQ/AQ) Certificates

As a condition of admission to an examination for subspecialty certification, an individual holding two or more subspecialty certificates (formerly special competence, special qualification, and/or added qualification) must surrender a sufficient number of certificates to reduce their number to one. If the individual fails the examination and the period of board qualification terminates, the surrendered certificate(s) will be restored. This action does not include subspecialty certificates (special qualification or special competence) in radioisotopic pathology or in dermatopathology.

Candidates with Disabilities

1. Policy. The ABP supports the intent of the Americans with Disabilities Act. The ABP will endeavor to provide qualified candidates who have documented disabilities the necessary auxiliary aids and services that do not fundamentally alter the measurement of the skills or knowledge the examination is intended to test or result in an undue burden.
2. Documentation of Disability. Candidates requesting accommodation due to a disability must provide documentation of the disability. Such documentation should include a specific diagnosis of the disability and include medical records or other documentation of the diagnosis of the disability by an appropriate medical professional. The ABP reserves the right to verify the disability and to request additional documentation as necessary. All required documentation acceptable to the ABP must be received no later than the application deadline.
3. Type of Accommodation. Candidates requesting accommodation must identify the type of accommodation requested. The ABP, however, will determine the type of accommodation to be made for a candidate with a verified disability. Accommodations that fundamentally alter the measurement of skills or knowledge the examination is intended to test will not be offered.
4. Application Deadline. Candidates requesting accommodations are urged to contact the ABP as far in advance of the examination as possible. Requests for accommodation and documentation of disability must be received no later than the application deadline.

Appeals Procedure

An individual who has received an unfavorable ruling regarding qualification to take an examination may initiate an appeal of such determination by making a written request for reconsideration to the ABP within 90 days of the date of the ruling.

A candidate who fails a certifying examination may request that the examination be rescored. The request my be made in writing within 90 days of the date the examination results were reported and must be accompanied by a fee of $50. There will be no further appeal from failure of an examination. There will be no discrimination in future dealings with the ABP against anyone who has requested an appeal.

American Board of Pediatrics

111 Silver Cedar Ct
Chapel Hill, NC 27514-1651
919 929-0461
919 929-9255 Fax
E-mail: abpeds@abpeds.org
Internet: http://www.abp.org

(These criteria are subject to change. All applicants are advised to consult the American Board of Pediatrics [ABP] to ascertain whether any changes have been made, especially before undertaking any variations in the training program.)

Examination Admission Requirements

An applicant for examination for certification (*Note:* The term "candidate" will be synonymous with applicant throughout the document) must meet the following general requirements:

The applicant must be a graduate of an accredited medical school in the United States or Canada or of a foreign medical school that is listed by the World Health Organization (WHO). A valid (current), unrestricted license to practice medicine in one of the states, districts, or territories of the United States or a province of Canada is a requirement for admission to the examination, but it may be submitted separately from the initial application.

A candidate who is reregistering for the examination must submit the license with the reregistration material. If an applicant has any action pending regarding the right to have an unrestricted license to practice medicine, admission to the examination may be denied.

The applicant must complete 3 years of pediatric training in programs accredited by the Accreditation Council for Graduate Medical Education (ACGME) on the advice of the Residency Review Committee (RRC) for Pediatrics (*Note:* Hereafter, accreditation will refer to accreditation by the RRC) or in programs in Canada accredited by the Royal College of Physicians and Surgeons of Canada (RCPSC).

The ABP requires program directors to verify satisfactory completion of training and to evaluate the acceptability of the applicant as a practitioner of pediatrics.

Graduation from Medical School

The applicant must be a graduate of a medical school that has been accredited by the Liaison Committee on Medical Education (LCME) in the United States, the RCPSC in Canada, or the American Osteopathic Association (AOA) in the United States.

An applicant who is a graduate of a medical school that has not been accredited by the LCME, RCPSC, or AOA but is listed by WHO may apply for examination if he or she has a standard certificate either from the Educational Commission for Foreign Medical Graduates (ECFMG) or the Medical Council of Canada.

The graduate of a foreign medical school must submit a photocopy of the medical school diploma showing the medical degree and the date it was awarded. A certificate showing that the applicant has passed a final examination is not acceptable.

License Requirement

The applicant must have a valid (current), unrestricted license to practice medicine in one of the states, districts, or territories of the United States or a province of Canada or unrestricted privileges to practice medicine in the US Armed Forces. A copy of the valid license must be received by October 1, 1999. Reregistrants must submit the license with the reregistration material.

Foreign nationals practicing abroad may be exempted from this policy upon presentation of proof of licensure equivalency in the country in which they reside. This proof must be received by October 1, 1999. Candidates who practice or plan to practice abroad must submit a letter, in addition to the licensure equivalency, stating that they will not practice in the United States or Canada.

The license requirement may be waived if, during the academic year 1999-2000, the applicant is in pediatric subspecialty training, nonpediatric specialty training, or is serving as a chief resident (PL-4) in a state, province, or district in which the medical licensing board does not require an unrestricted license. In order to obtain a waiver the program director of that training must submit written confirmation of the applicant's training to the ABP by October 1, 1999.

An applicant who takes the certifying examination but who does not meet the October 1, 1999, deadline for licensure will have the examination invalidated, will be disapproved, and will not receive a refund of the examination fee.

Training Requirements

An applicant must complete 3 years of postgraduate pediatric training in programs accredited by the RRC or, in Canada, by the RCPSC. (*Note:* The training requirements for individuals who graduated from medical school before July 1, 1978, are different from these requirements. Such applicants should contact the ABP for details.) The training curriculum must be compatible with the Program Requirements for Residency Education in Pediatrics, which are published annually in the *Graduate Medical Education Directory*. During this period of training, the applicant is expected to assume progressive responsibility for the care of patients. Credit will not be given for training completed before the medical degree is awarded.

A year of supervisory experience must be an integral part of the total 3-year program; this year must include 6 months of direct supervisory responsibility in general pediatrics (5 months for those beginning training after February 1, 1997).

The ABP recognizes four levels of pediatric training (PL-1 through PL-4) and defines these levels as follows:

PL-1: The first postgraduate year in general comprehensive pediatric training in an accredited program.

PL-2: The second postgraduate year in general comprehensive pediatric training in an accredited program following PL-1 but with increased responsibility for patient care and for the supervision of junior house staff and medical students.

PL-3: The third postgraduate year in general comprehensive pediatric training in an accredited program but with increasing responsibility for patient care and supervision of junior house staff and medical students.

PL-4: The fourth postgraduate year in general pediatric training in an accredited program when the applicant is designated as a chief resident.

Credit for Training in Accredited Programs Other Than Pediatrics

A physician transferring to pediatric residency training from another accredited residency, eg, family practice, internal medicine, transitional year, must correspond with the ABP to determine whether partial credit may be awarded for this training. Requests for credit must be submitted either by the candidate or the pediatric residency program director before the candidate enters pediatric residency training.

Credit for Pediatric Training in Nonaccredited Programs

The ABP has established requirements for a physician who has had at least 3 years of general comprehensive pediatric training in programs not accredited by the RRC or RCPSC (ie, international training or training in accredited osteopathic programs in the United States) and who wishes to apply for training credit. The interested physician, department chair, or program director *must* write to the ABP *before* training begins to be sure that the physician meets the requirements.

Special Alternative Pathway

The ABP recognizes that occasionally there will be an exceptional candidate who should be given special consideration to begin pediatric subspecialty training after the completion of the PL-2 year of general comprehensive pediatrics. Before the start of the PL-2 year, the department chair or program director *must* petition that a resident be considered for the Special Alternative Pathway (SAP), indicating that the candidate has superior overall competence. The subspecialty program director must also provide a letter outlining the clinical and research training proposed, including special requirements to be met during the PL-2 and PL-3 years. In addition, such candidates will be required to take a screening examination. The application material and the score on the screening examination will be reviewed by the Credentials Committee. An applicant who is approved for the SAP may not take the certifying examination until all training (no less than 5 years) is completed. Guidelines for the SAP are available from the ABP. Residents who wish to enter another specialty are not eligible for the SAP.

Special Programs

Medicine/Pediatrics (Med/Ped) Program

A special agreement exists with the American Board of Internal Medicine (ABIM) whereby an applicant may fulfill the training requirements of both the ABP and ABIM by completing 2 years of accredited training in general comprehensive pediatrics and 2 years of accredited training in general comprehensive internal medicine in an integrated approved program. The 4 years should be completed in the same combined training program; any deviation *must* be approved prospectively by both the ABP and the ABIM. Continuity clinics in each specialty must be provided throughout the 4 years. Guidelines for combined training have been approved by both the ABP and ABIM and are available by contacting either board. A list of institutions offering combined programs is published in the *Graduate Medical Education Directory*. An applicant may not take the certifying examination of the ABP until all 4 years of training have been completed.

Pediatrics/Neurology Program

A special agreement exists with the American Board of Psychiatry and Neurology (ABPN) whereby an applicant who completes at least 2 years of accredited training in general comprehensive pediatrics and the neurology training necessary to meet the requirements for certification in neurology with special qualifications in child neurology fulfills the training requirements of both the ABP and the ABPN. An applicant may not take the certifying examination of the ABP until all training has been completed.

Pediatrics/Physical Medicine and Rehabilitation Program

A special agreement exists with the American Board of Physical Medicine and Rehabilitation (ABPMR) whereby a physician interested in pediatric rehabilitation can qualify for admission to the certifying examinations of both the ABP and ABPMR. The residency training can be completed in 5 years in programs accredited by the RRCs of the ABP and the ABPMR. Proposed programs must be submitted to the ABP and ABPMR for approval before a candidate can be accepted into the joint training program. All training should be completed at one academic institution; any deviation *must* be approved *prospectively* by both the ABP and the ABPMR. Guidelines for combined training have been approved by both the ABP and the ABPMR and are available by contacting either board. An applicant may not take the certifying examination of the ABP until all training has been completed.

Pediatrics/Emergency Medicine Program

A special agreement exists with the American Board of Emergency Medicine (ABEM) whereby an applicant may fulfill the training requirements of both the ABP and the ABEM by completing joint training in 5 years. All 5 years should be completed in the same combined training program; any deviation *must* be approved *prospectively* by both the ABP and the ABEM. Training programs must also be approved *prospectively* by both the ABP and the ABEM. Guidelines for combined training have been approved by both the ABP and the ABEM and are available by contacting either board. An applicant may not take the certifying examination of the ABP until all training has been completed.

Pediatrics/Medical Genetics Program

A special agreement exists with the American Board of Medical Genetics (ABMG) whereby an applicant may fulfill the training requirements of both the ABP and ABMG by completing joint training in 5 years. All 5 years should be completed in the same combined training program; any deviation must be approved *prospectively* by both the ABP and ABMG. Training programs must also be approved *prospectively* by both the ABP and ABMG. Guidelines for combined training have been approved by both the ABP and ABMG and are available by contacting either board. An applicant may not take the certifying examination of the ABP until all training in both programs has been completed.

Pediatrics/Psychiatry/Child and Adolescent Psychiatry Program

A special agreement exists with the American Board of Psychiatry and Neurology (ABPN), whereby an applicant may fulfill the training requirements for certification in pediatrics, psychiatry, and special qualifications in child and adolescent psychiatry by completing joint training in 5 years. Training includes 24 months of general comprehensive pediatrics, 18 months of child and adolescent psychiatry, and 18 months of adult psychiatry. Physicians pursuing training in these programs may take the certifying examination of the ABP in the fall of the fifth year of training, provided that all pediatric training (except continuity clinics) is completed by the date of the examination. Credit for training via this route may be obtained only by training in one of the approved programs. Guidelines for combined training have been approved by the ABP and ABPN.

Further information concerning these combined training programs may be obtained by contacting the ABPN, 500 Lake Cook Rd, Ste 335, Deerfield, IL 60015, 847 945-7900.

Training Programs

The ABP approves applicants for admission to its certifying process. The ABP does not accredit training programs. Information regarding accreditation should be addressed to Executive Secretary, Residency Review Committee for Pediatrics, 515 N State St, Chicago, IL 60610, 312 464-4947.

Graduate School Courses

A fundamental concept of the ABP is that a residency training program should provide for properly organized, progressive responsibility for the care of children. The ABP believes that this can be accomplished through continuity of clinical experience under the supervision of attending physicians who are responsible for the care of these children. The substitution of a formal graduate or postgraduate school course that does not carry the essential ingredient of responsibility for patient care is inconsistent with this principle. Accordingly, the ABP will not accept such courses in fulfillment of its training requirements.

Military Service

Military service, unless as a resident in a military hospital that is accredited by the RRC, cannot be substituted for training requirements.

Special Situations

The ABP recognizes that situations may arise that are not explained by the preceding information. A physician may have worked in a pediatric field for many years yet be deficient in the formal training requirements for examination, or a physician may have completed specialized training not explained in the above requirements. In such cases, the individual should present his or her credentials to the ABP, which may ask the Credentials Committee to review them and to decide whether permission should be given to enter the certification process.

Tracking and Evaluation

The ABP regards the evaluation of trainee competency as a continuum that begins during training and concludes with the certifying examination following formal training. The ABP believes that the program director(s) and faculty play significant roles in the certification process and are the keys to a responsible system of determining which applicants should be admitted to the certifying examination. The program director is able to provide a meaningful overview of the resident's professional competence, especially in skills such as clinical judgment, moral and ethical behavior, professional attitudes and behavior, procedural skills, and humanistic qualities.

The ABP resident tracking and evaluation program is part of the certifying process of the ABP. The program director is required to indicate annually whether each resident's performance is satisfactory, marginal, or unsatisfactory. If a resident's performance is unsatisfactory, the resident will not receive credit for that period of training. A marginal evaluation indicates a need for remediation. If a resident receives a marginal rating for 2 consecutive years of training (eg, PL-1 and PL-2), he/she will not receive credit for the second marginal year and will have to repeat that entire year of training. If a resident receives a marginal rating for 1 year (eg, PL-1) and receives a satisfactory rating for the following year (eg, PL-2), then both the marginal year and the satisfactory year will be considered to be satisfactory. The resident who receives a marginal rating in the final year of training (eg, PL-3) will be reviewed by the ABP Credentials Committee before being allowed to take the certifying examination in general pediatrics.

The tracking system also identifies residents who transfer from one program to another or to a new specialty and ensures that the new program director recognizes those residents who need remediation.

Verification of Training by Directors of Pediatric Training Programs

Program directors will be sent Verification of Clinical Competence Forms for residents in their last year of training. (*Note:* The form will be sent to the program directors of pediatrics/psychiatry/child and adolescent psychiatry programs for residents in their fourth year of training.) The ABP requires the program director to verify completion of training and to sign either Statement A or Statement B on the Verification of Clinical Competence Form. Statement A is as follows: "I certify that the above-named applicant has demonstrated the necessary attitudes, knowledge, clinical judgment, technical skills, and interpersonal skills and is judged to be fully prepared for independent responsibility as a general pediatrician; to my knowledge he or she has moral and ethical integrity. The applicant is recommended for examination."

In recommending an applicant for the certifying examination, a program director should keep in mind the definition of a qualified applicant as determined by the ABP:

An applicant shall demonstrate the following abilities as they pertain to infants, children, and adolescents:

1. Assessment of the clinical issues and formulation of a management plan for any medical or health maintenance problem
2. Execution of the management plan with the patient and family, without further medical consultation, for all common problems of disease and health maintenance and for all medically life-threatening situations
3. Consultation, when appropriate, with physicians and other professionals regarding common problems and life-threatening situations
4. Arrangement for help for the patient and knowledge of what to anticipate from the consultant, being prepared personally to guide further management with assistance, when appropriate, for unusual problems requiring subspecialty, surgical, or other specialized skills.

Each applicant must have verification of training and verification of clinical competence on file in the ABP office to be admitted to the certifying examination. The applicant is responsible for ensuring that the program director submits all the required documents by the appropriate deadline.

When an applicant has not attained the appropriate knowledge and skills, the program director should sign Statement B on the Verification of Clinical Competence Form. By signing this statement, the program director is recommending that the applicant not be admitted to the certifying examination.

If an applicant's training is not verified and/or he/she is not recommended for admission to the certifying examination, the applicant will be required to complete an additional period of training in general comprehensive pediatrics in an accredited program in the United States or Canada before reapplying to the ABP. The director of the program where the additional training occurred *must* complete a separate Verification of Clinical Competence Form. Alternatively, the applicant may appeal to the Credentials Committee of the ABP. The Credentials Committee will gather additional information about the applicant and decide if permission to take the examination should be given. If the applicant appeals the decision, he/she will be asked to submit copies of certificates of satisfactory completion of training. If the applicant has been denied such certificates, then admission will be refused on the basis of incomplete training. However, possession of such certificates will not automatically admit the person to the ABP's certification process. Most training certificates attest to the achievement of a minimal level of competence or to the fulfillment of an employment contract. Therefore, the program director's statement on the Verification of Clinical Competence Form will take precedence over the certificate from the hospital. The ABP must have the program director's assurance that an applicant meets the standards expected of a certified pediatrician. Program directors are urged not to issue certificates of successful completion of training when the resident is deemed not to have met those standards.

The duration of training is 36 months. Absences in excess of 3 months, eg, vacation, sick leave, maternity leave, must be made up unless the program director believes that an absence of more than 3 months is justified, in which case a letter of explanation must be sent for review by the Credentials Committee.

The program director is required to provide further information about the applicant. The program director is asked to evaluate the applicant on a nine-point scale in the following areas: gathering data by history, by physical examination, and by laboratory studies; assessing data and arriving at a diagnosis; managing problems and maintaining health; interpersonal relationships with patients and families; interpersonal relationships with other members of the health team; and work habits and personal qualities.

The program director is asked to rate the applicant's overall clinical competency by indicating which of the following phrases best describes the applicant's ability to care for children in the United States or Canada. In these phrases, the word "manage" is defined as identifying the nature of the problem, determining methods of resolving or alleviating the problem, and carrying out management plans, including the appropriate and timely use of consultants.

1 Unable to manage many pediatric problems, including the most routine ones
2
3 Able to manage only the most routine problems of pediatrics
4
5 Able to manage the common problems of pediatrics adequately
6
7 Able to manage most pediatric problems in an effective way
8
9 Able to manage almost any pediatric problem in a highly effective manner

If the program director signs Statement A but gives a *rating of 3 or less in any single area or a rating of 4 or less for overall clinical competency*, the Credentials Committee will ask the program director to submit supporting documentation with the completed Verification of Clinical Competence Form. If the Credentials Committee concludes that the low ratings are substantiated, the applicant must complete an additional period of training in general comprehensive pediatrics in an accredited program either in the United States or Canada before reapplying to the ABP. The director of the program where the additional training occurred must complete a separate Verification of Clinical Competence Form. Alternatively, the applicant may appeal to the Credentials Committee.

Program directors are encouraged to have all residents in their programs take the In-Training Examination (ITE). The results of the ITE can provide valuable information for both the resident and the program.

To be compliant with the Program Requirements for Residency Education in Pediatrics established by the ACGME, the program director and the faculty must develop evaluation procedures for assessment of physician performance. Examples are medical record audits, rating scales for assessment of work habits, observational checklists for assessment of technical skills, oral examinations, and consumer questionnaires.

Certifying Examinations

Applicants for certifying examinations must complete all training by the first day of the month of the examination. A written request for waiver of this policy will be considered on a case-by-case basis.

After an application has been accepted, the candidate is expected to take the next examination offered. A candidate who withdraws from the examination by the published withdrawal deadline will be issued a refund of the examination fee. A candidate who withdraws after the published withdrawal deadline will forfeit all fees paid. To register for a future examination, payment of the reregistration fee will be required.

The names of certified pediatricians, but not their scores, will be sent to appropriate organizations, directories, and journals. The certificate will reflect the candidate's medical degree awarded at the time of graduation from medical school (eg, MD, MB, BS, or DO). Degrees awarded either before or after graduation from medical school will not be included on the certificate.

The ABP does not sponsor or maintain records about any courses that claim to be review courses in preparation for its certifying examinations, nor does the ABP track continuing medical education credits.

The validity of the performance of candidates on the certifying examination of the ABP is secured by every means available. The ABP should be contacted in the event of irregular behavior such as giving or obtaining unauthorized information or aid before, during, or after the examination or offering financial or other benefit to a proctor, employee, or agent of the ABP.

The ABP reserves the right to withhold permission for applicants to take its examinations and/or certification in the event of circumstances demonstrating that an applicant is not capable of performing the role of physician and advocate for infants, children, and adolescents. In such instances, the applicant will be notified; the applicant may appeal the decision to the Credentials Committee of the ABP.

For failing candidates who are concerned that their answer sheets were not scored correctly, hand scoring is available for a fee of $60. However, candidates are *not* encouraged to request this service since neither mechanical nor computer errors have ever been found. Requests should be made in writing accompanied by check or money order. Hand scoring is available for 11 months following the date of the examination.

General Pediatrics Certifying Examination

The certifying examination is given once a year in the fall in a number of locations throughout the United States. The dates of examinations and other information may be found on the ABP web site.

The examination lasts 2 days. Each day there are two sessions, each of 3 hours' duration, with a luncheon break between sessions. The 1999 certifying examination will be administered October 18-19. Applicants for the certifying examination *must* complete all their training by the first day of the month of the examination.

The content of the examination for certification is appropriate for the practice of general comprehensive pediatrics. Emphasis is placed on practical aspects; however, good practice is founded on sound scientific knowledge, and the candidate should be prepared to demonstrate an understanding of basic science.

The examination consists of multiple-choice questions. Examples of the types of questions to be used are mailed to registered candidates before the administration of the examination. Some questions are included in the examination for experimental purposes only. These questions will not contribute to the score.

Each candidate's examination score will be reported to his or her general pediatric program director. Periodically, the ABP conducts research utilizing data it has compiled; the candidate's anonymity is guaranteed in all such cases.

Application, Registration, and Fees

Application material for admission to the certifying examination of the ABP may be obtained by contacting the ABP. Residents in their last year of training are sent an application through their residency programs in early December 1998; residents should contact the ABP office if the application is not received by December 20. It is the applicant's responsibility to be aware of and to meet registration deadlines. (*Note:* Residents in a pediatrics/psychiatry/child and adolescent psychiatry program will be sent the material in December of the fourth year of training.)

For new applicants, the regular registration period begins December 1, 1998, and extends through February 27, 1999. An application *postmarked* by February 27 must be accompanied by the application fee of $1,180. Late registration for new applicants begins March 1 and extends through April 30, 1999. It is the applicant's responsibility to be aware of and to meet registration deadlines. A nonrefundable penalty fee of $225 is required for an application postmarked March 1 through April 30; thus, the late registration fee is $1,405. New applications that are postmarked after April 30, 1999, will not be accepted.

Regular reregistration begins February 15 and extends through April 30, 1999. Reregistration material postmarked by April 30 must be accompanied by the reregistration fee of $1,080. Late reregistration begins May 1 and extends through May 31, 1999. A nonrefundable penalty fee of $225 is required for all reregistration material postmarked May 1 through May 31, 1999; thus, the late registration fee is $1,305. Reregistration material that is postmarked after May 31, 1999, will not be accepted. A copy of a valid (current), unrestricted license to practice medicine must be included in this material.

Many deadlines set by the ABP are postmark deadlines. If there is a discrepancy between a metered postmark and an official US Postal Service postmark, the latter will be considered official.

Acknowledgment of *receipt* of the application will be sent promptly. The ABP should be contacted if acknowledgment of receipt is not received within 30 days of submission of the application. Applications received by the deadlines will be processed and evaluated, and the ABP will request directors of general pediatric training programs to verify successful completion of training.

Applicants who meet the training requirements of the ABP and who are recommended by their program director(s) will be accepted and registered for the certifying examination.

An applicant who does not receive notification of the acceptance or rejection of his or her application by August 10 should contact the ABP to inquire about the status of the application.

The cost of certification includes the following fees, payable only in United States (US) dollars:

Fees for New Applicants

Processing and Evaluation	$335
Examination	$845
Total New Candidate Fees	$1,180
Late Registration Fee (nonrefundable)	$225
Late Registration	*$1,405*

Fees for Reregistrants

Processing and Evaluation	$235
Examination	$845
Total Reregistrant Fees	$1,080
Late Registration Fee (nonrefundable)	$225
Late Registration	*$1,305*

Applicants can pay the total application fee by credit card, using either Visa or MasterCard, or by check.

For applicants not using US banks, the fee must be paid in US dollars using one of the following vehicles: (1) money order, (2) cashier's check, or (3) certified check. To be accepted for payment, these vehicles must be payable through a US bank. *The ABP cannot accept electronic transfer of funds from any organization, eg, US military, Western Union.*

Applicants should retain their acknowledgment letters, canceled checks, or credit card statements as proof of payment. *No other receipts will be issued.*

If an applicant is not accepted to take the ABP certifying examination, the examination fee will be refunded. Neither the processing and evaluation fee nor the penalty fee are refundable. If the applicant wishes to pursue certification in the future, he or she will be required to complete a new application and submit the full fee again.

After the ABP has accepted an application, the applicant is expected to take the next certifying examination offered. However, an applicant may withdraw by submitting a written notice *postmarked* no later than August 16, 1999. The applicant will be issued a refund of the examination fee ($845). An applicant whose withdrawal letter is postmarked after August 16 or who does not appear for the examination will forfeit all fees paid and will be required to submit a reregistration fee before being admitted to a future examination. Reregistration material for the next year's examination will be sent to the last address on file for the applicants who have previously been accepted to take the examination.

The ABP reserves the right to withhold permission for applicants to take its examinations and/or certification in the event of circumstances demonstrating that an applicant is not capable of performing the role of physician and advocate for infants, children, and adolescents. In such instances, the applicant will be notified; the applicant may appeal the decision to the Credentials Committee of the ABP.

Certification in the Pediatric Subspecialties

The ABP issues a Certificate of Special Qualifications in the following subspecialties: adolescent medicine, pediatric cardiology, pediatric critical care medicine, pediatric emergency medicine, pediatric endocrinology, pediatric gastroenterology, pediatric hematology-oncology, pediatric infectious diseases, neonatal-perinatal medicine, pediatric nephrology, pediatric pulmonology, and pediatric rheumatology.

The ABP, in conjunction with the ABIM and their Conjoint Board, the American Board of Allergy and Immunology (ABAI), offers a Certificate of Added Qualifications in clinical and laboratory immunology. Further information may be obtained by contacting the ABAI, 510 Walnut St, Ste 1701, Philadelphia, PA 19106-3619.

A Certificate of Added Qualifications in sports medicine is offered by the American Board of Family Practice (ABFP), the ABEM, the ABIM, and the ABP. Further information may be obtained by contacting the ABP.

A Certificate of Added Qualifications in medical toxicology is offered by the ABEM, the ABP, and the American Board of Preventive Medicine. Further information may be obtained by contacting the ABP.

Examination Admission Requirements

The applicant must be currently certified in pediatrics by the ABP. Applicants whose time-limited certification will expire before the examination must attain recertification at least 4 months before the examination date.

For candidates who began subspecialty training after January 1, 1995, 3 years of training is required. (The training requirements for candidates who began subspecialty training before January 1, 1995, may differ. Such individuals should contact the ABP for further information.) The program director(s) will be required to verify completion of training and sign a statement indicating whether the candidate is recommended to take the certifying examination. In addition, the program director(s) must verify clinical competence and meaningful accomplishment in research by completing the Verification of Competence Form.

The applicant must have a valid (current), unrestricted license to practice medicine in one of the states, districts, or territories of the United States or a province of Canada or unrestricted privileges to practice medicine in the US Armed Forces. A copy of the license may be submitted separately from the initial application, but it must be submitted by the deadline stated in the application packet. A candidate who is reregistering for the examination must submit the license with the reregistration material.

If an applicant has any action pending regarding the right to have an unrestricted license to practice medicine, admission to the examination may be denied. An applicant who is practicing the subspecialty abroad must provide proof of licensure equivalency in the country in which he or she resides. This information must be submitted by the deadline stated in the application packet. Candidates who practice or plan to practice abroad must submit a letter, in addition to the licensure equivalency, stating that they will not practice in the United States or Canada.

A subspecialty fellow who is believed to have demonstrated meaningful accomplishment in research, either before or during residency, may have a part of the training requirement waived. Evidence of such accomplishment might include a PhD degree or sustained research achievement culminating in the first-authored publication of a research paper in a peer-reviewed journal. The subspecialty program director may ask the Subboard to waive the research requirements and to reduce the time of subspecialty training by as much as 1 year. This petition must be made either before the beginning of training or during the first year of training. A candidate for this pathway must have completed 3 core years of general pediatrics in an accredited program in the United States or Canada and would not have the option of the SAP. Furthermore, a subspecialty fellow who receives a waiver by the Subboard must complete at least 2 years of training in the subspecialty with at least 1 year of broad-based clinical training. The training period requirement may be shortened for a candidate with extensive clinical experience by as much as 1 year by approval of the Credentials Committee. The candidate must meet the research requirements.

No credit toward subspecialty qualification will be granted for elective time spent in the subspecialty during the years of general pediatric training.

The RRC currently reviews and accredits pediatric subspecialty programs in all the certified subspecialties except adolescent medicine and pediatric emergency medicine, whose program requirements have been approved but whose programs have just begun the accreditation process.

A list of accredited programs is published in the *Graduate Medical Education Directory*.

General Criteria for Certification in the Pediatric Subspecialties

In addition to the training requirements, which are specific to each of the pediatric subspecialties, the following are required of candidates seeking certification in the pediatric subspecialties of adolescent medicine, cardiology, critical care medicine, emergency medicine, endocrinology, gastroenterology, hematology-oncology, infectious diseases, neonatal-perinatal medicine, nephrology, pulmonology, and rheumatology. Each candidate must be familiar with specific subspecialty training requirements as well as the policies stated in the current Booklet of Information.

A. Certification by the American Board of Pediatrics (ABP)

An applicant must take and pass the certifying examination in general pediatrics and must maintain a valid (current) certificate before being permitted to take a pediatric subspecialty certifying examination.

B. Licensure

An applicant must have a valid (current), unrestricted license to practice medicine in any of the states, districts, or territories of the United States or provinces of Canada in which he/she practices or have unrestricted privileges to practice medicine in the US armed forces. A copy of the unrestricted license must accompany the application material. An applicant who is practicing the subspecialty abroad may be exempted from this policy upon presentation of proof of licensure equivalency in the country in which he or she resides. Candidates who practice or plan to practice abroad must submit a letter, in addition to the licensure equivalency, stating that they will not practice in the United States or Canada.

C. Verification of Training

An applicant will be asked to list the program(s) where fellowship training occurred as well as the name(s) of the program director(s). The ABP will send a Verification of Competence Form to the program director(s) for completion. (*Note:* For new subspecialties, alternatives to the usual training requirements, such as practice experience, will be acceptable for a limited period as criteria for admission to the examination. Candidates should refer to the specific subspecialty eligibility criteria for details.) The role of the program director in the certification process is to verify completion of training and to sign the following statement on the Verification of Competence Form:

"I certify that the above-named applicant has demonstrated the necessary attitudes, knowledge, clinical judgment, research abilities, technical skills, and interpersonal skills and is judged to be fully prepared for independent responsibility as a pediatric subspecialist; to my knowledge, he/she has moral and ethical integrity. The applicant is recommended for examination."

An applicant must have the Verification Form(s) on file at the ABP in order to be admitted to the pediatric subspecialty examination. If an applicant's training is not verified and/or he/she is not recommended for admission, the applicant will be required to complete additional subspecialty fellowship training before reapplying. Alternatively, the applicant may appeal to the Credentials Committee of the Subboard. The Credentials Committee will gather additional information about the applicant and decide if he/she should be approved to take the examination. For an appeal, the applicant will be asked to submit copies of certificates of satisfactory completion of training. If the applicant has been denied such a certificate, then admission will be refused on the basis of incomplete training. A certificate of completion of training, as a basis for appeal, will be superseded by the program director's statement on the Verification of Competence Form because the certificate usually attests to the fulfillment of an employment contract or to the achievement of a minimal level of competence.

An applicant must satisfactorily complete all subspecialty training by the first day of the month of the examination.

No credit toward subspecialty qualification will be allowed for elective time spent in subspecialty areas during the general pediatric residency years (PL-1, 2, 3) or as a chief resident (PL-4).

An applicant seeking certification in another pediatric subspecialty or a non-ABP specialty (eg, allergy/immunology) on the basis of practice and/or training may not apply the same period of time toward fulfillment of these requirements.

D. Principles Regarding the Assessment of Meaningful Accomplishment in Research

1. Research experience is an essential part of the training of subspecialists. The general requirements for research in pediatric subspecialties approved by the ACGME for program accreditation must be met as evidence of research experience. These are as follows: "Within the institution, the subspecialty trainee must be exposed to, and take part in, research projects that are conducive to a questioning attitude, to protocol development, and to critical analysis of new therapies and of medical literature. Research experience should begin in the first year and continue for the entire period of training in order to allow adequate time for the development of research skills and to bring a project to completion. The trainees must help design, conduct, evaluate, and prepare for publication a clinical or laboratory research project in the subspecialty area. They should also be required to conduct research seminars and prepare a written report of their research activities. Instruction in related basic sciences and associated disciplines, such as research design, biostatistics, and epidemiology, must be offered through courses, workshops, and seminars."
2. Additional evidence of meaningful accomplishment in research must be submitted, including one or more of the following:
   a. First author of a research paper accepted for publication in a peer-reviewed journal deemed acceptable by the Subboard. A reprint of the paper, or a copy of the letter of acceptance by the journal and a copy of the manuscript, must be submitted.
   b. A research progress report (signed by both the applicant and mentor) of no more than five pages to include (a) a statement of hypothesis, (b) delineation of methodology, (c) results and analysis, and (d) significance of the research. An explanation must be provided by the program director/mentor if a research paper has not been submitted for publication within 2 years of completion of fellowship training.
   c. Submission of a research grant proposal that has been approved by an extramural organization with a critical review process acceptable to the Subboard. A copy of the approval letter must be included. A grant proposal will no longer meet the research requirement for fellows entering subspecialty training on or after January 1, 1998.
   d. A PhD degree in a field of science.
   e. A thesis accepted as partial fulfillment of the requirements for a postgraduate degree in a field relevant to the subspecialty. The thesis or a research progress report as described in 2(b) above must be submitted for review.
   f. First author of a research paper that has been submitted but not yet accepted for publication in a peer-reviewed journal deemed acceptable by the Subboard. A letter confirming the submission must be included as well as a copy of the submitted manuscript.
3. The program director is responsible for notifying all residents of the research requirements necessary for certification upon entry to the subspecialty training program. Furthermore, in the description of the candidate's research performance on the Verification of Competence Form, the program director must provide a detailed description of the experiences on which the acceptable evidence of meaningful research is based.
4. Research should be performed in a laboratory that best suits the candidate's interests. For example, the ABP is strongly supportive of the Pediatric Scientist Development Program that has been initiated by the Association of Medical School Pediatric Department Chairs.

Program Requirements for Residency Education in the Subspecialties of Pediatrics

Program Requirements for Residency Education in adolescent medicine, pediatric cardiology, pediatric critical care medicine, pediatric emergency medicine, pediatric endocrinology, pediatric gastroenterology, pediatric hematology-oncology, pediatric infectious diseases, medical toxicology, neonatal-perinatal medicine, pediatric nephrology, pediatric pulmonology, pediatric rheumatology, and sports medicine have been approved by the ACGME or by the RCPSC. Copies of the Program Requirements and lists of accredited programs are available from the office of the Residency Review Committee for Pediatrics, 515 N State St, Chicago, IL 60610 or the Office of Training and Evaluation, the Royal College of Physicians and Surgeons of Canada, 74 Stanley, Ottawa, Ontario, K1M 1P4. This information is published in the *Graduate Medical Education Directory* or in the RCPSC booklets of general information.

Training Leading to Dual Pediatric Subspecialty Certification

If an individual is certified in one subspecialty, he/she can become eligible to take another subspecialty examination after 2 years of additional training, of which at least 1 year must be broad-based clinical training.

An individual may petition the Credentials Committees of two pediatric subspecialties with a proposal for a 4-year integrated training program that would meet the eligibility requirements for certification in both subspecialties. This petition must be approved before subspecialty training begins or early in the first year of subspecialty training. Guidelines for dual subspecialty training may be obtained from the ABP.

Subspecialty "Fast-Tracking"

A subspecialty fellow who is believed to have demonstrated meaningful accomplishment in research, either before or during residency, may have a part of the training requirement waived. Evidence of such accomplishment might include a PhD degree or sustained research achievement culminating in the first-authored publication of a research paper in a peer-reviewed journal. The subspecialty program director may ask the Subboard to waive the research requirements and to reduce the time of subspecialty training by as much as 1 year. This petition must be made either before the beginning of training or during the first year of training. A candidate for this pathway must have completed 3 core years of pediatrics in an accredited program in the United States or Canada and would not have the option of the SAP. Furthermore, a subspecialty fellow who receives a waiver by the Subboard must complete at least 2 years of training in the subspecialty with at least 1 year of broad-based clinical training. The training period requirement may be shortened for a candidate with extensive clinical experience by as much as 1 year by approval of the Credentials Committee. The candidate must meet the research requirements.

It should be noted that these criteria and conditions are subject to change without notice. All applicants should be familiar with the current Booklet of Information. Applicants are advised to contact the ABP to ascertain whether the information they have is current.

Eligibility Criteria for Certification in Adolescent Medicine

The ABP has established a procedure for certification in adolescent medicine. In addition to the specific admission requirements listed below, there are general eligibility criteria that must be fulfilled to be eligible for certification. A copy of the general eligibility criteria is available upon request to the ABP.

Admission Requirements

To qualify for admission to the examination, an applicant must have completed one of the following:

A. Training

A subspecialty fellow entering adolescent medicine training before January 1, 1995, may apply for admission on the basis of completion of 2 years of subspecialty fellowship training in adolescent medicine.

Three years of full-time, broad-based fellowship training in adolescent medicine is required for fellows entering training on or after January 1, 1995. The period of training must be at least 33 months. Extended absences, whether for vacation, maternity leave, illness, etc, must be made up. If the program director believes that an extended absence of more than 3 months is justified, a letter of explanation should be sent by the director for review by the Credentials Committee.

For a fellow beginning adolescent medicine training on or after January 1, 1995, the following must be accomplished in order to become certified in the subspecialty: a Verification of Competence Form must be completed by the program director(s) stating satisfactory completion of the required training as well as verification of clinical competence and meaningful accomplishment in research; the fellow must meet the criteria stated in the "Principles Regarding the Assessment of Meaningful Accomplishment in Research"; and he/she must pass the subspecialty certifying examination. Verification of meaningful accomplishment in research will not be required for individuals who began training before January 1, 1995.

A fellow beginning part-time training after January 1, 1995, may complete the required training on a part-time basis not to exceed 6 years. No continuous absence of more than 1 year will be permitted.

Only those adolescent medicine training programs that are operated in association with general comprehensive residency programs in pediatrics or internal medicine accredited by the ACGME or by the RCPSC are acceptable. All subspecialty training must be completed in the United States or Canada unless the Credentials Committee of the Subboard has given approval for foreign subspecialty training to an applicant before he/she enrolls in such a program. An applicant wishing to obtain such approval should contact the ABP.

No credit will be given for subspecialty training during the core residency.

For an individual using the adolescent medicine fellowship training route (A), a Verification of Competence Form(s) will be required from the director(s) of the fellow's adolescent medicine training program(s).

B. Practice Experience

Five years of broad-based practice experience in adolescent medicine is required. A minimum of 50% of full-time, focused professional activity (and a minimum of 20 hours a week) must have been spent in the practice of adolescent medicine to receive credit. It is assumed that night and weekend time would be distributed in the same manner as regular time. These 5 years should be of such type and quality that they substitute for the clinical exposure one might have encountered during subspecialty fellowship training. All adolescent medicine experience must be accrued before December 31, 1998. No foreign adolescent medicine experience will be accepted by the Credentials Committee in fulfillment of the requirements.

For an individual utilizing the adolescent medicine practice experience route (B), an evaluation form(s) will be required from the adolescent medicine program director (if there is a subspecialty training program) or the pediatric department chair or the chief of pediatrics in the hospital(s) where the applicant is now or has been practicing adolescent medicine.

C. Partial Subspecialty Training and Practice

A combination of subspecialty fellowship training and practice experience equal to 5 years as outlined below may be utilized.

1. A fellow completing less than 12 months of fellowship training in adolescent medicine may receive practice credit on a month-for-month basis. For example, a 9-month subspecialty fellowship would be credited for 9 months of experience; this, added to 4 years and 3 months of adolescent medicine experience, would total 60 months or 5 years. These 5 years must be accrued before December 31, 1998.
2. A fellow completing 12 to 23 months of subspecialty fellowship training in adolescent medicine may receive credit on a two-for-one basis. For example, an 18-month subspecialty fellowship would be credited for 36 months of experience; this, added to 24 months of adolescent medicine experience, would total 60 months or 5 years. These 5 years must be accrued before December 31, 1998. No credit for partial training will be given for fellowship training that began on or after January 1, 1995.

For an individual utilizing the combination of training and practice experience route (C), a verification form(s) will be required from the director(s) of the applicant's adolescent medicine training program(s), and an evaluation form(s) will be required from the adolescent medicine program director (if there is a subspecialty training program) or the pediatric department chair or the chief of pediatrics in the hospital(s) where the applicant is now or has been practicing adolescent medicine.

The completed verification and evaluation form(s) should be sent directly to the ABP.

Accredited Training

The RRC has begun the process of accrediting training programs in adolescent medicine. A fellow entering subspecialty training in adolescent medicine before completion of the accreditation process by the RRC is advised to enter those programs in which the director or senior faculty of the program is certified in adolescent medicine or possesses equivalent credentials.

It should be noted that these criteria are subject to change without notice. All applicants are advised to contact the ABP to ascertain whether the information they have is current.

Eligibility Criteria for Certification in Pediatric Cardiology

The ABP has established a procedure for certification in pediatric cardiology. In addition to the specific admission requirements listed below, there are general eligibility criteria that must be fulfilled to be eligible for certification. A copy of the general eligibility criteria is available upon request to the ABP.

Admission Requirements

Physicians who entered training in pediatric cardiology on or after January 1, 1965, are required to complete their training in a program accredited for training in pediatric cardiology by the RRC for Pediatrics in the United States or the RCPSC in Canada.

A subspecialty fellow who entered pediatric cardiology training before January 1, 1988, may apply for admission on the basis of completion of 2 years of subspecialty fellowship training in pediatric cardiology.

Three years of full-time, broad-based subspecialty fellowship training in pediatric cardiology is required for fellows entering training on or after January 1, 1988. The period of training must be at least 33 months. Extended absences, whether for vacation, maternity leave, illness, etc, must be made up. If the program director believes that an extended absence of more than 3 months is justified, a letter of explanation should be sent by the director for review by the Credentials Committee.

For a fellow who began pediatric cardiology training on or after January 1, 1988, the following must be accomplished in order to become certified in the subspecialty: a Verification of Competence

Form must be completed by the program director(s) stating satisfactory completion of the required training as well as verification of clinical competence and meaningful accomplishment in research; the fellow must meet the criteria stated in the "Principles Regarding the Assessment of Meaningful Accomplishment in Research"; and he/she must pass the subspecialty certifying examination.

A fellow beginning part-time training after January 1, 1988, may complete the required training on a part-time basis not to exceed 6 years. No continuous absence of more than 1 year will be permitted.

Only those pediatric cardiology training programs that are operated in association with general comprehensive pediatric residency programs accredited by the RRC or by the RCPSC are acceptable. All subspecialty training must be completed in the United States or Canada unless the Credentials Committee of the Subboard has given approval for foreign subspecialty training to an applicant before he/she enrolls in such a program. An applicant wishing to obtain such approval should contact the ABP.

No credit will be given for subspecialty training during the core residency.

Dual Subcertification in Cardiology (Internal Medicine and Pediatrics)

There is no change in the usual training requirements in pediatric cardiology for graduates of combined medicine/pediatrics programs.

It should be noted that these criteria and conditions are subject to change without notice. All applicants are advised to contact the ABP to ascertain whether the information they have is current.

Eligibility Criteria for Certification in Pediatric Critical Care Medicine

The ABP has established a procedure for certification in pediatric critical care medicine. In addition to the specific admission requirements listed below, there are general eligibility criteria that must be fulfilled to be eligible for certification. A copy of the general eligibility criteria is available upon request to the ABP.

Admission Requirements

Physicians who entered training in pediatric critical care medicine on or after January 1, 1992, are required to complete their training in a program accredited for training in pediatric critical care medicine by the RRC for Pediatrics in the United States or the RCPSC in Canada.

A subspecialty fellow who entered pediatric critical care medicine training before January 1, 1988, may apply for admission on the basis of completion of 2 years of subspecialty fellowship training in pediatric critical care medicine. A subspecialty fellow who is certified in anesthesiology by the American Board of Anesthesiology may apply for admission on the basis of completion of 2 years of subspecialty fellowship training in pediatric critical care medicine.

Three years of full-time, broad-based subspecialty fellowship training in pediatric critical care medicine is required for fellows entering training on or after January 1, 1988. The period of training must be at least 33 months. Extended absences, whether for vacation, maternity leave, illness, etc, must be made up. If the program director believes that an extended absence of more than 3 months is justified, a letter of explanation should be sent by the director for review by the Credentials Committee.

For a fellow who began pediatric critical care medicine training on or after January 1, 1988, the following must be accomplished in order to become certified in the subspecialty: a Verification of Competence Form must be completed by the program director(s) stating satisfactory completion of the required training as well as verification of clinical competence and meaningful accomplishment in research; the fellow must meet the criteria stated in the "Principles Regarding the Assessment of Meaningful Accomplishment in Research"; and he/she must pass the subspecialty certifying examination.

A fellow beginning part-time training after January 1, 1988, may complete the required training on a part-time basis not to exceed 6 years. No continuous absence of more than 1 year will be permitted.

Only those pediatric critical care medicine training programs that are operated in association with general comprehensive pediatric residency programs accredited by the RRC or by the RCPSC are acceptable. All subspecialty training must be completed in the United States or Canada unless the Credentials Committee of the Subboard has given approval for foreign subspecialty training to an applicant before he/she enrolls in such a program. An applicant wishing to obtain such approval should contact the ABP.

No credit will be given for subspecialty training during the core residency.

Dual Subcertification in Critical Care Medicine (Internal Medicine and Pediatrics)

Individuals who are graduates of combined training programs in internal medicine and general pediatrics should contact both boards regarding dual subcertification opportunities.

It should be noted that these criteria and conditions are subject to change without notice. All applicants are advised to contact the ABP to ascertain whether the information they have is current.

Eligibility Criteria for Certification in Pediatric Emergency Medicine

The ABP and the ABEM have established a procedure for certification in pediatric emergency medicine. To be eligible for this subspecialty examination, a physician must be certified in either pediatrics by the ABP or emergency medicine by the ABEM. In addition to the specific admission requirements listed below, there are general eligibility criteria for all ABP subspecialties that must be fulfilled to be eligible for certification (a copy is available upon request to the ABP). The ABEM also has general requirements that must be fulfilled and are available from the ABEM.

Admission Requirements

To qualify for admission to the examination, an applicant must have completed one of the following:

A. Training

A subspecialty fellow entering pediatric emergency medicine training before January 1, 1995, may apply for admission on the basis of completion of 2 years of subspecialty fellowship training in pediatric emergency medicine. The program and the training must conform to the Program Requirements for Residency Education in Pediatric Emergency Medicine.

1. Requirements for candidates applying to the ABP for certification are as follows:

   Three years of broad-based fellowship training in pediatric emergency medicine is required for fellows entering training on or after January 1, 1995. The period of training must be at least 33 months. Extended absences, whether for vacation, maternity leave, illness, etc, must be made up. If the program director believes that an extended absence of more than 3 months is justified, a letter of explanation should be sent by the director for review by the Credentials Committee.

   For a fellow beginning pediatric emergency medicine training on or after January 1, 1995, the following must be accomplished in order to become certified in the subspecialty: a Verification of Competence Form must be completed by the program director(s) stating satisfactory completion of the required training as well as verification of clinical competence and meaningful accomplishment in research; the fellow must meet the criteria stated in the "Principles Regarding the Assessment of Meaningful Accomplishment in Research"; and he/she must pass the subspecialty certifying examination. Verification of meaningful accomplishment in research will not be required for individuals who began training before January 1, 1995.

A fellow beginning training after January 1, 1995, may complete the required training on a part-time basis not to exceed 6 years. No continuous absence of more than 1 year will be permitted.

2. Candidates whose primary certificate is in emergency medicine should contact the ABEM for certification requirements.

Only those pediatric emergency medicine training programs that are operated in association with general comprehensive pediatric or emergency medicine residency programs accredited by the ACGME or the RCPSC are acceptable. All subspecialty training must be completed in the United States or Canada unless the Credentials Committee of the Subboard has given approval for foreign subspecialty training to an applicant before he/she enrolls in such a program. An applicant wishing to obtain such approval should contact the ABP or the ABEM.

No credit will be given for subspecialty training during the core residency.

B. Dual Certification

A candidate who is certified by the ABP and the ABEM may apply via this pathway. A candidate who has completed training to meet the certification requirements of the ABP and the ABEM before January 1, 1999, may apply via this pathway.

Verification of Training

1. For a candidate utilizing the subspecialty fellowship training route, a Verification of Competence Form(s) from the director(s) of the applicant's pediatric emergency medicine training program(s) is required.
2. For a candidate utilizing the dual certification pathway, the certificate number and year of certification for each board must be provided.

Certification shall be time-limited for the number of years that the primary board currently grants certification (7 years for ABP and 10 years for ABEM).

Description of the Institution/Emergency Department

The individual(s) responsible for completion of the Verification of Competence Form(s) or the evaluation form(s) must provide a description of the institution and the ED.

Accredited Training

The RRC has begun the process of accrediting training programs in pediatric emergency medicine. An individual entering fellowship in pediatric emergency medicine before completion of the accreditation process by the RRC is advised to enter those programs in which the director or senior faculty of the program is certified in pediatric emergency medicine by the ABP and/or ABEM or possesses equivalent credentials.

It should be noted that these criteria and conditions are subject to change without notice. All applicants are advised to contact the ABP and the ABEM to ascertain whether the information they have is current.

Eligibility Criteria for Certification in Pediatric Endocrinology

The ABP has established a procedure for certification in pediatric endocrinology. In addition to the specific admission requirements listed below, there are general eligibility criteria that must be fulfilled to be eligible for certification. A copy of the general eligibility criteria is available upon request to the ABP.

Admission Requirements

Physicians who entered training in pediatric endocrinology on or after January 1, 1987, are required to complete their training in a program accredited for training in pediatric endocrinology by the RRC for Pediatrics in the United States or the RCPSC in Canada.

A subspecialty fellow who entered pediatric endocrinology before January 1, 1988, may apply for admission on the basis of completion of 2 years of subspecialty fellowship training in pediatric endocrinology.

Three years of full-time, broad-based fellowship training in pediatric endocrinology is required for fellows entering training on or after January 1, 1988. The period of training must be at least 33 months. Extended absences, whether for vacation, maternity leave, illness, etc, must be made up. If the program director believes that an extended absence of more than 3 months is justified, a letter of explanation should be sent by the director for review by the Credentials Committee.

For a fellow who began pediatric endocrinology training on or after January 1, 1988, the following must be accomplished in order to become certified in the subspecialty: a Verification of Competence Form must be completed by the program director(s) stating satisfactory completion of the required training as well as verification of clinical competence and meaningful accomplishment in research; the fellow must meet the criteria stated in the "Principles Regarding the Assessment of Meaningful Accomplishment in Research"; and he/she must pass the subspecialty certifying examination.

A fellow beginning part-time training after January 1, 1988, may complete the required training on a part-time basis not to exceed 6 years. No continuous absence of more than 1 year will be permitted.

Only those pediatric endocrinology training programs that are operated in association with general comprehensive pediatric residency programs accredited by the RRC or by the RCPSC are acceptable. All subspecialty training must be completed in the United States or Canada unless the Credentials Committee of the Subboard has given approval for foreign subspecialty training to an applicant before he/she enrolls in such a program. An applicant wishing to obtain such approval should contact the ABP.

No credit will be given for subspecialty training during the core residency.

Dual Subcertification in Endocrinology (Internal Medicine and Pediatrics)

Individuals who are graduates of combined training programs in internal medicine and general pediatrics should contact both boards regarding dual subcertification opportunities.

It should be noted that these criteria and conditions are subject to change without notice. All applicants are advised to contact the ABP to ascertain whether the information they have is current.

Eligibility Criteria for Certification in Pediatric Gastroenterology

The ABP has established a procedure for certification in pediatric gastroenterology. In addition to the specific admission requirements listed below, there are general eligibility criteria that must be fulfilled to be eligible for certification. A copy of the general eligibility criteria is available upon request to the ABP.

Admission Requirements

Physicians who entered training in pediatric gastroenterology on or after January 1, 1996, are required to complete their training in a program accredited for training in pediatric gastroenterology by the RRC for Pediatrics in the United States or the RCPSC in Canada.

A subspecialty fellow who entered pediatric gastroenterology training before January 1, 1990, may apply for admission on the basis of completion of 2 years of fellowship training in pediatric gastroenterology.

Three years of full-time, broad-based fellowship training in pediatric gastroenterology is required for fellows entering training on or after January 1, 1990. The period of training must be at least 33 months. Extended absences, whether for vacation, maternity leave, illness, etc, must be made up. If the program director believes that an extended absence of more than 3 months is justified, a letter of explanation should be sent by the director for review by the Credentials Committee.

For a fellow who began pediatric gastroenterology training on or after January 1, 1990, the following must be accomplished in order to become certified in the subspecialty: a Verification of Competence Form must be completed by the program director(s) stating satisfactory completion of the required training as well as verification of clinical competence and meaningful accomplishment in research; the fellow must meet the criteria stated in the "Principles Regarding the Assessment of Meaningful Accomplishment in Research"; and he/she must pass the subspecialty certifying examination.

A fellow beginning part-time training after January 1, 1990, may complete the required training on a part-time basis not to exceed 6 years. No continuous absence of more than 1 year will be permitted.

Only those pediatric gastroenterology training programs that are operated in association with general comprehensive pediatric residency programs accredited by the RRC or the RCPSC are acceptable. All subspecialty training must be completed in the United States or Canada unless the Credentials Committee of the Subboard has given approval for foreign subspecialty training to an applicant before he/she enrolls in such a program. An applicant wishing to obtain such approval should contact the ABP.

No credit will be given for subspecialty training during the core residency.

Dual Subcertification in Gastroenterology (Internal Medicine and Pediatrics)

Individuals who are graduates of combined training programs in internal medicine and general pediatrics should contact both boards regarding dual subcertification opportunities.

It should be noted that these criteria and conditions are subject to change without notice. All applicants are advised to contact the ABP to ascertain whether the information they have is current.

Eligibility Criteria for Certification in Pediatric Hematology-Oncology

The ABP has established a procedure for certification in pediatric hematology-oncology. In addition to the specific admission requirements listed below, there are general eligibility criteria that must be fulfilled to be eligible for certification. A copy of the general eligibility criteria is available upon request to the ABP.

Admission Requirements

Physicians who entered training in pediatric hematology-oncology on or after January 1, 1987, are required to complete their training in a program accredited for training in pediatric hematology-oncology by the RRC for Pediatrics in the United States or the RCPSC in Canada.

A subspecialty fellow who entered pediatric hematology-oncology training before January 1, 1986, may apply for admission on the basis of completion of 2 years of fellowship training in pediatric hematology-oncology.

Three years of full-time, broad-based fellowship training in pediatric hematology-oncology is required for fellows entering training on or after January 1, 1986. The period of training must be at least 33 months. Extended absences, whether for vacation, maternity leave, illness, etc, must be made up. If the program director believes that an extended absence of more than 3 months is justified, a letter of explanation should be sent by the director for review by the Credentials Committee.

For a fellow who began pediatric hematology-oncology training on or after January 1, 1988, the following must be accomplished in order to become certified in the subspecialty: a Verification of Competence Form must be completed by the program director(s) stating satisfactory completion of the required training as well as verification of clinical competence and meaningful accomplishment in research; the fellow must meet the criteria stated in the "Principles Regarding the Assessment of Meaningful Accomplishment in Research"; and he/she must pass the subspecialty certifying examination.

A fellow beginning part-time training after January 1, 1988, may complete the required training on a part-time basis not to exceed 6 years. No continuous absence of more than 1 year will be permitted.

Only those pediatric hematology-oncology training programs that are operated in association with general comprehensive pediatric residency programs accredited by the RRC or by the RCPSC are acceptable. All subspecialty training must be completed in the United States or Canada unless the Credentials Committee of the Subboard has given approval for foreign subspecialty training to an applicant before he/she enrolls in such a program. An applicant wishing to obtain such approval should contact the ABP.

No credit will be given for subspecialty training during the core residency.

Dual Subcertification in Hematology-Oncology (Internal Medicine and Pediatrics)

There is no change in the usual training requirements in pediatric hematology-oncology for graduates of combined medicine/pediatrics programs.

It should be noted that these criteria and conditions are subject to change without notice. All applicants are advised to contact the ABP to ascertain whether the information they have is current.

Eligibility Criteria for Certification in Pediatric Infectious Diseases

The ABP has established a procedure for certification in pediatric infectious diseases. In addition to the specific admission requirements listed below, there are general eligibility criteria that must be fulfilled to be eligible for certification. A copy of the general eligibility criteria is available upon request to the ABP.

Admission Requirements

To qualify for admission to the examination, an applicant must have completed one of the following:

A. Training

Physicians who enter training in pediatric infectious diseases on or after January 1, 2000, are required to complete their training in a program accredited for training in pediatric infectious diseases by the RRC for Pediatrics in the United States or the RCPSC in Canada.

A subspecialty fellow entering pediatric infectious diseases training before January 1, 1995, may apply for admission on the basis of completion of 2 years of fellowship training in pediatric infectious diseases.

Three years of full-time, broad-based fellowship training in pediatric infectious diseases is required for fellows entering training on or after January 1, 1995. The period of training must be at least 33 months. Extended absences, whether for vacation, maternity leave, illness, etc, must be made up. If the program director believes that an extended absence of more than 3 months is justified, a letter of explanation should be sent by the director for review by the Credentials Committee.

For a fellow beginning pediatric infectious diseases training on or after January 1, 1995, the following must be accomplished in order to become certified in the subspecialty: a Verification of Competence Form must be completed by the program director(s) stating satisfactory completion of the required training as well as verification of clinical competence and meaningful accomplishment in research; the fellow must meet the criteria stated in the "Principles Regarding the Assessment of Meaningful Accomplishment in Research"; and he/she must pass the subspecialty certifying examination. Verification of meaningful accomplishment in research will not be required for individuals who began training before January 1, 1995.

A fellow beginning part-time training after January 1, 1995, may complete the required training on a part-time basis not to exceed 6 years. No continuous absence of more than 1 year will be permitted.

Only those pediatric infectious diseases training programs that are operated in association with general comprehensive pediatric residency programs accredited by the RRC or the RCPSC are acceptable. All subspecialty training must be completed in the United States or Canada unless the Credentials Committee of the Subboard has given approval for foreign subspecialty training to an applicant before he/she enrolls in such a program. An applicant wishing to obtain such approval should contact the ABP.

No credit will be given for subspecialty training during the core residency.

For an individual using the pediatric infectious diseases fellowship training route (A), a Verification of Competence Form(s) will be required from the director(s) of the fellow's pediatric infectious diseases training program(s).

B. Practice Experience

Five years of broad-based practice experience in pediatric infectious diseases is required. A minimum of 50% of full-time professional activity must have been spent in the practice of pediatric infectious diseases to receive credit. It is assumed that night and weekend time would be distributed in the same manner as regular time. These 5 years should be of such type and quality that they substitute for the clinical exposure one might have encountered during subspecialty fellowship training. All pediatric infectious diseases experience must be accrued by December 31, 1998. No foreign pediatric infectious diseases experience will be accepted by the Credentials Committee in fulfillment of the requirements.

For an individual utilizing the pediatric infectious diseases practice experience route (B), an Evaluation Form(s) will be required from the pediatric infectious diseases program director (if there is a subspecialty training program) or the pediatric department chair or the chief of pediatrics in the hospital(s) where the applicant is now or has been practicing pediatric infectious diseases.

C. Partial Subspecialty Training and Practice

A combination of training and practice in pediatric infectious diseases equal to 5 years as outlined below may be utilized:

1. A fellow completing less than 12 months of fellowship training in pediatric infectious diseases may receive practice credit on a month-for-month basis. For example, a 9-month fellowship would be credited for 9 months of experience; this, added to 4 years and 3 months of pediatric infectious diseases experience, would total 60 months or 5 years. These 5 years must be accrued before December 31, 1998.
2. A fellow completing 12 to 23 months of fellowship training in pediatric infectious diseases may receive credit on a two-for-one basis. For example, an 18-month fellowship would be credited for 36 months of experience; this, added to 24 months of pediatric infectious diseases experience, would total 60 months or 5 years. These 5 years must be accrued before December 31, 1998. No credit for partial training will be given to a subspecialty fellow who begins training on or after January 1, 1995.

For an individual utilizing the combination subspecialty fellowship training and practice experience route (C), a Verification Form(s) will be required from the director(s) of the applicant's pediatric infectious diseases training program(s), and an Evaluation Form(s) will be required from the pediatric infectious diseases program director (if there is a subspecialty training program) or the pediatric department chair or the chief of pediatrics in the hospital(s) where the applicant is now or has been practicing pediatric infectious diseases.

The completed Verification and Evaluation Form(s) should be sent directly to the ABP.

Dual Subcertification in Infectious Diseases (Internal Medicine and Pediatrics)

Individuals who are graduates of combined training programs in internal medicine and general pediatrics should contact both boards regarding dual subcertification opportunities.

It should be noted that these criteria are subject to change without notice. All applicants are advised to contact the ABP to ascertain whether the information they have is current.

Eligibility Criteria for Certification in Medical Toxicology

The ABP in collaboration with the American Boards of Emergency Medicine and Preventive Medicine offers a certificate of added qualifications in medical toxicology. This document provides the requirements of the ABP. (*Note:* A candidate who has a primary certificate from one of the other two boards should contact that board office for its eligibility criteria.)

Admission Requirements

A. Certification by the ABP

An applicant must take and pass the certifying examination in general pediatrics and must maintain a valid (current) certificate before being permitted to take a pediatric subspecialty certifying examination.

B. Licensure

An applicant must have a valid (current), unrestricted license to practice medicine in any of the states, districts, or territories of the United States or provinces of Canada in which he/she practices or have unrestricted privileges to practice medicine in the US armed forces. A copy of the unrestricted license must accompany the application material.

C. Pathways

For admission to the certification examination in medical toxicology, the applicant must have completed one of four eligibility pathways. The pathways are: 1) medical toxicology training; 2) diplomate of American Board of Medical Toxicology (ABMT); 3) medical toxicology practice; 4) medical toxicology training plus practice.

1. Medical Toxicology Subspecialty Training Pathway

   An applicant must complete a fellowship in medical toxicology of 24 months' duration. The training program should be sponsored by and be based within reasonable geographical proximity to an accredited residency program in emergency medicine, pediatrics, preventive medicine, or any combination of these programs. An institution is discouraged from sponsoring more than one accredited medical toxicology program.

   The applicant must satisfactorily complete the subspecialty training by the first day of the month of the examination.

   Applicants seeking certification in more than one subspecialty on the basis of training may not apply the same training period toward fulfillment of requirements of more than one specialty or subspecialty.

The ABP will request verification of subspecialty training directly from the program director.

2. Diplomate of ABMT Pathway
ABMT diplomates who are also diplomates of an ABMS board may apply.

On June 30, 1999, the ABMT pathway will expire. To apply under the ABMT pathway an applicant must have fulfilled the requirements of this pathway by that date.

3. Medical Toxicology Practice Pathway
The practice pathway is available to physicians who, through study and focused practice experience, have developed qualifications in medical toxicology. The criteria for this category consist of all the following:

a. During a minimum of 60 months, which must have occurred during the most recent 7 years prior to the date the application is submitted, the applicant (a) must show a demonstrated commitment to teaching, scholarly activities, research, or administration and patient care in the specialty of medical toxicology and (b) must accumulate a minimum of 2,500 hours of direct patient care activities.

Direct patient care activities include primary or consultative care, exposure evaluation, screening and preventive services, and epidemiologic and health investigations. Telephone consultations are not considered a direct patient care activity.

b. Documented affiliation and activity with a poison control center certified by the American Association of Poison Control Centers (AAPCC) or the Canadian Association of Poison Control Centers (CAPCC) or their equivalent.

Applicants seeking certification in more than one specialty or subspecialty may not apply the same practice hours toward fulfillment of the requirements of more than one certifying specialty or subspecialty.

On June 30, 1999, the practice pathway will expire. To apply under the practice pathway an applicant must have fulfilled the requirements of the practice pathway by that date.

For each medical toxicology activity submitted to fulfill the eligibility criteria, a verification form must be completed. The verification forms are included with the application material, and it is the applicant's responsibility to provide the form to the appropriate individual for completion and return it to the ABP.

4. Partial Medical Toxicology Training Plus Practice Pathway
A combination of partial training and practice experience may be utilized to fulfill the eligibility requirements. This pathway will be utilized by physicians who have completed less than 2 years in a medical toxicology training program and/or have preceptorship training in medical toxicology and who have maintained a medical toxicology practice as outlined in Pathway 3 above.

Practice credit may be granted for partially completed subspecialty training or preceptorship training. The combination for training credit and medical toxicology practice must equal the requirements of the practice category of application (see Section C, items 1 and 2).

An applicant who has completed 1 to 11 months of subspecialty training in medical toxicology will receive practice credit toward the 60-month requirement on a month-for-month basis. An applicant who has completed 12 to 23 months of acceptable subspecialty training in medical toxicology will receive practice credit toward the 60-month requirement on a two-for-one basis for each month of training completed.

Preceptorship training will be reviewed for possible practice credit toward the 60-month requirement on a month-for-month basis, up to a maximum of 24 months credit.

Patient care hours accumulated during the subspecialty training and/or preceptorship will be reviewed for credit on an hour-for-hour basis toward fulfilling the minimum 2,500-hour direct patient care requirement.

On June 30, 1999, the medical toxicology training plus practice pathway will expire. To apply under this pathway, an applicant must have fulfilled the requirements of the practice pathway by that date.

It should be noted that these criteria are subject to change without notice. All applicants are advised to contact the ABP to ascertain whether the information they have is current.

Eligibility Criteria for Certification in Neonatal-Perinatal Medicine

The ABP has established a procedure for certification in neonatal-perinatal medicine. In addition to the specific admission requirements listed below, there are general eligibility criteria that must be fulfilled to be eligible for certification. A copy of the general eligibility criteria is available upon request to the ABP.

Admission Requirements

Physicians who entered training in neonatal-perinatal medicine on or after January 1, 1986, are required to complete their training in a program accredited for training in neonatal-perinatal medicine by the RRC for Pediatrics in the United States or the RCPSC in Canada. Only those programs that are a part of an institution that offers residency or fellowship training in obstetrics and gynecology and include experience in fetal-maternal-perinatal medicine will be considered.

A subspecialty fellow who entered neonatal-perinatal medicine training before January 1, 1989, may apply for admission on the basis of completion of 2 years of fellowship training in neonatal-perinatal medicine.

Three years of full-time, broad-based fellowship training in neonatal-perinatal medicine is required for fellows entering training on or after January 1, 1989. The period of training must be at least 33 months. Extended absences, whether for vacation, maternity leave, illness, etc, must be made up. If the program director believes that an extended absence of more than 3 months is justified, a letter of explanation should be sent by the director for review by the Credentials Committee.

For a fellow who began neonatal-perinatal medicine training on or after January 1, 1989, the following must be accomplished in order to become certified in the subspecialty: a Verification of Competence Form must be completed by the program director(s) stating satisfactory completion of the required training as well as verification of clinical competence and meaningful accomplishment in research; the fellow must meet the criteria stated in the "Principles Regarding the Assessment of Meaningful Accomplishment in Research"; and he/she must pass the subspecialty certifying examination.

A fellow beginning part-time training after January 1, 1989, may complete the required training on a part-time basis not to exceed 6 years. No continuous absence of more than 1 year will be permitted.

Only those neonatal-perinatal medicine training programs that are operated in association with general comprehensive pediatric residency programs accredited by the RRC or by the RCPSC are acceptable. All subspecialty training must be completed in the United States or Canada unless the Credentials Committee of the Subboard has given approval for foreign subspecialty training to an applicant before he/she enrolls in such a program. An applicant wishing to obtain such approval should contact the ABP.

No credit will be given for subspecialty training during the core residency.

It should be noted that these criteria and conditions are subject to change without notice. All applicants are advised to contact the ABP to ascertain whether the information they have is current.

Eligibility Criteria for Certification in Pediatric Nephrology

The ABP has established a procedure for certification in pediatric nephrology. In addition to the specific admission requirements listed below, there are general eligibility criteria that must be fulfilled to be eligible for certification. A copy of the general eligibility criteria is available upon request to the ABP.

Admission Requirements

Physicians who entered training in pediatric nephrology on or after January 1, 1987, are required to complete their training in a program accredited for training in pediatric nephrology by the RRC for Pediatrics in the United States or the RCPSC in Canada.

A subspecialty fellow who entered pediatric nephrology training before January 1, 1987, may apply for admission on the basis of completion of 2 years of fellowship training in pediatric nephrology.

Three years of full-time, broad-based fellowship training in pediatric nephrology is required for fellows entering training on or after January 1, 1987. The period of training must be at least 33 months. Extended absences, whether for vacation, maternity leave, illness, etc, must be made up. If the program director believes that an extended absence of more than 3 months is justified, a letter of explanation should be sent by the director for review by the Credentials Committee.

For a fellow who began pediatric nephrology training on or after January 1, 1988, the following must be accomplished in order to become certified in the subspecialty: a Verification of Competence Form must be completed by the program director(s) stating satisfactory completion of the required training as well as verification of clinical competence and meaningful accomplishment in research; the fellow must meet the criteria stated in the "Principles Regarding the Assessment of Meaningful Accomplishment in Research"; and he/she must pass the subspecialty certifying examination.

A fellow beginning part-time training after January 1, 1988, may complete the required training on a part-time basis not to exceed 6 years. No continuous absence of more than 1 year will be permitted.

Only those pediatric nephrology training programs that are operated in association with general comprehensive pediatric residency programs accredited by the RRC or the RCPSC are acceptable. All subspecialty training must be completed in the United States or Canada unless the Credentials Committee of the Subboard has given approval for foreign subspecialty training to an applicant before he/she enrolls in such a program. An applicant wishing to obtain such approval should contact the ABP.

No credit will be given for subspecialty training during the core residency.

Dual Subcertification in Nephrology (Internal Medicine and Pediatrics)

Individuals who are graduates of combined training programs in internal medicine and general pediatrics should contact both boards regarding dual subcertification opportunities.

It should be noted that these criteria and conditions are subject to change without notice. All applicants are advised to contact the ABP to ascertain whether the information they have is current.

Eligibility Criteria for Certification in Pediatric Pulmonology

The ABP has established a procedure for certification in pediatric pulmonology. In addition to the specific admission requirements listed below, there are general eligibility criteria that must be fulfilled to be eligible for certification. A copy of the general eligibility criteria is available upon request to the ABP.

Admission Requirements

Physicians who entered training in pediatric pulmonology on or after January 1, 1992, are required to complete their training in a program accredited for training in pediatric pulmonology by the RRC for Pediatrics in the United States or the RCPSC in Canada.

A subspecialty fellow who entered pediatric pulmonology training before January 1, 1986, may apply for admission on the basis of completion of 2 years of fellowship training in pediatric pulmonology.

Three years of full-time, broad-based fellowship training in pediatric pulmonology is required for fellows entering training on or after January 1, 1986. The period of training must be at least 33 months. Extended absences, whether for vacation, maternity leave, illness, etc, must be made up. If the program director believes that an extended absence of more than 3 months is justified, a letter of explanation should be sent by the director for review by the Credentials Committee.

For a fellow who began pediatric pulmonology training on or after January 1, 1988, the following must be accomplished in order to become certified in the subspecialty: a Verification of Competence Form must be completed by the program director(s) stating satisfactory completion of the required training as well as verification of clinical competence and meaningful accomplishment in research; the fellow must meet the criteria stated in the "Principles Regarding the Assessment of Meaningful Accomplishment in Research"; and he/she must pass the subspecialty certifying examination.

A fellow beginning part-time training after January 1, 1988, may complete the required training on a part-time basis not to exceed 6 years. No continuous absence of more than 1 year will be permitted.

Only those pediatric pulmonology training programs that are operated in association with general comprehensive pediatric residency programs accredited by the RRC or by the RCPSC are acceptable. All subspecialty training must be completed in the United States or Canada unless the Credentials Committee of the Subboard has given approval for foreign subspecialty training to an applicant before he/she enrolls in such a program. An applicant wishing to obtain such approval should contact the ABP.

No credit will be given for subspecialty training during the core residency.

Dual Subcertification in Pulmonology (Internal Medicine and Pediatrics)

Individuals who are graduates of combined training programs in internal medicine and general pediatrics should contact both boards regarding dual subcertification opportunities.

Subcertification in Pediatric Pulmonology and Allergy/Immunology

The intent of this route is to outline a mechanism whereby residents already certified in pediatrics may qualify for subcertification in both pediatric pulmonology and allergy/immunology in a shorter total period of time than that presently required (3 years pediatric pulmonology plus 2 years allergy/immunology). This can be accomplished by successfully completing research training relating to the requirements of both the Subboard of Pediatric Pulmonology and the Conjoint Board of Allergy/Immunology.

The total training program would require no less than 4 years (48 months) with at least 1 year spent in clinical pulmonology training and 1 year in clinical training for allergy/immunology. The minimum research requirement is 12 months in an environment and project relevant to both pulmonology and allergy/ immunology. The fourth year would be spent in training acceptable to the Subboard of Pediatric Pulmonology and may be in clinical training or relevant additional research training.

1. Training in pediatric pulmonology may precede or follow training in allergy/immunology.
2. The candidate must train in pediatric pulmonology and allergy/immunology programs accredited by the RRC; the two programs do not necessarily have to be at the same institution. The research project selected by the trainee must be discussed with and approved by both training program directors.
3. The trainee must supply written details of any research project for which he/she plans to seek joint approval of both the Subboard of Pediatric Pulmonology and the Conjoint Board of Allergy/ Immunology before or early in the course of his/her first year in a subspecialty program. The Subboard and Conjoint Board, in turn, will provide a preliminary written opinion to the trainee concerning the acceptability of the research project. This early approval is no guarantee of acceptance of the final research product.
4. The trainee is required to satisfy both the General Eligibility Requirements for Certification in Pediatric Subspecialties and the eligibility criteria specific to the Subboard and Conjoint Board as listed in the *Graduate Medical Education Directory*. Final admission to either certification examination is granted by the Credentials Committees after completion of training, fulfillment of the research competence requirements, and review of all application materials submitted by the candidate.

It should be noted that these criteria and conditions are subject to change without notice. All applicants are advised to contact the ABP to ascertain whether the information they have is current.

Eligibility Criteria for Certification in Pediatric Rheumatology

The ABP has established a procedure for certification in pediatric rheumatology. In addition to the specific admission requirements listed below, there are general eligibility criteria that must be fulfilled to be eligible for certification. A copy of the general eligibility criteria is available upon request to the ABP.

Admission Requirements

To qualify for admission to the examination, an applicant must have completed one of the following:

A. Training

Physicians who enter training in pediatric rheumatology on or after January 1, 1999, must complete their training in a program accredited for training in pediatric rheumatology by the RRC for Pediatrics in the United States or the RCPSC in Canada.

A subspecialty fellow who entered pediatric rheumatology training before January 1, 1992, may apply for admission on the basis of completion of 2 years of fellowship training in pediatric rheumatology.

Three years of full-time, broad-based fellowship training in pediatric rheumatology is required for fellows entering training on or after January 1, 1992. The period of training must be at least 33 months. Extended absences, whether for vacation, maternity leave, illness, etc, must be made up. If the program director believes that an extended absence of more than 3 months is justified, a letter of explanation should be sent by the director for review by the Credentials Committee.

For a fellow who began pediatric rheumatology training on or after January 1, 1992, the following must be accomplished in order to become certified in the subspecialty: a Verification of Competence Form must be completed by the program director(s) stating satisfactory completion of the required training as well as verification of clinical competence and meaningful accomplishment in research; the fellow must meet the criteria stated in the "Principles Regarding the Assessment of Meaningful Accomplishment in Research"; and he/she must pass the subspecialty certifying examination.

A fellow beginning part-time training after January 1, 1992, may complete the required training on a part-time basis not to exceed 6 years. No continuous absence of more than 1 year will be permitted.

All subspecialty training must be completed in the United States or Canada unless the Credentials Committee of the Subboard has given approval for foreign subspecialty training to an applicant before he/she enrolls in such a program. An applicant wishing to obtain such approval should contact the ABP.

No credit will be given for subspecialty training during the core residency.

For an individual using the pediatric rheumatology fellowship training route (A), a Verification of Competence Form(s) will be required from the director(s) of the fellow's pediatric rheumatology training program(s).

B. Practice Experience

Five years of broad-based practice experience in pediatric rheumatology is required. A minimum of 50% of full-time professional activity must be spent in the practice of pediatric rheumatology to receive credit. It is assumed that night and weekend time would be distributed in the same manner as regular time. These 5 years should be of such type and quality that they substitute for the clinical exposure one might have encountered during subspecialty residency training. All pediatric rheumatology experience must be accrued before December 31, 1996. No foreign pediatric rheumatology experience will be accepted by the Credentials Committee in fulfillment of the requirements.

For an individual utilizing the pediatric rheumatology practice experience route (B), an evaluation form(s) will be required from the pediatric rheumatology program director (if there is a subspecialty training program) or the pediatric department chair or the chief of pediatrics in the hospital(s) where the applicant is now or has been practicing pediatric rheumatology.

C. Partial Subspecialty Training and Practice

A combination of partial subspecialty fellowship training and practice experience in pediatric rheumatology equal to 5 years as outlined below may be utilized:

1. A fellow completing less than 12 months of fellowship training in pediatric rheumatology may receive practice credit on a month-for-month basis. For example, a 9-month fellowship would be credited for 9 months of experience; this, added to 4 years and 3 months of pediatric rheumatology experience, would total 60 months or 5 years. These 5 years must be accrued before December 31, 1996.
2. A fellow completing 12 to 23 months of fellowship training in pediatric rheumatology may receive credit on a two-for-one basis. For example, an 18-month fellowship would be credited for 36 months of experience; this, added to 24 months of pediatric rheumatology experience, would total 60 months or 5 years. These 5 years must be accrued before December 31, 1996. No credit for partial training will be given for a subspecialty fellow who began training on or after January 1, 1992.

For an individual utilizing the combination partial subspecialty fellowship training and practice experience route (C), a Verification Form(s) will be required from the director(s) of the applicant's pediatric rheumatology training program(s), and an Evaluation Form(s) will be required from the pediatric rheumatology program director (if there is a subspecialty training program) or the pediatric department chair or the chief of pediatrics in the hospital(s) where the applicant is now or has been practicing pediatric rheumatology.

The completed verification and evaluation form(s) should be sent directly to the ABP.

Dual Subcertification in Rheumatology (Internal Medicine and Pediatrics)

Individuals who are graduates of combined training programs in internal medicine and general pediatrics should contact both boards regarding dual subcertification opportunities.

Subcertification in Pediatric Rheumatology and Allergy/Immunology

A candidate who is certified in pediatrics may qualify for subcertification in both pediatric rheumatology and allergy/immunology in a shorter total period of training than that presently required (3 years of pediatric rheumatology plus 2 years of allergy/immunology). This compression of training by 1 year can be accomplished by successfully completing research training relating to the requirements of both the Subboard of Pediatric Rheumatology and the Conjoint Board of Allergy/Immunology.

The total training program would require no less than 4 years (48 months) with at least 1 year spent in clinical rheumatology training and 1 year in clinical training for allergy/immunology. The clinical rheumatology training should also include at least another 2 years of at least one-half day/week of an outpatient rheumatology experience plus 1 month/year of inpatient rheumatology service to assure longitudinal exposure to rheumatologic problems in children. The minimum research requirement is 24 months in an environment and project relevant to both rheumatology and allergy/immunology, particularly immunologically related research.

1. Although training in clinical pediatric rheumatology may precede or follow training in allergy/ immunology, such training should occur at latest in the second year of this combined fellowship. An integrated training program may be developed that must be prospectively approved by both boards.
2. The candidate must train in pediatric rheumatology and allergy/immunology programs accredited by the RRC. The two programs should preferably be in the same institution, but programs in the same city may be acceptable.
3. The research project selected by the trainee must be discussed with and approved by both training program directors. The trainee must supply written details of any research project for which he/she plans to seek joint approval of both the Subboard of Pediatric Rheumatology and the Conjoint Board of Allergy/Immunology before or early in the course of his/her first year in a subspecialty program. The Subboard and Conjoint Board, in turn, will provide a preliminary written opinion to the trainee concerning the acceptability of the research project. This early approval is no guarantee of the acceptance of the final research product.
4. The trainee is required to satisfy both the General Eligibility Requirements for Certification in Pediatric Subspecialties and the eligibility criteria specific to the Subboard and Conjoint Board as listed in the *Graduate Medical Education Directory*. Final admission to either certification examination is granted by the Credentials Committees after completion of training, fulfillment of the research competence requirements, and review of all application materials submitted by the candidate.

It should be noted that these criteria and conditions are subject to change without notice. All applicants are advised to contact the ABP to ascertain whether the information they have is current.

Eligibility Criteria for Certification in Sports Medicine

The ABP in collaboration with the American Boards of Family Practice, Internal Medicine, and Emergency Medicine offers a certificate of added qualifications in sports medicine. This document provides the requirements of the ABP. (*Note:* A candidate who has a primary certificate from one of the other three boards should contact that board office for its eligibility criteria.)

Admission Requirements

A. Certification by the American Board of Pediatrics (ABP)

An applicant must take and pass the certifying examination in general pediatrics and must maintain a valid (current) certificate before being permitted to take a pediatric subspecialty certifying examination.

B. Licensure

An applicant must have a valid (current), unrestricted license to practice medicine in any of the states, districts, or territories of the United States or provinces of Canada in which he/she practices or have unrestricted privileges to practice medicine in the US armed forces. A copy of the unrestricted license must accompany the application material.

C. Training or Practice Experience

To qualify for admission to the examination, an applicant must have completed one of the following:

1. Training

   An applicant must have completed a minimum of 1 year in a sports medicine training program that is associated with an accredited residency program in family practice, emergency medicine, internal medicine, or pediatrics.

   The applicant must satisfactorily complete the subspecialty training by the first day of the month of the examination.

   A Verification of Competence Form must be completed by the program director stating satisfactory completion of the required training as well as verification of clinical competence. The ABP will send this form to the program director for completion.
2. Practice Experience

   Five years of practice experience in sports medicine is required. This experience must consist of at least 20% of total professional time devoted to sports medicine. The activities that qualify a candidate are one or more of the following:

   a. Field supervision of athletes
   b. Emergency assessment and care of acutely injured athletes
   c. Diagnosis, treatment, management, and disposition of common sports injuries and illnesses
   d. Management of medical problems in the athlete
   e. Rehabilitation of the ill or injured athlete
   f. Exercise as treatment

Partial training in sports medicine (ie, less than 12 months) will be credited on a month-by-month basis as practice experience.

An evaluation form must be completed by an individual to verify that at least 20% of professional time is devoted to sports medicine in one or more of the six activities cited above. The form must be completed by a physician who is knowledgeable about the applicant's practice, such as the pediatric department chair, the chief of pediatrics, chief of staff, or the medical director of a hospital where the applicant has admitting privileges. A partner or practice associate is not acceptable.

Practice experience accrued before 1987 will not be considered. All sports medicine experience must be accrued by June 30, 1999.

It should be noted that these criteria are subject to change without notice. All applicants are advised to contact the ABP to ascertain whether the information they have is current.

1999 Subspecialty Certifying Examinations

Each subspecialty certifying examination is administered every 2 years. Dates of the examinations and other information may be found on the ABP web site. Application material for admission to a subspecialty examination may be obtained by contacting the ABP. Application forms are available only during the registration period for that examination.

The examinations last one-half day with a time limit of 4½ hours and consist of multiple-choice questions. Examples of the types of questions to be used are mailed to registered candidates before the administration of each examination. Some questions are included in the examination for experimental purposes only. These questions will not contribute to the score. A content outline is available on the ABP web site.

Each candidate's examination score will be reported to the subspecialty program director where training occurred. The names of those certified are sent to the ABMS for publication in the *Directory of Certified Pediatricians* and to various pediatric journals. Periodically, the ABP conducts research utilizing data it has compiled; the candidate's anonymity is guaranteed in all such cases.

Subspecialty examinations will be administered on August 9, 1999, in endocrinology, gastroenterology, and infectious diseases and on November 15, 1999, in adolescent medicine, nephrology, and neonatal-perinatal medicine. The certifying examination in sports medicine will be administered on April 16, 1999. It is the applicant's responsibility to be aware of and to meet registration deadlines.

The fees (in US dollars) for all subspecialty examinations are:

Fees for New Subspecialty Applicants	
Processing and evaluation	$375
Examination	$1,000
Regular Registration	*$1,375*
Late registration fee	$225
Late registration	*$1,600*
Fees for Subspecialty Reregistrants	
Processing and evaluation	$275
Examination	$1,000
Regular Registration	*$1,275*
Late registration fee	$225
Late registration	*$1,500*

A nonrefundable penalty fee of $225 is required for late registration.

Applicants can pay the total application fee by credit card, using either Visa or MasterCard, or by check.

For applicants not using US banks, the fee must be paid in US dollars using one of the following vehicles: (1) money order, (2) cashier's check or (3) certified check. To be accepted for payment, these vehicles must be payable through a US bank.

The ABP cannot accept electronic transfer of funds from any organization, eg, US military, Western Union.

Registration Dates for Subspecialty Examinations

For subspecialty examinations given on August 9, 1999:

New applicants	
Regular	October 1—November 30, 1998
Late	December 1—December 31, 1998
Reregistrants	
Regular	December 15, 1998—February 16, 1999
Late	Feburary 17—March 16, 1999

For subspecialty examinations given on November 15, 1999:

New applicants	
Regular	February 1—March 31, 1999
Late	April 1—April 30, 1999
Reregistrants	
Regular	March 15, 1999—May 15, 1999
Late	May 16—June 15, 1999

Applications will not be accepted after the appropriate postmarked date.

Recertification

General Pediatric Recertification

In November 1985, the ABP established a policy of time-limited certification. This policy became effective for those individuals certified in general pediatrics and in the pediatric subspecialties after May 1, 1988. Initial certificates will expire after 7 years.

The Program for Renewal of Certification in Pediatrics (PRCP) is the process by which the ABP recertifies diplomates in general pediatrics. Diplomates who wish to be issued a new certificate after the 7-year period must successfully complete the PRCP for renewal of certification in pediatrics.

Diplomates certified before May 1, 1988, will not be affected by the policy of time-limited certification; however, those who choose to achieve certification renewal on a voluntary basis may do so by completing the PRCP. Their certification will not be affected if they are not successful in completing the PRCP.

Subspecialty Recertification

The Program for Renewal of Certification in Pediatric Subspecialties (PRCP-S) is the process by which the ABP recertifies diplomates in the pediatric subspecialties. Diplomates who wish to be issued a new Certificate of Special Qualifications or Added Qualifications in a subspecialty of pediatrics after the 7-year period must successfully complete the PRCP-S.

A diplomate who holds a Certificate of Special Qualifications does not have to be recertified in general pediatrics in order to recertify in the subspecialty. However, a subspecialist who has been certified or recertified within the previous 7 years in the subspecialty may become recertified in general pediatrics by successfully completing a modified version of PRCP called PRCP-MS Program for Renewal of Certification in Pediatrics Modified for Subspecialists (PRCP-MS).

Since Certificates of Added Qualifications are based upon a continuing working knowledge of the broad discipline of general comprehensive pediatrics, candidates will be required to hold a permanent or unexpired time-limited certificate in general pediatrics to be recertified in an ABP subspecialty in which a Certificate of Added Qualifications (eg, sports medicine) has been given.

Diplomates certified in a pediatric subspecialty before May 2, 1988, except for pediatric pulmonology (1986) and pediatric critical care medicine (1987), will not be affected by the policy of time-limited certification; however, those who choose to achieve certification renewal on a voluntary basis may do so by completing the PRCP-S. Their certification will not be affected if they are not successful in completing the PRCP-S.

Policies

Board Status

The ABP has decided to follow the longstanding recommendations of the ABMS to its member boards not to use the term "Board eligible" because of continuing confusion about the term.

If an inquiry is made to the Board regarding the status of an individual, the response will be only whether the individual has been certified or not. Upon receipt of a signed release form, provided by the Board, information will be released regarding whether an individual's application to take a general or subspecialty certifying examination was accepted and when.

The allegation by an applicant that he or she has completed the required training and, therefore, is board eligible, without review and approval by the ABP, is not acceptable.

Time Limit to Certification

Candidates who have met the training requirements and whose applications to take the certifying examinations have been accepted by the ABP have unlimited time to become certified, subject to their continued compliance with Board policies and requirements, which are subject to change.

Disability

An applicant who wishes to request special accommodations to take a certifying examination due to a disability is urged to notify the Board in writing of the need for accommodations as early as possible during the application period. The applicant will be sent the ABP policy on disabilities. The deadline for notifying the ABP is the registration deadline (postmarked).

Maintenance of an Active State License

A diplomate's certificate will remain valid and effective only so long as the diplomate maintains an active license to practice medicine from the state in which the diplomate practices or lives. This requirement will be waived only under the following two circumstances:

Fellowship: This requirement will be waived only during the pendency of fellowship, for fellows for whom the licensure requirement was waived at the time of certification.

Practicing abroad: This requirement will be waived for a diplomate who is practicing abroad but only while they are practicing abroad.

Revocation of Certificates

All certificates issued by the ABP are subject to the provisions of the articles of incorporation and the bylaws of the ABP. Each certificate is subject to possible revocation in the event that

1. the issuance of such certificate or its receipt by the physician so certified shall have been contrary to or in violation of any of the provisions of the ABP's articles of incorporation or bylaws; or
2. the physician so certified shall not have been eligible to receive such certificate, irrespective of whether the facts constituting him or her so ineligible were known to any or all of the members of the ABP at the time of the issuance of such certificate; or
3. the physician so certified shall have made any misstatement of fact in his/her application for such certificate or in any other statement or representation to the ABP, its members, representatives, or agents.

If the ABP obtains probable cause to believe that a certificate should be revoked for any of the reasons set forth above, it may institute proceedings for revocation thereof by mailing written notice to the holder of such certificate that a hearing will be held to determine whether the certificate should be revoked. The steps to be taken are outlined in the Rules of Appellate Procedure of the ABP, which may be obtained by writing to the ABP.

Reinstatement of Certificates

When a certificate issued by the ABP has been revoked, the certificate may be restored once the physician has submitted a request for reinstatement and the Credentials Committee's recommendation for reinstatement is approved by the Board of Directors.

Additional Information and Inquiries

Please address all inquiries concerning examination applications to

American Board of Pediatrics
111 Silver Cedar Ct
Chapel Hill, NC 27514-1651
919 929-0461
919 929-9255 Fax
E-mail: abpeds@abpeds.org
http://www.abp.org

American Board of Physical Medicine and Rehabilitation

21 First St SW/Ste 674
Rochester MN 55902
507 282-1776
507 282-9142 Fax

Nicolas E Walsh, MD, Chairman, San Antonio, Texas
Bruce M Gans, MD, Vice Chairman, Detroit, Michigan
Gerald Felsenthal, MD, Treasurer, Baltimore, Maryland
Murray E Brandstater, MBBS, PhD, Secretary, Loma Linda, California
Robert P Christopher, MD, Memphis, Tennessee
Joel A DeLisa, MD, MS, Newark, New Jersey
Margaret C Hammond, MD, Seattle, Washington
Joseph C Honet, MD, Detroit, Michigan
F Patrick Maloney, MD, Little Rock, Arkansas
Malcolm C McPhee, MD, Scottsdale, Arizona
Stephen F Noll, MD, Rochester, Minnesota
William E Staas, Jr, MD, Philadelphia, Pennsylvania
Jay V S Subbarao, MD, MS, Chicago, Illinois
Margaret A Turk, MD, Syracuse, New York

(These criteria and conditions are subject to change without notice. All applicants are advised to contact the American Board of Physical Medicine and Rehabilitation [ABPMR] to ascertain whether the information below is current.)

General Requirements

A. Requirements for graduates of educational institutions in the United States or Canada
   1. Graduation from a US or Canadian medical school approved by the Liaison Committee on Medical Education (LCME) or graduation from an osteopathic medical school approved by the American Osteopathic Association (AOA).
   2. Possession of a current, valid, unrestricted license to practice medicine or osteopathy in a US licensing jurisdiction or Puerto Rico or licensure in Canada. Evidence of licensure or an acceptable equivalent will be required prior to issuance of the certificate.
   3. Satisfactory completion of the requirements of the Board for graduate education and experience in physical medicine and rehabilitation (PM&R) as set forth below. A resident is expected to complete training in PM&R in a single program, except when significant extenuating circumstances make a change advisable.
   4. Satisfactory compliance with rules and regulations of the Board pertaining to the completion and filing of the application for examination and payment of required fees.

B. Requirements for graduates of educational institutions outside the United States or Canada
   1. Possession of a valid certificate from the Educational Council for Foreign Medical Graduates (ECFMG) prior to entry into a PM&R residency training program.
   2. Possession of a current, valid, unrestricted license to practice medicine or osteopathy in a US licensing jurisdiction or Puerto Rico or licensure in Canada will be required prior to issuance of the certificate.
   3. Satisfactory completion of the Board's requirements for graduate education and experience in PM&R as set forth below. A resident is expected to complete training in a single program except when significant extenuating circumstances make a change advisable.

4. Satisfactory compliance with rules and regulations of the Board pertaining to the completion and filing of the application for examination and the payment of required fees.

Residency Training Requirements

Applicants for the certification examinations must have satisfactorily completed 48 months (4 years) of training in a PM&R residency approved by the ACGME. Twelve of the 48 months must consist of a coordinated program of experience in fundamental clinical skills such as an accredited transitional year or include 6 months or more in accredited training in family practice, internal medicine, pediatrics, or surgery or any combination of these patient care experiences. The remaining months of this year may include any combination of accredited specialties or subspecialties.

Accredited training in any of the specialties or subspecialties must be for a period of at least 4 weeks. No more than 8 weeks may be in nondirect patient care experiences. Training in fundamental clinical skills must be completed within the first 2 years of the 4-year training program.

The program director and the Credentials Committee of the Board, at the beginning of the residency, will make the decision regarding the acceptability for credit of the 12 months of training in fundamental clinical skills approved by the ACGME, or the Royal College of Physicians and Surgeons of Canada (RCPSC), or the AOA.

The program must include 36 months in PM&R in a training program accredited by the ACGME or the RCPSC. This format is mandatory for all residents who entered training in 1985 or subsequently. A resident is expected to complete training in a single program except when significant extenuating circumstances make a change advisable. In the event of a transfer, the resident is expected to complete all the PM&R program requirements as outlined by the Residency Review Committee (RRC).

All required training and experience as stated above must be taken in the United States, Puerto Rico, or Canada.

The training program must include a significant amount of time spent in primary responsibility for the direct patient care management of hospitalized patients on the PM&R service. Residents must devote at least one third of their residency experience to the care of these hospitalized PM&R patients. They must spend at least one third of the training in the care of outpatients, including a significant experience in the care of musculoskeletal problems.

During PM&R training, the resident must develop comprehensive basic and clinical knowledge, skills, experience, and measurable competencies in areas such as

- history and physical examination pertinent to PM&R;
- assessment of neurological, musculoskeletal, and cardiovascular-pulmonary systems;
- determining impairment and disability;
- data gathering and interpreting of psychosocial and vocational factors;
- achievement of basic qualifications in the performance and interpretation of electrodiagnostic evaluations;
- physiatric therapeutic and diagnostic injection techniques;
- prescriptions for orthotics, prosthetics, wheelchair and ambulatory devices, special beds, and other assistive devices;
- prescriptions with specific details appropriate to the patient for therapeutic modalities and therapeutic exercises;
- understanding of coordinated psychologic and vocational interventions and tests;
- familiarity with the safety, maintenance, and actual use of medical equipment common to the various therapy areas and laboratories;
- formal experience in evaluation and application of cardiac and pulmonary rehabilitation as related to physiatric responsibilities;
- inpatient and outpatient pediatric rehabilitation;
- collaboration with other medical professionals and members of the allied health team, including management techniques consistent with the resident's team leadership role and the treatment program management role of the physiatrist;
- geriatric rehabilitation;
- sports medicine rehabilitation; and
- injury, illness, and disability prevention.

Also, the resident must achieve the ability to accept progressive responsibility in diagnosing, assessing, and managing the conditions commonly encountered by the physiatrist in the rehabilitative management of conditions such as:

- acute musculoskeletal pain syndromes;
- chronic pain management;
- congenital or acquired myopathies, peripheral neuropathies, and motor neuron and motor system diseases;
- rehabilitative care of traumatic brain injury;
- hereditary, developmental, and acquired central nervous system disorders;
- rehabilitation care of spinal cord trauma and diseases;
- rehabilitative care of patients with amputations for both congenital and acquired conditions in patients of all ages;
- sexual dysfunction common to the physically impaired;
- postfracture care and rehabilitation of postoperative joint arthroplasty;
- pulmonary, cardiac, oncologic, and other common medical conditions seen in persons with physical disabilities;
- geriatric diseases and impairments and functional limitations;
- rheumatologic disorders treated by the physiatrist;
- medical conditions or complications commonly seen and managed in the physiatric patient; medical conditioning, reconditioning, and fitness; and
- soft tissue disorders.

The program requirements section on PM&R in the current *Graduate Medical Education Directory* provides additional details of PM&R residencies. This book, published annually by the American Medical Association (AMA), cites specific programming by the individual residency and its institutional base.

Credit for Other Specialty Training

Physicians who have had 1 or more years of training (up to and including certification) in a program approved by the ACGME, the RCPSC, or the AOA in related relevant specialties may receive up to a maximum of 12 months of non-PM&R training credit on recommendation of the program director and at the discretion of the Board. These relevant specialties include internal medicine, neurology, orthopedics, pediatrics, family practice, and surgery. *Completion of 36 months of training in an ACGME-approved PM&R residency is mandatory.*

The non-PM&R training credit will be considered for approval by the Board only upon recommendation of the residency training program director. Alternatively, upon the recommendation of the program director, the Board may accept a noncoordinated ACGME-approved "transitional" year or an ACGME-approved year of training. This alternative training may be in family practice, internal medicine, pediatrics, neurology, orthopedics, or surgery.

No credit will be given toward shortening the basic required 4-year program for non-ACGME-approved residencies, fellowships, or internships; for Fifth Pathway in a United States AMA-designated training institution; or for hospital house physician experience. No credit will be allowed for fellowships prior to or during residency training.

All the required training and experience as stated above must have been taken in the United States, Puerto Rico, or Canada. If a candidate wishes to complete an elective rotation at an international site or at any other location not accredited by the ACGME, the RCPSC, or the AOA, this must be accomplished during the 6 weeks of leave time allowed for each resident.

Absence from Training

A resident should not be absent from the residency training for more than 6 weeks (30 working days) yearly. Regardless of institutional policies regarding absences, any leave time beyond 6 weeks would need to be made up by arrangement with the program director.

Leave time is defined as sick leave, vacation, maternity leave, leave for locum tenens, or work in another program that is not ACGME-accredited. A candidate may not accumulate leave time or vacation to reduce the overall duration of training.

Dual Specialty Certification

Residents may elect to pursue integrated training in PM&R and another specialty by enrolling in a combined training program. The ABPMR currently approves three types of combined training: pediatrics and PM&R, internal medicine and PM&R, or neurology and PM&R. All three programs require completion of at least 36 months of accredited training in general comprehensive PM&R.

The proposed program agreed to by the respective residency training program directors should be submitted by the program directors to both Boards for approval. Admissibility to Part I of the PM&R certification examination may be sought during the last year of training.

A full year of clinical practice, fellowship, research, or a combination of these activities, consisting of at least 6 months of clinical practice in PM&R, is required for admissibility to the Part II certification examination in PM&R.

Guidelines for program directors interested in developing such a program are available through the ABPMR office.

Combined Training in Pediatrics and PM&R

A special agreement exists between the American Board of Pediatrics (ABP) and the ABPMR whereby a physician interested in dual specialty certification in pediatrics and in PM&R can qualify for admission to the certification examinations of both boards. The individual residency curriculum must be submitted prospectively by the program directors to both boards no later than the end of the R-2 year of the combined program and may be designed to be completed in a minimum of 60 months. The non-PM&R 12-month segment of the 4-year PM&R residency will be credited on the basis of satisfactory completion of the regular first year of pediatric residency.

The ABP requires a minimum of 36 months of general comprehensive pediatric training with 6 months' credit for pediatric rehabilitation within the PM&R training. The ABPMR requires a minimum of 36 months accredited PM&R residency with 6 months' credit for related rotations during the pediatric training. These rotations could include developmental pediatrics, neonatology, pediatric neurology, pediatric neurosurgery, or pediatric orthopedics.

Six months full-time equivalent (FTE) of pediatric rehabilitation is required. Twenty-four months of the 36 months PM&R training must be in adult PM&R.

It is recommended that all training be completed at one academic institution; any deviation will require prospective approval by both boards. When two separate institutions are involved, there should be evidence of adequate coordination to provide an appropriate educational experience.

Before the end of the R-2 year of training in either specialty, the ABPMR must approve the training plan for the given resident. After the program is approved, the resident's registration form is submitted. Vacation is shared pro rata between the training time spent in pediatrics and that spent in PM&R.

Combined Training in Internal Medicine and PM&R

A special agreement exists between the American Board of Internal Medicine (ABIM) and the ABPMR whereby a prospective resident interested in dual specialty certification in internal medicine and in PM&R can qualify to apply for admission to the certification examination of each Board by satisfactory completion of a preplanned, combined, and integrated program that could be designed to be completed in a minimum of 60 months.

The non-PM&R 12-month segment of the 48 months of PM&R residency concerned with basic fundamental clinical skills will be credited on the basis of satisfactory completion of the regular first year of internal medicine residency. In addition, the ABPMR requires a minimum of 36 months of accredited PM&R residency with 6 months' credit for internal medicine rotations in such areas as rheumatology, endocrinology, cardiovascular, or pulmonary subspecialties of internal medicine.

During the 30 months in PM&R, the resident must satisfactorily complete 24 months of hospital and outpatient clinical management of patients receiving PM&R services. Physical medicine and rehabilitation training includes basic and advanced knowledge of musculoskeletal and neuromuscular anatomy and physiology as related to kinesiology, exercise, and functional activities as well as to immobilization and inactivity. Applications and prescription of therapeutic exercise, orthotics, prosthetics, and assistive and supportive devices for ambulation and mobility are essential.

The following segments of training in PM&R are also required:

- experience with inpatient or outpatient pediatric rehabilitation
- adequate training to achieve basic qualifications in electromyography and electrodiagnosis
- opportunities to achieve understanding of special aspects of rehabilitation of patients in geriatric age groups

The 3-year internal medicine residency requirements are met in part by the ABIM's recognizing 6 months' credit for PM&R residency training involving PM&R management of patients with problems related to internal medicine. Such problems include those occurring in patients with rheumatologic, cardiovascular, pulmonary, stroke, and oncologic conditions.

It is recommended that all training be completed at one academic institution. If two separate institutions are involved, there should be evidence of adequate coordination to provide an appropriate educational experience. Any deviation requires prospective approval by both boards. Before the end of the R-2 level of training in either specialty, the ABPMR prospectively requires approval of a detailed curricular plan for a given resident signed by both program directors. After the program is approved, the resident's registration form is submitted. Vacation is shared pro rata between the two training programs.

Combined Training in Neurology and PM&R

The American Board of Psychiatry and Neurology (ABPN) and the ABPMR have approved the proposal that residents interested in dual certification in neurology and in PM&R can qualify to apply for admission to the certification examinations of each Board. This is accomplished by satisfactory completion of an integrated program planned and approved by both boards prior to the end of the R-2 year, designed to be completed in a minimum of 72 months.

For purposes of this dual certification, both specialty boards require a 12-month basic clinical skills segment in internal medicine. The ABPMR requires a minimum of 36 months of accredited PM&R

residency, and the ABPN requires 36 months of accredited neurology residency.

In order to decrease the total training time to 72 months (a reduction of 1 year), 12 months of training in areas that satisfy the special requirements in neurology and in PM&R must consist of 6 months of training in PM&R acceptable to the program director in neurology, and 6 months of training in neurology acceptable to the program director in PM&R.

It is recommended that all training be completed at one academic institution. If two institutions are involved, adequate coordination should provide an appropriate educational experience that meets the requirements and approval of each board. Before the end of the R-2 year of training in either specialty, both program directors sign and submit a training plan for a given resident to the ABPMR for approval. After the program is approved, the resident's registration form is submitted. Vacation is shared pro rata between the two training programs.

Clinical Investigator Pathway

The ABPMR provides an opportunity for interested residents to participate in a Clinical Investigator Pathway (CIP) during their training. The ABPMR's criteria for certification as a Clinical Investigator requires that a resident complete a 5-year residency program that integrates training in PM&R and clinical research.

The purpose of the CIP is to increase both the quality and capacity of physiatric research nationally by enabling a select group of clinically- and research-minded residents to become well-trained in physiatric practice and research. The CIP is intended for PM&R residents in PM&R programs that have a strong emphasis on physiatric research.

The first year of the 5-year CIP is devoted to fundamental clinical skills required in general medicine. The following 4 years of residency training combine clinical and investigative training. Within any 4-year PM&R residency program, 6 months are allowed for research. The additional fifth year in the CIP allows for more in-depth research to occur with a total of 18 months of research. In addition to these required 18 months of research training, 6 more months of combined experience in clinical and research areas may be included. However, there should be enough overlap between clinical training and clinical research that sufficient time is available to achieve competence in both areas.

Interested candidates should contact their residency program director for additional information.

Examination Admissibility Requirements

Part I

To be admissible to Part I of the Board certification examination, candidates are required to satisfactorily complete at least 48 months of postgraduate residency training, of which at least 36 months should be spent in supervised education and clinical practice in PM&R as part of an ACGME-accredited training program.

Satisfactory completion of the educational and training requirements in force at the beginning of the resident's training in an accredited program will be considered acceptable for application for admissibility to the certification examinations.

Final admissibility is contingent upon receipt of the final-year evaluation by the program director, due May 1 in the examination year. If a resident is placed on probationary status during the final year of the residency program, this status must be rescinded by the program director before May 1 for the resident to be admissible.

In order to have the application considered for examination, the applicant must be scheduled to complete the graduate medical education requirements on or before August 31 following the scheduled examination date for which he or she has applied.

Residents in approved PM&R programs in Canada, upon satisfactory completion of all the requirements for certification in that country, may apply for admissibility to Part I of the certification examination.

Part II

At least 1 full-time or equivalent year of PM&R clinical practice, PM&R-related fellowship, PM&R-related research, or a combination of these activities is required after satisfactory completion of an accredited PM&R residency training program.

The clinical practice must provide evidence of acceptable professional, ethical, and humanistic conduct attested to by two Board-certified physiatrists in the candidate's local or regional area. In rare instances in which a physiatrist is not geographically available, two licensed physicians in the area may support the candidate's application for Part II.

Alternatively, a candidate may take Part I and II in the same year if all residency training and practice time requirements have been completed. However, if the candidate does not pass Part I, the results of Part II will not count or be recognized in any way.

Also required is the candidate's possession of a current, valid, unrestricted license to practice medicine or osteopathy in a US licensing jurisdiction or Puerto Rico or licensure in Canada. Evidence of this licensure or an acceptable equivalent must be submitted with the application for certification examinations.

In order to have the application considered for examination, the applicant must be scheduled to complete the clinical practice requirements on or before August 31 following the scheduled examination date for which he or she has applied.

Application Requirements and Fees

Application Documentation - Part I

The application form for Part I that must be submitted by an applicant for the examination leading to certification can be obtained only by writing to the Board. The completed application must contain

- a copy of the medical degree diploma or certificate;
- the program director's statement that the applicant has or is anticipated to have satisfactorily completed an approved graduate program; and
- the names of three or more physiatrists or other physicians to whom the Board can write for professional and character references.

The applicant must submit a form, received from the Board, to the residency training program director; this form requests the rating of the professional ability of the applicant. The program director should promptly return the completed form to the Board office.

No decision regarding an applicant's admissibility to the examinations will be made until the physicians from whom references are requested have replied. All information submitted to the Board by a physician from whom a reference has been requested will remain confidential and will not be disclosed to the applicant without the permission of the said physician. Strict confidentiality of references submitted is required to ensure that the Board will receive complete and accurate evaluations of all applicants.

Application Documentation - Part II

An applicant applying for Part II must write a letter to the Board describing the professional time spent during his or her 1 full-time or equivalent year of PM&R clinical practice, PM&R-related fellowship, PM&R-related research, or combination of these.

The applicant must also submit statements from two physicians (from the applicant's local or regional area), preferably Board-certified physiatrists, verifying the applicant's 1 year in clinical practice, fellowship, research, or combination of these according to acceptable professional, ethical, and humanistic standards. Acceptable verification statements and/or references will be from individuals unrelated to the candidate, whether family member, spouse, or significant other.

Applicants are required to submit a notarized copy of their current, valid, unrestricted license to practice medicine or osteopathy in a US licensing jurisdiction or Puerto Rico or licensure in Canada, or evidence of possession of an acceptable equivalent.

Accommodations for Persons with Disabilities

The ABPMR supports the Americans with Disabilities Act (ADA) and makes reasonable accommodations in examination procedures for individuals with documented disabilities. Applicants with disabilities may request modifications in the administration of the examination. The Board will grant such requests unless the modifications would place undue burden on the ABPMR or would fundamentally alter the measurement of the knowledge or skills the examination is intended to test.

Applicants considering the need for modifications are urged to obtain from the Board a copy of Procedures for Requesting Accommodations under the ADA. This publication outlines the documentation required of applicants with disabilities who request examination modifications.

All required documentation must be submitted to the Board office by January 1 of the year of the scheduled examination. Applicants anticipating the need for accommodations should contact the Board office well in advance of January 1 to allow sufficient time to submit any required documentation by the January 1 deadline.

Fees

All fees must accompany the application for examination.

Part I

An applicant who plans to take Part I only must submit a fee of $850. Of this amount, $200 covers an initial processing fee and an application processing fee and is not refundable. (See "Site Fee" below)

Part I Reapplication

An applicant who reapplies to take Part I only must submit a fee of $750. This amount includes a $100 nonrefundable reapplication processing fee. (See "Site Fee" below)

Part II

An applicant who plans to take Part II only must submit a fee of $950 along with the required documentation for Part II application. Of this amount, $100 is an application processing fee and is not refundable.

Part II Reapplication

An applicant who reapplies to take Part II only must submit a fee of $950. This amount includes a $100 nonrefundable reapplication processing fee.

Parts I and II

An applicant who plans to take both Part I and Part II initially in the same year must submit a fee of $1800 with the application. Of this amount, $300 covers an initial processing fee and an application processing fee and is not refundable.

Part I Reapplication and II

An applicant reapplying to take Part I and applying to take Part II for the first time must submit a fee of $1700. This amount includes a $100 nonrefundable reapplication processing fee for Part I and a $100 nonrefundable application processing fee for Part II.

Part I Reapplication and Part II Reapplication

An applicant reapplying to take both Parts I and II the same year must submit a $1700 fee. This amount includes a $100 nonrefundable reapplication processing fee for each Part I and Part II.

Site Fee

There is an additional $100 charge for those candidates selecting either Dallas, Texas, or Philadelphia, Pennsylvania, as an optional Part I examination site.

Late Fee

An additional $200 is required after the November 15 deadline.

Reexamination

Physicians who have failed Part I or Part II can apply for admissibility for reexamination during any subsequent examination period. As indicated in the earlier fee schedule, fees for reexamination are $750 for Part I, or $950 for Part II; if both Parts I and II are retaken the same year, the fee is $1700. A $100 nonrefundable processing fee, which is required for each Part I or Part II application for reexamination, is included in these fees. Currently, there is no limit to the number of times a physician may apply for repeat examinations.

Deadline

The appropriate fees and the completed application materials for admissibility must be postmarked and mailed by November 15 of the year before the scheduled examination. This applies to

- Part I only;
- Part II only;
- Parts I and II of the examination in the same year;
- Applications for reexamination.

An additional $200 penalty fee will be required for consideration of applications postmarked after November 15 and before December 15.

Refunds and Forfeiture of Fees

Except as hereafter provided, no fees paid will be refunded. The Board will return the refundable portion of the fee only in the event that

- an applicant withdraws the application prior to the meeting of the Board to act thereon; or
- an applicant is declared not admissible to the examination.

Once an applicant has been declared admissible and is a candidate, the fees will be forfeited if the candidate withdraws for any reason or does not appear for the scheduled examination for which he or she applied.

The Board is a nonprofit organization, and the candidates' fees are used solely for defraying the actual expenses of the Board. The directors of the Board serve without remuneration. The Board reserves the right to change the fees when necessary.

Examination Policies and Procedures

Designation of Admissibility

"Board admissible" is a term used by the Board to define the status of an applicant who has been accepted by the Board as a candidate to take the examination for which he or she has applied. Designation of "Board admissible" does not continue beyond the date such an examination is given, regardless of results. The Board does not accept any use of the term "Board eligible" in lieu of documented admissibility.

A. For applicants who have not previously applied, or who have previously applied and have withdrawn their application, or who have previously applied and have been declared not admissible

The procedures required for these applicants toward becoming admissible to Board examination are as follows:

1. Timely filing of the completed application form, license, and educational credentials
2. Payment of the fees for the examination (see earlier fee structure)
3. Submission of requested references
4. Confirmation from the Board office verifying Board action regarding the applicant's admissibility status

B. For applicants who are reapplying for Part I, having failed Part I, or having applied but not sat for Part I of the examination

The procedures required for these applicants toward becoming admissible to Board examination are as follows:

1. Submission of a letter from the applicant to the Board requesting admissibility for reexamination
2. Payment of the fees for the examination (see earlier fee structure)
3. Confirmation from the Board office verifying Board action regarding the applicant's admissibility status

C. For applicants who are applying for Part II, having successfully completed Part I, or who are reapplying for Part II, having failed Part II but having successfully completed Part I

The procedures required for these applicants toward being designated Board admissible are as follows:

1. Submission by the applicant to the Board of a letter of application for the examination or, if required, the resubmission of an application form. The letter should contain a statement describing the required PM&R clinical practice, PM&R-related fellowship, PM&R-related research, or a combination of these.
2. Payment of the fees for the examination (see earlier fee structure).
3. Provision by applicant to the Board of a notarized copy of the current, valid, unrestricted license;
4. Timely filing of completed forms from two physicians (preferably Board-certified physiatrists) verifying 1 year of clinical practice, fellowship, research, or a combination of these.
5. Board office verification of Board action regarding the applicant's admissibility status.

Following the establishment of Board admissibility, the candidate will be notified of the time and place for the examination.

Note: Due to the large volume of documentation that the Board office will be receiving and processing on or before November 15, we ask that applicants do not call to verify receipt of their mailing. Applicants should check with their training director to see if documentation was sent to the Board office. An applicant who does not receive any notification from the Board regarding his/her application by December 15 should then contact the Board office.

Statement of Nondiscrimination

The ABPMR does not discriminate among applicants on the basis of age, sex, race, religion, national origin, disability, or marital status.

The Examination

As part of the requirements for certification by the ABPMR, candidates must demonstrate satisfactory performance in an examination conducted by the Board covering the field of PM&R. The examination for certification is given in two parts, written (Part I) and oral (Part II).

Part I and Part II of the Board examination are given once each year, usually in May at such times and places as the Board designates. While Part I of the examination is administered the same day and time at Dallas, Texas, and Philadelphia, Pennsylvania, in addition to Rochester, Minnesota, Part II is administered only at the Rochester test site.

Candidates should not bring cellular phones, pagers, laptop computers, recording devices, books, or study materials into the examination room.

Part I

The written examination is divided into morning and afternoon periods of approximately 4 hours each. The questions are designed to test the candidate's knowledge of basic sciences and clinical management as related to PM&R and will be in the form of objective testing.

If a candidate believes the scoring of his or her written examination is inaccurate, a request may be made to have the examination scored manually. The request must be filed in writing to the Board office within 30 days of notification of test results with an explanation of reasons for concern and with payment of a $100 fee for the manual rescoring.

Part II

The oral examinations are given by the directors of the Board, with the assistance of selected guest examiners. The candidate is examined by three examiners, each of whom conducts a 40-minute segment of the total 120-minute examination. Two 5-minute breaks divide the three portions of the oral examination.

Candidates will be expected to present in a concise, orderly fashion evidence of their proficiency in the management of various clinical conditions that come within the field of PM&R. During the oral examination, the examiner will ask questions about diagnostic procedures, therapeutic procedures, and patient management.

The candidate should be prepared to demonstrate familiarity with the literature of basic and clinical research, as well as recent significant literature pertinent to PM&R. Conciseness and clarity of statements are expected. Evidence of the professional maturity of the candidate in clinical procedures and of factual knowledge will be sought.

In the event a candidate taking both Parts I and II examinations in the same year fails Part I of the examination, the results of Part II will not count or be recognized in any way. Both Parts I and II would need to be retaken for certification.

In addition to clinical PM&R, both the written and the oral portions of the examination will cover certain aspects of the basic sciences. The basic science components of the examinations may include:

- Anatomy: kinesiology and functional anatomy, biomechanics, neuroanatomy, and musculoskeletal anatomy
- Physics: electricity, mechanics, and biophysics of physical agents
- Physiology: physiology and pathophysiology of nerve, muscle, and bone, and of the cardiovascular, pulmonary, genitourinary, and central nervous systems; effects of physical and pharmacological agents used in PM&R; exercise and inactivity
- Pathology: pathology of muscles, nerves, bones, joints, soft tissues, and of the central nervous system
- Other fundamental clinical sciences: use of clinical knowledge, skills, experience, and competencies as listed under "Residency Training Requirements" above

The Certificate

Upon approval of the application and the candidate's successful completion of the examinations, the Board will grant a certificate to the effect that the candidate has met the requirements of the Board. The recipient of a certificate will be known as a diplomate, or a certificant, of the American Board of Physical Medicine and Rehabilitation.

The Board began issuing 10-year, time-limited diplomate certificates in 1993. The expiration date for these certificates is June 30 of the given year. Recertification procedures and requirements are described briefly in a following section and in depth in a separate *Booklet of Information* available upon request from the Board office. Certificates issued prior to 1993 have no time-limited stipulations; holders of these pre-1993 certificates have no Board-based requirements for recertification.

Residents entering a training program are hereby informed and must be aware that time-limited certification for PM&R began in 1993 for all diplomates certified thereafter.

A certificate granted by this Board does not of itself confer or purport to confer any degree or legal qualifications, privileges, or license to practice PM&R. The Board does not limit or interfere with the professional activity of any duly licensed physician who is not certified by this Board. Privileges granted physicians in the practice of PM&R in any hospital or clinic are the prerogatives of that hospital or clinic, not of this Board.

The names of consenting diplomates of the Board appear in *The Official ABMS Directory of Board Certified Medical Specialists* published by Marquis Who's Who, of New Providence, New Jersey.

Special Policies And Procedures

Unethical and Irregular Behavior

Candidates who apply to take an examination must certify that the information they provide in their applications is true and accurate. Examples of unethical or irregular behavior include, but are not limited to, situations where:

1. any misrepresentation is discovered in the candidate's application, in any other information submitted to the Board, or in the identity of a person applying to take or sitting for the examination; or
2. any financial or other benefit is offered by a candidate to any director, officer, employee, proctor, or other agent or representative of the Board in order to obtain a right, privilege, or benefit not usually granted by the Board to similarly situated candidates; or
3. any irregular behavior during the examination such as copying answers, sharing information, using notes, or otherwise giving or receiving aid is discovered by observation, statistical analysis, or answer sheets (score sheets), or otherwise; or
4. the chief proctor of the written examination or the oral examiner deems any portion of the candidate's absence from the designated examination room for whatever reason and any duration as unexcused or otherwise impermissible.

The candidate in question shall be given written notice of the charges and an opportunity to respond in accordance with the appeals procedures set forth in the rules and regulations of the Board.

If the Board determines that a violation has occurred, the Board may permanently bar the person(s) involved in the violation from all future examinations, invalidate the results of or refuse to score prior examinations taken by the person(s), withhold or revoke the certificate(s) of the person(s), and/or take other appropriate action. If sanctions are imposed pursuant to the rules and regulations of the Board, the Board may notify legitimately interested third parties of its action.

If the Board determines that irregular behavior has occurred during an examination, the Board will make every effort to withhold the scores of only those candidates directly implicated in the irregularity. In some instances, the evidence of irregularity, though sufficiently strong enough to cast doubt on the validity of scores, may not enable the Board to identify the specific candidates involved in the irregularity. In such circumstances, the Board may withhold the scores of candidates not directly implicated in the irregularity and, if necessary, may require those candidates to take an additional examination at a later date to ensure the validity of all scores.

The examination booklets are copyrighted as the sole property of the Board and must not be removed by the candidate from the test area or reproduced in any way. Any reproduction of the test booklet, in whole or in part, is a federal offense and also may subject the candidate to the sanctions listed above. No notes, textbooks, other reference materials, scratch paper, or electronic devices may be taken into either the written or oral certification examination.

Misrepresentation

Misrepresentation or alleged misrepresentation of a person as a diplomate of the American Board of Physical Medicine and Rehabilitation or as having obtained a status of eligibility to take the certification examination will be investigated and acted upon by the ABPMR. The Board will seek verifiable evidence of such misrepresentation from the individual in question and other sources. Once sufficient evidence for reasonable verification of such misrepresentation has been obtained, the Board will notify the individual and each related licensing agency of the evidence it has been able to obtain.

Such misrepresentation may include, but is not limited to, inclusion of an uncertified physician's name in a listing of other certified physicians, whether in newspapers, telephone yellow pages, or other means of soliciting patients, with the inference that all so listed are certified in PM&R.

Substance Abuse

If a history of substance abuse exists, candidates must provide documentation that they can safely and effectively perform the duties and responsibilities of a Board diplomate. The Board treats this information as confidential. Such documentation may consist of

1. evidence of a successful completion of a supervised treatment program,
2. evidence of a documented period of abstinence, or
3. evidence of current participation in a supervised rehabilitation program combined with evidence that the candidate is no longer engaged in the illegal use of drugs.

Appeals

The Board has adopted appeal procedures and an appellate review process. The procedures are available to individuals who disagree with the Board's decisions regarding applications for certification and admissibility to examinations, requests for accommodations due to disabilities, written examination, the oral examination process and procedures, the oral examination results, and other matters.

A copy of the appeal procedures and appellate review process is available upon request from the Board office. Failure to comply with the appeal procedures, including the requirement that appeals be instituted within 30 days after notice was given of the decision or action to be appealed, results in a waiver of appeal rights.

Revocation of Certification

A certificate is issued by the Board with the understanding that it remains the property of the Board. Any certificate issued by the Board shall be subject to revocation at any time if the Board determines, in its sole judgment, that the diplomate holding the certificate was in some respect not properly qualified to receive or retain it.

Reasons for Revocation

The Board may at its discretion revoke a certificate for due cause, including, but not limited to, the following:

1. The diplomate made any material misstatement or omission to the Board.
2. The diplomate did not possess the necessary qualifications and requirements to receive the certificate at the time it was issued, whether or not such deficiency was known to the Board.
3. The diplomate engaged in irregular behavior in connection with an examination of the ABPMR, whether or not such practice had an effect on the performance of the candidate on that examination. Examples of irregular behavior may include, but are not limited to, copying answers from or knowingly giving answers to

another individual, using notes during an examination, attempting to copy or distribute examination questions, or failing to return an examination booklet in the prescribed manner to the ABPMR or its representatives.

4. The diplomate misrepresented his or her status with regard to board certification, including any misstatement of fact about being board certified in any specialty or subspecialty.
5. The diplomate engaged in conduct that violated the moral or ethical standards of medical practice accepted by organized medicine in the locality where the diplomate is practicing, resulting in a revocation, suspension, qualification, or other limitation of his or her license to practice medicine, or the expulsion, suspension, disqualification or other limitation from membership in a local, regional, national, or other organization of his or her professional peers.
6. The diplomate's license to practice medicine has been revoked, suspended, qualified, or limited in any jurisdiction.

The holder of the revoked certificate will be given written notice of the reasons for its revocation. The notice will be sent by registered or certified mail to the last address that the holder has provided to the Board. Revocation will be considered final upon mailing of the notification.

Upon revocation of certification, the holder shall return the ABPMR certificate and other evidence of certification to the executive director of the Board and his or her name shall be removed from the list of certified physiatrists.

Individuals may appeal by complying with the appeal procedure. Failure to make a timely appeal will result in a loss of appeal rights. (Contact the ABPMR office for the Board's appeal procedure.)

Certificate Reinstatement

Should the circumstances that justified revocation of the certificate be corrected, the Board may, at its discretion, reinstate the certificate after appropriate review of the individual's licensure and performance, using the same standards and requirements applied to the applicants for certification.

Recertification

Beginning in 1993, the Board began issuing time-limited certificates that are valid for 10 years. To maintain certification beyond the 10-year period, diplomates certified since 1993 must participate in the recertification program. The guiding principle of the recertification program of the ABPMR is to foster the continuing development of excellence in patient care and all aspects of the practice of PM&R by its diplomates. Through its recertification program, the ABPMR seeks to encourage, stimulate, and support its diplomates in a program of self-directed, lifelong learning through the pursuit of continuing medical education (CME).

The recertification process permits diplomates to demonstrate that they continue to meet the requirements of the ABPMR. Recertification also provides patients and their families, funding agencies, and the public in general with assurance of the continuing up-to-date knowledge of PM&R diplomates.

To participate in the recertification program, an ABPMR diplomate must

- hold a current, valid, unrestricted license to practice medicine or osteopathy in a US licensing jurisdiction or Puerto Rico, licensure in Canada, or evidence of possession of an acceptable equivalent;
- pay an annual $75 fee;
- provide evidence of an average of 50 CME credits annually, for a total of 500 CME hours over the 10-year period; and
- successfully complete a written examination.

Diplomates are automatically enrolled in the recertification program upon issuance of their time-limited certificates. Those who do not pay their fees or do not report CME credits for 4 or more years are considered nonparticipants.

The Board office will notify nonparticipants when their certificates have expired. Delayed participation in the recertification process may require completion of the requirements for initial certification, so diplomates are advised to monitor their participation carefully.

The recertification examination is an open-book, take-home test consisting of 200 multiple-choice questions. Diplomates have 10 weeks to complete the examination and return it to the ABPMR. The examination content is organized into modules. A core module is completed by all participants. The participants then select two additional modules from specific subspecialty areas in PM&R.

For complete information on the recertification process and requirements, please request a copy of the current *Recertification Booklet of Information* from the Board office.

Certificate of Subspecialization in Spinal Cord Injury (SCI) Medicine

The application and information on the examination process for Subspecialization in Spinal Cord Injury Medicine are available to all diplomates of American Board of Medical Specialties' member boards. The first examination is scheduled for October 1998. The *Subspecialty Certification in Spinal Cord Injury Medicine Booklet of Information*, which summarizes the training and/or practice requirements and the application process, including deadlines and fees, is available from the ABPMR office.

American Board of Plastic Surgery

Seven Penn Center/Ste 400
1635 Market St
Philadelphia, PA 19103-2204
215 587-9322
215 587-9622 Fax
E-mail: abps@p3.net
Internet: http://www.abplsurg.org

(These criteria and conditions are subject to change without notice. All applicants are advised to contact the American Board of Plastic Surgery, Inc [ABPS], to ascertain whether the information below is correct.)

Introduction

The ABPS, which was organized in June 1937 by representatives of various groups interested in this type of surgery, received recognition as a subsidiary of the American Board of Surgery (ABS) in May 1938. The ABPS was given the status of a major specialty board in May 1941 by action of the Advisory Board for Medical Specialties as approved by the Council on Medical Education of the American Medical Association (AMA), which has designated certain specialty fields as being suitable to be represented by specialty boards.

The Board is organized under the laws of the State of Illinois for charitable, scientific, and educational purposes. No part of its net earnings shall inure to the benefit of any private member, director, officer, or other individual, nor shall the Board ever declare or make to any such persons any dividend or other distribution. Nothing herein, however, shall prevent the payment of reasonable compensation for services rendered or the reimbursement of reasonable expenses incurred in connection with the Board's affairs.

Plastic surgeons certified by the Board are listed in the *Official ABMS Directory of Board Certified Medical Specialists,* published by Marquis Who's Who in cooperation with the American Board of Medical Specialties (ABMS).

Mission Statement

The mission of the ABPS is to promote safe, ethical, efficacious plastic surgery to the public by maintaining high standards for the examination and certification of plastic surgeons as specialists and subspecialists.

Description of Plastic Surgery

Plastic surgery deals with the repair, reconstruction, or replacement of physical defects of form or function involving the skin, musculoskeletal system, cranio-maxillofacial structures, hand, extremities, breast and trunk, and external genitalia. It uses aesthetic surgical principles not only to improve undesirable qualities of normal structures but also in all reconstructive procedures as well.

Special knowledge and skill in the design and surgery of grafts, flaps, free tissue transfer, and replantation is necessary. Competence in the management of complex wounds, in the use of implantable materials, and in tumor surgery is required. Plastic surgery has been prominent in the development of innovative techniques such as microvascular and cranio-maxillofacial surgery, liposuction, and tissue transfer. The foundation of surgical anatomy, physiology, pathology, and other basic sciences is fundamental to this specialty.

Competency in plastic surgery implies a special combination of basic knowledge, surgical judgment, technical expertise, ethics, and interpersonal skills in order to achieve satisfactory patient relationships and problem resolution.

Sponsoring Organizations

The ABPS consists of 20 directors who manage the affairs of the organization. Nineteen directors are elected by the Board from names submitted by the following sponsoring organizations:

- The Aesthetic Surgery Education & Research Foundation, Inc.
- American Association for Accreditation of Ambulatory Surgical Facilities, Inc
- Association of Academic Chairmen of Plastic Surgery
- The American Association for Hand Surgery
- The American Association of Plastic Surgeons
- The American Association of Pediatric Plastic Surgeons
- The American Burn Association
- The American Head and Neck Society
- American Society Cleft-Palate Craniofacial Association
- American Association for the Peripheral Nerve
- The American Society for Reconstructive Microsurgery
- The American College of Surgeons (ACS)
- The American Society for Aesthetic Plastic Surgery, Inc
- The American Society for Surgery of the Hand
- The American Society of Maxillofacial Surgeons
- The American Society of Plastic and Reconstructive Surgeons, Inc (ASPRS)
- The American Surgical Association
- The Canadian Society of Plastic Surgeons
- The Council of Regional Societies of Plastic and Reconstructive Surgery
- The Plastic Surgery Research Council
- Plastic Surgery Education Foundation

Once elected to the Board, that person's obligation will be primarily to the Board and not to the sponsoring organization.

In addition, one director is elected by the Board from names submitted by the ABS.

These 20 individuals are the directors of the Board. Surgeons who fulfill the requirements of the Board and who are granted certification by the Board are known as diplomates of the ABPS.

Purposes

The essential purposes of the Board are

1. to establish requirements for the qualifications of applicants who request a certificate of their ability in the field of plastic surgery in its broadest sense;
2. to conduct examinations of approved candidates who seek certification by the Board;
3. to issue certificates to those who meet the Board's requirements and pass the respective examinations;
4. to do and engage in any and all lawful activities that may be incidental or reasonably related to any of the foregoing purposes.

The Board is not an educational institution, and certificates issued by the Board are not to be considered degrees. The certificate does not confer on any person legal qualifications, privileges, or license to practice medicine or the specialty of plastic surgery.

Standards of certification are clearly distinct from those of licensure; possession of a Board certificate does not indicate total qualification for practice privileges, nor does it imply exclusion of others not so certified. The Board does not purport in any way to interfere with or limit the professional activities of any licensed physician, nor does it desire to interfere with practitioners of medicine or any of their regular or legitimate activities.

It is not the intent nor has it been the function of the Board to define requirements for membership on the staff of hospitals or to define who shall or shall not perform plastic surgical operations. The Board is not a primary source of censure or primary review of ethical problems.

Policies

It is the Board's prerogative to determine the professional, ethical, moral, physical, and mental fitness of any candidate for its certificate.

The Board will consider opinions expressed concerning an individual's credentials only if they are in writing and signed.

It is the policy of the Board to maintain its autonomy and independence from political and economical considerations that might affect plastic surgery.

The Board recognizes the role of legitimate advertising in the changing medical scene, but it does not approve of advertising that arouses unrealistic expectations, is false or misleading, minimizes the magnitude and possible risks of surgery, or solicits patients for operations that they might not otherwise consider.

Such advertising is improper and inconsistent with the high standards of professional and ethical behavior implied by certification by the ABPS. The Board takes statements regarding Board status seriously and may penalize persons misstating their status.

General Requirements

The following requirements for admissibility are in agreement with those promulgated by the ABMS:

1. The Board will accept only those persons whose major professional activity is limited to the field of plastic surgery.
2. The person must maintain an ethical standing in the profession and moral status in the community acceptable to the ABPS in conformity with the Code of Ethics of the ASPRS. Moral and ethical practices that do not conform with the ASPRS Code of Ethics may result in rejection of an application or in deferral of examination until such matters have been resolved satisfactorily.

The Board may deny a candidate the privilege of sitting for an examination, or may refuse issuance of a certificate, if it is found by additional disclosures or a recent change in status that the candidate no longer meets the general or professional requirements.

Professional Requirements

The Board considers the requirements detailed in the sections on prerequisite training and training requirements to be minimal. Candidates are encouraged to take advantage of broadening experiences in other fields.

The Board reserves the right to

1. request lists of operations performed solely by the candidate for 1 or more years;
2. request special and extra examinations: written, oral, or practical;
3. request any specific data concerning the candidate that may be deemed necessary before making a final decision for certification;
4. consider evidence that a candidate's practice after completion of training is not in accord with generally accepted medical or ethical standards, which may result in rejection of the application or deferral of the examination until such time as the matter has been satisfactorily resolved.

Undergraduate Medical or Osteopathic Education

Before prerequisite training, candidates must have graduated from a medical school in a state or jurisdiction of the United States that is accredited at the date of graduation by the Liaison Committee for Medical Education (LCME), a Canadian medical school accredited by the Committee on Accreditation of Canadian Medical Schools (CACMS), or a US osteopathic school accredited by the American Osteopathic Association (AOA).

Graduates of medical schools located outside the jurisdiction of the United States and Canada must possess a currently valid standard certificate from the Educational Commission for Foreign Medical Graduates (ECFMG) or have completed a Fifth Pathway program in an accredited school of medicine in the United States.

Official Evaluation of Prerequisite Training

Official evaluation of prerequisite training by the Board is required prior to the initiation of residency training in plastic surgery. This simple preliminary step will prevent later disappointment. It is the responsibility of all prospective trainees in plastic surgery to secure this evaluation. Each prospective trainee must obtain a Request for Evaluation of Training Form from the Board office prior to completion of prerequisite training. Along with the completed Request for Evaluation of Training Form, prospective candidates are required to submit a $150 nonrefundable processing fee (made payable to The American Board of Plastic Surgery, Inc, in US funds) and a copy of their medical school diploma.

Directors of accredited residency training programs in plastic surgery must require all prospective trainees to have an official evaluation and approval of their prerequisite training by the Board before they begin plastic surgery training.

Approval for residency training in plastic surgery will be provided to those individuals who clearly meet the Board's established training requirements. Further information for detailed credential review will be obtained on all other individuals where training was in other than accredited programs.

Official evaluations will be made by the Credentials and Requirements Committee. Individual officers or members of the Board cannot and will not make such estimates or rulings. It should be emphasized that the answers to many questions require a decision by one or more of the committees of the Board. This applies particularly to evaluation of training and questions of admissibility. Decisions are referred to the entire Board at the next scheduled Board meeting.

The process of reaching a final decision may require several months, since the full Board meets only twice annually. March 1 and September 1 are the last postmarked dates for submission of written special requests and documentation for consideration by the Credentials and Requirements Committee.

The Board will issue neither a letter verifying prerequisite training nor an Application for Examination and Certification Form until the Request for Evaluation of Training Form has been received and approved.

Training Requirements

There are two major pathways toward obtaining acceptable graduate level training in plastic surgery: the independent model and the integrated model.

In an independent model, the candidate must complete both (1) prerequisite training and (2) requisite training (plastic surgery). In an integrated model, no such distinction exists.

Residents may transfer, prior to the last 2 years, from an independent type of program to another independent program and from an integrated type of program to another integrated program, but they may not exchange accredited years of training between the two different models.

The minimum acceptable residency year, for both prerequisite and requisite training, must include at least 48 weeks of full-time experience.

Independent Model

This consists of at least 3 years of general surgery residency training followed by 2 or 3 years of plastic surgery residency training.

Prerequisite Training

For United States or Canadian doctors of medicine or osteopathy with their medical degree or osteopathic degree granted in the United States or Canada, and international medical graduates, one of the following pathways must be taken:

1. A minimum of 3 years of clinical training in general surgery with progressive responsibility in the same program is required. Rotating internships will not be accepted in lieu of a clinical year in general surgery. Broad surgical training experience is required. Therefore, no more than 6 months of training may be spent on any single subspecialty surgical service during the 3 years. This program must be approved by the Residency Review Committee (RRC) for Surgery and accredited in the United States by the Accreditation Council for Graduate Medical Education (ACGME) or in Canada by the Royal College of Physicians and Surgeons (RCPSC) for full training. The minimum of 3 years of clinical training with progressive responsibility in the same program in general surgery must be completed before the candidate enters a plastic surgery residency. The satisfactory completion of this requirement must be verified in writing by the general surgery program director (see "Verification of Prerequisite Training," below). Or
2. An accredited residency training program in neurological surgery, orthopedic surgery, otolaryngology, or urology. Prospective candidates may initiate residency training in plastic surgery following satisfactory completion of the entire course of training in the United States or Canada, as prescribed for certification by the American Board of Neurological Surgery, the American Board of Orthopaedic Surgery, the American Board of Otolaryngology, or the American Board of Urology. They must meet and comply with the most current requirements in these specialties. Satisfactory completion of training must be verified in writing by the training program director (see "Verification of Prerequisite Training," below) and evidence of current admissibility to the respective specialty board's examination process in the United States is required.

For prospective candidates with an MD degree obtained in the United States or Canada combined with a DMD or DDS degree

Satisfactory completion of a residency program in oral and maxillofacial surgery approved by the American Dental Association (ADA) is an alternate pathway for prerequisite training prior to plastic surgery residency. The satisfactory completion of this training must be verified in writing by the oral and maxillofacial surgery program director. This program must include the integration of a medical school component resulting in a doctor of medicine (MD) degree.

This combined training must also include a minimum of 24 months of progressive responsibility on surgical rotations under the direction of the general surgery program director after receipt of the MD degree. The general surgery program director must verify in writing the completion of 24 months of general surgery training, the level of responsibility held, inclusive dates, and specific content of rotation. Rotations in general surgery during medical school, prior to the MD degree, will not be considered as fulfilling any part of the 24-month minimum requirement. If the general surgery component is completed at an institution other than the sponsoring institution of the oral and maxillofacial surgery residency, then this training must be completed consecutively, with all 24 months spent in the same general surgery program that has been reviewed by the RRC for Surgery and is accredited by the ACGME in the United States.

Verification of Prerequisite Training

To ensure written verification from the program director under whom the candidate completed prerequisite training, the Board office will mail a verification form for completion and return by the program director. It is the candidate's responsibility to determine that the form has been completed and returned to the Board office.

Requisite Training

Graduate Education in Plastic Surgery

Two years of plastic surgery training is required, and the final year must be at the senior level. Residents entering a plastic surgery residency accredited for 3 years of training must complete the entire 3 years, including 1 year of senior responsibility.

Candidates beginning plastic surgery residency on or after July 1, 1995, will be required to complete both years of a 2-year program in the same institution or the last 2 years of a 3-year program in the same institution. In either instance, the final year must be at the senior level.

Training in plastic surgery must be obtained in either the United States or Canada. The Board recognizes training in those programs in the United States that have been reviewed by the RRC for Plastic Surgery and accredited by the ACGME or those programs in Canada approved by the RCPSC.

Content of Training

Candidates must hold positions of increasing responsibility for the care of patients during these years of training. For this reason, major operative experience and senior responsibility are essential to surgical education and training.

An important factor in the development of a surgeon is an opportunity to grow, under guidance and supervision, by progressive and succeeding stages to eventually assume complete responsibility for the surgical care of the patient.

It is imperative that a resident hold positions of increasing responsibility when obtaining training in more than one institution, and 1 full year of experience must be at the senior level. The normal training year for the program must be completed. No credit is granted for part of a year of training.

The Board considers a residency in plastic surgery to be a full-time endeavor and looks with disfavor upon any other arrangement. The minimum acceptable training year is 48 weeks. Should absence exceed 4 weeks per annum for any reason, the circumstances and possible makeup time of this irregular training arrangement must be approved by the RRC for Plastic Surgery, and documentation of this approval must be provided to the Board by the program director.

Training in plastic surgery must cover the entire spectrum of plastic surgery. It should include experience in both the functional and aesthetic (cosmetic) management of congenital and acquired defects of the head and neck, trunk, and extremities. Sufficient material of a diversified nature should be available to prepare the trainee to pass the examination(s) of the Board after the prescribed period of training.

This period of specialized training should emphasize the relationship of basic science—anatomy, pathology, physiology, biochemistry, and microbiology—to surgical principles fundamental to all branches of surgery and especially to plastic surgery. In addition, the training program must provide in-depth exposure to the following subjects: the care of emergencies, shock, wound healing, blood replacement, fluid and electrolyte balance, pharmacology, anesthetics, and chemotherapy.

Accredited Residency Programs

Information concerning accredited training programs for the independent model may be found in the *Graduate Medical Education Directory* (the "Green Book") published by the American Medical Association (AMA) under the aegis of the ACGME. Copies of this directory are available at many medical schools and libraries, or candidates may order the directory directly from the AMA by calling toll-free 800 621-8335, or by writing to the American Medical Association, PO Box 7046, Dover, DE 19903-7046.

The Board does not inspect or approve residencies. The RRC for Plastic Surgery inspects and makes recommendations for or against approval of a residency training program in plastic surgery only after the director of the residency has filed an application for approval with the Secretary of the Residency Review Committee for Plastic Surgery (Doris A Stoll, PhD), 515 N State Street, Chicago, IL 60610; 312 464-5504.

The RRC consists of nine members, three representatives from each of the following: the ABPS, the ACS, and the AMA.

Neither the Board nor its individual members can be responsible for the placement of applicants for training. The Board does not maintain a list of available openings in programs. Prospective candidates seeking accredited training in plastic surgery should correspond directly with the directors of those training programs in which they are interested.

Most plastic surgery residencies participate in a special Plastic Surgery Matching Program. For information, contact Plastic Surgery Matching Program, PO Box 7999, San Francisco, CA 94120; 415 923-3907.

Nonapproved Residencies

No other residencies in the United States, Canada, or other countries are acceptable in lieu of those specified above. This in no way implies that quality training cannot be acquired elsewhere, but the Board has no method of evaluating the quality of such programs and must be consistent in its requirements.

The Board grants no credit for training, residency, and/or experience in disciplines other than those named.

Integrated Model

United States Program

Candidates must have a medical or osteopathic degree granted in the United States or Canada by an institution accredited by the LCME or the AOA.

Accreditation by the ACGME is required for all years of the training program.

Training of no less than 5 years of clinical residency under the authority and direction of the plastic surgery program director is required. No less than 24 months of this program must be concentrated plastic surgery training, and the final 12 months must entail senior clinical plastic surgery responsibility. The last 2 years of training must be completed in the same program.

Canadian Combined Program

This requirement will pertain to all those applying for admission to the ABPS examination process beginning in the year 2000, but candidates may begin such a course of training before then if they so desire.

The third year of training in the Canadian 5-year combined program must consist of varied rotations of a general surgery nature demonstrating progressive responsibility at a third-year level. This program must be approved by the RCPSC for full training.

Rotations may include the alimentary tract; the abdomen and its contents; the breast, skin, and soft tissue; the head and neck, including trauma, vascular, endocrine, congenital, and oncologic disorders, particularly tumors of the skin, salivary glands, thyroid, parathyroid, and oral cavity; the vascular system, excluding the intracranial vessels, the heart, and those vessels intrinsic and immediately adjacent thereto; the endocrine system; surgical oncology, including coordinated multimodality management of the cancer patient by screening surveillance, surgical adjunctive therapy, rehabilitation, and follow-up; comprehensive management of trauma, including musculoskeletal, hand, and head injuries (responsibility for all phases of care of the injured patient is an essential component of general surgery); and complete care of critically ill patients with underlying surgical conditions in the emergency room, intensive care unit, and trauma/burn units. No more than 6 months of this training may be spent on any single subspecialty surgical service, such as a burn unit, during the 3 years.

A Request for Evaluation of Training Form must be completed and returned by the candidate to the Board office along with a $100 nonrefundable processing fee in US funds (made payable to The American Board of Plastic Surgery, Inc).

A Verification Form must be completed and signed by both the director of postgraduate education for the university's department of surgery and the director of the university's training program in plastic surgery. After completion of plastic surgery training, the director of postgraduate surgical education and the plastic surgery program director will be required to complete and sign the last page of the Application for Examination and Certification Form.

Applying for Examination and Certification

The prime purpose of the Board is to pass judgment on the education, training, and knowledge of broadly competent and responsible plastic surgeons. Certification by the Board indicates qualification of a specialist at a superior level of excellence. The quality of training of surgeons, as shown by their successful completion of the Board examinations, will be reflected in their ability to achieve good results in practice.

The Board will issue no letters attesting to admissibility for its examinations to any person, institution, or organization until this formal application, along with the required supporting documents, has been received and approved.

The Application Process

In order to be admitted to the examination process leading to Board certification, prospective candidates should write to the Board office requesting application materials no later than December of the final year of their residency. An Application for Examination and Certification request card may also be obtained from the residency program director, who will receive these yellow post cards in December. Upon this written request, an Application for Examination and Certification Form will be provided and should be completed and submitted to the Board office by the deadline indicated in the Application cover letter.

Prospective candidates must submit a completed Application for Examination and Certification Form to the Board office within 2 years after completion of their residency in plastic surgery in order to be considered for admission to the examinations leading to Board certification.

Deadline for Submission of Application Material
Applications for admission to the written examination must be received in the Board office by the deadlines listed in the *Booklet of Information*.

Licensure
All candidates must have a currently valid, registered, full, and unrestricted license to practice medicine in a state, territory, or possession of the United States or in a Canadian province, and they must continue to be licensed throughout the certification process. A temporary limited license, such as an educational, institutional, or house permit, is not acceptable. A photocopy of an active registration certificate bearing a date that will be valid at the time of examination(s) must be submitted by the candidate.

Commissioned officers of the medical service of the armed forces of the United States or Canada on active duty need not present evidence of current registration of licensure but must provide appropriate information regarding their status.

Letters of Recommendation
If a candidate has completed training in more than one program in plastic surgery, the program director of the first year of training must verify to the Board, in writing, the satisfactory completion of that year of training. Additionally, the Board may require favorable evaluations and verification from other surgeons.

Residency Graduation Form (US Programs)
A Residency Graduation Form will be mailed by the Board office directly to the plastic surgery program director for completion at the end of the resident's training in plastic surgery. A single form will be sent for each resident and will require signatures in two places. The first signature, by the program director, will signify that to the best of his/her knowledge, the individual has fulfilled all of the prerequisite and requisite graduate medical education requirements prescribed by the Board. The second signature will (1) attest that the individual has completed a residency training program in plastic surgery accredited by the RRC for Plastic Surgery under his/her direction and that the accredited number of years included a year of senior responsibility; and (2) recommend the individual for admission to the examination process of the Board. The corresponding boxes to each of these statements must be checked, as applicable, in addition to the program director signing the form.

The Board requires each program director to complete a Residency Graduation Form for each resident by July 15.

If the program director elects not to sign either statement, the director is required to provide a full written explanation of the reason the required signature(s) is not provided. The individual's application cannot be processed, nor will the individual be admitted to the examination process of the Board, without both required signatures.

The program director must record any deficiencies that were responsible for the lack of signature(s) and discuss these with the individual. This written communication must be given to the individual and a copy must be forwarded to the Board office. If further educational training or experience is completed, the program director should request, within 30 days, that another Residency Graduation Form be sent for the required signature(s). If the individual is still felt to be deficient and not recommended for admission to the examination process of the Board, the program director again must communicate the cause for the lack of signature(s) to the Board office.

Failure on the part of the program director to complete the Residency Graduation Form within the stipulated framework will be considered an abrogation of the responsibility of the program director, and the RRC for Plastic Surgery shall be so notified.

Required Signatures (Canadian Programs)
Plastic surgery residents who complete their training in Canada will be sent an Application for Examination and Certification Form that must be completed accurately and signed by them. It must also be completed and signed by both the director of postgraduate surgical education and the plastic surgery program director responsible for the resident's senior year. The signature of the director of postgraduate surgical education will signify that the resident has fulfilled all of the prerequisite and requisite graduate medical education requirements prescribed by the ABPS to the best of his/her knowledge. The two signatures by the plastic surgery program director will (1) attest that the resident has completed a plastic surgery residency accredited by the RCPSC and has included a senior year of responsibility under his/her direction; and (2) recommend the resident for admission to the examination process of the ABPS.

Notification of Admissibility

A candidate whose Application for Examination and Certification Form is approved will be notified in writing. An Information Form and Identification Form will be sent with this notification. They are to be completed and returned to the Board office within 30 days of notification. Failure to complete and return these forms will prevent the candidate from receiving further information pertaining to the Written Examination.

If it appears that the stated requirements have not been met, further details may be requested. This information will be reviewed by the Credentials and Requirements Committee. The committee meets twice yearly (spring and fall), and decisions are not rendered at any other time.

Until the application has been received and approved, the Board will not inform any person, institution, or organization that a candidate is admissible to the examination process.

Admissibility to the Examination Process
Each approved candidate shall be entitled to take an examination(s) as required by the Board.

All candidates must comply with the current regulations in effect for the year in which the examination is taken, regardless of the time the original application was approved. It is the responsibility of candidates to seek information concerning the current requirements for certification by the Board. The Board does not assume responsibility for notifying candidates of changing requirements or the impending loss of admissibility to take an examination. A new *Booklet of Information* is published yearly in July.

All candidates taking an examination of the ABPS must complete the entire examination.

Certification by any other specialty Board does not exempt candidates from any part of the examination process.

Written Examination

The Written Examination will be conducted in the fall each year or at any other time deemed suitable by the Board. The examination will be given on the dates specified and at the time specified. No exceptions will be made, and special examinations will be given only under unusual circumstances (see "Examination of Candidates with Disabilities" under "Special Situations").

Admissibility to the Written Examination

Candidates admissible to the examination process may take the Written Examination in the spring of the year following successful completion of residency in plastic surgery, provided the Application for Examination and Certification Form is approved.

Candidates approved for admission to the Written Examination on or after July 1, 1991, will be offered five consecutive opportunities to appear for the Written Examination. Candidates may take the Written Examination three times during this 5-year period. Candidates who have not passed the Written Examination during this period will no longer be candidates for examination.

In either situation, the satisfactory completion of an additional year of training is required before a candidate can be considered for readmission to the Written Examination. This additional year of training can be taken in a formal residency or a suitable plastic surgery preceptorship. This additional year of training must be approved in advance by the Credentials and Requirements Committee of the Board. Evidence of satisfactory completion of this year of training is required before further consideration for examination will be made.

If the Board approves the candidate's request for readmission to the Written Examination, two more consecutive opportunities to appear for the Written Examination will be offered. Once approval is received, the candidate must sit for examination at the first available opportunity. Candidates who do not successfully pass the Written Examination within these two consecutive opportunities will be required to repeat an entire plastic surgery residency to again be admissible to the examination process.

Announcement Information

Candidates who are admissible to the Written Examination will be sent annually, throughout their period of admissibility, an Announcement Packet including an Announcement Letter, *Booklet of Information*, reply card (green), and a hotel reservation card. Candidates may use the hotel reservation card if they wish to stay in the hotel at which the examination is to be given. When the reply card (green) is received, candidates must signify their intent to take the examination by completing and returning the reply card and examination fee immediately to the Board office.

Both sides of the reply card (green) must be completed. Otherwise, candidates will not be scheduled for examination. Hospital or academic appointments must recorded on the reply card (green).

Candidates are responsible for their own travel, hotel accommodations, and expenses.

Admission to Examination

If the returned Reply Card (green) and examination fee for the Written Examination are not received by the date indicated in the Announcement Letter, the candidate may not be accepted for admission to that Written Examination.

Reply Card and Examination Fee Deadline

An Announcement Mailing will be sent in January 1999 for candidates approved for the examination process on or before December 31, 1998. The Reply Card (green) deadline for the Fall Written Examination is the close of the business day on March 1, 1999. The examination fee of $900 must accompany the Reply Card (green) in order to be scheduled for the Written Examination. A late penalty fee of $500 must accompany the Reply Card and examination fee if received by the Board office from March 2, 1999, up to and including the close of the business day on March 15, 1999. Reply cards and examination fees received March 2 up to March 15 will be considered only on a space available basis.

An Announcement Mailing and Approval Packet will be sent in July 1999 for candidates approved for the process after December 31, 1998. The Reply Card deadline for the Fall Written Examination is the close of the business day on August 3, 1999. The examination fee of $900 must accompany the Reply Card in order to be scheduled for the Written Examination. The August 3, 1999, deadline for candidates completing residency on June 30, 1999, is absolute. No late Reply Cards will be accepted.

Reply Cards and examination fees received in the Board office after the close of the business day on March 15 or August 3, as noted above, will not be accepted for admission to the September 15, 1999, Written Examination.

Admission Cards

For candidates approved for the examination process before December 31, 1998: Candidates will be mailed an Admission Card (white) in July or not later than 1 month before the Examination.

For candidates approved for the examination process after December 31, 1998: Candidates will be provided with an admission card when they register for the morning session of the examination. Printed on this card will be the candidate's name and current address; candidate number; the date, time, and location of the examination; the specific room in which the candidate is to take the examination; and the "Result Mailing Date." Candidates must use their candidate number, which is printed on the card, throughout the examination.

Late arrival may result in denial of admission to the examination.

Advise the Board office immediately by telephone (215 587-9322) if the admission card (white) is lost prior to the examination.

Withdrawal from Examination

Candidates wishing to withdraw from the examination must send written notification postmarked at least 30 calendar days before the date of the examination. The examination fee will be refunded, less a processing charge of $700. Candidates who withdraw from the examination after this date or who fail to appear for the examination will forfeit the entire fee. The Board may waive this rule if the circumstances warrant.

Registration and Administration of the Examination

All candidates must take the entire examination on the same day and at the same time.

Candidates must register for the morning and afternoon sessions on the date, time, and location specified on their admission cards (white). If for any reason candidates are delayed or cannot arrive on time, they must notify the proctor or the Board office. If candidates are unable to attend the examination, they must notify the Board office either by letter or by telephone prior to the time of registration for the morning session. Anyone who is more than 30 minutes late will not be admitted to the examination.

The Board office will provide each candidate with lead pencils for use during the examination. No other writing implements may be used.

Candidates are not permitted to bring any notes, textbooks, or other reference materials into the examination. Scratch paper is not permitted, but space for notes and calculations is provided in the Question Book.

Question Books are prepared by and/or at the direction of the ABPS, are the sole and exclusive property of the ABPS, and said books are protected under the copyright laws of the United States and other countries. The Question Books may only be used for such purposes as are designated from time to time by the ABPS, and other than such designated purposes, all other rights are reserved by the ABPS.

Copying, by any means, of all or any part of such Question Books or removal from the examination room or unauthorized use in any way whatsoever of said Question Books are strictly prohibited.

Change of Address
If a candidate's address, as it appears on the admission card (white), is incorrect or will change before the "Result Mailing Date," please enter the corrected or new address on the back of the admission card (white) in the space provided before turning it in to a proctor at the end of the afternoon session. Admission cards (white) will be collected from all candidates at the conclusion of the examination.

Examination Schedule
The Written Examination will consist of a morning session and an afternoon session. The sessions are not separate examinations but are graded together as one examination and will not be separately administered.

The morning session is 3 hours and 15 minutes in duration, and the afternoon session is 3 hours in duration. Both sessions consist of two types of questions, multiple choice (one best answer) and true/false (multiple answers).

In general, each test item consists of a question, a case history, or a situation followed by a list of possible answers. Instructions for completion of each type are given in the Question Book that candidates will receive at the examination. Included in each Question Book is an Answer Sheet upon which candidates must record their answers by filling in the appropriate circles (in pencil).

Content of the Examination

The subjects covered in the examination are listed below, and both sessions will cover the entire field of plastic surgery, with no differentiation in content between the morning and afternoon sessions:

1. Basic techniques, wound healing, microsurgery, transplantation
2. Burns, sepsis, metabolism, trauma, resuscitation, nutrition, endocrinology, shock, hematology
3. Pre- and postoperative care, anesthesia, cardiorespiratory care, complications, clinical pharmacology
4. Tumors of the head and neck, skin, and breast, including treatment by radiation therapy, immunotherapy, chemotherapy, and surgery
5. Trunk, lower extremity, musculoskeletal system, pressure ulcers, rehabilitation
6. Hand, peripheral nerves, rehabilitation
7. Maxillofacial and craniofacial surgery and microsurgery
8. Congenital anomalies, genetics, teratology, facial deformity, speech pathology, gynecology, and genitourinary problems
9. Aesthetic (cosmetic) surgery, psychiatry, and legal medicine
10. Basic knowledge of pathology (eg, the biologic behavior of neoplasms, inflammation, and repair)
11. Gross and functional anatomy, embryology

The questions for the examination cover subjects considered to be of fundamental importance to competent performance in the field of plastic surgery. Every effort is made to avoid "trick" questions, ambiguity, and questions involving irrelevant facts. All questions are analyzed by psychometric techniques to ensure their quality.

Candidates will pass or fail on the strength of their performance on the entire Written Examination.

Results

Letters of notification of the results (pass or fail) of the Written Examination will be mailed on the date indicated on the admission card (white). The time period between administration of the examination and notification is necessary to allow for extensive analysis and to ensure that individual results are reliable and accurate.

Results of the examination will be divulged to no one until after the Board result letter has had time to reach candidates. If a week has elapsed after the "Result Mailing Date" and candidates still have not received the letter from the Board, they may then call for information. Information will be given to no one but a candidate personally. The Board staff will verify candidates' identity prior to releasing results to them.

Each candidate will receive a single final grade (pass or fail) for the entire examination. To complete the Written Examination successfully, candidates must achieve a passing grade for the entire examination.

The score (pass or fail) on the examination will be determined by the total number of alternatives answered correctly. Therefore, candidates are encouraged to answer all items.

Pass
If a candidate passes the Written Examination, he/she will be informed of this fact.

Fail
If a candidate fails the Written Examination, he/she will be informed of this fact.

In case of failure, the candidate must repeat the entire Written Examination.

Hand Scoring ($200)
Hand scoring of the Written Examination will be performed upon written request. To request hand scoring, candidates must write to the Board office within 30 days from notification of the results. Candidates will be responsible for an extra charge for hand scoring of the examination. This charge will be determined by the secretary-treasurer of the Board. Currently, that fee is $200.

Cancellation of Examination
Should the ABPS, in its sole discretion, cancel the Written Examination, or as a result of events beyond its control be unable to administer the Written Examination at the appointed date, time, and location, or should ABPS fail to conclude a candidate's Written Examination, the ABPS is not responsible for any expenses the candidate may have incurred in connection with the cancelled Written Examination, nor for any expenses the candidate may incur for any substitute Written Examination.

Oral Examination

Candidates who are admissible to the Oral Examination will be sent annually, throughout their period of admissibility, an Information Letter including the program disks and instructions for case list compilation.

Note: 1999 is an exceptional year in that the Oral Examination will be held in March and September. Only one examination is offered to each candidate. Admissibility is determined by the Board office based on the approval date of the Application for Examination and Certification Form and, for those whose Application Material was approved to the Examination process prior to July 1, 1997, the satisfaction of the 2-year practice requirement.

Prior to becoming admissible to the Oral Examination, candidates must have passed the Written Examination. Candidates admissible to the examination process before July 1, 1997, must have fulfilled the 2-year independent practice requirement.

Admissibility to the March 1999 Oral Examination

Only those candidates who submit a 7-month case list collected during the period beginning January 1, 1998, through July 31, 1998, along with the $500 nonrefundable fee, will be sent an Announcement Packet for the March 1999 Oral Examination.

Admissibility to the September 1999 Oral Examination

Only those candidates who submit a 7-month case list collected during the period beginning July 1, 1998, through January 31, 1999, along with the $500 nonrefundable fee, will be sent an Announcement Packet for the September 1999 Oral Examination.

Candidates approved for admission to the examination process *before* July 1, 1991, will be offered five opportunities in 7 calendar years to appear for the Oral Examination. Candidates who do not pass the Oral Examination during this period will no longer be candidates for examination.

Candidates approved for admission to the examination process, *on or after* July 1, 1991, will be offered three opportunities in 5 calendar years to appear for the Oral Examination. Candidates who do not pass the Oral Examination during this period will no longer be candidates for examination.

In both situations, the satisfactory completion of an additional year of full-time training is required before candidates can be considered for readmission to the Oral Examination. This additional year of training can be taken in a formal residency or a suitable plastic surgery preceptorship. This additional year of training must be approved in advance by the Credentials and Requirements Committee of the Board. Evidence of satisfactory completion of this year of training is required before further consideration for examination will be made.

If the Board approves the candidate's request for readmission to the Oral Examination, two more consecutive opportunities to appear for the Oral Examination will be offered. Once approval is received, the candidate must sit for the examination at the first available opportunity. Candidates who do not successfully pass the Oral Examination within these two consecutive opportunities will be required to repeat an entire plastic surgery residency to again be admissible to the examination process.

Practice Requirement

1. Candidates approved for admission to the examination process before July 1, 1986, and *after* July 1, 1997, do not have a practice requirement.
2. Candidates approved for admission to the examination process between July 1, 1986, and June 30, 1997, must have been in the independent practice of plastic surgery for at least 2 years. The 2 years of practice need not be consecutive, but the candidate must be in practice during all or part of the 7-month period required for compilation of the case list. *Note:* That period begins on January 1, 1998, and ends on July 31, 1998, for the March 1999 Examination and begins on July 1, 1998, and ends on January 31, 1999, for the September 1999 Examination.
3. A fellowship is not considered independent practice.
4. Candidates must be actively engaged primarily in the practice of plastic surgery.
5. Candidates must hold active operating privileges in a United States, Canadian, or foreign hospital.

Case List Compilation

Candidates for the March 1999 Oral Examination will be required to provide the Board with a compilation of operative cases and hospitalized patients during all or part of the 7-month period beginning with January 1, 1998, and ending July 31, 1998. Case Lists are due in the Board office before the close of the business day on September 1, 1998.

Candidates for the September 1999 Oral Examination are required to provide the Board with a compilation of operative cases and hospitalized patients during all or part of the 7-month period beginning July 1, 1998, and ending January 31, 1999. Case Lists are due in the Board office before the close of the business day on March 1, 1999.

Although the Board recognizes volunteer surgical activity in developing countries, these cases may not be included in compilation of case list materials for the Oral Examination because of the lack of continuum of care.

An Information Packet including the program disk and program instructions for compiling the 7-month case list will be sent to candidates. Disks will be available for the September 1999 Oral Examination up to and including December 1, 1998. No disk requests will be honored after this date.

The Case List compilation method is a Board-provided computerized program available on an IBM-, Mac-, or Power Mac-compatible 3 1/2-inch disk. The computerized program provides a standardized Case List that facilitates the Board's review. Candidates with IBM-, Mac-, or Power Mac-compatible office equipment or those desiring to rent such services will find the menu driven program easy to complete.

The printed case list will be in chronological order for each institution (hospital, office-based surgery, etc.) and include: patient's initials, hospital (or other) identifying number, age in months and days, sex, date of operation, case classification, diagnosis, procedure(s) performed (if any), CPT codes plus modifiers (identical to those used for billing on that case), and outcome including complications.

Using the Board-provided program, the Case List may be prepared, selected and printed from the menu options. A "landscape compatible" (horizontal) laser printer is required to print in the correct format. A vertically oriented printout (for presubmission review) may be obtained from a simple dot-matrix printer. Offices not having IBM-, Mac-, or Power Mac-compatible equipment may choose to have their raw data transferred to this form by renting stenographic service. After generation of the Case Lists and preparation of the additional material, the disks must be returned to the Board office with the original and a copy of the Candidate Case Summary Sheet (obtainable via the Board program) and completed Case Lists (affidavits for each institution are automatically printed out on the last page of each institution's Case List).

Instructions for Data Compilation

The Board recommends that candidates begin compiling the Case List on a weekly or monthly basis, rather than waiting until the last month of the compilation period to begin Case List compilation on the disk program. The "missing data report" on the reports menu will assist in reviewing entered data—including CPT codes. A trial printing well in advance of the deadline will also help in troubleshooting problems.

1. Providing complete diagnosis and procedure information is essential. From the operative notes, give an accurate written description of the diagnosis and the operative procedure(s). *Do not use ICD-9 and CPT codes in place of the written description of the diagnosis and procedure(s).* If the case was nonoperative, include a discharge summary diagnosis. Include all CPT codes plus modifiers used for insurance billing purposes, as well as all cases that were not billed to insurance (eg, aesthetic/cosmetic cases). CPT cases starting with 99 (office visits, consultations, etc) do not need to be included. Properly documented managed care relationships; military, Veterans Administration, Kaiser Permanente, and Shriners Hospitals; and candidates practicing in Canada and foreign countries are exempt from using CPT codes. For these exemptions mark the CPT code waver field as "yes."
2. Do not list assistant cases, namely cases billed by the candidate as an assistant surgeon. This exclusion does not cover cases done by a resident and attended by the candidate, or cases billed as co-surgeon; such cases should be included on the case list.

   Do not list voluntary surgical activity in developing countries. Although the Board recognizes volunteer surgical activity in developing countries, these cases may not be included in compilation of case list materials for the Oral Examination because of the lack of continuum of care.

3. Providing "outcome" information is essential. A short statement with respect to the outcome of each case will help guide the Board. Not all cases "heal without complications." Examples include "necrosis of tip of flap" or "normal sensation returned, but index finger stiff after tendon repair." The computer program allows outcome recording by number selection—only numbers 3, 4, and 5 require written explanation.
4. The list must include multiple operative procedures performed on the same patient. This inclusion allows automatic cross-referencing by the computer program. However, hospital number (or other) identifying numbers and patient initials (do not use full names) must be consistent for the patient with multiple procedures (eg, if a patient is listed at more than one institution, the same identifying number must be used to identify the patient).
5. All operative procedures must be included, whether inpatient, outpatient, or office-based surgery. All patients hospitalized by the candidate as the admitting physician must also be included, even if the patient is managed nonoperatively. Office-based surgery that does not require a dictated note (eg, nevi) does not need to be included. However, the Board suggests that the candidate err in the direction of inclusion of cases rather than exclusion. Do not include inpatient consultations on other services that did not culminate in a surgical procedure.
6. All emergency room patients who required an operative note must be included.
7. The completed lists must be signed by the medical record librarian/administrator of each institution (hospital, ambulatory surgery center, etc) and properly notarized as a complete list of the candidate's operative experience. Operations done by the candidate in the office must also be listed and notarized by the appropriate office personnel who can attest to the completeness. The institution's affidavit sheet prints out in sequence as the last page of each institution's Case List.
8. Two Candidate Case Summary Sheets (original and copy) must be submitted. This form facilitates the Board's review. The computer program generates the form directly by menu selection.

Preparation for Submission of Data

1. Print your 7-month Case List, using landscape format.
2. Obtain notarized affidavits from the medical record librarian/administrator of each institution (see "Instructions for Data Compilation," #7 above).
3. Make a copy of the entire case list only after you have proofread the accuracy of the list including the notarized affidavits.
4. Place the original 7-month Case List, including the signed and notarized affidavits for each institution, in a separate numerical compilation. Make a separate numerical compilation for each of the copies. The end of each institution's Case List is noted by the respective Candidate Affidavit Sheet, which includes the six-digit candidate number, name, address, telephone number(s), and notarized affidavit signed by the candidate. Staple each institution's Case List together.

Take the stapled Case List for the first institution (case list starts with page 1) and staple the "Candidate Affidavit Sheet" to the top of this section only. Follow the same procedure for the copy.

Place all stapled original 7-month Case Lists together, including the signed and notarized affidavits. Place the Candidate Case Summary Sheet on the bottom. Bind the entire 7-month Case List using a binder clip or a rubber band. Follow the same procedure for your stapled copies of the 7-month Case List. Do not place this material in binders or notebooks.

Submitting Material to the Board Office

Note that the deadline date for submission of case list materials for the March 1999 Examination is September 1, 1998.

For the September 1999 Examination, case lists must be submitted by March 1, 1999.

Candidates are required to submit the following items to the Board office:

Checklist for Case List submission to the Board

- One original Case List—including signed and notarized affidavits
- One copy of Case List—including signed and notarized affidavits
- One original and one copy of Candidate Case Summary Sheet
- Candidate Affidavit Sheet
- One copy of Candidate Affidavit Sheet
- Original Board program disks
- Most recent backup disks containing all files. Please label the disk with your name and Board six-digit candidate number. Examine contents of the disk for all required information
- Check in the amount of $500 (nonrefundable, US currency only) made payable to The American Board of Plastic Surgery, Inc. This fee provides for review of the Case List and selection of cases for preparation for Case Reports

The Board strongly recommends candidates send materials by a guaranteed delivery carrier, thus providing assurance and receipt of delivery. Use of a guaranteed delivery carrier, which often can verify receipt of delivery within 30 minutes, minimizes the need to call the Board office concerning your materials and allows the Board staff to process the large volume of received material.

Reminder

Candidates who do not provide the required items in the manner outlined will not be considered for admission to the Oral Examination.

Submitted items will be returned to the candidate. No exceptions will be made regarding late, incomplete, incorrect, or missing data from the Case Lists.

No lists or other material will be accepted after the September 1, 1998, or March 1, 1999, deadline dates.

Each candidate is responsible for keeping copies of all materials submitted to the Board. This includes a copy of the backup disk and the Board-provided program on your computer. The Board staff can not make copies of incomplete information or make corrections for candidates.

Make sure that all materials have been proofread, placed in numerical orders, and properly collated. Check to be sure that the backup disk has all of the required information.

Photographic Documentation

Particular emphasis should be placed on the necessity of photographic documentation. Preoperative and postoperative photographs are mandatory for all cases selected for case reports, and intraoperative photographs may aid in further illustration of the clinical problem. The candidate must provide a signed notarized affidavit attesting that all submitted photographs are the original and unaltered documentation of the patient cases presented for the Oral Examination. Digital photographs will be accepted beginning with the September 1999 Oral Examination.

The Board advises candidates who have not acquired the habit of routine photographic documentation of all patients to do so immediately. Any cases from the collection period may be selected and must have photographic documentation, including all hand cases (ie, carpal tunnel cases, etc). Transparencies are not acceptable.

Board Review and Selection Process

The Board reviews the Candidate's 7-month Case List and the Candidate Case Summary Sheet to determine if the candidate's operative list reflects sufficient diversity, complexity, and volume to demonstrate adequate maturity of practice of plastic surgery to permit examination of the candidate for certification as an expert in the specialty. In the event that the case list submitted is not adequate to allow selection of cases, the candidate will be deemed ineligible for the 1999 Oral Examination. This will constitute one of the five calendar year opportunities to appear for the Oral Examination, but will not count as an unsatisfactory performance (ie, one of the three opportunities to sit for the Oral Examination).

The candidate will be allowed to submit another case list for the following year for the duration of his/her period of admissibility. Candidates are notified in writing regarding Case Lists that the Board has found to be inadequate to allow for selection of Case Reports. This decision is final and not subject to appeal.

The Board selects cases from the candidate's Case List and requests the candidate to prepare Case Reports for these selected cases. The selected Case Reports will be prepared in the same format and with similar requirements as in past years.

For the March 24, 25, 26, 1999, Oral Examination:
The Announcement Packet will be mailed to candidates by December 31, 1998. It includes the list of Board-selected cases for preparation as Case Reports, a *Booklet of Information*, Reply Card (green), and a hotel reservation card. Candidates are asked not to contact the Board office prior to that date with respect to the submitted case list.

For the September 16, 17, 18, 1999, Oral Examination:
The Announcement Packet will be mailed to candidates by June 1, 1999. It includes the list of Board-selected cases for preparation as Case Reports, a *Booklet of Information*, Reply Card (green), and a hotel reservation card. Candidates are asked not to contact the Board office prior to that date with respect to the submitted case list.

Instructions and Information Pertaining to the March 24, 25, 26, 1999, and September 16, 17, 18, 1999, Oral Examination

The Oral Examination will be conducted each fall or at such other time as deemed suitable by the Board. The examination will be given on the dates and at the times specified. No exceptions will be made.

Announcement Information and Admission to the Oral Examination

Those candidates admissible to the Oral Examination will receive an Announcement Packet approximately 2 months in advance of the date of the examination. It includes a *Booklet of Information*, Reply Card (green), a hotel reservation card, and the list of cases for preparation as Case Reports.

When the Reply Card (green) is received, candidates must signify their intent to take the examination by completing both sides and returning the Reply Card (green) and balance of the examination fee of $1,000 to the Board office by the deadline date indicated in the Announcement Letter and on the Reply Card.

Candidates must complete both sides of the Reply Card (green) including all hospital or academic appointments. Otherwise, candidates will not be scheduled for examination.

Candidates are responsible for their own travel, hotel accommodations, and expenses.

Admission to Examination

The returned Reply Card (green) and balance of the examination fee of $1,000 for the Oral Examination must be received in the Board office by the close of the business day on February 1, 1999, in order to be scheduled for the March 1999 examination and by the close of the business day on July 1, 1999, for the September 1999 examination.

Reply cards (green) and Examination Fees ($1,000) received from February 2 to February 8, 1999 (March Oral Examination) or July 2 to July 8, 1999 (September Oral Examination) will require a late penalty fee of $700.

Reply cards (green) and Examination Fees ($1,000) received in the Board office after the close of the business day February 8, 1999, or July 8, 1999, will not be accepted for admission to the respective March or September Examination.

Once scheduled for the Oral Examination, the candidate receives preparation materials for the Case Reports. These materials include five folders for the examination, tab indices, a Photographic Affidavit Sheet, and labels for assembling and binding the selected Case Reports. It is essential that candidates place the candidate number, which appears on the Admission Card (white), on each label to be affixed to the cover of each case report, along with the other required information.

Once scheduled for the Oral Examination, the candidate also receives a candidate Admission Card (white). The Admission Card lists the candidate's name, current address, candidate number, date and location of the examination, and the specific room to which candidates are to report.

Advise the Board office immediately by telephone if the Admission Card (white) is lost prior to the examination.

Withdrawal from Examination

Candidates wishing to withdraw from the examination must provide written notification to the Board office at least 30 calendar days before the examination date. The examination fee will be refunded less a processing charge of $700. Candidates who withdraw from the examination after this date or who fail to appear for the examination will forfeit the entire examination fee. The Board may waive this rule only if the circumstances warrant.

Requirements for Case Reports

Note the 7-month case collection periods for the 1999 Oral Examinations:

For the March 1999 Examination—January 1, 1998, through July 31, 1998

For the September 1999 Examination—July 1, 1998, through January 31, 1999

The following materials, collated in the order below, must be present in each of the submitted case reports. Candidates are required to use Board-supplied folders and tab indices to assemble each of their Case Reports. This will facilitate review of your Case Reports by the Examiners. The required materials are:

Before the First Tab:
Selected Case List Summary Sheet (Before Case Report #1 only)
Photographic Affidavit Sheet
Title Page
Tabs:
A Narrative Summary
Photographs with a signed affidavit that these are unaltered
Copies of the operative notes
Copies of the anesthesia records
Copies of pertinent laboratory data
Copies of pertinent pathology reports
Photographs of the pertinent radiographs
Progress Notes: Copies of hospital progress notes and office/clinic notes (separate office/clinic from hospital notes with divider sheet provided)
Copies of bills including CPT codes
Other if needed (eg, information from patient case before or after the 7-month case collection period if needed)

Candidates must use the 10 tab indices (provided by the Board) to divide the material compiled when assembling Case Reports for the required sections above.

See the detailed explanation of the requirements for each section below. The candidate is encouraged to read this section carefully. Improper or disorganized preparation of this material is sufficient cause to disqualify a candidate for continued examination.

Please note, in the event that more than one procedure is performed on the patient during the 7-month case list collection period, include all procedures and hospitalization(s) that fall within the 7-month collection period. Candidates are not required to document procedures that fall prior to or after the 7-month case collection period. However, if these procedures increase the understanding of the case, they may be included at the candidate's discretion. Documentation for procedures falling outside the 7-month case collection period does not have to be complete—the candidate may be selective.

Note: If the records are not in English, an accurate and complete English translation must accompany them.

Explanation of Requirements

Before the First Tab:

- Selected Case List Summary Sheet
  (Before Case Report #1 only)

Candidates must provide a Selected Case List Summary Sheet. Type each summary page on white bond paper. If necessary, copy multiple pages as a double-sided list on white bond paper. Bind the summary sheet(s) before Tab 1, at the beginning of the folder for Case Report #1. The list must be identified with the candidate name and candidate number.

- Photographic Affidavit Sheet

Affidavit Sheet must be signed and properly notarized, attesting that all photographs are the original and unaltered documentation of the patient cases presented for the Oral Examination.

Place the Photographic Affidavit immediately behind the Selected Case List Summary Sheet prior to the first Tab in Case Report #1.

- Title Page

Each report must be typed or reproduced on standard, letter-sized white paper (8 1/2-inch x 11-inch) with the candidate's full name, candidate number, the number of the case, the hospital or other identifying number, the principal diagnosis, and the primary operation listed on the title page. Categorize cases exactly as was done on the 7-month case list compilation.

For each case, include the following title page information in front of the first Tab:

January 1, 1998, through July 31, 1998, for the March 1999 Examination

July 1, 1998, through January 31, 1999, for the September 1999 Examination

Board Case Number

CATEGORY	ANATOMY
Aesthetic	Head and Neck
Burn	Breast
Cancer	Hand
Congenital	Upper Extremity
Skin	Trunk
Trauma	Lower Extremity
Other	Genitalia

Patient's hospital (or other) identifying number

Primary diagnosis

Procedure(s) done by the candidate

- Tabs
- Narrative Summary (First Tab)

A brief (one-page) narrative summary of the preoperative, operative, and postoperative course of the patient is required. Include a final separate paragraph entitled "outcome." Indicate here the outcome of the treatment and the final condition of the patient.

- Photographs

Pre-and postoperative photographs, approximately 4-inch x 6-inch color or black-and-white prints glued on 8 ½-inch x 11-inch white bond paper are preferred. The Board strongly recommends intraoperative photographs when they provide clarifying information. Digital photographs will be accepted starting with the September 1999 Oral Examination. Note the Photographic Affidavit Sheet (placed behind the Selected Case List Summary Sheet) applies to all submitted photographs. It must be signed and properly notarized attesting that all photographs are original and unaltered documentation of patient cases presented for Oral Examination. Diagrams or simple drawings may be substituted for intraoperative photographs. Descriptive legends and dates of the photographs must be placed adjacent to or below each photograph.

- Operative Report

This should include photocopies of originals for all operative reports for procedure performed by the candidate on this specific patient during the 7-month period. Operative reports of minor procedures performed by the candidate in the office during the 7-month collection period should also be included. You may include copies of the operative reports of procedures performed outside the 7-month collection period or those that were performed by another surgeon if they clarify the patient's course. Group all operative notes together in chronological order.

- Anesthetic Report

Photocopies of the original anesthetic records are required. This should include all anesthetic records for procedures performed by the candidate during the 7-month collection period. You may include copies of the anesthetic reports of procedures performed outside the 7-month collection period or those that were performed by another surgeon if they clarify the patient's course. Group all anesthetic records in chronological order.

- Laboratory

Photocopies of pertinent laboratory data are required. Group the data together in chronological order. Candidates are encouraged to use their judgment when including this material.

- Pathology

Photocopies of any pertinent pathology reports are required. Group all pathology reports together in chronological order.

- Radiology

Photographs of pertinent x-rays or scans are required. (Actual x-rays are unacceptable.) Date each x-ray or scan in a manner that is easily visible. Photocopies of corresponding reports from the radiologist for each x-ray should be included in this section. Compile this material in chronological order, with reports placed adjacent to the corresponding reproduction of the radiograph.

- Progress Notes—Hospital Progress Records and Office/Clinic Notes

Photocopies of the original progress notes including the patient's history and physical examination, discharge summaries, and all postoperative and post-discharge progress notes, both in the hospital and from the office/clinic records, including the initial consultation. If legibility is a problem, also include a typewritten copy. Copies of physician orders, vital signs, and nursing notes are not necessary and may be included only if they are needed to clarify the patient's course. Organize all notes in chronological order. Separate Hospital notes and Office/Clinic progress notes with divider sheet provided by the Board.

When excessively long hospitalizations resulted in progress note sections of such thickness that they cannot be bound in one case folder, this section may be debrided of nonpertinent notes, bound separately, and brought to the examination. The candidate retains the notes and does not turn them in with the Case Reports. A notation regarding the debriding must appear at the beginning of the progress note section. The candidate will produce this extra material only upon the examiners' request.

- Billing—including CPT Codes

Photocopies of the actual bill(s) submitted to the patient, or a printed copy of bill(s) generated by electronic billing, are required. Delete the actual dollar amount of the fee.

Note: Include a printed copy of the bill for bills that were electronically generated. The printed copy must be accompanied by a signed and notarized statement from the billing company or billing representative stating that this copy represents what was electronically billed to the insurance company or patient.

Candidates who have a computerized billing system and do not have or keep a copy of the Health Insurance Claim Form (HICF) sheets may substitute a computer generated report at the time of examination for inclusion in the presentation of their Case Reports. *Note:* The actual procedure typed out must be included on the billing statement even though this is not a part of the HICF sheet.

Candidates who did not keep a copy of the actual bill submitted to the patient or insurance company, or have misplaced it, may submit a computer generated bill in its place and must include a notarized affidavit from the administrator in charge of billing to attest to the factual representation of the original bill.

If a bill was generated, but it was not sent to the patient, candidates must submit a copy of that bill.

For a cosmetic procedure where no bill is generated, candidates must provide a notarized affidavit to the effect that no bill was sent, and it must be signed by the billing representative.

Report all CPT codes for each procedure in the case list if the candidate was responsible for generating a code to document the procedure performed or for the purpose of third party billing. If coding was not generated for a particular procedure(s), a notarized affidavit, signed by the administrator of the responsible institution or agency, must be submitted to verify that coding or billing was not required.

CPT codes for VA patients and services performed gratis, such as those on an individual in their office, should be coded exactly as any other case.

- Other

Any additional material such as procedures performed on the patient before or after the case collection period may be added here. Do not include debrided material from long hospitalizations here.

Disqualification on Case Reports

If a candidate is disqualified for continuation in the examination process because the case reports are judged unacceptable (for whatever reason) it will not be recorded as a failure but is counted as one of the five opportunities to appear for the Oral Examination. However, because the Board has incurred expenses to provide a candidate with an examination, the examination fee less the processing charge of $700 will be refunded.

Presentation of Case Reports

During the 40-minute examination, candidates must be prepared to defend the choice of operation and to present alternate treatment plans considered. Hospital and office records must clearly identify the candidate as the attending physician and surgeon. However, the candidate need not necessarily be the admitting physician, so long as he/she is clearly the attending plastic surgeon. Cases done by a resident under the candidate's supervision may be chosen by the Board and will be considered in the same way as cases done personally.

The Board regards the Case Reports submitted as important evidence of the candidate's basic ability to carry out plastic surgical procedures and to organize and present information in a succinct and complete fashion. Improper or disorganized preparation of this material will be sufficient cause to disqualify a candidate for continued examination.

Examination Schedule

The Oral Examination will occupy 3 full days. A detailed schedule is included in the Announcement Letter. Candidates are required to be present for each day of the examination at the times listed in the Announcement Letter. Late arrival may result in denial of admission to the examination.

Instructions and Procedures

Candidates will receive specific instructions concerning the examination at the Registration and Orientation Sessions on each morning of the examination. On each examination day, candidates will also be given a schedule showing the time and the room location for the Case Report Session and the two Theory and Practice Sessions of the examination. Failure to appear on time for any session of the examination will lead to a failing grade on that section. Candidates should be outside the examination room 5 minutes before the scheduled time. It is not necessary for candidates to announce their presence. If, however, a candidate has not been invited into the examination room by the examiners by 10 minutes after the scheduled time, candidates should notify the temporary Board office immediately.

The Board has made every effort to assign candidates to examiners whose knowledge of the candidate's background would not bias their evaluation of performance. If a candidate finds that an examiner to whom he/she has been assigned played a role in the candidate's training, is a close friend or relative, is a close professional associate, or has examined the candidate previously, the temporary Board office must be notified immediately. However, unless conflicts are identified in advance of the actual examination, the conduct and grades of that session cannot be contested based on prior contact or knowledge.

Description of the Examination

Each examination session is designed to evaluate the candidate's breadth and depth of knowledge, the ability to apply it in the solution of a wide range of clinical problems, and matters related to ethics. Each session is structured in that the examiners are given a schema to be followed. This approach assures uniformity and prevents duplication. Each of the examiners on each team is expected to pose problems and questions to candidates.

The examination consists of one Case Report Session and two Theory and Practice Sessions.

Oral Examination Examiners

All examiners are diplomates of the ABPS, are active in the practice and/or teaching of plastic surgery, and have been certified by the Board for no less than 5 years. They are respected members of the profession and are known for their surgical knowledge, expertise, and scientific contributions. They have been instructed in the technique and purposes of the examination process. Each team includes a Senior Examiner and a Guest Examiner.

The Case Report and Theory Practice Sessions are considered as one total examination. Candidates will pass or fail on the strength of their combined performance on all portions of the Oral Examination.

At the conclusion of each examination session, candidates may be offered an opportunity to add to earlier answers, modify them, or simply comment on the examination process.

Three teams of two examiners will examine each candidate. All six examiners will give grades and all six grades combined will determine the passing or failing status of each candidate.

The Board is determined that the examination shall be as comprehensive and objective as practical. The intention is that every candidate be provided an equal opportunity to become Board certified. The same standard is applied to each candidate insofar as is possible.

Change of Address

If a candidate's address, as it appears on the Admission Card (white), is incorrect, the corrected or new address must be indicated on the back of the Admission Card (white) in the space provided. This card is required when receiving the Result Letter on the last day of the Oral Examination.

Debriefing Session

On the evening of the last examination day, there will be a voluntary debriefing session, which the Board encourages candidates to attend for the purpose of evaluating the examination.

Distribution of Result Letters to Candidates

Result letters will be distributed after the conclusion of the last session on the third day of the examination. Candidates are required to present the Admission Card (white) or photo identification to the proctors in order to receive their Result Letter. Candidates not present for distribution of the Result Letters will have their letter mailed from the Board office the week following the Examination.

Examination Performance Critique ($200)

Candidates receiving a failing grade who desire information concerning performance on their Oral Examination may request a critique by writing to the Board office. Requests must be received within 30 days of the date on the result letter. Candidates will be responsible for a charge of $200 for information concerning their performance.

Cancellation of Examination

Should the ABPS, in its sole discretion, cancel the Oral Examination, or as a result of events beyond its control be unable to administer the Oral Examination at the appointed date, time, and location, or should ABPS fail to conclude a candidate's Oral Examination, the ABPS is not responsible for any expense the candidate may have incurred in connection with the cancelled Oral Examination, nor for any expense the candidate may incur for any substitute Oral Examination.

Fee Schedule

Processing **$150**

The processing fee of $150 must be submitted with the Request for Evaluation of Training Form and is nonrefundable.

Registration **$500**

The registration fee of $500 must be submitted with the Application for Examination and Certification Form and is nonrefundable.

Written Examination **$900**

The Written Examination fee of $900 is a separate fee in addition to the Registration Fee of $500 submitted with the Application for Examination and Certification Form. This Examination fee of $900 must be submitted when the Reply Card (green) requesting examination is returned to the Board office. The fee for the Written Examination must accompany the Reply Card in order for the candidate to be scheduled for the examination.

Written Examination and Registration Late Penalty Fees **$500**

Oral Examination **$1,500 (Total amount)**

Case List Review Fee **$500**

The Review Fee of $500 must be enclosed with the case list to provide for review and selection of cases for preparation as Case Reports. This fee is nonrefundable.

Oral Examination Fee **$1,000**

The balance of the examination fee of $1,000 must be submitted with the Reply Card (green) in order to be scheduled for the examination.

Oral Examination Late Penalty Fee **$700**

Written and Oral Examination Withdrawal Fee **$700**

A withdrawal fee of $700 will be deducted from the Written or Oral Examination Fee for candidates who provide written notice of withdrawal at least 30 days before the date of the examination. Candidates who withdraw from the examination less than 30 days before the date of the examination will forfeit the entire examination fee.

Credentialing Fee **$150**

A Crendentialing Fee of $150 must be submitted with requests for special consideration by the Board for the Credentials and Requirements Committee.

Certificate Fee **$100**

A new Certificate fee of $100 must be submitted to the Board with all requests for each additional certificate by Diplomates.

Verification of Status Fee **$25**

A Verification Fee of $25 is required from all institutions and/or organizations who submit more than three requests within 1 month for written verification on the status of individuals. The $25 fee applies to each additional request over and above three in 1 month.

Checks Returned for Insufficient Funds **$50**

A charge of $50 is applicable whenever a check received in payment of a fee is returned to the Board office from the bank for nonpayment due to insufficient funds. This charge must be included with the original fee when a new check is resubmitted to the Board.

Fees must be submitted in United States currency only. Foreign currencies, including Canadian, are unacceptable.

Fees are subject to change by the Board. The fee schedule applicable to current examinations will apply regardless of when a candidate is approved for admission to the examination process.

The Board is a nonprofit organization, and the fees of candidates are used solely for defraying the actual expenses of the Board. The directors of the Board serve without remuneration. Because of the limited number of plastic surgeons certified by this Board, it may be necessary for the Board to request a voluntary annual contribution from its diplomates.

Repeat Examination Fee

Fees for repeat examinations are the same as for the current original examinations.

Refunds

For the Written Examination, a refund of the examination fee (less a processing charge of $700) will be granted provided the candidate submits a written request for withdrawal received in the Board office at least 30 calendar days prior to the date of the examination.

For the Oral Examination, a refund of the examination fee (less a processing charge of $700) will be granted provided the candidate submits a written request for withdrawal received in the Board office at least 30 calendar days prior to the date of the examination.

For either the Written or Oral Examination, candidates who notify the Board office in writing less than 30 calendar days prior to the examination date of their intent to withdraw, or who fail to appear for examination, will forfeit the entire examination fee. The Board may waive this rule only if the circumstances warrant.

Special Situations

Appeals Policy

The Board has established a policy relative to resolution of questions or disagreements regarding its decisions on admissibility to examination; the form, content, administration, or results of the Written Examination; the administration of the Oral Examination; and the revocation of certificates. If an individual has a concern in any of these areas, it should be expressed in writing to the Board office, and a copy of the Appeals Policy will be sent to that individual.

Examination of Candidates with Disabilities

The ABPS has established a policy regarding examination of candidates with disabilities. If a candidate is requesting an accommodation based on a disability, the request should be expressed in writing to the Board office when submitting the Application for Examination and Certification Form. A copy of the policy regarding Examination of Candidates with Disabilities will be sent to that candidate. The ABPS complies with the Americans with Disabilities Act (ADA) and will provide reasonable accommodations to candidates with proven disabilities.

All materials submitted to document a disability must be received in the Board office in a timely fashion but no later than the deadline for all other documents required for admission to the examination for which accommodation is sought.

Examination Irregularities

The validity of scores on the Board's examinations is protected by every means available. The Board will not report a score which it has determined to be invalid, ie, which does not represent a reasonable assessment of the candidate's knowledge or competence sampled by the examination. The performance of all candidates is monitored and may be analyzed for the purposes of detecting invalid scores.

The Written Examination is supervised by proctors to ensure that the examination is properly conducted. If evidence by observation or analysis suggests that a candidate's scores may be invalid because of irregular behavior, the Board will withhold those scores pending further investigation and the affected candidate will be notified.

Examples of irregularities affecting the validity of scores would include (but not be limited to) the following: 1) using notes; 2) sharing information or discussing the examination in progress; 3) copying answers from another candidate; 4) permitting one's answers to be copied; or 5) unauthorized possession, reproduction, or disclosure of examination questions or other specific information regarding the content of the examination, before, during, or after the examination.

In such circumstances, upon analysis of all available information, the Board will make a determination as to the validity of the scores in question. If the Board determines that the scores are invalid, it will not release them, and notification of that determination may be made to legitimately interested third parties.

Candidates or other persons who are directly implicated in an irregularity are subject to additional sanctions. For example, the Board may bar such persons permanently from all future examinations, terminate a candidate's participation in an ongoing examination, invalidate the results of the candidate's examination, and withhold or revoke a certificate or take other appropriate action. Candidates or other persons subject to additional sanctions will be provided with a written notice of the charges and an opportunity to respond to such charges in accordance with the reconsideration and appeal procedure established by the Board.

Substance Abuse or Chemical Dependency

Candidates with a history of abuse of a controlled substance or chemical dependency will not be admitted to any examination unless they present evidence satisfactory to the Board that they have successfully completed the program of treatment prescribed for their condition and the Board is satisfied that they are currently free of such substance abuse or chemical dependency.

Certification

After candidates have met the requirements for admissibility and passed the examinations, the Board will issue certificates attesting to their qualifications in plastic surgery. A surgeon granted certification by the Board is known as a diplomate of the Board.

It shall be the prerogative of the Board to determine the fitness, professionally and ethically, of any candidate for a certificate, and the Board, for cause, may defer or deny certification to any candidate.

Certificates

Certificates issued by the Board shall be in such form as the Directors may from time to time determine. Certificates are signed by the chair, vice-chair, and secretary-treasurer of the Board and shall have placed upon them the official seal of the Board.

Certificates of the Board shall state that the holder has met the requirements of the Board and is certified by the Board as a medical specialist in plastic surgery and is entitled to be known as a "Diplomate of the American Board of Plastic Surgery, Inc." The names of all diplomates will be submitted to the American Board of Medical Specialties (ABMS) for publication in its directory. Diplomates should notify the Board in advance if they do not wish to be listed.

Additional certificates are available upon written request. A fee of $100 for each certificate ordered should be included with the request. The diplomate's name should be listed, as it should appear on the certificate.

Recertification Examination

The Recertification Examination will be first offered in the year 2002. Effective 1995, certificates issued by the Board are dated and will be valid for 10 years. Revalidation will be accomplished by the Board's recertification process. Certificates issued prior to 1995 are valid indefinitely. A diplomate may take the recertification examination 3 years prior to the diplomate's original expiration date. The date of recertification will be 10 years from the date of the diplomate's original expiration date.

Revocation

Any certificate issued by the Board shall be subject to revocation at any time that the Board determines that a diplomate was not properly qualified to receive it.

Each certificate issued by the Board shall be subject to revocation if the diplomate so certified has made any misstatement of material fact, or has failed to make any statement of material fact, in his or her application for such certificate or in any other statement or representation to the Board or its representatives, or has otherwise acquired the certificate by deception. Upon revocation, the certificate shall be returned to the Board.

The Board shall have the jurisdiction and right to determine whether or not the information placed before it is sufficient to constitute grounds for the revocation of any certificate. The diplomate will be provided with a copy of the appeals policy of the Board, and this policy will be observed in pursuing resolution of the problem.

Certification of Added Qualifications in Surgery of the Hand (CAQSH) and CAQSH Recertification

The Board offers an examination for Certification and Recertification of Added Qualifications in Surgery of the Hand (CAQSH). The examination is described in a separate CAQSH *Booklet of Information* that may be obtained from the Board office upon request.

Foreign Certificates

A physician holding a foreign certificate issued by the Board between 1960 and 1973 must relinquish the certificate to the Board in the event that the individual returns to the United States for the purpose of practicing plastic surgery. A foreign certificate is not valid in the United States. Such individuals may apply for examination and certification in the manner described herein.

Inquiries as to Status

The Board does not consider a candidate's record to be in the public domain. When an inquiry is received by the Board regarding a candidate's status with the Board, a general, but factual, statement is provided which indicates that candidate's status within the process of certification. The Board provides this information only to individuals, organizations, and institutions with a reasonably valid "need to know" for professional reasons. Only written requests for verification of a candidate's status during the process of certification are accepted.

A charge of $25 will apply to all institutions and/or organizations that submit more than three requests within 1 month, for written information on the status of individuals. The $25 fee will apply to each additional request received over and above the allocated number of three requests per month.

A candidate who has fulfilled the established prerequisite and requisite training requirements and has submitted an Application for Examination and Certification Form that has been approved and who is currently admissible to the examination process of the ABPS may use the term "Board admissible," but only for such length of time as such candidate is still admissible.

The Directors may adopt such further rules and regulations governing requirements, examinations, and issuance and revocation of certification as they may from time to time determine.

American Board of Preventive Medicine

9950 W Lawrence Ave/Ste 106
Schiller Park, IL 60176
847 671-1750
847 671-1751 Fax
E-mail: abpm@abprevmed.org
Internet: http://www.abprevmed.org

Requirements for Admission to Examinations

Each applicant for a certificate in aerospace medicine, occupational medicine, or public health and general preventive medicine must meet certain requirements to be admitted to the certifying examination. Such requirements are determined by the American Board of Preventive Medicine (ABPM).

Approval for admission to the examination can only be established after the review of a complete application by the full Board. No individual member of the Board is authorized to give an opinion on the admissibility of candidates, nor does the Board do preliminary credential reviews.

For the information of applicants, such requirements are summarized below. An applicant worksheet is available from the ABPM website at http://www.abprevmed.org for use in comparing the ABPM requirements to an applicant's training and experience.

General Requirements

1. *Medical School:* Graduation from a medical school in the United States which at the time of the applicant's graduation was accredited by the Liaison Committee on Medical Education, a school of osteopathic medicine approved by the American Osteopathic Association, an accredited medical school in Canada, or a medical school located outside the United States and Canada that is deemed satisfactory to the Board.

2. *Current License(s)*: Unrestricted and currently valid license(s) to practice medicine in a state, the District of Columbia, or a territory, commonwealth, or possession of the United States or province of Canada. No license may be restricted, revoked, or suspended or currently under such notice.
3. *Clinical Year:* A year of supervised postgraduate clinical training provided as part of a graduate medical education program accredited by the Accreditation Council for Graduate Medical Education (ACGME). Clinical training accredited by the Royal College of Physicians and Surgeons of Canada or the College of Family Physicians of Canada is also acceptable. The training must include at least 6 months of direct patient care comprising ambulatory and inpatient experience.
4. *Academic Year:* Successful completion of a course of graduate academic study and award of a Master of Public Health or equivalent masters degree, the course content of which shall include biostatistics, epidemiology, health services management and administration, and environmental health.
5. *Practicum Year:* Residency practicum of not less than 1 year that is accredited by the ACGME in the specialty area for which certification is being sought and that shall have provided supervised experience in the practice of that specialty area of preventive medicine and planned instruction, observation, and active participation in a comprehensive organized program.
6. *Current Practice:* The applicant must have been engaged in essentially full-time training for, or practice in, the specialty area for which certification is being sought for at least 2 of the 5 years preceding application for certification.

Special Requirements in Aerospace Medicine

1. A period of not less than 1 year of supervised training and instruction, accredited by the ACGME in the specialty area of aerospace medicine, is required. (See 5 under "General Requirements," above.)
2. The applicant must have been engaged in training for, or the practice of, aerospace medicine for at least 2 of the 5 years preceding application for certification. (See 6 under "General Requirements," above.)

Special Requirements in Occupational Medicine

1. A period of not less than 1 year of supervised training and instruction, accredited by the ACGME in the specialty area of occupational medicine, is required. (See 5 under "General Requirements," above.)
2. The applicant must have been engaged in training for, or the practice of, occupational medicine for at least 2 of the 5 years preceding application for certification. (See 6 under "General Requirements," above.)

Special Requirements in Public Health and General Preventive Medicine

1. A period of not less than 1 year of supervised training and instruction, accredited by the ACGME in the specialty area of public health and/or general preventive medicine, is required. (See 5 under "General Requirements," above.)
2. The applicant must have been engaged in training for, or the practice of, public health and general preventive medicine for at least 2 of the 5 years preceding application for certification. (See 6 under "General Requirements," above.)

Equivalencies for Accredited Training

Persons graduating from a school of medicine or school of osteopathic medicine prior to January 1, 1984, who have not formally completed all of the components previously described may be considered for admission to the examination if their training and experience are judged by the Board to provide suitable equivalency for formal training.

The Board will consider granting equivalency credit toward satisfying training requirements for such factors as:

1. Teaching or completion of three-credit hour, postgraduate-level academic course work in each of the four core areas: epidemiology, biostatistics, health services management and administration, and environmental health; and
2. Periods of full-time practice, research, or teaching in the specialty area of preventive medicine in which certification is sought. A total of 8 years of full-time practice is required if no other specialty certification is held, but may be reduced to 6 years if certification is held in another specialty recognized by the American Board of Medical Specialties (ABMS). For those with an MPH or equivalent masters degree but no practicum year, a period of 4 years of full-time practice is required in the specialty area of preventive medicine for which certification is being sought, a period that can be reduced to 3 years if other ABMS specialty certification is held.

Each applicant is considered individually by the Board in accordance with the existing guidelines. An applicant worksheet is available from the ABPM web site at http://www.abprevmed.org for use in comparing the ABPM requirements to an applicant's training and experience. Practice time needed for the equivalency pathway is summarized on this worksheet. Applications must be received by June 1 of each year. Requirements must be completed by August 1 of the year in which the applicant wishes to sit for the examination.

Persons graduating from a school of medicine or school of osteopathic medicine after January 1, 1984, will be admissible to the examination only after completing ACGME-accredited residency training in preventive medicine. No equivalency pathways will be considered for such graduates.

Special Pathway for ABPM Diplomates

Diplomates of ABPM who have graduated from medical school after January 1, 1984, may request consideration through a special pathway. In order to qualify for this special pathway, applicants must have completed an ACGME-accredited residency in a specialty area of preventive medicine, been certified in that specialty area, be applying for certification by ABPM in an additional preventive medicine specialty area, and have sufficient practice time to meet the requirements. A total of 2 years of essentially full-time practice is required in the specialty area for which the additional certification is sought. In addition, the applicant must have been engaged in essentially full-time training for, or practice in, the specialty area for which the second certification is being sought for at least 2 of the last 5 years.

Internet Web Site

http://www.abprevmed.org

The ABPM has a web site on the internet that includes the latest version of the application and other publications. Please refer to this site for current information about the ABPM.

Application

Individuals seeking to apply for admission to the examination should write to the executive director of the Board for application forms, or the application may be downloaded from the ABPM web site on the internet (see above).

Examination

The examination is a 1-day written examination given in the late fall of each year. It is a multiple-choice examination, with the morning portion covering the core knowledge of preventive medicine and the afternoon portion covering aerospace medicine, occupational medicine, or public health and general preventive medicine.

Applicants requiring special examination accommodations due to a disability should contact the Board office for assistance at least 1 month prior to the examination.

Reapplication and Reexamination

An applicant approved for admission to the examination who does not take the examination, or who fails to pass the examination within the 3-year approval period, is required to file a new application and pay a new application fee.

Applicants not approved for admission to the examination may request reconsideration of their applications on the basis of new or additional information within 2 years of the filing date of the original application, with payment of the re-review fee.

Candidates not passing the examination may, upon timely registration and payment of appropriate fee, be admitted to reexamination during their approval period.

A candidate who has failed the examination on two or more occasions may be required to have additional training, in accordance with recommendations from the full Board, before being admitted to further examination.

Multiple Certification

An individual may apply sequentially for admission to examination in more than one specialty area of preventive medicine. Applicants may not apply in more than one specialty area in a given year. An applicant must fulfill the individual requirements of each specialty area in which application is made and cannot double-count the same periods for practice time.

Certification

Upon satisfactory completion of the examination, a certificate will be issued stating that the applicant has been found to possess special knowledge in the specified specialty area of preventive medicine. The certificate will be signed by the officers of the Board and will have the seal of the Board affixed. Each certificate remains the property of the Board, but the person to whom it is issued is entitled to its possession unless it is revoked.

Any certificate issued by the Board may be revoked if evidence, satisfactory to the Board, is presented that the applicant was not eligible to receive it at the time of issuance, that any pertinent fact had been misstated, misrepresented, or concealed, or that any license to practice medicine has been suspended or revoked. *Note:* The issuance of a certificate to a person does not constitute membership on the Board.

Time-Limited Certificates

Note: By action of the Board in August 1994, ABPM now issues 10-year, time-limited certificates. The first time-limited certificates were issued in 1998 to candidates who passed the certifying examination given in November 1997.

Notice of Certification

The examination results, without individual identifiers, are reviewed by the full Board during its January meeting. Final determination of candidates' certification status is made at that time.

Candidates who have taken the examination may expect to be notified of results by mail within 3 months after taking the examination.

Fees

The members of the Board serve without compensation. Fees are based on the actual expenses incurred in review of applications; examination development, administration, and scoring; and office administration.

A nonrefundable application fee of $300* is required if the applicant holds an MPH or equivalent masters degree and has completed an ACGME-accredited residency in the specialty area of preventive medicine in which certification is sought.

A nonrefundable application fee of $550* is required if the applicant is applying through the equivalency pathway.

A nonrefundable application fee of $450* is required if the applicant is applying through the special pathway for ABPM diplomates.

A nonrefundable re-review fee of $100* is required to reactivate an application within 2 years of the original review.

The examination fee of $1,250* is due 45 days prior to the examination. The examination fee is nonrefundable within 45 days of the examination.

* *Note:* All fees are reviewed annually and are subject to change at the direction of the Board.

Please contact the Board office for the current fee schedule.

Listing of Individuals Certified

A list, current to the date of publication, of persons to whom certificates have been issued by the Board may be found in *The Official ABMS Directory of Board Certified Medical Specialists.*

Reporting of Changes of Address

Once certified, physicians should notify the following offices of any changes of address:

1. The American Board of Preventive Medicine, Inc
2. The Physician Biographic Records Department, American Medical Association, 515 North State Street, Chicago, IL 60610, the office that maintains a master file of all physicians in the US
3. Marquis Who's Who, 121 Chanlon Road, New Providence, NJ 07974, publisher of *The Official ABMS Directory of Board Certified Medical Specialists*

Important Dates

April 15: Deadline for receipt of action plans from candidates failing examinations on two or more occasions.

June 1: Deadline for completed application forms, application fees, and reapplication requests to be received in the Board office for the November examination.

July 15: Deadline for receipt of additional information not included with the June 1 application. Deadline for receipt of re-review requests and fees.

August 1: Deadline for completion of requirements to sit for the November examination.

August: Meeting of the Board to determine admissibility of applicants to November examination. Letters of notification of admissibility for November examination are mailed to candidates after the August Board meeting. Notification is not given by telephone.

September/October: Deadline for examination fee 45 days prior to the examination. Date varies from year to year and is stated in the letter of admissibility.

November: Annual 1-day written examination in Chicago, Illinois. For the next two years the dates are November 8, 1999, and November 13, 2000. Future examination dates are not available at this time.

January: Meeting of the Board to determine the pass/non-pass score for the previous November examination.

February: Results of November certifying examination are mailed to candidates after the January Board meeting. Notification is not given by telephone.

American Board of Psychiatry and Neurology

500 Lake Cook Rd/Ste 335
Deerfield, IL 60015
847 945-7900
847 945-1146 Fax
Internet: http://www.abpn.com

(Please note that this is not an official document of the American Board of Psychiatry and Neurology. The Board cannot accept responsibility for errors made in the printing of this material. Please contact the Board's executive office for official policies and procedures of the board.)

Throughout this section, the American Board of Psychiatry and Neurology may be referred to as the "Board" or as "ABPN."

The information in the ABPN section is effective for the November 3, 1999, Part I examination only. Contact the Board office for the most current information.

Deadlines for the November 3, 1999, Part I Exam

Part I Application	February 1, 1999
Part I Late Application	March 1, 1999
Completion of residency training	June 30, 1999
Written confirmation of completion of residency training	July 15, 1999
Part I Reexamination Fee	Board will notify applicant

(Contact the Board office if you have not received a billing statement by February 15, 2000)

Part I Reexamination Late Fee	30 days after reexamination fee deadline

Fee Schedule (Effective February 1999)

Part I Application Fee	$425
Part I Examination Fee	$450
Part I Late Application Fee *(in addition to the above)*	$250
Part I Reexamination Fee	$450
Part I Reexamination Late Application Fee *(in addition to the above)*	$75
Part II Examination Fee	$1,025
Psychiatry Part II Reexamination Fee	$1,025
Neurology/Child Neurology Part II Reexamination Fee:	
One section	$700
Two or three sections	$1,025
Application/Licensure Appeal Fee	$350
Part I Appeal Fee	$300
Part II Feedback Fee	$100
Part II Appeal Fee	Same as reexamination fee *(see above)*
Duplicate certificate fee	$50
Returned check charge	$50

All fees must be submitted in US currency. The ABPN reserves the right to revise fee schedules.

I. General Information

A. Certificates

The Board currently issues the following eight types of certificates:
1. Psychiatry
2. Neurology
3. Neurology with special qualification in child neurology
4. Child and adolescent psychiatry
5. Geriatric psychiatry
6. Clinical neurophysiology
7. Addiction psychiatry
8. Forensic psychiatry

In addition, the Board will begin issuing certificates in pain management in the year 2000.

An applicant may be certified in more than one area and will receive a separate certificate for each area in which he or she qualifies. Each certificate shall be in such form and for such period of time as may be specified by the Board.

B. Recertification

As of October 1, 1994, all individuals achieving Board certification by the American Board of Psychiatry and Neurology, Inc, are issued 10-year, time-limited certificates. Certificates issued in the subspecialties of geriatric psychiatry, clinical neurophysiology, addiction psychiatry, and forensic psychiatry, including those issued prior to October 1, 1994, are 10-year, time-limited certificates.

C. Revocation of Certificates

The Board shall have authority to revoke any certificate issued by it or to place a certificate holder on probation for a fixed or indefinite period of time if (1) the certificate was issued contrary to, or in violation of, the bylaws or any rule or regulation of the Board, or (2) the person to whom the certificate was issued made any material misstatement or omission of fact to the Board in his or her application or otherwise.

Certification shall continue in force only so long as the holder has an unlimited license to practice medicine in a state, commonwealth, territory, or possession of the United States or province of Canada. A full and unrestricted medical license must be maintained even if a physician is out of the country for extended periods of time. Restrictions include but are not limited to conditions, contingencies, probation, and stipulated agreements. It is the responsibility of the candidate/diplomate to inform the Board immediately upon a change in licensure status.

D. Irregular Behavior Including Unethical Behavior of Candidates

The Board believes that the ethics of candidates for certification are of concern. The following rules apply:
1. Falsification of credentials will be cause for the Board's refusal to admit a candidate to examination for up to 5 years.
2. The Board will consider legal action against anyone who forges an ABPN certificate, copies ABPN examinations or otherwise uses them in conflict with copyright laws, or in any other way violates

the legal prerogatives of the Board. Such activities will also be cause for the Board's refusal to admit a candidate to examination for up to 5 years.

3. Scores on the Part I examination may be invalidated for reasons of irregular behavior. Statistical analyses may be used to confirm suspected cheating. If an examination score is invalidated, the candidate may submit a written appeal within 30 days of notice of invalidation. An appeal fee of $300 must accompany the written appeal. The Committee to Review Appeals will review the materials and make a recommendation to the Board. The Board will review the materials and make a decision that, in all cases, will be final and binding on the Board and on the candidate. All correspondence or other materials should be sent to the Board office. If an examination score is invalidated because of irregular behavior, the Board will not consider the candidate for examination for a period of up to 5 years, depending on the irregular behavior. A repeat application and Part I examination fee will be required.
4. Irregular behavior on the Part II examination may be considered sufficient reason to invalidate a candidate's score. If the examination score is invalidated, the candidate may submit a written appeal within 30 days of notice of invalidation. An appeal fee of $300 must accompany the written appeal. The Committee on Irregular Behavior will review the materials and make a recommendation to the Board. The Board will review the materials and make a decision that, in all cases, will be final and binding on the Board and on the candidate. All correspondence or other materials should be sent to the Board office. If an examination score is invalidated because of irregular behavior, the Board will not consider the candidate for examination for a period of up to 5 years, depending on the irregular behavior. A repeat Part II application and Part II examination fee will be required.
5. "Irregular behavior" shall include, but not be limited to, the following conduct: (a) copying of answers from another candidate's examination; (b) knowingly permitting another candidate to copy one's answers on an examination; (c) unauthorized possession, reproduction, or disclosure (via oral, written, or electronic media) of examination materials or content, at any time; (d) use of audio equipment to record any part of the Part II examination; (e) offering any financial or other benefit to any director, officer, employee, proctor, diplomate, or other agent or representative of the Board in return for any right, privilege, or benefit that is not granted by the Board to other similarly situated candidates or persons; (f) not complying with proctors' or examiners' instructions; (g) disregarding time limits; and (h) any other form of disruptive behavior.
6. Notification of the Board's action may be sent to legitimately interested third parties, including the American Medical Association, state medical societies, medical licensing boards, and appropriate specialty societies.

E. Board Eligibility

The ABPN, in accordance with the policy of the American Board of Medical Specialties (ABMS), does not recognize or use the term "Board eligible" and does not issue statements concerning "Board eligibility." The Board informs an applicant of admissibility to examination only when the applicant has an active, approved application on file in the Board office.

F. Conflict of Interest

In order to maintain the confidence of the public and the medical profession in the integrity of the Board, it is important for those doing its work to avoid certain activities that could provide the opportunity for an actual conflict of interest or the appearance thereof. A conflict of interest is defined as an instance wherein a competing outside activity or holding could influence or appear to influence the Board's activities in the area of policy development, evaluation of training programs, or examination development. Examples of such competing outside interests are compensated direct employment, paid advisory or consultant positions, significant personal investments, or other affiliations as an officer and/or director in a pharmaceutical or medical supply company.

As an alternative to regulating investment or employment, the Board has chosen to manage matters related to the appearance of a conflict of interest by encouraging disclosure of significant financial interests or relationships and abstention from participation in decision making related to a matter that could give rise to a conflict of interest (due to a material financial interest or relationship).

Annually, Board members, subspecialty committee members, test committee members, written examination proctors, the Executive Vice President, and staff members of the Board are required to complete a form disclosing the following general information:

1. License restrictions to practice medicine
2. Participation in board review courses or publication of materials in any media format, including the Internet, regarding board review in psychiatry or neurology
3. Significant financial holdings in any pharmaceutical or medical supply company
4. An affiliation in the capacity of trustee, officer, director, or other major capacity with any pharmaceutical or medical supply company
5. Any other affiliations that would present a potential or apparent conflict of interest or commitment

Any individual who participates in any review course that is publicized as being a Board review course, or in any course that could be construed as a Board review course, or who has edited or provided written or audiovisual materials for publications identified as preparation for Board examinations, or who copies, reproduces, or discloses (via oral, written, or electronic media) examination materials or content should not participate as an examiner in any Part II or child and adolescent psychiatry examination, or as a member of any Board committee, for at least 12 months subsequent to the course or publication of any written or audiovisual materials.

II. Requirements for Admission to Examination

A. General Requirements for All Applicants

In order to be eligible for examination, an applicant must:

1. Be a graduate of an accredited medical school in the United States or Canada or of an international medical school listed by the World Health Organization.
2. Have an *unlimited license* to practice medicine in a state, commonwealth, territory, or possession of the United States or province of Canada. Applicants are required to submit a copy of their unlimited licenses with their Part I applications. Any candidate submitting a temporary (education or training) license at the time of application for Part I will be required to submit a copy of his/her current unlimited license, as described above, no later than December 31 of the year in which the candidate passed the Part I examination.

   Candidates in possession of restricted, suspended, or revoked licenses in any state will not be scheduled for examination. Restrictions include but are not limited to conditions, contingencies, probation, and stipulated agreements.
3. Have satisfactorily completed the Board's specialized training requirements in psychiatry, neurology, neurology with special qualification in child neurology, or any of its subspecialties. Training requirements for the primary specialties are explained in the sections that follow.
4. Submit a completed official application form including all required attachments and the appropriate application and exami-

nation fees by the specified deadline. *(See the beginning of the ABPN section for the fee schedule and application deadlines. See Section III for a complete description of the application process.)*

B. General Training Requirements

References to "residency" refer to entry at the graduate year 2 level unless otherwise stated. Residency training must be in the specialty in which the applicant seeks certification, except for residents who are in an approved combined training program. *(See Section VI.D for more information about combined training programs.)*

Training programs approved by the Residency Review Committees and accredited by the Accreditation Council for Graduate Medical Education (ACGME) can be found in the current edition of the *Graduate Medical Education Directory* published by the American Medical Association. This directory includes the "Essentials of Accredited Residencies in Graduate Medical Education: Institutional and Program Requirements."

To ensure continuity of training, the Board requires that 2 of the 3 years of residency training, excluding the GY1, be spent in a single program. Training may be completed on a part-time basis, provided that it is no less than half-time, and credit will not be given for less than 1-year blocks of training except under special circumstances, which must be approved by the ABPN Credentials Committee. In such cases, it is the responsibility of the applicant to provide detailed documentation from the respective training directors outlining training content, duties, and responsibilities. Each case will be considered on an individual basis.

Training programs may develop individual leave or vacation time for residents in accordance with the overall institutional policy. Leave or vacation time may not be utilized to reduce the total amount of required residency training or to make up deficiencies in training.

C. Psychiatry: Specific Training Requirements

Unless otherwise specified (see sections on Canadian and other international training below), all training must be completed in programs accredited by the ACGME).

An applicant seeking admission to examination for certification in psychiatry must have satisfactorily completed an ACGME-accredited GY1 *(see below)* and 3 full years of postgraduate, specialized residency training in a psychiatry program accredited by the ACGME. See the sections below for information regarding Canadian and other international training requirements. Different requirements apply for applicants who began training in psychiatry prior to 1986. These candidates should call the Board office if they have any questions.

The following two patterns of training are acceptable:

1. *Three-year psychiatry residency program*
   A broad-based clinical year of ACGME-accredited training in internal medicine, family practice, or pediatrics; or an ACGME-accredited transitional year program that included a minimum of 4 months of primary care; or an ACGME-accredited residency in a clinical specialty requiring comprehensive and continuous patient care.
   and
   Three full years of postgraduate, specialized residency training in a psychiatry program accredited by the ACGME.
   or
2. *Four-year psychiatry residency program*
   Four years of training in an ACGME-accredited program in psychiatry is acceptable providing that no fewer than 4 months during one of the years of training was spent in an approved program in which the resident had direct, supervised responsibility for the general medical care of children and/or adults.

Canadian training programs

Applicants who entered a Canadian residency program on or after July 1, 1997, will not be granted training credit. Applicants entering Canadian residency training before July 1, 1997, may be granted training credit if their residency training was completed in a Canadian program accredited by the Royal College of Physicians and Surgeons of Canada (RCPSC). Applicants entering Canadian residency training before July 1, 1986, should contact the Board office for program requirements.

Effective January 1, 1994, physicians who trained in accredited programs in Canada must have completed an approved GY1 as described in section II.C.1 plus 4 years of postgraduate, specialized residency training in a psychiatry program accredited by the RCPSC.

Other international training

Physicians entering psychiatry residency training on or after July 1, 1997, will not be granted credit for international training. Physicians entering psychiatry residency training prior to July 1, 1997, may be granted credit for international training *only* if they:

1. Achieve a national certificate accepted by the ABPN by the year 2005. The only certificates accepted by the ABPN are MRCPsych, FRANZCP, FF Psych (SA), and Israel's Specialty Certification of the Scientific Council of the Israel Medical Association. If a physician's training was not completed in its entirety (internship and residency training) in the country issuing the certificate, the physician must complete an additional year of approved primary care training in the United States.
   and
2. Initiate the ABPN certification process by the year 2007.

Physicians who entered residency training in the United Kingdom prior to July 1, 1986, should contact the Board office for training credit information.

D. Neurology: Specific Training Requirements

Unless otherwise specified (see sections on Canadian and other international training below), all training must be completed in programs accredited by the ACGME.

An applicant seeking admission to examination for certification in neurology must have satisfactorily completed an ACGME-accredited GY1 *(see below)* and 3 full years of postgraduate, specialized residency training in a neurology program accredited by the ACGME. See the sections below for information regarding Canadian and other international training requirements. Different requirements apply for applicants who began training in neurology prior to 1991. These candidates should call the Board office if they have any questions.

Two patterns of training are acceptable.

1. *Three-year neurology residency program*
   A full year of ACGME-accredited training in internal medicine, or as an acceptable alternative, a full year in an ACGME-accredited program in which a minimum of 6 months of training must be in internal medicine, the details of which must be documented by the training director. The composition of these 6 months *cannot* include rotations in neurology or emergency medicine. To ensure that these 6 months constitute a high quality experience, they should emphasize progressive responsibility for the resident. At least 2 of the additional 6 months must be spent in internal medicine, pediatrics, and/or emergency medicine. No more than 2 of the remaining 4 months may be spent in neurology.
   and
   Three full years of postgraduate, specialized residency training in a neurology program accredited by the ACGME.
   or
2. *Four-year neurology residency training*
   Four years of training in a neurology residency program accredited by the ACGME.

Canadian training programs
Applicants who entered a Canadian residency program on or after July 1, 1997, will not be granted training credit. Applicants entering Canadian residency training before July 1, 1997, may be granted training credit if their residency training was completed in a Canadian program accredited by the RCPSC.

Effective January 1, 1994, physicians who trained in accredited programs in Canada must have successfully completed an approved GY1 as described in section II.D.1 plus *4* years of postgraduate, specialized residency training in a neurology program accredited by the RCPSC.

Other international training
Physicians entering neurology residency training on or after July 1, 1997, will not be granted credit for international training. Physicians entering neurology residency training prior to July 1, 1997, may be granted GY1 credit for training completed in an international program *only* if they:

1. Achieve a national certificate accepted by the ABPN in internal medicine by the year 2005. The only internal medicine certificates accepted by the ABPN are MRCP(UK), MRACP, FCP, and MRCP(I).
 and
2. Initiate the ABPN certification process by the year 2007.

E. Neurology With Special Qualification in Child Neurology: Specific Training Requirements

Proper preparation for the practice of child neurology requires that the practitioner be a qualified neurologist who has had additional training in pediatrics and child neurology. To qualify for this certificate a different type of preparation and certifying examination are required. The same diploma will be used, the only difference being that instead of certifying qualification in "neurology," it certifies qualification in "neurology with special qualification in child neurology."

Unless otherwise specified (see sections on Canadian and Other international training, below), all training must be completed in programs accredited by the ACGME. Different requirements apply for applicants who began training in child neurology prior to 1991. These candidates should call the Board office if they have any questions.

Three patterns of training are acceptable for 2 of the 5 years of training.

1. *General pediatrics*
 The usual pathway is 2 years of training in general pediatrics in an ACGME-accredited program. This is the only pathway that allows the applicant admission for examination by both the American Board of Pediatrics and the American Board of Psychiatry and Neurology.
 or
2. *General pediatrics/basic neurosciences research*
 One year of training in general pediatrics in an ACGME-accredited program and 1 year of research in the basic neurosciences. The basic neurosciences pathway was created as an alternative track for residents who are planning a research career in academic child neurology. The year of basic neurosciences must provide training in a research discipline related to child neurology and is intended to increase the trainee's knowledge base and competitiveness for federal and nonfederal grant support. The trainee must make at least an 80% time commitment to basic neurosciences during this year of training.
 For the purpose of this training track, basic neurosciences is defined as laboratory research related to the cellular or molecular basis of neurologic diseases. Examples of relevant basic disciplines include molecular neurogenetics, neurochemistry, neuropharmacology, neurophysiology, neuroanatomy, neuroimmunology, developmental neurobiology, biophysics, and cell biology.
 This track of training must be approved by the Board prior to completion of the 5 years of training.
 or
3. *General pediatrics/internal medicine*
 One year of training in general pediatrics and 1 year of training in internal medicine in ACGME-accredited programs. An acceptable alternative to the 1 year of internal medicine is a full year of ACGME-accredited training that includes a minimum of 6 months of internal medicine, the details of which must be documented by the training director. The composition of these 6 months *cannot* include rotations in neurology, pediatrics, or emergency medicine. To ensure that these 6 months constitute a high quality experience, they should emphasize progressive responsibility for the resident. At least 2 of the additional 6 months must be spent in internal medicine, pediatrics, and/or emergency medicine. No more than 2 of the remaining 4 months may be spent in neurology.
 and

In addition, all candidates will be required to complete 3 full years of postgraduate, specialized residency training in a child neurology program accredited by the ACGME.

Canadian training programs
Applicants who entered a Canadian residency program on or after July 1, 1998, will not be granted training credit. Applicants entering Canadian residency training before July 1, 1998, may be granted training credit if their residency training was completed in a Canadian program accredited by the RCPSC.

Other international training
Physicians entering child neurology residency training on or after July 1, 1998, will not be granted credit for international training. Physicians entering child neurology residency training prior to July 1, 1998, may be granted up to 2 years of general pediatrics and/or 1 year of internal medicine credit for training completed in an international program *only* if they:

1. Achieve a national certificate accepted by the ABPN in pediatrics and/or internal medicine by the year 2005. The only certificates accepted by the ABPN for pediatrics and/or internal medicine are MRCP(UK), MRACP, FCP(SA), and MRCP(I).
 and
2. Initiate the ABPN certification process by the year 2007.

III. Application for Certification

A. General Information

A physician who wishes to be examined by the Board shall complete, sign, and file with the Executive Vice President an application on the current official application form. The *Information for Applicants* booklet and *Application for Certification* are revised each year and may be obtained from the Board office. *Only applications submitted on the current application form will be accepted. Photocopies or faxed copies of applications will not be accepted.*

An acknowledgment postcard accompanies each application. This card, when stamped, self-addressed, and enclosed with the application, will be returned to the applicant as acknowledgment that the application has been received by the Board office. Once the card is returned to the applicant, it may take up to 16 weeks for the applicant to receive further information regarding the status of the application. Applications are reviewed in order of receipt. An applicant who does not receive *any* notification from the Board regarding his/her application by August 1, 1999, should contact the Board office.

Certification Requirements

B. Deadlines and Fees

Deadline for receipt of completed applications in the Board office for the November 3, 1999, Part I examination is February 1, 1999. There is a nonrefundable late fee of $250 for applications received in the Board office between February 1, 1999, and March 1, 1999. Applications received after March 1, 1999, will be returned. A complete list of fees appears at the beginning of this document.

Applications submitted without the appropriate fees will not be accepted. Fees received without applications will be returned. Part I application and examination fees are neither refundable nor transferable.

C. Completing the Application and Supporting Documentation

Indicate the specialty in which you are seeking certification.

Social Security Number
Provide your social security number.

Candidate Name
If your name differs from that indicated on your supporting documentation, you must include certified documentation (marriage license, name change determination, etc) of the change. If your name changes at any time subsequent to the application, certified documentation of the name change must be submitted to the Board office.

Mailing Address
This is an address at which the Board can contact you; therefore, do not use a temporary address. *Candidates are responsible for keeping the Board informed about any change of address.*

Office and Home Telephone and Fax Numbers
Provide your *primary* office phone number, home telephone number, and fax number.

1. Date of birth
Provide your birth date.

2. Medical education
Include the complete name of each medical school attended, along with accurate and complete attendance and graduation dates. Be certain to include the degree obtained (MD or DO).

3. Licensure
All questions regarding licensure must be answered. Do not leave any blanks.

In addition, enclose with the application a copy of either your unlimited medical license or the current renewal registration card for your unlimited license, *whichever shows the license expiration date.* If you have a temporary (education or training) license at the time of application, you must submit a copy of your current unlimited license in a state, commonwealth, territory, or possession of the United States or province of Canada in order to take the Part II examination. Candidates who do not submit copies of their licenses by December 31 of the year in which they pass the Part I examination will not be scheduled for the Part II examination. *If you have a temporary (education or training) license, please indicate this on the application form.*

A candidate in possession of a restricted, suspended, or revoked license will not be accepted for any examination. Restrictions include but are not limited to conditions, contingencies, probation, and stipulated agreements.

4. Have you ever applied to this Board before?
Indicate the name under which you applied.

5. Do you currently have another application on file with this Board?
A candidate may *not* have more than one application for certification in the same specialty or subspecialty on file with the Board office at any one time.

6. Applicants with disabilities
Please refer to Section VII.

7. First postgraduate year (First 2 years for child neurology)
Enclose with the application a letter of verification from the training director describing the exact length and content of rotations completed during GY1. All documentation must include exact dates (month/day/year) of training.

Psychiatry candidates only:
If the GY1 was a full year of internal medicine, pediatrics, or family practice, a photocopy of the certificate of completion, *including the exact dates*, may be submitted in lieu of the letter from the training director.

Neurology candidates only:
If the GY1 was a full year of internal medicine, a photocopy of the certificate of completion, *including the exact dates*, may be submitted in lieu of the letter from the training director.

Neurology with special qualification in child neurology candidates only:
If either of the first 2 years was a full year of internal medicine or pediatrics, a photocopy of the certificate(s) of completion, *including the exact dates*, may be submitted in lieu of the letter from the training director.

Reapplicants only:
If you are reapplying for examination and were previously accepted for examination, you do not need to include the GY1 and residency training documentation with this reapplication.

8. Residency training
List all residency training in chronological order, including exact dates (month/day/year).

In addition, enclose with the application a copy of certificate(s) of training including exact dates, or a letter of verification of training from the training director(s), including exact dates of training. If training was completed in child and adolescent psychiatry, the training director of the child and adolescent psychiatry program must document the child and adolescent psychiatry training.

If you are still in training, a letter from the training director must be submitted *with the application* documenting that you are in the final year of training and that training will be completed by June 30, 1999. *This letter must include the date on which you started training.* Immediately after you have completed training, the training director must submit to the Board a letter verifying successful completion of training or a copy of the certificate of training. All documentation must include exact dates of training.

In order to be eligible for the November 3, 1999, Part I examination, candidates must have fulfilled all training requirements by June 30, 1999. If documentation of successful completion of training is not received in the Board office by July 15, 1999, the candidate will be removed from the Part I roster.

Due to the large volume of documentation that the Board office will be receiving on or before July 15, we ask that applicants *do not call* to verify that the Board received documentation from their residency program. Applicants should check with their training director to see if documentation was sent to the Board office.

Reapplicants only:
If you are reapplying for examination and were previously accepted for examination, you do not need to include the GY1 and residency training documentation with this reapplication.

Application Statement
Read, sign, and date the application statement. Applications with altered or unsigned application statements will not be accepted and will be returned.

9. Examination Site
From the list provided, select your top four preferences for examination site.

Part I sites are assigned based on the order in which applications are received and approved in the Board office. If a site is filled to capacity, the second choice will be assigned. If the second choice site is filled to capacity, the third choice will be assigned, etc.

10. Other Diplomate Information (if any)
List any other Board certifications.

D. Appeal Procedure for Negative Determinations Regarding Applications or Licensure

The rejection of credentials for admission to an examination is considered a "negative determination." An applicant who has submitted a formal application and receives a negative determination regarding his/her application may appeal by complying with the following procedures:

Within 30 days after date of notice of a negative determination, the applicant may indicate, in writing, his/her request for a formal appeal of his/her application rejection. An appeal fee of $350 and any additional written information tending to rebut the negative determination must accompany this request. All correspondence and other materials should be sent to the Board office.

For psychiatry applicants, the Committee on Credentials for Psychiatry will review the materials and recommend action to the Psychiatry Council, which consists of all current psychiatry directors. The Psychiatry Council will review the materials and make a decision that, in all events, will be final and binding on the Council, on the Board, and on the applicant.

For neurology and neurology with special qualification in child neurology applicants, the Committee on Credentials for Neurology will review the materials and recommend action to the Neurology Council, which consists of all current neurology directors. The Neurology Council will review the materials and make a decision that, in all events, will be final and binding on the Council, on the Board, and on the applicant.

Any applicant who does not satisfy the Board's licensure requirement may submit a letter of appeal to the Board office. The appeal materials will be sent to the respective Credentials Committee, which will review the materials and make a recommendation to the respective Council. The Council will vote on the recommendation of the Committee.

IV. Examinations

A. General Information Pertaining to All Examinations

The Board does not endorse or recommend any texts or other teaching aids identified as "Board preparation" material. Furthermore, the Board does not have any affiliation with, or responsibility for, programs identifying themselves as "Board Review Courses." Although the purpose of the examination is to test the qualifications of the candidate in psychiatry, neurology, or both, it must not be forgotten that these medical disciplines constitute part of the broad field of general medicine. The Board requires proficiency in neurology on the part of those it certifies in psychiatry and vice versa, but examines the candidate in accordance with the certificate he or she seeks.

The Board may conduct examinations at such times and places as it deems appropriate. The Board reserves the right to limit the number of candidates admitted to any scheduled examination. The administration and grading of all examinations shall be at the sole discretion of the Board. After completion of such examinations, the executive vice president will notify candidates in writing as to the results.

To become Board certified, each candidate must pass both Part I and Part II of the examination given by the Board. There is no limit on the number of times a candidate may apply for the Part I examination. A passing grade on the Part I examination will be valid for a period of 6 years, or three attempts to pass the Part II examination, whichever comes first. Candidates who are unsuccessful in the Part II examination during the allotted time period will be required to retake the Part I examination.

Each examination shall cover such subjects as the Board may determine. The ABPN currently uses *DSM-IV* as the primary authority on psychiatric diagnostic nomenclature for its examinations.

The Board will send the names of all those achieving certification or recertification to the ABMS for publication.

The Board is not liable for candidate travel and/or other related expenses incurred as a result of an examination cancellation.

General questions about requirements and logistics of ABPN examinations may be asked of ABPN staff by telephone or on site. Verbal complaints to staff, directors, proctors, or examiners that continue after explanation of ABPN policy may rise to the level of harassment, in which case they will constitute irregular behavior *(see Section I.D)*. At no time should a candidate discuss the administration or the grading of an examination with the examiners.

Candidates are required to bring government-issued photo identification to the examination. They will be asked to present this ID at registration. Government-issued photo identification includes military IDs, passports, valid driver's licenses, and state IDs. If the name on the admission slip is different from the name that appears on the photo ID, certified documentation verifying a name change must also be presented.

Candidates may not bring food, drink, cellular phones, pagers, books, or study materials into the examination.

B. Part I Examination Procedures

Successful completion of the Part I written examination in psychiatry and neurology is required of candidates seeking certification in psychiatry, neurology, or neurology with special qualification in child neurology. In order to successfully complete the Part I examination, a candidate must pass both parts of the two-part written examination at the same examination administration.

1. *Scheduling*

The Part I examination is given once a year on a regional basis throughout the United States and Canada, as well as in selected sites outside North America. The Board will advise an applicant, in writing, of acceptance for examination.

Applicants will be expected to indicate, in order of preference, their choice of four examination sites. Every effort is made to accommodate candidates in the locale of their choice. Request for transfer to another site must be made in writing at least 90 days prior to the Part I examination. Changes will be made subject to space availability. One month prior to the examination candidates will receive an admission notice specifying their examination site and time to report for examination.

All applicants are required to sit for the Part I examination for which they have applied. Applicants who fail to do so will be required to submit a new application, copy of unlimited license, and the application and Part I examination fees. *Candidates who are unable to sit for their scheduled Part I examination owing to an emergency should contact the Board office in writing no later than 30 days after the date of the examination.*

2. *Reexamination*

A candidate who fails the initial Part I examination may, upon payment of the Part I reexamination fee, repeat the examination the following year. There is no limit on the number of times an applicant may apply to take the Part I examination. Two negative determinations necessitate reapplication (new application, copy of unlimited license, and payment of application and Part I examination fees). Reexaminees who do not sit for reexamination as scheduled will also be required to submit a new application, copy of unlimited license, and payment of the application and Part I examination fees. Candidates applying for reexamination do not need to include another copy of their GY1 and residency documentation if the Board approved their original application.

C. Psychiatry Part I Examination Content

The psychiatric portion of the examination will include questions in the following areas:

- Development and the life cycle
- Neurobiological and psychosocial aspects of psychopathology
- Diagnostic procedures
- Psychiatric disorders and comorbid disorders
- Pharmacological and nonpharmacological treatments
- Special topics in psychiatry (suicide, dangerousness, ethics, mental health delivery systems, history of psychiatry, and community, consultation-liaison, emergency, and forensic psychiatry)

The neurologic portion of the examination will include questions in the following areas:

- Basic science aspects of neurological disorders (cellular and molecular neurobiology, neuroanatomy, neuropathology, and neurophysiology)
- Incidence/risk of neurological disorders
- Diagnostic procedures (history, neurological examination, neurochemistry, neuroelectrophysiology, neuroradiology, neuropsychological testing)
- Clinical evaluation and management of neurological disorders

D. Neurology/Neurology with Special Qualification in Child Neurology Part I Examination Content

The neurologic portion of the examination will include questions in the following areas of adult and child neurology:

- Neuroanatomy
- Neuropathology
- Neurochemistry
- Neurophysiology
- Neuropharmacology
- Neuroimmunology/neurovirology
- Genetics
- Neuroendocrinology
- Neuroimaging
- Neuro-ophthalmology
- Neuro-otology
- Cerebrospinal fluid

The psychiatric portion of the examination will include questions in the following areas:

- Development and disorders of childhood
- Psychopathology and diagnostic criteria
- The doctor-patient relationship
- Behavioral and personality changes associated with structural changes
- Alcoholism and other substance abuse
- Altered states of consciousness
- Memory disorders and cortical changes with dysfunction
- Psychiatric problems associated with medical disease
- Diagnostic procedures
- Psychopharmacology and nonpharmacologic therapeutic modalities

E. Appeal Procedure for Negative Determinations Regarding Part I Examinations

A failing grade on the Part I examination is considered a "negative determination." A candidate who receives a negative determination may appeal by complying with the procedures detailed below.

Within 30 days after date of notice of a negative determination, the unsuccessful candidate may indicate, in writing, his/her request to have his/her examination hand scored. The appeal fee of $300 must accompany the request. The candidate will be informed of the results of the hand scoring in writing that, in all events, will be final and binding on the Board and on the candidate. All correspondence and other materials should be sent to the Board office.

F. Part II Examination Procedures

1. *Assignment and Scheduling*

All successful Part I candidates will receive a notice of assignment to a Part II examination (Part II billing statement), together with a request to submit the required examination fee. Candidates will be asked to sign a statement that they possess a current, unlimited license to practice medicine in a state, commonwealth, territory, or possession of the United States or province of Canada. Candidates who submitted a temporary (education or training) license at the time of application to Part I will be required to submit a copy of their unlimited licenses by December 31 of the year in which they passed the Part I examination. *Candidates who do not submit copies of their licenses by this deadline will not be scheduled for the Part II examination.*

Any candidate in possession of a restricted, suspended, or revoked license will not be scheduled for the Part II examination. Restrictions include but are not limited to conditions, contingencies, probation, and stipulated agreements.

Scheduling for the Part II examination will be made on a regional basis as often as possible. The limited space available and the complicated logistics involved in administering the Part II examination make it extremely difficult for the Board to allow candidates to select either the site or the date for examination. Candidates who do not attend the Part II examination for which they are initially scheduled must submit a Part II application to be put on a waiting list for future examinations (see Section IV.F.2).

Candidates who have submitted a Part II application will be scheduled for examination within 1 year from the date the Part II application is received in the Board office whenever possible. Due to space limitations a wait longer than 1 year may be necessary. Candidates will be scheduled for examination based on space availability and order of receipt of application.

Candidates who have submitted a Part II application may choose to decline two invitations to Part II examinations. If the third invitation is declined, the candidate will be required to submit a new Part II application and will be placed at the end of the waiting list once the application is received in the Board office. Although it is the candidate's privilege to decline the invitation, there is no guarantee that another date or location will be available within the year's examination cycle.

One month prior to the date of the assigned Part II examination, a candidate will receive informational materials and an admission notice specifying the date, time, and place to report for registration. Candidates are requested to report for registration only on the day and at the time indicated on the admission notice. Registration schedules are arranged to accommodate candidates in accordance with their examination schedules.

2. *Fees and Applications*

Candidates who do not pay the Part II examination fee for their scheduled examination by the deadline specified will be removed from the roster of candidates for that examination. Such candidates will be required to request and submit a Part II application in order to be scheduled for a future Part II examination. The examination fee should not be sent with the application. The Board will request the examination fee when the new assignment is made.

A candidate who is unable to attend the Part II examination to which he/she has been admitted and who fails to notify the Executive Vice President in writing at least 60 days before the date of such examination shall forfeit the examination fee. Such candidates will be required to request and submit a Part II application in order to be scheduled for a future Part II examination and must again pay the required Part II examination fee when a new assignment is made.

3. *Reexamination*

A passing grade on the Part I examination dated on or after March 1, 1987, will be valid for a period of 6 years or three attempts to complete the Part II examination successfully, whichever comes first. Candidates who are unsuccessful in the Part II examination during the allotted time period will be required to retake the Part I examination. These candidates must request and submit a new Part I application and the application and Part I examination fees.

Psychiatry candidates must pass both sections of the Part II examination. A candidate who fails one or both sections of the examination must repeat both sections at each subsequently scheduled examination until he/she passes both sections at the same examination.

Neurology candidates must pass all three (two adult and one child) sections of the Part II examination. A candidate must repeat the section or sections he/she failed at each subsequently scheduled examination until he/she passes all the sections.

Child Neurology candidates must pass all three (two child and one adult) sections of the Part II examination. A candidate must repeat the section or sections he/she failed at each subsequently scheduled examination until he/she passes all the sections.

Candidates who fail the Part II examination are automatically assigned to another Part II examination and are required to be present as scheduled. Candidates who fail to take the reexamination at the time specified, as well as candidates who do not pay their reexamination fee by the specified deadline, are required to request and submit a Part II application.

4. *Grade letters and certificates*

Candidates will receive written notification as to whether they passed or failed approximately 30 days after the Part II examination. Successful candidates will receive their certificates within 90 days of receiving their grade letters. It is the candidate's responsibility to notify the Board office, in writing, if he or she does not receive the certificate within the time frame specified in the grade letter. If a candidate does not do so, he/she will have to request a duplicate certificate and pay a $50 processing fee.

5. *Duplicate certificates*

Requests for duplicates of ABPN certificates must include your name, address, phone number, birthdate, signature, and indication of how you want your name printed on the certificate. You must include with your request copies of (1) your current unlimited medical license stating the expiration date and (2) for security purposes, government-issued photo identification, such as a driver's license or passport. Also include a check in the amount of $50 for each duplicate certificate ordered, payable to the American Board of Psychiatry and Neurology, Inc. Certificates are printed approximately five times per year. Depending on when a duplicate certificate is requested, it may be 2 to 4 months until the diplomate receives the duplicate certificate.

G. Part II Examination Format

Part II, an oral examination, will include the examination of patients under the supervision of one or more examiners. The manner of examining patients and the reasoning and deductions therefrom will constitute an important part of the examination. Knowledge of basic science principles, special diagnostic procedures, management recommendations, and assessment of risk are also essential parts of the examination, which focuses on evaluation of clinical skills.

Candidates are expected to discuss their findings with their examiners. Questions frequently cover such areas as diagnosis, differential diagnosis, evaluation, treatment, prognosis, and management. Reference to the basic sciences of psychiatry and neurology may be made.

Note taking is permitted during oral examinations provided that only blank paper is used. All notes must be left in the examination room at the conclusion of the examination. Notes will not be used in the assignment of grades and will be destroyed. Failure to adhere to this policy will constitute irregular behavior *(see section I.D)*.

1. *Psychiatry*

Psychiatry candidates will take two examinations:

- One 1-hour examination in clinical psychiatry (patient)
- One 1-hour examination in clinical psychiatry (audiovisual)

In the patient section, the psychiatry candidate will be given approximately 30 minutes to examine a patient under the supervision of one or more examiners. Following the examination of the patient, the discussion with the examiner(s), which will be approximately 30 minutes in length, will focus on physician-patient interaction, conduct of the clinical examination, capacity to elicit clinical data, formulation, differential diagnosis and prognosis, therapeutic management, and knowledge of therapies. Additional questions may be addressed to the basic science of psychiatry.

The audiovisual section will consist of a videotaped psychiatric examination of approximately 25 minutes, which the candidate will observe. Candidates will then be individually examined by one or more examiners with particular reference to the content of the tape. This discussion may also include other clinical topics.

2. *Neurology and Child Neurology*

Neurology candidates will take three examinations:

- One 1-hour examination in clinical neurology (patient)
- One 1-hour examination in clinical neurology (vignette)
- One 1-hour examination in clinical child neurology (vignette)

Child Neurology candidates will take three examinations:

- One 1-hour examination in clinical child neurology (patient)
- One 1-hour examination in clinical child neurology (vignette)
- One 1-hour examination in clinical neurology (vignette)

In the neurology and child neurology patient sections, the candidate will be given approximately 30 minutes to examine the patient under the supervision of one or more examiners. During the patient examination, the candidate's ability to obtain an adequate history and perform a neurologic examination will be observed. Following the examination of the patient, the discussion with the examiner(s), which will be approximately 30 minutes, will focus on the evaluation of the findings and discussion of the diagnosis, treatment, and management. This discussion may not be limited to the patient examined and may also include other clinical topics. The examiners may also ask additional questions concerning the basic science of neurology.

Multiple written vignettes of patient encounters will be utilized as a basis for discussion of diagnosis and treatment in those sections in which there is no patient present.

Since candidates in child neurology are to be certified in "neurology with special qualification in child neurology," it is agreed that those candidates will be expected to pass a 1-hour oral examination in clinical neurology (vignette), which is set at the same level of difficulty established for neurology candidates. The pass/fail standards for that hour in clinical neurology (vignette) will be the same whether the candidate is seeking certification in neurology or in neurology with special qualification in child neurology.

H. Feedback and Appeal Procedures for Negative Determinations Regarding Part II Examinations

A failing grade on a Part II examination is considered a "negative determination." Within 30 days after date of notice of a negative determination, the unsuccessful candidate may indicate, in writing, his/her request for feedback. The fee for providing feedback is $100 and must accompany the written request. After such request, the candidate will be provided a checklist concerning his/her performance on sections not passed. All correspondence or other materials should be sent to the Board office.

A candidate who receives a negative determination may *appeal* by complying with the procedures detailed below.

Within 60 days after date of notice of a negative determination, the unsuccessful candidate may indicate, in writing, his/her request for a formal appeal of the examination results. An appeal fee equal to the candidate's reexamination fee and written information tending to rebut the negative determination must accompany this request. All correspondence and other materials should be sent to the Board office.

For psychiatry candidates the Committee to Review Appeals for Psychiatry will review the materials and recommend action to the Psychiatry Council, which consists of all current psychiatry directors. The Psychiatry Council will review the material and make a decision that, in all events, will be final and binding on the Council, on the Board, and on the candidate.

For neurology and neurology with special qualification in child neurology candidates, the Committee to Review Appeals for Neurology will review the materials and recommend action to the Neurology Council, which consists of all current neurology directors. The Neurology Council will review the materials and make a decision that, in all events, will be final and binding on the Council, on the Board, and on the candidate.

V. Subspecialization

For complete information about subspecialty certification, please contact the Board office to request the current editions of the following ABPN publications:

- *Information for Applicants for Certification in Child and Adolescent Psychiatry*
- *Information for Applicants for Certification in the Subspecialties of Geriatric Psychiatry, Clinical Neurophysiology, Addiction Psychiatry, and Forensic Psychiatry*

A. The Committee on Certification in Child and Adolescent Psychiatry

In February 1959, the ABPN, in concurrence with the Advisory Board for Medical Specialties, established a Committee on Certification in Child Psychiatry. This was done to establish officially the field of child psychiatry as a definite area of subspecialization in psychiatry and to provide a means of identifying the properly trained and experienced child psychiatrist as distinguished from those who claim proficiency in this field without adequate background and qualifications. In November 1987, the name of the committee was changed to the Committee on Certification in Child and Adolescent Psychiatry.

The actual mechanics of certification of qualified candidates and the establishment of basic policies have been delegated by the Board to the Committee, which operates under the supervision of, and in accordance with, the policies of the Board. The Committee presently consists of six members certified in child and adolescent psychiatry, one Board director certified in psychiatry by the ABPN, and one member certified by the American Board of Pediatrics. The Committee holds meetings each year for the purpose of examining candidates and transacting business.

Each applicant for certification in child and adolescent psychiatry must be certified by the Board in the specialty of psychiatry prior to applying for examination in child and adolescent psychiatry. Training must be completed by the application deadline. The general policies regarding training, application, and examination in child and adolescent psychiatry are contained in the pamphlet *Information for Applicants for Certification in Child and Adolescent Psychiatry*, which is available from the Board office.

Please note that applicants may submit application for examination in psychiatry after successful completion of the GY1, 2 years of residency training in psychiatry, and 1 year of residency training in child and adolescent psychiatry.

B. The Committee on Certification in the Subspecialty of Geriatric Psychiatry

In November 1989, the ABPN, in concurrence with the ABMS, established a Committee on Certification for Added Qualifications in Geriatric Psychiatry. This was done to establish officially the field of geriatric psychiatry as a definite area of subspecialization in psychiatry and to provide a means of identifying the properly trained and experienced geriatric psychiatrist. In 1997 the name of the committee was changed to the Committee on Certification in the Subspecialty of Geriatric Psychiatry.

The actual mechanics of certification of qualified candidates have been delegated by the Board to the Committee, which operates under the supervision of, and in accordance with, policies of the Board.

Each applicant for certification in geriatric psychiatry must be certified by the Board in the specialty of psychiatry prior to applying for examination for subspecialty certification in geriatric psychiatry. The general policies regarding training, application, and examination in geriatric psychiatry are contained in the pamphlet *Information for Applicants for Certification in the Subspecialties of Geriatric Psychiatry, Clinical Neurophysiology, Addiction Psychiatry, and Forensic Psychiatry*, which is available from the Board office.

C. The Committee on Certification in the Subspecialty of Clinical Neurophysiology

In October 1990, the ABPN, in concurrence with the ABMS, established a Committee on Certification for Added Qualifications in Clinical Neurophysiology. This was done to establish officially the field of clinical neurophysiology as a definite area of subspecialization in neurology and psychiatry and to provide a means of identifying the properly trained and experienced clinical neurophysiologist. In 1997 the name of the committee was changed to the Committee on Certification in the Subspecialty of Clinical Neurophysiology.

The actual mechanics of certification of qualified candidates have been delegated by the Board to the Committee, which operates under the supervision of, and in accordance with, the policies of the Board.

Each applicant for certification in clinical neurophysiology must be certified by the Board in the specialty of neurology, neurology with special qualification in child neurology, or psychiatry prior to applying for examination for subspecialty certification in clinical neurophysiology. The general policies regarding training, application, and examination in clinical neurophysiology are contained in the pamphlet *Information for Applicants for Certification in the Subspecialties of Geriatric Psychiatry, Clinical Neurophysiology,*

Addiction Psychiatry, and Forensic Psychiatry, which is available from the Board office.

D. The Committee on Certification in the Subspecialty of Addiction Psychiatry

In October 1991, the ABPN, in concurrence with the ABMS, established a Committee on Certification for Added Qualifications in Addiction Psychiatry. This was done to establish officially the field of addiction psychiatry as a definite area of subspecialization in psychiatry and to provide a means of identifying the properly trained and experienced addiction psychiatrist. In 1997 the name of the committee was changed to the Committee on Certification in the Subspecialty of Addiction Psychiatry.

The actual mechanics of certification of qualified candidates have been delegated by the Board to the Committee, which operates under the supervision of, and in accordance with, the policies of the Board.

Each applicant for certification in addiction psychiatry must be certified by the Board in the specialty of psychiatry prior to applying for examination for subspecialty certification in addiction psychiatry. The general policies regarding training, application, and examination in addiction psychiatry are contained in the pamphlet *Information for Applicants for Certification in the Subspecialties of Geriatric Psychiatry, Clinical Neurophysiology, Addiction Psychiatry, and Forensic Psychiatry*, which is available from the Board office.

E. The Committee on Certification in the Subspecialty of Forensic Psychiatry

In November 1992, the ABPN, in concurrence with the ABMS, established a Committee on Certification for Added Qualifications in Forensic Psychiatry. This was done to establish officially the field of forensic psychiatry as a definite area of subspecialization in psychiatry and to provide a means of identifying the properly trained and experienced forensic psychiatrist. In 1997 the name of the committee was changed to the Committee on Certification in the Subspecialty of Forensic Psychiatry.

The actual mechanics of certification of qualified candidates have been delegated by the Board to the Committee, which operates under the supervision of, and in accordance with, the policies of the Board.

Each applicant for certification in forensic psychiatry must be certified by the Board in the specialty of psychiatry prior to applying for examination for subspecialty certification in forensic psychiatry. The general policies regarding training, application, and examination in forensic psychiatry are contained in the pamphlet *Information for Applicants for Certification in the Subspecialties of Geriatric Psychiatry, Clinical Neurophysiology, Addiction Psychiatry, and Forensic Psychiatry*, which is available from the Board office.

VI. Special Programs

A. Supplementary Certification

A candidate who has been certified in psychiatry, neurology, or neurology with special qualification in child neurology may apply for supplementary certification in another primary specialty upon submission of a new Part I application and Part I examination fee. The candidate will be scheduled for the next available Part I examination in the supplementary specialty. The credentials for such other certificate must be acceptable to the Board.

A candidate may have more than one application on file with the Board at any one time if the applications are for certification in different specialties or subspecialties. It is the responsibility of the applicant to contact the Board office to avoid possible conflicts in examination scheduling.

1. *Dual certification in psychiatry and neurology*

Unless otherwise specified (see section on Canadian training programs below), all training must be completed in programs accredited by the ACGME.

Applicants seeking certification both in psychiatry and neurology who began residency training prior to January 1, 1988, must have completed 5 years of the following ACGME-accredited postgraduate training:

a. A GY1 that meets requirements for either psychiatry or neurology *(see sections II.C and II.D)*
and
b. Two years of ACGME-accredited residency training in psychiatry in a single training program
and
c. Two years of ACGME-accredited residency training in neurology in a single training program.

Applicants seeking certification both in psychiatry and neurology who began residency training on or after January 1, 1988, must have completed one of the following training tracks:

1. An ABPN-approved combined psychiatry/neurology training program *(recommended)*
A GY1 that meets the requirements for entry into a *neurology* program *(see section II.D)*.
and
Five years of residency training in an ABPN-approved combined psychiatry/neurology training program.
or

2. Individual psychiatry and neurology programs
A GY1 that meets the requirements for entry into a *neurology* program *(see section II.D)*
and
Six full years of postgraduate residency training in ACGME-accredited programs, including 3 full years in psychiatry and 3 full years in neurology.
or

3. Non-ABPN-approved combined training programs
A GY1 that meets the requirements for entry into a *neurology* program *(see section II.D)*
and
At the discretion and approval of both training directors, and in accordance with Residency Review Committee requirements, applicants may complete 5 full years of postgraduate training in ACGME-accredited programs including 2 full years of residency training in psychiatry in a single program, 2 full years of residency training in neurology in a single program, and a full year that is jointly sponsored and coordinated by the psychiatry and neurology training directors to allow the resident to successfully complete all the essentials for an approved residency program in psychiatry and an approved residency program in neurology.

The 5 years of residency training are usually taken at one institution but may be taken at no more than two institutions. An application for examination may be submitted after completion of the GY1, the 2 full years of residency training in one specialty, and the full year of jointly sponsored residency training.

For residents entering residency training on or after July 1, 1999: Program directors must contact the Board office for a copy of the combined psychiatry/neurology guidelines and must submit to the Board for review, *no later than the beginning of the GY3*, a proposal for a resident to train in psychiatry and neurology that conforms to these guidelines.

Canadian training programs

Applicants who entered a Canadian residency program on or after July 1, 1997, will not be granted training credit. Applicants entering Canadian residency before July 1, 1997, may be granted training credit if their residency training was completed in a Canadian program accredited by the RCPSC.

2. *Dual certification in neurology and neurology with special qualification in child neurology*

Applicants who have achieved certification in neurology and who wish to be certified in neurology with special qualification in child neurology will need to obtain the additional training described below. *Unless otherwise specified (see section on Canadian training below), all training must be completed in programs accredited by the ACGME.*

Training requirements include:

a. A minimum of 12 months of approved training in general pediatrics

and

b. A minimum of 12 months of approved training in clinical child neurology

A maximum of 3 months of child neurology training obtained during a neurology residency may be applied toward the required 12 months of child neurology training only if the 3 months took place in an ACGME-accredited child neurology program, which must be documented by the neurology program director.

Candidates will be required to request and submit a new completed Part I application and the application fee. Such candidates will not be required to retake the Part I examination in neurology. The Part II examination fee will be requested after the application has been approved. Two 1-hour examinations in child neurology will be taken during the Part II examination.

Canadian training programs

Applicants who entered a Canadian residency program on or after July 1, 1998, will not be granted training credit. Applicants entering Canadian residency before July 1, 1998, may be granted training credit if their residency training was completed in a Canadian program accredited by the RCPSC.

3. *Dual certification in child and adolescent psychiatry and in neurology with special qualification in child neurology*

An applicant who wishes to obtain certificates both in child and adolescent psychiatry and in neurology with special qualification in child neurology must meet the following requirements:

a. Certification by the Board in the specialty of general psychiatry prior to applying for examination in child and adolescent psychiatry (a minimum of 2 years of approved residency training in general psychiatry is required);

b. Completion of the requirements for certification in child and adolescent psychiatry;

and

c. Completion of the requirements for certification in neurology with special qualification in child neurology.

B. Joint Training in Pediatrics/Psychiatry/Child and Adolescent Psychiatry

The American Board of Pediatrics, the ABPN, and the Committee on Certification in Child and Adolescent Psychiatry of the ABPN have approved programs for combined pediatrics/psychiatry/child and adolescent psychiatry residency training. This training consists of 24 months of pediatrics, 18 months of adult psychiatry, and 18 months of child and adolescent psychiatry. Completion of the program will satisfy the training requirements for certification in all three areas. Physicians pursuing training in these programs may not apply for examination until all training has been completed.

C. Joint Training in Neurology/Radiology/Neuroradiology

The American Board of Radiology and the ABPN have approved programs for combined training in neurology/radiology/neuroradiology. Completion of the program will satisfy the training requirements for certification in all three areas. In order to be certified in neuroradiology, a resident must have completed certification in both diagnostic radiology and neurology.

D. Combined Training Leading to Certification by Two Boards

Approved combined/joint training programs are listed in the *Graduate Medical Education Directory.* A list of programs approved since the last edition of the *Graduate Medical Education Directory* may be obtained by writing the ABPN or by calling the ABPN's faxback service at (847) 945-7900 x229. The Board currently has the following programs:

1. *Dual certification in psychiatry/family practice*

The American Board of Family Practice and the ABPN have approved guidelines for combined psychiatry/family practice residency training. In order to satisfy training requirements in psychiatry, a resident who resigns from the combined psychiatry/family practice training program must complete 36 months of residency training, of which 30 months of training must be completed in psychiatry. In addition, the program requirements for psychiatry as defined in the *Graduate Medical Education Directory* must be satisfied.

2. *Dual certification in psychiatry/internal medicine*

The American Board of Internal Medicine and the ABPN have approved programs for combined psychiatry/internal medicine residency. In order to satisfy training requirements in psychiatry, a resident who resigns from the combined psychiatry/internal medicine training program must complete 36 months of residency training, of which 30 months of training must be completed in psychiatry. In addition, the program requirements for psychiatry as defined in the *Graduate Medical Education Directory* must be satisfied.

3. *Dual certification in neurology/internal medicine*

The American Board of Internal Medicine and the ABPN have approved programs for combined neurology/internal medicine residency training. In order to satisfy training requirements in neurology, a resident who resigns from the combined neurology/internal medicine training program must complete 36 months of residency training, of which 30 months of training must be completed in neurology. In addition, the program requirements for neurology as defined in the *Graduate Medical Education Directory* must be satisfied.

4. *Dual certification in neurology/physical medicine and rehabilitation*

The American Board of Physical Medicine and Rehabilitation and the ABPN have approved programs for combined neurology/physical medicine and rehabilitation residency training. In order to satisfy training requirements in neurology, a resident who resigns from the combined training program must complete 36 months of residency training, of which 30 months of training must be completed in neurology. In addition, the program requirements for neurology as defined in the *Graduate Medical Education Directory* must be satisfied.

VII. Applicants with Disabilities and Qualifications for Testing Accommodations

A. General Information

The Board recognizes that physicians with disabilities may wish to take the certifying examinations and will attempt to make accommodations for applicants with verified disabilities. The Board supports the intent of the *Americans with Disabilities Act (ADA).* You are reminded, however, that "auxiliary aids (and services) can only be offered if they do not fundamentally alter the measurement of skills or knowledge the examination is intended to test" (*Americans with Disabilities Act*, Public Law 101-336 (§309 [b][3]). To this extent, the Board will provide reasonable accommodations during testing to provide equal opportunity for persons with disabilities. The documentation requesting reasonable accommodations must identify a disability and provide a rationale for specified modifications to standard testing procedures.

Applicants who request accommodations because of a disability must advise the Board in writing no later than the deadline for submitting applications for examination. All documentation and other evidence substantiating the disability must be submitted to the Board no later than 30 days after the deadline for filing an application for examination. Required documentation includes completion of the *Application for Testing Accommodations* and appropriate checklists at the end of this section. If the Board deems it necessary, an independent assessment may be requested at the expense of the Board.

Documentation and other evidence substantiating the disability includes, but is not limited to, each of the following:

- A report diagnosing the applicant's disability written by a professional appropriately qualified for evaluating the disability. The report must be printed on the certified examiner's letterhead, with the examiner's credentials, address, and telephone number given in the letterhead or title. The report must include the candidate's name, date of birth, and date of testing, and it must be signed by the examiner.
- A history of the disability, including previous settings in which accommodations have been granted. Having had prior accommodations granted does not necessarily influence the decision of the Board to grant or deny a current request for accommodation. If there is no history of prior accommodations, the examiner must explain why current circumstances necessitate accommodations.
- Diagnostic information about the specified disability using standard nomenclature from sources such as the *International Classification of Diseases* and the American Psychiatric Association *Diagnostic and Statistical Manual of Mental Disorders*.
- Specific recommended accommodations, with a rationale for why each accommodation is needed. A description of any functional limitations associated with the disability is important to the Board's evaluation of the request.

B. Requirements for Applicants with Learning Disabilities

Documentation submitted to the Board must include the following:

- A psychoeducational evaluation of the applicant as an adult prepared by a certified psychologist or learning disabilities specialist.
- A complete cognitive assessment using the Wechsler Adult Intelligence Scale-III, the Kaufman Adolescent and Adult Intelligence Test, the Woodcock-Johnson Cognitive Battery-Revised, as well as other formal tests that measure information processing and achievement. The test instruments must be statistically valid, reliable, and standardized for adult populations. Test performance must be reported in standard scores or percentiles.
- A comprehensive achievement battery in relevant areas such as reading, written language, and mathematics. Informal methods of assessment and analysis that are useful include direct observation, error analysis, and diagnostic teaching.
- Evaluation of information processing skills that include, but are not limited to, short- and long-term memory, auditory processing, motor skills, executive functioning, and phonological awareness skills. Typical instruments include, but are not limited to, Woodcock-Johnson Psychoeducational Test
- Battery-Revised, Tests of Cognitive Abilities, the Detroit Tests of Learning Aptitudes-Adult, and the Wechsler Memory Scales-III.
- A history of the candidate's educational performance documenting the nature of school difficulties. Information about learning difficulties in elementary, secondary, and postsecondary settings, as well as documentation of prior accommodations, should be included. The Board recognizes that diagnostic practices vary considerably and prefers to base decisions on as much information as possible. The evaluation must provide evidence of cognitive, information processing, and achievement deficits that relate to the requested test accommodations.

C. Requirements for Applicants with Attention-Deficit/Hyperactivity Disorder

- The diagnostic evaluation process should be multidimensional and involve one or more certified professionals (physician, psychologist, neuropsychologist, learning specialist) in order to include historical, observational, medical, neuropsychological, and educational testing information.
- In most cases, the report should be done within 3 years of the candidate's request for accommodations. A description of current functional limitations relative to the requested accommodations must be included.
- The report must include a summary of clinical interviews, observations, and results of information from checklists completed by the candidate and parents, teachers, professionals, or supervisors. Complete family, developmental, educational, and medical histories are needed to complement neuropsychological and educational assessments that provide intellectual, cognitive, information processing, and educational data. A differential diagnosis should be discussed.
- Each test must be listed and results must be reported using standard scores or percentiles.
- Based upon the particular disabilities of the candidate, the report must delineate recommendations with a rationale for treatment (medication and/or behavior modification) and academic accommodations backed up by a rationale for why specified test accommodations are needed. It is particularly important to document prior accommodations.

D. Review of Documentation

A letter detailing the specific accommodations requested because of a disability must be submitted for each examination and/or reexamination. Documentation should be marked "ADA Materials" and mailed to the attention of the executive vice president at the Board office.

Each report is reviewed carefully before accommodations are provided. If the Board does not find appropriate and sufficient evidence to grant accommodations, the applicant will be informed that the request has been denied.

Any applicant whose request for accommodations because of a disability is denied may submit a letter of appeal. All requests for appeal should be submitted to the Board office within 30 days of the original notice of denial and must be accompanied by the required $400 appeal fee as well as any further information that rebuts the Board's original decision. The Disabilities Accommodations Committee will then review the materials and make a decision that will be final and binding for the Committee, the Board, and the applicant.

E. Examination Formats and Test Accommodations

The ABPN administers examinations with the following formats:

Examination	Format
Part I examination Subspecialty examinations Child and adolescent psychiatry written examinations	Written, multiple-choice, proctored examinations
Part II examinations Child and adolescent psychiatry examinations	Oral examination: Interview of live patient (all oral examinations) Videotape (Psychiatry Part II; Child and adolescent psychiatry) Vignette (Neurology/Child neurology Part II; Child and adolescent psychiatry)

Test accommodations may include, but are not limited to, the following:

Written Examinations

- Assistance in completing answer sheets
- Extended testing time
- Large print examination
- Separate examination room
- Reader
- Use of assistive devices

Oral Examinations

- Infrared headphones during videotaped examinations
- Use of assistive devices

American Board of Radiology

5255 E Williams Cir/Ste 3200
Tucson, AZ 85711-7409
520 790-2900
520 790-3200 Fax
E-mail: info@theabr.org
Internet: http://www.theabr.org

(These criteria and conditions are subject to change without notice. All applicants are advised to contact the American Board of Radiology [ABR] to ascertain whether the information below is current.)

Certificates

A certificate will be issued to each candidate who has finished a prescribed and approved period of training and study and has passed written and oral examinations demonstrating an adequate level of knowledge and ability in diagnostic radiology or radiation oncology in accordance with the definitions as stated in the Bylaws and Rules and Regulations of the ABR.

A certificate granted by the Board does not of itself confer, or purport to confer, any degree or legal qualifications, privileges, or license to practice radiology.

Definitions

1. Diagnostic radiology is that branch of radiology that deals with the utilization of all modalities of radiant energy in medical diagnosis and therapeutic procedures utilizing radiologic guidance. This includes, but is not restricted to, imaging techniques and methodologies utilizing radiations emitted by x-ray tubes, radionuclides, ultrasonographic devices, and radiofrequency electromagnetic radiation emitted by atoms.
2. Radiation oncology is that branch of radiology that deals with the therapeutic applications of radiant energy and its modifiers and the study and management of cancer and other diseases.

Diagnostic Radiology Training Requirements

Candidates beginning their graduate medical education after January 1, 1997, will be required to have 5 years of approved training with a minimum of 4 years in diagnostic radiology. These 4 years must be spent in a department approved for training in diagnostic radiology by the Residency Review Committee (RRC) for Diagnostic Radiology of the Accreditation Council for Graduate Medical Education (ACGME), or by the Royal College of Physicians and Surgeons of Canada (RCPSC). A minimum of 6 months, but not more than 12 months, must be spent in nuclear radiology in the 4-year program. Candidates may spend no more than 8 months in rotations outside the parent institutions.

The other year must be accredited clinical training in internal medicine, pediatrics, surgery or surgical specialties, obstetrics and gynecology, neurology, family practice, emergency medicine, or any combination of these. This clinical year will usually be the first postgraduate year. No more than a total of 3 months may be spent in radiology, radiation oncology, and/or pathology. All clinical training must be in an ACGME, American Osteopathic Association (AOA), or equivalent approved program.

Residents must have basic cardiac life support certification; advanced cardiac life support certification is encouraged.

It is not the intent of the ABR for programs to use any of the 4 years for traditional fellowship training. The designation of "fellowship" is reserved for training beyond the 4-year residency.

In a 4-year approved residency program, not more than 12 months may be spent in a single discipline (research is considered a discipline).

In a 4-year program, the resident is expected to remain in that program for all 4 years. If a transfer to another program is necessary or desired, that transfer must have the agreement of both program directors and the prospective notification to the ABR.

Candidates will be considered for the physics portion of the written examination only when they have completed 12 months of diagnostic radiology training. After 24 months of diagnostic radiology training and having passed the physics examination, the candidate will be allowed to sit for the clinical examination. If the candidate has not already passed the physics examination, he/she may take both the clinical and physics examinations together.

A candidate who has passed the written examination and will complete 60 months of approved training by September 30 in the year in which the exam is given will be considered for the oral examination. Admissibility to the oral examination is determined by the executive committee.

First-time applicants completing 5 years of training by the year 2001 will be issued a lifetime certificate in diagnostic radiology upon successful completion of the oral examination.

Residents completing 5 years of training by the year 2002 will be issued a 10-year-limited certificate in diagnostic radiology upon successful completion of the oral examination.

Radiation Oncology

Candidates beginning their graduate medical education after December 1995 will be required to have 5 years of approved training with a minimum of 4 years in radiation oncology. These 4 years must be spent in a department approved to train in radiation oncology by the RRC for Radiation Oncology for the ACGME, or by the RCPSC. The 4-year residency training period must include 36 months of clinical radiation oncology with exposure to pathology and medical oncology. A maximum of 3 months' training in diagnostic radiology will be allowed. Candidates may spend no more than 8 months in rotations outside the parent institution.

The other year, which must precede the radiation oncology training, must be ACGME-, AOA-, or RCPSC-accredited clinical training in internal medicine, surgery or surgical specialties, pediatrics, family practice, obstetrics and gynecology, transitional, or categorical radiation oncology, or any combination of these. Specialties other than those listed, including pathology, do not satisfy the PG1 requirement of the ABR.

Candidates will be admissible to the written examination only after they have completed 4 years of approved training or if they will complete this amount of training by September 30 of the year in which the examination is given. This must include a PGY1 clinical year of training in the United States or Canada. Requests for credit for this training in other English-speaking countries must be submitted to the executive committee.

Residents must have current basic cardiac life support certification. Advanced cardiac life support certification is encouraged.

The resident is expected to remain in a training program for its duration. If a transfer to another program is necessary or desired, that transfer must have the agreement of both program directors and the prospective notification of the ABR.

A candidate who has passed the written examination and will complete 60 months of approved training by September 30 in the year in which the exam is given will be considered for the oral examination. Admissibility to the oral examination is determined by the executive committee.

Effective in 1995, successful candidates will be issued a 10-year, time-limited certificate in radiation oncology.

Certificate of Added Qualifications (CAQs) and Certificate of Special Competence

A 10-year limited certificate will be issued to each diplomate certified in either radiology or diagnostic radiology who has finished a prescribed and approved period of training and study and has passed an oral examination demonstrating an adequate level of knowledge and ability in the area of expertise for which he/she has applied in accordance with the definitions stated in the Bylaws and Rules and Regulations of the ABR.

Definitions

1. Neuroradiology is that branch of radiology dealing with (1) the brain and its coverings, (2) the skull base and ENT, and (3) the spine.
2. Pediatric radiology is the branch of radiology dealing with children.
3. Vascular and interventional radiology is the branch of radiology dealing with the diagnosis and treatment of diseases using percutaneous methods guided by various radiologic imaging modalities.
4. Nuclear radiology is the branch of radiology that involves the use of radionuclides and radiolabeled substances for diagnostic imaging and related in vivo techniques.

Certificates of Added Qualifications in Neuroradiology, Pediatric Radiology, and Vascular/Interventional Radiology

For the years 1995-1999, there are two ways of meeting the requirements:

1. Have a minimum of 1 year full-time training (fellowship) following the completion of residency training and must have completed at least 1 year of practice or additional training (one third of that time) in the subspecialty. Fellowship training must be documented by letter from the program director. Practice experience must be verified by letter from the chief of service or department chairman; or
2. Have completed at least 5 years of active recent practice experience with a minimum of one third time (based on a 45-hour work week, 15 hours per week) devoted exclusively to all aspects of the subspecialty. This encompasses actual participation and interpretation of examinations and procedures as well as time devoted to consultation with referring physician, attendance at related con-

ferences, and pre- and post-procedure visits with patients. This experience must be attested to by the chief of service. This 5 years of practice experience will be acceptable only for the first 5 years of examination (1995-1999).

A summary of experience data must be submitted with the neuroradiology and vascular and interventional applications.

Candidates finishing their fellowship in 1999 will not be required to have received their training in an accredited fellowship program.

After 1999, candidates will be required to have successfully completed 1 year of fellowship training after residency in a program approved for such training and accredited by the ACGME and 1 year of practice or additional approved training.

Diagnostic Radiology with Special Competence in Nuclear Radiology

Candidates will be required to have a minimum of 1 year of full-time training in nuclear radiology in a department approved for training in nuclear radiology by the RRC for diagnostic radiology or nuclear medicine by the RRC for Nuclear Medicine and accredited by the ACGME. Credit will not be given for any training obtained during the 4 years of diagnostic radiology residency.

Qualifications of Applicants for Certification by the ABR

Each applicant for admission to an examination for a certificate to be issued by the ABR in diagnostic radiology or radiation oncology shall be required to present evidence satisfactory to the Board that the applicant has met the following standards:

1. General Qualifications: That the applicant is a specialist in diagnostic radiology or radiation oncology as outlined in Article II, Section 2, of the Rules and Regulations and is recognized by his/her peers to have high moral and ethical standards in his/her profession.
2. General Professional Education: Graduation from a medical school accredited at the date of graduation by the Liaison Committee on Medical Education of the American Medical Association, the RCPSC, or from a college of osteopathic medicine approved by the AOA. If the applicant is a graduate of a medical school outside the United States or Canada, the applicant must be screened with approval by an agency acceptable to the Board of Trustees.
3. Special Training: The period of special training shall be as the Board of Trustees, by resolution or motion, shall determine from time to time. The Board of Trustees requires a written statement from the applicant's current program director, attesting that the applicant will have satisfactorily completed the required special training and will have achieved adequate professional qualifications for the examination in diagnostic radiology or radiation oncology by the appointed time and is prepared to take that examination.
4. In special instances these requirements may be modified by majority vote of the entire Board of Trustees or by the executive committee acting in its stead.
5. If the program director fails to indicate in writing that the applicant will have the required special training and will have achieved adequate professional qualifications, documentation of the reason(s) must be submitted along with evidence that the candidate has been appropriately apprised of his/her deficiencies. The executive committee of the Board will notify the applicant in writing that an appeals mechanism exists as outlined in paragraphs 6 and 7 below.
6. In utilizing the appeals mechanism, the applicant must provide the executive committee of the Board with a written statement supporting the appeal. The executive committee may ask the program director to submit a written response to the applicant's appeal.
7. The executive committee must reach a final decision without delay in determining the candidate's admissibility to the examination.

Application and Fee

Application for examination must be made in exact duplicate (two original copies on prescribed forms that may be obtained from the ABR office). No photocopy or any other kind of copy will be accepted. These forms should be submitted with photographs, autographed on the front, and the current application fee (US currency) by the deadline established for filing. Applications for the written examination to be given in any year will not be accepted prior to July 1 of the preceding year and must be filed no later than the deadline of September 30 of the preceding year. There is a nonrefundable penalty fee for any application postmarked between October 1 and October 31. No application will be accepted after October 31.

Incomplete applications will not be accepted. The postmark affixed to the last item received to complete the application must be on or before the deadline date.

In the event of withdrawal of an application, only a portion of the fee can be refunded.

A candidate will have three consecutive opportunities to appear for and pass the written examination, beginning with the written examination for which he/she is first declared admissible. If a candidate fails to accomplish this, he/she must submit a new application and fee in effect at that time. Failure to accept an appointment, cancellation of an appointment, or failure to appear for a scheduled written examination will be regarded as one of the three opportunities.

A candidate who has passed the written examination will have three consecutive opportunities to appear for and pass the oral examination, beginning with the oral examination for which he/she is first declared admissible. If a candidate fails to accomplish this, he/she must submit a new application and the fee in effect at that time and reinitiate the examination process, including the written examination. Failure to accept an appointment, cancellation of an appointment, or failure to appear for a scheduled oral examination will be regarded as one of the three opportunities.

A candidate who finds it necessary for any reason to cancel after acceptance of an appointment for either the written or oral examination shall be required to submit an additional fee. This amount represents administrative costs to the Board. A candidate who fails to appear for an examination without notifying the office of the ABR at least 20 days prior to the first date of the examination will be charged the full application fee in existence at the time of payment. (Under certain circumstances, the ABR, entirely at its discretion, may excuse such a candidate from this penalty, provided the reason for such absence is substantiated in writing.)

Objectives of the Written Examination

In 1965 it became apparent to the Board of Trustees of the ABR that the then current oral examination could not cover the entire burgeoning field of radiology without the addition of more segments and, in turn, more examiners. This would impose a further burden not only on candidates but also on the Board itself. It was decided, therefore, to search for other methods of examination. At that time, it was agreed to adopt a written examination to be given annually as a prerequisite for the oral examination. The content of the examination was to include the basic sciences of anatomy, pathology, physiology, and pharmacology as these subjects relate to clinical practice.

Also to be included were radiologic techniques, radiologic physics, and radiation biology.

Thus, the content of the examination in radiation oncology now includes the basic sciences of physics, radiation biology, and clinical oncology, as well as anatomy, pathology, physiology, and chemotherapy as these subjects relate to the clinical practice of radiation oncology.

A pool of multiple-choice questions was developed, and the first examination was given in 1969 to all candidates seeking certification in diagnostic radiology or radiation oncology.

Content of Written Examination in Each Field

Each examination consists of approximately 450 multiple-choice questions to be administered over a period of approximately 8 hours. About one half of the questions are distributed on the afternoon of one day, and the other half distributed on the morning of the following day.

New written examinations are formulated each year in all categories of radiology, and the content of the examinations is carefully evaluated in order to keep pace with new information and developments. The number of questions in each category may be changed as necessity dictates from year to year.

Beginning in 1984, a candidate who takes the written examination in diagnostic radiology and fails the diagnostic portion but passes physics must repeat the diagnostic portion but will not be required to repeat physics.

Beginning in 1998, a candidate who takes the written examination in radiation oncology and passes two of the three portions, either clinical, physics, or radiation biology, must repeat only the portion that he/she failed. Those candidates who fail the physics and the radiation biology portions of the examination or the clinical oncology portion of the examination must repeat the entire examination.

Beginning in 1987, a candidate who passes the diagnostic portion but fails physics must repeat and pass the physics portion before admission to the oral examination.

Candidates in diagnostic radiology may expect to be asked questions on magnetic resonance imaging in the written and oral examinations.

Oral Examination

Oral examinations are given at a time designated by the Board of Trustees. At the present time, the oral examinations are conducted yearly in May or June.

Admissibility to the oral examination is determined by the executive committee. Experience has shown that to delay taking the oral examination does not benefit the candidate.

No recording device of any kind may be brought to the examination.

A certificate will not be issued until verification has been received from the program director that all requirements have been fulfilled in the training program.

Content of Oral Examination for Diagnostic Radiology

Candidates applying for examination in diagnostic radiology will be examined for a period of 25 minutes each by ten examiners. The categories to be covered are musculoskeletal, cardiopulmonary, gastrointestinal tract, genitourinary tract, neuroradiology, vascular and interventional radiology, nuclear radiology, ultrasound, pediatric radiology, and breast radiology.

Content of Oral Examination for Radiation Oncology

Candidates applying for examination in radiation oncology will be examined for a period of 30 minutes each by eight examiners. The subject matter of this examination concerns the clinical management of malignant disease and is usually presented according to the anatomical site of the primary tumor. The anatomical sites are divided into the following eight categories: gastrointestinal tract; gynecologic malignancies; genitourinary tract; reticuloendothelial system; head, neck, and skin; breast; central nervous system and pediatric malignancies; and lung and mediastinum, soft tissue, and bone.

Reexaminations

Failures

A candidate who fails the oral examination in diagnostic radiology or in radiation oncology may be scheduled for reexamination. The reexamination fee in effect at that time must be submitted.

A candidate who fails to pass the oral examination after three consecutive opportunities must start the examination procedure from the beginning with the submission of a new application and fee in effect at that time, and retake the entire written examination.

Conditions

Candidates in diagnostic radiology who have conditioned one, two, or three categories in the oral examination will be reexamined by two examiners in each conditioned category. Candidates in radiation oncology who have conditioned one or two categories in the oral examination will be reexamined by two examiners in each conditioned category. Candidates must pass the reexamination by both examiners in each category to remove the condition. Candidates conditioning in the oral examination will have three consecutive opportunities to appear for and pass the examination. If after three opportunities the candidate fails to pass the examination, he/she must submit a new application and fee in effect at that time and will be required to repeat the entire oral examination at the next opportunity.

Status of a Physician

The Board will reply to an inquiry concerning the status of a physician with one of the following statements:

1. The physician is Board certified.
2. The physician is in the examination process, that is, has an approved application on file but has not passed the examination.
3. The physician is neither certified nor in the examination process.

Note: No official status of Board qualified or Board eligible is recognized by the Board.

Final Action of the Board

The final action of the Board is based on the applicant's professional record, training, and attainment in the field of diagnostic radiology or in radiation oncology, as well as on the results of his/her examination. This Board has been organized, not to prevent qualified radiologists from obtaining certification, but to assist them in becoming recognized in their communities as men and women competent to practice diagnostic radiology or radiation oncology.

Revocation of Certificates

Certificates issued by this Board are subject to the provisions of Articles of Incorporation and the Bylaws. According to Article IX, Section 4, of the Bylaws, any certificate issued by the Board of Trustees shall be subject to revocation in the event that

1. the issuance of such certificate, or its receipt by the individual so certified, shall have been contrary to, or in violation of, any provision of the Certificate of Incorporation of this, the ABR, or of these Bylaws or rules and regulations adopted by the Board of Trustees; or
2. the individual so certified shall not have been eligible in fact to receive such certificate; or

3. the individual so certified shall have made any misstatement of fact in the application, or in any other communication, to the corporation or its representatives; or
4. the individual so certified shall have been convicted by a court of competent jurisdiction of a felony or of any misdemeanor involving, in the opinion of the Board of Trustees, moral turpitude; or
5. the license to practice medicine of the individual so certified shall be revoked.

Before any such certificate shall be revoked, a notice shall be sent by registered or certified mail to the last known address of the holder of such certificate, as it appears on the records of this corporation, setting forth the act, omission, or conduct alleged or complained of and giving the holder of such certificate a reasonable opportunity to answer in writing thereto. Such certificate holder shall have not less than 30 days in which to reply thereto. The Board of Trustees may, at its discretion, make such further investigation as it deems necessary and proper.

The Board of Trustees of this corporation shall have the sole power, jurisdiction, and right to determine and decide whether the evidence or information before it is sufficient to constitute one of the grounds for revocation of any certificate issued by this corporation, and the decision of such Board of Trustees in the premise shall be final.

All correspondence should be addressed to the executive director:

M Paul Capp, MD
American Board of Radiology, Inc
5255 E Williams Cir/Ste 3200
Tucson, AZ 85711
520 790-2900
520 790-3200 Fax

American Board of Surgery

1617 John F Kennedy Blvd/Ste 860
Philadelphia, PA 19103-1847
215 568-4000
215 563-5718 Fax
Internet: http://www.absurgery.org

(The material that follows is revised annually. All applicants are advised to contact the American Board of Surgery to obtain current information.)

Specialty of Surgery (General Surgery) Defined

The Board interprets the term "general surgery" in a comprehensive but specific manner, as a discipline having a central core of knowledge embracing anatomy, physiology, metabolism, immunology, nutrition, pathology, wound healing, shock and resuscitation, intensive care, and neoplasia, which are common to all surgical specialties.

A general surgeon is one who has acquired specialized knowledge and experience related to the diagnosis, preoperative, operative, and postoperative management, including the management of complications, in nine primary components of surgery, all of which are essential to the education of a broadly based surgeon

- Alimentary tract.
- Abdomen and its contents.
- Breast, skin, and soft tissue.

- Head and neck, including trauma, vascular, endocrine, congenital and oncologic disorders—particularly tumors of the skin, salivary glands, thyroid, parathyroid, and the oral cavity.
- Vascular system, excluding the intracranial vessels and heart.
- Endocrine system, including thyroid, parathyroid, adrenal, and endocrine pancreas.
- Surgical oncology, including coordinated multimodality management of the cancer patient by screening, surveillance, surgical adjunctive therapy, rehabilitation, and follow-up.
- Comprehensive management of trauma, including musculoskeletal, hand, and head injuries. The responsibility for all phases of care of the injured patient is an essential component of general surgery.
- Complete care of critically ill patients with underlying surgical conditions, in the emergency room, intensive care unit and trauma/burn units.

Additionally, the general surgeon is expected to have significant preoperative, operative, and postoperative experience in pediatric, plastic, general thoracic, and transplant surgery. Also, the surgeon must have understanding of the management of the more common problems in cardiac, gynecologic, neurologic, orthopedic, and urologic surgery, and of the administration of anesthetic agents.

The general surgeon must be capable of employing endoscopic techniques, particularly proctosigmoidoscopy, colonoscopy, esophagogastroduodenoscopy, laparoscopy, and operative choledochoscopy, and must have experience in other relevant diagnostic and therapeutic techniques including laryngoscopy, bronchoscopy, and fine needle aspiration. The general surgeon should also have the opportunity to become familiar with evolving diagnostic and therapeutic methods, including the following:

- Investigation and manipulation of the distal common bile duct (including sphincterotomy)
- Stereotactic breast biopsy techniques, including advanced breast biopsy instrumentation (ABBI), core needle biopsy, and mammotome techniques
- Physiologic testing and evaluation of the gastrointestinal tract
- Diagnostic ultrasonography of the following areas: Head and neck, breast, abdomen, including intraoperative and laparoscopic ultrasound, and endorectal
- Noninvasive diagnostic evaluation of the vascular system and invasive vascular interventional techniques
- Sentinel lymph node mapping and biopsy techniques for breast cancer and melanoma

The Meaning of Certification

The Board considers certification to be based upon a process that includes the education and evaluation phases and an examination phase. It holds that undergraduate and graduate education are of the utmost importance and requires the program director's endorsement and attestation that the applicant has had an appropriate educational experience and has attained a sufficiently high level of knowledge, judgment, and skills to be prepared for designation by the Board's Certificate as a Specialist in Surgery, upon successful completion of the examinations, and to enter into independent practice of the specialty.

Graduate Education in Surgery

I. General Information

The purpose of graduate education in surgery is to provide the opportunity to acquire a broad understanding of human biology as it relates to disorders of a surgical nature and the technical knowledge and skills appropriate to be applied by a specialist in surgery. This goal can best be attained by means of a progressively graded curriculum of study and clinical experience under guidance and supervision of senior surgeons and that provides progression through succeeding stages of responsibility for patient care up to the final one of complete management. Major operative experience and senior/chief responsibility at the final stage of the program are essential components of surgical education. The Board will not accept into the process of certification anyone who has not had such an experience in the specialty of surgery, as previously defined, regardless of the number of years spent in educational programs.

The graduate educational requirements set forth on these pages are considered to be the minimal requirements of the Board and should not be interpreted to be restrictive in nature. The Board recognizes that the time required for the total educational process should be sufficient to provide adequate clinical experience for the development of sound surgical judgment and adequate technical skill. These requirements do not preclude additional desirable educational experience, and program directors are encouraged to retain residents in a program as long as is required to achieve the necessary level of qualifications.

The integration of basic sciences with clinical experience is considered to be superior to formal courses in such subjects. Accordingly, while recognizing the value of formal courses in the study of surgery and the basic sciences at approved graduate schools of medicine, the Board will not accept such courses in lieu of any part of the required clinical years of surgical education.

The Board may at its discretion require that a member of the Board or a designated diplomate observe and report upon the clinical performance of an applicant before establishing admissibility to examination or awarding certification.

While a program may develop its own vacation, illness and other leave policies for the resident, one year of approved residency toward the Board's requirements must be 52 weeks in duration and must include at least 48 weeks of full-time surgical experience. Furthermore, unused vacation and other leave time may not be accumulated to reduce the overall duration of residency expected by the Board.

All phases of the graduate educational process must be completed in a manner satisfactory to the Board.

II. Acceptable Programs

The residency programs in surgery in the United States that are reviewed and approved by the Residency Review Committee for Surgery and the Accreditation Council for Graduate Medical Education (ACGME) are acceptable to the Board as an adequate educational experience.

In Canada, those university residency programs in surgery that are accredited by the Royal College of Physicians and Surgeons of Canada (RCPSC) offer an acceptable educational experience. Applicants from such programs must meet the Board's specific requirements and cannot receive credit for postgraduate education in countries other than the United States or Canada.

Except as mentioned above, participation in postgraduate surgical programs in countries other than the United States is not creditable toward the Board's educational requirements unless under the specific conditions set forth in the section "Credit for Foreign Graduate Education."

Listings of accredited programs in the United States may be found in the *Graduate Medical Education Directory*, published annually under the auspices of the ACGME.

Requirements for Certification in Surgery

I. General

A. Must have demonstrated to the satisfaction of the authorities of his or her graduate educational program in surgery, to their peers, and to the Board that one has attained the level of qualifications in surgery required by the Board.

B. Must have a moral and ethical standing satisfactory to the Board and in conformity with the Statements on Principles of the American College of Surgeons, and its interpretations.

C. Must be actively engaged in the practice of surgery as indicated by holding admitting privileges to a surgical service in an accredited health care organization, or be currently engaged in pursuing additional graduate education in a component of surgery or one of the other recognized surgical specialties.

D. Must hold a permanent, unconditional, unrestricted and unexpired license to practice allopathic or osteopathic medicine in a state or jurisdiction of the United States or province of Canada. The applicant must inform the Board of any conditions or restrictions in force on any active medical license he or she holds. When there is a restriction or condition in force on any of the applicant's medical licenses, the Credentials Committee of the Board will determine whether the applicant satisfies the licensure requirement of the Board.

II. Educational

A. Undergraduate Medical

1. Must have graduated from an accredited school of allopathic or osteopathic medicine in the United States or Canada.
2. Graduates of schools of medicine from countries other than the United States or Canada must present evidence of Final Certification by the Educational Commission for Foreign Medical Graduates (ECFMG).

B. Graduate Education in Surgery

1. Must have satisfactorily completed a minimum of 5 years of progressive education, following graduation from medical school in a program in surgery accredited by the ACGME or the RCPSC.
2. Must have completed all phases of graduate education in surgery in a program in surgery so accredited. Experience obtained in accredited programs in other recognized specialties, although containing some exposure to surgery, is not acceptable. A flexible or transitional first year is not creditable toward the Board's requirements as a PGY1 unless it is accomplished in an institution having an accredited program in surgery and at least 6 months of the year is spent in surgical disciplines.
3. Candidates entering programs on or after July 1, 1995, must have, in a program accredited for a minimum of 5 years, at least 54 months of clinical surgical experience with progressively increasing levels of responsibility. There must be no less than 36 months devoted to the primary components of surgery (general surgery) as previously defined. The entire chief resident experience must be devoted to the primary components of the specialty of surgery. No more than 4 months of the chief residency may be devoted to any one of the primary components of surgery. During junior years, a total of 6 months may be assigned to nonclinical or nonsurgical disciplines that are clearly supportive of the needs of the individual resident and appropriate to the overall goals of the general surgical training program. Experience in surgical pathology and endoscopy is considered to be clinical surgery, but obstetrics and ophthalmology are not. No more than a total of 12 months during junior years may be allocated to any one surgical specialty other than general surgery.
4. Must have 12 months in the capacity of chief resident in general surgery. The Board considers the terms chief resident and senior resident to be synonymous and to mean the 12 months in the program in which the resident assumes the ultimate clinical responsibilities for patient care under the supervision of the teaching staff. The majority of the twelve months of chief residency must be served in the final year. However, to take advantage of a unique educational opportunity in a program during a resident's final year, a portion of the chief residency may be served in the next to the last year, provided it is no earlier than the fourth clinical year and has been approved by the Residency Review Committee for Surgery followed by notification to the Board. The chief residency must be spent only in the parent or an integrated institution unless rotation to an affiliated institution has been approved by the Residency Review Committee for Surgery.
5. The Board expects a residency year to include no less than 48 weeks of full-time surgical experience. In order to provide programs with flexibility, the Board will accept as creditable a total of 144 weeks of experience during the first 3 clinical years and a total of 96 weeks during the last 2 clinical years.
6. All phases of the graduate educational process must be in accordance with the Program Requirements for Residency Education in General Surgery as promulgated by the ACGME and approved by the RRC for Surgery.
7. The Board believes that for optimal surgical education the resident should spend at least the final 2 residency years in the same program.

III. Operative Experience

Applicants for examination must meet the criteria established by the RRC, ie, a minimum of 500 procedures in 5 years and a minimum of 150 procedures in the chief/senior year. This must include operative experience in each of the areas of primary responsibility in the "Specialty of Surgery (General Surgery) Defined" set forth previously.

Each applicant must submit a tabulation of the operative procedures performed as surgeon, and those performed as first assistant or teaching assistant. The Board provides an Operative Experience form for this purpose when application material is obtained by the applicant. The Resident's Record form, available to program directors for residents' use through the RRC for Surgery, may be submitted in lieu of the Board's Operative Experience form.

In tabulating cases toward Board requirements, credit may be claimed "As Surgeon" when the resident has actively participated in the patient's care; has made or confirmed the diagnosis; participated in selection of the appropriate operative procedure; has either performed or been responsibly involved in performing the critical portions of the operative procedure; and has been a responsible participant in both pre- and postoperative care.

When previous personal operative experience justifies a teaching role, residents may act as teaching assistants and list such cases for the fourth and fifth year only. You may claim credit as a teaching assistant when you have actually been present and scrubbed and acted as an assistant to guide a more junior trainee through the procedure. All this must be accomplished under the supervision of the responsible member of the senior staff. An individual cannot claim credit as both responsible surgeon and teaching assistant.

Applicants must also list the number of patients with multiple organ trauma for whom operation was not required and the number of patients with critical surgical problems for whom they had primary responsibility. Failure to submit a complete and properly authenticated list of operative procedures will constitute an incomplete application.

Applicants are advised to keep a copy of the lists of operative work they submit, for their records, as the Board cannot furnish copies.

IV. Special Information for Program Directors

A. Program directors are cautioned that appointment of residents at advanced levels without being certain that their previous training is in accordance with the Board's requirements may result in the affected residents not being accepted by the Board upon completion of the program. In any case in which there is question, program directors should make inquiry of the Board prior to taking action.

B. According to the Program Requirements for Residency Education in General Surgery promulgated by the ACGME, special approval of the RRC for Surgery must be obtained (1) if a chief resident is assigned to an institution other than the parent one or an "integrated" one; (2) if rotations to any one approved "affiliate" exceed 6 months; (3) if more than 1 year of the total program is spent away from the parent and integrated institutions; or (4) if more than 6 months' total is spent in any assignment outside the parent, the integrated, or approved affiliated institutions. The Board concurs in this and deviations from these stipulations will be considered unacceptable training.

C. Since the RRC does not act upon the adequacy of postgraduate surgical education outside the United States, program directors must request the Board's approval, in advance, if they wish periods of training abroad to be creditable toward the Board's requirements. The Board will rule on individual requests.

Credit for Military Service

Credit will not be granted toward the minimum requirements of the Board for service in the Armed Forces, the Public Health Service, the National Institutes of Health, or other governmental agencies unless the service was as a duly appointed resident in an accredited program in surgery.

Credit for Foreign Graduate Education

Acceptance for examination and certification by the American Board of Surgery is based upon satisfactory completion of the stated requirements in accredited residency programs in surgery in the United States. Regardless of an individual's professional attainments here or abroad, no credit will be granted directly to an applicant for surgical education in a foreign country. The Board will consider granting partial credit only upon the request of the program director of an accredited program who has observed the applicant as a junior resident for 9 to 12 months and wishes to advance the applicant to a higher level in that program. The credit granted will not be valid until the applicant has successfully completed that program. If the applicant moves to another program the credit is not transferable and must again be requested by the new program director.

Applicants from accredited Canadian programs must have completed all of the requirements in the Canadian program or in combination with an accredited US program. No credit for postgraduate surgical education outside the US and Canada will be granted to those applicants seeking certification who completed a Canadian program. Applicants from Canadian programs must complete the Board's stipulated requirements.

Requirements Governing Admissibility to Examinations for Certification in Surgery

1. An applicant is admissible to the examinations only when all of the preliminary and graduate educational requirements of the Board, currently in force at the time of receipt of the formal application, have been satisfactorily fulfilled; the operative experience has been reviewed and deemed acceptable; the general credentials are in order; the program director has certified to the Board in writing that the applicant has attained the required clinical skills; and the formal application has been reviewed and approved. The applicant then must successfully complete the Qualifying Examination before becoming admissible to the Certifying Examination.

2. Applicants will be offered five opportunities to take the Qualifying Examination within the 5-year period following approval of the formal application, at centers designated by the Board in accord with their last recorded address. For those applicants who entered a surgery residency on July 1, 1995, and thereafter, those who do not submit their application to the Board within 3 years of completing a program accredited by the ACGME or who do not take the Qualifying Examination within 2 years following approval of their application will no longer have any status with the Board and will not be reconsidered for admission to examination.

   If applicants are not successful in completing the Qualifying Examination within the stated admissibility period, the satisfactory completion of an additional year of education in general surgery will be required in order to be considered for readmission to examination under the same conditions as listed in (2) above. This must be in a general surgery program accredited by the ACGME that has agreed to structure the additional year according to the Board's guidelines. The Board's approval of the proposed additional experience must be secured in advance.

3. The Certifying Examination will be offered to those who have passed the Qualifying Examination and have thus become "Candidates for Certification" at the earliest time consistent with the Board's geographical examination schedule.

   Candidates will be offered three and only three opportunities to appear for examination during the 5 academic years after completion of the Qualifying Examination. The admissibility expiration date shall be established as June 30 of the fifth calendar year after passing the Qualifying Examination. An opportunity offered which is refused or not taken will be counted as one of the three available. Failure to respond in writing to the reply card is considered an opportunity offered that is not taken and will therefore be counted as one of the three opportunities.

   After three opportunities (ie, failure at Certifying Examinations and/or opportunities refused—including failure to appear for a scheduled examination), a candidate will no longer be admissible to examination, regardless of the original expiration date for admissibility. Satisfactory completion of an additional year of education in general surgery in an accredited program that has agreed to structure the additional year according to the Board's guidelines, with a favorable endorsement to the Board from the program director, will be required in order to be considered for readmission to examination. This year must be approved in advance by the Board.

   If the Board approves the candidate's application for readmission to the Certifying Examination upon completion of the specified additional year of education in general surgery, the candidate will then be offered three further opportunities within the ensuing 5 years. If not successful within that time, the candidate cannot again be considered until completion of a minimum of 3 years of residency in general surgery, including a chief year, in an accredited program, and favorable endorsement to the Board by the program director. The candidate must then reapply as a new applicant. This necessitates submission of a Reapplication for Admission to Examination and all supporting documents, payment of the established fees, and successful completion again of the Qualifying Examination before advancing to the status of "Candidate for Certification."

4. Those who, 10 years after approval of their original application or reapplication, have not become certified and from whom there has been no written communication will no longer be considered active applicants. If they wish to reapply later they will be considered "New Applicants" and must fulfill the requirements then in place.

5. The Board, on the basis of its judgment, may deny or grant an "applicant" or "Candidate for Certification" the privilege of examination whenever the facts in the case are deemed by the Board to so warrant.

   The Board does not use or sanction the terms "Board eligible" or "Board qualified." The standing of an individual with the Board varies according to the current status of credentials and will be so reported.

Special Certification in Surgical Subspecialties

The Board has been authorized by the American Board of Medical Specialties to award Certification in certain disciplines related to the overall specialty of surgery to those diplomates of this Board who meet the defined requirements. These disciplines include general vascular surgery, pediatric surgery, surgery of the hand, and surgical critical care.

The Board considers all of the above disciplines to be an integral part of the specialty of surgery and expects that all surgeons certified in surgery by this Board may practice in these areas if they so desire and demonstrate the capability, even though they may not have obtained additional certification. Subspecialty certification is designed to recognize those diplomates who have advanced education, experience, and other activities beyond that of the well-trained general surgeon.

Those seeking the American Board of Surgery's Subspecialty Certification must have a currently valid Certificate in Surgery issued by the Board; must have completed the required additional education in the discipline beyond that required for General Certification; must demonstrate operative experience and/or patient care data acceptable to the Board; must show evidence of dedication to the discipline by the means specified by the Board; and must receive favorable endorsement by the director of the residency program in the particular discipline. Finally, successful completion of the prescribed examinations is required.

Those who are interested in obtaining information regarding Certification in general vascular surgery, pediatric surgery, surgery of the hand, or surgical critical care may obtain it from the Board upon request.

Examinations Offered by the Board

The Board offers examinations leading to certification in surgery, general vascular surgery, pediatric surgery, surgery of the hand, and in surgical critical care; also, in-training examinations in general surgery and in pediatric surgery.

The examinations for certification are offered to individuals, but the in-training examinations are offered to program directors for their use as an educational assessment of the individual resident's grasp of surgical fundamentals.

The Board notifies candidates for general and subspecialty certification of their performance on examinations. The Board also reports examinee performance to the director of the program in which the candidate completed the final year of residency. All reports pertaining to in-training examinations are provided only to program directors.

All examinations are developed by directors of the American Board of Surgery with contributions by examination consultants.

I. Examinations for Certification in Surgery

A. The Qualifying Examination

This examination is written and is offered once a year in the fall. It is given simultaneously in a number of locations in the United States.

Applicants whose applications have been approved by the Board are sent annually, throughout their period of admissibility, an announcement of the examination. With the announcement is a reply card that must be returned to the Board with other specified material if the applicant wishes to be scheduled for this examination. Shortly before the date of an examination an admission card is sent to the applicant indicating the specific location of the examination center and reporting times, with a pamphlet describing the examination and the types of questions to be expected.

The 1-day Qualifying Examination consists of multiple-choice questions designed to evaluate knowledge of general surgical principles and the basic sciences applicable to surgery.

Successful completion of the Qualifying Examination is a requirement for all, to attain the status of "Candidate for Certification" and admission to the Certifying Examination.

Those unsuccessful on the Qualifying Examination may review the examination at the Board office if such a request is made and the review is completed within 90 days after examination results are mailed. The review requires an appointment and payment of a fee.

B. The Certifying Examination

Examinations are held six times a year within the continental United States. Candidates for Certification will receive an announcement of the examination to which they may be assigned, based on their geographic location, approximately 2 months prior to the examination session, with a reply card that must be returned at once if a candidate wishes to be included in that examination. Failure to return or late return of a card will result in that examination being counted as one of the three opportunities to be offered. If the Board cannot accommodate a candidate at that particular examination it will not be counted as an opportunity. A candidate assigned to an examination will be sent an Admission Card indicating the specific time and place to report for examination.

The examinations are conducted by members of the American Board of Surgery and selected associate examiners who are diplomates of the Board and usually from the local geographic area.

The examinations consist of three oral sessions conducted by teams of two examiners, directed toward determining the candidate's understanding of clinical entities, level of surgical judgment, problem solving ability, and sensitivity to moral and ethical issues. During all sessions the ability to apply knowledge of anatomy, physiology, pathology, biochemistry, and bacteriology to clinical problems is also evaluated.

II. Examinations for Subspecialty Certification

The Board offers examinations for Subspecialty Certification in general vascular surgery, pediatric surgery, surgery of the hand, and surgical critical care. These examinations are described in separate pamphlets pertaining to the respective disciplines, which may be obtained from the Board office upon request.

III. In-Training Examinations

The Board offers annually to directors of accredited residency programs in surgery and in pediatric surgery written in-training examinations that are designed to measure the general level of knowledge attained by residents regarding the fundamentals of the basic sciences and management of clinical problems related to surgery and to pediatric surgery. The In-Training Examination in Surgery is constructed to evaluate the knowledge of the resident who has completed 2 years of graduate education in surgery, but, at the program director's discretion, may be administered to anyone. It is also designed to meet the first milestone required by the *Essentials* for residencies in general surgery. Directors of accredited programs in pediatric surgery should find the Pediatric Surgery In-Training Examination useful in the evaluation of all residents in their programs.

The Board will normally furnish pertinent information to the directors of all accredited programs in surgery and in pediatric surgery several months in advance of each year's examination and ascertain the number of test booklets desired. The examinations, administered by the participating program directors, take place each winter.

Program directors should take note of the fact that the Board does not contact each integrated or affiliated institution in which residents are located but depends upon the director of the program to order an adequate number of test booklets for all residents in the total program, which includes not only the parent institution but also all those included under the program designation in the *Graduate Medical Education Directory*.

It is important to note that the In-Training Examinations are not offered to individuals, but only to program directors. The In-Training Examinations are not required by the Board as part of the certification process.

The In-Training Examinations are prepared by the Board as an evaluation instrument for program directors, to be used as an assessment of residents' progress and not as a pool of questions for study or other purposes. Duplication and improper use of the examination material defeats the purpose of the examinations and will not be tolerated by the Board. The examinations are protected by copyright.

Application for Examination for Certification in Surgery

In the early spring the Board will mail a Booklet of Information and a Preliminary Evaluation Form to all residents who, according to the Board's records, will be expected to complete their residency that summer in surgery programs accredited by the ACGME. This form must be completed precisely and be received in the Board office no later than May 1. Applicants should not submit documents, testimonials, letters of recommendation, case reports, or other information unless requested to do so by the Board.

If, after review of the information submitted on the Preliminary Evaluation Form, it is determined by the Board that applicants have met or will meet the educational requirements for admission to examination in the past or current year, a formal Application for Admission to Examination will be sent to the Applicant.

The Application for Admission to Examination must be completed and returned to be received in the Board Office by *no later than* July 15. An application is not considered to be complete unless the form is accompanied by all required documents including an identification form with a photograph attached, a completed American Board of Surgery Operative Experience Form or a copy of the Resident's Record, and a check for $200.

If the completed application is received between July 15 and August 15, a late fee will be charged. No applications will be accepted after August 15.

Applicants who complete the educational requirements after September 30 will not be considered for admission to the Qualifying Examination in that year, but must wait until the following year.

The acceptability of an applicant does not depend solely upon the completion of an approved program of education but also upon information available to the Board regarding professional maturity, surgical judgment, technical capabilities, and ethical standing.

Applicants who have submitted an Application for Examination form will be notified regarding admissibility to examination.

Fees

Registration (Prior to July 15)
(payable with application form and nonrefundable) US $200
Registration (Late—July 15 to August 15)
(payable with application form and nonrefundable) US $450
Qualifying Examination (payable with Reply Card) US $400
Certifying Examination (payable with Reply Card) US $600

Fees for reexamination are the same as shown above for each examination.

Each fee for examination or reexamination includes a US $200 processing charge, which is not refunded if an individual withdraws after being scheduled for an examination.

To withdraw, one must notify the Board Office at least 15 business days before a scheduled examination. Failure to appear for examination, or withdrawal without giving at least 15 business days' notice, will result in forfeiture of the entire fee for examination.

Fees are subject to change as directed by the Board.

The Board is a nonprofit organization. The directors of the Board, except those on the executive staff, serve without remuneration.

Issuance of Certificates

A candidate who has met all requirements and has successfully completed the examinations of the American Board of Surgery in one or another of the areas of certification will then be issued a certificate by this Board, signed by its officers, attesting to qualifications in that area.

The Board issues certificates in surgery, general vascular surgery, pediatric surgery, surgery of the hand, and surgical critical care.

Those certified in surgery prior to December 31, 1975, were issued a certificate with no indication of time limited validity. All certificates issued on or after January 1, 1976, bear a limiting date of 10 years, after which they are no longer valid.

Those whose certificates have expired and who have not achieved recertification will no longer be listed in the ABMS *Directory of Board-Certified Medical Specialists as diplomates in the discipline concerned.*

Recertification

The American Board of Surgery offers recertification in surgery to its diplomates and in all the disciplines in which it offers Subspecialty Certification. The Board considers recertification to be voluntary in the same connotation as is original certification.

The purpose of recertification is to demonstrate to the profession and the public, through periodic evaluations, that the surgical specialist has maintained continuing qualifications on a currently acceptable level in the diplomate's chosen area of practice. The American Board of Surgery believes that such periodic evaluation of its diplomates is in their own interest as well as in the public interest.

A diplomate can initiate the recertification process when certification has been held at least 7 years. Pamphlets outlining requirements for recertification in the various disciplines may be obtained from the Board upon request. To facilitate receiving the Board's mailings pertaining to the recertification process, it is important for all diplomates to notify the Board promptly whenever their addresses change.

Recertification in Surgical Subspecialties

Surgical subspecialty recertification is offered to diplomates holding certificates in general vascular surgery, pediatric surgery, surgery of the hand, and surgical critical care.

Details concerning requirements for recertification in the disciplines mentioned above are similar to those for recertification in surgery, and pertinent pamphlets may be obtained from the Board upon request.

Inquiry as to Status

The Board considers an individual's record not to be in the public domain. When a written inquiry is received by the Board regarding an individual's status, a general but factual statement is provided that indicates the person's location within the examination process.

Special Situations

Irregularities

The furnishing of false information to the Board or examination irregularities may result in the rejection of an application, the barring of an applicant from examination, the denial or revocation of a certificate, or other appropriate sanctions, as set forth more fully in the Application For Admission to Examination and Instructions to Examinees.

Substance Abuse

Applicants with a history of substance abuse will not be admitted to any examination unless they present evidence satisfactory to the Board that they have successfully completed the program of treatment prescribed for their condition. Further, the Board must be satisfied that they are currently free of substance abuse.

Disabilities

The American Board of Surgery complies with the Americans with Disabilities Act by making a reasonable effort to provide Board applicants who have documented disabilities with modifications in its examination process that are appropriate for such disabilities but that do not alter the measurement of the skills or knowledge that the examination process is intended to test. Any disability that an applicant believes requires such a modification in the Board's examination must be identified and documented by the applicant within 60 days after the applicant is notified of admissibility to examination or within 60 days after the applicant learns of such disability, whichever is later.

Reconsideration and Appeals

The Board has adopted a policy with regard to reconsideration and appeals of decisions adverse to applicants regarding their individual credentials and admissibility to the examinations and questions regarding the form, administration, and results of examinations. A copy of that policy is available from the Board office to anyone considering a request for reconsideration or an appeal. A request for reconsideration, which is the first step, must be made in writing to the Board office within 90 days of receipt of notice from the Board of the action in question.

Revocation of Certificate

Any certificate issued by the American Board of Surgery, Inc, shall be subject to revocation at any time that the directors shall determine, in their sole judgment, that a candidate who has received the certificate falsified any part of the application or the required documentation, or was in some other respect not properly qualified to receive it.

American Board of Thoracic Surgery

Richard J Cleveland, MD, Secretary
One Rotary Ctr/Ste 803
Evanston, IL 60201
847 475-1520
847 475-6240 Fax
E-mail: abts_evanston@msn.com

(These criteria and conditions are subject to change without notice. All applicants are advised to contact the American Board of Thoracic Surgery [ABTS] to ascertain whether the information below is current.)

General Requirements

Certification by the ABTS may be achieved by fulfilling the following requirements:

1. Certification by the American Board of Surgery (for information, the applicant should see the current *Booklet of Information* available from the American Board of Surgery, 1617 John F Kennedy Blvd, Philadelphia, PA 19103).
2. Completion of a thoracic surgical residency accredited by the Residency Review Committee (RRC) for Thoracic Surgery that provides adequate education and operative experience in cardiovascular and general thoracic surgery.
3. An ethical standing in the profession and a moral status in the community that are acceptable to the Board.
4. A satisfactory performance on the ABTS examinations.
5. A currently registered full and unrestricted license to practice medicine granted by a state or other United States jurisdiction. The license must be valid at the time of application for admission to examination. A temporary limited license such as an educational, institutional, or house staff permit is not acceptable to the Board.

Residency Requirements

Candidates must have fulfilled all of the residency requirements of the Board in force at the time their applications are received.

Candidates for certification must complete a minimum of 24 months of residency training in thoracic and cardiovascular surgery in a program accredited by the RRC for Thoracic Surgery. This must include 12 months of senior responsibility. The director of the thoracic training program is required to approve the application form by signature, certifying that the candidate has satisfactorily completed the residency in thoracic surgery as described above. Once an application is received, it is considered the official and only record. The Board assumes that the appropriate signatures authenticate the accuracy of the case lists and all other information submitted on the application.

Education and adequate operative experience in both general thoracic surgery and cardiovascular surgery are essential parts of any approved thoracic surgery residency program, irrespective of the area of thoracic surgery in which a candidate may choose to practice.

Operative Case Criteria

The operative experience requirement of the ABTS has two parts. One is concerned with the intensity or volume of cases, and the other with the distribution of cases (index cases).

1. Surgical Volume (Intensity)

The Board's operative experience requirements include an annual average of 125 major operations performed by each resident for each year that the program is approved by the RRC for Thoracic Surgery. In a 2-year program, this requirement is met if a resident performs a total of 250 major cases over the course of his/her residency; in a 3-year program, the resident must perform 375 major cases.

This guideline on intensity of cases conforms to the Program Requirements for Residency Education in Thoracic Surgery as published by the Accreditation Council for Graduate Medical Education (ACGME) and the RRC for Thoracic Surgery.

The application of any candidate whose supervised operative experience fails to meet the requirement of an annual average of 125 major operations with a minimal number of 100 in any 1 year will be referred to the Credentials Committee for review.

2. Index Cases (Distribution)

Index cases are full-credit cases only. The applications of candidates whose operative experience does not include the required number of index cases as listed below will be sent to the Credentials Committee for review. The number of index cases required to meet the minimal acceptable standards in the various areas are:

- Lungs, pleura, chest wall — 50
  - Pneumonectomy, lobectomy, segmentectomy — 30
  - Other — 20
- Esophagus, mediastinum, diaphragm — 15
  - Esophageal operations — 8
  - Other — 7
- Congenital heart — 20
- Acquired valvular heart — 20
- Myocardial revascularization — 35
- Pacemaker implantations/closed EP —10
- Bronchoscopy and esophagoscopy — 25

Endoscopic procedures may be counted for credit whether they are performed as independent procedures or immediately preceding a thoracic operation.

Major vascular operations outside the thorax should be listed.

The Board recognizes that supervised operative experience in a well-organized teaching setting that is approved by the RRC for Thoracic Surgery protects the patient, who, in most instances, is the personal and identifiable responsibility of a faculty surgeon. This supervised experience optimally prepares the candidate to begin the independent practice of cardiothoracic surgery after the completion of residency.

The Credentials Committee has been authorized by the Board to reject a candidate if his/her operative experience during the thoracic surgery residency is considered to be inadequate. The candidate, the program director, and the RRC for Thoracic Surgery will be notified if such action is taken. If the Credentials Committee finds the applicant's operative experience inadequate and additional training is required, the additional training must be approved in advance. Should the program director determine that a resident needs additional training beyond the number of years that have been approved by the ACGME and the RRC for Thoracic Surgery, before submitting an application, this additional training must also be approved by the Board in advance.

Even though emphasis on one or another facet of thoracic surgery (pulmonary, cardiovascular, esophageal, thoracic trauma, etc) may have characterized a candidate's residency experience, the candidate is nevertheless held accountable for knowledge concerning all phases of the field, including extracorporeal perfusion (physiological concepts, techniques, and complications), cardiac devices, management of dysrhythmias, and thoracic oncology. In addition, a candidate should have had responsibility for the care of pediatric general thoracic surgical patients and be competent in video-assisted thoracoscopic surgery. The candidate should also have an in-depth knowledge of the management of acutely ill patients in the intensive care unit. This requires an understanding of cardiorespiratory physiology, respirators, blood gases, metabolic alterations, cardiac output, hyperalimentation, and many other areas. By virtue of his/her residency in thoracic surgery, the candidate is expected to be fully qualified in the surgical care of critically ill patients.

Operative Experience Credit

Credit will be allowed for supervised operative experience in a well-organized teaching setting only when the following criteria are met:

1. The resident participated in the diagnosis, preoperative planning, surgical indications, and selection of the appropriate operation.
2. The resident performed under appropriate supervision in a well-organized teaching setting approved by the RRC for Thoracic Surgery those technical manipulations that constituted the essential parts of the procedure itself.
3. The resident was substantially involved in postoperative care.

Supervision and active participation by thoracic surgery faculty are required in preoperative, intraoperative, and postoperative care.

The Board also emphasizes that first-assisting at operations is an important part of resident experience, particularly in complex or relatively uncommon cases.

Applications

Before applying for examination, prospective candidates should consider whether they are able to meet the minimum requirements of the Board, which include certification by the American Board of Surgery. They should then submit a letter to the office of the secretary of the Board, briefly outlining their thoracic surgery residency experience and requesting an application.

An application will be sent to candidates who have completed residency programs that have been approved by the RRC for Thoracic Surgery. Each applicant should consult with his/her program director regarding the correct way to complete the operative case list forms.

The deadline for submitting the completed application is August 1. Failure to meet that deadline will result in a delay of at least 1 year.

The ABTS takes particular note of the problems facing those with a disability and stands ready to alter its examination procedures in such a way that individuals who are competent to practice thoracic surgery have the opportunity to take the Board's examination under circumstances that accommodate the individual's disability. Individuals requiring special consideration because of a disability should notify the Board at least 60 days before the August 1 deadline for submitting an application.

Candidates are notified of their eligibility for examination when their applications have been approved.

Examinations

It is the policy of the ABTS to consider a candidate for examination only after he/she has completed a thoracic surgery residency program approved by the RRC for Thoracic Surgery.

Separate written and oral examinations are held annually at times and places determined by the Board. Information regarding the dates and places of the examinations is published in the Examination and Licensure column of the *Journal of the American Medical Association*, the *Journal of Thoracic and Cardiovascular Surgery*, and the *Annals of Thoracic Surgery*.

Part I—Written Examination

The examination consists of a written examination designed primarily to assess cognitive skills.

Part II—Oral Examination

Successful completion of the Part I (written) examination is a requirement for admission to the Part II (oral) examination. The oral examination is designed to test the candidate's knowledge, judgment, and ability to correlate information in the management of clinical problems in general thoracic and cardiovascular surgery.

Examination Sequence

Candidates should apply for the examination within 5 years of the satisfactory completion of their thoracic surgery residency. Any candidates applying for the examination 5 years or more after the satisfactory completion of residency will be considered individually, and recommendations for additional training will be made before they will be eligible to apply for examination.

After a candidate is declared eligible for the written examination (Part I), he/she must pass Part I within 4 years. The candidate who successfully completes Part I of the examination then must pass Part II within the succeeding 4 years.

Candidates who fail an examination (Part I or Part II) are eligible to repeat the examination the following year.

Candidates who fail either Part I or Part II of the examination three times, or do not pass either part of the examination within the allotted time period of 4 years, will be required to complete an additional thoracic surgical educational program, which must be approved in advance by the Board, before they will be permitted to retake the examination. Candidates who complete the required additional training must file an addendum to their application, have their eligibility for examination reviewed by the Credentials Committee, and pay a new registration fee. They will be given two more opportunities to take the examination (Part I or Part II) within the succeeding 2 years.

Candidates who fail either Part I or Part II a fifth time will be required to complete another approved thoracic surgery residency before they will be eligible to reapply for examination by the Board.

Fees

Registration fee (not refundable)	$400
Part I examination fee	$945
Part I reexamination fee	$945
Part II examination fee	$1,000
Part II reexamination fee	$1,000

Candidates who do not appear for their scheduled examination (Part I or Part II) or who cancel less than 6 weeks prior to either examination may forfeit their examination fee.

The Board is a nonprofit corporation, and the fees from candidates are used solely to defray actual expenses incurred in conducting examinations and carrying out the business of the Board. The directors of the Board serve without remuneration.

Appeals

Individuals who receive an unfavorable ruling from a committee of the Board may appeal such determination by mailing a notice of appeal to the office of the ABTS within 30 days of the date such ruling was mailed. A copy of the appeals procedure will be mailed to the candidate.

The only appeal permitted if an applicant fails the written examination is a request for a hand rescoring to verify the accuracy of the score as reported. This request must be made within 30 days of the time the examination results are received by the candidate.

The only appeal with respect to the oral examination is the opportunity to request immediate reexamination following the completion of the oral examination. A candidate who believes that any of his/her examiners has been unfair or biased during a portion of the oral examination may request reexamination by another examiner. The grade on reexamination will be the final grade of the candidate for that portion of the examination.

Chemical Dependency

Qualified applicants who have a history of chemical dependency that has been reported to the Board and who submit documentation suitable to the Board that their dependency has been under control for a period of at least 2 years will be admitted to the examination process.

For candidates who are already in the examination process and develop a chemical dependency as reported to the Board, the process will be suspended until the candidate can provide documentation suitable to the Board that the condition has been under control for a period of 2 years. At that time, the candidate will be readmitted to the examination process. The requirement to be accepted for examination within 5 years of completion of an approved thoracic surgery residency will not be waived.

Certification

After a candidate has met the requirements for eligibility and passed the examination, a certificate attesting to the candidate's qualifications in thoracic surgery will be issued by the Board. The certificate is valid for 10 years.

Recertification

Applicants who are certified in thoracic surgery are issued certificates that are valid for 10 years from the date of certification, after which the certificates will no longer be valid. Certificates can be renewed before expiration by fulfilling the requirements for recertification specified by the ABTS at that time. A Recertification Booklet is available upon request.

Denial or Revocation of Certificate

No certificate shall be issued or a certificate may be revoked by the Board if it determines that

a. the candidate for certification or diplomate did not possess the required qualifications and requirements for examination, whether such deficiency was known to the Board or any committee thereof before examination or at the time of issuance of the certificate, as the case may be;

b. the candidate for certification or diplomate withheld information in his/her application or made a material misstatement or any other misrepresentation to the Board or any committee thereof, whether intentional or unintentional.

c. the candidate for certification or diplomate was convicted by a court of competent jurisdiction of any felony or misdemeanor involving moral turpitude and, in the opinion of the Board, having a material relationship to the practice of medicine;
d. the candidate for certification or diplomate had his/her license to practice medicine revoked or was disciplined or censured by any court or other body having proper jurisdiction and authority because of any act or omission arising from the practice of medicine; or
e. the candidate for certification or diplomate had a history of chemical dependency or developed such during the certification process and failed to report same to the Board.

American Board of Urology

Stuart S Howards, MD, Executive Secretary
2216 Ivy Rd/Ste 210
Charlottesville, VA 22903
804 979-0059
804 979-0266 Fax

(These criteria and conditions are subject to change without notice. All applicants are advised to contact the American Board of Urology to ascertain whether the information they have is current.)

Purpose

The American Board of Urology, Inc, hereinafter sometimes referred to as "the Board," is organized to encourage study, improve standards, and promote competency in the practice of urology. The objective of the Board is to identify for the public's knowledge those physicians who have satisfied the Board's criteria for certification and recertification in the specialty of urology. Certification by the Board does not guarantee competence in practice but does indicate that the physician has completed basic training requirements and has demonstrated at the time of examination a fund of knowledge and expertise in the care of those patients whose cases were reviewed by the Board, as described elsewhere in this booklet.

Functions of the Board

The Board arranges and conducts examinations testing the qualifications of voluntary candidates, and it grants and issues certificates to accepted candidates duly licensed to practice medicine. The Board holds the power to revoke such a certificate.

The Board endeavors to serve the public, hospitals, medical schools, medical societies, and practitioners of medicine by preparing a list of urologists whom it has certified. Lists of diplomates of this Board are published annually in *The Official ABMS Directory of Board Certified Medical Specialists* and in the *Directory of Physicians in the United States*, published by the American Medical Association (AMA).

The Board is not responsible for opinions expressed concerning an individual's credentials for the examinations or status in the certification process unless they are expressed in writing and signed by the president or executive secretary of the Board.

Associations of the Board

The nominating societies of this Board and sponsors of its activities are the American Urological Association, the American Association of Genito-Urinary Surgeons, the American Association of Clinical Urologists, the Society of University Urologists, the American College of Surgeons, and the Section on Urology of the American Academy of Pediatrics.

The American Board of Urology and 23 other medical specialty boards are members of the American Board of Medical Specialties

(ABMS), which includes as associate members the Association of American Medical Colleges, the American Hospital Association, the AMA, the Federation of State Medical Boards of the United States, the National Board of Medical Examiners, and the Council of Medical Specialty Societies.

Limitations of Functions of the Board

Application for certification is entirely voluntary.

Only one certificate for each qualified individual is issued by the Board.

The Board makes no attempt to control the practice of urology by license or legal regulation and in no way interferes with or limits the professional activities of any duly licensed physician.

Requirements

An applicant may initiate application for certification by the Board during the final year of his or her residency training or at some point thereafter. For details of the certification process see "The Certification Process." Every applicant, however, must meet certain basic requirements, as follows:

A. Prerequisites

1. Education and residency: Except as noted in the requirements for international medical graduates, the applicant must be a graduate of a medical school approved by the Liaison Committee on Medical Education or a school of osteopathy approved by the Bureau of Professional Education of the American Osteopathic Association and have completed a urology residency program accredited by the Accreditation Council for Graduate Medical Education (ACGME) or Royal College of Physicians and Surgeons of Canada (RCPSC). The ACGME training programs in urology are described in the AMA's *Graduate Medical Education Directory*, Section II, "The Essentials of Accredited Residencies in Graduate Medical Education."
2. Postgraduate training requirements: The American Board of Urology mandates a minimum of 5 clinical years of postgraduate medical training, of which 12 months must be spent in general surgery with guidelines provided for preferred rotations, and 36 months must be spent in clinical urology. The remaining 12 months must be spent in general surgery, urology, or other clinical disciplines relevant to urology and acceptable to the Board. Suggested guidelines for the general surgery years include 24-36 weeks of abdominal surgery, 4-8 weeks of transplantation, 4-8 weeks of trauma, 4-8 weeks of vascular, and 0-8 weeks of other specialties such as pediatric surgery, gynecology, and plastic surgery. Dedicated research rotations are permitted only in 6-year programs. Scholarly endeavors are permitted during primary clinical rotations within a 5-year program, (2+3 or 1+4).

   All the above training must be in ACGME-approved programs. Regardless of the training format provided, the final 12 months of training must be spent as a chief resident in urology. The chief residency should be part of a planned program curriculum as outlined in a preapproved rotation provided to the Board. A minimum of 12 months must be served as a chief resident in urology with appropriate clinical responsibility under supervision in institutions that are part of the ACGME-approved program.

   For a program requiring more than 36 months of urology training, the candidate must complete the program as defined by the Residency Review Committee for Urology. Variances shall not be granted for an individual to take preurology training out of sequence after the completion of his or her urology residency. Preurology credit will be given only to an individual who has trained in ACGME-approved or RCPSC-approved training programs. Lesser degrees of training shall not receive such approval. Any resident who intends to transfer to another urology residency program during the urologic portion of the training must obtain the approval of the Board prior to the change. The resident must petition the Board in advance for said approval. The Board also requires the written acknowledgment and approval of both program directors.

   In regard to leaves of absence for parental leave, illness, injury, disability, alcohol or substance abuse, and vacation during residency training in urology, no more than 10% of the time allocated to the clinical training portion of the residency program can be omitted.

   To be admissible to the certification process of the Board, the resident must have completed in a satisfactory manner the training requirements of his or her specific program in effect at the time of acceptance in the program, as established by the Residency Review Committee for Urology or the Accreditation Committee of the RCPSC.
3. Requirements for Canadian trainees: To meet the requirements for admissibility to the certification process of the Board, a Canadian-trained urologist must have graduated from a US or Canadian medical school approved by the Liaison Committee for Medical Education and have completed the previously described preurology and urology requirements, with the final year as chief resident, in programs approved by the ACGME or the Accreditation Committee of the RCPSC. Upon successful completion of this training, the candidate may sit for the Qualifying (Part 1) Examination of the American Board of Urology. To be admissible to the Certifying (Part 2) Examination, the Canadian-trained candidate must be certified by the RCPSC.
4. Requirements for international medical graduates: International medical graduates from schools outside the United States providing an equivalent medical background who have completed an ACGME-approved urology residency and the prerequisite ACGME-approved preurology training in the United States may qualify for examination by the American Board of Urology. All such applicants must have a valid certificate from the Education Committee for Foreign Medical Graduates.
5. Licensure requirements: Applicants seeking certification by the American Board of Urology must also have a valid medical license that is not subject to any restrictions, conditions, or limitations. The applicant must inform the Board of any conditions or restrictions in force on any active medical license he or she holds. When there is a restriction or condition in force on any of the applicant's medical licenses, the Credentials Committee of the American Board of Urology will determine whether the applicant satisfies the licensure requirement of the Board.
6. Clinical competency requirements: In addition to the training and licensure requirements, the applicant must demonstrate competence in clinical practice. The Board will obtain evidence of this through a review of logs of cases performed by the applicant and by direct communication with the applicant's peers.
7. Misrepresentation and nonresponse procedure: Applicants for certification who misrepresent or do not respond to questions on the application will be, at a minimum, deferred from the process for 1 year.
8. Requirements for applicants with a history of chemical dependency: Such applicants will not be admitted to the Qualifying (Part 1) or Certifying (Part 2) Examination unless they present evidence to the Board that they have satisfactorily completed the program of treatment prescribed for their condition. In addition, any such applicants for the Certifying (Part 2) Examination may have a site visit of their practices by a representative of the Board.

B. Application

1. A special application form provided by the Executive Secretary shall be completed by the applicant and returned to the Board office by overnight courier for guaranteed receipt. Applications must be in the Board office by November 1 in order to permit the applicant to be admitted for the Qualifying (Part 1) Examination the following May or June. Applications and documentation material postmarked before but not received in the Board office by November 1 will incur a late fee of $300. No applications will be accepted after December 1. No application will be considered by the Credentials Committee or the Board unless it is submitted by the deadline set forth and is complete and includes all required supporting documentation. The Executive Secretary will determine if an application is complete.
2. The application must be accompanied by a notarized copy of a graduation certificate from a medical school approved by the Liaison Committee on Medical Education or from a school of osteopathy approved by the Bureau of Professional Education of the American Osteopathic Association.
3. The candidate must provide specific verification (such as a notarized certificate or an original letter from the director of the program(s) where the applicant completed graduate year 1 and 2) of successful completion of the preurology postgraduate training requirement in a program approved by the ACGME. Preurology training must be documented separately from urology training.

   Graduates of medical schools not approved by the Liaison Committee on Medical Education, the Bureau of Professional Education of the American Osteopathic Association, or the Accreditation Committee of the RCPSC must furnish a notarized copy of a valid Education Committee for Foreign Medical Graduates Certificate (or Fifth Pathway certificate).
4. Examination fees and dates for the Qualifying (Part 1) Examination are described under "Fees and Deadlines."
5. For each applicant, the director of the program where the applicant is finishing residency training must provide a letter to the Board office by January 1 confirming that the applicant is expected to have successfully completed 1 year of training in the capacity of chief resident during the calendar year in which the Qualifying (Part I) Examination is to be taken. The program director must also complete an evaluation form supplied by the Board. This evaluation must be received in the Board office by March 1 preceding the Qualifying (Part 1) Examination to be given the following May or June.
6. Applicants for certification must be approved by the Credentials Committee and the Board. Additional information may be requested by the executive secretary. No duty or obligation to assist any applicant in completing the application is implied. The applicant is responsible for ensuring that all supporting documents are received in the Board office at the indicated time.
7. As a condition of application to the certification process, applicants must sign a waiver releasing, discharging, and exonerating the Board, its directors, officers, members, examiners, employees, and agents from any and all claims, losses, costs, expenses, damages, and judgments (including reasonable attorneys' fees) alleged to have arisen from, out of, or in connection with the certification process.
8. As a condition of application to the certification process, the applicant must sign a waiver allowing the Board to release examination results achieved in the qualifying and certifying examinations to the residency program director and to the Residency Review Committee for Urology.
9. Any applicant who requires special aids or assistance due to a physical or mental disability during the Board examinations should indicate this on the application. You will be expected to submit appropriate documentation substantiating your disability. The Board reserves the right to verify your disability.

C. Fees and Deadlines

1. The current examination fee may be changed without notice. This fee reimburses the Board for expenses incurred in preparing and processing the applications and examinations of the candidate. No fees are refundable.

   Unused fees will be credited for the next available examination only. If the credit is not used at the first available opportunity, it will be forfeited.
2. Payment of $875 must accompany the initial application for the Qualifying (Part 1) Examination except in the case of chief residents, who shall pay $600 as the fee for the initial application. Chief residents only may delay the fee payment until January 5. An additional fee of $875 must accompany application for the Certifying (Part 2) Examination. An applicant or candidate secures no vested right to certification as a result of paying an examination fee.
3. Cancellation fees are as follows:
   $500 for failure to appear
   $300 for unexcused absence
   $200 for excused absence (in cases of personal or family illness/death).
4. Only one excused absence is permitted at the discretion of the Board and extends the period of admissibility for 1 year. The excused absence fee of $200 will be assessed. Following one excused absence, any subsequent absences are classified as unexcused. There will be no further extensions of admissibility, and an unexcused absence fee and reinstatement fee, if any, will be assessed. Applications will be considered inactive if two successive examination appointments are canceled by the applicant. A reinstatement fee is assessed after two consecutive absences. If the candidate does not already exceed the 5-year time limit, he or she may regain active status by paying the reinstatement fee of $600 plus an additional fee for an unexcused absence or for a nonappearance.
5. A $300 late fee will be assessed for any application and/or documentation and/or fees not received in the Board office by the prescribed deadlines. Overnight courier for guaranteed receipt is recommended. A $100 fee will be assessed for all returned checks.
6. The fee for the Preliminary Examination is $400. If a Preliminary Examination appointment is canceled, a $150 cancellation fee will be assessed.
7. The application fee for recertification is $950.
8. The fee for a site visit by a Board representative is $2,000 plus expenses.
9. A $50 administrative fee will be assessed for processing the application of any candidate subsequently deferred from an examination. The balance of the fee will be returned.

The Certification Process

Applicants approved by the Board to enter the certification process must complete both a written Qualifying (Part 1) Examination and, after passing this examination, a subsequent Certifying (Part 2) Examination. Assessment of clinical competence through review of practice logs and peer review will also be carried out prior to admission to the Certifying (Part 2) Examination. Applicants who have not applied to take the Qualifying (Part 1) Examination within 5 years of the completion of their urological residency will be required to pass a written Preliminary Examination before being permitted to enter the certification process. The Preliminary Examination is given each November during the annual In-Service

Examination. Contact the Board office before August 15 for information.

Applicants who have not completed certification within 5 years of the first scheduled Qualifying (Part 1) Examination to which the candidate has applied will be required to pass a written Preliminary Examination before being allowed to reenter the certification process at the Part 1 level (see paragraph above).

Certification must be achieved within 5 years of the first scheduled Qualifying (Part 1) Examination after entering the certification process.

A. The Qualifying (Part 1) Examination

The Qualifying (Part 1) Examination is a written examination given in May or June of each year simultaneously at several different locations. An applicant failing the Qualifying (Part 1) Examination must repeat it the next year unless the absence is excused by the Board office (see "Fees and Deadlines," above). Failure to retake the examination at the first available opportunity will result in assessment of an unexcused absence fee on subsequent applications. The applicant must pass the Qualifying (Part I) Examination in sufficient time to allow for completion of the certification process within the 5 years of active candidacy allotted (see "The Certification Process," above).

The Qualifying (Part I) Examination is designed to assess knowledge of the entire field of urology and allied subjects. This includes, but may not be limited to, andrology (including infertility), calculus disease (including endourology and shock wave lithotripsy), congenital anomalies, pediatric urology, urologic disorders of females, infectious diseases, neurourology and urodynamics, obstructive diseases, psychological disorders, renovascular hypertension and renal transplantation, sexuality and impotence, adrenal diseases and endocrinology, trauma, and urologic oncology.

B. The Certifying (Part 2) Examination

Candidates for the Certifying (Part 2) Examination must have met all training requirements and have passed the Qualifying (Part 1) Examination. The Certifying (Part 2) Examination includes assessment of clinical competence through review of practice logs and peer review and three practical examinations (an oral examination and written examinations in urologic imaging and pathology). In addition, the candidate must have engaged in a minimum of 18 months of urological practice with primary patient responsibility in a single community, an academic institution, or in the Armed Forces.

A yearly extension of the period of admissibility may be granted for fellowships relevant to urology of 1 year or longer. Credit is subject to Board approval; fellowship training must be documented. Six months credit toward the 18-month practice period requirement may be awarded to an individual for fellowship training approved by the Board, effective with successful completion of the fellowship. Applicants must notify the Board office in writing if they spend 1 or more years in postresidency fellowship training.

Application for admission to the Certifying (Part 2) Examination is made by completing the Supplemental Application form available from the Board office. This application must be returned by overnight courier for guaranteed receipt and be received in the Board office by July 1 prior to the Certifying (Part 2) Examination of the following year. In addition, a surgical log of all major and minor cases performed as the primary surgeon, including narrative descriptions of deaths, complications, and errant diagnoses, prepared in accordance with the formats provided by the American Board of Urology, must be received in the Board office by November 15 prior to the next Certifying (Part 2) Examination the following year. Each log must document no less than 12 and no more than 18 consecutive months. This log must be verified by the candidate and notarized. Overnight courier for guaranteed receipt is recommended.

Applicants will be assessed $300 for logs received between November 15 and December 1. No surgical logs will be accepted after December 1.

The oral, urologic imaging, and pathology examinations are all regarded as separate examinations. In the event of failure of any one of the three, only the failed examination need be repeated.

Extensions of the period to complete certification are granted by the Board because of extenuating circumstances (eg, involvement in a fellowship of 1 or more years duration, subject to Board approval, and deferral for an inadequate surgical log). The candidate should request such extensions in writing, including the reason.

The candidate must successfully complete all three parts of the Certifying (Part 2) Examination within 5 years of the first scheduled Qualifying (Part 1) Examination after entering the certification process. To re-enter the process, it is necessary to pass a written Preliminary Examination and reenter the certification process at the Qualifying (Part 1) Examination level.

C. Steps in the Certifying (Part 2) Examination

1. Assessment of Clinical Competence

Urology is the specialty that deals with the medical and surgical disorders of the genitourinary tract, including the adrenal gland. Candidates must demonstrate knowledge, competence, and surgical experience in the broad domains of urology such as infertility, impotence, calculus disease, endourology, extracorporeal shock wave lithotripsy, neurourology, urodynamics, urologic imaging, uropathology, female urology, pediatric urology, infectious disease, obstructive disease, psychologic disorders, renovascular disease, transplantation, genitourinary sexuality, trauma, and oncology.

Candidates for the Certifying (Part 2) Examination must be in the full-time practice of urology and must be licensed to practice medicine in the area of current practice activity.

The candidate must sign a waiver authorizing any and all third parties contacted by the Board to furnish to the Board such records and information, including confidential information related to the candidate's abilities and reputation as a urologist, as the Board (in its sole discretion) may deem necessary or advisable.

Under no circumstances will the source of peer review letters be revealed to any person other than to members of the American Board of Urology.

The candidate will be required to release, discharge, and exonerate the Board, its directors, officers, members, examiners, employees, and agents (including any and all third parties furnishing information to the Board) from any and all claims, losses, costs, expenses, damages, and judgments (including reasonable attorneys' fees) alleged to have arisen from, out of, or in connection with the certification process.

As evidence of competency, the candidate must submit a log of his/her cases performed as surgeon that is to be no less than 12 consecutive months and no more than 18 consecutive months in length. Logs should reflect the most recent 12-18 months in the area of current practice as described earlier in this section.

Photostatic copies of patient records from the patient care facility and/or office records of any one or more of the above cases may be requested by the Board. The candidate shall be responsible for obtaining patient consent for the disclosure of patient records to the Board or for ensuring that the patient records disclosed to the Board do not contain any patient-identifying information. The candidate is expected to furnish such records within 1 month of the request. Surgical log review is an important component of the certification process. While there is no minimum number of cases established for an acceptable log, a surgical experience well below the norm for the peer group may be cause for the trustees to delay the certification process until there is sufficient experience to assess adequately a candidate's practice pattern and management abilities.

In the case of military or public health physicians subject to unexpected changes of assignment, the Board may accept cases from the previous assignment.

The Board will review the surgical logs of urologic subspecialists in the context of the expected sub-specialty experience. The 5-year period of admissibility for completing certification will be extended one time by 1 year for candidates whose certification is delayed because of an inadequate surgical log.

To further ascertain and document the candidate's qualifications for certification, the American Board of Urology will solicit information and comments from appropriate individuals, such as fellow practitioners, or from organizations, such as medical societies and licensing agencies.

Upon receipt of the practice logs and peer review information, the credentials of the candidate will be reviewed by the Credentials Committee of the Board. Evidence of ethical, moral, and professional behavior and an appropriate pattern of urologic practice, including experience with an adequate volume and variety of clinical material, will be sought. Areas of inadequacy may be cause for deferment or discontinuation of the certifying process until these areas are clarified or corrected. Actions of the Board to achieve clarification may include

a. inquiry into practice irregularities by the Credentials Committee of the Board;
b. request for certified copies of candidate's health care facility and/or office records for review;
c. invitation to appear before the Board for a personal interview;
d. a site visit to the candidate's community at the candidate's expense; and/or
e. other appropriate measures that may be deemed necessary to assess apparent deviations from standard urologic practice.

The candidate will not be permitted to continue the certification process until the Board has satisfied itself of the appropriateness of the candidate's practice pattern and professional behavior. The Board may elect to defer continuation of the certification process pending investigation and resolution of any inadequacies or deviations. It may deny certification when serious practice deviations or unethical conduct are involved. These include, but are not limited to, cheating on or improper or disruptive conduct during any examination conducted by the Board, the solicitation or distribution of examination materials, and misrepresentation of an applicant's or candidate's status in the certification process.

2. The Oral, Pathology, and Urologic Imaging Examinations
These examinations are given annually in January or February at a single site. The pathology and urologic imaging examinations are written and are based on projected photographic slide material. The oral examination is an interactive process between examiner and candidate, during which an assessment is made of the ability to diagnose and manage urologic problems. Since the candidate has passed the Qualifying (Part 1) Examination, the examiner presumes in the oral examination that the candidate has a satisfactory degree of cognitive knowledge of urology. Therefore, the oral examination will concentrate upon the following:

a. Problem-solving ability. Evaluation is made of the candidate's ability to collect pertinent information systematically, integrate it, assess the problem, and propose an appropriate solution.
b. Response to a change in a clinical situation. The candidate's ability to manage changing clinical conditions is evaluated through the flexible interaction between the examiner and the candidate. Changed clinical conditions may be posed by the examiner in order to assess various responses by the candidate or may be developed by the examiner from the outcome of management recommendations offered by the candidate during the interview.
c. Professional behavior in the role of a urologist. The candidate's attitude, interaction with the examiner, and expression of patient management concerns contribute to the assessment of professional behavior.

Unforeseeable Events

Certain unforeseeable events such as a natural disaster, war, government regulations, strikes, civil disorders, curtailment of transportation, and the like may make it inadvisable, illegal, or impossible for the Board to administer an examination to a candidate at the scheduled date, time, and location. In any such circumstance, the Board is not responsible for any expense the candidate may have incurred to be present for the examination or may incur for any future or substitute examination.

Final Action of the Board

Final action regarding each applicant is the sole prerogative of the Board and is based upon the applicant's training, professional record, performance in clinical practice, and the results of the examinations given by the Board.

Regardless of the sequence by which the various steps of certification may have been accomplished, the process itself is not considered complete until the Board's final action. At any point in the process, the Board may delay or even deny certification upon consideration of information that appears to the Board to justify such action.

The activities described in "Requirements" and "The Certification Process" of this guidebook proceed from the Certificate of Incorporation and Bylaws, which state the nature of the business, objects, and purposes proposed to be transacted and carried out by this corporation.

Appeals Procedure

The Board has established an appeals process for candidates denied certification or for diplomates with time-limited certificates denied recertification. A copy of the appeals process may be obtained from the Board office upon written request by the affected party.

An appeal must be initiated by a candidate or diplomate within 30 days after the mailing by the Board of the adverse decision. The candidate or diplomate must provide written notice requesting a hearing to appeal the Board's decision and cite the specific reasons given by the Board that are alleged to be erroneous.

Board Eligible Status

The American Board of Urology does not recognize or use the term "Board eligible" in reference to its applicants or candidates. A candidate is not certified (ie, does not become a diplomate) until all components of the certification process are successfully completed. Active candidacy for Board certification shall begin when the candidate first makes application for the Qualifying (Part 1) Examination (which must occur within 5 years of completing the residency) and the candidate must have passed the Certifying (Part 2) Examination within 5 years of active candidacy. When the 5-year period of candidacy has expired the individual is no longer a candidate for certification.

Inquiry as to Status

The Board considers a candidate's record not to be in the public domain. When a written inquiry is received by the Board regarding a candidate's status, a general but factual statement is provided that indicates the person's status within the examination process. The Board provides this information only to individuals, organizations, and institutions supplying a signed release of information from the candidate, and a charge of $35 per request will apply.

Recertification

Certificates issued by the American Board of Urology on or after January 1, 1985, expire on the anniversary of the date of issue and are valid for 10 years only. A physician who fails to be recertified by the expiration date is no longer a diplomate of the Board, and his or her name is deleted from *The Official ABMS Directory of Board Certified Medical Specialists*. It is recommended, therefore, that diplomates possessing a time-limited certificate make plans to obtain recertification beginning up to 3 years before the expiration date of their current certificate.

The Board endorses the concept of lifelong learning in urology for its diplomates. Candidates for recertification must demonstrate their involvement in continuing urologic education by documenting 90 urology-related credits, 30 hours of which must be Category I, within a 3-year period by September 1 of the year the Recertification Examination is to be taken. The office of the American Board of Urology will notify diplomates holding a time-limited certificate 3 years prior to its expiration. At that time a handbook detailing the recertification process titled *Information for Applicants for Recertification* will be provided. This handbook is also available on request from the Board office.

Diplomates are responsible for keeping the Board office informed of address changes.

Revocation of Certificate

Certificates issued by this Board are the property of the Board and are issued pursuant to the rules and regulations of the Board. Each certificate is issued to an individual physician who, by signature, agrees to revocation of the certificate in the event that:

a. the issuance of such certificate or its receipt by the physician so certified shall have been contrary to, or in violation of, any provision of the Certificate of Incorporation, Bylaws, or rules and regulations of the Board in force at the time of issuance; or
b. the physician or party certified shall not have been eligible to receive such certificate, regardless of whether or not the facts constituting ineligibility were known to, or could have been ascertained by, the directors of the Board at the time of issuance of such certificate; or
c. the physician or party so certified shall have made a material misstatement of fact in application for such certificate or in any other statement or representation to the Board or its representatives; or
d. the physician so certified shall at any time have neglected to maintain the degree of competency in the practice of the specialty of urology as set up by the Board and shall refuse to submit to reexamination by the Board; or
e. the physician so certified has been found by the Board to be guilty of unethical practices or immoral conduct or of conduct leading to revocation of license. These objective standards include conduct that violates state medical laws, rules and regulations of local and state medical boards, and relevant AMA guidelines, and conduct leading to revocation of license to practice medicine in any state, regardless of continuing licensure in any other state.

The Board of Trustees of this corporation shall have the sole power, jurisdiction, and right to determine and decide whether the evidence and information before it is sufficient to constitute one of the grounds for revocation of any certificate issued by this Board.

When the Board is made aware of facts possibly constituting grounds for revocation, the Board will give the physician written notification identifying the specific facts that have come to its attention. The Board may require any physician so certified to appear before the Board of Trustees or before any one or more of them, or before an individual designated by the Board, upon not less than 20 days written notice, and to show cause at that time and place specified in the notice why the certificate may not be revoked on any one of the grounds specified in such notice. The diplomate may bring to this hearing persons or documents in defense of any actions.

The failure of any physician so notified to appear as required in such notice, without due excuse deemed sufficient to the Board of Trustees, shall constitute *ipso facto* cause for revocation of the certificate. The decisions of the Board of Trustees relating to all matters under this section shall be final and binding.

The diplomate will be required to attest that he/she has read and understands the above provisions regarding the grounds for revocation of certificate issued and the procedures to be followed in determining whether or not a certificate should be revoked and to release, discharge, and exonerate the Board, its directors, officers, members, employees, and agents from any and all loss, damage, claim, or complaint by reason of any act or omission.

Trademark and Seal

The trademark and seal of the American Board of Urology are registered. Any unauthorized use of the trademark and seal is prohibited without express permission of the Board.

Summary of Fees

Checks should be made payable to the American Board of Urology. All checks must be in US dollars. A $100 fee will be assessed for all checks returned by the bank.

Qualifying (Part I) Examination	
Residents	$575
Practitioners	$825
Certifying (Part II) Examination	$825
Reexamination (Part I)	$825
Reexamination (Part II)—Each section, subsequent year	$300
Cancellation Fees	
Excused absence	$200
Unexcused absence	$300
Failure to appear	$500
Reinstatement after two successive absences	$600 (plus cancellation fees)
Denial of admissibility to Part II Examination for inadequate surgical log	$175 (remaining balance of money returned)
Recertification	$900
Preliminary Examination	$400
Preliminary Examination cancellation fee	$150
Late fee—(application, documentation, fees)	$300
ANSF@ fee	$100
Site visit (plus expenses)	$2,000
Official verification of status	$35

Examination Dates for 1998-1999

Qualifying (Part 1) Examination

June 3, 1999
June 1, 2000
June 7, 2001 (tentative)

Certifying (Part 2) Examination

February 17-19, 2000
February 16-18, 2001

Appendix C Medical Licensure Information

This section contains two articles on the basics of medical licensure and the United States Medical Licensing Examination, as published in *Licensing and Credentialing: What Physicians Need to Know,* in addition to information on the licensure policies of state medical boards, published in *US Medical Licensure Statistics and Requirements by State, 1998-1999*. To order these books, call the AMA at 800 621-8335.

Important Note

It is strongly recommended that candidates contact the medical licensing board in a given US state or jurisdiction for the most current information on that licensing jurisdiction's requirements.

Obtaining a Medical License: The Basics

By the Federation of State Medical Boards

[Reprinted from *Licensing and Credentialing: What Physicians Need to Know*, pages 1-4]

Increasing public demand for protection, coupled with the growth in the number and sophistication of fraudulent practitioners over the past 2 decades, has resulted in stronger and more complex licensing boards and licensing statutes throughout the country. As might be expected, the rate of change differs widely among the states' licensing boards, depending on each jurisdiction's resources and Medical Practice Act, as well as on legislative, media, and public expectations. All medical boards have continued to improve licensure processes, and a trend toward uniformity among licensing boards exists to enhance both the initial licensure process and licensure portability.

Many states have expanded what is considered to be the practice of medicine to address new trends in the medical field that need to be regulated by medical boards. For example, a number of states have passed legislation in recent years that empower medical boards to have jurisdiction over the practice of medicine across state boundaries or treatment decisions made by medical directors of managed care organizations.

Within this context, a physician seeking initial licensure or subsequently applying for a license in other states should anticipate the possibility of delays due to the necessary investigation of credentials and past practice, as well as the need to comply with necessary licensing standards. To assist a physician in the quest for licensure, this article attempts to provide some ground rules. These suggestions will not apply in all cases but generally will help most physicians applying for licensure as well as benefit the licensing board of the state in which the physician wishes to practice.

When contacting a licensing board for the first time, ask for a copy of its current licensing requirements and the average time it takes to process applications. This will provide the physician with a solid idea of when to consider closing an existing practice and/or plan a move as well as with information about the potential problem areas to be addressed in completing an application. While initial licensure requirements for domestic and international medical graduates differ somewhat among states, all states will require proof of prior education and training and proof of the completion of a rigorous licensure examination approved by the board. Specifically, all physicians must submit proof of successful completion of all three steps of the United States Medical Licensing Examination (USMLE). However, because some medical students and physicians had completed portions of the National Board of Medical Examiners and Federation Licensing Examination (FLEX) sequences before the implementation of USMLE in 1994, certain combinations of ex-

Licensure Requirements

aminations may be considered by medical licensing authorities as comparable to the USMLE. The USMLE program recommends that such combinations be accepted for medical licensure only if completed prior to the year 2000. For information on the USMLE, physicians should contact the USMLE Office of the Secretariat at

215 590-9600, 3750 Market St, Philadelphia, PA 19104-3910.

At the initial contact, the physician should provide the licensing board with a resume or curriculum vitae. This will allow a licensing board to evaluate potential problem areas early in the process. In short, the initial contact should be used to develop a set of reasonable expectations about the duration and complexity of the licensing process in a state to avoid frustration about the time required to obtain licensure. Unreasonable expectations can result in financial jeopardy due to the premature closing of a practice or failure to meet a starting date with an employer in the new state.

A physician should never try to hide derogatory information from a licensing board. It is much better to come forward with the information, assist the board in obtaining records and other necessary data, and provide information about mitigating circumstances that would prevent license denial. Full and frank disclosure of all information requested is by far the best approach to successful licensure. A physician should remember that in most states, making a false statement on an application for licensure is grounds for denial or future restriction.

A physician who is actively involved in the licensing process can often shorten the length of time it takes to obtain a license. Personally contacting and following up with the medical schools, training programs, and appropriate hospitals will motivate these institutions to verify credentials more expeditiously. Following up with the licensing boards in other states where the physician holds or has held a license also may assist in shortening the time for licensure. It is important to note a difference between follow-up and excessive use of phone contact, which often delays the processing of requested verification materials, since the physician's application or request may need to be pulled from the "stack" to answer an inquiry. A short note to the organization processing the request for information 30 days after the initial letter or form was mailed may be a better course to follow than frequent phone contact. Another option for physicians applying for licensure is the Federation Credentials Verification Service (FCVS). The FCVS was created in 1996 by the Federation of State Medical Boards of the United States to provide a centralized, uniform process for state medical boards—as well as private, governmental and commercial entities—to obtain a verified, primary source record of a physician's core credentials. The FCVS repository of information allows a physician to establish a confidential, lifetime professional portfolio that can be forwarded, at the physician's request, to any entity that has established an agreement with FCVS. Currently, the majority of licensing authorities accept FCVS-verified documents for licensure. For more information on FCVS, call toll free, 1-888-ASK-FCVS (1-888-275-3287).

A wise physician will exercise patience and courtesy in the licensing process. State licensing boards and their staff, in most cases, do the best job possible to protect the public with the resources provided them. This requires taking the necessary time to fairly evaluate each application for licensure. In that same context, all actively practicing physicians should be cognizant of state laws; they may be providing care or performing acts that might not, until recently, have required them to hold a license.

Even for physicians with uncomplicated histories who submit complete and accurate applications, delays in obtaining a medical license may be encountered. Physicians should plan for at least a 60-day period from the time they submit a completed application for license and the actual date licensure is granted. Physicians who are graduates of a medical school outside the United States should anticipate a slightly longer period. All physicians should be cognizant of the fact that, in general, the highest volume of licensure applications is received between the months of April and September. This is the peak period because physicians with families want to relocate before the academic school year starts for their children, residents want and need licensure to begin practicing, and state employees with school-age children often take their earned vacation time during this period. Finally, it is important to remember that hospital credentialing and qualification for medical malpractice insurance are based on possession of full and unrestricted licensure. This too may mean additional time before a physician can actually begin practicing.

Physicians informed about the process and working cooperatively with the licensing board need not find licensing an unpleasant experience. Members of the medical profession should always remember that the business of medical licensing boards is to protect the public from unqualified and unfit physicians. However, licensing boards also strive to ensure a process that protects the legal rights and privileges of physicians. While maintaining this balance often appears bureaucratic and cumbersome, the end result is improved health care for the people of the United States.

This article was provided by the Federation of State Medical Boards as an update to the original, authored by the late Douglas N. Cerf.

Federation of State Medical Boards
400 Fuller Wiser Road, Suite 300
Euless, TX 76039
817 868-4000
817 868-4099 Fax
http://www.fsmb.org

Examinations Used for Entry to Residency Education and the Practice of Medicine

By Arthur Osteen, PhD

[Reprinted from *Licensing and Credentialing: What Physicians Need to Know*, pages 5-11]

Introduction

A single examination for licensure of physicians, other than osteopathic physicians, was a long time in coming. Prior to the development of the Federation Licensing Examination (FLEX) by the Federation of State Medical Boards (FSMB) in 1968, each licensing jurisdiction had its own official examination. Because licensing jurisdictions did not always accept scores on examinations given by other jurisdictions, moving from one state to another could easily involve passing a licensing examination in the new state. The private, nongovernmental National Board of Medical Examiners (NBME) provided the NBME examination, which was adopted by most, but not all, licensing boards. Over several years following the development of FLEX, the number of state examinations gradually dwindled until there were only two examinations in use for licensing purposes—FLEX and the NBME examination.

Even this degree of uniformity did not completely simplify the medical examination process. During the time when FLEX, particularly the three-part FLEX, was in use, individual states had different rules about what constituted passing marks, as well as other rules related to passing the examination. Was the FLEX weighted-average

(FWA) used—a system of determining a passing score that gave greater emphasis to clinical questions than to basic science questions—or did the candidate have to receive a passing score on all parts of the examination? And did the candidate have to pass all parts of the examination at a single sitting, or could separate parts of the examination be passed at different administrations of the examination? The fact that states had conflicting rules on these matters meant that frequently a physician passing the FLEX could have a license in one jurisdiction but be denied a license in a neighboring one.

The issues raised by these differing state rules have been resolved by the implementation of the United States Medical Licensure Examination (USMLE) and a standard set of rules for what constitutes passing scores. But some questions still remain with regard to the use of the current examination, and a new set of issues has arisen with the introduction of a clinical skills assessment (CSA) by the Educational Commission for Foreign Medical Graduates (ECFMG). The following comments are intended to describe the current debate about the USMLE and to suggest that progress is being made in finding equitable solutions. When the current questions are resolved, it is likely that a new and different set will appear.

United States Medical Licensing Examination

The USMLE has replaced the two earlier licensing examinations, the NBME examination and the FLEX, sponsored by the FSMB. The first two steps of the USMLE, the three-step examination prepared by the NBME and in use since 1991, are administered on the same day in examination centers in the United States and abroad. It is used by many medical schools for promotion and graduation. These two steps are also used by the ECFMG as part of its requirement for certification of international medical graduates (IMGs), replacing the ECFMG's Foreign Medical Graduates Examination in the Medical Sciences (FMGEMS).

Factors Leading to the Development of the USMLE

Prior to development of the USMLE, the majority of US medical school graduates (USMGs) took the earlier NBME examination for licensure, while the rest took either the two-part or the three-part FLEX. The NBME examination was administered to USMGs on site at medical schools during the academic year. All IMGs took either the three-part FLEX or its successor examination, the two-part FLEX. The examinations were administered to IMGs by individual state licensing boards. In spite of the fact that the IMGs who achieved licensure through the FLEX were outnumbered by the USMGs who achieved licensure through that route, some members of the IMG community believed that requiring IMGs to take FLEX was discriminatory and that it was in fact more difficult than the NBME examination, which only USMGs were allowed to select.

FMGEMS Not Equivalent to FLEX or USMLE

The IMGs were also concerned that they were required to pass an additional examination. The Health Professions Educational Assistance Act of 1976 (PL 94-484) required IMGs coming to the United States to either practice medicine or as exchange visitors for graduate medical education (GME) to pass an examination "equivalent" to the NBME examination, Parts I and II. The FMGEMS was determined as equivalent by the Secretary of the Department of Health and Human Services *only for the purposes of PL 94-484, but not in all respects.* In fact, the FMGEMS did not cover all of the NBME examination content areas and was not the same length. Furthermore, and of even more importance, the FMGEMS was never officially adopted by licensing boards as a licensing examination. Therefore, *IMGs who passed FMGEMS but did not pass the FLEX when it was available must now pass the USMLE to gain a license to practice medicine in the United States.*

Reporting Combination Scores from FLEX and USMLE

The USMLE was phased into use over a 4-year period from 1991 to 1994; the last complete FLEX was given in 1993. Combinations of scores from the FLEX and USMLE can be submitted for licensing purposes until 2000. The various acceptable combinations are generally described in *US Medical Licensure Statistics and Requirements by State*. More specific information is available each year in the NBME's *Bulletin of Information* about the USMLE.

The USMLE as a Prerequisite for GME: Pros and Cons

Some Program Directors Require IMGs to Pass USMLE Steps 1 and 2

Most GME programs in the United States accept ECFMG certificates based on pre-USMLE ECFMG examinations as fulfilling the requirements for entering a residency program. However, some GME program directors reportedly will not appoint IMGs unless they have passed USMLE Steps 1 and 2. These program directors may be in states where the licensing board requires that all graduates pass USMLE Steps 1 and 2 in order to be appointed. Some program directors may believe that the USMLE provides a better evaluation than the FMGEMS. Those who remember GME before PL 94-484 was passed recall that a large number of IMGs admitted to the US before that time were not able to qualify for appointment to residency training and were, consequently, unable to practice medicine in the US.

Requiring USMGs and IMGs to Pass USMLE Steps 1 and 2 Versus Requiring only IMGs to Do So

As noted above, program directors in some states are able to appoint only residents who have passed Steps 1 and 2 of the USMLE. In those states, USMGs will have had to pass Steps 1 and 2 to be appointed. In the majority of states, USMGs can be appointed without having passed Steps 1 and 2. The argument is made that requiring USMGs to take USMLE Steps 1 and 2 prior to entering GME is not justified, because the content and quality of US medical schools is known to program directors, and they do not need additional assessment of knowledge and skills.

Moreover, requiring USMGs to complete the first two USMLE steps prior to being accepted to a GME program can cause timing problems. The USMLE Step 2 is given in August and March, and scores are not available for several weeks. If medical students take the examination in August *before* their senior year in order to receive scores in time to apply for a residency, some will not have completed all of the subject matter covered in Step 2. If they wait until March of their senior year, when they will have covered most of the subject matter, their scores will not be available in time for applying for residency.

The problems related to timely access to Step 2 by USMGs will be alleviated when the NBME completes its arrangements to provide a computer-based USMLE on a less rigid schedule at examination centers throughout the United States, making it possible for US medical students to take the examination during their senior year, but in time to apply for residency education.

Fifty-one Medical Schools Require USMGs to Pass the USMLE to Graduate

Data from the Liaison Committee for Medical Education (LCME) surveys for 1997-1998 indicate that 114 of the 125 LCME-accredited medical schools require students to take USMLE Step 1; 99 of these schools require students to pass Step 1. Ninety-six of the 125 schools require students to take Step 2; 59 of these schools require students to pass. Fifty-seven of the 125 schools require students to pass both Steps 1 and 2 in order to graduate. While 2%-4% of USMGs fail the USMLE after the maximum allowable number of attempts, 7%-10% fail on the first attempt and would not be able to enter a GME program on schedule if passing were a requirement. It is the perception that the percentage of students passing the examination on the first attempt increases when a school requires it for graduation.

Many medical educators, supported by current American Medical Association policy, argue against a requirement that USMGs pass USMLE Steps 1 and 2 prior to being accepted into a residency program. They contend that the faculty of a medical school function more reliably than a written examination in determining who is qualified to enter a residency. Those medical educators arguing for a universal requirement for USMLE Steps 1 and 2 contend that a requirement to pass the examination is justified to prevent those few USMGs unable to pass the USMLE from entering a residency. A resident who is unable to pass the examination causes problems for the program, since virtually all residents need a license at some point in residency education. Losing a resident, particularly in a small program, causes administrative problems, including that of providing care to patients.

Increasing Numbers of USMGs Voluntarily Taking USMLE Steps 1 and 2

Even when no requirements exist, increasing numbers of USMGs are electing to take USMLE Steps 1 and 2 before applying to a GME program, believing that their chances of being appointed are increased by having passed the first two steps. Data from the NBME indicate that in 1996-1997 the number of individuals taking USMLE Step 2 for the first time (18,168) was higher than the number of US graduates (15,887) for that academic year. While the larger number includes individuals who postponed their examination until after graduation as well as Canadian medical students, it appears that, even without a universal requirement, more USMGs are taking Step 2 than are required to do so by the 95 medical schools mentioned above. The NBME reports that, in recent years, more students are taking Step 1 in August than in March, which also indicates that more USMGs are taking the examination in preparation for application to residency programs.

FSMB Proposal for USMLE Steps 1 and 2 Requirement Prior to GME Adopted by Nine States

In 1996, the FSMB adopted the "Report on Licensure of Physicians Enrolled in Postgraduate Training Programs," which recommended that all state medical boards "develop mechanisms to allow resident physicians to be brought under the jurisdiction of the medical boards." The report recommended that all applicants for a resident educational permit or license be required to pass USMLE steps 1 and 2 or the examination of the National Board of Osteopathic Medical Examinations. Nine states have adopted such a requirement; 17 other states require full licensure at some point during residency (usually the second year), and it is likely that additional states will adopt similar rules.

At its June 1998 Annual Meeting, the AMA House of Delegates adopted a report that called for a meeting of representatives from organizations involved in medical education and licensure to discuss this issue and, if possible, to reach an agreement concerning appropriate policy. Like the AMA, the Association of American Medical Colleges (AAMC) opposes requiring US graduates to pass a licensing examination to gain eligibility for appointment to residency. The AAMC's concern, like that of the AMA, is that such a requirement would infringe on the responsibilities of medical faculty to determine readiness for entry to GME. The AAMC is also concerned that the requirement could influence faculty to "teach to" the examination, thereby weakening the medical curriculum.

While it was hoped that replacing three examinations for medical education and licensing purposes with a multipurpose, single examination would alleviate IMG perceptions of inequitable treatment, it is likely that this perception will remain as long as some program directors continue to appoint only IMGs who have passed USMLE Steps 1 and 2.

Clinical Skills Assessment: A New Controversy

The ECFMG Clinical Skills Assessment

Since July 1, 1998, the ECFMG has required IMGs seeking ECFMG certification to pass a clinical skills assessment (CSA). At present, USMGs are not required to pass a national examination of this kind. Some US medical schools administer a similar examination, and all US schools assess the core clinical skills and behaviors of students, including their ability to interview patients.

The USMLE Steps 1 and 2 will continue to be accepted as the ECFMG medical science examination. The new CSA will incorporate the English language proficiency test, providing a direct measure of the examinee's ability to gather and interpret data and communicate effectively in a physician-patient relationship.

The IMGs express concern that the CSA is inequitable, not only in that IMGs are burdened with an examination not required of USMGs, but also because all IMG examinees are required to travel to Philadelphia and to pay the $1,200 fee. At its June 1998 Annual Meeting, the AMA House of Delegates adopted a resolution proposing that the CSA be offered at multiple sites and at the lowest cost feasible. It is possible that the examination will be offered at multiple sites after ECFMG has had more experience with it.

The NBME Clinical Skills Assessment

The IMGs may not feel at a disadvantage in this regard for too long. The NBME is well advanced in its development of a clinical skills assessment instrument to be used as part of the regular administration of the USMLE. It is anticipated that this assessment will be implemented by 2003.

A Look Back—and Ahead

For the past 21 years, I have been a member of the staff of the Continuing Medical Education Division of the AMA. In this capacity, I have worked with the Council on Medical Education, which is concerned with AMA policies regarding licensure, and have assisted in preparing various AMA reports and publications dealing with licensure matters.

It appears to me that during those 21 years, many of the inequities relating to the use of licensing examinations have been resolved. There is only one examination in use now. It has a single pass rate and a single set of rules concerning what is an acceptable score. It appears likely that the few remaining differences between examination requirements for USMGs and IMGs will be resolved, either through the adoption of the same rules for both or through development of a consensus on why different rules for the two groups are desirable.

Those who are concerned should continue to debate. They should keep in mind, however, that considerable progress has already been made in unifying the medical examination process, which has been of benefit to physicians and to the public.

Arthur Osteen, PhD, is Director of the Office of Physician Credentials and Qualifications, Division of Continuing Medical Education, American Medical Association. He may be reached at

AMA
515 N State St
Chicago, IL 60610
312 464-4677
312 464-5830 Fax

Licensure Policies and Regulations of State Medical Boards

[Summarized from *US Medical Licensure Statistics and Requirements by State, 1998-1999*]

State Medical Board Standards for Administration of the United States Medical Licensing Examination

In 1990, the Federation of State Medical Boards (FSMB) and the National Board of Medical Examiners (NBME) established the United States Medical Licensing Examination (USMLE), a single examination for assessment of US and international medical school students or graduates seeking initial licensure by US licensing jurisdictions. The USMLE replaced the Federation Licensing Examination (FLEX) and the certification examination of the NBME, as well as the Foreign Medical Graduate Examination in the Medical Sciences (FMGEMS), which was formerly used by the Educational Commission for Foreign Medical Graduates (ECFMG) for certification purposes.

The USMLE is a single examination program with three steps. Each step is complementary to the others; no step can stand alone in the assessment of readiness for medical licensure. Each USMLE step is composed of multiple-choice questions, requires 2 days of testing, and is administered semiannually.

Many states require US or Canadian medical school graduates to have from 6 months to 1 year of accredited US or Canadian graduate medical education (GME) to take USMLE Step 3. Graduates of foreign medical schools are generally required to have completed more GME (as much as 3 years in several states). California, Maryland, Nebraska, Nevada, New York, Tennessee, Utah, and West Virginia do not require completion of GME to take Step 3.

Nearly all medical licensing authorities require completion of Steps 1, 2, and 3 within a 7-year period (exceptions are Michigan and Rhode Island, which require passage in 5 and 6 years, respectively; California, which allows 10 years; and Nevada, New York, and North Carolina, which do not impose a time limit). This 7-year period begins when the medical student or graduate first passes Step 1 or Step 2. Many licensing authorities also limit the number of attempts allowed to pass each step.

Endorsement Policies of State Boards

Policies of medical licensing boards for endorsements of medical licensing examinations taken before and after the development of the Federation Licensing Examination (FLEX) vary from state to state. Each state board created its own licensing examination before FLEX, which may partially explain the sizable variation in endorsement policies from one state to another. Some boards will endorse scores on state licensing examinations in use prior to the development of FLEX, which may be endorsed in connection with a passing score on the Special Purpose Examination (SPEX). Endorsement of a certificate of the National Board of Medical Examiners (NBME) or of an examination refers to issuance of a license based on an acceptable score on the NBME or the state's board exam.

Endorsement relates to the issuance of licenses to physicians who hold licenses in other states or jurisdictions. Each state has strict endorsement requirements.

Thirty-seven state medical boards require some or all candidates for licensure endorsement to appear for an interview; six (California, Idaho, Maine, North Carolina, Wisconsin, and Wyoming) require some or all candidates to appear for an oral examination.

Fifteen boards require that a license be endorsed within a certain period after examination (usually 10 years, but 3 months in Delaware and 6 months in New Mexico). In most of these 15 states, SPEX is required if the time limit is not met.

All medical boards will accept or consider for endorsement the national board certificate of the NBME or the United States Medical Licensing Examination (USMLE), except the Virgin Islands, which does not accept endorsements. Texas will not endorse the NBME certificate held by a candidate who has never been licensed. Forty-four boards will endorse the Licentiate of the Medical Council of Canada (LMCC); 14 will endorse a state board examination from another jurisdiction, occasionally in combination with a certificate from an American Board of Medical Specialties (ABMS) specialty board; 10 will endorse an ABMS board certificate; and four (Alaska, Minnesota, Rhode Island, and Texas) will endorse the certificates of the National Board of Osteopathic Medical Examiners (NBOME). (Endorsement of these credentials is subject to any specific requirements in effect in that state.)

Additional Requirements for Endorsement of Licenses Held by International Medical Graduates

In all states, international medical graduates (IMGs) seeking licensure by endorsement must meet the same requirements as US graduates, in addition to the requirements described below.

All states except Oklahoma require that IMGs seeking licensure endorsement hold a certificate from the Educational Commission for Foreign Medical Graduates (ECFMG). In lieu of holding that certificate, a candidate for licensure in Louisiana or Maine may have passed a certification examination of an American Board of Medical Specialties (ABMS) board or the Visa Qualifying Examination; in North Dakota, a specialty board examination; and in Wisconsin, the Foreign Medical Graduate Examination in the Medical Sciences (FMGEMS).

About half of the boards require IMG candidates to have graduated from a state-approved foreign medical school; some also require 3 years of US or Canadian graduate medical education (GME). A majority of jurisdictions also may require an interview or oral examination prior to endorsement.

Policies of State Medical Boards About the Special Purpose Examination (SPEX)

The Special Purpose Examination (SPEX), a 1-day, computer-administered examination with approximately 420 multiple-choice questions, assesses knowledge required of all physicians, regardless of specialty. SPEX is used to assess physicians who have held a valid, unrestricted license in a US or Canadian jurisdiction who are

a) required by the state medical board to demonstrate current medical knowledge,

b) seeking endorsement licensure some years beyond initial examination, or

c) seeking license reinstatement after a period of professional inactivity. Physicians holding a valid, unrestricted license may also apply for SPEX, independent of any request or approval from a medical licensing board.

Forty-six jurisdictions use SPEX to assess current competence or if a candidate has not taken a written licensure exam or the American Board of Medical Specialties (ABMS) board certification examination within a specified number of years (usually 10). In 22 states, SPEX scores are valid for an unlimited length of time. Forty jurisdictions will accept SPEX scores from other licensing jurisdictions.

Nine US jurisdictions do not have SPEX policies—Guam, Massachusetts, New Hampshire, New Jersey, Oklahoma, Puerto Rico, Rhode Island, South Dakota, and Vermont. Of these, however, Oklahoma and Puerto Rico will accept SPEX scores from other jurisdictions for licensure endorsement.

Policies of State Medical Boards for Initial Medical Licensure of US Medical School Graduates

All states require a written examination for initial licensure—generally the three-step United States Medical Licensing Examination (USMLE), which has replaced the Federation Licensing Examination (FLEX) and the national board examination of the National Board of Medical Examiners (NBME).

More than half of the state medical boards require graduates of US medical schools to have completed 1 year of graduate medical education (GME) to take USMLE Step 3. Sixteen boards do not require completion of any GME to take Step 3 (although in some cases a candidate must be enrolled in a GME program). All boards require completion of at least 1 year of GME before issuing a full, unrestricted license. Forty-two jurisdictions require 1 year; Connecticut, Maine, Michigan, New Hampshire, New Mexico, Pennsylvania, South Dakota, Utah, and Washington require 2 years; Nevada requires 3 years.

Policies for Initial Medical Licensure of Canadian Citizens Who Are Graduates of Accredited Canadian Medical Schools

When considering applications for licensure, all state medical boards consider Canadian citizens who have graduated from an accredited Canadian medical school on the same basis as graduates of accredited US medical schools.

Forty-four licensing boards endorse the Licentiate of the Medical Council of Canada (LMCC) as evidence of passing an acceptable licensing examination (applicants must also pass all other board requirements for licensure).

With the exception of the District of Columbia and Guam, all medical boards accept Canadian graduation medical education (GME) as equivalent to GME in a US program accredited by the Accreditation Council for Graduate Medical Education (ACGME). These rules do not uniformly apply to international medical graduates (IMGs), who should refer to the following section.

Policies of State Medical Boards for Initial Licensure of International Medical Graduates

All international medical graduates (IMGs) must hold a certificate from the Educational Commission for Foreign Medical Graduates (ECFMG) before taking Step 3 of the United States Medical Licensing Examination (USMLE). For IMGs seeking licensure, Oklahoma is the only state that does not require an ECFMG certificate.

Thirty-seven states will endorse for licensure the Licentiate of the Medical Council of Canada (LMCC) when held by an IMG.

Thirteen state boards allow IMGs to take USMLE Step 3 before they have had GME in a US or Canadian hospital. All states, however, require at least 1 year of GME for licensure, and 28 states require 3 years. Candidates are not awarded a license until they undertake the required GME in the United States and meet other board requirements (eg, an ECFMG certificate, personal interview, payment of fees).

Medical Student Clerkship Regulations of State Medical Boards

For purposes of this publication, a clerkship is defined as clinical education provided to medical students. Twenty-three states evaluate the quality of clinical clerkships in connection with an application for licensure. In most states, clerkships for US medical students must take place in hospitals affiliated with medical schools accredited by the Liaison Committee on Medical Education (LCME). Fourteen states have additional and/or more specific bases for evaluation.

Twenty-one boards regulate clerkships provided in their states to students of foreign medical schools (including US citizens studying medicine in foreign schools). Of these, Pennsylvania and Puerto Rico forbid such clerkships. For purposes of licensure, 18 states accept only those clerkships completed in hospital departments with GME programs accredited by the Accreditation Council for Graduate Medical Education (ACGME). Seven states have additional unspecified regulations.

Additional Graduate Medical Education and Specialty Certificate Policies of State Medical Boards

A number of state medical boards have additional graduate medical education (GME) and specialty certificate policies for international medical graduates (IMGs). Fourteen states have requirements for appointment to GME programs other than requiring an Educational Commission for Foreign Medical Graduates (ECFMG) certificate or a limited license—California, Connecticut, Iowa, Kansas, Kentucky, Louisiana, Michigan, Minnesota, Nevada, New Jersey, New Mexico, Pennsylvania, Texas, and Vermont.

Three boards—Connecticut, Maine, and Nebraska—indicated that GME completed in foreign countries other than Canada may be considered for credit toward a license. Specialty certificates of foreign boards, such as the Royal College of Physicians in the United Kingdom, are accepted for credit toward a license in seven states—Connecticut, Maine, New York, Oklahoma, Oregon, Rhode Island, and Vermont.

Thirty-seven medical boards accept GME accredited by the Accreditation Council for Graduate Medical Education (ACGME) for licensure of osteopathic medical graduates.

Accredited Subspecialties and Nonaccredited Fellowships That Satisfy GME Requirements for Licensure

Both the AMA and the ACGME define a residency as GME that takes place in any of the more than 100 specialties or subspecialties that have ACGME Program Requirements (eg, the specialty of internal medicine, the subspecialty of cardiovascular disease). A fellowship is defined as clinical or research-oriented GME in an area of medicine that does not have ACGME Program Requirements.

All state medical boards accept GME in specialties accredited by the ACGME as satisfying their GME requirements for licensure. Forty-six jurisdictions—all except Alaska, Arkansas, Guam, Montana, Oklahoma, Pennsylvania, Puerto Rico, and Tennessee—accept residency education in subspecialties accredited by ACGME as satisfying their GME requirements for licensure.

Eight boards accept clinical fellowships not accredited by ACGME, and two boards—New York and North Carolina—accept research fellowships not accredited by ACGME to satisfy the GME requirement for licensure.

Licensure Requirement Exemptions for Eminent Physicians and Medical School Faculty

Nine boards license physicians through recognition of eminence in medical education or medical practice. Physicians appointed to a medical school faculty are excused from the GME requirement for licensure in 14 states and from the examination requirement for limited licensure or teaching certification in 12 states. These faculty appointees would, however, receive a limited license or similar credential.

Temporary or Limited Licenses, Permits, Certificates, and Registration Issued by State Medical Boards

Forty-three states issue educational licenses, permits, certificates, or registration to resident physicians in GME programs. (The GME program director generally provides a list of residents and any other required information directly to the licensing jurisdiction.) In 23 of those states, residents must obtain a new permit/ license when changing residency programs within the state. In seven states—California, Indiana, Kentucky, Massachusetts, Mississippi, New Hampshire, and New Mexico—prospective residents must have passed United States Medical Licensing Examination (USMLE) Step 1 to receive a permit/license.

Forty-four boards issue temporary and educational permits, limited and temporary licenses, or other certificates for the practice of medicine. The terms for the issuance of such certificates vary, but in general they must be renewed once a year with a stipulated maximum number of renewals allowed (usually 5 years).

Some states permit state institutions to hire unlicensed physicians to work under the supervision of licensed physicians. In many instances, the state departments of mental health and public health that operate these hospitals will not hire physicians who have not had at least 1 year of GME in an English-speaking hospital. International medical graduates are generally not considered for these positions unless they are in the United States with a permanent resident visa. An unlicensed physician employed by a state hospital is required in most states to register with the state board of medical examiners, which may issue a limited permit to practice within the institution.

Thirty-one states issue teaching (visiting professor) licenses, 15 issue locum tenens permits, and 22 issue inactive licenses (for physicians who want to maintain licensure in that state although they are currently practicing in another state).

Contact Information for State Medical Boards

Larry Dixon, Executive Director
Alabama State Board of Medical Examiners
PO Box 946
848 Washington Ave
Montgomery, AL 36101-0946
334 242-4116
334 242-4155 Fax

Leslie Abel, Executive Administrator
Alaska State Medical Board
Division of Occupational Licensing
3601 C St, Ste 722
Anchorage, AK 99503-5986
907 269-8160
907 269-8156 Fax
Leslie_Abel@commerce.state.ak.us

Claudia Foutz, Executive Director
Arizona Board of Medical Examiners
1651 E Morten, Ste 210
Phoenix, AZ 85020
602 255-3751
602 255-1848 Fax

Peggy Pryor-Cryer, Executive Secretary
Arkansas State Medical Board
2100 River Front Dr, Ste 200
Little Rock, AR 72202-1793
501 296-1802
501 296-1805 Fax

Ronald Joseph, Executive Director
Medical Board of California
1426 Howe Ave, Ste 56
Sacramento, CA 95825-3236
916 263-2389
916 263-2387 Fax

Susan Miller, Program Administrator
Colorado Board of Medical Examiners
1560 Broadway, Ste 1300
Denver, CO 80202-5140
303 894-7690
303 894-7692 Fax
susan.miller@dora.state.co.us

Debra Johnson, Health Program Supervisor
State of Connecticut, Department of Public Health
Physician Licensure Unit
PO Box 340308, 410 Capital Ave, MS #12APP
Hartford, CT 06134-0308
860 509-7586
860 509-8457 Fax

Brenda Petty-Ball, Executive Director
Delaware Board of Medical Practice
PO Box 1401
861 Silver Lake Blvd, Ste 203
Dover, DE 19903
302 739-4522 x229
302 739-2711 Fax

James Granger, Executive Director
District of Columbia Board of Medicine
614 H St NW, Rm 108
Washington, DC 20001
202 727-5365
202 727-4087 Fax

Tonya Williams, EdD, Executive Director
Florida Board of Medicine
1940 N Monroe St
Tallahassee, FL 32399-0770
850 488-0595
850 922-3040 Fax

Greg Schuder, Acting Executive Director
Georgia Composite State Board of Medical Examiners
166 Pryor St SW, Rm 424
Atlanta, GA 30303-3465
404 656-3913
404 656-9723 Fax

Teofilia P Cruz, RN MS, Executive Director
Guam Board of Medical Examiners
PO Box 2816
1304 E Sunset Blvd
Agana, GU 96910-2816
671 475-0251 or 0252
671 477-4733 Fax
tcruz@ncsbn.org

Constance Cabral-Makanani, Executive Director
Hawaii Board of Medical Examiners
1010 Richards St
Honolulu, HI 96813
808 586-2708
808 586-2874 Fax

Darleene Thorsted, Executive Director
Idaho State Board of Medicine
280 N 8th St, Ste 202
Boise, ID 83702
208 334-2822
208 334-2801 Fax

Pat Eubanks, Manager, Medical Unit
Illinois Board of Medical Examiners
Department of Professional Regulations
320 W Washington, 3rd Fl
Springfield, IL 62786
217 785-0820
217 524-2470 Fax

Laura Langford, RN, Executive Director
Indiana Health Professions Bureau
402 W Washington St, Rm 041
Indianapolis, IN 46204
317 232-2960
317 233-4236 Fax

Ann Martino, PhD, Executive Director
Iowa State Board of Medical Examiners
Executive Hills West
1209 E Court Ave
Des Moines, IA 50319-0180
515 281-5171
515 242-5908 Fax
amartino@idpn.state.ia.us

Lawrence Buening, Executive Director
Kansas Board of Healing Arts
235 SW Topeka Blvd
Topeka, KS 66603-3068
785 296-7413
785 296-8052 Fax

C William Schmidt, Executive Director
Kentucky Board of Medical Licensure
310 Whittington Pkwy, Ste 1B
Louisville, KY 40222
502 429-8046
502 429-9923 Fax

Delmar Rorison, Executive Director
Louisiana State Board of Medical Examiners
PO Box 30250
630 Camp St
New Orleans, LA 70130-0250
504 524-6763
504 568-8893 Fax

Randal Manning, Executive Director
Maine Board of Licensure in Medicine
137 State House Station
Two Bangor St
Augusta, ME 04333
207 287-3601
207 287-6590 Fax

J Compton, Executive Director
Maryland Board of Physician Quality Assurance
PO Box 2571
4201 Patterson Ave, 3rd Fl
Baltimore, MD 21215-0095
410 764-4777
410 358-2252 Fax
bpqa@erols.com

Alexander Fleming, JD, Executive Director
Massachusetts Board of Registration in Medicine
10 West St, 3rd Fl
Boston, MA 02111
617 727-3086
617 451-9568 Fax

Carol Engle, Director of Licensing
Michigan Board of Medical Licensure
611 W Ottawa St
Lansing, MI 48933
517 335-7222
517 335-4478 Fax

Robert Leach, JD, Executive Director
Minnesota Board of Medical Practice
University Park Plaza
2829 University Ave SE, Ste 400
Minneapolis, MN 55414-3246
612 617-2130
612 617-2166 Fax

Thomas Stevens, MD, Executive Officer
Mississippi State Board of Medical Licensure
2600 Insurance Center Dr, Ste 200B
Jackson, MS 39216
601 354-6645
601-987-4159 Fax

Tina Steinman, Executive Director
Missouri State Board of Registration for the Healing Arts
Department of Professional Regulation
PO Box 4, 3605 Missouri Blvd
Jefferson City, MO 65102-0004
573 751-0098
573 751-3166 Fax

Patricia England, JD, Executive Secretary
Montana Board of Medical Examiners
PO Box 200513
111 N Jackson
Helena, MT 59620-0513
406 444-1988
406 444-9396 Fax

Katherine Brown, Team Leader
Nebraska Health and Human Services System
Department of Regulation and Licensure, Credentialing Div.
301 Centennial Mall South, PO Box 94986
Lincoln, NE 68509-4986
402 471-2118
402 471-3577 Fax
doh6131@vmhost.cdp.state.ne.us

Larry Lessly, JD, Executive Director
Nevada State Board of Medical Examiners
PO Box 7238
1105 Terminal Way, Ste 301
Reno, NV 89502
702 688-2559
702 688-2321 Fax
nsbme@govmail.state.nv.us

Karen Lamourex, Administrator
New Hampshire Board of Registration in Medicine
2 Industrial Park Dr, Ste 8
Concord, NH 03301-8520
603 271-1205
603 271-6702 Fax

Judith Gleason, Executive Director
New Jersey State Board of Medical Examiners
140 E Front Street, 2nd Fl
Trenton, NJ 08608
609 826-7100
609 777-0956 Fax

Kristen Hedrick, Executive Director
New Mexico Board of Medical Examiners
Lamy Bldg, 2nd Fl
491 Old Santa Fe Trail
Santa Fe, NM 87501
505 827-7363
505 827-7377 Fax

Thomas Monahan, Executive Secretary
New York State Education Department
Cultural Education Center, Rm 3023
Empire State Plaza
Albany, NY 12230
518 474-3841
518 486-4846 Fax
medbd@mail.nysed.gov

Andy Watry, Executive Director
North Carolina Board of Medical Examiners
PO Box 20007
Raleigh, NC 27619-0007
919 828-1212
919 828-1295 Fax

Rolf Sletten, JD, Executive Secretary and Treasurer
North Dakota Board of Medical Examiners
418 E Broadway Ave, Ste 12
Bismarck, ND 58501
701 328-6500
701 328-6505 Fax
bomex@tic.bisman.com

Ray Bumgarner, JD, Executive Director
Ohio State Medical Board
77 S High St, 17th Fl
Columbus, OH 43266-0315
614 466-3934
614 728-5946 Fax
med_bumgarn@ohio.gov

Lyle Kelsey, Executive Director
Oklahoma State Board of Licensure & Supervision
PO Box 18256
Oklahoma City, OK 73154-0256
405 848-2189
405 848-8240 Fax
osbmls@osbmls.state.ok.us

Kathleen Haley, JD, Executive Director
Oregon Board of Medical Examiners
620 Crown Plaza
1500 SW First Ave
Portland, OR 97201-5826
503 229-5770
503 229-6543 Fax

Cindy Warner, Administrative Officer
Pennsylvania State Board of Medicine
PO Box 2649, 116 Pine St
Harrisburg, PA 17101
717 787-2381
717 787-7769 Fax

Ivonne Fernandez Colon, Executive Director
Puerto Rico Board of Medical Examiners
Department of Health
PO Box 13969
San Juan, PR 00908
787 782-8989
787 782-8733 Fax

Milton Hamolsky, MD, Chief Administrative Officer
Rhode Island Board of Medicine and Discipline
Joseph E Cannon Bldg, Rm 205
Three Capitol Hill
Providence, RI 02908-5097
401 222-3855
401 222-2158 Fax

Aaron Kozloski, JD, Board Administrator
South Carolina Department of Labor, Licensing & Regulation
PO Box 11289
110 Centerview Dr, Ste 202
Columbia, SC 29211-1289
803-896-4500
803 896-4515 Fax
medboard@zip.llr.sc.edu

Robert Johnson, Executive Secretary
South Dakota State Board of Medical & Osteopathic Examiners
1323 S Minnesota Ave
Sioux Falls, SD 57105
605 334-8343
605 336-0270 Fax

Kathy Riggs, PhD, Administrator
Tennessee Department of Health
First Floor, Cordell Hull Bldg
426 Fifth Ave N
Nashville, TN 37247-1010
615 532-4384
615 532-5164 Fax

Bruce Levy, JD MD, Executive Director
Texas State Board of Medical Examiners
PO Box 2029
Austin, TX 78768-2029
512 305-7010
512 305-7006 Fax

Douglas Borba, Executive Director
State of Utah Department of Commerce
Division of Occupational & Professional Licensing
PO Box 146741, 160 East 300 South
Salt Lake City, UT 84114-6741
801 530-6628
801 530-6511 Fax

Barbara Neuman, JD, Executive Director
Vermont Board of Medical Practice
109 State St
Montpelier, VT 05609-1106
802 828-2673
802 828-5450 Fax

Lydia Scott, Executive Assistant
Virgin Islands Board of Medical Examiners
Office of the Commissioner, Department of Health
48 Sugar Estate
St Thomas, VI 00802
809 774-0117
809 777-4001 Fax

Warren Koontz, MD, Executive Director
Virginia State Board of Medicine
6606 W Broad St, 4th Fl
Richmond, VA 23230-1717
804 662-9960
804 662-9943 Fax

Bonnie King, Executive Director
Washington State Department of Public Health
Medical Quality Assurance Commission
PO Box 47866, 1300 SE Quince St
Olympia, WA 98504-7866
360 664-8480
360 586-8480 Fax
blk0303@hub.doh.wa.gov

Ronald Walton, Executive Director
West Virginia Board of Medicine
101 Dee Dr
Charleston, WV 25311
304 558-2921
304 558-2084 Fax

Patrick Braatz, Bureau Director
State of Wisconsin Medical Examining Board
Bureau of Health Professions, Dept of Regulation & Licensing
PO Box 8935, 1400 E Washington Ave
Madison, WI 53708-8935
608 266-0483
608 267-1803 Fax

Carole Shotwell, JD, Executive Secretary
Wyoming Board of Medicine
Colony Bldg, 2nd Fl
211 W 19th St
Cheyenne, WY 82002
307 778-7053
307 778-2069 Fax
wyobom@aol.com

Appendix D

Medical Schools in the United States

Alabama

00102 University of Alabama School of Medicine
Birmingham, AL 35294

00106 University of South Alabama College of Medicine
Mobile, AL 37788

Arizona

00301 University of Arizona College of Medicine
Tucson, AZ 85724

Arkansas

00401 University of Arkansas College of Medicine
Little Rock, AR 77205

California

00502 University of California, San Francisco School of Medicine
San Francisco, CA 94143

00506 University of Southern California School of Medicine
Los Angeles, CA 90033

00511 Stanford University School of Medicine
Palo Alto, CA 94305

00512 Loma Linda University School of Medicine
Loma Linda, CA 92350

00514 University of California, Los Angeles School of Medicine
Los Angeles, CA 90024

00515 University of California, California College of Medicine
Irvine, CA 92717

00518 University of California, San Diego School of Medicine
La Jolla, CA 92093

00519 University of California, Davis School of Medicine
Davis, CA 95616

Colorado

00702 University of Colorado School of Medicine
Denver, CO 80262

Connecticut

00801 Yale University School of Medicine
New Haven, CT 06510

00802 University of Connecticut School of Medicine
Farmington, CT 06032

District of Columbia

01001 George Washington University School of Medicine
Washington, DC 20037

01002 Georgetown University School of Medicine
Washington, DC 20007

01003 Howard University College of Medicine
Washington, DC 20059

Florida

01102 University of Miami School of Medicine
Miami, FL 33101

01103 University of Florida College of Medicine
Gainesville, FL 32610

01104 University of South Florida College of Medicine
Tampa, FL 33612

Georgia

01201 Medical College of Georgia
Augusta, GA 30912

01205 Emory University School of Medicine
Atlanta, GA 30322

01221 Morehouse School of Medicine
Atlanta, GA 30314

01222 Mercer University School of Medicine
Macon, GA 31207

Hawaii

01401 University of Hawaii John A Burns School of Medicine
Honolulu, HI 96822

Illinois

01601 Rush Medical College of Rush University
Chicago, IL 60612

01602 University of Chicago, Pritzker School of Medicine
Chicago, IL 60637

01606 Northwestern University Medical School
Chicago, IL 60611

01611 University of Illinois College of Medicine
Chicago, IL 60612

01642 Finch University of Health Sciences/The Chicago Medical School
North Chicago, IL 60064

01643 Loyola University of Chicago, Stritch School of Medicine
Maywood, IL 60153

01645 Southern Illinois University School of Medicine
Springfield, IL 62708

Indiana

01720 Indiana University School of Medicine
Indianapolis, IN 46223

Iowa

01803 University of Iowa College of Medicine
Iowa City, IA 52242

Kansas

01902 University of Kansas School of Medicine
Kansas City, KS 66103

Kentucky

02002 University of Louisville School of Medicine
Louisville, KY 40292

02012 University of Kentucky College of Medicine
Lexington, KY 40536

Louisiana

02101 Tulane University School of Medicine
New Orleans, LA 70112

02105 Louisiana State University School of Medicine in New Orleans
New Orleans, LA 70112

02106 Louisiana State University School of Medicine in Shreveport
Shreveport, LA 71130

Maryland

02301 University of Maryland School of Medicine
Baltimore, MD 21201

02307 Johns Hopkins University School of Medicine
Baltimore, MD 21205

02312 Uniformed Services University of the Health Sciences, F Edward Hebert School of Medicine
Bethesda, MD 20014

Massachusetts

02401 Harvard Medical School
Boston, MA 02115

02405 Boston University School of Medicine
Boston, MA 02118

02407 Tufts University School of Medicine
Boston, MA 02111

02416 University of Massachusetts Medical School
Worcester, MA 01605

Michigan

02501 University of Michigan Medical School
Ann Arbor, MI 48109

02507 Wayne State University School of Medicine
Detroit, MI 48201

02512 Michigan State University College of Human Medicine
East Lansing, MI 48824

Minnesota

02604 University of Minnesota Medical School
Minneapolis, MN 55455

02607 University of Minnesota, Duluth School of Medicine
Duluth, MN 55812

02608 Mayo Medical School
Rochester, MN 55905

Mississippi

02701 University of Mississippi School of Medicine
Jackson, MS 39216

Missouri

02802 Washington University School of Medicine
St Louis, MO 63110

02803 University of Missouri, Columbia School of Medicine
Columbia, MO 65212

02834 Saint Louis University School of Medicine
St Louis, MO 63104

02846 University of Missouri, Kansas City School of Medicine
Kansas City, MO 64108

Nebraska

03005 University of Nebraska College of Medicine
Omaha, NE 68105

03006 Creighton University School of Medicine
Omaha, NE 68178

Nevada

03101 University of Nevada School of Medicine
Reno, NV 89557

New Hampshire

03201 Dartmouth Medical School
Hanover, NH 03756

New Jersey

03305 UMDNJ-New Jersey Medical School
Newark, NJ 07103

03306 UMDNJ-Robert Wood Johnson Medical School
Piscataway, NJ 08854

New Mexico

03401 University of New Mexico School of Medicine
Albuquerque, NM 87131

New York

03501 Columbia University College of Physicians and Surgeons
New York, NY 10032

03503 Albany Medical College
Albany, NY 12208

03506 State University of New York at Buffalo School of Medicine
Buffalo, NY 14214

03508 State University of New York Health Science Center at Brooklyn College of Medicine
Brooklyn, NY 12203

03509 New York Medical College
Valhalla, NY 10595

03515 State University of New York Health Science Center at Syracuse College of Medicine
Syracuse, NY 13210

03519 New York University School of Medicine
New York, NY 10016

03520 Cornell University Joan and Sanford I. Weill Medical College
New York, NY 10021

03545 University of Rochester School of Medicine and Dentistry
Rochester, NY 14642

03546 Albert Einstein College of Medicine of Yeshiva University
New York, NY 10461

03547 Mount Sinai School of Medicine of City University of New York
New York, NY 10029

03548 State University of New York at Stony Brook, School of Medicine
Stony Brook, NY 11794

North Carolina

03601 University of North Carolina at Chapel Hill School of Medicine
Chapel Hill, NC 27514

03605 Wake Forest University School of Medicine
Winston-Salem, NC 27103

03607 Duke University School of Medicine
Durham, NC 27710

03608 East Carolina University School of Medicine
Greenville, NC 27834

North Dakota

03701 University of North Dakota School of Medicine and Health Sciences
Grand Forks, ND 58202

Ohio

03806 Case Western Reserve University School of Medicine
Cleveland, OH 44206

03840 Ohio State University College of Medicine
Columbus, OH 43210

03841 University of Cincinnati College of Medicine
Cincinnati, OH 45267

03843 Medical College of Ohio at Toledo
Toledo, OH 43699

03844 Northeastern Ohio Universities College of Medicine
Rootstown, OH 44272

03845 Wright State University School of Medicine
Dayton, OH 45401

Oklahoma

03901 University of Oklahoma College of Medicine
Oklahoma City, OK 73190

Oregon

04002 Oregon Health Sciences University School of Medicine
Portland, OR 97201

Pennsylvania

04101 University of Pennsylvania School of Medicine
Philadelphia, PA 19104

04102 Jefferson Medical College of Thomas Jefferson University
Philadelphia, PA 19107

04112 University of Pittsburgh School of Medicine
Pittsburgh, PA 15261

04113 Temple University School of Medicine
Philadelphia, PA 19140

04114 Pennsylvania State University College of Medicine
Hershey, PA 17033

04115 MCP-Hahnemann School of Medicine
Philadelphia, PA 19102

Puerto Rico

04201 University of Puerto Rico School of Medicine
San Juan, PR 00936

04202 Ponce School of Medicine
Ponce, PR 00732

04203 Universidad Central del Caribe Escuela de Medicina
Bayamon, PR 00960-6032

Rhode Island

04301 Brown University Program in Medicine
Providence, RI 02912

South Carolina

04501 Medical University of South Carolina College of Medicine
Charleston, SC 29425

04504 University of South Carolina School of Medicine
Columbia, SC 29208

South Dakota

04601 University of South Dakota School of Medicine
Vermillion, SD 57069

Tennessee

04705 Vanderbilt University School of Medicine
Nashville, TN 37232

04706 University of Tennessee College of Medicine
Memphis, TN 38163

04707 Meharry Medical College School of Medicine
Nashville, TN 37208

04720 East Tennessee State University, James H Quillen College of Medicine
Johnson City, TN 37614

Texas

04802 University of Texas Medical Branch at Galveston
Galveston, TX 77550

04804 Baylor College of Medicine
Houston, TX 77030

04812 University of Texas Southwestern Medical School at Dallas
Dallas, TX 75235

04813 University of Texas Medical School at San Antonio
San Antonio, TX 78284

04814 University of Texas Medical School at Houston
Houston, TX 77225

04815 Texas Tech University Health Science Center School of Medicine
Lubbock, TX 79430

04816 Texas A & M University College of Medicine
College Station, TX 77843

Utah

04901 University of Utah School of Medicine
Salt Lake City, UT 84132

Vermont

05002 University of Vermont College of Medicine
Burlington, VT 05405

Virginia

05101 University of Virginia School of Medicine
Charlottesville, VA 22908

05104 Virginia Commonwealth University, Medical College of Virginia
Richmond, VA 23298

05107 Eastern Virginia Medical School of the Medical College of Hampton Roads
Norfolk, VA 23501

Washington

05404 University of Washington School of Medicine
Seattle, WA 98195

West Virginia

05501 West Virginia University School of Medicine
Morgantown, WV 26506

05502 Marshall University School of Medicine
Huntington, WV 25701

Wisconsin

05605 University of Wisconsin Medical School
Madison, WI 53706

05606 Medical College of Wisconsin
Milwaukee, WI 53226

Appendix E

Graduate Medical Education Glossary

Accreditation Council for Graduate Medical Education (ACGME)—An accrediting agency composed of representatives from five national associations interested in graduate medical education (each of which appoints four representatives) in addition to a federal government representative, two public representatives chosen by the ACGME, and a resident physician representative. The chair of the Residency Review Committee Council, an ACGME advisory body, participates in ACGME meetings in a nonvoting capacity. The ACGME, through its 27 review committees (26 Residency Review Committees, or RRCs, and the Transitional Year Review Committee), accredits graduate medical education programs.

Affiliated institution (see "major participating institution")—Term no longer used by the AMA or ACGME; it has been replaced by "major participating institution."

Annual Survey of Graduate Medical Education Programs—Conducted by the AMA Department of Data Collection. All programs accredited by the ACGME and combined specialty programs approved by their respective boards receive the survey, which collects data on program characteristics such as clinical and research facilities and the work and learning environment residents can expect. Data collected from the survey are used to produce the following products:

- Graduate Medical Education Directory
- Graduate Medical Education Directory on CD-ROM
- FREIDA Online (Fellowship and Residency Electronic Interactive Database Access system)
- State-level Data for Accredited Graduate Medical Education Programs in the US
- Medical Education issue of the Journal of the American Medical Association
- AMA Physician Masterfile
- AMA Physician Select

Categorical positions (see also "Graduate Year 1")—Positions for residents who remain in a given program or specialty until completion of the year(s) required for admission to specialty board examination.

Combined specialty programs—Programs recognized by two or more separate specialty boards to provide GME in a particular combined specialty (listed below). Each combined specialty program is made up of two programs, accredited separately by the ACGME, at the same institution. Neither the ACGME nor the Residency Review Committees reviews the combined program as a single entity. Resident physicians completing these programs are eligible for board certification.

Internal medicine/emergency medicine
Internal medicine/family practice
Internal medicine/neurology
Internal medicine/pediatrics
Internal medicine/physical medicine and rehabilitation
Internal medicine/preventive medicine
Internal medicine/psychiatry
Neurology/physical medicine and rehabilitation
Neurology/diagnostic radiology/neuroradiology
Pediatrics/emergency medicine
Pediatrics/medical genetics
Pediatrics/physical medicine and rehabilitation
Pediatrics/psychiatry/child and adolescent psychiatry
Psychiatry/family practice
Psychiatry/neurology

Consortium—A group of healthcare organizations established to pursue joint objectives. If a consortium is formally established as an ongoing organizational entity with a commitment to graduate

Glossary

medical education, it may serve as a sponsoring institution of a GME program.

Core discipline program (see "General specialty program")—Term still appears, but is being replaced by "general specialty program."

Chief resident—A position in the final year of the residency (eg, surgery) or in the year after the residency is completed (eg, internal medicine and pediatrics); the individual in this position plays a significant administrative or teaching role in guiding new residents.

ECFMG number—The number assigned by the Educational Commission for Foreign Medical Graduates (ECFMG) to each international medical graduate physician who applies for certification from ECFMG. Almost all graduates of foreign medical schools must have an ECFMG certificate to participate in GME in the US.

Fellow (see "Resident or resident physician")—An individual undertaking post-residency training in a field of research that is not accredited by the ACGME. Some specialties also use "fellow" to designate resident physicians in subspecialty GME programs, but both the AMA and ACGME prefer "resident" or "resident physician" to designate individuals in all ACGME-accredited programs.

Fellowship and Residency Electronic Interactive Database Access (FREIDA Online)—An electronic information resource maintained by the AMA that assists medical students and residents in selecting GME programs. It includes all ACGME-accredited residency programs, with expanded listings for the more than 85% of programs that provide such information as program benefits (including compensation), resident-to-faculty ratio, work schedule, policies, and educational environment. FREIDA became available on-line in a Beta test version in 1996 and became fully operational in 1997; it is currently available through the AMA home page at http://www.ama-assn.org. The last DOS version of FREIDA was produced in 1996.

Fifth pathway—One of several ways that individuals who obtain their undergraduate medical education abroad can enter GME in the United States. The fifth pathway is a period of supervised clinical training for students who obtained their premedical education in the United States, received undergraduate medical education abroad, and passed Step 1 of the United States Medical Licensing Examination. After these students successfully complete a year of clinical training sponsored by an LCME-accredited US medical school and pass USMLE Step 2, they become eligible for an ACGME-accredited residency as an international medical graduate.

General specialty program (see also "Core discipline program")—The primary specialty (eg, anesthesiology, family practice, internal medicine) to which subspecialty programs are attached. Provides resident physicians, under supervision, with the knowledge and skills needed to be practitioners in a specified area of medical practice. General specialty programs function within an institution and are subject to all ACGME accreditation actions, policies, and procedures. Completing an ACGME-accredited residency in a general specialty program is one of the requirements of certification by a specialty board.

GME—Graduate medical education.

Graduate Medical Education Directory—Annual publication recognized as the official list of programs accredited by the ACGME. Known informally as the "Green Book," the Directory lists all ACGME-accredited programs in 95 specialties and subspecialties, current educational standards ("Program Requirements") for 101 areas, and the certification requirements of 24 medical specialty boards.

Graduate Year (see also "Program year")—Refers to an individual's current year of accredited GME; this may not correspond to the program year, since a resident could be in the third year of the current program but in his/her fifth year of GME.

Graduate Year 1 (GY1)—Used in connection with residents and with residency positions to indicate the first year of training after medical school. Individuals in GY1 positions who plan to complete the entire program are counted as enrolled in Graduate Year 1 (GY1), Categorical. Individuals in GY1 positions who are using their first year in a residency program as a prerequisite to enter another specialty or subspecialty program are counted as enrolled in Graduate Year 1 (GY1), Preliminary. Not all specialties offer GY1 positions; in those specialties approved for GY1 positions, some programs do not offer them. Furthermore, although by definition residents in GY1 positions are not required to have prior GME, some residents who fill such positions may have had previous training.

Health care organizations/structures

- An *academic medical center* (or *academic health center*) is composed of a medical school, a teaching hospital, and one or more health professions schools. There may be both inpatient and outpatient (ambulatory) sites for training within an academic medical center.
- *An ambulatory care site*—such as a physician's office, outpatient or ambulatory clinic, or emergency room—provides care on an outpatient basis (ie, does not require an overnight stay in a licensed hospital or nursing home bed).
- A *group practice* involves physicians working in systematic association, with the joint use of equipment and technical personnel and with centralized administration and financial organization. Group practices may be multispecialty or single specialty, open panel or closed panel.
  1. A *multispecialty group practice* is made up of physicians practicing various specialties/subspecialties who work together.
  2. In a *closed-panel system*, a managed care organization (MCO) employs a select group of physicians—either directly (ie, staff-model HMO) or through a contract arrangement with a physician group (ie, group-model HMO)—who agree to provide care only to patients enrolled in the MCO.
- A *health maintenance organization* (HMO) handles the financing and the delivery of a broad range of health services to an enrolled population in exchange for a prepaid fee. Four common types of HMOs are:
  1. Staff model—owns and operates its own facilities and directly employs its physicians.
  2. Group model—contracts with an outside physician group practice to provide health care services to HMO enrollees.
  3. Network model—contracts with two or more outside physician groups.
  4. IPA model—contracts with physicians in independent practice (IPAs) to provide health care services to enrollees.

Institution—An organization having the primary purpose of providing educational and/or health care services (eg, a university, a medical school, a hospital, a school of public health, a health department, a public health agency, an organized health care delivery system, a medical examiner's office, a consortium, or an educational foundation). A *sponsoring institution* is the institution that assumes the ultimate responsibility for a GME program. A *major participating institution* is an institution to which residents rotate for a required experience of long duration and/or those that require explicit approval by the appropriate RRC prior to utilization. Major participating institutions are listed as part of an accredited program in the *Graduate Medical Education Directory*.

Note: Hospitals and other institutions that provide rotations of less than one-sixth of the program length or less than a total of 6 months are not listed in the *Directory*.

Intern (see "Resident or resident physician")—No longer used by the AMA or ACGME; replaced by "resident" or "resident physician." Historically, "intern" was used to designate individuals in the first post-MD year of hospital training; less commonly, it designated individuals in the first year of any residency program. Since 1975, the *Graduate Medical Education Directory* and the ACGME have used "resident" or "resident physician" to designate all individuals in ACGME-accredited programs.

International medical graduate (IMG)—A graduate from a medical school not accredited by the Liaison Committee on Medical Education (LCME).

In-training examination (also known as "in-service examination")—Examinations to gauge residents' progress toward meeting a residency program's educational objectives. Certification boards of the American Board of Medical Specialties (ABMS) and medical specialty societies offer in-training examinations on a periodic basis.

LCME—Liaison Committee on Medical Education.

Major participating institution—See "Institution."

Match—See "NRMP."

Medical school affiliation—Institutions that sponsor an accredited program are not required to have a formal relationship with a medical school. Where such a relationship exists, the affiliation is identified by the dean of the medical school as major (M), graduate only (G), or limited (L). Major affiliation signifies that an institution is an important part of the teaching program of the medical school and is a significant unit in the clinical clerkship program. Graduate only affiliation indicates that the institution is affiliated with the medical school only for its graduate programs. Limited affiliation signifies that the institution is affiliated with the medical school's teaching program only for brief, occasional, and/or unique rotations of students or residents.

Medical school number—Unique 5-digit identifier for each medical school.

Medical Student Section (MSS)— A section of the AMA House of Delegates, the AMA-MSS represents 36,000 medical student members of the AMA.

National Resident Matching Program (NRMP)—Informally referred to as the "Match," this process matches GME programs and applicants to those programs. Managed by the Association of American Medical Colleges (AAMC), the NRMP system was developed to provide both applicants and residency program directors an opportunity to consider their options for accepting and offering appointments to residency programs, respectively, and to have their decisions announced at a specific time.

Preliminary positions (see also "Graduate Year 1")—Positions for residents who are obtaining training required to enter another program or specialty. Some residents in preliminary positions may move into permanent positions in the second year. Preliminary positions are usually one year in length and usually offered for Graduate Year 1. Internal medicine, surgery, and transitional year programs commonly offer preliminary positions.

Program—The unit of GME specialty training, comprising a series of learning experiences, which is evaluated for accreditation.

Program Accreditation System (PAS)—A database system developed by the ACGME to maintain information on programs, institutions, survey dates, accreditation status, codes, etc.

Program director—The official responsible for maintaining the quality of a GME program so that it meets ACGME accreditation standards. Other duties of the program director include preparing a written statement outlining the program's educational goals; providing an accurate statistical and narrative description of the program as requested by the Residency Review Committee (RRC); and providing for the selection, supervision, and evaluation of residents for appointment to and completion of the program.

Program merge/split/absorption—In a merge, two programs combine to create one new program; the new program becomes the accredited unit and accreditation is voluntarily withdrawn from both former programs. In a split, one program divides into two separate programs and each program receives accreditation. In an absorption, one program takes over the other program; the absorbed program is granted voluntary withdrawal status, while the other program remains accredited.

Program year (see also "Graduate Year")—Refers to the current year of training within a specific program; this may not correspond to the graduate year, since a resident could be in the third year of the current program but in his/her fifth year of GME.

Resident and Fellow Section (RFS)—A section of the AMA House of Delegates, the AMA-RFS represents 40,000 resident members of the AMA.

Residency review committees (RRCs)—The 26 committees within the ACGME system that meet periodically to review programs within their specialty and/or subspecialty, propose program requirements for new specialties/subspecialties, and revise requirements for existing specialties/subspecialties.

Resident or resident physician—Any individual at any level in an ACGME-accredited GME program, including subspecialty programs. Local usage might refer to these individuals as interns, house officers, house staff, trainees, fellows, junior faculty, or other comparable terminology.

Section on Medical Schools—A section of the AMA House of Delegates with representation from the 125 accredited US medical schools.

Sponsoring institution—See "Institution."

Subspecialty program—Provides advanced GME in a narrow field of study within a medical specialty, eg, geriatric medicine within the field of internal medicine. Most subspecialty programs are subject to ACGME accreditation actions, policies, and procedures. Completing an ACGME-accredited residency in a particular subspecialty program may qualify the physician to seek certification by the related subspecialty board. Some subspecialty programs are accredited independently of the related general specialty program and are not dependent on a general specialty program. Other subspecialty programs function only in conjunction with an accredited general specialty program, and the subspecialty program's accreditation status is related to the status of the accredited general specialty program. The Residency Review Committee (RRC) determines whether accreditation of a given subspecialty program is dependent on accreditation of the related general specialty program.

Teaching staff—Any individual who has received a formal assignment to teach resident physicians. In some institutions appointment to the medical staff of the hospital constitutes appointment to the teaching staff.

Transitional year program—Broad-based clinical training in an ACGME-accredited residency program that provides a balanced GME curriculum in multiple clinical disciplines. Developed for the year between medical school graduation and a specialty residency program, the transitional year is designed to facilitate the choice of and/or preparation for a specific specialty; it is not meant to prepare participants for the independent practice of medicine. In order to sponsor a transitional year program, an institution and its affiliate must conduct two or more ACGME-accredited programs that participate in the transitional year.

USMLE (see also "ECMFG")—United States Medical Licensing Examination.

USMLE number—Refer to "ECFMG number."